BNF for Children

2026 2027

September 2026 – 27

BMJ Group

PHARMACEUTICAL PRESS
Essential Knowledge

RCPCH
Royal College of Paediatrics and Child Health
Leading the way in Children's Health

NPPG
Neonatal & Paediatric Pharmacy Group

Published jointly by
BMJ
Tavistock Square
London
WC1H 9JP
UK

and
Pharmaceutical Press Ltd
66-68 East Smithfield
London
E1W 1AW
UK

Pharmaceutical Press Ltd is the Royal College of Pharmacy's knowledge business.

and
RCPCH Publications Ltd
5–11 Theobalds Road
London
WC1X 8SH
UK

BNFC 2026-27 ISBN: 978 0 85711 497 6

Printed by GGP Media GmbH, Pößneck, Germany

Typeset by Data Standards Ltd, UK

Text design by Peter Burgess

A catalogue record for this book is available from the British Library.

Requesting copies of BNF and BNFC

Paper copies may be obtained through any bookseller or direct from:
Pharmaceutical Press Ltd
c/o Macmillan Distribution (MDL)
Hampshire International Business Park
Lime Tree Way
Basingstoke
Hampshire
RG24 8YJ
Tel: +44 (0) 1256 302 699
Fax: +44 (0) 1256 812 521
direct@macmillan.co.uk

or via our website www.PharmaceuticalPress.com/shop/.

For all bulk orders of more than 20 copies:
Tel: +44 (0) 207 572 2266
CustomerSupport@PharmaceuticalPress.com

BNFC is available as a mobile app, online (bnfc.nice.org.uk/) and also through MedicinesComplete. In addition, BNFC content can be integrated into a local formulary by using BNFC on FormularyComplete; see www.bnf.org for details.

About BNFC content

BNFC is for rapid reference by UK health professionals engaged in prescribing, dispensing, and administering medicines to children.

BNFC has been constructed using robust procedures for gathering, assessing and assimilating information on paediatric drug treatment, but may not always include all the information necessary for prescribing and dispensing. It is expected that the reader will be relying on appropriate professional knowledge and expertise to interpret the contents in the context of the circumstances of the individual child. BNFC should be used in conjunction with other appropriate and up-to-date literature and, where necessary, supplemented by expert advice. Information is also available from Medicines Information Services.

Special care is required in managing childhood conditions with unlicensed medicines or with licensed medicines for unlicensed uses. Responsibility for the appropriate use of medicines lies solely with the individual health professional.

Please refer to digital versions of BNFC for the most up-to-date content. BNFC is published in print but interim updates are issued and published in the digital versions of BNFC. The publishers work to ensure that the information is as accurate and up-to-date as possible at the date of publication, but knowledge and best practice in this field change regularly. BNFC's accuracy and currency cannot be guaranteed and neither the publishers nor the authors accept any responsibility for errors or omissions. While considerable efforts have been made to check the material in this publication, it should be treated as a guide only. Prescribers, pharmacists and other healthcare professionals are advised to check www.bnf.org for information about key updates and corrections.

Preface

BNFC aims to provide prescribers, pharmacists, and other healthcare professionals with sound up-to-date information on the use of medicines for treating children.

A joint publication of BMJ Group, Pharmaceutical Press, the Royal College of Paediatrics and Child Health, and the Neonatal and Paediatric Pharmacy Group, BNFC is published under the authority of a Paediatric Formulary Committee which comprises representatives of these bodies, the Department of Health for England, and the Medicines and Healthcare products Regulatory Agency.

Many areas of paediatric practice have suffered from inadequate information on effective medicines. BNFC addresses this significant knowledge gap by providing practical information on the use of medicines in children of all ages from birth to adolescence. Information in BNFC has been validated against emerging evidence, best-practice guidelines, and crucially, advice from a network of clinical experts.

Drawing information from manufacturers' literature where appropriate, BNFC also includes a great deal of advice that goes beyond marketing authorisations (product licences). This is necessary because licensed indications frequently do not cover the clinical needs of children; in some cases, products for use in children need to be specially manufactured or imported. Careful consideration has been given to establishing the clinical need for unlicensed interventions with respect to the evidence and experience of their safety and efficacy; local paediatric formularies, clinical literature and national information resources have been invaluable in this process.

BNFC has been designed for rapid reference and the information presented has been carefully selected to aid decisions on prescribing, dispensing and administration of medicines. Less detail is given on areas such as malignant disease and the very specialist use of medicines generally undertaken in tertiary centres. BNFC should be interpreted in the light of professional knowledge and it should be supplemented as necessary by specialised publications. Information is also available from Medicines Information Services (see inside front cover).

It is **important** to use the most recent BNFC information for making clinical decisions. The print edition of BNFC is updated in September each year. Monthly updates are provided online via MedicinesComplete and NICE (www.nice.org.uk). The more important changes listed under Changes p. xvii are cumulative (from one print edition to the next), and can be printed off each month to show the main changes since the last print edition as an aide memoire for those using print copies.

The BNF website (www.bnf.org) includes additional information of relevance to healthcare professionals. Other digital formats of BNFC are also available.

BNF Partnership welcomes comments from healthcare professionals. Comments and constructive criticism should be sent to:

British National Formulary
Pharmaceutical Press Limited
66–68 East Smithfield
London
E1W 1AW
editor@bnf.org

The contact email for manufacturers or pharmaceutical companies wishing to contact BNF is manufacturerinfo@bnf.org

Contents

Acknowledgements

The Paediatric Formulary Committee is grateful to individuals and organisations that have provided advice and information to BNF for Children (BNFC).

Contributors for this update were:

S. Bailey, G.D.L. Bates, H. Bedford, M.W. Beresford, R.M. Bingham, L. Brook, K.G. Brownlee, I.F. Burgess, A. Cant, R. Carr, T.D. Cheetham, A.G. Cleary, A.J. Cotgrove, A. Dhawan, P.N. Durrington, A.B. Edgar, J.A. Edge, D.A.C. Elliman, N.D. Embleton, A. Freyer, P.J. Goadsby, J. Gray, J.W. Gregory, P. Gringras, C. Hendriksz, R.F. Howard, R.G. Hull, S. Jones, B.A. Judd, E. Junaid, P.T. Khaw, J.M.W. Kirk, E.G.H. Lyall, P.S. Malone, S.D. Marks, D.F. Marsh, P. McHenry, P.J. McKiernan, L.M. Melvin, E. Miller, S. Moledina, R.E. Morton, P. Mulholland, C. Nelson-Piercy, J.M. Neuberger, K.K. Nischal, C.Y. Ng, J.Y. Paton, G.A. Pearson, J. Puntis, J. Rogers, K.E. Rogstad, J.W. Sander, N.J. Scolding, M.R. Sharland, N.J. Shaw, O.F.W Stumper, A.G. Sutcliffe, E.A. Taylor, S. Thomas, J.A. Vale, S. Vijay, J.O. Warner, N.J.A. Webb, A.D. Weeks, R. Welbury, Z. Zaiwalla, and S.M. Zuberi.

Valuable advice has been provided by the following expert groups: Association of British Paediatric Nurses, British Association of Dermatologists' Therapy & Guidelines Sub-committee, British Association for Paediatric Nephrology, British Association for Sexual Health and HIV, British Oncology Pharmacy Association, British Paediatric Allergy, Immunisation & Infection Group, British Paediatric Neurology Association, British Pain Society, British Society for Allergy & Clinical Immunology, British Society for Antimicrobial Chemotherapy, British Society of Gastroenterology, British Society for Haematology, British Society for Paediatric Endocrinology and Diabetes, British Society of Paediatric Gastroenterology, Hepatology and Nutrition, British Society of Rheumatology, British Thoracic Society, College of Mental Health Pharmacy, College of Sexual and Reproductive Healthcare, ENT UK, National Poisons Information Service & TOXBASE, Neonatal and Paediatric Pharmacy Group, Royal College of Anaesthetists, Royal College of Obstetricians and Gynaecologists, Royal College of Ophthalmologists, Royal College of Paediatrics and Child Health, Royal College of Pathologists, Royal College of Physicians, Royal College of Psychiatrists, UK Drugs in Lactation Advisory Service, UKHSA, UK Malaria Expert Advisory Group, UK Paediatric Antimicrobial Stewardship, UK Teratology Information Service.

We also value the contribution made by clinical pharmacology trainee M. Amran from University College London Hospitals NHS Foundation Trust.

The BNF and BNFC Editorial Team includes specialist pharmacists from the Evelina London Children's Hospital, who bring valuable experience in the use of medicines in paediatric care.

The MHRA have provided valuable assistance.

Correspondents in the pharmaceutical industry have provided information on new products and commented on products in BNFC.

Numerous doctors, pharmacists, nurses, and others have sent comments and suggestions.

The BNF and BNFC Editorial Team are grateful for the support and access to in-house expertise at Pharmaceutical Press and acknowledge the assistance of K. Baxter, A. Chester, N. Potter, D. Wright and their teams.

M. Bhudoye, M. Bradbury, T. Chaney, C. Choi, A. Devanand, O. Ekhuemelo, A. Greenwood, E. Hong, V. Inneh, S. Khan, C. Lam, T. Tahmasi, and Z. Toma provided considerable assistance during the production of this update of BNFC.

BNF Staff

CONTENT DIRECTOR

Kate Towers *BPharm (AU), GCClinPharm (AU)*

HEAD OF CONTENT (BNF AND BNFC)

Kristina Fowlie *MPharm, PGCertPharmPract*

SENIOR EDITORIAL STAFF

Hannah Arnold *BPharm (NZ)*

Rosalind Barker *BMus, MA*

Natasha Bell-Asher *BPharm (NZ), PGDipClinPharm (NZ)*

Alison Brayfield *BPharm, MRCPharm*

Catherine Cadart *BPharm (AU), BA(Hons), GradDipHospPharm (AU), MRCPharm*

Darren Chan *BSc, MSc*

Leah Hamilton *BPharm (NZ)*

Mahinaz Harrison *BPharm, DipPharmPract, IP*

Emily Henderson *BPharm (NZ), PGCertClinPharm (NZ)*

Jannah Jansz *BSc(Hons)*

Florence Ma *BPharm (HK), MClinPharm (HK), MSc*

Jean MacKershan *BSc, PgDip*

Angela McFarlane *BSc, DipClinPharm*

Laura Pham *BPharm(Hons) (AU)*

Claire Preston *BPharm, PGDipMedMan, MRCPharm*

India Smith *MPharm, PGCert*

EDITORIAL STAFF

Sharnee Breingan *BPharm(Hons) (NZ)*

Adam Brelsford *MPharm, PhD*

Anneka Brown *MPharm, PGDipClinPharm, IP, MRCPharm*

Charlotte Clark *MPharm, IP*

Molly Dennis *MPharm, PGDipClinPharm, IP*

Faye Gardner *MPharm, PGCertClinPharm*

Hannah George *MPharm*

Sue Wend Ho *BPharm (AU), MRCPharm*

Emma Jones *MPharm*

Elizabeth King *MAPharmT*

Julia Lacey *BPharm, PGDipClinPharm, PharmD*

Anne Lee *MPhil, FRCPharm*

Sorcha McCann *MPharm, PGDipClinPharm, IPresc, MRCPharm*

Marie McIlwain *MPharm, PGDipPharmPrac, MRCPharm*

Lona Mehta *MPharm, MRCPharm*

Navpreet Mittal *MPharm, PGCert*

Nalwenga Mutambo *MPharm*

Sophie Odeyale *MPharm, PhD*

Barbara Okpala *MPharm, PGDipGPP*

Bhavini Patel *MPharm(Hons), PGDipClinPharm, IP*

Dipesh Patel *MPharm, PGDipClinPharm, IP*

Heenaben Patel *MPharm, PGDipClinPharm, MRCPharm*

Punam Solanki *MPharm, PGCertClinPharm*

Renee Spriggs *BPharm (NZ), PGCertClinPharm (NZ)*

Miranda Stuart *BPharm(Hons) (NZ), PGCertClinPharm (NZ)*

Paula Sutton *BPharm (NZ), PGCertPharm (NZ)*

Shaunagh Swain *BPharm(Hons) (AU)*

Jodie-Anne Swatton *BSc(Hons)*

Harpreet Takhar *MPharm, MRCPharm*

Iris Yapp *MPharm, PGClinDip, GDL*

Jennifer Yick *MPharm*

SUPPORT STAFF

Libby Achilles *BSc(Hons)*

Sophia Aldwinckle *BSc(Hons)*

Lauren Cheetham *BA(Hons)*

Clare Dunne *BSc(Hons), PhD, DIC, ARCS, MRSC*

Melanie Eustace

Ella Farrelly *BSc(Hons), MSc*

Rebecca Harwood *BSc(Hons), MRSB*

Rhiann Jhaj *MPharm*

Jonathan Law *BSc(Hons), MSc*

Philip Lee *BSc(Hons), PhD*

Rebecca Luckhurst *BSc(Hons), MSc*

Hang Nguyen *BSc(Hons)*

Jessica Nguyen *BPharm(Hons) (AU), GradCertPharmPrac (AU)*

Yvette Palmer *BSc(Hons)*

Najwa Zaman *BSc(Hons), MSc*

Paediatric Formulary Committee

CHAIR

David Tuthill
MB BCh, FRCPCH

DEPUTY CHAIR

Neil A. Caldwell
BSc, MSc, IP, MRCPharm, FFRPS

COMMITTEE MEMBERS

Mya Aye
MBBS, MMedSc (Paediatrics), FRCPCH, PG Dip Paediatric Palliative Care

Will Carroll
MD FRCPCH

Emily Lam (lay member)

James H. Larcombe
MB, ChB, PhD, FRCGP, DipAdvGP

Alison Lockley (lay member)
Cert Ed, MA, MA (Econ)

Poonam Lumb
MPharm(Hons), PGDipGPP, IP, MRPharmS

E. David G. McIntosh
MB BS, MPH, LLM, PhD, FAFPHM, FRACP, FRCPCH, FFPM, DRCOG, DCH, DipPharmMed

David Quine
BSc, MB ChB, MRCPCH, MD

Shiva Ramroop
MBBS, MRCPCH

Emma Sturgess
BSc(Hons), MSc, RN(child), PGC (NMP)

Andrew Wignell
MPharm, PGDipClinPharm, IP, MRPharmS

Dental Advisory Group

CHAIR

Sarah Manton
BDS, FDSRCS Ed, FHEA, PhD, FDFTEd

COMMITTEE MEMBERS

Natasha Bell-Asher
BPharm (NZ), PGDipClinPharm (NZ)

Elaine Boylan (observer)
PhD

Andrew K. Brewer
BSc, BchD, MFDS (Glas)

Alexander Crighton
BDS, MB, ChB, FDS, OM

Kristina Fowlie
MPharm, PGCertPharmPract

Faye Gardner
MPharm, PGCertClinPharm

Monica Neil
BDS, MFDS RCS, MSc, MPaed Dent RCS, FDS RCS, MBA

Suzanne Sykes
BDS (Hons), MSc Adv HCP (Open), MFGDP (UK) MJDF, PG Cert Dental Sedation and Pain Management (UCL), Dip FMS (FMS), Dip Spec Care Dent RCSEd

Adrian Thorp
BDS, LLB (Hons), MFDS RCS (Eng), M Surg Dent RCS (Eng), MAcadMEd, FDS RCSEd, FDTFEd, FFGDP (UK), FCGDent, PG Cert

ADVICE ON DENTAL PRACTICE

The **British Dental Association** has contributed to the advice on medicines for dental practice through its representatives on the Dental Advisory Group.

Nurse Prescribers' Advisory Group

COMMITTEE MEMBERS

Kristina Fowlie
MPharm, PGCertPharmPract

Matt Griffiths
BA(Hons), FAETC, RGN, Cert A&E, NISP, PHECC

Tracy Hall
MSc, BSc(Hons), RN, DN, NIP, Dip N, Cert N, QN

Stacey Moss
BSc, RGN

Fiona Peniston-Bird
BSc(Hons), NIP, RHV, RGN

Kathy Radley
BSc, RGN

Neil Thomas (representative of Chief Nursing Officer for Wales)

How BNF and BNF for Children are constructed

Overview

BNFC is an independent professional publication that addresses the day-to-day prescribing information needs of healthcare professionals involved in the care of children. Use of this resource throughout the health service helps to ensure that medicines are used safely, effectively, and appropriately.

Hundreds of changes are made between print editions, and are published monthly in a number of digital formats. The most clinically significant updates are listed under Changes p. xvii.

BNFC is unique in bringing together authoritative, independent guidance on best practice with clinically validated drug information.

Information in BNFC has been validated against emerging evidence, best-practice guidelines, and advice from a network of clinical experts. BNFC includes a great deal of advice that goes beyond marketing authorisations (product licences or summaries of product characteristics). This is necessary because licensed indications frequently do not cover the clinical needs of children; in some cases, products for use in children need to be specially manufactured or imported. Careful consideration has been given to establishing the clinical need for unlicensed interventions with respect to the evidence and experience of their safety and efficacy.

Validation of information follows a standardised process. Where the evidence base is weak, further validation may be undertaken through a process of peer review. The process and its governance are outlined in greater detail in the sections that follow.

Paediatric Formulary Committee

The Paediatric Formulary Committee (PFC) is responsible for the content of BNFC. The PFC comprises pharmacy, medical, and nursing representatives with a paediatric background, and lay representatives who have worked with children or acted as a carer of a paediatric patient; there are also representatives from the Medicines and Healthcare products Regulatory Agency (MHRA) and the Department of Health for England. The PFC decides on matters of policy and reviews amendments to BNFC in the light of new complex or contentious evidence and expert advice.

Dental Advisory Group

The Dental Advisory Group oversees the preparation of advice on the drug management of dental and oral conditions; the group includes representatives from the British Dental Association and a representative from the UK Health Departments.

Nurse Prescribers' Advisory Group

The Nurse Prescribers' Advisory Group oversees the list of drugs approved for inclusion in the Nurse Prescribers' Formulary; the group includes representatives from a range of nursing disciplines and stakeholder organisations.

Expert advisers

BNFC uses representatives from expert groups (professional societies and advisory bodies) to provide expert advice on clinical content. These expert advisers are practice-based healthcare professionals (including doctors, pharmacists, nurses, and dentists), and are regarded as specialists in their field. The role of these expert advisers is to provide independent advice on their area of expertise by reviewing existing text and commenting on amendments drafted by the clinical writers. These clinical experts help to ensure that BNFC remains reliable by:

- commenting on the relevance of the text in the context of best clinical practice in the UK;
- checking draft amendments for appropriate interpretation of any new evidence;
- providing expert opinion in areas of controversy or when reliable evidence is lacking;
- advising on the use of unlicensed medicines or of licensed medicines for unlicensed uses ('off-label' use).

BNFC may also call on other clinical specialists for specific developments when particular expertise is required.

BNFC works closely with a number of expert bodies that produce clinical guidelines. Drafts or pre-publication copies of guidelines are often received for comment and for assimilation into BNFC.

BNF and BNFC Editorial Team

Clinical writers have worked as pharmacists or possess a pharmacy degree and many have a further, relevant post-graduate qualification; they therefore have a sound understanding of how drugs are used in clinical practice. A number of the clinical writers have specific experience of paediatric practice. As a team, the clinical writers are responsible for editing, maintaining, and updating content. They follow a systematic prioritisation process in response to updates to the evidence base in order to ensure the most clinically important topics are reviewed as quickly as possible. In addition, review of content is carried out proactively, with the aim of considering all recommendations for review every 3 to 4 years.

Amendments to the text are drafted when the clinical writers are satisfied that any new information is reliable and relevant. A set of standard criteria defines when content is referred to expert advisers, the Paediatric Formulary Committee or other advisory groups, or submitted for peer review.

Clinical writers prepare the text for publication and undertake a number of validation checks at various stages of the content creation process.

Sources of BNFC information

BNFC uses a variety of sources for its information; the main ones are shown below.

Summaries of product characteristics

BNFC reviews the summaries of product characteristics (SPCs) of all new products as well as revised SPCs for existing products. The SPCs are a key source of product information and are carefully processed. Such processing involves:

- verifying the approved names of all relevant ingredients including 'non-active' ingredients (BNFC is committed to using approved names and descriptions as laid down by the Human Medicines Regulations 2012);
- comparing the indications, cautions, contra-indications, and side-effects with similar existing drugs. Where these are different from the expected pattern, justification is sought for their inclusion or exclusion;
- seeking independent data on the use of drugs in pregnancy and breast-feeding;
- incorporating the information into BNFC using established criteria for the presentation and inclusion of the data;
- checking interpretation of the information by a second clinical writer before submitting to a content approver; changes relating to doses receive a further check;
- identifying potential clinical problems or omissions and seeking further information from manufacturers or from expert advisers;
- constructing, with the help of expert advisers, a comment on the role of the drug in the context of similar drugs.

Much of this processing is applicable to the following sources as well.

Literature

Clinical writers monitor and process various sources of information on a regular basis. When a difference between the advice in BNFC and the source is noted, the new information is assessed for reliability (using tools based on Scottish Intercollegiate Guidelines Network (SIGN) methodology if appropriate) and relevance to UK clinical practice. If necessary, new text is drafted and discussed with expert advisers and the Paediatric Formulary Committee. BNFC enjoys a close working relationship with a number of national information providers.

In addition to the routine process, which is used to identify 'triggers' for changing the content, systematic literature searches are used to identify the best quality evidence available to inform an update. Clinical writers receive training in critical appraisal, literature evaluation, and search strategies.

Consensus guidelines

The advice in BNFC is checked against consensus guidelines produced by expert bodies. The quality of the guidelines is assessed using adapted versions of the AGREE II tool. A number of bodies make drafts or pre-publication copies of the guidelines available to BNFC; it is therefore possible to ensure that a consistent message is disseminated. BNFC routinely processes guidelines from the National Institute for Health and Care Excellence (NICE), the All Wales Medicines Strategy Group (AWMSG), the Scottish Medicines Consortium (SMC), and SIGN.

Reference sources

Paediatric formularies and reference sources are used to provide background information for the review of existing text or for the construction of new text. The BNF and BNFC Editorial Team works closely with the editorial team that produces *Martindale: The Complete Drug Reference* and has access to *Martindale* information resources. Each team keeps the other informed of significant developments and shifts in the trends of drug usage.

Peer review

Although every effort is made to identify the most robust data available, inevitably there are areas where the evidence base is weak or contradictory. While BNFC has the valuable support of expert advisers and the Paediatric Formulary Committee, the recommendations made may be subject to a further level of scrutiny through peer review to ensure they reflect best practice.

Content for open peer review is posted on bnf.org and interested parties are notified via a number of channels, including the BNF and BNFC newsletter.

Statutory information

BNFC routinely processes relevant information from various Government bodies including Statutory Instruments and regulations affecting the Prescription Only Medicines Order. Official compendia such as the British Pharmacopoeia and its addenda are processed routinely to ensure that BNFC complies with the relevant sections of the Human Medicines Regulations 2012.

BNFC maintains close links with the Home Office (in relation to controlled drug regulations) and the Medicines and Healthcare products Regulatory Agency (including the British Pharmacopoeia Commission). Safety warnings issued by the Commission on Human Medicines (CHM) and guidelines on drug use issued by the UK health departments are processed as a matter of routine.

Relevant professional statements issued by the Royal College of Pharmacy are included in BNFC as are guidelines from bodies such as the Royal College of Paediatrics and Child Health.

Medicines and devices

NHS Prescription Services (from the NHS Business Services Authority) provides non-clinical, categorical information (including prices) on the medicines and devices included in BNFC.

Comments from readers

Readers of BNFC are invited to send in comments. Numerous letters and emails are received by the BNF and BNFC Editorial Team. Such feedback helps to ensure that BNFC provides practical and clinically relevant information. Many changes in the presentation and scope of BNFC have resulted from comments sent in by users.

Comments from industry

Close scrutiny of BNFC by the manufacturers provides an additional check and allows them an opportunity to raise issues about BNFC's presentation of the role of various drugs; this is yet another check on the balance of BNFC's advice. All comments are looked at with care and, where necessary, additional information and expert advice are sought.

Market research

Market research is conducted at regular intervals to gather feedback on specific areas of development.

Assessing the evidence

From January 2016, recommendations made in BNFC have been evidence graded to reflect the strength of the recommendation. The addition of evidence grading is to support clinical decision-making based on the best available evidence.

Recommendations from summaries of product characteristics

Recommendations from summaries of product characteristics (SPCs) and other product literature are either preceded by "manufacturer advises" or have the symbol M (manufacturer information) displayed next to the recommendation within the text.

Grading system

BNFC has adopted a five-level grading system from A to E, based on the former SIGN grading system. This grade is displayed next to the recommendation within the text.

Evidence used to make a recommendation is assessed for validity using standardised methodology tools based on AGREE II or SIGN and then assigned a level of evidence. The recommendation is given a grade that is extrapolated from the level of evidence, and an assessment of the body of evidence and its applicability.

Evidence assigned a level 1- or 2- score has an unacceptable level of bias or confounding and is not used to form recommendations.

Levels of evidence

- **Level 1++**
  High quality meta-analyses, systematic reviews of randomised controlled trials (RCTs), or RCTs with a very low risk of bias.
- **Level 1+**
  Well-conducted meta-analyses, systematic reviews, or RCTs with a low risk of bias.
- **Level 1–**
  Meta-analyses, systematic reviews, or RCTs with a high risk of bias.
- **Level 2++**
  High quality systematic reviews of case control or cohort studies; or high quality case control or cohort studies with a very low risk of confounding or bias and a high probability that the relationship is causal.
- **Level 2+**
  Well-conducted case control or cohort studies with a low risk of confounding or bias and a moderate probability that the relationship is causal.
- **Level 2–**
  Case control or cohort studies with a high risk of confounding or bias and a significant risk that the relationship is not causal.
- **Level 3**
  Non-analytic studies, e.g. case reports, case series.
- **Level 4**
  Expert advice or clinical experience from respected authorities.

Grades of recommendation

- **Grade A: High strength**
  NICE-accredited guidelines; or other guidelines, assessed using AGREE II, that meet the grade A threshold; or at least one meta-analysis, systematic review, or RCT rated as 1++, and directly applicable to the target population; or a body of evidence consisting principally of studies rated as 1+, directly applicable to the target population, and demonstrating overall consistency of results.
- **Grade B: Moderate strength**
  Guidelines, assessed using AGREE II, that meet the grade B threshold; or a body of evidence including studies rated as 2++, directly applicable to the target population, and demonstrating overall consistency of results; or extrapolated evidence from studies rated as 1++ or 1+.
- **Grade C: Low strength**
  Guidelines, assessed using AGREE II, that meet the grade C threshold; or a body of evidence including studies rated as 2+, directly applicable to the target population and demonstrating overall consistency of results; or extrapolated evidence from studies rated as 2++.

- **Grade D: Very low strength**
  Guidelines, assessed using AGREE II, that meet the grade D threshold; or evidence level 3; or extrapolated evidence from studies rated as 2+; or tertiary reference source created by a transparent, defined methodology, where the basis for recommendation is clear.
- **Grade E: Practice point**
  Evidence level 4.

How to use BNF and BNFC in print

Introduction

In order to achieve the safe, effective, and appropriate use of medicines, healthcare professionals must be able to use BNFC effectively, and keep up to date with significant changes in BNFC that are relevant to their clinical practice. This *How to Use BNFC* is key to understanding the structure of BNFC for all healthcare professionals involved with prescribing, monitoring, supplying, and administering medicines, as well as supporting the learning of students training to join these professions.

BNFC provides information on the use of medicines in children ranging from neonates (including preterm neonates) to adolescents. The terms infant, child, and adolescent are not used consistently in the literature; to avoid ambiguity actual ages are used in the dose statements in BNFC. The term neonate is used to describe a newborn infant aged 0–28 days. The terms child or children are used generically to describe the entire range from infant to adolescent in BNFC.

Structure of BNFC

The BNFC print edition is structured as follows:

Front matter, comprising information on how to use BNFC, the significant content changes in each edition, and guidance on various prescribing matters (e.g. prescription writing, the use of intravenous drugs, particular considerations for special patient populations).

Chapters, containing drug monographs describing the uses, safety issues and other considerations involved in the use of drugs; drug class monographs; and treatment summaries, covering guidance on the selection of drugs. Monographs and treatment summaries are divided into chapters based on specific aspects of medical care, such as Chapter 5, Infections, or Chapter 16, Emergency treatment of poisoning; or drug use related to a particular system of the body, such as Chapter 2, Cardiovascular.

Within each chapter, content is organised alphabetically by therapeutic use (e.g. Airways disease, obstructive), with the treatment summaries first, (e.g. Asthma, acute p. 174), followed by the monographs of the drugs used to manage the conditions discussed in the treatment summary. Within each therapeutic use, the drugs are organised alphabetically by classification (e.g. Antimuscarinics, Beta$_2$-agonist bronchodilators) and then alphabetically within each classification (e.g. Formoterol fumarate, Salbutamol, Salmeterol, Terbutaline sulfate).

Appendices, covering interactions, borderline substances, and cautionary and advisory labels.

Back matter, covering the lists of medicines approved by the NHS for Dental and Nurse Practitioner prescribing, proprietary and specials manufacturers' contact details, and the index. Quick reference guides for life support and key drug doses in medical emergencies are also included, for ease of access.

Navigating BNFC

The contents page provides the high-level layout of information within BNFC; and in addition, each chapter begins with a small contents section, describing the therapeutic uses covered within that chapter. Once in a chapter, location is guided by the side of the page showing the chapter number (the *thumbnail*), alongside the chapter title. The top of the page includes the therapeutic use (the *running head*) alongside the page number.

Once on a page, visual cues aid navigation: treatment summary information is in black type, with therapeutic use titles similarly styled in black, whereas the use of colour indicates drug-related information, including drug classification titles, drug class monographs, and drug monographs.

Although navigation is possible by browsing, primarily access to the information is via the index, which covers the titles of drug class monographs, drug monographs and treatment summaries. The index also includes the names of branded medicines and other topics of relevance, such as abbreviations, guidance sections, tables, and images.

Content types

Treatment summaries

Treatment summaries are of three main types;

- an overview of delivering a drug to a particular body system (e.g. Skin conditions, management p. 886),
- a comparison between a group or groups of drugs (e.g. Beta-adrenoceptor blocking drugs p. 120),
- an overview of the drug management or prophylaxis of common conditions intended to facilitate rapid appraisal of options (e.g. Hypertension p. 116, or Malaria, prophylaxis p. 476).

In order to select safe and effective medicines for individual children, information in the treatment summaries must be used in conjunction with other prescribing details about the drugs and knowledge of the child's medical and drug history.

Monographs

Overview

All of the information for the systemic use of a drug is contained within one monograph. Where a drug has systemic and local uses, for example, chloramphenicol, and the considerations around drug use are markedly different according to the route of administration, the monograph is split into the relevant chapters.

Monographs used within specialist settings (such as drugs used for malignancy and drugs given via intravitreal injection) contain less detail than regular monographs within BNFC since it is expected that those undertaking treatment will have specialist knowledge and access to specialist literature. These monographs include the words [Specialist drug] alongside the monograph title, and so are easily identifiable in content. Specialist monographs will continue to include information to support patient safety and non-specialist patient care (allergy and cross-sensitivity, conception and contraception, contra-indications, important safety information, indications (high-level), interactions, medicinal forms, patient and carer advice, side-effects, synonyms, and unlicensed use), but will not contain information which is within the remit of specialist care (breast feeding, cautions, directions for administration, doses, drug action, effects on laboratory tests, exception to legal category, handling and storage, hepatic impairment, less suitable for prescribing, monitoring requirements, palliative care, pregnancy, prescribing and dispensing information, pre-treatment screening, profession-specific information, renal impairment, and treatment cessation). The current level of additional prescribing information has been retained for drug monographs that have a mix of specialist and non-specialist uses (such as methotrexate that is used for both malignancy and rheumatological conditions), although specialist indications within these monographs will no longer include doses.

Monographs may include over 20 sections; the number of sections included within an individual monograph is dependent on whether relevant information has been identified and whether it is used within specialist settings. The following information describes these sections and their uses in more detail.

Nomenclature

Monograph titles follow the convention of recommended international non-proprietary names (rINNs), or, in the absence of a rINN, British Approved Names. Relevant synonyms are included below the title and, in some instances a brief description of the drug action is included.

In some monographs, immediately below the nomenclature or drug action, there are a number of cross references used to signpost the user to any additional information they need to consider about a drug. This is most common for drugs formulated in combinations, where users will be signposted to the monographs for the individual ingredients to access full prescribing information for the combination drug (e.g. senna with ispaghula husk p. 52) or for drugs that are related to a drug class monograph (see Drug class monographs, below).

Indication and dose

User feedback has highlighted that one of the main uses of BNFC is identifying indications and doses of drugs. Therefore, indication and dose information appears towards the top of the monograph and highlighted by a coloured panel to aid quick reference.

The indication and dose section is highly structured, giving clarity around which doses should be used for which indications and by which route. Where a dose varies with a specific preparation or formulation, dosing information appears under a heading of the preparation name.

Doses are either expressed in terms of a definite frequency (e.g. 1 g 4 times daily) or in the total daily dose format (e.g. 6 g daily in 3 divided doses); the total daily dose should be divided into individual doses (in the second example, the child should receive 2 g 3 times daily).

Doses for specific patient groups (e.g. neonates) may be included if they are different to the standard dose. Doses for children can be identified by the relevant age range and may vary according to their age or body-weight.

Selecting the dose

The dose of a drug may vary according to different indications, routes of administration, age, body-weight, and body surface area. The right dose should be selected for the right age and body-weight (or body surface area) of the child, as well as for the right indication, route of administration, and preparation.

Wherever possible age and weight ranges do not overlap. When interpreting age ranges it is important to understand that a child is considered to be 11 up until the point of their 12th birthday, meaning that an age range of child 12 to 17 years is applicable to a child from the day of their 12th birthday until the day before their 18th birthday. All age ranges should be interpreted in this way. Similarly, when interpreting weight ranges, it should be understood that a weight of up to 30 kg is applicable to a child up to, but not including, the point that they tip the scales at 30 kg and a weight range of 35 to 59 kg is applicable to a child as soon as they tip the scales at 35 kg right up until, but not including, the point that they tip the scales at 60 kg. All weight ranges should be interpreted in this way.

A pragmatic approach should be applied to these cut-off points depending on the child's physiological development, condition, and if weight is appropriate for the child's age.

For some drugs (e.g. vancomycin p. 398) the neonatal dose varies according to the *corrected gestational* age of the neonate. Corrected gestational age is the neonate's total age expressed in weeks from the start of the mother's last menstrual period. For example, a 3 week old baby born at 27 weeks gestation is treated as having a corrected gestational age of 30 weeks. A term baby has a corrected gestational age of 37–42 weeks when born. For most other drugs, the dose can be based on the child's actual date of birth irrespective of corrected gestational age. However, the degree of prematurity, the maturity of renal and hepatic function, and the clinical properties of the drug need to be considered on an individual basis.

Many children's doses in BNFC are standardised by *body-weight*. To calculate the dose for a given child the weight-standardised dose is multiplied by the child's weight (or occasionally by the child's ideal weight for height). The calculated dose should not normally exceed the maximum recommended dose for an adult. For example, if the dose is 8 mg/kg (max. 300 mg), a child of 10 kg body-weight should receive 80 mg, but a child of 40 kg body-weight should receive 300 mg (rather than 320 mg). Calculation by body-weight in the overweight child may result in much higher doses being administered than necessary; in such cases, the dose should be calculated from an ideal weight for height.

Occasionally, some doses in BNFC are standardised by *body surface area* because many physiological phenomena correlate better with body surface area. In these cases, to calculate the dose for a given child, the body surface area-standardised dose is multiplied by the child's body surface area. The child's body surface area can be estimated from his or her weight using the tables for Body surface area in children (image) p. 1478.

Wherever possible, doses are expressed in terms of a definite frequency (e.g. if the dose is 1 mg/kg twice daily, a child of body-weight 9 kg would receive 9 mg twice daily). Occasionally, it is necessary to include doses in the total daily dose format (e.g. 10 mg/kg daily in 3 divided doses); in these cases the total daily dose should be divided into individual doses (in this example a child of body-weight 9 kg would receive 30 mg 3 times daily).

Most drugs can be administered at slightly irregular intervals during the day. Some drugs, e.g. antimicrobials, are best given at regular intervals. Some flexibility should be allowed in children to avoid waking them during the night. For example, the night-time dose may be given at the child's bedtime.

Special care should be taken when converting doses from one metric unit to another, and when calculating infusion rates or the volume of a preparation to administer. Where possible, doses should be rounded to facilitate administration of suitable volumes of liquid preparations, or an appropriate strength of tablet or capsule.

Other information relevant to Indication and dose

The dose panel also contains, where known, an indication of **pharmacokinetic considerations** that may affect the choice of dose, and **dose equivalence** information, which may aid the selection of dose when switching between drugs or preparations.

BNFC includes **unlicensed use** of medicines when the clinical need cannot be met by licensed medicines; such use should be supported by appropriate evidence and experience. When BNFC recommends an unlicensed medicine or the 'off-label' use of a licensed medicine, this is shown below the indication and dose panel in the unlicensed use section.

Minimising harm and drug safety

The drug chosen to treat a particular condition should minimise the patient's susceptibility to adverse effects and, where co-morbidities exist, have minimal detrimental effects on the patient's other diseases. To achieve this, the *Contra-indications*, *Cautions* and *Side-effects* of the relevant drug should be reviewed.

The information under Cautions can be used to assess the risks of using a drug in a patient who has co-morbidities that are also included in the Cautions for that drug—if a safer alternative cannot be found, the drug may be prescribed while monitoring the patient for adverse effects or deterioration in the co-morbidity. Contra-indications are far more restrictive than Cautions and mean that the drug should be avoided in a patient with a condition that is contra-indicated.

The impact that potential side-effects may have on a patient's quality of life should also be assessed. For instance, in a child who has constipation, it may be preferable to avoid a drug that frequently causes constipation.

The *Important safety information* section in BNFC, delineated by a coloured outline box, highlights important safety concerns, often those raised by regulatory authorities or guideline producers. Safety warnings issued by the Commission on Human Medicines (CHM) or Medicines and Healthcare products Regulatory Agency (MHRA) are found here.

Drug selection should aim to minimise drug interactions. If it is necessary to prescribe a potentially serious combination of drugs, patients should be monitored appropriately. The mechanisms underlying drug interactions are explained in Appendix 1, followed by details of drug interactions.

Use of drugs in specific patient populations

Drug selection should aim to minimise the potential for drug accumulation, adverse drug reactions, and exacerbation of pre-existing hepatic or renal disease. If it is necessary to prescribe drugs whose effect is altered by hepatic or renal disease, appropriate drug dose adjustments should be made, and patients should be monitored adequately. The general principles for prescribing are outlined under Prescribing in hepatic impairment p. 16, and Prescribing in renal impairment p. 16. Information about drugs that should be avoided or used with caution in hepatic disease or renal impairment can be found in drug monographs under *Hepatic impairment* and *Renal impairment* (e.g. fluconazole p. 463).

Similarly, drug selection should aim to minimise harm to the fetus, nursing infant, and mother. The infant should be monitored for potential side-effects of drugs used by the mother during pregnancy or breast-feeding. The general principles for prescribing are outlined under Prescribing in pregnancy p. 19 and Prescribing in breast-feeding p. 19. The Treatment summaries provide guidance on the drug treatment of common conditions that can occur during pregnancy or breast-feeding (e.g. Venous thromboembolism p. 101). Information about the use of specific drugs during pregnancy and breast feeding can be found in their drug monographs under *Pregnancy*, and *Breast feeding* (e.g. fluconazole p. 463).

The section *Conception and contraception* contains information around considerations for females of childbearing potential or men who might father a child (e.g. isotretinoin p. 937).

Administration and monitoring

When selecting the most appropriate drug, it may be necessary to screen the patient for certain genetic markers or metabolic states. This information is included within a section called *Pre-treatment screening* (e.g. abacavir p. 513). This section covers one-off tests required to assess the suitability of a patient for a particular drug.

Once the drug has been selected, it needs to be given in the most appropriate manner. The *Directions for administration* section provides practical information on the preparation of intravenous drug infusions, including compatibility of drugs with standard intravenous infusion fluids, method of dilution or reconstitution, and administration rates. In addition, general advice relevant to other routes of administration is provided within this section (e.g. fentanyl p. 334) and further details, such as masking the bitter taste of some medicines.

Whenever possible, intramuscular injections should be **avoided** in children because they are painful.

After selecting and administering the most appropriate drug by the most appropriate route, patients should be monitored to ensure they are achieving the expected benefits from drug treatment without any unwanted side-effects. The *Monitoring* section specifies any special monitoring requirements, including information on monitoring the plasma concentration of drugs with a narrow therapeutic index (e.g. theophylline p. 196). Monitoring may, in certain cases, be affected by the impact of a drug on laboratory tests (e.g. hydroxocobalamin p. 711), and this information is included in *Effects on laboratory tests*.

In some cases, when a drug is withdrawn, further monitoring or precautions may be advised (e.g. clonidine hydrochloride p. 120); these are covered under *Treatment cessation*.

Choice and supply

The prescriber, the child's carer, and the child (if appropriate) should agree on the health outcomes desired and on the strategy for achieving them. Taking the time to explain to the child (and the child's carer if appropriate) the rationale and the potential adverse effects of treatment may improve adherence. For some medicines there is a special need for counselling (e.g. appropriate posture during administration of doxycycline p. 434, or recognising signs of blood, liver, or skin disorders with carbamazepine p. 234); this is shown in *Patient and carer advice*.

Other information contained in the latter half of the monograph also helps prescribers and those dispensing medicines choose medicinal forms (by indicating information such as flavour or when branded products are not interchangeable e.g. modified-release theophylline p. 196), assess the suitability of a drug for prescribing, understand the NHS funding status for a drug (e.g. sildenafil p. 139), or assess when a patient may be able to purchase a drug without prescription (e.g. loperamide hydrochloride p. 55).

Medicinal forms

In BNFC, preparations follow immediately after the monograph for the drug that is their main ingredient.

The medicinal forms section provides information on the type of formulation (e.g. tablet), the amount of active drug in a solid dosage form, and the concentration of active drug in a liquid dosage form. The legal status is shown for prescription-only medicines and controlled drugs, as well as pharmacy medicines and medicines on the general sales list. Practitioners are reminded, by a statement under the heading of "Medicinal Form" that not all products containing a specific drug ingredient may be similarly licensed. To be clear on the precise licensing status of specific medicinal forms, practitioners should check the product literature for the particular product being prescribed or dispensed.

Details of all medicinal forms available on the dm+d for each drug in BNFC appears in this section. In print editions, due to space constraints, only certain branded products are included in detail. Where medicinal forms are listed they should not be inferred as equivalent to the other brands listed under the same form heading. For example, all the products listed under a heading of "Modified release capsule" will be available as modified release capsules, however, the brands listed under that form heading may have different release profiles, the available strengths may vary and/or the products may have different licensing information. Practitioners must ensure that the particular product being prescribed or dispensed is appropriate.

Children should be prescribed a preparation that complements their daily routine, and that provides the right dose of drug for the right indication and route of administration. When dispensing liquid preparations, a sugar-free preparation should always be used in preference to one containing sugar. Patients receiving medicines containing cariogenic sugars should be advised of appropriate dental hygiene measures to prevent caries.

Typical layout of a monograph and associated medicinal forms

❶ Class monographs and Drug monographs
In most cases, all information that relates to an individual drug is contained within its drug monograph

Some drugs formulated in combinations include cross reference links that signpost to component drug monographs. Cross reference links are preceded by the following statement, which appears below the title of relevant monographs: The properties listed below are those particular to the combination only. For the properties of the components please consider, ...

Class monographs have been created where substantial amounts of information are common to all drugs in a drug class; these are indicated by a flag symbol in a circle:

Drug monographs with a corresponding class monograph are indicated by a tab with a flag symbol; the tab includes the page number of the corresponding class monograph: 1234

Drug monographs that are used within specialist settings include [Specialist drug] alongside the monograph title. These monographs contain less detail, however, information to support patient safety and non-specialist patient care is included where relevant information has been identified

For further information, see How to use BNF Publications

❷ Drug classifications
Used to inform users of the class of a drug and to assist in finding other drugs of the same class. May be based on pharmacological class (e.g. opioids) but can also be associated with the use of the drug (e.g. cough suppressants)

❸ Review date
The date of last review of the content

❹ Specific preparation name
If the dose varies with a specific preparation or formulation it appears under a heading of the preparation name

Class monograph ❶

CLASSIFICATION ❷

1234

Drug monograph ❶

❸ 01-Sep-2023

(Synonym) another name by which a drug may be known

- **DRUG ACTION** how a drug exerts its effect in the body
- **INDICATIONS AND DOSE**
  Indications are the clinical reasons a drug is used. The dose of a drug will often depend on the indications
  Indication
  ▸ ROUTE
  ▸ Age groups: [Neonate/Child]
  Dose and frequency of administration (max. dose)
  SPECIFIC PREPARATION NAME ❹
  Indication
  ▸ ROUTE
  ▸ Age groups: [Neonate/Child]
  Dose and frequency of administration (max. dose)
  DOSE ADJUSTMENTS DUE TO INTERACTIONS dosing information when used concurrently with other drugs
  DOSES AT EXTREMES OF BODY-WEIGHT dosing information for patients who are overweight or underweight
  DOSE EQUIVALENCE AND CONVERSION information around the bioequivalence between formulations of the same drug, or equivalent doses of drugs that are members of the same class
  PHARMACOKINETICS how the body affects a drug (absorption, distribution, metabolism, and excretion)
  POTENCY a measure of drug activity expressed in terms of the concentration required to produce an effect of given intensity
- **UNLICENSED USE** describes the use of medicines outside the terms of their UK licence (off-label use), or use of medicines that have no licence for use in the UK

IMPORTANT SAFETY INFORMATION
Information produced and disseminated by drug regulators often highlights serious risks associated with the use of a drug, and may include advice that is mandatory

- **CONTRA-INDICATIONS** circumstances when a drug should be avoided
- **CAUTIONS** details of precautions required
- **INTERACTIONS** when one drug changes the effects of another drug; the mechanisms underlying drug interactions are explained in Appendix 1
- **SIDE-EFFECTS** listed in order of frequency, where known, and arranged alphabetically
- **ALLERGY AND CROSS-SENSITIVITY** for drugs that carry an increased risk of hypersensitivity reactions
- **CONCEPTION AND CONTRACEPTION** potential for a drug to have harmful effects on an unborn child when prescribing for a woman of childbearing age or for a man trying to father a child; information on the effect of drugs on the efficacy of latex condoms or diaphragms

- PREGNANCY advice on the use of a drug during pregnancy
- BREAST FEEDING [EvGr] advice on the use of a drug during breast feeding ⟨A⟩ ❺
- HEPATIC IMPAIRMENT advice on the use of a drug in hepatic impairment
- RENAL IMPAIRMENT advice on the use of a drug in renal impairment
- PRE-TREATMENT SCREENING covers one off tests required to assess the suitability of a patient for a particular drug
- MONITORING REQUIREMENTS specifies any special monitoring requirements, including information on monitoring the plasma concentration of drugs with a narrow therapeutic index
- EFFECTS ON LABORATORY TESTS for drugs that can interfere with the accuracy of seemingly unrelated laboratory tests
- TREATMENT CESSATION specifies whether further monitoring or precautions are advised when the drug is withdrawn
- DIRECTIONS FOR ADMINISTRATION practical information on the preparation of intravenous drug infusions; general advice relevant to other routes of administration
- PRESCRIBING AND DISPENSING INFORMATION practical information around how a drug can be prescribed and dispensed including details of when brand prescribing is necessary
- HANDLING AND STORAGE includes information on drugs that can cause adverse effects to those who handle them before they are taken by, or administered to, a patient; advice on storage conditions
- PATIENT AND CARER ADVICE for drugs with a special need for counselling
- PROFESSION SPECIFIC INFORMATION provides details of the restrictions certain professions such as dental practitioners or nurse prescribers need to be aware of when prescribing on the NHS
- NATIONAL FUNDING/ACCESS DECISIONS references to NICE Technology Appraisals, SMC advice and AWMSG advice
- LESS SUITABLE FOR PRESCRIBING preparations that are considered by the Paediatric Formulary Committee to be less suitable for prescribing
- EXCEPTION TO LEGAL CATEGORY advice and information on drugs which may be sold without a prescription under specific conditions

---

- MEDICINAL FORMS

  Form

  CAUTIONARY AND ADVISORY LABELS if applicable

  EXCIPIENTS clinically important but not comprehensive [consult manufacturer information for full details]

  ELECTROLYTES if clinically significant quantities occur

  ▸ **Preparation name** (Manufacturer/Non-proprietary)

  Drug name and strength pack sizes [PoM] ❻ Prices

  Combinations available this indicates a combination preparation is available and a cross reference page number is provided to locate this preparation

❺ Evidence grading

Evidence grading to reflect the strengths of recommendations will be applied as content goes through the revalidation process. A five level evidence grading system based on the former SIGN grading system has been adopted. The grades ⟨A⟩ ⟨B⟩ ⟨C⟩ ⟨D⟩ ⟨E⟩ are displayed next to the recommendations within the text, and are preceded by the symbol: [EvGr]

The symbol ⟨M⟩ indicates manufacturer information

For further information, see How BNF Publications are constructed

❻ Legal categories

[PoM] This symbol has been placed against those preparations that are available only on a prescription issued by an appropriate practitioner. For more detailed information see *Medicines, Ethics and Practice*, London, Pharmaceutical Press (always consult latest edition)

[CD1] [CD2] [CD3] [CD4-1] [CD4-2] [CD5] These symbols indicate that the preparations are subject to the prescription requirements of the Misuse of Drugs Act

For regulations governing prescriptions for such preparations, see Controlled Drugs and Drug Dependence

Not all monographs include all possible sections; sections are only included when relevant information has been identified

Information on possible inclusion of excipients and electrolytes is covered at the level of the dose form (e.g. tablet). It is not possible to keep abreast of all of the generic products available on the UK market, and so this information serves as a reminder to the healthcare professional that, if the presence of a particular excipient is of concern, they should check the product literature for the particular product being prescribed or dispensed.

Cautionary and advisory labels that pharmacists are recommended to add when dispensing are included in the medicinal forms section. Details of these labels can be found in Appendix 3, Guidance for cautionary and advisory labels p. 1433.

In the case of compound preparations, the prescribing information for all constituents should be taken into account.

Prices in BNFC

Basic NHS **net prices** are given in BNFC to provide an indication of relative cost. Where there is a choice of suitable preparations for a particular disease or condition the relative cost may be used in making a selection. Cost-effective prescribing must, however, take into account other factors (such as dose frequency and duration of treatment) that affect the total cost. The use of more expensive drugs is justified if it will result in better treatment of the patient, or a reduction of the length of an illness, or the time spent in hospital.

Prices are regularly updated using the Drug Tariff and proprietary price information published by the NHS dictionary of medicines and devices (dm+d, www.nhsbsa.nhs.uk/pharmacies-gp-practices-and-appliance-contractors/nhs-dictionary-medicines-and-devices-dmd). The weekly updated dm+d data (including prices) can be accessed using the dm+d browser of the NHS Business Services Authority (dmd-browser.nhsbsa.nhs.uk/). Prices have been calculated from the net cost used in pricing NHS prescriptions and generally reflect whole dispensing packs. Prices for extemporaneously prepared preparations are not provided in BNFC as prices vary between different manufacturers.

BNFC prices are not suitable for quoting to patients seeking private prescriptions or contemplating over-the-counter purchases because they do not take into account VAT, professional fees, and other overheads.

A fuller explanation of costs to the NHS may be obtained from the Drug Tariff. Separate drug tariffs are applicable to England and Wales (www.nhsbsa.nhs.uk/pharmacies-gp-practices-and-appliance-contractors/drug-tariff), Scotland (publichealthscotland.scot/resources-and-tools/medical-practice-and-pharmaceuticals/scottish-drug-tariff/), and Northern Ireland (bso.hscni.net/directorates/operations/family-practitioner-services/pharmacy/contractor-information/drug-tariff-and-related-materials/drug-tariff-2/); prices in the different tariffs may vary.

Drug class monographs

Drug class monographs contain information relating to a class of drugs sharing the same properties (e.g. tetracyclines p. 433); this ensures such information is easier to find, and has a regularised structure.

For consistency and ease of use, the class monograph follows the same structure as a drug monograph. Class monographs are indicated by the presence of a flag (e.g. beta-adrenoceptor blockers (systemic) p. 121). If a drug monograph has a corresponding class monograph, that needs to be considered in tandem, in order to understand the full information about a drug, the monograph is also indicated by a flag 1234 (e.g. metoprolol tartrate p. 126). Within this flag, the page number of the drug class monograph is provided (e.g. 1234), to help navigate the user to this information. This is particularly useful where occasionally, due to differences in therapeutic use, the drug monograph may not directly follow the drug class monograph (e.g. sotalol hydrochloride p. 90).

Other content

Nutrition

Appendix 2 includes tables of ACBS-approved enteral feeds and nutritional supplements based on their energy and protein content. Sections on foods for special diets, specialised formulae for specific clinical conditions, and nutritional supplements for metabolic diseases are also included.

Other useful information

Finding significant changes in BNFC

- ***Changes***, provides a list of significant changes, dose changes, classification changes, new names, and new preparations that have been incorporated into BNFC, as well as a list of preparations that have been discontinued and removed from BNFC. Changes listed online are cumulative (from one print edition to the next), and can be printed off each month to show the main changes since the last print edition as an aide memoire for those using print copies. So many changes are made for each update of BNFC, that not all of them can be accommodated in the *Changes* section. We encourage healthcare professionals to review regularly the prescribing information on drugs that they encounter frequently;
- ***Changes to the Dental Practitioners' Formulary***, are located at the end of the Dental List;
- ***BNF and BNFC newsletter***, is available free of charge. It alerts healthcare professionals to details of significant changes in the clinical content of these publications and to the way that this information is delivered. It also provides tips on using these publications effectively, and highlights forthcoming changes to the publications. To sign up for the BNF and BNFC newsletter go to www.bnf.org.

Using other sources for medicines information

BNFC is designed as a digest for rapid reference. Less detail is given on areas such as malignant disease and anaesthesia. BNFC should be interpreted in the light of professional knowledge and supplemented as necessary by specialised publications and by reference to the product literature. Information is also available from medicines information services.

Changes

Monthly updates are provided online via Medicines Complete and the NICE BNFC website. The changes listed below are cumulative (from one print edition to the next).

Significant changes

Significant changes that appear in the print edition of BNFC 2026 – 2027:

- Aciclovir p. 500: new dosing for post-exposure prophylaxis of varicella zoster infection.
- Adrenaline/epinephrine: name change to adrenaline p. 159.
- Albumin solution: name change to albumin p. 736.
- Amoxicillin p. 417: updated indications and dose for prophylaxis of recurrent urinary-tract infection.
- Antibacterials, principles of therapy p. 358: updated guidance on notifiable diseases.
- Antibacterials, use for prophylaxis p. 359: updated guidance for endoscopic retrograde cholangiopancreatography.
- Antibacterials, use for prophylaxis p. 359: updated guidance for *Haemophilus influenzae* type b infection: prevention of secondary disease.
- Anti-D (Rh0) immunoglobulin: name change to anti-D immunoglobulins p. 953.
- Antidiabetic drugs and drugs with neuromuscular blocking effects: pharmacodynamic effects drug groups deleted from Interactions.
- Asthma, acute p. 174: update to criteria for severity of acute asthma attacks.
- Azithromycin p. 402: new indication and dose for prevention of secondary case of *Haemophilus influenzae* type b disease.
- Azithromycin p. 402: updated indication and dose for uncomplicated gonorrhoea and new indication and dose for gonococcal conjunctivitis.
- Bee venom extract: name change to bee venom extracts p. 209.
- Birch bark extract: name change to birch bark extracts p. 895.
- Budesonide with formoterol p. 187 (*Symbicort* 100/6 Turbohaler®): updated dosing for asthma, maintenance and reliever therapy.
- Cefalexin p. 385: updated indications and dose for prophylaxis of recurrent urinary-tract infection.
- Cefixime p. 389: updated indications and dose for uncomplicated gonorrhoea and disseminated gonococcal infection.
- Cefotaxime p. 389: deleted indication and dose for disseminated gonococcal infection.
- Ceftriaxone p. 391: updated indication for uncomplicated gonorrhoea and updated indications and dose for disseminated gonococcal infections.
- Cefuroxime p. 388: new indication and dose for gonococcal conjunctivitis.
- Charcoal, activated: name change to activated charcoal p. 1043.
- Ciprofloxacin p. 429: new indication and dose for prevention of secondary case of *Haemophilus influenzae* type b disease.
- Ciprofloxacin p. 429: updated indication and dose for disseminated gonococcal infection.
- COVID-19 p. 490: update to guidance for symptomatic management of cough, and anxiety and agitation.
- COVID-19 vaccine p. 988: monograph updated to reflect current guidance.
- COVID-19 vaccines p. 964: updated guidance for immunisation.
- COVID-19 vaccines p. 964: updated guidance on the Spring 2026 immunisation campaign.
- Digoxin-specific antibody: name change to digoxin-specific antibody fragments p. 1046.
- Diphtheria vaccine p. 965: updated guidance for immunisation.
- Diphtheria with tetanus and pertussis vaccine: name change to diphtheria, tetanus, and pertussis vaccine p. 988.
- Diphtheria with tetanus and poliomyelitis vaccine: name change to diphtheria, tetanus, and poliomyelitis vaccine p. 989.
- Diphtheria with tetanus, pertussis and poliomyelitis vaccine: name change to diphtheria, tetanus, pertussis, and poliomyelitis vaccine p. 989.
- Diphtheria with tetanus, pertussis, poliomyelitis and haemophilus influenzae type b vaccine: name change to diphtheria, tetanus, pertussis, poliomyelitis, and haemophilus influenzae type b vaccine p. 990.
- Dried prothrombin complex: name change to prothrombin complex p. 98.
- Drugs with anticoagulant effects and drugs with antiplatelet effects: pharmacodynamic effects drug groups combined and renamed as drugs that cause bleeding; see Appendix 1 Interactions p. 1053.
- Epilepsy p. 227: updated guidance on management.
- Factor VIII fraction, dried: name change to factor VIII p. 95.
- Factor VIIa (recombinant): name change to factor VIIa p. 95.
- Factor XIII A-subunit (recombinant): name change to factor XIII A-subunit p. 97.
- Factor XIII fraction, dried: name change to factor XIII p. 97.
- Fenfluramine p. 238: new indication and dose for Lennox-Gastaut syndrome and update to structure of existing dosing for Dravet syndrome.
- Fibrinogen, dried: name change to fibrinogen p. 97.
- Genital system infections, antibacterial therapy p. 368: updated guidance for management of gonorrhoea: uncomplicated.
- Givinostat p. 811: new important safety information.
- GLP-1 receptor agonists and dual GLP-1/GIP receptor agonists: strengthened warnings on acute pancreatitis, including necrotising and fatal cases [MHRA/CHM advice] (advice in dulaglutide, liraglutide, semaglutide; see example in dulaglutide p. 560).
- Grass pollen extract: name change to grass pollen extracts p. 209.
- Guidance included on biotin interference with laboratory tests (advice in biotin, levothyroxine sodium, liothyronine sodium, parenteral nutrition supplements, vitamins with minerals and trace elements; see example in levothyroxine sodium p. 599).
- Haemophilus influenzae type b conjugate vaccine p. 966: updated guidance for immunisation.
- Haemophilus influenzae type b with meningococcal group C vaccine: name change to haemophilus influenzae type b and meningococcal group C vaccine p. 990.
- Helminth infections p. 473: updated guidance for roundworm and hookworm infections.
- Heparin (unfractionated): name change to heparin p. 111.
- Hepatitis B vaccine p. 968: updated guidance for immunisation.
- Hepatitis B vaccine p. 968: updated guidance for post-exposure prophylaxis of neonates.
- Herpesvirus infections p. 498: updated guidance for post-exposure prophylaxis against chickenpox or shingles.
- House dust mite extract: name change to house-dust mite extracts p. 210.
- Hydroxyethylcellulose: name change to hyetellose p. 841.

- Immunisation schedule p. 961: updated guidance.
- Immunisation schedule p. 961: updated guidance for immunisation against respiratory syncytial virus.
- Immunoglobulins p. 951: updated guidance for uses of normal immunoglobulin and varicella-zoster immunoglobulin.
- Improving information supplied with Gabapentinoids (pregabalin/gabapentin), Benzodiazepines and Z-drugs [MHRA/CHM advice] (advice in gabapentin, all benzodiazepines; see Benzodiazepines p. 266).
- Influenza p. 525: updated guidance on management.
- Influenza vaccine p. 971: updated guidance for immunisation.
- Influenza vaccine (inactivated) p. 994: update to ovalbumin content.
- Influenza vaccine (live) p. 1001: update to cautions.
- Isotretinoin p. 937: changes to prescribing guidance and additional risk minimisation measures [MHRA/CHM advice].
- Isotretinoin p. 937: updates to prescribing guidance and survey of services [MHRA/CHM advice].
- Ivacaftor with tezacaftor and elexacaftor p. 220 (*Kaftrio*®): risk of psychological side effects [MHRA/CHM advice].
- Levamisole p. 645: indications and dosing for roundworm infections and hookworm infections removed, and important safety information updated.
- Life support algorithm (image) p. inside back pages: newborn life support algorithm, paediatric basic life support algorithm, paediatric out-of-hospital basic life support algorithm, and paediatric advanced life support algorithm images updated.
- Liraglutide p. 562: monograph updated to incorporate new preparations.
- Malaria, treatment p. 482: updated guidance.
- Measles, mumps and rubella vaccine: name change to measles, mumps, and rubella vaccine p. 1002.
- Measles, Mumps and Rubella vaccine p. 972: updated guidance for immunisation.
- Meningococcal group B vaccine (rDNA, component, adsorbed): name change to meningococcal group B vaccine p. 995.
- Meningococcal groups A with C and W135 and Y vaccine: name change to meningococcal groups A, C, W135, and Y vaccine p. 996.
- Meningococcal vaccines p. 973: updated guidance for immunisation.
- Mesalazine p. 33 and idiopathic intracranial hypertension [MHRA/CHM advice].
- Nitrofurantoin p. 458: updated indications and dose for prophylaxis of recurrent urinary-tract infection.
- Noradrenaline/norepinephrine: name change to noradrenaline p. 145.
- Normal immunoglobulin p. 955: new dosing for post-exposure prophylaxis of varicella-zoster infection.
- Ocular corticosteroids: cautions updated (advice in betamethasone, dexamethasone, fluorometholone, prednisolone; see example in fluorometholone p. 836).
- Ocular NSAIDs: cautions updated (advice in diclofenac sodium, ketorolac trometamol; see example in diclofenac sodium p. 818).
- Ofloxacin p. 846: deleted indication and dose for disseminated gonococcal infection.
- Omeprazole p. 64: new advice in cautions and renal impairment for oral suspension.
- Paracetamol p. 325: reminder that taking paracetamol during pregnancy remains safe [MHRA/CHM advice].
- Paraffin, yellow, soft: name change to yellow soft paraffin p. 843.
- Penicillamine p. 768: harm from incorrect recording of a penicillin allergy as a penicillamine allergy [National Patient Safety Alert advice].
- Penicillins: harm from incorrect recording of a penicillin allergy as a penicillamine allergy [National Patient Safety Alert advice] (advice in all penicillins; see Penicillins p. 411).
- Pertussis vaccine p. 974: updated guidance for immunisation.
- Pneumococcal polysaccharide conjugate vaccine (adsorbed): name change to pneumococcal polysaccharide conjugate vaccine p. 996.
- Pneumococcal vaccine p. 975: updated guidance for immunisation.
- Poliomyelitis vaccine p. 976: updated guidance for immunisation.
- Protein C concentrate: name change to protein C p. 98.
- Rasburicase p. 684: harm from delayed administration of rasburicase for tumour lysis syndrome [National Patient Safety Alert advice].
- Rasburicase p. 684: update to indication and dosing.
- Respiratory syncytial virus immunisation p. 979: updated guidance.
- Respiratory syncytial virus immunisation p. 979: updated guidance for immunisation of infants and children.
- Respiratory syncytial virus (RSV) vaccine: name change to respiratory syncytial virus vaccine p. 998.
- Respiratory syncytial virus vaccine p. 998 (*Abrysvo*®): be alert to a small risk of Guillain-Barré syndrome following vaccination in older adults [MHRA/CHM advice].
- Respiratory system infections, antibacterial therapy p. 371: updated guidance on community-acquired pneumonia.
- Respiratory system infections, antibacterial therapy p. 371: updated guidance on hospital-acquired pneumonia.
- Salbutamol p. 181: reminder of the risks from overuse in asthma and to be aware of changes in the SABA prescribing guidelines [MHRA/CHM advice].
- Semaglutide p. 77 (*Wegovy*®, *Ozempic*®, and *Rybelsus*®): risk of non-arteritic anterior ischaemic optic neuropathy (NAION) [MHRA/CHM advice].
- Sepsis p. 362: updated guidance on intravenous fluids and vasopressors.
- Silver sulfadiazine: name change to sulfadiazine silver p. 899.
- Sodium clodronate: name change to clodronate disodium p. 534.
- Sodium valproate p. 252: update to important safety information.
- Supply of medicines p. 6: updated guidance on labelling of prescribed medicines.
- Terbutaline sulfate p. 183: reminder of the risks from overuse in asthma and to be aware of changes in the SABA prescribing guidelines [MHRA/CHM advice].
- Tetanus vaccine p. 981: updated guidance for immunisation.
- Thiopurines and intrahepatic cholestasis of pregnancy [MHRA/CHM advice] (advice in azathioprine, mercaptopurine, tioguanine; see example in azathioprine p. 638).
- Tree pollen extract: name change to tree pollen extracts p. 211.
- Trimethoprim p. 443: updated indications and dose for prophylaxis of recurrent urinary-tract infection.
- Ulipristal acetate p. 626: updated breast-feeding advice.
- Urea (13C) p. 67: name change to urea (^{13}C).
- Vaccination, general principles p. 959: updated guidance for vaccines and asplenia, splenic dysfunction, or complement disorders.
- Vaccination, general principles p. 959: updated guidance on vaccination in pregnancy.
- Valproate (*Belvo*®, *Convulex*®, *Depakote*®, *Dyzantil*®, *Epilim*®, *Epilim Chrono*® or *Chronosphere*®, *Episenta*®, *Epival*®, and *Syonell*®): updated safety and educational

materials to support patient discussion on reproductive risks [MHRA/CHM advice] (advice in sodium valproate, valproic acid; see example in sodium valproate p. 252).
- Valproic acid p. 259: update to important safety information.
- Varicella-zoster vaccines p. 983: updated guidance for pre-exposure prophylaxis against varicella (chickenpox).
- Vitamins p. 780: updated guidance for management of vitamin D deficiency.
- Wasp venom extract: name change to wasp venom extracts p. 212.
- Zanamivir p. 528: deleted indication and dose for treatment of influenza [uncomplicated, resistant to other treatments, and inhaled formulation unsuitable].
- Zanamivir p. 528: update to indications for prophylaxis and treatment of influenza.

Dose changes

Changes in dose statements that appear in the print edition of BNFC 2026 — 2027:
- Aciclovir p. 500 [update to neonate dose for varicella zoster (chickenpox), treatment].
- Amiodarone hydrochloride p. 88 [update to dose for ventricular fibrillation or pulseless ventricular tachycardia refractory to defibrillation [for cardiopulmonary resuscitation]].
- Amoxicillin p. 417 [update to age ranges and duration of treatment for community-acquired pneumonia in children].
- Baloxavir marboxil p. 527 [update to age ranges and dosing for post-exposure prophylaxis of influenza and treatment of influenza].
- Clarithromycin p. 403 [update to age ranges and duration of treatment for community-acquired pneumonia in children].
- Dexamethasone p. 543 [new indication and dose for congenital adrenal hyperplasia replaces previous indication and dose for physiological replacement].
- Erythromycin p. 406 [update to age ranges and duration of treatment for community-acquired pneumonia in children].
- Evinacumab p. 157 [update to age range].
- Fludrocortisone acetate p. 544 [new indications for primary adrenal insufficiency and congenital adrenal hyperplasia replace previous indication for mineralocorticoid replacement in adrenocortical insufficiency; updates to structure of dosing].
- Oseltamivir p. 527 [update to indication for post-exposure prophylaxis of influenza, and update to dosing for neonates in post-exposure prophylaxis of influenza].
- Palivizumab p. 986 [update to indications and dose].
- Pimecrolimus p. 919 [update to dosing for short-term treatment of mild to moderate atopic eczema (including flares) when topical corticosteroids cannot be used].
- Prednisolone p. 548 [new indications and doses for adrenal insufficiency and congenital adrenal hyperplasia replace previous indication and dose for corticosteroid replacement therapy].
- Vancomycin p. 398 [update to indications and dose for neonates].
- Varicella-zoster immunoglobulin p. 958 [update to indications and dose].
- Varicella-zoster vaccine p. 1004 [update to dose interval for immunisation against varicella infection (chickenpox) for children aged 1 year and older].

Classification changes

Classification changes that appear in the print edition of BNFC 2026 — 2027:
- Levamisole p. 645 [primary classification changed to Immunosuppressants].

New monographs

New monographs that appear in the print edition of BNFC 2026 — 2027:
- *Abrysvo*® [respiratory syncytial virus vaccine p. 998].
- *Adtralza*® [tralokinumab p. 924].
- *Alyftrek*® [deutivacaftor with tezacaftor and vanzacaftor p. 218].
- *Andembry*® [garadacimab p. 215].
- Artesunate p. 484.
- Baricitinib p. 802.
- *Beyfortus*® [nirsevimab p. 985].
- *Hympavzi*® [marstacimab p. 94].
- *Imvanex*® [smallpox and mpox vaccines p. 998].
- *Jakavi*® [ruxolitinib p. 692].
- *Nemluvio*® [nemolizumab p. 923].
- *Noxafil*® [posaconazole p. 466].
- *Nulibry*® [fosdenopterin p. 756].
- Piperaquine phosphate with artenimol p. 487.
- *Skyclarys*® [omaveloxolone p. 755].
- *Tzield*® [teplizumab p. 567].
- *Vimkunya*® [chikungunya vaccine (inactivated) p. 987].
- *Voranigo*® [vorasidenib p. 695].
- *Zavicefta*® [ceftazidime with avibactam p. 395].

New preparations

New preparations that appear in the print edition of BNFC 2026 — 2027:
- *EURneffy*® [adrenaline p. 159].
- Fludrocortisone acetate 0.1 mg/mL oral solution p. 544.
- *Pedmarqsi*® [sodium thiosulfate p. 1044].
- *Varitect CP*® [varicella-zoster immunoglobulin p. 958].

Deleted monographs

Deleted monographs since the print edition of BNFC 2025 — 2026:
- Castor oil with collodion and colophony.
- Colestipol hydrochloride.
- Hepatitis A with typhoid vaccine.
- Macrogol 3350 with anhydrous sodium sulfate, potassium chloride, sodium bicarbonate and sodium chloride.
- Potassium bicarbonate with potassium acid tartrate.
- Ranitidine.
- Sotrovimab.

Deleted preparations

Deleted preparations since the print edition of BNFC 2025 — 2026:
- Varicella-zoster immunoglobulin solution for injection (Bio Products Laboratory).
- *Victoza*® [liraglutide p. 562].

Guidance on prescribing

General guidance

Medicines should be given to children only when they are necessary, and in all cases the potential benefit of administering the medicine should be considered in relation to the risk involved. This is particularly important during pregnancy, when the risk to both mother and fetus must be considered.

It is important to discuss treatment options carefully with the child and the child's carer. In particular, the child and the child's carer should be helped to distinguish the adverse effects of prescribed drugs from the effects of the medical disorder. When the beneficial effects of the medicine are likely to be delayed, this should be highlighted.

For guidance on medicines optimisation, see Medicines optimisation p. 24.

Never Events Never events are serious and avoidable medical errors for which there should be preventative measures in place to stop their occurrence.

The NHS Never Events policy and framework can be viewed at: www.england.nhs.uk/publication/never-events/.

For never events related to single drugs or drug classes, BNFC contain information within the monographs, in the important safety information section.

Prescribing competency framework The Royal College of Pharmacy has published a Prescribing Competency Framework that includes a common set of competencies that form the basis for prescribing, regardless of professional background. The competencies have been developed to help healthcare professionals be safe and effective prescribers with the aim of supporting patients to get the best outcomes from their medicines. It is available at www.rcpharm.org/professional-standards/a-competency-framework-for-all-prescribers/.

Transitional services for chronic conditions

The process of moving from paediatric to adult services can lead to a loss of continuity in care and provoke anxiety in children and their carers. EvGr Practitioners should start planning for adult care when the child reaches the age of 13 or 14 at the latest and a child-centred approach should be taken. Consider designating a named practitioner among those providing care to the child to take a coordinating role and to act as an advocate for the child, maintaining a link between the various practitioners involved in care (including a named GP). (A)

Drug treatment in children

Children, and particularly neonates, differ from adults in their response to drugs. Special care is needed in the neonatal period (first 28 days of life) and doses should always be calculated with care; the risk of toxicity is increased by a reduced rate of drug clearance and differing target organ sensitivity. The terms infant, child and adolescent are used inconsistently in the literature. However, **for reference purposes only**, the terms generally used to describe the paediatric stages of development are:

Preterm neonate	Born at < 37 weeks gestation
Term neonate	Born at 37 to 42 weeks gestation
Post-term neonate	Born at ≥42 weeks gestation
Neonate	From 0 up to 28 days of age (or first 4 weeks of life)
Infant	From 28 days up to 24 months of age
Child	From 2 years up to 12 years of age
Adolescent	From 12 years up to 18 years of age

In BNFC, the term neonate is used to describe a newborn infant aged 0 up to 28 days. The terms child or children are used generically to describe the entire range from infant to adolescent (1 month–17 years). An age range is specified when the dose information applies to a narrower age range than a child from 1 month–17 years.

Administration of medicines to children

Children should be involved in decisions about taking medicines and encouraged to take responsibility for using them correctly. The degree of such involvement will depend on the child's age, understanding, and personal circumstances.

Occasionally a medicine or its taste has to be disguised or masked with small quantities of food. However, unless specifically permitted (e.g. some formulations of pancreatin p. 56), a medicine should **not** be mixed with large quantities of food because the full dose might not be taken and the child might develop an aversion to food if the medicine imparts an unpleasant taste. Medicines should not be mixed or administered in a baby's feeding bottle.

Children under 5 years (and some older children) find a liquid formulation more acceptable than tablets or capsules. However, for long-term treatment it may be possible for a child to be taught to take tablets or capsules.

An oral syringe should be used for accurate measurement and controlled administration of an oral liquid medicine. The unpleasant taste of an oral liquid can be disguised by flavouring it or by giving a favourite food or drink immediately afterwards, but the potential for food-drug interactions should be considered.

Advice should be given on dental hygiene to those receiving medicines containing cariogenic sugars for long-term treatment; sugar-free medicines should be provided whenever possible.

Children with nasal feeding tubes in place for prolonged periods should be encouraged to take medicines by mouth if possible; enteric feeding should generally be interrupted before the medicine is given (particularly if enteral feeds reduce the absorption of a particular drug). Oral liquids can be given through the tube provided that precautions are taken to guard against blockage; the dose should be washed down with warm water. When a medicine is given through a nasogastric tube to a neonate, **sterile water** must be used to accompany the medicine or to wash it down.

The intravenous route is generally chosen when a medicine cannot be given by mouth; reliable access, often a central vein, should be used for children whose treatment involves irritant or inotropic drugs or who need to receive the medicine over a long period or for home therapy. The subcutaneous route is used most commonly for insulin administration. Intramuscular injections should preferably be **avoided** in children, particularly neonates, infants, and young children. However, the intramuscular route may be advantageous for administration of single doses of medicines when intravenous cannulation would be more problematic or painful to the child. Certain drugs, e.g. some vaccines, are only administered intramuscularly.

The intrathecal, epidural and intraosseous routes should be used **only** by staff specially trained to administer medicines by these routes. Local protocols for the management of intrathecal injections must be in place.

Managing medicines in school

Administration of a medicine during schooltime should be avoided if possible; medicines should be prescribed for once or twice-daily administration whenever practicable. If the medicine needs to be taken in school, this should be discussed with parents or carers and the necessary arrangements made in advance; where appropriate, involvement of a school nurse should be sought. *Managing Medicines in Schools and Early Years Settings* produced by the Department of Health and Social Care provides guidance on using medicines in schools (www.gov.uk/government/organisations/department-of-health-and-social-care).

Patient information leaflets

Manufacturers' patient information leaflets that accompany a medicine, cover only the licensed use of the medicine. Therefore, when a medicine is used outside its licence, it may be appropriate to advise the child and the child's parent or carer that some of the information in the leaflet might not apply to the child's treatment. Where necessary, inappropriate advice in the patient information leaflet should be identified and reassurance provided about the correct use in the context of the child's condition.

Biological medicines

Biological medicines are medicines that are made by or derived from a biological source using biotechnology processes, such as recombinant DNA technology. The size and complexity of biological medicines, as well as the way they are produced, may result in a degree of natural variability in molecules of the same active substance, particularly in different batches of the medicine. This variation is maintained within strict acceptable limits. Examples of biological medicines include insulins and monoclonal antibodies. EvGr Biological medicines must be prescribed by brand name and the brand name specified on the prescription should be dispensed in order to avoid inadvertent switching. Automatic substitution of brands at the point of dispensing is not appropriate for biological medicines. Ⓐ

Biosimilar medicines

A **biosimilar medicine** is a biological medicine that is highly similar and clinically equivalent (in terms of quality, safety, and efficacy) to an existing biological medicine that has already been authorised in the European Union (known as the reference biological medicine or originator medicine). The active substance of a biosimilar medicine is similar, but not identical, to the originator biological medicine. Once the patent for a biological medicine has expired, a biosimilar medicine may be authorised by the European Medicines Agency (EMA). A biosimilar medicine is not the same as a generic medicine, which contains a simpler chemical structure and a molecular structure that is identical to the originator medicine.

Therapeutic equivalence EvGr Biosimilar medicines should be considered to be therapeutically equivalent to the originator biological medicine within their authorised indications. Ⓐ Biosimilar medicines are usually licensed for all the indications of the originator biological medicine, but this depends on the evidence submitted to the EMA for authorisation and must be scientifically justified on the basis of demonstrated or extrapolated equivalence.

Prescribing and dispensing The choice of whether to prescribe a biosimilar medicine or the originator biological medicine rests with the clinician in consultation with the patient. EvGr Biological medicines (including biosimilar medicines) must be prescribed by brand name and the brand name specified on the prescription should be dispensed in order to avoid inadvertent switching. Automatic substitution of brands at the point of dispensing is not appropriate for biological medicines. Ⓐ

Safety monitoring Biosimilar medicines are subject to a black triangle status (▼) at the time of initial authorisation. EvGr It is important to report suspected adverse reactions using the Yellow Card scheme (see Adverse reactions to drugs p. 11). For all biological medicines, adverse reaction reports should clearly state the brand name and the batch number of the suspected medicine. Ⓐ

National funding/access decisions The Department of Health and Social Care has confirmed that, in England, NICE can decide to apply the same remit, and the resulting technology appraisal guidance, to relevant biosimilar medicines which appear on the market subsequent to their originator biological medicine.

National information In England, see www.nice.org.uk/About/What-we-do/Our-Programmes/NICE-guidance/NICE-technology-appraisal-guidance.

In Northern Ireland, see niformulary.hscni.net/managed-entry/biosimilars/.

In Scotland, see www.scottishmedicines.org.uk/about-us/policies-publications/.

In Wales, see awttc.nhs.wales/accessing-medicines/make-a-submission/pharmaceutical-industry-submissions/submit-for-awmsg-appraisal/invisible/appraisal-of-biosimilar-medicines-cell-therapies-and-gene-therapies/.

Availability The following are examples of drugs available as a biosimilar medicine (this list is not exhaustive):

- Adalimumab p. 806
- Enoxaparin sodium p. 110
- Epoetin alfa p. 699
- Epoetin zeta p. 701
- Etanercept p. 808
- Filgrastim p. 716
- Infliximab p. 39
- Insulin glargine p. 573
- Insulin lispro p. 571
- Rituximab p. 659
- Somatropin p. 586

Complementary and alternative medicine

An increasing amount of information on complementary and alternative medicine is becoming available. Where appropriate, the child and the child's carers should be asked about the use of their medicines, including dietary supplements and topical products. The scope of BNFC is restricted to the discussion of conventional medicines but reference is made to complementary treatments if they affect conventional therapy (e.g. interactions with St John's wort). Further information on herbal medicines is available at www.gov.uk/government/organisations/medicines-and-healthcare-products-regulatory-agency.

BNFC and marketing authorisation

Where appropriate the *doses, indications, cautions, contra-indications,* and *side-effects* in BNFC reflect those in the manufacturers' Summaries of Product Characteristics (SPCs) which, in turn, reflect those in the corresponding marketing authorisations (formerly known as Product Licences). BNFC does not generally include proprietary medicines that are not supported by a valid Summary of Product Characteristics or when the marketing authorisation holder has not been able to supply essential information. When a preparation is available from more than one manufacturer, BNFC reflects advice that is the most clinically relevant regardless of any variation in the marketing authorisation. Unlicensed products can be obtained from 'special-order' manufacturers or specialist importing companies.

As far as possible, medicines should be prescribed within the terms of the marketing authorisation. However, many children require medicines not specifically licensed for paediatric use. Although medicines cannot be promoted outside the limits of the licence, the Human Medicines Regulations 2012 do not prohibit the use of unlicensed medicines.

BNFC includes advice involving the use of unlicensed medicines or of licensed medicines for unlicensed uses ('off-label' use). Such advice reflects careful consideration of the options available to manage a given condition and the weight of evidence and experience of the unlicensed intervention, and limitations of the marketing authorisation should not preclude unlicensed use where clinically appropriate. Where an unlicensed drug or 'off-label' use is included, this is indicated in the unlicensed use section of the drug monograph.

Prescribing unlicensed medicines Prescribing unlicensed medicines or medicines outside the recommendations of their marketing authorisation alters (and probably increases) the prescriber's professional responsibility and potential liability. The prescriber should be able to justify and feel competent in using such medicines, and also inform the patient or the patient's carer that the prescribed medicine is unlicensed.

Drugs and driving

Prescribers and other healthcare professionals should advise children and their carers if treatment is likely to affect their ability to perform skilled tasks (e.g. driving). This applies especially to drugs with sedative effects; patients should be warned that these effects are increased by alcohol. General information about a patient's fitness to drive is available from the Driver and Vehicle Licensing Agency at www.gov.uk/government/organisations/driver-and-vehicle-licensing-agency.

A new offence of driving, attempting to drive, or being in charge of a vehicle, with certain specified controlled drugs in excess of specified limits, came into force on 2nd March 2015. This offence is an addition to the existing rules on drug impaired driving and fitness to drive, and applies to two groups of drugs—commonly abused drugs, including amfetamines, cannabis, cocaine, and ketamine p. 1023, and drugs used mainly for medical reasons, such as opioids and benzodiazepines. Anyone found to have any of the drugs (including related drugs, for example, apomorphine hydrochloride) above specified limits in their blood will be guilty of an offence, whether their driving was impaired or not. This also includes prescribed drugs which metabolise to those included in the offence, for example, selegiline hydrochloride. However, the legislation provides a statutory "medical defence" for patients taking drugs for medical reasons in accordance with instructions, *if their driving was not impaired*—it continues to be an offence to drive if actually impaired. Patients should therefore be advised to continue taking their medicines as prescribed, and when driving, to carry suitable evidence that the drug was prescribed, or sold, to treat a medical or dental problem, and that it was taken according to the instructions given by the prescriber, or information provided with the medicine (e.g. a repeat prescription form or the medicine's patient information leaflet). Further information is available from the Department for Transport at www.gov.uk/government/collections/drug-driving.

Oral syringes

An **oral syringe** is supplied when oral liquid medicines are prescribed in doses other than multiples of 5 mL. The oral syringe is marked in 0.5-mL divisions from 1 to 5 mL to measure doses of less than 5 mL (other sizes of oral syringe may also be available). It is provided with an adaptor and an instruction leaflet. The 5-*mL spoon* is used for doses of 5 mL (or multiples thereof).

Excipients

Branded oral liquid preparations that do not contain *fructose, glucose,* or *sucrose* are described as 'sugar-free' in BNFC. Preparations containing hydrogenated glucose syrup, mannitol, maltitol, sorbitol, or xylitol are also marked 'sugar-free' since they do not cause dental caries. Children receiving medicines containing cariogenic sugars, or their carers, should be advised of dental hygiene measures to prevent caries. Sugar-free preparations should be used whenever possible, particularly if treatment is required for a long period.

Where information on the presence of *ethanol (alcohol), aspartame, gluten, sulfites, tartrazine, arachis (peanut) oil* or *sesame oil* is available, this is indicated in BNFC against the relevant preparation.

Information is provided on *selected excipients* in skin preparations, in vaccines, and on *selected preservatives* and *excipients* in eye drops and injections.

The presence of *benzyl alcohol* and *polyoxyl castor oil* (polyethoxylated castor oil) in injections is indicated in BNFC. Benzyl alcohol has been associated with a fatal toxic syndrome in preterm neonates, and therefore, parenteral preparations containing the preservative should not be used in neonates. Polyoxyl castor oils, used as vehicles in intravenous injections, have been associated with severe anaphylactoid reactions.

The presence of *propylene glycol* in oral or parenteral medicines is indicated in BNFC; it can cause adverse effects if its elimination is impaired, e.g. in renal failure, in neonates and young children, and in slow metabolisers of the substance. It may interact with metronidazole p. 409.

The *lactose* content in most medicines is too small to cause problems in most lactose-intolerant children. However in severe lactose intolerance, the lactose content should be determined before prescribing. The amount of lactose varies according to manufacturer, product, formulation, and strength.

The Neonatal & Paediatric Pharmacy Group has produced a position statement on how to choose a suitable oral liquid medicine for a child. This statement, which has been endorsed by the Royal College of Paediatrics and Child Health, includes practical advice on assessing excipient content, in addition to other key considerations. For further information, see: nppg.org.uk/choosing-an-oral-liquid-for-a-child/

Electrolytes

The *sodium* content of medicines should be considered for all patients, especially those with cardiovascular disease or on a reduced sodium diet, or those requiring long-term or regular medication.

Some formulations of medicines, especially those that are effervescent, dispersible or soluble, can contain high levels of sodium as an excipient and this may be associated with an increased risk of cardiovascular events, including hypertension.

The sodium content of a medicine is provided in the product literature for all medicines containing $\geq$ 1 mmol sodium per dose; below this level is considered essentially sodium-free. Medicines containing $\geq$ 17 mmol sodium in the total daily dose are considered to have a high sodium content and this is highlighted for medicines intended to be taken regularly (repeated use for more than 2 days every week) or long-term (continuous daily use for more than 1 month). 17 mmol sodium is approximately 20% of the WHO recommended maximum daily dietary intake of sodium for an adult.

Important In the absence of information on excipients or electrolytes in BNFC and in the product literature (available at www.medicines.org.uk/emc/), contact the manufacturer if it is essential to check details.

Health and safety

When handling chemical or biological materials particular attention should be given to the possibility of allergy, fire, explosion, radiation, or poisoning. Care is required to avoid sources of heat (including hair dryers) when flammable substances are used on the skin or hair. Substances, such as corticosteroids, some antimicrobials, phenothiazines, and many cytotoxics, are irritant or very potent and should be handled with caution; contact with the skin and inhalation of dust should be avoided. Healthcare professionals and carers should guard against exposure to sensitising, toxic or irritant substances if it is necessary to crush tablets or open capsules.

EEA and Swiss prescriptions

Pharmacists can dispense prescriptions issued by doctors, dentists, and nurse prescribers from the European Economic Area (EEA) or Switzerland (except prescriptions for controlled drugs in Schedules 1, 2, or 3, or for drugs without a UK marketing authorisation). Prescriptions should be written in ink or otherwise so as to be indelible, should be dated, should state the name of the patient, should state the address of the prescriber, should contain particulars indicating whether the prescriber is a doctor, dentist, or nurse, and should be signed by the prescriber.

Security and validity of prescriptions

The Councils of the British Medical Association and the Royal Pharmaceutical Society have issued a joint statement on the security and validity of prescriptions.

In particular, prescription forms should:

- not be left unattended at reception desks;
- not be left in a car where they may be visible;
- when not in use, be kept in a locked drawer within the surgery and at home.

Where there is any doubt about the authenticity of a prescription, the pharmacist should contact the prescriber. If this is done by telephone, the number should be obtained from the directory rather than relying on the information on the prescription form, which may be false.

Patient group direction (PGD)

In most cases, the most appropriate clinical care will be provided on an individual basis by a prescriber to a specific child. However, a Patient Group Direction for supply and administration of medicines by other healthcare professionals can be used where it would benefit the child's care without compromising safety.

A Patient Group Direction is a written direction relating to the supply and administration (or administration only) of a licensed prescription-only medicine (including some Controlled Drugs in specific circumstances) by certain classes of healthcare professionals; the Direction is signed by a doctor (or dentist) and by a pharmacist. Further information on Patient Group Directions is available in Health Service Circular HSC 2000/026 (England), HDL (2001) 7 (Scotland), and WHC (2000) 116 (Wales); see also the Human Medicines Regulations 2012.

NICE, Scottish Medicines Consortium and All Wales Medicines Strategy Group

Advice issued by the National Institute for Health and Care Excellence (NICE), the Scottish Medicines Consortium (SMC) and the All Wales Medicines Strategy Group (AWMSG) is referenced in BNFC when relevant. Full details of this advice together with updates can be obtained from the funding body websites: www.nice.org.uk, www.scottishmedicines.org.uk and awttc.nhs.wales/.

Specialised commissioning decisions

NHS England develops specialised commissioning policies that define access to specialised services for particular groups of patients to ensure consistency in access to treatments nationwide. For further information, see www.england.nhs.uk/specialised-commissioning-document-library/routinely-commissioned-policies/.

NHS England also commissions treatments for patients aged less than 18 years where specific commissioning conditions within a NICE Technology Appraisal or NHS England policy are met, see www.england.nhs.uk/publication/commissioning-medicines-for-children-specialised-services/.

National genomic test directory

The *National genomic test directory* specifies which genomic tests are commissioned by the NHS in England, the technology by which they are available, and the patients who will be eligible to access a test. For further information, see www.england.nhs.uk/publication/national-genomic-test-directories/.

Prescription writing

Shared care

In its guidelines on responsibility for prescribing (circular EL (91) 127) between hospitals and general practitioners, the Department of Health has advised that legal responsibility for prescribing lies with the doctor who signs the prescription.

Requirements

Prescriptions should be written legibly in ink or otherwise so as to be indelible (it is permissible to issue carbon copies of NHS prescriptions as long as they are signed in ink), should be dated, should state the name and address of the patient, the address of the prescriber, an indication of the type of prescriber, and should be signed in ink by the prescriber (computer-generated facsimile signatures do not meet the legal requirement). The age and the date of birth of the patient should preferably be stated, and it is a legal requirement in the case of prescription-only medicines to state the age for children under 12 years. These recommendations are acceptable for **prescription-only medicines**. Prescriptions for controlled drugs have additional legal requirements.

Wherever appropriate the prescriber should state the current weight of the child to enable the dose prescribed to be checked. Consideration should also be given to including the dose per unit mass e.g. mg/kg or the dose per m^2 body-surface area e.g. mg/m^2 where this would reduce error.

The following should be noted:

- The strength or quantity to be contained in capsules, lozenges, tablets etc. should be stated by the prescriber. In particular, strength of liquid preparations should be clearly stated (e.g. 125 mg/5 mL).
- Quantities of 1 gram or more should be written as 1 g, 1.5 g etc. Quantities less than 1 gram should be written in milligrams, e.g. 500 mg, not 0.5 g. Quantities less than 1 mg should be written in micrograms, e.g. 100 micrograms, not 0.1 mg. The unnecessary use of decimal points should be avoided, e.g. 3 mg, not 3.0 mg. When decimals are unavoidable a zero should be written in front of the decimal point where there is no other figure, e.g. 0.5 mL, not .5 mL. Use of the decimal point is acceptable to express a range, e.g. 0.5 to 1 g.
- 'Micrograms' and 'nanograms' should **not** be abbreviated. Similarly 'units' should **not** be abbreviated.
- The term 'millilitre' (ml or mL) is used in medicine and pharmacy, and cubic centimetre, c.c., or cm^3 should not be used. (The use of capital 'L' in mL is a printing

convention throughout BNFC; both 'mL' and 'ml' are recognised SI abbreviations).

- Dose and dose frequency should be stated; in the case of preparations to be taken 'as required' a **minimum dose interval** should be specified. Care should be taken to ensure children receive the correct dose of the active drug. Therefore, the dose should normally be stated in terms of the mass of the active drug (e.g. '125 mg 3 times daily'); terms such as '5 mL' or '1 tablet' should be avoided except for compound preparations. When doses other than multiples of 5 mL are prescribed for *oral liquid preparations* the dose-volume will be provided by means of an **oral syringe**, (except for preparations intended to be measured with a pipette). Suitable quantities:
  - Elixirs, Linctuses, and Paediatric Mixtures (5-mL dose), 50, 100, or 150 mL
  - Adult Mixtures (10 mL dose), 200 or 300 mL
  - Ear Drops, Eye drops, and Nasal Drops, 10 mL (or the manufacturer's pack)
  - Eye Lotions, Gargles, and Mouthwashes, 200 mL
- The names of drugs and preparations should be written clearly and **not** abbreviated, using approved titles **only**; **avoid** creating generic titles for modified-release preparations.
- The quantity to be supplied may be stated by indicating the number of days of treatment required in the box provided on NHS forms. In most cases the exact amount will be supplied. This does not apply to items directed to be used as required—if the dose and frequency are not given then the quantity to be supplied needs to be stated. When several items are ordered on one form the box can be marked with the number of days of treatment provided the quantity is added for any item for which the amount cannot be calculated.
- Although directions should preferably be in **English without abbreviation**, it is recognised that some Latin abbreviations are used.

Sample prescription

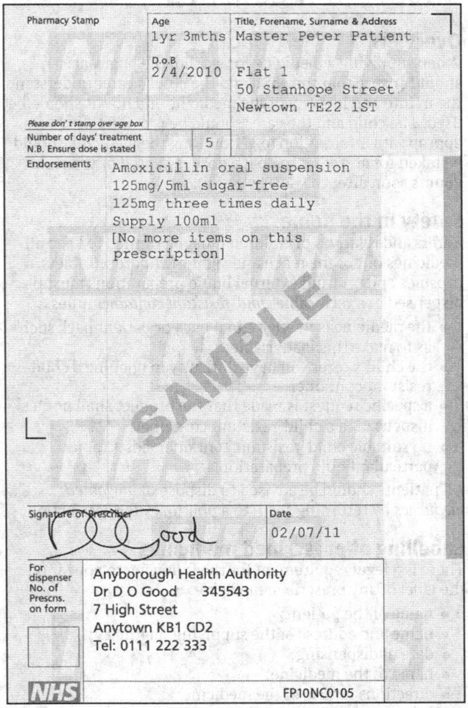
Pharmacy Stamp

Age: 1yr 3mths

D.o.B: 2/4/2010

Title, Forename, Surname & Address: Master Peter Patient, Flat 1, 50 Stanhope Street, Newtown TE22 1ST

Please don't stamp over age box

Number of days' treatment N.B. Ensure dose is stated: 5

Endorsements

Amoxicillin oral suspension
125mg/5ml sugar-free
125mg three times daily
Supply 100ml
[No more items on this prescription]

SAMPLE

Signature of Prescriber — Date: 02/07/11

For dispenser No. of Prescns. on form

Anyborough Health Authority
Dr D O Good 345543
7 High Street
Anytown KB1 CD2
Tel: 0111 222 333

NHS FP10NC0105

Abbreviation of titles In general, titles of drugs and preparations should be written *in full*. Unofficial abbreviations should **not** be used as they may be misinterpreted.

Non-proprietary titles Where non-proprietary ('generic') titles are given, they should be used for prescribing. This will enable any suitable product to be dispensed, thereby saving delay to the patient and sometimes expense to the health service. The only exception is where there is a demonstrable difference in clinical effect between each manufacturer's version of the formulation, making it important that the child should always receive the same brand; in such cases, the brand name or the manufacturer should be stated.

Non-proprietary names of compound preparations Non-proprietary names of **compound preparations** which appear in BNFC are those that have been compiled by the British Pharmacopoeia Commission or another recognised body; whenever possible they reflect the names of the active ingredients. Prescribers should avoid creating their own compound names for the purposes of generic prescribing; such names do not have an approved definition and can be misinterpreted.

Special care should be taken to avoid errors when prescribing compound preparations; in particular the hyphen in the prefix 'co-' should be retained. Special care should also be taken to avoid creating generic names for **modified-release** preparations where the use of these names could lead to confusion between formulations with different duration of action.

Supply of medicines

Overview

When supplying a medicine for a child, the pharmacist should ensure that the child and the child's carer understand the nature and identity of the medicine and how it should be used. The child and the carer should be provided with appropriate information (e.g. how long the medicine should be taken for and what to do if a dose is missed or the child vomits soon after the dose is given).

Safety in the home

Carers and relatives of children must be warned to keep all medicines out of the reach and sight of children. Tablets, capsules and oral and external liquid preparations must be dispensed in a reclosable *child-resistant container* unless:

- the medicine is in an original pack or patient pack such as to make this inadvisable;
- the child's carer will have difficulty in opening a child-resistant container;
- a specific request is made that the product shall not be dispensed in a child-resistant container;
- no suitable child-resistant container exists for a particular liquid preparation.

All patients should be advised to dispose of *unwanted medicines* by returning them to a pharmacy for destruction.

Labelling of prescribed medicines

There is a legal requirement for the following to appear on the label of any prescribed medicine:

- name of the patient;
- name and address of the supplying pharmacy;
- date of dispensing;
- name of the medicine;
- directions for use of the medicine;
- precautions relating to the use of the medicine.

The Royal College of Pharmacy recommends that the following also appears on the label:

- the words 'Keep out of the reach and sight of children';
- where applicable, the words 'Use this medicine only on your skin'.

A pharmacist can exercise professional skill and judgement to amend or include more appropriate wording for the name of the medicine, the directions for use, or the precautions relating to the use of the medicine.

The Neonatal and Paediatric Pharmacy Group advises that doses of oral liquid medicines should be expressed in terms of millilitres only e.g. 'give 5 mL once daily.' Detailed guidance on Labelling of Dispensed Oral Medicines for Children is available at: nppg.org.uk/labelling-position-statement/.

Unlicensed medicines

A drug or formulation that is not covered by a marketing authorisation may be obtained from a pharmaceutical company, imported by a specialist importer, manufactured by a commercial or hospital licensed manufacturing unit, or prepared extemporaneously against a prescription.

The safeguards that apply to products with marketing authorisation should be extended, as far as possible, to the use of unlicensed medicines. The safety, efficacy, and quality (including labelling) of unlicensed medicines should be assured by means of clear policies on their prescribing, purchase, supply, and administration. Extra care is required with unlicensed medicines because less information may be available on the drug and any formulation of the drug.

The following should be agreed with the supplier when ordering an unlicensed or extemporaneously prepared medicine:

- the specification of the formulation;
- documentation confirming the specification and quality of the product supplied (e.g. a certificate of conformity or of analysis);
- for imported preparations product and licensing information should be supplied in English.

Extemporaneous preparations

A product should be dispensed extemporaneously only when no product with a marketing authorisation is available. Every effort should be made to ensure that an extemporaneously prepared product is stable and that it delivers the requisite dose reliably; the child should be provided with a consistent formulation regardless of where the medicine is supplied to minimise variations in quality. Where there is doubt about the formulation, advice should be sought from a medicines information centre, the pharmacy at a children's hospital, a hospital production unit, a hospital quality control department, or the manufacturer.

In many cases it is preferable to give a licensed product by an unlicensed route (e.g. an injection solution given by mouth) than to prepare a special formulation. When tablets or capsules are cut, dispersed, or used for preparing liquids immediately before administration, it is important to confirm uniform dispersal of the active ingredient, especially if only a portion of the solid content (e.g. a tablet segment) is used or if only an aliquot of the liquid is to be administered.

In some cases the child's clinical condition may require a dose to be administered in the absence of full information on the method of administration. It is important to ensure that the appropriate supporting information is available at the earliest opportunity.

Preparation of products that produce harmful dust (e.g. cytotoxic drugs, hormones, or potentially sensitising drugs such as neomycin sulfate p. 898) should be **avoided** or undertaken with appropriate precautions to protect staff and carers.

The BP direction that a preparation must be *freshly prepared* indicates that it must be made not more than 24 hours before it is issued for use. The direction that a preparation should be *recently prepared* indicates that deterioration is likely if the preparation is stored for longer than about 4 weeks at 15–25°C.

The term **water** used without qualification means either potable water freshly drawn direct from the public supply and suitable for drinking or freshly boiled and cooled purified water. The latter should be used if the public supply is from a local storage tank or if the potable water is unsuitable for a particular preparation.

Emergency supply of medicines

Emergency supply requested by member of the public

Pharmacists are sometimes called upon by members of the public to make an emergency supply of medicines. The Human Medicines Regulations 2012 allows exemptions from the Prescription Only requirements for emergency supply to be made by a person lawfully conducting a retail pharmacy business provided:

a) that the pharmacist has interviewed the person requesting the prescription-only medicine and is satisfied:
   i) that there is immediate need for the prescription-only medicine and that it is impracticable in the circumstances to obtain a prescription without undue delay;
   ii) that treatment with the prescription-only medicine has on a previous occasion been prescribed for the person requesting it;
   iii) as to the dose that it would be appropriate for the person to take;
b) that no greater quantity shall be supplied than will provide 5 days' treatment of phenobarbital p. 264, *phenobarbital sodium*, or Controlled Drugs in Schedules 4 or 5 (doctors, dentists, or nurse prescribers from the European Economic Area and Switzerland, or their patients, cannot request an emergency supply of Controlled Drugs in Schedules 1, 2, or 3, or drugs that do not have a UK marketing authorisation) or 30 days' treatment for other prescription-only medicines, except when the prescription-only medicine is:
   i) insulin, an ointment or cream, or a preparation for the relief of asthma in an aerosol dispenser when the smallest pack can be supplied;
   ii) an oral contraceptive when a full cycle may be supplied;
   iii) an antibiotic in liquid form for oral administration when the smallest quantity that will provide a full course of treatment can be supplied;
c) that an entry shall be made by the pharmacist in the prescription book stating:
   i) the date of supply;
   ii) the name, quantity and, where appropriate, the pharmaceutical form and strength;
   iii) the name and address of the patient;
   iv) the nature of the emergency;
d) that the container or package must be labelled to show:
   i) the date of supply;
   ii) the name, quantity and, where appropriate, the pharmaceutical form and strength;
   iii) the name of the patient;
   iv) the name and address of the pharmacy;
   v) the words 'Emergency supply';
   vi) the words 'Keep out of the reach of children' (or similar warning);
e) that the prescription-only medicine is not a substance specifically excluded from the emergency supply provision, and does not contain a Controlled Drug specified in Schedules 1, 2, or 3 to the Misuse of Drugs Regulations 2001 except for phenobarbital p. 264 or *phenobarbital sodium* for the treatment of epilepsy: for details see *Medicines, Ethics and Practice*, London, Pharmaceutical Press (always consult latest edition). Doctors, dentists, or nurse prescribers from the European Economic Area and Switzerland, or their patients, cannot request an emergency supply of Controlled Drugs in Schedules 1, 2, or 3, or drugs that do not have a UK marketing authorisation.

Emergency supply requested by prescriber

Emergency supply of a prescription-only medicine may also be made at the request of a doctor, a dentist, a supplementary prescriber, a community practitioner nurse prescriber, a nurse, pharmacist, physiotherapist, therapeutic radiographer, optometrist, podiatrist or paramedic independent prescriber; or a doctor, dentist, or nurse prescriber from the European Economic Area or Switzerland, provided:

a) that the pharmacist is satisfied that the prescriber by reason of some emergency is unable to furnish a prescription immediately;
b) that the prescriber has undertaken to furnish a prescription within 72 hours;
c) that the medicine is supplied in accordance with the directions of the prescriber requesting it;
d) that the medicine is not a Controlled Drug specified in Schedules 1, 2, or 3 to the Misuse of Drugs Regulations 2001 except for phenobarbital p. 264 or *phenobarbital sodium* for the treatment of epilepsy: for details see *Medicines, Ethics and Practice*, London, Pharmaceutical Press (always consult latest edition); (Doctors, dentists, or nurse prescribers from the European Economic Area and Switzerland, or their patients, cannot request an emergency supply of Controlled Drugs in Schedules 1, 2, or 3, or drugs that do not have a UK marketing authorisation).
e) that an entry shall be made in the prescription book stating:
   i) the date of supply;
   ii) the name, quantity and, where appropriate, the pharmaceutical form and strength;
   iii) the name and address of the practitioner requesting the emergency supply;
   iv) the name and address of the patient;
   v) the date on the prescription;
   vi) when the prescription is received the entry should be amended to include the date on which it is received.

Royal College of Pharmacy's guidelines

1. The pharmacist should consider the medical consequences of not supplying a medicine in an emergency.
2. If the pharmacist is unable to make an emergency supply of a medicine the pharmacist should advise the patient how to obtain essential medical care.

For conditions that apply to supplies made at the request of a patient see Medicines, Ethics and Practice, London Pharmaceutical Press, (always consult latest edition).

Controlled drugs and drug dependence

Regulations and classification

The Misuse of Drugs Act, 1971 as amended prohibits certain activities in relation to 'Controlled Drugs', in particular their manufacture, supply, and possession (except where permitted by the 2001 Regulations or under licence from the Secretary of State). The penalties applicable to offences involving the different drugs are graded broadly according to the *harmfulness attributable to a drug when it is misused* and for this purpose the drugs are defined in the following three classes:

- **Class A** includes: alfentanil p. 1022, cocaine, diamorphine hydrochloride p. 332 (heroin), dipipanone hydrochloride, fentanyl p. 334, lysergide (LSD), methadone hydrochloride p. 357, 3,4-methylenedioxymethamfetamine (MDMA, 'ecstasy'), morphine p. 338, opium, oxycodone hydrochloride p. 340, pethidine hydrochloride p. 342, phencyclidine, remifentanil p. 1022, and class B substances when prepared for injection.
- **Class B** includes: oral amfetamines, barbiturates, cannabis, *Sativex*®, codeine phosphate p. 331, dihydrocodeine tartrate p. 333, ethylmorphine, glutethimide, ketamine p. 1023, nabilone p. 313, pentazocine, phenmetrazine, and pholcodine.
- **Class C** includes: certain drugs related to the amfetamines such as benzfetamine and chlorphentermine, buprenorphine p. 329, mazindol, meprobamate, pemoline, pipradrol, most benzodiazepines, tramadol hydrochloride p. 343, zaleplon, zolpidem tartrate, zopiclone, androgenic and anabolic steroids, clenbuterol, chorionic gonadotrophin (HCG), non-human chorionic gonadotrophin, somatotropin, somatrem, somatropin p. 586, gabapentin p. 240, pregabalin and nitrous oxide.

The Misuse of Drugs (Safe Custody) Regulations 1973 as amended details the storage and safe custody requirements for Controlled Drugs.

The Misuse of Drugs Regulations 2001 (and subsequent amendments) defines the classes of person who are authorised to supply and possess Controlled Drugs while acting in their professional capacities and lays down the conditions under which these activities may be carried out. In the 2001 regulations, drugs are divided into five Schedules, each specifying the requirements governing such activities as import, export, production, supply, possession, prescribing, and record keeping which apply to them.

- **Schedule 1** includes drugs not used medicinally such as hallucinogenic drugs (e.g. LSD), ecstasy-type substances, raw opium, and cannabis. A Home Office licence is generally required for their production, possession, or supply. A Controlled Drug register must be used to record details of any Schedule 1 Controlled Drugs received or supplied by a pharmacy.
- **Schedule 2** includes opiates (e.g. diamorphine hydrochloride p. 332 (heroin), morphine p. 338, methadone hydrochloride p. 357, oxycodone hydrochloride p. 340, pethidine hydrochloride p. 342), major stimulants (e.g. amfetamines), quinalbarbitone (secobarbital), cocaine, ketamine p. 1023, and cannabis-based products for medicinal use in humans. Schedule 2 Controlled Drugs are subject to the full Controlled Drug requirements relating to prescriptions, safe custody (except for quinalbarbitone (secobarbital) and some liquid preparations), and the need to keep a Controlled Drug register, (unless exempted in Schedule 5). Possession, supply and procurement is authorised for pharmacists and other classes of persons named in the 2001 Regulations.
- **Schedule 3** includes the barbiturates (except secobarbital, now Schedule 2), buprenorphine p. 329, gabapentin p. 240, mazindol, meprobamate, midazolam p. 273, pentazocine, phentermine, pregabalin, temazepam p. 1024, and tramadol hydrochloride p. 343. They are subject to the special prescription requirements. Safe custody requirements do apply, except for any 5,5 disubstituted barbituric acid (e.g. phenobarbital), gabapentin p. 240, mazindol, meprobamate, midazolam p. 273, pentazocine, phentermine, pregabalin, tramadol hydrochloride p. 343, or any stereoisomeric form or salts of the above. Records in registers do not need to be kept (although there are requirements for the retention of invoices for 2 years).
- **Schedule 4** includes in Part I drugs that are subject to minimal control, such as benzodiazepines (except temazepam p. 1024 and midazolam p. 273, which are in Schedule 3), non-benzodiazepine hypnotics (zaleplon, zolpidem tartrate, and zopiclone) and *Sativex*®. Part II includes androgenic and anabolic steroids, clenbuterol, chorionic gonadotrophin (HCG), non-human chorionic gonadotrophin, somatotropin, somatrem, and somatropin p. 586. Controlled drug prescription requirements do not apply and Schedule 4 Controlled Drugs are not subject to safe custody requirements. Records in registers do not need to be kept (except in the case of *Sativex*®).
- **Schedule 5** includes preparations of certain Controlled Drugs (such as codeine, pholcodine, or morphine p. 338) which due to their low strength, are exempt from virtually all Controlled Drug requirements other than retention of invoices for two years, and nitrous oxide.

Since the Responsible Pharmacist Regulations were published in 2008, standing operation procedures for the management of Controlled Drugs, are required in registered pharmacies.

The Health Act 2006 introduced the concept of the 'accountable officer' with responsibility for the management of Controlled Drugs and related governance issues in their organisation. Most recently, in 2013 The Controlled Drugs (Supervision of Management and Use) Regulations were published to ensure good governance concerning the safe management and use of Controlled Drugs in England and Scotland.

Prescriptions

Preparations in Schedules 1, 2, 3, 4 and 5 of the Misuse of Drugs Regulations 2001 (and subsequent amendments) are identified throughout BNF and BNFC using the following symbols:

CD1	for preparations in Schedule 1
CD2	for preparations in Schedule 2
CD3	for preparations in Schedule 3
CD4-1	for preparations in Schedule 4 (Part I)
CD4-2	for preparations in Schedule 4 (Part II)
CD5	for preparations in Schedule 5

The principal legal requirements relating to medical prescriptions are listed below (see also Department of Health Guidance at www.gov.uk/dh).

Prescription requirements Prescriptions for Controlled Drugs that are subject to prescription requirements (all preparations in Schedules 2 and 3) must be indelible, must be *signed* by the prescriber, include the *date* on which they were signed, and specify the prescriber's *address* (must be within the UK). A computer-generated prescription is acceptable, but the prescriber's signature must be handwritten. Advanced electronic signatures can be accepted for Schedule 2 and 3 Controlled Drugs where the Electronic Prescribing Service (EPS) is used. All prescriptions for Controlled Drugs that are subject to the prescription requirements must always state:

- the name and address of the patient (use of a PO Box is acceptable);
- in the case of a preparation, the form (the dosage form e.g. tablets must be included on a Controlled Drugs prescription irrespective of whether it is implicit in the proprietary name e.g. *MST Continus*, or whether only one form is available), and, where appropriate, the strength of the preparation (when more than one strength of a preparation exists the strength required must be specified); to avoid ambiguity, where a prescription requests multiple strengths of a medicine, each strength should be prescribed separately (i.e. separate dose, total quantity, etc);
- for liquids, the total volume in millilitres (in both words and figures) of the preparation to be supplied; for dosage units (tablets, capsules, ampoules), state the total number (in both words and figures) of dosage units to be supplied (e.g. 10 tablets [of 10 mg] rather than 100 mg total quantity);
- the dose, which must be clearly defined (i.e. the instruction 'one as directed' constitutes a dose but 'as directed' does not); it is not necessary that the dose is stated in both words and figures;
- the words 'for dental treatment only' if issued by a dentist.

A pharmacist is **not** allowed to dispense a Controlled Drug unless all the information required by law is given on the prescription. In the case of a prescription for a Controlled Drug in Schedule 2 or 3, a pharmacist can amend the prescription *if* it specifies the total quantity only in words or in figures or if it contains minor typographical errors, provided that such amendments are indelible and clearly attributable to the pharmacist (e.g. name, date, signature and GPhC registration number). The prescription should be marked with the date of supply at the time the Controlled Drug supply is made.

The Department of Health and the Scottish Government have issued a strong recommendation that the maximum quantity of Schedule 2, 3 or 4 Controlled Drugs prescribed should not exceed 30 days; exceptionally, to cover a justifiable clinical need and after consideration of any risk, a prescription can be issued for a longer period, but the reasons for the decision should be recorded on the patient's notes.

A prescription for a Controlled Drug in Schedules 2, 3, or 4 is valid for 28 days after the date stated thereon (the prescriber may forward-date the prescription; the start date may also be specified in the body of the prescription). Schedule 5 prescriptions are valid for 6 months from the appropriate date.

See sample prescription:

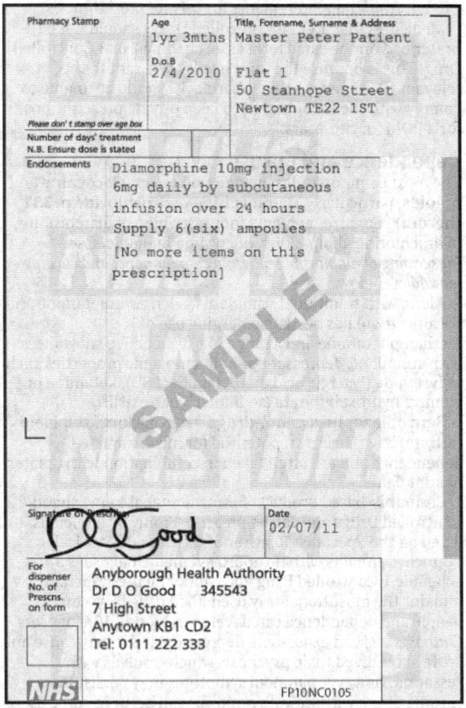

Pharmacy Stamp

Age
1yr 3mths

D.o.B
2/4/2010

Title, Forename, Surname & Address
Master Peter Patient
Flat 1
50 Stanhope Street
Newtown TE22 1ST

Please don't stamp over age box

Number of days' treatment
N.B. Ensure dose is stated

Endorsements

Diamorphine 10mg injection
6mg daily by subcutaneous
infusion over 24 hours
Supply 6(six) ampoules
[No more items on this
prescription]

SAMPLE

Signature of Prescriber

Date
02/07/11

For dispenser
No. of Prescns. on form

Anyborough Health Authority
Dr D O Good 345543
7 High Street
Anytown KB1 CD2
Tel: 0111 222 333

NHS

FP10NC0105

Instalments and repeatable prescriptions Prescriptions for Schedule 2 or 3 Controlled Drugs can be dispensed by instalments. An instalment prescription must have an instalment direction including both the dose and the instalment amount specified separately on the prescription, and it must also state the interval between each time the medicine can be supplied.

The first instalment must be dispensed no later than 28 days after the appropriate day (i.e. date of signing unless the prescriber indicates a date before which the Controlled Drug should not be dispensed) and the remainder should be dispensed in accordance with the instructions on the prescription. The prescription must be marked with the date of each supply.

The instalment direction is a legal requirement and needs to be complied with, however, for certain situations (e.g. if a pharmacy is closed on the day an instalment is due) the Home Office has approved specific wording which provides pharmacists some flexibility for supply. For details, see Medicines, Ethics and Practice, London, Pharmaceutical Press (always consult latest edition) or see Home Office approved wording for instalment prescribing (Circular 027/2015), available at www.gov.uk/.

Repeatable prescriptions are prescriptions which contain a direction that they can be dispensed more than once (e.g. repeat × 3). Only Schedule 4 and 5 Controlled Drugs are permitted on repeatable prescriptions.

Private prescriptions Private prescriptions for Controlled Drugs in Schedules 2 and 3 must be written on specially designated forms which are provided by local NHS England area teams in England (form FP10PCD), local NHS Health Boards in Scotland (form PPCD) and Wales (form W10PCD); in addition, prescriptions must specify the *prescriber's identification number* (or a NHS prescriber code in Scotland).

Prescriptions to be supplied by a pharmacist in hospital are exempt from the requirements for private prescriptions.

Medicines that are not Controlled Drugs should not be prescribed on the same form as a Schedule 2 or 3 Controlled Drug. This is because the form needs to be sent to the relevant NHS agency so the pharmacist would be unable to comply with the requirement to keep private prescriptions for a POM for two years.

Dependence and misuse

The most common drugs of addiction are **crack cocaine** and **opioids**, particularly **diamorphine hydrochloride** **p. 332** **(heroin)** . For arrangements for prescribing of diamorphine hydrochloride, dipipanone, or cocaine for addicts, see *Prescribing of diamorphine (heroin), dipipanone, and cocaine for addicts* below.

Along with traditional stimulants, such as amfetamine and cocaine, there has been an emerging use of methamphetamine and a range of psychoactive substances with stimulant, depressant or hallucinogenic properties such as lysergide (lysergic acid diethylamide, LSD), ketamine or gamma-hydroxybutyrate (sodium oxybate, GHB).

Benzodiazepines and Z-drugs (i.e. zopiclone, zolpidem tartrate) have their own potential for misuse and dependence and are often taken in combination with opiates or stimulants.

Cannabis-based products for medicinal use are Schedule 2 Controlled Drugs and can be prescribed only by clinicians listed on the Specialist Register of the General Medical Council. Cannabis with no approved medicinal use is a Schedule 1 Controlled Drug and cannot be prescribed. It remains the most frequently used illicit drug by young people and dependence can develop in around 10% of users. Cannabis use can exacerbate depression and it may cause an acute short-lived toxic psychosis which resolves with cessation, however paranoid symptoms may persist in chronic users; withdrawal symptoms can occur in some users and these can contribute to sleep problems, agitation and risk of self-harm.

Supervised consumption

Supervised consumption is not a legal requirement under the 2001 Regulations. Nevertheless, when supervised consumption is directed on the prescription, the Department of Health recommends that any deviation from the prescriber's intended method of supply should be documented and the justification for this recorded.

Individuals prescribed opioid substitution therapy can take their daily dose under the supervision of a doctor, nurse, or pharmacist during the dose stabilisation phase (usually the first 3 months of treatment), after a relapse or period of instability, or if there is a significant increase in the dose of methadone. Supervised consumption should continue (in accordance with local protocols) until the prescriber is confident that the patient is compliant with their treatment. It is good practice for pharmacists to alert the prescriber when a patient has missed consecutive daily doses.

Prescribing drugs likely to cause dependence or misuse

The prescriber has three main responsibilities:

- To avoid creating dependence by introducing drugs to patients without sufficient reason. In this context, the proper use of the morphine-like drugs is well understood. The dangers of other Controlled Drugs are less clear because recognition of dependence is not easy and its effects, and those of withdrawal, are less obvious.
- To see that the patient does not gradually increase the dose of a drug, given for good medical reasons, to the point where dependence becomes more likely. This tendency is seen especially with hypnotics and anxiolytics. The prescriber should keep a close eye on the amount prescribed to prevent patients from accumulating stocks. A minimal amount should be prescribed in the first instance, or when seeing a patient for the first time.
- To avoid being used as an unwitting source of supply for addicts and being vigilant to methods for obtaining medicines. Methods include visiting more than one doctor, fabricating stories, and forging prescriptions.

Patients under temporary care should be given only small supplies of drugs unless they present an unequivocal letter from their own doctor. Doctors should also remember that their own patients may be attempting to collect prescriptions from other prescribers, especially in hospitals. It is sensible to reduce dosages steadily or to issue weekly or even daily prescriptions for small amounts if it is apparent that dependence is occurring.

Prescribers are responsible for the security of prescription forms once issued to them. The stealing and misuse of prescription forms could be minimised by the following precautions:

- records of serial numbers received and issued should be retained for at least three years;
- blank prescriptions should never be pre-signed;
- prescription forms should not be left unattended and should be locked in a secure drawer, cupboard, or carrying case when not in use;
- doctors', dentists' and surgery stamps should be kept in a secure location separate from the prescription forms;
- alterations are best avoided but if any are made and the prescription is to be used, best practice is for the prescriber to cross out the error, initial and date the error, then write the correct information;
- if an error made in a prescription cannot be corrected, best practice for the prescriber is to put a line through the script and write 'spoiled' on the form, or destroy the form and start writing a new prescription;
- prescribers and pharmacists dispensing drugs prone to abuse should ensure compliance with all relevant legal requirements specially when dealing with prescriptions for Controlled Drugs (see *Prescription requirements* and *Instalments* above);
- at the time of dispensing, prescriptions should be stamped with the pharmacy stamp and endorsed by the pharmacist or pharmacy technician with what has been supplied; where loss or theft is suspected, the police should be informed immediately.

Travelling abroad

Prescribed drugs listed in Schedule 4 Part II (CD Anab) for self-administration and Schedule 5 of the Misuse of Drugs Regulations 2001 (and subsequent amendments) are not subject to export or import licensing. A personal import/export licence is required for patients travelling abroad with Schedules 2, 3, or 4 Part I (CD Benz) and Part II (CD Anab) Controlled Drugs if, they are carrying more than 3 months' supply or are travelling for 3 calendar months or more. A Home Office licence is required for any amount of a Schedule 1 Controlled Drug imported into the UK for personal use regardless of the duration of travel. Further details can be obtained at www.gov.uk/guidance/controlled-drugs-licences-fees-and-returns or from the Home Office by contacting DFLU.ie@homeoffice.gsi.gov.uk. In cases of emergency, telephone (020) 7035 6330.

Applications for obtaining a licence must be supported by a cover letter signed by the prescribing doctor or drug worker, which must confirm:

- the patient's name and address;
- the travel itinerary;
- the names of the prescribed Controlled Drug(s), doses and total amounts to be carried.

Applications for licences should be sent to the Home Office, Drugs & Firearms Licensing Unit, Fry Building, 2 Marsham Street, London, SW1P 4DF.

Alternatively, completed application forms can be emailed to DFLU.ie@homeoffice.gsi.gov.uk. A minimum of 10 days should be allowed for processing the application.

Patients travelling for less than 3 months or carrying less than 3 months supply of Controlled Drugs do not require a personal export/import licence, but are advised to carry a cover letter signed by the prescribing doctor or drug worker. Those travelling for more than 3 months are advised to make arrangements to have their medication prescribed by a practitioner in the country they are visiting.

Doctors who want to take Controlled Drugs abroad while accompanying patients may similarly be issued with licences. Licences are not normally issued to doctors who want to take Controlled Drugs abroad solely in case a family emergency should arise.

Personal export/import licences do not have any legal status outside the UK and are issued only to comply with the Misuse of Drugs Act 2001 and to facilitate passage through UK Customs and Excise control. For clearance in the country to be visited it is necessary to approach that country's consulate in the UK.

Notification of patients receiving structured drug treatment for substance dependence

In **England**, doctors should report cases where they are providing structured drug treatment for substance dependence to their local National Drug Treatment Monitoring System (NDTMS) Team. General information about NDTMS can be found at www.gov.uk/government/collections/alcohol-and-drug-misuse-prevention-and-treatment-guidance.

Enquiries about NDTMS, and how to submit data, should initially be directed to:

- EvidenceApplicationteam@phe.gov.uk

In **Scotland**, doctors should report cases to the Substance Drug Misuse Database. General information about the Scottish Drug Misuse Database can be found in www.isdscotland.org/Health-Topics/Drugs-and-Alcohol-Misuse/Drugs-Misuse/Scottish-Drug-Misuse-Database/. Enquiries about reporting can be directed to:

- nss.isdsubstancemisuse@nhs.net

In **Northern Ireland**, the Misuse of Drugs (Notification of and Supply to Addicts) (Northern Ireland) Regulations 1973 require doctors to send particulars of persons whom they consider to be addicted to certain Controlled Drugs to the Chief Medical Officer of the Ministry of Health and Social Services. The Northern Ireland contact is:

Public Health Information & Research Branch
Department of Health
Annexe 2
Castle Buildings
Stormont
Belfast
BT4 3SQ
028 9052 2340
phirb@health-ni.gov.uk

Public Health Information & Research Branch also maintains the Northern Ireland Drug Misuse Database (NIDMD) which collects detailed information on those presenting for treatment, on drugs misused and injecting behaviour; participation is not a statutory requirement.

In **Wales**, doctors should report cases where they are providing structured drug treatment for substance dependence on the Welsh National Database for Substance Misuse; enquiries should be directed to:

- substancemisuse-queries@wales.nhs.uk

Prescribing of diamorphine (heroin), dipipanone, and cocaine for addicts

The Misuse of Drugs (Supply to Addicts) Regulations 1997 require that **only** medical practitioners who hold a special licence issued by the Home Secretary (or Scottish Government's Chief Medical Officer) may prescribe, administer, or supply diamorphine hydrochloride p. 332, dipipanone, or cocaine for *the treatment of drug addiction*. Medical prescribers, pharmacists independent prescribers, nurses independent prescribers and supplementary prescribers do not require a special licence for prescribing diamorphine hydrochloride p. 332, dipipanone, or cocaine for patients (including addicts) for relieving pain from organic disease or injury.

Adverse reactions to drugs

Yellow Card scheme

Any drug may produce unwanted or unexpected adverse reactions. Rapid detection and recording of adverse drug reactions is of vital importance so that unrecognised hazards are identified promptly and appropriate regulatory action is taken to ensure that medicines are used safely. Healthcare professionals and coroners are urged to report suspected adverse drug reactions directly to the Medicines and Healthcare products Regulatory Agency (MHRA) through the Yellow Card scheme using the online form on the Yellow Card website (yellowcard.mhra.gov.uk), or by downloading and using the Yellow Card app. Reporting is also integrated into some clinical systems such as EMIS, SystmOne, Vision, MiDatabank, and Ulysses.

Suspected adverse drug reactions to any therapeutic agent should be reported, including drugs (*self-medication* as well as those *prescribed*), blood products, vaccines, radiographic contrast media, complementary, homeopathic and herbal products. This includes suspected adverse drug reactions associated with misuse, overdose, medication errors or from use of unlicensed and off-label medicines. For biological or biosimilar medicines and vaccines, adverse reaction reports should clearly state the brand name and the batch number of the suspected medicine or vaccine.

The Yellow Card scheme can also be used to report medical device adverse incidents, defective medicines, suspected falsified (fake) medicines, as well as safety concerns associated with e-cigarettes and their refill containers (e-liquids).

Report all suspected adverse drug reactions that are:

- **serious, medically significant or result in harm.** Serious events are fatal, life-threatening, a congenital abnormality, disabling or incapacitating, or resulting in hospitalisation;
- associated with **newer drugs and vaccines**; the most up to date list of black triangle medicines is available at: www.gov.uk/guidance/the-yellow-card-scheme-guidance-for-healthcare-professionals#black-triangle-scheme.

If in doubt whether to report a suspected adverse drug reaction, please complete a Yellow Card.

The identification and reporting of adverse reactions to drugs in children and neonates is particularly important because:

- the action of the drug and its pharmacokinetics in children (especially in the very young) may be different from that in adults;
- drugs may not have been extensively tested in children;

- many drugs are not specifically licensed for use in children and are used either 'off-label' or as unlicensed products;
- drugs may affect the way a child grows and develops or may cause delayed adverse reactions which do not occur in adults;
- suitable formulations may not be available to allow precise dosing in children or they may contain excipients that should be used with caution in children;
- the nature and course of illnesses and adverse drug reactions may differ between adults and children.

Even if reported through the British Paediatric Surveillance Unit's Orange Card scheme, any identified suspected adverse drug reactions should also be submitted through the Yellow Card scheme at yellowcard.mhra.gov.uk.

Spontaneous reporting is particularly valuable for recognising possible new hazards rapidly. An adverse reaction should be reported even if it is not certain that the drug has caused it, or if the reaction is well recognised, or if other drugs have been given at the same time. Reports of overdoses (deliberate or accidental) can complicate the assessment of adverse drug reactions, but provide important information on the potential toxicity of drugs.

A freephone service is available to all parts of the UK for advice and information on suspected adverse drug reactions; contact the National Yellow Card Information Service at the MHRA on 0800 731 6789 (9am to 5pm Monday to Friday only). Outside office hours a telephone-answering machine will take messages.

The MHRA commissions six regional Yellow Card Centres to increase awareness as well as to educate and promote the reporting of suspected side-effects to the Yellow Card scheme from healthcare professionals, patients, and their representative organisations. The following Yellow Card Centres can be contacted for further information:

Yellow Card Centre Northwest
2nd Floor
70 Pembroke Place
Liverpool
L69 3GF
0151 794 8122
yccnorthwest@rlbuht.nhs.net

Yellow Card Centre Northern & Yorkshire
Regional Drug and Therapeutics Centre
16/17 Framlington Place
Newcastle upon Tyne
NE2 4AB
0191 213 7855
yccnorthernandyorkshire@nuth.nhs.uk

Yellow Card Centre West Midlands
City Hospital
Dudley Road
Birmingham
B18 7QH
0121 507 5672
swb-tr.swbh-team-yccwestmidlands@nhs.net

Yellow Card Centre Northern Ireland
Northern Ireland Medicines and Poisons Advice Service
Belfast Health and Social Care Trust
Pharmacy Department
Building 36
Knockbracken Clinic
Knockbracken Healthcare Park
Saintfield Road
Belfast
BT8 8BH
028 9504 0558
medicineinfo@belfasttrust.hscni.net

Yellow Card Centre Scotland
51 Little France Crescent
Old Dalkeith Road
Edinburgh
EH16 4SA
0131 242 2919
yccscotland@nhslothian.scot.nhs.uk

Yellow Card Centre Wales
All Wales Therapeutics and Toxicology Centre
Academic Building
University Hospital Llandough
Penlan Road
Penarth
Vale of Glamorgan
CF64 2XX
029 2074 5831
yccwales@wales.nhs.uk

The MHRA's database facilitates the monitoring of adverse drug reactions. More detailed information on reporting and a list of products currently under additional monitoring can be found on the MHRA website: www.gov.uk/government/organisations/medicines-and-healthcare-products-regulatory-agency.

MHRA Drug Safety Update *Drug Safety Update* is a monthly newsletter from the MHRA and the Commission on Human Medicines (CHM); it is available at www.gov.uk/drug-safety-update. Drug Safety Update is also available to access from the Yellow Card app, which allows users to create a watchlist of medicines.

Interactive Drug Analysis Profiles *interactive Drug Analysis Profiles* (iDAPs) are available on the Yellow Card website (yellowcard.mhra.gov.uk) under *What is being reported*. Each iDAP contains complete data for all spontaneous suspected adverse drug reactions, or side-effects, which have been reported on that drug substance to the MHRA via the Yellow Card scheme, from healthcare professionals and members of the public. iDAPs are also available to access from the Yellow Card app.

Yellow Card biobank Yellow Card biobank is a collaboration between the MHRA and Genomics England that aims to improve understanding of how a patient's genetic makeup may increase their risk of harm from side-effects. Through the collection of genetic samples from patients who have experienced suspected side-effects, the Yellow Card biobank will create a repository of genetic information that can be used to help determine whether a suspected side-effect was caused by a specific genetic trait. Further information (including current topics) can be found on the Yellow Card website (yellowcard.mhra.gov.uk).

Self-reporting

Patients and their carers can also report suspected adverse drug reactions to the MHRA. Healthcare professionals are encouraged to discuss side-effects with patients and carers and encourage them to self-report if side-effects occur.

Reports can be submitted directly to the MHRA through the Yellow Card scheme using the online form, by downloading a copy of the form from the Yellow Card website, using the Yellow Card app, or by freephone on 0800 731 6789. Alternatively, patient Yellow Cards may be available from pharmacies and GP surgeries. Information for patients and carers about the Yellow Card scheme is available in other languages from the Yellow Card website (yellowcard.mhra.gov.uk).

Prescription-event monitoring

In addition to the MHRA's Yellow Card scheme, an independent scheme monitors the safety of new medicines using a different approach. The Drug Safety Research Unit identifies patients who have been prescribed selected new medicines and collects data on clinical events in these patients. The data are submitted on a voluntary basis by general practitioners on green forms. More information about the scheme and the Unit's educational material is available from www.dsru.org.

Newer drugs and vaccines

Only limited information is available from clinical trials on the safety of new medicines. Further understanding about the safety of medicines depends on the availability of information from routine clinical practice.

The black triangle symbol (▼) identifies newly licensed medicines that require additional monitoring, such as new active substances and biosimilar medicines. The black triangle symbol also appears in the Patient Information Leaflets for relevant medicines, with a brief explanation of what it means. Products usually retain a black triangle for 5 years, but this can be extended if required.

Spontaneous reporting is particularly valuable for recognising possible new hazards rapidly. For medicines showing the black triangle symbol, the MHRA asks that all suspected reactions (including those considered not to be serious) are reported through the Yellow Card scheme. An adverse reaction should be reported even if it is not certain that the drug has caused it, or if the reaction is well recognised, or if other drugs have been given at the same time.

A list of products under additional monitoring can be found on the MHRA's website (www.gov.uk/guidance/the-yellow-card-scheme-guidance-for-healthcare-professionals#black-triangle-scheme).

Established drugs and vaccines

Healthcare professionals and coroners are asked to report all suspected reactions to established drugs (including over-the-counter, herbal, homeopathic, and unlicensed medicines and medicines used off-label) and vaccines that are **serious, medically significant, or result in harm**. Serious reactions include those that are fatal, life-threatening, disabling, incapacitating, or which result in or prolong hospitalisation, or a congenital abnormality; they should be reported even if the effect is well recognised. Examples include anaphylaxis, blood disorders, endocrine disturbances, effects on fertility, haemorrhage from any site, renal impairment, jaundice, ophthalmic disorders, severe CNS effects, severe skin reactions, reactions in pregnant females, and any drug interactions. Reports of serious adverse reactions are required to enable comparison with other drugs of a similar class. Reports of overdoses (deliberate or accidental) can complicate the assessment of adverse drug reactions, but provide important information on the potential toxicity of drugs.

For established drugs there is no need to report well-known, relatively minor side-effects, such as dry mouth with tricyclic antidepressants or constipation with opioids.

Medication errors

Adverse drug reactions where harm occurs as a result of a medication error are reportable through the Yellow Card scheme or through a local risk management system (LRMS).

In England, medication errors reported via a LRMS are uploaded to the national Learn From Patient Safety Events service (LFPSE); if a LRMS is not available, medication errors can also be reported directly via the LFPSE online service (record.learn-from-patient-safety-events.nhs.uk). If incidents are uploaded into LFPSE, these will be shared with the MHRA. (This service is being rolled out across England, Wales, and Northern Ireland—speak to your local safety team about which system you should currently be using.) If LFPSE is not available and harm occurs, report through the Yellow Card scheme.

In Scotland, local incident/event management systems with a focus on quality improvement and learning are promoted. The Healthcare Improvement Scotland *Adverse Events National Framework: Learning from adverse events through reporting and review - A national framework for Scotland: December* 2019 (www.healthcareimprovementscotland.org/our_work/governance_and_assurance/learning_from_adverse_events/national_framework.aspx) provides useful context to the management of adverse events.

Adverse reactions to medical devices

Suspected adverse reactions to medical devices including dental or surgical materials, intra-uterine devices, and contact lens fluids should be reported. Information about reporting medical device adverse incidents can be found at: yellowcard.mhra.gov.uk/medicaldevices.

Side-effects in the BNF for Children

The BNF for Children includes clinically relevant side-effects for most drugs; an exhaustive list is not included for drugs that are used by specialists (e.g. cytotoxic drugs and drugs used in anaesthesia). Where causality has not been established, side-effects in the manufacturers' literature may be omitted from the BNF for Children.

Recognising that hypersensitivity reactions (including anaphylactic and anaphylactoid reactions) can occur with virtually all drugs, this effect is not generally listed, unless the drug carries an increased risk of such reactions or specific management advice is provided by the manufacturer. Administration site reactions have been omitted from the BNF for Children (e.g. pain at injection site). The BNF for Children also omits effects that are likely to have little clinical consequence (e.g. transient increase in liver enzymes). Drugs that are applied locally or topically carry a theoretical or low risk of systemic absorption and therefore systemic side-effects for these drugs are not listed in the BNF for Children unless they are associated with a high risk to patient safety. Infections are a known complication of treatment with drugs that affect the immune system (e.g. corticosteroids or immunosuppressants); this side-effect is listed in the BNF for Children as 'increased risk of infection'. Symptoms of drug withdrawal reactions are not individually listed, but are collectively termed 'withdrawal syndrome'.

Description of the frequency of side-effects	
Very common	greater than 1 in 10
Common	1 in 100 to 1 in 10
Uncommon [formerly 'less commonly' in BNF publications]	1 in 1000 to 1 in 100
Rare	1 in 10 000 to 1 in 1000
Very rare	less than 1 in 10 000
Frequency not known	frequency is not defined by product literature or the side-effect has been reported from post-marketing surveillance data

The BNF for Children might not use the same wording as manufacturers' literature because, for consistency, the terms used to describe side-effects are standardised using a defined vocabulary across all of the drug monographs in the BNF for Children (e.g. postural hypotension is used for the term orthostatic hypotension). In addition, individual side-effects are often grouped together in the BNF for Children where there are two or more similar side-effects (e.g. hepatitis, hepatic failure, and jaundice are grouped together as 'hepatic disorders').

Some drug monographs in the BNF for Children include information that is common across the drug class. If a side-effect is associated with at least 60% of the drugs in a class then it will appear as a class side-effect for all drugs in the class, and the frequency of the side-effect will be the highest of all the drugs in that class.

Special problems

Symptoms Children may be poor at expressing the symptoms of an adverse drug reaction and parental opinion may be required.

Delayed drug effects Some reactions (e.g. cancers and effects on development) may become manifest months or years after exposure. Any suspicion of such an association should be reported through the Yellow Card scheme.

Congenital abnormalities When an infant is born with a congenital abnormality or there is a malformed aborted fetus doctors are asked to consider whether this might be an adverse reaction to a drug and to report all drugs (including self-medication) taken during pregnancy.

Prevention of adverse reactions

Adverse reactions may be prevented as follows:

- never use any drug unless there is a good indication. If the patient is pregnant do not use a drug unless the need for it is imperative;
- allergy and idiosyncrasy are important causes of adverse drug reactions. Ask if the child has had previous reactions to the drug or formulation;
- prescribe as few drugs as possible and give very clear instructions to the child, parent, or carer;
- whenever possible use a familiar drug; with a new drug be particularly alert for adverse reactions or unexpected events;
- consider if excipients (e.g. colouring agents) may be contributing to the adverse reaction. If the reaction is minor, a trial of an alternative formulation of the same drug may be considered before abandoning the drug;
- obtain a full drug history including asking if the child is already taking other drugs *including over-the-counter medicines*; interactions may occur;
- age and hepatic or renal disease may alter the metabolism or excretion of drugs, particularly in neonates, which can affect the potential for adverse effects. Genetic factors may also be responsible for variations in metabolism, and therefore for the adverse effects of the drug;
- warn the child, parent, or carer if serious adverse reactions are liable to occur.

The MHRA has produced guidance on risk minimisation measures for medicines to ensure their safe and effective use. These measures are intended to prevent or reduce the risk of an adverse event, or to reduce the severity or impact should an adverse event occur, as well as supporting informed decision making. For more information, see www.gov.uk/government/publications/risk-minimisation-measures-for-medicines.

Drug allergy (suspected or confirmed)

Suspected drug allergy is any reaction caused by a drug with clinical features compatible with an immunological mechanism. All drugs have the potential to cause adverse drug reactions, but not all of these are allergic in nature. A reaction is more likely to be caused by drug allergy if:

- The reaction occurred while the child was being treated with the drug, or
- The drug is known to cause this pattern of reaction, or
- The child has had a similar reaction to the same drug or drug-class previously.

A suspected reaction is less likely to be caused by a drug allergy if there is a possible non-drug cause or if there are only gastro-intestinal symptoms present.

The following signs, allergic patterns and timing of onset can be used to help decide whether to suspect drug allergy:
Immediate, rapidly-evolving reactions (onset usually less than 1 hour after drug exposure)

- Anaphylaxis, with erythema, urticaria or angioedema, and hypotension and/or bronchospasm. See also Antihistamines, allergen immunotherapy and allergic emergencies p. 199
- Urticaria or angioedema without systemic features
- Exacerbation of asthma e.g. with non-steroidal anti-inflammatory drugs (NSAIDs)

*Non-immediate reactions, **without** systemic involvement* (onset usually 6–10 days after first drug exposure or 3 days after second exposure)

- Cutaneous reactions, e.g. widespread red macules and/or papules, or, fixed drug eruption (localised inflamed skin)

*Non-immediate reactions, **with** systemic involvement* (onset may be variable, usually 3 days to 6 weeks after first drug exposure, depending on features, or 3 days after second exposure)

- Cutaneous reactions with systemic features, e.g. drug reaction with eosinophilia and systemic signs (DRESS) or drug hypersensitivity syndrome (DHS), characterised by widespread red macules, papules or erythroderma, fever, lymphadenopathy, liver dysfunction or eosinophilia
- Toxic epidermal necrolysis or Stevens–Johnson syndrome
- Acute generalised exanthematous pustulosis (AGEP)

EvGr Suspected drug allergy information should be clearly and accurately documented in clinical notes and prescriptions, and shared among all healthcare professionals. Children and parents or carers should be given information about which drugs and drug-classes to avoid and encouraged to share the drug allergy status.

If a drug allergy is suspected, consider stopping the suspected drug and advising the child and parent or carer to avoid this drug in future. Symptoms of the acute reaction should be treated, in hospital if severe. Children presenting with a suspected anaphylactic reaction, or a severe or non-immediate cutaneous reaction, should be referred to a specialist drug allergy service. Children presenting with a suspected drug allergic reaction or anaphylaxis to NSAIDs, and local and general anaesthetics may also need to be referred to a specialist drug allergy service, e.g. in cases of anaphylactoid reactions or to determine future treatment options. Children presenting with a suspected drug allergic reaction or anaphylaxis associated with beta-lactam antibiotics should be referred to a specialist drug allergy service if their disease or condition can only be treated by a beta-lactam antibiotic or they are likely to need beta-lactam antibiotics frequently in the future (e.g. immunodeficient children). ⟨A⟩ For further information see Drug allergy: diagnosis and management. NICE Clinical Guideline 183 (September 2014) www.nice.org.uk/guidance/cg183.

Defective medicines

During the manufacture or distribution of a medicine an error or accident may occur whereby the finished product does not conform to its specification. While such a defect may impair the therapeutic effect of the product and could adversely affect the health of a patient, it should **not** be confused with an adverse drug reaction where the product conforms to its specification. Reports of a defective medicine can be made online through the Yellow Card scheme.

The Defective Medicines Report Centre (DMRC) assists with the investigation of problems arising from licensed medicinal products thought to be defective and co-ordinates any necessary protective action. Reports on suspect defective medicinal products should include the brand or the non-proprietary name, the name of the manufacturer or supplier, the strength and dosage form of the product, the product licence number, the batch number or numbers of the product, the nature of the defect, and an account of any action already taken in consequence. The Centre can be contacted at:

The Defective Medicines Report Centre
Medicines and Healthcare products Regulatory Agency
10 South Colonnade
Canary Wharf
London
E14 4PU
dmrc@mhra.gov.uk

During office hours (8:45am to 4:45pm Monday to Friday), contact DMRC on 020 3080 6574.

Out of hours (urgent reports outside of normal working hours, at weekends or on public holidays), contact DMRC on 07795 641 532.

Guidance on intravenous infusions

Intravenous infusions for neonatal intensive care

Intravenous policy A local policy on the dilution of drugs with intravenous fluids should be drawn up by a multi-disciplinary team and issued as a document to the members of staff concerned.

Centralised additive services are provided in a number of hospital pharmacy departments and should be used in preference to making additions on wards.

The information that follows should be read in conjunction with local policy documents.

Guidelines

- Drugs should only be diluted with infusion fluid when constant plasma concentrations are needed or when the administration of a more concentrated solution would be harmful.
- In general, only one drug should be mixed with an infusion fluid in a syringe and the components should be compatible. Ready-prepared solutions should be used whenever possible. Drugs should not normally be added to blood products, mannitol, or sodium bicarbonate. Only specially formulated additives should be used with fat emulsions or amino-acid solutions.
- Solutions should be thoroughly mixed by shaking and checked for absence of particulate matter before use.
- Strict asepsis should be maintained throughout and in general the giving set should not be used for more than 24 hours (for drug admixtures).
- The infusion syringe should be labelled with the neonate's name and hospital number, the name and quantity of drug, the infusion fluid, and the expiry date and time. If a problem occurs during administration, containers should be retained for a period after use in case they are needed for investigation.
- Administration using a suitable motorised syringe driver is advocated for preparations where strict control over administration is required.
- It is good practice to examine intravenous infusions from time to time while they are running. If cloudiness, crystallisation, change of colour, or any other sign of interaction or contamination is observed the infusion should be discontinued.

Problems

Microbial contamination The accidental entry and subsequent growth of micro-organisms converts the infusion fluid pathway into a potential vehicle for infection with micro-organisms, particularly species of Candida, Enterobacter, and Klebsiella. Ready-prepared infusions containing the additional drugs, or infusions prepared by an additive service (when available) should therefore be used in preference to making extemporaneous additions to infusion containers on wards etc. However, when this is necessary strict aseptic procedure should be followed.

Incompatibility Physical and chemical incompatibilities may occur with loss of potency, increase in toxicity, or other adverse effect. The solutions may become opalescent or precipitation may occur, but in many instances there is no visual indication of incompatibility. Interaction may take place at any point in the infusion fluid pathway, and the potential for incompatibility is increased when more than one substance is added to the infusion fluid.

Common incompatibilities Precipitation reactions are numerous and varied and may occur as a result of pH, concentration changes, 'salting-out' effects, complexation or other chemical changes. Precipitation or other particle formation must be avoided since, apart from lack of control of dosage on administration, it may initiate or exacerbate adverse effects. This is particularly important in the case of drugs which have been implicated in either thrombophlebitis (e.g. diazepam) or in skin sloughing or necrosis caused by extravasation (e.g. sodium bicarbonate and parenteral nutrition). It is also especially important to effect solution of colloidal drugs and to prevent their subsequent precipitation in order to avoid a pyrogenic reaction (e.g. amphotericin B).

It is considered undesirable to mix beta-lactam antibiotics, such as semi-synthetic penicillins and cephalosporins, with proteinaceous materials on the grounds that immunogenic and allergenic conjugates could be formed.

A number of preparations undergo significant loss of potency when added singly or in combination to large volume infusions. Examples include ampicillin in infusions that contain glucose or lactates.

Blood Because of the large number of incompatibilities, drugs should not be added to blood and blood products for infusion purposes. Examples of incompatibility with blood include hypertonic mannitol solutions (irreversible crenation of red cells), dextrans (rouleaux formation and interference with cross-matching), glucose (clumping of red cells), and oxytocin (inactivated).

If the giving set is not changed after the administration of blood, but used for other infusion fluids, a fibrin clot may form which, apart from blocking the set, increases the likelihood of microbial growth.

Intravenous fat emulsion These may break down with coalescence of fat globules and separation of phases when additions such as antibacterials or electrolytes are made, thus increasing the possibility of embolism. Only specially formulated products such as *Vitlipid N®* may be added to appropriate intravenous fat emulsions.

Other infusions Infusions that frequently give rise to incompatibility include amino acids, mannitol, and sodium bicarbonate.

Method

Ready-prepared infusions should be used whenever available. When dilution of drugs is required to be made extemporaneously, any product reconstitution instructions such as those relating to concentration, vehicle, mixing, and handling precautions should be strictly followed using an aseptic technique throughout. Once the product has been reconstituted, further dilution with the infusion fluid should be made immediately in order to minimise microbial contamination and, with certain products, to prevent degradation or other formulation change which may occur; e.g. reconstituted ampicillin injection degrades rapidly on standing, and also may form polymers which could cause sensitivity reactions.

It is also important in certain instances that an infusion fluid of specific pH be used (e.g. **furosemide** injection requires dilution in infusions of pH greater than 5.5).

When drug dilutions are made it is important to mix thoroughly; additions should not be made to an infusion container that has been connected to a giving set, as mixing is hampered. If the solutions are not thoroughly mixed, a concentrated layer of the drug may form owing to differences in density. **Potassium chloride** is particularly prone to this 'layering' effect when added without adequate mixing to infusions; if such a mixture is administered it may have a serious effect on the heart.

A time limit between dilution and completion of administration must be imposed for certain admixtures to guarantee satisfactory drug potency and compatibility. For admixtures in which degradation occurs without the formation of toxic substances, an acceptable limit is the time taken for 10% decomposition of the drug. When toxic substances are produced stricter limits may be imposed. Because of the risk of microbial contamination a maximum time limit of 24 hours may be appropriate for additions made elsewhere than in hospital pharmacies offering central additive service.

Certain injections must be protected from light during continuous infusion to minimise oxidation, e.g. sodium nitroprusside.

Drugs given by continuous intravenous infusion to neonates

The information provided in BNFC covers dilution with *Glucose intravenous infusion* 5% and 10% and *Sodium chloride intravenous infusion* 0.9%. Compatibility with glucose 5% and with sodium chloride 0.9% indicates compatibility with *Sodium chloride and glucose intravenous infusion*. Infusion of a large volume of hypotonic solution should be avoided, therefore care should be taken if water for injections is used.

Prescribing in hepatic impairment

Overview

Children have a large reserve of hepatic metabolic capacity and modification of the choice and dosage of drugs is usually unnecessary even in apparently severe liver disease. However, special consideration is required in the following situations:

- liver failure characterised by severe derangement of liver enzymes and profound jaundice; the use of sedative drugs, opioids, and drugs such as diuretics and amphotericin B p. 462 which produce hypokalaemia may precipitate hepatic encephalopathy;
- impaired coagulation, which can affect response to oral anticoagulants;
- in cholestatic jaundice elimination may be impaired of drugs such as fusidic acid p. 441 and rifampicin p. 449 which are excreted in the bile;
- in hypoproteinaemia, the effect of highly protein-bound drugs such as phenytoin p. 249, prednisolone p. 548, warfarin sodium p. 115, and benzodiazepines may be increased;
- use of hepatotoxic drugs is more likely to cause toxicity in children with liver disease; such drugs should be avoided if possible;
- in neonates, particularly preterm neonates, and also in infants metabolic pathways may differ from older children and adults because liver enzyme pathways may be immature.

Where care is needed when prescribing in hepatic impairment, this is indicated under the relevant drug in BNFC.

Prescribing in renal impairment

Issues encountered in renal impairment

The use of drugs in children with reduced renal function can give rise to problems for several reasons:

- reduced renal excretion of a drug or its metabolites may produce toxicity;
- sensitivity to some drugs is increased even if elimination is unimpaired;
- many side-effects are tolerated poorly by children with renal impairment;
- some drugs are not effective when renal function is reduced;
- neonates, particularly preterm, may have immature renal function.

Many of these problems can be avoided by reducing the dose or by using alternative drugs.

If even mild renal impairment is considered likely on clinical grounds, renal function should be checked before prescribing any drug which requires dose modification.

General Guidance

Drugs eliminated via the kidneys can accumulate during acute kidney injury (AKI) or chronic kidney disease (CKD) and this can lead to further renal impairment or adverse effects. EvGr A review of these drugs is therefore required; any drug which can cause or exacerbate renal impairment should be avoided in AKI, and the appropriateness reviewed in CKD. (E)

Where care is needed when prescribing in renal impairment, this is indicated under the relevant drug in BNFC. Dose recommendations are based on the severity of renal impairment.

When both efficacy and toxicity are closely related to plasma-drug concentration, recommended regimens should be regarded only as a guide to initial treatment; subsequent doses must be adjusted according to clinical response and plasma-drug concentration.

The total daily maintenance dose of a drug can be reduced either by reducing the size of the individual doses or by increasing the interval between doses.

For some drugs, although the size of the maintenance dose is reduced it is important to give a loading dose if an immediate effect is required. This is because it takes about five times the half-life of the drug to achieve steady-state plasma concentration. Because the plasma half-life of drugs excreted by the kidney is prolonged in renal impairment, it can take many doses at the reduced dosage to achieve a therapeutic plasma concentration. The loading dose should usually be the same as the initial dose for a child with normal renal function.

For information and advice on the prevention, detection, and management of acute kidney injury, see NICE clinical guideline: **Acute Kidney Injury** (www.nice.org.uk/guidance/ng148).

Important: dosage adjustment advice in BNFC The information on dose adjustment in BNFC may be expressed in terms of estimated glomerular filtration rate (mL/minute/1.73 m^2). However, in product literature, the effects of renal impairment on drug elimination is usually stated in terms of *creatinine clearance* (CrCl). EvGr Although these two measures of renal function are not interchangeable, for most drugs and for most children of average build and height, estimated glomerular filtration rate (using the modified Bedside Schwartz equation) rather than CrCl can be used to determine dosage adjustments. If clinicians have any concerns, they should discuss with these with their local paediatric nephrology department. ⟨E⟩

Renal function in adults is routinely reported by clinical laboratories based on estimated glomerular filtration rate (eGFR) normalised to a body surface area of 1.73 m^2; however, eGFR is derived from either the Chronic Kidney Disease Epidemiology Collaboration (CKD-EPI) formula or the Modification of Diet in Renal Disease (MDRD) formula which are not validated for use in children. EvGr eGFR derived from the CKD-EPI or MDRD formula should **not** be used to adjust drug doses in children with renal impairment. ⟨E⟩

In BNFC, values for measures of renal function are included where possible. However, where such values are not available, BNFC reflects the terms used in the published information.

Estimating renal function

Glomerular filtration rate is low at birth and increases rapidly during the first 6 months. Thereafter, glomerular filtration rate increases gradually to reach adult levels by 1–2 years of age, when standardised to a typical adult body surface area (1.73 m^2). In the first weeks after birth, serum creatinine falls; a single measure of serum creatinine provides only a crude estimate of renal function and observing the change over days is of more use. In the neonate, a sustained rise in serum creatinine or a lack of the expected postnatal decline, is indicative of a reduced glomerular filtration rate.

The serum-creatinine concentration is sometimes used as a measure of renal function but is only a **rough guide** even when corrected for age, weight, and sex.

Estimated glomerular filtration rate EvGr Estimated glomerular filtration rate should be used with caution in very malnourished children or those with liver disease. ⟨E⟩

Modified Bedside Schwartz EvGr The following equations are a guide to calculating estimated glomerular filtration rate in children: ⟨E⟩

Child over 1 month:
Estimated glomerular filtration rate (mL/minute/1.73 m^2)= 35 $\times$ height (cm)/serum creatinine (micromol/litre)

Neonate:
Estimated glomerular filtration rate (mL/minute/1.73 m^2)= 30 $\times$ height (cm)/serum creatinine (micromol/litre)

The values used in these formulas may differ according to locality or laboratory.

Chronic kidney disease

For guidance on the management of children with, or who are at risk of, chronic kidney disease, see NICE guideline: **Chronic kidney disease: assessment and management** (available at: www.nice.org.uk/guidance/ng203).

Classification of chronic kidney disease using GFR and ACR categories (in adults) Chronic kidney disease **in adults** is classified using a combination of GFR and albumin: creatinine ratio (ACR). A decreased GFR and an increased ACR is associated with an increased risk of adverse outcomes.

For example, an adult with an eGFR of 25 ml/min/1.73 m^2 and an ACR of 15 mg/mmol has a CKD classification of G4A2.

Dialysis

For prescribing in children on renal replacement therapy consult specialist literature.

Classification of chronic kidney disease using GFR and ACR categories (in adults)

GFR and ACR categories and risk of adverse outcomes		ACR categories (mg/mmol), description and range		
		<3 Normal to mild increase	3–30 Moderate increase	>30 Severe increase
		A1	A2	A3
GFR categories (ml/min/1.73m^2), description and range: ≥90 Normal or high	G1	No CKD in the absence of markers of kidney damage		
60–89 Mild reduction relative to normal range for a young adult	G2			
45–59 Mild-moderate reduction	G3a			
30–44 Moderate-severe reduction	G3b			
15–29 Severe reduction	G4			
<15 Kidney failure	G5			

Increasing risk (from A1 to A3)

Increasing risk (from G1 to G5)

Abbreviations: ACR, albumin:creatinine ratio; CKD, chronic kidney disease; GFR, glomerular filtration rate

Adapted with the kind permission of the Kidney Disease: Improving Global Outcomes (KDIGO) CKD Work Group, 2013.

Prescribing in pregnancy

Overview

Drugs can have harmful effects on the embryo or fetus at any time during pregnancy. It is important to bear this in mind when prescribing for a woman of *childbearing age* or for men *trying* to *father* a child.

During the *first trimester* drugs can produce congenital malformations (teratogenesis), and the period of greatest risk is from the third to the eleventh week of pregnancy.

During the *second* and *third trimesters* drugs can affect the growth or functional development of the fetus, or they can have toxic effects on fetal tissues.

Drugs given shortly before term or during labour can have adverse effects on labour or on the neonate after delivery.

Not all the damaging effects of intra-uterine exposure to drugs are obvious at birth, some may only manifest later in life. Such late-onset effects include malignancy, e.g. adenocarcinoma of the vagina after puberty in females exposed to diethylstilbestrol in the womb, and adverse effects on intellectual, social, and functional development.

BNF and BNFC identify drugs which:

- may have harmful effects in pregnancy and indicate the trimester of risk
- are not known to be harmful in pregnancy

The information is based on human data, but information from *animal* studies has been included for some drugs when its omission might be misleading. Maternal drug doses may require adjustment during pregnancy due to changes in maternal physiology but this is beyond the scope of BNF and BNFC.

Where care is needed when prescribing in pregnancy, this is indicated under the relevant drug in BNF and BNFC.

Important

Drugs should be prescribed in pregnancy only if the expected benefit to the mother is thought to be greater than the risk to the fetus, and all drugs should be avoided if possible during the first trimester. Drugs which have been extensively used in pregnancy and appear to be usually safe should be prescribed in preference to new or untried drugs; and the smallest effective dose should be used. Few drugs have been shown conclusively to be teratogenic in humans, but no drug is safe beyond all doubt in early pregnancy. Screening procedures are available when there is a known risk of certain defects.

Absence of information does not imply safety. It should be noted that BNF and BNFC provide independent advice and may not always agree with the product literature.

Information on drugs and pregnancy is also available from the UK Teratology Information Service at: www.uktis.org.

MHRA/CHM advice: Medicines in pregnancy and breastfeeding: new initiative for consistent guidance; report on optimising data for medicines used during pregnancy (February 2021)

The Safer Medicines in Pregnancy and Breastfeeding Consortium, formed of the MHRA and partner organisations, aims to improve the health information available to women who are thinking about becoming pregnant, are pregnant, or are breast-feeding, and ensure that they can make informed decisions about their healthcare, particularly about medicines. To support this, healthcare professionals are requested to report inconsistencies in UK advice on the use of individual or classes of medicines during pregnancy or breast-feeding via the consortium at: www.gov.uk/government/publications/safer-medicines-in-pregnancy-and-breastfeeding-consortium.

The Report of the CHM Expert Working Group on Optimising Data on Medicines used During Pregnancy provides recommendations on ways in which data on medicines used during pregnancy and breast-feeding can be better collected and made available for analysis. This will enable more robust evidence to be generated through research and will help to develop clear and consistent advice about medicines used during pregnancy and breast-feeding. The report is available at: www.gov.uk/government/publications/report-of-the-commission-on-human-medicines-expert-working-group-on-optimising-data-on-medicines-used-during-pregnancy.

Prescribing in breast-feeding

Overview

Breast-feeding is beneficial; the immunological and nutritional value of breast milk to the infant is greater than that of formula feeds.

Although there is concern that drugs taken by the mother might affect the infant, there is very little information on this. In the absence of evidence of an effect, the potential for harm to the infant can be inferred from:

- the amount of drug or active metabolite of the drug delivered to the infant (dependent on the pharmacokinetic characteristics of the drug in the mother);
- the efficiency of absorption, distribution, and elimination of the drug by the infant (infant pharmacokinetics);
- the nature of the effect of the drug on the infant (pharmacodynamic properties of the drug in the infant).

Most medicines given to a mother cause no harm to breast-fed infants and there are few contra-indications to breast-feeding when maternal medicines are necessary. However, administration of some drugs to nursing mothers can harm the infant. In the first week of life, some such as preterm or jaundiced infants are at a slightly higher risk of toxicity.

Toxicity to the infant can occur if the drug enters the milk in pharmacologically significant quantities. The concentration in milk of some drugs (e.g. fluvastatin p. 155) may exceed the concentration in maternal plasma so that therapeutic doses in the mother can cause toxicity to the infant. Some drugs inhibit the infant's sucking reflex (e.g. phenobarbital p. 264) while others can affect lactation (e.g. bromocriptine). Drugs in breast milk may, at least theoretically, cause hypersensitivity in the infant even when concentration is too low for a pharmacological effect. BNFC identifies drugs:

- which should be used with caution or which are contra-indicated in breast-feeding for the reasons given above;
- which, on present evidence, may be given to the mother during breast-feeding, because they appear in milk in amounts which are too small to be harmful to the infant;
- which are not known to be harmful to the infant although they are present in milk in significant amounts.

Where care is needed when prescribing in breast-feeding, this is indicated under the relevant drug in BNFC.

Important

For many drugs insufficient evidence is available to provide guidance and it is advisable to administer only essential drugs to a mother during breast-feeding. Because of the inadequacy of information on drugs in breast-feeding, absence of information does not imply safety.

MHRA/CHM advice: Medicines in pregnancy and breastfeeding: new initiative for consistent guidance; report on optimising data for medicines used during pregnancy (February 2021)

The Safer Medicines in Pregnancy and Breastfeeding Consortium, formed of the MHRA and partner organisations, aims to improve the health information available to women who are thinking about becoming pregnant, are pregnant, or are breast-feeding, and ensure that they can make informed decisions about their healthcare, particularly about medicines. To support this, healthcare professionals are requested to report inconsistencies in UK advice on the use of individual or classes of medicines during pregnancy or breast-feeding via the consortium at: www.gov.uk/government/publications/safer-medicines-in-pregnancy-and-breastfeeding-consortium.

The Report of the CHM Expert Working Group on Optimising Data on Medicines used During Pregnancy provides recommendations on ways in which data on medicines used during pregnancy and breast-feeding can be better collected and made available for analysis. This will enable more robust evidence to be generated through research and will help to develop clear and consistent advice about medicines used during pregnancy and breast-feeding. The report is available at: www.gov.uk/government/publications/report-of-the-commission-on-human-medicines-expert-working-group-on-optimising-data-on-medicines-used-during-pregnancy.

Prescribing in palliative care

Overview

Palliative care is the active and total approach to the care of children and young adults with life-limiting and life-threatening conditions, embracing physical, emotional, social, and spiritual elements of their care. It focuses on enhancing the quality of life for the child and support for their family, and includes the management of distressing symptoms, provision of respite, and care following death and bereavement.

Effective palliative care requires a broad multidisciplinary approach that includes the whole family, and ideally should start as soon as possible after diagnosis or recognition of a life-threatening condition.

Drug treatment The number of drugs should be as few as possible. Oral medication is usually appropriate unless there is severe nausea and vomiting, dysphagia, weakness, or coma, when parenteral medication may be necessary.

For further information on the use of medicines in paediatric palliative care, see the Association for Paediatric Palliative Medicine (APPM) Master Formulary available at www.appm.org.uk/formulary/.

Pain

Pain management in palliative care is focused on achieving control of pain by administering the right drug in the right dose at the right time. Analgesics can be divided into three broad classes: non-opioid (paracetamol p. 325, NSAID), opioid (e.g. codeine phosphate p. 331 'weak', morphine p. 338 'strong') and adjuvant (e.g. antidepressants, antiepileptics). Drugs from the different classes are used alone or in combination according to the type of pain and response to treatment. Analgesics are more effective in preventing pain than in the relief of established pain; it is important that they are given regularly.

Paracetamol or a NSAID given regularly will often be sufficient to manage mild pain. If non-opioid analgesics alone are not sufficient, then an opioid analgesic alone or in combination with a non-opioid analgesic at an adequate dosage, may be helpful in the control of moderate pain. Codeine phosphate or tramadol hydrochloride p. 343 can be considered for moderate pain. If these preparations do not control the pain then morphine is the most useful opioid analgesic. Alternatives to morphine, including transdermal buprenorphine p. 329, transdermal fentanyl p. 334, hydromorphone hydrochloride p. 337, methadone hydrochloride p. 357, or oxycodone hydrochloride p. 340, should be initiated by those with experience in palliative care. Initiation of an opioid analgesic should not be delayed by concern over a theoretical likelihood of psychological dependence (addiction).

Bone metastases In addition to the above approach, radiotherapy and bisphosphonates may be useful for pain due to bone metastases.

Neuropathic pain Patients with neuropathic pain may benefit from a trial of a tricyclic antidepressant, most commonly amitriptyline hydrochloride p. 289, for several weeks. An antiepileptic such as carbamazepine p. 234, may be added or substituted if pain persists. Ketamine p. 1023 is sometimes used under specialist supervision for neuropathic pain that responds poorly to opioid analgesics. Pain due to nerve compression may be reduced by a corticosteroid such as dexamethasone p. 543, which reduces oedema around the tumour, thus reducing compression. Nerve blocks can be considered when pain is localised to a specific area. Transcutaneous electrical nerve stimulation (TENS) may also help.

Pain management with opioids

Oral route Treatment with morphine p. 338 is given by mouth as immediate-release or modified-release preparations. During the titration phase the initial dose is based on the previous medication used, the severity of the pain, and other factors such as presence of renal impairment or frailty. The dose is given either as an immediate-release preparation 4-hourly (for starting doses, see Morphine), or as a 12-hourly modified-release preparation, in addition to rescue doses. If replacing a weaker opioid analgesic (such as codeine phosphate p. 331), starting doses are usually higher.

If pain occurs between regular doses of morphine ('breakthrough pain'), an additional dose ('rescue dose') of immediate-release morphine should be given. An additional dose should also be given 30 minutes before an activity that causes pain, such as wound dressing. The standard dose of a strong opioid for breakthrough pain is usually one-tenth to one-sixth of the regular 24-hour dose, repeated every 2–4 hours as required (up to hourly may be needed if pain is severe or in the last days of life). Review pain management if rescue analgesic is required frequently (twice daily or more). Each child should be assessed on an individual basis. Formulations of fentanyl p. 334 that are administered nasally, buccally or sublingually are not licensed for use in children; their usefulness in children is also limited by dose availability.

Children often require a higher dose of morphine in proportion to their body-weight compared to adults. Children are more susceptible to certain adverse effects of opioids such as urinary retention (which can be eased by bethanechol chloride), and opioid-induced pruritus.

When adjusting the dose of morphine, the number of rescue doses required and the response to them should be taken into account; increments of morphine should not exceed one-third to one-half of the total daily dose every 24 hours. Thereafter, the dose should be adjusted with careful assessment of the pain, and the use of adjuvant analgesics should also be considered. Upward titration of the dose of morphine stops when either the pain is relieved or unacceptable adverse effects occur, after which it is necessary to consider alternative measures.

Once their pain is controlled, children started on 4-hourly immediate-release morphine can be transferred to the same total 24-hour dose of morphine given as the modified-release preparation for 12-hourly or 24-hourly administration. The first dose of the modified-release preparation is given with, or within 4 hours of the last dose of the immediate-release preparation. For preparations suitable for 12-hourly or 24-hourly administration see modified-release preparations under morphine. Increments should be made to the dose, not to the frequency of administration. The patient must be monitored closely for efficacy and side-effects, particularly constipation, and nausea and vomiting. A suitable laxative should be prescribed routinely.

Oxycodone hydrochloride p. 340 can be used in children who require an opioid but cannot tolerate morphine. If the child is already receiving an opioid, oxycodone hydrochloride should be started at a dose equivalent to the current analgesic. Oxycodone hydrochloride immediate-release preparations can be given for breakthrough pain.

Equivalent doses of opioid analgesics.

This table is only an **approximate** guide (doses may not correspond with those given in clinical practice); children should be carefully monitored after any change in medication and dose titration may be required.

Analgesic/Route	Dose
Codeine: PO	100 mg
Diamorphine: IM, IV, SC	3 mg
Dihydrocodeine: PO	100 mg
Hydromorphone: PO	2 mg
Morphine: PO	10 mg
Morphine: IM, IV, SC	5 mg
Oxycodone: PO	6.6 mg
Tramadol: PO	100 mg

PO = by mouth; IM = intramuscular; IV = intravenous; SC = subcutaneous

Parenteral route Diamorphine hydrochloride p. 332 is preferred for injection because, being more soluble, it can be given in a smaller volume. The equivalent subcutaneous dose is approximately a third of the oral dose of morphine p. 338. Subcutaneous infusion of diamorphine hydrochloride via a continuous infusion device can be useful (for details, see Continuous subcutaneous infusions).

If the child can resume taking medicines by mouth, then oral morphine may be substituted for subcutaneous infusion of diamorphine hydrochloride. See the table *Approximate equivalent doses of morphine and diamorphine*.

Rectal route Morphine p. 338 is also available for rectal administration as suppositories.

Transdermal route Transdermal preparations of fentanyl p. 334 and buprenorphine p. 329 [not licensed for use in children] are available; they are not suitable for acute pain or in those children whose analgesic requirements are changing rapidly because the long time to steady state prevents rapid titration of the dose. Prescribers should ensure that they are familiar with the correct use of transdermal preparations (see under fentanyl) because inappropriate use has caused fatalities.

The following 24-hour oral doses of morphine p. 338 are considered to be *approximately* equivalent to the buprenorphine and fentanyl patches shown, however when switching due to possible opioid-induced hyperalgesia, reduce the calculated equivalent dose of the new opioid by one-quarter to one-half.

Buprenorphine patches are *approximately* equivalent to the following 24-hour doses of oral morphine

morphine salt 12 mg daily	≡ buprenorphine '5' patch
morphine salt 24 mg daily	≡ buprenorphine '10' patch
morphine salt 36 mg daily	≡ buprenorphine '15' patch
morphine salt 48 mg daily	≡ buprenorphine '20' patch
morphine salt 84 mg daily	≡ buprenorphine '35' patch
morphine salt 126 mg daily	≡ buprenorphine '52.5' patch
morphine salt 168 mg daily	≡ buprenorphine '70' patch

Formulations of transdermal patches are available as 72-hourly, 96-hourly and 7-day patches, for further information see buprenorphine in BNF. Conversion ratios vary and these figures are a guide only. Morphine equivalences for transdermal opioid preparations have been approximated to allow comparison with available preparations of oral morphine.

72-hour Fentanyl patches are *approximately* equivalent to the following 24-hour doses of oral morphine

morphine salt 30 mg daily	≡ fentanyl '12' patch
morphine salt 60 mg daily	≡ fentanyl '25' patch
morphine salt 120 mg daily	≡ fentanyl '50' patch
morphine salt 180 mg daily	≡ fentanyl '75' patch
morphine salt 240 mg daily	≡ fentanyl '100' patch

Fentanyl equivalences in this table are for children on well-tolerated opioid therapy for long periods; fentanyl patches should not be used in opioid naive children. Conversion ratios vary and these figures are a guide only. Morphine equivalences for transdermal opioid preparations have been approximated to allow comparison with available preparations of oral morphine.

Symptom control

Unlicensed indications or routes Several recommendations in this section involve unlicensed indications or routes.

Anorexia Anorexia may be helped by prednisolone p. 548 or dexamethasone p. 543.

Anxiety Anxiety can be treated with a long-acting benzodiazepine such as diazepam p. 270, or by continuous infusion of the short-acting benzodiazepine midazolam p. 273. Interventions for more acute episodes of anxiety (such as panic attacks) include short-acting benzodiazepines such as lorazepam p. 272 given sublingually or midazolam given subcutaneously. Temazepam p. 1024 provides useful night-time sedation in some children.

Capillary bleeding Capillary bleeding can be treated with tranexamic acid p. 92 by mouth; treatment is usually continued for one week after the bleeding has stopped but it can be continued at a reduced dose if bleeding persists. Alternatively, gauze soaked in tranexamic acid 100 mg/mL or adrenaline solution 1 mg/mL (1 in 1000) p. 159 can be applied to the affected area.

Vitamin K may be useful for the treatment and prevention of bleeding associated with prolonged clotting in liver disease. In severe chronic cholestasis, absorption of vitamin K may be impaired; either parenteral or water-soluble oral vitamin K should be considered.

Constipation Constipation is a common cause of distress and is almost invariable after administration of an opioid analgesic. It should be prevented if possible by the regular administration of laxatives. Suitable laxatives include osmotic laxatives (such as lactulose p. 46 or macrogols), stimulant laxatives (such as co-danthramer p. 51 and senna p. 52) or the combination of lactulose and a senna preparation. Naloxone hydrochloride p. 1047 given by mouth may help relieve opioid-induced constipation; it is poorly absorbed but opioid withdrawal reactions have been reported.

Convulsions Intractable seizures are relatively common in children dying from non-malignant conditions. Phenobarbital p. 264 by mouth or as a continuous subcutaneous infusion may be beneficial; continuous infusion of midazolam p. 273 is an alternative. Both cause drowsiness, but this is rarely a concern in the context of intractable seizures. For breakthrough convulsions diazepam p. 270 given rectally (as a solution), buccal midazolam, or paraldehyde p. 269 as an enema may be appropriate.

See *Continuous subcutaneous infusions*, below, for the use of midazolam by subcutaneous infusion using a continuous infusion device.

Dry mouth Dry mouth may be caused by certain medications including opioid analgesics, antimuscarinic drugs (e.g. hyoscine), antidepressants and some antiemetics; if possible, an alternative preparation should be considered. Dry mouth may be relieved by good mouth care and measures such as chewing sugar-free gum, sucking ice or pineapple chunks, or the use of artificial saliva, dry mouth associated with candidiasis can be treated by oral preparations of nystatin p. 885 or miconazole p. 884, alternatively, fluconazole p. 463 can be given by mouth.

Dysphagia A corticosteroid such as dexamethasone p. 543 may help, temporarily, if there is an obstruction due to tumour. See also *Dry mouth*, above.

Dyspnoea Breathlessness at rest may be relieved by regular oral morphine p. 338 in carefully titrated doses. Diazepam p. 270 may be helpful for dyspnoea associated with anxiety. Sublingual lorazepam p. 272 or subcutaneous or buccal midazolam p. 273 are alternatives. A nebulised short-acting beta$_2$ agonist or a corticosteroid, such as dexamethasone p. 543 or prednisolone p. 548, may also be helpful for bronchospasm or partial obstruction.

Excessive respiratory secretion Excessive respiratory secretion (death rattle) may be reduced by hyoscine hydrobromide patches p. 320 or by subcutaneous or intravenous injection of hyoscine hydrobromide p. 320, however, care must be taken to avoid the discomfort of dry mouth. Alternatively, glycopyrronium bromide p. 1014 may be given.

Hyoscine hydrobromide can be administered by subcutaneous or intravenous infusion using a continuous infusion device.

Fungating tumours Fungating tumours can be treated by regular dressing and antibacterial drugs; systemic treatment with metronidazole p. 409 is often required to reduce malodour, but topical metronidazole is also used.

Gastro-intestinal pain The pain of bowel colic may be reduced by loperamide hydrochloride p. 55. Hyoscine hydrobromide p. 320 may also be helpful in reducing the frequency of spasms; it is given sublingually as *Kwells*® tablets and also by subcutanous infusion.

Gastric distension pain due to pressure on the stomach may be helped by a preparation incorporating an antacid with an antiflatulent and a prokinetic such as domperidone before meals.

Hiccup Hiccup due to gastric distension may be helped by a preparation incorporating an antacid with an antiflatulent.

Insomnia Children with advanced cancer may not sleep because of discomfort, cramps, night sweats, joint stiffness, or fear. There should be appropriate treatment of these problems before hypnotics are used. Benzodiazepines, such as temazepam p. 1024, may be useful.

Intractable cough Intractable cough may be relieved by moist inhalations or by regular administration of oral morphine p. 338 every 4 hours. Methadone hydrochloride linctus p. 357 should be avoided because it has a long duration of action and tends to accumulate.

Mucosal bleeding Mucosal bleeding from the mouth and nose occurs commonly in the terminal phase, particularly in a child suffering from haemopoeitic malignancy. Bleeding from the nose caused by a single bleeding point can be arrested by cauterisation or by dressing it. Tranexamic acid p. 92 may be effective applied topically or given systemically.

Muscle spasm The pain of muscle spasm can be helped by a muscle relaxant such as diazepam p. 270 or baclofen p. 814.

Nausea and vomiting Nausea and vomiting are common in children with advanced cancer. Ideally, the cause should be determined before treatment with an antiemetic is started.

Nausea and vomiting with opioid therapy are less common in children than in adults but may occur particularly in the initial stages and can be prevented by giving an antiemetic. An antiemetic is usually necessary only for the first 4 or 5 days and therefore combined preparations containing an opioid with an antiemetic are not recommended because they lead to unnecessary antiemetic therapy (and associated side-effects when used long-term).

Metoclopramide hydrochloride p. 315 has a prokinetic action and is used by mouth for nausea and vomiting associated with gastritis, gastric stasis, and functional bowel obstruction. Drugs with antimuscarinic effects antagonise prokinetic drugs and, if possible, should not therefore be used concurrently.

Haloperidol p. 296 is used by mouth or by continuous intravenous or subcutaneous infusion for most metabolic causes of vomiting (e.g. hypercalcaemia, renal failure).

Cyclizine p. 313 is used for nausea and vomiting due to mechanical bowel obstruction, raised intracranial pressure, and motion sickness.

Ondansetron p. 317 is most effective when the vomiting is due to damaged or irritated gut mucosa (e.g. after chemotherapy or radiotherapy).

Antiemetic therapy should be reviewed every 24 hours; it may be necessary to substitute the antiemetic or to add another one.

Levomepromazine p. 321 can be used if first-line antiemetics are inadequate. Dexamethasone p. 543 by mouth can be used as an adjunct.

See *Continuous subcutaneous infusions*, below, for the administration of antiemetics by subcutaneous infusion using a continuous infusion device.

Pruritus Pruritus, even when associated with obstructive jaundice, often responds to simple measures such as application of emollients. Ondansetron p. 317 may be effective in some children. Where opioid analgesics cause pruritus it may be appropriate to review the dose or to switch to an alternative opioid analgesic. In the case of obstructive jaundice, further measures include administration of colestyramine p. 151.

Raised intracranial pressure Headache due to raised intracranial pressure often responds to a high dose of a corticosteroid, such as dexamethasone p. 543, for 4 to 5 days, subsequently reduced if possible; dexamethasone should be given before 6 p.m. to reduce the risk of insomnia. Treatment of headache and of associated nausea and vomiting should also be considered.

Restlessness and confusion Restlessness and confusion may require treatment with haloperidol p. 296. Levomepromazine p. 321 is also used occasionally for restlessness.

Continuous subcutaneous infusions

Although drugs can usually be administered *by mouth* to control symptoms in palliative care, the parenteral route may sometimes be necessary. Repeated administration of *intramuscular injections* should be avoided in children, particularly if cachectic. This has led to the use of portable continuous infusion devices such as syringe drivers to give a *continuous subcutaneous infusion*, which can provide good control of symptoms with little discomfort or inconvenience to the patient.

Indications for the **parenteral route** are:

- inability to take medicines by mouth owing to *nausea and vomiting*, *dysphagia*, *severe weakness*, or *coma*;
- *malignant bowel obstruction* for which surgery is inappropriate (avoiding the need for an intravenous infusion or for insertion of a nasogastric tube);
- refusal by the child to take regular medication by mouth.

Syringe driver rate settings Staff using syringe drivers should be **adequately trained** and different rate settings should be **clearly identified** and **differentiated**; incorrect use of syringe drivers is a common cause of medication errors.

Bowel colic and excessive respiratory secretions Hyoscine hydrobromide p. 320 effectively reduces respiratory secretions and is sedative (but occasionally causes paradoxical agitation); it is given in a *subcutaneous* or *intravenous infusion*. Glycopyrronium bromide p. 1014 may also be used.

Hyoscine butylbromide p. 68 is effective in bowel colic, is less sedative than hyoscine hydrobromide, but is not always adequate for the control of respiratory secretions; it is given by *subcutaneous infusion* (**important**: *hyoscine butylbromide* must not be confused with *hyoscine hydrobromide*, above).

Confusion and restlessness Haloperidol p. 296 has little sedative effect. Levomepromazine p. 321 has a sedative effect. Midazolam p. 273 is a sedative and an antiepileptic that may be suitable for a very restless patient.

Convulsions If a child has previously been receiving an antiepileptic drug *or* has a primary or secondary cerebral tumour *or* is at risk of convulsion (e.g. owing to uraemia) antiepileptic medication should not be stopped. Midazolam p. 273 is the benzodiazepine antiepileptic of choice for *continuous subcutaneous infusion*.

Nausea and vomiting Levomepromazine p. 321 causes sedation in about 50% of patients. Haloperidol p. 296 has little sedative effect.

Cyclizine p. 313 is particularly likely to precipitate if mixed with diamorphine hydrochloride p. 332 or other drugs (see under *Mixing and compatibility*); it is given by *subcutaneous infusion*.

Pain control Diamorphine hydrochloride p. 332 is the preferred opioid since its high solubility permits a large dose to be given in a small volume (see under *Mixing and compatibility*). The table shows approximate equivalent doses of morphine p. 338 and diamorphine hydrochloride.

Mixing and compatibility The general principle that injections should be given into separate sites (and should not be mixed) does not apply to the use of syringe drivers in palliative care. Provided that there is evidence of compatibility, selected injections can be mixed in syringe drivers. Not all types of medication can be used in a subcutaneous infusion. In particular, chlorpromazine hydrochloride p. 295, prochlorperazine p. 322, and diazepam p. 270 are **contra-indicated** as they cause skin reactions at the injection site; to a lesser extent cyclizine p. 313 and levomepromazine p. 321 also sometimes cause local irritation.

In theory injections dissolved in water for injections are more likely to be associated with pain (possibly owing to their hypotonicity). The use of physiological saline (sodium chloride 0.9% p. 728) however increases the likelihood of precipitation when more than one drug is used; moreover subcutaneous infusion rates are so slow (0.1– 0.3 mL/hour) that pain is not usually a problem when water is used as a diluent.

Compatibility with diamorphine Diamorphine can be given by *subcutaneous infusion* in a strength of up to 250 mg/mL; up to a strength of 40 mg/mL either *water for injections* or *physiological saline* (sodium chloride 0.9%) is a suitable diluent—above that strength only *water for injections* is used (to avoid precipitation).

The following can be mixed with *diamorphine*:

- **Cyclizine**, may precipitate at concentrations above 10 mg/mL *or* in the presence of sodium chloride 0.9% *or* as the concentration of diamorphine relative to cyclizine increases; mixtures of diamorphine and cyclizine are also likely to precipitate after 24 hours.
- **Dexamethasone**, special care is needed to avoid precipitation of dexamethasone when preparing it.
- **Haloperidol**, mixtures of haloperidol and diamorphine are likely to precipitate after 24 hours if haloperidol concentration is above 2 mg/mL.
- **Hyoscine butylbromide**
- **Hyoscine hydrobromide**
- **Levomepromazine**
- **Metoclopramide**, under some conditions infusions containing metoclopramide become discoloured; such solutions should be discarded.
- **Midazolam**

Subcutaneous infusion solution should be monitored regularly both to check for precipitation (and discolouration) and to ensure that the infusion is running at the correct rate.

Problems encountered with syringe drivers The following are problems that may be encountered with syringe drivers and the action that should be taken:

- if the subcutaneous infusion runs *too quickly* check the rate setting and the calculation;
- if the subcutaneous infusion runs *too slowly* check the start button, the battery, the syringe driver, the cannula, and make sure that the injection site is not inflamed;
- if there is an *injection site reaction* make sure that the site does not need to be changed—firmness or swelling at the site of injection is not in itself an indication for change, but pain or obvious inflammation is.

Equivalent doses of morphine sulfate and diamorphine hydrochloride given over 24 hours

These equivalences are *approximate only* and should be adjusted according to response

ORAL MORPHINE	PARENTERAL MORPHINE	PARENTERAL DIAMORPHINE
Oral morphine sulfate **over 24 hours**	Subcutaneous infusion of morphine sulfate **over 24 hours**	Subcutaneous infusion of diamorphine hydrochloride **over 24 hours**
30 mg	15 mg	10 mg
60 mg	30 mg	20 mg
90 mg	45 mg	30 mg
120 mg	60 mg	40 mg
180 mg	90 mg	60 mg
240 mg	120 mg	80 mg
360 mg	180 mg	120 mg
480 mg	240 mg	160 mg
600 mg	300 mg	200 mg
780 mg	390 mg	260 mg
960 mg	480 mg	320 mg
1200 mg	600 mg	400 mg

If breakthrough pain occurs give a subcutaneous injection equivalent to one-tenth to one-sixth of the total 24-hour subcutaneous infusion dose. With an intermittent subcutaneous injection absorption is smoother so that the risk of adverse effects at peak absorption is avoided (an even better method is to use a subcutaneous butterfly needle). To minimise the risk of infection no individual subcutaneous infusion solution should be used for longer than 24 hours.

Drugs and sport

Anti-doping

UK Anti-Doping, the national body responsible for the UK's anti-doping policy, advises that athletes are personally responsible should a prohibited substance be detected in their body. Information regarding the use of medicines in sport is available from:

UK Anti-doping
Fleetbank House
2-6 Salisbury Square
London
EC4Y 8AE
(020) 7842 3450
ukad@ukad.org.uk
www.ukad.org.uk

Information about the prohibited status of specific medications based on the current World Anti-Doping Agency Prohibited List is available from Global Drug Reference Online: www.globaldro.com/UK/search

General Medical Council's advice

Doctors who prescribe or collude in the provision of drugs or treatment with the intention of improperly enhancing an individual's performance in sport contravene the GMC's guidance, and such actions would usually raise a question of a doctor's continued registration. This does not preclude the provision of any care or treatment where the doctor's intention is to protect or improve the patient's health.

Medicines optimisation

Overview

Medicines are the most common intervention in healthcare for the prevention, treatment and/or management of many illnesses. As life expectancy increases and as the population ages, more people are living with several long-term conditions that are being managed with an increasing number of medicines. Medicines use can be complex and how patients can take their medicines safely and effectively is a challenge for the health service.

Multimorbidity (the presence of 2 or more long-term conditions) is associated with a greater use of health services, higher mortality, higher treatment burden (due to polypharmacy or multiple appointments), and reduced quality of life. The risk of patients suffering harm from their medicines increases with polypharmacy, and treatment regimens (including non-pharmacological treatments) can very easily become burdensome for patients with multimorbidity and can lead to care becoming fragmented and uncoordinated. Prescribers should consider the risks and benefits of treatments recommended from guidance for single health conditions, as the evidence for these recommendations is regularly drawn from patients without multimorbidity and who are taking fewer prescribed regular medicines. The management of risk factors for future disease can also be a major treatment burden for patients with multimorbidity and should be taken into consideration.

Medicines optimisation encompasses many aspects of medicines use and helps to ensure that they are taken as intended, thus supporting the management of long-term conditions, multimorbidities, and appropriate polypharmacy. It focuses on actions taken by all health and social care practitioners, and requires greater patient engagement and professional collaboration across health and social care settings. Through the adoption of a patient-focused approach to safe and effective medicines use, medicines optimisation changes the way patients are supported to get the best possible outcomes from their medicines. The use of shared decision-making informed by the best available evidence to guide decisions, ensures all patients have the opportunity to be involved in decisions about their medicines, taking into account their needs, preferences and values.

Overprescribing in the NHS has been reviewed by the Department of Health and Social Care in order to reduce the risk of harm, manage the spend on medicines, and ensure patients taking multiple medicines are receiving the most appropriate treatments for their needs. The national overprescribing review report is available at: www.gov.uk/government/publications/national-overprescribing-review-report.

Optimisation tools

Medicines optimisation includes aspects of care such as clinical assessment, clinical audits, disease prevention, health education, individual reviews and monitoring, and risk management. Having effective processes and systems in place can minimise the risk of preventable medicines-related problems (such as interactions with other medicines or comorbidities, and side-effects). Health and social care organisations should consider the use of multiple methods for identifying medicines-related patient safety incidents; learning from these incidents is important for guiding practice and minimising patient harm.

When optimising patient care, areas of intervention to consider include: deprescribing; medicines reconciliation, reviews and repeat prescribing; problematic polypharmacy; reducing medication waste and errors; and self-management plans. Self-management plans can be led by the child and their parents/carers or health professional, and vary in their content depending on the individual needs of the child, with the aim of supporting both them and their parents/carers involvement and empowerment in managing their condition.

Medicines optimisation services such as Structured Medication Reviews (SMRs), the Discharge Medicines Service (DMS), and New Medicines Service (NMS) are available to support children with their medicines. These can be undertaken in different care settings, such as community pharmacies or Primary Care Networks, and should be led by an appropriate health professional with effective communication skills, technical knowledge in the processes for managing medicines, and therapeutic knowledge on medicines use. Further information about these services is available from the Pharmaceutical Services Negotiating Committee, available at: psnc.org.uk/services-commissioning/; NHS England, available at: www.england.nhs.uk/primary-care/pharmacy/community-pharmacy-contractual-framework/; Community Pharmacy Wales, available at: cpwales.org.uk/Services-and-commissioning-d54; Community Pharmacy Northern Ireland, available at: www.communitypharmacyni.co.uk/services/; and Community Pharmacy Scotland, available at: www.cps.scot/core.

To support the medicines optimisation agenda, good practice guidance for health professionals details four guiding principles for medicines optimisation. These are:

- Aim to understand the patient's experience;
- Evidence-based choice of medicines;
- Ensure medicines use is as safe as possible;
- Make medicines optimisation part of routine practice.

For further guidance around medicines optimisation and tools to use, NHS England have compiled useful links; NICE have produced guidelines on **Medicines optimisation** and **Multimorbidity**; and the Scottish Government have produced a guideline on **Polypharmacy**, see *Useful resources*.

Communication

As health professionals from various disciplines and specialties may be caring for the same child at the same time, good communication is required between health professionals in order to avoid fragmentation of care. Medication reviews may be carried out by health professionals other than the prescriber; therefore the prescriber should be informed of the review and its outcome—particularly if difficulties with adherence were discussed and further review is required.

There is a greater risk of poor communication and unintended medication changes when children transfer between different care providers (such as when a child is admitted to or discharged from hospital). To support high-quality care when moving from one care setting to another, relevant information about medicines should be shared with children, their parents/carers, and between health and social care practitioners using robust and transparent processes. Information should be securely shared between health and social care practitioners ideally within 24 hours of patient transfer.

Good communication between health professionals, children and their parents/carers is needed for shared decision-making and supporting adherence. Information about their condition and possible treatments should be provided in a format that meets the child's and their parent's/carer's individual needs and preferences. The use of patient decision aids during consultations can help support a shared decision-making approach, and ensure children and their parents/carers are able to make well-informed choices that are consistent with their values and preferences.

For further guidance around communication between health professionals, children and their parents/carers, NICE have produced guidelines on **Medicines optimisation** and **Babies, children and young people's experience of healthcare** (see *Useful resources*). For guidance on the transition from paediatric to adult services, see *Transitional services for chronic conditions* in Guidance on prescribing p. 1.

Organisations such as the 'NHS Specialist Pharmacy Service' help support medicines optimisation across the NHS by joining health professionals together through online networks (e.g. Regional Medicines Optimisation Committees and the English Deprescribing Network). This is available at: www.sps.nhs.uk/.

Useful resources

Medicines optimisation: the safe and effective use of medicines to enable the best possible outcomes. National Institute for Health and Care Excellence. NICE guideline 5. March 2015.
www.nice.org.uk/guidance/ng5

Multimorbidity: clinical assessment and management. National Institute for Health and Care Excellence. NICE guideline 56. September 2016.
www.nice.org.uk/guidance/ng56

Babies, children and young people's experience of healthcare. National Institute for Health and Care Excellence. NICE Guideline 204. August 2021.
www.nice.org.uk/guidance/ng204

Medicines Optimisation. NHS England.
www.england.nhs.uk/medicines-2/medicines-optimisation/

Polypharmacy Guidance, Realistic Prescribing. Scottish Government Polypharmacy Model of Care Group. 3rd Edition. 2018.
www.therapeutics.scot.nhs.uk/polypharmacy/

Medicines Optimisation: Helping patients to make the most of medicines. Royal Pharmaceutical Society. May 2013.
rcpharm.org/pharmacy-guides/medicines-optimisation/

Antimicrobial stewardship

Overview

Effective antimicrobials are required for preventive and curative measures, protecting patients from potentially fatal diseases, and ensuring that complex procedures can be provided at low risk of infection. Antimicrobial resistance (AMR) is the loss of antimicrobial effectiveness, and although it evolves naturally, this process is accelerated by the inappropriate or incorrect use of antimicrobials. Direct consequences of infection with resistant microorganisms can be severe and affect all areas of health, such as prolonged illnesses and hospital stays, increased costs and mortality, and reduced protection for patients undergoing operations or procedures. AMR is an international problem with an increasing prevalence that has consequences for the whole of society. The UK Government has recognised AMR as a significant area of concern and have committed global action to address this as a priority. For information and resources on the UK's plans for AMR, see the Public Health England (PHE) collection: **Antimicrobial resistance** (www.gov.uk/government/collections/antimicrobial-resistance-amr-information-and-resources).

Antimicrobial stewardship (AMS) refers to an organisational or healthcare system-wide approach to promoting and monitoring judicious use of antimicrobials to preserve their future effectiveness. Addressing AMR through improving stewardship is a national medicines optimisation priority, led by NHS England and supported by PHE.

AMR can be managed by a combination of interventions that address:

- A political commitment to prioritise AMR;
- Monitoring antimicrobial use and resistance in microbes;
- Development of new drugs, treatments, and diagnostics;
- Individuals' behaviour relating to infection prevention and control, antimicrobial use, and AMR;
- Healthcare professionals' prescribing decisions.

Guidance for organisations (commissioners and providers)

Commissioners (clinical commissioning groups and local authorities) and providers (e.g. hospitals, GPs, out-of-hours services, dentists, and social enterprises) of health or social care services should establish an AMS programme, taking into account the resources needed to support AMS across all care settings. An AMS programme should take into consideration monitoring and evaluating antimicrobial prescribing, regular feedback to individual prescribers, education and training for health and social care staff, and integrating audits into existing quality improvement programmes.

Commissioners should work collaboratively to provide consistent information and advice to the public and health professionals that reduces inappropriate antimicrobial demand and use, and limits the spread of infection. Local authority public health teams should ensure that information and resources (such as posters, leaflets and digital resources) are made available through multiple routes to provide a coordinated system of information. Information should include simple and practical steps such as scrupulous personal and safe food hygiene practices.

Organisations should involve lead health and social care staff in establishing processes for developing, reviewing, updating, and implementing local antimicrobial guidelines in line with national guidance and informed by local prescribing data and resistance patterns.

Organisations should also consider establishing processes for reviewing national horizon scanning to plan for the availability of new antimicrobials and to use an existing local decision-making group to consider the introduction of new antimicrobials locally.

Guidance for health and social care staff

Health and social care staff should assist with the implementation of local or national guidelines and recognise the significance of them for AMS.

Health professionals should be familiar with current AMS campaigns and programmes. For further information, see PHE and Health Education England's e-learning session **All Our Health: Antimicrobial Resistance** (portal.e-lfh.org.uk/Component/Details/571263), PHE guidance **Health matters: antimicrobial resistance** (www.gov.uk/government/publications/health-matters-antimicrobial-resistance), and the PHE campaigns **Antibiotic Guardian** (antibioticguardian.com/) and **Keep Antibiotics Working** (campaignresources.phe.gov.uk/resources/campaigns/58-keep-antibiotics-working).

Health professionals should be aware of resources and services that can help individuals minimise infections such as travel vaccination clinics, screening programmes, sexual health services, immunisation programmes, and other local referral pathways or schemes. The benefits of good hygiene, vaccination, and other preventative measures to reduce the risk of acquiring infections should be discussed with individuals, and individuals referred to further information or services if necessary.

Those involved in providing care should be educated about the standard principles of infection prevention and control. They should be trained in hand decontamination, the use of personal protective equipment, and the safe use and disposal of sharps. For further information, see NICE guideline: **Healthcare-associated infections** (see *Useful resources*).

Guidance on antimicrobial prescribing

National antimicrobial prescribing and stewardship competencies have been developed to improve the quality of antimicrobial treatment and stewardship. For further information, see Antimicrobial Resistance and Healthcare Associated Infections and PHE guidance: **Antimicrobial prescribing and stewardship competencies** (see *Useful resources*).

National toolkits to support the implementation of AMS best practice include the Royal College of General Practitioners' **TARGET antibiotics toolkit** (www.rcgp.org.uk/TARGETantibiotics) for primary care, and PHE's **Start smart – then focus** (www.gov.uk/government/publications/antimicrobial-stewardship-start-smart-then-focus) for secondary care, and **Dental antimicrobial stewardship: toolkit** (www.gov.uk/guidance/dental-antimicrobial-stewardship-toolkit) for dentists.

Clinical syndrome-specific guidance and advice to help slow the development of AMR have been developed by NICE, in collaboration with PHE, and are available at www.nice.org.uk/.

Considerations for antimicrobial prescribing When deciding whether or not to prescribe an antimicrobial, undertake a clinical assessment and consider the risk of AMR for individual patients and the population as a whole. An immediate antimicrobial prescription for a patient who is likely to have a self-limiting condition is not recommended.

Document in the patient's records (electronically wherever possible) the decisions related to antimicrobial use, including the plan as discussed with the patient, and their family and/or carers (if appropriate), and reason for prescribing/not prescribing an antimicrobial.

In hospital, microbiological samples should be taken before initiating an antimicrobial for patients with suspected infection. In primary care, consider taking microbiological samples when prescribing an antimicrobial for patients with recurrent or persistent infections. The choice of antimicrobial should be reviewed when microbiological results are available. For non-severe infections, consider taking microbiological samples before making a decision about prescribing an antimicrobial, providing it is safe to withhold treatment until the results are available.

Follow local or national guidelines on prescribing the shortest effective course and most appropriate dose and route of administration. Review intravenous antimicrobials within 48 hours (taking into account response to treatment and microbiological results) and consider stepping down to oral antimicrobials where possible. If prescribing outside of local or national guidelines, document in the patient's records the reasons for the decision.

Patients on antimicrobial treatment should be appropriately monitored to reduce side-effects and be assessed on the continued need for treatment. Repeat antimicrobial prescriptions are not recommended, unless needed for a particular clinical condition or indication. Avoid issuing a repeat prescription for longer than 6 months without review.

Advice for patients and their family and/or carers Prescribers, primary care and community pharmacy teams should provide patients with resources educating them about not asking for antimicrobials as a preventive measure against becoming ill or as a stand-by measure, unless the patient has a specific condition or a specific risk that requires antimicrobial prophylaxis.

Prescribers should discuss with patients, and their family and/or carers (if appropriate) the likely nature of the condition, their views on antimicrobials, benefits and harms of antimicrobial prescribing, and why prescribing an antimicrobial may not always be the best option. Information should be provided about what to do if their symptoms worsen or if problems arise as a result of treatment. Written information should be provided if needed.

If antimicrobial treatment is not the most appropriate option, prescribers should advise patients, and their family and/or carers (if appropriate) about other options (as appropriate), such as self-care with over-the-counter preparations, back-up (delayed) prescribing, or other non-pharmacological interventions. Prescribers, primary care and community pharmacy teams should verbally emphasise and provide written advice about managing self-limiting infections.

If antimicrobials are prescribed or supplied, prescribers, primary care and community pharmacy teams should provide patients with verbal and written information on the correct use of antimicrobials. Advice should encourage people to:

- Take, or use antimicrobials only when recommended by a suitably qualified health professional;
- Obtain antimicrobials only from a health professional;
- Take, or use antimicrobials as instructed (right dose for the duration specified and via the right route);
- Return any unused antimicrobials to a pharmacy for safe disposal.

Useful resources

Antimicrobial prescribing and stewardship competencies. Antimicrobial Resistance and Healthcare Associated Infections (ARHAI) and Public Health England guideline. October 2013.

www.gov.uk/government/publications/antimicrobial-prescribing-and-stewardship-competencies

Antimicrobial resistance (AMR): applying All Our Health. Public Health England guideline. April 2015 (updated June 2019).

www.gov.uk/government/publications/antimicrobial-resistance-amr-applying-all-our-health

Antimicrobial stewardship: systems and processes for effective antimicrobial medicine use. National Institute for Health and Care Excellence. NICE guideline 15. August 2015.

www.nice.org.uk/guidance/NG15

Antimicrobial stewardship: changing risk-related behaviours in the general population. National Institute for Health and Care Excellence. NICE guideline 63. January 2017.

www.nice.org.uk/guidance/NG63

Healthcare-associated infections: prevention and control in primary and community care. National Institute for Health and Care Excellence. Clinical guideline 139. March 2012 (updated February 2017).

www.nice.org.uk/guidance/cg139

Prescribing in dental practice

General guidance

Advice on the drug management of dental and oral conditions has been integrated into the main text. For ease of access, guidance on such conditions is usually identified by means of a relevant heading (e.g. Dental and Orofacial Pain) in the appropriate sections.

The following is a list of topics of particular relevance to dentists.

- Prescribing by dentists, see Prescription writing p. 4
- Oral side-effects of drugs, see Adverse reactions to drugs p. 11
- Medical emergencies in dental practice, see BNF
- Medical problems in dental practice, see BNF

Drug management of dental and oral conditions

Dental and orofacial pain, see Analgesics p. 323

- Neuropathic pain p. 348
- Non-opioid analgesics and compound analgesic preparations, see Analgesics p. 323
- Opioid analgesics, see Analgesics p. 323
- Non-steroidal anti-inflammatory drugs p. 816

Oral infections

Bacterial infections, see Antibacterials, principles of therapy p. 358

- Phenoxymethylpenicillin p. 416
- Broad-spectrum penicillins (amoxicillin p. 417 and ampicillin p. 419)
- Cephalosporins (cefalexin p. 385 and cefradine p. 387)
- Tetracyclines p. 433
- Macrolides (clarithromycin p. 403, erythromycin p. 406 and azithromycin p. 402)
- Clindamycin p. 400
- Metronidazole p. 409
- Fusidic acid p. 441

Fungal infections

- Local treatment, see Oropharyngeal fungal infections p. 883
- Systemic treatment, see Antifungals, systemic use p. 459

Viral infections

- Herpetic gingivostomatitis, local treatment, see Oropharyngeal viral infections p. 885
- Herpetic gingivostomatitis, systemic treatment, see Oropharyngeal viral infections p. 885 and Herpesvirus infections p. 498
- Herpes labialis, see Skin infections p. 895

Anaesthetics, anxiolytics and hypnotics

- Sedation, anaesthesia, and resuscitation in dental practice p. 1007
- Hypnotics, see Hypnotics and anxiolytics p. 350
- Sedation for dental procedures, see Hypnotics and anxiolytics p. 350
- Anaesthesia (local) p. 1025

Minerals

- Fluoride p. 879

Oral ulceration and inflammation

- See Oral ulceration and inflammation p. 880

Mouthwashes, gargles and dentifrices

- See Mouthwashes and other preparations for oropharyngeal use p. 877

Dry mouth

- See Dry mouth p. 875

Aromatic inhalations

- See Aromatic inhalations, cough preparations and systemic nasal decongestants p. 223

Nasal decongestants

- See Aromatic inhalations, cough preparations and systemic nasal decongestants p. 223

Dental Practitioners' Formulary

- See Dental Practitioners' Formulary p. 1437

Chapter 1
Gastro-intestinal system

CONTENTS

1 Chronic bowel disorders

1.1 Coeliac disease

Coeliac disease

25-Jul-2016

Description of condition

Coeliac disease is an autoimmune condition which is associated with chronic inflammation of the small intestine. Dietary proteins known as gluten, which are present in wheat, barley and rye, activate an abnormal immune response in the intestinal mucosa, which can lead to malabsorption of nutrients.

Aims of treatment

The management of coeliac disease is aimed at eliminating symptoms (such as diarrhoea, bloating and abdominal pain) and reducing the risk of complications, including those resulting from malabsorption.

Non-drug treatment

EvGr The only effective treatment for coeliac disease is a strict, life-long, gluten-free diet. A range of gluten-free products is available for prescription (see *Borderline substances*). (A)

Drug treatment

EvGr Children who have coeliac disease are at an increased risk of malabsorption of key nutrients (such as calcium and vitamin D). Supplementation of key nutrients may be required if dietary intake is insufficient.

Carers of children who have coeliac disease should be advised **not** to medicate with over-the-counter vitamin or mineral supplements. Initiation of supplementation should involve a discussion with a member of the child's healthcare team in order to identify the individual needs of the patient and to allow for appropriate ongoing monitoring. (A)

Useful Resources

Coeliac disease: recognition, assessment and management. National Institute for Health and Care Excellence. Clinical guideline 20. September 2015.
www.nice.org.uk/guidance/ng20

1.2 Inflammatory bowel disease

Crohn's disease

25-Sep-2023

Description of condition

Crohn's disease is a chronic, inflammatory bowel disease that mainly affects the gastro-intestinal tract. It is characterised by thickened areas of the gastro-intestinal wall with inflammation extending through all layers, deep ulceration and fissuring of the mucosa, and the presence of granulomas; affected areas may occur in any part of the gastro-intestinal tract, interspersed with areas of relatively normal tissue. Crohn's disease may present as recurrent attacks, with acute exacerbations combined with periods of remission or less active disease. Symptoms depend on the site of disease but may include abdominal pain, diarrhoea, fever, weight loss, and rectal bleeding.

Complications of Crohn's disease include intestinal strictures, abscesses in the wall of the intestine or adjacent structures, fistulae, anaemia, malnutrition, colorectal and small bowel cancers, and growth failure and delayed puberty in children. Crohn's disease may also be associated with extra-intestinal manifestation: the most common are arthritis and abnormalities of the joints, eyes, liver and skin. Crohn's disease is also a cause of secondary osteoporosis and those at greatest risk should be monitored for osteopenia and assessed for the risk of fractures.

Up to a third of patients with Crohn's disease are diagnosed before the age of 21 years but there is a lack of evidence regarding treatment for children. Paediatric practice is often based on extrapolation from adult studies.

Fistulating Crohn's disease

Fistulating Crohn's disease is a complication that involves the formation of a fistula between the intestine and adjacent structures, such as perianal skin, bladder, and vagina. It occurs in about one quarter of patients, mostly when the disease involves the ileocolonic area.

Aims of treatment

Treatment is largely directed at the induction and maintenance of remission and the relief of symptoms. Active treatment of acute Crohn's disease should be distinguished from preventing relapse. The aims of drug treatment are to reduce symptoms and maintain or improve quality of life, while minimising toxicity related to drugs over both the short and long term. Drug treatment should always be initiated by a paediatric gastroenterologist.

In fistulating Crohn's disease, surgery and medical treatment aim to close and maintain closure of the fistula.

Non-drug treatment

EvGr In addition to drug treatment, management options for Crohn's disease include Smoking cessation p. 353 and attention to nutrition, which plays an important role in supportive care. Surgery may be considered in certain children with early disease limited to the distal ileum and in severe or chronic active disease. (A)

Drug treatment

Treatment of acute disease

Monotherapy

EvGr A corticosteroid (either prednisolone p. 548 or methylprednisolone p. 547 or intravenous hydrocortisone p. 544), is used to induce remission in children with a first presentation or a single inflammatory exacerbation of Crohn's disease in a 12-month period.

Enteral nutrition is an alternative to a corticosteroid when there is concern about growth or side effects.

In children with distal ileal, ileocaecal or right-sided colonic disease, in whom a conventional corticosteroid is unsuitable or contra-indicated, budesonide p. 36 [unlicensed] may be considered. Budesonide is less effective but may cause fewer side-effects than other corticosteroids, as systemic exposure is limited. Aminosalicylates (such as sulfasalazine p. 35 and mesalazine p. 33) are an alternative option in these children. They are less effective than a corticosteroid or budesonide [unlicensed], but may be preferred because they have fewer side-effects. Aminosalicylates and budesonide are not appropriate for severe presentations or exacerbations. (A)

Add-on treatment

EvGr Add on treatment is prescribed if there are two or more inflammatory exacerbations in a 12-month period, or the corticosteroid dose cannot be reduced.

Azathioprine p. 638 or mercaptopurine p. 671 [unlicensed indications] can be added to a corticosteroid or budesonide to induce remission. In children who cannot tolerate azathioprine or mercaptopurine or in whom thiopurine methyltransferase (TPMT) activity is deficient, methotrexate p. 672 can be added to a corticosteroid.

Under specialist care, certain tumour necrosis factor alpha inhibitors may be used for the treatment of severe, active Crohn's disease, and for moderate to severely active disease, certain interleukin inhibitors may be used. (A)

Maintenance of remission

EvGr Children, and their parents or carers, should be made aware of the risk of relapse with and without drug treatment, and symptoms that may suggest a relapse (most frequently unintended weight loss, abdominal pain, diarrhoea and general ill-health). For those who choose not to receive maintenance treatment during remission, a suitable follow up plan should be agreed upon and information provided on how to access healthcare if a relapse should occur.

Azathioprine or mercaptopurine [unlicensed indications] as monotherapy can be used to maintain remission when previously used with a corticosteroid to induce remission. They may also be used in children who have not previously received these drugs (particularly those with adverse prognostic factors such as early age of onset, perianal disease, corticosteroid use at presentation, and severe presentations). Methotrexate [unlicensed] can be used to maintain remission only in children who required methotrexate to induce remission, or who are intolerant of or are not suitable for azathioprine or mercaptopurine for maintenance. Corticosteroids or budesonide should not be used. (A)

Maintaining remission following surgery

EvGr Azathioprine in combination with up to 3 months' postoperative metronidazole p. 409 [unlicensed indication] should be considered to maintain remission in children with ileocolonic Crohn's disease who have had complete macroscopic resection within the previous 3 months. Azathioprine alone should be considered for patients who cannot tolerate metronidazole p. 409. (A) Aminosalicylates are no longer recommended due to the lack of clinical efficacy. NICE do not consider mercaptopurine to be a cost-effective treatment and do not recommend its use.

EvGr Biologic therapies should no longer be used to maintain remission after complete macroscopic resection of ileocolonic Crohn's disease because of limited evidence. Budesonide should also not be used in these patients. (A)

Other treatments

EvGr Loperamide hydrochloride p. 55 can be used to manage diarrhoea associated with Crohn's disease in children who do not have colitis. (A) Colestyramine p. 151 is licensed for the relief of diarrhoea associated with Crohn's disease. See also Diarrhoea (acute) p. 54.

Fistulating Crohn's disease

Perianal fistulae are the most common occurrence in children with fistulating Crohn's disease. EvGr Treatment may not be necessary for simple, asymptomatic perianal fistulae. When fistulae are symptomatic, local drainage and surgery may be required in conjunction with medical therapy.

Metronidazole p. 409 or ciprofloxacin p. 429 [unlicensed indications], alone or in combination, can improve symptoms of fistulating Crohn's disease but complete healing occurs rarely. Metronidazole should be given for at least 6 weeks but no longer than 3 months because of concerns about peripheral neuropathy. Other antibacterials should be given if specifically indicated (e.g. in sepsis associated with fistulae and perianal disease) and for managing bacterial overgrowth in the small bowel.

Either azathioprine p. 638 or mercaptopurine p. 671 [unlicensed indications] is used to control the inflammation in perianal and enterocutaneous fistulating Crohn's disease and they are continued for maintenance.

Infliximab p. 39 is recommended for children with perianal and enterocutaneous active fistulating Crohn's disease who have not responded to conventional therapy (including antibacterials, drainage and immunosuppressive treatments), or who are intolerant of or have contra-indications to conventional therapy. Infliximab should be used after ensuring that all sepsis is actively draining.

Abscess drainage, fistulotomy, and seton insertion may be appropriate, particularly before infliximab treatment.

Azathioprine, mercaptopurine or infliximab should be continued as maintenance treatment for at least one year.

For the management of non-perianal fistulating Crohn's disease (including entero-gynaecological and enterovesical fistulae) surgery is the only recommended approach. (A)

Useful Resources

Crohn's disease: management. National Institute for Health and Care Excellence. Clinical guideline 129. May 2019.
www.nice.org.uk/guidance/ng129

Ulcerative colitis

03-May-2024

Description of condition

Ulcerative colitis is a chronic inflammatory condition, characterised by diffuse mucosal inflammation—it has a relapsing-remitting pattern. It is a life-long disease that is associated with significant morbidity. Ulcerative colitis is more common in adults; however in children it predominately presents between the ages of 5 and 16 years.

The pattern of inflammation is continuous, extending from the rectum upwards to a varying degree. Inflammation of the rectum is referred to as **proctitis**, and inflammation of the rectum and sigmoid colon as **proctosigmoiditis**. **Left-sided colitis** refers to disease involving the colon distal to the splenic flexure. **Extensive colitis** affects the colon proximal to the splenic flexure, and includes pan-colitis, where the whole colon is involved. Child-onset ulcerative colitis is classified as extensive in 60–80% of all cases. Common symptoms of active disease or relapse include bloody diarrhoea, an urgent need to defaecate, and abdominal pain.

Complications associated with ulcerative colitis include an increased risk of colorectal cancer, secondary osteoporosis, venous thromboembolism, and toxic megacolon. Growth and pubertal development can be affected in children.

Aims of treatment

Treatment is focused on treating active disease to manage symptoms and to induce and maintain remission.

Drug treatment

Overview

Management of ulcerative colitis is dependent on factors such as clinical severity, extent of disease, and the child's preference. As limited distal disease is uncommon in children, paediatric treatment strategy depends mainly on disease severity rather than the extent of disease. Clinical and laboratory investigations are used to determine the extent and severity of disease and to guide treatment. Severity is classified as mild, moderate or severe (or in remission) by using the Paediatric Ulcerative Colitis Activity Index to assess bowel movement, limitations on daily activity and the presence of abdominal pain or melaena—see the NICE guideline for Ulcerative Colitis for further information (see *Useful resources*).

EvGr The extent of disease should be considered when choosing the route of administration for aminosalicylates and corticosteroids; whether oral treatment, topical treatment or both are to be used. ⟨A⟩

If the inflammation is distal, a rectal preparation is adequate, but if the inflammation is extended, systemic medication is required. Either suppositories or enemas can be offered, taking into account the child's preferences.

EvGr Rectal foam preparations and suppositories can be used when children have difficulty retaining liquid enemas.

Diarrhoea that is associated with active ulcerative colitis is sometimes treated with anti-diarrhoeal drugs (such as loperamide hydrochloride p. 55 [unlicensed under 4 years]) on the advice of a specialist; however their use is contra-indicated in acute ulcerative colitis as they can increase the risk of toxic megacolon.

A macrogol-containing osmotic laxative (such as macrogol 3350 with potassium chloride, sodium bicarbonate and sodium chloride p. 47) may be useful for proximal faecal loading in proctitis. ⟨E⟩

Oral aminosalicylates for the treatment of ulcerative colitis are available in different preparations and release forms. EvGr The preparation and dosing schedule should be chosen taking into account the delivery characteristics and suitability for the patient. When used to maintain remission, single daily doses of oral aminosalicylates can be more effective than multiple daily dosing, but may result in more side-effects.

The duration of corticosteroid course (usually 4 to 8 weeks) depends on the corticosteroid chosen. ⟨A⟩

Treatment of acute mild-to-moderate ulcerative colitis

Proctitis

EvGr A topical aminosalicylate is recommended as first-line treatment for children with a mild-to-moderate initial presentation or inflammatory exacerbation of proctitis. If remission is not achieved within 4 weeks, adding an oral aminosalicylate should be considered. If the response remains inadequate, consider adding a topical or an oral corticosteroid for 4 to 8 weeks.

Monotherapy with an oral aminosalicylate can be considered in children who prefer not to use enemas or suppositories, although this may not be as effective. If remission is not achieved within 4 weeks, adding a topical or an oral corticosteroid for 4 to 8 weeks should be considered.

A topical or an oral corticosteroid for 4 to 8 weeks should be considered for children in whom aminosalicylates are unsuitable. ⟨A⟩

Proctosigmoiditis and left-sided ulcerative colitis

EvGr A topical aminosalicylate is recommended as first-line treatment for children with a mild-to-moderate initial presentation or inflammatory exacerbation of proctosigmoiditis or left-sided ulcerative colitis. If remission is not achieved within 4 weeks, consider adding a high-dose oral aminosalicylate, or switching to a high-dose oral aminosalicylate and 4 to 8 weeks of a topical corticosteroid. If response remains inadequate, stop topical treatment and offer an oral aminosalicylate and 4 to 8 weeks of an oral corticosteroid.

Monotherapy with a high-dose oral aminosalicylate can be considered for children who prefer not to use enemas or suppositories, although this may not be as effective. If remission is not achieved within 4 weeks, an oral corticosteroid for 4 to 8 weeks in addition to the high-dose aminosalicylate should be offered.

A topical or an oral corticosteroid for 4 to 8 weeks should be considered for children in whom aminosalicylates are unsuitable. ⟨A⟩

Extensive ulcerative colitis

EvGr A topical aminosalicylate and a high-dose oral aminosalicylate is recommended as first-line treatment for children with a mild-to-moderate initial presentation or inflammatory exacerbation of extensive ulcerative colitis. If remission is not achieved within 4 weeks, stop topical aminosalicylate treatment and offer a high-dose oral aminosalicylate and 4 to 8 weeks of an oral corticosteroid. An oral corticosteroid for 4 to 8 weeks should be considered for children in whom aminosalicylates are unsuitable. ⟨A⟩

Treatment of acute moderate-to-severe ulcerative colitis

EvGr Under specialist care, certain sphingosine-1-phosphate receptor modulators may be used for the treatment of moderate-to-severe active ulcerative colitis. ⟨A⟩

Treatment of acute severe ulcerative colitis

Acute severe ulcerative colitis of any extent can be life-threatening and is regarded as a medical emergency. EvGr Immediate hospital admission is required for treatment.

Intravenous corticosteroids (such as hydrocortisone p. 544 or methylprednisolone p. 547) should be given to induce remission in children with acute severe ulcerative colitis (whether it is a first presentation or an inflammatory exacerbation) while assessing the need for surgery. If intravenous corticosteroids are contra-indicated, declined or cannot be tolerated, then intravenous ciclosporin p. 640 [unlicensed indication], or surgery should be considered. A combination of intravenous ciclosporin with intravenous corticosteroids, or surgery is second line therapy for children who have little or no improvement within 72 hours of starting intravenous corticosteroids or in children whose symptoms worsen despite treatment with a corticosteroid. (A)

EvGr Alternatively, infliximab p. 39 can be used on specialist advice in children over 6 years, if there is little or no improvement within 72 hours of starting intravenous corticosteroids or in children whose symptoms worsen despite treatment with a corticosteroid.

In patients who experience an initial response to steroids followed by deterioration, stool cultures should be taken to exclude pathogens; cytomegalovirus activation should be considered. (E)

Infliximab for ulcerative colitis

EvGr Infliximab can be used to treat acute severe active ulcerative colitis in children over 6 years who have had an inadequate response to conventional treatment (including corticosteroids and azathioprine p. 638 or mercaptopurine p. 671) or if conventional treatment is not tolerated or contra-indicated. Treatment with these agents is continued into the maintenance phase if effective and tolerated.

Infliximab can also be used to treat acute exacerbations of severely active ulcerative colitis in children over 6 years, if ciclosporin p. 640 is contra-indicated or clinically inappropriate. (A)

Maintaining remission in mild, moderate or severe ulcerative colitis

EvGr To reduce the chances of relapse occurring, maintenance therapy with an aminosalicylate is recommended in most children. Corticosteroids are **not** suitable for maintenance treatment because of their side-effects.

After a mild-to-moderate inflammatory exacerbation of *proctitis* or *proctosigmoiditis*, a rectal aminosalicylate can be started alone or in combination with an oral aminosalicylate, administered daily or as part of an intermittent regimen (such as twice to three times weekly or the first seven days of each month). An oral aminosalicylate can be used alone in children who prefer not to use enemas or suppositories, although this may not be as effective.

A low dose of oral aminosalicylate is given to maintain remission in children after a mild-to-moderate inflammatory exacerbation of *left-sided or extensive* ulcerative colitis.

When used to maintain remission, single daily dosing of oral aminosalicylates can be more effective than multiple daily dosing, but may result in more side-effects.

Oral azathioprine or mercaptopurine [unlicensed indications] can be considered to maintain remission, if there has been two or more inflammatory exacerbations in a 12-month period that require treatment with systemic corticosteroids or if remission is not maintained by aminosalicylates, or following a single acute severe episode. (A) EvGr Oral azathioprine or mercaptopurine is usually required in these cases as an aminosalicylate alone may be ineffective in more severe disease. (E)

There is no evidence to support the use of methotrexate p. 672 to induce or maintain remission in ulcerative colitis though its use is common in clinical practice.

Treatment with certain tumor necrosis factor alpha (TNF-a) inhibitors and sphingosine-1-phosphate receptor modulators may be continued into the maintenance phase.

Non-drug treatment

EvGr Surgery may be necessary as emergency treatment for severe ulcerative colitis that does not respond to drug treatment. Patients can also choose to have elective surgery for unresponsive or frequently relapsing disease that is affecting their quality of life. (A)

Useful Resources

Ulcerative colitis: management. National Institute for Health and Care Excellence. Clinical guideline 130. May 2019.
www.nice.org.uk/guidance/NG130

Other drugs used for Inflammatory bowel disease
Adalimumab, p. 806 · Risankizumab, p. 38

AMINOSALICYLATES

Aminosalicylates

● **SIDE-EFFECTS**

- **Common or very common** Arthralgia · cough · diarrhoea · dizziness · fever · gastrointestinal discomfort · headache · leucopenia · myalgia · nausea · proteinuria · skin reactions · vomiting
- **Uncommon** Alopecia · depression · dyspnoea · face oedema · pancreatitis · paraesthesia · photosensitivity reaction · tachycardia · thrombocytopenia · vertigo
- **Rare or very rare** Agranulocytosis · angioedema · blood disorder · bone marrow disorders · cardiac inflammation · hepatic disorders · interstitial lung disease · lupus-like syndrome · nephritis tubulointerstitial · nephrotic syndrome · neutropenia · peripheral neuropathy · renal impairment · respiratory disorders
- **Frequency not known** Cholelithiasis · eosinophilia · haematuria · haemolytic anaemia · oligozoospermia (reversible) · severe cutaneous adverse reactions (SCARs) · ulcerative colitis aggravated

SIDE-EFFECTS, FURTHER INFORMATION A blood count should be performed and the drug stopped immediately if there is suspicion of a blood dyscrasia.

● **ALLERGY AND CROSS-SENSITIVITY** EvGr Contra-indicated in salicylate hypersensitivity (M).

● **MONITORING REQUIREMENTS** Renal function should be monitored before starting an oral aminosalicylate, at 3 months of treatment, and then annually during treatment.

● **PATIENT AND CARER ADVICE**
Blood disorders Patients receiving aminosalicylates, and their carers, should be advised to report any unexplained bleeding, bruising, purpura, sore throat, fever or malaise that occurs during treatment.

above

Balsalazide sodium

24-Jun-2021

● **INDICATIONS AND DOSE**

Treatment of mild to moderate ulcerative colitis, acute attack

▶ BY MOUTH

▶ Child 12–17 years: 2.25 g 3 times a day until remission occurs or for up to maximum of 12 weeks

Maintenance of remission of ulcerative colitis

▶ BY MOUTH

▶ Child 12–17 years: 1.5 g twice daily (max. per dose 3 g), adjusted according to response; maximum 6 g per day

● **UNLICENSED USE** Not licensed for use in children under 18 years.

● **CAUTIONS** History of asthma

● **INTERACTIONS** → Appendix 1: balsalazide

● **PREGNANCY** Manufacturer advises avoid.

● **BREAST FEEDING** Diarrhoea may develop in the infant.
Monitoring Monitor breast-fed infants for diarrhoea.

● **HEPATIC IMPAIRMENT** Manufacturer advises caution; avoid in severe impairment (no information available).

● **RENAL IMPAIRMENT** EvGr Use with caution in mild impairment; avoid in moderate to severe impairment. (M)

● **MEDICINAL FORMS** There can be variation in the licensing of different medicines containing the same drug.

Oral capsule

CAUTIONARY AND ADVISORY LABELS 21, 25

▸ **Colazide** (Almirall Ltd)
Balsalazide disodium 750 mg Colazide 750mg capsules | 130 capsule [PoM] £30.42 DT = £30.42

F 32

Mesalazine

17-Dec-2025

● **INDICATIONS AND DOSE**

DOSE EQUIVALENCE AND CONVERSION

▶ There is no evidence to show that any one oral preparation of mesalazine is more effective than another; however, the delivery characteristics of oral mesalazine preparations may vary.

ASACOL ® MR 400MG TABLETS

Treatment of mild to moderate ulcerative colitis, acute attack

▶ BY MOUTH
▸ Child 12–17 years: 800 mg 3 times a day

Maintenance of remission of ulcerative colitis and Crohn's ileo-colitis

▶ BY MOUTH
▸ Child 12–17 years: 400–800 mg 2–3 times a day

ASACOL ® FOAM ENEMA

Treatment of acute attack of mild to moderate ulcerative colitis affecting the rectosigmoid region

▶ BY RECTUM
▸ Child 12–17 years: 1 g daily for 4–6 weeks, to be administered into the rectum

Treatment of acute attack of mild to moderate ulcerative colitis, affecting the descending colon

▶ BY RECTUM
▸ Child 12–17 years: 2 g once daily for 4–6 weeks, to be administered into the rectum

ASACOL ® SUPPOSITORIES

Treatment and maintenance of remission of ulcerative colitis affecting the rectosigmoid region

▶ BY RECTUM
▸ Child 12–17 years: 250–500 mg 3 times a day, last dose to be administered at bedtime

OCTASA ® MR 400MG AND 800MG TABLETS

Treatment of mild to moderate ulcerative colitis, acute attack

▶ BY MOUTH
▸ Child 6–17 years (body-weight up to 40 kg): Initially 30–50 mg/kg daily in divided doses, increased if necessary up to 75 mg/kg daily in divided doses
▸ Child 6–17 years (body-weight 40 kg and above): 2.4 g once daily, alternatively 2.4–4 g daily in divided doses

Maintenance of remission of ulcerative colitis and Crohn's ileo-colitis

▶ BY MOUTH
▸ Child 6–17 years (body-weight up to 40 kg): 15–30 mg/kg daily in divided doses
▸ Child 6–17 years (body-weight 40 kg and above): 1.2–2 g once daily, alternatively 1.2–2 g daily in divided doses

PENTASA ® GRANULES

Treatment of mild to moderate ulcerative colitis, acute attack

▶ BY MOUTH
▸ Child 5–17 years (body-weight up to 40 kg): 10–20 mg/kg 3 times a day
▸ Child 5–17 years (body-weight 40 kg and above): 1–2 g twice daily, alternatively 2–4 g daily in 3–4 divided doses

Maintenance of remission of ulcerative colitis

▶ BY MOUTH
▸ Child 5–17 years (body-weight up to 40 kg): 7.5–15 mg/kg twice daily, alternatively 15–30 mg/kg daily in 3 divided doses
▸ Child 5–17 years (body-weight 40 kg and above): 2 g once daily

PENTASA ® RETENTION ENEMA

Treatment of acute attack of mild to moderate ulcerative colitis affecting the rectosigmoid region

▶ BY RECTUM
▸ Child 12–17 years: 1 g once daily, dose to be administered at bedtime

PENTASA ® SUPPOSITORIES

Treatment of acute attack, ulcerative proctitis

▶ BY RECTUM
▸ Child 12–17 years: 1 g daily for 2–4 weeks

Maintenance, ulcerative proctitis

▶ BY RECTUM
▸ Child 12–17 years: 1 g daily

PENTASA ® TABLETS

Treatment of mild to moderate ulcerative colitis, acute attack

▶ BY MOUTH
▸ Child 5–17 years (body-weight up to 40 kg): 10–20 mg/kg 3 times a day
▸ Child 5–17 years (body-weight 40 kg and above): 1–2 g twice daily, alternatively 2–4 g daily in 3 divided doses

Maintenance of remission of ulcerative colitis

▶ BY MOUTH
▸ Child 5–17 years (body-weight up to 40 kg): 7.5–15 mg/kg twice daily, alternatively 15–30 mg/kg daily in 3 divided doses
▸ Child 5–17 years (body-weight 40 kg and above): 2 g once daily

SALOFALK ® ENEMA

Treatment of acute attack of mild to moderate ulcerative colitis or maintenance of remission

▶ BY RECTUM
▸ Child 12–17 years: 2 g once daily, dose to be administered at bedtime

SALOFALK ® GRANULES

Treatment of mild to moderate ulcerative colitis, acute attack

▶ BY MOUTH
▸ Child 5–17 years (body-weight up to 40 kg): 30–50 mg/kg once daily, dose preferably given in the morning, alternatively 10–20 mg/kg 3 times a day
▸ Child 5–17 years (body-weight 40 kg and above): 1.5–3 g once daily, dose preferably given in the morning, alternatively 0.5–1 g 3 times a day

Maintenance of remission of ulcerative colitis

▶ BY MOUTH
▸ Child 5–17 years (body-weight up to 40 kg): 7.5–15 mg/kg twice daily, alternatively 15–30 mg/kg daily in 3 divided doses
▸ Child 5–17 years (body-weight 40 kg and above): 500 mg 3 times a day

SALOFALK ® RECTAL FOAM

Treatment of mild ulcerative colitis affecting sigmoid colon and rectum

▶ BY RECTUM
▸ Child 12–17 years: 2 g once daily, dose to be administered into the rectum at bedtime, alternatively 2 g daily in 2 divided doses

continued →

SALOFALK ® SUPPOSITORIES

Treatment of acute attack of mild to moderate ulcerative colitis affecting the rectum, sigmoid colon, and descending colon

▶ BY RECTUM

▸ Child 12–17 years: 0.5–1 g 2–3 times a day, to be given using 500 mg suppositories, dose to be adjusted according to response

SALOFALK ® TABLETS

Treatment of mild to moderate ulcerative colitis, acute attack

▶ BY MOUTH

▸ Child 5–17 years (body-weight up to 40 kg): 10–20 mg/kg 3 times a day

▸ Child 5–17 years (body-weight 40 kg and above): 0.5–1 g 3 times a day

Maintenance of remission of ulcerative colitis

▶ BY MOUTH

▸ Child 5–17 years (body-weight up to 40 kg): 7.5–15 mg/kg twice daily, alternatively 15–30 mg/kg daily in 3 divided doses

▸ Child 5–17 years (body-weight 40 kg and above): 500 mg 3 times a day

● UNLICENSED USE

▸ With oral use *Asacol®* (all preparations) not licensed for use in children under 18 years. *Pentasa®* tablets not licensed for use in children under 15 years. *Pentasa®* granules and *Salofalk®* tablets and granules not licensed for use in children under 6 years.

▸ With rectal use *Asacol®* (all preparations) and *Salofalk®* enema not licensed for use in children under 18 years. *Salofalk®* suppositories and *Pentasa®* suppositories not licensed for use in children. *Salofalk®* rectal foam no dose recommendations for children (age range not specified by manufacturer).

IMPORTANT SAFETY INFORMATION

MHRA/CHM ADVICE: MESALAZINE AND IDIOPATHIC INTRACRANIAL HYPERTENSION (DECEMBER 2025)

A European review of safety data found very rare reports of idiopathic intracranial hypertension (IIH) associated with mesalazine therapy. Healthcare professionals are advised to exercise caution when prescribing for patients with previously diagnosed or suspected IIH, and to monitor for signs and symptoms during treatment. If IIH occurs, symptoms should be managed immediately and discontinuation of mesalazine therapy considered.

Patients and their carers should be counselled to seek immediate medical attention if signs or symptoms of IIH develop.

● CONTRA-INDICATIONS

▸ With oral use Blood clotting abnormalities

● CAUTIONS Maintain adequate fluid intake · pulmonary disease

● INTERACTIONS → Appendix 1: mesalazine

● SIDE-EFFECTS

GENERAL SIDE-EFFECTS

▶ **Rare or very rare** Anaemia · constipation · drug fever · hypersensitivity · nephritis · pulmonary fibrosis

▶ **Frequency not known** Nephrolithiasis

SPECIFIC SIDE-EFFECTS

▶ **Common or very common**

▸ With oral use Asthenia · gastrointestinal disorders · hypertension · pain

▸ With rectal use Flatulence

▶ **Uncommon**

▸ With oral use Chest pain · drowsiness · ear pain · hypotension · laryngeal pain · tremor

▶ **Rare or very rare**

▸ With oral use Intracranial pressure increased · pericardial effusion

▶ **Frequency not known**

▸ With oral use Condition aggravated · increased risk of infection · ketonuria · minimal change disease · weight decreased

▸ With rectal use Idiopathic intracranial hypertension

SIDE-EFFECTS, FURTHER INFORMATION Discontinue immediately if symptoms of acute intolerance syndrome occur such as cramping, abdominal pain, bloody diarrhoea, fever, severe headache, and rash. Worsening abdominal pain and diarrhoea may be difficult to distinguish from an exacerbation of inflammatory bowel disease.

● PREGNANCY Negligible quantities cross placenta.

● BREAST FEEDING Diarrhoea reported in breast-fed infants, but negligible amounts of mesalazine detected in breast milk.

Monitoring Monitor breast-fed infant for diarrhoea.

● HEPATIC IMPAIRMENT Manufacturer advises caution in mild to moderate impairment; avoid in severe impairment.

● RENAL IMPAIRMENT [EvGr] Use with caution in mild to moderate impairment (risk of toxicity including crystalluria); avoid in severe impairment. ⟨M⟩

● DIRECTIONS FOR ADMINISTRATION

PENTASA ® GRANULES Manufacturer advises granules should be placed on tongue and washed down with water or orange juice without chewing.

Expert sources advise contents of one sachet should be weighed and divided immediately before use; discard any remaining granules.

PENTASA ® TABLETS Manufacturer advises tablets may be halved, quartered, or dispersed in water, but should not be chewed.

SALOFALK ® GRANULES Manufacturer advises granules should be placed on tongue and washed down with water without chewing.

● PRESCRIBING AND DISPENSING INFORMATION There is no evidence to show that any one oral preparation of mesalazine is more effective than another; however, the delivery characteristics of oral mesalazine preparations may vary.

Flavours of granule formulations of *Salofalk®* may include vanilla.

● PATIENT AND CARER ADVICE If it is necessary to switch a patient to a different brand of mesalazine, the patient should be advised to report any changes in symptoms. Some products may require special administration advice; patients and carers should be informed.

Medicines for Children leaflet: Mesalazine (oral) for inflammatory bowel disease www.medicinesforchildren.org.uk/medicines/mesalazine-oral-for-inflammatory-bowel-disease/

Medicines for Children leaflet: Mesalazine foam enema for inflammatory bowel disease www.medicinesforchildren.org.uk/medicines/mesalazine-foam-enema-for-inflammatory-bowel-disease/

Medicines for Children leaflet: Mesalazine liquid enema for inflammatory bowel disease www.medicinesforchildren.org.uk/medicines/mesalazine-liquid-enema-for-inflammatory-bowel-disease/

Medicines for Children leaflet: Mesalazine suppositories for inflammatory bowel disease www.medicinesforchildren.org.uk/medicines/mesalazine-suppositories-for-inflammatory-bowel-disease/

- **MEDICINAL FORMS** There can be variation in the licensing of different medicines containing the same drug.

Modified-release tablet

CAUTIONARY AND ADVISORY LABELS 21(does not apply to Pentasa ® tablets), 25 (does not apply to Pentasa ® tablets)

▸ **Pentasa** (Ferring Pharmaceuticals Ltd)
Mesalazine 500 mg Pentasa 500mg modified-release tablets | 100 tablet PoM £30.74 DT = £30.74
Mesalazine 1 gram Pentasa 1g modified-release tablets | 60 tablet PoM £36.89 DT = £36.89

Gastro-resistant tablet

CAUTIONARY AND ADVISORY LABELS 5, 25

▸ **Octasa MR** (Tillotts Pharma UK Ltd)
Mesalazine 400 mg Octasa 400mg MR gastro-resistant tablets | 90 tablet PoM £19.50 DT = £19.50 | 120 tablet PoM £26.00 DT = £26.00
Mesalazine 800 mg Octasa 800mg MR gastro-resistant tablets | 90 tablet PoM £40.38 | 180 tablet PoM £80.75 DT = £80.75

▸ **Salofalk** (Dr. Falk Pharma UK Ltd)
Mesalazine 500 mg Salofalk 500mg gastro-resistant tablets | 100 tablet PoM £32.38 DT = £32.38

Suppository

▸ **Pentasa** (Ferring Pharmaceuticals Ltd)
Mesalazine 1 gram Pentasa 1g suppositories | 28 suppository PoM £40.01 DT = £40.01

▸ **Salofalk** (Dr. Falk Pharma UK Ltd)
Mesalazine 500 mg Salofalk 500mg suppositories | 30 suppository PoM £14.81 DT = £14.81
Mesalazine 1 gram Salofalk 1g suppositories | 30 suppository PoM £29.62

Rectal foam

EXCIPIENTS: May contain Cetostearyl alcohol (including cetyl and stearyl alcohol), disodium edetate, hydroxybenzoates (parabens), polysorbates, propylene glycol, sodium metabisulfite

▸ **Salofalk** (Dr. Falk Pharma UK Ltd)
Mesalazine 1 gram per 1 application Salofalk 1g/application foam enema | 14 actuation PoM £30.17 DT = £30.17

Modified-release granules

CAUTIONARY AND ADVISORY LABELS 25 (does not apply to Pentasa ® granules)

EXCIPIENTS: May contain Aspartame

▸ **Pentasa** (Ferring Pharmaceuticals Ltd)
Mesalazine 1 gram Pentasa 1g modified-release granules sachets | 50 sachet PoM £30.74 DT = £30.74 SF
Mesalazine 2 gram Pentasa 2g modified-release granules sachets | 60 sachet PoM £73.78 DT = £73.78 SF

▸ **Salofalk** (Dr. Falk Pharma UK Ltd)
Mesalazine 1 gram Salofalk 1g gastro-resistant modified-release granules sachets | 50 sachet PoM £28.74 DT = £28.74 SF
Mesalazine 1.5 gram Salofalk 1.5g gastro-resistant modified-release granules sachets | 60 sachet PoM £48.85 DT = £48.85 SF
Mesalazine 3 gram Salofalk 3g gastro-resistant modified-release granules sachets | 60 sachet PoM £97.70 DT = £97.70 SF

Enema

▸ **Pentasa** (Ferring Pharmaceuticals Ltd)
Mesalazine 10 mg per 1 ml Pentasa Mesalazine 1g/100ml enema | 7 enema PoM £17.73 DT = £17.73

▸ **Salofalk** (Dr. Falk Pharma UK Ltd)
Mesalazine 33.9 mg per 1 ml Salofalk 2g/59ml enema | 7 enema PoM £29.92 DT = £29.92

F 32

Olsalazine sodium

24-Jun-2021

- **INDICATIONS AND DOSE**

Treatment of acute attack of mild ulcerative colitis

▶ BY MOUTH

▸ Child 2–17 years: 500 mg twice daily, dose to be taken after food, then increased if necessary up to 1 g 3 times a day, dose to be increased over 1 week

Maintenance of remission of mild ulcerative colitis

▶ BY MOUTH

▸ Child 2–17 years: Maintenance 250–500 mg twice daily, dose to be taken after food

- **UNLICENSED USE** Not licensed for use in children under 12 years.
- **SIDE-EFFECTS** Palpitations · vision blurred
- **PREGNANCY** Manufacturer advises avoid unless potential benefit outweighs risk.
- **BREAST FEEDING**
  Monitoring Monitor breast-fed infants for diarrhoea.
- **RENAL IMPAIRMENT** EvGr Use with caution in mild to moderate impairment; avoid in significant impairment. ⟨M⟩
- **DIRECTIONS FOR ADMINISTRATION** Expert sources advise capsules can be opened and contents sprinkled on food.

- **MEDICINAL FORMS** There can be variation in the licensing of different medicines containing the same drug. Forms available from special-order manufacturers include: oral suspension, oral solution

Oral tablet

CAUTIONARY AND ADVISORY LABELS 21

▸ **Olsalazine sodium (Non-proprietary)**
Olsalazine sodium 500 mg Olsalazine 500mg tablets | 60 tablet PoM £161.00 DT = £161.00

Oral capsule

CAUTIONARY AND ADVISORY LABELS 21

▸ **Olsalazine sodium (Non-proprietary)**
Olsalazine sodium 250 mg Olsalazine 250mg capsules | 112 capsule PoM £144.00 DT = £144.00

F 32

Sulfasalazine

24-Jun-2021

(Sulphasalazine)

- **INDICATIONS AND DOSE**

Treatment of acute attack of mild to moderate and severe ulcerative colitis | Active Crohn's disease

▶ BY MOUTH

▸ Child 2–11 years: 10–15 mg/kg 4–6 times a day (max. per dose 1 g) until remission occurs; increased if necessary up to 60 mg/kg daily in divided doses

▸ Child 12–17 years: 1–2 g 4 times a day until remission occurs

▶ BY RECTUM

▸ Child 5–7 years: 500 mg twice daily

▸ Child 8–11 years: 500 mg, dose to be administered in the morning and 1 g, dose to be administered at night

▸ Child 12–17 years: 0.5–1 g twice daily

Maintenance of remission of mild to moderate and severe ulcerative colitis

▶ BY MOUTH

▸ Child 2–11 years: 5–7.5 mg/kg 4 times a day (max. per dose 500 mg)

▸ Child 12–17 years: 500 mg 4 times a day

▶ BY RECTUM

▸ Child 5–7 years: 500 mg twice daily

▸ Child 8–11 years: 500 mg, dose to be administered in the morning and 1 g, dose to be administered at night

▸ Child 12–17 years: 0.5–1 g twice daily

Juvenile idiopathic arthritis

▶ BY MOUTH

▸ Child 2–11 years: Initially 5 mg/kg twice daily for 1 week, then 10 mg/kg twice daily for 1 week, then 20 mg/kg twice daily for 1 week; maintenance 20–25 mg/kg twice daily; maximum 2 g per day

▸ Child 12–17 years: Initially 5 mg/kg twice daily for 1 week, then 10 mg/kg twice daily for 1 week, then 20 mg/kg twice daily for 1 week; maintenance 20–25 mg/kg twice daily; maximum 3 g per day

- **UNLICENSED USE** Not licensed for use in children for juvenile idiopathic arthritis.

> **IMPORTANT SAFETY INFORMATION**
> SAFE PRACTICE
> Sulfasalazine has been confused with sulfadiazine; care must be taken to ensure the correct drug is prescribed and dispensed.

- **CONTRA-INDICATIONS** Child under 2 years of age
- **CAUTIONS** Acute porphyrias p. 745 · G6PD deficiency · history of allergy · history of asthma · maintain adequate fluid intake · risk of haematological toxicity · risk of hepatic toxicity · slow acetylator status
- **INTERACTIONS** → Appendix 1: sulfasalazine
- **SIDE-EFFECTS**

GENERAL SIDE-EFFECTS
- **Common or very common** Insomnia · stomatitis · taste altered · tinnitus
- **Uncommon** Seizure · vasculitis
- **Frequency not known** Anaemia · appetite decreased · ataxia · crystalluria · cyanosis · encephalopathy · hallucination · hypoprothrombinaemia · lymphadenopathy · macrocytosis · meningitis aseptic · methaemoglobinaemia · parotitis · periorbital oedema · pseudomembranous enterocolitis · serum sickness · smell disorders · systemic lupus erythematosus (SLE) · yellow discolouration of body fluids

SPECIFIC SIDE-EFFECTS
- With oral use Urine discolouration

SIDE-EFFECTS, FURTHER INFORMATION Incidence of side-effects increases with higher doses.

Blood disorders Haematological abnormalities occur usually in the first 3 to 6 months of treatment—discontinue if these occur.

- **PREGNANCY** Theoretical risk of neonatal haemolysis in third trimester; adequate folate supplements should be given to mother.
- **BREAST FEEDING** Small amounts in milk (1 report of bloody diarrhoea); theoretical risk of neonatal haemolysis especially in G6PD-deficient infants.
- **HEPATIC IMPAIRMENT** Manufacturer advises caution.
- **RENAL IMPAIRMENT** [EvGr] Use with caution in mild to moderate impairment (risk of toxicity including crystalluria); avoid in severe impairment. ⟨M⟩
- **MONITORING REQUIREMENTS**
  - Blood disorders Close monitoring of full blood counts (including differential white cell count and platelet count) is necessary initially, and at monthly intervals during the first 3 months.
  - Renal function Although the manufacturer recommends renal function tests in rheumatic diseases, evidence of practical value is unsatisfactory.
  - Liver function Liver function tests should be performed at monthly intervals for first 3 months.
- **PATIENT AND CARER ADVICE**

Contact lenses Some soft contact lenses may be stained.

- **MEDICINAL FORMS** There can be variation in the licensing of different medicines containing the same drug. Forms available from special-order manufacturers include: oral suspension

Oral tablet

CAUTIONARY AND ADVISORY LABELS 14
- **Sulfasalazine (Non-proprietary)**

  Sulfasalazine 500 mg Sulfasalazine 500mg tablets | 112 tablet [PoM] £14.42 DT = £7.02

Oral suspension

CAUTIONARY AND ADVISORY LABELS 14

EXCIPIENTS: May contain Alcohol
- **Sulfasalazine (Non-proprietary)**

  Sulfasalazine 50 mg per 1 ml Sulfasalazine 250mg/5ml oral suspension sugar free | 500 ml [PoM] £63.56–£151.41 DT = £151.41 [SF]

Gastro-resistant tablet

CAUTIONARY AND ADVISORY LABELS 5, 14, 25
- **Sulfasalazine (Non-proprietary)**

  Sulfasalazine 500 mg Sulfasalazine 500mg gastro-resistant tablets | 112 tablet [PoM] £15.50 DT = £8.68

Suppository

CAUTIONARY AND ADVISORY LABELS 14
- **Sulfasalazine (Non-proprietary)**

  Sulfasalazine 500 mg Sulfasalazine 500mg suppositories | 10 suppository [PoM] £3.30 DT = £3.30

CORTICOSTEROIDS

F 540

Budesonide

26-Feb-2026

- **DRUG ACTION** Budesonide is a glucocorticoid, which exerts significant local anti-inflammatory effects.

- **INDICATIONS AND DOSE**

Mild to moderate Crohn's disease affecting the ileum and/or ascending colon
- BY MOUTH USING MODIFIED-RELEASE CAPSULES
  - Child 12–17 years: 9 mg once daily for up to 8 weeks, to be taken in the morning, when stopping treatment, reduce dose for the last 2–4 weeks of therapy

BUDENOFALK ® CAPSULES

Mild to moderate Crohn's disease affecting the ileum and/or ascending colon
- BY MOUTH
  - Child 12–17 years: 3 mg 3 times a day for up to 8 weeks, reduce dose gradually over 2 weeks following treatment course before stopping

ENTOCORT ® ENEMA

Ulcerative colitis involving rectal and recto-sigmoid disease
- BY RECTUM
  - Child 12–17 years: 1 enema once daily for 4 weeks, to be administered at bedtime

- **UNLICENSED USE** Not licensed for use in children for Crohn's disease or ulcerative colitis.
- **INTERACTIONS** → Appendix 1: corticosteroids
- **SIDE-EFFECTS**
  - **Common or very common**
  - With oral use Fatigue · muscle twitching · oedema · oral disorders
  - With rectal use Depression · gastrointestinal disorders
  - **Uncommon**
  - With rectal use Akathisia · insomnia
  - **Rare or very rare**
  - With oral use Malaise
  - With rectal use Adrenal hypofunction

SIDE-EFFECTS, FURTHER INFORMATION Systemic absorption can follow rectal administration, therefore also consider the side-effects of systemic corticosteroids.

- **HEPATIC IMPAIRMENT** For *Budenofalk®* manufacturer advises avoid in cirrhosis (risk of increased exposure, limited information available).
- **DIRECTIONS FOR ADMINISTRATION**
  - With oral use Expert sources advise capsules can be opened and the contents mixed with apple or orange juice.
- **PRESCRIBING AND DISPENSING INFORMATION**
  - With oral use Dispense modified-release capsules in original container (contains desiccant).

● **MEDICINAL FORMS** There can be variation in the licensing of different medicines containing the same drug.

Gastro-resistant capsule

CAUTIONARY AND ADVISORY LABELS 5, 10, 22, 25

▸ **Budenofalk** (Dr. Falk Pharma UK Ltd)

Budesonide 3 mg Budenofalk 3mg gastro-resistant capsules | 100 capsule PoM £75.05 DT = £75.05

Modified-release capsule

CAUTIONARY AND ADVISORY LABELS 10, 25

▸ **Budesonide (Non-proprietary)**

Budesonide 3 mg Budesonide 3mg gastro-resistant modified-release capsules | 100 capsule PoM £75.05 DT = £75.05

Enema

▸ **Entocort** (Tillotts Pharma UK Ltd)

Budesonide 20 microgram per 1 ml Entocort 2mg/100ml enema | 7 enema PoM £33.66 DT = £33.66

IMMUNOSUPPRESSANTS › IMMUNOMODULATING DRUGS

Etrasimod

25-Jun-2024

● **DRUG ACTION** Etrasimod is a sphingosine-1-phosphate receptor modulator, which prevents movement of lymphocytes out of lymph nodes, thereby limiting inflammation in the intestine.

● **INDICATIONS AND DOSE**

Ulcerative colitis (initiated under specialist supervision)

▶ BY MOUTH

▸ Child 16–17 years: 2 mg once daily

● **CONTRA-INDICATIONS** Active malignancy · decompensated heart failure (requiring inpatient treatment) in the previous 6 months · heart failure (New York Heart Association class III or IV) in the previous 6 months · immunodeficiency · myocardial infarction in the previous 6 months · phototherapy with UV-B radiation or PUVA-photochemotherapy (increased risk of cutaneous neoplasm) · posterior reversible encephalopathy syndrome (suspected or confirmed) · progressive multifocal leukoencephalopathy · second-degree Mobitz type II AV block, third-degree AV block, sick sinus syndrome or sino-atrial block, if the patient does not have a pacemaker · severe active infection · stroke (including transient ischaemic attack) in the previous 6 months · unstable angina in the previous 6 months

● **CAUTIONS** Administration of vaccinations · arrhythmias requiring treatment with Class Ia or Class III anti-arrhythmic drugs · asthma · body-weight less than 40 kg (increased risk of exposure) · cerebrovascular disease · chronic obstructive pulmonary disease · diabetes mellitus (increased risk of macular oedema) · heart failure · immunosuppression or other risk factors for infection · myocardial infarction · patients receiving QT-prolonging or heart rate-lowering drugs, including beta-blockers and heart rate-lowering calcium-channel blockers · pulmonary fibrosis · recurrent syncope · retinal disease (increased risk of macular oedema) · second-degree Mobitz type I AV block · severe respiratory disease · severe untreated sleep apnoea · significant QT prolongation (QTc equal to or greater than 470 milliseconds in females, or QTc equal to or greater than 450 milliseconds in males) · sinus bradycardia (heart rate below 50 beats per minute) · uncontrolled hypertension · uveitis (increased risk of macular oedema)

CAUTIONS, FURTHER INFORMATION

▸ Bradycardia and cardiac rhythm disturbance EvGr Etrasimod may cause transient bradycardia, AV conduction delays and heart block after the first dose. It is not recommended in patients with a history of cardiac arrest, cerebrovascular disease, symptomatic bradycardia or recurrent syncope, unstable ischaemic heart disease, uncontrolled hypertension, severe untreated sleep apnoea, or significant QT prolongation or other risk factors for QT prolongation unless the anticipated benefits outweigh the potential risks, and advice from a cardiologist (including monitoring advice) is sought before initiation. ⟨M⟩

▸ Vaccinations EvGr Vaccination may be less effective during and for up to 2 weeks after stopping treatment. Live attenuated vaccines should be avoided during and for 2 weeks after stopping treatment; if they are required they should be given at least 1 month prior to initiation. ⟨M⟩

● **INTERACTIONS** → Appendix 1: etrasimod

● **SIDE-EFFECTS**

▶ **Common or very common** Arrhythmias · cystitis · dizziness · headache · hypercholesterolaemia · hypertension · increased risk of infection · lymphopenia · neutropenia · visual impairment

▶ **Uncommon** Atrioventricular block · macular oedema

▶ **Frequency not known** Hepatic disorders

● **CONCEPTION AND CONTRACEPTION** EvGr Exclude pregnancy before treatment; females of childbearing potential should use effective contraception during treatment and for at least 14 days after last dose. ⟨M⟩

● **PREGNANCY** EvGr Avoid (toxicity in *animal* studies and limited human data suggests increased risk of abnormal pregnancy outcomes). ⟨M⟩

● **BREAST FEEDING** Specialist sources indicate use with caution, especially if breast-feeding a newborn or preterm infant (no information available). High plasma-protein binding suggests limited excretion into milk.

● **HEPATIC IMPAIRMENT** EvGr Caution when history of significant liver disease (no information available); avoid in severe impairment. ⟨M⟩

● **MONITORING REQUIREMENTS**

▸ EvGr ECG should be obtained for all patients prior to treatment initiation. Patients with certain pre-existing cardiac conditions should be monitored for bradycardia for 4 hours after the first dose, and another ECG obtained after this 4-hour period ⟨M⟩—consult product literature for further information.

▸ EvGr Monitor blood pressure regularly during treatment.

▸ Monitor hepatic transaminases and bilirubin before initiation of treatment and then at months 1, 3, 6, 9, 12, and periodically thereafter (interrupt treatment if significant liver injury occurs: liver transaminases above 3 times the upper limit of normal and total bilirubin above 2 times the upper limit of normal).

▸ Monitor full blood count before initiation and periodically during treatment (interrupt treatment if lymphocyte count reduced) ⟨M⟩—consult product literature.

▸ EvGr Eye examination recommended in all patients at initiation of treatment and then as clinically indicated (interrupt treatment if macular oedema occurs); patients with history of diabetes or uveitis or retinal disease to have eye examination periodically during treatment. ⟨M⟩

● **DIRECTIONS FOR ADMINISTRATION** EvGr Tablet should be taken with food for the first 3 days of treatment to reduce potential transient heart rate lowering effects, after which it can be taken with or without food. ⟨M⟩

● **PRESCRIBING AND DISPENSING INFORMATION** The manufacturer of *Velsipity*® has provided a *Checklist for Prescribers*.

● **PATIENT AND CARER ADVICE** Patients and carers should be given advice on how to administer etrasimod tablets. Patients and carers should be advised to avoid exposure to sunlight without protection. Patients and carers should be advised to promptly report symptoms of infection during and for up to 2 weeks after stopping treatment.

Patient card and guide Patients and carers should be given a *Patient/Caregiver Guide*.

Female patients of childbearing potential should be given a *Patient card*.

Missed doses If treatment is interrupted for 7 or more consecutive days, resume treatment with food for the first 3 doses.

Driving and skilled tasks Patients and carers should be counselled on the effects on driving and performance of skilled tasks—increased risk of dizziness.

- **NATIONAL FUNDING/ACCESS DECISIONS** For full details see funding body website

NICE decisions

- **Etrasimod for treating moderately to severely active ulcerative colitis in people aged 16 and over (March 2024)** NICE TA956 Recommended

Scottish Medicines Consortium (SMC) decisions

- **Etrasimod (*Velsipity*®) for the treatment of patients 16 years of age and older with moderately to severely active ulcerative colitis who have had an inadequate response, lost response, or were intolerant to either conventional therapy, or a biological agent (June 2024)** SMC No. SMC2655 Recommended

- **MEDICINAL FORMS** There can be variation in the licensing of different medicines containing the same drug.

Oral tablet

EXCIPIENTS: May contain Tartrazine

- **Velsipity** (Pfizer Ltd) ▼
  Etrasimod (as Etrasimod arginine) 2 mg Velsipity 2mg tablets | 28 tablet [PoM] £843.84 (Hospital only)

IMMUNOSUPPRESSANTS › INTERLEUKIN INHIBITORS

Risankizumab

14-Jan-2025

- **DRUG ACTION** Risankizumab is a humanised monoclonal antibody that binds selectively to interleukin-23 and blocks the activity of pro-inflammatory cytokines.

- **INDICATIONS AND DOSE**

Crohn's disease (under expert supervision)

- INITIALLY BY INTRAVENOUS INFUSION
  - Child 16–17 years: Initially 600 mg every 4 weeks for 3 doses, to be given on weeks 0, 4, and 8, then (by subcutaneous injection) maintenance 360 mg every 8 weeks, first subcutaneous dose to be given on week 12, consider discontinuation if no response after 24 weeks

- **CONTRA-INDICATIONS** Clinically significant active infection
- **CAUTIONS** Chronic infection · history of recurrent infection · risk of infection

CAUTIONS, FURTHER INFORMATION

- Risk of infection Manufacturer advises consider anti-tuberculosis therapy before initiation of risankizumab in patients with a history of latent or active tuberculosis in whom an adequate course of treatment cannot be confirmed.

Manufacturer advises consider completion of immunisations according to current guidelines before initiating treatment (consult product literature for appropriate interval between vaccination and administration of risankizumab).

- **INTERACTIONS** → Appendix 1: monoclonal antibodies
- **SIDE-EFFECTS**
  - **Common or very common** Asthenia · headaches · increased risk of infection · malaise · skin reactions
- **CONCEPTION AND CONTRACEPTION** Manufacturer advises effective contraception in women of childbearing potential during treatment and for at least 21 weeks after treatment.
- **PREGNANCY** Manufacturer advises avoid (limited information available).
- **BREAST FEEDING** Manufacturer advises avoid (no information available).
- **PRE-TREATMENT SCREENING** Manufacturer advises patients should be evaluated for tuberculosis infection before treatment.
- **MONITORING REQUIREMENTS** Manufacturer advises monitor for signs and symptoms of active tuberculosis during treatment.
- **DIRECTIONS FOR ADMINISTRATION** For *cartridge*, take carton out of the refrigerator at least 45 minutes before administration.

For *subcutaneous injection*, inject into the thigh or abdomen and avoid injecting into areas of the skin that are tender, bruised, erythematous, or hardened. Patients may self-administer *Skyrizi*® after appropriate training in subcutaneous injection technique.

For *intermittent intravenous infusion*, dilute to a concentration of approximately 1.2–6 mg/mL with Glucose 5% and give over at least 1 hour.

- **PRESCRIBING AND DISPENSING INFORMATION** Risankizumab is a biological medicine. Biological medicines must be prescribed and dispensed by brand name, see *Biological medicines* and *Biosimilar medicines*, under Guidance on prescribing p. 1; manufacturer advises to record the brand name and batch number after each administration.
- **HANDLING AND STORAGE** Manufacturer advises store in a refrigerator (2–8°C) and protect from light.
- **PATIENT AND CARER ADVICE** Patients and their carers should be advised to seek medical attention if signs or symptoms of infection occur.

Self-administration If appropriate, patients and their carers should be given training in subcutaneous injection technique.

- **NATIONAL FUNDING/ACCESS DECISIONS** For full details see funding body website

NICE decisions

- **Risankizumab for previously treated moderately to severely active Crohn's disease (May 2023)** NICE TA888 Recommended with restrictions

Scottish Medicines Consortium (SMC) decisions

- **Risankizumab (*Skyrizi*®) for the treatment of patients 16 years and older with moderately to severely active Crohn's disease who have had an inadequate response to, lost response to, or were intolerant to conventional therapy or a biologic therapy, or if such therapies are not advisable (November 2023)** SMC No. SMC2534 Recommended

- **MEDICINAL FORMS** There can be variation in the licensing of different medicines containing the same drug.

Solution for injection

EXCIPIENTS: May contain Polysorbates

- **Skyrizi** (AbbVie Ltd)
  Risankizumab 150 mg per 1 ml Skyrizi 180mg/1.2ml solution for injection cartridges | 1 cartridge [PoM] £3,326.09 (Hospital only)
  Skyrizi 360mg/2.4ml solution for injection cartridges | 1 cartridge [PoM] £3,326.09
  Skyrizi 150mg/1ml solution for injection pre-filled pens | 1 pre-filled disposable injection [PoM] £3,326.09 (Hospital only)
  Skyrizi 150mg/1ml solution for injection pre-filled syringes | 1 pre-filled disposable injection [PoM] £3,326.09 (Hospital only)

Solution for infusion

EXCIPIENTS: May contain Polysorbates

- **Skyrizi** (AbbVie Ltd)
  Risankizumab 60 mg per 1 ml Skyrizi 600mg/10ml concentrate for solution for infusion vials | 1 vial [PoM] £3,326.09 (Hospital only)

IMMUNOSUPPRESSANTS › TUMOR NECROSIS FACTOR ALPHA (TNF-α) INHIBITORS

Infliximab

29-Oct-2025

● **INDICATIONS AND DOSE**

Active Crohn's disease (under expert supervision)

▶ BY INTRAVENOUS INFUSION

▶ Child 6–17 years: Initially 5 mg/kg, then 5 mg/kg, to be taken at week 2 and 6 after initial dose, then maintenance 5 mg/kg every 8 weeks, interval between maintenance doses adjusted according to response; discontinue if no response within 10 weeks of initial infusion (after 3 doses)

Fistulating Crohn's disease (under expert supervision)

▶ BY INTRAVENOUS INFUSION

▶ Child 6–17 years: Initially 5 mg/kg, then 5 mg/kg after 2 weeks, followed by 5 mg/kg after 4 weeks, if condition has responded consult product literature for guidance on further doses

Active ulcerative colitis (under expert supervision)

▶ BY INTRAVENOUS INFUSION

▶ Child 6–17 years: Initially 5 mg/kg, then 5 mg/kg, to be taken at week 2 and 6 after initial dose, then 5 mg/kg every 8 weeks, discontinue if no response within 8 weeks of initial infusion (after 3 doses)

● **UNLICENSED USE** Not licensed for fistulating Crohn's disease in children.

IMPORTANT SAFETY INFORMATION

Adequate resuscitation facilities must be available when infliximab is used.

● **CONTRA-INDICATIONS** Moderate or severe heart failure · severe infections

● **CAUTIONS** Demyelinating disorders (risk of exacerbation) · dermatomyositis · development of malignancy · hepatitis B virus—monitor for active infection · history of malignancy · history of prolonged immunosuppressant or PUVA treatment in patients with psoriasis · mild heart failure (discontinue if symptoms develop or worsen) · predisposition to infection (discontinue if new serious infection develops) · risk of delayed hypersensitivity reactions if drug-free interval exceeds 16 weeks (re-administration after interval exceeding 16 weeks not recommended)

CAUTIONS, FURTHER INFORMATION

▶ Infection Manufacturer advises patients should be up-to-date with current immunisation schedule before initiating treatment.

▶ Tuberculosis Manufacturer advises to evaluate patients for active and latent tuberculosis before treatment. Active tuberculosis should be treated with standard treatment for at least 2 months before starting infliximab. If latent tuberculosis is diagnosed, treatment should be started before commencing treatment with infliximab. Patients who have previously received adequate treatment for tuberculosis can start infliximab but should be monitored every 3 months for possible recurrence. In patients without active tuberculosis but who were previously not treated adequately, chemoprophylaxis should ideally be completed before starting infliximab. In patients at high risk of tuberculosis who cannot be assessed by tuberculin skin test, chemoprophylaxis can be given concurrently with infliximab. Patients should be advised to seek medical attention if symptoms suggestive of tuberculosis develop (e.g. persistent cough, weight loss and fever).

▶ Hypersensitivity reactions Hypersensitivity reactions (including fever, chest pain, hypotension, hypertension, dyspnoea, transient visual loss, pruritus, urticaria, serum sickness-like reactions, angioedema, anaphylaxis) reported during or within 1–2 hours after infusion (risk greatest during first or second infusion or in patients who discontinue other immunosuppressants). Manufacturer advises prophylactic antipyretics, antihistamines, or hydrocortisone may be administered.

● **INTERACTIONS** → Appendix 1: monoclonal antibodies

● **SIDE-EFFECTS**

▶ **Common or very common** Abscess · alopecia · anaemia · arrhythmias · arthralgia · chest pain · chills · constipation · decreased leucocytes · depression · diarrhoea · dizziness · dyspnoea · eye inflammation · fatigue · fever · gastrointestinal discomfort · gastrointestinal disorders · haemorrhage · headache · hepatic disorders · hyperhidrosis · hypertension · hypotension · increased risk of infection · infusion related reaction · insomnia · lymphadenopathy · myalgia · nausea · neutropenia · oedema · pain · palpitations · respiratory disorders · sensation abnormal · sepsis · skin reactions · vasodilation · vertigo

▶ **Uncommon** Anxiety · cheilitis · cholecystitis · confusion · drowsiness · dyslipidaemia · healing impaired · heart failure · hypersensitivity · lupus erythematosus · lymphocytosis · memory loss · neoplasms · nerve disorders · pancreatitis · peripheral ischaemia · pulmonary oedema · seborrhoea · seizure · syncope · thrombocytopenia · thrombophlebitis · weight increased

▶ **Rare or very rare** Agranulocytosis · circulatory collapse · cyanosis · demyelinating disorders · granuloma · haemolytic anaemia · hepatitis B reactivation · interstitial lung disease · meningitis · pancytopenia · pericardial effusion · pulmonary fibrosis · sarcoid-like reaction · severe cutaneous adverse reactions (SCARs) · transverse myelitis · vasculitis · vasospasm

▶ **Frequency not known** Bone fracture · dermatomyositis exacerbated · hepatosplenic T-cell lymphoma (increased risk in inflammatory bowel disease) · myocardial infarction · myocardial ischaemia · sarcoidosis · stroke · ulcerative colitis aggravated · vision loss

● **CONCEPTION AND CONTRACEPTION** Manufacturer advises adequate contraception during and for at least 6 months after last dose.

● **PREGNANCY** Use only if essential.

● **BREAST FEEDING** Specialist sources indicate amount present in milk probably too small to be harmful.

● **PRE-TREATMENT SCREENING**

Tuberculosis Manufacturer advises patients should be evaluated for tuberculosis before treatment.

● **MONITORING REQUIREMENTS**

▶ Monitor for infection before, during, and for 6 months after treatment.

▶ All patients should be observed carefully for 1–2 hours after infusion and resuscitation equipment should be available for immediate use (risk of hypersensitivity reactions).

▶ Monitor for symptoms of delayed hypersensitivity if re-administered after a prolonged period.

▶ Manufacturer advises periodic skin examination for non-melanoma skin cancer, particularly in patients with risk factors.

● **DIRECTIONS FOR ADMINISTRATION** EvGr For *intermittent intravenous infusion*, dilute reconstituted solution with Sodium Chloride 0.9%. Reconstitute each 100 mg vial with 10 mL Water for Injections using a 21-gauge or smaller needle and gently swirl vial without shaking to dissolve; allow to stand for 5 minutes. Dilute requisite dose with infusion fluid to a usual final volume of 250 mL (maximum concentration 4 mg/mL). Give over 2 hours through a low protein-binding filter (1.2 micron or less). Start infusion within 3 hours of reconstitution. Ⓜ

● **PRESCRIBING AND DISPENSING INFORMATION** Infliximab is a biological medicine. Biological medicines must be prescribed and dispensed by brand name, see *Biological medicines* and *Biosimilar medicines*, under Guidance on prescribing p. 1.

- **HANDLING AND STORAGE** Store in a refrigerator (2–8°C)—consult product literature for further information regarding storage outside refrigerator.
- **PATIENT AND CARER ADVICE**
  Tuberculosis Patients and carers should be advised to seek medical attention if symptoms suggestive of tuberculosis (e.g. persistent cough, weight loss, and fever) develop.
  Blood disorders Patients and carers should be advised to seek medical attention if symptoms suggestive of blood disorders (such as fever, sore throat, bruising, or bleeding) develop.
  Hypersensitivity reactions Patients and carers should be advised to keep Alert card with them at all times and seek medical advice if symptoms of delayed hypersensitivity develop.
  Alert card An alert card should be provided.
  Driving and skilled tasks Manufacturer advises patients and carers should be counselled on the effects on driving and performance of skilled tasks—increased risk of dizziness.
- **NATIONAL FUNDING/ACCESS DECISIONS**
  For full details see funding body website
  NICE decisions
  - **Infliximab for Crohn's disease (May 2010)** NICE TA187 Recommended with restrictions
  - **Infliximab, adalimumab and golimumab for treating moderately to severely active ulcerative colitis after the failure of conventional therapy (February 2015)** NICE TA329 Recommended with restrictions

- **MEDICINAL FORMS** There can be variation in the licensing of different medicines containing the same drug.
  Powder for solution for infusion
  CAUTIONARY AND ADVISORY LABELS 10
  EXCIPIENTS: May contain Polysorbates
  - **Flixabi** (Biogen Idec Ltd)
    Infliximab 100 mg Flixabi 100mg powder for concentrate for solution for infusion vials | 1 vial [PoM] £377.00 (Hospital only)
  - **Remicade** (Janssen-Cilag Ltd)
    Infliximab 100 mg Remicade 100mg powder for concentrate for solution for infusion vials | 1 vial [PoM] £419.62 (Hospital only)
  - **Remsima** (Celltrion Healthcare UK Ltd)
    Infliximab 100 mg Remsima 100mg powder for concentrate for solution for infusion vials | 1 vial [PoM] £377.66 (Hospital only)
  - **Zessly** (Sandoz Ltd) ▼
    Infliximab 100 mg Zessly 100mg powder for concentrate for solution for infusion vials | 1 vial [PoM] £377.66 (Hospital only)

1.3 Irritable bowel syndrome

Irritable bowel syndrome

02-May-2020

Description of condition

Irritable bowel syndrome (IBS) is a gastrointestinal disorder characterised by abdominal pain or discomfort that may be relieved by defaecation. It can also be associated with the passage of mucus, bloating, and disordered defaecation; either diarrhoea, constipation, or alternating diarrhoea and constipation. Constipation presents with straining, urgency, and a sensation of incomplete evacuation. Before a diagnosis of IBS is made, the symptoms should be present at least once per week for at least 2 months and other potential pathological causes of the symptoms should be excluded. IBS symptoms are often aggravated by psychological factors, such as anxieties, emotional stress, and fear.

Aims of treatment

Treatment of IBS is focused on symptom control in order to improve quality of life, including minimising abdominal pain and normalising the frequency and consistency of stools.

Non-drug treatment

[EvGr] There is no evidence of the effectiveness of any form of dietary advice or increased fibre intake in children and it is not known whether dietary advice recommended to adult patients is of benefit to children. ⟨A⟩

[EvGr] Eating regularly, limiting fresh fruit intake, and, reducing intake of 'resistant starch' and insoluble fibre (e.g. bran) can be recommended. If an increase in dietary fibre is required, soluble fibre such as oats, ispaghula husk p. 45, or sterculia p. 46 can be recommended. Ensuring a sufficient intake of fluids can also be recommended. ⟨E⟩

Drug treatment

[EvGr] Clinicians should only prescribe drugs for children with IBS in cases of severe symptoms that have not responded to non-drug approaches. Treatment options include laxatives, antimotility drugs or antispasmodic drugs. ⟨A⟩

[EvGr] A laxative can be used to treat abdominal pain if the underlying cause is suspected to be constipation. An osmotic laxative, such as a macrogol or lactulose p. 46, is preferred; lactulose may cause flatulence during the first few days of treatment. Loperamide hydrochloride p. 55 may relieve diarrhoea and antispasmodic drugs may relieve pain. ⟨E⟩

ANTISPASMODICS

Mebeverine with ispaghula husk

09-Nov-2020

The properties listed below are those particular to the combination only. For the properties of the components please consider, mebeverine hydrochloride p. 69, ispaghula husk p. 45.

- **INDICATIONS AND DOSE**
  Irritable bowel syndrome
  ▶ BY MOUTH
  - Child 12–17 years: 1 sachet twice daily, in water, morning and evening, 30 minutes before food and 1 sachet daily if required, taken 30 minutes before midday meal

- **DIRECTIONS FOR ADMINISTRATION** Manufacturer advises contents of one sachet should be stirred into a glass (approx. 150 mL) of cold water and drunk immediately.
- **PATIENT AND CARER ADVICE** Patients or carers should be given advice on how to administer ispaghula husk with mebeverine granules.

- **MEDICINAL FORMS** There can be variation in the licensing of different medicines containing the same drug.
  Effervescent granules
  CAUTIONARY AND ADVISORY LABELS 13, 22
  EXCIPIENTS: May contain Aspartame
  ELECTROLYTES: May contain Potassium
  - **Fybogel Mebeverine** (Reckitt Benckiser Healthcare (UK) Ltd)
    Mebeverine hydrochloride 135 mg, Ispaghula husk 3.5 gram Fybogel Mebeverine effervescent granules sachets orange | 10 sachet [P] £10.64 DT = £10.64 [SF]

Peppermint oil

19-Nov-2020

● **INDICATIONS AND DOSE**

COLPERMIN®

Relief of abdominal colic and distension, particularly in irritable bowel syndrome

▶ BY MOUTH

▶ Child 15–17 years: 1–2 capsules 3 times a day for up to 3 months if necessary, capsule to be swallowed whole with water

● **CAUTIONS** Sensitivity to menthol

● **INTERACTIONS** → Appendix 1: peppermint

● **SIDE-EFFECTS** Ataxia · bradycardia · gastrointestinal discomfort · gastrooesophageal reflux disease · headache · nausea · paraesthesia · rash erythematous · tremor · vomiting

● **PREGNANCY** Not known to be harmful.

● **BREAST FEEDING** Significant levels of menthol in breast milk unlikely.

● **DIRECTIONS FOR ADMINISTRATION** Manufacturer advises capsules should not be broken or chewed because peppermint oil may irritate mouth or oesophagus.

● **MEDICINAL FORMS** There can be variation in the licensing of different medicines containing the same drug.

Modified-release capsule

CAUTIONARY AND ADVISORY LABELS 5, 22, 25

EXCIPIENTS: May contain Arachis (peanut) oil

▶ Colpermin (McNeil Products Ltd)

Peppermint oil 200 microlitre Colpermin IBS Relief gastro-resistant modified-release capsules | 20 capsule GSL £5.07 | 100 capsule GSL £17.48 DT = £17.48

1.4 Short bowel syndrome

Short bowel syndrome

31-Aug-2016

Description of condition

Children with a shortened bowel due to large surgical resection (with or without stoma formation) may require medical management to ensure adequate absorption of nutrients and fluid. Absorption of oral medication is also often impaired.

Aims of treatment

The management of short bowel syndrome focuses on ensuring adequate nutrition and drug absorption, thereby reducing the risk of complications resulting from these effects.

Drug treatment

Nutritional deficiencies

EvGr Children with a short bowel may require replacement of vitamins and minerals depending on the extent and position of the bowel resection. Deficiencies in vitamins A, B_{12}, D, E, and K, essential fatty acids, zinc and selenium can occur.

Hypomagnesaemia is common and is treated with oral or intravenous magnesium supplementation (see Magnesium imbalance p. 737), though administration of oral magnesium may cause diarrhoea. Occasionally the use of oral alfacalcidol p. 787 and correction of sodium depletion may be useful. Nutritional support can range from oral supplements to parenteral nutrition, depending on the severity of intestinal failure. Ⓐ

Diarrhoea and high output stomas

Diarrhoea is a common symptom of short bowel syndrome and can be due to multiple factors. EvGr The use of oral rehydration salts can be considered in order to promote adequate hydration. Oral intake influences the volume of stool passed, so reducing food intake will lessen diarrhoea, but will also exacerbate the problems of undernutrition. A child may require parenteral nutrition to allow them to eat less if the extent of diarrhoea is unacceptable.

Pharmacological treatment may be necessary, with the choice of drug depending on the potential for side-effects and the degree of resection. Ⓐ

Antimotility drugs

EvGr Loperamide hydrochloride p. 55 reduces intestinal motility and thus exerts antidiarrhoeal actions. Loperamide hydrochloride is preferred over other antimotility drugs as it is not sedative and does not cause dependence or fat malabsorption. High doses of loperamide hydrochloride [unlicensed] may be required in children with a short bowel due to disrupted enterohepatic circulation and a rapid gastro-intestinal transit time.

Co-phenotrope p. 54 has traditionally been used alone or in combination with other medications to help decrease faecal output. Co-phenotrope crosses the blood–brain barrier and can produce central nervous system side-effects, which may limit its use; the potential for dependence and anticholinergic effects may also restrict its use. Ⓐ

Colestyramine

EvGr In children with an intact colon and less than 100 cm of ileum resected, colestyramine p. 151 can be used to bind the unabsorbed bile salts, which reduces diarrhoea. When colestyramine is given to these children, it is important to monitor for evidence of fat malabsorption (steatorrhoea) or fat-soluble vitamin deficiencies. Ⓐ

Antisecretory drugs

EvGr Drugs that reduce gastric acid secretion reduce jejunostomy output. Omeprazole p. 64 is readily absorbed in the duodenum and upper small bowel, but if less than 50 cm of jejunum remains, it may need to be given intravenously. Use of a proton pump inhibitor alone does not eliminate the need for further intervention for fluid control (such as antimotility agents, intravenous fluids, or oral rehydration salts). Ⓐ

Growth factors

Growth factors can be used to facilitate intestinal adaptation after surgery in children with short bowel syndrome, thus enhancing fluid, electrolyte, and micronutrient absorption.

Teduglutide p. 42 is an analogue of endogenous human glucagon-like peptide 2 (GLP-2) which is licensed for use in the management of short bowel syndrome in children aged one year and over. It may be considered after a period of stabilisation following surgery, during which intravenous fluids and nutritional support should have been optimised.

Drug absorption

For *Prescribing in children with stoma* see Stoma care p. 84.

EvGr Many drugs are incompletely absorbed by children with a short bowel and may need to be prescribed in much higher doses than usual (such as levothyroxine, warfarin, oral contraceptives, and digoxin) or may need to be given intravenously. Ⓐ

Several factors can alter the absorption of drugs taken by mouth in children with a compromised gastrointestinal system. The most important factors are the length of intestine available for drug absorption, and which section has been removed. The small intestine, with its large surface area and high blood flow, is the most important site of drug absorption. The larger the amount of the small intestine that has been removed, the higher the possibility that drug absorption will be affected. Other factors such as gastric emptying and gastric transit time also affect drug handling.

EvGr Enteric-coated and modified-release preparations are unsuitable for use in patients with short bowel syndrome, particularly in children with an ileostomy, as there may not be sufficient release of the active ingredient.

Dosage forms with quick dissolution (such as soluble tablets) should be used. Uncoated tablets and liquid formulations may also be suitable. (A) EvGr Before prescribing liquid formulations, prescribers should consider the osmolarity, excipient content, and volume required. Hyperosmolar liquids and some excipients (such as sorbitol) can result in fluid loss. The calorie density of oral supplements should also be considered, as it will influence the volume to be taken. (E)

AMINO ACIDS AND DERIVATIVES

Teduglutide

07-Jul-2022

● **DRUG ACTION** Teduglutide is an analogue of human glucagon-like peptide-2 (GLP-2), which preserves mucosal integrity by promoting growth and repair of the intestine.

● **INDICATIONS AND DOSE**

Short bowel syndrome (initiated under specialist supervision)

▶ BY SUBCUTANEOUS INJECTION

▶ Child 1–17 years: 0.05 mg/kg once daily, dose to be administered to alternating quadrants of the abdomen; alternatively the thigh can be used, for optimal injection volume per body weight and when to review treatment, consult product literature

● **CONTRA-INDICATIONS** Active or suspected malignancy · history of gastro-intestinal malignancy (in previous 5 years)

● **CAUTIONS** Abrupt withdrawal of parenteral support (reduce gradually with concomitant monitoring of fluid status) · cardiac insufficiency · cardiovascular disease · colo-rectal polyps · hypertension

CAUTIONS, FURTHER INFORMATION

▶ Colo-rectal polyps Manufacturer advises faecal occult blood testing before initiation of treatment and yearly thereafter; colonoscopy or sigmoidoscopy should be performed if unexplained blood in stool. Manufacturer also advises colonoscopy or sigmoidoscopy after 1 year of treatment and then every 5 years thereafter.

● **SIDE-EFFECTS**

▶ **Common or very common** Anxiety · appetite decreased · congestive heart failure · cough · dyspnoea · fluid imbalance · gallbladder disorders · gastrointestinal discomfort · gastrointestinal disorders · gastrointestinal stoma complication · headache · influenza like illness · insomnia · nausea · pancreatitis · peripheral oedema · respiratory tract infection · vomiting

▶ **Uncommon** Syncope

● **ALLERGY AND CROSS-SENSITIVITY** Manufacturer advises caution in patients with tetracycline hypersensitivity.

● **PREGNANCY** EvGr Specialist sources indicate use if necessary—no human data available. (D)

● **BREAST FEEDING** Manufacturer advises avoid—toxicity in *animal* studies.

● **RENAL IMPAIRMENT**

Dose adjustments EvGr Use half the daily dose if creatinine clearance is less than 50 mL/minute, (M) see p. 16.

● **MONITORING REQUIREMENTS** Manufacturer advises monitoring of small bowel function, gall bladder, bile ducts and pancreas during treatment.

● **TREATMENT CESSATION** Caution when discontinuing treatment—risk of dehydration.

● **PATIENT AND CARER ADVICE** Patients with cardiovascular disease should seek medical attention if they notice sudden weight gain, swollen ankles or dyspnoea—may indicate increased fluid absorption.

● **NATIONAL FUNDING/ACCESS DECISIONS**
For full details see funding body website

NICE decisions

▶ **Teduglutide for treating short bowel syndrome (June 2022)**
NICE TA804 Recommended

Scottish Medicines Consortium (SMC) decisions

▶ **Teduglutide (*Revestive*®) for the treatment of patients aged 1 year to 17 years with short bowel syndrome (April 2018)**
SMC No. 1139/16 Recommended with restrictions

● **MEDICINAL FORMS** There can be variation in the licensing of different medicines containing the same drug.

Powder and solvent for solution for injection

▶ Revestive (Takeda UK Ltd) ▼

Teduglutide 1.25 mg Revestive 1.25mg powder and solvent for solution for injection vials | 28 vial PoM £7,307.70 (Hospital only)

Teduglutide 5 mg Revestive 5mg powder and solvent for solution for injection vials | 28 vial PoM £14,615.39 (Hospital only)

2 Constipation and bowel cleansing

2.1 Bowel cleansing

Other drugs used for Bowel cleansing Bisacodyl, p. 50 · Docusate sodium, p. 49

DIAGNOSTIC AGENTS > RADIOGRAPHIC CONTRAST MEDIA

Meglumine amidotrizoate with sodium amidotrizoate

05-Oct-2021

(Diatrizoates)

● **DRUG ACTION** Meglumine amidotrizoate with sodium amidotrizoate is a radiological contrast medium with high osmolality.

● **INDICATIONS AND DOSE**

Uncomplicated meconium ileus

▶ BY RECTUM

▶ Neonate: 15–30 mL for 1 dose.

Distal intestinal obstruction syndrome in children with cystic fibrosis

▶ BY MOUTH, OR BY RECTUM

▶ Child 1–23 months: 15–30 mL for 1 dose

▶ Child (body-weight 15–25 kg): 50 mL for 1 dose

▶ Child (body-weight 26 kg and above): 100 mL for 1 dose

Radiological investigations

▶ Child: Dose to be recommended by radiologist

● **UNLICENSED USE** Not licensed for use in distal intestinal obstruction syndrome.

● **CONTRA-INDICATIONS** Hyperthyroidism

● **CAUTIONS** Asthma · benign nodular goitre · dehydration · electrolyte disturbance (correct first) · enteritis · history of allergy · in children with oesophageal fistulae (aspiration may lead to pulmonary oedema) · latent hyperthyroidism · risk of anaphylactoid reactions increased by concomitant administration of beta-blockers

● **SIDE-EFFECTS**

GENERAL SIDE-EFFECTS Abdominal pain · cardiac arrest · consciousness impaired · diarrhoea · dizziness · dyspnoea · electrolyte imbalance · face oedema · fever · fluid imbalance · gastrointestinal disorders · headache · hyperhidrosis · hypersensitivity · hyperthyroidism ·

hypotension · nausea · pneumonia aspiration · pulmonary oedema · respiratory disorders · shock · skin reactions · tachycardia · toxic epidermal necrolysis · vomiting

SPECIFIC SIDE-EFFECTS
- With oral use Oral blistering

- **ALLERGY AND CROSS-SENSITIVITY** EvGr Contra-indicated if hypersensitivity to iodine. (M)
- **PREGNANCY** Manufacturer advises caution.
- **BREAST FEEDING** Amount probably too small to be harmful.
- **DIRECTIONS FOR ADMINISTRATION** Expert sources advise intravenous prehydration is essential in neonates and infants. Fluid intake should be encouraged for 3 hours after administration. *By mouth*, for child bodyweight 25 kg and under, expert sources advise dilute *Gastrografin*® with 3 times its volume of water or fruit juice; for child bodyweight over 25 kg, dilute *Gastrografin*® with twice its volume of water or fruit juice. *By rectum*, administration must be carried out slowly under radiological supervision to ensure required site is reached. For child under 5 years, expert sources advise dilute *Gastrografin*® with 5 times its volume of water; for child over 5 years dilute *Gastrografin*® with 4 times its volume of water.
- **MEDICINAL FORMS** There can be variation in the licensing of different medicines containing the same drug.

Oral solution

EXCIPIENTS: May contain Disodium edetate

- **Meglumine amidotrizoate with sodium amidotrizoate (Non-proprietary)**
 Sodium amidotrizoate 100 mg per 1 ml, Meglumine amidotrizoate 660 mg per 1 ml Meglumine amidotrizoate 3.3g/5ml / Sodium amidotrizoate 500mg/5ml oral solution sugar free | 30 ml PoM SF

LAXATIVES > OSMOTIC LAXATIVES

Citric acid with magnesium carbonate

09-May-2024

- **DRUG ACTION** Formulated as a bowel cleansing preparation

- **INDICATIONS AND DOSE**

Bowel evacuation for surgery, colonoscopy or radiological examination

▸ BY MOUTH
- Child 5–9 years: One-third of a sachet to be given at 8 a.m. the day before the procedure and, one-third of a sachet to be given between 2 and 4 p.m. the day before the procedure
- Child 10–17 years: 0.5–1 sachet, given at 8 a.m. the day before the procedure and 0.5–1 sachet, given between 2 and 4 p.m. the day before the procedure

- **CONTRA-INDICATIONS** Acute intestinal or gastric ulceration · acute severe colitis · gastric retention · gastro-intestinal obstruction · gastro-intestinal perforation · toxic megacolon
- **CAUTIONS** Debilitated · hypovolaemia (should be corrected before administration of bowel cleansing preparations) · patients with fluid and electrolyte disturbances

CAUTIONS, FURTHER INFORMATION Adequate hydration should be maintained during treatment.
- **INTERACTIONS** → Appendix 1: bowel cleansing preparations
- **SIDE-EFFECTS**
- **Common or very common** Gastrointestinal discomfort · nausea · vomiting
- **Uncommon** Dehydration · dizziness · electrolyte imbalance · headache

SIDE-EFFECTS, FURTHER INFORMATION Abdominal pain is usually transient and can be reduced by taking preparation more slowly.
- **PREGNANCY** Use with caution.
- **BREAST FEEDING** Use with caution.
- **RENAL IMPAIRMENT** EvGr Caution in mild to moderate impairment; avoid in severe impairment (risk of hypermagnesaemia). (M)
- **MONITORING REQUIREMENTS** Renal function should be measured before starting treatment in patients at risk of fluid and electrolyte disturbances.
- **DIRECTIONS FOR ADMINISTRATION** Manufacturer advises one sachet should be reconstituted with 200 mL of hot water; the solution should be allowed to cool for approx. 30 minutes before drinking.
- **PRESCRIBING AND DISPENSING INFORMATION** Reconstitution of one sachet containing 11.57 g magnesium carbonate and 17.79 g anhydrous citric acid produces a solution containing magnesium citrate with 118 mmol Mg^{2+}.

 Flavours of oral powders may include lemon and lime.
- **PATIENT AND CARER ADVICE** Low residue or fluid only diet (e.g. water, fruit squash, clear soup, black tea or coffee) recommended before procedure (according to prescriber's advice) and copious intake of clear fluids recommended until procedure. Patient or carers should be given advice on how to administer oral powder.
- **MEDICINAL FORMS** There can be variation in the licensing of different medicines containing the same drug.

Effervescent powder

CAUTIONARY AND ADVISORY LABELS 13, 10

ELECTROLYTES: May contain Magnesium

- **Citramag** (Cambridge Healthcare Supplies Ltd)
 Magnesium carbonate heavy 11.57 gram, Citric acid anhydrous 17.79 gram Citramag effervescent powder sachets | 10 sachet P £20.50 DT = £20.50 SF

LAXATIVES > STIMULANT LAXATIVES

Magnesium citrate with sodium picosulfate

09-May-2024

- **DRUG ACTION** Formulated as a bowel cleansing preparation

- **INDICATIONS AND DOSE**

PICOLAX® SACHETS

Bowel evacuation on day before radiological procedure, endoscopy, or surgery

▸ BY MOUTH
- Child 1 year: 0.25 sachet taken before 8 a.m, then 0.25 sachet after 6–8 hours
- Child 2–3 years: 0.5 sachet taken before 8 a.m, then 0.5 sachet after 6–8 hours
- Child 4–8 years: 1 sachet taken before 8 a.m, then 0.5 sachet after 6–8 hours
- Child 9–17 years: 1 sachet taken before 8 a.m, then 1 sachet after 6–8 hours

PHARMACOKINETICS
- For *Picolax*®: Acts within 3 hours of first dose.

- **CONTRA-INDICATIONS** Acute severe colitis · ascites · congestive cardiac failure · gastric retention · gastro-intestinal obstruction · gastro-intestinal perforation · gastro-intestinal ulceration · toxic megacolon
- **CAUTIONS** Cardiac disease · children · colitis · debilitated patients · fluid and electrolyte disturbances (avoid in severe dehydration or hypermagnesaemia) · hypovolaemia (should be corrected before administration) · recent gastro-intestinal surgery

- **INTERACTIONS** → Appendix 1: bowel cleansing preparations
- **SIDE-EFFECTS**
  - ▶ **Common or very common** Gastrointestinal discomfort · headache · nausea
  - ▶ **Uncommon** Confusion · electrolyte imbalance · gastrointestinal disorders · seizures · skin reactions · vomiting
- **PREGNANCY** Caution.
- **BREAST FEEDING** Caution.
- **HEPATIC IMPAIRMENT** Avoid in hepatic coma if risk of renal failure.
- **RENAL IMPAIRMENT** EvGr Caution in mild to moderate impairment; avoid in severe impairment (risk of hypermagnesaemia). (M)
- **DIRECTIONS FOR ADMINISTRATION** Manufacturer advises one sachet of sodium picosulfate with magnesium citrate powder should be reconstituted with 150 mL (approx. half a glass) of cold water; patients should be warned that heat is generated during reconstitution and that the solution should be allowed to cool before drinking.
- **PRESCRIBING AND DISPENSING INFORMATION** Flavours of oral powder formulations may include lemon.

PICOLAX® SACHETS One reconstituted sachet contains K^+ 5 mmol and Mg^{2+} 87 mmol.

- **PATIENT AND CARER ADVICE** Low residue diet recommended on the day before procedure and copious intake of water or other clear fluids recommended during treatment. Patients and carers should be given advice on how to administer oral powder; they should be warned that heat is generated during reconstitution and that the solution should be allowed to cool before drinking.

- **MEDICINAL FORMS** There can be variation in the licensing of different medicines containing the same drug.

Powder for oral solution

CAUTIONARY AND ADVISORY LABELS 10, 13

ELECTROLYTES: May contain Magnesium, potassium

▶ **Picolax** (Ferring Pharmaceuticals Ltd)

Sodium picosulfate 10 mg, Magnesium oxide 3.5 gram, Citric acid anhydrous 12 gram Picolax oral powder 16.1g sachets | 20 sachet PoM £33.90 SF

2.2 Constipation

Constipation

14-Nov-2025

Description of condition

Constipation is defaecation that is unsatisfactory because of infrequent stools, difficult stool passage, or seemingly incomplete defaecation. It can occur at any age and is common in childhood.

Overview

Before prescribing laxatives it is important to be sure that the child *is* constipated and that the constipation is not secondary to an underlying undiagnosed complaint. Early identification of constipation and effective treatment can improve outcomes for children. Without early diagnosis and treatment, an acute episode of constipation can lead to anal fissure and become chronic. In children with secondary constipation caused by a drug, the drug should be reviewed.

Laxatives

Bulk-forming laxatives

Bulk-forming laxatives include bran, ispaghula husk p. 45, methylcellulose and sterculia p. 46. They are of particular value in children with small hard stools if fibre cannot be increased in the diet. EvGr They relieve constipation by increasing faecal mass, which stimulates peristalsis; children and their carers should be advised that the full effect may take some days to develop. Adequate fluid intake must be maintained to avoid intestinal obstruction, though this may be difficult for children. (A)

Methylcellulose, ispaghula husk and sterculia may be used in patients who cannot tolerate bran. Methylcellulose also acts as a faecal softener.

Stimulant laxatives

Stimulant laxatives include bisacodyl p. 50, sodium picosulfate p. 53, and members of the anthraquinone group, senna p. 52, co-danthramer p. 51 and co-danthrusate p. 51. Stimulant laxatives increase intestinal motility and often cause abdominal cramp; they should be avoided in intestinal obstruction.

The use of co-danthramer and co-danthrusate is limited to constipation in terminally ill patients because of potential carcinogenicity (based on animal studies) and evidence of genotoxicity.

Docusate sodium p. 49 is believed to act as both a stimulant laxative and as a faecal softener (below). Glycerol suppositories act as a lubricant and as a rectal stimulant by virtue of the mildly irritant action of glycerol.

Faecal softeners

Faecal softeners are claimed to act by decreasing surface tension and increasing penetration of intestinal fluid into the faecal mass. Docusate sodium, and glycerol suppositories p. 51 have softening properties. Enemas containing arachis oil p. 49 (ground-nut oil, peanut oil) lubricate and soften impacted faeces and promote a bowel movement. Liquid paraffin has also been used as a lubricant for the passage of stool but manufacturer advises that it should be used with caution because of its adverse effects, which include anal seepage and the risks of granulomatous disease of the gastro-intestinal tract or of lipoid pneumonia on aspiration.

Osmotic laxatives

Osmotic laxatives increase the amount of water in the large bowel, either by drawing fluid from the body into the bowel or by retaining the fluid they were administered with. Lactulose p. 46 is a semi-synthetic disaccharide which is not absorbed from the gastro-intestinal tract. It produces an osmotic diarrhoea of low faecal pH, and discourages the proliferation of ammonia-producing organisms. It is therefore useful in the treatment of hepatic encephalopathy. Macrogols (such as macrogol 3350 with potassium chloride, sodium bicarbonate and sodium chloride p. 47) are inert polymers of ethylene glycol which sequester fluid in the bowel; giving fluid with macrogols may reduce the dehydrating effect sometimes seen with osmotic laxatives.

Macrogols are an effective non-traumatic means of evacuation in children with faecal impaction and can be used in the long-term management of chronic constipation.

Bowel cleansing preparations

Bowel cleansing preparations are used before colonic surgery, colonoscopy, or radiological examination to ensure the bowel is free of solid contents; examples include citric acid with magnesium carbonate p. 43, magnesium citrate with sodium picosulfate p. 43, and sodium acid phosphate with sodium phosphate p. 48. Bowel cleansing preparations are not treatments for constipation.

Management

EvGr The first-line treatment for children with constipation requires the use of a laxative in combination with dietary modification and behavioural interventions. Diet modification alone is not recommended as first-line treatment.

In children, an increase in dietary fibre, adequate fluid intake, and exercise is advised. Diet should be balanced and contain fruits, vegetables, high-fibre bread, baked beans, and wholegrain breakfast cereals. Unprocessed bran (which may cause bloating and flatulence and reduces the absorption of micronutrients) is **not** recommended.

If faecal impaction is not present (or has been treated), the child should be treated promptly with a laxative. A macrogol (such as macrogol 3350 with potassium chloride, sodium bicarbonate and sodium chloride) is preferred as first-line management, with the dose adjusted according to symptoms and response. If the response is inadequate add a stimulant laxative, or change to a stimulant laxative if the first-line therapy is not tolerated. If stools remain hard, lactulose or another laxative with softening effects, such as docusate sodium should be added.

In children with chronic constipation, laxatives should be continued for several weeks after a regular pattern of bowel movements or toilet training is established. The dose of laxatives should then be tapered gradually, over a period of months, according to response. Some children may require laxative therapy for several years.

A shorter duration of laxative treatment may be possible in some children with a very short history of constipation, but they should be carefully monitored for a relapse of constipation.

Laxatives should be administered at a time that produces an effect that is likely to fit in with the child's toilet routine. ⟨A⟩

Faecal impaction

EvGr Treatment of faecal impaction may initially increase symptoms of soiling and abdominal pain. An oral preparation containing a macrogol (such as macrogol 3350 with potassium chloride, sodium bicarbonate and sodium chloride) is used first-line for all children to clear faecal mass and to establish and maintain soft well-formed stools. In children over 1 year of age with faecal impaction, an escalating dose regimen should be used. If disimpaction does not occur after 2 weeks of macrogol treatment, a stimulant laxative should be added. If macrogol therapy is not tolerated, change to a stimulant laxative alone or, if stools are hard, use in combination with an osmotic laxative such as lactulose. Long-term regular use of laxatives is essential to maintain well-formed stools and prevent recurrence of faecal impaction; intermittent use may provoke relapses.

Suppositories and enemas should not be used in primary care unless all oral medications have failed and preferably only then following specialist advice. If all oral medication for treatment of impaction has failed, a sodium citrate enema p. 49 can be administered. Sodium acid phosphate with sodium phosphate enema may be administered under specialist supervision if disimpaction does not occur with a sodium citrate enema. Although rectal administration of laxatives may be effective, this route is frequently distressing for the child and may lead to persistence of withholding. Manual evacuation under anaesthetic may be necessary if disimpaction does not occur after oral and rectal treatment. Children undergoing disimpaction should be reviewed within one week. Maintenance treatment should be started as soon as the bowel is disimpacted. ⟨A⟩

Useful Resources

Constipation in children and young people: Diagnosis and management. National Institute for Health and Care Excellence. Clinical guideline 99. May 2010, updated July 2017.
www.nice.org.uk/guidance/cg99

LAXATIVES › BULK-FORMING LAXATIVES

Ispaghula husk

27-Jul-2020

- **DRUG ACTION** Bulk-forming laxatives relieve constipation by increasing faecal mass which stimulates peristalsis.

- **INDICATIONS AND DOSE**

Constipation

▶ BY MOUTH

- ▶ Child 1 month–5 years: 2.5–5 mL twice daily, dose to be taken only when prescribed by a doctor, as half or whole level spoonful in water, preferably after meals, morning and evening
- ▶ Child 6–11 years: 2.5–5 mL twice daily, dose to be given as a half or whole level spoonful in water, preferably after meals, morning and evening
- ▶ Child 12–17 years: 1 sachet twice daily, dose to be given in water preferably after meals, morning and evening

Constipation (dose approved for use by community practitioner nurse prescribers)

▶ BY MOUTH

- ▶ Child 6–11 years: 2.5–5 mL twice daily, dose to be given as a half or whole level spoonful in water, preferably after meals, morning and evening
- ▶ Child 12–17 years: 1 sachet twice daily, dose to be given in water preferably after meals, morning and evening

DOSE EQUIVALENCE AND CONVERSION

- ▶ 1 sachet equivalent to 2 level 5 ml spoonsful.

- **CONTRA-INDICATIONS** Colonic atony · faecal impaction · intestinal obstruction · reduced gut motility · sudden change in bowel habit that has persisted more than two weeks · undiagnosed rectal bleeding
- **CAUTIONS** Adequate fluid intake should be maintained to avoid oesophageal or intestinal obstruction
- **SIDE-EFFECTS** Abdominal distension · bronchospasm · conjunctivitis · gastrointestinal disorders · hypersensitivity · rhinitis · skin reactions
- **DIRECTIONS FOR ADMINISTRATION** Manufacturer advises dose to be taken with at least 150 mL liquid.
- **PRESCRIBING AND DISPENSING INFORMATION** Flavours of soluble granules formulations may include plain, lemon, or orange.
- **HANDLING AND STORAGE** Ispaghula husk contains potent allergens. Individuals exposed to the product (including those handling the product) can develop hypersensitivity reactions such as rhinitis, conjunctivitis, bronchospasm and in some cases, anaphylaxis.
- **PATIENT AND CARER ADVICE** Manufacturer advises that preparations that swell in contact with liquid should always be carefully swallowed with water and should not be taken immediately before going to bed. Patients and their carers should be advised that the full effect may take some days to develop and should be given advice on how to administer ispaghula husk.

- **MEDICINAL FORMS** There can be variation in the licensing of different medicines containing the same drug.

Effervescent granules

CAUTIONARY AND ADVISORY LABELS 13

EXCIPIENTS: May contain Aspartame

- ▶ **Fybogel** (Reckitt Benckiser Healthcare (UK) Ltd)
  Ispaghula husk 3.5 gram Fybogel 3.5g effervescent granules sachets plain SF | 30 sachet GSL £6.32 DT = £6.32 SF
  Fybogel Orange 3.5g effervescent granules sachets SF | 30 sachet GSL £6.32 DT = £6.32 SF
  Fybogel Lemon 3.5g effervescent granules sachets SF | 30 sachet GSL £6.32 DT = £6.32 SF
- ▶ **Fybogel Hi-Fibre** (Reckitt Benckiser Healthcare (UK) Ltd)
  Ispaghula husk 3.5 gram Fybogel Hi-Fibre Orange 3.5g effervescent granules sachets | 10 sachet GSL £3.55 DT = £3.55 SF | 30 sachet GSL £9.70 DT = £6.32 SF

Fybogel Hi-Fibre Lemon 3.5g effervescent granules sachets | 10 sachet GSL £3.55 DT = £3.55 SF

▸ **Ispagel** (Bristol Laboratories Ltd)

Ispaghula husk 3.5 gram Ispagel Orange 3.5g effervescent granules sachets | 10 sachet GSL £4.50 DT = £3.55 SF | 30 sachet GSL £6.50 DT = £6.32 SF

Granules for oral suspension

CAUTIONARY AND ADVISORY LABELS 13

EXCIPIENTS: May contain Aspartame

▸ **Ispaghula husk (Non-proprietary)**

Ispaghula husk 3.5 gram Ispaghula husk 3.5g granules for oral suspension sachets gluten free sugar free | 30 sachet GSL SF

Combinations available: ***Senna with ispaghula husk***, p. 52

Sterculia

12-Aug-2020

- **DRUG ACTION** Sterculia is a bulk-forming laxative. It relieves constipation by increasing faecal mass which stimulates peristalsis.

- **INDICATIONS AND DOSE**

Constipation

▶ BY MOUTH

▸ Child 6–11 years: 0.5–1 sachet 1–2 times a day, alternatively, half to one heaped 5-mL spoonful once or twice a day; washed down without chewing with plenty of liquid after meals

▸ Child 12–17 years: 1–2 sachets 1–2 times a day, alternatively, one to two heaped 5-mL spoonfuls once or twice a day; washed down without chewing with plenty of liquid after meals

- **CONTRA-INDICATIONS** Colonic atony · difficulty swallowing · faecal impaction · intestinal obstruction
- **CAUTIONS** Adequate fluid intake should be maintained to avoid oesophageal or intestinal obstruction

  CAUTIONS, FURTHER INFORMATION It may be necessary to supervise debilitated patients or those with intestinal narrowing or decreased motility to ensure adequate fluid intake.
- **SIDE-EFFECTS** Diarrhoea · gastrointestinal discomfort · gastrointestinal disorders · nausea
- **DIRECTIONS FOR ADMINISTRATION** Manufacturer advises may be mixed with soft food (e.g. yoghurt) before swallowing, followed by plenty of liquid.
- **PATIENT AND CARER ADVICE** Patients and their carers should be advised that the full effect may take some days to develop. Preparations that swell in contact with liquid should always be carefully swallowed with water and should not be taken immediately before going to bed.

- **MEDICINAL FORMS** No licensed medicines listed.

Sterculia with frangula

The properties listed below are those particular to the combination only. For the properties of the components please consider, sterculia above.

- **INDICATIONS AND DOSE**

Constipation

▶ BY MOUTH

▸ Child 6–11 years: 0.5–1 sachet 1–2 times a day, alternatively, 0.5–1 heaped 5-mL spoonful once or twice a day; washed down without chewing with plenty of liquid after meals

▸ Child 12–17 years: 1–2 sachets 1–2 times a day, alternatively, 1–2 heaped 5 mL spoonfuls once or twice a day; washed down without chewing with plenty of liquid after meals

- **PREGNANCY** Manufacturer advises avoid.
- **BREAST FEEDING** Manufacturer advises avoid.
- **PATIENT AND CARER ADVICE** Patients and their carers should be advised that the full effect may take some days to develop. Preparations that swell in contact with liquid should always be carefully swallowed with water and should not be taken immediately before going to bed.

- **MEDICINAL FORMS** No licensed medicines listed.

LAXATIVES › OSMOTIC LAXATIVES

Lactulose

10-Nov-2021

- **INDICATIONS AND DOSE**

Constipation

▶ BY MOUTH

▸ Child 1–11 months: 2.5 mL twice daily, to be adjusted according to response

▸ Child 1–4 years: 2.5–10 mL twice daily, to be adjusted according to response

▸ Child 5–17 years: 5–20 mL twice daily, to be adjusted according to response

Hepatic encephalopathy (portal systemic encephalopathy)

▶ BY MOUTH

▸ Child 12–17 years: 30–50 mL 3 times a day, dose subsequently adjusted to produce 2–3 soft stools per day

Constipation (dose approved for use by community practitioner nurse prescribers)

▶ BY MOUTH

▸ Child 1–11 months: 2.5 mL twice daily, to be adjusted according to response

▸ Child 1–4 years: 5 mL twice daily, to be adjusted according to response

▸ Child 5–10 years: 10 mL twice daily, to be adjusted according to response

▸ Child 11–17 years: Initially 15 mL twice daily, to be adjusted according to response

PHARMACOKINETICS

▸ Lactulose may take up to 48 hours to act.

- **UNLICENSED USE** Not licensed for use in children for hepatic encephalopathy.
- **CONTRA-INDICATIONS** Galactosaemia · gastro-intestinal obstruction · gastro-intestinal perforation · risk of gastro-intestinal perforation
- **CAUTIONS** Lactose intolerance
- **SIDE-EFFECTS**

▶ **Common or very common** Abdominal pain · diarrhoea · flatulence · nausea · vomiting

▶ **Uncommon** Electrolyte imbalance

- **PREGNANCY** Not known to be harmful.
- **PATIENT AND CARER ADVICE**

Medicines for Children leaflet: Lactulose for constipation www.medicinesforchildren.org.uk/medicines/lactulose-for-constipation/

- **MEDICINAL FORMS** There can be variation in the licensing of different medicines containing the same drug.

Oral solution

▸ **Lactulose (Non-proprietary)**

Lactulose 666.667 mg per 1 ml Lactulose 10g/15ml oral solution 15ml sachets sugar free | 10 sachet P £3.43 DT = £3.76 SF

Lactulose 10g/15ml oral solution 15ml sachets sugar free unflavoured | 10 sachet P £2.50 DT = £3.76 SF

Lactulose 680 mg per 1 ml Lactulose 3.1-3.7g/5ml oral solution | 300 ml P £2.69–£7.80 | 500 ml P £12.00 DT = £7.10

Macrogol 3350 with potassium chloride, sodium bicarbonate and sodium chloride

27-Jan-2025

● **INDICATIONS AND DOSE**

Chronic constipation (dose for 'paediatric' sachets) | Prevention of faecal impaction (dose for 'paediatric' sachets)

▶ BY MOUTH

- Child 1–11 months: 0.5–1 sachet daily
- Child 12–23 months: 1 sachet daily in 1–2 divided doses, adjust dose to produce regular soft stools; maximum 4 sachets per day
- Child 2–5 years: 1 sachet daily in 1–2 divided doses, adjust dose to produce regular soft stools; maximum 4 sachets per day
- Child 6–11 years: 2 sachets daily in 1–2 divided doses, adjust dose to produce regular soft stools; maximum 4 sachets per day

Faecal impaction (dose for 'paediatric' sachets)

▶ BY MOUTH

- Child 1–11 months: 0.5–1 sachet daily
- Child 12–23 months: 2 sachets on first day, dose then increased to 4 sachets per day for 2 days, then 6 sachets per day for 2 days, then 8 sachets per day, total daily dose to be taken within a 12-hour period, after disimpaction, switch to maintenance laxative therapy
- Child 2–4 years: 2 sachets on first day, dose then increased to 4 sachets per day for 2 days, then 6 sachets per day for 2 days, then 8 sachets per day, total daily dose to be taken within a 12-hour period, after disimpaction, switch to maintenance laxative therapy
- Child 5–11 years: 4 sachets on first day, dose then increased in steps of 2 sachets per day up to maximum 12 sachets per day, total daily dose to be taken within a 12-hour period, after disimpaction, switch to maintenance laxative therapy

Chronic constipation (dose for 'half-strength' sachets)

▶ BY MOUTH

- Child 12–17 years: 2 sachets 1–3 times a day usually for up to 2 weeks; maintenance 2 sachets 1–2 times a day

Faecal impaction (dose for 'half-strength' sachets)

▶ BY MOUTH

- Child 12–17 years: 8 sachets on first day, dose then increased in steps of 4 sachets per day up to maximum 16 sachets per day, total daily dose to be taken within a 6-hour period, after disimpaction, switch to maintenance laxative therapy if required

Chronic constipation (dose for 'full-strength' sachets)

▶ BY MOUTH

- Child 12–17 years: 1 sachet 1–3 times a day usually for up to 2 weeks; maintenance 1 sachet 1–2 times a day

Faecal impaction (dose for 'full-strength' sachets)

▶ BY MOUTH

- Child 12–17 years: 4 sachets on first day, dose then increased in steps of 2 sachets per day up to maximum 8 sachets per day, total daily dose to be taken within a 6-hour period, after disimpaction, switch to maintenance laxative therapy if required

DOSE EQUIVALENCE AND CONVERSION

- Each 'paediatric' sachet contains 6.563 g of macrogol 3350; each 'half-strength' sachet contains 6.563 g of macrogol 3350; each 'full-strength' sachet contains 13.125 g of macrogol 3350.

MOVICOL ® READY TO TAKE SACHETS

Chronic constipation

▶ BY MOUTH

- Child 12–17 years: 1 sachet 1–3 times a day usually for up to 2 weeks; maintenance 1 sachet 1–2 times a day

Faecal impaction

▶ BY MOUTH

- Child 12–17 years: 4 sachets on first day, dose then increased in steps of 2 sachets per day up to maximum 8 sachets per day, total daily dose to be taken within a 6-hour period; patients should also take an additional 1 litre of fluid daily, after disimpaction, switch to maintenance laxative therapy if required

MOVICOL ® LIQUID

Chronic constipation

▶ BY MOUTH

- Child 12–17 years: 25 mL 1–3 times a day usually for up to 2 weeks; maintenance 25 mL 1–2 times a day

● **UNLICENSED USE** Macrogol 3350 with potassium chloride, sodium bicarbonate and sodium chloride may be used as detailed below, although these situations are considered outside the scope of its licence:

- EvGr chronic constipation/prevention of faecal impaction in children aged under 1 year;
- dose for chronic constipation/prevention of faecal impaction in children aged 6 years;
- faecal impaction in children aged under 5 years;
- dose titration schedule for faecal impaction in children aged 12–17 years (A).

IMPORTANT SAFETY INFORMATION

MHRA/CHM ADVICE: POLYETHYLENE GLYCOL (PEG) LAXATIVES AND STARCH-BASED THICKENERS: POTENTIAL INTERACTIVE EFFECT WHEN MIXED, LEADING TO AN INCREASED RISK OF ASPIRATION (APRIL 2021)

Addition of a macrogol (PEG)-based laxative to a liquid that has been thickened with a starch-based thickener may counteract the thickening action, resulting in a thin watery liquid that, when swallowed, increases the risk of potentially fatal aspiration in patients with dysphagia. Healthcare professionals are advised to avoid directly mixing macrogol-based laxatives with starch-based thickeners, especially for patients with dysphagia who are considered at risk of aspiration.

● **CONTRA-INDICATIONS** Intestinal obstruction · intestinal perforation · paralytic ileus · severe inflammatory conditions of the intestinal tract (including Crohn's disease, ulcerative colitis and toxic megacolon) · use of 'paediatric' sachets for faecal impaction in impaired cardiovascular function (no information available)

● **CAUTIONS** Cardiovascular impairment (should not take more than 2 'full-strength' sachets or 4 'half-strength' sachets in any one hour) · impaired consciousness (with high doses) · impaired gag reflex (with high doses) · reflux oesophagitis (with high doses)

● **INTERACTIONS** → Appendix 1: macrogol 3350

● **SIDE-EFFECTS** Allergic dermatitis · gastrointestinal discomfort · gastrointestinal disorders · headache · nausea · peripheral oedema · vomiting

● **PREGNANCY** Manufacturers advise may be used—limited data available.

● **RENAL IMPAIRMENT** Manufacturers advise avoid use of 'paediatric' sachets for faecal impaction—no information available.

● **DIRECTIONS FOR ADMINISTRATION** Manufacturers advise dissolve contents of each 'half-strength' sachet of oral powder in 62.5 mL of water, and each 'full-strength' sachet of oral powder in 125 mL of water; after reconstitution the solution should be kept in a refrigerator—for further information consult product literature.

Manufacturers advise dissolve contents of each 'paediatric' sachet of oral powder in 62.5 mL of water; after reconstitution the solution should be kept in a refrigerator—for further information consult product literature.

MOVICOL® LIQUID Manufacturer advises dilute 25 mL of oral concentrate with 100 mL of water; after dilution the solution should be discarded if unused after 24 hours.

- **PATIENT AND CARER ADVICE** Patients or carers should be counselled on how to take the oral powder and oral solution.

Medicines for Children leaflet: Movicol for constipation www.medicinesforchildren.org.uk/medicines/movicol-for-constipation/

- **MEDICINAL FORMS** There can be variation in the licensing of different medicines containing the same drug.

Oral solution

CAUTIONARY AND ADVISORY LABELS 13

ELECTROLYTES: May contain Bicarbonate, chloride, potassium, sodium

- Movicol (Forum Health Products Ltd)

Macrogol '3350' 13.125 gram, Potassium 27 mmol per 1 litre, Bicarbonate 85 mmol per 1 litre, Chloride 267 mmol per 1 litre, Sodium 325 mmol per 1 litre Movicol Ready to Take oral solution 25ml sachets | 30 sachet [P] £11.49 DT = £9.89 [SF]

Powder for oral solution

CAUTIONARY AND ADVISORY LABELS 10, 13

ELECTROLYTES: May contain Bicarbonate, chloride, potassium, sodium

- Macrogol 3350 with potassium chloride, sodium bicarbonate and sodium chloride (Non-proprietary)

Macrogol '3350' 105 gram per 1 litre, Potassium 5.4 mmol per 1 litre, Bicarbonate 17 mmol per 1 litre, Chloride 53 mmol per 1 litre, Sodium 65 mmol per 1 litre Macrogol compound oral powder sachets NPF sugar free | 30 sachet [P] [NHS] DT = £6.60 [SF]

- CosmoCol (Stirling Anglian Pharmaceuticals Ltd)

Macrogol '3350' 105 gram per 1 litre, Potassium 5.4 mmol per 1 litre, Bicarbonate 17 mmol per 1 litre, Chloride 53 mmol per 1 litre, Sodium 65 mmol per 1 litre CosmoCol Paediatric oral powder 6.9g sachets | 30 sachet [PoM] £4.32 DT = £4.38 [SF]
CosmoCol Orange Flavour oral powder sachets | 20 sachet [P] £4.60 DT = £4.60 [SF] | 30 sachet [P] £6.60 DT = £6.60 [SF]
CosmoCol Lemon and Lime Flavour oral powder sachets | 20 sachet [P] £4.60 DT = £4.60 [SF] | 30 sachet [P] £6.60 DT = £6.60 [SF]
CosmoCol Orange Lemon and Lime oral powder sachets | 30 sachet [P] £6.60 DT = £6.60 [SF]
CosmoCol Plain oral powder sachets | 30 sachet [P] £6.60 DT = £6.60 [SF]

- Laxido (Galen Ltd)

Macrogol '3350' 105 gram per 1 litre, Potassium 5.4 mmol per 1 litre, Bicarbonate 17 mmol per 1 litre, Chloride 53 mmol per 1 litre, Sodium 65 mmol per 1 litre Laxido Orange oral powder sachets sugar free | 20 sachet [P] £4.26 DT = £4.60 [SF] | 30 sachet [P] £6.09 DT = £6.60 [SF]
Laxido Paediatric Plain oral powder 6.9g sachets | 30 sachet [PoM] £4.38 DT = £4.38 [SF]

- Movicol (Norgine Pharmaceuticals Ltd, Forum Health Products Ltd)

Macrogol '3350' 105 gram per 1 litre, Potassium 5.4 mmol per 1 litre, Bicarbonate 17 mmol per 1 litre, Chloride 53 mmol per 1 litre, Sodium 65 mmol per 1 litre Movicol Paediatric Plain oral powder 6.9g sachets | 30 sachet [PoM] £4.38 DT = £4.38 [SF]
Movicol Paediatric Chocolate oral powder 6.8g sachets | 30 sachet [PoM] £4.38 DT = £4.38 [SF]
Movicol Chocolate oral powder 13.7g sachets | 30 sachet [P] £10.49 DT = £6.60 [SF]
Movicol Plain oral powder 13.7g sachets | 30 sachet [P] £10.49 DT = £6.60 [SF]
Movicol oral powder 13.7g sachets lemon & lime | 20 sachet [P] £7.35 DT = £4.60 [SF] | 30 sachet [P] £10.49 DT = £6.60 [SF] | 50 sachet [P] £15.89 [SF]

- Strigol (Strides Pharma UK Ltd)

Macrogol '3350' 105 gram per 1 litre, Potassium 5.4 mmol per 1 litre, Bicarbonate 17 mmol per 1 litre, Chloride 53 mmol per 1 litre, Sodium 65 mmol per 1 litre Strigol Paediatric oral powder 6.86g sachets | 30 sachet [PoM] £3.15 DT = £4.38 [SF]
Strigol oral powder 13.72g sachets lemon | 20 sachet [P] £3.50 DT = £4.60 [SF] | 30 sachet [P] £4.99 DT = £6.60 [SF]
Strigol oral powder 13.72g sachets orange | 30 sachet [P] £4.99 DT = £6.60 [SF]

Magnesium hydroxide

01-Dec-2021

- **INDICATIONS AND DOSE**

Constipation

- BY MOUTH
  - Child 3–11 years: 5–10 mL as required, dose to be given mixed with water at bedtime
  - Child 12–17 years: 30–45 mL as required, dose to be given mixed with water at bedtime

- **CONTRA-INDICATIONS** Acute gastro-intestinal conditions
- **CAUTIONS** Debilitated patients
- **INTERACTIONS** → Appendix 1: magnesium
- **HEPATIC IMPAIRMENT** Avoid in hepatic coma if risk of renal failure.
- **RENAL IMPAIRMENT** [EvGr] Caution (risk of hypermagnesaemia); avoid in severe renal failure. ⟨M⟩
- **PRESCRIBING AND DISPENSING INFORMATION** When prepared extemporaneously, the BP states Magnesium Hydroxide Mixture, BP consists of an aqueous suspension containing about 8% hydrated magnesium oxide.

- **MEDICINAL FORMS** There can be variation in the licensing of different medicines containing the same drug.

Oral suspension

- Phillips' Milk of Magnesia (Omega Pharma Ltd)

Magnesium hydroxide 79 mg per 1 ml Phillips' Milk of Magnesia 415mg/5ml oral suspension | 200 ml [GSL] £4.52 DT = £4.52

Sodium acid phosphate with sodium phosphate

18-Oct-2021

- **INDICATIONS AND DOSE**

Constipation (using Phosphates Enema BP Formula B) | Bowel evacuation before abdominal radiological procedures, endoscopy, and surgery (using Phosphates Enema BP Formula B)

- BY RECTUM
  - Child 3–6 years: 45–65 mL once daily
  - Child 7–11 years: 65–100 mL once daily
  - Child 12–17 years: 100–128 mL once daily

Constipation, using Phosphates Enema BP Formula B (dose approved for use by community practitioner nurse prescribers)

- BY RECTUM
  - Child 3–17 years: Reduced according to body-weight

Constipation, using Phosphates Enema (Cleen Ready-to-Use) (dose approved for use by community practitioner nurse prescribers)

- BY RECTUM
  - Child 3–11 years: On doctor's advice only
  - Child 12–17 years: 118 mL

FLEET® READY-TO-USE ENEMA

Constipation | Bowel evacuation before abdominal radiological procedures | Bowel evacuation before endoscopy | Bowel evacuation before surgery

- BY RECTUM
  - Child 3–6 years: 40–60 mL once daily
  - Child 7–11 years: 60–90 mL once daily
  - Child 12–17 years: 90–118 mL once daily

- **CONTRA-INDICATIONS** Conditions associated with increased colonic absorption · gastro-intestinal obstruction · inflammatory bowel disease

- **CAUTIONS** Ascites · congestive heart failure · debilitated patients · fluid and electrolyte disturbances · uncontrolled hypertension
- **INTERACTIONS** → Appendix 1: bowel cleansing preparations
- **SIDE-EFFECTS**
  - **Common or very common** Chills · dizziness · electrolyte imbalance · gastrointestinal discomfort · malaise · nausea · pain · vomiting
  - **Rare or very rare** Dehydration · metabolic acidosis · skin reactions
  - **Frequency not known** Syncope · tetany
- **RENAL IMPAIRMENT** EvGr Caution; avoid in significant impairment. (M)
- **PRESCRIBING AND DISPENSING INFORMATION** When prepared extemporaneously, the BP states Phosphates Enema BP Formula B consists of sodium dihydrogen phosphate dihydrate 12.8 g, disodium phosphate dodecahydrate 10.24 g, purified water, freshly boiled and cooled, to 128 mL.
- **MEDICINAL FORMS** There can be variation in the licensing of different medicines containing the same drug.

Enema

- Sodium acid phosphate with sodium phosphate (Non-proprietary)
  Disodium hydrogen phosphate dodecahydrate 80 mg per 1 ml, Sodium dihydrogen phosphate dihydrate 100 mg per 1 ml Phosphates enema (Formula B) 128ml long tube | 1 enema [P] £42.94–£79.12 DT = £83.70
  Phosphates enema (Formula B) 128ml standard tube | 1 enema [P] £61.50 DT = £61.99
- Fleet Ready-to-use (Recordati Pharmaceuticals Ltd)
  Disodium hydrogen phosphate dodecahydrate 80 mg per 1 ml, Sodium dihydrogen phosphate dihydrate 181 mg per 1 ml Cleen Ready-to-use 133ml enema | 1 enema [P] £4.49 DT = £4.49

Sodium citrate

18-Nov-2021

- **INDICATIONS AND DOSE**

Constipation (dose approved for use by community practitioner nurse prescribers)

- BY RECTUM
  - Child 3–17 years: 5 mL for 1 dose

MICOLETTE®

Constipation

- BY RECTUM
  - Child 3–17 years: 5–10 mL for 1 dose

MICRALAX®

Constipation

- BY RECTUM
  - Child 3–17 years: 5 mL for 1 dose

RELAXIT®

Constipation

- BY RECTUM
  - Child 1 month–2 years: 5 mL for 1 dose, insert only half the nozzle length
  - Child 3–17 years: 5 mL for 1 dose

- **CONTRA-INDICATIONS** Acute gastro-intestinal conditions
- **CAUTIONS** Sodium and water retention in susceptible individuals
- **INTERACTIONS** → Appendix 1: sodium citrate
- **SIDE-EFFECTS** Polyuria
- **MEDICINAL FORMS** There can be variation in the licensing of different medicines containing the same drug.

Enema

- Micralax Micro-enema (RPH Pharmaceuticals AB)
  Sodium citrate 90 mg per 1 ml Micralax Micro-enema 5ml | 12 enema [P] £9.99

LAXATIVES › SOFTENING LAXATIVES

Arachis oil

18-Nov-2020

- **INDICATIONS AND DOSE**

To soften impacted faeces

- BY RECTUM
  - Child 3–6 years (under close medical supervision): 45–65 mL as required
  - Child 7–11 years (under close medical supervision): 65–100 mL as required
  - Child 12–17 years (under close medical supervision): 100–130 mL as required

- **UNLICENSED USE** Licensed for use in children (age range not specified by manufacturer).
- **CONTRA-INDICATIONS** Inflammatory bowel disease (except under medical supervision)
- **CAUTIONS** Hypersensitivity to soya · intestinal obstruction
- **ALLERGY AND CROSS-SENSITIVITY** EvGr Contra-indicated if history of hypersensitivity to arachis oil or peanuts. (M)
- **DIRECTIONS FOR ADMINISTRATION** Manufacturer advises warm enema in warm water before use.
- **MEDICINAL FORMS** There can be variation in the licensing of different medicines containing the same drug.

Enema

- Arachis oil (Non-proprietary)
  Arachis oil 1 ml per 1 ml Arachis oil 130ml enema | 1 enema [P] £57.39 DT = £57.39

Docusate sodium

12-Apr-2023

(Dioctyl sodium sulphosuccinate)

- **INDICATIONS AND DOSE**

Chronic constipation

- BY MOUTH
  - Child 6–23 months: 12.5 mg 3 times a day, use paediatric oral solution, dose to be adjusted according to response
  - Child 2–11 years: 12.5–25 mg 3 times a day, use paediatric oral solution, dose to be adjusted according to response
  - Child 12–17 years: 100 mg 3 times a day, dose can be increased if necessary up to maximum 500 mg daily in divided doses
- BY RECTUM
  - Child 12–17 years: 120 mg for 1 dose

Adjunct in abdominal radiological procedures

- BY MOUTH
  - Child 12–17 years: 400 mg for 1 dose, to be administered with barium meal
- BY RECTUM
  - Child 12–17 years: 120 mg for 1 dose

PHARMACOKINETICS

- Oral preparations act within 1–2 days; response to rectal administration usually occurs within 20 minutes.

- **UNLICENSED USE** *Adult oral solution and capsules* not licensed for use in children under 12 years.
- **CONTRA-INDICATIONS** Avoid in intestinal obstruction
- **CAUTIONS** Do not give with liquid paraffin · excessive use of stimulant laxatives can cause diarrhoea and related

effects such as hypokalaemia · rectal preparations not indicated if haemorrhoids or anal fissure

- **INTERACTIONS** → Appendix 1: docusates
- **SIDE-EFFECTS**
  - **Rare or very rare**
  - With oral use Abdominal cramps · nausea · rash
- **PREGNANCY** Not known to be harmful—manufacturer advises caution.
- **BREAST FEEDING** Manufacturer advises caution—present in milk following oral administration. Rectal administration not known to be harmful.
- **DIRECTIONS FOR ADMINISTRATION** For administration *by mouth*, manufacturer advises solution may be mixed with milk or squash.
- **MEDICINAL FORMS** There can be variation in the licensing of different medicines containing the same drug.

Oral solution

- **Docusate sodium (Non-proprietary)**
  - **Docusate sodium 2.5 mg per 1 ml** Docusate 12.5mg/5ml oral solution sugar free | 300 ml [P] £21.20–£34.99 DT = £33.24 [SF]
  - **Docusate sodium 10 mg per 1 ml** Docusate 50mg/5ml oral solution sugar free | 300 ml [P] £28.00 DT = £16.36 [SF]
  - **Docusate sodium 20 mg per 1 ml** Docusate 100mg/5ml oral solution sugar free | 150 ml [P] £29.40 DT = £29.40 [SF] | 300 ml [P] £35.01 DT = £35.01 [SF]
- **Docusol** (Typharm Ltd)
  - **Docusate sodium 2.5 mg per 1 ml** Docusol Paediatric 12.5mg/5ml oral solution | 125 ml [P] £4.46 [SF]

Oral capsule

- **Docusate sodium (Non-proprietary)**
  - **Docusate sodium 100 mg** Docusate 100mg capsules | 30 capsule [P] £3.23 DT = £3.25 | 100 capsule [P] £11.37 DT = £11.39
- **Dioctyl** (Teofarma S.r.l.)
  - **Docusate sodium 100 mg** Dioctyl 100mg capsules | 30 capsule [P] £3.25 DT = £3.25 | 100 capsule [P] £11.39 DT = £11.39

Enema

- **Norgalax** (Essential Pharma Ltd)
  - **Docusate sodium 12 mg per 1 gram** Norgalax 120mg/10g enema | 6 enema [P] £28.00 DT = £28.00

Combinations available: ***Co-danthrusate***, p. 51

LAXATIVES > STIMULANT LAXATIVES

Bisacodyl

10-Sep-2020

- **INDICATIONS AND DOSE**

Constipation

- BY MOUTH
  - Child 4–17 years: 5–20 mg once daily, dose to be taken at night, dose to be adjusted according to response
- BY RECTUM
  - Child 2–17 years: 5–10 mg once daily, dose to be adjusted according to response

Bowel clearance before radiological procedures and surgery

- INITIALLY BY MOUTH
  - Child 4–9 years: 5 mg for 1 dose, dose to be taken 2 days before procedure at bedtime, then (by mouth) 5 mg for 1 dose, dose to be taken 1 day before procedure at bedtime, then (by rectum) 5 mg for 1 dose, dose to be administered 1 hour before procedure if required
  - Child 10–17 years: 10 mg for 1 dose, dose to be taken 2 days before procedure at bedtime, then (by mouth) 10 mg for 1 dose, dose to be taken 1 day before procedure at bedtime, then (by rectum) 10 mg for 1 dose, dose to be administered 1 hour before procedure if required

Constipation (dose approved for use by community practitioner nurse prescribers)

- BY MOUTH
  - Child 4–17 years: 5–20 mg once daily, dose to be taken at night, dose to be adjusted according to response (on doctor's advice only)
- BY RECTUM
  - Child 4–9 years: 5 mg once daily, dose to be adjusted according to response
  - Child 10–17 years: 10 mg once daily, dose to be taken in the morning

PHARMACOKINETICS
- Tablets act in 10–12 hours; suppositories act in 20–60 minutes.

- **UNLICENSED USE**
  - With rectal use [EvGr] Bisacodyl may be used in children aged under 10 years for the management of constipation, (A) but the higher dose option is not licensed in this age group.
  - With oral use [EvGr] Bisacodyl may be used in children for the management of constipation, (A) but the higher dose option is not licensed.

IMPORTANT SAFETY INFORMATION

MHRA/CHM ADVICE: STIMULANT LAXATIVES (BISACODYL, SENNA AND SENNOSIDES, SODIUM PICOSULFATE) AVAILABLE OVER-THE-COUNTER: NEW MEASURES TO SUPPORT SAFE USE (AUGUST 2020)

Following a national safety review and concerns over misuse and abuse, the MHRA has introduced new pack size restrictions, revised recommended ages for use, and new safety warnings for over-the-counter stimulant laxatives (administered orally and rectally). Patients should be advised that dietary and lifestyle measures should be used first-line for relieving short-term occasional constipation, and that stimulant laxatives should only be used if these measures and other laxatives (bulk-forming and osmotic) are ineffective.

Smaller packs will remain available for general sale for the treatment of short-term, occasional constipation in adults only, and will be limited to a pack size of two short treatment courses. Stimulant laxatives should not be used in children under 12 years of age without advice from a prescriber; in children aged 12 to 17 years, products can be supplied under the supervision of a pharmacist.

- **CONTRA-INDICATIONS** Acute abdominal conditions · acute inflammatory bowel disease · intestinal obstruction · severe dehydration
- **CAUTIONS** Excessive use of stimulant laxatives can cause diarrhoea and related effects such as hypokalaemia · prolonged use may harm intestinal function · risk of electrolyte imbalance with prolonged use
- **SIDE-EFFECTS**
  - **Common or very common** Gastrointestinal discomfort · nausea
  - **Uncommon** Haematochezia · vomiting
  - **Rare or very rare** Angioedema · colitis · dehydration
- **PREGNANCY** May be suitable for constipation in pregnancy, if a stimulant effect is necessary.
- **MEDICINAL FORMS** There can be variation in the licensing of different medicines containing the same drug. Forms available from special-order manufacturers include: oral suspension, suppository

Gastro-resistant tablet

CAUTIONARY AND ADVISORY LABELS 5, 25

- **Bisacodyl (Non-proprietary)**
  - **Bisacodyl 5 mg** Bisacodyl 5mg gastro-resistant tablets | 60 tablet [P] £6.50 DT = £2.19 | 100 tablet [P] £3.65–£10.83

- **Dulco-Lax (bisacodyl)** (Opella Healthcare UK Ltd)
  Bisacodyl 5 mg Dulcolax Twelve Plus 5mg gastro-resistant tablets | 40 tablet P £3.39 | 100 tablet P £8.41

Suppository

- **Dulco-Lax (bisacodyl)** (Opella Healthcare UK Ltd, Opella POM UK Ltd)
  Bisacodyl 5 mg Dulcolax 5mg suppositories | 5 suppository PoM £1.11 DT = £1.11
  Bisacodyl 10 mg Dulcolax Twelve Plus 10mg suppositories | 12 suppository P £3.43 DT = £3.43

Co-danthramer

16-Mar-2020

● **INDICATIONS AND DOSE**

Constipation in palliative care (standard strength capsules)

▶ BY MOUTH USING CAPSULES

- Child 6–11 years: 1 capsule once daily, dose should be taken at night
- Child 12–17 years: 1–2 capsules once daily, dose should be taken at night

Constipation in palliative care (strong capsules)

▶ BY MOUTH USING CAPSULES

- Child 12–17 years: 1–2 capsules once daily, dose should be given at night

Constipation in palliative care (standard strength suspension)

▶ BY MOUTH USING ORAL SUSPENSION

- Child 2–11 years: 2.5–5 mL once daily, dose should be taken at night
- Child 12–17 years: 5–10 mL once daily, dose should be taken at night

Constipation in palliative care (strong suspension)

▶ BY MOUTH USING ORAL SUSPENSION

- Child 12–17 years: 5 mL once daily, dose should be taken at night

DOSE EQUIVALENCE AND CONVERSION

- Co-danthramer (standard strength) capsules contain dantron 25 mg with poloxamer '188' 200 mg per capsule.
- Co-danthramer (standard strength) oral suspension contains dantron 25 mg with poloxamer '188' 200 mg per 5 mL.
- Co-danthramer **strong** capsules contain dantron 37.5 mg with poloxamer '188' 500 mg.
- Co-danthramer **strong** oral suspension contains dantron 75 mg with poloxamer '188' 1 g per 5 mL.
- Co-danthramer suspension 5 mL = one co-danthramer capsule, **but** strong co-danthramer suspension 5 mL = two strong co-danthramer capsules.

● **CONTRA-INDICATIONS** Acute abdominal conditions · acute inflammatory bowel disease · intestinal obstruction · severe dehydration

● **CAUTIONS** Excessive use of stimulant laxatives can cause diarrhoea and related effects such as hypokalaemia · may cause local irritation · *rodent* studies indicate potential carcinogenic risk

CAUTIONS, FURTHER INFORMATION

- Local irritation Avoid prolonged contact with skin (incontinent patients or infants wearing nappies—risk of irritation and excoriation).

● **SIDE-EFFECTS** Abdominal cramps · asthenia · gastrointestinal disorders · hypermagnesaemia · skin reactions · urine discolouration

● **PREGNANCY** Manufacturers advise avoid—limited information available.

● **BREAST FEEDING** Manufacturers advise avoid—no information available.

● **PRESCRIBING AND DISPENSING INFORMATION**

Palliative care For further information on the use of co-danthramer in palliative care, see www.medicinescomplete.com/#/content/palliative/stimulant-laxatives.

● **MEDICINAL FORMS** There can be variation in the licensing of different medicines containing the same drug.

Oral suspension

CAUTIONARY AND ADVISORY LABELS 14 (urine red)

- **Co-danthramer (Non-proprietary)**
  Dantron 5 mg per 1 ml, Poloxamer 188 40 mg per 1 ml Co-danthramer 25mg/200mg/5ml oral suspension sugar free | 300 ml PoM [CD] SF
  Dantron 15 mg per 1 ml, Poloxamer 188 200 mg per 1 ml Co-danthramer 75mg/1000mg/5ml oral suspension sugar free | 300 ml PoM £503.98 SF

Co-danthrusate

16-Mar-2020

● **INDICATIONS AND DOSE**

Constipation in palliative care

▶ BY MOUTH USING ORAL SUSPENSION

- Child 6–11 years: 5 mL once daily, to be taken at night
- Child 12–17 years: 5–15 mL once daily, to be taken at night

DOSE EQUIVALENCE AND CONVERSION

- Co-danthrusate suspension contains dantron 50 mg and docusate sodium 60 mg per 5 mL.

● **CONTRA-INDICATIONS** Acute abdominal conditions · acute inflammatory bowel disease · intestinal obstruction · severe dehydration

● **CAUTIONS** Excessive use of stimulant laxatives can cause diarrhoea and related effects such as hypokalaemia · may cause local irritation · *rodent* studies indicate potential carcinogenic risk

CAUTIONS, FURTHER INFORMATION

- Local irritation Avoid prolonged contact with skin (incontinent patients—risk of irritation and excoriation).

● **INTERACTIONS** → Appendix 1: docusates

● **SIDE-EFFECTS** Gastrointestinal disorders · skin reactions · urine discolouration

● **PREGNANCY** Manufacturers advise avoid—limited information available.

● **BREAST FEEDING** Manufacturers advise avoid—no information available.

● **MEDICINAL FORMS** No licensed medicines listed.

Glycerol
(Glycerin)

10-Nov-2021

● **INDICATIONS AND DOSE**

Constipation

▶ BY RECTUM

- Child 1–11 months: 1 g as required
- Child 1–11 years: 2 g as required
- Child 12–17 years: 4 g as required

● **DIRECTIONS FOR ADMINISTRATION** Manufacturer advises moisten suppositories with water before insertion.

● **PRESCRIBING AND DISPENSING INFORMATION** When prepared extemporaneously, the BP states Glycerol Suppositories, BP consists of gelatin 140 mg, glycerol 700 mg, purified water to 1 g.

● **PATIENT AND CARER ADVICE**

Medicines for Children leaflet: Glycerin (glycerol) suppositories for constipation www.medicinesforchildren.org.uk/medicines/glycerin-glycerol-suppositories-for-constipation/

- **MEDICINAL FORMS** There can be variation in the licensing of different medicines containing the same drug. Forms available from special-order manufacturers include: suppository

Suppository

- Glycerol (Non-proprietary)
  Glycerol 700 mg Glycerol 1g suppositories | 12 suppository GSL £4.32 DT = £3.02
  Glycerol 1400 mg Glycerol 2g suppositories | 12 suppository GSL £3.14 DT = £3.16
  Glycerol 2800 mg Glycerol 4g suppositories | 12 suppository GSL £3.31 DT = £1.92

Senna

03-May-2023

- **DRUG ACTION** Senna is a stimulant laxative. After metabolism of sennosides in the gut the anthrone component stimulates peristalsis thereby increasing the motility of the large intestine.

- **INDICATIONS AND DOSE**

Constipation

▶ BY MOUTH USING TABLETS
- Child 2-3 years: 3.75–15 mg once daily, to be adjusted according to response
- Child 4-5 years: 3.75–30 mg once daily, to be adjusted according to response
- Child 6-17 years: 7.5–30 mg once daily, to be adjusted according to response

▶ BY MOUTH USING SYRUP
- Child 1 month-3 years: 3.75–15 mg once daily, to be adjusted according to response
- Child 4-17 years: 3.75–30 mg once daily, to be adjusted according to response

Constipation (dose approved for use by community practitioner nurse prescribers)

▶ BY MOUTH USING TABLETS
- Child 6-17 years: 7.5–30 mg once daily, to be adjusted according to response

▶ BY MOUTH USING SYRUP
- Child 2-3 years: 3.75–15 mg once daily, to be adjusted according to response
- Child 4-17 years: 3.75–30 mg once daily, to be adjusted according to response

PHARMACOKINETICS
- Onset of action 8–12 hours.

- **UNLICENSED USE** *Tablets* and *syrup* not licensed for use in children under 12 years.
  Doses in BNF Publications adhere to national guidelines and may differ from those in product literature.

IMPORTANT SAFETY INFORMATION

MHRA/CHM ADVICE: STIMULANT LAXATIVES (BISACODYL, SENNA AND SENNOSIDES, SODIUM PICOSULFATE) AVAILABLE OVER-THE-COUNTER: NEW MEASURES TO SUPPORT SAFE USE (AUGUST 2020)

Following a national safety review and concerns over misuse and abuse, the MHRA has introduced new pack size restrictions, revised recommended ages for use, and new safety warnings for over-the-counter stimulant laxatives (administered orally and rectally). Patients should be advised that dietary and lifestyle measures should be used first-line for relieving short-term occasional constipation, and that stimulant laxatives should only be used if these measures and other laxatives (bulk-forming and osmotic) are ineffective.

Smaller packs will remain available for general sale for the treatment of short-term, occasional constipation in adults only, and will be limited to a pack size of two short treatment courses. Stimulant laxatives should not be used in children under 12 years of age without advice from a prescriber; in children aged 12 to 17 years, products can be supplied under the supervision of a pharmacist.

- **CONTRA-INDICATIONS** Atony · intestinal obstruction · undiagnosed abdominal pain
- **SIDE-EFFECTS** Albuminuria · diarrhoea · electrolyte imbalance · fluid imbalance · gastrointestinal discomfort · haematuria · pseudomelanosis coli · skin reactions · urine discolouration

  SIDE-EFFECTS, FURTHER INFORMATION Prolonged or excessive use can cause hypokalaemia.
- **PREGNANCY** EvGr Specialist sources indicate suitable for use in pregnancy. ⟨D⟩
- **BREAST FEEDING** EvGr Specialist sources indicate suitable for use in breast-feeding in infants over 1 month. ⟨D⟩
- **PATIENT AND CARER ADVICE**
  Medicines for Children leaflet: Senna for constipation www.medicinesforchildren.org.uk/medicines/senna-for-constipation/
- **NATIONAL FUNDING/ACCESS DECISIONS**
  NHS restrictions *Senokot*® tablets are not prescribable in NHS primary care.
- **EXCEPTIONS TO LEGAL CATEGORY** Senna is on sale to the public for use in children over 12 years; doses on packs may vary from those in BNF Publications.

- **MEDICINAL FORMS** There can be variation in the licensing of different medicines containing the same drug.

Oral tablet

- Senna (Non-proprietary)
  Sennoside B (as Sennosides) 7.5 mg Sennosides 7.5mg tablets Adult | 20 tablet P £0.44
  Sennosides 7.5mg tablets 12 Years Plus | 60 tablet P £1.31
- Cenlax (Manx Healthcare Ltd)
  Sennoside B (as Sennosides) 7.5 mg Cenlax 7.5mg tablets 12 Years Plus | 20 tablet P £0.80 | 60 tablet P £1.70
- Senease Twelve Years Plus (RX Farma)
  Sennoside B (as Sennosides) 7.5 mg Senease Twelve Years Plus 7.5mg tablets | 60 tablet P £2.99 | 100 tablet P £4.98
- Senokot (Reckitt Benckiser Healthcare (UK) Ltd)
  Sennoside B (as Senna fruit) 7.5 mg Senokot 7.5mg tablets 12 Years Plus | 500 tablet PoM £12.50
  Sennoside B (as Senna fruit) 15 mg Senokot Max Strength tablets 12 Years Plus | 24 tablet P £4.52 DT = £4.52 | 48 tablet P £7.43 DT = £7.43

Oral solution

- Senease Twelve Years Plus (RX Farma)
  Sennoside B (as Sennosides) 1.5 mg per 1 ml Senease Twelve Years Plus 7.5mg/5ml syrup | 150 ml P £5.37 SF
- Senokot (Reckitt Benckiser Healthcare (UK) Ltd)
  Sennoside B (as Sennosides) 1.5 mg per 1 ml Senokot 7.5mg/5ml Syrup 12 Years Plus | 150 ml P £5.36 SF | 500 ml P £11.14 DT = £11.14 SF

Senna with ispaghula husk

11-Nov-2020

The properties listed below are those particular to the combination only. For the properties of the components please consider, senna above, ispaghula husk p. 45.

- **INDICATIONS AND DOSE**

Constipation

▶ BY MOUTH
- Child 12-17 years: 5–10 g once daily, to be taken at night, up to 2–3 times a week

DOSE EQUIVALENCE AND CONVERSION
- 5 g equivalent to one level spoonful of granules.

- **PREGNANCY** Manufacturer advises avoid during first trimester. To be used only intermittently and only if dietary and lifestyle changes fail.
- **DIRECTIONS FOR ADMINISTRATION** EvGr Take at night with at least 150 mL liquid. ⟨M⟩

- **MEDICINAL FORMS** There can be variation in the licensing of different medicines containing the same drug.

Oral granules

CAUTIONARY AND ADVISORY LABELS 25

EXCIPIENTS: May contain Sucrose

▸ **Manevac** (Ceuta Healthcare Ltd)
Senna fruit 124 mg per 1 gram, Ispaghula 542 mg per 1 gram Manevac granules | 400 gram [PoM] £9.50

Sodium acid phosphate with sodium bicarbonate

03-Dec-2020

The properties listed below are those particular to the combination only. For the properties of the components please consider, sodium bicarbonate p. 725.

- **INDICATIONS AND DOSE**

LECICARBON A ®

Constipation | Bowel evacuation [before diagnostic or therapeutic procedures in the rectum]

▶ BY RECTUM

▸ Child 12–17 years: 1 suppository as required, dose may be repeated after 30–60 minutes

PHARMACOKINETICS

▸ Onset of action 15–30 minutes.

LECICARBON C ®

Constipation | Bowel evacuation [before diagnostic or therapeutic procedures in the rectum]

▶ BY RECTUM

▸ Child 1–11 years: 1 suppository as required, dose may be repeated after 30–60 minutes

PHARMACOKINETICS

▸ Onset of action 15–30 minutes.

- **CONTRA-INDICATIONS** Anal and rectal region diseases (risk of excessive absorption of carbon dioxide, particularly in infants and children) · ileus · toxic megacolon (except with explicit permission of the physician)
- **INTERACTIONS** → Appendix 1: bowel cleansing preparations · sodium bicarbonate
- **ALLERGY AND CROSS-SENSITIVITY** [EvGr] Contra-indicated in patients with peanut or soya hypersensitivity. ⟨M⟩
- **PREGNANCY** [EvGr] Use only if potential benefit outweighs risk—effect of the expanding volume of carbon dioxide may be negligible. ⟨M⟩
- **BREAST FEEDING** [EvGr] Suitable for use in breast-feeding—the developed carbon dioxide will not be excreted in milk. ⟨M⟩
- **DIRECTIONS FOR ADMINISTRATION** [EvGr] Moisten suppositories with water before insertion if needed. ⟨M⟩
- **MEDICINAL FORMS** No licensed medicines listed.

Sodium picosulfate

11-Nov-2021

(Sodium picosulphate)

- **DRUG ACTION** Sodium picosulfate is a stimulant laxative. After metabolism in the colon it stimulates the mucosa thereby increasing the motility of the large intestine.

- **INDICATIONS AND DOSE**

Constipation

▶ BY MOUTH

▸ Child 1 month–3 years: 2.5–10 mg once daily, dose to be adjusted according to response

▸ Child 4–17 years: 2.5–20 mg once daily, dose to be adjusted according to response

Constipation (dose approved for use by community practitioner nurse prescribers)

▶ BY MOUTH

▸ Child 1 month–3 years: 250 micrograms/kg once daily (max. per dose 5 mg), dose to be taken at night, dose to be adjusted according to response (on doctor's advice only)

▸ Child 4–10 years: 2.5–5 mg once daily, dose to be taken at night, dose to be adjusted according to response (on doctor's advice only)

▸ Child 11–17 years: 5–10 mg once daily, dose to be taken at night, dose to be adjusted according to response

PHARMACOKINETICS

▸ Onset of action 6–12 hours.

- **UNLICENSED USE** Sodium picosulfate doses in BNF Publications adhere to national guidelines and may differ from those in product literature.

IMPORTANT SAFETY INFORMATION

MHRA/CHM ADVICE: STIMULANT LAXATIVES (BISACODYL, SENNA AND SENNOSIDES, SODIUM PICOSULFATE) AVAILABLE OVER-THE-COUNTER: NEW MEASURES TO SUPPORT SAFE USE (AUGUST 2020)

Following a national safety review and concerns over misuse and abuse, the MHRA has introduced new pack size restrictions, revised recommended ages for use, and new safety warnings for over-the-counter stimulant laxatives (administered orally and rectally). Patients should be advised that dietary and lifestyle measures should be used first-line for relieving short-term occasional constipation, and that stimulant laxatives should only be used if these measures and other laxatives (bulk-forming and osmotic) are ineffective.

Smaller packs will remain available for general sale for the treatment of short-term, occasional constipation in adults only, and will be limited to a pack size of two short treatment courses. Stimulant laxatives should not be used in children under 12 years of age without advice from a prescriber; in children aged 12 to 17 years, products can be supplied under the supervision of a pharmacist.

- **CONTRA-INDICATIONS** Intestinal obstruction · undiagnosed abdominal pain
- **INTERACTIONS** → Appendix 1: sodium picosulfate
- **SIDE-EFFECTS**
  - ▶ **Common or very common** Diarrhoea · gastrointestinal discomfort
  - ▶ **Uncommon** Dizziness · nausea · vomiting
  - ▶ **Frequency not known** Angioedema · skin reactions · syncope

  SIDE-EFFECTS, FURTHER INFORMATION Prolonged or excessive use can cause diarrhoea and related effects such as hypokalaemia.
- **PREGNANCY** Manufacturer states evidence limited but not known to be harmful.
- **BREAST FEEDING** [EvGr] Specialist sources indicate suitable for use in breast-feeding in infants over 1 month—not known to be present in milk. ⟨D⟩
- **PATIENT AND CARER ADVICE**
Medicines for Children leaflet: Sodium picosulfate for constipation www.medicinesforchildren.org.uk/medicines/sodium-picosulfate-for-constipation/
- **MEDICINAL FORMS** There can be variation in the licensing of different medicines containing the same drug.

Oral solution

EXCIPIENTS: May contain Alcohol

▸ **Sodium picosulfate (Non-proprietary)**
Sodium picosulfate 1 mg per 1 ml Sodium picosulfate 5mg/5ml oral solution sugar free | 100 ml [P] £1.56–£14.50 [SF] | 300 ml [P] £45.00 DT = £17.00 [SF]

▸ **Dulco-Lax (sodium picosulfate)** (Opella Healthcare UK Ltd)
Sodium picosulfate 1 mg per 1 ml Dulcolax Pico Twelve Plus 5mg/5ml liquid | 300 ml [P] £7.51 DT = £17.00 [SF]

3 Diarrhoea

Diarrhoea (acute)

08-Mar-2022

Description of condition

Diarrhoea is the abnormal passing of loose or liquid stools, with increased frequency, increased volume, or both. Acute diarrhoea is that which lasts less than 14 days, but symptoms usually spontaneously resolve within 2–4 days. It can result from infection, as a side-effect of a drug, or as an acute symptom of a chronic gastro-intestinal disorder (such as Crohn's disease p. 29, Irritable bowel syndrome p. 40, or Ulcerative colitis p. 31). It may also occur when intestinal motility or morphology is altered.

Prompt investigation is required to identify or exclude any serious underlying cause if the child has any red flag symptoms as such unexplained weight loss, rectal bleeding, persistent diarrhoea, a systemic illness, has received recent hospital treatment or antibiotic treatment, or following foreign travel (other than to Western Europe, North America, Australia or New Zealand).

Aims of treatment

The priority in acute diarrhoea treatment, as in gastro-enteritis, is the prevention or reversal of fluid and electrolyte depletion and the management of dehydration when it is present. This is particularly important in infants, when excessive water and electrolyte loss and dehydration can be life-threatening.

Treatment

Most episodes of acute diarrhoea will settle spontaneously without the need for any medical treatment. [EvGr] Oral rehydration therapy (ORT, such as disodium hydrogen citrate with glucose, potassium chloride and sodium chloride p. 731; potassium chloride with sodium chloride p. 728; potassium chloride with rice powder, sodium chloride and sodium citrate p. 732) is the mainstay of treatment to prevent or correct diarrhoeal dehydration and to maintain the appropriate fluid intake once rehydration is achieved—see Fluids and electrolytes p. 722.

However, in children with severe dehydration and in those unable to drink, immediate admission to hospital and urgent replacement treatment with an intravenous rehydration fluid is recommended—see Fluids and electrolytes p. 722.

ORT is recommended for children at *increased risk of dehydration* and for those *with clinical dehydration* (including hypernatraemic dehydration). If the child is unable to drink the ORT, or vomits persistently, consider giving the solution via a nasogastric tube.

In infants, after rehydration, encourage breast-feeding, other milk feeds and fluid intake. In older children, after rehydration, give full-strength milk straight away, reintroduce the child's usual solid food, and avoid giving fruit juices and carbonated drinks until the diarrhoea has stopped.

In children with gastroenteritis, but *without clinical dehydration*, encourage fluid intake, continue breast-feeding and other milk feeds, and discourage the drinking of fruit juices and carbonated drinks.

In general, antidiarrhoeal drugs have no practical benefit for children with acute or persistent diarrhoea and their use is generally not recommended (side-effects include drowsiness, abdominal distension and ileus). ⟨A⟩

Racecadotril is licensed, as an adjunct to rehydration, for the symptomatic treatment of uncomplicated acute diarrhoea in children over 3 months; it should only be used when supportive measures, including oral rehydration, are insufficient to control the condition.

Antibacterial drugs for acute diarrhoea

[EvGr] Antibacterial treatment is **not** recommended *routinely* for children with acute diarrhoea. Antibacterial treatment is recommended in cases of extra-intestinal spread of bacterial infection; *Clostridioides difficile*-associated pseudomembranous colitis; giardiasis, dysenteric shigellosis, dysenteric amoebiasis, or cholera; in children under 6 months with salmonella gastroenteritis; in children who are malnourished or immunocompromised; and in children with suspected or confirmed septicaemia. For children who have recently been abroad, seek specialist advice about antibacterial therapy. ⟨A⟩ For guidance on antibacterial treatment for some infections that cause acute diarrhoea, see Gastro-intestinal system infections, antibacterial therapy p. 367.

Related drugs

Other drugs used for diarrhoea: codeine phosphate p. 331, co-phenotrope below, methylcellulose.

Other drugs used for Diarrhoea Colestyramine, p. 151

ANTIDIARRHOEALS › ANTIPROPULSIVES

Co-phenotrope

F 327

25-Nov-2020

● **INDICATIONS AND DOSE**

Adjunct to rehydration in acute diarrhoea

▶ BY MOUTH
- Child 2–3 years: 0.5 tablet 3 times a day
- Child 4–8 years: 1 tablet 3 times a day
- Child 9–11 years: 1 tablet 4 times a day
- Child 12–15 years: 2 tablets 3 times a day
- Child 16–17 years: Initially 4 tablets, followed by 2 tablets every 6 hours until diarrhoea controlled

Control of faecal consistency after colostomy or ileostomy

▶ BY MOUTH
- Child 2–3 years: 0.5 tablet 3 times a day
- Child 4–8 years: 1 tablet 3 times a day
- Child 9–11 years: 1 tablet 4 times a day
- Child 12–15 years: 2 tablets 3 times a day
- Child 16–17 years: Initially 4 tablets, then 2 tablets 4 times a day

● **UNLICENSED USE** Not licensed for use in children under 4 years.

● **CONTRA-INDICATIONS** Antibiotic-associated colitis · gastro-intestinal obstruction · intestinal atony · myasthenia gravis (but some antimuscarinics may be used to decrease muscarinic side-effects of anticholinesterases) · paralytic ileus · pyloric stenosis · severe ulcerative colitis · significant bladder outflow obstruction · toxic megacolon · urinary retention

● **CAUTIONS** Presence of subclinical doses of atropine may give rise to atropine side-effects in susceptible individuals or in overdosage · young children are particularly susceptible to **overdosage**—symptoms may be delayed and observation is needed for at least 48 hours after ingestion

● **INTERACTIONS** → Appendix 1: atropine · opioids

● **SIDE-EFFECTS** Abdominal discomfort · angioedema · angle closure glaucoma · appetite decreased · cardiac disorder · depression · dysuria · fever · gastrointestinal disorders · malaise · mucosal dryness · mydriasis · restlessness · vision disorders

● **PREGNANCY** Manufacturer advises caution.

- **BREAST FEEDING** May be present in milk.
- **HEPATIC IMPAIRMENT** Manufacturer advises caution; avoid in jaundice.
- **DIRECTIONS FOR ADMINISTRATION** Expert sources advise for administration *by mouth* tablets may be crushed.
- **PRESCRIBING AND DISPENSING INFORMATION** A mixture of diphenoxylate hydrochloride and atropine sulfate in the mass proportions 100 parts to 1 part respectively.
- **EXCEPTIONS TO LEGAL CATEGORY** Co-phenotrope 2.5/0.025 can be sold to the public for adults and children over 16 years (provided packs do not contain more than 20 tablets) as an adjunct to rehydration in acute diarrhoea (max. daily dose 10 tablets).

- **MEDICINAL FORMS** There can be variation in the licensing of different medicines containing the same drug. Forms available from special-order manufacturers include: oral tablet

Oral tablet

- Co-phenotrope (Non-proprietary)
  Atropine sulfate 25 microgram, Diphenoxylate hydrochloride 2.5 mg Lomotil 2.5mg/25microgram tablets | 100 tablet PoM CD5
  Lofenoxal 2.5mg/25microgram tablets | 20 tablet PoM DT = £31.64 CD5

Loperamide hydrochloride

10-Nov-2021

- **INDICATIONS AND DOSE**

Symptomatic treatment of acute diarrhoea

- BY MOUTH
- Child 4–7 years: 1 mg 3–4 times a day for up to 3 days only
- Child 8–11 years: 2 mg 4 times a day for up to 5 days
- Child 12–17 years: Initially 4 mg, followed by 2 mg for up to 5 days, dose to be taken after each loose stool; usual dose 6–8 mg daily; maximum 16 mg per day

Chronic diarrhoea

- BY MOUTH
- Child 1–11 months: 100–200 micrograms/kg twice daily, to be given 30 minutes before feeds; increased if necessary up to 2 mg/kg daily in divided doses
- Child 1–11 years: 100–200 micrograms/kg 3–4 times a day (max. per dose 2 mg), increased if necessary up to 1.25 mg/kg daily in divided doses; maximum 16 mg per day
- Child 12–17 years: 2–4 mg 2–4 times a day; maximum 16 mg per day

- **UNLICENSED USE** Not licensed for use in children for chronic diarrhoea. *Capsules* not licensed for use in children under 8 years. *Syrup* not licensed for use in children under 4 years.

IMPORTANT SAFETY INFORMATION

MHRA/CHM ADVICE: REPORTS OF SERIOUS CARDIAC ADVERSE REACTIONS WITH HIGH DOSES OF LOPERAMIDE ASSOCIATED WITH ABUSE OR MISUSE (SEPTEMBER 2017)

Serious cardiovascular events (such as QT prolongation, torsades de pointes, and cardiac arrest), including fatalities, have been reported in association with large overdoses of loperamide.

Healthcare professionals are reminded that if symptoms of overdose occur, naloxone can be given as an antidote. The duration of action of loperamide is longer than that of naloxone (1–3 hours), so repeated treatment with naloxone might be indicated; patients should be monitored closely for at least 48 hours to detect possible CNS depression.

Pharmacists should remind patients not to take more than the recommended dose on the label.

- **CONTRA-INDICATIONS** Active ulcerative colitis · antibiotic-associated colitis · bacterial enterocolitis · conditions where abdominal distension develops · conditions where inhibition of peristalsis should be avoided
- **CAUTIONS** Not recommended for children under 12 years
- **INTERACTIONS** → Appendix 1: loperamide
- **SIDE-EFFECTS**
  - **Common or very common** Gastrointestinal disorders · headache · nausea
  - **Uncommon** Dizziness · drowsiness · dry mouth · gastrointestinal discomfort · skin reactions · vomiting
  - **Rare or very rare** Angioedema · consciousness impaired · coordination abnormal · fatigue · miosis · muscle tone increased · severe cutaneous adverse reactions (SCARs) · urinary retention
- **PREGNANCY** Manufacturers advise avoid—no information available.
- **BREAST FEEDING** Amount probably too small to be harmful.
- **HEPATIC IMPAIRMENT** Manufacturer advises caution—risk of reduced first pass metabolism leading to central nervous system toxicity.
- **PATIENT AND CARER ADVICE**
  Medicines for Children leaflet: Loperamide for diarrhoea www.medicinesforchildren.org.uk/medicines/loperamide-for-diarrhoea/
- **EXCEPTIONS TO LEGAL CATEGORY** Loperamide can be sold to the public, for use in adults and children over 12 years, provided it is licensed and labelled for the treatment of acute diarrhoea.

- **MEDICINAL FORMS** There can be variation in the licensing of different medicines containing the same drug. Forms available from special-order manufacturers include: oral suspension, oral solution

Oral tablet

- Loperamide hydrochloride (Non-proprietary)
  Loperamide hydrochloride 2 mg Loperamide 2mg tablets | 30 tablet PoM £2.34 DT = £1.91
- Norimode (Tillomed Laboratories Ltd)
  Loperamide hydrochloride 2 mg Norimode 2mg tablets | 30 tablet PoM £2.15 DT = £1.91

Oral capsule

- Loperamide hydrochloride (Non-proprietary)
  Loperamide hydrochloride 2 mg Loperamide 2mg capsules | 30 capsule PoM £1.44 DT = £0.72

Oral lyophilisate

- Loperamide hydrochloride (Non-proprietary)
  Loperamide hydrochloride 2 mg Loperamide 2mg oral lyophilisates sugar free | 12 tablet P £5.19–£8.00 DT = £5.19 SF

Orodispersible tablet

- Imodium (McNeil Products Ltd)
  Loperamide hydrochloride 2 mg Imodium Instant Melts 2mg orodispersible tablets | 12 tablet P £5.21 DT = £5.21 SF

Loperamide with simeticone

24-Apr-2020

The properties listed below are those particular to the combination only. For the properties of the components please consider, loperamide hydrochloride above, simeticone p. 60.

- **INDICATIONS AND DOSE**

Acute diarrhoea with abdominal colic

- BY MOUTH
- Child 12–17 years: Initially 1 tablet, then 1 tablet, after each loose stool, for up to 2 days; maximum 4 tablets per day

- **INTERACTIONS** → Appendix 1: loperamide

- **MEDICINAL FORMS** There can be variation in the licensing of different medicines containing the same drug.

Oral tablet

- **Imodium Plus** (McNeil Products Ltd)
  Loperamide hydrochloride 2 mg, Dimeticone (as Simeticone) 125 mg Imodium Dual Action Relief tablets | 12 tablet P £5.94 DT = £5.94

4 Exocrine pancreatic insufficiency

Exocrine pancreatic insufficiency

20-Aug-2024

Description of condition

Exocrine pancreatic insufficiency is characterised by reduced secretion of pancreatic enzymes into the duodenum.

The main clinical manifestations are maldigestion and malnutrition, associated with low circulating levels of micronutrients, fat-soluble vitamins and lipoproteins. Children also present with gastro-intestinal symptoms, such as diarrhoea, abdominal cramps and steatorrhoea.

Exocrine pancreatic insufficiency can result from cystic fibrosis, coeliac disease, Zollinger-Ellison syndrome, and gastro-intestinal or pancreatic surgical resection.

Aims of treatment

The aim of treatment is to relieve gastro-intestinal symptoms and to achieve a normal nutritional status.

Drug treatment

EvGr Pancreatic enzyme replacement therapy with pancreatin below is the mainstay of treatment for children with exocrine pancreatic insufficiency. (A)

Pancreatin contains the three main groups of digestive enzymes: lipase, amylase and protease. These enzymes respectively digest fats, carbohydrates and proteins into their basic components so that they can be absorbed and utilised by the body. EvGr Pancreatin should be administered with meals and snacks. The dose should be adjusted, as necessary, to the lowest effective dose according to the symptoms of maldigestion and malabsorption. (A)

Fibrosing colonopathy has been reported in children with cystic fibrosis taking high dose pancreatic enzyme replacement therapy (in excess of 10 000 units/kg/day of lipase). Possible risk factors are sex (boys are at greater risk than girls), more severe cystic fibrosis, and concomitant use of laxatives. The peak age for developing fibrosing colonopathy is between 2 and 8 years. The manufacturer of *Nutrizym 22*® recommend that the total dose of pancreatin used in patients with cystic fibrosis should not usually exceed 10 000 units/kg/day of lipase. Manufacturers recommend that if a patient taking pancreatin develops new abdominal symptoms (or any change in existing abdominal symptoms) the patient should be reviewed to exclude the possibility of colonic damage.

There is limited evidence that acid suppression may improve the effectiveness of pancreatin. EvGr Acid-suppressing drugs (proton pump inhibitors or H_2-receptor antagonists) may be trialled in children who continue to experience symptoms despite high doses of pancreatin.

Levels of fat-soluble vitamins and micronutrients (such as zinc and selenium) should be routinely assessed and supplementation recommended whenever necessary. (A)

Pancreatin preparations

Preparation	Protease units	Amylase units	Lipase units
Creon® 10 000 capsule, e/c granules	600	8000	10 000
Creon® Micro e/c granules (per 100 mg)	200	3600	5000
Pancrex V® capsule, powder	430	9000	8000
Pancrex V '125'® capsule, powder	160	3300	2950
Pancrex V® powder (per gram)	1400	30 000	25 000

Higher-strength pancreatin preparations

Preparation	Protease units	Amylase units	Lipase units
Creon® 25 000 capsule, e/c pellets	1000	18 000	25 000
Nutrizym 22® capsule, e/c minitablets	1100	19 800	22 000

Non-drug treatment

EvGr Dietary advice should be provided. Food intake should be distributed between three main meals per day, and two or three snacks. Food that is difficult to digest should be avoided, such as legumes (peas, beans, lentils) and high-fibre foods. Alcohol should be avoided completely. Reduced fat diets are not recommended. (A)

Medium-chain triglycerides (see MCT oil, in *Borderline substances*), which are directly absorbed by the intestinal mucosa, were thought to be useful in some children. However evidence has shown that MCT-enriched preparations offer no advantage over a normal balanced diet.

PANCREATIC ENZYMES

Pancreatin

15-Aug-2024

- **DRUG ACTION** Supplements of pancreatin are given to compensate for reduced or absent exocrine secretion. They assist the digestion of starch, fat, and protein.

- **INDICATIONS AND DOSE**

CREON® 10000

Pancreatic insufficiency

▶ BY MOUTH

- Child: Initially 1–2 capsules, dose to be taken with each meal either taken whole or contents mixed with acidic fluid or soft food (then swallowed immediately without chewing)

CREON® 25000

Pancreatic insufficiency

▶ BY MOUTH

- Child 2-17 years: Initially 1–2 capsules, dose to be taken with each meal either taken whole or contents mixed with acidic fluid or soft food (then swallowed immediately without chewing)

CREON® MICRO

Pancreatic insufficiency

▶ BY MOUTH

- Neonate: Initially 100 mg, for administration advice, see *Directions for administration*.
- Child: Initially 100 mg, for administration advice, see *Directions for administration*

DOSE EQUIVALENCE AND CONVERSION

- For *Creon® Micro*: 100 mg granules = one measured scoopful (scoop supplied with product).

NUTRIZYM 22® GASTRO-RESISTANT CAPSULES

Pancreatic insufficiency

▶ BY MOUTH

▸ Child 15–17 years: Initially 1–2 capsules, dose to be taken with meals and 1 capsule as required, dose to be taken with snacks, doses should be swallowed whole or contents taken with water, or mixed with acidic fluid or soft food (then swallowed immediately without chewing)

PANCREX® V

Pancreatic insufficiency

▶ BY MOUTH

▸ Child 1–11 months: 1–2 capsules, contents of capsule to be mixed with feeds

▸ Child 1–17 years: 2–6 capsules, dose to be taken with each meal either swallowed whole or sprinkled on food

PANCREX® V CAPSULES '125'

Pancreatic insufficiency

▶ BY MOUTH

▸ Neonate: 1–2 capsules, contents of capsule to be given in each feed (or mixed with feed and given by spoon).

PANCREX® V POWDER

Pancreatic insufficiency

▶ BY MOUTH

▸ Neonate: 250–500 mg, dose to be taken with each feed.

▸ Child: 0.5–2 g, to be taken before or with meals, washed down or mixed with milk or water

● CONTRA-INDICATIONS

NUTRIZYM 22® GASTRO-RESISTANT CAPSULES Should not be used in children aged 15 years or less with cystic fibrosis

● CAUTIONS Can irritate the perioral skin and buccal mucosa if retained in the mouth · excessive doses can cause perianal irritation

● INTERACTIONS → Appendix 1: pancreatin

● SIDE-EFFECTS

▶ **Common or very common** Abdominal distension · constipation · nausea · vomiting

▶ **Uncommon** Skin reactions

▶ **Frequency not known** Fibrosing colonopathy

● PREGNANCY Not known to be harmful.

● DIRECTIONS FOR ADMINISTRATION Pancreatin is inactivated by gastric acid therefore manufacturer advises pancreatin preparations are best taken with food (or immediately before or after food). Since pancreatin is inactivated by heat, excessive heat should be avoided if preparations are mixed with liquids or food; manufacturer advises the resulting mixtures should not be kept for more than one hour and any left-over food or liquid containing pancreatin should be discarded. Enteric-coated preparations deliver a higher enzyme concentration in the duodenum (provided the capsule contents are swallowed whole without chewing). Manufacturer advises gastro-resistant granules should be mixed with slightly acidic soft food or liquid such as apple juice, and then swallowed immediately without chewing. Capsules containing enteric-coated granules can be opened and the granules administered in the same way. For infants, *Creon® Micro* granules can be mixed with a small amount of milk on a spoon and administered immediately—granules should not be added to the baby's bottle. Manufacturer advises *Pancrex® V* powder may be administered via nasogastric tube or gastrostomy tube—consult local and national official guidelines.

● PRESCRIBING AND DISPENSING INFORMATION Preparations may contain pork pancreatin—consult product literature.

● HANDLING AND STORAGE Hypersensitivity reactions have occasionally occurred in those handling the powder.

● PATIENT AND CARER ADVICE Patients or carers should be given advice on administration. It is important to ensure adequate hydration at all times in patients receiving higher-strength pancreatin preparations.
Medicines for Children leaflet: Pancreatin for pancreatic insufficiency www.medicinesforchildren.org.uk/medicines/pancreatin-for-pancreatic-insufficiency/

● MEDICINAL FORMS There can be variation in the licensing of different medicines containing the same drug.

Gastro-resistant capsule

▸ **Creon** (Viatris UK Healthcare Ltd)

Protease 600 unit, Amylase 8000 unit, Lipase 10000 unit Creon 10000 gastro-resistant capsules | 100 capsule [P] £12.93

Protease 1000 unit, Amylase 18000 unit, Lipase 25000 unit Creon 25000 gastro-resistant capsules | 100 capsule [PoM] £28.25

▸ **Nutrizym** (Zentiva Pharma UK Ltd)

Protease 1100 unit, Amylase 19800 unit, Lipase 22000 unit Nutrizym 22 gastro-resistant capsules | 100 capsule [PoM] £39.80

Gastro-resistant granules

CAUTIONARY AND ADVISORY LABELS 25

▸ **Creon** (Viatris UK Healthcare Ltd)

Protease 200 unit, Amylase 3600 unit, Lipase 5000 unit Creon Micro Pancreatin 60.12mg gastro-resistant granules | 20 gram [P] £31.50

Oral capsule

▸ **Pancrex** (Essential Pharmaceuticals Ltd)

Protease 160 unit, Lipase 2950 unit, Amylase 3300 unit Pancrex V 125mg capsules | 300 capsule [P] £44.17

Protease 430 unit, Lipase 8000 unit, Amylase 9000 unit Pancrex V capsules | 300 capsule [P] £55.86

Powder for gastroenteral or oral liquid

▸ **Pancrex** (Essential Pharmaceuticals Ltd)

Protease 1400 unit, Lipase 25000 unit, Amylase 30000 unit Pancrex V oral powder | 300 gram [P] £246.40 [SF]

5 Food allergy

Food allergy

02-Aug-2022

Description of condition

Food allergy is an adverse immune response to a food, commonly associated with cutaneous and gastro-intestinal reactions, and less frequently associated with respiratory reactions and anaphylaxis. It is distinct from food intolerance which is non-immunological. Cow's milk, hen's eggs, soy, wheat, peanuts, tree nuts, fish, and shellfish are the most common allergens. Cross-reactivity between similar foods can occur (e.g. allergy to other mammalian milk in patients with cow's milk allergy).

Management of food allergy

[EvGr] Allergy caused by specific foods should be managed by strict avoidance of the causal food. Educating the child or their carer about appropriate nutrition, food preparation, and the risks of accidental exposure is recommended, such as food and drinks to avoid, ensuring adequate nutritional intake, and interpreting food labels. For children in whom elimination diets might affect growth, a consultation with a nutritionist is recommended to identify alternative dietary sources. ⟨A⟩

Sodium cromoglicate p. 58 is licensed as an adjunct to dietary avoidance in children with food allergy.

[EvGr] Peanut protein p. 210 may be offered as an adjunct to dietary avoidance to certain children with peanut allergy, and treatment can be continued into adulthood. ⟨A⟩

Drug treatment

EvGr There is low quality evidence to support the use of antihistamines to treat acute, **non-life-threatening** symptoms (such as flushing and urticaria) if accidental ingestion of allergenic food has occurred. Chlorphenamine maleate p. 205 is licensed for the symptomatic control of food allergy. In case of food-induced anaphylaxis, intramuscular adrenaline p. 159 is the first-line immediate treatment. Carers and children (of an appropriate age) who are at risk of anaphylaxis should be trained to use self-injectable adrenaline. ⟨A⟩ For further guidance, see Antihistamines, allergen immunotherapy and allergic emergencies p. 199.

Cow's milk allergy

EvGr Parents of infants with suspected allergy to cow's milk should be informed about the most appropriate hypoallergenic formula or milk substitute. Cow's milk avoidance is recommended for the mothers of breast-fed infants who have cow's milk allergy. Children who are allergic to milk should receive alternative dietary sources of calcium and vitamin D. ⟨A⟩

Useful Resources

Food allergy in under 19s: assessment and diagnosis. National Institute for Health and Care Excellence. Clinical guideline 116. February 2011
www.nice.org.uk/guidance/cg116

MAST-CELL STABILISERS

Sodium cromoglicate

03-Aug-2023

(Sodium cromoglycate)

● **INDICATIONS AND DOSE**

Food allergy (in conjunction with dietary restriction)

▶ BY MOUTH

▶ Child 2–13 years: Initially 100 mg 4 times a day for 2–3 weeks, to be taken before meals, dose then increased if necessary up to 40 mg/kg per day, then reduced according to response

▶ Child 14–17 years: Initially 200 mg 4 times a day for 2–3 weeks, to be taken before meals, dose then increased if necessary up to 40 mg/kg per day, then reduced according to response

● **SIDE-EFFECTS** Arthralgia · nausea · rash

● **PREGNANCY** Not known to be harmful.

● **BREAST FEEDING** Unlikely to be present in milk.

● **DIRECTIONS FOR ADMINISTRATION** Expert sources advise capsules may be swallowed whole or the contents dissolved in hot water and diluted with cold water before taking.

● **PATIENT AND CARER ADVICE** Patient counselling is advised for sodium cromoglicate capsules (administration).

● **MEDICINAL FORMS** There can be variation in the licensing of different medicines containing the same drug. Forms available from special-order manufacturers include: oral solution

Oral solution

▶ **Sodium cromoglicate (Non-proprietary)**

Sodium cromoglicate 20 mg per 1 ml Sodium cromoglicate 100mg/5ml oral solution 5ml unit dose ampoules sugar free | 96 unit dose PoM £121.86 DT = £121.86 SF

Oral capsule

CAUTIONARY AND ADVISORY LABELS 22

▶ **Sodium cromoglicate (Non-proprietary)**

Sodium cromoglicate 100 mg Sodium cromoglicate 100mg capsules | 100 capsule PoM £262.00 DT = £164.74

6 Gastric acid disorders and ulceration

6.1 Dyspepsia

Dyspepsia

03-Jan-2019

Description of condition

Dyspepsia covers upper abdominal pain, fullness, early satiety, bloating, and nausea. It can occur with gastric and duodenal ulceration, gastro-oesophageal reflux disease, gastritis, and upper gastro-intestinal motility disorders, but most commonly it is of uncertain origin.

Non-drug treatment

Patients with dyspepsia should be advised about lifestyle changes (avoidance of excess alcohol and of aggravating foods such as fats); other measures include weight reduction, Smoking cessation p. 353, and raising the head of the bed.

Drug treatment

Some medications may cause dyspepsia—these should be stopped, if possible.

A compound alginate preparation may provide relief from dyspepsia; persistent dyspepsia requires investigation. Treatment with a H_2-receptor antagonist or a proton pump inhibitor should be initiated only on the advice of a hospital specialist.

Helicobacter pylori may be present in children with dyspepsia. *H. pylori* eradication therapy should be considered for persistent dyspepsia if it is ulcer-like. However, most children with functional (investigated, non-ulcer) dyspepsia do not benefit symptomatically from *H. pylori* eradication.

ANTACIDS › ALGINATE

Alginic acid

09-Nov-2021

● **INDICATIONS AND DOSE**

GAVISCON INFANT ® POWDER SACHETS

Management of gastro-oesophageal reflux disease

▶ BY MOUTH

▶ Neonate (body-weight up to 4.5 kg): 1 sachet as required, to be mixed with feeds (or water, for breast-fed infants); maximum 6 sachets per day.

▶ Neonate (body-weight 4.5 kg and above): 2 sachets as required, to be mixed with feeds (or water, for breast-fed infants); maximum 12 sachets per day.

▶ Child 1–23 months (body-weight up to 4.5 kg): 1 sachet as required, to be mixed with feeds (or water, for breast-fed infants); maximum 6 sachets per day

▶ Child 1–23 months (body-weight 4.5 kg and above): 2 sachets as required, to be mixed with feeds (or water, for breast-fed infants); maximum 12 sachets per day

● **CONTRA-INDICATIONS** Intestinal obstruction · preterm neonates · where excessive water loss likely (e.g. fever, diarrhoea, vomiting, high room temperature)

GAVISCON INFANT ® POWDER SACHETS Concurrent use of preparations containing thickening agents

● **RENAL IMPAIRMENT** EvGr Avoid (risk of hypernatraemia). ⟨M⟩

- **MEDICINAL FORMS** There can be variation in the licensing of different medicines containing the same drug.

Oral powder

ELECTROLYTES: May contain Sodium

- **Gaviscon Infant** (Reckitt Benckiser Healthcare (UK) Ltd)
  Magnesium alginate 87.5 mg, Sodium alginate 225 mg Gaviscon Infant oral powder sachets | 30 sachet [P] £7.64 DT = £7.64 [SF]

Sodium alginate with potassium bicarbonate

The properties listed below are those particular to the combination only. For the properties of the components please consider, alginic acid p. 58.

- **INDICATIONS AND DOSE**

Management of mild symptoms of dyspepsia and gastro-oesophageal reflux disease

- BY MOUTH USING CHEWABLE TABLETS
  - Child 6–11 years (under medical advice only): 1 tablet, to be chewed after meals and at bedtime
  - Child 12–17 years: 1–2 tablets, to be chewed after meals and at bedtime
- BY MOUTH USING ORAL SUSPENSION
  - Child 2–11 years (under medical advice only): 2.5–5 mL, to be taken after meals and at bedtime
  - Child 12–17 years: 5–10 mL, to be taken after meals and at bedtime

- **PRESCRIBING AND DISPENSING INFORMATION** Flavours of oral liquid formulations may include aniseed or peppermint.

- **MEDICINAL FORMS** There can be variation in the licensing of different medicines containing the same drug.

Oral suspension

ELECTROLYTES: May contain Potassium, sodium

- **Acidex Advance** (Wockhardt UK Ltd)
  Potassium bicarbonate 20 mg per 1 ml, Sodium alginate 100 mg per 1 ml Acidex Advance oral suspension peppermint | 250 ml [P] £3.26 DT = £4.36 [SF] | 500 ml [P] £6.52 DT = £8.72 [SF]
  Acidex Advance oral suspension aniseed | 250 ml [P] £3.26 DT = £4.36 [SF] | 500 ml [P] £6.52 DT = £8.72 [SF]
- **Gaviscon Advance** (Reckitt Benckiser Healthcare (UK) Ltd)
  Potassium bicarbonate 20 mg per 1 ml, Sodium alginate 100 mg per 1 ml Gaviscon Advance oral suspension aniseed | 250 ml [P] £4.36 DT = £4.36 [SF] | 500 ml [P] £8.72 DT = £8.72 [SF]
  Gaviscon Advance oral suspension peppermint | 250 ml [P] £4.36 DT = £4.36 [SF] | 500 ml [P] £8.72 DT = £8.72 [SF]

Chewable tablet

EXCIPIENTS: May contain Aspartame

ELECTROLYTES: May contain Potassium, sodium

- **Gaviscon Advance** (Reckitt Benckiser Healthcare (UK) Ltd)
  Potassium bicarbonate 100 mg, Sodium alginate 500 mg Gaviscon Advance Mint chewable tablets | 24 tablet [GSL] £5.17 [SF] | 60 tablet [GSL] £6.32 DT = £6.32 [SF]

ANTACIDS > ALUMINIUM AND MAGNESIUM

Co-magaldrox

15-Dec-2020

The properties listed below are those particular to the combination only. For the properties of the components please consider, magnesium hydroxide p. 48.

- **INDICATIONS AND DOSE**

MAALOX®

Dyspepsia

- BY MOUTH
  - Child 14–17 years: 10–20 mL, to be taken 20–60 minutes after meals, and at bedtime or when required

MUCOGEL®

Dyspepsia

- BY MOUTH
  - Child 12–17 years: 10–20 mL 3 times a day, to be taken 20–60 minutes after meals, and at bedtime, or when required

- **INTERACTIONS** → Appendix 1: aluminium hydroxide · magnesium
- **SIDE-EFFECTS**
  - **Uncommon** Constipation · diarrhoea
  - **Rare or very rare** Electrolyte imbalance
  - **Frequency not known** Abdominal pain · hyperaluminaemia
- **RENAL IMPAIRMENT** There is a risk of accumulation and aluminium toxicity with antacids containing aluminium salts. Absorption of aluminium from aluminium salts is increased by citrates, which are contained in many effervescent preparations (such as effervescent analgesics).
- **PRESCRIBING AND DISPENSING INFORMATION** Co-magaldrox is a mixture of aluminium hydroxide and magnesium hydroxide; the proportions are expressed in the form x/y where x and y are the strengths in milligrams per unit dose of magnesium hydroxide and aluminium hydroxide respectively.
  MAALOX® *Maalox®* suspension is low in sodium.
  MUCOGEL® *Mucogel®* suspension is low in sodium.

- **MEDICINAL FORMS** There can be variation in the licensing of different medicines containing the same drug.

Oral suspension

- **Mucogel** (Rosemont Pharmaceuticals Ltd)
  Magnesium hydroxide 39 mg per 1 ml, Aluminium hydroxide gel dried 44 mg per 1 ml Mucogel oral suspension | 500 ml [GSL] £2.99 DT = £2.99 [SF]

Simeticone with aluminium hydroxide and magnesium hydroxide

04-May-2020

The properties listed below are those particular to the combination only. For the properties of the components please consider, simeticone p. 60.

- **INDICATIONS AND DOSE**

Dyspepsia

- BY MOUTH
  - Child 2–4 years: 5 mL 3 times a day, to be taken after meals and at bedtime, or when required
  - Child 5–11 years: 5 mL 3–4 times a day, to be taken after meals and at bedtime, or when required
  - Child 12–17 years: 5–10 mL 4 times a day, to be taken after meals and at bedtime, or when required

- **INTERACTIONS** → Appendix 1: aluminium hydroxide · antacids · magnesium
- **SIDE-EFFECTS**
  - **Uncommon** Constipation · diarrhoea
  - **Rare or very rare** Electrolyte imbalance
  - **Frequency not known** Abdominal pain · hyperaluminaemia
- **RENAL IMPAIRMENT** There is a risk of accumulation and aluminium toxicity with antacids containing aluminium salts. Absorption of aluminium from aluminium salts is increased by citrates, which are contained in many effervescent preparations (such as effervescent analgesics).

- **MEDICINAL FORMS** There can be variation in the licensing of different medicines containing the same drug.

Oral suspension

- Maalox Plus (Opella Healthcare UK Ltd)
  Simeticone 5 mg per 1 ml, Aluminium hydroxide gel dried 35 mg per 1 ml, Magnesium hydroxide 40 mg per 1 ml Maalox Plus oral suspension | 250 ml GSL £3.84 SF

ANTACIDS > MAGNESIUM

Magnesium trisilicate with magnesium carbonate and sodium bicarbonate

30-Nov-2021

The properties listed below are those particular to the combination only. For the properties of the components please consider, magnesium trisilicate, magnesium carbonate, sodium bicarbonate p. 725.

- **INDICATIONS AND DOSE**

Dyspepsia

▶ BY MOUTH

- Child 5-11 years: 5–10 mL 3 times a day, alternatively as required, dose to be made up with water
- Child 12-17 years: 10–20 mL 3 times a day, alternatively as required, dose to be made up with water

- **CONTRA-INDICATIONS** Hypophosphataemia · severe renal failure
- **CAUTIONS** Heart failure · hypermagnesaemia · hypertension · metabolic alkalosis · respiratory alkalosis
- **INTERACTIONS** → Appendix 1: magnesium · sodium bicarbonate
- **HEPATIC IMPAIRMENT** In patients with fluid retention avoid antacids containing large amounts of sodium. Avoid antacids containing magnesium salts in hepatic coma if there is a risk of renal failure.
- **RENAL IMPAIRMENT** EvGr Extreme caution (high sodium content); avoid in severe renal failure. (M)
- **PRESCRIBING AND DISPENSING INFORMATION** When prepared extemporaneously, the BP states Magnesium Trisilicate Mixture, BP consists of 5% each of magnesium trisilicate, light magnesium carbonate, and sodium bicarbonate in a suitable vehicle with a peppermint flavour.
- **MEDICINAL FORMS** No licensed medicines listed.

ANTIFOAMING DRUGS

Simeticone

05-Jun-2020

(Activated dimeticone)

- **DRUG ACTION** Simeticone (activated dimeticone) is an antifoaming agent.

- **INDICATIONS AND DOSE**

DENTINOX®

Colic | Wind pains

▶ BY MOUTH

- Neonate: 2.5 mL, to be taken with or after each feed; may be added to bottle feed; maximum 6 doses per day.
- Child 1 month–1 year: 2.5 mL, to be taken with or after each feed; may be added to bottle feed; maximum 6 doses per day

INFACOL®

Colic | Wind pains

▶ BY MOUTH

- Neonate: 0.5–1 mL, to be taken before feeds.
- Child 1 month–1 year: 0.5–1 mL, to be taken before feeds

- **PRESCRIBING AND DISPENSING INFORMATION**
  DENTINOX® The brand name *Dentinox®* is also used for other preparations including teething gel.
- **PATIENT AND CARER ADVICE**
  INFACOL® Patients or carers should be given advice on use of the *Infacol®* dropper.
- **LESS SUITABLE FOR PRESCRIBING**
  DENTINOX® *Dentinox®* colic drops are less suitable for prescribing (evidence of benefit in infantile colic uncertain).
  INFACOL® *Infacol®* is less suitable for prescribing (evidence of benefit in infantile colic uncertain).
- **MEDICINAL FORMS** There can be variation in the licensing of different medicines containing the same drug.

Oral suspension

- Infacol (Dendron Brands Ltd)
  Simeticone 40 mg per 1 ml Infacol 40mg/ml oral suspension | 55 ml GSL £4.64 DT = £4.64 SF | 85 ml GSL £6.78 DT = £6.78 SF

Oral drops

- Dentinox Infant (Dendron Brands Ltd)
  Simeticone 8.4 mg per 1 ml Dentinox Infant colic drops | 100 ml GSL £2.19 DT = £2.19

Combinations available: ***Simeticone with aluminium hydroxide and magnesium hydroxide,*** **p. 59**

6.2 Gastric and duodenal ulceration

Peptic ulceration

Overview

Peptic ulceration commonly involves the stomach, duodenum, and lower oesophagus; after gastric surgery it involves the gastro-enterostomy stoma. Healing can be promoted by general measures, Smoking cessation p. 353 and taking antacids and by antisecretory drug treatment, but relapse is common when treatment ceases. Nearly all duodenal ulcers and most gastric ulcers not associated with NSAIDs are caused by *Helicobacter pylori*.

Helicobacter pylori infection

Eradication of *Helicobacter pylori* reduces the recurrence of gastric and duodenal ulcers and the risk of rebleeding. The presence of *H. pylori* should be confirmed before starting eradication treatment. If possible, the antibacterial sensitivity of the organism should be established at the time of endoscopy and biopsy. Acid inhibition combined with antibacterial treatment is highly effective in the eradication of *H. pylori*; reinfection is rare. Antibiotic-associated colitis is an uncommon risk.

Treatment to eradicate *H. pylori* infection in children should be initiated under specialist supervision. One week triple-therapy regimens that comprise omeprazole p. 64, amoxicillin p. 417, and either clarithromycin p. 403 or metronidazole p. 409 are recommended. Resistance to clarithromycin or to metronidazole is much more common than to amoxicillin and can develop during treatment. A regimen containing amoxicillin and clarithromycin is therefore recommended for initial therapy and one containing amoxicillin and metronidazole is recommended for eradication failure or for a child who has been treated with a macrolide for other infections. There is usually no need to continue antisecretory treatment (with a proton pump inhibitor or H_2-receptor antagonist); however, if the ulcer is large, or complicated by haemorrhage or perforation then antisecretory treatment is continued for a further 3 weeks. Lansoprazole p. 63 may be considered if omeprazole is unsuitable. Treatment failure usually indicates antibacterial resistance or poor compliance.

Two-week triple-therapy regimens offer the possibility of higher eradication rates compared to one-week regimens, but adverse effects are common and poor compliance is likely to offset any possible gain.

Two-week dual-therapy regimens using a proton pump inhibitor and a single antibacterial produce low rates of *H. pylori* eradication and are **not** recommended.

See under *NSAID-associated ulcers* for the role of *H. pylori* eradication therapy in children starting or taking NSAIDs.

Test for *Helicobacter pylori*

Urea (^{13}C) breath test kits are available for confirming the presence of gastro-duodenal infection with *Helicobacter pylori*. The test involves collection of breath samples before and after ingestion of an oral solution of urea (^{13}C); the samples are sent for analysis by an appropriate laboratory. The test should not be performed within 4 weeks of treatment with an antibacterial or within 2 weeks of treatment with an antisecretory drug. A specific urea (^{13}C) breath test kit for children is available (*Helicobacter Test INFAI for children of the age* 3–11®). However the appropriateness of testing for *H. pylori* infection in children has not been established. Breath, saliva, faecal, and urine tests for *H. pylori* are frequently unreliable in children; the most accurate method of diagnosis is endoscopy with biopsy.

NSAID-associated ulcers

Gastro-intestinal bleeding and ulceration can occur with NSAID use. Whenever possible, NSAIDs should be **withdrawn** if an ulcer occurs.

Children at high risk of developing gastro-intestinal complications with a NSAID include those with a history of peptic ulcer disease or serious upper gastro-intestinal complication, those taking other medicines that increase the risk of upper gastro-intestinal side-effects, or those with serious co-morbidity. In children at risk of ulceration, a proton pump inhibitor can be considered for protection against gastric and duodenal ulcers associated with non-selective NSAIDs; high dose ranitidine is an alternative.

NSAID use and *H. pylori* infection are independent risk factors for gastro-intestinal bleeding and ulceration. In children already taking a NSAID, eradication of *H. pylori* is unlikely to reduce the risk of NSAID-induced bleeding or ulceration. However, in children about to start long-term NSAID treatment who are *H. pylori* positive and have dyspepsia or a history of gastric or duodenal ulcer, eradication of *H. pylori* may reduce the overall risk of ulceration.

If the NSAID can be *discontinued* in a child who has developed an ulcer, a proton pump inhibitor usually produces the most rapid healing; alternatively the ulcer can be treated with an H_2-receptor antagonist.

If *NSAID treatment needs to continue*, the ulcer is treated with a proton pump inhibitor.

GASTROPROTECTIVE COMPLEXES AND CHELATORS

Sucralfate

19-Nov-2021

● **DRUG ACTION** Sucralfate is a complex of aluminium hydroxide and sulfated sucrose which forms a barrier to protect the mucosa from acid, pepsin and bile attack in gastric and duodenal ulcers.

● **INDICATIONS AND DOSE**

Benign gastric ulceration | Benign duodenal ulceration

▶ BY MOUTH
- Child 1 month–1 year: 250 mg 4–6 times a day
- Child 2–11 years: 500 mg 4–6 times a day
- Child 12–14 years: 1 g 4–6 times a day
- Child 15–17 years: 2 g twice daily, dose to be taken on rising and at bedtime, alternatively 1 g 4 times a day for 4–6 weeks, or in resistant cases up to 12 weeks, dose to be taken 1 hour before meals and at bedtime; maximum 8 g per day

Prophylaxis of stress ulceration in child under intensive care

▶ BY MOUTH
- Child 1 month–1 year: 250 mg 4–6 times a day
- Child 2–11 years: 500 mg 4–6 times a day
- Child 12–14 years: 1 g 4–6 times a day
- Child 15–17 years: 1 g 6 times a day; maximum 8 g per day

● **UNLICENSED USE** Not licensed for use in children under 15 years. Tablets not licensed for prophylaxis of stress ulceration.

● **CAUTIONS** Patients under intensive care (**Important:** reports of bezoar formation)

CAUTIONS, FURTHER INFORMATION
- Bezoar formation Following reports of bezoar formation associated with sucralfate, caution is advised in seriously ill patients, especially those receiving concomitant enteral feeds or those with predisposing conditions such as delayed gastric emptying.

● **INTERACTIONS** → Appendix 1: sucralfate

● **SIDE-EFFECTS**
- **Common or very common** Constipation
- **Uncommon** Dry mouth · nausea
- **Rare or very rare** Bezoar · rash
- **Frequency not known** Back pain · bone disorders · diarrhoea · dizziness · drowsiness · encephalopathy · flatulence · headache · vertigo

● **PREGNANCY** No evidence of harm; absorption from gastro-intestinal tract negligible.

● **BREAST FEEDING** Amount probably too small to be harmful.

● **RENAL IMPAIRMENT** EvGr Caution (aluminium is absorbed and may accumulate). (M)

● **DIRECTIONS FOR ADMINISTRATION** Expert sources advise administration of sucralfate and enteral feeds should be separated by 1 hour. EvGr For administration by *mouth*, sucralfate should be given 1 hour before meals. (M) *Oral suspension* blocks fine-bore feeding tubes. Expert sources advise crushed *tablets* may be dispersed in water.

● **PRESCRIBING AND DISPENSING INFORMATION** Flavours of oral liquid formulations may include aniseed and caramel.

- **MEDICINAL FORMS** There can be variation in the licensing of different medicines containing the same drug. Forms available from special-order manufacturers include: oral tablet, oral suspension

Oral tablet

CAUTIONARY AND ADVISORY LABELS 5

▸ **Sucralfate (Non-proprietary)**

Sucralfate 1 gram Sulcrate 1g tablets | 100 tablet ☒
Carafate 1g tablets | 100 tablet ☒

Oral suspension

CAUTIONARY AND ADVISORY LABELS 5

▸ **Sucralfate (Non-proprietary)**

Sucralfate 100 mg per 1 ml Carafate 1g/10ml oral suspension | 420 ml PoM ☒ (Hospital only) SF

Sucralfate 200 mg per 1 ml Sucralfate 1g/5ml oral suspension sugar free | 200 ml PoM £288.48–£548.12 DT = £288.48 SF

PROTON PUMP INHIBITORS

Proton pump inhibitors

Overview

Omeprazole p. 64 is an effective short-term treatment for *gastric* and *duodenal ulcers*; it is also used in combination with antibacterials for the eradication of *Helicobacter pylori*. An initial short course of omeprazole is the treatment of choice in *gastro-oesophageal reflux disease* with severe symptoms; children with endoscopically confirmed *erosive, ulcerative, or stricturing oesophagitis* usually need to be maintained on omeprazole.

Omeprazole is also used for the prevention and treatment of NSAID-associated ulcers. In children who need to continue NSAID treatment after an ulcer has healed, the dose of omeprazole should not normally be reduced because asymptomatic ulcer deterioration may occur.

Omeprazole is effective in the treatment of the *Zollinger-Ellison syndrome* (including cases resistant to other treatment). It is also used to reduce the degradation of pancreatic enzyme supplements in children with cystic fibrosis.

Lansoprazole p. 63 is not licensed for use in children, but may be considered when the available formulations of omeprazole are unsuitable.

Esomeprazole below can be used for the management of gastro-oesophageal reflux disease when the available formulations of omeprazole and lansoprazole are unsuitable.

Proton pump inhibitors

- **DRUG ACTION** Proton pump inhibitors inhibit gastric acid secretion by blocking the hydrogen-potassium adenosine triphosphatase enzyme system (the 'proton pump') of the gastric parietal cell.

IMPORTANT SAFETY INFORMATION

MHRA ADVICE: PROTON PUMP INHIBITORS (PPIS): VERY LOW RISK OF SUBACUTE CUTANEOUS LUPUS ERYTHEMATOSUS (SEPTEMBER 2015)

Very infrequent cases of subacute cutaneous lupus erythematosus (SCLE) have been reported in patients taking PPIs. Drug-induced SCLE can occur weeks, months or even years after exposure to the drug.

If a patient treated with a PPI develops lesions—especially in sun-exposed areas of the skin—and it is accompanied by arthralgia:

- advise them to avoid exposing the skin to sunlight;
- consider SCLE as a possible diagnosis;
- consider discontinuing PPI treatment unless it is imperative for a serious acid-related condition; a patient who develops SCLE with a particular PPI may be at risk of the same reaction with another;
- in most cases, symptoms resolve on PPI withdrawal; topical or systemic steroids might be necessary for treatment of SCLE only if there are no signs of remission after a few weeks or months.

- **CAUTIONS** May increase the risk of gastro-intestinal infections (including *Clostridioides difficile* infection) · may reduce absorption of vitamin B_{12} with long-term treatment · patients at risk of osteoporosis

CAUTIONS, FURTHER INFORMATION

▸ Risk of osteoporosis Patients at risk of osteoporosis should maintain an adequate intake of calcium and vitamin D, and if necessary, receive other preventative therapy.

- **SIDE-EFFECTS**
  - ▶ **Common or very common** Abdominal pain · constipation · diarrhoea · dizziness · dry mouth · gastrointestinal disorders · headache · insomnia · nausea · skin reactions · vomiting
  - ▶ **Uncommon** Arthralgia · bone fractures · confusion · depression · drowsiness · leucopenia · malaise · myalgia · paraesthesia · peripheral oedema · thrombocytopenia · vertigo · vision disorders
  - ▶ **Rare or very rare** Agranulocytosis · alopecia · gynaecomastia · hallucination · hepatic disorders · hyperhidrosis · hyponatraemia · nephritis tubulointerstitial · pancytopenia · photosensitivity reaction · severe cutaneous adverse reactions (SCARs) · stomatitis · taste altered
  - ▶ **Frequency not known** Gastrointestinal infection · hypomagnesaemia (more common after 1 year of treatment, but sometimes after 3 months of treatment) · subacute cutaneous lupus erythematosus
- **MONITORING REQUIREMENTS** Measurement of serum-magnesium concentrations should be considered before and during prolonged treatment with a proton pump inhibitor, especially when used with other drugs that cause hypomagnesaemia or with digoxin.
- **PRESCRIBING AND DISPENSING INFORMATION** A proton pump inhibitor should be prescribed for appropriate indications at the lowest effective dose for the shortest period; the need for long-term treatment should be reviewed periodically.

above

Esomeprazole

10-Apr-2024

- **INDICATIONS AND DOSE**

Gastro-oesophageal reflux disease (in the presence of erosive reflux oesophagitis)

▶ BY MOUTH

- ▸ Child 1–11 years (body-weight 10–19 kg): 10 mg once daily for 8 weeks
- ▸ Child 1–11 years (body-weight 20 kg and above): 10–20 mg once daily for 8 weeks
- ▸ Child 12–17 years: 40 mg once daily for 4 weeks, continued for further 4 weeks if not fully healed or symptoms persist; maintenance 20 mg once daily

▶ BY INTRAVENOUS INJECTION, OR BY INTRAVENOUS INFUSION

- ▸ Child 1–11 years (body-weight up to 20 kg): 10 mg once daily until oral administration possible
- ▸ Child 1–11 years (body-weight 20 kg and above): 10–20 mg once daily until oral administration possible
- ▸ Child 12–17 years: 40 mg once daily until oral administration possible

Gastro-oesophageal reflux disease (in the absence of oesophagitis)

▶ BY MOUTH

- ▸ Child 1–11 years (body-weight 10 kg and above): 10 mg once daily for up to 8 weeks
- ▸ Child 12–17 years: 20 mg once daily for up to 4 weeks

- ▶ BY INTRAVENOUS INJECTION, OR BY INTRAVENOUS INFUSION
- ▸ Child 1–11 years: 10 mg once daily until oral administration possible
- ▸ Child 12–17 years: 20 mg once daily until oral administration possible

● **INTERACTIONS** → Appendix 1: proton pump inhibitors

● **SIDE-EFFECTS**

GENERAL SIDE-EFFECTS

▶ **Rare or very rare** Aggression · agitation · bronchospasm · gastrointestinal candidiasis · muscle weakness · renal failure

SPECIFIC SIDE-EFFECTS

▶ **Rare or very rare**

▸ With parenteral use Encephalopathy

● **PREGNANCY** Manufacturer advises caution—no information available.

● **BREAST FEEDING** Specialist sources indicate use with caution—limited human data available. Likely to be present in milk, but amount probably too small to be harmful.

● **HEPATIC IMPAIRMENT** Manufacturer advises caution in severe impairment.

Dose adjustments Manufacturer advises in children 1–11 years, max. 10 mg daily in severe impairment.

Manufacturer advises in children 12–17 years, max. 20 mg daily in severe impairment.

● **RENAL IMPAIRMENT** Manufacturer advises caution in severe renal insufficiency.

● **DIRECTIONS FOR ADMINISTRATION**

▸ With intravenous use For *intravenous injection*, give over at least 3 minutes. [EvGr] For *intravenous infusion*, dilute reconstituted solution to a concentration not exceeding 800 micrograms/mL with Sodium Chloride 0.9%; give over 10–30 minutes. ⟨M⟩

▸ With oral use [EvGr] Do not chew or crush capsules; swallow whole *or* mix capsule contents in water and drink within 30 minutes. Do not crush or chew tablets; swallow whole *or* disperse in water and drink within 30 minutes. Disperse the contents of each sachet of gastro-resistant granules in approx. 15 mL water. Stir and leave to thicken for a few minutes; stir again before administration and use within 30 minutes; rinse container with 15 mL water to obtain full dose. ⟨M⟩ For administration through a gastric tube, consult product literature.

● **PATIENT AND CARER ADVICE** Counselling on administration of gastro-resistant capsules, tablets, and granules advised.

● **MEDICINAL FORMS** There can be variation in the licensing of different medicines containing the same drug. Forms available from special-order manufacturers include: oral suspension

Gastro-resistant capsule

▸ **Esomeprazole (Non-proprietary)**

Esomeprazole 20 mg Esomeprazole 20mg gastro-resistant capsules | 28 capsule [PoM] £6.80 DT = £2.21

Esomeprazole 40 mg Esomeprazole 40mg gastro-resistant capsules | 28 capsule [PoM] £7.15 DT = £2.41

▸ **Emozul** (Krka UK Ltd)

Esomeprazole 20 mg Emozul 20mg gastro-resistant capsules | 28 capsule [PoM] £5.30 DT = £2.21

Esomeprazole 40 mg Emozul 40mg gastro-resistant capsules | 28 capsule [PoM] £6.37 DT = £2.41

Gastro-resistant tablet

▸ **Esomeprazole (Non-proprietary)**

Esomeprazole 20 mg Esomeprazole 20mg gastro-resistant tablets | 28 tablet [PoM] £7.40 DT = £1.76

Esomeprazole 40 mg Esomeprazole 40mg gastro-resistant tablets | 28 tablet [PoM] £10.00 DT = £1.68

▸ **Nexium** (Grunenthal Ltd)

Esomeprazole 20 mg Nexium 20mg gastro-resistant tablets | 28 tablet [PoM] £18.50 DT = £1.76

Esomeprazole 40 mg Nexium 40mg gastro-resistant tablets | 28 tablet [PoM] £25.19 DT = £1.68

Powder for solution for injection

▸ **Esomeprazole (Non-proprietary)**

Esomeprazole (as Esomeprazole sodium) 40 mg Esomeprazole 40mg powder for solution for injection vials | 1 vial [PoM] £2.53–£4.25 (Hospital only)

▸ **Nexium** (Grunenthal Ltd)

Esomeprazole (as Esomeprazole sodium) 40 mg Nexium I.V 40mg powder for solution for injection vials | 10 vial [PoM] £42.50 (Hospital only)

Gastro-resistant granules

CAUTIONARY AND ADVISORY LABELS 25

▸ **Esomeprazole (Non-proprietary)**

Esomeprazole (as Esomeprazole magnesium trihydrate) 10 mg Esomeprazole 10mg gastro-resistant granules sachets | 28 sachet [PoM] £35.35 DT = £35.35

▸ **Nexium** (Grunenthal Ltd)

Esomeprazole (as Esomeprazole magnesium trihydrate) 10 mg Nexium 10mg gastro-resistant granules sachets | 28 sachet [PoM] £25.19 DT = £35.35

62

Lansoprazole

17-Apr-2024

● **INDICATIONS AND DOSE**

Benign gastric ulcer

▶ BY MOUTH

- ▸ Child (body-weight up to 30 kg): 0.5–1 mg/kg once daily (max. per dose 15 mg), dose to be taken in the morning
- ▸ Child (body-weight 30 kg and above): 15–30 mg once daily, dose to be taken in the morning

Duodenal ulcer

▶ BY MOUTH

- ▸ Child (body-weight up to 30 kg): 0.5–1 mg/kg once daily (max. per dose 15 mg), dose to be taken in the morning
- ▸ Child (body-weight 30 kg and above): 15–30 mg once daily, dose to be taken in the morning

NSAID-associated duodenal ulcer | NSAID-associated gastric ulcer

▶ BY MOUTH

- ▸ Child (body-weight up to 30 kg): 0.5–1 mg/kg once daily (max. per dose 15 mg), dose to be taken in the morning
- ▸ Child (body-weight 30 kg and above): 15–30 mg once daily, dose to be taken in the morning

Gastro-oesophageal reflux disease

▶ BY MOUTH

- ▸ Child (body-weight up to 30 kg): 0.5–1 mg/kg once daily (max. per dose 15 mg), dose to be taken in the morning
- ▸ Child (body-weight 30 kg and above): 15–30 mg once daily, dose to be taken in the morning

Acid-related dyspepsia

▶ BY MOUTH

- ▸ Child (body-weight up to 30 kg): 0.5–1 mg/kg once daily (max. per dose 15 mg), dose to be taken in the morning
- ▸ Child (body-weight 30 kg and above): 15–30 mg once daily, dose to be taken in the morning

Fat malabsorption despite pancreatic enzyme replacement therapy in cystic fibrosis

▶ BY MOUTH

- ▸ Child (body-weight up to 30 kg): 0.5–1 mg/kg once daily (max. per dose 15 mg), dose to be taken in the morning
- ▸ Child (body-weight 30 kg and above): 15–30 mg once daily, dose to be taken in the morning

● **UNLICENSED USE** Not licensed for use in children.

● **INTERACTIONS** → Appendix 1: proton pump inhibitors

● **SIDE-EFFECTS**

▶ **Common or very common** Dry throat · fatigue

▶ **Uncommon** Eosinophilia · oedema

▶ **Rare or very rare** Anaemia · angioedema · appetite decreased · erectile dysfunction · fever · glossitis ·

oesophageal candidiasis · pancreatitis · restlessness · tremor

- **PREGNANCY** Manufacturer advises avoid.
- **BREAST FEEDING** Specialist sources indicate use with caution—no human data available. Likely to be present in milk, but amount probably too small to be harmful.
- **HEPATIC IMPAIRMENT** Manufacturer advises caution in moderate to severe impairment (risk of increased exposure).

  Dose adjustments Manufacturer advises dose reduction of 50% in moderate to severe impairment.
- **DIRECTIONS FOR ADMINISTRATION** Manufacturer advises orodispersible tablets should be placed on the tongue, allowed to disperse and swallowed, or may be swallowed whole with a glass of water. Alternatively, tablets can be dispersed in a small amount of water and administered by an oral syringe or nasogastric tube.
- **PATIENT AND CARER ADVICE** Counselling on administration of orodispersible tablet advised.

  Medicines for Children leaflet: Lansoprazole for gastro-oesophageal reflux disease (GORD) and ulcers www.medicinesforchildren.org.uk/medicines/lansoprazole-for-gastro-oesophageal-reflux-disease-gord-and-ulcers/

- **MEDICINAL FORMS** There can be variation in the licensing of different medicines containing the same drug. Forms available from special-order manufacturers include: oral suspension, oral solution, oral powder

Gastro-resistant capsule

CAUTIONARY AND ADVISORY LABELS 5, 22, 25

▸ **Lansoprazole (Non-proprietary)**

Lansoprazole 15 mg Lansoprazole 15mg gastro-resistant capsules | 28 capsule [PoM] £15.79 DT = £0.76 | 100 capsule [PoM] £2.64

Lansoprazole 30 mg Lansoprazole 30mg gastro-resistant capsules | 28 capsule [PoM] £28.36 DT = £1.01 | 56 capsule [PoM] £1.48–£2.03 | 100 capsule [PoM] £3.43–£6.40

Orodispersible tablet

CAUTIONARY AND ADVISORY LABELS 5, 22

EXCIPIENTS: May contain Aspartame

▸ **Lansoprazole (Non-proprietary)**

Lansoprazole 15 mg Lansoprazole 15mg orodispersible tablets | 28 tablet [PoM] £3.20 DT = £1.81

Lansoprazole 30 mg Lansoprazole 30mg orodispersible tablets | 28 tablet [PoM] £6.20 DT = £3.66

▸ **Zoton FasTab** (Pfizer Ltd)

Lansoprazole 15 mg Zoton FasTab 15mg | 28 tablet [PoM] £2.99 DT = £1.81

Lansoprazole 30 mg Zoton FasTab 30mg | 28 tablet [PoM] £5.50 DT = £3.66

F 62

Omeprazole

04-Mar-2026

- **INDICATIONS AND DOSE**

***Helicobacter pylori* eradication in combination with amoxicillin and clarithromycin; or in combination with amoxicillin and metronidazole; or in combination with clarithromycin and metronidazole**

▸ BY MOUTH
- Child 1–5 years: 1–2 mg/kg once daily (max. per dose 40 mg)
- Child 6–11 years: 1–2 mg/kg once daily (max. per dose 40 mg)
- Child 12–17 years: 40 mg once daily

Treatment of duodenal ulcers including those complicating NSAID therapy | Treatment of benign gastric ulcers including those complicating NSAID therapy

▸ BY MOUTH
- Neonate: 700 micrograms/kg once daily for 7–14 days, then increased if necessary to 1.4–2.8 mg/kg once daily.
- Child 1 month–1 year: 700 micrograms/kg once daily, increased if necessary to 3 mg/kg once daily (max. per dose 20 mg)
- Child 2–17 years (body-weight 10–19 kg): 10 mg once daily, increased if necessary to 20 mg once daily
- Child 2–17 years (body-weight 20 kg and above): 20 mg once daily, increased if necessary to 40 mg once daily

▸ BY INTRAVENOUS INFUSION
- Child 1 month–11 years: Initially 500 micrograms/kg once daily (max. per dose 20 mg), increased if necessary to 2 mg/kg once daily (max. per dose 40 mg)
- Child 12–17 years: 40 mg once daily

Zollinger–Ellison syndrome

▸ BY MOUTH
- Neonate: 700 micrograms/kg once daily for 7–14 days, then increased if necessary to 1.4–2.8 mg/kg once daily.
- Child 1 month–1 year: 700 micrograms/kg once daily, increased if necessary to 3 mg/kg once daily (max. per dose 20 mg)
- Child 2–17 years (body-weight 10–19 kg): 10 mg once daily, increased if necessary to 20 mg once daily
- Child 2–17 years (body-weight 20 kg and above): 20 mg once daily, increased if necessary to 40 mg once daily

▸ BY INTRAVENOUS INFUSION
- Child 1 month–11 years: Initially 500 micrograms/kg once daily (max. per dose 20 mg), increased if necessary to 2 mg/kg once daily (max. per dose 40 mg)
- Child 12–17 years: 40 mg once daily

Gastro-oesophageal reflux disease

▸ BY MOUTH
- Neonate: 700 micrograms/kg once daily for 7–14 days, then increased if necessary to 1.4–2.8 mg/kg once daily.
- Child 1 month–1 year: 700 micrograms/kg once daily, increased if necessary to 3 mg/kg once daily (max. per dose 20 mg)
- Child 2–17 years (body-weight 10–19 kg): 10 mg once daily, increased if necessary to 20 mg once daily, in severe ulcerating reflux oesophagitis, maximum 12 weeks at higher dose
- Child 2–17 years (body-weight 20 kg and above): 20 mg once daily, increased if necessary to 40 mg once daily, in severe ulcerating reflux oesophagitis, maximum 12 weeks at higher dose

▸ BY INTRAVENOUS INFUSION
- Child 1 month–11 years: Initially 500 micrograms/kg once daily (max. per dose 20 mg), increased if necessary to 2 mg/kg once daily (max. per dose 40 mg)
- Child 12–17 years: 40 mg once daily

Acid-related dyspepsia

▸ BY MOUTH
- Neonate: 700 micrograms/kg once daily for 7–14 days, then increased if necessary to 1.4–2.8 mg/kg once daily.
- Child 1 month–1 year: 700 micrograms/kg once daily, increased if necessary to 3 mg/kg once daily (max. per dose 20 mg)
- Child 2–17 years (initiated by a specialist) (body-weight 10–19 kg): 10 mg once daily, increased if necessary to 20 mg once daily
- Child 2–17 years (initiated by a specialist) (body-weight 20 kg and above): 20 mg once daily, increased if necessary to 40 mg once daily

▸ BY INTRAVENOUS INFUSION
- Child 1 month–11 years: Initially 500 micrograms/kg once daily (max. per dose 20 mg), increased if necessary to 2 mg/kg once daily (max. per dose 40 mg)
- Child 12–17 years: 40 mg once daily

Fat malabsorption despite pancreatic enzyme replacement therapy in cystic fibrosis

▶ BY MOUTH

- ▶ Neonate: 700 micrograms/kg once daily for 7–14 days, then increased if necessary to 1.4–2.8 mg/kg once daily.
- ▶ Child 1 month–1 year: 700 micrograms/kg once daily, increased if necessary to 3 mg/kg once daily (max. per dose 20 mg)
- ▶ Child 2–17 years (body-weight 10–19 kg): 10 mg once daily, increased if necessary to 20 mg once daily
- ▶ Child 2–17 years (body-weight 20 kg and above): 20 mg once daily, increased if necessary to 40 mg once daily

▶ BY INTRAVENOUS INFUSION

- ▶ Child 1 month–11 years: Initially 500 micrograms/kg once daily (max. per dose 20 mg), increased if necessary to 2 mg/kg once daily (max. per dose 40 mg)
- ▶ Child 12–17 years: 40 mg once daily

● **UNLICENSED USE** Omeprazole *capsules*, *tablets* and *oral suspension* may be used in neonates, but they are not licensed for this age group. Omeprazole *capsules*, *tablets* and *oral suspension* may be used in children as detailed below, although these situations are considered unlicensed:

- *Helicobacter pylori* eradication in combination with antibiotics in children aged under 4 years;
- treatment of duodenal ulcers including those complicating NSAID therapy;
- treatment of benign gastric ulcers including those complicating NSAID therapy;
- Zollinger-Ellison syndrome;
- gastro-oesophageal reflux disease and acid-related dyspepsia in children aged under 1 year and under 10 kg for *capsules* and *tablets*, and in children aged under 1 month for *oral suspension*;
- fat malabsorption despite pancreatic enzyme replacement therapy in cystic fibrosis.

Omeprazole for *intravenous infusion* may be used in children aged 12–17 years, but it is not licensed for this age group.

● **CAUTIONS** Potassium-restricted diet (*oral suspension* may contain potassium—consult product literature)

● **INTERACTIONS** → Appendix 1: proton pump inhibitors

● **SIDE-EFFECTS**

▶ **Rare or very rare** Aggression · agitation · bronchospasm · gastrointestinal candidiasis · muscle weakness

● **PREGNANCY** Not known to be harmful.

● **BREAST FEEDING** Specialist sources indicate amount in milk is small and not known to be harmful; EvGr therapeutic doses unlikely to affect infant. ⟨M⟩

● **HEPATIC IMPAIRMENT**

Dose adjustments No more than 700 micrograms/kg (max. 20 mg) once daily.

● **RENAL IMPAIRMENT** EvGr Caution (*oral suspension* may contain potassium—consult product literature). ⟨M⟩

● **DIRECTIONS FOR ADMINISTRATION** For administration by *mouth* using tablets or capsules:

- Tablets (*Losec MUPS*®, *Mezzopram*®) or capules (*Losec*®) containing enteric-coated pellets can be dispersed in non-carbonated water or a slightly acidic liquid e.g. fruit juice or apple sauce; do **not** use milk or carbonated water. The dispersion should be stirred just before drinking and taken immediately, rinsed down with half a glass of water. The enteric-coated pellets must not be chewed.
- Enteric-coated tablets (*Dexcel*®) must be swallowed whole and not chewed or crushed.

For instructions on reconstitution of oral suspension, consult product literature.

For administration through an *enteral feeding tube*, expert sources advise use *Losec MUPS*® or suspend the contents of a capsule containing omeprazole in 10 mL Sodium Bicarbonate 8.4% (1 mmol Na^+/mL). Allow to stand for 10 minutes before administration.

EvGr For *intermittent intravenous infusion*, dilute reconstituted solution to a concentration of 400 micrograms/mL with Glucose 5% or Sodium Chloride 0.9%; give over 20–30 minutes. ⟨M⟩

● **PATIENT AND CARER ADVICE**

▶ With oral use Counselling on administration advised.

Medicines for Children leaflet: Omeprazole for gastro-oesophageal reflux disease (GORD) www.medicinesforchildren.org.uk/medicines/omeprazole-for-gastro-oesophageal-reflux-disease-gord/

● **PROFESSION SPECIFIC INFORMATION**

Dental practitioners' formulary Gastro-resistant omeprazole capsules may be prescribed.

● **MEDICINAL FORMS** There can be variation in the licensing of different medicines containing the same drug. Forms available from special-order manufacturers include: oral suspension, oral solution

Gastro-resistant capsule

CAUTIONARY AND ADVISORY LABELS 25

▶ **Omeprazole (Non-proprietary)**

Omeprazole 10 mg Omeprazole 10mg gastro-resistant capsules | 28 capsule PoM £7.44 DT = £0.82

Omeprazole 20 mg Omeprazole 20mg gastro-resistant capsules | 28 capsule PoM £11.14 DT = £0.78 | 56 capsule PoM £1.52–£1.90 | 100 capsule PoM £3.07 | 250 capsule PoM £6.43–£10.80

Omeprazole 40 mg Omeprazole 40mg gastro-resistant capsules | 7 capsule PoM £4.93 DT = £0.60 | 28 capsule PoM £1.88–£19.72

▶ **Losec** (Neon Healthcare Ltd)

Omeprazole 10 mg Losec 10mg gastro-resistant capsules | 28 capsule PoM £11.16 DT = £0.82

Omeprazole 20 mg Losec 20mg gastro-resistant capsules | 28 capsule PoM £16.70 DT = £0.78

Omeprazole 40 mg Losec 40mg gastro-resistant capsules | 7 capsule PoM £8.35 DT = £0.60

Gastro-resistant tablet

CAUTIONARY AND ADVISORY LABELS 25

▶ **Omeprazole (Non-proprietary)**

Omeprazole 10 mg Omeprazole 10mg gastro-resistant tablets | 28 tablet PoM £18.91 DT = £9.88

Omeprazole 20 mg Omeprazole 20mg gastro-resistant tablets | 28 tablet PoM £28.56 DT = £5.92

Omeprazole 40 mg Omeprazole 40mg gastro-resistant tablets | 7 tablet PoM £14.28 DT = £10.41

▶ **Losec MUPS** (Neon Healthcare Ltd)

Omeprazole (as Omeprazole magnesium) 10 mg Losec MUPS 10mg gastro-resistant tablets | 28 tablet PoM £9.30 DT = £9.44

Omeprazole (as Omeprazole magnesium) 20 mg Losec MUPS 20mg gastro-resistant tablets | 28 tablet PoM £13.92 DT = £14.04

Omeprazole (as Omeprazole magnesium) 40 mg Losec MUPS 40mg gastro-resistant tablets | 7 tablet PoM £6.96 DT = £6.92

▶ **Mezzopram** (Sandoz Ltd)

Omeprazole (as Omeprazole magnesium) 10 mg Mezzopram 10mg dispersible gastro-resistant tablets | 28 tablet PoM £6.58 DT = £9.44

Omeprazole (as Omeprazole magnesium) 20 mg Mezzopram 20mg dispersible gastro-resistant tablets | 28 tablet PoM £9.86 DT = £14.04

Omeprazole (as Omeprazole magnesium) 40 mg Mezzopram 40mg dispersible gastro-resistant tablets | 7 tablet PoM £4.93 DT = £6.92

Oral suspension

EXCIPIENTS: May contain Hydroxybenzoates (parabens)

ELECTROLYTES: May contain Potassium, sodium

▶ **Omeprazole (Non-proprietary)**

Omeprazole 1 mg per 1 ml Omeprazole 1mg/ml oral suspension sugar free | 75 ml PoM £120.05 DT = £120.05 SF

Omeprazole 2 mg per 1 ml Omeprazole 10mg/5ml oral suspension sugar free | 75 ml PoM £134.11 DT = £134.11 SF

Omeprazole 4 mg per 1 ml Omeprazole 20mg/5ml oral suspension sugar free | 75 ml PoM £253.07 DT = £253.07 SF

Oral solution

EXCIPIENTS: May contain Disodium edetate, polysorbates, propylene glycol

ELECTROLYTES: May contain Sodium

▸ **Omeprazole (Non-proprietary)**

Omeprazole 670 microgram per 1 ml Omeprazole 10mg/15ml oral solution unit dose sugar free | 14 unit dose [PoM] £115.73–£183.18 DT = £115.73 [SF]

Omeprazole 1.33 mg per 1 ml Omeprazole 20mg/15ml oral solution unit dose sugar free | 14 unit dose [PoM] £218.40–£349.44 DT = £218.40 [SF]

Powder for solution for infusion

▸ **Omeprazole (Non-proprietary)**

Omeprazole (as Omeprazole sodium) 40 mg Omeprazole 40mg powder for solution for infusion vials | 5 vial [PoM] £26.00–£29.23 (Hospital only) | 5 vial [PoM] £27.50 | 10 vial [PoM] £55.08 (Hospital only)

6.3 Gastro-oesophageal reflux disease

Gastro-oesophageal reflux disease

29-Oct-2025

Description of condition

Gastro-oesophageal reflux is the passage of gastric contents into the oesophagus and occurs as a result of transient lower oesophageal sphincter relaxation. It is considered physiological in infants when symptoms are absent or not troublesome. Regurgitation is the voluntary or involuntary movement of part or all of the stomach contents up the oesophagus at least as far as the mouth and often emerging from the mouth. It is common in infants under the age of 1 year and considered normal, and usually resolves without treatment before 1 year of age. Gastro-oesophageal reflux disease (GORD) occurs when reflux results in complications, or symptoms are severe enough to require medical treatment.

In infants up to 1 year of age symptoms suggestive of GORD include excessive crying, crying when feeding, unusual neck posture, hoarseness, chronic cough, faltering growth and feeding difficulties such as gagging, choking or refusal. In older children symptoms include heartburn, retrosternal and epigastric pain.

Risk factors for developing GORD include premature birth, hiatus hernia and neurodisability. Complications that might occur include reflux oesophagitis, aspiration pneumonia, dental erosions and recurrent otitis media.

In children with vomiting and regurgitation problems, look for 'red flag symptoms' such as frequent and forceful vomiting, bile-stained vomit, or blood in vomit or stools, that may suggest disorders other than GORD.

Aims of treatment

The aim of treatment is to manage symptoms of GORD in children and raise awareness of symptoms that need investigating.

Non-drug treatment

[EvGr] Parents and carers of well infants should be reassured that most symptoms of uncomplicated gastro-oesophageal reflux are common and resolve without treatment before 1 year of age.

In breast-fed infants with frequent regurgitation and marked distress, ensure that a person with appropriate expertise and training carries out a breastfeeding assessment.

In formula-fed infants with frequent regurgitation and marked distress use a stepped care approach with review of feeding history, reduction of feed volumes if excessive for the infant's weight, and then a 1–2 week trial of smaller and more frequent feeds. If symptoms are still not improving give a trial of thickened formula for another 1–2 weeks.

Children and adolescents who are obese should be advised that weight reduction may help with their symptoms.

Surgery may be considered under specialist advice for children with severe, intractable GORD where medical treatment has been unsuccessful, or feeding regimens to manage symptoms have proved impractical. ⟨A⟩

Drug treatment

Initial management

[EvGr] If non-pharmacological methods fail for breast-fed infants, consider alginic acid p. 58 for 1–2 weeks. If successful, this should be continued but consider withholding it at intervals to see if the infant has recovered.

If non-pharmacological methods fail for formula-fed infants, the thickened formula should be stopped and a trial of alginic acid for 1–2 weeks should be used. If successful, it should be continued, but consider withholding it at intervals to see if the infant has recovered.

Acid-suppressing drugs, such as Proton pump inhibitors p. 62 or histamine$_2$-receptor antagonists (H_2-receptor antagonists) should not be used to treat regurgitation in children occurring as an isolated symptom. ⟨A⟩

Follow up management

[EvGr] For children who are unable to communicate about their symptoms (e.g. infants, young children and those with communication difficulties), a 4-week trial of a proton pump inhibitor (PPI) or H_2-receptor antagonist should be considered in those who have regurgitation with one or more of the following symptoms: unexplained feeding difficulties, distressed behaviour or faltering growth.

For children and young people with persistent heartburn, retrosternal or epigastric pain, a 4-week trial of a PPI or H_2-receptor antagonist should be considered.

When choosing between a PPI or H_2-receptor antagonist availability of age-appropriate preparations, patient/carer preference should be taken into account.

Response to treatment should be reviewed after 4 weeks and referral for endoscopy considered if the symptoms did not resolve, or recur after stopping treatment.

Treatment of gastro-oesophageal reflux or GORD with metoclopramide hydrochloride p. 315 (unlicensed), domperidone p. 314 (unlicensed), or erythromycin p. 406 (unlicensed) should only be offered when the benefits outweigh the risk of side-effects, other interventions have been tried, and there is specialist paediatric agreement for its use.

Infants, children and young people with endoscopy-proven reflux oesophagitis should be offered treatment with a PPI or H_2-receptor antagonist, and repeat endoscopic examination performed as necessary to guide subsequent treatment. ⟨A⟩

Enteral tube feeding

[EvGr] Enteral tube feeding should only be considered as an option to promote weight gain in infants and children with regurgitation and faltering growth if other pathologies have been ruled out, and/or the recommended feeding and medical management is unsuccessful.

A specific and individualised nutrition plan must be in place for these children with a strategy to reduce it as soon as possible. Oral stimulation is encouraged by continuing oral feeding as tolerated, ensuring that the intended target weight is achieved and sustained. Enteral tube feeding should be reduced and stopped as soon as possible.

Jejunal feeding can be considered in patients who need enteral tube feeding but cannot tolerate intragastric feeds because of regurgitation or if reflux-related pulmonary aspiration is a concern. ⟨A⟩

For advice on specialised formula feeds, see Enteral nutrition p. 777.

GORD in pregnancy

EvGr Heartburn and acid reflux are symptoms of Dyspepsia p. 58 in pregnancy commonly caused by GORD. Dietary and lifestyle advice should be given as first-line management. If this approach fails to control symptoms, an antacid or an alginate can be used. If this is ineffective or symptoms are severe, omeprazole p. 64 may help to control symptoms. (A)

Useful Resources

Gastro-oesophageal reflux disease in children and young people: diagnosis and management. National Institute for Health and Care Excellence. NICE guideline 1. January 2015, updated October 2019.
www.nice.org.uk/guidance/ng1

Other drugs used for Gastro-oesophageal reflux disease
Esomeprazole, p. 62 · Lansoprazole, p. 63

ANTACIDS > ALGINATE

Sodium alginate with calcium carbonate and sodium bicarbonate

11-Nov-2021

The properties listed below are those particular to the combination only. For the properties of the components please consider, alginic acid p. 58, sodium bicarbonate p. 725, calcium carbonate p. 733.

● **INDICATIONS AND DOSE**

Gastro-oesophageal reflux disease

▶ BY MOUTH

▸ Child 6-11 years: 5–10 mL, to be taken after meals and at bedtime

▸ Child 12-17 years: 10–20 mL, to be taken after meals and at bedtime

● **INTERACTIONS** → Appendix 1: calcium compounds · sodium bicarbonate

● **PRESCRIBING AND DISPENSING INFORMATION** Flavours of oral liquid formulations may include aniseed or peppermint.

● **PATIENT AND CARER ADVICE**
Medicines for Children leaflet: Gaviscon for gastro-oesophageal reflux disease www.medicinesforchildren.org.uk/medicines/gaviscon-for-gastro-oesophageal-reflux-disease/

● **MEDICINAL FORMS** There can be variation in the licensing of different medicines containing the same drug.

Oral suspension

ELECTROLYTES: May contain Sodium

▸ **Sodium alginate with calcium carbonate and sodium bicarbonate (Non-proprietary)**
Calcium carbonate 16 mg per 1 ml, Sodium bicarbonate 26.7 mg per 1 ml, Sodium alginate 50 mg per 1 ml Care Heartburn Relief oral suspension | 500 ml GSL £4.69 DT = £4.69 SF

▶ Brands may include Peptac, Rennie

6.4 Helicobacter pylori infection

DIAGNOSTIC AGENTS

Urea (^{13}C)

06-Mar-2026

● **INDICATIONS AND DOSE**

Diagnosis of gastro-duodenal *Helicobacter pylori* infection

▶ BY MOUTH

▸ Child: (consult product literature)

● **MEDICINAL FORMS** There can be variation in the licensing of different medicines containing the same drug.

Oral tablet

▸ **Diabact UBT** (Mayoly UK Ltd)
Urea [13-C] 50 mg diabact UBT 50mg tablets | 1 tablet PoM £21.25 DT = £21.25 | 10 tablet PoM £78.75 (Hospital only)

Powder for oral solution

▸ **Helicobacter Test INFAI** (INFAI UK Ltd)
Urea [13-C] 45 mg Helicobacter Test INFAI for children breath test kit | 1 kit PoM £19.20 DT = £19.20 SF
Urea [13-C] 75 mg Helicobacter Test INFAI breath test kit | 1 kit PoM £21.70 DT = £21.70 SF | 50 kit PoM £950.00 SF

7 Gastro-intestinal smooth muscle spasm

Antispasmodics

02-May-2020

Antimuscarinics

Antimuscarinics (formerly termed 'anticholinergics') reduce intestinal motility and are used for gastro-intestinal smooth muscle spasm. They include the tertiary amine dicycloverine hydrochloride p. 68, and the quaternary ammonium compounds propantheline bromide p. 69 and hyoscine butylbromide p. 68. The quaternary ammonium compounds are less lipid soluble than tertiary amines and are less likely to cross the blood-brain barrier; therefore have a lower risk for central nervous system side-effects. They are also less well absorbed from the gastro-intestinal tract.

Dicycloverine hydrochloride may also have some direct action on smooth muscle. Hyoscine butylbromide is advocated as a gastro-intestinal antispasmodic, but is poorly absorbed.

Other antispasmodics

Alverine citrate p. 69, mebeverine hydrochloride p. 69, and peppermint oil p. 41 are direct-acting intestinal smooth muscle relaxants and may relieve abdominal pain or spasm in Irritable bowel syndrome p. 40.

Motility stimulants

Domperidone is a dopamine receptor antagonist which accelerates gastric emptying, improves gastroduodenal motility, and enhances the strength of lower oesophageal sphincter pressure. The MHRA and CHM have released important safety information and restrictions regarding the use of domperidone, and a reminder of contra-indications. For further information, see *Important safety information* for domperidone p. 314.

A low dose of erythromycin p. 406 stimulates gastro-intestinal motility. Expert sources advise that erythromycin may help some neonates with gut motility problems; its value in speeding up full enteral feeding and reduction in total parenteral nutrition (TPN)-associated cholestasis must be weighed against possible occurrence of pyloric stenosis after high-dose use.

ANTIMUSCARINICS

603

Dicycloverine hydrochloride
23-Apr-2020

(Dicyclomine hydrochloride)

● **INDICATIONS AND DOSE**

Symptomatic relief of gastro-intestinal disorders characterised by smooth muscle spasm

▶ BY MOUTH
- Child 6–23 months: 5–10 mg 3–4 times a day, dose to be taken 15 minutes before feeds
- Child 2–11 years: 10 mg 3 times a day
- Child 12–17 years: 10–20 mg 3 times a day

● **CONTRA-INDICATIONS** Child under 6 months

● **INTERACTIONS** → Appendix 1: dicycloverine

● **SIDE-EFFECTS** Appetite decreased · fatigue · thirst

● **PREGNANCY** Not known to be harmful; manufacturer advises use only if essential.

● **BREAST FEEDING** Avoid—present in milk; apnoea reported in infant.

● **EXCEPTIONS TO LEGAL CATEGORY** Dicycloverine hydrochloride can be sold to the public provided that max. single dose is 10 mg and max. daily dose is 60 mg.

● **MEDICINAL FORMS** There can be variation in the licensing of different medicines containing the same drug.

Oral tablet

▸ Dicycloverine hydrochloride (Non-proprietary)
Dicycloverine hydrochloride 10 mg Dicycloverine 10mg tablets | 100 tablet PoM £212.24 DT = £11.20
Dicycloverine hydrochloride 20 mg Dicycloverine 20mg tablets | 84 tablet PoM £226.57 DT = £9.85

Oral solution

▸ Dicycloverine hydrochloride (Non-proprietary)
Dicycloverine hydrochloride 2 mg per 1 ml Dicycloverine 10mg/5ml oral solution sugar free | 120 ml PoM [X] SF
Dicycloverine 10mg/5ml oral solution | 120 ml PoM £174.11 DT = £174.11

Dicycloverine hydrochloride with aluminium hydroxide, magnesium oxide and simeticone
28-Apr-2020

The properties listed below are those particular to the combination only. For the properties of the components please consider, dicycloverine hydrochloride above, simeticone p. 60.

● **INDICATIONS AND DOSE**

Symptomatic relief of gastro-intestinal disorders characterised by smooth muscle spasm

▶ BY MOUTH
- Child 12–17 years: 10–20 mL every 4 hours as required

● **INTERACTIONS** → Appendix 1: aluminium hydroxide · antacids · dicycloverine · magnesium

● **SIDE-EFFECTS** Anticholinergic syndrome

● **RENAL IMPAIRMENT** There is a risk of accumulation and aluminium toxicity with antacids containing aluminium salts. Absorption of aluminium from aluminium salts is increased by citrates, which are contained in many effervescent preparations (such as effervescent analgesics).

● **MEDICINAL FORMS** No licensed medicines listed.

603

Hyoscine butylbromide
03-Apr-2024

● **INDICATIONS AND DOSE**

Symptomatic relief of gastro-intestinal or genito-urinary disorders characterised by smooth muscle spasm

▶ BY MOUTH
- Child 6–11 years: 10 mg 3 times a day
- Child 12–17 years: 20 mg 4 times a day

Acute spasm | Spasm in diagnostic procedures

▶ BY INTRAMUSCULAR INJECTION, OR BY SLOW INTRAVENOUS INJECTION
- Child 2–5 years: 5 mg for 1 dose, dose can be repeated after 30 minutes if required (may be repeated more frequently in endoscopy); maximum 15 mg per day
- Child 6–11 years: 5–10 mg for 1 dose, dose can be repeated after 30 minutes if required (may be repeated more frequently in endoscopy); maximum 30 mg per day
- Child 12–17 years: 20 mg for 1 dose, dose can be repeated after 30 minutes if required (may be repeated more frequently in endoscopy); maximum 80 mg per day

Excessive respiratory secretions in palliative care

▶ BY MOUTH
- Child 1 month–1 year: 300–500 micrograms/kg 3–4 times a day (max. per dose 5 mg)
- Child 2–4 years: 5 mg 3–4 times a day
- Child 5–11 years: 10 mg 3–4 times a day
- Child 12–17 years: 10–20 mg 3–4 times a day

▶ BY INTRAMUSCULAR INJECTION, OR BY SLOW INTRAVENOUS INJECTION
- Child 1 month–4 years: 300–500 micrograms/kg 3–4 times a day (max. per dose 5 mg)
- Child 5–11 years: 5–10 mg 3–4 times a day
- Child 12–17 years: 10–20 mg 3–4 times a day

Bowel colic in palliative care

▶ BY MOUTH
- Child 1 month–1 year: 300–500 micrograms/kg 3–4 times a day (max. per dose 5 mg)
- Child 2–4 years: 5 mg 3–4 times a day
- Child 5–11 years: 10 mg 3–4 times a day
- Child 12–17 years: 10–20 mg 3–4 times a day

▶ BY INTRAMUSCULAR INJECTION, OR BY SLOW INTRAVENOUS INJECTION
- Child 1 month–4 years: 300–500 micrograms/kg 3–4 times a day (max. per dose 5 mg)
- Child 5–11 years: 5–10 mg 3–4 times a day
- Child 12–17 years: 10–20 mg 3–4 times a day

PHARMACOKINETICS
- Administration by mouth is associated with poor absorption.

● **UNLICENSED USE** *Tablets* not licensed for use in children under 6 years. *Injection* not licensed for use in children (age range not specified by manufacturer).

IMPORTANT SAFETY INFORMATION

MHRA/CHM ADVICE: HYOSCINE BUTYLBROMIDE (*BUSCOPAN*®) INJECTION: RISK OF SERIOUS ADVERSE EFFECTS IN PATIENTS WITH UNDERLYING CARDIAC DISEASE (FEBRUARY 2017)

The MHRA advises that hyoscine butylbromide injection can cause serious adverse effects including tachycardia, hypotension, and anaphylaxis; several reports have noted that anaphylaxis is more likely to be fatal in patients with underlying coronary heart disease. Hyoscine butylbromide injection is contra-indicated in patients with tachycardia and should be used with caution in patients with cardiac disease; the MHRA recommends that these patients are monitored and that resuscitation equipment and trained personnel are readily available.

INTRAVENOUS ADMINISTRATION
Healthcare professionals are reminded that intravenous hyoscine butylbromide must be given slowly to reduce the risk of marked hypotension and anaphylactic shock.

- CONTRA-INDICATIONS
  - With intramuscular use or intravenous use Tachycardia
- INTERACTIONS → Appendix 1: hyoscine
- SIDE-EFFECTS
  GENERAL SIDE-EFFECTS Dyspnoea
  SPECIFIC SIDE-EFFECTS
  - With parenteral use Anaphylactic reaction · feeling hot · hypotension · mydriasis · sweat changes
- PREGNANCY Manufacturer advises avoid.
- BREAST FEEDING Amount too small to be harmful.
- DIRECTIONS FOR ADMINISTRATION For *slow intravenous injection*, expert sources advise may be diluted with Glucose 5% or Sodium Chloride 0.9%.
  For administration by *mouth*, expert sources advise injection solution may be used; content of ampoule may be stored in a refrigerator for up to 24 hours after opening.
- PRESCRIBING AND DISPENSING INFORMATION
  Palliative care For further information on the use of hyoscine butylbromide in palliative care, see www.medicinescomplete.com/#/content/palliative/hyoscine-butylbromide.
- EXCEPTIONS TO LEGAL CATEGORY Hyoscine butylbromide tablets can be sold to the public for medically confirmed irritable bowel syndrome, provided single dose does not exceed 20 mg, daily dose does not exceed 80 mg, and pack does not contain a total of more than 240 mg.

- MEDICINAL FORMS There can be variation in the licensing of different medicines containing the same drug. Forms available from special-order manufacturers include: oral suspension, oral solution

Solution for injection
- Hyoscine butylbromide (Non-proprietary)
  Hyoscine butylbromide 20 mg per 1 ml Hyoscine butylbromide 20mg/1ml solution for injection ampoules | 10 ampoule [PoM] £2.92 DT = £4.19 (Hospital only)
- Buscopan (Opella POM UK Ltd)
  Hyoscine butylbromide 20 mg per 1 ml Buscopan 20mg/1ml solution for injection ampoules | 10 ampoule [PoM] £4.19 DT = £4.19

Oral tablet
- Hyoscine butylbromide (Non-proprietary)
  Hyoscine butylbromide 10 mg Hyoscine butylbromide 10mg tablets | 56 tablet [PoM] £4.02–£7.00 DT = £6.79 | 100 tablet [PoM] £7.06–£12.09
  Hyoscine butylbromide 20 mg Hyoscine butylbromide 20mg tablets | 56 tablet [PoM] £6.43–£11.84 | 100 tablet [PoM] £20.76 DT = £15.95
- Buscopan (Opella POM UK Ltd)
  Hyoscine butylbromide 10 mg Buscopan 10mg tablets | 56 tablet [PoM] £4.11 DT = £6.79
- Sigmopan (Ria Generics Ltd)
  Hyoscine butylbromide 10 mg Sigmopan 10mg tablets | 100 tablet [PoM] £5.90

F 603

Propantheline bromide

27-Apr-2021

- INDICATIONS AND DOSE

Symptomatic relief of gastro-intestinal disorders characterised by smooth muscle spasm

▶ BY MOUTH
- Child 1 month–11 years: 300 micrograms/kg 3–4 times a day (max. per dose 15 mg), dose to be taken at least one hour before food
- Child 12–17 years: 15 mg 3 times a day, dose to be taken at least one hour before food and 30 mg, dose to be taken at night; maximum 120 mg per day

- UNLICENSED USE Not licensed for use in children.
- INTERACTIONS → Appendix 1: propantheline
- SIDE-EFFECTS Arrhythmias · bronchial secretion decreased · mydriasis
- PREGNANCY Manufacturer advises avoid unless essential—no information available.
- BREAST FEEDING May suppress lactation.
- HEPATIC IMPAIRMENT Manufacturer advises caution.
- RENAL IMPAIRMENT Manufacturer advises caution.

- MEDICINAL FORMS There can be variation in the licensing of different medicines containing the same drug. Forms available from special-order manufacturers include: oral suspension, oral solution

Oral tablet
CAUTIONARY AND ADVISORY LABELS 23
- Propantheline bromide (Non-proprietary)
  Propantheline bromide 15 mg Propantheline bromide 15mg tablets | 112 tablet [PoM] £104.99–£195.14 DT = £20.74
- Pro-Banthine (Grunenthal Ltd)
  Propantheline bromide 15 mg Pro-Banthine 15mg tablets | 112 tablet [PoM] £20.74 DT = £20.74

ANTISPASMODICS

Alverine citrate

28-Aug-2020

- INDICATIONS AND DOSE

Symptomatic relief of gastro-intestinal disorders characterised by smooth muscle spasm | Dysmenorrhoea

▶ BY MOUTH
- Child 12–17 years: 60–120 mg 1–3 times a day

- CONTRA-INDICATIONS Intestinal obstruction · paralytic ileus
- SIDE-EFFECTS Dizziness · dyspnoea · headache · hepatitis · jaundice (discontinue) · nausea · skin reactions · wheezing
- PREGNANCY Manufacturer advises avoid—limited information available
- BREAST FEEDING Manufacturer advises avoid—limited information available.
- PATIENT AND CARER ADVICE
  Driving and skilled tasks Dizziness may affect performance of skilled tasks (e.g. driving).

- MEDICINAL FORMS There can be variation in the licensing of different medicines containing the same drug.

Oral capsule
- Alverine citrate (Non-proprietary)
  Alverine citrate 60 mg Alverine 60mg capsules | 100 capsule [P] £16.45 DT = £5.19
  Alverine citrate 120 mg Alverine 120mg capsules | 60 capsule [P] £19.42 DT = £5.79

Mebeverine hydrochloride

10-Nov-2021

- INDICATIONS AND DOSE

Adjunct in gastro-intestinal disorders characterised by smooth muscle spasm

▶ BY MOUTH USING IMMEDIATE-RELEASE MEDICINES
- Child 3 years: 25 mg 3 times a day, dose preferably taken 20 minutes before meals
- Child 4–7 years: 50 mg 3 times a day, dose preferably taken 20 minutes before meals
- Child 8–9 years: 100 mg 3 times a day, dose preferably taken 20 minutes before meals
- Child 10–17 years: 135–150 mg 3 times a day, dose preferably taken 20 minutes before meals

Irritable bowel syndrome

▶ BY MOUTH USING MODIFIED-RELEASE MEDICINES
- Child 12–17 years: 200 mg twice daily

- **UNLICENSED USE** *Suspension* not licensed for use in children under 10 years. *Tablets* and *modified-release capsules* not licensed for use in children.
- **CONTRA-INDICATIONS** Paralytic ileus
- **SIDE-EFFECTS** Angioedema · face oedema · skin reactions
- **PREGNANCY** Not known to be harmful—manufacturers advise avoid.
- **BREAST FEEDING** Manufacturers advise avoid—no information available.
- **PATIENT AND CARER ADVICE** Patients or carers should be given advice on the timing of administration of mebeverine hydrochloride tablets and oral suspension.
Medicines for Children leaflet: Mebeverine hydrochloride for intestinal spasm www.medicinesforchildren.org.uk/medicines/mebeverine-hydrochloride-for-intestinal-spasm/

- **MEDICINAL FORMS** There can be variation in the licensing of different medicines containing the same drug. Forms available from special-order manufacturers include: oral suspension

Oral tablet

- ▸ **Mebeverine hydrochloride (Non-proprietary)**
Mebeverine hydrochloride 135 mg Mebeverine 135mg tablets | 100 tablet PoM £9.02 DT = £2.13
- ▸ **Colofac** (Ceuta Healthcare Ltd)
Mebeverine hydrochloride 135 mg Colofac 135mg tablets | 100 tablet PoM £9.02 DT = £2.13

Oral suspension

- ▸ **Mebeverine hydrochloride (Non-proprietary)**
Mebeverine hydrochloride (as Mebeverine pamoate) 10 mg per 1 ml Mebeverine 50mg/5ml oral suspension sugar free | 300 ml PoM £205.70 DT = £146.49 SF

Modified-release capsule

CAUTIONARY AND ADVISORY LABELS 25

- ▸ **Mebeverine hydrochloride (Non-proprietary)**
Mebeverine hydrochloride 200 mg Mebeverine 200mg modified-release capsules | 60 capsule PoM £9.22 DT = £11.08
- ▸ **Aurobeverine MR** (Milpharm Ltd)
Mebeverine hydrochloride 200 mg Aurobeverine MR 200mg capsules | 60 capsule PoM £6.92 DT = £11.08
- ▸ **Colofac MR** (Ceuta Healthcare Ltd)
Mebeverine hydrochloride 200 mg Colofac MR 200mg capsules | 60 capsule PoM £6.92 DT = £11.08

8 Liver disorders and related conditions

8.1 Biliary disorders

Cholestasis

14-Sep-2020

Description of condition

Cholestasis is an impairment of bile formation and/or bile flow, which may clinically present with fatigue, pruritus, dark urine, pale stools and, in its most overt form, jaundice and signs of fat soluble vitamin deficiencies.

Treatment

EvGr Ursodeoxycholic acid p. 72 [unlicensed] and colestyramine p. 151 [unlicensed under 6 years] are used to relieve cholestatic pruritus in children, even if evidence to support their use is limited.

Colestyramine is an anion-exchange resin that is not absorbed from the gastro-intestinal tract. It relieves pruritus by forming an insoluble complex in the intestine with bile acids and other compounds—the reduction of serum bile acid levels reduces excess deposition in the dermal tissue with a resultant decrease in pruritus.

Alternative drugs for **intractable** cholestatic pruritus should be used with caution and **under specialist supervision** as these children usually have severe liver disease—careful monitoring is required. Drugs that may be considered include rifampicin p. 449 [unlicensed indication], opioid antagonists [unlicensed indication], and phenobarbital p. 264 [unlicensed indication]. (E) The MHRA/CHM have released important safety information on the use of antiepileptic drugs and the risk of suicidal thoughts and behaviour. For further information, see Epilepsy p. 227.

Inborn errors of primary bile acid synthesis

27-Apr-2018

Description of condition

Inborn errors of primary bile acid synthesis are a group of diseases in which the liver does not produce enough primary bile acids due to enzyme deficiencies. These acids are the main components of the bile, and include cholic acid and chenodeoxycholic acid.

Treatment

Cholic acid p. 71 is licensed for the treatment of inborn errors of primary bile acid synthesis due to an inborn deficiency of two specific liver enzymes. It acts by replacing some of the missing bile acids, therefore relieving the symptoms of the disease.

Chenodeoxycholic acid p. 71 is licensed for the treatment of inborn errors of primary bile acid synthesis due to a deficiency of one specific enzyme in the bile acid synthesis pathway when presenting as cerebrotendinous xanthomatosis.

Ursodeoxycholic acid p. 72 [unlicensed indication] has been used to treat inborn errors in primary bile acid synthesis, but there is an absence of evidence to recommend its use.

Primary biliary cholangitis

30-May-2017

Description of condition

Primary biliary cholangitis (or primary biliary cirrhosis) is a chronic cholestatic disease which develops due to progressive destruction of small and intermediate bile ducts within the liver, subsequently evolving to fibrosis and cirrhosis.

Treatment

EvGr Ursodeoxycholic acid p. 72 is recommended for the management of primary biliary cholangitis, including those with asymptomatic disease. It slows disease progression, but the effect on overall survival is uncertain. (A)

Smith-Lemli-Opitz syndrome

30-May-2017

Description of condition

Smith-Lemli-Opitz syndrome is an inborn error of cholesterol synthesis. It is characterised by multiple congenital anomalies, intellectual deficit, growth delay, microcephaly, and behavioural problems. The disease is present at birth, but may be detected in later childhood or adulthood in mild forms. Hypoglycaemia due to adrenal insufficiency can present as an acute manifestation.

Aims of treatment

There is currently no cure for Smith-Lemli-Opitz syndrome. Management is aimed at symptom relief and alleviation of functional disabilities.

Treatment

EvGr Children with Smith-Lemli-Opitz syndrome are treated with dietary cholesterol supplementation, including high cholesterol foods (such as egg yolks) or a suspension of pharmaceutical grade cholesterol p. 73 (available from Special-order manufacturers p. 1448 or specialist importing companies) to help improve growth failure and photosensitivity. ⟨E⟩ However, it is not clear who will benefit most from cholesterol treatment or how long it should continue.

EvGr In some cases bile acid supplements, such as chenodeoxycholic acid below [unlicensed] and ursodeoxycholic acid p. 72 [unlicensed indication] have been also used for this condition, but their use is not generally recommended. ⟨E⟩

BILE ACIDS

Chenodeoxycholic acid

05-Apr-2018

- **INDICATIONS AND DOSE**

Cerebrotendinous xanthomatosis (specialist use only)

▶ BY MOUTH

▸ Child: Initially 5 mg/kg daily in 3 divided doses, adjusted according to response; maximum 15 mg/kg per day; maximum 1000 mg per day

Defective synthesis of bile acid (specialist use only)

▶ BY MOUTH

▸ Neonate: Initially 5 mg/kg 3 times a day, reduced to 2.5 mg/kg 3 times a day.

▸ Child: Initially 5 mg/kg 3 times a day, reduced to 2.5 mg/kg 3 times a day

Smith-Lemli-Opitz syndrome (specialist use only)

▶ BY MOUTH

▸ Neonate: 7 mg/kg once daily, alternatively 7 mg/kg daily in divided doses.

▸ Child: 7 mg/kg once daily, alternatively 7 mg/kg daily in divided doses

- **UNLICENSED USE** Not licensed for defective synthesis of bile acid. Not licensed for Smith-Lemli-Opitz syndrome.
- **CONTRA-INDICATIONS** Non-functioning gall bladder · radio-opaque stones
- **INTERACTIONS** → Appendix 1: chenodeoxycholic acid
- **SIDE-EFFECTS** Constipation
- **PREGNANCY** Manufacturer advises avoid—fetotoxicity reported in *animal* studies.
- **HEPATIC IMPAIRMENT** Manufacturer advises monitor—no information available.
- **RENAL IMPAIRMENT** Manufacturer advises monitor—no information available.
- **MONITORING REQUIREMENTS** Manufacturer advises to monitor serum cholestanol levels and/or urine bile alcohols every 3 months during the initiation of therapy and dose adjustment, and then at least annually; liver function should also be monitored during initiation of therapy and then at least annually; additional or more frequent investigations may need to be undertaken to monitor therapy during periods of fast growth or concomitant disease.
- **DIRECTIONS FOR ADMINISTRATION** For administration *by mouth* in patients who are unable to swallow capsules and/or need to take a dose below 250 mg, manufacturer advises to add capsule contents to sodium bicarbonate solution 8.4%—for further information, consult product literature.
- **MEDICINAL FORMS** There can be variation in the licensing of different medicines containing the same drug.

Oral capsule

▸ Chenodeoxycholic acid (non-proprietary) ▼
Chenodeoxycholic acid 250 mg Chenodeoxycholic acid 250mg capsules | 100 capsule PoM £14,000.00 (Hospital only)

Cholic acid

04-Sep-2020

- **DRUG ACTION** Cholic acid is the predominant primary bile acid in humans, which can be used to provide a source of bile acid in patients with inborn deficiencies in bile acid synthesis.
- **INDICATIONS AND DOSE**

Inborn errors of primary bile acid synthesis (initiated by a specialist)

▶ BY MOUTH

▸ Child (body-weight up to 10 kg): 50 mg daily, then increased in steps of 50 mg daily in divided doses; usual dose 5–15 mg/kg daily in divided doses, dose to be given with food at the same time each day

▸ Child (body-weight 10 kg and above): Usual dose 5–15 mg/kg daily; increased in steps of 50 mg daily in divided doses if required, dose to be given with food at the same time each day; Usual maximum 500 mg/24 hours

- **INTERACTIONS** → Appendix 1: cholic acid
- **SIDE-EFFECTS** Cholelithiasis (long term use) · diarrhoea · pruritus

SIDE-EFFECTS, FURTHER INFORMATION Patients presenting with pruritus and/or persistent diarrhoea should be investigated for potential overdose by a serum and/or urine bile acid assay.
- **PREGNANCY** Limited data available—not known to be harmful, manufacturer advises continue treatment.
Monitoring Manufacturer advises monitor patient parameters more frequently in pregnancy.
- **BREAST FEEDING** Present in milk but not known to be harmful.
- **HEPATIC IMPAIRMENT** Manufacturer advises caution and stop treatment if there are signs of severe hepatic failure—limited information available (no experience with impairment from causes not related to inborn errors of primary bile acid synthesis).
Dose adjustments Manufacturer advises adjust dose as the degree of impairment improves during treatment.
- **MONITORING REQUIREMENTS** Manufacturer advises monitor serum and/or urine bile-acid concentrations every 3 months for the first year, then every 6 months for three years, then annually; monitor liver function tests at the same or greater frequency.
- **DIRECTIONS FOR ADMINISTRATION** Manufacturer advises capsules may be opened and the content added to infant formula, juice, fruit compote, or yoghurt for administration.
- **PATIENT AND CARER ADVICE** Counselling advised on administration.
- **MEDICINAL FORMS** There can be variation in the licensing of different medicines containing the same drug.

Oral capsule

CAUTIONARY AND ADVISORY LABELS 25

▸ Orphacol (Abacus Medicine Pharma Services Ltd) ▼
Cholic acid 50 mg Orphacol 50mg capsules | 30 capsule PoM £1,860.00
Cholic acid 250 mg Orphacol 250mg capsules | 30 capsule PoM £6,630.00

Ursodeoxycholic acid
03-Jul-2025

• **INDICATIONS AND DOSE**

Cholestasis

▶ BY MOUTH

▸ Neonate: 5 mg/kg 3 times a day, increased if necessary up to 10 mg/kg 3 times a day, dose to be adjusted according to response.

▸ Child 1–23 months: 5 mg/kg 3 times a day, increased if necessary up to 10 mg/kg 3 times a day, dose to be adjusted according to response

Improvement of hepatic metabolism of essential fatty acids and bile flow, in children with cystic fibrosis

▶ BY MOUTH

▸ Child: 20–30 mg/kg daily in 2–3 divided doses

Cholestasis associated with total parenteral nutrition

▶ BY MOUTH

▸ Neonate: 10 mg/kg 3 times a day.

▸ Child: 10 mg/kg 3 times a day

Sclerosing cholangitis

▶ BY MOUTH

▸ Child: 5–10 mg/kg 2–3 times a day, increased if necessary up to 15 mg/kg 3 times a day, dose to be adjusted according to response

• **UNLICENSED USE** Not licensed for use in children for the treatment of cholestasis, sclerosing cholangitis, cholestasis associated with total parenteral nutrition or the improvement of hepatic metabolism of essential fatty acids and bile flow in cystic fibrosis.

• **CONTRA-INDICATIONS** Acute inflammation of the gall bladder · frequent episodes of biliary colic · inflammatory diseases and other conditions of the colon, liver or small intestine which interfere with enterohepatic circulation of bile salts · non-functioning gall bladder · radio-opaque stones

• **INTERACTIONS** → Appendix 1: ursodeoxycholic acid

• **SIDE-EFFECTS**

▶ **Common or very common** Diarrhoea · pale faeces

▶ **Rare or very rare** Abdominal pain upper · cholelithiasis calcification · hepatic cirrhosis exacerbated · skin reactions

▶ **Frequency not known** Nausea · vomiting

• **CONCEPTION AND CONTRACEPTION** [EvGr] Females of childbearing potential should use effective contraception during treatment; low-oestrogen containing oral contraceptives or non-hormonal methods are recommended. ⟨M⟩

• **PREGNANCY** [EvGr] Avoid unless essential (toxicity in *animal* studies). ⟨M⟩

• **BREAST FEEDING** Not known to be harmful but manufacturer advises avoid.

• **HEPATIC IMPAIRMENT** Avoid in chronic liver disease (but used in primary biliary cirrhosis).

• **PATIENT AND CARER ADVICE** Patients should be given dietary advice (including avoidance of excessive cholesterol and calories).

Medicines for Children leaflet: Ursodeoxycholic acid for cholestasis and sclerosing cholangitis www.medicinesforchildren.org.uk/medicines/ursodeoxycholic-acid-for-cholestasis-and-sclerosing-cholangitis/

• **MEDICINAL FORMS** There can be variation in the licensing of different medicines containing the same drug. Forms available from special-order manufacturers include: oral suspension, oral solution

Oral tablet

CAUTIONARY AND ADVISORY LABELS 21

▸ Ursodeoxycholic acid (Non-proprietary)

Ursodeoxycholic acid 150 mg Ursodeoxycholic acid 150mg tablets | 60 tablet [PoM] £117.18 DT = £110.55

Ursodeoxycholic acid 300 mg Ursodeoxycholic acid 300mg tablets | 60 tablet [PoM] £91.25 DT = £87.44

▸ Cholurso (Mayoly UK Ltd)

Ursodeoxycholic acid 250 mg Cholurso 250mg tablets | 60 tablet [PoM] £18.00 DT = £18.00

Ursodeoxycholic acid 500 mg Cholurso 500mg tablets | 60 tablet [PoM] £45.00

▸ Ursofalk (Dr. Falk Pharma UK Ltd)

Ursodeoxycholic acid 500 mg Ursofalk 500mg tablets | 100 tablet [PoM] £80.00 DT = £69.07

▸ Ursonorm (PRO.MED.CS Praha a.s.)

Ursodeoxycholic acid 500 mg Ursonorm 500mg tablets | 60 tablet [PoM] £45.00 | 100 tablet [PoM] £79.00 DT = £69.07

Oral suspension

CAUTIONARY AND ADVISORY LABELS 21

▸ Deoxxa (Eclosix Ltd)

Ursodeoxycholic acid 50 mg per 1 ml Deoxxa 250mg/5ml oral suspension | 250 ml [PoM] £26.95 DT = £26.98 [SF]

▸ Ursofalk (Dr. Falk Pharma UK Ltd)

Ursodeoxycholic acid 50 mg per 1 ml Ursofalk 250mg/5ml oral suspension | 250 ml [PoM] £26.98 DT = £26.98 [SF]

Oral capsule

CAUTIONARY AND ADVISORY LABELS 21

▸ Ursodeoxycholic acid (Non-proprietary)

Ursodeoxycholic acid 250 mg Ursodeoxycholic acid 250mg capsules | 60 capsule [PoM] £29.00 DT = £12.88 | 100 capsule [PoM] £45.00

Ursodeoxycholic acid 500 mg Ursodeoxycholic acid 500mg capsules | 60 capsule [PoM] £24.00–£38.40 DT = £24.00

▸ Ursofalk (Dr. Falk Pharma UK Ltd)

Ursodeoxycholic acid 250 mg Ursofalk 250mg capsules | 60 capsule [PoM] £30.17 DT = £12.88 | 100 capsule [PoM] £31.88

▸ Ursonorm (PRO.MED.CS Praha a.s.)

Ursodeoxycholic acid 250 mg Ursonorm 250mg capsules | 60 capsule [PoM] £29.00 DT = £12.88

ILEAL BILE ACID TRANSPORTER INHIBITORS

Maralixibat
12-Dec-2025

• **DRUG ACTION** Maralixibat is an inhibitor of the ileal bile acid transporter that acts locally in the ileum to reduce re-uptake of bile acids from the intestines into the liver, thereby preventing their accumulation.

• **INDICATIONS AND DOSE**

Cholestatic pruritus [associated with Alagille syndrome] (under expert supervision)

▶ BY MOUTH

▸ Child 2 months–17 years: Initially 190 micrograms/kg once daily (max. per dose 14.25 mg) for 7 days, dose to be taken up to 30 minutes before or with a meal in the morning, then increased to 380 micrograms/kg once daily (max. per dose 28.5 mg), dose to be taken up to 30 minutes before or with a meal in the morning, reduce dose to 190 micrograms/kg once daily or interrupt treatment if poor tolerability; consider alternative treatment if no benefit after 3 months

• **SIDE-EFFECTS**

▶ **Common or very common** Abdominal pain · diarrhoea

• **PREGNANCY** [EvGr] Avoid (no information available). ⟨M⟩

• **BREAST FEEDING** [EvGr] Present in milk but amount probably too small to be harmful ⟨M⟩ (recommendation also supported by tertiary sources).

● **MONITORING REQUIREMENTS**
- EvGr Monitor liver function tests before starting and during treatment.
- Monitor INR and fat-soluble vitamin levels before starting treatment. ⟨M⟩

● **HANDLING AND STORAGE** Protect from light and discard within 130 days after first opening.

● **PATIENT AND CARER ADVICE**
Missed doses If a dose is more than 12 hours late, the missed dose should not be taken and the next dose should be taken at the normal time.

● **NATIONAL FUNDING/ACCESS DECISIONS**
For full details see funding body website
Scottish Medicines Consortium (SMC) decisions
- **Maralixibat (*Livmarli*®) for the treatment of cholestatic pruritus in patients with Alagille syndrome (ALGS) 2 months of age and older (December 2025) SMC No. SMC2806** Recommended with restrictions

● **MEDICINAL FORMS** There can be variation in the licensing of different medicines containing the same drug.
Oral solution
EXCIPIENTS: May contain Disodium edetate, propylene glycol
- Livmarli (Mirum Pharmaceuticals International BV) ▼
Maralixibat (as Maralixibat chloride) 9.5 mg per 1 ml Livmarli 9.5mg/ml oral solution | 30 ml PoM £43,970.00 (Hospital only) SF

Odevixibat 22-Jul-2022

● **DRUG ACTION** Odevixibat is an inhibitor of the ileal bile acid transporter that acts locally in the ileum to reduce re-uptake of bile acids from the intestines into the liver, thereby preventing their accumulation and resultant damage to liver tissue.

● **INDICATIONS AND DOSE**
Progressive familial intrahepatic cholestasis (under expert supervision)
- BY MOUTH
- Child 6 months–17 years: 40 micrograms/kg once daily (max. per dose 2.4 mg), to be taken in the morning, increased if necessary up to 120 micrograms/kg once daily (max. per dose 7.2 mg), to be taken in the morning, dose to be increased if adequate clinical response not achieved after 3 months at initial dose. Consider alternative treatment if no benefit after 6 months

● **CAUTIONS** Impaired gastrointestinal motility or enterohepatic circulation (potential for reduced efficacy)

● **SIDE-EFFECTS**
- **Common or very common** Diarrhoea · diarrhoea haemorrhagic · faeces soft · gastrointestinal discomfort · hepatomegaly

● **CONCEPTION AND CONTRACEPTION** EvGr Effective contraception required during treatment in females of childbearing potential (important: effectiveness of some oral contraceptives may be reduced; barrier contraception should be used). ⟨M⟩

● **PREGNANCY** EvGr Avoid—reproductive toxicity in *animal* studies. ⟨M⟩

● **BREAST FEEDING** EvGr Avoid—no information available. ⟨M⟩

● **MONITORING REQUIREMENTS** EvGr Monitor liver function tests, INR and fat-soluble vitamins before starting treatment, and then as clinically indicated. ⟨M⟩

● **DIRECTIONS FOR ADMINISTRATION** EvGr Capsules may be swallowed whole with water. Alternatively, capsules may be opened and the contents mixed into approximately 2 tablespoons of soft food (e.g. yoghurt, apple sauce) at or below room temperature, and administered immediately. ⟨M⟩

● **PATIENT AND CARER ADVICE** Patients or carers should be given advice on how to administer *Bylvay*® capsules.

● **NATIONAL FUNDING/ACCESS DECISIONS**
For full details see funding body website
NICE decisions
- **Odevixibat for treating progressive familial intrahepatic cholestasis (February 2022) NICE HST17** Recommended

● **MEDICINAL FORMS** There can be variation in the licensing of different medicines containing the same drug.
Oral capsule
- Bylvay (Ipsen Ltd) ▼
Odevixibat (as Odevixibat sesquihydrate) 200 microgram Bylvay 200microgram capsules | 30 capsule PoM £3,085.00 (Hospital only)
Odevixibat (as Odevixibat sesquihydrate) 400 microgram Bylvay 400microgram capsules | 30 capsule PoM £6,170.00 (Hospital only)
Odevixibat (as Odevixibat sesquihydrate) 600 microgram Bylvay 600microgram capsules | 30 capsule PoM £9,255.00 (Hospital only)
Odevixibat (as Odevixibat sesquihydrate) 1.2 mg Bylvay 1200microgram capsules | 30 capsule PoM £18,510.00 (Hospital only)

LIPIDS › STEROLS

Cholesterol 12-Aug-2020

● **INDICATIONS AND DOSE**
Smith-Lemli-Opitz syndrome
- BY MOUTH
- Neonate: 5–10 mg/kg 3–4 times a day.
- Child: 5–10 mg/kg 3–4 times a day, doses up to 15 mg/kg 4 times daily have been used

● **UNLICENSED USE** Not licensed.

● **CONTRA-INDICATIONS** For contra-indications, consult product literature.

● **CAUTIONS** For advice on cautions, consult product literature.

● **DIRECTIONS FOR ADMINISTRATION** Expert sources advise cholesterol powder can be mixed with a vegetable oil before administration.

● **MEDICINAL FORMS** Forms available from special-order manufacturers include: oral suspension, oral powder

8.2 Oesophageal varices

Other drugs used for Oesophageal varices Carvedilol, p. 146 · Propranolol hydrochloride, p. 123 · Vasopressin, p. 74

PITUITARY AND HYPOTHALAMIC HORMONES AND ANALOGUES › VASOPRESSIN AND ANALOGUES

Terlipressin acetate 14-Apr-2023

● **INDICATIONS AND DOSE**
GLYPRESSIN® INJECTION
Adjunct in acute massive haemorrhage of gastro-intestinal tract or oesophageal varices (under expert supervision)
- BY INTRAVENOUS INJECTION
- Child 12–17 years (body-weight up to 50 kg): Initially 2 mg every 4 hours until bleeding controlled, then reduced to 1 mg every 4 hours if required, maximum duration 48 hours

continued →

- Child 12-17 years (body-weight 50 kg and above): Initially 2 mg every 4 hours until bleeding controlled, reduced if not tolerated to 1 mg every 4 hours, maximum duration 48 hours

VARIQUEL® INJECTION

Adjunct in acute massive haemorrhage of gastro-intestinal tract or oesophageal varices (under expert supervision)

▶ BY INTRAVENOUS INJECTION
- Child 12-17 years (body-weight up to 50 kg): Initially 1 mg, then 1 mg every 4–6 hours for up to 72 hours
- Child 12-17 years (body-weight 50-69 kg): Initially 1.5 mg, then 1 mg every 4–6 hours for up to 72 hours
- Child 12-17 years (body-weight 70 kg and above): Initially 2 mg, then 1 mg every 4–6 hours for up to 72 hours

- **UNLICENSED USE** Unlicensed for use in children.
- **CAUTIONS** Arrhythmia · electrolyte and fluid disturbances · heart disease · history of QT-interval prolongation · respiratory disease · septic shock · uncontrolled hypertension · vascular disease
- **SIDE-EFFECTS**

▶ **Common or very common** Abdominal cramps · arrhythmias · diarrhoea · headache · hypertension · hypotension · nausea · pallor · peripheral ischaemia · vasoconstriction

▶ **Uncommon** Chest pain · cyanosis · fluid overload · heart failure · hot flush · hyponatraemia · injection site necrosis · intestinal ischaemia · ischaemic heart disease · lymphangitis · myocardial infarction · pulmonary oedema · respiratory disorders · seizure · skin reactions · uterine ischaemia · vomiting

▶ **Rare or very rare** Dyspnoea · stroke

▶ **Frequency not known** QT interval prolongation

- **PREGNANCY** Avoid unless benefits outweigh risk—uterine contractions and increased intra-uterine pressure in early pregnancy, and decreased uterine blood flow reported.
- **BREAST FEEDING** Avoid unless benefits outweigh risk—no information available.
- **RENAL IMPAIRMENT** [EvGr] Use with caution in chronic renal failure. ⟨M⟩
- **DIRECTIONS FOR ADMINISTRATION**

VARIQUEL® INJECTION For *intravenous injection*, give undiluted over at least 1 minute.

- **HANDLING AND STORAGE** Store solutions for injection in a refrigerator (2–8°C) and protect from light.

- **MEDICINAL FORMS** There can be variation in the licensing of different medicines containing the same drug.

Solution for injection

▸ Terlipressin acetate (Non-proprietary)

Terlipressin acetate 120 microgram per 1 ml Terlipressin 1mg/8.5ml solution for injection vials | 5 vial [PoM] £95.00 (Hospital only)

Terlipressin 1mg/8.5ml solution for injection ampoules | 5 ampoule [PoM] £96.95 (Hospital only)

Terlipressin acetate 200 microgram per 1 ml Terlipressin 1mg/5ml solution for injection vials | 5 vial [PoM] £96.95 (Hospital only)

Powder and solvent for solution for injection

▸ Terlipressin acetate (Non-proprietary)

Terlipressin acetate 1 mg Terlipressin 1mg powder and solvent for solution for injection vials | 5 vial [PoM] £92.33 (Hospital only)

▸ Glypressin (Ipsen Ltd)

Terlipressin acetate 1 mg Glypressin 1mg powder and solvent for solution for injection vials | 5 vial [PoM] £92.33

Vasopressin

17-Sep-2024

(ADH; Antidiuretic hormone)

- **DRUG ACTION** Vasopressin is an endogenous hormone with a direct antidiuretic effect on the kidney; it is given in the synthetic form of argipressin.

- **INDICATIONS AND DOSE**

Adjunct in acute massive haemorrhage of gastrointestinal tract or oesophageal varices (specialist use only)

▶ BY CONTINUOUS INTRAVENOUS INFUSION
- Child: (consult local protocol)

DOSE EQUIVALENCE AND CONVERSION
- Argipressin 1 unit is equivalent to vasopressin 1 unit.

- **UNLICENSED USE** Not licensed for use in children.
- **CONTRA-INDICATIONS** Chronic nephritis (until reasonable blood nitrogen concentrations attained) · vascular disease (especially disease of coronary arteries) unless extreme caution
- **CAUTIONS** Asthma · avoid fluid overload · conditions which might be aggravated by water retention · epilepsy · heart failure · hypertension · migraine
- **INTERACTIONS** → Appendix 1: vasopressin
- **SIDE-EFFECTS** Abdominal pain · angina pectoris · bronchospasm · cardiac arrest · chest pain · diarrhoea · flatulence · fluid imbalance · gangrene · headache · hyperhidrosis · hypertension · musculoskeletal chest pain · nausea · pallor · peripheral ischaemia · tremor · urticaria · vertigo · vomiting
- **PREGNANCY** Oxytocic effect in third trimester.
- **BREAST FEEDING** Not known to be harmful.

- **MEDICINAL FORMS** There can be variation in the licensing of different medicines containing the same drug. Forms available from special-order manufacturers include: solution for injection

Solution for injection

▸ Vasopressin (Non-proprietary)

Argipressin 20 unit per 1 ml Argipressin 20units/1ml solution for injection ampoules | 10 ampoule [PoM] £750.00–£754.86 (Hospital only)

9 Obesity

Obesity

29-Nov-2023

Description of condition

Overweight, obesity, or increased central adiposity are associated with an increased risk of developing a number of health conditions, including type 2 diabetes, hypertension, dyslipidaemia, and respiratory and musculoskeletal conditions. They are also associated with psychological and psychiatric morbidities. Children living with obesity are more likely to be obese as adults, and have a higher risk of morbidity, disability and premature mortality in adulthood.

BMI and waist-to-height ratio are measures of obesity and central adiposity, respectively. Both these measures aid the evaluation of health risks in overweight and obese children, although BMI alone should be interpreted with caution as it is not a direct measure of central adiposity. Assessing the BMI of children is more complicated than for adults because it changes as they grow and mature, with different growth patterns seen between boys and girls.

The following growth reference charts are recommended to determine the weight status of children: the Royal College of Paediatrics and Child Health UK WHO growth charts, available at: www.rcpch.ac.uk/resources/uk-who-growth-charts-2-18-years and BMI charts, available at: www.rcpch.ac.uk/resources/body-mass-index-bmi-chart.

Overweight and obesity in children are defined as follows:

- overweight: BMI 91st centile (+1.34 standard deviations (SDs) above the mean)
- clinical obesity: BMI 98th centile (+2.05 SDs above the mean)
- severe obesity: BMI 99.6th centile (+2.68 SDs above the mean)

Clinical judgement should be used when interpreting BMI below the 91st centile, especially as children in the healthy weight category may nevertheless have increased central adiposity.

Central adiposity based on waist-to-height ratio in children aged 5 years and over is defined as follows:

- increased central adiposity: waist-to-height ratio 0.5 to 0.59
- high central adiposity: waist-to-height ratio 0.6 or more

Aims of treatment

Children who are overweight or obese and are no longer growing taller will ultimately need to lose weight and maintain weight loss to improve their BMI. Preventing further weight gain while making lifestyle changes may be an appropriate short-term aim for children who are still growing taller.

Overview

EvGr Weight management interventions should be delivered by staff experienced in the management of overweight and obesity, and the goals of management agreed with the child and their parents/carers. (A)

An initial assessment should consider potential underlying causes (e.g. hypothyroidism) and a review of the appropriateness of current medications which are known to cause weight gain, e.g. atypical antipsychotics, beta-adrenoceptor blocking drugs, insulin (when used in the treatment of type 2 diabetes), sodium valproate, and tricyclic antidepressants. Children should be assessed for comorbidities such as hypertension, hyperinsulinaemia, dyslipidaemia, type 2 diabetes, psychosocial dysfunction, and exacerbation of conditions such as asthma.

Lifestyle changes

EvGr Children who are overweight or obese should be encouraged to engage in a sustainable weight management programme which includes behavioural change strategies to increase physical activity and improve diet and eating behaviour. These changes should be encouraged within the whole family. Any dietary changes should be age appropriate and consistent with healthy eating recommendations. (A)

Drug treatment

EvGr Drug treatment should **never** be used as the sole element of treatment and should be used as part of an overall weight management plan. Drug treatment is not generally recommended for children younger than 12 years, unless there are exceptional circumstances, such as severe comorbidities. In children aged over 12 years, orlistat below [unlicensed use] may be considered if physical comorbidities, such as orthopaedic problems or sleep apnoea, or severe psychological comorbidities are present. Treatment should be started and monitored in a specialist paediatric setting by experienced multidisciplinary teams. An initial 6–12 month trial is recommended, with regular reviews to assess effectiveness, side-effects and adherence. Treatment may also be used to maintain weight loss rather than to continue to lose weight.

Under expert supervision, setmelanotide p. 76 may be considered in children with specific genetic conditions. (A)

Surgery

EvGr Surgical intervention is not generally recommended in children, but may be considered in exceptional circumstances and where physiological maturity has been achieved or is nearly achieved. (A)

Useful Resources

Obesity: identification, assessment and management. National Institute for Health and Care Excellence. Clinical guideline 189. November 2014 (updated July 2023). www.nice.org.uk/guidance/cg189

ANTIOBESITY DRUGS

Orlistat

11-Nov-2022

- **DRUG ACTION** Orlistat, a lipase inhibitor, reduces the absorption of dietary fat.
- **INDICATIONS AND DOSE**

Adjunct in obesity

▶ BY MOUTH

▶ Child 12–17 years (initiated by a specialist): 120 mg up to 3 times a day, dose to be taken immediately before, during, or up to 1 hour after each main meal, continue treatment beyond 12 weeks only under specialist supervision, if a meal is missed or contains no fat, the dose of orlistat should be omitted

- **UNLICENSED USE** Not licensed for use in children.
- **CONTRA-INDICATIONS** Cholestasis · chronic malabsorption syndrome
- **CAUTIONS** Chronic kidney disease · may impair absorption of fat-soluble vitamins · volume depletion

CAUTIONS, FURTHER INFORMATION Vitamin supplementation (especially of vitamin D) may be considered if there is concern about deficiency of fat-soluble vitamins.

- **INTERACTIONS** → Appendix 1: orlistat
- **SIDE-EFFECTS**

▶ **Common or very common** Abdominal pain (may be minimised by reduced fat intake) · anxiety · diarrhoea · gastrointestinal disorders

▶ **Frequency not known** Anorectal haemorrhage · bullous dermatitis · cholelithiasis · diverticulitis · hepatitis · oxalate nephropathy · pancreatitis · renal failure

- **PREGNANCY** Use with caution.
- **BREAST FEEDING** Avoid—no information available.
- **MEDICINAL FORMS** There can be variation in the licensing of different medicines containing the same drug.

Oral capsule

▶ Orlistat (Non-proprietary)

Orlistat 120 mg Orlistat 120mg capsules | 84 capsule PoM £31.21 DT = £13.61

▶ Alli (Haleon UK Trading Ltd)

Orlistat 60 mg Alli 60mg capsules | 84 capsule P £33.77 DT = £33.77

▶ Orlos (Crescent Pharma Ltd)

Orlistat 60 mg Orlos 60mg capsules | 84 capsule P £24.56 DT = £33.77

▶ Xenical (Neon Healthcare Ltd)

Orlistat 120 mg Xenical 120mg capsules | 84 capsule PoM £31.63 DT = £13.61

Setmelanotide

05-Aug-2024

● **DRUG ACTION** Setmelanotide is a centrally-acting selective melanocortin-4 receptor agonist that regulates hunger, satiety, and energy expenditure, thereby promoting weight loss.

● **INDICATIONS AND DOSE**

Obesity with underlying genetic aetiology [pro-opiomelanocortin (POMC), proprotein convertase subtilisin/kexin type 1 (PCSK1), or leptin receptor (LEPR) deficiency] (under expert supervision)

▶ BY SUBCUTANEOUS INJECTION

▸ Child 6–11 years: 0.5 mg once daily for 2 weeks, to be administered in the morning, then increased if tolerated to 1 mg once daily for 2 weeks, to be administered in the morning; increased if tolerated to 2 mg once daily, to be administered in the morning, then increased if necessary up to 2.5 mg once daily, to be administered in the morning

▸ Child 12–17 years: 1 mg once daily for 2 weeks, to be administered in the morning, then increased if tolerated to 2 mg once daily, to be administered in the morning; increased if necessary to 2.5 mg once daily, to be administered in the morning, then increased if necessary up to 3 mg once daily, to be administered in the morning

Obesity with underlying genetic aetiology [Bardet-Biedl syndrome (BBS)] (under expert supervision)

▶ BY SUBCUTANEOUS INJECTION

▸ Child 6–15 years: 1 mg once daily for 1 week, to be administered in the morning, if not tolerated, reduce dose to 0.5 mg once daily; then if tolerated, increase dose to 1 mg once daily, then increased if tolerated to 2 mg once daily for 1 week, to be administered in the morning, then increased if tolerated to 3 mg once daily, to be administered in the morning

▸ Child 16–17 years: 2 mg once daily for 2 weeks, to be administered in the morning, if not tolerated, reduce dose to 1 mg once daily; then if tolerated, increase dose to 2 mg once daily, then increased if tolerated to 3 mg once daily, to be administered in the morning

● **CAUTIONS** Contains benzyl alcohol as an excipient (risk of allergic reactions, and of metabolic acidosis due to accumulation over time)

● **SIDE-EFFECTS**

▶ **Common or very common** Alopecia · asthenia · constipation · depression · diarrhoea · dizziness · dry mouth · gastrointestinal discomfort · headaches · hot flush · hyperhidrosis · muscle complaints · nausea · neoplasms · pain · sexual dysfunction · skin reactions · sleep disorders · vertigo · vomiting

▶ **Uncommon** Altered smell sensation · anxiety · arthralgia · chest pain · chills · cough · drowsiness · eye naevus · gastrointestinal disorders · genital abnormalities · genital disorder female · hair colour changes · hyperaesthesia · jaundice ocular · mood altered · nail discolouration · nail disorder · oral disorders · rhinorrhoea · scleral discolouration · taste altered · temperature sensation altered · yawning

▶ **Frequency not known** Hyperpigmentation disorders · tongue discolouration

● **PREGNANCY** EvGr No evidence of teratogenicity in *animal* studies, but lack of information in pregnant women. Avoid initiation during pregnancy—weight loss during pregnancy may cause fetal harm. If pregnancy occurs during treatment in a patient who is still losing weight, consider reducing dose or discontinuing treatment. If pregnancy occurs during treatment in a patient who has reached a stable weight, consider continuing treatment. Ⓜ

Monitoring EvGr Monitor weight against recommended weight gain if treatment is continued during pregnancy. Ⓜ

● **BREAST FEEDING** EvGr Avoid—present in milk in *animal* studies. Ⓜ

● **HEPATIC IMPAIRMENT** EvGr Avoid (no information available). Ⓜ

● **RENAL IMPAIRMENT** EvGr Avoid in end-stage renal disease (no information available). Ⓜ

Dose adjustments EvGr Start with reduced dose in severe impairment (risk of increased exposure—consult product literature). Ⓜ

● **MONITORING REQUIREMENTS**

▶ EvGr Full body examination of pre-existing and new skin pigmentary lesions is advised at baseline and annually during treatment.

▶ Monitor heart rate and blood pressure at least every 6 months during treatment.

▶ Monitor patients with depression during treatment for signs of suicidal thoughts or behaviours.

▶ Monitor height and weight against growth charts to evaluate the impact of treatment-related weight loss on growth and maturation. Ⓜ

● **DIRECTIONS FOR ADMINISTRATION** EvGr Allow the vial to reach room temperature prior to administration. Inject into the abdomen (except for the 5 cm around the navel); rotate injection site and avoid skin that is red, swollen, or irritated. Ⓜ Patients may self-administer *Imcivree*® after appropriate training in preparation and administration.

● **HANDLING AND STORAGE** Store unopened vials in a refrigerator (2–8°C) and protect from light; may be stored at room temperature (below 30°C) for up to 30 days. Once opened, vials may be stored for a maximum of 28 days at 2–30°C.

● **PATIENT AND CARER ADVICE** Patients who have a penile erection lasting longer than 4 hours should be advised to seek emergency medical attention for potential priapism.

Self-administration Patients and their carers should be given training in subcutaneous injection technique.

Missed doses If a dose is missed, the missed dose should be omitted and the next dose administered at the normal time.

● **NATIONAL FUNDING/ACCESS DECISIONS**

For full details see funding body website

NICE decisions

▶ **Setmelanotide for treating obesity caused by LEPR or POMC deficiency (July 2022)** NICE HST21 Recommended

▶ **Setmelanotide for treating obesity and hyperphagia in Bardet-Biedl syndrome (May 2024)** NICE HST31 Recommended with restrictions

● **MEDICINAL FORMS** There can be variation in the licensing of different medicines containing the same drug.

Solution for injection

EXCIPIENTS: May contain Benzyl alcohol, disodium edetate

▸ **Imcivree** (Rhythm Pharmaceuticals UK Ltd) ▼

Setmelanotide 10 mg per 1 ml Imcivree 10mg/1ml solution for injection vials | 1 vial PoM £2,376.00 (Hospital only)

BLOOD GLUCOSE LOWERING DRUGS › GLUCAGON-LIKE PEPTIDE-1 RECEPTOR AGONISTS

Semaglutide

26-Feb-2026

● **DRUG ACTION** Semaglutide binds to, and activates, the GLP-1 (glucagon-like peptide-1) receptor to increase insulin secretion, suppress glucagon secretion, and slow gastric emptying.

● **INDICATIONS AND DOSE**

WEGOVY®

Weight management [in conjunction with dietary measures and increased physical activity in individuals with a BMI in the 95th percentile or more, and body-weight above 60 kg]

▶ BY SUBCUTANEOUS INJECTION

▶ Child 12–17 years: Initially 0.25 mg once weekly for at least 4 weeks, then increased if tolerated to 0.5 mg once weekly for at least 4 weeks, then increased if tolerated to 1 mg once weekly for at least 4 weeks, then increased if tolerated to 1.7 mg once weekly for at least 4 weeks, then maintenance 2.4 mg once weekly

DOSE ADJUSTMENTS DUE TO INTERACTIONS

▶ Dose of concomitant insulin or sulfonylurea may need to be reduced.

IMPORTANT SAFETY INFORMATION

MHRA/CHM ADVICE: GLP-1 RECEPTOR AGONISTS: REPORTS OF DIABETIC KETOACIDOSIS WHEN CONCOMITANT INSULIN WAS RAPIDLY REDUCED OR DISCONTINUED (JUNE 2019)

Serious and life-threatening cases of diabetic ketoacidosis have been reported in patients with type 2 diabetes mellitus on a combination of insulin and the glucagon-like peptide-1 (GLP-1) receptor agonist exenatide, liraglutide, or dulaglutide, particularly after discontinuation or rapid dose reduction of concomitant insulin. The MHRA has not currently received any UK reports of diabetic ketoacidosis with the GLP-1 receptor agonists lixisenatide and semaglutide but this risk cannot be excluded. Healthcare professionals are advised that any dose reduction of insulin should be done in a stepwise manner with careful blood glucose self-monitoring, particularly when GLP-1 receptor agonist therapy is initiated. Patients should be informed of the risk factors for and signs and symptoms of diabetic ketoacidosis, and advised to seek immediate medical attention if these develop.

MHRA/CHM ADVICE: *OZEMPIC®* (SEMAGLUTIDE): VIGILANCE REQUIRED DUE TO POTENTIALLY HARMFUL FALSIFIED PRODUCTS (NOVEMBER 2023)

Falsified *Ozempic®* preparations, some containing insulin, have been found in the UK. Healthcare professionals are advised to remind patients to always obtain prescription medicines from qualified healthcare providers, and not to use preparations they suspect are falsified as this may lead to serious harm. Healthcare professionals should remain vigilant for symptoms associated with hypoglycaemia in patients who may have obtained a falsified preparation containing insulin; patients should be advised to seek immediate medical attention if such symptoms occur. Suspected falsified preparations should be quarantined and reported to the Yellow Card scheme.

MHRA/CHM ADVICE: GLP-1 RECEPTOR AGONISTS: REMINDER OF THE POTENTIAL SIDE EFFECTS AND TO BE AWARE OF THE POTENTIAL FOR MISUSE (OCTOBER 2024)

The MHRA reminds healthcare professionals to ensure that patients are aware of potential side-effects associated with glucagon-like peptide-1 (GLP-1) receptor agonists following anecdotal evidence and Yellow Card reports suggesting misuse of these medicines for weight management outside of their licence. The only GLP-1 receptor agonists licensed for weight management are liraglutide p. 562 (*Saxenda®*), semaglutide above (*Wegovy®*), and tirzepatide (*Mounjaro®*; licensed in adults only), which is also a glucose-dependent insulinotropic polypeptide (GIP) receptor agonist. The benefits and risks of these medicines for weight loss in individuals who are not obese, or who are not overweight with weight-related co-morbidities, have not been studied.

Healthcare professionals should inform patients and carers upon initial prescription and at any dose increase about the common risk of gastro-intestinal side-effects (including nausea, vomiting, diarrhoea, and constipation) associated with GLP-1 receptor agonists; these are usually non-serious but can persist for several days and may lead to serious complications such as severe dehydration and kidney damage, resulting in hospitalisation. For this reason, patients should be advised to stay well hydrated by drinking plenty of fluids throughout treatment. They should also be informed of other serious but less common side-effects, including acute gallstone disease, pancreatitis, and serious allergic reactions. Healthcare professionals are advised that hypoglycaemia can occur in non-diabetic patients using semaglutide for weight management and therefore to ensure patients and carers know the signs and symptoms to be aware of, and to seek immediate medical attention if these occur.

Patients and carers should be advised to ensure that prescriptions are only obtained from registered healthcare professionals and that private prescriptions are dispensed from authorised sources to avoid the risk of receiving falsified pens (see also advice issued in November 2023, above). Patients and carers should consult the patient information leaflet for instructions on the use of GLP-1 receptor agonists, and be advised to only administer the prescribed dose.

MHRA/CHM ADVICE: GLP-1 AND DUAL GIP/GLP-1 RECEPTOR AGONISTS: POTENTIAL RISK OF PULMONARY ASPIRATION DURING GENERAL ANAESTHESIA OR DEEP SEDATION (JANUARY 2025)

An EU review has concluded that glucagon-like peptide-1 (GLP-1) and dual glucose-dependent insulinotropic polypeptide (GIP)/GLP-1 receptor agonists are associated with a potential risk of pulmonary aspiration in patients undergoing surgery or procedures requiring general anaesthesia or deep sedation. These medicines are known to slow gastric emptying, thereby increasing the risk of residual gastric contents despite preoperative fasting, which could lead to pulmonary aspiration and other severe complications, such as aspiration pneumonia.

The MHRA advises healthcare professionals to identify the increased risk of aspiration as early as possible, ideally at the pre-assessment clinic before surgery, in patients using GLP-1 or dual GIP/GLP-1 receptor agonists. Anaesthetists should complete an individualised preoperative risk assessment and consider the following:

- patients with underlying diabetic gastroparesis, as well as other co-morbidities such as obesity or gastroesophageal reflux disease, and symptoms of delayed gastric emptying (such as nausea, vomiting and abdominal pain) may have a higher risk of aspiration;
- directly asking patients or their carers about their use of GLP-1 or dual GIP/GLP-1 receptor agonists, as private prescriptions may not be included in the patient's medical notes or drug history, and patients who may have purchased these medications for use in aesthetic weight loss may not readily disclose this

information (see also advice issued in October 2024, above).

There is limited evidence to support any recommendations on a time frame to withhold GLP-1 or dual GIP/GLP-1 receptor agonists prior to anaesthesia, new fasting guidelines, or an appropriate medical procedure to confirm an empty stomach. Anaesthetists should manage aspiration risk in line with usual anaesthetic practice and retain flexibility to provide individualised assessment.

Healthcare professionals should counsel patients or their carers to continue taking their prescribed medicines and not stop treatment without first discussing with their doctor. They should also be advised regarding the risk of aspiration and that there may be a need to modify pre-procedure instruction and anaesthetic technique.

MHRA/CHM ADVICE: GLP-1 RECEPTOR AGONISTS AND DUAL GLP-1/GIP RECEPTOR AGONISTS: STRENGTHENED WARNINGS ON ACUTE PANCREATITIS, INCLUDING NECROTISING AND FATAL CASES (JANUARY 2026)

Following rare reports of necrotising and fatal pancreatitis associated with glucagon-like peptide-1 (GLP-1) and dual GLP-1/glucose-dependent insulinotropic polypeptide (GIP) receptor agonists, healthcare professionals are advised to:

- remain vigilant to the risk, and signs and symptoms of acute pancreatitis;
- use these drugs with caution in patients with a history of pancreatitis;
- enquire about privately prescribed GLP-1 or dual GLP-1/GIP receptor agonists if a patient presents with suspected symptoms, as such use may not appear in their medical history;
- discontinue treatment immediately if pancreatitis is suspected, and not to restart treatment if confirmed;
- counsel patients or their carers to seek urgent medical attention if they develop persistent severe abdominal pain that may radiate to the back, and may be accompanied by nausea and vomiting.

MHRA/CHM ADVICE: SEMAGLUTIDE (*WEGOVY*®, *OZEMPIC*®, AND *RYBELSUS*®): RISK OF NON-ARTERITIC ANTERIOR ISCHAEMIC OPTIC NEUROPATHY (NAION) (FEBRUARY 2026)

Semaglutide therapy has been associated with very rare reports of non-arteritic anterior ischaemic optic neuropathy (NAION), a condition that can cause sudden, painless vision loss, typically in one eye, often described as a blurring or cloudiness of vision. Healthcare professionals are advised to:

- enquire about privately prescribed semaglutide if a patient presents with suspected symptoms, as such use may not appear in their medical history;
- urgently refer patients with suspected symptoms for an ophthalmological examination;
- discontinue treatment immediately if NAION is confirmed;
- counsel patients or their carers to seek urgent medical attention if signs and symptoms of NAION, including rapidly worsening eyesight in one or both eyes, occur.

- **CAUTIONS** Diabetic retinopathy (in patients treated with insulin) · general anaesthesia or deep sedation (risk of pulmonary aspiration due to delayed gastric emptying) · history of pancreatitis · severe congestive heart failure (no information available)
- **INTERACTIONS** → Appendix 1: glucagon-like peptide-1 receptor agonists
- **SIDE-EFFECTS**
- ▶ **Common or very common** Alopecia · burping · cholelithiasis · constipation · diabetic retinopathy (in patients with type 2 diabetes) · diarrhoea · dizziness · dysaesthesia · fatigue · gastrointestinal discomfort · gastrointestinal disorders · headache · hypoglycaemia · nausea · taste altered · vomiting
- ▶ **Uncommon** Hypotension · pancreatitis acute (discontinue)
- ▶ **Rare or very rare** Angioedema · optic neuropathy (discontinue)
- ▶ **Frequency not known** Necrotising pancreatitis (discontinue)

SIDE-EFFECTS, FURTHER INFORMATION Discontinue if symptoms of acute pancreatitis occur, such as persistent, severe abdominal pain; fatal cases reported. If pancreatitis confirmed, do not restart treatment.

- **CONCEPTION AND CONTRACEPTION** EvGr Females of childbearing potential should use effective contraception during and for at least 2 months after stopping treatment. Discontinue treatment at least 2 months before planned pregnancy. ⟨M⟩
- **PREGNANCY** Manufacturer advises avoid—toxicity in *animal* studies.
- **BREAST FEEDING** Manufacturer advises avoid—present in milk in *animal* studies.
- **HEPATIC IMPAIRMENT** Manufacturer advises caution (limited information in severe impairment).
- **RENAL IMPAIRMENT** Manufacturer advises avoid in end-stage renal disease.
- **DIRECTIONS FOR ADMINISTRATION** For *subcutaneous injection*, inject into the abdomen, thigh, or upper arm.
- **PRESCRIBING AND DISPENSING INFORMATION** Semaglutide is a biological medicine. Biological medicines must be prescribed and dispensed by brand name, see *Biological medicines* and *Biosimilar medicines*, under Guidance on prescribing p. 1; record the brand name and batch number after each administration.

WEGOVY® EvGr Discontinue treatment if BMI has not reduced by at least 5% after 12 weeks on maintenance dose or maximum tolerated dose. ⟨M⟩

- **HANDLING AND STORAGE** Store injection pens in a refrigerator (2–8°C)—after first use can also be stored at room temperature (below 30°C) for up to 6 weeks; keep cap on pen to protect from light.
- **PATIENT AND CARER ADVICE** Patients and their carers should be advised that glucagon-like peptide-1 (GLP-1) receptor agonists should only be used if they have been prescribed by a healthcare professional and should not be switched, including between brands containing the same GLP-1 receptor agonist, without prior consultation, in order to reduce the risk of adverse effects or loss of treatment efficacy.

Patients and their carers should be given advice on how to administer semaglutide injection and when to discard it, including not attempting to extract any remaining medicine.

Acute pancreatitis Patients and their carers should be told how to recognise signs and symptoms of acute pancreatitis and advised to seek immediate medical attention if symptoms such as persistent, severe abdominal pain develop.

Dehydration Patients and their carers should be informed of the potential risk of dehydration in relation to gastro-intestinal side-effects and advised to take precautions to avoid fluid depletion.

Information for patients The MHRA has produced guidance for patients on GLP-1 medicines for weight loss: www.gov.uk/government/publications/glp-1-medicines-for-weight-loss-and-diabetes-what-you-need-to-know/glp-1-medicines-for-weight-loss-and-diabetes-what-you-need-to-know.

Missed doses If a dose is more than 5 days late, the missed dose should not be administered and the next dose should be administered at the normal time. If more doses are missed, consider re-starting at a reduced dose.

Driving and skilled tasks Patients and carers should be counselled on the effects on driving and performance of skilled tasks—increased risk of dizziness, particularly during the dose escalation period.

● MEDICINAL FORMS There can be variation in the licensing of different medicines containing the same drug.

Solution for injection

EXCIPIENTS: May contain Propylene glycol

▸ Wegovy FlexTouch (Novo Nordisk Ltd) ▼

Semaglutide 676 microgram per 1 ml Wegovy FlexTouch 0.25mg/0.37ml solution for injection 1.5ml pre-filled pens | 1 pre-filled disposable injection PoM £73.25 DT = £73.25

Semaglutide 1.34 mg per 1 ml Wegovy FlexTouch 1mg/0.75ml solution for injection 3ml pre-filled pens | 1 pre-filled disposable injection PoM £73.25 DT = £73.25

Wegovy FlexTouch 0.5mg/0.37ml solution for injection 1.5ml pre-filled pens | 1 pre-filled disposable injection PoM £73.25 DT = £73.25

Semaglutide 2.27 mg per 1 ml Wegovy FlexTouch 1.7mg/0.75ml solution for injection 3ml pre-filled pens | 1 pre-filled disposable injection PoM £124.53 DT = £124.53

Semaglutide 3.2 mg per 1 ml Wegovy FlexTouch 2.4mg/0.75ml solution for injection 3ml pre-filled pens | 1 pre-filled disposable injection PoM £175.80 DT = £175.80

10 Rectal and anal disorders

10.1 Anal fissures

Anal fissure

31-Aug-2016

Description of condition

An anal fissure is a tear or ulcer in the lining of the anal canal, immediately within the anal margin. Clinical features of anal fissure include bleeding and persistent pain on defecation, and a linear split in the anal mucosa. Constipation (passage of hard stools) is the most common cause in children. The majority of anal fissures are posterior, and an underlying cause should be considered (secondary anal fissure) if fissures are multiple, occur laterally, and are refractory to treatment.

EvGr Suspect sexual abuse if a child has an anal fissure, and if constipation, Crohn's disease or passing hard stools have been excluded as the cause (see also *Useful resources* below). Ⓐ

Aims of treatment

The aim of treatment is to relieve pain and promote healing of the fissure.

Drug treatment

EvGr Initial management of acute anal fissures should focus on ensuring that stools are soft and easily passed. Osmotic laxatives, such as lactulose p. 46 or macrogols (macrogol 3350 with potassium chloride, sodium bicarbonate and sodium chloride p. 47), are recommended. A simple analgesic (such as paracetamol p. 325 or ibuprofen p. 821, may be offered for prolonged burning pain following defecation.

Children should be referred to a paediatric specialist if the anal fissure has not healed following two weeks of initial management, or earlier if there is significant pain. Ⓐ

Useful Resources

Child maltreatment: when to suspect maltreatment in under 18s. National Institute for Health and Care Excellence. Clinical guideline 89. July 2009.
www.nice.org.uk/guidance/cg89

10.2 Haemorrhoids

Haemorrhoids

05-Feb-2024

Description of condition

Haemorrhoids, or piles, are abnormal swellings of the vascular mucosal anal cushions around the anus. Internal haemorrhoids arise above the dentate line and are usually painless unless they become strangulated. External haemorrhoids originate below the dentate line and can be itchy or painful. Haemorrhoids in children are rare but may occur in infants with portal hypertension.

Aims of treatment

The aims of treatment are to reduce the symptoms (pain, bleeding and swelling), promote healing, and prevent recurrence.

Non-drug treatment

EvGr Stools should be kept soft and easy to pass (to minimise straining) by increasing dietary fibre and fluid intake. Advice about perianal hygiene is helpful to aid healing and reduce irritation and itching. Ⓐ

Drug treatment

EvGr If constipation is present, it should be treated, see Constipation p. 44.

A simple analgesic, such as paracetamol p. 325, can be used for pain relief. NSAIDs should be avoided if rectal bleeding is present.

Symptomatic treatment with a locally applied preparation is appropriate for short periods. Ⓔ Manufacturer advises preparations containing local anaesthetics (lidocaine, cinchocaine, and pramocaine [unlicensed]) should only be used for a few days as they may cause sensitisation of the anal skin—local anaesthetic ointments can be absorbed through the rectal mucosa (with a theoretical risk of systemic effects) and very rarely may cause increased irritation; excessive application should be **avoided** in infants and children.

Topical preparations combining corticosteroids with local anaesthetics and soothing agents are available for the management of haemorrhoids. Manufacturer advises long-term use of corticosteroid creams can cause ulceration and permanent damage due to thinning of the perianal skin and should be avoided. Continuous or excessive use carries a risk of adrenal suppression and systemic corticosteroid effects (particularly in infants).

EvGr Topical preparations containing corticosteroids must not be used if infection is present (such as perianal streptococcal infection, *herpes simplex* or perianal thrush).

Recurrent symptoms should be referred to secondary care for further investigation and management. Ⓔ

Related drugs

Topical preparations used for haemorrhoids: lidocaine hydrochloride p. 1029, benzyl benzoate with bismuth oxide, bismuth subgallate, hydrocortisone acetate, peru balsam and zinc oxide p. 80, cinchocaine with hydrocortisone p. 81, cinchocaine with prednisolone p. 82.

CORTICOSTEROIDS

Benzyl benzoate with bismuth oxide, bismuth subgallate, hydrocortisone acetate, peru balsam and zinc oxide

26-Jul-2025

● **INDICATIONS AND DOSE**

Haemorrhoids | Pruritus ani

▶ BY RECTUM USING OINTMENT

▶ Child 12–17 years: Apply twice daily for no longer than 7 days, to be applied morning and night, an additional dose should be applied after a bowel movement

▶ BY RECTUM USING SUPPOSITORIES

▶ Child 12–17 years: 1 suppository twice daily for no longer than 7 days, to be inserted night and morning, additional dose after a bowel movement

IMPORTANT SAFETY INFORMATION

MHRA/CHM ADVICE: CORTICOSTEROIDS: RARE RISK OF CENTRAL SEROUS CHORIORETINOPATHY WITH LOCAL AS WELL AS SYSTEMIC ADMINISTRATION (AUGUST 2017)

See Corticosteroids, general use p. 537.

MHRA/CHM ADVICE: TOPICAL CORTICOSTEROIDS: INFORMATION ON THE RISK OF TOPICAL STEROID WITHDRAWAL REACTIONS (SEPTEMBER 2021)

Rarely, long-term continuous or inappropriate use of topical corticosteroids, particularly those of moderate to high potency, can result in the development of rebound flares, reported as dermatitis with intense redness, stinging, and burning that can spread beyond the initial treatment area.

The MHRA advises that the lowest potency topical corticosteroid needed should be used. For patients who are currently on long-term topical corticosteroid treatment, consider reducing potency or frequency of application (or both). Healthcare professionals should also be vigilant for the signs and symptoms of topical corticosteroid withdrawal reactions and review the position statement from the National Eczema Society, the British Dermatological Nursing Group, and the British Association of Dermatologists: www.bad.org.uk/topical-steroid-withdrawal-joint-statement/.

Healthcare professionals should inform patients:

- how much should be applied, as under-use can prolong treatment duration;
- how long they should use a topical corticosteroid for, especially on sensitive areas such as the face and genitals;
- to always apply topical corticosteroids as instructed and consult the patient information leaflet provided;
- to seek medical advice before using a topical corticosteroid on a new body area, as some areas of the body are more prone to side-effects;
- to return for medical advice if their skin condition worsens while using topical corticosteroid, and advise them when it would be appropriate to re-treat without a consultation and;
- if their skin worsens within 2 weeks of stopping a topical corticosteroid, treatment should not be started again without consulting their doctor unless they have previously been advised to do so.

The MHRA advises healthcare professionals to report any suspected adverse effects, via the Yellow Card Scheme, even when the adverse affects occur after stopping corticosteroid treatment.

ADRENAL INSUFFICIENCY CARD (APRIL 2023)

The British Society for Paediatric Endocrinology and Diabetes (BSPED) has developed an Adrenal Insufficiency Card which should be issued to children with adrenal insufficiency and steroid dependence. The card includes a management summary for the emergency treatment of adrenal crisis and sick day dosing, and can be issued by any healthcare professional managing such patients. The BSPED Adrenal Insufficiency Card is available at: www.bsped.org.uk/adrenal-insufficiency.

MHRA/CHM ADVICE: TOPICAL STEROIDS: INTRODUCTION OF NEW LABELLING AND A REMINDER OF THE POSSIBILITY OF SEVERE SIDE EFFECTS, INCLUDING TOPICAL STEROID WITHDRAWAL REACTIONS (MAY 2024)

The risk of serious side-effects, such as Topical Steroid Withdrawal Reactions (TSW), thinning of the skin, and systemic effects, increases with prolonged use of higher potency topical corticosteroids. Regulatory action has resulted in new labelling for topical corticosteroids with information on their potency to assist with patient counselling and correct selection. The MHRA continue to receive reports regarding TSW, particularly associated with eczema treatment; healthcare professionals are reminded to continue to follow the advice issued in 2021 (see above). In addition, healthcare professionals are advised that alternative treatments should be considered if previous discontinuation of a topical corticosteroid was associated with a reaction suspicious of TSW, and that they should support patients living with symptoms of TSW and review treatment plans alongside them.

Healthcare professionals should review the position statement from the National Eczema Society, the British Dermatological Nursing Group, and the British Association of Dermatologists: www.bad.org.uk/topical-steroid-withdrawal-joint-statement/.

The MHRA Patient Safety Leaflet on topical corticosteroids and withdrawal reactions can be used to aid patient counselling: www.gov.uk/guidance/topical-corticosteroids-and-withdrawal-reactions.

● **CONTRA-INDICATIONS** Infection—consult product literature

● **SIDE-EFFECTS** Skin reactions · vision disorders

● **PREGNANCY** Manufacturer advises avoid—toxicity in animal studies.

● **BREAST FEEDING** Manufacturer advises avoid.

● **PRESCRIBING AND DISPENSING INFORMATION** A proprietary brand *Anusol Plus HC*® (ointment and suppositories) is on sale to the public.

● **PATIENT AND CARER ADVICE** If systemic absorption occurs following topical or local use, side-effects applicable to systemic corticosteroids may apply; a patient information leaflet should be supplied and the need for a Steroid Treatment Card considered, see Corticosteroids, general use p. 537.

● **MEDICINAL FORMS** There can be variation in the licensing of different medicines containing the same drug.

Rectal ointment

▸ Anusol-Hc (Church & Dwight UK Ltd)
Hydrocortisone acetate 2.5 mg per 1 gram, Bismuth oxide 8.75 mg per 1 gram, Benzyl benzoate 12.5 mg per 1 gram, Peru Balsam 18.75 mg per 1 gram, Bismuth subgallate 22.5 mg per 1 gram, Zinc oxide 107.5 mg per 1 gram Anusol HC ointment | 30 gram [PoM] £6.40

Suppository

▸ Anusol-Hc (Church & Dwight UK Ltd)
Hydrocortisone acetate 10 mg, Bismuth oxide 24 mg, Benzyl benzoate 33 mg, Peru Balsam 49 mg, Bismuth subgallate 59 mg, Zinc oxide 296 mg Anusol HC suppositories | 12 suppository [PoM] £4.52

Cinchocaine with hydrocortisone

26-Jul-2025

● **INDICATIONS AND DOSE**

PROCTOSEDYL ® OINTMENT

Haemorrhoids | Pruritus ani

▶ TO THE SKIN, OR BY RECTUM

▸ Child: Apply twice daily, to be administered morning and night and after a bowel movement. Apply externally or by rectum. Do not use for longer than 7 days

PROCTOSEDYL ® SUPPOSITORIES

Haemorrhoids | Pruritus ani

▶ BY RECTUM

▸ Child 12–17 years: 1 suppository, insert suppository night and morning and after a bowel movement. Do not use for longer than 7 days

UNIROID-HC ® OINTMENT

Haemorrhoids | Pruritus ani

▶ TO THE SKIN, OR BY RECTUM

▸ Child 1 month–11 years (under medical advice only): Apply twice daily, and apply after a bowel movement, apply externally or by rectum, do not use for longer than 7 days

▸ Child 12–17 years: Apply twice daily, and apply after a bowel movement, apply externally or by rectum, do not use for longer than 7 days

UNIROID-HC ® SUPPOSITORIES

Haemorrhoids | Pruritus ani

▶ BY RECTUM

▸ Child 12–17 years: 1 suppository, insert twice daily and after a bowel movement. Do not use for longer than 7 days

IMPORTANT SAFETY INFORMATION

MHRA/CHM ADVICE: CORTICOSTEROIDS: RARE RISK OF CENTRAL SEROUS CHORIORETINOPATHY WITH LOCAL AS WELL AS SYSTEMIC ADMINISTRATION (AUGUST 2017)

See Corticosteroids, general use p. 537.

MHRA/CHM ADVICE: TOPICAL CORTICOSTEROIDS: INFORMATION ON THE RISK OF TOPICAL STEROID WITHDRAWAL REACTIONS (SEPTEMBER 2021)

Rarely, long-term continuous or inappropriate use of topical corticosteroids, particularly those of moderate to high potency, can result in the development of rebound flares, reported as dermatitis with intense redness, stinging, and burning that can spread beyond the initial treatment area.

The MHRA advises that the lowest potency topical corticosteroid needed should be used. For patients who are currently on long-term topical corticosteroid treatment, consider reducing potency or frequency of application (or both). Healthcare professionals should also be vigilant for the signs and symptoms of topical corticosteroid withdrawal reactions and review the position statement from the National Eczema Society, the British Dermatological Nursing Group, and the British Association of Dermatologists: www.bad.org.uk/topical-steroid-withdrawal-joint-statement/.

Healthcare professionals should inform patients:

- how much should be applied, as under-use can prolong treatment duration;
- how long they should use a topical corticosteroid for, especially on sensitive areas such as the face and genitals;
- to always apply topical corticosteroids as instructed and consult the patient information leaflet provided;
- to seek medical advice before using a topical corticosteroid on a new body area, as some areas of the body are more prone to side-effects;
- to return for medical advice if their skin condition worsens while using topical corticosteroid, and advise them when it would be appropriate to re-treat without a consultation and;
- if their skin worsens within 2 weeks of stopping a topical corticosteroid, treatment should not be started again without consulting their doctor unless they have previously been advised to do so

The MHRA advises healthcare professionals to report any suspected adverse effects, via the Yellow Card Scheme, even when the adverse affects occur after stopping corticosteroid treatment.

ADRENAL INSUFFICIENCY CARD (APRIL 2023)

The British Society for Paediatric Endocrinology and Diabetes (BSPED) has developed an Adrenal Insufficiency Card which should be issued to children with adrenal insufficiency and steroid dependence. The card includes a management summary for the emergency treatment of adrenal crisis and sick day dosing, and can be issued by any healthcare professional managing such patients. The BSPED Adrenal Insufficiency Card is available at: www.bsped.org.uk/adrenal-insufficiency.

MHRA/CHM ADVICE: TOPICAL STEROIDS: INTRODUCTION OF NEW LABELLING AND A REMINDER OF THE POSSIBILITY OF SEVERE SIDE EFFECTS, INCLUDING TOPICAL STEROID WITHDRAWAL REACTIONS (MAY 2024)

The risk of serious side-effects, such as Topical Steroid Withdrawal Reactions (TSW), thinning of the skin, and systemic effects, increases with prolonged use of higher potency topical corticosteroids. Regulatory action has resulted in new labelling for topical corticosteroids with information on their potency to assist with patient counselling and correct selection. The MHRA continue to receive reports regarding TSW, particularly associated with eczema treatment; healthcare professionals are reminded to continue to follow the advice issued in 2021 (see above). In addition, healthcare professionals are advised that alternative treatments should be considered if previous discontinuation of a topical corticosteroid was associated with a reaction suspicious of TSW, and that they should support patients living with symptoms of TSW and review treatment plans alongside them.

Healthcare professionals should review the position statement from the National Eczema Society, the British Dermatological Nursing Group, and the British Association of Dermatologists: www.bad.org.uk/topical-steroid-withdrawal-joint-statement/.

The MHRA Patient Safety Leaflet on topical corticosteroids and withdrawal reactions can be used to aid patient counselling: www.gov.uk/guidance/topical-corticosteroids-and-withdrawal-reactions.

● **CONTRA-INDICATIONS** Infection—consult product literature

● **CAUTIONS** Local anaesthetic component can be absorbed through the rectal mucosa (avoid excessive application, particularly in children and infants) · local anaesthetic component may cause sensitisation (use for short periods only—no longer than a few days)

● **SIDE-EFFECTS** Adrenal suppression · skin reactions · vision disorders

● **PATIENT AND CARER ADVICE** If systemic absorption occurs following topical and local use, side-effects applicable to systemic corticosteroids may apply; a patient information leaflet should be supplied and the need for a Steroid Treatment Card considered, see Corticosteroids, general use p. 537.

● MEDICINAL FORMS There can be variation in the licensing of different medicines containing the same drug.

Rectal ointment

▸ Proctosedyl (Phoenix Labs Ltd)
Cinchocaine hydrochloride 5 mg per 1 gram, Hydrocortisone 5 mg per 1 gram Proctosedyl ointment | 30 gram PoM £10.34 DT = £10.34

▸ Uniroid HC (Essential Generics Ltd)
Cinchocaine hydrochloride 5 mg per 1 gram, Hydrocortisone 5 mg per 1 gram Uniroid HC ointment | 30 gram PoM £5.91 DT = £10.34

Suppository

▸ Proctosedyl (Phoenix Labs Ltd)
Cinchocaine hydrochloride 5 mg, Hydrocortisone 5 mg Proctosedyl suppositories | 12 suppository PoM £5.08 DT = £4.31

▸ Uniroid HC (Essential Generics Ltd)
Cinchocaine hydrochloride 5 mg, Hydrocortisone 5 mg Uniroid HC suppositories | 12 suppository PoM £2.67 DT = £4.31

Cinchocaine with prednisolone

26-Jul-2025

● INDICATIONS AND DOSE

Haemorrhoids | Pruritus ani

▶ BY RECTUM USING OINTMENT

▸ Child: Apply twice daily for 5–7 days, apply 3–4 times a day on the first day if necessary, then apply once daily for a few days after symptoms have cleared

▶ BY RECTUM USING SUPPOSITORIES

▸ Child 12-17 years: 1 suppository daily for 5–7 days, to be inserted after a bowel movement

Haemorrhoids (severe cases) | Pruritus ani (severe cases)

▶ BY RECTUM USING SUPPOSITORIES

▸ Child 12-17 years: Initially 1 suppository 2–3 times a day, then 1 suppository daily for a total of 5–7 days, to be inserted after a bowel movement

IMPORTANT SAFETY INFORMATION

MHRA/CHM ADVICE: CORTICOSTEROIDS: RARE RISK OF CENTRAL SEROUS CHORIORETINOPATHY WITH LOCAL AS WELL AS SYSTEMIC ADMINISTRATION (AUGUST 2017)

See Corticosteroids, general use p. 537.

MHRA/CHM ADVICE: TOPICAL CORTICOSTEROIDS: INFORMATION ON THE RISK OF TOPICAL STEROID WITHDRAWAL REACTIONS (SEPTEMBER 2021)

Rarely, long-term continuous or inappropriate use of topical corticosteroids, particularly those of moderate to high potency, can result in the development of rebound flares, reported as dermatitis with intense redness, stinging, and burning that can spread beyond the initial treatment area.

The MHRA advises that the lowest potency topical corticosteroid needed should be used. For patients who are currently on long-term topical corticosteroid treatment, consider reducing potency or frequency of application (or both). Healthcare professionals should also be vigilant for the signs and symptoms of topical corticosteroid withdrawal reactions and review the position statement from the National Eczema Society, the British Dermatological Nursing Group, and the British Association of Dermatologists: www.bad.org.uk/topical-steroid-withdrawal-joint-statement/.

Healthcare professionals should inform patients:

- how much should be applied, as under-use can prolong treatment duration;
- how long they should use a topical corticosteroid for, especially on sensitive areas such as the face and genitals;
- to always apply topical corticosteroids as instructed and consult the patient information leaflet provided;
- to seek medical advice before using a topical corticosteroid on a new body area, as some areas of the body are more prone to side-effects;
- to return for medical advice if their skin condition worsens while using topical corticosteroid, and advise them when it would be appropriate to re-treat without a consultation and;
- if their skin worsens within 2 weeks of stopping a topical corticosteroid, treatment should not be started again without consulting their doctor unless they have previously been advised to do so

The MHRA advises healthcare professionals to report any suspected adverse effects, via the Yellow Card Scheme, even when the adverse affects occur after stopping corticosteroid treatment.

ADRENAL INSUFFICIENCY CARD (APRIL 2023)

The British Society for Paediatric Endocrinology and Diabetes (BSPED) has developed an Adrenal Insufficiency Card which should be issued to children with adrenal insufficiency and steroid dependence. The card includes a management summary for the emergency treatment of adrenal crisis and sick day dosing, and can be issued by any healthcare professional managing such patients. The BSPED Adrenal Insufficiency Card is available at: www.bsped.org.uk/adrenal-insufficiency.

MHRA/CHM ADVICE: TOPICAL STEROIDS: INTRODUCTION OF NEW LABELLING AND A REMINDER OF THE POSSIBILITY OF SEVERE SIDE EFFECTS, INCLUDING TOPICAL STEROID WITHDRAWAL REACTIONS (MAY 2024)

The risk of serious side-effects, such as Topical Steroid Withdrawal Reactions (TSW), thinning of the skin, and systemic effects, increases with prolonged use of higher potency topical corticosteroids. Regulatory action has resulted in new labelling for topical corticosteroids with information on their potency to assist with patient counselling and correct selection. The MHRA continue to receive reports regarding TSW, particularly associated with eczema treatment; healthcare professionals are reminded to continue to follow the advice issued in 2021 (see above). In addition, healthcare professionals are advised that alternative treatments should be considered if previous discontinuation of a topical corticosteroid was associated with a reaction suspicious of TSW, and that they should support patients living with symptoms of TSW and review treatment plans alongside them.

Healthcare professionals should review the position statement from the National Eczema Society, the British Dermatological Nursing Group, and the British Association of Dermatologists: www.bad.org.uk/topical-steroid-withdrawal-joint-statement/.

The MHRA Patient Safety Leaflet on topical corticosteroids and withdrawal reactions can be used to aid patient counselling: www.gov.uk/guidance/topical-corticosteroids-and-withdrawal-reactions.

● CONTRA-INDICATIONS Infection—consult product literature

● CAUTIONS Local anaesthetic component can be absorbed through the rectal mucosa (avoid excessive application) · local anaesthetic component may cause sensitisation (use for short periods only—no longer than a few days)

● PATIENT AND CARER ADVICE If systemic absorption occurs following topical and local use, side-effects applicable to systemic corticosteroids may apply; a patient information leaflet should be supplied and the need for a Steroid Treatment Card considered, see Corticosteroids, general use p. 537.

● **MEDICINAL FORMS** There can be variation in the licensing of different medicines containing the same drug.

Rectal ointment

▸ Scheriproct (Karo Healthcare UK Ltd)
Prednisolone hexanoate 1.9 mg per 1 gram, Cinchocaine hydrochloride 5 mg per 1 gram Scheriproct ointment | 30 gram [PoM] £3.23 DT = £3.23

Suppository

▸ Scheriproct (Karo Healthcare UK Ltd)
Cinchocaine hydrochloride 1 mg, Prednisolone hexanoate 1.3 mg Scheriproct suppositories | 12 suppository [PoM] £1.52 DT = £1.52

Hydrocortisone with lidocaine

26-Jul-2025

● **INDICATIONS AND DOSE**

Haemorrhoids | Pruritus ani

▶ BY RECTUM USING AEROSOL SPRAY

▸ Child 2–13 years (under medical advice only): 1 spray up to 3 times a day, spray once over the affected area

▸ Child 14–17 years: 1 spray up to 3 times a day for no longer than 7 days without medical advice, spray once over the affected area

▶ BY RECTUM USING OINTMENT

▸ Child: Apply several times daily, for short term use only

IMPORTANT SAFETY INFORMATION

MHRA/CHM ADVICE: CORTICOSTEROIDS: RARE RISK OF CENTRAL SEROUS CHORIORETINOPATHY WITH LOCAL AS WELL AS SYSTEMIC ADMINISTRATION (AUGUST 2017)

See Corticosteroids, general use p. 537.

MHRA/CHM ADVICE: TOPICAL CORTICOSTEROIDS: INFORMATION ON THE RISK OF TOPICAL STEROID WITHDRAWAL REACTIONS (SEPTEMBER 2021)

Rarely, long-term continuous or inappropriate use of topical corticosteroids, particularly those of moderate to high potency, can result in the development of rebound flares, reported as dermatitis with intense redness, stinging, and burning that can spread beyond the initial treatment area.

The MHRA advises that the lowest potency topical corticosteroid needed should be used. For patients who are currently on long-term topical corticosteroid treatment, consider reducing potency or frequency of application (or both). Healthcare professionals should also be vigilant for the signs and symptoms of topical corticosteroid withdrawal reactions and review the position statement from the National Eczema Society, the British Dermatological Nursing Group, and the British Association of Dermatologists www.bad.org.uk/topical-steroid-withdrawal-joint-statement/.

Healthcare professionals should inform patients:

- how much should be applied, as under-use can prolong treatment duration;
- how long they should use a topical corticosteroid for, especially on sensitive areas such as the face and genitals;
- to always apply topical corticosteroids as instructed and consult the patient information leaflet provided;
- to seek medical advice before using a topical corticosteroid on a new body area, as some areas of the body are more prone to side-effects;
- to return for medical advice if their skin condition worsens while using topical corticosteroid, and advise them when it would be appropriate to re-treat without a consultation and;
- if their skin worsens within 2 weeks of stopping a topical corticosteroid, treatment should not be started again without consulting their doctor unless they have previously been advised to do so.

The MHRA advises healthcare professionals to report any suspected adverse effects, via the Yellow Card Scheme, even when the adverse affects occur after stopping corticosteroid treatment.

ADRENAL INSUFFICIENCY CARD (APRIL 2023)

The British Society for Paediatric Endocrinology and Diabetes (BSPED) has developed an Adrenal Insufficiency Card which should be issued to children with adrenal insufficiency and steroid dependence. The card includes a management summary for the emergency treatment of adrenal crisis and sick day dosing, and can be issued by any healthcare professional managing such patients. The BSPED Adrenal Insufficiency Card is available at: www.bsped.org.uk/adrenal-insufficiency.

MHRA/CHM ADVICE: TOPICAL STEROIDS: INTRODUCTION OF NEW LABELLING AND A REMINDER OF THE POSSIBILITY OF SEVERE SIDE EFFECTS, INCLUDING TOPICAL STEROID WITHDRAWAL REACTIONS (MAY 2024)

The risk of serious side-effects, such as Topical Steroid Withdrawal Reactions (TSW), thinning of the skin, and systemic effects, increases with prolonged use of higher potency topical corticosteroids. Regulatory action has resulted in new labelling for topical corticosteroids with information on their potency to assist with patient counselling and correct selection. The MHRA continue to receive reports regarding TSW, particularly associated with eczema treatment; healthcare professionals are reminded to continue to follow the advice issued in 2021 (see above). In addition, healthcare professionals are advised that alternative treatments should be considered if previous discontinuation of a topical corticosteroid was associated with a reaction suspicious of TSW, and that they should support patients living with symptoms of TSW and review treatment plans alongside them.

Healthcare professionals should review the position statement from the National Eczema Society, the British Dermatological Nursing Group, and the British Association of Dermatologists: www.bad.org.uk/topical-steroid-withdrawal-joint-statement/.

The MHRA Patient Safety Leaflet on topical corticosteroids and withdrawal reactions can be used to aid patient counselling: www.gov.uk/guidance/topical-corticosteroids-and-withdrawal-reactions.

● **CONTRA-INDICATIONS** Infection—consult product literature

● **CAUTIONS** Local anaesthetic component can be absorbed through the rectal mucosa (avoid excessive application) · local anaesthetic component may cause sensitisation (use for short periods only—no longer than a few days)

● **SIDE-EFFECTS** Adrenal suppression · paraesthesia · seizure (with high doses) · skin reactions · vision disorders

● **PATIENT AND CARER ADVICE** If systemic absorption occurs following topical and local use, side-effects applicable to systemic corticosteroids may apply; a patient information leaflet should be supplied and the need for a Steroid Treatment Card considered, see Corticosteroids, general use p. 537.

● **MEDICINAL FORMS** There can be variation in the licensing of different medicines containing the same drug.

Cutaneous ointment

▸ Xyloproct (Aspen Pharma Trading Ltd)
Hydrocortisone acetate 2.75 mg per 1 gram, Lidocaine 50 mg per 1 gram Xyloproct 5%/0.275% ointment | 20 gram [PoM] £4.19 DT = £4.19

11 Stoma care

Stoma care

17-Mar-2021

Description of condition

A stoma is an artificial opening on the abdomen to divert flow of faeces or urine into an external pouch located outside of the body. This procedure may be temporary or permanent. Colostomy and ileostomy are the most common forms of stoma but a gastrostomy, jejunostomy, duodenostomy, or caecostomy may also be performed. Understanding the type and extent of surgical intervention in each patient is crucial in managing the patient's pharmaceutical needs correctly.

Prescribing in patients with stoma

Prescribing for patients with a stoma calls for special care due to modifications in drug delivery, resulting in a higher risk of sub-optimal absorption. The following is a brief account of some of the main points to be borne in mind.

Enteric-coated and modified-release medicines are **unsuitable**, particularly in patients with an ileostomy, as there may be insufficient release of the active ingredient. Preparation forms with quick dissolution and absorption should be used. Liquids, capsules, and uncoated or soluble tablets are usually well absorbed. When a solid-dose form such as a capsule or a tablet is given, the contents of the stoma bag should be checked for any remnants.

Preparations containing sorbitol as an excipient may have a laxative effect.

Opioid **analgesics** may cause constipation in colostomy patients. Aspirin and NSAIDs may cause gastric irritation and bleeding; faecal output should be monitored for traces of blood.

The effect of **antacids** in patients with a stoma is dependent on the class of antacids and the type of stoma. Calcium-containing antacids can cause constipation and magnesium-containing antacids can cause diarrhoea, especially in patients with an ileostomy as they can cause osmotic diarrhoea. The aluminium hydroxide antacids can cause constipation and may be of concern in colostomy patients.

The **antidiarrhoeal** drugs, loperamide hydrochloride p. 55 and codeine phosphate p. 331, reduce intestinal motility and decrease water and sodium output from an ileostomy. Loperamide hydrochloride circulates through the enterohepatic circulation, which is disrupted in patients with a short bowel.

Patients with a stoma are particularly susceptible to fluid and sodium depletion which can often lead to hypokalaemia; potassium supplements are not usually required. Hypokalaemia may cause an increased sensitivity to digoxin p. 91.

Diuretics may cause excessive dehydration in patients with an ileostomy or with urostomy and potassium depletion may easily occur; potassium-sparing diuretics are available.

Iron preparations may cause diarrhoea in ileostomy patients, constipation in colostomy patients, and sore skin if output leaks; stools may also appear black. Parenteral iron is licensed for use in patients who are unable to tolerate gastro-intestinal adverse effects of oral iron.

Laxatives may cause rapid and severe loss of water and electrolytes in ileostomy patients and are, therefore, used with caution. In colostomy patients, bulk-forming laxatives may provide more benefit than a stimulant laxative; they aid in the formation of solid stools and promote regularity. Stool softeners can also help with constipation.

Liquid formulations of potassium supplements are preferred to modified-release formulations; to avoid osmotic diarrhoea, the daily dose is split into divided doses.

Care of stoma

Patients and their carers are usually given advice about the use of cleansing agents, protective creams, lotions, deodorants, or sealants whilst in hospital, either by the surgeon or by stoma care nurses. Voluntary organisations offer help and support to patients with stoma.

Chapter 2
Cardiovascular system

CONTENTS

1 Arrhythmias

Arrhythmias

10-Aug-2022

Overview

Management of an arrhythmia requires precise diagnosis of the type of arrhythmia; electrocardiography and referral to a paediatric cardiologist is essential; underlying causes such as heart failure require appropriate treatment.

Bradycardia

Adrenaline p. 159 is useful in the treatment of symptomatic bradycardia in an infant or child.

Supraventricular tachycardia

In supraventricular tachycardia adenosine p. 89 is given by rapid intravenous injection. If adenosine is ineffective, intravenous amiodarone hydrochloride p. 88, flecainide acetate p. 87, or a beta-blocker (such as esmolol hydrochloride p. 125) can be tried; verapamil hydrochloride p. 129 can also be considered in children aged over 1 year. Atenolol p. 125, sotalol hydrochloride p. 90, and flecainide acetate are used for the prophylaxis of paroxysmal supraventricular tachycardias.

The use of d.c. shock and vagal stimulation also have a role in the treatment of supraventricular tachycardia.

Syndromes associated with accessory conducting pathways

Amiodarone hydrochloride, flecainide acetate, or a beta-blocker is used to prevent recurrence of supraventricular tachycardia in infants and young children with these syndromes (e.g. Wolff-Parkinson-White syndrome).

Atrial flutter

In atrial flutter without structural heart defects, sinus rhythm is restored with d.c. shock or cardiac pacing; drug treatment is usually not necessary. Amiodarone hydrochloride is used in atrial flutter when structural heart defects are present or after heart surgery. Sotalol hydrochloride may also be considered.

Atrial fibrillation

Atrial fibrillation is very rare in children. To restore sinus rhythm d.c. shock is used; beta-blockers, alone or together with digoxin p. 91 may be useful for ventricular rate control.

Ectopic tachycardia

Intravenous amiodarone hydrochloride is used in conjunction with body cooling and synchronised pacing in postoperative junctional ectopic tachycardia. Oral amiodarone hydrochloride or flecainide acetate is used in congenital junctional ectopic tachycardia.

Amiodarone hydrochloride, flecainide acetate, or a beta-blocker is used in atrial ectopic tachycardia; amiodarone hydrochloride is preferred in those with poor ventricular function.

Ventricular tachycardia and ventricular fibrillation

Pulseless ventricular tachycardia or ventricular fibrillation require resuscitation, see Paediatric Advanced Life Support Algorithm in Life support algorithm (image) Inside back pages. Amiodarone hydrochloride is used in resuscitation for pulseless ventricular tachycardia or ventricular fibrillation unresponsive to defibrillation; lidocaine hydrochloride p. 86 can be used as an alternative.

Amiodarone hydrochloride is also used in a haemodynamically stable child when drug treatment is required; lidocaine hydrochloride can be used as an alternative only if amiodarone hydrochloride is not available.

Torsade de pointes

Torsade de pointes is a form of ventricular tachycardia associated with long QT syndrome, which may be congenital or drug induced. Episodes may be self-limiting, but are frequently recurrent and can cause impairment or loss of consciousness. If not controlled, the arrhythmia can progress to ventricular fibrillation and sometimes death. Intravenous magnesium sulfate can be used to treat torsade de pointes (dose recommendations vary—consult local guidelines). Anti-arrhythmics can further prolong the QT interval, thus worsening the condition.

Anti-arrhythmic drugs

Anti-arrhythmic drugs can be classified clinically into those that act on supraventricular arrhythmias (e.g. verapamil hydrochloride), those that act on both supraventricular and ventricular arrhythmias (e.g. amiodarone hydrochloride), and those that act on ventricular arrhythmias (e.g. lidocaine hydrochloride).

Anti-arrhythmic drugs can also be classified according to their effects on the electrical behaviour of myocardial cells during activity (the Vaughan Williams classification) although this classification is of less clinical significance:

- Class I: membrane stabilising drugs (e.g. lidocaine, flecainide)
- Class II: beta-blockers
- Class III: amiodarone; sotalol (also Class II)
- Class IV: calcium-channel blockers (includes verapamil but not dihydropyridines)

The negative inotropic effects of anti-arrhythmic drugs tend to be additive. Therefore special care should be taken if two or more are used, especially if myocardial function is impaired. Most drugs that are effective in countering arrhythmias can also provoke them in some circumstances; moreover, hypokalaemia enhances the arrhythmogenic (pro-arrhythmic) effect of many drugs.

Adenosine is the treatment of choice for terminating supraventricular tachycardias, including those associated with accessory conducting pathways (e.g. Wolff-Parkinson-White syndrome). It is also used in the diagnosis of supraventricular arrhythmias. It is not negatively inotropic and does not cause significant hypotension. The injection should be administered by rapid intravenous injection into a central or large peripheral vein.

Amiodarone hydrochloride is useful in the management of both supraventricular and ventricular tachyarrhythmias. It can be given by intravenous infusion and by mouth, and causes little or no myocardial depression. Unlike oral amiodarone hydrochloride, intravenous amiodarone hydrochloride acts relatively rapidly. Intravenous amiodarone hydrochloride is also used in cardiopulmonary resuscitation for ventricular fibrillation or pulseless ventricular tachycardia unresponsive to defibrillation.

Amiodarone hydrochloride has a very long half-life (extending to several weeks) and only needs to be given once daily (but high doses may cause nausea unless divided). Many weeks or months may be required to achieve steady state plasma-amiodarone concentration; this is particularly important when drug interactions are likely.

Beta-blockers act as anti-arrhythmic drugs principally by attenuating the effects of the sympathetic system on automaticity and conductivity within the heart. Sotalol hydrochloride has a role in the management of ventricular arrhythmias.

Oral administration of digoxin slows the ventricular rate in atrial fibrillation and in atrial flutter. However, intravenous infusion of digoxin is rarely effective for rapid control of ventricular rate.

Flecainide acetate is useful for the treatment of resistant re-entry supraventricular tachycardia, ventricular tachycardia, ventricular ectopic beats, arrhythmias associated with accessory conducting pathways (e.g. Wolff-Parkinson-White syndrome), and paroxysmal atrial fibrillation. Flecainide acetate crosses the placenta and can be used to control fetal supraventricular arrhythmias.

Lidocaine hydrochloride can be used as an alternative to amiodarone hydrochloride for cardiopulmonary resuscitation in children with ventricular fibrillation or pulseless ventricular tachycardia unresponsive to defibrillation. Doses may need to be reduced in children with persistently poor cardiac output and hepatic or renal failure.

Verapamil hydrochloride can cause severe haemodynamic compromise (refractory hypotension and cardiac arrest) when used for the acute treatment of arrhythmias in neonates and infants; it is contra-indicated in children aged under 1 year. It is also contra-indicated in those with congestive heart failure, syndromes associated with accessory conducting pathways (e.g. Wolff-Parkinson-White syndrome), and in most receiving concomitant beta-blockers. It can be useful in older children with supraventricular tachycardia.

Other drugs used for Arrhythmias Metoprolol tartrate, p. 126

ANTIARRHYTHMICS › CLASS IB

Lidocaine hydrochloride

20-Nov-2025

(Lignocaine hydrochloride)

● **INDICATIONS AND DOSE**

Ventricular arrhythmias | Pulseless ventricular tachycardia | Ventricular fibrillation

▶ INITIALLY BY INTRAVENOUS INJECTION, OR BY INTRAOSSEOUS INJECTION

▸ Neonate: Initially 0.5–1 mg/kg, followed immediately by (by intravenous infusion) 0.6–3 mg/kg/hour, alternatively (by intravenous injection or by intraosseous injection) 0.5–1 mg/kg repeated at intervals of not less than 5 minutes if infusion is not immediately available following initial injection, until infusion can be initiated; maximum 3 mg/kg per course.

▸ Child 1 month–11 years: Initially 0.5–1 mg/kg, followed immediately by (by intravenous infusion) 0.6–3 mg/kg/hour, alternatively (by intravenous injection or by intraosseous injection) 0.5–1 mg/kg repeated at intervals of not less than 5 minutes if infusion is not immediately available following initial injection, until infusion can be initiated; maximum 3 mg/kg per course

▸ Child 12–17 years: Initially 50–100 mg, followed by (by intravenous infusion) 120 mg, dose to be given over 30 minutes, then (by intravenous infusion) 240 mg, dose to be given over 2 hours, then (by intravenous infusion) 60 mg/hour, reduce dose further if infusion is continued beyond 24 hours, if infusion not immediately available following initial injection, the initial injection dose may be repeated at intervals of not less than 5 minutes (to a maximum 300 mg dose in 1 hour) until infusion can be initiated

Neonatal seizures

▶ BY INTRAVENOUS INFUSION

▸ Neonate: Initially 2 mg/kg, dose to be given over 10 minutes, followed by 6 mg/kg/hour for 6 hours; reduced to 4 mg/kg/hour for 12 hours, then reduced to 2 mg/kg/hour for a further 12 hours, preterm neonates may require lower doses.

● **UNLICENSED USE** Not licensed for use in children under 1 year.

● **CONTRA-INDICATIONS** All grades of atrioventricular block · severe myocardial depression · sino-atrial disorders

● **CAUTIONS** Acute porphyrias p. 745 (consider infusion with glucose for its anti-porphyrinogenic effects) · congestive cardiac failure (consider lower dose) · post cardiac surgery (consider lower dose)

● **INTERACTIONS** → Appendix 1: antiarrhythmics

● **SIDE-EFFECTS** Anxiety · arrhythmias · atrioventricular block · cardiac arrest · circulatory collapse · confusion · dizziness · drowsiness · euphoric mood · headache · hypotension (may lead to cardiac arrest) · loss of consciousness · methaemoglobinaemia · muscle twitching · myocardial contractility decreased · nausea · neurological effects · nystagmus · pain · psychosis · respiratory disorders · seizure · sensation abnormal · temperature sensation altered · tinnitus · tremor · vision blurred · vomiting

SIDE-EFFECTS, FURTHER INFORMATION Methylthioninium chloride can be used for the acute symptomatic treatment of drug-induced methaemoglobinaemia.

● **PREGNANCY** Crosses the placenta but not known to be harmful in *animal* studies—use if benefit outweighs risk.

- **BREAST FEEDING** Present in milk but amount too small to be harmful.
- **HEPATIC IMPAIRMENT** Manufacturer advises caution (risk of increased exposure).
  Dose adjustments Manufacturer advises slower infusion rate.
- **RENAL IMPAIRMENT** Possible accumulation of lidocaine and active metabolite; caution in severe impairment.
- **MONITORING REQUIREMENTS** Monitor ECG and have resuscitation facilities available.
- **DIRECTIONS FOR ADMINISTRATION** For *intravenous infusion*, expert sources advise dilute with Glucose 5% or Sodium Chloride 0.9%.

- **MEDICINAL FORMS** There can be variation in the licensing of different medicines containing the same drug. Forms available from special-order manufacturers include: solution for injection

Solution for injection

▸ Lidocaine hydrochloride (Non-proprietary)

Lidocaine hydrochloride 5 mg per 1 ml Lidocaine 50mg/10ml (0.5%) solution for injection ampoules | 10 ampoule PoM £10.00 DT = £10.00

Lidocaine hydrochloride 10 mg per 1 ml Lidocaine 100mg/10ml (1%) solution for injection Mini-Plasco ampoules | 20 ampoule PoM £13.80

Lidocaine 100mg/10ml (1%) solution for injection ampoules | 10 ampoule PoM £6.30–£7.00 DT = £8.10 | 20 ampoule PoM £14.60–£234.00 (Hospital only)

Lidocaine 200mg/20ml (1%) solution for injection vials | 10 vial PoM £26.40

Lidocaine 200mg/20ml (1%) solution for injection ampoules | 1 ampoule PoM £25.07 (Hospital only) | 10 ampoule PoM £12.60–£14.00 DT = £14.00 | 20 ampoule PoM £20.00–£501.40 (Hospital only)

Lidocaine 50mg/5ml (1%) solution for injection ampoules | 1 ampoule PoM £8.28 (Hospital only) | 10 ampoule PoM £4.00–£6.06 DT = £6.95 | 20 ampoule PoM £13.00–£165.60 (Hospital only)

Lidocaine 20mg/2ml (1%) solution for injection ampoules | 10 ampoule PoM £5.17 DT = £5.17

Lidocaine 50mg/5ml (1%) solution for injection Mini-Plasco ampoules | 20 ampoule PoM £8.05

Lidocaine hydrochloride 20 mg per 1 ml Lidocaine 100mg/5ml (2%) solution for injection ampoules | 10 ampoule PoM £5.40–£6.00 DT = £7.60 | 20 ampoule PoM £16.40–£165.00 (Hospital only)

Lidocaine 40mg/2ml (2%) solution for injection ampoules | 10 ampoule PoM £5.84 DT = £5.88

Lidocaine 100mg/5ml (2%) solution for injection Mini-Plasco ampoules | 20 ampoule PoM £12.00

Lidocaine 200mg/10ml (2%) solution for injection ampoules | 20 ampoule PoM £14.95–£382.80 (Hospital only)

Lidocaine 400mg/20ml (2%) solution for injection ampoules | 10 ampoule PoM £13.50–£15.00 DT = £15.00 | 20 ampoule PoM £32.60–£521.80 (Hospital only)

ANTIARRHYTHMICS › CLASS IC

Flecainide acetate

03-Apr-2025

- **INDICATIONS AND DOSE**

Resistant re-entry supraventricular tachycardia (initiated under direction of hospital consultant) | Ventricular ectopic beats or ventricular tachycardia (initiated under direction of hospital consultant) | Arrhythmias associated with accessory conduction pathways (e.g. Wolff-Parkinson-White syndrome) (initiated under direction of hospital consultant) | Paroxysmal atrial fibrillation (initiated under direction of hospital consultant)

▸ BY MOUTH

- ▸ Neonate: 2 mg/kg 2–3 times a day, dose to be adjusted according to response and plasma-flecainide concentration.
- ▸ Child 1 month–5 years: 2 mg/kg 2–3 times a day, dose to be adjusted according to response and plasma-flecainide concentration; maximum 8 mg/kg per day
- ▸ Child 6–11 years: 2 mg/kg 2–3 times a day, dose to be adjusted according to response and plasma-flecainide concentration; maximum 8 mg/kg per day or 300 mg per day (whichever is lower)
- ▸ Child 12–17 years: Initially 50–100 mg twice daily, dose can be increased if necessary up to 300 mg per day (maximum dose of 400 mg per day can be used for ventricular arrhythmias in heavily built children)

DOSE ADJUSTMENTS DUE TO INTERACTIONS

- ▸ Manufacturer advises reduce dose by half with concurrent use of amiodarone.

- **UNLICENSED USE** Not licensed for use in children under 12 years.
- **CONTRA-INDICATIONS** Abnormal left ventricular function · atrial conduction defects (unless pacing rescue available) · bundle branch block (unless pacing rescue available) · distal block (unless pacing rescue available) · haemodynamically significant valvular heart disease · heart failure · history of myocardial infarction and either asymptomatic ventricular ectopics or asymptomatic non-sustained ventricular tachycardia · long-standing atrial fibrillation where conversion to sinus rhythm not attempted · second-degree or greater AV block (unless pacing rescue available) · sinus node dysfunction (unless pacing rescue available)
- **CAUTIONS** Atrial fibrillation following heart surgery · patients with pacemakers (especially those who may be pacemaker dependent because stimulation threshold may rise appreciably)
- **INTERACTIONS** → Appendix 1: antiarrhythmics
- **SIDE-EFFECTS**
  - ▸ **Common or very common** Arrhythmias · asthenia · dizziness · dyspnoea · fever · oedema · vision disorders
  - ▸ **Uncommon** Alopecia · appetite decreased · constipation · diarrhoea · flatulence · gastrointestinal discomfort · nausea · skin reactions · vomiting
  - ▸ **Rare or very rare** Anxiety · confusion · corneal deposits · depression · drowsiness · flushing · hallucination · headache · hepatic disorders · hyperhidrosis · inflammation · insomnia · interstitial lung disease · memory loss · movement disorders · peripheral neuropathy · photosensitivity reaction · seizure · sensation abnormal · syncope · tinnitus · tremor · vertigo
  - ▸ **Frequency not known** Altered pacing threshold · atrioventricular block · cardiac arrest · chest pain · heart failure · hypotension · palpitations · pulmonary fibrosis · QT interval prolongation
- **PREGNANCY** Used in pregnancy to treat maternal and fetal arrhythmias in specialist centres; toxicity reported in *animal* studies; infant hyperbilirubinaemia also reported.
- **BREAST FEEDING** Significant amount present in milk but not known to be harmful.
- **HEPATIC IMPAIRMENT**
  Dose adjustments Avoid or reduce dose in severe impairment.
  Monitoring Monitor plasma-flecainide concentration.
- **RENAL IMPAIRMENT**
  Dose adjustments Reduce dose by 25–50% if estimated glomerular filtration rate less than 35 mL/minute/1.73 m^2.
  Monitoring Monitor plasma-flecainide concentration.
- **MONITORING REQUIREMENTS**
  - ▸ Plasma-flecainide concentration for optimal response 200–800 micrograms/litre; blood sample should be taken immediately before next dose.
- **DIRECTIONS FOR ADMINISTRATION** EvGr For administration *by mouth*, take on an empty stomach; milk,

infant formula, and dairy products may reduce absorption of flecainide. (M) Liquid has a local anaesthetic effect. Do not store liquid in refrigerator.

- **PATIENT AND CARER ADVICE**
Medicines for Children leaflet: Flecainide for arrhythmias www.medicinesforchildren.org.uk/medicines/flecainide-for-arrhythmias/

- **MEDICINAL FORMS** There can be variation in the licensing of different medicines containing the same drug. Forms available from special-order manufacturers include: oral suspension, oral solution

Oral tablet

▸ Flecainide acetate (Non-proprietary)

Flecainide acetate 50 mg Flecainide 50mg tablets | 60 tablet PoM £7.68 DT = £2.10

Flecainide acetate 100 mg Flecainide 100mg tablets | 60 tablet PoM £8.06 DT = £3.00

Oral solution

▸ Flecainide acetate (Non-proprietary)

Flecainide acetate 5 mg per 1 ml Flecainide 25mg/5ml oral solution sugar free | 300 ml PoM £375.00 SF

Flecainide acetate 10 mg per 1 ml Flecainide 50mg/5ml oral solution sugar free | 150 ml PoM £300.00 SF

ANTIARRHYTHMICS › CLASS III

Amiodarone hydrochloride 20-Nov-2025

- **INDICATIONS AND DOSE**

Supraventricular and ventricular arrhythmias (initiated in hospital or under specialist supervision)

▸ BY MOUTH

▸ Neonate: Initially 5–10 mg/kg twice daily for 7–10 days, then reduced to 5–10 mg/kg daily.

▸ Child 1 month–11 years: Initially 5–10 mg/kg twice daily (max. per dose 200 mg) for 7–10 days, then reduced to 5–10 mg/kg once daily; maximum 200 mg per day

▸ Child 12–17 years: 200 mg 3 times a day for 1 week, then 200 mg twice daily for 1 week, then usually 200 mg daily adjusted according to response

▸ BY INTRAVENOUS INFUSION

▸ Neonate: 5 mg/kg every 12–24 hours, dose to be given over 30 minutes.

▸ INITIALLY BY INTRAVENOUS INFUSION

▸ Child: Initially 5 mg/kg, dose to be given slowly, over longer than 20 minutes, to avoid bradycardia and cardiac arrest, then (by continuous intravenous infusion) 300 micrograms/kg/hour, dose to be adjusted according to response, increased if necessary up to 1.5 milligrams/kg/hour; maximum 1.2 g per day

Ventricular fibrillation or pulseless ventricular tachycardia refractory to defibrillation [for cardiopulmonary resuscitation]

▸ BY INTRAVENOUS INJECTION

▸ Neonate: 5 mg/kg for 1 dose, dose can be repeated **once** if required. Consult Resuscitation Council (UK) guidelines for further details.

▸ Child: 5 mg/kg for 1 dose (max. per dose 300 mg), then 5 mg/kg for 1 dose (max. per dose 150 mg), dose to be given if required. Consult Resuscitation Council (UK) guidelines for further details

- **UNLICENSED USE** Not licensed for use in children under 3 years.

IMPORTANT SAFETY INFORMATION

MHRA/CHM ADVICE: SOFOSBUVIR WITH DACLATASVIR; SOFOSBUVIR AND LEDIPASVIR (MAY 2015); SIMEPREVIR WITH SOFOSBUVIR (AUGUST 2015): RISK OF SEVERE BRADYCARDIA AND HEART BLOCK WHEN TAKEN WITH AMIODARONE

Avoid concomitant use unless other antiarrhythmics cannot be given.

MHRA/CHM ADVICE: AMIODARONE (*CORDARONE X*®): REMINDER OF RISKS OF TREATMENT AND NEED FOR PATIENT MONITORING AND SUPERVISION (MARCH 2022)

Healthcare professionals are reminded that amiodarone can cause serious adverse reactions affecting the eyes, heart, lung, liver, thyroid gland, skin, and peripheral nervous system that may persist for a month or longer after treatment discontinuation. Some of these reactions may be life-threatening but onset can be delayed; patients should be supervised and reviewed regularly, especially those on long-term treatment. Liver and thyroid function tests should be performed—see *Monitoring requirements*.

Patients and carers should be counselled to seek medical advice if new or worsening respiratory symptoms develop; healthcare professionals should consider using computerised tomography (CT) scans if pulmonary toxicity is suspected. Patients and carers should also be advised to seek immediate medical attention if other symptoms of serious adverse reactions develop during or after stopping treatment.

- **CONTRA-INDICATIONS**

GENERAL CONTRA-INDICATIONS Avoid in severe conduction disturbances (unless pacemaker fitted) · avoid in sinus node disease (unless pacemaker fitted) · avoid rapid loading after cardiac surgery · iodine sensitivity · sino-atrial heart block (except in cardiac arrest) · sinus bradycardia (except in cardiac arrest) · thyroid dysfunction

SPECIFIC CONTRA-INDICATIONS

▸ With intravenous use Avoid bolus injection in cardiomyopathy · avoid bolus injection in congestive heart failure · avoid in circulatory collapse · avoid in severe arterial hypotension · avoid in severe respiratory failure

- **CAUTIONS**

GENERAL CAUTIONS Acute porphyrias p. 745 · conduction disturbances (in excessive dosage) · heart failure · hypokalaemia · severe bradycardia (in excessive dosage)

SPECIFIC CAUTIONS

▸ With intravenous use Avoid benzyl alcohol containing injections in neonates · moderate and transient fall in blood pressure (circulatory collapse precipitated by rapid administration or overdosage) · severe hepatocellular toxicity

- **INTERACTIONS** → Appendix 1: antiarrhythmics

- **SIDE-EFFECTS**

GENERAL SIDE-EFFECTS

▸ **Common or very common** Arrhythmias · hepatic disorders · hyperthyroidism · nausea · pulmonary fibrosis · skin reactions

▸ **Rare or very rare** Bronchospasm (in patients with severe respiratory failure) · headache · idiopathic intracranial hypertension · nerve disorders · SIADH

▸ **Frequency not known** Angioedema · confusion · delirium · pancreatitis · severe cutaneous adverse reactions (SCARs)

SPECIFIC SIDE-EFFECTS

▸ **Common or very common**

▸ With oral use Constipation · corneal deposits · hypothyroidism · interstitial lung disease · movement disorders · photosensitivity reaction · respiratory disorders · sleep disorders · taste altered · vomiting

- With parenteral use Hypotension (following rapid injection)
- **Uncommon**
- With oral use Cardiac conduction disorders · dry mouth · myopathy (usually reversible on discontinuation) · peripheral neuropathy (usually reversible on discontinuation)
- **Rare or very rare**
- With oral use Alopecia · aplastic anaemia · epididymo-orchitis · erectile dysfunction · haemolytic anaemia · pulmonary haemorrhage · thrombocytopenia · vertigo
- With parenteral use Hot flush · hyperhidrosis · interstitial pneumonitis · pulmonary toxicity
- **Frequency not known**
- With oral use Altered smell sensation · appetite decreased · parkinsonism · vasculitis
- With parenteral use Agranulocytosis · libido decreased · neutropenia

SIDE-EFFECTS, FURTHER INFORMATION Side-effects can occur at any time during treatment with, or in the months after stopping amiodarone.

Corneal microdeposits Patients taking amiodarone may develop corneal microdeposits (reversible on withdrawal of treatment). However, if vision is impaired or if optic neuritis or optic neuropathy occur, amiodarone must be stopped to prevent blindness and expert advice sought.

Thyroid function Amiodarone contains iodine and can cause disorders of thyroid function; both hypothyroidism and hyperthyroidism can occur. Hypothyroidism can be treated with replacement therapy without withdrawing amiodarone if it is essential; careful supervision is required.

Hepatotoxicity Amiodarone is also associated with hepatotoxicity and treatment should be discontinued if severe liver function abnormalities or clinical signs of liver disease develop.

Pulmonary toxicity If new or progressive shortness of breath or cough develops in patients taking amiodarone (or recently stopped), pulmonary toxicity should always be suspected. Pulmonary toxicity is usually reversible following early withdrawal of amiodarone.

- **PREGNANCY** Possible risk of neonatal goitre; use only if no alternative.
- **BREAST FEEDING** Avoid; present in milk in significant amounts; theoretical risk of neonatal hypothyroidism from release of iodine.
- **MONITORING REQUIREMENTS**
- EvGr Liver function tests required before treatment and then every 6 months.
- Serum potassium concentration should be measured before treatment.
- Chest x-ray required before treatment.
- Pulmonary function tests required before treatment.
- Thyroid function tests should be performed before treatment, then at 6-monthly intervals, and for several months after stopping treatment. Thyroid stimulating hormone levels should be measured if thyroid dysfunction is suspected. ⟨M⟩ Consult specialist if thyroid function is abnormal.
- With intravenous use EvGr ECG monitoring and resuscitation facilities must be available. Monitor liver transaminases closely. ⟨M⟩
- **DIRECTIONS FOR ADMINISTRATION**
- With intravenous use EvGr Intravenous infusion via central venous catheter recommended if repeated or continuous infusion required, as infusion via peripheral veins may cause pain and inflammation. In emergency use for cardiopulmonary resuscitation, a peripheral venous route can be used if central venous access is not available; the peripheral line should be flushed liberally. ⟨M⟩ For *intravenous infusion*, manufacturer advises dilute to a concentration of not less than 600 micrograms/mL with Glucose 5%. Incompatible with Sodium Chloride infusion fluids; avoid equipment containing the plasticizer di-2-ethylhexphthalate (DEHP).
- With oral use For administration *by mouth*, expert sources advise tablets may be crushed and dispersed in water; injection solution should **not** be given orally (irritant).
- **PATIENT AND CARER ADVICE**

Phototoxicity Because of the possibility of phototoxic reactions, patients should be advised to shield the skin from light during treatment and for several months after discontinuing amiodarone; a wide-spectrum sunscreen to protect against both long-wave ultraviolet and visible light should be used.

Concurrent sofosbuvir-containing regimens If taking amiodarone with concurrent sofosbuvir-containing regimens, patients and their carers should be told how to recognise signs and symptoms of bradycardia and heart block and advised to seek immediate medical attention if symptoms such as shortness of breath, light-headedness, palpitations, fainting, unusual tiredness or chest pain develop.

Medicines for Children leaflet: Amiodarone for abnormal heart rhythms www.medicinesforchildren.org.uk/medicines/amiodarone-for-abnormal-heart-rhythms/

Driving and skilled tasks Patients and carers should be cautioned on the effects on driving and performance of skilled tasks—corneal microdeposits may be associated with blurred vision (see *Side-effects, further information*).

- **MEDICINAL FORMS** There can be variation in the licensing of different medicines containing the same drug. Forms available from special-order manufacturers include: oral suspension, oral solution

Oral tablet

CAUTIONARY AND ADVISORY LABELS 11

- Amiodarone hydrochloride (Non-proprietary)

Amiodarone hydrochloride 100 mg Amiodarone 100mg tablets | 28 tablet PoM £9.90 DT = £8.56

Amiodarone hydrochloride 200 mg Amiodarone 200mg tablets | 28 tablet PoM £14.50 DT = £8.68

Solution for injection

EXCIPIENTS: May contain Benzyl alcohol

- Amiodarone hydrochloride (Non-proprietary)

Amiodarone hydrochloride 30 mg per 1 ml Amiodarone 300mg/10ml solution for injection pre-filled syringes | 1 pre-filled disposable injection PoM £39.39–£74.06

Amiodarone hydrochloride 50 mg per 1 ml Amiodarone 150mg/3ml concentrate for solution for injection ampoules | 5 ampoule PoM £7.75 (Hospital only) | 10 ampoule PoM £25.00

ANTIARRHYTHMICS › OTHER

Adenosine

28-Jul-2020

- **INDICATIONS AND DOSE**

Used in conjunction with radionuclide myocardial perfusion imaging in patients who cannot exercise adequately or for whom exercise is inappropriate

- BY INTRAVENOUS INFUSION
- Child: (consult product literature)

Termination of supraventricular tachycardias, including those associated with accessory conducting pathways (e.g. Wolff-Parkinson-White syndrome) | Diagnosis of supraventricular arrhythmias

- BY RAPID INTRAVENOUS INJECTION
- Neonate: Initially 150 micrograms/kg, then increased in steps of 50–100 micrograms/kg every 1–2 minutes if required, dose to be repeated until tachycardia terminated or maximum single dose of 300 micrograms/kg given.

continued →

- Child 1–11 months: Initially 150 micrograms/kg, then increased in steps of 50–100 micrograms/kg every 1–2 minutes if required, dose to be repeated until tachycardia terminated or maximum single dose of 500 micrograms/kg given
- Child 1–11 years: Initially 100 micrograms/kg, then increased in steps of 50–100 micrograms/kg every 1–2 minutes if required, dose to be repeated until tachycardia terminated or maximum single dose of 500 micrograms/kg (max.12 mg) given
- Child 12–17 years: Initially 3 mg, followed by 6 mg after 1–2 minutes if required, followed by 12 mg after 1–2 minutes if required, in some children over 12 years 3 mg dose ineffective (e.g. if a small peripheral vein is used for administration) and higher initial dose sometimes used; however, those with *heart transplant* are **very sensitive** to the effects of adenosine, and should **not** receive higher initial doses

- **UNLICENSED USE** *Adenocor*® licensed for treatment of paroxysmal supraventricular tachycardia in children; not licensed for diagnosis in children; *Adenoscan*® not licensed in children.
- **CONTRA-INDICATIONS** Asthma · decompensated heart failure · long QT syndrome · second- or third-degree AV block and sick sinus syndrome (unless pacemaker fitted) · severe hypotension
- **CAUTIONS** Atrial fibrillation · atrial fibrillation with accessory pathway (conduction down anomalous pathway may increase) · atrial flutter · atrial flutter with accessory pathway (conduction down anomalous pathway may increase) · autonomic dysfunction · bundle branch block · first-degree AV block · heart transplant · left main coronary artery stenosis · left to right shunt · pericardial effusion · pericarditis · QT-interval prolongation · recent myocardial infarction · severe heart failure · stenotic carotid artery disease with cerebrovascular insufficiency · stenotic valvular heart disease · uncorrected hypovolaemia
- **INTERACTIONS** → Appendix 1: antiarrhythmics
- **SIDE-EFFECTS**
  - **Common or very common** Abdominal discomfort · arrhythmias · atrioventricular block · chest discomfort · chest pain (discontinue) · dizziness · dry mouth · dyspnoea · flushing · headache · hypotension (discontinue if severe) · pain · paraesthesia · throat discomfort
  - **Uncommon** Asthenia · back discomfort · bradycardia (discontinue if asystole or severe bradycardia occur) · hyperhidrosis · limb discomfort · nervousness · taste metallic
  - **Rare or very rare** Drowsiness · nasal congestion · nipple tenderness · respiratory disorders · respiratory failure (discontinue) · tinnitus · tremor · urinary urgency · vision blurred
  - **Frequency not known** Apnoea · cardiac arrest · loss of consciousness · nausea · seizure · syncope · vomiting
- **PREGNANCY** Large doses may produce fetal toxicity; manufacturer advises use only if potential benefit outweighs risk.
- **BREAST FEEDING** No information available—unlikely to be present in milk owing to short half-life.
- **MONITORING REQUIREMENTS** Monitor ECG and have resuscitation facilities available.
- **DIRECTIONS FOR ADMINISTRATION** For *rapid intravenous injection*, expert sources advise give over 2 seconds into central or large peripheral vein followed by rapid Sodium Chloride 0.9% flush; injection solution may be diluted with Sodium Chloride 0.9% if required.
- **MEDICINAL FORMS** There can be variation in the licensing of different medicines containing the same drug. Forms available from special-order manufacturers include: solution for injection, infusion, solution for infusion

Solution for injection

ELECTROLYTES: May contain Sodium

- **Adenosine (Non-proprietary)**

  Adenosine 3 mg per 1 ml Adenosine 6mg/2ml solution for injection vials | 5 vial PoM £33.00 (Hospital only) | 6 vial PoM £26.70–£29.24 (Hospital only)

  Adenosine 6mg/2ml solution for injection ampoules | 10 ampoule PoM £44.50 (Hospital only)

Solution for infusion

ELECTROLYTES: May contain Sodium

- **Adenosine (Non-proprietary)**

  Adenosine 3 mg per 1 ml Adenosine 30mg/10ml solution for infusion vials | 5 vial PoM £93.50 (Hospital only) | 6 vial PoM £70.00–£85.57 (Hospital only)

BETA-ADRENOCEPTOR BLOCKERS › NON-SELECTIVE

F 121

Sotalol hydrochloride

26-Jul-2021

- **INDICATIONS AND DOSE**

Life-threatening arrhythmias including ventricular tachyarrhythmias

▶ BY MOUTH

- Child 12–17 years: Initially 80 mg once daily, alternatively initially 40 mg twice daily, then increased to 80–160 mg twice daily, dose to be increased gradually at intervals of 2–3 days; higher doses of 480–640 mg daily may be required for life-threatening ventricular arrhythmias (under specialist supervision)

Ventricular arrhythmias, life-threatening ventricular tachyarrhythmia and supraventricular arrhythmias (initiated under specialist supervision)

▶ BY MOUTH

- Neonate: Initially 1 mg/kg twice daily, increased if necessary up to 4 mg/kg twice daily, dose to be increased at intervals of 3–4 days.

Atrial flutter, ventricular arrhythmias, life-threatening ventricular tachyarrhythmia and supraventricular arrhythmias (initiated under specialist supervision)

▶ BY MOUTH

- Child 1 month–11 years: Initially 1 mg/kg twice daily, then increased if necessary up to 4 mg/kg twice daily (max. per dose 80 mg twice daily), dose to be increased at intervals of 2–3 days
- Child 12–17 years: Initially 80 mg once daily, alternatively initially 40 mg twice daily, increased to 80–160 mg twice daily, dose to be increased gradually at intervals of 2–3 days

- **UNLICENSED USE** Not licensed for use in children under 12 years.

IMPORTANT SAFETY INFORMATION

Sotalol may prolong the QT interval, and it occasionally causes life threatening ventricular arrhythmias (**important**: manufacturer advises particular care is required to avoid hypokalaemia in patients taking sotalol—electrolyte disturbances, particularly hypokalaemia and hypomagnesaemia should be corrected before sotalol started and during use).

Manufacturer advises reduce dose or discontinue if corrected QT interval exceeds 550 msec.

- **CONTRA-INDICATIONS** Long QT syndrome (congenital or acquired) · torsade de pointes
- **CAUTIONS** Diarrhoea (severe or prolonged)

- **INTERACTIONS** → Appendix 1: beta blockers, non-selective
- **SIDE-EFFECTS**
  - ▶ **Common or very common** Anxiety · arrhythmia · chest pain · dyspepsia · fever · flatulence · hearing impairment · mood altered · muscle spasms · oedema · palpitations · sexual dysfunction · taste altered · torsade de pointes (increased risk in females)
- **BREAST FEEDING** Water soluble beta-blockers such as sotalol are present in breast milk in greater amounts than other beta blockers.
- **RENAL IMPAIRMENT** Expert sources advise avoid if estimated glomerular filtration rate less than 10 mL/minute/1.73 m^2.

  Dose adjustments See p. 16.

  Expert sources advise halve normal dose if estimated glomerular filtration rate 30–60 mL/minute/1.73 m^2; use one-quarter normal dose if estimated glomerular filtration rate 10–30 mL/minute/1.73 m^2.
- **MONITORING REQUIREMENTS** Measurement of corrected QT interval, and monitoring of ECG and electrolytes required; correct hypokalaemia, hypomagnesaemia, or other electrolyte disturbances.
- **DIRECTIONS FOR ADMINISTRATION** For administration *by mouth*, expert sources advise tablets may be crushed and dispersed in water.

- **MEDICINAL FORMS** There can be variation in the licensing of different medicines containing the same drug. Forms available from special-order manufacturers include: oral suspension, oral solution

Oral tablet

CAUTIONARY AND ADVISORY LABELS 8

▶ **Sotalol hydrochloride (Non-proprietary)**

Sotalol hydrochloride 40 mg Sotalol 40mg tablets | 28 tablet PoM £6.74 DT = £0.95

Sotalol hydrochloride 80 mg Sotalol 80mg tablets | 28 tablet PoM £10.00 DT = £1.43

Sotalol hydrochloride 160 mg Sotalol 160mg tablets | 28 tablet PoM £16.46 DT = £7.47

CARDIAC GLYCOSIDES

Cardiac glycosides

16-Sep-2025

Digoxin-specific antibody fragments

Serious cases of digoxin toxicity should be discussed with the National Poisons Information Service (see further information, under Poisoning, emergency treatment p. 1036). Digoxin-specific antibody fragments p. 1046 are indicated for the treatment of known or strongly suspected life-threatening digoxin toxicity associated with ventricular arrhythmias or bradyarrhythmias unresponsive to atropine sulfate p. 1013 and when measures beyond the withdrawal of digoxin below and correction of any electrolyte abnormalities are considered necessary.

Digoxin

Digoxin is most useful in the treatment of supraventricular tachycardias, especially for controlling ventricular response in persistent atrial fibrillation. Digoxin has a limited role in children with chronic heart failure.

For the management of atrial fibrillation, the maintenance dose of digoxin is determined on the basis of the ventricular rate at rest, which should not be allowed to fall below an acceptable level for the child.

Digoxin is now rarely used for rapid control of heart rate, even with intravenous administration, response may take many hours; persistence of tachycardia is therefore not an indication for exceeding the recommended dose. The intramuscular route is **not** recommended.

In children with heart failure who are in sinus rhythm, a loading dose may not be required.

Unwanted effects depend both on the concentration of digoxin in the plasma and on the sensitivity of the conducting system or of the myocardium, which is often increased in heart disease. It can sometimes be difficult to distinguish between toxic effects and clinical deterioration because the symptoms of both are similar. The plasma-digoxin concentration alone cannot indicate toxicity reliably, but the likelihood of toxicity increases progressively through the range 1.5 to 3 micrograms/litre for digoxin. Renal function is very important in determining digoxin dosage.

Hypokalaemia predisposes the child to digitalis toxicity and should be avoided; it is managed by giving a potassium-sparing diuretic or, if necessary, potassium supplements.

If toxicity occurs, digoxin should be withdrawn; serious manifestations require urgent specialist management. Digoxin-specific antibody fragments are available for reversal of life-threatening overdosage.

Digoxin

15-Apr-2024

- **DRUG ACTION** Digoxin is a cardiac glycoside that increases the force of myocardial contraction and reduces conductivity within the atrioventricular (AV) node.

- **INDICATIONS AND DOSE**

Supraventricular arrhythmias | Chronic heart failure

▶ BY MOUTH

- ▶ Neonate (body-weight up to 1.5 kg): Initially 25 micrograms/kg in 3 divided doses for 24 hours, then 4–6 micrograms/kg daily in 1–2 divided doses.
- ▶ Neonate (body-weight 1.5–2.5 kg): Initially 30 micrograms/kg in 3 divided doses for 24 hours, then 4–6 micrograms/kg daily in 1–2 divided doses.
- ▶ Neonate (body-weight 2.6 kg and above): Initially 45 micrograms/kg in 3 divided doses for 24 hours, then 10 micrograms/kg daily in 1–2 divided doses.
- ▶ Child 1 month–1 year: Initially 45 micrograms/kg in 3 divided doses for 24 hours, then 10 micrograms/kg daily in 1–2 divided doses
- ▶ Child 2–4 years: Initially 35 micrograms/kg in 3 divided doses for 24 hours, then 10 micrograms/kg daily in 1–2 divided doses
- ▶ Child 5–9 years: Initially 25 micrograms/kg in 3 divided doses for 24 hours, maximum 750 micrograms per day, then 6 micrograms/kg daily in 1–2 divided doses, maximum 250 micrograms per day
- ▶ Child 10–17 years: Initially 0.75–1.5 mg in 3 divided doses for 24 hours, then 62.5–250 micrograms daily in 1–2 divided doses, higher doses may be necessary

▶ BY INTRAVENOUS INFUSION

- ▶ Neonate (body-weight up to 1.5 kg): Initially 20 micrograms/kg in 3 divided doses for 24 hours, then 4–6 micrograms/kg daily in 1–2 divided doses.
- ▶ Neonate (body-weight 1.5–2.5 kg): Initially 30 micrograms/kg in 3 divided doses for 24 hours, then 4–6 micrograms/kg daily in 1–2 divided doses.
- ▶ Neonate (body-weight 2.6 kg and above): Initially 35 micrograms/kg in 3 divided doses for 24 hours, then 10 micrograms/kg daily in 1–2 divided doses.
- ▶ Child 1 month–1 year: Initially 35 micrograms/kg in 3 divided doses for 24 hours, then 10 micrograms/kg daily in 1–2 divided doses

continued →

- Child 2–4 years: Initially 35 micrograms/kg in 3 divided doses for 24 hours, then 10 micrograms/kg daily in 1–2 divided doses
- Child 5–9 years: Initially 25 micrograms/kg in 3 divided doses for 24 hours, maximum 500 micrograms per day, then 6 micrograms/kg daily in 1–2 divided doses, maximum 250 micrograms per day
- Child 10–17 years: Initially 0.5–1 mg in 3 divided doses for 24 hours, then 62.5–250 micrograms daily in 1–2 divided doses, higher doses may be necessary

DOSE ADJUSTMENTS DUE TO INTERACTIONS
- Manufacturer advises reduce dose by half with concurrent use of amiodarone, dronedarone and quinine.

DOSE EQUIVALENCE AND CONVERSION
- Dose may need to be reduced if digoxin (or another cardiac glycoside) has been given in the preceding 2 weeks.
- When switching from intravenous to oral route may need to increase dose by 20–33% to maintain the same plasma-digoxin concentration.

- **UNLICENSED USE** Digoxin is licensed for use in heart failure and supraventricular arrhythmias.
- **CONTRA-INDICATIONS** Constrictive pericarditis (unless to control atrial fibrillation or improve systolic dysfunction—but use with caution) · hypertrophic cardiomyopathy (unless concomitant atrial fibrillation and heart failure—but use with caution) · intermittent complete heart block · myocarditis · second degree AV block · supraventricular arrhythmias associated with accessory conducting pathways e.g. Wolff-Parkinson-White syndrome (although can be used in infancy) · ventricular tachycardia or fibrillation
- **CAUTIONS** Hypercalcaemia (risk of digitalis toxicity) · hypokalaemia (risk of digitalis toxicity) · hypomagnesaemia (risk of digitalis toxicity) · hypoxia (risk of digitalis toxicity) · recent myocardial infarction · severe respiratory disease · sick sinus syndrome · thyroid disease
- **INTERACTIONS** → Appendix 1: digoxin
- **SIDE-EFFECTS**
  - **Common or very common** Arrhythmias · cardiac conduction disorder · cerebral impairment · diarrhoea · dizziness · eosinophilia · nausea · skin reactions · vision disorders · vomiting
  - **Uncommon** Depression
  - **Rare or very rare** Appetite decreased · asthenia · confusion · gastrointestinal disorders · gynaecomastia · headache · malaise · psychosis · thrombocytopenia

  Overdose If toxicity occurs, digoxin should be withdrawn; serious manifestations require urgent specialist management.
- **PREGNANCY**
  Dose adjustments May need dosage adjustment.
- **BREAST FEEDING** Amount too small to be harmful.
- **RENAL IMPAIRMENT**
  Dose adjustments Expert sources advise use half normal dose if estimated glomerular filtration rate is 10–50 mL/minute/1.73 m^2 and use a quarter normal dose if estimated glomerular filtration rate is less than 10 mL/minute/1.73 m^2. See p. 16.
- **MONITORING REQUIREMENTS**
  - For plasma-digoxin concentration assay, blood should be taken at least 6 hours after a dose.
  - Plasma-digoxin concentration should be maintained in the range 0.8–2 micrograms/litre.
  - Monitor serum electrolytes and renal function. Toxicity increased by electrolyte disturbances.
- **DIRECTIONS FOR ADMINISTRATION**
  - With intravenous use Avoid rapid intravenous administration (risk of hypertension and reduced coronary flow). For *intravenous infusion*, dilute with Sodium Chloride 0.9% or Glucose 5% to a max. concentration of 62.5 micrograms/mL; loading doses should be given over 30–60 minutes and maintenance dose over 10–20 minutes.
  - With oral use For *oral* administration, oral solution must **not** be diluted.
- **PATIENT AND CARER ADVICE** Patient counselling is advised for digoxin elixir (use pipette).
- **MEDICINAL FORMS** There can be variation in the licensing of different medicines containing the same drug. Forms available from special-order manufacturers include: oral suspension, oral solution, solution for injection

Oral tablet
- Digoxin (Non-proprietary)
  Digoxin 62.5 microgram Digoxin 62.5microgram tablets | 28 tablet PoM £2.35 DT = £1.09 | 30 tablet PoM £1.17–£2.45
  Digoxin 125 microgram Digoxin 125microgram tablets | 28 tablet PoM £2.38 DT = £1.06 | 30 tablet PoM £1.14–£2.45
  Digoxin 250 microgram Digoxin 250microgram tablets | 28 tablet PoM £2.28 DT = £1.06 | 30 tablet PoM £1.14–£2.45

Solution for injection
EXCIPIENTS: May contain Alcohol, propylene glycol
- Digoxin (Non-proprietary)
  Digoxin 100 microgram per 1 ml Lanoxin Injection Pediatric 100micrograms/1ml solution for injection ampoules | 10 ampoule PoM 🅇

Solution for infusion
- Digoxin (Non-proprietary)
  Digoxin 250 microgram per 1 ml Digoxin 500micrograms/2ml solution for infusion ampoules | 5 ampoule PoM £4.95 (Hospital only)

Oral solution
- Digoxin (Non-proprietary)
  Digoxin 50 microgram per 1 ml Digoxin 50micrograms/ml oral solution | 60 ml PoM £6.95 DT = £6.95

2 Bleeding disorders

ANTIHAEMORRHAGICS > ANTIFIBRINOLYTICS

Tranexamic acid

05-Jan-2024

- **DRUG ACTION** Tranexamic acid is an antifibrinolytic that prevents or reduces bleeding by impairing fibrin dissolution.
- **INDICATIONS AND DOSE**

Inhibition of fibrinolysis
- BY MOUTH
  - Child: 15–25 mg/kg 2–3 times a day (max. per dose 1.5 g)
- BY SLOW INTRAVENOUS INJECTION
  - Child: 10 mg/kg 2–3 times a day (max. per dose 1 g), dose to be given over at least 10 minutes
- BY CONTINUOUS INTRAVENOUS INFUSION
  - Child: 45 mg/kg/24 hours

Menorrhagia
- BY MOUTH
  - Child 12–17 years: 1 g 3 times a day for up to 4 days, to be initiated when menstruation has started, dose can be increased if necessary up to maximum 4 g per day

Hereditary angioedema
- BY MOUTH
  - Child: 15–25 mg/kg 2–3 times a day (max. per dose 1.5 g), for short-term prophylaxis of hereditary angioedema, tranexamic acid is started several days before planned procedures which may trigger an acute

attack of hereditary angioedema (e.g. dental work) and continued for 2–5 days afterwards

- ▶ BY SLOW INTRAVENOUS INJECTION
- ▸ Child: 10 mg/kg 2–3 times a day (max. per dose 1 g), dose to be given over at least 10 minutes
- ▶ BY CONTINUOUS INTRAVENOUS INFUSION
- ▸ Child: 45 mg/kg/24 hours

Prevention of excessive bleeding after dental procedures (e.g. in haemophilia)

- ▶ BY INTRAVENOUS INJECTION
- ▸ Child 6–17 years: 10 mg/kg for 1 dose (max. per dose 1.5 g), to be given pre-operatively
- ▶ BY MOUTH
- ▸ Child 6–17 years: 15–25 mg/kg for 1 dose (max. per dose 1.5 g), to be given pre-operatively, then 15–25 mg/kg 2–3 times a day (max. per dose 1.5 g) for up to 8 days, to be given postoperatively

Prevention of excessive bleeding after dental procedures (e.g. in haemophilia) with mouthwash 5% solution (specialist use only)

- ▶ BY OROMUCOSAL ADMINISTRATION
- ▸ Child 6–17 years: 5–10 mL 4 times a day for 2 days, rinse mouth with solution; the solution should not be swallowed

Reduction of blood loss during cardiac surgery

- ▶ BY SLOW INTRAVENOUS INJECTION, OR BY INTRAVENOUS INFUSION
- ▸ Child: (consult local protocol)

Haemorrhage following major trauma

- ▶ INITIALLY BY SLOW INTRAVENOUS INJECTION
- ▸ Child: Loading dose 15 mg/kg (max. per dose 1 g), given as soon as possible within 3 hours of the injury, followed by (by continuous intravenous infusion) 2 mg/kg/hour (max. per dose 1 g) for at least 8 hours or until bleeding stops

Prevention and treatment of haemorrhage following head injury [Glasgow Coma Scale score of 12 or less, and without active extracranial bleeding]

- ▶ BY SLOW INTRAVENOUS INJECTION
- ▸ Neonate: 15–30 mg/kg for 1 dose, given as soon as possible within 2 hours of the injury.
- ▸ Child 1 month–15 years: 15–30 mg/kg for 1 dose (max. per dose 2 g), given as soon as possible within 2 hours of the injury
- ▸ Child 16–17 years: 2 g for 1 dose, given as soon as possible within 2 hours of the injury

● **UNLICENSED USE** Not licensed for reduction of blood loss during cardiac surgery; injection not licensed for use in children under 1 year or for administration by intravenous infusion.

▸ With intravenous use Advanced Paediatric Life Support (APLS) guidance advises tranexamic acid is used for haemorrhage following major trauma, but this is unlicensed. [EvGr] Tranexamic acid is used for prevention and treatment of haemorrhage following head injury, ⟨A⟩ but this is unlicensed.

● **CONTRA-INDICATIONS** Fibrinolytic conditions following disseminated intravascular coagulation (unless predominant activation of fibrinolytic system with severe bleeding) · history of convulsions · thromboembolic disease

● **CAUTIONS** Irregular menstrual bleeding (establish cause before initiating therapy) · massive haematuria (avoid if risk of ureteric obstruction) · patients receiving oral contraceptives (increased risk of thrombosis)

CAUTIONS, FURTHER INFORMATION

▸ Menorrhagia Before initiating treatment for menorrhagia, exclude structural or histological causes or fibroids causing distortion of uterine cavity.

● **SIDE-EFFECTS**

GENERAL SIDE-EFFECTS

- ▶ **Common or very common** Diarrhoea (reduce dose) · nausea · vomiting
- ▶ **Uncommon** Allergic dermatitis
- ▶ **Rare or very rare** Colour vision change (discontinue) · embolism and thrombosis
- ▶ **Frequency not known** Seizure (more common at high doses) · visual impairment (discontinue)

SPECIFIC SIDE-EFFECTS

▸ With intravenous use Hypotension · malaise (on rapid intravenous injection)

● **PREGNANCY** No evidence of teratogenicity in *animal* studies; manufacturer advises use only if potential benefit outweighs risk—crosses the placenta.

● **BREAST FEEDING** Small amount present in milk—antifibrinolytic effect in infant unlikely.

● **RENAL IMPAIRMENT** Avoid in severe impairment.
Dose adjustments Reduce dose in mild to moderate impairment.

● **MONITORING REQUIREMENTS** Regular liver function tests in long-term treatment of hereditary angioedema.

● **DIRECTIONS FOR ADMINISTRATION** [EvGr] Give by slow intravenous injection or infusion at a maximum rate of 100 mg/minute; can be diluted in Glucose 5% *or* Sodium Chloride 0.9%. ⟨M⟩

● **PATIENT AND CARER ADVICE**
Medicines for Children leaflet: Tranexamic acid for heavy bleeding during periods www.medicinesforchildren.org.uk/medicines/tranexamic-acid-for-heavy-bleeding-during-periods/
Medicines for Children leaflet: Tranexamic acid for the treatment or prevention of bleeding in haemophilia and other clotting problems www.medicinesforchildren.org.uk/medicines/tranexamic-acid-for-the-treatment-or-prevention-of-bleeding-in-haemophilia-and-other-clotting-problems/

● **MEDICINAL FORMS** There can be variation in the licensing of different medicines containing the same drug. Forms available from special-order manufacturers include: oral suspension, oral solution

Oral tablet

▸ **Tranexamic acid (Non-proprietary)**
Tranexamic acid 500 mg Tranexamic acid 500mg tablets | 60 tablet [PoM] £13.95 DT = £3.25

▸ **Cyklokapron** (Viatris UK Healthcare Ltd)
Tranexamic acid 500 mg Cyklokapron 500mg tablets | 60 tablet [PoM] £14.30 DT = £3.25

Solution for injection

▸ **Tranexamic acid (Non-proprietary)**
Tranexamic acid 100 mg per 1 ml Tranexamic acid 500mg/5ml solution for injection ampoules | 5 ampoule [PoM] £7.50 DT = £7.50 (Hospital only) | 10 ampoule [PoM] £15.47 DT = £15.47 (Hospital only)
Tranexamic acid 1g/10ml solution for injection ampoules | 5 ampoule [PoM] £15.00 (Hospital only)

▸ **Cyklokapron** (Pfizer Ltd)
Tranexamic acid 100 mg per 1 ml Cyklokapron 500mg/5ml solution for injection ampoules | 10 ampoule [PoM] £15.47 DT = £15.47 (Hospital only)

2.1 Coagulation factor deficiencies

ANTIHAEMORRHAGICS > HAEMOSTATICS

Emicizumab

22-Aug-2025

- **DRUG ACTION** Emicizumab is a monoclonal antibody that bridges activated factor IX and factor X to restore function of missing activated factor VIII, which is needed for haemostasis.

- **INDICATIONS AND DOSE**

Prophylaxis of haemorrhage in haemophilia A (initiated by a specialist)

▶ BY SUBCUTANEOUS INJECTION

▶ Child: Initially 3 mg/kg once weekly for 4 weeks, then maintenance 1.5 mg/kg once weekly, alternatively maintenance 3 mg/kg every 2 weeks, alternatively maintenance 6 mg/kg every 4 weeks

- **CAUTIONS** Children under 1 year · concomitant bypassing agent · risk factors for thrombotic microangiopathy

CAUTIONS, FURTHER INFORMATION

▶ Concomitant bypassing agent Manufacturer advises discontinue bypassing agents the day before starting emicizumab; if a bypassing agent is required—consult product literature.

- **SIDE-EFFECTS**

▶ **Common or very common** Arthralgia · diarrhoea · fever · headache · myalgia

▶ **Uncommon** Cavernous sinus thrombosis · embolism and thrombosis · skin necrosis · thrombotic microangiopathy

- **CONCEPTION AND CONTRACEPTION** Manufacturer advises effective contraception during and for 6 months after treatment in women of childbearing potential.
- **PREGNANCY** Manufacturer advises use only if potential benefit outweighs risk—no information available.
- **BREAST FEEDING** Manufacturer advises avoid—no information available.
- **EFFECT ON LABORATORY TESTS** Manufacturer advises to avoid intrinsic pathway clotting-based laboratory tests or use with caution as results may be misinterpreted—consult product literature.
- **DIRECTIONS FOR ADMINISTRATION** Manufacturer advises max. 2 mL per injection site; rotate injection site and avoid skin that is tender, damaged or scarred. Patients or their caregivers may self-administer *Hemlibra*® after appropriate training.
- **PRESCRIBING AND DISPENSING INFORMATION** Emicizumab is a biological medicine. Biological medicines must be prescribed and dispensed by brand name, see *Biological medicines* and *Biosimilar medicines*, under Guidance on prescribing p. 1; manufacturer advises to record the brand name and batch number after each administration.
- **PATIENT AND CARER ADVICE**

Missed doses Manufacturer advises if a dose is missed, the missed dose may be taken up to a day before the next scheduled dose. The next dose should then be taken on the usual scheduled dosing day.

- **MEDICINAL FORMS** There can be variation in the licensing of different medicines containing the same drug.

Solution for injection

▶ **Hemlibra** (Roche Products Ltd)

Emicizumab 30 mg per 1 ml Hemlibra 12mg/0.4ml solution for injection vials | 1 vial PoM £966.12 (Hospital only)
Hemlibra 30mg/1ml solution for injection vials | 1 vial PoM £2,415.30 (Hospital only)

Emicizumab 150 mg per 1 ml Hemlibra 150mg/1ml solution for injection vials | 1 vial PoM £12,076.50 (Hospital only)
Hemlibra 105mg/0.7ml solution for injection vials | 1 vial PoM £8,453.55 (Hospital only)
Hemlibra 60mg/0.4ml solution for injection vials | 1 vial PoM £4,830.60 (Hospital only)

Marstacimab

06-Feb-2026

- **DRUG ACTION** Marstacimab is a recombinant human monoclonal antibody that binds to tissue factor pathway inhibitor, thereby preventing inhibition of the extrinsic coagulation pathway and promoting haemostasis.

- **INDICATIONS AND DOSE**

Haemophilia A (initiated by a specialist) | Haemophilia B (initiated by a specialist)

▶ BY SUBCUTANEOUS INJECTION

▶ Child 12–17 years (body-weight 35–49 kg): Loading dose 300 mg for 1 dose, then 150 mg once weekly

▶ Child 12–17 years (body-weight 50 kg and above): Loading dose 300 mg for 1 dose, then 150 mg once weekly, increased if necessary up to 300 mg once weekly, increased dose used if control of bleeding events is inadequate

- **CAUTIONS** Increased risk of thromboembolic events · major surgery (interrupt treatment—consult product literature)

CAUTIONS, FURTHER INFORMATION

▶ Increased risk of thromboembolic events EvGr Consider benefits versus risks of treatment in patients that may be at increased risk of thromboembolic events, such as those with a history of coronary artery disease, venous or arterial thrombosis, or ischaemic disease, and in those with acute severe illness with increased tissue factor expression (such as serious infection, sepsis, trauma, crush injuries, or cancer). Monitor patients for early signs of thrombosis and offer thromboprophylaxis; interrupt treatment if thromboembolism occurs. ⟨M⟩

- **SIDE-EFFECTS**

▶ **Common or very common** Headache · hypertension · skin reactions

- **CONCEPTION AND CONTRACEPTION** EvGr Females of childbearing potential should use effective contraception during and for at least 1 month after last treatment. ⟨M⟩
- **PREGNANCY** EvGr Use only if potential benefit outweighs risk (no information available). ⟨M⟩
- **BREAST FEEDING** Specialist sources indicate use with caution, especially if breast-feeding a neonate or preterm infant (no information available). Large molecular weight suggests limited excretion into milk and drug molecule likely to be partially destroyed in the infant's gastro-intestinal tract; waiting for at least 2 weeks postpartum to resume treatment may minimise transfer to infant.
- **DIRECTIONS FOR ADMINISTRATION** For *subcutaneous injection*, remove prefilled pen from the refrigerator 15 to 30 minutes before administration. Inject into the abdomen or thigh, or buttocks (if not self-administered); rotate injection site and avoid skin that is bruised, red, tender, hard, scarred, or where there are stretch marks. *Hympavzi*® may be self-administered or administered by a carer after appropriate training in subcutaneous injection technique. A 300 mg dose should be administered as two consecutive 150 mg injections at separate injection sites.
- **PRESCRIBING AND DISPENSING INFORMATION** Marstacimab is a biological medicine. Biological medicines must be prescribed and dispensed by brand name, see *Biological medicines* and *Biosimilar medicines*, under Guidance on prescribing p. 1; record the brand name and batch number after each administration.

- **HANDLING AND STORAGE** Store in a refrigerator (2–8°C) and protect from light; may be stored at room temperature (below 30°C) for up to 7 days.
- **PATIENT AND CARER ADVICE**
Hypersensitivity reactions Patients and carers should be advised to discontinue treatment and seek immediate medical attention if a severe hypersensitivity reaction develops.
Breakthrough bleeding Patients and carers should be advised on the management of breakthrough bleeding using clotting factors, as marstacimab should not be used for treatment of such events—consult product literature.
Self-administration Patients and carers should be given training in subcutaneous injection technique if appropriate.
Missed doses If a dose is missed, administer as soon as possible before the day of the next scheduled dose, and resume the usual weekly dosing schedule. If the missed dose is more than 13 days after the last dose, restart treatment with loading dose.
- **NATIONAL FUNDING/ACCESS DECISIONS**
For full details see funding body website

NICE decisions
- **Marstacimab for treating severe haemophilia A or B in people 12 years and over without anti-factor antibodies [for haemophilia B] (June 2025)** NICE TA1073 Recommended
- **Marstacimab for treating severe haemophilia A or B in people 12 years and over without anti-factor antibodies [for haemophilia A] (June 2025)** NICE TA1073 Not recommended

Scottish Medicines Consortium (SMC) decisions
- **Marstacimab (*Hympavzi*®) for routine prophylaxis of bleeding episodes in patients 12 years of age and older, weighing at least 35 kg, with severe haemophilia A without factor VIII inhibitors, or severe haemophilia B without factor IX inhibitors (January 2026)** SMC No. SMC2759 Recommended with restrictions

- **MEDICINAL FORMS** There can be variation in the licensing of different medicines containing the same drug.

Solution for injection
EXCIPIENTS: May contain Disodium edetate, polysorbates
- Hympavzi (Pfizer Ltd) ▼
Marstacimab 150 mg per 1 ml Hympavzi 150mg/1ml solution for injection pre-filled pens | 1 pre-filled disposable injection PoM £9,299.00 (Hospital only)

BLOOD AND RELATED PRODUCTS › COAGULATION PROTEINS

Factor VIIa [Specialist drug] 10-Oct-2025

- **INDICATIONS AND DOSE**

Congenital haemophilia [with inhibitors to, or high anamnestic response to, factors VIII or IX] | Acquired haemophilia | Congenital factor VII deficiency | Glanzmann's thrombasthenia
- BY INTRAVENOUS INJECTION
- Child: Specialist drug – access specialist resources for dosing information

- **SIDE-EFFECTS**
- **Common or very common** Dizziness · headache · injection related reaction
- **Uncommon** Embolism and thrombosis · fever · hepatic disorders · intestinal ischaemia · skin reactions
- **Rare or very rare** Angina pectoris · cerebrovascular insufficiency · coagulation disorders · myocardial infarction · nausea · peripheral ischaemia
- **Frequency not known** Angioedema · flushing
- **ALLERGY AND CROSS-SENSITIVITY** For *Cevenfacta*®, contra-indicated if hypersensitivity to rabbits or rabbit protein. For *NovoSeven*®, contra-indicated if hypersensitivity to mouse, hamster or bovine protein.
- **PREGNANCY**
NOVOSEVEN ® EvGr Avoid (limited information available). (M)
- **BREAST FEEDING**
NOVOSEVEN ® Specialist source suggest probably safe in breast-feeding; unlikely to enter milk or be absorbed from infants gastro-intestinal tract.
- **MEDICINAL FORMS** There can be variation in the licensing of different medicines containing the same drug.

Powder and solvent for solution for injection
EXCIPIENTS: May contain Polysorbates
- Cevenfacta (LFB Biopharmaceuticals Ltd) ▼
Eptacog beta activated 1 mg Cevenfacta 1mg (45,000units) powder and solvent for solution for injection vials | 1 vial PoM £525.20
Eptacog beta activated 2 mg Cevenfacta 2mg (90,000units) powder and solvent for solution for injection vials | 1 vial PoM £1,050.40
Eptacog beta activated 5 mg Cevenfacta 5mg (225,000units) powder and solvent for solution for injection vials | 1 vial PoM £2,626.00
- NovoSeven (Novo Nordisk Ltd)
Eptacog alfa activated 1 mg NovoSeven 1mg (50,000units) powder and solvent for solution for injection pre-filled syringes | 1 pre-filled disposable injection PoM £525.20 (Hospital only)
Eptacog alfa activated 2 mg NovoSeven 2mg (100,000units) powder and solvent for solution for injection pre-filled syringes | 1 pre-filled disposable injection PoM £1,050.40 (Hospital only)
Eptacog alfa activated 5 mg NovoSeven 5mg (250,000units) powder and solvent for solution for injection pre-filled syringes | 1 pre-filled disposable injection PoM £2,626.00 (Hospital only)

Factor VIII [Specialist drug] 16-Sep-2025

- **INDICATIONS AND DOSE**

Congenital factor VIII deficiency (haemophilia A), acquired factor VIII deficiency | Von Willebrand's disease
- BY INTRAVENOUS INJECTION, OR BY INTRAVENOUS INFUSION, OR BY CONTINUOUS INTRAVENOUS INFUSION
- Child: Specialist drug – access specialist resources for dosing information

- **SIDE-EFFECTS**
- **Common or very common** Anamnestic reaction · cough · device thrombosis · diarrhoea · factor VIII inhibition · fever · flushing · haemorrhage · headaches · infusion related reaction · joint disorders · nausea · pain · skin reactions · thrombophlebitis · vomiting
- **Uncommon** Dizziness · fatigue · feeling hot · hyperaemia · hypersensitivity · hypertension · insomnia · lymphoedema · musculoskeletal stiffness · myocardial infarction · peripheral oedema · sinus tachycardia
- **NATIONAL FUNDING/ACCESS DECISIONS**
For full details see funding body website

NICE decisions
- **Efanesoctocog alfa for treating and preventing bleeding episodes in haemophilia A in people 2 years and over (April 2025)** NICE TA1051 Recommended with restrictions

- **MEDICINAL FORMS** There can be variation in the licensing of different medicines containing the same drug.

Powder and solvent for solution for injection
EXCIPIENTS: May contain Polysorbates, sucrose
- Factor viii (Non-proprietary)
Dried Factor VIII Fraction type 8Y 250unit powder and solvent for solution for injection vials | 1 vial PoM £137.00
Factor VIII 500 unit, von Willebrand factor 1000 unit Dried Factor VIII Fraction type 8Y 500unit powder and solvent for solution for injection vials | 1 vial PoM £274.00
- Advate (Takeda UK Ltd)
Octocog alfa 250 unit Advate 250unit powder and 2ml solvent for solution for injection vials | 1 vial PoM £177.50

Advate 250unit powder and 5ml solvent for solution for injection vials | 1 vial PoM £177.50

Octocog alfa 500 unit Advate 500unit powder and 5ml solvent for solution for injection vials | 1 vial PoM £355.00

Advate 500unit powder and 2ml solvent for solution for injection vials | 1 vial PoM £355.00

Octocog alfa 1000 unit Advate 1,000unit powder and solvent for solution for injection vials | 1 vial PoM £710.00

Octocog alfa 2000 unit Advate 2,000unit powder and solvent for solution for injection vials | 1 vial PoM £1,420.00

- **Altuvoct** (Swedish Orphan Biovitrum Ltd) ▼

Efanesoctocog alfa 250 unit Altuvoct 250unit powder and solvent for solution for injection vials | 1 vial PoM £600.00 (Hospital only)

Efanesoctocog alfa 500 unit Altuvoct 500unit powder and solvent for solution for injection vials | 1 vial PoM £1,200.00 (Hospital only)

Efanesoctocog alfa 1000 unit Altuvoct 1,000unit powder and solvent for solution for injection vials | 1 vial PoM £2,400.00 (Hospital only)

Efanesoctocog alfa 2000 unit Altuvoct 2,000unit powder and solvent for solution for injection vials | 1 vial PoM £4,800.00 (Hospital only)

Efanesoctocog alfa 3000 unit Altuvoct 3,000unit powder and solvent for solution for injection vials | 1 vial PoM £7,200.00 (Hospital only)

Efanesoctocog alfa 4000 unit Altuvoct 4,000unit powder and solvent for solution for injection vials | 1 vial PoM £9,600.00 (Hospital only)

- **Elocta** (Swedish Orphan Biovitrum Ltd)

Efmoroctocog alfa 250 unit Elocta 250unit powder and solvent for solution for injection vials | 1 vial PoM £212.50 (Hospital only)

Efmoroctocog alfa 500 unit Elocta 500unit powder and solvent for solution for injection vials | 1 vial PoM £425.00 (Hospital only)

Efmoroctocog alfa 750 unit Elocta 750unit powder and solvent for solution for injection vials | 1 vial PoM £637.50 (Hospital only)

Efmoroctocog alfa 1000 unit Elocta 1,000unit powder and solvent for solution for injection vials | 1 vial PoM £850.00 (Hospital only)

Efmoroctocog alfa 1500 unit Elocta 1,500unit powder and solvent for solution for injection vials | 1 vial PoM £1,275.00 (Hospital only)

Efmoroctocog alfa 2000 unit Elocta 2,000unit powder and solvent for solution for injection vials | 1 vial PoM £1,700.00 (Hospital only)

Efmoroctocog alfa 3000 unit Elocta 3,000unit powder and solvent for solution for injection vials | 1 vial PoM £2,550.00 (Hospital only)

- **Esperoct** (Novo Nordisk Ltd) ▼

Turoctocog alfa pegol 500 unit Esperoct 500unit powder and solvent for solution for injection vials | 1 vial PoM £425.00 (Hospital only)

Turoctocog alfa pegol 1000 unit Esperoct 1,000unit powder and solvent for solution for injection vials | 1 vial PoM £850.00 (Hospital only)

Turoctocog alfa pegol 1500 unit Esperoct 1,500unit powder and solvent for solution for injection vials | 1 vial PoM £1,275.00 (Hospital only)

Turoctocog alfa pegol 2000 unit Esperoct 2,000unit powder and solvent for solution for injection vials | 1 vial PoM £1,700.00 (Hospital only)

Turoctocog alfa pegol 3000 unit Esperoct 3,000unit powder and solvent for solution for injection vials | 1 vial PoM £2,550.00 (Hospital only)

- **Haemoctin** (Grifols UK Ltd)

Factor VIII high purity 1000 unit Haemoctin 1,000unit powder and solvent for solution for injection vials | 1 vial PoM £600.00 (Hospital only)

- **Nuwiq** (Octapharma Ltd)

Simoctocog alfa 250 unit Nuwiq 250unit powder and solvent for solution for injection vials | 1 vial PoM £190.00 (Hospital only)

Simoctocog alfa 500 unit Nuwiq 500unit powder and solvent for solution for injection vials | 1 vial PoM £380.00 (Hospital only)

Simoctocog alfa 1000 unit Nuwiq 1,000unit powder and solvent for solution for injection vials | 1 vial PoM £760.00 (Hospital only)

Simoctocog alfa 1500 unit Nuwiq 1,500unit powder and solvent for solution for injection vials | 1 vial PoM £1,140.00 (Hospital only)

Simoctocog alfa 2000 unit Nuwiq 2,000unit powder and solvent for solution for injection vials | 1 vial PoM £1,520.00 (Hospital only)

- **Obizur** (Takeda UK Ltd) ▼

Susoctocog alfa 500 unit Obizur 500unit powder and solvent for solution for injection vials | 1 vial PoM £1,145.00 (Hospital only)

- **Octanate LV** (Octapharma Ltd)

von Willebrand factor 600 unit, Factor VIII 1000 unit Octanate LV 1,000unit powder and solvent for solution for injection vials | 1 vial PoM £600.00 (Hospital only)

- **ReFacto** (Pfizer Ltd)

Moroctocog alfa 250 unit ReFacto AF 250unit powder and solvent for solution for injection vials | 1 vial PoM £125.55 (Hospital only)

ReFacto AF 250unit powder and solvent for solution for injection pre-filled syringes | 1 pre-filled disposable injection PoM £125.55 (Hospital only)

Moroctocog alfa 500 unit ReFacto AF 500unit powder and solvent for solution for injection vials | 1 vial PoM £251.10 (Hospital only)

ReFacto AF 500unit powder and solvent for solution for injection pre-filled syringes | 1 pre-filled disposable injection PoM £251.10 (Hospital only)

Moroctocog alfa 1000 unit ReFacto AF 1,000unit powder and solvent for solution for injection vials | 1 vial PoM £502.20 (Hospital only)

ReFacto AF 1,000unit powder and solvent for solution for injection pre-filled syringes | 1 pre-filled disposable injection PoM £502.20 (Hospital only)

Moroctocog alfa 2000 unit ReFacto AF 2,000unit powder and solvent for solution for injection pre-filled syringes | 1 pre-filled disposable injection PoM £1,004.40 (Hospital only)

ReFacto AF 2,000unit powder and solvent for solution for injection vials | 1 vial PoM £1,004.40 (Hospital only)

Moroctocog alfa 3000 unit ReFacto AF 3,000unit powder and solvent for solution for injection pre-filled syringes | 1 pre-filled disposable injection PoM £1,506.60 (Hospital only)

- **Voncento** (CSL Behring UK Ltd)

Factor VIII 500 unit, von Willebrand factor 1200 unit Voncento 500unit/1,200unit powder and solvent for solution for injection vials | 1 vial PoM £385.00

Factor VIII 1000 unit, von Willebrand factor 2400 unit Voncento 1,000unit/2,400unit powder and solvent for solution for injection vials | 1 vial PoM £770.00

Powder and solvent for solution for infusion

- **Advate** (Takeda UK Ltd)

Octocog alfa 1500 unit Advate 1,500unit powder and solvent for solution for infusion vials | 1 vial PoM £1,065.00

Octocog alfa 3000 unit Advate 3,000unit powder and solvent for solution for infusion vials | 1 vial PoM £2,130.00

- **Wilate 1000** (Octapharma Ltd)

Factor VIII 1000 unit, von Willebrand factor 1000 unit Wilate 1000 powder and solvent for solution for infusion vials | 1 vial PoM £500.00 (Hospital only)

- **Wilate 500** (Octapharma Ltd)

Factor VIII 500 unit, von Willebrand factor 500 unit Wilate 500 powder and solvent for solution for infusion vials | 1 vial PoM £250.00 (Hospital only)

Factor IX [Specialist drug]

22-Nov-2023

● **INDICATIONS AND DOSE**

Congenital factor IX deficiency (haemophilia B)

- BY INTRAVENOUS INJECTION, OR BY INTRAVENOUS INFUSION
- Child: Specialist drug – access specialist resources for dosing information

● **CONTRA-INDICATIONS** Disseminated intravascular coagulation

● **SIDE-EFFECTS**

- **Common or very common** Anxiety · dizziness · dyspnoea · ear pruritus · factor IX inhibition · fatigue · feeling cold · headache · hot flush · hyperaesthesia · hypersensitivity · nausea · oral disorders · pain · skin reactions · taste altered · urinary tract obstruction
- **Uncommon** Appetite decreased · haematuria · hypotension · palpitations · renal colic
- **Frequency not known** Disseminated intravascular coagulation · embolism and thrombosis · myocardial infarction · nephrotic syndrome

● **ALLERGY AND CROSS-SENSITIVITY** EvGr For *BeneFIX*®, *Idelvion*®, *Refixia*®, and *Rixubis*®, contra-indicated if hypersensitivity to hamster protein. ⟨M⟩

● **MEDICINAL FORMS** There can be variation in the licensing of different medicines containing the same drug.

Powder and solvent for solution for injection

EXCIPIENTS: May contain Polysorbates

▸ Alprolix (Swedish Orphan Biovitrum Ltd)

Eftrenonacog alfa 250 unit Alprolix 250unit powder and solvent for solution for injection vials | 1 vial PoM £300.00 (Hospital only)

Eftrenonacog alfa 500 unit Alprolix 500unit powder and solvent for solution for injection vials | 1 vial PoM £600.00 (Hospital only)

Eftrenonacog alfa 1000 unit Alprolix 1,000unit powder and solvent for solution for injection vials | 1 vial PoM £1,200.00 (Hospital only)

Eftrenonacog alfa 2000 unit Alprolix 2,000unit powder and solvent for solution for injection vials | 1 vial PoM £2,400.00 (Hospital only)

Eftrenonacog alfa 3000 unit Alprolix 3,000unit powder and solvent for solution for injection vials | 1 vial PoM £3,600.00 (Hospital only)

▸ Idelvion (CSL Behring UK Ltd)

Albutrepenonacog alfa 250 unit Idelvion 250unit powder and solvent for solution for injection vials | 1 vial PoM £522.50 (Hospital only)

Albutrepenonacog alfa 500 unit Idelvion 500unit powder and solvent for solution for injection vials | 1 vial PoM £1,045.00 (Hospital only)

Albutrepenonacog alfa 1000 unit Idelvion 1,000unit powder and solvent for solution for injection vials | 1 vial PoM £2,090.00 (Hospital only)

Albutrepenonacog alfa 2000 unit Idelvion 2,000unit powder and solvent for solution for injection vials | 1 vial PoM £4,180.00 (Hospital only)

▸ Refixia (Novo Nordisk Ltd) ▼

Nonacog beta pegol 500 unit Refixia 500unit powder and solvent for solution for injection vials | 1 vial PoM £1,221.50 (Hospital only)

Nonacog beta pegol 1000 unit Refixia 1,000unit powder and solvent for solution for injection vials | 1 vial PoM £2,443.00 (Hospital only)

Nonacog beta pegol 2000 unit Refixia 2,000unit powder and solvent for solution for injection vials | 1 vial PoM £4,886.00 (Hospital only)

Nonacog beta pegol 3000 unit Refixia 3,000unit powder and solvent for solution for injection vials | 1 vial PoM £7,329.00 (Hospital only)

▸ Replenine-VF (Bio Products Laboratory Ltd)

Factor IX high purity 500 unit Replenine-VF 500unit powder and solvent for solution for injection vials | 1 vial PoM £265.00 (Hospital only)

Factor IX high purity 1000 unit Replenine-VF 1,000unit powder and solvent for solution for injection vials | 1 vial PoM £530.00 (Hospital only)

▸ Rixubis (Takeda UK Ltd)

Nonacog gamma 1000 unit Rixubis 1,000unit powder and solvent for solution for injection vials | 1 vial PoM £607.20 (Hospital only)

Nonacog gamma 2000 unit Rixubis 2,000unit powder and solvent for solution for injection vials | 1 vial PoM £1,214.40 (Hospital only)

Powder and solvent for solution for infusion

EXCIPIENTS: May contain Polysorbates

▸ BeneFIX (Pfizer Ltd)

Nonacog alfa 250 unit BeneFIX 250unit powder and solvent for solution for infusion vials | 1 vial PoM £151.80 (Hospital only)

Nonacog alfa 500 unit BeneFIX 500unit powder and solvent for solution for infusion vials | 1 vial PoM £303.60 (Hospital only)

Nonacog alfa 1000 unit BeneFIX 1,000unit powder and solvent for solution for infusion vials | 1 vial PoM £607.20 (Hospital only)

Nonacog alfa 2000 unit BeneFIX 2,000unit powder and solvent for solution for infusion vials | 1 vial PoM £1,214.40 (Hospital only)

Nonacog alfa 3000 unit BeneFIX 3,000unit powder and solvent for solution for infusion vials | 1 vial PoM £1,821.60 (Hospital only)

Factor XIII [Specialist drug] 16-Sep-2025

(Fibrin-stabilising factor)

● **INDICATIONS AND DOSE**

Congenital factor XIII deficiency

▸ BY INTRAVENOUS INJECTION, OR BY INTRAVENOUS INFUSION

▸ Child: Specialist drug – access specialist resources for dosing information

● **SIDE-EFFECTS**

▸ **Rare or very rare** Anaphylactoid reaction · dyspnoea · skin reactions

● **MEDICINAL FORMS** There can be variation in the licensing of different medicines containing the same drug.

Powder and solvent for solution for injection

▸ Fibrogammin P (CSL Behring UK Ltd)

Factor XIII 250 unit Fibrogammin 250unit powder and solvent for solution for injection vials | 1 vial PoM £152.50

Factor XIII 1250 unit Fibrogammin 1,250unit powder and solvent for solution for injection vials | 1 vial PoM £762.50

Factor XIII A-subunit [Specialist drug]

10-Oct-2025

(Catridecacog)

● **INDICATIONS AND DOSE**

Congenital factor XIII A-subunit deficiency

▸ BY INTRAVENOUS INJECTION

▸ Child: Specialist drug – access specialist resources for dosing information

● **SIDE-EFFECTS**

▸ **Common or very common** Headache · leucopenia · neutropenia · pain in extremity

● **MEDICINAL FORMS** There can be variation in the licensing of different medicines containing the same drug.

Powder and solvent for solution for injection

EXCIPIENTS: May contain Polysorbates

▸ NovoThirteen (Novo Nordisk Ltd)

Catridecacog 2500 unit NovoThirteen 2,500unit powder and solvent for solution for injection vials | 1 vial PoM £15,918.13

Fibrinogen [Specialist drug] 10-Oct-2025

(Human fibrinogen)

● **INDICATIONS AND DOSE**

Hypofibrinogenaemia or afibrinogenaemia

▸ BY INTRAVENOUS INJECTION, OR BY INTRAVENOUS INFUSION

▸ Child: Specialist drug – access specialist resources for dosing information

● **SIDE-EFFECTS**

▸ **Common or very common** Chills · cough · headache · hypersensitivity · pallor · skin reactions · vomiting

▸ **Uncommon** Asthma · dizziness · embolism and thrombosis · feeling hot · night sweats · tinnitus

● **MEDICINAL FORMS** There can be variation in the licensing of different medicines containing the same drug.

Powder for solution for infusion

▸ Riastap (CSL Behring UK Ltd)

Human fibrinogen 1 gram Riastap 1g powder for solution for infusion vials | 1 vial PoM £400.00 (Hospital only)

Powder and solvent for solution for infusion

ELECTROLYTES: May contain Sodium

▸ FibCLOT (LFB Biopharmaceuticals Ltd)

Human fibrinogen 1.5 gram FibCLOT 1.5g powder and solvent for solution for infusion vials | 1 vial PoM £600.00 (Hospital only)

▸ Fibryga (Octapharma Ltd)

Human fibrinogen 1 gram Fibryga 1g powder and solvent for solution for infusion bottles | 1 bottle PoM £400.00 (Hospital only)

Protein C [Specialist drug]

10-Oct-2025

● **INDICATIONS AND DOSE**

Congenital protein C deficiency

▶ BY INTRAVENOUS INJECTION

▸ Child: Specialist drug – access specialist resources for dosing information

● **SIDE-EFFECTS**

▶ **Rare or very rare** Dizziness · fever · skin reactions

▶ **Frequency not known** Haemothorax · hyperhidrosis · restlessness

● **MEDICINAL FORMS** There can be variation in the licensing of different medicines containing the same drug.

Powder and solvent for solution for injection

▸ Ceprotin (Takeda UK Ltd)

Protein C human 500 unit Ceprotin 500unit powder and solvent for solution for injection vials | 1 vial PoM £1,000.00

Protein C human 1000 unit Ceprotin 1000unit powder and solvent for solution for injection vials | 1 vial PoM £2,000.00

Prothrombin complex [Specialist drug]

15-Apr-2026

(Human prothrombin complex)

● **INDICATIONS AND DOSE**

Congenital deficiency of factors II, VII, IX, or X if purified specific coagulation factors not available | Acquired deficiency of factors II, VII, IX, or X (e.g. during warfarin treatment)

▶ BY INTRAVENOUS INFUSION

▸ Child: Specialist drug – access specialist resources for dosing information

● **CONTRA-INDICATIONS** History of heparin induced thrombocytopenia · myocardial infarction within the last 3 months (no information available) · unstable angina within the last 3 months (no information available)

● **SIDE-EFFECTS**

▶ **Common or very common** Embolism and thrombosis

▶ **Uncommon** Anxiety · device thrombosis · haemorrhage · hepatic function abnormal · hypertension · respiratory disorders

▶ **Frequency not known** Cardiac arrest · chills · circulatory collapse · disseminated intravascular coagulation · dyspnoea · heparin-induced thrombocytopenia · hypotension · nausea · skin reactions · tachycardia · tremor

● **MEDICINAL FORMS** There can be variation in the licensing of different medicines containing the same drug.

Powder and solvent for solution for injection

▸ Beriplex P/N (CSL Behring UK Ltd)

Factor VII 175 unit, Protein S 195 unit, Factor IX 255 unit, Protein C 300 unit, Factor II 340 unit, Factor X 410 unit Beriplex P/N 250 powder and solvent for solution for injection vials | 1 vial PoM £150.00 (Hospital only)

Factor VII 350 unit, Protein S 390 unit, Factor IX 510 unit, Protein C 600 unit, Factor II 680 unit, Factor X 820 unit Beriplex P/N 500 powder and solvent for solution for injection vials | 1 vial PoM £300.00 (Hospital only)

Factor VII 700 unit, Protein S 1000 unit, Factor IX 1020 unit, Protein C 1200 unit, Factor II 1360 unit, Factor X 1640 unit Beriplex P/N 1,000 powder and solvent for solution for injection vials | 1 vial PoM £600.00 (Hospital only)

Powder and solvent for solution for infusion

▸ Octaplex (Octapharma Ltd)

Factor VII 330 unit, Protein C 380 unit, Protein S 390 unit, Factor X 480 unit, Factor II 490 unit, Factor IX 500 unit Octaplex 500unit powder and solvent for solution for infusion vials | 1 vial PoM £245.00 (Hospital only)

Octaplex 1,000unit powder and solvent for solution for infusion vials | 1 vial PoM £490.00 (Hospital only)

Von Willebrand factor [Specialist drug]

03-Mar-2021

● **INDICATIONS AND DOSE**

von Willebrand disease

▶ BY SLOW INTRAVENOUS INJECTION

▸ Child: Specialist drug – access specialist resources for dosing information

● **SIDE-EFFECTS**

▶ **Uncommon** Angioedema · chest tightness · chills · flushing · headache · hypotension · lethargy · nausea · paraesthesia · restlessness · tachycardia · urticaria generalised · vomiting · wheezing

▶ **Rare or very rare** Fever

▶ **Frequency not known** Thromboembolism

● **MEDICINAL FORMS** There can be variation in the licensing of different medicines containing the same drug.

Powder and solvent for solution for injection

EXCIPIENTS: May contain Polysorbates

ELECTROLYTES: May contain Sodium

▸ Veyvondi (Takeda UK Ltd)

Vonicog alfa 650 unit Veyvondi 650unit powder and solvent for solution for injection vials | 1 vial PoM £598.00 (Hospital only)

Vonicog alfa 1300 unit Veyvondi 1,300unit powder and solvent for solution for injection vials | 1 vial PoM £1,196.00 (Hospital only)

▸ Willfact (LFB Biopharmaceuticals Ltd)

von Willebrand factor 1000 unit Willfact 1,000unit powder and solvent for solution for injection vials | 1 vial PoM £922.00 (Hospital only)

BLOOD AND RELATED PRODUCTS ›
HAEMOSTATIC PRODUCTS

Factor VIII inhibitor bypassing fraction [Specialist drug]

30-Jan-2020

● **INDICATIONS AND DOSE**

Congenital factor VIII deficiency (haemophilia A) and factor VIII inhibitors | Non-haemophiliac patients with acquired factor VIII inhibitors

▶ BY INTRAVENOUS INFUSION, OR BY INTRAVENOUS INJECTION

▸ Child: Specialist drug – access specialist resources for dosing information

● **CONTRA-INDICATIONS** Disseminated intravascular coagulation

● **SIDE-EFFECTS**

▶ **Common or very common** Dizziness · headache · hypersensitivity · hypotension · skin reactions

▶ **Frequency not known** Abdominal discomfort · anamnestic reaction · angioedema · chest discomfort · chills · cough · diarrhoea · disseminated intravascular coagulation · drowsiness · dyspnoea · embolism and thrombosis · fever · flushing · hypertension · ischaemic stroke · malaise · myocardial infarction · nausea · paraesthesia · respiratory disorders · restlessness · tachycardia · taste altered · vomiting

● **MEDICINAL FORMS** There can be variation in the licensing of different medicines containing the same drug.

Powder and solvent for solution for infusion

▸ FEIBA Imuno (Takeda UK Ltd)

Factor VIII inhibitor bypassing fraction 500 unit FEIBA 100units/ml (500unit) powder and 5ml solvent for solution for infusion vials | 1 vial PoM £390.00 (Hospital only)

Factor VIII inhibitor bypassing fraction 1000 unit FEIBA 100units/ml (1,000unit) powder and 10ml solvent for solution for infusion vials | 1 vial PoM £780.00 (Hospital only)

BLOOD AND RELATED PRODUCTS › PLASMA PRODUCTS

Fresh frozen plasma [Specialist drug]

15-Apr-2026

● **INDICATIONS AND DOSE**

Replacement of coagulation factors or other plasma proteins

▶ BY INTRAVENOUS INFUSION

▸ Child: Specialist drug – access specialist resources for dosing information

● **CONTRA-INDICATIONS** Avoid use as a volume expander · IgA deficiency with confirmed antibodies to IgA

● **SIDE-EFFECTS**

▶ **Common or very common** Skin reactions

▶ **Uncommon** Fever · hypersensitivity · hypoxia · nausea · sensation abnormal · vomiting

▶ **Rare or very rare** Abdominal pain · anxiety · arrhythmias · back pain · cardiac arrest · chest discomfort · chills · circulatory collapse · citrate toxicity · dizziness · dyspnoea · flushing · haemolytic anaemia · haemorrhage · hyperhidrosis · hypertension · hypotension · localised oedema · malaise · procedural complications · pulmonary oedema · respiratory disorders · thromboembolism

● **MEDICINAL FORMS** There can be variation in the licensing of different medicines containing the same drug.

Infusion

▸ **OctaplasLG** (Octapharma Ltd)

Human plasma proteins 57.5 mg per 1 ml OctaplasLG Blood Group A infusion 200ml bags | 1 bag PoM £75.00 (Hospital only)
OctaplasLG Blood Group B infusion 200ml bags | 1 bag PoM £75.00 (Hospital only)
OctaplasLG Blood Group AB infusion 200ml bags | 1 bag PoM £75.00 (Hospital only)
OctaplasLG Blood Group O infusion 200ml bags | 1 bag PoM £75.00 (Hospital only)

2.2 Subarachnoid haemorrhage

CALCIUM-CHANNEL BLOCKERS

F 126

Nimodipine

01-Dec-2021

● **DRUG ACTION** Nimodipine is a dihydropyridine calcium-channel blocker.

● **INDICATIONS AND DOSE**

Treatment of vasospasm following subarachnoid haemorrhage (specialist use only)

▶ BY INTRAVENOUS INFUSION

▸ Child 1 month–11 years: Initially 15 micrograms/kg/hour (max. per dose 500 micrograms/hour), increased after 2 hours if no severe decrease in blood pressure; increased to 30 micrograms/kg/hour (max. per dose 2 mg/hour), continue for at least 5 days (max. 14 days), use initial dose of 7.5 micrograms/kg/hour if blood pressure unstable

▸ Child 12–17 years (body-weight up to 70 kg): Initially 0.5 mg/hour, increased after 2 hours if no severe decrease in blood pressure; increased to 1–2 mg/hour, continue for at least 5 days (max. 14 days)

▸ Child 12–17 years (body-weight 70 kg and above): Initially up to 1 mg/hour, use dose if blood pressure stable; increased after 2 hours if no severe decrease in blood pressure; increased to 1–2 mg/hour, continue for at least 5 days (max. 14 days)

Prevention of vasospasm following subarachnoid haemorrhage

▶ BY MOUTH

▸ Child: 0.9–1.2 mg/kg 6 times a day (max. per dose 60 mg), started within 4 days of haemorrhage and continued for 21 days

● **UNLICENSED USE** Not licensed for use in children.

> **IMPORTANT SAFETY INFORMATION**
>
> **SAFE PRACTICE**
>
> Nimodipine has been confused with amlodipine; care must be taken to ensure the correct drug is prescribed and dispensed.

● **CAUTIONS** Cerebral oedema · hypotension · severely raised intracranial pressure

● **INTERACTIONS** → Appendix 1: calcium-channel blockers

● **SIDE-EFFECTS**

▶ **Uncommon** Thrombocytopenia · vasodilation

▶ **Rare or very rare** Bradycardia · ileus

● **PREGNANCY** Manufacturer advises use only if potential benefit outweighs risk.

● **BREAST FEEDING** Manufacturer advises avoid—present in milk.

● **HEPATIC IMPAIRMENT**

▸ With oral use Manufacturer advises consider avoiding in severe impairment.

Dose adjustments

▸ With oral use In adults, manufacturer advises dose reduction—consult product literature.

● **DIRECTIONS FOR ADMINISTRATION** EvGr Avoid concomitant administration of nimodipine infusion and tablets. ⟨M⟩

▸ With oral use For administration *by mouth*, expert sources advise tablets may be crushed but are light sensitive.

▸ With intravenous use EvGr For *continuous intravenous infusion*, administer undiluted via an infusion pump and three-way stopcock on a central venous catheter connected to a running infusion of Glucose 5%, or Sodium Chloride 0.9% (consult product literature); not to be added to an infusion container; incompatible with polyvinyl chloride giving sets or containers; protect infusion from light. ⟨M⟩ Polyethylene, polypropylene, or glass apparatus should be used.

● **MEDICINAL FORMS** There can be variation in the licensing of different medicines containing the same drug. Forms available from special-order manufacturers include: oral suspension

Solution for infusion

▸ **Nimotop** (Laboratoire X.O)

Nimodipine 200 microgram per 1 ml Nimotop 0.02% solution for infusion 50ml vials | 1 vial PoM £13.60 (Hospital only)

Oral tablet

▸ **Nimotop** (Laboratoire X.O)

Nimodipine 30 mg Nimotop 30mg tablets | 100 tablet PoM £40.00 DT = £40.00

3 Blood clots

3.1 Blocked catheters and lines

Other drugs used for Blocked catheters and lines Heparin, p. 111

ANTITHROMBOTIC DRUGS › TISSUE PLASMINOGEN ACTIVATORS

Fibrinolytic drugs

Overview

Alteplase below, streptokinase below and urokinase p. 101 are used in children to dissolve intravascular thrombi and unblock occluded arteriovenous shunts, catheters, and indwelling central lines blocked with fibrin clots. Treatment should be started as soon as possible after a clot has formed and discontinued once a pulse in the affected limb is detected, or the shunt or catheter unblocked.

The safety and efficacy of treatment remains uncertain, especially in neonates. A fibrinolytic drug is probably only appropriate where arterial occlusion threatens ischaemic damage; an anticoagulant may stop the clot getting bigger. Alteplase is the preferred fibrinolytic in children and neonates; there is less risk of adverse effects including allergic reactions.

Fibrinolytics

- **DRUG ACTION** Fibrinolytic drugs act as thrombolytics by activating plasminogen to form plasmin, which degrades fibrin and so breaks up thrombi.
- **CONTRA-INDICATIONS** Acute pancreatitis · aneurysm · aortic dissection · arteriovenous malformation · bacterial endocarditis · bleeding diatheses · coagulation defects · coma · history of cerebrovascular disease (especially recent events or with any residual disability) · neoplasm with risk of haemorrhage · oesophageal varices · pericarditis · recent gastro-intestinal ulceration · recent haemorrhage · recent surgery (including dental extraction) · recent trauma · severe hypertension
- **CAUTIONS** Conditions in which thrombolysis might give rise to embolic complications such as enlarged left atrium with atrial fibrillation (risk of dissolution of clot and subsequent embolisation) · external chest compression · hypertension · risk of bleeding (including that from venepuncture or invasive procedures)
- **SIDE-EFFECTS**
  - **Common or very common** Anaphylactic reaction · angina pectoris · cardiac arrest · cardiogenic shock · chills · CNS haemorrhage · ecchymosis · fever · haemorrhage · heart failure · ischaemia recurrent (when used in myocardial infarction) · nausea · pulmonary oedema · vomiting
  - **Uncommon** Mitral valve incompetence · reperfusion arrhythmia (when used in myocardial infarction)
  - **Rare or very rare** Seizure

  SIDE-EFFECTS, FURTHER INFORMATION Serious bleeding calls for discontinuation of the thrombolytic and may require administration of coagulation factors and antifibrinolytic drugs.
- **PREGNANCY** Thrombolytic drugs can possibly lead to premature separation of the placenta in the first 18 weeks of pregnancy. There is also a risk of maternal haemorrhage throughout pregnancy and post-partum, and also a theoretical risk of fetal haemorrhage throughout pregnancy.
- **HEPATIC IMPAIRMENT** Manufacturers advise avoid in severe impairment.

above

Alteplase

27-Jul-2023

(rt-PA; Tissue-type plasminogen activator)

- **INDICATIONS AND DOSE**

Intravascular thrombosis

▶ BY INTRAVENOUS INFUSION

- Neonate: 100–500 micrograms/kg/hour for 3–6 hours, use ultrasound assessment to monitor effect before considering a second course of treatment (consult local protocol).
- Child: 100–500 micrograms/kg/hour for 3–6 hours, use ultrasound assessment to monitor effect before considering a second course of treatment; maximum 100 mg per day

ACTILYSE CATHFLO®

Thrombolytic treatment of occluded central venous access devices (including those used for haemodialysis)

▶ BY INTRAVENOUS INJECTION

- Child: (consult product literature)

- **UNLICENSED USE** *Actilyse®* not licensed for use in children.
- **CONTRA-INDICATIONS** Recent delivery
- **INTERACTIONS** → Appendix 1: alteplase
- **SIDE-EFFECTS**
  - **Common or very common** Haemorrhagic stroke · hypotension
  - **Uncommon** Haemothorax
  - **Rare or very rare** Agitation · confusion · delirium · depression · epilepsy · psychosis · speech impairment
  - **Frequency not known** Brain oedema (caused by reperfusion)
- **ALLERGY AND CROSS-SENSITIVITY** EvGr Contra-indicated if history of hypersensitivity to gentamicin (residue from manufacturing process). Ⓜ
- **DIRECTIONS FOR ADMINISTRATION** For *intravenous infusion* (*Actilyse®*), manufacturer advises dissolve in Water for Injections to a concentration of 1 mg/mL or 2 mg/mL and infuse intravenously; alternatively dilute further in Sodium Chloride 0.9% to a concentration of not less than 200 micrograms/mL; not to be diluted in Glucose.
- **MEDICINAL FORMS** There can be variation in the licensing of different medicines containing the same drug. Forms available from special-order manufacturers include: solution for injection

Powder and solvent for solution for injection

- **Actilyse** (Boehringer Ingelheim Ltd)

  Alteplase 10 mg Actilyse 10mg powder and solvent for solution for injection vials | 1 vial PoM £172.80

  Alteplase 20 mg Actilyse 20mg powder and solvent for solution for injection vials | 1 vial PoM £259.20

Powder and solvent for solution for infusion

- **Actilyse** (Boehringer Ingelheim Ltd)

  Alteplase 50 mg Actilyse 50mg powder and solvent for solution for infusion vials | 1 vial PoM £432.00

above

Streptokinase

13-Apr-2021

- **INDICATIONS AND DOSE**

Intravascular thrombosis

▶ INITIALLY BY INTRAVENOUS INFUSION

- Child 1 month–11 years: Initially 2500–4000 units/kg, dose to be given over 30 minutes, followed by (by continuous intravenous infusion) 500–1000 units/kg/hour for up to 3 days until reperfusion occurs

- Child 12–17 years: Initially 250 000 units, dose to be given over 30 minutes, followed by (by continuous intravenous infusion) 100 000 units/hour for up to 3 days until reperfusion occurs

- **UNLICENSED USE** Not licensed for use in children.
- **CAUTIONS** Cavernous pulmonary disease · recent streptococcal infections
- **INTERACTIONS** → Appendix 1: streptokinase
- **SIDE-EFFECTS**
- ▶ **Common or very common** Arrhythmias · asthenia · diarrhoea · epigastric pain · headache · malaise · pain · pericarditis
- ▶ **Uncommon** Myocardial rupture · pericardial disorders · respiratory arrest · splenic rupture
- ▶ **Rare or very rare** Arthritis · eye inflammation · hypersensitivity · nephritis · nerve disorders · neurological effects · pulmonary oedema non-cardiogenic (caused by reperfusion) · shock · vasculitis
- **ALLERGY AND CROSS-SENSITIVITY** Contra-indicated if previous allergic reaction to either streptokinase or anistreplase (no longer available). Prolonged persistence of antibodies to streptokinase and anistreplase (no longer available) can reduce the effectiveness of subsequent treatment; therefore, streptokinase should not be used again beyond 4 days of first administration of either streptokinase or anistreplase.
- **DIRECTIONS FOR ADMINISTRATION** For *intravenous infusion*, manufacturer advises reconstitute with Sodium Chloride 0.9%, then dilute further with Glucose 5% or Sodium Chloride 0.9% after reconstitution. Expert sources advise monitor fibrinogen concentration closely; if fibrinogen concentration less than 1 g/litre, stop streptokinase infusion and start heparin; restart streptokinase once fibrinogen concentration reaches 1 g/litre.

- **MEDICINAL FORMS** There can be variation in the licensing of different medicines containing the same drug.

Powder for solution for infusion

▶ Streptokinase (Non-proprietary)

Streptokinase 1.5 mega unit Streptokinase 1.5million unit powder for solution for infusion vials | 1 vial PoM £195.00 (Hospital only)

Streptokinase 250000 unit Streptokinase 250,000unit powder for solution for infusion vials | 1 vial PoM £97.50 (Hospital only)

F 100

Urokinase

04-Jan-2022

- **INDICATIONS AND DOSE**

Occluded arteriovenous shunts, catheters, and indwelling central lines

▶ TO THE DEVICE AS A FLUSH

- Neonate: 5000–25 000 units, instil directly into occluded catheter or central line **only**, dilute dose in Sodium Chloride 0.9% to fill catheter dead space. Leave for 20–60 minutes then aspirate the lysate and flush with Sodium Chloride 0.9%.
- Child: 5000–25 000 units, instil directly into occluded catheter or central line **only**, dilute dose in Sodium Chloride 0.9% to fill catheter dead space. Leave for 20–60 minutes then aspirate the lysate and flush with Sodium Chloride 0.9%

- **CAUTIONS** Cavernous pulmonary disease
- **INTERACTIONS** → Appendix 1: urokinase
- **SIDE-EFFECTS**
- ▶ **Common or very common** Artery dissection · embolism and thrombosis · stroke
- ▶ **Uncommon** Renal failure
- ▶ **Rare or very rare** Vascular pseudoaneurysm
- **BREAST FEEDING** Manufacturer advises avoid—no information available.

- **MEDICINAL FORMS** There can be variation in the licensing of different medicines containing the same drug.

Powder for solution for injection

▶ Syner-KINASE (Syner-Med (Pharmaceutical Products) Ltd)

Urokinase 10000 unit Syner-KINASE 10,000unit powder for solution for injection vials | 1 vial PoM £35.95 (Hospital only)

Urokinase 25000 unit Syner-KINASE 25,000unit powder for solution for injection vials | 1 vial PoM £45.95 (Hospital only)

Urokinase 100000 unit Syner-KINASE 100,000unit powder for solution for injection vials | 1 vial PoM £112.95 (Hospital only)

Urokinase 250000 unit Syner-KINASE 250,000unit powder for solution for injection vials | 1 vial PoM £140.00 (Hospital only)

Urokinase 500000 unit Syner-KINASE 500,000unit powder for solution for injection vials | 1 vial PoM £270.00 (Hospital only)

3.2 Thromboembolism

Venous thromboembolism

10-Aug-2022

Venous thromboembolism prophylaxis

For guidance on reducing the risk of venous thromboembolism (VTE) in children with COVID-19, see NICE rapid guideline: **Managing COVID-19** (available at: www.nice.org.uk/guidance/ng191), and SIGN rapid guideline: **Prevention and management of venous thromboembolism in patients with COVID-19** (available at: www.sign.ac.uk/our-guidelines/prevention-and-management-of-venous-thromboembolism-in-covid-19/). For further information on COVID-19, see COVID-19 p. 490.

Low-dose heparin p. 111 by subcutaneous injection is used to prevent thrombotic episodes in 'high-risk' patients; laboratory monitoring of APTT or anti-Factor Xa concentration is also required in prophylactic regimens in children. Low molecular weight heparins, aspirin p. 104 (antiplatelet dose), and warfarin sodium p. 115 can also be used for prophylaxis.

The following guidance on reducing the risk of VTE applies to children aged over 16 years and is based on the NICE guideline: **Venous thromboembolism in over 16s** (see *Useful resources*).

EvGr All children over 16 years old should undergo a risk assessment to identify their risk of VTE and bleeding on admission to hospital. ⟨A⟩ Commonly used risk assessment tools can be found at: www.nice.org.uk/guidance/ng89/resources. Children over 16 years old considered to be at high risk of VTE include those who are anticipated to have a substantial reduction in mobility, those with obesity, malignant disease, history of VTE and thrombophilic disorder. Pregnancy and the postpartum period are also risk factors for VTE.

There are two methods of thromboprophylaxis: mechanical and pharmacological. Options for mechanical prophylaxis are anti-embolism stockings that provide graduated compression and produce a calf pressure of 14–15 mmHg, and intermittent pneumatic compression. EvGr Anti-embolism stockings should be worn day and night until the child is sufficiently mobile; they should not be offered to children over 16 years old admitted with conditions such as severe leg oedema, or local conditions (e.g. gangrene, dermatitis).

When using pharmacological prophylaxis, in most cases, it should start as soon as possible or within 14 hours of admission. Children over 16 years of age with risk factors for bleeding (e.g. thrombocytopenia, acquired or untreated inherited bleeding disorders) should *only* receive pharmacological prophylaxis when their risk of VTE outweighs their risk of bleeding. Children over 16 years of age receiving anticoagulant treatment who are at high risk of

VTE should be considered for prophylaxis if their anticoagulant treatment is interrupted, for example during the peri-operative period. (A)

Surgical patients

EvGr To reduce the risk of VTE in surgical patients over 16 years old, regional anaesthesia over general anaesthesia should be used if possible.

Mechanical prophylaxis (e.g. anti-embolism stockings or intermittent pneumatic compression) should be offered to children over 16 years old with major trauma, or undergoing cranial, abdominal, bariatric, thoracic, maxillofacial, ear, nose, and throat, cardiac or elective spinal surgery. Prophylaxis should continue until the child is sufficiently mobile or discharged from hospital (or for 30 days in spinal injury, elective spinal surgery or cranial surgery). (A) Choice of mechanical prophylaxis depends on factors such as the type of surgery, suitability for the child, and their condition.

EvGr Pharmacological prophylaxis should be considered in children over 16 years old undergoing general or orthopaedic surgery when the risk of VTE outweighs the risk of bleeding. (A) The choice of prophylaxis will depend on the type of surgery, suitability for the patient, and local policy. EvGr A low molecular weight heparin is suitable in all types of general and orthopaedic surgery; heparin is preferred in patients with renal impairment. Fondaparinux sodium [unlicensed] is an option for children over 16 years old undergoing abdominal, bariatric, thoracic or cardiac surgery, or for patients with lower limb immobilisation or fragility fractures of the pelvis, hip or proximal femur.

Pharmacological prophylaxis in general surgery should usually continue for at least 7 days post-surgery, or until sufficient mobility has been re-established. Pharmacological prophylaxis should be extended to 28 days after major cancer surgery in the abdomen, and to 30 days in spinal surgery.

Mechanical prophylaxis with intermittent pneumatic compression should be considered when pharmacological prophylaxis is contra-indicated in children over 16 years old undergoing lower limb amputation, or those with major trauma or fragility fractures of the pelvis, hip or proximal femur. (A)

Medical patients

The choice of prophylaxis will depend on the medical condition, suitability for the patient, and local policy. EvGr Acutely ill medical patients over 16 years old who are at high risk of VTE should be offered pharmacological prophylaxis. Children over 16 years old should be given either a low molecular weight heparin as a first-line option, or fondaparinux sodium [unlicensed] as an alternative, for a minimum of 7 days. Children over 16 years old with renal impairment should be given either a low molecular weight heparin or heparin and the dose should be adjusted as necessary.

Mechanical prophylaxis can be considered when pharmacological prophylaxis is contra-indicated; their use should be continued until the child is sufficiently mobile. (A)

Thromboprophylaxis in pregnancy

EvGr All pregnant young women over 16 years old (who are not in active labour), or young women over 16 years old who have given birth, had a miscarriage or termination of pregnancy during the past 6 weeks, with a risk of VTE that outweighs the risk of bleeding should be considered for pharmacological prophylaxis with a low molecular weight heparin during hospital admission. In pregnant young women over 16 years old, prophylaxis should be continued until there is no longer a risk of VTE, or until discharge from hospital. Young women over 16 years old who have given birth, had a miscarriage or termination of pregnancy during the past 6 weeks, should start thromboprophylaxis with a low molecular weight heparin 4–8 hours after the event, unless contra-indicated, and continue for a minimum of 7 days.

Additional mechanical prophylaxis should be considered for young women over 16 years old who are likely to be immobilised or have significantly reduced mobility and continued until the young woman is sufficiently mobile or discharged from hospital. Intermittent pneumatic compression should be used as the first-line option and anti-embolism stockings as an alternative. (A)

Venous thromboembolism treatment

For guidance on the management of venous thromboembolism in children aged 16 years and over with COVID-19, see SIGN rapid guideline: **Prevention and management of venous thromboembolism in patients with COVID-19** (available at: www.sign.ac.uk/our-guidelines/prevention-and-management-of-venous-thromboembolism-in-covid-19/). For further information on COVID-19, see COVID-19 p. 490.

For the initial treatment of thrombotic episodes heparin p. 111 is given as an intravenous loading dose, followed by continuous intravenous infusion (using an infusion pump) or by intermittent subcutaneous injection; the use of intermittent intravenous injection is no longer recommended. Alternatively, a low molecular weight heparin may be given for initial treatment. If oral anticoagulation with warfarin sodium p. 115 [unlicensed] is also required, it may be started at the same time as the heparin (the heparin needs to be continued for at least 5 days and until the INR has been in the therapeutic range for 2 consecutive days). Laboratory monitoring of coagulation activity, preferably on a daily basis, involves determination of the activated partial thromboplastin time (APTT) (for heparin only) or of the anti-Factor Xa concentration (for low molecular weight heparins). Local guidelines on recommended APTT for neonates and children should be followed; monitoring of APTT should be discussed with a specialist prior to treatment for thrombotic episodes in neonates.

Treatment of venous thromboembolism in pregnancy

Heparins are used for the management of venous thromboembolism in pregnancy because they do not cross the placenta. Low molecular weight heparins are preferred because they have a lower risk of osteoporosis and of heparin-induced thrombocytopenia. Low molecular weight heparins are eliminated more rapidly in pregnancy, requiring alteration of the dosage regimen for drugs such as dalteparin sodium p. 109, enoxaparin sodium p. 110 and tinzaparin sodium p. 112; see also under individual drugs. Treatment should be stopped at the onset of labour and advice sought from a specialist on continuing therapy after birth.

Extracorporeal circuits

Heparin is also used in the maintenance of extracorporeal circuits in cardiopulmonary bypass and haemodialysis.

Haemorrhage

If haemorrhage occurs, it is usually sufficient to withdraw heparin or low molecular weight heparin, but if rapid reversal of the effects of the heparin is required, protamine sulfate p. 1046 is a specific antidote (but only partially reverses the effects of low molecular weight heparins).

For information on the management of haemorrhage in patients on oral anticoagulants, see Oral anticoagulants p. 103.

Useful Resources

Venous thromboembolism in over 16s: reducing the risk of hospital-acquired deep vein thrombosis or pulmonary embolism. National Institute for Health and Care Excellence. NICE guideline 89. March 2018 (updated August 2019). www.nice.org.uk/guidance/ng89

Oral anticoagulants

10-Aug-2022

Overview

The main use of anticoagulants is to prevent thrombus formation or extension of an existing thrombus in the slower-moving venous side of the circulation, where the thrombus consists of a fibrin web enmeshed with platelets and red cells.

Anticoagulants are of less use in preventing thrombus formation in arteries, for in faster-flowing vessels thrombi are composed mainly of platelets with little fibrin.

Children prescribed an anticoagulant and their parents or carers should be provided with verbal and written information about the child's treatment, including how and when to seek medical attention. Immediate medical attention is required in certain children, such as in those with bleeding that is severe, does not stop or recurs, or who have other signs or symptoms of concern; in particular, children who have sustained a head injury should be referred to a hospital emergency department.

Vitamin K antagonists, such as warfarin, antagonise the effects of vitamin K and take at least 48 to 72 hours for the anticoagulant effect to develop fully; if an immediate effect is required, heparin or a low molecular weight heparin must be given concomitantly.

Uses

Warfarin sodium p. 115 [unlicensed] is the drug of choice for the treatment of systemic thromboembolism in children (not neonates) after initial heparinisation. It may also be used occasionally for the treatment of intravascular or intracardiac thrombi. Warfarin sodium is used prophylactically in those with chronic atrial fibrillation, dilated cardiomyopathy, certain forms of reconstructive heart surgery, mechanical prosthetic heart valves, and some forms of hereditary thrombophilia (e.g. homozygous protein C deficiency).

Heparin or a low molecular weight heparin (see under Parenteral anticoagulants p. 104) is usually preferred for the prophylaxis of venous thromboembolism in children undergoing surgery; alternatively warfarin sodium can be continued in selected children currently taking warfarin sodium and who are at a high risk of thromboembolism (seek expert advice).

Dose

The base-line prothrombin time should be determined but the initial dose should not be delayed whilst awaiting the result.

An induction dose is usually given over 4 days. The subsequent maintenance dose depends on the prothrombin time, reported as INR (international normalised ratio) and should be taken at the same time each day.

Target INR

The following indications and target INRs for adults for warfarin take into account recommendations of the British Society for Haematology Guidelines on Oral Anticoagulation with warfarin—fourth edition. *Br J Haematol* 2011; **154**: 311–324:

An INR which is within 0.5 units of the target value is generally satisfactory; larger deviations require dosage adjustment. Target values (rather than ranges) are now recommended.

INR 2.5 for:

- treatment of deep-vein thrombosis or pulmonary embolism (including those associated with antiphospholipid syndrome or for recurrence in patients no longer receiving warfarin sodium)
- atrial fibrillation
- cardioversion—target INR should be achieved at least 3 weeks before cardioversion and anticoagulation should continue for at least 4 weeks after the procedure (higher target values, such as an INR of 3, can be used for up to 4 weeks before the procedure to avoid cancellations due to low INR)
- dilated cardiomyopathy
- mitral stenosis or regurgitation in patients with either atrial fibrillation, a history of systemic embolism, a left atrial thrombus, or an enlarged left atrium
- bioprosthetic heart valves in the mitral position (treat for 3 months), or in patients with a history of systemic embolism (treat for at least 3 months), or with a left atrial thrombus at surgery (treat until clot resolves), or with other risk factors (e.g. atrial fibrillation or a low ventricular ejection fraction)
- acute arterial embolism requiring embolectomy (consider long-term treatment)
- myocardial infarction

INR 3.5 for:

- recurrent deep-vein thrombosis or pulmonary embolism in patients currently receiving anticoagulation and with an INR above 2;

Mechanical prosthetic heart valves:

- the recommended target INR depends on the type and location of the valve, and patient-related risk factors
- consider increasing the INR target or adding an antiplatelet drug, if an embolic event occurs whilst anticoagulated at the target INR.

Haemorrhage

The main adverse effect of all oral anticoagulants is haemorrhage. Checking the INR and omitting doses when appropriate is essential; if the anticoagulant is stopped but not reversed, the INR should be measured 2–3 days later to ensure that it is falling. The cause of an elevated INR should be investigated. The following recommendations (which take into account the recommendations of the British Society for Haematology Guidelines on Oral Anticoagulation with Warfarin—fourth edition. *Br J Haematol* 2011; **154**: 311–324) are based on the result of the INR and whether there is major or minor bleeding; the recommendations apply to adults taking warfarin:

- Major bleeding—stop warfarin sodium; give phytomenadione p. 795 (vitamin K_1) by slow intravenous injection; give prothrombin complex p. 98 (factors II, VII, IX, and X); if prothrombin complex unavailable, fresh frozen plasma can be given but is less effective; recombinant factor VIIa is not recommended for emergency anticoagulation reversal
- INR >8.0, minor bleeding—stop warfarin sodium; give phytomenadione (vitamin K_1) by slow intravenous injection; repeat dose of phytomenadione if INR still too high after 24 hours; restart warfarin sodium when INR <5.0
- INR >8.0, no bleeding—stop warfarin sodium; give phytomenadione (vitamin K_1) by mouth using the intravenous preparation orally [unlicensed use]; repeat dose of phytomenadione if INR still too high after 24 hours; restart warfarin sodium when INR <5.0
- INR 5.0–8.0, minor bleeding—stop warfarin sodium; give phytomenadione (vitamin K_1) by slow intravenous injection; restart warfarin sodium when INR <5.0
- INR 5.0–8.0, no bleeding—withhold 1 or 2 doses of warfarin sodium and reduce subsequent maintenance dose
- Unexpected bleeding at therapeutic levels—always investigate possibility of underlying cause e.g. unsuspected renal or gastro-intestinal tract pathology

Parenteral anticoagulants

19-Mar-2025

Anticoagulants

Although thrombotic episodes are uncommon in childhood, anticoagulants may be required in children with congenital heart disease; in children undergoing haemodialysis; for preventing thrombosis in children requiring chemotherapy and following surgery; and for systemic venous thromboembolism secondary to inherited thrombophilias, systemic lupus erythematosus, or indwelling central venous catheters.

Children prescribed an anticoagulant and their parents or carers should be provided with verbal and written information about the child's treatment, including how and when to seek medical attention. Immediate medical attention is required in certain children, such as in those with bleeding that is severe, does not stop or recurs, or who have other signs or symptoms of concern; in particular, children who have sustained a head injury should be referred to a hospital emergency department.

Heparin

Heparin initiates anticoagulation rapidly but has a short duration of action. It is often referred to as **'standard'** or **'unfractionated'** heparin p. 111 to distinguish it from the **low molecular weight heparins**, which have a longer duration of action. For children at high risk of bleeding, heparin is more suitable than low molecular weight heparin because its effect can be terminated rapidly by stopping the infusion.

Heparins are used in both the treatment and prophylaxis of thromboembolic disease, mainly to prevent further clotting rather than to lyse existing clots—surgery or a thrombolytic drug may be necessary if a thrombus obstructs major vessels.

Low molecular weight heparins

Dalteparin sodium p. 109, enoxaparin sodium p. 110, and tinzaparin sodium p. 112 are low molecular weight heparins used for treatment and prophylaxis of thrombotic episodes in children. Their duration of action is longer than that of heparin and in adults and older children *once-daily subcutaneous* dosage is sometimes possible; however, younger children require relatively higher doses (possibly due to larger volume of distribution, altered heparin pharmacokinetics, or lower plasma concentrations of antithrombin) and twice daily dosage is sometimes necessary. Low molecular weight heparins are convenient to use, especially in children with poor venous access.

Heparinoids

Danaparoid sodium p. 108 is a heparinoid that has a role in children who develop heparin-induced thrombocytopenia, providing they have no evidence of cross-reactivity.

Heparin flushes

The use of heparin flushes should be kept to a minimum. For maintaining patency of peripheral venous catheters, sodium chloride injection 0.9% is as effective as heparin flushes. The role of heparin flushes in maintaining patency of arterial and central venous catheters is unclear.

An NPSA alert was issued in 2008 regarding the risks associated with intravenous heparin flushes. Since the alert, subsequent safety incidents have been reported and there has been wide variation in local practices with the use of heparin flushes and locks. The National Infusion and Vascular Access Society (NIVAS) board have produced guidance for the flushing and locking of vascular access devices in children, which aims to provide advice to standardise practice nationally. The guidance advises that:

- When maintaining the patency of a device, preferably use sodium chloride 0.9% as a flush;
- When flushing an IV catheter after medication administration, use sodium chloride 0.9% or a compatible fluid;
- Pre-filled sodium chloride 0.9% syringes should be used where possible to enhance patient safety;
- If using heparin as a locking solution, use products that are clearly labelled "for maintenance of patency of intravenous devices" to reduce the risk of inadvertent administration of an overdose of heparin.

For further information, see the National Infusion and Vascular Access Society **Guidance for vascular access device flushing and locking for paediatric patients** (available at: nivas.org.uk/).

Epoprostenol

Epoprostenol p. 140 (prostacyclin) can be given to inhibit platelet aggregation during renal dialysis when heparins are unsuitable or contra-indicated. It is a potent vasodilator and therefore its side-effects include flushing, headache and hypotension.

Other drugs used for Thromboembolism Alteplase, p. 100 · Streptokinase, p. 100

ANTITHROMBOTIC DRUGS › ANTIPLATELET DRUGS

Antiplatelet drugs

10-Aug-2022

Overview

Antiplatelet drugs decrease platelet aggregation and inhibit thrombus formation in the arterial circulation, because in faster-flowing vessels, thrombi are composed mainly of platelets with little fibrin.

Aspirin below has limited use in children because it has been associated with Reye's syndrome. Aspirin-containing preparations should not be given to children and adolescents under 16 years, unless specifically indicated, such as for Kawasaki disease, for prophylaxis of clot formation after cardiac surgery, or for prophylaxis of stroke in children at high risk.

If aspirin causes dyspepsia, or if the child is at a high risk of gastro-intestinal bleeding, a proton pump inhibitor or a H_2-receptor antagonist can be added.

Dipyridamole p. 105 is also used as an antiplatelet drug to prevent clot formation after cardiac surgery and may be used with specialist advice for treatment of persistent coronary artery aneurysms in Kawasaki disease.

Kawasaki disease

Initial treatment is with high dose aspirin and a single dose of intravenous normal immunoglobulin; this combination has an additive anti-inflammatory effect resulting in faster resolution of fever and a decreased incidence of coronary artery complications. After the acute phase, when the patient is afebrile, aspirin is continued at a lower dose to prevent coronary artery abnormalities.

Aspirin

15-Apr-2024

(Acetylsalicylic Acid)

● **INDICATIONS AND DOSE**

Antiplatelet | Prevention of thrombus formation after cardiac surgery

▶ BY MOUTH

▶ Neonate: 1–5 mg/kg once daily.

- ▸ Child 1 month–11 years: 1–5 mg/kg once daily (max. per dose 75 mg)
- ▸ Child 12–17 years: 75 mg once daily

Kawasaki disease

▶ BY MOUTH

- ▸ Neonate: Initially 8 mg/kg 4 times a day for 2 weeks *or* until afebrile, followed by 5 mg/kg once daily for 6–8 weeks, if no evidence of coronary lesions after 8 weeks, discontinue treatment or seek expert advice.
- ▸ Child 1 month–11 years: Initially 7.5–12.5 mg/kg 4 times a day for 2 weeks *or* until afebrile, then 2–5 mg/kg once daily for 6–8 weeks, if no evidence of coronary lesions after 8 weeks, discontinue treatment or seek expert advice

Mild to moderate pain (dose approved for use by community practitioner nurse prescribers) | Pyrexia (dose approved for use by community practitioner nurse prescribers)

▶ BY MOUTH

- ▸ Child 16–17 years: 300–600 mg every 4–6 hours as required, maximum 2.4 g per day without doctor's advice

● **UNLICENSED USE** Not licensed for use in children under 16 years.

● **CONTRA-INDICATIONS** Active peptic ulceration · bleeding disorders · children under 16 years (risk of Reye's syndrome) · haemophilia · previous peptic ulceration (analgesic dose) · severe cardiac failure (analgesic dose)

CONTRA-INDICATIONS, FURTHER INFORMATION

▸ Reye's syndrome Owing to an association with Reye's syndrome, manufacturer advises aspirin-containing preparations should not be given to children under 16 years, unless specifically indicated, e.g. for Kawasaki disease.

● **CAUTIONS** Allergic disease · anaemia · asthma · dehydration · G6PD deficiency · history of gout · hypertension · may mask symptoms of infection · preferably avoid during fever or viral infection in children (risk of Reye's syndrome) · previous peptic ulceration (but manufacturers may advise avoidance of aspirin in history of peptic ulceration) · thyrotoxicosis

● **INTERACTIONS** → Appendix 1: aspirin

● **SIDE-EFFECTS**

- ▶ **Common or very common** Dyspepsia · haemorrhage
- ▶ **Uncommon** Dyspnoea · rhinitis · severe cutaneous adverse reactions (SCARs) · skin reactions
- ▶ **Rare or very rare** Aplastic anaemia · asthmatic attack · bronchospasm · erythema nodosum · gastrointestinal haemorrhage (severe) · granulocytosis · haemorrhagic vasculitis · intracranial haemorrhage · menorrhagia · nausea · thrombocytopenia · vomiting
- ▶ **Frequency not known** Fluid retention · gastrointestinal disorders · headache · hearing loss · hepatic failure · hyperuricaemia · iron deficiency anaemia · renal impairment · sodium retention · tinnitus · vertigo

Overdose The main features of salicylate poisoning are hyperventilation, tinnitus, deafness, vasodilatation, and sweating. Coma is uncommon but indicates very severe poisoning.

For specific details on the management of poisoning, see Aspirin, under Emergency treatment of poisoning p. 1036.

● **ALLERGY AND CROSS-SENSITIVITY** EvGr Aspirin is **contra-indicated** in history of hypersensitivity to aspirin or any other NSAID—which includes those in whom attacks of asthma, angioedema, urticaria, or rhinitis have been precipitated by aspirin or any other NSAID. Ⓜ

● **PREGNANCY** Use antiplatelet doses with caution during third trimester; impaired platelet function and risk of haemorrhage; delayed onset and increased duration of labour with increased blood loss; avoid analgesic doses if possible in last few weeks (low doses probably not harmful); high doses may be related to intra-uterine growth restriction, teratogenic effects, closure of fetal ductus arteriosus in utero and possibly persistent pulmonary hypertension of newborn; kernicterus may occur in jaundiced neonates.

● **BREAST FEEDING** Avoid—possible risk of Reye's syndrome; regular use of high doses could impair platelet function and produce hypoprothrombinaemia in infant if neonatal vitamin K stores low.

● **HEPATIC IMPAIRMENT** Manufacturer advises use with caution in mild-to-moderate impairment; avoid in severe impairment.

● **RENAL IMPAIRMENT** EvGr Caution in mild to moderate impairment (risk of fluid retention, further renal impairment, and gastro-intestinal bleeding); avoid in severe impairment. Ⓜ

● **PATIENT AND CARER ADVICE**

Medicines for Children leaflet: Aspirin for prevention of blood clots www.medicinesforchildren.org.uk/medicines/aspirin-for-prevention-of-blood-clots/

● **MEDICINAL FORMS** There can be variation in the licensing of different medicines containing the same drug. Forms available from special-order manufacturers include: oral capsule, oral suspension, oral solution

Oral tablet

CAUTIONARY AND ADVISORY LABELS 21, 32

▸ Aspirin (Non-proprietary)

Aspirin 75 mg Aspirin 75mg tablets | 28 tablet PoM £3.80 DT = £0.65

Aspirin 300 mg Aspirin 300mg tablets | 28 tablet P £1.70 | 32 tablet P £0.79 DT = £0.80

Gastro-resistant tablet

CAUTIONARY AND ADVISORY LABELS 5, 25, 32

▸ Aspirin (Non-proprietary)

Aspirin 75 mg Aspirin 75mg gastro-resistant tablets | 28 tablet P £2.15 DT = £0.92 | 56 tablet P £2.40–£4.30

▸ Nu-Seals (Alliance Pharmaceuticals Ltd)

Aspirin 75 mg Nu-Seals 75 gastro-resistant tablets | 56 tablet P £3.12

Dispersible tablet

CAUTIONARY AND ADVISORY LABELS 13, 21, 32

▸ Aspirin (Non-proprietary)

Aspirin 75 mg Aspirin 75mg dispersible tablets | 1000 tablet PoM ☒

Aspirin 300 mg Aspirin 300mg dispersible tablets | 32 tablet P £0.93 DT = £0.82

Dipyridamole

15-Apr-2024

● **INDICATIONS AND DOSE**

Kawasaki disease (initiated under specialist supervision)

▶ BY MOUTH USING IMMEDIATE-RELEASE MEDICINES

- ▸ Child 1 month–11 years: 1 mg/kg 3 times a day

Prevention of thrombus formation after cardiac surgery

▶ BY MOUTH USING IMMEDIATE-RELEASE MEDICINES

- ▸ Child 1 month–11 years: 2.5 mg/kg twice daily
- ▸ Child 12–17 years: 100–200 mg 3 times a day

● **UNLICENSED USE** Not licensed for use in children.

● **CAUTIONS** Coagulation disorders · heart failure · hypotension · left ventricular outflow obstruction · myasthenia gravis (risk of exacerbation) · rapidly worsening angina · recent myocardial infarction · severe coronary artery disease

● **INTERACTIONS** → Appendix 1: dipyridamole

- **SIDE-EFFECTS**
  - **Common or very common** Angina pectoris · diarrhoea · dizziness · headache · myalgia · nausea · skin reactions · vomiting
  - **Frequency not known** Angioedema · bronchospasm · haemorrhage · hot flush · hypotension · tachycardia · thrombocytopenia
- **PREGNANCY** Not known to be harmful.
- **BREAST FEEDING** Manufacturers advise use only if essential—small amount present in milk.

- **MEDICINAL FORMS** There can be variation in the licensing of different medicines containing the same drug. Forms available from special-order manufacturers include: oral suspension, oral solution

Oral tablet

CAUTIONARY AND ADVISORY LABELS 22

- Dipyridamole (Non-proprietary)
  - **Dipyridamole 25 mg** Dipyridamole 25mg tablets | 84 tablet PoM £12.28 DT = £8.67
  - **Dipyridamole 100 mg** Dipyridamole 100mg tablets | 84 tablet PoM £50.86 DT = £45.66

Oral suspension

- Dipyridamole (Non-proprietary)
  - **Dipyridamole 10 mg per 1 ml** Dipyridamole 50mg/5ml oral suspension sugar free | 150 ml PoM £217.61 DT = £217.61 SF

ANTITHROMBOTIC DRUGS > FACTOR Xa INHIBITORS

Rivaroxaban

15-Apr-2024

- **DRUG ACTION** Rivaroxaban is a direct inhibitor of activated factor X (factor Xa).

- **INDICATIONS AND DOSE**

Treatment of venous thromboembolism | Prophylaxis of recurrent venous thromboembolism

► BY MOUTH

- Neonate (body-weight 2.6 kg and above): (consult product literature).
- Child (body-weight 2.6–2.9 kg): 0.8 mg 3 times a day for at least 3 months, to be given following completion of at least 5 days of initial parenteral anticoagulant treatment, review dose and body-weight regularly, for dose adjustments before and after invasive procedures, surgical intervention and for duration of treatment for catheter related thrombosis—consult product literature, treatment can be extended up to 12 months if required, taking into account the risk for recurrent thrombosis versus the potential bleeding risk
- Child (body-weight 3–3.9 kg): 0.9 mg 3 times a day for at least 3 months, to be given following completion of at least 5 days of initial parenteral anticoagulant treatment, review dose and body-weight regularly, for dose adjustments before and after invasive procedures, surgical intervention and for duration of treatment for catheter related thrombosis—consult product literature, treatment can be extended up to 12 months if required, taking into account the risk for recurrent thrombosis versus the potential bleeding risk
- Child (body-weight 4–4.9 kg): 1.4 mg 3 times a day for at least 3 months, to be given following completion of at least 5 days of initial parenteral anticoagulant treatment, review dose and body-weight regularly, for dose adjustments before and after invasive procedures, surgical intervention and for duration of treatment for catheter related thrombosis—consult product literature, treatment can be extended up to 12 months if required, taking into account the risk for recurrent thrombosis versus the potential bleeding risk
- Child (body-weight 5–6.9 kg): 1.6 mg 3 times a day for at least 3 months, to be given following completion of at least 5 days of initial parenteral anticoagulant treatment, review dose and body-weight regularly, for dose adjustments before and after invasive procedures, surgical intervention and for duration of treatment for catheter related thrombosis—consult product literature, treatment can be extended up to 12 months if required, taking into account the risk for recurrent thrombosis versus the potential bleeding risk
- Child (body-weight 7–7.9 kg): 1.8 mg 3 times a day for at least 3 months, to be given following completion of at least 5 days of initial parenteral anticoagulant treatment, review dose and body-weight regularly, for dose adjustments before and after invasive procedures, surgical intervention and for duration of treatment for catheter related thrombosis—consult product literature, treatment can be extended up to 12 months if required, taking into account the risk for recurrent thrombosis versus the potential bleeding risk
- Child (body-weight 8–8.9 kg): 2.4 mg 3 times a day for at least 3 months, to be given following completion of at least 5 days of initial parenteral anticoagulant treatment, review dose and body-weight regularly, for dose adjustments before and after invasive procedures, surgical intervention and for duration of treatment for catheter related thrombosis—consult product literature, treatment can be extended up to 12 months if required, taking into account the risk for recurrent thrombosis versus the potential bleeding risk
- Child (body-weight 9–9.9 kg): 2.8 mg 3 times a day for at least 3 months, to be given following completion of at least 5 days of initial parenteral anticoagulant treatment, review dose and body-weight regularly, for dose adjustments before and after invasive procedures, surgical intervention and for duration of treatment for catheter related thrombosis—consult product literature, treatment can be extended up to 12 months if required, taking into account the risk for recurrent thrombosis versus the potential bleeding risk
- Child (body-weight 10–11.9 kg): 3 mg 3 times a day for at least 3 months, to be given following completion of at least 5 days of initial parenteral anticoagulant treatment, review dose and body-weight regularly, for dose adjustments before and after invasive procedures, surgical intervention and for duration of treatment for catheter related thrombosis—consult product literature, treatment can be extended up to 12 months if required, taking into account the risk for recurrent thrombosis versus the potential bleeding risk
- Child (body-weight 12–29.9 kg): 5 mg twice daily for at least 3 months, to be given following completion of at least 5 days of initial parenteral anticoagulant treatment, for dose adjustments before and after invasive procedures, surgical intervention and for duration of treatment for catheter related thrombosis—consult product literature, treatment can be extended up to 12 months if required, taking into account the risk for recurrent thrombosis versus the potential bleeding risk
- Child (body-weight 30–49.9 kg): 15 mg once daily for at least 3 months, to be given following completion of at least 5 days of initial parenteral anticoagulant treatment, for dose adjustments before and after invasive procedures, surgical intervention and for duration of treatment for catheter related thrombosis—consult product literature, treatment can be extended up to 12 months if required, taking into account the risk for recurrent thrombosis versus the potential bleeding risk
- Child (body-weight 50 kg and above): 20 mg once daily for at least 3 months, to be given following completion of

at least 5 days of initial parenteral anticoagulant treatment, for dose adjustments before and after invasive procedures, surgical intervention and for duration of treatment for catheter related thrombosis—consult product literature, treatment can be extended up to 12 months if required, taking into account the risk for recurrent thrombosis versus the potential bleeding risk

DOSE EQUIVALENCE AND CONVERSION

- For information on changing from, or to, other anticoagulants—consult product literature.

IMPORTANT SAFETY INFORMATION

MHRA/CHM ADVICE: NEW ORAL ANTICOAGULANTS APIXABAN (*ELIQUIS®*), DABIGATRAN (*PRADAXA®*) AND RIVAROXABAN (*XARELTO®*) (OCTOBER 2013)

The following contra-indications now apply to all new oral anticoagulants, for all indications and doses:

- a lesion or condition, if considered a significant risk factor for major bleeding—see *Contra-indications* for further information;
- concomitant treatment with any other anticoagulant agent—see *Contra-indications* for further information.

Healthcare professionals are advised to take caution when deciding to prescribe these anticoagulants to patients with other conditions, undergoing other procedures, and on other treatments, which may increase the risk of major bleeding. The renal function of patients should also be considered.

MHRA/CHM ADVICE: RIVAROXABAN (*XARELTO®*) AFTER TRANSCATHETER AORTIC VALVE REPLACEMENT: INCREASE IN ALL-CAUSE MORTALITY, THROMBOEMBOLIC AND BLEEDING EVENTS IN A CLINICAL TRIAL (OCTOBER 2018)

A phase 3 clinical trial showed that the risk of all-cause death and bleeding after transcatheter aortic valve replacement (TAVR) approximately doubled in patients assigned to a rivaroxaban-based anticoagulation strategy compared with those receiving an antiplatelet-based strategy (clopidogrel and aspirin). The MHRA reminds healthcare professionals that rivaroxaban should not be used for thromboprophylaxis in patients with prosthetic heart valves, including patients who have undergone TAVR. Rivaroxaban treatment in patients who undergo TAVR should be stopped and switched to standard care.

MHRA/CHM ADVICE: DIRECT-ACTING ORAL ANTICOAGULANTS (DOACS): INCREASED RISK OF RECURRENT THROMBOTIC EVENTS IN PATIENTS WITH ANTIPHOSPHOLIPID SYNDROME (JUNE 2019)

A clinical trial has shown an increased risk of recurrent thrombotic events associated with rivaroxaban compared with warfarin, in patients with antiphospholipid syndrome and a history of thrombosis. There may be a similar risk associated with other DOACs. Healthcare professionals are advised that DOACs are not recommended in patients with antiphospholipid syndrome, particularly high-risk patients who test positive for all three antiphospholipid tests—lupus anticoagulant, anticardiolipin antibodies, and anti-beta$_2$ glycoprotein I antibodies. Continued treatment should be reviewed in these patients to determine if appropriate, and switching to a vitamin K antagonist such as warfarin should be considered.

MHRA/CHM ADVICE: RIVAROXABAN (*XARELTO®*): REMINDER THAT 15 MG AND 20 MG TABLETS SHOULD BE TAKEN WITH FOOD (JULY 2019)

The MHRA has received a small number of reports suggesting a lack of efficacy (thromboembolic events) in patients taking 15 mg or 20 mg rivaroxaban tablets on an empty stomach. Healthcare professionals are advised to remind patients to take rivaroxaban 15 mg or 20 mg tablets with food. In those who have difficulty swallowing, these tablets can be crushed and mixed with water or apple puree immediately before, and followed by food immediately after, ingestion.

MHRA/CHM ADVICE: DIRECT-ACTING ORAL ANTICOAGULANTS (DOACS): REMINDER OF BLEEDING RISK, INCLUDING AVAILABILITY OF REVERSAL AGENTS (JUNE 2020)

The MHRA reminds healthcare professionals to remain vigilant for signs and symptoms of bleeding complications during treatment with rivaroxaban after ongoing reports of serious, potentially fatal bleeds associated with the use of DOACs. Healthcare professionals are also advised to use rivaroxaban with caution in patients with increased bleeding risk, and to ensure that those with renal impairment are dosed appropriately and their renal function monitored during treatment. Patients and their carers should be counselled on the signs and symptoms of bleeding, and encouraged to read the patient information leaflet.

MHRA/CHM ADVICE: WARFARIN AND OTHER ANTICOAGULANTS: MONITORING OF PATIENTS DURING THE COVID-19 PANDEMIC (OCTOBER 2020)

Healthcare professionals are reminded that:

- direct-acting oral anticoagulants (DOACs), such as rivaroxaban, may interact with other medicines (including antibacterials and antivirals)—advice in product literature should be followed to minimise the risk of potential interactions;
- if patients are switched from warfarin to rivaroxaban, warfarin treatment should be stopped before rivaroxaban treatment is started to reduce the risk of over-anticoagulation and bleeding.

MHRA/CHM ADVICE: DIRECT-ACTING ORAL ANTICOAGULANTS (DOACS): PAEDIATRIC FORMULATIONS (MAY 2023)

Rivaroxaban (*Xarelto®*) is available as granules for oral suspension for use in children. Patients and their carers should be counselled on its preparation and dosing, to read and follow the *Instructions for Use* booklet provided, and on the availability of an educational video.

- **CONTRA-INDICATIONS** Active bleeding · antiphospholipid syndrome (increased risk of recurrent thrombotic events) · arteriovenous malformation · less than 6 months of age with less than 10 days of oral feeding and who at birth had less than 37 weeks of gestation · major intraspinal or intracerebral vascular abnormalities · malignant neoplasms at high risk of bleeding · oesophageal varices · prosthetic heart valve (efficacy not established) · recent brain or spinal injury · recent brain surgery · recent gastro-intestinal ulcer · recent intracranial haemorrhage · recent ophthalmic surgery · recent spine surgery · significant risk of major bleeding · use with any other anticoagulant · vascular aneurysm

CONTRA-INDICATIONS, FURTHER INFORMATION

- Use with any other anticoagulant [EvGr] Concomitant use with any other anticoagulant is contra-indicated, except when switching therapy, or when heparin is given at doses necessary to maintain an open central venous or arterial catheter or for catheter ablation—use with caution. ⟨M⟩

- **CAUTIONS** Anaesthesia with postoperative indwelling epidural catheter (risk of paralysis—monitor neurological signs and consider placement or removal of a catheter when the anticoagulant effect of rivaroxaban is estimated to be low) · bronchiectasis · cerebral vein and sinus thrombosis in CNS infection · risk of bleeding · severe hypertension · vascular retinopathy
- **INTERACTIONS** → Appendix 1: factor XA inhibitors
- **SIDE-EFFECTS**

- **Common or very common** Anaemia · asthenia · constipation · diarrhoea · dizziness · fever · gastrointestinal discomfort · haemorrhage · headache · hypotension · menorrhagia · nausea · oedema · pain in extremity · post procedural

anaemia · renal impairment · skin reactions · tachycardia · vomiting · wound complications
- **Uncommon** Angioedema · dry mouth · hepatic disorders · hypersensitivity · intracranial haemorrhage · malaise · syncope · thrombocytopenia · thrombocytosis
- **Rare or very rare** Severe cutaneous adverse reactions (SCARs) · vascular pseudoaneurysm

- **PREGNANCY** Manufacturer advises avoid—toxicity in *animal* studies.
- **BREAST FEEDING** Manufacturer advises avoid—present in milk in *animal* studies.
- **HEPATIC IMPAIRMENT** Manufacturer advises avoid in hepatic disease with coagulopathy and clinically-relevant bleeding risk including patients with moderate to severe cirrhosis.
- **RENAL IMPAIRMENT** See p. 16. EvGr Use with caution if concomitant use of drugs that increase plasma-rivaroxaban concentration (consult product literature). Avoid in children 1 year or older if estimated glomerular filtration rate less than 50 ml/min/1.73 m^2 and in children under 1 year with serum creatinine results above 97.5th percentile—consult product literature. ⟨M⟩
- **MONITORING REQUIREMENTS**
  - Patients should be monitored for signs of bleeding or anaemia; treatment should be stopped if severe bleeding occurs.
  - No routine anticoagulant monitoring required (INR tests are unreliable).
- **DIRECTIONS FOR ADMINISTRATION** Manufacturer advises tablets may be crushed and mixed with water or apple puree just before administration.

  For *Xarelto*® granules for oral suspension, the appropriate blue syringes (1 mL, 5 mL or 10 mL) should be used to ensure accurate dosing. Each dose should be immediately followed by one typical serving of liquid; this may include the liquid volume used for feeding. Reconstituted oral suspension should be discarded after 14 days.

  Once reconstituted, *Xarelto*® granules for oral suspension may be given through a nasogastric or gastric feeding tube—consult product literature.
- **PRESCRIBING AND DISPENSING INFORMATION** The manufacturer of *Xarelto*® has provided a *Prescriber Guide*.

  Xarelto® granules for oral suspension should be used in patients with a body-weight of at least 2.6 kg to less than 30 kg. Do not split or use lower strength *Xarelto*® tablets to provide doses for children with body-weight below 30 kg; only *Xarelto*® 15 mg tablets and *Xarelto*® 20 mg tablets are licensed for use in children and adolescents aged less than 18 years.

  Xarelto® granules for oral suspension contains sodium benzoate which may increase jaundice in newborn infants (up to four weeks old).
- **PATIENT AND CARER ADVICE** Patients and their carers should be given advice on how to administer *Xarelto*® granules for oral suspension.

  Vomiting If vomiting occurs within 30 minutes after receiving the dose, a new dose should be given. The dose should not be re-administered if vomiting occurs after 30 minutes.

  Patients and their carers should be provided with an alert card and advised to keep it with them at all times.
- **NATIONAL FUNDING/ACCESS DECISIONS**
  For full details see funding body website

  All Wales Medicines Strategy Group (AWMSG) decisions
  - **Rivaroxaban (*Xarelto*®) for the treatment of venous thromboembolism (VTE) and prevention of VTE recurrence in term neonates, infants and toddlers, children, and adolescents aged less than 18 years after at least 5 days of initial parenteral anticoagulation treatment (December 2021)** AWMSG No. 3875 Recommended

- **MEDICINAL FORMS** There can be variation in the licensing of different medicines containing the same drug.

Oral tablet

CAUTIONARY AND ADVISORY LABELS 10, 21 (15 and 20 mg tablets)
- **Rivaroxaban (non-proprietary)** ▼
  - **Rivaroxaban 2.5 mg** Rivaroxaban 2.5mg tablets | 56 tablet PoM £60.48 DT = £1.00 | 56 tablet PoM £3.18 DT = £1.00 (Hospital only)
  - **Rivaroxaban 10 mg** Rivaroxaban 10mg tablets | 10 tablet PoM £0.47–£18.00 | 30 tablet PoM £54.00 DT = £1.32 | 100 tablet PoM £4.40–£180.00
  - **Rivaroxaban 15 mg** Rivaroxaban 15mg tablets | 14 tablet PoM £0.55–£25.20 | 28 tablet PoM £50.40 DT = £0.90 | 42 tablet PoM £1.66–£75.60 | 100 tablet PoM £3.21–£180.00
  - **Rivaroxaban 20 mg** Rivaroxaban 20mg tablets | 28 tablet PoM £50.40 DT = £0.89 | 100 tablet PoM £4.39–£180.00
- **Xarelto** (Bayer Plc)
  - **Rivaroxaban 2.5 mg** Xarelto 2.5mg tablets | 56 tablet PoM £50.40 DT = £1.00
  - **Rivaroxaban 10 mg** Xarelto 10mg tablets | 10 tablet PoM £18.00 | 30 tablet PoM £54.00 DT = £1.32 | 100 tablet PoM £180.00
  - **Rivaroxaban 15 mg** Xarelto 15mg tablets | 14 tablet PoM £25.20 | 28 tablet PoM £50.40 DT = £0.90 | 42 tablet PoM £75.60 | 100 tablet PoM £180.00
  - **Rivaroxaban 20 mg** Xarelto 20mg tablets | 28 tablet PoM £50.40 DT = £0.89 | 100 tablet PoM £180.00

Granules for oral suspension

CAUTIONARY AND ADVISORY LABELS 10, 21

EXCIPIENTS: May contain Propylene glycol
- **Xarelto** (Bayer Plc)
  - **Rivaroxaban 1 mg per 1 ml** Xarelto 1mg/ml granules for oral suspension | 51.7 ml PoM £9.00 (Hospital only) SF | 103.4 ml PoM £18.00 DT = £18.00 SF

ANTITHROMBOTIC DRUGS › HEPARINOIDS

Danaparoid sodium

13-Jan-2021

- **INDICATIONS AND DOSE**

Thromboembolic disease in patients with history of heparin-induced thrombocytopenia
- INITIALLY BY INTRAVENOUS INJECTION
  - Neonate: Initially 30 units/kg, then (by continuous intravenous infusion) 1.2–2 units/kg/hour, infusion dose to be adjusted according to coagulation activity.
  - Child 1 month–15 years (body-weight up to 55 kg): Initially 30 units/kg (max. per dose 1250 units), then (by continuous intravenous infusion) 1.2–2 units/kg/hour, infusion dose to be adjusted according to coagulation activity
  - Child 1 month–15 years (body-weight 55 kg and above): Initially 30 units/kg (max. per dose 2500 units), then (by continuous intravenous infusion) 1.2–2 units/kg/hour, infusion dose to be adjusted according to coagulation activity
  - Child 16–17 years (body-weight up to 55 kg): Initially 1250 units, then (by continuous intravenous infusion) 400 units/hour for 2 hours, then (by continuous intravenous infusion) 300 units/hour for 2 hours, then (by continuous intravenous infusion) 200 units/hour for 5 days, infusion dose to be adjusted according to coagulation activity
  - Child 16–17 years (body-weight 55–90 kg): Initially 2500 units, then (by continuous intravenous infusion) 400 units/hour for 2 hours, then (by continuous intravenous infusion) 300 units/hour for 2 hours, then (by continuous intravenous infusion) 200 units/hour for 5 days, infusion dose to be adjusted according to coagulation activity
  - Child 16–17 years (body-weight 91 kg and above): Initially 3750 units, then (by continuous intravenous infusion)

400 units/hour for 2 hours, then (by continuous intravenous infusion) 300 units/hour for 2 hours, then (by continuous intravenous infusion) 200 units/hour for 5 days, infusion dose to be adjusted according to coagulation activity

- **UNLICENSED USE** Not licensed for use in children.
- **CONTRA-INDICATIONS** Active peptic ulcer (unless this is the reason for operation) · acute bacterial endocarditis · diabetic retinopathy · epidural anaesthesia (with treatment doses) · haemophilia and other haemorrhagic disorders · recent cerebral haemorrhage · severe uncontrolled hypertension · spinal anaesthesia (with treatment doses) · thrombocytopenia (unless patient has heparin-induced thrombocytopenia)
- **CAUTIONS** Antibodies to heparins (risk of antibody-induced thrombocytopenia) · body-weight over 90 kg · recent bleeding · risk of bleeding
- **INTERACTIONS** → Appendix 1: danaparoid
- **SIDE-EFFECTS**
  - **Common or very common** Haemorrhage · heparin-induced thrombocytopenia · skin reactions · thrombocytopenia
  - **Uncommon** Post procedural haematoma
  - **Rare or very rare** Anastomotic haemorrhage
- **PREGNANCY** Manufacturer advises avoid—limited information available but not known to be harmful.
- **BREAST FEEDING** Amount probably too small to be harmful but manufacturer advises avoid.
- **HEPATIC IMPAIRMENT** Manufacturer advises caution in moderate impairment with impaired haemostasis—increased risk of bleeding; avoid in severe hepatic failure unless patient has heparin-induced thrombocytopenia and no alternative available.
- **RENAL IMPAIRMENT** Use with caution in moderate impairment. Avoid in severe impairment unless patient has heparin-induced thrombocytopenia and no alternative available.
  Monitoring Increased risk of bleeding in renal impairment, monitor anti-Factor Xa activity.
- **MONITORING REQUIREMENTS** Monitor anti factor Xa activity in patients with body-weight over 90 kg.
- **DIRECTIONS FOR ADMINISTRATION** Manufacturer advises for *intravenous infusion*, dilute with Glucose 5% or Sodium Chloride 0.9%.

- **MEDICINAL FORMS** There can be variation in the licensing of different medicines containing the same drug.

Solution for injection

- **Danaparoid sodium (Non-proprietary)**
  Danaparoid sodium 1250 unit per 1 ml Danaparoid sodium 750units/0.6ml solution for injection ampoules | 10 ampoule PoM £599.99 (Hospital only)

ANTITHROMBOTIC DRUGS › HEPARINS

Heparins

- **CONTRA-INDICATIONS** Acute bacterial endocarditis · after major trauma · avoid injections containing benzyl alcohol in neonates · epidural anaesthesia with treatment doses · haemophilia or other haemorrhagic disorders · peptic ulcer · recent cerebral haemorrhage · recent surgery to eye · recent surgery to nervous system · spinal anaesthesia with treatment doses · thrombocytopenia (including history of heparin-induced thrombocytopenia)
- **CAUTIONS** Risk of bleeding · severe hypertension
- **SIDE-EFFECTS**
  - **Common or very common** Haemorrhage · heparin-induced thrombocytopenia · skin reactions
  - **Rare or very rare** Alopecia · hyperkalaemia · osteoporosis (following long term use) · spinal haematoma

SIDE-EFFECTS, FURTHER INFORMATION **Haemorrhage** If haemorrhage occurs it is usually sufficient to withdraw heparin or a low molecular weight heparin, but if rapid reversal of the effects of the heparin is required, protamine sulfate is a specific antidote (but only partially reverses the effects of low molecular weight heparins).

Heparin-induced thrombocytopenia Clinically important heparin-induced thrombocytopenia is immune-mediated and can be complicated by thrombosis. Signs of heparin-induced thrombocytopenia include a 30% reduction of platelet count, thrombosis, or skin allergy. If heparin-induced thrombocytopenia is strongly suspected or confirmed, the heparin should be stopped and an alternative anticoagulant, such as danaparoid, should be given. Ensure platelet counts return to normal range in those who require warfarin.

Hyperkalaemia Inhibition of aldosterone secretion by heparin or a low molecular weight heparin can result in hyperkalaemia; patients with diabetes mellitus, chronic renal failure, acidosis, raised plasma potassium or those taking potassium-sparing drugs seem to be more susceptible. The risk appears to increase with duration of therapy.

- **MONITORING REQUIREMENTS**
  - Heparin-induced thrombocytopenia Platelet counts should be measured just before treatment with heparin or low molecular weight heparin, and regular monitoring of platelet counts may be required if given for longer than 4 days. See the British Society for Haematology's Guidelines on the diagnosis and management of heparin-induced thrombocytopenia: second edition. *Br J Haematol* 2012; **159**: 528–540.
  - Hyperkalaemia Plasma-potassium concentration should be measured in patients at risk of hyperkalaemia before starting the heparin and monitored regularly thereafter, particularly if treatment is to be continued for longer than 7 days.

above

Dalteparin sodium

29-Sep-2025

- **DRUG ACTION** Dalteparin sodium is a low molecular weight heparin that acts as an anticoagulant by enhancing the effect of antithrombin III to primarily inhibit activated factor X (factor Xa), with a lesser effect on thrombin.

- **INDICATIONS AND DOSE**

Treatment of venous thromboembolism | Treatment of arterial thromboembolism

▶ BY SUBCUTANEOUS INJECTION

- Neonate: Initially 150 units/kg twice daily, dose adjusted in increments of 25 units/kg according to anti-Factor Xa plasma concentration.
- Child 1–23 months: Initially 150 units/kg twice daily, dose adjusted in increments of 25 units/kg according to anti-Factor Xa plasma concentration
- Child 2–7 years: Initially 125 units/kg twice daily, dose adjusted in increments of 25 units/kg according to anti-Factor Xa plasma concentration
- Child 8–17 years: Initially 100 units/kg twice daily, dose adjusted in increments of 25 units/kg according to anti-Factor Xa plasma concentration

Treatment of venous thromboembolism in pregnancy

▶ BY SUBCUTANEOUS INJECTION

- Child 12–17 years (body-weight up to 50 kg): 5000 units twice daily, use body-weight in early pregnancy to calculate the dose

continued →

- Child 12–17 years (body-weight 50–69 kg): 6000 units twice daily, use body-weight in early pregnancy to calculate the dose
- Child 12–17 years (body-weight 70–89 kg): 8000 units twice daily, use body-weight in early pregnancy to calculate the dose
- Child 12–17 years (body-weight 90 kg and above): 10 000 units twice daily, use body-weight in early pregnancy to calculate the dose

Prophylaxis of thromboembolism

▶ BY SUBCUTANEOUS INJECTION

- Neonate: 100 units/kg once daily.
- Child 1 month–11 years: 100 units/kg once daily
- Child 12–17 years: 2500–5000 units once daily

- **UNLICENSED USE** Dalteparin sodium may be used as detailed below, although these situations are considered unlicensed:
  - EvGr treatment of venous thromboembolism in neonates;
  - treatment of arterial thromboembolism (E);
  - treatment of venous thromboembolism in pregnancy;
  - EvGr prophylaxis of thromboembolism (E).
- **CONTRA-INDICATIONS** Mechanical prosthetic heart valve
- **INTERACTIONS** → Appendix 1: low molecular-weight heparins
- **SIDE-EFFECTS** Epidural haematoma · hypoaldosteronism · intracranial haemorrhage · prosthetic cardiac valve thrombosis
- **ALLERGY AND CROSS-SENSITIVITY** EvGr Contra-indicated in hypersensitivity to heparin or low molecular weight heparin. (M)
- **PREGNANCY** Not known to be harmful, low molecular weight heparins do not cross the placenta. Multidose vial contains benzyl alcohol—manufacturer advises avoid.
- **BREAST FEEDING** Due to the relatively high molecular weight and inactivation in the gastro-intestinal tract, passage into breast-milk and absorption by the nursing infant are likely to be negligible, however manufacturers advise avoid.
- **HEPATIC IMPAIRMENT** Manufacturer advises caution in severe impairment (increased risk of bleeding complications).

  Dose adjustments Manufacturer advises consider dose reduction in severe impairment.
- **RENAL IMPAIRMENT** Use of heparin may be preferable.

  Dose adjustments Risk of bleeding may be increased—dose reduction may be required.
- **MONITORING REQUIREMENTS**
  - EvGr Monitoring of anti-Factor Xa activity is required during the treatment of venous thromboembolism or arterial thromboembolism in neonates and children (see below) (M). Local policies on monitoring for prophylaxis of thromboembolism may vary—seek advice from a haematologist.
  - When used for Treatment of venous thromboembolism or Treatment of arterial thromboembolism EvGr Anti-Factor Xa plasma concentration should initially be monitored after the first, second or third dose—after the first dose in neonates and young children. For all ages, blood samples should be taken 4 hours after administration. Doses should be adjusted to achieve target anti-Factor Xa plasma concentration between 0.5–1 unit/mL; monitoring should be undertaken after each dose adjustment and continued until an adequate maintenance dose is established, then periodically thereafter. (M) See also *Unlicensed use*.
- **DIRECTIONS FOR ADMINISTRATION** For *subcutaneous injection*, administration into the anterolateral or posterolateral aspect of the abdomen, or the lateral part of the thigh is preferred. For recommended concentrations and instructions on dilution—consult product literature.
- **MEDICINAL FORMS** There can be variation in the licensing of different medicines containing the same drug.

Solution for injection

EXCIPIENTS: May contain Benzyl alcohol

▶ **Fragmin** (Pfizer Ltd)

Dalteparin sodium 2500 unit per 1 ml Fragmin 10,000units/4ml solution for injection ampoules | 10 ampoule PoM £51.22 DT = £51.22

Fragmin 10,000units/4ml solution for injection vials | 10 vial PoM £51.22 (Hospital only)

Dalteparin sodium 10000 unit per 1 ml Fragmin Graduated Syringe 10,000units/1ml solution for injection pre-filled syringes | 5 pre-filled disposable injection PoM £33.49 DT = £33.49

Dalteparin sodium 12500 unit per 1 ml Fragmin 2,500units/0.2ml solution for injection pre-filled syringes | 10 pre-filled disposable injection PoM £23.67 DT = £23.67

Dalteparin sodium 25000 unit per 1 ml Fragmin 18,000units/0.72ml solution for injection pre-filled syringes | 5 pre-filled disposable injection PoM £50.82 DT = £50.82

Fragmin 15,000units/0.6ml solution for injection pre-filled syringes | 5 pre-filled disposable injection PoM £43.31 DT = £43.31

Fragmin 5,000units/0.2ml solution for injection pre-filled syringes | 10 pre-filled disposable injection PoM £36.03 DT = £36.03

Fragmin 12,500units/0.5ml solution for injection pre-filled syringes | 5 pre-filled disposable injection PoM £36.70 DT = £36.70

Fragmin 7,500units/0.3ml solution for injection pre-filled syringes | 10 pre-filled disposable injection PoM £45.00 DT = £45.00

Fragmin 100,000units/4ml solution for injection vials | 1 vial PoM £48.66 DT = £48.66

Fragmin 10,000units/0.4ml solution for injection pre-filled syringes | 5 pre-filled disposable injection PoM £33.49 DT = £33.49

F 109

Enoxaparin sodium

29-Sep-2025

- **DRUG ACTION** Enoxaparin sodium is a low molecular weight heparin that acts as an anticoagulant by enhancing the effect of antithrombin III to primarily inhibit activated factor X (factor Xa), with a lesser effect on thrombin.
- **INDICATIONS AND DOSE**

Treatment of thrombotic episodes

▶ BY SUBCUTANEOUS INJECTION

- Neonate: 1.5–2 mg/kg twice daily.
- Child 1 month: 1.5 mg/kg twice daily
- Child 2 months–17 years: 1 mg/kg twice daily

Treatment of venous thromboembolism in pregnancy

▶ BY SUBCUTANEOUS INJECTION

- Child 12–17 years (body-weight up to 50 kg): 40 mg twice daily, dose based on early pregnancy body-weight
- Child 12–17 years (body-weight 50–69 kg): 60 mg twice daily, dose based on early pregnancy body-weight
- Child 12–17 years (body-weight 70–89 kg): 80 mg twice daily, dose based on early pregnancy body-weight
- Child 12–17 years (body-weight 90 kg and above): 100 mg twice daily, dose based on early pregnancy body-weight

Prophylaxis of thrombotic episodes

▶ BY SUBCUTANEOUS INJECTION

- Neonate: 750 micrograms/kg twice daily.
- Child 1 month: 750 micrograms/kg twice daily
- Child 2 months–17 years: 500 micrograms/kg twice daily (max. per dose 20 mg)

DOSE EQUIVALENCE AND CONVERSION

- 1 mg equivalent to 100 units.

- **UNLICENSED USE** Not licensed for treatment of venous thromboembolism in pregnancy.

  Not licensed for use in children.
- **CONTRA-INDICATIONS** Mechanical prosthetic heart valve
- **CAUTIONS** Obesity (increased risk of thromboembolism)

- **INTERACTIONS** → Appendix 1: low molecular-weight heparins
- **SIDE-EFFECTS**
  - **Common or very common** Haemorrhagic anaemia · headache · hypersensitivity · thrombocytopenia · thrombocytosis
  - **Uncommon** Hepatic disorders · injection site necrosis · intracranial haemorrhage
  - **Rare or very rare** Cutaneous vasculitis · eosinophilia
  - **Frequency not known** Acute generalised exanthematous pustulosis (AGEP)
- **ALLERGY AND CROSS-SENSITIVITY** EvGr Contra-indicated in hypersensitivity to heparin or low molecular weight heparin. (M)
- **PREGNANCY** Not known to be harmful, low molecular weight heparins do not cross the placenta. Multidose vial contains benzyl alcohol—avoid.
- **BREAST FEEDING** Manufacturer advises suitable for use during breast feeding—passage into breast milk and absorption by the nursing infant considered to be negligible due to the relatively high molecular weight of enoxaparin and inactivation in the gastro-intestinal tract.
- **HEPATIC IMPAIRMENT**
  Dose adjustments Reduce dose in severe impairment—risk of bleeding may be increased.
- **RENAL IMPAIRMENT** Risk of bleeding increased; use of heparin may be preferable. Consult specialist sources.
- **MONITORING REQUIREMENTS** Routine monitoring of anti-Factor Xa activity is not usually required during treatment with enoxaparin, except in neonates; monitoring may also be necessary in severely ill children and those with renal or hepatic impairment.
- **PRESCRIBING AND DISPENSING INFORMATION** Enoxaparin sodium is a biological medicine. Biological medicines must be prescribed and dispensed by brand name, see *Biological medicines* and *Biosimilar medicines*, under Guidance on prescribing p. 1.

- **MEDICINAL FORMS** There can be variation in the licensing of different medicines containing the same drug.

Solution for injection

EXCIPIENTS: May contain Benzyl alcohol

- **Arovi** (ROVI Biotech Ltd)
  Enoxaparin sodium 100 mg per 1 ml Arovi 20mg/0.2ml solution for injection pre-filled syringes | 10 pre-filled disposable injection PoM £15.49 DT = £20.86
  Arovi 60mg/0.6ml solution for injection pre-filled syringes | 10 pre-filled disposable injection PoM £29.16 DT = £39.26
  Arovi 40mg/0.4ml solution for injection pre-filled syringes | 10 pre-filled disposable injection PoM £22.47 DT = £30.27
  Arovi 80mg/0.8ml solution for injection pre-filled syringes | 10 pre-filled disposable injection PoM £40.94 DT = £55.13
  Arovi 100mg/1ml solution for injection pre-filled syringes | 10 pre-filled disposable injection PoM £53.69 DT = £72.30
  Enoxaparin sodium 150 mg per 1 ml Arovi 150mg/1ml solution for injection pre-filled syringes | 10 pre-filled disposable injection PoM £74.18 DT = £99.91
  Arovi 120mg/0.8ml solution for injection pre-filled syringes | 10 pre-filled disposable injection PoM £65.29 DT = £87.93
- **Clexane** (Sanofi)
  Enoxaparin sodium 100 mg per 1 ml Clexane 60mg/0.6ml solution for injection pre-filled syringes | 10 pre-filled disposable injection PoM £39.26 DT = £39.26
  Clexane 300mg/3ml solution for injection multidose vials | 1 vial PoM £21.33 DT = £21.33
  Clexane 80mg/0.8ml solution for injection pre-filled syringes | 10 pre-filled disposable injection PoM £55.13 DT = £55.13
  Clexane 40mg/0.4ml solution for injection pre-filled syringes | 10 pre-filled disposable injection PoM £30.27 DT = £30.27
  Clexane 100mg/1ml solution for injection pre-filled syringes | 10 pre-filled disposable injection PoM £72.30 DT = £72.30
  Clexane 20mg/0.2ml solution for injection pre-filled syringes | 10 pre-filled disposable injection PoM £20.86 DT = £20.86
  Enoxaparin sodium 150 mg per 1 ml Clexane Forte 120mg/0.8ml solution for injection pre-filled syringes | 10 pre-filled disposable injection PoM £87.93 DT = £87.93
  Clexane Forte 150mg/1ml solution for injection pre-filled syringes | 10 pre-filled disposable injection PoM £99.91 DT = £99.91
- **Inhixa** (Techdow Pharma England Ltd)
  Enoxaparin sodium 100 mg per 1 ml Inhixa 40mg/0.4ml solution for injection pre-filled syringes | 10 pre-filled disposable injection PoM £20.43 DT = £30.27
  Inhixa 80mg/0.8ml solution for injection pre-filled syringes | 10 pre-filled disposable injection PoM £37.22 DT = £55.13
  Inhixa 60mg/0.6ml solution for injection pre-filled syringes | 10 pre-filled disposable injection PoM £26.51 DT = £39.26
  Inhixa 100mg/1ml solution for injection pre-filled syringes | 10 pre-filled disposable injection PoM £48.81 DT = £72.30
  Inhixa 20mg/0.2ml solution for injection pre-filled syringes | 10 pre-filled disposable injection PoM £14.09 DT = £20.86
  Enoxaparin sodium 150 mg per 1 ml Inhixa 120mg/0.8ml solution for injection pre-filled syringes | 10 pre-filled disposable injection PoM £59.36 DT = £87.93
  Inhixa 150mg/1ml solution for injection pre-filled syringes | 10 pre-filled disposable injection PoM £67.44 DT = £99.91
- **Ledraxen** (Venipharm Ltd) ▼
  Enoxaparin sodium 100 mg per 1 ml Ledraxen 20mg/0.2ml solution for injection pre-filled syringes | 10 pre-filled disposable injection PoM £15.65 DT = £20.86
  Ledraxen 40mg/0.4ml solution for injection pre-filled syringes | 10 pre-filled disposable injection PoM £22.70 DT = £30.27
  Ledraxen 100mg/1ml solution for injection pre-filled syringes | 10 pre-filled disposable injection PoM £54.23 DT = £72.30
  Ledraxen 60mg/0.6ml solution for injection pre-filled syringes | 10 pre-filled disposable injection PoM £29.45 DT = £39.26
  Ledraxen 80mg/0.8ml solution for injection pre-filled syringes | 10 pre-filled disposable injection PoM £41.35 DT = £55.13

109

Heparin

29-Sep-2025

(Heparin (unfractionated))

- **DRUG ACTION** Heparin is an anticoagulant that enhances the effect of antithrombin III, which inhibits thrombin and activated factor X (factor Xa).

- **INDICATIONS AND DOSE**

Prevention of clotting in extracorporeal circuits

- TO THE DEVICE AS A FLUSH
  - Child: (consult product literature)

Maintenance of neonatal umbilical arterial catheter

- Neonate: 0.5 unit/hour.

Treatment of thombotic episodes

- INITIALLY BY INTRAVENOUS INJECTION
  - Neonate up to 35 weeks corrected gestational age: Initially 50 units/kg for 1 dose, then (by continuous intravenous infusion) 25 units/kg/hour, dose adjusted according to APTT.
  - Neonate: Initially 75 units/kg for 1 dose, then (by continuous intravenous infusion) 25 units/kg/hour, dose adjusted according to APTT.
  - Child 1–11 months: Initially 75 units/kg for 1 dose, then (by continuous intravenous infusion) 25 units/kg/hour, dose adjusted according to APTT
  - Child 1–17 years: Initially 75 units/kg for 1 dose, then (by continuous intravenous infusion) 20 units/kg/hour, dose adjusted according to APTT
- BY SUBCUTANEOUS INJECTION
  - Child: 250 units/kg twice daily, dose adjusted according to APTT

Prophylaxis of thrombotic episodes

- BY SUBCUTANEOUS INJECTION
  - Child: 100 units/kg twice daily (max. per dose 5000 units), dose adjusted according to APTT

continued →

Maintenance of cardiac shunts and critical stents
▶ TO THE DEVICE AS A FLUSH
▸ Child: (consult local protocol)

- **UNLICENSED USE** Check product literature for licensed use in children.
- **INTERACTIONS** → Appendix 1: heparin
- **SIDE-EFFECTS** Adrenal hypofunction · hypokalaemia · priapism · rebound hyperlipidaemia · thrombocytopenia
- **ALLERGY AND CROSS-SENSITIVITY** EvGr Caution in hypersensitivity to low molecular weight heparin. (M)
- **PREGNANCY** Does not cross the placenta; maternal osteoporosis reported after prolonged use; multidose vials may contain benzyl alcohol—some manufacturers advise avoid.
- **BREAST FEEDING** Not excreted into milk due to high molecular weight.
- **HEPATIC IMPAIRMENT** Manufacturer advises caution; consider avoiding in severe impairment (increased risk of bleeding complications).
Dose adjustments Manufacturer advises consider dose reduction if used in severe impairment.
- **RENAL IMPAIRMENT** EvGr Use with caution. (M)
Dose adjustments EvGr Consider dose reduction in severe impairment (increased risk of bleeding). (M)
- **DIRECTIONS FOR ADMINISTRATION** For *continuous intravenous infusion*, dilute with Glucose 5% or Sodium Chloride 0.9%.
▸ In neonates For *maintenance of neonatal umbilical arterial catheter*, dilute 50 units to a final volume of 50 mL with Sodium Chloride 0.45% or use ready-made bag containing 500 units in 500 mL Sodium Chloride 0.9%; infuse at 0.5 mL/hour. For *neonatal intensive care (treatment of thrombosis)*, dilute 1250 units/kg body-weight to a final volume of 50 mL with infusion fluid; an intravenous infusion rate of 1 mL/hour provides a dose of 25 units/kg/hour.

- **MEDICINAL FORMS** There can be variation in the licensing of different medicines containing the same drug. Forms available from special-order manufacturers include: solution for injection, solution for infusion

Solution for injection
EXCIPIENTS: May contain Benzyl alcohol
▸ **Heparin (Non-proprietary)**
Heparin sodium 1000 unit per 1 ml Heparin sodium 1,000units/1ml solution for injection ampoules | 10 ampoule PoM £20.05
Heparin sodium 5,000units/5ml solution for injection vials | 10 vial PoM £16.50–£49.76 | 10 vial PoM £16.50 (Hospital only)
Heparin sodium 20,000units/20ml solution for injection ampoules | 10 ampoule PoM £99.94 | 10 ampoule PoM £99.94 (Hospital only)
Heparin sodium 5,000units/5ml solution for injection ampoules | 10 ampoule PoM £52.46 | 10 ampoule PoM £52.46 (Hospital only)
Heparin sodium 10,000units/10ml solution for injection ampoules | 10 ampoule PoM £93.66 | 10 ampoule PoM £93.66 (Hospital only)
Heparin sodium 5000 unit per 1 ml Heparin sodium 25,000units/5ml solution for injection ampoules | 10 ampoule PoM £98.51 | 10 ampoule PoM £98.51 (Hospital only)
Heparin sodium 5,000units/1ml solution for injection ampoules | 10 ampoule PoM £28.90–£39.20
Heparin sodium 25,000units/5ml solution for injection vials | 10 vial PoM £45.00–£114.21 | 10 vial PoM £45.00 (Hospital only)
Heparin calcium 25000 unit per 1 ml Heparin calcium 5,000units/0.2ml solution for injection ampoules | 10 ampoule PoM £64.82
Heparin sodium 25000 unit per 1 ml Heparin sodium 25,000units/1ml solution for injection ampoules | 10 ampoule PoM £111.58
Heparin sodium 5,000units/0.2ml solution for injection ampoules | 10 ampoule PoM £54.16

Form unstated
EXCIPIENTS: May contain Benzyl alcohol
▸ **Heparin (Non-proprietary)**
Heparin sodium 10 unit per 1 ml Heparin sodium 50units/5ml patency solution ampoules | 10 ampoule PoM £20.20 DT = £20.20
Heparin sodium 50units/5ml I.V. flush solution ampoules | 10 ampoule PoM £20.20 DT = £20.20 | 10 ampoule PoM £20.20 DT = £20.20 (Hospital only)
Heparin sodium 100 unit per 1 ml Heparin sodium 200units/2ml I.V. flush solution ampoules | 10 ampoule PoM £21.17 DT = £21.17 (Hospital only) | 10 ampoule PoM £21.17 DT = £21.17
Heparin sodium 200units/2ml patency solution ampoules | 10 ampoule PoM £21.17 DT = £21.17

Infusion
▸ **Heparin (Non-proprietary)**
Heparin sodium 1 unit per 1 ml Heparin sodium 500units/500ml infusion Viaflex bags | 1 bag PoM £13.44 (Hospital only) | 20 bag PoM £268.80 (Hospital only)
Heparin sodium 2 unit per 1 ml Heparin sodium 1,000units/500ml infusion Viaflex bags | 1 bag PoM £13.44 (Hospital only) | 20 bag PoM £268.80 (Hospital only)
Heparin sodium 2,000units/1litre infusion Viaflex bags | 1 bag PoM £13.44 (Hospital only) | 10 bag PoM £134.40 (Hospital only)
Heparin sodium 5 unit per 1 ml Heparin sodium 5,000units/1litre infusion Viaflex bags | 1 bag PoM £12.79 (Hospital only) | 10 bag PoM £127.90 (Hospital only)

F 109

Tinzaparin sodium

29-Sep-2025

- **DRUG ACTION** Tinzaparin sodium is a low molecular weight heparin that acts as an anticoagulant by enhancing the effect of antithrombin III to primarily inhibit activated factor X (factor Xa), with a lesser effect on thrombin.

- **INDICATIONS AND DOSE**

Treatment of thrombotic episodes
▶ BY SUBCUTANEOUS INJECTION
▸ Child 1 month: 275 units/kg once daily
▸ Child 2–11 months: 250 units/kg once daily
▸ Child 1–4 years: 240 units/kg once daily
▸ Child 5–9 years: 200 units/kg once daily
▸ Child 10–17 years: 175 units/kg once daily

Treatment of venous thromboembolism in pregnancy
▶ BY SUBCUTANEOUS INJECTION
▸ Child 12–17 years: 175 units/kg once daily, dose based on early pregnancy body-weight

Prophylaxis of thrombotic episodes
▶ BY SUBCUTANEOUS INJECTION
▸ Child: 50 units/kg once daily

- **UNLICENSED USE** Not licensed for the treatment of venous thromboembolism in pregnancy.
Not licensed for use in children.
- **CONTRA-INDICATIONS** Mechanical prosthetic heart valve
- **INTERACTIONS** → Appendix 1: low molecular-weight heparins
- **SIDE-EFFECTS**
▶ **Common or very common** Anaemia
▶ **Rare or very rare** Angioedema · priapism · Stevens-Johnson syndrome · thrombocytosis
- **ALLERGY AND CROSS-SENSITIVITY** EvGr Contra-indicated in hypersensitivity to heparin or low molecular weight heparin. (M)
- **PREGNANCY** Not known to be harmful, low molecular weight heparins do not cross the placenta. Vials contain benzyl alcohol—manufacturer advises avoid.
- **BREAST FEEDING** Due to the relatively high molecular weight of tinzaparin and inactivation in the gastro-intestinal tract, passage into breast-milk and absorption by the nursing infant are likely to be negligible; however manufacturer advise avoid.
- **RENAL IMPAIRMENT** Risk of bleeding may be increased. Heparin may be preferable. Manufacturer advises caution if estimated glomerular filtration rate less than 30 mL/minute/1.73 m^2.
Monitoring In renal impairment monitoring of anti-Factor Xa may be required if estimated glomerular filtration rate less than 30 mL/minute/1.73 m^2.

● **MONITORING REQUIREMENTS** Routine monitoring of anti-Factor Xa activity is not usually required except in neonates; monitoring may also be necessary in severely ill children and those with renal or hepatic impairment.

● **MEDICINAL FORMS** There can be variation in the licensing of different medicines containing the same drug.

Solution for injection

EXCIPIENTS: May contain Benzyl alcohol, sulfites

▸ **Tinzaparin sodium (Non-proprietary)**

Tinzaparin sodium 10000 unit per 1 ml Tinzaparin sodium 3,500units/0.35ml solution for injection pre-filled syringes | 10 pre-filled disposable injection [PoM] £29.79 DT = £29.79

Tinzaparin sodium 4,500units/0.45ml solution for injection pre-filled syringes | 10 pre-filled disposable injection [PoM] £38.30 DT = £38.30

Tinzaparin sodium 2,500units/0.25ml solution for injection pre-filled syringes | 10 pre-filled disposable injection [PoM] £21.29 DT = £21.29

Tinzaparin sodium 20,000units/2ml solution for injection vials | 10 vial [PoM] £110.94 DT = £110.94

Tinzaparin sodium 20000 unit per 1 ml Tinzaparin sodium 8,000units/0.4ml solution for injection pre-filled syringes | 10 pre-filled disposable injection [PoM] £49.98 DT = £49.98

Tinzaparin sodium 14,000units/0.7ml solution for injection pre-filled syringes | 10 pre-filled disposable injection [PoM] £87.36 DT = £87.36

Tinzaparin sodium 16,000units/0.8ml solution for injection pre-filled syringes | 10 pre-filled disposable injection [PoM] £99.96 DT = £99.96

Tinzaparin sodium 40,000units/2ml solution for injection vials | 10 vial [PoM] £359.10 DT = £359.10

Tinzaparin sodium 12,000units/0.6ml solution for injection pre-filled syringes | 10 pre-filled disposable injection [PoM] £74.97 DT = £74.97

Tinzaparin sodium 10,000units/0.5ml solution for injection pre-filled syringes | 10 pre-filled disposable injection [PoM] £62.48 DT = £62.48

Tinzaparin sodium 18,000units/0.9ml solution for injection pre-filled syringes | 10 pre-filled disposable injection [PoM] £112.46 DT = £112.46

ANTITHROMBOTIC DRUGS › THROMBIN INHIBITORS, DIRECT

Dabigatran etexilate

10-May-2024

● **DRUG ACTION** Dabigatran etexilate is a direct thrombin inhibitor with a rapid onset of action.

● **INDICATIONS AND DOSE**

Treatment of venous thromboembolism | Prophylaxis of recurrent venous thromboembolism

▶ BY MOUTH USING GRANULES

- Child 4–11 months (body-weight 2.5 kg and above): Doses are based on body-weight and age in months—consult product literature, to be given following at least 5 days treatment with a parenteral anticoagulant
- Child 1–11 years (body-weight 5 kg and above): Doses are based on body-weight and age in years—consult product literature, to be given following at least 5 days treatment with a parenteral anticoagulant

▶ BY MOUTH USING CAPSULES

- Child 8 years (body-weight 11–12 kg): 75 mg twice daily, to be given following at least 5 days treatment with a parenteral anticoagulant
- Child 8–13 years (body-weight 13–20 kg): 110 mg twice daily, to be given following at least 5 days treatment with a parenteral anticoagulant
- Child 8–17 years (body-weight 21–30 kg): 150 mg twice daily, to be given following at least 5 days treatment with a parenteral anticoagulant
- Child 8–17 years (body-weight 31–40 kg): 185 mg twice daily, to be given following at least 5 days treatment with a parenteral anticoagulant
- Child 8–17 years (body-weight 41–50 kg): 220 mg twice daily, to be given following at least 5 days treatment with a parenteral anticoagulant
- Child 8–17 years (body-weight 51–60 kg): 260 mg twice daily, to be given following at least 5 days treatment with a parenteral anticoagulant
- Child 8–17 years (body-weight 61 kg and above): 300 mg twice daily, to be given following at least 5 days treatment with a parenteral anticoagulant

DOSE EQUIVALENCE AND CONVERSION

- For information on changing between formulations, or changing from, or to, other anticoagulants—consult product literature.

IMPORTANT SAFETY INFORMATION

MHRA/CHM ADVICE: NEW ORAL ANTICOAGULANTS APIXABAN (*ELIQUIS*®), DABIGATRAN (*PRADAXA*®) AND RIVAROXABAN (*XARELTO*®) (OCTOBER 2013)

The following contra-indications now apply to all new oral anticoagulants, for all indications and doses:

- a lesion or condition, if considered a significant risk factor for major bleeding—see *Contra-indications* for further information;
- concomitant treatment with any other anticoagulant agent—see *Contra-indications* for further information.

Healthcare professionals are advised to take caution when deciding to prescribe these anticoagulants to patients with other conditions, undergoing other procedures, and on other treatments, which may increase the risk of major bleeding. The renal function of patients should also be considered.

MHRA/CHM ADVICE: DIRECT-ACTING ORAL ANTICOAGULANTS (DOACS): INCREASED RISK OF RECURRENT THROMBOTIC EVENTS IN PATIENTS WITH ANTIPHOSPHOLIPID SYNDROME (JUNE 2019)

A clinical trial has shown an increased risk of recurrent thrombotic events associated with rivaroxaban compared with warfarin, in patients with antiphospholipid syndrome and a history of thrombosis. There may be a similar risk associated with other DOACs. Healthcare professionals are advised that DOACs are not recommended in patients with antiphospholipid syndrome, particularly high-risk patients who test positive for all three antiphospholipid tests—lupus anticoagulant, anticardiolipin antibodies, and anti-beta$_2$ glycoprotein I antibodies. Continued treatment should be reviewed in these patients to determine if appropriate, and switching to a vitamin K antagonist such as warfarin should be considered.

MHRA/CHM ADVICE: DIRECT-ACTING ORAL ANTICOAGULANTS (DOACS): REMINDER OF BLEEDING RISK, INCLUDING AVAILABILITY OF REVERSAL AGENTS (JUNE 2020)

The MHRA reminds healthcare professionals to remain vigilant for signs and symptoms of bleeding complications during treatment with dabigatran after ongoing reports of serious, potentially fatal bleeds associated with the use of DOACs. Healthcare professionals are also advised to use dabigatran with caution in patients with increased bleeding risk, and to ensure that those with renal impairment are dosed appropriately and their renal function monitored during treatment. Patients and their carers should be counselled on the signs and symptoms of bleeding, and encouraged to read the patient information leaflet.

MHRA/CHM ADVICE: WARFARIN AND OTHER ANTICOAGULANTS: MONITORING OF PATIENTS DURING THE COVID-19 PANDEMIC (OCTOBER 2020)

Healthcare professionals are reminded that:

- direct-acting oral anticoagulants (DOACs), such as dabigatran, may interact with other medicines (including antibacterials and antivirals)—advice in product literature should be followed to minimise the risk of potential interactions;
- if patients are switched from warfarin to dabigatran, warfarin treatment should be stopped before dabigatran treatment is started to reduce the risk of over-anticoagulation and bleeding.

> **MHRA/CHM ADVICE: DIRECT-ACTING ORAL ANTICOAGULANTS (DOACS): PAEDIATRIC FORMULATIONS (MAY 2023)**
> Dabigatran (*Pradaxa*®) is available as coated granules for use in children. Patients and their carers should be counselled on its preparation and dosing, and to read and follow the *Instructions for administration* in the patient information leaflet.

- **CONTRA-INDICATIONS** Active bleeding · antiphospholipid syndrome (increased risk of recurrent thrombotic events) · arteriovenous malformation · do not use as anticoagulant for prosthetic heart valve · major intraspinal or intracerebral vascular abnormalities · malignant neoplasms at high risk of bleeding · oesophageal varices · recent brain or spinal injury · recent brain surgery · recent gastro-intestinal ulcer · recent intracranial haemorrhage · recent ophthalmic surgery · recent spine surgery · significant risk of major bleeding · use with any other anticoagulant · vascular aneurysm

CONTRA-INDICATIONS, FURTHER INFORMATION
- Use with any other anticoagulant [EvGr] Concomitant use with any other anticoagulant is contra-indicated, except when switching therapy, or when heparin is given at doses necessary to maintain an open central venous or arterial catheter or for catheter ablation—use with caution. ⟨M⟩

- **CAUTIONS** Anaesthesia with postoperative indwelling epidural catheter (risk of paralysis—give initial dose at least 2 hours after catheter removal and monitor neurological signs) · bacterial endocarditis · bleeding disorders · encephalitis · gastritis · gastro-oesophageal reflux · intracranial abscess · meningitis (active) · oesophagitis · recent biopsy · recent major trauma · risk of bleeding · small bowel disease where absorption may be affected (consider parenteral anticoagulant) · thrombocytopenia
- **INTERACTIONS** → Appendix 1: thrombin inhibitors
- **SIDE-EFFECTS**
  - **Common or very common** Alopecia · anaemia · diarrhoea · gastrointestinal discomfort · gastrointestinal disorders · haemorrhage · nausea · skin reactions · thrombocytopenia · vomiting
  - **Uncommon** Dysphagia · hyperbilirubinaemia · intracranial haemorrhage · neutropenia
  - **Frequency not known** Agranulocytosis · angioedema · bronchospasm · hepatic function abnormal
- **PREGNANCY** Manufacturer advises avoid unless essential—toxicity in *animal* studies.
- **BREAST FEEDING** Manufacturer advises avoid—no information available.
- **HEPATIC IMPAIRMENT** Manufacturer advises avoid in severe impairment; consider avoiding in those with liver enzymes greater than 2 times the upper limit of normal (no information available).
- **RENAL IMPAIRMENT** See p. 16. [EvGr] Avoid if estimated glomerular filtration rate less than 50 mL/min/1.73m². ⟨M⟩
- **MONITORING REQUIREMENTS**
  - Patients should be monitored for signs of bleeding or anaemia; treatment should be stopped if severe bleeding occurs.
  - No routine anticoagulant monitoring required (INR tests are unreliable).
  - Assess renal function (manufacturer recommends Schwartz formula to calculate estimated glomerular filtration rate) before treatment in all patients and thereafter when clinically indicated.
- **DIRECTIONS FOR ADMINISTRATION** [EvGr] *Granules* should be mixed with apple juice or soft food (e.g. mashed banana or carrots, or apple sauce) that is at room temperature and administered immediately or within 30 minutes. Do **not** mix granules with milk or milk-containing products. ⟨M⟩
- **PRESCRIBING AND DISPENSING INFORMATION** Patients should be assessed for their ability to swallow capsules before starting treatment. *Pradaxa*® capsules should not be given to patients unable or unwilling to swallow the capsule whole; *Pradaxa*® granules may be used in children as soon as they can swallow soft food.
  The manufacturer of *Pradaxa*® has provided *Prescriber Guides*.
- **PATIENT AND CARER ADVICE** Patients and their carers should be advised to contact their doctor if gastro-intestinal symptoms such as dyspepsia develop during treatment.
  Administration Patients and their carers should be given advice on how to administer *Pradaxa*® granules.
  Alert card Patients and their carers should be provided with a patient alert card and advised to keep it with them at all times.
  Missed doses If a dose is more than 6 hours late, the missed dose should not be taken and the next dose should be taken at the normal time.
- **NATIONAL FUNDING/ACCESS DECISIONS**
  For full details see funding body website

All Wales Medicines Strategy Group (AWMSG) decisions
- **Dabigatran etexilate (*Pradaxa*®) for the treatment of venous thromboembolic events (VTE) and prevention of recurrent VTE in paediatric patients from 8 years to less than 18 years of age (December 2021)** AWMSG No. 2293 Recommended

- **MEDICINAL FORMS** There can be variation in the licensing of different medicines containing the same drug.

Oral capsule

CAUTIONARY AND ADVISORY LABELS 10, 25

- **Dabigatran etexilate (Non-proprietary)**
  Dabigatran etexilate (as Dabigatran etexilate mesilate) 75 mg Dabigatran etexilate 75mg capsules | 10 capsule [PoM] £8.49 DT = £8.50 | 60 capsule [PoM] £50.99–£65.60 DT = £51.00
  Dabigatran etexilate (as Dabigatran etexilate mesilate) 110 mg Dabigatran etexilate 110mg capsules | 10 capsule [PoM] £5.05–£8.50 DT = £0.89 | 60 capsule [PoM] £51.00 DT = £5.34
  Dabigatran etexilate (as Dabigatran etexilate mesilate) 150 mg Dabigatran etexilate 150mg capsules | 60 capsule [PoM] £51.00 DT = £5.48
- **Pradaxa** (Boehringer Ingelheim Ltd)
  Dabigatran etexilate (as Dabigatran etexilate mesilate) 75 mg Pradaxa 75mg capsules | 10 capsule [PoM] £8.50 DT = £8.50 | 60 capsule [PoM] £51.00 DT = £51.00
  Dabigatran etexilate (as Dabigatran etexilate mesilate) 110 mg Pradaxa 110mg capsules | 10 capsule [PoM] £8.50 DT = £0.89 | 60 capsule [PoM] £51.00 DT = £5.34
  Dabigatran etexilate (as Dabigatran etexilate mesilate) 150 mg Pradaxa 150mg capsules | 60 capsule [PoM] £51.00 DT = £5.48

Oral granules

CAUTIONARY AND ADVISORY LABELS 10

- **Pradaxa** (Boehringer Ingelheim Ltd)
  Dabigatran etexilate (as Dabigatran etexilate mesilate) 20 mg Pradaxa 20mg granules sachets | 60 sachet [PoM] £270.00 DT = £270.00 [SF]
  Dabigatran etexilate (as Dabigatran etexilate mesilate) 30 mg Pradaxa 30mg granules sachets | 60 sachet [PoM] £270.00 DT = £270.00 [SF]
  Dabigatran etexilate (as Dabigatran etexilate mesilate) 40 mg Pradaxa 40mg granules sachets | 60 sachet [PoM] £270.00 DT = £270.00 [SF]
  Dabigatran etexilate (as Dabigatran etexilate mesilate) 50 mg Pradaxa 50mg granules sachets | 60 sachet [PoM] £270.00 DT = £270.00 [SF]
  Dabigatran etexilate (as Dabigatran etexilate mesilate) 110 mg Pradaxa 110mg granules sachets | 60 sachet [PoM] £270.00 DT = £270.00 [SF]
  Dabigatran etexilate (as Dabigatran etexilate mesilate) 150 mg Pradaxa 150mg granules sachets | 60 sachet [PoM] £270.00 DT = £270.00 [SF]

ANTITHROMBOTIC DRUGS › VITAMIN K ANTAGONISTS

Vitamin K antagonists

IMPORTANT SAFETY INFORMATION

MHRA/CHM ADVICE: DIRECT-ACTING ANTIVIRALS TO TREAT CHRONIC HEPATITIS C: RISK OF INTERACTION WITH VITAMIN K ANTAGONISTS AND CHANGES IN INR (JANUARY 2017)

A EU-wide review has identified that changes in liver function, secondary to hepatitis C treatment with direct-acting antivirals, may affect the efficacy of vitamin K antagonists; the MHRA has advised that INR should be monitored closely in patients receiving concomitant treatment.

MHRA/CHM ADVICE: WARFARIN AND OTHER ANTICOAGULANTS: MONITORING OF PATIENTS DURING THE COVID-19 PANDEMIC (OCTOBER 2020)

Healthcare professionals are reminded that:
- acute illness (including COVID-19 infection) may exaggerate the effect of warfarin and necessitate a dose reduction;
- continued INR monitoring is important in patients taking warfarin or other vitamin K antagonists if they have suspected or confirmed COVID-19 infection, so they can be clinically managed at an early stage to reduce the risk of bleeding;
- vitamin K antagonists may interact with other medicines (including antibacterials and antivirals)—advice in product literature, such as INR monitoring in patients taking vitamin K antagonists who have recently started new medicines, should be followed to minimise the risk of potential interactions.

Patients on vitamin K antagonists (and their carers) should be reminded to carefully follow instructions for use (including the patient information leaflet) and advised to notify their GP or healthcare team if they:
- have symptoms of, or confirmed, COVID-19 infection;
- are otherwise unwell with sickness or diarrhoea, or have lost their appetite;
- have changed their diet, smoking habits, or alcohol consumption;
- are taking any new medicines or supplements;
- are unable to attend their next scheduled blood test for any reason.

● **CONTRA-INDICATIONS** Avoid use within 48 hours postpartum · haemorrhagic stroke · significant bleeding

● **CAUTIONS** Bacterial endocarditis (use only if warfarin otherwise indicated) · conditions in which risk of bleeding is increased · history of gastro-intestinal bleeding · hyperthyroidism · hypothyroidism · peptic ulcer · recent ischaemic stroke · recent surgery · uncontrolled hypertension

● **SIDE-EFFECTS**
- **Common or very common** Haemorrhage
- **Rare or very rare** Alopecia · nausea · vomiting
- **Frequency not known** Blue toe syndrome · CNS haemorrhage · diarrhoea · fever · haemothorax · jaundice · pancreatitis · skin necrosis (increased risk in patients with protein C or protein S deficiency) · skin reactions

● **CONCEPTION AND CONTRACEPTION** Women of child-bearing age should be warned of the danger of teratogenicity.

● **PREGNANCY** Should not be given in the first trimester of pregnancy. Warfarin, acenocoumarol, and phenindione cross the placenta with risk of congenital malformations, and placental, fetal, or neonatal haemorrhage, especially during the last few weeks of pregnancy and at delivery. Therefore, if at all possible, they should be avoided in pregnancy, especially in the first and third trimesters (difficult decisions may have to be made, particularly in women with prosthetic heart valves, atrial fibrillation, or with a history of recurrent venous thrombosis or pulmonary embolism). Stopping these drugs before the sixth week of gestation may largely avoid the risk of fetal abnormality.

● **HEPATIC IMPAIRMENT** In general, manufacturers advise caution in mild to moderate impairment; avoid in severe impairment.

● **MONITORING REQUIREMENTS**
- The base-line prothrombin time should be determined but the initial dose should not be delayed whilst awaiting the result.
- It is essential that the INR be determined daily or on alternate days in early days of treatment, *then* at longer intervals (depending on response), *then* up to every 12 weeks.
- Change in patient's clinical condition, particularly associated with liver disease, intercurrent illness, or drug administration, necessitates more frequent testing.

● **PATIENT AND CARER ADVICE** Anticoagulant treatment booklets should be issued to all patients or their carers; these booklets include advice for patients on anticoagulant treatment, an alert card to be carried by the patient at all times, and a section for recording of INR results and dosage information. In **England**, **Wales**, and **Northern Ireland**, they are available for purchase from:

3M Security Print and Systems Limited
Gorse Street, Chadderton
Oldham
OL9 9QH
Tel: 0845 610 1112

GP practices can obtain supplies through their Local Area Team stores. NHS Trusts can order supplies from cmswebshop.corp.xerox.com/NHS/Login.aspx.

In **Scotland**, treatment booklets and starter information packs can be obtained by emailing stockorders.DPPAS@apsgroup.co.uk or by fax on (0131) 6299 967

Electronic copies of the warfarin anticoagulant alert card and record booklet are also available as risk minimisation materials at www.medicines.org.uk/emc/rmm-directory/.

above

Warfarin sodium

07-Aug-2024

● **INDICATIONS AND DOSE**

Treatment and prophylaxis of thrombotic episodes (induction)

▶ BY MOUTH
- Neonate (initiated under specialist supervision): Initially 200 micrograms/kg for 1 dose on day 1, then reduced to 100 micrograms/kg once daily for the following 3 days, subsequent doses dependent on INR levels, induction dose may need to be altered according to condition (e.g. abnormal liver function tests, cardiac failure), concomitant interacting drugs, and if baseline INR above 1.3.
- Child: Initially 200 micrograms/kg (max. per dose 10 mg) for 1 dose on day 1, then reduced to 100 micrograms/kg once daily (max. per dose 5 mg) for the following 3 days, subsequent doses adjusted according to INR levels, induction dose may need to be altered according to condition (e.g. abnormal liver function tests, cardiac failure), concomitant interacting drugs, and if baseline INR above 1.3

continued →

Treatment and prophylaxis of thrombotic episodes following induction dose (if INR still below 1.4)
▶ BY MOUTH
▸ Neonate (under expert supervision): 200 micrograms/kg once daily.
▸ Child: 200 micrograms/kg once daily (max. per dose 10 mg)

Treatment and prophylaxis of thrombotic episodes following induction dose (if INR above 3.0)
▶ BY MOUTH
▸ Neonate (under expert supervision): 50 micrograms/kg once daily.
▸ Child: 50 micrograms/kg once daily (max. per dose 2.5 mg)

Treatment and prophylaxis of thrombotic episodes following induction dose (if INR above 3.5)
▶ BY MOUTH
▸ Neonate (under expert supervision): Dose to be omitted.
▸ Child: Dose to be omitted

Treatment and prophylaxis of thrombotic episodes (usual maintenance)
▶ BY MOUTH
▸ Neonate (under expert supervision): Maintenance 100–300 micrograms/kg once daily, doses up to 400 micrograms/kg once daily may be required especially if bottle fed, to be adjusted according to INR.
▸ Child: Maintenance 100–300 micrograms/kg once daily, doses up to 400 micrograms/kg once daily may be required especially if bottle fed, to be adjusted according to INR

● **UNLICENSED USE** Not licensed for use in children.

IMPORTANT SAFETY INFORMATION

MHRA/CHM ADVICE: WARFARIN: REPORTS OF CALCIPHYLAXIS (JULY 2016)

An EU-wide review has concluded that on rare occasions, warfarin use may lead to calciphylaxis—patients should be advised to consult their doctor if they develop a painful skin rash; if calciphylaxis is diagnosed, appropriate treatment should be started and consideration should be given to stopping treatment with warfarin. The MHRA has advised that calciphylaxis is most commonly observed in patients with known risk factors such as end-stage renal disease, however cases have also been reported in patients with normal renal function.

MHRA/CHM ADVICE: WARFARIN: BE ALERT TO THE RISK OF DRUG INTERACTIONS WITH TRAMADOL (JUNE 2024)

The MHRA has received a Coroner's report regarding the death of a patient from a bleed on the brain after taking warfarin with tramadol. Healthcare professionals are reminded that:
- there is a risk of increased INR when warfarin and tramadol are taken together which can lead to potentially life-threatening bruising and bleeding;
- caution should be exercised when warfarin is prescribed alongside other drugs due to the risk of drug interactions;
- dose adjustments for warfarin and/or additional INR monitoring should be considered when starting concomitant tramadol or other medicines.

Patients and carers should be advised of the increased risk of bleeding due to drug interactions with warfarin, to inform their healthcare professional that they are on warfarin treatment before taking any new medicines, and to discuss with their healthcare professional before stopping treatment. They should also be counselled to seek medical treatment and have an urgent INR test if any signs or symptoms of a major bleeding event occur.

● **CAUTIONS** Postpartum (delay warfarin until risk of haemorrhage is low—usually 5–7 days after delivery)

● **INTERACTIONS** → Appendix 1: coumarins

● **SIDE-EFFECTS** Calciphylaxis · hepatic function abnormal

● **PREGNANCY** Babies of mothers taking warfarin at the time of delivery need to be offered immediate prophylaxis with intramuscular phytomenadione (vitamin K_1).

● **BREAST FEEDING** Not present in milk in significant amounts and appears safe. Risk of haemorrhage which is increased by vitamin K deficiency.

● **RENAL IMPAIRMENT** Use with caution in mild to moderate impairment.

Monitoring In severe renal impairment, monitor INR more frequently.

● **PRESCRIBING AND DISPENSING INFORMATION**

Dietary differences Infant formula is supplemented with vitamin K, which makes formula-fed infants resistant to warfarin; they may therefore need higher doses. In contrast breast milk contains low concentrations of vitamin K making breast-fed infants more sensitive to warfarin.

● **PATIENT AND CARER ADVICE** Anticoagulant card to be provided.

Medicines for Children leaflet: Warfarin for the treatment and prevention of thrombosis www.medicinesforchildren.org.uk/medicines/warfarin-for-the-treatment-and-prevention-of-thrombosis/

● **MEDICINAL FORMS** There can be variation in the licensing of different medicines containing the same drug. Forms available from special-order manufacturers include: oral suspension, oral solution

Oral tablet

CAUTIONARY AND ADVISORY LABELS 10

▸ Warfarin sodium (Non-proprietary)

Warfarin sodium 500 microgram Warfarin 500microgram tablets | 28 tablet [PoM] £1.70 DT = £1.54

Warfarin sodium 1 mg Warfarin 1mg tablets | 28 tablet [PoM] £1.48 DT = £0.82

Warfarin sodium 3 mg Warfarin 3mg tablets | 28 tablet [PoM] £1.81 DT = £0.82

Warfarin sodium 4 mg Coumadin 4mg tablets | 100 tablet [PoM] [X]

Warfarin sodium 5 mg Warfarin 5mg tablets | 28 tablet [PoM] £3.39 DT = £0.98

Oral suspension

CAUTIONARY AND ADVISORY LABELS 10

▸ Warfarin sodium (Non-proprietary)

Warfarin sodium 1 mg per 1 ml Warfarin 1mg/ml oral suspension sugar free | 150 ml [PoM] £202.24 DT = £202.24 [SF]

4 Blood pressure conditions

4.1 Hypertension

Hypertension

10-Aug-2022

Overview

Hypertension in children and adolescents can have a substantial effect on long-term health. Possible causes of hypertension (e.g. congenital heart disease, renal disease and endocrine disorders) and the presence of any complications (e.g. left ventricular hypertrophy) should be established. Treatment should take account of contributory factors and any factors that increase the risk of cardiovascular complications.

Serious hypertension is rare in *neonates* but it can present with signs of congestive heart failure; the cause is often renal and can follow embolic arterial damage.

Children (or their parents or carers) should be given advice on lifestyle changes to reduce blood pressure or cardiovascular risk; these include weight reduction (in obese children), reduction of dietary salt, reduction of total and saturated fat, increasing exercise, increasing fruit and vegetable intake, and not smoking (for guidance on stopping smoking, see Smoking cessation p. 353).

Indications for antihypertensive therapy in children include symptomatic hypertension, secondary hypertension, hypertensive target-organ damage, diabetes mellitus, persistent hypertension despite lifestyle measures, and pulmonary hypertension. The effect of antihypertensive treatment on growth and development is not known; treatment should be started only if benefits are clear.

Antihypertensive therapy should be initiated with a single drug at the lowest recommended dose; the dose can be increased until the target blood pressure is achieved. Once the highest recommended dose is reached, or sooner if the patient begins to experience side-effects, a second drug may be added if blood pressure is not controlled. If more than one drug is required, these should be given as separate products to allow dose adjustment of individual drugs, but fixed-dose combination products may be useful in adolescents if compliance is a problem.

Acceptable drug classes for use in children with hypertension include **ACE inhibitors**, **alpha-blockers**, **beta-blockers**, **calcium-channel blockers**, and **thiazide diuretics**. There is limited information on the use of **angiotensin-II receptor antagonists** in children. Diuretics and beta-blockers have a long history of safety and efficacy in children. The newer classes of antihypertensive drugs, including ACE inhibitors and calcium-channel blockers have been shown to be safe and effective in short-term studies in children. Refractory hypertension may require additional treatment with agents such as minoxidil p. 136 or clonidine hydrochloride p. 120.

Cardiovascular risk reduction

Aspirin p. 104 may be used to reduce the risk of cardiovascular events; however, concerns about an increased risk of bleeding and Reye's syndrome need to be considered.

A **statin** can be of benefit in older children who have a high risk of cardiovascular disease and have hypercholesterolaemia.

Hypertension in diabetes

Hypertension can occur in type 2 diabetes and treatment prevents both macrovascular and microvascular complications. ACE inhibitors may be considered in children with diabetes and microalbuminaemia or proteinuric renal disease. Beta-blockers are best avoided in children with, or at a high risk of developing, diabetes, especially when combined with a thiazide diuretic.

Hypertension in renal disease

ACE inhibitors may be considered in children with microalbuminuria or proteinuric renal disease. High doses of loop diuretics may be required. Specific cautions apply to the use of ACE inhibitors in renal impairment, but ACE inhibitors may be effective. Dihydropyridine calcium-channel blockers may be added.

Hypertension in pregnancy

High blood pressure in pregnancy may usually be due to pre-existing essential hypertension or to pre-eclampsia. Methyldopa is safe in pregnancy. Beta-blockers are effective and safe in the third trimester. Modified-release preparations of nifedipine p. 128 [unlicensed] are also used for hypertension in pregnancy. Intravenous administration of labetalol hydrochloride p. 122 can be used to control hypertensive crises; alternatively hydralazine hydrochloride p. 136 can be given by the intravenous route.

Hypertensive emergencies

Hypertensive emergencies in children may be accompanied by signs of hypertensive encephalopathy, including seizures. Controlled reduction in blood pressure over 72–96 hours is essential; rapid reduction can reduce perfusion leading to organ damage. Treatment should be initiated with intravenous drugs; once blood pressure is controlled, oral therapy can be started. It may be necessary to infuse fluids particularly during the first 12 hours to expand plasma volume should the blood pressure drop too rapidly.

Controlled reduction of blood pressure is achieved by intravenous administration of labetalol hydrochloride or sodium nitroprusside p. 138. Esmolol hydrochloride p. 125 is useful for short-term use and has a short duration of action. Nicardipine hydrochloride p. 127 can be administered as a continuous intravenous infusion for life-threatening hypertension in paediatric intensive care settings. In less severe cases, nifedipine capsules can be used.

Other antihypertensive drugs which can be given intravenously include hydralazine hydrochloride and clonidine hydrochloride.

Hypertension in acute nephritis occurs as a result of sodium and water retention; it should be treated with sodium and fluid restriction, and with furosemide p. 163; antihypertensive drugs may be added if necessary.

Also see advice on short-term management of hypertensive episodes in phaeochromocytoma.

Phaeochromocytoma

Long-term management of phaeochromocytoma involves surgery. However, surgery should not take place until there is adequate blockade of both alpha- and beta-adrenoceptors. Alpha-blockers are used in the short-term management of hypertensive episodes in phaeochromocytoma. Once alpha blockade is established, tachycardia can be controlled by the cautious addition of a beta-blocker; a cardioselective beta-blocker is preferred. There is no nationwide consensus on the optimal drug regimen or doses used for the management of phaeochromocytoma.

Phenoxybenzamine hydrochloride p. 137, a powerful alpha-blocker, is effective in the management of phaeochromocytoma but it has many side-effects.

Pulmonary hypertension

Only pulmonary *arterial* hypertension is currently suitable for drug treatment. Pulmonary arterial hypertension includes persistent pulmonary hypertension of the newborn, idiopathic pulmonary arterial hypertension in children, and pulmonary hypertension related to congenital heart disease and cardiac surgery.

Some types of pulmonary hypertension are treated with vasodilator antihypertensive therapy and oxygen. Diuretics may also have a role in children with right-sided heart failure.

Initial treatment of *persistent pulmonary hypertension of the newborn* involves the administration of **nitric oxide**; epoprostenol p. 140 can be used until nitric oxide is available. Oral sildenafil p. 139 may be helpful in less severe cases. Epoprostenol and sildenafil can cause profound systemic hypotension. In rare circumstances either tolazoline p. 142 or magnesium sulfate p. 739 can be given by intravenous infusion when nitric oxide and epoprostenol have failed.

Treatment of *idiopathic pulmonary arterial hypertension* is determined by acute vasodilator testing; drugs used for treatment include calcium-channel blockers (usually nifedipine), long-term intravenous epoprostenol, nebulised iloprost p. 141, bosentan p. 139, or sildenafil.

Anticoagulation (usually with warfarin sodium p. 115) may also be required to prevent secondary thrombosis.

Inhaled nitric oxide is a potent and selective pulmonary vasodilator. It acts on cyclic guanosine monophosphate (cGMP) resulting in smooth muscle relaxation. Inhaled nitric oxide is used in the treatment of persistent pulmonary hypertension of the newborn, and may also be useful in other forms of arterial pulmonary hypertension. Dependency can occur with high doses and prolonged use; to avoid rebound pulmonary hypertension the drug should be withdrawn gradually, often with the aid of sildenafil p. 139.

Excess nitric oxide can cause methaemoglobinaemia; therefore, methaemoglobin concentration should be measured regularly, particularly in neonates.

Nitric oxide increases the risk of haemorrhage by inhibiting platelet aggregation, but it does not usually cause bleeding.

Epoprostenol p. 140 (prostacyclin) is a prostaglandin and a potent vasodilator. It is used in the treatment of persistent pulmonary hypertension of the newborn, idiopathic pulmonary arterial hypertension, and in the acute phase following cardiac surgery. It is given by continuous 24-hour intravenous infusion.

Epoprostenol is a powerful inhibitor of platelet aggregation and there is a possible risk of haemorrhage. It is sometimes used as an antiplatelet in renal dialysis when heparins are unsuitable or contra-indicated. It can also cause serious systemic hypotension and, if withdrawn suddenly, can cause pulmonary hypertensive crisis.

Children on prolonged treatment can become tolerant to epoprostenol, and therefore require an increase in dose.

Iloprost p. 141 is a synthetic analogue of epoprostenol and is efficacious when nebulised in adults with pulmonary arterial hypertension, but experience in children is limited. It is more stable than epoprostenol and has a longer half-life.

Bosentan p. 139 is a dual endothelin receptor antagonist used orally in the treatment of pulmonary arterial hypertension. The concentration of endothelin, a potent vasoconstrictor, is raised in sustained pulmonary hypertension.

Sildenafil, a vasodilator developed for the treatment of erectile dysfunction, is also used for pulmonary arterial hypertension. It is used either alone or as an adjunct to other drugs.

Sildenafil is a selective phosphodiesterase type-5 inhibitor. Inhibition of this enzyme in the lungs enhances the vasodilatory effects of nitric oxide and promotes relaxation of vascular smooth muscle.

Sildenafil has also been used in pulmonary hypertension for weaning children off inhaled nitric oxide following cardiac surgery, and less successfully in idiopathic pulmonary arterial hypertension.

Tolazoline p. 142 is now rarely used to correct pulmonary artery vasospasm in pulmonary hypertension of the newborn as better alternatives are available. Tolazoline is an alpha-blocker and produces both pulmonary and systemic vasodilation.

Antihypertensive drugs

Vasodilator antihypertensive drugs

Vasodilators have a potent hypotensive effect, especially when used in combination with a beta-blocker and a thiazide. **Important:** see Hypertension (hypertensive emergencies) for a warning on the hazards of a very rapid fall in blood pressure.

Hydralazine hydrochloride p. 136 is given by mouth as an adjunct to other antihypertensives for the treatment of resistant hypertension but is rarely used; when used alone it causes tachycardia and fluid retention.

Sodium nitroprusside p. 138 is given by intravenous infusion to control severe hypertensive crisis when parenteral treatment is necessary. At low doses it reduces systemic vascular resistance and increases cardiac output; at high doses it can produce profound systemic hypotension—continuous blood pressure monitoring is therefore essential. Sodium nitroprusside may also be used to control paradoxical hypertension after surgery for coarctation of the aorta.

Minoxidil p. 136 should be reserved for the treatment of severe hypertension resistant to other drugs. Vasodilatation is accompanied by increased cardiac output and tachycardia and children develop fluid retention. For this reason the addition of a beta-blocker and a diuretic (usually furosemide p. 163, in high dosage) are mandatory. Hypertrichosis is troublesome and renders this drug unsuitable for females.

Prazosin p. 119 and doxazosin p. 606 have alpha-blocking and vasodilator properties.

Centrally acting antihypertensive drugs

Methyldopa, a centrally acting antihypertensive, is of little value in the management of refractory sustained hypertension in infants and children. On prolonged use it is associated with fluid retention (which may be alleviated by concomitant use of diuretics).

Methyldopa is also effective for the management of hypertension in pregnancy.

Clonidine hydrochloride p. 120 is also a centrally acting antihypertensive but has the disadvantage that sudden withdrawal may cause a hypertensive crisis. Clonidine hydrochloride is also used under specialist supervision for pain management, sedation, and opioid withdrawal, attention deficit hyperactivity disorder, and Tourette syndrome.

Adrenergic neurone blocking drugs

Adrenergic neurone blocking drugs prevent the release of noradrenaline from postganglionic adrenergic neurones. These drugs do not control supine blood pressure and may cause postural hypotension. For this reason they have largely fallen from use in adults and are rarely used in children.

Alpha-adrenoceptor blocking drugs

Doxazosin and prazosin have post-synaptic alpha-blocking and vasodilator properties and rarely cause tachycardia. They can, however, reduce blood pressure rapidly after the first dose and should be introduced with caution.

Alpha-blockers can be used with other antihypertensive drugs in the treatment of resistant hypertension.

Drugs affecting the renin-angiotensin system

02-Mar-2026

Angiotensin-converting enzyme inhibitors

Angiotensin-converting enzyme inhibitors (ACE inhibitors) inhibit the conversion of angiotensin I to angiotensin II. The main indications of ACE inhibitors in children are shown below. In infants and young children, captopril p. 131 is often considered first.

Initiation under specialist supervision

Treatment with ACE inhibitors should be initiated under specialist supervision and with careful clinical monitoring in children.

Heart failure

ACE inhibitors have a valuable role in all grades of heart failure. Profound first-dose hypotension can occur when ACE inhibitors are introduced to children with heart failure who are already taking a high dose of a loop diuretic.

Temporary withdrawal of the loop diuretic reduces the risk, but can cause severe rebound pulmonary oedema.

Hypertension

ACE inhibitors may be considered for hypertension when thiazides and beta-blockers are contra-indicated, not tolerated, or fail to control blood pressure; they may be considered for hypertension in children with type 1 diabetes with nephropathy. ACE inhibitors can reduce blood pressure very rapidly in some patients particularly in those receiving diuretic therapy.

Diabetic nephropathy

ACE inhibitors also have a role in the management of diabetic nephropathy.

Renal effects

Renal function and electrolytes should be checked before starting ACE inhibitors (or increasing the dose) and monitored during treatment (more frequently if features mentioned below are present). Hyperkalaemia and other side-effects of ACE inhibitors are more common in children with impaired renal function and the dose may need to be reduced.

Concomitant treatment with NSAIDs increases the risk of renal damage, and potassium-sparing diuretics (or potassium-containing salt substitutes) increase the risk of hyperkalaemia.

In children with severe bilateral renal artery stenosis (or severe stenosis of the artery supplying a single functioning kidney), ACE inhibitors reduce or abolish glomerular filtration and are likely to cause severe and progressive renal failure. They are therefore contra-indicated in children known to have these forms of critical renovascular disease.

ACE inhibitor treatment is unlikely to have an adverse effect on overall renal function in children with severe unilateral renal artery stenosis and a normal contralateral kidney, but glomerular filtration is likely to be reduced (or even abolished) in the affected kidney and the long-term consequences are unknown.

ACE inhibitors are therefore best avoided in those with known or suspected renovascular disease, unless the blood pressure cannot be controlled by other drugs. If they are used in these circumstances renal function needs to be monitored.

ACE inhibitors should also be used with particular caution in children who may have undiagnosed and clinically silent renovascular disease. ACE inhibitors are useful for the management of hypertension and proteinuria in children with nephritis. They are thought to have a beneficial effect by reducing intra-glomerular hypertension and protecting the glomerular capillaries and membrane.

ACE inhibitors in combination with other drugs

Concomitant diuretics

ACE inhibitors can cause a very rapid fall in blood pressure in volume-depleted children; treatment should therefore be initiated with very low doses. In some children the diuretic dose may need to be reduced or the diuretic discontinued at least 24 hours beforehand (may not be possible in heart failure—risk of pulmonary oedema). If high-dose diuretic therapy cannot be stopped, close observation is recommended after administration of the first dose of ACE inhibitor, for at least 2 hours or until the blood pressure has stabilised.

Angiotensin-II receptor antagonists

Candesartan cilexetil p. 135, losartan potassium p. 135 and valsartan p. 135 are specific angiotensin-II receptor antagonists with many properties similar to those of the ACE inhibitors. However, unlike ACE inhibitors, they do not inhibit the breakdown of bradykinin and other kinins, and thus are less likely to cause the persistent dry cough which can complicate ACE inhibitor therapy. They are therefore a useful alternative for children who have to discontinue an ACE inhibitor because of persistent cough.

Candesartan cilexetil, losartan potassium or valsartan can be used as an alternative to an ACE inhibitor in the management of hypertension.

Renal effects

Angiotensin-II receptor antagonists should be used with caution in renal artery stenosis (see also Renal effects under ACE Inhibitors, above).

Neonates

The neonatal response to treatment with ACE inhibitors is very variable, and some neonates develop profound hypotension with even small doses; a test-dose should be used initially and increased cautiously. Adverse effects such as apnoea, seizures, renal failure, and severe unpredictable hypotension are very common in the first month of life and it is therefore recommended that ACE inhibitors are avoided whenever possible, particularly in preterm neonates.

Other drugs used for Hypertension Chlortalidone, p. 165

ALPHA-ADRENOCEPTOR BLOCKERS

Prazosin

15-Apr-2024

● **INDICATIONS AND DOSE**

Hypertension

▶ BY MOUTH

▸ Child 1 month–11 years: Initially 10–15 micrograms/kg 2–4 times a day, initial dose to be taken at bedtime, then increased to 500 micrograms/kg daily in divided doses, dose to be increased gradually; maximum 20 mg per day

▸ Child 12–17 years: Initially 500 micrograms 2–3 times a day for 3–7 days, initial dose to be taken at bedtime, then increased to 1 mg 2–3 times a day for a further 3–7 days, then increased if necessary up to 20 mg daily in divided doses, dose should be increased gradually

Congestive heart failure (rarely used)

▶ BY MOUTH

▸ Child 1 month–11 years: 5 micrograms/kg twice daily, initial dose to be taken at bedtime, then increased to 100 micrograms/kg daily in divided doses, doses should be increased gradually

▸ Child 12–17 years: 500 micrograms 2–4 times a day, initial dose to be taken at bedtime, then increased to 4 mg daily in divided doses; maintenance 4–20 mg daily in divided doses

● **UNLICENSED USE** Not licensed for use in children under 12 years.

● **CONTRA-INDICATIONS** History of postural hypotension · not recommended for congestive heart failure due to mechanical obstruction (e.g. aortic stenosis)

● **CAUTIONS** Cataract surgery (risk of intra-operative floppy iris syndrome) · first dose hypotension

● **INTERACTIONS** → Appendix 1: alpha blockers

● **SIDE-EFFECTS**

▶ **Common or very common** Asthenia · constipation · depression · diarrhoea · dizziness · drowsiness · dry mouth · dyspnoea · headache · nasal congestion · nausea · nervousness · oedema · palpitations · postural hypotension · sexual dysfunction · skin reactions · syncope · urinary disorders · vertigo · vision blurred · vomiting

▶ **Uncommon** Angina pectoris · arrhythmias · arthralgia · epistaxis · eye pain · eye redness · gastrointestinal discomfort · hyperhidrosis · paraesthesia · sleep disorders · tinnitus

- ▶ **Rare or very rare** Alopecia · fever · flushing · gynaecomastia · hallucination · hepatic function abnormal · pain · pancreatitis · vasculitis
- **PREGNANCY** No evidence of teratogenicity; manufacturers advise use only when potential benefit outweighs risk.
- **BREAST FEEDING** Present in milk, amount probably too small to be harmful; manufacturer advises use with caution.
- **HEPATIC IMPAIRMENT** Manufacturer advises caution (no information available).
  Dose adjustments In children 12 years and above, manufacturer advises initial dose reduction to 500 micrograms daily; increased with caution.
- **RENAL IMPAIRMENT**
  Dose adjustments In children 12 years and above, manufacturer advises initial dose reduction to 500 micrograms daily in moderate to severe impairment; increase with caution.
- **DIRECTIONS FOR ADMINISTRATION** Expert sources advise for administration *by mouth*, tablets may be dispersed in water.
- **PATIENT AND CARER ADVICE**
  First dose effect First dose may cause collapse due to hypotensive effect (therefore should be taken on retiring to bed).
  Driving and skilled tasks May affect performance of skilled tasks e.g. driving.

- **MEDICINAL FORMS** There can be variation in the licensing of different medicines containing the same drug. Forms available from special-order manufacturers include: oral tablet, oral suspension, oral solution

Oral tablet

- ▶ Prazosin (Non-proprietary)
  Prazosin (as Prazosin hydrochloride) 2 mg Minipress 2mg tablets | 100 tablet PoM ✗ DT = £83.39
  Prazosin (as Prazosin hydrochloride) 5 mg Minipress 5mg tablets | 100 tablet PoM ✗ DT = £51.18
- ▶ Hypovase (Pfizer Ltd)
  Prazosin (as Prazosin hydrochloride) 500 microgram Hypovase 500microgram tablets | 60 tablet PoM £2.69 DT = £2.69

ANTIHYPERTENSIVES, CENTRALLY ACTING

Clonidine hydrochloride

15-Apr-2024

- **INDICATIONS AND DOSE**

Severe hypertension

▶ BY MOUTH

- ▶ Child 2–17 years: Initially 0.5–1 microgram/kg 3 times a day, dose can be gradually increased if necessary up to 25 micrograms/kg daily in divided doses; maximum 1.2 mg per day

▶ BY SLOW INTRAVENOUS INJECTION

- ▶ Child 2–17 years: 2–6 micrograms/kg for 1 dose (max. per dose 300 micrograms)

- **UNLICENSED USE** Not licensed for use in children.
- **CONTRA-INDICATIONS** Severe bradyarrhythmia secondary to second- or third-degree AV block or sick sinus syndrome
- **CAUTIONS** Cerebrovascular disease · constipation · heart failure · history of depression · mild to moderate bradyarrhythmia · polyneuropathy · Raynaud's syndrome or other occlusive peripheral vascular disease
- **INTERACTIONS** → Appendix 1: clonidine
- **SIDE-EFFECTS**
- ▶ **Common or very common** Constipation · depression · dizziness · dry mouth · fatigue · headache · nausea · postural hypotension · salivary gland pain · sedation · sexual dysfunction · sleep disorders · vomiting
- ▶ **Uncommon** Delusions · hallucination · malaise · paraesthesia · Raynaud's phenomenon · skin reactions
- ▶ **Rare or very rare** Alopecia · atrioventricular block · dry eye · gynaecomastia · intestinal pseudo-obstruction · nasal dryness
- ▶ **Frequency not known** Accommodation disorder · arrhythmias · confusion
- **PREGNANCY** May lower fetal heart rate. Avoid oral use unless potential benefit outweighs risk. Avoid using injection.
- **BREAST FEEDING** Avoid—present in milk.
- **RENAL IMPAIRMENT** Manufacturer advises caution.
  Dose adjustments In adults, manufacturer advises adjust dose according to response (consult product literature).
- **TREATMENT CESSATION** Must be withdrawn gradually to avoid hypertensive crisis.
- **DIRECTIONS FOR ADMINISTRATION** For *intravenous injection*, manufacturer advises give over 10–15 minutes; compatible with Sodium Chloride 0.9% *or* Glucose 5%.
  For administration *by mouth*, expert sources advise *Catapres*® tablets may be crushed and dissolved in water.
- **PATIENT AND CARER ADVICE**
  Driving and skilled tasks Drowsiness may affect performance of skilled tasks (e.g. driving); effects of alcohol may be enhanced.
- **LESS SUITABLE FOR PRESCRIBING** Clonidine is less suitable for prescribing.

- **MEDICINAL FORMS** There can be variation in the licensing of different medicines containing the same drug. Forms available from special-order manufacturers include: oral suspension, oral solution, solution for injection

Oral tablet

CAUTIONARY AND ADVISORY LABELS 3, 8

- ▶ Clonidine hydrochloride (Non-proprietary)
  Clonidine hydrochloride 25 microgram Clonidine 25microgram tablets | 112 tablet PoM £18.00 DT = £5.94
  Clonidine hydrochloride 100 microgram Clonidine 100microgram tablets | 100 tablet PoM £10.05 DT = £8.04

Solution for injection

- ▶ Clonidine hydrochloride (Non-proprietary)
  Clonidine hydrochloride 150 microgram per 1 ml Clonidine 150micrograms/1ml solution for injection ampoules | 5 ampoule PoM £4.18 DT = £4.18 (Hospital only) | 5 ampoule PoM £15.00 DT = £4.18

Oral solution

- ▶ Clonidine hydrochloride (Non-proprietary)
  Clonidine hydrochloride 10 microgram per 1 ml Clonidine 50micrograms/5ml oral solution sugar free | 100 ml PoM £290.00 DT = £255.46 SF
  Clonidine hydrochloride 20 microgram per 1 ml Clonidine 100micrograms/5ml oral solution sugar free | 150 ml PoM £300.00 SF

BETA-ADRENOCEPTOR BLOCKERS

Beta-adrenoceptor blocking drugs

11-Oct-2023

Overview

Beta-adrenoceptor blocking drugs (beta-blockers) block the beta-adrenoceptors in the heart, peripheral vasculature, bronchi, pancreas, and liver.

Many beta-blockers are available but experience in children is limited to the use of only a few.

Differences between beta-blockers may affect choice. Water-soluble beta-blockers (such as atenolol p. 125 and sotalol hydrochloride p. 90) are less likely to enter the brain and may therefore cause less sleep disturbance and nightmares. Water-soluble beta-blockers are excreted by the kidneys and dosage reduction is often necessary in renal impairment.

Some beta-blockers, such as atenolol, have an intrinsically longer duration of action and need to be given only once daily. Carvedilol p. 146 and labetalol hydrochloride p. 122 are beta-blockers which have, in addition, an arteriolar vasodilating action and thus lower peripheral resistance. Although carvedilol and labetalol hydrochloride possess both alpha- and beta-blocking properties, these drugs have no important advantages over other beta-blockers in the treatment of hypertension.

Beta-blockers slow the heart and can depress the myocardium; they are contra-indicated in children with second- or third-degree heart block.

Beta-blockers can precipitate asthma and should usually be avoided in children with a history of asthma or bronchospasm. If there is no alternative, a child with well-controlled asthma can be treated for a co-existing condition (e.g. arrhythmia) with a cardioselective beta-blocker, which should be initiated with caution at a low dose by a specialist and the child monitored closely for adverse effects. Atenolol and metoprolol tartrate p. 126 have less effect on the $beta_2$ (bronchial) receptors and are, therefore, relatively *cardioselective*, but they are not *cardiospecific*; they have a lesser effect on airways resistance but are not free of this side-effect.

Beta-blockers are also associated with fatigue, coldness of the extremities, and sleep disturbances with nightmares (may be less common with the water-soluble beta-blockers).

Beta-blockers can affect carbohydrate metabolism causing hypoglycaemia or hyperglycaemia in children with or without diabetes; they can also interfere with metabolic and autonomic responses to hypoglycaemia thereby masking symptoms such as tachycardia. However, beta-blockers are not contra-indicated in diabetes, although the cardioselective beta-blockers (e.g. atenolol and metoprolol tartrate) may be preferred. Beta-blockers should be avoided altogether in those with frequent episodes of hypoglycaemia.

Hypertension

Beta-blockers are effective for reducing blood pressure, but their mode of action is not understood; they reduce cardiac output, alter baroceptor reflex sensitivity, and block peripheral adrenoceptors. Some beta-blockers depress plasma renin secretion. It is possible that a central effect may also partly explain their mode of action. Blood pressure can usually be controlled with relatively few side-effects. In general the dose of beta-blocker does not have to be high.

Labetalol hydrochloride may be given intravenously for *hypertensive emergencies* in children; however, care is needed to avoid dangerous hypotension or beta-blockade, particularly in neonates. Esmolol hydrochloride p. 125 is also used intravenously for the treatment of hypertension particularly in the peri-operative period.

Beta-blockers can be used to control the pulse rate in children with *phaeochromocytoma*. However, they should never be used alone as beta-blockade without concurrent alpha-blockade may lead to a hypertensive crisis; phenoxybenzamine hydrochloride p. 137 should always be used together with the beta-blocker.

Arrhythmias

In arrhythmias, beta-blockers act principally by attenuating the effects of the sympathetic system on automaticity and conductivity within the heart. They can be used alone or in conjunction with digoxin p. 91 to control the ventricular rate in *atrial fibrillation*. Beta-blockers are also useful in the management of *supraventricular tachycardias* and *ventricular tachycardias* particularly to prevent recurrence of the tachycardia.

Esmolol hydrochloride is a relatively cardioselective beta-blocker with a very short duration of action, used intravenously for the short-term treatment of supraventricular arrhythmias and sinus tachycardia, particularly in the peri-operative period.

Sotalol hydrochloride is a non-cardioselective beta-blocker with additional class III anti-arrhythmic activity. Atenolol and sotalol hydrochloride suppress ventricular ectopic beats and non-sustained ventricular tachycardia. However, the pro-arrhythmic effects of sotalol hydrochloride, particularly in children with sick sinus syndrome, may prolong the QT interval and induce torsade de pointes.

Heart failure

Beta-blockers may produce benefit in heart failure by blocking sympathetic activity and the addition of a beta-blocker such as carvedilol to other treatment for heart failure may be beneficial. Treatment should be initiated by those experienced in the management of heart failure.

Thyrotoxicosis

Beta-blockers are used in the management of *thyrotoxicosis* including neonatal thyrotoxicosis; propranolol hydrochloride p. 123 can reverse clinical symptoms within 4 days. Beta-blockers are also used for the pre-operative preparation for thyroidectomy; the thyroid gland is rendered less vascular, thus facilitating surgery.

Other uses

In tetralogy of Fallot, esmolol hydrochloride or propranolol hydrochloride may be given intravenously in the initial management of *cyanotic spells*; propranolol hydrochloride is given by mouth for preventing cyanotic spells. If a severe cyanotic spell in a child with congenital heart disease persists despite optimal use of 100% oxygen, propranolol hydrochloride is given by intravenous infusion. If cyanosis is still present after 10 minutes, sodium bicarbonate intravenous infusion p. 725 is given in a dose to correct acidosis (or dose calculated according to arterial blood gas results); sodium bicarbonate 4.2% intravenous infusion is appropriate for a child under 1 year and sodium bicarbonate 8.4% intravenous infusion in children over 1 year. If blood-glucose concentration is less than 3 mmol/litre, glucose 10% intravenous infusion is given, followed by intravenous or intramuscular injection of morphine p. 338.

Beta-blockers are also used in the *prophylaxis of migraine*. Betaxolol p. 851, levobunolol hydrochloride p. 852, and timolol maleate p. 852 are used topically in *glaucoma*.

EvGr Carvedilol [unlicensed use] and propranolol hydrochloride [unlicensed use] may be used for primary prevention of decompensated cirrhosis; carvedilol is considered first-choice as it has fewer side-effects and a greater effect on portal vein pressure. Carvedilol [unlicensed use] and propranolol hydrochloride [unlicensed use] are also used to prevent bleeding from oesophageal varices. (A) For further guidance see NICE guideline **Cirrhosis in over 16s: assessment and management** (available at: www.nice.org.uk/guidance/ng50).

Beta-adrenoceptor blockers (systemic)

- **CONTRA-INDICATIONS** Asthma · cardiogenic shock · hypotension · marked bradycardia · metabolic acidosis · phaeochromocytoma (apart from specific use with alpha-blockers) · second-degree AV block · severe peripheral arterial disease · sick sinus syndrome · third-degree AV block · uncontrolled heart failure

CONTRA-INDICATIONS, FURTHER INFORMATION

- Bronchospasm Beta-blockers, including those considered to be cardioselective, should usually be avoided in patients with a history of asthma, bronchospasm or a history of obstructive airways disease. However, when there is no alternative, a cardioselective beta-blocker can be given to these patients with caution and under specialist supervision. In such cases the risk of inducing bronchospasm should be appreciated and appropriate precautions taken.

- **CAUTIONS** Diabetes · first-degree AV block · history of obstructive airways disease (introduce cautiously) · myasthenia gravis · portal hypertension (risk of deterioration in liver function) · psoriasis · symptoms of thyrotoxicosis may be masked
- **SIDE-EFFECTS**
  - **Common or very common** Abdominal discomfort · bradycardia · confusion · depression · diarrhoea · dizziness · dry eye (reversible on discontinuation) · dyspnoea · erectile dysfunction · fatigue · headache · heart failure · nausea · paraesthesia · peripheral coldness · rash (reversible on discontinuation) · Raynaud's phenomenon · sleep disorders · syncope · visual impairment · vomiting
  - **Uncommon** Alopecia · atrioventricular block · bronchospasm
  - **Rare or very rare** Hallucination · psoriasis exacerbated

  SIDE-EFFECTS, FURTHER INFORMATION With administration by intravenous injection, excessive bradycardia can occur and may be countered with **intravenous injection** of atropine sulfate.

  Overdose Therapeutic overdosages with beta-blockers may cause lightheadedness, dizziness, and possibly syncope as a result of bradycardia and hypotension; heart failure may be precipitated or exacerbated. With administration by intravenous injection, excessive bradycardia can occur and may be countered with intravenous injection of atropine sulfate.

  For details on the management of poisoning, see Beta-blockers, under Emergency treatment of poisoning p. 1036.
- **ALLERGY AND CROSS-SENSITIVITY** EvGr Caution is advised in patients with a history of hypersensitivity—may increase sensitivity to allergens and result in more serious hypersensitivity response. ⟨M⟩ Furthermore, beta-adrenoceptor blockers may reduce response to adrenaline.
- **PREGNANCY** Beta-blockers may cause intra-uterine growth restriction, neonatal hypoglycaemia, and bradycardia; the risk is greater in severe hypertension.
- **BREAST FEEDING** With systemic use in the mother, infants should be monitored as there is a risk of possible toxicity due to beta-blockade. However, the amount of most beta-blockers present in milk is too small to affect infants.
- **MONITORING REQUIREMENTS** Monitor lung function (in patients with a history of obstructive airway disease).
- **TREATMENT CESSATION** Avoid abrupt withdrawal.

BETA-ADRENOCEPTOR BLOCKERS › ALPHA- AND BETA-ADRENOCEPTOR BLOCKERS

F 121

Labetalol hydrochloride

13-May-2021

- **INDICATIONS AND DOSE**

Hypertensive emergencies

▶ BY INTRAVENOUS INFUSION

- Neonate: Initially 0.5 mg/kg/hour (max. per dose 4 mg/kg/hour), dose to be adjusted according to response at intervals of at least 15 minutes.
- Child 1 month–11 years: Initially 0.5–1 mg/kg/hour (max. per dose 3 mg/kg/hour), dose to be adjusted according to response at intervals of at least 15 minutes
- Child 12–17 years: Initially 30–120 mg/hour, dose to be adjusted according to response at intervals of at least 15 minutes

Hypertension

▶ BY MOUTH

- Child 1 month–11 years: 1–2 mg/kg 3–4 times a day
- Child 12–17 years: Initially 50–100 mg twice daily, dose to be increased if required at intervals of 3–14 days; usual dose 200–400 mg twice daily, higher doses to be given in 3–4 divided doses; maximum 2.4 g per day

▶ BY INTRAVENOUS INJECTION

- Child 1 month–11 years: 250–500 micrograms/kg (max. per dose 20 mg) for 1 dose
- Child 12–17 years: 50 mg, dose to be given over at least 1 minute, then 50 mg after 5 minutes if required; maximum 200 mg per course

- **UNLICENSED USE** Not licensed for use in children.

> **IMPORTANT SAFETY INFORMATION**
>
> ▶ With intravenous use
>
> Consult local guidelines. In hypertensive encephalopathy reduce blood pressure to normotensive level over 24–48 hours (more rapid reduction may lead to cerebral infarction, blindness, and death). If child fitting, reduce blood pressure rapidly, but not to normal levels.

- **CAUTIONS** Liver damage
- **INTERACTIONS** → Appendix 1: beta blockers, non-selective
- **SIDE-EFFECTS**

  GENERAL SIDE-EFFECTS
  - **Common or very common** Drug fever · ejaculation failure · hypersensitivity · urinary disorders
  - **Rare or very rare** Hepatic disorders · systemic lupus erythematosus (SLE) · toxic myopathy · tremor
  - **Frequency not known** Cyanosis · hyperhidrosis · hyperkalaemia · interstitial lung disease · lethargy · lichenoid keratosis · muscle cramps · nasal congestion · peripheral oedema · postural hypotension · psychosis · thrombocytopenia

  SPECIFIC SIDE-EFFECTS
  - **Rare or very rare**
    - With oral use Peripheral vascular disease
  - **Frequency not known**
    - With intravenous use Fever · hypoglycaemia masked · intermittent claudication exacerbated · thyrotoxicosis masked
    - With oral use Photosensitivity reaction
- **PREGNANCY** The use of labetalol in maternal hypertension is not known to be harmful, except possibly in the first trimester. If labetalol is used close to delivery, infants should be monitored for signs of alpha-blockade (as well as beta blockade).
- **BREAST FEEDING** Infants should be monitored as there is a risk of possible toxicity due to alpha-blockade (in addition to beta-blockade).
- **HEPATIC IMPAIRMENT** Manufacturer advises caution (risk of slow metabolism).

  Dose adjustments In adults, manufacturer advises consider dose reduction.
- **RENAL IMPAIRMENT**

  Dose adjustments In adults, manufacturer advises consider dose reduction.
- **MONITORING REQUIREMENTS**
  - Liver damage Severe hepatocellular damage reported after both short-term and long-term treatment. Appropriate laboratory testing needed at first symptom of liver dysfunction and if laboratory evidence of damage (or if jaundice) labetalol should be stopped and not restarted.

- **EFFECT ON LABORATORY TESTS** Interferes with laboratory tests for catecholamines.
- **DIRECTIONS FOR ADMINISTRATION** EvGr For *intravenous infusion*, dilute to a concentration of 1 mg/mL in Glucose 5% or Sodium Chloride and Glucose 5%; (M) expert sources advise if fluid restricted may be given undiluted, preferably through a central venous catheter. EvGr Avoid upright position during and for 3 hours after intravenous administration. (M)

  For administration *by mouth*, expert sources advise injection may be given orally with squash or juice.
- **PATIENT AND CARER ADVICE**
  Medicines for Children leaflet: Labetalol hydrochloride for hypertension www.medicinesforchildren.org.uk/medicines/labetalol-hydrochloride-for-hypertension/

- **MEDICINAL FORMS** There can be variation in the licensing of different medicines containing the same drug. Forms available from special-order manufacturers include: oral suspension, oral solution

Solution for injection

▸ Labetalol hydrochloride (Non-proprietary)

Labetalol hydrochloride 5 mg per 1 ml Labetalol 50mg/10ml solution for injection ampoules | 5 ampoule PoM £60.00 (Hospital only) | 10 ampoule PoM £125.00 (Hospital only)
Labetalol 100mg/20ml solution for injection ampoules | 5 ampoule PoM £69.00–£148.82 (Hospital only)

Oral tablet

CAUTIONARY AND ADVISORY LABELS 8, 21

▸ Labetalol hydrochloride (Non-proprietary)

Labetalol hydrochloride 100 mg Labetalol 100mg tablets | 56 tablet PoM £22.50 DT = £4.34

Labetalol hydrochloride 200 mg Labetalol 200mg tablets | 56 tablet PoM £30.00 DT = £14.19

Labetalol hydrochloride 400 mg Labetalol 400mg tablets | 56 tablet PoM £35.90 DT = £21.12

▸ Trandate (RPH Pharmaceuticals AB)

Labetalol hydrochloride 100 mg Trandate 100mg tablets | 56 tablet PoM £4.87 DT = £4.34

Labetalol hydrochloride 200 mg Trandate 200mg tablets | 56 tablet PoM £8.72 DT = £14.19

BETA-ADRENOCEPTOR BLOCKERS › NON-SELECTIVE

121

Propranolol hydrochloride

03-Apr-2024

- **INDICATIONS AND DOSE**

Hyperthyroidism with autonomic symptoms

▸ BY MOUTH

▸ Neonate: Initially 250–500 micrograms/kg every 6–8 hours, adjusted according to response.

▸ Child: Initially 250–500 micrograms/kg every 8 hours, adjusted according to response; increased if necessary up to 1 mg/kg every 8 hours (max. per dose 40 mg every 8 hours)

▸ BY INTRAVENOUS INJECTION

▸ Neonate: Initially 20–50 micrograms/kg every 6–8 hours, adjusted according to response, to be given over 10 minutes.

▸ Child: Initially 25–50 micrograms/kg every 6–8 hours (max. per dose 5 mg), adjusted according to response, to be given over 10 minutes

Thyrotoxicosis (adjunct)

▸ BY MOUTH

▸ Neonate: Initially 250–500 micrograms/kg every 6–8 hours, adjusted according to response.

▸ Child: Initially 250–500 micrograms/kg every 8 hours, adjusted according to response; increased if necessary up to 1 mg/kg every 8 hours (max. per dose 40 mg every 8 hours)

▸ BY INTRAVENOUS INJECTION

▸ Neonate: Initially 20–50 micrograms/kg every 6–8 hours, adjusted according to response, to be given over 10 minutes.

▸ Child: Initially 25–50 micrograms/kg every 6–8 hours (max. per dose 5 mg), adjusted according to response, to be given over 10 minutes

Thyrotoxic crisis

▸ BY MOUTH

▸ Neonate: Initially 250–500 micrograms/kg every 6–8 hours, adjusted according to response.

▸ Child: Initially 250–500 micrograms/kg every 8 hours, adjusted according to response; increased if necessary up to 1 mg/kg every 8 hours (max. per dose 40 mg every 8 hours)

▸ BY INTRAVENOUS INJECTION

▸ Neonate: Initially 20–50 micrograms/kg every 6–8 hours, adjusted according to response, to be given over 10 minutes.

▸ Child: Initially 25–50 micrograms/kg every 6–8 hours (max. per dose 5 mg), adjusted according to response, to be given over 10 minutes

Hypertension

▸ BY MOUTH

▸ Neonate: Initially 250 micrograms/kg 3 times a day, then increased if necessary up to 2 mg/kg 3 times a day.

▸ Child 1 month–11 years: Initially 0.25–1 mg/kg 3 times a day, then increased to 5 mg/kg daily in divided doses, dose should be increased at weekly intervals

▸ Child 12–17 years: Initially 80 mg twice daily, then increased if necessary up to 160–320 mg daily, dose should be increased at weekly intervals, slow-release preparations may be used for once daily administration

Prevention of bleeding from medium or large oesophageal varices [in patients with cirrhosis]

▸ BY MOUTH

▸ Child 16–17 years: 40 mg twice daily, increased if necessary up to 160 mg twice daily, dose to be adjusted gradually according to heart rate and blood pressure

Primary prevention of decompensated cirrhosis [in patients with clinically significant portal hypertension]

▸ BY MOUTH

▸ Child 16–17 years: 40 mg twice daily, dose to be adjusted gradually according to heart rate and blood pressure

Migraine prophylaxis

▸ BY MOUTH

▸ Child 2–11 years: Initially 200–500 micrograms/kg twice daily; usual dose 10–20 mg twice daily (max. per dose 2 mg/kg twice daily)

▸ Child 12–17 years: Initially 20–40 mg twice daily; usual dose 40–80 mg twice daily (max. per dose 120 mg); maximum 4 mg/kg per day

Arrhythmias

▸ BY MOUTH

▸ Neonate: 250–500 micrograms/kg 3 times a day, adjusted according to response.

▸ Child: 250–500 micrograms/kg 3–4 times a day (max. per dose 1 mg/kg 4 times a day), adjusted according to response; maximum 160 mg per day

▸ BY SLOW INTRAVENOUS INJECTION

▸ Neonate: 20–50 micrograms/kg, then 20–50 micrograms/kg every 6–8 hours if required, eCG monitoring required.

continued →

- Child: 25–50 micrograms/kg, then 25–50 micrograms/kg every 6–8 hours if required, eCG monitoring required

Tetralogy of Fallot

- BY MOUTH
- Neonate: 0.25–1 mg/kg 2–3 times a day (max. per dose 2 mg/kg 3 times a day).
- Child 1 month–11 years: 0.25–1 mg/kg 3–4 times a day, maximum dose to be given in divided doses; maximum 5 mg/kg per day
- BY SLOW INTRAVENOUS INJECTION
- Neonate: Initially 15–20 micrograms/kg (max. per dose 100 micrograms/kg), then 15–20 micrograms/kg every 12 hours if required, eCG monitoring is required with administration.
- Child 1 month–11 years: Initially 15–20 micrograms/kg (max. per dose 100 micrograms/kg), higher doses are rarely necessary, then 15–20 micrograms/kg every 6–8 hours if required, eCG monitoring is required with administration

Infantile haemangioma [proliferating, with ulceration, risk of disfigurement, or functional impairment] (initiated under specialist supervision)

- BY MOUTH
- Child: Initially 1 mg/kg daily in 3 divided doses, to be increased after at least 24 hours, usual maintenance 2 mg/kg daily in 2–3 divided doses, dosing to be given using 5mg/5mL oral solution. Review treatment after 2–3 months and adjust dosing for weight gain. Most patients do not need treatment beyond 17 months of age, for neonates, preterm infants, patients with comorbidities, or those with segmental infantile haemangioma and suspected PHACES syndrome, reduced dosing is required, as determined by the supervising specialist; maximum 3 mg/kg per day

● **UNLICENSED USE** Not licensed for treatment of hypertension in children under 12 years. Propranolol hydrochloride may be used as detailed below, although these situations are considered unlicensed:
- EvGr prevention of bleeding from medium or large oesophageal varices;
- primary prevention of decompensated cirrhosis;
- treatment of infantile haemangioma. (A)

IMPORTANT SAFETY INFORMATION

SAFE PRACTICE

Propranolol has been confused with prednisolone; care must be taken to ensure the correct drug is prescribed and dispensed.

HEALTH SERVICES SAFETY INVESTIGATIONS BODY (HSSIB) PATIENT SAFETY INVESTIGATIONS: POTENTIAL UNDER-RECOGNISED RISK OF HARM FROM THE USE OF PROPRANOLOL (FEBRUARY 2020)

A review of reported incidents identified an increase in deaths due to propranolol overdose between 2012 and 2017. To minimise the risk of harm from toxicity and rapid deterioration due to propranolol overdose, the HSSIB has issued advice: www.hssib.org.uk/patient-safety-investigations/potential-under-recognised-risk-of-harm-from-the-use-of-propranolol/.

● **CONTRA-INDICATIONS**
- When used for Infantile haemangioma Hypoglycaemic episodes (recent or ongoing; interrupt treatment if significantly reduced oral intake)

● **INTERACTIONS** → Appendix 1: beta blockers, non-selective

● **SIDE-EFFECTS**
- **Rare or very rare** Intermittent claudication · memory loss · mood altered · neuromuscular dysfunction · postural hypotension · psychosis · skin reactions · thrombocytopenia
- **Frequency not known** Hypoglycaemia

Overdose Severe overdosages with propranolol may cause cardiovascular collapse, CNS depression, and convulsions.

● **HEPATIC IMPAIRMENT** EvGr Caution (increased risk of hepatic encephalopathy; risk of increased half-life). (M)
- When used for Prevention of bleeding from medium or large oesophageal varices or Primary prevention of decompensated cirrhosis EvGr Caution (may have greater effect on heart rate and blood pressure). (A)

Dose adjustments
- With oral use EvGr Consider dose reduction. (M)

● **RENAL IMPAIRMENT** EvGr Use with caution (risk of increased half-life). (M)

Dose adjustments EvGr Consider dose reduction. (M)

● **TREATMENT CESSATION**
- When used for Infantile haemangioma EvGr Treatment can be stopped abruptly during or at the end of therapy. (A)

● **DIRECTIONS FOR ADMINISTRATION** For *slow intravenous injection*, expert sources advise give over at least 3–5 minutes; may be diluted with Sodium Chloride 0.9% or Glucose 5%; incompatible with bicarbonate. Manufacturer advises rate of administration should not exceed 1 mg/minute.

● **PRESCRIBING AND DISPENSING INFORMATION** Modified-release preparations can be used for once daily administration.

● **PATIENT AND CARER ADVICE**
- When used for Infantile haemangioma Parents and carers should be provided with a drug dosing card to record dose adjustments, and a patient information leaflet such as that produced by the British Association of Dermatologists. tinyurl.com/yhb3ecr9

● **MEDICINAL FORMS** There can be variation in the licensing of different medicines containing the same drug. Forms available from special-order manufacturers include: oral suspension, oral solution

Oral tablet

CAUTIONARY AND ADVISORY LABELS 8

- **Propranolol hydrochloride (Non-proprietary)**
  - **Propranolol hydrochloride 10 mg** Propranolol 10mg tablets | 28 tablet PoM £1.54 DT = £0.64 | 1000 tablet PoM £23.57–£24.63
  - **Propranolol hydrochloride 40 mg** Propranolol 40mg tablets | 28 tablet PoM £3.52 DT = £0.98 | 1000 tablet PoM £33.50–£40.00
  - **Propranolol hydrochloride 80 mg** Propranolol 80mg tablets | 28 tablet PoM £2.50 | 56 tablet PoM £7.54 DT = £2.19
  - **Propranolol hydrochloride 160 mg** Propranolol 160mg tablets | 56 tablet PoM £6.50 DT = £5.87

Oral solution

CAUTIONARY AND ADVISORY LABELS 8

- **Propranolol hydrochloride (Non-proprietary)**
  - **Propranolol hydrochloride 1 mg per 1 ml** Propranolol 5mg/5ml oral solution sugar free | 150 ml PoM £23.50 DT = £16.11 SF
  - **Propranolol hydrochloride 2 mg per 1 ml** Propranolol 10mg/5ml oral solution sugar free | 150 ml PoM £28.45 DT = £20.52 SF
  - **Propranolol hydrochloride 8 mg per 1 ml** Propranolol 40mg/5ml oral solution sugar free | 150 ml PoM £36.50 DT = £22.30 SF
  - **Propranolol hydrochloride 10 mg per 1 ml** Propranolol 50mg/5ml oral solution sugar free | 150 ml PoM £38.50 DT = £26.60 SF

Modified-release capsule

CAUTIONARY AND ADVISORY LABELS 8, 25

- **Propranolol hydrochloride (Non-proprietary)**
  - **Propranolol hydrochloride 80 mg** Propranolol 80mg modified-release capsules | 1 capsule PoM ⊠
  - **Propranolol hydrochloride 160 mg** Propranolol 160mg modified-release capsules | 1 capsule PoM ⊠
- **Bedranol SR** (Sandoz Ltd, Almus Pharmaceuticals Ltd)
  - **Propranolol hydrochloride 80 mg** Bedranol SR 80mg capsules | 28 capsule PoM £4.16 DT = £4.95
  - **Propranolol hydrochloride 160 mg** Bedranol SR 160mg capsules | 28 capsule PoM £4.59 DT = £4.88

BETA-ADRENOCEPTOR BLOCKERS › SELECTIVE

F 121

Atenolol

01-Dec-2023

● **INDICATIONS AND DOSE**

Hypertension

▶ BY MOUTH

▶ Neonate: 0.5–2 mg/kg daily in 1–2 divided doses.

▶ Child 1 month–11 years: 0.5–2 mg/kg daily in 1–2 divided doses, doses higher than 50 mg per day are rarely necessary

▶ Child 12–17 years: 25–50 mg daily in 1–2 divided doses, higher doses are rarely necessary

Arrhythmias

▶ BY MOUTH

▶ Neonate: 0.5–2 mg/kg daily in 1–2 divided doses.

▶ Child 1 month–11 years: 0.5–2 mg/kg daily in 1–2 divided doses; maximum 100 mg per day

▶ Child 12–17 years: 50–100 mg daily in 1–2 divided doses

● **UNLICENSED USE** Not licensed for use in children under 12 years.

IMPORTANT SAFETY INFORMATION

SAFE PRACTICE

Atenolol has been confused with amlodipine; care must be taken to ensure the correct drug is prescribed and dispensed.

● **INTERACTIONS** → Appendix 1: beta blockers, selective

● **SIDE-EFFECTS**

▶ **Common or very common** Gastrointestinal disorder

▶ **Rare or very rare** Dry mouth · hepatic disorders · intermittent claudication · mood altered · postural hypotension · psychosis · skin reactions · thrombocytopenia

▶ **Frequency not known** Hypersensitivity · lupus-like syndrome

● **BREAST FEEDING** Water soluble beta-blockers such as atenolol are present in breast milk in greater amounts than other beta blockers.

● **RENAL IMPAIRMENT**

Dose adjustments Initially use 50% of usual dose if estimated glomerular filtration rate 10–35 mL/minute/1.73 m^2; initially use 30–50% of usual dose if estimated glomerular filtration rate less than 10 mL/minute/1.73 m^2.

● **PATIENT AND CARER ADVICE**

Medicines for Children leaflet: Atenolol for hypertension www.medicinesforchildren.org.uk/medicines/atenolol-for-hypertension/

● **MEDICINAL FORMS** There can be variation in the licensing of different medicines containing the same drug. Forms available from special-order manufacturers include: oral suspension, oral solution

Oral tablet

CAUTIONARY AND ADVISORY LABELS 8

▶ Atenolol (Non-proprietary)

Atenolol 25 mg Atenolol 25mg tablets | 28 tablet [PoM] £5.11 DT = £0.51

Atenolol 50 mg Atenolol 50mg tablets | 28 tablet [PoM] £10.22 DT = £0.54

Atenolol 100 mg Atenolol 100mg tablets | 28 tablet [PoM] £14.67 DT = £0.69

▶ Tenormin (Atnahs Pharma UK Ltd)

Atenolol 50 mg Tenormin LS 50mg tablets | 28 tablet [PoM] £10.22 DT = £0.54

Oral solution

CAUTIONARY AND ADVISORY LABELS 8

▶ Atenolol (Non-proprietary)

Atenolol 5 mg per 1 ml Atenolol 25mg/5ml oral solution sugar free | 300 ml [PoM] £10.48 DT = £5.54 [SF]

Oral suspension

CAUTIONARY AND ADVISORY LABELS 8

F 121

Esmolol hydrochloride

05-May-2021

● **INDICATIONS AND DOSE**

Arrhythmias | Hypertensive emergencies

▶ INITIALLY BY INTRAVENOUS INJECTION

▶ Child: Loading dose 500 micrograms/kg, to be given over 1 minute, then (by intravenous infusion) maintenance 50 micrograms/kg/minute for 4 minutes (rate reduced if low blood pressure or low heart rate), if inadequate response, repeat loading dose and increase maintenance infusion, (by intravenous injection) loading dose 500 micrograms/kg, given over 1 minute, then (by intravenous infusion) maintenance 100 micrograms/kg/minute for 4 minutes, if response still inadequate, repeat loading dose and increase maintenance infusion, (by intravenous injection) loading dose 500 micrograms/kg, given over 1 minute, then (by intravenous infusion) maintenance 150 micrograms/kg/minute for 4 minutes, if response still inadequate, repeat loading dose and increase maintenance infusion, (by intravenous injection) loading dose 500 micrograms/kg, given over 1 minute, then (by intravenous infusion) maintenance 200 micrograms/kg/minute for 4 minutes, doses over 300 micrograms/kg/minute not recommended

Tetralogy of Fallot

▶ INITIALLY BY INTRAVENOUS INJECTION

▶ Neonate: Initially 600 micrograms/kg, dose to be given over 1–2 minutes, then (by intravenous infusion) 300–900 micrograms/kg/minute if required.

● **UNLICENSED USE** Not licensed for use in children.

● **INTERACTIONS** → Appendix 1: beta blockers, selective

● **SIDE-EFFECTS**

▶ **Common or very common** Anxiety · appetite decreased · concentration impaired · drowsiness · hyperhidrosis

▶ **Uncommon** Arrhythmias · chills · constipation · costochondritis · dry mouth · dyspepsia · fever · flushing · nasal congestion · oedema · pain · pallor · peripheral vascular disease · pulmonary oedema · respiratory disorders · seizure · skin reactions · speech disorder · taste altered · thinking abnormal · urinary retention

▶ **Rare or very rare** Cardiac arrest · extravasation necrosis · thrombophlebitis

▶ **Frequency not known** Angioedema · coronary vasospasm · hyperkalaemia · metabolic acidosis

● **BREAST FEEDING** Manufacturer advises avoidance.

● **RENAL IMPAIRMENT** Manufacturer advises caution.

● **DIRECTIONS FOR ADMINISTRATION** Incompatible with bicarbonate.

● **MEDICINAL FORMS** There can be variation in the licensing of different medicines containing the same drug.

Solution for injection

▶ Esmolol hydrochloride (Non-proprietary)

Esmolol hydrochloride 10 mg per 1 ml Esmolol 100mg/10ml solution for injection ampoules | 5 ampoule [PoM] £50.00 (Hospital only)

Esmolol 100mg/10ml solution for injection vials | 5 vial [PoM] £38.95 (Hospital only) | 10 vial [PoM] £100.00 (Hospital only)

▸ **Brevibloc** (Baxter Healthcare Ltd)
Esmolol hydrochloride 10 mg per 1 ml Brevibloc Premixed 100mg/10ml solution for injection vials | 5 vial PoM £38.95 (Hospital only)

Infusion

▸ **Brevibloc** (Baxter Healthcare Ltd)
Esmolol hydrochloride 10 mg per 1 ml Brevibloc Premixed 2.5g/250ml infusion bags | 1 bag PoM £89.69 (Hospital only)

F 121

Metoprolol tartrate

02-Feb-2023

● **INDICATIONS AND DOSE**

Hypertension

▸ BY MOUTH USING IMMEDIATE-RELEASE MEDICINES
▸ Child 1 month–11 years: Initially 1 mg/kg twice daily, increased if necessary up to 8 mg/kg daily in 2–4 divided doses (max. per dose 400 mg)
▸ Child 12–17 years: Initially 50–100 mg daily, increased if necessary to 200 mg daily in 1–2 divided doses, high doses are rarely necessary; maximum 400 mg per day

▸ BY MOUTH USING MODIFIED-RELEASE MEDICINES
▸ Child 12–17 years: 200 mg once daily

Arrhythmias

▸ BY MOUTH USING IMMEDIATE-RELEASE MEDICINES
▸ Child 12–17 years: Usual dose 50 mg 2–3 times a day, then increased if necessary up to 300 mg daily in divided doses

● **UNLICENSED USE** Not licensed for use in children.

● **INTERACTIONS** → Appendix 1: beta blockers, selective

● **SIDE-EFFECTS**

▸ **Common or very common** Postural disorders
▸ **Rare or very rare** Alertness decreased · arrhythmia · arthritis · auditory disorder · chest pain · constipation · drowsiness · dry mouth · dystrophic skin lesion · eye irritation · gangrene · hyperhidrosis · muscle cramps · oedema · palpitations · personality disorder · rhinitis · sexual dysfunction · skin reactions · thrombocytopenia · weight increased
▸ **Frequency not known** Conjunctivitis · hepatitis · Peyronie's disease · retroperitoneal fibrosis

● **HEPATIC IMPAIRMENT** Manufacturer advises caution in severe impairment (bioavailability may be increased in patients with liver cirrhosis).
Dose adjustments In adults, manufacturer advises consider dose reduction in severe impairment.

● **MEDICINAL FORMS** There can be variation in the licensing of different medicines containing the same drug. Forms available from special-order manufacturers include: oral capsule, oral suspension, oral solution

Oral tablet

CAUTIONARY AND ADVISORY LABELS 8

▸ **Metoprolol tartrate (Non-proprietary)**
Metoprolol tartrate 25 mg Metoprolol 25mg tablets | 28 tablet PoM £18.75–£35.05 DT = £35.54
Metoprolol tartrate 50 mg Metoprolol 50mg tablets | 28 tablet PoM £2.36 DT = £1.42 | 56 tablet PoM £2.90
Metoprolol tartrate 100 mg Metoprolol 100mg tablets | 28 tablet PoM £3.98 DT = £2.26

CALCIUM-CHANNEL BLOCKERS

Calcium-channel blockers

Overview

Calcium-channel blockers differ in their predilection for the various possible sites of action and, therefore, their therapeutic effects are disparate, with much greater variation than those of beta-blockers. There are important differences between verapamil hydrochloride p. 129, diltiazem hydrochloride p. 168, and the dihydropyridine calcium-channel blockers (amlodipine p. 127, nicardipine hydrochloride p. 127, nifedipine p. 128, and nimodipine p. 99). Verapamil hydrochloride and diltiazem hydrochloride should usually be **avoided** in heart failure because they may further depress cardiac function and cause clinically significant deterioration.

Verapamil hydrochloride is used for the treatment of hypertension and arrhythmias. However, it is no longer first-line treatment for arrhythmias in children because it has been associated with fatal collapse especially in infants under 1 year; adenosine p. 89 is now recommended for first-line use.

Verapamil hydrochloride is a highly negatively inotropic calcium channel-blocker and it reduces cardiac output, slows the heart rate, and may impair atrioventricular conduction. It may precipitate heart failure, exacerbate conduction disorders, and cause hypotension at high doses and should **not** be used with beta-blockers. Constipation is the most common side-effect.

Nifedipine relaxes vascular smooth muscle and dilates coronary and peripheral arteries. It has more influence on vessels and less on the myocardium than does verapamil hydrochloride and unlike verapamil hydrochloride has no anti-arrhythmic activity. It rarely precipitates heart failure because any negative inotropic effect is offset by a reduction in left ventricular work. Short-acting formulations of nifedipine may be used if a modified-release preparation delivering the appropriate dose is not available or if a child is unable to swallow (a liquid preparation may be prepared using capsules). Nifedipine may also be used for the management of angina due to coronary artery disease in Kawasaki disease or progeria and in the management of Raynaud's syndrome.

Nicardipine hydrochloride has similar effects to those of nifedipine and may produce less reduction of myocardial contractility; it should only be used for the treatment of life-threatening hypertension in paediatric intensive care settings and in postoperative hypertension.

Amlodipine also resembles nifedipine and nicardipine hydrochloride in its effects and does not reduce myocardial contractility or produce clinical deterioration in heart failure. It has a longer duration of action and can be given once daily. Nifedipine and amlodipine are used for the treatment of hypertension. Side-effects associated with vasodilatation such as flushing and headache (which become less obtrusive after a few days), and ankle swelling (which may respond only partially to diuretics) are common.

Nimodipine is related to nifedipine but the smooth muscle relaxant effect preferentially acts on cerebral arteries. Its use is confined to prevention and treatment of vascular spasm following aneurysmal subarachnoid haemorrhage.

Diltiazem hydrochloride is a peripheral vasodilator and also has mild depressor effects on the myocardium. It is used in the treatment of Raynaud's syndrome.

Calcium-channel blockers

● **DRUG ACTION** Calcium-channel blockers (less correctly called 'calcium-antagonists') interfere with the inward displacement of calcium ions through the slow channels of active cell membranes. They influence the myocardial cells, the cells within the specialised conducting system of the heart, and the cells of vascular smooth muscle. Thus, myocardial contractility may be reduced, the formation and propagation of electrical impulses within the heart may be depressed, and coronary or systemic vascular tone may be diminished.

● **SIDE-EFFECTS**

▸ **Common or very common** Abdominal pain · dizziness · drowsiness · fatigue · flushing · headache · hypotension · nausea · palpitations · peripheral oedema · skin reactions · tachycardia · vomiting

- **Uncommon** Angioedema · depression · erectile dysfunction · gingival hyperplasia · myalgia · paraesthesia · syncope

Overdose Features of calcium-channel blocker poisoning include nausea, vomiting, dizziness, agitation, confusion, and coma in severe poisoning. Metabolic acidosis and hyperglycaemia may occur. In overdose, the dihydropyridine calcium-channel blockers cause severe hypotension secondary to profound peripheral vasodilatation. For details on the management of poisoning, see Calcium-channel blockers, under Emergency treatment of poisoning.

- **HEPATIC IMPAIRMENT** In general, manufacturers advise caution (risk of increased exposure).
- **TREATMENT CESSATION** There is some evidence that sudden withdrawal of calcium-channel blockers may be associated with an exacerbation of myocardial ischaemia.

F 126

Amlodipine

03-Mar-2022

- **DRUG ACTION** Amlodipine is a dihydropyridine calcium-channel blocker.

- **INDICATIONS AND DOSE**

Hypertension

- BY MOUTH
  - Child 1 month–11 years: Initially 100–200 micrograms/kg once daily; increased if necessary up to 400 micrograms/kg once daily, adjusted at intervals of 1–2 weeks; maximum 10 mg per day
  - Child 12–17 years: Initially 5 mg once daily; increased if necessary up to 10 mg once daily, adjusted at intervals of 1–2 weeks

DOSE EQUIVALENCE AND CONVERSION
- Tablets from various suppliers may contain different salts (e.g. amlodipine besilate, amlodipine maleate, and amlodipine mesilate) but the strength is expressed in terms of amlodipine (base); tablets containing different salts are considered interchangeable.

- **UNLICENSED USE** Not licensed for use in children under 6 years.

IMPORTANT SAFETY INFORMATION

SAFE PRACTICE

Amlodipine has been confused with nimodipine and atenolol; care must be taken to ensure the correct drug is prescribed and dispensed.

- **CONTRA-INDICATIONS** Cardiogenic shock · significant aortic stenosis · unstable angina
- **INTERACTIONS** → Appendix 1: calcium-channel blockers
- **SIDE-EFFECTS**
  - **Common or very common** Asthenia · constipation · diarrhoea · dyspepsia · dyspnoea · gastrointestinal disorders · joint disorders · muscle cramps · oedema · vision disorders
  - **Uncommon** Alopecia · anxiety · arrhythmias · chest pain · cough · dry mouth · gynaecomastia · hyperhidrosis · insomnia · malaise · mood altered · numbness · pain · rhinitis · taste altered · tinnitus · tremor · urinary disorders · weight changes
  - **Rare or very rare** Confusion · hepatic disorders · hyperglycaemia · leucopenia · muscle tone increased · myocardial infarction · pancreatitis · peripheral neuropathy · photosensitivity reaction · severe cutaneous adverse reactions (SCARs) · thrombocytopenia · vasculitis
  - **Frequency not known** Extrapyramidal symptoms · pulmonary oedema
- **PREGNANCY** No information available—manufacturer advises avoid, but risk to fetus should be balanced against risk of uncontrolled maternal hypertension.
- **BREAST FEEDING** Manufacturer advises avoid—no information available.
- **HEPATIC IMPAIRMENT**

Dose adjustments Manufacturer advises initiate at low dose and titrate slowly (limited information available).

- **DIRECTIONS FOR ADMINISTRATION** Expert sources advise tablets may be dispersed in water.
- **PATIENT AND CARER ADVICE**

Medicines for Children leaflet: Amlodipine for high blood pressure www.medicinesforchildren.org.uk/medicines/amlodipine-for-high-blood-pressure/

- **MEDICINAL FORMS** There can be variation in the licensing of different medicines containing the same drug. Forms available from special-order manufacturers include: oral suspension, oral solution

Oral tablet

- **Amlodipine (Non-proprietary)**

Amlodipine 2.5 mg Amlodipine 2.5mg tablets | 28 tablet PoM £10.53 DT = £3.55

Amlodipine 5 mg Amlodipine 5mg tablets | 28 tablet PoM £9.42 DT = £0.55 | 500 tablet PoM £9.82–£10.35

Amlodipine 10 mg Amlodipine 10mg tablets | 28 tablet PoM £14.07 DT = £0.58 | 500 tablet PoM £10.17–£11.06

- **Istin** (Viatris UK Healthcare Ltd)

Amlodipine 5 mg Istin 5mg tablets | 28 tablet PoM £11.08 DT = £0.55

Amlodipine 10 mg Istin 10mg tablets | 28 tablet PoM £16.55 DT = £0.58

Oral solution

- **Amlodipine (Non-proprietary)**

Amlodipine 1 mg per 1 ml Amlodipine 5mg/5ml oral solution sugar free | 150 ml PoM £72.00 DT = £56.24 SF

Amlodipine 2 mg per 1 ml Amlodipine 10mg/5ml oral solution sugar free | 150 ml PoM £110.00 DT = £84.76 SF

Oral suspension

- **Amlodipine (Non-proprietary)**

Amlodipine 1 mg per 1 ml Amlodipine 5mg/5ml oral suspension sugar free | 150 ml PoM £70.00 DT = £70.00 SF

F 126

Nicardipine hydrochloride

04-Jan-2022

- **DRUG ACTION** Nicardipine is a dihydropyridine calcium-channel blocker.

- **INDICATIONS AND DOSE**

Life-threatening hypertension (specialist use only) | Post-operative hypertension (specialist use only)

- BY CONTINUOUS INTRAVENOUS INFUSION
  - Neonate: Initially 500 nanograms/kg/minute (max. per dose 5 micrograms/kg/minute), adjusted according to response; maintenance 1–4 micrograms/kg/minute.
  - Child: Initially 500 nanograms/kg/minute (max. per dose 5 micrograms/kg/minute), adjusted according to response; maintenance 1–4 micrograms/kg/minute (max. per dose 250 micrograms/minute)

- **CONTRA-INDICATIONS** Acute porphyrias p. 745 · avoid within 8 days of myocardial infarction · cardiogenic shock · compensatory hypertension · significant or advanced aortic stenosis · unstable or acute attacks of angina
- **CAUTIONS** Congestive heart failure · elevated intracranial pressure · increased risk of serious hypotension · ischaemic heart disease · portal hypertension · pulmonary oedema · significantly impaired left ventricular function · stroke
- **INTERACTIONS** → Appendix 1: calcium-channel blockers
- **SIDE-EFFECTS** Atrioventricular block · hepatic disorders · ischaemic heart disease · paralytic ileus · pulmonary oedema · thrombocytopenia

SIDE-EFFECTS, FURTHER INFORMATION Systemic hypotension and reflex tachycardia with rapid reduction of blood pressure may occur — during intravenous use consider stopping infusion or decreasing dose by half.

- **PREGNANCY** May inhibit labour. Not to be used in multiple pregnancy (twins or more) unless there is no other acceptable alternative. Toxicity in *animal* studies. Risk of severe maternal hypotension and fatal fetal hypoxia—avoid excessive decrease in blood pressure.
- **BREAST FEEDING** Manufacturer advises avoid—present in breast milk.
- **HEPATIC IMPAIRMENT**
  Dose adjustments In adults, manufacturer advises dose reduction—consult product literature.
- **RENAL IMPAIRMENT** EvGr Caution (increased risk of serious hypotension). (M)
  Dose adjustments EvGr Use lowest dose. (M)
- **MONITORING REQUIREMENTS** Monitor blood pressure and heart rate at least every 5 minutes during intravenous infusion, and then until stable, and continue monitoring for at least 12 hours after end of infusion.
- **DIRECTIONS FOR ADMINISTRATION** Intravenous nicardipine should only be administered under the supervision of a specialist and in a hospital or intensive care setting in which patients can be closely monitored.
  For *continuous intravenous infusion*, manufacturer advises dilute to a concentration of 100–200 micrograms/mL with Glucose 5% and give *via* volumetric infusion pump or syringe driver; protect from light; risk of adsorption on to plastic in the presence of saline solutions; incompatible with bicarbonate or alkaline solutions—consult product literature. To minimise peripheral venous irritation, expert sources advise change site of infusion every 12 hours.

- **MEDICINAL FORMS** There can be variation in the licensing of different medicines containing the same drug.

Solution for infusion

- Nicardipine hydrochloride (Non-proprietary)
  Nicardipine hydrochloride 1 mg per 1 ml Nicardipine 10mg/10ml solution for infusion ampoules | 5 ampoule PoM £85.00 (Hospital only)
  Nicardipine hydrochloride 2.5 mg per 1 ml Cardene I.V. 25mg/10ml solution for infusion ampoules | 10 ampoule PoM (Hospital only)

126

Nifedipine

24-Jul-2020

- **INDICATIONS AND DOSE**

Hypertensive crisis | Acute angina in Kawasaki disease or progeria

- BY MOUTH USING IMMEDIATE-RELEASE MEDICINES
  - Child: Initially 250–500 micrograms/kg (max. per dose 10 mg), then repeat once if necessary, may cause unpredictable and severe reduction of blood pressure—monitor closely following administration; if ineffective consider alternative treatment and seek specialist advice

Hypertension | Angina in Kawasaki disease or progeria

- BY MOUTH USING IMMEDIATE-RELEASE MEDICINES
  - Child 1 month–11 years: 200–300 micrograms/kg 3 times a day, dose frequency depends on preparation used; maximum 3 mg/kg per day; maximum 90 mg per day
  - Child 12–17 years: 5–20 mg 3 times a day, dose frequency depends on preparation used; maximum 90 mg per day

Raynaud's syndrome

- BY MOUTH USING IMMEDIATE-RELEASE MEDICINES
  - Child 2–17 years: 2.5–10 mg 2–4 times a day, start with low doses at night and increase gradually to avoid postural hypotension, dose frequency depends on preparation used

Persistent hyperinsulinaemic hypoglycaemia

- BY MOUTH USING IMMEDIATE-RELEASE MEDICINES
  - Neonate: 100–200 micrograms/kg 4 times a day (max. per dose 600 micrograms/kg).

- **UNLICENSED USE** Not licensed for use in children.
- **CONTRA-INDICATIONS** Cardiogenic shock · significant aortic stenosis · within 1 month of myocardial infarction
- **CAUTIONS** Diabetes mellitus · heart failure · poor cardiac reserve · severe hypotension · short-acting formulations are not recommended for angina or long-term management of hypertension (their use may be associated with large variations in blood pressure and reflex tachycardia) · significantly impaired left ventricular function (heart failure deterioration observed)
- **INTERACTIONS** → Appendix 1: calcium-channel blockers
- **SIDE-EFFECTS**
  - **Common or very common** Constipation · malaise · oedema · vasodilation
  - **Uncommon** Allergic oedema · anxiety · chills · diarrhoea · dry mouth · epistaxis · gastrointestinal discomfort · gastrointestinal disorders · joint disorders · laryngeal oedema · migraine · muscle complaints · nasal congestion · pain · sleep disorders · tremor · urinary disorders · vertigo · vision disorders
  - **Rare or very rare** Appetite decreased · burping · cardiovascular disorder · fever · hyperhidrosis · mood altered · sensation abnormal
  - **Frequency not known** Agranulocytosis · bezoar · cerebral ischaemia · chest pain · dysphagia · dyspnoea · eye pain · gingival disorder · gynaecomastia (following long term use) · hepatic disorders · hyperglycaemia · ischaemic heart disease · leucopenia · myasthenia gravis aggravated · photoallergic reaction · pulmonary oedema · telangiectasia · toxic epidermal necrolysis · weight decreased
- **PREGNANCY** May inhibit labour; manufacturer advises avoid before week 20, but risk to fetus should be balanced against risk of uncontrolled maternal hypertension. Use only if other treatment options are not indicated or have failed.
- **BREAST FEEDING** Amount too small to be harmful but manufacturers advise avoid.
- **HEPATIC IMPAIRMENT**
  Dose adjustments In adults, manufacturer advises consider dose reduction—consult product literature.
- **DIRECTIONS FOR ADMINISTRATION** For rapid effect in *hypertensive crisis* or *acute angina*, bite capsules and swallow liquid or use liquid preparation if 5 mg or 10 mg dose inappropriate. If liquid unavailable, extract contents of capsule via a syringe and use immediately—cover syringe with foil to protect contents from light; capsule contents may be diluted with water if necessary.
- **PATIENT AND CARER ADVICE**
  Medicines for Children leaflet: Nifedipine for high blood pressure www.medicinesforchildren.org.uk/medicines/nifedipine-for-high-blood-pressure/

- **MEDICINAL FORMS** There can be variation in the licensing of different medicines containing the same drug. Forms available from special-order manufacturers include: oral suspension, oral drops

Oral capsule

- Nifedipine (Non-proprietary)
  Nifedipine 5 mg Nifedipine 5mg capsules | 90 capsule PoM £82.88 DT = £45.93
  Nifedipine 10 mg Nifedipine 10mg capsules | 90 capsule PoM £104.20 DT = £56.82

Oral drops

- Nifedipine (Non-proprietary)
  Nifedipine 20 mg per 1 ml Nifedipin-ratiopharm 20mg/ml oral drops | 30 ml PoM DT = £20.08

126

Verapamil hydrochloride

15-Apr-2024

- **INDICATIONS AND DOSE**

Treatment of supraventricular arrhythmias

▶ BY SLOW INTRAVENOUS INJECTION

▶ Child 1–17 years (administered on expert advice): 100–300 micrograms/kg (max. per dose 5 mg) for 1 dose, to be given over 2–3 minutes (with ECG and blood-pressure monitoring), dose can be repeated after 30 minutes if necessary

Hypertension

▶ BY MOUTH USING IMMEDIATE-RELEASE MEDICINES

▶ Child 12–23 months (administered on expert advice): 20 mg 2–3 times a day

▶ Child 2–17 years (administered on expert advice): 40–120 mg 2–3 times a day

Prophylaxis of supraventricular arrhythmias (administered on expert advice)

▶ BY MOUTH USING IMMEDIATE-RELEASE MEDICINES

▶ Child 12–23 months: 20 mg 2–3 times a day

▶ Child 2–17 years: 40–120 mg 2–3 times a day

- **CONTRA-INDICATIONS** Acute porphyrias p. 745 · atrial flutter or fibrillation associated with accessory conducting pathways (e.g. Wolff-Parkinson-White-syndrome) · bradycardia · cardiogenic shock · heart failure (with reduced ejection fraction) · history of significantly impaired left ventricular function (even if controlled by therapy) · hypotension · second- and third-degree AV block · sick sinus syndrome · sino-atrial block
- **CAUTIONS** Acute phase of myocardial infarction (avoid if bradycardia, hypotension, left ventricular failure) · first-degree AV block · neuromuscular disorders
- **INTERACTIONS** → Appendix 1: calcium-channel blockers
- **SIDE-EFFECTS**

GENERAL SIDE-EFFECTS Atrioventricular block · extrapyramidal symptoms · Stevens-Johnson syndrome · vertigo

SPECIFIC SIDE-EFFECTS

▶ **Common or very common**

▶ With intravenous use Bradycardia

▶ **Frequency not known**

▶ With intravenous use Cardiac arrest · hepatic impairment · hyperhidrosis · myocardial contractility decreased · nervousness · seizure

▶ With oral use Abdominal discomfort · alopecia · arrhythmias · arthralgia · constipation · erythromelalgia · galactorrhoea · heart failure · ileus · muscle weakness · tinnitus · tremor

Overdose In overdose, verapamil has a profound cardiac depressant effect causing hypotension and arrhythmias, including complete heart block and asystole.

- **PREGNANCY** May reduce uterine blood flow with fetal hypoxia. Manufacturer advises avoid in first trimester unless absolutely necessary. May inhibit labour.
- **BREAST FEEDING** Amount too small to be harmful.
- **HEPATIC IMPAIRMENT**

Dose adjustments

▶ With oral use Manufacturer advises dose reduction.

- **DIRECTIONS FOR ADMINISTRATION** For *intravenous injection*, expert sources advise may be diluted with Glucose 5% *or* Sodium Chloride 0.9%. Incompatible with solutions of pH greater than 6.
- **MEDICINAL FORMS** There can be variation in the licensing of different medicines containing the same drug. Forms available from special-order manufacturers include: oral suspension, oral solution

Oral tablet

▶ Verapamil hydrochloride (Non-proprietary)

Verapamil hydrochloride 40 mg Verapamil 40mg tablets | 84 tablet PoM £2.19 DT = £1.49

Verapamil hydrochloride 80 mg Verapamil 80mg tablets | 84 tablet PoM £3.44 DT = £2.42

Verapamil hydrochloride 120 mg Verapamil 120mg tablets | 28 tablet PoM £4.01 DT = £3.09

Verapamil hydrochloride 160 mg Verapamil 160mg tablets | 56 tablet PoM £44.20 DT = £31.53

Solution for injection

▶ Verapamil hydrochloride (Non-proprietary)

Verapamil hydrochloride 2.5 mg per 1 ml Verapamil 5mg/2ml solution for injection ampoules | 5 ampoule PoM £5.41 DT = £5.41 (Hospital only)

▶ Securon (Viatris UK Healthcare Ltd)

Verapamil hydrochloride 2.5 mg per 1 ml Securon IV 5mg/2ml solution for injection ampoules | 5 ampoule PoM £5.41 DT = £5.41

Oral solution

▶ Verapamil hydrochloride (Non-proprietary)

Verapamil hydrochloride 8 mg per 1 ml Verapamil 40mg/5ml oral solution sugar free | 150 ml PoM £158.85 DT = £158.85 SF

DIURETICS › THIAZIDES AND RELATED DIURETICS

Thiazides and related diuretics

- **CONTRA-INDICATIONS** Addison's disease · hypercalcaemia · hyponatraemia · refractory hypokalaemia · symptomatic hyperuricaemia
- **CAUTIONS** Diabetes · gout · risk of hypokalaemia · systemic lupus erythematosus

CAUTIONS, FURTHER INFORMATION

▶ Existing conditions Thiazides and related diuretics can exacerbate diabetes, gout, and systemic lupus erythematosus.

▶ Potassium loss Hypokalaemia can occur with thiazides and related diuretics.

Hypokalaemia is particularly dangerous in children being treated with cardiac glycosides. In hepatic impairment, hypokalaemia caused by diuretics can precipitate encephalopathy.

The use of potassium-sparing diuretics avoids the need to take potassium supplements.

- **SIDE-EFFECTS**

▶ **Common or very common** Alkalosis hypochloraemic · constipation · diarrhoea · dizziness · electrolyte imbalance · erectile dysfunction · fatigue · headache · hyperglycaemia · hyperuricaemia · nausea · postural hypotension · skin reactions · vomiting

▶ **Uncommon** Agranulocytosis · aplastic anaemia · leucopenia · pancreatitis · photosensitivity reaction · thrombocytopenia

▶ **Rare or very rare** Paraesthesia

- **PREGNANCY** Thiazides and related diuretics should not be used to treat gestational hypertension. They may cause neonatal thrombocytopenia, bone marrow suppression, jaundice, electrolyte disturbances, and hypoglycaemia; placental perfusion may also be reduced. Stimulation of labour, uterine inertia, and meconium staining have also been reported.
- **HEPATIC IMPAIRMENT** In general, manufacturer advises caution in mild to moderate impairment; avoid in severe impairment.
- **RENAL IMPAIRMENT** In general, manufacturers advise caution in mild to moderate impairment (risk of electrolyte imbalance and reduced renal function); avoid in severe impairment (ineffective if creatinine clearance less than 30 mL/minute). See p. 16.

- **MONITORING REQUIREMENTS** Electrolytes should be monitored, particularly with high doses and long-term use.

F 129

Bendroflumethiazide (Bendrofluazide)

10-Jul-2023

- **INDICATIONS AND DOSE**

Hypertension

▶ BY MOUTH

- Child 1 month–1 year: 50–100 micrograms/kg once daily, dose to be adjusted according to response
- Child 2–11 years: Initially 50–400 micrograms/kg once daily (max. per dose 10 mg), then maintenance 50–100 micrograms/kg once daily (max. per dose 10 mg), dose to be adjusted according to response
- Child 12–17 years: 2.5 mg once daily, dose to be taken as a single dose in the morning, higher doses are rarely necessary

Oedema in heart failure, renal disease and hepatic disease | Pulmonary oedema

▶ BY MOUTH

- Child 1 month–1 year: 50–100 micrograms/kg once daily, dose to be adjusted according to response
- Child 2–11 years: Initially 50–400 micrograms/kg once daily (max. per dose 10 mg), then maintenance 50–100 micrograms/kg once daily (max. per dose 10 mg), dose to be adjusted according to response
- Child 12–17 years: Initially 5–10 mg once daily or on alternate days, dose to be taken as a single dose in the morning, dose to be adjusted according to response; maximum 10 mg per day

- **INTERACTIONS** → Appendix 1: thiazide diuretics
- **SIDE-EFFECTS** Blood disorder · cholestasis · gastrointestinal disorder · gout · neutropenia · pneumonitis · pulmonary oedema · severe cutaneous adverse reactions (SCARs)
- **BREAST FEEDING** The amount present in milk is too small to be harmful. Large doses may suppress lactation.
- **MEDICINAL FORMS** There can be variation in the licensing of different medicines containing the same drug. Forms available from special-order manufacturers include: oral suspension, oral solution

Oral tablet

▶ **Bendroflumethiazide (Non-proprietary)**

Bendroflumethiazide 2.5 mg Bendroflumethiazide 2.5mg tablets | 28 tablet PoM £0.72 DT = £0.58

Bendroflumethiazide 5 mg Bendroflumethiazide 5mg tablets | 28 tablet PoM £0.98 DT = £0.74

F 129

Chlorothiazide

23-Sep-2020

- **INDICATIONS AND DOSE**

Heart failure | Hypertension | Ascites

▶ BY MOUTH

- Neonate: 10–20 mg/kg twice daily.
- Child 1–5 months: 10–20 mg/kg twice daily
- Child 6 months–11 years: 10 mg/kg twice daily (max. per dose 500 mg)
- Child 12–17 years: 0.25–1 g once daily, alternatively 125–500 mg twice daily

Reduction of diazoxide-induced sodium and water retention in the management of chronic hypoglycaemia | Potentiating the glycaemic effect of diazoxide in the management of chronic hypoglycaemia

▶ BY MOUTH

- Child: 3–5 mg/kg twice daily

Nephrogenic and partial pituitary diabetes insipidus

▶ BY MOUTH

- Child: 10–20 mg/kg twice daily (max. per dose 500 mg)

- **UNLICENSED USE** Not licensed.
- **CAUTIONS** Neonate (theoretical risk of kernicterus if very jaundiced)
- **INTERACTIONS** → Appendix 1: thiazide diuretics
- **BREAST FEEDING** The amount present in milk is too small to be harmful. Large doses may suppress lactation.
- **MEDICINAL FORMS** There can be variation in the licensing of different medicines containing the same drug. Forms available from special-order manufacturers include: oral tablet, oral suspension, oral solution

Oral tablet

▶ **Chlorothiazide (Non-proprietary)**

Chlorothiazide 250 mg Diuril 250mg tablets | 100 tablet PoM ☒

DRUGS ACTING ON THE RENIN-ANGIOTENSIN SYSTEM › ACE INHIBITORS

Angiotensin-converting enzyme inhibitors

IMPORTANT SAFETY INFORMATION

MHRA/CHM ADVICE: ACE INHIBITORS AND ANGIOTENSIN II RECEPTOR ANTAGONISTS: NOT FOR USE IN PREGNANCY (DECEMBER 2014)

See *Conception and contraception* and *Pregnancy*.

MHRA/CHM ADVICE: ACE INHIBITORS AND ANGIOTENSIN II RECEPTOR ANTAGONISTS: RECOMMENDATIONS ON HOW TO USE FOR BREASTFEEDING (DECEMBER 2014)

See *Breast feeding*.

- **CONTRA-INDICATIONS** Bilateral renovascular disease · hereditary or idiopathic angioedema · history of angioedema associated with prior ACE inhibitor therapy
- **CAUTIONS** Concomitant diuretics · diabetes (may lower blood glucose; increased risk of hyperkalaemia) · first dose hypotension (especially in patients taking high doses of diuretics, on a low-sodium diet, on dialysis, dehydrated, or with cerebrovascular disease, ischaemic heart disease, or heart failure) · neonates · patients of black African or African-Caribbean origin (may respond less well to ACE inhibitors) · primary aldosteronism (patients may respond less well to ACE inhibitors) · the risk of agranulocytosis is possibly increased in collagen vascular disease (blood counts recommended) · use with care in patients with aortic or mitral valve stenosis (risk of hypotension) · use with care in patients with hypertrophic cardiomyopathy

CAUTIONS, FURTHER INFORMATION

▶ Anaphylactoid reactions EvGr To prevent anaphylactoid reactions, ACE inhibitors should be avoided during dialysis with high-flux membranes (e.g. polyacrylonitrile) and during low-density lipoprotein apheresis with dextran sulfate; they should also be withheld before desensitisation with wasp or bee venom. ⟨M⟩

- **SIDE-EFFECTS**

▶ **Common or very common** Alopecia · angina pectoris · angioedema (can be delayed; more common in black patients) · arrhythmias · asthenia · chest pain · constipation · cough · depression · diarrhoea · dizziness · drowsiness · dry mouth · dyspnoea · electrolyte imbalance · gastrointestinal discomfort · headache · hypotension · myalgia · nausea · palpitations · paraesthesia · renal impairment · rhinitis · skin reactions · sleep disorder · syncope · taste altered · tinnitus · vertigo · vomiting

▶ **Uncommon** Arthralgia · confusion · eosinophilia · erectile dysfunction · fever · haemolytic anaemia · hyperhidrosis ·

myocardial infarction · pancreatitis · peripheral oedema · photosensitivity reaction · respiratory disorders · stroke
- **Rare or very rare** Agranulocytosis · hepatitis · leucopenia · neutropenia · pancytopenia · Stevens-Johnson syndrome · thrombocytopenia

SIDE-EFFECTS, FURTHER INFORMATION In light of reports of cholestatic jaundice, hepatitis, fulminant hepatic necrosis, and hepatic failure, ACE inhibitors should be discontinued if marked elevation of hepatic enzymes or jaundice occur.

- **ALLERGY AND CROSS-SENSITIVITY** EvGr ACE inhibitors are contra-indicated in patients with hypersensitivity to ACE inhibitors (including angioedema). ⟨M⟩
- **CONCEPTION AND CONTRACEPTION** EvGr Females planning pregnancy should be switched to alternative treatments that have an established safety profile for use in pregnancy, unless continued treatment with an angiotensin-converting enzyme inhibitor is considered essential ⟨M⟩(recommendation also supported by specialist sources).
- **PREGNANCY** EvGr Avoid (risk of teratogenicity in first trimester cannot be excluded; known risk of fetotoxicity (decreased renal function, oligohydramnios, skull ossification retardation) and neonatal toxicity (renal failure, hypotension, hyperkalaemia) in second and third trimesters); ⟨M⟩ recommendation also supported by specialist sources.
- **BREAST FEEDING** Information on the use of ACE inhibitors in breast-feeding is limited.
- **RENAL IMPAIRMENT** EvGr Caution (hyperkalaemia and other side-effects of ACE inhibitors are more common in those with impaired renal function). ⟨M⟩
  Dose adjustments EvGr Start with low dose and adjust according to response. ⟨M⟩
- **MONITORING REQUIREMENTS** Renal function and electrolytes should be checked before starting ACE inhibitors (or increasing the dose) and monitored during treatment (more frequently if side effects mentioned are present).
- **DIRECTIONS FOR ADMINISTRATION** For hypertension the first dose should preferably be given at bedtime.

130

Captopril

08-Jun-2021

- **INDICATIONS AND DOSE**

Hypertension

▶ BY MOUTH

- Preterm neonate (initiated under specialist supervision): Test dose 10 micrograms/kg, monitor blood pressure carefully for 1–2 hours; usual dose 10–50 micrograms/kg 2–3 times a day, then increased if necessary up to 300 micrograms/kg daily in divided doses, ongoing doses should only be given if test dose tolerated.
- Neonate (initiated under specialist supervision): Test dose 10–50 micrograms/kg, monitor blood pressure carefully for 1–2 hours; usual dose 10–50 micrograms/kg 2–3 times a day, then increased if necessary up to 2 mg/kg daily in divided doses, ongoing doses should only be given if test dose tolerated.
- Child 1-11 months (initiated under specialist supervision): Test dose 100 micrograms/kg (max. per dose 6.25 mg), monitor blood pressure carefully for 1–2 hours; usual dose 100–300 micrograms/kg 2–3 times a day, then increased if necessary up to 4 mg/kg daily in divided doses, ongoing doses should only be given if test dose tolerated
- Child 1-11 years (initiated under specialist supervision): Test dose 100 micrograms/kg (max. per dose 6.25 mg), monitor blood pressure carefully for 1–2 hours; usual dose 100–300 micrograms/kg 2–3 times a day, then increased if necessary up to 6 mg/kg daily in divided doses, ongoing doses should only be given if test dose tolerated
- Child 12-17 years (initiated under specialist supervision): Test dose 100 micrograms/kg, alternatively test dose 6.25 mg, monitor blood pressure carefully for 1–2 hours; usual dose 12.5–25 mg 2–3 times a day, then increased if necessary up to 150 mg daily in divided doses, ongoing doses should only be given if test dose tolerated

Heart failure

▶ BY MOUTH

- Preterm neonate (initiated under specialist supervision): Test dose 10 micrograms/kg, monitor blood pressure carefully for 1–2 hours; usual dose 10–50 micrograms/kg 2–3 times a day, then increased if necessary up to 300 micrograms/kg daily in divided doses, ongoing doses should only be given if test dose tolerated.
- Neonate (initiated under specialist supervision): Test dose 10–50 micrograms/kg, monitor blood pressure carefully for 1–2 hours; usual dose 10–50 micrograms/kg 2–3 times a day, then increased if necessary up to 2 mg/kg daily in divided doses, ongoing doses should only be given if test dose tolerated.
- Child 1-11 months (initiated under specialist supervision): Test dose 100 micrograms/kg (max. per dose 6.25 mg), monitor blood pressure carefully for 1–2 hours; usual dose 100–300 micrograms/kg 2–3 times a day, then increased if necessary up to 4 mg/kg daily in divided doses, ongoing doses should only be given if test dose tolerated
- Child 1-11 years (initiated under specialist supervision): Test dose 100 micrograms/kg (max. per dose 6.25 mg), monitor blood pressure carefully for 1–2 hours; usual dose 100–300 micrograms/kg 2–3 times a day, then increased if necessary up to 6 mg/kg daily in divided doses, ongoing doses should only be given if test dose tolerated
- Child 12-17 years (initiated under specialist supervision): Test dose 100 micrograms/kg, alternatively test dose 6.25 mg, monitor blood pressure carefully for 1–2 hours; usual dose 12.5–25 mg 2–3 times a day, then increased if necessary up to 150 mg daily in divided doses, ongoing doses should only be given if test dose tolerated

Proteinuria in nephritis (under expert supervision)

▶ BY MOUTH

- Preterm neonate: Test dose 10 micrograms/kg, monitor blood pressure carefully for 1–2 hours; usual dose 10–50 micrograms/kg 2–3 times a day, then increased if necessary up to 300 micrograms/kg daily in divided doses, ongoing doses should only be given if test dose tolerated.
- Neonate: Test dose 10–50 micrograms/kg, monitor blood pressure carefully for 1–2 hours; usual dose 10–50 micrograms/kg 2–3 times a day, then increased if necessary up to 2 mg/kg daily in divided doses, ongoing doses should only be given if test dose tolerated.
- Child 1-11 months: Test dose 100 micrograms/kg (max. per dose 6.25 mg), monitor blood pressure carefully for 1–2 hours; usual dose 100–300 micrograms/kg 2–3 times a day, then increased if necessary

continued →

up to 4 mg/kg daily in divided doses, ongoing doses should only be given if test dose tolerated
- Child 1–11 years: Test dose 100 micrograms/kg (max. per dose 6.25 mg), monitor blood pressure carefully for 1–2 hours; usual dose 100–300 micrograms/kg 2–3 times a day, then increased if necessary up to 6 mg/kg daily in divided doses, ongoing doses should only be given if test dose tolerated
- Child 12–17 years: Test dose 100 micrograms/kg, alternatively test dose 6.25 mg, monitor blood pressure carefully for 1–2 hours; usual dose 12.5–25 mg 2–3 times a day, then increased if necessary up to 150 mg daily in divided doses, ongoing doses should only be given if test dose tolerated

Diabetic nephropathy in type 1 diabetes mellitus

▶ BY MOUTH
- Child 12–17 years (under expert supervision): Test dose 100 micrograms/kg, alternatively test dose 6.25 mg, monitor blood pressure carefully for 1– 2 hours; usual dose 12.5–25 mg 2–3 times a day, increased if necessary up to 100 mg daily in divided doses, ongoing doses should only be given if test dose tolerated

● **UNLICENSED USE** Not licensed for proteinuria in nephritis. Captopril doses in BNF Publications differ from product licence.

● **CAUTIONS** Children (efficacy and safety not fully established)

● **INTERACTIONS** → Appendix 1: ACE inhibitors

● **SIDE-EFFECTS**
- ▶ **Common or very common** Insomnia · peptic ulcer
- ▶ **Uncommon** Appetite decreased · flushing · malaise · pallor · Raynaud's phenomenon
- ▶ **Rare or very rare** Alveolitis allergic · anaemia · aplastic anaemia · autoimmune disorder · cardiac arrest · cardiogenic shock · cerebrovascular insufficiency · gynaecomastia · hepatic disorders · hypoglycaemia · lymphadenopathy · nephrotic syndrome · oral disorders · proteinuria · urinary disorders · vision blurred

● **BREAST FEEDING** Avoid in first few weeks after delivery, particularly in preterm infants—risk of profound neonatal hypotension; can be used in mothers breast-feeding older infants if essential but monitor infant's blood pressure.

● **DIRECTIONS FOR ADMINISTRATION** Administer under close supervision. Expert sources advise give test dose whilst child supine. Tablets can be dispersed in water.

● **PATIENT AND CARER ADVICE**
Medicines for Children leaflet: Captopril for heart failure www.medicinesforchildren.org.uk/medicines/captopril-for-heart-failure/

● **MEDICINAL FORMS** There can be variation in the licensing of different medicines containing the same drug. Forms available from special-order manufacturers include: oral tablet, oral capsule, oral suspension, oral solution

Oral tablet

- Captopril (Non-proprietary)
 Captopril 12.5 mg Captopril 12.5mg tablets | 56 tablet [PoM] £202.50 DT = £21.41
 Captopril 25 mg Captopril 25mg tablets | 56 tablet [PoM] £211.00 DT = £25.60
 Captopril 50 mg Captopril 50mg tablets | 56 tablet [PoM] £220.00 DT = £27.78

Oral solution

ELECTROLYTES: May contain Sodium
- Captopril (Non-proprietary)
 Captopril 1 mg per 1 ml Captopril 5mg/5ml oral solution sugar free | 100 ml [PoM] £98.21 DT = £93.30 [SF]
 Captopril 5 mg per 1 ml Captopril 25mg/5ml oral solution sugar free | 100 ml [PoM] £108.94 DT = £101.00 [SF]

F 130

Enalapril maleate

30-May-2024

● **INDICATIONS AND DOSE**

Hypertension

▶ BY MOUTH USING TABLETS, OR BY MOUTH USING ORAL SOLUTION
- Neonate (under expert supervision): Initially 10 micrograms/kg once daily, monitor blood pressure carefully for 1–2 hours, increased if necessary up to 500 micrograms/kg daily in 1–3 divided doses, limited information.
- Child 1 month–11 years (under expert supervision): Initially 100 micrograms/kg once daily, monitor blood pressure carefully for 1–2 hours, then increased if necessary up to 1 mg/kg daily in 1–2 divided doses
- Child 12–17 years (under expert supervision) (body-weight up to 50 kg): Initially 2.5 mg once daily, monitor blood pressure carefully for 1–2 hours, maintenance 10–20 mg daily in 1–2 divided doses
- Child 12–17 years (under expert supervision) (body-weight 50 kg and above): Initially 2.5 mg once daily, monitor blood pressure carefully for 1–2 hours, maintenance 10–20 mg daily in 1–2 divided doses; maximum 40 mg per day

Heart failure

▶ BY MOUTH USING TABLETS, OR BY MOUTH USING ORAL SOLUTION
- Neonate (under expert supervision): Initially 10 micrograms/kg once daily, monitor blood pressure carefully for 1–2 hours, increased if necessary up to 500 micrograms/kg daily in 1–3 divided doses, limited information.
- Child 1 month–11 years (under expert supervision): Initially 100 micrograms/kg once daily, monitor blood pressure carefully for 1–2 hours, then increased if necessary up to 1 mg/kg daily in 1–2 divided doses
- Child 12–17 years (under expert supervision) (body-weight up to 50 kg): Initially 2.5 mg once daily, monitor blood pressure carefully for 1–2 hours, maintenance 10–20 mg daily in 1–2 divided doses
- Child 12–17 years (under expert supervision) (body-weight 50 kg and above): Initially 2.5 mg once daily, monitor blood pressure carefully for 1–2 hours, maintenance 10–20 mg daily in 1–2 divided doses; maximum 40 mg per day

Proteinuria in nephritis (under expert supervision)

▶ BY MOUTH USING TABLETS, OR BY MOUTH USING ORAL SOLUTION
- Neonate: Initially 10 micrograms/kg once daily, monitor blood pressure carefully for 1–2 hours, increased if necessary up to 500 micrograms/kg daily in 1–3 divided doses, limited information.
- Child 1 month–11 years: Initially 100 micrograms/kg once daily, monitor blood pressure carefully for 1–2 hours, then increased if necessary up to 1 mg/kg daily in 1–2 divided doses
- Child 12–17 years (body-weight up to 50 kg): Initially 2.5 mg once daily, monitor blood pressure carefully for 1–2 hours, maintenance 10–20 mg daily in 1–2 divided doses
- Child 12–17 years (body-weight 50 kg and above): Initially 2.5 mg once daily, monitor blood pressure carefully for 1–2 hours, maintenance 10–20 mg daily in 1–2 divided doses; maximum 40 mg per day

Diabetic nephropathy (under expert supervision)
▶ BY MOUTH USING TABLETS, OR BY MOUTH USING ORAL SOLUTION
- Child 12–17 years (body-weight up to 50 kg): Initially 2.5 mg once daily, monitor blood pressure carefully for 1–2 hours; maintenance 10–20 mg daily in 1–2 divided doses
- Child 12–17 years (body-weight 50 kg and above): Initially 2.5 mg once daily, monitor blood pressure carefully for 1–2 hours; maintenance 10–20 mg daily in 1–2 divided doses; maximum 40 mg per day

AQUMELDI ®

Heart failure (initiated by a specialist)
▶ BY MOUTH USING ORODISPERSIBLE TABLET
- Neonate: Test dose 10–40 micrograms/kg for 1 dose, test dose at the lower end of the recommended range should be used, monitor blood pressure carefully for 1–2 hours, then maintenance 150–300 micrograms/kg daily in 1–2 divided doses, to be started 8 hours after test dose, adjusted according to response.
- Child: Test dose 10–40 micrograms/kg for 1 dose (max. per dose 2 mg), monitor blood pressure carefully for 1–2 hours, then maintenance 150–300 micrograms/kg daily in 1–2 divided doses, to be started 8 hours after test dose, adjusted according to response; maximum 20 mg per day

- **UNLICENSED USE** Enalapril maleate oral *tablets* and *solution* may be used as detailed below, although these situations are considered unlicensed:
  - hypertension in children with body-weight under 20 kg;
  - heart failure;
  - proteinuria in nephritis;
  - diabetic nephropathy.
- **INTERACTIONS** → Appendix 1: ACE inhibitors
- **SIDE-EFFECTS**
  - **Common or very common** Hypersensitivity · urine abnormalities · vision blurred
  - **Uncommon** Anaemia · appetite decreased · asthma · bone marrow disorders · flushing · gastrointestinal disorders · hoarseness · hypoglycaemia · malaise · muscle cramps · nervousness · rhinorrhoea · sleep disorders · throat pain
  - **Rare or very rare** Alveolitis allergic · autoimmune disorder · gynaecomastia · hepatic disorders · lymphadenopathy · oral disorders · Raynaud's phenomenon · toxic epidermal necrolysis
  - **Frequency not known** SIADH
- **BREAST FEEDING** Avoid in first few weeks after delivery, particularly in preterm infants—risk of profound neonatal hypotension; can be used in mothers breast-feeding older infants if essential but monitor infant's blood pressure.
- **HEPATIC IMPAIRMENT** Enalapril is a prodrug.

  AQUMELDI ® EvGr Caution (no information available). Ⓜ
  - In neonates EvGr Avoid (no information available). Ⓜ
- **RENAL IMPAIRMENT** EvGr Avoid if estimated glomerular filtration rate less than 30 mL/minute/1.73 m² (no information available). Ⓜ See p. 16.

  AQUMELDI ® EvGr Caution if estimated glomerular filtration rate 30–49 mL/minute/1.73 m² or on dialysis. Avoid if estimated glomerular filtration rate less than 30 mL/minute/1.73 m². Ⓜ

  Dose adjustments EvGr Start with 50% of the test dose, then 50% of the maintenance dose, administer at 12-hour intervals and adjust dose according to response if estimated glomerular filtration rate 30–49 mL/minute/1.73 m²; the feasibility of measuring an accurate low dose should be considered.

  Start with 25% of the test dose, then 25% of the maintenance dose, administer at 12-hour intervals and adjust dose according to response if on dialysis; the feasibility of measuring an accurate low dose should be considered. Ⓜ

  See p. 16.
- **DIRECTIONS FOR ADMINISTRATION** Expert sources advise oral tablets may be crushed and suspended in water immediately before use.

  AQUMELDI ® Orodispersible tablets should be placed on the tongue or in the buccal cavity and allowed to disperse.

  For administration of doses less than 250 micrograms, or via an enteral feeding tube—consult product literature.
- **PATIENT AND CARER ADVICE**

  Medicines for Children leaflet: Enalapril for high blood pressure www.medicinesforchildren.org.uk/medicines/enalapril-for-high-blood-pressure/

  AQUMELDI ® Patients or carers should be given advice on how to administer orodispersible tablets.

- **MEDICINAL FORMS** There can be variation in the licensing of different medicines containing the same drug. Forms available from special-order manufacturers include: oral solution

Oral tablet

▶ **Enalapril maleate (Non-proprietary)**

Enalapril maleate 2.5 mg Enalapril 2.5mg tablets | 28 tablet PoM £7.00 DT = £4.47

Enalapril maleate 5 mg Enalapril 5mg tablets | 28 tablet PoM £4.13 DT = £0.81

Enalapril maleate 10 mg Enalapril 10mg tablets | 28 tablet PoM £5.64 DT = £0.78

Enalapril maleate 20 mg Enalapril 20mg tablets | 28 tablet PoM £6.63 DT = £0.84

▶ **Innovace** (Organon Pharma (UK) Ltd)

Enalapril maleate 2.5 mg Innovace 2.5mg tablets | 28 tablet PoM £5.35 DT = £4.47

Enalapril maleate 5 mg Innovace 5mg tablets | 28 tablet PoM £7.51 DT = £0.81

Enalapril maleate 10 mg Innovace 10mg tablets | 28 tablet PoM £10.53 DT = £0.78

Enalapril maleate 20 mg Innovace 20mg tablets | 28 tablet PoM £12.51 DT = £0.84

Oral solution

▶ **Enalapril maleate (Non-proprietary)**

Enalapril maleate 1 mg per 1 ml Enalapril 5mg/5ml oral solution sugar free | 150 ml PoM £245.14 DT = £245.14 SF

Orodispersible tablet

▶ **Aqumeldi** (Proveca Ltd)

Enalapril maleate 250 microgram Aqumeldi 0.25mg orodispersible tablets | 50 tablet PoM £34.25 DT = £34.25 SF | 100 tablet PoM £68.48 SF

Enalapril maleate 1 mg Aqumeldi 1mg orodispersible tablets | 50 tablet PoM £68.48 SF | 100 tablet PoM £136.97 SF

⚑ 130

Lisinopril

08-Aug-2023

- **INDICATIONS AND DOSE**

Hypertension
▶ BY MOUTH
- Child 6–11 years (under expert supervision): Initially 70 micrograms/kg once daily (max. per dose 5 mg), increased to up to 600 micrograms/kg once daily, alternatively increased to up to 40 mg once daily, dose to be increased in intervals of 1–2 weeks
- Child 12–17 years (under expert supervision): Initially 5 mg once daily; usual maintenance 10–20 mg once daily; maximum 80 mg per day

Proteinuria in nephritis (under expert supervision)
▶ BY MOUTH
- Child 6–11 years: Initially 70 micrograms/kg once daily (max. per dose 5 mg), increased to up to 600 micrograms/kg once daily, alternatively increased to up to 40 mg once daily, dose to be increased in intervals of 1–2 weeks

continued →

- Child 12–17 years: Initially 5 mg once daily; usual maintenance 10–20 mg once daily; maximum 80 mg per day

Diabetic nephropathy (under expert supervision)

- BY MOUTH
  - Child 12–17 years: Initially 5 mg once daily; usual maintenance 10–20 mg once daily; maximum 80 mg per day

Heart failure (adjunct) (under close medical supervision)

- BY MOUTH
  - Child 12–17 years: Initially 2.5 mg once daily; increased in steps of up to 10 mg at least every 2 weeks; maximum 35 mg per day

- **UNLICENSED USE** Not licensed for use in children.
- **INTERACTIONS** → Appendix 1: ACE inhibitors
- **SIDE-EFFECTS**
  - **Common or very common** Postural disorders
  - **Uncommon** Hallucination · mood altered · Raynaud's phenomenon
  - **Rare or very rare** Alveolitis allergic · anaemia · autoimmune disorder · azotaemia · bone marrow depression · gynaecomastia · hepatic disorders · hypersensitivity · hypoglycaemia · lymphadenopathy · olfactory nerve disorder · SIADH · sinusitis · toxic epidermal necrolysis
  - **Frequency not known** Leucocytosis · vasculitis
- **BREAST FEEDING** Not recommended; alternative treatment options, with better established safety information during breast-feeding, are available.
- **RENAL IMPAIRMENT** EvGr Avoid if estimated glomerular filtration rate less than 30 mL/minute/1.73 m². (M) See p. 16.
- **PRESCRIBING AND DISPENSING INFORMATION** The RCPCH and NPPG recommend that, when a liquid formulation of lisinopril is required, the following strength is used: 5 mg/5 mL.
- **PATIENT AND CARER ADVICE**
  Medicines for Children leaflet: Lisinopril for high blood pressure www.medicinesforchildren.org.uk/medicines/lisinopril-for-high-blood-pressure/

- **MEDICINAL FORMS** There can be variation in the licensing of different medicines containing the same drug. Forms available from special-order manufacturers include: oral suspension, oral solution

Oral tablet

- **Lisinopril (Non-proprietary)**
  - **Lisinopril 2.5 mg** Lisinopril 2.5mg tablets | 28 tablet PoM £8.02 DT = £0.61 | 500 tablet PoM £11.84–£11.92
  - **Lisinopril 5 mg** Lisinopril 5mg tablets | 28 tablet PoM £9.02 DT = £0.68 | 500 tablet PoM £10.93–£18.88
  - **Lisinopril 10 mg** Lisinopril 10mg tablets | 28 tablet PoM £11.81 DT = £0.73 | 500 tablet PoM £10.78–£21.44
  - **Lisinopril 20 mg** Lisinopril 20mg tablets | 28 tablet PoM £12.02 DT = £0.92 | 500 tablet PoM £12.75–£20.80
- **Zestril** (Atnahs Pharma UK Ltd)
  - **Lisinopril 5 mg** Zestril 5mg tablets | 28 tablet PoM £9.42 DT = £0.68
  - **Lisinopril 10 mg** Zestril 10mg tablets | 28 tablet PoM £14.76 DT = £0.73
  - **Lisinopril 20 mg** Zestril 20mg tablets | 28 tablet PoM £13.02 DT = £0.92

Oral solution

- **Lisinopril (Non-proprietary)**
  - **Lisinopril 1 mg per 1 ml** Lisinopril 5mg/5ml oral solution sugar free | 150 ml PoM £228.90–£235.77 DT = £235.77 SF

DRUGS ACTING ON THE RENIN-ANGIOTENSIN SYSTEM › ANGIOTENSIN II RECEPTOR ANTAGONISTS

Angiotensin II receptor antagonists

> **IMPORTANT SAFETY INFORMATION**
>
> **MHRA/CHM ADVICE: ACE INHIBITORS AND ANGIOTENSIN II RECEPTOR ANTAGONISTS: NOT FOR USE IN PREGNANCY (DECEMBER 2014)**
>
> See *Conception and contraception* and *Pregnancy*.
>
> **MHRA/CHM ADVICE: ACE INHIBITORS AND ANGIOTENSIN II RECEPTOR ANTAGONISTS: RECOMMENDATIONS ON HOW TO USE FOR BREASTFEEDING (DECEMBER 2014)**
>
> See *Breast feeding*.

- **CAUTIONS** Aortic or mitral valve stenosis · hypertrophic cardiomyopathy · patients of black African or African-Caribbean origin · patients with a history of angioedema · patients with primary aldosteronism (may not benefit from an angiotensin-II receptor antagonist) · renal artery stenosis
- **SIDE-EFFECTS**
  - **Common or very common** Abdominal pain · asthenia · back pain · cough · diarrhoea · dizziness · headache · hyperkalaemia · nausea · postural hypotension (more common in patients with intravascular volume depletion, e.g. those taking high-dose diuretics) · renal impairment · skin reactions · vertigo · vomiting
  - **Uncommon** Hepatic function abnormal · hypotension · myalgia · thrombocytopenia
  - **Rare or very rare** Angioedema · arthralgia
- **CONCEPTION AND CONTRACEPTION** EvGr Females planning pregnancy should be switched to alternative treatments that have an established safety profile for use in pregnancy, unless continued treatment with an angiotensin II receptor antagonist is considered essential (M) (recommendation also supported by specialist sources).
- **PREGNANCY** EvGr Avoid (risk of teratogenicity in first trimester cannot be excluded; known risk of fetotoxicity (decreased renal function, oligohydramnios, skull ossification retardation) and neonatal toxicity (renal failure, hypotension, hyperkalaemia) in second and third trimesters); (M) recommendation also supported by specialist sources.
- **BREAST FEEDING** EvGr Information on the use of angiotensin-II receptor antagonists in breast-feeding is limited. They are not recommended in breast-feeding. Alternative treatment options, with better established safety profile during breast-feeding, are preferable (M) (recommendation also supported by specialist sources).
- **HEPATIC IMPAIRMENT** In general, manufacturers advise caution in mild to moderate impairment (limited information available); avoid in severe impairment (no information available).
- **RENAL IMPAIRMENT**
  Dose adjustments In general, manufacturers advise start with low dose and adjust according to response.
- **MONITORING REQUIREMENTS** Monitor plasma-potassium concentration, particularly in children with renal impairment.

134

Candesartan cilexetil

28-Jan-2025

- **INDICATIONS AND DOSE**

Hypertension

▶ BY MOUTH

- Child 6–17 years (under expert supervision) (body-weight up to 50 kg): Initially 4 mg once daily, lower dose may be used in intravascular volume depletion; increased if necessary up to 8 mg once daily
- Child 6–17 years (under expert supervision) (body-weight 50 kg and above): Initially 4 mg once daily, lower dose may be used in intravascular volume depletion; increased if necessary up to 16 mg once daily

- **CONTRA-INDICATIONS** Cholestasis
- **INTERACTIONS** → Appendix 1: angiotensin-II receptor antagonists
- **SIDE-EFFECTS**
  - ▶ **Common or very common** Fever · increased risk of infection · oropharyngeal pain · sinus arrhythmia
  - ▶ **Uncommon** Hyponatraemia
  - ▶ **Rare or very rare** Agranulocytosis · hepatitis · leucopenia · neutropenia
- **HEPATIC IMPAIRMENT** Manufacturer advises avoid in severe impairment or cholestasis.
  Dose adjustments In adults, manufacturer advises dose reduction—consult product literature.
- **RENAL IMPAIRMENT** See p. 16. EvGr Caution if estimated glomerular filtration rate is less than 30 mL/minute/1.73 m^2 (no information available). Ⓜ

- **MEDICINAL FORMS** There can be variation in the licensing of different medicines containing the same drug. Forms available from special-order manufacturers include: oral suspension, oral solution

Oral tablet

▶ **Candesartan cilexetil (Non-proprietary)**

Candesartan cilexetil 2 mg Candesartan 2mg tablets | 7 tablet PoM £2.86 DT = £0.60 | 28 tablet PoM £2.28–£11.46

Candesartan cilexetil 4 mg Candesartan 4mg tablets | 7 tablet PoM £3.10 DT = £0.51 | 28 tablet PoM £0.49–£11.74

Candesartan cilexetil 8 mg Candesartan 8mg tablets | 28 tablet PoM £11.87 DT = £0.81

Candesartan cilexetil 16 mg Candesartan 16mg tablets | 28 tablet PoM £15.26 DT = £0.91

Candesartan cilexetil 32 mg Candesartan 32mg tablets | 28 tablet PoM £19.36 DT = £1.24

▶ **Amias** (Neon Healthcare Ltd)

Candesartan cilexetil 2 mg Amias 2mg tablets | 7 tablet PoM £3.58 DT = £0.60

Candesartan cilexetil 4 mg Amias 4mg tablets | 28 tablet PoM £9.78

Candesartan cilexetil 8 mg Amias 8mg tablets | 28 tablet PoM £9.89 DT = £0.81

Candesartan cilexetil 16 mg Amias 16mg tablets | 28 tablet PoM £12.72 DT = £0.91

Candesartan cilexetil 32 mg Amias 32mg tablets | 28 tablet PoM £16.13 DT = £1.24

134

Losartan potassium

10-Jun-2021

- **INDICATIONS AND DOSE**

Hypertension

▶ BY MOUTH

- Child 6–17 years (under expert supervision) (body-weight 20–49 kg): Initially 700 micrograms/kg once daily (max. per dose 25 mg), lower initial dose may be used in intravascular volume depletion, adjusted according to response to 50 mg once daily
- Child 6–17 years (under expert supervision) (body-weight 50 kg and above): Initially 50 mg once daily, adjusted according to response to 1.4 mg/kg once daily (max. per dose 100 mg)

Hypertension with intravascular volume depletion

▶ BY MOUTH

- Child 6–17 years (under expert supervision) (body-weight 50 kg and above): Initially 25 mg once daily; adjusted according to response to up to 1.4 mg/kg once daily (max. per dose 100 mg)

- **CAUTIONS** Severe heart failure
- **INTERACTIONS** → Appendix 1: angiotensin-II receptor antagonists
- **SIDE-EFFECTS**
  - ▶ **Common or very common** Anaemia · hypoglycaemia · postural disorders
  - ▶ **Uncommon** Angina pectoris · constipation · drowsiness · dyspnoea · oedema · palpitations · sleep disorder
  - ▶ **Rare or very rare** Atrial fibrillation · hepatitis · hypersensitivity · paraesthesia · stroke · syncope · vasculitis
  - ▶ **Frequency not known** Depression · erectile dysfunction · hyponatraemia · influenza like illness · malaise · migraine · pancreatitis · photosensitivity reaction · rhabdomyolysis · taste altered · tinnitus · urinary tract infection
- **HEPATIC IMPAIRMENT** Manufacturer advises avoid in all degrees of impairment (no information available).
- **RENAL IMPAIRMENT** EvGr Avoid if estimated glomerular filtration rate is less than 30 mL/minute/1.73 m^2 (no information available). Ⓜ See p. 16.
- **PRESCRIBING AND DISPENSING INFORMATION** Flavours of oral liquid formulations may include berry-citrus.

- **MEDICINAL FORMS** There can be variation in the licensing of different medicines containing the same drug. Forms available from special-order manufacturers include: oral suspension, oral solution

Oral tablet

▶ **Losartan potassium (Non-proprietary)**

Losartan potassium 12.5 mg Losartan 12.5mg tablets | 28 tablet PoM £36.00 DT = £1.22

Losartan potassium 25 mg Losartan 25mg tablets | 28 tablet PoM £19.42 DT = £0.63

Losartan potassium 50 mg Losartan 50mg tablets | 28 tablet PoM £15.36 DT = £0.66 | 100 tablet PoM £1.88–£3.99 | 500 tablet PoM £11.79–£12.86

Losartan potassium 100 mg Losartan 100mg tablets | 28 tablet PoM £19.42 DT = £0.76 | 100 tablet PoM £4.29–£4.60 | 250 tablet PoM £8.38

▶ **Cozaar** (Organon Pharma (UK) Ltd)

Losartan potassium 12.5 mg Cozaar 12.5mg tablets | 28 tablet PoM £9.70 DT = £1.22

Losartan potassium 25 mg Cozaar 25mg tablets | 28 tablet PoM £16.18 DT = £0.63

Losartan potassium 50 mg Cozaar 50mg tablets | 28 tablet PoM £12.80 DT = £0.66

Losartan potassium 100 mg Cozaar 100mg tablets | 28 tablet PoM £16.18 DT = £0.76

Oral solution

▶ **Losartan potassium (Non-proprietary)**

Losartan potassium 10 mg per 1 ml Losartan 50mg/5ml oral solution sugar free | 150 ml PoM £218.00 SF

134

Valsartan

10-Jun-2021

- **INDICATIONS AND DOSE**

Hypertension

▶ BY MOUTH

- Child 6–17 years (under expert supervision) (body-weight 18–34 kg): Initially 40 mg once daily, adjusted according to response; maximum 80 mg per day
- Child 6–17 years (under expert supervision) (body-weight 35–79 kg): Initially 80 mg once daily, adjusted according to response; maximum 160 mg per day

continued →

- Child 6–17 years (under expert supervision) (body-weight 80 kg and above): Initially 80 mg once daily, adjusted according to response; maximum 320 mg per day

- **UNLICENSED USE** Capsules not licensed for use in children.
- **CONTRA-INDICATIONS** Biliary cirrhosis · cholestasis
- **INTERACTIONS** → Appendix 1: angiotensin-II receptor antagonists
- **SIDE-EFFECTS** Appetite decreased · hyponatraemia · neutropenia · respiratory disorders · serum sickness · vasculitis
- **HEPATIC IMPAIRMENT**
Dose adjustments Manufacturer advises maximum 80 mg daily in mild to moderate impairment.
- **RENAL IMPAIRMENT** See p. 16. EvGr Avoid if creatinine clearance is less than 30 mL/minute (no information available). ◈
- **MEDICINAL FORMS** There can be variation in the licensing of different medicines containing the same drug. Forms available from special-order manufacturers include: oral suspension, oral solution

Oral tablet

- **Valsartan (Non-proprietary)**
Valsartan 40 mg Valsartan 40mg tablets | 7 tablet PoM £7.54 DT = £4.46 | 28 tablet PoM £9.54–£17.84
Valsartan 80 mg Valsartan 80mg tablets | 28 tablet PoM £13.69 DT = £13.69
Valsartan 160 mg Valsartan 160mg tablets | 28 tablet PoM £14.69 DT = £8.84
Valsartan 320 mg Valsartan 320mg tablets | 28 tablet PoM £20.23 DT = £5.32

Oral solution

- **Diovan** (Novartis Pharmaceuticals UK Ltd)
Valsartan 3 mg per 1 ml Diovan 3mg/1ml oral solution | 160 ml PoM £7.20 DT = £7.20

Oral capsule

- **Valsartan (Non-proprietary)**
Valsartan 40 mg Valsartan 40mg capsules | 28 capsule PoM £13.97 DT = £1.98
Valsartan 80 mg Valsartan 80mg capsules | 28 capsule PoM £13.97 DT = £3.37
Valsartan 160 mg Valsartan 160mg capsules | 28 capsule PoM £18.41 DT = £8.95

VASODILATORS › POTASSIUM-CHANNEL OPENERS

Minoxidil 08-Nov-2021

- **INDICATIONS AND DOSE**

Severe hypertension

▶ BY MOUTH

- Child 1 month–11 years: Initially 200 micrograms/kg daily in 1–2 divided doses, then increased in steps of 100–200 micrograms/kg, increased at intervals of at least 3 days; maximum 1 mg/kg per day
- Child 12–17 years: Initially 5 mg daily in 1–2 divided doses, then increased in steps of 5–10 mg daily, increased at intervals of at least 3 days; maximum 100 mg per day

- **CONTRA-INDICATIONS** Phaeochromocytoma
- **CAUTIONS** Acute porphyrias p. 745 · after myocardial infarction (until stabilised) · angina
- **INTERACTIONS** → Appendix 1: minoxidil
- **SIDE-EFFECTS**
▶ **Common or very common** Fluid retention · hair changes · oedema · pericardial disorders · pericarditis · tachycardia
▶ **Rare or very rare** Leucopenia · skin reactions · Stevens-Johnson syndrome · thrombocytopenia
▶ **Frequency not known** Angina pectoris · breast tenderness · gastrointestinal disorder · pleural effusion · sodium retention · weight increased
- **PREGNANCY** Avoid—possible toxicity including reduced placental perfusion. Neonatal hirsutism reported.
- **BREAST FEEDING** Present in milk but not known to be harmful.
- **RENAL IMPAIRMENT** EvGr Caution in significant impairment. ◈
Dose adjustments EvGr Smaller doses may be required in renal failure. ◈
- **MEDICINAL FORMS** There can be variation in the licensing of different medicines containing the same drug.

Oral tablet

- **Minoxidil (Non-proprietary)**
Minoxidil 2.5 mg Minoxidil 2.5mg tablets | 60 tablet PoM £8.88 DT = £8.88
Minoxidil 5 mg Minoxidil 5mg tablets | 60 tablet PoM £21.60 DT = £21.60
Minoxidil 10 mg Minoxidil 10mg tablets | 60 tablet PoM £30.68 DT = £30.68
- **Loniten** (Pfizer Ltd)
Minoxidil 2.5 mg Loniten 2.5mg tablets | 60 tablet PoM £8.88 DT = £8.88
Minoxidil 5 mg Loniten 5mg tablets | 60 tablet PoM £15.83 DT = £21.60
Minoxidil 10 mg Loniten 10mg tablets | 60 tablet PoM £30.68 DT = £30.68

VASODILATORS › VASODILATOR ANTIHYPERTENSIVES

Hydralazine hydrochloride 08-Dec-2021

- **INDICATIONS AND DOSE**

Resistant hypertension (adjunct)

▶ BY MOUTH

- Neonate: 250–500 micrograms/kg every 8–12 hours, increased if necessary to 2–3 mg/kg every 8 hours.
- Child 1 month–11 years: 250–500 micrograms/kg every 8–12 hours, increased if necessary to 7.5 mg/kg daily; maximum 200 mg per day
- Child 12–17 years: 25 mg twice daily, increased to 50–100 mg twice daily

▶ BY SLOW INTRAVENOUS INJECTION

- Neonate: 100–500 micrograms/kg, dose may be repeated if necessary every 4–6 hours; maximum 3 mg/kg per day.
- Child 1 month–11 years: 100–500 micrograms/kg, dose may be repeated if necessary every 4–6 hours; maximum 3 mg/kg per day; maximum 60 mg per day
- Child 12–17 years: 5–10 mg, dose may be repeated if necessary every 4–6 hours

▶ BY CONTINUOUS INTRAVENOUS INFUSION

- Neonate: 12.5–50 micrograms/kg/hour, continuous intravenous infusion is the preferred route in cardiac patients; maximum 2 mg/kg per day.
- Child 1 month–11 years: 12.5–50 micrograms/kg/hour, continuous intravenous infusion is the preferred route in cardiac patients; maximum 3 mg/kg per day
- Child 12–17 years: 3–9 mg/hour, continuous intravenous infusion is the preferred route in cardiac patients; maximum 3 mg/kg per day

- **UNLICENSED USE** Not licensed for use in children.
- **CONTRA-INDICATIONS** Acute porphyrias p. 745 · cor pulmonale · dissecting aortic aneurysm · high output heart failure · idiopathic systemic lupus erythematosus ·

myocardial insufficiency due to mechanical obstruction · severe tachycardia

- **CAUTIONS** Cerebrovascular disease · coronary artery disease (may provoke angina, avoid after myocardial infarction until stabilised) · occasionally blood pressure reduction too rapid even with low parenteral doses
- **INTERACTIONS** → Appendix 1: hydralazine
- **SIDE-EFFECTS**
  - **Common or very common** Angina pectoris · diarrhoea · dizziness · flushing · gastrointestinal disorders · headache · hypotension · joint disorders · lupus-like syndrome (after long-term therapy (more common in slow acetylator individuals)) · myalgia · nasal congestion · nausea · palpitations · tachycardia · vomiting
  - **Rare or very rare** Acute kidney injury · agranulocytosis · anaemia · anxiety · appetite decreased · conjunctivitis · depression · dyspnoea · eosinophilia · eye disorders · fever · glomerulonephritis · haematuria · haemolytic anaemia · hallucination · heart failure · hepatic disorders · leucocytosis · leucopenia · lymphadenopathy · malaise · nerve disorders · neutropenia · oedema · pancytopenia · paradoxical pressor response · paraesthesia · pleuritic pain · proteinuria · skin reactions · splenomegaly · thrombocytopenia · urinary retention · vasculitis · weight decreased

  SIDE-EFFECTS, FURTHER INFORMATION The incidence of side-effects is lower if the dose is kept low, but systemic lupus erythematosus should be suspected if there is unexplained weight loss, arthritis, or any other unexplained ill health.
- **PREGNANCY** Neonatal thrombocytopenia reported, but risk should be balanced against risk of uncontrolled maternal hypertension. Manufacturer advises avoid before third trimester.
- **BREAST FEEDING** Present in milk but not known to be harmful.

  Monitoring Monitor infant in breast-feeding.
- **HEPATIC IMPAIRMENT** Manufacturer advises caution (risk of accumulation).

  Dose adjustments Manufacturer advises adjust dose or dosing interval according to clinical response.
- **RENAL IMPAIRMENT**

  Dose adjustments See p. 16.

  In adults, manufacturer advises adjust dose or dosing interval according to clinical response if creatinine clearance less than 30 mL/minute (consult product literature).
- **MONITORING REQUIREMENTS** Manufacturer advises test for antinuclear factor and for proteinuria every 6 months and check acetylator status before increasing dose, but evidence of clinical value unsatisfactory.
- **DIRECTIONS FOR ADMINISTRATION** For administration *by mouth*, diluted injection may be given orally.

  For *continuous intravenous infusion*, initially reconstitute 20 mg with 1 mL Water for Injections, then dilute with Sodium Chloride 0.9%. Incompatible with Glucose intravenous infusion. For *intravenous injection*, initially reconstitute 20 mg with 1 mL Water for Injections, then dilute to a concentration of 0.5–1 mg/mL with Sodium Chloride 0.9% and administer over 5–20 minutes.

- **MEDICINAL FORMS** There can be variation in the licensing of different medicines containing the same drug. Forms available from special-order manufacturers include: oral tablet, oral suspension, oral solution

Oral tablet

EXCIPIENTS: May contain Gluten, propylene glycol

- Hydralazine hydrochloride (Non-proprietary)

  Hydralazine hydrochloride 10 mg Apo-Hydralazine 10mg tablets | 100 tablet [PoM] [X]

  Hydralazine hydrochloride 25 mg Hydralazine 25mg tablets | 56 tablet [PoM] £16.00 DT = £2.86 | 84 tablet [PoM] £14.00

  Hydralazine hydrochloride 50 mg Hydralazine 50mg tablets | 56 tablet [PoM] £15.46 DT = £3.04

Powder for solution for injection

- Hydralazine hydrochloride (Non-proprietary)

  Hydralazine hydrochloride 20 mg Hydralazine 20mg powder for concentrate for solution for injection ampoules | 5 ampoule [PoM] £74.17

4.1a Hypertension associated with phaeochromocytoma

VASODILATORS › PERIPHERAL VASODILATORS

Phenoxybenzamine hydrochloride

20-Sep-2021

- **INDICATIONS AND DOSE**

  Hypertension in phaeochromocytoma

  - BY MOUTH
    - Child: 0.5–1 mg/kg twice daily, adjusted according to response
- **UNLICENSED USE** Not licensed for use in children.
- **CONTRA-INDICATIONS** During recovery period after myocardial infarction (usually 3–4 weeks) · history of cerebrovascular accident
- **CAUTIONS** Avoid in Acute porphyrias p. 745 · carcinogenic in *animals* · cerebrovascular disease · congestive heart failure · severe ischaemic heart disease
- **SIDE-EFFECTS** Abdominal distress · dizziness · ejaculation failure · fatigue · miosis · nasal congestion · postural hypotension · reflex tachycardia
- **PREGNANCY** Hypotension may occur in newborn.
- **BREAST FEEDING** May be present in milk.
- **RENAL IMPAIRMENT** [EvGr] Use with caution. (M)
- **DIRECTIONS FOR ADMINISTRATION** For administration *by mouth*, expert sources advise capsules may be opened.
- **HANDLING AND STORAGE** Owing to risk of contact sensitisation healthcare professionals should avoid contamination of hands.

- **MEDICINAL FORMS** There can be variation in the licensing of different medicines containing the same drug. Forms available from special-order manufacturers include: oral suspension, oral solution

Oral capsule

- Phenoxybenzamine hydrochloride (Non-proprietary)

  Phenoxybenzamine hydrochloride 10 mg Phenoxybenzamine 10mg capsules | 30 capsule [PoM] £129.21 DT = £129.21

4.1b Hypertensive crises

Other drugs used for Hypertensive crises Labetalol hydrochloride, p. 122

VASODILATORS › VASODILATOR ANTIHYPERTENSIVES

Sodium nitroprusside

05-Oct-2021

● **INDICATIONS AND DOSE**

Hypertensive emergencies

▶ BY CONTINUOUS INTRAVENOUS INFUSION

▶ Neonate: Initially 500 nanograms/kg/minute, then increased in steps of 200 nanograms/kg/minute (max. per dose 8 micrograms/kg/minute) as required, max. 4 micrograms/kg/minute if used for longer than 24 hours.

▶ Child: Initially 500 nanograms/kg/minute, then increased in steps of 200 nanograms/kg/minute (max. per dose 8 micrograms/kg/minute) as required, max. 4 micrograms/kg/minute if used for longer than 24 hours

● **UNLICENSED USE** Not licensed for use in the UK.

● **CONTRA-INDICATIONS** Compensatory hypertension · impaired cerebral circulation · Leber's optic atrophy · severe vitamin B_{12} deficiency

● **CAUTIONS** Hyponatraemia · hypothermia · hypothyroidism · ischaemic heart disease

● **INTERACTIONS** → Appendix 1: nitroprusside

● **SIDE-EFFECTS** Abdominal pain · anaemia · arrhythmias · chest discomfort · cyanide toxicity · dizziness · flushing · headache · hyperhidrosis · hypothyroidism · hypovolaemia · ileus · intracranial pressure increased · methaemoglobinaemia · muscle twitching · nausea · palpitations · rash · thiocyanate toxicity

SIDE-EFFECTS, FURTHER INFORMATION Side-effects associated with over rapid reduction in blood pressure: Headache, dizziness, nausea, retching, abdominal pain, perspiration, palpitation, anxiety, retrosternal discomfort—reduce infusion rate if any of these side-effects occur.

Overdose Side-effects caused by excessive plasma concentration of the cyanide metabolite include tachycardia, sweating, hyperventilation, arrhythmias, marked metabolic acidosis (discontinue and give antidote, see cyanide in Emergency treatment of poisoning p. 1036).

● **PREGNANCY** Avoid prolonged use—potential for accumulation of cyanide in fetus.

● **BREAST FEEDING** No information available. Caution advised due to thiocyanate metabolite.

● **HEPATIC IMPAIRMENT** Use with caution. Avoid in hepatic failure—cyanide or thiocyanate metabolites may accumulate.

● **RENAL IMPAIRMENT** Avoid prolonged use—cyanide or thiocyanate metabolites may accumulate.

● **MONITORING REQUIREMENTS** Monitor blood pressure (including intra-arterial blood pressure) and blood-cyanide concentration, and if treatment exceeds 3 days, also blood thiocyanate concentration.

● **TREATMENT CESSATION** Avoid sudden withdrawal—terminate infusion over 15–30 minutes.

● **DIRECTIONS FOR ADMINISTRATION** For *continuous intravenous infusion* in Glucose 5%, manufacturer advises infuse *via* infusion device to allow precise control. For further details, consult product literature. Protect infusion from light.

● **MEDICINAL FORMS** There can be variation in the licensing of different medicines containing the same drug.

Powder and solvent for solution for infusion

▶ **Sodium nitroprusside (Non-proprietary)**

Sodium nitroprusside dihydrate 50 mg Nitroprussiat Fides 50mg powder and solvent for solution for infusion vials | 1 vial PoM ⊠ (Hospital only)

Sodium nitroprusside 50mg powder and solvent for solution for infusion vials | 1 vial PoM ⊠ (Hospital only)

4.1c Pulmonary hypertension

ENDOTHELIN RECEPTOR ANTAGONISTS

Ambrisentan

14-Apr-2023

● **INDICATIONS AND DOSE**

Pulmonary arterial hypertension (initiated by a specialist)

▶ BY MOUTH

▶ Child 8–17 years (body-weight 20–34 kg): 2.5 mg once daily, increased if necessary to 5 mg once daily

▶ Child 8–17 years (body-weight 35–49 kg): 5 mg once daily, increased if necessary to 7.5 mg once daily

▶ Child 8–17 years (body-weight 50 kg and above): 5 mg once daily, increased if necessary to 10 mg once daily

DOSE ADJUSTMENTS DUE TO INTERACTIONS

▶ EvGr With concurrent use of ciclosporin, max. dose 2.5 mg once daily in those weighing 20–49 kg, and max. dose 5 mg once daily in those weighing ≥ 50 kg. ⟨M⟩

● **CONTRA-INDICATIONS** Idiopathic pulmonary fibrosis

● **CAUTIONS** Not to be initiated in significant anaemia · pulmonary veno-occlusive disease

● **INTERACTIONS** → Appendix 1: endothelin receptor antagonists

● **SIDE-EFFECTS**

▶ **Common or very common** Abdominal pain · anaemia · asthenia · chest discomfort · constipation · diarrhoea · dizziness · dyspnoea · epistaxis · fluid retention · flushing · headaches · heart failure · hypersensitivity · hypotension · increased risk of infection · nasal congestion · nausea · palpitations · peripheral oedema · skin reactions · syncope · tinnitus · upper respiratory tract congestion · vision disorders · vomiting

▶ **Uncommon** Hepatic disorders · sudden hearing loss

● **ALLERGY AND CROSS-SENSITIVITY** EvGr Contra-indicated in patients with soya or peanut hypersensitivity (film-coating contains soya lecithin). ⟨M⟩

● **CONCEPTION AND CONTRACEPTION** Exclude pregnancy before treatment and ensure effective contraception during treatment. Monthly pregnancy tests advised.

● **PREGNANCY** Avoid (teratogenic in *animal* studies).

● **BREAST FEEDING** Manufacturer advises avoid—no information available.

● **HEPATIC IMPAIRMENT** Manufacturer advises avoid in severe impairment or if baseline serum transaminases exceed 3 times the upper limit of normal.

● **RENAL IMPAIRMENT** EvGr Use with caution if creatinine clearance less than 30 mL/minute. ⟨M⟩ See p. 16.

● **MONITORING REQUIREMENTS**

▶ Monitor haemoglobin concentration or haematocrit after 1 month and 3 months of starting treatment, and periodically thereafter (reduce dose or discontinue treatment if significant decrease in haemoglobin concentration or haematocrit observed).

▶ Monitor liver function before treatment, and monthly thereafter—discontinue if liver enzymes raised significantly or if symptoms of liver impairment develop.

- **PATIENT AND CARER ADVICE**
Alert card A patient alert card should be provided.
Driving and skilled tasks Patients and carers should be cautioned on the effects on driving and performance of skilled tasks—increased risk of dizziness, blurred vision, syncope, and fatigue.

- **NATIONAL FUNDING/ACCESS DECISIONS**
For full details see funding body website

All Wales Medicines Strategy Group (AWMSG) decisions

- **Ambrisentan (*Volibris*®) for the treatment of pulmonary arterial hypertension in adults, adolescents and children (aged 8 to less than 18 years) of WHO Functional Class II to III including use in combination treatment (November 2022)** AWMSG No. 4819 Recommended

- **MEDICINAL FORMS** There can be variation in the licensing of different medicines containing the same drug.

Oral tablet

EXCIPIENTS: May contain Lecithin

- **Ambrisentan (Non-proprietary)**
  - **Ambrisentan 5 mg** Ambrisentan 5mg tablets | 30 tablet PoM £1,375.37 DT = £1,618.08 | 30 tablet PoM £1,365.08–£1,618.00 DT = £1,618.08 (Hospital only)
  - **Ambrisentan 10 mg** Ambrisentan 10mg tablets | 30 tablet PoM £1,375.37 DT = £1,618.08 | 30 tablet PoM £1,365.08–£1,618.00 DT = £1,618.08 (Hospital only)
- **Volibris** (GlaxoSmithKline UK Ltd)
  - **Ambrisentan 2.5 mg** Volibris 2.5mg tablets | 30 tablet PoM £1,618.08 (Hospital only)
  - **Ambrisentan 5 mg** Volibris 5mg tablets | 30 tablet PoM £1,618.08 DT = £1,618.08 (Hospital only)
  - **Ambrisentan 10 mg** Volibris 10mg tablets | 30 tablet PoM £1,618.08 DT = £1,618.08 (Hospital only)

Bosentan

05-Feb-2020

- **INDICATIONS AND DOSE**

Pulmonary arterial hypertension (initiated under specialist supervision)

- BY MOUTH
  - Child 2–17 years (body-weight 10–20 kg): Initially 31.25 mg once daily for 4 weeks, then increased to 31.25 mg twice daily
  - Child 2–17 years (body-weight 20–40 kg): Initially 31.25 mg twice daily for 4 weeks, then increased to 62.5 mg twice daily
  - Child 12–17 years (body-weight 40 kg and above): Initially 62.5 mg twice daily for 4 weeks, then increased to 125 mg twice daily (max. per dose 250 mg)

- **CONTRA-INDICATIONS** Acute porphyrias p. 745
- **CAUTIONS** Not to be initiated if systemic systolic blood pressure is below 85 mmHg · pulmonary veno-occlusive disease
- **INTERACTIONS** → Appendix 1: endothelin receptor antagonists
- **SIDE-EFFECTS**
  - **Common or very common** Anaemia · diarrhoea · erythema · fluid retention · flushing · gastrooesophageal reflux disease · headache · hypotension · nasal congestion · oedema · palpitations · syncope
  - **Uncommon** Hepatic disorders · leucopenia · neutropenia · thrombocytopenia
  - **Rare or very rare** Angioedema
  - **Frequency not known** Abdominal pain · fever · increased risk of infection · pulmonary oedema · vision blurred · vomiting
- **CONCEPTION AND CONTRACEPTION** Effective contraception required during administration (hormonal contraception not considered effective). Monthly pregnancy tests advised.
- **PREGNANCY** Avoid (teratogenic in *animal* studies).
- **BREAST FEEDING** Manufacturer advises avoid—no information available.
- **HEPATIC IMPAIRMENT** Manufacturer advises avoid in moderate-to-severe impairment or if baseline serum transaminases exceed 3 times the upper limit of normal.
- **MONITORING REQUIREMENTS**
  - Monitor haemoglobin before and during treatment (monthly for first 4 months, then 3-monthly).
  - Monitor liver function before treatment, at monthly intervals during treatment, and 2 weeks after dose increase (reduce dose or suspend treatment if liver enzymes raised significantly)—discontinue if symptoms of liver impairment.
- **TREATMENT CESSATION** Avoid abrupt withdrawal—withdraw treatment gradually.

- **MEDICINAL FORMS** There can be variation in the licensing of different medicines containing the same drug.

Oral tablet

- **Bosentan (Non-proprietary)**
  - **Bosentan (as Bosentan monohydrate) 62.5 mg** Bosentan 62.5mg tablets | 56 tablet PoM £1,510.21 (Hospital only) | 56 tablet PoM £1,359.19
  - **Bosentan (as Bosentan monohydrate) 125 mg** Bosentan 125mg tablets | 56 tablet PoM £1,510.21 (Hospital only) | 56 tablet PoM £1,359.19–£1,510.21

PHOSPHODIESTERASE TYPE-5 INHIBITORS

Sildenafil

15-Apr-2024

- **INDICATIONS AND DOSE**

Pulmonary arterial hypertension (initiated under specialist supervision)

- BY MOUTH
  - Neonate: Initially 250–500 micrograms/kg every 4–8 hours, adjusted according to response, start with the lower dose and frequency, especially if used with other vasodilators; maximum 30 mg per day.
  - Child 1–11 months: Initially 250–500 micrograms/kg every 4–8 hours, adjusted according to response, start with the lower dose and frequency, especially if used with other vasodilators; maximum 30 mg per day
  - Child 1–17 years (body-weight up to 20 kg): 10 mg 3 times a day
  - Child 1–17 years (body-weight 20 kg and above): 20 mg 3 times a day

DOSE ADJUSTMENTS DUE TO INTERACTIONS

- Manufacturer advises reduce dose with concurrent use of moderate and potent inhibitors of CYP3A4 (avoid with ketoconazole, itraconazole and ritonavir)—no specific recommendation made for children.

- **UNLICENSED USE** Not licensed for use in children under 1 year.
- **CONTRA-INDICATIONS** Hereditary degenerative retinal disorders · history of non-arteritic anterior ischaemic optic neuropathy · recent history of myocardial infarction · recent history of stroke · sickle-cell anaemia
- **CAUTIONS** Active peptic ulceration · anatomical deformation of the penis (e.g. angulation, cavernosal fibrosis, Peyronie's disease) · autonomic dysfunction · bleeding disorders · cardiovascular disease · hypotension (avoid if severe) · intravascular volume depletion · left ventricular outflow obstruction · predisposition to priapism (e.g. in sickle-cell disease, multiple myeloma, or leukaemia) · pulmonary veno-occlusive disease
- **INTERACTIONS** → Appendix 1: phosphodiesterase type-5 inhibitors

● **SIDE-EFFECTS**

- **Common or very common** Alopecia · anaemia · anxiety · cough · diarrhoea · dizziness · fluid retention · gastrointestinal discomfort · gastrointestinal disorders · headaches · increased risk of infection · insomnia · nasal complaints · nausea · night sweats · pain · skin reactions · tremor · vasodilation · vision disorders
- **Uncommon** Arrhythmias · chest pain · drowsiness · dry eye · dry mouth · eye discomfort · eye disorders · eye inflammation · fatigue · feeling hot · gynaecomastia · haemorrhage · hypertension · hypotension · myalgia · numbness · palpitations · sinus congestion · tinnitus · vertigo · vomiting
- **Rare or very rare** Acute coronary syndrome · arteriosclerotic retinopathy · cerebrovascular insufficiency · glaucoma · haematospermia · hearing impairment · irritability · optic neuropathy (discontinue if sudden visual impairment occurs) · oral hypoaesthesia · priapism · retinal occlusion · scleral discolouration · seizure · severe cutaneous adverse reactions (SCARs) · sudden cardiac death · syncope · throat tightness

● **PREGNANCY** Use only if potential benefit outweighs risk—no evidence of harm in *animal* studies.

● **BREAST FEEDING** Manufacturer advises avoid—no information available.

● **HEPATIC IMPAIRMENT** Manufacturer advises caution in mild to moderate impairment; avoid in severe impairment (no information available).

Dose adjustments Manufacturer advises if not tolerated, consider dose reduction in mild to moderate impairment—consult product literature.

● **RENAL IMPAIRMENT**

Dose adjustments [EvGr] If usual dose not tolerated, consider dose reduction (consult product literature). (M)

● **TREATMENT CESSATION** Avoid abrupt withdrawal.

● **PATIENT AND CARER ADVICE**

Medicines for Children leaflet: Sildenafil for pulmonary hypertension www.medicinesforchildren.org.uk/medicines/sildenafil-for-pulmonary-hypertension/

● **NATIONAL FUNDING/ACCESS DECISIONS**

For full details see funding body website

Scottish Medicines Consortium (SMC) decisions

- **Sildenafil (*Revatio*®) for the treatment of paediatric patients aged 1 year to 17 years old with pulmonary arterial hypertension (December 2012)** SMC No. 809/12 Recommended with restrictions

● **MEDICINAL FORMS** There can be variation in the licensing of different medicines containing the same drug. Forms available from special-order manufacturers include: oral suspension, oral solution

Oral tablet

- **Sildenafil (Non-proprietary)**
  Sildenafil (as Sildenafil citrate) 20 mg Sildenafil 20mg tablets | 90 tablet [PoM] £446.33 DT = £446.33
- **Granpidam** (Accord-UK Ltd)
  Sildenafil (as Sildenafil citrate) 20 mg Granpidam 20mg tablets | 90 tablet [PoM] £424.01 DT = £446.33
- **Revatio** (Viatris UK Healthcare Ltd)
  Sildenafil (as Sildenafil citrate) 20 mg Revatio 20mg tablets | 90 tablet [PoM] £446.33 DT = £446.33

Oral suspension

- **Sildenafil (Non-proprietary)**
  Sildenafil (as Sildenafil citrate) 10 mg per 1 ml Sildenafil 10mg/ml oral suspension sugar free | 122 ml [PoM] £186.75 DT = £186.75 [SF]
- **Revatio** (Viatris UK Healthcare Ltd)
  Sildenafil (as Sildenafil citrate) 10 mg per 1 ml Revatio 10mg/ml oral suspension | 90 ml [PoM] £186.75 DT = £186.75 [SF]

PROSTAGLANDINS AND RELATED SUBSTANCES

Epoprostenol
25-Jan-2021

(Prostacyclin)

● **DRUG ACTION** Epoprostenol is a prostaglandin and a potent vasodilator. It is also a powerful inhibitor of platelet aggregation.

● **INDICATIONS AND DOSE**

Persistent pulmonary hypertension of the newborn

- BY CONTINUOUS INTRAVENOUS INFUSION
  - Neonate: Initially 2 nanograms/kg/minute, increased if necessary up to 20 nanograms/kg/minute, dose adjusted according to response, rarely doses up to 40 nanograms/kg/minute are used.

Idiopathic pulmonary arterial hypertension

- BY CONTINUOUS INTRAVENOUS INFUSION
  - Child: Initially 2 nanograms/kg/minute, increased if necessary up to 40 nanograms/kg/minute

PHARMACOKINETICS

- Short half-life of approximately 3 minutes, therefore it must be administered by continuous intravenous infusion.

● **UNLICENSED USE** Not licensed for use in children.

● **CONTRA-INDICATIONS** Severe left ventricular dysfunction

● **CAUTIONS** Avoid abrupt withdrawal (risk of rebound pulmonary hypertension/pulmonary hypertensive crisis) · extreme caution in coronary artery disease · haemorrhagic diathesis · pulmonary veno-occlusive disease · reconstituted solution highly alkaline—avoid extravasation (irritant to tissues) · risk of pulmonary oedema (dose titration for pulmonary hypertension should be in hospital)

● **INTERACTIONS** → Appendix 1: epoprostenol

● **SIDE-EFFECTS**

- **Common or very common** Abdominal pain · anxiety · arrhythmias · arthralgia · chest discomfort · diarrhoea · flushing · haemorrhage · headache · intracranial haemorrhage · nausea · pain · rash · sepsis · vomiting
- **Uncommon** Dry mouth · hyperhidrosis
- **Rare or very rare** Fatigue · hyperthyroidism · intravenous catheter occlusion · local infection · pallor
- **Frequency not known** Ascites · pulmonary oedema (avoid chronic use if occurs during dose titration) · spleen abnormalities

● **PREGNANCY** Manufacturer advises caution—no information available.

● **BREAST FEEDING** Manufacturer advises avoid—no information available.

● **MONITORING REQUIREMENTS**

- Anticoagulant monitoring required when given with anticoagulants.
- Monitor blood pressure.

● **TREATMENT CESSATION** Avoid abrupt withdrawal (risk of rebound pulmonary hypertension and pulmonary hypertensive crisis).

● **DIRECTIONS FOR ADMINISTRATION** Directions for administration vary depending on the preparation used—for instructions *in adults*, consult product literature. For *neonatal intensive care*—consult local protocols.

● **MEDICINAL FORMS** There can be variation in the licensing of different medicines containing the same drug.

Powder for solution for infusion

- **Epoprostenol (Non-proprietary)**
  Epoprostenol (as Epoprostenol sodium) 1.5 mg Epoprostenol 1.5mg powder (pH12) for solution for infusion vials | 1 vial [PoM] [H] (Hospital only)

▸ **Veletri** (Janssen-Cilag Ltd)
Epoprostenol (as Epoprostenol sodium) 500 microgram Veletri 500microgram powder for solution for infusion vials | 1 vial PoM £24.44 (Hospital only)
Epoprostenol (as Epoprostenol sodium) 1.5 mg Veletri 1.5mg powder for solution for infusion vials | 1 vial PoM £49.24

Powder and solvent for solution for infusion
ELECTROLYTES: May contain Sodium
▸ **Flolan** (GlaxoSmithKline UK Ltd)
Epoprostenol (as Epoprostenol sodium) 500 microgram Flolan 500microgram powder and solvent for solution for infusion vials | 1 vial PoM £22.22
Epoprostenol (as Epoprostenol sodium) 1.5 mg Flolan 1.5mg powder and solvent for solution for infusion vials | 1 vial PoM £44.76 (Hospital only)

Iloprost

13-Jan-2021

● **INDICATIONS AND DOSE**

Idiopathic or familial pulmonary arterial hypertension (initiated under specialist supervision)

▶ BY INHALATION OF NEBULISED SOLUTION
▸ Child 8–17 years: Initially 2.5 micrograms for 1 dose, increased to 5 micrograms for 1 dose, increased if tolerated to 5 micrograms 6–9 times a day, adjusted according to response; reduced if not tolerated to 2.5 micrograms 6–9 times a day, reduce to lower maintenance dose if high dose not tolerated

Raynaud's syndrome

▶ BY INTRAVENOUS INFUSION
▸ Child 12–17 years: Initially 0.5 nanogram/kg/minute, increased to 1–2 nanograms/kg/minute given over 6 hours daily for 3–5 days, dose increase should be performed gradually

● **UNLICENSED USE** Not licensed for use in children.

● **CONTRA-INDICATIONS**
GENERAL CONTRA-INDICATIONS Conditions which increase risk of haemorrhage · congenital or acquired valvular defects with myocardial function disorders (not related to pulmonary hypertension) · decompensated heart failure (unless under close medical supervision) · severe arrhythmias · severe coronary heart disease · unstable angina · within 3 months of cerebrovascular events · within 6 months of myocardial infarction
SPECIFIC CONTRA-INDICATIONS
▸ When used by inhalation Pulmonary veno-occlusive disease · systolic blood pressure below 85 mmHg · unstable pulmonary hypertension with advanced right heart failure
▸ With intravenous use Acute or chronic congestive heart failure (NYHA II-IV) · pulmonary oedema

● **CAUTIONS**
GENERAL CAUTIONS Hypotension
SPECIFIC CAUTIONS
▸ When used by inhalation Acute pulmonary infection · severe asthma
▸ With intravenous use Significant heart disease

● **INTERACTIONS** → Appendix 1: iloprost

● **SIDE-EFFECTS**
GENERAL SIDE-EFFECTS
▶ **Common or very common** Cough · diarrhoea · dizziness · dyspnoea · haemorrhage · hypotension · nausea · pain · palpitations · syncope · vomiting
▶ **Uncommon** Taste altered · thrombocytopenia
SPECIFIC SIDE-EFFECTS
▶ **Common or very common**
▸ When used by inhalation Chest discomfort · headache · oral disorders · rash · tachycardia · throat complaints · vasodilation
▸ With intravenous use Angina pectoris · anxiety · appetite decreased · arrhythmias · arthralgia · asthenia · bradyphrenia · chills · confusion · drowsiness · feeling hot · fever · flushing · gastrointestinal discomfort · headaches · hyperhidrosis · muscle complaints · sensation abnormal · thirst · vertigo
▶ **Uncommon**
▸ With intravenous use Asthma · cerebrovascular insufficiency · constipation · depression · dry mouth · dysphagia · dysuria · embolism and thrombosis · eye discomfort · hallucination · heart failure · hepatic impairment · myocardial infarction · pruritus · pulmonary oedema · renal pain · seizure · tetany · tremor · vision blurred
▶ **Frequency not known**
▸ When used by inhalation Respiratory disorders

● **PREGNANCY**
▸ When used by inhalation Use if potential benefit outweighs risk.
▸ With intravenous use Manufacturer advises avoid—toxicity in *animal* studies.

● **BREAST FEEDING** Manufacturer advises avoid—no information available.

● **HEPATIC IMPAIRMENT** Manufacturer advises caution (risk of increased exposure).
Dose adjustments In adults, manufacturer advises initial dose reduction—consult product literature.

● **MONITORING REQUIREMENTS**
▸ With intravenous use Manufacturer advises monitor blood pressure and heart rate at the start of the infusion and at every dose increase.

● **DIRECTIONS FOR ADMINISTRATION** For *intravenous infusion* dilute to a concentration of 200 nanograms/mL with Glucose 5% or Sodium Chloride 0.9%; alternatively, may be diluted to a concentration of 2 micrograms/mL and given via syringe driver.
For *inhaled treatment*, to minimise accidental exposure use only with nebulisers listed in product literature in a well ventilated room.

● **PRESCRIBING AND DISPENSING INFORMATION**
▸ When used by inhalation Delivery characteristics of nebuliser devices may vary—only switch devices under medical supervision.
▸ With intravenous use Concentrate for infusion available on a named patient basis from Bayer Schering in 0.5 mL and 1 mL ampoules.

● **HANDLING AND STORAGE** Manufacturer advises avoid contact with skin and eyes.

● **PATIENT AND CARER ADVICE**
Driving and skilled tasks Manufacturer advises patients and carers should be counselled on the effects on driving and performance of skilled tasks—increased risk of dizziness.

● **MEDICINAL FORMS** There can be variation in the licensing of different medicines containing the same drug.

Solution for infusion
EXCIPIENTS: May contain Ethanol
▸ **Iloprost (Non-proprietary)**
Iloprost (as Iloprost trometamol) 100 microgram per 1 ml Ilomedin 100micrograms/1ml solution for infusion ampoules | 1 ampoule PoM ⊠
Iloprost 50micrograms/0.5ml concentrate for solution for infusion ampoules | 1 ampoule PoM £58.00–£75.00 (Hospital only) | 5 ampoule PoM £300.00 (Hospital only)

Nebuliser liquid
EXCIPIENTS: May contain Ethanol
▸ **Iloprost (Non-proprietary)**
Iloprost (as Iloprost trometamol) 10 microgram per 1 ml Iloprost 10micrograms/1ml nebuliser liquid ampoules | 30 ampoule PoM £300.00
▸ **Ventavis** (Bayer Plc)
Iloprost (as Iloprost trometamol) 10 microgram per 1 ml Ventavis 10micrograms/ml nebuliser solution 1ml ampoules | 42 ampoule PoM £560.27 (Hospital only) | 168 ampoule PoM £2,241.08 (Hospital only)

Ventavis 10micrograms/ml nebuliser solution 1ml ampoules with Breelib | 168 ampoule [PoM] £2,241.08

Iloprost (as Iloprost trometamol) 20 microgram per 1 ml Ventavis 20micrograms/ml nebuliser solution 1ml ampoules with Breelib | 168 ampoule [PoM] £2,241.08

Ventavis 20micrograms/ml nebuliser solution 1ml ampoules | 42 ampoule [PoM] £560.27

VASODILATORS > PERIPHERAL VASODILATORS

Tolazoline

- **DRUG ACTION** Tolazoline is an alpha-blocker and produces both pulmonary and systemic vasodilation.

- **INDICATIONS AND DOSE**

Correction of pulmonary vasospasm in neonates

▶ INITIALLY BY INTRAVENOUS INJECTION

▶ Neonate: Initially 1 mg/kg, to be given over 2–5 minutes, followed by (by continuous intravenous infusion) maintenance 200 micrograms/kg/hour if required, careful blood pressure monitoring should be carried out, doses above 300 micrograms/kg/hour associated with cardiotoxicity and renal failure.

▶ BY ENDOTRACHEAL TUBE

▶ Neonate: 200 micrograms/kg.

- **UNLICENSED USE** Not licensed for use in children.
- **CONTRA-INDICATIONS** Peptic ulcer disease
- **CAUTIONS** Cardiotoxic accumulation may occur with continuous infusion (particularly in renal impairment) · mitral stenosis
- **SIDE-EFFECTS** Arrhythmias · blood disorder · chills · diarrhoea · epigastric pain · flushing · haematuria · haemorrhage (with high doses) · headache · hyperhidrosis · hypertension (with high doses) · hypotension (severe; with high doses) · metabolic alkalosis · nausea · oliguria · rash macular · renal failure (with high doses) · thrombocytopenia · vomiting
- **RENAL IMPAIRMENT** Accumulates in renal impairment. Risk of cardiotoxicity.
  Dose adjustments Lower doses may be necessary.
- **MONITORING REQUIREMENTS** Monitor blood pressure regularly for sustained systemic hypotension.
- **DIRECTIONS FOR ADMINISTRATION** For *continuous intravenous infusion*, dilute with Glucose 5% or Sodium Chloride 0.9%. Prepare a fresh solution every 24 hours. For *endotracheal administration*, dilute with 0.5–1 mL of Sodium Chloride 0.9%.
- **MEDICINAL FORMS** Forms available from special-order manufacturers include: solution for injection

4.2 Hypotension and shock

Sympathomimetics

15-Jan-2025

Overview

The properties of sympathomimetics vary according to whether they act on alpha or on beta adrenergic receptors. Response to sympathomimetics can also vary considerably in children, particularly neonates. It is important to titrate the dose to the desired effect and to monitor the child closely.

Inotropic sympathomimetics

Dopamine hydrochloride p. 143 has a variable, unpredictable, and dose dependent impact on vascular tone. Low dose infusion normally causes vasodilatation, but there is little evidence that this is clinically beneficial; moderate doses increase myocardial contractility and cardiac output in older children, but in neonates moderate doses may cause a reduction in cardiac output. High doses cause vasoconstriction and increase vascular resistance, and should therefore be used with caution following cardiac surgery, or where there is co-existing neonatal pulmonary hypertension.

In neonates the response to inotropic sympathomimetics varies considerably, particularly in those born prematurely; careful dose titration and monitoring are necessary.

Shock

Shock is a medical emergency associated with a high mortality. The underlying causes of shock such as haemorrhage, sepsis or myocardial insufficiency should be corrected. Additional treatment is dependent on the type of shock.

Septic shock is associated with severe hypovolaemia (due to fluid loss, vasodilation and capillary leak) which must be corrected promptly to prevent tissue hypoxia and organ failure. If hypotension persists despite volume replacement, a vasoactive agent such as noradrenaline p. 145, adrenaline p. 159 or dopamine hydrochloride can be used. The use of further vasoactive therapy such as vasopressin p. 74 or inodilators, should be driven by individual patient physiology on specialist advice.

In *cardiogenic shock*, the aim is to improve cardiac output and to reduce the afterload on the heart. If central venous pressure is low, cautious volume expansion with a colloid or crystalloid can be used. An inotrope such as adrenaline or dopamine hydrochloride should be given to increase cardiac output. Dobutamine p. 143 is a peripheral vasodilator and is an alternative if hypotension is not significant.

Milrinone p. 150 has both inotropic and vasodilatory effects and can be used when vascular resistance is high. Alternatively, glyceryl trinitrate p. 158 or sodium nitroprusside p. 138 (on specialist advice only) can be used to reduce vasoconstriction.

Hypovolaemic shock should be treated with a crystalloid or colloid solution (or whole or reconstituted blood if source of hypovolaemia is haemorrhage) and further steps to improve cardiac output and decrease vascular resistance can be taken, as in cardiogenic shock.

The use of sympathomimetic inotropes and vasoconstrictors should preferably be confined to the intensive care setting and undertaken with invasive haemodynamic monitoring.

See also advice on the management of anaphylactic shock in Antihistamines, allergen immunotherapy and allergic emergencies p. 199.

Vasoconstrictor sympathomimetics

Vasoconstrictor sympathomimetics raise blood pressure transiently by acting on alpha-adrenergic receptors to constrict peripheral vessels. They are sometimes used as an emergency method of elevating blood pressure where other measures have failed.

The danger of vasoconstrictors is that although they raise blood pressure they also reduce perfusion of vital organs such as the kidney.

Ephedrine hydrochloride p. 144 is used to reverse hypotension caused by spinal and epidural anaesthesia.

Metaraminol p. 144 is used as a vasopressor during cardiopulmonary bypass.

Phenylephrine hydrochloride p. 145 causes peripheral vasoconstriction and increases arterial pressure.

Ephedrine hydrochloride, metaraminol and phenylephrine hydrochloride are rarely needed in children and should be used under specialist supervision.

Noradrenaline is reserved for children with low systemic vascular resistance that is unresponsive to fluid resuscitation following septic shock, spinal shock, and anaphylaxis.

Adrenaline is mainly used for its inotropic action. Low doses (acting on beta receptors) cause systemic and pulmonary vasodilation, with some increase in heart rate and stroke volume and also an increase in contractility; high doses act predominantly on alpha receptors causing intense systemic vasoconstriction.

SYMPATHOMIMETICS › INOTROPIC

Dobutamine

30-May-2023

- **DRUG ACTION** Dobutamine is a cardiac stimulant which acts on $beta_1$ receptors in cardiac muscle, and increases contractility.

- **INDICATIONS AND DOSE**

Inotropic support in low cardiac output states, after cardiac surgery, cardiomyopathies, shock

▶ BY CONTINUOUS INTRAVENOUS INFUSION

▸ Neonate: Initially 5 micrograms/kg/minute, then adjusted according to response to 2–20 micrograms/kg/minute, doses as low as 0.5–1 microgram/kg/minute have been used.

▸ Child: Initially 5 micrograms/kg/minute, then adjusted according to response to 2–20 micrograms/kg/minute, doses as low as 0.5–1 microgram/kg/minute have been used

- **CONTRA-INDICATIONS** Phaeochromocytoma
- **CAUTIONS** Acute heart failure · acute myocardial infarction · arrhythmias · correct hypercapnia before starting and during treatment · correct hypovolaemia before starting and during treatment · correct hypoxia before starting and during treatment · correct metabolic acidosis before starting and during treatment · diabetes mellitus · extravasation may cause tissue necrosis · extreme caution or avoid in marked obstruction of cardiac ejection (such as idiopathic hypertrophic subaortic stenosis) · hyperthyroidism · ischaemic heart disease · occlusive vascular disease · severe hypotension · susceptibility to angle-closure glaucoma · tachycardia · tolerance may develop with continuous infusions longer than 72 hours
- **INTERACTIONS** → Appendix 1: sympathomimetics, inotropic
- **SIDE-EFFECTS**

▶ **Common or very common** Arrhythmias · bronchospasm · chest pain · dyspnoea · eosinophilia · fever · inflammation localised · ischaemic heart disease · nausea · palpitations · platelet aggregation inhibition (on prolonged administration) · skin reactions · urinary urgency · vasoconstriction

▶ **Uncommon** Myocardial infarction

▶ **Rare or very rare** Atrioventricular block · cardiac arrest · coronary vasospasm · hypertension · hypokalaemia · hypotension

▶ **Frequency not known** Anxiety · cardiomyopathy · feeling hot · headache · myoclonus · paraesthesia · tremor

- **PREGNANCY** No evidence of harm in *animal* studies—manufacturers advise use only if potential benefit outweighs risk.
- **BREAST FEEDING** Manufacturers advise avoid—no information available.
- **DIRECTIONS FOR ADMINISTRATION** Manufacturer advises dobutamine *injection* should be diluted before use or given undiluted with syringe pump. Dobutamine *concentrate* for intravenous infusion should be diluted before use.

For *continuous intravenous infusion*, manufacturer advises using infusion pump, dilute to a concentration of 0.5–1 mg/mL (max. 5 mg/mL if fluid restricted) with Glucose 5% *or* Sodium Chloride 0.9%; infuse higher concentration solutions through central venous catheter only. Incompatible with bicarbonate and other strong alkaline solutions.

For *neonatal intensive care*, manufacturer advises dilute 30 mg/kg body-weight to a final volume of 50 mL with Glucose 5% *or* Sodium Chloride 0.9%; an intravenous infusion rate of 0.5 mL/hour provides a dose of 5 micrograms/kg/minute; max. concentration of 5 mg/mL; infuse higher concentration solutions through central venous catheter only. Incompatible with bicarbonate and other strong alkaline solutions.

- **MEDICINAL FORMS** There can be variation in the licensing of different medicines containing the same drug. Forms available from special-order manufacturers include: solution for infusion

Solution for infusion

EXCIPIENTS: May contain Sulfites

▸ **Dobutamine (Non-proprietary)**

Dobutamine (as Dobutamine hydrochloride) 5 mg per 1 ml Dobutamine 250mg/50ml solution for infusion vials | 1 vial [PoM] £11.20

Dobutamine 250mg/50ml solution for infusion pre-filled syringes | 1 pre-filled disposable injection [PoM] £15.00 (Hospital only)

Dobutamine (as Dobutamine hydrochloride) 12.5 mg per 1 ml Dobutamine 250mg/20ml concentrate for solution for infusion ampoules | 10 ampoule [PoM] £63.50 | 10 ampoule [PoM] £52.50-£63.50 (Hospital only)

Dopamine hydrochloride

22-Feb-2021

- **DRUG ACTION** Dopamine is a cardiac stimulant which acts on $beta_1$ receptors in cardiac muscle, and increases contractility with little effect on rate.

- **INDICATIONS AND DOSE**

To correct the haemodynamic imbalance due to acute hypotension, shock, cardiac failure, adjunct following cardiac surgery

▶ BY CONTINUOUS INTRAVENOUS INFUSION

▸ Neonate: Initially 3 micrograms/kg/minute, increased if necessary up to 20 micrograms/kg/minute, dose to be adjusted according to response.

▸ Child: Initially 5 micrograms/kg/minute, increased if necessary up to 20 micrograms/kg/minute, dose to be adjusted according to response

- **UNLICENSED USE** Not licensed for use in children under 12 years.
- **CONTRA-INDICATIONS** Phaeochromocytoma · tachyarrhythmia
- **CAUTIONS** Correct hypovolaemia · hypertension (may raise blood pressure) · hyperthyroidism
- **INTERACTIONS** → Appendix 1: sympathomimetics, inotropic
- **SIDE-EFFECTS** Angina pectoris · anxiety · arrhythmias · azotaemia · cardiac conduction disorder · dyspnoea · gangrene · headache · hypertension · mydriasis · nausea · palpitations · piloerection · polyuria · tremor · vasoconstriction · vomiting
- **PREGNANCY** No evidence of harm in *animal* studies—manufacturer advises use only if potential benefit outweighs risk.
- **BREAST FEEDING** May suppress lactation—not known to be harmful.
- **DIRECTIONS FOR ADMINISTRATION** [EvGr] Dopamine concentrate for intravenous infusion to be diluted before use; give via a large vein.

For *continuous intravenous infusion*, dilute to a max. concentration of 3.2 mg/mL with Glucose 5% *or* Sodium Chloride 0.9%. ⟨M⟩ Expert sources advise infuse higher concentrations through central venous catheter using a syringe pump to avoid extravasation. Incompatible with bicarbonate and other alkaline solutions.

Neonatal intensive care, expert sources advise dilute 30 mg/kg body-weight to a final volume of 50 mL with infusion fluid; an intravenous infusion rate of 0.3 mL/hour provides a dose of 3 micrograms/kg/minute. EvGr Max. concentration of 3.2 mg/mL. ⟨M⟩ Expert sources advise infuse higher concentrations through central venous catheter using a syringe pump. Incompatible with bicarbonate and other alkaline solutions.

- **MEDICINAL FORMS** There can be variation in the licensing of different medicines containing the same drug. Forms available from special-order manufacturers include: solution for infusion

Solution for infusion

- **Dopamine hydrochloride (Non-proprietary)**
  Dopamine hydrochloride 40 mg per 1 ml Dopamine 200mg/5ml solution for infusion ampoules | 10 ampoule PoM £14.78 | 10 ampoule PoM £14.78 (Hospital only)
  Dopamine 200mg/5ml concentrate for solution for infusion ampoules | 5 ampoule PoM £14.75 (Hospital only) | 10 ampoule PoM £20.00 (Hospital only)
- **Neoatricon** (Piramal Critical Care Ltd)
  Dopamine hydrochloride 1.5 mg per 1 ml Neoatricon 45mg/30ml solution for infusion vials | 1 vial PoM £480.00 (Hospital only)
  Dopamine hydrochloride 4.5 mg per 1 ml Neoatricon 225mg/50ml solution for infusion vials | 1 vial PoM £576.00 (Hospital only)

SYMPATHOMIMETICS › VASOCONSTRICTOR

Ephedrine hydrochloride

29-Mar-2022

- **INDICATIONS AND DOSE**

Reversal of hypotension from spinal or epidural anaesthesia

▶ BY SLOW INTRAVENOUS INJECTION

- Child 1 month–11 years: 500–750 micrograms/kg every 3–4 minutes (max. per dose 9 mg), adjusted according to response, injection solution to contain ephedrine hydrochloride 30 mg/mL, alternatively 17–25 mg/m^2 every 3–4 minutes (max. per dose 9 mg), adjusted according to response, injection solution to contain ephedrine hydrochloride 30 mg/mL; maximum 30 mg per course
- Child 12–17 years: 3–7.5 mg every 3–4 minutes (max. per dose 9 mg), adjusted according to response; maximum 30 mg per course

- **CAUTIONS** Diabetes mellitus · hypertension · hyperthyroidism · susceptibility to angle-closure glaucoma
- **INTERACTIONS** → Appendix 1: sympathomimetics, vasoconstrictor
- **SIDE-EFFECTS**

▶ **Common or very common** Anxiety · arrhythmias · asthenia · confusion · depression · dyspnoea · headache · hyperhidrosis · insomnia · irritability · nausea · palpitations · vomiting

▶ **Rare or very rare** Acute urinary retention

▶ **Frequency not known** Acute angle closure glaucoma · angina pectoris · appetite decreased · cardiac arrest · dizziness · hypokalaemia · intracranial haemorrhage · psychotic disorder · pulmonary oedema · tremor

- **PREGNANCY** Increased fetal heart rate reported with parenteral ephedrine.
- **BREAST FEEDING** Present in milk; manufacturer advises avoid—irritability and disturbed sleep reported.
- **MEDICINAL FORMS** There can be variation in the licensing of different medicines containing the same drug. Forms available from special-order manufacturers include: solution for injection

Solution for injection

- **Ephedrine hydrochloride (Non-proprietary)**
  Ephedrine hydrochloride 3 mg per 1 ml Ephedrine 30mg/10ml solution for injection ampoules | 10 ampoule PoM £124.09–£185.73
  Ephedrine 30mg/10ml solution for injection pre-filled syringes | 1 pre-filled disposable injection PoM £9.50 | 10 pre-filled disposable injection PoM £95.00
  Ephedrine hydrochloride 30 mg per 1 ml Ephedrine 30mg/1ml solution for injection ampoules | 10 ampoule PoM £172.76–£387.80

Metaraminol

28-Apr-2020

- **INDICATIONS AND DOSE**

Emergency treatment of acute hypotension

▶ INITIALLY BY INTRAVENOUS INJECTION

- Child 12–17 years: Initially 0.5–5 mg, then (by intravenous infusion) 15–100 mg, adjusted according to response

Acute hypotension

▶ BY INTRAVENOUS INFUSION

- Child 12–17 years: 15–100 mg, adjusted according to response

- **CAUTIONS** Cirrhosis · coronary vascular thrombosis · diabetes mellitus · extravasation at injection site may cause necrosis · following myocardial infarction · hypercapnia · hypertension · hyperthyroidism · hypoxia · mesenteric vascular thrombosis · peripheral vascular thrombosis · Prinzmetal's variant angina · susceptibility to angle-closure glaucoma · uncorrected hypovolaemia

CAUTIONS, FURTHER INFORMATION

- Hypertensive response Metaraminol has a longer duration of action than noradrenaline, and an excessive vasopressor response may cause a prolonged rise in blood pressure.

- **INTERACTIONS** → Appendix 1: sympathomimetics, vasoconstrictor
- **SIDE-EFFECTS**

▶ **Common or very common** Headache · hypertension

▶ **Rare or very rare** Skin exfoliation · soft tissue necrosis

▶ **Frequency not known** Abscess · arrhythmias · nausea · palpitations · peripheral ischaemia

- **PREGNANCY** May reduce placental perfusion—manufacturer advises use only if potential benefit outweighs risk.
- **BREAST FEEDING** Manufacturer advises caution—no information available.
- **MONITORING REQUIREMENTS** Monitor blood pressure and rate of flow frequently.
- **DIRECTIONS FOR ADMINISTRATION** For *intravenous infusion*, dilute to a concentration of 30–200 micrograms/mL with Glucose 5% or Sodium Chloride 0.9% and give through a central venous catheter.
- **MEDICINAL FORMS** There can be variation in the licensing of different medicines containing the same drug. Forms available from special-order manufacturers include: solution for injection

Solution for injection

- **Metaraminol (Non-proprietary)**
  Metaraminol (as Metaraminol tartrate) 500 microgram per 1 ml Metaraminol 2.5mg/5ml solution for injection ampoules | 10 ampoule PoM £62.90 (Hospital only)
  Metaraminol 5mg/10ml solution for injection ampoules | 10 ampoule PoM £127.60 (Hospital only)
  Metaraminol 2.5mg/5ml solution for injection pre-filled syringes | 10 pre-filled disposable injection PoM £95.00 (Hospital only)
  Metaraminol 5mg/10ml solution for injection vials | 10 vial PoM £55.00 (Hospital only)

Metaraminol (as Metaraminol tartrate) 10 mg per 1 ml Metaraminol 10mg/1ml solution for injection vials | 10 vial [PoM] £20.50 (Hospital only)
Metaraminol 10mg/1ml solution for injection ampoules | 5 ampoule [PoM] £25.00 | 10 ampoule [PoM] £83.90 | 10 ampoule [PoM] £25.00 (Hospital only)

Noradrenaline

13-Apr-2026

(Norepinephrine)

- **DRUG ACTION** Noradrenaline (norepinephrine) is a sympathomimetic which acts predominantly on alpha adrenergic receptors, which causes peripheral vasoconstriction, leading to increased blood pressure.

- **INDICATIONS AND DOSE**

Acute hypotension (septic shock) | Shock secondary to excessive vasodilation

▶ BY CONTINUOUS INTRAVENOUS INFUSION

- Neonate: 20–100 nanograms/kg/minute (max. per dose 1 microgram/kg/minute), adjusted according to response, dilute the 1 mg/mL concentrate for infusion for this dose.
- Child: 20–100 nanograms/kg/minute (max. per dose 1 microgram/kg/minute), adjusted according to response, dilute the 1 mg/mL concentrate for infusion for this dose

DOSE EQUIVALENCE AND CONVERSION

- 1 mg of noradrenaline base is equivalent to 2 mg of noradrenaline acid tartrate. **Doses expressed as the base.**

- **UNLICENSED USE** Not licensed for use in children.

IMPORTANT SAFETY INFORMATION

ASSOCIATION OF NORADRENALINE 0.08 MG/ML (4 MG IN 50 ML) AND 0.16 MG/ML (8 MG IN 50 ML) SOLUTION FOR INFUSION WITH POTENTIAL RISK OF MEDICATION ERRORS

Healthcare professionals should be aware of the differences in strength and presentation between noradrenaline products—manufacturer advises noradrenaline 0.08 mg/mL solution for infusion and noradrenaline 0.16 mg/mL solution for infusion must **not** be diluted before use and should only be used for the on-going treatment of patients already established on noradrenaline therapy, whose dose requirements are clinically confirmed to be escalating.

- **CONTRA-INDICATIONS** Hypertension
- **CAUTIONS** Coronary vascular thrombosis · diabetes mellitus · extravasation at injection site may cause necrosis · following myocardial infarction · hypercapnia · hyperthyroidism · hypoxia · mesenteric vascular thrombosis · peripheral vascular thrombosis · Prinzmetal's variant angina · susceptibility to angle-closure glaucoma · uncorrected hypovolaemia
- **INTERACTIONS** → Appendix 1: sympathomimetics, vasoconstrictor
- **SIDE-EFFECTS** Acute glaucoma · anxiety · arrhythmias · asthenia · cardiomyopathy · confusion · dyspnoea · extravasation necrosis · gangrene · headache · heart failure · hypovolaemia · hypoxia · injection site necrosis · insomnia · ischaemia · myocardial contractility increased · nausea · palpitations · peripheral ischaemia · psychotic disorder · respiratory failure · tremor · urinary retention · vomiting
- **PREGNANCY** Manufacturer advises use if potential benefit outweighs risk—may reduce placental perfusion and induce fetal bradycardia.
- **MONITORING REQUIREMENTS** Monitor blood pressure and rate of flow frequently.
- **DIRECTIONS FOR ADMINISTRATION** For *continuous intravenous infusion*, using 1 mg/mL concentrate for infusion, dilute to a max. concentration of noradrenaline (base) 40 micrograms/mL (higher concentrations can be used if fluid-restricted) with Glucose 5% or Sodium Chloride and Glucose. Infuse through central venous catheter; discard if discoloured. Incompatible with bicarbonate or alkaline solutions.
  For *neonatal intensive care*, using 1 mg/mL concentrate for infusion, dilute 600 micrograms (base)/kg body-weight to a final volume of 50 mL with infusion fluid; an intravenous infusion rate of 0.1 mL/hour provides a dose of 20 nanograms (base)/kg/minute; infuse through central venous catheter; max. concentration of noradrenaline (base) 40 micrograms/mL (higher concentrations can be used if fluid-restricted). Discard if discoloured. Incompatible with bicarbonate or alkaline solutions.
- **PRESCRIBING AND DISPENSING INFORMATION** For a period of time, preparations on the UK market may be described as either noradrenaline base or noradrenaline acid tartrate; doses in BNF Publications are expressed as the base.

- **MEDICINAL FORMS** There can be variation in the licensing of different medicines containing the same drug. Forms available from special-order manufacturers include: infusion, solution for infusion

Solution for infusion

▶ Noradrenaline (Non-proprietary)

Noradrenaline (as Noradrenaline acid tartrate) 80 microgram per 1 ml Noradrenaline (base) 4mg/50ml solution for infusion vials | 10 vial [PoM] £111.00 (Hospital only)

Noradrenaline (as Noradrenaline acid tartrate) 1 mg per 1 ml Noradrenaline (base) 1mg/1ml concentrate for solution for infusion ampoules | 10 ampoule [PoM] [X] (Hospital only)
Noradrenaline (base) 8mg/8ml concentrate for solution for infusion ampoules | 10 ampoule [PoM] £116.00–£145.30 (Hospital only)
Noradrenaline (base) 2mg/2ml solution for infusion ampoules | 5 ampoule [PoM] £12.00 (Hospital only)
Noradrenaline (base) 2mg/2ml concentrate for solution for infusion ampoules | 10 ampoule [PoM] £22.00 (Hospital only)
Noradrenaline (base) 4mg/4ml concentrate for solution for infusion ampoules | 5 ampoule [PoM] £22.00 (Hospital only) | 10 ampoule [PoM] £44.00–£72.00 (Hospital only)
Noradrenaline (base) 10mg/10ml concentrate for solution for infusion ampoules | 10 ampoule [PoM] [X] (Hospital only)

▶ Sinora (Sandoz Ltd)

Noradrenaline (as Noradrenaline acid tartrate) 160 microgram per 1 ml Sinora 8mg/50ml solution for infusion vials | 1 vial [PoM] £14.22 (Hospital only)

Phenylephrine hydrochloride

- **INDICATIONS AND DOSE**

Acute hypotension

▶ BY SUBCUTANEOUS INJECTION, OR BY INTRAMUSCULAR INJECTION

- Child 1–11 years: 100 micrograms/kg every 1–2 hours (max. per dose 5 mg) as required
- Child 12–17 years: Initially 2–5 mg (max. per dose 5 mg), followed by 1–10 mg, after at least 15 minutes if required

▶ BY SLOW INTRAVENOUS INJECTION

- Child 1–11 years: Initially 5–20 micrograms/kg (max. per dose 500 micrograms), repeated as necessary after at least 15 minutes
- Child 12–17 years: 100–500 micrograms, repeated as necessary after at least 15 minutes

continued →

- ▶ BY INTRAVENOUS INFUSION
  - ▶ Child 1–15 years: Initially 100–500 nanograms/kg/minute, adjusted according to response
  - ▶ Child 16–17 years: Initially up to 180 micrograms/minute, reduced to 30–60 micrograms/minute, adjusted according to response

- **UNLICENSED USE** Not licensed for use in children by intravenous infusion or injection.
- **CONTRA-INDICATIONS** Hypertension · severe hyperthyroidism
- **CAUTIONS** Coronary disease · coronary vascular thrombosis · diabetes · extravasation at injection site may cause necrosis · following myocardial infarction · hypercapnia · hyperthyroidism · hypoxia · mesenteric vascular thrombosis · peripheral vascular thrombosis · Prinzmetal's variant angina · susceptibility to angle-closure glaucoma · uncorrected hypovolaemia

  CAUTIONS, FURTHER INFORMATION
  - ▶ Hypertensive response Phenylephrine has a longer duration of action than noradrenaline, and an excessive vasopressor response may cause a prolonged rise in blood pressure.
- **INTERACTIONS** → Appendix 1: sympathomimetics, vasoconstrictor
- **SIDE-EFFECTS** Anxiety · arrhythmias · cardiac arrest · confusion · dizziness · dyspnoea · extravasation necrosis · flushing · glaucoma exacerbated · glucose tolerance impaired · headache · hyperhidrosis · hypersalivation · hypertensive crisis · hypotension · insomnia · intracranial haemorrhage · ischaemic heart disease · metabolic change · muscle weakness · mydriasis · nausea · pallor · palpitations · paraesthesia · peripheral coldness · piloerection · psychotic disorder · pulmonary oedema · soft tissue necrosis · syncope · tremor · urinary disorders · vomiting
- **PREGNANCY** Avoid if possible; malformations reported following use in first trimester; fetal hypoxia and bradycardia reported in late pregnancy and labour.
- **MONITORING REQUIREMENTS** Contra-indicated in hypertension—monitor blood pressure and rate of flow frequently.
- **DIRECTIONS FOR ADMINISTRATION** For *intravenous injection*, dilute to a concentration of 1 mg/mL with Water for Injections and administer slowly. For *intravenous infusion*, dilute to a concentration of 20 micrograms/mL with Glucose 5% or Sodium Chloride 0.9% and administer as a continuous infusion via a central venous catheter using a controlled infusion device.
- **PRESCRIBING AND DISPENSING INFORMATION** Intravenous administration preferred when managing acute hypotension in children.

- **MEDICINAL FORMS** There can be variation in the licensing of different medicines containing the same drug. Forms available from special-order manufacturers include: solution for injection

Solution for injection

▶ **Phenylephrine hydrochloride (Non-proprietary)**

Phenylephrine (as Phenylephrine hydrochloride) 50 microgram per 1 ml Phenylephrine 500micrograms/10ml solution for injection pre-filled syringes | 10 pre-filled disposable injection PoM £150.00 (Hospital only)

Phenylephrine hydrochloride 100 microgram per 1 ml Phenylephrine 1mg/10ml solution for injection ampoules | 10 ampoule PoM £50.45 (Hospital only)

Phenylephrine 2mg/20ml solution for injection vials | 10 vial PoM £150.00 (Hospital only)

Phenylephrine hydrochloride 10 mg per 1 ml Phenylephrine 10mg/1ml solution for injection ampoules | 10 ampoule PoM £99.12 (Hospital only)

Phenylephrine 10mg/1ml concentrate for solution for injection ampoules | 10 ampoule PoM £108.22 (Hospital only)

5 Heart failure

Other drugs used for Heart failure Bendroflumethiazide, p. 130 · Captopril, p. 131 · Chlorothiazide, p. 130 · Chlortalidone, p. 165 · Digoxin, p. 91 · Enalapril maleate, p. 132 · Glyceryl trinitrate, p. 158 · Lisinopril, p. 133 Prazosin, p. 119

BETA-ADRENOCEPTOR BLOCKERS › ALPHA- AND BETA-ADRENOCEPTOR BLOCKERS

F 121

Carvedilol

18-Mar-2026

- **INDICATIONS AND DOSE**

Adjunct in heart failure (limited information available)
- ▶ BY MOUTH
  - ▶ Child 2–17 years: Initially 50 micrograms/kg twice daily (max. per dose 3.125 mg) for at least 2 weeks, then increased to 100 micrograms/kg twice daily for at least 2 weeks, then increased to 200 micrograms/kg twice daily, then increased if necessary up to 350 micrograms/kg twice daily (max. per dose 25 mg)

Prevention of bleeding from medium or large oesophageal varices [in patients with cirrhosis]
- ▶ BY MOUTH
  - ▶ Child 16–17 years: 6.25 mg once daily, increased if necessary up to 12.5 mg once daily, dose to be adjusted gradually according to heart rate and blood pressure

Primary prevention of decompensated cirrhosis [in patients with clinically significant portal hypertension]
- ▶ BY MOUTH
  - ▶ Child 16–17 years: 6.25 mg once daily, dose to be adjusted gradually according to heart rate and blood pressure

- **UNLICENSED USE** Not licensed for use in children under 18 years.
- **CONTRA-INDICATIONS** Acute or decompensated heart failure requiring intravenous inotropes
- **INTERACTIONS** → Appendix 1: beta blockers, non-selective
- **SIDE-EFFECTS**
  - ▶ **Common or very common** Anaemia · asthma · dyspepsia · eye irritation · fluid imbalance · genital oedema · hypercholesterolaemia · hyperglycaemia · hypoglycaemia · increased risk of infection · oedema · peripheral vascular disease · postural hypotension · pulmonary oedema · renal impairment · urinary disorders · weight increased
  - ▶ **Uncommon** Angina pectoris · constipation · hyperhidrosis · skin reactions
  - ▶ **Rare or very rare** Dry mouth · hypersensitivity · leucopenia · nasal congestion · severe cutaneous adverse reactions (SCARs) · thrombocytopenia
- **PREGNANCY** Information on the safety of carvedilol during pregnancy is lacking. If carvedilol is used close to delivery, infants should be monitored for signs of alpha-blockade (as well as beta-blockade).
- **BREAST FEEDING** Infants should be monitored as there is a risk of possible toxicity due to alpha-blockade (in addition to beta-blockade).
- **HEPATIC IMPAIRMENT** EvGr Avoid in severe impairment. (M)
  - ▶ When used for Prevention of bleeding from medium or large oesophageal varices or Primary prevention of decompensated cirrhosis EvGr Caution in mild to moderate impairment (may have greater effect on heart rate and blood pressure). (A)

  Dose adjustments EvGr Dose adjustment may be required in moderate impairment. (M)

- **MONITORING REQUIREMENTS** Monitor renal function during dose titration in patients with heart failure who also have renal impairment, low blood pressure, ischaemic heart disease, or diffuse vascular disease.
- **PATIENT AND CARER ADVICE**
Medicines for Children leaflet: Carvedilol for heart failure
www.medicinesforchildren.org.uk/medicines/carvedilol-for-heart-failure/

- **MEDICINAL FORMS** There can be variation in the licensing of different medicines containing the same drug. Forms available from special-order manufacturers include: oral suspension

Oral tablet

CAUTIONARY AND ADVISORY LABELS 8

- Carvedilol (Non-proprietary)
  - **Carvedilol 3.125 mg** Carvedilol 3.125mg tablets | 28 tablet PoM £2.13 DT = £0.72
  - **Carvedilol 6.25 mg** Carvedilol 6.25mg tablets | 28 tablet PoM £3.66 DT = £1.07
  - **Carvedilol 12.5 mg** Carvedilol 12.5mg tablets | 28 tablet PoM £4.05 DT = £1.05
  - **Carvedilol 25 mg** Carvedilol 25mg tablets | 28 tablet PoM £4.75 DT = £1.07

DIURETICS › POTASSIUM-SPARING DIURETICS › MINERALOCORTICOID RECEPTOR ANTAGONISTS

Potassium canrenoate

11-Dec-2020

- **INDICATIONS AND DOSE**

Short-term diuresis for oedema in heart failure and in ascites

▶ BY INTRAVENOUS INJECTION, OR BY INTRAVENOUS INFUSION

- Neonate: 1–2 mg/kg twice daily.
- Child 1 month–11 years: 1–2 mg/kg twice daily
- Child 12–17 years: 1–2 mg/kg twice daily (max. per dose 200 mg)

DOSE EQUIVALENCE AND CONVERSION

- To convert to equivalent oral spironolactone dose, multiply potassium canrenoate dose by 0.7.

- **UNLICENSED USE** Not licensed for use in the UK.
- **CONTRA-INDICATIONS** Hyperkalaemia · hyponatraemia
- **CAUTIONS** Acute porphyrias p. 745 · hypotension · *rodent* studies indicate potential carcinogenic risk
- **INTERACTIONS** → Appendix 1: potassium canrenoate
- **SIDE-EFFECTS**
  - **Common or very common** Ataxia · drowsiness · headache · hyperuricaemia · menstruation irregular
  - **Uncommon** Electrolyte imbalance · eosinophilia · thrombocytopenia
  - **Rare or very rare** Agranulocytosis · alopecia · hepatotoxicity · hypersensitivity · osteomalacia · skin reactions · voice alteration
  - **Frequency not known** Acidosis hyperchloraemic · breast pain · confusion (transient; with high doses) · gastrointestinal disorder · gynaecomastia · hirsutism · hypotension
- **PREGNANCY** Crosses placenta. Feminisation and undescended testes in male fetus in *animal* studies—manufacturer advises avoid.
- **BREAST FEEDING** Present in breast milk—manufacturer advises avoid.
- **RENAL IMPAIRMENT** Use with caution if estimated glomerular filtration rate 30–60 mL/minute/1.73 m^2. Avoid if estimated glomerular filtration rate less than 30 mL/minute/1.73 m^2.
Monitoring Monitor plasma-potassium concentration if estimated glomerular filtration rate 30–60 mL/minute/1.73 m^2.
- **MONITORING REQUIREMENTS** Monitor electrolytes (discontinue if hyperkalaemia occurs).
- **DIRECTIONS FOR ADMINISTRATION** For *intravenous injection*, manufacturer advises give over 2–3 minutes (consult product literature).
- **PRESCRIBING AND DISPENSING INFORMATION** Potassium canrenoate injection is available from 'special-order' manufacturers or specialist importing companies.

- **MEDICINAL FORMS** There can be variation in the licensing of different medicines containing the same drug.

Solution for injection

- Potassium canrenoate (Non-proprietary)
  - **Potassium canrenoate 20 mg per 1 ml** Potassium canrenoate 200mg/10ml solution for injection ampoules | 1 ampoule PoM ⊠ Aldactone 200mg/10ml solution for injection ampoules | 10 ampoule PoM ⊠

Spironolactone

14-May-2025

- **INDICATIONS AND DOSE**

Oedema in heart failure and in ascites | Nephrotic syndrome

▶ BY MOUTH

- Neonate: Initially 1–2 mg/kg daily in 1–2 divided doses, dose increased if necessary up to 7 mg/kg per day in resistant ascites.
- Child 1 month–11 years: Initially 1–3 mg/kg daily in 1–2 divided doses, dose increased if necessary up to 9 mg/kg per day in resistant ascites
- Child 12–17 years: Initially 50–100 mg daily in 1–2 divided doses, dose increased if necessary up to 9 mg/kg per day in resistant ascites; maximum 400 mg per day

Reduction of hypokalaemia induced by diuretics or amphotericin B

▶ BY MOUTH

- Neonate: Initially 1–2 mg/kg daily in 1–2 divided doses.
- Child 1 month–11 years: Initially 1–3 mg/kg daily in 1–2 divided doses
- Child 12–17 years: Initially 50–100 mg daily in 1–2 divided doses

- **UNLICENSED USE** Not licensed for reduction of hypokalaemia induced by diuretics or amphotericin B.
- **CONTRA-INDICATIONS** Addison's disease · anuria · hyperkalaemia
- **CAUTIONS** Acute porphyrias p. 745 · *rodent* studies indicate potential carcinogenic risk
- **INTERACTIONS** → Appendix 1: mineralocorticoid receptor antagonists
- **SIDE-EFFECTS** Acidosis hyperchloraemic · acute kidney injury · agranulocytosis · alopecia · breast neoplasm benign · breast pain · confusion · dizziness · electrolyte imbalance · gastrointestinal disorder · gynaecomastia · hepatic function abnormal · hyperkalaemia (discontinue) · hypertrichosis · leg cramps · leucopenia · libido disorder · malaise · menstrual disorder · nausea · severe cutaneous adverse reactions (SCARs) · skin reactions · thrombocytopenia
- **PREGNANCY** Use only if potential benefit outweighs risk—feminisation of male fetus in *animal* studies.
- **BREAST FEEDING** Metabolites present in milk, but amount probably too small to be harmful.
- **RENAL IMPAIRMENT** Avoid in acute renal insufficiency or severe impairment.
Monitoring Monitor plasma-potassium concentration (high risk of hyperkalaemia in renal impairment).

- **MONITORING REQUIREMENTS** Monitor electrolytes—discontinue if hyperkalaemia occurs.
- **PRESCRIBING AND DISPENSING INFORMATION** The RCPCH and NPPG recommend that, when a liquid formulation of spironolactone is required, the following strength is used: 50 mg/5 mL.
- **PATIENT AND CARER ADVICE**
Medicines for Children leaflet: Spironolactone for heart failure www.medicinesforchildren.org.uk/medicines/spironolactone-for-heart-failure/

- **MEDICINAL FORMS** There can be variation in the licensing of different medicines containing the same drug. Forms available from special-order manufacturers include: oral suspension, oral solution

Oral tablet

CAUTIONARY AND ADVISORY LABELS 21

▸ **Spironolactone (Non-proprietary)**
Spironolactone 12.5 mg Spironolactone 12.5mg tablets | 28 tablet PoM £24.00 DT = £23.19
Spironolactone 25 mg Spironolactone 25mg tablets | 28 tablet PoM £1.34 DT = £0.91
Spironolactone 50 mg Spironolactone 50mg tablets | 28 tablet PoM £4.26 DT = £1.70
Spironolactone 100 mg Spironolactone 100mg tablets | 28 tablet PoM £4.38 DT = £1.69

▸ **Aldactone** (Pfizer Ltd)
Spironolactone 25 mg Aldactone 25mg tablets | 100 tablet PoM £8.89
Spironolactone 50 mg Aldactone 50mg tablets | 100 tablet PoM £17.78
Spironolactone 100 mg Aldactone 100mg tablets | 28 tablet PoM £9.96 DT = £1.69

Oral solution

▸ **Spironolactone (Non-proprietary)**
Spironolactone 5 mg per 1 ml Spironolactone 25mg/5ml oral solution sugar free | 125 ml PoM £119.87–£180.00 SF

▸ **Urospir** (Rosemont Pharmaceuticals Ltd)
Spironolactone 5 mg per 1 ml Urospir 25mg/5ml oral solution | 150 ml PoM £123.93 SF
Spironolactone 10 mg per 1 ml Urospir 50mg/5ml oral solution | 150 ml PoM £247.85 SF

Oral suspension

CAUTIONARY AND ADVISORY LABELS 21

▸ **Qaialdo** (Nova Laboratories Ltd)
Spironolactone 10 mg per 1 ml Qaialdo 10mg/ml oral suspension | 150 ml PoM £247.85

DRUGS ACTING ON THE RENIN-ANGIOTENSIN SYSTEM › ANGIOTENSIN II RECEPTOR ANTAGONISTS

Sacubitril with valsartan

03-Sep-2024

The properties listed below are those particular to the combination only. For the properties of the components please consider, valsartan p. 135.

- **DRUG ACTION** Sacubitril (a prodrug) inhibits the breakdown of natriuretic peptides resulting in varied effects including increased diuresis, natriuresis, and vasodilation.

- **INDICATIONS AND DOSE**

Symptomatic chronic heart failure with left ventricular systolic dysfunction [in patients not currently taking an ACE inhibitor or angiotensin II receptor antagonist, or stabilised on low doses of either of these agents] (dose rounded to the closest combination of full 6/6 mg and/or 15/16 mg strength capsules containing granules)

▶ BY MOUTH USING GRANULES
▸ Child 1–17 years (body-weight up to 40 kg): Initially 0.8 mg/kg twice daily for 3–4 weeks, increased if tolerated to 1.6 mg/kg twice daily (max. per dose 50 mg) for 3–4 weeks, increased if tolerated to 2.3 mg/kg twice daily for 3–4 weeks, then increased if tolerated to 3.1 mg/kg twice daily

Symptomatic chronic heart failure with left ventricular systolic dysfunction [in patients not currently taking an ACE inhibitor or angiotensin II receptor antagonist, or stabilised on low doses of either of these agents]

▶ BY MOUTH
▸ Child 1–17 years (body-weight 40–49 kg): Initially 0.8 mg/kg twice daily for 3–4 weeks, dose rounded to the closest combination of full 6/6 mg or 15/16 mg strength capsules containing granules, increased if tolerated to 50 mg twice daily for 3–4 weeks, dose to be given using 24/26 mg strength tablet, increased if tolerated to 100 mg twice daily for 3–4 weeks, dose to be given using 49/51 mg strength tablet, then increased if tolerated to 150 mg twice daily, dose to be given using 24/26 mg plus 49/51 mg strength tablets
▸ Child 1–17 years (body-weight 50 kg and above): Initially 50 mg twice daily for 3–4 weeks, dose to be given using 24/26 mg strength tablet, increased if tolerated to 100 mg twice daily for 3–4 weeks, dose to be given using 49/51 mg strength tablet, increased if tolerated to 150 mg twice daily for 3–4 weeks, dose to be given using 24/26 mg plus 49/51 mg strength tablets, then increased if tolerated to 200 mg twice daily, dose to be given using 97/103 mg strength tablet

Symptomatic chronic heart failure with left ventricular systolic dysfunction [in patients currently stabilised on an ACE inhibitor or angiotensin II receptor antagonist] (dose rounded to the closest combination of full 6/6 mg or 15/16 mg strength capsules containing granules)

▶ BY MOUTH USING GRANULES
▸ Child 1–17 years (body-weight up to 40 kg): Initially 1.6 mg/kg twice daily (max. per dose 50 mg) for 2–4 weeks, increased if tolerated to 2.3 mg/kg twice daily for 2–4 weeks, then increased if tolerated to 3.1 mg/kg twice daily

Symptomatic chronic heart failure with left ventricular systolic dysfunction [in patients currently stabilised on an ACE inhibitor or angiotensin II receptor antagonist]

▶ BY MOUTH
▸ Child 1–17 years (body-weight 40–49 kg): Initially 50 mg twice daily for 2–4 weeks, dose to be given using 24/26 mg strength tablet, increased if tolerated to 100 mg twice daily for 2–4 weeks, dose to be given using 49/51 mg strength tablet, then increased if tolerated to 150 mg twice daily, dose to be given using 24/26 mg plus 49/51 mg strength tablets
▸ Child 1–17 years (body-weight 50 kg and above): Initially 100 mg twice daily for 2–4 weeks, dose to be given using 49/51 mg strength tablet, increased if tolerated to 150 mg twice daily for 2–4 weeks, dose to be given using 24/26 mg plus 49/51 mg strength tablets, then increased if tolerated to 200 mg twice daily, dose to be given using 97/103 mg strength tablet

DOSE EQUIVALENCE AND CONVERSION
▸ *Entresto*® tablets and granules contain *x*/*y* mg of sacubitril and valsartan, respectively.
▸ Doses in BNF Publications are expressed as the total of both drug strengths.
▸ For *Entresto*® tablets, used in patients weighing 40 kg or more, the 24/26 mg strength equates to a dose of 50 mg, the 49/51 mg strength equates to a dose of 100 mg, and the 97/103 mg strength equates to a dose of 200 mg.
▸ For *Entresto*® granules in capsules for opening, used in children weighing less than 40 kg, the 6/6 mg strength equates to a dose of 12 mg and the 15/16 mg strength equates to a dose of 31 mg.
▸ Valsartan in *Entresto*® is more bioavailable than other tablet formulations—26 mg, 51 mg, and 103 mg

valsartan in *Entresto*® is equivalent to 40 mg, 80 mg, and 160 mg, respectively, in other valsartan tablet formulations.

- **CONTRA-INDICATIONS** Concomitant use with an ACE inhibitor (risk of angioedema—do not initiate until at least 36 hours after the last dose when switching treatment) · concomitant use with an angiotensin II receptor antagonist · hereditary or idiopathic angioedema · known history of angioedema related to previous ACE inhibitor or angiotensin II receptor antagonist
- **CAUTIONS** Serum-potassium concentration above 5.3 mmol/litre (do not initiate—may increase risk of hyperkalaemia) · systolic BP less than 5th percentile for the age of the child (do not initiate—limited data available)
- **INTERACTIONS** → Appendix 1: angiotensin-II receptor antagonists · sacubitril
- **SIDE-EFFECTS**
  - **Common or very common** Anaemia · asthenia · cough · diarrhoea · dizziness · electrolyte imbalance · gastritis · headache · hypoglycaemia · hypotension · nausea · renal impairment · syncope · vertigo
  - **Uncommon** Angioedema · skin reactions
  - **Rare or very rare** Hallucinations · paranoia · sleep disorder
  - **Frequency not known** Psychiatric disorder
- **PREGNANCY** EvGr Avoid—toxicity with sacubitril in *animal* studies. (M)
- **BREAST FEEDING** EvGr Avoid—present in milk in *animal* studies. (M)
- **HEPATIC IMPAIRMENT** EvGr Caution in moderate impairment or if hepatic transaminases exceed 2 times the upper limit of normal (limited information available); avoid in severe impairment, biliary cirrhosis, or cholestasis (no information available). (M)

  Dose adjustments EvGr In moderate impairment or if hepatic transaminases exceed 2 times the upper limit of normal, start with 50 mg twice daily (dose to be given using 24/26 mg strength tablet) in those weighing at least 50 kg, or 0.8 mg/kg twice daily (dose rounded to the closest combination of full 6/6 mg or 15/16 mg strength capsules containing granules) in those weighing less than 50 kg. (M)
- **RENAL IMPAIRMENT** EvGr Caution (increased risk of hypotension; limited information available in severe impairment); avoid in end-stage renal disease (no information available). (M)

  Dose adjustments EvGr If estimated glomerular filtration rate less than 30 mL/minute/1.73m^2,start with 50 mg twice daily (dose to be given using 24/26 mg strength tablet) in those weighing at least 50 kg, or 0.8 mg/kg twice daily (dose rounded to the closest combination of full 6/6 mg or 15/16 mg strength capsules containing granules) in those weighing less than 50 kg. Also consider these starting doses if estimated glomerular filtration rate 30–60 mL/minute/1.73m^2. (M) See p. 16.
- **DIRECTIONS FOR ADMINISTRATION** EvGr *Entresto*® oral granules are administered by opening the capsule and sprinkling the granules onto a small amount (1 to 2 teaspoons) of soft food, then given immediately. Capsules should not be swallowed whole. (M)
- **PATIENT AND CARER ADVICE** Patients and their carers should be given advice on how to administer *Entresto*® oral granules.

- **MEDICINAL FORMS** There can be variation in the licensing of different medicines containing the same drug.

Oral tablet

- **Entresto** (Novartis Pharmaceuticals UK Ltd)
  - **Sacubitril 24 mg, Valsartan 26 mg** Entresto 24mg/26mg tablets | 28 tablet PoM £45.78 DT = £45.78
  - **Sacubitril 49 mg, Valsartan 51 mg** Entresto 49mg/51mg tablets | 28 tablet PoM £45.78 | 56 tablet PoM £91.56 DT = £91.56
  - **Sacubitril 97 mg, Valsartan 103 mg** Entresto 97mg/103mg tablets | 56 tablet PoM £91.56 DT = £91.56

Oral granules

- **Entresto** (Novartis Pharmaceuticals UK Ltd)
  - **Sacubitril 6 mg, Valsartan 6 mg** Entresto 6mg/6mg granules in capsules for opening | 60 capsule PoM £10.14
  - **Sacubitril 15 mg, Valsartan 16 mg** Entresto 15mg/16mg granules in capsules for opening | 60 capsule PoM £25.36

PHOSPHODIESTERASE TYPE-3 INHIBITORS

Enoximone

24-Jun-2021

- **DRUG ACTION** Enoximone is a phosphodiesterase type-3 inhibitor that exerts most effect on the myocardium; it has positive inotropic properties and vasodilator activity.
- **INDICATIONS AND DOSE**

Congestive heart failure, low cardiac output following cardiac surgery

- INITIALLY BY SLOW INTRAVENOUS INJECTION
  - Neonate: Loading dose 500 micrograms/kg, followed by (by continuous intravenous infusion) 5–20 micrograms/kg/minute, adjusted according to response, infusion to be given over 24 hours; maximum 24 mg/kg per day.
  - Child: Loading dose 500 micrograms/kg, followed by (by continuous intravenous infusion) 5–20 micrograms/kg/minute, adjusted according to response, infusion dose to be given over 24 hours; maximum 24 mg/kg per day

- **UNLICENSED USE** Not licensed for use in children.
- **CAUTIONS** Heart failure associated with hypertrophic cardiomyopathy, stenotic or obstructive valvular disease or other outlet obstruction
- **SIDE-EFFECTS**
  - **Common or very common** Headache · hypotension · insomnia
  - **Uncommon** Arrhythmias · diarrhoea · dizziness · nausea · vomiting
  - **Rare or very rare** Chills · fever · fluid retention · myalgia · oliguria · urinary retention
- **PREGNANCY** Manufacturer advises use only if potential benefit outweighs risk.
- **BREAST FEEDING** Manufacturer advises caution—no information available.
- **RENAL IMPAIRMENT**

  Dose adjustments In adults, manufacturer advises consider dose reduction (consult product literature).
- **MONITORING REQUIREMENTS** Monitor blood pressure, heart rate, ECG, central venous pressure, fluid and electrolyte status, renal function, platelet count and hepatic enzymes.
- **DIRECTIONS FOR ADMINISTRATION** Incompatible with glucose solutions. Use only plastic containers or syringes; crystal formation if glass used. Avoid extravasation.

  For *intravenous administration*, dilute to concentration of 2.5 mg/mL with Sodium Chloride 0.9% or Water for Injections; the initial loading dose should be given by slow intravenous injection over at least 15 minutes.
- **PRESCRIBING AND DISPENSING INFORMATION** Phosphodiesterase type-3 inhibitors possess positive inotropic and vasodilator activity and are useful in infants and children with low cardiac output especially after cardiac surgery. Phosphodiesterase type-3 inhibitors should be limited to short-term use because long-term oral administration has been associated with increased mortality in adults with congestive heart failure.

● **PATIENT AND CARER ADVICE**
Medicines for Children leaflet: Enoximone for pulmonary hypertension www.medicinesforchildren.org.uk/medicines/enoximone-for-pulmonary-hypertension/

● **MEDICINAL FORMS** There can be variation in the licensing of different medicines containing the same drug.

Solution for injection

EXCIPIENTS: May contain Alcohol, propylene glycol

▸ **Perfan** (Macure Pharma UK Ltd)
Enoximone 5 mg per 1 ml Perfan 100mg/20ml solution for injection ampoules | 10 ampoule PoM £150.15 (Hospital only)

Milrinone

27-Jan-2020

● **DRUG ACTION** Milrinone is a phosphodiesterase type-3 inhibitor that exerts most effect on the myocardium; it has positive inotropic properties and vasodilator activity.

● **INDICATIONS AND DOSE**

Congestive heart failure, low cardiac output following cardiac surgery, shock

▶ INITIALLY BY INTRAVENOUS INFUSION

▸ Neonate: Initially 50–75 micrograms/kg, given over 30-60 minutes, reduce or omit initial dose if at risk of hypotension, then (by continuous intravenous infusion) 30–45 micrograms/kg/hour for 2–3 days (usually for 12 hours after cardiac surgery).

▸ Child: Initially 50–75 micrograms/kg, given over 30-60 minutes, reduce or omit initial dose if at risk of hypotension, then (by continuous intravenous infusion) 30–45 micrograms/kg/hour for 2–3 days (usually for 12 hours after cardiac surgery)

● **UNLICENSED USE** Not licensed for use in children under 18 years.

● **CONTRA-INDICATIONS** Severe hypovolaemia

● **CAUTIONS** Correct hypokalaemia · heart failure associated with hypertrophic cardiomyopathy, stenotic or obstructive valvular disease or other outlet obstruction

● **SIDE-EFFECTS**

▶ **Common or very common** Arrhythmia supraventricular (increased risk in patients with pre-existing arrhythmias) · arrhythmias · headache · hypotension

▶ **Uncommon** Angina pectoris · chest pain · hypokalaemia · thrombocytopenia · tremor

▶ **Rare or very rare** Anaphylactic shock · bronchospasm · skin eruption

▶ **Frequency not known** Intraventricular haemorrhage · renal failure

● **PREGNANCY** Manufacturer advises use only if potential benefit outweighs risk.

● **BREAST FEEDING** Manufacturer advises avoid—no information available.

● **RENAL IMPAIRMENT**

Dose adjustments Use half to three-quarters normal dose and monitor response if estimated glomerular filtration rate less than 50 mL/minute/1.73 m^2.

● **MONITORING REQUIREMENTS** Monitor blood pressure, heart rate, ECG, central venous pressure, fluid and electrolyte status, renal function, platelet count and hepatic enzymes.

● **DIRECTIONS FOR ADMINISTRATION** Avoid extravasation.

For *intravenous infusion* dilute with Glucose 5% or Sodium Chloride 0.9% *or* Sodium Chloride and Glucose intravenous infusion to a concentration of 200 micrograms/mL (higher concentrations of 400 micrograms/mL have been used).

Loading dose may be given undiluted if fluid-restricted.

● **PRESCRIBING AND DISPENSING INFORMATION**
Phosphodiesterase type-3 inhibitors possess positive inotropic and vasodilator activity and are useful in infants and children with low cardiac output especially after cardiac surgery. Phosphodiesterase type-3 inhibitors should be limited to short-term use because long-term oral administration has been associated with increased mortality in adults with congestive heart failure.

● **MEDICINAL FORMS** There can be variation in the licensing of different medicines containing the same drug. Forms available from special-order manufacturers include: solution for infusion

Solution for injection

▸ **Milrinone (Non-proprietary)**
Milrinone (as Milrinone lactate) 1 mg per 1 ml Milrinone 10mg/10ml solution for injection vials | 10 vial PoM £179.06 (Hospital only)

Solution for infusion

▸ **Milrinone (Non-proprietary)**
Milrinone 1 mg per 1 ml Milrinone 10mg/10ml solution for infusion ampoules | 10 ampoule PoM £149.50–£199.06 (Hospital only)
Milrinone 10mg/10ml concentrate for solution for infusion ampoules | 10 ampoule PoM ⊠ (Hospital only)

▸ **Primacor** (Sanofi)
Milrinone 1 mg per 1 ml Primacor 10mg/10ml solution for injection ampoules | 10 ampoule PoM £199.06 (Hospital only)

6 Hyperlipidaemia

Dyslipidaemias

06-Jul-2021

Cardiovascular disease risk factors

Atherosclerosis begins in childhood and raised serum cholesterol in children is associated with cardiovascular disease in adulthood. Lowering the cholesterol, without hindering growth and development in children and adolescents, should reduce the risk of cardiovascular disease in later life.

The risk factors for developing cardiovascular disease include raised serum cholesterol concentration, smoking, hypertension, impaired glucose tolerance, male sex, ethnicity, obesity, triglyceride concentration, chronic kidney disease, and a family history of cardiovascular disease. Heterozygous familial hypercholesterolaemia is the most common cause of raised serum cholesterol in children; homozygous familial hypercholesterolaemia is very rare and its specialised management is not covered in BNFC. EvGr Familial hypercholesterolaemia can lead to a greater risk of early coronary heart disease and should be managed by a specialist. Ⓐ

Secondary causes of hypercholesterolaemia should be addressed, these include obesity, diet, diabetes mellitus, hypothyroidism, nephrotic syndrome, obstructive biliary disease, glycogen storage disease, and drugs such as corticosteroids.

Management

The aim of management of hypercholesterolaemia is to reduce the risk of atherosclerosis while ensuring adequate growth and development. Children with hypercholesterolaemia (or their carers) should receive advice on appropriate lifestyle changes such as improved diet, increased exercise, weight reduction, and Smoking cessation p. 353; Hypertension p. 116 should also be managed appropriately. Drug therapy may also be necessary.

Hypothyroidism

Children with hypothyroidism should receive adequate thyroid replacement therapy before their requirement for lipid-regulating treatment is assessed because correction of hypothyroidism itself may resolve the lipid abnormality.

Untreated hypothyroidism increases the risk of myositis with lipid-regulating drugs.

Heterozygous familial hypercholesterolaemia

In heterozygous familial hypercholesterolaemia, drug treatment is often required as lifestyle modifications alone are unlikely to sufficiently lower cholesterol concentration. EvGr Treatment with lipid-regulating drugs should be considered by the age of 10 years, although the decision to initiate or defer treatment will depend on the child's age, the age of onset of coronary heart disease within the family, and the presence of other cardiovascular risk factors. Lipid-regulating drug treatment before the age of 10 years, or a higher dose of statin than licensed for use in the appropriate age group, or a combination of lipid-regulating drugs should be considered in children with a family history of coronary heart disease in early adulthood.

Statins are the lipid-regulating drug of choice and treatment should be life-long. In children who are intolerant to statins, ezetimibe p. 152, fibrates, or bile acid sequestrants should be considered as alternative options. Vitamins A, D and K, and folic acid supplementation can be given to patients on long-term bile acid sequestrants. Ⓐ

Secondary hypercholesterolaemia

Drug treatment may be indicated in children 10 years and older (rarely necessary in younger children) who are at a high risk of developing cardiovascular disease if 6–12 months of dietary and other lifestyle interventions have failed to lower cholesterol concentration adequately.

Lipid-regulating drugs

Experience in the use of lipid-regulating drugs in children is limited and they should be initiated on specialist advice.

Statins are more effective than other classes of drugs in lowering LDL-cholesterol but less effective than the fibrates in reducing triglycerides. Statins also increase concentrations of HDL-cholesterol. Statins reduce cardiovascular disease events and total mortality in adults, irrespective of the initial cholesterol concentration. They are the drugs of first choice in children and are generally well tolerated; atorvastatin p. 154 and simvastatin p. 156 are the preferred statins. Other lipid-regulating drugs can be used if statins are ineffective or are not tolerated.

Ezetimibe can be used alone when statins are not tolerated, or in combination with a statin when a high dose statin fails to control cholesterol concentration adequately.

Bile acid sequestrants are also available but tolerability of and compliance with these drugs is poor, and their use is declining.

Fibrates may reduce the risk of coronary heart disease in those with low HDL-cholesterol or with raised triglycerides. Evidence for the use of a fibrate (bezafibrate p. 152 or fenofibrate p. 153) in children is limited; fibrates should be considered only if dietary intervention and treatment with a statin and a bile acid sequestrant is unsuccessful or contra-indicated.

Evolocumab p. 157 is licensed for the treatment of homozygous familial hypercholesterolaemia; it is used in combination with other lipid-lowering therapies.

In hypertriglyceridaemia which cannot be controlled by very strict diet, omega-3 fatty acid compounds can be considered.

LIPID MODIFYING DRUGS › BILE ACID SEQUESTRANTS

Bile acid sequestrants

- **DRUG ACTION** Bile acid sequestrants act by binding bile acids, preventing their reabsorption; this promotes hepatic conversion of cholesterol into bile acids; the resultant increased LDL-receptor activity of liver cells increases the clearance of LDL-cholesterol from the plasma.
- **CAUTIONS** Interference with the absorption of fat-soluble vitamins (supplements of vitamins A, D, K, and folic acid may be required when treatment is prolonged).
- **SIDE-EFFECTS**
  - **Common or very common** Constipation · dyspepsia · nausea · vomiting
  - **Rare or very rare** Intestinal obstruction
- **PREGNANCY** Bile acid sequestrants should be used with caution as although the drugs are not absorbed, they may cause fat-soluble vitamin deficiency on prolonged use.
- **BREAST FEEDING** Bile acid sequestrants should be used with caution as although the drugs are not absorbed, they may cause fat-soluble vitamin deficiency on prolonged use.
- **MONITORING REQUIREMENTS** A child's growth and development should be monitored.

above

Colestyramine
(Cholestyramine)

20-Jul-2020

- **INDICATIONS AND DOSE**

Familial hypercholesterolaemia

▸ BY MOUTH

- Child 6–11 years: Initially 4 g once daily, then increased to 4 g up to 3 times a day, adjusted according to response
- Child 12–17 years: Initially 4 g once daily, then increased in steps of 4 g every week; increased to 12–24 g daily in 1–4 divided doses, adjusted according to response; maximum 36 g per day

Pruritus associated with partial biliary obstruction and primary biliary cirrhosis

▸ BY MOUTH

- Child 1–11 months: 1 g once daily, adjusted according to response, total daily dose may alternatively be given in 2–4 divided doses; maximum 9 g per day
- Child 1–5 years: 2 g once daily, adjusted according to response, total daily dose may alternatively be given in 2–4 divided doses; maximum 18 g per day
- Child 6–11 years: 4 g once daily, adjusted according to response, total daily dose may alternatively be given in 2–4 divided doses; maximum 24 g per day
- Child 12–17 years: 4–8 g once daily, adjusted according to response, total daily dose may alternatively be given in 2–4 divided doses; maximum 36 g per day

Diarrhoea associated with Crohn's disease, ileal resection, vagotomy, diabetic vagal neuropathy, and radiation

▸ BY MOUTH

- Child 1–11 months: 1 g once daily, adjusted according to response, total daily dose may alternatively be given in 2–4 divided doses, if no response within 3 days an alternative therapy should be initiated; maximum 9 g per day
- Child 1–5 years: 2 g once daily, adjusted according to response, total daily dose may alternatively be given in 2–4 divided doses, if no response within 3 days an alternative therapy should be initiated; maximum 18 g per day

continued →

- ▸ Child 6–11 years: 4 g once daily, adjusted according to response, total daily dose may alternatively be given in 2–4 divided doses, if no response within 3 days an alternative therapy should be initiated; maximum 24 g per day
- ▸ Child 12–17 years: 4–8 g once daily, adjusted according to response, total daily dose may alternatively be given in 2–4 divided doses, if no response within 3 days an alternative therapy should be initiated; maximum 36 g per day

- **CONTRA-INDICATIONS** Complete biliary obstruction (not likely to be effective)
- **INTERACTIONS** → Appendix 1: colestyramine
- **SIDE-EFFECTS**
  - ▶ **Uncommon** Acidosis hyperchloraemic · appetite decreased · bleeding tendency · diarrhoea · gastrointestinal discomfort · gastrointestinal disorders · hypoprothrombinaemia · night blindness · osteoporosis · skin reactions · tongue irritation · vitamin deficiencies
- **DIRECTIONS FOR ADMINISTRATION** Manufacturer advises the contents of each sachet should be mixed with at least 150 mL of water or other suitable liquid such as fruit juice, skimmed milk, thin soups, and pulpy fruits with a high moisture content.
- **PATIENT AND CARER ADVICE** Patient counselling on administration is advised for colestyramine powder (avoid other drugs at same time).

- **MEDICINAL FORMS** There can be variation in the licensing of different medicines containing the same drug. Forms available from special-order manufacturers include: oral suspension, oral solution

Powder for oral suspension

CAUTIONARY AND ADVISORY LABELS 13

EXCIPIENTS: May contain Aspartame, sucrose

▸ **Colestyramine (Non-proprietary)**
Colestyramine anhydrous 4 gram Colestyramine 4g oral powder sachets sugar free | 50 sachet PoM £35.64 DT = £32.84 SF

▸ **Questran Light** (Neon Healthcare Ltd)
Colestyramine anhydrous 4 gram Questran Light 4g oral powder sachets | 50 sachet PoM £16.15 DT = £32.84 SF

LIPID MODIFYING DRUGS › CHOLESTEROL ABSORPTION INHIBITORS

Ezetimibe

02-Jan-2024

- **DRUG ACTION** Ezetimibe inhibits the intestinal absorption of cholesterol.

- **INDICATIONS AND DOSE**

Adjunct to dietary measures and statin treatment in primary hypercholesterolaemia | Adjunct to dietary measures and statin in homozygous familial hypercholesterolaemia | Primary hypercholesterolaemia (if statin inappropriate or not tolerated) | Adjunct to dietary measures in homozygous sitosterolaemia

▶ BY MOUTH
- ▸ Child 10–17 years: 10 mg once daily

- **INTERACTIONS** → Appendix 1: ezetimibe
- **SIDE-EFFECTS**
  - ▶ **Common or very common** Asthenia · diarrhoea · gastrointestinal discomfort · gastrointestinal disorders · headache · muscle complaints
  - ▶ **Uncommon** Appetite decreased · arthralgia · chest pain · cough · dry mouth · hot flush · hypertension · muscle weakness · nausea · pain · paraesthesia · peripheral oedema · skin reactions
  - ▶ **Frequency not known** Constipation · depression · dizziness · dyspnoea · hepatitis · myopathy · pancreatitis · thrombocytopenia
- **PREGNANCY** Manufacturer advises use only if potential benefit outweighs risk—no information available.
- **BREAST FEEDING** Manufacturer advises avoid—present in milk in *animal* studies.
- **HEPATIC IMPAIRMENT** Manufacturer advises avoid in moderate to severe impairment.

- **MEDICINAL FORMS** There can be variation in the licensing of different medicines containing the same drug.

Oral tablet

▸ **Ezetimibe (Non-proprietary)**
Ezetimibe 10 mg Ezetimibe 10mg tablets | 28 tablet PoM £29.50 DT = £0.94

▸ **Ezetrol** (Organon Pharma (UK) Ltd)
Ezetimibe 10 mg Ezetrol 10mg tablets | 28 tablet PoM £26.31 DT = £0.94

Combinations available: *Simvastatin with ezetimibe*, p. 157

LIPID MODIFYING DRUGS › FIBRATES

Bezafibrate

09-Aug-2021

- **DRUG ACTION** Fibrates act by decreasing serum triglycerides; they have variable effect on LDL-cholesterol.

- **INDICATIONS AND DOSE**

Hyperlipidaemia including familial hypercholesterolaemia (administered on expert advice)

▶ BY MOUTH USING IMMEDIATE-RELEASE MEDICINES
- ▸ Child 10–17 years: 200 mg once daily, increased if necessary up to 200 mg 3 times a day, to be adjusted according to response

- **UNLICENSED USE** Not licensed for use in children.
- **CONTRA-INDICATIONS** Gall bladder disease · hypoalbuminaemia · nephrotic syndrome · photosensitivity to fibrates
- **CAUTIONS** Correct hypothyroidism before initiating treatment · risk factors for myopathy
- **INTERACTIONS** → Appendix 1: fibrates
- **SIDE-EFFECTS**
  - ▶ **Common or very common** Appetite decreased · gastrointestinal disorder
  - ▶ **Uncommon** Acute kidney injury · alopecia · cholestasis · constipation · diarrhoea · dizziness · erectile dysfunction · gastrointestinal discomfort · headache · muscle complaints · muscle weakness · nausea · photosensitivity reaction · skin reactions
  - ▶ **Rare or very rare** Cholelithiasis · depression · insomnia · interstitial lung disease · pancreatitis · pancytopenia · paraesthesia · peripheral neuropathy · rhabdomyolysis (increased risk in renal impairment) · severe cutaneous adverse reactions (SCARs) · thrombocytopenic purpura
- **PREGNANCY** Manufacturers advise avoid—no information available.
- **BREAST FEEDING** Manufacturer advises avoid—no information available.
- **HEPATIC IMPAIRMENT** Manufacturer advises avoid in significant impairment (except in fatty liver disease).
- **RENAL IMPAIRMENT** Manufacturer advises avoid *immediate-release* preparations if creatinine clearance less than 15 mL/minute. Manufacturer advises avoid *modified-release* preparations if creatinine clearance less than 60 mL/minute.

  Myotoxicity Manufacturer advises special care needed in patients with renal disease, as progressive increases in serum creatinine concentration or failure to follow dosage guidelines may result in myotoxicity (rhabdomyolysis); discontinue if myotoxicity suspected or creatine kinase concentration increases significantly.

Dose adjustments See p. 16.

In adults, manufacturer advises reduce dose if creatinine clearance 15–60 mL/minute (consult product literature).

- **MONITORING REQUIREMENTS** Consider monitoring of liver function and creatine kinase when fibrates used in combination with a statin.
- **PRESCRIBING AND DISPENSING INFORMATION** Fibrates are mainly used in those whose serum-triglyceride concentration is greater than 10 mmol/litre or in those who cannot tolerate a statin (specialist use).

- **MEDICINAL FORMS** There can be variation in the licensing of different medicines containing the same drug. Forms available from special-order manufacturers include: oral suspension

Oral tablet

CAUTIONARY AND ADVISORY LABELS 21

▸ **Bezafibrate (Non-proprietary)**
Bezafibrate 200 mg Bezafibrate 200mg tablets | 100 tablet PoM £9.00 DT = £9.92

Fenofibrate

09-Aug-2021

- **DRUG ACTION** Fibrates act by decreasing serum triglycerides; they have variable effect on LDL-cholesterol.

- **INDICATIONS AND DOSE**

Hyperlipidaemias including familial hypercholesterolaemia (administered on expert advice)

▸ BY MOUTH USING CAPSULES

▸ Child 4–14 years: One 67 mg (micronised) capsule per 20 kg body-weight daily, maximum four 67 mg capsules daily, or max. three 67 mg capsules daily with concomitant statin

▸ Child 15–17 years: Initially 3 capsules daily, then increased if necessary to 4 capsules daily, max. 3 capsules daily with concomitant statin, dose relates to 67 mg (micronised) capsules

DOSE ADJUSTMENTS DUE TO INTERACTIONS

▸ Manufacturer advises max. dose 200 mg daily with concurrent use of a statin—no specific recommendation made for children.

- **UNLICENSED USE** 200 mg and 267 mg capsules not licensed in children. Tablets not licensed in children.
- **CONTRA-INDICATIONS** Gall bladder disease · pancreatitis (unless due to severe hypertriglyceridaemia) · photosensitivity to fibrates · photosensitivity to ketoprofen
- **CAUTIONS** Correct hypothyroidism before initiating treatment · risk factors for myopathy
- **INTERACTIONS** → Appendix 1: fibrates
- **SIDE-EFFECTS**

▸ **Common or very common** Abdominal pain · diarrhoea · flatulence · nausea · vomiting

▸ **Uncommon** Cholelithiasis · embolism and thrombosis · headache · muscle complaints · muscle weakness · myopathy · pancreatitis · sexual dysfunction · skin reactions

▸ **Rare or very rare** Alopecia · hepatic disorders · photosensitivity reaction

▸ **Frequency not known** Fatigue · interstitial lung disease · rhabdomyolysis (increased risk in renal impairment) · severe cutaneous adverse reactions (SCARs)

- **PREGNANCY** Avoid—embryotoxicity in *animal* studies.
- **BREAST FEEDING** Manufacturers advise avoid—no information available.
- **HEPATIC IMPAIRMENT** Manufacturer advises avoid —no information available.
- **RENAL IMPAIRMENT** EvGr Use with caution in mild-to-moderate impairment; avoid if estimated glomerular filtration rate less than 30 mL/minute/1.73 m^2. (M)

Myotoxicity EvGr Special care needed in patients with renal disease, as progressive increases in serum creatinine concentration or failure to follow dosage guidelines may result in myotoxicity (rhabdomyolysis); discontinue if myotoxicity suspected or creatine kinase concentration increases significantly. (M)

Dose adjustments See p. 16.

EvGr Max. 67 mg daily if estimated glomerular filtration rate 30–59 mL/minute/1.73 m^2. (M)

- **MONITORING REQUIREMENTS** Manufacturer advises monitor hepatic transaminases every 3 months during the first 12 months of treatment and periodically thereafter—discontinue treatment if levels increase to more than 3 times the upper limit of normal; monitor serum creatinine levels during the first 3 months of treatment and periodically thereafter—interrupt treatment if creatinine level is 50% above the upper limit of normal.
- **PRESCRIBING AND DISPENSING INFORMATION** Fibrates are mainly used in those whose serum-triglyceride concentration is greater than 10 mmol/litre or in those who cannot tolerate a statin (specialist use).

- **MEDICINAL FORMS** There can be variation in the licensing of different medicines containing the same drug.

Oral capsule

CAUTIONARY AND ADVISORY LABELS 21

▸ **Fenofibrate (Non-proprietary)**
Fenofibrate micronised 67 mg Fenofibrate micronised 67mg capsules | 90 capsule PoM £23.30 DT = £20.39
Fenofibrate micronised 200 mg Fenofibrate micronised 200mg capsules | 28 capsule PoM £5.00 DT = £3.28
Fenofibrate micronised 267 mg Fenofibrate micronised 267mg capsules | 28 capsule PoM £34.00 DT = £17.67

▸ **Lipantil Micro** (Viatris UK Healthcare Ltd)
Fenofibrate micronised 67 mg Lipantil Micro 67 capsules | 90 capsule PoM £23.30 DT = £20.39
Fenofibrate micronised 200 mg Lipantil Micro 200 capsules | 28 capsule PoM £14.23 DT = £3.28
Fenofibrate micronised 267 mg Lipantil Micro 267 capsules | 28 capsule PoM £21.75 DT = £17.67

LIPID MODIFYING DRUGS › STATINS

Statins

- **DRUG ACTION** Statins competitively inhibit 3-hydroxy-3-methylglutaryl coenzyme A (HMG CoA) reductase, an enzyme involved in cholesterol synthesis, especially in the liver.

IMPORTANT SAFETY INFORMATION

MHRA/CHM ADVICE: STATINS: VERY INFREQUENT REPORTS OF MYASTHENIA GRAVIS (SEPTEMBER 2023)

There has been a very small number of reports of new-onset, or exacerbation of pre-existing, myasthenia gravis or ocular myasthenia associated with statin use, albeit very infrequent and no reported fatalities. In most cases, patients recovered after stopping statin treatment. However, a minority continued to experience symptoms, some of which recurred on rechallenge with the same, or an alternative, statin. Symptom onset ranged from a few days to 3 months after starting statin treatment.

Healthcare professionals are advised to refer patients who present with suspected new-onset myasthenia gravis symptoms, after starting a statin, to a neurologist—the statin may need to be discontinued if its risks outweigh the benefits. Healthcare professionals are also advised to counsel patients and their carers to:

- inform their doctor, before taking a statin, if they have a history of myasthenia gravis or ocular myasthenia as it may exacerbate their symptoms;
- continue taking their statin unless they are advised to stop;

- inform their doctor if they experience symptoms such as weakness in the arms or legs that worsens after activity, double vision, drooping of the eyelids, difficulty swallowing, or shortness of breath;
- seek immediate medical attention if they develop severe breathing or swallowing problems.

● **CAUTIONS** Risk factors for muscle toxicity, including myopathy or rhabdomyolysis

CAUTIONS, FURTHER INFORMATION

▸ Muscle effects EvGr Muscle toxicity can occur with all statins, however the likelihood increases with higher doses and in certain patients. Statins should be used with caution in patients at increased risk of muscle toxicity. This includes those with a personal or family history of muscular disorders, history of muscular toxicity or unexplained persistent muscle pain, history of liver disease, known genetic polymorphisms—consult product literature, renal impairment, hypothyroidism, or those who undertake strenuous exercise. (M) See also *Monitoring requirements*.

▸ Hypothyroidism Hypothyroidism should be managed adequately before starting treatment with a statin.

● **SIDE-EFFECTS**

▶ **Common or very common** Arthralgia · asthenia · constipation · diarrhoea · dizziness · flatulence · gastrointestinal discomfort · headache · muscle complaints · nausea · sleep disorders · thrombocytopenia

▶ **Uncommon** Alopecia · hepatic disorders · memory loss · pancreatitis · paraesthesia · sexual dysfunction · skin reactions · vomiting

▶ **Rare or very rare** Lupus-like syndrome · myopathy · peripheral neuropathy · tendon disorders

▶ **Frequency not known** Depression · diabetes mellitus (in those at risk) · interstitial lung disease · neuromuscular dysfunction

SIDE-EFFECTS, FURTHER INFORMATION **Muscle effects** Although myalgia has been reported commonly in patients receiving statins, muscle toxicity truly attributable to statin use is rare. The risk of myopathy, myositis, and rhabdomyolysis associated with statin use is also rare. If muscle pain, weakness, or cramps occur during treatment, creatine kinase concentrations should be measured; if the concentration is more than 5 times the ULN (in the absence of strenuous exercise), treatment should be discontinued. If muscular symptoms are severe and cause daily discomfort, treatment discontinuation should be considered, even if creatine kinase concentrations are less than 5 times the ULN. If symptoms resolve and creatine kinase concentrations return to normal, the statin can be reintroduced, or introduction of an alternative statin can be considered, at the lowest dose and the patient monitored closely.

Interstitial lung disease If patients develop symptoms such as dyspnoea, cough, and weight loss, they should seek medical attention.

● **CONCEPTION AND CONTRACEPTION** Adequate contraception is required during treatment and for 1 month afterwards.

● **PREGNANCY** Statins should be avoided in pregnancy (discontinue 3 months before attempting to conceive) as congenital anomalies have been reported and the decreased synthesis of cholesterol possibly affects fetal development.

● **HEPATIC IMPAIRMENT** In general, manufacturers advise caution (risk of increased exposure); avoid in active disease or unexplained persistent elevations in serum transaminases.

● **MONITORING REQUIREMENTS**

▶ EvGr Before starting treatment with statins, at least one full lipid profile should be measured, including total cholesterol, triglycerides, HDL-cholesterol, non-HDL-cholesterol and LDL-cholesterol concentrations, and repeated 2–3 months after starting or changing treatment. Baseline thyroid-stimulating hormone (in patients with symptoms of underactive or overactive thyroid), and renal function should also be assessed. (A)

▶ Liver function EvGr Liver transaminases should be measured before starting treatment with statins, repeated 2–3 months after starting or changing treatment, and then at 12 months, unless indicated at other times by signs or symptoms suggestive of hepatotoxicity. Patients with serum transaminases that are raised, but less than 3 times the upper limit of normal (ULN), should **not** be routinely excluded from statin therapy. (A) EvGr Those with serum transaminases of more than 3 times the ULN should discontinue statin therapy. (M)

▶ Muscle effects Creatine kinase concentration should be measured in children before treatment and if unexplained muscle pain occurs.

● **PATIENT AND CARER ADVICE** Advise patients to report promptly unexplained muscle pain, tenderness, or weakness.

153

Atorvastatin

12-Sep-2024

● **INDICATIONS AND DOSE**

Hyperlipidaemia including familial hypercholesterolaemia

▶ BY MOUTH

▸ Child 10–17 years: Initially 10 mg once daily, then increased if necessary up to 20 mg once daily, dose to be adjusted at intervals of at least 4 weeks

Homozygous familial hypercholesterolaemia

▶ BY MOUTH

▸ Child 10–17 years: Initially 10 mg once daily, then increased if necessary up to 80 mg once daily, dose to be adjusted at intervals of at least 4 weeks

DOSE ADJUSTMENTS DUE TO INTERACTIONS

▸ Manufacturer advises if concurrent use of ciclosporin is unavoidable, max. dose cannot exceed 10 mg daily.

● **CAUTIONS** Haemorrhagic stroke

● **INTERACTIONS** → Appendix 1: statins

● **SIDE-EFFECTS**

▶ **Common or very common** Epistaxis · hyperglycaemia · hypersensitivity · joint swelling · laryngeal pain · nasopharyngitis · pain

▶ **Uncommon** Appetite decreased · burping · chest pain · fever · hypoglycaemia · malaise · numbness · peripheral oedema · taste altered · tinnitus · vision disorders · weight increased

▶ **Rare or very rare** Angioedema · gynaecomastia · hearing loss · severe cutaneous adverse reactions (SCARs)

● **BREAST FEEDING** Manufacturer advises avoid—no information available.

● **PATIENT AND CARER ADVICE** Patient counselling is advised for atorvastatin tablets (muscle effects).
Medicines for Children leaflet: Atorvastatin for high cholesterol
www.medicinesforchildren.org.uk/medicines/atorvastatin-for-high-cholesterol/

● **MEDICINAL FORMS** There can be variation in the licensing of different medicines containing the same drug. Forms available from special-order manufacturers include: oral suspension, oral solution

Oral tablet

▸ Atorvastatin (Non-proprietary)

Atorvastatin (as Atorvastatin calcium trihydrate)
10 mg Atorvastatin 10mg tablets | 28 tablet PoM £15.60 DT = £0.55 | 90 tablet PoM £35.52

Atorvastatin (as Atorvastatin calcium trihydrate)
20 mg Atorvastatin 20mg tablets | 28 tablet PoM £29.57 DT = £0.61 | 56 tablet PoM £0.83–£0.96 | 90 tablet PoM £3.85

Atorvastatin (as Atorvastatin calcium trihydrate) 30 mg Atorvastatin 30mg tablets | 28 tablet PoM £29.40 DT = £3.26
Atorvastatin (as Atorvastatin calcium trihydrate) 40 mg Atorvastatin 40mg tablets | 28 tablet PoM £29.57 DT = £0.69 | 90 tablet PoM £67.32
Atorvastatin (as Atorvastatin calcium trihydrate) 60 mg Atorvastatin 60mg tablets | 28 tablet PoM £33.60 DT = £3.78
Atorvastatin (as Atorvastatin calcium trihydrate) 80 mg Atorvastatin 80mg tablets | 28 tablet PoM £33.85 DT = £1.14

▶ **Lipitor** (Viatris UK Healthcare Ltd)
Atorvastatin (as Atorvastatin calcium trihydrate) 10 mg Lipitor 10mg tablets | 28 tablet PoM £13.00 DT = £0.55
Atorvastatin (as Atorvastatin calcium trihydrate) 20 mg Lipitor 20mg tablets | 28 tablet PoM £24.64 DT = £0.61
Atorvastatin (as Atorvastatin calcium trihydrate) 40 mg Lipitor 40mg tablets | 28 tablet PoM £24.64 DT = £0.69
Atorvastatin (as Atorvastatin calcium trihydrate) 80 mg Lipitor 80mg tablets | 28 tablet PoM £28.21 DT = £1.14

Oral suspension

▶ **Atorvastatin (Non-proprietary)**
Atorvastatin (as Atorvastatin calcium trihydrate) 4 mg per 1 ml Atorvastatin 20mg/5ml oral suspension sugar free | 150 ml PoM £233.60 DT = £233.60 SF

Chewable tablet

CAUTIONARY AND ADVISORY LABELS 24

▶ **Lipitor** (Viatris UK Healthcare Ltd)
Atorvastatin (as Atorvastatin calcium trihydrate) 10 mg Lipitor 10mg chewable tablets | 30 tablet PoM £13.80 DT = £13.80 SF
Atorvastatin (as Atorvastatin calcium trihydrate) 20 mg Lipitor 20mg chewable tablets | 30 tablet PoM £26.40 DT = £26.40 SF

F 153

Fluvastatin

20-Jul-2021

● **INDICATIONS AND DOSE**

Heterozygous familial hypercholesterolaemia

▶ BY MOUTH USING IMMEDIATE-RELEASE MEDICINES

▶ Child 9–17 years: Initially 20 mg daily, dose to be taken in the evening, then adjusted in steps of 20 mg daily (max. per dose 40 mg twice daily), adjusted at intervals of at least 6 weeks; maximum 80 mg per day

▶ BY MOUTH USING MODIFIED-RELEASE MEDICINES

▶ Child 9–17 years: 80 mg daily, dose form is not appropriate for initial dose titration

● **INTERACTIONS** → Appendix 1: statins

● **SIDE-EFFECTS**

▶ **Rare or very rare** Angioedema · face oedema · muscle weakness · sensation abnormal · vasculitis

● **BREAST FEEDING** Manufacturer advises avoid—no information available.

● **RENAL IMPAIRMENT**

Dose adjustments EvGr Doses above 40 mg daily should be initiated with caution if creatinine clearance less than 30 mL/minute (limited information available), Ⓜ see p. 16.

● **PATIENT AND CARER ADVICE** Patient counselling is advised for fluvastatin tablets/capsules (muscle effects).

● **NATIONAL FUNDING/ACCESS DECISIONS**

For full details see funding body website

Scottish Medicines Consortium (SMC) decisions

▶ **Fluvastatin (*Lescol*®) for the secondary prevention of coronary events after percutaneous coronary intervention (February 2004)** SMC No. 76/04 Recommended with restrictions

● **MEDICINAL FORMS** There can be variation in the licensing of different medicines containing the same drug.

Modified-release tablet

CAUTIONARY AND ADVISORY LABELS 25

▶ **Fluvastatin (Non-proprietary)**
Fluvastatin (as Fluvastatin sodium) 80 mg Fluvastatin 80mg modified-release tablets | 28 tablet PoM £19.20–£37.00 DT = £19.20

Oral capsule

▶ **Fluvastatin (Non-proprietary)**
Fluvastatin (as Fluvastatin sodium) 20 mg Fluvastatin 20mg capsules | 28 capsule PoM £6.25 DT = £4.09
Fluvastatin (as Fluvastatin sodium) 40 mg Fluvastatin 40mg capsules | 28 capsule PoM £8.40 DT = £7.97

F 153

Pravastatin sodium

26-Apr-2021

● **INDICATIONS AND DOSE**

Hyperlipidaemia including familial hypercholesterolaemia

▶ BY MOUTH

▶ Child 8–13 years: 10 mg once daily, to be taken at night, then increased if necessary up to 20 mg once daily, to be taken at night, dose to be adjusted at intervals of at least 4 weeks

▶ Child 14–17 years: 10 mg once daily, to be taken at night, then increased if necessary up to 40 mg once daily, to be taken at night, dose to be adjusted at intervals of at least 4 weeks

DOSE ADJUSTMENTS DUE TO INTERACTIONS

▶ Manufacturer advises reduce maximum daily dose with concurrent use of glecaprevir with pibrentasvir—consult product literature.

● **INTERACTIONS** → Appendix 1: statins

● **SIDE-EFFECTS**

▶ **Uncommon** Hair abnormal · scalp abnormal · urinary disorders · vision disorders

▶ **Frequency not known** Muscle weakness · musculoskeletal pain

● **BREAST FEEDING** Manufacturer advises avoid—small amount of drug present in breast milk.

● **HEPATIC IMPAIRMENT**

Dose adjustments Manufacturer advises initial dose reduction to 10 mg daily; adjust according to response.

● **RENAL IMPAIRMENT**

Dose adjustments Manufacturer advises initial dose of 10 mg once daily in moderate to severe impairment.

● **PATIENT AND CARER ADVICE** Patient counselling is advised for pravastatin tablets (muscle effects).

● **MEDICINAL FORMS** There can be variation in the licensing of different medicines containing the same drug. Forms available from special-order manufacturers include: oral suspension, oral solution

Oral tablet

▶ **Pravastatin sodium (Non-proprietary)**
Pravastatin sodium 10 mg Pravastatin 10mg tablets | 28 tablet PoM £1.60 DT = £0.99
Pravastatin sodium 20 mg Pravastatin 20mg tablets | 28 tablet PoM £1.38 DT = £1.03
Pravastatin sodium 40 mg Pravastatin 40mg tablets | 28 tablet PoM £1.68 DT = £1.26

F 153

Rosuvastatin

24-Mar-2025

● **INDICATIONS AND DOSE**

Heterozygous familial hypercholesterolaemia (specialist use only)

▶ BY MOUTH

▶ Child 6–9 years: Initially 5 mg once daily, then increased if necessary up to 10 mg once daily, dose to be increased gradually at intervals of at least 4 weeks

▶ Child 10–17 years: Initially 5 mg once daily, then increased if necessary up to 20 mg once daily, dose to be increased gradually at intervals of at least 4 weeks, use lower max. dose in children with risk factors for myopathy or rhabdomyolysis (including personal or family history of muscular disorders or toxicity)

continued →

Homozygous familial hypercholesterolaemia (specialist use only)

▶ BY MOUTH

▸ Child 6–17 years: Initially 5–10 mg once daily, then increased if necessary up to 20 mg once daily, dose to be increased gradually at intervals of at least 4 weeks, use lower max. dose in children with risk factors for myopathy or rhabdomyolysis (including personal or family history of muscular disorders or toxicity)

▸ Child 6–17 years (patients of Asian origin): Initially 5 mg once daily, then increased if necessary up to 20 mg once daily, dose to be increased gradually at intervals of at least 4 weeks, use lower max. dose in children with risk factors for myopathy or rhabdomyolysis (including personal or family history of muscular disorders or toxicity).

DOSE ADJUSTMENTS DUE TO INTERACTIONS

▸ EvGr Initially 5 mg daily with concurrent use of elbasvir with grazoprevir—max. dose 10 mg daily.

▸ Initially 5 mg daily with concurrent use of sofosbuvir with velpatasvir—max. dose 10 mg daily.

▸ Initially 5 mg daily, or reduce dose by half with concurrent use of teriflunomide.

▸ Max. dose 5 mg daily with concurrent use of glecaprevir with pibrentasvir.

▸ Initially 5 mg daily with concurrent use of atazanavir boosted with ritonavir—max. dose 10 mg daily.

▸ Initially 5 mg daily with concurrent use of lopinavir boosted with ritonavir; for max. daily dose—consult product literature.

▸ Max. dose 10 mg daily with concurrent use of atazanavir boosted with cobicistat. ⟨M⟩

● **INTERACTIONS** → Appendix 1: statins

● **SIDE-EFFECTS**

▶ **Rare or very rare** Gynaecomastia · haematuria · polyneuropathy

▶ **Frequency not known** Cough · dyspnoea · oedema · proteinuria · severe cutaneous adverse reactions (SCARs)

● **BREAST FEEDING** Manufacturer advises avoid—no information available.

● **RENAL IMPAIRMENT** EvGr Avoid if creatinine clearance less than 30 mL/minute. ⟨M⟩

Dose adjustments See p. 16.

EvGr Reduce initial dose if creatinine clearance 30–60 mL/minute. ⟨M⟩

● **MONITORING REQUIREMENTS** Manufacturer advises consider routine monitoring of renal function when using 40 mg daily dose.

● **DIRECTIONS FOR ADMINISTRATION** Capsules may be swallowed whole. Alternatively, capsules may be opened and the contents mixed into 1 teaspoonful of soft food (e.g. apple sauce) and swallowed within 1 hour without chewing, followed with a glass of water.

● **PATIENT AND CARER ADVICE** Patient counselling is advised for rosuvastatin tablets/capsules (muscle effects).

● **MEDICINAL FORMS** There can be variation in the licensing of different medicines containing the same drug. Forms available from special-order manufacturers include: oral suspension

Oral tablet

▸ Rosuvastatin (Non-proprietary)

Rosuvastatin (as Rosuvastatin calcium) 5 mg Rosuvastatin 5mg tablets | 28 tablet PoM £21.64 DT = £0.66 | 250 tablet PoM £4.14–£6.43

Rosuvastatin (as Rosuvastatin calcium) 10 mg Rosuvastatin 10mg tablets | 28 tablet PoM £21.64 DT = £0.78 | 250 tablet PoM £6.12–£8.04

Rosuvastatin (as Rosuvastatin calcium) 15 mg Rosuvastatin 15mg tablets | 28 tablet PoM £4.97–£5.56 DT = £4.97

Rosuvastatin (as Rosuvastatin calcium) 20 mg Rosuvastatin 20mg tablets | 28 tablet PoM £31.22 DT = £0.86 | 250 tablet PoM £6.99–£8.74

Rosuvastatin (as Rosuvastatin calcium) 30 mg Rosuvastatin 30mg tablets | 28 tablet PoM £5.97–£7.16 DT = £5.97

Rosuvastatin (as Rosuvastatin calcium) 40 mg Rosuvastatin 40mg tablets | 28 tablet PoM £35.63 DT = £1.24

▸ Crestor (AstraZeneca UK Ltd)

Rosuvastatin (as Rosuvastatin calcium) 5 mg Crestor 5mg tablets | 28 tablet PoM £18.03 DT = £0.66

Rosuvastatin (as Rosuvastatin calcium) 10 mg Crestor 10mg tablets | 28 tablet PoM £18.03 DT = £0.78

Rosuvastatin (as Rosuvastatin calcium) 20 mg Crestor 20mg tablets | 28 tablet PoM £26.02 DT = £0.86

Rosuvastatin (as Rosuvastatin calcium) 40 mg Crestor 40mg tablets | 28 tablet PoM £29.69 DT = £1.24

Oral capsule

▸ Rosuvastatin (Non-proprietary)

Rosuvastatin (as Rosuvastatin calcium) 5 mg Rosuvastatin 5mg capsules | 28 capsule PoM £8.52 DT = £8.52

Rosuvastatin (as Rosuvastatin calcium) 10 mg Rosuvastatin 10mg capsules | 28 capsule PoM £9.54 DT = £9.54

Rosuvastatin (as Rosuvastatin calcium) 20 mg Rosuvastatin 20mg capsules | 28 capsule PoM £12.72 DT = £12.72

Rosuvastatin (as Rosuvastatin calcium) 40 mg Rosuvastatin 40mg capsules | 28 capsule PoM £15.12 DT = £15.12

F 153

Simvastatin

20-Jul-2021

● **INDICATIONS AND DOSE**

Hyperlipidaemia including familial hypercholesterolaemia

▶ BY MOUTH

▸ Child 5–9 years: Initially 10 mg once daily, dose to be taken at night, then increased if necessary up to 20 mg once daily, dose to be taken at night, increased at intervals of at least 4 weeks

▸ Child 10–17 years: Initially 10 mg once daily, dose to be taken at night, then increased if necessary up to 40 mg once daily, dose to be taken at night, increased at intervals of at least 4 weeks

DOSE ADJUSTMENTS DUE TO INTERACTIONS

▸ Manufacturer advises max. dose 10 mg daily with concurrent use of bezafibrate—no specific recommendation made for children.

▸ Manufacturer advises max. dose 20 mg daily with concurrent use of amiodarone or amlodipine—no specific recommendation made for children.

▸ Manufacturer advises reduce dose with concurrent use of some moderate inhibitors of CYP3A4 (max. 20 mg daily with verapamil and diltiazem)—no specific recommendation made for children.

● **UNLICENSED USE** Not licensed for use in children under 10 years.

● **INTERACTIONS** → Appendix 1: statins

● **SIDE-EFFECTS**

▶ **Rare or very rare** Acute kidney injury · anaemia

▶ **Frequency not known** Cognitive impairment

● **BREAST FEEDING** Manufacturer advises avoid—no information available.

● **RENAL IMPAIRMENT**

Dose adjustments EvGr Doses above 10 mg daily should be used with caution if creatinine clearance less than 30 mL/minute, ⟨M⟩ see p. 16.

● **PATIENT AND CARER ADVICE** Patient counselling is advised for simvastatin tablets/oral suspension (muscle effects).

● **MEDICINAL FORMS** There can be variation in the licensing of different medicines containing the same drug. Forms available from special-order manufacturers include: oral suspension, oral solution

Oral tablet

▸ Simvastatin (Non-proprietary)

Simvastatin 10 mg Simvastatin 10mg tablets | 28 tablet PoM £14.42 DT = £0.59 | 500 tablet PoM £10.54–£13.04

Simvastatin 20 mg Simvastatin 20mg tablets | 28 tablet [PoM] £23.75 DT = £0.69 | 500 tablet [PoM] £11.96–£14.99
Simvastatin 40 mg Simvastatin 40mg tablets | 28 tablet [PoM] £23.75 DT = £0.79 | 500 tablet [PoM] £13.39–£16.95
Simvastatin 80 mg Simvastatin 80mg tablets | 28 tablet [PoM] £6.00 DT = £1.30

▸ **Zocor** (Organon Pharma (UK) Ltd)
Simvastatin 20 mg Zocor 20mg tablets | 28 tablet [PoM] £29.69 DT = £0.69
Simvastatin 40 mg Zocor 40mg tablets | 28 tablet [PoM] £29.69 DT = £0.79

Oral suspension

EXCIPIENTS: May contain Propylene glycol

▸ **Simvastatin (Non-proprietary)**
Simvastatin 4 mg per 1 ml Simvastatin 20mg/5ml oral suspension sugar free | 150 ml [PoM] £219.54 DT = £219.54 [SF]
Simvastatin 8 mg per 1 ml Simvastatin 40mg/5ml oral suspension sugar free | 150 ml [PoM] £308.23 DT = £308.23 [SF]

Simvastatin with ezetimibe

10-Dec-2020

The properties listed below are those particular to the combination only. For the properties of the components please consider, simvastatin p. 156, ezetimibe p. 152.

● **INDICATIONS AND DOSE**

Homozygous familial hypercholesterolaemia, primary hypercholesterolaemia, and mixed hyperlipidaemia in patients over 10 years stabilised on the individual components in the same proportions, or for patients not adequately controlled by statin alone

▶ BY MOUTH

▸ Child (initiated by a specialist): (consult product literature)

● **INTERACTIONS** → Appendix 1: ezetimibe · statins

● **MEDICINAL FORMS** There can be variation in the licensing of different medicines containing the same drug.

Oral tablet

▸ **Simvastatin with ezetimibe (Non-proprietary)**
Ezetimibe 10 mg, Simvastatin 20 mg Simvastatin 20mg / Ezetimibe 10mg tablets | 28 tablet [PoM] £33.42 DT = £33.42
Ezetimibe 10 mg, Simvastatin 40 mg Simvastatin 40mg / Ezetimibe 10mg tablets | 28 tablet [PoM] £38.98 DT = £38.98
Ezetimibe 10 mg, Simvastatin 80 mg Simvastatin 80mg / Ezetimibe 10mg tablets | 28 tablet [PoM] £41.21 DT = £41.21

▸ **Inegy** (Organon Pharma (UK) Ltd)
Ezetimibe 10 mg, Simvastatin 20 mg Inegy 10mg/20mg tablets | 28 tablet [PoM] £33.42 DT = £33.42
Ezetimibe 10 mg, Simvastatin 40 mg Inegy 10mg/40mg tablets | 28 tablet [PoM] £38.98 DT = £38.98
Ezetimibe 10 mg, Simvastatin 80 mg Inegy 10mg/80mg tablets | 28 tablet [PoM] £41.21 DT = £41.21

LIPID MODIFYING DRUGS › OTHER

Evinacumab

19-Jun-2025

● **DRUG ACTION** Evinacumab is a recombinant human monoclonal antibody that binds to and blocks the angiopoeitin-like 3 protein (ANGPTL3) to prevent its inhibition of lipoprotein and endothelial lipase, thereby lowering triglycerides and cholesterol.

● **INDICATIONS AND DOSE**

Homozygous familial hypercholesterolaemia (under expert supervision)

▶ BY INTRAVENOUS INFUSION

▸ Child 6 months–17 years: 15 mg/kg every 4 weeks

● **SIDE-EFFECTS**

▶ **Common or very common** Abdominal pain · asthenia · constipation · dizziness · increased risk of infection · influenza like illness · infusion related reaction · nausea · pain · rhinorrhoea

▶ **Uncommon** Hypersensitivity

● **CONCEPTION AND CONTRACEPTION** [EvGr] Females of childbearing potential should use effective contraception during treatment and for at least 5 months after last treatment. ◆M◆

● **PREGNANCY** [EvGr] Avoid unless potential benefit outweighs risk (toxicity in *animal* studies). ◆M◆

● **BREAST FEEDING** Specialist sources indicate use with caution, especially if breast-feeding a neonate or pre-term infant (no information available). Large molecular weight suggests limited excretion into milk and drug molecule likely to be partially destroyed in the infant's gastro-intestinal tract.

● **DIRECTIONS FOR ADMINISTRATION** For *intravenous infusion* (*Evkeeza*®), dilute requisite dose in Glucose 5% or Sodium Chloride 0.9% to a final concentration of 0.5–20 mg/mL (gently invert, do not shake); give over 60 minutes through an in-line or add-on filter (0.2–5 micron).

● **PRESCRIBING AND DISPENSING INFORMATION** Evinacumab is a biological medicine. Biological medicines must be prescribed and dispensed by brand name, see *Biological medicines* and *Biosimilar medicines*, under Guidance on prescribing p. 1; record the brand name and batch number after each administration.

● **HANDLING AND STORAGE** Store in a refrigerator (2–8°C) and protect from light—consult product literature about storage after dilution.

● **PATIENT AND CARER ADVICE**

Driving and skilled tasks Patients and carers should be cautioned on the effects on driving and performance of skilled tasks—increased risk of dizziness, fatigue and asthenia.

● **NATIONAL FUNDING/ACCESS DECISIONS**

For full details see funding body website

NICE decisions

▶ **Evinacumab for treating homozygous familial hypercholesterolaemia in people 12 years and over (September 2024)** NICE TA1002 Recommended

● **MEDICINAL FORMS** There can be variation in the licensing of different medicines containing the same drug.

Solution for infusion

EXCIPIENTS: May contain Polysorbates

▸ **Evkeeza** (Ultragenyx UK Ltd) ▼
Evinacumab 150 mg per 1 ml Evkeeza 345mg/2.3ml concentrate for solution for infusion vials | 1 vial [PoM] £6,432.75 (Hospital only)

Evolocumab

14-Oct-2021

● **DRUG ACTION** Evolocumab binds to a pro-protein involved in the regulation of LDL receptors on liver cells; receptor numbers are increased, which results in increased uptake of LDL-cholesterol from the blood.

● **INDICATIONS AND DOSE**

Homozygous familial hypercholesterolaemia (in combination with other lipid-lowering therapies)

▶ BY SUBCUTANEOUS INJECTION

▸ Child 12–17 years: Initially 420 mg every month; increased if necessary to 420 mg every 2 weeks, if inadequate response after 12 weeks of treatment, to be administered into the thigh, abdomen or upper arm

Homozygous familial hypercholesterolaemia in patients on apheresis (in combination with other lipid-lowering therapies)

▶ BY SUBCUTANEOUS INJECTION

▸ Child 12–17 years: 420 mg every 2 weeks, to correspond with apheresis schedule, to be administered into the thigh, abdomen or upper arm

- **SIDE-EFFECTS**
- ▶ **Common or very common** Arthralgia · back pain · hypersensitivity · increased risk of infection · nausea · skin reactions
- ▶ **Uncommon** Influenza like illness
- ▶ **Rare or very rare** Angioedema
- **PREGNANCY** Manufacturer advises avoid unless essential—limited information available.
- **BREAST FEEDING** Manufacturer advises avoid—no information available.
- **HEPATIC IMPAIRMENT** Manufacturer advises caution in moderate to severe impairment (risk of reduced efficacy; no information available in severe impairment).
- **HANDLING AND STORAGE** Manufacturer advises store in a refrigerator (2–8°C)—consult product literature for further information regarding storage outside refrigerator.
- **PATIENT AND CARER ADVICE** Patients and their carers should be given training in subcutaneous injection technique.

- **MEDICINAL FORMS** There can be variation in the licensing of different medicines containing the same drug.

Solution for injection

▸ Repatha SureClick (Amgen Ltd)
Evolocumab 140 mg per 1 ml Repatha SureClick 140mg/1ml solution for injection pre-filled pens | 2 pre-filled disposable injection PoM £340.20 DT = £340.20

7 Myocardial ischaemia

NITRATES

Nitrates

16-Sep-2021

Overview

Nitrates (such as glyceryl trinitrate below) are potent coronary vasodilators, but their principal benefit follows from a reduction in venous return which reduces left ventricular work. Unwanted effects (such as flushing, headache, and postural hypotension) may limit therapy, especially if the child is unusually sensitive to the effects of nitrates or is hypovolaemic. Glyceryl trinitrate is also used in extravasation.

Nitrates

- **CONTRA-INDICATIONS** Aortic stenosis · cardiac tamponade · constrictive pericarditis · hypertrophic cardiomyopathy · hypotensive conditions · hypovolaemia · marked anaemia · mitral stenosis · raised intracranial pressure due to cerebral haemorrhage · raised intracranial pressure due to head trauma · toxic pulmonary oedema
- **CAUTIONS** Heart failure due to obstruction · hypothermia · hypothyroidism · hypoxaemia · malnutrition · metal-containing transdermal systems should be removed before magnetic resonance imaging procedures, cardioversion, or diathermy · recent history of myocardial infarction · susceptibility to angle-closure glaucoma · tolerance · ventilation and perfusion abnormalities

CAUTIONS, FURTHER INFORMATION

▸ **Tolerance** Children receiving nitrates continuously throughout the day can develop tolerance (with reduced therapeutic effects). Reduction of blood-nitrate concentrations to low levels for 4 to 8 hours each day usually maintains effectiveness in such patients.

- **SIDE-EFFECTS**
- ▶ **Common or very common** Arrhythmias · asthenia · cerebral ischaemia · dizziness · drowsiness · flushing · headache · hypotension · nausea
- ▶ **Uncommon** Circulatory collapse · diarrhoea · skin reactions · syncope · vomiting
- **ALLERGY AND CROSS-SENSITIVITY** EvGr Contra-indicated in nitrate hypersensitivity. ⟨M⟩
- **BREAST FEEDING** No information available—manufacturers advise use only if potential benefit outweighs risk.
- **HEPATIC IMPAIRMENT** In general, manufacturers advise caution in severe impairment.
- **RENAL IMPAIRMENT** In general, manufacturers advise caution in severe impairment.
- **MONITORING REQUIREMENTS** Monitor blood pressure and heart rate during intravenous infusion.
- **TREATMENT CESSATION** Avoid abrupt withdrawal.

above

Glyceryl trinitrate

07-Jan-2025

- **INDICATIONS AND DOSE**

Hypertension during and after cardiac surgery | Heart failure after cardiac surgery | Coronary vasoconstriction in myocardial ischaemia | Vasoconstriction in shock

▶ BY CONTINUOUS INTRAVENOUS INFUSION

▸ Neonate: 0.2–0.5 microgram/kg/minute, adjusted according to response, maintenance 1–3 micrograms/kg/minute (max. per dose 10 micrograms/kg/minute).

▸ Child: Initially 0.2–0.5 microgram/kg/minute, adjusted according to response, maintenance 1–3 micrograms/kg/minute (max. per dose 10 micrograms/kg/minute); maximum 200 micrograms/minute

- **UNLICENSED USE** Not licensed for use in children.
- **INTERACTIONS** → Appendix 1: nitrates
- **SIDE-EFFECTS**
- ▶ **Uncommon** Cardiac disorder · cyanosis
- ▶ **Rare or very rare** Methaemoglobinaemia · respiratory disorder · restlessness
- ▶ **Frequency not known** Hyperhidrosis
- **PREGNANCY** Not known to be harmful.
- **DIRECTIONS FOR ADMINISTRATION** For *continuous intravenous infusion*, dilute to max. concentration of 400 micrograms/mL (but concentration of 1 mg/mL has been used via a central venous catheter) with Glucose 5% or Sodium Chloride 0.9%. *Neonatal intensive care*, dilute 3 mg/kg body-weight to a final volume of 50 mL with Glucose 5% or Sodium Chloride 0.9%; an intravenous infusion rate of 1 mL/hour provides a dose of 1 microgram/kg/minute; max. concentration of 400 micrograms/mL (but concentration of 1 mg/mL has been used via a central venous catheter).

Glass or polyethylene apparatus is preferable; loss of potency will occur if PVC is used. Glyceryl trinitrate 1 mg/mL to be diluted before use or given undiluted with syringe pump. Glyceryl trinitrate 5 mg/mL to be diluted before use.

- **MEDICINAL FORMS** There can be variation in the licensing of different medicines containing the same drug. Forms available from special-order manufacturers include: solution for infusion

Solution for infusion

EXCIPIENTS: May contain Ethanol, propylene glycol

▸ Glyceryl trinitrate (Non-proprietary)
Glyceryl trinitrate 1 mg per 1 ml Glyceryl trinitrate 10mg/10ml solution for infusion ampoules | 10 ampoule PoM £34.80

Glyceryl trinitrate 50mg/50ml solution for infusion vials | 1 vial [PoM] £21.00 (Hospital only) | 10 vial [PoM] £250.00

Glyceryl trinitrate 5 mg per 1 ml Glyceryl trinitrate 50mg/10ml solution for infusion ampoules | 5 ampoule [PoM] £64.90 (Hospital only)

Glyceryl trinitrate 25mg/5ml solution for infusion ampoules | 5 ampoule [PoM] £32.45 (Hospital only)

▸ **Nitronal** (Beaumont Pharma Ltd)

Glyceryl trinitrate 1 mg per 1 ml Nitronal 50mg/50ml solution for infusion vials | 1 vial [PoM] £17.40

7.1 Cardiac arrest

Cardiopulmonary resuscitation

05-May-2021

Overview

The algorithms for cardiopulmonary resuscitation (Life support algorithm (image) Inside back pages) reflect the recommendations of the Resuscitation Council (UK) and cover paediatric out-of-hospital basic life support, paediatric basic life support, paediatric advanced life support, and newborn life support; these have been reproduced with the kind permission of the Resuscitation Council (UK). The guidelines are available at www.resus.org.uk.

Paediatric advanced life support

Cardiopulmonary (cardiac) arrest in children occurs less frequently than adults and mostly represents the terminal event of circulatory failure or respiratory failure.

During cardiopulmonary arrest in children without intravenous access, the intraosseous route is an alternative.

For the management of acute anaphylaxis, see allergic emergencies under Antihistamines, allergen immunotherapy and allergic emergencies p. 199.

SYMPATHOMIMETICS › VASOCONSTRICTOR

Adrenaline

13-Apr-2026

(Epinephrine)

● **DRUG ACTION** Adrenaline (epinephrine) acts on both alpha and beta receptors and increases both heart rate and contractility ($beta_1$ effects); it can cause peripheral vasodilation (a $beta_2$ effect) or vasoconstriction (an alpha effect).

● **INDICATIONS AND DOSE**

Cardiopulmonary resuscitation (specialist use only)

▸ BY SLOW INTRAVENOUS INJECTION

▸ Neonate up to 1 days: Consult Resuscitation Council (UK) guidance on newborn resuscitation or local protocols.

▸ Neonate 1 days to 28 days: 10 micrograms/kg every 3–5 minutes as required, a 1 in 10 000 (100 micrograms/mL) solution is recommended, suitable syringe to be used for measuring small volume.

▸ Child: 10 micrograms/kg every 3–5 minutes (max. per dose 1 mg) as required, a 1 in 10 000 (100 micrograms/mL) solution is recommended, suitable syringe to be used for measuring small volume

Acute hypotension

▸ BY CONTINUOUS INTRAVENOUS INFUSION

▸ Neonate: Initially 100 nanograms/kg/minute, to be adjusted according to response, higher doses up to 1.5 micrograms/kg/minute have been used in acute hypotension.

▸ Child: Initially 100 nanograms/kg/minute, to be adjusted according to response, higher doses up to 1.5 micrograms/kg/minute have been used in acute hypotension

Croup (when not effectively controlled with corticosteroid treatment)

▸ BY INHALATION OF NEBULISED SOLUTION

▸ Child 1 month–11 years: 400 micrograms/kg for 1 dose (max. per dose 5 mg), dose to be repeated after 30 minutes if necessary

PHARMACOKINETICS

▸ The effects of nebulised adrenaline for the treatment of croup lasts for 2–3 hours.

Emergency treatment of acute anaphylaxis (under expert supervision)

▸ BY INTRAMUSCULAR INJECTION

▸ Child up to 6 months: 100–150 micrograms, using adrenaline 1 in 1000 (1 mg/mL) injection, repeat dose after 5 minutes if no response; if life-threatening features persist, further doses can be given every 5 minutes until specialist critical care available, suitable syringe to be used for measuring small volume; injected preferably into the anterolateral aspect of the middle third of the thigh

▸ Child 6 months–5 years: 150 micrograms, using adrenaline 1 in 1000 (1 mg/mL) injection, repeat dose after 5 minutes if no response; if life-threatening features persist, further doses can be given every 5 minutes until specialist critical care available, suitable syringe to be used for measuring small volume; injected preferably into the anterolateral aspect of the middle third of the thigh

▸ Child 6–11 years: 300 micrograms, using adrenaline 1 in 1000 (1 mg/mL) injection, repeat dose after 5 minutes if no response; if life-threatening features persist, further doses can be given every 5 minutes until specialist critical care available, to be injected preferably into the anterolateral aspect of the middle third of the thigh

▸ Child 12–17 years: 500 micrograms, using adrenaline 1 in 1000 (1 mg/mL) injection, repeat dose after 5 minutes if no response; if life-threatening features persist, further doses can be given every 5 minutes until specialist critical care available, to be injected preferably into the anterolateral aspect of the middle third of the thigh, 300 micrograms to be administered if child is small or prepubertal

Refractory anaphylaxis [persistent symptoms despite at least 2 appropriate doses of intramuscular adrenaline] (specialist use only)

▸ BY INTRAVENOUS INFUSION

▸ Child: Consult Resuscitation Council (UK) emergency treatment of anaphylaxis guideline or local protocols

EURNEFFY® NASAL SPRAY

Acute anaphylaxis (for self-administration at the first signs of anaphylaxis)

▸ BY INTRANASAL ADMINISTRATION

▸ Child (body-weight 30 kg and above): 2 mg, then 2 mg after 5 minutes as required

DOSE EQUIVALENCE AND CONVERSION

▸ For *EURneffy®* nasal spray: 2 mg is approx. equivalent to 300 micrograms by intramuscular injection with an auto-injector.

EPIPEN® AUTO-INJECTOR 300 MICROGRAMS

Acute anaphylaxis (for self-administration at the first signs of anaphylaxis)

▸ BY INTRAMUSCULAR INJECTION

▸ Child (body-weight 25 kg and above): 300 micrograms, then 300 micrograms after 5 minutes as required

continued →

EPIPEN ® JR AUTO-INJECTOR 150 MICROGRAMS

Acute anaphylaxis (for self-administration at the first signs of anaphylaxis)

▶ BY INTRAMUSCULAR INJECTION

- Child (body-weight up to 15 kg): 150 micrograms, then 150 micrograms after 5 minutes as required
- Child (body-weight 15–24 kg): 150 micrograms, then 150 micrograms after 5 minutes as required, on the basis of a dose of 10 micrograms/kg, 300 micrograms may be more appropriate for some children

JEXT ® AUTO-INJECTOR 150 MICROGRAMS

Acute anaphylaxis (for self-administration at the first signs of anaphylaxis)

▶ BY INTRAMUSCULAR INJECTION

- Child (body-weight up to 15 kg): 150 micrograms, then 150 micrograms after 5 minutes as required
- Child (body-weight 15–24 kg): 150 micrograms, then 150 micrograms after 5 minutes as required, on the basis of a dose of 10 micrograms/kg, 300 micrograms may be more appropriate for some children

JEXT ® AUTO-INJECTOR 300 MICROGRAMS

Acute anaphylaxis (for self-administration at the first signs of anaphylaxis)

▶ BY INTRAMUSCULAR INJECTION

- Child (body-weight 25 kg and above): 300 micrograms, then 300 micrograms after 5 minutes as required

● **UNLICENSED USE**

- With intramuscular use for Acute anaphylaxis (for self-administration at the first signs of anaphylaxis) EvGr Adrenaline, given via an auto-injector, is used in the doses provided in BNF Publications, but these may differ from those licensed. ⟨E⟩
- With intravenous use EvGr Adrenaline is used for cardiopulmonary resuscitation in neonates and infants with body-weight under 5 kg, ⟨A⟩ but it is not licensed for this age group.
- With intravenous use for Acute hypotension Adrenaline 1 in 1000 (1 mg/mL) solution is not licensed for intravenous administration.
- With intramuscular use EvGr Adrenaline is used in the doses provided in BNF Publications for the emergency treatment of acute anaphylaxis in children up to 6 months, ⟨A⟩ but these may differ from those licensed.
- When used for Croup Expert sources advise adrenaline 1 in 1000 (1 mg/mL) solution may be used, but it is not licensed for this indication.

IMPORTANT SAFETY INFORMATION

SAFE PRACTICE

Intravenous route should be used with **extreme care** by specialists only.

MHRA/CHM ADVICE: ADRENALINE AUTO-INJECTORS: UPDATED ADVICE AFTER EUROPEAN REVIEW (AUGUST 2017)

Following a European review of all adrenaline auto-injectors approved in the EU, the MHRA recommend that 2 adrenaline auto-injectors are prescribed, which patients should carry at all times. This is particularly important for patients with allergic asthma, who are at increased risk of a severe anaphylactic reaction. Patients with allergies and their carers should be trained to use the particular auto-injector they have been prescribed and encouraged to practise using a trainer device. Patients are advised to check the expiry date of the adrenaline auto-injectors and obtain replacements before they expire.

NATIONAL PATIENT SAFETY ALERT: RECALL OF *EMERADE* ® 500 MICROGRAMS AND *EMERADE* ® 300 MICROGRAMS AUTO-INJECTORS DUE TO THE POTENTIAL FOR DEVICE FAILURE (MAY 2023)

All unexpired batches of *Emerade* ® 500 micrograms and *Emerade* ® 300 micrograms adrenaline auto-injectors (also referred to as pens) have been recalled as a precautionary measure due to an issue identified by the manufacturer where some auto-injectors failed to deliver adrenaline or activated prematurely after being dropped. Future production of these preparations is on hold and no further supplies will be available; patients should be switched to an equivalent strength adrenaline auto-injector in an alternative brand—*EpiPen* ® **300 micrograms** or *Jext* ® **300 micrograms** are appropriate alternatives to *Emerade* ® **500 micrograms.** This recall also applies to schools, and to adrenaline auto-injectors held by healthcare professionals, such as in emergency anaphylaxis kits and dental kits; anaphylaxis kits in the healthcare setting should be restocked with adrenaline ampoules (together with dosing charts for use of intramuscular adrenaline to treat anaphylaxis, needles and syringes) and **not** auto-injectors. Patients and their carers should be advised:

- to carry 2 in-date adrenaline auto-injectors with them at all times in case a second dose needs to be administered before the arrival of emergency services;
- that they need to receive training so that they are confident in using any new devices—instructions for use can be found in patient information leaflets and training videos on respective manufacturers' websites;
- of the signs and symptoms of anaphylaxis and the actions they should take immediately;
- that the risk of mishandling or failure exists with all adrenaline auto-injectors, and that a second adrenaline auto-injector should be used immediately if the first fails to activate, despite pressing firmly against the thigh. If the patient is not improving, further attempts to activate a failed auto-injector should be made even if one auto-injector has worked, as this may suggest a need for further doses while waiting for emergency services.

Healthcare professionals and patients are strongly recommended to order a trainer device from the manufacturer to ensure they are familiar with use and prepared for an emergency.

For further information, refer to the National Patient Safety Alert available at: www.gov.uk/drug-device-alerts/national-patient-safety-alert-class-1-medicines-recall-notification-recall-of-emerade-500-micrograms-and-emerade-300-micrograms-auto-injectors-due-to-the-potential-for-device-failure-natpsa-slash-2023-slash-004-slash-mhra.

● **CAUTIONS** Arrhythmias · cerebrovascular disease · cor pulmonale · diabetes mellitus · hypercalcaemia · hyperreflexia · hypertension · hyperthyroidism · hypokalaemia · ischaemic heart disease · obstructive cardiomyopathy · occlusive vascular disease · organic brain damage · phaeochromocytoma · prostate disorders · psychoneurosis · severe angina · susceptibility to angle-closure glaucoma

CAUTIONS, FURTHER INFORMATION Cautions listed are only for non-life-threatening situations.

● **INTERACTIONS** → Appendix 1: sympathomimetics, vasoconstrictor

● **SIDE-EFFECTS**

GENERAL SIDE-EFFECTS

- ▶ **Common or very common** Anxiety · palpitations · tremor
- ▶ **Uncommon** Asthenia · dizziness · nausea

SPECIFIC SIDE-EFFECTS

- **Common or very common**
- With intranasal use Feeling jittery · headaches · nasal complaints · throat complaints
- **Uncommon**
- With intranasal use Chest discomfort · epistaxis · euphoric mood · excessive tearing · feeling hot · oral disorders · oropharyngeal pain · paraesthesia · paranasal sinus discomfort · pruritus
- **Rare or very rare**
- With parenteral use Cardiomyopathy
- **Frequency not known**
- With intramuscular use Muscle necrosis · necrotising fasciitis · peripheral ischaemia
- With intravenous use Hemiplegia · muscle rigidity
- With parenteral use Angina pectoris · angle closure glaucoma · appetite decreased · arrhythmias · CNS haemorrhage · confusion · dry mouth · dyspnoea · headache · hepatic necrosis · hyperglycaemia · hyperhidrosis · hypersalivation · hypertension (increased risk of cerebral haemorrhage) · hypokalaemia · injection site necrosis · insomnia · intestinal necrosis · metabolic acidosis · mydriasis · myocardial infarction · pallor · peripheral coldness · psychosis · pulmonary oedema (on excessive dosage or extreme sensitivity) · renal necrosis · soft tissue necrosis · urinary disorders · vomiting

● **PREGNANCY**

- With intranasal use or parenteral use May reduce placental perfusion and cause tachycardia, cardiac irregularities, and extrasystoles in fetus. Can delay second stage of labour. Manufacturers advise use only if benefit outweighs risk.

● **BREAST FEEDING**

- With intranasal use or parenteral use Present in milk but unlikely to be harmful as poor oral bioavailability.

● **RENAL IMPAIRMENT** Manufacturers advise use with caution in severe impairment.

● **MONITORING REQUIREMENTS** Monitor blood pressure and ECG.

● **DIRECTIONS FOR ADMINISTRATION**

- With intravenous use for Acute hypotension For *continuous intravenous infusion*, expert sources advise dilute with Glucose 5% or Sodium Chloride 0.9% and give through a central venous catheter. Incompatible with bicarbonate and alkaline solutions. *Neonatal intensive care*, expert sources advise dilute 3 mg/kg body-weight to a final volume of 50 mL with infusion fluid; an intravenous infusion rate of 0.1 mL/hour provides a dose of 100 nanograms/kg/minute; infuse through a central venous catheter. Incompatible with bicarbonate and alkaline solutions. Expert sources advise these infusions are usually made up with adrenaline 1 in 1000 (1 mg/mL) solution.
- When used for Croup For nebulisation, expert sources advise adrenaline 1 in 1000 solution may be diluted with sterile sodium chloride 0.9% solution.

● **PRESCRIBING AND DISPENSING INFORMATION**

- When used for Acute anaphylaxis (for self-administration at the first signs of anaphylaxis) Patients and their carers should be instructed in the administration of adrenaline by *intramuscular injection* or by *nasal spray*.
- With intramuscular use It is important, in acute anaphylaxis where intramuscular injection might still succeed, time should not be wasted seeking intravenous access. Great vigilance is needed to ensure that the *correct strength* of adrenaline injection is used; anaphylactic shock kits need to make a *very clear distinction* between the 1 in 10 000 strength and the 1 in 1000 strength. Packs for self-administration need to be **clearly labelled with instructions** on how to administer adrenaline (intramuscularly, preferably at the midpoint of the outer thigh, through light clothing if necessary) so that in the case of rapid collapse someone else is able to give it. Adrenaline for administration by intramuscular injection is available in 'auto-injectors' (e.g. *EpiPen*® or *Jext*®), pre-assembled syringes fitted with a needle suitable for very rapid administration (if necessary by a bystander or a healthcare provider if it is the only preparation available); injection technique is device specific. To ensure patients receive the auto-injector device that they have been trained to use, prescribers should specify the brand to be dispensed. If switching between brands, patients should receive full training in use of the new auto-injector device. Licensed doses differ between brands of adrenaline auto-injectors. Adrenaline bioavailability has the potential to be influenced by a number of factors including formulation, propulsive force of the device, needle length, and patient specific factors—consult product literature for further information.

● **PATIENT AND CARER ADVICE**

- With intramuscular use Patients and carers should be advised on the safe and effective use of adrenaline auto-injector devices in advance and to sign up for expiry alert services—see also *Important safety information*. For further information, see MHRA guidance: Adrenaline Auto-Injectors (AAIs) Safety Campaign at: www.gov.uk/government/publications/adrenaline-auto-injectors-aais-safety-campaign.

At the first signs of anaphylaxis

- With intramuscular use or intranasal use Patients and carers should be advised the following:
  - Use your adrenaline *auto-injector* or *nasal spray* immediately if you have any signs of anaphylaxis. Use even if in doubt of severity, don't delay;
  - Call 999 and say anaphylaxis ("ana-fill-axis")—straight after using your adrenaline *auto-injector* or *nasal spray*;
  - Lie down and raise your legs;
  - Use a second adrenaline *auto-injector* or *nasal spray* if your symptoms haven't improved after 5 minutes. Both doses of the *nasal spray* should be administered into the same nostril;
  - Lying down is important to keep blood flowing to your organs; you can sit up if you are struggling to breathe, but keep your legs elevated as far as possible and lie back down again as soon as you can. Young children may need to lie down first to help assist *injection* administration by carer;
  - An ambulance should be called even if symptoms appear to be improving after using an adrenaline *auto-injector* or *nasal spray* and the individual should not be left alone. The purpose of adrenaline *auto-injectors* or *nasal sprays* is to start treatment for anaphylaxis that is continued by the emergency services.

Medicines for Children leaflet: Adrenaline auto-injector for anaphylaxis www.medicinesforchildren.org.uk/medicines/adrenaline-auto-injector-for-anaphylaxis/

EPIPEN® AUTO-INJECTOR 300 MICROGRAMS 1.7 mL of the solution remains in the auto-injector device after use.

EPIPEN® JR AUTO-INJECTOR 150 MICROGRAMS 1.7 mL of the solution remains in the auto-injector device after use.

JEXT® AUTO-INJECTOR 150 MICROGRAMS 1.25 mL of the solution remains in the auto-injector device after use.

JEXT® AUTO-INJECTOR 300 MICROGRAMS 1.1 mL of the solution remains in the auto-injector device after use.

● **EXCEPTIONS TO LEGAL CATEGORY** POM restriction does not apply to the intramuscular administration of up to 1 mg of adrenaline injection 1 in 1000 (1 mg/mL) for the emergency treatment of anaphylaxis.

- **MEDICINAL FORMS** There can be variation in the licensing of different medicines containing the same drug. Forms available from special-order manufacturers include: solution for injection

Solution for injection

EXCIPIENTS: May contain Sulfites

▸ **Adrenaline (Non-proprietary)**

Adrenaline 100 microgram per 1 ml Adrenaline (base) 100micrograms/1ml (1 in 10,000) dilute solution for injection ampoules | 10 ampoule PoM £166.53 DT = £166.53

Adrenaline (base) 1mg/10ml (1 in 10,000) dilute solution for injection pre-filled syringes | 1 pre-filled disposable injection PoM £7.21-£18.00 (Hospital only) | 10 pre-filled disposable injection PoM £180.00 (Hospital only)

Adrenaline (as Adrenaline acid tartrate) 100 microgram per 1 ml Adrenaline (base) 1mg/10ml (1 in 10,000) dilute solution for injection ampoules | 10 ampoule PoM £189.07 DT = £189.07

Adrenaline (base) 500micrograms/5ml (1 in 10,000) dilute solution for injection ampoules | 10 ampoule PoM £157.65

Adrenaline 1 mg per 1 ml Adrenaline (base) 10mg/10ml (1 in 1,000) solution for injection ampoules | 10 ampoule PoM £172.76-£324.78 DT = £172.76

Adrenaline (base) for anaphylaxis 1mg/1ml (1 in 1,000) solution for injection pre-filled syringes | 1 pre-filled disposable injection PoM £15.77 DT = £15.77

Adrenaline (base) 1mg/1ml (1 in 1,000) solution for injection pre-filled syringes | 1 pre-filled disposable injection PoM £15.77 DT = £15.77

Adrenaline (as Adrenaline acid tartrate) 1 mg per 1 ml Adrenaline (base) 5mg/5ml (1 in 1,000) solution for injection ampoules | 10 ampoule PoM £211.89 DT = £211.89

Adrenaline (base) 500micrograms/0.5ml (1 in 1,000) solution for injection ampoules | 10 ampoule PoM £364.07-£684.44 DT = £364.07

Adrenaline (base) 1mg/1ml (1 in 1,000) solution for injection ampoules | 10 ampoule PoM £11.81 DT = £11.81 (Hospital only) | 10 ampoule PoM £6.00-£11.81 DT = £11.81

▸ **EpiPen** (Viatris UK Healthcare Ltd)

Adrenaline 500 microgram per 1 ml EpiPen Jr. 150micrograms/0.3ml (1 in 2,000) solution for injection auto-injectors | 1 pre-filled disposable injection PoM £60.69 DT = £60.69 | 2 pre-filled disposable injection PoM £121.38 DT = £121.38

Adrenaline 1 mg per 1 ml EpiPen 300micrograms/0.3ml (1 in 1,000) solution for injection auto-injectors | 1 pre-filled disposable injection PoM £60.69 DT = £60.69 | 2 pre-filled disposable injection PoM £121.38

▸ **Jext** (ALK-Abello Ltd)

Adrenaline 1 mg per 1 ml Jext 300micrograms/0.3ml (1 in 1,000) solution for injection auto-injectors | 1 pre-filled disposable injection PoM £60.69 DT = £60.69

Adrenaline (as Adrenaline acid tartrate) 1 mg per 1 ml Jext 150micrograms/0.15ml (1 in 1,000) solution for injection auto-injectors | 1 pre-filled disposable injection PoM £60.69 DT = £60.69

Spray

EXCIPIENTS: May contain Benzalkonium chloride, disodium edetate, sodium metabisulfite

▸ **EURneffy** (ALK-Abello Ltd)

Adrenaline 20 mg per 1 ml EURneffy 2mg/100microlitres nasal spray unit dose | 2 unit dose PoM £182.10

8 Oedema

Diuretics

07-Mar-2026

Overview

Diuretics are used for a variety of conditions in children including pulmonary oedema (caused by conditions such as respiratory distress syndrome and bronchopulmonary dysplasia), congestive heart failure, and hypertension. Hypertension in children is often resistant to therapy and may require the use of several drugs in combination. Maintenance of fluid and electrolyte balance can be difficult in children on diuretics, particularly neonates whose renal function may be immature.

Loop diuretics are used for pulmonary oedema, congestive heart failure, and in renal disease.

Thiazides are used less commonly than loop diuretics but are often used in combination with loop diuretics or spironolactone p. 147 in the management of pulmonary oedema and, in lower doses, for hypertension associated with cardiac disease.

Aminophylline **infusion** p. 195 has been used with intravenous furosemide p. 163 to relieve fluid overload in critically ill children.

Thiazides and related diuretics

Thiazides and related compounds are moderately potent diuretics; they inhibit sodium reabsorption at the beginning of the distal convoluted tubule. They are usually administered early in the day so that the diuresis does not interfere with sleep.

In the management of *hypertension* a low dose of a thiazide produces a maximal or near-maximal blood pressure lowering effect, with very little biochemical disturbance. Higher doses cause more marked changes in plasma potassium, sodium, uric acid, glucose, and lipids, with little advantage in blood pressure control. Thiazides also have a role in chronic heart failure.

Bendroflumethiazide p. 130 is licensed for use in children; chlorothiazide p. 130 is also used.

Chlortalidone p. 165, a thiazide-related compound, has a longer duration of action than the thiazides and may be given on alternate days in younger children.

Metolazone p. 166 is particularly effective when combined with a loop diuretic (even in renal failure) and is most effective when given 30–60 minutes before furosemide. Profound diuresis can occur and the child should therefore be monitored carefully to avoid potentially dangerous electrolyte disturbance.

Loop diuretics

Loop diuretics inhibit reabsorption of sodium, potassium, and chloride from the ascending limb of the loop of Henlé in the renal tubule and are powerful diuretics.

Furosemide and bumetanide p. 163 are similar in activity; they produce dose-related diuresis. Furosemide is used extensively in children. It can be used for pulmonary oedema (e.g. in respiratory distress syndrome and bronchopulmonary dysplasia), congestive heart failure, and in renal disease.

Potassium-sparing diuretics and mineralocorticoid receptor antagonists

Spironolactone is the most commonly used potassium sparing diuretic in children; it is a mineralocorticoid receptor antagonist and enhances potassium retention and sodium excretion in the distal tubule. Spironolactone is combined with other diuretics to reduce urinary potassium loss. It is also used in nephrotic syndrome, the long-term management of Bartter's syndrome, and high doses can help to control ascites in babies with chronic neonatal hepatitis. The clinical value of spironolactone in the management of pulmonary oedema in preterm neonates with chronic lung disease is uncertain.

Potassium canrenoate p. 147 given intravenously, is an alternative mineralocorticoid receptor antagonist that may be useful if a potassium-sparing diuretic is required and the child is unable to take oral medication. It is metabolised to canrenone, which is also a metabolite of spironolactone.

Amiloride hydrochloride p. 165 on its own is a weak diuretic. It causes retention of potassium and is therefore given with thiazide or loop diuretics as an alternative to giving potassium supplements.

A potassium-sparing diuretic such as spironolactone or amiloride hydrochloride may also be used in the management of amphotericin B-induced hypokalaemia.

Potassium supplements must **not** be given with potassium-sparing diuretics. Administration of a potassium-sparing diuretic to a child receiving an ACE inhibitor or an angiotensin-II receptor antagonist can also cause severe hyperkalaemia.

Potassium-sparing diuretics with other diuretics

Although it is preferable to prescribe diuretics separately in children, the use of fixed combinations may be justified in older children if compliance is a problem. (Some preparations may not be licensed for use in children—consult product literature).

Other diuretics

Mannitol p. 164 is used to treat cerebral oedema, raised intraocular pressure, peripheral oedema, and ascites.

The carbonic anhydrase inhibitor acetazolamide p. 852 is a weak diuretic although it is little used for its diuretic effect.

Eye drops of dorzolamide p. 854 and brinzolamide p. 853 inhibit the formation of aqueous humour and are used in glaucoma.

Diuretics with potassium

Diuretics and potassium supplements should be prescribed separately.

DIURETICS › LOOP DIURETICS

Loop diuretics

- **DRUG ACTION** Loop diuretics inhibit reabsorption from the ascending limb of the loop of Henlé in the renal tubule and are powerful diuretics.
- **CONTRA-INDICATIONS** Anuria · renal failure due to nephrotoxic or hepatotoxic drugs · severe hypokalaemia · severe hyponatraemia
- **CAUTIONS** Can cause acute urinary retention in children with obstruction of urinary outflow · can exacerbate diabetes (but hyperglycaemia less likely than with thiazides) · can exacerbate gout · comatose and precomatose states associated with liver cirrhosis · hypotension should be corrected before initiation of treatment · hypovolaemia should be corrected before initiation of treatment

  CAUTIONS, FURTHER INFORMATION
  - Potassium loss Hypokalaemia can occur with loop diuretics.
    Hypokalaemia is particularly dangerous in children being treated with cardiac glycosides. In hepatic impairment, hypokalaemia caused by diuretics can precipitate encephalopathy.
    The use of potassium-sparing diuretics avoids the need to take potassium supplements.
  - Urinary retention Loop diuretics can cause acute urinary retention in children with obstruction of urinary outflow, therefore manufacturer advises adequate urinary output should be established before initiating treatment.
- **SIDE-EFFECTS**
  - **Common or very common** Dizziness · electrolyte imbalance · fatigue · headache · metabolic alkalosis · muscle spasms · nausea
  - **Uncommon** Diarrhoea
  - **Rare or very rare** Bone marrow depression · photosensitivity reaction
  - **Frequency not known** Deafness (more common in renal impairment) · leucopenia · paraesthesia · rash · severe cutaneous adverse reactions (SCARs) · thrombocytopenia · tinnitus (more common with rapid intravenous administration, and in renal impairment) · vomiting
- **HEPATIC IMPAIRMENT** Hypokalaemia induced by loop diuretics may precipitate hepatic encephalopathy and coma—potassium-sparing diuretics can be used to prevent this.
- **RENAL IMPAIRMENT** High doses or rapid intravenous administration can cause tinnitus and deafness.
  Dose adjustments High doses of loop diuretics may occasionally be needed in renal impairment.
- **MONITORING REQUIREMENTS** Monitor electrolytes during treatment.

F above

Bumetanide

- **INDICATIONS AND DOSE**

Oedema in heart failure, renal disease, and hepatic disease | Pulmonary oedema

▶ BY MOUTH
- Child 1 month–11 years: 15–50 micrograms/kg 1–4 times a day (max. per dose 2 mg); maximum 5 mg per day
- Child 12–17 years: Initially 1 mg, dose to be taken in the morning, then 1 mg after 6–8 hours if required

Oedema in heart failure, renal disease, and hepatic disease (severe cases) | Pulmonary oedema (severe cases)

▶ BY MOUTH
- Child 12–17 years: Initially 5 mg daily, increased in steps of 5 mg every 12–24 hours, adjusted according to response

- **UNLICENSED USE** Not licensed for use in children under 12 years.
- **INTERACTIONS** → Appendix 1: loop diuretics
- **SIDE-EFFECTS**
  - **Common or very common** Dehydration · hypotension · skin reactions
  - **Uncommon** Breast pain · chest discomfort · ear pain · vertigo
  - **Rare or very rare** Hearing impairment
  - **Frequency not known** Arthralgia · encephalopathy · gastrointestinal discomfort · gynaecomastia · hyperglycaemia · hyperuricaemia · muscle cramps · musculoskeletal pain (with high doses in renal failure)
- **PREGNANCY** Bumetanide should not be used to treat gestational hypertension because of the maternal hypovolaemia associated with this condition.
- **BREAST FEEDING** No information available. May inhibit lactation.

- **MEDICINAL FORMS** There can be variation in the licensing of different medicines containing the same drug. Forms available from special-order manufacturers include: oral suspension

Oral tablet
- **Bumetanide (Non-proprietary)**
  Bumetanide 1 mg Bumetanide 1mg tablets | 28 tablet PoM £6.00 DT = £4.48
  Bumetanide 5 mg Bumetanide 5mg tablets | 28 tablet PoM £64.00 DT = £67.75

Oral solution
- **Bumetanide (Non-proprietary)**
  Bumetanide 200 microgram per 1 ml Bumetanide 1mg/5ml oral solution sugar free | 150 ml PoM £279.03 DT = £279.03 SF

F above

Furosemide

10-Nov-2025

(Frusemide)

- **INDICATIONS AND DOSE**

Oedema in heart failure, renal disease, and hepatic disease | Pulmonary oedema

▶ BY MOUTH
- Neonate up to 31 weeks corrected gestational age: 0.5–2 mg/kg every 24 hours.

continued →

- Neonate: 0.5–2 mg/kg every 12–24 hours.
- Child 1 month–11 years: 0.5–2 mg/kg 2–3 times a day, alternatively 0.5–2 mg/kg every 24 hours, if corrected gestational age of under 31 weeks, higher doses may be required in resistant oedema; maximum 80 mg per day; maximum 12 mg/kg per day
- Child 12–17 years: 20–40 mg once daily, increased to 80–120 mg per day in resistant oedema

▶ BY SLOW INTRAVENOUS INJECTION

- Neonate up to 31 weeks corrected gestational age: 0.5–1 mg/kg every 24 hours.
- Neonate: 0.5–1 mg/kg every 12–24 hours.
- Child 1 month–11 years: 0.5–1 mg/kg every 8 hours (max. per dose 40 mg) as required, increased if necessary up to 2 mg/kg every 8 hours (max. per dose 40 mg)
- Child 12–17 years: 20–40 mg every 8 hours as required, higher doses may be required in resistant cases

▶ BY CONTINUOUS INTRAVENOUS INFUSION

- Child 1 month–11 years: 0.1–2 mg/kg/hour
- Child 12–17 years: 0.1–2 mg/kg/hour

Oedema in heart failure, renal disease, and hepatic disease following cardiac surgery | Pulmonary oedema following cardiac surgery

▶ BY CONTINUOUS INTRAVENOUS INFUSION

- Child: Initially 100 micrograms/kg/hour, dose to be doubled every 2 hours until urine output exceeds 1 mL/kg/hour

Oliguria due to acute or chronic renal insufficiency [GFR below 20 mL/minute]

▶ BY MOUTH

- Child 12–17 years: Initially 250 mg for 1 dose, then increased in steps of 250 mg every 4–6 hours (max. per dose 2 g) if required

▶ BY INTRAVENOUS INFUSION

- Child 1 month–11 years: 2–5 mg/kg up to 4 times a day; maximum 1 g per day
- Child 12–17 years: Initially 250 mg, dose to be administered over 1 hour, increased to 500 mg administered over 2 hours if satisfactory urine output not obtained; then increased to 1 g administered over 4 hours if satisfactory response not obtained within subsequent hour; effective dose of up to 1 g given at a maximum rate of 4 mg/minute can be repeated every 24 hours; if no response obtained dialysis probably required

● **CAUTIONS** Effect may be prolonged in neonates · hepatorenal syndrome · hypoproteinaemia may reduce diuretic effect and increase risk of side-effects

● **INTERACTIONS** → Appendix 1: loop diuretics

● **SIDE-EFFECTS**

GENERAL SIDE-EFFECTS Agranulocytosis · aplastic anaemia · auditory disorder (more common with rapid intravenous administration, and in renal impairment) · diabetes mellitus · eosinophilia · fever · gout · haemolytic anaemia · malaise · mucosal reaction · nephritis tubulointerstitial · nephrocalcinosis (with long-term use in preterm infants) · nephrolithiasis (with long-term use in preterm infants) · pancreatitis acute · shock · skin eruption · tetany · vasculitis

SPECIFIC SIDE-EFFECTS

- With oral use Acute kidney injury · hepatic disorders · metabolic acidosis · psychiatric disorder · urinary disorders
- With parenteral use Acute urinary retention · cholestasis

● **PREGNANCY** Furosemide should not be used to treat gestational hypertension because of the maternal hypovolaemia associated with this condition.

● **BREAST FEEDING** Amount too small to be harmful. May inhibit lactation.

● **DIRECTIONS FOR ADMINISTRATION** For *intravenous injection*, give over 5–10 minutes at a usual rate of 100 micrograms/kg/minute (not exceeding 500 micrograms/kg/minute), max. 4 mg/minute; lower rate of infusion may be necessary in renal impairment. For *intravenous infusion*, dilute with Sodium Chloride 0.9% to a concentration of 1–2 mg/mL. Glucose solutions unsuitable (infusion pH must be above 5.5).

For administration by *mouth*, tablets can be crushed and mixed with water or injection solution diluted and given by mouth. Risk of ototoxicity may be reduced by giving high oral doses in 2 or more divided doses.

● **PRESCRIBING AND DISPENSING INFORMATION**

- With oral use Some liquid preparations contain alcohol, caution especially in neonates.

● **MEDICINAL FORMS** There can be variation in the licensing of different medicines containing the same drug. Forms available from special-order manufacturers include: oral suspension, oral solution

Oral tablet

▶ **Furosemide (Non-proprietary)**

Furosemide 20 mg Furosemide 20mg tablets | 28 tablet PoM £0.68 DT = £0.60

Furosemide 40 mg Furosemide 40mg tablets | 28 tablet PoM £1.00 DT = £0.76 | 250 tablet PoM £5.89

Furosemide 500 mg Furosemide 500mg tablets | 28 tablet PoM £27.00 DT = £18.11

Solution for injection

▶ **Furosemide (Non-proprietary)**

Furosemide 10 mg per 1 ml Furosemide 250mg/25ml solution for injection ampoules | 10 ampoule PoM £40.00 DT = £40.00
Furosemide 40mg/4ml solution for injection ampoules | 10 ampoule PoM £14.67 | 10 ampoule PoM £12.19 (Hospital only)
Furosemide 50mg/5ml solution for injection ampoules | 10 ampoule PoM £15.40–£17.00 DT = £15.40 | 10 ampoule PoM £15.40–£18.70 DT = £15.40 (Hospital only)
Furosemide 20mg/2ml solution for injection ampoules | 5 ampoule PoM £6.60 (Hospital only) | 10 ampoule PoM £12.15–£13.20 DT = £13.20 | 10 ampoule PoM £12.15–£16.50 DT = £13.20 (Hospital only)

Oral solution

EXCIPIENTS: May contain Alcohol

▶ **Furosemide (Non-proprietary)**

Furosemide 4 mg per 1 ml Furosemide 20mg/5ml oral solution sugar free | 150 ml PoM £14.35 DT = £8.53 SF

Furosemide 8 mg per 1 ml Furosemide 40mg/5ml oral solution sugar free | 150 ml PoM £18.78 DT = £17.83 SF

Furosemide 10 mg per 1 ml Furosemide 50mg/5ml oral solution sugar free | 150 ml PoM £19.36 DT = £17.80 SF

▶ **Frusol** (Rosemont Pharmaceuticals Ltd)

Furosemide 4 mg per 1 ml Frusol 20mg/5ml oral solution | 150 ml PoM £12.07 DT = £8.53 SF

Furosemide 8 mg per 1 ml Frusol 40mg/5ml oral solution | 150 ml PoM £15.58 DT = £17.83 SF

Furosemide 10 mg per 1 ml Frusol 50mg/5ml oral solution | 150 ml PoM £16.84 DT = £17.80 SF

DIURETICS > OSMOTIC DIURETICS

Mannitol

15-Oct-2021

● **INDICATIONS AND DOSE**

Cerebral oedema

▶ BY INTRAVENOUS INFUSION

- Child 1 month–11 years: 0.25–1.5 g/kg, repeated if necessary, to be administered over 30–60 minutes, dose may be repeated 1–2 times after 4–8 hours
- Child 12–17 years: 0.25–2 g/kg, repeated if necessary, to be administered over 30-60 minutes, dose may be repeated 1–2 times after 4–8 hours

Peripheral oedema and ascites

▶ BY INTRAVENOUS INFUSION

- Child: 1–2 g/kg, to be given over 2–6 hours

- **UNLICENSED USE** Not licensed for use in children under 12 years.
- **CONTRA-INDICATIONS** Anuria · intracranial bleeding (except during craniotomy) · severe cardiac failure · severe dehydration · severe pulmonary oedema
- **CAUTIONS** Extravasation causes inflammation and thrombophlebitis
- **INTERACTIONS** → Appendix 1: mannitol
- **SIDE-EFFECTS**
  - **Common or very common** Cough · headache · vomiting
  - **Uncommon** Dizziness · fever · malaise · nausea · pain · skin reactions
  - **Frequency not known** Arrhythmia · asthenia · azotaemia · chest pain · chills · coma · compartment syndrome · confusion · congestive heart failure · dry mouth · electrolyte imbalance · fluid imbalance · hyperhidrosis · hypersensitivity · hypertension · lethargy · metabolic acidosis · muscle complaints · musculoskeletal stiffness · nephrotic syndrome · neurotoxicity · peripheral oedema · pulmonary oedema · rebound intracranial pressure increase · renal impairment · rhinitis · seizure · thirst · urinary disorders · vision blurred
- **PREGNANCY** Manufacturer advises avoid unless essential— no information available.
- **BREAST FEEDING** Manufacturer advises avoid unless essential—no information available.
- **RENAL IMPAIRMENT** EvGr Caution in severe impairment (consult product literature). Ⓜ
- **PRE-TREATMENT SCREENING** Assess cardiac function before treatment.
- **MONITORING REQUIREMENTS** Monitor fluid and electrolyte balance, serum osmolality, and cardiac, pulmonary and renal function.
- **DIRECTIONS FOR ADMINISTRATION** Examine infusion for crystals. If crystals present, dissolve by warming infusion fluid (allow to cool to body temperature before administration).

  An in-line filter is recommended.

- **MEDICINAL FORMS** There can be variation in the licensing of different medicines containing the same drug. Forms available from special-order manufacturers include: infusion, solution for infusion

Infusion

- Mannitol (Non-proprietary)
  - **Mannitol 100 mg per 1 ml** Mannitol 50g/500ml (10%) infusion Viaflo bags | 1 bag PoM
  - **Mannitol 150 mg per 1 ml** Mannitol 75g/500ml (15%) infusion Viaflo bags | 20 bag PoM (Hospital only)
  - **Mannitol 200 mg per 1 ml** Polyfusor mannitol 20% infusion 500ml bottles | 12 bottle PoM £203.88

DIURETICS > POTASSIUM-SPARING DIURETICS

Amiloride hydrochloride

09-Apr-2026

- **INDICATIONS AND DOSE**

Adjunct to thiazide or loop diuretics for oedema in heart failure, and hepatic disease (where potassium conservation desirable)

- BY MOUTH
  - Neonate: 100–200 micrograms/kg twice daily.
  - Child 1 month–11 years: 100–200 micrograms/kg twice daily (max. per dose 10 mg)
  - Child 12–17 years: 5–10 mg twice daily

- **UNLICENSED USE** Not licensed for use in children.
- **CONTRA-INDICATIONS** Addison's disease · anuria · hyperkalaemia
- **CAUTIONS** Diabetes mellitus
- **INTERACTIONS** → Appendix 1: potassium-sparing diuretics
- **SIDE-EFFECTS** Alopecia · angina pectoris · aplastic anaemia · appetite decreased · arrhythmia · arthralgia · asthenia · atrioventricular block exacerbated · bladder spasm · chest pain · confusion · constipation · cough · depression · diarrhoea · dizziness · drowsiness · dry mouth · dyspnoea · dysuria · electrolyte imbalance · encephalopathy · gastrointestinal discomfort · gastrointestinal disorders · gastrointestinal haemorrhage · gout · headache · insomnia · jaundice · muscle cramps · nasal congestion · nausea · nervousness · neutropenia · pain · palpitations · paraesthesia · postural hypotension · sexual dysfunction · skin reactions · tinnitus · tremor · vertigo · visual impairment · vomiting
- **PREGNANCY** Not to be used to treat gestational hypertension.
- **BREAST FEEDING** Manufacturer advises avoid—no information available.
- **RENAL IMPAIRMENT** Manufacturers advise avoid in severe impairment.

  Monitoring Monitor plasma-potassium concentration (high risk of hyperkalaemia in renal impairment).
- **MONITORING REQUIREMENTS** Monitor electrolytes.

- **MEDICINAL FORMS** There can be variation in the licensing of different medicines containing the same drug. Forms available from special-order manufacturers include: oral suspension, oral solution

Oral tablet

- Amiloride hydrochloride (Non-proprietary)
  - **Amiloride hydrochloride 5 mg** Amiloride 5mg tablets | 28 tablet PoM £39.82 DT = £14.05

Oral solution

EXCIPIENTS: May contain Propylene glycol

- Amiloride hydrochloride (Non-proprietary)
  - **Amiloride hydrochloride 1 mg per 1 ml** Amiloride 5mg/5ml oral solution sugar free | 150 ml PoM £158.85 DT = £158.85 SF

DIURETICS > THIAZIDES AND RELATED DIURETICS

129

Chlortalidone

(Chlorthalidone)

- **INDICATIONS AND DOSE**

Ascites | Oedema in nephrotic syndrome

- BY MOUTH
  - Child 5–11 years: 0.5–1 mg/kg every 48 hours (max. per dose 1.7 mg/kg every 48 hours), dose to be taken in the morning
  - Child 12–17 years: Up to 50 mg daily

Hypertension

- BY MOUTH
  - Child 5–11 years: 0.5–1 mg/kg every 48 hours (max. per dose 1.7 mg/kg every 48 hours), dose to be taken in the morning
  - Child 12–17 years: 25 mg daily, dose to be taken in the morning, then increased if necessary to 50 mg daily

Stable heart failure

- BY MOUTH
  - Child 5–11 years: 0.5–1 mg/kg every 48 hours (max. per dose 1.7 mg/kg every 48 hours), dose to be taken in the morning
  - Child 12–17 years: 25–50 mg daily, dose to be taken in the morning, then increased if necessary to 100–200 mg daily, reduce to lowest effective dose for maintenance

- **INTERACTIONS** → Appendix 1: thiazide diuretics

Cardiovascular system 2

- **SIDE-EFFECTS**
  - **Common or very common** Appetite decreased · gastrointestinal discomfort
  - **Uncommon** Gout
  - **Rare or very rare** Arrhythmia · diabetes mellitus exacerbated · eosinophilia · glycosuria · hepatic disorders · nephritis tubulointerstitial · pulmonary oedema · respiratory disorder
- **BREAST FEEDING** The amount present in milk is too small to be harmful. Large doses may suppress lactation.
- **MEDICINAL FORMS** There can be variation in the licensing of different medicines containing the same drug. Forms available from special-order manufacturers include: oral suspension

Oral tablet

- **Chlortalidone (Non-proprietary)**
  - **Chlortalidone 25 mg** Chlortalidone 25mg tablets | 100 tablet PoM ☒ (Hospital only)
  - **Chlortalidone 50 mg** Chlortalidone 50mg tablets | 30 tablet PoM £88.04 DT = £20.90
- **Hylaton** (Morningside Healthcare Ltd)
  - **Chlortalidone 12.5 mg** Hylaton 12.5mg tablets | 30 tablet PoM £42.00 DT = £42.00
  - **Chlortalidone 50 mg** Hylaton 50mg tablets | 30 tablet PoM £59.00 DT = £20.90

F 129

Metolazone

27-Mar-2025

- **INDICATIONS AND DOSE**

Oedema resistant to loop diuretics in heart failure, renal disease and hepatic disease (under expert supervision) | Pulmonary oedema (under expert supervision) | Adjunct to loop diuretics to induce diuresis (under expert supervision)

- BY MOUTH
  - Child 1 month–11 years: 100–200 micrograms/kg 1–2 times a day, dosing recommendations for children are based on metolazone preparations with different bioavailability to *Xaqua*® tablets (licensed for use in adults).
  - Child 12–17 years: 5–10 mg once daily, dose to be taken in the morning, dose can be increased to twice daily in resistant oedema, if necessary. Dosing recommendations for children are based on metolazone preparations with different bioavailability to *Xaqua*® tablets (licensed for use in adults).

DOSE EQUIVALENCE AND CONVERSION

- Metolazone preparations are not interchangeable due to differences in bioavailability.

- **UNLICENSED USE** Not licensed for use in children.

IMPORTANT SAFETY INFORMATION

MHRA/CHM ADVICE: *XAQUA*® (METOLAZONE) 5 MG TABLETS: EXERCISE CAUTION WHEN SWITCHING PATIENTS BETWEEN METOLAZONE PREPARATIONS (JANUARY 2023)

The MHRA advises caution if switching patients between different metolazone preparations because of potential differences in bioavailability and dosing instructions. Healthcare professionals are advised to:

- consider prescribing the licensed formulation (*Xaqua*®) over unlicensed imported preparations for new patients;
- assess individual patient factors before switching from unlicensed preparations to *Xaqua*®;
- consider adjusting the dose and monitor patients when switching to *Xaqua*®;
- only split *Xaqua*® tablets into halves using the tablet score-line;
- prescribe and supply metolazone by brand name, or manufacturer name, and document this clearly.

Healthcare professionals are advised to counsel patients or their carers:

- not to use different metolazone preparations at the same time;
- to be aware of the brand name, or manufacturer of the preparation prescribed, and specific dosing instructions;
- on the signs and symptoms of electrolyte imbalance that may occur when switching preparations, and to contact a healthcare professional if they develop;
- on the signs and symptoms of an inadequate dose, and to contact a healthcare professional if they occur;
- not to stop taking metolazone without discussion with their doctor.

- **CAUTIONS** Acute porphyrias p. 745
- **INTERACTIONS** → Appendix 1: thiazide diuretics
- **SIDE-EFFECTS**
  - **Common or very common** Azotaemia · glycosuria · hypotension · muscle complaints
  - **Uncommon** Arthralgia · gout · vasculitis
  - **Rare or very rare** Apathy · appetite decreased · asthenia · chest pain · chills · confusion · dehydration · drowsiness · gastrointestinal discomfort · haemoconcentration · hepatic disorders · hepatic encephalopathy · hypoplastic anaemia · palpitations · peripheral neuropathy · psychotic depression · renal impairment · restlessness · seizure · severe cutaneous adverse reactions (SCARs) · syncope · tachycardia · venous thrombosis · vertigo · vision blurred
- **BREAST FEEDING** Specialist sources indicate that levels in milk have not been determined, but are likely to be too low to affect the infant. Large doses may suppress lactation.
- **RENAL IMPAIRMENT** See p. 16. Manufacturer advises metolazone remains effective if estimated glomerular filtration rate is less than 30 mL/minute/1.73 m^2 but is associated with a risk of excessive diuresis.
- **MEDICINAL FORMS** Forms available from special-order manufacturers include: oral suspension, oral solution

9 Patent ductus arteriosus

Drugs affecting the ductus arteriosus

Closure of the ductus arteriosus

Patent ductus arteriosus is a frequent problem in premature neonates with respiratory distress syndrome. Substantial left-to-right shunting through the ductus arteriosus may increase the risk of intraventricular haemorrhage, necrotising enterocolitis, bronchopulmonary dysplasia, and possibly death.

Indometacin p. 824 or ibuprofen p. 821 can be used to close the ductus arteriosus. Indometacin has been used for many years and is effective but it reduces cerebral blood flow, and causes a transient fall in renal and gastro-intestinal blood flow. Ibuprofen may also be used; it has little effect on renal function (there may be a small reduction in sodium excretion) when used in doses for closure of the ductus arteriosus; gastro-intestinal problems are uncommon.

If drug treatment fails to close the ductus arteriosus, surgery may be indicated.

Maintenance of patency

In the newborn with duct-dependent congenital heart disease it is often necessary to maintain the patency of the ductus arteriosus whilst awaiting surgery.

Alprostadil p. 167 (prostaglandin E1) and dinoprostone p. 167 (prostaglandin E2) are potent vasodilators that are effective for maintaining the patency of the ductus arteriosus. They are usually given by continuous intravenous infusion, but oral dosing of dinoprostone is still used in some centres.

During the infusion of a prostaglandin, the newborn requires careful monitoring of heart rate, blood pressure, respiratory rate, and core body temperature. In the event of complications such as apnoea, profound bradycardia, or severe hypotension, the infusion should be temporarily stopped and the complication dealt with; the infusion should be restarted at a lower dose. Recurrent or prolonged apnoea may require ventilatory support in order for the prostaglandin infusion to continue.

PROSTAGLANDINS AND RELATED SUBSTANCES

Alprostadil
20-Jul-2020

- **INDICATIONS AND DOSE**

Maintaining patency of the ductus arteriosus

▶ BY CONTINUOUS INTRAVENOUS INFUSION

▸ Neonate: Initially 5 nanograms/kg/minute, adjusted according to response, adjusted in steps of 5 nanograms/kg/minute (max. per dose 100 nanograms/kg/minute), maximum dose associated with increased side-effects.

- **UNLICENSED USE** Alprostadil doses in BNFC may differ from those in product literature.
- **CONTRA-INDICATIONS** Avoid in hyaline membrane disease
- **CAUTIONS** History of haemorrhage
- **INTERACTIONS** → Appendix 1: alprostadil
- **SIDE-EFFECTS**

▶ **Common or very common** Apnoea (more common in neonates under 2 kg) · arrhythmias · diarrhoea · fever · hypotension · seizure · vasodilation

▶ **Uncommon** Exostosis · gastrointestinal disorders · vascular fragility

▶ **Frequency not known** Cardiac arrest · disseminated intravascular coagulation · hypokalaemia · oedema · sepsis

- **MONITORING REQUIREMENTS**

▶ During the infusion of a prostaglandin, the newborn requires careful monitoring of heart rate, blood pressure, respiratory rate, and core body temperature.

▶ Monitor arterial pressure, respiratory rate, heart rate, temperature, and venous blood pressure in arm and leg; facilities for intubation and ventilation must be immediately available

- **DIRECTIONS FOR ADMINISTRATION** Expert sources advise dilute 150 micrograms/kg body-weight to a final volume of 50 mL with Glucose 5% or Sodium Chloride 0.9%; an intravenous infusion rate of 0.1 mL/hour provides a dose of 5 nanograms/kg/minute. Manufacturer advises undiluted solution must not come into contact with the barrel of the plastic syringe; add the required volume of alprostadil to a volume of infusion fluid in the syringe and then make up to final volume.

- **MEDICINAL FORMS** There can be variation in the licensing of different medicines containing the same drug.

Solution for infusion

▸ Neupedix (Sovereign Medical Ltd)

Alprostadil 500 microgram per 1 ml Neupedix 500micrograms/1ml concentrate for solution for infusion ampoules | 5 ampoule PoM £325.00 (Hospital only)

▸ Prostin VR (Pfizer Ltd)

Alprostadil 500 microgram per 1 ml Prostin VR 500micrograms/1ml concentrate for solution for infusion ampoules | 5 ampoule PoM £375.96 (Hospital only)

Dinoprostone
24-Jun-2021

- **INDICATIONS AND DOSE**

Maintaining patency of the ductus arteriosus

▶ BY CONTINUOUS INTRAVENOUS INFUSION

▸ Neonate: Initially 5 nanograms/kg/minute, then increased in steps of 5 nanograms/kg/minute as required; increased to 20 nanograms/kg/minute, doses up to 100 nanogram/kg/minute have been used but are associated with increased side-effects.

▶ BY MOUTH

▸ Neonate: 20–25 micrograms/kg every 1–2 hours, then increased if necessary to 40–50 micrograms/kg every 1–2 hours, if treatment continues for more than 1 week gradually reduce the dose.

- **UNLICENSED USE** Not licensed for use in children.
- **CONTRA-INDICATIONS** Avoid in hyaline membrane disease
- **CAUTIONS** History of haemorrhage
- **SIDE-EFFECTS**

▶ **Rare or very rare** Disseminated intravascular coagulation

▶ **Frequency not known** Asthma · back pain · bronchospasm · cardiac arrest · chills · diarrhoea · dizziness · fever · flushing · headache · hypertension · infection · nausea · uterine rupture · vomiting

- **HEPATIC IMPAIRMENT** Manufacturer advises avoid.
- **RENAL IMPAIRMENT** EvGr Avoid. (M)
- **MONITORING REQUIREMENTS** Monitor arterial oxygenation, heart rate, temperature, and blood pressure in arm and leg; facilities for intubation and ventilation must be immediately available. During infusion of dinoprostone, the newborn requires careful monitoring of heart rate, blood pressure, respiratory rate and core body temperature.
- **DIRECTIONS FOR ADMINISTRATION** For *continuous intravenous infusion*, dilute to a concentration of 1 microgram/mL with Glucose 5% or Sodium Chloride 0.9%. For administration by *mouth*, injection solution can be given orally; dilute with water.

- **MEDICINAL FORMS** There can be variation in the licensing of different medicines containing the same drug.

Solution for infusion

▸ Prostin E2 (Pfizer Ltd)

Dinoprostone 1 mg per 1 ml Prostin E2 750micrograms/0.75ml solution for infusion ampoules | 1 ampoule PoM £8.52 (Hospital only)

Dinoprostone 10 mg per 1 ml Prostin E2 5mg/0.5ml solution for infusion ampoules | 1 ampoule PoM £18.40 (Hospital only)

10 Vascular disease

Peripheral vascular disease
10-Aug-2022

Classification and management

Raynaud's phenomenon, a vasospastic peripheral vascular disease, consists of episodic vasospasm of the fingers and toes often associated with exposure to cold. EvGr Referral to a rheumatologist is recommended for children aged 12 years and under with Raynaud's phenomenon.

Management of Raynaud's phenomenon includes avoidance of exposure to cold and Smoking cessation p. 353 (if appropriate). If lifestyle modifications fail and symptoms are having a significant negative impact, a trial of nifedipine p. 128 as prophylaxis can be considered. (A) Expert sources advise diltiazem hydrochloride p. 168 [unlicensed use] may be used in the treatment of Raynaud's phenomenon. In very severe cases, where digital infarction is likely, expert sources advise intravenous infusion of the prostacyclin analogue iloprost p. 141 [unlicensed use] may be considered.

The evidence for drug treatment in *chilblains* is limited and does not support its routine use.

CALCIUM-CHANNEL BLOCKERS

F 126

Diltiazem hydrochloride

15-Apr-2024

- **INDICATIONS AND DOSE**

Raynaud's syndrome

▶ BY MOUTH

▸ Child 12-17 years: 30–60 mg 2–3 times a day

- **UNLICENSED USE** Not licensed for use in Raynaud's syndrome.
- **CONTRA-INDICATIONS** Acute porphyrias p. 745 · cardiogenic shock · heart failure (with reduced ejection fraction) · left ventricular failure with pulmonary congestion · second- or third-degree AV block (unless pacemaker fitted) · severe bradycardia · sick sinus syndrome · significant aortic stenosis
- **CAUTIONS** Bradycardia (avoid if severe) · first degree AV block · prolonged PR interval · significantly impaired left ventricular function
- **INTERACTIONS** → Appendix 1: calcium-channel blockers
- **SIDE-EFFECTS**

▶ **Common or very common** Cardiac conduction disorders · constipation · gastrointestinal discomfort · malaise

▶ **Uncommon** Arrhythmias · diarrhoea · insomnia · nervousness

▶ **Rare or very rare** Dry mouth

▶ **Frequency not known** Asthma exacerbated · bronchospasm · cardiac arrest · congestive heart failure · extrapyramidal symptoms · fever · gynaecomastia · hepatitis · hyperglycaemia · hyperhidrosis · lupus-like syndrome · mood altered · photosensitivity reaction · severe cutaneous adverse reactions (SCARs) · thrombocytopenia · vasculitis

Overdose In overdose, diltiazem has a profound cardiac depressant effect causing hypotension and arrhythmias, including complete heart block and asystole.

- **PREGNANCY** Avoid.
- **BREAST FEEDING** Significant amount present in milk—no evidence of harm but avoid unless no safer alternative.
- **HEPATIC IMPAIRMENT**

Dose adjustments In adults, manufacturers advise dose reduction—consult product literature.

- **RENAL IMPAIRMENT**

Dose adjustments In adults, manufacturers advise reduced initial dose (consult product literature).

- **MEDICINAL FORMS** There can be variation in the licensing of different medicines containing the same drug. Forms available from special-order manufacturers include: oral suspension, oral solution

Modified-release tablet

CAUTIONARY AND ADVISORY LABELS 25

▸ **Diltiazem hydrochloride (Non-proprietary)**

Diltiazem hydrochloride 60 mg Diltiazem 60mg modified-release tablets | 84 tablet PoM £10.45 DT = £4.15 | 90 tablet PoM £6.49 | 100 tablet PoM £29.01

▸ **Retalzem** (Kent Pharma (UK) Ltd)

Diltiazem hydrochloride 60 mg Retalzem 60 modified-release tablets | 84 tablet PoM £7.43 DT = £4.15

▸ **Tildiem** (Sanofi)

Diltiazem hydrochloride 60 mg Tildiem 60mg modified-release tablets | 90 tablet PoM £7.96

▸ **Tildiem Retard** (Sanofi)

Diltiazem hydrochloride 90 mg Tildiem Retard 90mg tablets | 56 tablet PoM £7.27 DT = £7.27

Diltiazem hydrochloride 120 mg Tildiem Retard 120mg tablets | 56 tablet PoM £7.15 DT = £7.15

▸ **Zeyam** (Ennogen Healthcare International Ltd)

Diltiazem hydrochloride 60 mg Zeyam 60mg modified-release tablets | 84 tablet PoM £6.45 DT = £4.15

Chapter 3 Respiratory system

CONTENTS

Respiratory system, inhaled drug delivery

26-Jul-2025

Overview

The inhaled route delivers the drug directly to the airways; the dose required is smaller than when given by mouth and side-effects are reduced.

Inhaler devices

Different types of inhaler devices are available, these include *pressurised metered-dose inhalers, breath-actuated metered-dose inhalers, dry powder inhalers*, and *soft mist inhalers*. Their administration techniques vary and good technique is essential in ensuring optimum use of inhaler devices. Pressurised metered-dose inhalers (pMDIs) require dexterity and the ability to coordinate actuation with inhalation; a spacer device, with or without a face mask, should usually be used in children (for information on spacers, see *Spacer devices*). Dry powder inhalers or breath-actuated metered-dose inhalers require a minimum inspiratory effort to be able to generate enough inspiratory flow to allow effective drug delivery, which may not be achievable for some children, particularly younger ones. A child's ability to achieve an effective technique with the inhaler device will therefore influence choice, as will the suitability of the inhaler device for the child and their parent's/carer's lifestyle, their preference, the environmental impact of the device, the presence of an integral dose counter, concomitant prescribed inhaler devices, and the range of available inhaler device types for a specific drug.

The number and different types of inhalers given to a child should be minimised. To help reduce confusion and ensure children receive inhalers they have been given training for, the brand and inhaler device should be specified when prescribing. The strength of inhaler device should be considered and the one that uses the least amount of puffs to deliver the required dose is favourable.

Children, and their parents or carers should be instructed carefully on the use of the inhaler and be able to demonstrate satisfactory technique. It is important to check that the inhaler continues to be used correctly because inadequate inhalation technique may be mistaken for a lack of response to the drug. For guidance on the correct use of inhaler devices, see Asthma and Lung UK: **How to use your inhaler** (see *Useful resources*).

On changing from a pMDI to a dry powder inhaler, the child may notice a lack of sensation in the mouth and throat previously associated with each actuation; coughing may also occur.

EvGr For children aged under 5 years with chronic stable asthma, corticosteroid and bronchodilator treatment should routinely be delivered by a pMDI and a spacer with a face mask where necessary, until the child is able to breath reproducibly using the spacer mouthpiece. Ⓐ

In children over the age of 5 years with mild or moderate acute asthma attacks, a pMDI with a spacer is at least as effective as nebulisation.

Advice to be given to children and their family or carers
Children and their family or carers should be advised on how to check the number of medication doses in their inhaler device. For metered-dose inhalers, they should be informed that these inhaler devices deliver a fixed number of medication doses per canister, and that after these doses have been used up, the inhaler will continue to actuate, expelling propellant gas but no active ingredient. This may lead to children inadvertently using 'empty' inhalers and inhaling propellant only instead of medication, which could lead to exacerbation and destabilisation of their condition, as well as unnecessary expulsion of harmful propellant gas into the environment. An inhaler with an integral dose counter which alerts children and their parents or carers when all therapeutic doses have been delivered should be used where possible. For inhalers without a dose counter there is no accurate way to gauge the remaining number of effective doses other than by either recording every actuation used, or by calculating when the inhaler is likely to become 'empty' according to their standard usage. Shaking, weighing, or floating the inhaler device, or using it until it no longer actuates are inaccurate and not recommended.

Children and their family/carers should also be advised to follow manufacturers' instructions on the care and cleaning of their inhaler device, and to return empty or expired inhalers to pharmacies for correct disposal (and recycling where available).

For information on inhalers and their environmental impact, see British Thoracic Society, NICE, and SIGN patient decision aid: **Asthma inhalers and climate change** (see *Useful resources*).

MHRA/CHM advice: Pressurised metered dose inhalers (pMDI): risk of airway obstruction from aspiration of loose objects (July 2018)
The MHRA have received reports of patients who have inhaled objects into the back of the throat—in some cases objects were aspirated, causing airway obstruction. Patients should be reminded to remove the mouthpiece cover fully, shake the inhaler device and check that both the outside and inside of the mouthpiece are clear and undamaged before inhaling a dose, and to store the inhaler with the mouthpiece cover on.

Spacer devices

Spacer devices remove the need for coordination between actuation of a pMDI and inhalation. They reduce the velocity of the aerosol and subsequent impaction on the oropharynx and allow more time for evaporation of the propellant so that a larger proportion of the particles can be inhaled and deposited in the lungs. A spacer device (with or without a face mask) should usually be prescribed for use with a pMDI in children, particularly those requiring high doses of inhaled corticosteroids, and for children who are prone to candidiasis with inhaled corticosteroids. Smaller-volume spacers may be more manageable for pre-school children and infants. The spacer device used should be compatible with the prescribed inhaler. Spacer devices should not be regarded as interchangeable; children and their parents or carers should be advised not to switch between spacer devices. For information on the different types of spacers available, see Spacers p. 198.

Use and care of spacer devices

The suitability of the spacer device should be carefully assessed; opening the one-way valve is dependent on the child's inspiratory flow. Some spacer devices can be tipped at an angle to open the valve during inhaler actuation and inspiration to assist the child.

Children should inhale from the spacer device as soon as possible after actuation because the drug aerosol is very short-lived. Single puffs should be inhaled (i.e. one puff at a time) using either the tidal (or multiple) breathing method or the single breath and hold method, until the total dose (which may be more than a single puff) has been administered. Tidal breathing is as effective as single breaths. The choice of breathing method is dependent on factors such as the child's ability, inspiratory flow, and age. Children and their parents or carers should be counselled appropriately on the chosen breathing method.

The spacer device should be cleaned once a month by washing in mild detergent and allowed to air-dry; the mouthpiece should be wiped clean of detergent before use. Some manufacturers recommend more frequent cleaning, but this should be avoided since any electrostatic charge may affect drug delivery. Spacer devices should be replaced every 6–12 months.

For more information on the use of spacer devices, see Asthma and Lung UK: **Spacers** (see *Useful resources*).

Nebulisers

A nebuliser converts a solution of a drug into an aerosol for inhalation via a face mask or a mouthpiece. It delivers higher doses of drug to the airways than is usual with standard inhalers. Nebulisers may be used undiluted or may require dilution; the usual diluent is sterile sodium chloride 0.9% (physiological saline). Indications for use of a nebuliser include:

- to deliver a beta$_2$ agonist or ipratropium bromide p. 177 to a child with an *acute exacerbation* of asthma or of airways obstruction;
- to deliver medication to a child unable to use other inhalational devices;
- to deliver an antibacterial (such as colistimethate sodium p. 426 or tobramycin p. 380) or a mucolytic to a child with cystic fibrosis;
- to deliver budesonide p. 186 to a child with severe croup;
- to deliver pentamidine isetionate p. 472 for the prophylaxis of pneumocystis pneumonia.

A National Patient Safety Alert (NatPSA) was issued by NHS England regarding the inadvertent use of piped medical air via a flowmeter to drive the administration of nebulised medication. For further information, see NHS England NatPSA: **Eliminating the risk of inadvertent connection to medical air via a flowmeter** (available at: www.england.nhs.uk/publication/national-patient-safety-alert-eliminating-the-risk-of-inadvertent-connection-to-medical-air-via-a-flowmeter/).

The proportion of nebuliser solution that reaches the lungs depends on the type of nebuliser. The extent to which the nebulised solution is deposited in the airways or alveoli depends on the particle size, pattern of breath inhalation, and lung disease severity. Particles with a mass median diameter of 1–5 microns are deposited in the airways, and a particle size of 1–2 microns is needed for alveolar deposition. The type of nebuliser is therefore chosen according to the deposition required and according to the viscosity of the solution.

When a nebuliser is prescribed, the child or child's parent/carer must:

- have clear instructions on how to use the nebuliser, and maintain and clean it;
- be instructed not to treat acute attacks without also seeking medical help;
- have regular reviews as appropriate.

Due to the serious risks associated with the use of nebulised asthma rescue medications without adequate medical supervision, the home use of nebulisers for the acute treatment of asthma should only be initiated and managed by asthma specialists. For further information, see *Important safety information* in individual bronchodilator monographs such as salbutamol p. 181.

Jet nebulisers

Jet nebulisers are more widely used than ultrasonic nebulisers. Most jet nebulisers require an optimum flow rate of 6–8 litres/minute and can be driven by air or oxygen. Domiciliary oxygen cylinders do not provide an adequate flow rate therefore an electrical compressor is required for domiciliary use.

Some jet nebulisers are able to increase drug output during inspiration and hence increase efficiency.

Tubing

The Department of Health and Social Care has reminded users of the need to use the correct grade of tubing when connecting a nebuliser to a medical gas supply or compressor.

Ultrasonic nebulisers

Ultrasonic nebulisers produce an aerosol by ultrasonic vibration of the drug solution and therefore do not require a gas flow; they are not suitable for the nebulisation of some drugs, such as dornase alfa p. 218 or nebulised suspensions.

Vibrating mesh nebulisers

Vibrating mesh nebulisers produce an aerosol of consistently small sized particles by using the vibration of the mesh to act as a pump to push the liquid drug through the holes of the mesh. They do not require a compressed air source, can be battery operated, and are silent, small, and portable.

Peak flow meters

Peak flow meters may be used to assess lung function in children aged over 5 years with asthma, but symptom monitoring is the most reliable assessment of asthma control. They are best used for short periods to assess the severity of asthma and to monitor response to treatment; continuous use of peak flow meters may detract from compliance with inhalers. Peak flow diaries are available for children to use to record their peak flow scores.

For information on the types of peak flow meters available, see Peak flow meters: low range p. 198, and Peak flow meters: standard range p. 198.

Useful Resources

Patient decision aid: Asthma inhalers and climate change. British Thoracic Society, National Institute for Health and Care Excellence, and Scottish Intercollegiate Guidelines Network. NICE guideline NG245. November 2024.
www.nice.org.uk/guidance/ng245/resources

Spacers. Asthma and Lung UK. January 2024.
www.asthmaandlung.org.uk/symptoms-tests-treatments/treatments/spacers

How to use your inhaler. Asthma and Lung UK.
www.asthmaandlung.org.uk/living-with/inhaler-videos

Resources for families and children, young people with asthma, schools, primary healthcare professionals, secondary healthcare professionals. Beat asthma. www.beatasthma.co.uk/resources/

1 Airways disease, obstructive

Asthma, chronic

10-Nov-2025

Description of condition

Asthma is a common chronic inflammatory condition of the airways, associated with airway hyperresponsiveness and variable airflow obstruction. The most frequent symptoms of asthma are cough, wheeze, chest tightness, and breathlessness. Asthma symptoms vary over time and in intensity and can gradually or suddenly worsen, provoking an acute asthma attack that, if severe, may require hospitalisation.

Aims of treatment

The aim of treatment is to achieve control of asthma. Complete control of asthma is defined as no daytime symptoms, no night-time awakening due to asthma, no asthma attacks, no need for rescue medication, no limitations on activity including exercise, normal lung function (in practical terms forced expiratory volume in 1 second (FEV_1) and/or peak expiratory flow (PEF) > 80% predicted or best), and minimal side-effects from treatment. Uncontrolled asthma refers to asthma symptoms that impact a person's lifestyle or restrict their normal activities; it includes any asthma exacerbation needing treatment with oral corticosteroids and/or frequent regular symptoms such as needing a reliever inhaler 3 or more days per week, or night-time awakening due to asthma symptoms at least once a week. For effective asthma management, the patient's/carer's concerns and expectations should also be considered as these may differ from clinical goals.

Lifestyle changes

EvGr Weight loss in overweight or obese patients may lead to an improvement in asthma symptoms and control. Patients/carers should be advised on approaches for minimising exposure to air pollution and any other personal triggers which cause asthma symptoms and exacerbations. Patients with asthma and parents of children with asthma should also be advised about the dangers of smoking, to themselves and to their children, and be offered appropriate support to stop smoking. Ⓐ For further information, see Smoking cessation p. 353.

Principles of pharmacological management

EvGr A stepwise approach aims to stop symptoms quickly and to improve peak flow. Treatment should be started at the level most appropriate to initial severity of asthma. The aim is to achieve early control and to maintain it by stepping up treatment as necessary and decreasing treatment when control is good. Possible reasons for uncontrolled asthma (such as alternative diagnoses or co-morbidities, suboptimal adherence or inhaler technique, active or passive smoking, and psychosocial, seasonal, or environmental factors) should be taken into account or addressed before starting or adjusting treatment. The response should be reviewed 8 to 12 weeks after starting or adjusting asthma treatment.

Short-acting $beta_2$ agonists (SABAs) such as salbutamol or terbutaline should not be prescribed to children with asthma without a concomitant prescription of an inhaled corticosteroid (ICS) as clinical outcomes are poorer when a SABA is used alone.

A self-management programme comprising of a written personalised action plan and education should be offered to all children with asthma (and/or their family or carers), and should be supported with regular review by a healthcare professional. Ⓐ

The following terms may be used in *Drug treatment for children aged 12 years and over*, *Drug treatment for children aged 5 to 11 years*, and *Decreasing treatment*:

- **Anti-inflammatory reliever (AIR) therapy (for children aged 12 years and over)**
  - AIR therapy is treatment with a reliever inhaler that contains a combination of an ICS and the fast-onset long-acting $beta_2$ agonist (LABA) formoterol. When this is used in response to symptoms without regular maintenance therapy, it is called **as-needed AIR** therapy. Currently, only budesonide with formoterol p. 187 is licensed for as-needed AIR therapy in mild asthma.
- **Maintenance and reliever therapy (MART) (for children aged 5 years and over)**
  - MART refers to treatment with a combination inhaler containing an ICS and formoterol used for daily maintenance therapy *and* the relief of symptoms as needed. The terms low-dose MART and moderate-dose MART refer to the ICS dosage of the maintenance component of MART, see budesonide with formoterol.

For information on devices used for the delivery of inhaled medicines, see Respiratory system, inhaled drug delivery p. 169.

Drug treatment for children aged 12 years and over

For definitions of terms used in the treatment pathways, see *Principles of pharmacological management*, and for guidance on ICS doses, see *Inhaled corticosteroid (ICS) doses for children aged 12 years and over* table.

Initial treatment

EvGr The recommended first-line treatment for newly-diagnosed asthma is as-needed AIR therapy with a low-dose ICS and formoterol combination inhaler such as budesonide with formoterol. If the child presents as highly symptomatic or with a severe exacerbation, start treatment with low-dose MART (a course of oral corticosteroids may also be needed to treat acute symptoms); consider stepping down to as-needed AIR therapy at a later date if their asthma is controlled. Ⓐ

Further treatment

EvGr Offer low-dose MART to children with asthma not controlled on as-needed AIR therapy.

If asthma is not controlled on low-dose MART, offer moderate-dose MART. Ⓐ

For children not controlled on moderate-dose MART despite good adherence:

- EvGr check their fractional exhaled nitric oxide (FeNO) level if available, and blood eosinophil count. If either of these is raised, refer to a specialist in asthma care;
- if neither FeNO nor eosinophil count is raised, consider a trial of either a leukotriene receptor antagonist (LTRA) such as montelukast p. 194 or a long-acting muscarinic receptor antagonist (LAMA) such as tiotropium p. 178 in addition to moderate-dose MART. Review after 8–12 weeks and:
  - if asthma is controlled, continue treatment;
  - if asthma control is improved, but still inadequate, continue the treatment and start a trial of the other drug (LTRA or LAMA);
  - if control has not improved, stop the LTRA or LAMA and start a trial of the alternative drug (LAMA or LTRA).

If asthma is not controlled despite treatment with moderate-dose MART and trials of an LTRA and a LAMA, refer the child to a specialist in asthma care. Ⓐ

Specialist treatments for severe or difficult asthma may include theophylline, high-dose ICS, continuous oral corticosteroids, immunotherapy, or monoclonal antibodies. For further information, see British Thoracic Society (BTS)/NICE/SIGN guidance NG244: **Asthma pathway** (available at: www.nice.org.uk/guidance/ng244), and BTS/SIGN guideline 158: **British guideline on the management of asthma** (see *Useful resources*).

Treatment pathways for children with existing asthma

Many children with existing asthma will be on treatment pathways recommended in previous BTS/SIGN and NICE asthma guidelines.

EvGr For children with confirmed asthma who are currently receiving treatment with a SABA only, change to as-needed AIR therapy with a low-dose ICS and formoterol combination inhaler such as budesonide with formoterol p. 187.

Children with asthma that is well controlled on their current regimen which includes an ICS can remain on their current treatment pathway.

For children with uncontrolled asthma, consider changing treatment as follows: (A)

Transferring children aged 12 years and over with uncontrolled asthma from other treatment pathways

Current treatment	Consider changing to
Regular low-dose ICS plus as-needed SABA	Low-dose MART
Regular low-dose ICS/LABA combination inhaler plus as-needed SABA	Low-dose MART
Regular low-dose ICS and LTRA plus as-needed SABA	Low-dose MART, +/- LTRA
Regular low-dose ICS/LABA combination inhaler and LTRA plus as-needed SABA	Low-dose MART, +/- LTRA
Regular moderate-dose ICS plus as-needed SABA	Moderate-dose MART
Regular moderate-dose ICS/LABA combination inhaler plus as-needed SABA	Moderate-dose MART
Regular moderate-dose ICS and LTRA or LAMA, or both, plus as-needed SABA	Moderate-dose MART, +/- LTRA, +/- LAMA
Regular moderate-dose ICS/LABA combination inhaler and LTRA or LAMA, or both, plus as-needed SABA	Moderate-dose MART, +/- LTRA, +/- LAMA
Any regimen including high-dose ICS	Refer to asthma specialist

Note: When changing from a regimen containing an LTRA or a LAMA, or both, to MART, consider whether to stop or continue the LAMA and/or LTRA based on the degree of benefit achieved when first introduced.

EvGr If asthma is still not controlled despite treatment with moderate-dose MART and trials of an LTRA and a LAMA, refer the child to a specialist in asthma care. (A)

Drug treatment for children aged 5 to 11 years

For definitions of terms used in the treatment pathways, see *Principles of pharmacological management*, and for guidance on ICS doses, see *Inhaled corticosteroid (ICS) doses for children aged 5 to 11 years* table.

Initial treatment

EvGr Offer a twice-daily paediatric low-dose ICS, plus a SABA as needed. (A)

Further treatment

MART pathway

EvGr Consider paediatric low-dose MART [unlicensed use] for children with asthma that is not controlled on twice-daily paediatric low-dose ICS plus SABA as needed, as long as they are assessed to have the ability to manage a MART regimen (otherwise, see *Conventional pathway (if MART regimen is unsuitable)*).

Consider increasing to paediatric moderate-dose MART [unlicensed use] if asthma is not controlled on paediatric low-dose MART.

Children on MART do not normally need a SABA separately, however, an additional metered-dose SABA inhaler plus a spacer may be provided for emergency use in children aged under 12 years who may be unable to activate a dry powder inhaler during an acute asthma attack.

Refer children to a specialist in asthma care if asthma is not controlled on paediatric moderate-dose MART. (A)

Conventional pathway (if MART regimen is unsuitable)

EvGr In children with uncontrolled asthma, consider adding a leukotriene receptor antagonist (LTRA) such as montelukast p. 194 to twice-daily paediatric low-dose ICS plus SABA as needed. Stop the LTRA if it is ineffective after 8–12 weeks.

If asthma is not controlled on twice-daily paediatric low-dose ICS, plus SABA as needed, offer a twice-daily paediatric low-dose ICS and LABA combination inhaler plus SABA as needed (with or without an LTRA depending on previous response).

If asthma is not controlled on twice-daily paediatric low-dose ICS and LABA combination inhaler, plus SABA as needed, offer a twice-daily paediatric moderate-dose ICS and LABA combination inhaler plus SABA as needed (with or without an LTRA depending on previous response).

Refer children to a specialist in asthma care if asthma is not controlled on twice-daily paediatric moderate-dose ICS and LABA combination inhaler (with or without an LTRA depending on previous response). (A)

Drug treatment for children aged under 5 years

Differentiating asthma symptoms from those caused by recurrent viral infections in children aged under 5 years is challenging; children with recurrent wheeze and features suggesting asthma should be treated empirically as outlined below. EvGr Any pre-school child with an admission to hospital, or 2 or more admissions to an emergency department, with wheeze in a 12-month period should be referred to a specialist respiratory paediatrician.

For children with suspected asthma and symptoms that indicate the need for maintenance therapy or who have severe acute episodes of difficulty breathing and wheeze, consider an 8 to 12 week trial of twice-daily paediatric low-dose ICS plus SABA as needed. (A)

If symptoms do not resolve during the trial period:

- EvGr check inhaler technique and adherence;
- check if there is an environmental source for their symptoms (e.g. mould in the home, cold housing, smokers, or indoor air pollution);
- review whether an alternative diagnosis is likely;
- refer the child to a specialist in asthma care if none of these explain the failure to respond to treatment.

If symptoms do resolve after 8 to 12 weeks, consider stopping the ICS and SABA treatment, and review the symptoms after a further 3 months. If symptoms recur by the 3-month review, or if the child has an acute episode requiring systemic corticosteroids or hospitalisation, restart twice-daily paediatric low-dose ICS with as-needed SABA. Titrate up to twice-daily paediatric moderate-dose ICS if needed. Consider a further trial without treatment after reviewing the child within 12 months.

If suspected asthma is uncontrolled on paediatric moderate-dose ICS plus SABA as needed, consider adding a leukotriene receptor antagonist (LTRA) such as montelukast. Review after 8–12 weeks and stop the LTRA if ineffective.

If suspected asthma is uncontrolled on paediatric moderate-dose ICS and a trial of an LTRA has been unsuccessful or not tolerated, stop the LTRA and refer the child to a specialist in asthma care for further investigation and management. Ⓐ

Decreasing treatment

For definitions of terms used, see *Principles of pharmacological management.*

EvGr When the patient's asthma has been well controlled and maintained, the potential risks and benefits of decreasing their current maintenance treatment should be discussed. When deciding which drug to decrease first and at what rate, the severity of asthma, the side-effects of treatment, duration on current dose, the beneficial effect achieved, and the patient's preference should be considered. Patients should be regularly reviewed when decreasing treatment. Allow at least 8 to 12 weeks before considering further treatment reduction.

If considering step-down treatment for patients aged 12 years and over who are using low-dose regular ICS plus a SABA as needed or low-dose MART, step down to as-needed AIR therapy. Ⓐ

Pregnancy

EvGr Patients with asthma should be closely monitored during pregnancy. It is important that asthma is well controlled during pregnancy to avoid maternal or fetal complications.

Patients should be counselled about the importance and safety of taking their asthma medication during pregnancy to maintain good control. Patients who smoke should be advised about the dangers to themselves and to their baby and be offered appropriate support to stop smoking. Ⓐ For further information, see Smoking cessation p. 353.

EvGr Short- and long-acting beta$_2$ agonists, inhaled corticosteroids, and oral theophylline can be used as normal during pregnancy. Oral corticosteroids should be offered if necessary as the benefits outweigh the risks. If leukotriene receptor antagonists or long-acting muscarinic receptor antagonists are required to achieve adequate control, they should not be withheld. Ⓐ

Inhaled corticosteroid dosages

Inhaled corticosteroid (ICS) doses for children aged 12 years and over

Dose type	Corticosteroid and form (MDI = metered dose inhaler; DPI = dry powder inhaler)	Dose
Low dose	Beclometasone dipropionate standard particle MDI and DPI	200-500 micrograms per day in 2 divided doses
	Beclometasone dipropionate extra-fine particle MDI	100-200 micrograms per day in 2 divided doses
	Budesonide DPI	200-400 micrograms per day as a single dose or in 2 divided doses
	Ciclesonide MDI	80-160 micrograms per day as a single dose
	Fluticasone propionate MDI and DPI	100-250 micrograms per day in 2 divided doses
	Mometasone furoate DPI	200 micrograms per day as a single dose
	Mometasone furoate inhalation powder capsules	80 micrograms per day as a single dose
Moderate dose	Beclometasone dipropionate standard particle MDI and DPI	600-800 micrograms per day in 2 divided doses
	Beclometasone dipropionate extra-fine particle MDI	300-400 micrograms per day in 2 divided doses
	Budesonide DPI	600-800 micrograms per day as a single dose or in 2 divided doses
	Ciclesonide MDI	240-320 micrograms per day as a single dose or in 2 divided doses
	Fluticasone propionate MDI and DPI	300-500 micrograms per day in 2 divided doses
	Fluticasone furoate DPI	100 micrograms per day as a single dose
	Mometasone furoate DPI	400 micrograms per day as a single dose or in 2 divided doses
	Mometasone furoate inhalation powder capsules	160 micrograms per day as a single dose

Dose type	Corticosteroid and form (MDI = metered dose inhaler; DPI = dry powder inhaler)	Dose
High dose	Beclometasone dipropionate standard particle MDI and DPI	1–2 mg per day in 2 divided doses
	Beclometasone dipropionate extra-fine particle MDI	500–800 micrograms per day in 2 divided doses
	Budesonide DPI	1–1.6 mg per day in 2 divided doses
	Ciclesonide MDI	400–640 micrograms per day in 2 divided doses
	Fluticasone propionate MDI and DPI	600–1000 micrograms per day in 2 divided doses
	Fluticasone furoate DPI	200 micrograms per day as a single dose
	Mometasone furoate DPI	600–800 micrograms per day in 2 divided doses
	Mometasone furoate inhalation powder capsules	320 micrograms per day as a single dose

Notes: The dose relates to the metered ICS dose, which may be different to the dose that leaves the mouthpiece (delivered dose) and the labelled strength. If an ICS/LABA inhaler is used in a MART regimen, the dose relates to the regular ICS maintenance dose. Dosages in the table are not strict dose equivalences but a guide to similar clinical effectiveness; the smallest dosage should be used to obtain optimal control. Not all inhalers are licensed for use at all dosages or for all ages (see the respective drug monographs for further information). The dosages in this table are based on BTS/NICE/SIGN guidance NG245: Asthma: diagnosis, monitoring and chronic asthma management.

Inhaled corticosteroid (ICS) doses for children aged 5 to 11 years

Dose type	Corticosteroid and form (MDI = metered dose inhaler; DPI = dry powder inhaler)	Dose
Paediatric low dose	Beclometasone dipropionate standard particle MDI	100–200 micrograms per day in 2 divided doses
	Beclometasone dipropionate extra-fine particle MDI	100 micrograms per day in 2 divided doses
	Budesonide DPI	100–200 micrograms per day as a single dose or in 2 divided doses
	Ciclesonide MDI	80 micrograms per day as a single dose
	Fluticasone propionate MDI and DPI	100 micrograms per day in 2 divided doses
Paediatric moderate dose	Beclometasone dipropionate standard particle MDI	300–400 micrograms per day in 2–4 divided doses
	Beclometasone dipropionate extra-fine particle MDI	150–200 micrograms per day in 2 divided doses
	Budesonide DPI	300–400 micrograms per day as a single dose or in 2 divided doses
	Ciclesonide MDI	160 micrograms per day as a single dose or in 2 divided doses
	Fluticasone propionate MDI and DPI	150–200 micrograms per day in 2 divided doses
Paediatric high dose	Beclometasone dipropionate standard particle MDI	500–800 micrograms per day in 2–4 divided doses
	Beclometasone dipropionate extra-fine particle MDI	300–400 micrograms per day in 2 divided doses
	Budesonide DPI	500–800 micrograms per day in 2 divided doses
	Ciclesonide MDI	240–320 micrograms per day in 2 divided doses
	Fluticasone propionate MDI and DPI	250–400 micrograms per day in 2 divided doses

Notes: The dose relates to the metered ICS dose, which may be different to the dose that leaves the mouthpiece (delivered dose) and the labelled strength. If an ICS/LABA inhaler is used in a MART regimen, the dose relates to the regular ICS maintenance dose. Dosages in the table are not strict dose equivalences but a guide to similar clinical effectiveness; the smallest dosage should be used to obtain optimal control. Not all inhalers are licensed for use at all dosages or for all ages (see the respective drug monographs for further information). The dosages in this table are based on BTS/NICE/SIGN guidance NG245: Asthma: diagnosis, monitoring and chronic asthma management.

Useful Resources

Asthma: diagnosis, monitoring and chronic asthma management. British Thoracic Society, National Institute for Health and Care Excellence, and Scottish Intercollegiate Guidelines Network. NICE guideline NG245. November 2024.
www.nice.org.uk/guidance/ng245

British guideline on the management of asthma. British Thoracic Society and Scottish Intercollegiate Guidelines Network. A national clinical guideline SIGN158. November 2024.
www.sign.ac.uk/sign-158-british-guideline-on-the-management-of-asthma

Asthma, acute

12-Jun-2025

Description of condition

Acute asthma is the progressive worsening of asthma symptoms, including breathlessness, wheeze, cough, and chest tightness. An acute exacerbation is marked by a reduction in baseline objective measures of pulmonary function, such as peak expiratory flow rate and FEV_1.

Most asthma attacks severe enough to require hospitalisation develop relatively slowly over a period of six hours or more. In children, intermittent wheezing attacks are usually triggered by viral infections and response to asthma medication may be inconsistent. Low birth weight and/or prematurity may be risk factors for recurrent wheeze.

An asthma care bundle is available to inform the management of patients discharged from hospital following an acute asthma attack. It aims to reduce the number of hospital admissions and improve patient outcomes. For more information, see British Thoracic Society: **Asthma care bundles** (available at: www.brit-thoracic.org.uk/quality-improvement/clinical-resources/asthma/bts-asthma-care-bundles/).

Aims of treatment

The aim of treatment is to relieve airflow obstruction and prevent future relapses. Early treatment is most advantageous.

Levels of severity

Children

EvGr An acute exacerbation of asthma should be correctly differentiated from poor asthma control and its severity categorised in order to be appropriately treated. The categories are described as follows: (A)

Moderate acute asthma

- Able to talk in sentences;
- Arterial oxygen saturation (SpO_2) $\geq$ 92%;
- Peak expiratory flow (PEF) $\geq$ 50% best or predicted;
- Heart rate $\leq$ 140/minute in children aged 1–5 years; heart rate $\leq$ 125/minute in children aged over 5 years;
- Respiratory rate $\leq$ 40/minute in children aged 1–5 years; respiratory rate $\leq$ 30/minute in children aged over 5 years.

Severe acute asthma

- Can't complete sentences in one breath or too breathless to talk or feed;
- SpO_2 < 92%;
- PEF 33–50% best or predicted;
- Heart rate > 140/minute in children aged 1–5 years; heart rate > 125/minute in children aged over 5 years;
- Respiratory rate > 40/minute in children aged 1–5 years; respiratory rate > 30/minute in children aged over 5 years.

Life-threatening acute asthma

SpO_2 < 92%, plus any one of the following in a child with severe asthma:

- PEF < 33% best or predicted;
- Silent chest;
- Cyanosis;
- Poor respiratory effort;
- Hypotension;
- Exhaustion;
- Confusion.

Management in children aged 2 years and over

EvGr Children with features of **severe** or **life-threatening** acute asthma should start treatment as soon as possible and be referred to hospital immediately following initial assessment.

Any child who fails to respond to treatment adequately at any time should also be referred to hospital immediately.

Supplementary high flow oxygen (via a tight-fitting face mask or nasal cannula) should be given to all children with life-threatening acute asthma or SpO_2 < 94% to achieve normal saturations of 94–98%.

First-line treatment for acute asthma is an inhaled short-acting beta$_2$ agonist (such as salbutamol p. 181) given as soon as possible. For children with mild to moderate acute asthma, a pressurised metered-dose inhaler and spacer device is the preferred option. The dose given should be individualised according to severity and adjusted based on response. Parents/carers of children with acute asthma at home, should seek urgent medical attention if initial symptoms are not controlled with up to 10 puffs of salbutamol via a spacer; if symptoms are severe, additional bronchodilator doses should be given as needed whilst awaiting medical attention. Urgent medical attention should also be sought if a child's symptoms return within 3–4 hours; if symptoms return within this time, a further or larger dose (maximum of 10 puffs of salbutamol via a spacer) should be given whilst awaiting medical attention. For children with acute severe or life-threatening symptoms, administration via an oxygen-driven nebuliser is recommended, if available. (A) Home use of nebulisers for the treatment of acute asthma in children should be initiated and managed by an appropriate specialist.

EvGr In all cases of acute asthma, children should be prescribed an adequate dose of oral prednisolone p. 548. Treatment for up to 3 days is usually sufficient, but the length of the course should be tailored to the number of days necessary to bring about recovery. Repeat the dose in children who vomit and consider the intravenous route in those who are unable to retain oral medication. It is considered good practice that inhaled corticosteroids are continued at their usual maintenance dose whilst receiving additional treatment for the attack, but they should not be used as a replacement for the oral corticosteroid. (A)

For information on the general use and side-effects of corticosteroids, see Corticosteroids, general use p. 537. For information on the cessation of oral corticosteroid treatment, see *Treatment cessation* for systemic corticosteroids (such as prednisolone).

EvGr Nebulised ipratropium bromide p. 177 can be combined with a nebulised beta$_2$ agonist for children with a poor initial response to beta$_2$ agonist therapy to provide greater bronchodilation. Consider adding magnesium sulfate p. 739 [unlicensed use] to each nebulised salbutamol and ipratropium bromide in the first hour in children with a short duration of severe acute asthma symptoms presenting with an oxygen saturation less than 92%.

Children with continuing severe acute asthma despite frequent nebulised beta$_2$ agonists and ipratropium bromide plus oral corticosteroids, and those with life-threatening features, need urgent review by a specialist with a view to transfer to a high dependency unit or paediatric intensive care unit (PICU) to receive second-line intravenous therapies.

In children who respond poorly to first-line treatments, intravenous magnesium sulfate [unlicensed use] may be considered as first-line intravenous treatment. In a severe asthma attack where the child has not responded to initial inhaled therapy, early addition of a single bolus dose of intravenous salbutamol may be an option. Continuous intravenous infusion of salbutamol, administered under specialist supervision with continuous ECG and electrolyte monitoring, should be considered in children with unreliable inhalation or severe refractory asthma. Intravenous aminophylline p. 195 may be considered in children with severe or life-threatening acute asthma unresponsive to maximal doses of bronchodilators and corticosteroids. (A)

Management in children aged under 2 years

EvGr Acute asthma treatment for all children aged under 2 years should be given in the hospital setting. Treatment of children aged under 1 year should be under the direct guidance of a respiratory paediatrician.

For moderate and severe acute asthma attacks, immediate treatment with oxygen via a tight-fitting face mask or nasal prongs should be given to achieve normal SpO_2 saturations of 94-98%. Trial an inhaled short-acting beta$_2$ agonist and if response is poor, combine nebulised ipratropium bromide p. 177 to each nebulised beta$_2$ agonist dose. Consider oral prednisolone daily for up to 3 days, early in the management of severe asthma attacks.

In children not responsive to first-line treatments or have life-threatening features, discuss management with a senior paediatrician or the PICU team. ⟨A⟩

Follow up in all cases

EvGr Episodes of acute asthma may be a failure of preventative therapy, review is required to prevent further episodes. A careful history should be taken to establish the reason for the asthma attack. Inhaler technique should be checked and regular treatment should be reviewed. Children and their parents or carers should be given a written asthma action plan aimed at preventing relapse, optimising treatment, and preventing delay in seeking assistance in future attacks. It is essential that the child's GP practice is informed within 24 hours of discharge from the emergency department or hospital following an asthma attack, and the child be reviewed by their GP within 2 working days. Children who have had a near-fatal asthma attack should be kept under specialist supervision indefinitely. A respiratory specialist should follow up all children admitted with a severe asthma attack for at least one year after the admission. ⟨A⟩

Useful Resources

British guideline on the management of asthma. British Thoracic Society and Scottish Intercollegiate Guidelines Network. A national clinical guideline SIGN 158. July 2019, updated May 2025.
www.sign.ac.uk/sign-158-british-guideline-on-the-management-of-asthma

Oxygen

Overview

Oxygen should be regarded as a drug. It is prescribed for hypoxaemic patients to increase alveolar oxygen tension and decrease the work of breathing. The concentration of oxygen required depends on the condition being treated; administration of an inappropriate concentration of oxygen may have serious or even fatal consequences. High concentrations of oxygen can cause pulmonary epithelial damage (bronchopulmonary dysplasia), convulsions, and retinal damage, especially in preterm neonates.

Oxygen is probably the most common drug used in medical emergencies. It should be prescribed initially to achieve a normal or near-normal oxygen saturation. In most acutely ill children with an expected or known normal or low arterial carbon dioxide ($P_a\,CO_2$), oxygen saturation should be maintained above 92%; some clinicians may aim for a target of 94–98%. In some clinical situations, such as carbon monoxide poisoning, it is more appropriate to aim for the highest possible oxygen saturation until the child is stable. Hypercapnic respiratory failure is rare in children; in those children at risk, a lower oxygen saturation target of 88–92% is indicated.

High concentration oxygen therapy is safe in uncomplicated cases of conditions such as pneumonia, pulmonary thromboembolism, pulmonary fibrosis, shock, severe trauma, sepsis, or anaphylaxis. In such conditions low arterial oxygen ($P_a\,O_2$) is usually associated with low or normal arterial carbon dioxide ($P_a\,CO_2$), and therefore there is little risk of hypoventilation and carbon dioxide retention.

In severe acute asthma, the arterial carbon dioxide ($P_a\,CO_2$) is usually subnormal but as asthma deteriorates it may rise steeply (particularly in children). These patients usually require high concentrations of oxygen and if the arterial carbon dioxide ($P_a\,CO_2$) remains high despite other treatment, intermittent positive-pressure ventilation needs to be considered urgently.

Oxygen should not be given to neonates except under expert supervision. Particular care is required in preterm neonates because of the risk of hyperoxia.

Low concentration oxygen therapy (controlled oxygen therapy) is reserved for children at risk of hypercapnic respiratory failure, which is more likely in children with:

- advanced cystic fibrosis;
- advanced non-cystic fibrosis bronchiectasis;
- severe kyphoscoliosis or severe ankylosing spondylitis;
- severe lung scarring caused by tuberculosis;
- musculoskeletal disorders with respiratory weakness, especially if on home ventilation;
- an overdose of opioids, benzodiazepines, or other drugs causing respiratory depression.

Until blood gases can be measured, initial oxygen should be given using a controlled concentration of 28% or less, titrated towards a target concentration of 88–92%. The aim is to provide the child with enough oxygen to achieve an acceptable arterial oxygen tension without worsening carbon dioxide retention and respiratory acidosis. Patients may carry an *oxygen alert card*.

The oxygen alert card template is available at www.brit-thoracic.org.uk.

Domiciliary oxygen

Oxygen should only be prescribed for use in the home after careful evaluation in hospital by a respiratory care specialist. Carers and children who smoke should be advised of the risks of smoking when receiving oxygen, including the risk of fire. Smoking cessation p. 353 therapy should be recommended before home oxygen prescription.

Long-term oxygen therapy

The aim of long-term oxygen therapy is to maintain oxygen saturation of at least 92%. Children (especially those with chronic neonatal lung disease) often require supplemental oxygen, either for 24-hours a day or during periods of sleep; many children are eventually weaned off long-term oxygen therapy as their condition improves.

Long-term oxygen therapy should be considered for children with conditions such as:

- bronchopulmonary dysplasia (chronic neonatal lung disease);
- congenital heart disease with pulmonary hypertension;
- pulmonary hypertension secondary to pulmonary disease;
- idiopathic pulmonary hypertension;
- sickle-cell disease with persistent nocturnal hypoxia;
- interstitial lung disease and obliterative bronchiolitis;
- cystic fibrosis;
- obstructive sleep apnoea syndrome;
- neuromuscular or skeletal disease requiring non-invasive ventilation;
- pulmonary malignancy or other terminal disease with disabling dyspnoea.

Increased respiratory depression is seldom a problem in children with stable respiratory failure treated with low concentrations of oxygen although it may occur during exacerbations; children and their carers should be warned to call for medical help if drowsiness or confusion occurs.

Short-burst oxygen therapy

Oxygen is occasionally prescribed for short-burst (intermittent) use for episodes of breathlessness.

Ambulatory oxygen therapy

Ambulatory oxygen is prescribed for children on long-term oxygen therapy who need to be away from home on a regular basis.

Oxygen therapy equipment

Under the NHS oxygen may be supplied as **oxygen cylinders**. Oxygen flow can be adjusted as the cylinders are equipped with an oxygen flow meter. Oxygen delivered from a cylinder should be passed through a humidifier if used for long periods.

Oxygen concentrators are more economical for children who require oxygen for long periods, and in England and Wales can be ordered on the NHS on a regional tendering basis. A concentrator is recommended for a child who requires oxygen for more than 8 hours a day (or 21 cylinders per month). Exceptionally, if a higher concentration of oxygen is required the output of 2 oxygen concentrators can be combined using a 'Y' connection.

A nasal cannula is usually preferred to a face mask for long-term oxygen therapy from an oxygen concentrator. Nasal cannulas can, however, cause dermatitis and mucosal drying in sensitive individuals.

Giving oxygen by nasal cannula allows the child to talk, eat, and drink, but the concentration of oxygen is not controlled and the method may not be appropriate for acute respiratory failure. When oxygen is given through a nasal cannula at a rate of 1–2 litres/minute the inspiratory oxygen concentration is usually low, but it varies with ventilation and can be high if the patient is underventilating.

Arrangements for supplying oxygen

The following oxygen services may be ordered in England and Wales:

- emergency oxygen;
- short-burst (intermittent) oxygen therapy;
- long-term oxygen therapy;
- ambulatory oxygen.

The type of oxygen service (or combination of services) should be ordered on a Home Oxygen Order Form (HOOF); the amount of oxygen required (hours per day) and flow rate should be specified. The clinician will determine the appropriate equipment to be provided. Special needs or preferences should be specified on the HOOF.

The clinician should obtain the consent of the child or carers to pass on the child's details to the supplier, the fire brigade, and other relevant organisations. The supplier will contact the child or carer to make arrangements for delivery, installation, and maintenance of the equipment. The supplier will also train the child or carer to use the equipment.

The clinician should send the HOOF to the supplier who will continue to provide the service until a revised HOOF is received, or until notified that the child no longer requires the home oxygen service.

- East of England, North East: BOC Medical: Tel: 0800 136 603 Fax: 0800 169 9989
- South West: Air Liquide: Tel: 0808 202 2229 Fax: 0191 497 4340
- London East, Midlands, North West: Air Liquide: Tel: 0500 823 773 Fax: 0800 781 4610
- Yorkshire and Humberside, West Midlands, Wales: Air Products: Tel: 0800 373 580 Fax: 0800 214 709
- South East Coast, South Central: Dolby Vivisol: Tel: 08443 814 402 Fax: 0800 781 4610

In **Scotland** refer the child for assessment by a paediatric respiratory consultant. If the need for a concentrator is confirmed the consultant will arrange for the provision of a concentrator through the Common Services Agency. Prescribers should complete a Scottish Home Oxygen Order Form (SHOOF) and email it to Health Facilities Scotland. Health Facilities Scotland will then liaise with their contractor to arrange the supply of oxygen. Further information can be obtained at www.dolbyvivisol.com/services/healthcare-professionals/.

In **Northern Ireland** oxygen concentrators and cylinders should be prescribed on form HS21; oxygen concentrators are supplied by a local contractor. Prescriptions for oxygen cylinders and accessories can be dispensed by pharmacists contracted to provide domiciliary oxygen services.

Croup

21-Oct-2020

Management

EvGr Mild croup is largely self-limiting, but treatment with a single dose of a corticosteroid (e.g. dexamethasone p. 543) by mouth may be of benefit.

Moderate to severe croup (or mild croup that might cause complications such as in those with chronic lung disease, immunodeficiency, impending respiratory failure, or in children aged under 3 months) calls for hospital admission; a single dose of a corticosteroid (e.g. dexamethasone or prednisolone p. 548 by mouth) should be administered while awaiting hospital admission. If the child is too unwell to receive oral medication, dexamethasone (by intramuscular injection) or budesonide p. 186 (by nebulisation) are suitable alternatives while awaiting hospital admission.

For severe croup not effectively controlled with corticosteroid treatment, nebulised adrenaline solution 1 in 1000 (1 mg/mL) p. 159 should be given with close clinical monitoring; (A) the clinical effects of nebulised adrenaline last at least 1 hour, but usually subside 2 hours after administration. EvGr The child needs to be monitored carefully for recurrence of severe respiratory distress. (A)

Other drugs used for Airways disease, obstructive
Dupilumab, p. 920

ANTIMUSCARINICS

Antimuscarinics (inhaled)

09-Feb-2016

- **CAUTIONS** Bladder outflow obstruction · paradoxical bronchospasm · prostatic hyperplasia · susceptibility to angle-closure glaucoma
- **SIDE-EFFECTS**
  - **Common or very common** Arrhythmias · constipation · cough · dizziness · dry mouth · headache · nausea
  - **Uncommon** Dysphonia · glaucoma · palpitations · skin reactions · stomatitis · urinary disorders · vision blurred

F above

Ipratropium bromide

13-Mar-2025

- **INDICATIONS AND DOSE**

Reversible airways obstruction
- BY INHALATION OF AEROSOL
  - Child 1 month–5 years: 20 micrograms 3 times a day
  - Child 6–11 years: 20–40 micrograms 3 times a day
  - Child 12–17 years: 20–40 micrograms 3–4 times a day

Acute bronchospasm
- BY INHALATION OF NEBULISED SOLUTION
  - Child 1 month–5 years: 125–250 micrograms as required; maximum 1 mg per day
  - Child 6–11 years: 250 micrograms as required; maximum 1 mg per day
  - Child 12–17 years: 500 micrograms as required, doses higher than max. can be given under medical supervision; maximum 2 mg per day

Severe or life-threatening acute asthma
- BY INHALATION OF NEBULISED SOLUTION
  - Child 1 month–11 years: 250 micrograms every 20–30 minutes for the first 2 hours, then 250 micrograms every 4–6 hours as required
  - Child 12–17 years: 500 micrograms every 4–6 hours as required

PHARMACOKINETICS
- The maximal effect of inhaled ipratropium occurs 30–60 minutes after use; its duration of

continued →

action is 3 to 6 hours and bronchodilation can usually be maintained with treatment 3 times a day.

- **UNLICENSED USE** [EvGr] The dose of ipratropium for severe or life-threatening acute asthma is unlicensed. ⟨A⟩ *Inhalvent*® not licensed for use in children under 6 years.

IMPORTANT SAFETY INFORMATION

MHRA/CHM ADVICE: PRESSURISED METERED DOSE INHALERS (PMDI): RISK OF AIRWAY OBSTRUCTION FROM ASPIRATION OF LOOSE OBJECTS (JULY 2018)

See Respiratory system, inhaled drug delivery p. 169.

MHRA/CHM ADVICE: NEBULISED ASTHMA RESCUE THERAPY IN CHILDREN: HOME USE OF NEBULISERS IN PAEDIATRIC ASTHMA SHOULD BE INITIATED AND MANAGED ONLY BY SPECIALISTS (AUGUST 2022)

The MHRA has reviewed the evidence regarding a number of deaths in children with asthma, where the clinically unsupervised use of a nebuliser to deliver asthma rescue medication was a potential contributory factor.

Healthcare professionals are advised that home use of nebulisers for the acute treatment of asthma in children and adolescents should only be initiated and managed by asthma specialists. Home use of nebulisers for this purpose, without adequate medical supervision, can mask a deterioration in the underlying disease, which could result in delays in seeking medical attention and be fatal or have serious consequences. The purchase of nebulisers for this purpose, outside of medical advice, is not recommended.

Patients and their carers should be advised to seek urgent medical attention if worsening asthma symptoms are not relieved by prescribed rescue medication, even if there is short-term recovery following its use. They should receive training from a healthcare professional on the usage and maintenance of the nebuliser, and be given advice on when to seek medical attention, so that deterioration in asthma control can be treated without delay. Patients (or their carers) who have been using a nebuliser at home without specialist management should contact their GP about referral to a specialist.

The MHRA has produced videos to support this advice—guidance for healthcare professionals is available at: www.youtube.com/watch?v=qfppzpdeYmk and guidance for patients, parents, and carers is available at: www.youtube.com/watch?v=NO0ir0i043Q.

- **CAUTIONS** Avoid spraying near eyes · cystic fibrosis

CAUTIONS, FURTHER INFORMATION

- Glaucoma *Acute angle-closure glaucoma* has been reported with nebulised ipratropium, particularly when given with nebulised salbutamol (and possibly other beta$_2$ agonists); care needed to protect the patient's eyes from nebulised drug or drug powder.

- **INTERACTIONS** → Appendix 1: ipratropium
- **SIDE-EFFECTS**
  - **Common or very common** Gastrointestinal motility disorder · throat complaints
  - **Uncommon** Corneal oedema · diarrhoea · eye disorders · eye pain · respiratory disorders · vision disorders · vomiting
- **ALLERGY AND CROSS-SENSITIVITY** Contra-indicated in patients with hypersensitivity to atropine or its derivatives.
- **PREGNANCY**
  - When used for Asthma Inhaled drugs can be taken as normal during pregnancy.
  - When used for Reversible airways obstruction [EvGr] Use only if potential benefit outweighs the risk. ⟨M⟩
- **BREAST FEEDING** No information available—manufacturer advises only use if potential benefit outweighs risk.
- **DIRECTIONS FOR ADMINISTRATION** Manufacturer advises if dilution of ipratropium bromide nebuliser solution is necessary use only sterile sodium chloride 0.9%.
- **PRESCRIBING AND DISPENSING INFORMATION**
  - When used for Asthma For choice of therapy, see Asthma, acute p. 174 and Asthma, chronic p. 171.
- **PATIENT AND CARER ADVICE** Patients or carers should be counselled on appropriate administration technique and warned against accidental contact with the eye (due to risk of ocular complications).

Driving and skilled tasks Manufacturer advises patients and carers should be counselled on the effects on driving and performance of skilled tasks—increased risk of dizziness and vision disorders.

- **MEDICINAL FORMS** There can be variation in the licensing of different medicines containing the same drug.

Nebuliser liquid

- **Ipratropium bromide (Non-proprietary)**

  Ipratropium bromide 250 microgram per 1 ml Ipratropium bromide 500micrograms/2ml nebuliser liquid unit dose vials | 20 unit dose [PoM] £7.70 DT = £7.70

  Ipratropium bromide 250micrograms/1ml nebuliser liquid unit dose vials | 20 unit dose [PoM] £10.70 DT = £10.70

  Ipratropium 250micrograms/1ml nebuliser liquid Steri-Neb unit dose vials | 20 unit dose [PoM] £8.99 DT = £10.70

  Ipratropium 500micrograms/2ml nebuliser liquid Steri-Neb unit dose vials | 20 unit dose [PoM] £5.94 DT = £7.70
- **Atrovent UDV** (Boehringer Ingelheim Ltd)

  Ipratropium bromide 250 microgram per 1 ml Atrovent 500micrograms/2ml nebuliser liquid UDVs | 20 unit dose [PoM] £4.87 DT = £7.70

  Atrovent 250micrograms/1ml nebuliser liquid UDVs | 20 unit dose [PoM] £4.14 DT = £10.70

Pressurised inhalation

- **Atrovent** (Boehringer Ingelheim Ltd)

  Ipratropium bromide 20 microgram per 1 dose Atrovent 20micrograms/dose inhaler CFC free | 200 dose [PoM] £5.56 DT = £5.56
- **Inhalvent** (Alissa Healthcare Research Ltd)

  Ipratropium bromide 20 microgram per 1 dose Inhalvent 20micrograms/dose inhaler | 200 dose [PoM] £5.56 DT = £5.56

F 177

Tiotropium

13-Mar-2025

- **INDICATIONS AND DOSE**

SPIRIVA RESPIMAT®

Severe asthma [add-on to inhaled corticosteroid (over 400 micrograms budesonide daily or equivalent) and 1 controller, or inhaled corticosteroid (200–400 micrograms budesonide daily or equivalent) and 2 controllers, in patients who have suffered one or more severe exacerbations in the last year]

- BY INHALATION
  - Child 6–11 years: 5 micrograms once daily

Severe asthma [add-on to inhaled corticosteroid (over 800 micrograms budesonide daily or equivalent) and 1 controller, or inhaled corticosteroid (400–800 micrograms budesonide daily or equivalent) and 2 controllers, in patients who have suffered one or more severe exacerbations in the last year]

- BY INHALATION
  - Child 12–17 years: 5 micrograms once daily

DOSE EQUIVALENCE AND CONVERSION

- For *Spiriva Respimat*®: 2 puffs of inhalation solution is equivalent to 5 micrograms tiotropium.

IMPORTANT SAFETY INFORMATION

MHRA/CHM ADVICE: PRESSURISED METERED DOSE INHALERS (PMDI): RISK OF AIRWAY OBSTRUCTION FROM ASPIRATION OF LOOSE OBJECTS (JULY 2018)

See Respiratory system, inhaled drug delivery p. 169.

- **CAUTIONS** Arrhythmia (unstable, life-threatening or requiring intervention in the previous 12 months) · heart failure (hospitalisation for moderate to severe heart failure in the previous 12 months) · myocardial infarction in the previous 6 months
- **INTERACTIONS** → Appendix 1: tiotropium
- **SIDE-EFFECTS**
  - **Uncommon** Gastrointestinal disorders · increased risk of infection · taste altered
  - **Rare or very rare** Bronchospasm · dysphagia · epistaxis · insomnia · oral disorders
  - **Frequency not known** Dehydration · joint swelling · skin ulcer
- **PREGNANCY** Inhaled drugs can be taken as normal during pregnancy.
- **BREAST FEEDING** Manufacturer advises avoid—no information available.
- **RENAL IMPAIRMENT** Manufacturer advises use only if potential benefit outweighs risk if creatinine clearance less than or equal to 50 mL/minute—plasma-tiotropium concentration raised. See p. 16.
- **PRESCRIBING AND DISPENSING INFORMATION** For choice of therapy, see Asthma, acute p. 174 and Asthma, chronic p. 171.
- **PATIENT AND CARER ADVICE** Patients or carers should be advised that the *Respimat*® inhaler device is re-usable and can be used with a total of 6 cartridges before it needs to be replaced. Refer patients or carers to the Instructions for Use for information on how and when to replace the cartridge.

  Patients or carers should be given advice on appropriate inhaler technique.
- **NATIONAL FUNDING/ACCESS DECISIONS**
  For full details see funding body website

  Scottish Medicines Consortium (SMC) decisions
  - **Tiotropium (*Spiriva Respimat*®) as add-on maintenance bronchodilator treatment in patients aged 6 years and older with severe asthma who experienced one or more severe asthma exacerbations in the preceding year (January 2019)** SMC No. SMC2118 Recommended

  All Wales Medicines Strategy Group (AWMSG) decisions
  - **Tiotropium (*Spiriva Respimat*®) as add-on maintenance bronchodilator treatment in patients aged 6 years and older with severe asthma who experienced one or more severe asthma exacerbations in the preceding year (December 2018)** AWMSG No. 1882 Recommended

- **MEDICINAL FORMS** There can be variation in the licensing of different medicines containing the same drug.

  Inhalation solution
  - **Spiriva Respimat** (Boehringer Ingelheim Ltd)
    Tiotropium (as Tiotropium bromide) 2.5 microgram per 1 dose Spiriva Respimat 2.5micrograms/dose inhalation solution refill cartridge | 60 dose PoM £23.00 DT = £23.00
    Spiriva Respimat 2.5micrograms/dose inhalation solution cartridge with device | 60 dose PoM £23.00 DT = £23.00

BETA$_2$-ADRENOCEPTOR AGONISTS, SELECTIVE

Beta$_2$-adrenoceptor agonists, selective

12-Feb-2016

- **CAUTIONS** Arrhythmias · cardiovascular disease · diabetes (risk of hyperglycaemia and ketoacidosis, especially with intravenous use) · hypertension · hyperthyroidism · hypokalaemia · susceptibility to QT-interval prolongation

  CAUTIONS, FURTHER INFORMATION
  - Hypokalaemia Potentially serious hypokalaemia may result from beta$_2$ agonist therapy. EvGr Particular caution is required in severe asthma or COPD, because this effect may be potentiated by concomitant treatment with theophylline and its derivatives, corticosteroids, diuretics, and by hypoxia. ⟨M⟩
- **SIDE-EFFECTS**
  - **Common or very common** Arrhythmias · dizziness · headache · hyperglycaemia · palpitations · tremor
  - **Rare or very rare** Bronchospasm paradoxical (sometimes severe)
- **PREGNANCY** Inhaled drugs for asthma can be taken as normal during pregnancy.
- **MONITORING REQUIREMENTS**
  - In severe asthma, plasma-potassium concentration should be monitored (risk of hypokalaemia).
  - In patients with diabetes, monitor blood glucose (risk of hyperglycaemia and ketoacidosis, especially when beta$_2$ agonist given intravenously).
- **PATIENT AND CARER ADVICE** The **dose**, the frequency, and the maximum number of inhalations in 24 hours of the beta$_2$ agonist should be **stated explicitly** to the patient or their carer. The patient or their carer should be advised to seek medical advice when the prescribed dose of beta$_2$ agonist fails to provide the usual degree of symptomatic relief because this usually indicates a worsening of the asthma and the patient may require a prophylactic drug. Patients or their carers should be advised to follow manufacturers' instructions on the care and cleansing of inhaler devices.

BETA$_2$-ADRENOCEPTOR AGONISTS, SELECTIVE › LONG-ACTING

above

Formoterol fumarate

17-Jan-2023

(Eformoterol fumarate)

- **INDICATIONS AND DOSE**

  Reversible airways obstruction in patients requiring long-term regular bronchodilator therapy | Nocturnal asthma in patients requiring long-term regular bronchodilator therapy | Prophylaxis of exercise-induced bronchospasm in patients requiring long-term regular bronchodilator therapy | Chronic asthma in patients who regularly use an inhaled corticosteroid
  - BY INHALATION OF POWDER
    - Child 6–11 years: 12 micrograms twice daily, a daily dose of 24 micrograms of formoterol should be sufficient for the majority of children, particularly for younger age-groups; higher doses should be used rarely, and only when control is not maintained on the lower dose
    - Child 12–17 years: 12 micrograms twice daily, dose may be increased in more severe airway obstruction; increased to 24 micrograms twice daily, a daily dose of 24 micrograms of formoterol should be sufficient for the majority of children, particularly for younger age-groups; higher doses should be used rarely, and only when control is not maintained on the lower dose
  - BY INHALATION OF AEROSOL
    - Child 12–17 years: 12 micrograms twice daily, dose may be increased in more severe airway obstruction; increased to 24 micrograms twice daily, a daily dose of 24 micrograms of formoterol should be sufficient for the majority of children, particularly for younger age-groups; higher doses should be used rarely, and only when control is not maintained on the lower dose

  OXIS®

  Chronic asthma
  - BY INHALATION OF POWDER
    - Child 6–17 years: 6–12 micrograms 1–2 times a day (max. per dose 12 micrograms), occasionally doses up to the maximum daily may be needed, reassess

continued →

3 Respiratory system

treatment if additional doses required on more than 2 days a week; maximum 48 micrograms per day

Relief of bronchospasm

- BY INHALATION OF POWDER
  - Child 6–17 years: 6–12 micrograms

Prophylaxis of exercise-induced bronchospasm

- BY INHALATION OF POWDER
  - Child 6–17 years: 6–12 micrograms, dose to be taken before exercise

PHARMACOKINETICS

- At recommended inhaled doses, the duration of action of formoterol is about 12 hours.

IMPORTANT SAFETY INFORMATION

CHM ADVICE

To ensure safe use, the CHM has advised that for the management of chronic asthma, long-acting beta$_2$ agonist (formoterol) should:

- be added only if regular use of standard-dose inhaled corticosteroids has failed to control asthma adequately;
- not be initiated in patients with rapidly deteriorating asthma;
- be introduced at a low dose and the effect properly monitored before considering dose increase;
- be discontinued in the absence of benefit;
- not be used for the relief of exercise-induced asthma symptoms unless regular inhaled corticosteroids are also used;
- be reviewed as clinically appropriate: stepping down therapy should be considered when good long-term asthma control has been achieved.

MHRA/CHM ADVICE: PRESSURISED METERED DOSE INHALERS (PMDI): RISK OF AIRWAY OBSTRUCTION FROM ASPIRATION OF LOOSE OBJECTS (JULY 2018)

See Respiratory system, inhaled drug delivery p. 169.

- **INTERACTIONS** → Appendix 1: beta$_2$ agonists
- **SIDE-EFFECTS**
  - **Common or very common** Muscle cramps · nausea
  - **Uncommon** Angina pectoris · hypokalaemia · sleep disorder · taste altered
  - **Rare or very rare** Anxiety · QT interval prolongation
- **PREGNANCY** Inhaled drugs for asthma can be taken as normal during pregnancy.
- **BREAST FEEDING** Inhaled drugs for asthma can be taken as normal during breast-feeding.
- **PRESCRIBING AND DISPENSING INFORMATION**
  - When used for Asthma For choice of therapy, see Asthma, acute p. 174 and Asthma, chronic p. 171.
- **PATIENT AND CARER ADVICE** Advise patients not to exceed prescribed dose, and to follow manufacturer's directions; if a previously effective dose of inhaled formoterol fails to provide adequate relief, a doctor's advice should be obtained as soon as possible. Patients should be advised to report any deterioration in symptoms following initiation of treatment with a long-acting beta$_2$ agonist. Patient or carer should be given advice on how to administer formoterol fumarate inhalers.
- **MEDICINAL FORMS** There can be variation in the licensing of different medicines containing the same drug.

Inhalation powder

- **Easyhaler (formoterol)** (Orion Pharma (UK) Ltd)
  Formoterol fumarate dihydrate 12 microgram per 1 dose Formoterol Easyhaler 12micrograms/dose dry powder inhaler | 120 dose PoM £23.75 DT = £23.75
- **Oxis Turbohaler** (AstraZeneca UK Ltd)
  Formoterol fumarate dihydrate 6 microgram per 1 dose Oxis 6 Turbohaler | 60 dose PoM £24.80 DT = £24.80
  Formoterol fumarate dihydrate 12 microgram per 1 dose Oxis 12 Turbohaler | 60 dose PoM £24.80 DT = £24.80

Pressurised inhalation

EXCIPIENTS: May contain Alcohol

- **Atimos Modulite** (Chiesi Ltd)
  Formoterol fumarate dihydrate 12 microgram per 1 dose Atimos Modulite 12micrograms/dose inhaler | 100 dose PoM £30.06 DT = £30.06

Combinations available: ***Budesonide with formoterol***, p. 187 · ***Fluticasone with formoterol***, p. 190

F 179

Salmeterol

17-Jan-2023

- **INDICATIONS AND DOSE**

Reversible airways obstruction in patients requiring long-term regular bronchodilator therapy | Nocturnal asthma in patients requiring long-term regular bronchodilator therapy | Prevention of exercise-induced bronchospasm in patients requiring long-term regular bronchodilator therapy | Chronic asthma only in patients who regularly use an inhaled corticosteroid (not for immediate relief of acute asthma)

- BY INHALATION OF AEROSOL, OR BY INHALATION OF POWDER
  - Child 5–11 years: 50 micrograms twice daily
  - Child 12–17 years: 50 micrograms twice daily, dose may be increased in more severe airway obstruction; increased to 100 micrograms twice daily

PHARMACOKINETICS

- At recommended inhaled doses, the duration of action of salmeterol is about 12 hours.

- **UNLICENSED USE** *Neovent*® not licensed for use in children under 12 years.

IMPORTANT SAFETY INFORMATION

CHM ADVICE

To ensure safe use, the CHM has advised that for the management of chronic asthma, long-acting beta$_2$ agonist (salmeterol) should:

- be added only if regular use of standard-dose inhaled corticosteroids has failed to control asthma adequately;
- not be initiated in patients with rapidly deteriorating asthma;
- be introduced at a low dose and the effect properly monitored before considering dose increase;
- be discontinued in the absence of benefit;
- not be used for the relief of exercise-induced asthma symptoms unless regular inhaled corticosteroids are also used;
- be reviewed as clinically appropriate: stepping down therapy should be considered when good long-term asthma control has been achieved.

MHRA/CHM ADVICE: PRESSURISED METERED DOSE INHALERS (PMDI): RISK OF AIRWAY OBSTRUCTION FROM ASPIRATION OF LOOSE OBJECTS (JULY 2018)

See Respiratory system, inhaled drug delivery p. 169.

- **INTERACTIONS** → Appendix 1: beta$_2$ agonists
- **SIDE-EFFECTS**
  - **Common or very common** Muscle cramps
  - **Uncommon** Nervousness · skin reactions
  - **Rare or very rare** Arthralgia · bronchospasm · chest pain · hypokalaemia · insomnia · nausea · oedema · oropharyngeal irritation
- **PREGNANCY** Inhaled drugs for asthma can be taken as normal during pregnancy.
- **BREAST FEEDING** Inhaled drugs for asthma can be taken as normal during breast-feeding.

- **PRESCRIBING AND DISPENSING INFORMATION**
  - When used for Asthma For choice of therapy, see Asthma, acute p. 174 and Asthma, chronic p. 171.
- **PATIENT AND CARER ADVICE** Advise patients that salmeterol should **not** be used for relief of acute attacks, not to exceed prescribed dose, and to follow manufacturer's directions; if a previously effective dose of inhaled salmeterol fails to provide adequate relief, a doctor's advice should be obtained as soon as possible. Patients should be advised to report any deterioration in symptoms following initiation of treatment with a long-acting beta$_2$ agonist.
  Medicines for Children leaflet: Salmeterol inhaler for asthma www.medicinesforchildren.org.uk/medicines/salmeterol-inhaler-for-asthma/
- **MEDICINAL FORMS** There can be variation in the licensing of different medicines containing the same drug.

Inhalation powder

- **Serevent Accuhaler** (GlaxoSmithKline UK Ltd)
  Salmeterol (as Salmeterol xinafoate) 50 microgram per 1 dose Serevent 50micrograms/dose Accuhaler | 60 dose PoM £35.11 DT = £35.11

Pressurised inhalation

- **Serevent Evohaler** (GlaxoSmithKline UK Ltd)
  Salmeterol (as Salmeterol xinafoate) 25 microgram per 1 dose Serevent 25micrograms/dose Evohaler | 120 dose PoM £29.26 DT = £29.26
- **Soltel** (Cipla EU Ltd)
  Salmeterol (as Salmeterol xinafoate) 25 microgram per 1 dose Soltel 25micrograms/dose inhaler CFC free | 120 dose PoM £19.95 DT = £29.26

Combinations available: ***Fluticasone with salmeterol,*** p. 190

BETA$_2$-ADRENOCEPTOR AGONISTS, SELECTIVE › SHORT-ACTING

F 179

Salbutamol

01-May-2025

(Albuterol)

- **INDICATIONS AND DOSE**

Chronic asthma [in line with management advice for chronic asthma]

▶ BY INHALATION OF AEROSOL
- Child 1-17 years: 100–200 micrograms, to be taken when required for symptomatic relief, review prevention medication if salbutamol usage is 3 or more days per week, or if nocturnal symptoms occur

▶ BY INHALATION OF POWDER
- Child 6-17 years: 100–200 micrograms, to be taken when required for symptomatic relief, review prevention medication if salbutamol usage is 3 or more days per week, or if nocturnal symptoms occur

▶ BY INHALATION OF NEBULISED SOLUTION
- Child 1-4 years (initiated by a specialist): 2.5 mg, to be taken when required for symptomatic relief, review prevention medication if salbutamol usage is 3 or more days per week, or if nocturnal symptoms occur
- Child 5-17 years (initiated by a specialist): 2.5–5 mg, to be taken when required for symptomatic relief, review prevention medication if salbutamol usage is 3 or more days per week, or if nocturnal symptoms occur

Acute asthma [in line with management advice for acute asthma]

▶ BY INHALATION OF AEROSOL
- Child 1-2 years: 100 micrograms every 0.5–1 minute for up to 10 doses, each dose to be inhaled separately via a spacer and a close-fitting face mask; repeat every 10–20 minutes or when required
- Child 3-17 years: 100 micrograms every 0.5–1 minute for up to 10 doses, each dose to be inhaled separately via a spacer; repeat every 10–20 minutes or when required

▶ BY INHALATION OF POWDER
- Child 6-17 years: 100 micrograms every 0.5–1 minute for up to 10 doses, each dose to be inhaled separately; repeat every 10–20 minutes or when required, alternatively 200 micrograms every 0.5–1 minute for up to 5 doses, each dose to be inhaled separately; repeat every 10–20 minutes or when required

▶ BY INHALATION OF NEBULISED SOLUTION
- Child 1-4 years: 2.5 mg, repeat every 20–30 minutes or when required, give via oxygen-driven nebuliser if available
- Child 5-17 years: 2.5–5 mg, repeat every 20–30 minutes or when required, give via oxygen-driven nebuliser if available

▶ BY SLOW INTRAVENOUS INJECTION
- Child 12-23 months: 5 micrograms/kg for 1 dose, to be administered over 5–10 minutes
- Child 2-17 years: 15 micrograms/kg for 1 dose (max. per dose 250 micrograms), to be administered over 5–10 minutes

▶ BY CONTINUOUS INTRAVENOUS INFUSION
- Child: 1–2 micrograms/kg/minute, to be adjusted according to response and tolerance, increased if necessary up to 5 micrograms/kg/minute, doses above 2 micrograms/kg/minute should be given in a high dependency or intensive care setting

Prophylaxis of allergen- or exercise-induced bronchospasm

▶ BY INHALATION OF AEROSOL
- Child: 100–200 micrograms, to be taken 10–15 minutes before challenge

▶ BY INHALATION OF POWDER
- Child 6-11 years: 100–200 micrograms, to be taken 10–15 minutes before challenge
- Child 12-17 years: 200 micrograms, to be taken 10–15 minutes before challenge

Exacerbation of reversible airways obstruction

▶ BY INHALATION OF AEROSOL
- Child: 100–200 micrograms, to be taken up to 4 times a day for persistent symptoms

Severe hyperkalaemia

▶ BY SLOW INTRAVENOUS INJECTION
- Neonate: 4 micrograms/kg, to be administered over 5 minutes, dose can be repeated if necessary.
- Child: 4 micrograms/kg, to be administered over 5 minutes, dose can be repeated if necessary

▶ BY INHALATION OF NEBULISED SOLUTION
- Neonate: 2.5–5 mg, dose can be repeated if necessary, intravenous injection route preferred over inhalation of nebulised solution.
- Child: 2.5–5 mg, dose can be repeated if necessary, intravenous injection route preferred over inhalation of nebulised solution

PHARMACOKINETICS
- When used by inhalation At recommended inhaled doses, the duration of action of salbutamol is about 3 to 5 hours.

- **UNLICENSED USE**
  - When used for Asthma or Prophylaxis of allergen- or exercise-induced bronchospasm or Exacerbation of reversible airways obstruction National guidelines and expert advice recommend that salbutamol is used as detailed within the indications and dose section, but this may differ from licensed product information.
  - When used for Severe hyperkalaemia Not licensed for use.
  - With intravenous use Injection and solution for intravenous infusion not licensed for use in children under 12 years.

Administration of undiluted salbutamol injection through a central venous catheter is not licensed.

IMPORTANT SAFETY INFORMATION

MHRA/CHM ADVICE: PRESSURISED METERED DOSE INHALERS (PMDI): RISK OF AIRWAY OBSTRUCTION FROM ASPIRATION OF LOOSE OBJECTS (JULY 2018)

See Respiratory system, inhaled drug delivery p. 169.

MHRA/CHM ADVICE: NEBULISED ASTHMA RESCUE THERAPY IN CHILDREN: HOME USE OF NEBULISERS IN PAEDIATRIC ASTHMA SHOULD BE INITIATED AND MANAGED ONLY BY SPECIALISTS (AUGUST 2022)

The MHRA has reviewed the evidence regarding a number of deaths in children with asthma, where the clinically unsupervised use of a nebuliser to deliver asthma rescue medication was a potential contributory factor. Healthcare professionals are advised that home use of nebulisers for the acute treatment of asthma in children and adolescents should only be initiated and managed by asthma specialists. Home use of nebulisers for this purpose, without adequate medical supervision, can mask a deterioration in the underlying disease, which could result in delays in seeking medical attention and be fatal or have serious consequences. The purchase of nebulisers for this purpose, outside of medical advice, is not recommended. Patients and their carers should be advised to seek urgent medical attention if worsening asthma symptoms are not relieved by prescribed rescue medication, even if there is short-term recovery following its use. They should receive training from a healthcare professional on the usage and maintenance of the nebuliser, and be given advice on when to seek medical attention, so that deterioration in asthma control can be treated without delay. Patients (or their carers) who have been using a nebuliser at home without specialist management should contact their GP about referral to a specialist. The MHRA has produced videos to support this advice—guidance for healthcare professionals is available at: www.youtube.com/watch?v=qfppzpdeYmk and guidance for patients, parents, and carers is available at: www.youtube.com/watch?v=NO0ir0i043Q.

MHRA/CHM ADVICE: SHORT-ACTING BETA 2 AGONISTS (SABA) (SALBUTAMOL): REMINDER OF THE RISKS FROM OVERUSE IN ASTHMA AND TO BE AWARE OF CHANGES IN THE SABA PRESCRIBING GUIDELINES (APRIL 2025)

A review by the MHRA and the EMA's Pharmacovigilance Risk Assessment Committee (PRAC) found that the overuse of short-acting beta$_2$ agonists (SABA) was associated with an increased risk of severe asthma exacerbations, hospitalisations, and mortality, irrespective of disease severity or concomitant anti-inflammatory maintenance therapy. Healthcare professionals are reminded that excessive use of SABA to relieve acute symptoms may mask progression of the underlying disease and contribute to an increased risk of severe and life-threatening exacerbations, and are therefore advised to:

- avoid prescribing SABA to any asthma patient without a concomitant inhaled corticosteroid;
- ensure all asthma patients receive optimal anti-inflammatory maintenance therapy, even when well controlled, and their treatment is individualised;
- review and adjust treatment in those who use as-needed SABA more than twice weekly;
- urgently review patients who have increased their SABA prescription requests or have failed to collect their prescribed anti-inflammatory maintenance therapy;
- consider the recommended alternatives (i.e. anti-inflammatory reliever (AIR) therapy and maintenance and reliever therapy (MART)) in patients aged over 12 years with poorly-controlled asthma.

Healthcare professionals should counsel patients and carers to use their inhalers as prescribed and follow their agreed asthma plan if available. Additionally, patients and carers should be reminded when to request an asthma review and when to seek urgent medical assistance. See also *Prescribing and dispensing information* and *Patient and carer advice*.

- **INTERACTIONS** → Appendix 1: beta$_2$ agonists
- **SIDE-EFFECTS**

GENERAL SIDE-EFFECTS
- **Uncommon** Myocardial ischaemia
- **Rare or very rare** Akathisia · hypokalaemia (with high doses) · vasodilation

SPECIFIC SIDE-EFFECTS
- **Common or very common**
- When used by inhalation Anxiety
- With oral or parenteral use Muscle cramps
- **Uncommon**
- When used by inhalation Muscle complaints · oral disorders · taste altered · throat irritation
- With parenteral use Pulmonary oedema
- **Rare or very rare**
- When used by inhalation Dry mouth · hallucination · lactic acidosis (with high doses) · nausea · pruritus · sleep disorders · vomiting
- With parenteral use Nausea
- **Frequency not known**
- With oral use Metabolic change
- With parenteral use Lactic acidosis (with high doses) · metabolic change · vomiting

- **BREAST FEEDING** Inhaled drugs for asthma can be taken as normal during breast-feeding.
- **DIRECTIONS FOR ADMINISTRATION** For *continuous intravenous infusion*, dilute to a concentration of 200 micrograms/mL with Glucose 5% *or* Sodium Chloride 0.9%. If fluid-restricted, can be given undiluted through central venous catheter [unlicensed]. For *intravenous injection*, dilute to a concentration of 50 micrograms/mL with Glucose 5%, Sodium Chloride 0.9%, *or* Water for injections.
  For *nebulisation*, dilute nebuliser solution with a suitable volume of sterile Sodium Chloride 0.9% solution according to nebuliser type and duration of administration; salbutamol and ipratropium bromide solutions are compatible and can be mixed for nebulisation.
- **PRESCRIBING AND DISPENSING INFORMATION** For information on devices used for the delivery of inhaled medicines, see Respiratory system, inhaled drug delivery p. 169.
  - When used for Asthma For choice of therapy, see Asthma, acute p. 174 and Asthma, chronic p. 171.
- **PATIENT AND CARER ADVICE** *For inhalation by aerosol or dry powder*, advise patients and carers not to exceed prescribed dose and to follow manufacturer's directions; if a previously effective dose of inhaled salbutamol fails to provide at least 3 hours relief, a doctor's advice should be obtained as soon as possible. *For inhalation by nebuliser*, the dose given by nebuliser is substantially higher than that given by inhaler. Patients should therefore be warned that it is dangerous to exceed the prescribed dose and they should seek medical advice if they fail to respond to the usual dose of the respirator solution.
  Medicines for Children leaflet: Salbutamol inhaler for asthma and wheeze www.medicinesforchildren.org.uk/medicines/salbutamol-inhaler-for-asthma-and-wheeze/

● **MEDICINAL FORMS** There can be variation in the licensing of different medicines containing the same drug.

Inhalation powder

- **Easyhaler (salbutamol)** (Orion Pharma (UK) Ltd)
  Salbutamol 100 microgram per 1 dose Easyhaler Salbutamol sulfate 100micrograms/dose dry powder inhaler | 200 dose [PoM] £3.31 DT = £3.31
  Salbutamol 200 microgram per 1 dose Easyhaler Salbutamol sulfate 200micrograms/dose dry powder inhaler | 200 dose [PoM] £6.63 DT = £6.63
- **Salbulin Novolizer** (Viatris UK Healthcare Ltd)
  Salbutamol (as Salbutamol sulfate) 100 microgram per 1 dose Salbulin Novolizer 100micrograms/dose inhalation powder | 200 dose [PoM] £4.95 DT = £4.95
  Salbulin Novolizer 100micrograms/dose inhalation powder refill | 200 dose [PoM] £2.75 DT = £2.75
- **Ventolin Accuhaler** (GlaxoSmithKline UK Ltd)
  Salbutamol 200 microgram per 1 dose Ventolin 200micrograms/dose Accuhaler | 60 dose [PoM] £3.60 DT = £3.60

Solution for injection

- **Ventolin** (GlaxoSmithKline UK Ltd)
  Salbutamol (as Salbutamol sulfate) 500 microgram per 1 ml Ventolin 500micrograms/1ml solution for injection ampoules | 5 ampoule [PoM] £1.91 DT = £1.91

Solution for infusion

- **Ventolin** (GlaxoSmithKline UK Ltd)
  Salbutamol (as Salbutamol sulfate) 1 mg per 1 ml Ventolin 5mg/5ml solution for infusion ampoules | 10 ampoule [PoM] £24.81 DT = £24.81

Pressurised inhalation

- **Asthalin** (Cipla EU Ltd)
  Salbutamol (as Salbutamol sulfate) 100 microgram per 1 dose Asthalin 100micrograms/dose inhaler | 200 dose [PoM] £1.50 DT = £1.50
- **Salamol** (Teva UK Ltd)
  Salbutamol (as Salbutamol sulfate) 100 microgram per 1 dose Salamol 100micrograms/dose inhaler CFC free | 200 dose [PoM] £1.46 DT = £1.50
- **Salamol Easi-Breathe** (Teva UK Ltd)
  Salbutamol (as Salbutamol sulfate) 100 microgram per 1 dose Salamol 100micrograms/dose Easi-Breathe inhaler | 200 dose [PoM] £6.30 DT = £6.30
- **Ventolin Evohaler** (GlaxoSmithKline UK Ltd)
  Salbutamol (as Salbutamol sulfate) 100 microgram per 1 dose Ventolin 100micrograms/dose Evohaler | 200 dose [PoM] £1.50 DT = £1.50

Nebuliser liquid

- **Salbutamol (Non-proprietary)**
  Salbutamol (as Salbutamol sulfate) 830 microgram per 1 ml Salbutamol 2.5mg/3ml nebuliser liquid unit dose vials | 25 unit dose [PoM] (Hospital only)
  Salbutamol (as Salbutamol sulfate) 1 mg per 1 ml Salbutamol 2.5mg/2.5ml nebuliser liquid unit dose ampoules | 20 unit dose [PoM] £6.40–£22.86 DT = £16.25 | 30 unit dose [PoM] £14.00–£25.50
  Salbutamol (as Salbutamol sulfate) 2 mg per 1 ml Salbutamol 5mg/2.5ml nebuliser liquid unit dose ampoules | 20 unit dose [PoM] £19.00–£24.81 DT = £22.00 | 30 unit dose [PoM] £30.00–£31.92
- **Ventolin** (GlaxoSmithKline UK Ltd)
  Salbutamol (as Salbutamol sulfate) 5 mg per 1 ml Ventolin 5mg/ml respirator solution | 20 ml [PoM] £2.18 DT = £2.18

179

Terbutaline sulfate

01-May-2025

● **INDICATIONS AND DOSE**

Acute asthma

▶ BY SUBCUTANEOUS INJECTION, OR BY SLOW INTRAVENOUS INJECTION

- Child 2–14 years: 10 micrograms/kg up to 4 times a day (max. per dose 300 micrograms), reserve intravenous beta$_2$ agonists for those in whom inhaled therapy cannot be used reliably or there is no current effect
- Child 15–17 years: 250–500 micrograms up to 4 times a day, reserve intravenous beta$_2$ agonists for those in whom inhaled therapy cannot be used reliably or there is no current effect

▶ BY CONTINUOUS INTRAVENOUS INFUSION

- Child: Loading dose 2–4 micrograms/kg, then 1–10 micrograms/kg/hour, dose to be adjusted according to response and heart rate, close monitoring is required for doses above 10 micrograms/kg/hour, reserve intravenous beta$_2$ agonists for those in whom inhaled therapy cannot be used reliably or there is no current effect

Moderate, severe, or life-threatening acute asthma

▶ BY INHALATION OF NEBULISED SOLUTION

- Child 1 month–4 years: 5 mg, repeat every 20–30 minutes or when required, give via oxygen-driven nebuliser if available
- Child 5–11 years: 5–10 mg, repeat every 20–30 minutes or when required, give via oxygen-driven nebuliser if available
- Child 12–17 years: 10 mg, repeat every 20–30 minutes or when required, give via oxygen-driven nebuliser if available

Exacerbation of reversible airways obstruction (including nocturnal asthma) | Prevention of exercise-induced bronchospasm

▶ BY INHALATION OF POWDER

- Child 5–17 years: 500 micrograms up to 4 times a day, for occasional use only

▶ BY MOUTH

- Child 1 month–6 years: 75 micrograms/kg 3 times a day (max. per dose 2.5 mg), administration by mouth is not recommended
- Child 7–14 years: 2.5 mg 2–3 times a day, administration by mouth is not recommended
- Child 15–17 years: Initially 2.5 mg 3 times a day, then increased if necessary to 5 mg 3 times a day, administration by mouth is not recommended

PHARMACOKINETICS

- At recommended inhaled doses, the duration of action of terbutaline is about 3 to 5 hours.

● **UNLICENSED USE** Tablets not licensed for use in children under 7 years. Injection not licensed for use in children under 2 years.

IMPORTANT SAFETY INFORMATION

MHRA/CHM ADVICE: NEBULISED ASTHMA RESCUE THERAPY IN CHILDREN: HOME USE OF NEBULISERS IN PAEDIATRIC ASTHMA SHOULD BE INITIATED AND MANAGED ONLY BY SPECIALISTS (AUGUST 2022)

The MHRA has reviewed the evidence regarding a number of deaths in children with asthma, where the clinically unsupervised use of a nebuliser to deliver asthma rescue medication was a potential contributory factor. Healthcare professionals are advised that home use of nebulisers for the acute treatment of asthma in children and adolescents should only be initiated and managed by asthma specialists. Home use of nebulisers for this purpose, without adequate medical supervision, can mask a deterioration in the underlying disease, which could result in delays in seeking medical attention and be fatal or have serious consequences. The purchase of nebulisers for this purpose, outside of medical advice, is not recommended. Patients and their carers should be advised to seek urgent medical attention if worsening asthma symptoms are not relieved by prescribed rescue medication, even if there is short-term recovery following its use. They should receive training from a healthcare professional on the usage and maintenance of the nebuliser, and be given advice on when to seek medical attention, so that deterioration in asthma control can be treated without delay. Patients (or their carers) who have been using a nebuliser at home without specialist management should contact their GP about referral to a specialist. The MHRA has produced videos to support this advice—guidance for healthcare professionals is available at: www.youtube.com/watch?v=qfppzpdeYmk and guidance for patients, parents, and carers is available at: www.youtube.com/watch?v=NO0ir0i043Q.

MHRA/CHM ADVICE: SHORT-ACTING BETA 2 AGONISTS (SABA) (TERBUTALINE): REMINDER OF THE RISKS FROM OVERUSE IN ASTHMA AND TO BE AWARE OF CHANGES IN THE SABA PRESCRIBING GUIDELINES (APRIL 2025)

A review by the MHRA and the EMA's Pharmacovigilance Risk Assessment Committee (PRAC) found that the overuse of short-acting beta$_2$ agonists (SABA) was associated with an increased risk of severe asthma exacerbations, hospitalisations, and mortality, irrespective of disease severity or concomitant anti-inflammatory maintenance therapy. Healthcare professionals are reminded that excessive use of SABA to relieve acute symptoms may mask progression of the underlying disease and contribute to an increased risk of severe and life-threatening exacerbations, and are therefore advised to:

- avoid prescribing SABA to any asthma patient without a concomitant inhaled corticosteroid;
- ensure all asthma patients receive optimal anti-inflammatory maintenance therapy, even when well controlled, and their treatment is individualised;
- review and adjust treatment in those who use as-needed SABA more than twice weekly;
- urgently review patients who have increased their SABA prescription requests or have failed to collect their prescribed anti-inflammatory maintenance therapy;
- consider the recommended alternatives (i.e. anti-inflammatory reliever (AIR) therapy and maintenance and reliever therapy (MART)) in patients aged over 12 years with poorly-controlled asthma.

Healthcare professionals should counsel patients and carers to use their inhalers as prescribed and follow their agreed asthma plan if available. Additionally, patients and carers should be reminded when to request an asthma review and when to seek urgent medical assistance. See also *Prescribing and dispensing information* and *Patient and carer advice*.

- **INTERACTIONS** → Appendix 1: beta$_2$ agonists
- **SIDE-EFFECTS**

GENERAL SIDE-EFFECTS

- **Common or very common** Hypokalaemia · hypotension · muscle spasms · nausea
- **Rare or very rare** Myocardial ischaemia · vasodilation
- **Frequency not known** Angioedema · anxiety · behaviour abnormal · bronchospasm · circulatory collapse · oral irritation · skin reactions · sleep disorder · throat irritation

SPECIFIC SIDE-EFFECTS

- **Uncommon**
  - With parenteral use Pulmonary oedema
- **Rare or very rare**
  - With parenteral use Lactic acidosis
- **Frequency not known**
  - When used by inhalation Lactic acidosis (with high doses)
  - With parenteral use Akathisia · bleeding tendency

- **PREGNANCY** Inhaled drugs for asthma can be taken as normal during pregnancy.
- **BREAST FEEDING** Inhaled drugs for asthma can be taken as normal during breast-feeding.
- **DIRECTIONS FOR ADMINISTRATION** EvGr For *continuous intravenous infusion*, dilute to a concentration of 3–5 micrograms/mL with Glucose 5% *or* Sodium Chloride 0.9%. (M) If fluid-restricted, expert sources advise dilute to a concentration of 100 micrograms/mL; give via a syringe pump.

EvGr For *nebulisation*, dilute nebuliser solution with sterile Sodium Chloride 0.9% solution, if required, according to nebuliser type and duration of administration; terbutaline and ipratropium bromide solutions are compatible and may be mixed for nebulisation. (M)

- **PRESCRIBING AND DISPENSING INFORMATION**
  - When used for Asthma For choice of therapy, see Asthma, acute p. 174 and Asthma, chronic p. 171.
- **PATIENT AND CARER ADVICE** *For inhalation by dry powder*, advise patients and carers not to exceed prescribed dose and to follow manufacturer's directions; if a previously effective dose of inhaled terbutaline fails to provide at least 3 hours relief, a doctor's advice should be obtained as soon as possible. *For inhalation by nebuliser*, the dose given by nebuliser is substantially higher than that given by inhaler. Patients should therefore be warned that it is dangerous to exceed the prescribed dose and they should seek medical advice if they fail to respond to the usual dose of the respirator solution.

- **MEDICINAL FORMS** There can be variation in the licensing of different medicines containing the same drug.

Solution for injection

- **Bricanyl** (AstraZeneca UK Ltd)
  Terbutaline sulfate 500 microgram per 1 ml Bricanyl 2.5mg/5ml solution for injection ampoules | 10 ampoule PoM £20.09 DT = £20.09

Inhalation powder

- **Bricanyl Turbohaler** (AstraZeneca UK Ltd)
  Terbutaline sulfate 500 microgram per 1 dose Bricanyl 500micrograms/dose Turbohaler | 120 dose PoM £8.30 DT = £8.30

Nebuliser liquid

- **Terbutaline sulfate (Non-proprietary)**
  Terbutaline sulfate 2.5 mg per 1 ml Terbutaline 5mg/2ml nebuliser liquid unit dose vials | 20 unit dose PoM £8.91–£12.50 DT = £11.64
- **Bricanyl Respules** (AstraZeneca UK Ltd)
  Terbutaline sulfate 2.5 mg per 1 ml Bricanyl 5mg/2ml Respules | 20 unit dose PoM £11.64 DT = £11.64

CORTICOSTEROIDS

Corticosteroids (inhaled)

IMPORTANT SAFETY INFORMATION

MHRA/CHM ADVICE: CORTICOSTEROIDS: RARE RISK OF CENTRAL SEROUS CHORIORETINOPATHY WITH LOCAL AS WELL AS SYSTEMIC ADMINISTRATION (AUGUST 2017)

Central serous chorioretinopathy is a retinal disorder that has been linked to the systemic use of corticosteroids. Recently, it has also been reported after local administration of corticosteroids via inhaled and intranasal, epidural, intra-articular, topical dermal, and periocular routes. The MHRA recommends that patients should be advised to report any blurred vision or other visual disturbances with corticosteroid treatment given by any route; consider referral to an ophthalmologist for evaluation of possible causes if a patient presents with vision problems.

ADRENAL INSUFFICIENCY CARD (APRIL 2023)

The British Society for Paediatric Endocrinology and Diabetes (BSPED) has developed an Adrenal Insufficiency Card which should be issued to children with adrenal insufficiency and steroid dependence. The card includes a management summary for the emergency treatment of adrenal crisis and sick day dosing, and can be issued by any healthcare professional managing such patients. The BSPED Adrenal Insufficiency Card is available at: www.bsped.org.uk/adrenal-insufficiency.

- **SIDE-EFFECTS**
- **Common or very common** Headache · oral candidiasis · taste altered · voice alteration
- **Uncommon** Bronchospasm paradoxical · cataract · vision blurred
- **Rare or very rare** Adrenal suppression · anxiety · behaviour abnormal · glaucoma · growth retardation · sleep disorder
- **Frequency not known** Pneumonia (in patients with COPD)

SIDE-EFFECTS, FURTHER INFORMATION Systemic absorption may follow inhaled administration particularly if high doses are used or if treatment is prolonged. Therefore also consider the side-effects of systemic corticosteroids.

Candidiasis The risk of oral candidiasis can be reduced by using a spacer device with the corticosteroid inhaler; rinsing the mouth with water after inhalation of a dose may also be helpful. An anti-fungal oral suspension or oral gel can be used to treat oral candidiasis without discontinuing corticosteroid therapy.

Paradoxical bronchospasm The potential for paradoxical bronchospasm (calling for discontinuation and alternative therapy) should be borne in mind. Mild bronchospasm may be prevented by inhalation of a short-acting $beta_2$ agonist beforehand (or by transfer from an aerosol inhalation to a dry powder inhalation).

- **PREGNANCY** Inhaled drugs for asthma can be taken as normal during pregnancy.
- **BREAST FEEDING** Inhaled corticosteroids for asthma can be taken as normal during breast-feeding.
- **MONITORING REQUIREMENTS** The height and weight of children receiving prolonged treatment with inhaled corticosteroids should be monitored annually; if growth is slowed, referral to a paediatrician should be considered.
- **PATIENT AND CARER ADVICE** If systemic absorption occurs following inhaled use, side-effects applicable to systemic corticosteroids may apply.
- **NATIONAL FUNDING/ACCESS DECISIONS**

For full details see funding body website

NICE decisions

- **Inhaled corticosteroids for the treatment of chronic asthma in children under 12 years (November 2007)** NICE TA131 Recommended
- **Inhaled corticosteroids for the treatment of chronic asthma in adults and children over 12 years (March 2008)** NICE TA138 Recommended

F 184

Beclometasone dipropionate

26-Jul-2025

(Beclomethasone dipropionate)

- **INDICATIONS AND DOSE**

Prophylaxis of asthma

- BY INHALATION OF POWDER
- Child 5-11 years: 100–200 micrograms twice daily, dose to be adjusted as necessary
- Child 12-17 years: 200–400 micrograms twice daily; increased if necessary up to 800 micrograms twice daily, dose to be adjusted as necessary

DOSE EQUIVALENCE AND CONVERSION

- Dose adjustments may be required for some inhaler devices, see under individual preparations.

CLENIL MODULITE ®

Prophylaxis of asthma

- BY INHALATION OF AEROSOL
- Child 2-11 years: 100–200 micrograms twice daily
- Child 12-17 years: 200–400 micrograms twice daily; increased if necessary up to 1 mg twice daily

QVAR ® PREPARATIONS

Prophylaxis of asthma

- BY INHALATION OF AEROSOL
- Child 5-11 years: 50–100 micrograms twice daily, using Autohaler or MDI device
- Child 12-17 years: 50–200 micrograms twice daily, using Autohaler, MDI, or Easi-Breathe device; increased if necessary up to 400 micrograms twice daily

POTENCY

- *Qvar*® has extra-fine particles, is more potent than traditional beclometasone dipropionate CFC-containing inhalers and is approximately twice as potent as *Clenil Modulite*®.

SOPROBEC ®

Prophylaxis of asthma

- BY INHALATION OF AEROSOL
- Child: 100 micrograms twice daily; increased if necessary up to 400 micrograms daily in 2–4 divided doses

- **UNLICENSED USE** *Easyhaler*® *Beclometasone Dipropionate* is not licensed for use in children. *Clenil Modulite*® 200 and 250 are not licensed for use in children.

IMPORTANT SAFETY INFORMATION

MHRA/CHM ADVICE (JULY 2008)

Beclometasone dipropionate CFC-free pressurised metered-dose inhalers (*Qvar*® and *Clenil Modulite*®) are **not** interchangeable and should be prescribed by brand name; *Qvar*® has extra-fine particles, is more potent than traditional beclometasone dipropionate CFC-containing inhalers, and is approximately twice as potent as *Clenil Modulite*®.

MHRA/CHM ADVICE: PRESSURISED METERED DOSE INHALERS (PMDI): RISK OF AIRWAY OBSTRUCTION FROM ASPIRATION OF LOOSE OBJECTS (JULY 2018)

See Respiratory system, inhaled drug delivery p. 169.

- **INTERACTIONS** → Appendix 1: corticosteroids
- **SIDE-EFFECTS**
- **Common or very common** Throat irritation
- **Rare or very rare** Wheezing
- **PRESCRIBING AND DISPENSING INFORMATION** For choice of therapy, see Asthma, acute p. 174 and Asthma, chronic p. 171. The MHRA has advised (July 2008) that beclometasone dipropionate CFC-free inhalers should be prescribed by brand name. Pressurised metered-doses inhalers with extra-fine particles (*Qvar*® and *Kelhale*®) are more potent than, and not interchangeable with, traditional CFC-containing and CFC-free inhalers (*Clenil Modulite*® and *Soprobec*®).

QVAR ® PREPARATIONS When switching a patient with well-controlled asthma from another corticosteroid inhaler, initially a 100-microgram metered dose of *Qvar*® should be prescribed for 200–250 micrograms of beclometasone dipropionate or budesonide and for 100 micrograms of fluticasone propionate. When switching a patient with poorly controlled asthma from another corticosteroid inhaler, initially a 100-microgram metered dose of *Qvar*® should be prescribed for 100 micrograms of beclometasone dipropionate, budesonide, or fluticasone propionate; the dose of *Qvar*® should be adjusted according to response.

- **PROFESSION SPECIFIC INFORMATION**

Dental practitioners' formulary *Clenil Modulite*® 50 micrograms/metered inhalation may be prescribed.

● **MEDICINAL FORMS** There can be variation in the licensing of different medicines containing the same drug.

Inhalation powder

CAUTIONARY AND ADVISORY LABELS 8, 10

▸ **Easyhaler (beclometasone)** (Orion Pharma (UK) Ltd)

Beclometasone dipropionate 200 microgram per 1 dose Easyhaler Beclometasone 200micrograms/dose dry powder inhaler | 200 dose [PoM] £14.93 DT = £14.93

Pressurised inhalation

CAUTIONARY AND ADVISORY LABELS 8, 10

▸ **Clenil Modulite** (Chiesi Ltd)

Beclometasone dipropionate 50 microgram per 1 dose Clenil Modulite 50micrograms/dose inhaler | 200 dose [PoM] £3.70 DT = £3.70

Beclometasone dipropionate 100 microgram per 1 dose Clenil Modulite 100micrograms/dose inhaler | 200 dose [PoM] £7.42 DT = £7.42

Beclometasone dipropionate 200 microgram per 1 dose Clenil Modulite 200micrograms/dose inhaler | 200 dose [PoM] £16.17 DT = £16.17

Beclometasone dipropionate 250 microgram per 1 dose Clenil Modulite 250micrograms/dose inhaler | 200 dose [PoM] £16.29 DT = £16.29

▸ **Kelhale** (Cipla EU Ltd)

Beclometasone dipropionate 50 microgram per 1 dose Kelhale 50micrograms/dose inhaler | 200 dose [PoM] £5.20 DT = £3.70

Beclometasone dipropionate 100 microgram per 1 dose Kelhale 100micrograms/dose inhaler | 200 dose [PoM] £5.20 DT = £7.42

▸ **Qvar** (Teva UK Ltd)

Beclometasone dipropionate 50 microgram per 1 dose Qvar 50 inhaler | 200 dose [PoM] £7.87 DT = £3.70

Beclometasone dipropionate 100 microgram per 1 dose Qvar 100 inhaler | 200 dose [PoM] £17.21 DT = £7.42

▸ **Qvar Autohaler** (Teva UK Ltd)

Beclometasone dipropionate 50 microgram per 1 dose Qvar 50 Autohaler | 200 dose [PoM] £7.87 DT = £7.87

Beclometasone dipropionate 100 microgram per 1 dose Qvar 100 Autohaler | 200 dose [PoM] £17.21 DT = £17.21

▸ **Qvar Easi-Breathe** (Teva UK Ltd)

Beclometasone dipropionate 50 microgram per 1 dose Qvar 50micrograms/dose Easi-Breathe inhaler | 200 dose [PoM] £7.74 DT = £7.87

Beclometasone dipropionate 100 microgram per 1 dose Qvar 100micrograms/dose Easi-Breathe inhaler | 200 dose [PoM] £16.95 DT = £17.21

▸ **Soprobec** (Glenmark Pharmaceuticals Europe Ltd)

Beclometasone dipropionate 50 microgram per 1 dose Soprobec 50micrograms/dose inhaler | 200 dose [PoM] £2.41 DT = £3.70

Beclometasone dipropionate 100 microgram per 1 dose Soprobec 100micrograms/dose inhaler | 200 dose [PoM] £4.82 DT = £7.42

Beclometasone dipropionate 200 microgram per 1 dose Soprobec 200micrograms/dose inhaler | 200 dose [PoM] £10.51 DT = £16.17

Beclometasone dipropionate 250 microgram per 1 dose Soprobec 250micrograms/dose inhaler | 200 dose [PoM] £10.59 DT = £16.29

184

Budesonide

26-Feb-2026

● **DRUG ACTION** Budesonide is a glucocorticoid, which exerts significant local anti-inflammatory effects.

● **INDICATIONS AND DOSE**

Bronchopulmonary dysplasia with spontaneous respiration

▸ BY INHALATION OF NEBULISED SUSPENSION

▸ Neonate: 500 micrograms twice daily.

▸ Child 1–4 months: 500 micrograms twice daily

Bronchopulmonary dysplasia with spontaneous respiration (severe symptoms)

▸ BY INHALATION OF NEBULISED SUSPENSION

▸ Child 1–4 months (body-weight 2.5 kg and above): 1 mg twice daily

Prophylaxis of mild to moderate asthma (in patients stabilised on twice daily dose)

▸ BY INHALATION OF POWDER

▸ Child 6–11 years: 200–400 micrograms once daily, to be taken in the evening

▸ Child 12–17 years: 200–400 micrograms once daily, to be taken in the evening, increased if necessary up to 800 micrograms once daily, to be taken in the evening

Prophylaxis of asthma

▸ BY INHALATION OF POWDER

▸ Child 6–11 years: 100–400 micrograms twice daily, dose to be adjusted as necessary

▸ Child 12–17 years: 100–800 micrograms twice daily, dose to be adjusted as necessary

▸ BY INHALATION OF NEBULISED SUSPENSION

▸ Child 6 months–11 years: 125–500 micrograms twice daily, dose adjusted according to response up to maximum 2 mg per day

▸ Child 12–17 years: Initially 0.25–1 mg twice daily, dose adjusted according to response up to maximum 2 mg per day, doses higher than recommended max. may be used in severe disease

POTENCY

▸ Dose adjustments may be required for some inhaler devices, see under individual preparations.

BUDELIN NOVOLIZER®

Prophylaxis of asthma

▸ BY INHALATION OF POWDER

▸ Child 6–11 years: 200–400 micrograms twice daily, dose to be adjusted as necessary

▸ Child 12–17 years: 200–800 micrograms twice daily, dose to be adjusted as necessary

Alternative in mild to moderate asthma, for patients previously stabilised on a twice daily dose

▸ BY INHALATION OF POWDER

▸ Child 6–11 years: 200–400 micrograms once daily, to be taken in the evening

▸ Child 12–17 years: 200–400 micrograms once daily, to be taken in the evening, increased if necessary up to 800 micrograms once daily, to be taken in the evening

PULMICORT® RESPULES

Prophylaxis of asthma

▸ BY INHALATION OF NEBULISED SUSPENSION

▸ Child 3 months–11 years: Initially 0.5–1 mg twice daily, reduced to 250–500 micrograms twice daily

▸ Child 12–17 years: Initially 1–2 mg twice daily, reduced to 0.5–1 mg twice daily

Croup

▸ BY INHALATION OF NEBULISED SUSPENSION

▸ Child: 2 mg for 1 dose, dose may be repeated every 12 hours until clinical improvement, alternatively 1 mg for 2 doses separated by a 30 minute interval, dose may be repeated every 12 hours until clinical improvement

PULMICORT® TURBOHALER

Prophylaxis of asthma

▸ BY INHALATION OF POWDER

▸ Child 5–11 years: 100–400 micrograms twice daily, dose to be adjusted as necessary

▸ Child 12–17 years: 100–800 micrograms twice daily, dose to be adjusted as necessary

Alternative in mild to moderate asthma, for patients previously stabilised on a twice daily dose

▸ BY INHALATION OF POWDER

▸ Child 5–11 years: 200–400 micrograms once daily, to be taken in the evening

▸ Child 12–17 years: 200–400 micrograms once daily, to be taken in the evening, increased if necessary up to 800 micrograms once daily, to be taken in the evening

- **UNLICENSED USE** *Pulmicort® nebuliser solution* not licensed for use in children under 3 months; not licensed for use in bronchopulmonary dysplasia.
- **INTERACTIONS** → Appendix 1: corticosteroids
- **SIDE-EFFECTS**
  - **Common or very common** Cough · throat irritation
  - **Uncommon** Muscle spasms · tremor
  - **Rare or very rare** Akathisia
- **DIRECTIONS FOR ADMINISTRATION** Budesonide nebuliser suspension is not suitable for use in ultrasonic nebulisers.
- **PRESCRIBING AND DISPENSING INFORMATION**
  - When used for Asthma For choice of therapy, see Asthma, acute p. 174 and Asthma, chronic p. 171.
- **PATIENT AND CARER ADVICE** Patients or carers should be given advice on how to administer budesonide dry powder inhaler and nebuliser suspension.
  Medicines for Children leaflet: Budesonide inhaler for asthma prevention www.medicinesforchildren.org.uk/medicines/budesonide-inhaler-for-asthma-prevention/
  BUDELIN NOVOLIZER® Patients or carers should be given advice on administration of *Budelin Novolizer®*.

- **MEDICINAL FORMS** There can be variation in the licensing of different medicines containing the same drug.

Inhalation powder

CAUTIONARY AND ADVISORY LABELS 8, 10

- **Budelin Novolizer** (Viatris UK Healthcare Ltd)
  Budesonide 200 microgram per 1 dose Budelin Novolizer 200micrograms/dose inhalation powder | 100 dose [PoM] £14.86 DT = £14.86
  Budelin Novolizer 200micrograms/dose inhalation powder refill | 100 dose [PoM] £9.59 DT = £9.59
- **Easyhaler (budesonide)** (Orion Pharma (UK) Ltd)
  Budesonide 100 microgram per 1 dose Easyhaler Budesonide 100micrograms/dose dry powder inhaler | 200 dose [PoM] £8.86 DT = £14.25
  Budesonide 200 microgram per 1 dose Easyhaler Budesonide 200micrograms/dose dry powder inhaler | 200 dose [PoM] £17.71
  Budesonide 400 microgram per 1 dose Easyhaler Budesonide 400micrograms/dose dry powder inhaler | 100 dose [PoM] £17.71
- **Pulmicort Turbohaler** (AstraZeneca UK Ltd)
  Budesonide 100 microgram per 1 dose Pulmicort 100 Turbohaler | 200 dose [PoM] £14.25 DT = £14.25
  Budesonide 200 microgram per 1 dose Pulmicort 200 Turbohaler | 100 dose [PoM] £14.25 DT = £14.25
  Budesonide 400 microgram per 1 dose Pulmicort 400 Turbohaler | 50 dose [PoM] £14.25 DT = £14.25

Nebuliser liquid

CAUTIONARY AND ADVISORY LABELS 8, 10

- **Budesonide (Non-proprietary)**
  Budesonide 250 microgram per 1 ml Budesonide 500micrograms/2ml nebuliser suspension unit dose ampoules | 20 unit dose [PoM] £30.12 DT = £30.12
  Budesonide 500micrograms/2ml nebuliser liquid unit dose vials | 20 unit dose [PoM] £30.12 DT = £20.94
  Budesonide 500 microgram per 1 ml Budesonide 1mg/2ml nebuliser suspension unit dose ampoules | 20 unit dose [PoM] £45.60 DT = £45.60
  Budesonide 1mg/2ml nebuliser liquid unit dose vials | 20 unit dose [PoM] £45.60 DT = £22.44
- **Pulmicort Respules** (AstraZeneca UK Ltd)
  Budesonide 250 microgram per 1 ml Pulmicort 0.5mg Respules | 20 unit dose [PoM] £31.70 DT = £20.94
  Budesonide 500 microgram per 1 ml Pulmicort 1mg Respules | 20 unit dose [PoM] £48.00 DT = £22.44

Budesonide with formoterol

13-Nov-2025

The properties listed below are those particular to the combination only. For the properties of the components please consider, budesonide p. 186, formoterol fumarate p. 179.

- **INDICATIONS AND DOSE**

DUORESP SPIROMAX® 160MICROGRAMS/4.5MICROGRAMS

Asthma, maintenance therapy
- BY INHALATION OF POWDER
  - Child 12-17 years: Initially 1–2 inhalations twice daily; reduced to 1 inhalation daily, dose reduced only if control is maintained

Asthma, maintenance and reliever therapy
- BY INHALATION OF POWDER
  - Child 12-17 years: Maintenance 2 inhalations daily in 1–2 divided doses, increased if necessary to 2 inhalations twice daily; 1 inhalation as required, for relief of symptoms, increased if necessary up to 6 inhalations as required, max. 8 inhalations per day; up to 12 inhalations daily can be used for a limited time but medical assessment is recommended

Mild asthma, reliever therapy
- BY INHALATION OF POWDER
  - Child 12-17 years: 1 inhalation as required, for relief of symptoms, increased if necessary up to 6 inhalations as required, max. 8 inhalations per day; up to 12 inhalations daily can be used for a limited time but medical assessment is recommended

DUORESP SPIROMAX® 320MICROGRAMS/9MICROGRAMS

Asthma, maintenance therapy
- BY INHALATION OF POWDER
  - Child 12-17 years: Initially 1 inhalation twice daily; reduced to 1 inhalation daily, dose reduced only if control is maintained

FOBUMIX® 160/4.5 EASYHALER

Asthma, maintenance therapy
- BY INHALATION OF POWDER
  - Child 12-17 years: Initially 1–2 inhalations twice daily; reduced to 1 inhalation daily, dose reduced only if control is maintained

Asthma, maintenance and reliever therapy
- BY INHALATION OF POWDER
  - Child 12-17 years: Maintenance 2 inhalations daily in 1–2 divided doses, increased if necessary to 2 inhalations twice daily; 1 inhalation as required, for relief of symptoms, increased if necessary up to 6 inhalations as required, max. 8 inhalations per day; up to 12 inhalations daily can be used for a limited time but medical assessment is recommended

Mild asthma, reliever therapy
- BY INHALATION OF POWDER
  - Child 12-17 years: 1 inhalation as required, for relief of symptoms, increased if necessary up to 6 inhalations as required, max. 8 inhalations per day; up to 12 inhalations daily can be used for a limited time but medical assessment is recommended

FOBUMIX® 320/9 EASYHALER

Asthma, maintenance therapy
- BY INHALATION OF POWDER
  - Child 12-17 years: Initially 1 inhalation twice daily; reduced to 1 inhalation daily, dose reduced only if control is maintained

continued →

FOBUMIX ® 80/4.5 EASYHALER

Asthma, maintenance therapy

▶ BY INHALATION OF POWDER

▸ Child 6–17 years: Initially 1–2 inhalations twice daily; reduced to 1 inhalation daily, dose reduced only if control is maintained

Asthma, maintenance and reliever therapy

▶ BY INHALATION OF POWDER

▸ Child 12–17 years: Maintenance 2 inhalations daily in 1–2 divided doses; 1 inhalation as required, for relief of symptoms, increased if necessary up to 6 inhalations as required, max. 8 inhalations per day; up to 12 inhalations daily can be used for a limited time but medical assessment is recommended

SYMBICORT 100/6 TURBOHALER ®

Asthma, maintenance therapy

▶ BY INHALATION OF POWDER

▸ Child 6–17 years: Initially 1–2 inhalations twice daily; reduced to 1 inhalation daily, dose reduced only if control is maintained

Asthma, maintenance and reliever therapy

▶ BY INHALATION OF POWDER

▸ Child 6–11 years: Maintenance 1 inhalation daily; 1 inhalation as required, for relief of symptoms, increased if necessary up to 4 inhalations as required, usual max. 4 inhalations per day; up to 8 inhalations daily can be used for a limited time but medical assessment is recommended, alternatively maintenance 1 inhalation twice daily; 1 inhalation as required, for relief of symptoms, increased if necessary up to 4 inhalations as required, usual max. 4 inhalations per day; up to 8 inhalations daily can be used for a limited time but medical assessment is recommended

▸ Child 12–17 years: Maintenance 2 inhalations daily in 1–2 divided doses; 1 inhalation as required, for relief of symptoms, increased if necessary up to 6 inhalations as required, max. 8 inhalations per day; up to 12 inhalations daily can be used for a limited time but medical assessment is recommended

SYMBICORT 200/6 TURBOHALER ®

Asthma, maintenance therapy

▶ BY INHALATION OF POWDER

▸ Child 12–17 years: Initially 1–2 inhalations twice daily; reduced to 1 inhalation daily, dose reduced only if control is maintained

Asthma, maintenance and reliever therapy

▶ BY INHALATION OF POWDER

▸ Child 12–17 years: Maintenance 2 inhalations daily in 1–2 divided doses, increased if necessary to 2 inhalations twice daily; 1 inhalation as required, for relief of symptoms, increased if necessary up to 6 inhalations as required, max. 8 inhalations per day; up to 12 inhalations daily can be used for a limited time but medical assessment is recommended

Mild asthma, reliever therapy

▶ BY INHALATION OF POWDER

▸ Child 12–17 years: 1 inhalation as required, for relief of symptoms, increased if necessary up to 6 inhalations as required, max. 8 inhalations per day; up to 12 inhalations daily can be used for a limited time but medical assessment is recommended

SYMBICORT 400/12 TURBOHALER ®

Asthma, maintenance therapy

▶ BY INHALATION OF POWDER

▸ Child 12–17 years: Initially 1 inhalation twice daily; reduced to 1 inhalation daily, dose reduced only if control is maintained

SYMBICORT ® 100/3 PRESSURISED INHALER

Asthma, maintenance therapy

▶ BY INHALATION OF AEROSOL

▸ Child 12–17 years: Initially 2–4 inhalations twice daily; reduced to 1 inhalation daily, dose reduced only if control is maintained

Asthma, maintenance and reliever therapy

▶ BY INHALATION OF AEROSOL

▸ Child 12–17 years: Maintenance 4 inhalations daily in 1–2 divided doses, increased if necessary up to 4 inhalations twice daily; 2 inhalations as required for relief of symptoms, increased if necessary up to 12 inhalations as required, usual max. 16 inhalations per day; up to 24 inhalations daily can be used for a limited time but medical assessment is recommended

WOCKAIR ® 160MICROGRAMS/4.5MICROGRAMS

Asthma, maintenance therapy

▶ BY INHALATION OF POWDER

▸ Child 12–17 years: Initially 1–2 inhalations twice daily; reduced to 1 inhalation daily, dose reduced only if control is maintained

Asthma, maintenance and reliever therapy

▶ BY INHALATION OF POWDER

▸ Child 12–17 years: Maintenance 2 inhalations daily in 1–2 divided doses, increased if necessary to 2 inhalations twice daily; 1 inhalation as required, for relief of symptoms, increased if necessary up to 6 inhalations as required, max. 8 inhalations per day; up to 12 inhalations daily can be used for a limited time but medical assessment is recommended

Mild asthma, reliever therapy

▶ BY INHALATION OF POWDER

▸ Child 12–17 years: 1 inhalation as required, for relief of symptoms, increased if necessary up to 6 inhalations as required, max. 8 inhalations per day; up to 12 inhalations daily can be used for a limited time but medical assessment is recommended

WOCKAIR ® 320MICROGRAMS/9MICROGRAMS

Asthma, maintenance therapy

▶ BY INHALATION OF POWDER

▸ Child 12–17 years: Initially 1 inhalation twice daily; reduced to 1 inhalation daily, dose reduced only if control is maintained

● **INTERACTIONS** → Appendix 1: beta$_2$ agonists · corticosteroids

● **PATIENT AND CARER ADVICE** Patient counselling is advised for budesonide with formoterol inhalation (administration).

● **NATIONAL FUNDING/ACCESS DECISIONS**
For full details see funding body website

Scottish Medicines Consortium (SMC) decisions

▸ **Budesonide/formoterol 100/6, 200/6 inhalation powder turbohaler (*Symbicort*® SMART ®) for asthma in adolescents aged 12 years and over (June 2017)** SMC No. 1244/17 Recommended

▸ **Budesonide/formoterol 200/6 inhalation powder (*Symbicort*® Turbohaler ®) as reliever therapy for adults and adolescents 12 years and older with mild asthma (May 2024)** SMC No. SMC2622 Recommended with restrictions

● **MEDICINAL FORMS** There can be variation in the licensing of different medicines containing the same drug.

Inhalation powder

CAUTIONARY AND ADVISORY LABELS 8, 10 (high doses)

▸ DuoResp Spiromax (Teva UK Ltd)

Formoterol fumarate dihydrate 6 microgram per 1 dose, Budesonide 200 microgram per 1 dose DuoResp Spiromax 160micrograms/dose / 4.5micrograms/dose dry powder inhaler | 120 dose [PoM] £27.97 DT = £28.00

Formoterol fumarate dihydrate 12 microgram per 1 dose, Budesonide 400 microgram per 1 dose DuoResp Spiromax 320micrograms/dose / 9micrograms/dose dry powder inhaler | 60 dose PoM £27.97 DT = £28.00

▸ **Fobumix Easyhaler** (Orion Pharma (UK) Ltd)

Formoterol fumarate dihydrate 6 microgram per 1 dose, Budesonide 100 microgram per 1 dose Fobumix Easyhaler 80micrograms/dose / 4.5micrograms/dose dry powder inhaler | 120 dose PoM £21.50 DT = £28.00

Formoterol fumarate dihydrate 6 microgram per 1 dose, Budesonide 200 microgram per 1 dose Fobumix Easyhaler 160micrograms/dose / 4.5micrograms/dose dry powder inhaler | 60 dose PoM £10.75 | 120 dose PoM £21.50 DT = £28.00

Formoterol fumarate dihydrate 12 microgram per 1 dose, Budesonide 400 microgram per 1 dose Fobumix Easyhaler 320micrograms/dose / 9micrograms/dose dry powder inhaler | 60 dose PoM £21.50 DT = £28.00

▸ **Symbicort Turbohaler** (AstraZeneca UK Ltd)

Formoterol fumarate dihydrate 6 microgram per 1 dose, Budesonide 100 microgram per 1 dose Symbicort 100/6 Turbohaler | 120 dose PoM £28.00 DT = £28.00

Formoterol fumarate dihydrate 6 microgram per 1 dose, Budesonide 200 microgram per 1 dose Symbicort 200/6 Turbohaler | 120 dose PoM £28.00 DT = £28.00

Formoterol fumarate dihydrate 12 microgram per 1 dose, Budesonide 400 microgram per 1 dose Symbicort 400/12 Turbohaler | 60 dose PoM £28.00 DT = £28.00

▸ **WockAIR** (Wockhardt UK Ltd)

Formoterol fumarate dihydrate 6 microgram per 1 dose, Budesonide 200 microgram per 1 dose WockAIR 160micrograms/dose / 4.5micrograms/dose dry powder inhaler | 120 dose PoM £19.00 DT = £28.00

Formoterol fumarate dihydrate 12 microgram per 1 dose, Budesonide 400 microgram per 1 dose WockAIR 320micrograms/dose / 9micrograms/dose dry powder inhaler | 60 dose PoM £19.00 DT = £28.00

Pressurised inhalation

CAUTIONARY AND ADVISORY LABELS 8, 10 (high doses)

▸ **Symbicort** (AstraZeneca UK Ltd)

Formoterol fumarate dihydrate 3 microgram per 1 dose, Budesonide 100 microgram per 1 dose Symbicort 100micrograms/dose / 3micrograms/dose pressurised inhaler | 120 dose PoM £14.00 DT = £14.00

184

Ciclesonide

26-Jul-2025

● **INDICATIONS AND DOSE**

Prophylaxis of asthma

▸ BY INHALATION OF AEROSOL

▸ Child 12–17 years: 160 micrograms once daily, increased if necessary up to 320 micrograms twice daily, dose increased in severe asthma; reduced to 80 micrograms once daily, dose reduced only if control is maintained

IMPORTANT SAFETY INFORMATION

MHRA/CHM ADVICE: PRESSURISED METERED DOSE INHALERS (PMDI): RISK OF AIRWAY OBSTRUCTION FROM ASPIRATION OF LOOSE OBJECTS (JULY 2018)

See Respiratory system, inhaled drug delivery p. 169.

● **INTERACTIONS** → Appendix 1: corticosteroids

● **SIDE-EFFECTS** Cushing's syndrome

● **HEPATIC IMPAIRMENT** Manufacturer advises caution in severe impairment (risk of increased exposure, no information available).

● **PRESCRIBING AND DISPENSING INFORMATION** For choice of therapy, see Asthma, acute p. 174 and Asthma, chronic p. 171.

● **PATIENT AND CARER ADVICE** Patients or carers should be given advice on how to administer ciclesonide aerosol inhaler.

● **MEDICINAL FORMS** There can be variation in the licensing of different medicines containing the same drug.

Pressurised inhalation

CAUTIONARY AND ADVISORY LABELS 8

▸ **Ciclesonide (Non-proprietary)**

Ciclesonide 80 microgram per 1 dose Ciclesonide 80micrograms/dose inhaler CFC free | 120 dose PoM £29.55–£42.00 DT = £32.83

Ciclesonide 160 microgram per 1 dose Ciclesonide 160micrograms/dose inhaler CFC free | 120 dose PoM £32.83–£48.00 DT = £38.62

▸ **Alvesco** (Covis Pharma GmbH)

Ciclesonide 80 microgram per 1 dose Alvesco 80 inhaler | 120 dose PoM £32.83 DT = £32.83

Ciclesonide 160 microgram per 1 dose Alvesco 160 inhaler | 120 dose PoM £38.62 DT = £38.62

184

Fluticasone

26-Jul-2025

● **INDICATIONS AND DOSE**

Prophylaxis of asthma

▸ BY INHALATION OF POWDER

▸ Child 5–15 years: Initially 50–100 micrograms twice daily, increased if necessary up to 200 micrograms twice daily, dose to be adjusted as necessary

▸ Child 16–17 years: Initially 100–500 micrograms twice daily, increased if necessary up to 1 mg twice daily, doses above 500 micrograms twice daily to be initiated by a specialist, dose to be adjusted as necessary

▸ BY INHALATION OF AEROSOL

▸ Child 4–15 years: Initially 50–100 micrograms twice daily, increased if necessary up to 200 micrograms twice daily, dose to be adjusted as necessary

▸ Child 16–17 years: Initially 100–500 micrograms twice daily, increased if necessary up to 1 mg twice daily, doses above 500 micrograms twice daily to be initiated by a specialist, dose to be adjusted as necessary

▸ BY INHALATION OF NEBULISED SUSPENSION

▸ Child 4–15 years: 1 mg twice daily

▸ Child 16–17 years: 0.5–2 mg twice daily

IMPORTANT SAFETY INFORMATION

MHRA/CHM ADVICE: PRESSURISED METERED DOSE INHALERS (PMDI): RISK OF AIRWAY OBSTRUCTION FROM ASPIRATION OF LOOSE OBJECTS (JULY 2018)

See Respiratory system, inhaled drug delivery p. 169.

● **INTERACTIONS** → Appendix 1: corticosteroids

● **SIDE-EFFECTS**

▸ **Rare or very rare** Dyspepsia

● **DIRECTIONS FOR ADMINISTRATION** EvGr Fluticasone nebuliser liquid may be diluted with sterile sodium chloride 0.9%. It is not suitable for use in ultrasonic nebulisers. Ⓜ

● **PRESCRIBING AND DISPENSING INFORMATION** For choice of therapy, see Asthma, acute p. 174 and Asthma, chronic p. 171.

● **PATIENT AND CARER ADVICE** Patients or carers should be given advice on how to administer all fluticasone inhalation preparations.

Medicines for Children leaflet: Fluticasone inhaler for asthma prevention (prophylaxis) www.medicinesforchildren.org.uk/medicines/fluticasone-inhaler-for-asthma-prevention-prophylaxis/

● **MEDICINAL FORMS** There can be variation in the licensing of different medicines containing the same drug.

Inhalation powder

CAUTIONARY AND ADVISORY LABELS 8, 10

▸ **Flixotide Accuhaler** (GlaxoSmithKline UK Ltd)

Fluticasone propionate 50 microgram per 1 dose Flixotide 50micrograms/dose Accuhaler | 60 dose PoM £4.00 DT = £4.00

Fluticasone propionate 100 microgram per 1 dose Flixotide 100micrograms/dose Accuhaler | 60 dose PoM £8.00 DT = £8.00
Fluticasone propionate 250 microgram per 1 dose Flixotide 250micrograms/dose Accuhaler | 60 dose PoM £25.51 DT = £25.51
Fluticasone propionate 500 microgram per 1 dose Flixotide 500micrograms/dose Accuhaler | 60 dose PoM £43.37 DT = £43.37

Pressurised inhalation

CAUTIONARY AND ADVISORY LABELS 8, 10

▸ Flixotide Evohaler (GlaxoSmithKline UK Ltd)
Fluticasone propionate 50 microgram per 1 dose Flixotide 50micrograms/dose Evohaler | 120 dose PoM £6.53 DT = £6.53
Fluticasone propionate 125 microgram per 1 dose Flixotide 125micrograms/dose Evohaler | 120 dose PoM £21.26 DT = £21.26
Fluticasone propionate 250 microgram per 1 dose Flixotide 250micrograms/dose Evohaler | 120 dose PoM £36.14 DT = £36.14

Fluticasone with formoterol

20-Apr-2021

The properties listed below are those particular to the combination only. For the properties of the components please consider, fluticasone p. 189, formoterol fumarate p. 179.

● **INDICATIONS AND DOSE**

FLUTIFORM® 125

Prophylaxis of asthma

▶ BY INHALATION OF AEROSOL

▸ Child 12–17 years: 2 puffs twice daily

FLUTIFORM® 50

Prophylaxis of asthma

▶ BY INHALATION OF AEROSOL

▸ Child 5–17 years: 2 puffs twice daily

FLUTIFORM® K-HALER 125

Prophylaxis of asthma

▶ BY INHALATION OF AEROSOL

▸ Child 12–17 years: 2 puffs twice daily

FLUTIFORM® K-HALER 50

Prophylaxis of asthma

▶ BY INHALATION OF AEROSOL

▸ Child 12–17 years: 2 puffs twice daily

● **INTERACTIONS** → Appendix 1: $beta_2$ agonists · corticosteroids

● **SIDE-EFFECTS**

▶ **Uncommon** Dry mouth · rash · sleep disorders

▶ **Rare or very rare** Asthenia · cough · diarrhoea · dyspepsia · hypertension · muscle spasms · oral fungal infection · peripheral oedema · vertigo

● **PATIENT AND CARER ADVICE** Patients or carers should be given advice on how to administer fluticasone with formoterol aerosol inhalation.

● **NATIONAL FUNDING/ACCESS DECISIONS** For full details see funding body website

Scottish Medicines Consortium (SMC) decisions

▶ **Fluticasone propionate with formoterol fumarate (*Flutiform*®) for the regular treatment of asthma (October 2012)** SMC No. 736/11 Recommended

▶ **Fluticasone propionate with formoterol fumarate (*Flutiform*® 50/5 metered dose inhaler) for the regular treatment of asthma in children aged 5 to 12 years (June 2019)** SMC No. SMC2178 Recommended

● **MEDICINAL FORMS** There can be variation in the licensing of different medicines containing the same drug.

Pressurised inhalation

CAUTIONARY AND ADVISORY LABELS 8, 10 (high doses)

▸ Flutiform (Napp Pharmaceuticals Ltd)
Formoterol fumarate dihydrate 5 microgram per 1 dose, Fluticasone propionate 50 microgram per 1 dose Flutiform 50micrograms/dose / 5micrograms/dose inhaler | 120 dose PoM £14.40 DT = £14.40
Formoterol fumarate dihydrate 5 microgram per 1 dose, Fluticasone propionate 125 microgram per 1 dose Flutiform 125micrograms/dose / 5micrograms/dose inhaler | 120 dose PoM £28.00 DT = £28.00

Fluticasone with salmeterol

13-Oct-2022

The properties listed below are those particular to the combination only. For the properties of the components please consider, fluticasone p. 189, salmeterol p. 180.

● **INDICATIONS AND DOSE**

AVENOR® 25/125

Prophylaxis of asthma

▶ BY INHALATION OF AEROSOL

▸ Child 12–17 years: 2 inhalations twice daily

AVENOR® 25/250

Prophylaxis of asthma

▶ BY INHALATION OF AEROSOL

▸ Child 12–17 years: 2 inhalations twice daily

AVENOR® 25/50

Prophylaxis of asthma

▶ BY INHALATION OF AEROSOL

▸ Child 4–17 years: 2 inhalations twice daily, reduced to 2 inhalations once daily, use reduced dose only if control maintained

COMBISAL® 25/125

Prophylaxis of asthma

▶ BY INHALATION OF AEROSOL

▸ Child 12–17 years: 2 inhalations twice daily

COMBISAL® 25/250

Prophylaxis of asthma

▶ BY INHALATION OF AEROSOL

▸ Child 12–17 years: 2 inhalations twice daily

COMBISAL® 25/50

Prophylaxis of asthma

▶ BY INHALATION OF AEROSOL

▸ Child 4–17 years: 2 inhalations twice daily, reduced to 2 inhalations once daily, use reduced dose only if control maintained

FIXKOH AIRMASTER® 50/100

Prophylaxis of asthma

▶ BY INHALATION OF POWDER

▸ Child 12–17 years: 1 inhalation twice daily, reduced to 1 inhalation once daily, use reduced dose only if control maintained

FIXKOH AIRMASTER® 50/250

Prophylaxis of asthma

▶ BY INHALATION OF POWDER

▸ Child 12–17 years: 1 inhalation twice daily

FIXKOH AIRMASTER® 50/500

Prophylaxis of asthma

▶ BY INHALATION OF POWDER

▸ Child 12–17 years: 1 inhalation twice daily

FUSACOMB 50/250 EASYHALER®

Prophylaxis of asthma

▶ BY INHALATION OF POWDER

▸ Child 12–17 years: 1 inhalation twice daily, reduced to 1 inhalation once daily, use reduced dose only if control maintained

FUSACOMB 50/500 EASYHALER®

Prophylaxis of asthma

▶ BY INHALATION OF POWDER

▸ Child 12–17 years: 1 inhalation twice daily

SEFFALAIR SPIROMAX® 12.75/100

Prophylaxis of asthma

▶ BY INHALATION OF POWDER

- Child 12–17 years: 1 inhalation twice daily

SEFFALAIR SPIROMAX® 12.75/202

Prophylaxis of asthma

▶ BY INHALATION OF POWDER

- Child 12–17 years: 1 inhalation twice daily

SEREFLO CIPHALER® 50/250

Prophylaxis of asthma

▶ BY INHALATION OF POWDER

- Child 12–17 years: 1 inhalation twice daily, reduced to 1 inhalation once daily, use reduced dose only if control maintained

SERETIDE 100 ACCUHALER®

Prophylaxis of asthma

▶ BY INHALATION OF POWDER

- Child 4–17 years: 1 inhalation twice daily, reduced to 1 inhalation once daily, use reduced dose only if control maintained

SERETIDE 125 EVOHALER®

Prophylaxis of asthma

▶ BY INHALATION OF AEROSOL

- Child 12–17 years: 2 puffs twice daily

SERETIDE 250 ACCUHALER®

Prophylaxis of asthma

▶ BY INHALATION OF POWDER

- Child 12–17 years: 1 inhalation twice daily

SERETIDE 250 EVOHALER®

Prophylaxis of asthma

▶ BY INHALATION OF AEROSOL

- Child 12–17 years: 2 puffs twice daily

SERETIDE 50 EVOHALER®

Prophylaxis of asthma

▶ BY INHALATION OF AEROSOL

- Child 4–17 years: 2 puffs twice daily, reduced to 2 puffs once daily, use reduced dose only if control maintained

SERETIDE 500 ACCUHALER®

Prophylaxis of asthma

▶ BY INHALATION OF POWDER

- Child 12–17 years: 1 inhalation twice daily

STALPEX® 50/500

Prophylaxis of severe asthma

▶ BY INHALATION OF POWDER

- Child 12–17 years: 1 inhalation twice daily

IMPORTANT SAFETY INFORMATION

EvGr *Seffalair Spiromax®* 12.75/100 and 12.75/202 *dry powder inhalers* are not interchangeable with other fluticasone with salmeterol preparations, as the delivered doses differ. Ⓜ

● **INTERACTIONS** → Appendix 1: beta$_2$ agonists · corticosteroids

● **PRESCRIBING AND DISPENSING INFORMATION**

EvGr *Volumatic®* spacer devices are compatible with *Seretide Evohaler®* pressurised metered-dose inhalers.

Only the *AeroChamber Plus®* spacer device is compatible with *Avenor®* and *Combisal®* pressurised metered-dose inhalers. Ⓜ

● **PATIENT AND CARER ADVICE** Patients or carers should be given advice on how to administer fluticasone with salmeterol dry powder inhalation and aerosol inhalation.

● **MEDICINAL FORMS** There can be variation in the licensing of different medicines containing the same drug.

Inhalation powder

CAUTIONARY AND ADVISORY LABELS 8, 10

▶ **Fixkoh Airmaster** (Genus Pharmaceuticals Holdings Ltd)

Salmeterol (as Salmeterol xinafoate) 50 microgram per 1 dose, Fluticasone propionate 100 microgram per 1 dose Fixkoh Airmaster 50micrograms/dose / 100micrograms/dose dry powder inhaler | 60 dose PoM £14.47 DT = £17.46

Salmeterol (as Salmeterol xinafoate) 50 microgram per 1 dose, Fluticasone propionate 250 microgram per 1 dose Fixkoh Airmaster 50micrograms/dose / 250micrograms/dose dry powder inhaler | 60 dose PoM £19.29 DT = £33.95

Salmeterol (as Salmeterol xinafoate) 50 microgram per 1 dose, Fluticasone propionate 500 microgram per 1 dose Fixkoh Airmaster 50micrograms/dose / 500micrograms/dose dry powder inhaler | 60 dose PoM £16.12 DT = £32.74

▶ **Fusacomb Easyhaler** (Orion Pharma (UK) Ltd)

Salmeterol (as Salmeterol xinafoate) 50 microgram per 1 dose, Fluticasone propionate 250 microgram per 1 dose Fusacomb Easyhaler 50micrograms/dose / 250micrograms/dose dry powder inhaler | 60 dose PoM £21.50 DT = £33.95

Salmeterol (as Salmeterol xinafoate) 50 microgram per 1 dose, Fluticasone propionate 500 microgram per 1 dose Fusacomb Easyhaler 50micrograms/dose / 500micrograms/dose dry powder inhaler | 60 dose PoM £26.99 DT = £32.74

▶ **Sereflo Ciphaler** (Cipla EU Ltd)

Salmeterol (as Salmeterol xinafoate) 50 microgram per 1 dose, Fluticasone propionate 250 microgram per 1 dose Sereflo Ciphaler 50micrograms/dose / 250micrograms/dose dry powder inhaler | 60 dose PoM £10.99 DT = £33.95

▶ **Seretide Accuhaler** (GlaxoSmithKline UK Ltd)

Salmeterol (as Salmeterol xinafoate) 50 microgram per 1 dose, Fluticasone propionate 100 microgram per 1 dose Seretide 100 Accuhaler | 60 dose PoM £17.46 DT = £17.46

Salmeterol (as Salmeterol xinafoate) 50 microgram per 1 dose, Fluticasone propionate 250 microgram per 1 dose Seretide 250 Accuhaler | 60 dose PoM £33.95 DT = £33.95

Salmeterol (as Salmeterol xinafoate) 50 microgram per 1 dose, Fluticasone propionate 500 microgram per 1 dose Seretide 500 Accuhaler | 60 dose PoM £32.74 DT = £32.74

▶ **Stalpex** (Glenmark Pharmaceuticals Europe Ltd)

Salmeterol (as Salmeterol xinafoate) 50 microgram per 1 dose, Fluticasone propionate 500 microgram per 1 dose Stalpex 50micrograms/dose / 500micrograms/dose dry powder inhaler | 60 dose PoM £16.12 DT = £32.74

Pressurised inhalation

CAUTIONARY AND ADVISORY LABELS 8, 10

▶ **Avenor** (Zentiva Pharma UK Ltd)

Salmeterol (as Salmeterol xinafoate) 25 microgram per 1 dose, Fluticasone propionate 50 microgram per 1 dose Avenor 25micrograms/dose / 50micrograms/dose inhaler | 120 dose PoM £12.99 DT = £17.46

Salmeterol (as Salmeterol xinafoate) 25 microgram per 1 dose, Fluticasone propionate 125 microgram per 1 dose Avenor 25micrograms/dose / 125micrograms/dose inhaler | 120 dose PoM £10.33 DT = £23.45

Salmeterol (as Salmeterol xinafoate) 25 microgram per 1 dose, Fluticasone propionate 250 microgram per 1 dose Avenor 25micrograms/dose / 250micrograms/dose inhaler | 120 dose PoM £13.66 DT = £29.32

▶ **Combisal** (Aspire Pharma Ltd)

Salmeterol (as Salmeterol xinafoate) 25 microgram per 1 dose, Fluticasone propionate 50 microgram per 1 dose Combisal 25micrograms/dose / 50micrograms/dose inhaler | 120 dose PoM £13.50 DT = £17.46

Salmeterol (as Salmeterol xinafoate) 25 microgram per 1 dose, Fluticasone propionate 125 microgram per 1 dose Combisal 25micrograms/dose / 125micrograms/dose inhaler | 120 dose PoM £10.48 DT = £23.45

Salmeterol (as Salmeterol xinafoate) 25 microgram per 1 dose, Fluticasone propionate 250 microgram per 1 dose Combisal 25micrograms/dose / 250micrograms/dose inhaler | 120 dose PoM £13.99 DT = £29.32

▶ **Seretide Evohaler** (GlaxoSmithKline UK Ltd)

Salmeterol (as Salmeterol xinafoate) 25 microgram per 1 dose, Fluticasone propionate 50 microgram per 1 dose Seretide 50 Evohaler | 120 dose PoM £17.46 DT = £17.46

Salmeterol (as Salmeterol xinafoate) 25 microgram per 1 dose, Fluticasone propionate 125 microgram per 1 dose Seretide 125 Evohaler | 120 dose [PoM] £23.45 DT = £23.45
Salmeterol (as Salmeterol xinafoate) 25 microgram per 1 dose, Fluticasone propionate 250 microgram per 1 dose Seretide 250 Evohaler | 120 dose [PoM] £29.32 DT = £29.32

F 179

Fluticasone with vilanterol
20-Apr-2021

The properties listed below are those particular to the combination only. For the properties of the components please consider, fluticasone p. 189.

- **INDICATIONS AND DOSE**

RELVAR ELLIPTA® 184 MICROGRAMS/22 MICROGRAMS

Prophylaxis of asthma
- BY INHALATION OF POWDER
- Child 12–17 years: 1 inhalation once daily

RELVAR ELLIPTA® 92 MICROGRAMS/22 MICROGRAMS

Prophylaxis of asthma
- BY INHALATION OF POWDER
- Child 12–17 years: 1 inhalation once daily

- **INTERACTIONS** → Appendix 1: beta$_2$ agonists · corticosteroids
- **SIDE-EFFECTS**
  - **Common or very common** Abdominal pain · arthralgia · back pain · bone fracture · cough · dysphonia · fever · increased risk of infection · muscle spasms · oropharyngeal pain
  - **Uncommon** Vision blurred
  - **Rare or very rare** Angioedema · anxiety
- **PREGNANCY** Manufacturer advises use only if potential benefit outweighs risk.
- **BREAST FEEDING** Manufacturer advises avoid—no information available.
- **HEPATIC IMPAIRMENT** Manufacturer advises caution.
  Dose adjustments Manufacturer advises maximum dose of 92 microgram/22 microgram once daily in moderate to severe impairment.
- **PATIENT AND CARER ADVICE** Patients or carers should be given advice on how to administer fluticasone with vilanterol powder for inhalation.
- **MEDICINAL FORMS** There can be variation in the licensing of different medicines containing the same drug.

Inhalation powder

CAUTIONARY AND ADVISORY LABELS 8, 10

- **Relvar Ellipta** (GlaxoSmithKline UK Ltd)
  Vilanterol 22 microgram per 1 dose, Fluticasone furoate 92 microgram per 1 dose Relvar Ellipta 92micrograms/dose / 22micrograms/dose dry powder inhaler | 30 dose [PoM] £22.00 DT = £22.00
  Vilanterol 22 microgram per 1 dose, Fluticasone furoate 184 microgram per 1 dose Relvar Ellipta 184micrograms/dose / 22micrograms/dose dry powder inhaler | 30 dose [PoM] £29.50 DT = £29.50

F 184

Mometasone furoate
26-Jul-2025

- **INDICATIONS AND DOSE**

Prophylaxis of asthma
- BY INHALATION OF POWDER
- Child 12–17 years: Initially 400 micrograms once daily, to be inhaled in the evening, alternatively initially 200 micrograms twice daily; reduced to 200 micrograms once daily, to be inhaled in the evening, dose to be reduced if control maintained

Prophylaxis of severe asthma
- BY INHALATION OF POWDER
- Child 12–17 years: Initially 400 micrograms twice daily, reduce to the lowest effective dose when control achieved

- **INTERACTIONS** → Appendix 1: corticosteroids
- **SIDE-EFFECTS**
  - **Common or very common** Candida infection
- **PRESCRIBING AND DISPENSING INFORMATION** For choice of therapy, see Asthma, acute p. 174 and Asthma, chronic p. 171.
- **PATIENT AND CARER ADVICE** Patients or carers should be given advice on how to administer mometasone by inhaler.
  Medicines for Children leaflet: Mometasone furoate inhaler for asthma prevention (prophylaxis) www.medicinesforchildren.org.uk/medicines/mometasone-furoate-inhaler-for-asthma-prevention-prophylaxis/
- **NATIONAL FUNDING/ACCESS DECISIONS**
  For full details see funding body website
  Scottish Medicines Consortium (SMC) decisions
  - **Mometasone furoate (*Asmanex® Twisthaler®*) for asthma (November 2003)** SMC No. 79/03 Recommended with restrictions
- **MEDICINAL FORMS** No licensed medicines listed.

IMMUNOSUPPRESSANTS › MONOCLONAL ANTIBODIES

Mepolizumab
06-Jun-2025

- **DRUG ACTION** Mepolizumab is a humanised anti-interleukin-5 (anti-IL-5) monoclonal antibody; it reduces the production and survival of eosinophils.
- **INDICATIONS AND DOSE**

Add on treatment for severe refractory eosinophilic asthma (under expert supervision)
- BY SUBCUTANEOUS INJECTION
- Child 6–11 years: 40 mg every 4 weeks
- Child 12–17 years: 100 mg every 4 weeks

- **CAUTIONS** Helminth infection
  CAUTIONS, FURTHER INFORMATION Manufacturer advises pre-existing helminth infections should be treated before initiation of therapy; if patients become infected during treatment and do not respond to anti-helminth treatment, consider treatment interruption.
- **SIDE-EFFECTS**
  - **Common or very common** Abdominal pain upper · administration related reaction · back pain · fever · headache · hypersensitivity · increased risk of infection · nasal congestion · skin reactions
  - **Frequency not known** Angioedema
- **PREGNANCY** Manufacturer advises avoid unless potential benefit outweighs risk—limited data available.
- **BREAST FEEDING** Manufacturer advises avoid—present in milk in *animal* studies.
- **DIRECTIONS FOR ADMINISTRATION** Manufacturer advises injection is given into the thigh, abdomen, or upper arm. Patients may self-administer *Nucala®* pre-filled devices into the thigh or abdomen after appropriate training in preparation and administration.
- **PRESCRIBING AND DISPENSING INFORMATION** Mepolizumab is a biological medicine. Biological medicines must be prescribed and dispensed by brand name, see *Biological medicines* and *Biosimilar medicines*, under Guidance on prescribing p. 1; record the brand name and batch number after each administration.

For choice of therapy, see Asthma, acute p. 174 and Asthma, chronic p. 171.

- **PATIENT AND CARER ADVICE** Patients and their carers should be advised to seek medical advice if their asthma remains uncontrolled or worsens after initiation of treatment.
- **NATIONAL FUNDING/ACCESS DECISIONS**
For full details see funding body website

Scottish Medicines Consortium (SMC) decisions

- **Mepolizumab (*Nucala*®) as an add-on treatment for severe refractory eosinophilic asthma in adults, adolescents and children aged 6 years and older (May 2025)** SMC No. SMC2765 Recommended with restrictions

All Wales Medicines Strategy Group (AWMSG) decisions

- **Mepolizumab (*Nucala*®) as add-on treatment for severe refractory eosinophilic asthma in patients aged 6 years and older (April 2019)** AWMSG No. 3750 Recommended with restrictions

- **MEDICINAL FORMS** There can be variation in the licensing of different medicines containing the same drug.

Solution for injection

EXCIPIENTS: May contain Edetic acid (edta), polysorbates

- **Nucala** (GlaxoSmithKline UK Ltd)
Mepolizumab 100 mg per 1 ml Nucala 100mg/1ml solution for injection pre-filled pens | 1 pre-filled disposable injection PoM £840.00
Nucala 40mg/0.4ml solution for injection pre-filled syringes | 1 pre-filled disposable injection PoM £336.00 (Hospital only)
Nucala 100mg/1ml solution for injection pre-filled syringes | 1 pre-filled disposable injection PoM £840.00

Omalizumab

17-May-2021

- **INDICATIONS AND DOSE**

Prophylaxis of severe persistent allergic asthma

- BY SUBCUTANEOUS INJECTION
- Child 6–17 years: Dose according to immunoglobulin E concentration and body-weight (consult product literature)

Add-on therapy for chronic spontaneous urticaria in patients who have had an inadequate response to H_1 antihistamine treatment

- BY SUBCUTANEOUS INJECTION
- Child 12–17 years: 300 mg every 4 weeks

- **CAUTIONS** Autoimmune disease · susceptibility to helminth infection—discontinue if infection does not respond to anthelmintic
- **SIDE-EFFECTS**
- **Common or very common** Fever · gastrointestinal discomfort · headache · skin reactions
- **Uncommon** Cough · diarrhoea · dizziness · drowsiness · fatigue · flushing · increased risk of infection · influenza like illness · limb swelling · nausea · paraesthesia · photosensitivity reaction · postural hypotension · respiratory disorders · syncope · weight increased
- **Rare or very rare** Angioedema · hypersensitivity · systemic lupus erythematosus (SLE)
- **Frequency not known** Alopecia · eosinophilic granulomatosis with polyangiitis · immune thrombocytopenic purpura · joint disorders · lymphadenopathy · myalgia

SIDE-EFFECTS, FURTHER INFORMATION **Eosinophilic granulomatosis with polyangiitis (Churg-Strauss syndrome)** Churg-Strauss syndrome has occurred rarely in patients given omalizumab; the reaction is usually associated with the reduction of oral corticosteroid therapy. Churg-Strauss syndrome can present as eosinophilia, vasculitic rash, cardiac complications, worsening pulmonary symptoms, or peripheral neuropathy.

Hypersensitivity reactions Hypersensitivity reactions can also occur immediately following treatment with omalizumab or sometimes more than 24 hours after the first injection.

- **PREGNANCY** Manufacturer advises avoid unless essential—crosses the placenta.
- **BREAST FEEDING** Manufacturer advises avoid—present in milk in *animal* studies.
- **HEPATIC IMPAIRMENT** Manufacturer advises caution (no information available).
- **RENAL IMPAIRMENT** Manufacturer advises caution—no information available.
- **PRESCRIBING AND DISPENSING INFORMATION** Omalizumab is a biological medicine. Biological medicines must be prescribed and dispensed by brand name, see *Biological medicines* and *Biosimilar medicines*, under Guidance on prescribing p. 1; record the brand name and batch number after each administration.
- When used for Asthma For choice of therapy, see Asthma, acute p. 174 and Asthma, chronic p. 171.
- **NATIONAL FUNDING/ACCESS DECISIONS**
For full details see funding body website

NICE decisions

- **Omalizumab for severe persistent allergic asthma (April 2013)** NICE TA278 Recommended
- **Omalizumab for previously treated chronic spontaneous urticaria (June 2015)** NICE TA339 Recommended with restrictions

Scottish Medicines Consortium (SMC) decisions

- **Omalizumab (*Xolair*®) as add-on therapy for the treatment of chronic spontaneous urticaria in adult and adolescent (12 years and above) patients with inadequate response to H_1-antihistamine treatment (January 2015)** SMC No. 1017/14 Recommended with restrictions

- **MEDICINAL FORMS** There can be variation in the licensing of different medicines containing the same drug.

Solution for injection

- **Omlyclo** (Celltrion Healthcare UK Ltd) ▼
Omalizumab 150 mg per 1 ml Omlyclo 75mg/0.5ml solution for injection pre-filled pens | 1 pre-filled disposable injection PoM £115.25 (Hospital only)
Omlyclo 75mg/0.5ml solution for injection pre-filled syringes | 1 pre-filled disposable injection PoM £115.25 (Hospital only)
Omlyclo 150mg/1ml solution for injection pre-filled syringes | 1 pre-filled disposable injection PoM £230.54 (Hospital only)
Omlyclo 150mg/1ml solution for injection pre-filled pens | 1 pre-filled disposable injection PoM £230.54 (Hospital only)
- **Xolair** (Novartis Pharmaceuticals UK Ltd)
Omalizumab 150 mg per 1 ml Xolair 300mg/2ml solution for injection pre-filled pens | 1 pre-filled disposable injection PoM £512.30 (Hospital only)
Xolair 150mg/1ml solution for injection pre-filled syringes | 1 pre-filled disposable injection PoM £256.15
Xolair 75mg/0.5ml solution for injection pre-filled pens | 1 pre-filled disposable injection PoM £128.07 (Hospital only)
Xolair 150mg/1ml solution for injection pre-filled pens | 1 pre-filled disposable injection PoM £256.15 (Hospital only)
Xolair 300mg/2ml solution for injection pre-filled syringes | 1 pre-filled disposable injection PoM £512.30 (Hospital only)
Xolair 75mg/0.5ml solution for injection pre-filled syringes | 1 pre-filled disposable injection PoM £128.07

Tezepelumab 21-Aug-2023

- **DRUG ACTION** Tezepelumab is a monoclonal antibody that interferes with thymic stromal lymphopoietin (TSLP) binding, thereby reducing the production of inflammatory biomarkers and cytokines.

- **INDICATIONS AND DOSE**

Severe asthma [add-on maintenance therapy] (initiated by a specialist)

▶ BY SUBCUTANEOUS INJECTION

▶ Child 12–17 years: 210 mg every 4 weeks

PHARMACOKINETICS

▶ The half-life of tezepelumab is approx. 26 days.

- **CAUTIONS** Helminth infections · serious infections

CAUTIONS, FURTHER INFORMATION [EvGr] Pre-existing helminth infections and serious infections should be treated before starting tezepelumab. During tezepelumab therapy, if a helminth infection develops and does not respond to anti-helminth treatment, or a serious infection develops, discontinue tezepelumab until the infection is resolved. ⟨M⟩

- **INTERACTIONS** → Appendix 1: monoclonal antibodies
- **SIDE-EFFECTS**

▶ **Common or very common** Arthralgia · increased risk of infection · skin reactions

▶ **Frequency not known** Hypersensitivity

- **PREGNANCY** [EvGr] Avoid unless potential benefit outweighs risk—limited information available. ⟨M⟩
- **BREAST FEEDING** [EvGr] Avoid during first few days after birth—risk of transfer to infant cannot be excluded; present in milk in *animal* studies. ⟨M⟩
- **DIRECTIONS FOR ADMINISTRATION** [EvGr] Inject into the thigh or abdomen (except for the 5 cm around the navel), or upper arm (if not self-administered); rotate injection site and avoid skin that is tender, bruised, erythematous, or hardened. ⟨M⟩ Patients may self-administer *Tezspire*® after appropriate training in preparation and administration.
- **PRESCRIBING AND DISPENSING INFORMATION** Tezepelumab is a biological medicine. Biological medicines must be prescribed and dispensed by brand name, see *Biological medicines* and *Biosimilar medicines*, under Guidance on prescribing p. 1; record the brand name and batch number after each administration.

For choice of therapy, see Asthma, acute p. 174 and Asthma, chronic p. 171.

- **HANDLING AND STORAGE** Store in a refrigerator (2–8°C) and protect from light; may be kept at room temperature (max. 25°C) for max. 30 days.
- **PATIENT AND CARER ADVICE** Patients and their carers should be instructed to seek medical advice if their asthma remains uncontrolled or worsens after initiation of treatment. Patients and their carers should be advised of the signs and symptoms of a cardiac event and to seek immediate medical attention if they occur.

Self-administration Patients or their carers should be given training in subcutaneous injection technique.

A patient leaflet and user manual should be provided.

- **NATIONAL FUNDING/ACCESS DECISIONS**

For full details see funding body website

NICE decisions

▶ **Tezepelumab for treating severe asthma (April 2023)** NICE TA880 Recommended with restrictions

Scottish Medicines Consortium (SMC) decisions

▶ **Tezepelumab (*Tezspire*®) as add-on maintenance treatment in adults and adolescents 12 years and older with severe asthma who are inadequately controlled despite high dose inhaled corticosteroids plus another medicinal product for maintenance treatment (August 2023)** SMC No. SMC2541 Recommended with restrictions

- **MEDICINAL FORMS** There can be variation in the licensing of different medicines containing the same drug.

Solution for injection

EXCIPIENTS: May contain L-proline, polysorbates

▶ Tezspire (AstraZeneca UK Ltd) ▼

Tezepelumab 110 mg per 1 ml Tezspire 210mg/1.91ml solution for injection pre-filled pens | 1 pre-filled disposable injection [PoM] £1,265.00 (Hospital only)

Tezspire 210mg/1.91ml solution for injection pre-filled syringes | 1 pre-filled disposable injection [PoM] £1,265.00 (Hospital only)

LEUKOTRIENE RECEPTOR ANTAGONISTS

Montelukast 02-May-2024

- **INDICATIONS AND DOSE**

Prophylaxis of asthma

▶ BY MOUTH

▶ Child 6 months–5 years: 4 mg once daily, dose to be taken in the evening

▶ Child 6–14 years: 5 mg once daily, dose to be taken in the evening

▶ Child 15–17 years: 10 mg once daily, dose to be taken in the evening

Symptomatic relief of seasonal allergic rhinitis in patients with asthma

▶ BY MOUTH

▶ Child 15–17 years: 10 mg once daily, dose to be taken in the evening

IMPORTANT SAFETY INFORMATION

MHRA/CHM ADVICE: MONTELUKAST (*SINGULAIR*®): REMINDER OF THE RISK OF NEUROPSYCHIATRIC REACTIONS (SEPTEMBER 2019)

Healthcare professionals are advised to be alert for neuropsychiatric reactions, including speech impairment and obsessive-compulsive symptoms, in adults, adolescents, and children taking montelukast. Patients should be advised to read the list of neuropsychiatric reactions in the information leaflet and seek immediate medical attention if they occur.

For further details, see: www.gov.uk/drug-safety-update/montelukast-singulair-reminder-of-the-risk-of-neuropsychiatric-reactions.

MHRA/CHM ADVICE: MONTELUKAST: REMINDER OF THE RISK OF NEUROPSYCHIATRIC REACTIONS (APRIL 2024)

Following a review of the available evidence, warnings about the risk of neuropsychiatric reactions associated with montelukast have been strengthened and highlighted in product literature to increase awareness. Such reactions include new or worsening changes in mood, sleep, or behaviour (e.g. nightmares, aggression, anxiety, depression, or thoughts of self-injury), and have been reported in adults, adolescents, and children. In addition to advice issued in 2019, healthcare professionals are advised to discontinue montelukast in patients who develop new or worsening neuropsychiatric symptoms.

The MHRA has produced videos to support this advice—guidance for healthcare professionals is available at: www.youtube.com/watch?v=rpFog4QNf4k and guidance for patients, parents, and carers is available at: www.youtube.com/watch?v=e5hv96JGjtw.

For further details, see: www.gov.uk/drug-safety-update/montelukast-reminder-of-the-risk-of-neuropsychiatric-reactions.

- **INTERACTIONS** → Appendix 1: montelukast

● **SIDE-EFFECTS**
- **Common or very common** Diarrhoea · fever · gastrointestinal discomfort · headache · nausea · skin reactions · upper respiratory tract infection · vomiting
- **Uncommon** Akathisia · anxiety · arthralgia · asthenia · behaviour abnormal · depression · dizziness · drowsiness · dry mouth · haemorrhage · malaise · mood altered · muscle complaints · oedema · seizure · sensation abnormal · sleep disorders
- **Rare or very rare** Angioedema · concentration impaired · disorientation · eosinophilic granulomatosis with polyangiitis · erythema nodosum · hallucination · hepatic disorders · memory impairment · palpitations · psychiatric disorders · pulmonary eosinophilia · speech disorder · suicidal behaviours · tremor

SIDE-EFFECTS, FURTHER INFORMATION Eosinophilic granulomatosis with polyangiitis (Churg-Strauss syndrome) has occurred very rarely in association with the use of montelukast; in many of the reported cases the reaction followed the reduction or withdrawal of oral corticosteroid therapy. Prescribers should be alert to the development of eosinophilia, vasculitic rash, worsening pulmonary symptoms, cardiac complications, or peripheral neuropathy.

● **PREGNANCY** Manufacturer advises avoid unless essential. There is limited evidence for the safe use of montelukast during pregnancy; however, it can be taken as normal in women who have shown a significant improvement in asthma not achievable with other drugs before becoming pregnant.

● **BREAST FEEDING** Manufacturer advises avoid unless essential.

● **DIRECTIONS FOR ADMINISTRATION** Manufacturer advises granules may be swallowed or mixed with cold, soft food (not liquid) and taken immediately.

● **PRESCRIBING AND DISPENSING INFORMATION**
- When used for Asthma For choice of therapy, see Asthma, acute p. 174 and Asthma, chronic p. 171.

Flavours of chewable tablet formulations may include cherry.

● **PATIENT AND CARER ADVICE**
Administration Patients or carers should be given advice on how to administer montelukast granules.
Risk of neuropsychiatric reactions Patients and carers should be advised to seek medical attention if changes in behaviour occur—see also *Important safety information*.
Medicines for Children leaflet: Montelukast for asthma www.medicinesforchildren.org.uk/medicines/montelukast-for-asthma/

● **NATIONAL FUNDING/ACCESS DECISIONS**
SINGULAIR ® CHEWABLE TABLETS For full details see funding body website

Scottish Medicines Consortium (SMC) decisions
- Montelukast (*Singulair® Paediatric*) chewable tablets for asthma in children aged 2–14 years (July 2007) SMC No. 383/07 Recommended with restrictions

SINGULAIR ® GRANULES For full details see funding body website

Scottish Medicines Consortium (SMC) decisions
- Montelukast (*Singulair® Paediatric*) for asthma in children aged 2–14 years SMC No. 383/07 Recommended with restrictions

● **MEDICINAL FORMS** There can be variation in the licensing of different medicines containing the same drug.

Oral tablet
- **Montelukast (Non-proprietary)**
 Montelukast (as Montelukast sodium) 10 mg Montelukast 10mg tablets | 28 tablet [PoM] £32.36 DT = £0.82
- **Singulair** (Organon Pharma (UK) Ltd)
 Montelukast (as Montelukast sodium) 10 mg Singulair 10mg tablets | 28 tablet [PoM] £26.97 DT = £0.82

Oral granules
- **Montelukast (Non-proprietary)**
 Montelukast (as Montelukast sodium) 4 mg Montelukast 4mg granules sachets sugar free | 28 sachet [PoM] £5.32–£8.79 DT = £5.20 [SF]

Chewable tablet
CAUTIONARY AND ADVISORY LABELS 23, 24
EXCIPIENTS: May contain Aspartame
- **Montelukast (Non-proprietary)**
 Montelukast (as Montelukast sodium) 4 mg Montelukast 4mg chewable tablets sugar free | 28 tablet [PoM] £30.83 DT = £0.87 [SF]
 Montelukast (as Montelukast sodium) 5 mg Montelukast 5mg chewable tablets sugar free | 28 tablet [PoM] £30.83 DT = £0.95 [SF]
- **Singulair** (Organon Pharma (UK) Ltd)
 Montelukast (as Montelukast sodium) 5 mg Singulair Paediatric 5mg chewable tablets | 28 tablet [PoM] £25.69 DT = £0.95 [SF]

XANTHINES

Aminophylline

03-Aug-2023

● **INDICATIONS AND DOSE**

Severe acute asthma in patients not previously treated with theophylline
- BY SLOW INTRAVENOUS INJECTION
- Child: 5 mg/kg (max. per dose 500 mg), to be followed by intravenous infusion

Severe acute asthma
- BY INTRAVENOUS INFUSION
- Child 1 month–11 years: 1 mg/kg/hour, adjusted according to plasma-theophylline concentration
- Child 12–17 years: 500–700 micrograms/kg/hour, adjusted according to plasma-theophylline concentration

DOSE ADJUSTMENTS DUE TO INTERACTIONS
- Dose adjustment may be necessary if smoking started or stopped during treatment.

DOSES AT EXTREMES OF BODY-WEIGHT
- To avoid excessive dosage in obese patients, dose should be calculated on the basis of ideal weight for height.

PHARMACOKINETICS
- Aminophylline is a stable mixture or combination of theophylline and ethylenediamine; the ethylenediamine confers greater solubility in water.
- Theophylline is metabolised in the liver. The plasma-theophylline concentration is increased in heart failure, hepatic impairment, and in viral infections. The plasma-theophylline concentration is decreased in smokers, and by alcohol consumption. Differences in the half-life of aminophylline are important because the toxic dose is close to the therapeutic dose.

● **UNLICENSED USE** Aminophylline injection not licensed for use in children under 6 months.

● **CAUTIONS** Arrhythmias following rapid intravenous injection · cardiac arrhythmias or other cardiac disease · epilepsy · fever · hypertension · peptic ulcer · risk of hypokalaemia · thyroid disorder

● **INTERACTIONS** → Appendix 1: aminophylline

● **SIDE-EFFECTS** Abdominal pain · anxiety · arrhythmia (more common when given too rapidly by intravenous injection) · confusion · delirium · diarrhoea · dizziness · electrolyte imbalance · gastrointestinal haemorrhage · gastrooesophageal reflux disease · headache · hyperthermia · hyperventilation · hypotension (more common when given too rapidly by intravenous injection) · insomnia · mania · metabolic disorder · nausea · pain · palpitations · seizure (more common when given too rapidly by intravenous injection) · skin reactions · tachycardia (more common when given too rapidly by intravenous injection) · thirst · tremor · vertigo · visual impairment · vomiting

SIDE-EFFECTS, FURTHER INFORMATION Potentially serious hypokalaemia may result from $beta_2$-agonist therapy. Particular caution is required in severe asthma, because this effect may be potentiated by concomitant treatment with theophylline and its derivatives, corticosteroids, and diuretics, and by hypoxia. Plasma-potassium concentration should therefore be monitored in severe asthma.

Overdose Theophylline and related drugs in overdose can cause vomiting (which may be severe and intractable), agitation, restlessness, dilated pupils, sinus tachycardia, and hyperglycaemia. More serious effects are haematemesis, convulsions, and supraventricular and ventricular arrhythmias. Severe hypokalaemia may develop rapidly.

For specific details on the management of poisoning, see *Theophylline*, under Emergency treatment of poisoning p. 1036.

- **ALLERGY AND CROSS-SENSITIVITY** Allergy to ethylenediamine can cause urticaria, erythema, and exfoliative dermatitis.
- **PREGNANCY** Neonatal irritability and apnoea have been reported. Theophylline can be taken as normal during pregnancy as it is particularly important that asthma should be well controlled during pregnancy.
- **BREAST FEEDING** Present in milk—irritability in infant reported. Theophylline can be taken as normal during breast-feeding.
- **HEPATIC IMPAIRMENT** Manufacturer advises caution (risk of reduced clearance).

  Dose adjustments Manufacturer advises maintenance dose reduction—consult product literature.
- **MONITORING REQUIREMENTS**
  - Aminophylline is monitored therapeutically in terms of plasma-theophylline concentrations; a blood sample should be taken 4–6 hours after starting treatment.
  - Measurement of plasma-theophylline concentration may be helpful and is **essential** if a loading dose of intravenous aminophylline is to be given to patients who are already taking theophylline, because serious side-effects such as convulsions and arrhythmias can occasionally precede other symptoms of toxicity.
  - In most individuals, a plasma-theophylline concentration of 10–20 mg/litre (55–110 micromol/litre) is required for satisfactory bronchodilation, although a lower plasma-theophylline concentration of 5–15 mg/litre may be effective. Adverse effects can occur within the range 10–20 mg/litre and both the frequency and severity increase at concentrations above 20 mg/litre.
- **DIRECTIONS FOR ADMINISTRATION** For *intravenous injection*, manufacturer advises give **very slowly** over at least 20 minutes (with close monitoring).

  For *intravenous infusion*, expert sources advise dilute to a concentration of 1 mg/mL with Glucose 5% *or* Sodium Chloride 0.9%.
- **PRESCRIBING AND DISPENSING INFORMATION** Patients taking oral theophylline should not normally receive a loading dose of intravenous aminophylline.

  For choice of therapy, see Asthma, acute p. 174 and Asthma, chronic p. 171. Consider intravenous aminophylline for treatment of severe and life-threatening acute asthma only after consultation with senior medical staff.
- **MEDICINAL FORMS** There can be variation in the licensing of different medicines containing the same drug. Forms available from special-order manufacturers include: solution for infusion

Solution for injection

- **Aminophylline (Non-proprietary)**

  Aminophylline 25 mg per 1 ml Aminophylline 250mg/10ml solution for injection ampoules | 10 ampoule PoM £13.50–£15.00 DT = £15.00

Theophylline

15-Apr-2024

- **INDICATIONS AND DOSE**

UNIPHYLLIN CONTINUS®

Chronic asthma

- BY MOUTH USING MODIFIED-RELEASE MEDICINES
  - Child 2–11 years: 9 mg/kg every 12 hours (max. per dose 200 mg), dose may be increased in some children with chronic asthma; increased to 10–16 mg/kg every 12 hours (max. per dose 400 mg), may be appropriate to give larger evening or morning dose to achieve optimum therapeutic effect when symptoms most severe; in patients whose night or daytime symptoms persist despite other therapy, who are not currently receiving theophylline, total daily requirement may be added as single evening or morning dose
  - Child 12–17 years: 200 mg every 12 hours, adjusted according to response to 400 mg every 12 hours, may be appropriate to give larger evening or morning dose to achieve optimum therapeutic effect when symptoms most severe; in patients whose night or daytime symptoms persist despite other therapy, who are not currently receiving theophylline, total daily requirement may be added as single evening or morning dose

DOSE ADJUSTMENTS DUE TO INTERACTIONS

- Dose adjustment may be necessary if smoking started or stopped during treatment.

PHARMACOKINETICS

- Theophylline is metabolised in the liver. The plasma-theophylline concentration is increased in heart failure, hepatic impairment, and in viral infections. The plasma-theophylline concentration is decreased in smokers, and by alcohol consumption. Differences in the half-life of theophylline are important because the toxic dose is close to the therapeutic dose.

- **CAUTIONS** Cardiac arrhythmias or other cardiac disease · epilepsy · fever · hypertension · peptic ulcer · risk of hypokalaemia · thyroid disorder
- **INTERACTIONS** → Appendix 1: theophylline
- **SIDE-EFFECTS** Anxiety · arrhythmias · diarrhoea · dizziness · gastrointestinal discomfort · gastrooesophageal reflux disease · headache · hyperuricaemia · nausea · palpitations · seizure · skin reactions · sleep disorders · tremor · urinary disorders · vomiting

  SIDE-EFFECTS, FURTHER INFORMATION Potentially serious hypokalaemia may result from $beta_2$-agonist therapy. Particular caution is required in severe asthma, because this effect may be potentiated by concomitant treatment with theophylline and its derivatives, corticosteroids, and diuretics, and by hypoxia. Plasma-potassium concentration should therefore be monitored in severe asthma.

  Overdose Theophylline in overdose can cause vomiting (which may be severe and intractable), agitation, restlessness, dilated pupils, sinus tachycardia, and hyperglycaemia. More serious effects are haematemesis, convulsions, and supraventricular and ventricular arrhythmias. Severe hypokalaemia may develop rapidly.

For details on the management of poisoning, see Theophylline, under Emergency treatment of poisoning p. 1036.

- **PREGNANCY** Neonatal irritability and apnoea have been reported. Theophylline can be taken as normal during pregnancy as it is particularly important that asthma should be well controlled during pregnancy.
- **BREAST FEEDING** Present in milk—irritability in infant reported; modified-release preparations preferable. Theophylline can be taken as normal during breast-feeding.
- **HEPATIC IMPAIRMENT** Manufacturer advises caution (risk of increased exposure).
  Dose adjustments Manufacturer advises consider dose reduction.
- **MONITORING REQUIREMENTS**
  - In most individuals, a plasma-theophylline concentration of 10–20 mg/litre (55–110 micromol/litre) is required for satisfactory bronchodilation, although a lower plasma-theophylline concentration of 5–15 mg/litre may be effective. Adverse effects can occur within the range 10–20 mg/litre and both the frequency and severity increase at concentrations above 20 mg/litre.
  - Plasma-theophylline concentration is measured 5 days after starting oral treatment and at least 3 days after any dose adjustment. A blood sample should usually be taken 4–6 hours after an oral dose of a modified-release preparation (sampling times may vary—consult local guidelines).
- **PRESCRIBING AND DISPENSING INFORMATION** For choice of therapy, see Asthma, acute p. 174 and Asthma, chronic p. 171.
  The rate of absorption from modified-release preparations can vary between brands. If a prescription for a modified-release oral theophylline preparation does not specify a brand name, the pharmacist should contact the prescriber and agree the brand to be dispensed. Additionally, it is essential that a patient discharged from hospital should be maintained on the brand on which that patient was stabilised as an in-patient.

- **MEDICINAL FORMS** There can be variation in the licensing of different medicines containing the same drug.

Modified-release tablet

CAUTIONARY AND ADVISORY LABELS 25

- **Uniphyllin Continus** (Ennogen Healthcare International Ltd)
  Theophylline 200 mg Uniphyllin 200mg prolonged-release tablets | 56 tablet [P] £29.80 DT = £29.80
  Theophylline 300 mg Uniphyllin 300mg prolonged-release tablets | 56 tablet [P] £29.80 DT = £29.80
  Theophylline 400 mg Uniphyllin 400mg prolonged-release tablets | 56 tablet [P] £29.80 DT = £29.80

Nebuliser solutions

- **HYPERTONIC SODIUM CHLORIDE SOLUTIONS**

MUCOCLEAR® 3%

- **INDICATIONS AND DOSE**

Mobilise lower respiratory tract secretions in mucous consolidation (e.g. cystic fibrosis) | Mild to moderate acute viral bronchiolitis in infants

- BY INHALATION OF NEBULISED SOLUTION
  - Child: 4 mL 2–4 times a day, temporary irritation, such as coughing, hoarseness, or reversible bronchoconstriction may occur; an inhaled bronchodilator can be used before treatment with hypertonic sodium chloride to reduce the risk of these adverse effects

MucoClear 3% inhalation solution 4ml ampoules (Pari Medical Ltd) **Sodium chloride 30 mg per 1 ml** 20 ampoule • NHS indicative price = £12.98 • Drug Tariff (Part IXa) | 60 ampoule • NHS indicative price = £27.00 • Drug Tariff (Part IXa)

MUCOCLEAR® 6%

- **INDICATIONS AND DOSE**

Mobilise lower respiratory tract secretions in mucous consolidation (e.g. cystic fibrosis)

- BY INHALATION OF NEBULISED SOLUTION
  - Child: 4 mL twice daily, temporary irritation, such as coughing, hoarseness, or reversible bronchoconstriction may occur; an inhaled bronchodilator can be used before treatment with hypertonic sodium chloride to reduce the risk of these adverse effects

MucoClear 6% inhalation solution 4ml ampoules (Pari Medical Ltd) **Sodium chloride 60 mg per 1 ml** 20 ampoule • NHS indicative price = £12.98 • Drug Tariff (Part IXa) | 60 ampoule • NHS indicative price = £27.00 • Drug Tariff (Part IXa)

NEBUSAL®

- **INDICATIONS AND DOSE**

Mobilise lower respiratory tract secretions in mucous consolidation (e.g. cystic fibrosis)

- BY INHALATION OF NEBULISED SOLUTION
  - Child: 4 mL up to twice daily, temporary irritation, such as coughing, hoarseness, or reversible bronchoconstriction may occur; an inhaled bronchodilator can be used before treatment with hypertonic sodium chloride to reduce the risk of these adverse effects

Nebusal 7% inhalation solution 4ml vials (Accord-UK Ltd) **Sodium chloride 70 mg per 1 ml** 60 vial • NHS indicative price = £27.00 • Drug Tariff (Part IXa)

PULMOCLEAR®

- **INDICATIONS AND DOSE**

Mobilise lower respiratory tract secretions and prevent drying of bronchial mucous.

- BY INHALATION OF NEBULISED SOLUTION
  - Child: (consult product literature)

PulmoClear 6% inhalation solution 4ml vials (TriOn Pharma Ltd) 60 vial • NHS indicative price = £16.59 • Drug Tariff (Part IXa)

PulmoClear 3% inhalation solution 4ml vials (TriOn Pharma Ltd) **Sodium chloride 30 mg per 1 ml** 60 vial • NHS indicative price = £16.47 • Drug Tariff (Part IXa)

PulmoClear 7% inhalation solution 4ml vials (TriOn Pharma Ltd) **Sodium chloride 70 mg per 1 ml** 60 vial • NHS indicative price = £16.59 • Drug Tariff (Part IXa)

RESP-EASE®

- **INDICATIONS AND DOSE**

Mobilise lower respiratory tract secretions and prevent drying of bronchial mucous.

- BY INHALATION OF NEBULISED SOLUTION
  - Child: (consult product literature)

Resp-Ease 3% inhalation solution 4ml ampoules (Venture Healthcare Ltd) **Sodium chloride 30 mg per 1 ml** 60 ampoule • NHS indicative price = £21.60 • Drug Tariff (Part IXa)

Resp-Ease 6% inhalation solution 4ml ampoules (Venture Healthcare Ltd) **Sodium chloride 60 mg per 1 ml** 60 ampoule • NHS indicative price = £21.60 • Drug Tariff (Part IXa)

Resp-Ease 7% inhalation solution 4ml vials (Venture Healthcare Ltd) **Sodium chloride 70 mg per 1 ml** 60 vial • NHS indicative price = £21.60 • Drug Tariff (Part IXa)

Peak flow meters: low range

● LOW RANGE PEAK FLOW METERS

MEDI® LOW RANGE

Range 40–420 litres/minute.
Compliant to standard EN ISO 23747:2007 except for scale range.

Medi peak flow meter low range (Medicareplus International Ltd)
1 device • NHS indicative price = £6.50 • Drug Tariff (Part IXa) price = £4.50

MINI-WRIGHT® LOW RANGE

Range 30–400 litres/minute.
Compliant to standard EN ISO 23747:2007 except for scale range.

Mini-Wright peak flow meter low range (Clement Clarke International Ltd)
1 device • NHS indicative price = £7.55 • Drug Tariff (Part IXa) price = £4.50

POCKETPEAK® LOW RANGE

Range 50–400 litres/minute.
Compliant to standard EN ISO 23747:2007 except for scale range.

nSpire Pocket Peak peak flow meter low range (nSpire Health Ltd)
1 device • NHS indicative price = £6.53 • Drug Tariff (Part IXa) price = £4.50

Peak flow meters: standard range

● STANDARD RANGE PEAK FLOW METERS

AIRZONE®

Range 60–720 litres/minute.
Conforms to standard EN ISO 23747:2007.

AirZone peak flow meter standard range (Clement Clarke International Ltd)
1 device • NHS indicative price = £4.19 • Drug Tariff (Part IXa) price = £4.25

MEDI® STANDARD RANGE

Range 60–800 litres/minute.
Conforms to standard EN ISO 23747:2007.

Medi peak flow meter standard range (Medicareplus International Ltd)
1 device • NHS indicative price = £4.50 • Drug Tariff (Part IXa) price = £4.25

MICROPEAK®

Range 60–900 litres/minute.
Conforms to standard EN ISO 23747:2007.

MicroPeak peak flow meter standard range (Micro Medical Ltd)
1 device • NHS indicative price = £6.50 • Drug Tariff (Part IXa) price = £4.25

MINI-WRIGHT® STANDARD RANGE

Range 60–800 litres/minute.
Conforms to standard EN ISO 23747:2007.

Mini-Wright peak flow meter standard range (Clement Clarke International Ltd)
1 device • NHS indicative price = £7.50 • Drug Tariff (Part IXa) price = £4.25

PIKO-1®

Range 15–999 litres/minute.
Conforms to standard EN ISO 23747:2007.

nSpire PiKo-1 peak flow meter standard range (nSpire Health Ltd)
1 device • NHS indicative price = £9.50 • Drug Tariff (Part IXa) price = £4.25

PINNACLE®

Range 60–900 litres/minute.
Conforms to standard EN ISO 23747:2007.

Fyne Dynamics Pinnacle peak flow meter standard range (Fyne Dynamics Ltd)
1 device • NHS indicative price = £6.50 • Drug Tariff (Part IXa) price = £4.25

POCKETPEAK® STANDARD RANGE

Range 60–800 litres/minute.
Conforms to standard EN ISO 23747:2007.

nSpire Pocket Peak peak flow meter standard range (nSpire Health Ltd)
1 device • NHS indicative price = £6.53 • Drug Tariff (Part IXa) price = £4.25

VITALOGRAPH®

Range 50–800 litres/minute.
Conforms to standard EN ISO 23747:2007.

Vitalograph peak flow meter standard range (Vitalograph Ltd)
1 device • NHS indicative price = £4.83 • Drug Tariff (Part IXa) price = £4.25

Spacers

● SPACERS

A2A SPACER®

For use with all pressurised (aerosol) inhalers.

A2A Spacer (Clement Clarke International Ltd)
1 device • NHS indicative price = £4.15 • Drug Tariff (Part IXa)

A2A Spacer with medium mask (Clement Clarke International Ltd)
1 device • NHS indicative price = £6.68 • Drug Tariff (Part IXa)

A2A Spacer with small mask (Clement Clarke International Ltd)
1 device • NHS indicative price = £6.68 • Drug Tariff (Part IXa)

ABLE SPACER®

Small-volume device. For use with all pressurised (aerosol) inhalers.

Able Spacer 2 (Clement Clarke International Ltd)
1 device • NHS indicative price = £4.39 • Drug Tariff (Part IXa)

Able Spacer 2 with medium mask (Clement Clarke International Ltd)
1 device • NHS indicative price = £7.16 • Drug Tariff (Part IXa)

Able Spacer 2 with small mask (Clement Clarke International Ltd)
1 device • NHS indicative price = £7.16 • Drug Tariff (Part IXa)

AEROCHAMBER PLUS®

Medium-volume device. For use with all pressurised (aerosol) inhalers.

AeroChamber Plus (Trudell Medical UK Ltd)
1 device • NHS indicative price = £5.22 • Drug Tariff (Part IXa)

AeroChamber Plus with adult mask (Trudell Medical UK Ltd)
1 device • NHS indicative price = £8.72 • Drug Tariff (Part IXa)

AeroChamber Plus with child mask (Trudell Medical UK Ltd)
1 device • NHS indicative price = £8.72 • Drug Tariff (Part IXa)

AeroChamber Plus with infant mask (Trudell Medical UK Ltd)
1 device • NHS indicative price = £8.72 • Drug Tariff (Part IXa)

BABYHALER®

For paediatric use with *Flixotide*®, and *Ventolin*® inhalers.

● PRESCRIBING AND DISPENSING INFORMATION

Not available for NHS prescription.

Babyhaler (GlaxoSmithKline UK Ltd)
1 device • No NHS indicative price available • Drug Tariff (Part IXa)

EASYCHAMBER® SPACER

For use with all pressurised (aerosol) inhalers.

EasyChamber Spacer (TriOn Pharma Ltd)
1 device • NHS indicative price = £3.98 • Drug Tariff (Part IXa)

EasyChamber Spacer with adult mask 6 years - adult (TriOn Pharma Ltd)
1 device • NHS indicative price = £6.59 • Drug Tariff (Part IXa)

EasyChamber Spacer with child mask 2-6 years (TriOn Pharma Ltd)
1 device • NHS indicative price = £6.55 • Drug Tariff (Part IXa)

EasyChamber Spacer with infant mask 0-24 months (TriOn Pharma Ltd)
1 device • NHS indicative price = £6.53 • Drug Tariff (Part IXa)

OPTICHAMBER®

For use with all pressurised (aerosol) inhalers.

OptiChamber (Respironics (UK) Ltd)
1 device • NHS indicative price = £4.28 • Drug Tariff (Part IXa)

OPTICHAMBER® DIAMOND

For use with all pressurised (aerosol) inhalers.

OptiChamber Diamond (Respironics (UK) Ltd)
1 device • NHS indicative price = £4.49 • Drug Tariff (Part IXa)

OptiChamber Diamond with large LiteTouch mask 5 years-adult (Respironics (UK) Ltd)
1 device • NHS indicative price = £7.49 • Drug Tariff (Part IXa)

OptiChamber Diamond with medium LiteTouch mask 1-5 years (Respironics (UK) Ltd)
1 device • NHS indicative price = £7.49 • Drug Tariff (Part IXa)

OptiChamber Diamond with small LiteTouch mask 0-18 months (Respironics (UK) Ltd)
1 device • NHS indicative price = £7.49 • Drug Tariff (Part IXa)

POCKET CHAMBER®
Small volume device. For use with all pressurised (aerosol) inhalers.

Pocket Chamber (nSpire Health Ltd)
1 device • NHS indicative price = £4.18 • Drug Tariff (Part IXa)

Pocket Chamber with adult mask (nSpire Health Ltd)
1 device • NHS indicative price = £9.75 • Drug Tariff (Part IXa)

Pocket Chamber with child mask (nSpire Health Ltd)
1 device • NHS indicative price = £9.75 • Drug Tariff (Part IXa)

Pocket Chamber with infant mask (nSpire Health Ltd)
1 device • NHS indicative price = £9.75 • Drug Tariff (Part IXa)

Pocket Chamber with teenager mask (nSpire Health Ltd)
1 device • NHS indicative price = £9.75 • Drug Tariff (Part IXa)

SPACE CHAMBER PLUS®
For use with all pressurised (aerosol) inhalers.

Space Chamber Plus (Medical Developments International Ltd)
1 device • NHS indicative price = £4.34 • Drug Tariff (Part IXa)

Space Chamber Plus with large mask (Medical Developments International Ltd)
1 device • NHS indicative price = £7.10 • Drug Tariff (Part IXa)

Space Chamber Plus with medium mask (Medical Developments International Ltd)
1 device • NHS indicative price = £7.10 • Drug Tariff (Part IXa)

Space Chamber Plus with small mask (Medical Developments International Ltd)
1 device • NHS indicative price = £7.10 • Drug Tariff (Part IXa)

VOLUMATIC®
Large-volume device. For use with *Clenil Modulite®*, *Flixotide®*, *Seretide®*, *Serevent®*, and *Ventolin®* inhalers.

Volumatic (GlaxoSmithKline UK Ltd)
1 device • NHS indicative price = £3.88 • Drug Tariff (Part IXa)

Volumatic with paediatric mask (GlaxoSmithKline UK Ltd)
1 device • NHS indicative price = £6.83 • Drug Tariff (Part IXa)

VORTEX®
Medium-volume device. For use with all pressurised (aerosol) inhalers.

2 Allergic conditions

Antihistamines, allergen immunotherapy and allergic emergencies

18-Dec-2025

Antihistamines

Antihistamines (histamine H_1-receptor antagonists) are classified as *sedating* or *non-sedating*, according to their relative potential for CNS depression. Antihistamines differ in their duration of action, incidence of drowsiness, and antimuscarinic effects; the response to an antihistamine may vary from child to child. Either a sedating or a non-sedating antihistamine may be used to treat an acute allergic reaction; for conditions with more persistent symptoms which require regular treatment, a non-sedating anti-histamine should be used to minimise the risk of sedation and psychomotor impairment associated with sedating antihistamines.

Oral antihistamines are used in the treatment of nasal allergies, particularly seasonal allergic rhinitis (hay fever), and may be of some value in vasomotor rhinitis; rhinorrhoea and sneezing is reduced, but antihistamines are usually less effective for nasal congestion. Antihistamines are used topically to treat allergic reactions in the eye and in the nose. Topical application of antihistamines to the skin is not recommended.

An oral antihistamine may be used to prevent urticaria, and for the treatment of acute urticarial rashes, pruritus, insect bites, and stings.

Antihistamines are also used in the management of nausea and vomiting, and migraine. In addition, antihistamines may be given in anaphylaxis following initial stabilisation of the child, especially in children with persistent cutaneous symptoms—for further information, see *Anaphylaxis*.

The *non-sedating* antihistamine cetirizine hydrochloride p. 202 is safe and effective in children. Other non-sedating antihistamines that are used include acrivastine p. 201, bilastine p. 201, desloratadine p. 202 (an active metabolite of loratadine p. 204), fexofenadine hydrochloride p. 203 (an active metabolite of terfenadine), levocetirizine hydrochloride p. 203 (an isomer of cetirizine hydrochloride), loratadine, and mizolastine p. 204. Most non-sedating antihistamines are long-acting (usually 12–24 hours). There is little evidence that desloratadine or levocetirizine hydrochloride confer any additional benefit—they should be reserved for children who cannot tolerate other therapies.

Sedating antihistamines are occasionally useful when insomnia is associated with urticaria and pruritus. Most of the sedating antihistamines are relatively short-acting, but promethazine may be effective for up to 12 hours. Alimemazine tartrate p. 205 and **promethazine** have a more sedative effect than chlorphenamine maleate p. 205 and cyclizine p. 313.

Allergen immunotherapy

Immunotherapy using allergen vaccines containing house dust mite, animal dander (cat or dog), or grass pollen extracts p. 209 and tree pollen extracts p. 211 can improve symptoms of asthma and allergic rhinoconjunctivitis in children. Vaccines containing bee venom extracts p. 209 or wasp venom extracts p. 212 may be used to reduce the risk of severe anaphylaxis and systemic reactions in children with hypersensitivity to wasp and bee stings. An oral preparation of grass pollen extracts p. 209 is licensed for disease-modifying treatment of grass pollen-induced rhinitis and conjunctivitis, and an oral preparation of house-dust mite extracts p. 210 is licensed for disease-modifying treatment of house dust mite allergic rhinitis in certain children. EvGr Desensitisation treatment with peanut protein p. 210 may be offered to certain children with peanut allergy, and treatment can be continued into adulthood. Ⓐ Children requiring immunotherapy must be referred to a hospital specialist for accurate diagnosis, assessment, and treatment.

Omalizumab p. 193 is a monoclonal antibody that binds to immunoglobulin E (IgE). It is licensed for use as additional therapy in children over 6 years with proven IgE-mediated sensitivity to inhaled allergens, whose severe persistent allergic asthma cannot be controlled adequately with high-dose inhaled corticosteroid together with a long-acting beta$_2$ agonist. Omalizumab should be initiated by physicians experienced in the treatment of severe persistent asthma. Omalizumab is also indicated as add-on therapy for the treatment of chronic spontaneous urticaria in patients who have had an inadequate response to H_1 antihistamine treatment.

Anaphylaxis and allergic emergencies

Anaphylaxis

Anaphylaxis is a severe, life-threatening, generalised or systemic hypersensitivity reaction. It is characterised by rapidly developing airway and/or breathing and/or circulation problems, and is usually associated with skin and mucosal changes; prompt treatment is required.

The most common allergens that cause anaphylaxis

include food (e.g. peanuts, sesame, soy, tree nuts, shellfish, and cow's milk—see Food allergy p. 57), drugs (e.g. antibacterials, aspirin and other NSAIDs, neuromuscular blocking drugs, chlorhexidine, contrast media, and vaccines), venom (e.g. insect stings), and latex. In the case of drugs, anaphylaxis is more likely after parenteral administration; resuscitation facilities must always be available for injections associated with special risk. Refined arachis (peanut) oil, which may be present in some medicinal products, is unlikely to cause an allergic reaction—nevertheless it is wise to check the full formula of preparations which may contain allergens.

Certain children may be at higher risk of anaphylaxis, either because of an existing comorbidity (such as asthma) or because of an increased likelihood of repeated exposure to the same allergen (such as those with venom or food allergies).

Recommendations on the management of anaphylaxis reflect the *Resuscitation Council (UK)—Emergency treatment of anaphylaxis: Guidelines for healthcare providers (May* 2021*)* and *NICE—Anaphylaxis: assessment and referral after emergency treatment guidelines (CG*134*, updated August* 2020*)*.

Initial treatment of anaphylaxis

Cardiopulmonary arrest may follow an anaphylactic reaction—start cardiopulmonary resuscitation (CPR) immediately. For guidance on CPR, see Life support algorithm (image) Inside back pages.

EvGr Immediately call for an ambulance or the resuscitation team and begin initial treatment for anaphylaxis.

Remove the trigger causing the anaphylactic reaction (e.g. stopping the suspected drug or removing the stinger after an insect sting). Place the child in a comfortable position taking into account their presenting signs and symptoms—lay the child flat (with or without legs raised) to aid in the restoration of blood pressure, or in a semi-recumbent position for children with airway and breathing problems (and no evidence of cardiovascular instability) to make breathing easier, or in the recovery position for unconscious children who are breathing normally; pregnant females should lie on their left side to prevent aortocaval compression.

Intramuscular adrenaline p. 159 should be given as first line treatment for anaphylaxis. If there is doubt about the diagnosis, give intramuscular adrenaline and seek expert advice. Adrenaline provides physiological reversal of the immediate symptoms associated with hypersensitivity reactions. Assess response to treatment by monitoring vital signs (such as blood pressure, pulse, respiratory function, and level of consciousness) and auscultate for wheeze.

A repeat dose of intramuscular adrenaline should be given after a 5-minute interval if there is no improvement in the child's condition. Children who have no improvement in respiratory and/or cardiovascular problems despite 2 appropriate doses of intramuscular adrenaline, should have their care escalated quickly and managed as having refractory anaphylaxis. Ⓐ For further information, see *Refractory anaphylaxis*.

EvGr Nebulised adrenaline may be effective as an adjunct to treat upper airways obstruction caused by laryngeal oedema, but only after treatment with intramuscular adrenaline and not as an alternative.

High-flow oxygen should be given as soon as it is available.

Intravenous fluids should be given to children with hypotension/shock, or if there is poor response to an initial dose of adrenaline.

Antihistamines are not recommended as part of the initial emergency treatment of anaphylaxis. Following stabilisation of the child, a non-sedating oral antihistamine such as cetirizine hydrochloride p. 202 (in preference to chlorphenamine maleate) may be considered, especially in children with persistent cutaneous symptoms (urticaria and/or angioedema). If oral administration is not possible, intramuscular or intravenous chlorphenamine maleate p. 205 can be given.

The routine use of corticosteroids for the emergency treatment of anaphylaxis is not recommended. Consider corticosteroids after initial resuscitation for refractory reactions or ongoing asthma/shock; corticosteroids must not be given preferentially to adrenaline p. 159. Corticosteroids should be given via the oral route where possible.

Inhaled bronchodilator therapy with salbutamol p. 181 and/or ipratropium bromide p. 177 may also be considered for children with persisting respiratory problems, but should not be used as an alternative to further treatment with adrenaline. Ⓐ For guidance on the management of bronchospasm in severe asthma, see Asthma, acute p. 174.

For further guidance on the initial management of anaphylaxis, see Resuscitation Council (UK) guideline: **Emergency treatment of anaphylaxis** (available at: www.resus.org.uk/library/additional-guidance/guidance-anaphylaxis/emergency-treatment).

Refractory anaphylaxis

Refractory anaphylaxis is defined as anaphylaxis that requires ongoing treatment due to persisting respiratory and/or cardiovascular problems despite 2 appropriate doses of intramuscular adrenaline— EvGr seek early critical care support.

Children should be treated with an intravenous adrenaline infusion. Intravenous adrenaline should only be given by experienced specialists and in a setting where children can be carefully monitored. If an intravenous infusion cannot be administered safely (e.g. due to a child being outside a hospital setting), continue to give intramuscular adrenaline at 5-minute intervals while life-threatening cardiovascular and/or respiratory features persist. Adrenaline therapy should be supported with intravenous fluid therapy. Ⓐ For further guidance on intravenous adrenaline and other treatment options in refractory anaphylaxis (such as nebulised adrenaline, bronchodilators, vasopressors, corticosteroids, and glucagon (for children on beta-blockers)), see Resuscitation Council (UK) guideline: **Emergency treatment of anaphylaxis** (available at: www.resus.org.uk/library/additional-guidance/guidance-anaphylaxis/emergency-treatment).

Discharge and follow-up

EvGr Prior to discharge from hospital, children (or their family or carers) should be provided with 2 adrenaline auto-injectors, trained on their correct use, and advised to carry these with them at all times. The provision of adrenaline auto-injectors are appropriate for all children who have had anaphylaxis, with the exception of those with a drug-induced reaction (unless future exposure to the trigger drug will be difficult to avoid). Children who are provided with auto-injectors should have appropriate follow-up including contact with their general practitioner.

Children and their family or carers should also be provided with information about anaphylaxis, the risk of a biphasic reaction (with clear instructions to return to hospital if symptoms return), avoidance of suspected triggers, and what to do if an anaphylactic reaction occurs. An emergency management or action plan should be provided, and referral to a specialist allergy clinic made. Ⓐ

Angioedema

Allergic angioedema

Angioedema can be caused by an allergic reaction. It involves the swelling of deeper tissues, most commonly in the eyelids and lips, and sometimes the tongue and throat. Allergic angioedema that occurs with life-threatening airway and/or breathing and/or circulatory problems should be managed as **anaphylaxis**. For further guidance, see *Anaphylaxis*.

Hereditary angioedema
The treatment of hereditary angioedema should be under specialist supervision. Unlike allergic angioedema, adrenaline, corticosteroids, and antihistamines should not be used for the treatment of acute attacks (including attacks involving laryngeal oedema) as they are ineffective and may delay appropriate treatment—intubation may be necessary. The administration of C1-esterase inhibitor p. 212 (in fresh frozen plasma or in partially purified form) can terminate acute attacks of *hereditary angioedema*; it can also be used for short-term prophylaxis before dental, medical, or surgical procedures. Tranexamic acid p. 92 is used for short-term or long-term prophylaxis of hereditary angioedema; short-term prophylaxis is started several days before planned procedures which may trigger an acute attack of hereditary angioedema (e.g. dental work) and continued for 2–5 days afterwards. Danazol [unlicensed indication] is best avoided in children because of its androgenic effects, but it can be used for short-term prophylaxis of hereditary angioedema.

Berotralstat p. 214, garadacimab p. 215, or lanadelumab p. 214 may be an option for the prevention of recurrent attacks of hereditary angioedema.

Dose of intramuscular injection of adrenaline for the emergency treatment of anaphylaxis by healthcare professionals

Age	Dose	Volume of adrenaline
Child up to 6 months	100-150 micrograms	0.1-0.15 mL 1 in 1000 (1 mg/mL) adrenaline[1]
Child 6 months-5 years	150 micrograms	0.15 mL 1 in 1000 (1 mg/mL) adrenaline[2]
Child 6-11 years	300 micrograms	0.3 mL 1 in 1000 (1 mg/mL) adrenaline
Child 12-17 years	500 micrograms	0.5 mL 1 in 1000 (1 mg/mL) adrenaline[3]

Repeat dose after 5 minutes if no response. If life-threatening features persist, further doses can be given every 5 minutes until specialist critical care available.

1. Use suitable syringe for measuring small volume
2. Use suitable syringe for measuring small volume
3. 300 micrograms (0.3 mL) if child is small or prepubertal

ANTIHISTAMINES › NON-SEDATING

Acrivastine

23-Apr-2021

- **INDICATIONS AND DOSE**

Symptomatic relief of allergy such as hayfever, chronic idiopathic urticaria
▸ BY MOUTH
▸ Child 12-17 years: 8 mg 3 times a day

- **CONTRA-INDICATIONS** Avoid in Acute porphyrias p. 745
- **INTERACTIONS** → Appendix 1: antihistamines, non-sedating
- **SIDE-EFFECTS**
▸ **Common or very common** Drowsiness · dry mouth
▸ **Frequency not known** Dizziness · rash
SIDE-EFFECTS, FURTHER INFORMATION Non-sedating antihistamines such as acrivastine cause less sedation and psychomotor impairment than the older antihistamines, but can still occur; sedation is generally minimal. This is because non-sedating antihistamines penetrate the blood brain barrier to a much lesser extent.
- **ALLERGY AND CROSS-SENSITIVITY** EvGr Contra-indicated if history of hypersensitivity to triprolidine. (M)
- **PREGNANCY** Most manufacturers of antihistamines advise avoiding their use during pregnancy; however, there is no evidence of teratogenicity.
- **BREAST FEEDING** Most antihistamines are present in breast milk in varying amounts; although not known to be harmful, most manufacturers advise avoiding their use in mothers who are breast-feeding.
- **RENAL IMPAIRMENT** EvGr Avoid in severe impairment. (M)
- **PATIENT AND CARER ADVICE**
Driving and skilled tasks Patients and their carers should be advised that drowsiness can occur and may affect performance of skilled tasks (e.g. cycling or driving).

- **MEDICINAL FORMS** There can be variation in the licensing of different medicines containing the same drug.

Oral capsule
▸ Acrivastine (Non-proprietary)
Acrivastine 8 mg Acrivastine 8mg capsules | 24 capsule P £4.45-£8.74
▸ Benadryl Allergy Relief (McNeil Products Ltd)
Acrivastine 8 mg Benadryl Allergy Relief 8mg capsules | 48 capsule P £10.75

Bilastine

14-Dec-2020

- **INDICATIONS AND DOSE**

Symptomatic relief of allergic rhinoconjunctivitis and urticaria
▸ BY MOUTH
▸ Child 12-17 years: 20 mg once daily

- **CONTRA-INDICATIONS** Avoid in Acute porphyrias p. 745
- **INTERACTIONS** → Appendix 1: antihistamines, non-sedating
- **SIDE-EFFECTS**
▸ **Common or very common** Drowsiness · headache
▸ **Uncommon** Anxiety · appetite increased · asthenia · bundle branch block · diarrhoea · dry mouth · dyspnoea · fever · gastritis · gastrointestinal discomfort · insomnia · nasal complaints · nausea · oral herpes · pre-existing condition improved · pruritus · QT interval prolongation · sinus arrhythmia · thirst · tinnitus · vertigo · weight increased
SIDE-EFFECTS, FURTHER INFORMATION Non-sedating antihistamines such as bilastine cause less sedation and psychomotor impairment than the older antihistamines, but can still occur; sedation is generally minimal. This is because non-sedating antihistamines penetrate the blood brain barrier to a much lesser extent.
- **PREGNANCY** Avoid—limited information available. Most manufacturers of antihistamines advise avoiding their use during pregnancy; however, there is no evidence of teratogenicity.
- **BREAST FEEDING** Avoid—no information available. Most antihistamines are present in breast milk in varying amounts; although not known to be harmful, most manufacturers advise avoiding their use in mothers who are breast-feeding.
- **DIRECTIONS FOR ADMINISTRATION** Manufacturer advises tablet should be taken 1 hour before or 2 hours after food or fruit juice.
- **PATIENT AND CARER ADVICE** Patients or carers should be given advice on how to administer bilastine tablets.
Driving and skilled tasks Patients and their carers should be advised that drowsiness can occur and may affect performance of skilled tasks (e.g. cycling or driving).

● **MEDICINAL FORMS** There can be variation in the licensing of different medicines containing the same drug.

Oral tablet

CAUTIONARY AND ADVISORY LABELS 23

▸ Bilastine (Non-proprietary)

Bilastine 20 mg Bilastine 20mg tablets | 30 tablet PoM DT = £6.00

▸ Ilaxten (A. Menarini Farmaceutica Internazionale SRL)

Bilastine 20 mg Ilaxten 20mg tablets | 30 tablet PoM £6.00 DT = £6.00

Cetirizine hydrochloride

10-Nov-2021

● **INDICATIONS AND DOSE**

Symptomatic relief of allergy such as hay fever, chronic idiopathic urticaria, atopic dermatitis

▸ BY MOUTH

▸ Child 1 year: 250 micrograms/kg twice daily
▸ Child 2–5 years: 2.5 mg twice daily
▸ Child 6–11 years: 5 mg twice daily
▸ Child 12–17 years: 10 mg once daily

● **UNLICENSED USE** Not licensed for use in children under 2 years.

● **CAUTIONS** Epilepsy

● **INTERACTIONS** → Appendix 1: antihistamines, non-sedating

● **SIDE-EFFECTS**

▸ **Uncommon** Agitation · asthenia · diarrhoea · malaise · paraesthesia · skin reactions

▸ **Rare or very rare** Aggression · angioedema · confusion · cough · depression · eye disorders · eye swelling · feeling abnormal · hallucination · hepatic disorders · movement disorders · nausea · oedema · seizure · sleep disorders · syncope · tachycardia · taste altered · thrombocytopenia · tic · tremor · urinary disorders · vision disorders · weight increased

▸ **Frequency not known** Acute generalised exanthematous pustulosis (AGEP) · appetite increased · arthralgia · drowsiness · dry mouth · erectile dysfunction · eye pain · memory impairment · myalgia · suicidal ideation · vertigo

SIDE-EFFECTS, FURTHER INFORMATION **Pruritus** New-onset pruritus has been reported after stopping long-term treatment with cetirizine.

Sedation and psychomotor impairment Non-sedating antihistamines such as cetirizine hydrochloride cause less sedation and psychomotor impairment than the older antihistamines, but can still occur; sedation is generally minimal. This is because non-sedating antihistamines penetrate the blood brain barrier to a much lesser extent.

● **PREGNANCY** Most manufacturers of antihistamines advise avoiding their use during pregnancy; however, there is no evidence of teratogenicity.

● **BREAST FEEDING** Most antihistamines are present in breast milk in varying amounts; although not known to be harmful, most manufacturers advise avoiding their use in mothers who are breast-feeding.

● **RENAL IMPAIRMENT** Avoid if estimated glomerular filtration rate less than 10 mL/minute/1.73 m^2.

Dose adjustments Use half normal dose if estimated glomerular filtration rate 30–50 mL/minute/1.73 m^2.

Use half normal dose and reduce dose frequency to alternate days if estimated glomerular filtration rate 10–30 mL/minute/1.73 m^2.

● **PATIENT AND CARER ADVICE**

Medicines for Children leaflet: Cetirizine for hayfever
www.medicinesforchildren.org.uk/medicines/cetirizine-for-hayfever/

Driving and skilled tasks Patients and their carers should be advised that drowsiness can occur and may affect performance of skilled tasks (e.g. cycling or driving).

● **PROFESSION SPECIFIC INFORMATION**

Dental practitioners' formulary Cetirizine Tablets 10 mg may be prescribed.

Cetirizine Oral Solution 5 mg/5 mL may be prescribed.

● **MEDICINAL FORMS** There can be variation in the licensing of different medicines containing the same drug.

Oral tablet

▸ Cetirizine hydrochloride (Non-proprietary)

Cetirizine hydrochloride 10 mg Cetirizine 10mg tablets | 30 tablet PoM £0.66 DT = £0.70

Oral solution

EXCIPIENTS: May contain Propylene glycol

▸ Cetirizine hydrochloride (Non-proprietary)

Cetirizine hydrochloride 1 mg per 1 ml Cetirizine 1mg/ml oral solution sugar free | 200 ml PoM £17.50 DT = £7.52 SF

Desloratadine

23-Apr-2021

● **INDICATIONS AND DOSE**

Symptomatic relief of allergy such as allergic rhinitis, urticaria, chronic idiopathic urticaria

▸ BY MOUTH

▸ Child 1–5 years: 1.25 mg once daily
▸ Child 6–11 years: 2.5 mg once daily
▸ Child 12–17 years: 5 mg once daily

PHARMACOKINETICS

▸ Desloratadine is a metabolite of loratadine.

● **INTERACTIONS** → Appendix 1: antihistamines, non-sedating

● **SIDE-EFFECTS**

▸ **Common or very common** Asthenia · dry mouth · headache

▸ **Rare or very rare** Akathisia · arrhythmias · diarrhoea · dizziness · drowsiness · gastrointestinal discomfort · hallucination · hepatic disorders · insomnia · myalgia · nausea · palpitations · seizure · vomiting

▸ **Frequency not known** Behaviour abnormal · photosensitivity reaction · QT interval prolongation

SIDE-EFFECTS, FURTHER INFORMATION Non-sedating antihistamines such as desloratadine cause less sedation and psychomotor impairment than the older antihistamines, but can still occur; sedation is generally minimal. This is because non-sedating antihistamines penetrate the blood brain barrier to a much lesser extent.

● **ALLERGY AND CROSS-SENSITIVITY** EvGr Contra-indicated if history of hypersensitivity to loratadine. (M)

● **PREGNANCY** Most manufacturers of antihistamines advise avoiding their use during pregnancy; however, there is no evidence of teratogenicity.

● **BREAST FEEDING** Most antihistamines are present in breast milk in varying amounts; although not known to be harmful, most manufacturers advise avoiding their use in mothers who are breast-feeding.

● **RENAL IMPAIRMENT** EvGr Use with caution in severe impairment. (M)

● **PRESCRIBING AND DISPENSING INFORMATION** Flavours of oral liquid formulations may include bubblegum.

● **PATIENT AND CARER ADVICE**

Driving and skilled tasks Patients and their carers should be advised that drowsiness can occur and may affect performance of skilled tasks (e.g. cycling or driving).

● **MEDICINAL FORMS** There can be variation in the licensing of different medicines containing the same drug.

Oral tablet

▸ Desloratadine (Non-proprietary)

Desloratadine 5 mg Desloratadine 5mg tablets | 30 tablet [PoM] £6.60 DT = £1.73

▸ Neoclarityn (Organon Pharma (UK) Ltd)

Desloratadine 5 mg Neoclarityn 5mg tablets | 30 tablet [PoM] £6.77 DT = £1.73

Oral solution

EXCIPIENTS: May contain Propylene glycol, sorbitol

▸ Desloratadine (Non-proprietary)

Desloratadine 500 microgram per 1 ml Desloratadine 2.5mg/5ml oral solution sugar free | 150 ml [PoM] £8.12 DT = £10.15 [SF]

▸ Neoclarityn (Organon Pharma (UK) Ltd)

Desloratadine 500 microgram per 1 ml Neoclarityn 2.5mg/5ml oral solution | 100 ml [PoM] £6.77 DT = £6.77 [SF] | 150 ml [PoM] £10.15 DT = £10.15 [SF]

Fexofenadine hydrochloride

14-Dec-2020

● **INDICATIONS AND DOSE**

Symptomatic relief of seasonal allergic rhinitis

▶ BY MOUTH

▸ Child 6–11 years: 30 mg twice daily

▸ Child 12–17 years: 120 mg once daily

Symptomatic relief of chronic idiopathic urticaria

▶ BY MOUTH

▸ Child 12–17 years: 180 mg once daily

PHARMACOKINETICS

▸ Fexofenadine is a metabolite of terfenadine.

● **INTERACTIONS** → Appendix 1: antihistamines, non-sedating

● **SIDE-EFFECTS**

▶ **Common or very common** Dizziness · drowsiness · headache · nausea

▶ **Uncommon** Fatigue

▶ **Frequency not known** Diarrhoea · nervousness · palpitations · skin reactions · sleep disorders · tachycardia

SIDE-EFFECTS, FURTHER INFORMATION Non-sedating antihistamines such as fexofenadine cause less sedation and psychomotor impairment than the older antihistamines, but can still occur; sedation is generally minimal. This is because non-sedating antihistamines penetrate the blood brain barrier to a much lesser extent.

● **PREGNANCY** Most manufacturers of antihistamines advise avoiding their use during pregnancy; however, there is no evidence of teratogenicity.

● **BREAST FEEDING** Most antihistamines are present in breast milk in varying amounts; although not known to be harmful, most manufacturers advise avoiding their use in mothers who are breast-feeding.

● **PATIENT AND CARER ADVICE**

Driving and skilled tasks Patients and their carers should be advised that drowsiness can occur and may affect performance of skilled tasks (e.g. cycling or driving).

● **MEDICINAL FORMS** There can be variation in the licensing of different medicines containing the same drug. Forms available from special-order manufacturers include: oral suspension, oral solution

Oral tablet

CAUTIONARY AND ADVISORY LABELS 5

▸ Fexofenadine hydrochloride (Non-proprietary)

Fexofenadine hydrochloride 120 mg Fexofenadine 120mg tablets | 30 tablet [PoM] £7.15 DT = £1.07

Fexofenadine hydrochloride 180 mg Fexofenadine 180mg tablets | 30 tablet [PoM] £9.65 DT = £3.30

▸ Telfast (Opella POM UK Ltd)

Fexofenadine hydrochloride 30 mg Telfast 30mg tablets | 60 tablet [PoM] £5.46 DT = £5.46

Fexofenadine hydrochloride 180 mg Telfast 180mg tablets | 30 tablet [PoM] £7.58 DT = £3.30

Levocetirizine hydrochloride

14-Dec-2020

● **INDICATIONS AND DOSE**

Symptomatic relief of allergy such as hay fever, urticaria

▶ BY MOUTH

▸ Child 2–5 years: 1.25 mg twice daily

▸ Child 6–17 years: 5 mg once daily

PHARMACOKINETICS

▸ Levocetirizine is an isomer of cetirizine.

● **CONTRA-INDICATIONS** Avoid in Acute porphyrias p. 745

● **INTERACTIONS** → Appendix 1: antihistamines, non-sedating

● **SIDE-EFFECTS**

▶ **Uncommon** Abdominal pain · asthenia

▶ **Frequency not known** Aggression · agitation · angioedema · appetite increased · arthralgia · constipation · depression · diarrhoea · dizziness · drowsiness · dyspnoea · hallucination · hepatitis · myalgia · nausea · oculogyration · oedema · palpitations · paraesthesia · seizure · skin reactions · sleep disorders · suicidal ideation · syncope · tachycardia · taste altered · tremor · urinary disorders · vertigo · vision disorders · vomiting · weight increased

SIDE-EFFECTS, FURTHER INFORMATION **Pruritus** New-onset pruritus has been reported after stopping long-term treatment with levocetirizine.

Sedation and psychomotor impairment Non-sedating antihistamines such as levocetirizine cause less sedation and psychomotor impairment than the older antihistamines, but can still occur; sedation is generally minimal. This is because non-sedating antihistamines penetrate the blood brain barrier to a much lesser extent.

● **PREGNANCY** Most manufacturers of antihistamines advise avoiding their use during pregnancy; however, there is no evidence of teratogenicity.

● **BREAST FEEDING** Most antihistamines are present in breast milk in varying amounts; although not known to be harmful, most manufacturers advise avoiding their use in mothers who are breast-feeding.

● **RENAL IMPAIRMENT** Avoid if estimated glomerular filtration rate less than 10 mL/minute/1.73 m^2.

Dose adjustments Reduce dose frequency to alternate days if estimated glomerular filtration rate 30–50 mL/minute/1.73 m^2.

Reduce dose frequency to every 3 days if estimated glomerular filtration rate 10–30 mL/minute/1.73 m^2.

● **PATIENT AND CARER ADVICE**

Driving and skilled tasks Patients and their carers should be advised that drowsiness can occur and may affect performance of skilled tasks (e.g. cycling or driving).

● **MEDICINAL FORMS** There can be variation in the licensing of different medicines containing the same drug.

Oral tablet

▸ Levocetirizine hydrochloride (Non-proprietary)

Levocetirizine dihydrochloride 5 mg Levocetirizine 5mg tablets | 30 tablet [PoM] £5.10 DT = £4.85

▸ Xyzal (UCB Pharma Ltd)

Levocetirizine dihydrochloride 5 mg Xyzal 5mg tablets | 30 tablet [PoM] £4.39 DT = £4.85

Oral solution

▸ Xyzal (UCB Pharma Ltd)

Levocetirizine dihydrochloride 500 microgram per 1 ml Xyzal 0.5mg/ml oral solution | 200 ml [PoM] £6.00 DT = £6.00 [SF]

Loratadine

10-Nov-2021

- **INDICATIONS AND DOSE**

Symptomatic relief of allergy such as hay fever, chronic idiopathic urticaria

▶ BY MOUTH

▶ Child 2–11 years (body-weight up to 31 kg): 5 mg once daily

▶ Child 2–11 years (body-weight 31 kg and above): 10 mg once daily

▶ Child 12–17 years: 10 mg once daily

- **INTERACTIONS** → Appendix 1: antihistamines, non-sedating
- **SIDE-EFFECTS**

▶ **Common or very common** Drowsiness · fatigue · headache · nervousness

▶ **Uncommon** Appetite increased · insomnia

▶ **Rare or very rare** Alopecia · angioedema · dizziness · dry mouth · gastritis · hepatic function abnormal · nausea · palpitations · rash · seizure · tachycardia

SIDE-EFFECTS, FURTHER INFORMATION Non-sedating antihistamines such as loratadine cause less sedation and psychomotor impairment than the older antihistamines, but can still occur; sedation is generally minimal. This is because non-sedating antihistamines penetrate the blood brain barrier to a much lesser extent.

- **PREGNANCY** Most manufacturers of antihistamines advise avoiding their use during pregnancy; however, there is no evidence of teratogenicity.
- **BREAST FEEDING** Most antihistamines are present in breast milk in varying amounts; although not known to be harmful, most manufacturers advise avoiding their use in mothers who are breast-feeding.
- **HEPATIC IMPAIRMENT** Manufacturer advises caution in severe impairment (risk of increased exposure).

Dose adjustments Manufacturer advises initial dose reduction to alternate days in severe impairment.

- **PATIENT AND CARER ADVICE**

Medicines for Children leaflet: Loratadine for allergy symptoms www.medicinesforchildren.org.uk/medicines/loratadine-for-allergy-symptoms/

Driving and skilled tasks Patients and their carers should be advised that drowsiness can occur and may affect performance of skilled tasks (e.g. cycling or driving).

- **PROFESSION SPECIFIC INFORMATION**

Dental practitioners' formulary Loratadine 10 mg tablets may be prescribed.

Loratadine syrup 5 mg/5 mL may be prescribed.

- **MEDICINAL FORMS** There can be variation in the licensing of different medicines containing the same drug.

Oral tablet

▶ Loratadine (Non-proprietary)

Loratadine 10 mg Loratadine 10mg tablets | 30 tablet [PoM] [S] DT = £0.67

Oral solution

EXCIPIENTS: May contain Propylene glycol

▶ Loratadine (Non-proprietary)

Loratadine 1 mg per 1 ml Loratadine 5mg/5ml oral solution | 100 ml [PoM] £1.91 DT = £1.91

Loratadine 5mg/5ml oral solution sugar free | 100 ml [P] £3.78 DT = £3.78 [SF]

Mizolastine

14-Dec-2020

- **INDICATIONS AND DOSE**

Symptomatic relief of allergy such as hay fever, urticaria

▶ BY MOUTH

▶ Child 12–17 years: 10 mg once daily

- **CONTRA-INDICATIONS** Cardiac disease · susceptibility to QT-interval prolongation
- **INTERACTIONS** → Appendix 1: antihistamines, non-sedating
- **SIDE-EFFECTS**

▶ **Common or very common** Appetite increased · asthenia · diarrhoea · dizziness · drowsiness · dry mouth · gastrointestinal discomfort · headache · nausea · weight increased

▶ **Uncommon** Anxiety · arrhythmias · arthralgia · depression · myalgia · palpitations

▶ **Rare or very rare** Hypersensitivity

▶ **Frequency not known** Asthma exacerbated · bronchospasm · QT interval prolongation

SIDE-EFFECTS, FURTHER INFORMATION Non-sedating antihistamines such as mizolastine cause less sedation and psychomotor impairment than the older antihistamines, but can still occur; sedation is generally minimal. This is because non-sedating antihistamines penetrate the blood brain barrier to a much lesser extent.

- **PREGNANCY** Most manufacturers of antihistamines advise avoiding their use during pregnancy; however, there is no evidence of teratogenicity.
- **BREAST FEEDING** Most antihistamines are present in breast milk in varying amounts; although not known to be harmful, most manufacturers advise avoiding their use in mothers who are breast-feeding.
- **HEPATIC IMPAIRMENT** Manufacturer advises avoid in significant impairment.
- **PATIENT AND CARER ADVICE**

Driving and skilled tasks Patients and their carers should be advised that drowsiness can occur and may affect performance of skilled tasks (e.g. cycling or driving).

- **MEDICINAL FORMS** No licensed medicines listed.

Rupatadine

29-Apr-2019

- **DRUG ACTION** Rupatadine is a second generation non-sedating antihistamine.
- **INDICATIONS AND DOSE**

Symptomatic relief of allergic rhinitis and urticaria

▶ BY MOUTH USING TABLETS

▶ Child 12–17 years: 10 mg once daily

▶ BY MOUTH USING ORAL SOLUTION

▶ Child 2–11 years (body-weight 10–24 kg): 2.5 mg once daily

▶ Child 2–11 years (body-weight 25 kg and above): 5 mg once daily

- **CAUTIONS** History of QT-interval prolongation · predisposition to arrhythmia · uncorrected hypokalaemia
- **INTERACTIONS** → Appendix 1: antihistamines, non-sedating
- **SIDE-EFFECTS**

▶ **Common or very common** Asthenia · dizziness · drowsiness · dry mouth · headache

▶ **Uncommon** Appetite increased · arthralgia · back pain · concentration impaired · constipation · cough · diarrhoea · dry throat · eosinophilia · epistaxis · fever · gastrointestinal discomfort · increased risk of infection · irritability · malaise · myalgia · nasal dryness · nausea · neutropenia · night sweats · oropharyngeal pain · skin reactions · thirst · vomiting · weight increased

▶ **Rare or very rare** Palpitations · tachycardia

SIDE-EFFECTS, FURTHER INFORMATION Non-sedating antihistamines such as rupatadine cause less sedation and psychomotor impairment than the older antihistamines, but can still occur; sedation is generally minimal. This is because non-sedating antihistamines penetrate the blood brain barrier to a much lesser extent.

- **PREGNANCY** Most manufacturers of antihistamines advise avoiding their use during pregnancy; however, there is no evidence of teratogenicity.
- **BREAST FEEDING** Most antihistamines are present in breast milk in varying amounts; although not known to be harmful, most manufacturers advise avoiding their use in mothers who are breast-feeding.
- **HEPATIC IMPAIRMENT** Manufacturer advises avoid (no information available).
- **RENAL IMPAIRMENT** Manufacturer advises avoid—no information available.

- **MEDICINAL FORMS** There can be variation in the licensing of different medicines containing the same drug.

Oral tablet

- ▸ Rupatadine (Non-proprietary)
  Rupatadine (as Rupatadine fumarate) 10 mg Rupatadine 10mg tablets | 30 tablet [PoM] £75.82 DT = £75.82

Oral solution

- ▸ Rupatadine (Non-proprietary)
  Rupatadine (as Rupatadine fumarate) 1 mg per 1 ml Rupatadine 1mg/ml oral solution | 120 ml [PoM] £9.95–£15.92 DT = £9.95

ANTIHISTAMINES › SEDATING

Alimemazine tartrate

27-Jun-2023

(Trimeprazine tartrate)

- **INDICATIONS AND DOSE**

Urticaria | Pruritus

▶ BY MOUTH

- ▸ Child 6 months–1 year (specialist use only): 250 micrograms/kg 3–4 times a day (max. per dose 2.5 mg)
- ▸ Child 2–4 years: 2.5 mg 3–4 times a day
- ▸ Child 5–11 years: 5 mg 3–4 times a day
- ▸ Child 12–17 years: 10 mg 2–3 times a day, in severe cases doses up to 100 mg per day have been used

Premedication to anaesthesia

▶ BY MOUTH

- ▸ Child 2–6 years: Up to 2 mg/kg for 1 dose, to be given 1–2 hours before operation

- **UNLICENSED USE** Expert sources advise alimemazine tartrate is used in children from the age of 6 months to 2 years for the treatment of urticaria and pruritus, but it is not licensed for this age group.
- **CONTRA-INDICATIONS** Children under 2 years except on specialist advice (risk of respiratory depression) · epilepsy · hepatic dysfunction · history of narrow angle glaucoma · hypothyroidism · myasthenia gravis · neonate (due to significant antimuscarinic activity) · Parkinson's disease · phaeochromocytoma · renal dysfunction
- **CAUTIONS** Cardiovascular diseases (due to tachycardia-inducing and hypotensive effects of phenothiazines) · exposure to sunlight should be avoided during treatment with high doses · pyloroduodenal obstruction · susceptibility to QT interval prolongation · urinary retention · volume depleted patients who are more susceptible to orthostatic hypotension
- **INTERACTIONS** → Appendix 1: antihistamines, sedating
- **SIDE-EFFECTS** Accommodation disorder · agitation · arrhythmias · atrioventricular block · bile thrombus · constipation · drowsiness · dry mouth · eosinophilia · hepatic disorders · hyperprolactinaemia · insomnia · leucopenia (on prolonged high dose) · movement disorders · nasal congestion · parkinsonism · QT interval prolongation · seizure · tardive dyskinesia (more common after long term high doses) · urinary retention · ventricular fibrillation (increased risk with hypokalaemia and cardiac disease) · ventricular tachycardia (increased risk with hypokalaemia and cardiac disease)

SIDE-EFFECTS, FURTHER INFORMATION Drowsiness may diminish after a few days.

Children are more susceptible to side-effects.

- **PREGNANCY** Most manufacturers of antihistamines advise avoiding their use during pregnancy; however, there is no evidence of teratogenicity. Use in the latter part of the third trimester may cause adverse effects in neonates such as irritability, paradoxical excitability, and tremor.
- **BREAST FEEDING** Most antihistamines are present in breast milk in varying amounts; although not known to be harmful, most manufacturers advise avoiding their use in mothers who are breast-feeding.
- **HEPATIC IMPAIRMENT** Manufacturer advises avoid—no information available.
- **RENAL IMPAIRMENT** [EvGr] Avoid. ⟨M⟩
- **PATIENT AND CARER ADVICE**

Driving and skilled tasks Drowsiness may affect performance of skilled tasks (e.g. cycling or driving); sedating effects enhanced by alcohol.

- **MEDICINAL FORMS** There can be variation in the licensing of different medicines containing the same drug. Forms available from special-order manufacturers include: oral solution

Oral tablet

CAUTIONARY AND ADVISORY LABELS 2

- ▸ Alimemazine tartrate (Non-proprietary)
  Alimemazine tartrate 10 mg Alimemazine 10mg tablets | 28 tablet [PoM] £106.10 DT = £37.48

Oral solution

CAUTIONARY AND ADVISORY LABELS 2

- ▸ Alimemazine tartrate (Non-proprietary)
  Alimemazine tartrate 1.5 mg per 1 ml Alimemazine 7.5mg/5ml oral solution | 100 ml [PoM] £179.55 DT = £135.00
  Alimemazine 7.5mg/5ml oral solution sugar free | 100 ml [PoM] £107.74–£168.00 DT = £168.00 [SF]
  Alimemazine tartrate 2 mg per 1 ml Alimemazine 10mg/5ml oral solution sugar free | 100 ml [PoM] £196.83 DT = £196.83 [SF]
  Alimemazine tartrate 6 mg per 1 ml Alimemazine 30mg/5ml oral solution sugar free | 100 ml [PoM] £146.10–£230.00 DT = £230.00 [SF]
  Alimemazine 30mg/5ml oral solution | 100 ml [PoM] £243.51 DT = £231.63
- ▸ Alfresed (SyriMed)
  Alimemazine tartrate 1.5 mg per 1 ml Alfresed 7.5mg/5ml syrup | 100 ml [PoM] £89.00 DT = £135.00
  Alimemazine tartrate 6 mg per 1 ml Alfresed 30mg/5ml syrup | 100 ml [PoM] £99.00 DT = £231.63
- ▸ Itzenal (Zentiva Pharma UK Ltd)
  Alimemazine tartrate 1.5 mg per 1 ml Itzenal 7.5mg/5ml oral solution sugar free | 100 ml [PoM] £89.00 DT = £168.00 [SF]
  Alimemazine tartrate 6 mg per 1 ml Itzenal 30mg/5ml oral solution sugar free | 100 ml [PoM] £99.00 DT = £230.00 [SF]

Chlorphenamine maleate

10-Oct-2023

(Chlorpheniramine maleate)

- **INDICATIONS AND DOSE**

Symptomatic relief of allergy such as hay fever, urticaria, food allergy, drug reactions | Relief of itch associated with chickenpox

▶ BY MOUTH

- ▸ Child 1–23 months: 1 mg twice daily
- ▸ Child 2–5 years: 1 mg every 4–6 hours
- ▸ Child 6–11 years: 2 mg every 4–6 hours
- ▸ Child 12–17 years: 4 mg every 4–6 hours

continued →

Symptomatic relief of allergy such as hay fever, urticaria, food allergy, drug reactions

▶ BY INTRAMUSCULAR INJECTION, OR BY INTRAVENOUS INJECTION

- Child 1–5 months: 250 micrograms/kg for 1 dose (max. per dose 2.5 mg), to be repeated if necessary; maximum 4 doses per day
- Child 6 months–5 years: 2.5 mg for 1 dose, to be repeated if necessary; maximum 4 doses per day
- Child 6–11 years: 5 mg for 1 dose, to be repeated if necessary; maximum 4 doses per day
- Child 12–17 years: 10 mg for 1 dose, to be repeated if necessary; maximum 4 doses per day

Emergency treatment of anaphylactic reactions

▶ BY INTRAMUSCULAR INJECTION, OR BY INTRAVENOUS INJECTION

- Child 1–5 months: 250 micrograms/kg for 1 dose (max. per dose 2.5 mg), to be repeated if necessary; maximum 4 doses per day
- Child 6 months–5 years: 2.5 mg for 1 dose, to be repeated if necessary; maximum 4 doses per day
- Child 6–11 years: 5 mg for 1 dose, to be repeated if necessary; maximum 4 doses per day
- Child 12–17 years: 10 mg for 1 dose, to be repeated if necessary; maximum 4 doses per day

● **UNLICENSED USE** Expert sources advise that chlorphenamine may be used in children under 1 year of age for the treatment of allergies and of itch associated with chickenpox, but it is not licensed for this age group.

IMPORTANT SAFETY INFORMATION

MHRA/CHM ADVICE: OVER-THE-COUNTER COUGH AND COLD MEDICINES FOR CHILDREN (APRIL 2009)

Children under 6 years should not be given over-the-counter cough and cold medicines containing chlorphenamine.

● **CONTRA-INDICATIONS** Neonate (due to significant antimuscarinic activity)

● **CAUTIONS** Epilepsy · pyloroduodenal obstruction · susceptibility to angle-closure glaucoma · urinary retention

● **INTERACTIONS** → Appendix 1: antihistamines, sedating

● **SIDE-EFFECTS**

GENERAL SIDE-EFFECTS

▶ **Common or very common** Concentration impaired · coordination abnormal · dizziness · dry mouth · fatigue · headache · nausea · vision blurred

▶ **Frequency not known** Agitation · appetite decreased · blood disorder · bronchial secretion viscosity increased · depression · diarrhoea · haemolytic anaemia · hypotension · irritability · muscle twitching · muscle weakness · nightmare · palpitations · photosensitivity reaction · skin reactions · tinnitus · urinary retention · vomiting

SPECIFIC SIDE-EFFECTS

▶ **Common or very common**

▸ With oral use Drowsiness

▶ **Frequency not known**

▸ With oral use Angioedema · arrhythmias · chest tightness · confusion · gastrointestinal discomfort · hepatic disorders

▸ With parenteral use Central nervous system stimulation · dyspepsia · gastrointestinal disorder · hepatitis · sedation

SIDE-EFFECTS, FURTHER INFORMATION Children are more susceptible to side-effects.

● **PREGNANCY** Most manufacturers of antihistamines advise avoiding their use during pregnancy; however, there is no evidence of teratogenicity. Use in the latter part of the third trimester may cause adverse effects in neonates such as irritability, paradoxical excitability, and tremor.

● **BREAST FEEDING** Most antihistamines are present in breast milk in varying amounts; although not known to be harmful, most manufacturers advise avoiding their use in mothers who are breast-feeding.

● **HEPATIC IMPAIRMENT** Manufacturer advises caution.

● **DIRECTIONS FOR ADMINISTRATION** For *intravenous injection*, manufacturer advises give over 1 minute; if small dose required, dilute with Sodium Chloride 0.9%.

● **PATIENT AND CARER ADVICE**

Medicines for Children leaflet: Chlorphenamine maleate for allergy www.medicinesforchildren.org.uk/medicines/chlorphenamine-maleate-for-allergy/

Driving and skilled tasks Drowsiness may affect performance of skilled tasks (e.g. cycling or driving); sedating effects enhanced by alcohol.

● **PROFESSION SPECIFIC INFORMATION**

Dental practitioners' formulary Chlorphenamine tablets may be prescribed.

Chlorphenamine oral solution may be prescribed.

● **EXCEPTIONS TO LEGAL CATEGORY**

▸ With intramuscular use or intravenous use Prescription only medicine restriction does not apply to chlorphenamine injection where administration is for saving life in emergency.

● **MEDICINAL FORMS** There can be variation in the licensing of different medicines containing the same drug. Forms available from special-order manufacturers include: oral solution

Solution for injection

▸ Chlorphenamine maleate (Non-proprietary)

Chlorphenamine maleate 10 mg per 1 ml Chlorphenamine 10mg/1ml solution for injection ampoules | 5 ampoule [PoM] £22.50 DT = £25.49 (Hospital only) | 5 ampoule [PoM] £25.49 DT = £25.49

Oral tablet

CAUTIONARY AND ADVISORY LABELS 2

▸ Chlorphenamine maleate (Non-proprietary)

Chlorphenamine maleate 4 mg Chlorphenamine 4mg tablets | 28 tablet [P] £8.05 DT = £0.70 | 60 tablet [P] £1.95

▸ Allerief (Crescent Pharma Ltd)

Chlorphenamine maleate 4 mg Allerief 4mg tablets | 28 tablet [P] £3.07 DT = £0.70

▸ Hayleve (Genesis Pharmaceuticals Ltd)

Chlorphenamine maleate 4 mg Hayleve 4mg tablets | 28 tablet [P] £2.47 DT = £0.70

▸ Piriton (Haleon UK Trading Ltd)

Chlorphenamine maleate 4 mg Piriton 4mg tablets | 500 tablet [P] £22.37

Piriton Allergy 4mg tablets | 30 tablet [P] £3.63 | 60 tablet [P] £5.59

Oral solution

CAUTIONARY AND ADVISORY LABELS 2

▸ Chlorphenamine maleate (Non-proprietary)

Chlorphenamine maleate 400 microgram per 1 ml Chlorphenamine 2mg/5ml oral solution sugar free | 150 ml [P] £31.58 DT = £31.58 [SF]

▸ Allerief (Crescent Pharma Ltd)

Chlorphenamine maleate 400 microgram per 1 ml Allerief 2mg/5ml oral solution | 150 ml [P] £2.21 DT = £31.58 [SF]

▸ Piriton (Haleon UK Trading Ltd)

Chlorphenamine maleate 400 microgram per 1 ml Piriton 2mg/5ml syrup | 150 ml [P] £4.05 DT = £4.05

Hydroxyzine hydrochloride

27-Apr-2021

● **DRUG ACTION** Hydroxyzine is a sedating antihistamine which exerts its actions by antagonising the effects of histamine.

● **INDICATIONS AND DOSE**

Pruritus

▶ BY MOUTH

- Child 6 months–5 years: 5–15 mg daily in divided doses, dose adjusted according to weight; maximum 2 mg/kg per day

- Child 6–17 years (body-weight up to 40 kg): Initially 15–25 mg daily in divided doses, dose increased as necessary, adjusted according to weight; maximum 2 mg/kg per day
- Child 6–17 years (body-weight 40 kg and above): Initially 15–25 mg daily in divided doses, increased if necessary to 50–100 mg daily in divided doses, dose adjusted according to weight

IMPORTANT SAFETY INFORMATION

MHRA/CHM ADVICE: RISK OF QT-INTERVAL PROLONGATION AND TORSADE DE POINTES (APRIL 2015)

Following concerns of heart rhythm abnormalities, the safety and efficacy of hydroxyzine has been reviewed by the European Medicines Agency. The review concludes that hydroxyzine is associated with a small risk of QT-interval prolongation and torsade de pointes; these events are most likely to occur in patients who have risk factors for QT prolongation, e.g. concomitant use of drugs that prolong the QT-interval, cardiovascular disease, family history of sudden cardiac death, significant electrolyte imbalance (low plasma-potassium or plasma-magnesium concentrations), or significant bradycardia.

To minimise the risk of such adverse effects, the following dose restrictions have been made and new cautions and contra-indications added:

- Hydroxyzine is contra-indicated in patients with prolonged QT-interval or who have risk factors for QT-interval prolongation;
- Consider the risks of QT-interval prolongation and torsade de pointes before prescribing to patients taking drugs that lower heart rate or plasma-potassium concentration;
- In children with body-weight up to 40 kg, the maximum daily dose is 2 mg/kg;
- The lowest effective dose for the shortest period of time should be prescribed.

- **CONTRA-INDICATIONS** Acquired or congenital QT interval prolongation · predisposition to QT interval prolongation

CONTRA-INDICATIONS, FURTHER INFORMATION Risk factors for QT interval prolongation include significant electrolyte imbalance, bradycardia, cardiovascular disease, and family history of sudden cardiac death.

- **CAUTIONS** Bladder outflow obstruction · breathing problems · cardiovascular disease · children · decreased gastrointestinal motility · dementia · epilepsy · hypertension · hyperthyroidism · myasthenia gravis · pyloroduodenal obstruction · stenosing peptic ulcer · susceptibility to angle-closure glaucoma · urinary retention

CAUTIONS, FURTHER INFORMATION Children have an increased susceptibility to side-effects, particularly CNS effects.

- **INTERACTIONS** → Appendix 1: antihistamines, sedating
- **SIDE-EFFECTS**
  - **Rare or very rare** Alopecia · hyperhidrosis · severe cutaneous adverse reactions (SCARs) · skin reactions
  - **Frequency not known** Agranulocytosis · anticholinergic syndrome · anxiety · appetite decreased · arrhythmias · asthenia · blood disorder · bronchial secretion viscosity increased · chest tightness · chills · coma · concentration impaired · confusion · constipation · depression · diarrhoea · dizziness · drowsiness · dry mouth · dry throat · dyskinesia (with high doses) · epigastric pain · fever · flushing · gastrointestinal disorders · haemolytic anaemia · hallucination · headache · hepatic function abnormal · hypotension · irritability · labyrinthitis · leucopenia · malaise · menstruation irregular · movement disorders · myalgia · nasal congestion · nausea · palpitations · paraesthesia · QT interval prolongation · respiratory disorders · respiratory tract dryness · seizure (with high doses) · sexual dysfunction · sleep disorders · speech slurred · taste bitter · thrombocytopenia · tinnitus · tremor (with high doses) · urinary disorders · vertigo · vision disorders · vomiting · weight increased

SIDE-EFFECTS, FURTHER INFORMATION Paradoxical stimulation may occur rarely, especially with high doses. Drowsiness may diminish after a few days of treatment.

- **ALLERGY AND CROSS-SENSITIVITY** Manufacturer advises hydroxyzine should be avoided in patients with previous hypersensitivity to cetirizine or other piperazine derivatives, and aminophylline.
- **PREGNANCY** Manufacturers advise avoid—toxicity in *animal* studies with higher doses. Use in the latter part of the third trimester may cause irritability, paradoxical excitability, and tremor in the neonate.
- **BREAST FEEDING** Manufacturer advises avoid—expected to be present in milk but effect unknown.
- **HEPATIC IMPAIRMENT** Manufacturer advises caution in mild to moderate impairment (increased risk of accumulation); avoid in severe impairment.

Dose adjustments Manufacturer advises dose reduction of 33% in mild to moderate impairment.

- **RENAL IMPAIRMENT** EvGr Use with caution. (M)

Dose adjustments EvGr Reduce daily dose by half in moderate to severe renal impairment. (M)

- **EFFECT ON LABORATORY TESTS** May interfere with methacholine test—manufacturer advises stop treatment 96 hours prior to test. May interfere with skin testing for allergy—manufacturer advises stop treatment one week prior to test.
- **PATIENT AND CARER ADVICE**

Driving and skilled tasks Drowsiness may affect performance of skilled tasks (e.g. cycling or driving); sedating effects enhanced by alcohol.

- **MEDICINAL FORMS** There can be variation in the licensing of different medicines containing the same drug. Forms available from special-order manufacturers include: oral suspension, oral solution

Oral tablet

CAUTIONARY AND ADVISORY LABELS 2

- **Hydroxyzine hydrochloride (Non-proprietary)**

Hydroxyzine hydrochloride 10 mg Hydroxyzine 10mg tablets | 84 tablet PoM £2.80 DT = £2.45

Hydroxyzine hydrochloride 25 mg Hydroxyzine 25mg tablets | 28 tablet PoM £1.50 DT = £0.80

Oral solution

CAUTIONARY AND ADVISORY LABELS 2

EXCIPIENTS: May contain Alcohol, sucrose

Ketotifen

14-Dec-2020

- **INDICATIONS AND DOSE**

Allergic rhinitis

- BY MOUTH
  - Child 3–17 years: 1 mg twice daily

- **CONTRA-INDICATIONS** Avoid in Acute porphyrias p. 745
- **CAUTIONS** Epilepsy · pyloroduodenal obstruction · susceptibility to angle-closure glaucoma · urinary retention
- **INTERACTIONS** → Appendix 1: antihistamines, sedating
- **SIDE-EFFECTS**
  - **Common or very common** Anxiety · insomnia · irritability
  - **Uncommon** Cystitis · dizziness · dry mouth · skin reactions
  - **Rare or very rare** Hepatitis · sedation · seizure · Stevens-Johnson syndrome · weight increased

SIDE-EFFECTS, FURTHER INFORMATION Drowsiness is a significant side-effect with most of the older antihistamines although paradoxical stimulation may occur rarely, especially with high doses. Drowsiness may diminish after a few days of treatment and is considerably less of a problem with the newer antihistamines.

- **PREGNANCY** Most manufacturers of antihistamines advise avoiding their use during pregnancy; however, there is no evidence of teratogenicity. Use in the latter part of the third trimester may cause adverse effects in neonates such as irritability, paradoxical excitability, and tremor.
- **BREAST FEEDING** Most antihistamines are present in breast milk in varying amounts; although not known to be harmful, most manufacturers advise avoiding their use in mothers who are breast-feeding.
- **PATIENT AND CARER ADVICE**
  Driving and skilled tasks Drowsiness may affect performance of skilled tasks (e.g. driving or cycling); sedating effects enhanced by alcohol.

- **MEDICINAL FORMS** There can be variation in the licensing of different medicines containing the same drug. Forms available from special-order manufacturers include: oral solution

Oral tablet

CAUTIONARY AND ADVISORY LABELS 2, 21

▸ Zaditen (CD Pharma Srl)

Ketotifen (as Ketotifen fumarate) 1 mg Zaditen 1mg tablets | 60 tablet [PoM] £19.95 DT = £19.95

Oral solution

CAUTIONARY AND ADVISORY LABELS 2, 21

▸ Zaditen (CD Pharma Srl)

Ketotifen (as Ketotifen fumarate) 200 microgram per 1 ml Zaditen 1mg/5ml elixir | 300 ml [PoM] £22.45 DT = £22.45 [SF]

Promethazine hydrochloride

27-Jun-2023

- **INDICATIONS AND DOSE**

Symptomatic relief of allergy such as hay fever and urticaria | Insomnia associated with urticaria and pruritus

▸ BY MOUTH

- Child 2–4 years: 5 mg twice daily, alternatively 5–15 mg once daily, dose to be taken at night
- Child 5–9 years: 5–10 mg twice daily, alternatively 10–25 mg once daily, dose to be taken at night
- Child 10–17 years: 10–20 mg 2–3 times a day, alternatively 25 mg once daily, dose to be taken at night, increased if necessary to 25 mg twice daily

Sedation (short-term use)

▸ BY MOUTH

- Child 2–4 years: 15–20 mg
- Child 5–9 years: 20–25 mg
- Child 10–17 years: 25–50 mg

Sedation in intensive care

▸ BY MOUTH, OR BY SLOW INTRAVENOUS INJECTION, OR BY DEEP INTRAMUSCULAR INJECTION

- Child 1 month–11 years: 0.5–1 mg/kg 4 times a day (max. per dose 25 mg), adjusted according to response
- Child 12–17 years: 25–50 mg 4 times a day, adjusted according to response

Nausea | Vomiting | Vertigo | Labyrinthine disorders | Motion sickness

▸ BY MOUTH

- Child 2–4 years: 5 mg, to be taken at bedtime on night before travel, repeat following morning if necessary
- Child 5–9 years: 10 mg, to be taken at bedtime on night before travel, repeat following morning if necessary
- Child 10–17 years: 20–25 mg, to be taken at bedtime on night before travel, repeat following morning if necessary

- **UNLICENSED USE** Not licensed for use for sedation in children under 2 years.

IMPORTANT SAFETY INFORMATION

MHRA/CHM ADVICE: OVER-THE-COUNTER COUGH AND COLD MEDICINES FOR CHILDREN (APRIL 2009)

Children under 6 years should not be given over-the-counter cough and cold medicines containing promethazine.

- **CONTRA-INDICATIONS** Neonate (due to significant antimuscarinic activity) · should not be given to children under 2 years, except on specialist advice, due to the potential for fatal respiratory depression
- **CAUTIONS**
  GENERAL CAUTIONS Epilepsy · pyloroduodenal obstruction · severe coronary artery disease · susceptibility to angle-closure glaucoma · susceptibility to QT interval prolongation · urinary retention
  SPECIFIC CAUTIONS Avoid extravasation with intravenous injection
- **INTERACTIONS** → Appendix 1: antihistamines, sedating
- **SIDE-EFFECTS**
  GENERAL SIDE-EFFECTS Arrhythmias · blood disorder · confusion · dizziness · drowsiness · dry mouth · headache · hypotension · jaundice · movement disorders · palpitations · photosensitivity reaction · QT interval prolongation · urinary retention · vision blurred
  SPECIFIC SIDE-EFFECTS
  ▸ With oral use Agranulocytosis · angle closure glaucoma · anticholinergic syndrome · anxiety · insomnia · leucopenia · nasal congestion · nausea · rash · seizure · thrombocytopenia · tinnitus · tremor · vomiting
  ▸ With parenteral use Appetite decreased · epigastric discomfort · fatigue · haemolytic anaemia · hypersensitivity · muscle spasms · nightmare · restlessness · skin reactions
- **PREGNANCY** Most manufacturers of antihistamines advise avoiding their use during pregnancy; however, there is no evidence of teratogenicity. Use in the latter part of the third trimester may cause adverse effects in neonates such as irritability, paradoxical excitability, and tremor.
- **BREAST FEEDING** Most antihistamines are present in breast milk in varying amounts; although not known to be harmful, most manufacturers advise avoiding their use in mothers who are breast-feeding.
- **HEPATIC IMPAIRMENT** Manufacturer advises caution.
- **RENAL IMPAIRMENT** [EvGr] Use with caution. ⟨M⟩
- **PATIENT AND CARER ADVICE**
  Driving and skilled tasks Drowsiness may affect the performance of skilled tasks (e.g. cycling or driving); sedating effects enhanced by alcohol.
- **PROFESSION SPECIFIC INFORMATION**
  Dental practitioners' formulary Promethazine Hydrochloride Tablets 10 mg or 25 mg may be prescribed.
  Promethazine Hydrochloride Oral Solution (elixir) 5 mg/5 mL may be prescribed.
- **LESS SUITABLE FOR PRESCRIBING** Promethazine is less suitable for prescribing for sedation.
- **EXCEPTIONS TO LEGAL CATEGORY** Prescription only medicine restriction does not apply to promethazine hydrochloride injection where administration is for saving life in emergency.

- **MEDICINAL FORMS** There can be variation in the licensing of different medicines containing the same drug. Forms available from special-order manufacturers include: oral suspension, oral solution

Solution for injection

EXCIPIENTS: May contain Sulfites

- **Phenergan** (Opella POM UK Ltd)
  Promethazine hydrochloride 25 mg per 1 ml Phenergan 25mg/1ml solution for injection ampoules | 10 ampoule [PoM] £6.74 DT = £6.74

Oral tablet

CAUTIONARY AND ADVISORY LABELS 2

- **Promethazine hydrochloride (Non-proprietary)**
  Promethazine hydrochloride 10 mg Promethazine hydrochloride 10mg tablets | 56 tablet [PoM] £2.20 DT = £1.85
  Promethazine hydrochloride 25 mg Promethazine hydrochloride 25mg tablets | 56 tablet [PoM] £34.19 DT = £2.03
- **Sominex** (Dexcel-Pharma Ltd)
  Promethazine hydrochloride 20 mg Sominex 20mg tablets | 8 tablet [P] £1.89 DT = £1.89 | 16 tablet [P] £2.69 DT = £2.69

Oral solution

CAUTIONARY AND ADVISORY LABELS 2
EXCIPIENTS: May contain Sulfites
ELECTROLYTES: May contain Sodium

- **Phenergan** (Opella Healthcare UK Ltd)
  Promethazine hydrochloride 1 mg per 1 ml Phenergan 5mg/5ml elixir | 100 ml [P] £4.08 DT = £4.08 [SF]

VACCINES > ALLERGEN-TYPE VACCINES

Bee venom extracts

23-Oct-2025

- **INDICATIONS AND DOSE**

Hypersensitivity to bee venom (under expert supervision)

▶ BY SUBCUTANEOUS INJECTION
- Child: (consult product literature)

IMPORTANT SAFETY INFORMATION

DESENSITISING VACCINES

In view of concerns about the safety of desensitising vaccines, it is recommended that they are used by specialists and only for licensed indications.

[EvGr] Desensitising vaccines should generally be avoided or used with particular care in patients with asthma. (M)

- **CONTRA-INDICATIONS** Consult product literature
- **CAUTIONS** Consult product literature
- **INTERACTIONS** → Appendix 1: bee venom extracts
- **SIDE-EFFECTS** Consult product literature.
  Hypersensitivity reactions Hypersensitivity reactions to immunotherapy can be life-threatening. Cardiopulmonary resuscitation must be immediately available and patients need to be monitored for at least 30 minutes after administration. If symptoms or signs of hypersensitivity develop (e.g. rash, urticaria, bronchospasm, faintness), **even when mild**, the patient should be observed until these have resolved completely.
- **PREGNANCY** [EvGr] Avoid initiating up-dosing treatment (no information available). If pregnancy occurs during maintenance treatment, *Alutard SQ Bee Venom*® may be continued after the general condition of the patient is evaluated, including reactions to previous injections. (M)
- **BREAST FEEDING** Specialist sources indicate probably compatible (no information available). High molecular weight makes excretion into milk unlikely and inactivation in the gastrointestinal tract suggests limited absorption by the infant.
- **DIRECTIONS FOR ADMINISTRATION** [EvGr] For *subcutaneous injection* (*Alutard SQ Bee Venom*®), the vial must be turned slowly upside down 10 to 20 times to make a homogenous suspension before use. Administer slowly, either laterally in the distal part of the upper arm or dorsally in the proximal part of the forearm. (M)
- **PRESCRIBING AND DISPENSING INFORMATION** Each set of allergen extracts usually contains vials for the administration of graded amounts of allergen to patients undergoing hyposensitisation. Maintenance sets containing vials at the highest strength are also available. Product literature must be consulted for details of allergens, vial strengths, and administration.
- **HANDLING AND STORAGE** Store unopened vials in a refrigerator (2–8°C) and protect from light. Once opened, vials may be stored for a maximum of 6 months in a refrigerator (2–8°C) when used for one individual patient.
- **PATIENT AND CARER ADVICE** Patients and carers should be counselled to avoid physical exercise, hot baths, and alcohol on the day of injection—potential amplification of anaphylactic reaction. They should also be advised to seek immediate medical attention if severe delayed systemic reactions develop, and to inform their doctor before the next injection of any local or systemic reactions that occur subsequently.
  Asthma Patients and carers should be advised to seek immediate medical attention if their asthma deteriorates suddenly during treatment.
  Driving and skilled tasks Patients and carers should be counselled on the effects on driving and performance of skilled tasks—increased risk of dizziness or vertigo.
- **NATIONAL FUNDING/ACCESS DECISIONS**
  For full details see funding body website
  NICE decisions
  ▶ ***Pharmalgen*® for the treatment of bee and wasp venom allergy (February 2012)** NICE TA246 Recommended with restrictions
- **MEDICINAL FORMS** There can be variation in the licensing of different medicines containing the same drug.

Suspension for injection

- **Alutard SQ Bee Venom** (ALK-Abello Ltd)
  Bee venom 100 SQ-U per 1 ml Alutard SQ Bee Venom 500 SQ-U/5ml suspension for injection vials | 1 vial [PoM] [X] (Hospital only)
  Bee venom 1000 SQ-U per 1 ml Alutard SQ Bee Venom 5,000 SQ-U/5ml suspension for injection vials | 1 vial [PoM] [X] (Hospital only)
  Bee venom 10000 SQ-U per 1 ml Alutard SQ Bee Venom 50,000 SQ-U/5ml suspension for injection vials | 1 vial [PoM] [X] (Hospital only)
  Bee venom 100000 SQ-U per 1 ml Alutard SQ Bee Venom maintenance pack suspension for injection vials | 1 vial [PoM] £462.61 (Hospital only)

Grass pollen extracts

23-Oct-2025

- **INDICATIONS AND DOSE**

Treatment of seasonal allergic hay fever due to grass pollen in patients who have failed to respond to anti-allergy drugs

▶ BY SUBCUTANEOUS INJECTION
- Child: (consult product literature)

Treatment of seasonal allergic hay fever due to grass pollen in patients who have failed to respond to anti-allergy drugs (initiated under specialist supervision)

▶ BY MOUTH
- Child 5–17 years: 1 tablet daily, treatment to be started at least 4 months before start of pollen season and continue for up to 3 years

IMPORTANT SAFETY INFORMATION

DESENSITISING VACCINES

In view of concerns about the safety of desensitising vaccines, it is recommended that they are used by

specialists and only for licensed indications.
EvGr Desensitising vaccines should generally be avoided or used with particular care in patients with asthma. (M)

- **CONTRA-INDICATIONS** Consult product literature
- **CAUTIONS** Consult product literature
- **INTERACTIONS** → Appendix 1: grass pollen extracts
- **SIDE-EFFECTS** Consult product literature.
  Hypersensitivity reactions Hypersensitivity reactions to immunotherapy can be life-threatening. Cardiopulmonary resuscitation must be immediately available and patients need to be monitored for at least 30 minutes (oral) or 1 hour (subcutaneous) after administration. If symptoms or signs of hypersensitivity develop (e.g. rash, urticaria, bronchospasm, faintness), **even when mild**, the patient should be observed until these have resolved completely.
- **PREGNANCY** Should be avoided in pregnant women—consult product literature.
- **MONITORING REQUIREMENTS** The first dose of grass pollen extract (*Grazax*®) should be taken under medical supervision and the patient should be monitored for 20–30 minutes.
- **DIRECTIONS FOR ADMINISTRATION** Manufacturer advises oral lyophilisates should be placed under the tongue and allowed to disperse. Advise patient not to swallow for 1 minute, or eat or drink for 5 minutes after taking the tablet. The first should be taken under medical supervision and the patient should be monitored for 20–30 minutes.
- **PRESCRIBING AND DISPENSING INFORMATION** Each set of allergen extracts usually contains vials for the administration of graded amounts of allergen to patients undergoing hyposensitisation. Maintenance sets containing vials at the highest strength are also available. Product literature must be consulted for details of allergens, vial strengths, and administration.
- **PATIENT AND CARER ADVICE** Patients or carers should be given advice on how to administer oral lyophilisates.
- **MEDICINAL FORMS** There can be variation in the licensing of different medicines containing the same drug.

Form unstated

- Pollinex Grasses + Rye (Allergy Therapeutics (UK) Ltd)
  Pollinex Grasses + Rye suspension for injection treatment and extension course vials | 4 vial PoM £450.00

Oral lyophilisate

- Grazax (ALK-Abello Ltd)
  Timothy grass (Phleum pratense) pollen allergen extract 75000 SQ-T Grazax 75,000 SQ-T oral lyophilisates | 30 tablet PoM £94.73 DT = £94.73 SF

House-dust mite extracts

23-Oct-2025

- **INDICATIONS AND DOSE**

Moderate to severe house dust mite allergic rhinitis [in patients who have failed to respond to anti-allergy drugs] (initiated by a specialist)

▶ BY MOUTH

- Child 12–17 years: 1 tablet daily for up to 18 months, consider discontinuation of treatment if no improvement during the first 12 months

IMPORTANT SAFETY INFORMATION

DESENSITISING VACCINES

In view of concerns about the safety of desensitising vaccines, it is recommended that they are used by specialists and only for licensed indications.

EvGr Desensitising vaccines should generally be avoided or used with particular care in patients with asthma. (M)

- **CONTRA-INDICATIONS** Consult product literature
- **CAUTIONS** Consult product literature
- **INTERACTIONS** → Appendix 1: house-dust mite extracts
- **SIDE-EFFECTS** Consult product literature.
  Hypersensitivity reactions Hypersensitivity reactions to immunotherapy can be life-threatening. Cardiopulmonary resuscitation must be immediately available and patients need to be monitored for at least 30 minutes after administration. If symptoms or signs of hypersensitivity develop (e.g. rash, urticaria, bronchospasm, faintness), **even when mild**, the patient should be observed until these have resolved completely.
- **PREGNANCY** EvGr Avoid initiation during pregnancy—limited information available. If pregnancy occurs during treatment, *Acarizax*® may be continued after the general condition and lung function of the patient are evaluated, including reactions to previous doses—close supervision of patients with pre-existing asthma is recommended. (M)
- **DIRECTIONS FOR ADMINISTRATION** EvGr Oral lyophilisates should be placed under the tongue and allowed to disperse. Advise patient not to swallow for 1 minute, or eat or drink for 5 minutes after taking the tablet. The first dose should be taken under medical supervision and the patient should be monitored for at least 30 minutes. (M)
- **PATIENT AND CARER ADVICE**
  Administration Patients or carers should be given advice on how to administer oral lyophilisates.
  Asthma Patients or carers should be advised to seek immediate medical attention if their asthma deteriorates suddenly during treatment.
  Eosinophilic oesophagitis Patients or carers should be advised to seek medical attention if severe or persistent gastro-oesophageal symptoms (such as dysphagia or dyspepsia) develop during treatment.
  Missed doses If treatment is interrupted for more than 7 days, patients or carers should be advised to seek medical advice before resuming treatment.
- **NATIONAL FUNDING/ACCESS DECISIONS**
  For full details see funding body website

NICE decisions

▶ **12 SQ-HDM SLIT for treating allergic rhinitis and allergic asthma caused by house dust mites [in patients with allergic rhinitis] (March 2025)** NICE TA1045 Recommended

- **MEDICINAL FORMS** There can be variation in the licensing of different medicines containing the same drug.

Oral lyophilisate

- Acarizax (ALK-Abello Ltd)
  Acarizax 12 SQ-HDM oral lyophilisates | 30 tablet PoM £80.12 SF

Peanut protein

20-Oct-2022

- **INDICATIONS AND DOSE**

Peanut allergy [in conjunction with dietary restriction] (under expert supervision)

▶ BY MOUTH

- Child 4–17 years: (consult product literature)

IMPORTANT SAFETY INFORMATION

DESENSITISING VACCINES

In view of concerns about the safety of desensitising vaccines, it is recommended that they are used by specialists and only for licensed indications.

EvGr Desensitising vaccines should generally be avoided or used with particular care in patients with asthma. ⟨M⟩

- **CONTRA-INDICATIONS** Consult product literature
- **CAUTIONS** Consult product literature
- **INTERACTIONS** → Appendix 1: peanut protein
- **SIDE-EFFECTS** Consult product literature.

Hypersensitivity reactions Allergic reactions mostly occur during the first 2 hours after ingestion of the dose and are usually mild or moderate; however severe reactions including life-threatening anaphylaxis may occur. Severe reactions such as difficulty swallowing, difficulty breathing, vomiting, diarrhoea, or severe flushing or itching of the skin require immediate treatment. Self-injectable adrenaline must be available to the patient at all times. Patients need to be monitored for at least 1 hour after the last dose.

Eosinophilic oesophagitis In patients who experience severe or persistent gastrointestinal symptoms, including dysphagia, gastroesophageal reflux, chest pain, or abdominal pain, the manufacturer advises treatment must be discontinued and a diagnosis of eosinophilic oesophagitis should be considered.

- **PREGNANCY** EvGr Avoid initiation during pregnancy—no information available. If pregnancy occurs during treatment, discontinue *Palforzia*® unless potential benefit outweighs risk of anaphylactic reaction to continuing treatment. ⟨M⟩
- **BREAST FEEDING** EvGr Use with caution—no information available; peanut allergens present in milk after maternal consumption of peanuts. ⟨M⟩
- **PRESCRIBING AND DISPENSING INFORMATION** *Palforzia*® is a biological medicine. Biological medicines must be prescribed and dispensed by brand name, see *Biological medicines* and *Biosimilar medicines*, under Guidance on prescribing p. 1; record the brand name and batch number after each administration.

Palforzia® contains peanut protein as defatted powder of *Arachis hypogaea L.*, semen (peanuts) which desensitises patients with peanut allergy.

The manufacturer of *Palforzia*® has provided a user manual for healthcare professionals.

- **PATIENT AND CARER ADVICE** Patients or carers should be instructed on the potential risk factors for systemic allergic reactions and how to recognise their signs and symptoms. Patients should be advised to carry self-injectable adrenaline at all times; if use is necessary, immediate medical care should be sought and treatment stopped until the patient has been assessed.

A safety booklet for patients and caregivers, and a patient alert card should be provided.

Driving and skilled tasks Patients and carers should be counselled on the effects on driving and performance of skilled tasks—exercise caution for 2 hours after a dose in case of allergic reaction.

- **NATIONAL FUNDING/ACCESS DECISIONS**

For full details see funding body website

NICE decisions

- ***Palforzia*® for treating peanut allergy in children and young people (February 2022)** NICE TA769 Recommended

Scottish Medicines Consortium (SMC) decisions

- **Defatted powder of *Arachis hypogaea L.*, semen (*Palforzia*®) for the treatment of patients aged 4 to 17 years with a confirmed diagnosis of peanut allergy (October 2022)** SMC No. SMC2487 Not recommended

- **MEDICINAL FORMS** There can be variation in the licensing of different medicines containing the same drug.

Form unstated

CAUTIONARY AND ADVISORY LABELS 21

- **Palforzia** (Diagenics Ltd) ▼
  - Palforzia Level 3 (12mg daily) 2 week up-dosing pack | 48 capsule PoM £141.68 (Hospital only)
  - Palforzia initial dose escalation pack | 13 capsule PoM £10.12 (Hospital only)
  - Palforzia Level 7 (120mg daily) 2 week up-dosing pack | 32 capsule PoM £141.68 (Hospital only)
  - Palforzia Level 8 (160mg daily) 2 week up-dosing pack | 64 capsule PoM £141.68 (Hospital only)
  - Palforzia Level 10 (240mg daily) 2 week up-dosing pack | 64 capsule PoM £141.68 (Hospital only)

Oral powder

CAUTIONARY AND ADVISORY LABELS 21

- **Palforzia** (Diagenics Ltd) ▼

Peanut protein (as defatted powder of Arachis hypogaea L., semen [peanuts]) 500 microgram Palforzia 0.5mg oral powder in capsules for opening | 2 capsule PoM ⊠ (Hospital only)

Peanut protein (as defatted powder of Arachis hypogaea L., semen [peanuts]) 1 mg Palforzia Level 1 (3mg daily) 2 week up-dosing pack | 48 capsule PoM £141.68 (Hospital only)
Palforzia Level 2 (6mg daily) 2 week up-dosing pack | 96 capsule PoM £141.68 (Hospital only)
Palforzia 1mg oral powder in capsules for opening | 11 capsule PoM ⊠ (Hospital only)

Peanut protein (as defatted powder of Arachis hypogaea L., semen [peanuts]) 10 mg Palforzia 10mg oral powder in capsules for opening | 16 capsule PoM ⊠ (Hospital only)

Peanut protein (as defatted powder of Arachis hypogaea L., semen [peanuts]) 20 mg Palforzia Level 4 (20mg daily) 2 week up-dosing pack | 16 capsule PoM £141.68 (Hospital only)
Palforzia 20mg oral powder in capsules for opening | 16 capsule PoM ⊠ (Hospital only)
Palforzia Level 5 (40mg daily) 2 week up-dosing pack | 32 capsule PoM £141.68 (Hospital only)
Palforzia Level 6 (80mg daily) 2 week up-dosing pack | 64 capsule PoM £141.68 (Hospital only)

Peanut protein (as defatted powder of Arachis hypogaea L., semen [peanuts]) 100 mg Palforzia Level 9 (200mg daily) 2 week up-dosing pack | 32 capsule PoM £141.68 (Hospital only)
Palforzia 100mg oral powder in capsules for opening | 16 capsule PoM ⊠ (Hospital only)

Peanut protein (as defatted powder of Arachis hypogaea L., semen [peanuts]) 300 mg Palforzia Level 11 (300mg daily) 2 week up-dosing pack | 15 sachet PoM £141.68 (Hospital only)
Palforzia maintenance pack 300mg oral powder sachets | 30 sachet PoM £303.60 (Hospital only)

Tree pollen extracts

23-Oct-2025

- **INDICATIONS AND DOSE**

Treatment of seasonal allergic hay fever due to tree pollen in patients who have failed to respond to anti-allergy drugs (under expert supervision)

- BY SUBCUTANEOUS INJECTION
- Child: (consult product literature)

IMPORTANT SAFETY INFORMATION

DESENSITISING VACCINES

In view of concerns about the safety of desensitising vaccines, it is recommended that they are used by specialists and only for licensed indications.

EvGr Desensitising vaccines should generally be avoided or used with particular care in patients with asthma. ⟨M⟩

- **CONTRA-INDICATIONS** Consult product literature
- **CAUTIONS** Consult product literature
- **INTERACTIONS** → Appendix 1: tree pollen extracts
- **SIDE-EFFECTS** Consult product literature.

Hypersensitivity reactions Hypersensitivity reactions

to immunotherapy can be life-threatening. Cardiopulmonary resuscitation must be immediately available and patients need to be monitored for at least 30 minutes (oral) or 1 hour (subcutaneous) after administration. If symptoms or signs of hypersensitivity develop (e.g. rash, urticaria, bronchospasm, faintness), **even when mild**, the patient should be observed until these have resolved completely.

- **PREGNANCY** EvGr Avoid (no information available). Ⓜ
- **BREAST FEEDING** Specialist sources indicate probably compatible (no information available). High molecular weight makes excretion into milk unlikely and inactivation in the gastrointestinal tract suggests limited absorption by the infant.
- **PRESCRIBING AND DISPENSING INFORMATION** Each set of allergen extracts usually contains vials for the administration of graded amounts of allergen to patients undergoing hyposensitisation. Maintenance sets containing vials at the highest strength are also available. Product literature must be consulted for details of allergens, vial strengths, and administration.

- **MEDICINAL FORMS** There can be variation in the licensing of different medicines containing the same drug.

Form unstated

- **Pollinex Trees** (Allergy Therapeutics (UK) Ltd)
  Pollinex Trees suspension for injection treatment and extension course vials | 4 vial PoM £450.00

Suspension for injection

- **Pollinex Trees** (Allergy Therapeutics (UK) Ltd)
  Pollinex Trees No 3 suspension for injection 1ml vials | 1 vial PoM ☒
  Pollinex Trees No 2 suspension for injection 1ml vials | 1 vial PoM ☒
  Pollinex Trees No 1 suspension for injection 1ml vials | 1 vial PoM ☒

Wasp venom extracts

23-Oct-2025

- **INDICATIONS AND DOSE**

Hypersensitivity to wasp venom (under expert supervision)

▶ BY SUBCUTANEOUS INJECTION
▶ Child: (consult product literature)

IMPORTANT SAFETY INFORMATION

DESENSITISING VACCINES

In view of concerns about the safety of desensitising vaccines, it is recommended that they are used by specialists and only for licensed indications.

EvGr Desensitising vaccines should generally be avoided or used with particular care in patients with asthma. Ⓜ

- **CONTRA-INDICATIONS** Consult product literature
- **CAUTIONS** Consult product literature
- **INTERACTIONS** → Appendix 1: wasp venom extracts
- **SIDE-EFFECTS** Consult product literature.
  Hypersensitivity reactions Hypersensitivity reactions to immunotherapy can be life-threatening. Cardiopulmonary resuscitation must be immediately available and patients need to be monitored for at least 30 minutes after administration. If symptoms or signs of hypersensitivity develop (e.g. rash, urticaria, bronchospasm, faintness), **even when mild**, the patient should be observed until these have resolved completely.
- **PREGNANCY** EvGr Avoid initiating up-dosing treatment (no information available). If pregnancy occurs during maintenance treatment, *Alutard SQ Wasp Venom*® may be continued after the general condition of the patient is evaluated, including reactions to previous injections. Ⓜ
- **BREAST FEEDING** Specialist sources indicate probably compatible (no information available). High molecular weight makes excretion into milk unlikely and inactivation in the gastrointestinal tract suggests limited absorption by the infant.
- **DIRECTIONS FOR ADMINISTRATION** EvGr For *subcutaneous injection* (*Alutard SQ Wasp Venom*®), the vial must be turned slowly upside down 10 to 20 times to make a homogenous suspension before use. Administer slowly, either laterally in the distal part of the upper arm or dorsally in the proximal part of the forearm. Ⓜ
- **PRESCRIBING AND DISPENSING INFORMATION** Each set of allergen extracts usually contains vials for the administration of graded amounts of allergen to patients undergoing hyposensitisation. Maintenance sets containing vials at the highest strength are also available. Product literature must be consulted for details of allergens, vial strengths, and administration.
- **HANDLING AND STORAGE** Store unopened vials in a refrigerator (2–8°C) and protect from light. Once opened, vials may be stored for a maximum of 6 months in a refrigerator (2–8°C) when used for one individual patient.
- **PATIENT AND CARER ADVICE** Patients and carers should be counselled to avoid physical exercise, hot baths, and alcohol on the day of injection—potential amplification of anaphylactic reaction. They should also be advised to seek immediate medical attention if severe delayed systemic reactions develop, and to inform their doctor before the next injection of any local or systemic reactions that occur subsequently.
  Asthma Patients and carers should be advised to seek immediate medical attention if their asthma deteriorates suddenly during treatment.
  Driving and skilled tasks Patients and carers should be counselled on the effects on driving and performance of skilled tasks—increased risk of dizziness or vertigo.
- **NATIONAL FUNDING/ACCESS DECISIONS**
  For full details see funding body website

NICE decisions

▶ ***Pharmalgen***® **for bee and wasp venom allergy (February 2012)** NICE TA246 Recommended with restrictions

- **MEDICINAL FORMS** There can be variation in the licensing of different medicines containing the same drug.

Suspension for injection

- **Alutard SQ Wasp Venom** (ALK-Abello Ltd)
  Wasp venom 100 SQ-U per 1 ml Alutard SQ Wasp Venom 500 SQ-U/5ml suspension for injection vials | 1 vial PoM ☒ (Hospital only)
  Wasp venom 1000 SQ-U per 1 ml Alutard SQ Wasp Venom 5,000 SQ-U/5ml suspension for injection vials | 1 vial PoM ☒ (Hospital only)
  Wasp venom 10000 SQ-U per 1 ml Alutard SQ Wasp Venom 50,000 SQ-U/5ml suspension for injection vials | 1 vial PoM ☒ (Hospital only)
  Wasp venom 100000 SQ-U per 1 ml Alutard SQ Wasp Venom maintenance pack suspension for injection vials | 1 vial PoM £462.61 (Hospital only)

2.1 Angioedema

DRUGS USED IN HEREDITARY ANGIOEDEMA ›
COMPLEMENT REGULATORY PROTEINS

C1-esterase inhibitor

30-Oct-2020

- **INDICATIONS AND DOSE**

BERINERT®

Acute attacks of hereditary angioedema (under expert supervision)

▶ BY SLOW INTRAVENOUS INJECTION, OR BY INTRAVENOUS INFUSION
▶ Child: 20 units/kg

Short-term prophylaxis of hereditary angioedema before dental, medical, or surgical procedures (under expert supervision)
▸ BY SLOW INTRAVENOUS INJECTION, OR BY INTRAVENOUS INFUSION
▸ Child: 15–30 units/kg (max. per dose 1000 units) for 1 dose, to be administered less than 6 hours before procedure

CINRYZE®

Acute attacks of hereditary angioedema (under expert supervision)
▸ BY SLOW INTRAVENOUS INJECTION
▸ Child 2–11 years (body-weight 10–25 kg): 500 units for 1 dose, dose may be repeated if necessary after 60 minutes
▸ Child 2–11 years (body-weight 26 kg and above): 1000 units for 1 dose, dose may be repeated if necessary after 60 minutes
▸ Child 12–17 years: 1000 units for 1 dose, dose may be repeated if necessary after 60 minutes (or sooner for patients experiencing laryngeal attacks or if treatment initiation is delayed)

Short-term prophylaxis of hereditary angioedema before dental, medical, or surgical procedures (under expert supervision)
▸ BY SLOW INTRAVENOUS INJECTION
▸ Child 2–11 years (body-weight 10–25 kg): 500 units for 1 dose, to be administered up to 24 hours before procedure
▸ Child 2–11 years (body-weight 26 kg and above): 1000 units for 1 dose, to be administered up to 24 hours before procedure
▸ Child 12–17 years: 1000 units for 1 dose, to be administered up to 24 hours before procedure

Long-term prophylaxis of severe, recurrent attacks of hereditary angioedema where acute treatment is inadequate, or when oral prophylaxis is inadequate or not tolerated (under expert supervision)
▸ BY SLOW INTRAVENOUS INJECTION
▸ Child 6–11 years: 500 units every 3–4 days, dose and dosing interval to be adjusted according to response
▸ Child 12–17 years: 1000 units every 3–4 days, interval between doses to be adjusted according to response

● **CAUTIONS** Vaccination against hepatitis A and hepatitis B may be required

● **SIDE-EFFECTS**
▸ **Rare or very rare** Dizziness · dyspnoea · flushing · headache · hypersensitivity · hypertension · hypotension · nausea · tachycardia · thrombosis (with high doses) · urticaria

● **PREGNANCY** Manufacturer advises avoid unless essential.

● **DIRECTIONS FOR ADMINISTRATION**
CINRYZE® For *slow intravenous injection*, manufacturer advises reconstitute (with solvent provided) to a concentration of 100 units/mL; give at a rate of 1 mL/minute.

● **PRESCRIBING AND DISPENSING INFORMATION** C1-esterase inhibitor is prepared from human plasma.

● **NATIONAL FUNDING/ACCESS DECISIONS**
CINRYZE® For full details see funding body website

All Wales Medicines Strategy Group (AWMSG) decisions
▸ **C1 inhibitor (human) (*Cinryze*®) for the treatment and pre-procedure prevention of attacks of hereditary angioedema (HAE) in patients 2 years old and above; routine prevention of angioedema attacks in patients 6 years old and above with severe and recurrent attacks of HAE, where acute treatment is inadequate, or when oral prophylaxis is inadequate or not tolerated (October 2017)** AWMSG No. 3295 Recommended

● **MEDICINAL FORMS** There can be variation in the licensing of different medicines containing the same drug.

Powder and solvent for solution for injection
ELECTROLYTES: May contain Sodium
▸ **Berinert P** (CSL Behring UK Ltd)
C1-esterase inhibitor human 500 unit Berinert 500unit powder and solvent for solution for injection vials | 1 vial [PoM] £670.00
C1-esterase inhibitor human 1500 unit Berinert 1,500unit powder and solvent for solution for injection vials | 1 vial [PoM] £2,010.00
▸ **Cinryze** (Takeda UK Ltd)
C1-esterase inhibitor human 500 unit Cinryze 500unit powder and solvent for solution for injection vials | 2 vial [PoM] £1,336.00

Conestat alfa

15-Jun-2021

● **INDICATIONS AND DOSE**

Acute attacks of hereditary angioedema in patients with C1-esterase inhibitor deficiency (under expert supervision)
▸ BY SLOW INTRAVENOUS INJECTION
▸ Child 2–11 years (body-weight up to 84 kg): 50 units/kg for 1 dose, to be administered over 5 minutes, dose may be repeated if there has been an inadequate response after 60 minutes; maximum 2 doses per day
▸ Child 2–11 years (body-weight 84 kg and above): 4200 units for 1 dose, to be administered over 5 minutes, dose may be repeated if there has been an inadequate response after 60 minutes; maximum 2 doses per day
▸ Child 12–17 years (body-weight up to 84 kg): 50 units/kg for 1 dose, to be administered over 5 minutes, dose may be repeated if there has been an inadequate response after 120 minutes; maximum 2 doses per day
▸ Child 12–17 years (body-weight 84 kg and above): 4200 units for 1 dose, to be administered over 5 minutes, dose may be repeated if there has been an inadequate response after 120 minutes; maximum 2 doses per day

● **CONTRA-INDICATIONS** Rabbit allergy

● **SIDE-EFFECTS**
▸ **Common or very common** Nausea
▸ **Uncommon** Abdominal discomfort · auricular swelling · diarrhoea · dizziness · headache · numbness · oral paraesthesia · throat irritation · urticaria · vertigo

● **ALLERGY AND CROSS-SENSITIVITY** [EvGr] Caution—possible risk of hypersensitivity reaction in presence of a clinical allergy to cows' milk. ⟨M⟩

● **PREGNANCY** Use only if potential benefit outweighs risk—toxicity in *animal* studies.

● **BREAST FEEDING** Use only if potential benefit outweighs risk—no information available.

● **PRESCRIBING AND DISPENSING INFORMATION** Conestat alfa is a biological medicine. Biological medicines must be prescribed and dispensed by brand name, see *Biological medicines* and *Biosimilar medicines*, under Guidance on prescribing p. 1; record the brand name and batch number after each administration.

● **PATIENT AND CARER ADVICE**
Driving and skilled tasks Patients and carers should be counselled on the effects on driving and performance of skilled tasks—increased risk of headache, vertigo or dizziness.

● **NATIONAL FUNDING/ACCESS DECISIONS**
For full details see funding body website

Scottish Medicines Consortium (SMC) decisions
▸ **Conestat alfa (*Ruconest*®) for the treatment of acute angioedema attacks in adults and adolescents with hereditary angioedema (HAE) due to C1-esterase inhibitor deficiency (August 2018)** SMC No. 745/11 Recommended

All Wales Medicines Strategy Group (AWMSG) decisions

- **Conestat alfa (*Ruconest*®) for the treatment of acute angioedema attacks in adults, adolescents and children (aged 2 years and above) with hereditary angioedema (HAE) due to C1-esterase inhibitor deficiency (May 2021)** AWMSG No. 4519 Recommended

● **MEDICINAL FORMS** No licensed medicines listed.

DRUGS USED IN HEREDITARY ANGIOEDEMA › KALLIKREIN INHIBITORS

Berotralstat 01-Apr-2022

● **DRUG ACTION** Berotralstat is a plasma kallikrein inhibitor, which limits the production of bradykinin, a potent vasodilator associated with angioedema attacks.

● **INDICATIONS AND DOSE**

Prevention of recurrent attacks of hereditary angioedema

▶ BY MOUTH

▶ Child 12–17 years (body-weight 40 kg and above): 150 mg once daily, dose to be taken with food

● **CONTRA-INDICATIONS** Body-weight less than 40 kg · not a treatment for acute attacks of angioedema—initiate individualised treatment for breakthrough attacks

● **CAUTIONS** Risk factors for QT prolongation

CAUTIONS, FURTHER INFORMATION

▶ QT prolongation EvGr If treatment with berotralstat is unavoidable, monitoring is recommended—consult product literature. ⟨M⟩

● **INTERACTIONS** → Appendix 1: berotralstat

● **SIDE-EFFECTS**

▶ **Common or very common** Diarrhoea · gastrointestinal discomfort · gastrointestinal disorders · headaches · rash · vomiting

▶ **Frequency not known** Nausea

● **CONCEPTION AND CONTRACEPTION** EvGr Females of childbearing potential should use effective contraception during and for at least 1 month after last treatment. Efficacy of desogestrel-containing contraceptives may be reduced—consult product literature. ⟨M⟩

● **PREGNANCY** EvGr Avoid—limited information available. ⟨M⟩

● **BREAST FEEDING** EvGr Avoid—present in milk in *animal* studies. ⟨M⟩

● **HEPATIC IMPAIRMENT** EvGr Avoid in moderate or severe impairment (risk of increased exposure). ⟨M⟩

● **RENAL IMPAIRMENT** EvGr Avoid in severe impairment (increased risk of prolonged QT); if treatment is unavoidable, monitoring is required—consult product literature. ⟨M⟩

● **PATIENT AND CARER ADVICE**

Missed doses If a dose is missed or not taken at the usual time, the missed dose should be taken as soon as possible on the same day. The next dose should be taken at the usual time.

● **NATIONAL FUNDING/ACCESS DECISIONS**

For full details see funding body website

NICE decisions

- **Berotralstat for preventing recurrent attacks of hereditary angioedema (October 2021)** NICE TA738 Recommended with restrictions

Scottish Medicines Consortium (SMC) decisions

- **Berotralstat (*Orladeyo*®) for the routine prevention of recurrent attacks of hereditary angioedema (HAE) in adult and adolescent patients aged 12 years and older (March 2022)** SMC No. SMC2405 Recommended with restrictions

● **MEDICINAL FORMS** There can be variation in the licensing of different medicines containing the same drug.

Oral capsule

CAUTIONARY AND ADVISORY LABELS 21

EXCIPIENTS: May contain Gelatin

▶ **Orladeyo** (BioCryst Ireland Ltd) ▼

Berotralstat (as Berotralstat dihydrochloride) 150 mg Orladeyo 150mg capsules | 28 capsule PoM £10,205.00 (Hospital only)

Lanadelumab 09-Nov-2020

● **DRUG ACTION** Lanadelumab is a humanised monoclonal antibody which inhibits plasma kallikrein activity, thereby limiting the production of bradykinin, a potent vasodilator associated with angioedema attacks in patients with hereditary angioedema.

● **INDICATIONS AND DOSE**

Prevention of recurrent attacks of hereditary angioedema (initiated under specialist supervision)

▶ BY SUBCUTANEOUS INJECTION

▶ Child 12–17 years: 300 mg every 2 weeks, reduced to 300 mg every 4 weeks, in those stable and attack free—consult product literature

● **CONTRA-INDICATIONS** Not a treatment for acute attacks of angioedema—initiate individualised treatment for breakthrough attacks

● **SIDE-EFFECTS**

▶ **Common or very common** Dizziness · hypersensitivity · myalgia · oral disorders · skin reactions

● **PREGNANCY** Manufacturer advises preferable to avoid—limited or no information available; *animal* studies do not indicate toxicity.

● **BREAST FEEDING** Manufacturer advises avoid during first few days after birth—possible risk from transfer of antibodies to infant. After this time, use during breast-feeding only if clinically needed.

● **EFFECT ON LABORATORY TESTS** Manufacturer advises may increase activated partial thromboplastin time (aPTT) due to an interaction with the aPTT assay—consult product literature.

● **DIRECTIONS FOR ADMINISTRATION** Manufacturer advises to withdraw dose from the vial into a syringe with an 18 gauge needle and inject, using a suitable gauge needle, into the abdomen, thigh, or upper outer arm within 2 hours—consult product literature for further information. *Takhzyro*® may be self-administered or administered by a carer after appropriate training in subcutaneous injection technique.

● **PRESCRIBING AND DISPENSING INFORMATION** Lanadelumab is a biological medicine. Biological medicines must be prescribed and dispensed by brand name, see *Biological medicines* and *Biosimilar medicines*, under Guidance on prescribing p. 1; manufacturer advises to record the brand name and batch number after each administration.

● **HANDLING AND STORAGE** Manufacturer advises store in a refrigerator (2–8°C) and protect from light—consult product literature for further information regarding storage outside refrigerator.

● **PATIENT AND CARER ADVICE**

Self-administration Manufacturer advises patients and their carers should be given training in subcutaneous injection technique if appropriate.

Missed doses Manufacturer advises if a dose is missed, it should be taken as soon as possible ensuring at least 10 days between doses.

- **NATIONAL FUNDING/ACCESS DECISIONS** For full details see funding body website

NICE decisions

- **Lanadelumab for preventing recurrent attacks of hereditary angioedema (October 2019)** NICE TA606 Recommended with restrictions

Scottish Medicines Consortium (SMC) decisions

- **Lanadelumab (*Takhzyro*®) for routine prevention of recurrent attacks of hereditary angioedema (HAE) in patients aged 12 years and older (December 2019)** SMC No. SMC2206 Recommended with restrictions

- **MEDICINAL FORMS** There can be variation in the licensing of different medicines containing the same drug.

Solution for injection

EXCIPIENTS: May contain Polysorbates

- **Takhzyro** (Takeda UK Ltd)

Lanadelumab 150 mg per 1 ml Takhzyro 150mg/1ml solution for injection pre-filled syringes | 1 pre-filled disposable injection PoM £12,420.00 (Hospital only)
Takhzyro 300mg/2ml solution for injection pre-filled syringes | 1 pre-filled disposable injection PoM £12,420.00 (Hospital only)
Takhzyro 300mg/2ml solution for injection pre-filled pens | 1 pre-filled disposable injection PoM £12,420.00

DRUGS USED IN HEREDITARY ANGIOEDEMA ›

SELECTIVE BRADYKININ B_2 ANTAGONISTS

Icatibant

22-Oct-2020

- **INDICATIONS AND DOSE**

Acute attacks of hereditary angioedema in patients with C1-esterase inhibitor deficiency

- BY SUBCUTANEOUS INJECTION
- Child 2–17 years (body-weight 12 kg and above): (consult product literature)

- **CAUTIONS** Ischaemic heart disease · stroke
- **INTERACTIONS** → Appendix 1: icatibant
- **SIDE-EFFECTS**
  - **Common or very common** Dizziness · fever · headache · nausea · skin reactions
- **PREGNANCY** Manufacturer advises use only if potential benefit outweighs risk—toxicity in *animal* studies.
- **BREAST FEEDING** Manufacturer advises avoid for 12 hours after administration.
- **NATIONAL FUNDING/ACCESS DECISIONS** For full details see funding body website

Scottish Medicines Consortium (SMC) decisions

- **Icatibant (*Firazyr*®) for the symptomatic treatment of acute attacks of hereditary angioedema in adolescents and children aged 2 years and older (with C1-esterase-inhibitor deficiency) (May 2018)** SMC No. 1332/18 Recommended

All Wales Medicines Strategy Group (AWMSG) decisions

- **Icatibant acetate (*Firazyr*®) for the symptomatic treatment of acute attacks of hereditary angioedema (HAE) in adults, adolescents and children aged 2 years and older, with C1 esterase-inhibitor deficiency (June 2018)** AWMSG No. 3293 Recommended

- **MEDICINAL FORMS** There can be variation in the licensing of different medicines containing the same drug.

Solution for injection

- **Icatibant (Non-proprietary)**

Icatibant (as Icatibant acetate) 10 mg per 1 ml Icatibant 30mg/3ml solution for injection pre-filled syringes | 1 pre-filled disposable injection PoM £1,395.00 | 1 pre-filled disposable injection PoM £837.00–£1,395.00 (Hospital only) | 3 pre-filled disposable injection PoM £4,185.00 (Hospital only)

FACTOR XIIA INHIBITORS

Garadacimab

05-Nov-2025

- **DRUG ACTION** Garadacimab is a fully human recombinant monoclonal antibody which binds to factor XIIa, thereby inhibiting the kallikrein cascade and the production of bradykinin, a potent vasodilator associated with inflammation and swelling in hereditary angioedema.

- **INDICATIONS AND DOSE**

Prevention of recurrent attacks of hereditary angioedema (initiated under specialist supervision)

- BY SUBCUTANEOUS INJECTION
- Child 12–17 years: Loading dose 400 mg for 1 dose, then maintenance 200 mg every month, maintenance dose to be started 1 month after initial loading dose, consider discontinuing treatment if insufficient response after 3 months

- **CONTRA-INDICATIONS** Not a treatment for acute attacks of angioedema (initiate individualised treatment for breakthrough attacks)
- **SIDE-EFFECTS**
  - **Common or very common** Abdominal pain · headache
- **PREGNANCY** EvGr Preferable to avoid (limited or no information available; *animal* studies do not indicate toxicity). ⟨M⟩
- **BREAST FEEDING** EvGr Use only if potential benefit outweighs risk (possible risk from transfer of antibodies to infant during first few days after birth). ⟨M⟩
- **EFFECT ON LABORATORY TESTS** May decrease D-dimer concentrations—consult product literature. May increase activated partial thromboplastin time (aPTT) due to an interaction with the aPTT assay—consult product literature.
- **DIRECTIONS FOR ADMINISTRATION** Take the syringe out of the refrigerator at least 30 minutes before administration and inject into the abdomen (except for 2 cm around the navel), thigh, or upper arm (if not self-administered); rotate injection site and avoid moles and skin that is tender, bruised, injured, scarred, red, or hard. *Andembry*® may be self-administered or administered by a carer after appropriate training in subcutaneous injection technique.
- **PRESCRIBING AND DISPENSING INFORMATION** Garadacimab is a biological medicine. Biological medicines must be prescribed and dispensed by brand name, see *Biological medicines* and *Biosimilar medicines*, under Guidance on prescribing p. 1; record the brand name and batch number after each administration.
- **HANDLING AND STORAGE** Store in a refrigerator (2–8°C) and protect from light. Once removed from refrigerator, may be stored at room temperature (up to 25°C) for up to 2 months.
- **PATIENT AND CARER ADVICE**
Self-administration Patients and carers should be given training in subcutaneous injection technique if appropriate.
- **NATIONAL FUNDING/ACCESS DECISIONS** For full details see funding body website

NICE decisions

- **Garadacimab for preventing recurrent attacks of hereditary angioedema in people 12 years and over (October 2025)** NICE TA1101 Recommended with restrictions

- **MEDICINAL FORMS** There can be variation in the licensing of different medicines containing the same drug.

Solution for injection

EXCIPIENTS: May contain L-proline, polysorbates

▸ **Andembry** (CSL Behring UK Ltd) ▼

Garadacimab 167 mg per 1 ml Andembry 200mg/1.2ml solution for injection pre-filled pens | 1 pre-filled disposable injection PoM £20,625.00 (Hospital only)

3 Conditions affecting sputum viscosity

MUCOLYTICS

Carbocisteine 02-Jan-2024

- **INDICATIONS AND DOSE**

Reduction of sputum viscosity

▸ BY MOUTH

▸ Child 2–4 years: 62.5–125 mg 4 times a day

▸ Child 5–11 years: 250 mg 3 times a day

▸ Child 12–17 years: Initially 2.25 g daily in divided doses, then reduced to 1.5 g daily in divided doses, dose to be reduced as condition improves

IMPORTANT SAFETY INFORMATION

Mucodyne Paediatric® syrup 250 mg/5 mL has replaced the 125 mg/5 mL formulation—take care to ensure the appropriate dose is administered.

- **CONTRA-INDICATIONS** Active peptic ulceration
- **CAUTIONS** History of peptic ulceration (may disrupt the gastric mucosal barrier)
- **SIDE-EFFECTS** Gastrointestinal haemorrhage · skin reactions · Stevens-Johnson syndrome · vomiting
- **PREGNANCY** Manufacturer advises avoid in first trimester.
- **BREAST FEEDING** No information available.
- **PRESCRIBING AND DISPENSING INFORMATION** Flavours of oral liquid formulations may include cherry, raspberry, cinnamon, or rum.
- **MEDICINAL FORMS** There can be variation in the licensing of different medicines containing the same drug.

Oral solution

▸ **Carbocisteine (Non-proprietary)**

Carbocisteine 50 mg per 1 ml Carbocisteine 250mg/5ml oral solution sugar free | 300 ml PoM £8.39 DT = £6.16 SF
Carbocisteine 250mg/5ml oral solution | 300 ml PoM £7.55 DT = £7.55

Carbocisteine 75 mg per 1 ml Carbocisteine 750mg/10ml oral solution 10ml sachets sugar free | 15 sachet PoM £3.85 DT = £5.81 SF

Carbocisteine 150 mg per 1 ml Carbocisteine 750mg/5ml oral solution sugar free | 100 ml PoM £20.19 SF | 200 ml PoM £39.29 DT = £39.29 SF

Oral capsule

▸ **Carbocisteine (Non-proprietary)**

Carbocisteine 375 mg Carbocisteine 375mg capsules | 120 capsule PoM £18.98 DT = £2.82

Carbocisteine 750 mg Carbocisteine 750mg capsules | 60 capsule PoM £30.00 DT = £18.98

3.1 Cystic fibrosis

Cystic fibrosis 07-Aug-2024

Description of condition

Cystic fibrosis is a genetic disorder affecting the lungs, pancreas, liver, intestine, and reproductive organs. The main clinical signs are pulmonary disease, with recurrent infections and the production of copious viscous sputum, and malabsorption due to pancreatic insufficiency. Other complications include hepatobiliary disease, osteoporosis, cystic fibrosis-related diabetes, and distal intestinal obstruction syndrome.

Aims of treatment

The aim of treatment includes preventing and managing lung infections, loosening and removing thick, sticky mucus from the lungs, preventing or treating intestinal obstruction, and providing sufficient nutrition and hydration.

Lung function is a key predictor of life expectancy in people with cystic fibrosis and optimising lung function is a major aim of care.

Non-drug treatment

Specialist physiotherapists should assess patients with cystic fibrosis and provide advice on airway clearance, nebuliser use, musculoskeletal disorders, physical activity, and urinary incontinence. The importance of airway clearance techniques should be discussed with patients and their parents or carers and appropriate training provided. Patients should be advised that regular exercise improves both lung function and overall fitness.

Drug treatment

Treatment for cystic fibrosis lung disease is based on the prevention of lung infection and the maintenance of lung function. EvGr In patients with cystic fibrosis, who have clinical evidence of lung disease, the frequency of routine review should be based on their clinical condition, but children should be reviewed at least every 8 weeks. More frequent review is required immediately after diagnosis and during early life. Ⓐ

Cystic fibrosis transmembrane conductance regulator (CFTR) modulators

EvGr CFTR modulators can be used for the treatment of cystic fibrosis in certain patients (specialist use). Ⓐ

Mucolytics

EvGr Patients with cystic fibrosis who have evidence of lung disease should be offered a mucolytic. Dornase alfa p. 218 is the first choice mucolytic [unlicensed in children under 5 years of age]. If there is an inadequate response, dornase alfa p. 218 and hypertonic sodium chloride p. 728, or hypertonic sodium chloride p. 728 alone should be considered.

Mannitol dry powder for inhalation p. 164 should be considered for children [unlicensed indication] who cannot use dornase alfa p. 218 and hypertonic sodium chloride p. 728 because of ineligibility, intolerance, or inadequate response. Ⓐ

Pulmonary infection

Staphylococcus aureus

EvGr Flucloxacillin p. 424 [unlicensed indication] should be offered for prophylaxis against respiratory *Staphylococcus aureus* infection in children from the point of diagnosis up to 3 years of age. Continuing prophylaxis in children up to 6 years of age should also be considered. An alternative oral antibacterial should be given in children allergic to penicillin.

In children who are already taking prophylaxis and have a respiratory sample culture that is positive for *Staph. aureus*, prophylaxis adherence should be reviewed and antibacterial treatment started. A prophylactic antibacterial should be restarted after treatment (consult local protocol).

Patients who are not taking prophylaxis and have a new *Staph. aureus* infection can be given an oral anti-*Staph. aureus* antibacterial, if they are clinically well. If they are clinically unwell and have pulmonary disease, oral or intravenous (depending on infection severity) broad-spectrum antibacterials with activity against *Staph. aureus* should be given (consult local protocol).

A long-term antibacterial should be considered to suppress **chronic** *Staph. aureus* respiratory infection in patients whose pulmonary disease is stable. In patients with chronic *Staph. aureus* respiratory infection who become clinically unwell with pulmonary disease, oral or intravenous (depending on infection severity) broad-spectrum antibacterials with activity against *Staph. aureus* should be given. In those patients with new evidence of **meticillin-resistant *Staphylococcus aureus* (MRSA)** respiratory infection (with or without pulmonary exacerbation), specialist microbiological advice should be sought.

Antibacterials should not be routinely used to suppress chronic MRSA in patients with stable pulmonary disease.

If a patient with cystic fibrosis and chronic MRSA respiratory infection becomes unwell with a pulmonary exacerbation or shows a decline in pulmonary function, specialist microbiological advice should be sought. (A)

Pseudomonas aeruginosa

EvGr If a patient with cystic fibrosis develops a new *Pseudomonas aeruginosa* infection, eradication therapy with a course of oral antibacterial should be started (by intravenous injection, if they are clinically unwell), in combination with an inhaled antibacterial. An extended course of oral and inhaled antibacterial should follow (consult local protocol).

If eradication therapy is not successful, sustained treatment with an inhaled antibacterial should be offered. Nebulised colistimethate sodium p. 426 should be considered as first-line treatment (but see also colistimethate sodium p. 426 by dry powder inhalation National funding/access decisions).

In patients with **chronic** *Ps. aeruginosa* infection (when treatment has not eradicated the infection) who become clinically unwell with pulmonary exacerbations, an oral antibacterial or a combination of two intravenous antibacterial drugs of different classes (depending on infection severity) should be used. Changing antibacterial regimens should be considered to treat exacerbations (consult local protocol).

Nebulised aztreonam p. 408, nebulised tobramycin p. 380, or tobramycin dry powder for inhalation p. 380 [unlicensed indication in child under 6 years] (see tobramycin p. 380 National funding/access decisions) should be considered for those who are deteriorating despite regular inhaled colistimethate sodium p. 426. (A)

Burkholderia cepacia complex

EvGr Patients who develop a new *Burkholderia cepacia* complex infection, should be given eradication therapy with a combination of intravenous antibacterial drugs (specialist microbiological advice should be sought on the choice of antibacterials). (A) There is no evidence to support using antibacterials to suppress **chronic** *Burkholderia cepacia* complex infection in patients with cystic fibrosis who have stable pulmonary status.

EvGr Specialist microbiological advice should be sought for patients with chronic *Burkholderia cepacia* complex infection (when treatment has not eradicated the infection) and who become clinically unwell with a pulmonary disease exacerbation.

An inhaled antibacterial should be considered for those who have chronic *Burkholderia cepacia* complex infection and declining pulmonary status; treatment should be stopped if there is no observed benefit. (A)

Haemophilus influenzae

EvGr *Haemophilus influenzae* infection in the absence of clinical evidence of pulmonary infection should be treated with an appropriate oral antibacterial drug. In those who are unwell with clinical evidence of pulmonary infection, an appropriate antibacterial should be given by mouth or intravenously depending on the severity of the illness (consult local protocol). (A)

Non-tuberculous mycobacteria

EvGr Non-tuberculous mycobacterial eradication therapy should be considered for patients with cystic fibrosis who are clinically unwell and whose pulmonary disease has not responded to other recommended treatments. Specialist microbiological advice should be sought on the choice of antibacterial and on the duration of treatment. (A)

Aspergillus fumigatus complex

EvGr Treatment with an antifungal drug should only be considered to suppress **chronic** *Aspergillus fumigatus* complex respiratory infection in patients with declining pulmonary status. Specialist microbiological advice should be sought on the choice of antifungal drug. (A)

Unidentified infections

EvGr An oral or intravenous (depending on the exacerbation severity) broad-spectrum antibacterial should be used for patients who have a pulmonary disease exacerbation and no clear cause. If a causative pathogen is identified, an appropriate treatment should be selected (consult local protocol). (A)

Immunomodulatory drugs

EvGr Long-term treatment with azithromycin p. 402 [unlicensed indication], at an immunomodulatory dose, should be offered to patients with deteriorating lung function or repeated pulmonary exacerbations. In those patients with continued deterioration in lung function or continuing pulmonary exacerbations, azithromycin p. 402 should be discontinued and the use of an oral corticosteroid considered. (A)

Nutrition and exocrine pancreatic insufficiency

EvGr A cystic fibrosis specialist dietitian should offer advice on optimal nutrition.

Pancreatin p. 56 should be offered to patients with exocrine pancreatic insufficiency. Dose should be adjusted as needed to minimise any symptoms or signs of malabsorption (see Exocrine pancreatic insufficiency p. 56). An acid-suppressing drug, such as an H_2 receptor antagonist or a proton pump inhibitor [unlicensed indications] can be considered for patients who have persistent symptoms or signs of malabsorption. (A)

Distal intestinal obstruction syndrome

EvGr Oral or intravenous fluids should be offered to ensure adequate hydration for patients with distal intestinal obstruction syndrome. Meglumine amidotrizoate with sodium amidotrizoate solution p. 42 (orally or via an enteral tube) should be considered as first-line treatment for distal intestinal obstruction syndrome. An iso-osmotic polyethylene glycol and electrolyte solution (macrogols) (orally or via an enteral tube) can be considered as a second-line treatment. Surgery is a last resort, if prolonged treatment with a polyethylene glycol solution is not effective. Suspected distal intestinal obstruction syndrome should be managed in a specialist cystic fibrosis centre. (A)

Liver disease

EvGr If liver function blood tests are abnormal in patients with cystic fibrosis, ursodeoxycholic acid p. 72 [unlicensed indication] can be given until liver function is restored. (A)

Bone mineral density

EvGr Patients should be monitored for cystic fibrosis-related low bone mineral density. (A)

Cystic fibrosis-related diabetes

EvGr Patients should be monitored for cystic fibrosis-related diabetes. (A)

Useful Resources

Cystic fibrosis: diagnosis and management. National Institute for Health and Care Excellence. NICE guideline 78. October 2017
www.nice.org.uk/guidance/NG78

MUCOLYTICS

Deutivacaftor with tezacaftor and vanzacaftor

20-Mar-2026

- **INDICATIONS AND DOSE**

Cystic fibrosis [using tablets containing 50/20/4 mg deutivacaftor/tezacaftor/vanzacaftor] (specialist use only)

▶ BY MOUTH

▸ Child 6–11 years (body-weight up to 40 kg): 3 tablets once daily

Cystic fibrosis [using tablets containing 125/50/10 mg deutivacaftor/tezacaftor/vanzacaftor] (specialist use only)

▶ BY MOUTH

▸ Child 6–11 years (body-weight 40 kg and above): 2 tablets once daily

▸ Child 12–17 years: 2 tablets once daily

DOSE ADJUSTMENTS DUE TO INTERACTIONS

▸ EvGr *For children aged* 6–11 *years (body-weight up to* 40 *kg)*, with concurrent use of potent CYP3A4 inhibitors reduce dose to 2 *tablets* of 50/20/4 mg once a week.

▸ *For children aged* 6–11 *years (body-weight up to* 40 *kg)*, with concurrent use of moderate CYP3A4 inhibitors reduce dose to 2 *tablets* of 50/20/4 mg on alternate days.

▸ *For children aged* 6–11 *years (body-weight* 40 *kg and above)*, with concurrent use of potent CYP3A4 inhibitors reduce dose to 1 *tablet* of 125/50/10 mg once a week.

▸ *For children aged* 6–11 *years (body-weight* 40 *kg and above)*, with concurrent use of moderate CYP3A4 inhibitors reduce dose to 1 *tablet* of 125/50/10 mg on alternate days.

▸ *For children aged* 12–17 *years*, with concurrent use of potent CYP3A4 inhibitors reduce dose to 1 *tablet* of 125/50/10 mg once a week.

▸ *For children aged* 12–17 *years*, with concurrent use of moderate CYP3A4 inhibitors reduce dose to 1 *tablet* of 125/50/10 mg on alternate days. (M)

DOSE EQUIVALENCE AND CONVERSION

▸ Dose expressed as *x/y/z* mg of deutivacaftor/tezacaftor/vanzacaftor.

- **INTERACTIONS** → Appendix 1: deutivacaftor · tezacaftor · vanzacaftor
- **SIDE-EFFECTS**

▶ **Common or very common** Diarrhoea · headache · rash

SIDE-EFFECTS, FURTHER INFORMATION Manufacturer advises interrupt treatment if transaminase levels more than 5 times the upper limit of normal *or* transaminase levels more than 3 times the upper limit of normal **and** blood bilirubin more than twice the upper limit of normal—consult product literature.

- **PREGNANCY** EvGr Avoid unless potential benefit outweighs risk (limited information available). (M)
- **BREAST FEEDING** EvGr Avoid (present in milk in *animal* studies). (M)
- **HEPATIC IMPAIRMENT** EvGr Avoid in severe impairment; use with caution only if benefit outweighs risk in moderate impairment (limited information available). (M)
- **RENAL IMPAIRMENT** EvGr Use with caution in severe impairment or end-stage renal disease (no information available). (M)
- **MONITORING REQUIREMENTS**

▶ EvGr Monitor liver function before treatment, every 3 months during the first year of treatment, then annually thereafter (more frequent monitoring should be considered in patients with a history of liver disease or transaminase elevations).

▶ Baseline and follow-up ophthalmic examinations are recommended. (M)

- **DIRECTIONS FOR ADMINISTRATION** EvGr *Tablets* should be taken with fat-containing food. (M)
- **PATIENT AND CARER ADVICE**

Missed doses If a dose is more than 6 hours late, the missed dose should not be taken and the next dose should be taken at the normal time.

- **NATIONAL FUNDING/ACCESS DECISIONS**

For full details see funding body website

NICE decisions

▶ **Vanzacaftor-tezacaftor-deutivacaftor for treating cystic fibrosis with 1 or more F508del mutations in the CFTR gene in people 6 years and over (July 2025)** NICE TA1085 Recommended

Scottish Medicines Consortium (SMC) decisions

▶ **Vanzacaftor/tezacaftor/deutivacaftor (*Alyftrek*®) for the treatment of cystic fibrosis in people aged 6 years and older who have at least one F508del mutation or another responsive mutation in the cystic fibrosis transmembrane conductance regulator gene (March 2026)** SMC No. SMC2800 Recommended with restrictions

- **MEDICINAL FORMS** There can be variation in the licensing of different medicines containing the same drug.

Oral tablet

▸ **Alyftrek** (Vertex Pharmaceuticals (Europe) Ltd) ▼

Vanzacaftor (as Vanzacaftor calcium dihydrate) 4 mg, Tezacaftor 20 mg, Deutivacaftor 50 mg Alyftrek 50mg/20mg/4mg tablets | 84 tablet PoM £16,110.00 (Hospital only)

Vanzacaftor (as Vanzacaftor calcium dihydrate) 10 mg, Tezacaftor 50 mg, Deutivacaftor 125 mg Alyftrek 125mg/50mg/10mg tablets | 56 tablet PoM £16,110.00 (Hospital only)

Dornase alfa

17-Aug-2020

(Phosphorylated glycosylated recombinant human deoxyribonuclease 1 (rhDNase))

- **DRUG ACTION** Dornase alfa is a genetically engineered version of a naturally occurring human enzyme which cleaves extracellular deoxyribonucleic acid (DNA).

- **INDICATIONS AND DOSE**

Management of cystic fibrosis patients with a forced vital capacity (FVC) of greater than 40% of predicted to improve pulmonary function

▶ BY INHALATION OF NEBULISED SOLUTION

▸ Child 5–17 years: 2500 units once daily, administered by jet nebuliser

DOSE EQUIVALENCE AND CONVERSION

▸ Dornase alfa 1000 units is equivalent to 1 mg.

- **SIDE-EFFECTS** Chest pain · conjunctivitis · dyspepsia · dysphonia · dyspnoea · fever · increased risk of infection · skin reactions
- **PREGNANCY** No evidence of teratogenicity; manufacturer advises use only if potential benefit outweighs risk.
- **BREAST FEEDING** Amount probably too small to be harmful—manufacturer advises caution.
- **DIRECTIONS FOR ADMINISTRATION** Dornase alfa is administered undiluted by inhalation using a jet nebuliser; ultrasonic nebulisers are unsuitable. Expert sources advise usually once daily at least 1 hour before physiotherapy.
- **PRESCRIBING AND DISPENSING INFORMATION** Not all children benefit from treatment with dornase alfa; improvement occurs within 2 weeks, but in more severely affected children a trial of 6–12 weeks may be required.
- **PATIENT AND CARER ADVICE**
Medicines for Children leaflet: Dornase alfa for cystic fibrosis www.medicinesforchildren.org.uk/medicines/dornase-alfa-for-cystic-fibrosis/

- **MEDICINAL FORMS** There can be variation in the licensing of different medicines containing the same drug.

Nebuliser liquid

- Pulmozyme (Roche Products Ltd)
Dornase alfa 1 mg per 1 ml Pulmozyme 2.5mg nebuliser liquid 2.5ml ampoules | 30 ampoule PoM £496.43 DT = £496.43

Ivacaftor

06-Aug-2024

- **DRUG ACTION** Ivacaftor is a cystic fibrosis transmembrane conductance regulator (CFTR) protein potentiator that increases chloride transport in the abnormal CFTR protein.

- **INDICATIONS AND DOSE**

Cystic fibrosis (specialist use only)

- BY MOUTH USING GRANULES
- Child 1-2 months (body-weight 3 kg and above): 13.4 mg every 12 hours
- Child 3-5 months (body-weight 3 kg and above): 25 mg every 12 hours
- Child 6 months-17 years (body-weight 5-6 kg): 25 mg every 12 hours
- Child 6 months-17 years (body-weight 7-13 kg): 50 mg every 12 hours
- Child 6 months-17 years (body-weight 14-24 kg): 75 mg every 12 hours
- Child 6-17 years (body-weight 25 kg and above): Use tablets

Cystic fibrosis (specialist use only)

- BY MOUTH USING TABLETS
- Child 6-17 years (body-weight 25 kg and above): 150 mg every 12 hours

DOSE ADJUSTMENTS DUE TO INTERACTIONS

- EvGr *For tablets,* reduce dose to 150 mg twice a week with concurrent use of potent CYP3A4 inhibitors; the evening dose of ivacaftor should not be taken.
- *For tablets,* reduce dose to 150 mg once daily with concurrent use of moderate CYP3A4 inhibitors; the evening dose of ivacaftor should not be taken.
- *For children aged* 1–3 *months,* avoid concurrent use of potent and moderate CYP3A4 inhibitors.
- *For children aged* 4–5 *months (body-weight* 3 *kg and above),* if the benefit of concurrent use with a potent or moderate CYP3A4 inhibitor outweighs the risk, reduce dose of *granules* to 25 mg twice weekly or less frequently, adjust dosing interval according to clinical response and tolerability; the evening dose of ivacaftor should not be taken.
- *For children aged* 6 *months to* 17 *years (body-weight* 5–6 *kg),* reduce dose of *granules* to 25 mg twice weekly with concurrent use of potent CYP3A4 inhibitors; the evening dose of ivacaftor should not be taken.
- *For children aged* 6 *months to* 17 *years (body-weight* 7–13 *kg),* reduce dose of *granules* to 50 mg twice weekly with concurrent use of potent CYP3A4 inhibitors; the evening dose of ivacaftor should not be taken.
- *For children aged* 6 *months to* 17 *years (body-weight* 14–24 *kg),* reduce dose of *granules* to 75 mg twice weekly with concurrent use of potent CYP3A4 inhibitors; the evening dose of ivacaftor should not be taken.
- *For children aged* 6 *months to* 17 *years,* reduce dose frequency of *granules* to once daily with concurrent use of moderate CYP3A4 inhibitors; the evening dose of ivacaftor should not be taken. Ⓜ

IMPORTANT SAFETY INFORMATION

MHRA/CHM ADVICE: IVACAFTOR, TEZACAFTOR, ELEXACAFTOR (*KAFTRIO*®) IN COMBINATION WITH IVACAFTOR (*KALYDECO*®): RISK OF SERIOUS LIVER INJURY; UPDATED ADVICE ON LIVER FUNCTION TESTING (FEBRUARY 2022)

A European review of safety data identified a case of liver failure requiring transplantation in an adult patient, with pre-existing cirrhosis and portal hypertension, taking ivacaftor/tezacaftor/elexacaftor (*Kaftrio*®) in combination with ivacaftor (*Kalydeco*®). Other cases of serious liver injury, characterised by elevations in alanine aminotransferase (ALT), aspartate aminotransferase (AST), and total bilirubin, were also identified in 2 adult patients, with no history of liver disease, taking this combination.

Healthcare professionals are advised to:

- measure total bilirubin levels in addition to ALT and AST levels before initiating treatment, every 3 months during the first year of treatment, and annually thereafter; more frequent monitoring should be considered in patients with a history of liver disease or transaminase elevations;
- use with caution and close monitoring in patients with advanced pre-existing liver disease, and only if the benefits outweigh the risks;
- promptly evaluate and measure liver function in patients who report symptoms that may indicate liver injury;
- discontinue treatment if significant elevation of liver enzymes occurs (see *Side-effects*), or signs and symptoms of liver injury develop; once liver abnormalities have resolved, consider the benefits and risks before resuming treatment.

Patients and carers should be counselled to seek immediate medical advice if signs of liver problems develop.

- **CAUTIONS** Organ transplantation (no information available)
- **INTERACTIONS** → Appendix 1: ivacaftor
- **SIDE-EFFECTS**
- **Common or very common** Breast abnormalities · diarrhoea · dizziness · ear discomfort · flatulence · gastrointestinal discomfort · headache · hypoglycaemia · increased risk of infection · nasal complaints · nausea · oropharyngeal pain · ototoxicity · respiratory disorders · skin reactions · throat erythema · tympanic membrane hyperaemia
- **Uncommon** Gynaecomastia
- **Frequency not known** Cataract · hepatic disorders

SIDE-EFFECTS, FURTHER INFORMATION Manufacturer advises interrupt treatment if transaminase levels more than 5 times the upper limit of normal *or* transaminase levels more than 3 times the upper limit of normal **and** blood bilirubin more than twice the upper limit of normal—consult product literature.

3 Respiratory system

- **PREGNANCY** Manufacturer advises avoid—limited information available.
- **BREAST FEEDING** Manufacturer advises avoid—present in milk in *animal* studies.
- **HEPATIC IMPAIRMENT** EvGr *For children aged* 1–3 *months (body-weight* 3 *kg and above),* avoid in all degrees of impairment.

  For children aged 4–5 *months (body-weight* 3 *kg and above),* avoid unless benefit outweighs risk in all degrees of impairment (variability in hepatic metabolism).

  For children aged 6 *months to* 17 *years,* avoid unless benefit outweighs risk in severe impairment (risk of increased exposure–serious liver injury reported). ⟨M⟩

  Dose adjustments EvGr *For tablets,* reduce dose to 150 mg once daily in moderate impairment; in severe impairment reduce starting dose to 150 mg on alternate days or less frequently, adjust dosing interval according to clinical response and tolerability. The evening dose of ivacaftor should not be taken.

  For children aged 4–5 *months (body-weight* 3 *kg and above),* reduce dose of *granules* to 25 mg once daily or less frequently in moderate to severe impairment, adjust dosing interval according to clinical response and tolerability.

  For children aged 6 *months to* 17 *years (body-weight* 5–6 *kg),* reduce dose of *granules* to 25 mg once daily (omit evening dose) in moderate impairment; in severe impairment, reduce starting dose to 25 mg on alternate days, adjust dosing interval according to clinical response and tolerability.

  For children aged 6 *months to* 17 *years (body-weight* 7–13 *kg),* reduce dose of *granules* to 50 mg once daily (omit evening dose) in moderate impairment; in severe impairment, reduce starting dose to 50 mg on alternate days, adjust dosing interval according to clinical response and tolerability.

  For children aged 6 *months to* 17 *years (body-weight* 14–24 *kg),* reduce dose of *granules* to 75 mg once daily (omit evening dose) in moderate impairment; in severe impairment, reduce starting dose to 75 mg on alternate days, adjust dosing interval according to clinical response and tolerability. ⟨M⟩
- **RENAL IMPAIRMENT** Manufacturer advises caution in severe impairment or end-stage renal disease—limited information available.
- **MONITORING REQUIREMENTS**
  - EvGr Monitor liver function before treatment, every 3 months during the first year of treatment, then annually thereafter (more frequent monitoring should be considered in patients with a history of liver disease or transaminase elevations).
  - Baseline and follow-up ophthalmic examinations are advised in children. ⟨M⟩
- **DIRECTIONS FOR ADMINISTRATION** EvGr *Tablets* should be taken with fat-containing food.

  Granules should be mixed into 5 mL of soft food or liquid (at room temperature or below) and consumed immediately; if not immediately consumed, the mixture should be ingested within one hour. Fat-containing food should be consumed just before or after the dose is taken. ⟨M⟩
- **PRESCRIBING AND DISPENSING INFORMATION** Ivacaftor should be prescribed by a physician experienced in the treatment of cystic fibrosis.
- **PATIENT AND CARER ADVICE**

  Missed doses EvGr If a dose is more than 6 hours late, the missed dose should not be taken and the next dose should be taken at the normal time. ⟨M⟩

  Driving and skilled tasks EvGr Patients and their carers should be counselled on the effects on driving and skilled tasks—increased risk of dizziness. ⟨M⟩
- **MEDICINAL FORMS** There can be variation in the licensing of different medicines containing the same drug.

Oral tablet

CAUTIONARY AND ADVISORY LABELS 25

- **Kalydeco** (Vertex Pharmaceuticals (Europe) Ltd)

  Ivacaftor 75 mg Kalydeco 75mg tablets | 28 tablet PoM £7,000.00 (Hospital only)

  Ivacaftor 150 mg Kalydeco 150mg tablets | 28 tablet PoM £7,000.00 (Hospital only) | 56 tablet PoM £14,000.00 (Hospital only)

Oral granules

- **Kalydeco** (Vertex Pharmaceuticals (Europe) Ltd)

  Ivacaftor 13.4 mg Kalydeco 13.4mg granules sachets | 56 sachet PoM £14,000.00 (Hospital only) SF

  Ivacaftor 25 mg Kalydeco 25mg granules sachets | 56 sachet PoM £14,000.00 (Hospital only) SF

  Ivacaftor 50 mg Kalydeco 50mg granules sachets | 56 sachet PoM £14,000.00 (Hospital only) SF

  Ivacaftor 59.5 mg Kalydeco 59.5mg granules sachets | 28 sachet PoM £7,000.00 (Hospital only) SF

  Ivacaftor 75 mg Kalydeco 75mg granules sachets | 28 sachet PoM £7,000.00 (Hospital only) SF | 56 sachet PoM £14,000.00 (Hospital only) SF

Ivacaftor with tezacaftor and elexacaftor

09-May-2025

The properties listed below are those particular to the combination only. For the properties of the components please consider, ivacaftor p. 219, tezacaftor with ivacaftor p. 223.

- **INDICATIONS AND DOSE**

Cystic fibrosis (in combination with ivacaftor) [using tablets containing 37.5/25/50 mg ivacaftor/tezacaftor/elexacaftor] (specialist use only)

▶ BY MOUTH

- Child 6–11 years (body-weight up to 30 kg): 2 tablets, to be taken in the morning and, *Ivacaftor* 75 mg to be taken in the evening (about 12 hours apart)

Cystic fibrosis (in combination with ivacaftor) [using tablets containing 75/50/100 mg ivacaftor/tezacaftor/elexacaftor] (specialist use only)

▶ BY MOUTH

- Child 6–11 years (body-weight 30 kg and above): 2 tablets, to be taken in the morning and, *Ivacaftor* 150 mg to be taken in the evening (about 12 hours apart)
- Child 12–17 years: 2 tablets, to be taken in the morning and, *Ivacaftor* 150 mg to be taken in the evening (about 12 hours apart)

Cystic fibrosis (in combination with ivacaftor) [using granules containing 60/40/80 mg ivacaftor/tezacaftor/elexacaftor] (specialist use only)

▶ BY MOUTH

- Child 2–5 years (body-weight up to 14 kg): 1 sachet, to be taken in the morning and, *Ivacaftor* 59.5 mg sachet to be taken in the evening (about 12 hours apart)

Cystic fibrosis (in combination with ivacaftor) [using granules containing 75/50/100 mg ivacaftor/tezacaftor/elexacaftor] (specialist use only)

▶ BY MOUTH

- Child 2–5 years (body-weight 14 kg and above): 1 sachet, to be taken in the morning and, *Ivacaftor* 75 mg sachet to be taken in the evening (about 12 hours apart)

DOSE ADJUSTMENTS DUE TO INTERACTIONS

- EvGr With concurrent use of potent CYP3A4 inhibitors, reduce dose to 2 *tablets* or 1 sachet of *granules* twice a week, taken approximately 3–4 days apart; the evening dose of ivacaftor should not be taken.
- With concurrent use of moderate CYP3A4 inhibitors, reduce dose to 2 *tablets* or 1 sachet of *granules* every other morning, with ivacaftor taken in the mornings

alternate to ivacaftor/tezacaftor/elexacaftor; the evening dose of ivacaftor should not be taken. ⟨M⟩

IMPORTANT SAFETY INFORMATION

MHRA/CHM ADVICE: IVACAFTOR, TEZACAFTOR, ELEXACAFTOR (*KAFTRIO*®) IN COMBINATION WITH IVACAFTOR (*KALYDECO*®): RISK OF SERIOUS LIVER INJURY; UPDATED ADVICE ON LIVER FUNCTION TESTING (FEBRUARY 2022)

A European review of safety data identified a case of liver failure requiring transplantation in an adult patient, with pre-existing cirrhosis and portal hypertension, taking ivacaftor/tezacaftor/elexacaftor (*Kaftrio*®) in combination with ivacaftor (*Kalydeco*®). Other cases of serious liver injury, characterised by elevations in alanine aminotransferase (ALT), aspartate aminotransferase (AST), and total bilirubin, were also identified in 2 adult patients, with no history of liver disease, taking this combination.

Healthcare professionals are advised to:

- measure total bilirubin levels in addition to ALT and AST levels before initiating treatment, every 3 months during the first year of treatment, and annually thereafter; more frequent monitoring should be considered in patients with a history of liver disease or transaminase elevations;
- use with caution and close monitoring in patients with advanced pre-existing liver disease, and only if the benefits outweigh the risks;
- promptly evaluate and measure liver function in patients who report symptoms that may indicate liver injury;
- discontinue treatment if significant elevation of liver enzymes occurs (see *Side-effects* of ivacaftor p. 219), or signs and symptoms of liver injury develop; once liver abnormalities have resolved, consider the benefits and risks before resuming treatment.

Patients and carers should be counselled to seek immediate medical advice if signs of liver problems develop.

MHRA/CHM ADVICE: *KAFTRIO*® (IVACAFTOR, TEZACAFTOR, ELEXACAFTOR): RISK OF PSYCHOLOGICAL SIDE EFFECTS (MAY 2025)

The MHRA and CHM have advised that there is a small increase in risk of psychological side-effects associated with *Kaftrio*® in a minority of patients. However, this risk may also be related to patients adjusting to improvements in their physical health and quality of life from taking *Kaftrio*®. Additionally, patients with life-limiting conditions, such as cystic fibrosis, are already at increased risk of developing poor mental health.

Healthcare professionals are advised to counsel patients and carers:

- to be alert to the development of psychological side-effects (e.g. anxiety, low mood, sleep disturbance, poor concentration, or forgetfulness), which usually occur within the first 3 months of treatment;
- that these side-effects may manifest as persistent changes in behaviour, such as being more disruptive or difficult to manage;
- that these symptoms may be short-lived for many patients, but some patients will continue to experience them whilst taking *Kaftrio*®;
- to seek prompt medical advice if they notice signs or symptoms of psychological side-effects.

Healthcare professionals should also discuss the benefit-risk balance of *Kaftrio*® treatment with patients and carers, and consider treatment discontinuation if these signs or symptoms develop.

● **INTERACTIONS** → Appendix 1: elexacaftor · ivacaftor · tezacaftor

● **SIDE-EFFECTS**

▶ **Common or very common** Breast abnormalities · diarrhoea · dizziness · ear discomfort · flatulence · gastrointestinal discomfort · headache · hypoglycaemia · increased risk of infection · nasal complaints · nausea · oropharyngeal pain · ototoxicity · respiratory disorders · skin reactions · throat erythema · tympanic membrane hyperaemia

▶ **Uncommon** Gynaecomastia

▶ **Frequency not known** Anxiety · behaviour abnormal · cataract · concentration impaired · depressed mood · liver injury · memory impairment · mood altered · sleep disorder

SIDE-EFFECTS, FURTHER INFORMATION Manufacturer advises interrupt treatment if transaminase levels more than 5 times the upper limit of normal *or* transaminase levels more than 3 times the upper limit of normal **and** blood bilirubin more than twice the upper limit of normal—consult product literature.

● **HEPATIC IMPAIRMENT** EvGr Avoid in severe impairment; use with caution only if benefit outweighs risk in moderate impairment (risk of increased exposure–serious liver injury reported). ⟨M⟩

Dose adjustments EvGr In moderate impairment, alternate dose between 1 and 2 *tablets* in the mornings, and omit evening dose of ivacaftor.

In moderate impairment, reduce dose to 1 sachet of *granules* daily on days 1–3, omit dose on day 4, 1 sachet daily on days 5–6, omit dose on day 7, and omit every evening dose of ivacaftor; repeat weekly. ⟨M⟩

● **DIRECTIONS FOR ADMINISTRATION** EvGr *Tablets* and *granules* should be taken with fat-containing food. The contents of each sachet of *granules* should be mixed with 1 teaspoon (5 mL) of soft food or liquid (e.g. puréed fruits, yoghurt, milk, or juice), at room temperature or below, and consumed within an hour. ⟨M⟩

● **PATIENT AND CARER ADVICE**

Missed doses Manufacturer advises if the morning dose is more than 6 hours late, the missed dose should be taken and the evening dose of ivacaftor omitted; the next morning dose should be taken at the normal time. If the evening dose of ivacaftor is more than 6 hours late, the missed dose should **not** be taken and the next morning dose should be taken at the normal time.

● **NATIONAL FUNDING/ACCESS DECISIONS**

For full details see funding body website

NICE decisions

▶ **Ivacaftor–tezacaftor–elexacaftor, tezacaftor–ivacaftor and lumacaftor–ivacaftor for treating cystic fibrosis (July 2024)** NICE TA988 Recommended

Scottish Medicines Consortium (SMC) decisions

▶ **Ivacaftor with tezacaftor and elexacaftor (*Kaftrio*®) in combination with ivacaftor for the treatment of cystic fibrosis in patients aged 2 years and older who have at least one F508del mutation in the cystic fibrosis transmembrane conductance regulator gene (July 2024)** SMC No. SMC2713 Recommended

● **MEDICINAL FORMS** There can be variation in the licensing of different medicines containing the same drug.

Oral tablet

CAUTIONARY AND ADVISORY LABELS 25

▶ **Kaftrio** (Vertex Pharmaceuticals (Europe) Ltd)

Tezacaftor 25 mg, Ivacaftor 37.5 mg, Elexacaftor 50 mg Kaftrio 37.5mg/25mg/50mg tablets | 56 tablet PoM £8,346.30 (Hospital only)

Tezacaftor 50 mg, Ivacaftor 75 mg, Elexacaftor 100 mg Kaftrio 75mg/50mg/100mg tablets | 56 tablet PoM £8,346.30 (Hospital only)

Oral granules

▶ **Ivacaftor with tezacaftor and elexacaftor (Non-proprietary)**

Tezacaftor 40 mg, Ivacaftor 60 mg, Elexacaftor 80 mg Kaftrio 60mg/40mg/80mg granules sachets | 28 sachet PoM £8,346.30 (Hospital only) SF

Tezacaftor 50 mg, Ivacaftor 75 mg, Elexacaftor 100 mg Kaftrio 75mg/50mg/100mg granules sachets | 28 sachet PoM £8,346.30 (Hospital only) SF

Lumacaftor with ivacaftor

12-Aug-2024

The properties listed below are those particular to the combination only. For the properties of the components please consider, ivacaftor p. 219.

- **INDICATIONS AND DOSE**

Cystic fibrosis (specialist use only)

▶ BY MOUTH USING GRANULES
- Child 12–23 months (body-weight 7–8 kg): 75/94 mg every 12 hours
- Child 12–23 months (body-weight 9–13 kg): 100/125 mg every 12 hours
- Child 12–23 months (body-weight 14 kg and above): 150/188 mg every 12 hours
- Child 2–5 years (body-weight up to 14 kg): 100/125 mg every 12 hours
- Child 2–5 years (body-weight 14 kg and above): 150/188 mg every 12 hours

▶ BY MOUTH USING TABLETS
- Child 6–11 years: 200/250 mg every 12 hours
- Child 12–17 years: 400/250 mg every 12 hours

DOSE ADJUSTMENTS DUE TO INTERACTIONS
- EvGr *For children aged 12–23 months (body-weight 7–8 kg)*, reduce initial dose to 75/94 mg on alternate days for the first week in those already taking a potent CYP3A4 inhibitor.
- *For children aged 12–23 months (body-weight 9–13 kg)*, reduce initial dose to 100/125 mg on alternate days for the first week in those already taking a potent CYP3A4 inhibitor.
- *For children aged 12–23 months (body-weight 14 kg and above)*, reduce initial dose to 150/188 mg on alternate days for the first week in those already taking a potent CYP3A4 inhibitor.
- *For children aged 2–5 years (body-weight up to 14 kg)*, reduce initial dose to 100/125 mg on alternate days for the first week in those already taking a potent CYP3A4 inhibitor.
- *For children aged 2–5 years (body-weight 14 kg and above)*, reduce initial dose to 150/188 mg on alternate days for the first week in those already taking a potent CYP3A4 inhibitor.
- *For children aged 6–11 years*, reduce initial dose to 100/125 mg once daily for the first week in those already taking a potent CYP3A4 inhibitor.
- *For children aged 12–17 years*, reduce initial dose to 200/125 mg once daily for the first week in those already taking a potent CYP3A4 inhibitor. (M)

DOSE EQUIVALENCE AND CONVERSION
- Dose expressed as *x*/*y* mg of lumacaftor/ivacaftor.

- **CAUTIONS** Forced expiratory volume in 1 second (FEV_1) less than 40% of the predicted normal value—additional monitoring recommended at initiation of treatment · pulmonary exacerbation—no information available
- **INTERACTIONS** → Appendix 1: ivacaftor · lumacaftor
- **SIDE-EFFECTS**

▶ **Common or very common** Breast abnormalities · diarrhoea · dizziness · dyspnoea · ear discomfort · flatulence · gastrointestinal discomfort · headache · increased risk of infection · menstrual cycle irregularities · nasal complaints · nausea · oropharyngeal pain · ototoxicity · productive cough · rash · respiratory disorders · sputum increased · throat erythema · tympanic membrane hyperaemia · vomiting

▶ **Uncommon** Gynaecomastia · hepatic encephalopathy · hepatitis cholestatic · hypertension

▶ **Frequency not known** Cataract

SIDE-EFFECTS, FURTHER INFORMATION Manufacturer advises interrupt treatment if transaminase levels more than 5 times the upper limit of normal *or* transaminase levels more than 3 times the upper limit of normal **and** blood bilirubin more than twice the upper limit of normal—consult product literature.

- **HEPATIC IMPAIRMENT** EvGr Use with caution only if benefit outweighs risk in severe impairment (risk of increased exposure–serious liver injury reported). (M)

Dose adjustments EvGr *For children aged 12–23 months (body-weight 7–8 kg)*, omit evening dose on alternate days in moderate impairment; in severe impairment, reduce dose to 75/94 mg every 24 hours or less frequently.

For children aged 12–23 months (body-weight 9–13 kg), omit evening dose on alternate days in moderate impairment; in severe impairment, reduce dose to 100/125 mg every 24 hours or less frequently.

For children aged 12–23 months (body-weight 14 kg and above), omit evening dose on alternate days in moderate impairment; in severe impairment, reduce dose to 150/188 mg every 24 hours or less frequently.

For children aged 2–5 years (body-weight up to 14 kg), omit evening dose on alternate days in moderate impairment; in severe impairment, reduce dose to 100/125 mg every 24 hours or less frequently.

For children aged 2–5 years (body-weight 14 kg and above), omit evening dose on alternate days in moderate impairment; in severe impairment, reduce dose to 150/188 mg every 24 hours or less frequently.

For children aged 6–11 years, reduce evening dose to 100/125 mg in moderate impairment; in severe impairment, reduce dose to 100/125 mg every 12 hours or less frequently.

For children aged 12–17 years, reduce evening dose to 200/125 mg in moderate impairment; in severe impairment, reduce dose to 200/125 mg every 12 hours or less frequently. (M)

- **PRE-TREATMENT SCREENING** If the patient's genotype is unknown, a validated genotyping method should be performed to confirm the presence of the F508del mutation on both alleles of the CFTR gene before starting treatment.
- **MONITORING REQUIREMENTS** Manufacturer advises monitor blood pressure periodically during treatment.
- **EFFECT ON LABORATORY TESTS** False positive urine screening tests for tetrahydrocannabinol have been reported—manufacturer advises consider alternative confirmatory method.
- **DIRECTIONS FOR ADMINISTRATION** Manufacturer advises *tablets* and *granules* should be taken with fat-containing food. For *granules*, the contents of each sachet should be mixed with 1 teaspoon (5 mL) of soft food or liquid (e.g. puréed fruits, yoghurt, milk, or juice), at room temperature or below, and consumed within an hour.
- **PATIENT AND CARER ADVICE**

Missed doses If a dose is more than 6 hours late, the missed dose should not be taken and the next dose should be taken at the normal time.

- **NATIONAL FUNDING/ACCESS DECISIONS**

For full details see funding body website

NICE decisions

▶ **Ivacaftor-tezacaftor-elexacaftor, tezacaftor-ivacaftor and lumacaftor-ivacaftor for treating cystic fibrosis (July 2024)** NICE TA988 Recommended

Scottish Medicines Consortium (SMC) decisions

▶ **Lumacaftor with ivacaftor (*Orkambi*®) for the treatment of cystic fibrosis in patients aged 1 year and older who are homozygous for the F508del mutation in the cystic fibrosis**

transmembrane conductance regulator gene (July 2024)
SMC No. SMC2712 Recommended

- **MEDICINAL FORMS** There can be variation in the licensing of different medicines containing the same drug.

Oral tablet

CAUTIONARY AND ADVISORY LABELS 25

EXCIPIENTS: May contain Propylene glycol

- **Orkambi** (Vertex Pharmaceuticals (Europe) Ltd)
  Lumacaftor 100 mg, Ivacaftor 125 mg Orkambi 100mg/125mg tablets | 112 tablet [PoM] £8,000.00 (Hospital only)
  Ivacaftor 125 mg, Lumacaftor 200 mg Orkambi 200mg/125mg tablets | 112 tablet [PoM] £8,000.00 (Hospital only)

Tezacaftor with ivacaftor

01-Aug-2024

The properties listed below are those particular to the combination only. For the properties of the components please consider, ivacaftor p. 219.

- **INDICATIONS AND DOSE**

Cystic fibrosis (in combination with ivacaftor) (specialist use only)

- BY MOUTH
- Child 6–11 years (body-weight up to 30 kg): 50/75 mg, to be taken in the morning and, *Ivacaftor* 75 mg to be taken in the evening (about 12 hours apart)
- Child 6–11 years (body-weight 30 kg and above): 100/150 mg, to be taken in the morning and, *Ivacaftor* 150 mg to be taken in the evening (about 12 hours apart)
- Child 12–17 years: 100/150 mg, to be taken in the morning and, *Ivacaftor* 150 mg to be taken in the evening (about 12 hours apart)

DOSE ADJUSTMENTS DUE TO INTERACTIONS

- [EvGr] *For children aged* 6 –11 *years (body-weight up to* 30 *kg)*, with concurrent use of potent CYP3A4 inhibitors, reduce dose to 50/75 mg tezacaftor/ivacaftor twice a week, taken approximately 3–4 days apart; the evening dose of ivacaftor should not be taken. With concurrent use of moderate CYP3A4 inhibitors, reduce dose to 50/75 mg tezacaftor/ivacaftor every other morning, with ivacaftor 75 mg taken in the mornings alternate to tezacaftor/ivacaftor; the evening dose of ivacaftor should not be taken.
- *For children aged* 6 –17 *years (body-weight* 30 *kg and above)*, with concurrent use of potent CYP3A4 inhibitors, reduce dose to 100/150 mg tezacaftor/ivacaftor twice a week, taken approximately 3–4 days apart; the evening dose of ivacaftor should not be taken. With concurrent use of moderate CYP3A4 inhibitors, reduce dose to 100/150 mg tezacaftor/ivacaftor every other morning, with ivacaftor 150 mg taken in the mornings alternate to tezacaftor/ivacaftor; the evening dose of ivacaftor should not be taken. ⟨M⟩

DOSE EQUIVALENCE AND CONVERSION

- Combination dose expressed as *x*/*y* mg of tezacaftor/ivacaftor.

- **INTERACTIONS** → Appendix 1: ivacaftor · tezacaftor
- **SIDE-EFFECTS**
- **Common or very common** Abdominal pain · breast abnormalities · diarrhoea · dizziness · ear discomfort · headache · increased risk of infection · nasal congestion · nausea · oropharyngeal pain · ototoxicity · rash · sinus congestion · throat erythema · tympanic membrane hyperaemia
- **Uncommon** Gynaecomastia
- **Frequency not known** Hepatic function abnormal · lens opacity

SIDE-EFFECTS, FURTHER INFORMATION Manufacturer advises interrupt treatment if transaminase levels more than 5 times the upper limit of normal *or* transaminase levels more than 3 times the upper limit of normal **and** blood bilirubin more than twice the upper limit of normal—consult product literature.

- **HEPATIC IMPAIRMENT** [EvGr] Use with caution only if benefit outweighs risk in severe impairment (risk of increased exposure—serious liver injury reported). ⟨M⟩
  Dose adjustments [EvGr] Omit evening dose of ivacaftor in moderate or severe impairment; in severe impairment, tezacaftor/ivacaftor should be taken once daily or less frequently, adjust dosing interval according to clinical response and tolerability. ⟨M⟩
- **DIRECTIONS FOR ADMINISTRATION** [EvGr] Doses should be taken with fat-containing food. ⟨M⟩
- **PATIENT AND CARER ADVICE**
  Missed doses Manufacturer advises if a dose is more than 6 hours late, the missed dose should not be taken and the next dose should be taken at the normal time.
- **NATIONAL FUNDING/ACCESS DECISIONS**
  For full details see funding body website

NICE decisions

- **Ivacaftor–tezacaftor–elexacaftor, tezacaftor–ivacaftor and lumacaftor–ivacaftor for treating cystic fibrosis (July 2024)** NICE TA988 Recommended

Scottish Medicines Consortium (SMC) decisions

- **Tezacaftor with ivacaftor (*Symkevi*®) in combination with ivacaftor for the treatment of patients with cystic fibrosis aged 6 years and older who are homozygous for the F508del mutation or who are heterozygous for the F508del mutation and have one of the following mutations in the cystic fibrosis transmembrane conductance regulator gene: P67L, R117C, L206W, R352Q, A455E, D579G, 711+3A→G, S945L, S977F, R1070W, D1152H, 2789+5G→A, 3272-26A→G, and 3849 +10kbC→T (July 2024)** SMC No. SMC2711 Recommended

- **MEDICINAL FORMS** There can be variation in the licensing of different medicines containing the same drug.

Oral tablet

CAUTIONARY AND ADVISORY LABELS 25

- **Symkevi** (Vertex Pharmaceuticals (Europe) Ltd)
  Tezacaftor 50 mg, Ivacaftor 75 mg Symkevi 50mg/75mg tablets | 28 tablet [PoM] £6,293.91 (Hospital only)
  Tezacaftor 100 mg, Ivacaftor 150 mg Symkevi 100mg/150mg tablets | 28 tablet [PoM] £6,293.91 (Hospital only)

4 Cough and congestion

Aromatic inhalations, cough preparations and systemic nasal decongestants

03-May-2024

Aromatic inhalations

Inhalations containing volatile substances such as eucalyptus oil are traditionally used to relieve congestion and ease breathing. Although the vapour may contain little of the additive it encourages deliberate inspiration of warm moist air which is often comforting. Boiling water should not be used owing to the risk of scalding.

Strong aromatic decongestants (applied as rubs or to pillows) are not recommended for infants under the age of 3 months. Sodium chloride 0.9% solution given as nasal drops can be used to liquefy mucous secretions and relieve nasal congestion in infants and young children; administration before feeds may ease feeding difficulties caused by nasal congestion.

Cough preparations

Cough suppressants

Cough may be a symptom of an underlying disorder such as asthma, gastro-oesophageal reflux disease, or rhinitis, which should be addressed before prescribing cough suppressants. Cough may be associated with smoking or environmental pollutants. Cough can also result from bronchiectasis including that associated with cystic fibrosis; cough can also have a significant habit component. There is little evidence of any significant benefit from the use of cough suppressants in children with acute cough in ambulatory settings. Cough suppressants may cause sputum retention and this can be harmful in children with bronchiectasis.

The use of cough suppressants containing opioid analgesics is not generally recommended in children and should be avoided in children under 6 years; the use of over-the-counter cough suppressants containing codeine phosphate p. 331 should be avoided in children under 12 years and in children of any age known to be CYP2D6 ultra-rapid metabolisers.

Sedating antihistamines are used as the cough suppressant component of many compound cough preparations on sale to the public; all tend to cause drowsiness which may reflect their main mode of action.

MHRA/CHM advice: Pholcodine-containing cough and cold medicines: withdrawal from UK market as a precautionary measure (March 2023)

Following a review of cumulative safety information, the MHRA has found that pholcodine use in the 12 months preceding anaesthesia was significantly associated with an increased risk of peri-anaesthetic anaphylaxis to neuromuscular blocking agents (NMBAs). Although the absolute risk is very small, pholcodine-containing preparations are being withdrawn because their benefits do not outweigh this risk.

Healthcare professionals are advised to ask patients scheduled to receive general anaesthesia with NMBAs if they have taken pholcodine, particularly in the past 12 months. Patients or carers should be advised of this risk, and that there is no increased risk of allergic reactions, including anaphylaxis, with other allergens following pholcodine use.

Demulcent and expectorant cough preparations

Simple linctus and other demulcent cough preparations containing soothing substances, such as syrup or glycerol, may temporarily relieve a dry irritating cough. These preparations have the advantage of being harmless and inexpensive and sugar-free versions are available.

Expectorants are claimed to promote expulsion of bronchial secretions, but there is no evidence that any drug can specifically facilitate expectoration.

EvGr An over-the-counter cough medicine containing the expectorant guaifenesin may be used for acute cough in children aged over 12 years; there is some evidence to suggest it may reduce symptoms. (A)

Compound cough preparations for children are on sale to the public but should not be used in children under 6 years; the rationale for some is dubious. Care should be taken to give the correct dose and to not use more than one preparation at a time.

MHRA/CHM advice: Over-the-counter cough and cold medicines for children (March 2008 and February 2009)

Children under 6 years should not be given over-the-counter cough and cold medicines containing the following ingredients:

- brompheniramine, chlorphenamine maleate p. 205, diphenhydramine, doxylamine, promethazine, or triprolidine (antihistamines);
- dextromethorphan (cough suppressant);
- guaifenesin or ipecacuanha (expectorants);
- phenylephrine hydrochloride, pseudoephedrine hydrochloride p. 869, ephedrine hydrochloride p. 869, oxymetazoline, or xylometazoline hydrochloride p. 870 (decongestants).

Over-the-counter cough and cold medicines can be considered for children aged 6–12 years after basic principles of best care have been tried, but treatment should be restricted to five days or less. Children should not be given more than 1 cough or cold preparation at a time because different brands may contain the same active ingredient; care should be taken to give the correct dose.

Nasal decongestants, systemic

Nasal congestion in children due to allergic or vasomotor rhinitis should be treated with oral antihistamines, topical nasal preparations containing corticosteroids, or topical decongestants.

There is little evidence to support the use of systemic decongestants in children.

Pseudoephedrine hydrochloride is commonly combined with other ingredients (including antihistamines) in preparations intended for the relief of cough and cold symptoms; it has few sympathomimetic effects but is only recommended for short-term use.

COUGH AND COLD PREPARATIONS

Citric acid

17-Jul-2024

- **DRUG ACTION** Formulated as simple linctus

- **INDICATIONS AND DOSE**

Cough

▶ BY MOUTH

▶ Child 1 month–11 years: 5–10 mL 3–4 times a day, this dose is for Simple Linctus, Paediatric, BP (0.625%)

Cough

▶ BY MOUTH

▶ Child 12-17 years: 5 mL 3–4 times a day, this dose is for Simple Linctus, BP (2.5%)

- **PRESCRIBING AND DISPENSING INFORMATION** Flavours of oral liquid formulations may include anise.

When prepared extemporaneously, the BP states Simple Linctus, Paediatric, BP consists of citric acid monohydrate 0.625% and Simple Linctus, BP consists of citric acid monohydrate 2.5%, both in a suitable vehicle with an anise flavour.

- **PATIENT AND CARER ADVICE**

Medicines for Children leaflet: Simple linctus for cough www.medicinesforchildren.org.uk/medicines/simple-linctus-for-cough/

- **MEDICINAL FORMS** There can be variation in the licensing of different medicines containing the same drug.

Oral solution

▶ Citric acid (Non-proprietary)

Citric acid monohydrate 6.25 mg per 1 ml Care Simple linctus paediatric sugar free | 200 ml GSL £1.75 DT = £1.75 SF
Bell's Children's Cough Relief | 200 ml GSL £1.27 DT = £2.15
Simple linctus paediatric | 200 ml GSL £1.52–£2.15 DT = £2.15

Citric acid monohydrate 25 mg per 1 ml Simple linctus sugar free | 200 ml GSL £2.68 DT = £2.69 SF | 2000 ml GSL £26.80 SF
Simple linctus | 200 ml GSL £1.27–£1.49 DT = £2.07

MENTHOL AND DERIVATIVES

Eucalyptus with menthol

18-Mar-2020

- **INDICATIONS AND DOSE**

Aromatic inhalation for relief of nasal congestion

▶ BY INHALATION

▶ Child 3 months–17 years: Add one teaspoonful to a pint of hot, **not** boiling, water and inhale the vapour; repeat after 4 hours if necessary

- **PRESCRIBING AND DISPENSING INFORMATION** When prepared extemporaneously, the BP states Menthol and Eucalyptus Inhalation, BP 1980 consists of racementhol or levomenthol 2 g, eucalyptus oil 10 mL, light magnesium carbonate 7 g, water to 100 mL.

  Not recommended (applied as a rub or to pillows) for infants under the age of 3 months.

- **PROFESSION SPECIFIC INFORMATION**

Dental practitioners' formulary Menthol and Eucalyptus Inhalation BP, 1980 may be prescribed.

- **MEDICINAL FORMS** No licensed medicines listed.

5 Respiratory depression, respiratory distress syndrome and apnoea

Respiratory stimulants

Respiratory stimulants

Respiratory stimulants (analeptic drugs), such as caffeine citrate p. 226, reduce the frequency of neonatal apnoea, and the need for mechanical ventilation during the first 7 days of treatment. They are typically used in the management of very preterm neonates, and continued until a corrected gestational age of 34 to 35 weeks is reached (or longer if necessary). They should only be given under **expert supervision** in hospital; it is important to rule out any underlying disorder, such as seizures, hypoglycaemia, or infection, causing respiratory exhaustion before starting treatment with a respiratory stimulant.

Pulmonary surfactants

Pulmonary surfactants derived from animal lungs, beractant below and poractant alfa below are used to prevent and treat respiratory distress syndrome (hyaline membrane disease) in neonates and preterm neonates. Prophylactic use of a pulmonary surfactant may reduce the need for mechanical ventilation and is more effective than 'rescue treatment' in preterm neonates of 29 weeks or less corrected gestational age. Pulmonary surfactants may also be of benefit in neonates with meconium aspiration syndrome or intrapartum streptococcal infection. Pulmonary immaturity with surfactant deficit is the commonest reason for respiratory failure in the neonate, especially in those of less than 30 weeks corrected gestational age. Betamethasone p. 542 given to the mother (at least 12 hours but preferably 48 hours) before delivery substantially enhances pulmonary maturity in the neonate.

PULMONARY SURFACTANTS

Beractant

29-Apr-2020

- **INDICATIONS AND DOSE**

Treatment of respiratory distress syndrome in preterm neonates, birth-weight over 700 g (specialist use only)

▶ BY ENDOTRACHEAL TUBE

▶ Preterm neonate: 100 mg/kg, preferably administer within 8 hours of birth; dose may be repeated within 48 hours at intervals of at least 6 hours for up to 4 doses.

Prophylaxis of respiratory distress syndrome in preterm neonates (specialist use only)

▶ BY ENDOTRACHEAL TUBE

▶ Neonate up to 32 weeks corrected gestational age: 100 mg/kg, preferably administer within 15 minutes of birth; dose may be repeated within 48 hours at intervals of at least 6 hours for up to 4 doses.

DOSE EQUIVALENCE AND CONVERSION

▶ Phospholipid 100 mg/kg is equivalent to a volume of 4 mL/kg.

- **CAUTIONS** Consult product literature
- **SIDE-EFFECTS**

▶ **Uncommon** Endotracheal tube obstruction

▶ **Frequency not known** Bradycardia · hypoxia

- **MEDICINAL FORMS** There can be variation in the licensing of different medicines containing the same drug.

Suspension for endotracheopulmonary instillation

▶ Survanta (AbbVie Ltd)

Phospholipids (as Beractant) 25 mg per 1 ml Survanta 200mg/8ml endotracheopulmonary suspension bottles | 1 bottle PoM £306.43 (Hospital only)

Poractant alfa

29-Apr-2020

- **INDICATIONS AND DOSE**

Treatment of respiratory distress syndrome in neonates, birth weight over 700 g (specialist use only)

▶ BY ENDOTRACHEAL TUBE

▶ Neonate: 100–200 mg/kg, then 100 mg/kg every 12 hours if required, maximum 300–400 mg/kg per course.

Prophylaxis of respiratory distress syndrome (specialist use only)

▶ BY ENDOTRACHEAL TUBE

▶ Neonate 24 weeks to 31 weeks corrected gestational age: 100–200 mg/kg, administer soon after birth, preferably within 15 minutes, then 100 mg/kg after 6–12 hours if required, then 100 mg/kg after 12 hours if required, and if neonate still intubated. Max 300–400 mg/kg per course.

- **CAUTIONS** Consult product literature
- **SIDE-EFFECTS**

▶ **Rare or very rare** Bradycardia · hypotension

▶ **Frequency not known** Hyperoxia

- **MEDICINAL FORMS** There can be variation in the licensing of different medicines containing the same drug.

Suspension for endotracheopulmonary instillation

▶ Curosurf (Chiesi Ltd)

Poractant alfa 80 mg per 1 ml Curosurf 240mg/3ml endotracheopulmonary suspension vials | 1 vial PoM £547.40 (Hospital only)

Curosurf 120mg/1.5ml endotracheopulmonary suspension vials | 1 vial PoM £281.64 (Hospital only)

5.1 Neonatal apnoea

XANTHINES

Caffeine citrate

11-Mar-2026

● **INDICATIONS AND DOSE**

Neonatal apnoea (specialist supervision in hospital)

▶ BY MOUTH, OR BY INTRAVENOUS INFUSION

▸ Neonate: Loading dose 20 mg/kg, then maintenance 5 mg/kg once daily, started 24 hours after the loading dose; increased if necessary up to 20 mg/kg daily, a maintenance dose above 20 mg/kg daily can be considered if therapeutic efficacy is not achieved—the plasma-caffeine concentration should be monitored to ensure that a safe level is maintained.

DOSE EQUIVALENCE AND CONVERSION

▸ Caffeine citrate 2 mg ≡ caffeine base 1 mg

PHARMACOKINETICS

▸ Caffeine citrate is well absorbed when given orally.

● **UNLICENSED USE** EvGr Higher maintenance doses differ from product literature and adhere to national guidelines. ⟨A⟩

● **CAUTIONS** Cardiovascular disease · gastro-oesophageal reflux · rhythm disorder · seizure disorders

● **INTERACTIONS** → Appendix 1: caffeine citrate

● **SIDE-EFFECTS**

▶ **Common or very common** Arrhythmias · hyperglycaemia

▶ **Uncommon** Seizure

▶ **Frequency not known** Brain injury · deafness · failure to thrive · feeding intolerance · feeling jittery · gastrointestinal disorders · hypoglycaemia · increased cardiac output · irritability · regurgitation · restlessness

● **HEPATIC IMPAIRMENT** Manufacturer advises caution (risk of increased frequency of side-effects).

Dose adjustments Manufacturer advises consider dose adjustment according to plasma-caffeine concentration.

● **RENAL IMPAIRMENT** EvGr Use with caution (potential for accumulation). ⟨M⟩

Dose adjustments EvGr Reduced daily maintenance dose required (consult product literature). ⟨M⟩

● **MONITORING REQUIREMENTS**

▶ EvGr The therapeutic range for plasma-caffeine concentration is usually 10–20 mg/litre (50–100 micromol/litre), but a concentration of 25–35 mg/litre (130–180 micromol/litre) may be required. Signs of toxicity only normally occur at concentrations greater than 50 mg/litre (260 micromol/litre). ⟨D⟩

▶ Monitor for recurrence of apnoea for 1 week after stopping treatment.

● **DIRECTIONS FOR ADMINISTRATION** Caffeine citrate injection may be administered *by mouth* or *by intravenous infusion*. For *intravenous infusion*, manufacturer advises give loading dose over 30 minutes and maintenance doses over 10 minutes.

● **PRESCRIBING AND DISPENSING INFORMATION** The MHRA advises that to minimise the risk of dosing errors, when prescribing, doses should be expressed as caffeine citrate.

Care should be taken when prescribing and dispensing as preparations with different strengths may be available.

● **NATIONAL FUNDING/ACCESS DECISIONS**

For full details see funding body website

Scottish Medicines Consortium (SMC) decisions

▶ **Caffeine citrate (*Peyona*®) for the treatment of primary apnoea of premature newborns (September 2013)**
SMC No. 814/12 Recommended

● **MEDICINAL FORMS** There can be variation in the licensing of different medicines containing the same drug. Forms available from special-order manufacturers include: oral suspension, oral solution

Solution for infusion

▸ Caffeine citrate (Non-proprietary)
Caffeine citrate 10 mg per 1 ml Caffeine citrate 10mg/1ml solution for infusion ampoules | 10 ampoule PoM £48.82

▸ Fenapin (Galvany Pharma Ltd)
Caffeine citrate 20 mg per 1 ml Fenapin 20mg/1ml solution for infusion ampoules | 5 ampoule PoM £19.50

▸ Gencebok (Gennisium Pharma)
Caffeine citrate 10 mg per 1 ml Gencebok 10mg/1ml solution for infusion ampoules | 10 ampoule PoM £66.00 (Hospital only) | 50 ampoule PoM £330.00 (Hospital only)

▸ Peyona (Chiesi Ltd)
Caffeine citrate 20 mg per 1 ml Peyona 20mg/1ml solution for infusion ampoules | 10 ampoule PoM £172.50 (Hospital only)

Oral solution

▸ Caffeine citrate (Non-proprietary)
Caffeine citrate 10 mg per 1 ml Caffeine citrate 50mg/5ml oral solution | 5 ml PoM £25.99 DT = £25.99

Chapter 4
Nervous system

CONTENTS

1 Epilepsy and other seizure disorders

Epilepsy

21-Nov-2025

Epilepsy control

The objective of treatment is to prevent the occurrence of seizures by maintaining an effective dose of one or more antiepileptic drugs. Careful adjustment of doses is necessary, usually starting with low doses and increasing gradually until seizures are controlled or there are significant side-effects.

When choosing an antiepileptic drug, the seizure type, epilepsy syndrome, need for treatment, risks and benefits of treatment with antiepileptic drugs (including their importance in reducing the risk of epilepsy-related death), and the child's age, sex, comorbidities, concomitant medication, preference, and personal circumstances (such as education, employment, likelihood of pregnancy, or planning a family) should be taken into account.

The frequency of administration is often determined by the plasma-drug half-life, and should be kept as low as possible to encourage better adherence. Most antiepileptics, when used in usual dosage, can be given twice daily. Lamotrigine, perampanel, phenobarbital and phenytoin, which have long half-lives, can be given as a daily dose at bedtime. However, with large doses, some antiepileptics may need to be given three times daily to avoid side-effects associated with high peak plasma-drug concentrations. Young children metabolise some antiepileptics more rapidly than adults and therefore may require more frequent doses and a higher amount per kilogram body-weight.

Management

EvGr A single antiepileptic drug should be prescribed wherever possible and will achieve seizure control for the majority of children. When monotherapy with a first-line antiepileptic drug is unsuccessful (does not reduce or stop seizures, or if side-effects are intolerable), monotherapy with an alternative drug should be tried; the diagnosis should be checked before starting an alternative drug if the first drug showed lack of efficacy. The change from one antiepileptic drug to another should be cautious, slowly withdrawing the first drug only when the new regimen has been established. Combination (adjunctive) therapy with two or more antiepileptic drugs may be necessary, but the concurrent use of antiepileptic drugs increases the risk of side-effects and drug interactions. If combination therapy does not reduce seizures, revert to the regimen (monotherapy or combination therapy) that provided the best balance between tolerability and efficacy. Ⓐ

For guidance on when to refer children to tertiary epilepsy services, see NICE guideline: **Epilepsies in children, young people and adults** (see *Useful resources*).

Monitoring

Routine measurement of plasma concentrations of antiepileptic drugs is not usually necessary, however, monitoring of plasma-drug concentrations may be considered in children with uncontrolled seizures, suspected poor adherence to medication, side-effects, or a specific clinical condition needing closer supervision (such as renal failure).

Plasma concentrations of some medications may change during pregnancy and monitoring may be required (see *Reproductive risks*).

Withdrawal

EvGr The decision to withdraw antiepileptic drugs from a seizure-free child may be considered after the child has been seizure-free for at least two years, depending on their individual circumstances. An assessment to determine the risk of seizure recurrence if antiepileptic drugs are discontinued should be carried out. If there is any doubt or concern, the assessment should be done by an epilepsy specialist. Ⓐ Even in children who have been seizure-free for several years, there is a significant risk of seizure recurrence on drug withdrawal.

EvGr In children receiving several antiepileptic drugs, only one drug should be withdrawn at a time. Avoid abrupt withdrawal, particularly of barbiturates and benzodiazepines, because this can precipitate severe rebound seizures. Reduction in dosage should be gradual and for most drugs, this would usually be over at least three months. In the case of barbiturates and benzodiazepines, withdrawal of the drug would typically be over a longer period to reduce the risk of drug-related withdrawal symptoms.

If seizures recur during or after discontinuation of an antiepileptic drug, the last dose reduction should be reversed and guidance sought from an epilepsy specialist. Ⓐ

Safety considerations and MHRA advice

Reproductive risks

Due to safety data showing a significant risk of serious harm to babies after exposure to valproate during pregnancy, evidence of potential male infertility, and a possible association with neurodevelopmental disorders in children born to males treated with valproate in the 3 months prior to conception, a National Patient Safety Alert and additional regulatory measures have been issued by the MHRA.

Valproate-containing medicines (including sodium valproate and valproic acid) should not be initiated in individuals (male or female) aged under 55 years unless 2 specialists have independently agreed and documented that there is no other effective and tolerated treatment, or that there are compelling reasons that reproductive risks do not apply. If valproate is initiated or continued in females who are able to have children (including young females who are likely to need treatment when they are old enough to have children), the potential risks and benefits of treatment should be discussed and the likelihood of pregnancy considered. The Pregnancy Prevention Programme must be put in place, if appropriate. The MHRA also advises that as a precaution, all male patients being treated with valproate who may father children should use effective contraception (condoms plus contraception used by their female partner) during treatment and for 3 months after stopping treatment. Males taking valproate who are planning a family within the following year should be informed of the potential fertility risks and treatment options. For further information, see *Important safety information*, *Conception and contraception*, and *Pregnancy* in sodium valproate p. 252 and valproic acid p. 259.

The MHRA also advises that topiramate must not be used in females of childbearing potential unless the conditions of the Pregnancy Prevention Programme are met. Topiramate must not be used during pregnancy unless there is no other suitable alternative. For further information, see *Important safety information*, *Conception and contraception*, and *Pregnancy* in topiramate p. 257.

The MHRA has also issued advice on the use of antiepileptic drugs in pregnancy due to the associated risk of teratogenicity.

MHRA/CHM advice: Antiepileptic drugs in pregnancy: updated advice following comprehensive safety review (January 2021)

Valproate, in particular, is highly teratogenic and evidence supports that use in pregnancy leads to congenital malformations (approximately 10% risk) and neurodevelopmental disorders (approximately 30–40% risk). Prescribers are reminded that valproate must **not** be used in females of childbearing potential unless the conditions of the Pregnancy Prevention Programme are met and alternative treatments are ineffective or not tolerated. Valproate must not be used during pregnancy unless there is no other suitable alternative. For further information, see sodium valproate p. 252 and valproic acid p. 259.

In the context of the known harms associated with valproate, the CHM initiated a safety review on the use of other key antiepileptic drugs in pregnancy for the risk of major congenital malformations, neurodevelopmental disorders or delay, and other effects on the child. Safety data for carbamazepine, gabapentin, lamotrigine, levetiracetam, oxcarbazepine, phenobarbital, phenytoin, pregabalin, topiramate, and zonisamide were reviewed. Much of the evidence base related to epilepsy, and as such, the review focused on the risks and decisions for epilepsy treatment.

The review confirmed that lamotrigine and levetiracetam are the safer of the drugs reviewed; large studies of pregnancies exposed to lamotrigine or levetiracetam monotherapy did not suggest an increased risk of major congenital malformations (at usual maintenance doses). Data for neurodevelopmental outcomes were more limited; available studies did not suggest an increased risk of neurodevelopmental disorders or delay associated with *in-utero* exposure to either lamotrigine or levetiracetam, however the data were inadequate to completely rule out the possibility of an increased risk. Lamotrigine and levetiracetam were not associated with an increased risk of fetal loss, intra-uterine growth restriction, or preterm birth.

For carbamazepine, phenobarbital, phenytoin, and topiramate, the data showed that use during pregnancy was associated with an increased risk of major congenital malformations; the risk for carbamazepine, phenobarbital, and topiramate was shown to be dose dependent. There is the possibility of adverse effects on neurodevelopment associated with the use of phenobarbital and phenytoin, and an increased risk of intra-uterine growth restriction with phenobarbital, topiramate, and zonisamide. The available data for carbamazepine did not suggest an increased risk of neurodevelopmental disorders or delay associated with in-utero exposure; however, the data were inadequate to completely rule out the possibility of an increased risk. For information on other antiepileptic drugs, see *Pregnancy* in the individual drug monographs.

Specialists should discuss the risks associated with antiepileptic drugs and untreated epilepsy during pregnancy with female patients when initiating treatment and during annual reviews; a safety information leaflet is available to aid discussion. Treatment should be reviewed according to the patient's clinical condition and circumstance. Female patients should be advised not to stop their antiepileptic treatment without discussing this with their doctor, and to seek urgent medical advice if they are on antiepileptic drugs and think they could be pregnant. Those who are planning a pregnancy should be urgently referred to a specialist for advice on antiepileptic treatment and offered folic acid.

With any antiepileptic drug used during pregnancy, monotherapy and use of the lowest effective dose are recommended where possible. Plasma concentrations of antiepileptic drugs (particularly lamotrigine and phenytoin) can be affected by physiological changes during pregnancy and post-partum. Prescribers should consult product literature and relevant clinical guidance for dosing and monitoring recommendations. For further information, also see *Monitoring in Pregnancy* in individual drug monographs.

Other considerations

Prescribers should also carefully consider the choice of antiepileptic therapy in pre-pubescent girls who may later become pregnant. Females of childbearing potential who take antiepileptic drugs should be given advice about the need for a highly effective contraception method to avoid unplanned pregnancy—for further information, see *Contraception in patients taking medication with teratogenic potential* in Contraceptives, hormonal p. 609. Some antiepileptic drugs can reduce the efficacy of hormonal contraceptives, and the efficacy of some antiepileptics may be affected by hormonal contraceptives.

Once an unplanned pregnancy is discovered, specialist advice should be sought; the risk of harm to the mother and fetus from convulsive seizures outweighs the risk of continued therapy. The likelihood of a female who is taking antiepileptic drugs having a baby with no malformations is approximately 90%, and it is important that female patients do not stop taking essential treatment because of concern over harm to the fetus. To reduce the risk of neural tube defects, folate supplementation is advised throughout the first trimester.

Female patients who have seizures in the second half of pregnancy should be assessed for eclampsia before any change is made to antiepileptic treatment. Status epilepticus should be treated according to the standard protocol.

Routine injection of vitamin K at birth minimises the risk of neonatal haemorrhage associated with antiepileptics.

Withdrawal effects in the newborn may occur with some antiepileptic drugs.

Epilepsy and Pregnancy Register
All pregnant females with epilepsy, whether taking medication or not, should be encouraged to notify the UK Epilepsy and Pregnancy Register (available at: www.epilepsyandpregnancy.co.uk).

Breast-feeding
Young females taking antiepileptic monotherapy should generally be encouraged to breast-feed; if a female is on combination therapy or if there are other risk factors, such as premature birth, close monitoring is recommended. Patients and their family should be made aware of signs of toxicity in the infant and advised to seek medical advice if these occur.

All infants should be monitored for sedation, feeding difficulties, adequate weight gain, and developmental milestones. Infants should also be monitored for side-effects associated with the antiepileptic drug particularly with newer antiepileptics, if the antiepileptic is readily transferred into breast-milk causing high infant serum-drug concentrations (e.g. ethosuximide, lamotrigine, primidone, and zonisamide), or if slower metabolism in the infant causes drugs to accumulate (e.g. phenobarbital and lamotrigine). Serum-drug concentration monitoring should be undertaken in breast-fed infants if suspected side-effects develop; if toxicity develops it may be necessary to introduce formula feeds to limit the infant's drug exposure, or to wean the infant off breast-milk altogether.

Primidone, phenobarbital, and the benzodiazepines are associated with an established risk of drowsiness in breast-fed babies and caution is required.

Withdrawal effects may occur in infants if a mother suddenly stops breast-feeding, particularly if she is taking phenobarbital, primidone, or lamotrigine.

MHRA/CHM advice: Antiepileptics: risk of suicidal thoughts and behaviour (August 2008)
A Europe-wide review concluded that all antiepileptic drugs may be associated with a small increased risk of suicidal thoughts and behaviour; symptoms may occur as early as 1 week after starting treatment. The MHRA has recommended that children and their parents or carers should be advised to seek medical advice if any mood changes, distressing thoughts, or feelings about suicide or self-harming develop, and that the child should be referred for appropriate treatment if necessary. They should also be advised not to stop or switch antiepileptic treatment and to seek advice from a healthcare professional if concerned.

MHRA/CHM advice: Antiepileptic drugs: updated advice on switching between different manufacturers' products (November 2017)
The CHM has reviewed spontaneous adverse reactions received by the MHRA and publications that reported potential harm arising from switching of antiepileptic drugs in patients previously stabilised on a branded product to a generic. The CHM concluded that reports of loss of seizure control and/or worsening of side-effects around the time of switching between products could be explained as chance associations, but that a causal role of switching could not be ruled out in all cases. The following guidance has been issued to help minimise risk:

- Different antiepileptic drugs vary considerably in their characteristics, which influences the risk of whether switching between different manufacturers' products of a particular drug may cause adverse effects or loss of seizure control;
- Antiepileptic drugs have been divided into three risk-based categories to help healthcare professionals decide whether it is necessary to maintain continuity of supply of a specific manufacturer's product. These categories are listed below;
- If it is felt desirable for a patient to be maintained on a specific manufacturer's product this should be prescribed either by specifying a brand name, or by using the generic drug name and name of the manufacturer (otherwise known as the Marketing Authorisation Holder);
- This advice relates only to antiepileptic drug use for treatment of epilepsy; it does not apply to their use in other indications (e.g. mood stabilisation, neuropathic pain);
- Please report on a Yellow Card any suspected adverse reactions to antiepileptic drugs;
- Dispensing pharmacists should ensure the continuity of supply of a particular product when the prescription specifies it. If the prescribed product is unavailable, it may be necessary to dispense a product from a different manufacturer to maintain continuity of treatment of that antiepileptic drug. Such cases should be discussed and agreed with both the prescriber and patient (or carer);
- Usual dispensing practice can be followed when a specific product is not stated.

Category 1
Carbamazepine **p. 234**, **phenobarbital** **p. 264**, **phenytoin** **p. 249**, **primidone** **p. 265**. For these drugs, doctors are advised to ensure that their patient is maintained on a specific manufacturer's product.

Category 2
Clobazam **p. 267**, **clonazepam** **p. 268**, **eslicarbazepine acetate** **p. 236**, **lamotrigine** **p. 243**, **oxcarbazepine** **p. 246**, **perampanel** **p. 247**, **rufinamide** **p. 250**, **topiramate** **p. 257**, **valproate**, **zonisamide** **p. 263**. For these drugs, the need for continued supply of a particular manufacturer's product should be based on clinical judgement and consultation with the patient and/or carer taking into account factors such as seizure frequency, treatment history, and potential implications to the patient of having a breakthrough seizure. Non-clinical factors as for Category 3 drugs should also be considered.

Category 3
Brivaracetam **p. 232**, **ethosuximide** **p. 237**, **gabapentin** **p. 240**, **lacosamide** **p. 241**, **levetiracetam** **p. 245**, **pregabalin**, **tiagabine** **p. 256**, **vigabatrin** **p. 261**. For these drugs, it is usually unnecessary to ensure that patients are maintained on a specific manufacturer's product as therapeutic equivalence can be assumed, however, other factors are important when considering whether switching is appropriate. Differences between alternative products (e.g. product name, packaging, appearance, and taste) may be perceived negatively by patients and/or carers, and may lead to dissatisfaction, anxiety, confusion, dosing errors, and reduced adherence. In addition, difficulties for patients with co-morbid autism, mental health problems, or learning disability should also be considered.

Antiepileptic hypersensitivity syndrome
Antiepileptic hypersensitivity syndrome is a rare but potentially fatal syndrome associated with some antiepileptic drugs (carbamazepine, lacosamide, lamotrigine, oxcarbazepine, phenobarbital, phenytoin, primidone, and rufinamide); rarely cross-sensitivity occurs between some of these antiepileptic drugs. Some other antiepileptics (eslicarbazepine acetate, stiripentol p. 256, and zonisamide) have a theoretical risk. The symptoms usually start between 1 and 8 weeks of exposure; fever, rash, and lymphadenopathy are most commonly seen. Other systemic signs include liver dysfunction, haematological, renal, and pulmonary abnormalities, vasculitis, and multi-organ failure. If signs or symptoms of hypersensitivity syndrome occur, the drug should be withdrawn immediately, the child should not be re-exposed, and expert advice should be sought.

Driving
If a driver has a seizure (of any type) they must stop driving immediately and inform the Driver and Vehicle Licensing Agency (DVLA).

Patients who have had a first unprovoked epileptic seizure

or a single isolated seizure must not drive for 6 months; driving may then be resumed, provided the patient has been assessed by a specialist as fit to drive and investigations do not suggest a risk of further seizures.

Patients with established epilepsy may drive a motor vehicle provided they are not a danger to the public and are compliant with treatment and follow up. To continue driving, these patients must be seizure-free for at least one year (or have a pattern of seizures established for one year where there is no influence on their level of consciousness or the ability to act); also, they must not have a history of unprovoked seizures.

Patients who have had a *seizure while asleep* are not permitted to drive for one year from the date of each seizure unless:

- a history or pattern of sleep seizures occurring **only** ever while asleep has been established over the course of at least one year from the date of the first sleep seizure; or
- an established pattern of purely asleep seizures can be demonstrated over the course of three years if the patient has previously had seizures whilst awake (or awake and asleep).

The DVLA recommends that patients should not drive during medication changes or withdrawal of antiepileptic drugs, and for 6 months after their last dose. If a seizure occurs due to a prescribed change or withdrawal of epilepsy treatment, the patient will have their driving license revoked for 1 year; relicensing may be considered earlier if treatment has been reinstated for 6 months and no further seizures have occurred.

Focal seizures with or without secondary generalisation

The MHRA regulatory measures and advice on the reproductive risks associated with sodium valproate p. 252 and topiramate, and the use of antiepileptic drugs in pregnancy should be followed—see *Safety considerations and MHRA advice*.

Focal seizures with or without secondary generalisation is also referred to as focal seizures with or without evolution to bilateral tonic-clonic seizures.

EvGr Consider lamotrigine or levetiracetam as first-line options for treating focal seizures. If monotherapy with either lamotrigine or levetiracetam is unsuccessful, the other of these options should be considered. If monotherapy with these drugs is unsuccessful, consider carbamazepine p. 234, oxcarbazepine p. 246, or zonisamide p. 263 [unlicensed use] as second-line monotherapy options. Lacosamide p. 241 should be considered as third-line monotherapy.

If monotherapy is unsuccessful, adjunctive treatment should be considered. First-line options for adjunctive treatment include carbamazepine, lacosamide, lamotrigine, levetiracetam, oxcarbazepine, topiramate p. 257, or zonisamide. Second-line options include brivaracetam p. 232, eslicarbazepine acetate p. 236, perampanel p. 247, or pregabalin [unlicensed use]. Third-line options include phenobarbital p. 264, phenytoin p. 249, sodium valproate p. 252, tiagabine p. 256, or vigabatrin p. 261. (A)

Generalised seizures

The MHRA regulatory measures and advice on the reproductive risks associated with sodium valproate and topiramate, and the use of antiepileptic drugs in pregnancy should be followed—see *Safety considerations and MHRA advice*.

Tonic-clonic seizures

EvGr Offer lamotrigine p. 243, levetiracetam p. 245, or sodium valproate as first-line monotherapy for generalised tonic-clonic seizures. If monotherapy with lamotrigine, levetiracetam, or sodium valproate is unsuccessful, the other of these options should be tried.

If monotherapy is unsuccessful, adjunctive treatment should be considered. First-line options for adjunctive treatment include clobazam p. 267, lamotrigine, levetiracetam, perampanel, sodium valproate, or topiramate. Second-line options include brivaracetam [unlicensed use], lacosamide, phenobarbital, primidone p. 265, or zonisamide [unlicensed use]. (A)

Absence seizures

EvGr Offer ethosuximide p. 237 as first-line treatment for absence seizures. If treatment with ethosuximide is unsuccessful, consider lamotrigine, levetiracetam [unlicensed use], or sodium valproate as second-line monotherapy or adjunctive treatment. If treatment with lamotrigine, levetiracetam, or sodium valproate is unsuccessful, the other of these options should be considered as monotherapy or adjunctive treatment. (A)

Offer lamotrigine, levetiracetam [unlicensed use], or sodium valproate as first-line monotherapy for absence seizures with, or at risk of, other seizure types. If monotherapy with lamotrigine, levetiracetam, or sodium valproate is unsuccessful, the other of these options should be tried as monotherapy or adjunctive treatment. If first-line treatments tried are unsuccessful, consider ethosuximide as a second-line adjunctive treatment.

Children with absence seizures may have their seizures exacerbated if treated with carbamazepine, gabapentin, oxcarbazepine, phenobarbital, phenytoin, pregabalin, tiagabine, or vigabatrin.

Myoclonic seizures

Myoclonic seizures (myoclonic jerks) occur in a variety of syndromes, and response to treatment varies considerably.

EvGr For children aged under 4 years with myoclonic seizures, either seek guidance on treatment from, or refer to, a tertiary paediatric neurologist.

Offer levetiracetam [unlicensed use] or sodium valproate as first-line treatment for myoclonic seizures. If treatment with levetiracetam or sodium valproate is unsuccessful, the other of these options should be offered as monotherapy or adjunctive treatment.

If first-line treatment is unsuccessful, consider monotherapy or adjunctive treatment with brivaracetam [unlicensed use], clobazam, clonazepam p. 268, lamotrigine, phenobarbital, piracetam [unlicensed use], topiramate [unlicensed use], or zonisamide [unlicensed use].

In children with myoclonic seizures, the use of carbamazepine, gabapentin, oxcarbazepine, phenytoin, pregabalin, tiagabine, or vigabatrin is not recommended because they may exacerbate seizures. (A) Lamotrigine may also occasionally exacerbate myoclonic seizures.

Atonic or tonic seizures

EvGr Offer lamotrigine or sodium valproate as first-line treatment for atonic or tonic seizures. If treatment with lamotrigine or sodium valproate is unsuccessful, the other of these options should be offered as monotherapy or adjunctive treatment.

If first-line treatment is unsuccessful, consider monotherapy or adjunctive treatment with clobazam, rufinamide p. 250 [unlicensed use], or topiramate [unlicensed use].

If all other treatments are unsuccessful, consider felbamate [unlicensed] as adjunctive treatment under the supervision of a neurologist with expertise in epilepsy. (A)

Children with atonic or tonic seizures may have their seizures exacerbated if treated with carbamazepine, gabapentin, oxcarbazepine, pregabalin, tiagabine, or vigabatrin.

Epilepsy syndromes

Some drugs are licensed for use in particular epilepsy syndromes. The epilepsy syndromes are specific types of epilepsy that are characterised according to a number of features including seizure type, age of onset, and EEG characteristics. Children with an epilepsy syndrome that is likely to be drug-resistant (failure of adequate trials of two antiepileptic drugs (whether as monotherapy or in combination) to achieve sustained seizure freedom) should be referred to a tertiary epilepsy service. For further guidance on epilepsy syndromes, see NICE guideline: **Epilepsies in children, young people and adults** (see *Useful resources*).

The MHRA regulatory measures and advice on the reproductive risks associated with sodium valproate and topiramate, and the use of antiepileptic drugs in pregnancy should be followed—see ***Safety considerations and MHRA advice.***

Idiopathic generalised epilepsies

EvGr Offer lamotrigine, levetiracetam, or sodium valproate as first-line monotherapy for idiopathic generalised epilepsies. If treatment with lamotrigine, levetiracetam, or sodium valproate is unsuccessful, the other of these options should be offered as monotherapy or adjunctive treatment.

If first-line options are unsuccessful, consider perampanel or topiramate as second-line adjunctive treatment options. Ⓐ

Infantile spasms

EvGr A tertiary paediatric neurologist with expertise in epilepsy should be involved in decisions regarding the treatment of infantile spasms.

Vigabatrin monotherapy is the treatment of choice for infantile spasms associated with tuberous sclerosis. If vigabatrin is ineffective, prednisolone p. 548 should be added after 1 week. In spasms of other causes, a combination of vigabatrin and prednisolone should be offered as first-line treatment, unless the child is at high risk of steroid-related side-effects, in which case vigabatrin monotherapy should be considered. Levetiracetam [unlicensed use], nitrazepam [unlicensed use], sodium valproate, or topiramate [unlicensed use] may be considered for second-line treatment options following advice from tertiary paediatric epilepsy specialists. Ⓐ

Dravet syndrome

EvGr A neurologist with expertise in epilepsy should be involved in decisions regarding the treatment of Dravet syndrome.

Sodium valproate should be considered as first-line treatment for all children with Dravet syndrome, including females, because of the severity of the syndrome and the lack of evidence for other effective first-line options.

If monotherapy with sodium valproate is unsuccessful, consider triple therapy with clobazam and stiripentol p. 256 as first-line adjunctive treatment.

If triple therapy with sodium valproate, clobazam, and stiripentol is unsuccessful, cannabidiol p. 233 with clobazam, or fenfluramine p. 238 may be considered as second-line adjunctive treatment options in certain children.

Under the supervision of a neurologist with expertise in epilepsy, further adjunctive treatment options include topiramate [unlicensed use] or levetiracetam [unlicensed use]; or if all other treatments are unsuccessful, potassium bromide [unlicensed] may be considered. Ⓐ

Children with Dravet syndrome may have their seizures exacerbated if treated with carbamazepine, gabapentin, lacosamide, lamotrigine, oxcarbazepine, phenobarbital, pregabalin, tiagabine, or vigabatrin.

Lennox-Gastaut syndrome

EvGr A neurologist with expertise in epilepsy should be involved in decisions regarding the treatment of Lennox-Gastaut syndrome.

Sodium valproate should be considered as first-line treatment for all children with Lennox-Gastaut syndrome, including females, because of the severity of the syndrome and the lack of evidence for other effective first-line options.

If monotherapy with sodium valproate is unsuccessful, consider lamotrigine as second-line monotherapy or adjunctive treatment. Third-line adjunctive treatment options include cannabidiol with clobazam, fenfluramine, clobazam, rufinamide p. 250, or topiramate p. 257.

Felbamate [unlicensed] may be considered as adjunctive therapy under the supervision of a neurologist with expertise in epilepsy when all other treatment options are unsuccessful. Ⓐ

Children with Lennox-Gastaut syndrome may have their seizures exacerbated if treated with carbamazepine, gabapentin, lacosamide, lamotrigine, oxcarbazepine, phenobarbital, pregabalin, tiagabine, or vigabatrin.

Landau-Kleffner syndrome and epilepsy with myoclonic-atonic seizures (Doose syndrome)

Always discuss with or refer to tertiary epilepsy specialists.

Neonatal seizures

Seizures can occur before delivery, but they are most common up to 24 hours after birth. Seizures in neonates occur as a result of biochemical disturbances, inborn errors of metabolism, hypoxic ischaemic encephalopathy, drug withdrawal, meningitis, stroke, cerebral haemorrhage or malformation, or severe jaundice (kernicterus).

Seizures caused by biochemical imbalance and those in neonates with inherited abnormal pyridoxine or biotin metabolism should be corrected by treating the underlying cause. Seizures caused by drug withdrawal following intra-uterine exposure are treated with a drug withdrawal regimen.

Phenobarbital p. 264 can be used to manage neonatal seizures where there is a risk of recurrence; phenytoin p. 249 is an alternative. Midazolam p. 273 and **rectal** paraldehyde p. 269 may also be useful in the management of acute neonatal seizures. Lidocaine hydrochloride p. 86 may be used if other treatments are unsuccessful; lidocaine hydrochloride should not be given to neonates who have received phenytoin infusion because of the risk of cardiac toxicity.

Repeated or cluster seizures, prolonged seizures, and status epilepticus

Repeated or cluster seizures (typically 3 or more self-terminating seizures in 24 hours), prolonged convulsive seizures (a seizure that lasts less than 5 minutes, but more than 2 minutes longer than a child's usual seizure), and convulsive status epilepticus (a seizure that lasts 5 minutes or longer, or recurrent seizures without recovery in between) should be managed as a medical emergency.

For further guidance on the management of convulsive status epilepticus, see Status epilepticus p. 269, and for a quick reference resource with doses of benzodiazepines for use in convulsive status epilepticus, see *Seizures* in Medical emergencies in the community p. 1480.

Repeated or cluster seizures, or prolonged seizures

EvGr The child's individualised emergency management plan should be followed, if immediately available. If an individualised emergency management plan is not available, treatment with a benzodiazepine (such as clobazam p. 267 or midazolam) should be urgently considered for children with repeated or cluster seizures, or prolonged convulsive seizures. For convulsive seizures that last 5 minutes or longer, or recurrent seizures without recovery in between, follow the recommendations for convulsive status epilepticus, see Status epilepticus p. 269.

If there is concern that repeated or cluster seizures, or prolonged seizures (convulsive or non-convulsive) may recur, an emergency management plan should be agreed with the child (and/or their parents/carers) if they do not have one already.

Expert guidance should be sought if the child has further episodes of repeated or cluster seizures. (A)

Febrile convulsions

Brief febrile convulsions need no specific treatment. *Prolonged febrile convulsions* (those lasting 5 minutes or longer), or *recurrent febrile convulsions* without recovery must be treated actively as for convulsive status epilepticus, see Status epilepticus p. 269.

Long-term anticonvulsant prophylaxis for febrile convulsions is rarely indicated.

Useful resources

Epilepsies in children, young people and adults. National Institute for Health and Care Excellence. NICE guideline 217. January 2025.

www.nice.org.uk/guidance/ng217

Epilepsies in children and young people: Investigative procedures and management. Scottish Intercollegiate Guidelines Network. SIGN guideline 159. May 2021.

www.sign.ac.uk/our-guidelines/epilepsies-in-children-and-young-people-investigative-procedures-and-management/

Other drugs used for Epilepsy and other seizure disorders Acetazolamide, p. 852

ANTIEPILEPTICS

Brivaracetam

04-Aug-2022

● **INDICATIONS AND DOSE**

Adjunctive therapy of focal seizures with or without secondary generalisation

▸ BY MOUTH, OR BY INTRAVENOUS INJECTION, OR BY INTRAVENOUS INFUSION

▸ Child 2–17 years (body-weight 10–19 kg): Initially 0.5–1.25 mg/kg twice daily, adjusted according to response; usual maintenance 1.25 mg/kg twice daily (max. per dose 2.5 mg/kg twice daily)

▸ Child 2–17 years (body-weight 20–49 kg): Initially 0.5–1 mg/kg twice daily, adjusted according to response; usual maintenance 1 mg/kg twice daily (max. per dose 2 mg/kg twice daily)

▸ Child 2–17 years (body-weight 50 kg and above): Initially 25–50 mg twice daily, adjusted according to response; usual maintenance 50 mg twice daily (max. per dose 100 mg twice daily)

IMPORTANT SAFETY INFORMATION

MHRA/CHM ADVICE: ANTIEPILEPTICS: RISK OF SUICIDAL THOUGHTS AND BEHAVIOUR (AUGUST 2008)

See Epilepsy p. 227.

MHRA/CHM ADVICE: ANTIEPILEPTIC DRUGS: UPDATED ADVICE ON SWITCHING BETWEEN DIFFERENT MANUFACTURERS' PRODUCTS (NOVEMBER 2017)

See Epilepsy p. 227.

MHRA/CHM ADVICE: ANTIEPILEPTIC DRUGS IN PREGNANCY: UPDATED ADVICE FOLLOWING COMPREHENSIVE SAFETY REVIEW (JANUARY 2021)

See Epilepsy p. 227.

● **INTERACTIONS** → Appendix 1: antiepileptics

● **SIDE-EFFECTS**

▸ **Common or very common** Anxiety · appetite decreased · constipation · cough · depression · dizziness · drowsiness · fatigue · increased risk of infection · insomnia · irritability · nausea · vertigo · vomiting

▸ **Uncommon** Behaviour abnormal · neutropenia · psychotic disorder

▸ **Frequency not known** Akathisia · severe cutaneous adverse reactions (SCARs) · suicidal behaviours

● **PREGNANCY** Manufacturer advises avoid unless potential benefit outweighs risk—limited information available. See also *Pregnancy* in Epilepsy p. 227.

● **BREAST FEEDING** Manufacturer advises avoid—present in milk in *animal* studies.

● **HEPATIC IMPAIRMENT** EvGr Caution (risk of increased exposure). (M)

Dose adjustments EvGr Initial dose of 25 mg twice daily, max. maintenance dose of 75 mg twice daily in children with body-weight 50 kg and above (no information available).

Initial dose of 0.5 mg/kg twice daily, max. maintenance dose of 1.5 mg/kg twice daily in children with body-weight from 20 kg to 49 kg (no information available).

Initial dose of 0.5 mg/kg twice daily, max. maintenance dose of 2 mg/kg twice daily in children with body-weight from 10 kg to 19 kg (no information available). (M)

● **TREATMENT CESSATION** EvGr Avoid abrupt withdrawal. In children 16 years and older, reduce daily dose in steps of 50 mg at weekly intervals, then reduce to 20 mg daily for a final week. In children younger than 16 years, reduce dose by a maximum of half the daily dose every week until either a dose of 1 mg/kg daily (in children with body-weight up to 50 kg) or 50 mg daily (in children with body-weight 50 kg or more) is reached and given for 1 week, then reduce to 20 mg daily for a final week. (M)

● **DIRECTIONS FOR ADMINISTRATION**

▸ With intravenous use For intermittent *intravenous infusion*, manufacturer advises dilute in Glucose 5% *or* Sodium Chloride 0.9% *or* Lactated Ringer's solution; give over 15 minutes.

▸ With oral use Manufacturer advises oral solution can be diluted in water or juice shortly before swallowing.

● **PRESCRIBING AND DISPENSING INFORMATION** Manufacturer advises if switching between oral therapy and intravenous therapy (for those temporarily unable to take oral medication), the total daily dose and the frequency of administration should be maintained.

● **PATIENT AND CARER ADVICE**

Missed doses Manufacturer advises if one or more doses are missed, a single dose should be taken as soon as possible and the next dose should be taken at the usual time.

Driving and skilled tasks Manufacturer advises patients and carers should be cautioned on the effects on driving and performance of skilled tasks—increased risk of dizziness.

● **NATIONAL FUNDING/ACCESS DECISIONS**

For full details see funding body website

Scottish Medicines Consortium (SMC) decisions

▸ **Brivaracetam (*Briviact*®) as adjunctive therapy in the treatment of partial-onset seizures with or without secondary generalisation in adult and adolescent patients from 16 years of age with epilepsy (July 2016)** SMC No. 1160/16 Recommended with restrictions

▸ **Brivaracetam (*Briviact*®) for the treatment of partial-onset seizures with or without secondary generalisation in children from 4 years of age to 15 with epilepsy (December 2018)** SMC No. SMC2113 Recommended with restrictions

All Wales Medicines Strategy Group (AWMSG) decisions

▸ **Brivaracetam (*Briviact*®) as adjunctive therapy in the treatment of partial-onset seizures with or without secondary generalisation in patients from 2 years of age with epilepsy (July 2022)** AWMSG No. 4614 Recommended with restrictions

- **MEDICINAL FORMS** There can be variation in the licensing of different medicines containing the same drug.

Solution for injection

CAUTIONARY AND ADVISORY LABELS 2
ELECTROLYTES: May contain Sodium

- **Briviact** (UCB Pharma Ltd)
  Brivaracetam 10 mg per 1 ml Briviact 50mg/5ml solution for injection vials | 10 vial PoM £222.75 (Hospital only)

Oral tablet

CAUTIONARY AND ADVISORY LABELS 2, 8, 25

- **Briviact** (UCB Pharma Ltd)
  Brivaracetam 10 mg Briviact 10mg tablets | 14 tablet PoM £34.64 DT = £34.64
  Brivaracetam 25 mg Briviact 25mg tablets | 56 tablet PoM £129.64 DT = £129.64
  Brivaracetam 50 mg Briviact 50mg tablets | 56 tablet PoM £129.64 DT = £129.64
  Brivaracetam 75 mg Briviact 75mg tablets | 56 tablet PoM £129.64 DT = £129.64
  Brivaracetam 100 mg Briviact 100mg tablets | 56 tablet PoM £129.64 DT = £129.64

Oral solution

CAUTIONARY AND ADVISORY LABELS 2, 8
EXCIPIENTS: May contain Sorbitol
ELECTROLYTES: May contain Sodium

- **Briviact** (UCB Pharma Ltd)
  Brivaracetam 10 mg per 1 ml Briviact 10mg/ml oral solution | 300 ml PoM £115.83 DT = £115.83 SF

Cannabidiol (CBD)

06-Mar-2026

- **DRUG ACTION** Cannabidiol (CBD) is a cannabinoid agent. Although the exact mechanism of action is unknown, it is thought to modulate intracellular calcium levels and adenosine-mediated signalling, which reduces neuronal activity.

- **INDICATIONS AND DOSE**

Seizures associated with Lennox-Gastaut syndrome [adjunctive treatment with clobazam] (specialist use only) | Seizures associated with Dravet syndrome [adjunctive treatment with clobazam] (specialist use only)

▶ BY MOUTH

- Child 2–17 years: Initially 2.5 mg/kg twice daily for 1 week, then increased to 5 mg/kg twice daily, then increased in steps of 2.5 mg/kg twice daily if required, dose to be adjusted according to response at weekly intervals, food may affect absorption (take at the same time with respect to food); maximum 20 mg/kg per day

Seizures associated with tuberous sclerosis complex [adjunctive treatment] (specialist use only)

▶ BY MOUTH

- Child 2–17 years: Initially 2.5 mg/kg twice daily for 1 week, then increased to 5 mg/kg twice daily, then increased in steps of 2.5 mg/kg twice daily if required, dose to be adjusted according to response at weekly intervals, food may affect absorption (take at the same time with respect to food); maximum 25 mg/kg per day

IMPORTANT SAFETY INFORMATION

MHRA/CHM ADVICE: ANTIEPILEPTICS: RISK OF SUICIDAL THOUGHTS AND BEHAVIOUR (AUGUST 2008)
See Epilepsy p. 227.

MHRA/CHM ADVICE: ANTIEPILEPTIC DRUGS: UPDATED ADVICE ON SWITCHING BETWEEN DIFFERENT MANUFACTURERS' PRODUCTS (NOVEMBER 2017)
See Epilepsy p. 227.

MHRA/CHM ADVICE: ANTIEPILEPTIC DRUGS IN PREGNANCY: UPDATED ADVICE FOLLOWING COMPREHENSIVE SAFETY REVIEW (JANUARY 2021)
See Epilepsy p. 227.

- **INTERACTIONS** → Appendix 1: cannabidiol
- **SIDE-EFFECTS**
  - ▶ **Common or very common** Aggression · appetite decreased · cough · diarrhoea · drowsiness · fatigue · fever · increased risk of infection · irritability · nausea · rash · seizure · vomiting · weight decreased
  - ▶ **Frequency not known** Anaemia · suicidal behaviours
- **PREGNANCY** Manufacturer advises avoid unless potential benefit outweighs risk—toxicity in *animal* studies. See also *Pregnancy* in Epilepsy p. 227.
- **BREAST FEEDING** Manufacturer advises avoid—limited information available.
- **HEPATIC IMPAIRMENT** Manufacturer advises caution in moderate to severe impairment (risk of increased exposure).
  Dose adjustments Manufacturer advises dose reduction in moderate to severe impairment—consult product literature.
- **MONITORING REQUIREMENTS** Manufacturer advises monitor liver function at baseline, at 1 month, 3 months, and 6 months of treatment, then periodically thereafter; more frequent monitoring is recommended in patients with raised baseline ALT or AST or taking valproate. Restart monitoring schedule if dose increased above 10 mg/kg/day. If transaminase or bilirubin levels increase significantly or symptoms of hepatic dysfunction occur, treatment should be withheld or permanently discontinued based on severity—consult product literature.
- **TREATMENT CESSATION** Manufacturer advises avoid abrupt withdrawal—withdraw treatment gradually.
- **DIRECTIONS FOR ADMINISTRATION** For administration advice via nasogastric or gastrostomy tube—consult product literature.
- **PATIENT AND CARER ADVICE** Oral solution should be discarded 12 weeks after first opening.
  Missed doses If doses are missed for more than 7 days, dose titration should be re-started.
  Driving and skilled tasks Patients and carers should be counselled on the effects on driving and performance of skilled tasks—increased risk of somnolence and sedation. Effects of alcohol increased.
  For information on 2015 legislation regarding driving whilst taking certain controlled drugs, including cannabis, see Drugs and driving under Guidance on prescribing p. 1.
- **NATIONAL FUNDING/ACCESS DECISIONS**
  For full details see funding body website

NICE decisions

- ▶ **Cannabidiol with clobazam for treating seizures associated with Dravet syndrome (December 2019)** NICE TA614 Recommended with restrictions
- ▶ **Cannabidiol with clobazam for treating seizures associated with Lennox-Gastaut syndrome (December 2019)** NICE TA615 Recommended with restrictions
- ▶ **Cannabidiol for treating seizures caused by tuberous sclerosis complex (March 2023)** NICE TA873 Recommended with restrictions

Scottish Medicines Consortium (SMC) decisions

- ▶ **Cannabidiol (*Epidyolex*®) as adjunctive therapy of seizures associated with Dravet syndrome (DS) in conjunction with clobazam, for patients 2 years of age and older (September 2020)** SMC No. SMC2262 Recommended
- ▶ **Cannabidiol (*Epidyolex*®) as adjunctive therapy of seizures associated with Lennox-Gastaut syndrome (LGS) in**

conjunction with clobazam, for patients 2 years of age and older (September 2020) SMC No. SMC2263 Recommended

- Cannabidiol (*Epidyolex*®) as adjunctive therapy of seizures associated with tuberous sclerosis complex (TSC) for patients 2 years of age and older (February 2022) SMC No. SMC2402 Recommended

- **MEDICINAL FORMS** There can be variation in the licensing of different medicines containing the same drug. Forms available from special-order manufacturers include: oral solution

Oral solution

CAUTIONARY AND ADVISORY LABELS 2, 8

EXCIPIENTS: May contain Benzyl alcohol, ethanol, sesame oil

- Epidyolex (Jazz Pharmaceuticals Operations UK Ltd)
  Cannabidiol 100 mg per 1 ml Epidyolex 100mg/ml oral solution | 100 ml PoM £850.29 DT = £850.29 CD5 SF

Carbamazepine

16-Jul-2024

- **INDICATIONS AND DOSE**

Trigeminal neuralgia

▶ BY MOUTH USING IMMEDIATE-RELEASE MEDICINES

- Child 1 month–11 years: Initially 5 mg/kg once daily, dose to be taken at night, alternatively initially 2.5 mg/kg twice daily, then increased in steps of 2.5–5 mg/kg every 3–7 days as required; maintenance 5 mg/kg 2–3 times a day, increased if necessary up to 20 mg/kg daily
- Child 12–17 years: Initially 100–200 mg 1–2 times a day, then increased to 200–400 mg 2–3 times a day, increased if necessary up to 1.8 g daily, dose should be increased slowly

Prophylaxis of bipolar disorder

▶ BY MOUTH USING IMMEDIATE-RELEASE MEDICINES

- Child 1 month–11 years: Initially 5 mg/kg once daily, dose to be taken at night, alternatively initially 2.5 mg/kg twice daily, then increased in steps of 2.5–5 mg/kg every 3–7 days as required; maintenance 5 mg/kg 2–3 times a day, increased if necessary up to 20 mg/kg daily
- Child 12–17 years: Initially 100–200 mg 1–2 times a day, then increased to 200–400 mg 2–3 times a day, increased if necessary up to 1.8 g daily, dose should be increased slowly

Focal and generalised tonic-clonic seizures

▶ BY MOUTH USING IMMEDIATE-RELEASE MEDICINES

- Child 1 month–11 years: Initially 5 mg/kg once daily, dose to be taken at night, alternatively initially 2.5 mg/kg twice daily, then increased in steps of 2.5–5 mg/kg every 3–7 days as required; maintenance 5 mg/kg 2–3 times a day, increased if necessary up to 20 mg/kg daily
- Child 12–17 years: Initially 100–200 mg 1–2 times a day, then increased to 200–400 mg 2–3 times a day, increased if necessary up to 1.8 g daily, dose should be increased slowly

▶ BY RECTUM

- Child: Up to 250 mg up to 4 times a day, to be used for short-term use (max. 7 days) when oral therapy temporarily not possible, use approx. 25% more than the oral dose

DOSE EQUIVALENCE AND CONVERSION

- Suppositories of 125 mg may be considered to be approximately equivalent in therapeutic effect to tablets of 100 mg but final adjustment should always depend on clinical response (plasma concentration monitoring recommended).

CARBAGEN® SR

Trigeminal neuralgia

▶ BY MOUTH

- Child 5–11 years: Initially 5 mg/kg daily in 1–2 divided doses, then increased in steps of 2.5–5 mg/kg every 3–7 days as required; maintenance 10–15 mg/kg daily in 1–2 divided doses, increased if necessary up to 20 mg/kg daily in 1–2 divided doses
- Child 12–17 years: Initially 100–400 mg daily in 1–2 divided doses, then increased to 400–1200 mg daily in 1–2 divided doses, increased if necessary up to 1.8 g daily in 1–2 divided doses, dose should be increased slowly

Focal and generalised tonic-clonic seizures | Prophylaxis of bipolar disorder

▶ BY MOUTH

- Child 5–11 years: Initially 5 mg/kg daily in 1–2 divided doses, then increased in steps of 2.5–5 mg/kg every 3–7 days as required, dose should be increased slowly; maintenance 10–15 mg/kg daily in 1–2 divided doses, increased if necessary up to 20 mg/kg daily in 1–2 divided doses
- Child 12–17 years: Initially 100–400 mg daily in 1–2 divided doses, then increased to 400–1200 mg daily in 1–2 divided doses, increased if necessary up to 1.8 g daily in 1–2 divided doses, dose should be increased slowly

TEGRETOL® PROLONGED RELEASE

Focal and generalised tonic-clonic seizures | Prophylaxis of bipolar disorder

▶ BY MOUTH

- Child 5–11 years: Initially 5 mg/kg daily in 2 divided doses, then increased in steps of 2.5–5 mg/kg every 3–7 days as required; maintenance 10–15 mg/kg daily in 2 divided doses, increased if necessary up to 20 mg/kg daily in 2 divided doses
- Child 12–17 years: Initially 100–400 mg daily in 2 divided doses, dose should be increased slowly; maintenance 400–1200 mg daily in 2 divided doses, increased if necessary up to 1.8 g daily in 2 divided doses

Trigeminal neuralgia

▶ BY MOUTH

- Child 5–11 years: Initially 5 mg/kg daily in 2 divided doses, then increased in steps of 2.5–5 mg/kg every 3–7 days as required; maintenance 10–15 mg/kg daily in 2 divided doses, increased if necessary up to 20 mg/kg daily in 2 divided doses
- Child 12–17 years: Initially 100–400 mg daily in 2 divided doses, dose should be increased slowly; maintenance 400–1200 mg daily in 2 divided doses, increased if necessary up to 1.8 g daily in 2 divided doses, dose should be increased slowly

- **UNLICENSED USE** Not licensed for use in trigeminal neuralgia or prophylaxis of bipolar disorder.

IMPORTANT SAFETY INFORMATION

MHRA/CHM ADVICE: *TEGRETOL*® 100 MG/5 ML LIQUID (CARBAMAZEPINE): TEMPORARY STOCK-OUT AND UPDATE TO POSOLOGY (REDUCTION OF MAXIMUM DAILY DOSE) (APRIL 2024)

Tegretol® 100 mg/5 mL liquid/oral suspension will imminently be out of stock due to manufacturing constraints associated with the excipient sorbitol, therefore the maximum dose of *Tegretol*® liquid has been reduced to 1200 mg per day. Patients that require *Tegretol*® liquid should be switched to alternative oral formulations of *Tegretol*®, such as immediate-release or prolonged-release tablets, where possible. If this is not feasible, other antiepileptic medicines should be considered. Patients requiring more than the maximum daily dose of *Tegretol*® liquid should be permanently switched to an appropriate alternative. For treatment guidelines and advice on switching antiepileptic medicines, see Epilepsy p. 227.

MHRA/CHM ADVICE: ANTIEPILEPTICS: RISK OF SUICIDAL THOUGHTS AND BEHAVIOUR (AUGUST 2008)

See Epilepsy p. 227.

MHRA/CHM ADVICE: ANTIEPILEPTIC DRUGS: UPDATED ADVICE ON SWITCHING BETWEEN DIFFERENT MANUFACTURERS' PRODUCTS (NOVEMBER 2017)

See Epilepsy p. 227 and see also *Prescribing and dispensing information*.

MHRA/CHM ADVICE: ANTIEPILEPTIC DRUGS IN PREGNANCY: UPDATED ADVICE FOLLOWING COMPREHENSIVE SAFETY REVIEW (JANUARY 2021)

See Epilepsy p. 227.

- **CONTRA-INDICATIONS** Acute porphyrias p. 745 · AV conduction abnormalities (unless paced) · history of bone-marrow depression
- **CAUTIONS** Cardiac disease · history of haematological reactions to other drugs · presence of HLA-B*1502 or HLA-A*3101 allele · seizures (may be exacerbated) · skin reactions · susceptibility to angle-closure glaucoma

CAUTIONS, FURTHER INFORMATION MHRA advises consider vitamin D supplementation in patients who are immobilised for long periods or who have inadequate sun exposure or dietary intake of calcium.

▸ **Blood, hepatic, or skin disorders** EvGr Carbamazepine should be withdrawn immediately in cases of aggravated liver dysfunction or acute liver disease. Leucopenia that is severe, progressive, or associated with clinical symptoms requires withdrawal (if necessary under cover of a suitable alternative). ⟨M⟩

▸ **HLA allele** EvGr The presence of HLA-B*1502 allele, particularly in individuals of Han Chinese or Thai origin, is strongly associated with an increased risk of Stevens-Johnson syndrome—see also *Pre-treatment screening*.

The presence of HLA-A*3101 allele, particularly in individuals of European or Japanese origin, is associated with an increased risk of cutaneous adverse reactions but there are insufficient data to support pre-treatment screening. Consider use if potential benefit outweighs risk. ⟨M⟩

▸ **Seizure exacerbation** EvGr Carbamazepine may exacerbate seizures in patients with absence or myoclonic seizures (including juvenile myoclonic epilepsy), tonic or atonic seizures, Dravet syndrome, Lennox-Gastaut syndrome, and myoclonic-atonic seizures. ⟨A⟩

- **INTERACTIONS** → Appendix 1: antiepileptics
- **SIDE-EFFECTS**

▸ **Common or very common** Dizziness · drowsiness · dry mouth · eosinophilia · fatigue · fluid imbalance · gastrointestinal discomfort · headache · hyponatraemia · leucopenia · movement disorders · nausea · oedema · skin reactions · thrombocytopenia · vision disorders · vomiting · weight increased

▸ **Uncommon** Constipation · diarrhoea · eye disorders · tic · tremor

▸ **Rare or very rare** Aggression · agranulocytosis · albuminuria · alopecia · anaemia · angioedema · anxiety · appetite decreased · arrhythmias · arthralgia · azotaemia · bone disorders · bone marrow disorders · cardiac conduction disorders · circulatory collapse · confusion · congestive heart failure · conjunctivitis · coronary artery disease aggravated · depression · dyspnoea · embolism and thrombosis · erythema nodosum · fever · folate deficiency · galactorrhoea · gynaecomastia · haematuria · haemolytic anaemia · hallucinations · hearing impairment · hepatic disorders · hirsutism · hyperacusia · hyperhidrosis · hypersensitivity · hypertension · hypogammaglobulinaemia · hypotension · lens opacity · leucocytosis · lymphadenopathy · meningitis aseptic · muscle complaints · muscle weakness · nephritis tubulointerstitial · nervous system disorder · neuroleptic malignant syndrome (discontinue—potentially fatal) · oral disorders · pancreatitis · paraesthesia · paresis · peripheral neuropathy · photosensitivity reaction · pneumonia · pneumonitis · pseudolymphoma · psychosis · red blood cell abnormalities · renal impairment · severe cutaneous adverse reactions (SCARs) · sexual dysfunction · speech impairment · spermatogenesis abnormal · syncope · systemic lupus erythematosus (SLE) · taste altered · tinnitus · urinary disorders · vanishing bile duct syndrome · vasculitis

▸ **Frequency not known** Bone fracture · colitis · human herpesvirus 6 infection reactivation · memory loss · nail loss · suicidal behaviours

SIDE-EFFECTS, FURTHER INFORMATION Some side-effects (such as headache, ataxia, drowsiness, nausea, vomiting, blurring of vision, dizziness and allergic skin reactions) are dose-related, and may be dose-limiting. These side-effects are more common at the start of treatment.

Overdose For details on the management of poisoning, see Active elimination techniques, under Emergency treatment of poisoning p. 1036.

- **ALLERGY AND CROSS-SENSITIVITY** Antiepileptic hypersensitivity syndrome associated with carbamazepine. See under Epilepsy p. 227 for more information. EvGr Caution—cross-sensitivity reported with oxcarbazepine, phenytoin, primidone, and phenobarbital. ⟨M⟩
- **PREGNANCY** An increased risk of major congenital malformations has been seen with carbamazepine, see *Pregnancy* in Epilepsy p. 227 for further details.

Monitoring EvGr Plasma-drug concentration should be monitored and may be maintained on the lower side of the therapeutic range provided seizure control is maintained. ⟨M⟩

- **BREAST FEEDING** Amount probably too small to be harmful.

Monitoring Monitor infant for possible adverse reactions.

- **HEPATIC IMPAIRMENT** Manufacturer advises caution and close monitoring—no information available.
- **RENAL IMPAIRMENT** EvGr Use with caution. ⟨M⟩
- **PRE-TREATMENT SCREENING** EvGr Test for HLA-B*1502 allele in individuals of Han Chinese or Thai origin, and consider testing in other at-risk Asian populations such as individuals of Filipino or Malaysian origin (avoid unless no alternative). ⟨M⟩
- **MONITORING REQUIREMENTS**

▸ Plasma concentration for optimum response 4–12 mg/litre (20–50 micromol/litre) measured after 1–2 weeks.

▸ Manufacturer recommends blood counts and hepatic and renal function tests (but evidence of practical value uncertain).

- **TREATMENT CESSATION** When stopping treatment with carbamazepine for bipolar disorder, reduce the dose gradually over a period of at least 4 weeks.
- **DIRECTIONS FOR ADMINISTRATION** Expert sources advise oral liquid has been used rectally—should be retained for at least 2 hours (but may have laxative effect).

TEGRETOL® PROLONGED RELEASE Manufacturer advises *Tegretol® Prolonged Release* tablets can be halved but should not be chewed.

- **PRESCRIBING AND DISPENSING INFORMATION**

Switching between formulations Different formulations of oral preparations may vary in bioavailability. Patients being treated for epilepsy should be maintained on a specific manufacturer's product.

Patients requiring *Tegretol®* 100 mg/5 mL liquid should

be switched to an appropriate alternative—see *Important safety information.*

- **PATIENT AND CARER ADVICE**

Blood, hepatic, or skin disorders Patients or their carers should be told how to recognise signs of blood, liver, or skin disorders, and advised to seek immediate medical attention if symptoms such as fever, rash, mouth ulcers, bruising, or bleeding develop.

Medicines for Children leaflet: Carbamazepine (oral) for preventing seizures www.medicinesforchildren.org.uk/medicines/carbamazepine-oral-for-preventing-seizures/

- **PROFESSION SPECIFIC INFORMATION**

Dental practitioners' formulary Carbamazepine Tablets may be prescribed.

- **MEDICINAL FORMS** There can be variation in the licensing of different medicines containing the same drug. Forms available from special-order manufacturers include: oral suspension, oral solution

Oral tablet

CAUTIONARY AND ADVISORY LABELS 3, 8

▸ Carbamazepine (Non-proprietary)

Carbamazepine 100 mg Carbamazepine 100mg tablets | 84 tablet PoM £3.10 DT = £2.07

Carbamazepine 200 mg Carbamazepine 200mg tablets | 84 tablet PoM £4.50 DT = £3.83

Carbamazepine 400 mg Carbamazepine 400mg tablets | 56 tablet PoM £6.00 DT = £5.02

▸ Tegretol (Novartis Pharmaceuticals UK Ltd)

Carbamazepine 100 mg Tegretol 100mg tablets | 84 tablet PoM £2.07 DT = £2.07

Carbamazepine 200 mg Tegretol 200mg tablets | 84 tablet PoM £3.83 DT = £3.83

Carbamazepine 400 mg Tegretol 400mg tablets | 56 tablet PoM £5.02 DT = £5.02

Modified-release tablet

CAUTIONARY AND ADVISORY LABELS 3, 8, 25

▸ Curatil Prolonged Release (Tillomed Laboratories Ltd)

Carbamazepine 200 mg Curatil Prolonged Release 200mg tablets | 56 tablet PoM £3.83 DT = £5.20 (Hospital only)

▸ Tegretol Retard (Novartis Pharmaceuticals UK Ltd)

Carbamazepine 200 mg Tegretol Prolonged Release 200mg tablets | 56 tablet PoM £5.20 DT = £5.20

Carbamazepine 400 mg Tegretol Prolonged Release 400mg tablets | 56 tablet PoM £10.24 DT = £10.24

Suppository

CAUTIONARY AND ADVISORY LABELS 3, 8

▸ Carbamazepine (Non-proprietary)

Carbamazepine 125 mg Carbamazepine 125mg suppositories | 5 suppository PoM £123.60 DT = £123.60

Carbamazepine 250 mg Carbamazepine 250mg suppositories | 5 suppository PoM £190.87 DT = £190.87

Oral suspension

CAUTIONARY AND ADVISORY LABELS 3, 8

▸ Carbamazepine (Non-proprietary)

Carbamazepine 20 mg per 1 ml Carbamazepine 100mg/5ml oral suspension sugar free | 300 ml PoM £12.92 DT = £12.02 SF

▸ Tegretol (Novartis Pharmaceuticals UK Ltd)

Carbamazepine 20 mg per 1 ml Tegretol 100mg/5ml liquid | 300 ml PoM £6.12 DT = £12.02 SF

Oral solution

CAUTIONARY AND ADVISORY LABELS 3, 8

Eslicarbazepine acetate

17-Oct-2022

- **INDICATIONS AND DOSE**

Adjunctive therapy of focal seizures with or without secondary generalisation

▸ BY MOUTH

▸ Child 6–17 years (body-weight up to 60 kg): Initially 10 mg/kg once daily, then increased in steps of 10 mg/kg daily, every 1–2 weeks, increased if necessary up to 30 mg/kg daily (max. per dose 1.2 g)

▸ Child 6–17 years (body-weight 60 kg and above): Initially 400 mg once daily for 1–2 weeks, then increased to 800 mg once daily (max. per dose 1.2 g)

IMPORTANT SAFETY INFORMATION

MHRA/CHM ADVICE: ANTIEPILEPTICS: RISK OF SUICIDAL THOUGHTS AND BEHAVIOUR (AUGUST 2008)

See Epilepsy p. 227.

MHRA/CHM ADVICE: ANTIEPILEPTIC DRUGS: UPDATED ADVICE ON SWITCHING BETWEEN DIFFERENT MANUFACTURERS' PRODUCTS (NOVEMBER 2017)

See Epilepsy p. 227 and see also *Prescribing and dispensing information.*

MHRA/CHM ADVICE: ANTIEPILEPTIC DRUGS IN PREGNANCY: UPDATED ADVICE FOLLOWING COMPREHENSIVE SAFETY REVIEW (JANUARY 2021)

See Epilepsy p. 227.

- **CONTRA-INDICATIONS** Second- or third-degree AV block
- **CAUTIONS** Hyponatraemia · PR-interval prolongation · presence of HLA-B*1502 or HLA-A*3101 allele

CAUTIONS, FURTHER INFORMATION

▸ HLA allele EvGr The presence of HLA-B*1502 allele, particularly in individuals of Han Chinese or Thai origin, is strongly associated with an increased risk of carbamazepine-induced Stevens-Johnson syndrome; this may also occur with eslicarbazepine acetate, a structurally-related antiepileptic—see also *Pre-treatment screening.*

The presence of HLA-A*3101 allele, particularly in individuals of European or Japanese origin, is associated with an increased risk of carbamazepine-induced cutaneous adverse reactions. This may also occur with eslicarbazepine acetate, a structurally-related antiepileptic, but there are insufficient data to support pre-treatment screening. Consider use if potential benefit outweighs risk. Ⓜ

- **INTERACTIONS** → Appendix 1: antiepileptics
- **SIDE-EFFECTS**

▸ **Common or very common** Anxiety · appetite decreased · asthenia · concentration impaired · diarrhoea · dizziness · drowsiness · gait abnormal · gastrointestinal discomfort · headaches · movement disorders · nausea · skin reactions · sleep disorders · tremor · vertigo · vision disorders · vomiting · weight changes

▸ **Uncommon** Alopecia · altered smell sensation · anaemia · bone metabolism disorder · bradycardia · cerebellar syndrome · chest pain · chills · confusion · constipation · crying · dehydration · depression · dry mouth · electrolyte imbalance · eye disorders · flushing · gastritis · haemorrhage · hearing impairment · hyperhidrosis · hypertension · hypotension · hypothyroidism · increased risk of infection · liver disorder · malaise · memory impairment · mood altered · muscle weakness · myalgia · pain in extremity · palpitations · peripheral coldness · peripheral neuropathy · peripheral oedema · psychomotor retardation · psychotic disorder · sensation abnormal · speech impairment · tinnitus · toothache

▸ **Frequency not known** Angioedema · inappropriate antidiuretic hormone secretion like-syndrome · leucopenia · pancreatitis · severe cutaneous adverse reactions (SCARs) · suicidal behaviours · thrombocytopenia

- **ALLERGY AND CROSS-SENSITIVITY** Antiepileptic hypersensitivity syndrome theoretically associated with eslicarbazepine. See under Epilepsy p. 227 for more information.
- **PREGNANCY** EvGr Caution—reproductive toxicity in *animal* studies. Ⓜ See also *Pregnancy* in Epilepsy p. 227.
- **BREAST FEEDING** Manufacturer advises avoid—present in milk in *animal* studies.

- **HEPATIC IMPAIRMENT** Manufacturer advises caution in mild to moderate impairment—limited information; avoid in severe impairment—no information available.
- **RENAL IMPAIRMENT** Manufacturer advises avoid if creatinine clearance less than 30 mL/minute.

Dose adjustments See p. 16.

Manufacturer advises *child 6–17 years (body-weight up to 60 kg)*, reduce initial dose to 5 mg/kg once daily or 10 mg/kg every other day for 2 weeks, then increase to 10 mg/kg once daily if creatinine clearance 30–60 mL/minute. The dose may be further increased based on individual response.

Manufacturer advises *child 6–17 years (body-weight 60 kg and above)*, reduce initial dose to 200 mg once daily or 400 mg every other day for 2 weeks, then increase to 400 mg once daily if creatinine clearance 30–60 mL/minute. The dose may be further increased based on individual response.

- **PRE-TREATMENT SCREENING** EvGr Test for HLA-B*1502 allele in individuals of Han Chinese or Thai origin, and consider testing in other at-risk Asian populations such as individuals of Filipino or Malaysian origin (consider use if potential benefit outweighs risk). (M)
- **MONITORING REQUIREMENTS** Monitor plasma-sodium concentration in patients at risk of hyponatraemia and discontinue treatment if hyponatraemia occurs.
- **PRESCRIBING AND DISPENSING INFORMATION**

Switching between formulations Care should be taken when switching between oral formulations. The need for continued supply of a particular manufacturer's product should be based on clinical judgement and consultation with the patient or their carer, taking into account factors such as seizure frequency and treatment history.

- **PATIENT AND CARER ADVICE**

Driving and skilled tasks Manufacturer advises patients and carers should be cautioned on the effects on driving and performance of skilled tasks—increased risk of dizziness, somnolence and visual disorders.

- **NATIONAL FUNDING/ACCESS DECISIONS**

For full details see funding body website

Scottish Medicines Consortium (SMC) decisions

- **Eslicarbazepine acetate (*Zebinix*®) for adjunctive therapy in adolescents and children aged above 6 years with partial-onset seizures with or without secondary generalisation (February 2019)** SMC No. SMC2087 Recommended with restrictions

All Wales Medicines Strategy Group (AWMSG) decisions

- **Eslicarbazepine acetate (*Zebinix*®) as adjunctive therapy in adults, adolescents and children aged above six years, with partial-onset seizures with or without secondary generalisation (June 2019)** AWMSG No. 1214 Recommended with restrictions

---

- **MEDICINAL FORMS** There can be variation in the licensing of different medicines containing the same drug.

Oral tablet

CAUTIONARY AND ADVISORY LABELS 8

- **Eslicarbazepine acetate (Non-proprietary)**
  - **Eslicarbazepine acetate 200 mg** Eslicarbazepine 200mg tablets | 60 tablet PoM £68.00 DT = £68.00
  - **Eslicarbazepine acetate 800 mg** Eslicarbazepine 800mg tablets | 30 tablet PoM £129.20 DT = £39.03
- **Arupsan** (Accord-UK Ltd)
  - **Eslicarbazepine acetate 200 mg** Arupsan 200mg tablets | 60 tablet PoM £68.00 DT = £68.00
  - **Eslicarbazepine acetate 800 mg** Arupsan 800mg tablets | 30 tablet PoM £44.69 DT = £39.03
- **Zebinix** (BIAL Pharma UK Ltd)
  - **Eslicarbazepine acetate 200 mg** Zebinix 200mg tablets | 60 tablet PoM £68.00 DT = £68.00
  - **Eslicarbazepine acetate 800 mg** Zebinix 800mg tablets | 30 tablet PoM £136.00 DT = £39.03

Oral suspension

CAUTIONARY AND ADVISORY LABELS 8

- **Zebinix** (BIAL Pharma UK Ltd)
  - **Eslicarbazepine acetate 50 mg per 1 ml** Zebinix 50mg/1ml oral suspension | 200 ml PoM £56.67 DT = £56.67 SF

Ethosuximide

26-Oct-2021

- **INDICATIONS AND DOSE**

Absence seizures | Atypical absence seizures (adjunct) | Myoclonic seizures

▶ BY MOUTH

- Child 1 month–5 years: Initially 5 mg/kg twice daily (max. per dose 125 mg), dose to be increased every 5–7 days; maintenance 10–20 mg/kg twice daily (max. per dose 500 mg), total daily dose may rarely be given in 3 divided doses
- Child 6–17 years: Initially 250 mg twice daily, then increased in steps of 250 mg every 5–7 days; usual dose 500–750 mg twice daily, increased if necessary up to 1 g twice daily

IMPORTANT SAFETY INFORMATION

MHRA/CHM ADVICE: ANTIEPILEPTICS: RISK OF SUICIDAL THOUGHTS AND BEHAVIOUR (AUGUST 2008)

See Epilepsy p. 227.

MHRA/CHM ADVICE: ANTIEPILEPTIC DRUGS: UPDATED ADVICE ON SWITCHING BETWEEN DIFFERENT MANUFACTURERS' PRODUCTS (NOVEMBER 2017)

See Epilepsy p. 227.

MHRA/CHM ADVICE: ANTIEPILEPTIC DRUGS IN PREGNANCY: UPDATED ADVICE FOLLOWING COMPREHENSIVE SAFETY REVIEW (JANUARY 2021)

See Epilepsy p. 227.

- **CAUTIONS** Avoid in Acute porphyrias p. 745
- **INTERACTIONS** → Appendix 1: antiepileptics
- **SIDE-EFFECTS**
  - **Common or very common** Appetite decreased · dizziness · drowsiness · gastrointestinal discomfort · gastrointestinal disorder · headache · movement disorders · nausea · skin reactions · vomiting
  - **Uncommon** Aggression · agranulocytosis · bone marrow disorders · concentration impaired · depression · diarrhoea · eosinophilia · fatigue · haemorrhage · hiccups · leucopenia · lupus erythematosus · mood altered · myopia · oral disorders · psychotic disorder · severe cutaneous adverse reactions (SCARs) · sleep disorders · suicidal behaviours · weight decreased
  - **Frequency not known** Generalised tonic-clonic seizure · libido increased · thrombocytopenia

SIDE-EFFECTS, FURTHER INFORMATION Blood counts required if features of fever, sore throat, mouth ulcers, bruising or bleeding.

- **PREGNANCY** See also *Pregnancy* in Epilepsy p. 227.

Monitoring EvGr Plasma-drug concentration should be regularly monitored during pregnancy; lowest effective dose must not be exceeded. (M)

- **BREAST FEEDING** Present in milk. Hyperexcitability and sedation reported.
- **HEPATIC IMPAIRMENT** Use with caution.
- **RENAL IMPAIRMENT** EvGr Use with caution—monitor drug concentration. (M)
- **PATIENT AND CARER ADVICE**

Blood disorders Patients or their carers should be told how to recognise signs of blood disorders, and advised to seek immediate medical attention if symptoms such as fever, mouth ulcers, bruising, or bleeding develop.

- **MEDICINAL FORMS** There can be variation in the licensing of different medicines containing the same drug.

Oral solution

CAUTIONARY AND ADVISORY LABELS 8

- **Ethosuximide (Non-proprietary)**
  Ethosuximide 50 mg per 1 ml Ethosuximide 250mg/5ml syrup | 200 ml [PoM] £173.00 DT = £93.05
  Ethosuximide 250mg/5ml oral solution sugar free | 125 ml [PoM] £108.13 DT = £108.13 [SF] | 200 ml [PoM] £173.00 DT = £173.00 [SF] | 250 ml [PoM] £216.25 DT = £216.25 [SF]
  Ethosuximide 100 mg per 1 ml Ethosuximide 500mg/5ml oral solution sugar free | 200 ml [PoM] £155.00 [SF]
- **Emeside** (Fontus Health Ltd)
  Ethosuximide 50 mg per 1 ml Emeside 250mg/5ml syrup | 200 ml [PoM] £91.43 DT = £93.05

Oral capsule

CAUTIONARY AND ADVISORY LABELS 8

- **Ethosuximide (Non-proprietary)**
  Ethosuximide 250 mg Ethosuximide 250mg capsules | 56 capsule [PoM] £210.68 DT = £23.80
- **Emeside** (Fontus Health Ltd)
  Ethosuximide 250 mg Emeside 250mg capsules | 56 capsule [PoM] £88.50 DT = £23.80
- **Epesri** (Strides Pharma UK Ltd)
  Ethosuximide 250 mg Epesri 250mg capsules | 56 capsule [PoM] £100.41 DT = £23.80

Fenfluramine

23-Sep-2025

- **DRUG ACTION** Fenfluramine is a serotonin-releasing agent that stimulates multiple 5-HT receptor subtypes; this action on serotonin receptors in the brain may contribute to its anti-seizure activity.

- **INDICATIONS AND DOSE**

Adjunctive therapy of seizures associated with Dravet syndrome [without concomitant stiripentol] (under expert supervision)

▶ BY MOUTH

- Child 2–17 years: Initially 0.1 mg/kg twice daily (max. per dose 13 mg) for 1 week, then increased if necessary to 0.2 mg/kg twice daily (max. per dose 13 mg) for 1 week, for patients who require more rapid titration the dose may be increased every 4 days; increased if necessary to 0.35 mg/kg twice daily (max. per dose 13 mg)

Adjunctive therapy of seizures associated with Dravet syndrome [with concomitant stiripentol] (under expert supervision)

▶ BY MOUTH

- Child 2–17 years: Initially 0.1 mg/kg twice daily (max. per dose 8.6 mg) for 1 week, then increased if necessary to 0.2 mg/kg twice daily (max. per dose 8.6 mg)

Adjunctive therapy of seizures associated with Lennox-Gastaut syndrome (under expert supervision)

▶ BY MOUTH

- Child 2–17 years: Initially 0.1 mg/kg twice daily (max. per dose 13 mg) for 1 week, then increased if tolerated to 0.2 mg/kg twice daily (max. per dose 13 mg) for 1 week, for patients who require more rapid titration the dose may be increased every 4 days, dose to be further increased if tolerated to the recommended maintenance dose; maintenance 0.35 mg/kg twice daily (max. per dose 13 mg)

IMPORTANT SAFETY INFORMATION

MHRA/CHM ADVICE: ANTIEPILEPTICS: RISK OF SUICIDAL THOUGHTS AND BEHAVIOUR (AUGUST 2008)

See Epilepsy p. 227.

MHRA/CHM ADVICE: ANTIEPILEPTIC DRUGS: UPDATED ADVICE ON SWITCHING BETWEEN DIFFERENT MANUFACTURERS' PRODUCTS (NOVEMBER 2017)

See Epilepsy p. 227.

MHRA/CHM ADVICE: ANTIEPILEPTIC DRUGS IN PREGNANCY: UPDATED ADVICE FOLLOWING COMPREHENSIVE SAFETY REVIEW (JANUARY 2021)

See Epilepsy p. 227.

- **CONTRA-INDICATIONS** Pulmonary arterial hypertension · valvular heart disease (aortic or mitral)
- **CAUTIONS** History of anorexia nervosa · history of bulimia nervosa
- **INTERACTIONS** → Appendix 1: fenfluramine
- **SIDE-EFFECTS**
  - **Common or very common** Agitation · appetite decreased · asthenia · ataxia · behaviour abnormal · constipation · diarrhoea · drowsiness · fall · fever · hypersalivation · increased risk of infection · insomnia · mood altered · muscle tone decreased · status epilepticus · tremor · vomiting · weight decreased
  - **Frequency not known** Angle closure glaucoma · mydriasis · pulmonary arterial hypertension · suicidal behaviours
- **PREGNANCY** [EvGr] Avoid—limited information available. ⟨M⟩ See also *Pregnancy* in Epilepsy p. 227.
- **BREAST FEEDING** [EvGr] Avoid—present in milk in *animal* studies. ⟨M⟩
- **HEPATIC IMPAIRMENT**
  - When used for Adjunctive therapy of seizures associated with Dravet syndrome [without concomitant stiripentol] or Adjunctive therapy of seizures associated with Lennox-Gastaut syndrome [EvGr] Caution. ⟨M⟩
  - When used for Adjunctive therapy of seizures associated with Dravet syndrome [with concomitant stiripentol] [EvGr] Avoid in moderate to severe impairment (no information available). ⟨M⟩

  Dose adjustments
  - When used for Adjunctive therapy of seizures associated with Dravet syndrome [without concomitant stiripentol] or Adjunctive therapy of seizures associated with Lennox-Gastaut syndrome [EvGr] Consider slower dose titration in all degrees of impairment. Maximum dose 0.2 mg/kg twice daily (maximum 17 mg per day) in severe impairment. ⟨M⟩
  - When used for Adjunctive therapy of seizures associated with Dravet syndrome [with concomitant stiripentol] [EvGr] Consider slower dose titration in mild impairment. ⟨M⟩
- **RENAL IMPAIRMENT**
  - When used for Adjunctive therapy of seizures associated with Dravet syndrome [without concomitant stiripentol] or Adjunctive therapy of seizures associated with Lennox-Gastaut syndrome [EvGr] Caution. ⟨M⟩
  - When used for Adjunctive therapy of seizures associated with Dravet syndrome [with concomitant stiripentol] [EvGr] Avoid (no information available). ⟨M⟩

  Dose adjustments
  - When used for Adjunctive therapy of seizures associated with Dravet syndrome [without concomitant stiripentol] or Adjunctive therapy of seizures associated with Lennox-Gastaut syndrome [EvGr] Consider slower dose titration. ⟨M⟩
- **MONITORING REQUIREMENTS**
  - [EvGr] An echocardiogram should be performed before starting treatment, then every 6 months for the first 2 years, and annually thereafter; if pathological valvular changes or pulmonary arterial hypertension develop, a follow-up echocardiogram should be performed at an earlier timeframe—consult product literature. An echocardiogram should also be performed 3–6 months after discontinuation of treatment for any reason.
  - Monitor body-weight during treatment. ⟨M⟩
- **PRESCRIBING AND DISPENSING INFORMATION** *Fintepla*® should be prescribed and dispensed according to the controlled access programme.

  The manufacturer has provided a *Prescriber Guide*.

● **PATIENT AND CARER ADVICE** The manufacturer of *Fintepla*® has provided a *Patient and Caregiver Guide*.

● **NATIONAL FUNDING/ACCESS DECISIONS**
For full details see funding body website

NICE decisions

▶ **Fenfluramine for treating seizures associated with Dravet syndrome (July 2022)** NICE TA808 Recommended with restrictions

▶ **Fenfluramine for treating seizures associated with Lennox-Gastaut syndrome in people 2 years and over (March 2025)** NICE TA1050 Recommended with restrictions

Scottish Medicines Consortium (SMC) decisions

▶ **Fenfluramine (*Fintepla*®) for the treatment of seizures associated with Dravet syndrome as an add-on therapy to other antiepileptic medicines for patients 2 years of age and older (October 2023)** SMC No. SMC2569 Recommended with restrictions

▶ **Fenfluramine (*Fintepla*®) for the treatment of seizures associated with Lennox-Gastaut syndrome as an add-on therapy to other antiepileptic medicines for patients 2 years of age and older (February 2025)** SMC No. SMC2723 Recommended with restrictions

● **MEDICINAL FORMS** There can be variation in the licensing of different medicines containing the same drug.

Oral solution

CAUTIONARY AND ADVISORY LABELS 2, 8

EXCIPIENTS: May contain Glucose, hydroxybenzoates (parabens)

▶ **Fintepla** (UCB Pharma Ltd) ▼
Fenfluramine (as Fenfluramine hydrochloride) 2.2 mg per 1 ml Fintepla 2.2mg/ml oral solution | 120 ml [PoM] £1,802.88 (Hospital only) [SF] | 360 ml [PoM] £5,408.65 (Hospital only) [SF]

Fosphenytoin sodium

10-May-2021

● **DRUG ACTION** Fosphenytoin is a pro-drug of phenytoin.

● **INDICATIONS AND DOSE**

Status epilepticus

▶ BY INTRAVENOUS INFUSION

▶ Child 5–17 years: Initially 20 mg(PE)/kg, dose to be administered at a rate of 2–3 mg(PE)/kg/minute, maximum 150 mg(PE)/minute, then 4–5 mg(PE)/kg daily in 1–4 divided doses, dose to be administered at a rate of 1–2 mg(PE)/kg/minute, maximum 100 mg(PE)/minute, dose to be adjusted according to response and trough plasma-phenytoin concentration

Prophylaxis or treatment of seizures associated with neurosurgery or head injury

▶ BY INTRAVENOUS INFUSION

▶ Child 5–17 years: Initially 10–15 mg(PE)/kg, then 4–5 mg(PE)/kg daily in 1–4 divided doses, dose to be administered at a rate of 1–2 mg(PE)/kg/minute, maximum 100 mg(PE)/minute, dose to be adjusted according to response and trough plasma-phenytoin concentration

Temporary substitution for oral phenytoin

▶ BY INTRAVENOUS INFUSION

▶ Child 5–17 years: Same dose and same dosing frequency as oral phenytoin therapy, intravenous infusion to be administered at a rate of 1–2 mg(PE)/kg/minute, maximum 100 mg(PE)/minute

DOSE EQUIVALENCE AND CONVERSION

▶ Doses are expressed as phenytoin sodium equivalent (PE); fosphenytoin sodium 1.5 mg ≡ phenytoin sodium 1 mg.

● **UNLICENSED USE** Fosphenytoin sodium doses in BNFC may differ from those in product literature.

IMPORTANT SAFETY INFORMATION

MHRA/CHM ADVICE: ANTIEPILEPTICS: RISK OF SUICIDAL THOUGHTS AND BEHAVIOUR (AUGUST 2008)
See Epilepsy p. 227.

MHRA/CHM ADVICE: ANTIEPILEPTIC DRUGS: UPDATED ADVICE ON SWITCHING BETWEEN DIFFERENT MANUFACTURERS' PRODUCTS (NOVEMBER 2017)
See Epilepsy p. 227.

MHRA/CHM ADVICE: ANTIEPILEPTIC DRUGS IN PREGNANCY: UPDATED ADVICE FOLLOWING COMPREHENSIVE SAFETY REVIEW (JANUARY 2021)
See Epilepsy p. 227.

● **CONTRA-INDICATIONS** Acute porphyrias p. 745 · second-degree heart block · sino-atrial block · sinus bradycardia · Stokes-Adams syndrome · third-degree heart block

● **CAUTIONS** Heart failure · hypotension · injection solutions alkaline (irritant to tissues) · respiratory depression · resuscitation facilities must be available

● **INTERACTIONS** → Appendix 1: antiepileptics

● **SIDE-EFFECTS**

▶ **Common or very common** Asthenia · chills · dizziness · drowsiness · dry mouth · dysarthria · euphoric mood · headache · hypotension · movement disorders · nausea · nystagmus · sensation abnormal · skin reactions · stupor · taste altered · tinnitus · tremor · vasodilation · vertigo · vision disorders · vomiting

▶ **Uncommon** Cardiac arrest · confusion · hearing impairment · muscle complaints · muscle weakness · nervousness · oral disorders · reflexes abnormal · severe cutaneous adverse reactions (SCARs) · systemic lupus erythematosus (SLE) · thinking abnormal

▶ **Frequency not known** Acute psychosis · agranulocytosis · appetite disorder · atrial conduction depression (more common if injection too rapid) · atrioventricular block · bone disorders · bone fracture · bone marrow disorders · bradycardia · cardiotoxicity · cerebrovascular insufficiency · circulatory collapse (more common if injection too rapid) · coarsening of the facial features · constipation · delirium · Dupuytren's contracture · encephalopathy · granulocytopenia · groin tingling · hair changes · hepatic disorders · hyperglycaemia · hypersensitivity · insomnia · leucopenia · lymphadenopathy · nephritis tubulointerstitial · Peyronie's disease · pneumonitis · polyarteritis nodosa · polyarthritis · purple glove syndrome · respiratory disorders · sensory peripheral polyneuropathy · suicidal behaviours · thrombocytopenia · tonic seizure · ventricular conduction depression (more common if injection too rapid) · ventricular fibrillation (more common if injection too rapid)

SIDE-EFFECTS, FURTHER INFORMATION Fosphenytoin has been associated with severe cardiovascular reactions including asystole, ventricular fibrillation, and cardiac arrest. Hypotension, bradycardia, and heart block have also been reported. The following are recommended: monitor heart rate, blood pressure, and respiratory function for duration of infusion; observe patient for at least 30 minutes after infusion; if hypotension occurs, reduce infusion rate or discontinue; reduce dose or infusion rate in renal or hepatic impairment.

● **ALLERGY AND CROSS-SENSITIVITY** Cross-sensitivity reported with carbamazepine.

● **PREGNANCY** An increased risk of major congenital malformations and possibility of adverse effects on neurodevelopment have been seen with phenytoin, see *Pregnancy* in Epilepsy p. 227.

Monitoring Changes in plasma-protein binding make interpretation of plasma-phenytoin concentrations difficult—monitor unbound fraction.

EvGr Doses should be adjusted on the basis of plasma-drug concentration monitoring—phenytoin pharmacokinetics altered during pregnancy. (M)

- **BREAST FEEDING** Small amounts present in milk, but not known to be harmful.
- **HEPATIC IMPAIRMENT** Manufacturer advises caution—monitor free plasma-phenytoin concentration (rather than total plasma-phenytoin concentration) in hepatic impairment or hypoalbuminaemia and in hyperbilirubinaemia.

Dose adjustments Manufacturer advises consider a 10–25% reduction in dose or infusion rate (except in the treatment of status epilepticus) in hepatic impairment or hypoalbuminaemia.

- **RENAL IMPAIRMENT** EvGr Caution—monitor free plasma-phenytoin concentration (rather than total plasma-phenytoin concentration) in renal impairment or hypoalbuminaemia. (M)

Dose adjustments EvGr Consider a 10–25% reduction in dose or infusion rate (except in the treatment of status epilepticus) in renal impairment or hypoalbuminaemia. (M)

- **PRE-TREATMENT SCREENING** HLA-B* 1502 allele in individuals of Han Chinese or Thai origin—avoid unless essential (increased risk of Stevens-Johnson syndrome).
- **MONITORING REQUIREMENTS**
  - Manufacturer recommends blood counts (but evidence of practical value uncertain).
  - Monitor heart rate, blood pressure, ECG, and respiratory function for during infusion.
- **DIRECTIONS FOR ADMINISTRATION** For *intermittent intravenous infusion* (*Pro-Epanutin*®), manufacturer advises give *in* Glucose 5% *or* Sodium Chloride 0.9%; dilute to a concentration of 1.5–25 mg (phenytoin sodium equivalent (PE))/mL.
- **PRESCRIBING AND DISPENSING INFORMATION** Prescriptions for fosphenytoin sodium should state the dose in terms of phenytoin sodium equivalent (PE); fosphenytoin sodium 1.5 mg ≡ phenytoin sodium 1 mg.

- **MEDICINAL FORMS** There can be variation in the licensing of different medicines containing the same drug.

Solution for injection

ELECTROLYTES: May contain Phosphate

- **Pro-Epanutin** (Pfizer Ltd)

Fosphenytoin sodium 75 mg per 1 ml Pro-Epanutin 750mg/10ml concentrate for solution for injection vials | 10 vial PoM £400.00 (Hospital only)

Gabapentin

04-Feb-2026

- **INDICATIONS AND DOSE**

Adjunctive treatment of focal seizures with or without secondary generalisation

- BY MOUTH
  - Child 2–5 years: 10 mg/kg once daily on day 1, then 10 mg/kg twice daily on day 2, then 10 mg/kg 3 times a day on day 3, then increased to 30–70 mg/kg daily in 3 divided doses, adjusted according to response, some children may not tolerate daily increments; longer intervals (up to weekly) may be more appropriate
  - Child 6–11 years: 10 mg/kg once daily (max. per dose 300 mg) on day 1, then 10 mg/kg twice daily (max. per dose 300 mg) on day 2, then 10 mg/kg 3 times a day (max. per dose 300 mg) on day 3; usual dose 25–35 mg/kg daily in 3 divided doses, some children may not tolerate daily increments; longer intervals (up to weekly) may be more appropriate, daily dose maximum to be given in 3 divided doses; maximum 70 mg/kg per day
  - Child 12–17 years: Initially 300 mg once daily on day 1, then 300 mg twice daily on day 2, then 300 mg 3 times a day on day 3, alternatively initially 300 mg 3 times a day on day 1, then increased in steps of 300 mg every 2–3 days in 3 divided doses, adjusted according to response; usual dose 0.9–3.6 g daily in 3 divided doses (max. per dose 1.6 g 3 times a day), some children may not tolerate daily increments; longer intervals (up to weekly) may be more appropriate

Monotherapy for focal seizures with or without secondary generalisation

- BY MOUTH
  - Child 12–17 years: Initially 300 mg once daily on day 1, then 300 mg twice daily on day 2, then 300 mg 3 times a day on day 3, alternatively initially 300 mg 3 times a day on day 1, then increased in steps of 300 mg every 2–3 days in 3 divided doses, adjusted according to response; usual dose 0.9–3.6 g daily in 3 divided doses (max. per dose 1.6 g 3 times a day), some children may not tolerate daily increments; longer intervals (up to weekly) may be more appropriate

- **UNLICENSED USE** Not licensed for use in children under 6 years. Not licensed at doses over 50 mg/kg daily in children under 12 years.

IMPORTANT SAFETY INFORMATION

The levels of propylene glycol, acesulfame K and saccharin sodium may exceed the recommended WHO daily intake limits if high doses of gabapentin oral solution (Rosemont brand) are given to adolescents or adults with low body-weight (39–50 kg)—consult product literature.

MHRA/CHM ADVICE: ANTIEPILEPTICS: RISK OF SUICIDAL THOUGHTS AND BEHAVIOUR (AUGUST 2008)

See Epilepsy p. 227.

MHRA/CHM ADVICE: GABAPENTIN (*NEURONTIN*®): RISK OF SEVERE RESPIRATORY DEPRESSION (OCTOBER 2017)

Gabapentin has been associated with a rare risk of severe respiratory depression even without concomitant opioid medicines. Patients with compromised respiratory function, respiratory or neurological disease, renal impairment, and concomitant use of central nervous system (CNS) depressants might be at higher risk of experiencing severe respiratory depression and dose adjustments may be necessary in these patients.

MHRA/CHM ADVICE: ANTIEPILEPTIC DRUGS: UPDATED ADVICE ON SWITCHING BETWEEN DIFFERENT MANUFACTURERS' PRODUCTS (NOVEMBER 2017)

See Epilepsy p. 227.

MHRA/CHM ADVICE: GABAPENTIN (*NEURONTIN*®) AND RISK OF ABUSE AND DEPENDENCE: NEW SCHEDULING REQUIREMENTS FROM 1 APRIL (APRIL 2019)

Following concerns about abuse, gabapentin has been reclassified as a Class C controlled substance and is now a Schedule 3 drug, but is exempt from safe custody requirements. Healthcare professionals should evaluate patients carefully for a history of drug abuse before prescribing gabapentin, and observe patients for signs of abuse and dependence. Patients should be informed of the potentially fatal risks of interactions between gabapentin and alcohol, and with other medicines that cause CNS depression, particularly opioids.

MHRA/CHM ADVICE: ANTIEPILEPTIC DRUGS IN PREGNANCY: UPDATED ADVICE FOLLOWING COMPREHENSIVE SAFETY REVIEW (JANUARY 2021)

See Epilepsy p. 227.

MHRA/CHM ADVICE: IMPROVING INFORMATION SUPPLIED WITH GABAPENTINOIDS (PREGABALIN/GABAPENTIN), BENZODIAZEPINES AND Z-DRUGS (JANUARY 2026)

An MHRA review concluded that warnings regarding addiction, dependence, withdrawal, and tolerance need to be strengthened, to better inform healthcare professionals and patients of these known risks. Specialist use of these medicines for conditions such as epilepsy or sedation during medical procedures were not included as part of this review. Healthcare professionals are advised to create a strategy with patients for reducing or ending treatment prior to treatment initiation and provide an individually tailored dose reduction schedule, as well as counselling on the risk of drug withdrawal syndrome. All patients should be closely monitored for signs of misuse, abuse, addiction or tolerance, and regular support provided, especially to those at increased risk of drug withdrawal syndrome.

- **CAUTIONS** Diabetes mellitus · high doses of oral solution in adolescents and adults with low body-weight · history of substance abuse · respiratory depression, see *Important safety information* · seizures (may be exacerbated)

CAUTIONS, FURTHER INFORMATION

- Seizure exacerbation EvGr Gabapentin may exacerbate seizures in patients with absence or myoclonic seizures (including juvenile myoclonic epilepsy), tonic or atonic seizures, Dravet syndrome, Lennox-Gastaut syndrome, and myoclonic-atonic seizures. (A)

- **INTERACTIONS** → Appendix 1: antiepileptics
- **SIDE-EFFECTS**
  - **Common or very common** Anxiety · appetite abnormal · arthralgia · asthenia · behaviour abnormal · confusion · constipation · cough · depression · diarrhoea · dizziness · drowsiness · dry mouth · dry throat · dysarthria · dyspnoea · emotional lability · fever · flatulence · gait abnormal · gastrointestinal discomfort · headache · hypertension · increased risk of infection · insomnia · leucopenia · malaise · memory loss · movement disorders · muscle complaints · nausea · nystagmus · oedema · pain · reflexes abnormal · sensation abnormal · sexual dysfunction · skin reactions · thinking abnormal · tooth disorder · tremor · vasodilation · vertigo · visual impairment · vomiting · weight increased
  - **Uncommon** Cognitive impairment · dysphagia · hyperglycaemia · palpitations
  - **Rare or very rare** Hypoglycaemia · loss of consciousness · respiratory depression
  - **Frequency not known** Acute kidney injury · alopecia · angioedema · breast enlargement · chest pain · drug dependence · gynaecomastia · hallucination · hepatic disorders · hyponatraemia · pancreatitis · rhabdomyolysis · severe cutaneous adverse reactions (SCARs) · suicidal behaviours · thrombocytopenia · tinnitus · urinary incontinence · withdrawal syndrome
- **PREGNANCY** Manufacturer advises avoid unless benefit outweighs risk — toxicity reported. See also *Pregnancy* in Epilepsy p. 227.
- **BREAST FEEDING** Present in milk—manufacturer advises use only if potential benefit outweighs risk. See also *Breast-feeding* in Epilepsy p. 227.
- **RENAL IMPAIRMENT**

Dose adjustments See p. 16.

Manufacturer advises reduce dose if creatinine clearance less than 80 mL/minute (consult product literature).

- **EFFECT ON LABORATORY TESTS** False positive readings with some urinary protein tests.
- **TREATMENT CESSATION** The MHRA advises avoid abrupt treatment cessation—reduce dose gradually to minimise symptoms of withdrawal (specialist use such as epilepsy or sedation during medical procedures not included in MHRA review—see also *Important safety information*).
- **DIRECTIONS FOR ADMINISTRATION** Expert sources advise capsules can be opened but the bitter taste is difficult to mask.
- **PATIENT AND CARER ADVICE**

Medicines for Children leaflet: Gabapentin for preventing seizures www.medicinesforchildren.org.uk/medicines/gabapentin-for-preventing-seizures/

Patient leaflet NHS England has produced a patient leaflet with information on the reclassification of gabapentin.

- **MEDICINAL FORMS** There can be variation in the licensing of different medicines containing the same drug. Forms available from special-order manufacturers include: oral suspension, oral solution

Oral tablet

CAUTIONARY AND ADVISORY LABELS 3, 5, 8, 25

- **Gabapentin (Non-proprietary)**
  - **Gabapentin 600 mg** Gabapentin 600mg tablets | 100 tablet PoM £52.50 DT = £4.09 CD3
  - **Gabapentin 800 mg** Gabapentin 800mg tablets | 100 tablet PoM £78.00 DT = £10.20 CD3
- **Neurontin** (Viatris UK Healthcare Ltd)
  - **Gabapentin 600 mg** Neurontin 600mg tablets | 100 tablet PoM £84.80 DT = £4.09 CD3
  - **Gabapentin 800 mg** Neurontin 800mg tablets | 100 tablet PoM £98.13 DT = £10.20 CD3

Oral capsule

CAUTIONARY AND ADVISORY LABELS 3, 5, 8, 25

- **Gabapentin (Non-proprietary)**
  - **Gabapentin 100 mg** Gabapentin 100mg capsules | 100 capsule PoM £18.29 DT = £1.10 CD3
  - **Gabapentin 300 mg** Gabapentin 300mg capsules | 100 capsule PoM £42.40 DT = £1.63 CD3
  - **Gabapentin 400 mg** Gabapentin 400mg capsules | 100 capsule PoM £49.06 DT = £1.96 CD3
- **Neurontin** (Viatris UK Healthcare Ltd)
  - **Gabapentin 100 mg** Neurontin 100mg capsules | 100 capsule PoM £18.29 DT = £1.10 CD3
  - **Gabapentin 300 mg** Neurontin 300mg capsules | 100 capsule PoM £42.40 DT = £1.63 CD3
  - **Gabapentin 400 mg** Neurontin 400mg capsules | 100 capsule PoM £49.06 DT = £1.96 CD3

Oral solution

CAUTIONARY AND ADVISORY LABELS 3, 5, 8

EXCIPIENTS: May contain Propylene glycol

ELECTROLYTES: May contain Potassium, sodium

- **Gabapentin (Non-proprietary)**
  - **Gabapentin 50 mg per 1 ml** Neurontin 250mg/5ml oral solution | 470 ml PoM (S) CD3
  - Gabapentin 50mg/ml oral solution sugar free | 150 ml PoM £67.29 DT = £13.79 Schedule 3 (CD No Register Exempt Safe Custody) SF

Lacosamide

11-Nov-2022

- **INDICATIONS AND DOSE**

Monotherapy of focal seizures with or without secondary generalisation

▶ BY MOUTH, OR BY INTRAVENOUS INFUSION

- Child (body-weight 50 kg and above): Initially 50 mg twice daily, then increased to 100 mg twice daily after 1 week, alternatively initially 100 mg twice daily; increased in steps of 50 mg twice daily (max. per dose 300 mg twice daily) if necessary and if tolerated, dose to be increased at weekly intervals
- Child 2–17 years (body-weight 10–39 kg): Initially 1 mg/kg twice daily, then increased to 2 mg/kg twice daily after 1 week; increased in steps of 1 mg/kg twice daily (max. per dose 6 mg/kg twice daily) if necessary and if tolerated, dose to be increased at weekly intervals
- Child 2–17 years (body-weight 40–49 kg): Initially 1 mg/kg twice daily, then increased to 2 mg/kg twice daily after 1 week; increased in steps of 1 mg/kg twice daily (max. per dose 5 mg/kg twice daily) if necessary and if tolerated, dose to be increased at weekly intervals

continued →

Monotherapy of focal seizures with or without secondary generalisation (alternative loading dose regimen when it is necessary to rapidly attain therapeutic plasma concentrations) (under close medical supervision)

▶ BY MOUTH, OR BY INTRAVENOUS INFUSION

▸ Child (body-weight 50 kg and above): Loading dose 200 mg, followed by 100 mg twice daily, to be given 12 hours after initial dose; increased in steps of 50 mg twice daily (max. per dose 300 mg twice daily) if necessary and if tolerated, dose to be increased at weekly intervals

Adjunctive treatment of focal seizures with or without secondary generalisation

▶ BY MOUTH, OR BY INTRAVENOUS INFUSION

▸ Child (body-weight 50 kg and above): Initially 50 mg twice daily, then increased to 100 mg twice daily after 1 week; increased in steps of 50 mg twice daily (max. per dose 200 mg twice daily) if necessary and if tolerated, dose to be increased at weekly intervals

▸ Child 2–17 years (body-weight 10–19 kg): Initially 1 mg/kg twice daily, then increased to 2 mg/kg twice daily after 1 week; increased in steps of 1 mg/kg twice daily (max. per dose 6 mg/kg twice daily) if necessary and if tolerated, dose to be increased at weekly intervals

▸ Child 2–17 years (body-weight 20–29 kg): Initially 1 mg/kg twice daily, then increased to 2 mg/kg twice daily after 1 week; increased in steps of 1 mg/kg twice daily (max. per dose 5 mg/kg twice daily) if necessary and if tolerated, dose to be increased at weekly intervals

▸ Child 2–17 years (body-weight 30–49 kg): Initially 1 mg/kg twice daily, then increased to 2 mg/kg twice daily after 1 week; increased in steps of 1 mg/kg twice daily (max. per dose 4 mg/kg twice daily) if necessary and if tolerated, dose to be increased at weekly intervals

Adjunctive treatment of primary generalised tonic-clonic seizures

▶ BY MOUTH, OR BY INTRAVENOUS INFUSION

▸ Child (body-weight 50 kg and above): Initially 50 mg twice daily, then increased to 100 mg twice daily after 1 week; increased in steps of 50 mg twice daily (max. per dose 200 mg twice daily) if necessary and if tolerated, dose to be increased at weekly intervals

▸ Child 4–17 years (body-weight 10–19 kg): Initially 1 mg/kg twice daily, then increased to 2 mg/kg twice daily after 1 week; increased in steps of 1 mg/kg twice daily (max. per dose 6 mg/kg twice daily) if necessary and if tolerated, dose to be increased at weekly intervals

▸ Child 4–17 years (body-weight 20–29 kg): Initially 1 mg/kg twice daily, then increased to 2 mg/kg twice daily after 1 week; increased in steps of 1 mg/kg twice daily (max. per dose 5 mg/kg twice daily) if necessary and if tolerated, dose to be increased at weekly intervals

▸ Child 4–17 years (body-weight 30–49 kg): Initially 1 mg/kg twice daily, then increased to 2 mg/kg twice daily after 1 week; increased in steps of 1 mg/kg twice daily (max. per dose 4 mg/kg twice daily) if necessary and if tolerated, dose to be increased at weekly intervals

Adjunctive treatment of focal seizures with or without secondary generalisation (alternative loading dose regimen when it is necessary to rapidly attain therapeutic plasma concentrations) (under close medical supervision) | Adjunctive treatment of primary generalised tonic-clonic seizures (alternative loading dose regimen when it is necessary to rapidly attain therapeutic plasma concentrations) (under close medical supervision)

▶ BY MOUTH, OR BY INTRAVENOUS INFUSION

▸ Child (body-weight 50 kg and above): Loading dose 200 mg, followed by 100 mg twice daily, to be given 12 hours after initial dose; increased in steps of 50 mg twice daily (max. per dose 200 mg twice daily) if necessary and if tolerated, dose to be increased at weekly intervals

IMPORTANT SAFETY INFORMATION

MHRA/CHM ADVICE: ANTIEPILEPTICS: RISK OF SUICIDAL THOUGHTS AND BEHAVIOUR (AUGUST 2008)

See Epilepsy p. 227.

MHRA/CHM ADVICE: ANTIEPILEPTIC DRUGS: UPDATED ADVICE ON SWITCHING BETWEEN DIFFERENT MANUFACTURERS' PRODUCTS (NOVEMBER 2017)

See Epilepsy p. 227.

MHRA/CHM ADVICE: ANTIEPILEPTIC DRUGS IN PREGNANCY: UPDATED ADVICE FOLLOWING COMPREHENSIVE SAFETY REVIEW (JANUARY 2021)

See Epilepsy p. 227.

- **CONTRA-INDICATIONS** Second- or third-degree AV block
- **CAUTIONS** Conduction problems · risk of PR-interval prolongation · seizures (may be exacerbated) · severe cardiac disease

CAUTIONS, FURTHER INFORMATION

▸ **Seizure exacerbation** EvGr Lacosamide may exacerbate seizures in patients with Dravet syndrome and Lennox-Gastaut syndrome. (A)

- **INTERACTIONS** → Appendix 1: antiepileptics
- **SIDE-EFFECTS**

▶ **Common or very common** Asthenia · cognitive disorder · concentration impaired · confusion · constipation · depression · diarrhoea · dizziness · drowsiness · dry mouth · dysarthria · dyspepsia · feeling drunk · flatulence · gait abnormal · headache · insomnia · memory impairment · mood altered · movement disorders · muscle spasms · myoclonic seizure · nausea · nystagmus · sensation abnormal · skin reactions · tinnitus · tremor · vertigo · vision disorders · vomiting

▶ **Uncommon** Agitation · angioedema · arrhythmias · atrioventricular block · behaviour abnormal · hallucination · psychotic disorder · suicidal behaviours · syncope

▶ **Frequency not known** Agranulocytosis · appetite decreased · fever · increased risk of infection · severe cutaneous adverse reactions (SCARs)

- **ALLERGY AND CROSS-SENSITIVITY** Antiepileptic hypersensitivity syndrome associated with lacosamide. See under Epilepsy p. 227 for more information.
- **PREGNANCY** EvGr Avoid unless potential benefit outweighs risk—embryotoxic in *animal* studies. (M) See also *Pregnancy* in Epilepsy p. 227.
- **BREAST FEEDING** Specialist sources indicate use with caution only if no suitable alternative—present in milk; monitor infant neurodevelopment and monitor infant for adverse effects.
- **HEPATIC IMPAIRMENT** Manufacturer advises caution (risk of increased exposure), particularly in severe impairment (no information available).

  Dose adjustments Manufacturer advises consider dose reduction—consult product literature.
- **RENAL IMPAIRMENT**

  Dose adjustments EvGr Dose reduction may be required (consult product literature). (M)
- **DIRECTIONS FOR ADMINISTRATION** For *intermittent intravenous infusion*, manufacturer advises give undiluted or dilute with Glucose 5% *or* Sodium Chloride 0.9% *or* Lactated Ringer's Solution; give over 15–60 minutes—give doses greater than 200 mg over at least 30 minutes.
- **PRESCRIBING AND DISPENSING INFORMATION** Flavours of syrup may include strawberry.
- **PATIENT AND CARER ADVICE** Patients and carers should be counselled on the symptoms of cardiac arrhythmia and

advised to seek immediate medical advice if these occur.
Medicines for Children leaflet: Lacosamide for preventing seizures www.medicinesforchildren.org.uk/medicines/lacosamide-for-preventing-seizures/

Missed doses If a dose is more than 6 hours late, the missed dose should not be taken and the next dose should be taken at the normal time.

Driving and skilled tasks Patients and carers should be counselled on the effects on driving and performance of skilled tasks—increased risk of dizziness and blurred vision.

- **NATIONAL FUNDING/ACCESS DECISIONS**
For full details see funding body website

Scottish Medicines Consortium (SMC) decisions

- **Lacosamide (*Vimpat*®) as adjunctive therapy in the treatment of partial-onset seizures with or without secondary generalisation in patients with epilepsy aged 16 years or older (February 2009)** SMC No. 532/09 Recommended with restrictions
- **Lacosamide (*Vimpat*®) as adjunctive therapy in the treatment of partial-onset seizures with or without secondary generalisation in adolescents and children from 4 years of age with epilepsy (February 2018)** SMC No. 1301/18 Recommended with restrictions

All Wales Medicines Strategy Group (AWMSG) decisions

- **Lacosamide (*Vimpat*®) as adjunctive therapy in the treatment of partial-onset seizures with or without secondary generalisation in children from 2 years of age up to 15 years of age with epilepsy (October 2022)** AWMSG No. 4698 Recommended

- **MEDICINAL FORMS** There can be variation in the licensing of different medicines containing the same drug.

Solution for infusion

ELECTROLYTES: May contain Sodium

- Lacosamide (Non-proprietary)
Lacosamide 10 mg per 1 ml Lacosamide 200mg/20ml solution for infusion vials | 1 vial PoM £29.70 DT = £29.70 (Hospital only)
- Vimpat (UCB Pharma Ltd)
Lacosamide 10 mg per 1 ml Vimpat 200mg/20ml solution for infusion vials | 1 vial PoM £29.70 DT = £29.70

Oral tablet

CAUTIONARY AND ADVISORY LABELS 8

- Lacosamide (Non-proprietary)
Lacosamide 50 mg Lacosamide 50mg tablets | 14 tablet PoM £10.81 DT = £0.97
Lacosamide 100 mg Lacosamide 100mg tablets | 14 tablet PoM £1.14–£21.62 | 56 tablet PoM £86.50 DT = £2.35
Lacosamide 150 mg Lacosamide 150mg tablets | 14 tablet PoM £32.44 DT = £2.80 | 56 tablet PoM £129.74 DT = £11.20
Lacosamide 200 mg Lacosamide 200mg tablets | 56 tablet PoM £168.66 DT = £3.58
- Vimpat (UCB Pharma Ltd)
Lacosamide 50 mg Vimpat 50mg tablets | 14 tablet PoM £10.81 DT = £0.97
Lacosamide 100 mg Vimpat 100mg tablets | 14 tablet PoM £21.62 | 56 tablet PoM £86.50 DT = £2.35
Lacosamide 150 mg Vimpat 150mg tablets | 14 tablet PoM £32.44 DT = £2.80 | 56 tablet PoM £129.74 DT = £11.20
Lacosamide 200 mg Vimpat 200mg tablets | 56 tablet PoM £144.16 DT = £3.58

Oral solution

CAUTIONARY AND ADVISORY LABELS 8
EXCIPIENTS: May contain Aspartame, propylene glycol
ELECTROLYTES: May contain Sodium

- Lacosamide (Non-proprietary)
Lacosamide 10 mg per 1 ml Lacosamide 10mg/ml oral solution sugar free | 200 ml PoM £25.74 DT = £10.64 SF
- Vimpat (UCB Pharma Ltd)
Lacosamide 10 mg per 1 ml Vimpat 10mg/ml syrup | 200 ml PoM £25.74 DT = £10.64 SF

Lamotrigine

17-Oct-2022

- **INDICATIONS AND DOSE**

Monotherapy of focal seizures | Monotherapy of primary and secondary generalised tonic-clonic seizures | Monotherapy of seizures associated with Lennox-Gastaut syndrome

▶ BY MOUTH

- Child 12–17 years: Initially 25 mg once daily for 14 days, then increased to 50 mg once daily for further 14 days, then increased in steps of up to 100 mg every 7–14 days; maintenance 100–200 mg daily in 1–2 divided doses; increased if necessary up to 500 mg daily, dose titration should be repeated if restarting after interval of more than 5 days

Monotherapy of typical absence seizures

▶ BY MOUTH

- Child 2–11 years: Initially 300 micrograms/kg daily in 1–2 divided doses, for 14 days, then 600 micrograms/kg daily in 1–2 divided doses, for further 14 days, then increased in steps of up to 600 micrograms/kg every 7–14 days; maintenance 1–10 mg/kg daily in 1–2 divided doses, increased if necessary up to 15 mg/kg daily, dose titration should be repeated if restarting after interval of more than 5 days

Adjunctive therapy of focal seizures with valproate | Adjunctive therapy of primary and secondary generalised tonic-clonic seizures with valproate | Adjunctive therapy of seizures associated with Lennox-Gastaut syndrome with valproate

▶ BY MOUTH

- Child 2–11 years (body-weight up to 13 kg): Initially 2 mg once daily on alternate days for first 14 days, then 300 micrograms/kg once daily for further 14 days, then increased in steps of up to 300 micrograms/kg every 7–14 days; maintenance 1–5 mg/kg daily in 1–2 divided doses, dose titration should be repeated if restarting after interval of more than 5 days; maximum 200 mg per day
- Child 2–11 years (body-weight 13 kg and above): Initially 150 micrograms/kg once daily for 14 days, then 300 micrograms/kg once daily for further 14 days, then increased in steps of up to 300 micrograms/kg every 7–14 days; maintenance 1–5 mg/kg daily in 1–2 divided doses, dose titration should be repeated if restarting after interval of more than 5 days; maximum 200 mg per day
- Child 12–17 years: Initially 25 mg once daily on alternate days for 14 days, then 25 mg once daily for further 14 days, then increased in steps of up to 50 mg every 7–14 days; maintenance 100–200 mg daily in 1–2 divided doses, dose titration should be repeated if restarting after interval of more than 5 days

Adjunctive therapy of focal seizures (with enzyme inducing drugs) without valproate | Adjunctive therapy of primary and secondary generalised tonic-clonic seizures (with enzyme inducing drugs) without valproate | Adjunctive therapy of seizures associated with Lennox-Gastaut syndromes (with enzyme inducing drugs) without valproate

▶ BY MOUTH

- Child 2–11 years: Initially 300 micrograms/kg twice daily for 14 days, then 600 micrograms/kg twice daily for further 14 days, then increased in steps of up to 1.2 mg/kg every 7–14 days; maintenance 5–15 mg/kg daily in 1–2 divided doses, dose titration should be repeated if restarting after interval of more than 5 days; maximum 400 mg per day
- Child 12–17 years: Initially 50 mg once daily for 14 days, then 50 mg twice daily for further 14 days, then increased in steps of up to 100 mg every

continued →

7–14 days; maintenance 200–400 mg daily in 2 divided doses, increased if necessary up to 700 mg daily, dose titration should be repeated if restarting after interval of more than 5 days

Adjunctive therapy of focal seizures (without enzyme inducing drugs) without valproate | Adjunctive therapy of primary and secondary generalised tonic-clonic seizures (without enzyme inducing drugs) without valproate | Adjunctive therapy of seizures associated with Lennox-Gastaut syndromes (without enzyme inducing drugs) without valproate

- BY MOUTH
  - Child 2–11 years: Initially 300 micrograms/kg daily in 1–2 divided doses for 14 days, then 600 micrograms/kg daily in 1–2 divided doses for further 14 days, then increased in steps of up to 600 micrograms/kg every 7–14 days; maintenance 1–10 mg/kg daily in 1–2 divided doses, dose titration should be repeated if restarting after interval of more than 5 days; maximum 200 mg per day
  - Child 12–17 years: Initially 25 mg once daily for 14 days, then increased to 50 mg once daily for further 14 days, then increased in steps of up to 100 mg every 7–14 days; maintenance 100–200 mg daily in 1–2 divided doses, dose titration should be repeated if restarting after interval of more than 5 days

IMPORTANT SAFETY INFORMATION

MHRA/CHM ADVICE: ANTIEPILEPTICS: RISK OF SUICIDAL THOUGHTS AND BEHAVIOUR (AUGUST 2008)

See Epilepsy p. 227.

MHRA/CHM ADVICE: ANTIEPILEPTIC DRUGS: UPDATED ADVICE ON SWITCHING BETWEEN DIFFERENT MANUFACTURERS' PRODUCTS (NOVEMBER 2017)

See Epilepsy p. 227 and see also *Prescribing and dispensing information.*

MHRA/CHM ADVICE: ANTIEPILEPTIC DRUGS IN PREGNANCY: UPDATED ADVICE FOLLOWING COMPREHENSIVE SAFETY REVIEW (JANUARY 2021)

See Epilepsy p. 227.

- **CAUTIONS** Brugada syndrome · seizures (may be exacerbated)

  CAUTIONS, FURTHER INFORMATION
  - **Seizure exacerbation** EvGr Lamotrigine may exacerbate seizures in patients with myoclonic seizures (including juvenile myoclonic epilepsy), Dravet syndrome, and Lennox-Gastaut syndrome. (A)
- **INTERACTIONS** → Appendix 1: antiepileptics
- **SIDE-EFFECTS**
  - **Common or very common** Aggression · agitation · arthralgia · diarrhoea · dizziness · drowsiness · dry mouth · fatigue · headache · irritability · nausea · pain · rash · sleep disorders · tremor · vomiting
  - **Uncommon** Alopecia · movement disorders · vision disorders
  - **Rare or very rare** Confusion · conjunctivitis · disseminated intravascular coagulation · face oedema · fever · haemophagocytic lymphohistiocytosis · hallucination · hepatic disorders · lupus-like syndrome · lymphadenopathy · meningitis aseptic · multi organ failure · nystagmus · seizure · severe cutaneous adverse reactions (SCARs) · tic
  - **Frequency not known** Suicidal behaviours

  SIDE-EFFECTS, FURTHER INFORMATION Serious skin reactions including Stevens-Johnson syndrome and toxic epidermal necrolysis have developed; most rashes occur in the first 8 weeks. Rash is sometimes associated with hypersensitivity syndrome and is more common in patients with history of allergy or rash from other antiepileptic drugs. Consider withdrawal if rash or signs of hypersensitivity syndrome develop. Factors associated with increased risk of serious skin reactions include concomitant use of valproate, initial lamotrigine dosing higher than recommended, and more rapid dose escalation than recommended.
- **ALLERGY AND CROSS-SENSITIVITY** Antiepileptic hypersensitivity syndrome associated with lamotrigine. See under Epilepsy p. 227 for more information.
- **PREGNANCY** See also *Pregnancy* in Epilepsy p. 227.

  Monitoring EvGr Plasma-drug concentration should be monitored before, during, and after pregnancy, including shortly after birth, and doses adjusted according to response—plasma levels alter during pregnancy and may increase rapidly after birth. (M)
- **BREAST FEEDING** Present in milk, but limited data suggest no harmful effect on infant.
- **HEPATIC IMPAIRMENT** Manufacturer advises caution in moderate to severe impairment.

  Dose adjustments Manufacturer advises dose reduction of approx. 50% in moderate impairment, and approx. 75% in severe impairment; adjust according to response.
- **RENAL IMPAIRMENT** EvGr Caution in renal failure; metabolite may accumulate. (M)

  Dose adjustments EvGr Consider reducing maintenance dose in significant impairment. (M)
- **TREATMENT CESSATION** Avoid abrupt withdrawal (taper off over 2 weeks or longer) unless serious skin reaction occurs.
- **PRESCRIBING AND DISPENSING INFORMATION** Patients being treated for epilepsy may need to be maintained on a specific manufacturer's branded or generic lamotrigine product.

  Switching between formulations Care should be taken when switching between oral formulations in the treatment of epilepsy. The need for continued supply of a particular manufacturer's product should be based on clinical judgement and consultation with the patient or their carer, taking into account factors such as seizure frequency and treatment history.
- **PATIENT AND CARER ADVICE**

  Skin reactions Warn patients and carers to see their doctor immediately if rash or signs or symptoms of hypersensitivity syndrome develop.

  Blood disorders Patients and their carers should be alert for symptoms and signs suggestive of bone-marrow failure, such as anaemia, bruising, or infection. Aplastic anaemia, bone-marrow depression, and pancytopenia have been associated rarely with lamotrigine.

  Medicines for Children leaflet: Lamotrigine for preventing seizures www.medicinesforchildren.org.uk/medicines/lamotrigine-for-preventing-seizures/
- **MEDICINAL FORMS** There can be variation in the licensing of different medicines containing the same drug. Forms available from special-order manufacturers include: oral suspension, oral solution

Dispersible tablet

CAUTIONARY AND ADVISORY LABELS 8, 13

- **Lamotrigine (Non-proprietary)**

  Lamotrigine 5 mg Lamotrigine 5mg dispersible tablets sugar free | 28 tablet PoM £16.00 DT = £13.18 SF

  Lamotrigine 25 mg Lamotrigine 25mg dispersible tablets sugar free | 56 tablet PoM £20.00 DT = £19.70 SF

  Lamotrigine 100 mg Lamotrigine 100mg dispersible tablets sugar free | 56 tablet PoM £58.68 DT = £13.75 SF
- **Lamictal** (GlaxoSmithKline UK Ltd)

  Lamotrigine 2 mg Lamictal 2mg dispersible tablets | 30 tablet PoM £18.81 DT = £18.81 SF

  Lamotrigine 5 mg Lamictal 5mg dispersible tablets | 30 tablet PoM £10.05 SF

  Lamotrigine 25 mg Lamictal 25mg dispersible tablets | 56 tablet PoM £23.53 DT = £19.70 SF

  Lamotrigine 100 mg Lamictal 100mg dispersible tablets | 56 tablet PoM £69.04 DT = £13.75 SF

Oral tablet

CAUTIONARY AND ADVISORY LABELS 8

▸ **Lamotrigine (Non-proprietary)**
Lamotrigine 25 mg Lamotrigine 25mg tablets | 56 tablet [PoM] £4.00 DT = £0.90
Lamotrigine 50 mg Lamotrigine 50mg tablets | 56 tablet [PoM] £6.00 DT = £1.14
Lamotrigine 100 mg Lamotrigine 100mg tablets | 56 tablet [PoM] £8.00 DT = £1.27
Lamotrigine 200 mg Lamotrigine 200mg tablets | 56 tablet [PoM] £10.00 DT = £1.98

▸ **Lamictal** (GlaxoSmithKline UK Ltd)
Lamotrigine 25 mg Lamictal 25mg tablets | 56 tablet [PoM] £23.53 DT = £0.90
Lamotrigine 50 mg Lamictal 50mg tablets | 56 tablet [PoM] £40.02 DT = £1.14
Lamotrigine 100 mg Lamictal 100mg tablets | 56 tablet [PoM] £69.04 DT = £1.27
Lamotrigine 200 mg Lamictal 200mg tablets | 56 tablet [PoM] £117.35 DT = £1.98

Oral suspension

▸ **Lamotrigine (Non-proprietary)**
Lamotrigine 10 mg per 1 ml Lamotrigine 10mg/ml oral suspension sugar free | 300 ml [PoM] £43.87 [SF]

Levetiracetam

31-Jan-2025

● **INDICATIONS AND DOSE**

Monotherapy of focal seizures with or without secondary generalisation

▶ BY MOUTH, OR BY INTRAVENOUS INFUSION

▸ Child 16–17 years: Initially 250 mg once daily for 1 week, then increased to 250 mg twice daily, dose then increased in steps of 250 mg twice daily every 2 weeks up to maximum 1.5 g twice daily, to be adjusted according to response

Adjunctive therapy of focal seizures with or without secondary generalisation

▶ BY MOUTH

▸ Child 1–5 months: Initially 7 mg/kg once daily, dose then increased in steps of up to 7 mg/kg twice daily every 2 weeks up to maximum 21 mg/kg twice daily
▸ Child 6 months–17 years (body-weight up to 50 kg): Initially 10 mg/kg once daily, dose then increased in steps of up to 10 mg/kg twice daily every 2 weeks up to maximum 30 mg/kg twice daily
▸ Child 12–17 years (body-weight 50 kg and above): Initially 250 mg twice daily, dose then increased in steps of 500 mg twice daily every 2–4 weeks up to maximum 1.5 g twice daily

▶ BY INTRAVENOUS INFUSION

▸ Child 4–17 years (body-weight up to 50 kg): Initially 10 mg/kg once daily, dose then increased in steps of up to 10 mg/kg twice daily every 2 weeks up to maximum 30 mg/kg twice daily
▸ Child 12–17 years (body-weight 50 kg and above): Initially 250 mg twice daily, dose then increased in steps of 500 mg twice daily every 2 weeks up to maximum 1.5 g twice daily

Adjunctive therapy of myoclonic seizures and tonic-clonic seizures

▶ BY MOUTH, OR BY INTRAVENOUS INFUSION

▸ Child 12–17 years (body-weight up to 50 kg): Initially 10 mg/kg once daily, dose then increased in steps of up to 10 mg/kg twice daily every 2 weeks up to maximum 30 mg/kg twice daily
▸ Child 12–17 years (body-weight 50 kg and above): Initially 250 mg twice daily, dose then increased in steps of 500 mg twice daily every 2 weeks up to maximum 1.5 g twice daily

Convulsive status epilepticus (administered on expert advice)

▶ BY INTRAVENOUS INFUSION

▸ Child: 40 mg/kg for 1 dose (max. per dose 3 g), consult local protocols

● **UNLICENSED USE** [EvGr] Initial dosing recommendations for levetiracetam ⟨E⟩ in BNF Publications differ from product licence. [EvGr] Levetiracetam is used for the treatment of convulsive status epilepticus, ⟨A⟩ but is not licensed for this indication. [EvGr] *Granules* and *granules for oral solution* are not licensed for use in children aged under 6 years, for initial treatment in children with body-weight less than 25 kg, or for the administration of doses below 250 mg—*oral solution* should be used. ⟨M⟩

IMPORTANT SAFETY INFORMATION

MHRA/CHM ADVICE: ANTIEPILEPTICS: RISK OF SUICIDAL THOUGHTS AND BEHAVIOUR (AUGUST 2008)
See Epilepsy p. 227.

MHRA/CHM ADVICE: ANTIEPILEPTIC DRUGS: UPDATED ADVICE ON SWITCHING BETWEEN DIFFERENT MANUFACTURERS' PRODUCTS (NOVEMBER 2017)
See Epilepsy p. 227.

MHRA/CHM ADVICE: ANTIEPILEPTIC DRUGS IN PREGNANCY: UPDATED ADVICE FOLLOWING COMPREHENSIVE SAFETY REVIEW (JANUARY 2021)
See Epilepsy p. 227.

● **CAUTIONS** Risk factors for QT interval prolongation

● **INTERACTIONS** → Appendix 1: antiepileptics

● **SIDE-EFFECTS**

▶ **Common or very common** Anxiety · appetite decreased · asthenia · behaviour abnormal · cough · depression · diarrhoea · dizziness · drowsiness · gastrointestinal discomfort · headache · increased risk of infection · insomnia · mood altered · movement disorders · nausea · skin reactions · tremor · vertigo · vomiting

▶ **Uncommon** Alopecia · concentration impaired · confusion · hallucination · leucopenia · memory impairment · muscle weakness · myalgia · paraesthesia · psychotic disorder · suicidal behaviours · thrombocytopenia · vision disorders · weight changes

▶ **Rare or very rare** Acute kidney injury · agranulocytosis · bone marrow disorders · delirium · encephalopathy · gait abnormal · hepatic disorders · hyponatraemia · neutropenia · pancreatitis · personality disorder · QT interval prolongation · rhabdomyolysis · seizures exacerbated · severe cutaneous adverse reactions (SCARs) · thinking abnormal

▶ **Frequency not known** Neuroleptic malignant syndrome (discontinue—potentially fatal)

● **PREGNANCY** See also *Pregnancy* in Epilepsy p. 227.
Monitoring [EvGr] Clinical response should be monitored during pregnancy—plasma concentrations decrease during pregnancy (by up to 60% in the third trimester). ⟨M⟩

● **BREAST FEEDING** Present in milk—manufacturer advises avoid.

● **HEPATIC IMPAIRMENT** Manufacturer advises caution in severe impairment.
Dose adjustments Manufacturer advises maintenance dose reduction of 50% in severe impairment if creatinine clearance is less than 60 mL/minute/1.73 m^2—consult product literature.

● **RENAL IMPAIRMENT**
Dose adjustments Reduce dose if estimated glomerular filtration rate less than 80 mL/minute/1.73 m^2 (consult product literature).

● **DIRECTIONS FOR ADMINISTRATION**

▸ When used for Focal seizures or Myoclonic seizures or Tonic-clonic seizures [EvGr] When using *concentrate for solution for infusion,* dilute calculated dose with at least 100 mL Glucose 5% or Sodium Chloride 0.9%; give over 15 minutes. ⟨M⟩ If a smaller volume is required, local policies advise to dilute to a final concentration of 2.5–15 mg/mL.

- With intravenous use for Convulsive status epilepticus [EvGr] When using *concentrate for solution for infusion,* dilute calculated dose with Glucose 5% or Sodium Chloride 0.9% to a concentration of 50 mg/mL and give over 5 minutes. ⟨A⟩
- With oral use [EvGr] For administration of *oral solution,* dose may be diluted in a glass of water. ⟨M⟩

● **PRESCRIBING AND DISPENSING INFORMATION** If switching between oral therapy and intravenous therapy (for those temporarily unable to take oral medication), the intravenous dose should be the same as the established oral dose.

● **PATIENT AND CARER ADVICE** Patients and caregivers should be advised to seek medical advice if signs of depression or suicidal ideation emerge. Patients should consult their doctor immediately if seizures worsen.
Medicines for Children leaflet: Levetiracetam for preventing seizures www.medicinesforchildren.org.uk/medicines/levetiracetam-for-preventing-seizures/
Driving and skilled tasks Patients and carers should be cautioned on the effects on driving and performance of skilled tasks—increased risk of somnolence or other CNS side-effects.

● **MEDICINAL FORMS** There can be variation in the licensing of different medicines containing the same drug. Forms available from special-order manufacturers include: oral solution, infusion

Oral tablet

CAUTIONARY AND ADVISORY LABELS 3, 8

- **Levetiracetam (Non-proprietary)**
  Levetiracetam 250 mg Levetiracetam 250mg tablets | 60 tablet [PoM] £25.25 DT = £1.27
  Levetiracetam 500 mg Levetiracetam 500mg tablets | 60 tablet [PoM] £47.31 DT = £2.93 | 200 tablet [PoM] £17.70
  Levetiracetam 750 mg Levetiracetam 750mg tablets | 60 tablet [PoM] £81.25 DT = £2.77
  Levetiracetam 1 gram Levetiracetam 1g tablets | 60 tablet [PoM] £92.25 DT = £3.44
- **Keppra** (UCB Pharma Ltd)
  Levetiracetam 250 mg Keppra 250mg tablets | 60 tablet [PoM] £28.01 DT = £1.27
  Levetiracetam 500 mg Keppra 500mg tablets | 60 tablet [PoM] £49.32 DT = £2.93
  Levetiracetam 750 mg Keppra 750mg tablets | 60 tablet [PoM] £84.02 DT = £2.77
  Levetiracetam 1 gram Keppra 1g tablets | 60 tablet [PoM] £95.34 DT = £3.44

Solution for infusion

ELECTROLYTES: May contain Sodium

- **Levetiracetam (Non-proprietary)**
  Levetiracetam 100 mg per 1 ml Levetiracetam 500mg/5ml solution for infusion ampoules | 10 ampoule [PoM] £127.31 DT = £127.31 (Hospital only)
  Levetiracetam 500mg/5ml concentrate for solution for infusion vials | 10 vial [PoM] £127.50 DT = £127.31 (Hospital only)
- **Desitrend** (Desitin Pharma Ltd)
  Levetiracetam 100 mg per 1 ml Desitrend 500mg/5ml concentrate for solution for infusion ampoules | 10 ampoule [PoM] £127.31 DT = £127.31
- **Keppra** (UCB Pharma Ltd)
  Levetiracetam 100 mg per 1 ml Keppra 500mg/5ml concentrate for solution for infusion vials | 10 vial [PoM] £127.31 DT = £127.31 (Hospital only)

Oral solution

CAUTIONARY AND ADVISORY LABELS 3, 8

- **Levetiracetam (Non-proprietary)**
  Levetiracetam 100 mg per 1 ml Levetiracetam 100mg/ml oral solution sugar free | 150 ml [PoM] £26.40 [SF] | 300 ml [PoM] £66.95 DT = £3.45 [SF]
- **Eltam** (Medley Pharma Ltd)
  Levetiracetam 100 mg per 1 ml Eltam 100mg/ml oral solution | 150 ml [PoM] £23.30 [SF] | 300 ml [PoM] £48.95 DT = £3.45 [SF]
- **Keppra** (UCB Pharma Ltd)
  Levetiracetam 100 mg per 1 ml Keppra 100mg/ml oral solution | 150 ml [PoM] £33.48 [SF] | 300 ml [PoM] £66.95 DT = £3.45 [SF]

Granules for oral solution

CAUTIONARY AND ADVISORY LABELS 3, 8

- **Levetiracetam (Non-proprietary)**
  Levetiracetam 250 mg Levetiracetam 250mg granules for oral solution sachets sugar free | 60 sachet [PoM] £22.41–£29.20 [SF]
  Levetiracetam 500 mg Levetiracetam 500mg granules for oral solution sachets sugar free | 60 sachet [PoM] £39.46–£51.40 [SF]
  Levetiracetam 750 mg Levetiracetam 750mg granules for oral solution sachets sugar free | 60 sachet [PoM] £57.87–£101.28 [SF]
  Levetiracetam 1 gram Levetiracetam 1g granules for oral solution sachets sugar free | 60 sachet [PoM] £76.27–£99.20 [SF]
  Levetiracetam 1.5 gram Levetiracetam 1.5g granules for oral solution sachets sugar free | 60 sachet [PoM] £110.73–£193.78 [SF]

Oral granules

CAUTIONARY AND ADVISORY LABELS 3, 8

- **Desitrend** (Desitin Pharma Ltd)
  Levetiracetam 250 mg Desitrend 250mg granules sachets | 60 sachet [PoM] £22.41 DT = £22.41 [SF]
  Levetiracetam 500 mg Desitrend 500mg granules sachets | 60 sachet [PoM] £39.46 DT = £39.46 [SF]
  Levetiracetam 1 gram Desitrend 1000mg granules sachets | 60 sachet [PoM] £76.27 DT = £76.27 [SF]

Infusion

ELECTROLYTES: May contain Sodium

Oxcarbazepine

17-Oct-2022

● **INDICATIONS AND DOSE**

Monotherapy for the treatment of focal seizures with or without secondary generalised tonic-clonic seizures

▶ BY MOUTH

- Child 6–17 years: Initially 4–5 mg/kg twice daily (max. per dose 300 mg), then increased in steps of up to 5 mg/kg twice daily, adjusted according to response, dose to be adjusted at weekly intervals; maximum 46 mg/kg per day

Adjunctive therapy for the treatment of focal seizures with or without secondary generalised tonic-clonic seizures

▶ BY MOUTH

- Child 6–17 years: Initially 4–5 mg/kg twice daily (max. per dose 300 mg), then increased in steps of up to 5 mg/kg twice daily, adjusted according to response, dose to be adjusted at weekly intervals; maintenance 15 mg/kg twice daily; maximum 46 mg/kg per day

DOSE ADJUSTMENTS DUE TO INTERACTIONS

- In adjunctive therapy, the dose of concomitant antiepileptics may need to be reduced when using high doses of oxcarbazepine.

IMPORTANT SAFETY INFORMATION

MHRA/CHM ADVICE: ANTIEPILEPTICS: RISK OF SUICIDAL THOUGHTS AND BEHAVIOUR (AUGUST 2008)

See Epilepsy p. 227.

MHRA/CHM ADVICE: ANTIEPILEPTIC DRUGS: UPDATED ADVICE ON SWITCHING BETWEEN DIFFERENT MANUFACTURERS' PRODUCTS (NOVEMBER 2017)

See Epilepsy p. 227 and see also *Prescribing and dispensing information.*

MHRA/CHM ADVICE: ANTIEPILEPTIC DRUGS IN PREGNANCY: UPDATED ADVICE FOLLOWING COMPREHENSIVE SAFETY REVIEW (JANUARY 2021)

See Epilepsy p. 227.

● **CAUTIONS** Avoid in Acute porphyrias p. 745 · cardiac conduction disorders · heart failure · hyponatraemia ·

presence of HLA-B*1502 or HLA-A*3101 allele · seizures (may be exacerbated)

CAUTIONS, FURTHER INFORMATION

- HLA allele EvGr The presence of HLA-B*1502 allele, particularly in individuals of Han Chinese or Thai origin, is strongly associated with an increased risk of carbamazepine-induced Stevens-Johnson syndrome; this may also occur with oxcarbazepine, a structurally-related antiepileptic—see also *Pre-treatment screening*.

  The presence of HLA-A*3101 allele, particularly in individuals of European or Japanese origin, is associated with an increased risk of carbamazepine-induced cutaneous adverse reactions. This may also occur with oxcarbazepine, a structurally-related antiepileptic, but there are insufficient data to support pre-treatment screening. Consider use if potential benefit outweighs risk. (M)
- Seizure exacerbation EvGr Oxcarbazepine may exacerbate seizures in patients with absence or myoclonic seizures (including juvenile myoclonic epilepsy), tonic or atonic seizures, Dravet syndrome, Lennox-Gastaut syndrome, and myoclonic-atonic seizures. (A)

- **INTERACTIONS** → Appendix 1: antiepileptics
- **SIDE-EFFECTS**
  - **Common or very common** Abdominal pain · agitation · alopecia · asthenia · ataxia · concentration impaired · confusion · constipation · depression · diarrhoea · dizziness · drowsiness · emotional lability · headache · hyponatraemia · memory loss · nausea · nystagmus · skin reactions · speech impairment · tremor · vertigo · vision disorders · vomiting · weight increased
  - **Uncommon** Hypertension · hypothyroidism · leucopenia
  - **Rare or very rare** Agranulocytosis · angioedema · arrhythmia · atrioventricular block · bone disorders · bone fracture · bone marrow disorders · hepatitis · inappropriate antidiuretic hormone secretion like-syndrome · neutropenia · pancreatitis · severe cutaneous adverse reactions (SCARs) · systemic lupus erythematosus (SLE) · thrombocytopenia
  - **Frequency not known** Suicidal behaviours
- **ALLERGY AND CROSS-SENSITIVITY** Caution in patients with hypersensitivity to carbamazepine. Antiepileptic hypersensitivity syndrome associated with oxcarbazepine. See under Epilepsy p. 227 for more information.
- **PREGNANCY** See also *Pregnancy* in Epilepsy p. 227.
  Monitoring EvGr Clinical response should be monitored carefully during pregnancy, and plasma concentration monitoring of the active metabolite should be considered during and after pregnancy (if doses were increased during pregnancy)—plasma levels of the active metabolite may gradually decrease during pregnancy. (M)
- **BREAST FEEDING** Amount probably too small to be harmful but manufacturer advises avoid.
- **HEPATIC IMPAIRMENT** Manufacturer advises caution in severe impairment (no information available).
- **RENAL IMPAIRMENT**
  Dose adjustments EvGr Halve initial dose if creatinine clearance less than 30 mL/minute; increase according to response at intervals of at least 1 week. (M) See p. 16.
- **PRE-TREATMENT SCREENING** EvGr Test for HLA-B*1502 allele in individuals of Han Chinese or Thai origin, and consider testing in other at-risk Asian populations such as individuals of Filipino or Malaysian origin (consider use if potential benefit outweighs risk). (M)
- **MONITORING REQUIREMENTS**
  - Monitor plasma-sodium concentration in patients at risk of hyponatraemia.
  - Monitor body-weight in patients with heart failure.
- **PRESCRIBING AND DISPENSING INFORMATION** Patients may need to be maintained on a specific manufacturer's branded or generic oxcarbazepine product.
  Switching between formulations Care should be taken when switching between oral formulations. The need for continued supply of a particular manufacturer's product should be based on clinical judgement and consultation with the patient or their carer, taking into account factors such as seizure frequency and treatment history.
- **PATIENT AND CARER ADVICE**
  Blood, hepatic, or skin disorders Patients or their carers should be told how to recognise signs of blood, liver, or skin disorders, and advised to seek immediate medical attention if symptoms such as lethargy, confusion, muscular twitching, fever, rash, blistering, mouth ulcers, bruising, or bleeding develop.
  Medicines for Children: Oxcarbazepine for preventing seizures www.medicinesforchildren.org.uk/medicines/oxcarbazepine-for-preventing-seizures/
- **MEDICINAL FORMS** There can be variation in the licensing of different medicines containing the same drug. Forms available from special-order manufacturers include: oral suspension

Oral tablet

CAUTIONARY AND ADVISORY LABELS 3, 8

- **Oxcarbazepine (Non-proprietary)**
  Oxcarbazepine 150 mg Oxcarbazepine 150mg tablets | 50 tablet PoM £22.03 DT = £22.29
  Oxcarbazepine 300 mg Oxcarbazepine 300mg tablets | 50 tablet PoM £24.48 DT = £5.79
  Oxcarbazepine 600 mg Oxcarbazepine 600mg tablets | 50 tablet PoM £51.22 DT = £46.83
- **Trileptal** (Novartis Pharmaceuticals UK Ltd)
  Oxcarbazepine 150 mg Trileptal 150mg tablets | 50 tablet PoM £12.24 DT = £22.29
  Oxcarbazepine 300 mg Trileptal 300mg tablets | 50 tablet PoM £24.48 DT = £5.79
  Oxcarbazepine 600 mg Trileptal 600mg tablets | 50 tablet PoM £48.96 DT = £46.83

Oral suspension

CAUTIONARY AND ADVISORY LABELS 3, 8
EXCIPIENTS: May contain Propylene glycol

- **Trileptal** (Novartis Pharmaceuticals UK Ltd)
  Oxcarbazepine 60 mg per 1 ml Trileptal 60mg/ml oral suspension | 250 ml PoM £48.96 DT = £48.96 SF

Perampanel

22-Jun-2021

- **INDICATIONS AND DOSE**

Adjunctive treatment of focal seizures with or without secondary generalised seizures

- BY MOUTH
  - Child 4–11 years (body-weight up to 20 kg): Initially 1 mg once daily, dose to be taken before bedtime, then increased, if tolerated, in steps of 1 mg at intervals of at least every 2 weeks, adjusted according to response; maintenance 2–4 mg once daily, then increased, if tolerated, in steps of 0.5 mg at intervals of at least every 2 weeks, adjusted according to response; maximum 6 mg per day
  - Child 4–11 years (body-weight 20–29 kg): Initially 1 mg once daily, dose to be taken before bedtime, then increased, if tolerated, in steps of 1 mg at intervals of at least every 2 weeks, adjusted according to response; maintenance 4–6 mg once daily; maximum 8 mg per day
  - Child 4–11 years (body-weight 30 kg and above): Initially 2 mg once daily, dose to be taken before bedtime, then increased, if tolerated, in steps of 2 mg at intervals of at least every 2 weeks, adjusted according to response; maintenance 4–8 mg once daily; maximum 12 mg per day

continued →

- Child 12–17 years: Initially 2 mg once daily, dose to be taken before bedtime, then increased, if tolerated, in steps of 2 mg at intervals of at least every 2 weeks, adjusted according to response; maintenance 4–8 mg once daily; maximum 12 mg per day

Adjunctive treatment of primary generalised tonic-clonic seizures

- BY MOUTH
- Child 7–11 years (body-weight up to 20 kg): Initially 1 mg once daily, dose to be taken before bedtime, then increased, if tolerated, in steps of 1 mg at intervals of at least every 2 weeks, adjusted according to response; maintenance 2–4 mg once daily, then increased, if tolerated, in steps of 0.5 mg at intervals of at least every 2 weeks, adjusted according to response; maximum 6 mg per day
- Child 7–11 years (body-weight 20–29 kg): Initially 1 mg once daily, dose to be taken before bedtime, then increased in steps of 1 mg at intervals of at least every 2 weeks, adjusted according to response; maintenance 4–6 mg once daily; maximum 8 mg per day
- Child 7–11 years (body-weight 30 kg and above): Initially 2 mg once daily, dose to be taken before bedtime, then increased, if tolerated, in steps of 2 mg at intervals of at least every 2 weeks, adjusted according to response; maintenance 4–8 mg once daily; maximum 12 mg per day
- Child 12–17 years: Initially 2 mg once daily, dose to be taken before bedtime, then increased, if tolerated, in steps of 2 mg at intervals of at least every 2 weeks, adjusted according to response, maintenance up to 8 mg once daily; maximum 12 mg per day

DOSE ADJUSTMENTS DUE TO INTERACTIONS

- Titrate at intervals of at least 1 week with concomitant carbamazepine, fosphenytoin, oxcarbazepine, or phenytoin.

IMPORTANT SAFETY INFORMATION

MHRA/CHM ADVICE: ANTIEPILEPTICS: RISK OF SUICIDAL THOUGHTS AND BEHAVIOUR (AUGUST 2008)

See Epilepsy p. 227.

MHRA/CHM ADVICE: ANTIEPILEPTIC DRUGS: UPDATED ADVICE ON SWITCHING BETWEEN DIFFERENT MANUFACTURERS' PRODUCTS (NOVEMBER 2017)

See Epilepsy p. 227 and see also *Prescribing and dispensing information*.

MHRA/CHM ADVICE: ANTIEPILEPTIC DRUGS IN PREGNANCY: UPDATED ADVICE FOLLOWING COMPREHENSIVE SAFETY REVIEW (JANUARY 2021)

See Epilepsy p. 227.

- **INTERACTIONS** → Appendix 1: antiepileptics
- **SIDE-EFFECTS**
  - **Common or very common** Anxiety · appetite abnormal · back pain · behaviour abnormal · confusion · dizziness · drowsiness · dysarthria · fatigue · gait abnormal · irritability · movement disorders · nausea · vertigo · vision disorders · weight increased
  - **Uncommon** Suicidal behaviours
  - **Frequency not known** Homicidal ideation · severe cutaneous adverse reactions (SCARs)
- **PREGNANCY** EvGr Avoid—embryotoxic in *animal* studies. (M) See also *Pregnancy* in Epilepsy p. 227.
- **BREAST FEEDING** Avoid—present in milk in *animal* studies.
- **HEPATIC IMPAIRMENT** EvGr Caution in mild to moderate impairment; avoid in severe impairment. (M)
  Dose adjustments EvGr Maximum 8 mg per day in mild to moderate impairment. (M)
- **RENAL IMPAIRMENT** EvGr Avoid in moderate or severe impairment. (M)
- **PRESCRIBING AND DISPENSING INFORMATION**
  Switching between formulations Care should be taken when switching between oral formulations. The need for continued supply of a particular manufacturer's product should be based on clinical judgement and consultation with the patient or their carer, taking into account factors such as seizure frequency and treatment history.
  Patients may need to be maintained on a specific manufacturer's branded or generic perampanel product.
- **PATIENT AND CARER ADVICE**
  Driving and skilled tasks Manufacturer advises patients and carers should be cautioned on the effects on driving and performance of skilled tasks—increased risk of dizziness and drowsiness.
- **NATIONAL FUNDING/ACCESS DECISIONS**
  For full details see funding body website

Scottish Medicines Consortium (SMC) decisions

- **Perampanel (*Fycompa®*) for the adjunctive treatment of partial-onset seizures with or without secondary generalised seizures in patients with epilepsy aged 12 years and older (December 2012)** SMC No. 819/12 Recommended with restrictions
- **Perampanel oral suspension (*Fycompa®*) for the adjunctive treatment of partial-onset seizures with or without secondary generalised seizures in patients with epilepsy aged 12 years and older (August 2019)** SMC No. SMC2172 Recommended with restrictions

All Wales Medicines Strategy Group (AWMSG) decisions

- **Perampanel (*Fycompa®*) for the adjunctive treatment of partial-onset seizures with or without secondary generalised seizures in patients from 4 years of age up to 12 years of age (May 2021)** AWMSG No. 4770 Recommended with restrictions

- **MEDICINAL FORMS** There can be variation in the licensing of different medicines containing the same drug. Forms available from special-order manufacturers include: oral suspension

Oral tablet

CAUTIONARY AND ADVISORY LABELS 3, 8, 25

- **Perampanel (Non-proprietary)**
  Perampanel 2 mg Perampanel 2mg tablets | 7 tablet PoM £35.00 DT = £35.00 | 28 tablet PoM £140.00 DT = £140.00
  Perampanel 4 mg Perampanel 4mg tablets | 28 tablet PoM £140.00 DT = £140.00
  Perampanel 6 mg Perampanel 6mg tablets | 28 tablet PoM £140.00 DT = £140.00
  Perampanel 8 mg Perampanel 8mg tablets | 28 tablet PoM £140.00 DT = £140.00
  Perampanel 10 mg Perampanel 10mg tablets | 28 tablet PoM £140.00 DT = £140.00
  Perampanel 12 mg Perampanel 12mg tablets | 28 tablet PoM £140.00 DT = £140.00
- **Fycompa** (Eisai Ltd)
  Perampanel 2 mg Fycompa 2mg tablets | 7 tablet PoM £35.00 DT = £35.00 | 28 tablet PoM £140.00 DT = £140.00
  Perampanel 4 mg Fycompa 4mg tablets | 28 tablet PoM £140.00 DT = £140.00
  Perampanel 6 mg Fycompa 6mg tablets | 28 tablet PoM £140.00 DT = £140.00
  Perampanel 8 mg Fycompa 8mg tablets | 28 tablet PoM £140.00 DT = £140.00
  Perampanel 10 mg Fycompa 10mg tablets | 28 tablet PoM £140.00 DT = £140.00
  Perampanel 12 mg Fycompa 12mg tablets | 28 tablet PoM £140.00 DT = £140.00

Oral suspension

CAUTIONARY AND ADVISORY LABELS 3, 8

EXCIPIENTS: May contain Sorbitol

- **Perampanel (Non-proprietary)**
  Perampanel 500 microgram per 1 ml Perampanel 500micrograms/ml oral suspension sugar free | 340 ml PoM £127.50 DT = £127.50 SF

Phenytoin

13-Oct-2025

● **INDICATIONS AND DOSE**

Tonic-clonic seizures | Focal seizures

▶ BY MOUTH

- Child 1 month–11 years: Initially 1.5–2.5 mg/kg twice daily (max. per dose 150 mg), then adjusted according to response to 2.5–5 mg/kg twice daily (max. per dose 150 mg), dose also adjusted according to plasma-phenytoin concentration, increased if necessary up to 7.5 mg/kg twice daily (max. per dose 150 mg)
- Child 12–17 years: Initially 75–150 mg twice daily, then adjusted according to response to 150–200 mg twice daily, dose also adjusted according to plasma-phenytoin concentration, increased if necessary up to 300 mg twice daily

▶ INITIALLY BY SLOW INTRAVENOUS INJECTION

- Neonate: Loading dose 18 mg/kg for 1 dose, dose to be administered over 20–30 minutes, then (by mouth) adjusted according to response to 2.5–5 mg/kg twice daily, dose also adjusted according to plasma-phenytoin concentration, (by mouth) increased if necessary up to 7.5 mg/kg twice daily.

Prevention and treatment of seizures during or following neurosurgery or severe head injury

▶ BY MOUTH

- Child: Initially 2.5 mg/kg twice daily, then adjusted according to response to 4–8 mg/kg daily, dose also adjusted according to plasma-phenytoin concentration; maximum 300 mg per day

Status epilepticus | Acute symptomatic seizures associated with head trauma or neurosurgery

▶ INITIALLY BY SLOW INTRAVENOUS INJECTION, OR BY INTRAVENOUS INFUSION

- Neonate: Loading dose 20 mg/kg for 1 dose, then (by slow intravenous injection or by intravenous infusion) 2.5–5 mg/kg twice daily.
- Child 1 month–11 years: Loading dose 20 mg/kg for 1 dose, then (by slow intravenous injection or by intravenous infusion) 2.5–5 mg/kg twice daily
- Child 12–17 years: Loading dose 20 mg/kg for 1 dose, then (by intravenous infusion or by slow intravenous injection) up to 100 mg 3–4 times a day

DOSE EQUIVALENCE AND CONVERSION

- Preparations containing phenytoin sodium are **not** bioequivalent to those containing phenytoin base (such as *Epanutin Infatabs*® and *Epanutin*® suspension); 100 mg of phenytoin sodium is approximately equivalent in therapeutic effect to 92 mg phenytoin base. The dose is the same for all phenytoin products when initiating therapy. However, if switching between these products the difference in phenytoin content may be clinically significant. Care is needed when making changes between formulations and plasma-phenytoin concentration monitoring is recommended.

PHARMACOKINETICS

- Phenytoin has a narrow therapeutic index and the relationship between dose and plasma-drug concentration is non-linear; small dosage increases in some patients may produce large increases in plasma-drug concentration with acute toxic side-effects. Similarly, a few missed doses or a small change in drug absorption may result in a marked change in plasma-drug concentration. Monitoring of plasma-drug concentration improves dosage adjustment.

● **UNLICENSED USE**

- With oral use Licensed for use in children (age range not specified by manufacturer).
- With intravenous use Phenytoin doses in BNF publications may differ from those in product literature.

IMPORTANT SAFETY INFORMATION

MHRA/CHM ADVICE: ANTIEPILEPTICS: RISK OF SUICIDAL THOUGHTS AND BEHAVIOUR (AUGUST 2008)

See Epilepsy p. 227.

NHS ENGLAND PATIENT SAFETY ALERT: RISK OF DEATH AND SEVERE HARM FROM ERROR WITH INJECTABLE PHENYTOIN (NOVEMBER 2016)

Use of injectable phenytoin is error-prone throughout the prescribing, preparation, administration and monitoring processes; all relevant staff should be made aware of appropriate guidance on the safe use of injectable phenytoin to reduce the risk of error.

MHRA/CHM ADVICE: ANTIEPILEPTIC DRUGS: UPDATED ADVICE ON SWITCHING BETWEEN DIFFERENT MANUFACTURERS' PRODUCTS (NOVEMBER 2017)

See Epilepsy p. 227 and see also *Prescribing and dispensing information*.

MHRA/CHM ADVICE: ANTIEPILEPTIC DRUGS IN PREGNANCY: UPDATED ADVICE FOLLOWING COMPREHENSIVE SAFETY REVIEW (JANUARY 2021)

See Epilepsy p. 227.

● **CONTRA-INDICATIONS**

GENERAL CONTRA-INDICATIONS Acute porphyrias p. 745

SPECIFIC CONTRA-INDICATIONS

- With intravenous use Second- and third-degree heart block · sino-atrial block · sinus bradycardia · Stokes-Adams syndrome

● **CAUTIONS**

GENERAL CAUTIONS Enteral feeding (interrupt feeding for 2 hours before and after dose; more frequent monitoring may be necessary) · presence of HLA-B*1502 allele · seizures (may be exacerbated)

SPECIFIC CAUTIONS

- With intravenous use Heart failure · hypotension · injection solutions alkaline (irritant to tissues) · respiratory depression · resuscitation facilities must be available

CAUTIONS, FURTHER INFORMATION MHRA advises consider vitamin D supplementation in patients who are immobilised for long periods or who have inadequate sun exposure or dietary intake of calcium.

EvGr Intramuscular phenytoin should not be used (absorption is slow and erratic). (M)

- HLA allele EvGr Limited evidence suggests that the presence of HLA-B*1502 allele, particularly in individuals of Han Chinese or Thai origin, may be associated with an increased risk of Stevens-Johnson syndrome. Consider use if potential benefit outweighs risk. (M)
- Seizure exacerbation EvGr Phenytoin may exacerbate seizures in patients with absence or myoclonic seizures (including juvenile myoclonic epilepsy), and myoclonic-atonic seizures. (A)

● **INTERACTIONS** → Appendix 1: antiepileptics

● **SIDE-EFFECTS**

GENERAL SIDE-EFFECTS Agranulocytosis · bone disorders · bone fracture · bone marrow disorders · cerebrovascular insufficiency · coarsening of the facial features · confusion · constipation · dizziness · drowsiness · Dupuytren's contracture · dysarthria · eosinophilia · fever · gingival hyperplasia (maintain good oral hygiene) · granulocytopenia · hair changes · headache · hepatic disorders · hypersensitivity · insomnia · joint disorders · leucopenia · lip swelling · lymphatic abnormalities · macrocytosis · megaloblastic anaemia · movement disorders · muscle twitching · nausea · neoplasms ·

nephritis tubulointerstitial · nervousness · nystagmus · paraesthesia · Peyronie's disease · pneumonitis · polyarteritis nodosa · pseudolymphoma · sensory peripheral polyneuropathy · severe cutaneous adverse reactions (SCARs) · skin reactions · suicidal behaviours · systemic lupus erythematosus (SLE) · taste altered · thrombocytopenia · tremor · vertigo · vomiting

SPECIFIC SIDE-EFFECTS
- With oral use Electrolyte imbalance · vitamin D deficiency
- With parenteral use Arrhythmias · atrial conduction depression (more common if injection too rapid) · cardiac arrest · extravasation necrosis · hypotension · injection site necrosis · purple glove syndrome · respiratory arrest (more common if injection too rapid) · respiratory disorder · tonic seizure (more common if injection too rapid) · ventricular conduction depression (more common if injection too rapid) · ventricular fibrillation (more common if injection too rapid)

SIDE-EFFECTS, FURTHER INFORMATION **Rash** Discontinue; if mild re-introduce cautiously but discontinue immediately if recurrence.

Bradycardia and hypotension With intravenous use; reduce rate of administration if bradycardia or hypotension occurs.

Overdose Symptoms of phenytoin toxicity include nystagmus, diplopia, slurred speech, ataxia, confusion, and hyperglycaemia.

- **ALLERGY AND CROSS-SENSITIVITY** Cross-sensitivity reported with carbamazepine. Antiepileptic hypersensitivity syndrome associated with phenytoin. See under Epilepsy p. 227 for more information.
- **PREGNANCY** An increased risk of major congenital malformations and possibility of adverse effects on neurodevelopment have been seen with phenytoin, see *Pregnancy* in Epilepsy p. 227.

Monitoring Changes in plasma-protein binding make interpretation of plasma-phenytoin concentrations difficult—monitor unbound fraction.

EvGr Doses should be adjusted on the basis of plasma-drug concentration monitoring—phenytoin pharmacokinetics altered during pregnancy. (M)

- **BREAST FEEDING** Specialist sources indicate present in milk but amount probably too small to be harmful.
- **HEPATIC IMPAIRMENT** Manufacturer advises caution (increased risk of accumulation and toxicity due to decreased protein binding in hepatic impairment, hypoalbuminaemia, or hyperbilirubinaemia).

Dose adjustments
- With oral use Manufacturer advises consider dose reduction.
- With intravenous use Manufacturer advises consider maintenance dose reduction.

- **MONITORING REQUIREMENTS**
- Therapeutic plasma-phenytoin concentrations reduced in first 3 months of life because of reduced protein binding.
- Trough plasma concentration for optimum response: neonate–3 months, 6–15 mg/litre (25–60 micromol/litre); child 3 months–18 years, 10–20 mg/litre (40–80 micromol/litre).
- Blood counts Manufacturer recommends blood counts (but evidence of practical value uncertain).
- With intravenous use Monitor ECG and blood pressure.

- **DIRECTIONS FOR ADMINISTRATION** Manufacturer advises each injection or infusion should be preceded and followed by an injection of Sodium Chloride 0.9% through the same needle or catheter to avoid local venous irritation. EvGr For *intravenous injection*, give into a large vein at a rate not exceeding 1 mg/kg/minute (max. 50 mg/minute). (D) Manufacturer advises for *intravenous infusion*, dilute to a concentration not exceeding 10 mg/mL with Sodium Chloride 0.9% and give into a large vein through an in-line filter (0.22–0.50 micron). EvGr Give at a rate not exceeding 1 mg/kg/minute (max. 50 mg/minute). (D) Complete administration within 1 hour of preparation.
- **PRESCRIBING AND DISPENSING INFORMATION** Switching between formulations Different formulations of oral preparations may vary in bioavailability. Patients being treated for epilepsy should be maintained on a specific manufacturer's product.
- **PATIENT AND CARER ADVICE** Blood or skin disorders Patients or their carers should be told how to recognise signs of blood or skin disorders, and advised to seek immediate medical attention if symptoms such as fever, rash, mouth ulcers, bruising, or bleeding develop. Leucopenia that is severe, progressive, or associated with clinical symptoms requires withdrawal (if necessary under cover of a suitable alternative).

Medicines for Children leaflet: Phenytoin for preventing seizures www.medicinesforchildren.org.uk/medicines/phenytoin-for-preventing-seizures/

- **MEDICINAL FORMS** There can be variation in the licensing of different medicines containing the same drug. Forms available from special-order manufacturers include: chewable tablet, oral suspension, oral solution

Oral tablet
CAUTIONARY AND ADVISORY LABELS 8
- Phenytoin (Non-proprietary)

Phenytoin sodium 100 mg Phenytoin sodium 100mg tablets | 28 tablet PoM £12.26 DT = £10.18

Solution for injection
EXCIPIENTS: May contain Alcohol, propylene glycol
- Phenytoin (Non-proprietary)

Phenytoin sodium 50 mg per 1 ml Phenytoin sodium 250mg/5ml solution for injection ampoules | 5 ampoule PoM £24.40 (Hospital only) | 10 ampoule PoM £34.00 (Hospital only)

Oral suspension
CAUTIONARY AND ADVISORY LABELS 8
EXCIPIENTS: May contain Alcohol, polysorbates, sucrose
- Phenytoin (Non-proprietary)

Phenytoin 6 mg per 1 ml Dilantin-30 suspension | 250 ml PoM ⊠
- Epanutin (Viatris UK Healthcare Ltd)

Phenytoin 6 mg per 1 ml Epanutin 30mg/5ml oral suspension | 500 ml PoM £4.27 DT = £4.27

Oral capsule
CAUTIONARY AND ADVISORY LABELS 8
- Phenytoin (Non-proprietary)

Phenytoin sodium 25 mg Phenytoin sodium 25mg capsules | 28 capsule PoM £7.24 DT = £13.77
Phenytoin sodium 50 mg Phenytoin sodium 50mg capsules | 28 capsule PoM £7.07 DT = £7.07
Phenytoin sodium 100 mg Phenytoin sodium 100mg capsules | 84 capsule PoM £10.32 DT = £9.14
Phenytoin sodium 300 mg Phenytoin sodium 300mg capsules | 28 capsule PoM £9.11 DT = £16.92

Chewable tablet
CAUTIONARY AND ADVISORY LABELS 8, 24
EXCIPIENTS: May contain Sucrose
- Phenytoin (Non-proprietary)

Phenytoin 50 mg Dilantin Infatabs 50mg chewable tablets | 100 tablet PoM ⊠
- Epanutin (Viatris UK Healthcare Ltd)

Phenytoin 50 mg Epanutin Infatabs 50mg chewable tablets | 200 tablet PoM £13.18 DT = £13.18

Rufinamide
11-Nov-2021

- **INDICATIONS AND DOSE**

Adjunctive treatment of seizures in Lennox-Gastaut syndrome without valproate (initiated by a specialist)
- BY MOUTH
- Child 1-3 years: Initially 5 mg/kg twice daily, then increased in steps of up to 5 mg/kg twice daily (max. per dose 22.5 mg/kg twice daily), adjusted according to response, dose to be increased at intervals of not less

than 3 days to the target dose (maximum dose), each dose should be given to the nearest 0.5 mL
- Child 4–17 years (body-weight up to 30 kg): Initially 100 mg twice daily, then increased in steps of 100 mg twice daily (max. per dose 500 mg twice daily), adjusted according to response, dose to be increased at intervals of not less than 3 days
- Child 4–17 years (body-weight 30–50 kg): Initially 200 mg twice daily, then increased in steps of 200 mg twice daily (max. per dose 900 mg twice daily), adjusted according to response, dose to be increased at intervals of not less than 2 days
- Child 4–17 years (body-weight 50.1–70 kg): Initially 200 mg twice daily, then increased in steps of 200 mg twice daily (max. per dose 1.2 g twice daily), adjusted according to response, dose to be increased at intervals of not less than 2 days
- Child 4–17 years (body-weight 70.1 kg and above): Initially 200 mg twice daily, then increased in steps of 200 mg twice daily (max. per dose 1.6 g twice daily), adjusted according to response, dose to be increased at intervals of not less than 2 days

Adjunctive treatment of seizures in Lennox-Gastaut syndrome with valproate (initiated by a specialist)

- BY MOUTH
- Child 1–3 years: Initially 5 mg/kg twice daily, then increased in steps of up to 5 mg/kg twice daily (max. per dose 15 mg/kg twice daily), adjusted according to response, dose to be increased at intervals of not less than 3 days to the target dose (maximum dose), each dose should be given to the nearest 0.5 mL
- Child 4–17 years (body-weight up to 30 kg): Initially 100 mg twice daily, then increased in steps of 100 mg twice daily (max. per dose 300 mg twice daily), adjusted according to response, dose to be increased at intervals of not less than 2 days
- Child 4–17 years (body-weight 30–50 kg): Initially 200 mg twice daily, then increased in steps of 200 mg twice daily (max. per dose 600 mg twice daily), adjusted according to response, dose to be increased at intervals of not less than 2 days
- Child 4–17 years (body-weight 50.1–70 kg): Initially 200 mg twice daily, then increased in steps of 200 mg twice daily (max. per dose 800 mg twice daily), adjusted according to response, dose to be increased at intervals of not less than 2 days
- Child 4–17 years (body-weight 70.1 kg and above): Initially 200 mg twice daily, then increased in steps of 200 mg twice daily (max. per dose 1.1 g twice daily), adjusted according to response, dose to be increased at intervals of not less than 2 days

IMPORTANT SAFETY INFORMATION

MHRA/CHM ADVICE: ANTIEPILEPTICS: RISK OF SUICIDAL THOUGHTS AND BEHAVIOUR (AUGUST 2008)

See Epilepsy p. 227.

MHRA/CHM ADVICE: ANTIEPILEPTIC DRUGS: UPDATED ADVICE ON SWITCHING BETWEEN DIFFERENT MANUFACTURERS' PRODUCTS (NOVEMBER 2017)

See Epilepsy p. 227 and see also *Prescribing and dispensing information*.

MHRA/CHM ADVICE: ANTIEPILEPTIC DRUGS IN PREGNANCY: UPDATED ADVICE FOLLOWING COMPREHENSIVE SAFETY REVIEW (JANUARY 2021)

See Epilepsy p. 227.

- **CAUTIONS** Patients at risk of further shortening of QTc interval
- **INTERACTIONS** → Appendix 1: antiepileptics
- **SIDE-EFFECTS**
  - **Common or very common** Anxiety · appetite decreased · back pain · constipation · diarrhoea · dizziness · drowsiness · eating disorder · epistaxis · fatigue · gait abnormal · gastrointestinal discomfort · headache · increased risk of infection · insomnia · movement disorders · nausea · nystagmus · oligomenorrhoea · seizures · skin reactions · tremor · vertigo · vision disorders · vomiting · weight decreased
  - **Uncommon** Hypersensitivity
  - **Frequency not known** Suicidal behaviours
- **ALLERGY AND CROSS-SENSITIVITY** Antiepileptic hypersensitivity syndrome associated with rufinamide. See under Epilepsy p. 227 for more information.
- **PREGNANCY** Manufacturer advises avoid unless essential—toxicity in *animal* studies. See also *Pregnancy* in Epilepsy p. 227.
- **BREAST FEEDING** Manufacturer advises avoid—no information available.
- **HEPATIC IMPAIRMENT** Manufacturer advises caution in mild to moderate impairment; avoid in severe impairment (no information available).
  Dose adjustments Manufacturer advises cautious dose titration in mild to moderate impairment.
- **DIRECTIONS FOR ADMINISTRATION** Manufacturer advises tablets may be crushed and given in half a glass of water.
- **PRESCRIBING AND DISPENSING INFORMATION**
  Switching between formulations Care should be taken when switching between oral formulations. The need for continued supply of a particular manufacturer's product should be based on clinical judgement and consultation with the patient or their carer, taking into account factors such as seizure frequency and treatment history.
  Patients may need to be maintained on a specific manufacturer's branded or generic rufinamide product.
- **PATIENT AND CARER ADVICE** Counselling on antiepileptic hypersensitivity syndrome is advised.
  Medicines for Children leaflet: Rufinamide for preventing seizures www.medicinesforchildren.org.uk/medicines/rufinamide-for-preventing-seizures/
  Driving and skilled tasks Manufacturer advises patients and carers should be cautioned on the effects on driving and performance of skilled tasks—increased risk of dizziness, somnolence and blurred vision.
- **NATIONAL FUNDING/ACCESS DECISIONS**
  For full details see funding body website

Scottish Medicines Consortium (SMC) decisions

- **Rufinamide (*Inovelon*®) as adjunctive therapy in the treatment of seizures associated with Lennox-Gastaut syndrome in patients four years and older (November 2008)** SMC No. 416/07 Recommended with restrictions
- **Rufinamide 40 mg/mL oral suspension (*Inovelon*®) as adjunctive therapy in the treatment of seizures associated with Lennox-Gastaut syndrome (LGS) in patients 4 years of age or older (July 2012)** SMC No. 795/12 Recommended with restrictions
- **Rufinamide (*Inovelon*®) as adjunctive therapy in the treatment of seizures associated with Lennox-Gastaut syndrome in patients aged 1 year up to 4 years (April 2019)** SMC No. SMC2146 Recommended with restrictions

All Wales Medicines Strategy Group (AWMSG) decisions

- **Rufinamide 40 mg/mL oral suspension (*Inovelon*®) as adjunctive therapy in the treatment of seizures associated with Lennox-Gastaut syndrome in patients 1 year of age and older (June 2019)** AWMSG No. 991 Recommended with restrictions

● **MEDICINAL FORMS** There can be variation in the licensing of different medicines containing the same drug.

Oral tablet

CAUTIONARY AND ADVISORY LABELS 8, 21

▸ **Rufinamide (Non-proprietary)**

Rufinamide 100 mg Rufinamide 100mg tablets | 10 tablet PoM £5.15 DT = £5.15

Rufinamide 200 mg Rufinamide 200mg tablets | 60 tablet PoM £61.77 DT = £61.77

Rufinamide 400 mg Rufinamide 400mg tablets | 60 tablet PoM £102.96 DT = £102.96

▸ **Inovelon** (Eisai Ltd)

Rufinamide 100 mg Inovelon 100mg tablets | 10 tablet PoM £5.15 DT = £5.15

Oral suspension

CAUTIONARY AND ADVISORY LABELS 8, 21

EXCIPIENTS: May contain Propylene glycol

▸ **Rufinamide (Non-proprietary)**

Rufinamide 40 mg per 1 ml Rufinamide 40mg/ml oral suspension sugar free | 460 ml PoM £94.71 DT = £94.71 SF

Sodium valproate

24-Mar-2026

(Valproate sodium)

● **INDICATIONS AND DOSE**

All forms of epilepsy

▶ BY MOUTH USING IMMEDIATE-RELEASE MEDICINES

▸ Neonate: Initially 20 mg/kg once daily; maintenance 10 mg/kg twice daily.

▸ Child 1 month–11 years: Initially 10–15 mg/kg daily in 1–2 divided doses (max. per dose 600 mg); maintenance 25–30 mg/kg daily in 2 divided doses, doses up to 60 mg/kg daily in 2 divided doses may be used in infantile spasms; monitor clinical chemistry and haematological parameters if dose exceeds 40 mg/kg daily

▸ Child 12–17 years: Initially 600 mg daily in 1–2 divided doses, increased in steps of 150–300 mg every 3 days; maintenance 1–2 g daily in 2 divided doses; maximum 2.5 g per day

▶ BY RECTUM

▸ Neonate: Initially 20 mg/kg once daily; maintenance 10 mg/kg twice daily.

▸ Child 1 month–11 years: Initially 10–15 mg/kg daily in 1–2 divided doses (max. per dose 600 mg); maintenance 25–30 mg/kg daily in 2 divided doses, doses up to 60 mg/kg daily in 2 divided doses may be used in infantile spasms; monitor clinical chemistry and haematological parameters if dose exceeds 40 mg/kg daily

▸ Child 12–17 years: Initially 600 mg daily in 1–2 divided doses, increased in steps of 150–300 mg every 3 days; maintenance 1–2 g daily in 2 divided doses; maximum 2.5 g per day

Initiation of valproate treatment

▶ INITIALLY BY INTRAVENOUS INJECTION

▸ Neonate: 10 mg/kg twice daily.

▸ Child 1 month–11 years: Initially 10 mg/kg, then (by intravenous infusion or by intravenous injection) increased to 20–40 mg/kg daily in 2–4 divided doses, alternatively (by continuous intravenous infusion) increased to 20–40 mg/kg daily, monitor clinical chemistry and haematological parameters if dose exceeds 40 mg/kg daily

▸ Child 12–17 years: Initially 10 mg/kg, followed by (by intravenous infusion or by intravenous injection) up to 2.5 g daily in 2–4 divided doses, alternatively (by continuous intravenous infusion) up to 2.5 g daily; (by intravenous injection or by intravenous infusion or by continuous intravenous infusion) usual dose 1–2 g daily, alternatively (by intravenous injection or by intravenous infusion or by continuous intravenous infusion) usual dose 20–30 mg/kg daily, intravenous injection to be administered over 3–5 minutes

Continuation of valproate treatment

▶ BY INTRAVENOUS INJECTION, OR BY INTRAVENOUS INFUSION, OR BY CONTINUOUS INTRAVENOUS INFUSION

▸ Child: If switching from oral therapy to intravenous therapy give the same dose as current oral daily dose, give over 3–5 minutes by intravenous injection *or* in 2–4 divided doses by intravenous infusion

EPILIM CHRONOSPHERE ®

All forms of epilepsy

▶ BY MOUTH

▸ Child: Total daily dose to be given in 1–2 divided doses (consult product literature)

EPILIM CHRONO ®

All forms of epilepsy

▶ BY MOUTH

▸ Child (body-weight 20 kg and above): Total daily dose to be given in 1–2 divided doses (consult product literature)

EPISENTA ® CAPSULES

All forms of epilepsy

▶ BY MOUTH

▸ Child: Total daily dose to be given in 1–2 divided doses (consult product literature)

EPISENTA ® GRANULES

All forms of epilepsy

▶ BY MOUTH

▸ Child: Total daily dose to be given in 1–2 divided doses (consult product literature)

EPIVAL ®

All forms of epilepsy

▶ BY MOUTH

▸ Child: Total daily dose to be given in 1–2 divided doses (consult product literature)

IMPORTANT SAFETY INFORMATION

MHRA/CHM ADVICE: ANTIEPILEPTICS: RISK OF SUICIDAL THOUGHTS AND BEHAVIOUR (AUGUST 2008)

See Epilepsy p. 227.

MHRA/CHM ADVICE: ANTIEPILEPTIC DRUGS: UPDATED ADVICE ON SWITCHING BETWEEN DIFFERENT MANUFACTURERS' PRODUCTS (NOVEMBER 2017)

See Epilepsy p. 227 and see also *Prescribing and dispensing information*.

VALPROATE AND REPRODUCTIVE RISKS

Valproate is highly teratogenic and evidence shows that use in pregnancy can lead to neurodevelopmental disorders (approx. 30–40% risk) and congenital malformations (approx. 11% risk). It can also potentially cause infertility in males and neurodevelopmental disorders in children born to males treated with valproate in the 3 months prior to conception. Valproate must not be initiated in any patients under 55 years of age unless 2 specialists independently review and document that there is no other effective or tolerated treatment, or there are compelling reasons that the reproductive risks do not apply. Male patients under 55 years of age who are already taking valproate can continue to have it prescribed in accordance with standard clinical practice by a single prescriber. In females of childbearing potential, the conditions of the Pregnancy Prevention Programme must be met and a valproate risk acknowledgement form completed annually. Male patients (of any age) who may father a child must be counselled on using effective contraception during treatment and for 3 months after stopping.

Patients should be informed not to stop taking valproate without advice from a specialist because epilepsy or bipolar disorder may worsen without treatment.

For further information and resources, see MHRA/CHM advice below, *Conception and contraception*, *Pregnancy*, *Prescribing and dispensing information*, and *Patient and carer advice*; refer to the MHRA information page at: www.gov.uk/guidance/valproate-reproductive-risks.

MHRA/CHM ADVICE: ANTIEPILEPTIC DRUGS IN PREGNANCY: UPDATED ADVICE FOLLOWING COMPREHENSIVE SAFETY REVIEW (JANUARY 2021)

See Epilepsy p. 227.

MHRA/CHM ADVICE: FULL PACK DISPENSING OF VALPROATE-CONTAINING MEDICINES (OCTOBER 2023)

Valproate medicines have been dispensed to patients in alternative packaging because the prescribed amount was different to that of the manufacturer's original full pack. This resulted in patients not always receiving all the risk materials about the use of these medicines in pregnancy. Pharmacists are advised that all patients (male and female) must receive their valproate medicines in the manufacturer's original full pack (i.e. original pack dispensing) and the amount dispensed must be as close as possible to the amount stated on the prescription (NHS or private). Rarely, exceptions to this requirement can be made on an individual patient basis, provided a risk assessment is carried out on the need to dispense repackaged valproate medicines (e.g. in a monitored dosage system), whereby a patient information leaflet must be supplied.

MHRA/CHM ADVICE: VALPROATE (*DYZANTIL*®, *EPILIM*®, *EPILIM CHRONO*® OR *CHRONOSPHERE*®, *EPISENTA*®, AND *EPIVAL*®): NEW SAFETY AND EDUCATIONAL MATERIALS TO SUPPORT REGULATORY MEASURES IN MEN AND WOMEN UNDER 55 YEARS OF AGE (JANUARY 2024)

Healthcare professionals are advised to review, and integrate into their clinical practice, safety and educational materials that support new regulatory measures (see *Prescribing and dispensing information*). General practice and pharmacy teams should continue to prescribe and dispense valproate according to current safety measures. If required, patients should be referred to a specialist to discuss treatment options. Patients on valproate medicines should be fully informed of the potential risks and counselled on treatment options at initial prescribing and at all subsequent reviews.

Healthcare professionals should advise patients to:

- not stop taking valproate medicines without advice from a specialist as their epilepsy or bipolar disorder may worsen;
- attend any offered appointments to discuss their treatment plan and to talk to a healthcare professional if they have any concerns;
- consult the new Patient Guide and Patient Information Leaflet for information on the risks of valproate.

MHRA/CHM ADVICE: VALPROATE USE IN MEN: AS A PRECAUTION, MEN AND THEIR PARTNERS SHOULD USE EFFECTIVE CONTRACEPTION (SEPTEMBER 2024)

The MHRA has reviewed findings from a retrospective observational study that suggest a potential increased risk of neurodevelopmental disorders in children born to males taking valproate medicines in the 3 months before conception; however, causality is unconfirmed. In addition to current safety measures, healthcare professionals should advise male patients (of any age) who may father a child:

- about this risk at treatment initiation or at the next treatment review, irrespective of indication and also after intravenous valproate;
- to use effective contraception (i.e. condoms plus contraception used by their female partner) during and for 3 months after valproate treatment;
- to refrain from donating sperm during and for 3 months after valproate treatment.

Healthcare professionals are also advised that:

- male patients who are planning a family in the next year should be referred to a specialist to discuss alternative treatment;
- female partners of male patients taking valproate medicines who are pregnant or planning a pregnancy (including those undergoing IVF) should be referred for prenatal counselling.

MHRA/CHM ADVICE: VALPROATE (*DYZANTIL*®, *EPILIM*®, *EPILIM CHRONO*® OR *CHRONOSPHERE*®, *EPISENTA*®, AND *EPIVAL*®): REVIEW BY TWO SPECIALISTS IS REQUIRED FOR INITIATING VALPROATE BUT NOT FOR MALE PATIENTS ALREADY TAKING VALPROATE (FEBRUARY 2025)

Healthcare professionals are reminded that the current safety measure advising all patients under 55 years of age to be reviewed by two specialists before initiating valproate remains in place, however, the CHM has advised that this will not be required for male patients who are already taking valproate. Healthcare professionals are also reminded that all previously issued safety measures continue to apply.

The CHM has produced infographics to clarify the situations where review by two specialists may be required.

For female patients under 55 years of age, see: assets.publishing.service.gov.uk/media/67adf28c6e6c8d18118acd69/250213_MHRA_Valproate_Infographic_Female_under_55_CC_V7.pdf.

For male patients under 55 years of age, see: assets.publishing.service.gov.uk/media/67adf2aa6e6c8d18118acd6a/250213_MHRA_Valproate_Infographic_Male_under_55_CC_V7.pdf.

For male and female patients aged 55 years and older, see: assets.publishing.service.gov.uk/media/67adf2c62c594609b38acd71/250213_MHRA_Valproate_Infographic_55_or_older_CC_V7.pdf.

MHRA/CHM ADVICE: VALPROATE (*DYZANTIL*®, *EPILIM*®, *EPILIM CHRONO*® OR *CHRONOSPHERE*®, *EPISENTA*®, AND *EPIVAL*®): UPDATED SAFETY AND EDUCATIONAL MATERIALS TO SUPPORT PATIENT DISCUSSION ON REPRODUCTIVE RISKS (JUNE 2025)

The MHRA reminds healthcare professionals of the potential risk of neurodevelopmental disorders in children fathered by males taking valproate around the time of conception. Children exposed to valproate in utero also have a higher risk of being born with a low birth weight or being small for gestational age, compared to those unexposed to antiepileptic drugs or exposed to lamotrigine.

Safety and educational materials have therefore been updated in line with regulatory requirements and are available at: www.gov.uk/guidance/valproate-reproductive-risks#materials-and-resources. These should be reviewed and integrated into clinical practice for all patients being treated with valproate.

- **CONTRA-INDICATIONS** Acute porphyrias p. 745 · known or suspected mitochondrial disorders (higher rate of acute liver failure and liver-related deaths) · personal or family history of severe hepatic dysfunction · urea cycle disorders (risk of hyperammonaemia)
- **CAUTIONS** Systemic lupus erythematosus

CAUTIONS, FURTHER INFORMATION The MHRA advises consider vitamin D supplementation in patients that are immobilised for long periods or who have inadequate sun exposure or dietary intake of calcium.

▶ Liver toxicity Liver dysfunction (including fatal hepatic failure) has occurred in association with valproate (especially in children under 3 years and in those with metabolic or degenerative disorders, organic brain disease or severe seizure disorders associated with mental retardation) usually in first 6 months and usually involving multiple antiepileptic therapy. EvGr Raised liver enzymes during valproate treatment are usually transient but patients should be reassessed clinically and liver function (including prothrombin time) monitored until return to normal—discontinue if abnormally prolonged prothrombin time (particularly in association with other relevant abnormalities). Ⓜ

- **INTERACTIONS** → Appendix 1: antiepileptics
- **SIDE-EFFECTS**

GENERAL SIDE-EFFECTS

▶ **Common or very common** Abdominal pain · agitation · alopecia (regrowth may be curly) · anaemia · behaviour abnormal · concentration impaired · confusion · deafness · diarrhoea · drowsiness · haemorrhage · hallucination · headache · hepatic disorders · hypersensitivity · hyponatraemia · memory loss · menstrual cycle irregularities · movement disorders · nail disorder · nausea · nystagmus · oral disorders · seizures · stupor · thrombocytopenia · tremor · urinary disorders · vomiting · weight increased

▶ **Uncommon** Androgenetic alopecia · angioedema · bone disorders · bone fracture · bone marrow disorders · coma · encephalopathy · hair changes · hypothermia · leucopenia · pancreatitis · paraesthesia · parkinsonism · peripheral oedema · pleural effusion · renal failure · SIADH · skin reactions · vasculitis · virilism

▶ **Rare or very rare** Agranulocytosis · cerebral atrophy · cognitive disorder · dementia · diplopia · Fanconi syndrome acquired · gynaecomastia · hyperammonaemia · hypothyroidism · infertility male · learning disability · myelodysplastic syndrome · nephritis tubulointerstitial · obesity · polycystic ovaries · red blood cell abnormalities · rhabdomyolysis · severe cutaneous adverse reactions (SCARs) · systemic lupus erythematosus (SLE) · urine abnormalities

▶ **Frequency not known** Alertness increased · suicidal behaviours

SPECIFIC SIDE-EFFECTS

▶ **Common or very common**

▶ With intravenous use Dizziness

SIDE-EFFECTS, FURTHER INFORMATION

Hepatic dysfunction Withdraw treatment immediately if persistent vomiting and abdominal pain, anorexia, jaundice, oedema, malaise, drowsiness, or loss of seizure control.

Pancreatitis Discontinue treatment if symptoms of pancreatitis develop.

- **CONCEPTION AND CONTRACEPTION** The MHRA advises that all women and girls of childbearing potential being treated with valproate medicines must be supported on a Pregnancy Prevention Programme—pregnancy should be excluded before treatment initiation. Highly effective contraception must be used during treatment i.e. at least 1, preferably highly effective user-independent contraceptive method (such as an intra-uterine device or implant), or 2 complementary forms including a barrier method. The MHRA advises that all male patients being treated with valproate medicines and who may father children should use effective contraception (i.e. condoms plus contraception used by their female partner) during and for 3 months after treatment. The MHRA advises that male patients taking valproate medicines should be informed of the risk of infertility, and of data showing testicular toxicity in *animal* studies.
- **PREGNANCY** For *migraine prophylaxis*[unlicensed] and *bipolar disorder*, the MHRA advises that valproate medicines must not be used. For *epilepsy*, the MHRA advises valproate must not be used unless two specialists independently consider and document that there is no other effective or tolerated treatment (see also *Important safety information*). If valproate is to be used, the lowest effective dose should be prescribed in divided doses to be taken throughout the day; modified-release preparations may be preferable to avoid high peak plasma-valproate concentrations. There is no dose threshold considered to be without any risk, however, the risk of birth defects and neurodevelopmental disorders is greater at higher doses. EvGr Specialist prenatal monitoring should be instigated when valproate has been taken in pregnancy. Ⓜ Neonatal bleeding (related to hypofibrinaemia) reported. Neonatal hepatotoxicity also reported. See also *Pregnancy* in Epilepsy p. 227.
- **BREAST FEEDING** Present in milk—risk of haematological disorders in breast-fed newborns and infants.
- **HEPATIC IMPAIRMENT** Manufacturer advises avoid.
- **RENAL IMPAIRMENT**

Dose adjustments EvGr Consider dose reduction. Ⓜ

- **MONITORING REQUIREMENTS**

▶ Plasma-valproate concentrations are not a useful index of efficacy, therefore routine monitoring is unhelpful.

▶ Monitor liver function before therapy and during first 6 months especially in patients most at risk.

▶ Measure full blood count and ensure no undue potential for bleeding before starting and before surgery.

- **EFFECT ON LABORATORY TESTS** False-positive urine tests for ketones.
- **TREATMENT CESSATION** EvGr Avoid abrupt withdrawal; if treatment with valproate is stopped, reduce the dose gradually over at least 4 weeks. Ⓐ
- **DIRECTIONS FOR ADMINISTRATION** Manufacturer advises for *intravenous injection*, give over 3–5 minutes. For *intravenous infusion*, dilute with Glucose 5% *or* Sodium Chloride 0.9%. Reconstitute *Epilim*® with solvent provided then dilute with infusion fluid if required. Displacement value may be significant, consult local guidelines.

For *rectal administration*, expert sources advise sodium valproate oral solution may be given rectally and retained for 15 minutes (may require dilution with water to prevent rapid expulsion).

EPILIM CHRONOSPHERE® Manufacturer advises granules may be mixed with soft food or drink that is cold or at room temperature, and swallowed immediately without chewing.

EPILIM® **SYRUP** Manufacturer advises may be diluted, preferably in Syrup BP; use within 14 days.

EPISENTA® **CAPSULES** Manufacturer advises contents of capsule may be mixed with soft food or drink that is cold or at room temperature and swallowed immediately without chewing.

EPISENTA® **GRANULES** Manufacturer advises granules may be mixed with soft food or drink that is cold or at room temperature and swallowed immediately without chewing.

EPIVAL® Manufacturer advises tablets may be halved but not crushed or chewed.

- **PRESCRIBING AND DISPENSING INFORMATION** The Pregnancy Prevention Programme is supported by the following safety and educational materials: *Guide for Female Patients*, *Guide for Male Patients*, *Guide for Healthcare Professionals*, *Annual Risk Acknowledgement Form for Female Patients*, *Risk Acknowledgement Form for Male Patients Starting Valproate*, *Patient Card*, and *Pharmacy Poster*.

In addition, the MHRA advises that pharmacists must dispense valproate medicines in the manufacturer's original full pack.

Safety and educational materials, and resources for healthcare professionals are available from the MHRA guidance page on Valproate - reproductive risks, at: www.gov.uk/guidance/valproate-reproductive-risks.

The Royal College of Pharmacy has also produced a safe supply algorithm, available at: rcpharm.org/wp-content/uploads/2026/04/Valproate-safe-supply-community-pharmacy-FINAL.pdf.

Switching between formulations Care should be taken when switching between oral formulations in the treatment of *epilepsy*. The need for continued supply of a particular manufacturer's product should be based on clinical judgement and consultation with the patient or their carer, taking into account factors such as seizure frequency and treatment history.

Patients being treated for epilepsy may need to be maintained on a specific manufacturer's branded or generic oral sodium valproate product.

EPILIM CHRONOSPHERE® Prescribe dose to the nearest whole 50-mg sachet.

- **PATIENT AND CARER ADVICE** The MHRA advises that patients should **not** stop taking valproate without first discussing it with a specialist. Female patients or their carers should be advised to immediately contact their GP for an urgent referral to a specialist in case of suspected pregnancy. Female partners of male patients taking valproate medicines should be referred for prenatal counselling if pregnancy is suspected.

Blood or hepatic disorders Patients or their carers should be told how to recognise signs and symptoms of blood or liver disorders and advised to seek immediate medical attention if symptoms develop.

Pancreatitis Patients or their carers should be told how to recognise signs and symptoms of pancreatitis and advised to seek immediate medical attention if symptoms such as abdominal pain, nausea, or vomiting develop.

Suicidal ideation and behaviour Patients or their carers should be advised to seek immediate medical attention if any signs of suicidal thoughts or behaviour develop.

Patient guide A patient guide must be provided.

Pregnancy Prevention Programme Pharmacists must ensure that female patients have a patient card—see also *Important safety information*.

Decision aid NHS England has produced a patient decision aid for females of childbearing potential who are considering or are taking valproate medicines for epilepsy, available at: www.england.nhs.uk/publication/decision-support-tool-is-valproate-the-right-epilepsy-treatment-for-me/.

Medicines for Children leaflet: Sodium valproate for preventing seizures www.medicinesforchildren.org.uk/medicines/sodium-valproate-for-preventing-seizures/

EPILIM CHRONOSPHERE® Patients and carers should be counselled on the administration of granules.

EPISENTA® CAPSULES Patients and carers should be counselled on the administration of capsules.

EPISENTA® GRANULES Patients and carers should be counselled on the administration of granules.

- **MEDICINAL FORMS** There can be variation in the licensing of different medicines containing the same drug. Forms available from special-order manufacturers include: oral suspension, oral solution, suppository

Oral tablet

CAUTIONARY AND ADVISORY LABELS 8, 10, 21

- Epilim (Sanofi) ▼
  Sodium valproate 100 mg Epilim 100mg crushable tablets | 30 tablet [PoM] £1.68 DT = £1.68

Modified-release tablet

CAUTIONARY AND ADVISORY LABELS 8, 10, 21, 25

- Epilim Chrono (Sanofi) ▼
  Sodium valproate 200 mg Epilim Chrono 200 tablets | 30 tablet [PoM] £3.50 DT = £3.50
  Sodium valproate 300 mg Epilim Chrono 300 tablets | 30 tablet [PoM] £5.24 DT = £5.24
  Sodium valproate 500 mg Epilim Chrono 500 tablets | 30 tablet [PoM] £8.73 DT = £8.73
- Epival CR (G.L. Pharma UK Ltd) ▼
  Sodium valproate 300 mg Epival CR 300mg tablets | 30 tablet [PoM] £3.40 DT = £5.24
  Sodium valproate 500 mg Epival CR 500mg tablets | 30 tablet [PoM] £5.67 DT = £8.73

Gastro-resistant tablet

CAUTIONARY AND ADVISORY LABELS 5, 8, 10, 25

- Sodium valproate (non-proprietary) ▼
  Sodium valproate 200 mg Sodium valproate 200mg gastro-resistant tablets | 30 tablet [PoM] £2.51–£4.20 DT = £1.99
  Sodium valproate 500 mg Sodium valproate 500mg gastro-resistant tablets | 30 tablet [PoM] £5.78–£30.00 DT = £5.78
- Epilim (Sanofi) ▼
  Sodium valproate 200 mg Epilim 200 gastro-resistant tablets | 30 tablet [PoM] £1.99 DT = £1.99
  Sodium valproate 500 mg Epilim 500 gastro-resistant tablets | 30 tablet [PoM] £5.78 DT = £5.78

Powder and solvent for solution for injection

- Sodium valproate (non-proprietary) ▼
  Sodium valproate 400 mg Sodium valproate 400mg powder and solvent for solution for injection vials | 4 vial [PoM] £53.28 (Hospital only)
- Epilim (Sanofi) ▼
  Sodium valproate 400 mg Epilim Intravenous 400mg powder and solvent for solution for injection vials | 1 vial [PoM] £13.32 DT = £13.32

Solution for injection

- Sodium valproate (non-proprietary) ▼
  Sodium valproate 100 mg per 1 ml Sodium valproate 400mg/4ml solution for injection ampoules | 5 ampoule [PoM] £69.25 DT = £57.90
  Sodium valproate 400mg/4ml solution for injection vials | 5 vial [PoM] £60.00 (Hospital only)
  Sodium valproate 300mg/3ml solution for injection vials | 5 vial [PoM] £60.00 (Hospital only)
- Episenta (Desitin Pharma Ltd) ▼
  Sodium valproate 100 mg per 1 ml Episenta 300mg/3ml solution for injection ampoules | 5 ampoule [PoM] £35.00 DT = £35.00

Modified-release capsule

CAUTIONARY AND ADVISORY LABELS 8, 10, 21, 25

- Episenta (Desitin Pharma Ltd) ▼
  Sodium valproate 150 mg Episenta 150mg modified-release capsules | 30 capsule [PoM] £2.76 DT = £2.76
  Sodium valproate 300 mg Episenta 300mg modified-release capsules | 30 capsule [PoM] £4.56 DT = £4.56

Oral solution

CAUTIONARY AND ADVISORY LABELS 8, 10, 21

- Sodium valproate (non-proprietary) ▼
  Sodium valproate 40 mg per 1 ml Sodium valproate 200mg/5ml oral solution sugar free | 300 ml [PoM] £7.29–£14.67 DT = £13.96 [SF]
  Sodium valproate 200 mg per 1 ml Depakin 200mg/ml oral solution | 40 ml [PoM] [X]
- Epilim (Sanofi) ▼
  Sodium valproate 40 mg per 1 ml Epilim 200mg/5ml liquid | 300 ml [PoM] £7.78 DT = £13.96 [SF]
  Epilim 200mg/5ml syrup | 300 ml [PoM] £9.33 DT = £9.33

Modified-release granules

CAUTIONARY AND ADVISORY LABELS 8, 10, 21, 25

- Epilim Chronosphere MR (Sanofi) ▼
  Sodium valproate 50 mg Epilim Chronosphere MR 50mg granules sachets | 30 sachet [PoM] £30.00 DT = £30.00 [SF]
  Sodium valproate 100 mg Epilim Chronosphere MR 100mg granules sachets | 30 sachet [PoM] £30.00 DT = £30.00 [SF]
  Sodium valproate 250 mg Epilim Chronosphere MR 250mg granules sachets | 30 sachet [PoM] £30.00 DT = £30.00 [SF]
  Sodium valproate 500 mg Epilim Chronosphere MR 500mg granules sachets | 30 sachet [PoM] £30.00 DT = £30.00 [SF]
- Episenta (Desitin Pharma Ltd) ▼
  Sodium valproate 500 mg Episenta 500mg modified-release granules sachets | 30 sachet [PoM] £6.30 DT = £30.00 [SF]

Sodium valproate 1 gram Episenta 1000mg modified-release granules sachets | 30 sachet PoM £12.30 DT = £30.00 SF

Stripentol

16-Aug-2023

● **INDICATIONS AND DOSE**

Adjunctive therapy of refractory generalised tonic-clonic seizures in patients with severe myoclonic epilepsy in infancy (Dravet syndrome) in combination with clobazam and valproate (under expert supervision)

▶ BY MOUTH

▶ Child 1 month–5 years: Initially 20 mg/kg daily in 2–3 divided doses for 1 week, then increased to 30 mg/kg daily in 2–3 divided doses for 1 week, then increased to 50 mg/kg daily in 2–3 divided doses

▶ Child 6–11 years: Initially 20 mg/kg daily in 2–3 divided doses for 1 week, then increased in steps of 10 mg/kg daily in 2–3 divided doses, dose to be increased at intervals of 1 week to 50 mg/kg daily in 2–3 divided doses

▶ Child 12–17 years: Initially 20 mg/kg daily in 2–3 divided doses for 1 week, then increased to 30 mg/kg daily in 2–3 divided doses for 1 week, then increased in steps of 5 mg/kg daily in 2–3 divided doses, dose to be increased at intervals of 1 week, until the optimum dose is reached based on clinical judgement; maximum 50 mg/kg per day

DOSE EQUIVALENCE AND CONVERSION

▶ Stiripentol capsules and oral powder sachets are **not** bioequivalent. If a switch of formulation is required, manufacturer advises this is done under clinical supervision in case of intolerance.

IMPORTANT SAFETY INFORMATION

MHRA/CHM ADVICE: ANTIEPILEPTICS: RISK OF SUICIDAL THOUGHTS AND BEHAVIOUR (AUGUST 2008)

See Epilepsy p. 227.

MHRA/CHM ADVICE: ANTIEPILEPTIC DRUGS: UPDATED ADVICE ON SWITCHING BETWEEN DIFFERENT MANUFACTURERS' PRODUCTS (NOVEMBER 2017)

See Epilepsy p. 227.

MHRA/CHM ADVICE: ANTIEPILEPTIC DRUGS IN PREGNANCY: UPDATED ADVICE FOLLOWING COMPREHENSIVE SAFETY REVIEW (JANUARY 2021)

See Epilepsy p. 227.

● **CONTRA-INDICATIONS** History of psychosis in the form of episodes of delirium

● **CAUTIONS** Age under 3 years (limited information available)

● **INTERACTIONS** → Appendix 1: antiepileptics

● **SIDE-EFFECTS**

▶ **Common or very common** Agitation · appetite decreased · behaviour abnormal · drowsiness · irritability · movement disorders · muscle tone decreased · nausea · neutropenia · sleep disorders · vomiting · weight decreased

▶ **Uncommon** Diplopia · fatigue · photosensitivity reaction · skin reactions

▶ **Rare or very rare** Thrombocytopenia

▶ **Frequency not known** Suicidal behaviours

● **ALLERGY AND CROSS-SENSITIVITY** Antiepileptic hypersensitivity syndrome theoretically associated with stiripentol. See under Epilepsy p. 227 for more information.

● **PREGNANCY** See also *Pregnancy* in Epilepsy p. 227.

● **BREAST FEEDING** Present in milk in *animal* studies.

● **HEPATIC IMPAIRMENT** Manufacturer advises avoid (no information available).

● **RENAL IMPAIRMENT** EvGr Avoid—no information available. ⟨M⟩

● **MONITORING REQUIREMENTS**

▶ Perform full blood count and liver function tests prior to initiating treatment and every 6 months thereafter.

▶ Manufacturer advises monitor growth.

● **PATIENT AND CARER ADVICE**

Medicines for Children leaflet: Stiripentol for preventing seizures www.medicinesforchildren.org.uk/medicines/stiripentol-for-preventing-seizures/

● **NATIONAL FUNDING/ACCESS DECISIONS**

For full details see funding body website

Scottish Medicines Consortium (SMC) decisions

▶ Stiripentol (*Diacomit*®) for use in conjunction with clobazam and valproate as adjunctive therapy of refractory generalised tonic-clonic seizures in patients with severe myoclonic epilepsy in infancy (SMEI; Dravet' s syndrome) whose seizures are not adequately controlled with clobazam and valproate (September 2017) SMC No. 524/08 Recommended

All Wales Medicines Strategy Group (AWMSG) decisions

▶ Stiripentol (*Diacomit*®) for use in conjunction with clobazam and valproate as adjunctive therapy of refractory generalized tonic-clonic seizures in patients with severe myoclonic epilepsy in infancy (SMEI; Dravet syndrome) whose seizures are not adequately controlled with clobazam and valproate (November 2017) AWMSG No. 3468 Recommended

● **MEDICINAL FORMS** There can be variation in the licensing of different medicines containing the same drug.

Oral capsule

CAUTIONARY AND ADVISORY LABELS 1, 8, 21

▶ **Diacomit** (Alan Pharmaceuticals)

Stiripentol 250 mg Diacomit 250mg capsules | 60 capsule PoM £284.00 DT = £284.00

Stiripentol 500 mg Diacomit 500mg capsules | 60 capsule PoM £493.00 DT = £493.00

Powder for oral suspension

CAUTIONARY AND ADVISORY LABELS 1, 8, 13, 21

EXCIPIENTS: May contain Aspartame

▶ **Diacomit** (Alan Pharmaceuticals)

Stiripentol 250 mg Diacomit 250mg oral powder sachets | 60 sachet PoM £284.00 DT = £284.00

Stiripentol 500 mg Diacomit 500mg oral powder sachets | 60 sachet PoM £493.00 DT = £493.00

Tiagabine

17-Oct-2022

● **INDICATIONS AND DOSE**

Adjunctive treatment for focal seizures with or without secondary generalisation that are not satisfactorily controlled by other antiepileptics (with enzyme-inducing drugs)

▶ BY MOUTH

▶ Child 12–17 years: Initially 5–10 mg daily in 1–2 divided doses, then increased in steps of 5–10 mg/24 hours every week; maintenance 30–45 mg daily in 2–3 divided doses

Adjunctive treatment for focal seizures with or without secondary generalisation that are not satisfactorily controlled by other antiepileptics (without enzyme-inducing drugs)

▶ BY MOUTH

▶ Child 12–17 years: Initially 5–10 mg daily in 1–2 divided doses, then increased in steps of 5–10 mg/24 hours every week; maintenance 15–30 mg daily in 2–3 divided doses

IMPORTANT SAFETY INFORMATION

MHRA/CHM ADVICE: ANTIEPILEPTICS: RISK OF SUICIDAL THOUGHTS AND BEHAVIOUR (AUGUST 2008)

See Epilepsy p. 227.

MHRA/CHM ADVICE: ANTIEPILEPTIC DRUGS: UPDATED ADVICE ON SWITCHING BETWEEN DIFFERENT MANUFACTURERS' PRODUCTS (NOVEMBER 2017)

See Epilepsy p. 227.

MHRA/CHM ADVICE: ANTIEPILEPTIC DRUGS IN PREGNANCY: UPDATED ADVICE FOLLOWING COMPREHENSIVE SAFETY REVIEW (JANUARY 2021)

See Epilepsy p. 227.

- **CAUTIONS** Avoid in Acute porphyrias p. 745 · seizures (may be exacerbated)

CAUTIONS, FURTHER INFORMATION

- Seizure exacerbation EvGr Tiagabine may exacerbate seizures in patients with absence or myoclonic seizures (including juvenile myoclonic epilepsy), tonic or atonic seizures, Dravet syndrome, and Lennox-Gastaut syndrome. (A)

- **INTERACTIONS** → Appendix 1: antiepileptics
- **SIDE-EFFECTS**
  - **Common or very common** Abdominal pain · behaviour abnormal · concentration impaired · depression · diarrhoea · dizziness · emotional lability · fatigue · gait abnormal · insomnia · nausea · nervousness · speech disorder · tremor · vision disorders · vomiting
  - **Uncommon** Drowsiness · psychosis · skin reactions
  - **Rare or very rare** Delusions · hallucination
  - **Frequency not known** Suicidal behaviours
- **PREGNANCY** EvGr Avoid unless potential benefit outweighs risk—toxicity in *animal* studies. (M) See also *Pregnancy* in Epilepsy p. 227.
- **HEPATIC IMPAIRMENT** Manufacturer advises caution in mild to moderate impairment (risk of increased exposure); avoid in severe impairment.
  Dose adjustments Manufacturer advises dose reduction and/or longer dose interval with careful titration in mild to moderate impairment.
- **PATIENT AND CARER ADVICE**
  Medicines for Children leaflet: Tiagabine for epilepsy www.medicinesforchildren.org.uk/medicines/tiagabine-for-epilepsy/
  Driving and skilled tasks May impair performance of skilled tasks (e.g. driving).

- **MEDICINAL FORMS** There can be variation in the licensing of different medicines containing the same drug. Forms available from special-order manufacturers include: oral suspension

Oral tablet

CAUTIONARY AND ADVISORY LABELS 21

- **Gabitril** (Teva UK Ltd)
  Tiagabine (as Tiagabine hydrochloride monohydrate)
  5 mg Gabitril 5mg tablets | 100 tablet PoM £52.04 DT = £52.04
  Tiagabine (as Tiagabine hydrochloride monohydrate)
  10 mg Gabitril 10mg tablets | 100 tablet PoM £104.09 DT = £104.09
  Tiagabine (as Tiagabine hydrochloride monohydrate)
  15 mg Gabitril 15mg tablets | 100 tablet PoM £156.13 DT = £156.13

Topiramate

18-Sep-2024

- **INDICATIONS AND DOSE**

Monotherapy of generalised tonic-clonic seizures or focal seizures with or without secondary generalisation

- BY MOUTH
  - Child 6–17 years: Initially 0.5–1 mg/kg once daily (max. per dose 25 mg) for 1 week, dose to be taken at night, then increased in steps of 250–500 micrograms/kg twice daily, dose to be increased by a maximum of 25 mg twice daily at intervals of 1–2 weeks; usual dose 50 mg twice daily (max. per dose 7.5 mg/kg twice daily), if child cannot tolerate titration regimens recommended above then smaller steps or longer interval between steps may be used; maximum 500 mg per day

Adjunctive treatment of generalised tonic-clonic seizures or focal seizures with or without secondary generalisation | Adjunctive treatment for seizures associated with Lennox-Gastaut syndrome

- BY MOUTH
  - Child 2–17 years: Initially 1–3 mg/kg once daily (max. per dose 25 mg) for 1 week, dose to be taken at night, then increased in steps of 0.5–1.5 mg/kg twice daily, dose to be increased by a maximum of 25 mg twice daily at intervals of 1–2 weeks; usual dose 2.5–4.5 mg/kg twice daily (max. per dose 7.5 mg/kg twice daily), if child cannot tolerate recommended titration regimen then smaller steps or longer interval between steps may be used; maximum 400 mg per day

Migraine prophylaxis

- BY MOUTH
  - Child 16–17 years: Initially 25 mg once daily for 1 week, dose to be taken at night, then increased in steps of 25 mg every week; usual dose 50–100 mg daily in 2 divided doses, if child cannot tolerate recommended titration regimen then smaller steps or longer interval between steps may be used; maximum 200 mg per day

- **UNLICENSED USE** Not licensed for use in children for migraine prophylaxis.

IMPORTANT SAFETY INFORMATION

MHRA/CHM ADVICE: ANTIEPILEPTICS: RISK OF SUICIDAL THOUGHTS AND BEHAVIOUR (AUGUST 2008)

See Epilepsy p. 227.

MHRA/CHM ADVICE: ANTIEPILEPTIC DRUGS: UPDATED ADVICE ON SWITCHING BETWEEN DIFFERENT MANUFACTURERS' PRODUCTS (NOVEMBER 2017)

See Epilepsy p. 227 and see also *Prescribing and dispensing information*.

MHRA/CHM ADVICE: ANTIEPILEPTIC DRUGS IN PREGNANCY: UPDATED ADVICE FOLLOWING COMPREHENSIVE SAFETY REVIEW (JANUARY 2021)

See Epilepsy p. 227.

MHRA/CHM ADVICE: TOPIRAMATE (*TOPAMAX*®): START OF SAFETY REVIEW TRIGGERED BY A STUDY REPORTING AN INCREASED RISK OF NEURODEVELOPMENTAL DISABILITIES IN CHILDREN WITH PRENATAL EXPOSURE (JULY 2022)

The MHRA has started a new safety review of topiramate following a large observational study that found a dose-dependent association between prenatal exposure and an increased risk of autism spectrum disorders, intellectual disability, and neurodevelopmental disorders in children. Healthcare professionals are reminded that topiramate must be prescribed according to current guidance. In addition, females of childbearing potential or their carers should be counselled on the importance of avoiding pregnancy due to these emerging risks, as well as the established risks associated with topiramate use in pregnancy.

MHRA/CHM ADVICE: TOPIRAMATE (*TOPAMAX*®): INTRODUCTION OF NEW SAFETY MEASURES, INCLUDING A PREGNANCY PREVENTION PROGRAMME (JUNE 2024)

Following the safety review above, the MHRA concluded that the use of topiramate during pregnancy is associated with significant harm to the unborn child, including a higher risk of congenital malformations and low birth-weight, and a potential increased risk of intellectual disability, autism spectrum disorders, and ADHD.

Topiramate must not be used in females of childbearing potential unless the conditions of the Pregnancy Prevention Programme are met (see *Conception and contraception*). Use of topiramate in pregnancy is contra-indicated for migraine prophylaxis, and it must only be considered for epilepsy if there is no suitable alternative treatment (see *Pregnancy*).

Female patients (and their carers) must be fully informed of the risks associated with the use of topiramate during pregnancy; supporting materials have been provided to use in the implementation of the Pregnancy Prevention Programme (see *Prescribing and dispensing information*). The MHRA advises that:

- Prescribers must identify all new and existing females of childbearing potential on topiramate, explain clearly the conditions of the Pregnancy Prevention Programme, provide the Patient Guide, and complete and sign the Risk Awareness Form (at treatment initiation and at each annual review)—copies of the form must be given to the patient or carer and, if necessary, sent to their GP;
- Pharmacists must ensure topiramate is dispensed in whole packs whenever possible—all packs dispensed to females of childbearing potential should have a warning symbol either on the carton or via a sticker. They must also provide the Patient Card and check if the patient is using highly effective contraception, if they are not, patients should be advised to contact their GP for a follow-up appointment.

- **CAUTIONS** Avoid in Acute porphyrias p. 745 · risk of metabolic acidosis · risk of nephrolithiasis—ensure adequate hydration (especially in strenuous activity or warm environment)
- **INTERACTIONS** → Appendix 1: antiepileptics
- **SIDE-EFFECTS**

▸ **Common or very common** Alopecia · anaemia · anxiety · appetite abnormal · asthenia · behaviour abnormal · cognitive impairment · concentration impaired · confusion · constipation · cough · depression · diarrhoea · dizziness · drowsiness · dry mouth · dyspnoea · ear discomfort · eye disorders · feeling abnormal · fever · gait abnormal · gastrointestinal discomfort · gastrointestinal disorders · haemorrhage · hypersensitivity · joint disorders · malaise · memory loss · mood altered · movement disorders · muscle complaints · muscle weakness · nasal complaints · nasopharyngitis · nausea · oral disorders · pain · seizures · sensation abnormal · skin reactions · sleep disorders · speech impairment · taste altered · tinnitus · tremor · urinary disorders · urolithiases · vertigo · vision disorders · vomiting · weight changes

▸ **Uncommon** Abnormal sensation in eye · anhidrosis · arrhythmias · aura · cerebellar syndrome · consciousness impaired · crying · drooling · dry eye · dysgraphia · dysphonia · eosinophilia · facial swelling · hallucinations · hearing impairment · hyperthermia · hypokalaemia · hypotension · influenza like illness · learning disability · leucopenia · lymphadenopathy · metabolic acidosis · musculoskeletal stiffness · palpitations · pancreatitis · paranasal sinus hypersecretion · peripheral coldness · peripheral neuropathy · polydipsia · psychotic disorder · renal pain · sexual dysfunction · smell altered · suicidal behaviours · syncope · thinking abnormal · thirst · thrombocytopenia · vasodilation

▸ **Rare or very rare** Eye inflammation · face oedema · glaucoma · hepatic disorders · limb discomfort · neutropenia · Raynaud's phenomenon · renal tubular acidosis · severe cutaneous adverse reactions (SCARs) · unresponsive to stimuli

SIDE-EFFECTS, FURTHER INFORMATION Topiramate has been associated with acute myopia with secondary angle-closure glaucoma, typically occurring within 1 month of starting treatment. Choroidal effusions resulting in anterior displacement of the lens and iris have also been reported. If raised intra-ocular pressure occurs: seek specialist ophthalmological advice; use appropriate measures to reduce intra-ocular pressure and stop topiramate as rapidly as feasible.

- **CONCEPTION AND CONTRACEPTION** The MHRA advises that all females of childbearing potential being treated with topiramate must follow the requirements of the Pregnancy Prevention Programme—pregnancy should be excluded before treatment initiation. Highly effective contraception must be used during and for at least 4 weeks after stopping treatment.
- **PREGNANCY** For *migraine prophylaxis*, the MHRA advises that topiramate must not be used. For *epilepsy*, the MHRA advises that topiramate must not be used unless there is no suitable alternative treatment; in such cases, patients must be counselled about the risks (see *Important safety information*). EvGr If used during pregnancy, careful prenatal monitoring should be performed. ⟨M⟩ See also *Pregnancy* in Epilepsy p. 227.
- **BREAST FEEDING** Manufacturer advises avoid—present in milk.
- **HEPATIC IMPAIRMENT** Manufacturer advises caution (risk of decreased clearance).
- **RENAL IMPAIRMENT** EvGr Use with caution. ⟨M⟩

Dose adjustments EvGr Half usual starting and maintenance dose if creatinine clearance 70 mL/minute or less (reduced clearance and longer time to steady-state plasma concentration). ⟨M⟩ See p. 16.

- **DIRECTIONS FOR ADMINISTRATION**

TOPAMAX® CAPSULES Manufacturer advises swallow whole or sprinkle contents of capsule on soft food and swallow immediately without chewing.

- **PRESCRIBING AND DISPENSING INFORMATION** The Pregnancy Prevention Programme is supported by the following safety and educational materials: *Patient Guide*, *Guide for Healthcare Professionals*, *Risk Awareness Form*, *Patient Card*, and *Warning Stickers*.

In addition, the MHRA advises that pharmacists must dispense topiramate in whole packs—see also *Important safety information*.

Switching between formulations Care should be taken when switching between oral formulations in the treatment of epilepsy. The need for continued supply of a particular manufacturer's product should be based on clinical judgement and consultation with the patient or their carer, taking into account factors such as seizure frequency and treatment history.

Patients being treated for epilepsy may need to be maintained on a specific manufacturer's branded or generic topiramate product.

- **PATIENT AND CARER ADVICE**

Pregnancy Prevention Programme A patient card and patient guide must be provided to females of childbearing potential—see also *Important safety information*.

Medicines for Children leaflet: Topiramate for preventing seizures www.medicinesforchildren.org.uk/medicines/topiramate-for-preventing-seizures/

Driving and skilled tasks Patients and carers should be counselled on the effects on driving and performance of skilled tasks—increased risk of dizziness and visual disturbances.

TOPAMAX® CAPSULES Patients or carers should be given advice on how to administer *Topamax® Sprinkle* capsules.

- **MEDICINAL FORMS** There can be variation in the licensing of different medicines containing the same drug. Forms available from special-order manufacturers include: oral suspension, oral solution

Oral tablet

CAUTIONARY AND ADVISORY LABELS 2, 8

▸ **Topiramate (non-proprietary)** ▼

Topiramate 25 mg Topiramate 25mg tablets | 60 tablet PoM £16.40 DT = £1.18

Topiramate 50 mg Topiramate 50mg tablets | 60 tablet PoM £26.94 DT = £1.46

Topiramate 100 mg Topiramate 100mg tablets | 60 tablet PoM £48.25 DT = £1.79

Topiramate 200 mg Topiramate 200mg tablets | 60 tablet PoM £93.70 DT = £7.14

▸ Topamax (Janssen-Cilag Ltd) ▼

Topiramate 25 mg Topamax 25mg tablets | 60 tablet PoM £19.29 DT = £1.18

Topiramate 50 mg Topamax 50mg tablets | 60 tablet PoM £31.69 DT = £1.46

Topiramate 100 mg Topamax 100mg tablets | 60 tablet PoM £56.76 DT = £1.79

Topiramate 200 mg Topamax 200mg tablets | 60 tablet PoM £110.23 DT = £7.14

Oral solution

▸ Topiramate (non-proprietary) ▼

Topiramate 20 mg per 1 ml Topiramate 20mg/ml oral solution sugar free | 150 ml PoM £165.00–£305.00 SF | 280 ml PoM £330.72–£559.00 SF

Oral suspension

CAUTIONARY AND ADVISORY LABELS 2, 8

▸ Topiramate (non-proprietary) ▼

Topiramate 10 mg per 1 ml Topiramate 50mg/5ml oral suspension sugar free | 150 ml PoM £186.00–£235.83 DT = £235.83 SF

Topiramate 20 mg per 1 ml Topiramate 100mg/5ml oral suspension sugar free | 280 ml PoM £342.70 DT = £342.70 SF

Oral capsule

CAUTIONARY AND ADVISORY LABELS 2, 8

▸ Topamax (Janssen-Cilag Ltd) ▼

Topiramate 15 mg Topamax 15mg sprinkle capsules | 60 capsule PoM £14.79 DT = £14.79

Topiramate 25 mg Topamax 25mg sprinkle capsules | 60 capsule PoM £22.18 DT = £22.18

Topiramate 50 mg Topamax 50mg sprinkle capsules | 60 capsule PoM £36.45 DT = £36.45

Valproic acid

24-Mar-2026

● **INDICATIONS AND DOSE**

CONVULEX®

Epilepsy

▸ BY MOUTH

- Child 1 month–11 years: Initially 10–15 mg/kg daily in 2–4 divided doses, max. 600 mg daily; usual maintenance 25–30 mg/kg daily in 2–4 divided doses, doses up to 60 mg/kg daily in 2–4 divided doses in infantile spasms; monitor clinical chemistry and haematological parameters if dose exceeds 40 mg/kg daily
- Child 12–17 years: Initially 600 mg daily in 2–4 divided doses, increased in steps of 150–300 mg every 3 days; usual maintenance 1–2 g daily in 2–4 divided doses, max. 2.5 g daily in 2–4 divided doses

DOSE EQUIVALENCE AND CONVERSION

- *Convulex*® has a 1:1 dose relationship with products containing sodium valproate, but nevertheless care is needed if switching or making changes.

IMPORTANT SAFETY INFORMATION

MHRA/CHM ADVICE: ANTIEPILEPTICS: RISK OF SUICIDAL THOUGHTS AND BEHAVIOUR (AUGUST 2008)

See Epilepsy p. 227.

MHRA/CHM ADVICE: ANTIEPILEPTIC DRUGS: UPDATED ADVICE ON SWITCHING BETWEEN DIFFERENT MANUFACTURERS' PRODUCTS (NOVEMBER 2017)

See Epilepsy p. 227 and see also *Prescribing and dispensing information*.

VALPROATE AND REPRODUCTIVE RISKS

Valproate is highly teratogenic and evidence shows that use in pregnancy can lead to neurodevelopmental disorders (approx. 30–40% risk) and congenital malformations (approx. 11% risk). It can also potentially cause infertility in males and neurodevelopmental disorders in children born to males treated with valproate in the 3 months prior to conception. Valproate must not be initiated in any patients under 55 years of age unless 2 specialists independently review and document that there is no other effective or tolerated treatment, or there are compelling reasons that the reproductive risks do not apply. Male patients under 55 years of age who are already taking valproate can continue to have it prescribed in accordance with standard clinical practice by a single prescriber. In females of childbearing potential, the conditions of the Pregnancy Prevention Programme must be met and a valproate risk acknowledgement form completed annually. Male patients (of any age) who may father a child must be counselled on using effective contraception during treatment and for 3 months after stopping.

Patients should be informed not to stop taking valproate without advice from a specialist because epilepsy or bipolar disorder may worsen without treatment.

For further information and resources, see MHRA/CHM advice below, *Conception and contraception*, *Pregnancy*, *Prescribing and dispensing information*, and *Patient and carer advice*; refer to the MHRA information page at: www.gov.uk/guidance/valproate-reproductive-risks.

MHRA/CHM ADVICE: ANTIEPILEPTIC DRUGS IN PREGNANCY: UPDATED ADVICE FOLLOWING COMPREHENSIVE SAFETY REVIEW (JANUARY 2021)

See Epilepsy p. 227.

MHRA/CHM ADVICE: FULL PACK DISPENSING OF VALPROATE-CONTAINING MEDICINES (OCTOBER 2023)

Valproate medicines have been dispensed to patients in alternative packaging because the prescribed amount was different to that of the manufacturer's original full pack. This resulted in patients not always receiving all the risk materials about the use of these medicines in pregnancy. Pharmacists are advised that all patients (male and female) must receive their valproate medicines in the manufacturer's original full pack (i.e. original pack dispensing) and the amount dispensed must be as close as possible to the amount stated on the prescription (NHS or private). Rarely, exceptions to this requirement can be made on an individual patient basis, provided a risk assessment is carried out on the need to dispense repackaged valproate medicines (e.g. in a monitored dosage system), whereby a patient information leaflet must be supplied.

MHRA/CHM ADVICE: VALPROATE (*BELVO*®, *CONVULEX*®, *DEPAKOTE*®, AND *SYONELL*®): NEW SAFETY AND EDUCATIONAL MATERIALS TO SUPPORT REGULATORY MEASURES IN MEN AND WOMEN UNDER 55 YEARS OF AGE (JANUARY 2024)

Healthcare professionals are advised to review, and integrate into their clinical practice, safety and educational materials that support new regulatory measures (see *Prescribing and dispensing information*). General practice and pharmacy teams should continue to prescribe and dispense valproate according to current safety measures. If required, patients should be referred to a specialist to discuss treatment options. Patients on valproate medicines should be fully informed of the potential risks and counselled on treatment options at initial prescribing and at all subsequent reviews.

Healthcare professionals should advise patients to:

- not stop taking valproate medicines without advice from a specialist as their epilepsy or bipolar disorder may worsen;
- attend any offered appointments to discuss their treatment plan and to talk to a healthcare professional if they have any concerns;

- consult the new Patient Guide and Patient Information Leaflet for information on the risks of valproate.

MHRA/CHM ADVICE: VALPROATE USE IN MEN: AS A PRECAUTION, MEN AND THEIR PARTNERS SHOULD USE EFFECTIVE CONTRACEPTION (SEPTEMBER 2024)

The MHRA has reviewed findings from a retrospective observational study that suggest a potential increased risk of neurodevelopmental disorders in children born to males taking valproate medicines in the 3 months before conception; however, causality is unconfirmed. In addition to current safety measures, healthcare professionals should advise male patients (of any age) who may father a child:

- about this risk at treatment initiation or at the next treatment review, irrespective of indication and also after intravenous valproate;
- to use effective contraception (i.e. condoms plus contraception used by their female partner) during and for 3 months after valproate treatment;
- to refrain from donating sperm during and for 3 months after valproate treatment.

Healthcare professionals are also advised that:

- male patients who are planning a family in the next year should be referred to a specialist to discuss alternative treatment;
- female partners of male patients taking valproate medicines who are pregnant or planning a pregnancy (including those undergoing IVF) should be referred for prenatal counselling.

MHRA/CHM ADVICE: VALPROATE (*BELVO*®, *CONVULEX*®, *DEPAKOTE*®, AND *SYONELL*®): REVIEW BY TWO SPECIALISTS IS REQUIRED FOR INITIATING VALPROATE BUT NOT FOR MALE PATIENTS ALREADY TAKING VALPROATE (FEBRUARY 2025)

Healthcare professionals are reminded that the current safety measure advising all patients under 55 years of age to be reviewed by two specialists before initiating valproate remains in place, however, the CHM has advised that this will not be required for male patients who are already taking valproate. Healthcare professionals are also reminded that all previously issued safety measures continue to apply.

The CHM has produced infographics to clarify the situations where review by two specialists may be required.

For female patients under 55 years of age, see: assets.publishing.service.gov.uk/media/67adf28c6e6c8d18118acd69/250213_MHRA_Valproate_Infographic_Female_under_55_CC_V7.pdf.

For male patients under 55 years of age, see: assets.publishing.service.gov.uk/media/67adf2aa6e6c8d18118acd6a/250213_MHRA_Valproate_Infographic_Male_under_55_CC_V7.pdf.

For male and female patients aged 55 years and older, see: assets.publishing.service.gov.uk/media/67adf2c62c594609b38acd71/250213_MHRA_Valproate_Infographic_55_or_older_CC_V7.pdf.

MHRA/CHM ADVICE: VALPROATE (*BELVO*®, *CONVULEX*®, *DEPAKOTE*® AND *SYONELL*®): UPDATED SAFETY AND EDUCATIONAL MATERIALS TO SUPPORT PATIENT DISCUSSION ON REPRODUCTIVE RISKS (JUNE 2025)

The MHRA reminds healthcare professionals of the potential risk of neurodevelopmental disorders in children fathered by males taking valproate around the time of conception. Children exposed to valproate in utero also have a higher risk of being born with a low birth weight or being small for gestational age, compared to those unexposed to antiepileptic drugs or exposed to lamotrigine.

Safety and educational materials have therefore been updated in line with regulatory requirements and are available at: www.gov.uk/guidance/valproate-reproductive-risks#materials-and-resources. These should be reviewed and integrated into clinical practice for all patients being treated with valproate.

- **CONTRA-INDICATIONS** Acute porphyrias p. 745 · known or suspected mitochondrial disorders (higher rate of acute liver failure and liver-related deaths) · personal or family history of severe hepatic dysfunction · urea cycle disorders (risk of hyperammonaemia)
- **CAUTIONS** Systemic lupus erythematosus

CAUTIONS, FURTHER INFORMATION

▸ **Liver toxicity** Liver dysfunction (including fatal hepatic failure) has occurred in association with valproate (especially in children under 3 years and in those with metabolic or degenerative disorders, organic brain disease or severe seizure disorders associated with mental retardation) usually in first 6 months and usually involving multiple antiepileptic therapy. EvGr Raised liver enzymes during valproate treatment are usually transient but patients should be reassessed clinically and liver function (including prothrombin time) monitored until return to normal—discontinue if abnormally prolonged prothrombin time (particularly in association with other relevant abnormalities). Ⓜ

The MHRA advises consider vitamin D supplementation in patients who are immobilised for long periods or who have inadequate sun exposure or dietary intake of calcium.

- **INTERACTIONS** → Appendix 1: antiepileptics
- **SIDE-EFFECTS**

▸ **Common or very common** Abdominal pain · agitation · alopecia · anaemia · behaviour abnormal · concentration impaired · confusion · diarrhoea · drowsiness · haemorrhage · hallucination · headache · hearing loss · hepatic disorders · hypersensitivity · hyponatraemia · memory impairment · menstrual cycle irregularities · movement disorders · nail disorder · nausea · nystagmus · oral disorders · seizures · stupor · thrombocytopenia · tremor · urinary disorders · vomiting · weight increased

▸ **Uncommon** Angioedema · bone disorders · bone fracture · bone marrow disorders · coma · encephalopathy · eosinophilic pleural effusion · hair changes · hyperandrogenism · hypothermia · leucopenia · pancreatitis · paraesthesia · parkinsonism · peripheral oedema · renal failure · SIADH · skin reactions · vasculitis · virilism

▸ **Rare or very rare** Agranulocytosis · cerebral atrophy · cognitive disorder · dementia · diplopia · Fanconi syndrome acquired · hyperammonaemia · hypothyroidism · infertility male · learning disability · myelodysplastic syndrome · nephritis tubulointerstitial · obesity · polycystic ovarian syndrome · red blood cell abnormalities · rhabdomyolysis · severe cutaneous adverse reactions (SCARs) · systemic lupus erythematosus (SLE)

▸ **Frequency not known** Gynaecomastia · hypocarnitinaemia · suicidal behaviours

SIDE-EFFECTS, FURTHER INFORMATION

Hepatic dysfunction Withdraw treatment immediately if persistent vomiting and abdominal pain, anorexia, jaundice, oedema, malaise, drowsiness, or loss of seizure control.

Pancreatitis Discontinue treatment if symptoms of pancreatitis develop.

- **CONCEPTION AND CONTRACEPTION** The MHRA advises that all women and girls of childbearing potential being treated with valproate medicines must be supported on a Pregnancy Prevention Programme—pregnancy should be excluded before treatment initiation. Highly effective contraception must be used during treatment i.e. at least 1, preferably highly effective user-independent contraceptive method (such as an intra-uterine device or implant), or 2 complementary forms including a barrier method. The MHRA advises that all male patients being treated with valproate medicines and who may father children should use effective contraception (i.e. condoms plus contraception used by their female partner) during and for 3 months after treatment. The MHRA advises that male patients taking valproate medicines should be informed of the risk of infertility, and of data showing testicular toxicity in *animal* studies.

- **PREGNANCY** For *migraine prophylaxis* [unlicensed] and *bipolar disorder*, the MHRA advises that valproate medicines must not be used. For *epilepsy*, the MHRA advises valproate must not be used unless two specialists independently consider and document that there is no other effective or tolerated treatment (see also *Important safety information*). If valproate is to be used, the lowest effective dose should be prescribed in divided doses to be taken throughout the day; modified-release preparations may be preferable to avoid high peak plasma-valproate concentrations. There is no dose threshold considered to be without any risk, however, the risk of birth defects and neurodevelopmental disorders is greater at higher doses. EvGr Specialist prenatal monitoring should be instigated when valproate has been taken in pregnancy. ⟨M⟩ Neonatal bleeding (related to hypofibrinaemia). Neonatal hepatotoxicity also reported. See also *Pregnancy* in Epilepsy p. 227.
- **BREAST FEEDING** Present in milk—risk of haematological disorders in breast-fed newborns and infants.
- **HEPATIC IMPAIRMENT** Manufacturer advises avoid.
- **RENAL IMPAIRMENT**

Dose adjustments EvGr Consider dose reduction. ⟨M⟩

- **MONITORING REQUIREMENTS**
  - Monitor closely if dose greater than 45 mg/kg daily.
  - Monitor liver function before therapy and during first 6 months especially in patients most at risk.
  - Measure full blood count and ensure no undue potential for bleeding before starting and before surgery.
- **EFFECT ON LABORATORY TESTS** False-positive urine tests for ketones.
- **TREATMENT CESSATION** EvGr In bipolar disorder, avoid abrupt withdrawal; if treatment with valproate is stopped, reduce the dose gradually over at least 4 weeks. ⟨A⟩
- **PRESCRIBING AND DISPENSING INFORMATION** The Pregnancy Prevention Programme is supported by the following safety and educational materials: *Guide for Female Patients*, *Guide for Male Patients*, *Guide for Healthcare Professionals*, *Annual Risk Acknowledgement Form for Female Patients*, *Risk Acknowledgement Form for Male Patients Starting Valproate*, *Patient Card*, and *Pharmacy Poster*.

In addition, the MHRA advises that pharmacist must dispense valproate medicines in the manufacturer's original full pack.

Safety and educational materials, and resources for healthcare professionals are available from the MHRA guidance page on Valproate - reproductive risks, at: www.gov.uk/guidance/valproate-reproductive-risks.

The Royal College of Pharmacy has also produced a safe supply algorithm, available at: rcpharm.org/wp-content/uploads/2026/04/Valproate-safe-supply-community-pharmacy-FINAL.pdf.

CONVULEX® Patients being treated for epilepsy may need to be maintained on a specific manufacturer's branded or generic oral valproic acid product.

- **PATIENT AND CARER ADVICE** The MHRA advises that patients should **not** stop taking valproate without first discussing it with a specialist. Female patients or their carers should be advised to immediately contact their GP for an urgent referral to a specialist in case of suspected pregnancy. Female partners of male patients taking valproate medicines should be referred for prenatal counselling if pregnancy is suspected.

Blood or hepatic disorders Patients or their carers should be told how to recognise signs and symptoms of blood or liver disorders and advised to seek immediate medical attention if symptoms develop.

Pancreatitis Patients or their carers should be told how to recognise signs and symptoms of pancreatitis and advised to seek immediate medical attention if symptoms such as abdominal pain, nausea, or vomiting develop.

Suicidal ideation and behaviour Patients or their carers should be advised to seek immediate medical attention if any signs of suicidal thoughts or behaviour develop.

Patient guide A patient guide must be provided.

Pregnancy Prevention Programme Pharmacists must ensure that female patients have a patient card—see also *Important safety information*.

Decision aid NHS England has produced a patient decision aid for females of childbearing potential who are considering or are taking valproate medicines for epilepsy, available at: www.england.nhs.uk/publication/decision-support-tool-is-valproate-the-right-epilepsy-treatment-for-me/.

- **MEDICINAL FORMS** There can be variation in the licensing of different medicines containing the same drug.

Gastro-resistant capsule

CAUTIONARY AND ADVISORY LABELS 8, 10, 21, 25

- Convulex (G.L. Pharma UK Ltd) ▼
  - **Valproic acid 150 mg** Convulex 150mg gastro-resistant capsules | 30 capsule PoM £2.80 DT = £2.80
  - **Valproic acid 300 mg** Convulex 300mg gastro-resistant capsules | 30 capsule PoM £5.60 DT = £5.60
  - **Valproic acid 500 mg** Convulex 500mg gastro-resistant capsules | 30 capsule PoM £7.38 DT = £7.38

Vigabatrin

19-Mar-2024

- **INDICATIONS AND DOSE**

Adjunctive treatment of focal seizures with or without secondary generalisation not satisfactorily controlled with other antiepileptics (under expert supervision)

- BY MOUTH
  - Neonate: Initially 15–20 mg/kg twice daily, to be increased over 2–3 weeks to usual maintenance dose, usual maintenance 30–40 mg/kg twice daily (max. per dose 75 mg/kg).
  - Child 1–23 months: Initially 15–20 mg/kg twice daily (max. per dose 250 mg), to be increased over 2–3 weeks to usual maintenance dose, usual maintenance 30–40 mg/kg twice daily (max. per dose 75 mg/kg)
  - Child 2–11 years: Initially 15–20 mg/kg twice daily (max. per dose 250 mg), to be increased over 2–3 weeks to usual maintenance dose, usual maintenance 30–40 mg/kg twice daily (max. per dose 1.5 g)
  - Child 12–17 years: Initially 250 mg twice daily, to be increased over 2–3 weeks to usual maintenance dose, usual maintenance 1–1.5 g twice daily
- BY RECTUM
  - Child 1–23 months: Initially 15–20 mg/kg twice daily (max. per dose 250 mg), to be increased over 2–3 weeks to usual maintenance dose, usual maintenance 30–40 mg/kg twice daily (max. per dose 75 mg/kg)
  - Child 2–11 years: Initially 15–20 mg/kg twice daily (max. per dose 250 mg), to be increased over 2–3 weeks to usual maintenance dose, usual maintenance 30–40 mg/kg twice daily (max. per dose 1.5 g)
  - Child 12–17 years: Initially 250 mg twice daily, to be increased over 2–3 weeks to usual maintenance dose, usual maintenance 1–1.5 g twice daily

continued →

Infantile spasms [in combination with prednisolone or as monotherapy] (under expert supervision)
- ▶ BY MOUTH
- ▸ Child 1–23 months: Initially 25 mg/kg twice daily on day 1, followed by 50 mg/kg twice daily on days 2–4; increased if necessary up to 75 mg/kg twice daily from day 5 if spasms continue

● **UNLICENSED USE** Granules not licensed for rectal use. Tablets not licensed to be crushed and dispersed in liquid. Vigabatrin doses in BNF Publications may differ from those in product literature. EvGr Vigabatrin as combination therapy with prednisolone is used for the treatment of infantile spasms, (B) but such use is not licensed for this indication.

IMPORTANT SAFETY INFORMATION

MHRA/CHM ADVICE: ANTIEPILEPTICS: RISK OF SUICIDAL THOUGHTS AND BEHAVIOUR (AUGUST 2008)
See Epilepsy p. 227.

MHRA/CHM ADVICE: ANTIEPILEPTIC DRUGS: UPDATED ADVICE ON SWITCHING BETWEEN DIFFERENT MANUFACTURERS' PRODUCTS (NOVEMBER 2017)
See Epilepsy p. 227.

MHRA/CHM ADVICE: ANTIEPILEPTIC DRUGS IN PREGNANCY: UPDATED ADVICE FOLLOWING COMPREHENSIVE SAFETY REVIEW (JANUARY 2021)
See Epilepsy p. 227.

● **CONTRA-INDICATIONS** Visual field defects

● **CAUTIONS** History of behavioural problems · history of depression · history of psychosis · seizures (may be exacerbated)

CAUTIONS, FURTHER INFORMATION
- ▸ Seizure exacerbation EvGr Vigabatrin may exacerbate seizures in patients with absence or myoclonic seizures (including juvenile myoclonic epilepsy), tonic or atonic seizures, Dravet syndrome, Lennox-Gastaut syndrome, and myoclonic-atonic seizures. (A)
- ▸ Visual field defects Vigabatrin is associated with visual field defects. The onset of symptoms varies from 1 month to several years after starting. In most cases, visual field defects have persisted despite discontinuation, and further deterioration after discontinuation cannot be excluded. EvGr Visual field testing should be carried out before treatment and at 6-month intervals. Patients and their carers should be warned to report any new visual symptoms that develop and those with symptoms should be referred for an urgent ophthalmological opinion. Gradual withdrawal of vigabatrin should be considered. (M)

● **INTERACTIONS** → Appendix 1: antiepileptics

● **SIDE-EFFECTS**

GENERAL SIDE-EFFECTS
- ▶ **Rare or very rare** Suicidal behaviours

SPECIFIC SIDE-EFFECTS
- ▶ **Common or very common**
- ▸ With oral use Abdominal pain · alopecia · anaemia · anxiety · arthralgia · behaviour abnormal · concentration impaired · depression · dizziness · drowsiness · eye disorders · fatigue · headache · insomnia · memory loss · mood altered · nausea · oedema · paraesthesia · speech disorder · thinking abnormal · tremor · vision disorders · vomiting · weight increased
- ▶ **Uncommon**
- ▸ With oral use Movement disorders · psychotic disorder · seizure (patients with myoclonic seizures at greater risk) · skin reactions
- ▶ **Rare or very rare**
- ▸ With oral use Angioedema · encephalopathy · hallucination · hepatitis · optic neuritis
- ▶ **Frequency not known**
- ▸ With oral use Intramyelinic oedema (particularly in infants) · movement disorder (in infantile spasms) · muscle tone increased

SIDE-EFFECTS, FURTHER INFORMATION **Encephalopathic symptoms** Encephalopathic symptoms including marked sedation, stupor, and confusion with non-specific slow wave EEG can occur rarely -reduce dose or withdraw.

Visual field defects About one-third of patients treated with vigabatrin have suffered visual field defects; counselling and careful monitoring for this side-effect are required.

● **PREGNANCY** EvGr Avoid unless essential—toxicity in *animal* studies. (M) See also *Pregnancy* in Epilepsy p. 227.

● **BREAST FEEDING** Present in milk—manufacturer advises avoid.

● **RENAL IMPAIRMENT**

Dose adjustments EvGr Consider reduced dose or increased dose interval if creatinine clearance less than 60 mL/minute. (M) See p. 16.

● **MONITORING REQUIREMENTS**
- ▶ Closely monitor neurological function.
- ▸ When used for Infantile spasms EvGr Monitor closely for additive side-effects when used as combination therapy with prednisolone. (E)

● **DIRECTIONS FOR ADMINISTRATION**
- ▸ With oral use EvGr The contents of a sachet of granules should be dissolved in at least 100 mL of water, fruit juice, or milk immediately before taking. (M) Expert sources advise film-coated tablets may be crushed and dispersed in liquid. EvGr Soluble tablets should be dissolved in a small volume of water (approximately 5 or 10 mL) before administration. (M)
- ▸ With rectal use Expert sources advise contents of a sachet of granules should be dissolved in a small amount of water and administered rectally.

● **PATIENT AND CARER ADVICE** Patients and their carers should be warned to report any new visual symptoms that develop.

Medicines for Children leaflet: Vigabatrin for preventing seizures www.medicinesforchildren.org.uk/medicines/vigabatrin-for-preventing-seizures/

Driving and skilled tasks Patients and carers should be cautioned on the effects on driving and performance of skilled or hazardous tasks—increased risk of visual field defects.

● **NATIONAL FUNDING/ACCESS DECISIONS**

For full details see funding body website

Scottish Medicines Consortium (SMC) decisions
- ▶ **Vigabatrin (*Kigabeq*®) for children from 1 month to less than 7 years of age: as monotherapy for the treatment of infantile spasms (West's syndrome); in combination with other antiepileptic medicinal products for patients with resistant partial epilepsy (focal onset seizures) with or without secondary generalisation, where all other appropriate medicinal product combinations have proved inadequate or have not been tolerated (June 2021)** SMC No. SMC2352 Recommended with restrictions

● **MEDICINAL FORMS** There can be variation in the licensing of different medicines containing the same drug. Forms available from special-order manufacturers include: oral solution

Soluble tablet

CAUTIONARY AND ADVISORY LABELS 1, 8, 13
- ▸ **Kigabeq** (Alan Pharmaceuticals)

Vigabatrin 100 mg Kigabeq 100mg soluble tablets | 100 tablet PoM £66.47 DT = £66.47 SF

Vigabatrin 500 mg Kigabeq 500mg soluble tablets | 50 tablet PoM £148.72 DT = £148.72 SF

Oral tablet

CAUTIONARY AND ADVISORY LABELS 3, 8

▸ **Sabril** (Sanofi)

Vigabatrin 500 mg Sabril 500mg tablets | 100 tablet PoM £44.41 DT = £44.41

Oral solution

▸ **Vigabatrin (Non-proprietary)**

Vigabatrin 100 mg per 1 ml Vigabatrin 100mg/ml oral solution sugar free | 150 ml PoM £79.50–£147.10 SF

Granules for oral solution

CAUTIONARY AND ADVISORY LABELS 3, 8, 13

▸ **Sabril** (Sanofi)

Vigabatrin 500 mg Sabril 500mg granules for oral solution sachets | 50 sachet PoM £24.60 DT = £24.60 SF

Zonisamide

11-Nov-2021

● **INDICATIONS AND DOSE**

Adjunctive treatment for refractory focal seizures with or without secondary generalisation

▸ BY MOUTH

▸ Child 6–17 years (body-weight 20–54 kg): Initially 1 mg/kg once daily for 7 days, then increased in steps of 1 mg/kg every 7 days, usual maintenance 6–8 mg/kg once daily (max. per dose 500 mg once daily), dose to be increased at 2-week intervals in patients who are **not** receiving concomitant carbamazepine, phenytoin, phenobarbital or other potent inducers of cytochrome P450 enzyme CYP3A4

▸ Child 6–17 years (body-weight 55 kg and above): Initially 1 mg/kg once daily for 7 days, then increased in steps of 1 mg/kg every 7 days, usual maintenance 300–500 mg once daily, dose to be increased at 2-week intervals in patients who are **not** receiving concomitant carbamazepine, phenytoin, phenobarbital or other potent inducers of cytochrome P450 enzyme CYP3A4

IMPORTANT SAFETY INFORMATION

MHRA/CHM ADVICE: ANTIEPILEPTICS: RISK OF SUICIDAL THOUGHTS AND BEHAVIOUR (AUGUST 2008)

See Epilepsy p. 227.

MHRA/CHM ADVICE: ANTIEPILEPTIC DRUGS: UPDATED ADVICE ON SWITCHING BETWEEN DIFFERENT MANUFACTURERS' PRODUCTS (NOVEMBER 2017)

See Epilepsy p. 227 and see also *Prescribing and dispensing information*.

MHRA/CHM ADVICE: ANTIEPILEPTIC DRUGS IN PREGNANCY: UPDATED ADVICE FOLLOWING COMPREHENSIVE SAFETY REVIEW (JANUARY 2021)

See Epilepsy p. 227.

● **CAUTIONS** History of eye disorders · low body-weight or poor appetite—monitor weight throughout treatment (fatal cases of weight loss reported in children) · metabolic acidosis—monitor serum bicarbonate concentration in children and those with other risk factors (consider dose reduction or discontinuation if metabolic acidosis develops) · risk factors for renal stone formation (particularly predisposition to nephrolithiasis)

CAUTIONS, FURTHER INFORMATION EvGr Avoid overheating and ensure adequate hydration especially in children, during strenuous activity or if in warm environment (fatal cases of heat stroke reported in children). ⟨M⟩

● **INTERACTIONS** → Appendix 1: antiepileptics

● **SIDE-EFFECTS**

▸ **Common or very common** Alopecia · anxiety · appetite decreased · ataxia · bradyphrenia · concentration impaired · confusion · constipation · depression · diarrhoea · dizziness · drowsiness · fatigue · fever · gastrointestinal discomfort · hypersensitivity · influenza like illness · insomnia · memory loss · mood altered · nausea · nystagmus · paraesthesia · peripheral oedema · psychosis · rash (consider discontinuation) · skin reactions · speech disorder · tremor · urolithiases · vision disorders · vomiting · weight decreased

▸ **Uncommon** Behaviour abnormal · gallbladder disorders · hallucination · hypokalaemia · increased risk of infection · leucopenia · respiratory disorder · seizures · suicidal behaviours · thrombocytopenia

▸ **Rare or very rare** Agranulocytosis · alveolitis allergic · angle closure glaucoma · anhidrosis · bone marrow disorders · coma · dyspnoea · eye pain · heat stroke · hepatocellular injury · hydronephrosis · leucocytosis · lymphadenopathy · metabolic acidosis · myasthenic syndrome · neuroleptic malignant syndrome · pancreatitis · renal failure · renal tubular acidosis · rhabdomyolysis · severe cutaneous adverse reactions (SCARs) · urine abnormal

▸ **Frequency not known** Sudden unexplained death in epilepsy

● **ALLERGY AND CROSS-SENSITIVITY** Contra-indicated in sulfonamide hypersensitivity.

Antiepileptic hypersensitivity syndrome theoretically associated with zonisamide. See under Epilepsy p. 227 for more information.

● **CONCEPTION AND CONTRACEPTION** Manufacturer advises women of childbearing potential should use effective contraception during treatment and for one month after last dose—avoid in women of childbearing potential not using effective contraception unless clearly necessary and the potential benefit outweighs risk; patients should be fully informed of the risks related to the use of zonisamide during pregnancy.

● **PREGNANCY** An increased risk of intra-uterine growth restriction has been seen with zonisamide, see *Pregnancy* in Epilepsy p. 227.

● **BREAST FEEDING** Manufacturer advises avoid for 4 weeks after last dose.

● **HEPATIC IMPAIRMENT** Avoid in severe impairment.

Dose adjustments Initially increase dose at 2-week intervals if mild or moderate impairment.

● **RENAL IMPAIRMENT**

Dose adjustments Initially increase dose at 2-week intervals; discontinue if renal function deteriorates.

● **TREATMENT CESSATION** Avoid abrupt withdrawal (consult product literature for recommended withdrawal regimens in children).

● **PRESCRIBING AND DISPENSING INFORMATION**

Switching between formulations Care should be taken when switching between oral formulations. The need for continued supply of a particular manufacturer's product should be based on clinical judgement and consultation with the patient or their carer, taking into account factors such as seizure frequency and treatment history.

Patients may need to be maintained on a specific manufacturer's branded or generic zonisamide product.

● **PATIENT AND CARER ADVICE** Children and their carers should be made aware of how to prevent and recognise overheating and dehydration.

Medicines for Children leaflet: Zonisamide for preventing seizures www.medicinesforchildren.org.uk/medicines/zonisamide-for-preventing-seizures/

● **NATIONAL FUNDING/ACCESS DECISIONS**

For full details see funding body website

Scottish Medicines Consortium (SMC) decisions

▸ **Zonisamide (*Zonegran*®) as adjunctive therapy in the treatment of partial seizures, with or without secondary generalisation, in adolescents, and children aged 6 years and**

4 Nervous system

above (March 2014) SMC No. 949/14 Recommended with restrictions

- **MEDICINAL FORMS** There can be variation in the licensing of different medicines containing the same drug. Forms available from special-order manufacturers include: oral suspension, oral solution

Oral suspension

CAUTIONARY AND ADVISORY LABELS 3, 8, 10

▸ Zonisamide (Non-proprietary)

Zonisamide 20 mg per 1 ml Zonisamide 20mg/ml oral suspension sugar free | 150 ml [PoM] £109.14 [SF]

▸ Desizon (Desitin Pharma Ltd)

Zonisamide 20 mg per 1 ml Desizon 20mg/ml oral suspension | 250 ml [PoM] £181.90 DT = £181.90

Oral capsule

CAUTIONARY AND ADVISORY LABELS 3, 8, 10

▸ Zonisamide (Non-proprietary)

Zonisamide 25 mg Zonisamide 25mg capsules | 14 capsule [PoM] £15.18 DT = £2.91

Zonisamide 50 mg Zonisamide 50mg capsules | 56 capsule [PoM] £47.04 DT = £4.28

Zonisamide 100 mg Zonisamide 100mg capsules | 56 capsule [PoM] £62.72 DT = £4.87

Zonisamide 200 mg Zonisamide 200mg capsules | 28 capsule [PoM] £62.72–£106.62

▸ Zonegran (Advanz Pharma)

Zonisamide 25 mg Zonegran 25mg capsules | 14 capsule [PoM] £8.82 DT = £2.91

Zonisamide 50 mg Zonegran 50mg capsules | 56 capsule [PoM] £47.04 DT = £4.28

Zonisamide 100 mg Zonegran 100mg capsules | 56 capsule [PoM] £62.72 DT = £4.87

ANTIEPILEPTICS > BARBITURATES

Phenobarbital

17-Oct-2022

(Phenobarbitone)

- **INDICATIONS AND DOSE**

All forms of epilepsy except typical absence seizures

▸ BY MOUTH

- Child 1 month–11 years: Initially 1–1.5 mg/kg twice daily, then increased in steps of 2 mg/kg daily as required; maintenance 2.5–4 mg/kg 1–2 times a day
- Child 12–17 years: 60–180 mg once daily

▸ INITIALLY BY SLOW INTRAVENOUS INJECTION

- Neonate: Initially 20 mg/kg, then (by slow intravenous injection or by mouth) 2.5–5 mg/kg once daily, adjusted according to response.

Status epilepticus

▸ BY SLOW INTRAVENOUS INJECTION

- Neonate: Initially 20 mg/kg, then 2.5–5 mg/kg 1–2 times a day.
- Child 1 month–11 years: Initially 20 mg/kg, then 2.5–5 mg/kg 1–2 times a day
- Child 12–17 years: Initially 20 mg/kg (max. per dose 1 g), then 300 mg twice daily

DOSE EQUIVALENCE AND CONVERSION

- For therapeutic purposes phenobarbital and phenobarbital sodium may be considered equivalent in effect.

IMPORTANT SAFETY INFORMATION

MHRA/CHM ADVICE: ANTIEPILEPTICS: RISK OF SUICIDAL THOUGHTS AND BEHAVIOUR (AUGUST 2008)

See Epilepsy p. 227.

MHRA/CHM ADVICE: ANTIEPILEPTIC DRUGS: UPDATED ADVICE ON SWITCHING BETWEEN DIFFERENT MANUFACTURERS' PRODUCTS (NOVEMBER 2017)

See Epilepsy p. 227 and see also *Prescribing and dispensing information*.

MHRA/CHM ADVICE: ANTIEPILEPTIC DRUGS IN PREGNANCY: UPDATED ADVICE FOLLOWING COMPREHENSIVE SAFETY REVIEW (JANUARY 2021)

See Epilepsy p. 227.

- **CAUTIONS** Avoid in Acute porphyrias p. 745 · children · debilitated · history of alcohol abuse · history of drug abuse · respiratory depression (avoid if severe) · seizures (may be exacerbated)

CAUTIONS, FURTHER INFORMATION MHRA advises consider vitamin D supplementation in patients who are immobilised for long periods or who have inadequate sun exposure or dietary intake of calcium.

▸ Seizure exacerbation [EvGr] Phenobarbital may exacerbate seizures in patients with absence seizures, Dravet syndrome, and Lennox-Gastaut syndrome. ⟨A⟩

- **INTERACTIONS** → Appendix 1: antiepileptics
- **SIDE-EFFECTS**

GENERAL SIDE-EFFECTS Agitation · agranulocytosis · anticonvulsant hypersensitivity syndrome · behaviour abnormal · bone disorders · bone fracture · cognitive impairment · confusion · depression · drowsiness · folate deficiency · hepatic disorders · memory loss · movement disorders · nystagmus · respiratory depression · severe cutaneous adverse reactions (SCARs) · skin reactions · suicidal behaviours

SPECIFIC SIDE-EFFECTS

▸ With oral use Hallucination · hypotension · megaloblastic anaemia · thrombocytopenia

▸ With parenteral use Anaemia · aplastic anaemia · Dupuytren's contracture · hypocalcaemia · irritability

Overdose For details on the management of poisoning, see Active elimination techniques, under Emergency treatment of poisoning p. 1036.

- **ALLERGY AND CROSS-SENSITIVITY** Cross-sensitivity reported with carbamazepine. Antiepileptic hypersensitivity syndrome associated with phenobarbital. See under Epilepsy p. 227 for more information.
- **PREGNANCY** An increased risk of major congenital malformations and intra-uterine growth restriction, and possibility of adverse effects on neurodevelopment have been seen with phenobarbital, see *Pregnancy* in Epilepsy p. 227 for further details.
- **BREAST FEEDING** Avoid if possible; drowsiness may occur.
- **HEPATIC IMPAIRMENT** Manufacturer advises caution in mild to moderate impairment; avoid in severe impairment.
- **RENAL IMPAIRMENT** [EvGr] Use with caution in mild to moderate impairment; avoid in severe impairment. ⟨M⟩
- **MONITORING REQUIREMENTS**

▸ Plasma-phenobarbital concentration for optimum response is 15–40 mg/litre (60–180 micromol/litre); however, monitoring the plasma-drug concentration is less useful than with other drugs because tolerance occurs.

- **TREATMENT CESSATION** Avoid abrupt withdrawal (dependence with prolonged use).
- **DIRECTIONS FOR ADMINISTRATION** For administration by *mouth*, tablets may be crushed.

[EvGr] For *intravenous injection*, dilute injection solution 1 in 10 with Water for Injections; ⟨M⟩ give at a rate not more than 1 mg/kg/minute.

- **PRESCRIBING AND DISPENSING INFORMATION** The RCPCH and NPPG position statement *Choosing an Oral Liquid Medicine for Children* states that recommended practice in the UK is to use an ethanol-free unlicensed 50 mg/5 mL liquid for the oral administration of phenobarbital to children when an oral liquid is required. Phenobarbital Elixir BP (15 mg/5 mL) contains 38% v/v of ethanol (alcohol), and so there is potential for accumulation when ingested repeatedly, especially in young children with low or immature metabolic capacity.

Switching between formulations Different formulations of oral preparations may vary in bioavailability. Patients should be maintained on a specific manufacturer's product.

- **PATIENT AND CARER ADVICE**
Medicines for Children leaflet: Phenobarbital for preventing seizures www.medicinesforchildren.org.uk/medicines/phenobarbital-for-preventing-seizures/

- **MEDICINAL FORMS** There can be variation in the licensing of different medicines containing the same drug. Forms available from special-order manufacturers include: oral tablet, oral capsule, oral suspension

Oral tablet

CAUTIONARY AND ADVISORY LABELS 2, 8

▸ Phenobarbital (Non-proprietary)

Phenobarbital 15 mg Phenobarbital 15mg tablets | 28 tablet [PoM] £24.95 DT = £3.76 [CD3]

Phenobarbital 30 mg Phenobarbital 30mg tablets | 28 tablet [PoM] £5.89 DT = £0.77 [CD3]

Phenobarbital 60 mg Phenobarbital 60mg tablets | 28 tablet [PoM] £7.99 DT = £1.23 [CD3]

Solution for injection

EXCIPIENTS: May contain Propylene glycol

▸ Phenobarbital (Non-proprietary)

Phenobarbital sodium 30 mg per 1 ml Phenobarbital 30mg/1ml solution for injection ampoules | 10 ampoule [PoM] £181.74 DT = £181.74 [CD3]

Phenobarbital sodium 60 mg per 1 ml Phenobarbital 60mg/1ml solution for injection ampoules | 10 ampoule [PoM] £138.52–£197.01 DT = £197.01 [CD3]

Phenobarbital sodium 200 mg per 1 ml Phenobarbital 200mg/1ml solution for injection ampoules | 10 ampoule [PoM] £112.94–£149.15 DT = £149.15 [CD3]

Primidone

11-Aug-2022

- **DRUG ACTION** Primidone is partially converted to phenobarbital, but is also considered to have some antiepileptic action in its own right.

- **INDICATIONS AND DOSE**

All forms of epilepsy except typical absence seizures

▶ BY MOUTH

- Child 1 month–1 year: Initially 125 mg daily, dose to be taken at bedtime, then increased in steps of 125 mg every 3 days, adjusted according to response; maintenance 125–250 mg twice daily
- Child 2–4 years: Initially 125 mg once daily, dose to be taken at bedtime, then increased in steps of 125 mg every 3 days, adjusted according to response; maintenance 250–375 mg twice daily
- Child 5–8 years: Initially 125 mg once daily, dose to be taken at bedtime, then increased in steps of 125 mg every 3 days, adjusted according to response; maintenance 375–500 mg twice daily
- Child 9–17 years: Initially 125 mg once daily, dose to be taken at bedtime, then increased in steps of 125 mg every 3 days, increased to 250 mg twice daily, then increased in steps of 250 mg every 3 days (max. per dose 750 mg twice daily), adjusted according to response

IMPORTANT SAFETY INFORMATION

MHRA/CHM ADVICE: ANTIEPILEPTICS: RISK OF SUICIDAL THOUGHTS AND BEHAVIOUR (AUGUST 2008)

See Epilepsy p. 227.

MHRA/CHM ADVICE: ANTIEPILEPTIC DRUGS: UPDATED ADVICE ON SWITCHING BETWEEN DIFFERENT MANUFACTURERS' PRODUCTS (NOVEMBER 2017)

See Epilepsy p. 227 and see also *Prescribing and dispensing information*.

MHRA/CHM ADVICE: ANTIEPILEPTIC DRUGS IN PREGNANCY: UPDATED ADVICE FOLLOWING COMPREHENSIVE SAFETY REVIEW (JANUARY 2021)

See Epilepsy p. 227.

- **CAUTIONS** Avoid in Acute porphyrias p. 745 · children · debilitated · history of alcohol abuse · history of drug abuse · respiratory depression (consider dose reduction)

CAUTIONS, FURTHER INFORMATION MHRA advises consider vitamin D supplementation in patients who are immobilised for long periods or who have inadequate sun exposure or dietary intake of calcium.

- **INTERACTIONS** → Appendix 1: antiepileptics
- **SIDE-EFFECTS**

▶ **Common or very common** Apathy · movement disorders · nausea · nystagmus · visual impairment

▶ **Uncommon** Dizziness · headache · hypersensitivity · skin reactions · vomiting

▶ **Rare or very rare** Arthralgia · bone disorders · Dupuytren's contracture · leucopenia · lymphadenopathy · megaloblastic anaemia (may be treated with folic acid) · psychotic disorder · severe cutaneous adverse reactions (SCARs) · systemic lupus erythematosus (SLE) · thrombocytopenia

▶ **Frequency not known** Bone fracture · confusion · drowsiness · hallucination · suicidal behaviours

- **ALLERGY AND CROSS-SENSITIVITY** Cross-sensitivity reported with carbamazepine. Antiepileptic hypersensitivity syndrome associated with primidone. See under Epilepsy p. 227 for more information.
- **PREGNANCY** [EvGr] Caution—increased risk of congenital malformations following exposure during pregnancy. [M] See also *Pregnancy* in Epilepsy p. 227.
- **HEPATIC IMPAIRMENT** Manufacturer advises caution.

Dose adjustments Manufacturer advises consider dose reduction.

- **RENAL IMPAIRMENT** [EvGr] Use with caution. [M]

Dose adjustments [EvGr] Consider dose reduction. [M]

- **MONITORING REQUIREMENTS**

▶ Monitor plasma concentrations of derived phenobarbital; plasma concentration for optimum response is 15–40 mg/litre (60–180 micromol/litre).

- **TREATMENT CESSATION** Avoid abrupt withdrawal (dependence with prolonged use).
- **PRESCRIBING AND DISPENSING INFORMATION**

Switching between formulations Different formulations of oral preparations may vary in bioavailability. Patients being treated for epilepsy should be maintained on a specific manufacturer's product.

- **MEDICINAL FORMS** There can be variation in the licensing of different medicines containing the same drug. Forms available from special-order manufacturers include: oral capsule, oral suspension

Oral tablet

CAUTIONARY AND ADVISORY LABELS 2, 8

▸ Primidone (Non-proprietary)

Primidone 50 mg Primidone 50mg tablets | 100 tablet [PoM] £118.71 DT = £118.71

Primidone 125 mg Primidone 125mg tablets | 50 tablet [PoM] £65.00 DT = £65.00

Primidone 250 mg Primidone 250mg tablets | 30 tablet [PoM] £18.53 | 100 tablet [PoM] £105.99 DT = £47.10

▸ Enodama (Desitin Pharma Ltd)

Primidone 50 mg Enodama 50mg tablets | 100 tablet [PoM] £90.00 DT = £118.71

Oral suspension

▸ **Primidone (Non-proprietary)**
Primidone 25 mg per 1 ml Liskantin Saft 125mg/5ml oral suspension | 250 ml PoM (Hospital only)

CARBONIC ANHYDRASE INHIBITORS

Sultiame
31-Mar-2025

(Sulthiame)

- **DRUG ACTION** Sultiame is a carbonic anhydrase inhibitor which has an antiepileptic effect.

- **INDICATIONS AND DOSE**

Rolandic epilepsy (self-limited epilepsy with centrotemporal spikes) (under expert supervision)

▸ BY MOUTH

▸ Child (body-weight 12 kg and above): Initially 2.5 mg/kg daily in 3 divided doses, gradually increase dose over 1 week depending on individual response; usual maintenance 5–10 mg/kg daily in 3 divided doses, discontinue treatment if adequate response not achieved after 1–2 months

IMPORTANT SAFETY INFORMATION

MHRA/CHM ADVICE: ANTIEPILEPTICS: RISK OF SUICIDAL THOUGHTS AND BEHAVIOUR (AUGUST 2008)
See Epilepsy p. 227.

MHRA/CHM ADVICE: ANTIEPILEPTIC DRUGS: UPDATED ADVICE ON SWITCHING BETWEEN DIFFERENT MANUFACTURERS' PRODUCTS (NOVEMBER 2017)
See Epilepsy p. 227.

MHRA/CHM ADVICE: ANTIEPILEPTIC DRUGS IN PREGNANCY: UPDATED ADVICE FOLLOWING COMPREHENSIVE SAFETY REVIEW (JANUARY 2021)
See Epilepsy p. 227.

- **CONTRA-INDICATIONS** Acute porphyrias p. 745 · hypertension · hyperthyroidism
- **CAUTIONS** History of psychiatric disorders
- **INTERACTIONS** → Appendix 1: antiepileptics
- **SIDE-EFFECTS**

▸ **Common or very common** Angina pectoris · appetite decreased · diplopia · dizziness · dyspnoea · epigastric discomfort · headache · hiccups · paraesthesia · respiratory disorders · tachycardia · weight decreased

▸ **Uncommon** Anxiety · arthralgia · hallucination · lack of drive · myasthenic phenomena · status epilepticus

▸ **Frequency not known** Acute kidney injury · behaviour abnormal · cognitive impairment · depression · diarrhoea · hepatotoxicity · polyneuropathy · severe cutaneous adverse reactions (SCARs) · suicidal behaviours

- **ALLERGY AND CROSS-SENSITIVITY** EvGr Contra-indicated in patients with sulfonamide hypersensitivity. Ⓜ
- **PREGNANCY** EvGr Avoid unless essential (embryotoxic in *animal* studies). Ⓜ See also *Pregnancy* in Epilepsy p. 227.
- **BREAST FEEDING** EvGr Avoid (no information available). Ⓜ
- **RENAL IMPAIRMENT** EvGr Use with caution. Ⓜ
- **MONITORING REQUIREMENTS** EvGr Monitor full blood count, liver and renal function before treatment, repeat weekly for the first month of treatment, then monthly during the first 6 months, and then 2–4 times a year thereafter—discontinue treatment if persistent increase in serum creatinine, or progressive thrombocytopenia or leucopenia accompanied by clinical symptoms. Ⓜ
- **TREATMENT CESSATION** Avoid abrupt withdrawal.
- **DIRECTIONS FOR ADMINISTRATION** For *oral suspension*, each dose administered should be immediately followed by a glass of water, juice or milk to reduce bitter taste. Alternatively, each dose may be mixed, preferably with a small amount of water, or with orange juice, milk, yoghurt or wheat porridge just before administration. Do **not** administer with carbonated drinks or hot foods. *Oral suspension* may be administered via a feeding tube—consult product literature.
- **PATIENT AND CARER ADVICE** Patients and carers should be given advice on how to administer *Ospolot*® oral suspension. Patients and carers should be advised to seek immediate medical attention if fever, sore throat, allergic skin reactions with lymph node swelling, or flu-like symptoms occur during treatment.

Driving and skilled tasks Patients and carers should be cautioned on the effects on driving and performance of skilled tasks—increased risk of impaired reactions; effects enhanced by alcohol.

- **MEDICINAL FORMS** There can be variation in the licensing of different medicines containing the same drug.

Oral suspension

CAUTIONARY AND ADVISORY LABELS 2, 8
EXCIPIENTS: May contain Glucose, hydroxybenzoates (parabens), sucrose, sulfites

▸ **Ospolot** (Desitin Pharma Ltd)
Sultiame 20 mg per 1 ml Ospolot 20mg/ml oral suspension | 250 ml PoM £91.25

HYPNOTICS, SEDATIVES AND ANXIOLYTICS › BENZODIAZEPINES

Benzodiazepines

IMPORTANT SAFETY INFORMATION

MHRA/CHM ADVICE: BENZODIAZEPINES AND OPIOIDS: REMINDER OF RISK OF POTENTIALLY FATAL RESPIRATORY DEPRESSION (MARCH 2020)

The MHRA reminds healthcare professionals that benzodiazepines and benzodiazepine-like drugs co-prescribed with opioids can produce additive CNS depressant effects, thereby increasing the risk of sedation, respiratory depression, coma, and death. Healthcare professionals are advised to only co-prescribe if there is no alternative and, if necessary, the lowest possible doses should be given for the shortest duration. Patients should be closely monitored for signs of respiratory depression at initiation of treatment and when there is any change in prescribing, such as dose adjustments or new interactions. If methadone is co-prescribed with a benzodiazepine or benzodiazepine-like drug, the respiratory depressant effect of methadone may be delayed; patients should be monitored for at least 2 weeks after initiation or changes in prescribing. Patients should be informed of the signs and symptoms of respiratory depression and sedation, and advised to seek urgent medical attention should these occur.

MHRA/CHM ADVICE: IMPROVING INFORMATION SUPPLIED WITH GABAPENTINOIDS (PREGABALIN/GABAPENTIN), BENZODIAZEPINES AND Z-DRUGS (JANUARY 2026)

An MHRA review concluded that warnings regarding addiction, dependence, withdrawal, and tolerance need to be strengthened, to better inform healthcare professionals and patients of these known risks. Specialist use of these medicines for conditions such as epilepsy or sedation during medical procedures were not included as part of this review. Healthcare professionals are advised to create a strategy with patients for reducing or ending treatment prior to treatment initiation and provide an individually tailored dose reduction schedule, as well as counselling on the risk of drug withdrawal syndrome. All patients should be closely monitored for signs of misuse, abuse, addiction or tolerance, and regular support provided, especially to those at increased risk of drug withdrawal syndrome.

- **CONTRA-INDICATIONS** Acute pulmonary insufficiency · marked neuromuscular respiratory weakness · obsessional states · phobic states · sleep apnoea syndrome · unstable myasthenia gravis
- **CAUTIONS** Avoid prolonged use (and abrupt withdrawal thereafter) · history of alcohol dependence or abuse · history of drug dependence or abuse · myasthenia gravis · personality disorder (within the fearful group—dependent, avoidant, obsessive-compulsive) may increase risk of dependence · respiratory disease

CAUTIONS, FURTHER INFORMATION
- **Paradoxical effects** A paradoxical increase in hostility and aggression may be reported by patients taking benzodiazepines. The effects range from talkativeness and excitement to aggressive and antisocial acts. Adjustment of the dose (up or down) sometimes attenuates the impulses. Increased anxiety and perceptual disorders are other paradoxical effects.

- **SIDE-EFFECTS**
  - **Common or very common** Alertness decreased · anxiety · ataxia · confusion · depression · dizziness · drowsiness · dysarthria · fatigue · headache · hypotension · mood altered · muscle weakness · nausea · respiratory depression (particularly with high dose and intravenous use—facilities for its treatment are essential) · sleep disorders · tremor · vision disorders · withdrawal syndrome
  - **Uncommon** Agitation (more common in children) · anterograde amnesia · behaviour abnormal · hallucination · libido disorder · rash
  - **Rare or very rare** Aggression (more common in children) · blood disorder · delusions · jaundice · paradoxical drug reaction · restlessness (with sedative and peri-operative use) · urinary retention
  - **Frequency not known** Drug use disorders

  Overdose Benzodiazepines taken alone cause drowsiness, ataxia, dysarthria, nystagmus, and occasionally respiratory depression, and coma. For details on the management of poisoning, see Benzodiazepines, under Emergency treatment of poisoning p. 1036.

- **PREGNANCY** Risk of neonatal withdrawal symptoms when used during pregnancy. Avoid regular use and use only if there is a clear indication such as seizure control. High doses administered during late pregnancy or labour may cause neonatal hypothermia, hypotonia, and respiratory depression.
- **HEPATIC IMPAIRMENT** In general, manufacturers advise caution in mild to moderate impairment; avoid in severe impairment. Benzodiazepines with a shorter half-life are considered safer.

  Dose adjustments In general, manufacturers advise dose reduction in mild to moderate impairment, adjust dose according to response.
- **RENAL IMPAIRMENT** In general, manufacturers advise caution (risk of increased cerebral sensitivity to benzodiazepines).

  Dose adjustments In general, manufacturers advise to consider dose reduction.
- **TREATMENT CESSATION** The MHRA advises avoid abrupt treatment cessation—reduce dose gradually to minimise symptoms of withdrawal (specialist use such as epilepsy or sedation during medical procedures not included in MHRA review—see also *Important safety information*).
- **PATIENT AND CARER ADVICE**

  Driving and skilled tasks May cause drowsiness, impair judgement and increase reaction time, and so affect ability to drive or perform skilled tasks; effects of alcohol increased. Moreover the hangover effects of a night dose may impair performance on the following day.

  For information on 2015 legislation regarding driving whilst taking certain controlled drugs, including benzodiazepines, see *Drugs and driving* under Guidance on prescribing p. 1.

266

Clobazam

26-Oct-2021

- **INDICATIONS AND DOSE**

Adjunct in epilepsy
- BY MOUTH
  - Child 1 month–5 years: Initially 125 micrograms/kg twice daily, dose to be increased if necessary every 5 days, maintenance 250 micrograms/kg twice daily (max. per dose 500 micrograms/kg twice daily); maximum 30 mg per day
  - Child 6–17 years: Initially 5 mg daily, dose to be increased if necessary at intervals of 5 days, maintenance 0.3–1 mg/kg daily, daily doses of up to 30 mg may be given as a single dose at bedtime, higher doses should be divided; maximum 60 mg per day

Monotherapy for catamenial (menstruation) seizures (usually for 7–10 days each month, just before and during menstruation) (under expert supervision) | Cluster seizures
- BY MOUTH
  - Child 1 month–5 years: Initially 125 micrograms/kg twice daily, dose to be increased if necessary every 5 days, maintenance 250 micrograms/kg twice daily (max. per dose 500 micrograms/kg twice daily); maximum 30 mg per day
  - Child 6–17 years: Initially 5 mg daily, dose to be increased if necessary at intervals of 5 days, maintenance 0.3–1 mg/kg daily, daily doses of up to 30 mg may be given as a single dose at bedtime, higher doses should be divided; maximum 60 mg per day

- **UNLICENSED USE** Not licensed for use in children under 6 years. Not licensed as monotherapy.

IMPORTANT SAFETY INFORMATION

SAFE PRACTICE
Clobazam has been confused with clonazepam; care must be taken to ensure the correct drug is prescribed and dispensed.

MHRA/CHM ADVICE: ANTIEPILEPTICS: RISK OF SUICIDAL THOUGHTS AND BEHAVIOUR (AUGUST 2008)
See Epilepsy p. 227.

MHRA/CHM ADVICE: ANTIEPILEPTIC DRUGS: UPDATED ADVICE ON SWITCHING BETWEEN DIFFERENT MANUFACTURERS' PRODUCTS (NOVEMBER 2017)
See Epilepsy p. 227 and see also *Prescribing and dispensing information*.

MHRA/CHM ADVICE: ANTIEPILEPTIC DRUGS IN PREGNANCY: UPDATED ADVICE FOLLOWING COMPREHENSIVE SAFETY REVIEW (JANUARY 2021)
See Epilepsy p. 227.

- **CONTRA-INDICATIONS** Respiratory depression
- **CAUTIONS** Muscle weakness · organic brain changes

  CAUTIONS, FURTHER INFORMATION The effectiveness of clobazam may decrease significantly after weeks or months of continuous therapy.
- **INTERACTIONS** → Appendix 1: benzodiazepines
- **SIDE-EFFECTS** Appetite decreased · consciousness impaired · constipation · dry mouth · fall · gait unsteady · libido loss · movement disorders · muscle spasms · nystagmus · psychotic disorder · respiratory disorder · severe cutaneous adverse reactions (SCARs) · skin reactions · speech impairment · suicidal behaviours · weight increased
- **PREGNANCY** See *Pregnancy* in Epilepsy p. 227.

- **BREAST FEEDING** Benzodiazepines are present in milk, and should be avoided if possible during breast-feeding.
Monitoring All infants should be monitored for sedation, feeding difficulties, adequate weight gain, and developmental milestones.
- **MONITORING REQUIREMENTS** Routine measurement of plasma concentrations of antiepileptic drugs is not usually justified, because the target concentration ranges are arbitrary and often vary between individuals. However, plasma drug concentrations may be measured in children with worsening seizures, status epilepticus, suspected noncompliance, or suspected toxicity. Similarly, haematological and biochemical monitoring should not be undertaken unless clinically indicated.
- **PRESCRIBING AND DISPENSING INFORMATION**
Switching between formulations Care should be taken when switching between oral formulations in the treatment of epilepsy. The need for continued supply of a particular manufacturer's product should be based on clinical judgement and consultation with the patient or their carer, taking into account factors such as seizure frequency and treatment history.
Patients being treated for epilepsy may need to be maintained on a specific manufacturer's branded or generic clobazam product.
- **PATIENT AND CARER ADVICE**
Medicines for Children leaflet: Clobazam for preventing seizures www.medicinesforchildren.org.uk/medicines/clobazam-for-preventing-seizures/
- **NATIONAL FUNDING/ACCESS DECISIONS**
NHS restrictions Clobazam is not prescribable in NHS primary care except for the treatment of epilepsy; endorse prescription 'SLS'.

- **MEDICINAL FORMS** There can be variation in the licensing of different medicines containing the same drug. Forms available from special-order manufacturers include: oral capsule, oral suspension

Oral tablet

CAUTIONARY AND ADVISORY LABELS 2, 8

- **Clobazam (Non-proprietary)**
  - **Clobazam 10 mg** Clobazam 10mg tablets | 30 tablet [PoM] £5.99 DT = £2.28 [CD4-1]
  - **Clobazam 20 mg** Clobazam 20mg tablets | 30 tablet [PoM] £9.75 DT = £9.75 [CD4-1]
- **Frisium** (Atnahs Pharma UK Ltd)
  - **Clobazam 10 mg** Frisium 10mg tablets | 30 tablet [PoM] £2.51 DT = £2.28 [CD4-1]

Oral suspension

CAUTIONARY AND ADVISORY LABELS 2, 8

EXCIPIENTS: May contain Hydroxybenzoates (parabens), polysorbates, propylene glycol

- **Clobazam (Non-proprietary)**
  - **Clobazam 1 mg per 1 ml** Clobazam 5mg/5ml oral suspension sugar free | 150 ml [PoM] £90.00 DT = £30.52 [CD4-1] [SF] | 250 ml [PoM] £150.00–£276.00 [CD4-1] [SF]
  - **Clobazam 2 mg per 1 ml** Clobazam 10mg/5ml oral suspension sugar free | 150 ml [PoM] £95.00 DT = £25.24 [CD4-1] [SF] | 250 ml [PoM] £158.34–£291.34 [CD4-1] [SF]
- **Perizam** (Rosemont Pharmaceuticals Ltd)
  - **Clobazam 1 mg per 1 ml** Perizam 1mg/ml oral suspension | 150 ml [PoM] £90.00 DT = £30.52 [CD4-1] [SF]
  - **Clobazam 2 mg per 1 ml** Perizam 2mg/ml oral suspension | 150 ml [PoM] £95.00 DT = £25.24 [CD4-1] [SF]
- **Zacco** (SyriMed)
  - **Clobazam 1 mg per 1 ml** Zacco 5mg/5ml oral suspension | 150 ml [PoM] £50.00 DT = £30.52 [CD4-1] [SF]
  - **Clobazam 2 mg per 1 ml** Zacco 10mg/5ml oral suspension | 150 ml [PoM] £55.00 DT = £25.24 [CD4-1] [SF]

266

Clonazepam

26-Oct-2021

- **INDICATIONS AND DOSE**

All forms of epilepsy

- BY MOUTH
  - Child 1–11 months: Initially 250 micrograms once daily for 4 nights, dose to be increased over 2–4 weeks, usual dose 0.5–1 mg daily, dose to be taken at night; may be given in 3 divided doses if necessary
  - Child 1–4 years: Initially 250 micrograms once daily for 4 nights, dose to be increased over 2–4 weeks, usual dose 1–3 mg daily, dose to be taken at night; may be given in 3 divided doses if necessary
  - Child 5–11 years: Initially 500 micrograms once daily for 4 nights, dose to be increased over 2–4 weeks, usual dose 3–6 mg daily, dose to be taken at night; may be given in 3 divided doses if necessary
  - Child 12–17 years: Initially 1 mg once daily for 4 nights, dose to be increased over 2–4 weeks, usual dose 4–8 mg daily, dose usually taken at night; may be given in 3–4 divided doses if necessary

- **UNLICENSED USE** Clonazepam doses in BNFC may differ from those in product literature.

IMPORTANT SAFETY INFORMATION

SAFE PRACTICE

Clonazepam has been confused with clobazam; care must be taken to ensure the correct drug is prescribed and dispensed.

MHRA/CHM ADVICE: ANTIEPILEPTICS: RISK OF SUICIDAL THOUGHTS AND BEHAVIOUR (AUGUST 2008)

See Epilepsy p. 227.

MHRA/CHM ADVICE: ANTIEPILEPTIC DRUGS: UPDATED ADVICE ON SWITCHING BETWEEN DIFFERENT MANUFACTURERS' PRODUCTS (NOVEMBER 2017)

See Epilepsy p. 227 and see also *Prescribing and dispensing information.*

MHRA/CHM ADVICE: ANTIEPILEPTIC DRUGS IN PREGNANCY: UPDATED ADVICE FOLLOWING COMPREHENSIVE SAFETY REVIEW (JANUARY 2021)

See Epilepsy p. 227.

- **CONTRA-INDICATIONS** Coma · current alcohol abuse · current drug abuse · respiratory depression
- **CAUTIONS** Acute porphyrias p. 745 · airways obstruction · brain damage · cerebellar ataxia · depression · spinal ataxia · suicidal ideation
CAUTIONS, FURTHER INFORMATION The effectiveness of clonazepam may decrease significantly after weeks or months of continuous therapy.
- **INTERACTIONS** → Appendix 1: benzodiazepines
- **SIDE-EFFECTS**
  - **Common or very common** Nystagmus
  - **Frequency not known** Alopecia · bronchial secretion increased · cardiac arrest · concentration impaired · drooling · epigastric discomfort · gastrointestinal disorder · heart failure · hypersalivation · incomplete precocious puberty · movement disorders · muscle tone decreased · psychotic disorder · seizure presentation change · sexual dysfunction · skin reactions · speech impairment · suicidal behaviours · urinary incontinence
- **PREGNANCY** See *Pregnancy* in Epilepsy p. 227.
- **BREAST FEEDING** Present in milk, and should be avoided if possible during breast-feeding.
Monitoring All infants should be monitored for sedation, feeding difficulties, adequate weight gain, and developmental milestones.
- **MONITORING REQUIREMENTS** Routine measurement of plasma concentrations of antiepileptic drugs is not usually

justified, because the target concentration ranges are arbitrary and often vary between individuals. However, plasma drug concentrations may be measured in children with worsening seizures, status epilepticus, suspected noncompliance, or suspected toxicity. Similarly, haematological and biochemical monitoring should not be undertaken unless clinically indicated.

- **PRESCRIBING AND DISPENSING INFORMATION** The RCPCH and NPPG recommend that, when a liquid special of clonazepam is required, the following strength is used: 2 mg/5 mL.

Switching between formulations Care should be taken when switching between oral formulations in the treatment of epilepsy. The need for continued supply of a particular manufacturer's product should be based on clinical judgement and consultation with the patient or their carer, taking into account factors such as seizure frequency and treatment history.

Patients being treated for epilepsy may need to be maintained on a specific manufacturer's branded or generic oral clonazepam product.

- **PATIENT AND CARER ADVICE**

Medicines for Children leaflet: Clonazepam for preventing seizures www.medicinesforchildren.org.uk/medicines/clonazepam-for-preventing-seizures/

- **MEDICINAL FORMS** There can be variation in the licensing of different medicines containing the same drug. Forms available from special-order manufacturers include: orodispersible tablet, oral suspension, oral solution

Oral tablet

CAUTIONARY AND ADVISORY LABELS 2, 8

▸ Clonazepam (Non-proprietary)

Clonazepam 500 microgram Clonazepam 500microgram tablets | 100 tablet PoM £32.27 DT = £2.44 CD4-1

Clonazepam 1 mg Clonazepam 1mg tablets | 100 tablet PoM £41.95 DT = £41.95 CD4-1

Clonazepam 2 mg Clonazepam 2mg tablets | 100 tablet PoM £34.99 DT = £2.08 CD4-1

Oral solution

CAUTIONARY AND ADVISORY LABELS 2, 8

EXCIPIENTS: May contain Ethanol

▸ Clonazepam (Non-proprietary)

Clonazepam 100 microgram per 1 ml Clonazepam 500micrograms/5ml oral solution sugar free | 150 ml PoM £69.50 DT = £36.39 CD4-1 SF

Clonazepam 400 microgram per 1 ml Clonazepam 2mg/5ml oral solution sugar free | 150 ml PoM £90.30 DT = £49.79 CD4-1 SF

1.1 Status epilepticus

Status epilepticus

23-May-2024

Description of condition

Status epilepticus, defined as a seizure that lasts 5 minutes or longer, or recurrent seizures without recovery in between, should be managed as a medical emergency to prevent neurological injury and death. Status epilepticus may be convulsive or non-convulsive. Non-convulsive status epilepticus can be difficult to detect and its management requires specialist advice.

Causes of status epilepticus include poorly-controlled epilepsy (therapy non-adherence or withdrawal), eclampsia, metabolic abnormalities, alcohol or drug withdrawal, infection such as CNS infections, a tumour, airway obstruction, hypoxia, and shock.

Aims of treatment

The aim of treatment is to stop the seizure as soon as possible. After 5 minutes, seizures are unlikely to stop without medical intervention, and seizures become harder to stop the longer they last.

Convulsive status epilepticus

For a quick reference resource with doses of benzodiazepines for the management of convulsive status epilepticus, see *Seizures* in Medical emergencies in the community p. 1480.

The immediate management of convulsive status epilepticus includes securing the child's airway, giving oxygen, and monitoring cardiac and respiratory function. Underlying causes should be managed appropriately. In children with established epilepsy, obtaining serum-antiepileptic concentrations can determine if non-adherence is a cause, and may inform treatment choice and doses.

EvGr The individualised emergency management plan of children with epilepsy, if immediately available, should be followed. Where such a plan is unavailable or in those with other underlying causes, children in the community should immediately be given buccal midazolam p. 273 or rectal diazepam p. 270. If intravenous access and resuscitation facilities are immediately available, intravenous lorazepam p. 272 should be given. (A) EvGr Rectal paraldehyde below may also be considered as a treatment option, if intravenous access is unavailable. (E)

EvGr Where there is no response to the first benzodiazepine dose, emergency services should be called if in the community or expert advice sought if in hospital. The child's individualised emergency management plan, if immediately available, should continue to be followed; otherwise, a second benzodiazepine dose should be given if the seizure has not stopped within 5-10 minutes of the first dose.

If there is no response to two benzodiazepine doses, either levetiracetam p. 245 [unlicensed use] or phenytoin p. 249 may be given as second-line treatment, taking into account that levetiracetam may be quicker to give and has fewer side-effects. (A) EvGr Phenytoin should generally be avoided in children already taking it, but may be considered if the plasma-phenytoin concentration is significantly below the therapeutic range. (E) EvGr If there is no response, an alternative second-line treatment option should be considered under expert advice. Phenobarbital p. 264 may also be considered if these options are not effective or suitable.

If second-line treatment options are unsuccessful, consider general anaesthesia as third-line treatment under expert advice.

If there is concern that convulsive status epilepticus may recur, an emergency management plan should be agreed with the child (and/or their parents/carers) if they do not have one already. (A)

Useful Resources

Epilepsies in children, young people and adults. National Institute for Health and Care Excellence. NICE guideline 217. April 2022.
www.nice.org.uk/guidance/ng217

Other drugs used for Status epilepticus Fosphenytoin sodium, p. 239

ANTIEPILEPTICS

Paraldehyde

10-Mar-2020

- **INDICATIONS AND DOSE**

Status epilepticus

▸ BY RECTUM

▸ Neonate: 0.8 mL/kilogram for 1 dose, the dose is based on the use of a premixed solution of paraldehyde in olive oil in equal volumes.

▸ Child: 0.8 mL/kilogram for 1 dose (max. per dose 20 mL), the dose is based on the use of a premixed solution of paraldehyde in olive oil in equal volumes

- **UNLICENSED USE** Not licensed for use in children as an enema.
- **CONTRA-INDICATIONS** Gastric disorders · rectal administration in colitis
- **CAUTIONS** Bronchopulmonary disease
- **INTERACTIONS** → Appendix 1: antiepileptics
- **SIDE-EFFECTS** Rash
- **PREGNANCY** Avoid unless essential—crosses placenta. See also *Pregnancy* in Epilepsy p. 227.
- **BREAST FEEDING** Avoid unless essential—present in milk.
- **HEPATIC IMPAIRMENT** Manufacturer advises caution.
- **PATIENT AND CARER ADVICE**
Medicines for Children leaflet: Paraldehyde (rectal) for stopping seizures www.medicinesforchildren.org.uk/medicines/rectal-paraldehyde-for-stopping-seizures/

- **MEDICINAL FORMS** Forms available from special-order manufacturers include: enema

ANTIEPILEPTICS › BARBITURATES

Thiopental sodium
(Thiopentone sodium)

10-May-2021

- **INDICATIONS AND DOSE**

Prolonged status epilepticus

▶ INITIALLY BY SLOW INTRAVENOUS INJECTION

- Neonate: Initially up to 2 mg/kg, then (by continuous intravenous infusion) up to 8 mg/kg/hour, adjusted according to response.
- Child: Initially up to 4 mg/kg, then (by continuous intravenous infusion) up to 8 mg/kg/hour, adjusted according to response

Induction of anaesthesia

▶ BY SLOW INTRAVENOUS INJECTION

- Neonate: Initially up to 2 mg/kg, then 1 mg/kg, repeated if necessary; maximum 4 mg/kg per course.
- Child: Initially up to 4 mg/kg, then 1 mg/kg, repeated if necessary; maximum 7 mg/kg per course

- **UNLICENSED USE** Not licensed for use in status epilepticus. Not licensed for use by intravenous infusion.

IMPORTANT SAFETY INFORMATION
Thiopental sodium should only be administered by, or under the direct supervision of, personnel experienced in its use, with adequate training in anaesthesia and airway management, and when resuscitation equipment is available.

- **CONTRA-INDICATIONS** Acute porphyrias p. 745 · myotonic dystrophy
- **CAUTIONS** Acute circulatory failure (shock) · avoid intra-arterial injection · cardiovascular disease · hypovolaemia · reconstituted solution is highly alkaline (extravasation causes tissue necrosis and severe pain) · respiratory diseases (avoid in acute asthma)
- **INTERACTIONS** → Appendix 1: thiopental
- **SIDE-EFFECTS**
  - ▶ **Common or very common** Arrhythmia · myocardial contractility decreased
  - ▶ **Frequency not known** Appetite decreased · circulatory collapse · cough · electrolyte imbalance · extravasation necrosis · hypotension · respiratory disorders · skin eruption · sneezing
- **PREGNANCY** May depress neonatal respiration when used during delivery.
- **BREAST FEEDING** Breast-feeding can be resumed as soon as mother has recovered sufficiently from anaesthesia.
- **HEPATIC IMPAIRMENT** Manufacturer advises caution.
Dose adjustments Manufacturer advises dose reduction.
- **RENAL IMPAIRMENT** EvGr Caution in severe impairment. (M)
- **DIRECTIONS FOR ADMINISTRATION** EvGr For *intravenous injection*, reconstitute 500-mg vial with 20 mL Water for Injections to give 25 mg/mL solution; give over at least 10–15 seconds; for *intravenous infusion* reconstituted solution may be further diluted with Sodium Chloride 0.9%. (M)
- **PATIENT AND CARER ADVICE**
Driving and skilled tasks Patients given sedatives and analgesics during minor outpatient procedures should be very carefully warned about the risk of driving or undertaking skilled tasks afterwards. For a short general anaesthetic the risk extends to **at least 24 hours** after administration. Responsible persons should be available to take patients home. The dangers of taking **alcohol** should also be emphasised.

- **MEDICINAL FORMS** There can be variation in the licensing of different medicines containing the same drug. Forms available from special-order manufacturers include: solution for injection

Powder for solution for injection

▶ Thiopental sodium (Non-proprietary)

Thiopental sodium 500 mg Thiopental 500mg powder for solution for injection vials | 10 vial PoM £57.60 | 10 vial PoM £69.00 (Hospital only)

HYPNOTICS, SEDATIVES AND ANXIOLYTICS › BENZODIAZEPINES

266

Diazepam

16-Apr-2024

- **INDICATIONS AND DOSE**

Tetanus

▶ BY INTRAVENOUS INJECTION

- Child: 100–300 micrograms/kg every 1–4 hours

▶ BY CONTINUOUS INTRAVENOUS INFUSION

- Child: 3–10 mg/kg/24 hours, dose to be adjusted according to response

▶ BY NASODUODENAL TUBE

- Child: 3–10 mg/kg, dose to be given over 24 hours, dose to be adjusted according to response

Muscle spasm in cerebral spasticity or in postoperative skeletal muscle spasm

▶ BY MOUTH

- Child 1-11 months: Initially 250 micrograms/kg twice daily
- Child 1-4 years: Initially 2.5 mg twice daily
- Child 5-11 years: Initially 5 mg twice daily
- Child 12-17 years: Initially 10 mg twice daily, dose can be increased if necessary up to maximum 40 mg per day

Status epilepticus | Febrile convulsions | Convulsions due to poisoning

▶ BY INTRAVENOUS INJECTION

- Neonate: 300–400 micrograms/kg for 1 dose, then 300–400 micrograms/kg for 1 dose, to be administered 10 minutes after first dose if required.
- Child 1 month-11 years: 300–400 micrograms/kg for 1 dose (max. per dose 10 mg), then 300–400 micrograms/kg for 1 dose (max. per dose 10 mg), to be administered 10 minutes after first dose if required
- Child 12-17 years: 10 mg for 1 dose, then 10 mg for 1 dose, to be administered 10 minutes after first dose if required

▸ BY RECTUM

▸ Neonate: 1.25–2.5 mg for 1 dose, then 1.25–2.5 mg for 1 dose, to be administered 5–10 minutes after first dose if required.

▸ Child 1 month–1 year: 5 mg for 1 dose, then 5 mg for 1 dose, to be administered 5–10 minutes after first dose if required

▸ Child 2–11 years: 5–10 mg for 1 dose, then 5–10 mg for 1 dose, to be administered 5–10 minutes after first dose if required

▸ Child 12–17 years: 10–20 mg for 1 dose, then 10–20 mg for 1 dose, to be administered 5–10 minutes after first dose if required

Life-threatening acute drug-induced dystonic reactions

▸ BY INTRAVENOUS INJECTION

▸ Child 1 month–11 years: 100 micrograms/kg, dose can be repeated if necessary

▸ Child 12–17 years: 5–10 mg, dose can be repeated if necessary

● **UNLICENSED USE**

▸ With rectal use *Diazepam Desitin®*, *Diazepam Rectubes®*, and *Stesolid Rectal Tubes®* not licensed for use in children under 1 year.

IMPORTANT SAFETY INFORMATION

ANAESTHESIA

Benzodiazepines should only be administered for anaesthesia by, or under the direct supervision of, personnel experienced in their use, with adequate training in anaesthesia and airway management.

● **CONTRA-INDICATIONS** Avoid injections containing benzyl alcohol in neonates · CNS depression · compromised airway · hyperkinesis · respiratory depression

● **CAUTIONS**

GENERAL CAUTIONS Muscle weakness · organic brain changes · parenteral administration (close observation required until full recovery from sedation)

SPECIFIC CAUTIONS

▸ With intravenous use High risk of venous thrombophlebitis with intravenous use (reduced by using an emulsion formulation)

CAUTIONS, FURTHER INFORMATION

▸ Special precautions for intravenous injection When given intravenously facilities for reversing respiratory depression with mechanical ventilation must be immediately available.

● **INTERACTIONS** → Appendix 1: benzodiazepines

● **SIDE-EFFECTS**

GENERAL SIDE-EFFECTS

▸ **Common or very common** Appetite abnormal · gastrointestinal disorder · movement disorders · muscle spasms · palpitations · sensory disorder

▸ **Uncommon** Concentration impaired · constipation · diarrhoea · hypersalivation · skin reactions · speech slurred · vomiting

▸ **Rare or very rare** Bradycardia · bronchial secretion increased · cardiac arrest · dry mouth · gynaecomastia · heart failure · leucopenia · loss of consciousness · memory loss · psychosis · respiratory arrest · sexual dysfunction · syncope · urinary incontinence · vertigo

▸ **Frequency not known** Apnoea · nystagmus

SPECIFIC SIDE-EFFECTS

▸ **Rare or very rare**

▸ With intravenous or oral use Psychiatric disorder

● **PREGNANCY** Women who have seizures in the second half of pregnancy should be assessed for eclampsia before any change is made to antiepileptic treatment. Status epilepticus should be treated according to the standard protocol.

Epilepsy and Pregnancy Register All pregnant women with epilepsy, whether taking medication or not, should be encouraged to notify the UK Epilepsy and Pregnancy Register (Tel: 0800 389 1248).

● **BREAST FEEDING** Present in milk, and should be avoided if possible during breast-feeding.

● **DIRECTIONS FOR ADMINISTRATION**

▸ With intravenous use Diazepam is adsorbed by plastics of infusion bags and giving sets. Expert sources advise emulsion formulation preferred for intravenous use. [EvGr] For *continuous intravenous infusion* (emulsion) (*Diazemuls®*), dilute to a concentration of max. 400 micrograms/mL with Glucose 5% or 10%; max. 6 hours between addition and completion of infusion. For *continuous intravenous infusion* (solution) (*Diazepam*, Hameln), dilute to a concentration of max. 80 micrograms/mL with Glucose 5% or Sodium Chloride 0.9%. ⟨M⟩

▸ With intravenous use for Status epilepticus or Febrile convulsions or Convulsions due to poisoning or Life-threatening acute drug-induced dystonic reactions [EvGr] For *intravenous injection*, give over 3–5 minutes. ⟨M⟩

● **PATIENT AND CARER ADVICE** Patients or carers should be given advice on how and when to administer rectal diazepam. Patients given sedatives and analgesics during minor outpatient procedures should be very carefully warned about the risks of undertaking skilled tasks (e.g. driving) afterwards. For intravenous benzodiazepines the risk extends to **at least 24 hours** after administration. Responsible persons should be available to take patients home afterwards. The dangers of taking **alcohol** should be emphasised.

Medicines for Children leaflet: Diazepam (rectal) for stopping seizures www.medicinesforchildren.org.uk/medicines/diazepam-rectal-for-stopping-seizures/

Medicines for Children leaflet: Diazepam for muscle spasm www.medicinesforchildren.org.uk/medicines/diazepam-for-muscle-spasm/

● **PROFESSION SPECIFIC INFORMATION**

Dental practitioners' formulary Diazepam Tablets may be prescribed.

Diazepam Oral Solution 2 mg/5 mL may be prescribed.

● **MEDICINAL FORMS** There can be variation in the licensing of different medicines containing the same drug. Forms available from special-order manufacturers include: oral suspension, oral solution, suppository

Oral tablet

CAUTIONARY AND ADVISORY LABELS 2

▸ **Diazepam (Non-proprietary)**

Diazepam 2 mg Diazepam 2mg tablets | 28 tablet [PoM] £0.79 DT = £0.64 [CD4-1]

Diazepam 5 mg Diazepam 5mg tablets | 28 tablet [PoM] £0.81 DT = £0.65 [CD4-1]

Diazepam 10 mg Diazepam 10mg tablets | 28 tablet [PoM] £0.87 DT = £0.73 [CD4-1]

Solution for injection

EXCIPIENTS: May contain Benzyl alcohol, ethanol, propylene glycol

▸ **Diazepam (Non-proprietary)**

Diazepam 5 mg per 1 ml Diazepam 10mg/2ml solution for injection ampoules | 10 ampoule [PoM] £9.75–£40.30 DT = £40.30 [CD4-1]

Oral suspension

CAUTIONARY AND ADVISORY LABELS 2

EXCIPIENTS: May contain Ethanol, hydroxybenzoates (parabens), potassium sorbate, sucrose

Oral solution

CAUTIONARY AND ADVISORY LABELS 2

EXCIPIENTS: May contain Hydroxybenzoates (parabens), propylene glycol, sorbic acid, sorbitol

Enema

CAUTIONARY AND ADVISORY LABELS 2

EXCIPIENTS: May contain Benzyl alcohol, ethanol, propylene glycol

▸ **Diazepam (Non-proprietary)**

Diazepam 2 mg per 1 ml Diazepam 5mg/2.5ml rectal solution tube | 5 tube PoM £5.85 DT = £5.85 CD4-1

Diazepam 4 mg per 1 ml Diazepam 10mg/2.5ml rectal solution tube | 5 tube PoM £8.78 DT = £8.78 CD4-1

F 266

Lorazepam

11-Aug-2022

● **INDICATIONS AND DOSE**

Premedication

▶ BY MOUTH

▸ Child 1 month–11 years: 50–100 micrograms/kg (max. per dose 4 mg), to be given at least 1 hour before procedure, same dose may be given the night before procedure in addition to, or to replace, dose before procedure

▸ Child 12-17 years: 1–4 mg, to be given at least 1 hour before procedure, same dose may be given the night before procedure in addition to, or to replace, dose before procedure

▶ BY SLOW INTRAVENOUS INJECTION

▸ Child: 50–100 micrograms/kg for 1 dose (max. per dose 4 mg), to be administered 30–45 minutes before procedure

Status epilepticus | Febrile convulsions | Convulsions caused by poisoning

▶ BY SLOW INTRAVENOUS INJECTION

▸ Neonate: 100 micrograms/kg for 1 dose, then 100 micrograms/kg for 1 dose, to be given 5–10 minutes after first dose if required.

▸ Child 1 month–11 years: 100 micrograms/kg for 1 dose (max. per dose 4 mg), then 100 micrograms/kg for 1 dose (max. per dose 4 mg), to be given 5–10 minutes after first dose if required

▸ Child 12-17 years: 4 mg for 1 dose, then 4 mg for 1 dose, to be given 5–10 minutes after first dose if required

● **UNLICENSED USE** Not licensed for use in febrile convulsions. Not licensed for use in convulsions caused by poisoning. Not licensed for use as intravenous premedication in children under 12 years. Not licensed for use as oral premedication in children under 5 years.

IMPORTANT SAFETY INFORMATION

ANAESTHESIA

Benzodiazepines should only be administered for anaesthesia by, or under the direct supervision of, personnel experienced in their use, with adequate training in anaesthesia and airway management.

● **CONTRA-INDICATIONS** Avoid injections containing benzyl alcohol in neonates · CNS depression · compromised airway · respiratory depression

● **CAUTIONS** Muscle weakness · organic brain changes · parenteral administration

CAUTIONS, FURTHER INFORMATION

▸ Paradoxical effects A paradoxical increase in hostility and aggression may be reported by patients taking benzodiazepines. The effects range from talkativeness and excitement to aggressive and antisocial acts. Adjustment of the dose (up or down) sometimes attenuates the impulses. Increased anxiety and perceptual disorders are other paradoxical effects.

▸ Special precautions for parenteral administration When given parenterally, facilities for managing respiratory depression with mechanical ventilation must be available. Close observation required until full recovery from sedation.

● **INTERACTIONS** → Appendix 1: benzodiazepines

● **SIDE-EFFECTS**

GENERAL SIDE-EFFECTS

▶ **Common or very common** Apnoea · asthenia · coma · disinhibition · extrapyramidal symptoms · hypothermia · memory loss · speech slurred

▶ **Uncommon** Allergic dermatitis · constipation · sexual dysfunction

▶ **Rare or very rare** Agranulocytosis · hyponatraemia · pancytopenia · SIADH · thrombocytopenia

▶ **Frequency not known** Suicidal behaviours

SPECIFIC SIDE-EFFECTS

▶ **Common or very common**

▸ With parenteral use Vertigo

▶ **Rare or very rare**

▸ With oral use Saliva altered

▶ **Frequency not known**

▸ With oral use Psychosis

▸ With parenteral use Leucopenia

● **BREAST FEEDING** Benzodiazepines are present in milk, and should be avoided if possible during breast-feeding.

● **DIRECTIONS FOR ADMINISTRATION** For *intravenous injection*, dilute with an equal volume of Sodium Chloride 0.9% (for neonates, dilute injection solution to a concentration of 100 micrograms/mL). Give into a large vein over 3–5 minutes; max. rate 50 micrograms/kg over 3 minutes.

● **PATIENT AND CARER ADVICE**

Driving and skilled tasks Patients given sedatives and analgesics during minor outpatient procedures should be very carefully warned about the risks of undertaking skilled tasks (e.g. driving) afterwards. For intravenous benzodiazepines the risk extends to **at least 24 hours** after administration. Responsible persons should be available to take patients home afterwards. The dangers of taking **alcohol** should be emphasised.

● **MEDICINAL FORMS** There can be variation in the licensing of different medicines containing the same drug. Forms available from special-order manufacturers include: oral suspension, solution for injection

Oral tablet

CAUTIONARY AND ADVISORY LABELS 2

EXCIPIENTS: May contain Tartrazine

▸ **Lorazepam (Non-proprietary)**

Lorazepam 250 microgram Lorazepam 250microgram tablets | 28 tablet PoM £32.20–£56.00 DT = £32.20 CD4-1

Lorazepam 500 microgram Lorazepam 500microgram tablets | 28 tablet PoM £18.85 DT = £3.19 CD4-1

Lorazepam 1 mg Lorazepam 1mg tablets | 28 tablet PoM £28.00 DT = £1.65 CD4-1

Lorazepam 2.5 mg Lorazepam 2.5mg tablets | 28 tablet PoM £11.43 DT = £2.47 CD4-1

Solution for injection

EXCIPIENTS: May contain Benzyl alcohol, propylene glycol

▸ **Lorazepam (Non-proprietary)**

Lorazepam 2 mg per 1 ml Lorazepam 2mg/1ml solution for injection Carpuject cartridges | 10 cartridge PoM ⊠ (Hospital only) CD4-1
Lorazepam 2mg/1ml solution for injection vials | 10 vial PoM ⊠ CD4-1

Lorazepam 4 mg per 1 ml Ativan 4mg/1ml solution for injection vials | 25 vial PoM ⊠ (Hospital only) CD4-1
Lorazepam 4mg/1ml solution for injection ampoules | 10 ampoule PoM £199.00 DT = £199.00 CD4-1

266

Midazolam

01-Dec-2025

● **INDICATIONS AND DOSE**

Status epilepticus | Febrile convulsions

▶ BY BUCCAL ADMINISTRATION

- Neonate: 300 micrograms/kg for 1 dose, then 300 micrograms/kg for 1 dose, to be given 5–10 minutes after first dose if required.
- Child 1-2 months: 300 micrograms/kg for 1 dose (max. per dose 2.5 mg), then 300 micrograms/kg for 1 dose (max. per dose 2.5 mg), to be given 5–10 minutes after first dose if required
- Child 3-11 months: 2.5 mg for 1 dose, then 2.5 mg for 1 dose, to be given 5–10 minutes after first dose if required
- Child 1-4 years: 5 mg for 1 dose, then 5 mg for 1 dose, to be given 5–10 minutes after first dose if required
- Child 5-9 years: 7.5 mg for 1 dose, then 7.5 mg for 1 dose, to be given 5–10 minutes after first dose if required
- Child 10-17 years: 10 mg for 1 dose, then 10 mg for 1 dose, to be given 5–10 minutes after first dose if required

▶ INITIALLY BY INTRAVENOUS INJECTION

- Neonate: Initially 150–200 micrograms/kg for 1 dose, followed by (by continuous intravenous infusion) 60 micrograms/kg/hour, rate increased in steps of 60 micrograms/kg/hour every 15 minutes until seizure controlled; maximum 300 micrograms/kg/hour.
- Child: Initially 150–200 micrograms/kg for 1 dose, followed by (by continuous intravenous infusion) 60 micrograms/kg/hour, rate increased in steps of 60 micrograms/kg/hour every 15 minutes until seizure controlled; maximum 300 micrograms/kg/hour

Conscious sedation for procedures

▶ BY MOUTH

- Child: 500 micrograms/kg for 1 dose (max. per dose 20 mg), to be administered 30–60 minutes before procedure using a liquid special or injection solution given by mouth

▶ BY BUCCAL ADMINISTRATION

- Child 6 months-9 years: 200–300 micrograms/kg (max. per dose 5 mg)
- Child 10-17 years (body-weight up to 70 kg): 6–7 mg
- Child 10-17 years (body-weight 70 kg and above): 6–7 mg, (max. per dose 8 mg)

▶ BY RECTUM

- Child 6 months-11 years: 300–500 micrograms/kg for 1 dose, to be administered 15–30 minutes before procedure

▶ BY INTRAVENOUS INJECTION

- Child 1 month-5 years: Initially 25–50 micrograms/kg for 1 dose, to be administered over 2–3 minutes, 5–10 minutes before procedure, dose can be increased if necessary in small steps to maximum 6 mg per course
- Child 6-11 years: Initially 25–50 micrograms/kg for 1 dose, to be administered over 2–3 minutes, 5–10 minutes before procedure, dose can be increased if necessary in small steps to maximum 10 mg per course
- Child 12-17 years: Initially 25–50 micrograms/kg for 1 dose, to be administered over 2–3 minutes, 5–10 minutes before procedure, dose can be increased if necessary in small steps to maximum 7.5 mg per course

Premedication

▶ BY MOUTH

- Child: 500 micrograms/kg for 1 dose (max. per dose 20 mg), to be administered 15–30 minutes before the procedure using a liquid special or injection solution given by mouth

▶ BY RECTUM

- Child 6 months-11 years: 300–500 micrograms/kg for 1 dose, to be administered 15–30 minutes before induction

Induction of anaesthesia (but rarely used)

▶ BY SLOW INTRAVENOUS INJECTION

- Child 7-17 years: Initially 150 micrograms/kg (max. per dose 7.5 mg), dose to be given in steps of 50 micrograms/kg (max. 2.5 mg) over 2–5 minutes; wait for 2–5 minutes before subsequent dosing, then 50 micrograms/kg every 2 minutes (max. per dose 2.5 mg) if required; maximum 500 micrograms/kg per course; maximum 25 mg per course

Sedation of patient receiving intensive care

▶ INITIALLY BY SLOW INTRAVENOUS INJECTION

- Child 6 months-11 years: Initially 50–200 micrograms/kg, to be administered over at least 3 minutes, followed by (by continuous intravenous infusion) 30–120 micrograms/kg/hour, adjusted according to response, initial dose may not be required and lower maintenance doses needed if opioid analgesics also used; reduce dose (or reduce or omit initial dose) in hypovolaemia, vasoconstriction, or hypothermia
- Child 12-17 years: Initially 30–300 micrograms/kg, dose to be given in steps of 1–2.5 mg every 2 minutes, followed by (by continuous intravenous infusion) 30–200 micrograms/kg/hour, adjusted according to response, initial dose may not be required and lower maintenance doses needed if opioid analgesics also used; reduce dose (or reduce or omit initial dose) in hypovolaemia, vasoconstriction, or hypothermia

▶ BY CONTINUOUS INTRAVENOUS INFUSION

- Neonate up to 32 weeks corrected gestational age: 60 micrograms/kg/hour for 24 hours, then reduced to 30 micrograms/kg/hour, adjusted according to response for maximum treatment duration of 4 days.
- Neonate 32 weeks corrected gestational age and above: 60 micrograms/kg/hour, adjusted according to response for maximum treatment duration of 4 days.
- Child 1-5 months: 60 micrograms/kg/hour, adjusted according to response

MIPROSED ®

Conscious sedation for procedures | Premedication

▶ BY MOUTH

- Child 6 months-14 years: 250–500 micrograms/kg for 1 dose (max. per dose 20 mg), to be administered 15 to 30 minutes before procedure or anaesthesia

OZALIN ®

Conscious sedation for procedures | Premedication

▶ BY MOUTH

- Child 6 months-17 years: 250 micrograms/kg for 1 dose (max. per dose 20 mg), to be administered 30 minutes before procedure or anaesthesia

● **UNLICENSED USE** Oromucosal solution not licensed for use in children under 3 months. Unlicensed oromucosal formulations are also available and may have different doses—refer to product literature.

Injection not licensed for use in status epilepticus or febrile convulsions.

Injection not licensed for use by mouth for conscious sedation or premedication.

Not licensed for use by buccal administration for conscious sedation.

IMPORTANT SAFETY INFORMATION

ANAESTHESIA

Benzodiazepines should only be administered for anaesthesia by, or under the direct supervision of, personnel experienced in their use, with adequate training in anaesthesia and airway management.

NHS NEVER EVENT: MIS-SELECTION OF HIGH-STRENGTH MIDAZOLAM DURING CONSCIOUS SEDATION (JANUARY 2018).

In clinical areas performing conscious sedation, high-strength preparations (5 mg/mL in 2 mL and 10 mL ampoules, or 2 mg/mL in 5 mL ampoules) should **not** be selected in place of the 1 mg/mL preparation.

The areas where high-strength midazolam is used should be restricted to those performing general anaesthesia, intensive care, palliative care, or areas where its use has been formally risk-assessed in the organisation. In these situations the higher strength may be more appropriate to administer the prescribed dose.

It is advised that flumazenil is available when midazolam is used, to reverse the effects if necessary.

- **CONTRA-INDICATIONS** CNS depression · compromised airway · severe respiratory depression
- **CAUTIONS**

GENERAL CAUTIONS Cardiac disease · children (particularly if cardiovascular impairment) · debilitated patients (reduce dose) · hypothermia · hypovolaemia (risk of severe hypotension) · neonates · risk of airways obstruction and hypoventilation in children under 6 months (monitor respiratory rate and oxygen saturation) · vasoconstriction

SPECIFIC CAUTIONS

- With intravenous use Concentration of midazolam in children under 15 kg not to exceed 1 mg/mL

CAUTIONS, FURTHER INFORMATION

- Recovery when used for sedation Midazolam has a fast onset of action, recovery is faster than for other benzodiazepines such as diazepam, but may be significantly longer in the elderly, in patients with a low cardiac output, or after repeated dosing.

- **INTERACTIONS** → Appendix 1: benzodiazepines
- **SIDE-EFFECTS**

GENERAL SIDE-EFFECTS

- **Common or very common** Vomiting
- **Uncommon** Skin reactions
- **Rare or very rare** Dry mouth · dyspnoea · hiccups · movement disorders · respiratory disorders
- **Frequency not known** Disinhibition (severe; with sedative and peri-operative use) · vertigo

SPECIFIC SIDE-EFFECTS

- **Common or very common**
- With buccal use Level of consciousness decreased
- **Rare or very rare**
- With buccal use Apnoea · bradycardia · cardiac arrest · constipation · physical assault · vasodilation
- **Frequency not known**
- With buccal use Appetite increased · fall · gastrointestinal disorder · saliva altered · thrombosis · urinary incontinence
- With oral use Angioedema · arrhythmias · asthenia · enuresis · gait instability · hypersalivation · hypoxia · myopathy
- With parenteral or rectal use Angioedema · apnoea · appetite increased · bradycardia · cardiac arrest · constipation · drug withdrawal seizure · embolism and thrombosis · fall · gastrointestinal disorder · level of consciousness decreased · physical assault · saliva altered · urinary incontinence · vasodilation
- With rectal use Respiratory arrest (more common with high doses)

SIDE-EFFECTS, FURTHER INFORMATION Higher doses are associated with prolonged sedation and risk of hypoventilation. The co-administration of midazolam with other sedative, hypnotic, or CNS-depressant drugs results in increased sedation. Midazolam accumulates in adipose tissue, which can significantly prolong sedation, especially in patients with obesity, hepatic impairment or renal impairment.

Overdose There have been reports of overdosage when high strength midazolam has been used for conscious sedation. The use of high-strength midazolam (5mg/mL in 2mL and 10mL ampoules, or 2mg/mL in 5mL ampoules) should be restricted to general anaesthesia, intensive care, palliative care, or other situations where the risk has been assessed. It is advised that flumazenil is available when midazolam is used, to reverse the effects if necessary.

- **BREAST FEEDING** Small amount present in milk—avoid breast-feeding for 24 hours after administration (although amount probably too small to be harmful after single doses).
- **HEPATIC IMPAIRMENT** For *parenteral preparations* manufacturer advises caution in all degrees of impairment.

Dose adjustments For *parenteral preparations* manufacturer advises consider dose reduction in all degrees of impairment.

- **RENAL IMPAIRMENT** Manufacturer advises use with caution in chronic renal failure.
- **DIRECTIONS FOR ADMINISTRATION** For *intravenous infusion* (*Hypnovel*®), give continuously *in* Glucose 5% *or* Sodium chloride 0.9%. For *intravenous injection* in status epilepticus and febrile convulsions, dilute with Glucose 5% or Sodium Chloride 0.9%; rapid intravenous injection (less than 2 minutes) may cause seizure-like myoclonus in preterm neonate. For neonate and children under 15 kg dilute to a max. concentration of 1 mg/mL. *Neonatal intensive care*, dilute 15 mg/kg body-weight to a final volume of 50 mL with infusion fluid; an intravenous infusion rate of 0.1 mL/hour provides a dose of 30 micrograms/kg/hour.

For *buccal* administration, give the full dose slowly over 4–5 seconds into one buccal cavity (space between the gum and the cheek). Alternatively, give half the dose over 2–3 seconds into one side of the mouth, and then the other half into the other side of the mouth.

For administration *by mouth* for sedation and premedication, licensed oral solutions are available. Alternatively, injection solution may be diluted with apple or black currant juice, chocolate sauce, or cola.

MIPROSED® EvGr *Miprosed*® 5 mg/mL oral solution may be diluted with apple juice or blackcurrant cordial. M

OZALIN® *Ozalin*® 2 mg/mL oral solution is supplied in single-use glass ampoules and the dose must be measured using the graduated oral applicator and filter straw provided.

- **PRESCRIBING AND DISPENSING INFORMATION** The RCPCH and NPPG recommend that, when a liquid special of midazolam is required, the following strength is used: 10 mg/5 mL.
- **PATIENT AND CARER ADVICE** Patients or carers should be given advice on how and when to administer midazolam oromucosal solution.

Patients given sedatives and analgesics during minor outpatient procedures should be very carefully warned about the risks of undertaking skilled tasks (e.g. driving) afterwards. For intravenous benzodiazepines the risk extends to **at least 24 hours** after administration. Responsible persons should be available to take patients home afterwards. The dangers of taking **alcohol** should be emphasised.

Medicines for Children leaflet: Midazolam for stopping seizures www.medicinesforchildren.org.uk/medicines/midazolam-for-stopping-seizures/

- **NATIONAL FUNDING/ACCESS DECISIONS**

For full details see funding body website

Scottish Medicines Consortium (SMC) decisions

- **Midazolam oromucosal solution (*Epistatus*®) for the treatment of prolonged, acute, convulsive seizures in children and adolescents aged 10 to less than 18 years (November 2017)** SMC No. 1279/17 Recommended
- **Midazolam oral solution (*Ozalin*®) for moderate sedation before a therapeutic or diagnostic procedure, or as premedication before anaesthesia, in children from 6 months to 17 years of age (October 2021)** SMC No. SMC2392 Recommended

- **MEDICINAL FORMS** There can be variation in the licensing of different medicines containing the same drug. Forms available from special-order manufacturers include: oral solution, oromucosal solution, solution for injection, infusion, solution for infusion

Solution for injection

- **Midazolam (Non-proprietary)**

Midazolam (as Midazolam hydrochloride) 1 mg per 1 ml Midazolam 5mg/5ml solution for injection ampoules | 10 ampoule [PoM] £13.59–£16.89 DT = £13.59 [CD3]
Midazolam 5mg/5ml solution for injection pre-filled syringes | 1 pre-filled disposable injection [PoM] £11.53 (Hospital only) [CD3]
Midazolam 2mg/2ml solution for injection ampoules | 10 ampoule [PoM] £9.30 DT = £9.30 [CD3]

Midazolam (as Midazolam hydrochloride) 2 mg per 1 ml Midazolam 10mg/5ml solution for injection ampoules | 10 ampoule [PoM] £6.75–£9.80 DT = £9.80 [CD3]

Midazolam (as Midazolam hydrochloride) 5 mg per 1 ml Midazolam 50mg/10ml solution for injection ampoules | 10 ampoule [PoM] £33.00 DT = £33.00 (Hospital only) [CD3] | 10 ampoule [PoM] £33.00–£33.77 DT = £33.00 [CD3]
Midazolam 15mg/3ml solution for injection ampoules | 10 ampoule [PoM] £7.26 (Hospital only) [CD3]
Midazolam 10mg/2ml solution for injection ampoules | 10 ampoule [PoM] £4.68–£8.72 DT = £4.27 [CD3]

- **Hypnovel** (Neon Healthcare Ltd)

Midazolam (as Midazolam hydrochloride) 5 mg per 1 ml Hypnovel 10mg/2ml solution for injection ampoules | 10 ampoule [PoM] £7.11 DT = £4.27 [CD3]

Solution for infusion

- **Midazolam (Non-proprietary)**

Midazolam (as Midazolam hydrochloride) 1 mg per 1 ml Midazolam 50mg/50ml solution for infusion vials | 1 vial [PoM] £9.56–£13.20 [CD3]

Midazolam (as Midazolam hydrochloride) 2 mg per 1 ml Midazolam 100mg/50ml solution for infusion vials | 1 vial [PoM] £14.85 (Hospital only) [CD3] | 1 vial [PoM] £9.96 [CD3]

Oral solution

CAUTIONARY AND ADVISORY LABELS 2
EXCIPIENTS: May contain Ethanol, propylene glycol

- **Midazolam (Non-proprietary)**

Midazolam (as Midazolam hydrochloride) 2 mg per 1 ml Midazolam 2mg/ml oral solution sugar free | 118 ml [PoM] [X] Schedule 3 (CD No Register Exempt Safe Custody) [SF]

- **Miprosed** (SyriMed)

Midazolam 5 mg per 1 ml Miprosed 5mg/ml oral solution | 7.5 ml [PoM] £18.00 (Hospital only) Schedule 3 (CD No Register Exempt Safe Custody) [SF]

- **Ozalin** (Primex Pharmaceuticals Oy)

Midazolam (as Midazolam maleate) 2 mg per 1 ml Ozalin 2mg/ml oral solution 5ml unit dose ampoules | 10 ampoule [PoM] £187.00 (Hospital only) Schedule 3 (CD No Register Exempt Safe Custody) [SF]

Oromucosal solution

CAUTIONARY AND ADVISORY LABELS 2
EXCIPIENTS: May contain Ethanol

- **Midazolam (Non-proprietary)**

Midazolam (as Midazolam hydrochloride) 5 mg per 1 ml Midazolam 10mg/2ml oromucosal solution pre-filled oral syringes sugar free | 4 unit dose [PoM] £91.50 DT = £91.50 Schedule 3 (CD No Register Exempt Safe Custody) [SF]
Midazolam 5mg/1ml oromucosal solution pre-filled oral syringes sugar free | 4 unit dose [PoM] £85.80 DT = £85.50 Schedule 3 (CD No Register Exempt Safe Custody) [SF]
Midazolam 2.5mg/0.5ml oromucosal solution pre-filled oral syringes sugar free | 4 unit dose [PoM] £82.00 DT = £82.00 Schedule 3 (CD No Register Exempt Safe Custody) [SF]
Midazolam 7.5mg/1.5ml oromucosal solution pre-filled oral syringes sugar free | 4 unit dose [PoM] £89.00 DT = £89.00 Schedule 3 (CD No Register Exempt Safe Custody) [SF]

- **Buccolam** (Neuraxpharm UK Ltd)

Midazolam (as Midazolam hydrochloride) 5 mg per 1 ml Buccolam 7.5mg/1.5ml oromucosal solution pre-filled oral syringes | 4 unit dose [PoM] £89.00 DT = £89.00 Schedule 3 (CD No Register Exempt Safe Custody) [SF]
Buccolam 10mg/2ml oromucosal solution pre-filled oral syringes | 4 unit dose [PoM] £91.50 DT = £91.50 Schedule 3 (CD No Register Exempt Safe Custody) [SF]
Buccolam 5mg/1ml oromucosal solution pre-filled oral syringes | 4 unit dose [PoM] £85.50 DT = £85.50 Schedule 3 (CD No Register Exempt Safe Custody) [SF]
Buccolam 2.5mg/0.5ml oromucosal solution pre-filled oral syringes | 4 unit dose [PoM] £82.00 DT = £82.00 Schedule 3 (CD No Register Exempt Safe Custody) [SF]

- **Epistatus** (SERB)

Midazolam (as Midazolam maleate) 10 mg per 1 ml Epistatus 5mg/0.5ml oromucosal solution pre-filled oral syringes | 1 unit dose [PoM] £43.75 DT = £43.75 Schedule 3 (CD No Register Exempt Safe Custody) [SF]
Epistatus 10mg/1ml oromucosal solution pre-filled oral syringes | 1 unit dose [PoM] £45.76 DT = £45.76 Schedule 3 (CD No Register Exempt Safe Custody) [SF]
Epistatus 2.5mg/0.25ml oromucosal solution pre-filled oral syringes | 1 unit dose [PoM] £43.75 DT = £43.75 Schedule 3 (CD No Register Exempt Safe Custody) [SF]
Epistatus 7.5mg/0.75ml oromucosal solution pre-filled oral syringes | 1 unit dose [PoM] £43.75 DT = £43.75 Schedule 3 (CD No Register Exempt Safe Custody) [SF]

2 Mental health disorders

2.1 Attention deficit hyperactivity disorder

Attention deficit hyperactivity disorder

04-Aug-2018

Description of condition

Attention deficit hyperactivity disorder (ADHD) is a behavioural disorder characterised by hyperactivity, impulsivity and inattention, which can lead to functional impairment such as psychological, social, educational or occupational difficulties. While these symptoms tend to co-exist, some patients are predominantly hyperactive and impulsive, while others are principally inattentive. Symptoms typically appear in children aged 3–7 years, but may not be recognised until after 7 years of age, especially if hyperactivity is not present. ADHD is more commonly diagnosed in males than in females.

ADHD is usually a persisting disorder and some children continue to have symptoms throughout adolescence and into adulthood, where inattentive symptoms tend to persist, and hyperactive-impulsive symptoms tend to recede over time. ADHD is also associated with an increased risk of disorders such as oppositional defiant disorder (ODD), conduct disorder, and possibly mood disorders such as depression, mania, and anxiety, as well as substance misuse.

Aims of treatment

The aims of treatment are to reduce functional impairment, severity of symptoms, and to improve quality of life.

Non-drug treatment

EvGr Children and their parents, or carers should be advised about the importance of a balanced diet, good nutrition and regular exercise. If hyperactivity appears to be influenced by certain foods or drinks, parents or carers should be advised to keep a diary of food or drinks consumed and the associated behaviour. A referral to a dietician should be made where appropriate. Ⓐ

Environmental modifications are changes made to the physical environment that can help reduce the impact of ADHD symptoms on a child's day-to-day life. EvGr The modifications should be specific to the child's circumstances, and may involve changes to seating arrangements, lighting and noise, reducing distractions, optimising education by having shorter periods of focus with movement breaks, and the appropriate use of teaching assistants at school. These changes should form part of the discussion at the time of diagnosis of ADHD and be trialled and reviewed for effectiveness before drug treatment is started.

In children aged under 5 years, an ADHD-focused parent-training programme that teaches parents or carers behaviour therapy techniques is recommended as first-line treatment. Specialist advice should be sought if symptoms are still causing significant impairment after completion of the programme and implementation of environmental modifications.

In children aged 5 years and over, advice about ADHD and ADHD-focused support should be given to all parents or carers. In children with ADHD and symptoms of oppositional defiant disorder or conduct disorder, a training programme specific for the coexisting condition, involving either the parent or carer with or without the child is also recommended. Drug treatment should be reserved for children whose symptoms are causing persistent and significant impairment of at least one area of function (such as interpersonal relationships, education attainment, and risk awareness) despite environmental modifications.

In adolescents, a course of cognitive behavioural therapy (CBT) in combination with drug treatment should be considered for those who have had some benefit from drug treatment, but still have symptoms causing significant impairment in at least one area of function (such as social skills with peers, problem-solving, self-control, active listening skills, or dealing with and expressing feelings). Ⓐ

Drug treatment

Child aged under 5 years

EvGr Drug treatment should only be considered in children under 5 years of age on advice from a specialist ADHD service. Ⓐ

Child aged 5 years and over

EvGr Drug treatment should be initiated by a specialist trained in the diagnosis and management of ADHD. Following dose stabilisation, continuation and monitoring of drug treatment can be undertaken by the child's general practitioner under a shared care arrangement. Children with ADHD and anxiety disorder, tic disorder, or autism spectrum disorder should be offered the same treatment options as other children with ADHD. Ⓐ Treatment options for ADHD are not licensed for use in children under 6 years of age.

EvGr Methylphenidate hydrochloride p. 277 is recommended as first-line treatment. If a 6-week trial of methylphenidate hydrochloride p. 277 at the maximum tolerated dose does not reduce symptoms and associated impairment, consider switching to lisdexamfetamine mesilate p. 281. Dexamfetamine sulfate p. 280 can be given to children who are having a beneficial response to lisdexamfetamine mesilate but cannot tolerate its longer duration of effect.

Modified-release preparations of stimulants are preferred because of their pharmacokinetic profile, convenience, improved adherence, reduced risk of drug diversion (drugs being forwarded to others for non-prescription use or misuse), and the lack of need to be taken to school. Immediate-release preparations can be given when more flexible dosing regimens are required, or during initial dose titration. A combination of a modified-release and immediate-release preparation taken at different times of the day can be used to extend the duration of effect. The magnitude, duration of effect, and side-effects of stimulants vary between patients.

Atomoxetine below or guanfacine p. 281 can be given to children who are intolerant of both methylphenidate hydrochloride p. 277 and lisdexamfetamine mesilate, or if symptoms have not responded to separate 6-week trials of both drugs following adequate dose titration and consideration of alternative preparations. If sustained orthostatic hypotension or fainting episodes occur with guanfacine p. 281 treatment, the dose should be reduced or an alternative treatment offered.

Advice from, or referral to a tertiary specialist ADHD service should be considered if the child is unresponsive to one or more stimulant drugs (e.g. methylphenidate hydrochloride p. 277 and lisdexamfetamine mesilate) and one non-stimulant drug (e.g. atomoxetine below and guanfacine p. 281). A specialist service should also be consulted for advice before starting clonidine hydrochloride p. 120 [unlicensed] in children with ADHD and sleep disturbances, rages or tics, and before starting atypical antipsychotics in addition to stimulants in children with ADHD and co-existing pervasive aggression, rages or irritability. Ⓐ

Other treatment options such as bupropion hydrochloride, modafinil, and tricyclic antidepressants [all unlicensed] have been used in the management of ADHD, but due to limited evidence their use is not recommended without specialist advice.

EvGr Children should be monitored for effectiveness of treatment and side-effects, in addition to changes in sleep pattern, and the potential for stimulant diversion or misuse. If the child develops new, or has worsening of existing seizures, review drug treatment and stop any drug that might be contributing to the seizures; treatment can be cautiously reintroduced if it is unlikely to be the cause. Monitor children for the development of tics associated with stimulant use. If tics are stimulant related, consider a dose reduction, stopping treatment, or changing to a non-stimulant drug. If there is worsening of behaviour, consider adjusting drug treatment and reviewing the diagnosis.

Treatment should be reviewed by a specialist at least once a year and trials of treatment-free periods, or dose reductions considered where appropriate. Ⓐ

Useful Resources

Attention deficit hyperactivity disorder: diagnosis and management. National Institute for Health and Care Excellence. Clinical guideline 87. March 2018.
www.nice.org.uk/guidance/ng87

CNS STIMULANTS > CENTRALLY ACTING SYMPATHOMIMETICS

Atomoxetine

26-Oct-2021

● **INDICATIONS AND DOSE**

Attention deficit hyperactivity disorder (initiated by a specialist)

▶ BY MOUTH

▶ Child 6–17 years (body-weight up to 70 kg): Initially 500 micrograms/kg daily for 7 days, dose is increased according to response; maintenance 1.2 mg/kg daily, total daily dose may be given either as a single dose in

the morning or in 2 divided doses with last dose no later than early evening, high daily doses to be given under the direction of a specialist; maximum 1.8 mg/kg per day; maximum 120 mg per day
- Child 6–17 years (body-weight 70 kg and above): Initially 40 mg daily for 7 days, dose is increased according to response; maintenance 80 mg daily, total daily dose may be given either as a single dose in the morning or in 2 divided doses with last dose no later than early evening, high daily doses to be given under the direction of a specialist; maximum 120 mg per day

- **UNLICENSED USE** Atomoxetine doses in BNF Publications may differ from those in product literature.
  Doses above 100 mg daily not licensed.
- **CONTRA-INDICATIONS** Phaeochromocytoma · severe cardiovascular disease · severe cerebrovascular disease
- **CAUTIONS** Aggressive behaviour · cardiovascular disease · cerebrovascular disease · emotional lability · history of seizures · hostility · hypertension · mania · psychosis · QT-interval prolongation · structural cardiac abnormalities · susceptibility to angle-closure glaucoma · tachycardia
- **INTERACTIONS** → Appendix 1: atomoxetine
- **SIDE-EFFECTS**
- ▶ **Common or very common** Anxiety · appetite decreased · asthenia · chest pain · constipation · depression · dizziness · drowsiness · gastrointestinal discomfort · headaches · insomnia · mood altered · mydriasis · nausea · skin reactions · tic · vomiting · weight decreased
- ▶ **Uncommon** Behaviour abnormal · dyspnoea · hallucination · hyperhidrosis · hypersensitivity · palpitations · psychosis · QT interval prolongation · seizure · sensation abnormal · sinus tachycardia · suicidal behaviour · syncope · tremor · vision blurred
- ▶ **Rare or very rare** Genital pain · hepatic disorders · priapism · Raynaud's phenomenon · urinary disorders
- ▶ **Frequency not known** Sudden cardiac death
- **PREGNANCY** Manufacturer advises avoid unless potential benefit outweighs risk.
- **BREAST FEEDING** Avoid-present in milk in *animal* studies.
- **HEPATIC IMPAIRMENT**
  Dose adjustments Manufacturer advises halve dose in moderate impairment and quarter dose in severe impairment.
- **MONITORING REQUIREMENTS**
- ▶ Monitor for appearance or worsening of anxiety, depression or tics.
- ▶ Pulse, blood pressure, psychiatric symptoms, appetite, weight and height should be recorded at initiation of therapy, following each dose adjustment, and at least every 6 months thereafter.
- **PATIENT AND CARER ADVICE**
  Suicidal ideation Following reports of suicidal thoughts and behaviour, patients and their carers should be informed about the risk and told to report clinical worsening, suicidal thoughts or behaviour, irritability, agitation, or depression.
  Hepatic impairment Following rare reports of hepatic disorders, patients and carers should be advised of the risk and be told how to recognise symptoms; prompt medical attention should be sought in case of abdominal pain, unexplained nausea, malaise, darkening of the urine, or jaundice.
  Medicines for Children leaflet: Atomoxetine for ADHD
  www.medicinesforchildren.org.uk/medicines/atomoxetine-for-adhd/
- **NATIONAL FUNDING/ACCESS DECISIONS**
  For full details see funding body website
  Scottish Medicines Consortium (SMC) decisions
- ▶ **Atomoxetine oral solution (*Strattera*®) for treatment of attention-deficit/hyperactivity disorder (ADHD) in children of 6 years and older, in adolescents and in adults as part of a comprehensive treatment programme (December 2015)**
  SMC No. 1107/15 Recommended with restrictions
- **MEDICINAL FORMS** There can be variation in the licensing of different medicines containing the same drug. Forms available from special-order manufacturers include: oral suspension, oral solution

Oral solution

CAUTIONARY AND ADVISORY LABELS 3

- ▸ Atomoxetine (Non-proprietary)

  Atomoxetine (as Atomoxetine hydrochloride) 4 mg per 1 ml Atomoxetine 4mg/ml oral solution sugar free | 100 ml [PoM] £35.33–£60.06 DT = £35.33 [SF]

Oral capsule

CAUTIONARY AND ADVISORY LABELS 3, 25

- ▸ Atomoxetine (Non-proprietary)

  Atomoxetine (as Atomoxetine hydrochloride) 10 mg Atomoxetine 10mg capsules | 7 capsule [PoM] £9.12 | 28 capsule [PoM] £53.09 DT = £6.58

  Atomoxetine (as Atomoxetine hydrochloride) 18 mg Atomoxetine 18mg capsules | 7 capsule [PoM] £9.12 | 28 capsule [PoM] £53.09 DT = £7.32

  Atomoxetine (as Atomoxetine hydrochloride) 25 mg Atomoxetine 25mg capsules | 7 capsule [PoM] £9.18 | 28 capsule [PoM] £53.09 DT = £6.37

  Atomoxetine (as Atomoxetine hydrochloride) 40 mg Atomoxetine 40mg capsules | 7 capsule [PoM] £9.15 | 28 capsule [PoM] £53.09 DT = £4.31

  Atomoxetine (as Atomoxetine hydrochloride) 60 mg Atomoxetine 60mg capsules | 28 capsule [PoM] £53.09 DT = £6.27

  Atomoxetine (as Atomoxetine hydrochloride) 80 mg Atomoxetine 80mg capsules | 28 capsule [PoM] £70.79 DT = £6.82

  Atomoxetine (as Atomoxetine hydrochloride) 100 mg Atomoxetine 100mg capsules | 28 capsule [PoM] £70.79 DT = £6.59

Methylphenidate hydrochloride

07-Oct-2022

- **INDICATIONS AND DOSE**

Attention deficit hyperactivity disorder (initiated under specialist supervision)

▶ BY MOUTH USING IMMEDIATE-RELEASE MEDICINES

- Child 4–5 years: Initially 2.5 mg twice daily, increased in steps of 2.5 mg daily if required, at weekly intervals, increased if necessary up to 1.4 mg/kg daily in 2–3 divided doses, discontinue if no response after 1 month, if effect wears off in evening (with rebound hyperactivity) a dose at bedtime may be appropriate (establish need with trial bedtime dose). Treatment may be started using a modified-release preparation
- Child 6–17 years: Initially 5 mg 1–2 times a day, increased in steps of 5–10 mg daily if required, at weekly intervals, increased if necessary up to 60 mg daily in 2–3 divided doses, increased if necessary up to 2.1 mg/kg daily in 2–3 divided doses, the licensed maximum dose is 60 mg daily in 2–3 doses, higher dose (up to a maximum of 90 mg daily) under the direction of a specialist, discontinue if no response after 1 month, if effect wears off in evening (with rebound hyperactivity) a dose at bedtime may be appropriate (establish need with trial bedtime dose). Treatment may be started using a modified-release preparation

DOSE EQUIVALENCE AND CONVERSION

- ▸ When switching from *immediate-release* preparations to *modified-release* preparations—consult product literature.

continued →

CONCERTA® XL

Attention deficit hyperactivity disorder

▶ BY MOUTH

▶ Child 6–17 years: Initially 18 mg once daily, dose to be taken in the morning, increased in steps of 18 mg every week, adjusted according to response; increased if necessary up to 2.1 mg/kg daily, licensed max. dose is 54 mg once daily, to be increased to higher dose only under direction of specialist; discontinue if no response after 1 month; maximum 108 mg per day

DOSE EQUIVALENCE AND CONVERSION

▶ Total daily dose of 15 mg of standard-release formulation is considered equivalent to *Concerta®* XL 18 mg once daily.

DELMOSART® PROLONGED-RELEASE TABLET

Attention deficit hyperactivity disorder (under expert supervision)

▶ BY MOUTH

▶ Child 6–17 years: Initially 18 mg once daily, dose to be taken in the morning, then increased in steps of 18 mg every week if required, discontinue if no response after 1 month; maximum 54 mg per day

DOSE EQUIVALENCE AND CONVERSION

▶ Total daily dose of 15 mg of standard-release formulation is considered equivalent to *Delmosart®* 18 mg once daily.

EQUASYM® XL

Attention deficit hyperactivity disorder

▶ BY MOUTH

▶ Child 6–17 years: Initially 10 mg once daily, dose to be taken in the morning before breakfast; increased gradually at weekly intervals if necessary; increased if necessary up to 2.1 mg/kg daily, licensed max. dose is 60 mg daily, to be increased to higher dose only under direction of specialist; discontinue if no response after 1 month; maximum 90 mg per day

MEDIKINET® XL

Attention deficit hyperactivity disorder

▶ BY MOUTH

▶ Child 6–17 years: Initially 10 mg once daily, dose to be taken in the morning with breakfast; adjusted at weekly intervals according to response; increased if necessary up to 2.1 mg/kg daily, licensed max. dose is 60 mg daily, to be increased to higher dose only under direction of specialist; discontinue if no response after 1 month; maximum 90 mg per day

XAGGITIN® XL

Attention deficit hyperactivity disorder (under expert supervision)

▶ BY MOUTH

▶ Child 6–17 years: Initially 18 mg once daily, dose to be taken in the morning, increased in steps of 18 mg every week, adjusted according to response, discontinue if no response after 1 month; maximum 54 mg per day

DOSE EQUIVALENCE AND CONVERSION

▶ Total daily dose of 15 mg of standard-release formulation is considered equivalent to *Xaggitin®* XL 18 mg once daily.

- **UNLICENSED USE** Doses over 60 mg daily not licensed; doses of *Concerta® XL* over 54 mg daily not licensed.
  Not licensed for use in children under 6 years.

IMPORTANT SAFETY INFORMATION

MHRA/CHM ADVICE: METHYLPHENIDATE LONG-ACTING (MODIFIED-RELEASE) PREPARATIONS: CAUTION IF SWITCHING BETWEEN PRODUCTS DUE TO DIFFERENCES IN FORMULATIONS (SEPTEMBER 2022)

All long-acting preparations of methylphenidate contain an immediate-release component and a modified-release component. The biphasic-release profiles of different preparations are not all equivalent and contain different proportions of immediate-release and modified-release components. The MHRA has advised caution when switching between such preparations, due to differences in dosing frequency, administration with food, amount and timing of the modified-release component, and overall clinical effect.

Healthcare professionals are advised to:
- follow the specific dosage recommendations for each preparation;
- discuss the reasons for switching with patients or their carers, including any possible changes in symptoms and side-effects;
- take patient preferences into account when considering a switch;
- provide counselling on administration of the new preparation, especially with regards to food;
- follow current clinical guidance on prescribing by brand name, or by manufacturer name if generic;
- avoid frequent switching between different preparations.

- **CONTRA-INDICATIONS** Anorexia nervosa · arrhythmias · cardiomyopathy · cardiovascular disease · cerebrovascular disorders · heart failure · hyperthyroidism · mania · phaeochromocytoma · psychosis · severe depression · severe hypertension · structural cardiac abnormalities · suicidal tendencies · uncontrolled bipolar disorder · vasculitis
- **CAUTIONS** Agitation · alcohol dependence · anxiety · drug dependence · epilepsy (discontinue if increased seizure frequency) · family history of Tourette syndrome · susceptibility to angle-closure glaucoma · tics

  CONCERTA® XL Dysphagia (dose form not appropriate) · restricted gastro-intestinal lumen (dose form not appropriate)

  DELMOSART® PROLONGED-RELEASE TABLET Dysphagia (dose form not appropriate) · restricted gastro-intestinal lumen (dose form not appropriate)

  XAGGITIN® XL Dysphagia (dose form not appropriate)
- **INTERACTIONS** → Appendix 1: methylphenidate
- **SIDE-EFFECTS**

▶ **Common or very common** Aggression (or hostility) · alopecia · anxiety · appetite decreased · arrhythmias · arthralgia · asthenia · behaviour abnormal · cough · depression · diarrhoea · dizziness · drowsiness · dry mouth · feeling jittery · fever · gastrointestinal discomfort · growth retardation · headaches · hyperhidrosis · hypertension · increased risk of infection · laryngeal pain · mood altered · movement disorders · muscle complaints · nausea · oropharyngeal pain · palpitations · paraesthesia · sexual dysfunction · skin reactions · sleep disorders · thirst · tic · vertigo · vision disorders · vomiting · weight decreased

▶ **Uncommon** Angioedema · chest discomfort · constipation · dry eye · dyspnoea · haematuria · hallucinations · hot flush · psychotic disorder · speech impairment · suicidal behaviours · tremor · urinary disorders

▶ **Rare or very rare** Anaemia · angina pectoris · cardiac arrest · cerebrovascular insufficiency · confusion · gynaecomastia · hepatic coma · hepatic disorders · hyperfocus · leucopenia · mydriasis · myocardial infarction · neuroleptic malignant syndrome (discontinue—potentially fatal) · peripheral coldness · Raynaud's phenomenon · seizures · sudden cardiac death · thinking abnormal · thrombocytopenia

▶ **Frequency not known** Delusions · drug dependence · hyperpyrexia · intracranial haemorrhage · pancytopenia · vasculitis

- **PREGNANCY** Limited experience—avoid unless potential benefit outweighs risk.
- **BREAST FEEDING** Limited information available—avoid.

- **MONITORING REQUIREMENTS**
  - Monitor for psychiatric disorders.
  - Pulse, blood pressure, psychiatric symptoms, appetite, weight and height should be recorded at initiation of therapy, following each dose adjustment, and at least every 6 months thereafter.
- **TREATMENT CESSATION** Avoid abrupt withdrawal.
- **DIRECTIONS FOR ADMINISTRATION**

EQUASYM® XL Manufacturer advises contents of capsule can be sprinkled on a tablespoon of apple sauce (then swallowed immediately without chewing).

MEDIKINET® XL Manufacturer advises contents of capsule can be sprinkled on a tablespoon of apple sauce or yoghurt (then swallowed immediately without chewing).

- **PRESCRIBING AND DISPENSING INFORMATION** Different versions of modified-release preparations may not have the same clinical effect. To avoid confusion between these different formulations of methylphenidate, prescribers should specify the brand or manufacturer name, if generic, to be dispensed—see also *Important safety information*.

CONCERTA® XL Consists of an immediate-release component (22% of the dose) and a modified-release component (78% of the dose).

EQUASYM® XL Consists of an immediate-release component (30% of the dose) and a modified-release component (70% of the dose).

MEDIKINET® XL Consists of an immediate-release component (50% of the dose) and a modified-release component (50% of the dose).

- **PATIENT AND CARER ADVICE**

Medicines for Children leaflet: Methylphenidate for ADHD www.medicinesforchildren.org.uk/medicines/methylphenidate-for-adhd/

Driving and skilled tasks Prescribers and other healthcare professionals should advise patients if treatment is likely to affect their ability to perform skilled tasks (e.g. driving). This applies especially to drugs with sedative effects; patients should be warned that these effects are increased by alcohol. General information about a patient's fitness to drive is available from the Driver and Vehicle Licensing Agency at www.gov.uk/government/organisations/driver-and-vehicle-licensing-agency.

2015 legislation regarding driving whilst taking certain drugs, may also apply to methylphenidate, see *Drugs and driving* under Guidance on prescribing p. 1.

CONCERTA® XL Tablet membrane may pass through gastro-intestinal tract unchanged.

DELMOSART® PROLONGED-RELEASE TABLET Manufacturer advises tablet membrane may pass through gastro-intestinal tract unchanged.

- **MEDICINAL FORMS** There can be variation in the licensing of different medicines containing the same drug. Forms available from special-order manufacturers include: oral suspension, oral solution

Oral tablet

- **Methylphenidate hydrochloride (Non-proprietary)**
  - **Methylphenidate hydrochloride 5 mg** Methylphenidate 5mg tablets | 30 tablet [PoM] £7.50 DT = £3.03 [CD2]
  - **Methylphenidate hydrochloride 10 mg** Methylphenidate 10mg tablets | 30 tablet [PoM] £10.00 DT = £3.09 [CD2]
  - **Methylphenidate hydrochloride 20 mg** Methylphenidate 20mg tablets | 30 tablet [PoM] £16.38 DT = £6.50 [CD2]
- **Medikinet** (Medice UK Ltd)
  - **Methylphenidate hydrochloride 5 mg** Medikinet 5mg tablets | 30 tablet [PoM] £3.03 DT = £3.03 [CD2]
  - **Methylphenidate hydrochloride 10 mg** Medikinet 10mg tablets | 30 tablet [PoM] £5.49 DT = £3.09 [CD2]
  - **Methylphenidate hydrochloride 20 mg** Medikinet 20mg tablets | 30 tablet [PoM] £10.92 DT = £6.50 [CD2]
- **Ritalin** (InfectoPharm Ltd)
  - **Methylphenidate hydrochloride 10 mg** Ritalin 10mg tablets | 30 tablet [PoM] £6.68 DT = £3.09 [CD2]
- **Tranquilyn** (Genesis Pharmaceuticals Ltd)
  - **Methylphenidate hydrochloride 5 mg** Tranquilyn 5mg tablets | 30 tablet [PoM] £3.03 DT = £3.03 [CD2]
  - **Methylphenidate hydrochloride 10 mg** Tranquilyn 10mg tablets | 30 tablet [PoM] £5.49 DT = £3.09 [CD2]
  - **Methylphenidate hydrochloride 20 mg** Tranquilyn 20mg tablets | 30 tablet [PoM] £10.92 DT = £6.50 [CD2]

Modified-release tablet

CAUTIONARY AND ADVISORY LABELS 25

- **Concerta XL** (Janssen-Cilag Ltd)
  - **Methylphenidate hydrochloride 18 mg** Concerta XL 18mg tablets | 30 tablet [PoM] £31.19 DT = £31.19 [CD2]
  - **Methylphenidate hydrochloride 27 mg** Concerta XL 27mg tablets | 30 tablet [PoM] £36.81 DT = £36.81 [CD2]
  - **Methylphenidate hydrochloride 36 mg** Concerta XL 36mg tablets | 30 tablet [PoM] £42.45 DT = £42.45 [CD2]
  - **Methylphenidate hydrochloride 54 mg** Concerta XL 54mg tablets | 30 tablet [PoM] £73.62 DT = £36.80 [CD2]
- **Delmosart** (Accord-UK Ltd)
  - **Methylphenidate hydrochloride 18 mg** Delmosart 18mg modified-release tablets | 30 tablet [PoM] £15.57 DT = £31.19 [CD2]
  - **Methylphenidate hydrochloride 27 mg** Delmosart 27mg modified-release tablets | 30 tablet [PoM] £18.39 DT = £36.81 [CD2]
  - **Methylphenidate hydrochloride 36 mg** Delmosart 36mg modified-release tablets | 30 tablet [PoM] £21.21 DT = £42.45 [CD2]
  - **Methylphenidate hydrochloride 54 mg** Delmosart 54mg modified-release tablets | 30 tablet [PoM] £36.79 DT = £36.80 [CD2]
- **Xaggitin XL** (Ethypharm UK Ltd)
  - **Methylphenidate hydrochloride 18 mg** Xaggitin XL 18mg tablets | 30 tablet [PoM] £15.58 DT = £31.19 [CD2]
  - **Methylphenidate hydrochloride 27 mg** Xaggitin XL 27mg tablets | 30 tablet [PoM] £18.40 DT = £36.81 [CD2]
  - **Methylphenidate hydrochloride 36 mg** Xaggitin XL 36mg tablets | 30 tablet [PoM] £21.22 DT = £42.45 [CD2]
  - **Methylphenidate hydrochloride 54 mg** Xaggitin XL 54mg tablets | 30 tablet [PoM] £36.80 DT = £36.80 [CD2]

Modified-release capsule

CAUTIONARY AND ADVISORY LABELS 25

- **Equasym XL** (Takeda UK Ltd)
  - **Methylphenidate hydrochloride 10 mg** Equasym XL 10mg capsules | 30 capsule [PoM] £25.00 DT = £25.00 [CD2]
  - **Methylphenidate hydrochloride 20 mg** Equasym XL 20mg capsules | 30 capsule [PoM] £30.00 DT = £30.00 [CD2]
  - **Methylphenidate hydrochloride 30 mg** Equasym XL 30mg capsules | 30 capsule [PoM] £35.00 DT = £35.00 [CD2]
- **Medikinet XL** (Medice UK Ltd) ▼
  - **Methylphenidate hydrochloride 5 mg** Medikinet XL 5mg capsules | 30 capsule [PoM] £24.04 DT = £24.04 [CD2]
  - **Methylphenidate hydrochloride 10 mg** Medikinet XL 10mg capsules | 30 capsule [PoM] £24.04 DT = £25.00 [CD2]
  - **Methylphenidate hydrochloride 20 mg** Medikinet XL 20mg capsules | 30 capsule [PoM] £28.86 DT = £30.00 [CD2]
  - **Methylphenidate hydrochloride 30 mg** Medikinet XL 30mg capsules | 30 capsule [PoM] £33.66 DT = £35.00 [CD2]
  - **Methylphenidate hydrochloride 40 mg** Medikinet XL 40mg capsules | 30 capsule [PoM] £57.72 DT = £57.72 [CD2]
  - **Methylphenidate hydrochloride 50 mg** Medikinet XL 50mg capsules | 30 capsule [PoM] £62.52 DT = £62.52 [CD2]
  - **Methylphenidate hydrochloride 60 mg** Medikinet XL 60mg capsules | 30 capsule [PoM] £67.32 DT = £67.32 [CD2]

Oral solution

- **Methylphenidate hydrochloride (Non-proprietary)**
  - **Methylphenidate hydrochloride 2 mg per 1 ml** Methylphenidate 2mg/ml oral solution sugar free | 150 ml [PoM] £85.00 DT = £85.00 [CD2] [SF]

CNS STIMULANTS › CENTRALLY ACTING SYMPATHOMIMETICS › AMFETAMINES

Dexamfetamine sulfate

09-May-2024

(Dexamphetamine sulphate)

● **INDICATIONS AND DOSE**

Refractory attention deficit hyperactivity disorder (initiated under specialist supervision)

▶ BY MOUTH

▶ Child 6–17 years: Initially 2.5 mg 2–3 times a day, increased in steps of 5 mg once weekly if required, usual maximum 1 mg/kg daily, up to 20 mg daily (40 mg daily has been required in some children); maintenance dose to be given in 2–4 divided doses

● **CONTRA-INDICATIONS** Advanced arteriosclerosis · anorexia · arrhythmias (life-threatening) · cardiomyopathies · cardiovascular disease · cerebrovascular disorders · heart failure · history of alcohol abuse · history of drug abuse · hyperexcitability · hyperthyroidism · moderate hypertension · psychiatric disorders · psychosis · severe hypertension · structural cardiac abnormalities · suicidal tendencies

CONTRA-INDICATIONS, FURTHER INFORMATION

▶ Psychiatric disorders Psychiatric disorders include severe depression, schizophrenia, borderline personality disorder and uncontrolled bipolar disorder. Co-morbidity with psychiatric disorders is common in attention deficit hyperactivity disorder. Manufacturer advises if new psychiatric symptoms develop or exacerbation of psychiatric disorders occurs, continue use only if benefits outweigh risks.

● **CAUTIONS** History of epilepsy (discontinue if seizures occur) · mild hypertension · susceptibility to angle-closure glaucoma · tics · Tourette syndrome

CAUTIONS, FURTHER INFORMATION

▶ Tics and Tourette syndrome Discontinue use if tics occur.

▶ Growth restriction in children Monitor height and weight as growth restriction may occur during prolonged therapy (drug-free periods may allow catch-up in growth but withdraw slowly to avoid inducing depression or renewed hyperactivity).

● **INTERACTIONS** → Appendix 1: amfetamines

● **SIDE-EFFECTS**

▶ **Common or very common** Abdominal pain · anxiety · appetite decreased · arrhythmias · arthralgia · behaviour abnormal · depression · dry mouth · headache · mood altered · movement disorders · muscle cramps · nausea · palpitations · poor weight gain · sleep disorders · vertigo · vomiting · weight decreased

▶ **Rare or very rare** Anaemia · angina pectoris · cardiac arrest · central nervous system vasculitis · cerebrovascular insufficiency · fatigue · growth retardation · hallucination · hepatic coma · hepatic function abnormal · intracranial haemorrhage · leucopenia · mydriasis · psychosis · seizure · skin reactions · suicidal behaviours · thrombocytopenia · tic (in those at risk) · vision disorders

▶ **Frequency not known** Acidosis · alopecia · cardiomyopathy · chest pain · circulatory collapse · colitis ischaemic · concentration impaired · confusion · diarrhoea · dizziness · drug dependence · hyperhidrosis · hypermetabolism · hyperpyrexia · kidney injury · myocardial infarction · neuroleptic malignant syndrome (discontinue—potentially fatal) · obsessive-compulsive disorder · reflexes increased · rhabdomyolysis · sexual dysfunction · sudden death · taste altered · tremor

Overdose Amfetamines cause wakefulness, excessive activity, paranoia, hallucinations, and hypertension followed by exhaustion, convulsions, hyperthermia, and coma. See Stimulants under Emergency treatment of poisoning p. 1036.

● **PREGNANCY** Avoid (retrospective evidence of uncertain significance suggesting possible embryotoxicity).

● **BREAST FEEDING** Significant amount in milk—avoid.

● **RENAL IMPAIRMENT** EvGr Use with caution (no information available). ⟨M⟩

● **MONITORING REQUIREMENTS**

▶ Monitor growth in children.

▶ Monitor for aggressive behaviour or hostility during initial treatment.

▶ Pulse, blood pressure, psychiatric symptoms, appetite, weight and height should be recorded at initiation of therapy, following each dose adjustment, and at least every 6 months thereafter.

● **TREATMENT CESSATION** Avoid abrupt withdrawal.

● **DIRECTIONS FOR ADMINISTRATION** Manufacturer advises tablets can be halved.

● **PRESCRIBING AND DISPENSING INFORMATION** Data on safety and efficacy of long-term use not complete.

● **PATIENT AND CARER ADVICE**

Driving and skilled tasks Prescribers and other healthcare professionals should advise patients if treatment is likely to affect their ability to perform skilled tasks (e.g. driving). This applies especially to drugs with sedative effects; patients should be warned that these effects are increased by alcohol.

For information on 2015 legislation regarding driving whilst taking certain controlled drugs, including amfetamines, see *Drugs and driving* under Guidance on prescribing p. 1.

● **MEDICINAL FORMS** There can be variation in the licensing of different medicines containing the same drug. Forms available from special-order manufacturers include: modified-release capsule, oral suspension, oral solution

Oral tablet

▶ **Dexamfetamine sulfate (Non-proprietary)**

Dexamfetamine sulfate 5 mg Dexamfetamine 5mg tablets | 28 tablet PoM £19.85 DT = £19.85 CD2

▶ **Amfexa** (Medice UK Ltd)

Dexamfetamine sulfate 5 mg Amfexa 5mg tablets | 30 tablet PoM £19.89 CD2

Dexamfetamine sulfate 10 mg Amfexa 10mg tablets | 30 tablet PoM £39.78 DT = £39.78 CD2

Dexamfetamine sulfate 20 mg Amfexa 20mg tablets | 30 tablet PoM £79.56 DT = £79.56 CD2

Oral solution

▶ **Dexamfetamine sulfate (Non-proprietary)**

Dexamfetamine sulfate 1 mg per 1 ml Dexamfetamine 5mg/5ml oral solution sugar free | 150 ml PoM £183.86 DT = £183.86 CD2 SF

Modified-release capsule

▶ **Dexamfetamine sulfate (Non-proprietary)**

Dexamfetamine sulfate 5 mg Dexedrine 5mg Spansules | 100 capsule PoM ⊠ CD2

Dexamfetamine sulfate 10 mg Dexedrine 10mg Spansules | 100 capsule PoM ⊠ CD2

▶ **Dexedrine Spansules** (Imported (United States))

Dexamfetamine sulfate 15 mg Dexedrine 15mg Spansules | 100 capsule PoM ⊠ CD2

Lisdexamfetamine mesilate

29-Oct-2020

- **DRUG ACTION** Lisdexamfetamine is a prodrug of dexamfetamine.

- **INDICATIONS AND DOSE**

Attention deficit hyperactivity disorder (initiated by a specialist)

▶ BY MOUTH

▶ Child 6–17 years: Initially 30 mg once daily, alternatively initially 20 mg once daily, increased in steps of 10–20 mg every week if required, dose to be taken in the morning, discontinue if response insufficient after 1 month; maximum 70 mg per day

- **CONTRA-INDICATIONS** Advanced arteriosclerosis · agitated states · hyperthyroidism · moderate hypertension · severe hypertension · symptomatic cardiovascular disease
- **CAUTIONS** Bipolar disorder · history of cardiovascular disease · history of substance abuse · may lower seizure threshold (discontinue if seizures occur) · psychotic disorders · susceptibility to angle-closure glaucoma · tics · Tourette syndrome

CAUTIONS, FURTHER INFORMATION

▶ Cardiovascular disease Manufacturer advises caution in patients with underlying conditions that might be compromised by increases in blood pressure or heart rate; see also *Contra-indications*.

- **INTERACTIONS** → Appendix 1: amfetamines
- **SIDE-EFFECTS**

▶ **Common or very common** Abdominal pain upper · anxiety · appetite decreased · behaviour abnormal · constipation · depression · diarrhoea · dizziness · drowsiness · dry mouth · dyspnoea · fatigue · feeling jittery · fever · headache · insomnia · mood altered · nausea · palpitations · psychiatric disorders · skin reactions · tachycardia · tremor · vomiting · weight decreased

▶ **Uncommon** Cardiomyopathy · erectile dysfunction · hallucination · hyperhidrosis · logorrhea · movement disorders · mydriasis · Raynaud's phenomenon · taste altered · vision blurred

▶ **Frequency not known** Angioedema · drug dependence · hepatitis allergic · psychotic disorder · seizure · Stevens-Johnson syndrome

Overdose Amfetamines cause wakefulness, excessive activity, paranoia, hallucinations, and hypertension followed by exhaustion, convulsions, hyperthermia, and coma. See Stimulants under Emergency treatment of poisoning p. 1036.

- **PREGNANCY** Manufacturer advises use only if potential benefit outweighs risk.
- **BREAST FEEDING** Manufacturer advises avoid—present in human milk.
- **RENAL IMPAIRMENT**

Dose adjustments Manufacturer advises max. dose 50 mg daily in severe impairment.

- **MONITORING REQUIREMENTS**

▶ Manufacturer advises monitor for aggressive behaviour or hostility during initial treatment.

▶ Manufacturer advises monitor pulse, blood pressure, and for psychiatric symptoms before treatment initiation, following each dose adjustment, and at least every 6 months thereafter. Monitor weight in adults before treatment initiation and during treatment; in children, height and weight should be recorded before treatment initiation, and height, weight and appetite monitored at least every 6 months during treatment.

- **TREATMENT CESSATION** Avoid abrupt withdrawal.
- **DIRECTIONS FOR ADMINISTRATION** Manufacturer advises swallow whole or mix contents of capsule with soft food such as yoghurt or in a glass of water or orange juice; contents should be dispersed completely and consumed immediately.
- **PATIENT AND CARER ADVICE** Patients and carers should be counselled on the administration of capsules.

Driving and skilled tasks Prescribers and other healthcare professionals should advise patients if treatment is likely to affect their ability to perform skilled tasks (e.g. driving). This applies especially to drugs with sedative effects; patients should be warned that these effects are increased by alcohol. General information about a patient's fitness to drive is available from the Driver and Vehicle Licensing Agency at www.gov.uk/government/organisations/driver-and-vehicle-licensing-agency.

For information on 2015 legislation regarding driving whilst taking certain controlled drugs, including amfetamines, see *Drugs and driving* under Guidance on prescribing p. 1.

- **NATIONAL FUNDING/ACCESS DECISIONS**

For full details see funding body website

Scottish Medicines Consortium (SMC) decisions

▶ **Lisdexamfetamine dimesylate (*Elvanse*®) for use as part of a comprehensive treatment programme for attention deficit/hyperactivity disorder (ADHD) in children aged 6 years of age and over when response to previous methylphenidate treatment is considered clinically inadequate (May 2013)** SMC No. 863/13 Recommended

All Wales Medicines Strategy Group (AWMSG) decisions

▶ **Lisdexamfetamine dimesylate (*Elvanse*®) for use as part of a treatment programme for attention deficit/hyperactivity disorder (ADHD) in children aged 6 years and over when response to previous methylphenidate treatment is considered clinically inadequate. Treatment must be under the supervision of a specialist in childhood and/or adolescent behavioural disorders (December 2013)** AWMSG No. 188 Recommended

- **MEDICINAL FORMS** There can be variation in the licensing of different medicines containing the same drug.

Oral capsule

CAUTIONARY AND ADVISORY LABELS 3

▶ Elvanse (Takeda UK Ltd)

Lisdexamfetamine dimesylate 20 mg Elvanse 20mg capsules | 28 capsule PoM £54.62 DT = £54.62 CD2

Lisdexamfetamine dimesylate 30 mg Elvanse 30mg capsules | 28 capsule PoM £58.24 DT = £58.24 CD2

Lisdexamfetamine dimesylate 40 mg Elvanse 40mg capsules | 28 capsule PoM £62.82 DT = £62.82 CD2

Lisdexamfetamine dimesylate 50 mg Elvanse 50mg capsules | 28 capsule PoM £68.60 DT = £68.60 CD2

Lisdexamfetamine dimesylate 60 mg Elvanse 60mg capsules | 28 capsule PoM £75.18 DT = £75.18 CD2

Lisdexamfetamine dimesylate 70 mg Elvanse 70mg capsules | 28 capsule PoM £83.16 DT = £83.16 CD2

SYMPATHOMIMETICS › ALPHA$_2$-ADRENOCEPTOR AGONISTS

Guanfacine

06-Jun-2025

- **INDICATIONS AND DOSE**

Attention deficit hyperactivity disorder in children for whom stimulants are not suitable, not tolerated or ineffective (initiated under specialist supervision)

▶ BY MOUTH

▶ Child 6–12 years (body-weight 25 kg and above): Initially 1 mg once daily; adjusted in steps of 1 mg every week if necessary and if tolerated; maintenance 0.05–0.12 mg/kg once daily (max. per dose 4 mg), for optimal weight-adjusted dose titrations, consult product literature

continued →

- ▸ Child 13–17 years (body-weight 34–41.4 kg): Initially 1 mg once daily; adjusted in steps of 1 mg every week if necessary and if tolerated; maintenance 0.05–0.12 mg/kg once daily (max. per dose 4 mg), for optimal weight-adjusted dose titrations, consult product literature
- ▸ Child 13–17 years (body-weight 41.5–49.4 kg): Initially 1 mg once daily; adjusted in steps of 1 mg every week if necessary and if tolerated; maintenance 0.05–0.12 mg/kg once daily (max. per dose 5 mg), for optimal weight-adjusted dose titrations, consult product literature
- ▸ Child 13–17 years (body-weight 49.5–58.4 kg): Initially 1 mg once daily; adjusted in steps of 1 mg every week if necessary and if tolerated; maintenance 0.05–0.12 mg/kg once daily (max. per dose 6 mg), for optimal weight-adjusted dose titrations, consult product literature
- ▸ Child 13–17 years (body-weight 58.5 kg and above): Initially 1 mg once daily; adjusted in steps of 1 mg every week if necessary and if tolerated; maintenance 0.05–0.12 mg/kg once daily (max. per dose 7 mg), for optimal weight-adjusted dose titrations, consult product literature

DOSE ADJUSTMENTS DUE TO INTERACTIONS

- ▸ EvGr Reduce dose by half with concurrent use of moderate and potent inhibitors of CYP3A4 and ciprofloxacin; further titrate dose if needed.
- ▸ Consider increasing dose by 1 mg per week, up to max. 7 mg daily if needed, with concurrent use of potent inducers of CYP3A4. (M)

● **CAUTIONS** Bradycardia (risk of torsade de pointes) · heart block (risk of torsade de pointes) · history of cardiovascular disease · history of QT-interval prolongation · hypokalaemia (risk of torsade de pointes)

● **INTERACTIONS** → Appendix 1: guanfacine

● **SIDE-EFFECTS**

- ▸ **Common or very common** Anxiety · appetite decreased · arrhythmias · asthenia · constipation · depression · diarrhoea · dizziness · drowsiness · dry mouth · gastrointestinal discomfort · headache · hypotension · mood altered · nausea · skin reactions · sleep disorders · urinary disorders · vomiting · weight increased
- ▸ **Uncommon** Asthma · atrioventricular block · chest pain · hallucination · loss of consciousness · pallor · seizure · syncope
- ▸ **Rare or very rare** Hypertension · hypertensive encephalopathy · malaise
- ▸ **Frequency not known** Erectile dysfunction

SIDE-EFFECTS, FURTHER INFORMATION Somnolence and sedation may occur, predominantly during the first 2-3 weeks of treatment and with dose increases; manufacturer advises to consider dose reduction or discontinuation of treatment if symptoms are clinically significant or persistent.

Overdose Features may include hypotension, initial hypertension, bradycardia, lethargy, and respiratory depression. Manufacturer advises that patients who develop lethargy should be observed for development of more serious toxicity for up to 24 hours.

● **CONCEPTION AND CONTRACEPTION** Manufacturer recommends effective contraception in females of childbearing potential.

● **PREGNANCY** Manufacturer advises avoid—toxicity in *animal* studies.

● **BREAST FEEDING** Manufacturer advises avoid—present in milk in *animal* studies.

● **HEPATIC IMPAIRMENT** Manufacturer advises caution (pharmacokinetics have not been assessed in paediatric patients with hepatic impairment).

Dose adjustments Manufacturer advises consider dose reduction.

● **RENAL IMPAIRMENT**

Dose adjustments EvGr Dose reduction may be required in severe impairment and end-stage renal disease (no information available in children with renal impairment). (M)

● **MONITORING REQUIREMENTS**

- ▸ Manufacturer advises to conduct a baseline evaluation to identify patients at risk of somnolence, sedation, hypotension, bradycardia, QT-prolongation, and arrhythmia; this should include assessment of cardiovascular status. Monitor for signs of these adverse effects weekly during dose titration and then every 3 months during the first year of treatment, and every 6 months thereafter. Monitor BMI prior to treatment and then every 3 months for the first year of treatment, and every 6 months thereafter. More frequent monitoring is advised following dose adjustments.
- ▸ Monitor blood pressure and pulse during dose downward titration and following discontinuation of treatment.

● **TREATMENT CESSATION** Manufacturer advises avoid abrupt withdrawal; consider dose tapering to minimise potential withdrawal effects.

● **DIRECTIONS FOR ADMINISTRATION** Manufacturer advises avoid administration with high fat meals (may increase absorption).

● **PATIENT AND CARER ADVICE** Patients or carers should be counselled on administration of guanfacine modified-release tablets.

Missed doses Manufacturer advises that patients and carers should inform their prescriber if more than one dose is missed; consider dose re-titration.

Driving and skilled tasks Manufacturer advises patients and carers should be counselled about the effects on driving and performance of skilled tasks—increased risk of dizziness and syncope.

● **NATIONAL FUNDING/ACCESS DECISIONS**

For full details see funding body website

All Wales Medicines Strategy Group (AWMSG) decisions

- ▸ **Guanfacine (*Intuniv*®) for the treatment of attention deficit hyperactivity disorder (ADHD) in children and adolescents 6 to 17 years old for whom stimulants are not suitable, not tolerated or have been shown to be ineffective (May 2025)** AWMSG No. 6440 Recommended

---

● **MEDICINAL FORMS** There can be variation in the licensing of different medicines containing the same drug.

Modified-release tablet

CAUTIONARY AND ADVISORY LABELS 2, 25

▸ **Guanfacine (Non-proprietary)**

Guanfacine (as Guanfacine hydrochloride) 1 mg Guanfacine 1mg modified-release tablets | 28 tablet PoM £95.00 DT = £56.00

Guanfacine (as Guanfacine hydrochloride) 2 mg Guanfacine 2mg modified-release tablets | 28 tablet PoM £99.00 DT = £58.52

Guanfacine (as Guanfacine hydrochloride) 3 mg Guanfacine 3mg modified-release tablets | 28 tablet PoM £111.20 DT = £65.52

Guanfacine (as Guanfacine hydrochloride) 4 mg Guanfacine 4mg modified-release tablets | 28 tablet PoM £129.30 DT = £76.16

Guanfacine (as Guanfacine hydrochloride) 5 mg Guanfacine 5mg modified-release tablets | 28 tablet PoM £76.16

Guanfacine (as Guanfacine hydrochloride) 6 mg Guanfacine 6mg modified-release tablets | 28 tablet PoM £76.16

Guanfacine (as Guanfacine hydrochloride) 7 mg Guanfacine 7mg modified-release tablets | 28 tablet PoM £76.16

▸ **Intuniv** (Takeda UK Ltd) ▼

Guanfacine (as Guanfacine hydrochloride) 1 mg Intuniv 1mg modified-release tablets | 28 tablet PoM £56.00 DT = £56.00

Guanfacine (as Guanfacine hydrochloride) 2 mg Intuniv 2mg modified-release tablets | 28 tablet PoM £58.52 DT = £58.52

Guanfacine (as Guanfacine hydrochloride) 3 mg Intuniv 3mg modified-release tablets | 28 tablet PoM £65.52 DT = £65.52

Guanfacine (as Guanfacine hydrochloride) 4 mg Intuniv 4mg modified-release tablets | 28 tablet PoM £76.16 DT = £76.16

2.2 Bipolar disorder and mania

Mania and hypomania 02-Oct-2024

Overview

Antimanic drugs are used in bipolar disorder to manage acute episodes of mania or hypomania, and to prevent recurrence. Children with bipolar disorder should be under the care of specialist mental health services.

EvGr An antidepressant drug may also be required for the treatment of co-existing bipolar depression, but should be avoided in children with rapid-cycling bipolar disorder, a recent history of mania or hypomania, or with rapid mood fluctuations. Consider stopping the antidepressant drug if the child develops mania or hypomania. (A)

Antipsychotic drugs

Aripiprazole p. 300 is licensed for the treatment of moderate to severe manic episodes in adolescents with bipolar disorder.

EvGr Other antipsychotic drugs (such as olanzapine p. 303 [unlicensed use], quetiapine p. 304 [unlicensed use], and risperidone p. 306 [unlicensed use]) are used in the treatment of acute episodes of mania or hypomania in children; if the response to antipsychotic drugs is inadequate, lithium or valproate [unlicensed use] may be added. In children already taking prophylactic treatment with lithium or valproate, if there is no improvement despite optimising the dose of lithium or valproate, an antipsychotic drug may be added to treat an acute episode of mania or hypomania. An antipsychotic drug may also be used concomitantly with lithium or valproate in the initial treatment of severe acute episodes of mania. (A) Valproate is highly teratogenic; for information on regulatory measures issued by the MHRA/CHM to ensure appropriate and safe use, see *valproate* below.

EvGr Atypical antipsychotics may be used for the long-term management of bipolar disorder in children to prevent recurrence of acute episodes.

When discontinuing antipsychotic drugs, the dose should be reduced gradually over at least 4 weeks to minimise the risk of recurrence. (A)

Benzodiazepines

EvGr Use of benzodiazepines may be helpful in the initial stages of treatment for behavioural disturbance or agitation in children. (A) Benzodiazepines should not be used for long periods because of the risk of dependence.

Lithium

EvGr Lithium salts (lithium carbonate p. 284 and lithium citrate p. 285 [unlicensed use]) are used in children for the treatment of acute episodes of mania, and for the long-term management of bipolar disorder to prevent recurrence of acute episodes. (A)

The decision to give prophylactic lithium must be based on careful consideration of the likelihood of recurrence in the individual child, and the benefit of treatment weighed against the risks. The full prophylactic effect of lithium may not occur for six to twelve months after the initiation of therapy.

Valproate

EvGr Valproate (valproic acid (as the semisodium salt) and sodium valproate) [unlicensed use] is used in children for the treatment of acute episodes of mania, and for the long-term management of bipolar disorder to prevent recurrence of acute episodes. (A)

Safety measures around the use of valproate have been revised, and the MHRA/CHM has issued a National Patient Safety Alert. This outlines new regulatory measures for initiation of valproate in individuals (males or females) aged under 55 years, and continued use in females of childbearing potential. Due to the high teratogenic risk associated with valproate, it must not be used in females of childbearing potential unless the conditions of the Pregnancy Prevention Programme are met and alternative treatments are ineffective or not tolerated. Valproate must not be used during pregnancy in patients with bipolar disorder. In addition to these measures, further advice has been issued around the use in males and the need to use effective contraception. For further information, see *Important safety information*, *Conception and contraception*, and *Pregnancy* in valproic acid p. 259 and sodium valproate p. 252.

Carbamazepine

Expert sources advise carbamazepine p. 234 [unlicensed use] is used in children for the long-term management of bipolar disorder to prevent recurrence of acute episodes.

LITHIUM SALTS

Lithium salts 03-May-2023

- **CONTRA-INDICATIONS** Addison's disease · cardiac disease associated with rhythm disorder · cardiac insufficiency · dehydration · family history of Brugada syndrome · low sodium diets · personal history of Brugada syndrome · untreated hypothyroidism
- **CAUTIONS** Avoid abrupt withdrawal · cardiac disease · concurrent ECT (may lower seizure threshold) · diuretic treatment (risk of toxicity) · epilepsy (may lower seizure threshold) · myasthenia gravis · psoriasis (risk of exacerbation) · QT interval prolongation · review dose as necessary in diarrhoea · review dose as necessary in intercurrent infection (especially if sweating profusely) · review dose as necessary in vomiting · surgery
- **SIDE-EFFECTS**
  - ▶ **Common or very common** Electrolyte imbalance
  - ▶ **Rare or very rare** Nephrotic syndrome
  - ▶ **Frequency not known** Abdominal discomfort · alopecia · angioedema · appetite decreased · arrhythmias · atrioventricular block · cardiomyopathy · cerebellar syndrome · circulatory collapse · coma · confusion · consciousness impaired · delirium · diarrhoea · dizziness · drug reaction with eosinophilia and systemic symptoms (DRESS) · dry mouth · encephalopathy · feeling dazed · folliculitis · gastritis · goitre · hyperglycaemia · hyperparathyroidism · hypersalivation · hypotension · hypothyroidism · idiopathic intracranial hypertension · leucocytosis · memory impairment · movement disorders · muscle weakness · myasthenia gravis · nausea · neoplasms · nephrogenic diabetes insipidus · neuroleptic malignant syndrome (discontinue—potentially fatal) · nystagmus · parathyroid hyperplasia · peripheral neuropathy · peripheral oedema · polydipsia · polyuria · QT interval prolongation · reflexes abnormal · renal disorders · renal impairment · rhabdomyolysis · seizure · serotonin syndrome · sexual dysfunction · skin reactions · skin ulcer · speech impairment · taste altered · thyrotoxicosis · tremor · vertigo · vision disorders · vomiting · weight increased

  SIDE-EFFECTS, FURTHER INFORMATION **Overdose** Signs of intoxication require withdrawal of treatment and include increasing gastro-intestinal disturbances (vomiting, diarrhoea), visual disturbances, polyuria, muscle weakness, fine tremor increasing to coarse tremor, CNS disturbances (confusion and drowsiness increasing to lack of coordination, restlessness, stupor); abnormal reflexes, myoclonus, incontinence, hypernatraemia. With severe overdosage seizures, cardiac arrhythmias (including sino-atrial block, bradycardia and first-degree heart block), blood pressure changes, circulatory failure, renal failure, coma and sudden death reported.

  For details on the management of poisoning, see

Lithium, under Emergency treatment of poisoning p. 1036.

- **CONCEPTION AND CONTRACEPTION** Manufacturer advises effective contraception during treatment for women of child bearing potential.
- **PREGNANCY** Avoid if possible, particularly in the first trimester (risk of teratogenicity, including cardiac abnormalities). Close monitoring of serum-lithium concentration advised in pregnancy (risk of toxicity in neonate).
Dose adjustments Dose requirements increased during the second and third trimesters (but on delivery return abruptly to normal).
- **BREAST FEEDING** Present in milk and risk of toxicity in infant—avoid.
- **RENAL IMPAIRMENT** See p. 16. EvGr Caution in mild to moderate impairment; avoid in severe impairment. (M)
- **MONITORING REQUIREMENTS**
  - Serum concentrations Lithium salts have a narrow therapeutic/toxic ratio and should therefore not be prescribed unless facilities for monitoring serum-lithium concentrations are available.
EvGr Samples should be taken 12 hours post dose; for twice-daily dosing, morning dose to be withheld until sample taken. (E) EvGr Serum-lithium concentrations should be monitored 1 week after treatment initiation, and 1 week after each dose (or formulation) change, and then weekly until concentrations are stable. (A)
EvGr An initial serum-lithium concentration between 0.6–0.8 mmol/litre is recommended for the treatment and prophylaxis of bipolar disorder in lithium-naïve patients, and between 0.4–0.6 mmol/litre for the treatment and prophylaxis of recurrent major depressive disorder (unipolar depression). Where the effect of lithium is sub-optimal, specialists may advise increasing the dose to obtain a serum concentration of 0.8–1 mmol/litre in bipolar disorder and 0.6–0.8 mmol/litre in unipolar depression. (E)
EvGr When serum-lithium concentrations are stable, monitor every 3 months for the first year, and every 6 months thereafter. Serum-lithium concentrations should be monitored every 3 months if patients: are taking drugs that interact with lithium; are at risk of impaired renal or thyroid function, have raised calcium levels, or other complications; have poor symptom control or poor adherence; or whose last serum-lithium concentration was 0.8 mmol/litre or higher. (A) EvGr Additional monitoring is required if a patient develops significant intercurrent disease, if there is a significant change in a patient's sodium or fluid intake, or if signs of lithium toxicity occur. (M)
  - EvGr Before treatment initiation, assess body-weight or BMI, renal and thyroid function, urea and electrolytes (including calcium levels), and a full blood count. An ECG is recommended in patients with cardiovascular disease or risk factors for it.
  - Body-weight and BMI, renal and thyroid function, and urea and electrolytes (including calcium levels) should be monitored at least every 6 months during treatment, and more often if there is evidence of impaired renal or thyroid function, raised calcium levels, or an increase in mood symptoms that might be related to impaired thyroid function or altered calcium levels. Specialists may recommend regular monitoring of cardiac function for some patients. (E)
- **TREATMENT CESSATION** EvGr If lithium is to be discontinued, the dose should be reduced gradually over a period of at least 4 weeks (preferably over a period of up to 3 months). Patients should be monitored closely for early signs of mania or depression during dose reduction and for 3 months after discontinuation of lithium. (A)
- **PATIENT AND CARER ADVICE** Patients and carers should be advised to report signs and symptoms of lithium toxicity, hypothyroidism, renal dysfunction (including polyuria and polydipsia), and benign intracranial hypertension (persistent headache and visual disturbance); medical attention should be sought if any of these occur. Patients and carers should also be counselled on the signs of relapse. Maintain adequate fluid intake and avoid dietary changes which reduce or increase sodium intake. Patients and carers should be made aware of the risk of dehydration due to factors such as excessive alcohol intake, hot climates, and vomiting or diarrhoea. Medical attention should be sought if dehydration occurs.
Lithium treatment packs A lithium treatment pack should be given to patients on initiation of treatment with lithium. The pack consists of a patient information booklet, lithium alert card, and a record book for tracking serum-lithium concentration. Packs may be purchased from

3M
0845 610 1112

NHS trusts can order supplies from cmswebshop.corp.xerox.com/NHS/Login.aspx.
Driving and skilled tasks May impair performance of skilled tasks (e.g. driving, operating machinery).

F 283

Lithium carbonate

10-Sep-2024

- **INDICATIONS AND DOSE**

Treatment and prophylaxis of mania (initiated by a specialist) | Treatment and prophylaxis of bipolar disorder (initiated by a specialist) | Treatment and prophylaxis of recurrent major depressive disorder [unipolar depression] (initiated by a specialist) | Treatment and prophylaxis of aggressive or self-harming behaviour (initiated by a specialist)

- BY MOUTH
  - Child 12–17 years: Initially 200–250 mg daily in 1–2 divided doses, dose adjusted according to serum-lithium concentration

DOSE EQUIVALENCE AND CONVERSION
- There is no clinically significant difference between the pharmacokinetics of *Priadel*® and *Camcolit*® modified-release tablets; however, other preparations may not be bioequivalent. Lithium should be prescribed by brand name and formulation (tablets and liquids are not interchangeable)—changing the preparation or formulation requires the same monitoring of serum-lithium concentration as initiation of lithium.

- **UNLICENSED USE** EvGr Lithium carbonate is used in the doses provided in BNFC for the treatment and prophylaxis of mania, bipolar disorder, recurrent major depressive disorder (unipolar depression), and aggressive or self-harming behaviour (E), but these are not licensed.
- **INTERACTIONS** → Appendix 1: lithium
- **SIDE-EFFECTS** Cardiac arrest · hyperthyroidism · parkinsonism

- **MEDICINAL FORMS** There can be variation in the licensing of different medicines containing the same drug. Forms available from special-order manufacturers include: oral suspension

Oral tablet

CAUTIONARY AND ADVISORY LABELS 10
- **Lithium carbonate (Non-proprietary)**
Lithium carbonate 250 mg Lithium carbonate 250mg tablets | 100 tablet PoM £99.53 DT = £99.53

Modified-release tablet

CAUTIONARY AND ADVISORY LABELS 10, 25
- **Camcolit** (Essential Pharma Ltd)
Lithium carbonate 400 mg Camcolit 400 modified-release tablets | 100 tablet PoM £48.18 DT = £18.60

- ▸ **Liskonum** (Teofarma S.r.l.)
  Lithium carbonate 450 mg Liskonum 450mg modified-release tablets | 60 tablet PoM £11.84 DT = £11.84
- ▸ **Priadel (lithium carbonate)** (Essential Pharma Ltd)
  Lithium carbonate 200 mg Priadel 200mg modified-release tablets | 100 tablet PoM £16.42 DT = £16.42
  Lithium carbonate 400 mg Priadel 400mg modified-release tablets | 100 tablet PoM £18.60 DT = £18.60

283

Lithium citrate

10-Sep-2024

● **INDICATIONS AND DOSE**

LI-LIQUID®

Treatment and prophylaxis of mania (initiated by a specialist) | Treatment and prophylaxis of bipolar disorder (initiated by a specialist) | Treatment and prophylaxis of recurrent major depressive disorder [unipolar depression] (initiated by a specialist) | Treatment and prophylaxis of aggressive or self-harming behaviour (initiated by a specialist)

▸ BY MOUTH

▸ Child 12–17 years: Initially 509 mg daily in 1–2 divided doses, dose adjusted according to serum-lithium concentration

DOSE EQUIVALENCE AND CONVERSION

- ▸ *Li-Liquid*® containing lithium citrate 509 mg in 5 mL is equivalent to lithium carbonate 200 mg; *Li-Liquid*® containing lithium citrate 1.018 g in 5 mL is equivalent to lithium carbonate 400 mg.
- ▸ **Preparations may vary widely in bioavailability**; lithium should be prescribed by brand name and formulation (tablets and liquids are not interchangeable)—changing the preparation or formulation requires the same monitoring of serum-lithium concentration as initiation of lithium.

PRIADEL® LIQUID

Treatment and prophylaxis of mania (initiated by a specialist) | Treatment and prophylaxis of bipolar disorder (initiated by a specialist) | Treatment and prophylaxis of recurrent major depressive disorder [unipolar depression] (initiated by a specialist) | Treatment and prophylaxis of aggressive or self-harming behaviour (initiated by a specialist)

▸ BY MOUTH

▸ Child 12–17 years: Initially 520 mg daily in 1–2 divided doses, dose adjusted according to serum-lithium concentration

DOSE EQUIVALENCE AND CONVERSION

- ▸ *Priadel*® liquid containing lithium citrate 520 mg in 5 mL is equivalent to lithium carbonate 204 mg.
- ▸ **Preparations may vary widely in bioavailability**; lithium should be prescribed by brand name and formulation (tablets and liquids are not interchangeable)—changing the preparation or formulation requires the same monitoring of serum-lithium concentration as initiation of lithium.

● **UNLICENSED USE** EvGr Lithium citrate is used in the doses provided in BNFC for the treatment and prophylaxis of mania, bipolar disorder, recurrent major depressive disorder (unipolar depression), and aggressive or self-harming behaviour ⟨E⟩, but these are not licensed.

● **INTERACTIONS** → Appendix 1: lithium

● **SIDE-EFFECTS** Thirst

● **MEDICINAL FORMS** There can be variation in the licensing of different medicines containing the same drug.

Oral solution

CAUTIONARY AND ADVISORY LABELS 10

- ▸ **Li-Liquid** (Rosemont Pharmaceuticals Ltd)
  Lithium citrate 101.8 mg per 1 ml Li-Liquid 509mg/5ml oral solution | 150 ml PoM £5.79 DT = £5.79
  Lithium citrate 203.6 mg per 1 ml Li-Liquid 1.018g/5ml oral solution | 150 ml PoM £17.49 DT = £17.49
- ▸ **Priadel (lithium citrate)** (Essential Pharma Ltd)
  Lithium citrate 104 mg per 1 ml Priadel 520mg/5ml liquid | 150 ml PoM £12.11 DT = £12.11 SF

2.3 Depression

Depression

10-Jul-2019

Description of condition

Depression is characterised by persistent low mood which can present as irritability, fatigue, and/or a loss of interest or pleasure in most activities and may be accompanied by symptoms of anxiety.

Associated symptoms, which determine disease severity, are sleep and appetite disturbance, lack of concentration, low self-confidence, agitation, guilt or self-blame and suicidal thoughts or acts.

Based on the International Statistical Classification of Diseases (ICD-10), depression can be classified as mild (four symptoms), moderate (five to six symptoms) or severe (seven or more symptoms, with or without psychotic symptoms).

Depression in childhood is not common and can have a more gradual onset than in adults. Affecting twice as many adolescent females than males, depression often occurs with other behavioural disorders. In almost half of the cases it resolves spontaneously within the first year.

Non-drug treatment

EvGr When assessing a child or young person with depression, take into account family history of mood disorders, experience of bullying or abuse, any alcohol and drug misuse and the possibility of parental substance misuse as this may impact on disease severity or affect treatment efficacy.

Any comorbid diagnoses and developmental, social and educational problems should be assessed and managed, either in sequence or in parallel with the treatment for depression.

St John's wort is a herbal remedy available without prescription for treating mild depression in adults. It should not be used for the treatment of depression in children. ⟨A⟩

Lifestyle changes

EvGr Regular exercise (45 minutes to 1 hour per session, up to 3 times a week) following a structured programme for 10 to 12 weeks, should be encouraged. Give children, and their parents or carers, advice about good sleep hygiene, anxiety management, nutrition and the benefits of a balanced diet. ⟨A⟩

Psychological therapy

EvGr Offer 3 months of psychological therapy as first-line treatment from a therapist trained in child and adolescent mental health, or a healthcare practitioner specifically trained in the psychological therapy. Therapy options include cognitive behavioural therapy (CBT), interpersonal psychotherapy (IPT), IPT for adolescents (IPT-A), non-directive supportive therapy (NDST), psychodynamic psychotherapy, family therapy, brief psychosocial interventions, and intensive psychological therapy.

In mild depression, for those who do not meet referral criteria or who do not want an intervention, a period of watchful waiting and re-assessment of symptoms within

2 weeks should be arranged. (A) For further information on criteria for referral to Child and Adolescent Mental Health Services (CAMHS) see NICE guideline **Depression in children and young people** (see *Useful resources*).

Drug treatment

Child aged 5 years and over

EvGr Antidepressants should not be used for the initial treatment of children with mild depression. For cases refractory to psychological treatment, antidepressant therapy may be considered under specialist advice.

Drug treatment should only be prescribed following assessment and diagnosis by a child and adolescent psychiatrist.

When an antidepressant is prescribed, the SSRI fluoxetine p. 288 is the first-line treatment in children.

The use of fluoxetine in children aged 5 to 11 years should be cautiously considered as effectiveness in this age group is not established.

For moderate to severe depression, antidepressants should only be offered to children in combination with concurrent psychological therapy.

In children aged 12 years and over, following multidisciplinary review, combination therapy can be considered as an alternative to psychological monotherapy, or in cases refractory to psychological therapy.

Children should be carefully monitored at the start of treatment (for example weekly contact for the first 4 weeks or according to individual needs). Following remission (no symptoms and full functioning for at least 8 weeks), antidepressant treatment should be continued at the same dose for at least 6 months.

For children unresponsive to treatment with fluoxetine in combination with a psychological therapy, it is recommended to consider an alternative psychological therapy.

In children who present with severe depression and recurrent depressive episodes who do not respond to or cannot tolerate fluoxetine, citalopram p. 287 [unlicensed indication] or sertraline p. 289 [unlicensed indication] can be used as an alternative under specialist supervision.

Paroxetine, venlafaxine and tricyclic antidepressants should not be used for the treatment of depression in children and young people.

In children aged 12 years and over with very severe depression and life-threatening symptoms (such as suicidal behaviour), or who have not responded to other treatments, electroconvulsive therapy can be considered under specialist care. (A)

Psychotic depression

EvGr Augmenting existing antidepressant treatment with second generation antipsychotics (under specialist supervision) should be considered for children with psychotic depression, although the optimum dose and duration of treatment are unknown. (A)

Suicidal behaviour and antidepressant therapy

EvGr The use of antidepressant drugs has been linked with suicidal thoughts and behaviour, mainly in the early stages of treatment. Children should be monitored for suicidal behaviour, self-harm or hostility, particularly at the beginning of treatment, with medication changes and at times of increased personal stress. (A) For further information on SSRI use and safety, see MHRA/CHM guidance **Selective serotonin reuptake inhibitors (SSRIs) and serotonin and noradrenaline reuptake inhibitors (SNRIs)** (see *Useful resources*).

Useful Resources

Depression in children and young people: identification and management. National Institute for Health and Care Excellence. National Guideline 134. September 2005 (updated June 2019)
www.nice.org.uk/guidance/ng134

Depression in children. National Institute for Health and Care Excellence. Clinical Knowledge Summary. March 2016
cks.nice.org.uk/depression-in-children

Selective serotonin reuptake inhibitors (SSRIs) and serotonin and noradrenaline reuptake inhibitors (SNRIs): use and safety. Medicines and Healthcare products Regulatory Agency. Guidance. December 2014.
www.gov.uk/government/publications/ssris-and-snris-use-and-safety/selective-serotonin-reuptake-inhibitors-ssris-and-serotonin-and-noradrenaline-reuptake-inhibitors-snris-use-and-safety

ANTIDEPRESSANTS > SELECTIVE SEROTONIN RE-UPTAKE INHIBITORS

Selective serotonin re-uptake inhibitors

- **DRUG ACTION** Selectively inhibit the re-uptake of serotonin (5-hydroxytryptamine, 5-HT).

IMPORTANT SAFETY INFORMATION

MHRA/CHM ADVICE: SSRI/SNRI ANTIDEPRESSANT MEDICINES: SMALL INCREASED RISK OF POSTPARTUM HAEMORRHAGE WHEN USED IN THE MONTH BEFORE DELIVERY (JANUARY 2021)

SSRIs are known to increase the risk of bleeding due to their effect on platelet function. Observational data suggest that the use of SSRIs in the last month before delivery may increase the risk of postpartum haemorrhage. Healthcare professionals should continue to consider the benefits and risks of antidepressant use during pregnancy, and the risks of untreated depression in pregnancy.

Healthcare professionals should also consider this finding in the context of individual patient risk factors for bleeding or thrombotic events. Anticoagulant medication in women at high risk of thrombotic events should not be stopped but healthcare professionals should be aware of the risk identified.

- **CONTRA-INDICATIONS** Poorly controlled epilepsy · SSRIs should not be used if the patient enters a manic phase
- **CAUTIONS** Cardiac disease · concurrent electroconvulsive therapy · diabetes mellitus · epilepsy (discontinue if convulsions develop) · history of bleeding disorders (especially gastro-intestinal bleeding) · history of mania · susceptibility to angle-closure glaucoma
- **SIDE-EFFECTS**
  - **Common or very common** Anxiety · appetite abnormal · arrhythmias · arthralgia · asthenia · concentration impaired · confusion · constipation · depersonalisation · diarrhoea · dizziness · drowsiness · dry mouth · fever · gastrointestinal discomfort · haemorrhage · headache · hyperhidrosis · malaise · mania · memory loss · menstrual cycle irregularities · myalgia · mydriasis · nausea (dose-related) · palpitations · paraesthesia · QT interval prolongation · sexual dysfunction · skin reactions · sleep disorders · taste altered · tinnitus · tremor · urinary disorders · visual impairment · vomiting · weight changes · yawning
  - **Uncommon** Alopecia · angioedema · behaviour abnormal · hallucination · leucopenia · movement disorders · photosensitivity reaction · postural hypotension · seizure · suicidal behaviours · syncope
  - **Rare or very rare** Galactorrhoea · hepatitis · hyperprolactinaemia · hyponatraemia · serotonin syndrome · severe cutaneous adverse reactions (SCARs) · SIADH · thrombocytopenia
  - **Frequency not known** Increased risk of fracture · withdrawal syndrome

SIDE-EFFECTS, FURTHER INFORMATION Symptoms of sexual dysfunction may persist after treatment has stopped.

Overdose Symptoms of poisoning by selective serotonin re-uptake inhibitors include nausea, vomiting, agitation, tremor, nystagmus, drowsiness, and sinus tachycardia; convulsions may occur. Rarely, severe poisoning results in the serotonin syndrome, with marked neuropsychiatric effects, neuromuscular hyperactivity, and autonomic instability; hyperthermia, rhabdomyolysis, renal failure, and coagulopathies may develop.

For details on the management of poisoning, see Selective serotonin re-uptake inhibitors, under Emergency treatment of poisoning p. 1036.

- **PREGNANCY** Specialist sources indicate SSRIs may be suitable for use in pregnancy, but the risks and benefits of use must be considered, and the lowest effective dose should be used. The available data regarding malformation risk for all SSRIs are conflicting and confounded, and a causal association between the use of SSRIs in pregnancy, and spontaneous miscarriage, preterm delivery, low birth weight, and adverse effects on infant neurodevelopment remains unconfirmed. Published data on first trimester use of fluoxetine and paroxetine are contradictory. Some studies suggest a small increased risk of cardiovascular malformations with the use of fluoxetine, and congenital malformations (particularly cardiovascular) with the use of paroxetine, however other studies do not support an association. There may be a small increased risk of persistent pulmonary hypertension in the newborn with the use of SSRIs beyond 20 weeks' gestation, and use in the later stages of pregnancy may result in neonatal withdrawal syndrome—neonates should be monitored for associated central nervous system, motor, respiratory, and gastro-intestinal symptoms. There may also be a small increased risk of postpartum haemorrhage when used in the month before delivery (see *Important safety information*).
- **BREAST FEEDING** Specialist sources indicate that sertraline and paroxetine are the SSRIs of choice in breast-feeding based on passage into milk, half-life, and published evidence of safety. However, all SSRIs can be used in breast-feeding with caution, and since there are risks with switching an SSRI, it may be more clinically appropriate to continue treatment with an SSRI that has been effective, or restart treatment with an SSRI that has previously been effective. With all SSRIs, infants should be monitored for drowsiness, poor feeding, adequate weight gain, gastro-intestinal disturbances, irritability, and restlessness.
- **HEPATIC IMPAIRMENT** In general, manufacturers advise caution (prolonged half-life).
- **TREATMENT CESSATION** Gastro-intestinal disturbances, headache, anxiety, dizziness, paraesthesia, electric shock sensation in the head, neck, and spine, tinnitus, sleep disturbances, fatigue, influenza-like symptoms, and sweating are the most common features of abrupt withdrawal of an SSRI or marked reduction of the dose; palpitation and visual disturbances can occur less commonly. The dose should be tapered over at least a few weeks to avoid these effects. For some patients, it may be necessary to withdraw treatment over a longer period; consider obtaining specialist advice if symptoms persist.

  Withdrawal effects may occur within 5 days of stopping treatment with antidepressant drugs; they are usually mild and self-limiting, but in some cases may be severe. The risk of withdrawal symptoms is increased if the antidepressant is stopped suddenly after regular administration for 8 weeks or more.
- **PATIENT AND CARER ADVICE**
  Driving and skilled tasks May also impair performance of skilled tasks (e.g. driving, operating machinery).

F 286

Citalopram

14-May-2025

- **INDICATIONS AND DOSE**

Major depression

▶ BY MOUTH USING TABLETS

▸ Child 12–17 years: Initially 10 mg once daily, increased if necessary to 20 mg once daily, dose to be increased over 2–4 weeks, doses up to 40 mg per day may be considered

▶ BY MOUTH USING ORAL DROPS

▸ Child 12–17 years: Initially 8 mg once daily, increased if necessary to 16 mg once daily, dose to be increased over 2–4 weeks, doses up to 32 mg per day may be considered

DOSE EQUIVALENCE AND CONVERSION

▸ 4 oral drops (8 mg) is equivalent in therapeutic effect to 10 mg tablet.

- **UNLICENSED USE** Not licensed for use in children.
- **CONTRA-INDICATIONS** QT-interval prolongation
- **CAUTIONS** Known CYP2C19 poor metabolisers (exposure to citalopram is increased) · susceptibility to QT-interval prolongation
- **INTERACTIONS** → Appendix 1: SSRIs
- **SIDE-EFFECTS**
  - ▶ **Common or very common** Acute angle closure glaucoma · apathy · flatulence · hypersalivation · migraine · rhinitis
  - ▶ **Uncommon** Oedema
  - ▶ **Rare or very rare** Cough · generalised tonic-clonic seizure
  - ▶ **Frequency not known** Hypokalaemia
- **BREAST FEEDING** Specialist sources indicate use with caution. Present in milk in small to moderate amounts; long half-life increases risk of accumulation in the infant.
- **HEPATIC IMPAIRMENT**
  Dose adjustments For *tablets* manufacturer advises lower initial doses, may be increased to max. 20 mg daily; use with extra caution and careful dose titration in severe impairment.

  For *oral drops* manufacturer advises lower initial dose, may be increased to max. 16 mg daily; use with extra caution and careful dose titration in severe impairment.
- **RENAL IMPAIRMENT** [EvGr] Use with caution; no information available for creatinine clearance less than 20 mL/minute. (M) See p. 16.
- **TREATMENT CESSATION** The dose should preferably be reduced gradually over about 4 weeks, or longer if withdrawal symptoms emerge (6 months in patients who have been on long-term maintenance treatment).
- **DIRECTIONS FOR ADMINISTRATION** Manufacturer advises *Cipramil*® oral drops should be mixed with water, orange juice, or apple juice before taking.
- **PATIENT AND CARER ADVICE** Counselling on administration of oral drops is advised.
  Driving and skilled tasks Patients should be advised of the effects of citalopram on driving and skilled tasks.

- **MEDICINAL FORMS** There can be variation in the licensing of different medicines containing the same drug.

Oral tablet

▸ **Citalopram (Non-proprietary)**

Citalopram (as Citalopram hydrobromide) 10 mg Citalopram 10mg tablets | 28 tablet [PoM] £9.00 DT = £0.65 | 28 tablet [PoM] [X] DT = £0.65 (Hospital only) | 250 tablet [PoM] £4.65–£7.06

Citalopram (as Citalopram hydrobromide) 20 mg Citalopram 20mg tablets | 28 tablet [PoM] [X] DT = £0.68 (Hospital only) | 28 tablet [PoM] £7.16 DT = £0.68 | 250 tablet [PoM] £6.47–£8.79

Citalopram (as Citalopram hydrobromide) 30 mg Citalopram 30mg tablets | 28 tablet [PoM] £14.40–£25.20

Citalopram (as Citalopram hydrobromide) 40 mg Citalopram 40mg tablets | 28 tablet PoM ⊠ DT = £0.79 (Hospital only) | 28 tablet PoM £3.00 DT = £0.79

▸ **Cipramil** (Lundbeck Ltd)

Citalopram (as Citalopram hydrobromide) 20 mg Cipramil 20mg tablets | 28 tablet PoM £8.95 DT = £0.68

Oral drops

EXCIPIENTS: May contain Ethanol, hydroxybenzoates (parabens)

▸ **Citalopram (Non-proprietary)**

Citalopram (as Citalopram hydrochloride) 40 mg per 1 ml Citalopram 40mg/ml oral drops sugar free | 15 ml PoM £14.09 DT = £8.38 SF

▸ **Cipramil** (Lundbeck Ltd)

Citalopram (as Citalopram hydrochloride) 40 mg per 1 ml Cipramil 40mg/ml drops | 15 ml PoM £10.08 DT = £8.38 SF

286

Fluoxetine

01-May-2023

● **INDICATIONS AND DOSE**

Major depression

▸ BY MOUTH

▸ Child 5–17 years: Initially 10 mg once daily, daily dose may be administered as a divided dose, increased if necessary up to 20 mg once daily, daily dose may be administered as a divided dose; dose may be increased after 1–2 weeks of initial dose

PHARMACOKINETICS

▸ Consider the long half-life of fluoxetine when adjusting dosage (or in overdosage).

● **UNLICENSED USE** EvGr Fluoxetine may be used in children from the age of 5 to 7 years for the treatment of major depression ⟨A⟩, but it is not licensed for this age group

● **INTERACTIONS** → Appendix 1: SSRIs

● **SIDE-EFFECTS**

▸ **Common or very common** Chills · feeling abnormal · postmenopausal haemorrhage · uterine disorder · vasodilation · vision blurred

▸ **Uncommon** Cold sweat · dysphagia · dyspnoea · hypotension · mood altered · muscle twitching · self-injurious behaviour · temperature sensation altered · thinking abnormal

▸ **Rare or very rare** Atelectasis · buccoglossal syndrome · interstitial lung disease · neutropenia · oesophageal pain · pharyngitis · serum sickness · speech disorder · vasculitis

▸ **Frequency not known** Growth retardation

● **BREAST FEEDING** Specialist sources indicate use with caution. Present in milk in moderate to significant amounts; very long half-life increases risk of accumulation in the infant.

● **HEPATIC IMPAIRMENT**

Dose adjustments Manufacturer advises dose reduction or increasing dose interval.

● **DIRECTIONS FOR ADMINISTRATION** Manufacturer advises dispersible tablets can be dispersed in water for administration or swallowed whole with plenty of water.

● **PATIENT AND CARER ADVICE** Patients and carers should be counselled on the administration of dispersible tablets.

Medicines for Children leaflet: Fluoxetine for depression, obsessive compulsive disorder and bulimia nervosa
www.medicinesforchildren.org.uk/medicines/fluoxetine-for-obsessive-compulsive-disorder-ocd-depression-and-bulimia-nervosa/

Driving and skilled tasks Patients should be counselled about the effects on driving and skilled tasks.

● **MEDICINAL FORMS** There can be variation in the licensing of different medicines containing the same drug. Forms available from special-order manufacturers include: oral suspension, oral solution

Oral tablet

▸ **Fluoxetine (Non-proprietary)**

Fluoxetine (as Fluoxetine hydrochloride) 10 mg Fluoxetine 10mg tablets | 30 tablet PoM £104.98 DT = £61.73

Dispersible tablet

CAUTIONARY AND ADVISORY LABELS 10

▸ **Olena** (Advanz Pharma)

Fluoxetine (as Fluoxetine hydrochloride) 20 mg Olena 20mg dispersible tablets | 28 tablet PoM £3.44 DT = £3.44 SF

Oral capsule

▸ **Fluoxetine (Non-proprietary)**

Fluoxetine (as Fluoxetine hydrochloride) 10 mg Fluoxetine 10mg capsules | 30 capsule PoM £53.60 DT = £2.35

Fluoxetine (as Fluoxetine hydrochloride) 20 mg Fluoxetine 20mg capsules | 30 capsule PoM £9.00 DT = £0.82

Fluoxetine (as Fluoxetine hydrochloride) 30 mg Fluoxetine 30mg capsules | 30 capsule PoM £9.99 DT = £1.37

Fluoxetine (as Fluoxetine hydrochloride) 40 mg Fluoxetine 40mg capsules | 30 capsule PoM £4.50 DT = £1.62

Fluoxetine (as Fluoxetine hydrochloride) 60 mg Fluoxetine 60mg capsules | 30 capsule PoM £54.36 DT = £1.23

Oral solution

▸ **Fluoxetine (Non-proprietary)**

Fluoxetine (as Fluoxetine hydrochloride) 4 mg per 1 ml Fluoxetine 20mg/5ml oral solution | 70 ml PoM £20.00 DT = £2.01
Fluoxetine 20mg/5ml oral solution sugar free | 70 ml PoM £12.95 DT = £3.93 SF

▸ **Prozep** (Rosemont Pharmaceuticals Ltd)

Fluoxetine (as Fluoxetine hydrochloride) 4 mg per 1 ml Prozep 20mg/5ml oral solution | 70 ml PoM £12.95 DT = £3.93 SF

286

Fluvoxamine maleate

01-May-2023

● **INDICATIONS AND DOSE**

Obsessive-compulsive disorder

▸ BY MOUTH

▸ Child 8–17 years: Initially 25 mg daily, then increased in steps of 25 mg every 4–7 days (max. per dose 100 mg twice daily) if required, dose to be increased according to response, doses above 50 mg should be given in 2 divided doses, if no improvement in obsessive-compulsive disorder within 10 weeks, treatment should be reconsidered

● **INTERACTIONS** → Appendix 1: SSRIs

● **SIDE-EFFECTS**

▸ **Rare or very rare** Hepatic function abnormal (discontinue)

▸ **Frequency not known** Glaucoma · hypomania · neuroleptic malignant-like syndrome (discontinue—potentially fatal) · withdrawal syndrome neonatal

● **BREAST FEEDING** Specialist sources indicate use with caution. Present in milk in small amounts; long half-life increases risk of accumulation in the infant.

● **HEPATIC IMPAIRMENT**

Dose adjustments Manufacturer advises low initial dose.

● **RENAL IMPAIRMENT**

Dose adjustments EvGr Start with a low dose. ⟨M⟩

● **TREATMENT CESSATION** The dose should preferably be reduced gradually over about 4 weeks, or longer if withdrawal symptoms emerge (6 months in patients who have been on long-term maintenance treatment).

● **PATIENT AND CARER ADVICE**

Driving and skilled tasks Patients should be counselled about the effects on driving and skilled tasks.

- **MEDICINAL FORMS** There can be variation in the licensing of different medicines containing the same drug. Forms available from special-order manufacturers include: oral suspension

Oral tablet

- **Faverin** (Viatris UK Healthcare Ltd)
  Fluvoxamine maleate 50 mg Faverin 50mg tablets | 60 tablet [PoM] £17.10 DT = £17.10
  Fluvoxamine maleate 100 mg Faverin 100mg tablets | 30 tablet [PoM] £17.10 DT = £17.10

F 286

Sertraline

18-Aug-2023

- **INDICATIONS AND DOSE**

Obsessive-compulsive disorder

▶ BY MOUTH

- Child 6–12 years: Initially 25 mg once daily for 1 week, then increased if necessary to 50 mg once daily, dose may be further increased in steps of 50 mg at intervals of at least 1 week up to maximum 200 mg per day
- Child 13–17 years: Initially 50 mg once daily, dose may be increased in steps of 50 mg at intervals of at least 1 week up to maximum 200 mg per day

Major depression

▶ BY MOUTH

- Child 12–17 years: Initially 50 mg once daily, dose may be increased in steps of 50 mg at intervals of at least 1 week up to maximum 200 mg per day

- **UNLICENSED USE** Not licensed for use in children for depression.
- **INTERACTIONS** → Appendix 1: SSRIs
- **SIDE-EFFECTS**
  - **Common or very common** Chest pain · depression · gastrointestinal disorders · increased risk of infection · mood altered · neuromuscular dysfunction · vasodilation
  - **Uncommon** Albuminuria · anaemia · back pain · breast pain · burping · chills · cold sweat · cystitis · dysphagia · dyspnoea · ear pain · eye pain · hypertension · hypothyroidism · migraine · muscle complaints · muscle weakness · oedema · oral disorders · osteoarthritis · periorbital oedema · respiratory disorders · sensation abnormal · speech disorder · thinking abnormal · thirst
  - **Rare or very rare** Balanoposthitis · bone disorder · cardiac disorder · coma · conversion disorder · diabetes mellitus · drug dependence · dysphonia · eye disorders · gait abnormal · genital discharge · glaucoma · hair texture abnormal · hepatic disorders · hiccups · hypercholesterolaemia · hypoglycaemia · injury · lymphadenopathy · myocardial infarction · neoplasms · neuroleptic malignant syndrome · oliguria · peripheral ischaemia · psychotic disorder · rhabdomyolysis · vasodilation procedure · vision disorders · vulvovaginal atrophy
  - **Frequency not known** Cerebrovascular insufficiency · gynaecomastia · hyperglycaemia · interstitial lung disease · pancreatitis
- **BREAST FEEDING** Specialist sources indicate can be used. Present in milk in small amounts; long half-life increases risk of accumulation in the infant.
- **HEPATIC IMPAIRMENT** Manufacturer advises avoid in severe impairment (no information available).
  Dose adjustments Manufacturer advises dose reduction or increasing dose interval in mild to moderate impairment.
- **TREATMENT CESSATION** The dose should preferably be reduced gradually over about 4 weeks, or longer if withdrawal symptoms emerge (6 months in patients who have been on long-term maintenance treatment).
- **DIRECTIONS FOR ADMINISTRATION** [EvGr] Sertraline *concentrate for oral solution* must be diluted before use; the requisite dose is diluted with approximately 120 mL (one glass) of water, ginger ale, lemon/lime soda, lemonade, or orange juice only and taken immediately. ⟨M⟩
- **PATIENT AND CARER ADVICE** Patients or carers should be given advice on how to administer sertraline concentrate for oral solution.
  Medicines for Children leaflet: Sertraline for OCD (obsessive compulsive disorder) and depression www.medicinesforchildren.org.uk/medicines/sertraline-for-obsessive-compulsive-disorder-ocd-and-depression/
  Driving and skilled tasks Patients should be counselled on the effects on driving and skilled tasks.
- **MEDICINAL FORMS** There can be variation in the licensing of different medicines containing the same drug. Forms available from special-order manufacturers include: oral tablet, oral suspension

Oral tablet

- **Sertraline (Non-proprietary)**
  Sertraline (as Sertraline hydrochloride) 25 mg Sertraline 25mg tablets | 28 tablet [PoM] £30.35 DT = £5.52
  Sertraline (as Sertraline hydrochloride) 50 mg Sertraline 50mg tablets | 28 tablet [PoM] £17.82 DT = £0.81 | 250 tablet [PoM] £8.03 | 500 tablet [PoM] £270.48
  Sertraline (as Sertraline hydrochloride) 100 mg Sertraline 100mg tablets | 28 tablet [PoM] £29.16 DT = £0.96 | 250 tablet [PoM] £9.72 | 500 tablet [PoM] £442.61
  Sertraline (as Sertraline hydrochloride) 150 mg Sertraline 150mg tablets | 30 tablet [PoM] £17.82–£25.00 DT = £17.82
  Sertraline (as Sertraline hydrochloride) 200 mg Sertraline 200mg tablets | 30 tablet [PoM] £23.76–£34.00 DT = £23.76
- **Contulen** (HFA Healthcare Ltd)
  Sertraline (as Sertraline hydrochloride) 50 mg Contulen 50mg tablets | 28 tablet [PoM] £17.82 DT = £0.81
  Sertraline (as Sertraline hydrochloride) 100 mg Contulen 100mg tablets | 28 tablet [PoM] £29.16 DT = £0.96
- **Lustral** (Viatris UK Healthcare Ltd)
  Sertraline (as Sertraline hydrochloride) 50 mg Lustral 50mg tablets | 28 tablet [PoM] £17.82 DT = £0.81
  Sertraline (as Sertraline hydrochloride) 100 mg Lustral 100mg tablets | 28 tablet [PoM] £29.16 DT = £0.96

Oral suspension

- **Sertraline (Non-proprietary)**
  Sertraline (as Sertraline hydrochloride) 10 mg per 1 ml Sertraline 50mg/5ml oral suspension sugar free | 150 ml [PoM] £201.80 [SF]

Concentrate for oral solution

CAUTIONARY AND ADVISORY LABELS 13

EXCIPIENTS: May contain Alcohol, butylated hydroxytoluene

- **Sertraline (Non-proprietary)**
  Sertraline (as Sertraline hydrochloride) 20 mg per 1 ml Sertraline 100mg/5ml concentrate for oral solution sugar free | 60 ml [PoM] £78.95–£90.00 [SF] | 150 ml [PoM] £90.00 [SF]

ANTIDEPRESSANTS › TRICYCLIC ANTIDEPRESSANTS

Amitriptyline hydrochloride

20-Oct-2020

- **INDICATIONS AND DOSE**

Neuropathic pain

▶ BY MOUTH

- Child 2–11 years: Initially 200–500 micrograms/kg once daily (max. per dose 10 mg), dose to be taken at night, increased if necessary; maximum 1 mg/kg twice daily on specialist advice
- Child 12–17 years: Initially 10 mg once daily, increased if necessary to 75 mg once daily, dose to be taken at night, dose to be increased gradually, higher doses to be given on specialist advice

- **UNLICENSED USE** Not licensed for use in neuropathic pain.
- **CONTRA-INDICATIONS** Arrhythmias · during manic phase of bipolar disorder · heart block · immediate recovery period after myocardial infarction
- **CAUTIONS** Cardiovascular disease · chronic constipation · diabetes · epilepsy · history of bipolar disorder · history of

psychosis · hyperthyroidism (risk of arrhythmias) · increased intra-ocular pressure · patients with a significant risk of suicide · phaeochromocytoma (risk of arrhythmias) · pyloric stenosis · susceptibility to angle-closure glaucoma · urinary retention

CAUTIONS, FURTHER INFORMATION EvGr Treatment should be stopped if the patient enters a manic phase. (M)

- **INTERACTIONS** → Appendix 1: tricyclic antidepressants
- **SIDE-EFFECTS**
  - **Common or very common** Accommodation disorder · anxiety · arrhythmias · behaviour abnormal · cardiac conduction disorders · concentration impaired · confusion · constipation · dizziness · drowsiness · dry mouth · fatigue · headache · hyperhidrosis · hyponatraemia · movement disorders · mydriasis · nasal congestion · nausea · palpitations · paraesthesia · postural hypotension · QT interval prolongation · sexual dysfunction · speech impairment · taste altered · thirst · tremor · urinary disorders · weight changes
  - **Uncommon** Circulatory collapse · diarrhoea · face oedema · galactorrhoea · heart failure aggravated · hepatic disorders · hypertension · mood altered · oral disorders · seizure · skin reactions · sleep disorders · tinnitus · vomiting
  - **Rare or very rare** Acute glaucoma · agranulocytosis · alopecia · appetite decreased · bone marrow depression · cardiomyopathy · eosinophilia · fever · gynaecomastia · hallucination · interstitial lung disease · leucopenia · paralytic ileus · photosensitivity reaction · polyneuropathy · pulmonary eosinophilia · suicidal behaviours · thrombocytopenia
  - **Frequency not known** Angioedema · anticholinergic syndrome · dry eye · hypersensitivity myocarditis · hyperthermia · increased risk of fracture · severe cutaneous adverse reactions (SCARs)

  Overdose Overdosage with amitriptyline is associated with a relatively high rate of fatality. Symptoms of overdosage may include dry mouth, coma of varying degree, hypotension, hypothermia, hyperreflexia, extensor plantar responses, convulsions, respiratory failure, cardiac conduction defects, and arrhythmias. Dilated pupils and urinary retention also occur. For details on the management of poisoning, see Tricyclic and related antidepressants, under Emergency treatment of poisoning p. 1036.
- **PREGNANCY** Use only if potential benefit outweighs risk.
- **BREAST FEEDING** The amount secreted into breast milk is too small to be harmful.
- **HEPATIC IMPAIRMENT** Manufacturer advises use with caution in mild-to-moderate impairment; avoid in severe impairment.
- **TREATMENT CESSATION** Withdrawal effects may occur within 5 days of stopping treatment with antidepressant drugs; they are usually mild and self-limiting, but in some cases may be severe. The risk of withdrawal symptoms is increased if the antidepressant is stopped suddenly after regular administration for 8 weeks or more. The dose should preferably be reduced gradually over about 4 weeks, or longer if withdrawal symptoms emerge (6 months in patients who have been on long-term maintenance treatment). If possible tricyclic and related antidepressants should be withdrawn slowly.
- **PRESCRIBING AND DISPENSING INFORMATION** Limited quantities of tricyclic antidepressants should be prescribed at any one time because their cardiovascular and epileptogenic effects are dangerous in overdosage.
- **PATIENT AND CARER ADVICE**
  Medicines for Children leaflet: Amitriptyline for neuropathic pain www.medicinesforchildren.org.uk/medicines/amitriptyline-for-neuropathic-pain/

  Driving and skilled tasks Drowsiness may affect the performance of skilled tasks (e.g. driving).
  Effects of alcohol enhanced.
- **MEDICINAL FORMS** There can be variation in the licensing of different medicines containing the same drug. Forms available from special-order manufacturers include: oral suspension, oral solution

Oral tablet

CAUTIONARY AND ADVISORY LABELS 2

- **Amitriptyline hydrochloride (Non-proprietary)**
  Amitriptyline hydrochloride 10 mg Amitriptyline 10mg tablets | 28 tablet PoM £0.79 DT = £0.55
  Amitriptyline hydrochloride 25 mg Amitriptyline 25mg tablets | 28 tablet PoM £0.89 DT = £0.60
  Amitriptyline hydrochloride 50 mg Amitriptyline 50mg tablets | 28 tablet PoM £1.08 DT = £0.68

Oral solution

CAUTIONARY AND ADVISORY LABELS 2

- **Amitriptyline hydrochloride (Non-proprietary)**
  Amitriptyline hydrochloride 2 mg per 1 ml Amitriptyline 10mg/5ml oral solution sugar free | 150 ml PoM £122.76 DT = £38.17 SF
  Amitriptyline hydrochloride 5 mg per 1 ml Amitriptyline 25mg/5ml oral solution sugar free | 150 ml PoM £18.00 DT = £10.48 SF
  Amitriptyline hydrochloride 10 mg per 1 ml Amitriptyline 50mg/5ml oral solution sugar free | 150 ml PoM £24.00 DT = £15.75 SF

Doxepin

20-Apr-2021

- **INDICATIONS AND DOSE**

  Depressive illness (particularly where sedation is required)

  ▶ BY MOUTH
  - Child 12–17 years: Initially 75 mg daily in divided doses, alternatively 75 mg once daily, adjusted according to response, dose to be taken at bedtime; maintenance 25–300 mg daily, doses above 100 mg given in 3 divided doses
- **CONTRA-INDICATIONS** Acute porphyrias p. 745 · during manic phase of bipolar disorder
- **CAUTIONS** Arrhythmias · cardiovascular disease · chronic constipation · diabetes · epilepsy · heart block · history of bipolar disorder · history of psychosis · hyperthyroidism (risk of arrhythmias) · immediate recovery period after myocardial infarction · patients with significant risk of suicide · phaeochromocytoma (risk of arrhythmias) · susceptibility to angle-closure glaucoma · urinary retention

  CAUTIONS, FURTHER INFORMATION Treatment should be stopped if the patient enters a manic phase.
- **INTERACTIONS** → Appendix 1: tricyclic antidepressants
- **SIDE-EFFECTS** Agitation · agranulocytosis · alopecia · anticholinergic syndrome · appetite decreased · asthenia · asthma exacerbated · bone marrow depression · breast enlargement · cardiovascular effects · chills · confusion · constipation · diarrhoea · dizziness · drowsiness · dry mouth · dyspepsia · eosinophilia · face oedema · flushing · galactorrhoea · gynaecomastia · haemolytic anaemia · hallucination · headache · hyperhidrosis · hyperpyrexia · increased risk of fracture · jaundice · leucopenia · mania · movement disorders · nausea · oral ulceration · paranoid delusions · photosensitivity reaction · postural hypotension · psychosis · seizure · sensation abnormal · sexual dysfunction · SIADH · skin reactions · sleep disorders · suicidal behaviours · tachycardia · taste altered · testicular swelling · thrombocytopenia · tinnitus · tremor · urinary retention · vision blurred · vomiting · weight increased · withdrawal syndrome (in neonates)

  Overdose Tricyclic and related antidepressants cause dry mouth, coma of varying degree, hypotension, hypothermia, hyperreflexia, extensor plantar responses, convulsions, respiratory failure, cardiac conduction defects, and arrhythmias. Dilated pupils and urinary retention also occur. For details on the management of poisoning see Tricyclic and related antidepressants under Emergency treatment of poisoning p. 1036.

- **PREGNANCY** Use with caution—limited information available.
- **BREAST FEEDING** The amount secreted into breast milk is too small to be harmful. Accumulation of metabolite may cause sedation and respiratory depression in neonate.
- **HEPATIC IMPAIRMENT** Manufacturer advises caution in mild to moderate impairment; avoid in severe impairment.
  Dose adjustments Manufacturer advises consider dose reduction in mild to moderate impairment.
- **RENAL IMPAIRMENT** EvGr Use with caution. ⟨M⟩
  Dose adjustments EvGr Consider dose reduction. ⟨M⟩
- **TREATMENT CESSATION** Withdrawal effects may occur within 5 days of stopping treatment with antidepressant drugs; they are usually mild and self-limiting, but in some cases may be severe. The risk of withdrawal symptoms is increased if the antidepressant is stopped suddenly after regular administration for 8 weeks or more. The dose should preferably be reduced gradually over about 4 weeks, or longer if withdrawal symptoms emerge (6 months in patients who have been on long-term maintenance treatment). If possible tricyclic and related antidepressants should be withdrawn slowly.
- **PRESCRIBING AND DISPENSING INFORMATION** Limited quantities of tricyclic antidepressants should be prescribed at any one time because their cardiovascular and epileptogenic effects are dangerous in overdosage.
- **PATIENT AND CARER ADVICE**
  Driving and skilled tasks Drowsiness may affect performance of skilled tasks (e.g. driving).
  Effects of alcohol enhanced.

- **MEDICINAL FORMS** There can be variation in the licensing of different medicines containing the same drug. Forms available from special-order manufacturers include: oral suspension, oral solution

Oral capsule

CAUTIONARY AND ADVISORY LABELS 2

- Doxepin (Non-proprietary)
  Doxepin (as Doxepin hydrochloride) 10 mg Doxepin 10mg capsules | 28 capsule PoM £81.50–£146.70 DT = £81.50
  Doxepin (as Doxepin hydrochloride) 25 mg Doxepin 25mg capsules | 28 capsule PoM £97.00 DT = £5.00
  Doxepin (as Doxepin hydrochloride) 50 mg Doxepin 50mg capsules | 28 capsule PoM £154.00 DT = £6.19

Imipramine hydrochloride

10-Nov-2021

- **INDICATIONS AND DOSE**

Nocturnal enuresis

▶ BY MOUTH

- Child 6–7 years: 25 mg once daily, to be taken at bedtime, initial period of treatment (including gradual withdrawal) 3 months—full physical examination before further course
- Child 8–10 years: 25–50 mg once daily, to be taken at bedtime, initial period of treatment (including gradual withdrawal) 3 months—full physical examination before further course
- Child 11–17 years: 50–75 mg once daily, to be taken at bedtime, initial period of treatment (including gradual withdrawal) 3 months—full physical examination before further course

Attention deficit hyperactivity disorder (under expert supervision)

▶ BY MOUTH

- Child 6–17 years: 10–30 mg twice daily

- **UNLICENSED USE** Not licensed for use for attention deficit hyperactivity disorder.
- **CONTRA-INDICATIONS** Acute porphyrias p. 745 · arrhythmia · during the manic phase of bipolar disorder · heart block · immediate recovery period after myocardial infarction
- **CAUTIONS** Cardiovascular disease · chronic constipation · diabetes · epilepsy · history of bipolar disorder · history of psychosis · hyperthyroidism (risk of arrhythmias) · increased intra-ocular pressure · patients with a significant risk of suicide · phaeochromocytoma (risk of arrhythmias) · susceptibility to angle-closure glaucoma · urinary retention
  CAUTIONS, FURTHER INFORMATION EvGr Treatment should be stopped if the patient enters a manic phase. ⟨M⟩
- **INTERACTIONS** → Appendix 1: tricyclic antidepressants
- **SIDE-EFFECTS**
  - **Common or very common** Anxiety · appetite decreased · arrhythmias · asthenia · cardiac conduction disorders · confusion · delirium · depression · dizziness · drowsiness · epilepsy · hallucination · headache · hepatic disorders · mood altered · nausea · palpitations · paraesthesia · postural hypotension · sexual dysfunction · skin reactions · sleep disorder · tremor · vomiting · weight changes
  - **Uncommon** Psychosis
  - **Rare or very rare** Aggression · agranulocytosis · alopecia · bone marrow depression · enlarged mammary gland · eosinophilia · fever · galactorrhoea · gastrointestinal disorders · glaucoma · heart failure · interstitial lung disease · leucopenia · movement disorders · mydriasis · oedema · oral disorders · peripheral vasospastic reaction · photosensitivity reaction · SIADH · speech disorder · thrombocytopenia
  - **Frequency not known** Anticholinergic syndrome · cardiovascular effects · drug fever · hyponatraemia · increased risk of fracture · neurological effects · paranoid delusions exacerbated · psychiatric disorder · respiratory depression (in neonates) · suicidal behaviours · tinnitus · urinary disorder · withdrawal symptoms

  Overdose Tricyclic and related antidepressants cause dry mouth, coma of varying degree, hypotension, hypothermia, hyperreflexia, extensor plantar responses, convulsions, respiratory failure, cardiac conduction defects, and arrhythmias. Dilated pupils and urinary retention also occur. For details on the management of poisoning see Tricyclic and related antidepressants under Emergency treatment of poisoning p. 1036.
- **PREGNANCY** Colic, tachycardia, dyspnoea, irritability, muscle spasms, respiratory depression and withdrawal symptoms reported in neonates when used in the third trimester.
- **BREAST FEEDING** The amount secreted into breast milk is too small to be harmful.
- **HEPATIC IMPAIRMENT** Manufacturer advises caution in mild to moderate impairment; avoid in severe impairment.
- **RENAL IMPAIRMENT** EvGr Caution in severe impairment. ⟨M⟩
- **TREATMENT CESSATION** Withdrawal effects may occur within 5 days of stopping treatment with antidepressant drugs; they are usually mild and self-limiting, but in some cases may be severe. The risk of withdrawal symptoms is increased if the antidepressant is stopped suddenly after regular administration for 8 weeks or more. The dose should preferably be reduced gradually over about 4 weeks, or longer if withdrawal symptoms emerge (6 months in patients who have been on long-term maintenance treatment). If possible tricyclic antidepressants should be withdrawn slowly.
- **PRESCRIBING AND DISPENSING INFORMATION** Limited quantities of tricyclic antidepressants should be prescribed at any one time because their cardiovascular and

epileptogenic effects are dangerous in overdosage.

- **PATIENT AND CARER ADVICE**
Medicines for Children leaflet: Imipramine for various conditions www.medicinesforchildren.org.uk/medicines/imipramine/
Driving and skilled tasks Drowsiness may affect the performance of skilled tasks (e.g. driving).
Effects of alcohol enhanced.

- **MEDICINAL FORMS** There can be variation in the licensing of different medicines containing the same drug. Forms available from special-order manufacturers include: oral suspension, oral solution

Oral tablet

CAUTIONARY AND ADVISORY LABELS 2

▸ **Imipramine hydrochloride (Non-proprietary)**
Imipramine hydrochloride 10 mg Imipramine 10mg tablets | 28 tablet PoM £6.30 DT = £3.63
Imipramine hydrochloride 25 mg Imipramine 25mg tablets | 28 tablet PoM £5.72 DT = £2.38

Oral solution

CAUTIONARY AND ADVISORY LABELS 2

▸ **Imipramine hydrochloride (Non-proprietary)**
Imipramine hydrochloride 5 mg per 1 ml Imipramine 25mg/5ml oral solution sugar free | 150 ml PoM £250.00 DT = £250.00 SF

Nortriptyline

07-Nov-2020

- **INDICATIONS AND DOSE**

Depressive illness

▸ BY MOUTH

▸ Child 12–17 years: To be initiated at a low dose, then increased if necessary to 30–50 mg daily in divided doses, alternatively increased if necessary to 30–50 mg once daily; maximum 150 mg per day

- **CONTRA-INDICATIONS** Arrhythmias · during the manic phase of bipolar disorder · heart block · immediate recovery period after myocardial infarction
- **CAUTIONS** Cardiovascular disease · chronic constipation · diabetes · epilepsy · history of bipolar disorder · history of psychosis · hyperthyroidism (risk of arrhythmias) · increased intra-ocular pressure · patients with a significant risk of suicide · phaeochromocytoma (risk of arrhythmias) · susceptibility to angle-closure glaucoma · urinary retention

CAUTIONS, FURTHER INFORMATION EvGr Treatment should be stopped if the patient enters a manic phase. Ⓜ

- **INTERACTIONS** → Appendix 1: tricyclic antidepressants
- **SIDE-EFFECTS**

▸ **Common or very common** Hypotension

▸ **Frequency not known** Agranulocytosis · alopecia · anxiety · appetite decreased · arrhythmias · asthenia · atrioventricular block · bone marrow disorders · breast enlargement · confusion · constipation · delusions · diarrhoea · dizziness · drowsiness · drug cross-reactivity · drug fever · dry mouth · eosinophilia · fever · flushing · galactorrhoea · gastrointestinal discomfort · gynaecomastia · hallucination · headache · hepatic disorders · hyperhidrosis · hypertension · hypomania · increased risk of fracture · increased risk of infection · malaise · movement disorders · mydriasis · myocardial infarction · nausea · oedema · oral disorders · palpitations · paralytic ileus · peripheral neuropathy · photosensitivity reaction · psychosis exacerbated · seizure · sensation abnormal · sexual dysfunction · SIADH · skin reactions · sleep disorders · stroke · suicidal behaviours · taste altered · testicular swelling · thrombocytopenia · tinnitus · tremor · urinary disorders · urinary tract dilation · vision disorders · vomiting · weight changes

Overdose Tricyclic and related antidepressants cause dry mouth, coma of varying degree, hypotension, hypothermia, hyperreflexia, extensor plantar responses, convulsions, respiratory failure, cardiac conduction defects, and arrhythmias. Dilated pupils and urinary retention also occur. For details on the management of poisoning see Tricyclic and related antidepressants under Emergency treatment of poisoning p. 1036.

- **PREGNANCY** Use only if potential benefit outweighs risk.
- **BREAST FEEDING** The amount secreted into breast milk is too small to be harmful.
- **HEPATIC IMPAIRMENT** Manufacture advises avoid in severe impairment.
- **MONITORING REQUIREMENTS**

▸ Manufacturer advises plasma-nortriptyline concentration monitoring if dose above 100 mg daily, but evidence of practical value uncertain.

- **TREATMENT CESSATION** Withdrawal effects may occur within 5 days of stopping treatment with antidepressant drugs; they are usually mild and self-limiting, but in some cases may be severe. The risk of withdrawal symptoms is increased if the antidepressant is stopped suddenly after regular administration for 8 weeks or more. The dose should preferably be reduced gradually over about 4 weeks, or longer if withdrawal symptoms emerge (6 months in patients who have been on long-term maintenance treatment). If possible tricyclic and related antidepressants should be withdrawn slowly.
- **PRESCRIBING AND DISPENSING INFORMATION** Limited quantities of tricyclic antidepressants should be prescribed at any one time because their cardiovascular and epileptogenic effects are dangerous in overdosage.
- **PATIENT AND CARER ADVICE** Drowsiness may affect the performance of skilled tasks (e.g. driving). Effects of alcohol enhanced.

- **MEDICINAL FORMS** There can be variation in the licensing of different medicines containing the same drug. Forms available from special-order manufacturers include: oral suspension, oral solution

Oral tablet

CAUTIONARY AND ADVISORY LABELS 2

▸ **Nortriptyline (Non-proprietary)**
Nortriptyline (as Nortriptyline hydrochloride) 10 mg Nortriptyline 10mg tablets | 28 tablet PoM £2.14 | 84 tablet PoM £6.42 | 100 tablet PoM £33.41 DT = £2.74
Nortriptyline (as Nortriptyline hydrochloride) 25 mg Nortriptyline 25mg tablets | 28 tablet PoM £2.46 | 84 tablet PoM £7.38 | 100 tablet PoM £35.22 DT = £2.46
Nortriptyline (as Nortriptyline hydrochloride) 50 mg Nortriptyline 50mg tablets | 30 tablet PoM £84.50 DT = £46.48

2.4 Psychoses and schizophrenia

Psychoses and related disorders

15-Feb-2021

Overview

There is little information on the efficacy and safety of antipsychotic drugs in children and adolescents and much of the information available has been extrapolated from adult data; in particular, little is known about the long-term effects of antipsychotic drugs at a vulnerable phase of physical growth and development. Antipsychotic drugs should be initiated and managed under the close supervision of an appropriate specialist.

Antipsychotic drugs, formally called 'major tranquillisers', are also known as neuroleptics. They have varying effects and properties; these include sedative, anxiolytic, antimanic, mood stabilising, and antidepressant properties. Antipsychotic drugs are used for a number of mental health disorders, mainly schizophrenia, and mania and hypomania, but may also be used in severe or difficult to treat depression in young people.

Schizophrenia

Psychosis and the specific diagnosis of schizophrenia in children and young people represent a major psychiatric disorder, or cluster of disorders that alters a person's perception, thoughts, mood, and behaviour. The symptoms of psychosis are usually divided into 'positive symptoms' such as hallucinations and delusions, and 'negative symptoms' such as emotional apathy and social withdrawal. Each patient will have a unique combination of symptoms and experiences. Typically, in child and adolescent-onset psychosis and schizophrenia, there is a prodromal period lasting up to 12 months. This is characterised by a deterioration in personal functioning and the onset of transient mild negative symptoms; most children with these symptoms do not go on to develop psychosis or schizophrenia, although they may be at higher risk of developing psychosis and schizophrenia at a later date.

The initial aim of treatment is to reduce acute phase symptoms and return the child to their baseline level of functioning.

EvGr An oral antipsychotic drug should be offered to children and young patients with schizophrenia in combination with psychological therapy, under specialist supervision. The choice of drug depends on factors such as the potential to cause extrapyramidal symptoms (including akathisia), cardiovascular adverse effects, metabolic adverse effects (including weight gain and diabetes), hormonal adverse effects (including increase in prolactin concentration), and patient and carer preference. Treatment with an antipsychotic drug should be considered an explicit individual therapeutic trial; doses should be started low and slowly titrated up to the minimum effective dose according to patient response and tolerability. Children should receive an antipsychotic drug at optimum dose for 4–6 weeks before it is deemed ineffective.

Prescribing more than one antipsychotic drug at a time should be avoided except in exceptional circumstances (e.g. clozapine augmentation or when changing medication during titration) because of the increased risk of adverse effects such as extrapyramidal symptoms, QT-interval prolongation, and sudden cardiac death. It is important to record reasons for continuing, changing, and stopping treatment, and the effects of such changes, including side-effects experienced.

Clozapine p. 301 [unlicensed in children aged under 16 years] can be offered if schizophrenia is not controlled despite the sequential use of at least 2 different antipsychotic drugs, each used for 6–8 weeks. If symptoms do not respond adequately to an optimised dose of clozapine, consider other causes of non-response (e.g. adherence to therapy, concurrent use of other drugs), review diagnosis, and check plasma-clozapine concentration before adding a second antipsychotic drug to augment clozapine; allow 8–10 weeks' treatment to assess response. Ⓐ EvGr Children must be registered with a clozapine patient monitoring service. Ⓜ

Antipsychotic drugs

First-generation antipsychotic drugs

The first-generation antipsychotic drugs (also known as typical or conventional) act predominantly by blocking dopamine D_2 receptors in the brain. They are more likely to cause a range of side-effects, particularly acute extrapyramidal symptoms and hyperprolactinaemia.

First-generation antipsychotics include the **phenothiazine** derivatives (chlorpromazine hydrochloride p. 295, levomepromazine p. 321, pericyazine p. 297, prochlorperazine p. 322, and trifluoperazine p. 298), the **butyrophenones** (haloperidol p. 296), the **diphenylbutylpiperidines** (pimozide p. 297) and the **substituted benzamides** (sulpiride p. 298).

Second-generation antipsychotic drugs

The second-generation antipsychotic drugs (also referred to as atypical) act on a range of receptors in comparison to first-generation antipsychotic drugs and are generally associated with a lower risk for acute extrapyramidal symptoms and tardive dyskinesia; the extent varies between individual drugs. However, second-generation antipsychotic drugs are associated with several other important adverse effects, such as weight gain and glucose intolerance.

Prescribing high-dose antipsychotic drugs

A *high-dose* antipsychotic is defined as a total daily dose of a single antipsychotic drug which exceeds the maximum licensed dose with respect to the age of the patient and the indication being treated, or a total daily dose of two or more antipsychotic drugs which exceeds the maximum licensed dose using the percentage method.

For further information and advice on prescribing high-dose antipsychotic medication, see The Royal College of Psychiatrists consensus statement available at www.rcpsych.ac.uk/.

There is no robust evidence that high doses of antipsychotic drug treatment is any more effective than standard doses for the treatment of schizophrenia. The majority of adverse effects associated with antipsychotic treatment are dose-related and there is clear evidence for a greater side-effect burden with high-dose antipsychotic drug use. Antipsychotic polypharmacy and 'when required' antipsychotic treatment are strongly associated with high-dose prescribing.

Important: When prescribing an antipsychotic for administration in an emergency situation (e.g. for rapid tranquillisation), the aim of treatment is to calm and sedate the patient without inducing sleep. EvGr The initial prescription should be written as a single dose, and not repeated until the effects of the initial dose has been reviewed. Oral and intramuscular drugs should be prescribed separately. The patient must be monitored for side-effects and vital signs at least every hour until there are no further concerns about their physical health status. Monitor the patient every 15 minutes if a high-dose antipsychotic drug has been given. Ⓐ

Prescribing of antipsychotic drugs in children with learning disabilities

EvGr In children with learning disabilities who are taking antipsychotic drugs and not experiencing psychotic symptoms, the following considerations should be taken into account:

- a reduction in dose or the discontinuation of long-term antipsychotic treatment;
- review of the child's condition after dose reduction or discontinuation of an antipsychotic drug;
- referral to a psychiatrist experienced in working with children who have learning disabilities and mental health problems;
- annual documentation of the reasons for continuing a prescription if the antipsychotic drug is not reduced in dose or discontinued. Ⓐ

Side-effects and choice of antipsychotic drug

There is little difference in efficacy between each of the antipsychotic drugs (other than clozapine p. 301), and response and tolerability to each antipsychotic drug varies. EvGr There is no first-line antipsychotic drug which is suitable for all children and the properties of individual antipsychotic drugs should be considered and discussed with the child or carers when prescribing. Ⓐ

Both first-generation and second-generation antipsychotic drugs are associated with side-effects which are common and contribute significantly to non-adherence and treatment discontinuation.

Extrapyramidal symptoms

Extrapyramidal symptoms are dose-related and are most likely to occur with high doses of high-potency first-generation antipsychotics such as the piperazine phenothiazines (trifluoperazine p. 298), and the butyrophenones (haloperidol p. 296). They are less common with some second-generation antipsychotics which have a lower liability for both acute and late onset EPS; particularly clozapine, olanzapine p. 303, quetiapine p. 304, and aripiprazole p. 300. Extrapyramidal symptoms cannot be predicted accurately because they depend on the dose, the class of antipsychotic drug, and on individual susceptibility.

Extrapyramidal symptoms consist of:

- *parkinsonian symptoms* (including bradykinesia, tremor), which may occur more commonly in females and may appear gradually;
- *dystonia* (uncontrolled muscle spasm in any part of the body), which occurs more commonly in children or young males; acute dystonia can appear within hours of starting antipsychotics;
- *akathisia* (restlessness), which characteristically occurs within hours to weeks of starting antipsychotic treatment or on dose increase and may be mistaken for psychotic agitation;
- *tardive dyskinesia* (abnormal involuntary movements of lips, tongue, face, and jaw), which can develop on long-term or high-dose therapy, or even after discontinuation; in some patients it can be irreversible.

EvGr When *parkinsonian* symptoms are identified, treatment should be reviewed with the aim of reducing exposure to high-dose and high-potency antipsychotic drugs. Although antimuscarinic drugs can relieve symptom burden, they should not be routinely prescribed for prophylaxis with antipsychotic drugs. Ⓐ

Tardive dyskinesia is the most serious manifestation of late-onset extrapyramidal symptoms for which there is no satisfactory treatment. EvGr Antipsychotic treatment should be carefully and regularly reviewed; any changes to dose or drug should be made gradually, over weeks or months, to minimise the risk of withdrawal tardive dyskinesia. Ⓐ However, some manufacturers suggest that drug withdrawal at the earliest signs of tardive dyskinesia (fine vermicular movements of the tongue) may halt its full development.

Hyperprolactinaemia

Most antipsychotic drugs, both first- and second-generation, increase prolactin concentration to some extent because dopamine inhibits prolactin release. Aripiprazole reduces prolactin concentration in a dose-dependent manner because it is a dopamine-receptor partial agonist. Risperidone p. 306, amisulpride p. 299, sulpiride p. 298, and first-generation antipsychotic drugs are most likely to cause symptomatic hyperprolactinaemia. Hyperprolactinaemia is very rare with aripiprazole, clozapine, and quetiapine treatment.

The clinical symptoms of hyperprolactinaemia include sexual dysfunction, reduced bone mineral density, menstrual disturbances, breast enlargement, galactorrhoea, and a possible increased risk of breast cancer.

Sexual dysfunction

Sexual dysfunction is reported as a side-effect of all antipsychotic medication; physical illness, psychiatric illness, and substance misuse are contributing factors. Antipsychotic-induced sexual dysfunction is caused by more than one mechanism. Reduced dopamine transmission and hyperprolactinaemia decrease libido; antimuscarinic effects can cause disorders of arousal; and alpha$_1$-adrenoceptor antagonists are associated with erection and ejaculation problems in men. Risperidone, haloperidol and olanzapine have a higher prevalence to cause sexual dysfunction. The antipsychotic drugs with the lowest risk of sexual dysfunction are aripiprazole and quetiapine.

Expert sources advise to consider dose reduction or discontinuation (where appropriate), or switching medication if sexual dysfunction is thought to be antipsychotic-induced.

Cardiovascular side-effects

Antipsychotic drugs have been associated with cardiovascular side-effects such as tachycardia, arrhythmias, and hypotension. QT-interval prolongation is a particular concern with pimozide p. 297. Overall risk is probably dose-related but there is also a higher probability of QT-interval prolongation in patients using any intravenous antipsychotic drug, or any antipsychotic drug or combination of antipsychotic drugs with doses exceeding the recommended maximum.

Antipsychotic drugs with a low tendency to prolong QT interval include aripiprazole, clozapine, olanzapine, risperidone, and sulpiride.

Hypotension

Postural hypotension is a common cardiac side-effect of antipsychotics usually presenting acutely during the initial dose titration; however it can be a chronic problem. Postural hypotension can lead to syncope and dangerous falls. The second-generation antipsychotics most likely to cause postural hypotension are clozapine and quetiapine. Slow dose titration is commonly used to minimise postural hypotension.

Hyperglycaemia and diabetes

Schizophrenia is associated with insulin resistance and diabetes; the risk of diabetes is probably increased in children with schizophrenia who take antipsychotic drugs. Some evidence suggests first-generation antipsychotic drugs are less likely to cause diabetes than second-generation antipsychotic drugs, and of the first-generation antipsychotic drugs, haloperidol has the lowest risk. Amisulpride and aripiprazole have the lowest risk of diabetes of the second-generation antipsychotic drugs.

Weight gain

There is some concern that children may be more sensitive than adults to the potential of antipsychotic drugs to cause weight gain and metabolic effects. Clozapine and olanzapine commonly cause weight gain. Amisulpride, aripiprazole, haloperidol, sulpiride, and trifluoperazine are least likely to cause weight gain.

Olanzapine is associated with more weight gain than other second-generation antipsychotic drugs. Weight gain happens soon after treatment with olanzapine has started.

Neuroleptic malignant syndrome

Neuroleptic malignant syndrome (hyperthermia, fluctuating level of consciousness, muscle rigidity, and autonomic dysfunction with fever, tachycardia, labile blood pressure, and sweating) is a rare but potentially fatal side-effect of all antipsychotic drugs.

Expert sources advise discontinuation of the antipsychotic drug is essential for at least 5 days, preferably longer. The signs and symptoms of neuroleptic malignant syndrome should be allowed to resolve completely. Bromocriptine and dantrolene have been used for treatment.

Monitoring

Expert sources advise to monitor full blood counts, urea and electrolytes, and liver function test at the start of therapy with antipsychotic drugs, and then yearly thereafter.

EvGr Blood lipids, prolactin concentration, fasting blood glucose and HbA$_{1c}$ should be measured at baseline, at 12 weeks, and then every 6 months thereafter.

Weight should be measured at baseline, weekly during the first 6 weeks, at 12 weeks, and then every 6 months thereafter.

Before initiating antipsychotic drugs, an ECG may be required, particularly if physical examination identifies cardiovascular risk factors (e.g. high blood pressure), if there is a personal history of cardiovascular disease, or if the child is being admitted as an inpatient.

Blood pressure monitoring is advised before starting therapy, at 12 weeks and every 6 months thereafter; (A) expert sources advise to also monitor blood pressure during dose titration of antipsychotic drugs.

MHRA/CHM advice: Clozapine and other antipsychotics
The MHRA/CHM have released important safety information regarding antipsychotics and monitoring blood concentrations for toxicity. For further information, see *Important safety information* in the amisulpride p. 299, aripiprazole p. 300, clozapine p. 301, olanzapine p. 303, quetiapine p. 304, risperidone p. 306, and sulpiride p. 298 monographs.

ANTIPSYCHOTICS

Antipsychotic drugs

● **CAUTIONS** Blood dyscrasias · cardiovascular disease · conditions predisposing to seizures · depression · diabetes (may raise blood glucose) · epilepsy · history of jaundice · myasthenia gravis · photosensitisation (may occur with higher dosages) · severe respiratory disease · susceptibility to angle-closure glaucoma

CAUTIONS, FURTHER INFORMATION
- **Cardiovascular disease** An ECG may be required, particularly if physical examination identifies cardiovascular risk factors, personal history of cardiovascular disease, or if the patient is being admitted as an inpatient.

● **SIDE-EFFECTS**
- **Common or very common** Agitation · amenorrhoea · arrhythmias · constipation · dizziness · drowsiness · dry mouth · erectile dysfunction · fatigue · galactorrhoea · gynaecomastia · hyperglycaemia · hyperprolactinaemia · hypersalivation · hypotension (dose-related) · insomnia · leucopenia · movement disorders · muscle rigidity · neutropenia · parkinsonism · postural hypotension (dose-related) · QT interval prolongation · rash · seizure · tremor · urinary retention · vomiting · weight increased
- **Uncommon** Agranulocytosis · confusion · neuroleptic malignant syndrome (discontinue—potentially fatal)
- **Rare or very rare** Sudden death · withdrawal syndrome neonatal

Overdose Phenothiazines cause less depression of consciousness and respiration than other sedatives. Hypotension, hypothermia, sinus tachycardia, and arrhythmias may complicate poisoning. For details on the management of poisoning see Antipsychotics under Emergency treatment of poisoning p. 1036.

● **PREGNANCY** Extrapyramidal effects and withdrawal syndrome have been reported occasionally in the neonate when antipsychotic drugs are taken during the third trimester of pregnancy. Following maternal use of antipsychotic drugs in the third trimester, neonates should be monitored for symptoms including agitation, hypertonia, hypotonia, tremor, drowsiness, feeding problems, and respiratory distress.

● **BREAST FEEDING** There is limited information available on the short- and long-term effects of antipsychotic drugs on the breast-fed infant. *Animal studies* indicate possible adverse effects of antipsychotic medicines on the developing nervous system. Chronic treatment with antipsychotic drugs whilst breast-feeding should be avoided unless absolutely necessary. Phenothiazine derivatives are sometimes used in breast-feeding women for short-term treatment of nausea and vomiting.

● **MONITORING REQUIREMENTS**
- It is advisable to monitor prolactin concentration at the start of therapy, at 6 months, and then yearly. Patients taking antipsychotic drugs not normally associated with symptomatic hyperprolactinaemia should be considered for prolactin monitoring if they show symptoms of hyperprolactinaemia (such as breast enlargement and galactorrhoea).
- Patients with schizophrenia should have physical health monitoring (including cardiovascular disease risk assessment) at least once per year.
- Regular clinical monitoring of endocrine function should be considered when children are taking an antipsychotic drug known to increase prolactin levels; this includes measuring weight and height, assessing sexual maturation, and monitoring menstrual function.

● **TREATMENT CESSATION** There is a high risk of relapse if medication is stopped after 1–2 years. Withdrawal of antipsychotic drugs after long-term therapy should always be gradual and closely monitored to avoid the risk of acute withdrawal syndromes or rapid relapse. Patients should be monitored for 2 years after withdrawal of antipsychotic medication for signs and symptoms of relapse.

● **PATIENT AND CARER ADVICE** As photosensitisation may occur with higher dosages, patients should avoid direct sunlight.

Driving and skilled tasks Drowsiness may affect performance of skilled tasks (e.g. driving or operating machinery), especially at start of treatment; effects of alcohol are enhanced.

ANTIPSYCHOTICS > FIRST-GENERATION

above

Chlorpromazine hydrochloride

27-Jun-2023

● **INDICATIONS AND DOSE**

Childhood schizophrenia and other psychoses (under expert supervision)
- BY MOUTH
- Child 1-5 years: 500 micrograms/kg every 4–6 hours, adjusted according to response; maximum 40 mg per day
- Child 6-11 years: 10 mg 3 times a day, adjusted according to response; maximum 75 mg per day
- Child 12-17 years: Initially 25 mg 3 times a day, adjusted according to response, alternatively initially 75 mg once daily, adjusted according to response, dose to be taken at night; maintenance 75–300 mg daily, increased if necessary up to 1 g daily

Relief of acute symptoms of psychoses (under expert supervision)
- BY DEEP INTRAMUSCULAR INJECTION
- Child 1-5 years: 500 micrograms/kg every 6–8 hours; maximum 40 mg per day
- Child 6-11 years: 500 micrograms/kg every 6–8 hours; maximum 75 mg per day
- Child 12-17 years: 25–50 mg every 6–8 hours

Nausea and vomiting in palliative care (where other drugs have failed or are not available)
- BY MOUTH
- Child 1-5 years: 500 micrograms/kg every 4–6 hours; maximum 40 mg per day
- Child 6-11 years: 500 micrograms/kg every 4–6 hours; maximum 75 mg per day
- Child 12-17 years: 10–25 mg every 4–6 hours
- BY DEEP INTRAMUSCULAR INJECTION
- Child 1-5 years: 500 micrograms/kg every 6–8 hours; maximum 40 mg per day
- Child 6-11 years: 500 micrograms/kg every 6–8 hours; maximum 75 mg per day
- Child 12-17 years: Initially 25 mg, then 25–50 mg every 3–4 hours until vomiting stops

continued →

DOSE EQUIVALENCE AND CONVERSION
- For equivalent therapeutic effect 100 mg chlorpromazine base given *rectally* as a suppository ≡ 20–25 mg chlorpromazine hydrochloride *by intramuscular injection* ≡ 40–50 mg of chlorpromazine base or hydrochloride given *by mouth*.

- **CONTRA-INDICATIONS** CNS depression · comatose states · hypothyroidism · phaeochromocytoma
- **CAUTIONS** Susceptibility to QT interval prolongation
- **INTERACTIONS** → Appendix 1: phenothiazine antipsychotics
- **SIDE-EFFECTS**

GENERAL SIDE-EFFECTS
- **Common or very common** Anxiety · glucose tolerance impaired · mood altered · muscle tone increased
- **Frequency not known** Accommodation disorder · angioedema · atrioventricular block · cardiac arrest · embolism and thrombosis · eye deposit · eye disorders · gastrointestinal disorders · hepatic disorders · hypertriglyceridaemia · hyponatraemia · photosensitivity reaction · respiratory disorders · sexual dysfunction · SIADH · skin reactions · systemic lupus erythematosus (SLE) · temperature regulation disorder · trismus

SPECIFIC SIDE-EFFECTS
- With intramuscular use Nasal congestion

SIDE-EFFECTS, FURTHER INFORMATION Acute dystonic reactions may occur; children are particularly susceptible.

- **HEPATIC IMPAIRMENT** Manufacturer advises caution in severe hepatic failure (increased risk of accumulation).
- **RENAL IMPAIRMENT** EvGr Caution in severe renal failure (risk of accumulation). (M)
- **MONITORING REQUIREMENTS**
  - With intramuscular use Patients should remain supine, with blood pressure monitoring for 30 minutes after intramuscular injection.
- **PRESCRIBING AND DISPENSING INFORMATION**

Palliative care For further information on the use of chlorpromazine hydrochloride in palliative care, see www.medicinescomplete.com/#/content/palliative/antipsychotics.

- **HANDLING AND STORAGE** Owing to the risk of contact sensitisation, pharmacists, nurses, and other health workers should avoid direct contact with chlorpromazine; tablets should not be crushed and solutions should be handled with care.

- **MEDICINAL FORMS** There can be variation in the licensing of different medicines containing the same drug. Forms available from special-order manufacturers include: oral capsule, oral suspension, oral solution, suppository

Oral tablet

CAUTIONARY AND ADVISORY LABELS 2, 11
- Chlorpromazine hydrochloride (Non-proprietary)
  Chlorpromazine hydrochloride 10 mg Chlorpromazine 10mg tablets | 28 tablet PoM £36.22–£63.00 DT = £10.85
  Chlorpromazine hydrochloride 25 mg Chlorpromazine 25mg tablets | 28 tablet PoM £37.13 DT = £16.34
  Chlorpromazine hydrochloride 50 mg Chlorpromazine 50mg tablets | 28 tablet PoM £37.50 DT = £16.34
  Chlorpromazine hydrochloride 100 mg Chlorpromazine 100mg tablets | 28 tablet PoM £39.99 DT = £29.72

Suppository

CAUTIONARY AND ADVISORY LABELS 2, 11

Oral solution

CAUTIONARY AND ADVISORY LABELS 2, 11
- Chlorpromazine hydrochloride (Non-proprietary)
  Chlorpromazine hydrochloride 5 mg per 1 ml Chlorpromazine 25mg/5ml syrup | 150 ml PoM £6.00 DT = £6.00
  Chlorpromazine 25mg/5ml oral solution sugar free | 150 ml PoM £12.00 DT = £12.00 SF
  Chlorpromazine 25mg/5ml oral solution | 150 ml PoM £6.00 DT = £6.00
  Chlorpromazine hydrochloride 20 mg per 1 ml Chlorpromazine 100mg/5ml oral solution | 150 ml PoM £35.68 DT = £35.68

F 295

Haloperidol

10-Jul-2024

- **INDICATIONS AND DOSE**

Schizophrenia [when alternatives ineffective or not tolerated] (under expert supervision)
- BY MOUTH
  - Child 13–17 years: 0.25–1.5 mg twice daily, alternatively 0.16–1 mg 3 times a day, individual benefit-risk should be assessed when considering doses above 3 mg daily; maximum 5 mg per day

Persistent, severe aggression in autism or pervasive developmental disorders [when other treatments ineffective or not tolerated] (under expert supervision)
- BY MOUTH
  - Child 6–11 years: 0.25–1.5 mg twice daily, alternatively 0.16–1 mg 3 times a day, the need for continued treatment must be reassessed after a maximum of 6 weeks and regularly thereafter
  - Child 12–17 years: 0.25–2.5 mg twice daily, alternatively 0.16–1.6 mg 3 times a day, the need for continued treatment must be reassessed after a maximum of 6 weeks and regularly thereafter

Severe tic disorders, including Tourette's syndrome [when educational, psychological and other pharmacological treatments ineffective] (under expert supervision)
- BY MOUTH
  - Child 10–17 years: 0.25–1.5 mg twice daily, alternatively 0.16–1 mg 3 times a day, the need for continued treatment must be reassessed every 6–12 months

Nausea and vomiting in palliative care
- BY MOUTH
  - Child 12–17 years: 1.5 mg once daily, dose to be taken at night, increased if necessary to 1.5 mg twice daily, max. 5 mg twice daily
- BY CONTINUOUS INTRAVENOUS INFUSION, OR BY CONTINUOUS SUBCUTANEOUS INFUSION
  - Child 1 month–11 years: 25–85 micrograms/kg/24 hours
  - Child 12–17 years: 1.5–5 mg/24 hours

Restlessness and confusion in palliative care
- BY MOUTH
  - Child 1–17 years: 10–20 micrograms/kg every 8–12 hours

- **UNLICENSED USE** Not licensed for use in palliative care.
- **CONTRA-INDICATIONS** CNS depression · comatose states · congenital long QT syndrome · history of torsade de pointes · history of ventricular arrhythmia · QTc-interval prolongation · recent acute myocardial infarction · uncompensated heart failure · uncorrected hypokalaemia
- **CAUTIONS** Bradycardia · electrolyte disturbances (correct before treatment initiation) · family history of QTc-interval prolongation · history of heavy alcohol exposure · hyperthyroidism · hypotension (including orthostatic hypotension) · prolactin-dependent tumours · prolactinaemia
- **INTERACTIONS** → Appendix 1: haloperidol
- **SIDE-EFFECTS**

GENERAL SIDE-EFFECTS
- **Common or very common** Depression · eye disorders · headache · nausea · neuromuscular dysfunction · psychotic disorder · vision disorders · weight decreased
- **Uncommon** Breast abnormalities · dyspnoea · gait abnormal · hepatic disorders · hyperhidrosis · menstrual cycle irregularities · muscle complaints · musculoskeletal stiffness · oedema · photosensitivity reaction · restlessness

· sexual dysfunction · skin reactions · temperature regulation disorders
- **Rare or very rare** Hypoglycaemia · respiratory disorders · SIADH · trismus
- **Frequency not known** Hypersensitivity vasculitis · pancytopenia · rhabdomyolysis · thrombocytopenia

SPECIFIC SIDE-EFFECTS
- With oral use Angioedema
- With parenteral use Severe cutaneous adverse reactions (SCARs)

SIDE-EFFECTS, FURTHER INFORMATION Haloperidol is a less sedating antipsychotic.

● **PREGNANCY** Manufacturer advises it is preferable to avoid—moderate amount of data indicate no malformative or fetal/neonatal toxicity, however there are isolated case reports of birth defects following fetal exposure, mostly in combination with other drugs; reproductive toxicity shown in *animal* studies.

● **HEPATIC IMPAIRMENT** Manufacturer advises caution.
Dose adjustments Manufacturer advises halve initial dose and then adjust if necessary with smaller increments and at longer intervals.

● **RENAL IMPAIRMENT** Manufacturer advises use with caution.
Dose adjustments Manufacturer advises consider lower initial dose in severe impairment and then adjust if necessary with smaller increments and at longer intervals.

● **MONITORING REQUIREMENTS**
- Manufacturer advises monitor electrolytes before treatment initiation and periodically during treatment.
- [EvGr] A baseline ECG is recommended before treatment initiation and the need for further ECGs during treatment must be assessed on an individual basis. ⟨M⟩

● **PRESCRIBING AND DISPENSING INFORMATION**
Palliative care For further information on the use of haloperidol in palliative care, see www.medicinescomplete.com/#/content/palliative/haloperidol.

● **MEDICINAL FORMS** There can be variation in the licensing of different medicines containing the same drug. Forms available from special-order manufacturers include: oral suspension, oral solution

Solution for injection
- **Haloperidol (Non-proprietary)**
  Haloperidol 5 mg per 1 ml Haloperidol 5mg/1ml solution for injection ampoules | 5 ampoule [PoM] £16.50–£25.85 | 10 ampoule [PoM] £67.89 DT = £51.69

Oral tablet
CAUTIONARY AND ADVISORY LABELS 2
- **Haloperidol (Non-proprietary)**
  Haloperidol 500 microgram Haloperidol 500microgram tablets | 28 tablet [PoM] £500.00 DT = £300.37
  Haloperidol 1.5 mg Haloperidol 1.5mg tablets | 28 tablet [PoM] £8.99 DT = £4.40
  Haloperidol 5 mg Haloperidol 5mg tablets | 28 tablet [PoM] £9.06 DT = £4.55
  Haloperidol 10 mg Haloperidol 10mg tablets | 28 tablet [PoM] £18.11 DT = £17.87

Oral solution
CAUTIONARY AND ADVISORY LABELS 2
- **Haloperidol (Non-proprietary)**
  Haloperidol 200 microgram per 1 ml Haloperidol 200micrograms/ml oral solution sugar free | 100 ml [PoM] £185.00 DT = £185.00 [SF]
  Haloperidol 1 mg per 1 ml Haloperidol 5mg/5ml oral solution sugar free | 100 ml [PoM] £22.83 DT = £22.83 [SF]
  Haloperidol 2 mg per 1 ml Haloperidol 10mg/5ml oral solution sugar free | 100 ml [PoM] £9.20 DT = £4.45 [SF]
- **Haldol** (Essential Pharma Ltd)
  Haloperidol 2 mg per 1 ml Haldol 2mg/ml oral solution | 100 ml [PoM] £4.45 DT = £4.45 [SF]

F 295

Pericyazine
27-Jun-2023

(Periciazine)

● **INDICATIONS AND DOSE**

Schizophrenia (under expert supervision) | Psychoses (severe mental or behavioural disorders only) (under expert supervision)

▶ BY MOUTH
- Child 1–11 years: Initially 500 micrograms daily for 10-kg child, increased by 1 mg for each additional 5 kg; dose may be gradually increased according to response but maintenance should not exceed twice initial dose; maximum 10 mg per day
- Child 12–17 years: Initially 25 mg 3 times a day, increased in steps of 25 mg every week, adjusted according to response, increased if necessary up to 100 mg 3 times a day, total daily dose may alternatively be given in 2 divided doses

● **UNLICENSED USE** Tablets not licensed for use in children.

● **CONTRA-INDICATIONS** CNS depression · comatose states · phaeochromocytoma

● **CAUTIONS** Hypothyroidism · susceptibility to QT interval prolongation

● **INTERACTIONS** → Appendix 1: phenothiazine antipsychotics

● **SIDE-EFFECTS** Atrioventricular block · cardiac arrest · consciousness impaired · contact dermatitis · glucose tolerance impaired · hepatic disorders · hyperthermia · nasal congestion · priapism · respiratory depression

● **HEPATIC IMPAIRMENT** Can precipitate coma; phenothiazines are hepatotoxic.

● **RENAL IMPAIRMENT** [EvGr] Use with caution (risk of accumulation). ⟨M⟩

● **MEDICINAL FORMS** There can be variation in the licensing of different medicines containing the same drug. Forms available from special-order manufacturers include: oral suspension, oral solution

Oral tablet
CAUTIONARY AND ADVISORY LABELS 2
- **Pericyazine (Non-proprietary)**
  Pericyazine 2.5 mg Pericyazine 2.5mg tablets | 84 tablet [PoM] £52.75 DT = £55.03
  Pericyazine 10 mg Pericyazine 10mg tablets | 84 tablet [PoM] £135.27 DT = £135.27

Oral solution
CAUTIONARY AND ADVISORY LABELS 2
- **Pericyazine (Non-proprietary)**
  Pericyazine 2 mg per 1 ml Pericyazine 10mg/5ml oral solution | 100 ml [PoM] £82.80 DT = £82.80

F 295

Pimozide
28-Oct-2021

● **INDICATIONS AND DOSE**

Schizophrenia

▶ BY MOUTH
- Child 12–17 years (under expert supervision): Initially 1 mg daily, adjusted according to response, then increased in steps of 2–4 mg at intervals of not less than 1 week; usual dose 2–20 mg daily

Tourette syndrome (under expert supervision)

▶ BY MOUTH
- Child 2–11 years: 1–4 mg daily
- Child 12–17 years: 2–10 mg daily

● **UNLICENSED USE** Not licensed for use in Tourette syndrome.

- **CONTRA-INDICATIONS** CNS depression · comatose states · history of arrhythmias · history or family history of congenital QT prolongation · phaeochromocytoma
- **INTERACTIONS** → Appendix 1: pimozide
- **SIDE-EFFECTS**
  - **Common or very common** Appetite decreased · depression · headache · hyperhidrosis · restlessness · sebaceous gland overactivity · urinary disorders · vision blurred
  - **Uncommon** Dysarthria · face oedema · muscle spasms · oculogyric crisis · skin reactions
  - **Frequency not known** Cardiac arrest · generalised tonic-clonic seizure · glycosuria · hyponatraemia · libido decreased · neck stiffness · temperature regulation disorders
- **HEPATIC IMPAIRMENT** Manufacturer advises caution.
- **RENAL IMPAIRMENT** EvGr Caution in renal failure. (M)
- **MONITORING REQUIREMENTS**
  - **ECG monitoring** Following reports of sudden unexplained death, an ECG is recommended before treatment. It is also recommended that patients taking pimozide should have an annual ECG (if the QT interval is prolonged, treatment should be reviewed and either withdrawn or dose reduced under close supervision) and that pimozide should not be given with other antipsychotic drugs (including depot preparations), tricyclic antidepressants or other drugs which prolong the QT interval, such as certain antimalarials, antiarrhythmic drugs and certain antihistamines and should not be given with drugs which cause electrolyte disturbances (especially diuretics).

- **MEDICINAL FORMS** There can be variation in the licensing of different medicines containing the same drug. Forms available from special-order manufacturers include: oral suspension

Oral tablet

CAUTIONARY AND ADVISORY LABELS 2

- **Pimozide (Non-proprietary)**
  Pimozide 1 mg Orap 1mg tablets | 100 tablet PoM (Hospital only)
- **Orap** (Eumedica Pharma Ltd)
  Pimozide 4 mg Orap 4mg tablets | 100 tablet PoM £40.31 DT = £40.31

F 295

Sulpiride

21-Oct-2021

- **INDICATIONS AND DOSE**

Schizophrenia with predominantly negative symptoms
- BY MOUTH
  - Child 14–17 years (under expert supervision): 200–400 mg twice daily; maximum 800 mg per day

Schizophrenia with mainly positive symptoms
- BY MOUTH
  - Child 14–17 years (under expert supervision): 200–400 mg twice daily; maximum 2.4 g per day

Tourette syndrome (under expert supervision)
- BY MOUTH
  - Child 2–11 years: 50–400 mg twice daily
  - Child 12–17 years: 100–400 mg twice daily

- **UNLICENSED USE** Not licensed for use in Tourette syndrome.

IMPORTANT SAFETY INFORMATION

MHRA/CHM ADVICE: CLOZAPINE AND OTHER ANTIPSYCHOTICS: MONITORING BLOOD CONCENTRATIONS FOR TOXICITY (AUGUST 2020)

Following fatal cases involving toxicity of clozapine and other antipsychotic medicines, the MHRA advises that monitoring blood concentration of sulpiride may be helpful in certain circumstances, such as patients presenting symptoms suggestive of toxicity, or when concomitant medicines may interact to increase blood concentration of sulpiride.

- **CONTRA-INDICATIONS** CNS depression · comatose states · phaeochromocytoma
- **CAUTIONS** Aggressive patients (even low doses may aggravate symptoms) · agitated patients (even low doses may aggravate symptoms) · excited patients (even low doses may aggravate symptoms)
- **INTERACTIONS** → Appendix 1: sulpiride
- **SIDE-EFFECTS**
  - **Common or very common** Breast abnormalities
  - **Uncommon** Muscle tone increased · orgasm abnormal
  - **Rare or very rare** Oculogyric crisis
  - **Frequency not known** Cardiac arrest · dyspnoea · embolism and thrombosis · hyponatraemia · SIADH · trismus · urticaria
- **RENAL IMPAIRMENT**
  Dose adjustments EvGr Reduce dose or increase dose interval; increase in small steps. (M)
- **MONITORING REQUIREMENTS** Sulpiride does not affect blood pressure to the same extent as other antipsychotic drugs and so blood pressure monitoring is not mandatory for this drug.
- **PRESCRIBING AND DISPENSING INFORMATION** Flavours of oral liquid formulations may include lemon and aniseed.
- **PATIENT AND CARER ADVICE**
  Medicines for Children leaflet: Sulpiride for schizophrenia and Tourette's syndrome www.medicinesforchildren.org.uk/medicines/sulpiride-for-schizophrenia-and-tourettes-syndrome/

- **MEDICINAL FORMS** There can be variation in the licensing of different medicines containing the same drug. Forms available from special-order manufacturers include: oral suspension, oral solution

Oral tablet

CAUTIONARY AND ADVISORY LABELS 2

- **Sulpiride (Non-proprietary)**
  Sulpiride 200 mg Sulpiride 200mg tablets | 30 tablet PoM £12.20 DT = £6.98
  Sulpiride 400 mg Sulpiride 400mg tablets | 30 tablet PoM £28.00 DT = £24.76

Oral solution

CAUTIONARY AND ADVISORY LABELS 2

- **Sulpiride (Non-proprietary)**
  Sulpiride 40 mg per 1 ml Sulpiride 200mg/5ml oral solution sugar free | 150 ml PoM £101.13 DT = £101.13 SF

F 295

Trifluoperazine

27-Jun-2023

- **INDICATIONS AND DOSE**

Schizophrenia and other psychoses | Short-term adjunctive management of psychomotor agitation, excitement, and violent or dangerously impulsive behaviour
- BY MOUTH
  - Child 12–17 years (under expert supervision): Initially 5 mg twice daily, daily dose may be increased by 5 mg after 1 week. If necessary, dose may be further increased in steps of 5 mg at intervals of 3 days. When satisfactory control has been achieved, reduce gradually until an effective maintenance level has been established

Short-term adjunctive management of severe anxiety
- BY MOUTH
  - Child 3–5 years (under expert supervision): Up to 500 micrograms twice daily
  - Child 6–11 years (under expert supervision): Up to 2 mg twice daily

- Child 12–17 years (under expert supervision): 1–2 mg twice daily, increased if necessary to 3 mg twice daily

Severe nausea and vomiting unresponsive to other antiemetics

- BY MOUTH
- Child 3–5 years: Up to 500 micrograms twice daily
- Child 6–11 years: Up to 2 mg twice daily
- Child 12–17 years: 1–2 mg twice daily (max. per dose 3 mg twice daily)

- **CONTRA-INDICATIONS** CNS depression · comatose states · phaeochromocytoma
- **CAUTIONS** Susceptibility to QT interval prolongation
- **INTERACTIONS** → Appendix 1: phenothiazine antipsychotics
- **SIDE-EFFECTS** Alertness decreased · anxiety · appetite decreased · blood disorder · cardiac arrest · embolism and thrombosis · hyperpyrexia · jaundice cholestatic · lens opacity · muscle weakness · oedema · pancytopenia · photosensitivity reaction · skin reactions · thrombocytopenia · urinary hesitation · vision blurred · withdrawal syndrome

SIDE-EFFECTS, FURTHER INFORMATION Extrapyramidal symptoms are more frequent at doses exceeding 6 mg daily. Acute dystonias are more common with potent first generation antipsychotics. The risk is increased in men, young adults, children, antipsychotic-naïve patients, rapid dose escalation, and abrupt treatment discontinuation.

- **HEPATIC IMPAIRMENT** Manufacturer advises avoid.
- **MONITORING REQUIREMENTS** Trifluoperazine does not affect blood pressure to the same extent as other antipsychotic drugs and so blood pressure monitoring is not mandatory for this drug.

- **MEDICINAL FORMS** There can be variation in the licensing of different medicines containing the same drug.

Oral tablet

CAUTIONARY AND ADVISORY LABELS 2

- Trifluoperazine (Non-proprietary)

Trifluoperazine (as Trifluoperazine hydrochloride) 1 mg Trifluoperazine 1mg tablets | 112 tablet PoM £47.30–£59.12 DT = £110.47

Trifluoperazine (as Trifluoperazine hydrochloride) 5 mg Trifluoperazine 5mg tablets | 112 tablet PoM £107.91–£134.89 DT = £134.89

Oral solution

CAUTIONARY AND ADVISORY LABELS 2

- Trifluoperazine (Non-proprietary)

Trifluoperazine (as Trifluoperazine hydrochloride) 200 microgram per 1 ml Trifluoperazine 1mg/5ml oral solution sugar free | 200 ml PoM £136.88 DT = £136.88 SF

Trifluoperazine (as Trifluoperazine hydrochloride) 1 mg per 1 ml Trifluoperazine 5mg/5ml oral solution sugar free | 150 ml PoM £86.00 DT = £78.88 SF

ANTIPSYCHOTICS > SECOND-GENERATION

F 295

Amisulpride

06-Jul-2021

- **DRUG ACTION** Amisulpride is a selective dopamine receptor antagonist with high affinity for mesolimbic D_2 and D_3 receptors.

- **INDICATIONS AND DOSE**

Acute psychotic episode in schizophrenia

- BY MOUTH
- Child 15–17 years (under expert supervision): 200–400 mg twice daily, adjusted according to response; maximum 1.2 g per day

Schizophrenia with predominantly negative symptoms

- BY MOUTH
- Child 15–17 years (under expert supervision): 50–300 mg daily

- **UNLICENSED USE** Not licensed for use in children under 18 years.

IMPORTANT SAFETY INFORMATION

MHRA/CHM ADVICE: CLOZAPINE AND OTHER ANTIPSYCHOTICS: MONITORING BLOOD CONCENTRATIONS FOR TOXICITY (AUGUST 2020)

Following fatal cases involving toxicity of clozapine and other antipsychotic medicines, the MHRA advises that monitoring blood concentration of amisulpride may be helpful in certain circumstances, such as patients presenting symptoms suggestive of toxicity, or when concomitant medicines may interact to increase blood concentration of amisulpride.

- **CONTRA-INDICATIONS** CNS depression · comatose states · phaeochromocytoma · pre-pubertal children · prolactin-dependent tumours
- **INTERACTIONS** → Appendix 1: atypical antipsychotics
- **SIDE-EFFECTS**
  - **Common or very common** Anxiety · breast pain · nausea · oculogyric crisis · orgasm abnormal · trismus · vision blurred
  - **Uncommon** Bone disorders · dyslipidaemia · hepatic disorders · nasal congestion · pneumonia aspiration
  - **Rare or very rare** Angioedema · embolism and thrombosis · hyponatraemia · neoplasms · SIADH · urticaria
  - **Frequency not known** Photosensitivity reaction
- **PREGNANCY** Avoid.
- **BREAST FEEDING** Avoid—no information available.
- **RENAL IMPAIRMENT** Manufacturer advises caution if creatinine clearance less than 10 mL/minute (no information available).

Dose adjustments See p. 16.

In adults, manufacturer advises halve dose if creatinine clearance 30–60 mL/minute; use one-third dose if creatinine clearance 10–30 mL/minute (consult product literature).

- **MONITORING REQUIREMENTS** Amisulpride does not affect blood pressure to the same extent as other antipsychotic drugs and so blood pressure monitoring is not mandatory for this drug.
- **PRESCRIBING AND DISPENSING INFORMATION** Flavours of oral liquid formulations may include caramel.

- **MEDICINAL FORMS** There can be variation in the licensing of different medicines containing the same drug. Forms available from special-order manufacturers include: oral suspension, oral solution

Oral tablet

CAUTIONARY AND ADVISORY LABELS 2

- Amisulpride (Non-proprietary)

Amisulpride 50 mg Amisulpride 50mg tablets | 60 tablet PoM £13.09 DT = £3.56

Amisulpride 100 mg Amisulpride 100mg tablets | 60 tablet PoM £20.30 DT = £5.07

Amisulpride 200 mg Amisulpride 200mg tablets | 60 tablet PoM £33.93 DT = £9.71

Amisulpride 400 mg Amisulpride 400mg tablets | 60 tablet PoM £70.79 DT = £49.44

Oral solution

CAUTIONARY AND ADVISORY LABELS 2

- Amisulpride (Non-proprietary)

Amisulpride 100 mg per 1 ml Amisulpride 100mg/ml oral solution sugar free | 60 ml PoM £87.48 DT = £79.88 SF

295

Aripiprazole

12-Jun-2025

- **DRUG ACTION** Aripiprazole is a dopamine D_2 partial agonist with weak 5-HT_{1a} partial agonism and 5-HT_{2A} receptor antagonism.

- **INDICATIONS AND DOSE**

Schizophrenia

▶ BY MOUTH

▶ Child 15–17 years (under expert supervision): Initially 2 mg once daily for 2 days, increased to 5 mg once daily for 2 days, then increased to 10 mg once daily, then increased in steps of 5 mg if required; maximum 30 mg per day

Treatment of mania (under expert supervision)

▶ BY MOUTH

▶ Child 13–17 years: Initially 2 mg once daily for 2 days, increased to 5 mg once daily for 2 days, then increased to 10 mg once daily, increased in steps of 5 mg if required, maximum duration of treatment 12 weeks, doses above 10 mg daily should only be used in exceptional cases; maximum 30 mg per day

DOSE ADJUSTMENTS DUE TO INTERACTIONS

▶ For aripiprazole dose adjustments with concurrent use of potent or moderate inducers of CYP3A4, or potent inhibitors of CYP3A4 and/or CYP2D6—consult product literature.

IMPORTANT SAFETY INFORMATION

MHRA/CHM ADVICE: CLOZAPINE AND OTHER ANTIPSYCHOTICS: MONITORING BLOOD CONCENTRATIONS FOR TOXICITY (AUGUST 2020)

Following fatal cases involving toxicity of clozapine and other antipsychotic medicines, the MHRA advises that monitoring blood concentration of aripiprazole may be helpful in certain circumstances, such as patients presenting symptoms suggestive of toxicity, or when concomitant medicines may interact to increase blood concentration of aripiprazole.

MHRA/CHM ADVICE: ARIPIPRAZOLE (*ABILIFY*®) AND GENERIC BRANDS): RISK OF PATHOLOGICAL GAMBLING (DECEMBER 2023)

There has been an increase in reports, via the Yellow Card Scheme, of gambling disorder and pathological gambling associated with aripiprazole in patients with and without a history of such disorders; the majority were reported to resolve upon dose reduction or treatment discontinuation. In addition, concerns have been raised with the MHRA about a lack of awareness of this issue, especially when gambling is a recognised common risk factor linked to suicide. Healthcare professionals are advised to counsel patients and their carers about this risk and to be alert for the development of new or increased urges to gamble and other impulse control symptoms, such as excessive eating or spending, or hypersexuality. The prescriber should consider reducing the dose or stopping the drug if these symptoms occur.

- **CAUTIONS** Cerebrovascular disease · risk of aspiration pneumonia
- **INTERACTIONS** → Appendix 1: atypical antipsychotics
- **SIDE-EFFECTS**

▶ **Common or very common** Anxiety · appetite abnormal · diabetes mellitus · gastrointestinal discomfort · headache · nausea · vision disorders

▶ **Uncommon** Depression · hiccups · sexual dysfunction

▶ **Frequency not known** Aggression · alopecia · cardiac arrest · chest pain · diabetic hyperosmolar coma · diabetic ketoacidosis · diarrhoea · dysphagia · embolism and thrombosis · generalised tonic-clonic seizure · hepatic disorders · hyperhidrosis · hypertension · hyponatraemia · laryngospasm · musculoskeletal stiffness · myalgia · oropharyngeal spasm · pancreatitis · pathological gambling · peripheral oedema · photosensitivity reaction · pneumonia aspiration · rhabdomyolysis · serotonin syndrome · speech disorder · suicidal behaviours · syncope · temperature regulation disorder · thrombocytopenia · urinary incontinence · weight decreased

SIDE-EFFECTS, FURTHER INFORMATION Increased incidence of side-effects associated with doses of 30 mg daily; doses above 10 mg daily should only be used in exceptional cases and with close clinical monitoring.

- **PREGNANCY** Use only if potential benefit outweighs risk.
- **BREAST FEEDING** Manufacturer advises avoid—present in milk.
- **HEPATIC IMPAIRMENT** Manufacturer advises caution in severe impairment (oral treatment preferred to intramuscular administration; limited information available).
- **MONITORING REQUIREMENTS** Aripiprazole does not affect blood pressure to the same extent as other antipsychotic drugs and so blood pressure monitoring is not mandatory for this drug.
- **DIRECTIONS FOR ADMINISTRATION** Orodispersible tablets should be placed on the tongue and allowed to dissolve, or be dispersed in water and swallowed.
- **PATIENT AND CARER ADVICE** Patients or carers should be given advice on how to administer aripiprazole orodispersible tablets.

Medicines for Children leaflet: Aripiprazole for schizophrenia, bipolar disorder and tics www.medicinesforchildren.org.uk/medicines/aripiprazole-for-schizophrenia-bipolar-disorder-and-tics/

- **NATIONAL FUNDING/ACCESS DECISIONS**

For full details see funding body website

NICE decisions

▶ **Aripiprazole for the treatment of schizophrenia in people aged 15 to 17 years (January 2011)** NICE TA213 Recommended with restrictions

▶ **Aripiprazole for treating moderate to severe manic episodes in adolescents with bipolar I disorder (July 2013)** NICE TA292 Recommended

Scottish Medicines Consortium (SMC) decisions

▶ **Aripiprazole oral (*Abilify*®) for treatment up to 12 weeks of moderate to severe manic episodes in Bipolar I Disorder in adolescents aged 13 years and older (September 2013)** SMC No. 891/13 Recommended with restrictions

- **MEDICINAL FORMS** There can be variation in the licensing of different medicines containing the same drug. Forms available from special-order manufacturers include: oral solution

Oral tablet

CAUTIONARY AND ADVISORY LABELS 2

▶ Aripiprazole (Non-proprietary)

Aripiprazole 1 mg Aripiprazole 1mg tablets | 28 tablet PoM £29.50–£53.10

Aripiprazole 2.5 mg Aripiprazole 2.5mg tablets | 28 tablet PoM £29.50–£53.10 DT = £29.50

Aripiprazole 5 mg Aripiprazole 5mg tablets | 28 tablet PoM £115.25 DT = £0.97

Aripiprazole 10 mg Aripiprazole 10mg tablets | 28 tablet PoM £115.25 DT = £1.00

Aripiprazole 15 mg Aripiprazole 15mg tablets | 28 tablet PoM £115.25 DT = £1.00

Aripiprazole 30 mg Aripiprazole 30mg tablets | 28 tablet PoM £230.50 DT = £1.45

▶ Abilify (Otsuka Pharmaceuticals (U.K.) Ltd)

Aripiprazole 5 mg Abilify 5mg tablets | 28 tablet PoM £96.04 DT = £0.97

Aripiprazole 10 mg Abilify 10mg tablets | 28 tablet PoM £96.04 DT = £1.00

Aripiprazole 15 mg Abilify 15mg tablets | 28 tablet PoM £96.04 DT = £1.00

Aripiprazole 30 mg Abilify 30mg tablets | 28 tablet PoM £192.08 DT = £1.45

▸ **Arpoya** (Torrent Pharma (UK) Ltd)

Aripiprazole 5 mg Arpoya 5mg tablets | 28 tablet PoM £0.95 DT = £0.97

Aripiprazole 10 mg Arpoya 10mg tablets | 28 tablet PoM £1.00 DT = £1.00

Aripiprazole 15 mg Arpoya 15mg tablets | 28 tablet PoM £0.98 DT = £1.00

Oral solution

CAUTIONARY AND ADVISORY LABELS 2

EXCIPIENTS: May contain Disodium edetate, hydroxybenzoates (parabens), propylene glycol, sucrose

▸ **Aripiprazole (Non-proprietary)**

Aripiprazole 1 mg per 1 ml Aripiprazole 1mg/ml oral solution sugar free | 150 ml PoM £101.20 DT = £101.20 SF

Aripiprazole 1mg/ml oral solution | 150 ml PoM £101.22 DT = £8.85

▸ **Abilify** (Otsuka Pharmaceuticals (U.K.) Ltd)

Aripiprazole 1 mg per 1 ml Abilify 1mg/ml oral solution | 150 ml PoM £102.90 DT = £8.85

Orodispersible tablet

CAUTIONARY AND ADVISORY LABELS 2

EXCIPIENTS: May contain Aspartame

▸ **Aripiprazole (Non-proprietary)**

Aripiprazole 10 mg Aripiprazole 10mg orodispersible tablets sugar free | 28 tablet PoM £79.27 DT = £8.96 SF

Aripiprazole 15 mg Aripiprazole 15mg orodispersible tablets sugar free | 28 tablet PoM £79.27 DT = £9.43 SF

▸ **Abilify** (Otsuka Pharmaceuticals (U.K.) Ltd)

Aripiprazole 10 mg Abilify 10mg orodispersible tablets | 28 tablet PoM £96.04 DT = £8.96 SF

Aripiprazole 15 mg Abilify 15mg orodispersible tablets | 28 tablet PoM £96.04 DT = £9.43 SF

▸ **Elozar** (Novumgen Ltd)

Aripiprazole 10 mg Elozar 10mg orodispersible tablets | 28 tablet PoM £15.67 DT = £8.96 SF

Aripiprazole 15 mg Elozar 15mg orodispersible tablets | 28 tablet PoM £17.67 DT = £9.43 SF

295

Clozapine

19-Nov-2025

● **DRUG ACTION** Clozapine is a dopamine D_1, dopamine D_2, 5-HT_{2A}, alpha$_1$-adrenoceptor, and muscarinic-receptor antagonist.

● **INDICATIONS AND DOSE**

Schizophrenia in patients unresponsive to, or intolerant of, conventional antipsychotic drugs

▶ BY MOUTH

▸ Child 12–17 years (under expert supervision): 12.5 mg 1–2 times a day for day 1, then 25–50 mg for day 2, then increased, if tolerated, in steps of 25–50 mg daily, dose to be increased gradually over 14–21 days, increased to up to 300 mg daily in divided doses, larger dose to be taken at night, up to 200 mg daily may be taken as a single dose at bedtime; increased in steps of 50–100 mg 1–2 times a week if required, it is preferable to increase once a week; usual dose 200–450 mg daily, max. 900 mg per day, if restarting after interval of more than 48 hours, 12.5 mg once or twice on first day (but may be feasible to increase more quickly than on initiation)—extreme caution if previous respiratory or cardiac arrest with initial dosing

● **UNLICENSED USE** Not licensed for use in children under 16 years.

IMPORTANT SAFETY INFORMATION

MHRA/CHM ADVICE: CLOZAPINE: REMINDER OF POTENTIALLY FATAL RISK OF INTESTINAL OBSTRUCTION, FAECAL IMPACTION, AND PARALYTIC ILEUS (OCTOBER 2017)

Clozapine has been associated with varying degrees of impairment of intestinal peristalsis—see Cautions and Contra-indications for further information. Patients and their carers should be advised to seek immediate medical advice before taking the next dose of clozapine if constipation develops.

MHRA/CHM ADVICE: CLOZAPINE AND OTHER ANTIPSYCHOTICS: MONITORING BLOOD CONCENTRATIONS FOR TOXICITY (AUGUST 2020)

Following fatal cases involving toxicity of clozapine and other antipsychotic medicines, the MHRA recommends monitoring blood concentration of clozapine for toxicity in certain clinical situations such as when:

- a patient stops smoking or switches to an e-cigarette;
- concomitant medicines may interact to increase blood clozapine levels;
- a patient has pneumonia or other serious infection;
- reduced clozapine metabolism is suspected;
- toxicity is suspected.

Clozapine blood concentration monitoring should be carried out in addition to the required blood tests to manage the risk of agranulocytosis.

● **CONTRA-INDICATIONS** Alcoholic and toxic psychoses · bone-marrow disorders · coma · drug intoxication · history of agranulocytosis · history of circulatory collapse · history of neutropenia · paralytic ileus · severe cardiac disorders (e.g. myocarditis) · severe CNS depression · uncontrolled epilepsy

● **CAUTIONS** Susceptibility to angle-closure glaucoma · taper off other antipsychotics before starting

CAUTIONS, FURTHER INFORMATION

▸ Agranulocytosis Neutropenia and potentially fatal agranulocytosis reported. Leucocyte and differential blood counts must be normal before starting; monitor counts every week for 18 weeks then at least every 2 weeks and if clozapine continued and blood count stable after 1 year at least every 4 weeks (and 4 weeks after discontinuation); if leucocyte count below 3000 /mm^3 or if absolute neutrophil count below 1500 /mm^3 discontinue permanently and refer to haematologist. Patients who have a low white blood cell count because of benign ethnic neutropenia may be started on clozapine with the agreement of a haematologist. Avoid drugs which depress leucopoiesis; patients should report immediately symptoms of infection, especially influenza-like illness.

▸ Myocarditis and cardiomyopathy Fatal myocarditis (most commonly in first 2 months) and cardiomyopathy reported.

- Perform physical examination and take full medical history before starting
- Specialist examination required if cardiac abnormalities or history of heart disease found—clozapine initiated only in absence of severe heart disease and if benefit outweighs risk
- Persistent tachycardia especially in first 2 months should prompt observation for other indicators for myocarditis or cardiomyopathy
- If myocarditis or cardiomyopathy suspected clozapine should be stopped and patient evaluated urgently by cardiologist
- Discontinue permanently in clozapine-induced myocarditis or cardiomyopathy

▸ Intestinal obstruction Impairment of intestinal peristalsis, including constipation, intestinal obstruction, faecal impaction, and paralytic ileus, (including fatal cases) reported. Clozapine should be used with caution in patients receiving drugs that may cause constipation (e.g. antimuscarinic drugs) or in those with a history of colonic disease or lower abdominal surgery. It is essential that constipation is recognised and actively treated.

● **INTERACTIONS** → Appendix 1: atypical antipsychotics

● **SIDE-EFFECTS**

▶ **Common or very common** Appetite decreased · eosinophilia · fever · headache · hypertension · leucocytosis · nausea ·

speech impairment · sweating abnormal · syncope · temperature regulation disorders · urinary disorders · vision blurred

- **Uncommon** Fall
- **Rare or very rare** Anaemia · cardiac arrest · cardiac inflammation · cardiomyopathy · circulatory collapse · delirium · diabetes mellitus · diabetic hyperosmolar coma · dyslipidaemia · dysphagia · embolism and thrombosis · gastrointestinal disorders · glucose tolerance impaired · hepatic disorders · increased risk of infection · intestinal obstruction (including fatal cases) · ketoacidosis · nephritis tubulointerstitial · obesity · obsessive-compulsive disorder · pancreatitis · parotid gland enlargement · pericardial effusion · respiratory disorders · restlessness · sexual dysfunction · skin reactions · sleep apnoea · thrombocytopenia · thrombocytosis
- **Frequency not known** Angina pectoris · angioedema · chest pain · cholinergic syndrome · diarrhoea · gastrointestinal discomfort · hypersensitivity vasculitis · mitral valve incompetence · muscle complaints · muscle weakness · myocardial infarction · nasal congestion · palpitations · polyserositis · pseudophaeochromocytoma · renal failure · rhabdomyolysis · sepsis · systemic lupus erythematosus (SLE)

SIDE-EFFECTS, FURTHER INFORMATION Hypersalivation associated with clozapine therapy can be treated with hyoscine hydrobromide [unlicensed indication], provided that the patient is not at particular risk from the additive antimuscarinic side-effects of hyoscine and clozapine.

- **PREGNANCY** Use with caution.
- **BREAST FEEDING** Avoid.
- **HEPATIC IMPAIRMENT** Manufacturer advises caution—monitor liver function (discontinue if liver enzymes are greater than 3 times the upper limit of normal or jaundice occurs); avoid in symptomatic or progressive impairment and in hepatic failure.
- **RENAL IMPAIRMENT** [EvGr] Avoid in severe impairment. ⟨M⟩
- **MONITORING REQUIREMENTS**
  - Monitor leucocyte and differential blood counts. Clozapine requires differential white blood cell monitoring weekly for 18 weeks, then fortnightly for up to one year, and then monthly as part of the clozapine patient monitoring service.
  - Blood clozapine concentration should be monitored in certain clinical situations—consult product literature.
  - Close medical supervision during initiation (risk of collapse because of hypotension and convulsions).
  - Blood lipids and weight should be measured at baseline, at 3 months (weight should be measured at frequent intervals during the first 3 months), and then yearly with antipsychotics. Patients taking clozapine require more frequent monitoring of these parameters: every 3 months for the first year, then yearly.
  - Monitor blood-glucose regularly. [EvGr] Patients taking antipsychotics should have glycosylated haemoglobin (HbA_{1C}) or fasting blood glucose tested at baseline, after 12 weeks of treatment, then either 6 monthly or yearly. ⟨A⟩ [EvGr] For patients taking clozapine, specialist sources recommend more frequent testing: at baseline, after one months' treatment, then every 4–6 months, ideally by oral glucose tolerance test or fasting plasma glucose (HbA_{1C} if fasting not possible); at a minimum, testing urine glucose or random plasma glucose. ⟨D⟩
  - Patient, prescriber, and supplying pharmacist must be registered with the appropriate Patient Monitoring Service—it takes several days to do this.
- **TREATMENT CESSATION** On planned withdrawal reduce dose over 1–2 weeks to avoid risk of rebound psychosis. If abrupt withdrawal necessary observe patient carefully.
- **DIRECTIONS FOR ADMINISTRATION** Manufacturer advises shake oral suspension well for 90 seconds when dispensing or if visibly settled and stand for 24 hours before use; otherwise shake well for 10 seconds before use. May be diluted with water. Orodispersible tablets should be placed on the tongue, allowed to dissolve and swallowed.
- **PRESCRIBING AND DISPENSING INFORMATION** Clozapine has been used for psychosis in Parkinson's disease in children aged 16 years and over.
- **PATIENT AND CARER ADVICE** Patients or carers should be given advice on how to administer clozapine oral suspension and orodispersible tablets.

- **MEDICINAL FORMS** There can be variation in the licensing of different medicines containing the same drug. Forms available from special-order manufacturers include: oral suspension, oral solution

Oral tablet

CAUTIONARY AND ADVISORY LABELS 2, 10

- **Clozapine (Non-proprietary)**

Clozapine 25 mg Clozapine 25mg tablets | 28 tablet [PoM] £3.02 (Hospital only) | 84 tablet [PoM] £8.40 DT = £16.64 (Hospital only) | 100 tablet [PoM] £10.00 (Hospital only)

Clozapine 100 mg Clozapine 100mg tablets | 28 tablet [PoM] £12.07 (Hospital only) | 84 tablet [PoM] £33.60 DT = £66.53 (Hospital only) | 100 tablet [PoM] £39.00 (Hospital only)

Clozapine 200 mg Clozapine 200mg tablets | 30 tablet [PoM] £25.86 | 100 tablet [PoM] £86.21 DT = £158.40

- **Clozaril** (Viatris UK Healthcare Ltd)

Clozapine 25 mg Clozaril 25mg tablets | 28 tablet [PoM] £3.02 (Hospital only) | 84 tablet [PoM] £8.40 DT = £16.64 (Hospital only) | 100 tablet [PoM] £10.00 (Hospital only)

Clozapine 100 mg Clozaril 100mg tablets | 28 tablet [PoM] £12.07 (Hospital only) | 84 tablet [PoM] £33.60 DT = £66.53 (Hospital only) | 100 tablet [PoM] £39.00 (Hospital only)

Clozapine 200 mg Clozaril 200mg tablets | 30 tablet [PoM] £25.86 | 100 tablet [PoM] £86.21 DT = £158.40

- **Denzapine** (Britannia Pharmaceuticals Ltd)

Clozapine 25 mg Denzapine 25mg tablets | 84 tablet [PoM] £16.64 DT = £16.64 | 100 tablet [PoM] £19.80

Clozapine 50 mg Denzapine 50mg tablets | 100 tablet [PoM] £39.60 DT = £39.60

Clozapine 100 mg Denzapine 100mg tablets | 84 tablet [PoM] £66.53 DT = £66.53 | 100 tablet [PoM] £79.20

Clozapine 200 mg Denzapine 200mg tablets | 100 tablet [PoM] £158.40 DT = £158.40

- **Zaponex** (Leyden Delta B.V.)

Clozapine 25 mg Zaponex 25mg tablets | 84 tablet [PoM] £8.28 DT = £16.64 | 500 tablet [PoM] £48.39

Clozapine 100 mg Zaponex 100mg tablets | 84 tablet [PoM] £33.88 DT = £66.53 | 500 tablet [PoM] £196.43

Oral suspension

CAUTIONARY AND ADVISORY LABELS 2, 10

- **Denzapine** (Britannia Pharmaceuticals Ltd)

Clozapine 50 mg per 1 ml Denzapine 50mg/ml oral suspension | 100 ml [PoM] £77.73 DT = £77.73 [SF]

Orodispersible tablet

CAUTIONARY AND ADVISORY LABELS 2, 10

EXCIPIENTS: May contain Aspartame

- **Clozapine (Non-proprietary)**

Clozapine 12.5 mg Clozapine 12.5mg orodispersible tablets sugar free | 50 tablet [PoM] £5.39 [SF]

Clozapine 25 mg Clozapine 25mg orodispersible tablets sugar free | 84 tablet [PoM] £18.11 [SF] | 100 tablet [PoM] £21.55 [SF]

Clozapine 50 mg Clozapine 50mg orodispersible tablets sugar free | 84 tablet [PoM] £36.21 [SF]

Clozapine 100 mg Clozapine 100mg orodispersible tablets sugar free | 84 tablet [PoM] £72.42 [SF] | 100 tablet [PoM] £86.21 [SF]

Clozapine 200 mg Clozapine 200mg orodispersible tablets sugar free | 100 tablet [PoM] £172.43 [SF]

- **Clozaril** (Viatris UK Healthcare Ltd)

Clozapine 12.5 mg Clozaril 12.5mg orodispersible tablets | 50 tablet [PoM] £5.39 [SF]

Clozapine 25 mg Clozaril 25mg orodispersible tablets | 84 tablet [PoM] £18.11 [SF] | 100 tablet [PoM] £21.55 [SF]

Clozapine 50 mg Clozaril 50mg orodispersible tablets | 84 tablet [PoM] £36.21 [SF]

Clozapine 100 mg Clozaril 100mg orodispersible tablets | 84 tablet [PoM] £72.42 [SF] | 100 tablet [PoM] £86.21 [SF]

Clozapine 200 mg Clozaril 200mg orodispersible tablets | 100 tablet [PoM] £172.43 [SF]

▸ Zaponex (Leyden Delta B.V.)

Clozapine 12.5 mg Zaponex 12.5mg orodispersible tablets | 28 tablet [PoM] £2.77 [SF]

Clozapine 25 mg Zaponex 25mg orodispersible tablets | 28 tablet [PoM] £5.55 [SF]

Clozapine 50 mg Zaponex 50mg orodispersible tablets | 28 tablet [PoM] £11.09 [SF]

Clozapine 100 mg Zaponex 100mg orodispersible tablets | 28 tablet [PoM] £22.18 [SF]

Clozapine 200 mg Zaponex 200mg orodispersible tablets | 28 tablet [PoM] £44.35 [SF]

295

Lurasidone hydrochloride

08-Jul-2021

- **DRUG ACTION** Lurasidone is a dopamine D_2, 5-HT_{2A}, 5-HT_7, $alpha_{2A}$- and $alpha_{2C}$- adrenoceptor antagonist, and is a partial agonist at 5-HT_{1a} receptors.

- **INDICATIONS AND DOSE**

Schizophrenia

▸ BY MOUTH

▸ Child 13–17 years: Initially 37 mg once daily, increased if necessary up to 74 mg once daily, treatment should be prescribed by a specialist

Schizophrenia [when given with moderate CYP3A4 inhibitors (e.g. diltiazem, erythromycin, fluconazole, and verapamil)]

▸ BY MOUTH

▸ Child 13–17 years: Initially 18.5 mg once daily (max. per dose 74 mg once daily), treatment should be prescribed by a specialist

- **CAUTIONS** Susceptibility to QT-interval prolongation
- **INTERACTIONS** → Appendix 1: atypical antipsychotics
- **SIDE-EFFECTS**

▸ **Common or very common** Anxiety · appetite abnormal · asthenia · concentration impaired · depression · headaches · hyperhidrosis · irritability · nausea · oculogyric crisis · psychotic disorder · sleep disorders · weight decreased

▸ **Uncommon** Aggression · alopecia · arthralgia · autoimmune thyroiditis · breast pain · chills · diarrhoea · dyspnoea · fever · gait abnormal · gastrointestinal discomfort · hair growth abnormal · hallucinations · hyperacusia · hyperandrogenism · hyperinsulinaemia · hypertension · hypothyroidism · increased risk of infection · malaise · memory impairment · menstrual cycle irregularities · muscle complaints · musculoskeletal stiffness · oral disorders · oropharyngeal pain · pain · palpitations · paraesthesia · perception altered · psychiatric disorders · renal disorder · sexual dysfunction · suicidal behaviours · taste altered · urinary disorders · urine abnormalities · urticaria · vision disorders

- **PREGNANCY** [EvGr] Use only if potential benefit outweighs risk—limited information available. ⟨M⟩
- **BREAST FEEDING** [EvGr] Use only if potential benefit outweighs risk—present in milk in *animal* studies. ⟨M⟩
- **HEPATIC IMPAIRMENT** Manufacturer advises caution in moderate to severe impairment (risk of increased exposure).

Dose adjustments Manufacturer advises initially 18.5 mg once daily in moderate to severe impairment, increased if necessary up to 74 mg once daily in moderate impairment, or up to max. 37 mg once daily in severe impairment.

- **RENAL IMPAIRMENT** [EvGr] Use only if potential benefit outweighs risk if creatinine clearance less than 15 mL/minute. ⟨M⟩

Dose adjustments [EvGr] Initially 18.5 mg once daily, up to max. 74 mg once daily if creatinine clearance less than 50 mL/minute. ⟨M⟩ see p. 16.

- **NATIONAL FUNDING/ACCESS DECISIONS** For full details see funding body website

All Wales Medicines Strategy Group (AWMSG) decisions

▸ **Lurasidone (*Latuda*®) for the treatment of schizophrenia in adults and adolescents aged 13 years and over (March 2021)** AWMSG No. 4394 Recommended

- **MEDICINAL FORMS** There can be variation in the licensing of different medicines containing the same drug.

Oral tablet

CAUTIONARY AND ADVISORY LABELS 2, 21, 25

▸ Lurasidone hydrochloride (Non-proprietary)

Lurasidone (as Lurasidone hydrochloride) 18.5 mg Lurasidone 18.5mg tablets | 28 tablet [PoM] £80.00 DT = £67.74

Lurasidone (as Lurasidone hydrochloride) 37 mg Lurasidone 37mg tablets | 28 tablet [PoM] £80.00 DT = £69.63

Lurasidone (as Lurasidone hydrochloride) 74 mg Lurasidone 74mg tablets | 28 tablet [PoM] £80.00 DT = £80.00

▸ Latuda (CNX Therapeutics Ltd)

Lurasidone (as Lurasidone hydrochloride) 18.5 mg Latuda 18.5mg tablets | 28 tablet [PoM] £80.00 DT = £67.74

Lurasidone (as Lurasidone hydrochloride) 37 mg Latuda 37mg tablets | 28 tablet [PoM] £80.00 DT = £69.63

Lurasidone (as Lurasidone hydrochloride) 74 mg Latuda 74mg tablets | 28 tablet [PoM] £80.00 DT = £80.00

295

Olanzapine

19-Nov-2025

- **DRUG ACTION** Olanzapine is a dopamine D_1, D_2, D_4, 5-HT_2, histamine-1-, and muscarinic-receptor antagonist.

- **INDICATIONS AND DOSE**

Schizophrenia | Combination therapy for mania

▸ BY MOUTH

▸ Child 12–17 years (under expert supervision): Initially 5–10 mg daily, adjusted according to response, usual dose 5–20 mg daily, doses greater than 10 mg daily only after reassessment, when one or more factors present that might result in slower metabolism (e.g. females, non-smoker) consider lower initial dose and more gradual dose increase; maximum 20 mg per day

Monotherapy for mania

▸ BY MOUTH

▸ Child 12–17 years (under expert supervision): 15 mg daily, adjusted according to response, usual dose 5–20 mg daily, doses greater than 15 mg daily only after reassessment, when one or more factors present that might result in slower metabolism (e.g. females, non-smoker) consider lower initial dose and more gradual dose increase; maximum 20 mg per day

- **UNLICENSED USE** Not licensed for use in children.

IMPORTANT SAFETY INFORMATION

MHRA/CHM ADVICE: CLOZAPINE AND OTHER ANTIPSYCHOTICS: MONITORING BLOOD CONCENTRATIONS FOR TOXICITY (AUGUST 2020)

Following fatal cases involving toxicity of clozapine and other antipsychotic medicines, the MHRA advises that monitoring blood concentration of olanzapine may be helpful in certain circumstances, such as patients presenting symptoms suggestive of toxicity, or when concomitant medicines may interact to increase blood concentration of olanzapine.

- **CAUTIONS** Bone-marrow depression · hypereosinophilic disorders · low leucocyte count · low neutrophil count · myeloproliferative disease · paralytic ileus
- **INTERACTIONS** → Appendix 1: atypical antipsychotics
- **SIDE-EFFECTS**

▸ **Common or very common** Anticholinergic syndrome · appetite increased · arthralgia · asthenia · eosinophilia ·

fever · glycosuria · hypersomnia · oedema · sexual dysfunction
- **Uncommon** Abdominal distension · alopecia · breast enlargement · diabetes mellitus · diabetic coma · dysarthria · embolism and thrombosis · epistaxis · ketoacidosis · memory loss · oculogyration · photosensitivity reaction · urinary disorders
- **Rare or very rare** Hepatic disorders · hypothermia · pancreatitis · rhabdomyolysis · thrombocytopenia

● **PREGNANCY** Use only if potential benefit outweighs risk; neonatal lethargy, tremor, and hypertonia reported when used in third trimester.

● **BREAST FEEDING** Avoid—present in milk.

● **HEPATIC IMPAIRMENT** Manufacturer advises caution.
Dose adjustments In adults, manufacturer advises consider initial dose reduction—consult product literature.

● **RENAL IMPAIRMENT**
Dose adjustments In adults, manufacturer advises consider initial dose reduction (consult product literature).

● **MONITORING REQUIREMENTS**
- Blood lipids and weight should be measured at baseline, at 3 months (weight should be measured at frequent intervals during the first 3 months), and then yearly with antipsychotic drugs. Patients taking olanzapine require more frequent monitoring of these parameters: every 3 months for the first year, then yearly.
- Monitor blood-glucose regularly. EvGr Patients taking antipsychotics should have glycosylated haemoglobin (HbA_{1C}) or fasting blood glucose tested at baseline, after 12 weeks of treatment, then either 6 monthly or yearly. (A) EvGr For patients taking olanzapine, specialist sources recommend more frequent testing: at baseline, after one months' treatment, then every 4–6 months, ideally by oral glucose tolerance test or fasting plasma glucose (HbA_{1C} if fasting not possible); at a minimum, testing urine glucose or random plasma glucose. (D)

● **DIRECTIONS FOR ADMINISTRATION** Manufacturer advises olanzapine orodispersible tablet may be placed on the tongue and allowed to dissolve, or dispersed in water, orange juice, apple juice, milk, or coffee.

● **PATIENT AND CARER ADVICE** Patients or carers should be given advice on how to administer orodispersible tablets.
Medicines for Children leaflet: Olanzapine for schizophrenia, bipolar disorder, mania and agitation www.medicinesforchildren.org.uk/medicines/olanzapine-for-schizophrenia-bipolar-disorder-mania-and-agitation/

● **MEDICINAL FORMS** There can be variation in the licensing of different medicines containing the same drug. Forms available from special-order manufacturers include: oral suspension, oral solution

Oral tablet
CAUTIONARY AND ADVISORY LABELS 2
- **Olanzapine (Non-proprietary)**
  Olanzapine 2.5 mg Olanzapine 2.5mg tablets | 28 tablet PoM £22.28 DT = £1.42
  Olanzapine 5 mg Olanzapine 5mg tablets | 28 tablet PoM £44.57 DT = £1.71
  Olanzapine 7.5 mg Olanzapine 7.5mg tablets | 28 tablet PoM £8.24 DT = £1.90 | 56 tablet PoM £3.30–£133.72
  Olanzapine 10 mg Olanzapine 10mg tablets | 28 tablet PoM £89.15 DT = £2.05
  Olanzapine 15 mg Olanzapine 15mg tablets | 28 tablet PoM £121.56 DT = £2.28
  Olanzapine 20 mg Olanzapine 20mg tablets | 28 tablet PoM £162.07 DT = £2.52
- **Zyprexa** (Neon Healthcare Ltd)
  Olanzapine 2.5 mg Zyprexa 2.5mg tablets | 28 tablet PoM £21.85 DT = £1.42
  Olanzapine 5 mg Zyprexa 5mg tablets | 28 tablet PoM £43.70 DT = £1.71
  Olanzapine 7.5 mg Zyprexa 7.5mg tablets | 56 tablet PoM £131.10
  Olanzapine 10 mg Zyprexa 10mg tablets | 28 tablet PoM £87.40 DT = £2.05
  Olanzapine 15 mg Zyprexa 15mg tablets | 28 tablet PoM £119.18 DT = £2.28
  Olanzapine 20 mg Zyprexa 20mg tablets | 28 tablet PoM £158.90 DT = £2.52

Oral lyophilisate
- **Zyprexa** (Neon Healthcare Ltd)
  Olanzapine 5 mg Zyprexa 5mg Velotabs | 28 tablet PoM £48.07 DT = £48.07 SF
  Olanzapine 10 mg Zyprexa 10mg Velotabs | 28 tablet PoM £87.40 DT = £87.40 SF
  Olanzapine 15 mg Zyprexa 15mg Velotabs | 28 tablet PoM £131.10 DT = £131.10 SF
  Olanzapine 20 mg Zyprexa 20mg Velotabs | 28 tablet PoM £174.79 DT = £174.79 SF

Orodispersible tablet
CAUTIONARY AND ADVISORY LABELS 2
EXCIPIENTS: May contain Aspartame
- **Olanzapine (Non-proprietary)**
  Olanzapine 5 mg Olanzapine 5mg orodispersible tablets sugar free | 28 tablet PoM £4.63–£49.02 DT = £4.65 SF
  Olanzapine 5mg orodispersible tablets | 28 tablet PoM £30.00 DT = £5.69
  Olanzapine 10 mg Olanzapine 10mg orodispersible tablets | 28 tablet PoM £50.00 DT = £7.04
  Olanzapine 10mg orodispersible tablets sugar free | 28 tablet PoM £4.49–£89.04 DT = £5.52 SF
  Olanzapine 15 mg Olanzapine 15mg orodispersible tablets sugar free | 28 tablet PoM £7.80–£133.72 DT = £16.80 SF
  Olanzapine 20 mg Olanzapine 20mg orodispersible tablets sugar free | 28 tablet PoM £6.39–£178.28 DT = £6.43 SF
  Olanzapine 20mg orodispersible tablets | 28 tablet PoM £80.00 DT = £8.84

295

Quetiapine

22-Aug-2022

● **DRUG ACTION** Quetiapine is a dopamine D_1, dopamine D_2, $5\text{-}HT_2$, $alpha_1$-adrenoceptor, and histamine-1 receptor antagonist.

● **INDICATIONS AND DOSE**

Schizophrenia
- BY MOUTH USING IMMEDIATE-RELEASE MEDICINES
- Child 12–17 years (under expert supervision): Initially 25 mg twice daily, adjusted according to response. adjusted in steps of 25–50 mg; maximum 750 mg per day
- BY MOUTH USING MODIFIED-RELEASE MEDICINES
- Child 12–17 years (under expert supervision): Initially 50 mg once daily, adjusted according to response. adjusted in steps of 50 mg daily, usual dose 400–800 mg once daily; maximum 800 mg per day

Treatment of mania in bipolar disorder
- BY MOUTH USING IMMEDIATE-RELEASE MEDICINES
- Child 12–17 years (under expert supervision): 25 mg twice daily for day 1, then 50 mg twice daily for day 2, then 100 mg twice daily for day 3, then 150 mg twice daily for day 4, then 200 mg twice daily for day 5, then adjusted in steps of up to 100 mg daily, adjusted according to response, usual dose 400–600 mg daily in 2 divided doses

DOSE EQUIVALENCE AND CONVERSION
- Patients can be switched from immediate-release to modified-release tablets at the equivalent daily dose; to maintain clinical response, dose titration may be required.

● **UNLICENSED USE** Not licensed for use in children.

IMPORTANT SAFETY INFORMATION

MHRA/CHM ADVICE: CLOZAPINE AND OTHER ANTIPSYCHOTICS: MONITORING BLOOD CONCENTRATIONS FOR TOXICITY (AUGUST 2020)

Following fatal cases involving toxicity of clozapine and other antipsychotic medicines, the MHRA advises that monitoring blood concentration of quetiapine may be helpful in certain circumstances, such as patients presenting symptoms suggestive of toxicity, or when concomitant medicines may interact to increase blood concentration of quetiapine.

- **CAUTIONS** Cerebrovascular disease · history or risk factors for sleep apnoea · patients at risk of aspiration pneumonia · treatment of depression in patients under 25 years (increased risk of suicide)
- **INTERACTIONS** → Appendix 1: atypical antipsychotics
- **SIDE-EFFECTS**
  - **Common or very common** Appetite increased · asthenia · dysarthria · dyspepsia · dyspnoea · fever · headache · irritability · palpitations · peripheral oedema · rhinitis · sleep disorders · suicidal behaviours · syncope · vision blurred · withdrawal syndrome
  - **Uncommon** Anaemia · diabetes mellitus · dysphagia · hyponatraemia · hypothyroidism · sexual dysfunction · skin reactions · thrombocytopenia
  - **Rare or very rare** Angioedema · breast swelling · gastrointestinal disorders · hepatic disorders · hypothermia · menstrual disorder · metabolic syndrome · pancreatitis · rhabdomyolysis · severe cutaneous adverse reactions (SCARs) · SIADH · venous thromboembolism
  - **Frequency not known** Sleep apnoea
- **PREGNANCY** Use only if potential benefit outweighs risk.
- **BREAST FEEDING** Manufacturer advises avoid.
- **HEPATIC IMPAIRMENT** Manufacturer advises caution (risk of increased plasma concentrations).
  Dose adjustments In adults, manufacturer advises dose reduction—consult product literature.

- **MEDICINAL FORMS** There can be variation in the licensing of different medicines containing the same drug. Forms available from special-order manufacturers include: oral suspension, oral solution, oral powder

Oral tablet

CAUTIONARY AND ADVISORY LABELS 2

▸ **Quetiapine (Non-proprietary)**
Quetiapine (as Quetiapine fumarate) 25 mg Quetiapine 25mg tablets | 30 tablet PoM £24.30 | 60 tablet PoM £40.59 DT = £1.05
Quetiapine (as Quetiapine fumarate) 50 mg Quetiapine 50mg tablets | 60 tablet PoM £12.50–21.10 DT = £12.50
Quetiapine (as Quetiapine fumarate) 100 mg Quetiapine 100mg tablets | 60 tablet PoM £135.72 DT = £2.50
Quetiapine (as Quetiapine fumarate) 150 mg Quetiapine 150mg tablets | 60 tablet PoM £135.72 DT = £3.20
Quetiapine (as Quetiapine fumarate) 200 mg Quetiapine 200mg tablets | 60 tablet PoM £159.72 DT = £3.27
Quetiapine (as Quetiapine fumarate) 300 mg Quetiapine 300mg tablets | 60 tablet PoM £204.00 DT = £3.57
Quetiapine (as Quetiapine fumarate) 400 mg Quetiapine 400mg tablets | 60 tablet PoM £25.00–£40.00 DT = £25.00

▸ **Seroquel** (Luye Pharma Ltd)
Quetiapine (as Quetiapine fumarate) 25 mg Seroquel 25mg tablets | 60 tablet PoM £48.60 DT = £1.05
Quetiapine (as Quetiapine fumarate) 100 mg Seroquel 100mg tablets | 60 tablet PoM £135.72 DT = £2.50
Quetiapine (as Quetiapine fumarate) 200 mg Seroquel 200mg tablets | 60 tablet PoM £135.72 DT = £3.27
Quetiapine (as Quetiapine fumarate) 300 mg Seroquel 300mg tablets | 60 tablet PoM £204.00 DT = £3.57

Modified-release tablet

CAUTIONARY AND ADVISORY LABELS 2, 23, 25

▸ **Quetiapine (Non-proprietary)**
Quetiapine (as Quetiapine fumarate) 50 mg Quetiapine 50mg modified-release tablets | 1 tablet PoM ⊠
Quetiapine (as Quetiapine fumarate) 150 mg Quetiapine 150mg modified-release tablets | 1 tablet PoM ⊠
Quetiapine (as Quetiapine fumarate) 200 mg Quetiapine 200mg modified-release tablets | 1 tablet PoM ⊠
Quetiapine (as Quetiapine fumarate) 300 mg Quetiapine 300mg modified-release tablets | 1 tablet PoM ⊠
Quetiapine (as Quetiapine fumarate) 400 mg Quetiapine 400mg modified-release tablets | 1 tablet PoM ⊠

▸ **Atrolak XL** (Accord-UK Ltd)
Quetiapine (as Quetiapine fumarate) 50 mg Atrolak XL 50mg tablets | 60 tablet PoM £67.65 DT = £67.66
Quetiapine (as Quetiapine fumarate) 150 mg Atrolak XL 150mg tablets | 60 tablet PoM £107.45 DT = £113.10
Quetiapine (as Quetiapine fumarate) 200 mg Atrolak XL 200mg tablets | 60 tablet PoM £113.09 DT = £113.10
Quetiapine (as Quetiapine fumarate) 300 mg Atrolak XL 300mg tablets | 60 tablet PoM £169.99 DT = £170.00
Quetiapine (as Quetiapine fumarate) 400 mg Atrolak XL 400mg tablets | 60 tablet PoM £226.19 DT = £226.20

▸ **Biquelle XL** (Aspire Pharma Ltd)
Quetiapine (as Quetiapine fumarate) 50 mg Biquelle XL 50mg tablets | 30 tablet PoM £14.73 | 60 tablet PoM £29.45 DT = £67.66
Quetiapine (as Quetiapine fumarate) 150 mg Biquelle XL 150mg tablets | 30 tablet PoM £24.73 | 60 tablet PoM £49.45 DT = £113.10
Quetiapine (as Quetiapine fumarate) 200 mg Biquelle XL 200mg tablets | 30 tablet PoM £24.73 | 60 tablet PoM £49.45 DT = £113.10
Quetiapine (as Quetiapine fumarate) 300 mg Biquelle XL 300mg tablets | 30 tablet PoM £37.23 | 60 tablet PoM £74.45 DT = £170.00
Quetiapine (as Quetiapine fumarate) 400 mg Biquelle XL 400mg tablets | 30 tablet PoM £49.48 | 60 tablet PoM £98.95 DT = £226.20
Quetiapine (as Quetiapine fumarate) 600 mg Biquelle XL 600mg tablets | 30 tablet PoM £70.73 DT = £70.73

▸ **Mintreleq XL** (Aristo Pharma Ltd)
Quetiapine (as Quetiapine fumarate) 50 mg Mintreleq XL 50mg tablets | 60 tablet PoM £14.99 DT = £67.66
Quetiapine (as Quetiapine fumarate) 150 mg Mintreleq XL 150mg tablets | 60 tablet PoM £29.99 DT = £113.10
Quetiapine (as Quetiapine fumarate) 200 mg Mintreleq XL 200mg tablets | 60 tablet PoM £29.99 DT = £113.10
Quetiapine (as Quetiapine fumarate) 300 mg Mintreleq XL 300mg tablets | 60 tablet PoM £49.99 DT = £170.00
Quetiapine (as Quetiapine fumarate) 400 mg Mintreleq XL 400mg tablets | 60 tablet PoM £64.99 DT = £226.20

▸ **Seroquel XL** (Luye Pharma Ltd)
Quetiapine (as Quetiapine fumarate) 50 mg Seroquel XL 50mg tablets | 60 tablet PoM £67.66 DT = £67.66
Quetiapine (as Quetiapine fumarate) 150 mg Seroquel XL 150mg tablets | 60 tablet PoM £113.10 DT = £113.10
Quetiapine (as Quetiapine fumarate) 200 mg Seroquel XL 200mg tablets | 60 tablet PoM £113.10 DT = £113.10
Quetiapine (as Quetiapine fumarate) 300 mg Seroquel XL 300mg tablets | 60 tablet PoM £170.00 DT = £170.00
Quetiapine (as Quetiapine fumarate) 400 mg Seroquel XL 400mg tablets | 60 tablet PoM £226.20 DT = £226.20

▸ **Sondate XL** (Teva UK Ltd)
Quetiapine (as Quetiapine fumarate) 50 mg Sondate XL 50mg tablets | 60 tablet PoM £11.99 DT = £67.66
Quetiapine (as Quetiapine fumarate) 150 mg Sondate XL 150mg tablets | 60 tablet PoM £25.99 DT = £113.10
Quetiapine (as Quetiapine fumarate) 200 mg Sondate XL 200mg tablets | 60 tablet PoM £25.99 DT = £113.10
Quetiapine (as Quetiapine fumarate) 300 mg Sondate XL 300mg tablets | 60 tablet PoM £44.99 DT = £170.00
Quetiapine (as Quetiapine fumarate) 400 mg Sondate XL 400mg tablets | 60 tablet PoM £59.99 DT = £226.20

▸ **Zaluron XL** (Fontus Health Ltd)
Quetiapine (as Quetiapine fumarate) 50 mg Zaluron XL 50mg tablets | 60 tablet PoM £27.96 DT = £67.66
Quetiapine (as Quetiapine fumarate) 150 mg Zaluron XL 150mg tablets | 60 tablet PoM £46.96 DT = £113.10
Quetiapine (as Quetiapine fumarate) 200 mg Zaluron XL 200mg tablets | 60 tablet PoM £46.96 DT = £113.10
Quetiapine (as Quetiapine fumarate) 300 mg Zaluron XL 300mg tablets | 60 tablet PoM £70.71 DT = £170.00
Quetiapine (as Quetiapine fumarate) 400 mg Zaluron XL 400mg tablets | 60 tablet PoM £93.98 DT = £226.20

Oral suspension

CAUTIONARY AND ADVISORY LABELS 2

▸ **Quetiapine (Non-proprietary)**
Quetiapine (as Quetiapine fumarate) 20 mg per 1 ml Quetiapine 20mg/ml oral suspension sugar free | 150 ml PoM £215.22 DT = £215.22 SF

295

Risperidone

21-Jan-2025

- **DRUG ACTION** Risperidone is a dopamine D_2, 5-HT_{2A}, alpha$_1$-adrenoceptor, and histamine-1 receptor antagonist.

- **INDICATIONS AND DOSE**

Acute and chronic psychosis

▸ BY MOUTH

▸ Child 12–17 years (under expert supervision): 2 mg daily in 1–2 divided doses for day 1, then 4 mg daily in 1–2 divided doses for day 2, slower titration is appropriate in some patients; usual dose 4–6 mg daily, doses above 10 mg daily only if benefit considered to outweigh risk; maximum 16 mg per day

Short-term monotherapy of mania in bipolar disorder (under expert supervision)

▸ BY MOUTH

▸ Child 12–17 years: Initially 500 micrograms once daily, then adjusted in steps of 0.5–1 mg daily, adjusted according to response; usual dose 2.5 mg daily in 1–2 divided doses; maximum 6 mg per day

Short-term treatment (up to 6 weeks) of persistent aggression in conduct disorder (under expert supervision)

▸ BY MOUTH

▸ Child 5–17 years (body-weight up to 50 kg): Initially 250 micrograms once daily, then increased in steps of 250 micrograms once daily on alternate days, adjusted according to response; usual dose 500 micrograms once daily; maximum 750 micrograms per day

▸ Child 5–17 years (body-weight 50 kg and above): Initially 500 micrograms once daily, then increased in steps of 500 micrograms once daily on alternate days, adjusted according to response; usual dose 1 mg once daily; maximum 1.5 mg per day

Short-term treatment of severe aggression in autism (under expert supervision)

▸ BY MOUTH

▸ Child 5–17 years (body-weight 15–20 kg): Initially 250 micrograms daily for at least 4 days, then increased if necessary to 500 micrograms daily, then increased in steps of 250 micrograms daily, dose to be increased at intervals of 2 weeks, review effectiveness and any side-effects after 3–4 weeks; stop if no response at 6 weeks; maximum 1 mg per day

▸ Child 5–17 years (body-weight 20–45 kg): Initially 500 micrograms daily for at least 4 days, then increased if necessary to 1 mg daily, then increased in steps of 500 micrograms daily, dose to be increased at intervals of 2 weeks, review effectiveness and any side-effects after 3–4 weeks; stop if no response at 6 weeks; maximum 2.5 mg per day

▸ Child 5–17 years (body-weight 45 kg and above): Initially 500 micrograms daily for at least 4 days, then increased if necessary to 1 mg daily, then increased in steps of 500 micrograms daily, dose to be increased at intervals of 2 weeks, review effectiveness and any side-effects after 3–4 weeks; stop if no response at 6 weeks; maximum 3 mg per day

- **UNLICENSED USE** Not licensed for use in children for psychosis, mania, or autism.

IMPORTANT SAFETY INFORMATION

SAFE PRACTICE

Risperidone has been confused with ropinirole; care must be taken to ensure the correct drug is prescribed and dispensed.

MHRA/CHM ADVICE: CLOZAPINE AND OTHER ANTIPSYCHOTICS: MONITORING BLOOD CONCENTRATIONS FOR TOXICITY (AUGUST 2020)

Following fatal cases involving toxicity of clozapine and other antipsychotic medicines, the MHRA advises that monitoring blood concentration of risperidone may be helpful in certain circumstances, such as patients presenting symptoms suggestive of toxicity, or when concomitant medicines may interact to increase blood concentration of risperidone.

- **CAUTIONS** Avoid in Acute porphyrias p. 745 · cataract surgery (risk of intra-operative floppy iris syndrome) · dehydration · family history of sudden cardiac death (perform ECG) · prolactin-dependent tumours
- **INTERACTIONS** → Appendix 1: atypical antipsychotics
- **SIDE-EFFECTS**

▸ **Common or very common** Anxiety · appetite abnormal · asthenia · chest discomfort · conjunctivitis · cough · depression · diarrhoea · dyspnoea · epistaxis · fall · fever · gastrointestinal discomfort · headache · hypertension · increased risk of infection · joint disorders · laryngeal pain · muscle spasms · nasal congestion · nausea · oedema · oral disorders · pain · skin reactions · sleep disorders · urinary disorders · vision disorders

▸ **Uncommon** Alopecia · anaemia · breast abnormalities · cardiac conduction disorders · cerebrovascular insufficiency · chills · coma · concentration impaired · consciousness impaired · cystitis · diabetes mellitus · dry eye · dysarthria · dysphagia · dysphonia · ear pain · eye disorders · feeling abnormal · flushing · gait abnormal · gastrointestinal disorders · malaise · menstrual cycle irregularities · mood altered · muscle weakness · palpitations · polydipsia · posture abnormal · procedural pain · respiratory disorders · sensation abnormal · sexual dysfunction · syncope · taste altered · thirst · thrombocytopenia · tinnitus · vaginal discharge · vertigo · weight decreased

▸ **Rare or very rare** Angioedema · catatonia · dandruff · diabetic ketoacidosis · embolism and thrombosis · eyelid crusting · glaucoma · hypoglycaemia · hypothermia · induration · jaundice · pancreatitis · peripheral coldness · rhabdomyolysis · SIADH · sleep apnoea · water intoxication · withdrawal syndrome

▸ **Frequency not known** Cardiac arrest · severe cutaneous adverse reactions (SCARs)

- **PREGNANCY** Use only if potential benefit outweighs risk.
- **BREAST FEEDING** Use only if potential benefit outweighs risk—small amount present in milk.
- **HEPATIC IMPAIRMENT** EvGr Caution. (M)

Dose adjustments EvGr Dose reduction to half the usual dose, and slower dose titration. (M)

- **RENAL IMPAIRMENT** EvGr Caution. (M)

Dose adjustments EvGr Initial and subsequent doses should be halved, with slower dose titration. (M)

- **DIRECTIONS FOR ADMINISTRATION** Orodispersible tablets should be placed on the tongue, allowed to dissolve and swallowed. Manufacturer advises oral liquid may be diluted with any non-alcoholic drink, except tea.
- **PATIENT AND CARER ADVICE** Patients or carers should be given advice on how to administer risperidone orodispersible tablets and oral liquid (counselling on use of dose syringe advised).

Medicines for Children leaflet: Risperidone for psychological disorders www.medicinesforchildren.org.uk/medicines/risperidone-for-psychological-disorders/

- **MEDICINAL FORMS** There can be variation in the licensing of different medicines containing the same drug. Forms available from special-order manufacturers include: oral solution

Oral tablet

CAUTIONARY AND ADVISORY LABELS 2

▸ **Risperidone (Non-proprietary)**

Risperidone 250 microgram Risperidone 250microgram tablets | 20 tablet PoM £38.00–£56.00

Risperidone 500 microgram Risperidone 500microgram tablets | 20 tablet PoM £23.86 DT = £2.65

Risperidone 1 mg Risperidone 1mg tablets | 20 tablet PoM £10.16 DT = £0.78 | 60 tablet PoM £2.16–£14.93

Risperidone 2 mg Risperidone 2mg tablets | 60 tablet PoM £60.10 DT = £1.44

Risperidone 3 mg Risperidone 3mg tablets | 60 tablet PoM £88.38 DT = £1.57

Risperidone 4 mg Risperidone 4mg tablets | 60 tablet PoM £116.67 DT = £1.83

Risperidone 6 mg Risperidone 6mg tablets | 28 tablet PoM £82.50 DT = £8.19

Oral solution

CAUTIONARY AND ADVISORY LABELS 2

▸ **Risperidone (Non-proprietary)**

Risperidone 1 mg per 1 ml Risperidone 1mg/ml oral solution sugar free | 100 ml PoM £9.46 DT = £3.26 SF

Orodispersible tablet

CAUTIONARY AND ADVISORY LABELS 2

EXCIPIENTS: May contain Aspartame

▸ **Risperidone (Non-proprietary)**

Risperidone 500 microgram Risperidone 500microgram orodispersible tablets sugar free | 28 tablet PoM £7.35–£23.03 DT = £7.35 SF

Risperidone 1 mg Risperidone 1mg orodispersible tablets sugar free | 28 tablet PoM £25.31 DT = £10.65 SF

Risperidone 2 mg Risperidone 2mg orodispersible tablets sugar free | 28 tablet PoM £45.82 DT = £9.55 SF

Risperidone 3 mg Risperidone 3mg orodispersible tablets sugar free | 28 tablet PoM £43.48 DT = £43.48 SF

Risperidone 4 mg Risperidone 4mg orodispersible tablets sugar free | 28 tablet PoM £56.02 DT = £56.02 SF

3 Movement disorders

Cerebral palsy and spasticity

18-Jan-2022

Description of condition

Cerebral palsy is a group of permanent, non-progressive abnormalities of the developing fetal or neonatal brain that lead to movement and posture disorders, causing activity limitation and functional impact. There can be accompanying clinical and developmental comorbidities. These include disturbances of sensation, perception, cognition, communication and behaviour, epilepsy, and secondary musculoskeletal problems (such as muscle contracture and abnormal torsion). Cerebral palsy is not curable and the comorbidities can impact on many areas of participation and quality of life, particularly eating, drinking, comfort, and sleep.

Spasticity

Spasticity in children is most commonly associated with cerebral palsy, but can also be associated with other non-progressive brain disorders.

Aims of treatment

Treatment involves managing spasticity to optimise movement and posture, while minimising potential secondary musculoskeletal deformity, as well as managing developmental and clinical comorbidities.

Non-drug treatment

EvGr All children with spasticity should be offered physiotherapy and, where necessary, occupational therapy. They can also benefit from orthoses.

Orthopaedic surgery can be used, as an adjunct to other interventions, to prevent deterioration and improve function. (A)

Drug treatment

Spasticity

EvGr Oral diazepam p. 270 or oral baclofen p. 814 can be used to treat discomfort, pain, muscle spasm and functional disability. If oral diazepam is initially used because of its rapid onset of action, consider changing to oral baclofen if a sustained, longer duration of effect is required or if long-term treatment is necessary. If the response to diazepam or baclofen after 4–6 weeks is unsatisfactory, a trial of combined treatment using both drugs can be considered. Consider reducing the dose if adverse effects such as drowsiness occur. Treatment cessation should be considered when management is reviewed and at least every six months.

If **dystonia** is considered to contribute significantly to problems with posture, function and pain, a trial of treatment with oral trihexyphenidyl hydrochloride p. 309, levodopa, or baclofen [unlicensed indications] can be considered.

Treatment with botulinum toxin type A p. 311 [unlicensed under 2 years] should be considered for those in whom focal spasticity of the upper or lower limbs is inhibiting fine motor function, affecting care and hygiene, causing pain or disturbing sleep, impeding tolerance of other treatments (such as orthoses), or causing cosmetic concerns. A trial of botulinum toxin type A treatment can also be considered in those with spasticity when *focal dystonia* [unlicensed] is causing problems, such as postural or functional difficulties or pain. Ongoing assessment of muscle tone, range of movement and motor function is required. Botulinum toxin type A treatment should **not** be offered to children receiving treatment with Aminoglycosides p. 376.

Treatment with intrathecal baclofen [unlicensed under 4 years] (administered by continuous pump) can be considered in children with spasticity if (despite the use of non-invasive treatments) spasticity or dystonia are causing difficulties with pain, muscle spasm, posture, function or self-care. Before deciding to implant the intrathecal baclofen pump, an intrathecal baclofen test should be performed to assess the therapeutic effect and to check for adverse effects. (A)

Developmental and clinical comorbidities

EvGr Regular assessment and appropriate nutritional support should be provided, especially if there are concerns about oral intake, growth or nutritional status. Enteral tube feeding can be provided if oral intake is insufficient to provide adequate nutrition. (A)

Children with cerebral palsy are likely to have risk factors for low bone mineral density and can have an increased risk of low-impact fractures. EvGr Calcium and vitamin D supplementation (such as colecalciferol with calcium carbonate p. 791) may be required. Children with reduced bone density and a history of low-impact fracture can be considered for bisphosphonate therapy (under specialist guidance). (A)

Pain is common in children with cerebral palsy, especially those with more severe motor impairment. Condition-specific causes of pain and discomfort include musculoskeletal problems (for example, scoliosis, hip subluxation and dislocation), increased muscle tone (including dystonia and spasticity), muscle fatigue and immobility, constipation, vomiting, and gastro-oesophageal reflux disease. Reversible causes of pain should be treated as appropriate, see *Spasticity* (above), Constipation p. 44,

Gastro-oesophageal reflux disease p. 66, Urinary frequency, enuresis and incontinence p. 602, Nocturnal enuresis in children p. 602, and Urinary-tract infections p. 454.

Other types of pain include non-specific back pain, headache, non-specific abdominal pain, dental pain and dysmenorrhoea. EvGr Initially, a 'stepped approach' trial of simple analgesia (such as paracetamol p. 325, ibuprofen p. 821, or both) for mild-to-moderate pain can be considered. If such a trial is unsuccessful, the child should be referred to a specialist pain team. (A)

In children with cerebral palsy, sleep disturbances are common. EvGr If no treatable cause is found, a trial of melatonin p. 351 [unlicensed] can be considered to manage sleep disturbances, particularly for problems with falling asleep. Regular sedative medication should **not** be used to manage primary sleep disorders in children with cerebral palsy without seeking specialist advice. (A)

Epilepsy can be associated with cerebral palsy; for its management, see Epilepsy p. 227.

Children with cerebral palsy are at greater risk of mental health problems, in comparison with the general age comparison population. For management of these conditions, see Depression p. 285, Anxiety (Hypnotics and anxiolytics p. 350), and Attention deficit hyperactivity disorder p. 275.

Drooling

EvGr Drooling can be managed with an antimuscarinic drug, such as glycopyrronium bromide p. 1014 [unlicensed in under 3 years] (oral or by enteral tube) or hyoscine hydrobromide (transdermal) p. 320 [unlicensed]. For children with dyskinetic cerebral palsy, trihexyphenidyl hydrochloride [unlicensed] can be used (on specialist advice). If antimuscarinic drugs provide insufficient benefit or are not tolerated, botulinum toxin type A injections to the salivary glands can be considered. High-dose botulinum toxin type A injections to the salivary glands can, rarely, cause breathing and swallowing difficulties, which requires urgent hospital admission. Surgery can be an option in cases resistant to drug treatment. (A)

Related drugs

Other drugs used for Cerebral palsy and spasticity: co-careldopa p. 310, dantrolene sodium p. 1025.

Transition planning

For guidance on the patient's transition from paediatric to adult services, see *Transitional services for chronic conditions* in Guidance on prescribing p. 1.

Useful Resources

Cerebral palsy in under 25s: assessment and management. National Institute for Health and Care Excellence. Clinical guideline 62. January 2017.
www.nice.org.uk/guidance/ng62

Spasticity in under 19s: management. National Institute for Health and Care Excellence. Clinical guideline 145. July 2012 (updated November 2016).
www.nice.org.uk/guidance/cg145

3.1 Dystonias and other involuntary movements

Dystonias and related disorders

Dystonias

Dystonias may result from conditions such as cerebral palsy or may be related to a deficiency of the neurotransmitter dopamine as in Segawa syndrome.

Dopaminergic drugs used in dystonias

Levodopa, the amino-acid precursor of dopamine, acts by replenishing depleted striatal dopamine. It is given with an extracerebral **dopa-decarboxylase inhibitor**, which reduces the peripheral conversion of levodopa to dopamine, thereby limiting side-effects such as nausea, vomiting, and cardiovascular effects; additionally, effective brain-dopamine concentrations are achieved with lower doses of levodopa. The extracerebral dopa-decarboxylase inhibitor most commonly used in children is carbidopa (in co-careldopa p. 310).

Levodopa therapy should be initiated at a low dose and increased in small steps; the final dose should be as low as possible. Intervals between doses should be chosen to suit the needs of the individual child.

In severe dystonias related to cerebral palsy, improvement can be expected within 2 weeks. Children with Segawa syndrome are particularly sensitive to levodopa; they may even become symptom free on small doses. Levodopa also has a role in treating metabolic disorders such as defects in tetrahydrobiopterin synthesis and dihydrobiopterin reductase deficiency. Tetrahydrobiopterin may have a role in metabolic disorders.

Children may experience nausea within 2 hours of taking a dose; nausea and vomiting with co-careldopa is rarely dose-limiting.

In dystonic cerebral palsy, treatment with larger doses of levodopa is associated with the development of potentially troublesome motor complications (including response fluctuations and dyskinesias). Response fluctuations are characterised by large variations in motor performance, with normal function during the 'on' period, and weakness and restricted mobility during the 'off' period.

Antimuscarinic drugs used in dystonias

The antimuscarinic drugs procyclidine hydrochloride p. 309 and trihexyphenidyl hydrochloride p. 309 reduce the symptoms of dystonias, including those induced by antipsychotic drugs; there is no justification for giving them routinely in the absence of dystonic symptoms. Tardive dyskinesia is not improved by antimuscarinic drugs and may be made worse.

There are no important differences between the antimuscarinic drugs, but some children tolerate one better than another.

Procyclidine hydrochloride can be given parenterally and is effective emergency treatment for acute drug-induced dystonic reactions.

If treatment with an antimuscarinic is ineffective, intravenous diazepam p. 270 can be given for life-threatening acute drug-induced dystonic reactions.

Drugs used in essential tremor, chorea, tics, and related disorders

Haloperidol p. 296 can also improve motor tics and symptoms of Tourette syndrome and related choreas. Other treatments for Tourette syndrome include pimozide p. 297 [unlicensed indication] (**important**: ECG monitoring required), and sulpiride p. 298 [unlicensed indication].

Propranolol hydrochloride p. 123 or another beta-adrenoceptor blocking drug may be useful in treating essential tremor or tremor associated with anxiety or thyrotoxicosis.

Botulinum toxin type A p. 311 should be used under specialist supervision. Treatment with botulinum toxin type A can be considered after an acquired non-progressive brain injury if rapid-onset spasticity causes postural or functional difficulties, and in children with spasticity in whom focal dystonia causes postural or functional difficulties or pain.

ANTIMUSCARINICS

Procyclidine hydrochloride
25-Aug-2022

- **DRUG ACTION** Procyclidine exerts its antiparkinsonian action by reducing the effects of the relative central cholinergic excess that occurs as a result of dopamine deficiency.

- **INDICATIONS AND DOSE**

Acute dystonia

▶ BY INTRAMUSCULAR INJECTION, OR BY INTRAVENOUS INJECTION

- Child 1 month–1 year: 0.5–2 mg for 1 dose, dose usually effective in 5–10 minutes but may need 30 minutes for relief
- Child 2–9 years: 2–5 mg for 1 dose, dose usually effective in 5–10 minutes but may need 30 minutes for relief
- Child 10–17 years: 5–10 mg, occasionally, more than 10 mg, dose usually effective in 5–10 minutes but may need 30 minutes for relief

Dystonia

▶ BY MOUTH

- Child 7–11 years: 1.25 mg 3 times a day
- Child 12–17 years: 2.5 mg 3 times a day

- **UNLICENSED USE** Not licensed for use in children.
- **CONTRA-INDICATIONS** Gastro-intestinal obstruction
- **CAUTIONS** Cardiovascular disease · hypertension · liable to abuse · psychotic disorders · pyrexia · those susceptible to angle-closure glaucoma
- **INTERACTIONS** → Appendix 1: procyclidine
- **SIDE-EFFECTS**
  - ▶ **Common or very common** Constipation · dry mouth · urinary retention · vision blurred
  - ▶ **Uncommon** Anxiety · cognitive impairment · confusion · dizziness · gingivitis · hallucination · memory loss · nausea · rash · vomiting
  - ▶ **Rare or very rare** Psychotic disorder
- **PREGNANCY** Use only if potential benefit outweighs risk.
- **BREAST FEEDING** No information available.
- **HEPATIC IMPAIRMENT** Manufacturer advises caution.
- **RENAL IMPAIRMENT** EvGr Use with caution. (M)
- **TREATMENT CESSATION** Avoid abrupt withdrawal in patients taking long-term treatment.
- **PATIENT AND CARER ADVICE**

Driving and skilled tasks May affect performance of skilled tasks (e.g. driving).

- **MEDICINAL FORMS** There can be variation in the licensing of different medicines containing the same drug. Forms available from special-order manufacturers include: oral suspension, oral solution

Solution for injection

▶ **Procyclidine hydrochloride (Non-proprietary)**

Procyclidine hydrochloride 5 mg per 1 ml Procyclidine 10mg/2ml solution for injection ampoules | 5 ampoule PoM £72.50 DT = £72.50

Oral tablet

▶ **Procyclidine hydrochloride (Non-proprietary)**

Procyclidine hydrochloride 5 mg Procyclidine 5mg tablets | 28 tablet PoM £5.94 DT = £1.39 | 100 tablet PoM £3.96–£8.94 | 500 tablet PoM £19.82–£44.63

▶ **Kemadrin** (Aspen Pharma Trading Ltd)

Procyclidine hydrochloride 5 mg Kemadrin 5mg tablets | 100 tablet PoM £4.72 | 500 tablet PoM £23.62

Oral solution

▶ **Procyclidine hydrochloride (Non-proprietary)**

Procyclidine hydrochloride 500 microgram per 1 ml Procyclidine 2.5mg/5ml oral solution sugar free | 150 ml PoM £48.72 DT = £48.72 SF

Procyclidine hydrochloride 1 mg per 1 ml Procyclidine 5mg/5ml oral solution sugar free | 150 ml PoM £72.14 DT = £72.14 SF

Trihexyphenidyl hydrochloride
27-Apr-2021

(Benzhexol hydrochloride)

- **DRUG ACTION** Trihexyphenidyl exerts its effects by reducing the effects of the relative central cholinergic excess that occurs as a result of dopamine deficiency.

- **INDICATIONS AND DOSE**

Dystonia

▶ BY MOUTH

- Child 3 months–17 years: Initially 1–2 mg daily in 1–2 divided doses, then increased in steps of 1 mg every 3–7 days, dose to be adjusted according to response and side-effects; maximum 2 mg/kg per day

- **UNLICENSED USE** Not licensed for use in children.
- **CONTRA-INDICATIONS** Myasthenia gravis
- **CAUTIONS** Cardiovascular disease · gastro-intestinal obstruction · hypertension · liable to abuse · psychotic disorders · pyrexia · those susceptible to angle-closure glaucoma
- **INTERACTIONS** → Appendix 1: trihexyphenidyl
- **SIDE-EFFECTS** Anxiety · bronchial secretion decreased · confusion · constipation · delusions · dizziness · dry mouth · dysphagia · euphoric mood · fever · flushing · hallucination · insomnia · memory loss · myasthenia gravis aggravated · mydriasis · nausea · skin reactions · tachycardia · thirst · urinary disorders · vision disorders · vomiting
- **PREGNANCY** Use only if potential benefit outweighs risk.
- **BREAST FEEDING** Avoid.
- **HEPATIC IMPAIRMENT** Manufacturer advises caution.
- **RENAL IMPAIRMENT** EvGr Use with caution. (M)
- **TREATMENT CESSATION** Avoid abrupt withdrawal in patients taking long-term treatment.
- **DIRECTIONS FOR ADMINISTRATION** Manufacturer advises tablets should be taken with or after food.
- **PATIENT AND CARER ADVICE**

Medicines for Children leaflet: Trihexyphenidyl hydrochloride for dystonia www.medicinesforchildren.org.uk/medicines/trihexyphenidyl-hydrochloride-for-dystonia/

Driving and skilled tasks May affect performance of skilled tasks (e.g. driving).

- **MEDICINAL FORMS** There can be variation in the licensing of different medicines containing the same drug. Forms available from special-order manufacturers include: oral suspension, oral solution

Oral tablet

▶ **Trihexyphenidyl hydrochloride (Non-proprietary)**

Trihexyphenidyl hydrochloride 2 mg Trihexyphenidyl 2mg tablets | 84 tablet PoM £260.00 DT = £116.57

Trihexyphenidyl hydrochloride 5 mg Trihexyphenidyl 5mg tablets | 84 tablet PoM £260.00 DT = £195.95

Oral solution

EXCIPIENTS: May contain Propylene glycol

▶ **Trihexyphenidyl hydrochloride (Non-proprietary)**

Trihexyphenidyl hydrochloride 1 mg per 1 ml Trihexyphenidyl 5mg/5ml oral solution | 200 ml PoM £112.78 DT = £112.78
Trihexyphenidyl 5mg/5ml syrup | 200 ml PoM £112.78 DT = £112.78

DOPAMINERGIC DRUGS › DOPAMINE PRECURSORS

Co-careldopa

06-Nov-2024

- **INDICATIONS AND DOSE**

Dopamine-sensitive dystonias including Segawa syndrome and dystonias related to cerebral palsy (dose expressed as levodopa)

▶ BY MOUTH

▶ Child 3 months–17 years: Initially 250 micrograms/kg 2–3 times a day, dose to be increased according to response every 2–3 days, increased if necessary up to 1 mg/kg 3 times a day, preparation containing 1:4 ratio of carbidopa:levodopa is to be used

Treatment of defects in tetrahydrobiopterin synthesis and dihydrobiopterin reductase deficiency (dose expressed as levodopa)

▶ BY MOUTH

▶ Neonate: Initially 250–500 micrograms/kg 4 times a day, dose to be increased every 4–5 days according to response, a preparation containing 1:4 carbidopa: levodopa to be administered; maintenance 2.5–3 mg/kg 4 times a day, at higher doses consider preparation containing 1:10 carbidopa:levodopa, review regularly (every 3–6 months).

▶ Child: Initially 250–500 micrograms/kg 4 times a day, dose to be increased every 4–5 days according to response, a preparation containing 1:4 carbidopa: levodopa to be administered; maintenance 2.5–3 mg/kg 4 times a day, at higher doses consider preparation containing 1:10 carbidopa:levodopa, review regularly (every 3–6 months in early childhood)

DOSE EQUIVALENCE AND CONVERSION

▶ The proportions are expressed in the form x/y where x and y are the strengths in milligrams of carbidopa and levodopa respectively.

▶ 2 tablets *Sinemet*® 12.5 mg/50 mg is equivalent to 1 tablet *Sinemet*® Plus 25 mg/100 mg.

- **UNLICENSED USE** Not licensed for use in children.
- **CONTRA-INDICATIONS** Angle-closure glaucoma · suspicious undiagnosed skin lesions or history of skin melanoma (risk of activation)
- **CAUTIONS** Acute stroke · cardiovascular disease · diabetes mellitus · history of myocardial infarction with residual arrhythmia · history of peptic ulcer · open-angle glaucoma (monitor intra-ocular pressure) · osteomalacia · psychiatric illness (avoid if severe and discontinue if deterioration) · pulmonary disease
- **INTERACTIONS** → Appendix 1: carbidopa · levodopa
- **SIDE-EFFECTS**

▶ **Rare or very rare** Drowsiness · seizure · sudden onset of sleep (can occur without warning)

▶ **Frequency not known** Agranulocytosis · alertness decreased · alopecia · anaemia · angioedema · anxiety · appetite decreased · asthenia · cardiac disorder · chest pain · compulsions · confusion · constipation · delusions · depression · diarrhoea · dizziness · dry mouth · dyskinesia (may be dose-limiting) · dysphagia · dyspnoea · eating disorders · euphoric mood · eye disorders · fall · focal tremor · gait abnormal · gastrointestinal discomfort · gastrointestinal disorders · gastrointestinal haemorrhage · haemolytic anaemia · hallucination · headache · Henoch-Schönlein purpura · hiccups · hoarseness · Horner's syndrome exacerbated · hypertension · hypotension · leucopenia · malaise · malignant melanoma · movement disorders · muscle complaints · nausea · neuroleptic malignant syndrome (on abrupt discontinuation) · oedema · oral disorders · palpitations · pathological gambling · postural disorders · psychotic disorder · respiration abnormal · sensation abnormal · sexual dysfunction · skin reactions · sleep disorders · suicidal ideation · sweat changes · syncope · taste bitter · teeth grinding · thrombocytopenia · trismus · urinary disorders · urine dark · vasodilation · vision disorders · vomiting · weight changes

- **PREGNANCY** Use with caution—toxicity has occurred in *animal* studies.
- **BREAST FEEDING** May suppress lactation; present in milk—avoid.
- **HEPATIC IMPAIRMENT** Manufacturer advises use with caution in hepatic disease.
- **MONITORING REQUIREMENTS** In prolonged therapy, psychiatric, hepatic, haematological, renal, and cardiovascular monitoring is advisable; warn patients to resume normal activities gradually.
- **EFFECT ON LABORATORY TESTS** False positive tests for urinary ketones have been reported.
- **TREATMENT CESSATION** Avoid abrupt withdrawal.
- **PRESCRIBING AND DISPENSING INFORMATION** Co-careldopa is a mixture of carbidopa and levodopa; the proportions are expressed in the form x/y where x and y are the strengths in milligrams of carbidopa and levodopa respectively.
- **PATIENT AND CARER ADVICE** Warn patients to resume normal activity gradually.

Driving and skilled tasks

Sudden onset of sleep Excessive daytime sleepiness and sudden onset of sleep can occur with co-careldopa.

Patients starting treatment should be warned of the risk and of the need to exercise caution when driving or operating machinery. Those who have experienced excessive sedation or sudden onset of sleep should refrain from driving or operating machines until these effects have stopped occurring.

Management of excessive daytime sleepiness should focus on the identification of an underlying cause, such as depression or concomitant medication. Patients should be counselled on improving sleep behaviour.

- **MEDICINAL FORMS** There can be variation in the licensing of different medicines containing the same drug. Forms available from special-order manufacturers include: oral suspension, oral solution

Oral tablet

CAUTIONARY AND ADVISORY LABELS 10, 14

▶ Co-careldopa (Non-proprietary)

Carbidopa (as Carbidopa monohydrate) 12.5 mg, Levodopa 50 mg Co-careldopa 12.5mg/50mg tablets | 90 tablet PoM £19.31 DT = £4.89 | 100 tablet PoM £4.19–£11.00

Carbidopa (as Carbidopa monohydrate) 25 mg, Levodopa 100 mg Co-careldopa 25mg/100mg tablets | 100 tablet PoM £15.00 DT = £7.10

Carbidopa (as Carbidopa monohydrate) 10 mg, Levodopa 100 mg Co-careldopa 10mg/100mg tablets | 100 tablet PoM £14.00 DT = £14.00

Carbidopa (as Carbidopa monohydrate) 25 mg, Levodopa 250 mg Co-careldopa 25mg/250mg tablets | 100 tablet PoM £35.00 DT = £35.00

▶ Sinemet 110 (Organon Pharma (UK) Ltd)

Carbidopa (as Carbidopa monohydrate) 10 mg, Levodopa 100 mg Sinemet 10mg/100mg tablets | 100 tablet PoM £7.30 DT = £14.00

▶ Sinemet 275 (Organon Pharma (UK) Ltd)

Carbidopa (as Carbidopa monohydrate) 25 mg, Levodopa 250 mg Sinemet 25mg/250mg tablets | 100 tablet PoM £18.29 DT = £35.00

▶ Sinemet 62.5 (Organon Pharma (UK) Ltd)

Carbidopa (as Carbidopa monohydrate) 12.5 mg, Levodopa 50 mg Sinemet 12.5mg/50mg tablets | 90 tablet PoM £6.28 DT = £4.89

▶ Sinemet Plus (Organon Pharma (UK) Ltd)

Carbidopa (as Carbidopa monohydrate) 25 mg, Levodopa 100 mg Sinemet Plus 25mg/100mg tablets | 100 tablet PoM £12.88 DT = £7.10

MUSCLE RELAXANTS > PERIPHERALLY ACTING > NEUROTOXINS (BOTULINUM TOXINS)

Botulinum toxin type A

12-Apr-2022

- **INDICATIONS AND DOSE**

Dynamic equinus foot deformity caused by spasticity in ambulant paediatric cerebral palsy (specialist use only) | Upper limb spasticity in paediatric cerebral palsy (specialist use only)

▶ BY INTRAMUSCULAR INJECTION
- Child 2–17 years: (consult product literature)

Chronic sialorrhoea [due to neurological or neurodevelopmental disorders] (specialist use only)

▶ BY LOCAL INFILTRATION
- Child 2–17 years (body-weight 12 kg and above): (consult product literature)

DOSE EQUIVALENCE AND CONVERSION
- **Important**: information is specific to each individual preparation.

- **CONTRA-INDICATIONS** Infection at injection site
- **CAUTIONS** Atrophy in target muscle · chronic respiratory disorder · excessive weakness in target muscle · history of aspiration · history of dysphagia · inflammation in target muscle · neurological disorders · neuromuscular disorders · off-label use (fatal adverse events reported)

CAUTIONS, FURTHER INFORMATION Neuromuscular or neurological disorders can lead to increased sensitivity and exaggerated muscle weakness including dysphagia and respiratory compromise.

- **INTERACTIONS** → Appendix 1: botulinum toxins
- **SIDE-EFFECTS**

▶ **Common or very common** Alopecia · asthenia · brow ptosis · constipation · dizziness · drowsiness · dry eye · dry mouth · dysphagia (most common after injection into sternocleidomastoid muscle and salivary gland) · ecchymosis (minimised by applying gentle pressure at injection site immediately after injection) · eye disorders · eye inflammation · eye irritation · face oedema · facial paresis · fever · gait abnormal · haematuria · headache · hot flush · increased risk of infection · influenza like illness · leukocyturia · ligament sprain · malaise · muscle complaints · muscle weakness · musculoskeletal stiffness · nausea · pain · sensation abnormal · skin reactions · subcutaneous nodule · vision disorders

▶ **Uncommon** Arthropathy · dysphonia · dyspnoea · facial paralysis · speech impairment · taste altered · vertigo

▶ **Frequency not known** Abdominal pain · angioedema · angle closure glaucoma · appetite decreased · arrhythmia · diarrhoea · hearing impairment · hypersensitivity · myocardial infarction · myopathy · nerve disorders · neuromuscular dysfunction · oral disorders · pneumonia aspiration (potentially fatal) · respiratory disorders · seizure · syncope · tinnitus · vomiting

- **CONCEPTION AND CONTRACEPTION** Avoid in women of child-bearing age unless using effective contraception.
- **PREGNANCY** Avoid unless essential—toxicity in *animal* studies (manufacturer of *Botox®* advise avoid).
- **BREAST FEEDING** Low risk of systemic absorption but avoid unless essential.
- **PRESCRIBING AND DISPENSING INFORMATION** Preparations are not interchangeable.
- **PATIENT AND CARER ADVICE** Patients and carers should be warned of the signs and symptoms of toxin spread, such as muscle weakness and breathing difficulties; they should be advised to seek immediate medical attention if swallowing, speech or breathing difficulties occur.

Medicines for Children leaflet: Botulinum toxin for muscle spasticity www.medicinesforchildren.org.uk/medicines/botulinum-toxin-for-muscle-spasticity/

- **NATIONAL FUNDING/ACCESS DECISIONS**

For full details see funding body website

All Wales Medicines Strategy Group (AWMSG) decisions

▶ **Clostridium botulinum neurotoxin type A (*Xeomin®*) for the symptomatic treatment of chronic sialorrhoea due to neurological or neurodevelopmental disorders in children and adolescents aged 2 to 17 years and weighing 12 kg or more (December 2021)** AWMSG No. 3986 Recommended

▶ **Clostridium botulinum type A toxin-haemagglutinin complex (*Dysport®*) for the symptomatic treatment of focal spasticity of upper limbs in paediatric cerebral palsy patients, two years of age or older (February 2022)** AWMSG No. 2626 Recommended

- **MEDICINAL FORMS** There can be variation in the licensing of different medicines containing the same drug.

Powder for solution for injection

▶ **Azzalure** (Galderma (UK) Ltd)
Botulinum toxin type A 125 unit Azzalure 125unit powder for solution for injection vials | 2 vial PoM £126.99

▶ **Bocouture** (Merz Aesthetics UK Ltd)
Botulinum toxin type A 50 unit Bocouture 50unit powder for solution for injection vials | 1 vial PoM ⊠
Botulinum toxin type A 100 unit Bocouture 100unit powder for solution for injection vials | 1 vial PoM ⊠

▶ **Botox** (AbbVie Ltd)
Botulinum toxin type A 50 unit Botox 50unit powder for solution for injection vials | 1 vial PoM £77.50 (Hospital only)
Botulinum toxin type A 100 unit Botox 100unit powder for solution for injection vials | 1 vial PoM £138.20 (Hospital only)
Botulinum toxin type A 200 unit Botox 200unit powder for solution for injection vials | 1 vial PoM £276.40 (Hospital only)

▶ **Dysport** (Ipsen Ltd)
Botulinum toxin type A 300 unit Dysport 300unit powder for solution for injection vials | 1 vial PoM £92.40
Botulinum toxin type A 500 unit Dysport 500unit powder for solution for injection vials | 2 vial PoM £308.00

▶ **Letybo** (Croma-Pharma GmbH)
Botulinum toxin type A 50 unit Letybo 50unit powder for solution for injection vials | 1 vial PoM £65.00 | 2 vial PoM £120.00 | 6 vial PoM £350.00

▶ **Xeomin** (Merz Pharma UK Ltd)
Botulinum toxin type A 50 unit Xeomin 50unit powder for solution for injection vials | 1 vial PoM £72.00
Botulinum toxin type A 100 unit Xeomin 100unit powder for solution for injection vials | 1 vial PoM £129.90
Botulinum toxin type A 200 unit Xeomin 200unit powder for solution for injection vials | 1 vial PoM £259.80 (Hospital only)

4 Nausea and labyrinth disorders

Nausea and labyrinth disorders

27-Mar-2025

Drug treatment

Antiemetics are generally only prescribed when the cause of vomiting is known because otherwise, they may delay diagnosis, particularly in children. If antiemetic drug treatment is indicated, the drug is chosen according to the aetiology of vomiting.

Antihistamines (e.g. cinnarizine p. 319, cyclizine p. 313, promethazine hydrochloride p. 208, promethazine teoclate p. 319) are effective against nausea and vomiting resulting from many underlying conditions. The duration of action and incidence of adverse effects, such as drowsiness and antimuscarinic effects, differ between antihistamines.

The phenothiazines (e.g. chlorpromazine hydrochloride p. 295, prochlorperazine p. 322, trifluoperazine p. 298) are dopamine antagonists and act centrally by blocking the chemoreceptor trigger zone. Severe dystonic reactions sometimes occur with phenothiazines, especially in children. Prochlorperazine is less sedating and available as a buccal tablet for children aged 12 years and over, which can be useful in patients with persistent vomiting or with severe nausea.

EvGr Other antipsychotic drugs including haloperidol p. 296 [unlicensed use] and levomepromazine p. 321 are used for the relief of nausea and vomiting in palliative care. (A) For information on the use of antiemetics in palliative care, see Prescribing in palliative care p. 20.

Metoclopramide hydrochloride p. 315 is an effective antiemetic and its activity closely resembles that of the phenothiazines. Metoclopramide hydrochloride also acts directly on the gastric smooth muscle stimulating gastric emptying and it may be superior to the phenothiazines for emesis associated with gastro-intestinal and biliary disease. It is licensed for use in children only as a second-line option for the prevention of delayed chemotherapy-induced nausea and vomiting, and the treatment of established postoperative nausea and vomiting. There is an increased risk of neurological side-effects in children.

Domperidone p. 314 acts at the chemoreceptor trigger zone. It has the advantage over metoclopramide hydrochloride and the phenothiazines of being less likely to cause central effects, such as sedation and dystonic reactions, because it does not readily cross the blood-brain barrier.

EvGr The $5HT_3$-receptor antagonists, granisetron p. 317 and ondansetron p. 317, are used in the management of nausea and vomiting in children receiving cytotoxics.

Dexamethasone has antiemetic effects and is used in the management of chemotherapy-induced nausea and vomiting.

The neurokinin 1-receptor antagonist, aprepitant p. 316, is used to prevent nausea and vomiting associated with chemotherapy. It is usually given in combination with a $5HT_3$-receptor antagonist (with or without a corticosteroid). (A) For further information on the prevention of nausea and vomiting caused by chemotherapy, see Cytotoxic drugs p. 660.

Nabilone p. 313 is a synthetic cannabinoid with antiemetic properties. There is limited evidence for nabilone use in children for nausea and vomiting caused by cytotoxic chemotherapy unresponsive to conventional antiemetics.

Nausea and vomiting during pregnancy

Nausea and vomiting in the first trimester of pregnancy is common and will usually resolve spontaneously within 16 to 20 weeks. EvGr For pregnant females who have nausea and vomiting, offer appropriate self-care advice (such as rest, oral hydration and dietary changes), and inform them about other available support (e.g. self-help information and support groups) and when to seek urgent medical advice. Take into consideration that a number of interventions may have already been tried. Antiemetics should be considered for females with persistent symptoms where self-care measures have been ineffective. If a non-pharmacological option is preferred, ginger may be helpful for mild to moderate nausea.

For females who choose pharmacological treatment, offer an antiemetic considering the advantages and disadvantages of each drug, as well as patient preference, and their experience with treatments in previous pregnancies. Although few drug options are specifically licensed for nausea and vomiting associated with pregnancy, their use is established practice. Antiemetic options include: cyclizine, prochlorperazine, promethazine hydrochloride p. 208, promethazine teoclate p. 319, and ondansetron. For further information on antiemetic options, see NICE guideline: **Antenatal care** (available at: www.nice.org.uk/guidance/ng201). Assess response to treatment after 24 hours; if the response is inadequate, switch to an antiemetic from a different therapeutic class. Reassess after 24 hours and if symptoms have not settled, specialist opinion should be sought. For females who have moderate to severe nausea and vomiting, consider intravenous fluids and adjunctive treatment with acupressure.

Hyperemesis gravidarum is a more serious condition, which requires regular antiemetic therapy, intravenous fluid and electrolyte replacement, and sometimes nutritional support. For females with severe or persistent hyperemesis gravidarum, antiemetics given by the parenteral or rectal routes may be more suitable than the oral route. Supplementation with thiamine p. 785 must be considered in order to reduce the risk of Wernicke's encephalopathy. (A)

Postoperative nausea and vomiting

The incidence of postoperative nausea and vomiting depends on many factors including the anaesthetic used, and the type and duration of surgery. Other risk factors include post-pubertal female sex, over 3 years of age, a history or family history of postoperative nausea and vomiting or motion sickness, and postoperative use of opioids. Therapy to prevent postoperative nausea and vomiting should be based on the assessed risk of postoperative nausea and vomiting in each patient. EvGr A combination of antiemetic drugs that have different mechanisms of action is often indicated in those at moderate and high risk of postoperative nausea and vomiting. When a prophylactic antiemetic drug has failed, postoperative nausea and vomiting should be treated with an antiemetic drug from a different therapeutic class.

Drugs used include $5HT_3$-receptor antagonists (e.g. ondansetron), dexamethasone, and droperidol p. 321. (A) Cyclizine is licensed for the prevention and treatment of postoperative nausea and vomiting caused by opioids and general anaesthetics. Prochlorperazine is licensed for the prevention and treatment of nausea and vomiting.

Opioid-induced nausea and vomiting

Expert sources advise that cyclizine, ondansetron, and prochlorperazine are used to relieve opioid-induced nausea and vomiting; ondansetron has the advantage of not producing sedation.

Motion sickness

Antiemetics should be given to prevent motion sickness rather than after nausea or vomiting develop. Hyoscine hydrobromide p. 320 is licensed to prevent motion sickness symptoms such as nausea, vomiting, and vertigo. For children aged 10 years and over, a transdermal hyoscine patch provides prolonged activity but it needs to be applied several hours before travelling. Antihistamine drugs may also be effective; the less sedating antihistamines include cinnarizine and cyclizine, and the more sedating antihistamines include promethazine hydrochloride p. 208 and promethazine teoclate p. 319. Domperidone, metoclopramide hydrochloride, $5HT_3$-receptor antagonists, and the phenothiazines (except promethazine—an antihistamine phenothiazine) are **ineffective** in motion sickness.

Nausea and vomiting associated with migraine

For information on the use of antiemetics in migraine attacks, see Migraine p. 345.

ANTIEMETICS AND ANTINAUSEANTS ›
ANTIHISTAMINES

Cyclizine

27-Oct-2023

- **INDICATIONS AND DOSE**

Nausea and vomiting of known cause | Nausea and vomiting associated with vestibular disorders

▶ BY MOUTH, OR BY INTRAVENOUS INJECTION
- Child 1 month–5 years: 0.5–1 mg/kg up to 3 times a day (max. per dose 25 mg), for motion sickness, take 1–2 hours before departure
- Child 6–11 years: 25 mg up to 3 times a day, for motion sickness, take 1–2 hours before departure
- Child 12–17 years: 50 mg up to 3 times a day, for motion sickness, take 1–2 hours before departure

▶ BY RECTUM
- Child 2–5 years: 12.5 mg up to 3 times a day
- Child 6–11 years: 25 mg up to 3 times a day
- Child 12–17 years: 50 mg up to 3 times a day

▶ BY CONTINUOUS INTRAVENOUS INFUSION, OR BY CONTINUOUS SUBCUTANEOUS INFUSION
- Child 1–23 months: 3 mg/kg/24 hours
- Child 2–5 years: 50 mg/24 hours
- Child 6–11 years: 75 mg/24 hours
- Child 12–17 years: 150 mg/24 hours

Nausea and vomiting in palliative care

▶ BY CONTINUOUS SUBCUTANEOUS INFUSION
- Child 1–23 months: 3 mg/kg/24 hours
- Child 2–5 years: 50 mg/24 hours
- Child 6–11 years: 75 mg/24 hours
- Child 12–17 years: 150 mg/24 hours

▶ BY MOUTH
- Child 1 month–5 years: 0.5–1 mg/kg up to 3 times a day (max. per dose 25 mg)
- Child 6–11 years: 25 mg up to 3 times a day
- Child 12–17 years: 50 mg up to 3 times a day

▶ BY INTRAVENOUS INJECTION
- Child 1 month–5 years: 0.5–1 mg/kg up to 3 times a day (max. per dose 25 mg)
- Child 6–11 years: 25 mg up to 3 times a day
- Child 12–17 years: 50 mg up to 3 times a day

▶ BY CONTINUOUS INTRAVENOUS INFUSION
- Child 1–23 months: 3 mg/kg/24 hours
- Child 2–5 years: 50 mg/24 hours
- Child 6–11 years: 75 mg/24 hours
- Child 12–17 years: 150 mg/24 hours

▶ BY RECTUM
- Child 2–5 years: 12.5 mg up to 3 times a day
- Child 6–11 years: 25 mg up to 3 times a day
- Child 12–17 years: 50 mg up to 3 times a day

- **UNLICENSED USE** Tablets not licensed for use in children under 6 years. Injection not licensed for use in children.
- **CONTRA-INDICATIONS** Neonate (due to significant antimuscarinic activity)
- **CAUTIONS** Epilepsy · glaucoma · may counteract haemodynamic benefits of opioids · neuromuscular disorders—increased risk of transient paralysis with intravenous use · pyloroduodenal obstruction · severe heart failure—may cause fall in cardiac output and associated increase in heart rate, mean arterial pressure and pulmonary wedge pressure · urinary retention
- **INTERACTIONS** → Appendix 1: antihistamines, sedating
- **SIDE-EFFECTS**

GENERAL SIDE-EFFECTS

▶ **Rare or very rare** Agitation (more common at high doses) · angle closure glaucoma · depression

▶ **Frequency not known** Abdominal pain · agranulocytosis · angioedema · anxiety · apnoea · appetite decreased · arrhythmias · asthenia · bronchospasm · constipation · diarrhoea · disorientation · dizziness · drowsiness · dry mouth · dry throat · euphoric mood · haemolytic anaemia · hallucinations · headache · hepatic disorders · hypertension · hypotension · increased gastric reflux · insomnia · leucopenia · movement disorders · muscle complaints · nasal dryness · nausea · oculogyric crisis · palpitations · paraesthesia · photosensitivity reaction · seizure · skin reactions · speech disorder · thrombocytopenia · tinnitus · tremor · urinary retention · vision blurred · vomiting

SPECIFIC SIDE-EFFECTS

▶ With oral use Level of consciousness decreased

▶ With parenteral use Chills · consciousness impaired · injection site necrosis · pain · paralysis · sensation of pressure · thrombophlebitis

- **PREGNANCY** Manufacturer advises avoid; however, there is no evidence of teratogenicity. The use of sedating antihistamines in the latter part of the third trimester may cause adverse effects in neonates such as irritability, paradoxical excitability, and tremor.
- **BREAST FEEDING** No information available. Most antihistamines are present in breast milk in varying amounts; although not known to be harmful, most manufacturers advise avoiding their use in mothers who are breast-feeding.
- **HEPATIC IMPAIRMENT** Manufacturer advises caution.
- **DIRECTIONS FOR ADMINISTRATION** For administration *by mouth*, tablets may be crushed.

For *intravenous injection*, give over 3–5 minutes.

Mixing and compatibility for the use of syringe drivers in palliative care Cyclizine may precipitate at concentrations above 10 mg/mL or in the presence of Sodium Chloride 0.9% *or* as the concentration of diamorphine relative to cyclizine increases; mixtures of diamorphine and cyclizine are also likely to precipitate after 24 hours.

- **PRESCRIBING AND DISPENSING INFORMATION**

Palliative care For further information on the use of cyclizine in palliative care, see www.medicinescomplete.com/#/content/palliative/antihistaminic-antimuscarinic-anti-emetics.

- **PATIENT AND CARER ADVICE**

Driving and skilled tasks Drowsiness may affect performance of skilled tasks (e.g. cycling, driving); effects of alcohol enhanced.

- **MEDICINAL FORMS** There can be variation in the licensing of different medicines containing the same drug. Forms available from special-order manufacturers include: oral suspension, oral solution, suppository

Oral tablet

CAUTIONARY AND ADVISORY LABELS 2

▶ **Cyclizine (Non-proprietary)**

Cyclizine hydrochloride 50 mg Cyclizine 50mg tablets | 30 tablet [P] £1.82–£5.00 | 100 tablet [P] £16.60 DT = £3.23

Solution for injection

▶ **Cyclizine (Non-proprietary)**

Cyclizine lactate 50 mg per 1 ml Cyclizine 50mg/1ml solution for injection ampoules | 5 ampoule [PoM] £5.96–£16.25 DT = £3.23 | 10 ampoule [PoM] £10.28–£35.00

ANTIEMETICS AND ANTINAUSEANTS ›
CANNABINOIDS

Nabilone

21-Jan-2020

- **INDICATIONS AND DOSE**

Nausea and vomiting caused by cytotoxic chemotherapy, unresponsive to conventional antiemetics (preferably in hospital setting) (under close medical supervision)

▶ BY MOUTH
- Child: (consult local protocol)

- **UNLICENSED USE** Not licensed for use in children.
- **CAUTIONS** Adverse effects on mental state can persist for 48–72 hours after stopping · heart disease · history of psychiatric disorder · hypertension
- **INTERACTIONS** → Appendix 1: nabilone
- **SIDE-EFFECTS** Abdominal pain · appetite decreased · concentration impaired · confusion · depression · dizziness · drowsiness · drug dependence · dry mouth · euphoric mood · feeling of relaxation · hallucination · headache · hypotension · movement disorders · nausea · psychosis · sleep disorder · tachycardia · tremor · vertigo · visual impairment

  SIDE-EFFECTS, FURTHER INFORMATION Drowsiness and dizziness occur frequently with standard doses.
- **PREGNANCY** Avoid unless essential.
- **BREAST FEEDING** Avoid—no information available.
- **HEPATIC IMPAIRMENT** Manufacturer advises avoid in severe impairment (primarily biliary excretion).
- **PATIENT AND CARER ADVICE**

  Behavioural effects Patients should be made aware of possible changes of mood and other adverse behavioural effects.

  Driving and skilled tasks Drowsiness may affect performance of skilled tasks (e.g. driving).

  Effects of alcohol enhanced.

  For information on 2015 legislation regarding driving whilst taking certain controlled drugs, including nabilone, see *Drugs and skilled tasks* under Guidance on prescribing p. 1.

- **MEDICINAL FORMS** There can be variation in the licensing of different medicines containing the same drug. Forms available from special-order manufacturers include: oral capsule

Oral capsule

CAUTIONARY AND ADVISORY LABELS 2

- **Nabilone (Non-proprietary)**

  Nabilone 250 microgram Nabilone 250microgram capsules | 20 capsule PoM £172.50 DT = £172.50 CD2

  Nabilone 1 mg Nabilone 1mg capsules | 20 capsule PoM £225.40 DT = £225.40 CD2

ANTIEMETICS AND ANTINAUSEANTS › DOPAMINE RECEPTOR ANTAGONISTS

Domperidone

20-Apr-2026

- **INDICATIONS AND DOSE**

Relief of nausea and vomiting

- BY MOUTH
  - Child 12–17 years (body-weight 35 kg and above): 10 mg up to 3 times a day for a usual maximum of 1 week

Gastro-oesophageal reflux disease (but efficacy not proven) (specialist use only)

- BY MOUTH
  - Neonate: 250 micrograms/kg 3 times a day, dose can be increased if response inadequate, increased if necessary up to 400 micrograms/kg 3 times a day, discontinue if response inadequate at higher dose.
  - Child: 250 micrograms/kg 3 times a day (max. per dose 10 mg), dose can be increased if response inadequate, increased if necessary up to 400 micrograms/kg 3 times a day (max. per dose 20 mg), discontinue if response inadequate at higher dose

- **UNLICENSED USE** Domperidone is used for the treatment of gastro-oesophageal reflux disease, but is not licensed for this indication.

IMPORTANT SAFETY INFORMATION

MHRA/CHM ADVICE (UPDATED DECEMBER 2019): DOMPERIDONE FOR NAUSEA AND VOMITING: LACK OF EFFICACY IN CHILDREN; REMINDER OF CONTRA-INDICATIONS IN ADULTS AND ADOLESCENTS

Domperidone is no longer indicated for the relief of nausea and vomiting in children aged under 12 years or those weighing less than 35 kg. A European review concluded that domperidone is not as effective in this population as previously thought and alternative treatments should be considered. Healthcare professionals are advised to adhere to the licensed dose and to use the lowest effective dose for the shortest possible duration (max. treatment duration should not usually exceed 1 week).

Healthcare professionals are also reminded of the existing contra-indications for use of domperidone (see *Contra-indications*, *Hepatic impairment*, and *Interactions*).

- **CONTRA-INDICATIONS** Cardiac disease · conditions where cardiac conduction is, or could be, impaired · gastro-intestinal haemorrhage · gastro-intestinal mechanical obstruction · gastro-intestinal mechanical perforation · if increased gastro-intestinal motility harmful · phaeochromocytoma (suspected or confirmed) · prolactinoma
- **INTERACTIONS** → Appendix 1: domperidone
- **SIDE-EFFECTS**
  - **Common or very common** Dry mouth
  - **Uncommon** Anxiety · asthenia · breast abnormalities · diarrhoea · drowsiness · headache · lactation disorders · libido loss · movement disorders · skin reactions
  - **Frequency not known** Angioedema · arrhythmias · depression · gynaecomastia · menstrual cycle irregularities · oculogyric crisis · QT interval prolongation · seizure · sudden cardiac death · urinary retention
- **PREGNANCY** EvGr Use only if potential benefit outweighs risk (limited information available). ⟨M⟩
- **BREAST FEEDING** Specialist sources indicate probably compatible (present in milk but amount too small to be harmful).
- **HEPATIC IMPAIRMENT** Manufacturer advises avoid in moderate to severe impairment.
- **RENAL IMPAIRMENT**

  Dose adjustments EvGr For repeated doses, consider dose reduction and reduce frequency of administration (consult product literature). ⟨M⟩
- **DIRECTIONS FOR ADMINISTRATION** Orodispersible tablets should be placed on the tongue, allowed to disperse, and swallowed with or without water.
- **PRESCRIBING AND DISPENSING INFORMATION**
  - When used for Gastro-oesophageal reflux disease Interrupt treatment occasionally to assess recurrence—consider restarting if symptoms recur.
- **PATIENT AND CARER ADVICE**

  Arrhythmia Patients and their carers should be told how to recognise signs of arrhythmia and advised to seek medical attention if symptoms such as palpitation or syncope develop.

  Medicines for Children leaflet: Domperidone for gastro-oesophageal reflux www.medicinesforchildren.org.uk/medicines/domperidone-for-gastro-oesophageal-reflux/

- **MEDICINAL FORMS** There can be variation in the licensing of different medicines containing the same drug. Forms available from special-order manufacturers include: oral suspension

Oral tablet

CAUTIONARY AND ADVISORY LABELS 22

▸ **Domperidone (Non-proprietary)**
Domperidone (as Domperidone maleate) 10 mg Domperidone 10mg tablets | 30 tablet PoM £2.17 DT = £0.89 | 100 tablet PoM £7.23 DT = £2.97

Oral suspension

CAUTIONARY AND ADVISORY LABELS 22

EXCIPIENTS: May contain Hydroxybenzoates (parabens), polysorbates, sorbitol

▸ **Domperidone (Non-proprietary)**
Domperidone 1 mg per 1 ml Domperidone 1mg/ml oral suspension sugar free | 200 ml PoM £49.32 DT = £49.32 SF

Orodispersible tablet

CAUTIONARY AND ADVISORY LABELS 22

EXCIPIENTS: May contain Aspartame

▸ **Epzit** (Novumgen Ltd)
Domperidone 10 mg Epzit 10mg orodispersible tablets | 30 tablet PoM £15.00 SF

Metoclopramide hydrochloride 24-Feb-2025

- **INDICATIONS AND DOSE**

Second-line option for treatment of established postoperative nausea and vomiting

▸ BY MOUTH, OR BY INTRAMUSCULAR INJECTION, OR BY SLOW INTRAVENOUS INJECTION

▸ Child 1–17 years: 100–150 micrograms/kg up to 3 times a day (max. per dose 10 mg) for a maximum of 48 hours

Second-line option for prevention of delayed chemotherapy-induced nausea and vomiting

▸ BY MOUTH, OR BY INTRAMUSCULAR INJECTION, OR BY SLOW INTRAVENOUS INJECTION

▸ Child 1–17 years: 100–150 micrograms/kg up to 3 times a day (max. per dose 10 mg) for a maximum of 5 days

- **UNLICENSED USE** Metoclopramide is used in the doses provided in BNFC as a second-line option for treatment of established post-operative nausea and vomiting and for prevention of delayed chemotherapy-induced nausea and vomiting, but these may differ from those licensed.

IMPORTANT SAFETY INFORMATION

MHRA/CHM ADVICE—METOCLOPRAMIDE: RISK OF NEUROLOGICAL ADVERSE EFFECTS—RESTRICTED DOSE AND DURATION OF USE (AUGUST 2013)

The benefits and risks of metoclopramide have been reviewed by the European Medicines Agency's Committee on Medicinal Products for Human Use, which concluded that the risk of neurological effects such as extrapyramidal disorders and tardive dyskinesia outweigh the benefits in long-term or high-dose treatment. To help minimise the risk of potentially serious neurological adverse effects, the following restrictions to indications, dose and duration of use have been made:

- In children aged 1–18 years, metoclopramide should only be used as a second-line option for treatment of established postoperative nausea and vomiting and for prevention of delayed chemotherapy-induced nausea and vomiting;
- Use of metoclopramide is contra-indicated in children aged under 1 year;
- Metoclopramide should only be prescribed for short-term use (up to 5 days, depending on indication);
- Recommended dose is 100–150 micrograms/kg (max. 10 mg), repeated up to 3 times daily;
- Intravenous doses should be administered as a slow bolus over at least 3 minutes;
- Oral liquid formulations should be given via an appropriately designed, graduated oral syringe to ensure dose accuracy.

- **CONTRA-INDICATIONS** 3–4 days after gastrointestinal surgery · epilepsy · gastro-intestinal haemorrhage · gastro-intestinal obstruction · gastro-intestinal perforation · phaeochromocytoma
- **CAUTIONS** Asthma · atopic allergy · bradycardia · cardiac conduction disturbances · children · may mask underlying disorders such as cerebral irritation · uncorrected electrolyte imbalance · young adults
- **INTERACTIONS** → Appendix 1: metoclopramide
- **SIDE-EFFECTS**

GENERAL SIDE-EFFECTS

▸ **Common or very common** Asthenia · depression · diarrhoea · drowsiness · hypotension · menstrual cycle irregularities · movement disorders · parkinsonism

▸ **Uncommon** Arrhythmias · hallucination · hyperprolactinaemia · level of consciousness decreased

▸ **Rare or very rare** Confusion · galactorrhoea · seizure

▸ **Frequency not known** Atrioventricular block · blood disorders · cardiac arrest · gynaecomastia · hypertension · neuroleptic malignant syndrome (discontinue—potentially fatal) · QT interval prolongation · shock · syncope · tremor

SPECIFIC SIDE-EFFECTS

▸ With parenteral use Anxiety · dizziness · dyspnoea · oedema · skin reactions · visual impairment

SIDE-EFFECTS, FURTHER INFORMATION Metoclopramide can induce acute dystonic reactions involving facial and skeletal muscle spasms and oculogyric crises. These dystonic effects are more common in the young, especially girls and young women; they usually occur shortly after starting treatment with metoclopramide and subside within 24 hours of stopping it. Use of an antimuscarinic drug such as procyclidine will abort dystonic attacks.

- **PREGNANCY** Not known to be harmful.
- **BREAST FEEDING** Small amount present in milk; avoid.
- **HEPATIC IMPAIRMENT** Manufacturer advises caution in severe impairment (risk of accumulation).
Dose adjustments Manufacturer advises dose reduction of 50% in severe impairment.
- **RENAL IMPAIRMENT**
Dose adjustments EvGr Reduce daily dose by 75% in end-stage renal disease.
Reduce dose by 50% in moderate to severe impairment. (M)
- **DIRECTIONS FOR ADMINISTRATION** Manufacturer advises oral liquid preparation to be given via a graduated oral dosing syringe.
EvGr For *intravenous injection*, give over at least 3 minutes. (M)
- **PATIENT AND CARER ADVICE** Counselling on use of pipette advised with oral solution.

- **MEDICINAL FORMS** There can be variation in the licensing of different medicines containing the same drug. Forms available from special-order manufacturers include: oral solution

Solution for injection

▸ **Metoclopramide hydrochloride (Non-proprietary)**
Metoclopramide hydrochloride 5 mg per 1 ml Metoclopramide 10mg/2ml solution for injection ampoules | 5 ampoule PoM £1.31-£5.13 | 10 ampoule PoM £0.49-£4.84 DT = £5.22 (Hospital only) | 10 ampoule PoM £4.84 DT = £5.22

Oral tablet

▸ **Metoclopramide hydrochloride (Non-proprietary)**
Metoclopramide hydrochloride 5 mg Metoclopramide 5mg tablets | 28 tablet PoM £3.75–£6.00 DT = £3.75
Metoclopramide hydrochloride 10 mg Metoclopramide 10mg tablets | 28 tablet PoM £1.40 DT = £0.67

▸ **Maxolon** (Advanz Pharma)
Metoclopramide hydrochloride 10 mg Maxolon 10mg tablets | 84 tablet PoM £5.24

Oral solution

▸ **Metoclopramide hydrochloride (Non-proprietary)**
Metoclopramide hydrochloride 1 mg per 1 ml Metoclopramide 5mg/5ml oral solution sugar free | 150 ml PoM £19.77 DT = £8.05 SF

ANTIEMETICS AND ANTINAUSEANTS ›
NEUROKININ-1 RECEPTOR ANTAGONISTS

Aprepitant

11-Sep-2018

● **INDICATIONS AND DOSE**

Adjunct treatment to prevent nausea and vomiting associated with moderately and highly emetogenic chemotherapy

▸ BY MOUTH

▸ Child 6 months–11 years (body-weight 6 kg and above): (consult product literature)

▸ Child 12–17 years: Initially 125 mg, dose to be taken 1 hour before chemotherapy, then 80 mg once daily for 2 days, dose to be taken 1 hour before chemotherapy *or* in the morning if no chemotherapy is given, consult product literature for dose of concomitant $5HT_3$-antagonist (and corticosteroid if required)

● **CONTRA-INDICATIONS** Acute porphyrias p. 745

● **INTERACTIONS** → Appendix 1: neurokinin-1 receptor antagonists

● **SIDE-EFFECTS**

▸ **Common or very common** Appetite decreased · asthenia · constipation · gastrointestinal discomfort · headache · hiccups

▸ **Uncommon** Anaemia · anxiety · burping · dizziness · drowsiness · dry mouth · febrile neutropenia · gastrointestinal disorders · hot flush · malaise · nausea · palpitations · skin reactions · urinary disorders · vomiting

▸ **Rare or very rare** Bradycardia · cardiovascular disorder · chest discomfort · cognitive disorder · conjunctivitis · cough · disorientation · euphoric mood · gait abnormal · hyperhidrosis · increased risk of infection · muscle spasms · muscle weakness · oedema · oropharyngeal pain · photosensitivity reaction · polydipsia · seborrhoea · severe cutaneous adverse reactions (SCARs) · sneezing · stomatitis · taste altered · throat irritation · tinnitus · weight decreased

▸ **Frequency not known** Dysarthria · dyspnoea · insomnia · miosis · sensation abnormal · visual acuity decreased · wheezing

● **CONCEPTION AND CONTRACEPTION** Manufacturer advises effectiveness of hormonal contraceptives may be reduced—alternative non-hormonal methods of contraception necessary during treatment and for 2 months after stopping aprepitant.

● **PREGNANCY** Manufacturer advises avoid unless clearly necessary—no information available.

● **BREAST FEEDING** Manufacturer advises avoid—present in milk in *animal* studies.

● **HEPATIC IMPAIRMENT** Manufacturer advises caution in moderate to severe impairment—limited information available.

● **NATIONAL FUNDING/ACCESS DECISIONS**
For full details see funding body website

Scottish Medicines Consortium (SMC) decisions

▸ **Aprepitant (*Emend*®) as part of combination therapy, for the prevention of nausea and vomiting associated with moderately emetogenic cancer chemotherapy in infants, toddlers and children from the age of six months to less than 12 years (powder for oral suspension) and adolescents from the age of 12 years to 17 years (hard capsules) (June 2017)** SMC No. 1241/17 Recommended

▸ **Aprepitant (*Emend*®) as part of combination therapy, for the prevention of nausea and vomiting associated with highly emetogenic cancer chemotherapy in children, toddlers and infants from the age of six months to under 12 years (powder for oral suspension) and adolescents from the age of 12 years to 17 years (hard capsules) (July 2017)** SMC No. 1252/17 Recommended

● **MEDICINAL FORMS** There can be variation in the licensing of different medicines containing the same drug.

Oral capsule

▸ **Aprepitant (Non-proprietary)**
Aprepitant 80 mg Aprepitant 80mg capsules | 2 capsule PoM £31.61 DT = £31.61 | 2 capsule PoM £31.61 DT = £31.61 (Hospital only)
Aprepitant 125 mg Aprepitant 125mg capsules | 5 capsule PoM £79.03 DT = £79.03 | 5 capsule PoM £79.03 DT = £79.03 (Hospital only)

▸ **Emend** (Merck Sharp & Dohme (UK) Ltd)
Aprepitant 80 mg Emend 80mg capsules | 2 capsule PoM ⊠ DT = £31.61
Aprepitant 125 mg Emend 125mg capsules | 1 capsule PoM ⊠

Powder for oral suspension

CAUTIONARY AND ADVISORY LABELS 13

▸ **Emend** (Merck Sharp & Dohme (UK) Ltd)
Aprepitant 125 mg Emend 125mg oral powder sachets | 1 sachet PoM £15.81

Fosaprepitant

02-Nov-2020

● **DRUG ACTION** Fosaprepitant is a prodrug of aprepitant.

● **INDICATIONS AND DOSE**

Adjunct to $5HT_3$-receptor antagonist (with or without dexamethasone) in preventing nausea and vomiting associated with moderately and highly emetogenic chemotherapy

▸ BY INTRAVENOUS INFUSION

▸ Child 6 months–11 years (body-weight 6 kg and above): Initially 3 mg/kg (max. per dose 115 mg) on day 1 of cycle, then 2 mg/kg (max. per dose 80 mg) on days 2 and 3 of cycle, dose to be administered over 60 minutes and completed 30 minutes before chemotherapy, consult product literature for dose of concomitant corticosteroid and $5HT_3$-receptor antagonist and for information on alternative dosing for single and multi-day regimens

▸ Child 12–17 years: Initially 115 mg on day 1 of cycle, then 80 mg on days 2 and 3 of cycle, dose to be administered over 30 minutes and completed 30 minutes before chemotherapy, consult product literature for dose of concomitant corticosteroid and $5HT_3$-receptor antagonist and for information on alternative dosing for single and multi-day regimens

● **CONTRA-INDICATIONS** Acute porphyrias p. 745

● **INTERACTIONS** → Appendix 1: neurokinin-1 receptor antagonists

● **SIDE-EFFECTS**

▸ **Common or very common** Appetite decreased · asthenia · constipation · flushing · gastrointestinal discomfort · headache · hiccups

▸ **Uncommon** Anaemia · anxiety · burping · dizziness · drowsiness · dry mouth · febrile neutropenia · gastrointestinal disorders · malaise · nausea · palpitations · skin reactions · thrombophlebitis · urinary disorders · vomiting

▸ **Rare or very rare** Bradycardia · cardiovascular disorder · chest discomfort · cognitive disorder · conjunctivitis · cough · disorientation · euphoric mood · gait abnormal · hyperhidrosis · increased risk of infection · muscle spasms ·

muscle weakness · oedema · oropharyngeal pain · photosensitivity reaction · polydipsia · seborrhoea · severe cutaneous adverse reactions (SCARs) · sneezing · stomatitis · taste altered · throat irritation · tinnitus · weight decreased
- **Frequency not known** Dysarthria · dyspnoea · insomnia · miosis · sensation abnormal · visual acuity decreased · wheezing

- **CONCEPTION AND CONTRACEPTION** Effectiveness of hormonal contraceptives reduced—effective non-hormonal methods of contraception necessary during treatment and for 2 months after stopping fosaprepitant.
- **PREGNANCY** Avoid unless potential benefit outweighs risk—no information available.
- **BREAST FEEDING** Avoid—present in milk in *animal* studies.
- **HEPATIC IMPAIRMENT** Manufacturer advises caution in moderate to severe impairment—limited information available.
- **DIRECTIONS FOR ADMINISTRATION** For *intravenous infusion* (*Ivemend*®), manufacturer advises give intermittently *in* Sodium Chloride 0.9%; reconstitute each 150 mg vial with 5 mL Sodium Chloride 0.9% gently without shaking to avoid foaming, then dilute in 145 mL infusion fluid; for volumes less than 150 ml, transfer the required volume to a bag or syringe prior to infusion; infuse through central venous catheter.
- **NATIONAL FUNDING/ACCESS DECISIONS** For full details see funding body website

Scottish Medicines Consortium (SMC) decisions
- **Fosaprepitant (*Ivemend*®) for the prevention of nausea and vomiting associated with highly and moderately emetogenic cancer chemotherapy in patients aged 6 months to 17 years (November 2018)** SMC No. SMC2108 Recommended

All Wales Medicines Strategy Group (AWMSG) decisions
- **Fosaprepitant (*Ivemend*®) for the prevention of nausea and vomiting associated with highly and moderately emetogenic cancer chemotherapy in patients aged 6 months to less than 18 years of age (December 2018)** AWMSG No. 3789 Recommended

- **MEDICINAL FORMS** There can be variation in the licensing of different medicines containing the same drug.

Powder for solution for infusion
- Fosaprepitant (Non-proprietary)
  Fosaprepitant (as Fosaprepitant dimeglumine) 150 mg Fosaprepitant 150mg powder for solution for infusion vials | 1 vial PoM (Hospital only)
- Ivemend (Merck Sharp & Dohme (UK) Ltd)
  Fosaprepitant (as Fosaprepitant dimeglumine) 150 mg Ivemend 150mg powder for solution for infusion vials | 1 vial PoM £47.42 (Hospital only)

ANTIEMETICS AND ANTINAUSEANTS › SEROTONIN (5HT3) RECEPTOR ANTAGONISTS

Granisetron
16-Jul-2020

- **DRUG ACTION** Granisetron is a specific $5HT_3$-receptor antagonist which blocks $5HT_3$ receptors in the gastro-intestinal tract and in the CNS.

- **INDICATIONS AND DOSE**

Management of nausea and vomiting induced by cytotoxic chemotherapy
- BY MOUTH
  - Child 12–17 years: 1–2 mg, to be taken within 1 hour before start of treatment, then 2 mg daily in 1–2 divided doses for up to 1 week following chemotherapy
- BY INTRAVENOUS INFUSION
  - Child 2–17 years: 10–40 micrograms/kg (max. per dose 3 mg), repeated if necessary, to be given before start of chemotherapy, for treatment, dose may be repeated within 24 hours if necessary, not less than 10 minutes after initial dose; maximum 2 doses per day

- **UNLICENSED USE** Tablets not licensed in children (age range not specified by manufacturer).
- **CAUTIONS** Subacute intestinal obstruction · susceptibility to QT-interval prolongation (including electrolyte disturbances)
- **INTERACTIONS** → Appendix 1: 5-HT3-receptor antagonists
- **SIDE-EFFECTS**
  - **Common or very common** Constipation · diarrhoea · headache · insomnia
  - **Uncommon** Extrapyramidal symptoms · QT interval prolongation · serotonin syndrome
- **PREGNANCY** Manufacturer advises avoid.
- **BREAST FEEDING** Avoid—no information available.
- **HEPATIC IMPAIRMENT** Manufacturer advises caution.
- **DIRECTIONS FOR ADMINISTRATION** For *intravenous infusion*, manufacturer advises dilute up to 3 mL of granisetron injection in Glucose 5% or Sodium Chloride 0.9% to a total volume of 10–30 mL; give over 5 minutes.

- **MEDICINAL FORMS** There can be variation in the licensing of different medicines containing the same drug.

Solution for injection
- Granisetron (Non-proprietary)
  Granisetron (as Granisetron hydrochloride) 1 mg per 1 ml Granisetron 3mg/3ml concentrate for solution for injection ampoules | 10 ampoule PoM £72.00
  Granisetron 1mg/1ml concentrate for solution for injection ampoules | 10 ampoule PoM £24.20 DT = £24.20

Oral tablet
- Granisetron (Non-proprietary)
  Granisetron (as Granisetron hydrochloride) 1 mg Granisetron 1mg tablets | 10 tablet PoM £51.20 DT = £41.91
- Kytril (Atnahs Pharma UK Ltd)
  Granisetron (as Granisetron hydrochloride) 1 mg Kytril 1mg tablets | 10 tablet PoM £52.39 DT = £41.91

Ondansetron
12-Feb-2024

- **DRUG ACTION** Ondansetron is a specific $5HT_3$-receptor antagonist which blocks $5HT_3$ receptors in the gastro-intestinal tract and in the CNS.

- **INDICATIONS AND DOSE**

Gastro-enteritis, management of vomiting
- BY MOUTH
  - Child 6 months–17 years: 100–150 micrograms/kg every 8–12 hours (max. per dose 8 mg) as required
- BY SLOW INTRAVENOUS INJECTION
  - Child 6 months–17 years: 100 micrograms/kg every 8–12 hours (max. per dose 8 mg) as required, dose to be given over at least 30 seconds
- BY INTRAVENOUS INFUSION
  - Child 6 months–17 years: 150 micrograms/kg every 8–12 hours (max. per dose 8 mg) as required

Prevention of postoperative nausea and vomiting
- BY SLOW INTRAVENOUS INJECTION
  - Child: 100 micrograms/kg for 1 dose (max. per dose 4 mg), dose to be given over at least 30 seconds before, during, or after induction of anaesthesia

Treatment of postoperative nausea and vomiting
- BY SLOW INTRAVENOUS INJECTION
  - Child: 100 micrograms/kg for 1 dose (max. per dose 4 mg), dose to be given over at least 30 seconds

continued →

Prevention and treatment of chemotherapy- and radiotherapy-induced nausea and vomiting—initial dose

▶ BY INTRAVENOUS INFUSION

- Child 6 months–17 years (body surface area up to 1.3 m^2): 5 mg/m^2 for 1 dose, dose to be administered immediately before chemotherapy, then give orally, alternatively initially 150 micrograms/kg for 1 dose (max. per dose 8 mg), dose to be administered immediately before chemotherapy, then 150 micrograms/kg every 4 hours (max. per dose 8 mg) for 2 further doses then give orally
- Child 6 months–17 years (body surface area 1.3 m^2 and above): 8 mg for 1 dose, dose to be administered immediately before chemotherapy, then give orally, alternatively initially 150 micrograms/kg for 1 dose (max. per dose 8 mg), dose to be administered immediately before chemotherapy, then 150 micrograms/kg every 4 hours (max. per dose 8 mg) for 2 further doses then give orally

Prevention and treatment of chemotherapy- and radiotherapy-induced nausea and vomiting—(follow-on dose based on body surface area)

▶ BY MOUTH

- Child 6 months–17 years (body surface area up to 0.6 m^2): 2 mg every 12 hours for up to 5 days, dose can be started 12 hours after intravenous administration
- Child 6 months–17 years (body surface area 0.6–1.2 m^2): 4 mg every 12 hours for up to 5 days, dose can be started 12 hours after intravenous administration
- Child 6 months–17 years (body surface area 1.3 m^2 and above): 8 mg every 12 hours for up to 5 days, dose can be started 12 hours after intravenous administration

Prevention and treatment of chemotherapy- and radiotherapy-induced nausea and vomiting—(follow-on dose based on body-weight)

▶ BY MOUTH

- Child 6 months–17 years (body-weight up to 10.1 kg): 2 mg every 12 hours for up to 5 days, dose can be started 12 hours after intravenous administration
- Child 6 months–17 years (body-weight 10.1–40 kg): 4 mg every 12 hours for up to 5 days, dose can be started 12 hours after intravenous administration
- Child 6 months–17 years (body-weight 41 kg and above): 8 mg every 12 hours for up to 5 days, dose can be started 12 hours after intravenous administration

● **UNLICENSED USE** EvGr Ondansetron is used for the management of vomiting in children and young people with gastro-enteritis, (E) but is not licensed for this indication. Not licensed for radiotherapy-induced nausea and vomiting in children.

IMPORTANT SAFETY INFORMATION

MHRA/CHM ADVICE: ONDANSETRON: SMALL INCREASED RISK OF ORAL CLEFTS FOLLOWING USE IN THE FIRST 12 WEEKS OF PREGNANCY (JANUARY 2020)

Epidemiological studies have identified a small increased risk of cleft lip and/or cleft palate in babies born to women who used oral ondansetron during the first trimester of pregnancy. Healthcare professionals are advised that if there is a clinical need for ondansetron in pregnancy, patients should be counselled on the potential benefits and risks, and the final decision made jointly.

● **CONTRA-INDICATIONS** Congenital long QT syndrome

● **CAUTIONS** Adenotonsillar surgery · subacute intestinal obstruction · susceptibility to QT-interval prolongation (including electrolyte disturbances)

● **INTERACTIONS** → Appendix 1: 5-HT3-receptor antagonists

● **SIDE-EFFECTS**

GENERAL SIDE-EFFECTS

▶ **Common or very common** Constipation · feeling hot · headache · sensation abnormal

▶ **Uncommon** Arrhythmias · chest pain · hiccups · hypotension · movement disorders · oculogyric crisis · seizure

▶ **Rare or very rare** Dizziness · QT interval prolongation · vision disorders

▶ **Frequency not known** Myocardial ischaemia

SPECIFIC SIDE-EFFECTS

▶ **Rare or very rare**

- With oral use Skin toxicity · toxic epidermal necrolysis
- With parenteral use Abdominal pain · bullous dermatitis · depression · diarrhoea · severe cutaneous adverse reactions (SCARs)

● **PREGNANCY** Manufacturer advises avoid in first trimester—small increased risk of congenital abnormalities such as orofacial clefts, see *Important safety information*.

● **BREAST FEEDING** Present in milk in *animal* studies—avoid.

● **HEPATIC IMPAIRMENT** Manufacturer advises caution in moderate to severe impairment (decreased clearance).

Dose adjustments Manufacturer advises a reduced maximum daily dose in moderate to severe impairment—consult product literature.

● **DIRECTIONS FOR ADMINISTRATION**

- With intravenous use EvGr For *intravenous infusion*, dilute required dose in 25–50 mL Glucose 5% *or* Sodium Chloride 0.9%; give over at least 15 minutes. (M)
- With oral use Orodispersible films and lyophylisates should be placed on the tongue, allowed to disperse and swallowed.

● **PRESCRIBING AND DISPENSING INFORMATION** Flavours of oral liquid formulations may include strawberry.

● **PATIENT AND CARER ADVICE** Patients or carers should be given advice on how to administer orodispersible films and lyophilisates.

● **MEDICINAL FORMS** There can be variation in the licensing of different medicines containing the same drug. Forms available from special-order manufacturers include: oral suspension, oral solution

Oral tablet

▶ Ondansetron (Non-proprietary)

Ondansetron (as Ondansetron hydrochloride dihydrate) 4 mg Ondansetron 4mg tablets | 10 tablet PoM £11.70 DT = £1.48 | 30 tablet PoM £4.20–£86.33

Ondansetron (as Ondansetron hydrochloride dihydrate) 8 mg Ondansetron 8mg tablets | 10 tablet PoM £57.55 DT = £3.43

Solution for injection

▶ Ondansetron (Non-proprietary)

Ondansetron (as Ondansetron hydrochloride dihydrate) 2 mg per 1 ml Ondansetron 8mg/4ml solution for injection ampoules | 5 ampoule PoM £38.37–£61.60 (Hospital only) | 5 ampoule PoM £27.90–£70.14 | 10 ampoule PoM £54.00–£70.00

Ondansetron 4mg/2ml solution for injection pre-filled syringes | 1 pre-filled disposable injection PoM £29.97 (Hospital only)

Ondansetron 8mg/4ml solution for injection pre-filled syringes | 1 pre-filled disposable injection PoM £59.95 (Hospital only)

Ondansetron 4mg/2ml solution for injection ampoules | 5 ampoule PoM £13.90–£29.97 (Hospital only) | 5 ampoule PoM £14.00–£35.04 | 10 ampoule PoM £26.00–£59.94 DT = £20.00 (Hospital only) | 10 ampoule PoM £20.00–£38.50 DT = £20.00

Oral solution

▶ Ondansetron (Non-proprietary)

Ondansetron (as Ondansetron hydrochloride) 800 microgram per 1 ml Ondansetron 4mg/5ml oral solution sugar free | 50 ml PoM £38.37 DT = £6.44 SF

Ondansetron (as Ondansetron hydrochloride) 1.6 mg per 1 ml Ondansetron 8mg/5ml oral solution sugar free | 50 ml PoM £30.00 SF | 100 ml PoM £134.37 DT = £134.37 SF

Orodispersible film

▸ **Setofilm** (Norgine Pharmaceuticals Ltd)
Ondansetron 4 mg Setofilm 4mg orodispersible films | 10 film [PoM] £28.50 DT = £28.50 [SF]
Ondansetron 8 mg Setofilm 8mg orodispersible films | 10 film [PoM] £57.00 DT = £57.00 [SF]

Orodispersible tablet

▸ **Ondansetron (Non-proprietary)**
Ondansetron 4 mg Ondansetron 4mg orodispersible tablets | 10 tablet [PoM] £35.97 DT = £24.29
Ondansetron 8 mg Ondansetron 8mg orodispersible tablets | 10 tablet [PoM] £71.94 DT = £71.94

ANTIHISTAMINES > SEDATING

Cinnarizine

27-Apr-2021

● **INDICATIONS AND DOSE**

Relief of symptoms of vestibular disorders, such as vertigo, tinnitus, nausea, and vomiting in Ménière's disease

▶ BY MOUTH
▸ Child 5–11 years: 15 mg 3 times a day
▸ Child 12–17 years: 30 mg 3 times a day

Motion sickness

▶ BY MOUTH
▸ Child 5–11 years: Initially 15 mg, dose to be taken 2 hours before travel, then 7.5 mg every 8 hours if required, dose to be taken during journey
▸ Child 12–17 years: Initially 30 mg, dose to be taken 2 hours before travel, then 15 mg every 8 hours if required, dose to be taken during journey

● **CONTRA-INDICATIONS** Avoid in Acute porphyrias p. 745 · neonate (due to significant antimuscarinic activity)

● **CAUTIONS** Epilepsy · glaucoma · pyloroduodenal obstruction · urinary retention

● **INTERACTIONS** → Appendix 1: antihistamines, sedating

● **SIDE-EFFECTS**
▶ **Common or very common** Drowsiness · gastrointestinal discomfort · nausea · weight increased
▶ **Uncommon** Fatigue · hyperhidrosis · vomiting
▶ **Frequency not known** Dry mouth · gastrointestinal disorder · headache · jaundice cholestatic · movement disorders · muscle rigidity · parkinsonism · skin reactions · subacute cutaneous lupus erythematosus · tremor

● **PREGNANCY** Manufacturer advises avoid; however, there is no evidence of teratogenicity. The use of sedating antihistamines in the latter part of the third trimester may cause adverse effects in neonates such as irritability, paradoxical excitability, and tremor.

● **BREAST FEEDING** Most antihistamines are present in breast milk in varying amounts; although not known to be harmful, most manufacturers advise avoiding their use in mothers who are breast-feeding.

● **HEPATIC IMPAIRMENT** Manufacturer advises caution in hepatic insufficiency—no information available.

● **RENAL IMPAIRMENT** [EvGr] Use with caution (no information available). ⟨M⟩

● **PATIENT AND CARER ADVICE**
Driving and skilled tasks Drowsiness may affect performance of skilled tasks (e.g. cycling, driving); sedating effects enhanced by alcohol.

● **MEDICINAL FORMS** There can be variation in the licensing of different medicines containing the same drug. Forms available from special-order manufacturers include: oral suspension

Oral tablet

CAUTIONARY AND ADVISORY LABELS 2

▸ **Cinnarizine (Non-proprietary)**
Cinnarizine 15 mg Cinnarizine 15mg tablets | 84 tablet [P] £6.88 DT = £2.95

▸ **Stugeron** (McNeil Products Ltd)
Cinnarizine 15 mg Stugeron 15mg tablets | 15 tablet [P] £3.51

Promethazine teoclate

27-Jun-2023

● **INDICATIONS AND DOSE**

Nausea | Vomiting | Labyrinthine disorders

▶ BY MOUTH
▸ Child 5–9 years: 12.5–37.5 mg daily
▸ Child 10–17 years: 25–75 mg daily; maximum 100 mg per day

Motion sickness prevention

▶ BY MOUTH
▸ Child 5–9 years: 12.5 mg once daily, dose to be taken at bedtime on night before travel or 1–2 hours before travel
▸ Child 10–17 years: 25 mg once daily, dose to be taken at bedtime on night before travel or 1–2 hours before travel

Motion sickness treatment

▶ BY MOUTH
▸ Child 5–9 years: Initially 12.5 mg, dose to be taken at onset of motion sickness, then 12.5 mg for a further two doses, doses to be taken at bedtime, starting on the evening of onset
▸ Child 10–17 years: Initially 25 mg, dose to be taken at onset of motion sickness, then 25 mg for a further two doses, doses to be taken at bedtime, starting on the evening of onset

IMPORTANT SAFETY INFORMATION

MHRA/CHM ADVICE: OVER-THE-COUNTER COUGH AND COLD MEDICINES FOR CHILDREN (APRIL 2009)

Children under 6 years should not be given over-the-counter cough and cold medicines containing promethazine.

● **CONTRA-INDICATIONS** Neonate (due to significant antimuscarinic activity) · should not be given to children under 2 years, except on specialist advice (potential for fatal respiratory depression)

● **CAUTIONS** Asthma · bronchiectasis · bronchitis · epilepsy · pyloroduodenal obstruction · Reye's syndrome · severe coronary artery disease · susceptibility to angle-closure glaucoma · susceptibility to QT interval prolongation · urinary retention

● **INTERACTIONS** → Appendix 1: antihistamines, sedating

● **SIDE-EFFECTS** Anticholinergic syndrome · anxiety · appetite decreased · arrhythmia · blood disorder · bronchial secretion viscosity increased · confusion · dizziness · drowsiness · dry mouth · epigastric discomfort · fatigue · haemolytic anaemia · headache · hypotension · jaundice · movement disorders · muscle spasms · nightmare · palpitations · photosensitivity reaction · urinary retention · vision blurred

SIDE-EFFECTS, FURTHER INFORMATION Paradoxical stimulation may occur, especially with high doses.

● **PREGNANCY** Most manufacturers of antihistamines advise avoiding their use during pregnancy; however, there is no evidence of teratogenicity. Use in the latter part of the third trimester may cause adverse effects in neonates such as irritability, paradoxical excitability, and tremor.

● **BREAST FEEDING** Most antihistamines are present in breast milk in varying amounts; although not known to be harmful, most manufacturers advise avoiding their use in mothers who are breast-feeding.

● **HEPATIC IMPAIRMENT** Manufacturer advises caution.

● **RENAL IMPAIRMENT** [EvGr] Use with caution. ⟨M⟩

● **PATIENT AND CARER ADVICE**

Driving and skilled tasks Drowsiness may affect performance of skilled tasks (e.g. cycling or driving); sedating effects enhanced by alcohol.

● **MEDICINAL FORMS** There can be variation in the licensing of different medicines containing the same drug.

Oral tablet

CAUTIONARY AND ADVISORY LABELS 2

▸ Promethazine teoclate (Non-proprietary)

Promethazine teoclate 25 mg Promethazine teoclate 25mg tablets | 28 tablet PoM DT = £4.65

ANTIMUSCARINICS

603

Hyoscine hydrobromide

16-Jan-2024

(Scopolamine hydrobromide)

● **INDICATIONS AND DOSE**

Motion sickness

▶ BY MOUTH

- Child 4-9 years: 75–150 micrograms, dose to be taken up to 30 minutes before the start of journey, then 75–150 micrograms every 6 hours if required; maximum 450 micrograms per day
- Child 10-17 years: 150–300 micrograms, dose to be taken up to 30 minutes before the start of journey, then 150–300 micrograms every 6 hours if required; maximum 900 micrograms per day

▶ BY TRANSDERMAL APPLICATION

- Child 10-17 years: Apply 1 patch, apply behind ear 5–6 hours before journey, then apply 1 patch after 72 hours if required, remove old patch and site replacement patch behind the other ear

Hypersalivation associated with clozapine therapy

▶ BY MOUTH

- Child 12-17 years: 300 micrograms up to 3 times a day; maximum 900 micrograms per day

Excessive respiratory secretions

▶ BY MOUTH, OR BY SUBLINGUAL ADMINISTRATION

- Child 2-11 years: 10 micrograms/kg 4 times a day (max. per dose 300 micrograms)
- Child 12-17 years: 300 micrograms 4 times a day

▶ BY TRANSDERMAL APPLICATION

- Child 1 month-2 years: 250 micrograms every 72 hours, dose equates to a quarter patch
- Child 3-9 years: 500 micrograms every 72 hours, dose equates to a half patch
- Child 10-17 years: 1 mg every 72 hours, dose equates to one patch

Excessive respiratory secretion in palliative care

▶ BY SUBCUTANEOUS INJECTION, OR BY INTRAVENOUS INJECTION

- Child: 10 micrograms/kg every 4–8 hours (max. per dose 600 micrograms)

▶ BY CONTINUOUS SUBCUTANEOUS INFUSION, OR BY INTRAVENOUS INFUSION

- Child: 40–60 micrograms/kg over 24 hours

Bowel colic pain in palliative care

▶ BY MOUTH USING SUBLINGUAL TABLETS

- Child: 10 micrograms/kg 3 times a day (max. per dose 300 micrograms), as *Kwells*®.

Premedication

▶ BY SUBCUTANEOUS INJECTION, OR BY INTRAMUSCULAR INJECTION

- Child 1-11 years: 15 micrograms/kg (max. per dose 600 micrograms), to be administered 30–60 minutes before induction of anaesthesia
- Child 12-17 years: 200–600 micrograms, to be administered 30–60 minutes before induction of anaesthesia

▶ BY INTRAVENOUS INJECTION

- Child 1-11 years: 15 micrograms/kg (max. per dose 600 micrograms), to be administered immediately before induction of anaesthesia
- Child 12-17 years: 200–600 micrograms, to be administered immediately before induction of anaesthesia

● **UNLICENSED USE** Not licensed for use in excessive respiratory secretions or hypersalivation associated with clozapine therapy.

IMPORTANT SAFETY INFORMATION

Antimuscarinic drugs used for premedication to general anaesthesia should only be administered by, or under the direct supervision of, personnel experienced in their use.

MHRA/CHM ADVICE: HYOSCINE HYDROBROMIDE PATCHES (*SCOPODERM*® 1.5 MG PATCH OR *SCOPODERM*® TTS PATCH): RISK OF ANTICHOLINERGIC SIDE EFFECTS, INCLUDING HYPERTHERMIA (JULY 2023)

There has been a small number of reports of serious and life-threatening anticholinergic side-effects associated with the use of hyoscine hydrobromide patches, including a fatality from hyperthermia in a child, particularly with unlicensed use. These side-effects (which include hyperthermia, urinary retention, delirium, hallucinations, seizures, respiratory paralysis, and coma) may persist for 24 hours or longer after patch removal as the drug in the skin continues to enter the bloodstream. Healthcare professionals are reminded to:

- be alert for potential signs and symptoms of anticholinergic side-effects, particularly with unlicensed use, and to manage promptly if they occur;
- be aware that children and the elderly are more susceptible to anticholinergic toxicity;
- counsel patients and their carers to seek immediate medical attention and remove the patch if signs and symptoms of serious anticholinergic side-effects occur; immediate action should also be taken to reduce body heat if a high temperature develops.

● **CAUTIONS** Epilepsy

CAUTIONS, FURTHER INFORMATION

▸ Anticholinergic syndrome

▸ With systemic use In some children hyoscine may cause the central anticholinergic syndrome (excitement, ataxia, hallucinations, behavioural abnormalities, and drowsiness).

● **INTERACTIONS** → Appendix 1: hyoscine

● **SIDE-EFFECTS**

▶ **Common or very common**

▸ With transdermal use Eye disorders · eyelid irritation

▶ **Rare or very rare**

▸ With transdermal use Concentration impaired · glaucoma · hallucinations · memory impairment · restlessness

▶ **Frequency not known**

▸ With oral use Asthma · cardiovascular disorders · central nervous system stimulation · gastrointestinal disorder · hallucination · hypersensitivity · hyperthermia · hypohidrosis · mydriasis · oedema · respiratory tract reaction · restlessness · seizure

▸ With parenteral use Agitation · angle closure glaucoma · arrhythmias · delirium · dysphagia · dyspnoea · epilepsy exacerbated · hallucination · hypersensitivity · idiosyncratic drug reaction · loss of consciousness · mydriasis · neuroleptic malignant syndrome (discontinue—potentially fatal) · psychotic disorder · thirst

▸ With transdermal use Balance impaired · coma · delirium · hyperthermia · respiratory paralysis · seizure

SIDE-EFFECTS, FURTHER INFORMATION Since systemic absorption can follow transdermal use, also consider the side-effects of systemic antimuscarinics.

- **PREGNANCY** Use only if potential benefit outweighs risk. Injection may depress neonatal respiration.
- **BREAST FEEDING** Amount too small to be harmful.
- **HEPATIC IMPAIRMENT** Manufacturer advises caution.
- **RENAL IMPAIRMENT** EvGr Use with caution. (M)
- **DIRECTIONS FOR ADMINISTRATION**
  - With transdermal use Expert sources advise *patch* applied to hairless area of skin behind ear; if less than whole patch required **either** cut with scissors along full thickness ensuring membrane is not peeled away **or** cover portion to prevent contact with skin.
  - With oral use For administration by *mouth*, expert sources advise injection solution may be given orally.
- **PRESCRIBING AND DISPENSING INFORMATION**

Palliative care For further information on the use of hyoscine hydrobromide in palliative care, see www.medicinescomplete.com/#/content/palliative/hyoscine-hydrobromide.

- **PATIENT AND CARER ADVICE**
  - With transdermal use Explain accompanying instructions to patient and in particular emphasise advice to wash hands after handling and to wash application site after removing, and to use one patch at a time.

Medicines for Children leaflet: Hyoscine hydrobromide patches to reduce saliva production www.medicinesforchildren.org.uk/medicines/hyoscine-hydrobromide-patches-to-reduce-saliva-production/

Driving and skilled tasks
- With transdermal use Drowsiness may persist for up to 24 hours or longer after removal of patch; effects of alcohol enhanced.

- **MEDICINAL FORMS** There can be variation in the licensing of different medicines containing the same drug. Forms available from special-order manufacturers include: oral suspension, oral solution

Oral tablet

CAUTIONARY AND ADVISORY LABELS 2

- **Kwells** (Dexcel-Pharma Ltd)
  Hyoscine hydrobromide 150 microgram Kwells Kids 150microgram tablets | 12 tablet P £2.50 DT = £2.50
  Hyoscine hydrobromide 300 microgram Kwells 300microgram tablets | 12 tablet P £2.50 DT = £2.50
- **Travel Calm** (The Boots Company Plc)
  Hyoscine hydrobromide 300 microgram Travel Calm 300microgram tablets | 12 tablet P ⊠ DT = £2.50

Solution for injection

- **Hyoscine hydrobromide (Non-proprietary)**
  Hyoscine hydrobromide 400 microgram per 1 ml Hyoscine hydrobromide 400micrograms/1ml solution for injection ampoules | 10 ampoule PoM £53.49 DT = £28.51
  Hyoscine hydrobromide 600 microgram per 1 ml Hyoscine hydrobromide 600micrograms/1ml solution for injection ampoules | 10 ampoule PoM £224.13–£421.36 DT = £224.13

Transdermal patch

CAUTIONARY AND ADVISORY LABELS 19

- **Hyoscine hydrobromide (Non-proprietary)**
  Hyoscine 1 mg per 72 hour Hyoscine 1mg/72hours transdermal patches | 1 patch PoM ⊠

ANTIPSYCHOTICS › FIRST-GENERATION

F 295

Droperidol

04-May-2021

- **DRUG ACTION** Droperidol is a butyrophenone, structurally related to haloperidol, which blocks dopamine receptors in the chemoreceptor trigger zone.

- **INDICATIONS AND DOSE**

Prevention and treatment of postoperative nausea and vomiting

- BY INTRAVENOUS INJECTION
  - Child 2–17 years: 20–50 micrograms/kg (max. per dose 1.25 mg), dose to be given 30 minutes before end of surgery, then 20–50 micrograms/kg every 6 hours (max. per dose 1.25 mg) if required

- **CONTRA-INDICATIONS** Bradycardia · comatose states · hypokalaemia · hypomagnesaemia · phaeochromocytoma · QT-interval prolongation
- **CAUTIONS** Chronic obstructive pulmonary disease · CNS depression · electrolyte disturbances · history of alcohol abuse · respiratory failure
- **INTERACTIONS** → Appendix 1: droperidol
- **SIDE-EFFECTS**
  - **Uncommon** Anxiety · oculogyration
  - **Rare or very rare** Blood disorder · cardiac arrest · dysphoria
  - **Frequency not known** Coma · epilepsy · hallucination · oligomenorrhoea · respiratory disorders · SIADH · syncope
- **BREAST FEEDING** Limited information available—avoid repeated administration.
- **HEPATIC IMPAIRMENT** Manufacturer advises caution.

Dose adjustments Manufacturer advises maximum 625 micrograms repeated every 6 hours as required.

- **RENAL IMPAIRMENT**

Dose adjustments EvGr Maximum 625 micrograms repeated every 6 hours as required. (M)

- **MONITORING REQUIREMENTS** Continuous pulse oximetry required if risk of ventricular arrhythmia—continue for 30 minutes following administration.

- **MEDICINAL FORMS** There can be variation in the licensing of different medicines containing the same drug.

Solution for injection

- **Droperidol (Non-proprietary)**
  Droperidol 2.5 mg per 1 ml Droperidol 2.5mg/1ml solution for injection vials | 10 vial PoM £39.40 (Hospital only)
  Droperidol 2.5mg/1ml solution for injection ampoules | 10 ampoule PoM £80.00 (Hospital only)

F 295

Levomepromazine

29-Nov-2023

(Methotrimeprazine)

- **INDICATIONS AND DOSE**

Restlessness and confusion in palliative care

- BY CONTINUOUS SUBCUTANEOUS INFUSION
  - Child 1–11 years: 0.35–3 mg/kg, to be administered over 24 hours
  - Child 12–17 years: 12.5–200 mg, to be administered over 24 hours

Nausea and vomiting in palliative care

- BY CONTINUOUS INTRAVENOUS INFUSION, OR BY SUBCUTANEOUS INFUSION
  - Child 1 month–11 years: 100–400 micrograms/kg, to be administered over 24 hours
  - Child 12–17 years: 5–25 mg, to be administered over 24 hours

- **CONTRA-INDICATIONS** CNS depression · comatose states · phaeochromocytoma

4 Nervous system

- **CAUTIONS** Patients receiving large initial doses should remain supine · susceptibility to QT interval prolongation
- **INTERACTIONS** → Appendix 1: phenothiazine antipsychotics
- **SIDE-EFFECTS**
  - **Common or very common** Asthenia · heat stroke
  - **Rare or very rare** Cardiac arrest · hepatic disorders
  - **Frequency not known** Allergic dermatitis · delirium · embolism and thrombosis · gastrointestinal disorders · glucose tolerance impaired · hyponatraemia · photosensitivity reaction · priapism · SIADH
- **HEPATIC IMPAIRMENT** Manufacturer advises consider avoiding.
- **DIRECTIONS FOR ADMINISTRATION** For administration by *subcutaneous infusion*, manufacturer advises dilute with a suitable volume of Sodium Chloride 0.9%.
- **PRESCRIBING AND DISPENSING INFORMATION**
  Palliative care For further information on the use of levomepromazine in palliative care, see www.medicinescomplete.com/#/content/palliative/levomepromazine.

- **MEDICINAL FORMS** There can be variation in the licensing of different medicines containing the same drug.

Solution for injection

- **Levomepromazine (Non-proprietary)**
  Levomepromazine hydrochloride 25 mg per 1 ml Levomepromazine 25mg/1ml solution for injection ampoules | 10 ampoule PoM £20.13–£30.00 DT = £20.13
- **Nozinan** (Neuraxpharm UK Ltd)
  Levomepromazine hydrochloride 25 mg per 1 ml Nozinan 25mg/1ml solution for injection ampoules | 10 ampoule PoM £20.13 DT = £20.13

F 295

Prochlorperazine

15-Apr-2024

- **INDICATIONS AND DOSE**

Prevention and treatment of nausea and vomiting

- BY MOUTH
  - Child 1–11 years (body-weight 10 kg and above): 250 micrograms/kg 2–3 times a day
  - Child 12–17 years: 5–10 mg up to 3 times a day as required
- BY INTRAMUSCULAR INJECTION
  - Child 2–4 years: 1.25–2.5 mg up to 3 times a day as required
  - Child 5–11 years: 5–6.25 mg up to 3 times a day as required
  - Child 12–17 years: 12.5 mg up to 3 times a day as required

Nausea and vomiting in previously diagnosed migraine

- BY BUCCAL ADMINISTRATION
  - Child 12–17 years: 3–6 mg twice daily

DOSE EQUIVALENCE AND CONVERSION
- Doses are expressed as prochlorperazine maleate or mesilate; 1 mg prochlorperazine maleate ≡ 1 mg prochlorperazine mesilate.

- **UNLICENSED USE** Injection not licensed for use in children. *Buccastem M®* tablets not licensed for use in children.
- **CONTRA-INDICATIONS** Avoid oral route in child under 10 kg · CNS depression · comatose states · phaeochromocytoma
- **CAUTIONS** Hypotension (more likely after intramuscular injection) · susceptibility to QT interval prolongation
- **INTERACTIONS** → Appendix 1: phenothiazine antipsychotics
- **SIDE-EFFECTS**
  GENERAL SIDE-EFFECTS Glucose tolerance impaired · hyponatraemia · photosensitivity reaction · SIADH
  SPECIFIC SIDE-EFFECTS
  - **Rare or very rare**
    - With buccal use Blood disorder · hepatic disorders
  - **Frequency not known**
    - With buccal use Oral disorders · skin eruption · taste altered
    - With intramuscular use Atrioventricular block · cardiac arrest · jaundice · nasal congestion · oculogyric crisis · respiratory depression
    - With oral use Atrioventricular block · cardiac arrest · jaundice · nasal congestion · oculogyric crisis · respiratory depression

  SIDE-EFFECTS, FURTHER INFORMATION Acute dystonias are more common with potent first-generation antipsychotics. The risk is increased in men, young adults, children, antipsychotic-naïve patients, rapid dose escalation, and abrupt treatment discontinuation.
- **HEPATIC IMPAIRMENT** Manufacturer advises avoid.
- **RENAL IMPAIRMENT**
  Dose adjustments Start with small doses in severe renal impairment because of increased cerebral sensitivity.
- **DIRECTIONS FOR ADMINISTRATION** Manufacturer advises buccal tablets are placed high between upper lip and gum and left to dissolve.
- **PATIENT AND CARER ADVICE** Patients or carers should be given advice on how to administer prochlorperazine buccal tablets.

- **MEDICINAL FORMS** There can be variation in the licensing of different medicines containing the same drug.

Solution for injection

- **Stemetil** (Atnahs Pharma UK Ltd)
  Prochlorperazine mesilate 12.5 mg per 1 ml Stemetil 12.5mg/1ml solution for injection ampoules | 10 ampoule PoM £5.23 DT = £5.23

Oral tablet

CAUTIONARY AND ADVISORY LABELS 2

- **Prochlorperazine (Non-proprietary)**
  Prochlorperazine maleate 5 mg Prochlorperazine 5mg tablets | 28 tablet PoM £3.00 DT = £0.83 | 84 tablet PoM £2.31–£7.80
- **Stemetil** (Atnahs Pharma UK Ltd)
  Prochlorperazine maleate 5 mg Stemetil 5mg tablets | 28 tablet PoM £1.98 DT = £0.83 | 84 tablet PoM £5.94

Buccal tablet

CAUTIONARY AND ADVISORY LABELS 2

- **Prochlorperazine (Non-proprietary)**
  Prochlorperazine maleate 3 mg Prochlorperazine 3mg buccal tablets | 8 tablet PoM £3.05 | 50 tablet PoM £26.00 DT = £10.67

5 Pain

Pain, chronic

04-May-2022

Overview

Pain is defined as an unpleasant sensory and emotional experience associated with, or resembling that associated with, actual or potential tissue damage. Physiologically, it can be described as **neuropathic**, **nociceptive** or **nociplastic**, and be classified as either **acute** or **chronic** in nature. Acute nociceptive pain generally responds to treatment with conventional analgesics, whereas chronic, neuropathic, and nociplastic pain respond poorly to conventional analgesics and can be difficult to treat.

Pain that has been present for more than 12 weeks or beyond the expected time of wound healing is defined as chronic, and has a wide-ranging impact on the child and their family. Chronic pain can result from disease- or treatment-related effects (such as with cancer or arthritis). It may also occur where pain persists after surgical interventions, or be of idiopathic origin. In the management of chronic pain, both disease and illness (complex combination of biological, psychological and social factors) should be taken into account. Comorbid symptoms and behaviours often accompany chronic pain (such as fatigue, sleep disturbance, diminished physical functioning, anxiety and mood disorders, and reduced school attendance). These can add to overall suffering and discomfort, reduce quality of life, and can even prevent or delay recovery. If left untreated in childhood, the harmful effects of pain can extend into adulthood.

Aims of treatment

Treatment aims to reduce pain or the functional effects of pain, improve quality of life, and reduce the risk of longer-term harms.

Management of chronic pain

EvGr The management of chronic pain in children is limited by a lack of evidence for recommendations in practice. Children whose symptoms have not responded to initial treatment strategies used for acute pain episodes, should therefore be managed in conjunction with specialists in paediatric chronic pain. While there are pharmacological and non-pharmacological management strategies available for chronic pain, recommendations are largely based on limited evidence and expert consensus. When chronic pain is suspected, effective non-opioid treatment strategies can usually be continued on a case-by-case basis while awaiting specialist input. Ⓔ

Non-drug treatment

EvGr Early biopsychosocial assessment and psychological intervention should be considered, especially where the risk of disability or distress is high. Psychological interventions (such as acceptance and commitment therapy (ACT), cognitive behavioural therapy (CBT), narrative therapy, mindfulness, meditation, relaxation, and distraction) should be part of a multidisciplinary approach to chronic pain management, with face-to-face interventions provided by suitably trained and supervised practitioners. Online or computerised delivery of psychological strategies such as self-distraction, relaxation, and CBT can be considered if face-to-face delivery is unsuitable or unavailable, however there is limited evidence on the efficacy of psychological therapy delivered virtually.

Education of the child and their family/carers should include an explanation and reassurance on pain causation, a brief summary of relevant pain mechanisms, and the role of psychosocial and physical factors in maintaining chronic pain.

Encouraging movement and exercise (including physiotherapy and occupational therapy where appropriate) should be incorporated in the management of many types of chronic pain in children, with consideration of early interventions to increase movement, physical activity, and restore function. Play therapy (such as playful activities and expressive arts) facilitated by a trained play therapist may be considered in hospital or outpatient settings.

Transcutaneous electrical nerve stimulation (TENS) is a low risk intervention that should be considered in some cases.

Pain interventions such as local anaesthetic blockade should only be considered on a case-by-case basis in specialist centres. Ⓔ

Drug treatment

EvGr The pharmacological management of chronic pain in children should be part of a wider multidisciplinary approach and utilise supported self-management strategies. Careful assessment is required prior to starting analgesia, along with regular reviews (minimum of once a year) and planned reassessment of side-effects and ongoing benefit (such as pain relief, improvement in function, and/or quality of life). All drugs started for managing chronic pain should be on a trial basis, guided by specialists, limited to the shortest possible duration, and continued only if benefits outweigh risks. The availability of suitable formulations or products may also guide treatment choice. Ⓔ

For comparative information of pain relief medication, see Analgesics below.

Non-opioid analgesics

EvGr The non-opioid analgesics paracetamol p. 325 and NSAIDs may be appropriate on occasions. Topical non-opioid analgesic preparations may be useful for the management of chronic musculoskeletal pain. The use of anti-neuropathic drugs such as low dose tricyclic antidepressants or antiepileptics for treating chronic pain should only be initiated in consultation with a specialist. Ⓔ

Opioid analgesics

Due to their side-effect profile and risks of addiction, physical dependence and overdose, opioids and compound analgesics that contain opioids are mostly unsuitable and are therefore rarely used in children with chronic pain. EvGr Opioid treatment should only be initiated by a paediatric specialist and used under exceptional circumstances, such as presence of known life-limiting illness. For children currently on opioids when chronic pain is suspected, treatment doses should not be escalated and specialist advice should be sought. Ⓔ

Resources providing information around good practice for healthcare professionals when managing specialist-initiated opioids (based on adult evidence) have been produced by the Faculty of Pain Medicine in partnership with PHE, and are available at: fpm.ac.uk/opioids-aware. Applicability in children should be considered by the prescriber prior to use.

Analgesics

04-Jan-2023

Pain relief

The non-opioid drugs, paracetamol p. 325 and ibuprofen p. 821 (and other NSAIDs), are particularly suitable for pain in musculoskeletal conditions, whereas the opioid analgesics are more suitable for moderate to severe pain, particularly of visceral origin.

Pain in sickle-cell disease

The pain of mild sickle-cell crises is managed with paracetamol, an NSAID, codeine phosphate p. 331, or dihydrocodeine tartrate p. 333. Severe crises may require the use of morphine p. 338 or diamorphine hydrochloride p. 332; concomitant use of an NSAID may potentiate analgesia and allow lower doses of the opioid to be used. A mixture of nitrous oxide and oxygen (*Entonox*®, *Equanox*®) may also be used.

Dental and orofacial pain

Analgesics should be used judiciously in dental care as a **temporary** measure until the cause of the pain has been dealt with.

Dental pain of inflammatory origin, such as that associated with pulpitis, apical infection, localised osteitis or pericoronitis is usually best managed by treating the infection, providing drainage, restorative procedures, and other local measures. Analgesics provide temporary relief of pain (usually for about 1 to 7 days) until the causative factors have been brought under control. In the case of pulpitis, intra-osseous infection or abscess, reliance on analgesics alone is usually inappropriate.

Similarly the pain and discomfort associated with acute problems of the oral mucosa (e.g. acute herpetic gingivostomatitis, erythema multiforme) may be relieved by benzydamine hydrochloride p. 881 or topical anaesthetics until the cause of the mucosal disorder has been dealt with. However, where a child is febrile, the antipyretic action of paracetamol or ibuprofen is often helpful.

The *choice* of an analgesic for dental purposes should be based on its suitability for the child. Most dental pain is relieved effectively by non-steroidal anti-inflammatory drugs (NSAIDs) e.g. ibuprofen. Paracetamol has analgesic and antipyretic effects but no anti-inflammatory effect.

Opioid analgesics such as dihydrocodeine tartrate act on the central nervous system and are traditionally used for *moderate to severe pain*. However, opioid analgesics are relatively ineffective in dental pain and their side-effects can be unpleasant.

Combining a non-opioid with an opioid analgesic can provide greater relief of pain than either analgesic given alone. However, this applies only when an adequate dose of each analgesic is used. Most combination analgesic preparations have not been shown to provide greater relief of pain than an adequate dose of the non-opioid component given alone. Moreover, combination preparations have the disadvantage of an increased number of side-effects.

Any analgesic given before a dental procedure should have a low risk of increasing postoperative bleeding. In the case of pain after the dental procedure, taking an analgesic before the effect of the local anaesthetic has worn off can improve control. Postoperative analgesia with ibuprofen is usually continued for about 24 to 72 hours.

Dysmenorrhoea

Paracetamol or a NSAID will generally provide adequate relief of pain from dysmenorrhoea. Alternatively use of a combined hormonal contraceptive in adolescent girls may prevent the pain.

Non-opioid analgesics and compound analgesic preparations

Paracetamol has analgesic and antipyretic properties but no demonstrable anti-inflammatory activity; unlike opioid analgesics, it does not cause respiratory depression and is less irritant to the stomach than the NSAIDs. **Overdosage** with paracetamol is particularly dangerous as it may cause hepatic damage which is sometimes not apparent for 4 to 6 days.

Non-steroidal anti-inflammatory analgesics (NSAIDs) are particularly useful for the treatment of children with chronic disease accompanied by pain and inflammation. Some of them are also used in the short-term treatment of mild to moderate pain including transient musculoskeletal pain but paracetamol is now often preferred. They are also suitable for the relief of pain in *dysmenorrhoea* and to treat pain caused by *secondary bone tumours*, many of which produce lysis of bone and release prostaglandins. Due to an association with Reye's syndrome, aspirin p. 104 should be avoided in children under 16 years except in Kawasaki disease or for its antiplatelet action. Several NSAIDs are also used for postoperative analgesia.

Compound analgesic preparations

Compound analgesic preparations that contain a simple analgesic (such as paracetamol) with an opioid component reduce the scope for effective titration of the individual components in the management of pain of varying intensity.

Compound analgesic preparations containing paracetamol with a *low dose* of an opioid analgesic (e.g. 8 mg of codeine phosphate per compound tablet) may be used in older children but the advantages have not been substantiated. The low dose of the opioid may be enough to cause opioid side-effects (in particular, constipation) and can complicate the treatment of **overdosage** yet may not provide significant additional relief of pain.

A *full dose* of the opioid component (e.g. 60 mg codeine phosphate) in compound analgesic preparations effectively augments the analgesic activity but is associated with the full range of opioid side-effects (including nausea, vomiting, severe constipation, drowsiness, respiratory depression, and risk of dependence on long-term administration).

In general, when assessing pain, it is necessary to weigh up carefully whether there is a need for a non-opioid and an opioid analgesic to be taken simultaneously.

Opioid analgesics and dependence

Opioid analgesics are usually used to relieve moderate to severe pain particularly of visceral origin. Repeated administration may cause tolerance, but this is no deterrent in the control of pain in terminal illness. Regular use of a potent opioid may be appropriate for certain cases of chronic non-malignant pain.

For general guidance on the use of opioid analgesics in chronic pain, see Pain, chronic p. 322.

Strong opioids

Morphine remains the most valuable opioid analgesic for severe pain although it frequently causes nausea and vomiting. It is the standard against which other opioid analgesics are compared. In addition to relief of pain, morphine also confers a state of euphoria and mental detachment.

Morphine is the opioid of choice for the oral treatment of *severe pain in palliative care*. It is given regularly every 4 hours (or every 12 or 24 hours as modified-release preparations).

Buprenorphine p. 329 has both opioid agonist and antagonist properties and may precipitate withdrawal symptoms, including pain, in children dependent on other opioids. It has abuse potential and may itself cause dependence. It has a much longer duration of action than morphine and sublingually is an effective analgesic for 6 to 8 hours. Unlike most opioid analgesics, the effects of buprenorphine p. 329 are only partially reversed by naloxone hydrochloride p. 1047. It is rarely used in children.

Diamorphine hydrochloride (heroin) p. 332 is a powerful opioid analgesic. It may cause less nausea and hypotension than morphine p. 338. In *palliative care* the greater solubility of diamorphine hydrochloride allows effective doses to be injected in smaller volumes and this is important in the emaciated child. Diamorphine hydrochloride is sometimes given by the intranasal route to treat acute pain in children and is available as a nasal spray; intranasal administration of diamorphine injection has been used [unlicensed].

Alfentanil p. 1022, fentanyl p. 334 and remifentanil p. 1022 are used by injection for intra-operative analgesia. Fentanyl is available in a transdermal drug delivery system as a self-adhesive patch which is changed every 72 hours.

Methadone hydrochloride p. 357 is less sedating than morphine and acts for longer periods. In prolonged use, methadone hydrochloride should not be administered more often than twice daily to avoid the risk of accumulation and opioid overdosage. Methadone hydrochloride may be used instead of morphine when excitation (or exacerbation of pain) occurs with morphine. Methadone hydrochloride may also be used to treat children with neonatal abstinence syndrome.

Papaveretum should not be used in children; morphine is easier to prescribe and less prone to error with regard to the strength and dose.

Pethidine hydrochloride p. 342 produces prompt but short-lasting analgesia; it is less constipating than morphine, but even in high doses is a less potent analgesic. Its use in children is not recommended. Pethidine hydrochloride is used for analgesia in labour; however, other opioids, such as morphine or diamorphine hydrochloride, are often preferred for obstetric pain.

Tramadol hydrochloride p. 343 is used in older children and produces analgesia by two mechanisms: an opioid effect and an enhancement of serotonergic and adrenergic pathways. It has fewer of the typical opioid side-effects (notably, less respiratory depression, less constipation and less addiction potential); psychiatric reactions have been reported.

Weak opioids

Codeine phosphate p. 331 can be used for the relief of short-term acute moderate pain in children older than 12 years where other painkillers such as paracetamol below or ibuprofen p. 821 have proved ineffective.

Dihydrocodeine tartrate p. 333 has an analgesic efficacy similar to that of codeine phosphate.

Postoperative analgesia

A combination of opioid and non-opioid analgesics is used to treat postoperative pain. The use of intra-operative opioids affects the prescribing of postoperative analgesics. A postoperative opioid analgesic should be given with care since it may potentiate any residual respiratory depression.

Morphine is used most widely. Tramadol hydrochloride is not as effective in severe pain as other opioid analgesics. Buprenorphine may antagonise the analgesic effect of previously administered opioids and is generally not recommended. Pethidine hydrochloride is generally not recommended for postoperative pain because it is metabolised to norpethidine which may accumulate, particularly in neonates and in renal impairment; norpethidine stimulates the central nervous system and may cause convulsions.

Opioids are also given epidurally [unlicensed route] in the postoperative period but are associated with side-effects such as pruritus, urinary retention, nausea and vomiting; respiratory depression can be delayed, particularly with morphine.

Patient-controlled analgesia (PCA) and nurse-controlled analgesia (NCA) can be used to relieve postoperative pain—consult hospital protocols.

Pain management and opioid dependence

Although caution is necessary, patients who are dependent on opioids or have a history of drug dependence may be treated with opioid analgesics when there is a clinical need. Treatment with opioid analgesics in this patient group should normally be carried out with the advice of specialists. However, doctors do not require a special licence to prescribe opioid analgesics to patients with opioid dependence for relief of pain due to organic disease or injury.

Other drugs used for Pain Diclofenac potassium, p. 817 · Mefenamic acid, p. 825

ANALGESICS › NON-OPIOID

Paracetamol

03-Oct-2025

(Acetaminophen)

● **INDICATIONS AND DOSE**

Pain | Pyrexia with discomfort

▶ BY MOUTH

- Neonate 28 weeks to 32 weeks corrected gestational age: 20 mg/kg for 1 dose, then 10–15 mg/kg every 8–12 hours as required, maximum daily dose to be given in divided doses; maximum 30 mg/kg per day.
- Neonate 32 weeks corrected gestational age and above: 20 mg/kg for 1 dose, then 10–15 mg/kg every 6–8 hours as required, maximum daily dose to be given in divided doses; maximum 60 mg/kg per day.
- Child 1-2 months: 30–60 mg every 8 hours as required, maximum daily dose to be given in divided doses; maximum 60 mg/kg per day
- Child 3-5 months: 60 mg, every 4–6 hours; maximum 4 doses per day
- Child 6-23 months: 120 mg, every 4–6 hours; maximum 4 doses per day
- Child 2-3 years: 180 mg, every 4–6 hours; maximum 4 doses per day
- Child 4-5 years: 240 mg, every 4–6 hours; maximum 4 doses per day
- Child 6-7 years: 240–250 mg, every 4–6 hours; maximum 4 doses per day
- Child 8-9 years: 360–375 mg, every 4–6 hours; maximum 4 doses per day
- Child 10-11 years: 480–500 mg, every 4–6 hours; maximum 4 doses per day
- Child 12-15 years: 480–750 mg, every 4–6 hours; maximum 4 doses per day
- Child 16-17 years: 0.5–1 g, every 4–6 hours; maximum 4 doses per day

▶ BY RECTUM

- Neonate 28 weeks to 32 weeks corrected gestational age: 20 mg/kg for 1 dose, then 10–15 mg/kg every 12 hours as required, maximum daily dose to be given in divided doses; maximum 30 mg/kg per day.
- Neonate 32 weeks corrected gestational age and above: 30 mg/kg for 1 dose, then 15–20 mg/kg every 8 hours as required, maximum daily dose to be given in divided doses; maximum 60 mg/kg per day.
- Child 1-2 months: 30–60 mg every 8 hours as required, maximum daily dose to be given in divided doses; maximum 60 mg/kg per day
- Child 3-11 months: 60–125 mg every 4–6 hours as required, maximum 4 doses per day
- Child 1-4 years: 125–250 mg every 4–6 hours as required, maximum 4 doses per day
- Child 5-11 years: 250–500 mg every 4–6 hours as required, maximum 4 doses per day
- Child 12-17 years: 500 mg every 4–6 hours

▶ BY INTRAVENOUS INFUSION

- Neonate 32 weeks corrected gestational age and above: 7.5 mg/kg every 8 hours, dose to be administered over 15 minutes.
- Neonate: 10 mg/kg, every 4–6 hours, dose to be administered over 15 minutes; maximum 30 mg/kg per day.
- Child (body-weight up to 10 kg): 10 mg/kg, every 4–6 hours, dose to be administered over 15 minutes; maximum 30 mg/kg per day
- Child (body-weight 10-50 kg): 15 mg/kg, every 4–6 hours, dose to be administered over 15 minutes; maximum 60 mg/kg per day
- Child (body-weight 51 kg and above): 1 g, every 4–6 hours, dose to be administered over 15 minutes; maximum 4 g per day

Pain in children with risk factors for hepatotoxicity | Pyrexia with discomfort in children with risk factors for hepatotoxicity

▶ BY INTRAVENOUS INFUSION

- Neonate 32 weeks corrected gestational age and above: 7.5 mg/kg every 8 hours, dose to be administered over 15 minutes.
- Neonate: 10 mg/kg, every 4–6 hours, dose to be administered over 15 minutes; maximum 30 mg/kg per day.
- Child (body-weight up to 10 kg): 10 mg/kg, every 4–6 hours, dose to be administered over 15 minutes; maximum 30 mg/kg per day

continued →

- ▸ Child (body-weight 10-50 kg): 15 mg/kg, every 4–6 hours, dose to be administered over 15 minutes; maximum 60 mg/kg per day
- ▸ Child (body-weight 51 kg and above): 1 g, every 4–6 hours, dose to be administered over 15 minutes; maximum 3 g per day

Post-operative pain

▶ BY MOUTH

- ▸ Child 1 month-5 years: 20–30 mg/kg for 1 dose, then 15–20 mg/kg every 4–6 hours, maximum daily dose to be given in divided doses; maximum 75 mg/kg per day
- ▸ Child 6-11 years: 20–30 mg/kg (max. per dose 1 g) for 1 dose, then 15–20 mg/kg every 4–6 hours, maximum daily dose to be given in divided doses; maximum 75 mg/kg per day; maximum 4 g per day
- ▸ Child 12-17 years: 1 g, every 4–6 hours; maximum 4 doses per day

▶ BY RECTUM

- ▸ Child 1-2 months: 30 mg/kg for 1 dose, then 15–20 mg/kg every 4–6 hours, maximum daily dose to be given in divided doses; maximum 75 mg/kg per day
- ▸ Child 3 months-5 years: 30–40 mg/kg for 1 dose, then 15–20 mg/kg every 4–6 hours, maximum daily dose to be given in divided doses; maximum 75 mg/kg per day
- ▸ Child 6-11 years: 30–40 mg/kg (max. per dose 1 g) for 1 dose, then 15–20 mg/kg every 4–6 hours, maximum daily dose to be given in divided doses; maximum 75 mg/kg per day; maximum 4 g per day
- ▸ Child 12-17 years: 1 g, every 4–6 hours; maximum 4 doses per day

Prophylaxis of post-immunisation pyrexia following immunisation with meningococcal group B vaccine (Bexsero ®) given as part of the routine immunisation schedule

▶ BY MOUTH

- ▸ Child 2-3 months: 60 mg every 4–6 hours for 3 doses, first dose to be given at the time of or as soon as possible after vaccination, additional doses may be given every 4–6 hours for up to 48 hours after vaccination if fever persists after the third dose and the child is otherwise well; maximum 4 doses per day, use weight-based doses for preterm infants born at less than 32 weeks gestation and currently weighing less than 4 kg—see oral doses for pain and pyrexia with discomfort

Post-immunisation pyrexia in infants

▶ BY MOUTH

- ▸ Child 2-3 months: 60 mg for 1 dose, then 60 mg for 1 dose, to be given 4–6 hours after first dose if required
- ▸ Child 4 months: 60 mg for 1 dose, then 60 mg, to be given 4–6 hours after previous dose; maximum 4 doses per day

● **UNLICENSED USE** Paracetamol oral suspension 500 mg/5 mL not licensed for use in children under 16 years. Not licensed for use in children under 2 months by mouth; under 3 months by rectum. UKHSA advises paracetamol is used in the doses provided in BNFC for the prophylaxis of post-immunisation pyrexia following immunisation with meningococcal group B vaccine (*Bexsero*®), but these may differ from those licensed. Intravenous infusion not licensed in pre-term neonates. Intravenous infusion dose not licensed in children and neonates with body-weight under 10 kg.

IMPORTANT SAFETY INFORMATION

MHRA/CHM ADVICE: PARACETAMOL AND PREGNANCY - REMINDER THAT TAKING PARACETAMOL DURING PREGNANCY REMAINS SAFE (SEPTEMBER 2025)

The MHRA advises there is no evidence that taking paracetamol during pregnancy causes autism in children, and this is supported by recent studies. The MHRA regularly reviews the safety of paracetamol to ensure that the benefits to the patient and unborn baby outweigh the risks.

Healthcare professionals should advise patients and carers that paracetamol is recommended as first line treatment for pain and fever during pregnancy, when used at the lowest effective dose for the shortest time. Untreated pain and fever can pose risks to the unborn baby, so it is important that these symptoms are managed with the recommended treatment; if these symptoms do not resolve, patients and carers should seek advice from their healthcare professional. Patients and carers should be advised that they should not swap to alternative drugs such as NSAIDs, as these are not generally recommended during pregnancy.

● **CAUTIONS** Before administering, check when paracetamol last administered and cumulative paracetamol dose over previous 24 hours · body-weight under 50 kg · chronic alcohol consumption · chronic dehydration · chronic malnutrition · long-term use (especially in those who are malnourished)

CAUTIONS, FURTHER INFORMATION [EvGr] Some patients may be at increased risk of experiencing toxicity at therapeutic doses, particularly those with a body-weight under 50 kg and those with risk factors for hepatotoxicity. Clinical judgement should be used to adjust the dose of oral and intravenous paracetamol in these patients.

Co-administration of enzyme-inducing antiepileptic medications may increase toxicity; doses should be reduced. ⟨E⟩

● **INTERACTIONS** → Appendix 1: paracetamol

● **SIDE-EFFECTS**

GENERAL SIDE-EFFECTS

▶ **Rare or very rare** Thrombocytopenia

SPECIFIC SIDE-EFFECTS

▶ **Common or very common**
- ▸ With rectal use Anorectal erythema

▶ **Rare or very rare**
- ▸ With intravenous use Hypersensitivity · hypotension · leucopenia · malaise · neutropenia
- ▸ With rectal use Angioedema · liver injury · severe cutaneous adverse reactions (SCARs) · skin reactions

▶ **Frequency not known**
- ▸ With intravenous use Flushing · skin reactions · tachycardia
- ▸ With oral use Agranulocytosis · bronchospasm · hepatic function abnormal · rash · severe cutaneous adverse reactions (SCARs)
- ▸ With rectal use Agranulocytosis · blood disorder

Overdose Liver damage and less frequently renal damage can occur following overdose.

Nausea and vomiting, the only early features of poisoning, usually settle within 24 hours. Persistence beyond this time, often associated with the onset of right subcostal pain and tenderness, usually indicates development of hepatic necrosis.

For specific details on the management of poisoning, see Paracetamol, under Emergency treatment of poisoning p. 1036.

● **PREGNANCY** Not known to be harmful.

● **BREAST FEEDING** Amount too small to be harmful.

● **HEPATIC IMPAIRMENT** Manufacturer advises caution (increased risk of toxicity).

● **RENAL IMPAIRMENT** [EvGr] Caution in severe impairment (consult product literature). ⟨M⟩

Dose adjustments

▸ With intravenous use [EvGr] Increase infusion dose interval to at least every 6 hours if creatinine clearance 30 mL/minute or less. ⟨M⟩ See p. 16.

- **DIRECTIONS FOR ADMINISTRATION** For *intravenous infusion* (*Perfalgan*®), manufacturer advises give in Glucose 5% *or* Sodium Chloride 0.9%; dilute to a concentration of not less than 1 mg/mL and use within an hour; may also be given undiluted. For children under 33 kg, use 50 mL-vial.
- **PRESCRIBING AND DISPENSING INFORMATION** BP directs that when Paediatric Paracetamol Oral Suspension or Paediatric Paracetamol Mixture is prescribed Paracetamol Oral Suspension 120 mg/5 mL should be dispensed.
- **PATIENT AND CARER ADVICE**
Medicines for Children leaflet: Paracetamol for mild-to-moderate pain www.medicinesforchildren.org.uk/medicines/paracetamol/
- **PROFESSION SPECIFIC INFORMATION**
Dental practitioners' formulary Paracetamol Tablets may be prescribed.
Paracetamol Soluble Tablets 500 mg may be prescribed.
Paracetamol Oral Suspension may be prescribed.
- **EXCEPTIONS TO LEGAL CATEGORY** Paracetamol capsules or tablets can be sold to the public provided packs contain no more than 32 capsules or tablets; pharmacists can sell multiple packs up to a total quantity of 100 capsules or tablets in justifiable circumstances.

- **MEDICINAL FORMS** There can be variation in the licensing of different medicines containing the same drug. Forms available from special-order manufacturers include: oral suspension, oral solution, oral powder, suppository

Oral tablet

CAUTIONARY AND ADVISORY LABELS 29(500 mg tablets in adults), 30

▸ **Paracetamol (Non-proprietary)**
Paracetamol 500 mg Paracetamol 500mg caplets | 32 tablet [PoM] £0.64 DT = £0.61 | 100 tablet [PoM] £2.50 DT = £1.91
Paracetamol 500mg tablets | 32 tablet [PoM] [X] DT = £0.61 | 100 tablet [PoM] £3.00 DT = £1.91 | 1000 tablet [PoM] £20.00–£31.60
Paracetamol 1 gram Paracetamol 1g tablets | 50 tablet [PoM] £5.98–£6.50 | 100 tablet [PoM] £9.20 DT = £9.20

Suppository

CAUTIONARY AND ADVISORY LABELS 30

▸ **Paracetamol (Non-proprietary)**
Paracetamol 80 mg Paracetamol 80mg suppositories | 10 suppository [P] £10.00 DT = £10.00
Paracetamol 120 mg Paracetamol 120mg suppositories | 10 suppository [P] £41.04 DT = £20.10
Paracetamol 125 mg Paracetamol 125mg suppositories | 10 suppository [P] £15.00 DT = £13.80
Paracetamol 240 mg Paracetamol 240mg suppositories | 10 suppository [P] £66.05 DT = £66.05
Paracetamol 250 mg Paracetamol 250mg suppositories | 10 suppository [P] £15.00–£27.60 DT = £27.60
Paracetamol 500 mg Paracetamol 500mg suppositories | 10 suppository [P] £41.27 DT = £41.27
Paracetamol 1 gram Paracetamol 1g suppositories | 10 suppository [P] £59.50–£60.00 DT = £59.50

▸ **Alvedon** (Esteve Pharmaceuticals Ltd)
Paracetamol 60 mg Alvedon 60mg suppositories | 10 suppository [P] £11.95
Paracetamol 125 mg Alvedon 125mg suppositories | 10 suppository [P] £13.80 DT = £13.80
Paracetamol 250 mg Alvedon 250mg suppositories | 10 suppository [P] £27.60 DT = £27.60

Oral suspension

CAUTIONARY AND ADVISORY LABELS 30

▸ **Paracetamol (Non-proprietary)**
Paracetamol 24 mg per 1 ml Paracetamol 120mg/5ml oral suspension paediatric | 100 ml [P] £3.69–£6.28
Paracetamol 120mg/5ml oral suspension paediatric sugar free | 100 ml [P] £2.22 DT = £2.16 [SF] | 200 ml [P] £4.44–£4.84 [SF] | 500 ml [P] £11.10–£14.00 [SF]
Paracetamol 50 mg per 1 ml Paracetamol 250mg/5ml oral suspension | 100 ml [P] £6.40 DT = £3.77 | 200 ml [P] £2.35 | 500 ml [P] £18.85–£31.70
Paracetamol 250mg/5ml oral suspension sugar free | 100 ml [P] £2.10–£3.80 [SF] | 200 ml [P] £12.00 DT = £3.56 [SF] | 500 ml [P] £18.35–£18.60 [SF] | 1000 ml [P] £42.30 [SF]
Paracetamol 100 mg per 1 ml Paracetamol 500mg/5ml oral suspension sugar free | 150 ml [PoM] £93.02 DT = £84.74 [SF]

▸ **Calpol** (McNeil Products Ltd)
Paracetamol 24 mg per 1 ml Calpol Infant Original 120mg/5ml oral suspension | 200 ml [P] £4.78
Calpol Infant 120mg/5ml oral suspension 5ml sachets sugar free | 12 sachet [GSL] £3.09 DT = £3.09 [SF] | 20 sachet [GSL] £4.90 DT = £4.90 [SF]
Calpol Infant 120mg/5ml oral suspension sugar free | 200 ml [P] £4.78 [SF]
Paracetamol 50 mg per 1 ml Calpol Six Plus 250mg/5ml oral suspension 5ml sachets sugar free | 12 sachet [GSL] £3.70 DT = £3.70 [SF]
Calpol Six Plus 250mg/5ml oral suspension sugar free | 100 ml [P] £3.65 [SF] | 200 ml [P] £5.66 DT = £3.56 [SF]

Effervescent tablet

CAUTIONARY AND ADVISORY LABELS 13, 29(500 mg tablets in adults), 30

▸ **Paracetamol (Non-proprietary)**
Paracetamol 500 mg Paracetamol 500mg soluble tablets | 100 tablet [PoM] [X] DT = £24.80
Paracetamol 500mg effervescent tablets | 60 tablet [PoM] £3.68–£8.10 | 100 tablet [PoM] £5.10–£11.58 DT = £5.81

▸ **Altridexamol** (TriOn Pharma Ltd)
Paracetamol 1 gram Altridexamol 1000mg effervescent tablets | 50 tablet [PoM] £7.89 DT = £7.89 [SF]

Oral capsule

CAUTIONARY AND ADVISORY LABELS 29(500 mg capsules in adults), 30

▸ **Paracetamol (Non-proprietary)**
Paracetamol 500 mg Paracetamol 500mg capsules | 100 capsule [PoM] £3.49 DT = £2.53

Solution for infusion

▸ **Paracetamol (Non-proprietary)**
Paracetamol 10 mg per 1 ml Paracetamol 500mg/50ml solution for infusion vials | 10 vial [PoM] £22.60
Paracetamol 100mg/10ml solution for infusion ampoules | 20 ampoule [PoM] £106.00 (Hospital only)
Paracetamol 1g/100ml solution for infusion bottles | 10 bottle [PoM] £12.45 (Hospital only)
Paracetamol 1g/100ml solution for infusion vials | 10 vial [PoM] £17.50–£21.40 (Hospital only)

Oral solution

CAUTIONARY AND ADVISORY LABELS 30

▸ **Paracetamol (Non-proprietary)**
Paracetamol 24 mg per 1 ml Paracetamol 120mg/5ml oral solution paediatric sugar free | 500 ml [P] [X] [SF]
Paracetamol 100 mg per 1 ml Paracetamol 500mg/5ml oral solution sugar free | 200 ml [PoM] £18.00 [SF]

Orodispersible tablet

CAUTIONARY AND ADVISORY LABELS 30

▸ **Calpol Fastmelts** (McNeil Products Ltd)
Paracetamol 250 mg Calpol Six Plus Fastmelts 250mg tablets | 24 tablet [P] £5.42 DT = £5.42 [SF]

Combinations available: ***Co-codamol***, p. 330 · ***Dihydrocodeine with paracetamol***, p. 334 · ***Tramadol with paracetamol***, p. 344

ANALGESICS > OPIOIDS

Opioids

IMPORTANT SAFETY INFORMATION

MHRA/CHM ADVICE: BENZODIAZEPINES AND OPIOIDS: REMINDER OF RISK OF POTENTIALLY FATAL RESPIRATORY DEPRESSION (MARCH 2020)

The MHRA reminds healthcare professionals that opioids co-prescribed with benzodiazepines and benzodiazepine-like drugs can produce additive CNS depressant effects, thereby increasing the risk of sedation, respiratory depression, coma, and death. Healthcare professionals are advised to only co-prescribe if there is no alternative and, if necessary, the lowest possible doses should be given for the shortest duration. Patients should be closely monitored for signs of respiratory depression at initiation of treatment and when there is any change in prescribing, such as dose adjustments or new interactions. If methadone is co-prescribed with a benzodiazepine or benzodiazepine-like drug, the respiratory depressant effect of methadone may be delayed; patients should be monitored for at least 2 weeks after initiation or changes in prescribing. Patients should be informed of the signs and symptoms of respiratory depression and sedation, and advised to seek urgent medical attention should these occur.

MHRA/CHM ADVICE: OPIOIDS: RISK OF DEPENDENCE AND ADDICTION (SEPTEMBER 2020)

New safety recommendations have been issued following a review of the risks of dependence and addiction associated with prolonged use (longer than 3 months) of opioids for non-malignant pain.

Healthcare professionals are advised to:

- discuss with patients that prolonged use of opioids, even at therapeutic doses, may lead to dependence and addiction;
- agree a treatment strategy and plan for end of treatment with the patient before starting opioids;
- counsel patients and their carers on the risks of tolerance and potentially fatal unintentional overdose, as well as signs and symptoms of overdose;
- provide regular monitoring and support to patients at increased risk, such as those with current or history of substance use disorder (including alcohol misuse) or mental health disorders;
- taper dosage slowly at the end of treatment to reduce the risk of withdrawal effects associated with abrupt discontinuation (tapering high doses may take weeks or months);
- consider hyperalgesia in patients on long-term opioid treatment who present with increased pain sensitivity;
- consult product literature for the latest advice and warnings for opioid use during pregnancy (see also *Pregnancy*).

The MHRA has also issued a safety leaflet for patients—see *Patient and carer advice*.

MHRA/CHM ADVICE: PROLONGED-RELEASE OPIOIDS: REMOVAL OF INDICATION FOR RELIEF OF POST-OPERATIVE PAIN (MARCH 2025)

Following a safety review by the MHRA and advice from the CHM, treatment of postoperative pain will be removed from the licensed indications of modified-release morphine and modified-release oxycodone due to the potential for harm and increased risk of persistent postoperative opioid use (PPOU) and opioid-induced ventilatory impairment (OIVI). Modified-release opioids provide relief from chronic severe pain and should not be used for acute pain relief after surgery; transdermal patches are also not recommended for such use. Modified-release opioids are associated with PPOU, defined as continued opioid use beyond 90 days after surgery, and OIVI, a serious form of respiratory depression that causes central respiratory depression, sedation, and upper airway obstruction.

Before surgery, healthcare professionals should discuss with the patient:

- the risks of PPOU and dependence, and potential risk of addiction and withdrawal reactions;
- the risk of OIVI, especially in those with underlying respiratory conditions;
- that postoperative pain is normally short-lived and should only require short-term treatment with immediate-release opioids;
- pain management strategies involving immediate-release opioids and multimodal analgesia, and plan for end of treatment.

Healthcare professionals should review the treatment, before and after surgery, of patients whose pain is managed with opioids pre-operatively, in line with Consensus Best Practice Guidelines (available at: www.cpoc.org.uk/sites/cpoc/files/documents/2021-03/surgery-and-opioids-2021.pdf).

At discharge from hospital, healthcare professionals should:

- only prescribe and supply a sufficient amount of immediate-release opioids for acute postoperative pain relief to minimise the risk of PPOU, dependence, stockpiling of unused opioids, and potential for diversion;
- communicate the pain management plan with primary care practice taking over care in the community and document in the patient's clinical notes.

Healthcare professionals should advise patients to:

- talk to their doctor about pain management and ongoing needs if they are already on modified-release opioids before surgery, as the risk of respiratory depression and PPOU is higher;
- dial 999 if they notice new or increased trouble with breathing;
- contact their doctor if they feel unable to stop taking opioids as originally planned.

Patients or their carer who are concerned about using more opioids than prescribed should also be counselled to seek advice from the NHS website (available at: www.nhs.uk/live-well/pain/how-to-get-nhs-help-for-your-pain/), or in Northern Ireland, the Health and Social Care website (available at: online.hscni.net/our-work/pharmacy-and-medicines-management/patient-initiatives/long-term-pain/).

- **CONTRA-INDICATIONS** Acute respiratory depression · comatose patients · head injury (opioid analgesics interfere with pupillary responses vital for neurological assessment) · raised intracranial pressure (opioid analgesics interfere with pupillary responses vital for neurological assessment) · risk of paralytic ileus
- **CAUTIONS** Adrenocortical insufficiency (reduced dose is recommended) · asthma (avoid during an acute attack) · central sleep apnoea · convulsive disorders · current or history of mental health disorder · current or history of substance use disorder · diseases of the biliary tract · hypotension · hypothyroidism (reduced dose is recommended) · impaired respiratory function (avoid in chronic obstructive pulmonary disease) · inflammatory bowel disorders · myasthenia gravis · obstructive bowel disorders · shock · urethral stenosis

CAUTIONS, FURTHER INFORMATION

- Dependence and addiction Prolonged use of opioid analgesics may lead to drug dependence and addiction, even at therapeutic doses. There is an increased risk in individuals with current or history of substance use disorder or mental health disorders. See also *Important safety information*.
- Central sleep apnoea Opioids cause a dose-dependent increased risk of central sleep apnoea, EvGr consider total opioid dose reduction. ⟨M⟩
- Palliative care EvGr In the control of pain in terminal illness, the cautions listed should not necessarily be a deterrent to the use of opioid analgesics. ⟨M⟩

- **SIDE-EFFECTS**
  - **Common or very common** Arrhythmias · confusion · constipation · dizziness · drowsiness · dry mouth · euphoric mood · flushing · hallucination · headache · hyperhidrosis · hypotension (with high doses) · miosis · nausea (more common on initiation) · palpitations · respiratory depression (with high doses) · skin reactions · urinary retention · vertigo · visual impairment · vomiting (more common on initiation)
  - **Uncommon** Drug dependence · dysphoria · seizure · withdrawal syndrome

SIDE-EFFECTS, FURTHER INFORMATION **Respiratory depression** Respiratory depression is a major concern with opioid analgesics and it may be treated by artificial ventilation or be reversed by naloxone. Neonates (particularly if pre-term) may be more susceptible.

Dependence, addiction, and withdrawal Long term use of opioids in non-malignant pain (longer than 3 months) carries an increased risk of dependence and addiction, even at therapeutic doses. At the end of treatment the dosage should be tapered slowly to reduce the risk of withdrawal effects; tapering from a high dose may take weeks or months. See also *Important safety information*.

Overdose Opioids (narcotic analgesics) cause coma, respiratory depression, and pinpoint pupils. For details on the management of poisoning, see Opioids, under Emergency treatment of poisoning p. 1036 and consider the specific antidote, naloxone hydrochloride.

- **PREGNANCY** Respiratory depression and withdrawal symptoms can occur in the neonate if opioid analgesics are used during delivery; also gastric stasis and inhalation pneumonia has been reported in the mother if opioid analgesics are used during labour.
- **TREATMENT CESSATION** Avoid abrupt withdrawal after long-term treatment; they should be withdrawn gradually to avoid abstinence symptoms.
- **PRESCRIBING AND DISPENSING INFORMATION** The *Faculty of Pain Medicine* has produced resources for healthcare professionals around opioid prescribing: www.fpm.ac.uk/faculty-of-pain-medicine/opioids-aware
- **PATIENT AND CARER ADVICE**

MHRA safety leaflet: Opioid medicines and the risk of addiction www.gov.uk/guidance/opioid-medicines-and-the-risk-of-addiction

Driving and skilled tasks Drowsiness may affect performance of skilled tasks (e.g. driving); effects of alcohol enhanced. Driving at the start of therapy with opioid analgesics, and following dose changes, should be avoided.

For information on 2015 legislation regarding driving whilst taking certain controlled drugs, including opioids, see *Drugs and driving* under Guidance on prescribing p. 1.

F 327

Buprenorphine

09-Oct-2022

- **DRUG ACTION** Buprenorphine is an opioid-receptor partial agonist (it has opioid agonist and antagonist properties).
- **INDICATIONS AND DOSE**

Moderate to severe pain

- BY SUBLINGUAL ADMINISTRATION
  - Child (body-weight 16–25 kg): 100 micrograms every 6–8 hours
  - Child (body-weight 25–37.5 kg): 100–200 micrograms every 6–8 hours
  - Child (body-weight 37.5–50 kg): 200–300 micrograms every 6–8 hours
  - Child (body-weight 50 kg and above): 200–400 micrograms every 6–8 hours
- BY INTRAMUSCULAR INJECTION, OR BY SLOW INTRAVENOUS INJECTION
  - Child 6 months–11 years: 3–6 micrograms/kg every 6–8 hours (max. per dose 9 micrograms/kg)
  - Child 12–17 years: 300–600 micrograms every 6–8 hours

- **UNLICENSED USE** Sublingual tablets not licensed for use in children under 6 years.

  Injection not licensed for use in children under 6 months.
- **CAUTIONS** Impaired consciousness
- **INTERACTIONS** → Appendix 1: opioids
- **SIDE-EFFECTS**

GENERAL SIDE-EFFECTS
- **Rare or very rare** Angioedema · bronchospasm
- **Frequency not known** Hepatic disorders

SPECIFIC SIDE-EFFECTS
- **Common or very common**
  - With parenteral use Hypersensitivity · withdrawal syndrome neonatal
  - With sublingual use Fatigue · sleep disorders
- **Uncommon**
  - With sublingual use Anxiety · apnoea · appetite decreased · atrioventricular block · coma · conjunctivitis · coordination abnormal · cyanosis · depersonalisation · depression · diarrhoea · diplopia · dyspepsia · dyspnoea · hypertension · pallor · paraesthesia · psychosis · speech slurred · tinnitus · tremor · urinary disorder
- **Frequency not known**
  - With parenteral use Psychotic disorder · vision blurred
  - With sublingual use Cerebrospinal fluid pressure increased · circulation impaired · haemorrhagic diathesis · oral disorders · syncope

Overdose The effects of buprenorphine are only partially reversed by naloxone.

- **BREAST FEEDING** Present in low levels in breast milk.

  Monitoring Neonates should be monitored for drowsiness, adequate weight gain, and developmental milestones.
- **HEPATIC IMPAIRMENT** Manufacturer advises caution; avoid in severe impairment (limited information available).
- **RENAL IMPAIRMENT** Some manufacturers advise caution in severe impairment (risk of increased and prolonged effects; consult product literature).

  Dose adjustments For *sublingual tablets*, some manufacturers advise dose reduction may be required in severe impairment (consult product literature).
- **PRE-TREATMENT SCREENING** Documentation of viral hepatitis status is recommended before commencing therapy for opioid dependence.
- **MONITORING REQUIREMENTS** Monitor liver function; when used in opioid dependence baseline liver function test is recommended before commencing therapy, and regular liver function tests should be performed throughout treatment.
- **DIRECTIONS FOR ADMINISTRATION** Manufacturer advises *sublingual tablets* may be halved.
- **PATIENT AND CARER ADVICE** Patients or carers should be given advice on how to administer buprenorphine products.

- **MEDICINAL FORMS** There can be variation in the licensing of different medicines containing the same drug.

Sublingual tablet

CAUTIONARY AND ADVISORY LABELS 2, 26

- Buprenorphine (Non-proprietary)

  Buprenorphine (as Buprenorphine hydrochloride) 400 microgram Buprenorphine 400microgram sublingual tablets sugar free | 7 tablet PoM £1.70 DT = £1.60 CD3 SF

  Buprenorphine (as Buprenorphine hydrochloride) 2 mg Buprenorphine 2mg sublingual tablets sugar free | 7 tablet PoM £5.38 DT = £1.37 CD3 SF

  Buprenorphine (as Buprenorphine hydrochloride) 8 mg Buprenorphine 8mg sublingual tablets sugar free | 7 tablet PoM £16.15 DT = £2.84 CD3 SF
- Prefibin (Sandoz Ltd)

  Buprenorphine (as Buprenorphine hydrochloride) 400 microgram Prefibin 0.4mg sublingual tablets | 7 tablet PoM £1.60 DT = £1.60 CD3 SF

  Buprenorphine (as Buprenorphine hydrochloride) 2 mg Prefibin 2mg sublingual tablets | 7 tablet PoM £5.38 DT = £1.37 CD3 SF

  Buprenorphine (as Buprenorphine hydrochloride) 8 mg Prefibin 8mg sublingual tablets | 7 tablet PoM £16.15 DT = £2.84 CD3 SF

- **Temgesic** (Eumedica Pharma Ltd)
  Buprenorphine (as Buprenorphine hydrochloride) 200 microgram Temgesic 200microgram sublingual tablets | 50 tablet PoM £5.04 DT = £5.04 CD3 SF
  Buprenorphine (as Buprenorphine hydrochloride) 400 microgram Temgesic 400microgram sublingual tablets | 50 tablet PoM £10.07 DT = £10.07 CD3 SF
- **Tephine** (Sandoz Ltd)
  Buprenorphine (as Buprenorphine hydrochloride) 200 microgram Tephine 200microgram sublingual tablets | 50 tablet PoM £4.27 DT = £5.04 CD3 SF
  Buprenorphine (as Buprenorphine hydrochloride) 400 microgram Tephine 400microgram sublingual tablets | 50 tablet PoM £8.54 DT = £10.07 CD3 SF

F 327

Co-codamol

13-Nov-2020

The properties listed below are those particular to the combination only. For the properties of the components please consider, paracetamol p. 325.

● **INDICATIONS AND DOSE**

Short-term treatment of acute moderate pain [using co-codamol 8/500 preparations only]

▶ BY MOUTH USING TABLETS, OR BY MOUTH USING EFFERVESCENT TABLETS
- Child 12–15 years: 1 tablet every 6 hours as required for maximum 3 days; maximum 4 tablets per day
- Child 16–17 years: 1–2 tablets every 6 hours as required for maximum 3 days; maximum 8 tablets per day

▶ BY MOUTH USING CAPSULES
- Child 12–15 years: 1 capsule every 6 hours as required for maximum 3 days; maximum 4 capsules per day
- Child 16–17 years: 1–2 capsules every 6 hours as required for maximum 3 days; maximum 8 capsules per day

Short-term treatment of acute moderate pain [using co-codamol 15/500 preparations only]

▶ BY MOUTH USING TABLETS, OR BY MOUTH USING EFFERVESCENT TABLETS
- Child 12–15 years: 1 tablet every 6 hours as required for maximum 3 days; maximum 4 tablets per day
- Child 16–17 years: 1–2 tablets every 6 hours as required for maximum 3 days; maximum 8 tablets per day

▶ BY MOUTH USING CAPSULES
- Child 12–15 years: 1 capsule every 6 hours as required for maximum 3 days; maximum 4 capsules per day
- Child 16–17 years: 1–2 capsules every 6 hours as required for maximum 3 days; maximum 8 capsules per day

Short-term treatment of acute moderate pain [using co-codamol 30/500 preparations only]

▶ BY MOUTH USING TABLETS, OR BY MOUTH USING EFFERVESCENT TABLETS
- Child 12–15 years: 1 tablet every 6 hours as required for maximum 3 days; maximum 4 tablets per day
- Child 16–17 years: 1–2 tablets every 6 hours as required for maximum 3 days; maximum 8 tablets per day

▶ BY MOUTH USING CAPSULES
- Child 12–15 years: 1 capsule every 6 hours as required for maximum 3 days; maximum 4 capsules per day
- Child 16–17 years: 1–2 capsules every 6 hours as required for maximum 3 days; maximum 8 capsules per day

▶ BY MOUTH USING ORAL SOLUTION
- Child 12–15 years: 5 mL every 6 hours as required for maximum 3 days; maximum 20 mL per day
- Child 16–17 years: 5–10 mL every 6 hours as required for maximum 3 days; maximum 40 mL per day

KAPAKE ® 15/500

Short-term treatment of acute pain

▶ BY MOUTH
- Child 12–15 years: 1 tablet every 6 hours as required for maximum 3 days; maximum 4 tablets per day
- Child 16–17 years: 2 tablets every 6 hours as required for maximum 3 days; maximum 8 tablets per day

IMPORTANT SAFETY INFORMATION
See codeine phosphate p. 331 for MHRA/CHM advice for restrictions on the use of codeine as an analgesic in children.

● **CONTRA-INDICATIONS** Acute ulcerative colitis · antibiotic-associated colitis · children who undergo the removal of tonsils or adenoids for the treatment of obstructive sleep apnoea · conditions where abdominal distention develops · conditions where inhibition of peristalsis should be avoided · known ultra-rapid codeine metabolisers

● **CAUTIONS** Acute abdomen · alcohol dependence · avoid abrupt withdrawal after long-term treatment · cardiac arrhythmias · chronic alcoholism · chronic dehydration · chronic malnutrition · not recommended for adolescents aged 12–18 years with breathing problems

CAUTIONS, FURTHER INFORMATION
- Variation in metabolism The capacity to metabolise codeine to morphine can vary considerably between individuals; there is a marked increase in morphine toxicity in patients who are ultra-rapid codeine metabolisers (CYP2D6 ultra-rapid metabolisers) and a reduced therapeutic effect in poor codeine metabolisers.

● **INTERACTIONS** → Appendix 1: opioids · paracetamol

● **SIDE-EFFECTS** Abdominal pain · addiction · agranulocytosis · blood disorder · irritability · pancreatitis · restlessness · severe cutaneous adverse reactions (SCARs) · thrombocytopenia

Overdose Liver damage (and less frequently renal damage) following overdosage with paracetamol.

● **BREAST FEEDING** Manufacturer advises avoid (recommendation also supported by MHRA and specialist sources). Present in milk and mothers vary considerably in their capacity to metabolise codeine; risk of opioid toxicity in infant.

● **HEPATIC IMPAIRMENT** Manufacturer advises caution in mild to moderate impairment; avoid in severe impairment.
Dose adjustments Manufacturer advises consider dose reduction in mild to moderate impairment.

● **RENAL IMPAIRMENT** Reduce dose or avoid codeine; increased and prolonged effect; increased cerebral sensitivity.

● **PRESCRIBING AND DISPENSING INFORMATION** Co-codamol is a mixture of codeine phosphate and paracetamol; the proportions are expressed in the form x/y, where x and y are the strengths in milligrams of codeine phosphate and paracetamol respectively.

When co-codamol tablets, dispersible (or effervescent) tablets, or capsules are prescribed and **no strength is stated**, tablets, dispersible (or effervescent) tablets, or capsules, respectively, containing codeine phosphate 8 mg and paracetamol 500 mg should be dispensed.

The Drug Tariff allows tablets of co-codamol labelled 'dispersible' to be dispensed against an order for 'effervescent' and *vice versa*.

● **LESS SUITABLE FOR PRESCRIBING** Co-codamol is less suitable for prescribing.

● **EXCEPTIONS TO LEGAL CATEGORY** Co-codamol 8/500 can be sold to the public in certain circumstances; for exemptions see *Medicines, Ethics and Practice,* London, Pharmaceutical Press (always consult latest edition).

● **MEDICINAL FORMS** There can be variation in the licensing of different medicines containing the same drug. Forms available from special-order manufacturers include: oral solution

Oral tablet

CAUTIONARY AND ADVISORY LABELS 2(does not apply to the 8/500 tablet), 29, 30

▸ **Co-codamol (Non-proprietary)**
Codeine phosphate 8 mg, Paracetamol 500 mg Co-codamol 8mg/500mg tablets | 100 tablet [PoM] £5.10 DT = £3.43 [CD5]
Codeine phosphate 15 mg, Paracetamol 500 mg Co-codamol 15mg/500mg tablets | 100 tablet [PoM] £15.00 DT = £2.68 [CD5]
Codeine phosphate 30 mg, Paracetamol 500 mg Co-codamol 30mg/500mg caplets | 100 tablet [PoM] £13.00 DT = £5.07 [CD5]
Co-codamol 30mg/500mg tablets | 30 tablet [PoM] £3.01 DT = £1.52 [CD5] | 100 tablet [PoM] £7.53 DT = £5.07 [CD5]

▸ **Codipar** (Advanz Pharma)
Codeine phosphate 15 mg, Paracetamol 500 mg Codipar 15mg/500mg tablets | 100 tablet [PoM] £8.25 DT = £2.68 [CD5]

▸ **Emcozin** (GlucoRx Ltd)
Codeine phosphate 30 mg, Paracetamol 500 mg Emcozin 30mg/500mg tablets | 100 tablet [PoM] £2.94 DT = £5.07 [CD5]

▸ **Migraleve Yellow** (McNeil Products Ltd)
Codeine phosphate 8 mg, Paracetamol 500 mg Migraleve Yellow tablets | 16 tablet [PoM] [⊠] [CD5]

▸ **Solpadeine Max** (Omega Pharma Ltd)
Codeine phosphate 12.8 mg, Paracetamol 500 mg Solpadeine Max 12.8mg/500mg tablets | 24 tablet [P] £5.04 DT = £5.04 [CD5]

▸ **Solpadol** (Phoenix Labs Ltd)
Codeine phosphate 30 mg, Paracetamol 500 mg Solpadol 30mg/500mg caplets | 100 tablet [PoM] £6.74 DT = £5.07 [CD5]

▸ **Zapain** (Advanz Pharma)
Codeine phosphate 30 mg, Paracetamol 500 mg Zapain 30mg/500mg tablets | 50 tablet [PoM] £1.56 [CD5] | 100 tablet [PoM] £3.11 DT = £5.07 [CD5]

Effervescent tablet

CAUTIONARY AND ADVISORY LABELS 2(does not apply to the 8/500 tablet), 13, 29, 30
EXCIPIENTS: May contain Aspartame
ELECTROLYTES: May contain Sodium

▸ **Co-codamol (Non-proprietary)**
Codeine phosphate 8 mg, Paracetamol 500 mg Co-codamol 8mg/500mg effervescent tablets sugar free | 100 tablet [PoM] £10.25 DT = £10.25 [CD5] [SF]
Co-codamol 8mg/500mg effervescent tablets | 100 tablet [PoM] £9.37 DT = £6.81 [CD5]
Codeine phosphate 15 mg, Paracetamol 500 mg Co-codamol 15mg/500mg effervescent tablets sugar free | 100 tablet [PoM] £8.25-£13.20 DT = £8.25 [CD5] [SF]
Codeine phosphate 30 mg, Paracetamol 500 mg Co-codamol 30mg/500mg effervescent tablets | 32 tablet [PoM] £5.40 DT = £2.32 [CD5] | 100 tablet [PoM] £19.20 DT = £7.25 [CD5]
Co-codamol 30mg/500mg effervescent tablets sugar free | 100 tablet [PoM] £8.90 [CD5] [SF]

▸ **Solpadol** (Phoenix Labs Ltd)
Codeine phosphate 30 mg, Paracetamol 500 mg Solpadol 30mg/500mg effervescent tablets | 100 tablet [PoM] £8.90 DT = £7.25 [CD5]

Oral capsule

CAUTIONARY AND ADVISORY LABELS 2(does not apply to the 8/500 capsule), 29, 30
EXCIPIENTS: May contain Sulfites

▸ **Co-codamol (Non-proprietary)**
Codeine phosphate 8 mg, Paracetamol 500 mg Co-codamol 8mg/500mg capsules | 32 capsule [PoM] £11.38 DT = £6.98 [CD5] | 100 capsule [PoM] £51.56 DT = £21.80 [CD5]
Codeine phosphate 15 mg, Paracetamol 500 mg Co-codamol 15mg/500mg capsules | 100 capsule [PoM] £7.01-£7.32 DT = £7.25 [CD5]
Codeine phosphate 30 mg, Paracetamol 500 mg Co-codamol 30mg/500mg capsules | 100 capsule [PoM] £9.90 DT = £4.67 [CD5]

▸ **Codipar** (Advanz Pharma)
Codeine phosphate 15 mg, Paracetamol 500 mg Codipar 15mg/500mg capsules | 100 capsule [PoM] £7.25 DT = £7.25 [CD5]

▸ **Tylex** (UCB Pharma Ltd)
Codeine phosphate 30 mg, Paracetamol 500 mg Tylex 30mg/500mg capsules | 100 capsule [PoM] £7.93 DT = £4.67 [CD5]

▸ **Zapain** (Advanz Pharma)
Codeine phosphate 30 mg, Paracetamol 500 mg Zapain 30mg/500mg capsules | 50 capsule [PoM] £1.93 [CD5] | 100 capsule [PoM] £3.85 DT = £4.67 [CD5]

327

Codeine phosphate

28-Mar-2024

● **INDICATIONS AND DOSE**

Diarrhoea
▸ BY MOUTH
▸ Child 12–17 years: 15–60 mg 3–4 times a day

Short-term treatment of acute moderate pain
▸ BY MOUTH
▸ Child 12–17 years: 30–60 mg every 6 hours as required for maximum 3 days

IMPORTANT SAFETY INFORMATION

MHRA/CHM ADVICE (JULY 2013) CODEINE FOR ANALGESIA: RESTRICTED USE IN CHILDREN DUE TO REPORTS OF MORPHINE TOXICITY

Codeine should only be used to relieve acute moderate pain in children older than 12 years and only if it cannot be relieved by other painkillers such as paracetamol or ibuprofen alone. A significant risk of serious and life-threatening adverse reactions has been identified in children with obstructive sleep apnoea who received codeine after tonsillectomy or adenoidectomy:

- in children aged 12–18 years, the maximum daily dose of codeine should not exceed 240 mg. Doses may be taken up to four times a day at intervals of no less than 6 hours. The lowest effective dose should be used and duration of treatment should be limited to 3 days
- codeine is contra-indicated in all children (under 18 years) who undergo the removal of tonsils or adenoids for the treatment of obstructive sleep apnoea
- codeine is not recommended for use in children whose breathing may be compromised, including those with neuromuscular disorders, severe cardiac or respiratory conditions, respiratory infections, multiple trauma or extensive surgical procedures
- codeine is contra-indicated in patients of any age who are known to be ultra-rapid metabolisers of codeine (CYP2D6 ultra-rapid metabolisers)
- codeine should not be used in breast-feeding mothers because it can pass to the baby through breast milk
- parents and carers should be advised on how to recognise signs and symptoms of morphine toxicity, and to stop treatment and seek medical attention if signs or symptoms of toxicity occur (including reduced consciousness, lack of appetite, somnolence, constipation, respiratory depression, 'pin-point' pupils, nausea, vomiting)

MHRA/CHM ADVICE (APRIL 2015) CODEINE FOR COUGH AND COLD: RESTRICTED USE IN CHILDREN

Do not use codeine in children under 12 years as it is associated with a risk of respiratory side effects. Codeine is not recommended for adolescents (12–18 years) who have problems with breathing. When prescribing or dispensing codeine-containing medicines for cough and cold, consider that codeine is contra-indicated in:

- children younger than 12 years old
- patients of any age known to be CYP2D6 ultra-rapid metabolisers
- breastfeeding mothers

MHRA/CHM ADVICE: CODEINE LINCTUS (CODEINE ORAL SOLUTIONS): RECLASSIFICATION TO PRESCRIPTION-ONLY MEDICINE (FEBRUARY 2024)

Following the results of a public consultation, codeine linctus has been reclassified as a prescription-only medicine (POM) due to the risk of dependence, addiction, and overdose. Healthcare professionals are reminded that codeine linctus is only authorised for the treatment of dry cough, and only considered to be effective for chronic coughs lasting over 8 weeks.

- **CONTRA-INDICATIONS** Acute ulcerative colitis · antibiotic-associated colitis · children under 18 years who undergo the removal of tonsils or adenoids for the treatment of obstructive sleep apnoea · conditions where abdominal distension develops · conditions where inhibition of peristalsis should be avoided · known ultra-rapid codeine metabolisers
- **CAUTIONS** Acute abdomen · cardiac arrhythmias · gallstones · not recommended for adolescents aged 12–18 years with breathing problems

CAUTIONS, FURTHER INFORMATION

▸ Variation in metabolism The capacity to metabolise codeine to morphine can vary considerably between individuals; there is a marked increase in morphine toxicity in patients who are ultra-rapid codeine metabolisers (CYP2D6 ultra-rapid metabolisers) and a reduced therapeutic effect in poor codeine metabolisers.

- **INTERACTIONS** → Appendix 1: opioids
- **SIDE-EFFECTS** Abdominal cramps · addiction · appetite decreased · biliary spasm · depression · dyskinesia · dyspnoea · face oedema · fatigue · fever · hyperglycaemia · hypersensitivity · hypothermia · intracranial pressure increased · lymphadenopathy · malaise · mood altered · muscle rigidity (with high doses) · nightmare · pancreatitis · restlessness · sexual dysfunction · splenomegaly · ureteral spasm · urinary disorders · vision disorders
- **BREAST FEEDING** Manufacturer advises avoid (recommendation also supported by MHRA and specialist sources). Present in milk and mothers vary considerably in their capacity to metabolise codeine; risk of opioid toxicity in infant.
- **HEPATIC IMPAIRMENT** [EvGr] Caution in mild to moderate impairment; avoid in severe impairment. ⟨M⟩
  Dose adjustments [EvGr] Reduce dose in mild to moderate impairment. ⟨M⟩
- **RENAL IMPAIRMENT** Avoid use or reduce dose; opioid effects increased and prolonged and increased cerebral sensitivity occurs.
- **PRESCRIBING AND DISPENSING INFORMATION** BP directs that when Diabetic Codeine Linctus is prescribed, Codeine Linctus formulated with a vehicle appropriate for administration to diabetics, whether or not labelled 'Diabetic Codeine Linctus', shall be dispensed or supplied.
- **PATIENT AND CARER ADVICE**
  Medicines for Children leaflet: Codeine phosphate for pain
  www.medicinesforchildren.org.uk/medicines/codeine-phosphate-for-pain/

- **MEDICINAL FORMS** There can be variation in the licensing of different medicines containing the same drug. Forms available from special-order manufacturers include: oral suspension, oral solution

Oral tablet

CAUTIONARY AND ADVISORY LABELS 2

▸ **Codeine phosphate (Non-proprietary)**

Codeine phosphate 15 mg Codeine 15mg tablets | 28 tablet [PoM] £1.35 DT = £0.74 [CD5] | 100 tablet [PoM] £3.36 DT = £2.64 [CD5]

Codeine phosphate 30 mg Codeine 30mg tablets | 28 tablet [PoM] £1.35 DT = £0.96 [CD5] | 100 tablet [PoM] £5.74 DT = £3.43 [CD5] | 500 tablet [PoM] £15.55 [CD5]

Codeine phosphate 60 mg Codeine 60mg tablets | 28 tablet [PoM] £2.59 DT = £1.81 [CD5]

Oral solution

CAUTIONARY AND ADVISORY LABELS 2

▸ **Codeine phosphate (Non-proprietary)**

Codeine phosphate 3 mg per 1 ml Codeine 15mg/5ml linctus sugar free | 200 ml [PoM] £19.50 DT = £18.29 [CD5] [SF] | 2000 ml [PoM] £161.90 [CD5] [SF]

Codeine 15mg/5ml linctus | 200 ml [PoM] £19.50–£31.20 DT = £19.50 [CD5]

▸ **Galcodine** (Thornton & Ross Ltd)

Codeine phosphate 3 mg per 1 ml Galcodine 15mg/5ml linctus | 2000 ml [PoM] £9.90 [CD5] [SF]

327

Diamorphine hydrochloride

13-Nov-2020

(Heroin hydrochloride)

- **INDICATIONS AND DOSE**

Acute or chronic pain

▸ BY MOUTH
- Child 1 month–11 years: 100–200 micrograms/kg every 4 hours (max. per dose 10 mg), adjusted according to response
- Child 12–17 years: 5–10 mg every 4 hours, adjusted according to response

▸ BY CONTINUOUS INTRAVENOUS INFUSION
- Child 1 month–11 years: 12.5–25 micrograms/kg/hour, adjusted according to response

▸ BY INTRAVENOUS INJECTION
- Child 1–2 months: 20 micrograms/kg every 6 hours, adjusted according to response
- Child 3–5 months: 25–50 micrograms/kg every 6 hours, adjusted according to response
- Child 6–11 months: 75 micrograms/kg every 4 hours, adjusted according to response
- Child 1–11 years: 75–100 micrograms/kg every 4 hours (max. per dose 5 mg), adjusted according to response
- Child 12–17 years: 2.5–5 mg every 4 hours, adjusted according to response

▸ BY INTRAMUSCULAR INJECTION, OR BY SUBCUTANEOUS INJECTION
- Child 12–17 years: 5 mg every 4 hours, adjusted according to response

Acute or chronic pain in ventilated neonates

▸ INITIALLY BY INTRAVENOUS INJECTION
- Neonate: Initially 50 micrograms/kg, dose to be administered over 30 minutes, followed by (by continuous intravenous infusion) 15 micrograms/kg/hour, adjusted according to response.

Acute or chronic pain in non-ventilated neonates

▸ BY CONTINUOUS INTRAVENOUS INFUSION
- Neonate: 2.5–7 micrograms/kg/hour, adjusted according to response.

Acute severe nociceptive pain in an emergency setting (specialist supervision in hospital)

▸ BY INTRANASAL ADMINISTRATION
- Child 2–15 years (body-weight 12–17 kg): 1.44 mg for 1 dose, spray into alternate nostrils
- Child 2–15 years (body-weight 18–23 kg): 2.16 mg for 1 dose, spray into alternate nostrils
- Child 2–15 years (body-weight 24–29 kg): 2.88 mg for 1 dose, spray into alternate nostrils
- Child 2–15 years (body-weight 30–39 kg): 3.2 mg for 1 dose, spray into alternate nostrils
- Child 2–15 years (body-weight 40–50 kg): 4.8 mg for 1 dose, spray into alternate nostrils

- **CONTRA-INDICATIONS** Delayed gastric emptying · phaeochromocytoma
- **CAUTIONS** CNS depression · severe cor pulmonale · severe diarrhoea · toxic psychosis
- **INTERACTIONS** → Appendix 1: opioids
- **SIDE-EFFECTS**

▸ **Common or very common**

▸ With intranasal use Haemorrhage · laryngitis · nasal complaints · procedural pain · taste altered

▸ **Uncommon**

▸ With intranasal use Abdominal pain · anxiety · conjunctivitis · drug toxicity · eye pruritus · feeling hot · fever · hiccups · hypoxia · level of consciousness decreased · pallor · paraesthesia

- **Frequency not known**
  - With parenteral use Biliary spasm · circulatory depression · intracranial pressure increased · mood altered

● **BREAST FEEDING** Therapeutic doses unlikely to affect infant; withdrawal symptoms in infants of dependent mothers; breast-feeding not best method of treating dependence in offspring.

● **HEPATIC IMPAIRMENT** Manufacturer advises caution.
Dose adjustments Manufacturer advises dose reduction.

● **RENAL IMPAIRMENT** Avoid use or reduce dose; opioid effects increased and prolonged; increased cerebral sensitivity.

● **MONITORING REQUIREMENTS**
- With intranasal use Manufacturer advises monitor for at least 30 minutes following administration.

● **DIRECTIONS FOR ADMINISTRATION**
- With intravenous use For *intravenous infusion*, manufacturer advises dilute in Glucose 5% or Sodium Chloride 0.9%; Glucose 5% is preferable as an infusion fluid.
- With intranasal use Manufacturer advises spray should be directed at the nasal side wall whilst the patient is in a semi-recumbent position.

● **PRESCRIBING AND DISPENSING INFORMATION** Intranasal administration of diamorphine hydrochloride injection has been used [unlicensed]—no dose recommendation.

● **NATIONAL FUNDING/ACCESS DECISIONS**
For full details see funding body website

All Wales Medicines Strategy Group (AWMSG) decisions
- **Diamorphine hydrochloride (*Ayendi*®) for the treatment of acute severe nociceptive pain in children and adolescents 2 to 15 years of age in a hospital setting. Diamorphine hydrochloride nasal spray should be administered in the emergency setting by practitioners experienced in the administration of opioids in children and with appropriate monitoring (November 2019)** AWMSG No. 2406 Recommended

● **MEDICINAL FORMS** There can be variation in the licensing of different medicines containing the same drug. Forms available from special-order manufacturers include: oral capsule, oral solution, solution for injection, powder for solution for injection

Powder for solution for injection
- **Diamorphine hydrochloride (Non-proprietary)**
  Diamorphine hydrochloride 5 mg Diamorphine 5mg powder for solution for injection ampoules | 5 ampoule [PoM] £12.80 DT = £12.80 [CD2]
  Diamorphine hydrochloride 10 mg Diamorphine 10mg powder for solution for injection ampoules | 5 ampoule [PoM] £16.56 [CD2]
  Diamorphine hydrochloride 30 mg Diamorphine 30mg powder for solution for injection ampoules | 5 ampoule [PoM] £16.52 DT = £16.52 [CD2]
  Diamorphine hydrochloride 100 mg Diamorphine 100mg powder for solution for injection ampoules | 5 ampoule [PoM] £42.39 DT = £42.39 [CD2]

Oral capsule
CAUTIONARY AND ADVISORY LABELS 2

Oral solution
CAUTIONARY AND ADVISORY LABELS 2

327

Dihydrocodeine tartrate

16-Feb-2021

● **INDICATIONS AND DOSE**

Moderate to severe pain
- BY MOUTH USING IMMEDIATE-RELEASE MEDICINES
  - Child 1–3 years: 500 micrograms/kg every 4–6 hours
  - Child 4–11 years: 0.5–1 mg/kg every 4–6 hours (max. per dose 30 mg)
  - Child 12–17 years: 30 mg every 4–6 hours
- BY INTRAMUSCULAR INJECTION, OR BY SUBCUTANEOUS INJECTION
  - Child 1–3 years: 500 micrograms/kg every 4–6 hours
  - Child 4–11 years: 0.5–1 mg/kg every 4–6 hours (max. per dose 30 mg)
  - Child 12–17 years: 30 mg every 4–6 hours, increased if necessary up to 50 mg every 4–6 hours

Chronic severe pain
- BY MOUTH USING MODIFIED-RELEASE MEDICINES
  - Child 12–17 years: 60–120 mg every 12 hours

DF118 FORTE®

Severe pain
- BY MOUTH
  - Child 12–17 years: 40–80 mg 3 times a day

● **UNLICENSED USE** Most preparations not licensed for use in children under 4 years.

● **CAUTIONS** Pancreatitis · severe cor pulmonale

● **INTERACTIONS** → Appendix 1: opioids

● **SIDE-EFFECTS**
GENERAL SIDE-EFFECTS Dysuria · mood altered
SPECIFIC SIDE-EFFECTS
- With oral use Biliary spasm · bronchospasm · hypothermia · sexual dysfunction · ureteral spasm

● **BREAST FEEDING** Specialist sources indicate caution—use the lowest effective dose for the shortest possible duration; monitor infant for adverse effects, including sedation, breathing difficulties, constipation, difficulty feeding and poor weight gain.

● **HEPATIC IMPAIRMENT** Manufacturer advises caution; consider avoiding.
Dose adjustments Manufacturer advises dose reduction, if used.

● **RENAL IMPAIRMENT** Avoid use or reduce dose; opioid effects increased and prolonged and increased cerebral sensitivity occurs.

● **PROFESSION SPECIFIC INFORMATION**
Dental practitioners' formulary Dihydrocodeine tablets 30 mg may be prescribed.

● **MEDICINAL FORMS** There can be variation in the licensing of different medicines containing the same drug. Forms available from special-order manufacturers include: oral suspension, oral solution

Oral tablet
CAUTIONARY AND ADVISORY LABELS 2
- **Dihydrocodeine tartrate (Non-proprietary)**
  Dihydrocodeine tartrate 30 mg Dihydrocodeine 30mg tablets | 28 tablet [PoM] £3.30 DT = £1.64 [CD5] | 30 tablet [PoM] £1.85-£3.00 [CD5] | 84 tablet [PoM] £6.62 [CD5] | 100 tablet [PoM] £10.00 DT = £5.86 [CD5] | 112 tablet [PoM] £8.84 [CD5]

Oral solution
CAUTIONARY AND ADVISORY LABELS 2

Modified-release tablet
CAUTIONARY AND ADVISORY LABELS 2, 25
- **Dihydrocodeine tartrate (Non-proprietary)**
  Dihydrocodeine tartrate 60 mg Dihydrocodeine 60mg modified-release tablets | 56 tablet [PoM] £9.88 DT = £9.88 [CD5]
  Dihydrocodeine tartrate 90 mg Dihydrocodeine 90mg modified-release tablets | 56 tablet [PoM] £16.45 DT = £16.45 [CD5]
  Dihydrocodeine tartrate 120 mg Dihydrocodeine 120mg modified-release tablets | 56 tablet [PoM] £19.71 DT = £19.71 [CD5]

327

Dihydrocodeine with paracetamol

26-Jan-2023

The properties listed below are those particular to the combination only. For the properties of the components please consider, paracetamol p. 325.

- **INDICATIONS AND DOSE**

Mild to moderate pain [using 10/500 preparations only]

▶ BY MOUTH

▶ Child 12–17 years: 1–2 tablets every 4–6 hours as required, to be given using 10/500 mg strength tablet; maximum 8 tablets per day

Severe pain [using 20/500 preparations only]

▶ BY MOUTH

▶ Child 12–17 years: 1–2 tablets every 4–6 hours as required, to be given using 20/500 mg strength tablet; maximum 8 tablets per day

Severe pain [using 30/500 preparations only]

▶ BY MOUTH

▶ Child 12–17 years: 1–2 tablets every 4–6 hours as required, to be given using 30/500 mg strength tablet; maximum 8 tablets per day

DOSE EQUIVALENCE AND CONVERSION

▶ Tablets contain a mixture of dihydrocodeine tartrate and paracetamol; the proportions are expressed in the form x/y, where x and y are the strengths in milligrams of dihydrocodeine and paracetamol respectively.

IMPORTANT SAFETY INFORMATION

MHRA/CHM ADVICE: DIHYDROCODEINE WITH PARACETAMOL (CO-DYDRAMOL): PRESCRIBE AND DISPENSE BY STRENGTH TO MINIMISE RISK OF MEDICATION ERROR (JANUARY 2018)

The MHRA has advised that dihydrocodeine with paracetamol preparations are prescribed and dispensed by strength to minimise dispensing errors and the risk of accidental opioid overdose—see Prescribing and dispensing information.

- **CAUTIONS** Alcohol dependence · before administering, check when paracetamol last administered and cumulative paracetamol dose over previous 24 hours · chronic alcoholism · chronic dehydration · chronic malnutrition · pancreatitis · severe cor pulmonale
- **INTERACTIONS** → Appendix 1: opioids · paracetamol
- **SIDE-EFFECTS** Abdominal pain · blood disorder · leucopenia · malaise · neutropenia · pancreatitis · paraesthesia · paralytic ileus · severe cutaneous adverse reactions (SCARs) · thrombocytopenia

  Overdose Liver damage (and less frequently renal damage) following overdosage with paracetamol.
- **BREAST FEEDING** Specialist sources indicate caution—use the lowest effective dose for the shortest possible duration; monitor infant for adverse effects, including sedation, breathing difficulties, constipation, difficulty feeding and poor weight gain.
- **HEPATIC IMPAIRMENT** Manufacturer advises consider avoiding in mild to moderate impairment; avoid in severe impairment.

  Dose adjustments Manufacturer advises dose reduction in mild to moderate impairment, if used.
- **RENAL IMPAIRMENT** Reduce dose or avoid dihydrocodeine; increased and prolonged effect; increased cerebral sensitivity.
- **PRESCRIBING AND DISPENSING INFORMATION** The MHRA advises when prescribing dihydrocodeine with paracetamol, the tablet strength and dose must be clearly indicated; when dispensing dihydrocodeine with paracetamol, ensure the prescribed strength is supplied—contact the prescriber if in doubt.

  The BP defines *Co-dydramol* Tablets as containing dihydrocodeine tartrate 10 mg and paracetamol 500 mg.
- **LESS SUITABLE FOR PRESCRIBING** Dihydrocodeine with paracetamol is less suitable for prescribing.
- **MEDICINAL FORMS** There can be variation in the licensing of different medicines containing the same drug. Forms available from special-order manufacturers include: oral suspension, oral solution

Oral tablet

CAUTIONARY AND ADVISORY LABELS 2, 29, 30

▶ Dihydrocodeine with paracetamol (Non-proprietary)

Dihydrocodeine tartrate 10 mg, Paracetamol 500 mg Co-dydramol 10mg/500mg tablets | 30 tablet PoM £2.20 DT = £0.97 CD5 | 100 tablet PoM £9.45 DT = £3.23 CD5

Dihydrocodeine tartrate 20 mg, Paracetamol 500 mg Co-dydramol 20mg/500mg tablets | 56 tablet PoM ℞ DT = £5.87 CD5 | 112 tablet PoM ℞ DT = £11.13 CD5

Dihydrocodeine tartrate 30 mg, Paracetamol 500 mg Co-dydramol 30mg/500mg tablets | 56 tablet PoM ℞ DT = £6.82 CD5

▶ Remedeine (Crescent Pharma Ltd)

Dihydrocodeine tartrate 20 mg, Paracetamol 500 mg Remedeine tablets | 56 tablet PoM £5.87 DT = £5.87 CD5 | 112 tablet PoM £11.13 DT = £11.13 CD5

Dihydrocodeine tartrate 30 mg, Paracetamol 500 mg Remedeine Forte tablets | 56 tablet PoM £6.82 DT = £6.82 CD5

327

Fentanyl

04-May-2023

- **INDICATIONS AND DOSE**

Chronic severe pain currently treated with a weak opioid analgesic (administered on expert advice)

▶ BY TRANSDERMAL APPLICATION

▶ Child 16–17 years: Initially 12 micrograms/hour every 72 hours, when starting, evaluation of the analgesic effect should not be made before the system has been worn for 24 hours (to allow for the gradual increase in plasma-fentanyl concentration)—previous analgesic therapy should be phased out gradually from time of first patch application, dose should be adjusted at 72 hour intervals in steps of 12–25 micrograms/hour if necessary. After a dose increase, the system should be worn through two 72-hour applications before any further increase in dose, more than one patch may be used at a time (but applied at the same time to avoid confusion)—consider additional or alternative analgesic therapy if dose required exceeds 300 micrograms/hour (important: it takes 20 hours or more for the plasma-fentanyl concentration to decrease by 50%—replacement opioid therapy should be initiated at a low dose and increased gradually). For further information including opioid dose conversion and the management of breakthrough pain, see *Pain management with opioids* under Prescribing in palliative care p. 20.

Chronic severe pain currently treated with a strong opioid analgesic (administered on expert advice)

▶ BY TRANSDERMAL APPLICATION

▶ Child 2–17 years: Initial dose based on previous 24-hour opioid requirement—consult product literature, for evaluating analgesic efficacy and dose increments—consult product literature, for conversion from long term oral morphine to transdermal fentanyl, see *Pain management with opioids* under Prescribing in palliative care p. 20.

Spontaneous respiration: analgesia and enhancement of anaesthesia, during operation

▶ BY INTRAVENOUS INJECTION

▸ Child 1 month–11 years: Initially 1–3 micrograms/kg, then 1 microgram/kg as required, dose to be administered over at least 30 seconds

▸ Child 12–17 years: Initially 50–100 micrograms (max. per dose 200 micrograms), dose maximum on specialist advice, then 25–50 micrograms as required, dose to be administered over at least 30 seconds

Assisted ventilation: analgesia and enhancement of anaesthesia during operation

▶ BY INTRAVENOUS INJECTION

▸ Neonate: Initially 1–5 micrograms/kg, then 1–3 micrograms/kg as required, dose to be administered over at least 30 seconds.

▸ Child 1 month–11 years: Initially 1–5 micrograms/kg, then 1–3 micrograms/kg as required, dose to be administered over at least 30 seconds

▸ Child 12–17 years: Initially 1–5 micrograms/kg, then 50–200 micrograms as required, dose to be administered over at least 30 seconds

Assisted ventilation: analgesia and respiratory depression in intensive care

▶ INITIALLY BY INTRAVENOUS INJECTION

▸ Neonate: Initially 1–5 micrograms/kg, then (by intravenous infusion) 1.5 micrograms/kg/hour, adjusted according to response.

▸ Child: Initially 1–5 micrograms/kg, then (by intravenous infusion) 1–6 micrograms/kg/hour, adjusted according to response

Breakthrough pain in patients receiving opioid therapy for chronic cancer pain (administered on expert advice)

▶ BY BUCCAL ADMINISTRATION USING LOZENGES

▸ Child 16–17 years: Initially 200 micrograms, dose to be given over 15 minutes, then 200 micrograms after 15 minutes if required, no more than 2 dose units for each pain episode; if adequate pain relief not achieved with 1 dose unit for consecutive breakthrough pain episodes, increase the strength of the dose unit until adequate pain relief achieved with 4 lozenges or less daily, if more than 4 episodes of breakthrough pain each day, adjust background analgesia

DOSE EQUIVALENCE AND CONVERSION

▸ Fentanyl films are **not bioequivalent** to other fentanyl preparations.

▸ Fentanyl preparations for the treatment of breakthrough pain are not interchangeable; if patients are switched from another fentanyl-containing preparation, a new dose titration is required.

DOSES AT EXTREMES OF BODY-WEIGHT

▸ To avoid excessive dosage in obese patients, weight-based doses may need to be calculated on the basis of ideal bodyweight.

● **UNLICENSED USE**

▸ With intravenous use Not licensed for use in children under 2 years; infusion not licensed for use in children under 12 years.

IMPORTANT SAFETY INFORMATION

MHRA/CHM ADVICE: TRANSDERMAL FENTANYL PATCHES: LIFE-THREATENING AND FATAL OPIOID TOXICITY FROM ACCIDENTAL EXPOSURE, PARTICULARLY IN CHILDREN (OCTOBER 2018)

Accidental exposure to transdermal fentanyl can occur if a patch is swallowed or transferred to another individual. Always fully inform patients and their carers about directions for safe use of fentanyl patches, including the importance of:

- not exceeding the prescribed dose;
- following the correct frequency of patch application, avoiding touching the adhesive side of patches, and washing hands after application;
- not cutting patches and avoiding exposure of patches to heat including via hot water;
- ensuring that old patches are removed before applying a new one;
- following instructions for safe storage and properly disposing of used patches or those which are not needed.

Patients and carers should be advised to seek immediate medical attention if overdose is suspected—see *Side-effects* and *Patient and carer advice* for further information.

MHRA/CHM ADVICE: TRANSDERMAL FENTANYL PATCHES FOR NON-CANCER PAIN: DO NOT USE IN OPIOID-NAÏVE PATIENTS (SEPTEMBER 2020)

A review noted that serious harm, including fatalities, has been reported with the use of fentanyl patches in both opioid-naïve and opioid-tolerant patients. There is considerable risk of respiratory depression with the use of fentanyl, especially in opioid-naïve patients, and significant risk with too rapid an escalation of dose, even in long-term opioid-tolerant patients.

The MHRA advises healthcare professionals that the use of fentanyl transdermal patches is contra-indicated in opioid-naïve patients; other analgesics and other opioids for non-malignant pain should be used before prescribing fentanyl patches. Patients and their carers should be reminded about the directions for safe use of fentanyl patches (see above).

● **CONTRA-INDICATIONS**

▸ With transdermal use Opioid-naïve patients

● **CAUTIONS**

GENERAL CAUTIONS Bradyarrhythmias · cerebral tumour · diabetes mellitus (with *Actiq*® and *Cynril*® lozenges) · impaired consciousness

SPECIFIC CAUTIONS

▸ With buccal use Mucositis—absorption from oral preparations may be increased, caution during dose titration

CAUTIONS, FURTHER INFORMATION

▸ With transdermal use EvGr Transdermal fentanyl patches are not suitable for acute pain or in those patients whose analgesic requirements are changing rapidly because the long time to steady state prevents rapid titration of the dose. (M)

▸ With intravenous use EvGr Repeated intra-operative doses should be given with care since the resulting respiratory depression can persist postoperatively and occasionally it may become apparent for the first time postoperatively when monitoring of the patient might be less intensive. (M)

● **INTERACTIONS** → Appendix 1: opioids

● **SIDE-EFFECTS**

▶ **Common or very common**

▸ With parenteral use Apnoea · hypertension · movement disorders · muscle rigidity · post procedural complications · respiratory disorders · vascular pain

▸ With transdermal use Anxiety · appetite decreased · asthenia · depression · diarrhoea · dyspnoea · gastrointestinal discomfort · hypertension · insomnia · malaise · muscle complaints · peripheral oedema · sensation abnormal · temperature sensation altered · tremor

▶ **Uncommon**

▸ With parenteral use Airway complication of anaesthesia · chills · hiccups · hypothermia

▸ With transdermal use Consciousness impaired · cyanosis · fever · gastrointestinal disorders · influenza like illness · memory loss · respiratory disorders · seizures · sexual dysfunction · vision blurred

- **Rare or very rare**
- With transdermal use Apnoea
- **Frequency not known**
- With buccal use Adrenal insufficiency · androgen deficiency · anxiety · appetite decreased · asthenia · coma · depersonalisation · depression · diarrhoea · dyspnoea · emotional lability · fever · gait abnormal · gastrointestinal discomfort · gastrointestinal disorders · gingival haemorrhage · gingivitis · injury · loss of consciousness · malaise · myoclonus · oral disorders · peripheral oedema · sensation abnormal · sleep disorders · speech slurred · taste altered · thinking abnormal · throat oedema · vasodilation · vision disorders · weight decreased · withdrawal syndrome neonatal
- With parenteral use Biliary spasm · cardiac arrest · cough · hyperalgesia · loss of consciousness
- With transdermal use Myoclonus · withdrawal syndrome neonatal

SIDE-EFFECTS, FURTHER INFORMATION **Muscle rigidity** Intravenous administration of fentanyl can cause muscle rigidity, which may involve the thoracic muscles. Manufacturer advises administration by slow intravenous injection to avoid; higher doses may require premedication with benzodiazepines and muscle relaxants.

Transdermal use Monitor patients using patches for increased side-effects if fever is present (increased absorption possible); avoid exposing application site to external heat, for example a hot bath or sauna (may also increase absorption).

● **BREAST FEEDING**
- With buccal use or intranasal use or sublingual use Manufacturer advises avoid during treatment and for 5 days after last administration—present in milk.
- With intravenous use Manufacturer advises avoid during treatment and for 24 hours after last administration—present in milk.
- With transdermal use Manufacturer advises avoid during treatment and for 72 hours after removal of patch—present in milk.

● **HEPATIC IMPAIRMENT** Manufacturer advises caution (risk of accumulation).

Dose adjustments Manufacturer advises cautious dose titration.

● **RENAL IMPAIRMENT** Manufacturer advises caution (risk of increased and prolonged effects).

Dose adjustments
- With intravenous use Manufacturer advises consider dose reduction.

● **DIRECTIONS FOR ADMINISTRATION**
- With transdermal use [EvGr] For *patches*, apply to dry, non-irritated, non-irradiated, non-hairy skin on torso or upper arm, removing after 72 hours and siting replacement patch on a different area (avoid using the same area for several days). ⟨M⟩
- With intravenous use [EvGr] For *intravenous infusion*, injection solution may be diluted in Glucose 5% or Sodium Chloride 0.9%. ⟨M⟩
- With buccal use [EvGr] Patients should be advised to place the lozenge in the mouth against the cheek and move it around the mouth using the applicator; each lozenge should be sucked over a 15 minute period. In patients with a dry mouth, water may be used to moisten the buccal mucosa. Patients with diabetes should be advised each lozenge contains approximately 2 g glucose. ⟨M⟩

● **PRESCRIBING AND DISPENSING INFORMATION**
- With transdermal use Prescriptions for fentanyl patches can be written to show the strength in terms of the release rate and it is acceptable to write *'Fentanyl 25 patches'* to prescribe patches that release fentanyl 25 micrograms per hour. The dosage should be expressed in terms of the interval between applying a patch and replacing it with a new one, e.g. *'one patch to be applied every 72 hours'*. The total quantity of patches to be supplied should be written in words and figures.

● **PATIENT AND CARER ADVICE**
- With transdermal use Patients and carers should be informed about safe use, including correct administration and disposal, strict adherence to dosage instructions, and the symptoms and signs of opioid overdosage. Patches should be removed immediately in case of breathing difficulties, marked drowsiness, confusion, dizziness, or impaired speech, and patients and carers should seek prompt medical attention.

Patients or carers should be given advice on how to administer fentanyl lozenges.

Medicines for Children leaflet: Fentanyl lozenges for pain www.medicinesforchildren.org.uk/medicines/fentanyl-lozenges-for-pain/

Medicines for Children leaflet: Fentanyl patches for pain www.medicinesforchildren.org.uk/medicines/fentanyl-patches-for-pain/

● **MEDICINAL FORMS** There can be variation in the licensing of different medicines containing the same drug. Forms available from special-order manufacturers include: solution for injection, infusion, solution for infusion

Solution for injection

- **Fentanyl (Non-proprietary)**
  Fentanyl (as Fentanyl citrate) 50 microgram per 1 ml Fentanyl 100micrograms/2ml solution for injection ampoules | 10 ampoule [PoM] £14.33 DT = £16.24 (Hospital only) [CD2] | 10 ampoule [PoM] £11.50–£16.24 DT = £16.24 [CD2]
  Fentanyl 500micrograms/10ml solution for injection ampoules | 10 ampoule [PoM] £14.50–£18.30 [CD2] | 10 ampoule [PoM] £14.50 (Hospital only) [CD2]
- **Sublimaze** (Piramal Critical Care Ltd)
  Fentanyl (as Fentanyl citrate) 50 microgram per 1 ml Sublimaze 500micrograms/10ml solution for injection ampoules | 5 ampoule [PoM] £6.53 DT = £6.53 [CD2]

Solution for infusion

- **Fentanyl (Non-proprietary)**
  Fentanyl (as Fentanyl citrate) 50 microgram per 1 ml Fentanyl 2.5mg/50ml solution for infusion vials | 1 vial [PoM] £9.80 (Hospital only) [CD2]

Transdermal patch

CAUTIONARY AND ADVISORY LABELS 2

- **Durogesic DTrans** (Janssen-Cilag Ltd)
  Fentanyl 12 microgram per 1 hour Durogesic DTrans 12micrograms/hour transdermal patches | 5 patch [PoM] £12.59 DT = £7.53 [CD2]
  Fentanyl 25 microgram per 1 hour Durogesic DTrans 25micrograms/hour transdermal patches | 5 patch [PoM] £17.99 DT = £10.77 [CD2]
  Fentanyl 50 microgram per 1 hour Durogesic DTrans 50micrograms/hour transdermal patches | 5 patch [PoM] £33.66 DT = £20.13 [CD2]
  Fentanyl 75 microgram per 1 hour Durogesic DTrans 75micrograms/hour transdermal patches | 5 patch [PoM] £46.99 DT = £28.07 [CD2]
  Fentanyl 100 microgram per 1 hour Durogesic DTrans 100micrograms/hour transdermal patches | 5 patch [PoM] £57.86 DT = £34.60 [CD2]
- **Fencino** (Luye Pharma Ltd)
  Fentanyl 12 microgram per 1 hour Fencino 12micrograms/hour transdermal patches | 5 patch [PoM] £8.46 DT = £7.53 [CD2]
  Fentanyl 25 microgram per 1 hour Fencino 25micrograms/hour transdermal patches | 5 patch [PoM] £12.10 DT = £10.77 [CD2]
  Fentanyl 50 microgram per 1 hour Fencino 50micrograms/hour transdermal patches | 5 patch [PoM] £22.62 DT = £20.13 [CD2]
  Fentanyl 75 microgram per 1 hour Fencino 75micrograms/hour transdermal patches | 5 patch [PoM] £31.54 DT = £28.07 [CD2]
  Fentanyl 100 microgram per 1 hour Fencino 100micrograms/hour transdermal patches | 5 patch [PoM] £38.88 DT = £34.60 [CD2]
- **Fenylat** (Luye Pharma Ltd)
  Fentanyl 12 microgram per 1 hour Fenylat 12micrograms/hour transdermal patches | 5 patch [PoM] £8.46 DT = £7.53 [CD2]
  Fentanyl 25 microgram per 1 hour Fenylat 25micrograms/hour transdermal patches | 5 patch [PoM] £12.10 DT = £10.77 [CD2]

Fentanyl 50 microgram per 1 hour Fenylat 50micrograms/hour transdermal patches | 5 patch [PoM] £22.62 DT = £20.13 [CD2]
Fentanyl 75 microgram per 1 hour Fenylat 75micrograms/hour transdermal patches | 5 patch [PoM] £31.54 DT = £28.07 [CD2]
Fentanyl 100 microgram per 1 hour Fenylat 100micrograms/hour transdermal patches | 5 patch [PoM] £38.88 DT = £34.60 [CD2]

▸ **Matrifen** (Teva UK Ltd)
Fentanyl 12 microgram per 1 hour Matrifen 12micrograms/hour transdermal patches | 5 patch [PoM] £7.52 DT = £7.53 [CD2]
Fentanyl 25 microgram per 1 hour Matrifen 25micrograms/hour transdermal patches | 5 patch [PoM] £10.76 DT = £10.77 [CD2]
Fentanyl 50 microgram per 1 hour Matrifen 50micrograms/hour transdermal patches | 5 patch [PoM] £20.12 DT = £20.13 [CD2]
Fentanyl 75 microgram per 1 hour Matrifen 75micrograms/hour transdermal patches | 5 patch [PoM] £28.06 DT = £28.07 [CD2]
Fentanyl 100 microgram per 1 hour Matrifen 100micrograms/hour transdermal patches | 5 patch [PoM] £34.59 DT = £34.60 [CD2]

▸ **Mezolar Matrix** (Sandoz Ltd)
Fentanyl 12 microgram per 1 hour Mezolar Matrix 12micrograms/hour transdermal patches | 5 patch [PoM] £7.53 DT = £7.53 [CD2]
Fentanyl 25 microgram per 1 hour Mezolar Matrix 25micrograms/hour transdermal patches | 5 patch [PoM] £10.77 DT = £10.77 [CD2]
Fentanyl 37.5 microgram per 1 hour Mezolar Matrix 37.5microgram/hour transdermal patches | 5 patch [PoM] £15.46 DT = £15.46 [CD2]
Fentanyl 50 microgram per 1 hour Mezolar Matrix 50micrograms/hour transdermal patches | 5 patch [PoM] £20.13 DT = £20.13 [CD2]
Fentanyl 75 microgram per 1 hour Mezolar Matrix 75micrograms/hour transdermal patches | 5 patch [PoM] £28.07 DT = £28.07 [CD2]
Fentanyl 100 microgram per 1 hour Mezolar Matrix 100micrograms/hour transdermal patches | 5 patch [PoM] £34.60 DT = £34.60 [CD2]

▸ **Opiodur** (Zentiva Pharma UK Ltd)
Fentanyl 12 microgram per 1 hour Opiodur 12micrograms/hour transdermal patches | 5 patch [PoM] £5.64 DT = £7.53 [CD2]
Fentanyl 25 microgram per 1 hour Opiodur 25micrograms/hour transdermal patches | 5 patch [PoM] £8.07 DT = £10.77 [CD2]
Fentanyl 50 microgram per 1 hour Opiodur 50micrograms/hour transdermal patches | 5 patch [PoM] £15.09 DT = £20.13 [CD2]
Fentanyl 75 microgram per 1 hour Opiodur 75micrograms/hour transdermal patches | 5 patch [PoM] £21.05 DT = £28.07 [CD2]
Fentanyl 100 microgram per 1 hour Opiodur 100micrograms/hour transdermal patches | 5 patch [PoM] £25.94 DT = £34.60 [CD2]

▸ **Victanyl** (Accord-UK Ltd)
Fentanyl 12 microgram per 1 hour Victanyl 12micrograms/hour transdermal patches | 5 patch [PoM] £12.58 DT = £7.53 [CD2]
Fentanyl 25 microgram per 1 hour Victanyl 25micrograms/hour transdermal patches | 5 patch [PoM] £25.89 DT = £10.77 [CD2]
Fentanyl 50 microgram per 1 hour Victanyl 50micrograms/hour transdermal patches | 5 patch [PoM] £48.36 DT = £20.13 [CD2]
Fentanyl 75 microgram per 1 hour Victanyl 75micrograms/hour transdermal patches | 5 patch [PoM] £67.41 DT = £28.07 [CD2]
Fentanyl 100 microgram per 1 hour Victanyl 100micrograms/hour transdermal patches | 5 patch [PoM] £83.09 DT = £34.60 [CD2]

▸ **Yemex** (Sandoz Ltd)
Fentanyl 12 microgram per 1 hour Yemex 12micrograms/hour transdermal patches | 5 patch [PoM] £12.59 DT = £7.53 [CD2]
Fentanyl 25 microgram per 1 hour Yemex 25micrograms/hour transdermal patches | 5 patch [PoM] £17.99 DT = £10.77 [CD2]
Fentanyl 50 microgram per 1 hour Yemex 50micrograms/hour transdermal patches | 5 patch [PoM] £33.66 DT = £20.13 [CD2]
Fentanyl 75 microgram per 1 hour Yemex 75micrograms/hour transdermal patches | 5 patch [PoM] £46.99 DT = £28.07 [CD2]
Fentanyl 100 microgram per 1 hour Yemex 100micrograms/hour transdermal patches | 5 patch [PoM] £57.86 DT = £34.60 [CD2]

Lozenge

CAUTIONARY AND ADVISORY LABELS 2
EXCIPIENTS: May contain Propylene glycol

▸ **Actiq** (Teva UK Ltd)
Fentanyl (as Fentanyl citrate) 200 microgram Actiq 200microgram lozenges with integral oromucosal applicator | 30 lozenge [PoM] £210.41 DT = £210.41 [CD2]
Fentanyl (as Fentanyl citrate) 400 microgram Actiq 400microgram lozenges with integral oromucosal applicator | 30 lozenge [PoM] £210.41 DT = £210.41 [CD2]
Fentanyl (as Fentanyl citrate) 600 microgram Actiq 600microgram lozenges with integral oromucosal applicator | 30 lozenge [PoM] £210.41 DT = £210.41 [CD2]
Fentanyl (as Fentanyl citrate) 800 microgram Actiq 800microgram lozenges with integral oromucosal applicator | 30 lozenge [PoM] £210.41 DT = £210.41 [CD2]
Fentanyl (as Fentanyl citrate) 1.2 mg Actiq 1.2mg lozenges with integral oromucosal applicator | 30 lozenge [PoM] £210.41 DT = £210.41 [CD2]
Fentanyl (as Fentanyl citrate) 1.6 mg Actiq 1.6mg lozenges with integral oromucosal applicator | 30 lozenge [PoM] £210.41 DT = £210.41 [CD2]

▸ **Cynril** (Fontus Health Ltd)
Fentanyl (as Fentanyl citrate) 200 microgram Cynril 200microgram lozenges with integral oromucosal applicator | 3 lozenge [PoM] £17.75 DT = £17.75 [CD2]
Fentanyl (as Fentanyl citrate) 400 microgram Cynril 400microgram lozenges with integral oromucosal applicator | 3 lozenge [PoM] £17.75 DT = £17.75 [CD2]
Fentanyl (as Fentanyl citrate) 600 microgram Cynril 600microgram lozenges with integral oromucosal applicator | 3 lozenge [PoM] £17.75 DT = £17.75 [CD2]
Fentanyl (as Fentanyl citrate) 800 microgram Cynril 800microgram lozenges with integral oromucosal applicator | 3 lozenge [PoM] £17.75 DT = £17.75 [CD2]
Fentanyl (as Fentanyl citrate) 1.2 mg Cynril 1.2mg lozenges with integral oromucosal applicator | 3 lozenge [PoM] £17.75 DT = £17.75 [CD2]
Fentanyl (as Fentanyl citrate) 1.6 mg Cynril 1.6mg lozenges with integral oromucosal applicator | 3 lozenge [PoM] £17.75 DT = £17.75 [CD2]

F 327

Hydromorphone hydrochloride

11-May-2021

● **INDICATIONS AND DOSE**

Severe pain in cancer

▸ BY MOUTH USING IMMEDIATE-RELEASE MEDICINES
▸ Child 12–17 years: 1.3 mg every 4 hours, dose to be increased if necessary according to severity of pain
▸ BY MOUTH USING MODIFIED-RELEASE MEDICINES
▸ Child 12–17 years: 4 mg every 12 hours, dose to be increased if necessary according to severity of pain

● **CONTRA-INDICATIONS** Acute abdomen

● **CAUTIONS** Pancreatitis · toxic psychosis

● **INTERACTIONS** → Appendix 1: opioids

● **SIDE-EFFECTS**
▸ **Common or very common** Abdominal pain · anxiety · appetite decreased · asthenia · sleep disorders
▸ **Uncommon** Depression · diarrhoea · dyspnoea · erectile dysfunction · malaise · movement disorders · paraesthesia · peripheral oedema · taste altered · tremor
▸ **Frequency not known** Hyperalgesia · paralytic ileus · withdrawal syndrome neonatal

● **BREAST FEEDING** Avoid—no information available.

● **HEPATIC IMPAIRMENT** Manufacturer advises avoid.

● **RENAL IMPAIRMENT** [EvGr] Use with caution. ⟨M⟩
Dose adjustments [EvGr] Consider dose reduction (risk of increased and prolonged effects). ⟨M⟩

● **DIRECTIONS FOR ADMINISTRATION** For *immediate-release* capsules, manufacturer advises swallow whole capsule or sprinkle contents on soft food. For *modified-release* capsules, manufacturer advises swallow whole or open capsule and sprinkle contents on soft cold food (swallow the pellets within the capsule whole; do not crush or chew).

● **PATIENT AND CARER ADVICE** Patients or carers should be given advice on how to administer hydromorphone hydrochloride capsules and modified-release capsules.

● **MEDICINAL FORMS** There can be variation in the licensing of different medicines containing the same drug. Forms available from special-order manufacturers include: oral solution

Modified-release capsule

CAUTIONARY AND ADVISORY LABELS 2

▸ **Palladone SR** (Napp Pharmaceuticals Ltd)

Hydromorphone hydrochloride 2 mg Palladone SR 2mg capsules | 56 capsule PoM £20.98 DT = £20.98 CD2

Hydromorphone hydrochloride 4 mg Palladone SR 4mg capsules | 56 capsule PoM £28.75 DT = £28.75 CD2

Hydromorphone hydrochloride 8 mg Palladone SR 8mg capsules | 56 capsule PoM £56.08 DT = £56.08 CD2

Oral capsule

CAUTIONARY AND ADVISORY LABELS 2

▸ **Palladone** (Napp Pharmaceuticals Ltd)

Hydromorphone hydrochloride 1.3 mg Palladone 1.3mg capsules | 56 capsule PoM £8.82 DT = £8.82 CD2

327

Morphine

03-Apr-2024

● **INDICATIONS AND DOSE**

Pain

▸ BY SUBCUTANEOUS INJECTION

- Neonate: Initially 100 micrograms/kg every 6 hours, dose to be adjusted according to response.
- Child 1-5 months: Initially 100–200 micrograms/kg every 6 hours, dose to be adjusted according to response
- Child 6 months-1 year: Initially 100–200 micrograms/kg every 4 hours, dose to be adjusted according to response
- Child 2-11 years: Initially 200 micrograms/kg every 4 hours (max. per dose 10 mg), dose to be adjusted according to response
- Child 12-17 years: Initially 2.5–10 mg every 4 hours, dose to be adjusted according to response

▸ INITIALLY BY INTRAVENOUS INJECTION

- Neonate: 50 micrograms/kg every 6 hours, to be administered over at least 5 minutes, dose to be adjusted according to response, alternatively (by intravenous injection) initially 50 micrograms/kg for 1 dose, to be administered over at least 5 minutes, followed by (by continuous intravenous infusion) 5–20 micrograms/kg/hour, dose to be adjusted according to response.
- Child 1-5 months: 100 micrograms/kg every 6 hours, to be administered over at least 5 minutes, dose to be adjusted according to response, alternatively (by intravenous injection) initially 100 micrograms/kg for 1 dose, to be administered over at least 5 minutes, followed by (by continuous intravenous infusion) 10–30 micrograms/kg/hour, dose to be adjusted according to response
- Child 6 months-11 years: 100 micrograms/kg every 4 hours, to be administered over at least 5 minutes, dose to be adjusted according to response, alternatively (by intravenous injection) initially 100 micrograms/kg for 1 dose, to be administered over at least 5 minutes, followed by (by continuous intravenous infusion) 20–30 micrograms/kg/hour, dose to be adjusted according to response
- Child 12-17 years: 5 mg every 4 hours, to be administered over at least 5 minutes, dose to be adjusted according to response, alternatively (by intravenous injection) initially 5 mg for 1 dose, to be administered over at least 5 minutes, followed by (by continuous intravenous infusion) 20–30 micrograms/kg/hour, dose to be adjusted according to response

▸ BY MOUTH USING IMMEDIATE-RELEASE MEDICINES, OR BY RECTUM

- Child 1-2 months: Initially 50–100 micrograms/kg every 4 hours, dose to be adjusted according to response
- Child 3-5 months: 100–150 micrograms/kg every 4 hours, dose to be adjusted according to response
- Child 6-11 months: 200 micrograms/kg every 4 hours, dose to be adjusted according to response
- Child 1 year: Initially 200–300 micrograms/kg every 4 hours, dose to be adjusted according to response
- Child 2-11 years: Initially 200–300 micrograms/kg every 4 hours (max. per dose 10 mg), dose to be adjusted according to response
- Child 12-17 years: Initially 5–10 mg every 4 hours, dose to be adjusted according to response

▸ BY CONTINUOUS SUBCUTANEOUS INFUSION

- Child 1-2 months: 10 micrograms/kg/hour, dose to be adjusted according to response
- Child 3 months-17 years: 20 micrograms/kg/hour, dose to be adjusted according to response

Pain [with modified-release 12-hourly preparations]

▸ BY MOUTH USING MODIFIED-RELEASE MEDICINES

- Child: Every 12 hours, dose adjusted according to daily morphine requirements, dosage requirements should be reviewed if the brand is altered

Pain [with modified-release 24-hourly preparations]

▸ BY MOUTH USING MODIFIED-RELEASE MEDICINES

- Child: Every 24 hours, dose adjusted according to daily morphine requirements, dosage requirements should be reviewed if the brand is altered

Neonatal opioid withdrawal (under expert supervision)

▸ BY MOUTH USING IMMEDIATE-RELEASE MEDICINES

- Neonate: Initially 40 micrograms/kg every 4 hours until symptoms controlled, dose to be increased if necessary; reduce frequency gradually over 6–10 days, stop when 40 micrograms/kg once daily achieved, dose may vary—consult local guidelines.

Persistent cyanosis in congenital heart disease when blood glucose less than 3 mmol/litre [following glucose]

▸ BY INTRAVENOUS INJECTION, OR BY INTRAMUSCULAR INJECTION

- Child: 100 micrograms/kg

DOSE EQUIVALENCE AND CONVERSION

- The doses stated refer equally to morphine hydrochloride and sulfate.

● **UNLICENSED USE** *Oramorph*® solution and *MXL*® capsules not licensed for use in children aged under 1 year. *Sevredol*® tablets not licensed for use in children under 3 years. *MST Continus*® preparations licensed to treat children with cancer pain (age-range not specified by manufacturer). *Actimorph*® orodispersible tablets not licensed for use in children under 6 months.

Suppositories are not licensed for use.

IMPORTANT SAFETY INFORMATION

Do not confuse *modified-release* 12-hourly preparations with 24-hourly preparations, see *Prescribing and dispensing information*.

Different strengths of *oral solution*, such as 10 mg/5 mL and 20 mg/mL, are available. In addition, a 100 micrograms/mL oral solution is available as an unlicensed ‘specials’ product that is used in and supplied from secondary care settings. Care should be taken to ensure that the correct strength of oral solution is prescribed and dispensed, and the dose stated as both quantity and volume.

HEALTH SERVICES SAFETY INVESTIGATIONS BODY (HSSIB) PATIENT SAFETY INVESTIGATIONS: UNINTENTIONAL OVERDOSE OF MORPHINE SULFATE ORAL SOLUTION (APRIL 2022)

A review of an unintentional overdose of morphine sulfate 10 mg/5 mL *oral solution* identified that it may have contributed to a patient's death. The patient had not seen the dispensing label on the outer carton, and mistakenly thought the strength on the bottle was the prescribed dose. To minimise the risk of harm, the HSSIB has issued advice: www.hssib.org.uk/patient-safety-investigations/unintentional-overdose-of-morphine-sulfate-oral-solution/.

- **CONTRA-INDICATIONS** Acute abdomen · delayed gastric emptying · heart failure secondary to chronic lung disease · phaeochromocytoma
- **CAUTIONS** Cardiac arrhythmias · pancreatitis · severe cor pulmonale
- **INTERACTIONS** → Appendix 1: opioids
- **SIDE-EFFECTS**
  - **Common or very common**
  - With oral use Appetite decreased · asthenia · gastrointestinal discomfort · insomnia · malaise · neuromuscular dysfunction
  - **Uncommon**
  - With oral use Agitation · bronchospasm · ileus · mood altered · myoclonus · peripheral oedema · pulmonary oedema · sensation abnormal · syncope · taste altered
  - **Frequency not known**
  - With oral use Amenorrhoea · biliary pain · cough decreased · hyperalgesia · hypertension · pancreatitis exacerbated · sexual dysfunction · sleep apnoea · thinking abnormal · ureteral spasm · withdrawal syndrome neonatal
  - With parenteral use Alertness decreased · bile duct disorders · mood altered · myoclonus · sexual dysfunction · ureteral spasm · urinary disorders · vision disorders
- **BREAST FEEDING** Therapeutic doses unlikely to affect infant.
- **HEPATIC IMPAIRMENT** Manufacturer advises caution. Avoid *oral preparations* in acute impairment; for *injectable preparations*—consult product literature.
  Dose adjustments Manufacturer advises consider dose reduction—consult product literature.
- **RENAL IMPAIRMENT** Avoid use or reduce dose; opioid effects increased and prolonged; increased cerebral sensitivity.
- **MONITORING REQUIREMENTS** Possible association between acute chest syndrome in patients with sickle cell disease treated with morphine during a vaso-occlusive crisis—manufacturer advises close monitoring for acute chest syndrome symptoms during treatment.
- **DIRECTIONS FOR ADMINISTRATION**
  - With intravenous use For *continuous intravenous infusion*, dilute with Glucose 5% or 10% or Sodium Chloride 0.9%.
    Neonatal intensive care, dilute 2.5 mg/kg body-weight to a final volume of 50 mL with infusion fluid; an intravenous infusion rate of 0.1 mL/hour provides a dose of 5 micrograms/kg/hour.
  - With oral use For *modified release capsules*—swallow whole or open capsule and sprinkle contents on soft food. [EvGr] For *orodispersible tablets*— place on the tongue, allow to disperse and swallow. Alternatively, tablets can be placed in a spoon and dispersed in a small amount of water before administration. ⟨M⟩
- **PRESCRIBING AND DISPENSING INFORMATION** Prescriptions must specify the 'form'.
  - With oral use Modified-release preparations are available as 12-hourly or 24-hourly formulations; prescribers must ensure that the correct preparation is prescribed. Preparations that should be given 12-hourly include *MST Continus*®, *Morphgesic*® *SR*, and *Zomorph*®. Preparations that should be given 24-hourly include *MXL*®.
    Oral solutions are available in different strengths; prescribers must ensure that the correct preparation is prescribed—see *Important safety information* for details.
  - With rectal use Both the strength of the suppositories and the morphine salt contained in them must be specified by the prescriber.
- **PATIENT AND CARER ADVICE** Patients or carers should be given advice on how to administer morphine modified-release capsules and orodispersible tablets.
  Medicines for Children leaflet: Morphine for pain www.medicinesforchildren.org.uk/medicines/morphine-for-pain/
- **EXCEPTIONS TO LEGAL CATEGORY**
  Morphine Oral Solutions Prescription-only medicines or schedule 2 controlled drug. The proportion of morphine hydrochloride may be altered when specified by the prescriber; if above 13 mg per 5 mL the solution becomes a schedule 2 controlled drug. It is usual to adjust the strength so that the dose volume is 5 or 10 mL.
  Oral solutions of morphine can be prescribed by writing the formula:
  Morphine hydrochloride 5 mg
  Chloroform water to 5 mL

- **MEDICINAL FORMS** There can be variation in the licensing of different medicines containing the same drug. Forms available from special-order manufacturers include: oral capsule, oral solution, solution for injection, infusion, solution for infusion

Oral tablet

CAUTIONARY AND ADVISORY LABELS 2

- **Sevredol** (Napp Pharmaceuticals Ltd)
  - **Morphine sulfate 10 mg** Sevredol 10mg tablets | 56 tablet [PoM] £5.31 DT = £5.31 [CD2]
  - **Morphine sulfate 20 mg** Sevredol 20mg tablets | 56 tablet [PoM] £10.61 DT = £10.61 [CD2]
  - **Morphine sulfate 50 mg** Sevredol 50mg tablets | 56 tablet [PoM] £28.02 DT = £28.02 [CD2]

Modified-release tablet

CAUTIONARY AND ADVISORY LABELS 2, 25

- **MST Continus** (Napp Pharmaceuticals Ltd)
  - **Morphine sulfate 5 mg** MST Continus 5mg tablets | 60 tablet [PoM] £3.29 DT = £3.29 [CD2]
  - **Morphine sulfate 10 mg** MST Continus 10mg tablets | 60 tablet [PoM] £5.20 DT = £5.20 [CD2]
  - **Morphine sulfate 15 mg** MST Continus 15mg tablets | 60 tablet [PoM] £9.10 DT = £9.10 [CD2]
  - **Morphine sulfate 30 mg** MST Continus 30mg tablets | 60 tablet [PoM] £12.47 DT = £12.47 [CD2]
  - **Morphine sulfate 60 mg** MST Continus 60mg tablets | 60 tablet [PoM] £24.32 DT = £24.32 [CD2]
  - **Morphine sulfate 100 mg** MST Continus 100mg tablets | 60 tablet [PoM] £38.50 DT = £38.50 [CD2]
- **Morphgesic SR** (Advanz Pharma)
  - **Morphine sulfate 10 mg** Morphgesic SR 10mg tablets | 60 tablet [PoM] £3.85 DT = £5.20 [CD2]
  - **Morphine sulfate 30 mg** Morphgesic SR 30mg tablets | 60 tablet [PoM] £9.24 DT = £12.47 [CD2]
  - **Morphine sulfate 60 mg** Morphgesic SR 60mg tablets | 60 tablet [PoM] £18.04 DT = £24.32 [CD2]
  - **Morphine sulfate 100 mg** Morphgesic SR 100mg tablets | 60 tablet [PoM] £28.54 DT = £38.50 [CD2]

Solution for injection

- **Morphine (Non-proprietary)**
  - **Morphine sulfate 1 mg per 1 ml** Morphine sulfate 5mg/5ml solution for injection ampoules | 10 ampoule [PoM] £93.60 DT = £93.60 [CD2]
    Morphine sulfate 1mg/1ml solution for injection ampoules | 10 ampoule [PoM] £74.00 (Hospital only) [CD2]
    Morphine sulfate 10mg/10ml solution for injection ampoules | 10 ampoule [PoM] £15.00–£98.00 DT = £17.50 [CD2]
  - **Morphine sulfate 10 mg per 1 ml** Morphine sulfate 10mg/1ml solution for injection ampoules | 10 ampoule [PoM] £14.72 DT = £3.78 (Hospital only) [CD2] | 10 ampoule [PoM] £6.66–£19.27 DT = £3.78 [CD2]
  - **Morphine sulfate 15 mg per 1 ml** Morphine sulfate 15mg/1ml solution for injection ampoules | 10 ampoule [PoM] £10.74 DT =

£12.17 (Hospital only) CD2 | 10 ampoule PoM £12.17 DT = £12.17 CD2

Morphine sulfate 20 mg per 1 ml Morphine sulfate 20mg/1ml solution for injection ampoules | 10 ampoule PoM £254.73–£455.52 DT = £254.73 CD2

Morphine sulfate 30 mg per 1 ml Morphine sulfate 30mg/1ml solution for injection ampoules | 10 ampoule PoM £15.79 DT = £48.44 (Hospital only) CD2 | 10 ampoule PoM £48.44 DT = £48.44 CD2

Morphine sulfate 60mg/2ml solution for injection ampoules | 5 ampoule PoM £19.96 DT = £12.00 CD2

Modified-release capsule

CAUTIONARY AND ADVISORY LABELS 2

▸ **MXL** (Napp Pharmaceuticals Ltd)

Morphine sulfate 30 mg MXL 30mg capsules | 28 capsule PoM £10.91 CD2

Morphine sulfate 60 mg MXL 60mg capsules | 28 capsule PoM £14.95 CD2

Morphine sulfate 90 mg MXL 90mg capsules | 28 capsule PoM £22.04 DT = £22.04 CD2

Morphine sulfate 120 mg MXL 120mg capsules | 28 capsule PoM £29.15 DT = £29.15 CD2

Morphine sulfate 150 mg MXL 150mg capsules | 28 capsule PoM £36.43 DT = £36.43 CD2

Morphine sulfate 200 mg MXL 200mg capsules | 28 capsule PoM £46.15 CD2

▸ **Zomorph** (Ethypharm UK Ltd)

Morphine sulfate 10 mg Zomorph 10mg modified-release capsules | 60 capsule PoM £3.47 DT = £3.47 CD2

Morphine sulfate 30 mg Zomorph 30mg modified-release capsules | 60 capsule PoM £8.30 DT = £8.30 CD2

Morphine sulfate 60 mg Zomorph 60mg modified-release capsules | 60 capsule PoM £16.20 DT = £16.20 CD2

Morphine sulfate 100 mg Zomorph 100mg modified-release capsules | 60 capsule PoM £21.80 DT = £21.80 CD2

Morphine sulfate 200 mg Zomorph 200mg modified-release capsules | 60 capsule PoM £43.60 DT = £43.60 CD2

Solution for infusion

▸ **Morphine (Non-proprietary)**

Morphine sulfate 1 mg per 1 ml Morphine sulfate 50mg/50ml solution for infusion vials | 1 vial PoM £5.78–£9.23 CD2 | 10 vial PoM £87.00 CD2

Morphine sulfate 2 mg per 1 ml Morphine sulfate 100mg/50ml solution for infusion vials | 1 vial PoM £6.48–£10.00 CD2 | 10 vial PoM £141.80 CD2

Oral solution

CAUTIONARY AND ADVISORY LABELS 2

▸ **Morphine (Non-proprietary)**

Morphine sulfate 2 mg per 1 ml Morphine sulfate 10mg/5ml oral solution | 100 ml PoM £2.16–£3.00 CD5 | 300 ml PoM £9.00 DT = £6.48 CD5 | 500 ml PoM £10.80–£14.15 CD5

Morphine sulfate 20 mg per 1 ml Morphine sulfate 20mg/ml oral solution sugar free | 120 ml PoM £22.43 DT = £19.50 CD2 SF

▸ **Oramorph** (Glenwood GmbH)

Morphine sulfate 2 mg per 1 ml Oramorph 10mg/5ml oral solution | 100 ml PoM £1.89 CD5 | 300 ml PoM £5.45 DT = £6.48 CD5 | 500 ml PoM £8.50 CD5

Orodispersible tablet

CAUTIONARY AND ADVISORY LABELS 2

▸ **Actimorph** (Ethypharm UK Ltd)

Morphine sulfate 1 mg Actimorph 1mg orodispersible tablets | 56 tablet PoM £4.75 DT = £4.75 CD2 SF

Morphine sulfate 2.5 mg Actimorph 2.5mg orodispersible tablets | 56 tablet PoM £5.75 DT = £5.75 CD2 SF

Morphine sulfate 5 mg Actimorph 5mg orodispersible tablets | 56 tablet PoM £6.75 DT = £6.75 CD2 SF

Morphine sulfate 10 mg Actimorph 10mg orodispersible tablets | 56 tablet PoM £7.75 DT = £7.75 CD2 SF

Morphine sulfate 20 mg Actimorph 20mg orodispersible tablets | 56 tablet PoM £9.75 DT = £9.75 CD2 SF

Morphine sulfate 30 mg Actimorph 30mg orodispersible tablets | 56 tablet PoM £13.00 DT = £13.00 CD2 SF

Infusion

▸ **Sendolor** (Eurocept International bv)

Morphine hydrochloride 1 mg per 1 ml Sendolor 100mg/100ml infusion bags | 1 bag PoM £23.13 (Hospital only) CD2

327

Oxycodone hydrochloride

18-Nov-2025

● **INDICATIONS AND DOSE**

Severe pain

▸ BY MOUTH USING IMMEDIATE-RELEASE MEDICINES

▸ Child 12–17 years: Initially 5 mg every 4–6 hours, dose to be increased if necessary according to severity of pain, some patients might require higher doses than the maximum daily dose; maximum 400 mg per day

▸ BY MOUTH USING MODIFIED-RELEASE MEDICINES

▸ Child 12–17 years: Initially 10 mg every 12 hours (max. per dose 200 mg every 12 hours), dose to be increased if necessary according to severity of pain, some patients might require higher doses than the maximum daily dose, use 12-hourly modified-release preparations for this dose; see *Prescribing and dispensing information*

Moderate to severe pain in palliative care

▸ BY MOUTH USING IMMEDIATE-RELEASE MEDICINES

▸ Child 1 month–11 years: Initially 200 micrograms/kg every 4–6 hours (max. per dose 5 mg), dose to be increased if necessary according to severity of pain

▸ Child 12–17 years: Initially 5 mg every 4–6 hours, dose to be increased if necessary according to severity of pain

▸ BY MOUTH USING MODIFIED-RELEASE MEDICINES

▸ Child 8–11 years: Initially 5 mg every 12 hours, dose to be increased if necessary according to severity of pain, use 12-hourly modified-release preparations for this dose; see *Prescribing and dispensing information*

▸ Child 12–17 years: Initially 10 mg every 12 hours, dose to be increased if necessary according to severity of pain, use 12-hourly modified-release preparations for this dose; see *Prescribing and dispensing information*

ONEXILA XL®

Severe pain

▸ BY MOUTH

▸ Child 12–17 years: Initially 10 mg every 24 hours, dose to be increased if necessary according to severity of pain, some patients may require higher doses than the maximum daily dose; maximum 400 mg per day

● **UNLICENSED USE** Oxycodone preparations are not licensed for use in children under 12 years and some may not be licensed for use in children—further information can be found in the product literature of the individual preparations.

IMPORTANT SAFETY INFORMATION

Do not confuse modified-release 12-hourly preparations with 24-hourly preparations, see *Prescribing and dispensing information.*

● **CONTRA-INDICATIONS** Acute abdomen · chronic constipation · cor pulmonale · delayed gastric emptying

● **CAUTIONS** Pancreatitis · toxic psychosis

● **INTERACTIONS** → Appendix 1: opioids

● **SIDE-EFFECTS**

▸ **Common or very common** Anxiety · appetite abnormal · asthenic conditions · bronchospasm · cognitive impairment · depression · diarrhoea · dyspnoea · gastrointestinal discomfort · hiccups · insomnia · mood altered · movement disorders · psychiatric disorders · thinking abnormal · tremor · urinary frequency increased

▸ **Uncommon** Burping · chest pain · chills · cough · dehydration · dysphagia · gastrointestinal disorders · hyperacusia · increased risk of infection · injury · lacrimation disorder · malaise · memory loss · migraine · neuromuscular dysfunction · oedema · oral disorders · pain · sensation abnormal · sexual dysfunction · SIADH · speech disorder · syncope · taste altered · thirst · vasodilation · voice alteration

- **Rare or very rare** Haemorrhage · lymphadenopathy · muscle spasms · photosensitivity reaction · tooth discolouration · weight changes
- **Frequency not known** Aggression · amenorrhoea · biliary colic · cholestasis

- **BREAST FEEDING** Present in milk—avoid.
- **HEPATIC IMPAIRMENT** EvGr Caution in mild impairment; avoid in moderate to severe impairment (M).

 Dose adjustments In adults, manufacturer advises initial dose reduction in mild impairment—consult product literature.
- **RENAL IMPAIRMENT** EvGr Caution (risk of increased and prolonged effects). (M)

 Dose adjustments EvGr Initial dose reduction of 50%; adjust according to response. (M)
- **PRESCRIBING AND DISPENSING INFORMATION** Modified-release preparations are available as 12-hourly or 24-hourly formulations. Preparations that should be given 12-hourly include *Abtard*®, *Carexil*®, *Ixyldone*®, *Leveraxo*®, *Longtec*®, *Oxeltra*®, *OxyContin*®, *Oxypro*®, *Oxylan*®, *Reltebon*®, and *Renocontin*®. Preparations that should be given 24-hourly include *Onexila*® *XL*.

 Palliative care For further information on the use of oxycodone in palliative care, see www.medicinescomplete.com/#/content/palliative/oxycodone.

- **MEDICINAL FORMS** There can be variation in the licensing of different medicines containing the same drug. Forms available from special-order manufacturers include: oral solution

Oral tablet

CAUTIONARY AND ADVISORY LABELS 2
EXCIPIENTS: May contain Lecithin

▸ **Oxyact** (G.L. Pharma UK Ltd)
Oxycodone hydrochloride 5 mg Oxyact 5mg tablets | 20 tablet PoM £1.95 CD2 | 56 tablet PoM £5.15 DT = £5.15 CD2
Oxycodone hydrochloride 10 mg Oxyact 10mg tablets | 56 tablet PoM £10.29 DT = £10.29 CD2
Oxycodone hydrochloride 20 mg Oxyact 20mg tablets | 56 tablet PoM £20.57 DT = £20.57 CD2

Modified-release tablet

CAUTIONARY AND ADVISORY LABELS 2, 25

▸ **Ixyldone** (Morningside Healthcare Ltd)
Oxycodone hydrochloride 5 mg Ixyldone 5mg modified-release tablets | 28 tablet PoM £2.96 DT = £12.52 CD2
Oxycodone hydrochloride 10 mg Ixyldone 10mg modified-release tablets | 56 tablet PoM £5.94 DT = £25.04 CD2
Oxycodone hydrochloride 15 mg Ixyldone 15mg modified-release tablets | 56 tablet PoM £9.05 DT = £38.12 CD2
Oxycodone hydrochloride 20 mg Ixyldone 20mg modified-release tablets | 56 tablet PoM £11.88 DT = £50.08 CD2
Oxycodone hydrochloride 30 mg Ixyldone 30mg modified-release tablets | 56 tablet PoM £18.10 DT = £76.23 CD2
Oxycodone hydrochloride 40 mg Ixyldone 40mg modified-release tablets | 56 tablet PoM £23.79 DT = £100.19 CD2
Oxycodone hydrochloride 60 mg Ixyldone 60mg modified-release tablets | 56 tablet PoM £36.19 DT = £152.49 CD2
Oxycodone hydrochloride 80 mg Ixyldone 80mg modified-release tablets | 56 tablet PoM £47.58 DT = £200.39 CD2

▸ **Longtec** (Qdem Pharmaceuticals Ltd)
Oxycodone hydrochloride 5 mg Longtec 5mg modified-release tablets | 28 tablet PoM £4.69 DT = £12.52 CD2
Oxycodone hydrochloride 10 mg Longtec 10mg modified-release tablets | 56 tablet PoM £9.39 DT = £25.04 CD2
Oxycodone hydrochloride 15 mg Longtec 15mg modified-release tablets | 56 tablet PoM £14.30 DT = £38.12 CD2
Oxycodone hydrochloride 20 mg Longtec 20mg modified-release tablets | 56 tablet PoM £18.78 DT = £50.08 CD2
Oxycodone hydrochloride 30 mg Longtec 30mg modified-release tablets | 56 tablet PoM £28.58 DT = £76.23 CD2
Oxycodone hydrochloride 40 mg Longtec 40mg modified-release tablets | 56 tablet PoM £37.57 DT = £100.19 CD2
Oxycodone hydrochloride 60 mg Longtec 60mg modified-release tablets | 56 tablet PoM £57.18 DT = £152.49 CD2
Oxycodone hydrochloride 80 mg Longtec 80mg modified-release tablets | 56 tablet PoM £75.14 DT = £200.39 CD2
Oxycodone hydrochloride 120 mg Longtec 120mg modified-release tablets | 56 tablet PoM £114.38 DT = £114.38 CD2

▸ **Oxeltra** (Wockhardt UK Ltd)
Oxycodone hydrochloride 5 mg Oxeltra 5mg modified-release tablets | 28 tablet PoM £3.13 DT = £12.52 CD2
Oxycodone hydrochloride 10 mg Oxeltra 10mg modified-release tablets | 56 tablet PoM £6.26 DT = £25.04 CD2
Oxycodone hydrochloride 15 mg Oxeltra 15mg modified-release tablets | 56 tablet PoM £9.53 DT = £38.12 CD2
Oxycodone hydrochloride 20 mg Oxeltra 20mg modified-release tablets | 56 tablet PoM £12.52 DT = £50.08 CD2
Oxycodone hydrochloride 30 mg Oxeltra 30mg modified-release tablets | 56 tablet PoM £19.06 DT = £76.23 CD2
Oxycodone hydrochloride 40 mg Oxeltra 40mg modified-release tablets | 56 tablet PoM £25.05 DT = £100.19 CD2
Oxycodone hydrochloride 60 mg Oxeltra 60mg modified-release tablets | 56 tablet PoM £38.12 DT = £152.49 CD2
Oxycodone hydrochloride 80 mg Oxeltra 80mg modified-release tablets | 56 tablet PoM £50.10 DT = £200.39 CD2

▸ **OxyContin** (Napp Pharmaceuticals Ltd)
Oxycodone hydrochloride 5 mg OxyContin 5mg modified-release tablets | 28 tablet PoM £12.52 DT = £12.52 CD2
Oxycodone hydrochloride 10 mg OxyContin 10mg modified-release tablets | 56 tablet PoM £25.04 DT = £25.04 CD2
Oxycodone hydrochloride 15 mg OxyContin 15mg modified-release tablets | 56 tablet PoM £38.12 DT = £38.12 CD2
Oxycodone hydrochloride 20 mg OxyContin 20mg modified-release tablets | 56 tablet PoM £50.08 DT = £50.08 CD2
Oxycodone hydrochloride 30 mg OxyContin 30mg modified-release tablets | 56 tablet PoM £76.23 DT = £76.23 CD2
Oxycodone hydrochloride 40 mg OxyContin 40mg modified-release tablets | 56 tablet PoM £100.19 DT = £100.19 CD2
Oxycodone hydrochloride 60 mg OxyContin 60mg modified-release tablets | 56 tablet PoM £152.49 DT = £152.49 CD2
Oxycodone hydrochloride 80 mg OxyContin 80mg modified-release tablets | 56 tablet PoM £200.39 DT = £200.39 CD2

▸ **Oxylan** (G.L. Pharma UK Ltd)
Oxycodone hydrochloride 5 mg Oxylan 5mg prolonged-release tablets | 14 tablet PoM £1.95 CD2 | 28 tablet PoM £2.66 DT = £12.52 CD2
Oxycodone hydrochloride 10 mg Oxylan 10mg prolonged-release tablets | 14 tablet PoM £1.95 CD2 | 56 tablet PoM £5.32 DT = £25.04 CD2
Oxycodone hydrochloride 15 mg Oxylan 15mg prolonged-release tablets | 56 tablet PoM £7.82 DT = £38.12 CD2
Oxycodone hydrochloride 20 mg Oxylan 20mg prolonged-release tablets | 56 tablet PoM £9.84 DT = £50.08 CD2
Oxycodone hydrochloride 30 mg Oxylan 30mg prolonged-release tablets | 56 tablet PoM £16.18 DT = £76.23 CD2
Oxycodone hydrochloride 40 mg Oxylan 40mg prolonged-release tablets | 56 tablet PoM £21.17 DT = £100.19 CD2
Oxycodone hydrochloride 60 mg Oxylan 60mg prolonged-release tablets | 56 tablet PoM £32.43 DT = £152.49 CD2
Oxycodone hydrochloride 80 mg Oxylan 80mg prolonged-release tablets | 56 tablet PoM £42.62 DT = £200.39 CD2

▸ **Oxypro** (Ridge Pharma Ltd)
Oxycodone hydrochloride 5 mg Oxypro 5mg modified-release tablets | 28 tablet PoM £3.13 DT = £12.52 CD2
Oxycodone hydrochloride 10 mg Oxypro 10mg modified-release tablets | 56 tablet PoM £6.26 DT = £25.04 CD2
Oxycodone hydrochloride 15 mg Oxypro 15mg modified-release tablets | 56 tablet PoM £9.53 DT = £38.12 CD2
Oxycodone hydrochloride 20 mg Oxypro 20mg modified-release tablets | 56 tablet PoM £12.52 DT = £50.08 CD2
Oxycodone hydrochloride 30 mg Oxypro 30mg modified-release tablets | 56 tablet PoM £19.06 DT = £76.23 CD2
Oxycodone hydrochloride 40 mg Oxypro 40mg modified-release tablets | 56 tablet PoM £25.05 DT = £100.19 CD2
Oxycodone hydrochloride 60 mg Oxypro 60mg modified-release tablets | 56 tablet PoM £38.12 DT = £152.49 CD2
Oxycodone hydrochloride 80 mg Oxypro 80mg modified-release tablets | 56 tablet PoM £50.10 DT = £200.39 CD2

▸ **Reltebon** (Accord-UK Ltd)
Oxycodone hydrochloride 5 mg Reltebon 5mg modified-release tablets | 28 tablet PoM £6.26 DT = £12.52 CD2
Oxycodone hydrochloride 10 mg Reltebon 10mg modified-release tablets | 56 tablet PoM £12.52 DT = £25.04 CD2
Oxycodone hydrochloride 15 mg Reltebon 15mg modified-release tablets | 56 tablet PoM £19.06 DT = £38.12 CD2

Oxycodone hydrochloride 20 mg Reltebon 20mg modified-release tablets | 56 tablet [PoM] £25.04 DT = £50.08 [CD2]
Oxycodone hydrochloride 30 mg Reltebon 30mg modified-release tablets | 56 tablet [PoM] £38.11 DT = £76.23 [CD2]
Oxycodone hydrochloride 40 mg Reltebon 40mg modified-release tablets | 56 tablet [PoM] £50.09 DT = £100.19 [CD2]
Oxycodone hydrochloride 60 mg Reltebon 60mg modified-release tablets | 56 tablet [PoM] £76.24 DT = £152.49 [CD2]
Oxycodone hydrochloride 80 mg Reltebon 80mg modified-release tablets | 56 tablet [PoM] £100.19 DT = £200.39 [CD2]

Oral capsule

CAUTIONARY AND ADVISORY LABELS 2

▸ **Oxycodone hydrochloride (Non-proprietary)**
Oxycodone hydrochloride 5 mg Oxycodone 5mg capsules | 56 capsule [PoM] £9.92–£10.00 DT = £11.43 [CD2]
Oxycodone hydrochloride 10 mg Oxycodone 10mg capsules | 56 capsule [PoM] £18.59–£20.00 DT = £22.86 [CD2]
Oxycodone hydrochloride 20 mg Oxycodone 20mg capsules | 56 capsule [PoM] £34.69–£40.00 DT = £45.71 [CD2]

▸ **Lynlor** (Accord-UK Ltd)
Oxycodone hydrochloride 5 mg Lynlor 5mg capsules | 56 capsule [PoM] £6.86 DT = £11.43 [CD2]
Oxycodone hydrochloride 10 mg Lynlor 10mg capsules | 56 capsule [PoM] £13.72 DT = £22.86 [CD2]
Oxycodone hydrochloride 20 mg Lynlor 20mg capsules | 56 capsule [PoM] £27.43 DT = £45.71 [CD2]

▸ **OxyNorm** (Napp Pharmaceuticals Ltd)
Oxycodone hydrochloride 5 mg OxyNorm 5mg capsules | 56 capsule [PoM] £11.43 DT = £11.43 [CD2]
Oxycodone hydrochloride 10 mg OxyNorm 10mg capsules | 56 capsule [PoM] £22.86 DT = £22.86 [CD2]
Oxycodone hydrochloride 20 mg OxyNorm 20mg capsules | 56 capsule [PoM] £45.71 DT = £45.71 [CD2]

▸ **Shortec** (Qdem Pharmaceuticals Ltd)
Oxycodone hydrochloride 5 mg Shortec 5mg capsules | 56 capsule [PoM] £6.86 DT = £11.43 [CD2]
Oxycodone hydrochloride 10 mg Shortec 10mg capsules | 56 capsule [PoM] £13.72 DT = £22.86 [CD2]
Oxycodone hydrochloride 20 mg Shortec 20mg capsules | 56 capsule [PoM] £27.43 DT = £45.71 [CD2]

Oral solution

CAUTIONARY AND ADVISORY LABELS 2

▸ **Oxycodone hydrochloride (Non-proprietary)**
Oxycodone hydrochloride 1 mg per 1 ml Oxycodone 5mg/5ml oral solution sugar free | 250 ml [PoM] £7.22–£9.77 DT = £5.46 [CD2] [SF]
Oxycodone hydrochloride 10 mg per 1 ml Oxycodone 10mg/ml oral solution sugar free | 120 ml [PoM] £46.43–£46.63 DT = £46.63 [CD2] [SF]

▸ **OxyNorm** (Napp Pharmaceuticals Ltd)
Oxycodone hydrochloride 1 mg per 1 ml OxyNorm liquid 1mg/ml oral solution | 250 ml [PoM] £9.71 DT = £5.46 [CD2] [SF]
Oxycodone hydrochloride 10 mg per 1 ml OxyNorm 10mg/ml concentrate oral solution | 120 ml [PoM] £46.63 DT = £46.63 [CD2] [SF]

F 327

Pethidine hydrochloride (Meperidine)

01-Jun-2021

● **INDICATIONS AND DOSE**

Obstetric analgesia

▶ BY SUBCUTANEOUS INJECTION, OR BY INTRAMUSCULAR INJECTION
▸ Child 12–17 years: 1 mg/kg (max. per dose 100 mg), then 1 mg/kg after 1–3 hours if required; maximum 400 mg per day

● **CONTRA-INDICATIONS** Phaeochromocytoma

● **CAUTIONS** Accumulation of metabolites may result in toxicity · cardiac arrhythmias · not suitable for severe continuing pain · severe cor pulmonale

● **INTERACTIONS** → Appendix 1: opioids

● **SIDE-EFFECTS** Anxiety · asthenia · biliary spasm · coordination abnormal · delirium · dysuria · hypothermia · syncope · tremor

Overdose Convulsions reported in overdosage.

● **BREAST FEEDING** Present in milk but not known to be harmful.

● **HEPATIC IMPAIRMENT** Manufacturer advises caution in mild to moderate impairment; avoid in severe impairment.
Dose adjustments Manufacturer advises dose reduction in mild to moderate impairment.

● **RENAL IMPAIRMENT** [EvGr] Caution in mild to moderate impairment; avoid in severe impairment (risk of increased and prolonged effects). ⟨M⟩
Dose adjustments [EvGr] Reduce dose in mild to moderate impairment. ⟨M⟩

● **MEDICINAL FORMS** There can be variation in the licensing of different medicines containing the same drug. Forms available from special-order manufacturers include: solution for injection

Solution for injection

▸ **Pethidine hydrochloride (Non-proprietary)**
Pethidine hydrochloride 50 mg per 1 ml Pethidine 50mg/1ml solution for injection ampoules | 10 ampoule [PoM] £5.11–£6.00 DT = £5.11 [CD2]
Pethidine 100mg/2ml solution for injection ampoules | 10 ampoule [PoM] £4.66–£6.50 DT = £4.66 [CD2]

F 327

Tapentadol

01-Sep-2022

● **INDICATIONS AND DOSE**

Moderate to severe acute pain which can be managed only with opioid analgesics

▶ BY MOUTH USING ORAL SOLUTION
▸ Child 2–17 years (specialist supervision in hospital) (body-weight 16 kg and above): 1.25 mg/kg every 4 hours (max. per dose 100 mg) for up to 3 days, the dose for children with a high BMI must not exceed the calculated dose for a body-weight at the 97.5 percentile for the given age

IMPORTANT SAFETY INFORMATION

MHRA/CHM ADVICE: TAPENTADOL (*PALEXIA*®): RISK OF SEIZURES AND REPORTS OF SEROTONIN SYNDROME WHEN CO-ADMINISTERED WITH OTHER MEDICINES (JANUARY 2019)

Tapentadol can induce seizures and should be prescribed with caution in patients with a history of seizure disorders or epilepsy. Seizure risk may be increased in patients taking other medicines that lower seizure threshold, for example, antidepressants such as selective serotonin reuptake inhibitors (SSRIs), serotonin-noradrenaline reuptake inhibitors (SNRIs), tricyclic antidepressants, and antipsychotics.

Serotonin syndrome has been reported when tapentadol is used in combination with serotonergic antidepressants—withdrawal of the serotonergic medicine, together with supportive symptomatic care, usually brings about a rapid improvement in serotonin syndrome.

● **CAUTIONS** Obesity

● **INTERACTIONS** → Appendix 1: opioids

● **SIDE-EFFECTS**
▶ **Common or very common** Anxiety · appetite decreased · asthenia · concentration impaired · depressed mood · diarrhoea · dyspnoea · feeling of body temperature change · gastrointestinal discomfort · mucosal dryness · muscle contractions involuntary · muscle spasms · oedema · sleep disorders · tremor
▶ **Uncommon** Cognitive impairment · dysarthria · feeling abnormal · irritability · level of consciousness decreased · memory impairment · movement disorders · sensation abnormal · sexual dysfunction · syncope · urinary disorders · weight decreased

- ▶ **Rare or very rare** Impaired gastric emptying · thinking abnormal
- **BREAST FEEDING** Avoid—no information available.
- **HEPATIC IMPAIRMENT** [EvGr] Avoid (no information available). ⟨M⟩
- **RENAL IMPAIRMENT** Manufacturer advises avoid (no information available).

- **MEDICINAL FORMS** There can be variation in the licensing of different medicines containing the same drug.

Oral solution

CAUTIONARY AND ADVISORY LABELS 2

EXCIPIENTS: May contain Propylene glycol

▸ **Palexia** (Grunenthal Ltd)
Tapentadol (as Tapentadol hydrochloride) 20 mg per 1 ml Palexia 20mg/ml oral solution | 100 ml [PoM] £17.80 DT = £17.80 [CD2] [SF]

327

Tramadol hydrochloride

25-Aug-2022

- **INDICATIONS AND DOSE**

Moderate to severe pain

▶ BY INTRAMUSCULAR INJECTION, OR BY INTRAVENOUS INJECTION, OR BY INTRAVENOUS INFUSION, OR BY SUBCUTANEOUS INJECTION

▸ Child 12–17 years: 50–100 mg every 4–6 hours, intravenous injection to be given over 2–3 minutes; Usual maximum 400 mg/24 hours

Moderate to severe acute pain

▶ BY MOUTH USING IMMEDIATE-RELEASE MEDICINES

▸ Child 12–17 years: Initially 100 mg, then 50–100 mg every 4–6 hours; Usual maximum 400 mg/24 hours

Moderate to severe chronic pain

▶ BY MOUTH USING IMMEDIATE-RELEASE MEDICINES

▸ Child 12–17 years: Initially 50 mg, then, adjusted according to response; Usual maximum 400 mg/24 hours

Postoperative pain

▶ BY INTRAVENOUS INJECTION, OR BY INTRAMUSCULAR INJECTION, OR BY INTRAVENOUS INFUSION, OR BY SUBCUTANEOUS INJECTION

▸ Child 12–17 years: Initially 100 mg, then 50 mg every 10–20 minutes if required up to total maximum 250 mg (including initial dose) in first hour, then 50–100 mg every 4–6 hours, intravenous injection to be given over 2–3 minutes; Usual maximum 400 mg/24 hours

Moderate to severe pain (with modified-release 12-hourly preparations)

▶ BY MOUTH USING MODIFIED-RELEASE MEDICINES

▸ Child 12–17 years: 50–100 mg twice daily, increased if necessary to 150–200 mg twice daily, doses exceeding the usual maximum not generally required; Usual maximum 400 mg/24 hours

Moderate to severe pain (with modified-release 24-hourly preparations)

▶ BY MOUTH USING MODIFIED-RELEASE MEDICINES

▸ Child 12–17 years: Initially 100–150 mg once daily, increased if necessary up to 400 mg once daily; Usual maximum 400 mg/24 hours

IMPORTANT SAFETY INFORMATION

Do not confuse modified-release 12-hourly preparations with 24-hourly preparations, see *Prescribing and dispensing information*.

- **CONTRA-INDICATIONS** Acute intoxication with alcohol · acute intoxication with analgesics · acute intoxication with hypnotics · acute intoxication with opioids · compromised respiratory function · not suitable for narcotic withdrawal treatment · uncontrolled epilepsy
- **CAUTIONS** Excessive bronchial secretions · history of epilepsy—use tramadol only if compelling reasons · impaired consciousness · not suitable as a substitute in opioid-dependent patients · postoperative use · susceptibility to seizures—use tramadol only if compelling reasons · variation in metabolism

CAUTIONS, FURTHER INFORMATION

▸ Variation in metabolism The capacity to metabolise tramadol can vary considerably between individuals; there is a risk of developing side-effects of opioid toxicity in patients who are ultra-rapid tramadol metabolisers (CYP2D6 ultra-rapid metabolisers) and the therapeutic effect may be reduced in poor tramadol metabolisers.

▸ Postoperative use Manufacturer advises extreme caution when used for postoperative pain relief in children—reports of rare, but life threatening adverse events after tonsillectomy and/or adenoidectomy for obstructive sleep apnoea; if used, monitor closely for symptoms of opioid toxicity.

- **INTERACTIONS** → Appendix 1: opioids
- **SIDE-EFFECTS**

GENERAL SIDE-EFFECTS

▶ **Common or very common** Fatigue

▶ **Rare or very rare** Dyspnoea · epileptiform seizure · respiratory disorders · vision blurred

▶ **Frequency not known** Asthma exacerbated · hypoglycaemia

SPECIFIC SIDE-EFFECTS

▶ **Uncommon**

▸ With parenteral use Circulatory collapse · gastrointestinal discomfort

▶ **Rare or very rare**

▸ With parenteral use Angioedema · appetite change · behaviour abnormal · cognitive disorder · dysuria · hypersensitivity · mood altered · movement disorders · muscle weakness · perception disorders · psychiatric disorder · sensation abnormal · sleep disorders

▶ **Frequency not known**

▸ With oral use Blood disorder · hiccups · hypertension · hyponatraemia · nightmare · paraesthesia · serotonin syndrome · syncope · urinary disorder

- **PREGNANCY** Embryotoxic in *animal* studies—manufacturers advise avoid.
- **BREAST FEEDING** Amount probably too small to be harmful, but manufacturer advises avoid.
- **HEPATIC IMPAIRMENT** Manufacturers advise caution (risk of delayed elimination); some *oral preparations* should be avoided in severe impairment—consult product literature.
  Dose adjustments Manufacturers advise consider increasing dosage interval.
- **RENAL IMPAIRMENT** Avoid use or reduce dose; opioid effects increased and prolonged and increased cerebral sensitivity occurs. Caution (avoid for *oral drops*) in severe impairment.
- **TREATMENT CESSATION** Manufacturer advises consider tapering the dose gradually to prevent withdrawal symptoms.
- **DIRECTIONS FOR ADMINISTRATION** Manufacturer advises tramadol hydrochloride *orodispersible tablets* should be sucked and then swallowed. May also be dispersed in water. Manufacturers advise some tramadol hydrochloride modified-release capsule preparations may be opened and the contents swallowed immediately without chewing—check individual preparations.
  For *intravenous infusion*, manufacturer advises dilute in Glucose 5% or Sodium Chloride 0.9%.
- **PRESCRIBING AND DISPENSING INFORMATION** Modified-release preparations are available as 12-hourly or 24-hourly formulations. Non-proprietary preparations of modified-release tramadol may be available as either 12-hourly or 24-hourly formulations; prescribers and

dispensers must ensure that the correct formulation is prescribed and dispensed. Branded preparations that should be given 12-hourly include *Brimisol® PR*, *Marol®*, *Maxitram® SR*, *Tilodol® SR*, *Tramquel® SR*, *Tramulief® SR*, *Zamadol® SR*, and *Zydol SR®*. Preparations that should be given 24-hourly include *Tradorec XL®*, *Zamadol® 24hr*, and *Zydol XL®*.

● **PATIENT AND CARER ADVICE** Patients or carers should be given advice on how to administer tramadol hydrochloride orodispersible tablets.
Medicines for Children leaflet: Tramadol for pain
www.medicinesforchildren.org.uk/medicines/tramadol-for-pain/

● **MEDICINAL FORMS** There can be variation in the licensing of different medicines containing the same drug. Forms available from special-order manufacturers include: oral suspension

Modified-release tablet

CAUTIONARY AND ADVISORY LABELS 2, 25

▸ **Tramadol hydrochloride (Non-proprietary)**
Tramadol hydrochloride 100 mg Tramadol 100mg modified-release tablets | 60 tablet [PoM] £20.66 [CD3]
Tramadol hydrochloride 150 mg Tramadol 150mg modified-release tablets | 60 tablet [PoM] £27.94 [CD3]
Tramadol hydrochloride 200 mg Tramadol 200mg modified-release tablets | 60 tablet [PoM] £43.20 [CD3]

▸ **Brimisol PR** (Bristol Laboratories Ltd)
Tramadol hydrochloride 100 mg Brimisol PR 100mg tablets | 60 tablet [PoM] [~~£~~] [CD3]
Tramadol hydrochloride 200 mg Brimisol PR 200mg tablets | 60 tablet [PoM] £36.00 [CD3]

▸ **Marol** (Teva UK Ltd)
Tramadol hydrochloride 100 mg Marol 100mg modified-release tablets | 60 tablet [PoM] £6.94 [CD3]
Tramadol hydrochloride 150 mg Marol 150mg modified-release tablets | 60 tablet [PoM] £10.39 [CD3]
Tramadol hydrochloride 200 mg Marol 200mg modified-release tablets | 60 tablet [PoM] £14.19 [CD3]

▸ **Tilodol SR** (Sandoz Ltd)
Tramadol hydrochloride 100 mg Tilodol SR 100mg tablets | 60 tablet [PoM] £15.52 [CD3]
Tramadol hydrochloride 150 mg Tilodol SR 150mg tablets | 60 tablet [PoM] £23.28 [CD3]
Tramadol hydrochloride 200 mg Tilodol SR 200mg tablets | 60 tablet [PoM] £31.04 [CD3]

▸ **Tramulief SR** (Advanz Pharma)
Tramadol hydrochloride 100 mg Tramulief SR 100mg tablets | 60 tablet [PoM] £6.98 [CD3]
Tramadol hydrochloride 150 mg Tramulief SR 150mg tablets | 60 tablet [PoM] £10.48 [CD3]
Tramadol hydrochloride 200 mg Tramulief SR 200mg tablets | 60 tablet [PoM] £14.28 [CD3]

▸ **Zydol SR** (Grunenthal Ltd)
Tramadol hydrochloride 50 mg Zydol SR 50mg tablets | 60 tablet [PoM] £4.60 DT = £4.60 [CD3]
Tramadol hydrochloride 100 mg Zydol SR 100mg tablets | 60 tablet [PoM] £17.22 [CD3]
Tramadol hydrochloride 150 mg Zydol SR 150mg tablets | 60 tablet [PoM] £25.83 [CD3]
Tramadol hydrochloride 200 mg Zydol SR 200mg tablets | 60 tablet [PoM] £34.40 [CD3]

▸ **Zydol XL** (Grunenthal Ltd)
Tramadol hydrochloride 400 mg Zydol XL 400mg tablets | 30 tablet [PoM] £32.47 [CD3]

Soluble tablet

CAUTIONARY AND ADVISORY LABELS 2, 13

▸ **Zydol** (Grunenthal Ltd)
Tramadol hydrochloride 50 mg Zydol 50mg soluble tablets | 100 tablet [PoM] £13.33 DT = £13.33 Schedule 3 (CD No Register Exempt Safe Custody) [SF]

Solution for injection

▸ **Tramadol hydrochloride (Non-proprietary)**
Tramadol hydrochloride 50 mg per 1 ml Tramadol 100mg/2ml solution for injection ampoules | 5 ampoule [PoM] £4.00 DT = £4.00 (Hospital only) [CD3] | 10 ampoule [PoM] £11.00 [CD3]

▸ **Zydol** (Grunenthal Ltd)
Tramadol hydrochloride 50 mg per 1 ml Zydol 100mg/2ml solution for injection ampoules | 5 ampoule [PoM] £4.00 DT = £4.00 [CD3]

Modified-release capsule

CAUTIONARY AND ADVISORY LABELS 2, 25

▸ **Tramadol hydrochloride (Non-proprietary)**
Tramadol hydrochloride 50 mg Tramadol 50mg modified-release capsules | 60 capsule [PoM] £7.24 DT = £7.24 [CD3]
Tramadol hydrochloride 100 mg Tramadol 100mg modified-release capsules | 60 capsule [PoM] £14.47 DT = £14.47 [CD3]
Tramadol hydrochloride 150 mg Tramadol 150mg modified-release capsules | 60 capsule [PoM] £21.71 DT = £21.71 [CD3]
Tramadol hydrochloride 200 mg Tramadol 200mg modified-release capsules | 60 capsule [PoM] £28.93 DT = £28.93 [CD3]

▸ **Maxitram SR** (Chiesi Ltd)
Tramadol hydrochloride 50 mg Maxitram SR 50mg capsules | 60 capsule [PoM] £4.55 DT = £7.24 [CD3]
Tramadol hydrochloride 100 mg Maxitram SR 100mg capsules | 60 capsule [PoM] £12.14 DT = £14.47 [CD3]
Tramadol hydrochloride 150 mg Maxitram SR 150mg capsules | 60 capsule [PoM] £18.21 DT = £21.71 [CD3]
Tramadol hydrochloride 200 mg Maxitram SR 200mg capsules | 60 capsule [PoM] £24.28 DT = £28.93 [CD3]

▸ **Zamadol SR** (Viatris UK Healthcare Ltd)
Tramadol hydrochloride 50 mg Zamadol SR 50mg capsules | 60 capsule [PoM] £7.24 DT = £7.24 [CD3]
Tramadol hydrochloride 100 mg Zamadol SR 100mg capsules | 60 capsule [PoM] £14.47 DT = £14.47 [CD3]
Tramadol hydrochloride 150 mg Zamadol SR 150mg capsules | 60 capsule [PoM] £21.71 DT = £21.71 [CD3]
Tramadol hydrochloride 200 mg Zamadol SR 200mg capsules | 60 capsule [PoM] £28.93 DT = £28.93 [CD3]

Oral capsule

CAUTIONARY AND ADVISORY LABELS 2

▸ **Tramadol hydrochloride (Non-proprietary)**
Tramadol hydrochloride 50 mg Tramadol 50mg capsules | 30 capsule [PoM] £2.50 DT = £0.65 [CD3] | 100 capsule [PoM] £7.63 DT = £2.17 [CD3]

▸ **Zamadol** (Viatris UK Healthcare Ltd)
Tramadol hydrochloride 50 mg Zamadol 50mg capsules | 100 capsule [PoM] £8.00 DT = £2.17 [CD3]

▸ **Zydol** (Grunenthal Ltd)
Tramadol hydrochloride 50 mg Zydol 50mg capsules | 100 capsule [PoM] £7.63 DT = £2.17 [CD3]

Orodispersible tablet

CAUTIONARY AND ADVISORY LABELS 2

▸ **Zamadol Melt** (Viatris UK Healthcare Ltd)
Tramadol hydrochloride 50 mg Zamadol Melt 50mg tablets | 60 tablet [PoM] £7.12 DT = £7.12 Schedule 3 (CD No Register Exempt Safe Custody) [SF]

Tramadol with paracetamol

22-Feb-2018

The properties listed below are those particular to the combination only. For the properties of the components please consider, paracetamol p. 325, tramadol hydrochloride p. 343.

● **INDICATIONS AND DOSE**

Moderate to severe pain

▸ BY MOUTH

▸ Child 12–17 years: 75/650 mg every 6 hours as required

DOSE EQUIVALENCE AND CONVERSION

▸ The proportions are expressed in the form x/y, where x and y are the strengths in milligrams of tramadol and paracetamol respectively.

● **INTERACTIONS** → Appendix 1: opioids · paracetamol

● **MEDICINAL FORMS** There can be variation in the licensing of different medicines containing the same drug.

Oral tablet

CAUTIONARY AND ADVISORY LABELS 2, 25, 29, 30

▸ **Tramadol with paracetamol (Non-proprietary)**
Tramadol hydrochloride 37.5 mg, Paracetamol 325 mg Tramadol 37.5mg / Paracetamol 325mg tablets | 60 tablet [PoM] £11.62 DT = £4.42 [CD3]

▸ **Tramacet** (Grunenthal Ltd)
Tramadol hydrochloride 37.5 mg, Paracetamol 325 mg Tramacet 37.5mg/325mg tablets | 60 tablet [PoM] £9.68 DT = £4.42 [CD3]

5.1 Headache

Cluster headache and other trigeminal autonomic cephalalgias

01-Jun-2021

Management

Cluster headache rarely responds to standard analgesics. Sumatriptan p. 346 given by subcutaneous injection is the drug of choice for the treatment of cluster headache. If an injection is unsuitable, sumatriptan nasal spray or zolmitriptan nasal spray p. 347 may be used. Treatment should be initiated by a specialist. Alternatively, 100% oxygen at a rate of 10–15 litres/minute for 10–20 minutes is useful in aborting an attack.

The other trigeminal autonomic cephalalgias, paroxysmal hemicrania (sensitive to indometacin p. 824), and short-lasting unilateral neuralgiform headache attacks with conjunctival injection and tearing, are seen rarely and are best managed by a specialist.

5.1a Migraine

Migraine

09-Nov-2025

Treatment of acute migraine

EvGr Migraine in children often responds to conservative management with avoidance of triggers (e.g. missed meals, dehydration, and irregular sleep) and simple analgesia, such as paracetamol p. 325 or an NSAID, usually ibuprofen p. 821.

If treatment with a simple analgesic is inadequate, an attack may be treated with a $5HT_1$-receptor agonist (preferably intranasally), such as sumatriptan p. 346 or zolmitriptan p. 347 [unlicensed use]. If a child does not respond to one $5HT_1$-receptor agonist, an alternative $5HT_1$-receptor agonist can be tried.

If a $5HT_1$-receptor agonist alone is ineffective, consider combination therapy with an NSAID, or paracetamol. In addition to their use as antiemetics, metoclopramide hydrochloride [unlicensed use] or prochlorperazine [unlicensed use], can also be given at the onset of migraine symptoms for the treatment of headache. (A)

Medication-overuse headache is a complication of migraine; the frequent use of acute treatment for migraine (opioid and non-opioid analgesics, or $5HT_1$-receptor agonists) increases the frequency and intensity of headache, and can become the cause of the headache. Children and their carers should be advised of the risk of developing medication-overuse headache.

Antiemetics

EvGr Migraine is frequently accompanied by nausea and/or vomiting, and antiemetics can be considered for relief. (A)

Prochlorperazine p. 322 is licensed for the relief of nausea and vomiting associated with migraine attacks.

Domperidone p. 314 is licensed for the relief of nausea and vomiting.

Prophylaxis of migraine

Where migraine attacks are frequent, possible triggers such as stress, other medicines (e.g. combined oral contraceptives), or diet, should be identified and avoided.

Expert sources advise that prophylactic treatment can be considered when migraine attacks are frequent and severe, and interfere with school and social life. EvGr However, there is limited evidence of benefit for prophylactic treatment in children and specialist advice should be sought. Propranolol hydrochloride p. 123 and topiramate p. 257 [unlicensed use] can be used for migraine prophylaxis. (A) However, the MHRA has advised that topiramate must not be used in females of childbearing potential unless the conditions of the Pregnancy Prevention Programme are met; it must not be used during pregnancy for migraine prophylaxis. For further information, see *Important safety information*, *Conception and contraception*, and *Pregnancy* in topiramate.

Pizotifen p. 346 is licensed for prophylaxis of migraine, but its efficacy in children has not been clearly established.

EvGr The need for continuing migraine prophylaxis should be reviewed 3–6 months after starting treatment. (A) Expert sources advise that in children it is often possible to stop prophylaxis after a period of treatment.

Useful Resources

Headaches in over 12s: diagnosis and management. National Institute for Health and Care Excellence. NICE guideline 150. September 2012 (updated June 2025).
www.nice.org.uk/guidance/cg150

ANTIHISTAMINES › SEDATING

Paracetamol with buclizine hydrochloride and codeine phosphate

22-Nov-2019

The properties listed below are those particular to the combination only. For the properties of the components please consider, paracetamol p. 325, codeine phosphate p. 331.

● **INDICATIONS AND DOSE**

MIGRALEVE ®

Acute migraine

▶ BY MOUTH

▶ Child 12–15 years: Initially 1 tablet, (pink tablet) to be taken at onset of attack, or if it is imminent, followed by 1 tablet every 4 hours if required, (yellow tablet) to be taken following initial dose; maximum 1 pink and 3 yellow tablets in 24 hours

▶ Child 16–17 years: Initially 2 tablets, (pink tablets) to be taken at onset of attack or if it is imminent, followed by 2 tablets every 4 hours if required, (yellow tablets) to be taken following initial dose; maximum 2 pink and 6 yellow tablets in 24 hours

● **INTERACTIONS** → Appendix 1: antihistamines, sedating · opioids · paracetamol

● **PRESCRIBING AND DISPENSING INFORMATION** See co-codamol p. 330 for *Migraleve®* Yellow preparations.

● **LESS SUITABLE FOR PRESCRIBING** *Migraleve®* is less suitable for prescribing.

● **MEDICINAL FORMS** There can be variation in the licensing of different medicines containing the same drug.

Oral tablet

CAUTIONARY AND ADVISORY LABELS 2, 17, 30

▶ Migraleve Pink (McNeil Products Ltd)
Buclizine hydrochloride 6.25 mg, Codeine phosphate 8 mg, Paracetamol 500 mg Migraleve Pink tablets | 12 tablet P £5.31 CD5 | 24 tablet P £8.43 CD5

Pizotifen

21-May-2024

● **INDICATIONS AND DOSE**

Prophylaxis of migraine

▶ BY MOUTH

▸ Child 5–17 years: Initially 500 micrograms once daily, dose to be taken at night, then increased if necessary up to 1.5 mg daily in divided doses, dose to be increased gradually, max. single dose (at night) 1 mg

● **CONTRA-INDICATIONS** Acute porphyrias p. 745

● **CAUTIONS** Avoid abrupt withdrawal · history of epilepsy · susceptibility to angle-closure glaucoma · urinary retention

● **INTERACTIONS** → Appendix 1: antihistamines, sedating

● **SIDE-EFFECTS**

▶ **Common or very common** Appetite increased · dizziness · drowsiness · dry mouth · fatigue · nausea · weight increased

▶ **Uncommon** Constipation

▶ **Rare or very rare** Aggression · anxiety · arthralgia · central nervous system stimulation · depression · hallucination · muscle complaints · paraesthesia · seizure · skin reactions · sleep disorders

▶ **Frequency not known** Hepatic disorders

● **PREGNANCY** Avoid unless potential benefit outweighs risk.

● **BREAST FEEDING** Amount probably too small to be harmful, but manufacturer advises avoid.

● **HEPATIC IMPAIRMENT** Manufacturer advises caution.

Dose adjustments Manufacturer advises consider dose reduction.

● **RENAL IMPAIRMENT** EvGr Use with caution. Ⓜ

Dose adjustments EvGr Consider dose reduction. Ⓜ

● **PATIENT AND CARER ADVICE**

Medicines for Children leaflet: Pizotifen for migraine headaches www.medicinesforchildren.org.uk/medicines/pizotifen-for-migraine-headaches/

Driving and skilled tasks Drowsiness may affect performance of skilled tasks (e.g. driving); effects of alcohol enhanced.

● **MEDICINAL FORMS** There can be variation in the licensing of different medicines containing the same drug. Forms available from special-order manufacturers include: oral solution

Oral tablet

CAUTIONARY AND ADVISORY LABELS 2

▸ **Pizotifen (Non-proprietary)**

Pizotifen (as Pizotifen malate) 500 microgram Pizotifen 500microgram tablets | 28 tablet PoM £1.81 DT = £0.96

Pizotifen (as Pizotifen malate) 1.5 mg Pizotifen 1.5mg tablets | 28 tablet PoM £4.60 DT = £1.47

TRIPTANS

Sumatriptan

24-May-2021

● **INDICATIONS AND DOSE**

Treatment of acute migraine

▶ BY MOUTH

▸ Child 6–9 years: Initially 25 mg for 1 dose, followed by 25 mg after at least 2 hours if required, to be taken only if migraine recurs (patient not responding to initial dose should not take second dose for same attack)

▸ Child 10–11 years: Initially 50 mg for 1 dose, followed by 50 mg after at least 2 hours, to be taken only if migraine recurs (patient not responding to initial dose should not take second dose for same attack)

▸ Child 12–17 years: Initially 50–100 mg for 1 dose, followed by 50–100 mg after at least 2 hours if required, to be taken only if migraine recurs (patient not responding to initial dose should not take second dose for same attack)

▶ BY SUBCUTANEOUS INJECTION

▸ Child 10–17 years: Initially 6 mg for 1 dose, followed by 6 mg after at least 1 hour if required, to be taken only if migraine recurs (patient not responding to initial dose should not take second dose for same attack), dose to be administered using an auto-injector; maximum 12 mg per day

▶ BY INTRANASAL ADMINISTRATION

▸ Child 12–17 years: Initially 10–20 mg for 1 dose, followed by 10–20 mg after at least 2 hours if required, to be taken only if migraine recurs (patient not responding to initial dose should not take second dose for same attack); maximum 40 mg per day

Treatment of acute cluster headache

▶ BY SUBCUTANEOUS INJECTION

▸ Child 10–17 years (under expert supervision): Initially 6 mg for 1 dose, followed by 6 mg after at least 1 hour if required, to be taken only if headache recurs (patient not responding to initial dose should not take second dose for same attack), dose to be administered using auto-injector; maximum 12 mg per day

▶ BY INTRANASAL ADMINISTRATION

▸ Child 12–17 years (under expert supervision): Initially 10–20 mg for 1 dose, followed by 10–20 mg after at least 2 hours if required, to be taken only if headache recurs (patient not responding to initial dose should not take second dose for same attack); maximum 40 mg per day

● **UNLICENSED USE** Tablets and injection not licensed for use in children. Not licensed for treating cluster headache in children. Intranasal doses for treating acute migraine in children may differ from those in product literature.

● **CONTRA-INDICATIONS** Coronary vasospasm · ischaemic heart disease · mild uncontrolled hypertension · moderate and severe hypertension · peripheral vascular disease · previous cerebrovascular accident · previous myocardial infarction · previous transient ischaemic attack · Prinzmetal's angina

● **CAUTIONS** Conditions which predispose to coronary artery disease · history of seizures · mild, controlled hypertension · risk factors for seizures

● **INTERACTIONS** → Appendix 1: triptans

● **SIDE-EFFECTS**

GENERAL SIDE-EFFECTS

▶ **Common or very common** Asthenia · dizziness · drowsiness · dyspnoea · feeling abnormal · flushing · myalgia · nausea · pain · sensation abnormal · skin reactions · temperature sensation altered · vomiting

▶ **Frequency not known** Angina pectoris · anxiety · arrhythmias · arthralgia · colitis ischaemic · coronary vasospasm · diarrhoea · dystonia · hyperhidrosis · hypersensitivity · hypotension · myocardial infarction · nystagmus · palpitations · Raynaud's phenomenon · seizure · tremor · vision disorders

SPECIFIC SIDE-EFFECTS

▶ **Common or very common**

▸ With intranasal use Epistaxis · nasal irritation · taste altered · throat irritation

▸ With subcutaneous use Haemorrhage · swelling

▶ **Frequency not known**

▸ With oral use Dysphagia

SIDE-EFFECTS, FURTHER INFORMATION Discontinue if symptoms of heat, heaviness, pressure or tightness (including throat and chest) occur.

● **ALLERGY AND CROSS-SENSITIVITY** EvGr Caution in patients with sensitivity to sulfonamides. Ⓜ

- **PREGNANCY** There is limited experience of using $5HT_1$-receptor agonists during pregnancy; manufacturers advise that they should be avoided unless the potential benefit outweighs the risk.
- **BREAST FEEDING** Present in milk but amount probably too small to be harmful; withhold breast-feeding for 12 hours after treatment.
- **HEPATIC IMPAIRMENT** Manufacturer advises caution (reduced pre-systemic clearance increases exposure); avoid in severe impairment (no information available).

  Dose adjustments

  ▸ With oral use In adults, manufacturer advises consider dose reduction—consult product literature.
- **RENAL IMPAIRMENT** EvGr Use with caution. (M)
- **PATIENT AND CARER ADVICE**

  Medicines for Children leaflet: Sumatriptan for migraine headaches www.medicinesforchildren.org.uk/medicines/sumatriptan-for-migraine-headaches/

  Driving and skilled tasks Drowsiness may affect performance of skilled tasks (e.g. driving).

- **MEDICINAL FORMS** There can be variation in the licensing of different medicines containing the same drug.

Solution for injection

CAUTIONARY AND ADVISORY LABELS 3

▸ **Sumatriptan (Non-proprietary)**

Sumatriptan (as Sumatriptan succinate) 6 mg per 1 ml Sumatriptan 3mg/0.5ml solution for injection pre-filled pens | 2 pre-filled disposable injection PoM £39.50–£45.00 DT = £39.50

Sumatriptan (as Sumatriptan succinate) 12 mg per 1 ml Sumatriptan 6mg/0.5ml solution for injection pre-filled pens | 2 pre-filled disposable injection PoM £45.00 DT = £46.99

▸ **Imigran Subject** (GlaxoSmithKline UK Ltd)

Sumatriptan (as Sumatriptan succinate) 12 mg per 1 ml Imigran Subject 6mg/0.5ml solution for injection syringe refill pack | 2 pre-filled disposable injection PoM £48.49 DT = £48.49

Imigran Subject 6mg/0.5ml solution for injection pre-filled syringes with device | 2 pre-filled disposable injection PoM £50.96 DT = £50.96

Oral tablet

CAUTIONARY AND ADVISORY LABELS 3

▸ **Sumatriptan (Non-proprietary)**

Sumatriptan (as Sumatriptan succinate) 50 mg Sumatriptan 50mg tablets | 6 tablet PoM £24.85 DT = £0.72

Sumatriptan (as Sumatriptan succinate) 100 mg Sumatriptan 100mg tablets | 6 tablet PoM £41.18 DT = £0.86

▸ **Imigran** (GlaxoSmithKline UK Ltd)

Sumatriptan (as Sumatriptan succinate) 50 mg Imigran Radis 50mg tablets | 6 tablet PoM £23.90 DT = £0.72

Imigran 50mg tablets | 6 tablet PoM £31.85 DT = £0.72

Sumatriptan (as Sumatriptan succinate) 100 mg Imigran 100mg tablets | 6 tablet PoM £51.48 DT = £0.86

Imigran Radis 100mg tablets | 6 tablet PoM £42.90 DT = £0.86

Spray

CAUTIONARY AND ADVISORY LABELS 3

▸ **Imigran** (GlaxoSmithKline UK Ltd)

Sumatriptan 100 mg per 1 ml Imigran 10mg nasal spray | 2 unit dose PoM £14.16 DT = £14.16

Sumatriptan 200 mg per 1 ml Imigran 20mg nasal spray | 2 unit dose PoM £14.16 | 6 unit dose PoM £42.47 DT = £42.47

Zolmitriptan

03-Sep-2020

- **INDICATIONS AND DOSE**

Treatment of acute migraine

▸ BY MOUTH

▸ Child 12–17 years: 2.5 mg, followed by 2.5 mg after at least 2 hours if required, dose to be taken only if migraine recurs, if response unsatisfactory after 3 attacks consider increasing dose to 5 mg or switching to alternative treatment; maximum 10 mg per day

▸ BY INTRANASAL ADMINISTRATION

▸ Child 12–17 years: 5 mg, dose to be administered as soon as possible after onset into one nostril only, followed by 5 mg after at least 2 hours if required, dose to be administered only if migraine recurs; maximum 10 mg per day

Treatment of acute cluster headache

▸ BY INTRANASAL ADMINISTRATION

▸ Child 12–17 years: 5 mg, dose to be administered as soon as possible after onset into one nostril only, followed by 5 mg after at least 2 hours if required, dose to be administered only if migraine recurs; maximum 10 mg per day

DOSE ADJUSTMENTS DUE TO INTERACTIONS

▸ Manufacturer advises max. dose 5 mg in 24 hours with concurrent use of moderate and potent inhibitors of CYP1A2, cimetidine and moclobemide.

DOSE EQUIVALENCE AND CONVERSION

▸ 1 spray of *Zomig*® nasal spray = 5 mg zolmitriptan.

- **UNLICENSED USE** Not licensed for use in children.
- **CONTRA-INDICATIONS** Arrhythmias associated with accessory cardiac conduction pathways · coronary vasospasm · ischaemic heart disease · moderate to severe hypertension · peripheral vascular disease · previous cerebrovascular accident · previous myocardial infarction · Prinzmetal's angina · transient ischaemic attack · uncontrolled hypertension · Wolff-Parkinson-White syndrome
- **CAUTIONS** Conditions which predispose to coronary artery disease
- **INTERACTIONS** → Appendix 1: triptans
- **SIDE-EFFECTS**

  GENERAL SIDE-EFFECTS

  ▸ **Common or very common** Abdominal pain · asthenia · chest discomfort · dizziness · drowsiness · dry mouth · dysphagia · feeling hot · headache · limb discomfort · muscle weakness · nausea · pain · palpitations · sensation abnormal · vomiting

  ▸ **Uncommon** Tachycardia · urinary disorders

  ▸ **Rare or very rare** Angina pectoris · angioedema · coronary vasospasm · gastrointestinal disorders · gastrointestinal infarction · hypersensitivity · myocardial infarction · splenic infarction · urticaria

  SPECIFIC SIDE-EFFECTS

  ▸ **Common or very common**

  ▸ With intranasal use Feeling abnormal · haemorrhage · myalgia · nasal discomfort · taste altered · throat pain

  ▸ With oral use Muscle complaints · sensation of pressure · throat complaints

  ▸ **Rare or very rare**

  ▸ With oral use Diarrhoea

  SIDE-EFFECTS, FURTHER INFORMATION Discontinue if symptoms of heat, heaviness, pressure or tightness (including throat and chest) occur.
- **PREGNANCY** There is limited experience of using $5HT_1$-receptor agonists during pregnancy; manufacturers advise that they should be avoided unless the potential benefit outweighs the risk.
- **BREAST FEEDING** Use with caution—present in milk in *animal* studies.
- **HEPATIC IMPAIRMENT** Manufacturer advises caution in moderate to severe impairment (risk of increased exposure).

  Dose adjustments In adults, manufacturer advises maximum 5 mg in 24 hours in moderate to severe impairment.
- **DIRECTIONS FOR ADMINISTRATION** Zolmitriptan orodispersible tablets should be placed on the tongue, allowed to disperse and swallowed.

- **PATIENT AND CARER ADVICE** Patients or carers should be given advice on how to administer zolmitriptan orodispersible tablets.

- **MEDICINAL FORMS** There can be variation in the licensing of different medicines containing the same drug.

Oral tablet

- **Zolmitriptan (Non-proprietary)**
  Zolmitriptan 2.5 mg Zolmitriptan 2.5mg tablets | 6 tablet PoM £31.50 DT = £28.83 | 12 tablet PoM £51.00 DT = £57.67
  Zolmitriptan 5 mg Zolmitriptan 5mg tablets | 6 tablet PoM £36.00-£64.70 DT = £36.00 | 12 tablet PoM £72.00 DT = £72.00
- **Zomig** (Grunenthal Ltd)
  Zolmitriptan 2.5 mg Zomig 2.5mg tablets | 6 tablet PoM £23.94 DT = £28.83

Spray

- **Zolmitriptan (Non-proprietary)**
  Zolmitriptan 50 mg per 1 ml Zolmitriptan 5mg/0.1ml nasal spray unit dose | 6 unit dose PoM £40.15 DT = £40.15

Orodispersible tablet

EXCIPIENTS: May contain Aspartame

- **Zolmitriptan (Non-proprietary)**
  Zolmitriptan 2.5 mg Zolmitriptan 2.5mg orodispersible tablets sugar free | 6 tablet PoM £22.79 DT = £3.01 SF
  Zolmitriptan 5 mg Zolmitriptan 5mg orodispersible tablets sugar free | 6 tablet PoM £36.00 DT = £4.63 SF
- **Zomig Rapimelt** (Grunenthal Ltd)
  Zolmitriptan 2.5 mg Zomig Rapimelt 2.5mg orodispersible tablets | 6 tablet PoM £23.99 DT = £3.01 SF
  Zolmitriptan 5 mg Zomig Rapimelt 5mg orodispersible tablets | 6 tablet PoM £23.94 DT = £4.63 SF

5.2 Neuropathic pain

Neuropathic pain

06-Oct-2020

MHRA/CHM important safety information

When using antiepileptics for the management of neuropathic pain, see Epilepsy p. 227 for information on the use of antiepileptic drugs and the risk of suicidal thoughts and behaviour.

For information on the use of opioids and risk of dependence and addiction, see *Important safety information* in individual drug monographs.

Overview and management

Neuropathic pain, which occurs as a result of damage to neural tissue, includes *compression neuropathies*, *peripheral neuropathies* (e.g. due to Diabetic complications p. 556, HIV infection p. 505, chemotherapy), *trauma*, *idiopathic neuropathy*, *central pain* (e.g. pain following spinal cord injury and syringomyelia), *postherpetic neuralgia*, and *phantom limb pain*. The pain may occur in an area of sensory deficit and may be described as burning, shooting or scalding; it may be accompanied by pain that is evoked by a non-noxious stimulus (allodynia).

Children with chronic neuropathic pain require multidisciplinary management, which may include physiotherapy and psychological support. Neuropathic pain is generally managed with a **tricyclic antidepressant** such as amitriptyline hydrochloride p. 289 or **antiepileptic drugs** such as carbamazepine p. 234. Children with localised pain may benefit from **topical local anaesthetic** preparations, particularly while awaiting specialist review. Neuropathic pain may respond only partially to **opioid analgesics**. A corticosteroid may help to relieve pressure in compression neuropathy and thereby reduce pain.

Chronic facial pain

Chronic oral and facial pain including *persistent idiopathic facial pain* (also termed 'atypical facial pain') and *temporomandibular dysfunction* (previously termed temporomandibular joint pain dysfunction syndrome) may call for prolonged use of analgesics or for other drugs. **Tricyclic antidepressants** may be useful for facial pain [unlicensed indication], but are not on the Dental Practitioners' List. Disorders of this type require specialist referral and psychological support to accompany drug treatment. Children on long-term therapy need to be monitored both for progress and for side-effects.

6 Pyrexia

Fever

15-Jan-2025

Description of condition

Feverish illness occurs commonly in children, particularly in those aged under 5 years. Fever can be defined as an elevation of body temperature above the normal daily variation and is usually an indication of an underlying infection. In most cases fever is due to a self-limiting viral infection, but it may also be the presenting feature of a serious bacterial infection, such as meningitis or pneumonia. Fever can also be due to a non-infectious cause such as vaccinations, or caused by conditions such as Kawasaki disease and paediatric multisystem inflammatory syndrome. In some children there may be no obvious cause despite careful assessment; these children are of particular concern because it is difficult to distinguish between simple viral illnesses and life-threatening bacterial infections. A fever with no obvious cause is generally a problem in young children, and the younger the child the more difficult it is to establish a diagnosis and assess the severity of illness.

Children aged under 5 years

The following recommendations provide guidance for the initial assessment and early management of children presenting with a feverish illness.

Assessment

EvGr Children presenting with a feverish illness should be assessed for any immediate life-threatening features, including compromise of the airway, breathing or circulation, and decreased level of consciousness. In addition, consider sepsis for those with fever and signs or symptoms of possible sepsis, see NICE guideline: **Suspected sepsis: recognition, diagnosis and early management** (see *useful resources*).

The NICE traffic light system should be used in conjunction with other investigations to assess for the presence or absence of signs or symptoms that can be used to predict the risk of serious illness (with red being high risk, amber being intermediate risk, and green being low risk), and management directed by the level of risk. Children aged under 3 months with a temperature of 38°C or higher are at high risk of serious illness. The duration of fever should not be used to predict the likelihood of serious illness. However, children with a fever lasting 5 days or longer should be assessed for Kawasaki disease. (A) EvGr The child's vaccination status with regards to *Haemophilus influenzae*, *Neisseria meningitidis*, and *Streptococcus pneumoniae* should also be established and considered. (E) EvGr Assess for signs and symptoms of specific diseases such as meningococcal disease, bacterial meningitis, scarlet fever, invasive group A streptococcus disease, herpes simplex encephalitis, pneumonia, urinary-tract infection, septic arthritis/osteomyelitis, or Kawasaki disease. In addition, enquire about any recent travel abroad and consider the possibility of imported infections according to the region visited. (A) For further information on the NICE traffic light system, risk assessment for serious illness, referral, and signs and symptoms of specific illnesses, see NICE guideline: **Fever in under 5s** (see *Useful resources*).

EvGr If a diagnosis has been made, the child should be managed in accordance to guidance for the management of that condition. (A)

Management

EvGr Refer children with symptoms or a combination of signs and symptoms suggestive of a life-threatening illness immediately for emergency medical care. (A)

For guidance on urgent transfer to hospital, and administration of pre-hospital antibacterials in children with suspected sepsis, see Sepsis p. 362 and NICE guideline: **Suspected sepsis: recognition, diagnosis and early management** (see *Useful resources*).

EvGr Children with suspected bacterial meningitis or meningococcal disease should be urgently transferred to hospital. For children with strongly suspected bacterial meningitis, parenteral antibacterials should be given in the community if there is likely to be a clinically significant delay in transfer to hospital. For children with strongly suspected meningococcal disease, parenteral antibacterials should be given as soon as possible in the community prior to urgent transfer to hospital, unless this will delay transfer. (A) For further guidance, see Central nervous system infections, antibacterial therapy p. 365 and NICE guideline: **Meningitis (bacterial) and meningococcal disease: recognition, diagnosis and management** (available at: www.nice.org.uk/guidance/ng240

EvGr Children assessed as high risk on the NICE traffic light system but who are not considered to have an immediately life-threatening illness, should be urgently referred to a paediatric specialist. (A) For further information on the management of children with any 'red-high risk' features or for information on the management of children with 'amber-intermediate risk' or 'green-low risk' features, see NICE guideline: **Fever in under 5s** (see *Useful resources*).

EvGr Following initial contact with a healthcare professional, parents and/or carers who are caring for a feverish child at home should be advised to seek further advice if:

- the child has a convulsion, develops a non-blanching rash, or has a fever that has lasted for 5 days or more;
- parents and/or carers are more worried or feel that the child is less well than when they previously sought advice, or are distressed or concerned that they are unable to look after the child.

In addition, parents and/or carers should be advised to consider seeking further advice if signs of dehydration (such as reduced urine output, dry mouth, absence of tears, sunken fontanelle, sunken eyes, and poor overall appearance) occur. Advice should also be provided about ensuring regular fluid intake to avoid dehydration (where a child is breastfed, the most appropriate fluid is breast milk), and on how to manage the child's fever.

Children should be dressed appropriately to prevent overheating or shivering; tepid sponging is not recommended to reduce body temperature.

Antipyretic drugs are not recommended for the sole aim of reducing body temperature in children with fever or for prevention of a febrile convulsion. Consider either paracetamol p. 325 or ibuprofen p. 821 for children with fever who appear distressed. If the child's distress is not alleviated with paracetamol p. 325, consider switching treatment to ibuprofen p. 821, and vice versa. Consider alternating paracetamol p. 325 and ibuprofen p. 821 if the child's distress persists or recurs before the next dose is due, but both drugs should not be given simultaneously. Antipyretic drugs should only be continued for as long as the child with fever appears distressed. (A)

Children aged 5 years and over

The following recommendations provide guidance for the initial assessment and early management of children presenting with a feverish illness.

Assessment

EvGr Children presenting with a feverish illness should be assessed for any immediate life-threatening features, including compromise of the airway, breathing or circulation, and decreased level of consciousness. (E) For children with fever and signs or symptoms of possible sepsis, see NICE guideline: **Suspected sepsis: recognition, diagnosis and early management** (see *Useful resources*).

EvGr The risk of serious illness should be guided by the history of the child's feverish illness, clinical examination, and the presence or absence of features associated with serious illness. The duration of fever should not be used to predict the likelihood of serious illness. However, children with a fever lasting 5 days or longer should be assessed for Kawasaki disease. The child's vaccination status with regards to *Haemophilus influenzae*, *Neisseria meningitidis*, and *Streptococcus pneumoniae* should also be established and considered. Assess for signs or symptoms of other specific diseases such as meningococcal disease, bacterial meningitis, scarlet fever, invasive group A streptococcus disease, herpes simplex encephalitis, pneumonia, urinary-tract infection, septic arthritis/osteomyelitis, or Kawasaki disease. In addition, consider the child's medical history, drug history, and any recent travel abroad and the possibility of an imported infection. (E)

Management

EvGr Clinicians should use their clinical judgement on when to refer children with fever for emergency medical care or further assessment. (E)

For guidance on urgent transfer to hospital, and administration of pre-hospital antibacterials in children with suspected sepsis, see Sepsis p. 362 and NICE guideline: **Suspected sepsis: recognition, diagnosis and early management** (see *Useful resources*).

EvGr Children with suspected bacterial meningitis or meningococcal disease should be urgently transferred to hospital. For children with strongly suspected bacterial meningitis, parenteral antibacterials should be given in the community if there is likely to be a clinically significant delay in transfer to hospital. For children with strongly suspected meningococcal disease, parenteral antibacterials should be given as soon as possible in the community prior to urgent transfer to hospital, unless this will delay transfer. (A) For further guidance, see Central nervous system infections, antibacterial therapy p. 365 and NICE guideline: **Meningitis (bacterial) and meningococcal disease: recognition, diagnosis and management** (available at: www.nice.org.uk/guidance/ng240).

EvGr Following initial contact with a healthcare professional, children and their parents and/or carers who are managing the fever at home should be advised to seek further advice if a convulsion occurs, a non-blanching rash develops, the fever has lasted for 5 days or more, or the child is less well than when advice was previously sought.

In addition, children and their parents and/or carers should be advised to consider seeking further advice if signs of dehydration (such as reduced urine output, dry mouth, absence of tears, sunken eyes, and poor overall appearance) occur. Advice should also be provided about ensuring regular fluid intake to avoid dehydration and on how to manage the fever.

Children should be dressed appropriately to prevent overheating or shivering; tepid sponging is not recommended to reduce body temperature.

Antipyretic drugs are not recommended for the sole aim of reducing body temperature in children with fever or for prevention of a febrile convulsion. Consider either paracetamol p. 325 or ibuprofen p. 821 for children with fever who appear distressed. If the child's distress is not alleviated with paracetamol p. 325, consider switching treatment to ibuprofen p. 821, and vice versa. Consider alternating paracetamol p. 325 and ibuprofen p. 821 if the child's distress persists or recurs before the next dose is due, but both drugs should not be given simultaneously. Antipyretic drugs should only be continued for as long as the child with fever appears distressed. (E)

Useful Resources

Fever in under 5s: assessment and initial management. National Institute for Health and Care Excellence. NICE guideline 143. November 2019, updated March 2024. www.nice.org.uk/guidance/ng143

Suspected sepsis: recognition, diagnosis and early management. National Institute for Health and Care Excellence. NICE guideline 51. July 2016, updated March 2024. www.nice.org.uk/guidance/ng51

7 Sleep disorders

7.1 Insomnia

Hypnotics and anxiolytics

Overview

Most anxiolytics ('sedatives') will induce sleep when given at night and most hypnotics will sedate when given during the day. Hypnotics and anxiolytics should be reserved for short courses to alleviate acute conditions after causal factors have been established.

The role of drug therapy in the management of anxiety disorders in children and adolescents is uncertain; drug therapy should be initiated only by specialists after psychosocial interventions have failed. Benzodiazepines and tricyclic antidepressants have been used but adverse effects may be problematic.

Hypnotics

The prescribing of hypnotics to children, except for occasional use such as for sedation for procedures is not justified. There is a risk of habituation with prolonged use. Problems settling children at night should be managed with behavioural therapy.

Dental procedures

Some anxious children may benefit from the use of a hypnotic the night before a dental appointment.

Chloral and derivatives

Chloral hydrate below and derivatives were formerly popular hypnotics for children. Chloral hydrate is now mainly used for sedation during diagnostic procedures.

Antihistamines

Some **antihistamines** such as promethazine hydrochloride p. 208 are used for occasional insomnia in adults; their prolonged duration of action can often cause drowsiness the following day. The sedative effect of antihistamines may diminish after a few days of continued treatment; antihistamines are associated with headache, psychomotor impairment and antimuscarinic effects. The use of hypnotics in children is not usually justified.

Melatonin

Melatonin p. 351 is a pineal hormone that may affect sleep pattern. Clinical experience suggests that when appropriate behavioural sleep interventions fail, melatonin may be of value for treating sleep onset insomnia and delayed sleep phase syndrome in children with conditions such as visual impairment, cerebral palsy, autism, and learning difficulties. It is also sometimes used before magnetic resonance imaging (MRI), computed tomography (CT), or EEG investigations. Little is known about its long-term effects in children, and there is uncertainty as to the effect on other circadian rhythms including endocrine or reproductive hormone secretion. The need to continue melatonin therapy should be reviewed every 6 months.

Anxiolytics

Anxiolytic treatment should be used in children only to relieve acute anxiety (and related insomnia) caused by fear (e.g. before surgery). Anxiolytic treatment should be limited to the lowest possible dose for the shortest possible time.

Buspirone

Buspirone hydrochloride is thought to act at specific serotonin ($5HT_{1A}$) receptors; safety and efficacy in children have yet to be determined.

HYPNOTICS, SEDATIVES AND ANXIOLYTICS › NON-BENZODIAZEPINE

Chloral hydrate

27-Apr-2023

● **INDICATIONS AND DOSE**

Sedation for painless procedures

▶ BY MOUTH

- Neonate: 30–50 mg/kg, to be given 45–60 minutes before procedure, doses up to 100 mg/kg may be used with respiratory monitoring.
- Child 1 month–11 years: 30–50 mg/kg (max. per dose 1 g), to be given 45–60 minutes before procedure, dose may be increased if necessary up to 100 mg/kg (max. per dose 2 g)
- Child 12–17 years: 1–2 g, to be given 45–60 minutes before procedure

▶ BY RECTUM

- Neonate: 30–50 mg/kg, to be given 45–60 minutes before procedure, doses up to 100 mg/kg may be used with respiratory monitoring, administration by rectum only if oral route not available.
- Child 1 month–11 years: 30–50 mg/kg (max. per dose 1 g), to be given 45–60 minutes before procedure, dose may be increased if necessary up to 100 mg/kg (max. per dose 2 g), administration by rectum only if oral route not available
- Child 12–17 years: 1–2 g, to be given 45–60 minutes before procedure, administration by rectum only if oral route not available

Severe insomnia [short-term use in patients with a suspected or definite neurodevelopmental disorder when insomnia is interfering with daily life and other therapies have failed] (specialist use only)

▶ BY MOUTH USING ORAL SOLUTION

- Child 2–11 years: 30–50 mg/kg once daily (max. per dose 1 g) for a maximum of 2 weeks, dose to be taken with water or milk at bedtime, repeat courses are not recommended and can only be administered after reassessment by a specialist
- Child 12–17 years: 430–860 mg once daily for a maximum of 2 weeks, dose to be taken with water or milk at bedtime, dose may be increased if necessary up to maximum 2 g once daily, repeat courses are not recommended and can only be administered after reassessment by a specialist

Severe insomnia, using cloral betaine 707 mg (≡ 414 mg chloral hydrate) tablets [short-term use in patients with a suspected or definite neurodevelopmental disorder when insomnia is interfering with daily life and other therapies have failed] (specialist use only)

▶ BY MOUTH USING TABLETS

▸ Child 12–17 years: 1–2 tablets once daily for a maximum of 2 weeks, dose to be taken with water or milk at bedtime, repeat courses are not recommended and can only be administered after reassessment by a specialist, alternatively 414–828 mg once daily for a maximum of 2 weeks, dose to be taken with water or milk at bedtime, repeat courses are not recommended and can only be administered after reassessment by a specialist; maximum 4 tablets per day; maximum 2 g per day

● **UNLICENSED USE** Not licensed for sedation for painless procedures.

IMPORTANT SAFETY INFORMATION

MHRA/CHM ADVICE: CHLORAL HYDRATE, CLORAL BETAINE (*WELLDORM*®): RESTRICTION OF PAEDIATRIC INDICATION (OCTOBER 2021)

Following a national review of safety and efficacy data, the use of chloral hydrate and cloral betaine (previously chloral betaine) for the treatment of severe insomnia has been further restricted in children and adolescents, to only those with a suspected or definite neurodevelopmental disorder when insomnia is interfering with daily life and other therapies have failed. Healthcare professionals are advised that their use in children and adolescents is not generally recommended and should be under specialist supervision. Repeat courses are not recommended and can only be administered after reassessment by a specialist. Following prolonged treatment, the dose should be tapered slowly before discontinuation, as abrupt discontinuation can lead to delirium. Treatment in all patients should be for the shortest duration possible and not exceeding 2 weeks.

● **CONTRA-INDICATIONS** Acute porphyrias p. 745 · gastritis · severe cardiac disease

● **CAUTIONS** Avoid contact with mucous membranes · avoid contact with skin · avoid prolonged use (and abrupt withdrawal thereafter)

● **INTERACTIONS** → Appendix 1: chloral hydrate

● **SIDE-EFFECTS** Agitation · allergic dermatitis · ataxia · confusion · delirium (more common on abrupt discontinuation) · drug use disorders · gastrointestinal discomfort · gastrointestinal disorders · headache · injury · ketonuria · kidney injury

● **PREGNANCY** Avoid.

● **BREAST FEEDING** Risk of sedation in infant—avoid.

● **HEPATIC IMPAIRMENT** Manufacturer advises avoid in marked impairment.

● **RENAL IMPAIRMENT** EvGr Caution in mild to moderate impairment; avoid in severe impairment. ⟨M⟩

Dose adjustments EvGr Dose adjustment may be necessary in mild to moderate impairment. ⟨M⟩

● **DIRECTIONS FOR ADMINISTRATION** For administration *by mouth*, expert sources advise dilute liquid with plenty of water or juice to mask unpleasant taste.

● **PRESCRIBING AND DISPENSING INFORMATION** Flavours of oral liquid formulations may include black currant.

The RCPCH and NPPG recommend that, when a liquid formulation of chloral hydrate is required, the following strength is used: 500 mg/5 mL.

● **PATIENT AND CARER ADVICE**

Driving and skilled tasks Drowsiness may persist the next day and affect performance of skilled tasks (e.g. driving); effects of alcohol enhanced.

● **LESS SUITABLE FOR PRESCRIBING** Chloral hydrate is less suitable for prescribing in insomnia.

● **MEDICINAL FORMS** There can be variation in the licensing of different medicines containing the same drug. Forms available from special-order manufacturers include: oral suspension, oral solution, suppository, enema

Oral solution

CAUTIONARY AND ADVISORY LABELS 1(paediatric solution only), 19 (solution other than paediatric only), 27

EXCIPIENTS: May contain Glucose, propylene glycol

▸ **Chloral hydrate (Non-proprietary)**

Chloral hydrate 28.66 mg per 1 ml Chloral hydrate 143.3mg/5ml oral solution BP | 150 ml PoM £244.25 DT = £244.25

Chloral hydrate 100 mg per 1 ml Chloral hydrate 500mg/5ml oral solution | 150 ml PoM £244.25 DT = £244.25

Melatonin

14-Dec-2022

● **INDICATIONS AND DOSE**

Sleep onset insomnia (initiated under specialist supervision) | Delayed sleep phase syndrome (initiated under specialist supervision)

▶ BY MOUTH USING MODIFIED-RELEASE TABLETS

▸ Child: Initially 2–3 mg once daily for 1–2 weeks, dose to be taken before bedtime, then increased if necessary to 4–6 mg once daily, dose to be taken before bedtime, dose can be increased if necessary up to maximum 10 mg per day

Insomnia in patients with learning disabilities and behaviour that challenges [where sleep hygiene measures have been insufficient] (initiated under specialist supervision)

▶ BY MOUTH USING MODIFIED-RELEASE TABLETS

▸ Child: Initially 2 mg once daily, dose to be taken 30–60 minutes before bedtime, increased if necessary to 4–6 mg once daily, dose to be taken 30–60 minutes before bedtime, dose can be increased if necessary up to maximum 10 mg per day

Insomnia in patients with ADHD [where sleep hygiene measures have been insufficient] (initiated under specialist supervision)

▶ BY MOUTH USING IMMEDIATE-RELEASE MEDICINES

▸ Child 6–17 years: Initially 1–2 mg once daily, dose to be taken 30–60 minutes before bedtime, increased if necessary up to 5 mg once daily, dose to be taken 30–60 minutes before bedtime, dose to be increased in steps of 1 mg at weekly intervals

DOSE EQUIVALENCE AND CONVERSION

▸ Caution is advised when switching between *immediate-release* formulations as the peak plasma-melatonin concentration may be higher with the oral solution than with tablets.

PHARMACOKINETICS

▸ The intake of food with *immediate-release* formulations may increase the bioavailability of melatonin—see *Directions for administration*.

SLENYTO®

Insomnia with autism spectrum disorder [where sleep hygiene measures have been insufficient] | Insomnia with Smith-Magenis syndrome [where sleep hygiene measures have been insufficient]

▶ BY MOUTH USING MODIFIED-RELEASE TABLETS

▸ Child 2-17 years: Initially 2 mg once daily, dose to be taken 30-60 minutes before bedtime, increased if necessary to 5 mg once daily, dose to be taken

continued →

30-60 minutes before bedtime, dose can be increased if necessary up to maximum 10 mg per day

- **UNLICENSED USE** EvGr Melatonin is used for insomnia in patients with learning disabilities and behaviour that challenges, (E) but is not licensed for this indication.

  Melatonin is used for sleep onset insomnia and delayed sleep phase syndrome, but is not licensed for these indications.

- **CAUTIONS** Autoimmune disease · susceptibility to seizures (risk of increased seizure frequency)

  CAUTIONS, FURTHER INFORMATION

  - Autoimmune disease EvGr Avoid—limited information available in patients with autoimmune disease; exacerbation reported occasionally. (M)

- **INTERACTIONS** → Appendix 1: melatonin
- **SIDE-EFFECTS**
  - **Common or very common** Arthralgia · behaviour abnormal · drowsiness · feeling abnormal · increased risk of infection · mood altered · pain · sudden onset of sleep
  - **Uncommon** Anxiety · asthenia · chest pain · dizziness · dry mouth · gastrointestinal discomfort · headaches · hyperbilirubinaemia · hypertension · menopausal symptoms · movement disorders · nausea · night sweats · oral disorders · skin reactions · sleep disorders · urine abnormalities · weight increased
  - **Rare or very rare** Angina pectoris · arthritis · concentration impaired · crying · depression · disorientation · electrolyte imbalance · excessive tearing · gastrointestinal disorders · haemorrhage · hot flush · hypertriglyceridaemia · leucopenia · memory loss · muscle complaints · nail disorder · palpitations · paraesthesia · prostatitis · seizures · sexual dysfunction · syncope · thirst · thrombocytopenia · urinary disorders · vertigo · vision disorders · vomiting
  - **Frequency not known** Angioedema · appetite decreased · constipation · dyspnoea · galactorrhoea · hyperglycaemia · neutropenia
- **PREGNANCY** No information available—avoid.
- **BREAST FEEDING** Present in milk—avoid.
- **HEPATIC IMPAIRMENT** EvGr For *modified-release tablets*, avoid (risk of decreased clearance; limited information available). For *immediate-release formulations*, avoid in moderate or severe impairment (risk of decreased clearance; limited information available). (M)
- **RENAL IMPAIRMENT** EvGr For *modified-release tablets*, caution (no information available). For *immediate-release formulations*, caution (increased risk of exposure; limited information available); avoid in severe impairment. (M)
- **DIRECTIONS FOR ADMINISTRATION** EvGr Modified-release tablets should be taken with or after food. Licensed immediate-release formulations should be taken on an empty stomach, 2 hours before or 2 hours after food (ideally at least 3 hours after food in those with significantly impaired glucose tolerance or diabetes)—intake with carbohydrate-rich meals may impair blood glucose control. The immediate-release tablet *Adaflex*® may be crushed and mixed with water immediately before administration.

  The modified-release tablet *Slenyto*® may be mixed whole into food or drink (e.g. yoghurt, orange juice, or ice-cream) immediately before administration. (M)

- **PRESCRIBING AND DISPENSING INFORMATION** Treatment with melatonin should be initiated and supervised by a specialist, but may be continued by general practitioners. The need to continue melatonin therapy should be reviewed every 6 months.

  Licensed doses differ between preparations—further information can be found in the product literature for the individual preparations. Melatonin is available as a modified-release tablet (*Circadin*® and *Slenyto*®) and also as immediate-release formulations, including a tablet (*Adaflex*®, *Ceyesto*®, and *Syncrodin*®), hard capsule, and oral solution. *Circadin*® is licensed for the short-term treatment of primary insomnia in adults aged 55 years and over, and some immediate-release formulations, such as *Adaflex*®, *Ceyesto*®, and *Syncrodin*®, are licensed for the short-term treatment of jet lag in adults. *Adaflex*®, *Ceyesto*®, and *Slenyto*® are used for the treatment of insomnia associated with behavioural disorders in children and adolescents. Unlicensed preparations are also available, however, there is variability in clinical effect of unlicensed formulations.

  The RCPCH and NPPG recommend that, when a liquid special of melatonin is required, the following strength is used: 1 mg/mL.

- **PATIENT AND CARER ADVICE** Patients or their carers should be counselled on the administration of melatonin.

  Medicines for Children leaflet: Melatonin for sleep disorders www.medicinesforchildren.org.uk/medicines/melatonin-for-sleep-disorders/

- **NATIONAL FUNDING/ACCESS DECISIONS**

  For full details see funding body website

  Scottish Medicines Consortium (SMC) decisions

  - **Melatonin (*Slenyto*®) for the treatment of insomnia in children aged 2 years and over with autism spectrum disorder (ASD) and/or Smith-Magenis syndrome, where sleep hygiene measures have been insufficient (January 2021)** SMC No. SMC2306 Not recommended

  All Wales Medicines Strategy Group (AWMSG) decisions

  - **Melatonin (*Slenyto*®) for the treatment of insomnia in children aged 2 years and over with autism spectrum disorder (ASD) and/or Smith-Magenis syndrome, where sleep hygiene measures have been insufficient (March 2021)** AWMSG No. 4694 Recommended

- **MEDICINAL FORMS** There can be variation in the licensing of different medicines containing the same drug. Forms available from special-order manufacturers include: oral tablet, modified-release tablet, oral solution

Oral tablet

CAUTIONARY AND ADVISORY LABELS 2

- **Melatonin (Non-proprietary)**

  Melatonin 500 microgram VesPro Melatonin 500microgram tablets | 1000 tablet PoM ⊠

  Melatonin 1 mg Melatonin 1mg tablets | 90 tablet PoM ⊠

  Melatonin 3 mg Melatonin 3mg tablets | 30 tablet PoM £19.81 DT = £11.25

  Melatonin 5 mg Melatonin Extra Strength 5mg tablets | 60 tablet PoM ⊠

  Melatonin 5mg tablets | 30 tablet PoM £10.89 DT = £10.89

- **Adaflex** (AGB-Pharma)

  Melatonin 1 mg Adaflex 1mg tablets | 30 tablet PoM £10.89 DT = £10.89

  Melatonin 2 mg Adaflex 2mg tablets | 30 tablet PoM £10.89 DT = £10.89

  Melatonin 3 mg Adaflex 3mg tablets | 30 tablet PoM £10.89 DT = £11.25

  Melatonin 4 mg Adaflex 4mg tablets | 30 tablet PoM £10.89 DT = £10.89

  Melatonin 5 mg Adaflex 5mg tablets | 30 tablet PoM £10.89 DT = £10.89

- **Ceyesto** (Alturix Ltd)

  Melatonin 3 mg Ceyesto 3mg tablets | 30 tablet PoM £10.99 DT = £11.25

- **Mellozzan** (Medice UK Ltd)

  Melatonin 2 mg Mellozzan 2mg tablets | 30 tablet PoM £10.89 DT = £10.89

  Melatonin 3 mg Mellozzan 3mg tablets | 30 tablet PoM £10.89 DT = £11.25

  Melatonin 5 mg Mellozzan 5mg tablets | 30 tablet PoM £10.89 DT = £10.89

- **Syncrodin** (Pharma Nord (UK) Ltd)

  Melatonin 3 mg Syncrodin 3mg tablets | 30 tablet PoM £14.95 DT = £11.25

Modified-release tablet

CAUTIONARY AND ADVISORY LABELS 2, 21, 25

▸ **Melatonin (Non-proprietary)**

Melatonin 2 mg Melatonin 2mg modified-release tablets | 30 tablet [PoM] £15.39 DT = £1.42

Melatonin 3 mg Melatonin 3mg modified-release tablets | 120 tablet [PoM] [X]

▸ **Circadin** (Flynn Pharma Ltd)

Melatonin 2 mg Circadin 2mg modified-release tablets | 30 tablet [PoM] £15.39 DT = £1.42

▸ **Slenyto** (Flynn Pharma Ltd)

Melatonin 1 mg Slenyto 1mg modified-release tablets | 60 tablet [PoM] £32.96 DT = £32.96

Melatonin 5 mg Slenyto 5mg modified-release tablets | 30 tablet [PoM] £82.40 DT = £82.40

Oral solution

CAUTIONARY AND ADVISORY LABELS 2

EXCIPIENTS: May contain Propylene glycol, sorbitol

▸ **Melatonin (Non-proprietary)**

Melatonin 1 mg per 1 ml Melatonin 1mg/ml oral solution sugar free | 50 ml [PoM] £6.85–£7.53 [SF] | 60 ml [PoM] £19.77–£60.00 [SF] | 100 ml [PoM] £10.00–£86.67 [SF] | 150 ml [PoM] £9.31–£130.00 DT = £10.29 [SF]

Melatonin 2 mg per 1 ml Melatonin 2mg/ml oral solution sugar free | 25 ml [PoM] £55.00 DT = £55.00 [SF]

▸ **Ceyesto** (Alturix Ltd)

Melatonin 1 mg per 1 ml Ceyesto 1mg/ml oral solution | 100 ml [PoM] £17.10 [SF] | 150 ml [PoM] £25.65 DT = £10.29 [SF]

▸ **Neomel** (Neoceuticals Ltd)

Melatonin 1 mg per 1 ml Neomel 1mg/ml oral solution | 150 ml [PoM] £25.60 DT = £10.29 [SF]

8 Substance dependence

Substance dependence

Guidance on treatment of drug misuse

Treatment of alcohol or opioid dependence in children requires specialist management. The UK health departments have produced guidance on the treatment of drug misuse in the UK. *Drug Misuse and Dependence: UK Guidelines on Clinical Management (*2017) is available at www.gov.uk/government/publications/drug-misuse-and-dependence-uk-guidelines-on-clinical-management.

Nicotine dependence

See Smoking cessation below.

Neonatal abstinence syndrome

Neonatal abstinence syndrome occurs at birth as a result of intra-uterine exposure to opioids or high-dose benzodiazepines. Treatment is usually initiated if:

- feeding becomes a problem and tube feeding is required;
- there is profuse vomiting or watery diarrhoea;
- the baby remains very unsettled after two consecutive feeds despite gentle swaddling and the use of a pacifier.

Treatment involves weaning the baby from the drug on which it is dependent. Morphine p. 338 or methadone hydrochloride p. 357 can be used in babies of mothers who have been taking opioids. Morphine is widely used because the dose can be easily adjusted, but methadone hydrochloride may provide smoother control of symptoms. Weaning babies from opioids usually takes 7–10 days.

Weaning babies from benzodiazepines that have a long half-life is difficult to manage; chlorpromazine hydrochloride p. 295 may be used in these situations but excessive sedation may occur. For babies who are dependent on barbiturates, phenobarbital p. 264 may be tried, although it does not control gastro-intestinal symptoms.

8.1 Nicotine dependence

Smoking cessation

24-Jan-2022

Overview

Smoking tobacco is the main cause of preventable illness and premature death in the UK. It is linked to a number of diseases such as cancer (primarily lung cancer), chronic obstructive pulmonary disease, and cardiovascular disease, and can lead to complications during pregnancy. Smoking cessation reduces the risk of developing or worsening of smoking-related illnesses, and the benefits begin as soon as an individual stops smoking.

Smoking cessation may be associated with temporary withdrawal symptoms caused by nicotine dependence, making it difficult for people to stop. These symptoms include nicotine cravings, irritability, depression, restlessness, poor concentration, light-headedness, sleep disturbances, and increased appetite. Weight gain is a concern for many people who stop smoking, however it is less likely to occur when drug treatment is used to aid smoking cessation.

Alternative forms of tobacco (smokeless tobacco) that are placed in the nose or mouth and not burned, are also associated with significant health risks such as oropharyngeal cancers, cardiovascular disease, and periodontal disease. As with smoking cessation, smokeless tobacco cessation reduces the risk of tobacco-related health problems, but may cause withdrawal symptoms.

Management

[EvGr] Individuals who use smokeless tobacco should be advised to stop, and be offered referral to local specialist tobacco cessation services for interventions and support. ⟨A⟩ For further guidance on smokeless tobacco cessation, see NICE guideline: **Tobacco: preventing uptake, promoting quitting and treating dependence** (see *Useful resources*).

[EvGr] Individuals who smoke tobacco should be advised to stop smoking and be offered interventions and support to facilitate smoking cessation. They should also be advised that stopping in one step ('stop in one go') offers the best chance of lasting success, and that a combination of drug treatment and behavioural support is likely to be the most effective approach. The 'stop in one go' approach is when an individual makes a commitment to stop smoking on or before a particular date (the quit date), rather than by gradually reducing their smoking. Individuals who are unwilling, or not ready, to stop smoking in one go may benefit from a 'harm reduction approach' that includes cutting down before stopping smoking, reducing smoking (without intending to stop), or temporarily not smoking. Although existing evidence is not clear about the health benefits of smoking reduction, it may mean individuals are more likely to stop smoking altogether in the future.

Individuals who wish to stop or reduce their harm from smoking should be referred to local stop-smoking services, if appropriate, where they will be provided with advice, drug treatment, and behavioural support options such as individual counselling or group meetings. Individuals who decline referral to local stop-smoking services should be referred to a suitable healthcare professional who can also offer drug treatment and practical advice.

Follow-up appointments should be offered to individuals attempting to stop smoking and those reducing their harm. Individuals who do not achieve their quitting or harm-reduction goals, should be encouraged to try again and the various intervention options available should be discussed. ⟨A⟩

Drug treatment for children aged 12 years and over

For guidance on smoking cessation during pregnancy, see *Pregnancy*.

EvGr Nicotine replacement therapy (NRT) below is the only drug treatment that should be considered to aid smoking cessation in children aged 12 years and over, alongside behavioural support. A combination of long-acting NRT (transdermal patch) and short-acting NRT (lozenges, gum, sublingual tablets, inhalator, nasal spray and oral spray) is the most effective treatment option for smoking cessation in children. (A) Nicotine transdermal patches are generally applied for 16 hours, with the patch removed overnight; if the child experiences strong nicotine cravings upon waking, a 24 hour patch can be used instead. Short-acting nicotine preparations are used whenever the urge to smoke occurs or to prevent cravings. EvGr As all NRT preparations appear to be equally effective, the choice of preparation for each child should take into consideration the child's likely adherence, preferences, and previous experience of smoking-cessation aids, as well as contra-indications, and side-effects.

A quit date should be agreed when NRT is prescribed for smoking cessation, and treatment should be available before the child stops smoking. For those who have successfully stopped smoking, offer the opportunity for a further course of NRT to prevent a relapse to smoking.

Children who are unwilling or not ready to stop smoking may also benefit from the use of NRT as part of a 'harm reduction approach', because the amount of nicotine in NRT is much lower and the way these products deliver nicotine makes them less addictive than smoking tobacco. These children should be advised that NRT will make it easier to reduce how much they smoke and improve their chance of stopping in the long-term. NRT can be used for as long as needed to help prevent a return to previous levels of smoking. (A)

In the UK, sale of e-cigarettes is prohibited in children under 18 years of age.

Pregnancy

EvGr Pregnant females should always be advised to stop smoking completely, and be informed about the risks to the unborn child of smoking during pregnancy and the harmful effects of exposure to second-hand smoke for both mother and baby. All pregnant females who smoke or have stopped smoking in the last 2 weeks should be referred to local stop-smoking services, and ongoing intensive support should be offered during and following pregnancy. For pregnant females who are reluctant or unable to attend stop-smoking services, consider alternative options such as home visits, and providing details for telephone quitlines or online stop-smoking support. Smoking cessation should also be encouraged for all members of the household.

Nicotine replacement therapy (NRT) should be considered along with behavioural support at the earliest opportunity in pregnancy. Pregnant females should be advised that compared to smoking tobacco, using NRT has much lower risks and is less addictive because of the much lower amount of nicotine in NRT and the way these products deliver nicotine. NRT may be continued after pregnancy, if needed, to prevent a relapse to smoking. (A)

Concomitant drugs

Polycyclic aromatic hydrocarbons found in tobacco smoke increase the metabolism of some drugs by inducing hepatic enzymes, often requiring an increase in dose. Information about drugs interacting with tobacco smoke can be found under *Interactions* of the relevant drug monograph.

Useful Resources

Tobacco: preventing uptake, promoting quitting and treating dependence. National Institute for Health and Care Excellence guideline NG209. November 2021, updated February 2025.
www.nice.org.uk/guidance/ng209

National Centre for Smoking Cessation and Training.
www.ncsct.co.uk

NICOTINIC RECEPTOR AGONISTS

Nicotine

17-Mar-2022

● **INDICATIONS AND DOSE**

Nicotine replacement therapy in individuals who smoke fewer than 20 cigarettes each day

▶ BY MOUTH USING CHEWING GUM
- Child 12–17 years: 2 mg as required, chew 1 piece of gum when the urge to smoke occurs or to prevent cravings, if attempting smoking cessation, treatment should continue for 3 months before reducing the dose

▶ BY SUBLINGUAL ADMINISTRATION USING SUBLINGUAL TABLETS
- Child 12–17 years: 1 tablet every 1 hour, increased to 2 tablets every 1 hour if required, if attempting smoking cessation, treatment should continue for up to 3 months before reducing the dose; maximum 40 tablets per day

Nicotine replacement therapy in individuals who smoke more than 20 cigarettes each day or who require more than 15 pieces of 2-mg strength gum each day

▶ BY MOUTH USING CHEWING GUM
- Child 12–17 years: 4 mg as required, chew 1 piece of gum when the urge to smoke occurs or to prevent cravings, individuals should not exceed 15 pieces of 4-mg strength gum daily, if attempting smoking cessation, treatment should continue for 3 months before reducing the dose

Nicotine replacement therapy in individuals who smoke more than 20 cigarettes each day

▶ BY SUBLINGUAL ADMINISTRATION USING SUBLINGUAL TABLETS
- Child 12–17 years: 2 tablets every 1 hour, if attempting smoking cessation, treatment should continue for up to 3 months before reducing the dose; maximum 40 tablets per day

Nicotine replacement therapy

▶ BY INHALATION USING INHALATOR
- Child 12–17 years: As required, the cartridges can be used when the urge to smoke occurs or to prevent cravings, individuals should not exceed 12 cartridges of the 10-mg strength daily, or 6 cartridges of the 15-mg strength daily

▶ BY MOUTH USING LOZENGES
- Child 12–17 years: 1 lozenge every 1–2 hours as required, one lozenge should be used when the urge to smoke occurs, individuals who smoke less than 20 cigarettes each day should usually use the lower-strength lozenges; individuals who smoke more than 20 cigarettes each day and those who fail to stop smoking with the low-strength lozenges should use the higher-strength lozenges; If attempting smoking cessation, treatment should continue for 6–12 weeks before attempting a reduction in dose; maximum 15 lozenges per day

▶ BY MOUTH USING OROMUCOSAL SPRAY
- Child 12–17 years: 1–2 sprays as required, individuals can spray in the mouth when the urge to smoke occurs or to prevent cravings, individuals should not exceed 2 sprays per episode (up to 4 sprays every hour); maximum 64 sprays per day

▶ BY INTRANASAL ADMINISTRATION USING NASAL SPRAY
- Child 12–17 years: 1 spray as required, individuals can spray into each nostril when the urge to smoke occurs, up to twice every hour for 16 hours daily, if attempting smoking cessation, treatment should continue for

8 weeks before reducing the dose; maximum 64 sprays per day

▶ BY TRANSDERMAL APPLICATION USING PATCHES

▶ Child 12–17 years: Individuals who smoke more than 10 cigarettes daily should apply a high-strength patch daily for 6–8 weeks, followed by the medium-strength patch for 2 weeks, and then the low-strength patch for the final 2 weeks; individuals who smoke fewer than 10 cigarettes daily can usually start with the medium-strength patch for 6–8 weeks, followed by the low-strength patch for 2–4 weeks; a slower titration schedule can be used in individuals who are not ready to quit but want to reduce cigarette consumption before a quit attempt; if abstinence is not achieved, or if withdrawal symptoms are experienced, the strength of the patch used should be maintained or increased until the patient is stabilised; individuals using the high-strength patch who experience excessive side-effects, that do not resolve within a few days, should change to a medium-strength patch for the remainder of the initial period and then use the low-strength patch for 2–4 weeks

● **UNLICENSED USE** All preparations are licensed for children over 12 years (with the exception of *Nicotinell®* lozenges which are licensed for children under 18 years only when recommended by a doctor).

● **CAUTIONS**

GENERAL CAUTIONS Diabetes mellitus—blood-glucose concentration should be monitored closely when initiating treatment · haemodynamically unstable patients hospitalised with cerebrovascular accident · haemodynamically unstable patients hospitalised with myocardial infarction · haemodynamically unstable patients hospitalised with severe arrhythmias · phaeochromocytoma · uncontrolled hyperthyroidism

SPECIFIC CAUTIONS

▶ When used by inhalation Bronchospastic disease · chronic throat disease · obstructive lung disease

▶ With intranasal use Bronchial asthma (may exacerbate)

▶ With oral use Gastritis (can be aggravated by swallowed nicotine) · *gum* may also stick to and damage dentures · oesophagitis (can be aggravated by swallowed nicotine) · peptic ulcers (can be aggravated by swallowed nicotine)

▶ With transdermal use *patches* should not be placed on broken skin · patients with skin disorders

CAUTIONS, FURTHER INFORMATION Most warnings for nicotine replacement therapy also apply to continued cigarette smoking, but the risk of continued smoking outweighs any risks of using nicotine preparations.

Specific cautions for individual preparations are usually related to the local effect of nicotine.

● **SIDE-EFFECTS**

GENERAL SIDE-EFFECTS

▶ **Common or very common** Dizziness · headache · hyperhidrosis · nausea · palpitations · skin reactions · vomiting

▶ **Uncommon** Flushing

SPECIFIC SIDE-EFFECTS

▶ **Common or very common**

▶ When used by inhalation Asthenia · cough · dry mouth · flatulence · gastrointestinal discomfort · hiccups · hypersensitivity · nasal complaints · oral disorders · taste altered · throat complaints

▶ With intranasal use Chest discomfort · cough · dyspnoea · epistaxis · nasal complaints · paraesthesia · throat irritation

▶ With oral use Anxiety · appetite abnormal · burping · diarrhoea · dyspepsia (may be caused by swallowed nicotine) · gastrointestinal disorders · hiccups · increased risk of infection · mood altered · oral disorders · sleep disorders

▶ With sublingual use Asthenia · cough · dry mouth · flatulence · gastrointestinal discomfort · hiccups · hypersensitivity · oral disorders · rhinitis · taste altered · throat complaints

▶ **Uncommon**

▶ When used by inhalation Abnormal dreams · arrhythmias · bronchospasm · burping · chest discomfort · dysphonia · dyspnoea · hypertension · malaise

▶ With intranasal use Abnormal dreams · asthenia · hypertension · malaise

▶ With oral use Anger · asthma exacerbated · cough · dyspepsia aggravated · dysphagia · haemorrhage · laryngospasm · nasal complaints · nocturia · numbness · overdose · pain · palpitations exacerbated · peripheral oedema · tachycardia · taste altered · throat complaints · vascular disorders

▶ With sublingual use Abnormal dreams · arrhythmias · bronchospasm · burping · chest discomfort · dysphonia · dyspnoea · hypertension · malaise · nasal complaints

▶ With transdermal use Arrhythmias · asthenia · chest discomfort · dyspnoea · hypertension · malaise · myalgia · paraesthesia

▶ **Rare or very rare**

▶ When used by inhalation Dysphagia

▶ With intranasal use Arrhythmias

▶ With oral use Coagulation disorder · platelet disorder

▶ With sublingual use Dysphagia

▶ With transdermal use Abdominal discomfort · angioedema · pain in extremity

▶ **Frequency not known**

▶ When used by inhalation Angioedema · excessive tearing · vision blurred

▶ With intranasal use Abdominal discomfort · angioedema · excessive tearing · oropharyngeal complaints

▶ With sublingual use Excessive tearing · muscle tightness · vision blurred

SIDE-EFFECTS, FURTHER INFORMATION Some systemic effects occur on initiation of therapy, particularly if the patient is using high-strength preparations; however, the patient may confuse side-effects of the nicotine-replacement preparation with nicotine withdrawal symptoms. Common symptoms of nicotine withdrawal include malaise, headache, dizziness, sleep disturbance, coughing, influenza-like symptoms, depression, irritability, increased appetite, weight gain, restlessness, anxiety, drowsiness, aphthous ulcers, decreased heart rate, and impaired concentration.

● **PREGNANCY** [EvGr] The use of nicotine replacement therapy is preferable to the continuation of smoking. Nicotine replacement therapy should be considered alongside behavioural support, at the earliest opportunity in pregnancy and continued after pregnancy if needed. If patches are used, they should be removed before bed. (A)
See also *Pregnancy* in Smoking cessation p. 353.

● **BREAST FEEDING** Nicotine is present in milk; however, the amount to which the infant is exposed is small and less hazardous than second-hand smoke. Intermittent therapy is preferred.

● **HEPATIC IMPAIRMENT** Manufacturer advises caution in moderate to severe impairment (risk of decreased clearance).

● **RENAL IMPAIRMENT** [EvGr] Use with caution in severe renal impairment. (M)

● **DIRECTIONS FOR ADMINISTRATION** [EvGr] Acidic beverages, such as coffee or fruit juice, may decrease the absorption of nicotine through the buccal mucosa and should be avoided for 15 minutes before the use of oral nicotine replacement therapy. (M)

Administration by transdermal patch Patches should be applied on waking to dry, non-hairy skin on the hip, trunk, or upper arm and held in position for 10–20 seconds to ensure adhesion; place next patch on a different area and avoid using the same site for several days.

Administration by nasal spray [EvGr] Initially 1 spray should be used in both nostrils but when withdrawing from therapy, the dose can be gradually reduced to 1 spray in 1 nostril. ⟨M⟩

Administration by oral spray The oral spray should be released into the mouth, holding the spray as close to the mouth as possible and avoiding the lips. The patient should not inhale while spraying and avoid swallowing for a few seconds after use. If using the oral spray for the first time, or if unit not used for 2 or more days, prime the unit before administration.

Administration by sublingual tablet Each tablet should be placed under the tongue and allowed to dissolve.

Administration by lozenge Slowly allow each lozenge to dissolve in the mouth; periodically move the lozenge from one side of the mouth to the other. Lozenges last for 10–30 minutes, depending on their size.

Administration by inhalation Insert the cartridge into the device and draw in air through the mouthpiece; each session can last for approximately 5 minutes. The amount of nicotine from 1 puff of the cartridge is less than that from a cigarette, therefore it is necessary to inhale more often than when smoking a cigarette. A single 15 mg cartridge lasts for approximately 40 minutes of intense use.

Administration by medicated chewing gum Chew the gum until the taste becomes strong, then rest it between the cheek and gum; when the taste starts to fade, repeat this process. One piece of gum lasts for approximately 30 minutes.

- **PRESCRIBING AND DISPENSING INFORMATION** Flavours of chewing gum and lozenges may include mint, freshfruit, freshmint, icy white, or cherry.
- **PATIENT AND CARER ADVICE** Patient or carers should be given advice on how to administer nicotine chewing gum, inhalators, lozenges, sublingual tablets, oral spray, nasal spray and patches.

- **MEDICINAL FORMS** There can be variation in the licensing of different medicines containing the same drug.

Spray

EXCIPIENTS: May contain Ethanol

▸ **Nicorette** (McNeil Products Ltd)

Nicotine 500 microgram per 1 dose Nicorette 500micrograms/dose nasal spray | 10 ml [GSL] £21.89 DT = £21.89

▸ **Nicorette QuickMist** (McNeil Products Ltd)

Nicotine 1 mg per 1 dose Nicorette QuickMist SmartTrack 1mg/dose mouthspray | 13.2 ml [GSL] £15.57 DT = £15.57 [SF] | 26.4 ml [GSL] £24.22 [SF]
Nicorette QuickMist 1mg/dose mouthspray freshmint | 13.2 ml [GSL] £15.57 DT = £15.57 [SF] | 26.4 ml [GSL] £24.22 [SF]
Nicorette QuickMist 1mg/dose mouthspray cool berry | 13.2 ml [GSL] £15.57 DT = £15.57 [SF] | 26.4 ml [GSL] £24.22 [SF]
Nicorette QuickMist 1mg/dose mouthspray spearmint | 13.2 ml [GSL] £15.57 DT = £15.57 [SF] | 26.4 ml [GSL] £24.22 [SF]

▸ **Nicotinell Rapid Relief** (Dr Reddy's Laboratories (UK) Ltd)

Nicotine 1 mg per 1 dose Nicotinell Rapid Relief 1mg/dose oromucosal spray | 13.2 ml [GSL] £13.17 DT = £15.57 [SF] | 26.4 ml [GSL] £19.75 [SF]

Inhalation vapour impregnated plug

▸ **Nicorette** (McNeil Products Ltd)

Nicotine 15 mg Nicorette 15mg Inhalator | 4 cartridge [GSL] £6.86 DT = £6.86 | 20 cartridge [GSL] £24.60 DT = £24.60 | 36 cartridge [GSL] £38.20 DT = £38.20

Sublingual tablet

CAUTIONARY AND ADVISORY LABELS 26

▸ **Nicorette Microtab** (McNeil Products Ltd)

Nicotine (as Nicotine beta-cyclodextrin complex) 2 mg Nicorette Microtab 2mg sublingual tablets | 100 tablet [GSL] £19.90 DT = £19.90 [SF]

Transdermal patch

▸ **NiQuitin** (Omega Pharma Ltd)

Nicotine 7 mg per 24 hour NiQuitin 7mg patches | 7 patch [GSL] £11.48 DT = £10.49

Nicotine 14 mg per 24 hour NiQuitin 14mg patches | 7 patch [GSL] £11.48 DT = £10.82

Nicotine 21 mg per 24 hour NiQuitin 21mg patches | 7 patch [GSL] £11.48 DT = £11.48

▸ **NiQuitin Clear** (Omega Pharma Ltd)

Nicotine 7 mg per 24 hour NiQuitin Clear 7mg patches | 7 patch [GSL] £11.48 DT = £10.49

Nicotine 14 mg per 24 hour NiQuitin Clear 14mg patches | 7 patch [GSL] £11.48 DT = £10.82 | 14 patch [GSL] £18.79

Nicotine 21 mg per 24 hour NiQuitin Clear 21mg patches | 7 patch [GSL] £11.48 DT = £11.48 | 14 patch [GSL] £18.79
NiQuitin Pre-Quit Clear 21mg patches | 7 patch [GSL] £11.48 DT = £11.48

▸ **Nicorette invisi** (McNeil Products Ltd)

Nicotine 10 mg per 16 hour Nicorette invisi 10mg/16hours patches | 7 patch [GSL] £11.85 DT = £11.85

Nicotine 15 mg per 16 hour Nicorette invisi 15mg/16hours patches | 7 patch [GSL] £11.85 DT = £11.85

Nicotine 25 mg per 16 hour Nicorette invisi 25mg/16hours patches | 7 patch [GSL] £11.85 DT = £11.85 | 14 patch [GSL] £20.99

▸ **Nicotinell TTS** (Dr Reddy's Laboratories (UK) Ltd)

Nicotine 7 mg per 24 hour Nicotinell TTS 10 patches | 7 patch [GSL] £10.49 DT = £10.49

Nicotine 14 mg per 24 hour Nicotinell TTS 20 patches | 7 patch [GSL] £10.82 DT = £10.82

Nicotine 21 mg per 24 hour Nicotinell TTS 30 patches | 7 patch [GSL] £11.48 DT = £11.48 | 21 patch [GSL] £28.20

Medicated chewing-gum

▸ **Nicorette** (McNeil Products Ltd)

Nicotine 2 mg Nicorette Freshmint 2mg medicated chewing gum | 30 piece [GSL] £5.44 DT = £5.44 [SF] | 105 piece [GSL] £12.37 DT = £12.37 [SF] | 210 piece [GSL] £20.11 DT = £20.11 [SF]
Nicorette Fruitfusion 2mg medicated chewing gum | 30 piece [GSL] £5.44 DT = £5.44 [SF] | 105 piece [GSL] £12.37 DT = £12.37 [SF]
Nicorette Original 2mg medicated chewing gum | 105 piece [GSL] £12.37 DT = £12.37 [SF] | 210 piece [GSL] £20.11 DT = £20.11 [SF]

Nicotine 4 mg Nicorette Fruitfusion 4mg medicated chewing gum | 105 piece [GSL] £15.14 [SF]
Nicorette Original 4mg medicated chewing gum | 105 piece [GSL] £15.14 [SF] | 210 piece [GSL] £24.89 [SF]
Nicorette Freshmint 4mg medicated chewing gum | 105 piece [GSL] £15.14 [SF] | 210 piece [GSL] £24.89 [SF]

▸ **Nicorette Icy White** (McNeil Products Ltd)

Nicotine 2 mg Nicorette Icy White 2mg medicated chewing gum | 30 piece [GSL] £5.44 DT = £5.44 [SF] | 105 piece [GSL] £12.37 DT = £12.37 [SF] | 210 piece [GSL] £20.11 DT = £20.11 [SF]

Nicotine 4 mg Nicorette Icy White 4mg medicated chewing gum | 105 piece [GSL] £15.14 [SF]

▸ **Nicotinell** (Dr Reddy's Laboratories (UK) Ltd)

Nicotine 2 mg Nicotinell Mint 2mg medicated chewing gum | 96 piece [GSL] £10.93 DT = £10.93 [SF] | 204 piece [GSL] £18.00 [SF]
Nicotinell Fruit 2mg medicated chewing gum | 96 piece [GSL] £10.93 DT = £10.93 [SF] | 204 piece [GSL] £18.00 [SF]

Nicotine 4 mg Nicotinell Mint 4mg medicated chewing gum | 96 piece [GSL] £13.57 DT = £10.18 [SF]
Nicotinell Fruit 4mg medicated chewing gum | 96 piece [GSL] £13.57 DT = £10.18 [SF]

Lozenge

EXCIPIENTS: May contain Aspartame

ELECTROLYTES: May contain Sodium

▸ **NiQuitin** (Omega Pharma Ltd)

Nicotine 2 mg NiQuitin Mint 2mg lozenges | 72 lozenge [GSL] £7.40 DT = £7.40 [SF]
NiQuitin Minis Citrus 2mg lozenges | 60 lozenge [GSL] £12.56 [SF]
NiQuitin Minis Mint 2mg lozenges | 60 lozenge [GSL] £12.56 [SF] | 100 lozenge [GSL] £17.74 [SF]

Nicotine 4 mg NiQuitin Minis Citrus 4mg lozenges | 60 lozenge [GSL] £12.56 DT = £12.56 [SF]
NiQuitin Mint 4mg lozenges | 72 lozenge [GSL] £7.40 DT = £7.40 [SF]
NiQuitin Minis Mint 4mg lozenges | 60 lozenge [GSL] £12.56 DT = £12.56 [SF] | 100 lozenge [GSL] £17.74 [SF]

▸ **Nicorette** (McNeil Products Ltd)

Nicotine 2 mg Nicorette Fruit 2mg lozenges | 40 lozenge [GSL] £7.01 DT = £7.37 [SF] | 80 lozenge [GSL] £12.05 DT = £12.05 [SF] | 160 lozenge [GSL] £21.70 [SF]
Nicorette Cools 2mg lozenges | 40 lozenge [GSL] £7.01 DT = £7.37 [SF] | 80 lozenge [GSL] £12.05 DT = £12.05 [SF] | 160 lozenge [GSL] £21.70 [SF]

Nicotine 4 mg Nicorette Fruit 4mg lozenges | 160 lozenge GSL £21.70 SF
Nicorette Cools 4mg lozenges | 80 lozenge GSL £12.17 DT = £12.17 SF

▸ **Nicotinell** (Dr Reddy's Laboratories (UK) Ltd)
Nicotine (as Nicotine bitartrate) 1 mg Nicotinell 1mg lozenges | 96 lozenge GSL £12.06 DT = £12.06 SF | 144 lozenge GSL £15.19 DT = £15.19 SF | 204 lozenge GSL £16.89 SF
Nicotine (as Nicotine bitartrate) 2 mg Nicotinell 2mg lozenges | 96 lozenge GSL £14.02 DT = £14.02 SF | 144 lozenge GSL £17.86 DT = £17.86 SF | 204 lozenge GSL £19.76 DT = £19.76 SF

8.2 Opioid dependence

ANALGESICS › OPIOIDS

F 327

Methadone hydrochloride

23-Sep-2024

● **INDICATIONS AND DOSE**

Neonatal opioid withdrawal

▸ BY MOUTH

▸ Neonate: Initially 100 micrograms/kg, then increased in steps of 50 micrograms/kg every 6 hours until symptoms are controlled, doses may vary, consult local guidelines, for maintenance, total daily dose that controls symptoms to be given in 2 divided doses.

● **UNLICENSED USE** Not licensed for use in children.

IMPORTANT SAFETY INFORMATION
Many preparations of Methadone oral solution are licensed for opioid drug addiction only but some are also licensed for analgesia in severe pain.

● **CONTRA-INDICATIONS** Phaeochromocytoma

● **CAUTIONS** Risk factors for QT-interval prolongation

CAUTIONS, FURTHER INFORMATION EvGr ECG monitoring recommended in patients with the following risk factors for QT-interval prolongation while taking methadone: history of cardiac conduction abnormalities, family history of sudden death, heart or liver disease, electrolyte abnormalities, or concomitant treatment with drugs that can prolong QT interval; patients requiring more than 100 mg daily should also be monitored. ⟨M⟩

● **INTERACTIONS** → Appendix 1: opioids

● **SIDE-EFFECTS** Dry eye · dysuria · hyperprolactinaemia · hypothermia · intracranial pressure increased · mood altered · nasal dryness · QT interval prolongation

SIDE-EFFECTS, FURTHER INFORMATION Methadone is a long-acting opioid therefore effects may be cumulative.

Methadone, even in low doses is a special hazard for children.

Overdose Methadone has a very long duration of action; patients may need to be monitored for long periods following large overdoses.

● **HEPATIC IMPAIRMENT** Manufacturer advises caution; consider avoiding in severe impairment (risk of increased exposure).

Dose adjustments Manufacturer advises consider dose reduction.

● **RENAL IMPAIRMENT** Avoid use or reduce dose; opioid effects increased and prolonged and increased cerebral sensitivity occurs.

● **TREATMENT CESSATION** Avoid abrupt withdrawal.

When used for neonatal opioid withdrawal, reduce dose over 7–10 days.

● **PRESCRIBING AND DISPENSING INFORMATION** Flavours of oral liquid formulations may include tolu.

METHADOSE ® The final strength of the methadone mixture to be dispensed to the patient must be specified on the prescription.

Important—care is required in prescribing and dispensing the **correct strength** since any confusion could lead to an overdose; this preparation should be dispensed only **after dilution** as appropriate with *Methadose*® Diluent (life of diluted solution 3 months) and is for drug dependent persons.

● **LESS SUITABLE FOR PRESCRIBING** Methadone linctus is less suitable for prescribing for cough in terminal disease (has a tendency to accumulate).

● **MEDICINAL FORMS** There can be variation in the licensing of different medicines containing the same drug. Forms available from special-order manufacturers include: oral tablet, oral capsule, oral suspension, oral solution

Oral tablet

CAUTIONARY AND ADVISORY LABELS 2

▸ **Methadone hydrochloride (Non-proprietary)**
Methadone hydrochloride 5 mg Methadone 5mg tablets | 50 tablet PoM £19.93–£34.20 DT = £19.93 CD2

Oral solution

CAUTIONARY AND ADVISORY LABELS 2

▸ **Methadone hydrochloride (Non-proprietary)**
Methadone hydrochloride 1 mg per 1 ml Methadone 1mg/ml oral solution | 100 ml PoM £0.92–£1.20 DT = £0.89 CD2 | 500 ml PoM £3.85–£5.40 DT = £4.45 CD2 | 2500 ml PoM £22.25–£34.80 CD2
Methadone 1mg/ml oral solution sugar free | 50 ml PoM £1.00 CD2 SF | 100 ml PoM £1.20 DT = £0.86 CD2 SF | 500 ml PoM £3.85–£6.00 DT = £4.30 CD2 SF | 2500 ml PoM £21.50–£32.10 CD2 SF

▸ **Methadose** (Rosemont Pharmaceuticals Ltd)
Methadone hydrochloride 10 mg per 1 ml Methadose 10mg/ml oral solution concentrate | 150 ml PoM £12.01 DT = £12.01 CD2 SF

▸ **Metharose** (Rosemont Pharmaceuticals Ltd)
Methadone hydrochloride 1 mg per 1 ml Metharose 1mg/ml oral solution sugar free | 500 ml PoM £6.82 DT = £4.30 CD2 SF

▸ **Physeptone** (Martindale Pharmaceuticals Ltd)
Methadone hydrochloride 1 mg per 1 ml Physeptone 1mg/ml oral solution sugar free | 100 ml PoM £1.27 DT = £0.86 CD2 SF | 500 ml PoM £6.42 DT = £4.30 CD2 SF | 2500 ml PoM £32.10 CD2 SF
Physeptone 1mg/ml mixture | 500 ml PoM £6.42 DT = £4.45 CD2 | 2500 ml PoM £32.10 CD2

Chapter 5
Infection

CONTENTS

1 Bacterial infection

Antibacterials, principles of therapy

10-Jun-2025

Antibacterial drug choice

Before selecting an antibacterial the clinician must first consider three factors— the patient, the known or likely causative organism, and the risk of bacterial resistance with repeated courses.

Factors related to the patient which must be considered include history of allergy, renal and hepatic function, susceptibility to infection (i.e. whether immunocompromised), ability to tolerate drugs by mouth, severity of illness, risk of complications, ethnic origin, age, whether taking other medication and, if female, whether pregnant, breast-feeding or taking an oral contraceptive.

The known or likely organism and its antibacterial sensitivity, in association with the factors above, will provide one or more antibacterial option. EvGr In children receiving antibacterial prophylaxis, an antibacterial from a different class should be used. (A)

Some children may be at higher risk of treatment failure. They include those who have had repeated antibacterial courses, a previous or current culture with resistant bacteria, or those at higher risk of developing complications.

Antibacterials, considerations before starting therapy

The following precepts should be considered before starting:

- Viral infections should not be treated with antibacterials. However, antibacterials may be used to treat secondary bacterial infection (e.g. bacterial pneumonia secondary to influenza);
- Samples should be taken for culture and sensitivity testing as appropriate; '**blind**' antibacterial prescribing for unexplained pyrexia usually leads to further difficulty in establishing the diagnosis;
- Knowledge of **prevalent organisms** and their current sensitivity is of great help in choosing an antibacterial before bacteriological confirmation is available. Generally, narrow-spectrum antibacterials are preferred to broad-spectrum antibacterials unless there is a clear clinical indication (e.g. life-threatening sepsis);
- The **dose** of an antibacterial varies according to a number of factors including age, weight, hepatic function, renal function, and severity of infection. The prescribing of the so-called 'standard' dose in serious infections may result in failure of treatment or even death of the patient; therefore it is important to prescribe a dose appropriate to the condition. An inadequate dose may also increase the likelihood of antibacterial resistance. On the other hand, for an antibacterial with a narrow margin between the toxic and therapeutic dose (e.g. an aminoglycoside) it is also important to avoid an excessive dose and the concentration of the drug in the plasma may need to be monitored;
- The **route** of administration of an antibacterial often depends on the severity of the infection. Life-threatening infections often require intravenous therapy. Antibacterials that are well absorbed may be given by mouth even for some serious infections. Parenteral administration is also appropriate when the oral route cannot be used (e.g. because of vomiting) or if absorption is inadequate (e.g. in neonates and young children). Whenever possible, painful intramuscular injections should be avoided in children;
- **Duration** of therapy depends on the nature of the infection and the response to treatment. Courses should not be unduly prolonged because they encourage resistance, they may lead to side-effects and they are costly. However, in certain infections such as tuberculosis or osteomyelitis it may be necessary to treat for prolonged periods. The prescription for an antibacterial should specify the duration of treatment or the date when treatment is to be reviewed.

For further guidance on the appropriate and effective use of antibacterials, see Antimicrobial stewardship p. 26.

Advice to be given to children and their parents and/or carers

If an antibacterial is given, advice should be given about directions for correct use and possible side-effects using verbal and written information.

If an antibacterial is **not** given, advice should be given about an antibacterial not being needed currently—discuss alternative options as appropriate, such as self-care with over-the-counter preparations, back-up (delayed) prescribing, or other non-pharmacological interventions.

Children and their parents, or carers should be advised to seek medical help if symptoms worsen rapidly or significantly at any time, if symptoms do not start to improve within an agreed time, if problems arise as a result of treatment, or if the child becomes systemically very unwell.

For information on advice for children and their family and/or carers when deciding if antibacterial treatment is necessary, see *Advice for patients and their family and/or carers* in Antimicrobial stewardship p. 26.

Antibacterials, considerations during therapy

EvGr Review choice of antibacterial if susceptibility results indicate bacterial resistance and symptoms are not improving—consult local microbiologist as needed. ⟨A⟩ If no bacterium is cultured, the antibacterial can be continued or stopped on clinical grounds.

Superinfection

In general, broad-spectrum antibacterial drugs such as the cephalosporins are more likely to be associated with adverse reactions related to the selection of resistant organisms e.g. *fungal infections* or *antibiotic-associated colitis* (pseudomembranous colitis); other problems associated with superinfection include vaginitis and pruritus ani.

Antibacterials, switching from parenteral to oral treatment

EvGr The ongoing parenteral administration of an antibacterial should be reviewed within 48 hours of treatment initiation and a switch to oral treatment considered if appropriate. ⟨A⟩ In older children it may be possible to switch to an oral antibacterial; in neonates and infants this should be done more cautiously because of the relatively high incidence of bacteraemia and the possibility of variable oral absorption.

Antibacterials for prophylaxis

In most situations, only a short course of prophylactic antibacterial is needed. Longer-term antibacterial prophylaxis is appropriate in specific indications such as vesico-ureteric reflux.

Notifiable diseases

In England, registered medical practitioners must report a suspected case of a notifiable disease listed below, or any other suspected infectious disease that may present a significant risk to human health as soon as possible. Urgent notifiable diseases must be reported to the local health protection team by telephone within 24 hours, and all cases reported using the online notification service within 3 days. For further information on reporting notifiable diseases, including the online service, see: www.gov.uk/guidance/notifiable-diseases-and-how-to-report-them.

Acute encephalitis	Legionnaires' disease
Acute flaccid paralysis (AFP) or Acute flaccid myelitis (AFM)	Leprosy
Acute infectious hepatitis (A/B/C)	Malaria
Acute meningitis	Measles
Acute poliomyelitis	Meningococcal septicaemia
Anthrax	Middle East respiratory syndrome (MERS)
Botulism	Mpox (previously known as monkeypox)
Brucellosis	Mumps
Chickenpox (varicella)	Neonatal herpes
Cholera	Plague
Congenital syphilis	Rabies
COVID-19	Rubella
Creutzfeldt-Jakob disease (CJD)	Severe acute respiratory syndrome (SARS)
Disseminated gonococcal infection (DGI)	Scarlet fever
Diphtheria	Smallpox
Enteric fever (typhoid or paratyphoid fever)	Tetanus
Food poisoning	Tuberculosis
Haemolytic uraemic syndrome (HUS)	Typhus
Infectious bloody diarrhoea	Viral haemorrhagic fever (VHF)
Influenza of zoonotic origin	Whooping cough
Invasive group A streptococcal disease	Yellow fever

In Wales, information on notifiable diseases is available from Public Health Wales (publichealthwales.nhs.wales/services-and-teams/aware-health-protection-team/).

In Northern Ireland, information on notifiable diseases is available from the Public Health Agency (www.niinfectioncontrolmanual.net/notifiable-diseases/).

In Scotland, information on notifiable diseases is available from Public Health Scotland (publichealthscotland.scot/population-health/health-protection/notifiable-diseases-health-risk-states-and-infections/overview/).

Antibacterials, use for prophylaxis

11-Dec-2025

Rheumatic fever: prevention of recurrence

- Phenoxymethylpenicillin p. 416 by mouth *or* erythromycin p. 406 by mouth.

Invasive group A streptococcal infection: prevention of secondary cases

- Phenoxymethylpenicillin by mouth.
- If penicillin allergic: azithromycin p. 402 [unlicensed use] (child aged 6 months and over), *or* clarithromycin p. 403 [unlicensed use], *or* erythromycin (in pregnancy or within 28 days of giving birth) by mouth.

The local health protection team should be contacted for advice on who should receive chemoprophylaxis. For further information, see UKHSA guidance: **UK guidelines for the management of contacts of invasive group A streptococcus (iGAS) infection in community settings** (see *Useful resources*).

Meningococcal disease: prevention of secondary cases

Neisseria meningitidis (meningococcus) can cause invasive meningococcal disease (IMD), including meningitis and septicaemia, albeit rarely. The aim of giving antibacterial prophylaxis is to eliminate asymptomatic carriage of *Neisseria meningitidis* from close contacts of the index case (including those with conjunctivitis), thereby reducing onward transmission and secondary cases.

Advice regarding the management of close contacts of a case of meningococcal disease should be sought from the local health protection team.

The following recommendations on antibacterial prophylaxis reflect advice from UKHSA **Guidance for public health management of meningococcal disease in the UK** (see *Useful resources*):

- Irrespective of vaccination status, antibacterial prophylaxis should be offered as soon as possible (ideally within 24 hours) after the diagnosis of the index case, to individuals who have had:
  - Prolonged close contact with the index case (including conjunctivitis cases) in a household type setting during the 7 days before onset of illness.
  - Sexual or other intimate contact during the 7 days before onset of illness.
  - Transient close contact with the index case only if they have been directly exposed to large particle droplets or secretions from the respiratory tract of a case around the time of admission to hospital.

The health protection team will lead on contact tracing and advise on the need for antibacterial prophylaxis for individuals who do not clearly fall into these categories.

Index cases treated with cephalosporins (such as ceftriaxone or cefotaxime) do not require antibacterial prophylaxis. If the index case (including conjunctivitis cases) is treated with any other antibacterial drug, antibacterial prophylaxis should be offered when the individual is able to take oral medication, and ideally before discharge from hospital.

Vaccination against *Neisseria meningitidis* should also be considered for the index case and close contacts following a case of IMD. For information on vaccination, see Meningococcal vaccines p. 973 and UKHSA: **Guidance for public health management of meningococcal disease in the UK** (see *Useful resources*).

Choice of antibacterial prophylaxis

- *First line*:
  - Ciprofloxacin p. 429 [unlicensed use];
  - Alternative if ciprofloxacin unsuitable, or if recent travel to the Middle East or Asia: rifampicin p. 449.
- *In pregnancy*:
  - Ciprofloxacin [unlicensed use], ceftriaxone p. 391 [unlicensed use], *or* azithromycin [unlicensed use].

Haemophilus influenzae type b infection: prevention of secondary disease

Haemophilus influenzae type b (Hib) can cause severe life-threatening disease in healthy children. With invasive Hib disease, the index case has a small, but significant risk of secondary Hib infection, particularly within 6 months of the first episode. Close contacts of the index case (mainly in a household, or pre-school or primary school setting) are also at increased risk of developing invasive Hib disease, especially within the first week of the index case becoming ill. Antibacterial prophylaxis aims to reduce the risk of secondary disease in the index case and among close contacts by eliminating asymptomatic pharyngeal carriage of Hib.

The following recommendations on antibacterial prophylaxis reflect advice from UKHSA guidance: **Revised recommendations for the prevention of secondary *Haemophilus influenzae* type b (Hib) disease** (see *Useful resources*).

All confirmed cases of invasive Hib disease should be given antibacterial prophylaxis prior to hospital discharge. All household contacts should be offered antibacterial prophylaxis as soon as invasive Hib disease is confirmed in the index case.

For a pre-school or primary school setting that has an outbreak (2 or more cases of invasive Hib disease within 120 days), antibacterial prophylaxis is recommended for all room contacts, including staff.

For a pre-school or primary school setting where the levels of contact are similar to those in a household (e.g. a small number of children attending the same child-minder for several hours each day), antibacterial prophylaxis for the close contact group should be considered.

For all eligible contacts, antibacterial prophylaxis should be offered up to 4 weeks after illness onset in the index case.

In addition to antibacterial prophylaxis, unimmunised or partially immunised index cases, household members, and other contacts aged under 10 years should complete their routine immunisation against Hib. For information on routine immunisation, see Haemophilus influenzae type b conjugate vaccine p. 966.

Choice of antibacterial prophylaxis

- *First line*:
  - Rifampicin;
  - Alternative if rifampicin unsuitable: ceftriaxone [unlicensed use] (based on limited evidence), *or* ciprofloxacin [unlicensed use] *or* azithromycin [unlicensed use] (however effectiveness in healthy individuals has not been determined).

Diphtheria: prevention of secondary cases

The risk of infection with diphtheria is directly related to the closeness and duration of contact with diphtheria cases or asymptomatic carriers. Antibacterial prophylaxis aims to reduce the risk of secondary disease by treating incubating disease in recently exposed contacts and eliminating asymptomatic carriage of diphtheria.

Management of close contacts of confirmed or probable diphtheria cases or asymptomatic carriers is led by the local health protection teams.

The following recommendations on antibacterial prophylaxis reflect advice from UKHSA guidance: **Public health control and management of diphtheria in England** (see *Useful resources*).

Close contacts of a confirmed or probable case or asymptomatic carrier of diphtheria should be investigated immediately, kept under surveillance, and be given antibacterial prophylaxis. Close contacts include children who have contact with a case or known carrier in a household type of setting, or through kissing or sexual contact, or who have been exposed to respiratory droplets or an undressed wound of a cutaneous case where splash or droplet contamination has occurred (such as healthcare workers).

In addition to antibacterial prophylaxis, vaccination with a diphtheria-containing vaccine should be considered. For information on vaccination, see *Post-exposure management* in Diphtheria vaccine p. 965.

Choice of antibacterial prophylaxis

- *First line*:
  - Azithromycin [unlicensed use], *or* clarithromycin [unlicensed use], *or* erythromycin (in pregnancy);
  - Alternative if more easily administered: benzathine benzylpenicillin p. 414 [unlicensed use].

Pertussis: prevention of secondary cases

Pertussis is highly contagious and can spread rapidly from person-to-person through contact with infectious respiratory particles. Prolonged and close contact with an index case during their early catarrhal phase is typically required for significant risk of pertussis transmission to arise, but the index case can remain infectious for up to 21 days following the onset of coughing.

The following recommendations on antibacterial prophylaxis reflect advice from UKHSA: **Guidance on the**

management of cases of pertussis in England during the re-emergence of pertussis in 2024 (see *Useful resources*).

In households, healthcare and relevant community settings, antibacterial prophylaxis should be offered to close contacts of the index case if the onset of coughing in the index case was within the preceding 14 days, and the close contact is in a priority group for public health action. Group 1 priority group includes individuals at increased risk of severe complications from pertussis ('vulnerable'). Group 2 priority group includes individuals who are at increased risk of transmitting pertussis to a 'vulnerable' individual in group 1, and who have not received a pertussis-containing vaccine more than one week and less than 5 years ago.

For further information on priority groups for public health action and definitions of close contacts, see UKHSA: **Guidance on the management of cases of pertussis in England during the re-emergence of pertussis in 2024** (see *Useful resources*).

Choice of antibacterial prophylaxis

- *First line*:
  - Azithromycin p. 402 [unlicensed use], clarithromycin p. 403 (preferred in neonates), *or* erythromycin p. 406;
  - Alternative if macrolides contra-indicated or not tolerated co-trimoxazole p. 431 [unlicensed use].
- *In pregnancy*:
  - Erythromycin is the preferred macrolide, with azithromycin [unlicensed use] second line, and clarithromycin third line.

Pneumococcal infection in asplenia or in patients with sickle-cell disease, antibacterial prophylaxis

- Phenoxymethylpenicillin p. 416 by mouth.

If cover also needed for *H. influenzae* in child give amoxicillin p. 417 instead.

If penicillin-allergic, erythromycin by mouth.

Antibacterial prophylaxis is not fully reliable. Antibacterial prophylaxis may be discontinued in children over 5 years of age with sickle-cell disease who have received pneumococcal immunisation and who do not have a history of severe pneumococcal infection.

Staphylococcus aureus lung infection in cystic fibrosis, antibacterial prophylaxis

- *Primary prevention*, flucloxacillin p. 424 by mouth.
- *Secondary prevention*, flucloxacillin by mouth.

Tuberculosis antibacterial prophylaxis in susceptible close contacts or those who have become tuberculin positive

See *Close contacts* and *Treatment of latent tuberculosis* under Tuberculosis p. 446.

Human and animal bites, antibacterial prophylaxis

See *Human and animal bites* in Skin infections, antibacterial therapy p. 373.

Gastro-intestinal procedures, antibacterial prophylaxis

Operations on stomach or oesophagus

- Single dose of i/v gentamicin p. 378 *or* i/v cefuroxime p. 388 *or* i/v co-amoxiclav p. 420 (additional intra-operative or postoperative doses may be given for prolonged procedures or if there is major blood loss).

Intravenous antibacterial prophylaxis should be given up to 30 minutes before the procedure.

Add i/v teicoplanin p. 396 (*or* vancomycin p. 398) if high risk of meticillin-resistant *Staphylococcus aureus*.

Open biliary surgery

- Single dose of i/v cefuroxime + i/v metronidazole p. 409 *or* i/v gentamicin + i/v metronidazole *or* i/v co-amoxiclav alone (additional intra-operative or postoperative doses may be given for prolonged procedures or if there is major blood loss).

Intravenous antibacterial prophylaxis should be given up to 30 minutes before the procedure.

Where i/v metronidazole is suggested, it may alternatively be given by suppository but to allow adequate absorption, it should be given 2 hours before surgery.

Add i/v teicoplanin (*or* vancomycin) if high risk of meticillin-resistant *Staphylococcus aureus*.

Resections of colon and rectum, and resections in inflammatory bowel disease, and appendicectomy

- Single dose of i/v gentamicin + i/v metronidazole *or* i/v cefuroxime + i/v metronidazole *or* i/v co-amoxiclav alone (additional intra-operative or postoperative doses may be given for prolonged procedures or if there is major blood loss).

Intravenous antibacterial prophylaxis should be given up to 30 minutes before the procedure.

Where i/v metronidazole is suggested, it may alternatively be given by suppository but to allow adequate absorption, it should be given 2 hours before surgery.

Add i/v teicoplanin (*or* vancomycin) if high risk of meticillin-resistant *Staphylococcus aureus*.

Endoscopic retrograde cholangiopancreatography

Refer to local antimicrobial guidelines.

Percutaneous endoscopic gastrostomy or jejunostomy

- Single dose of i/v co-amoxiclav or i/v cefuroxime.

Intravenous antibacterial prophylaxis should be given up to 30 minutes before the procedure.

Use single dose of i/v teicoplanin (*or* vancomycin) if history of allergy to penicillins or cephalosporins, or if high risk of meticillin-resistant *Staphylococcus aureus*.

Orthopaedic surgery, antibacterial prophylaxis

Closed fractures

- Single dose of i/v cefuroxime *or* i/v flucloxacillin (additional intra-operative or postoperative doses may be given for prolonged procedures or if there is major blood loss).

Intravenous antibacterial prophylaxis should be given up to 30 minutes before the procedure.

If history of allergy to penicillins or to cephalosporins or if high risk of meticillin-resistant *Staphylococcus aureus*, use single dose of i/v teicoplanin (*or* vancomycin) (additional intra-operative or postoperative doses may be given for prolonged procedures or if there is major blood loss).

Open fractures

- Use i/v co-amoxiclav alone *or* i/v cefuroxime + i/v metronidazole (*or* i/v clindamycin p. 400 alone if history of allergy to penicillins or to cephalosporins).

Add i/v teicoplanin (*or* vancomycin) if high risk of meticillin-resistant *Staphylococcus aureus*. Start prophylaxis within 3 hours of injury and continue until soft tissue closure (max. 72 hours).

At first debridement also use a single dose of i/v cefuroxime + i/v metronidazole + i/v gentamicin *or* i/v co-amoxiclav + i/v gentamicin (*or* i/v clindamycin + i/v gentamicin if history of allergy to penicillins or to cephalosporins).

At time of skeletal stabilisation and definitive soft tissue closure use a single dose of i/v gentamicin and i/v teicoplanin (*or* vancomycin) (intravenous antibacterial prophylaxis should be given up to 30 minutes before the procedure.

High lower-limb amputation

- Use i/v co-amoxiclav alone *or* i/v cefuroxime + i/v metronidazole.

Intravenous antibacterial prophylaxis should be given up to 30 minutes before the procedure.

Continue antibacterial prophylaxis for at least 2 doses after procedure (max. duration of prophylaxis 5 days). If history of allergy to penicillin or to cephalosporins, or if high risk of meticillin-resistant *Staphylococcus aureus*, use i/v teicoplanin (*or* vancomycin) + i/v gentamicin + i/v metronidazole.

Where i/v metronidazole is suggested, it may alternatively be given by suppository but to allow adequate absorption, it should be given 2 hours before surgery.

Obstetric surgery, antibacterial prophylaxis

Termination of pregnancy

- Single dose of oral metronidazole (additional intra-operative or postoperative doses may be given for prolonged procedures or if there is major blood loss).

If genital chlamydial infection cannot be ruled out, give doxycycline p. 434 postoperatively.

Infective endocarditis, antibacterial prophylaxis

NICE guidance: Antimicrobial prophylaxis against infective endocarditis in adults and children undergoing interventional procedures (March 2008, updated 2016)

- Chlorhexidine mouthwash is **not** recommended for the prevention of infective endocarditis in at risk children undergoing dental procedures.

Antibacterial prophylaxis is **not** *routinely* recommended for the prevention of infective endocarditis in children undergoing the following procedures:

- dental;
- upper and lower respiratory tract (including ear, nose, and throat procedures and bronchoscopy);
- genito-urinary tract (including urological, gynaecological, and obstetric procedures);
- upper and lower gastro-intestinal tract.

While these procedures can cause bacteraemia, there is no clear association with the development of infective endocarditis. Prophylaxis may expose children to the adverse effects of antimicrobials when the evidence of benefit has not been proven.

Any infection in children at risk of endocarditis should be investigated promptly and treated appropriately to reduce the risk of endocarditis.

If children at risk of infective endocarditis are undergoing a gastro-intestinal or genito-urinary tract procedure at a site where infection is suspected, they should receive appropriate antibacterial therapy that includes cover against organisms that cause endocarditis.

Children at risk of infective endocarditis should be:

- advised to maintain good oral hygiene;
- told how to recognise signs of infective endocarditis, and advised when to seek expert advice.

Patients at risk of infective endocarditis include those with valve replacement, acquired valvular heart disease with stenosis or regurgitation, structural congenital heart disease (including surgically corrected or palliated structural conditions, but excluding isolated atrial septal defect, fully repaired ventricular septal defect, fully repaired patent ductus arteriosus, and closure devices considered to be endothelialised), hypertrophic cardiomyopathy, or a previous episode of infective endocarditis.

Dermatological procedures

Advice of a Working Party of the British Society for Antimicrobial Chemotherapy is that patients who undergo dermatological procedures do not require antibacterial prophylaxis against endocarditis.

The British Association of Dermatologists Therapy Guidelines and Audit Subcommittee advise that such dermatological procedures include skin biopsies and excision of moles or of malignant lesions.

Joint prostheses and dental treatment, antibacterial prophylaxis

Advice of a Working Party of the British Society for Antimicrobial Chemotherapy is that patients with prosthetic joint implants (including total hip replacements) do not require antibacterial prophylaxis for dental treatment. The Working Party considers that it is unacceptable to expose patients to the adverse effects of antibacterials when there is no evidence that such prophylaxis is of any benefit, but that those who develop any intercurrent infection require prompt treatment with antibacterials to which the infecting organisms are sensitive.

The Working Party has commented that joint infections have rarely been shown to follow dental procedures and are even more rarely caused by oral streptococci.

Immunosuppression and indwelling intraperitoneal catheters

Advice of a Working Party of the British Society for Antimicrobial Chemotherapy is that patients who are immunosuppressed (including transplant patients) and patients with indwelling intraperitoneal catheters do not require antibacterial prophylaxis for dental treatment provided there is no other indication for prophylaxis.

The Working Party has commented that there is little evidence that dental treatment is followed by infection in immunosuppressed and immunodeficient patients nor is there evidence that dental treatment is followed by infection in patients with indwelling intraperitoneal catheters.

Useful Resources

Revised recommendations for the prevention of secondary *Haemophilus influenzae* type b (Hib) disease. UK Health Security Agency. September 2024.

www.gov.uk/government/publications/haemophilus-influenzae-type-b-hib-revised-recommendations-for-the-prevention-of-secondary-cases

Public health control and management of diphtheria in England. UK Health Security Agency. November 2023.

www.gov.uk/government/publications/diphtheria-public-health-control-and-management-in-england-and-wales

UK guidelines for the management of contacts of invasive group A streptococcus (iGAS) infection in community settings. UK Health Security Agency. March 2023.

www.gov.uk/government/publications/invasive-group-a-streptococcal-disease-managing-community-contacts

Guidance for public health management of meningococcal disease in the UK. UK Health Security Agency. November 2024.

www.gov.uk/government/publications/meningococcal-disease-guidance-on-public-health-management

Guidance on the management of cases of pertussis in England during the re-emergence of pertussis in 2024. UK Health Security Agency. August 2024.

www.gov.uk/government/publications/pertussis-guidelines-for-public-health-management

Sepsis

26-Feb-2026

Overview

Sepsis is a clinical syndrome caused by activation of the body's immune and coagulation systems due to infection. It is defined as life-threatening organ dysfunction caused by a dysregulated host response to an infection. Septic shock is a subset of sepsis, which describes circulatory, cellular, and metabolic abnormalities, with raised serum lactate and persistent hypotension despite fluid replacement; it carries a greater risk of mortality than sepsis alone. Signs and symptoms of sepsis can be very non-specific and variable. The risk of sepsis should be considered in anyone presenting with possible infection; early recognition and prompt treatment is essential in improving outcomes in patients who are deteriorating and at risk of organ dysfunction and death.

The term 'recently pregnant' refers to females of any age who have given birth within the preceding 4 weeks, or who have undergone a termination of pregnancy or experienced a miscarriage within the last 24 hours. Clinical judgement should be exercised following miscarriage (particularly in the second trimester) or termination of pregnancy (particularly in the second or third trimester), as physiological parameters may not have returned to pre-pregnancy levels.

Initial management of suspected or confirmed sepsis

For additional guidance on the management of meningococcal septicaemia, including **choice of antibacterial therapy**, see Central nervous system infections, antibacterial therapy p. 365.

EvGr In children with suspected or confirmed sepsis, a systematic approach should be used to assess their risk of severe illness or death, and of deterioration due to sepsis. The risk should be re-evaluated at regular intervals depending on severity (alongside other clinical parameters), or if there is a deterioration or unexpected change in the child's condition. (A) For information on assessing the risk of severe illness or death using criteria for risk stratification *or* the National Early Warning Score 2 (NEWS2) as appropriate (alongside other considerations), and for guidance on urgent hospital transfer, monitoring and escalation of care, see the relevant NICE guideline: **Suspected sepsis in under 16s: recognition, diagnosis and early management** or **Suspected sepsis in people aged 16 or over: recognition, assessment and early management** or **Suspected sepsis in pregnant or recently pregnant people: recognition, diagnosis and early management** (see *Useful resources*).

EvGr Neutropenic sepsis should be suspected in unwell children who have received systemic anticancer treatment in the last 30 days, or who have received or are receiving immunosuppressant treatment for reasons unrelated to cancer. (A) For guidance on the management of neutropenic sepsis, see NICE guideline CG151: **Neutropenic sepsis: prevention and management in people with cancer** (available at: www.nice.org.uk/guidance/cg151).

Initial treatment of suspected or confirmed sepsis includes the use of intravenous antibacterials, fluid resuscitation, inotropes/vasopressors, and oxygen, as clinically indicated.

Antibacterial therapy

For guidance on antibacterial management of sepsis in neonates, see Neonatal infection, antibacterial therapy p. 369.

Pre-hospital antibacterial therapy

EvGr For children in remote or rural locations with suspected sepsis and high-risk criteria for severe illness or death, antibacterial treatment should be given prior to hospital transfer according to local policy/guidance if the combined transfer and handover time to the emergency department is likely to be longer than 1 hour. (A)

Antibacterial therapy in hospital

EvGr Microbiological and blood samples should be taken before administering antibacterial treatment. A thorough clinical examination should be carried out to identify sources of infection, including sources that might need drainage or other interventions. If there is a clear source of infection, treat in line with local antimicrobial guidance.

The time frame during which antibacterials should be administered depends on assessment of the child's risk of severe illness or death from sepsis. For children assessed as high-risk of severe illness or death, intravenous antibacterial treatment should be administered within 1 hour of severity assessment (if not already given prior to hospital transfer). (A) For guidance on timing of antibacterials for children not assessed as high-risk, see the relevant NICE guideline: **Suspected sepsis in under 16s** or **Suspected sepsis in people aged 16 or over** or **Suspected sepsis in pregnant or recently pregnant people** (see *Useful resources*).

Choice of empirical antibacterial therapy

EvGr When the source of infection is confirmed or microbiological results are available, the choice of antibacterial should be reviewed, and where appropriate changed to a narrower-spectrum antibacterial agent. (A)

For suspected community-acquired sepsis and no clear source of infection:

- ***Intravenous** first line for children aged 1–2 months*
  - EvGr Ceftriaxone p. 391 **plus** amoxicillin p. 417 or ampicillin p. 419.
  - *Alternative in children who are known to have previously been infected or colonised with ceftriaxone-resistant bacteria:* consult local guidelines for choice of antibacterial. (A)
- ***Intravenous** first line for children aged 3 months –17 years*
  - EvGr Ceftriaxone.
  - *Alternative in children who are known to have previously been infected or colonised with ceftriaxone-resistant bacteria or who are pregnant or recently pregnant:* consult local guidelines for antibacterial choice. (A)

For suspected hospital-acquired sepsis and no clear source of infection:

- EvGr Consult local guidelines for antibacterial choice. (A)

Intravenous fluids and inotropes/vasopressors

EvGr The need for intravenous fluids should be assessed without delay, taking into consideration the child's lactate concentration, the presence of acute kidney injury, systolic blood pressure, and their risk of severe illness or death. (A) For guidance on sodium content of crystalloids, see Fluids and electrolytes p. 722.

EvGr Where appropriate, children should also be assessed by a critical care specialist for the need for inotropic/vasopressor support. (A)

Neonates

EvGr If fluid resuscitation is indicated, use a glucose-free crystalloid with a sodium content in the range of 130–154 mmol/litre such as potassium chloride with calcium chloride, sodium chloride and sodium lactate (Hartmann's solution), or sodium chloride 0.9%. A bolus of 10–20 mL/kg should be administered over less than 10 minutes, ensuring it is given within 1 hour of the infant being identified as high risk. A second bolus may be given if there is no improvement. Seek a consultant in-person review if there is no improvement after the second bolus. (A)

For further guidance on assessing the need for and administration of intravenous fluids, see NICE guideline: **Suspected sepsis in under 16s** (see *Useful resources*).

Children aged 1 month up to 16 years (including pregnant or recently pregnant females)

EvGr If fluid resuscitation is indicated, use a glucose-free crystalloid with a sodium content in the range of 130–154 mmol/litre such as potassium chloride with calcium chloride, sodium chloride and sodium lactate (Hartmann's solution), or sodium chloride 0.9%. A bolus of 10 mL/kg (maximum 250 mL) should be administered over less than 10 minutes, ensuring it is given within 1 hour of a child being identified as high risk. A smaller fluid volume may be needed in the presence of pre-existing conditions such as cardiac disease or kidney disease. A second bolus may be given if there is no improvement. Seek a consultant in-person review if there is no improvement after the second bolus. (A)

For further guidance on assessing the need for and administration of intravenous fluids, see NICE guideline: **Suspected sepsis in under 16s** or **Suspected sepsis in pregnant or recently pregnant people** (see *Useful resources*).

Individuals aged 16 years and over (excluding pregnant and recently pregnant females)

EvGr If fluid resuscitation is indicated, use an isotonic balanced crystalloid solution such as potassium chloride with calcium chloride, sodium chloride and sodium lactate (Hartmann's solution), or sodium chloride 0.9% if a balanced solution is not available. An initial bolus of 250 mL should be administered over 10–15 minutes, ensuring it is given within 1 hour of an individual being identified as high risk, or if there is evidence of hypoperfusion. Further boluses of 250 mL should be given if there is no improvement with reassessment after each dose, up to a total of 1000 mL. If the patient has not improved enough after 1000 mL has been given, advice should be sought from a senior clinical decision maker.

Where appropriate, patients should also be assessed by a critical care specialist for vasopressor support. If considering peripheral administration of vasopressors [unlicensed use], local policies should be followed and the peripheral line and cannula site closely monitored. (A)

For further guidance on assessing the need for and administration of intravenous fluids, see NICE guideline: **Suspected sepsis in people aged 16 or over** (see *Useful resources*).

Females aged 16 years and over who are pregnant or have recently been pregnant

EvGr If fluid resuscitation is indicated, use a crystalloid solution with a sodium content in the range of 130–154 mmol/litre such as potassium chloride with calcium chloride, sodium chloride and sodium lactate (Hartmann's solution), or sodium chloride 0.9%. A bolus of 500 mL should be administered over less than 15 minutes, ensuring it is given within 1 hour of an individual being identified as high risk. A second bolus of 500 mL may be given if there is no improvement. Seek a consultant in-person review if there is no improvement after the second bolus.

Where appropriate, patients should also be assessed by a critical care specialist for inotropic/vasopressor support. (A)

For further guidance on assessing the need for and administration of intravenous fluids, see NICE guideline: **Suspected sepsis in pregnant or recently pregnant people** (see *Useful resources*).

Oxygen

EvGr Oxygen should be given to children with suspected sepsis who have signs of shock or oxygen saturation (SpO_2) of less than 92 % when breathing air. Treatment with oxygen should also be considered for children with an SpO_2 of greater than 92 %, as clinically indicated. (A)

Useful Resources

Suspected sepsis in people aged 16 or over: recognition, assessment and early management. National Institute for Health and Care Excellence. NICE guideline 253. November 2025.
www.nice.org.uk/guidance/ng253

Suspected sepsis in pregnant or recently pregnant people: recognition, diagnosis and early management. National Institute for Health and Care Excellence. NICE guideline 255. November 2025.
www.nice.org.uk/guidance/ng255

Suspected sepsis in under 16s: recognition, diagnosis and early management. National Institute for Health and Care Excellence. NICE guideline 254. November 2025.
www.nice.org.uk/guidance/ng254

Cardiovascular system infections, antibacterial therapy

Endocarditis: initial 'blind' therapy

- Flucloxacillin p. 424 (*or* benzylpenicillin sodium p. 415 if symptoms less severe) + gentamicin p. 378
- *If cardiac prostheses present, or if penicillin-allergic, or if meticillin-resistant Staphylococcus aureus suspected,* vancomycin p. 398 + rifampicin p. 449 + gentamicin

Endocarditis caused by staphylococci

- Flucloxacillin
  - Add rifampicin for at least 2 weeks in prosthetic valve endocarditis
  - *Suggested duration of treatment* at least 4 weeks (at least 6 weeks for prosthetic valve endocarditis)
- *If penicillin-allergic or if meticillin-resistant Staphylococcus aureus,* vancomycin + rifampicin
  - *Suggested duration of treatment* at least 4 weeks (at least 6 weeks for prosthetic valve endocarditis)

Endocarditis (native valve) caused by fully-sensitive streptococci e.g. viridans streptococci

- Benzylpenicillin sodium
  - *Suggested duration of treatment* 4 weeks
- *Alternative if a large vegetation, intracardial abscess, or infected emboli are absent,* benzylpenicillin sodium + gentamicin
  - *Suggested duration of treatment* 2 weeks
- *If penicillin-allergic,* vancomycin
  - *Suggested duration of treatment* 4 weeks

Endocarditis (native valve) caused by less-sensitive streptococci

- Benzylpenicillin sodium + gentamicin
  - *Suggested duration of treatment* 4–6 weeks (stop gentamicin after 2 weeks for micro-organisms moderately sensitive to penicillin)
- *If aminoglycoside cannot be used and if streptococci moderately sensitive to penicillin,* benzylpenicillin sodium
  - *Suggested duration of treatment* 4 weeks
- *If penicillin-allergic or highly penicillin-resistant,* vancomycin (*or* teicoplanin p. 396) + gentamicin
  - *Suggested duration of treatment* 4–6 weeks (stop gentamicin after 2 weeks for micro-organisms moderately sensitive to penicillin)

Endocarditis (prosthetic valve) caused by streptococci

- Benzylpenicillin sodium + gentamicin
  - *Suggested duration of treatment* at least 6 weeks (stop gentamicin after 2 weeks if micro-organisms fully sensitive to penicillin)
- *If penicillin-allergic or highly penicillin-resistant,* vancomycin (*or* teicoplanin) + gentamicin
  - *Suggested duration of treatment* at least 6 weeks (stop gentamicin after 2 weeks if micro-organisms fully sensitive to penicillin)

Endocarditis caused by enterococci (e.g. *Enterococcus faecalis*)

- Amoxicillin p. 417 (*or* ampicillin p. 419) + gentamicin
  - If gentamicin-resistant, substitute gentamicin with streptomycin p. 380
  - *Suggested duration of treatment* at least 4 weeks (at least 6 weeks for prosthetic valve endocarditis)
- *If penicillin-allergic or penicillin-resistant*, vancomycin (*or* teicoplanin) + gentamicin
  - If gentamicin-resistant, substitute gentamicin with streptomycin
  - *Suggested duration of treatment* at least 4 weeks (at least 6 weeks for prosthetic valve endocarditis)

Endocarditis caused by *Haemophilus*, *Actinobacillus*, *Cardiobacterium*, *Eikenella*, and *Kingella* species ('HACEK' micro-organisms)

- Amoxicillin (*or* ampicillin) + gentamicin
  - *Suggested duration of treatment* 4 weeks (6 weeks for prosthetic valve endocarditis); stop gentamicin after 2 weeks
- *If amoxicillin-resistant*, ceftriaxone p. 391 + gentamicin
  - *Suggested duration of treatment* 4 weeks (6 weeks for prosthetic valve endocarditis); stop gentamicin after 2 weeks

Central nervous system infections, antibacterial therapy

03-Jun-2024

Meningitis and meningococcal disease

Meningitis involves inflammation of the membranes covering the brain and spinal cord (meninges)—causes can be infective (bacterial, viral, or fungal) or non-infective (certain cancers, autoimmune disorders, injury, or drugs). The most common causative organisms of acute bacterial meningitis are *Neisseria meningitidis* (meningococcus), *Streptococcus pneumoniae* (pneumococcus), and *Haemophilus influenzae* type b (Hib). *Listeria monocytogenes* is a rare cause of meningitis, usually affecting adults aged over 60 years, very young children, and those with other risk factors including pregnancy, cancer, kidney or liver disease, diabetes, alcohol misuse, and immunosuppression. Meningococcal disease refers to invasive infection caused by *N. meningitidis*, which can result in meningococcal meningitis, meningococcal septicaemia, or more commonly, a combination of both.

EvGr Bacterial meningitis and meningococcal disease are medical emergencies that require prompt recognition and treatment. Bacterial meningitis should be strongly suspected in patients with all the symptoms in the 'red flag' combination (fever, headache, neck stiffness, and altered level of consciousness or cognition), however, bacterial meningitis can still be strongly suspected even in the absence of some of these symptoms. Meningococcal disease should be strongly suspected in patients with a non-blanching petechial or purpuric rash with or without the 'red flag' symptoms of meningitis, however, the absence of a rash does not rule out meningococcal disease. Ⓐ For further guidance on the recognition of bacterial meningitis and meningococcal disease, see NICE guideline: **Meningitis (bacterial) and meningococcal disease: recognition, diagnosis and management** (see *Useful resources*).

Acute bacterial meningitis and meningococcal septicaemia are notifiable diseases in the UK. For further information, see *Notifiable diseases* in Antibacterials, principles of therapy p. 358.

Management

For guidance on the management of suspected bacterial meningitis and meningococcal disease in neonates, see Neonatal infection, antibacterial therapy p. 369.

EvGr Patients with suspected bacterial meningitis or meningococcal disease should be transferred to hospital as an emergency.

Patients with strongly suspected meningococcal disease should be given intravenous or intramuscular antibacterials as soon as possible outside of hospital, unless this will delay transfer to hospital. Patients with strongly suspected bacterial meningitis should be given intravenous or intramuscular antibacterials if there is likely to be a clinically significant delay in transfer to hospital.

Advice from an infection specialist should be obtained for all cases of bacterial meningitis, particularly for individuals who have recently travelled outside of the UK and may be at risk of antimicrobial resistance, and for those who are colonised with cephalosporin-resistant *Enterobacterales*.

For suspected bacterial meningitis and meningococcal disease, antibacterials should be started within 1 hour of the patient arriving at hospital if an appropriate first dose has not already been given in the community. Microbiological samples should be taken prior to starting treatment in hospital if it is safe to do so and will not cause a clinically significant delay. Empirical antibacterial therapy for suspected bacterial meningitis should be continued until investigation results suggest that an alternative treatment is required. Ⓐ

For further guidance on the investigation of bacterial meningitis and meningococcal disease, treatment of bacterial meningitis once the causative organism is known, and the management of complications and long-term effects, see NICE guideline: **Meningitis (bacterial) and meningococcal disease: recognition, diagnosis and management** (see *Useful resources*).

Choice of antibacterial therapy for bacterial meningitis and meningococcal disease (in individuals aged 1 month and older)

Emergency treatment of strongly suspected bacterial meningitis or meningococcal disease prior to transfer to hospital

- EvGr Ceftriaxone p. 391 or benzylpenicillin sodium p. 415.
- Do not give antibacterials outside of hospital if the patient has a severe allergy to a beta-lactam antibacterial. Ⓐ

Empirical antibacterial therapy for suspected bacterial meningitis in hospital

- EvGr *First line (including patients with non-severe allergy to a beta-lactam antibacterial)* : ceftriaxone. If ceftriaxone is contra-indicated for reasons other than allergy, cefotaxime p. 389 may be used.
  - *Alternative in patients with severe allergy to a beta-lactam antibacterial* : consider chloramphenicol p. 437 and seek advice from an infection specialist. Ⓐ

Patients with risk factors for L. monocytogenes:

- EvGr *First line*: amoxicillin p. 417 in addition to ceftriaxone (or cefotaxime).
  - *Alternative in those with non-severe allergy to a beta-lactam antibacterial* : consider co-trimoxazole p. 431 [unlicensed use] in addition to ceftriaxone (or cefotaxime), and seek advice from an infection specialist.
  - *Alternative in those with severe allergy to a beta-lactam antibacterial*: consider co-trimoxazole [unlicensed use] and chloramphenicol, and seek advice from an infection specialist. Ⓐ

Antibacterial therapy for meningococcal disease in hospital

- EvGr *First line (including patients with non-severe allergy to a beta-lactam antibacterial)* : ceftriaxone.

- *Alternative in patients with severe allergy to a beta-lactam antibacterial* : consider chloramphenicol and seek advice from an infection specialist. Ⓐ

Corticosteroids

Corticosteroids for bacterial meningitis

For some causes of bacterial meningitis, there is evidence that corticosteroids may reduce mortality in adults, and reduce hearing impairment in both adults and children.

EvGr For patients aged 3 months and older with strongly suspected or confirmed bacterial meningitis, give dexamethasone p. 543.

For infants aged between 28 days and 3 months with strongly suspected or confirmed bacterial meningitis, seek advice on giving dexamethasone from an infection specialist.

The first dose of dexamethasone should be given with or before the first dose of antibacterial treatment if possible, however, antibacterial treatment should not be delayed to administer dexamethasone. If antibacterial treatment was started less than 12 hours ago, dexamethasone should be given as soon as possible. Otherwise, seek advice from an infection specialist to decide whether dexamethasone is still likely to provide benefit.

If *S. pneumoniae* or *H. influenzae* type b are found to be the cause, continue dexamethasone. For all other causative organisms, stop dexamethasone treatment. If no causative organism is found, seek advice from an infection specialist on whether to continue dexamethasone. Ⓐ

Corticosteroids for meningococcal disease

EvGr Corticosteroids are not routinely recommended for patients with meningococcal disease, however, low-dose replacement corticosteroids can be considered for those with meningococcal septic shock unresponsive to high-dose vasoactive agents. Ⓐ

Prevention of secondary cases

EvGr The local health protection team should be contacted as soon as a case of meningococcal disease is suspected to undertake a public health assessment and to consider antibacterial chemoprophylaxis of cases and close contacts. Ⓐ For further information on the prevention of secondary cases of meningococcal disease or invasive *H. influenzae* type b infection, see Antibacterials, use for prophylaxis p. 359. For guidance on the public health management of meningococcal disease in the UK, see UKHSA guideline: **Guidance for public health management of meningococcal disease in the UK** (see *Useful resources*).

Useful Resources

Guidance for public health management of meningococcal disease in the UK. UK Health Security Agency. 2018, updated November 2024.
www.gov.uk/government/publications/meningococcal-disease-guidance-on-public-health-management

Meningitis (bacterial) and meningococcal disease: recognition, diagnosis and management. National Institute for Health and Care Excellence. NICE guideline 240. March 2024.
www.nice.org.uk/guidance/ng240

Diabetic foot infections, antibacterial therapy

26-Jan-2023

Diabetic foot infection

Diabetic foot infection is defined as any type of skin, soft tissue or bone infection below the ankle in children with diabetes. It includes cellulitis, paronychia, abscesses, myositis, tendonitis, necrotising fasciitis, osteomyelitis, and septic arthritis. It is defined clinically by the presence of at least 2 of the following: local swelling or induration, erythema, local tenderness or pain, local warmth, or purulent discharge.

For guidance on classification of infection severity, see NICE guideline: **Diabetic foot problems** (see *Useful resources*).

Treatment

EvGr Refer children immediately to acute services and inform the multidisciplinary foot care service if they have a limb-threatening or life-threatening diabetic foot problem, such as ulceration with fever or any signs of sepsis, ulceration with limb ischaemia, or gangrene.

Antibacterial treatment should be started as soon as possible if diabetic foot infection is suspected. Samples (such as soft tissue, bone sample, or deep swab) should be taken for microbiological testing before, or as close as possible to, the start of antibacterial treatment.

Offer an antibacterial taking into account the severity of infection, risk of complications, previous microbiological results, recent antibacterial use, and patient preferences. Ⓐ

For other considerations such as switching from intravenous to oral antibacterials, and for advice to be given to children and their parents, or carers, see Antibacterials, principles of therapy p. 358.

Reassessment

EvGr Reassess if symptoms worsen rapidly or significantly at any time, do not start to improve within 1–2 days of starting antibacterial treatment, or the patient becomes systemically very unwell or has severe pain out of proportion to the infection. Take into account other diagnoses (such as pressure sores, gout, or non-infected ulcers), signs and symptoms of a more serious illness (such as limb ischaemia, osteomyelitis, necrotising fasciitis, or sepsis), and previous antibacterial use.

Review the choice of antibacterial when microbiological results are available and change according to the results, using a narrower-spectrum antibacterial if appropriate. Ⓐ

Choice of antibacterial therapy

EvGr Seek specialist advice if a diabetic foot infection is suspected or confirmed in children. Ⓐ

Useful Resources

Diabetic foot problems: prevention and management. National Institute for Health and Care Excellence. NICE guideline 19. August 2015, updated September 2024.
www.nice.org.uk/guidance/ng19

Ear infections, antibacterial therapy

03-May-2022

Otitis externa

Otitis externa is inflammation of the external ear canal; it can be triggered by a bacterial infection caused by *Pseudomonas aeruginosa* or *Staphylococcus aureus*. For further information, including use of topical treatments, see *Otitis externa* in Ear p. 859. Oral antibacterials are rarely indicated but if they are required, consider seeking specialist advice.

Choice of antibacterial therapy

If pseudomonas suspected

- EvGr Ciprofloxacin p. 429 (*or* an aminoglycoside). Ⓔ

No penicillin allergy

- EvGr Flucloxacillin p. 424. Ⓔ

Penicillin allergy or intolerance

- EvGr Clarithromycin p. 403 (*or* azithromycin p. 402 *or* erythromycin p. 406). Ⓔ

Otitis media

Acute otitis media is inflammation in the middle ear associated with effusion and accompanied by an ear infection. Acute otitis media is commonly seen in children and is generally caused by viruses (respiratory syncytial virus, rhinovirus, adenovirus, influenza virus, and parainfluenza virus) or bacteria (*Haemophilus influenzae*, *Streptococcus pneumoniae*, *Streptococcus pyogenes*, and *Moraxella catarrhalis*); both virus and bacteria often co-exist. For further information, see *Acute otitis media* in Ear p. 859.

Choice of antibacterial therapy in children

No penicillin allergy

- *First line*: EvGr amoxicillin p. 417. Ⓐ
- *Second line* (worsening symptoms despite 2 to 3 days of antibacterial treatment): EvGr co-amoxiclav p. 420. Ⓐ

Penicillin allergy or intolerance

- *First line*: EvGr clarithromycin p. 403 or erythromycin p. 406 (in pregnancy). Ⓐ
- *Second line* (worsening symptoms despite 2 to 3 days of antibacterial treatment): EvGr Consult local microbiologist. Ⓐ

Eye infections, antibacterial therapy

07-May-2024

Conjunctivitis (purulent)

- Chloramphenicol eye drops p. 846.

Gastro-intestinal system infections, antibacterial therapy

20-Jul-2021

Gastro-enteritis

Frequently self-limiting and may not be bacterial.

- Antibacterial not usually indicated.

Campylobacter enteritis

Frequently self-limiting; treat if immunocompromised or if severe infection.

- Clarithromycin p. 403 (*or* azithromycin p. 402 *or* erythromycin p. 406)
- *Alternative*, ciprofloxacin p. 429
  - Strains with decreased sensitivity to ciprofloxacin isolated frequently

Salmonella (non-typhoid)

Treat invasive or severe infection. Do not treat less severe infection unless there is a risk of developing invasive infection (e.g. immunocompromised patients, those with haemoglobinopathy, or children under 6 months of age).

- Ciprofloxacin *or* cefotaxime p. 389

Shigellosis

Antibacterial not indicated for mild cases.

- Ciprofloxacin *or* azithromycin
- *Alternatives if micro-organism sensitive*, amoxicillin p. 417 *or* trimethoprim p. 443

Typhoid fever

Infections from Middle-East, South Asia, and South-East Asia may be multiple-antibacterial-resistant and sensitivity should be tested.

- Cefotaxime (*or* ceftriaxone p. 391)
  - Azithromycin may be an alternative in mild or moderate disease caused by multiple-antibacterial-resistant micro-organisms
- *Alternative if micro-organism sensitive*, ciprofloxacin *or* chloramphenicol p. 437

Clostridioides difficile infection

Clostridioides difficile (*C. difficile*) infection occurs when normal gut microbiota are suppressed, allowing levels of toxin producing strains of *C. difficile* to flourish. The toxin damages the lining of the colon and causes diarrhoea. Infection can be mild, moderate, severe, or life-threatening; complications include pseudomembranous colitis, toxic megacolon, colonic perforation, sepsis, and death.

C. difficile infection is most common in patients who are currently taking or have recently taken antibacterials. Clindamycin, cephalosporins (especially third and fourth generation), fluoroquinolones, and broad-spectrum penicillins have been frequently associated with *C. difficile* infection. Infection risk increases with longer duration of antibacterial treatment, concurrent use of multiple antibacterials, or multiple antibacterial courses. Other risk factors for *C. difficile* infection include current use of acid suppressing drugs (such as proton pump inhibitors), prolonged hospitalisation, underlying comorbidity, exposure to other people with the infection, and previous history of *C. difficile* infection(s).

For guidance on classification of *C. difficile* infection severity and non-antibacterial management options, see NICE guideline: **Clostridioides difficile infection** (see *Useful resources*). For guidance on diagnosis, infection control, and the management of life-threatening disease, see UK Health Security Agency (UKHSA) collection: **Clostridioides difficile: guidance, data and analysis** (available at www.gov.uk/government/collections/clostridium-difficile-guidance-data-and-analysis).

Treatment

EvGr Seek specialist advice for antibacterial treatment in children with suspected or confirmed *C. difficile* infection.

Antibacterials are not recommended for preventing *C. difficile* infection. Ⓐ For other considerations such as advice to be given to children, and if appropriate their family or carers, see Antibacterials, principles of therapy p. 358.

EvGr Urgently refer children with life-threatening infection to hospital.

Refer children with suspected or confirmed *C. difficile* infection to hospital if they are severely unwell, or their signs or symptoms worsen rapidly or significantly at any time.

Consider referral to hospital if the risk of complications or recurrence could be high because of individual factors such as comorbidities. Ⓐ

Reassessment

EvGr Reassess if signs or symptoms worsen rapidly or significantly at any time, or do not improve as expected.

Consider stopping antibacterial therapy if subsequent stool sample tests do not confirm *C. difficile* infection.

Clinical judgement should be used to determine if antibacterial treatment is ineffective (not usually possible until day 7 because diarrhoea may take 1–2 weeks to resolve). Ⓐ

Choice of antibacterial therapy

EvGr For children who cannot take oral medicines, seek specialist advice about other enteral routes (such as nasogastric tube or rectal catheter). Ⓐ

First episode of mild, moderate, or severe C. difficile infection

- ***Oral*** *first line* :
  - EvGr Vancomycin p. 398. Ⓐ
- ***Oral*** *second line* :
  - EvGr Fidaxomicin p. 439. Ⓐ

5 Infection

- If first and second line antibacterials are ineffective: EvGr Seek specialist advice. (A)

Further episode of C. difficile infection

- ***Oral*** *first line* for infection within 12 weeks of symptom resolution (relapse):
- ▸ EvGr Fidaxomicin p. 439. (A)
- ***Oral*** *first line* for infection more than 12 weeks after symptom resolution (recurrence):
- ▸ EvGr Vancomycin p. 398 or fidaxomicin p. 439. (A)

Life-threatening C. difficile infection

- EvGr Specialist may offer oral vancomycin p. 398 **with** intravenous metronidazole p. 409. (A)

Peritonitis

- A cephalosporin + metronidazole *or* amoxicillin + gentamicin p. 378 + metronidazole *or* piperacillin with tazobactam p. 413 alone

Peritonitis: peritoneal dialysis-associated

- Vancomycin p. 398 (*or* teicoplanin p. 396) + ceftazidime p. 390 added to dialysis fluid *or* vancomycin added to dialysis fluid + ciprofloxacin by mouth
- ▸ *Suggested duration of treatment* 14 days or longer

Necrotising enterocolitis in neonates

- Benzylpenicillin sodium p. 415 + gentamicin + metronidazole *or* amoxicillin (*or* ampicillin p. 419) + gentamicin + metronidazole *or* amoxicillin (*or* ampicillin) + cefotaxime + metronidazole

Useful Resources

Clostridioides difficile infection: antimicrobial prescribing. National Institute for Health and Care Excellence. NICE guideline 199. July 2021.
www.nice.org.uk/guidance/ng199

Genital system infections, antibacterial therapy

12-Nov-2025

Overview

Management of sexually transmitted infections (STIs) in children aged 15 years and under requires specialist advice from a sexual health clinician, a paediatrician, and a pharmacist, particularly in children aged under 12 years where such infections are very rare. The possibility of sexual abuse and exploitation in children of all ages with an STI should be considered and thoroughly investigated. Guidance on the drug treatment of STIs within the BNF for Children applies to children aged 12 years and over. For guidance on options for drug treatment in children aged under 12 years, and for further information on the management of STIs in children of all ages (including other treatment options), see the British Association for Sexual Health and HIV guideline: **National guideline on the management of sexually transmitted infections and related conditions in children and young people** (see *Useful resources*).

Uncomplicated genital chlamydial infection and uncomplicated non-gonococcal urethritis (non-specific urethritis)

EvGr Contact tracing recommended. (A)

Child aged 12 years and over

- *First line*: EvGr doxycycline p. 434 (A)
- *Alternative if tetracycline allergy or unsuitable*: EvGr azithromycin p. 402 (A)

Gonorrhoea: uncomplicated

Gonococcal ophthalmia in neonates is an ophthalmic emergency—seek specialist advice.

EvGr Prior to treating gonococcal infection obtain cultures from all potentially exposed sites for antimicrobial susceptibility testing.

In sexually active young people, test of cure following treatment is recommended, but is not necessary in non-pregnant individuals treated with ceftriaxone for anogenital infection that is sensitive to ceftriaxone, unless there are persistent signs or symptoms. Contact tracing is recommended. For sexual contacts presenting within 14 days of exposure, epidemiological treatment should be considered, whereas for contacts presenting after 14 days of exposure, treatment is only recommended following a positive test. Sexual intercourse should be avoided until 7 days after patients and their partner(s) have completed treatment. (A)

Child aged 12 years and over

- *First line*:
- ▸ EvGr Ceftriaxone p. 391 (A)
- *Alternatives due to allergy, needle phobia or contra-indications*:
- ▸ EvGr Gentamicin p. 378 **plus** azithromycin
- ▸ If intramuscular administration is not possible and antimicrobial susceptibility results are known: cefixime p. 389 [unlicensed use] **plus** azithromycin
- ▸ If sensitivity has been confirmed: azithromycin
- ▸ If other treatment options are inappropriate and sensitivity has been confirmed: ciprofloxacin p. 429 [unlicensed use] (A)

Pelvic inflammatory disease

Contact tracing recommended.

Child aged 12 years and over

- Doxycycline + metronidazole p. 409 + single-dose of ceftriaxone
- ▸ If severely ill, seek specialist advice.
- ▸ *Suggested duration of treatment* 14 days (except ceftriaxone)

Syphilis

EvGr Contact tracing recommended. (A)

Congenital syphilis is a notifiable disease in England. For further information, see *Notifiable diseases* in Antibacterials, principles of therapy p. 358.

Early syphilis (primary, secondary, and early latent—less than 2 years since infection) and late latent syphilis (more than 2 years since infection)

Child aged 12 years and over

- *First line*: EvGr benzathine benzylpenicillin p. 414 (A)
- *Alternatives include*: EvGr Doxycycline (A)

Asymptomatic contacts of patients with infectious syphilis

Child aged 12 years and over

- *First line*: EvGr Benzathine benzylpenicillin (A)
- *Alternatives include*: EvGr Doxycycline (A)

Useful Resources

National guideline on the management of sexually transmitted infections and related conditions in children and young people. British Association for Sexual Health and HIV. March 2021.
www.bashh.org/resources/guidelines

Musculoskeletal system infections, antibacterial therapy

Osteomyelitis

For management of osteomyelitis below the ankle in individuals with diabetes mellitus, see Diabetic foot infections, antibacterial therapy p. 366.

Seek specialist advice if chronic infection or prostheses present.

- Flucloxacillin p. 424
  - Consider adding fusidic acid p. 441 or rifampicin p. 449 for initial 2 weeks.
  - *Suggested duration of treatment* 6 weeks for acute infection
- *If penicillin-allergic*, clindamycin p. 400
  - Consider adding fusidic acid or rifampicin for initial 2 weeks.
  - *Suggested duration of treatment* 6 weeks for acute infection
- *If meticillin-resistant Staphylococcus aureus suspected*, vancomycin p. 398 (*or* teicoplanin p. 396)
  - Consider adding fusidic acid or rifampicin for initial 2 weeks.
  - *Suggested duration of treatment* 6 weeks for acute infection

Septic arthritis

For management of septic arthritis below the ankle in individuals with diabetes mellitus, see Diabetic foot infections, antibacterial therapy p. 366.

Seek specialist advice if prostheses present.

- Flucloxacillin
  - *Suggested duration of treatment* 4–6 weeks (longer if infection complicated).
- *If penicillin-allergic*, clindamycin
  - *Suggested duration of treatment* 4–6 weeks (longer if infection complicated).
- *If meticillin-resistant Staphylococcus aureus suspected*, vancomycin (*or* teicoplanin)
  - *Suggested duration of treatment* 4–6 weeks (longer if infection complicated).
- *If gonococcal arthritis or Gram-negative infection suspected*, cefotaxime p. 389 (*or* ceftriaxone p. 391)
  - *Suggested duration of treatment* 4–6 weeks (longer if infection complicated; treat gonococcal infection for 2 weeks).

Neonatal infection, antibacterial therapy

20-Feb-2025

Neonatal bacterial infection

Neonatal bacterial infection is a significant cause of mortality and morbidity in newborns, and there can be unnecessary delays in recognising and treating unwell neonates. Infection can be acquired any time before birth from a maternal infection while in-utero or in the birth canal during delivery, or from an external source after birth. Neonatal infection, depending on the time of onset, can be classified as early-onset infection (occurs less than 72 hours after birth) or late-onset infection (occurs 72 hours or more after birth).

For guidance on the prevention of early-onset neonatal infection before birth (including intrapartum antibacterials), see NICE guideline: **Neonatal infection** (see *Useful resources*).

Pre-hospital antibacterial therapy

EvGr If meningococcal disease (fever and purpuric rash) is specifically suspected, intravenous or intramuscular benzylpenicillin sodium p. 415 should be given as soon as possible in the community prior to urgent transfer to hospital, unless this will delay transfer. (A)

Management of early-onset infection

For guidance on the risk factors and clinical indicators of possible early-onset infection before and after birth, including 'red flags', and for investigations to be carried out before starting antibacterials, see NICE guideline: **Neonatal infection** (see *Useful resources*).

EvGr Antibacterial therapy should be initiated in neonates with any 'red flags' **or** 2 or more 'non-red flag' risk factors or clinical indicators.

Clinical judgement should be used for neonates without any 'red flags' **and** only 1 risk factor or clinical indicator, to decide whether it is safe to withhold antibacterials and if monitoring is required.

Antibacterial therapy should be considered for neonates who are being monitored for possible early-onset infection.

If antibacterial therapy is required, this should be given as soon as possible and within 1 hour of the decision to treat. (A)

Choice of empirical antibacterial therapy

- ***Intravenous** first line* :
  - EvGr Benzylpenicillin sodium with gentamicin p. 378 (unless local bacterial resistance patterns indicate the need for a different antibacterial).
  - If Gram-negative bacterial sepsis suspected, **add** an antibacterial active against Gram-negative bacteria (e.g. cefotaxime p. 389); if Gram-negative infection confirmed, **stop** benzylpenicillin sodium. (A)

For guidance on investigations during, and decisions after starting antibacterial treatment (including antibacterial therapy duration), and advice on site-specific early-onset infections, see NICE guideline: **Neonatal infection** (see *Useful resources*).

Management of late-onset infection

EvGr Assess the neonate's risk factors for and clinical indicators of possible late-onset infection. Take into account that prematurity, mechanical ventilation, history of surgery, and presence of a central catheter are associated with greater risk of late-onset neonatal infection; consider the risk of infection in the other neonates when one neonate from a multiple birth has infection. (A) For further information on clinical indicators for possible late-onset neonatal infection and for guidance on investigations to be carried out before starting antibacterials, see NICE guideline: **Neonatal infection** (see *Useful resources*).

EvGr When late-onset infection is suspected in a non-inpatient setting, seek early advice from a paediatrician. (A)

For guidance on assessing neonates for late-onset infection who have been admitted to hospital from home, see NICE guideline: **Suspected sepsis: recognition, diagnosis and early management** (available at: www.nice.org.uk/guidance/ng51).

EvGr If antibacterial therapy is required, this should be given as soon as possible and within 1 hour of the decision to treat.

To prevent fungal infection during antibacterial therapy, neonates who have a birthweight of up to 1.5 kg or were born at less than 30 weeks' gestation should be given prophylactic oral nystatin p. 885. If oral administration of nystatin is not possible, intravenous fluconazole p. 463 [unlicensed] should be used. (A)

Choice of empirical antibacterial therapy

- ***Intravenous** first line for neonates admitted from home* :
  - EvGr If more than 40 weeks corrected gestational age: ceftriaxone p. 391 with either amoxicillin p. 417 or ampicillin p. 419, unless already receiving an intravenous calcium infusion.

- If 40 weeks corrected gestational age or below, or receiving an intravenous calcium infusion: cefotaxime with either amoxicillin or ampicillin. Ⓐ

For guidance on the choice of antibacterial therapy for neonates with suspected late-onset infection in a neonatal unit, and for information on investigations during, and decisions after starting antibacterial treatment (including antibacterial therapy duration), see NICE guideline: **Neonatal infection** (see *Useful resources*).

Useful Resources

Neonatal infection: antibiotics for prevention and treatment. National Institute for Health and Care Excellence. NICE guideline 195. March 2024.
www.nice.org.uk/guidance/ng195

Nose infections, antibacterial therapy

31-Oct-2017

Sinusitis (acute)

Acute sinusitis is generally triggered by a viral infection, although occasionally it may become complicated by a bacterial infection caused by *Streptococcus pneumoniae*, *Haemophylus influenzae*, *Moraxella catharrhalis*, or *Staphylococcus aureus*. For further information *see* Sinusitis (acute) p. 870.

Treatment

EvGr Antibacterial therapy should *only* be offered to children with acute sinusitis who are systemically very unwell, have signs and symptoms of a more serious illness, those who are at high-risk of complications due to pre-existing comorbidities, or whenever bacterial sinusitis is suspected. Ⓐ For further information *see* Sinusitis (acute) p. 870.

Choice of antibacterial therapy
No penicillin allergy

- *First line*:
  - EvGr Non-life threatening symptoms: phenoxymethylpenicillin p. 416.
  - Systemically very unwell, signs and symptoms of a more serious illness, or at high-risk of complications: co-amoxiclav p. 420. Ⓐ
- *Second line* (worsening symptoms despite 2 or 3 days of antibiotic treatment):
  - EvGr Non-life threatening symptoms: co-amoxiclav.
  - Systemically very unwell, signs and symptoms of a more serious illness or at high-risk of complications: consult local microbiologist. Ⓐ

Penicillin allergy or intolerance

- *First line*: EvGr clarithromycin p. 403, or doxycycline p. 434 (for children above 12 years old). Ⓐ
- *Second line* (worsening symptoms despite 2 or 3 days of antibiotic treatment): EvGr Consult local microbiologist. Ⓐ

Useful Resources

Sinusitis (acute): antimicrobial prescribing. National Institute for Health and Care Excellence. NICE guideline 79. October 2017.
www.nice.org.uk/guidance/ng79

Oral bacterial infections

03-Jan-2021

Antibacterial drugs

Antibacterial drugs should only be prescribed for the *treatment* of oral infections on the basis of defined need. They may be used in conjunction with (but not as an alternative to) other appropriate measures, such as providing drainage or extracting a tooth.

The 'blind' prescribing of an antibacterial for unexplained pyrexia, cervical lymphadenopathy, or facial swelling can lead to difficulty in establishing the diagnosis. In severe oral infections, a sample should always be taken for bacteriology.

Oral infections which may require antibacterial treatment include acute periapical or periodontal abscess, cellulitis, acutely created oral-antral communication (and acute sinusitis), severe pericoronitis, localised osteitis, acute necrotising ulcerative gingivitis, and destructive forms of chronic periodontal disease. Most of these infections are readily resolved by the early establishment of drainage and removal of the cause (typically an infected necrotic pulp). Antibacterials may be required if treatment has to be delayed, in immunocompromised patients, or in those with conditions such as diabetes. Certain rarer infections including bacterial sialadenitis, osteomyelitis, actinomycosis, and infections involving fascial spaces such as Ludwig's angina, require antibiotics and specialist hospital care.

Antibacterial drugs may also be useful after dental surgery in some cases of spreading infection. Infection may spread to involve local lymph nodes, to fascial spaces (where it can cause airway obstruction), or into the bloodstream (where it can lead to cavernous sinus thrombosis and other serious complications). Extension of an infection can also lead to maxillary sinusitis; osteomyelitis is a complication, which usually arises when host resistance is reduced.

If the oral infection fails to respond to antibacterial treatment within 48 hours the antibacterial should be changed, preferably on the basis of bacteriological investigation. Failure to respond may also suggest an incorrect diagnosis, lack of essential additional measures (such as drainage), poor host resistance, or poor patient compliance.

Combination of a penicillin (or a macrolide) with metronidazole p. 409 may sometimes be helpful for the treatment of severe oral infections or oral infections.

For information on antibacterials used for the treatment of pericoronitis, acute necrotising ulcerative gingivitis, dental abscess, and sore throat, see Oropharyngeal infections, antibacterial therapy p. 883.

Penicillins

Phenoxymethylpenicillin p. 416 is effective for dentoalveolar abscess.

Broad-spectrum penicillins
Amoxicillin p. 417 is as effective as phenoxymethylpenicillin but is better absorbed; however, it may encourage emergence of resistant organisms.

Like phenoxymethylpenicillin, amoxicillin is ineffective against bacteria that produce beta-lactamases.

Co-amoxiclav p. 420 is active against beta-lactamase-producing bacteria that are resistant to amoxicillin. Co-amoxiclav may be used for severe dental infection with spreading cellulitis or dental infection not responding to first-line antibacterial treatment.

Cephalosporins

The cephalosporins offer little advantage over the penicillins in dental infections, often being less active against anaerobes. Infections due to oral streptococci (often termed viridans streptococci) which become resistant to penicillin are usually also resistant to cephalosporins. This is of importance in the case of patients who have had rheumatic fever and are on long-term penicillin therapy. Cefalexin p. 385 and cefradine p. 387 have been used in the treatment of oral infections.

Tetracyclines

In children over 12 years of age, tetracyclines can be effective against oral anaerobes but the development of resistance (especially by oral streptococci) has reduced their usefulness for the treatment of acute oral infections; they may still have a role in the treatment of destructive (refractory) forms of periodontal disease on specialist advice. Doxycycline p. 434 has a longer duration of action than tetracycline p. 436 or oxytetracycline p. 436 and need only be given once daily; it is reported to be more active against anaerobes than some other tetracyclines.

Macrolides

The macrolides are an alternative for oral infections in penicillin-allergic patients or where a beta-lactamase producing organism is involved. However, many organisms are now resistant to macrolides or rapidly develop resistance; their use should therefore be limited to short courses.

Clindamycin

Clindamycin p. 400 should not be used routinely for the treatment of oral infections because it may be no more effective than penicillins against anaerobes and there may be cross-resistance with erythromycin-resistant bacteria.

Metronidazole

Metronidazole is an alternative to a penicillin for the treatment of many oral infections where the patient is allergic to penicillin or the infection is due to beta-lactamase-producing anaerobes.

Respiratory system infections, antibacterial therapy

12-May-2026

Epiglottitis (*Haemophilus influenzae*)

- Cefotaxime p. 389 (*or* ceftriaxone p. 391)
- *If history of immediate hypersensitivity reaction to penicillin or to cephalosporins*, chloramphenicol p. 437

Bronchiectasis (non-cystic fibrosis), acute exacerbation

Bronchiectasis is a persistent or progressive condition caused by chronic inflammatory damage to the airways and is characterised by thick-walled, dilated bronchi. Signs and symptoms may range from intermittent expectoration and infection, to chronic cough, persistent daily production of sputum, bacterial colonisation, and recurrent infections. An acute exacerbation is defined as sustained deterioration of the child's signs and symptoms from their baseline and presents with worsening local symptoms, with or without increased wheeze, breathlessness or haemoptysis and may be accompanied by fever or pleurisy.

Treatment

EvGr Obtain a sputum sample and send for culture and susceptibility testing. Antibacterial therapy should be given to all children with an acute exacerbation. (A)

For children receiving prophylactic antibacterial therapy, switching from intravenous to oral antibacterials, and for advice to be given to children and their parents, or carers, see Antibacterials, principles of therapy p. 358.

EvGr Refer children to hospital if they have signs or symptoms suggestive of a more serious illness such as cardiorespiratory failure or sepsis. (A)

Reassessment

EvGr Reassess if symptoms worsen rapidly or significantly at any time and consider:

- Other diagnoses such as pneumonia, or signs and symptoms of a more serious illness such as cardiorespiratory failure, or sepsis;
- Previous antibacterial use that may have led to resistance.

Review choice of antibacterial if susceptibility results indicate bacterial resistance and symptoms are not improving—consult local microbiologist as needed. (A)

Choice of antibacterial therapy

EvGr The recommended total duration of treatment is 7–14 days.

Treatment should be guided by the most recent sputum culture and susceptibility results when available.

Seek specialist advice for children whose symptoms are not improving with repeated courses, or who are resistant to, or cannot take oral antibacterials. (A)

- ***Oral** first line* :
  - EvGr Amoxicillin p. 417, clarithromycin p. 403, or doxycycline p. 434 (child over 12 years).
  - Alternative if at high risk of treatment failure (repeated courses of antibacterials, previous culture with resistant or atypical bacteria, or high risk of complications): co-amoxiclav p. 420, or ciprofloxacin p. 429 (only if co-amoxiclav is inappropriate, and under specialist advice). (A)
- ***Intravenous** first line* (severely unwell or unable to take oral treatment):
  - EvGr Co-amoxiclav, piperacillin with tazobactam p. 413, or ciprofloxacin (only if co-amoxiclav and piperacillin with tazobactam are inappropriate, and under specialist advice). (A)

Antibacterial prophylaxis

EvGr For children with repeated acute exacerbations, a trial of antibacterial prophylaxis may be given on specialist advice only. (A)

Cough, acute

Acute cough is usually self-limiting and often resolves within 3–4 weeks without antibacterials. It is most commonly caused by a viral upper respiratory tract infection, but can have other infective causes such as acute bronchitis or pneumonia, or non-infective causes such as interstitial lung disease or gastro-oesophageal reflux disease.

Treatment

EvGr Children and their parents, or carers should be advised that an acute cough is usually self-limiting and to manage symptoms using self-care treatments. These include honey (for children over the age of 1 year) and over-the-counter cough medicines containing expectorants or cough suppressants, however there is limited evidence to support the use of such products. For more information, see Aromatic inhalations, cough preparations and systemic nasal decongestants p. 223.

Children with an acute cough who are systemically very unwell should be offered immediate antibacterial treatment.

Do not routinely offer an antibacterial to treat an acute cough associated with an upper respiratory tract infection or acute bronchitis in children who are not systemically very unwell or at higher risk of complications.

Children with a pre-existing co-morbidity or young children who were born prematurely are considered to be at a higher risk of complications if they present with an acute cough. In these patients, the need for immediate antibacterial treatment should be considered based on the face-to-face clinical examination. (A)

For general advice to give to children and their parents, or carers, see Antibacterials, principles of therapy p. 358.

EvGr Seek specialist advice, or refer children with an acute cough to hospital if they have signs or symptoms of a more serious illness or condition. (A)

Reassessment

EvGr Reassess if symptoms worsen rapidly or significantly taking into account alternative diagnoses, signs or symptoms suggestive of a more serious condition, and previous antibacterial use which may have led to resistant bacteria. (A)

Choice of antibacterial therapy

EvGr The recommended duration of oral treatment is 5 days. (A)

- *First line*:
  - EvGr Amoxicillin.
  - Alternative *first line* choices: clarithromycin, erythromycin p. 406, or doxycycline (child over 12 years). (A)
- Choice during pregnancy:
  - EvGr Amoxicillin or erythromycin. (A)

Pneumonia, community-acquired

Pneumonia is an acute infection of the lung parenchyma that presents with symptoms such as cough, chest pain, dyspnoea, and fever. It is classified as community-acquired if acquired outside of hospital.

For recommendations on the management of suspected or confirmed pneumonia secondary to COVID-19 infection, see NICE rapid guideline: **Managing COVID-19** (available at: www.nice.org.uk/guidance/ng191). For further information on COVID-19, see COVID-19 p. 490.

Treatment

EvGr Offer an antibacterial taking into account the severity of signs or symptoms based on clinical judgement, risk of complications, local antimicrobial resistance and surveillance data, recent antibacterial use, and recent microbiological test results.

Antibacterial treatment should be started as soon as possible after establishing a diagnosis and within 4 hours of presentation to hospital (if the child has suspected sepsis, see Sepsis p. 362 and NICE guideline on suspected sepsis in individuals aged under 16 years (www.nice.org.uk/guidance/ng254) and those aged 16 years or over (www.nice.org.uk/guidance/ng253).

Consider referring children to hospital or seeking specialist paediatric advice on further investigation and management. (A)

In children with severe community-acquired pneumonia in hospital, consider obtaining blood (if there are additional clinical indications such as suspected sepsis) and sputum cultures.

For other considerations such as switching from intravenous to oral antibacterials, and for advice to be given to children and their parents, or carers, see Antibacterials, principles of therapy p. 358 and NICE guideline on pneumonia (see *Useful resources*).

Reassessment

EvGr Reassess if signs or symptoms do not improve or worsen rapidly or significantly, and consider other possible non-bacterial causes such as influenza.

Send a sample, e.g. sputum, for microbiological testing if there is no improvement after antibacterial therapy and this has not already been done. If a sample has been sent for testing, review the choice of antibacterial and consider changing according to the results, using a narrower-spectrum antibacterial if appropriate.

Refer children to hospital if symptoms do not improve as expected with antibacterial treatment. (A)

Choice of antibacterial therapy

EvGr Treatment should be based on clinical judgement, suspected micro-organism, and if severe signs or symptoms guided by microbiological results when available.

Offer oral antibacterials to children who are able to take oral treatment and the severity of their condition does not require intravenous treatment.

Consider referral to hospital or seeking specialist advice if bacteria are resistant to oral antibacterials. Children under 1 month should be referred to a paediatric specialist. (A)

Non-severe

- ***Oral** first line* in children aged 1 month and over:
  - EvGr Amoxicillin p. 417.
  - Alternative in penicillin allergy or amoxicillin unsuitable (e.g. atypical pathogens suspected): clarithromycin p. 403, doxycycline p. 434 (child over 12 years), or erythromycin p. 406 (in pregnancy). (A)

Severe

- ***Oral** or **Intravenous** first line* in children aged 1 month and over:
  - EvGr Co-amoxiclav p. 420.
  - If atypical pathogens suspected: co-amoxiclav **with** clarithromycin **or** oral erythromycin (in pregnancy).
  - For alternatives in penicillin allergy consult local microbiologist. (A)

Pneumonia, hospital-acquired

Pneumonia is an acute infection of the lung parenchyma that presents with symptoms such as cough, chest pain, dyspnoea, and fever. It is classified as hospital-acquired when it develops 48 hours or more after hospital admission and it was not incubating at hospital admission, or if the child presents to hospital with pneumonia but was discharged within the last 7–10 days.

For recommendations on the management of suspected or confirmed pneumonia secondary to COVID-19 infection, see NICE rapid guideline: **Managing COVID-19** (available at: www.nice.org.uk/guidance/ng191). For further information on COVID-19, see COVID-19 p. 490.

Treatment

EvGr In children with signs or symptoms of pneumonia starting within 48 hours of hospital admission, follow the recommendations for children with community-acquired pneumonia. (A)

Offer an antibacterial taking into account:

- EvGr The severity of signs or symptoms;
- The number of days in hospital before onset of symptoms;
- The risk of complications;
- Local hospital and ward-based antimicrobial resistance data;
- Recent antibacterial use;
- Recent microbiological test results;
- Recent contact with health or social care settings;
- Risk of adverse effects such as *Clostridioides difficile* infection.

Antibacterial treatment should be started as soon as possible after establishing a diagnosis and within 4 hours of presentation to hospital (if the child has suspected sepsis, see Sepsis p. 362 and NICE guideline on suspected sepsis in individuals aged under 16 years (www.nice.org.uk/guidance/ng254) and those aged 16 years or over (www.nice.org.uk/guidance/ng253).

A sample (for example, sputum sample, nasopharyngeal swab or tracheal aspirate) should be taken for microbiological testing. (A)

For other considerations such as switching from intravenous to oral antibacterials, and for advice to be given to children and their parents, or carers see Antibacterials, principles of therapy p. 358 and NICE guideline on pneumonia (see *Useful resources*).

Reassessment

EvGr Reassess if symptoms do not improve or worsen rapidly or significantly.

When microbiological results are available, review the choice of antibacterial and change according to the results, using a narrower-spectrum antibacterial if appropriate.

Seek advice from a microbiologist if symptoms do not improve as expected with treatment, or multidrug-resistant bacteria are present. Ⓐ

Choice of antibacterial therapy

EvGr For children with non-severe signs or symptoms and not at higher risk of resistance, treatment should be guided by microbiological results when available. For children with severe signs or symptoms or at higher risk of resistance, treatment should be based on specialist microbiological advice and local resistance data.

Higher risk of resistance includes signs or symptoms starting more than 5 days after hospital admission, relevant comorbidity, recent use of broad-spectrum antibacterials, colonisation with multidrug-resistant bacteria, and recent contact with a health or social care setting before the current admission.

In children with signs or symptoms of pneumonia starting within 3 to 5 days of hospital admission and not at higher risk of resistance, consider following the recommendations for community-acquired pneumonia for choice of antibacterial.

In children under 1 month obtain specialist microbiological advice and consider local resistance data. Ⓐ

Non-severe signs or symptoms and not at higher risk of resistance

- ***Oral** first line* in children aged 1 month and over:
  - EvGr Co-amoxiclav.
  - Alternative in penicillin allergy or co-amoxiclav unsuitable: clarithromycin. Other options can be considered based on specialist microbiological advice and local resistance data. Ⓐ

Severe signs or symptoms (such as signs or symptoms of sepsis) or at higher risk of resistance

- ***Intravenous** first line* in children aged 1 month and over:
  - EvGr Piperacillin with tazobactam p. 413, ceftazidime p. 390, or ceftriaxone p. 391.
  - If meticillin-resistant *Staphylococcus aureus* confirmed or suspected, **add** teicoplanin p. 396, or vancomycin p. 398, or linezolid p. 442 [unlicensed] (child over 3 months under specialist advice only if vancomycin cannot be used). Ⓐ

Useful resources

Bronchiectasis (non-cystic fibrosis), acute exacerbation: antimicrobial prescribing. National Institute for Health and Care Excellence. NICE guideline 117. December 2018, updated September 2024.
www.nice.org.uk/guidance/ng117

Cough (acute): antimicrobial prescribing. National Institute for Health and Care Excellence. NICE guideline 120. February 2019.
www.nice.org.uk/guidance/ng120

Pneumonia: diagnosis and management. National Institute for Health and Care Excellence. NICE guideline 250. September 2025.
www.nice.org.uk/guidance/ng250

Skin infections, antibacterial therapy

06-May-2021

Impetigo

Impetigo is a contagious, superficial bacterial infection of the skin that affects all age groups, but it is more common in young children. Transmission occurs directly through close contact with an infected individual or indirectly via contaminated objects such as toys, clothing, or towels.

Impetigo can develop as a primary infection or as a secondary complication of pre-existing skin conditions such as eczema, scabies, or chickenpox. The two main clinical forms are non-bullous impetigo (most common form) and bullous impetigo. Non-bullous impetigo is characterised by thin-walled vesicles or pustules that rupture quickly, forming a golden-brown crust, while bullous impetigo is characterised by the presence of fluid-filled vesicles and blisters that rupture, leaving a thin, flat, yellow-brown crust.

Initial treatment

EvGr Patients, and if appropriate their family or carers, should be advised on good hygiene measures to reduce the spread of impetigo to other body areas and to other people.

In patients with **localised non-bullous impetigo** who are not systemically unwell or at high risk of complications, consider hydrogen peroxide 1% cream p. 945; if unsuitable (e.g. if impetigo is around the eyes), offer a topical antibacterial.

In patients with **widespread non-bullous impetigo** who are not systemically unwell or at high risk of complications, offer a topical **or** oral antibacterial. Take into account that both routes of administration are effective; any previous use of topical antibacterials that could have led to resistance; and the preferences of the patient and, their family or carers (if appropriate), including the practicalities of administration (particularly to large areas).

In patients with **non-bullous impetigo** who are systemically unwell or at high risk of complications and in all patients with **bullous impetigo**, offer an oral antibacterial.

Combination treatment with a topical and oral antibacterial is not recommended. Ⓐ

For other considerations such as advice to be given to patients, and if appropriate their family or carers, see Antibacterials, principles of therapy p. 358.

EvGr Refer patients to hospital if they have any signs or symptoms suggestive of a more serious condition or illness, or if they have widespread impetigo and are immunocompromised.

Consider referral to hospital or seeking specialist advice for patients who are systemically unwell, have a higher risk of complications, or if impetigo is difficult to treat (such as bullous impetigo (particularly in children aged under 1 year) or frequently recurrent impetigo). Ⓐ

Reassessment and further treatment

EvGr Reassess if symptoms worsen rapidly or significantly at any time, or do not improve after completion of the treatment course. Take into consideration other possible diagnoses (such as herpes simplex infection), signs or symptoms suggesting a more serious illness or condition (such as cellulitis), and previous antibacterial use that might have led to resistance.

For patients whose impetigo is worsening or has not improved after treatment with hydrogen peroxide 1% cream, offer a topical antibacterial if the infection remains localised, or a topical **or** oral antibacterial if infection has become widespread.

Offer an oral antibacterial to patients whose impetigo is worsening or has not improved after completing a course of topical antibacterial.

For patients whose impetigo is worsening or has not improved after completing a course of topical or oral antibacterials, consider sending a skin swab for microbiological testing.

For patients with impetigo that recurs frequently, send a skin swab for microbiological testing and consider taking a nasal swab and starting treatment for decolonisation (using topical treatments and personal hygiene measures).

If a skin swab has been sent for microbiological testing, review the choice of antibacterial and change according to the results if symptoms are not improving, using a narrower-spectrum antibacterial if possible. Ⓐ

Choice of antibacterial therapy

EvGr Treatment should be based on infection severity and number of lesions, suspected micro-organism, local antibacterial resistance data, and be guided by microbiological results if available. (A)

- ***Topical** first line* if hydrogen peroxide unsuitable or ineffective:
  - EvGr Fusidic acid p. 441.
  - Alternative if fusidic acid resistance suspected or confirmed: mupirocin p. 899. (A)
- ***Oral** first line* :
  - EvGr Flucloxacillin p. 424.
  - Alternative if penicillin allergy or flucloxacillin unsuitable: clarithromycin p. 403 or erythromycin p. 406 (in pregnancy). (A)
- If meticillin-resistant *Staphylococcus aureus* (MRSA) infection suspected or confirmed: EvGr Consult local microbiologist. (A)

Cellulitis and erysipelas

Cellulitis and erysipelas are infections of the subcutaneous tissues, which usually result from contamination of a break in the skin. Both conditions are characterised by acute localised inflammation and oedema. Lesions are more superficial in erysipelas and have a well-defined, raised margin.

For management of infection below the ankle in children with diabetes, see Diabetic foot infections, antibacterial therapy p. 366.

Treatment

EvGr Consider taking a swab for microbiological testing **only** if the skin is broken and there is risk of infection by an uncommon pathogen (for example, after a penetrating injury, exposure to water-born organisms, or an infection acquired outside the UK).

Drawing around the extent of the infection to monitor progress prior to initiating antibacterial treatment can also be considered, taking into account that redness may be less visible on darker skin tones.

Offer an antibacterial taking into account the severity of symptoms, site of infection, risk of uncommon pathogens, previous microbiological results from a swab, and the patient's meticillin-resistant *Staphylococcus aureus* (MRSA) status if known. (A)

For other considerations such as switching from intravenous to oral antibacterials, and for advice to be given to children and their parents, or carers, see Antibacterials, principles of therapy p. 358.

EvGr Manage any underlying condition that may predispose to cellulitis or erysipelas, such as diabetes mellitus, venous insufficiency, eczema, and oedema.

Refer children to hospital if they have signs or symptoms suggestive of a more serious illness, such as orbital cellulitis, osteomyelitis, septic arthritis, necrotising fasciitis, or sepsis.

Consider referral to hospital or seeking specialist advice for patients who have lymphangitis, are severely unwell, are unable to take oral antibacterials, have infection near the eyes or nose, or that could be caused by an uncommon pathogen. (A)

Reassessment

EvGr Reassess if symptoms worsen rapidly or significantly at any time, do not improve within 2–3 days of starting an antibacterial, or the child becomes systemically very unwell, has severe pain out of proportion to the infection, or has redness or swelling spreading beyond the initial presentation (taking into account that some initial spreading may occur). Take into consideration other possible diagnoses (such as an inflammatory reaction to an insect bite or deep vein thrombosis), any underlying condition that may predispose to cellulitis or erysipelas, signs or symptoms suggesting a more serious illness, results from microbiological tests, and previous antibacterial use that might have led to resistance.

Consider taking a swab for testing if the skin is broken and this has not already been done.

If a swab has been sent for microbiological testing, review the choice of antibacterial and change according to the results if signs or symptoms are not improving, using a narrower-spectrum antibacterial if possible.

Consider referral to hospital or seeking specialist advice if the infection has spread and is not responding to oral antibacterials. (A)

Choice of antibacterial therapy

EvGr Treatment should be based on clinical assessment, infection severity, suspected micro-organism, and site of infection.

Offer oral antibacterials to children who are able to take oral treatment and the severity of their condition does not require intravenous treatment.

Consider referral to hospital or seeking specialist advice if bacteria are resistant to oral antibacterials, patients cannot take oral treatment, or have infection near the eyes or nose.

Antibacterial choice for children under 1 month should be based on specialist advice. (A)

First choice antibacterials in children aged 1 month and over

- ***Oral** or **Intravenous** first line* :
  - EvGr Flucloxacillin p. 424.
  - Alternative in penicillin allergy or if flucloxacillin unsuitable: co-amoxiclav p. 420 (**not** in penicillin allergy), clarithromycin p. 403, or oral erythromycin p. 406 (in pregnancy). (A)
- ***Oral** or **Intravenous** first line if infection near the eyes or nose* :
  - EvGr Co-amoxiclav.
  - Alternative in penicillin allergy or co-amoxiclav unsuitable: clarithromycin. If anaerobes suspected, **add** metronidazole p. 409. (A)

Alternative choice antibacterials for severe infection in children aged 1 month and over

- ***Oral** or **Intravenous**:*
  - EvGr Co-amoxiclav, clindamycin p. 400, or intravenous cefuroxime p. 388.
  - If meticillin-resistant *Staphylococcus aureus* confirmed or suspected, **add** intravenous vancomycin p. 398, intravenous teicoplanin p. 396, or linezolid p. 442 (specialist use only if vancomycin or teicoplanin cannot be used).
  - Other antibacterials may be appropriate based on microbiological results and specialist advice. (A)

Insect bites and stings

Redness, itchiness, or pain and swelling after an insect sting or bite (including bites from spiders and ticks) is often caused by a localised inflammatory or allergic reaction rather than an infection, especially when there is a rapid onset. Rarely, symptoms may last for up to 10 days.

For the management of patients with a known or suspected tick bite, see Lyme disease p. 444. EvGr Consider referral or seeking specialist advice for patients with fever or persistent lesions after an insect bite or sting from outside the UK, as this may indicate a more serious illness such as rickettsial infection or malaria.

Antibacterials are not recommended for an insect bite or sting unless the patient has signs or symptoms of an infection. For the management of patients with a suspected infection, see *Cellulitis and erysipelas*. (A)

Human and animal bites

Human and animal bites that cause a break in the skin are an infection risk. Contributing factors of infection include the species causing the bite, type and location of the wound, and the child's individual risk factors (such as comorbidities, and age (neonates and infants are at higher risk of infection)).

For guidance on the management of insect bites, see *Insects bites and stings*.

Management

EvGr Children with a human or an animal bite should be assessed for their risk of tetanus, rabies, or a blood-borne viral infection (such as HIV, and hepatitis B and C), and should be managed accordingly. ⟨A⟩ For guidance on the management of tetanus- and rabies-prone wounds, see Tetanus vaccine p. 981 or Rabies vaccine p. 977.

EvGr The child's wound should be cleaned by irrigation and debrided as necessary.

For bites from wild or exotic animals (including birds and non-traditional pets), advice should be sought from a microbiologist as the spectrum of bacteria involved may be different and there may be a risk of other serious non-bacterial infections. Consider seeking advice for bites from unfamiliar domestic animals (including farm animals).

Refer children to hospital if they have signs or symptoms suggesting a more serious illness or condition (such as severe cellulitis, abscess, osteomyelitis, septic arthritis, necrotising fasciitis, or sepsis), or a penetrating wound involving the arteries, joints, nerves, muscles, tendons, bones or the central nervous system.

Consider referral to hospital or seeking specialist advice for children who have lymphangitis, are systemically unwell, have a bite in an area of poor circulation, are at risk of a serious wound infection due to comorbidities, or are unable to take oral antibacterials. ⟨A⟩

For considerations such as switching from intravenous to oral antibacterials, and for advice to be given to children and their parents, or carers, see Antibacterials, principles of therapy p. 358.

Prophylaxis for an uninfected bite

EvGr Offer antibacterial prophylaxis to children with a:

- cat or human bite that has broken the skin and drawn blood; or
- dog or other traditional pet bite (excluding cat bites) that has broken the skin and drawn blood if it:
  - has penetrated bone, joint, tendon or vascular structures;
  - is deep, a puncture or crush wound, or has caused significant tissue damage; or
  - is visibly contaminated (for example if there is dirt or a tooth in the wound).

Consider antibacterial prophylaxis in children with:

- a cat bite that has broken the skin but **not** drawn blood and the wound could be deep; or
- a human bite that has broken the skin but **not** drawn blood, *or* a dog or other traditional pet bite (excluding cat bites) that has broken the skin and drawn blood, if it:
  - involves a high-risk area (such as the hands, feet, face, genitals, skin overlying cartilaginous structures, or an area of poor circulation), or
  - is in a child at risk of a serious wound infection because of a comorbidity (such as diabetes, immunosuppression, asplenia, or decompensated liver disease).

Consider referral to hospital or seeking specialist advice for children who develop an infection despite taking antibacterial prophylaxis. ⟨A⟩

Treatment for an infected bite

EvGr To guide treatment for wounds that have a purulent or non-purulent discharge, a swab should be taken for microbiological testing.

Antibacterial therapy should be offered to children if there are signs or symptoms of infection (such as increased pain, inflammation, fever, discharge, or an unpleasant smell). ⟨A⟩

Reassessment

EvGr Reassess the child's wound if either:

- signs or symptoms of infection develop, worsen rapidly or significantly at any time, or do not improve within 1–2 days of starting an antibacterial; or
- the child becomes systemically unwell or has severe pain out of proportion to the infection.

If a skin swab has been sent for microbiological testing, review the choice of antibacterial and change according to the results if needed, using a narrower-spectrum antibacterial if possible.

Consider referral or seeking specialist advice if the infected wound is not responding to oral antibacterial therapy. ⟨A⟩

Choice of antibacterial for prophylaxis and treatment

EvGr For bites from a human, cat, dog, or other traditional pet, offer oral antibacterials to children who are able to take medication orally and the severity of their condition does not require intravenous antibacterials.

Antibacterial choice for children aged under 1 month should be based on specialist advice. ⟨A⟩

- ***Oral*** *first line* in children aged 1 month and over:
  - EvGr Co-amoxiclav p. 420.
  - Alternative in penicillin allergy or co-amoxiclav unsuitable:
    - for children aged under 12 years: co-trimoxazole p. 431 [unlicensed];
    - for children aged 12 years and over: doxycycline p. 434 **with** metronidazole p. 409;
    - seek specialist advice in pregnancy. ⟨A⟩
- ***Intravenous*** *first line* in children aged 1 month and over:
  - EvGr Co-amoxiclav.
  - Alternative in penicillin allergy or co-amoxiclav unsuitable: cefuroxime p. 388 *or* ceftriaxone p. 391, **with** metronidazole; seek specialist advice if a cephalosporin is not appropriate. ⟨A⟩

Secondary bacterial infection of common skin conditions

Common skin conditions that cause breaks in the skin are an infection risk, as bacteria that live on the skin may infiltrate the damaged area. The most commonly infected skin conditions are chickenpox, eczema, psoriasis, scabies, and shingles. For guidance on the management of underlying skin conditions and non-antibacterial treatment, see Eczema p. 905, Herpesvirus infections p. 498, Psoriasis p. 906, and Skin infections p. 895.

EvGr For secondary bacterial infections of common skin conditions other than eczema (such as chickenpox, psoriasis, scabies, and shingles) there is no evidence available for antibacterial use—seek specialist advice if needed. ⟨A⟩

The following recommendations cover the management of children with secondary bacterial skin infection of **eczema**. Signs and symptoms of secondary bacterial infection of eczema can include weeping, pustules, crusts, no response to treatment, rapidly worsening eczema, fever, and malaise. Even if weeping and crusts are present, not all eczema flares are caused by a bacterial infection.

Treatment of secondary bacterial skin infection of eczema

EvGr Taking a routine skin swab for microbiological testing at initial presentation is not recommended as eczema is often colonised with bacteria but may not be clinically infected.

In children who are not systemically unwell, an antibacterial is not routinely recommended. Take into account the evidence of limited benefit of antibacterials when used in addition to topical corticosteroids, risk of antimicrobial resistance with repeated courses, extent and severity of signs or symptoms, and risk of developing complications (higher in children with underlying conditions such as immunosuppression).

If an antibacterial is offered to children who are not systemically unwell, the choice between a topical or oral antibacterial should take into account the preferences of the child (and their family/carers), previous use of topical antibacterials as resistance can develop rapidly with extended or repeated use, practicalities of administration (particularly to large areas), and the extent and severity of signs or symptoms. A topical antibacterial may be more appropriate for a localised infection that is not severe, whereas, an oral antibacterial may be more appropriate if the infection is widespread or severe.

Offer an oral antibacterial to children who are systemically unwell (such as with a fever or malaise).

Underlying eczema and flares should be managed with emollients and topical corticosteroids regardless of whether antibacterials are offered (see Eczema p. 905). Ⓐ

For other considerations such as advice to be given to children and their parents or carers, see Antibacterials, principles of therapy p. 358.

EvGr Refer children to hospital if they have signs or symptoms suggestive of a more serious illness, such as necrotising fasciitis or sepsis. For children with signs and symptoms of cellulitis, see *Cellulitis and erysipelas*.

Consider referral to hospital or seeking specialist advice for children who are systemically unwell or at high risk of complications, or have infections that recur often. Ⓐ

Reassessment

EvGr Reassess if symptoms worsen rapidly or significantly at any time, do not improve after completion of an antibacterial course, the child becomes systemically unwell, or has pain out of proportion to the infection. Take into consideration other possible diagnoses (such as eczema herpeticum), signs or symptoms suggesting a more serious illness, and previous antibacterial use that might have led to resistance.

For children whose infection is worsening or has not improved as expected, consider sending a skin swab for microbiological testing.

For children with secondary bacterial infection of eczema that recurs frequently, send a skin swab for microbiological testing, and consider taking a nasal swab and starting treatment for decolonisation.

If a skin swab has been sent for microbiological testing, review the choice of antibacterial and change according to the results if symptoms are not improving, using a narrower-spectrum antibacterial if possible.

Consider referral to hospital or seeking specialist advice if the infection has spread and is not responding to oral antibacterials. Ⓐ

Choice of antibacterial therapy

EvGr Treatment should be based on infection severity, suspected micro-organism, local antibacterial resistance data, and be guided by microbiological results if available.

Antibacterial choice for children aged under 1 month should be based on specialist advice. Ⓐ

- ***Topical*** *first line* :
  - ▸ EvGr Fusidic acid p. 441.
  - ▸ If fusidic acid unsuitable or ineffective: offer an oral antibacterial. Ⓐ
- ***Oral*** *first line* :
  - ▸ EvGr Flucloxacillin p. 424.
  - ▸ Alternative if penicillin allergy or flucloxacillin unsuitable: clarithromycin p. 403 or erythromycin p. 406 (in pregnancy). Ⓐ
- If meticillin-resistant *Staphylococcus aureus* (MRSA) infection suspected or confirmed: EvGr Consult a local microbiologist. Ⓐ

Staphylococcal scalded skin syndrome

- Flucloxacillin
  - ▸ *Suggested duration of treatment* 7–10 days.
- *If penicillin-allergic*, clarithromycin (*or* azithromycin p. 402 *or* erythromycin)
  - ▸ *Suggested duration of treatment* 7–10 days.

Surgical wound infection

- Flucloxacillin *or* co-amoxiclav

Paronychia or 'septic spots' in neonate

- Flucloxacillin
  - ▸ If systemically unwell, add an aminoglycoside.

Useful Resources

Cellulitis and erysipelas: antimicrobial prescribing. National Institute for Health and Care Excellence. NICE guideline 141. September 2019.
www.nice.org.uk/guidance/ng141

Human and animal bites: antimicrobial prescribing. National Institute for Health and Care Excellence. NICE guideline 184. November 2020.
www.nice.org.uk/guidance/ng184

Impetigo: antimicrobial prescribing. National Institute for Health and Care Excellence. NICE guideline 153. February 2020.
www.nice.org.uk/guidance/ng153

Insect bites and stings: antimicrobial prescribing. National Institute for Health and Care Excellence. NICE guideline 182. September 2020.
www.nice.org.uk/guidance/ng182

Secondary bacterial infection of eczema and other common skin conditions: antimicrobial prescribing. National Institute for Health and Care Excellence. NICE guideline 190. March 2021.
www.nice.org.uk/guidance/ng190

Other drugs used for Bacterial infection Rifabutin, p. 448

ANTIBACTERIALS > AMINOGLYCOSIDES

Aminoglycosides

15-May-2024

Overview

These include amikacin p. 377, gentamicin p. 378, neomycin sulfate p. 898, streptomycin p. 380, and tobramycin p. 380. All are bactericidal and active against some Gram-positive and many Gram-negative organisms. Amikacin, gentamicin, and tobramycin are also active against *Pseudomonas aeruginosa*; streptomycin is active against *Mycobacterium tuberculosis* and is now almost entirely reserved for tuberculosis.

The aminoglycosides are not absorbed from the gut (although there is a risk of absorption in inflammatory bowel disease and liver failure) and must therefore be given by injection for systemic infections.

Gentamicin is the aminoglycoside of choice in the UK and is used widely for the treatment of serious infections. It has a broad spectrum but is inactive against anaerobes and has poor activity against haemolytic streptococci and pneumococci. When used for the 'blind' therapy of undiagnosed serious infections it is usually given in conjunction with a penicillin or metronidazole p. 409 (or both). Gentamicin is used together with another antibiotic for the treatment of endocarditis. Streptomycin may be used as an alternative in gentamicin-resistant enterococcal endocarditis.

Loading and maintenance doses of gentamicin may be calculated on the basis of the patient's weight and renal function (e.g. using a nomogram); adjustments are then made according to serum-gentamicin concentrations. High doses are occasionally indicated for serious infections, especially in the neonate or in the immunocompromised patient. Whenever possible treatment should not exceed 7 days.

Amikacin is more stable than gentamicin to enzyme inactivation. Amikacin is used in the treatment of serious infections caused by gentamicin-resistant Gram-negative bacilli.

Tobramycin has similar activity to gentamicin but is more active against *Pseudomonas aeruginosa*.

Neomycin sulfate is too toxic for parenteral administration and can only be used for infections of the skin or mucous membranes or to reduce the bacterial population of the colon prior to bowel surgery or in hepatic failure. Oral administration may lead to malabsorption. Small amounts of neomycin sulfate may be absorbed from the gut in patients with hepatic failure and, as these patients may also be uraemic, cumulation may occur with resultant ototoxicity.

Cystic fibrosis

A higher dose of parenteral aminoglycoside is often required in children with cystic fibrosis because renal clearance of the aminoglycoside is increased. Tobramycin is the preferred aminoglycoside for the treatment of pseudomonal lung infections in cystic fibrosis. Tobramycin can also be administered by nebuliser or by inhalation of powder on a cyclical basis (28 days of tobramycin followed by a 28-day tobramycin-free interval) for the treatment of chronic pulmonary *Pseudomonas aeruginosa* infection in cystic fibrosis; however, resistance may develop and some patients do not respond to treatment.

Once daily dosage

Once daily administration of aminoglycosides is more convenient, provides adequate serum concentrations, and has largely superseded *multiple-daily dose regimens* (given in 2–3 divided doses during the 24 hours). Local guidelines on dosage and serum concentrations should be consulted. A once-daily, high-dose regimen of an aminoglycoside should be avoided in children with endocarditis or burns of more than 20% of the total body surface area. There is insufficient evidence to recommend a once daily, high-dose regimen of an aminoglycoside in pregnancy.

Serum concentrations

Serum concentration monitoring avoids both excessive and subtherapeutic concentrations thus preventing toxicity and ensuring efficacy. Serum-aminoglycoside concentrations should be monitored in patients receiving parenteral aminoglycosides and **must** be determined in obesity, and in cystic fibrosis, or if high doses are being given, or if there is renal impairment.

Neonates

As aminoglycosides are eliminated principally via the kidney, neonatal treatment must reflect the changes in glomerular filtration that occur with increasing gestational and postnatal age. The *extended interval dose regimen* is used in neonates, and serum-aminoglycoside concentrations **must** be measured. In patients on single daily dose regimens it may become necessary to prolong the dose interval to more than 24 hours if the trough concentration is high.

Aminoglycosides (by injection)

- **CONTRA-INDICATIONS** Myasthenia gravis (aminoglycosides may impair neuromuscular transmission)
- **CAUTIONS** Auditory disorder · care must be taken with dosage (the main side-effects of the aminoglycosides are dose-related) · conditions characterised by muscular weakness (aminoglycosides may impair neuromuscular transmission) · if possible, dehydration should be corrected before starting an aminoglycoside · vestibular disorder · whenever possible, parenteral treatment should not exceed 7 days
- **SIDE-EFFECTS**
  - **Common or very common** Dysphonia · tinnitus · vomiting
  - **Uncommon** Cough · increased risk of infection · nausea · skin reactions
  - **Rare or very rare** Anaemia · aphonia · appetite decreased · azotaemia · bronchospasm · chest discomfort · diarrhoea · dizziness · eosinophilia · fever · haemoptysis · headache · hearing impairment · hypomagnesaemia · paraesthesia · renal impairment · taste altered
  - **Frequency not known** Confusion · lethargy · leucopenia · muscle weakness · nephrotoxicity · oropharyngeal pain · peripheral neuropathy · thrombocytopenia · vertigo

  SIDE-EFFECTS, FURTHER INFORMATION Ototoxicity and nephrotoxicity are important side-effects to consider with aminoglycoside therapy. Nephrotoxicity occurs most commonly in patients with renal impairment
- **PREGNANCY** There is a risk of auditory or vestibular nerve damage in the infant when aminoglycosides are used in the second and third trimesters of pregnancy. The risk is greatest with streptomycin. The risk is probably very small with gentamicin and tobramycin, but their use should be avoided unless essential.

  Monitoring If given during pregnancy, serum-aminoglycoside concentration monitoring is essential.
- **RENAL IMPAIRMENT** EvGr Aminoglycosides are primarily renally excreted and accumulation can occur in renal impairment (increased risk of ototoxicity and nephrotoxicity)—serum-aminoglycoside concentrations **must** be frequently monitored in patients with renal impairment. (M)

  Dose adjustments EvGr Reduce dose and/or increase the dose interval according to impairment (consult product literature). (M)
- **MONITORING REQUIREMENTS**
  - Serum concentrations Serum concentration monitoring avoids both excessive and subtherapeutic concentrations thus preventing toxicity and ensuring efficacy.

    Serum-aminoglycoside concentrations should be measured in all patients receiving parenteral aminoglycosides and **must** be determined in obesity, if high doses are being given and in cystic fibrosis.

    Serum aminoglycoside concentrations **must** be determined in neonates.

    In children with normal renal function, aminoglycoside concentrations should be measured after 3 or 4 doses of a multiple daily dose regimen.

    Blood samples should be taken just before the next dose is administered ('trough' concentration). If the pre-dose ('trough') concentration is high, the interval between doses must be increased. For multiple daily dose regimens, blood samples should also be taken approximately 1 hour after intramuscular or intravenous administration ('peak' concentration). If the post-dose ('peak') concentration is high, the dose must be decreased.
  - Renal function should be assessed before starting an aminoglycoside and during treatment.
  - Auditory and vestibular function should also be monitored during treatment.

above

Amikacin

24-Jul-2025

- **INDICATIONS AND DOSE**

Serious Gram-negative infections resistant to gentamicin (multiple daily dose regimen)

- BY SLOW INTRAVENOUS INJECTION
  - Child 1 month–11 years: 7.5 mg/kg every 12 hours
  - Child 12–17 years: 7.5 mg/kg every 12 hours (max. per dose 750 mg) for up to 10 days, alternatively 7.5 mg/kg every 8 hours (max. per dose 500 mg) for up to 10 days, increased frequency to be used in severe infection; maximum 15 g per course

continued →

Serious Gram-negative infections resistant to gentamicin (once daily dose regimen)
- ▶ BY INTRAVENOUS INFUSION, OR BY SLOW INTRAVENOUS INJECTION
- ▸ Child 1 month–11 years: Initially 15 mg/kg once daily, not to be used for endocarditis or meningitis, dose to be adjusted according to serum-amikacin concentration
- ▸ Child 12–17 years: Initially 15 mg/kg once daily (max. per dose 1.5 g), not to be used for endocarditis or meningitis, dose to be adjusted according to serum-amikacin concentration

Neonatal sepsis (extended interval dose regimen)
- ▶ BY SLOW INTRAVENOUS INJECTION, OR BY INTRAVENOUS INFUSION
- ▸ Neonate: 15 mg/kg every 24 hours.

Neonatal sepsis (multiple daily dose regimen)
- ▶ BY INTRAMUSCULAR INJECTION, OR BY SLOW INTRAVENOUS INJECTION, OR BY INTRAVENOUS INFUSION
- ▸ Neonate: Loading dose 10 mg/kg for 1 dose, then 7.5 mg/kg every 12 hours.

Pulmonary infection with *Pseudomonas aeruginosa* in cystic fibrosis
- ▶ BY INTRAVENOUS INFUSION
- ▸ Child: Initially 30 mg/kg once daily (max. per dose 1.5 g), dose to be adjusted according to serum-amikacin concentration
- ▶ BY SLOW INTRAVENOUS INJECTION, OR BY INTRAVENOUS INFUSION
- ▸ Child: Initially 10 mg/kg every 8 hours (max. per dose 500 mg), dose to be adjusted according to serum-amikacin concentration

Acute pyelonephritis (once daily dose regimen) | Urinary tract infection (catheter-associated, once daily dose regimen)
- ▶ BY INTRAVENOUS INFUSION, OR BY SLOW INTRAVENOUS INJECTION
- ▸ Child 3 months–11 years: Initially 15 mg/kg once daily, dose to be adjusted according to serum-amikacin concentration
- ▸ Child 12–15 years: Initially 15 mg/kg once daily (max. per dose 1.5 g), dose to be adjusted according to serum-amikacin concentration
- ▸ Child 16–17 years: Initially 15 mg/kg once daily (max. per dose 1.5 g), dose to be adjusted according to serum-amikacin concentration; maximum 15 g per course

DOSES AT EXTREMES OF BODY-WEIGHT
- ▸ To avoid excessive dosage in obese patients, dose should be calculated on the basis of ideal body-weight for height.

● **UNLICENSED USE** Dose for cystic fibrosis not licensed.

IMPORTANT SAFETY INFORMATION

MHRA/CHM ADVICE: AMINOGLYCOSIDES (GENTAMICIN, AMIKACIN, TOBRAMYCIN, AND NEOMYCIN): INCREASED RISK OF DEAFNESS IN PATIENTS WITH MITOCHONDRIAL MUTATIONS (JANUARY 2021)

The use of aminoglycosides is associated with rare cases of ototoxicity. A safety review found an increased risk of deafness in patients with mitochondrial mutations (particularly the m.1555A>G mutation), including cases where the patient's aminoglycoside serum levels were within the recommended range. Nevertheless, these mitochondrial mutations are considered rare and penetrance is uncertain.

Healthcare professionals are advised to consider the need for aminoglycoside treatment versus alternative options in patients with susceptible mutations. The need for genetic testing especially in those requiring recurrent or long-term treatment with aminoglycosides should also be considered, however, urgent treatment should not be delayed. To minimise the risks of adverse effects, continuous monitoring of renal and auditory function, as well as hepatic and laboratory parameters, is recommended for all patients. Those with known mitochondrial mutations or a family history of ototoxicity are advised to inform their doctor or pharmacist before using an aminoglycoside.

● **INTERACTIONS** → Appendix 1: aminoglycosides

● **SIDE-EFFECTS**
- ▶ **Rare or very rare** Albuminuria · arthralgia · balance impaired · hypotension · muscle twitching · tremor
- ▶ **Frequency not known** Apnoea · neuromuscular blockade · paralysis

● **PRE-TREATMENT SCREENING** NHS England commissions genetic testing under the *National genomic test directory* indication: R65 - Aminoglycoside exposure posing risk to hearing. The testing criteria is significant exposure to aminoglycosides posing risk of ototoxicity. This testing is relevant to individuals with a predisposition to gram-negative infections or with hearing loss who have been exposed to aminoglycosides. For further information, see www.england.nhs.uk/publication/national-genomic-test-directories/.

● **MONITORING REQUIREMENTS**
- ▸ With intravenous use *Multiple daily dose regimen*: one-hour ('peak') serum concentration should not exceed 30 mg/litre; pre-dose ('trough') concentration should be less than 10 mg/litre. *Once daily dose regimen*: pre-dose ('trough') concentration should be less than 5 mg/litre.

● **DIRECTIONS FOR ADMINISTRATION** For *intravenous infusion*, manufacturer advises dilute with Glucose 5% *or* Sodium Chloride 0.9%; give over 30–60 minutes. [EvGr] For *slow intravenous injection*, give over 5 minutes. ⟨E⟩

● **PRESCRIBING AND DISPENSING INFORMATION** Local guidelines may vary in the dosing advice provided.

● **MEDICINAL FORMS** There can be variation in the licensing of different medicines containing the same drug. Forms available from special-order manufacturers include: solution for injection

Solution for injection
- ▸ **Amikacin (Non-proprietary)**
  Amikacin (as Amikacin sulfate) 250 mg per 1 ml Amikacin 500mg/2ml solution for injection ampoules | 5 ampoule [PoM] £60.00 (Hospital only)
  Amikacin 500mg/2ml solution for injection vials | 5 vial [PoM] £40.00–£60.00 (Hospital only) | 5 vial [PoM] £40.00–£60.00
- ▸ **Amikin** (Vianex S.A.)
  Amikacin (as Amikacin sulfate) 50 mg per 1 ml Amikin 100mg/2ml solution for injection vials | 5 vial [PoM] £10.33 (Hospital only)

377

Gentamicin

20-Jun-2025

● **INDICATIONS AND DOSE**

Septicaemia | Meningitis and other CNS infections | Biliary-tract infection | Endocarditis | Pneumonia in hospital patients | Adjunct in listerial meningitis
- ▶ BY INTRAVENOUS INFUSION
- ▸ Child: Initially 7 mg/kg, to be given in a once daily regimen (not suitable for endocarditis or meningitis), subsequent doses adjusted according to serum-gentamicin concentration
- ▶ BY INTRAMUSCULAR INJECTION, OR BY SLOW INTRAVENOUS INJECTION
- ▸ Child 1 month–11 years: 2.5 mg/kg every 8 hours, to be given in a multiple daily dose regimen, intravenous injection to be administered over at least 3 minutes
- ▸ Child 12–17 years: 2 mg/kg every 8 hours, to be given in a multiple daily dose regimen, intravenous injection to be administered over at least 3 minutes

Neonatal sepsis
▶ BY SLOW INTRAVENOUS INJECTION, OR BY INTRAVENOUS INFUSION
▸ Neonate up to 7 days: 5 mg/kg every 36 hours, to be given in an extended interval dose regimen.
▸ Neonate 7 days to 28 days: 5 mg/kg every 24 hours, to be given in an extended interval dose regimen.

Bacterial ventriculitis and CNS infection (supplement to systemic therapy) (administered on expert advice)
▶ BY INTRATHECAL INJECTION, OR BY INTRAVENTRICULAR INJECTION
▸ Neonate: (consult local protocol).
▸ Child: Initially 1 mg daily, then increased if necessary to 5 mg daily, seek specialist advice

Acute pyelonephritis (once daily dose regimen) | Urinary tract infection (catheter-associated, once daily dose regimen)
▶ BY INTRAVENOUS INFUSION
▸ Child 3 months–15 years: Initially 7 mg/kg once daily, subsequent doses adjusted according to serum-gentamicin concentration
▸ Child 16-17 years: Initially 5–7 mg/kg once daily, subsequent doses adjusted according to serum-gentamicin concentration

Uncomplicated gonorrhoea [anogenital and pharyngeal infection—in combination with azithromycin]
▶ BY INTRAMUSCULAR INJECTION
▸ Child 12-17 years (body-weight 45 kg and above): 240 mg for 1 dose

DOSES AT EXTREMES OF BODY-WEIGHT
▸ With intramuscular use or intravenous use To avoid excessive dosage in obese patients, use ideal weight for height to calculate parenteral dose and monitor serum-gentamicin concentration closely.

● **UNLICENSED USE** Gentamicin doses in BNF Publications may differ from those in product literature.
EvGr Gentamicin is used in the doses provided in BNF Publications for the treatment of uncomplicated gonorrhoea, (A) but these are not licensed.

IMPORTANT SAFETY INFORMATION

MHRA/CHM ADVICE: POTENTIAL FOR HISTAMINE-RELATED ADVERSE DRUG REACTIONS WITH SOME BATCHES (NOVEMBER 2017)
▸ With intramuscular use or intrathecal use or intravenous use Following reports that some batches of gentamicin sulphate active pharmaceutical ingredient (API) used to manufacture gentamicin may contain higher than expected levels of histamine, which is a residual from the manufacturing process, the MHRA advise to monitor patients for signs of histamine-related adverse reactions; particular caution is required in patients taking concomitant drugs known to cause histamine release, in children, and in patients with severe renal impairment.

MHRA/CHM ADVICE: AMINOGLYCOSIDES (GENTAMICIN, AMIKACIN, TOBRAMYCIN, AND NEOMYCIN): INCREASED RISK OF DEAFNESS IN PATIENTS WITH MITOCHONDRIAL MUTATIONS (JANUARY 2021)
The use of aminoglycosides is associated with rare cases of ototoxicity. A safety review found an increased risk of deafness in patients with mitochondrial mutations (particularly the m.1555A>G mutation), including cases where the patient's aminoglycoside serum levels were within the recommended range. Nevertheless, these mitochondrial mutations are considered rare and penetrance is uncertain. No cases were identified with topical preparations but, based on a shared mechanism of effect, there is a potential risk with gentamicin and other aminoglycosides administered at the site of toxicity i.e. the ear.
Healthcare professionals are advised to consider the need for aminoglycoside treatment versus alternative options in patients with susceptible mutations. The need for genetic testing especially in those requiring recurrent or long-term treatment with aminoglycosides should also be considered, however, urgent treatment should not be delayed. To minimise the risks of adverse effects, continuous monitoring of renal and auditory function, as well as hepatic and laboratory parameters, is recommended for all patients. Those with known mitochondrial mutations or a family history of ototoxicity are advised to inform their doctor or pharmacist before using an aminoglycoside.

● **INTERACTIONS** → Appendix 1: aminoglycosides

● **SIDE-EFFECTS**
▶ **Rare or very rare** Fanconi syndrome acquired
▶ **Frequency not known** Antibiotic associated colitis · blood disorder · central neuropathy · depression · encephalopathy · hallucination · hepatic function abnormal · neurotoxicity · pseudomembranous enterocolitis · seizure · severe cutaneous adverse reactions (SCARs) · stomatitis · vestibular damage

● **PRE-TREATMENT SCREENING** NHS England commissions genetic testing under the *National genomic test directory* indication: R65 - Aminoglycoside exposure posing risk to hearing. The testing criteria is significant exposure to aminoglycosides posing risk of ototoxicity. This testing is relevant to individuals with a predisposition to gram-negative infections or with hearing loss who have been exposed to aminoglycosides. For further information, see www.england.nhs.uk/publication/national-genomic-test-directories/.

● **MONITORING REQUIREMENTS**
▸ With intravenous use in neonates Extended interval dose regimen in neonates: pre-dose ('trough') concentration should be less than 2 mg/litre (less than 1 mg/litre if more than 3 doses administered); consider monitoring one hour ('peak') concentration in neonates with poor response to treatment, with oedema, with Gram-negative infection, or with birth-weight greater than 4.5 kg (consider increasing dose if 'peak' concentration less than 8 mg/litre in severe sepsis).
▸ With intravenous use Once daily dose regimen: pre-dose ('trough') concentration should be less than 1 mg/litre.
▸ With intramuscular use or intravenous use Multiple daily dose regimen: one hour ('peak') serum concentration should be 5–10 mg/litre; pre-dose ('trough') concentration should be less than 2 mg/litre. Multiple daily dose regimen for endocarditis: one hour ('peak') serum concentration should be 3–5 mg/litre; pre-dose ('trough') concentration should be less than 1 mg/litre. Serum-gentamicin concentration should be determined twice each week (more often in renal impairment).
▸ With intrathecal use or intraventricular use Intrathecal/intraventricular injection: cerebrospinal fluid concentration should not exceed 10 mg/litre.

● **DIRECTIONS FOR ADMINISTRATION** For *intrathecal* or *intraventricular* injection, use preservative-free intrathecal preparations only.
EvGr For *intravenous infusion*, dilute in Glucose 5% or Sodium Chloride 0.9%; give over 20–30 minutes (give over 60 minutes for once daily dose regimen). (M)

● **PRESCRIBING AND DISPENSING INFORMATION** For choice of antibacterial therapy, see Antibacterials, use for prophylaxis p. 359, Cardiovascular system infections, antibacterial therapy p. 364, Central nervous system infections, antibacterial therapy p. 365, Gastro-intestinal system infections, antibacterial therapy p. 367, Genital system infections, antibacterial therapy p. 368, Respiratory system infections, antibacterial therapy p. 371, Urinary-tract infections p. 454.

Local guidelines may vary in the dosing advice provided.

Only preservative-free intrathecal preparation should be used.

● **MEDICINAL FORMS** There can be variation in the licensing of different medicines containing the same drug. Forms available from special-order manufacturers include: solution for injection, infusion

Solution for injection

▸ **Gentamicin (Non-proprietary)**

Gentamicin (as Gentamicin sulfate) 5 mg per 1 ml Gentamicin Intrathecal 5mg/1ml solution for injection ampoules | 5 ampoule PoM £108.84 (Hospital only)

Gentamicin (as Gentamicin sulfate) 10 mg per 1 ml Gentamicin 20mg/2ml solution for injection ampoules | 5 ampoule PoM £11.25 DT = £11.25

Gentamicin Paediatric 20mg/2ml solution for injection vials | 5 vial PoM £11.25

Gentamicin (as Gentamicin sulfate) 40 mg per 1 ml Gentamicin 80mg/2ml solution for injection ampoules | 5 ampoule PoM £12.95 DT = £6.88 | 5 ampoule PoM £12.95 DT = £6.88 (Hospital only) | 10 ampoule PoM £12.00 | 10 ampoule PoM £13.76 (Hospital only)

▸ **Cidomycin** (Advanz Pharma)

Gentamicin (as Gentamicin sulfate) 40 mg per 1 ml Cidomycin 80mg/2ml solution for injection vials | 5 vial PoM £6.88 DT = £6.88 (Hospital only)

Cidomycin 80mg/2ml solution for injection ampoules | 5 ampoule PoM £6.88 DT = £6.88

Infusion

▸ **Gentamicin (Non-proprietary)**

Gentamicin (as Gentamicin sulfate) 1 mg per 1 ml Gentamicin 80mg/80ml infusion polyethylene bottles | 20 bottle PoM £57.00 (Hospital only)

Gentamicin (as Gentamicin sulfate) 3 mg per 1 ml Gentamicin 360mg/120ml infusion polyethylene bottles | 20 bottle PoM £249.00 (Hospital only)

Gentamicin 240mg/80ml infusion polyethylene bottles | 20 bottle PoM £175.00 (Hospital only)

377

Streptomycin

20-Jun-2025

● **INDICATIONS AND DOSE**

Tuberculosis, resistant to other treatment, in combination with other drugs

▸ BY DEEP INTRAMUSCULAR INJECTION

▸ Child: 15 mg/kg once daily (max. per dose 1 g)

Adjunct to doxycycline in brucellosis (administered on expert advice)

▸ BY DEEP INTRAMUSCULAR INJECTION

▸ Child: 5–10 mg/kg every 6 hours, total daily dose may alternatively be given in 2–3 divided doses

● **UNLICENSED USE** Not licensed for use in children.

IMPORTANT SAFETY INFORMATION

Side-effects increase after a cumulative dose of 100 g, which should only be exceeded in exceptional circumstances.

MHRA/CHM ADVICE: AMINOGLYCOSIDES (GENTAMICIN, AMIKACIN, TOBRAMYCIN, AND NEOMYCIN): INCREASED RISK OF DEAFNESS IN PATIENTS WITH MITOCHONDRIAL MUTATIONS (JANUARY 2021)

The use of aminoglycosides is associated with rare cases of ototoxicity. A safety review found an increased risk of deafness in patients with mitochondrial mutations (particularly the m.1555A>G mutation), including cases where the patient's aminoglycoside serum levels were within the recommended range. Nevertheless, these mitochondrial mutations are considered rare and penetrance is uncertain.

Healthcare professionals are advised to consider the need for aminoglycoside treatment versus alternative options in patients with susceptible mutations. The need for genetic testing especially in those requiring recurrent or long-term treatment with aminoglycosides should also be considered, however, urgent treatment should not be delayed. To minimise the risks of adverse effects, continuous monitoring of renal and auditory function, as well as hepatic and laboratory parameters, is recommended for all patients. Those with known mitochondrial mutations or a family history of ototoxicity are advised to inform their doctor or pharmacist before using an aminoglycoside.

● **INTERACTIONS** → Appendix 1: aminoglycosides

● **SIDE-EFFECTS** Amblyopia · angioedema · Clostridioides difficile colitis · haemolytic anaemia · ototoxicity · pancytopenia

● **PRE-TREATMENT SCREENING** NHS England commissions genetic testing under the *National genomic test directory* indication: R65 - Aminoglycoside exposure posing risk to hearing. The testing criteria is significant exposure to aminoglycosides posing risk of ototoxicity. This testing is relevant to individuals with a predisposition to gram-negative infections or with hearing loss who have been exposed to aminoglycosides. For further information, see www.england.nhs.uk/publication/national-genomic-test-directories/.

● **MONITORING REQUIREMENTS**

▸ One-hour ('peak') concentration should be 15–40 mg/litre; pre-dose ('trough') concentration should be less than 5 mg/litre (less than 1 mg/litre in renal impairment).

● **MEDICINAL FORMS** Forms available from special-order manufacturers include: powder for solution for injection

377

Tobramycin

20-Jun-2025

● **INDICATIONS AND DOSE**

Chronic *Pseudomonas aeruginosa* infection in patients with cystic fibrosis

▸ BY INHALATION OF NEBULISED SOLUTION

▸ Child 6–17 years: 300 mg every 12 hours for 28 days, subsequent courses repeated after 28-day interval without tobramycin nebuliser solution

▸ BY INHALATION OF POWDER

▸ Child 6–17 years: 112 mg every 12 hours for 28 days, subsequent courses repeated after 28-day interval without tobramycin inhalation powder

Pulmonary infection with *Pseudomonas aeruginosa* in cystic fibrosis

▸ BY INTRAVENOUS INFUSION

▸ Child: Initially 10 mg/kg once daily (max. per dose 660 mg), to be given over 30 minutes, subsequent doses adjusted according to serum-tobramycin concentration

▸ BY SLOW INTRAVENOUS INJECTION

▸ Child: Initially 8–10 mg/kg daily in 3 divided doses, to be given as a multiple daily dose regimen over 3–5 minutes, subsequent doses adjusted according to serum-tobramycin concentration

Septicaemia | Meningitis and other CNS infections | Biliary-tract infection | Acute pyelonephritis | Pneumonia in hospital patients

▸ BY SLOW INTRAVENOUS INJECTION

▸ Child 1 month–11 years: 2–2.5 mg/kg every 8 hours, to be given as a multiple daily dose regimen over 3–5 minutes

▸ Child 12–17 years: 1 mg/kg every 8 hours, to be given as a multiple daily dose regimen over 3–5 minutes; increased if necessary up to 5 mg/kg daily in 3–4 divided doses, to be given in severe infections as a multiple daily dose regimen over 3–5 minutes, dose to be reduced back to 3 mg/kg as soon as clinically indicated

▶ BY INTRAVENOUS INFUSION

▸ Child: Initially 7 mg/kg, to be given as a once daily dose regimen, subsequent doses adjusted according to serum-tobramycin concentration

Neonatal sepsis

▶ BY INTRAVENOUS INJECTION, OR BY INTRAVENOUS INFUSION

▸ Neonate up to 32 weeks corrected gestational age: 4–5 mg/kg every 36 hours, to be given as an extended interval dose regimen, intravenous injection to be given over 3–5 minutes.

▸ Neonate 32 weeks corrected gestational age and above: 4–5 mg/kg every 24 hours, to be given as an extended interval dose regimen, intravenous injection to be given over 3–5 minutes.

▶ BY SLOW INTRAVENOUS INJECTION, OR BY INTRAVENOUS INFUSION

▸ Neonate up to 7 days: 2 mg/kg every 12 hours, to be given as a multiple daily dose regimen.

▸ Neonate 7 days to 28 days: 2–2.5 mg/kg every 8 hours, to be given as a multiple daily dose regimen.

DOSES AT EXTREMES OF BODY-WEIGHT

▸ With intravenous use To avoid excessive dosage in obese patients, use ideal weight for height to calculate parenteral dose and monitor serum-tobramycin concentration closely.

VANTOBRA ® NEBULISER SOLUTION

Chronic pulmonary *Pseudomonas aeruginosa* infection in patients with cystic fibrosis

▶ BY INHALATION OF NEBULISED SOLUTION

▸ Child 6-17 years: 170 mg every 12 hours for 28 days, subsequent courses repeated after 28-day interval without tobramycin nebuliser solution

IMPORTANT SAFETY INFORMATION

MHRA/CHM ADVICE: AMINOGLYCOSIDES (GENTAMICIN, AMIKACIN, TOBRAMYCIN, AND NEOMYCIN): INCREASED RISK OF DEAFNESS IN PATIENTS WITH MITOCHONDRIAL MUTATIONS (JANUARY 2021)

The use of aminoglycosides is associated with rare cases of ototoxicity. A safety review found an increased risk of deafness in patients with mitochondrial mutations (particularly the m.1555A>G mutation), including cases where the patient's aminoglycoside serum levels were within the recommended range. Nevertheless, these mitochondrial mutations are considered rare and penetrance is uncertain. No cases were identified with topical preparations but, based on a shared mechanism of effect, there is a potential risk with aminoglycosides administered at the site of toxicity i.e. the ear.

Healthcare professionals are advised to consider the need for aminoglycoside treatment versus alternative options in patients with susceptible mutations. The need for genetic testing especially in those requiring recurrent or long-term treatment with aminoglycosides should also be considered, however, urgent treatment should not be delayed. To minimise the risks of adverse effects, continuous monitoring of renal and auditory function, as well as hepatic and laboratory parameters, is recommended for all patients. Those with known mitochondrial mutations or a family history of ototoxicity are advised to inform their doctor or pharmacist before using an aminoglycoside.

● CAUTIONS

▸ When used by inhalation Auditory disorder · conditions characterised by muscular weakness (may impair neuromuscular transmission) · history of prolonged previous or concomitant intravenous aminoglycosides (increased risk of ototoxicity) · renal impairment (limited information available) · severe haemoptysis (risk of further haemorrhage) · vestibular disorder

● INTERACTIONS → Appendix 1: aminoglycosides

● SIDE-EFFECTS

▶ **Common or very common**

▸ When used by inhalation Malaise · respiratory disorder · sputum discolouration

▶ **Rare or very rare**

▸ When used by inhalation Abdominal pain · asthenia · asthma · drowsiness · ear disorder · ear pain · epistaxis · hypoxia · lymphadenopathy · oral ulceration · pain

▶ **Frequency not known**

▸ With parenteral use Granulocytopenia · leucocytosis · nerve disorders · urine abnormalities

SIDE-EFFECTS, FURTHER INFORMATION Manufacturer advises to monitor serum-tobramycin concentration in patients with known or suspected signs of auditory dysfunction; if ototoxicity develops — discontinue treatment until serum concentration falls below 2 mg/litre.

With inhaled use Since systemic absorption can follow inhaled use, also consider the side-effects of systemic aminoglycosides.

● RENAL IMPAIRMENT

▸ When used by inhalation EvGr Monitor serum-tobramycin concentration; if nephrotoxicity develops—discontinue treatment until serum concentration falls below 2 mg/litre. (M)

● PRE-TREATMENT SCREENING NHS England commissions genetic testing under the *National genomic test directory* indication: R65 - Aminoglycoside exposure posing risk to hearing. The testing criteria is significant exposure to aminoglycosides posing risk of ototoxicity. This testing is relevant to individuals with a predisposition to gram-negative infections or with hearing loss who have been exposed to aminoglycosides. For further information, see www.england.nhs.uk/publication/national-genomic-test-directories/.

● MONITORING REQUIREMENTS

▸ With intravenous use in neonates *Extended interval dose regimen in neonates*: pre-dose ('trough') concentration should be less than 2 mg/litre.

▸ With intravenous use *Once daily dose regimen*: pre-dose ('trough') concentration should be less than 1 mg/litre. *Multiple daily dose regimen*: one-hour ('peak') serum concentration should not exceed 10 mg/litre (8–12 mg/litre in cystic fibrosis); pre-dose ('trough') concentration should be less than 2 mg/litre.

▸ When used by inhalation Measure lung function before and after initial dose of tobramycin and monitor for bronchospasm; if bronchospasm occurs in a patient not using a bronchodilator, repeat test using bronchodilator. Manufacturer advises monitor renal function before treatment and then annually.

● DIRECTIONS FOR ADMINISTRATION

▸ With intravenous use For *intravenous infusion*, manufacturer advises dilute with Glucose 5% or Sodium Chloride 0.9%; give over 20–60 minutes.

▸ When used by inhalation Manufacturer advises other inhaled drugs should be administered before tobramycin.

● PRESCRIBING AND DISPENSING INFORMATION Local guidelines may vary in dosing advice provided.

● PATIENT AND CARER ADVICE

▸ When used by inhalation Patient counselling is advised for Tobramycin dry powder for inhalation (administration).

VANTOBRA® NEBULISER SOLUTION

Missed doses

▸ When used by inhalation Manufacturer advises if a dose is more than 6 hours late, the missed dose should not be taken and the next dose should be taken at the normal time.

● **NATIONAL FUNDING/ACCESS DECISIONS** For full details see funding body website

NICE decisions

▸ **Tobramycin by dry powder inhalation for pseudomonal lung infection in cystic fibrosis (March 2013) NICE TA276** Recommended with restrictions

● **MEDICINAL FORMS** There can be variation in the licensing of different medicines containing the same drug.

Solution for injection

▸ **Tobramycin (Non-proprietary)**

Tobramycin 40 mg per 1 ml Tobramycin 80mg/2ml solution for injection vials | 1 vial PoM £5.37 DT = £5.37 | 5 vial PoM £20.80 DT = £20.80

Tobramycin 240mg/6ml solution for injection vials | 1 vial PoM £19.20 DT = £19.20

Inhalation powder

▸ **Tobi Podhaler** (Viatris UK Healthcare Ltd)

Tobramycin 28 mg Tobi Podhaler 28mg inhalation powder capsules with device | 224 capsule PoM £1,790.00 DT = £1,790.00

Nebuliser liquid

▸ **Tobramycin (Non-proprietary)**

Tobramycin 60 mg per 1 ml Tobramycin 300mg/5ml nebuliser liquid ampoules | 56 ampoule PoM £719.00–£1,187.00 DT = £1,187.00 | 56 ampoule PoM £1,075.79 DT = £1,187.00 (Hospital only)

▸ **Bramitob** (Chiesi Ltd)

Tobramycin 75 mg per 1 ml Bramitob 300mg/4ml nebuliser solution 4ml ampoules | 56 ampoule PoM £1,187.00 DT = £1,187.00

▸ **Munuza** (Aristo Pharma Ltd)

Tobramycin 60 mg per 1 ml Munuza 300mg/5ml nebuliser solution 5ml ampoules | 56 ampoule PoM £779.99 DT = £1,187.00

▸ **TOBI** (Viatris UK Healthcare Ltd)

Tobramycin 60 mg per 1 ml Tobi 300mg/5ml nebuliser solution 5ml ampoules | 56 ampoule PoM £1,305.92 DT = £1,187.00

▸ **Tymbrineb** (Teva UK Ltd)

Tobramycin 60 mg per 1 ml Tymbrineb 300mg/5ml nebuliser solution 5ml ampoules | 56 ampoule PoM £780.00 DT = £1,187.00

▸ **Vantobra** (Pari Medical Ltd)

Tobramycin 100 mg per 1 ml Vantobra 170mg/1.7ml nebuliser solution 1.7ml ampoules | 56 ampoule PoM £950.00

ANTIBACTERIALS › CARBAPENEMS

Carbapenems

29-Sep-2021

Overview

The carbapenems are beta-lactam antibacterials with a broad-spectrum of activity which includes many Gram-positive and Gram-negative bacteria, and anaerobes; imipenem (imipenem with cilastatin p. 383) and meropenem p. 383 have activity against *Pseudomonas aeruginosa* but emerging acquired resistance can be a problem. The carbapenems are not active against meticillin-resistant *Staphylococcus aureus* (MRSA) and *Enterococcus faecium*.

Imipenem (imipenem with cilastatin) and meropenem are used for the treatment of severe and complicated infections including hospital-acquired pneumonia, intra-abdominal infections, skin and soft-tissue infections, and urinary-tract infections.

Ertapenem below is licensed for treating abdominal and gynaecological infections and for community-acquired pneumonia, but it is not active against atypical respiratory pathogens and its activity against penicillin-resistant pneumococci is unknown. Unlike the other carbapenems, ertapenem is not active against *Pseudomonas* or against *Acinetobacter* spp.

Imipenem is partially inactivated in the kidney by enzymatic activity and is therefore administered in combination with cilastatin (imipenem with cilastatin), a specific enzyme inhibitor, which blocks its renal metabolism. Meropenem and ertapenem are stable to the renal enzyme which inactivates imipenem and therefore can be given without cilastatin.

Side-effects of imipenem with cilastatin are similar to those of other beta-lactam antibiotics. Meropenem has less seizure-inducing potential and can be used to treat central nervous system infection.

Ertapenem

25-Oct-2021

● **INDICATIONS AND DOSE**

Abdominal infections | Acute gynaecological infections | Community-acquired pneumonia

▸ BY INTRAVENOUS INFUSION

▸ Child 3 months–12 years: 15 mg/kg every 12 hours (max. per dose 500 mg)

▸ Child 13–17 years: 1 g once daily

Diabetic foot infections of the skin and soft-tissue

▸ BY INTRAVENOUS INFUSION

▸ Child 13–17 years: 1 g once daily

● **CAUTIONS** CNS disorders—risk of seizures

● **INTERACTIONS** → Appendix 1: carbapenems

● **SIDE-EFFECTS**

▸ **Common or very common** Diarrhoea · skin reactions

▸ **Uncommon** Faeces discoloured · headache · hot flush · hypertension · melaena

▸ **Frequency not known** Aggression · hallucination · psychiatric disorder

● **ALLERGY AND CROSS-SENSITIVITY** EvGr Avoid if history of **immediate hypersensitivity** reaction to beta-lactam antibacterials.

Use with caution in patients with sensitivity to beta-lactam antibacterials. ⟨M⟩

● **PREGNANCY** Manufacturer advises avoid unless potential benefit outweighs risk.

● **BREAST FEEDING** Present in milk—manufacturer advises avoid.

● **RENAL IMPAIRMENT** Use with caution (risk of seizures); avoid if estimated glomerular filtration rate less than 30 mL/minute/1.73 m^2.

● **DIRECTIONS FOR ADMINISTRATION** For *intravenous infusion* (*Invanz*®), manufacturer advises give intermittently *in* Sodium Chloride 0.9%. Reconstitute 1 g with 10 mL Water for Injections *or* Sodium Chloride 0.9%; dilute requisite dose in infusion fluid to a final concentration not exceeding 20 mg/mL; give over 30 minutes; incompatible with glucose solutions.

● **PRESCRIBING AND DISPENSING INFORMATION** For choice of antibacterial therapy, see Diabetic foot infections, antibacterial therapy p. 366, Gastro-intestinal system infections, antibacterial therapy p. 367, Respiratory system infections, antibacterial therapy p. 371.

● **MEDICINAL FORMS** There can be variation in the licensing of different medicines containing the same drug.

Powder for solution for infusion

ELECTROLYTES: May contain Sodium

▸ **Ertapenem (Non-proprietary)**

Ertapenem (as Ertapenem sodium) 1 gram Ertapenem 1g powder for concentrate for solution for infusion vials | 1 vial PoM £36.00 DT = £31.65 (Hospital only) | 10 vial PoM £316.50 | 10 vial PoM £284.00–£316.50 (Hospital only)

▸ **Invanz** (Merck Sharp & Dohme (UK) Ltd)

Ertapenem (as Ertapenem sodium) 1 gram Invanz 1g powder for solution for infusion vials | 1 vial PoM £31.65 DT = £31.65 (Hospital only)

Imipenem with cilastatin

24-Nov-2020

● **INDICATIONS AND DOSE**

Aerobic and anaerobic Gram-positive and Gram-negative infections (not indicated for CNS infections) | Hospital-acquired septicaemia

▶ BY INTRAVENOUS INFUSION

- Neonate up to 7 days: 20 mg/kg every 12 hours.
- Neonate 7 days to 20 days: 20 mg/kg every 8 hours.
- Neonate 21 days to 28 days: 20 mg/kg every 6 hours.
- Child 1–2 months: 20 mg/kg every 6 hours
- Child 3 months–17 years: 15 mg/kg every 6 hours (max. per dose 500 mg)

Infection caused by *Pseudomonas* or other less sensitive organisms | Empirical treatment of infection in febrile patients with neutropenia | Life-threatening infection

▶ BY INTRAVENOUS INFUSION

- Child 3 months–17 years: 25 mg/kg every 6 hours (max. per dose 1 g)

Cystic fibrosis

▶ BY INTRAVENOUS INFUSION

- Child: 25 mg/kg every 6 hours (max. per dose 1 g)

DOSE EQUIVALENCE AND CONVERSION

- Dose expressed in terms of imipenem.

● **UNLICENSED USE** Not licensed for use in children under 1 year.

● **CAUTIONS** CNS disorders · epilepsy

● **INTERACTIONS** → Appendix 1: carbapenems

● **SIDE-EFFECTS**

▶ **Common or very common** Diarrhoea · eosinophilia · nausea · skin reactions · thrombophlebitis · vomiting

▶ **Uncommon** Bone marrow disorders · confusion · dizziness · drowsiness · hallucination · hypotension · leucopenia · movement disorders · psychiatric disorder · seizure · thrombocytopenia · thrombocytosis

▶ **Rare or very rare** Agranulocytosis · anaphylactic reaction · angioedema · chest discomfort · colitis haemorrhagic · cyanosis · dyspnoea · encephalopathy · flushing · focal tremor · gastrointestinal discomfort · haemolytic anaemia · headache · hearing loss · hepatic disorders · hyperhidrosis · hyperventilation · increased risk of infection · myasthenia gravis aggravated · oral disorders · palpitations · paraesthesia · polyarthralgia · polyuria · pseudomembranous enterocolitis · renal impairment · severe cutaneous adverse reactions (SCARs) · spinal pain · tachycardia · taste altered · tinnitus · tongue discolouration · tooth discolouration · urine discolouration · vertigo

▶ **Frequency not known** Agitation · antibiotic associated colitis

● **ALLERGY AND CROSS-SENSITIVITY** [EvGr] Avoid if history of **immediate hypersensitivity** reaction to beta-lactam antibacterials.

Use with caution in patients with sensitivity to beta-lactam antibacterials. ⟨M⟩

● **PREGNANCY** Manufacturer advises avoid unless potential benefit outweighs risk (toxicity in *animal* studies).

● **BREAST FEEDING** [EvGr] Specialist sources indicate suitable for use in breast-feeding. ⟨D⟩

● **RENAL IMPAIRMENT** Clinical data are insufficient to recommend dosing for children with impairment (serum creatinine greater than 2 mg/dl)—in *adults*, manufacturer advises reduce dose (consult product literature).

● **EFFECT ON LABORATORY TESTS** Positive Coombs' test.

● **DIRECTIONS FOR ADMINISTRATION** For *intravenous infusion*, manufacturer advises dilute to a concentration of 5 mg (as imipenem)/mL in Sodium Chloride 0.9%; give up to 500 mg (as imipenem) over 20–30 minutes, give dose greater than 500 mg (as imipenem) over 40–60 minutes.

● **MEDICINAL FORMS** There can be variation in the licensing of different medicines containing the same drug.

Powder for solution for infusion

ELECTROLYTES: May contain Sodium

▶ **Imipenem with cilastatin (Non-proprietary)**
Cilastatin (as Cilastatin sodium) 500 mg, Imipenem (as Imipenem monohydrate) 500 mg Imipenem 500mg / Cilastatin 500mg powder for solution for infusion vials | 10 vial [PoM] £170.10

Meropenem

18-Aug-2021

● **INDICATIONS AND DOSE**

Aerobic and anaerobic Gram-positive and Gram-negative infections | Hospital-acquired septicaemia

▶ BY INTRAVENOUS INFUSION, OR BY INTRAVENOUS INJECTION

- Neonate up to 7 days: 20 mg/kg every 12 hours.
- Neonate 7 days to 28 days: 20 mg/kg every 8 hours.
- Child 1 month–11 years (body-weight up to 50 kg): 10–20 mg/kg every 8 hours
- Child 1 month–11 years (body-weight 50 kg and above): 0.5–1 g every 8 hours
- Child 12–17 years: 0.5–1 g every 8 hours

Severe aerobic and anaerobic Gram-positive and Gram-negative infections

▶ BY INTRAVENOUS INFUSION, OR BY INTRAVENOUS INJECTION

- Neonate up to 7 days: 40 mg/kg every 12 hours.
- Neonate 7 days to 28 days: 40 mg/kg every 8 hours.

Exacerbations of chronic lower respiratory-tract infection in cystic fibrosis

▶ BY INTRAVENOUS INFUSION

- Child 1 month–11 years (body-weight up to 50 kg): 40 mg/kg every 8 hours
- Child 1 month–11 years (body-weight 50 kg and above): 2 g every 8 hours
- Child 12–17 years: 2 g every 8 hours

Meningitis

▶ BY INTRAVENOUS INFUSION

- Neonate up to 7 days: 40 mg/kg every 12 hours.
- Neonate 7 days to 28 days: 40 mg/kg every 8 hours.
- Child 1 month–11 years (body-weight up to 50 kg): 40 mg/kg every 8 hours
- Child 1 month–11 years (body-weight 50 kg and above): 2 g every 8 hours
- Child 12–17 years: 2 g every 8 hours

● **UNLICENSED USE** Not licensed for use in children under 3 months.

● **INTERACTIONS** → Appendix 1: carbapenems

● **SIDE-EFFECTS**

▶ **Common or very common** Abdominal pain · diarrhoea · headache · inflammation · nausea · pain · skin reactions · thrombocytosis · vomiting

▶ **Uncommon** Agranulocytosis · antibiotic associated colitis · eosinophilia · haemolytic anaemia · increased risk of infection · leucopenia · neutropenia · paraesthesia · severe cutaneous adverse reactions (SCARs) · thrombocytopenia · thrombophlebitis

▶ **Rare or very rare** Seizure

▶ **Frequency not known** Pseudomembranous enterocolitis

- **ALLERGY AND CROSS-SENSITIVITY** EvGr Avoid if history of **immediate hypersensitivity** reaction to beta-lactam antibacterials.
  Use with caution in patients with sensitivity to beta-lactam antibacterials. ⟨M⟩
- **PREGNANCY** Use only if potential benefit outweighs risk—no information available.
- **BREAST FEEDING** Unlikely to be absorbed (however, manufacturer advises avoid).
- **RENAL IMPAIRMENT**
  Dose adjustments See p. 16.
  Expert sources advise use normal dose every 12 hours if estimated glomerular filtration rate 26–50 mL/minute/1.73 m^2; use half normal dose every 12 hours if estimated glomerular filtration rate 10–25 mL/minute/1.73 m^2; use half normal dose every 24 hours if estimated glomerular filtration rate less than 10 mL/minute/1.73 m^2.
- **MONITORING REQUIREMENTS** Manufacturer advises monitor liver function—risk of hepatotoxicity.
- **EFFECT ON LABORATORY TESTS** Positive Coombs' test.
- **DIRECTIONS FOR ADMINISTRATION** Manufacturer advises *intravenous injection* to be administered over 5 minutes.
  Displacement value may be significant when reconstituting injection, consult local guidelines. For *intravenous infusion*, manufacturer advises dilute reconstituted solution further to a concentration of 1–20 mg/mL *in* Glucose 5% *or* Sodium Chloride 0.9%; give over 15–30 minutes.

- **MEDICINAL FORMS** There can be variation in the licensing of different medicines containing the same drug.

Powder for solution for injection

ELECTROLYTES: May contain Sodium

▸ **Meropenem (Non-proprietary)**

Meropenem (as Meropenem trihydrate) 500 mg Meropenem 500mg powder for solution for injection vials | 10 vial PoM £121.80 DT = £121.80 (Hospital only)

Meropenem (as Meropenem trihydrate) 1 gram Meropenem 1g powder for solution for injection vials | 10 vial PoM £243.60 DT = £243.60 (Hospital only)

▸ **Meronem** (Pfizer Ltd)

Meropenem (as Meropenem trihydrate) 500 mg Meronem 500mg powder for solution for injection vials | 10 vial PoM £103.14 DT = £121.80 (Hospital only)

Meropenem (as Meropenem trihydrate) 1 gram Meronem 1g powder for solution for injection vials | 10 vial PoM £206.28 DT = £243.60 (Hospital only)

ANTIBACTERIALS > CEPHALOSPORINS

Cephalosporins

01-Dec-2025

Overview

The cephalosporins are broad-spectrum antibiotics which are used for the treatment of septicaemia, pneumonia, meningitis, biliary-tract infections, peritonitis, and urinary-tract infections. The pharmacology of the cephalosporins is similar to that of the penicillins, excretion being principally renal. Cephalosporins penetrate the cerebrospinal fluid poorly unless the meninges are inflamed; cefotaxime p. 389 and ceftriaxone p. 391 are suitable cephalosporins for infections of the CNS (e.g meningitis).

The principal side-effect of the cephalosporins is hypersensitivity. Cross-reactivity between penicillins and first and early second-generation cephalosporins has been reported to occur in up to 10%, and for third-generation cephalosporins in 2–3%, of penicillin-allergic patients.

The orally active 'first generation' cephalosporins, cefalexin p. 385, cefradine p. 387, and cefadroxil p. 385 and the 'second generation' cephalosporin, cefaclor p. 387 have a similar antimicrobial spectrum. They are useful for urinary-tract infections, respiratory-tract infections, otitis media, and skin and soft-tissue infections. Cefaclor has good activity against *H. influenzae*. Cefadroxil has a long duration of action and can be given twice daily; it has poor activity against *H. influenzae*. **Cefuroxime axetil**, an ester of the 'second generation' cephalosporin cefuroxime p. 388, has the same antibacterial spectrum as the parent compound; it is poorly absorbed and needs to be given with food to maximise absorption.

Cefixime p. 389 is an orally active 'third generation' cephalosporin. It has a longer duration of action than the other cephalosporins that are active by mouth. It is only licensed for acute infections.

Cefuroxime is a 'second generation' cephalosporin that is less susceptible than the earlier cephalosporins to inactivation by beta-lactamases. It is, therefore, active against certain bacteria which are resistant to the other drugs and has greater activity against *Haemophilus influenzae*.

Cefotaxime, ceftazidime p. 390 and ceftriaxone are 'third generation' cephalosporins with greater activity than the 'second generation' cephalosporins against certain Gram-negative bacteria. However, they are less active than cefuroxime against Gram-positive bacteria, most notably *Staphylococcus aureus*. Their broad antibacterial spectrum may encourage superinfection with resistant bacteria or fungi.

Ceftazidime has good activity against pseudomonas. It is also active against other Gram-negative bacteria.

Ceftriaxone has a longer half-life and therefore needs to be given only once daily. Indications include serious infections such as septicaemia, pneumonia, and meningitis. The calcium salt of ceftriaxone forms a precipitate in the gall bladder which may rarely cause symptoms but these usually resolve when the antibacterial is stopped. In neonates, ceftriaxone may displace bilirubin from plasma-albumin and should be avoided in neonates with unconjugated hyperbilirubinaemia, hypoalbuminaemia, acidosis or impaired bilirubin binding.

Cephalosporins

- **DRUG ACTION** Cephalosporins are antibacterials that attach to penicillin binding proteins to interrupt cell wall biosynthesis, leading to bacterial cell lysis and death.
- **SIDE-EFFECTS**
  - ▸ **Common or very common** Abdominal pain · diarrhoea · dizziness · eosinophilia · headache · leucopenia · nausea · neutropenia · pseudomembranous enterocolitis · skin reactions · thrombocytopenia · vomiting
  - ▸ **Uncommon** Anaphylactic reaction · angioedema
  - ▸ **Rare or very rare** Agranulocytosis · haemolytic anaemia · nephritis tubulointerstitial (reversible) · severe cutaneous adverse reactions (SCARs)
- **ALLERGY AND CROSS-SENSITIVITY** EvGr Contra-indicated in patients with cephalosporin hypersensitivity. ⟨M⟩
  - ▸ Cross-sensitivity with other beta-lactam antibacterials Cross-reactivity between penicillins and first and early second-generation cephalosporins has been reported to occur in up to 10%, and for third-generation cephalosporins in 2–3%, of penicillin-allergic patients. EvGr Patients with a history of **immediate hypersensitivity** to penicillin and other beta-lactams should not receive a cephalosporin. Cephalosporins should be used with caution in patients with sensitivity to penicillin and other beta-lactams. ⟨M⟩
- **EFFECT ON LABORATORY TESTS** False positive urinary glucose (if tested for reducing substances). False positive Coombs' test.

ANTIBACTERIALS > CEPHALOSPORINS, FIRST-GENERATION

F 384

Cefadroxil

● **INDICATIONS AND DOSE**

Susceptible infections due to sensitive Gram-positive and Gram-negative bacteria

▶ BY MOUTH

- Child 6–17 years (body-weight up to 40 kg): 0.5 g twice daily
- Child 6–17 years (body-weight 40 kg and above): 0.5–1 g twice daily

Skin infections | Soft-tissue infections | Uncomplicated urinary-tract infections

▶ BY MOUTH

- Child 6–17 years (body-weight 40 kg and above): 1 g once daily

● **INTERACTIONS** → Appendix 1: cephalosporins

● **SIDE-EFFECTS**

▶ **Common or very common** Dyspepsia · glossitis

▶ **Uncommon** Increased risk of infection

▶ **Rare or very rare** Arthralgia · drug fever · fatigue · hepatic disorders · insomnia · nervousness · serum sickness-like reaction

● **PREGNANCY** Not known to be harmful.

● **BREAST FEEDING** Present in milk in low concentration, but appropriate to use.

● **RENAL IMPAIRMENT**

Dose adjustments Reduce dose if estimated glomerular filtration rate less than 50 mL/minute/1.73 m^2.

● **MEDICINAL FORMS** There can be variation in the licensing of different medicines containing the same drug.

Oral capsule

CAUTIONARY AND ADVISORY LABELS 9

▶ **Cefadroxil (Non-proprietary)**

Cefadroxil (as Cefadroxil monohydrate) 500 mg Cefadroxil 500mg capsules | 20 capsule [PoM] £22.38 DT = £22.38

F 384

Cefalexin

15-Jul-2025

(Cephalexin)

● **INDICATIONS AND DOSE**

Susceptible infections due to sensitive Gram-positive and Gram-negative bacteria

▶ BY MOUTH

- Neonate up to 7 days: 25 mg/kg twice daily (max. per dose 125 mg).
- Neonate 7 days to 20 days: 25 mg/kg 3 times a day (max. per dose 125 mg).
- Neonate 21 days to 28 days: 25 mg/kg 4 times a day (max. per dose 125 mg).
- Child 1–11 months: 12.5 mg/kg twice daily, alternatively 125 mg twice daily
- Child 1–4 years: 12.5 mg/kg twice daily, alternatively 125 mg 3 times a day
- Child 5–11 years: 12.5 mg/kg twice daily, alternatively 250 mg 3 times a day
- Child 12–17 years: 500 mg 2–3 times a day

Serious susceptible infections due to sensitive Gram-positive and Gram-negative bacteria

▶ BY MOUTH

- Child 1 month–11 years: 25 mg/kg 2–4 times a day (max. per dose 1 g)
- Child 12–17 years: 1–1.5 g 3–4 times a day

Prophylaxis of recurrent urinary-tract infection in non-pregnant females [using single-dose antibacterial prophylaxis]

▶ BY MOUTH

- Child 16–17 years: 500 mg for 1 dose, dose to be taken following exposure to a trigger

Prophylaxis of recurrent urinary-tract infection [using daily antibacterial prophylaxis]

▶ BY MOUTH

- Child 16–17 years: 125 mg once daily, dose to be taken at night, seek specialist advice if considering use for prophylaxis during pregnancy, in male patients, or for recurrent upper urinary-tract infection or recurrent complicated lower urinary-tract infection

Prophylaxis of recurrent urinary-tract infection [using daily antibacterial prophylaxis] (initiated under specialist supervision)

▶ BY MOUTH

- Child 3 months–15 years: 12.5 mg/kg once daily (max. per dose 125 mg), dose to be taken at night

Acute pyelonephritis | Urinary-tract infection (catheter-associated)

▶ BY MOUTH

- Child 3–11 months: 125 mg twice daily for 7 to 10 days, alternatively 12.5 mg/kg twice daily for 7 to 10 days, alternatively 25 mg/kg 2–4 times a day (max. per dose 1 g) for 7 to 10 days, increased dose used in severe infections
- Child 1–4 years: 125 mg 3 times a day for 7 to 10 days, alternatively 12.5 mg/kg twice daily for 7 to 10 days, alternatively 25 mg/kg 2–4 times a day (max. per dose 1 g) for 7 to 10 days, increased dose used in severe infections
- Child 5–11 years: 250 mg 3 times a day for 7 to 10 days, alternatively 12.5 mg/kg twice daily for 7 to 10 days, alternatively 25 mg/kg 2–4 times a day (max. per dose 1 g) for 7 to 10 days, increased dose used in severe infections
- Child 12–17 years: 500 mg 2–3 times a day for 7 to 10 days, alternatively 1–1.5 g 3–4 times a day for 7 to 10 days, increased dose used in severe infections

Lower urinary-tract infection in pregnancy

▶ BY MOUTH

- Child 12–17 years: 500 mg twice daily for 7 days

Lower urinary-tract infection

▶ BY MOUTH

- Child 3–11 months: 12.5 mg/kg twice daily for 3 days, alternatively 125 mg twice daily for 3 days
- Child 1–4 years: 12.5 mg/kg twice daily for 3 days, alternatively 125 mg 3 times a day for 3 days
- Child 5–11 years: 12.5 mg/kg twice daily for 3 days, alternatively 250 mg 3 times a day for 3 days
- Child 12–15 years: 500 mg twice daily for 3 days

● **UNLICENSED USE** [EvGr] Cefalexin is used for prophylaxis of recurrent urinary-tract infection, ⟨A⟩ but is not licensed for this indication.

● **INTERACTIONS** → Appendix 1: cephalosporins

● **SIDE-EFFECTS** Agitation · arthritis · confusion · fatigue · gastrointestinal discomfort · genital pruritus · hallucination · hepatitis (transient) · hypersensitivity · increased risk of infection · jaundice cholestatic (transient) · joint disorders · vaginal discharge

● **PREGNANCY** Not known to be harmful.

● **BREAST FEEDING** Present in milk in low concentration, but appropriate to use.

- **RENAL IMPAIRMENT**
Dose adjustments Reduce dose in moderate impairment.
- **PRESCRIBING AND DISPENSING INFORMATION** For choice of antibacterial therapy, see Urinary-tract infections p. 454.
- **PATIENT AND CARER ADVICE**
Medicines for Children leaflet: Cefalexin for bacterial infections www.medicinesforchildren.org.uk/medicines/cefalexin-for-bacterial-infections/
- **PROFESSION SPECIFIC INFORMATION**
Dental practitioners' formulary Cefalexin Capsules may be prescribed. Cefalexin Tablets may be prescribed. Cefalexin Oral Suspension may be prescribed.

- **MEDICINAL FORMS** There can be variation in the licensing of different medicines containing the same drug.

Oral tablet
CAUTIONARY AND ADVISORY LABELS 9
- Cefalexin (Non-proprietary)
Cefalexin 250 mg Cefalexin 250mg tablets | 28 tablet PoM £4.40 DT = £4.30
Cefalexin 500 mg Cefalexin 500mg tablets | 21 tablet PoM £4.50 DT = £2.81
- Ceporex (Crescent Pharma Ltd)
Cefalexin 250 mg Ceporex 250mg tablets | 28 tablet PoM DT = £4.30

Oral suspension
CAUTIONARY AND ADVISORY LABELS 9
- Cefalexin (Non-proprietary)
Cefalexin 25 mg per 1 ml Cefalexin 125mg/5ml oral suspension sugar free | 100 ml PoM £2.92–£8.50 DT = £2.92 SF
Cefalexin 125mg/5ml oral suspension | 100 ml PoM £8.20 DT = £7.84
Cefalexin 50 mg per 1 ml Cefalexin 250mg/5ml oral suspension sugar free | 100 ml PoM £3.38–£9.00 DT = £3.38 SF
Cefalexin 250mg/5ml oral suspension | 100 ml PoM £8.80 DT = £8.96

Oral capsule
CAUTIONARY AND ADVISORY LABELS 9
- Cefalexin (Non-proprietary)
Cefalexin 250 mg Cefalexin 250mg capsules | 28 capsule PoM £2.50 DT = £1.61
Cefalexin 500 mg Cefalexin 500mg capsules | 21 capsule PoM £2.70 DT = £1.95

384

Cefazolin

25-Aug-2020

- **INDICATIONS AND DOSE**

Surgical prophylaxis
- BY SLOW INTRAVENOUS INJECTION, OR BY INTRAVENOUS INFUSION, OR BY DEEP INTRAMUSCULAR INJECTION
- Child 12–17 years (body-weight 40 kg and above): 1 g for 1 dose, to be administered 30–60 minutes before surgery, then 0.5–1 g, to be administered if required during surgery (in procedures lasting 2 hours or more)

Skin infection | Soft tissue infection | Bone infection | Joint infection
- BY SLOW INTRAVENOUS INJECTION, OR BY INTRAVENOUS INFUSION, OR BY DEEP INTRAMUSCULAR INJECTION
- Child (body-weight up to 40 kg): 25–50 mg/kg daily in 2–4 divided doses, to be used for sensitive bacteria; increased if necessary up to 100 mg/kg daily in 3–4 divided doses, to be used for moderately-sensitive bacteria, single doses greater than 1 g should be given by intravenous infusion
- Child 12–17 years (body-weight 40 kg and above): 1–2 g daily in 2–3 divided doses, to be used for sensitive bacteria; increased to 3–4 g daily in 3–4 divided doses, to be used for moderately-sensitive bacteria, single doses greater than 1 g should be given by intravenous infusion; increased if necessary up to 6 g daily in 3–4 divided doses, to be used for severe infections, single doses greater than 1 g should be given by intravenous infusion

- **INTERACTIONS** → Appendix 1: cephalosporins
- **SIDE-EFFECTS**
- **Common or very common** Appetite decreased
- **Uncommon** Drug fever · interstitial lung disease · oral candidiasis (particularly in long term use) · seizure (in renal impairment) · thrombophlebitis
- **Rare or very rare** Akathisia · anaemia · anal pruritus · anxiety · asthenia · bone marrow disorders · chest pain · coagulation disorder · colour vision change · confusion · cough · drowsiness · dyspnoea · epileptogenic activity · face oedema · genital pruritus · hepatitis (transient) · hot flush · hyperglycaemia · hypersensitivity · hypoglycaemia · increased leucocytes · increased risk of infection · jaundice cholestatic (transient) · lymphopenia · malaise · nephropathy · proteinuria · respiratory disorders · sleep disorders · tongue swelling · vertigo

SIDE-EFFECTS, FURTHER INFORMATION Blood disorders including: leucopenia, granulocytopenia, thrombocytopenia, lymphopenia, eosinophillia and increased leucocytes are reversible.
- **PREGNANCY** Manufacturer advises avoid unless essential—limited data available but not known to harmful in *animal* studies. EvGr Specialist sources indicate suitable for use in pregnancy. ⟨D⟩
- **BREAST FEEDING** Present in milk in low concentration, but appropriate to use.
- **RENAL IMPAIRMENT** See p. 16. Manufacturer advises caution if creatinine clearance 40 mL/minute or less (increased risk of convulsions).
Dose adjustments Manufacturer advises dose reduction in impairment—consult product literature.
- **DIRECTIONS FOR ADMINISTRATION** Displacement value may be significant when reconstituting injection, consult local guidelines or product literature.
For *intravenous injection*, manufacturer advises reconstitute with Water for Injection *or* Glucose 5 or 10% *or* Sodium Chloride 0.9%; give over 3 to 5 minutes—consult product literature.
For intermittent *intravenous infusion*, manufacturer advises dilute reconstituted solution with Water for Injection *or* Glucose 5% *or* Sodium Chloride 0.9% *or* Compound Sodium Lactate *or* Ringer's Solution; give over 30 to 60 minutes—consult product literature.
For *intramuscular injection* manufacturer advises reconstitute with Water for Injection *or* Glucose 10% *or* Sodium Chloride 0.9% *or* Lidocaine Hydrochloride 0.5% (in children over 30 months of age); give as a deep *intramuscular injection*—consult product literature. Maximum of 500 mg to be administered per injection site—for doses greater than 500 mg give as divided doses throughout the day or at different injection sites.
- **PRESCRIBING AND DISPENSING INFORMATION** For choice of antibacterial therapy, see Antibacterials, use for prophylaxis p. 359, Skin infections, antibacterial therapy p. 373, Musculoskeletal system infections, antibacterial therapy p. 369.

- **MEDICINAL FORMS** There can be variation in the licensing of different medicines containing the same drug.

Powder for solution for injection
ELECTROLYTES: May contain Sodium
- Cefazolin (Non-proprietary)
Cefazolin (as Cefazolin sodium) 1 gram Cefazolin 1g powder for solution for injection vials | 10 vial PoM £161.83
Cefazolin (as Cefazolin sodium) 2 gram Cefazolin 2g powder for solution for injection vials | 10 vial PoM £183.90

384

Cefradine

22-Jul-2021

(Cephradine)

● **INDICATIONS AND DOSE**

Susceptible infections due to sensitive Gram-positive and Gram-negative bacteria | Surgical prophylaxis

▶ BY MOUTH
- Child 7–11 years: 25–50 mg/kg daily in 2–4 divided doses
- Child 12–17 years: 250–500 mg 4 times a day, alternatively 0.5–1 g twice daily; increased if necessary up to 1 g 4 times a day, increased dose may be used in severe infections

Prevention of *Staphylococcus aureus* lung infection in cystic fibrosis

▶ BY MOUTH
- Child 7–17 years: 2 g twice daily

● **UNLICENSED USE** Not licensed for use in children for prevention of *Staphylococcus aureus* lung infection in cystic fibrosis.

● **INTERACTIONS** → Appendix 1: cephalosporins

● **SIDE-EFFECTS**
▶ **Rare or very rare** Antibiotic associated colitis
▶ **Frequency not known** Akathisia · aplastic anaemia · arthralgia · blood disorder · chest tightness · confusion · gastrointestinal discomfort · glossitis · hepatitis (transient) · hypersensitivity · increased risk of infection · jaundice cholestatic · muscle tone increased · nervousness · oedema · sleep disorder

● **PREGNANCY** Not known to be harmful.

● **BREAST FEEDING** Present in milk in low concentration, but appropriate to use.

● **RENAL IMPAIRMENT**
Dose adjustments See p. 16.
EvGr Reduce dose if creatinine clearance less than 20 mL/minute. (M)

● **PROFESSION SPECIFIC INFORMATION**
Dental practitioners' formulary Cefradine Capsules may be prescribed.

● **MEDICINAL FORMS** There can be variation in the licensing of different medicines containing the same drug.

Oral capsule

CAUTIONARY AND ADVISORY LABELS 9

▸ **Cefradine (Non-proprietary)**

Cefradine 250 mg Cefradine 250mg capsules | 20 capsule PoM £23.00 DT = £20.20

Cefradine 500 mg Cefradine 500mg capsules | 20 capsule PoM £24.00 DT = £12.50

ANTIBACTERIALS > CEPHALOSPORINS, SECOND-GENERATION

384

Cefaclor

12-Apr-2021

● **INDICATIONS AND DOSE**

Susceptible infections due to sensitive Gram-positive and Gram-negative bacteria

▶ BY MOUTH USING IMMEDIATE-RELEASE MEDICINES
- Child 1–11 months: 20 mg/kg daily in 3 divided doses, alternatively 62.5 mg 3 times a day
- Child 1–4 years: 20 mg/kg daily in 3 divided doses, alternatively 125 mg 3 times a day
- Child 5–11 years: 20 mg/kg daily in 3 divided doses, usual max. 1 g daily, alternatively 250 mg 3 times a day
- Child 12–17 years: 250 mg 3 times a day; maximum 4 g per day

▶ BY MOUTH USING MODIFIED-RELEASE MEDICINES
- Child 12–17 years: 375 mg every 12 hours, dose to be taken with food

Severe susceptible infections due to sensitive Gram-positive and Gram-negative bacteria

▶ BY MOUTH USING IMMEDIATE-RELEASE MEDICINES
- Child 1–11 months: 40 mg/kg daily in 3 divided doses, usual max. 1 g daily, alternatively 125 mg 3 times a day
- Child 1–4 years: 40 mg/kg daily in 3 divided doses, usual max. 1 g daily, alternatively 250 mg 3 times a day
- Child 5–11 years: 40 mg/kg daily in 3 divided doses, usual max. 1 g daily
- Child 12–17 years: 500 mg 3 times a day; maximum 4 g per day

Pneumonia

▶ BY MOUTH USING MODIFIED-RELEASE MEDICINES
- Child 12–17 years: 750 mg every 12 hours, dose to be taken with food

Lower urinary-tract infections

▶ BY MOUTH USING MODIFIED-RELEASE MEDICINES
- Child 12–17 years: 375 mg every 12 hours, dose to be taken with food

Asymptomatic carriage of *Haemophilus influenzae* or mild exacerbations in cystic fibrosis

▶ BY MOUTH USING IMMEDIATE-RELEASE MEDICINES
- Child 1–11 months: 125 mg every 8 hours
- Child 1–6 years: 250 mg 3 times a day
- Child 7–17 years: 500 mg 3 times a day

● **INTERACTIONS** → Appendix 1: cephalosporins

● **SIDE-EFFECTS** Akathisia · anxiety · aplastic anaemia · arthralgia · arthritis · asthenia · colitis · confusion · drowsiness · dyspnoea · fever · genital pruritus · hallucination · hepatitis (transient) · hypersensitivity · increased risk of infection · insomnia · jaundice cholestatic (transient) · lymphadenopathy · lymphocytosis · muscle tone increased · oedema · paraesthesia · proteinuria · syncope · vasodilation

SIDE-EFFECTS, FURTHER INFORMATION Cefaclor is associated with protracted skin reactions, especially in children.

● **PREGNANCY** Not known to be harmful.

● **BREAST FEEDING** Present in milk in low concentration, but appropriate to use.

● **RENAL IMPAIRMENT** EvGr Use with caution. (M)

● **MEDICINAL FORMS** There can be variation in the licensing of different medicines containing the same drug.

Oral suspension

CAUTIONARY AND ADVISORY LABELS 9

▸ **Cefaclor (Non-proprietary)**

Cefaclor (as Cefaclor monohydrate) 50 mg per 1 ml Cefaclor 250mg/5ml oral suspension | 100 ml PoM £8.26 DT = £8.26

▸ **Distaclor** (Flynn Pharma Ltd)

Cefaclor (as Cefaclor monohydrate) 25 mg per 1 ml Distaclor 125mg/5ml oral suspension | 100 ml PoM £4.13 DT = £4.13

Modified-release tablet

CAUTIONARY AND ADVISORY LABELS 9, 21, 25

▸ **Cefaclor (Non-proprietary)**

Cefaclor (as Cefaclor monohydrate) 375 mg Cefaclor 375mg modified-release tablets | 14 tablet PoM £9.10 DT = £9.10

Oral capsule

CAUTIONARY AND ADVISORY LABELS 9

▸ **Cefaclor (Non-proprietary)**

Cefaclor (as Cefaclor monohydrate) 500 mg Cefaclor 500mg capsules | 21 capsule PoM £7.50 DT = £7.50

384

Cefoxitin

21-Aug-2019

● **INDICATIONS AND DOSE**

Complicated urinary tract infection | Pyelonephritis

▶ BY SLOW INTRAVENOUS INJECTION

- Child 12–17 years: 2 g every 4–6 hours; maximum 12 g per day

● **INTERACTIONS** → Appendix 1: cephalosporins

● **SIDE-EFFECTS** Anaemia · bone marrow failure · encephalopathy · fever · hypersensitivity · local reaction · myasthenia gravis aggravated · overgrowth of nonsusceptible organisms · renal impairment · thrombophlebitis

● **PREGNANCY** Manufacturer advises not known to be harmful.

● **BREAST FEEDING** EvGr Specialist sources indicate present in milk in low concentrations, but appropriate to use. ⟨D⟩

● **RENAL IMPAIRMENT**

Dose adjustments Manufacturer advises increase dosing interval to every 8-12 hours if creatinine clearance 30-50 mL/minute, or every 12-24 hours if creatinine clearance 10-29 mL/minute. Consult product literature if creatinine clearance less than 10 mL/minute. See p. 16.

● **DIRECTIONS FOR ADMINISTRATION** For *slow intravenous injection*, reconstitute with 10 mL Water for Injections; give over 3 to 5 minutes.

● **MEDICINAL FORMS** There can be variation in the licensing of different medicines containing the same drug. Forms available from special-order manufacturers include: powder for solution for injection

Powder for solution for injection

ELECTROLYTES: May contain Sodium

- **Cefoxitin (Non-proprietary)**
  - **Cefoxitin (as Cefoxitin sodium) 1 gram** Cefoxitin 1g powder for solution for injection vials | 10 vial PoM ☒
  - **Cefoxitin (as Cefoxitin sodium) 2 gram** Cefoxitin 2g powder for solution for injection vials | 10 vial PoM ☒
- **Renoxitin** (Renascience Pharma Ltd)
  - **Cefoxitin (as Cefoxitin sodium) 1 gram** Renoxitin 1g powder for solution for injection vials | 10 vial PoM £163.80 (Hospital only)
  - **Cefoxitin (as Cefoxitin sodium) 2 gram** Renoxitin 2g powder for solution for injection vials | 10 vial PoM £282.45 (Hospital only)

384

Cefuroxime

26-Nov-2025

● **INDICATIONS AND DOSE**

Susceptible infections due to Gram-positive and Gram-negative bacteria

▶ BY MOUTH

- Child 3 months–1 year: 10 mg/kg twice daily (max. per dose 125 mg)
- Child 2–11 years: 15 mg/kg twice daily (max. per dose 250 mg)
- Child 12–17 years: 250 mg twice daily, dose may be doubled in severe lower respiratory-tract infections or if pneumonia is suspected

▶ BY INTRAVENOUS INFUSION, OR BY INTRAVENOUS INJECTION

- Neonate up to 7 days: 25 mg/kg every 12 hours, increased if necessary to 50 mg/kg every 12 hours, increased dose used in severe infection.
- Neonate 7 days to 20 days: 25 mg/kg every 8 hours, increased if necessary to 50 mg/kg every 8 hours, increased dose used in severe infection.
- Neonate 21 days to 28 days: 25 mg/kg every 6 hours, increased if necessary to 50 mg/kg every 6 hours, increased dose used in severe infection.

▶ BY INTRAVENOUS INFUSION, OR BY INTRAVENOUS INJECTION, OR BY INTRAMUSCULAR INJECTION

- Child: 20 mg/kg every 8 hours (max. per dose 750 mg); increased to 50–60 mg/kg every 6–8 hours (max. per dose 1.5 g), increased dose used for severe infection and cystic fibrosis

Cellulitis | Erysipelas

▶ BY INTRAVENOUS INJECTION, OR BY INTRAVENOUS INFUSION

- Child: 20 mg/kg every 8 hours (max. per dose 750 mg); increased if necessary up to 50–60 mg/kg every 6–8 hours (max. per dose 1.5 g)

Prophylaxis of infection from human bites [in combination with other drugs] | Prophylaxis of infection from animal bites [in combination with other drugs] | Treatment of infection from human bites [in combination with other drugs] | Treatment of infection from animal bites [in combination with other drugs]

▶ BY INTRAVENOUS INFUSION, OR BY INTRAVENOUS INJECTION

- Child: 20 mg/kg every 8 hours (max. per dose 750 mg); increased if necessary to 50–60 mg/kg every 6–8 hours (max. per dose 1.5 g), increased dose used for severe infections

Lyme disease

▶ BY MOUTH

- Child 3 months–11 years: 15 mg/kg twice daily (max. per dose 500 mg) for 14–21 days (for 28 days in Lyme arthritis)
- Child 12–17 years: 500 mg twice daily for 14–21 days (for 28 days in Lyme arthritis)

Surgical prophylaxis

▶ INITIALLY BY INTRAVENOUS INJECTION

- Child: 50 mg/kg for 1 dose (max. per dose 1.5 g), to be administered up to 30 minutes before the procedure, then (by intravenous injection or by intramuscular injection) 30 mg/kg every 8 hours (max. per dose 750 mg) if required for up to 3 doses (for high-risk procedures)

Urinary-tract infection (lower)

▶ BY MOUTH

- Child (body-weight up to 40 kg): 15 mg/kg twice daily (max. per dose 250 mg)
- Child (body-weight 40 kg and above): 250 mg twice daily

Urinary tract infection (catheter-associated)

▶ BY INTRAVENOUS INFUSION, OR BY INTRAVENOUS INJECTION

- Child 3 months–15 years: 20 mg/kg every 8 hours (max. per dose 750 mg); increased to 50–60 mg/kg every 6–8 hours (max. per dose 1.5 g), increased dose used for severe infection
- Child 16–17 years: 0.75–1.5 g every 6–8 hours

Acute pyelonephritis

▶ BY MOUTH

- Child (body-weight up to 40 kg): 15 mg/kg twice daily (max. per dose 250 mg)
- Child (body-weight 40 kg and above): 250 mg twice daily

▶ BY INTRAVENOUS INFUSION, OR BY INTRAVENOUS INJECTION

- Child 3 months–15 years: 20 mg/kg every 8 hours (max. per dose 750 mg); increased to 50–60 mg/kg every 6–8 hours (max. per dose 1.5 g), increased dose used for severe infection
- Child 16–17 years: 0.75–1.5 g every 6–8 hours

● **UNLICENSED USE** EvGr Cefuroxime is used for the treatment of cellulitis, ⟨A⟩ but the dose increase is not licensed for this indication.

EvGr Cefuroxime is used for the treatment of erysipelas, ⟨A⟩ but the dose increase is not licensed for this indication.

Not licensed for treatment of Lyme disease in children under 12 years.

Duration of treatment in Lyme disease is unlicensed.

- **INTERACTIONS** → Appendix 1: cephalosporins
- **SIDE-EFFECTS**

GENERAL SIDE-EFFECTS
- **Common or very common** Increased risk of infection
- **Frequency not known** Drug fever

SPECIFIC SIDE-EFFECTS
- **Uncommon**
- With parenteral use Gastrointestinal disorder
- **Frequency not known**
- With oral use Hepatic disorders · Jarisch-Herxheimer reaction · serum sickness
- With parenteral use Cutaneous vasculitis
- **PREGNANCY** Not known to be harmful.
- **BREAST FEEDING** Present in milk in low concentration, but appropriate to use.
- **RENAL IMPAIRMENT**

Dose adjustments Reduce parenteral dose if estimated glomerular filtration rate less than 20 mL/minute/1.73 m^2.
- **DIRECTIONS FOR ADMINISTRATION**
- With intramuscular use or intravenous use Manufacturer advises single doses over 750 mg should be administered by the intravenous route only.
- With intravenous use Displacement value may be significant when reconstituting injection, consult local guidelines. For *intermittent intravenous infusion*, manufacturer advises dilute reconstituted solution further in Glucose 5% *or* Sodium Chloride 0.9%; give over 30–60 minutes.
- **PRESCRIBING AND DISPENSING INFORMATION** For choice of antibacterial therapy, see Antibacterials, use for prophylaxis p. 359, Lyme disease p. 444, Skin infections, antibacterial therapy p. 373, Urinary-tract infections p. 454.

- **MEDICINAL FORMS** There can be variation in the licensing of different medicines containing the same drug. Forms available from special-order manufacturers include: solution for injection, infusion

Oral tablet

CAUTIONARY AND ADVISORY LABELS 9, 21, 25
- **Cefuroxime (Non-proprietary)**

Cefuroxime (as Cefuroxime axetil) 250 mg Cefuroxime 250mg tablets | 14 tablet PoM £25.98 DT = £9.11

Powder for solution for injection

ELECTROLYTES: May contain Sodium
- **Cefuroxime (Non-proprietary)**

Cefuroxime (as Cefuroxime sodium) 50 mg Cefuroxime 50mg powder for solution for injection vials | 10 vial PoM £49.95 (Hospital only)

Cefuroxime (as Cefuroxime sodium) 250 mg Cefuroxime 250mg powder for solution for injection vials | 10 vial PoM £9.25 (Hospital only)

Cefuroxime (as Cefuroxime sodium) 750 mg Cefuroxime 750mg powder for solution for injection vials | 10 vial PoM £25.20 | 10 vial PoM £25.20–£34.10 (Hospital only)

Cefuroxime (as Cefuroxime sodium) 1.5 gram Cefuroxime 1.5g powder for solution for injection vials | 10 vial PoM £50.50 | 10 vial PoM £50.50–£69.20 (Hospital only)
- **Zinacef** (Sandoz Ltd)

Cefuroxime (as Cefuroxime sodium) 250 mg Zinacef 250mg powder for solution for injection vials | 5 vial PoM £4.70 (Hospital only)

Cefuroxime (as Cefuroxime sodium) 750 mg Zinacef 750mg powder for solution for injection vials | 5 vial PoM £11.72 (Hospital only)

Cefuroxime (as Cefuroxime sodium) 1.5 gram Zinacef 1.5g powder for solution for injection vials | 1 vial PoM £4.70 (Hospital only)

ANTIBACTERIALS › CEPHALOSPORINS, THIRD-GENERATION

F 384

Cefixime

26-Nov-2025

- **INDICATIONS AND DOSE**

Acute infections due to sensitive Gram-positive and Gram-negative bacteria
- BY MOUTH
- Child 6–11 months: 75 mg daily
- Child 1–4 years: 100 mg daily
- Child 5–9 years: 200 mg daily
- Child 10–17 years: 200–400 mg daily, alternatively 100–200 mg twice daily

Uncomplicated gonorrhoea [anogenital and pharyngeal infection, when sensitivity confirmed—in combination with azithromycin]
- BY MOUTH
- Child 12–17 years (body-weight 45 kg and above): 400 mg for 2 doses, the second dose to be given 6–12 hours after the first dose

Disseminated gonococcal infection [arthritis and arthritis-dermatitis syndrome, when sensitivity confirmed]
- BY MOUTH
- Child 12–17 years (body-weight 45 kg and above): 800 mg twice daily, to be used following parenteral ceftriaxone treatment, starting 24–48 hours after symptoms improve, to give 7 days treatment in total

- **UNLICENSED USE** EvGr Cefixime is used for the treatment of uncomplicated gonorrhoea and disseminated gonococcal infection, ⟨A⟩ but is not licensed for these indications.
- **INTERACTIONS** → Appendix 1: cephalosporins
- **SIDE-EFFECTS** Acute kidney injury · arthralgia · drug fever · dyspepsia · dyspnoea · face oedema · flatulence · genital pruritus · hypereosinophilia · jaundice · serum sickness-like reaction · thrombocytosis · vulvovaginal infection
- **PREGNANCY** Not known to be harmful.
- **BREAST FEEDING** Manufacturer advises avoid unless essential—no information available.
- **RENAL IMPAIRMENT** EvGr Caution in severe impairment. ⟨M⟩

Dose adjustments See p. 16.

EvGr Reduce dose if creatinine clearance less than 20 mL/minute (should not exceed 200 mg once daily). ⟨M⟩
- **PRESCRIBING AND DISPENSING INFORMATION** For choice of antibacterial therapy, see Genital system infections, antibacterial therapy p. 368.

- **MEDICINAL FORMS** There can be variation in the licensing of different medicines containing the same drug.

Oral tablet

CAUTIONARY AND ADVISORY LABELS 9
- **Cefixime (Non-proprietary)**

Cefixime 200 mg Cefixime 200mg tablets | 1 tablet PoM ⊠
- **Suprax** (Advanz Pharma)

Cefixime 200 mg Suprax 200mg tablets | 7 tablet PoM £13.23 DT = £13.23

F 384

Cefotaxime

26-Nov-2025

- **INDICATIONS AND DOSE**

Uncomplicated gonorrhoea
- BY INTRAMUSCULAR INJECTION
- Child 12–17 years: 500–1000 mg for 1 dose

continued →

5 Infection

Severe exacerbations of *Haemophilus influenzae* infection in cystic fibrosis
- BY INTRAVENOUS INJECTION, OR BY INTRAVENOUS INFUSION
  - Child: 50 mg/kg every 8 hours (max. per dose 4 g), alternatively 50 mg/kg every 6 hours (max. per dose 3 g)

Infections due to sensitive Gram-positive and Gram-negative bacteria | Surgical prophylaxis | Haemophilus epiglottitis
- BY INTRAMUSCULAR INJECTION, OR BY INTRAVENOUS INJECTION, OR BY INTRAVENOUS INFUSION
  - Neonate up to 7 days: 25 mg/kg every 12 hours.
  - Neonate 7 days to 20 days: 25 mg/kg every 8 hours.
  - Neonate 21 days to 28 days: 25 mg/kg every 6–8 hours.
  - Child: 50 mg/kg every 8–12 hours

Severe susceptible infections due to sensitive Gram-positive and Gram-negative bacteria | Meningitis
- BY INTRAVENOUS INJECTION, OR BY INTRAVENOUS INFUSION
  - Neonate up to 7 days: 50 mg/kg every 12 hours.
  - Neonate 7 days to 20 days: 50 mg/kg every 8 hours.
  - Neonate 21 days to 28 days: 50 mg/kg every 6–8 hours.
  - Child: 50 mg/kg every 6 hours (max. per dose 3 g)

- **INTERACTIONS** → Appendix 1: cephalosporins
- **SIDE-EFFECTS**
  - **Uncommon** Drug fever · Jarisch-Herxheimer reaction · renal impairment · seizure
  - **Frequency not known** Arrhythmia (following rapid injection) · bronchospasm · encephalopathy · fungal infection · hepatic disorders
- **PREGNANCY** Not known to be harmful.
- **BREAST FEEDING** Present in milk in low concentration, but appropriate to use.
- **RENAL IMPAIRMENT**
  Dose adjustments See p. 16.
  EvGr Usual initial dose, then use half normal dose if estimated glomerular filtration rate less than 5 mL/minute/1.73 m^2. (M)
- **DIRECTIONS FOR ADMINISTRATION**
  - With intramuscular use For *intramuscular injection*, doses over 1 g should be divided between more than one site.
  - With intravenous use Displacement value may be significant, consult local guidelines. For intermittent *intravenous infusion*, manufacturer advises dilute reconstituted solution in Glucose 5% *or* Sodium Chloride 0.9%; administer over 20–60 minutes; incompatible with alkaline solutions.
- **PRESCRIBING AND DISPENSING INFORMATION** For choice of antibacterial therapy, see Central nervous system infections, antibacterial therapy p. 365, Genital system infections, antibacterial therapy p. 368, Respiratory system infections, antibacterial therapy p. 371.

- **MEDICINAL FORMS** There can be variation in the licensing of different medicines containing the same drug.

Powder for solution for injection
- **Cefotaxime (Non-proprietary)**
  Cefotaxime (as Cefotaxime sodium) 500 mg Cefotaxime 500mg powder for solution for injection vials | 10 vial PoM £21.00–£30.00 (Hospital only)
  Cefotaxime (as Cefotaxime sodium) 1 gram Cefotaxime 1g powder for solution for injection vials | 10 vial PoM £35.00–£42.00 | 10 vial PoM £35.00–£42.00 (Hospital only)
  Cefotaxime (as Cefotaxime sodium) 2 gram Cefotaxime 2g powder for solution for injection vials | 10 vial PoM £55.00–£56.25 (Hospital only)

384

Ceftazidime

29-Nov-2021

- **INDICATIONS AND DOSE**

Pseudomonal lung infection in cystic fibrosis
- BY INTRAVENOUS INFUSION, OR BY INTRAVENOUS INJECTION, OR BY DEEP INTRAMUSCULAR INJECTION
  - Child: 50 mg/kg every 8 hours (max. per dose 3 g)

Febrile neutropenia
- BY INTRAVENOUS INFUSION, OR BY INTRAVENOUS INJECTION
  - Child: 50 mg/kg every 8 hours (max. per dose 2 g)

Meningitis
- BY INTRAVENOUS INJECTION, OR BY INTRAVENOUS INFUSION
  - Neonate up to 7 days: 50 mg/kg every 24 hours.
  - Neonate 7 days to 20 days: 50 mg/kg every 12 hours.
  - Neonate 21 days to 28 days: 50 mg/kg every 8 hours.
  - Child: 50 mg/kg every 8 hours (max. per dose 2 g)

Susceptible infections due to sensitive Gram-positive and Gram-negative bacteria
- BY INTRAVENOUS INJECTION, OR BY INTRAVENOUS INFUSION
  - Neonate up to 7 days: 25 mg/kg every 24 hours.
  - Neonate 7 days to 20 days: 25 mg/kg every 12 hours.
  - Neonate 21 days to 28 days: 25 mg/kg every 8 hours.
  - Child: 25 mg/kg every 8 hours (max. per dose 2 g)

Severe susceptible infections due to sensitive Gram-positive and Gram-negative bacteria
- BY INTRAVENOUS INJECTION, OR BY INTRAVENOUS INFUSION
  - Neonate up to 7 days: 50 mg/kg every 24 hours.
  - Neonate 7 days to 20 days: 50 mg/kg every 12 hours.
  - Neonate 21 days to 28 days: 50 mg/kg every 8 hours.
  - Child: 50 mg/kg every 8 hours (max. per dose 2 g)

Chronic *Burkholderia cepacia* infection in cystic fibrosis
- BY INHALATION OF NEBULISED SOLUTION
  - Child: 1 g twice daily

- **UNLICENSED USE** Nebulised route unlicensed.
- **INTERACTIONS** → Appendix 1: cephalosporins
- **SIDE-EFFECTS**
  - **Common or very common** Thrombocytosis · thrombophlebitis
  - **Uncommon** Antibiotic associated colitis · increased risk of infection
  - **Rare or very rare** Acute kidney injury
  - **Frequency not known** Coma · encephalopathy · jaundice · lymphocytosis · myoclonus · neurological effects · paraesthesia · seizure · taste altered · tremor
- **PREGNANCY** Not known to be harmful.
- **BREAST FEEDING** Present in milk in low concentration, but appropriate to use.
- **HEPATIC IMPAIRMENT** Manufacturer advises caution in severe impairment (no information available).
- **RENAL IMPAIRMENT** EvGr Use with caution. (M)
  Dose adjustments EvGr Reduce dose if creatinine clearance 50 mL/minute or less—consult product literature. (M) See p. 16.
- **DIRECTIONS FOR ADMINISTRATION** Intramuscular administration used when intravenous administration not possible; single doses over 1 g by intravenous route only.
  - With intravenous use Displacement value may be significant, consult local guidelines. For intermittent intravenous infusion dilute reconstituted solution further to a

concentration of not more than 40 mg/mL in Glucose 5% or Glucose 10% *or* Sodium Chloride 0.9%; give over 20–30 minutes.
- When used by inhalation For nebulisation, dissolve dose in 3 mL of Water for Injection.

● **MEDICINAL FORMS** There can be variation in the licensing of different medicines containing the same drug. Forms available from special-order manufacturers include: infusion, solution for infusion

Powder for solution for injection
ELECTROLYTES: May contain Sodium
- **Ceftazidime (Non-proprietary)**
  Ceftazidime (as Ceftazidime pentahydrate) 500 mg Ceftazidime 500mg powder for solution for injection vials | 1 vial [PoM] £4.25–£6.42 (Hospital only)
  Ceftazidime (as Ceftazidime pentahydrate) 1 gram Ceftazidime 1g powder for solution for injection vials | 1 vial [PoM] £12.42 (Hospital only) | 10 vial [PoM] £79.00 (Hospital only)
  Ceftazidime (as Ceftazidime pentahydrate) 2 gram Ceftazidime 2g powder for solution for injection vials | 1 vial [PoM] £26.16 (Hospital only) | 10 vial [PoM] £218.80 | 10 vial [PoM] £176.00–£218.80 (Hospital only)

Combinations available: ***Ceftazidime with avibactam***, p. 395

384

Ceftriaxone

26-Feb-2026

● **INDICATIONS AND DOSE**

Community-acquired pneumonia | Intra-abdominal infections | Complicated urinary-tract infections

▶ BY INTRAVENOUS INFUSION
- Neonate up to 15 days: 20–50 mg/kg once daily, doses at the higher end of the recommended range used in severe cases.
- Neonate 15 days to 28 days: 50–80 mg/kg once daily, doses at the higher end of the recommended range used in severe cases.
- Child 1 month–11 years (body-weight up to 50 kg): 50–80 mg/kg once daily, doses at the higher end of the recommended range used in severe cases
- Child 9–11 years (body-weight 50 kg and above): 1–2 g once daily, 2 g dose to be used for severe cases
- Child 12–17 years: 1–2 g once daily, 2 g dose to be used for severe cases

▶ BY INTRAVENOUS INJECTION
- Child 9–11 years (body-weight 50 kg and above): 1–2 g once daily, 2 g dose to be used for severe cases
- Child 12–17 years: 1–2 g once daily, 2 g dose to be used for severe cases

▶ BY DEEP INTRAMUSCULAR INJECTION
- Child 1 month–11 years (body-weight up to 50 kg): 50–80 mg/kg daily, doses at the higher end of the recommended range used in severe cases
- Child 9–11 years (body-weight 50 kg and above): 1–2 g once daily, 2 g dose to be used for severe cases
- Child 12–17 years: 1–2 g once daily, 2 g dose to be used for severe cases

Hospital-acquired pneumonia

▶ BY INTRAVENOUS INFUSION
- Neonate up to 15 days: 20–50 mg/kg once daily, doses at the higher end of the recommended range used in severe cases.
- Neonate 15 days to 28 days: 50–80 mg/kg once daily, doses at the higher end of the recommended range used in severe cases.
- Child 1 month–11 years (body-weight up to 50 kg): 50–80 mg/kg once daily, doses at the higher end of the recommended range used in severe cases
- Child 9–11 years (body-weight 50 kg and above): 2 g once daily
- Child 12–17 years: 2 g once daily

▶ BY INTRAVENOUS INJECTION
- Child 9–11 years (body-weight 50 kg and above): 2 g once daily
- Child 12–17 years: 2 g once daily

▶ BY DEEP INTRAMUSCULAR INJECTION
- Child 1 month–11 years (body-weight up to 50 kg): 50–80 mg/kg daily, doses at the higher end of the recommended range used in severe cases
- Child 9–11 years (body-weight 50 kg and above): 2 g once daily
- Child 12–17 years: 2 g once daily

Prophylaxis of infection from human bites [in combination with other drugs] | Prophylaxis of infection from animal bites [in combination with other drugs] | Treatment of infection from human bites [in combination with other drugs] | Treatment of infection from animal bites [in combination with other drugs]

▶ BY INTRAVENOUS INFUSION
- Child 1 month–11 years (body-weight up to 50 kg): 50–80 mg/kg once daily
- Child 9–11 years (body-weight 50 kg and above): 1–2 g once daily
- Child 12–17 years: 1–2 g once daily

▶ BY INTRAVENOUS INJECTION
- Child 9–11 years (body-weight 50 kg and above): 1–2 g once daily
- Child 12–17 years: 1–2 g once daily

Complicated skin and soft tissue infections | Infections of bones and joints

▶ BY INTRAVENOUS INFUSION
- Neonate up to 15 days: 20–50 mg/kg once daily, doses at the higher end of the recommended range used in severe cases.
- Neonate 15 days to 28 days: 50–100 mg/kg once daily, doses at the higher end of the recommended range used in severe cases.
- Child 1 month–11 years (body-weight up to 50 kg): 50–100 mg/kg once daily (max. per dose 4 g), doses at the higher end of the recommended range used in severe cases
- Child 9–11 years (body-weight 50 kg and above): 2 g once daily
- Child 12–17 years: 2 g once daily

▶ BY INTRAVENOUS INJECTION
- Child 9–11 years (body-weight 50 kg and above): 2 g once daily
- Child 12–17 years: 2 g once daily

▶ BY DEEP INTRAMUSCULAR INJECTION
- Child 1 month–11 years (body-weight up to 50 kg): 50–100 mg/kg daily, doses at the higher end of the recommended range used in severe cases; maximum 4 g per day
- Child 9–11 years (body-weight 50 kg and above): 2 g once daily
- Child 12–17 years: 2 g once daily

Suspected bacterial infection in neutropenic patients

▶ BY INTRAVENOUS INFUSION
- Neonate up to 15 days: 20–50 mg/kg once daily, doses at the higher end of the recommended range used in severe cases.
- Neonate 15 days to 28 days: 50–100 mg/kg once daily, doses at the higher end of the recommended range used in severe cases.

continued →

- Child 1 month–11 years (body-weight up to 50 kg): 50–100 mg/kg once daily (max. per dose 4 g), doses at the higher end of the recommended range used in severe cases
- Child 9–11 years (body-weight 50 kg and above): 2–4 g once daily, doses at the higher end of the recommended range used in severe cases
- Child 12–17 years: 2–4 g once daily, doses at the higher end of the recommended range used in severe cases

▶ BY INTRAVENOUS INJECTION
- Child 9–11 years (body-weight 50 kg and above): 2–4 g once daily, doses at the higher end of the recommended range used in severe cases; doses of 50 mg/kg or more should be given by infusion
- Child 12–17 years: 2–4 g once daily, doses at the higher end of the recommended range used in severe cases

▶ BY DEEP INTRAMUSCULAR INJECTION
- Child 1 month–11 years (body-weight up to 50 kg): 50–100 mg/kg daily, doses at the higher end of the recommended range used in severe cases; maximum 4 g per day
- Child 9–11 years (body-weight 50 kg and above): 2 g once daily, increased if necessary up to 4 g daily in 2 divided doses, doses at the higher end of the recommended range used in severe cases
- Child 12–17 years: 2 g once daily, increased if necessary up to 4 g daily in 2 divided doses, doses at the higher end of the recommended range used in severe cases

Suspected meningococcal disease [pre-hospital treatment] | Suspected bacterial meningitis [pre-hospital treatment where there is likely to be a clinically significant delay in transfer to hospital]

▶ BY DEEP INTRAMUSCULAR INJECTION
- Child 1 month: 250 mg for 1 dose, administer prior to urgent transfer to hospital unless this will delay transfer. The actual dose given should be communicated to the receiving hospital, where the child's weight should be obtained as soon as possible and the remainder of the dose given if necessary (see dosing for *Bacterial meningitis* and *Meningococcal disease*)
- Child 2–11 months: 500 mg for 1 dose, administer prior to urgent transfer to hospital unless this will delay transfer. The actual dose given should be communicated to the receiving hospital, where the child's weight should be obtained as soon as possible and the remainder of the dose given if necessary (see dosing for *Bacterial meningitis* and *Meningococcal disease*)
- Child 1–4 years: 1 g for 1 dose, administer prior to urgent transfer to hospital unless this will delay transfer. The actual dose given should be communicated to the receiving hospital, where the child's weight should be obtained as soon as possible and the remainder of the dose given if necessary (see dosing for *Bacterial meningitis* and *Meningococcal disease*)
- Child 5–8 years: 1.5 g for 1 dose, administer prior to urgent transfer to hospital unless this will delay transfer. The actual dose given should be communicated to the receiving hospital, where the child's weight should be obtained as soon as possible and the remainder of the dose given if necessary (see dosing for *Bacterial meningitis* and *Meningococcal disease*)
- Child 9–11 years: 2 g for 1 dose, administer prior to urgent transfer to hospital unless this will delay transfer. The actual dose given should be communicated to the receiving hospital, where the child's weight should be obtained as soon as possible and the remainder of the dose given if necessary (see dosing for *Bacterial meningitis* and *Meningococcal disease*)

▶ BY INTRAVENOUS INJECTION, OR BY DEEP INTRAMUSCULAR INJECTION
- Child 12–17 years: 2 g for 1 dose, administer prior to urgent transfer to hospital unless this will delay transfer

Bacterial meningitis | Meningococcal disease

▶ BY INTRAVENOUS INFUSION
- Neonate up to 15 days: 50 mg/kg once daily.
- Neonate 15 days to 28 days: 100 mg/kg once daily.
- Child 1 month–11 years (body-weight up to 50 kg): 100 mg/kg once daily (max. per dose 4 g), if the *total* daily dose exceeds 2 g consider giving in 2 divided doses
- Child 9–11 years (body-weight 50 kg and above): 2 g every 12 hours, alternatively 4 g once daily
- Child 12–17 years: 2 g every 12 hours, alternatively 4 g once daily

▶ BY INTRAVENOUS INJECTION
- Child 9–11 years (body-weight 50 kg and above): 2 g every 12 hours, alternatively 4 g once daily, doses of 50 mg/kg or more should be given by intravenous infusion
- Child 12–17 years: 2 g every 12 hours, alternatively 4 g once daily

Bacterial endocarditis

▶ BY INTRAVENOUS INFUSION
- Neonate up to 15 days: 50 mg/kg once daily.
- Neonate 15 days to 28 days: 100 mg/kg once daily.
- Child 1 month–11 years (body-weight up to 50 kg): 100 mg/kg once daily (max. per dose 4 g)
- Child 9–11 years (body-weight 50 kg and above): 2–4 g once daily, doses at the higher end of the recommended range used in severe cases
- Child 12–17 years: 2–4 g once daily, doses at the higher end of the recommended range used in severe cases

▶ BY INTRAVENOUS INJECTION
- Child 9–11 years (body-weight 50 kg and above): 2–4 g once daily, doses at the higher end of the recommended range used in severe cases; doses of 50 mg/kg or more should be given by infusion
- Child 12–17 years: 2–4 g once daily, doses at the higher end of the recommended range used in severe cases

▶ BY DEEP INTRAMUSCULAR INJECTION
- Child 1 month–11 years (body-weight up to 50 kg): 100 mg/kg daily; maximum 4 g per day
- Child 9–11 years (body-weight 50 kg and above): 2 g once daily, increased if necessary up to 4 g daily in 2 divided doses, doses at the higher end of the recommended range used in severe cases
- Child 12–17 years: 2 g once daily, increased if necessary up to 4 g daily in 2 divided doses, doses at the higher end of the recommended range used in severe cases

Surgical prophylaxis

▶ BY INTRAVENOUS INFUSION
- Neonate up to 15 days: 20–50 mg/kg for 1 dose, dose to be administered 30–90 minutes before procedure.
- Neonate 15 days to 28 days: 50–80 mg/kg for 1 dose, dose to be administered 30–90 minutes before procedure.
- Child 1 month–11 years (body-weight up to 50 kg): 50–80 mg/kg for 1 dose (max. per dose 2 g), dose to be administered 30–90 minutes before procedure

- ▸ Child 9–11 years (body-weight 50 kg and above): 2 g for 1 dose, dose to be administered 30–90 minutes before procedure
- ▸ Child 12–17 years: 2 g for 1 dose, dose to be administered 30–90 minutes before procedure

▶ BY INTRAVENOUS INJECTION
- ▸ Child 9–11 years (body-weight 50 kg and above): 2 g for 1 dose, dose to be administered 30–90 minutes before procedure
- ▸ Child 12–17 years: 2 g for 1 dose, dose to be administered 30–90 minutes before procedure

▶ BY DEEP INTRAMUSCULAR INJECTION
- ▸ Child 1 month–11 years (body-weight up to 50 kg): 50–80 mg/kg for 1 dose (max. per dose 2 g), dose to be administered 30–90 minutes before procedure
- ▸ Child 9–11 years (body-weight 50 kg and above): 2 g for 1 dose, dose to be administered 30–90 minutes before procedure
- ▸ Child 12–17 years: 2 g for 1 dose, dose to be administered 30–90 minutes before procedure

Pelvic inflammatory disease

▶ BY DEEP INTRAMUSCULAR INJECTION
- ▸ Child 12–17 years (body-weight 45 kg and above): 1 g for 1 dose

Uncomplicated gonorrhoea [anogenital and pharyngeal infection]

▶ BY DEEP INTRAMUSCULAR INJECTION
- ▸ Child 12–17 years (body-weight 45 kg and above): 1 g for 1 dose

Gonococcal conjunctivitis

▶ BY DEEP INTRAMUSCULAR INJECTION
- ▸ Child 12–17 years (body-weight 45 kg and above): 1 g for 1 dose

Gonococcal epididymo-orchitis

▶ BY DEEP INTRAMUSCULAR INJECTION
- ▸ Child 12–17 years (body-weight 45 kg and above): 1 g for 1 dose, to be followed by an additional antibacterial course to treat epididymo-orchitis

Disseminated gonococcal infection

▶ BY DEEP INTRAMUSCULAR INJECTION, OR BY INTRAVENOUS INFUSION, OR BY INTRAVENOUS INJECTION
- ▸ Child 12–17 years (body-weight 45 kg and above): 1 g every 24 hours

Disseminated gonococcal infection [arthritis and arthritis-dermatitis syndrome]

▶ BY DEEP INTRAMUSCULAR INJECTION, OR BY INTRAVENOUS INFUSION, OR BY INTRAVENOUS INJECTION
- ▸ Child 12–17 years (body-weight 45 kg and above): 1 g every 24 hours for 7 days, may be switched 24–48 hours after symptoms improve to a suitable oral antibacterial

Disseminated gonococcal infection [gonococcal meningitis]

▶ BY INTRAVENOUS INFUSION, OR BY INTRAVENOUS INJECTION
- ▸ Child 12–17 years (body-weight 45 kg and above): 1–2 g every 12–24 hours for 10–14 days

Disseminated gonococcal infection [gonococcal endocarditis]

▶ BY INTRAVENOUS INFUSION, OR BY INTRAVENOUS INJECTION
- ▸ Child 12–17 years (body-weight 45 kg and above): 1–2 g every 12–24 hours for at least 4 weeks

Syphilis

▶ BY INTRAVENOUS INFUSION, OR BY INTRAVENOUS INJECTION, OR BY DEEP INTRAMUSCULAR INJECTION
- ▸ Child 12–17 years (body-weight 50 kg and above): 0.5–1 g once daily for 10–14 days, dose increased to 2 g once daily for neurosyphilis

Disseminated Lyme borreliosis (early [Stage II] and late [Stage III]) (administered on expert advice)

▶ BY INTRAVENOUS INFUSION
- ▸ Neonate 15 days to 28 days: 50–80 mg/kg once daily for 14–21 days, the recommended treatment durations vary and national or local guidelines should be taken into consideration.

Lyme disease [affecting central nervous system]

▶ BY INTRAVENOUS INFUSION
- ▸ Child 1 month–11 years (administered on expert advice) (body-weight up to 50 kg): 80 mg/kg once daily for 21 days
- ▸ Child 1 month–11 years (administered on expert advice) (body-weight 50 kg and above): 2 g twice daily for 21 days, alternatively 4 g once daily for 21 days
- ▸ Child 12–17 years (administered on expert advice): 2 g twice daily for 21 days, alternatively 4 g once daily for 21 days

▶ BY INTRAVENOUS INJECTION
- ▸ Child 1 month–11 years (administered on expert advice) (body-weight 50 kg and above): 2 g twice daily for 21 days
- ▸ Child 12–17 years (administered on expert advice): 2 g twice daily for 21 days, alternatively 4 g once daily for 21 days

Lyme arthritis | Acrodermatitis chronica atrophicans

▶ BY INTRAVENOUS INFUSION
- ▸ Child 1 month–11 years (administered on expert advice) (body-weight up to 50 kg): 80 mg/kg once daily (max. per dose 2 g) for 28 days

▶ BY INTRAVENOUS INFUSION, OR BY INTRAVENOUS INJECTION
- ▸ Child 1 month–11 years (administered on expert advice) (body-weight 50 kg and above): 2 g once daily for 28 days
- ▸ Child 12–17 years (administered on expert advice): 2 g once daily for 28 days

Lyme carditis

▶ BY INTRAVENOUS INFUSION
- ▸ Child 1 month–11 years (administered on expert advice) (body-weight up to 50 kg): 80 mg/kg once daily (max. per dose 2 g) for 21 days

▶ BY INTRAVENOUS INFUSION, OR BY INTRAVENOUS INJECTION
- ▸ Child 1 month–11 years (administered on expert advice) (body-weight 50 kg and above): 2 g once daily for 21 days
- ▸ Child 12–17 years (administered on expert advice): 2 g once daily for 21 days

Prevention of secondary case of meningococcal meningitis

▶ BY DEEP INTRAMUSCULAR INJECTION
- ▸ Child 1 month–11 years: 125 mg for 1 dose
- ▸ Child 12–17 years: 250 mg for 1 dose

Prevention of secondary case of *Haemophilus influenzae* type b disease

▶ BY INTRAVENOUS INFUSION
- ▸ Child 1 month–11 years: 50 mg/kg once daily (max. per dose 1 g) for 2 days

▶ BY DEEP INTRAMUSCULAR INJECTION, OR BY INTRAVENOUS INJECTION, OR BY INTRAVENOUS INFUSION
- ▸ Child 12–17 years: 1 g once daily for 2 days

Acute otitis media

▶ BY DEEP INTRAMUSCULAR INJECTION
- ▸ Child 1 month–11 years (body-weight up to 50 kg): 50 mg/kg for 1 dose (max. per dose 2 g), dose can be given for 3 days if severely ill or previous therapy failed
- ▸ Child 9–11 years (body-weight 50 kg and above): 1–2 g for 1 dose, dose can be given for 3 days if severely ill or previous therapy failed
- ▸ Child 12–17 years: 1–2 g for 1 dose, dose can be given for 3 days if severely ill or previous therapy failed

● **UNLICENSED USE** EvGr Ceftriaxone is used for the treatment of pelvic inflammatory disease, Ⓐ but is not licensed for this indication. EvGr Ceftriaxone is used in the doses provided in BNF Publications for the treatment of uncomplicated gonorrhoea, gonococcal conjunctivitis, gonococcal epididymo-orchitis, and disseminated gonococcal infection (including arthritis and arthritis-dermatitis syndrome, and gonococcal meningitis and endocarditis), ⟨A⟩ but these are not licensed. EvGr Ceftriaxone is used for Lyme disease affecting the central nervous system in children with body-weight 50 kg and over and in children aged 12 years and over, ⟨A⟩ but the dose is not licensed for this indication.

UKHSA advises that ceftriaxone is used for the prevention of secondary cases of *Haemophilus influenzae* type b disease, but is not licensed for this indication.

Not licensed for prophylaxis of meningococcal meningitis.

- **CONTRA-INDICATIONS** Concomitant treatment with intravenous calcium (including total parenteral nutrition containing calcium) in premature and full-term neonates—risk of precipitation in urine and lungs (fatal reactions) · full-term neonates with jaundice, hypoalbuminaemia, acidosis, unconjugated hyperbilirubinaemia, or impaired bilirubin binding—risk of developing bilirubin encephalopathy · premature neonates less than 41 weeks corrected gestational age (postmenstrual age)
- **CAUTIONS**

  GENERAL CAUTIONS History of hypercalciuria · history of kidney stones · use with caution in neonates

  SPECIFIC CAUTIONS
  - With intravenous use Concomitant treatment with intravenous calcium (including total parenteral nutrition containing calcium)
- **INTERACTIONS** → Appendix 1: cephalosporins
- **SIDE-EFFECTS**
  - **Uncommon** Anaemia · coagulation disorder · fungal infection
  - **Rare or very rare** Bronchospasm · glycosuria · haematuria · oedema
  - **Frequency not known** Antibiotic associated colitis · cholelithiasis · hypersensitivity · kernicterus (in neonates) · nephrolithiasis · oral disorders · pancreatitis · seizure · vertigo

  SIDE-EFFECTS, FURTHER INFORMATION Precipitates of calcium ceftriaxone can occur in the gall bladder and urine (particularly in very young, dehydrated or those who are immobilised)—consider discontinuation if symptomatic.
- **PREGNANCY** Manufacturer advises use only if benefit outweighs risk—limited data available but not known to be harmful in *animal* studies. EvGr Specialist sources indicate suitable for use in pregnancy. ⟨D⟩
- **BREAST FEEDING** EvGr Specialist sources advise ceftriaxone is compatible with breastfeeding—present in milk in low concentration but limited effects to breast-fed infant. ⟨D⟩
- **HEPATIC IMPAIRMENT** Manufacturer advises caution in severe impairment (no information available).
- **RENAL IMPAIRMENT**

  Dose adjustments See p. 16.

  Manufacturer advises a dose reduction may be required in severe renal impairment in combination with hepatic impairment (limited information available)—monitor for efficacy.

  Expert sources advise max. 50 mg/kg daily or max. 2 g daily if estimated glomerular filtration rate less than 10 mL/minute/1.73 m^2.
- **MONITORING REQUIREMENTS** Manufacturer advises to monitor full blood count regularly during prolonged treatment.
- **DIRECTIONS FOR ADMINISTRATION**
  - With intravenous use in neonates EvGr Dilute reconstituted solution with Glucose 5% *or* Sodium Chloride 0.9%; give over at least 60 minutes (may displace bilirubin from serum albumin). ⟨M⟩ EvGr Alternatively dilute reconstituted solution with Glucose 10%. ⟨E⟩ Displacement value may be significant, consult local guidelines. Not to be given simultaneously with parenteral nutrition or infusion fluids containing calcium, even by different infusion lines.
  - With intravenous use EvGr For doses greater than 2 g daily, consider giving in two divided doses. ⟨M⟩ Displacement value may be significant, consult local guidelines. EvGr For *intravenous infusion* (preferred route), dilute reconstituted solution with Glucose 5% *or* Sodium Chloride 0.9%; give over at least 30 minutes. ⟨M⟩ Not to be given simultaneously with parenteral nutrition or infusion fluids containing calcium, even by different infusion lines; may be infused sequentially with infusion fluids containing calcium if infusion lines at different sites are used, or if the infusion lines are replaced or thoroughly flushed between infusions with Sodium Chloride 0.9% to avoid precipitation—consult product literature. EvGr For *intravenous injection*, give over 5 minutes. ⟨M⟩ Local policies may advise that doses of 50 mg/kg can be given by intravenous injection over 5 minutes to children under 12 years, although this is not licensed.
  - With intramuscular use EvGr The maximum single intramuscular dose is 2 g. Doses over 1 g should be divided between more than one site. Doses greater than 2 g must be given in two divided doses 12 hours apart or by intravenous administration. For *intramuscular injection*, may be mixed with 1% Lidocaine Hydrochloride Injection to reduce pain at intramuscular injection site. Intramuscular injection should only be considered when the intravenous route is not possible or less appropriate. ⟨M⟩ If administered by intramuscular injection, the lower end of the dose range should be used for the shortest time possible; volume depends on the age and size of the child. Displacement value may be significant, consult local guidelines.
- **PRESCRIBING AND DISPENSING INFORMATION** For choice of antibacterial therapy, see Antibacterials, use for prophylaxis p. 359, Cardiovascular system infections, antibacterial therapy p. 364, Central nervous system infections, antibacterial therapy p. 365, Gastro-intestinal system infections, antibacterial therapy p. 367, Genital system infections, antibacterial therapy p. 368, Lyme disease p. 444, Musculoskeletal system infections, antibacterial therapy p. 369, Respiratory system infections, antibacterial therapy p. 371, Sepsis p. 362, Skin infections, antibacterial therapy p. 373, Urinary-tract infections p. 454.

- **MEDICINAL FORMS** There can be variation in the licensing of different medicines containing the same drug. Forms available from special-order manufacturers include: infusion

Powder for solution for injection

ELECTROLYTES: May contain Sodium

- **Ceftriaxone (Non-proprietary)**

  Ceftriaxone (as Ceftriaxone sodium) 250 mg Ceftriaxone 250mg powder for solution for injection vials | 1 vial PoM £2.30 (Hospital only) | 10 vial PoM £24.00 (Hospital only)

  Ceftriaxone (as Ceftriaxone sodium) 1 gram Ceftriaxone 1g powder for solution for injection vials | 1 vial PoM £6.50 DT = £9.58 | 5 vial PoM £45.00 (Hospital only) | 10 vial PoM £60.00 | 10 vial PoM £86.22–£95.80 (Hospital only)

  Ceftriaxone (as Ceftriaxone sodium) 2 gram Ceftriaxone 2g powder for solution for injection vials | 1 vial PoM £18.30 (Hospital only) | 10 vial PoM £191.80 (Hospital only)

ANTIBACTERIALS › CEPHALOSPORINS, THIRD-GENERATION WITH BETA-LACTAMASE INHIBITOR

F 384

Ceftazidime with avibactam

26-Feb-2026

The properties listed below are those particular to the combination only. For the properties of the components please consider, ceftazidime p. 390.

● **INDICATIONS AND DOSE**

Complicated intra-abdominal infection | Complicated urinary tract infection [including pyelonephritis]

▶ BY INTRAVENOUS INFUSION

▸ Neonate: 20/5 mg/kg every 8 hours for 5–14 days, for doses in preterm neonates—consult product literature.

▸ Child 1-2 months: 30/7.5 mg/kg every 8 hours for 5–14 days, for doses in preterm infants—consult product literature

▸ Child 3-5 months: 40/10 mg/kg every 8 hours for 5–14 days, for doses in preterm infants—consult product literature

▸ Child 6 months-17 years: 50/12.5 mg/kg every 8 hours (max. per dose 2/0.5 g) for 5–14 days

Hospital-acquired pneumonia [including ventilator-associated pneumonia]

▶ BY INTRAVENOUS INFUSION

▸ Neonate: 20/5 mg/kg every 8 hours for 7–14 days, for doses in preterm neonates—consult product literature.

▸ Child 1-2 months: 30/7.5 mg/kg every 8 hours for 7–14 days, for doses in preterm infants—consult product literature

▸ Child 3-5 months: 40/10 mg/kg every 8 hours for 7–14 days, for doses in preterm infants—consult product literature

▸ Child 6 months-17 years: 50/12.5 mg/kg every 8 hours (max. per dose 2/0.5 g) for 7–14 days

Aerobic Gram-negative infections [in patients with limited treatment options] (administered on expert advice)

▶ BY INTRAVENOUS INFUSION

▸ Neonate: 20/5 mg/kg every 8 hours, duration should be guided by infection severity, pathogen, and response, for doses in preterm neonates—consult product literature.

▸ Child 1-2 months: 30/7.5 mg/kg every 8 hours, duration should be guided by infection severity, pathogen, and response, for doses in preterm infants—consult product literature

▸ Child 3-5 months: 40/10 mg/kg every 8 hours, duration should be guided by infection severity, pathogen, and response, for doses in preterm infants—consult product literature

▸ Child 6 months-17 years: 50/12.5 mg/kg every 8 hours (max. per dose 2/0.5 g), duration should be guided by infection severity, pathogen, and response

DOSE EQUIVALENCE AND CONVERSION

▸ Dose expressed as either *x*/*y* mg/kg or *x*/*y* g ceftazidime/avibactam.

● **CAUTIONS** Low-sodium diet (*Zavicefta*® is high in sodium)

● **INTERACTIONS** → Appendix 1: cephalosporins

● **SIDE-EFFECTS**

▶ **Common or very common** Increased risk of infection · thrombocytosis

▶ **Uncommon** Acute kidney injury · Clostridioides difficile colitis · lymphocytosis · paraesthesia · taste altered

▶ **Frequency not known** Jaundice · Kounis syndrome

● **PREGNANCY** EvGr Avoid unless potential benefit outweighs risk (toxicity in *animal* studies with avibactam). ⟨M⟩

● **BREAST FEEDING** Specialist sources indicate probably compatible (no information available for avibactam).

● **RENAL IMPAIRMENT** EvGr Use with caution. ⟨M⟩

Dose adjustments EvGr Reduce dose if creatinine clearance 50 mL/minute or less—consult product literature. ⟨M⟩ See p. 16.

● **DIRECTIONS FOR ADMINISTRATION** For *intravenous infusion* (*Zavicefta*®), reconstitute each vial with 10 mL Water for Injections; dilute requisite dose (based on ceftazidime component only) in an infusion bag or syringe and give over 120 minutes—consult product literature for further information.

● **PATIENT AND CARER ADVICE**

Driving and skilled tasks Patients and carers should be counselled on the effects on driving and performance of skilled tasks—increased risk of dizziness.

● **MEDICINAL FORMS** There can be variation in the licensing of different medicines containing the same drug.

Powder for solution for infusion

ELECTROLYTES: May contain Sodium

▸ **Zavicefta** (Pfizer Ltd)

Avibactam (as Avibactam sodium) 500 mg, Ceftazidime (as Ceftazidime pentahydrate) 2 gram Zavicefta 2g/0.5g powder for concentrate for solution for infusion vials | 10 vial PoM £857.00 (Hospital only)

ANTIBACTERIALS › CEPHALOSPORINS, OTHER

F 384

Cefepime

19-Aug-2020

● **INDICATIONS AND DOSE**

Infections due to sensitive Gram-positive and Gram-negative bacteria

▶ BY INTRAVENOUS INJECTION, OR BY INTRAVENOUS INFUSION, OR BY INTRAMUSCULAR INJECTION

▸ Child 1 month: 30 mg/kg every 8–12 hours, experience in children aged less than 2 months is limited—consult product literature; intravenous route preferred in severe infections

▸ Child 2 months-17 years (body-weight up to 41 kg): 50 mg/kg every 12 hours (max. per dose 2 g), increased if necessary to 50 mg/kg every 8 hours (max. per dose 2 g), increased dose used for severe infections, experience of intramuscular use is limited; intravenous route preferred in severe infections

Mild to moderate urinary tract infections

▶ BY INTRAVENOUS INJECTION, OR BY INTRAVENOUS INFUSION, OR BY INTRAMUSCULAR INJECTION

▸ Child (body-weight 41 kg and above): 0.5–1 g every 12 hours, experience of intramuscular use is limited

Mild to moderate infections due to sensitive Gram-positive and Gram-negative bacteria

▶ BY INTRAVENOUS INJECTION, OR BY INTRAVENOUS INFUSION, OR BY INTRAMUSCULAR INJECTION

▸ Child (body-weight 41 kg and above): 1 g every 12 hours, experience of intramuscular use is limited

Severe infections due to sensitive Gram-positive and Gram-negative bacteria

▶ BY INTRAVENOUS INJECTION, OR BY INTRAVENOUS INFUSION

▸ Child (body-weight 41 kg and above): 2 g every 12 hours, increased if necessary to 2 g every 8 hours, increased dose used for very severe infections

● **INTERACTIONS** → Appendix 1: cephalosporins

● **SIDE-EFFECTS**

▶ **Common or very common** Anaemia

- **Uncommon** Gastrointestinal disorders · increased risk of infection
- **Rare or very rare** Constipation · dyspnoea · genital pruritus · paraesthesia · seizure · taste altered · vasodilation
- **Frequency not known** Anaphylactic shock · antibiotic associated colitis · aplastic anaemia · Clostridioides difficile colitis · coma · confusion · consciousness impaired · encephalopathy · haemorrhage · hallucination · myoclonus · nephrotoxicity · renal failure

- **PREGNANCY** Manufacturer advises caution—no data available but not known to be harmful in *animal* studies.
- **BREAST FEEDING** Manufacturer advises caution—present in milk in very low quantities.
- **RENAL IMPAIRMENT** Manufacturer advises use with caution.
 Dose adjustments Manufacturer advises reduce dose—consult product literature.
- **DIRECTIONS FOR ADMINISTRATION** After reconstitution the solution is yellow to yellow-brown. Displacement value may be significant when reconstituting injection, consult local guidelines. For *intravenous infusion*, manufacturer advises reconstitute with 50 mL Glucose 5% or 10% *or* Sodium Chloride 0.9%; give over 30 minutes. For *intravenous injection*, manufacturer advises reconstitute with 10 mL Glucose 5% or 10% *or* Sodium Chloride 0.9%. For *intramuscular injection*, manufacturer advises reconstitute with 3 mL Water for Injection.
- **NATIONAL FUNDING/ACCESS DECISIONS**
 For full details see funding body website
 All Wales Medicines Strategy Group (AWMSG) decisions
 - **Cefepime (*Renapime*®) for resistant pseudomonas infections (November 2019)** AWMSG No. 4129 Recommended with restrictions

- **MEDICINAL FORMS** There can be variation in the licensing of different medicines containing the same drug.

Powder for solution for injection
- **Renapime** (Renascience Pharma Ltd)
 Cefepime (as Cefepime dihydrochloride monohydrate)
 1 gram Renapime 1g powder for solution for injection vials | 10 vial PoM £70.00
 Cefepime (as Cefepime dihydrochloride monohydrate)
 2 gram Renapime 2g powder for solution for injection vials | 10 vial PoM £110.00

F 384

Ceftaroline fosamil

04-Nov-2020

- **INDICATIONS AND DOSE**

Community-acquired pneumonia
- BY INTRAVENOUS INFUSION
 - Neonate: 6 mg/kg every 8 hours for 5–7 days.
 - Child up to 2 months: 6 mg/kg every 8 hours for 5–7 days
 - Child 2-23 months: 8 mg/kg every 8 hours for 5–7 days
 - Child 2-11 years: 12 mg/kg every 8 hours (max. per dose 400 mg) for 5–7 days
 - Child 12-17 years (body-weight up to 33 kg): 12 mg/kg every 8 hours (max. per dose 400 mg) for 5–7 days
 - Child 12-17 years (body-weight 33 kg and above): 600 mg every 12 hours for 5–7 days

Complicated skin infections | Complicated soft-tissue infections
- BY INTRAVENOUS INFUSION
 - Neonate: 6 mg/kg every 8 hours for 5–14 days.
 - Child up to 2 months: 6 mg/kg every 8 hours for 5–14 days
 - Child 2-23 months: 8 mg/kg every 8 hours for 5–14 days, for high dose regimen consult product literature
 - Child 2-11 years: 12 mg/kg every 8 hours (max. per dose 400 mg) for 5–14 days, for high dose regimen consult product literature
 - Child 12-17 years (body-weight up to 33 kg): 12 mg/kg every 8 hours (max. per dose 400 mg) for 5–14 days, for high dose regimen consult product literature
 - Child 12-17 years (body-weight 33 kg and above): 600 mg every 12 hours for 5–14 days, for high dose regimen consult product literature

- **CAUTIONS** Seizure disorders
- **INTERACTIONS** → Appendix 1: cephalosporins
- **SIDE-EFFECTS**
 - **Uncommon** Anaemia · Clostridioides difficile colitis · hypersensitivity
 - **Frequency not known** Antibiotic associated colitis
- **PREGNANCY** Manufacturer advises avoid unless essential—limited information; *animal* studies do not indicate toxicity.
- **BREAST FEEDING** Manufacturer advises avoid—no information available.
- **RENAL IMPAIRMENT**
 Dose adjustments Manufacturer advises reduce dose if creatinine clearance less than 51 mL/minute—consult product literature. See p. 16.
- **DIRECTIONS FOR ADMINISTRATION** For *intravenous infusion*, give intermittently *in* Glucose 5% *or* Sodium Chloride 0.9%. Dilute reconstituted solution to 50, 100, or 250 mL with infusion fluid; give over 5 to 60 minutes. Consult product literature for administration of high-dose regimen.
- **NATIONAL FUNDING/ACCESS DECISIONS**
 For full details see funding body website
 Scottish Medicines Consortium (SMC) decisions
 - **Ceftaroline fosamil (*Zinforo*®) for the treatment of complicated skin and soft tissue infections (cSSTIs) (January 2013)** SMC No. 830/12 Recommended with restrictions

- **MEDICINAL FORMS** There can be variation in the licensing of different medicines containing the same drug.

Powder for solution for infusion
- **Zinforo** (Pfizer Ltd)
 Ceftaroline fosamil (as Ceftaroline fosamil acetic acid solvate monohydrate) 600 mg Zinforo 600mg powder for concentrate for solution for infusion vials | 10 vial PoM £375.00 (Hospital only)

ANTIBACTERIALS > GLYCOPEPTIDE ANTIBACTERIALS

Teicoplanin

29-Aug-2025

- **DRUG ACTION** The glycopeptide antibiotic teicoplanin has bactericidal activity against aerobic and anaerobic Gram-positive bacteria including multi-resistant staphylococci. However, there are reports of *Staphylococcus aureus* with reduced susceptibility to glycopeptides and increasing reports of glycopeptide-resistant enterococci. Teicoplanin is similar to vancomycin, but has a significantly longer duration of action, allowing once daily administration after the loading dose.

- **INDICATIONS AND DOSE**

***Clostridioides difficile* infection**
- BY MOUTH
 - Child 12-17 years: 100–200 mg twice daily for 7–14 days

Cellulitis | Erysipelas
- BY INTRAVENOUS INFUSION
 - Child 1 month: Initially 16 mg/kg for 1 dose, followed by 8 mg/kg once daily, subsequent dose to be administered 24 hours after initial dose

▶ BY INTRAVENOUS INJECTION, OR BY INTRAVENOUS INFUSION
▸ Child 2 months–11 years: Initially 10 mg/kg every 12 hours for 3 doses, then 6–10 mg/kg once daily
▸ Child 12–17 years: Initially 6 mg/kg every 12 hours for 3 doses, then 6 mg/kg once daily

Serious infections caused by Gram-positive bacteria (e.g. complicated skin and soft-tissue infections, pneumonia, complicated urinary tract infections)

▶ BY INTRAVENOUS INJECTION, OR BY INTRAVENOUS INFUSION, OR BY INTRAMUSCULAR INJECTION
▸ Child 12–17 years: Initially 6 mg/kg every 12 hours for 3 doses, then 6 mg/kg once daily

Streptococcal or enterococcal endocarditis (in combination with another antibacterial) | Bone and joint infections

▶ INITIALLY BY INTRAVENOUS INJECTION, OR BY INTRAVENOUS INFUSION
▸ Child 12–17 years: 12 mg/kg every 12 hours for 3–5 doses, then (by intravenous injection or by intravenous infusion or by intramuscular injection) 12 mg/kg once daily

Surgical prophylaxis

▶ BY INTRAVENOUS INJECTION
▸ Child: (consult local protocol)

Serious infections caused by Gram-positive bacteria (including endocarditis, complicated skin and soft-tissue infections, pneumonia, complicated urinary tract infections, bone and joint infections)

▶ BY INTRAVENOUS INFUSION
▸ Neonate: Initially 16 mg/kg for 1 dose, followed by 8 mg/kg once daily, subsequent dose to be administered 24 hours after initial dose.
▸ Child 1 month: Initially 16 mg/kg for 1 dose, followed by 8 mg/kg once daily, subsequent dose to be administered 24 hours after initial dose

▶ BY INTRAVENOUS INJECTION, OR BY INTRAVENOUS INFUSION
▸ Child 2 months–11 years: Initially 10 mg/kg every 12 hours for 3 doses, then 6–10 mg/kg once daily

Peritonitis associated with peritoneal dialysis (added to dialysis fluid)

▶ BY INTRAPERITONEAL INFUSION
▸ Child 12–17 years: (consult local protocol)

PHARMACOKINETICS
▸ With oral use Teicoplanin should **not** be given by mouth for systemic infections because it is not absorbed significantly.

● **UNLICENSED USE** Not licensed for surgical prophylaxis.

● **INTERACTIONS** → Appendix 1: teicoplanin

● **SIDE-EFFECTS**

GENERAL SIDE-EFFECTS
▶ **Common or very common** Fever · pain · skin reactions
▶ **Uncommon** Bronchospasm · diarrhoea · dizziness · eosinophilia · headache · hearing impairment · hypersensitivity · leucopenia · nausea · ototoxicity · thrombocytopenia · vomiting
▶ **Rare or very rare** Abscess
▶ **Frequency not known** Agranulocytosis · angioedema · chills · increased risk of infection · nephrotoxicity · neutropenia · pancytopenia · renal impairment · seizure · severe cutaneous adverse reactions (SCARs) · thrombophlebitis

SPECIFIC SIDE-EFFECTS
▶ **Rare or very rare**
▸ With parenteral use Vancomycin-like infusion reaction

SIDE-EFFECTS, FURTHER INFORMATION Teicoplanin is associated with a lower incidence of nephrotoxicity than vancomycin.

● **ALLERGY AND CROSS-SENSITIVITY** EvGr Caution if history of vancomycin sensitivity. (M)

● **PREGNANCY** Manufacturer advises use only if potential benefit outweighs risk.

● **BREAST FEEDING** Specialist sources indicate probably compatible (limited information available). High plasma-protein binding suggests limited excretion into milk and poor oral bioavailability suggests limited absorption by the infant.

● **RENAL IMPAIRMENT** EvGr Monitor auditory and renal function regularly during treatment (increased risk of ototoxicity and nephrotoxicity). (M)

Dose adjustments See p. 16.
▸ With intramuscular use or intravenous use EvGr For children over 12 years of age, use normal dose regimen on days 1–4, then if creatinine clearance is: (M)
— 30–80 mL/minute, use half the normal maintenance dose (either give the normal maintenance dose every 2 days, or half the normal maintenance dose once daily);
— less than 30 mL/minute, use one-third of the normal maintenance dose (either give the normal maintenance dose every 3 days, or one-third of the normal maintenance dose once daily).

For children aged 12 years or under—consult local guidelines.

For target serum-teicoplanin trough concentrations—consult product literature or local guidelines.

● **MONITORING REQUIREMENTS**
▸ With intramuscular use or intravenous use EvGr Monitor serum-teicoplanin trough concentration at steady state after completion of loading dose and during maintenance treatment—consult product literature. (M)
▸ With intramuscular use or intravenous use EvGr Monitor auditory and renal function regularly during treatment, especially in patients receiving high loading doses or prolonged treatment (increased risk of ototoxicity and nephrotoxicity). Monitor complete blood counts periodically during treatment (risk of thrombocytopenia). (M)

● **DIRECTIONS FOR ADMINISTRATION**
▸ With intravenous use For *intermittent intravenous infusion*, reconstitute with Water for Injections provided and dilute further in a compatible diluent; give over 30 minutes.
▸ With oral use Injection can be used to prepare solution for *oral* administration.

● **PRESCRIBING AND DISPENSING INFORMATION** For choice of antibacterial therapy, see Antibacterials, use for prophylaxis p. 359, Cardiovascular system infections, antibacterial therapy p. 364, Gastro-intestinal system infections, antibacterial therapy p. 367, Musculoskeletal system infections, antibacterial therapy p. 369, Respiratory system infections, antibacterial therapy p. 371, Skin infections, antibacterial therapy p. 373, Urinary-tract infections p. 454.

● **MEDICINAL FORMS** There can be variation in the licensing of different medicines containing the same drug. Forms available from special-order manufacturers include: solution for injection

Powder for solution for injection

ELECTROLYTES: May contain Sodium

▸ **Teicoplanin (Non-proprietary)**

Teicoplanin 200 mg Teicoplanin 200mg powder for solution for injection vials | 1 vial PoM £4.42–£5.30 (Hospital only) | 1 vial PoM £3.93–£4.42

Teicoplanin 400 mg Teicoplanin 400mg powder for solution for injection vials | 1 vial PoM £7.57–£9.00 (Hospital only) | 1 vial PoM £7.32–£8.21

Powder and solvent for solution for injection

ELECTROLYTES: May contain Sodium

▸ **Teicoplanin (Non-proprietary)**

Teicoplanin 200 mg Teicoplanin 200mg powder and solvent for solution for injection vials | 1 vial PoM £5.04 DT = £4.42 (Hospital only) | 1 vial PoM £5.34 DT = £4.42

Teicoplanin 400 mg Teicoplanin 400mg powder and solvent for solution for injection vials | 1 vial PoM £8.58 DT = £8.21 (Hospital only) | 1 vial PoM £9.08 DT = £8.21

▸ **Targocid** (Sanofi)

Teicoplanin 200 mg Targocid 200mg powder and solvent for solution for injection vials | 1 vial PoM £4.42 DT = £4.42

Teicoplanin 400 mg Targocid 400mg powder and solvent for solution for injection vials | 1 vial PoM £8.21 DT = £8.21

Vancomycin

09-Apr-2025

● **DRUG ACTION** The glycopeptide antibiotic vancomycin has bactericidal activity against aerobic and anaerobic Gram-positive bacteria including multi-resistant staphylococci. However, there are reports of *Staphylococcus aureus* with reduced susceptibility to glycopeptides. There are increasing reports of glycopeptide-resistant enterococci. Penetration into cerebrospinal fluid is poor.

● **INDICATIONS AND DOSE**

Neonatal Gram-positive bacterial infections | Late-onset neonatal sepsis

▸ BY INTRAVENOUS INFUSION

▸ Neonate up to 29 weeks corrected gestational age: 15 mg/kg every 24 hours, dose to be given over 60 minutes by intermittent intravenous infusion, dose to be adjusted according to serum-concentration monitoring, duration should be tailored to type and severity of infection and the individual clinical response—consult product literature for further information.

▸ Neonate 29 weeks to 35 weeks corrected gestational age: 15 mg/kg every 12 hours, dose to be given over 60 minutes by intermittent intravenous infusion, dose to be adjusted according to serum-concentration monitoring, duration should be tailored to type and severity of infection and the individual clinical response—consult product literature for further information.

▸ Neonate 35 weeks corrected gestational age and above: 15 mg/kg every 8 hours, dose to be given over 60 minutes by intermittent intravenous infusion, dose to be adjusted according to serum-concentration monitoring, duration should be tailored to type and severity of infection and the individual clinical response—consult product literature for further information.

Neonatal Gram-positive bacterial infections and serum creatinine < 40 micromol/litre | Late-onset neonatal sepsis and serum creatinine < 40 micromol/litre

▸ BY CONTINUOUS INTRAVENOUS INFUSION

▸ Neonate up to 40 weeks corrected gestational age: Loading dose 15 mg/kg for 1 dose, dose to be given over 60 minutes by intravenous infusion, followed by 40 mg/kg/24 hours, dose to be adjusted according to serum-concentration monitoring.

▸ Neonate 40 weeks corrected gestational age and above: Loading dose 15 mg/kg for 1 dose, dose to be given over 60 minutes by intravenous infusion, followed by 50 mg/kg/24 hours, dose to be adjusted according to serum-concentration monitoring.

Neonatal Gram-positive bacterial infections and serum creatinine 40-59 micromol/litre | Late-onset neonatal sepsis and serum creatinine 40-59 micromol/litre

▸ BY CONTINUOUS INTRAVENOUS INFUSION

▸ Neonate: Loading dose 15 mg/kg for 1 dose, dose to be given over 60 minutes by intravenous infusion, followed by 30 mg/kg/24 hours, dose to be adjusted according to serum-concentration monitoring.

Neonatal Gram-positive bacterial infections and serum creatinine ≥ 60 micromol/litre | Late-onset neonatal sepsis and serum creatinine ≥ 60 micromol/litre

▸ BY CONTINUOUS INTRAVENOUS INFUSION

▸ Neonate: Loading dose 15 mg/kg for 1 dose, dose to be given over 60 minutes by intravenous infusion, followed by 20 mg/kg/24 hours, dose to be adjusted according to serum-concentration monitoring.

***Clostridioides difficile* infection**

▸ BY MOUTH

▸ Neonate: 10 mg/kg every 6 hours for 10 days.

▸ Child 1 month–11 years: 10 mg/kg every 6 hours (max. per dose 500 mg) for 10 days

▸ Child 12-17 years: 125 mg every 6 hours for 10 days; increased if necessary to 500 mg every 6 hours for 10 days, increased dose to be used if life-threatening or refractory infection

Cellulitis | Erysipelas

▸ BY INTRAVENOUS INFUSION

▸ Child 1 month–11 years: 10–15 mg/kg every 6 hours, dose to be adjusted according to serum-concentration monitoring

▸ Child 12-17 years: 15–20 mg/kg every 8–12 hours (max. per dose 2 g), dose to be adjusted according to serum-concentration monitoring

Complicated skin and soft tissue infections | Bone infections | Joint infections | Community-acquired pneumonia | Hospital-acquired pneumonia [including ventilator-associated pneumonia] | Infective endocarditis | Acute bacterial meningitis | Bacteraemia [occurring in association with or suspected to be associated with the licensed indications]

▸ BY INTRAVENOUS INFUSION

▸ Child 1 month–11 years: 10–15 mg/kg every 6 hours, dose to be adjusted according to serum-concentration monitoring, duration should be tailored to type and severity of infection and the individual clinical response—consult product literature for further information, doses higher than 60 mg/kg/day cannot be generally recommended as the safety of increased dosing has not been fully assessed

▸ Child 12-17 years: 15–20 mg/kg every 8–12 hours (max. per dose 2 g), dose to be adjusted according to serum-concentration monitoring, duration should be tailored to type and severity of infection and the individual clinical response—consult product literature for further information, in seriously ill patients, a loading dose of 25–30 mg/kg (usual max. 2 g) can be used to facilitate rapid attainment of the target trough serum-vancomycin concentration

Perioperative prophylaxis of bacterial endocarditis [in patients at high risk of developing bacterial endocarditis when undergoing major surgical procedures]

▸ BY INTRAVENOUS INFUSION

▸ Neonate: 15 mg/kg for 1 dose, to be given prior to induction of anaesthesia, a second dose may be required depending on duration of surgery.

▸ Child: 15 mg/kg for 1 dose, to be given prior to induction of anaesthesia, a second dose may be required depending on duration of surgery

Surgical prophylaxis (when high risk of MRSA)

▸ BY INTRAVENOUS INFUSION

▸ Child: (consult local protocol)

CNS infection e.g. ventriculitis (administered on expert advice)

▶ BY INTRAVENTRICULAR ADMINISTRATION

▸ Neonate: 10 mg every 24 hours.

▸ Child: 10 mg every 24 hours, for all children reduce to 5 mg once daily if ventricular size reduced or increase to 15–20 mg once daily if ventricular size increased, adjust dose according to CSF concentration after 3–4 days; aim for pre-dose ('trough') concentration less than 10 mg/litre. If CSF not draining free reduce dose frequency to once every 2–3 days

Peritonitis associated with peritoneal dialysis

▶ BY INTRAPERITONEAL ADMINISTRATION

▸ Child: Add to each bag of dialysis fluid to achieve a concentration of 20–25 mg/litre

Eradication of meticillin-resistant *Staphylococcus aureus* from the respiratory tract in cystic fibrosis

▶ BY INHALATION OF NEBULISED SOLUTION

▸ Child: 4 mg/kg twice daily (max. per dose 250 mg) for 5 days, alternatively 4 mg/kg 4 times a day (max. per dose 250 mg) for 5 days

DOSE EQUIVALENCE AND CONVERSION

▸ With intravenous use in neonates EvGr When switching from intermittent to continuous infusion, the loading dose may be omitted or reduced, depending on the time since the last intermittent dose and serum-vancomycin concentration ⟨E⟩—consult local protocol or seek specialist advice. EvGr When switching from continuous to intermittent infusion, the continuous infusion may be stopped and the first intermittent dose given when the serum-vancomycin concentration is within the target trough concentration range for intermittent dosing ⟨E⟩—consult local protocol or seek specialist advice.

PHARMACOKINETICS

▸ With oral use Vancomycin should **not** be given by mouth for systemic infections because it is not absorbed significantly.

● UNLICENSED USE Vancomycin doses in BNF Publications may differ from those in product literature. Use of vancomycin (added to dialysis fluid) for the treatment of peritonitis associated with peritoneal dialysis is an unlicensed route. Not licensed for intraventricular use or inhalation.

EvGr Vancomycin is used for the treatment of late-onset neonatal sepsis ⟨E⟩, but is not licensed for this indication.

● CONTRA-INDICATIONS

▸ With intravenous use Previous hearing loss

● CAUTIONS

▸ With intravenous use Premature neonates (monitor serum-concentration carefully) · young infants (monitor serum-concentration carefully)

▸ With oral use Systemic absorption may be enhanced in patients with inflammatory disorders of the intestinal mucosa or with *Clostridioides difficile*-induced pseudomembranous colitis (increased risk of adverse reactions)

● INTERACTIONS → Appendix 1: vancomycin

● SIDE-EFFECTS

GENERAL SIDE-EFFECTS Agranulocytosis · dizziness · drug fever · eosinophilia · hypersensitivity · nausea · nephritis tubulointerstitial · neutropenia (more common after 1 week or cumulative dose of 25g) · renal failure · severe cutaneous adverse reactions (SCARs) · skin reactions · thrombocytopenia · tinnitus (discontinue) · vasculitis · vertigo

SPECIFIC SIDE-EFFECTS

▶ **Common or very common**

▸ With intravenous use Vancomycin infusion reaction

▶ **Rare or very rare**

▸ With intravenous use Pseudomembranous enterocolitis

▶ **Frequency not known**

▸ With intravenous use Back pain · bradycardia · cardiac arrest (on rapid intravenous injection) · cardiogenic shock (on rapid intravenous injection) · chest pain · diarrhoea · dyspnoea · hearing loss · hypotension · muscle complaints · wheezing

SIDE-EFFECTS, FURTHER INFORMATION Vancomycin is associated with a higher incidence of nephrotoxicity than teicoplanin.

● ALLERGY AND CROSS-SENSITIVITY EvGr Caution if teicoplanin sensitivity. ⟨M⟩

● PREGNANCY Manufacturer advises use only if potential benefit outweighs risk.

Monitoring Serum-vancomycin concentration monitoring essential to reduce risk of fetal toxicity.

● BREAST FEEDING Present in milk—significant absorption following oral administration unlikely.

● RENAL IMPAIRMENT Manufacturer advises serial monitoring of renal function.

▸ With intravenous use Manufacturer advises use with caution—increased risk of toxic effects with prolonged high blood concentration, see also *Monitoring requirements*.

Dose adjustments

▸ With oral use Manufacturer advises dose adjustment is unlikely to be required unless substantial oral absorption occurs in inflammatory disorders of the intestinal mucosa or with *Clostridioides difficile*-induced pseudomembranous colitis, see *Monitoring requirements*.

▸ With intravenous use Manufacturer advises initial dose must not be reduced—consult product literature.

● MONITORING REQUIREMENTS

▸ With intravenous use For *intermittent* intravenous infusion, the manufacturer advises initial doses should be based on body-weight; subsequent dose adjustments should be based on serum-vancomycin concentrations to achieve targeted therapeutic concentrations. All patients require serum-vancomycin measurement (on the second day of treatment, immediately before the next dose if renal function is normal or earlier if renally impaired—consult product literature). Frequency of monitoring depends on the clinical situation and response to treatment; regular monitoring is indicated in high-dose therapy and longer-term use, particularly in patients with impaired renal function, impaired hearing, or concurrent use of nephrotoxic or ototoxic drugs. Manufacturer advises pre-dose ('trough') concentration should normally be 10–20 mg/litre depending on the site of infection and the susceptibility of the pathogen; trough concentration of 15–20 mg/litre is usually recommended to cover susceptible pathogens with MIC greater than or equal to 1 mg/litre—consult product literature.

Manufacturer advises periodic testing of auditory function. Manufacturer advises monitor blood counts, urinalysis, hepatic and renal function periodically in all patients; monitor leucocyte count regularly in patients receiving long-term vancomycin or if given concurrently with other drugs that may cause neutropenia or agranulocytosis.

▸ With intravenous use in neonates For *intermittent* intravenous infusion, the manufacturer advises initial doses should be based on post-menstrual age (corrected gestational age) and body-weight; subsequent dose adjustments should be based on serum-vancomycin concentrations to achieve targeted therapeutic concentrations. All patients require serum-vancomycin measurement (on the second day of treatment, immediately before the next dose if renal function is normal or earlier if renally impaired—consult product literature). Frequency of monitoring depends on the clinical situation and response to treatment; regular monitoring is indicated in high-dose therapy and longer-term use, particularly in patients with impaired renal function, impaired hearing, or concurrent use of nephrotoxic or ototoxic drugs. Manufacturer advises pre-dose ('trough') concentration should normally be 10–20 mg/litre depending on the site of infection and the susceptibility of the pathogen; trough concentration of 15–20 mg/litre is usually recommended to cover susceptible pathogens with MIC greater than or equal to 1 mg/litre—consult product literature. EvGr For *continuous* intravenous infusion, the target steady-state serum-vancomycin concentration is 15–25 mg/litre. Measure the serum-vancomycin concentration 24 and 48 hours after starting the infusion, **and** after each dose change, noting that steady-state may not have been achieved within 24 hours of starting the infusion or adjusting the dose. Thereafter if the serum concentration is within the target range, it should be remeasured every 3 days. Monitor more frequently if clinically unstable or if there is a change in body-weight, impaired renal function, impaired hearing, or concurrent use of nephrotoxic or ototoxic drugs. ⟨E⟩ Serum-vancomycin concentrations generally increase proportionally with increasing dose; EvGr dose adjustments may be calculated as follows (dose adjustments should be based on steady-state concentrations): ⟨E⟩

$$\text{New continuous infusion dose (mg/kg/24 hours)} = \frac{\text{Previous dose (mg/kg/24 hours)} \times 20\ \text{mg/litre}}{\text{Current vancomycin concentration (mg/litre)}}$$

- With oral use Manufacturer advises monitoring serum-vancomycin concentration in inflammatory intestinal disorders.

  Manufacturer advises serial tests of auditory function may be helpful to minimise the risk of ototoxicity in patients with an underlying hearing loss, or who are receiving concomitant therapy with other ototoxic drugs.
- With intraventricular use Aim for pre-dose ('trough') concentration less than 10 mg/litre.
- When used by inhalation Measure lung function before and after initial dose of vancomycin and monitor for bronchospasm.

● DIRECTIONS FOR ADMINISTRATION

- With intravenous use Avoid rapid infusion (risk of anaphylactoid reactions) and rotate infusion sites. Displacement value may be significant—consult product literature and local guidelines.

  For *intermittent intravenous infusion*, the reconstituted preparation should be further diluted in Sodium Chloride 0.9% *or* Glucose 5% *or* another compatible diluent to a concentration of up to 5 mg/mL (10 mg/mL can be used if fluid restricted and if infused via a central venous catheter, but increased risk of infusion-related effects); give over at least 60 minutes (rate not to exceed 10 mg/minute for doses over 500 mg); use continuous infusion only if intermittent not available (limited evidence—consult product literature).
- With intravenous use in neonates For *intermittent intravenous infusion*, the reconstituted preparation should be further diluted in Sodium Chloride 0.9% *or* Glucose 5% *or* another compatible diluent to a concentration of up to 5 mg/mL (10 mg/mL can be used if fluid restricted and if infused via a central venous catheter, but increased risk of infusion-related effects); give over at least 60 minutes. For *continuous intravenous infusion*, the reconstituted preparation should be further diluted in Sodium Chloride 0.9% *or* Glucose 5% *or* another compatible diluent to a concentration of up to 5 mg/mL (10 mg/mL can be used if fluid restricted and if infused via a central venous catheter, but increased risk of infusion-related effects); the loading dose should be given over 60 minutes.
- With oral use Injection can be used to prepare solution for *oral* administration—consult product literature.
- When used by inhalation For *nebulisation*, administer required dose in 4 mL of Sodium Chloride 0.9% (or Water for Injections). Administer inhaled bronchodilator before vancomycin.

● PRESCRIBING AND DISPENSING INFORMATION For choice of antibacterial therapy, see Antibacterials, use for prophylaxis p. 359, Cardiovascular system infections, antibacterial therapy p. 364, Central nervous system infections, antibacterial therapy p. 365, Gastro-intestinal system infections, antibacterial therapy p. 367, Musculoskeletal system infections, antibacterial therapy p. 369, Respiratory system infections, antibacterial therapy p. 371, Skin infections, antibacterial therapy p. 373.

● MEDICINAL FORMS There can be variation in the licensing of different medicines containing the same drug. Forms available from special-order manufacturers include: oral suspension, oral solution, solution for injection, infusion

Oral capsule

CAUTIONARY AND ADVISORY LABELS 9

- Vancomycin (Non-proprietary)
  - **Vancomycin (as Vancomycin hydrochloride) 125 mg** Vancomycin 125mg capsules | 28 capsule PoM £132.49 DT = £83.32
  - **Vancomycin (as Vancomycin hydrochloride) 250 mg** Vancomycin 250mg capsules | 28 capsule PoM £131.75 DT = £131.74

Powder for solution for infusion

- Vancomycin (Non-proprietary)
  - **Vancomycin (as Vancomycin hydrochloride) 500 mg** Vancomycin 500mg powder for solution for infusion vials | 10 vial PoM £100.50 Vancomycin 500mg powder for concentrate for solution for infusion vials | 1 vial PoM £10.05 | 1 vial PoM £5.49–£14.47 (Hospital only) | 5 vial PoM £50.25 | 10 vial PoM £100.05 (Hospital only) | 10 vial PoM £100.05
  - **Vancomycin (as Vancomycin hydrochloride) 1 gram** Vancomycin 1g powder for solution for infusion vials | 5 vial PoM ⊠ (Hospital only)
    Vancomycin 1g powder for concentrate for solution for infusion vials | 1 vial PoM £17.25 | 1 vial PoM £11.25 (Hospital only) | 5 vial PoM £86.25 | 10 vial PoM £150.00–£172.50 (Hospital only) | 10 vial PoM £172.50

ANTIBACTERIALS › LINCOSAMIDES

Clindamycin

22-Mar-2024

● DRUG ACTION Clindamycin is active against Gram-positive cocci, including streptococci and penicillin-resistant staphylococci, and also against many anaerobes, especially *Bacteroides fragilis*. It is well concentrated in bone and excreted in bile and urine.

● INDICATIONS AND DOSE

Staphylococcal bone and joint infections such as osteomyelitis | Peritonitis | Intra-abdominal sepsis | Meticillin-resistant *Staphylococcus aureus* (MRSA) in bronchiectasis, bone and joint infections, and skin and soft-tissue infections

▶ BY MOUTH

- Neonate up to 14 days: 3–6 mg/kg 3 times a day.
- Neonate 14 days to 28 days: 3–6 mg/kg 4 times a day.
- Child: 3–6 mg/kg 4 times a day (max. per dose 450 mg)

▶ BY INTRAMUSCULAR INJECTION, OR BY INTRAVENOUS INFUSION

- Child 1 month–11 years: 3.75–6.25 mg/kg 4 times a day, dose can be increased if necessary up to 10 mg/kg 4 times a day (minimum dose regardless of body-weight is 75 mg 4 times a day) for severe infections; total daily dose may alternatively be given in 3 divided doses, single doses above 600 mg to be administered by intravenous infusion only

- Child 12–17 years: 3.75–6.25 mg/kg 4 times a day, dose can be increased if necessary up to 10 mg/kg 4 times a day (maximum dose is 1.2 g 4 times a day) for severe infections; total daily dose may alternatively be given in 3 divided doses, single doses above 600 mg to be administered by intravenous infusion only, single doses by intravenous infusion not to exceed 1.2 g

Cellulitis | Erysipelas

- BY MOUTH
- Child: 3–6 mg/kg 4 times a day (max. per dose 450 mg) for 7 days then review
- BY INTRAVENOUS INFUSION
- Child 1 month–11 years: 3.75–6.25 mg/kg 4 times a day, dose can be increased if necessary up to 10 mg/kg 4 times a day (minimum dose regardless of body-weight is 75 mg 4 times a day) in life-threatening infection; total daily dose may alternatively be given in 3 divided doses
- Child 12–17 years: 3.75–6.25 mg/kg 4 times a day, dose can be increased if necessary up to 10 mg/kg 4 times a day (maximum dose is 1.2 g 4 times a day) in life-threatening infection; total daily dose may alternatively be given in 3 divided doses, single doses not to exceed 1.2 g

Staphylococcal lung infection in cystic fibrosis

- BY MOUTH
- Child: 5–7 mg/kg 4 times a day (max. per dose 600 mg)

Treatment of falciparum malaria (to be given with or following quinine)

- BY MOUTH
- Child: 7–13 mg/kg every 8 hours (max. per dose 450 mg) for 7 days

- **UNLICENSED USE** Not licensed for treatment of falciparum malaria.
- **CONTRA-INDICATIONS** Avoid injections containing benzyl alcohol in neonates · diarrhoeal states
- **CAUTIONS** Avoid in Acute porphyrias p. 745
- **INTERACTIONS** → Appendix 1: clindamycin
- **SIDE-EFFECTS**

GENERAL SIDE-EFFECTS

- **Common or very common** Abdominal pain · diarrhoea (discontinue) · pseudomembranous enterocolitis · skin reactions
- **Uncommon** Nausea · vomiting
- **Frequency not known** Agranulocytosis · Clostridioides difficile colitis · eosinophilia · jaundice · leucopenia · neutropenia · severe cutaneous adverse reactions (SCARs) · taste altered · thrombocytopenia

SPECIFIC SIDE-EFFECTS

- **Frequency not known**
- With oral use Angioedema · gastrointestinal disorders · vulvovaginal infection
- With parenteral use Cardiac arrest · colitis · hypotension · increased risk of infection · thrombophlebitis

SIDE-EFFECTS, FURTHER INFORMATION Clindamycin has been associated with antibiotic-associated colitis, which may be fatal. Although antibiotic-associated colitis can occur with most antibacterials, it occurs more frequently with clindamycin. If *C. difficile* infection is suspected or confirmed, discontinue the antibiotic if appropriate. Seek specialist advice if the antibiotic cannot be stopped and the diarrhoea is severe.

- **PREGNANCY** Manufacturer advises not known to be harmful in the second and third trimesters; use with caution in the first trimester—limited data.
- **BREAST FEEDING** EvGr Specialist sources indicate use with caution—present in milk. Monitor infant for effects on the gastrointestinal flora such as diarrhoea, candidiasis, or rarely, blood in the stool indicating possible antibiotic-associated colitis. ⟨D⟩
- **MONITORING REQUIREMENTS**
  - Monitor liver and renal function if treatment exceeds 10 days.
  - Monitor liver and renal function in neonates and infants.
- **DIRECTIONS FOR ADMINISTRATION** Avoid rapid intravenous administration. For *intravenous infusion*, manufacturer advises dilute to a concentration of not more than 18 mg/mL with Glucose 5% *or* Sodium Chloride 0.9%. Expert sources advise give over 10–60 minutes at a max. rate of 20 mg/kg/hour.
- **PRESCRIBING AND DISPENSING INFORMATION** For choice of antibacterial therapy, see Gastro-intestinal system infections, antibacterial therapy p. 367, Malaria, treatment p. 482, Musculoskeletal system infections, antibacterial therapy p. 369, Respiratory system infections, antibacterial therapy p. 371, Skin infections, antibacterial therapy p. 373.
- **PATIENT AND CARER ADVICE** Patients and their carers should be advised to discontinue and contact a doctor immediately if severe, prolonged or bloody diarrhoea develops.

  Capsules should be swallowed with a glass of water.
- **PROFESSION SPECIFIC INFORMATION**

Dental practitioners' formulary Clindamycin capsules may be prescribed.

- **MEDICINAL FORMS** There can be variation in the licensing of different medicines containing the same drug. Forms available from special-order manufacturers include: oral suspension, oral solution

Solution for injection

EXCIPIENTS: May contain Benzyl alcohol

- Clindamycin (Non-proprietary)
  Clindamycin (as Clindamycin phosphate) 150 mg per 1 ml Clindamycin 600mg/4ml solution for injection ampoules | 5 ampoule PoM £61.75 (Hospital only) | 10 ampoule PoM £100.00 (Hospital only)
  Clindamycin 300mg/2ml solution for injection ampoules | 5 ampoule PoM £31.01 (Hospital only) | 10 ampoule PoM £55.00 (Hospital only)
- Dalacin C (Pfizer Ltd)
  Clindamycin (as Clindamycin phosphate) 150 mg per 1 ml Dalacin C Phosphate 300mg/2ml solution for injection ampoules | 5 ampoule PoM £31.01 (Hospital only)
  Dalacin C Phosphate 600mg/4ml solution for injection ampoules | 5 ampoule PoM £61.75 (Hospital only)

Oral capsule

CAUTIONARY AND ADVISORY LABELS 9, 27

- Clindamycin (Non-proprietary)
  Clindamycin (as Clindamycin hydrochloride) 75 mg Clindamycin 75mg capsules | 24 capsule PoM £7.45 DT = £7.45
  Clindamycin (as Clindamycin hydrochloride) 150 mg Clindamycin 150mg capsules | 24 capsule PoM £13.72 DT = £2.27 | 100 capsule PoM £8.83–£55.08
  Clindamycin (as Clindamycin hydrochloride) 300 mg Clindamycin 300mg capsules | 30 capsule PoM £42.00 DT = £6.58
- Dalacin C (Pfizer Ltd)
  Clindamycin (as Clindamycin hydrochloride) 75 mg Dalacin C 75mg capsules | 24 capsule PoM £7.45 DT = £7.45
  Clindamycin (as Clindamycin hydrochloride) 150 mg Dalacin C 150mg capsules | 24 capsule PoM £13.72 DT = £2.27 | 100 capsule PoM £55.08

ANTIBACTERIALS > MACROLIDES

Macrolides

12-Nov-2025

Overview

The macrolides have an antibacterial spectrum that is similar but not identical to that of penicillin; they are thus an alternative in penicillin-allergic patients. They are active against many-penicillin-resistant staphylococci, but some are now also resistant to the macrolides.

Indications for the macrolides include campylobacter enteritis, respiratory infections (including pneumonia, whooping cough, Legionella, chlamydia, and mycoplasma infection), and skin infections.

Erythromycin p. 406 may be used in the treatment of early syphilis, and uncomplicated genital chlamydial infection. Erythromycin has poor activity against *Haemophilus influenzae*. Erythromycin causes nausea, vomiting, and diarrhoea in some patients; in mild to moderate infections this can be avoided by giving a lower dose or the total dose in 4 divided doses, but if a more serious infection, such as Legionella pneumonia, is suspected higher doses are needed.

Azithromycin below is a macrolide with slightly less activity than erythromycin against Gram-positive bacteria, but enhanced activity against some Gram-negative organisms including *H. influenzae*. Plasma concentrations are very low, but tissue concentrations are much higher. It has a long tissue half-life and once daily dosage is recommended. Azithromycin is also used in the treatment of uncomplicated genital chlamydial infection, non-gonococcal urethritis, uncomplicated gonorrhoea, typhoid [unlicensed indication], trachoma [unlicensed indication], and Lyme disease [unlicensed indication].

Clarithromycin p. 403 is an erythromycin derivative with slightly greater activity than the parent compound. Tissue concentrations are higher than with erythromycin. Clarithromycin is also used in regimens for *Helicobacter pylori* eradication.

Spiramycin is also a macrolide which is used for the treatment of toxoplasmosis.

Macrolides

● **CAUTIONS**

- With intravenous use or oral use Electrolyte disturbances (predisposition to QT interval prolongation) · may aggravate myasthenia gravis · predisposition to QT interval prolongation

● **SIDE-EFFECTS**

- **Common or very common** Appetite decreased · diarrhoea · dizziness · gastrointestinal discomfort · gastrointestinal disorders · headache · hearing impairment · insomnia · nausea · pancreatitis · paraesthesia · skin reactions · taste altered · vasodilation · vision disorders · vomiting
- **Uncommon** Angioedema · anxiety · arrhythmias · candida infection · chest pain · constipation · drowsiness · eosinophilia · hepatic disorders · leucopenia · neutropenia · palpitations · QT interval prolongation · severe cutaneous adverse reactions (SCARs) · tinnitus · vertigo
- **Rare or very rare** Infantile hypertrophic pyloric stenosis · myasthenia gravis · nephritis tubulointerstitial · pseudomembranous enterocolitis
- **Frequency not known** Clostridioides difficile colitis · hallucination · hypotension · seizure · smell altered · thrombocytopenia · tongue discolouration

● **PATIENT AND CARER ADVICE**

- With systemic use Parents and carers should be advised to seek medical attention if vomiting or irritability with feeding occurs, due to the risk of infantile hypertrophic pyloric stenosis.

above

Azithromycin

26-Nov-2025

● **INDICATIONS AND DOSE**

Mild diphtheria [confirmed or probable]

▶ BY MOUTH

- Child 6 months–11 years: 12 mg/kg once daily (max. per dose 500 mg) for 7–10 days
- Child 12–17 years: 500 mg once daily for 7–10 days

Prevention of secondary case of diphtheria

▶ BY MOUTH

- Child 6 months–11 years: 12 mg/kg once daily (max. per dose 500 mg) for 6 days
- Child 12–17 years: 500 mg once daily for 6 days

Prevention of secondary case of *Haemophilus influenzae* type b disease

▶ BY MOUTH

- Child: 10 mg/kg once daily (max. per dose 500 mg) for 3 days

Prevention of secondary case of invasive group A streptococcal infection in patients who are allergic to penicillin

▶ BY MOUTH

- Child 6 months–11 years: 12 mg/kg once daily (max. per dose 500 mg) for 5 days
- Child 12–17 years: 500 mg once daily for 5 days

Respiratory-tract infections, otitis media, skin and soft-tissue infections

▶ BY MOUTH

- Child 6 months–17 years (body-weight up to 15 kg): 10 mg/kg once daily for 3 days
- Child 6 months–17 years (body-weight 15–25 kg): 10 mg/kg once daily for 3 days, alternatively 200 mg once daily for 3 days
- Child 6 months–17 years (body-weight 26–35 kg): 10 mg/kg once daily for 3 days, alternatively 300 mg once daily for 3 days
- Child 6 months–17 years (body-weight 36–45 kg): 10 mg/kg once daily for 3 days, alternatively 400 mg once daily for 3 days
- Child 6 months–17 years (body-weight 46 kg and above): 500 mg once daily for 3 days

Infection in cystic fibrosis

▶ BY MOUTH

- Child 6 months–17 years: 10 mg/kg once daily (max. per dose 500 mg) for 3 days, repeated after 1 week to complete course, treatment may be repeated as necessary

Chronic *Pseudomonas aeruginosa* infection in cystic fibrosis

▶ BY MOUTH

- Child 6–17 years (body-weight 25–40 kg): 250 mg 3 times a week
- Child 6–17 years (body-weight 41 kg and above): 500 mg 3 times a week

Uncomplicated genital chlamydia | Uncomplicated non-gonococcal urethritis

▶ BY MOUTH

- Child 12–17 years (body-weight 45 kg and above): 1 g once daily for 1 day, then 500 mg once daily for 2 days

Uncomplicated gonorrhoea [anogenital and pharyngeal infection]

▶ BY MOUTH

- Child 12–17 years (body-weight 45 kg and above): 2 g for 1 dose, alternatively 1 g for 2 doses, the second dose to be given 6–12 hours after the first dose, 2-dose regimen may be given to reduce gastro-intestinal side-effects

Lyme disease [erythema migrans and/or non-focal symptoms]

▶ BY MOUTH

- Child 1 month–11 years (administered on expert advice) (body-weight up to 50 kg): 10 mg/kg once daily for 17 days
- Child 1 month–11 years (administered on expert advice) (body-weight 50 kg and above): 500 mg once daily for 17 days
- Child 12–17 years (administered on expert advice): 500 mg once daily for 17 days

Mild to moderate typhoid due to multiple-antibacterial resistant organisms

▶ BY MOUTH

- Child 6 months–17 years: 10 mg/kg once daily (max. per dose 500 mg) for 7 days

● **UNLICENSED USE** UKHSA advises azithromycin may be used as detailed below, although these situations are considered outside the scope of its licence:
- treatment and prevention of diphtheria;
- prevention of secondary cases of *Haemophilus influenzae* type b disease;
- prevention of secondary cases of invasive group A streptococcal infection.

Azithromycin may be used as detailed below, although these situations are considered outside the scope of its licence:
- chronic *Pseudomonas aeruginosa* infection in cystic fibrosis;
- EvGr dose for uncomplicated genital chlamydia;
- uncomplicated non-gonococcal urethritis;
- 2-dose regimen for uncomplicated gonorrhoea;
- Lyme disease; (A)
- mild to moderate typhoid due to multiple-antibacterial resistant organisms.

● **INTERACTIONS** → Appendix 1: macrolides

● **SIDE-EFFECTS**
- ▶ **Common or very common** Arthralgia
- ▶ **Uncommon** Numbness · oedema · photosensitivity reaction
- ▶ **Frequency not known** Acute kidney injury · aggression · akathisia · haemolytic anaemia · syncope

● **PREGNANCY** Manufacturers advise use only if adequate alternatives not available.

● **BREAST FEEDING** Present in milk; use only if no suitable alternatives.

● **HEPATIC IMPAIRMENT** Manufacturer advises caution; consider avoiding in severe impairment (no information available).

● **RENAL IMPAIRMENT** See p. 16.
EvGr Use with caution if estimated glomerular filtration rate less than 10 mL/minute/1.73 m^2. (M)

● **PRESCRIBING AND DISPENSING INFORMATION** For choice of antibacterial therapy, see Antibacterials, use for prophylaxis p. 359, Ear infections, antibacterial therapy p. 366, Genital system infections, antibacterial therapy p. 368, Lyme disease p. 444, Respiratory system infections, antibacterial therapy p. 371, Skin infections, antibacterial therapy p. 373.

● **PATIENT AND CARER ADVICE**
Medicines for Children leaflet: Azithromycin for bacterial infection www.medicinesforchildren.org.uk/medicines/azithromycin-for-bacterial-infection/

● **PROFESSION SPECIFIC INFORMATION**
Dental practitioners' formulary Azithromycin Capsules may be prescribed. Azithromycin Tablets may be prescribed. Azithromycin Oral Suspension 200 mg/5 mL may be prescribed.

● **MEDICINAL FORMS** There can be variation in the licensing of different medicines containing the same drug. Forms available from special-order manufacturers include: oral suspension

Oral tablet

CAUTIONARY AND ADVISORY LABELS 5, 9

▶ **Azithromycin (Non-proprietary)**
Azithromycin 250 mg Azithromycin 250mg tablets | 4 tablet PoM £1.49 DT = £0.69 | 6 tablet PoM £1.04–£2.24
Azithromycin 500 mg Azithromycin 500mg tablets | 3 tablet PoM £1.29 DT = £0.78

Oral suspension

CAUTIONARY AND ADVISORY LABELS 5, 9

▶ **Azithromycin (Non-proprietary)**
Azithromycin 40 mg per 1 ml Azithromycin 200mg/5ml oral suspension | 15 ml PoM £6.18 DT = £4.06 | 30 ml PoM £19.88 DT = £11.04

▶ **Zithromax** (Pfizer Ltd)
Azithromycin 40 mg per 1 ml Zithromax 200mg/5ml oral suspension | 15 ml PoM £4.06 DT = £4.06 | 22.5 ml PoM £6.10 DT = £6.10 | 30 ml PoM £11.04 DT = £11.04

Oral capsule

CAUTIONARY AND ADVISORY LABELS 5, 9, 23

▶ **Azithromycin (Non-proprietary)**
Azithromycin (as Azithromycin dihydrate) 250 mg Azithromycin 250mg capsules | 4 capsule PoM £0.82–£3.58 | 6 capsule PoM £4.97 DT = £1.32

▶ **Zithromax** (Pfizer Ltd)
Azithromycin (as Azithromycin dihydrate) 250 mg Zithromax 250mg capsules | 4 capsule PoM £7.16 | 6 capsule PoM £10.74 DT = £1.32

F 402

Clarithromycin

16-Jan-2026

● **INDICATIONS AND DOSE**

Cellulitis | Erysipelas

▶ BY MOUTH USING IMMEDIATE-RELEASE MEDICINES

- Child 1 month–11 years (body-weight up to 8 kg): 7.5 mg/kg twice daily for 5–7 days then review (review after 7 days if infection near the eyes or nose)
- Child 1 month–11 years (body-weight 8–11 kg): 62.5 mg twice daily for 5–7 days then review (review after 7 days if infection near the eyes or nose)
- Child 1 month–11 years (body-weight 12–19 kg): 125 mg twice daily for 5–7 days then review (review after 7 days if infection near the eyes or nose)
- Child 1 month–11 years (body-weight 20–29 kg): 187.5 mg twice daily for 5–7 days then review (review after 7 days if infection near the eyes or nose)
- Child 1 month–11 years (body-weight 30–40 kg): 250 mg twice daily for 5–7 days then review (review after 7 days if infection near the eyes or nose)
- Child 12–17 years: 250–500 mg twice daily for 5–7 days then review (review after 7 days if infection near the eyes or nose)

▶ BY INTRAVENOUS INFUSION

- Child 1 month–11 years: 7.5 mg/kg every 12 hours (max. per dose 500 mg)
- Child 12–17 years: 500 mg every 12 hours

Impetigo | Secondary bacterial infection of eczema

▶ BY MOUTH USING IMMEDIATE-RELEASE MEDICINES

- Child 1 month–11 years (body-weight up to 8 kg): 7.5 mg/kg twice daily for 5–7 days
- Child 1 month–11 years (body-weight 8–11 kg): 62.5 mg twice daily for 5–7 days
- Child 1 month–11 years (body-weight 12–19 kg): 125 mg twice daily for 5–7 days
- Child 1 month–11 years (body-weight 20–29 kg): 187.5 mg twice daily for 5–7 days
- Child 1 month–11 years (body-weight 30–40 kg): 250 mg twice daily for 5–7 days
- Child 12–17 years: 250 mg twice daily for 5–7 days, alternatively 500 mg twice daily for 5–7 days, increased dose used in severe infections

continued →

Community-acquired pneumonia
- ▶ BY MOUTH USING IMMEDIATE-RELEASE MEDICINES
- ▸ Child 1–2 months (body-weight up to 8 kg): 7.5 mg/kg twice daily for 5 days
- ▸ Child 3 months–11 years (body-weight up to 8 kg): 7.5 mg/kg twice daily for 3 days (5 days in severe infection)
- ▸ Child 3 months–11 years (body-weight 8–11 kg): 62.5 mg twice daily for 3 days (5 days in severe infection)
- ▸ Child 3 months–11 years (body-weight 12–19 kg): 125 mg twice daily for 3 days (5 days in severe infection)
- ▸ Child 3 months–11 years (body-weight 20–29 kg): 187.5 mg twice daily for 3 days (5 days in severe infection)
- ▸ Child 3 months–11 years (body-weight 30–40 kg): 250 mg twice daily for 3 days (5 days in severe infection)
- ▸ Child 12–17 years: 250–500 mg twice daily for 5 days
- ▶ BY INTRAVENOUS INFUSION
- ▸ Child 1 month–11 years: 7.5 mg/kg every 12 hours (max. per dose 500 mg)
- ▸ Child 12–17 years: 500 mg every 12 hours

Hospital-acquired pneumonia
- ▶ BY MOUTH USING IMMEDIATE-RELEASE MEDICINES
- ▸ Child 1 month–11 years (body-weight up to 8 kg): 7.5 mg/kg twice daily for 5 days then review
- ▸ Child 1 month–11 years (body-weight 8–11 kg): 62.5 mg twice daily for 5 days then review
- ▸ Child 1 month–11 years (body-weight 12–19 kg): 125 mg twice daily for 5 days then review
- ▸ Child 1 month–11 years (body-weight 20–29 kg): 187.5 mg twice daily for 5 days then review
- ▸ Child 1 month–11 years (body-weight 30–40 kg): 250 mg twice daily for 5 days then review
- ▸ Child 12–17 years: 500 mg twice daily for 5 days then review

Respiratory-tract infections | Mild to moderate skin and soft-tissue infections
- ▶ BY MOUTH USING IMMEDIATE-RELEASE MEDICINES
- ▸ Neonate: 7.5 mg/kg twice daily.
- ▸ Child 1 month–11 years (body-weight up to 8 kg): 7.5 mg/kg twice daily
- ▸ Child 1 month–11 years (body-weight 8–11 kg): 62.5 mg twice daily
- ▸ Child 1 month–11 years (body-weight 12–19 kg): 125 mg twice daily
- ▸ Child 1 month–11 years (body-weight 20–29 kg): 187.5 mg twice daily
- ▸ Child 1 month–11 years (body-weight 30–40 kg): 250 mg twice daily
- ▸ Child 12–17 years: 250 mg twice daily usually for 7–14 days, alternatively 500 mg twice daily usually for 7–14 days, increased dose used if required in severe infections
- ▶ BY MOUTH USING MODIFIED-RELEASE MEDICINES
- ▸ Child 12–17 years: 500 mg once daily usually for 7–14 days, alternatively 1 g once daily usually for 7–14 days, increased dose used if required in severe infections
- ▶ BY INTRAVENOUS INFUSION
- ▸ Child 1 month–11 years: 7.5 mg/kg every 12 hours (max. per dose 500 mg) maximum duration 5 days, switch to oral route when appropriate, to be administered into a large proximal vein
- ▸ Child 12–17 years: 500 mg every 12 hours maximum duration 5 days, switch to oral route when appropriate, to be administered into a large proximal vein

Acute exacerbation of bronchiectasis
- ▶ BY MOUTH USING IMMEDIATE-RELEASE MEDICINES
- ▸ Child 1 month–11 years (body-weight up to 8 kg): 7.5 mg/kg twice daily for 7–14 days
- ▸ Child 1 month–11 years (body-weight 8–11 kg): 62.5 mg twice daily for 7–14 days
- ▸ Child 1 month–11 years (body-weight 12–19 kg): 125 mg twice daily for 7–14 days
- ▸ Child 1 month–11 years (body-weight 20–29 kg): 187.5 mg twice daily for 7–14 days
- ▸ Child 1 month–11 years (body-weight 30–40 kg): 250 mg twice daily for 7–14 days
- ▸ Child 12–17 years: 250–500 mg twice daily for 7–14 days

Acute cough [if systemically very unwell or at higher risk of complications] | Acute sore throat
- ▶ BY MOUTH USING IMMEDIATE-RELEASE MEDICINES
- ▸ Child 1 month–11 years (body-weight up to 8 kg): 7.5 mg/kg twice daily for 5 days (10 days for scarlet fever)
- ▸ Child 1 month–11 years (body-weight 8–11 kg): 62.5 mg twice daily for 5 days (10 days for scarlet fever)
- ▸ Child 1 month–11 years (body-weight 12–19 kg): 125 mg twice daily for 5 days (10 days for scarlet fever)
- ▸ Child 1 month–11 years (body-weight 20–29 kg): 187.5 mg twice daily for 5 days (10 days for scarlet fever)
- ▸ Child 1 month–11 years (body-weight 30–40 kg): 250 mg twice daily for 5 days (10 days for scarlet fever)
- ▸ Child 12–17 years: 250–500 mg twice daily for 5 days (10 days for scarlet fever)

Prevention of secondary case of invasive group A streptococcal infection
- ▶ BY MOUTH USING IMMEDIATE-RELEASE MEDICINES
- ▸ Neonate: 7.5 mg/kg twice daily for 10 days.
- ▸ Child 1 month–11 years (body-weight up to 8 kg): 7.5 mg/kg twice daily for 10 days
- ▸ Child 1 month–11 years (body-weight 8–11 kg): 62.5 mg twice daily for 10 days
- ▸ Child 1 month–11 years (body-weight 12–19 kg): 125 mg twice daily for 10 days
- ▸ Child 1 month–11 years (body-weight 20–29 kg): 187.5 mg twice daily for 10 days
- ▸ Child 1 month–11 years (body-weight 30–40 kg): 250 mg twice daily for 10 days
- ▸ Child 12–17 years: 250–500 mg twice daily for 10 days

Acute otitis media
- ▶ BY MOUTH USING IMMEDIATE-RELEASE MEDICINES
- ▸ Neonate: 7.5 mg/kg twice daily.
- ▸ Child 1 month–11 years (body-weight up to 8 kg): 7.5 mg/kg twice daily for 5–7 days
- ▸ Child 1 month–11 years (body-weight 8–11 kg): 62.5 mg twice daily for 5–7 days
- ▸ Child 1 month–11 years (body-weight 12–19 kg): 125 mg twice daily for 5–7 days
- ▸ Child 1 month–11 years (body-weight 20–29 kg): 187.5 mg twice daily for 5–7 days
- ▸ Child 1 month–11 years (body-weight 30–40 kg): 250 mg twice daily for 5–7 days
- ▸ Child 12–17 years: 250–500 mg twice daily for 5–7 days
- ▶ BY INTRAVENOUS INFUSION
- ▸ Child 1 month–11 years: 7.5 mg/kg every 12 hours (max. per dose 500 mg) maximum duration 5 days, switch to oral route when appropriate, to be administered into a large proximal vein
- ▸ Child 12–17 years: 500 mg every 12 hours maximum duration 5 days, switch to oral route when appropriate, to be administered into a large proximal vein

Mild diphtheria [confirmed or probable]
- ▶ BY MOUTH USING IMMEDIATE-RELEASE MEDICINES
- ▸ Child 1 month–11 years: 7.5 mg/kg twice daily (max. per dose 500 mg) for 14 days
- ▸ Child 12–17 years: 500 mg twice daily for 14 days

Prevention of secondary case of diphtheria
- ▶ BY MOUTH USING IMMEDIATE-RELEASE MEDICINES
- ▸ Child 1 month–11 years: 7.5 mg/kg twice daily (max. per dose 500 mg) for 7 days
- ▸ Child 12–17 years: 500 mg twice daily for 7 days

Prevention of pertussis
- ▶ BY MOUTH USING IMMEDIATE-RELEASE MEDICINES
- ▸ Neonate: 7.5 mg/kg twice daily for 7 days.
- ▸ Child 1 month–11 years (body-weight up to 8 kg): 7.5 mg/kg twice daily for 7 days
- ▸ Child 1 month–11 years (body-weight 8–11 kg): 62.5 mg twice daily for 7 days
- ▸ Child 1 month–11 years (body-weight 12–19 kg): 125 mg twice daily for 7 days
- ▸ Child 1 month–11 years (body-weight 20–29 kg): 187.5 mg twice daily for 7 days
- ▸ Child 1 month–11 years (body-weight 30–40 kg): 250 mg twice daily for 7 days
- ▸ Child 12–17 years: 500 mg twice daily for 7 days

***Helicobacter pylori* eradication in combination with omeprazole, and amoxicillin or metronidazole**
- ▶ BY MOUTH USING IMMEDIATE-RELEASE MEDICINES
- ▸ Child 1–5 years: 7.5 mg/kg twice daily
- ▸ Child 6–11 years: 7.5 mg/kg twice daily (max. per dose 500 mg)
- ▸ Child 12–17 years: 500 mg twice daily

Acute sinusitis
- ▶ BY MOUTH USING IMMEDIATE-RELEASE MEDICINES
- ▸ Child 1 month–11 years (body-weight up to 8 kg): 7.5 mg/kg twice daily for 5 days
- ▸ Child 1 month–11 years (body-weight 8–11 kg): 62.5 mg twice daily for 5 days
- ▸ Child 1 month–11 years (body-weight 12–19 kg): 125 mg twice daily for 5 days
- ▸ Child 1 month–11 years (body-weight 20–29 kg): 187.5 mg twice daily for 5 days
- ▸ Child 1 month–11 years (body-weight 30–40 kg): 250 mg twice daily for 5 days
- ▸ Child 12–17 years: 250 mg twice daily for 5 days, alternatively 500 mg twice daily for 5 days

● **UNLICENSED USE** UKHSA advises clarithromycin may be used as detailed below, although these situations are considered unlicensed:
- prevention of secondary cases of invasive group A streptococcal infection;
- treatment and prevention of diphtheria.

EvGr Duration of treatment for acute sinusitis differs from product literature and adheres to national guidelines. (A)
- ▸ With oral use EvGr Duration of treatment for acute otitis media differs from product literature and adheres to national guidelines. (A) Tablets not licensed for use in children under 12 years; oral suspension not licensed for use in infants under 6 months.
- ▸ With intravenous use Intravenous infusion not licensed for use in children under 12 years.

● **INTERACTIONS** → Appendix 1: macrolides

● **SIDE-EFFECTS**

GENERAL SIDE-EFFECTS
- ▶ **Uncommon** Burping · dry mouth · haemorrhage · muscle complaints · oral disorders · thrombocytosis · tremor
- ▶ **Frequency not known** Abnormal dreams · agranulocytosis · depersonalisation · depression · mania · myopathy · psychotic disorder · renal failure · tooth discolouration · urine discolouration

SPECIFIC SIDE-EFFECTS
- ▶ **Uncommon**
- ▸ With oral use Increased risk of infection
- ▸ With parenteral use Cardiac arrest · dyskinesia · loss of consciousness · pulmonary embolism
- ▶ **Frequency not known**
- ▸ With oral use Disorientation

● **PREGNANCY** Manufacturer advises avoid, particularly in the first trimester, unless potential benefit outweighs risk.

● **BREAST FEEDING** Manufacturer advises avoid unless potential benefit outweighs risk—present in milk.

● **HEPATIC IMPAIRMENT** Manufacturer advises caution; avoid in severe failure if renal impairment also present.

● **RENAL IMPAIRMENT** EvGr Avoid if severe hepatic impairment also present. For *modified-release* preparations, avoid if creatinine clearance less than 30 mL/minute. (M)

Dose adjustments EvGr For *immediate-release* preparations, use half normal dose if creatinine clearance less than 30 mL/minute, max. duration 14 days.

For *modified-release* preparations, use half normal dose if creatinine clearance 30–60 mL/minute. (M)

See p. 16.

● **DIRECTIONS FOR ADMINISTRATION** For *intravenous infusion*, manufacturer advises give intermittently in Glucose 5% *or* Sodium Chloride 0.9%; dissolve initially in Water for Injections (500 mg in 10 mL) then dilute to a concentration of 2 mg/mL; give into large proximal vein over 60 minutes.

● **PRESCRIBING AND DISPENSING INFORMATION** For choice of antibacterial therapy, see Antibacterials, use for prophylaxis p. 359, Ear infections, antibacterial therapy p. 366, Nose infections, antibacterial therapy p. 370, Oropharyngeal infections, antibacterial therapy p. 883, Peptic ulceration p. 60, Respiratory system infections, antibacterial therapy p. 371, Skin infections, antibacterial therapy p. 373.

● **PATIENT AND CARER ADVICE**
Medicines for Children leaflet: Clarithromycin for bacterial infections www.medicinesforchildren.org.uk/medicines/clarithromycin-for-bacterial-infections/

● **PROFESSION SPECIFIC INFORMATION**
Dental practitioners' formulary Clarithromycin Tablets may be prescribed. Clarithromycin Oral Suspension may be prescribed.

● **MEDICINAL FORMS** There can be variation in the licensing of different medicines containing the same drug. Forms available from special-order manufacturers include: infusion

Oral tablet

CAUTIONARY AND ADVISORY LABELS 9
- ▸ **Clarithromycin (Non-proprietary)**
  Clarithromycin 250 mg Clarithromycin 250mg tablets | 14 tablet PoM £5.51 DT = £1.23
  Clarithromycin 500 mg Clarithromycin 500mg tablets | 14 tablet PoM £11.96 DT = £2.01

Modified-release tablet

CAUTIONARY AND ADVISORY LABELS 9, 21, 25
- ▸ **Xetinin XL** (Morningside Healthcare Ltd)
  Clarithromycin 500 mg Xetinin XL 500mg tablets | 7 tablet PoM £6.72 DT = £6.72 | 14 tablet PoM £13.23 DT = £13.23

Oral suspension

CAUTIONARY AND ADVISORY LABELS 9
- ▸ **Clarithromycin (Non-proprietary)**
  Clarithromycin 25 mg per 1 ml Clarithromycin 125mg/5ml oral suspension | 70 ml PoM £26.30 DT = £10.77
  Clarithromycin 50 mg per 1 ml Clarithromycin 250mg/5ml oral suspension | 70 ml PoM £52.56 DT = £20.69

Powder for solution for infusion

ELECTROLYTES: May contain Sodium
- ▸ **Clarithromycin (Non-proprietary)**
  Clarithromycin 500 mg Clarithromycin 500mg powder for solution for infusion vials | 1 vial PoM £11.25 (Hospital only)
  Clarithromycin 500mg powder for concentrate for solution for infusion vials | 1 vial PoM £11.15 (Hospital only) | 10 vial PoM £111.50 | 10 vial PoM £112.50 (Hospital only)

402

Erythromycin

16-Jan-2026

● **INDICATIONS AND DOSE**

Susceptible infections in patients with penicillin hypersensitivity (e.g. respiratory-tract infections (including Legionella infection), skin and oral infections, and campylobacter enteritis)

▶ BY MOUTH

- Neonate: 12.5 mg/kg every 6 hours.
- Child 1–23 months: 125 mg 4 times a day, alternatively 250 mg twice daily, increased to 250 mg 4 times a day, increased dose may be used in severe infections
- Child 2–7 years: 250 mg 4 times a day, alternatively 500 mg twice daily, increased to 500 mg 4 times a day, increased dose may be used in severe infections
- Child 8–17 years: 250–500 mg 4 times a day, alternatively 500–1000 mg twice daily, increased to 500–1000 mg 4 times a day, increased dose may be used in severe infections

▶ BY INTRAVENOUS INFUSION

- Neonate: 10–12.5 mg/kg every 6 hours.
- Child: 12.5 mg/kg every 6 hours (max. per dose 1 g)

Impetigo | Secondary bacterial infection of eczema

▶ BY MOUTH

- Child 8–17 years: 250–500 mg 4 times a day for 5–7 days

Cellulitis | Erysipelas

▶ BY MOUTH

- Child 8–17 years: 250–500 mg 4 times a day for 5–7 days then review

Community-acquired pneumonia

▶ BY MOUTH

- Child 8–11 years: 250–500 mg 4 times a day for 3 days (5 days in severe infection)
- Child 12–17 years: 250–500 mg 4 times a day for 5 days

Acute cough [if systemically very unwell or at higher risk of complications]

▶ BY MOUTH

- Child 1–23 months: 125 mg 4 times a day for 5 days, alternatively 250 mg twice daily for 5 days
- Child 2–7 years: 250 mg 4 times a day for 5 days, alternatively 500 mg twice daily for 5 days
- Child 8–17 years: 250–500 mg 4 times a day for 5 days, alternatively 500–1000 mg twice daily for 5 days

Acute sore throat

▶ BY MOUTH

- Child 8–17 years: 250–500 mg 4 times a day for 5 days, alternatively 500–1000 mg twice daily for 5 days

Acute otitis media

▶ BY MOUTH

- Child 8–17 years: 250–500 mg 4 times a day for 5–7 days, alternatively 500–1000 mg twice daily for 5–7 days

Early syphilis

▶ BY MOUTH

- Child 12–17 years: 500 mg 4 times a day for 14 days

Uncomplicated genital chlamydia

▶ BY MOUTH

- Child 12–17 years: 500 mg twice daily for 14 days

Prevention and treatment of pertussis

▶ BY MOUTH

- Neonate: 12.5 mg/kg every 6 hours.
- Child 1–23 months: 125 mg 4 times a day, alternatively 250 mg twice daily, increased to 250 mg 4 times a day, increased dose may be used in severe infections
- Child 2–7 years: 250 mg 4 times a day, alternatively 500 mg twice daily, increased to 500 mg 4 times a day, increased dose may be used in severe infections
- Child 8–17 years: 250–500 mg 4 times a day, alternatively 500–1000 mg twice daily, increased to 500–1000 mg 4 times a day, increased dose may be used in severe infections

▶ BY INTRAVENOUS INFUSION

- Neonate: 10–12.5 mg/kg every 6 hours.
- Child: 12.5 mg/kg every 6 hours (max. per dose 1 g)

Mild diphtheria [confirmed or probable]

▶ BY MOUTH

- Neonate: 10–15 mg/kg 4 times a day for 14 days, alternatively 20–30 mg/kg twice daily for 14 days.
- Child 1 month–11 years: 10–15 mg/kg 4 times a day (max. per dose 500 mg) for 14 days, alternatively 20–30 mg/kg twice daily (max. per dose 1 g) for 14 days
- Child 12–17 years: 500 mg 4 times a day for 14 days, alternatively 1 g twice daily for 14 days

Prevention of secondary case of diphtheria

▶ BY MOUTH

- Neonate: 10–15 mg/kg 4 times a day for 7 days, alternatively 20–30 mg/kg twice daily for 7 days.
- Child 1 month–11 years: 10–15 mg/kg 4 times a day (max. per dose 500 mg) for 7 days, alternatively 20–30 mg/kg twice daily (max. per dose 1 g) for 7 days
- Child 12–17 years: 500 mg 4 times a day for 7 days, alternatively 1 g twice daily for 7 days

Prevention of secondary case of invasive group A streptococcal infection [penicillin-allergic patients who are pregnant or within 28 days of delivery]

▶ BY MOUTH

- Child 8–17 years: 250–500 mg every 6 hours for 10 days

Prevention of pneumococcal infection in asplenia or in patients with sickle-cell disease (if penicillin-allergic)

▶ BY MOUTH

- Child 1–23 months: 125 mg twice daily, antibiotic prophylaxis is not fully reliable
- Child 2–7 years: 250 mg twice daily, antibiotic prophylaxis is not fully reliable. It may be discontinued in those over 5 years of age with sickle-cell disease who have received pneumococcal immunisation and who do not have a history of severe pneumococcal infection
- Child 8–17 years: 500 mg twice daily, antibiotic prophylaxis is not fully reliable. It may be discontinued in those with sickle-cell disease who have received pneumococcal immunisation and who do not have a history of severe pneumococcal infection

Prevention of recurrence of rheumatic fever

▶ BY MOUTH

- Child 1–23 months: 125 mg twice daily
- Child 2–17 years: 250 mg twice daily

Infantile acne

▶ BY MOUTH

- Child 1–23 months: 250 mg once daily, alternatively 125 mg twice daily

Acne

▶ BY MOUTH

- Child 12–17 years: 500 mg twice daily

Gastro-intestinal stasis

▶ BY MOUTH

- Neonate: 3 mg/kg 4 times a day.
- Child: 3 mg/kg 4 times a day

▶ BY INTRAVENOUS INFUSION

- Neonate: 3 mg/kg 4 times a day.
- Child 1–11 months: 3 mg/kg 4 times a day

- **UNLICENSED USE** EvGr Duration of treatment for acute otitis media differs from product literature and adheres to national guidelines. ⟨A⟩

  UKHSA advises erythromycin is used in the doses provided in BNF Publications for the treatment and prevention of diphtheria, but these may differ from those licensed.

  Erythromycin may be used for gastro-intestinal stasis, but it is not licensed for this indication.

  EvGr Erythromycin is used in the doses provided in BNFC for the treatment of infantile acne, ⟨E⟩ but these may differ from those licensed.

IMPORTANT SAFETY INFORMATION

MHRA/CHM ADVICE: ERYTHROMYCIN: CAUTION REQUIRED DUE TO CARDIAC RISKS (QT INTERVAL PROLONGATION); DRUG INTERACTION WITH RIVAROXABAN (DECEMBER 2020)

A European review of safety data highlighted an increased risk of cardiotoxicity (i.e. QT interval prolongation) associated with erythromycin. Healthcare professionals are advised that erythromycin should not be given to patients with a history of QT interval prolongation or ventricular arrhythmia (including torsade de pointes), or those with electrolyte disturbances. The benefit-risk balance of treatment should be assessed in patients at increased risk of a cardiac event; caution is required in those with cardiac disease or heart failure, conduction disturbances or clinically relevant bradycardia, or if taking concomitant medicines associated with QT interval prolongation. Patients and carers should be directed to the patient information leaflet and advised to seek medical attention if signs or symptoms of a cardiac event develop. A potential drug interaction between rivaroxaban and erythromycin resulting in an increased risk of bleeding has also been identified—consult product literature.

MHRA/CHM ADVICE: ERYTHROMYCIN: UPDATE ON KNOWN RISK OF INFANTILE HYPERTROPHIC PYLORIC STENOSIS (DECEMBER 2020)

A European review of safety data suggested an overall two- to three-fold increase in the risk of infantile hypertrophic pyloric stenosis after exposure to erythromycin during infancy, in general, and found the risk to be highest in the first 14 days after birth. Healthcare professionals are advised to assess the benefit-risk balance of erythromycin therapy in infants. Parents and carers should be advised to seek medical attention if vomiting or irritability with feeding occurs in infants during treatment.

- **CAUTIONS** Avoid in Acute porphyrias p. 745 · neonate under 2 weeks (risk of hypertrophic pyloric stenosis)
- **INTERACTIONS** → Appendix 1: macrolides
- **SIDE-EFFECTS**

  GENERAL SIDE-EFFECTS
  - **Rare or very rare** Hearing loss (can occur after large doses)

  SPECIFIC SIDE-EFFECTS
  - With oral use Cerebral impairment
  - With parenteral use Atrioventricular block
- **PREGNANCY** EvGr Use only if potential benefit outweighs risk ⟨M⟩ (recommendation also supported by specialist sources).
  - When used for Early syphilis EvGr Avoid (drug may not reach fetus in adequate concentration to prevent congenital syphilis). ⟨A⟩
- **BREAST FEEDING** Only small amounts in milk—not known to be harmful.
- **HEPATIC IMPAIRMENT** Manufacturer advises caution.
- **RENAL IMPAIRMENT**

  Dose adjustments Some manufacturers advise consider dose reduction in moderate to severe impairment (ototoxicity) (consult product literature).
- **DIRECTIONS FOR ADMINISTRATION**
  - With intravenous use Dilute reconstituted solution further in Glucose 5% (neutralised with Sodium Bicarbonate) or Sodium Chloride 0.9% to a concentration of 1–5 mg/mL; give over 20–60 minutes. Concentration of up to 10 mg/mL may be used in fluid-restriction if administered via a central venous catheter.
- **PRESCRIBING AND DISPENSING INFORMATION** For choice of antibacterial therapy, see Antibacterials, use for prophylaxis p. 359, Ear infections, antibacterial therapy p. 366, Gastro-intestinal system infections, antibacterial therapy p. 367, Genital system infections, antibacterial therapy p. 368, Oropharyngeal infections, antibacterial therapy p. 883, Respiratory system infections, antibacterial therapy p. 371, Skin infections, antibacterial therapy p. 373.
- **PATIENT AND CARER ADVICE**

  Medicines for Children leaflet: Erythromycin for bacterial infections www.medicinesforchildren.org.uk/medicines/erythromycin-for-bacterial-infections/
- **PROFESSION SPECIFIC INFORMATION**

  Dental practitioners' formulary Erythromycin tablets e/c may be prescribed. Erythromycin ethyl succinate oral suspension may be prescribed. Erythromycin stearate tablets may be prescribed. Erythromycin ethyl succinate tablets may be prescribed.

- **MEDICINAL FORMS** There can be variation in the licensing of different medicines containing the same drug.

Oral tablet

CAUTIONARY AND ADVISORY LABELS 9

- **Erythromycin (Non-proprietary)**

  Erythromycin (as Erythromycin ethyl succinate) 500 mg Erythromycin ethyl succinate 500mg tablets | 28 tablet PoM £15.95 DT = £15.95
- **Erythrocin** (Advanz Pharma)

  Erythromycin (as Erythromycin stearate) 250 mg Erythrocin 250 tablets | 100 tablet PoM £18.20 DT = £18.20

  Erythromycin (as Erythromycin stearate) 500 mg Erythrocin 500 tablets | 100 tablet PoM £36.40 DT = £36.40

Gastro-resistant tablet

CAUTIONARY AND ADVISORY LABELS 5, 9, 25

- **Erythromycin (Non-proprietary)**

  Erythromycin 250 mg Erythromycin 250mg gastro-resistant tablets | 28 tablet PoM £6.95 DT = £2.05

Oral suspension

CAUTIONARY AND ADVISORY LABELS 9

- **Erythromycin (Non-proprietary)**

  Erythromycin (as Erythromycin ethyl succinate) 25 mg per 1 ml Erythromycin ethyl succinate 125mg/5ml oral suspension | 100 ml PoM £8.10 DT = £7.95

  Erythromycin ethyl succinate 125mg/5ml oral suspension sugar free | 100 ml PoM £8.10 DT = £7.76 SF

  Erythromycin (as Erythromycin ethyl succinate) 50 mg per 1 ml Erythromycin ethyl succinate 250mg/5ml oral suspension | 100 ml PoM £13.70 DT = £11.89

  Erythromycin ethyl succinate 250mg/5ml oral suspension sugar free | 100 ml PoM £13.70 DT = £13.39 SF

  Erythromycin (as Erythromycin ethyl succinate) 100 mg per 1 ml Erythromycin ethyl succinate 500mg/5ml oral suspension | 100 ml PoM £24.70

Powder for solution for infusion

- **Erythromycin (Non-proprietary)**

  Erythromycin (as Erythromycin lactobionate)

  1 gram Erythromycin 1g powder for solution for infusion vials | 1 vial PoM £22.00–£22.92 (Hospital only)

ANTIBACTERIALS > MONOBACTAMS

Aztreonam

04-Nov-2024

● **DRUG ACTION** Aztreonam is a monocyclic beta-lactam ('monobactam') antibiotic with an antibacterial spectrum limited to Gram-negative aerobic bacteria including *Pseudomonas aeruginosa*, *Neisseria meningitidis*, and *Haemophilus influenzae*; it should not be used alone for 'blind' treatment since it is not active against Gram-positive organisms. Aztreonam is also effective against *Neisseria gonorrhoeae* (but not against concurrent chlamydial infection).

● **INDICATIONS AND DOSE**

Gram-negative infections including *Pseudomonas aeruginosa, Haemophilus influenzae,* and *Neisseria meningitidis*

▶ BY INTRAVENOUS INJECTION, OR BY INTRAVENOUS INFUSION

- Neonate up to 7 days: 30 mg/kg every 12 hours.
- Neonate 7 days to 28 days: 30 mg/kg every 6–8 hours.
- Child 1 month–11 years: 30 mg/kg every 6–8 hours
- Child 12–17 years: 1 g every 8 hours, alternatively 2 g every 12 hours

Severe gram-negative infections including *Pseudomonas aeruginosa, Haemophilus influenzae, Neisseria meningitidis,* and lung infections in cystic fibrosis

▶ BY INTRAVENOUS INFUSION, OR BY INTRAVENOUS INJECTION

- Child 2–11 years: 50 mg/kg every 6–8 hours (max. per dose 2 g 4 times a day)
- Child 12–17 years: 2 g every 6–8 hours

Chronic pulmonary *Pseudomonas aeruginosa* infection in patients with cystic fibrosis

▶ BY INHALATION OF NEBULISED SOLUTION

- Child 6–17 years: 75 mg 3 times a day for 28 days, doses to be administered at least 4 hours apart, subsequent courses repeated after 28-day interval without aztreonam nebuliser solution

● **UNLICENSED USE**

- With systemic use Injection not licensed for use in children under 7 days.

● **CAUTIONS**

- When used by inhalation Haemoptysis— risk of further haemorrhage

● **SIDE-EFFECTS**

GENERAL SIDE-EFFECTS

▶ **Common or very common** Dyspnoea · respiratory disorders

SPECIFIC SIDE-EFFECTS

▶ **Common or very common**

- When used by inhalation Cough · haemoptysis · joint disorders · laryngeal pain · nasal complaints · rash

▶ **Rare or very rare**

- With parenteral use Anaemia · asthenia · breast tenderness · chest pain · confusion · diplopia · dizziness · eosinophilia · haemorrhage · headache · hepatic disorders · hypotension · insomnia · leucocytosis · myalgia · nasal congestion · neutropenia · oral disorders · pancytopenia · paraesthesia · pseudomembranous enterocolitis · seizure · thrombocytopenia · thrombocytosis · tinnitus · vertigo · vulvovaginal candidiasis

▶ **Frequency not known**

- With parenteral use Abdominal pain · angioedema · Clostridioides difficile colitis · diarrhoea · nausea · skin reactions · taste altered · toxic epidermal necrolysis · vomiting

● **ALLERGY AND CROSS-SENSITIVITY** [EvGr] Contra-indicated in aztreonam hypersensitivity.

Use with caution in patients with hypersensitivity to other beta-lactam antibiotics (although aztreonam may be less likely than other beta-lactams to cause hypersensitivity in penicillin-sensitive patients). ⟨M⟩

● **PREGNANCY**

- With systemic use No information available; manufacturer of injection advises avoid.
- When used by inhalation No information available; manufacturer of powder for nebuliser solution advises avoid unless essential.

● **BREAST FEEDING** Amount in milk probably too small to be harmful.

● **HEPATIC IMPAIRMENT**

- With systemic use Manufacturer advises caution in chronic impairment with cirrhosis.

Dose adjustments

- With systemic use Manufacturer advises dose reduction of 20—25% for long term treatment of patients with chronic impairment with cirrhosis, especially in alcoholic cirrhosis and concomitant renal impairment.

● **RENAL IMPAIRMENT**

Dose adjustments

- With systemic use If estimated glomerular filtration rate 10–30 mL/minute/1.73 m^2, usual initial dose of injection, then half normal dose. If estimated glomerular filtration rate less than 10 mL/minute/1.73 m^2, usual initial dose of injection, then one-quarter normal dose.

● **MONITORING REQUIREMENTS**

- When used by inhalation Measure lung function before and after initial dose of aztreonam and monitor for bronchospasm.

● **EFFECT ON LABORATORY TESTS**

- With systemic use False positive Coombs' test.

● **DIRECTIONS FOR ADMINISTRATION**

- With intravenous use For *intravenous injection*, manufacturer advises give over 3–5 minutes. Displacement value of injection may be significant, consult local guidelines. For intermittent *intravenous infusion*, manufacturer advises dilute reconstituted solution further in Glucose 5% *or* Sodium Chloride 0.9% to a concentration of less than 20 mg/mL; to be given over 20–60 minutes.
- When used by inhalation Manufacturer advises other inhaled drugs should be administered before aztreonam; a bronchodilator should be administered before each dose.

● **NATIONAL FUNDING/ACCESS DECISIONS**

For full details see funding body website

Scottish Medicines Consortium (SMC) decisions

▶ **Aztreonam lysine (*Cayston*®) for suppressive therapy of chronic pulmonary infections due to *Pseudomonas aeruginosa* in patients with cystic fibrosis aged six years and older (January 2015)** SMC No. 753/12 Recommended with restrictions

● **MEDICINAL FORMS** There can be variation in the licensing of different medicines containing the same drug.

Powder and solvent for nebuliser solution

- **Cayston** (Gilead Sciences Ltd)
  Aztreonam (as Aztreonam lysine) 75 mg Cayston 75mg powder and solvent for nebuliser solution vials with Altera Nebuliser Handset | 84 vial [PoM] £3,272.30

Powder for solution for injection

- **Aztreonam (Non-proprietary)**
  Aztreonam 1 gram Aztreonam 1g powder for solution for injection vials | 1 vial [PoM] £17.40 (Hospital only)
  Aztreonam 2 gram Aztreonam 2g powder for solution for injection vials | 1 vial [PoM] £34.80 (Hospital only)

ANTIBACTERIALS > NITROIMIDAZOLE DERIVATIVES

Metronidazole

31-Oct-2025

- **DRUG ACTION** Metronidazole is an antimicrobial drug with high activity against anaerobic bacteria and protozoa.

- **INDICATIONS AND DOSE**

Anaerobic infections

▶ BY MOUTH
- Child 1 month: 7.5 mg/kg every 12 hours usually treated for 7 days
- Child 2 months–11 years: 7.5 mg/kg every 8 hours (max. per dose 400 mg) usually treated for 7 days
- Child 12–17 years: 400 mg every 8 hours usually treated for 7 days

▶ BY RECTUM
- Child 1–11 months: 125 mg 3 times a day for 3 days, then 125 mg twice daily for usual total treatment duration of 7 days
- Child 1–4 years: 250 mg 3 times a day for 3 days, then 250 mg twice daily for usual total treatment duration of 7 days
- Child 5–9 years: 500 mg 3 times a day for 3 days, then 500 mg twice daily for usual total treatment duration of 7 days
- Child 10–17 years: 1 g 3 times a day for 3 days, then 1 g twice daily for usual total treatment duration of 7 days

▶ BY INTRAVENOUS INFUSION
- Neonate up to 26 weeks corrected gestational age: Loading dose 15 mg/kg for 1 dose, then 7.5 mg/kg every 24 hours usually treated for a total duration of 7 days (for 10 days in *Clostridioides difficile* infection).
- Neonate 26 weeks to 34 weeks corrected gestational age: Loading dose 15 mg/kg for 1 dose, then 7.5 mg/kg every 12 hours usually treated for a total duration of 7 days (for 10 days in *Clostridioides difficile* infection).
- Neonate 34 weeks corrected gestational age and above: Loading dose 15 mg/kg for 1 dose, then 7.5 mg/kg every 8 hours usually treated for a total duration of 7 days (for 10 days in *Clostridioides difficile* infection).
- Child 1 month: Loading dose 15 mg/kg for 1 dose, then 7.5 mg/kg every 8 hours usually treated for a total duration of 7 days (for 10 days in *Clostridioides difficile* infection)
- Child 2 months–17 years: 7.5 mg/kg every 8 hours (max. per dose 500 mg) usually treated for 7 days (for 10 days in *Clostridioides difficile* infection)

Cellulitis | Erysipelas

▶ BY MOUTH
- Child 1 month: 7.5 mg/kg every 12 hours for 7 days then review
- Child 2 months–11 years: 7.5 mg/kg every 8 hours (max. per dose 400 mg) for 7 days then review
- Child 12–17 years: 400 mg every 8 hours for 7 days then review

▶ BY INTRAVENOUS INFUSION
- Child 1 month: Loading dose 15 mg/kg for 1 dose, then 7.5 mg/kg every 8 hours
- Child 2 months–17 years: 7.5 mg/kg every 8 hours (max. per dose 500 mg)

Prophylaxis of infection from human bites [in combination with other drugs] | Prophylaxis of infection from animal bites [in combination with other drugs]

▶ BY MOUTH
- Child 12–17 years: 400 mg 3 times a day for 3 days

▶ BY INTRAVENOUS INFUSION
- Child 1 month: Loading dose 15 mg/kg for 1 dose, then 7.5 mg/kg every 8 hours
- Child 2 months–17 years: 7.5 mg/kg every 8 hours (max. per dose 500 mg)

Treatment of infection from human bites [in combination with other drugs] | Treatment of infection from animal bites [in combination with other drugs]

▶ BY MOUTH
- Child 12–17 years: 400 mg 3 times a day for 5–7 days

▶ BY INTRAVENOUS INFUSION
- Child 1 month: Loading dose 15 mg/kg for 1 dose, then 7.5 mg/kg every 8 hours
- Child 2 months–17 years: 7.5 mg/kg every 8 hours (max. per dose 500 mg)

***Helicobacter pylori* eradication; in combination with clarithromycin and omeprazole**

▶ BY MOUTH
- Child 1–5 years: 100 mg twice daily
- Child 6–11 years: 200 mg twice daily
- Child 12–17 years: 400 mg twice daily

***Helicobacter pylori* eradication; in combination with amoxicillin and omeprazole**

▶ BY MOUTH
- Child 1–5 years: 100 mg 3 times a day
- Child 6–11 years: 200 mg 3 times a day
- Child 12–17 years: 400 mg 3 times a day

Fistulating Crohn's disease

▶ BY MOUTH
- Child: 7.5 mg/kg 3 times a day usually given for 1 month but should not be used for longer than 3 months because of concerns about peripheral neuropathy

Bacterial vaginosis

▶ BY VAGINA USING VAGINAL GEL
- Child: 1 applicatorful once daily for 5 days, dose to be administered at night

DOSE EQUIVALENCE AND CONVERSION
- 1 applicatorful of vaginal gel delivers a 5 g dose of metronidazole 0.75%.

Pelvic inflammatory disease

▶ BY MOUTH
- Child 12–17 years: 400 mg twice daily for 14 days

Acute ulcerative gingivitis

▶ BY MOUTH
- Child 1–2 years: 50 mg every 8 hours for 3 days
- Child 3–6 years: 100 mg every 12 hours for 3 days
- Child 7–9 years: 100 mg every 8 hours for 3 days
- Child 10–17 years: 200–250 mg every 8 hours for 3 days

Acute oral infections

▶ BY MOUTH
- Child 1–2 years: 50 mg every 8 hours for 3–7 days
- Child 3–6 years: 100 mg every 12 hours for 3–7 days
- Child 7–9 years: 100 mg every 8 hours for 3–7 days
- Child 10–17 years: 200–250 mg every 8 hours for 3–7 days

Surgical prophylaxis

▶ BY MOUTH
- Child 1 month–11 years: 30 mg/kg for 1 dose (max. per dose 500 mg), to be administered 2 hours before surgery
- Child 12–17 years: 400–500 mg for 1 dose, to be administered 2 hours before surgery, then 400–500 mg every 8 hours if required for up to 3 doses (in high-risk procedures)

▶ BY RECTUM
- Child 5–9 years: 500 mg for 1 dose, to be administered 2 hours before surgery, then 500 mg every 8 hours if required for up to 3 doses (in high-risk procedures)

continued →

5 Infection

- Child 10–17 years: 1 g for 1 dose, to be administered 2 hours before surgery, then 1 g every 8 hours if required for up to 3 doses (in high-risk procedures)
- BY INTRAVENOUS INFUSION
- Neonate up to 40 weeks corrected gestational age: 10 mg/kg for 1 dose, to be administered up to 30 minutes before the procedure.
- Neonate 40 weeks corrected gestational age and above: 20–30 mg/kg for 1 dose, to be administered up to 30 minutes before the procedure.
- Child 1 month–11 years: 30 mg/kg for 1 dose (max. per dose 500 mg), to be administered up to 30 minutes before the procedure
- Child 12–17 years: 500 mg for 1 dose, to be administered up to 30 minutes before the procedure, then 500 mg every 8 hours if required for up to 3 doses (in high-risk procedures)

Invasive intestinal amoebiasis

- BY MOUTH
- Child 1–2 years: 200 mg 3 times a day for 5 days
- Child 3–6 years: 200 mg 4 times a day for 5 days
- Child 7–9 years: 400 mg 3 times a day for 5 days
- Child 10–17 years: 800 mg 3 times a day for 5 days

Extra-intestinal amoebiasis (including liver abscess)

- BY MOUTH
- Child 1–2 years: 200 mg 3 times a day for 5–10 days
- Child 3–6 years: 200 mg 4 times a day for 5–10 days
- Child 7–9 years: 400 mg 3 times a day for 5–10 days
- Child 10–17 years: 800 mg 3 times a day for 5–10 days

Urogenital trichomoniasis

- BY MOUTH
- Child 1–2 years: 50 mg 3 times a day for 7 days
- Child 3–6 years: 100 mg twice daily for 7 days
- Child 7–9 years: 100 mg 3 times a day for 7 days
- Child 10–17 years: 200 mg 3 times a day for 7 days, alternatively 400–500 mg twice daily for 5–7 days, alternatively 2 g for 1 dose

Giardiasis

- BY MOUTH
- Child 1–2 years: 500 mg once daily for 3 days
- Child 3–6 years: 600–800 mg once daily for 3 days
- Child 7–9 years: 1 g once daily for 3 days
- Child 10–17 years: 2 g once daily for 3 days, alternatively 400 mg 3 times a day for 5 days, alternatively 500 mg twice daily for 7–10 days

Established case of tetanus

- BY INTRAVENOUS INFUSION
- Child: (consult product literature)

UNLICENSED USE Metronidazole vaginal gel not licensed for use in children under 18 years.

CAUTIONS

- With intravenous use Evidence or history of blood dyscrasia
- With systemic use Active or chronic severe CNS disease (risk of neurological aggravation) · active or chronic severe peripheral nervous system disease (risk of neurological aggravation) · Cockayne syndrome
- With vaginal use Avoid intravaginal preparations (particularly those that require the use of an applicator) in young girls who are not sexually active, unless there is no alternative · not recommended during menstruation · some systemic absorption may occur with vaginal gel

CAUTIONS, FURTHER INFORMATION

- Cockayne syndrome
- With systemic use EvGr Severe hepatotoxicity in patients with Cockayne syndrome, including fatal cases with a very rapid onset after starting treatment, has been reported. Metronidazole should not be used unless potential benefit outweighs risk and alternative treatment is unavailable. Liver function tests (LFTs) must be performed before, during, and after treatment until liver function is within normal ranges or baseline values are achieved. Metronidazole should be discontinued if LFTs are markedly elevated during treatment. Patients should be advised to stop treatment and seek immediate medical attention if symptoms of liver injury occur. (M)
- Blood dyscrasia
- With intravenous use EvGr Regular clinical and laboratory monitoring (including full blood count) advised in patients with evidence or history of blood dyscrasia if high-dose or prolonged treatment exceeding 10 days. (M)

INTERACTIONS → Appendix 1: metronidazole

SIDE-EFFECTS

- **Common or very common**
- With systemic use Dry mouth · myalgia · nausea · oral disorders · taste metallic · vomiting
- With vaginal use Pelvic discomfort · vulvovaginal candidiasis · vulvovaginal disorders
- **Uncommon**
- With systemic use Asthenia · headache · leucopenia (with long term or intensive therapy)
- With vaginal use Menstrual cycle irregularities · vaginal haemorrhage
- **Rare or very rare**
- With systemic use Agranulocytosis · angioedema · appetite decreased · ataxia · cerebellar syndrome · confusion · diarrhoea · dizziness · drowsiness · encephalopathy · epigastric pain · epileptiform seizure (with long term or intensive therapy) · flushing · hallucination · hepatic disorders · meningitis aseptic · mucositis · nerve disorders · neutropenia · pancreatitis · pancytopenia · peripheral neuropathy (with long term or intensive therapy) · psychotic disorder · seizure · severe cutaneous adverse reactions (SCARs) · skin reactions · thrombocytopenia · urine dark · vision disorders
- **Frequency not known**
- With systemic use Depressed mood · gastrointestinal disorder · hearing impairment · taste altered · tinnitus · vertigo

PREGNANCY

- With systemic use Manufacturer advises avoidance of high-dose regimens; use only if potential benefit outweighs risk.

BREAST FEEDING

- With systemic use Significant amount in milk; manufacturer advises avoid large single doses though otherwise compatible; may give milk a bitter taste.

HEPATIC IMPAIRMENT

- With intravenous use or oral use EvGr Caution in hepatic encephalopathy (risk of decreased clearance). (M)
- With intravenous use EvGr Caution in severe impairment (risk of decreased clearance). (M)

Monitoring

- With intravenous use EvGr Regular clinical and laboratory monitoring (including full blood count) advised if high-dose or prolonged treatment exceeding 10 days in severe impairment. (M)

Dose adjustments

- With intravenous use or oral use EvGr Reduce dose to one-third of the daily dose in hepatic encephalopathy (may be given once daily). (M)
- With intravenous use EvGr Reduce dose in severe impairment. (M)

MONITORING REQUIREMENTS

- With oral use or rectal use Regular clinical and laboratory monitoring (particularly leucocyte count) advised if treatment exceeds 10 days; patients should also be monitored for peripheral or central neuropathy.
- With intravenous use Regular clinical and laboratory monitoring (including full blood count) advised if high-dose or prolonged treatment exceeding 10 days; patients

should also be monitored for peripheral or central neuropathy.

● **EFFECT ON LABORATORY TESTS**

▸ With systemic use False negative or abnormally low blood test determinations for alanine aminotransferase (ALT), aspartate aminotransferase (AST), lactate dehydrogenase (LDH), triglycerides, and glucose hexokinase—consult product literature.

● **DIRECTIONS FOR ADMINISTRATION** EvGr For *intravenous infusion*, give over 20–60 minutes. (M)

● **PRESCRIBING AND DISPENSING INFORMATION** For choice of antibacterial therapy, see Antibacterials, use for prophylaxis p. 359, Antiprotozoal drugs p. 476, Gastro-intestinal system infections, antibacterial therapy p. 367, Genital system infections, antibacterial therapy p. 368, Oropharyngeal infections, antibacterial therapy p. 883, Peptic ulceration p. 60, Skin infections, antibacterial therapy p. 373.

Metronidazole is well absorbed orally and the intravenous route is normally reserved for severe infections. Metronidazole by the rectal route is an effective alternative to the intravenous route when oral administration is not possible.

● **PATIENT AND CARER ADVICE**

▸ With systemic use Patients or their carers should be advised that metronidazole may darken urine (due to presence of metabolites).

Medicines for Children leaflet: Metronidazole for bacterial infections www.medicinesforchildren.org.uk/medicines/metronidazole-for-bacterial-infections/

Driving and skilled tasks

▸ With systemic use Patients and carers should be counselled on the effects on driving and performance of skilled tasks—increased risk of drowsiness, dizziness, vertigo, confusion, hallucinations, convulsions, or visual disorders.

● **PROFESSION SPECIFIC INFORMATION**

Dental practitioners' formulary Metronidazole Tablets may be prescribed. Metronidazole Oral Suspension may be prescribed.

● **MEDICINAL FORMS** There can be variation in the licensing of different medicines containing the same drug. Forms available from special-order manufacturers include: oral suspension, oral solution, suppository

Oral tablet

CAUTIONARY AND ADVISORY LABELS 3, 4, 9, 21, 25, 27

▸ **Metronidazole (Non-proprietary)**

Metronidazole 200 mg Metronidazole 200mg tablets | 21 tablet PoM £4.00 DT = £1.13

Metronidazole 400 mg Metronidazole 400mg tablets | 21 tablet PoM £7.66 DT = £1.10

Metronidazole 500 mg Metronidazole 500mg tablets | 21 tablet PoM £40.75 DT = £9.42

▸ **Flagyl** (Purple Orchid Health Ltd)

Metronidazole 400 mg Flagyl 400mg tablets | 14 tablet PoM £6.34

Suppository

CAUTIONARY AND ADVISORY LABELS 3, 4, 9

▸ **Flagyl** (Purple Orchid Health Ltd)

Metronidazole 500 mg Flagyl 500mg suppositories | 10 suppository PoM £15.18 DT = £15.18

Metronidazole 1 gram Flagyl 1g suppositories | 10 suppository PoM £23.06 DT = £23.06

Oral suspension

CAUTIONARY AND ADVISORY LABELS 3, 4, 9

EXCIPIENTS: May contain Hydroxybenzoates (parabens), polysorbates, propylene glycol, sorbitol, sucrose

▸ **Metronidazole (Non-proprietary)**

Metronidazole (as Metronidazole benzoate) 40 mg per 1 ml Metronidazole 200mg/5ml oral suspension | 100 ml PoM £67.30 DT = £48.43

Vaginal gel

EXCIPIENTS: May contain Disodium edetate, hydroxybenzoates (parabens), propylene glycol

▸ **Zidoval** (Medical Valley Invest AB)

Metronidazole 7.5 mg per 1 gram Zidoval 0.75% vaginal gel | 40 gram PoM £4.31 DT = £4.31

Infusion

ELECTROLYTES: May contain Sodium

▸ **Metronidazole (Non-proprietary)**

Metronidazole 5 mg per 1 ml Metronidazole 500mg/100ml infusion 100ml Viaflo bags | 60 bag PoM £288.60 (Hospital only)
Metronidazole 500mg/100ml infusion polyethylene bottles | 20 bottle PoM £84.00 (Hospital only)

ANTIBACTERIALS › PENICILLINS

Penicillins

14-Jul-2021

Benzylpenicillin and phenoxymethylpenicillin

Benzylpenicillin sodium p. 415 (Penicillin G) remains an important and useful antibiotic but is inactivated by bacterial beta-lactamases. It is effective for many streptococcal (including pneumococcal), gonococcal, and meningococcal infections and also for anthrax, diphtheria, tetanus, gas-gangrene, and leptospirosis. It is also used in combination with gentamicin p. 378 for the empirical treatment of neonates with suspected early-onset infection (infection less than 72 hours after birth) and neonates who are in hospital with suspected sepsis within 72 hours of birth. Pneumococci, meningococci, and gonococci which have decreased sensitivity to penicillin have been isolated; benzylpenicillin sodium **is no longer the drug of first choice for pneumococcal meningitis**. Benzylpenicillin sodium is inactivated by gastric acid and absorption from the gastro-intestinal tract is low; therefore it must be given by injection.

Benzathine benzylpenicillin p. 414 or **procaine benzylpenicillin** are used in the treatment of syphilis.

Phenoxymethylpenicillin p. 416 (Penicillin V) has a similar antibacterial spectrum to benzylpenicillin sodium, but is less active. It is gastric acid-stable, so is suitable for oral administration. It should not be used for serious infections because absorption can be unpredictable and plasma concentrations variable. It is indicated principally for respiratory-tract infections in children, for streptococcal tonsillitis, and for continuing treatment after one or more injections of benzylpenicillin sodium when clinical response has begun. It should not be used for meningococcal or gonococcal infections. Phenoxymethylpenicillin is used for prophylaxis against streptococcal infections following rheumatic fever and against pneumococcal infections following splenectomy or in sickle cell disease.

Penicillinase-resistant penicillins

Most staphylococci are now resistant to benzylpenicillin sodium because they produce penicillinases. Flucloxacillin p. 424, however, is not inactivated by these enzymes and is thus effective in infections caused by penicillin-resistant staphylococci, which is the main indication for its use. Flucloxacillin is acid-stable and can, therefore, be given by mouth as well as by injection. Flucloxacillin is well absorbed from the gut.

Broad-spectrum penicillins

Ampicillin p. 419 is active against certain Gram-positive and Gram-negative organisms but is inactivated by penicillinases including those produced by *Staphylococcus aureus* and by common Gram-negative bacilli such as *Escherichia coli*. Ampicillin is also active against *Listeria* spp. and enterococci. Almost all staphylococci, approx. 60% of *E. coli* strains and approx. 20% of *Haemophilus influenzae* strains are now resistant. The likelihood of resistance should therefore be considered before using ampicillin for the 'blind' treatment of infections; in particular, it should not be used for hospital patients without checking sensitivity.

Ampicillin can be given by mouth, but less than half the dose is absorbed and absorption is further decreased by the presence of food in the gut. Ampicillin is well excreted in the bile and urine.

Amoxicillin p. 417 is a derivative of ampicillin and has a similar antibacterial spectrum. It is better absorbed than ampicillin when given by mouth, producing higher plasma and tissue concentrations; unlike ampicillin, absorption is not affected by the presence of food in the stomach.

Amoxicillin or ampicillin are principally indicated for the treatment of community-acquired pneumonia and middle ear infections, both of which may be due to *Streptococcus pneumoniae* and *H. influenzae*, and for urinary-tract infections. They are also used in the treatment of endocarditis and listerial meningitis. Amoxicillin is also used for the treatment of Lyme disease.

Maculopapular rashes occur commonly with ampicillin (and amoxicillin) but are not usually related to true penicillin allergy. They often occur in children with glandular fever; broad-spectrum penicillins should not therefore be used for 'blind' treatment of a sore throat. The risk of rash is also increased in children with acute or chronic lymphocytic leukaemia or in cytomegalovirus infection.

Co-amoxiclav p. 420 consists of amoxicillin with the beta-lactamase inhibitor clavulanic acid. Clavulanic acid itself has no significant antibacterial activity but, by inactivating beta-lactamases, it makes the combination active against beta-lactamase-producing bacteria that are resistant to amoxicillin. These include resistant strains of *Staph. aureus*, *E. coli*, and *H. influenzae*, as well as many *Bacteroides* and *Klebsiella* spp. Co-amoxiclav should be reserved for infections likely, or known, to be caused by amoxicillin-resistant beta-lactamase-producing strains.

A combination of ampicillin with flucloxacillin (as co-fluampicil p. 420) is available to treat infections involving either streptococci or staphylococci.

Antipseudomonal penicillins

Piperacillin, a ureidopenicillin, is only available in combination with the beta-lactamase inhibitor tazobactam. **Ticarcillin**, a carboxypenicillin, is only available in combination with the beta-lactamase inhibitor clavulanic acid. Both preparations have a broad spectrum of activity against a range of Gram-positive and Gram-negative bacteria, and anaerobes. Piperacillin with tazobactam p. 413 has activity against a wider range of Gram-negative organisms than ticarcillin with clavulanic acid and it is more active against *Pseudomonas aeruginosa*. These antibacterials are not active against MRSA. They are used in the treatment of septicaemia, hospital-acquired pneumonia, and complicated infections involving the urinary-tract, skin and soft tissue, or intra-abdomen. They may be used for the empirical treatment of septicaemia in immunocompromised children but otherwise should generally be reserved for serious infections resistant to other antibacterials. For severe pseudomonas infections these antipseudomonal penicillins can be given with an aminoglycoside (e.g. gentamicin) since they have a synergistic effect.

Piperacillin with tazobactam is used in cystic fibrosis for the treatment of *Ps. aeruginosa* colonisation when ciprofloxacin p. 429 and nebulised colistimethate sodium p. 426 have been ineffective; it can also be used in infective exacerbations, when it is combined with an aminoglycoside.

Mecillinams

Pivmecillinam hydrochloride p. 424 has significant activity against many Gram-negative bacteria including *Escherichia coli*, klebsiella, enterobacter, and salmonellae. It is not active against *Pseudomonas aeruginosa* or enterococci. Pivmecillinam hydrochloride is hydrolysed to mecillinam, which is the active drug.

Penicillins

● **DRUG ACTION** The penicillins are bactericidal and act by interfering with bacterial cell wall synthesis. They diffuse well into body tissues and fluids, but penetration into the cerebrospinal fluid is poor except when the meninges are inflamed. They are excreted in the urine in therapeutic concentrations.

IMPORTANT SAFETY INFORMATION

NHS ENGLAND NATIONAL PATIENT SAFETY ALERT: HARM FROM INCORRECT RECORDING OF A PENICILLIN ALLERGY AS A PENICILLAMINE ALLERGY (NOVEMBER 2025)

A review of national incident data has identified cases of penicillin allergy being recorded as penicillamine allergy in electronic prescribing systems by healthcare staff. The review identified one patient death as a result of an anaphylactic reaction to a penicillin-based antibiotic, which was inadvertently prescribed due to their penicillin allergy being documented as a penicillamine allergy on their GP record. All other relevant incidents were recorded as low or no harm due to healthcare staff identifying issues before it became clinically significant. To help resolve this issue and prevent reoccurrence, the following actions should be completed as soon as possible but no later than 20 November 2026:

- primary and secondary care organisations must form working groups to identify affected patients records, clinically review the accuracy of the allergy status, and update allergy records accordingly;
- in secondary care, allergy guidance and training must cover safe recording of allergy status in electronic prescribing systems and related digital healthcare systems, including checking and correcting allergy status on admission and discharge;
- in primary care, additional checks should be implemented when inputting allergy status into GP systems, particularly if this is completed by non-clinical staff;
- all organisations should work with digital system suppliers and user groups to develop technical mitigations and safety features (e.g. adding alerts and modifying search terms) to reduce the likelihood of inadvertent recording of the wrong allergy, and prioritise safe deployment of these upgrades once developed;
- the working group should strongly consider producing regular reports on allergy status until the issue is resolved.

● **CAUTIONS** History of allergy

● **SIDE-EFFECTS**

▶ **Common or very common** Diarrhoea · hypersensitivity · nausea · skin reactions · thrombocytopenia · vomiting

▶ **Uncommon** Arthralgia · leucopenia

▶ **Rare or very rare** Agranulocytosis · angioedema · haemolytic anaemia · hepatic disorders · nephritis tubulointerstitial · neutropenia · pseudomembranous enterocolitis · seizure · severe cutaneous adverse reactions (SCARs)

SIDE-EFFECTS, FURTHER INFORMATION Diarrhoea frequently occurs during oral penicillin therapy. It is most common with broad-spectrum penicillins, which can cause antibiotic-associated colitis.

● **ALLERGY AND CROSS-SENSITIVITY** The most important side-effect of the penicillins is hypersensitivity which causes rashes and anaphylaxis and can be fatal. Allergic reactions to penicillins occur in 1–10% of exposed individuals; anaphylactic reactions occur in fewer than 0.05% of treated patients. Patients with a history of atopic allergy (e.g. asthma, eczema, hay fever) are at a higher risk of anaphylactic reactions to penicillins. Individuals with a history of anaphylaxis, urticaria, or rash immediately after penicillin administration are at risk of immediate hypersensitivity to a penicillin; these individuals should not receive a penicillin. Individuals with a history of a minor rash (i.e. non-confluent, non-pruritic rash restricted to a small area of the body) or a rash that occurs more than 72 hours after penicillin administration are probably not allergic to penicillin and in these individuals a penicillin should not be withheld unnecessarily for serious infections; the possibility of an allergic reaction should, however, be borne in mind. Other beta-lactam antibiotics (including cephalosporins) can be used in these patients.

Patients who are allergic to one penicillin will be allergic to all because the hypersensitivity is related to the basic penicillin structure. Patients with a history of immediate hypersensitivity to penicillins may also react to the cephalosporins and other beta-lactam antibiotics, they should not receive these antibiotics. If a penicillin (or another beta-lactam antibiotic) is essential in an individual with immediate hypersensitivity to penicillin then specialist advice should be sought on hypersensitivity testing or using a beta-lactam antibiotic with a different structure to the penicillin that caused the hypersensitivity.

ANTIBACTERIALS > PENICILLINS, ANTIPSEUDOMONAL WITH BETA-LACTAMASE INHIBITOR

F 412

Piperacillin with tazobactam

10-Feb-2025

- **INDICATIONS AND DOSE**

Hospital-acquired pneumonia | Septicaemia | Complicated infections involving the urinary-tract | Complicated infections involving the skin | Complicated infections involving the soft-tissues

▶ BY INTRAVENOUS INFUSION

- Neonate: 90 mg/kg every 8 hours.
- Child 1 month–11 years: 90 mg/kg every 6–8 hours (max. per dose 4.5 g)
- Child 12–17 years: 4.5 g every 8 hours; increased if necessary to 4.5 g every 6 hours, increased frequency may be used for severe infections

Complicated intra-abdominal infections

▶ BY INTRAVENOUS INFUSION

- Child 2–11 years: 112.5 mg/kg every 8 hours (max. per dose 4.5 g)
- Child 12–17 years: 4.5 g every 8 hours; increased if necessary to 4.5 g every 6 hours, increased frequency may be used for severe infections

Acute exacerbation of bronchiectasis

▶ BY INTRAVENOUS INFUSION

- Child 1 month–11 years: 90 mg/kg every 6–8 hours (max. per dose 4.5 g)
- Child 12–17 years: 4.5 g every 8 hours; increased if necessary to 4.5 g every 6 hours, increased frequency may be used for severe infections

Infections in neutropenic patients

▶ BY INTRAVENOUS INFUSION

- Child: 90 mg/kg every 6 hours (max. per dose 4.5 g)

DOSE EQUIVALENCE AND CONVERSION

- Doses are expressed as piperacillin with tazobactam: the total of piperacillin and tazobactam components (both as sodium salts) in a ratio of 8:1.
- Piperacillin with tazobactam 4.5 g consists of piperacillin 4 g and tazobactam 500 mg; piperacillin with tazobactam 2.25 g consists of piperacillin 2 g and tazobactam 250 mg.

- **UNLICENSED USE** Not licensed for use in children under 12 years (except for children 2–12 years with neutropenia and complicated intra-abdominal infections).

EvGr Piperacillin with tazobactam is used for the treatment of acute exacerbation of bronchiectasis, (A) but is not licensed for this indication.

- **CAUTIONS** High doses may lead to hypernatraemia (owing to sodium content of preparations)
- **INTERACTIONS** → Appendix 1: penicillins
- **SIDE-EFFECTS**

▶ **Common or very common** Anaemia · candida infection · constipation · gastrointestinal discomfort · headache · insomnia

▶ **Uncommon** Flushing · hypokalaemia · hypotension · myalgia · thrombophlebitis

▶ **Rare or very rare** Epistaxis · stomatitis

▶ **Frequency not known** Eosinophilia · pancytopenia · pneumonia eosinophilic · renal failure · thrombocytosis

- **PREGNANCY** Manufacturers advise use only if potential benefit outweighs risk.
- **BREAST FEEDING** Trace amount in milk, but appropriate to use.
- **RENAL IMPAIRMENT**

Dose adjustments See p. 16.

EvGr *Child up to 12 years* 78.75 mg/kg (max. 4.5 g) every 8 hours if creatinine clearance less than 50 mL/minute.

Child 12–17 years max. 4.5 g every 8 hours if creatinine clearance 20–40 mL/minute; max. 4.5 g every 12 hours if creatinine clearance less than 20 mL/minute. (M)

- **EFFECT ON LABORATORY TESTS** False-positive urinary glucose (if tested for reducing substances).
- **DIRECTIONS FOR ADMINISTRATION** Displacement value may be significant when reconstituting injection, consult local guidelines. For *intravenous infusion*, dilute reconstituted solution to a concentration of 15–90 mg/mL with Glucose 5% *or* Sodium Chloride 0.9%; give over 30 minutes.
- **PRESCRIBING AND DISPENSING INFORMATION** For choice of antibacterial therapy, see Gastro-intestinal system infections, antibacterial therapy p. 367, Respiratory system infections, antibacterial therapy p. 371, Skin infections, antibacterial therapy p. 373, Urinary-tract infections p. 454.

- **MEDICINAL FORMS** There can be variation in the licensing of different medicines containing the same drug. Forms available from special-order manufacturers include: infusion, powder for solution for infusion

Powder for solution for infusion

ELECTROLYTES: May contain Sodium

▶ **Piperacillin with tazobactam (Non-proprietary)**

Tazobactam (as Tazobactam sodium) 250 mg, Piperacillin (as Piperacillin sodium) 2 gram Piperacillin 2g / Tazobactam 250mg powder for solution for infusion vials | 1 vial PoM £7.85 (Hospital only) | 10 vial PoM £7.65–£108.90 (Hospital only)

Tazobactam (as Tazobactam sodium) 500 mg, Piperacillin (as Piperacillin sodium) 4 gram Piperacillin 4g / Tazobactam 500mg powder for solution for infusion vials | 1 vial PoM £15.75–£19.97 (Hospital only) | 10 vial PoM £48.00–£223.90 (Hospital only)

▶ **Tazocin** (Pfizer Ltd)

Tazobactam (as Tazobactam sodium) 250 mg, Piperacillin (as Piperacillin sodium) 2 gram Tazocin 2g/0.25g powder for solution for infusion vials | 1 vial PoM £7.65 (Hospital only)

Tazobactam (as Tazobactam sodium) 500 mg, Piperacillin (as Piperacillin sodium) 4 gram Tazocin 4g/0.5g powder for solution for infusion vials | 1 vial PoM £15.17 (Hospital only)

ANTIBACTERIALS > PENICILLINS, BETA-LACTAMASE SENSITIVE

412

Benzathine benzylpenicillin
07-Apr-2026

(Benzathine penicillin G)

● **INDICATIONS AND DOSE**

Erysipelas | Yaws | Pinta | Prevention of secondary case of diphtheria

▶ BY DEEP INTRAMUSCULAR INJECTION

- Child (body-weight up to 30 kg): 0.6 million units for 1 dose, mid-lateral thigh muscle is the preferred site of injection
- Child (body-weight 30 kg and above): 1.2 million units for 1 dose, mid-lateral thigh muscle is the preferred site of injection

Early syphilis [primary, secondary, and early latent—less than 2 years since infection] | Asymptomatic contacts of patients with infectious syphilis

▶ BY DEEP INTRAMUSCULAR INJECTION

- Child 12–17 years: 2.4 million units for 1 dose, outer quadrant of the gluteus maximus or Hochstetter's ventrogluteal field is the preferred site of injection, in the third trimester of pregnancy (week 28 onwards) the dose should be repeated after 7 days

Late latent syphilis [more than 2 years since infection]

▶ BY DEEP INTRAMUSCULAR INJECTION

- Child 12–17 years: 2.4 million units once weekly for 3 weeks, outer quadrant of the gluteus maximus or Hochstetter's ventrogluteal field is the preferred site of injection

Prophylaxis of rheumatic fever [without cardiac involvement] | Prophylaxis of poststreptococcal glomerulonephritis [without cardiac involvement] | Prophylaxis of erysipelas [without cardiac involvement]

▶ BY DEEP INTRAMUSCULAR INJECTION

- Child (body-weight up to 30 kg): 0.6 million units every 3–4 weeks for at least 5 years or up to 21 years of age (whichever is longer), mid-lateral thigh muscle is the preferred site of injection in children
- Child (body-weight 30 kg and above): 1.2 million units every 3–4 weeks for at least 5 years or up to 21 years of age (whichever is longer), mid-lateral thigh muscle is the preferred site of injection in children

Prophylaxis of rheumatic fever [transient cardiac involvement] | Prophylaxis of poststreptococcal glomerulonephritis [transient cardiac involvement] | Prophylaxis of erysipelas [transient cardiac involvement]

▶ BY DEEP INTRAMUSCULAR INJECTION

- Child (body-weight up to 30 kg): 0.6 million units every 3–4 weeks for at least 10 years or up to 21 years of age (whichever is longer), mid-lateral thigh muscle is the preferred site of injection in children
- Child (body-weight 30 kg and above): 1.2 million units every 3–4 weeks for at least 10 years or up to 21 years of age (whichever is longer), mid-lateral thigh muscle is the preferred site of injection in children

Prophylaxis of rheumatic fever [persistent cardiac involvement] | Prophylaxis of poststreptococcal glomerulonephritis [persistent cardiac involvement] | Prophylaxis of erysipelas [persistent cardiac involvement]

▶ BY DEEP INTRAMUSCULAR INJECTION

- Child (body-weight up to 30 kg): 0.6 million units every 3–4 weeks for at least 10 years or up to 40 years of age (whichever is longer); life-long prophylaxis may be necessary, mid-lateral thigh muscle is the preferred site of injection in children
- Child (body-weight 30 kg and above): 1.2 million units every 3–4 weeks for at least 10 years or up to 40 years of age (whichever is longer); life-long prophylaxis may be necessary, mid-lateral thigh muscle is the preferred site of injection in children

● **UNLICENSED USE** UKHSA advises benzathine benzylpenicillin is used for the prevention of diphtheria, but is not licensed for this indication.

IMPORTANT SAFETY INFORMATION

When prescribing, dispensing, or administering, check that this is the correct preparation—benzathine benzylpenicillin is a long-acting form of benzylpenicillin and is **not** interchangeable with benzylpenicillin sodium.

SAFE PRACTICE

Benzathine benzylpenicillin has been confused with benzylpenicillin sodium; care must be taken to ensure the correct drug is prescribed and dispensed.

● **INTERACTIONS** → Appendix 1: penicillins

● **SIDE-EFFECTS**

- **Common or very common** Candida infection
- **Uncommon** Oral disorders
- **Rare or very rare** Nephropathy
- **Frequency not known** Antibiotic associated colitis · Hoigne's syndrome

● **ALLERGY AND CROSS-SENSITIVITY** Contra-indicated in patients allergic to peanuts or soya (contains phospholipids from soya lecithin).

● **PREGNANCY** Manufacturer advises not known to be harmful.

● **BREAST FEEDING** Manufacturer advises present in milk in small amounts but not known to be harmful. Monitor infant for effects on the gastrointestinal flora; discontinue breast feeding if diarrhoea, candidiasis or rash in the infant occur.

● **HEPATIC IMPAIRMENT** Manufacturer advises caution in impairment (possible risk of delayed metabolism and excretion in severe impairment).

● **RENAL IMPAIRMENT** Manufacturer advises caution in impairment (possible risk of delayed metabolism and excretion in severe impairment).

Dose adjustments Manufacturer advises reduce daily dose by 25% and give as a single dose if creatinine clearance 15–59 mL/minute; reduce daily dose by 50–80% and give in 2–3 divided doses if creatinine clearance less than 15 mL/minute (maximum 1–3 million units per day). See p. 16.

● **MONITORING REQUIREMENTS**

- Manufacturer advises observe the patient for hypersensitivity reactions for at least 30 minutes after the injection.
- Manufacturer advises monitor renal, hepatic and haematopoietic function periodically in patients on long-term treatment.

● **EFFECT ON LABORATORY TESTS** False-positive direct Coombs' test. False-positive urinary glucose. False-positive urobilinogen. False-positive urinary protein using precipitation techniques, the Folin-Ciocalteu-Lowry method, or the biuret method. False-positive urinary amino acids using the ninhydrin method. Increased levels of urinary 17-ketosteriods using the Zimmermann reaction.

● **DIRECTIONS FOR ADMINISTRATION** For *deep intramuscular injection*, reconstitute with Water for Injections *or* Lidocaine Hydrochloride Injection 1% (to reduce pain at injection site); inject slowly with low pressure. No more than 5 mL should be administered per injection site and do not administer into tissues with reduced perfusion. Avoid rubbing the injection site after the injection. For further information on reconstitution and administration—consult product literature.

- **PRESCRIBING AND DISPENSING INFORMATION** For choice of antibacterial therapy, see Antibacterials, use for prophylaxis p. 359, Genital system infections, antibacterial therapy p. 368.

- **MEDICINAL FORMS** There can be variation in the licensing of different medicines containing the same drug.

Powder for suspension for injection

EXCIPIENTS: May contain Lecithin, polysorbates

- Benzathine benzylpenicillin (Non-proprietary)
  Benzathine benzylpenicillin 1.2 mega unit Benzathine benzylpenicillin 1.2million unit powder for suspension for injection vials | 1 vial PoM £9.30 (Hospital only)
  Benzathine benzylpenicillin 2.4 mega unit Benzathine benzylpenicillin 2.4million unit powder for suspension for injection vials | 1 vial PoM £9.50 (Hospital only)

412

Benzylpenicillin sodium

10-Feb-2025

(Penicillin G)

- **INDICATIONS AND DOSE**

Mild to moderate susceptible infections | Throat infections | Otitis media | Pneumonia | Cellulitis

▶ BY INTRAMUSCULAR INJECTION, OR BY SLOW INTRAVENOUS INJECTION, OR BY INTRAVENOUS INFUSION

- Neonate up to 7 days: 25 mg/kg every 12 hours; increased if necessary to 25 mg/kg every 8 hours, intravenous route recommended in neonates.
- Neonate 7 days to 28 days: 25 mg/kg every 8 hours; increased if necessary to 50 mg/kg every 8 hours in severe infection, intravenous route recommended in neonates.
- Child: 25 mg/kg every 6 hours; increased if necessary to 50 mg/kg every 4–6 hours (max. per dose 2.4 g) in severe infection, intravenous route recommended in infants

Endocarditis (in combination with other antibacterial if necessary)

▶ BY SLOW INTRAVENOUS INJECTION, OR BY INTRAVENOUS INFUSION

- Child: 25 mg/kg every 4 hours; increased if necessary to 50 mg/kg every 4 hours (max. per dose 2.4 g)

Meningitis | Meningococcal disease

▶ BY INTRAVENOUS INFUSION

- Neonate up to 7 days: 50 mg/kg every 12 hours.
- Neonate 7 days to 28 days: 50 mg/kg every 8 hours.
- Child: 50 mg/kg every 4–6 hours (max. per dose 2.4 g)

Suspected meningococcal disease [pre-hospital treatment]

▶ BY INTRAVENOUS INJECTION, OR BY INTRAMUSCULAR INJECTION

- Neonate: 300 mg for 1 dose, administer prior to urgent transfer to hospital unless this will delay transfer.
- Child 1-11 months: 300 mg for 1 dose, administer prior to urgent transfer to hospital unless this will delay transfer
- Child 1-9 years: 600 mg for 1 dose, administer prior to urgent transfer to hospital unless this will delay transfer
- Child 10-17 years: 1.2 g for 1 dose, administer prior to urgent transfer to hospital unless this will delay transfer

Suspected bacterial meningitis [pre-hospital treatment where there is likely to be a clinically significant delay in transfer to hospital]

▶ BY INTRAVENOUS INJECTION, OR BY INTRAMUSCULAR INJECTION

- Child 1-11 months: 300 mg for 1 dose, administer prior to transfer to hospital
- Child 1-9 years: 600 mg for 1 dose, administer prior to transfer to hospital
- Child 10-17 years: 1.2 g for 1 dose, administer prior to transfer to hospital

Neonatal sepsis

▶ BY INTRAMUSCULAR INJECTION, OR BY SLOW INTRAVENOUS INJECTION, OR BY INTRAVENOUS INFUSION

- Neonate up to 7 days: 25 mg/kg every 12 hours; increased if necessary to 25 mg/kg every 8 hours, intravenous route recommended in neonates.
- Neonate 7 days to 28 days: 25 mg/kg every 8 hours; increased if necessary to 50 mg/kg every 8 hours in severe infection, intravenous route recommended in neonates.

Severe diphtheria [confirmed or probable] (in combination with a macrolide)

▶ BY SLOW INTRAVENOUS INJECTION, OR BY INTRAVENOUS INFUSION

- Child: 25 mg/kg every 6 hours for 14 days; increased if necessary to 50 mg/kg every 4–6 hours (max. per dose 2.4 g)

- **UNLICENSED USE** UKHSA advises benzylpenicillin sodium is used in the doses provided in BNF Publications for the treatment of diphtheria, but these may differ from those licensed.

IMPORTANT SAFETY INFORMATION

Intrathecal injection of benzylpenicillin sodium is **not** recommended.

When prescribing, dispensing, or administering, check that this is the correct preparation—benzylpenicillin sodium is a short-acting form of benzylpenicillin and is **not** interchangeable with benzathine benzylpenicillin.

SAFE PRACTICE

Benzylpenicillin sodium has been confused with benzathine benzylpenicillin; care must be taken to ensure the correct drug is prescribed and dispensed.

- **CAUTIONS** Accumulation of sodium from injection can occur with high doses
- **INTERACTIONS** → Appendix 1: penicillins
- **SIDE-EFFECTS**
  - ▶ **Common or very common** Fever · Jarisch-Herxheimer reaction
  - ▶ **Rare or very rare** Neurotoxicity
  - ▶ **Frequency not known** Coma
- **PREGNANCY** Not known to be harmful.
- **BREAST FEEDING** Trace amounts in milk, but appropriate to use.
- **RENAL IMPAIRMENT** Accumulation of sodium from injection can occur in renal failure. High doses may cause neurotoxicity, including cerebral irritation, convulsions, or coma.
  Dose adjustments Expert sources advise use normal dose every 8–12 hours if estimated glomerular filtration rate 10–50 mL/minute/1.73 m^2; use normal dose every 12 hours if estimated glomerular filtration rate less than 10 mL/minute/1.73 m^2. See p. 16.
- **EFFECT ON LABORATORY TESTS** False-positive urinary glucose (if tested for reducing substances).

5 Infection

- **DIRECTIONS FOR ADMINISTRATION** Intravenous route recommended in neonates and infants. For *intravenous infusion*, dilute with Glucose 5% *or* Sodium Chloride 0.9%; give over 15–30 minutes. Longer administration time is particularly important when using doses of 50 mg/kg (or greater) to avoid CNS toxicity.
- **PRESCRIBING AND DISPENSING INFORMATION** For choice of antibacterial therapy, see Cardiovascular system infections, antibacterial therapy p. 364, Central nervous system infections, antibacterial therapy p. 365, Respiratory system infections, antibacterial therapy p. 371, Skin infections, antibacterial therapy p. 373.

- **MEDICINAL FORMS** There can be variation in the licensing of different medicines containing the same drug. Forms available from special-order manufacturers include: infusion

Powder for solution for injection

ELECTROLYTES: May contain Sodium

- **Benzylpenicillin sodium (Non-proprietary)**
  Benzylpenicillin sodium 600 mg Benzylpenicillin sodium 600mg powder for solution for injection vials | 1 vial PoM £2.56 | 2 vial PoM £6.01 | 10 vial PoM £22.50-£25.59 | 25 vial PoM £75.12
  Benzylpenicillin sodium 1.2 gram Benzylpenicillin sodium 1.2g powder for solution for injection vials | 25 vial PoM £109.49

412

Phenoxymethylpenicillin

11-Nov-2021

(Penicillin V)

- **INDICATIONS AND DOSE**

Oral infections | Otitis media

▶ BY MOUTH

- Child 1-11 months: 62.5 mg 4 times a day, increased if necessary up to 12.5 mg/kg 4 times a day
- Child 1-5 years: 125 mg 4 times a day, increased if necessary up to 12.5 mg/kg 4 times a day
- Child 6-11 years: 250 mg 4 times a day, increased if necessary up to 12.5 mg/kg 4 times a day
- Child 12-17 years: 500 mg 4 times a day, increased if necessary up to 1 g 4 times a day

Acute sore throat

▶ BY MOUTH

- Child 1-11 months: 62.5 mg 4 times a day for 5–10 days, alternatively 125 mg twice daily for 5–10 days
- Child 1-5 years: 125 mg 4 times a day for 5–10 days, alternatively 250 mg twice daily for 5–10 days
- Child 6-11 years: 250 mg 4 times a day for 5–10 days, alternatively 500 mg twice daily for 5–10 days
- Child 12-17 years: 500 mg 4 times a day for 5–10 days, alternatively 1000 mg twice daily for 5–10 days

Prevention of recurrence of rheumatic fever

▶ BY MOUTH

- Child 1 month–5 years: 125 mg twice daily
- Child 6-17 years: 250 mg twice daily

Prevention of secondary case of invasive group A streptococcal infection

▶ BY MOUTH

- Neonate: 12.5 mg/kg every 6 hours (max. per dose 62.5 mg) for 10 days.
- Child 1-11 months: 62.5 mg every 6 hours for 10 days
- Child 1-5 years: 125 mg every 6 hours for 10 days
- Child 6-11 years: 250 mg every 6 hours for 10 days
- Child 12-17 years: 250–500 mg every 6 hours for 10 days

Prevention of pneumococcal infection in asplenia or in patients with sickle-cell disease

▶ BY MOUTH

- Child 1-11 months: 62.5 mg twice daily
- Child 1-4 years: 125 mg twice daily
- Child 5-17 years: 250 mg twice daily

Acute sinusitis

▶ BY MOUTH

- Child 1-11 months: 62.5 mg 4 times a day for 5 days
- Child 1-5 years: 125 mg 4 times a day for 5 days
- Child 6-11 years: 250 mg 4 times a day for 5 days
- Child 12-17 years: 500 mg 4 times a day for 5 days

- **UNLICENSED USE** EvGr Duration of treatment for acute sinusitis adheres to national guidelines. (A) See Sinusitis (acute) p. 870 for further information.
  Phenoxymethylpenicillin doses in BNF Publications may differ from product literature.
- **INTERACTIONS** → Appendix 1: penicillins
- **SIDE-EFFECTS** Circulatory collapse · coagulation disorder · eosinophilia · faeces soft · fever · increased risk of infection · neurotoxicity · oral disorders · paraesthesia
- **PREGNANCY** Not known to be harmful.
- **BREAST FEEDING** Trace amounts in milk, but appropriate to use.
- **EFFECT ON LABORATORY TESTS** False-positive urinary glucose (if tested for reducing substances).
- **PRESCRIBING AND DISPENSING INFORMATION** For choice of antibacterial therapy, see Antibacterials, use for prophylaxis p. 359, Nose infections, antibacterial therapy p. 370, Oral bacterial infections p. 370, Oropharyngeal infections, antibacterial therapy p. 883.
- **PATIENT AND CARER ADVICE**
  Medicines for Children leaflet: Penicillin V for bacterial infections www.medicinesforchildren.org.uk/medicines/penicillin-v-for-bacterial-infections/
  Medicines for Children leaflet: Penicillin V for prevention of pneumococcal infection www.medicinesforchildren.org.uk/medicines/penicillin-v-for-prevention-of-pneumococcal-infection/
- **PROFESSION SPECIFIC INFORMATION**
  Dental practitioners' formulary Phenoxymethylpenicillin Tablets may be prescribed. Phenoxymethylpenicillin Oral Solution may be prescribed.

- **MEDICINAL FORMS** There can be variation in the licensing of different medicines containing the same drug.

Oral tablet

CAUTIONARY AND ADVISORY LABELS 9, 23

- **Phenoxymethylpenicillin (Non-proprietary)**
  Phenoxymethylpenicillin (as Phenoxymethylpenicillin potassium) 250 mg Phenoxymethylpenicillin 250mg tablets | 28 tablet PoM £5.99 DT = £1.27
  Phenoxymethylpenicillin (as Phenoxymethylpenicillin potassium) 500 mg Phenoxymethylpenicillin 500mg tablets | 20 tablet PoM £3.99-£6.60 DT = £3.99

Oral solution

CAUTIONARY AND ADVISORY LABELS 9, 23

- **Phenoxymethylpenicillin (Non-proprietary)**
  Phenoxymethylpenicillin (as Phenoxymethylpenicillin potassium) 25 mg per 1 ml Phenoxymethylpenicillin 125mg/5ml oral solution | 100 ml PoM £25.00 DT = £1.44
  Phenoxymethylpenicillin 125mg/5ml oral solution sugar free | 100 ml PoM £25.00 DT = £3.01 SF
  Phenoxymethylpenicillin (as Phenoxymethylpenicillin potassium) 50 mg per 1 ml Phenoxymethylpenicillin 250mg/5ml oral solution | 100 ml PoM £35.00 DT = £1.98
  Phenoxymethylpenicillin 250mg/5ml oral solution sugar free | 100 ml PoM £35.00 DT = £2.14 SF

ANTIBACTERIALS > PENICILLINS, BROAD-SPECTRUM

412

Amoxicillin
16-Jan-2026

(Amoxycillin)

● **INDICATIONS AND DOSE**

Susceptible infections (e.g. sinusitis, salmonellosis, oral infections)

▶ BY MOUTH

- Neonate 7 days to 28 days: 30 mg/kg 3 times a day (max. per dose 125 mg).
- Child 1-11 months: 125 mg 3 times a day, increased if necessary up to 30 mg/kg 3 times a day
- Child 1-4 years: 250 mg 3 times a day, increased if necessary up to 30 mg/kg 3 times a day
- Child 5-11 years: 500 mg 3 times a day, increased if necessary up to 30 mg/kg 3 times a day (max. per dose 1 g)
- Child 12-17 years: 500 mg 3 times a day, increased if necessary up to 1 g 3 times a day, use increased dose in severe infections

▶ BY INTRAVENOUS INJECTION, OR BY INTRAVENOUS INFUSION

- Neonate up to 7 days: 30 mg/kg every 12 hours, increased if necessary to 60 mg/kg every 12 hours, increased dose used in severe infection.
- Neonate 7 days to 28 days: 30 mg/kg every 8 hours, increased if necessary to 60 mg/kg every 8 hours, increased dose used in severe infection.
- Child: 20–30 mg/kg every 8 hours (max. per dose 500 mg), increased if necessary to 40–60 mg/kg every 8 hours (max. per dose 1 g), increased dose used in severe infection

Community-acquired pneumonia

▶ BY MOUTH

- Child 1-2 months: 125 mg 3 times a day for 5 days, increased if necessary up to 30 mg/kg 3 times a day
- Child 3-11 months: 125 mg 3 times a day for 3 days, increased if necessary up to 30 mg/kg 3 times a day
- Child 1-4 years: 250 mg 3 times a day for 3 days, increased if necessary up to 30 mg/kg 3 times a day
- Child 5-11 years: 500 mg 3 times a day for 3 days, increased if necessary up to 30 mg/kg 3 times a day (max. per dose 1 g)
- Child 12-17 years: 500 mg 3 times a day for 5 days, increased if necessary up to 1 g 3 times a day

Acute exacerbation of bronchiectasis

▶ BY MOUTH

- Child 1-11 months: 125 mg 3 times a day for 7–14 days
- Child 1-4 years: 250 mg 3 times a day for 7–14 days
- Child 5-17 years: 500 mg 3 times a day for 7–14 days

Acute cough [if systemically very unwell or at higher risk of complications]

▶ BY MOUTH

- Child 1-11 months: 125 mg 3 times a day for 5 days
- Child 1-4 years: 250 mg 3 times a day for 5 days
- Child 5-17 years: 500 mg 3 times a day for 5 days

Acute otitis media

▶ BY MOUTH

- Child 1-11 months: 125 mg 3 times a day for 5–7 days
- Child 1-4 years: 250 mg 3 times a day for 5–7 days
- Child 5-17 years: 500 mg 3 times a day for 5–7 days

Cystic fibrosis (treatment of asymptomatic *Haemophilus influenzae* carriage or mild exacerbation)

▶ BY MOUTH

- Neonate 7 days to 28 days: 30 mg/kg 3 times a day (max. per dose 125 mg).
- Child 1-11 months: 125 mg 3 times a day, increased if necessary up to 30 mg/kg 3 times a day
- Child 1-4 years: 250 mg 3 times a day, increased if necessary up to 30 mg/kg 3 times a day
- Child 5-11 years: 500 mg 3 times a day, increased if necessary up to 30 mg/kg 3 times a day (max. per dose 1 g)
- Child 12-17 years: 500 mg 3 times a day, increased if necessary up to 1 g 3 times a day, use increased dose in severe infections

▶ BY INTRAVENOUS INJECTION, OR BY INTRAVENOUS INFUSION

- Neonate up to 7 days: 30 mg/kg every 12 hours, increased if necessary to 60 mg/kg every 12 hours, increased dose used in severe infection.
- Neonate 7 days to 28 days: 30 mg/kg every 8 hours, increased if necessary to 60 mg/kg every 8 hours, increased dose used in severe infection.
- Child: 20–30 mg/kg every 8 hours (max. per dose 500 mg), increased if necessary to 40–60 mg/kg every 8 hours (max. per dose 1 g), increased dose used in severe infection

Lyme disease (under expert supervision)

▶ BY MOUTH

- Neonate 7 days to 28 days: 30 mg/kg 3 times a day (max. per dose 125 mg) usual duration 2–4 weeks.

Lyme disease [erythema migrans and/or non-focal symptoms] | Lyme disease [affecting cranial nerves or peripheral nervous system]

▶ BY MOUTH

- Child 1 month-11 years (administered on expert advice) (body-weight up to 34 kg): 30 mg/kg 3 times a day for 21 days
- Child 1 month-11 years (administered on expert advice) (body-weight 34 kg and above): 1 g 3 times a day for 21 days
- Child 12-17 years (administered on expert advice): 1 g 3 times a day for 21 days

Lyme arthritis | Acrodermatitis chronica atrophicans

▶ BY MOUTH

- Child 1 month-11 years (administered on expert advice) (body-weight up to 34 kg): 30 mg/kg 3 times a day for 28 days
- Child 1 month-11 years (administered on expert advice) (body-weight 34 kg and above): 1 g 3 times a day for 28 days
- Child 12-17 years (administered on expert advice): 1 g 3 times a day for 28 days

Anthrax (treatment and post-exposure prophylaxis)

▶ BY MOUTH

- Child (body-weight up to 20 kg): 80 mg/kg daily in 3 divided doses
- Child (body-weight 20 kg and above): 500 mg 3 times a day

Listerial meningitis

▶ BY INTRAVENOUS INFUSION

- Neonate up to 7 days: 50–100 mg/kg every 12 hours.
- Neonate 7 days to 28 days: 50–100 mg/kg every 8 hours.
- Child: 50 mg/kg every 4–6 hours (max. per dose 2 g)

continued →

Group B streptococcal infection | Enterococcal endocarditis (in combination with another antibiotic)
▶ BY INTRAVENOUS INFUSION
- Neonate up to 7 days: 50 mg/kg every 12 hours.
- Neonate 7 days to 28 days: 50 mg/kg every 8 hours.
- Child: 50 mg/kg every 4–6 hours (max. per dose 2 g)

Prevention of pneumococcal infection in asplenia or in patients with sickle-cell disease—if cover also needed for *Haemophilus influenzae*
▶ BY MOUTH
- Child 1 month–4 years: 125 mg twice daily
- Child 5–11 years: 250 mg twice daily
- Child 12–17 years: 500 mg twice daily

***Helicobacter pylori* eradication in combination with clarithromycin and omeprazole**
▶ BY MOUTH
- Child 1–5 years: 250 mg twice daily
- Child 6–11 years: 500 mg twice daily
- Child 12–17 years: 1 g twice daily

***Helicobacter pylori* eradication in combination with metronidazole and omeprazole**
▶ BY MOUTH
- Child 1–5 years: 125 mg 3 times a day
- Child 6–11 years: 250 mg 3 times a day
- Child 12–17 years: 500 mg 3 times a day

Prophylaxis of recurrent urinary-tract infection in non-pregnant females [using single-dose antibacterial prophylaxis]
▶ BY MOUTH
- Child 16–17 years: 500 mg for 1 dose, dose to be taken following exposure to a trigger

Prophylaxis of recurrent urinary-tract infection [using daily antibacterial prophylaxis]
▶ BY MOUTH
- Child 16–17 years: 250 mg once daily, dose to be taken at night, seek specialist advice if considering use for prophylaxis during pregnancy, in male patients, or for recurrent upper urinary-tract infection or recurrent complicated lower urinary-tract infection

Prophylaxis of recurrent urinary-tract infection [using daily antibacterial prophylaxis] (initiated under specialist supervision)
▶ BY MOUTH
- Child 3–11 months: 62.5 mg once daily, dose to be taken at night
- Child 1–4 years: 125 mg once daily, dose to be taken at night
- Child 5–15 years: 250 mg once daily, dose to be taken at night

Lower urinary-tract infection in pregnancy
▶ BY MOUTH
- Child 12–17 years: 500 mg 3 times a day for 7 days

Lower urinary-tract infection
▶ BY MOUTH
- Child 3–11 months: 125 mg 3 times a day for 3 days
- Child 1–4 years: 250 mg 3 times a day for 3 days
- Child 5–15 years: 500 mg 3 times a day for 3 days

Asymptomatic bacteriuria in pregnancy
▶ BY MOUTH
- Child (body-weight 40 kg and above): 250–500 mg 3 times a day, alternatively 750–1000 mg twice daily

Urinary-tract infection (catheter-associated)
▶ BY MOUTH
- Child 3–11 months: 125 mg 3 times a day for 7 to 10 days
- Child 1–4 years: 250 mg 3 times a day for 7 to 10 days
- Child 5–15 years: 500 mg 3 times a day for 7 to 10 days
- Child 16–17 years: 500 mg 3 times a day for 7 days

● **UNLICENSED USE** Amoxicillin doses in BNF Publications may differ from those in product literature.

EvGr Duration of treatment for acute otitis media differs from product literature and adheres to national guidelines. Amoxicillin is used for the treatment of acute exacerbation of bronchiectasis, Ⓐ but is not licensed for this indication.

EvGr Amoxicillin is used for prophylaxis of recurrent urinary-tract infection, Ⓐ but is not licensed for this indication.

● **CAUTIONS**

GENERAL CAUTIONS Acute lymphocytic leukaemia (increased risk of erythematous rashes) · chronic lymphocytic leukaemia (increased risk of erythematous rashes) · cytomegalovirus infection (increased risk of erythematous rashes) · glandular fever (erythematous rashes common) · maintain adequate hydration with high doses (particularly during parenteral therapy)

SPECIFIC CAUTIONS
- With intravenous use Accumulation of sodium can occur with high parenteral doses

● **INTERACTIONS** → Appendix 1: penicillins

● **SIDE-EFFECTS**

GENERAL SIDE-EFFECTS
▶ **Rare or very rare** Antibiotic associated colitis · colitis haemorrhagic · crystalluria · dizziness · hyperkinesia · hypersensitivity vasculitis · mucocutaneous candidiasis
▶ **Frequency not known** Enterocolitis · Jarisch-Herxheimer reaction

SPECIFIC SIDE-EFFECTS
▶ **Rare or very rare**
- With oral use Black hairy tongue

● **PREGNANCY** Not known to be harmful.

● **BREAST FEEDING** Trace amount in milk, but appropriate to use.

● **HEPATIC IMPAIRMENT** Manufacturer advises caution.

● **RENAL IMPAIRMENT** Increased risk of convulsions. Accumulation of sodium from injection can occur in patients with renal impairment. Risk of crystalluria with high doses (particularly during parenteral therapy).

Dose adjustments See p. 16.

EvGr Reduce dose if estimated glomerular filtration rate 30 mL/minute/1.73 m^2 or less (consult product literature). Ⓜ

● **DIRECTIONS FOR ADMINISTRATION** Displacement value may be significant when reconstituting injection, consult local guidelines. Dilute intravenous injection to a concentration of 50 mg/mL (100 mg/mL for neonates). May be further diluted with Glucose 5% *or* Glucose 10% *or* Sodium chloride 0.9% *or* 0.45% for intravenous infusion. Give intravenous infusion over 30 minutes when using doses over 30 mg/kg.

● **PRESCRIBING AND DISPENSING INFORMATION** For choice of antibacterial therapy, see Anthrax p. 444, Antibacterials, use for prophylaxis p. 359, Cardiovascular system infections, antibacterial therapy p. 364, Central nervous system infections, antibacterial therapy p. 365, Ear infections, antibacterial therapy p. 366, Gastro-intestinal system infections, antibacterial therapy p. 367, Lyme disease p. 444, Nose infections, antibacterial therapy p. 370, Oral bacterial infections p. 370, Oropharyngeal infections, antibacterial therapy p. 883, Peptic ulceration p. 60, Respiratory system infections, antibacterial therapy p. 371, Urinary-tract infections p. 454.

● **PATIENT AND CARER ADVICE** Patient counselling is advised for amoxicillin oral suspension (use of oral dosing syringe).

Medicines for Children leaflet: Amoxicillin for bacterial infections www.medicinesforchildren.org.uk/medicines/amoxicillin-for-bacterial-infections/

● **PROFESSION SPECIFIC INFORMATION**

Dental practitioners' formulary Amoxicillin capsules may be prescribed. Amoxicillin sachets may be prescribed as Amoxicillin Oral Powder. Amoxicillin Oral Suspension may be prescribed.

● **MEDICINAL FORMS** There can be variation in the licensing of different medicines containing the same drug.

Powder for solution for injection

ELECTROLYTES: May contain Sodium

▸ Amoxicillin (Non-proprietary)

Amoxicillin (as Amoxicillin sodium) 250 mg Amoxicillin 250mg powder for solution for injection vials | 10 vial [PoM] £7.50 | 10 vial [PoM] £7.50 (Hospital only)

Amoxicillin (as Amoxicillin sodium) 500 mg Amoxicillin 500mg powder for solution for injection vials | 10 vial [PoM] £12.00 DT = £9.60 (Hospital only) | 10 vial [PoM] £12.00 DT = £9.60

Amoxicillin (as Amoxicillin sodium) 1 gram Amoxicillin 1g powder for solution for injection vials | 1 vial [PoM] £1.92 | 10 vial [PoM] £19.20 | 10 vial [PoM] £16.50 (Hospital only)

Oral suspension

CAUTIONARY AND ADVISORY LABELS 9

EXCIPIENTS: May contain Sucrose

▸ Amoxicillin (Non-proprietary)

Amoxicillin (as Amoxicillin trihydrate) 25 mg per 1 ml Amoxicillin 125mg/5ml oral suspension sugar free | 100 ml [PoM] £25.00 DT = £0.83 [SF]

Amoxicillin 125mg/5ml oral suspension | 100 ml [PoM] £2.20 DT = £0.93

Amoxicillin (as Amoxicillin trihydrate) 50 mg per 1 ml Amoxicillin 250mg/5ml oral suspension sugar free | 100 ml [PoM] £35.00 DT = £1.21 [SF]

Amoxicillin 250mg/5ml oral suspension | 100 ml [PoM] £35.00 DT = £1.38

Amoxicillin (as Amoxicillin trihydrate) 100 mg per 1 ml Amoxicillin 500mg/5ml oral suspension sugar free | 100 ml [PoM] £5.75–£10.32 DT = £10.18 [SF]

Oral capsule

CAUTIONARY AND ADVISORY LABELS 9

▸ Amoxicillin (Non-proprietary)

Amoxicillin (as Amoxicillin trihydrate) 250 mg Amoxicillin 250mg capsules | 15 capsule [PoM] [NHS] DT = £0.66 | 21 capsule [PoM] £8.99 DT = £0.92 | 500 capsule [PoM] £28.00–£120.00

Amoxicillin (as Amoxicillin trihydrate) 500 mg Amoxicillin 500mg capsules | 15 capsule [PoM] £7.85 DT = £0.85 | 21 capsule [PoM] £15.00 DT = £1.19 | 100 capsule [PoM] £5.67–£75.00

Powder for oral suspension

CAUTIONARY AND ADVISORY LABELS 9, 13

▸ Amoxicillin (Non-proprietary)

Amoxicillin (as Amoxicillin trihydrate) 3 gram Amoxicillin 3g oral powder sachets sugar free | 2 sachet [PoM] £46.00 DT = £44.49 [SF]

Combinations available: ***Co-amoxiclav***, p. 420

412

Ampicillin

24-Jul-2024

● **INDICATIONS AND DOSE**

Susceptible infections (including bronchitis, urinary-tract infections, otitis media, sinusitis, uncomplicated community-acquired pneumonia, salmonellosis)

▶ BY MOUTH

▸ Neonate 7 days to 20 days: 30 mg/kg 3 times a day (max. per dose 125 mg).

▸ Neonate 21 days to 28 days: 30 mg/kg 4 times a day (max. per dose 125 mg).

▸ Child 1–11 months: 125 mg 4 times a day, increased if necessary up to 30 mg/kg 4 times a day

▸ Child 1–4 years: 250 mg 4 times a day, increased if necessary up to 30 mg/kg 4 times a day

▸ Child 5–11 years: 500 mg 4 times a day, increased if necessary up to 30 mg/kg 4 times a day (max. per dose 1 g)

▸ Child 12–17 years: 500 mg 4 times a day, increased if necessary to 1 g 4 times a day, use increased dose in severe infection

▶ BY INTRAVENOUS INJECTION, OR BY INTRAVENOUS INFUSION

▸ Neonate up to 7 days: 30 mg/kg every 12 hours, increased if necessary to 60 mg/kg every 12 hours, increased dose used in severe infection, community-acquired pneumonia or salmonellosis.

▸ Neonate 7 days to 20 days: 30 mg/kg every 8 hours, increased if necessary to 60 mg/kg every 8 hours, increased dose used in severe infection, community-acquired pneumonia or salmonellosis.

▸ Neonate 21 days to 28 days: 30 mg/kg every 6 hours, increased if necessary to 60 mg/kg every 6 hours, increased dose used in severe infection, community-acquired pneumonia or salmonellosis.

▸ Child: 25 mg/kg every 6 hours (max. per dose 500 mg), increased if necessary to 50 mg/kg every 6 hours (max. per dose 1 g), increased dose used in severe infection

Group B streptococcal infection | Enterococcal endocarditis (in combination with another antibacterial)

▶ BY INTRAVENOUS INFUSION

▸ Neonate up to 7 days: 50 mg/kg every 12 hours.

▸ Neonate 7 days to 20 days: 50 mg/kg every 8 hours.

▸ Neonate 21 days to 28 days: 50 mg/kg every 6 hours.

▸ Child: 50 mg/kg every 4–6 hours (max. per dose 2 g)

Listerial meningitis

▶ BY INTRAVENOUS INFUSION

▸ Neonate up to 7 days: 100 mg/kg every 12 hours.

▸ Neonate 7 days to 20 days: 100 mg/kg every 8 hours.

▸ Neonate 21 days to 28 days: 100 mg/kg every 6 hours.

▸ Child: 50 mg/kg every 4–6 hours (max. per dose 2 g)

● **UNLICENSED USE** Ampicillin doses in BNF Publications may differ from those in product literature.

● **CAUTIONS**

GENERAL CAUTIONS Acute lymphocytic leukaemia (increased risk of erythematous rashes) · chronic lymphocytic leukaemia (increased risk of erythematous rashes) · cytomegalovirus infection (increased risk of erythematous rashes) · glandular fever (erythematous rashes common)

SPECIFIC CAUTIONS

▸ With intravenous use Accumulation of electrolytes contained in parenteral preparations can occur with high doses

● **INTERACTIONS** → Appendix 1: penicillins

● **SIDE-EFFECTS** Colitis haemorrhagic

● **PREGNANCY** Not known to be harmful.

● **BREAST FEEDING** Trace amounts in milk, but appropriate to use.

● **RENAL IMPAIRMENT** Rashes more common in renal impairment. Accumulation of sodium from injection can occur in patients with renal failure.

Dose adjustments [EvGr] Consider dose reduction or increase dose interval if creatinine clearance less than 10 mL/minute. ⟨M⟩ see p. 16.

● **DIRECTIONS FOR ADMINISTRATION**

▸ With oral use Administer at least 30 minutes before food.

▸ With intravenous use Displacement value may be significant when reconstituting injection, consult local guidelines. Dilute intravenous injection to a concentration of

50–100 mg/mL. May be further diluted with Glucose 5% or 10% *or* Sodium Chloride 0.9% or 0.45% for infusion. Give over 30 minutes when using doses of greater than 50 mg/kg to avoid CNS toxicity including convulsions.

- **PATIENT AND CARER ADVICE**
Medicines for Children leaflet: Ampicillin for infection www.medicinesforchildren.org.uk/medicines/ampicillin-for-infection/

- **MEDICINAL FORMS** There can be variation in the licensing of different medicines containing the same drug.

Oral capsule
CAUTIONARY AND ADVISORY LABELS 9, 23
▸ **Ampicillin (Non-proprietary)**
Ampicillin 500 mg Ampicillin 500mg capsules | 28 capsule PoM £47.96 DT = £47.96

Powder for solution for injection
▸ **Ampicillin (Non-proprietary)**
Ampicillin (as Ampicillin sodium) 500 mg Ampicillin 500mg powder for solution for injection vials | 10 vial PoM £82.22

F 412

Co-fluampicil

06-Feb-2025

- **INDICATIONS AND DOSE**

Mixed infections involving beta-lactamase-producing staphylococci
▸ BY MOUTH
▸ Child 10–17 years: 250/250 mg every 6 hours

Severe mixed infections involving beta-lactamase-producing staphylococci
▸ BY MOUTH
▸ Child 10–17 years: 500/500 mg every 6 hours

IMPORTANT SAFETY INFORMATION
HEPATIC DISORDERS
Cholestatic jaundice and hepatitis may occur very rarely, up to two months after treatment with flucloxacillin has been stopped. Administration for more than 2 weeks and increasing age are risk factors. Manufacturer advises:
- flucloxacillin should not be used in patients with a history of hepatic dysfunction associated with flucloxacillin;
- flucloxacillin should be used with caution in patients with hepatic impairment;
- careful enquiry should be made about hypersensitivity reactions to beta-lactam antibacterials.

- **CAUTIONS** Acute lymphocytic leukaemia (increased risk of erythematous rashes) · chronic lymphocytic leukaemia (increased risk of erythematous rashes) · cytomegalovirus infection (increased risk of erythematous rashes) · glandular fever (erythematous rashes common)
- **INTERACTIONS** → Appendix 1: penicillins
- **SIDE-EFFECTS** Bronchospasm · coma · dyspnoea · electrolyte imbalance · eosinophilia · erythema nodosum · gastrointestinal disorder · hallucination · Jarisch-Herxheimer reaction · myalgia · purpura non-thrombocytopenic · vasculitis
- **PREGNANCY** Not known to be harmful.
- **BREAST FEEDING** Trace amount in milk, but appropriate to use.
- **HEPATIC IMPAIRMENT** Manufacturer advises caution.
- **RENAL IMPAIRMENT**
Dose adjustments EvGr Reduce dose or frequency if creatinine clearance less than 10 mL/minute, Ⓜ see p. 16.
- **EFFECT ON LABORATORY TESTS** False-positive urinary glucose (if tested for reducing substances).
- **PRESCRIBING AND DISPENSING INFORMATION** Dose expressed as a combination of equal parts by mass of flucloxacillin and ampicillin.
- **MEDICINAL FORMS** No licensed medicines listed.

ANTIBACTERIALS › PENICILLINS, BROAD-SPECTRUM WITH BETA-LACTAMASE INHIBITOR

F 412

Co-amoxiclav

26-Jan-2026

- **INDICATIONS AND DOSE**

Infections due to beta-lactamase-producing strains (where amoxicillin alone not appropriate) [doses for 375 mg (250/125 mg) or 625 mg (500/125 mg) tablets]
▸ BY MOUTH USING TABLETS
▸ Child 12–17 years: 375 mg 3 times a day, alternatively 625 mg 3 times a day

Infections due to beta-lactamase-producing strains (where amoxicillin alone not appropriate) [doses for 1 g (875/125 mg) tablets]
▸ BY MOUTH USING TABLETS
▸ Child 6–17 years (body-weight 25–39 kg): 1 g twice daily
▸ Child 6–17 years (body-weight 40 kg and above): 1 g twice daily, alternatively 1 g 3 times a day

Infections due to beta-lactamase-producing strains (where amoxicillin alone not appropriate) [doses for 125/31 mg per 5 mL suspension]
▸ BY MOUTH USING ORAL SUSPENSION
▸ Neonate: 0.25 mL/kilogram 3 times a day.
▸ Child 1–11 months: 0.25 mL/kilogram 3 times a day, dose doubled if necessary
▸ Child 1–5 years: 0.25 mL/kilogram 3 times a day, dose doubled if necessary, alternatively 5 mL 3 times a day, dose doubled if necessary

Infections due to beta-lactamase-producing strains (where amoxicillin alone not appropriate) [doses for 250/62 mg per 5 mL suspension]
▸ BY MOUTH USING ORAL SUSPENSION
▸ Child 6–11 years: 0.15 mL/kilogram 3 times a day, dose doubled if necessary, alternatively 5 mL 3 times a day, dose doubled if necessary

Infections due to beta-lactamase-producing strains (where amoxicillin alone not appropriate) [doses for 400/57 mg per 5 mL suspension]
▸ BY MOUTH USING ORAL SUSPENSION
▸ Child 2–23 months: 0.15 mL/kilogram twice daily, dose doubled if necessary
▸ Child 2–6 years (body-weight 13–21 kg): 2.5 mL twice daily, dose doubled if necessary
▸ Child 7–12 years (body-weight 22–40 kg): 5 mL twice daily, dose doubled if necessary
▸ Child 12–17 years (body-weight 41 kg and above): 10 mL twice daily, alternatively 10 mL 3 times a day

Infections due to beta-lactamase-producing strains (where amoxicillin alone not appropriate) [doses for 600 mg (500/100 mg) or 1.2 g (1000/200 mg) injection]
▸ BY INTRAVENOUS INJECTION, OR BY INTRAVENOUS INFUSION
▸ Neonate: 30 mg/kg every 12 hours, intravenous infusion recommended in children less than 3 months.
▸ Child 1–2 months: 30 mg/kg every 12 hours, intravenous infusion recommended in children less than 3 months
▸ Child 3 months–17 years: 30 mg/kg every 8 hours (max. per dose 1.2 g)

Infections due to beta-lactamase-producing strains (where amoxicillin alone not appropriate) [doses for 2.2 g (2000/200 mg) injection]
▸ BY INTRAVENOUS INFUSION
▸ Neonate: 55 mg/kg every 12 hours.

- Child 1–2 months: 55 mg/kg every 12 hours
- Child 3 months–17 years (body-weight 4–39 kg): 55 mg/kg every 8 hours
- Child 3 months–17 years (body-weight 40 kg and above): 1.1 g every 8 hours, alternatively 2.2 g every 12 hours, increased if necessary to 2.2 g every 8 hours

Cellulitis [doses for 375 mg (250/125 mg) or 625 mg (500/125 mg) tablets] | Erysipelas [doses for 375 mg (250/125 mg) or 625 mg (500/125 mg) tablets]

▶ BY MOUTH USING TABLETS
- Child 12–17 years: 375 mg 3 times a day for 5–7 days then review (review after 7 days in severe infection or if infection near the eyes or nose), alternatively 625 mg 3 times a day for 5–7 days then review (review after 7 days in severe infection or if infection near the eyes or nose)

Cellulitis [doses for 125/31 mg per 5 mL suspension] | Erysipelas [doses for 125/31 mg per 5 mL suspension]

▶ BY MOUTH USING ORAL SUSPENSION
- Child 1–11 months: 0.25 mL/kilogram 3 times a day for 5–7 days then review (review after 7 days in severe infection or if infection near the eyes or nose), dose doubled if necessary
- Child 1–5 years: 0.25 mL/kilogram 3 times a day for 5–7 days then review (review after 7 days in severe infection or if infection near the eyes or nose), dose doubled if necessary, alternatively 5 mL 3 times a day for 5–7 days then review (review after 7 days in severe infection or if infection near the eyes or nose), dose doubled if necessary

Cellulitis [doses for 250/62 mg per 5 mL suspension] | Erysipelas [doses for 250/62 mg per 5 mL suspension]

▶ BY MOUTH USING ORAL SUSPENSION
- Child 6–11 years: 0.15 mL/kilogram 3 times a day for 5–7 days then review (review after 7 days in severe infection or if infection near the eyes or nose), dose doubled if necessary, alternatively 5 mL 3 times a day for 5–7 days then review (review after 7 days in severe infection or if infection near the eyes or nose), dose doubled if necessary

Cellulitis [doses for 600 mg (500/100 mg) or 1.2 g (1000/200 mg) injection] | Erysipelas [doses for 600 mg (500/100 mg) or 1.2 g (1000/200 mg) injection]

▶ BY INTRAVENOUS INJECTION, OR BY INTRAVENOUS INFUSION
- Child 1–2 months: 30 mg/kg every 12 hours, intravenous infusion recommended in children less than 3 months
- Child 3 months–17 years: 30 mg/kg every 8 hours (max. per dose 1.2 g)

Prophylaxis of infection from human bites [doses for 375 mg (250/125 mg) or 625 mg (500/125 mg) tablets] | Prophylaxis of infection from animal bites [doses for 375 mg (250/125 mg) or 625 mg (500/125 mg) tablets]

▶ BY MOUTH USING TABLETS
- Child 12–17 years: 375 mg 3 times a day for 3 days, alternatively 625 mg 3 times a day for 3 days

Prophylaxis of infection from human bites [doses for 125/31 mg per 5 mL suspension] | Prophylaxis of infection from animal bites [doses for 125/31 mg per 5 mL suspension]

▶ BY MOUTH USING ORAL SUSPENSION
- Child 1–11 months: 0.25 mL/kilogram 3 times a day for 3 days
- Child 1–5 years: 0.25 mL/kilogram 3 times a day for 3 days, alternatively 5 mL 3 times a day for 3 days

Prophylaxis of infection from human bites [doses for 250/62 mg per 5 mL suspension] | Prophylaxis of infection from animal bites [doses for 250/62 mg per 5 mL suspension]

▶ BY MOUTH USING ORAL SUSPENSION
- Child 6–11 years: 0.15 mL/kilogram 3 times a day for 3 days, alternatively 5 mL 3 times a day for 3 days

Prophylaxis of infection from human bites [doses for 600 mg (500/100 mg) or 1.2 g (1000/200 mg) injection] | Prophylaxis of infection from animal bites [doses for 600 mg (500/100 mg) or 1.2 g (1000/200 mg) injection]

▶ BY INTRAVENOUS INJECTION, OR BY INTRAVENOUS INFUSION
- Child 1–2 months: 30 mg/kg every 12 hours, intravenous infusion recommended in children less than 3 months
- Child 3 months–17 years: 30 mg/kg every 8 hours (max. per dose 1.2 g)

Treatment of infection from human bites [doses for 375 mg (250/125 mg) or 625 mg (500/125 mg) tablets] | Treatment of infection from animal bites [doses for 375 mg (250/125 mg) or 625 mg (500/125 mg) tablets]

▶ BY MOUTH USING TABLETS
- Child 12–17 years: 375 mg 3 times a day for 5–7 days, alternatively 625 mg 3 times a day for 5–7 days

Treatment of infection from human bites [doses for 125/31 mg per 5 mL suspension] | Treatment of infection from animal bites [doses for 125/31 mg per 5 mL suspension]

▶ BY MOUTH USING ORAL SUSPENSION
- Child 1–11 months: 0.25 mL/kilogram 3 times a day for 5–7 days
- Child 1–5 years: 0.25 mL/kilogram 3 times a day for 5–7 days, alternatively 5 mL 3 times a day for 5–7 days

Treatment of infection from human bites [doses for 250/62 mg per 5 mL suspension] | Treatment of infection from animal bites [doses for 250/62 mg per 5 mL suspension]

▶ BY MOUTH USING ORAL SUSPENSION
- Child 6–11 years: 0.15 mL/kilogram 3 times a day for 5–7 days, alternatively 5 mL 3 times a day for 5–7 days

Treatment of infection from human bites [doses for 600 mg (500/100 mg) or 1.2 g (1000/200 mg) injection] | Treatment of infection from animal bites [doses for 600 mg (500/100 mg) or 1.2 g (1000/200 mg) injection]

▶ BY INTRAVENOUS INJECTION, OR BY INTRAVENOUS INFUSION
- Child 1–2 months: 30 mg/kg every 12 hours, intravenous infusion recommended in children less than 3 months
- Child 3 months–17 years: 30 mg/kg every 8 hours (max. per dose 1.2 g)

Severe dental infection with spreading cellulitis [doses for 375 mg (250/125 mg) tablets] | Dental infection not responding to first-line antibacterial [doses for 375 mg (250/125 mg) tablets]

▶ BY MOUTH USING TABLETS
- Child 12–17 years: 375 mg 3 times a day for 5 days

Community-acquired pneumonia [doses for 625 mg (500/125 mg) tablets]

▶ BY MOUTH USING TABLETS
- Child 12–17 years: 625 mg 3 times a day for 5 days

Community-acquired pneumonia [doses for 125/31 mg per 5 mL suspension]

▶ BY MOUTH USING ORAL SUSPENSION
- Child 1–11 months: 0.5 mL/kilogram 3 times a day for 5 days
- Child 1–5 years: 0.5 mL/kilogram 3 times a day for 5 days, alternatively 10 mL 3 times a day for 5 days

Community-acquired pneumonia [doses for 250/62 mg per 5 mL suspension]

▶ BY MOUTH USING ORAL SUSPENSION
- Child 6–11 years: 0.3 mL/kilogram 3 times a day for 5 days, alternatively 10 mL 3 times a day for 5 days

continued →

Community-acquired pneumonia [doses for 600 mg (500/100 mg) or 1.2 g (1000/200 mg) injection]
- ▶ BY INTRAVENOUS INJECTION, OR BY INTRAVENOUS INFUSION
  - Child 1–2 months: 30 mg/kg every 12 hours, intravenous infusion recommended in children less than 3 months
  - Child 3 months–17 years: 30 mg/kg every 8 hours (max. per dose 1.2 g)

Hospital-acquired pneumonia [doses for 625 mg (500/125 mg) tablets]
- ▶ BY MOUTH USING TABLETS
  - Child 12–17 years: 625 mg 3 times a day for 5 days then review

Hospital-acquired pneumonia [doses for 125/31 mg per 5 mL suspension]
- ▶ BY MOUTH USING ORAL SUSPENSION
  - Child 1–11 months: 0.5 mL/kilogram 3 times a day for 5 days then review
  - Child 1–5 years: 0.5 mL/kilogram 3 times a day for 5 days then review, alternatively 10 mL 3 times a day for 5 days then review

Hospital-acquired pneumonia [doses for 250/62 mg per 5 mL suspension]
- ▶ BY MOUTH USING ORAL SUSPENSION
  - Child 6–11 years: 0.3 mL/kilogram 3 times a day for 5 days then review, alternatively 10 mL 3 times a day for 5 days then review

Acute exacerbation of bronchiectasis [doses for 375 mg (250/125 mg) or 625 mg (500/125 mg) tablets]
- ▶ BY MOUTH USING TABLETS
  - Child 12–17 years: 375 mg 3 times a day for 7–14 days, alternatively 625 mg 3 times a day for 7–14 days

Acute exacerbation of bronchiectasis [doses for 125/31 mg per 5 mL suspension]
- ▶ BY MOUTH USING ORAL SUSPENSION
  - Child 1–11 months: 0.25 mL/kilogram 3 times a day for 7–14 days
  - Child 1–5 years: 0.25 mL/kilogram 3 times a day for 7–14 days, alternatively 5 mL 3 times a day for 7–14 days

Acute exacerbation of bronchiectasis [doses for 250/62 mg per 5 mL suspension]
- ▶ BY MOUTH USING ORAL SUSPENSION
  - Child 6–11 years: 0.15 mL/kilogram 3 times a day for 7–14 days, alternatively 5 mL 3 times a day for 7–14 days

Acute exacerbation of bronchiectasis [doses for 600 mg (500/100 mg) or 1.2 g (1000/200 mg) injection]
- ▶ BY INTRAVENOUS INJECTION, OR BY INTRAVENOUS INFUSION
  - Child 1–2 months: 30 mg/kg every 12 hours, intravenous infusion is recommended in children less than 3 months
  - Child 3 months–17 years: 30 mg/kg every 8 hours (max. per dose 1.2 g)

Acute sinusitis [doses for 375 mg (250/125 mg) or 625 mg (500/125 mg) tablets]
- ▶ BY MOUTH USING TABLETS
  - Child 12–17 years: 375 mg 3 times a day for 5 days, alternatively 625 mg 3 times a day for 5 days

Acute sinusitis [doses for 125/31 mg per 5 mL suspension]
- ▶ BY MOUTH USING ORAL SUSPENSION
  - Child 1–11 months: 0.25 mL/kilogram 3 times a day for 5 days
  - Child 1–5 years: 0.25 mL/kilogram 3 times a day for 5 days, alternatively 5 mL 3 times a day for 5 days

Acute sinusitis [doses for 250/62 mg per 5 mL suspension]
- ▶ BY MOUTH USING ORAL SUSPENSION
  - Child 6–11 years: 0.15 mL/kilogram 3 times a day for 5 days, alternatively 5 mL 3 times a day for 5 days

Acute otitis media [doses for 375 mg (250/125 mg) or 625 mg (500/125 mg) tablets]
- ▶ BY MOUTH USING TABLETS
  - Child 12–17 years: 375 mg 3 times a day for 5–7 days, alternatively 625 mg 3 times a day for 5–7 days

Acute otitis media [doses for 125/31 mg per 5 mL suspension]
- ▶ BY MOUTH USING ORAL SUSPENSION
  - Child 1–11 months: 0.25 mL/kilogram 3 times a day for 5–7 days
  - Child 1–5 years: 0.25 mL/kilogram 3 times a day for 5–7 days, alternatively 5 mL 3 times a day for 5–7 days

Acute otitis media [doses for 250/62 mg per 5 mL suspension]
- ▶ BY MOUTH USING ORAL SUSPENSION
  - Child 6–11 years: 0.15 mL/kilogram 3 times a day for 5–7 days, alternatively 5 mL 3 times a day for 5–7 days

Acute pyelonephritis [doses for 375 mg (250/125 mg) or 625 mg (500/125 mg) tablets] | Urinary-tract infection (catheter-associated) [doses for 375 mg (250/125 mg) or 625 mg (500/125 mg) tablets]
- ▶ BY MOUTH USING TABLETS
  - Child 12–15 years: 375 mg 3 times a day for 7–10 days, alternatively 625 mg 3 times a day for 7–10 days
  - Child 16–17 years: 625 mg 3 times a day for 7–10 days

Acute pyelonephritis [doses for 125/31 mg per 5 mL suspension] | Urinary-tract infection (catheter-associated) [doses for 125/31 mg per 5 mL suspension]
- ▶ BY MOUTH USING ORAL SUSPENSION
  - Child 3–11 months: 0.25 mL/kilogram 3 times a day for 7–10 days, dose doubled if necessary
  - Child 1–5 years: 0.25 mL/kilogram 3 times a day for 7–10 days, dose doubled if necessary, alternatively 5 mL 3 times a day for 7–10 days, dose doubled if necessary

Acute pyelonephritis [doses for 250/62 mg per 5 mL suspension] | Urinary-tract infection (catheter-associated) [doses for 250/62 mg per 5 mL suspension]
- ▶ BY MOUTH USING ORAL SUSPENSION
  - Child 6–11 years: 0.15 mL/kilogram 3 times a day for 7–10 days, dose doubled if necessary, alternatively 5 mL 3 times a day for 7–10 days, dose doubled if necessary

Acute pyelonephritis [doses for 600 mg (500/100 mg) or 1.2 g (1000/200 mg) injection] | Urinary-tract infection (catheter-associated) [doses for 600 mg (500/100 mg) or 1.2 g (1000/200 mg) injection]
- ▶ BY INTRAVENOUS INJECTION, OR BY INTRAVENOUS INFUSION
  - Child 3 months–15 years: 30 mg/kg every 8 hours (max. per dose 1.2 g)
  - Child 16–17 years: 1.2 g every 8 hours

DOSE EQUIVALENCE AND CONVERSION
- Doses are expressed as co-amoxiclav: the total of amoxicillin (as the trihydrate or as the sodium salt) and clavulanic acid (as potassium clavulanate) components.
- Co-amoxiclav preparations contain different ratios of amoxicillin and clavulanic acid to enable appropriate dosing of amoxicillin without exceeding the maximum daily dose of clavulanic acid.
- For *tablets*, co-amoxiclav 375 mg consists of amoxicillin 250 mg and clavulanic acid 125 mg (2:1); co-amoxiclav 625 mg consists of amoxicillin 500 mg and clavulanic acid 125 mg (4:1); co-amoxiclav 1 g consists of amoxicillin 875 mg and clavulanic acid 125 mg (7:1).
- For *oral suspension*, co-amoxiclav 125/31 mg per 5 mL consists of amoxicillin 125 mg and clavulanic acid 31 mg per 5 mL (4:1); co-amoxiclav 250/62 mg per 5 mL consists of amoxicillin 250 mg and clavulanic acid

62 mg per 5 mL (4:1); co-amoxiclav 400/57 mg per 5 mL consists of amoxicillin 400 mg and clavulanic acid 57 mg per 5 mL (7:1).
- For *injection*, co-amoxiclav 600 mg consists of amoxicillin 500 mg and clavulanic acid 100 mg (5:1); co-amoxiclav 1.2 g consists of amoxicillin 1 g and clavulanic acid 200 mg (5:1); co-amoxiclav 2.2 g consists of amoxicillin 2 g and clavulanic acid 200 mg (10:1).

- **UNLICENSED USE** Co-amoxiclav may be used as detailed below, although these situations are considered unlicensed:
  - EvGr treatment of acute exacerbation of bronchiectasis
  - treatment of hospital-acquired pneumonia
  - duration of treatment for acute sinusitis
  - duration of treatment for acute otitis media (A)

IMPORTANT SAFETY INFORMATION
Co-amoxiclav preparations contain different ratios of amoxicillin and clavulanic acid to enable appropriate dosing of amoxicillin without exceeding the maximum daily dose of clavulanic acid.

- **CONTRA-INDICATIONS** History of co-amoxiclav-associated jaundice or hepatic dysfunction · history of penicillin-associated jaundice or hepatic dysfunction
- **CAUTIONS**

GENERAL CAUTIONS Acute lymphocytic leukaemia (increased risk of erythematous rashes) · chronic lymphocytic leukaemia (increased risk of erythematous rashes) · cytomegalovirus infection (increased risk of erythematous rashes) · glandular fever (erythematous rashes common) · maintain adequate hydration with high doses (particularly during parental therapy)

SPECIFIC CAUTIONS
- With intravenous use Accumulation of electrolytes contained in parenteral preparations can occur with high doses

- **INTERACTIONS** → Appendix 1: penicillins
- **SIDE-EFFECTS**

GENERAL SIDE-EFFECTS
- **Common or very common** Increased risk of infection
- **Uncommon** Dizziness · dyspepsia · headache
- **Frequency not known** Acute kidney injury · antibiotic associated colitis · colitis haemorrhagic · crystalluria · enterocolitis · hypersensitivity vasculitis · Kounis syndrome · meningitis aseptic · pancreatitis acute

SPECIFIC SIDE-EFFECTS
- With oral use Akathisia · black hairy tongue

SIDE-EFFECTS, FURTHER INFORMATION Hepatic events have been rarely reported in children. Signs and symptoms usually occur during or shortly after treatment but in some cases may occur several weeks after discontinuation.

- **PREGNANCY** Specialist sources indicate not known to be harmful. Avoid in preterm prelabour rupture of the membranes (PPROM)—possible increased risk of necrotising enterocolitis in the neonate.
- **BREAST FEEDING** Trace amount in milk, but appropriate to use.
- **HEPATIC IMPAIRMENT** Manufacturer advises caution.
Monitoring Monitor liver function in liver disease.
- **RENAL IMPAIRMENT** Risk of crystalluria with high doses (particularly during parenteral therapy).
  - With intravenous use Accumulation of electrolytes contained in parenteral preparations can occur in patients with renal failure.

Dose adjustments See p. 16.
- With oral use *Co-amoxiclav 375 mg (250/125 mg) tablets, 625 mg (500/125 mg) tablets, 125/31 mg per 5 mL suspension, or 250/62 mg per 5 mL suspension* : use normal dose every 12 hours if estimated glomerular filtration rate 10–30 mL/minute/1.73 m^2. Use the normal dose recommended for mild or moderate infections every 12 hours if estimated glomerular filtration rate less than 10 mL/minute/1.73 m^2. EvGr *Co-amoxiclav 1 g (875/125 mg) tablets or 400/57 mg per 5 mL suspension*: avoid if creatinine clearance less than 30 mL/minute. (M)
- With intravenous use *Co-amoxiclav 600 mg (500/100 mg) injection or 1.2 g (1000/200 mg) injection* : use normal initial dose and then use half normal dose every 12 hours if estimated glomerular filtration rate 10–30 mL/minute/1.73 m^2; use normal initial dose and then use half normal dose every 24 hours if estimated glomerular filtration rate less than 10 mL/minute/1.73 m^2. EvGr *Co-amoxiclav 2.2 g (2000/200 mg) injection*: avoid if creatinine clearance less than 30 mL/minute. (M)

- **DIRECTIONS FOR ADMINISTRATION** For *intermittent intravenous infusion using 600 mg (500/100 mg) or 1.2 g (1000/200 mg) injection*, dilute reconstituted solution to a concentration of 10 mg/mL with Sodium Chloride 0.9%; give over 30–40 minutes. For *intermittent intravenous infusion using 2.2 g (2000/200 mg) injection*, reconstitute 2.2 g initially with 20 mL Water for Injections, then dilute with at least 100 mL Sodium Chloride 0.9%; give over 30–40 minutes. For *intravenous injection using 600 mg (500/100 mg) or 1.2 g (1000/200 mg) injection*, administer over 3–4 minutes.
- **PRESCRIBING AND DISPENSING INFORMATION** For choice of antibacterial therapy, see Antibacterials, principles of therapy p. 358, Antibacterials, use for prophylaxis p. 359, Ear infections, antibacterial therapy p. 366, Nose infections, antibacterial therapy p. 370, Respiratory system infections, antibacterial therapy p. 371, Skin infections, antibacterial therapy p. 373, Urinary-tract infections p. 454.
- **PATIENT AND CARER ADVICE**
Medicines for Children leaflet: Co-amoxiclav for bacterial infections www.medicinesforchildren.org.uk/medicines/co-amoxiclav-for-bacterial-infections/
- **PROFESSION SPECIFIC INFORMATION**

Dental practitioners' formulary Co-amoxiclav 375 mg (250/125 mg) Tablets may be prescribed. Co-amoxiclav 125/31 mg per 5 mL Suspension may be prescribed. Co-amoxiclav 250/62 mg per 5 mL Suspension may be prescribed.

- **MEDICINAL FORMS** There can be variation in the licensing of different medicines containing the same drug. Forms available from special-order manufacturers include: infusion

Oral tablet

CAUTIONARY AND ADVISORY LABELS 9
- **Co-amoxiclav (Non-proprietary)**
  - **Clavulanic acid (as Potassium clavulanate) 125 mg, Amoxicillin (as Amoxicillin trihydrate) 250 mg** Co-amoxiclav 250mg/125mg tablets | 21 tablet PoM £6.00 DT = £1.50
  - **Clavulanic acid (as Potassium clavulanate) 125 mg, Amoxicillin (as Amoxicillin trihydrate) 500 mg** Co-amoxiclav 500mg/125mg tablets | 15 tablet PoM £4.96–£6.84 | 21 tablet PoM £12.00 DT = £1.86
  - **Clavulanic acid (as Potassium clavulanate) 125 mg, Amoxicillin (as Amoxicillin trihydrate) 875 mg** Co-amoxiclav 875mg/125mg tablets | 14 tablet PoM £5.99 DT = £5.99
- **Augmentin** (GlaxoSmithKline UK Ltd)
  - **Clavulanic acid (as Potassium clavulanate) 125 mg, Amoxicillin (as Amoxicillin trihydrate) 250 mg** Augmentin 375mg tablets | 21 tablet PoM £5.03 DT = £1.50
  - **Clavulanic acid (as Potassium clavulanate) 125 mg, Amoxicillin (as Amoxicillin trihydrate) 500 mg** Augmentin 625mg tablets | 21 tablet PoM £9.60 DT = £1.86

Oral suspension

CAUTIONARY AND ADVISORY LABELS 9

EXCIPIENTS: May contain Aspartame

▸ **Co-amoxiclav (Non-proprietary)**

Clavulanic acid (as Potassium clavulanate) 6.25 mg per 1 ml, Amoxicillin (as Amoxicillin trihydrate) 25 mg per 1 ml Co-amoxiclav 125mg/31mg/5ml oral suspension | 100 ml [PoM] £7.94 DT = £3.54

Clavulanic acid (as Potassium clavulanate) 12.5 mg per 1 ml, Amoxicillin (as Amoxicillin trihydrate) 50 mg per 1 ml Co-amoxiclav 250mg/62mg/5ml oral suspension | 100 ml [PoM] £8.02 DT = £3.60

Co-amoxiclav 250mg/62mg/5ml oral suspension sugar free | 100 ml [PoM] £6.25 DT = £6.25 [SF]

Clavulanic acid (as Potassium clavulanate) 11.4 mg per 1 ml, Amoxicillin (as Amoxicillin trihydrate) 80 mg per 1 ml Co-amoxiclav 400mg/57mg/5ml oral suspension | 35 ml [PoM] £4.13 DT = £4.13 | 70 ml [PoM] £5.79 DT = £5.79

Co-amoxiclav 400mg/57mg/5ml oral suspension sugar free | 70 ml [PoM] £6.97 DT = £3.65 [SF]

▸ **Augmentin** (GlaxoSmithKline UK Ltd)

Clavulanic acid (as Potassium clavulanate) 6.25 mg per 1 ml, Amoxicillin (as Amoxicillin trihydrate) 25 mg per 1 ml Augmentin 125/31 oral suspension | 100 ml [PoM] £3.54 DT = £3.54

Clavulanic acid (as Potassium clavulanate) 12.5 mg per 1 ml, Amoxicillin (as Amoxicillin trihydrate) 50 mg per 1 ml Augmentin 250/62 oral suspension | 100 ml [PoM] £3.60 DT = £3.60

▸ **Augmentin-Duo** (GlaxoSmithKline UK Ltd)

Clavulanic acid (as Potassium clavulanate) 11.4 mg per 1 ml, Amoxicillin (as Amoxicillin trihydrate) 80 mg per 1 ml Augmentin-Duo 400/57 oral suspension | 35 ml [PoM] £4.13 DT = £4.13 | 70 ml [PoM] £5.79 DT = £5.79

Powder for solution for injection

ELECTROLYTES: May contain Potassium, sodium

▸ **Co-amoxiclav (Non-proprietary)**

Clavulanic acid (as Potassium clavulanate) 100 mg, Amoxicillin (as Amoxicillin sodium) 500 mg Co-amoxiclav 500mg/100mg powder for solution for injection vials | 10 vial [PoM] £10.60–£17.14 (Hospital only)

Clavulanic acid (as Potassium clavulanate) 200 mg, Amoxicillin (as Amoxicillin sodium) 1000 mg Co-amoxiclav 1000mg/200mg powder for solution for injection vials | 10 vial [PoM] £14.85–£50.00 (Hospital only)

ANTIBACTERIALS › PENICILLINS, MECILLINAM-TYPE

F 412

Pivmecillinam hydrochloride

29-Jun-2023

● **INDICATIONS AND DOSE**

Acute uncomplicated cystitis

▸ BY MOUTH

▸ Child (body-weight 40 kg and above): Initially 400 mg for 1 dose, then 200 mg every 8 hours for 8 tablets (total of 10 tablets per course)

Chronic or recurrent bacteriuria

▸ BY MOUTH

▸ Child (body-weight 40 kg and above): 400 mg every 6–8 hours

Urinary-tract infections

▸ BY MOUTH

▸ Child (body-weight up to 40 kg): 5–10 mg/kg every 6 hours, alternatively 20–40 mg/kg daily in 3 divided doses

● **UNLICENSED USE** Not licensed for use in children under 3 months.

● **CONTRA-INDICATIONS** Carnitine deficiency · gastro-intestinal obstruction · oesophageal strictures

● **CAUTIONS** Avoid in Acute porphyrias p. 745

● **INTERACTIONS** → Appendix 1: penicillins

● **SIDE-EFFECTS**

▸ **Common or very common** Vulvovaginal fungal infection

▸ **Uncommon** Clostridioides difficile colitis · dizziness · fatigue · gastrointestinal discomfort · gastrointestinal disorders · headache · oral ulceration · vertigo

SIDE-EFFECTS, FURTHER INFORMATION Carnitine deficiency can occur with long-term or frequently-repeated treatment. Symptoms of carnitine deficiency include muscle aches, fatigue, and confusion.

● **PREGNANCY** Not known to be harmful, but manufacturer advises avoid.

● **BREAST FEEDING** Trace amount in milk, but appropriate to use.

● **MONITORING REQUIREMENTS** Liver and renal function tests required in long-term use.

● **EFFECT ON LABORATORY TESTS** False positive urinary glucose (if tested for reducing substances). False positive newborn screening results for isovaleric acidaemia may occur in neonates born to mothers receiving pivmecillinam during late pregnancy.

● **DIRECTIONS FOR ADMINISTRATION** Manufacturer advises tablets should be swallowed whole with plenty of fluid during meals while sitting or standing.

● **PATIENT AND CARER ADVICE** Patient counselling is advised on administration of pivmecillinam hydrochloride tablets (posture).

● **MEDICINAL FORMS** There can be variation in the licensing of different medicines containing the same drug.

Oral tablet

CAUTIONARY AND ADVISORY LABELS 9, 21, 27

▸ **Pivmecillinam hydrochloride (Non-proprietary)**

Pivmecillinam hydrochloride 200 mg Pivmecillinam 200mg tablets | 10 tablet [PoM] £9.00 DT = £5.40

▸ **Selexid** (Karo Healthcare UK Ltd)

Pivmecillinam hydrochloride 200 mg Selexid 200mg tablets | 10 tablet [PoM] £5.40 DT = £5.40 | 18 tablet [PoM] £9.72

ANTIBACTERIALS › PENICILLINS, PENICILLINASE-RESISTANT

F 412

Flucloxacillin

29-Nov-2021

● **INDICATIONS AND DOSE**

Infections due to beta-lactamase-producing staphylococci including otitis externa | Adjunct in pneumonia

▸ BY MOUTH

▸ Neonate up to 7 days: 25 mg/kg twice daily.

▸ Neonate 7 days to 20 days: 25 mg/kg 3 times a day.

▸ Neonate 21 days to 28 days: 25 mg/kg 4 times a day.

▸ Child 1 month–1 year: 62.5–125 mg 4 times a day

▸ Child 2–9 years: 125–250 mg 4 times a day

▸ Child 10–17 years: 250–500 mg 4 times a day

▸ BY INTRAMUSCULAR INJECTION

▸ Child: 12.5–25 mg/kg every 6 hours (max. per dose 500 mg)

▸ BY SLOW INTRAVENOUS INJECTION, OR BY INTRAVENOUS INFUSION

▸ Neonate up to 7 days: 25 mg/kg every 12 hours.

▸ Neonate 7 days to 20 days: 25 mg/kg every 8 hours.

▸ Neonate 21 days to 28 days: 25 mg/kg every 6 hours.

▸ Child: 12.5–25 mg/kg every 6 hours (max. per dose 1 g)

Impetigo

▸ BY MOUTH

▸ Neonate up to 7 days: 25 mg/kg twice daily.

- Neonate 7 days to 20 days: 25 mg/kg 3 times a day.
- Neonate 21 days to 28 days: 25 mg/kg 4 times a day.
- Child 1 month–1 year: 62.5–125 mg 4 times a day for 5–7 days
- Child 2–9 years: 125–250 mg 4 times a day for 5–7 days
- Child 10–17 years: 250–500 mg 4 times a day for 5–7 days
- BY INTRAMUSCULAR INJECTION
- Child: 12.5–25 mg/kg every 6 hours (max. per dose 500 mg)
- BY SLOW INTRAVENOUS INJECTION, OR BY INTRAVENOUS INFUSION
- Neonate up to 7 days: 25 mg/kg every 12 hours.
- Neonate 7 days to 20 days: 25 mg/kg every 8 hours.
- Neonate 21 days to 28 days: 25 mg/kg every 6 hours.
- Child: 12.5–25 mg/kg every 6 hours (max. per dose 1 g)

Severe infections due to beta-lactamase-producing staphylococci including otitis externa | Adjunct in pneumonia (severe infection) | Adjunct in impetigo (severe infection)
- BY SLOW INTRAVENOUS INJECTION, OR BY INTRAVENOUS INFUSION
- Neonate up to 7 days: 50 mg/kg every 12 hours.
- Neonate 7 days to 20 days: 50 mg/kg every 8 hours.
- Neonate 21 days to 28 days: 50 mg/kg every 6 hours.
- Child: 25–50 mg/kg every 6 hours (max. per dose 2 g)

Cellulitis | Erysipelas
- BY MOUTH
- Child 1 month–1 year: 62.5–125 mg 4 times a day for 5–7 days then review
- Child 2–9 years: 125–250 mg 4 times a day for 5–7 days then review
- Child 10–17 years: 250–500 mg 4 times a day for 5–7 days then review
- BY SLOW INTRAVENOUS INJECTION, OR BY INTRAVENOUS INFUSION
- Child: 12.5–25 mg/kg every 6 hours (max. per dose 1 g)

Secondary bacterial infection of eczema
- BY MOUTH
- Child 1 month–1 year: 62.5–125 mg 4 times a day for 5–7 days
- Child 2–9 years: 125–250 mg 4 times a day for 5–7 days
- Child 10–17 years: 250–500 mg 4 times a day for 5–7 days

Endocarditis (in combination with other antibacterial if necessary)
- BY SLOW INTRAVENOUS INJECTION, OR BY INTRAVENOUS INFUSION
- Child: 50 mg/kg every 6 hours (max. per dose 2 g)

Osteomyelitis
- BY SLOW INTRAVENOUS INJECTION, OR BY INTRAVENOUS INFUSION
- Neonate up to 7 days: 50–100 mg/kg every 12 hours.
- Neonate 7 days to 20 days: 50–100 mg/kg every 8 hours.
- Neonate 21 days to 28 days: 50–100 mg/kg every 6 hours.
- Child: 50 mg/kg every 6 hours (max. per dose 2 g)

Cerebral abscess | Staphylococcal meningitis
- BY SLOW INTRAVENOUS INJECTION, OR BY INTRAVENOUS INFUSION
- Neonate up to 7 days: 50–100 mg/kg every 12 hours.
- Neonate 7 days to 20 days: 50–100 mg/kg every 8 hours.
- Neonate 21 days to 28 days: 50–100 mg/kg every 6 hours.
- Child: 50 mg/kg every 6 hours (max. per dose 2 g)

Staphylococcal lung infection in cystic fibrosis
- BY MOUTH
- Child (body-weight up to 40 kg): 25 mg/kg 4 times a day, alternatively 100 mg/kg daily in 3 divided doses
- Child (body-weight 40 kg and above): 1 g 4 times a day, alternatively 4 g daily in 3 divided doses
- BY SLOW INTRAVENOUS INJECTION, OR BY INTRAVENOUS INFUSION
- Child: 50 mg/kg every 6 hours (max. per dose 2 g)

Prevention of *Staphylococcus aureus* lung infection in cystic fibrosis—primary prevention
- BY MOUTH
- Neonate: 125 mg twice daily.
- Child 1 month–3 years: 125 mg twice daily

Prevention of *Staphylococcus aureus* lung infection in cystic fibrosis—secondary prevention
- BY MOUTH
- Child: 50 mg/kg twice daily (max. per dose 1 g)

● **UNLICENSED USE** Flucloxacillin doses in BNF Publications may differ from those in product literature.

IMPORTANT SAFETY INFORMATION

HEPATIC DISORDERS

Cholestatic jaundice and hepatitis may occur very rarely, up to two months after treatment with flucloxacillin has been stopped. Administration for more than 2 weeks and increasing age are risk factors. Manufacturer advises:
- flucloxacillin should not be used in patients with a history of hepatic dysfunction associated with flucloxacillin
- flucloxacillin should be used with caution in patients with hepatic impairment
- careful enquiry should be made about hypersensitivity reactions to beta-lactam antibacterials

● **CAUTIONS**
- With intravenous use Accumulation of electrolytes can occur with high doses · risk of kernicterus in jaundiced neonates when high doses given parenterally

● **INTERACTIONS** → Appendix 1: penicillins

● **SIDE-EFFECTS**

GENERAL SIDE-EFFECTS
- **Rare or very rare** Fever · myalgia

SPECIFIC SIDE-EFFECTS
- **Common or very common**
- With oral use Gastrointestinal disorders
- **Rare or very rare**
- With oral use Eosinophilia
- **Frequency not known**
- With oral use Hypokalaemia · oesophageal disorder · oral pain · oropharyngeal pain · throat irritation
- With parenteral use Bronchospasm · coma · dyspnoea · electrolyte imbalance · erythema nodosum · hallucination · Jarisch-Herxheimer reaction · nephropathy · neurotoxicity · oral candidiasis · platelet dysfunction · purpura non-thrombocytopenic · vasculitis

SIDE-EFFECTS, FURTHER INFORMATION Potentially life-threatening hypokalaemia can occur, especially in high doses. This can be resistant to potassium supplementation. Regular monitoring of serum potassium levels is recommended when using higher doses of flucloxacillin.

- **PREGNANCY** Not known to be harmful.
- **BREAST FEEDING** Trace amounts in milk, but appropriate to use.
- **HEPATIC IMPAIRMENT** Manufacturer advises caution; including in those with risk factors for hepatic reactions.
- **RENAL IMPAIRMENT** Accumulation of sodium from injection can occur in patients with renal failure.
  - With intravenous use High doses may cause nephrotoxicity or neurotoxicity.

  Dose adjustments See p. 16.

  Expert sources advise use normal dose every 8 hours if estimated glomerular filtration rate less than 10 mL/minute/1.73 m^2.
- **EFFECT ON LABORATORY TESTS** False-positive urinary glucose (if tested for reducing substances).
- **DIRECTIONS FOR ADMINISTRATION** For *intravenous infusion*, dilute reconstituted solution *in* Glucose 5% *or* Sodium Chloride 0.9% and give intermittently over 30–60 minutes.
- **PRESCRIBING AND DISPENSING INFORMATION** For choice of antibacterial therapy, see Antibacterials, use for prophylaxis p. 359, Cardiovascular system infections, antibacterial therapy p. 364, Ear infections, antibacterial therapy p. 366, Musculoskeletal system infections, antibacterial therapy p. 369, Respiratory system infections, antibacterial therapy p. 371, Skin infections, antibacterial therapy p. 373.
- **PATIENT AND CARER ADVICE**

  Medicines for Children leaflet: Flucloxacillin for bacterial infections www.medicinesforchildren.org.uk/medicines/flucloxacillin-for-bacterial-infections/

- **MEDICINAL FORMS** There can be variation in the licensing of different medicines containing the same drug. Forms available from special-order manufacturers include: infusion

Oral solution

CAUTIONARY AND ADVISORY LABELS 9, 23

- Flucloxacillin (Non-proprietary)

  Flucloxacillin (as Flucloxacillin sodium) 25 mg per 1 ml Flucloxacillin 125mg/5ml oral solution | 100 ml [PoM] £20.83 DT = £1.87

  Flucloxacillin 125mg/5ml oral solution sugar free | 100 ml [PoM] £8.50 DT = £3.68 [SF]

  Flucloxacillin (as Flucloxacillin sodium) 50 mg per 1 ml Flucloxacillin 250mg/5ml oral solution sugar free | 100 ml [PoM] £12.50 DT = £7.22 [SF]

  Flucloxacillin 250mg/5ml oral solution | 100 ml [PoM] £47.10 DT = £2.06

Oral capsule

CAUTIONARY AND ADVISORY LABELS 9, 23

- Flucloxacillin (Non-proprietary)

  Flucloxacillin (as Flucloxacillin sodium) 250 mg Flucloxacillin 250mg capsules | 28 capsule [PoM] £5.00 DT = £1.15 | 100 capsule [PoM] £6.85

  Flucloxacillin (as Flucloxacillin sodium) 500 mg Flucloxacillin 500mg capsules | 28 capsule [PoM] £10.50 DT = £2.31 | 100 capsule [PoM] £6.50–£37.50

Powder for solution for injection

- Flucloxacillin (Non-proprietary)

  Flucloxacillin (as Flucloxacillin sodium) 250 mg Flucloxacillin 250mg powder for solution for injection vials | 10 vial [PoM] £8.60–£178.00 DT = £8.60 (Hospital only)

  Flucloxacillin (as Flucloxacillin sodium) 500 mg Flucloxacillin 500mg powder for solution for injection vials | 10 vial [PoM] £17.20–£359.00 DT = £17.20 (Hospital only)

  Flucloxacillin (as Flucloxacillin sodium) 1 gram Flucloxacillin 1g powder for solution for injection vials | 10 vial [PoM] £34.50–£712.00 DT = £34.50 (Hospital only)

  Flucloxacillin (as Flucloxacillin sodium) 2 gram Flucloxacillin 2g powder for solution for injection vials | 1 vial [PoM] £6.00 (Hospital only)

Combinations available: ***Co-fluampicil***, p. 420

ANTIBACTERIALS › POLYMYXINS

Colistimethate sodium

26-Feb-2024

(Colistin sulfomethate sodium)

- **DRUG ACTION** The polymyxin antibiotic, colistimethate sodium (colistin sulfomethate sodium), is active against Gram-negative organisms including *Pseudomonas aeruginosa*, *Acinetobacter baumanii*, and *Klebsiella pneumoniae*. It is not absorbed by mouth and thus needs to be given by injection for a systemic effect.

- **INDICATIONS AND DOSE**

Serious infections due to selected aerobic Gram-negative bacteria in patients with limited treatment options

▶ BY INTRAVENOUS INFUSION

- Neonate: 25 000–50 000 units/kg 3 times a day, the data supporting the dose regimen are very limited—consult product literature for available information, including recommendation to use lean body-weight for dosing.
- Child (body-weight up to 41 kg): 25 000–50 000 units/kg 3 times a day, the data supporting the dose regimen are very limited—consult product literature for available information, including recommendation to use lean body-weight for dosing
- Child (body-weight 41 kg and above): 4.5 million units twice daily, the data supporting the dose regimen are very limited—consult product literature for available information, including recommendation to use lean body-weight for dosing, alternatively 3 million units 3 times a day, the data supporting the dose regimen are very limited—consult product literature for available information, including recommendation to use lean body-weight for dosing

Management of chronic pulmonary infections due to *Pseudomonas aeruginosa* in patients with cystic fibrosis

▶ BY INHALATION OF NEBULISED SOLUTION

- Child 1–23 months: 0.5–1 million units twice daily, for specific advice on administration using nebulisers—consult product literature; maximum 2 million units per day
- Child 2–17 years: 1–2 million units 2–3 times a day, for specific advice on administration using nebulisers—consult product literature; maximum 6 million units per day

▶ BY INHALATION OF POWDER

- Child 6–17 years: 1.66 million units twice daily

- **CONTRA-INDICATIONS** Myasthenia gravis
- **CAUTIONS**

  GENERAL CAUTIONS Children under 1 year of age (effects of immature renal and metabolic function on conversion to active colistin not known)

  SPECIFIC CAUTIONS
  - When used by inhalation Severe haemoptysis—risk of further haemorrhage
- **INTERACTIONS** → Appendix 1: colistimethate
- **SIDE-EFFECTS**
  - **Common or very common**
  - When used by inhalation Arthralgia · asthenia · asthma · balance impaired · chest discomfort · cough · dysphonia · dyspnoea · fever · haemorrhage · headache · lower respiratory tract infection · nausea · respiratory disorders · taste altered · throat complaints · tinnitus · vomiting

- **Uncommon**
  - When used by inhalation Anxiety · appetite decreased · diarrhoea · drowsiness · ear congestion · flatulence · oral disorders · proteinuria · seizure · sputum purulent · thirst · weight change
- **Rare or very rare**
  - With parenteral use Confusion · nephrotoxicity · presyncope · psychosis · speech slurred · visual impairment
- **Frequency not known**
  - With parenteral use Apnoea · neurological effects · neurotoxicity · renal disorder · sensory disorder

SIDE-EFFECTS, FURTHER INFORMATION Neurotoxicity and nephrotoxicity are dose-related.

● **PREGNANCY**
- When used by inhalation Clinical use suggests probably safe.
- With intravenous use Manufacturer advises use only if potential benefit outweighs risk.

● **BREAST FEEDING** Present in milk but poorly absorbed from gut; manufacturers advise avoid (or use only if potential benefit outweighs risk).

● **HEPATIC IMPAIRMENT**
- With intravenous use Manufacturer advises caution (no information available).

● **RENAL IMPAIRMENT**
- When used by inhalation Manufacturer advises caution.
- With intravenous use Consult product literature.

Monitoring
- With intravenous use In renal impairment, monitor plasma colistimethate sodium concentration during parenteral treatment—consult product literature. Recommended 'peak' plasma colistimethate sodium concentration (approx. 1 hour after intravenous injection or infusion) 5–15 mg/litre; pre-dose ('trough') concentration 2–6 mg/litre.

● **MONITORING REQUIREMENTS**
- With intravenous use Monitor renal function.
- When used by inhalation Measure lung function before and after initial dose of colistimethate sodium and monitor for bronchospasm; if bronchospasm occurs in a patient not using a bronchodilator, repeat test using a bronchodilator before the dose of colistimethate sodium.

● **DIRECTIONS FOR ADMINISTRATION**
- When used by inhalation Manufacturer advises if other treatments are being administered, they should be taken in the order recommended by the physician. For *nebulisation*, consult product literature for information on reconstitution and dilution.
- With intravenous use For *intravenous infusion*, dilute to a concentration of 40 000 units/mL with Sodium Chloride 0.9%; give over 30–60 minutes. Patients fitted with a totally implantable venous access device may tolerate an injection. For *slow intravenous injection* into a totally implantable venous access device, dilute to a concentration of 90 000 units/mL with Sodium Chloride 0.9% for child under 12 years (200 000 units/mL for child over 12 years); give over at least 5 minutes.

● **PRESCRIBING AND DISPENSING INFORMATION**
Colistimethate sodium is included in some preparations for topical application.

● **PATIENT AND CARER ADVICE**
- When used by inhalation Patient should be advised to rinse mouth with water after each dose of dry powder inhalation. Patients or carers should be given advice on how to administer colistimethate sodium; first dose should be given under medical supervision.

Driving and skilled tasks Manufacturer advises patients and carers should be counselled on the effects on driving and performance of skilled tasks—increased risk of dizziness, confusion and visual disturbances.

● **NATIONAL FUNDING/ACCESS DECISIONS**
For full details see funding body website

NICE decisions
- **Colistimethate sodium and tobramycin dry powders for inhalation for treating pseudomonas lung infection in cystic fibrosis (March 2013)** NICE TA276 Recommended with restrictions

● **MEDICINAL FORMS** There can be variation in the licensing of different medicines containing the same drug.

Inhalation powder
- **Colobreathe** (Essential Pharma Ltd)
  Colistimethate sodium 1662500 unit Colobreathe 1,662,500unit inhalation powder capsules | 56 capsule [PoM] £968.80 DT = £968.80

Powder for nebuliser solution
- **Colistimethate sodium (Non-proprietary)**
  Colistimethate sodium 1000000 unit Colistimethate 1million unit powder for nebuliser solution unit dose vials | 1 unit dose [PoM] £6.80 | 10 unit dose [PoM] £67.00–£68.00 | 30 unit dose [PoM] £199.00–£204.00
  Colistimethate sodium 2000000 unit Colistimethate 2million unit powder for nebuliser solution unit dose vials | 1 unit dose [PoM] £5.39–£12.84 | 10 unit dose [PoM] £52.11–£122.40
- **Colicym** (Kent Pharma (UK) Ltd)
  Colistimethate sodium 1000000 unit Colicym 1million unit powder for nebuliser solution unit dose vials | 1 unit dose [PoM] £6.80 (Hospital only) | 30 unit dose [PoM] £204.00 (Hospital only)

Powder for solution for injection
ELECTROLYTES: May contain Sodium
- **Colistimethate sodium (Non-proprietary)**
  Colistimethate sodium 1000000 unit Colistimethate 1million unit powder for solution for injection vials | 1 vial [PoM] £3.98 | 10 vial [PoM] £33.98 DT = £33.98
  Colistimethate sodium 2000000 unit Colistimethate 2million unit powder for solution for injection vials | 1 vial [PoM] £5.59 | 10 vial [PoM] £54.96 DT = £54.96
- **Colomycin** (Teva UK Ltd)
  Colistimethate sodium 1000000 unit Colomycin 1million unit powder for solution for injection vials | 10 vial [PoM] £33.98 DT = £33.98
  Colistimethate sodium 2000000 unit Colomycin 2million unit powder for solution for injection vials | 10 vial [PoM] £54.96 DT = £54.96

ANTIBACTERIALS > QUINOLONES

Quinolones

09-Feb-2021

MHRA/CHM advice: Systemic and inhaled fluoroquinolones

The MHRA and CHM have released important safety information regarding the use of systemic and inhaled fluoroquinolones. For restrictions and precautions, see *Important safety information* for all quinolones (ciprofloxacin p. 429).

Overview

In the UK, only fluoroquinolones are available; the recommendations below therefore refer to the use of fluoroquinolones.

Ciprofloxacin is active against both Gram-positive and Gram-negative bacteria. It is particularly active against Gram-negative bacteria, including *Salmonella*, *Shigella*, *Campylobacter*, *Neisseria*, and *Pseudomonas*. Ciprofloxacin has only moderate activity against Gram-positive bacteria such as *Streptococcus pneumoniae* and *Enterococcus faecalis*; it should not be used for pneumococcal pneumonia. It is active against *Chlamydia* and some mycobacteria. Most anaerobic organisms are not susceptible.

Many *Staphylococci* are resistant to quinolones and their use should be avoided in MRSA infections.

Ofloxacin eye drops are used in ophthalmic infections.

There is much less experience of the other quinolones in children; expert advice should be sought.

Quinolones

IMPORTANT SAFETY INFORMATION

▸ With systemic use

The CSM has warned that quinolones may induce **convulsions** in patients with or without a history of convulsions; taking NSAIDs at the same time may also induce them.

TENDON DAMAGE

▸ With systemic use

Tendon damage (including rupture) has been reported rarely in patients receiving quinolones. Tendon rupture may occur within 48 hours of starting treatment; cases have also been reported several months after stopping a quinolone. Healthcare professionals are reminded that:

- quinolones are contra-indicated in patients with a history of tendon disorders related to quinolone use;
- the risk of tendon damage is increased by the concomitant use of corticosteroids;
- if tendinitis is suspected, the quinolone should be discontinued immediately.

MHRA/CHM ADVICE: SYSTEMIC AND INHALED FLUOROQUINOLONES: SMALL INCREASED RISK OF AORTIC ANEURYSM AND DISSECTION; ADVICE FOR PRESCRIBING IN HIGH-RISK PATIENTS (NOVEMBER 2018)

▸ With systemic use

The MHRA advises that benefit-risk should be assessed and other therapeutic options considered before using fluoroquinolones in patients at risk of aortic aneurysm and dissection. Factors that increase the risk of aortic aneurysm and dissection include:

- family history of aneurysm disease;
- pre-existing aortic aneurysm and/or aortic dissection;
- other risk factors or conditions predisposing to aortic aneurysm and dissection (e.g. Marfan syndrome, vascular Ehlers-Danlos syndrome, Takayasu arteritis, giant cell arteritis, Behçet's disease, hypertension, and known atherosclerosis).

Patients (particularly those at risk) and their carers should be informed about rare events of aortic aneurysm and dissection, and advised to seek immediate medical attention if sudden-onset severe abdominal, chest, or back pain develops.

MHRA/CHM ADVICE: FLUOROQUINOLONE ANTIBIOTICS: NEW RESTRICTIONS AND PRECAUTIONS FOR USE DUE TO VERY RARE REPORTS OF DISABLING AND POTENTIALLY LONG-LASTING OR IRREVERSIBLE SIDE EFFECTS (MARCH 2019)

▸ With systemic use

Disabling, long-lasting, or potentially irreversible adverse reactions affecting musculoskeletal and nervous systems have been reported very rarely with fluoroquinolone antibiotics. Healthcare professionals are advised to inform patients to stop treatment at the first signs of a serious adverse reaction, such as tendinitis or tendon rupture, muscle pain, muscle weakness, joint pain, joint swelling, peripheral neuropathy, and CNS effects, and to contact their doctor immediately. Fluoroquinolones should not be prescribed for non-severe or self-limiting infections, or non-bacterial conditions. Unless other commonly recommended antibiotics are inappropriate, fluoroquinolones should not be prescribed for mild to moderate infections. Fluoroquinolones should be avoided in patients who have previously had serious adverse reactions. Use of fluoroquinolones with corticosteroids should also be avoided as it may exacerbate fluoroquinolone-induced tendinitis and tendon rupture. Fluoroquinolones should be prescribed with caution in patients with renal impairment or solid-organ transplants as they are at a higher risk of tendon injury.

MHRA/CHM ADVICE: SYSTEMIC AND INHALED FLUOROQUINOLONES: SMALL RISK OF HEART VALVE REGURGITATION; CONSIDER OTHER THERAPEUTIC OPTIONS FIRST IN PATIENTS AT RISK (DECEMBER 2020)

▸ With systemic use

A European review of worldwide data found an increased risk of heart valve regurgitation associated with systemic and inhaled fluoroquinolones. A case-control study suggested a two-fold increased relative risk with current oral fluoroquinolone use compared with amoxicillin or azithromycin use. Healthcare professionals are advised that fluoroquinolones are authorised for use in serious, life-threatening bacterial infections, and should only be used after careful benefit-risk assessment and consideration of other therapeutic options in patients with the following risk factors:

- congenital or pre-existing heart valve disease;
- connective tissue disorders (e.g. Marfan syndrome or Ehlers-Danlos syndrome);
- other risk factors or conditions predisposing to heart valve regurgitation (e.g. hypertension, Turner's syndrome, Behçet's disease, rheumatoid arthritis, and infective endocarditis).

Patients should be advised to seek immediate medical attention if they experience a rapid onset of shortness of breath (especially when lying down flat in bed), swelling of the ankles, feet, or abdomen, or new-onset heart palpitations.

MHRA/CHM ADVICE: FLUOROQUINOLONE ANTIBIOTICS: REMINDER OF THE RISK OF DISABLING AND POTENTIALLY LONG-LASTING OR IRREVERSIBLE SIDE EFFECTS (AUGUST 2023)

▸ With systemic use

The risk of disabling and potentially long-lasting or irreversible adverse reactions affecting different, sometimes multiple, body systems resulted in the introduction of restrictions and precautions for fluoroquinolone antibiotics in 2019. However, a study of prescribing data has found no evidence that these measures changed fluoroquinolone prescribing patterns in primary care, and the MHRA has continued to receive reports of such reactions. Healthcare professionals are reminded to be alert to this risk and to continue to follow the advice issued in 2019 (see above).

MHRA/CHM ADVICE: FLUOROQUINOLONE ANTIBIOTICS: SUICIDAL THOUGHTS AND BEHAVIOUR (SEPTEMBER 2023)

▸ With systemic use

Fluoroquinolones can cause psychiatric side-effects, including depression and psychosis, even after the first dose. In rare cases, these can lead to thoughts or attempts of suicide, and have been associated with the completed suicide of a patient without a history of psychiatric disorders. Fluoroquinolones can also worsen existing psychiatric symptoms and treatment should be stopped immediately if such side-effects, including new or worsening depression or psychosis, occur. Healthcare professionals are advised to counsel patients or their carers to:

- inform their healthcare professional if they are prescribed a fluoroquinolone and have pre-existing depression or psychosis;
- be alert to any changes in mood or behaviour, even after treatment has stopped for some time, and to inform friends and family about the risk and signs of psychiatric side-effects associated with fluoroquinolones—medical advice should be sought if these occur;
- stop taking the fluoroquinolone and seek immediate medical advice if suicidal thoughts or behaviour develop.

MHRA/CHM ADVICE: FLUOROQUINOLONE ANTIBIOTICS: MUST NOW ONLY BE PRESCRIBED WHEN OTHER COMMONLY RECOMMENDED ANTIBIOTICS ARE INAPPROPRIATE (JANUARY 2024)

▸ With systemic use

Following a review of the effectiveness of current measures to reduce the identified risk of disabling and potentially long-lasting or irreversible adverse reactions, the MHRA has further restricted the use of fluoroquinolones. These adverse reactions, which may affect multiple body systems including musculoskeletal, nervous, psychiatric and sensory systems, have been reported in patients irrespective of their age and potential risk factors, and may last for months or years; the updated reporting incidence suggested a minimum frequency of between 1 and 10 per 10 000 patients. In addition to advice issued in 2019 and 2023 (see above), healthcare professionals are advised that fluoroquinolones should only be used when other commonly recommended antibiotics are inappropriate i.e. in situations where:

- there is resistance to other first-line antibiotics recommended for the infection;
- other first-line antibiotics are contra-indicated in an individual patient;
- other first-line antibiotics have caused side-effects that required treatment to be stopped;
- treatment with other first-line antibiotics has failed.

Patients should be advised to stop fluoroquinolone treatment at the first signs of a serious musculoskeletal, neurological or psychiatric side effect and to contact their doctor immediately (see *Patient and carer advice*).

- **CONTRA-INDICATIONS**

▸ With systemic use or when used by inhalation History of tendon disorders related to quinolone use

- **CAUTIONS**

▸ With systemic use or when used by inhalation Can prolong the QT interval · conditions that predispose to seizures · diabetes (may affect blood glucose) · exposure to excessive sunlight and UV radiation should be avoided during treatment and for 48 hours after stopping treatment · G6PD deficiency · history of epilepsy · myasthenia gravis (risk of exacerbation) · psychiatric disorders

▸ With systemic use Children or adolescents (arthropathy has developed in weight-bearing joints in young *animals*)

CAUTIONS, FURTHER INFORMATION

▸ With systemic use Quinolones cause arthropathy in the weight-bearing joints of immature *animals* and are therefore generally not recommended in children and growing adolescents. However, the significance of this effect in humans is uncertain and in some specific circumstances use of ciprofloxacin may be justified in children.

- **SIDE-EFFECTS**

▸ **Common or very common** Diarrhoea · eye discomfort · eye disorders · fungal infection · headache · nausea · skin reactions · taste altered · vision disorders · vomiting

▸ **Uncommon** Altered smell sensation · anxiety · appetite decreased · arrhythmias · arthralgia · asthenia · chest pain · confusion · constipation · cough · dizziness · dry eye · dyspnoea · eosinophilia · eye inflammation · fever · flatulence · gastrointestinal discomfort · hallucination · hearing impairment · hyperglycaemia · hyperhidrosis · hypersensitivity · hypoglycaemia · hypotension · muscle weakness · myalgia · pain · palpitations · peripheral neuropathy (sometimes irreversible) · renal impairment · seizure · sensation abnormal · sleep disorders · stomatitis · tendon disorders · thrombocytopenia · tinnitus · vertigo

▸ **Rare or very rare** Agranulocytosis · anaemia · angioedema · arthritis · coordination abnormal · depression · gait abnormal · haemolytic anaemia · hepatitis · idiopathic intracranial hypertension · leucopenia · myasthenia gravis aggravated · neutropenia · pancreatitis · pancytopenia · photosensitivity reaction · psychotic disorder · severe cutaneous adverse reactions (SCARs) · suicidal behaviours · syncope · tremor · vasculitis

▸ **Frequency not known** Drowsiness · heart valve incompetence · hypoglycaemic coma · increased risk of aortic aneurysm · increased risk of aortic dissection · memory impairment · polyneuropathy · QT interval prolongation

SIDE-EFFECTS, FURTHER INFORMATION The drug should be discontinued if neurological, psychiatric, tendon disorders or hypersensitivity reactions (including severe rash) occur. For more information regarding the safety of fluoroquinolones, please see Important Safety Information.

- **ALLERGY AND CROSS-SENSITIVITY** EvGr Use of quinolones contra-indicated in quinolone hypersensitivity. ⟨M⟩

- **PREGNANCY**

▸ With systemic use or when used by inhalation Avoid in pregnancy—shown to cause arthropathy in *animal* studies; safer alternatives are available.

- **PATIENT AND CARER ADVICE**

▸ With systemic use Patients and their carers should be advised to stop fluoroquinolone treatment at the first signs of a serious musculoskeletal, neurological or psychiatric side effect and to contact their doctor immediately. The MHRA has produced a patient advice sheet on fluoroquinolones and serious adverse reactions affecting tendons, muscles, joints, and nerves, which should be provided to patients and their carers: assets.publishing.service.gov.uk/media/65aa9125c69eea0010883840/FQ_Patient_Information_Sheet_-_TO_PUBLISH.pdf.

F 428

Ciprofloxacin

26-Nov-2025

- **INDICATIONS AND DOSE**

Fistulating Crohn's disease

▸ BY MOUTH

▸ Child: 5 mg/kg twice daily (max. per dose 500 mg)

Severe respiratory-tract infections, gastro-intestinal infection

▸ BY MOUTH

▸ Neonate: 15 mg/kg twice daily.

▸ Child: 20 mg/kg twice daily (max. per dose 750 mg)

▸ BY INTRAVENOUS INFUSION

▸ Neonate: 10 mg/kg every 12 hours, to be given over 60 minutes.

▸ Child: 10 mg/kg every 8 hours (max. per dose 400 mg), to be given over 60 minutes

Acute exacerbation of bronchiectasis (administered on expert advice)

▸ BY MOUTH

▸ Child 1–17 years: 20 mg/kg twice daily (max. per dose 750 mg) for 7–14 days

▸ BY INTRAVENOUS INFUSION

▸ Child 1–17 years: 10 mg/kg every 8 hours (max. per dose 400 mg), to be given over 60 minutes

Pseudomonal lower respiratory-tract infection in cystic fibrosis

▸ BY MOUTH

▸ Child: 20 mg/kg twice daily (max. per dose 750 mg)

▸ BY INTRAVENOUS INFUSION

▸ Child: 10 mg/kg every 8 hours (max. per dose 400 mg), to be given over 60 minutes

continued →

Complicated urinary-tract infections
▶ BY MOUTH
▸ Neonate: 10 mg/kg twice daily.
▸ Child: 10 mg/kg twice daily (max. per dose 750 mg); increased to 20 mg/kg twice daily (max. per dose 750 mg), increased dose used in severe infection
▶ BY INTRAVENOUS INFUSION
▸ Neonate: 6 mg/kg every 12 hours, to be given over 60 minutes.
▸ Child: 6 mg/kg every 8 hours (max. per dose 400 mg); increased to 10 mg/kg every 8 hours (max. per dose 400 mg), increased dose used in severe infection

Uncomplicated gonorrhoea [anogenital and pharyngeal infection, when sensitivity confirmed]
▶ BY MOUTH
▸ Child 12–17 years (body-weight 45 kg and above): 500 mg for 1 dose

Disseminated gonococcal infection [arthritis and arthritis-dermatitis syndrome, when sensitivity confirmed]
▶ BY MOUTH
▸ Child 12–17 years (body-weight 45 kg and above): 500 mg twice daily, to be used following parenteral ceftriaxone treatment, starting 24–48 hours after symptoms improve, to give 7 days treatment in total

Anthrax (treatment and post-exposure prophylaxis)
▶ BY MOUTH
▸ Child: 15 mg/kg twice daily (max. per dose 500 mg)
▶ BY INTRAVENOUS INFUSION
▸ Child: 10 mg/kg every 12 hours (max. per dose 400 mg)

Prevention of secondary case of *Haemophilus influenzae* type b disease
▶ BY MOUTH
▸ Child 2–4 years: 125 mg twice daily for 5 days
▸ Child 5–12 years: 250 mg twice daily for 5 days
▸ Child 13–17 years: 500 mg twice daily for 5 days

Prevention of secondary case of meningococcal disease
▶ BY MOUTH
▸ Neonate: 30 mg/kg for 1 dose (max. per dose 125 mg).
▸ Child 1–11 months: 30 mg/kg for 1 dose (max. per dose 125 mg)
▸ Child 1–4 years: 125 mg for 1 dose
▸ Child 5–11 years: 250 mg for 1 dose
▸ Child 12–17 years: 500 mg for 1 dose

Acute pyelonephritis | Urinary tract infection (catheter-associated)
▶ BY MOUTH
▸ Child 16–17 years: 500 mg twice daily for 7 days
▶ BY INTRAVENOUS INFUSION
▸ Child 16–17 years: 400 mg every 8–12 hours

● **UNLICENSED USE** EvGr Ciprofloxacin is used for the treatment of disseminated gonococcal infection, (A) but is not licensed for this indication. UKHSA advises that ciprofloxacin is used for the prevention of secondary cases of *Haemophilus influenzae* type b disease, but is not licensed for this indication. EvGr Ciprofloxacin is used for the treatment of uncomplicated gonorrhoea, (A) but is not licensed for this indication. UKHSA advises that ciprofloxacin is used for the prevention of secondary cases of meningococcal disease, but is not licensed for this indication.

Not licensed for use in children under 1 year of age. Licensed for use in children over 1 year for complicated urinary-tract infections, for pseudomonal lower respiratory-tract infections in cystic fibrosis, for prophylaxis and treatment of inhalational anthrax. Licensed for use in children over 1 year for other infections where the benefit is considered to outweigh the potential risks. Not licensed for use in children for gastro-intestinal anthrax.

● **CAUTIONS** Acute myocardial infarction (risk factor for QT interval prolongation) · avoid excessive alkalinity of urine (risk of crystalluria) · bradycardia (risk factor for QT interval prolongation) · congenital long QT syndrome (risk factor for QT interval prolongation) · electrolyte disturbances (risk factor for QT interval prolongation) · ensure adequate fluid intake (risk of crystalluria) · heart failure with reduced left ventricular ejection fraction (risk factor for QT interval prolongation) · history of symptomatic arrhythmias (risk factor for QT interval prolongation)

● **INTERACTIONS** → Appendix 1: quinolones

● **SIDE-EFFECTS**
▶ **Common or very common** Arthropathy
▶ **Uncommon** Akathisia · fungal superinfection · hepatic disorders · oedema · thrombocytosis · vasodilation
▶ **Rare or very rare** Antibiotic associated colitis · asthma · bone marrow depression · crystalluria · erythema nodosum · haematuria · intracranial pressure increased · leucocytosis · migraine · muscle cramps · muscle tone increased · nephritis tubulointerstitial · olfactory nerve disorder · status epilepticus
▶ **Frequency not known** Mood altered · self-injurious behaviour

● **PREGNANCY** UKHSA advises a single dose of ciprofloxacin may be used for prevention of secondary case of meningococcal disease.

● **BREAST FEEDING** Amount too small to be harmful but manufacturer advises avoid.

● **RENAL IMPAIRMENT**
Dose adjustments Reduce dose if estimated glomerular filtration rate less than 30 mL/minute/1.73 m^2—consult product literature.

● **PRESCRIBING AND DISPENSING INFORMATION** For choice of antibacterial therapy, see Antibacterials, use for prophylaxis p. 359, Anthrax p. 444, Gastro-intestinal system infections, antibacterial therapy p. 367, Genital system infections, antibacterial therapy p. 368, Respiratory system infections, antibacterial therapy p. 371, Urinary-tract infections p. 454.

● **PATIENT AND CARER ADVICE** Granules present in the oral suspension should not be chewed.
Medicines for Children leaflet: Ciprofloxacin for bacterial infection www.medicinesforchildren.org.uk/medicines/ciprofloxacin-for-bacterial-infection/
Driving and skilled tasks May impair performance of skilled tasks (e.g. driving); effects enhanced by alcohol.

● **MEDICINAL FORMS** There can be variation in the licensing of different medicines containing the same drug. Forms available from special-order manufacturers include: oral suspension

Oral tablet
CAUTIONARY AND ADVISORY LABELS 7, 9, 25
▸ **Ciprofloxacin (Non-proprietary)**
Ciprofloxacin (as Ciprofloxacin hydrochloride)
100 mg Ciprofloxacin 100mg tablets | 20 tablet PoM £48.00 DT = £48.00
Ciprofloxacin (as Ciprofloxacin hydrochloride)
250 mg Ciprofloxacin 250mg tablets | 10 tablet PoM £1.17 DT = £0.64 | 20 tablet PoM £1.28–£2.34
Ciprofloxacin (as Ciprofloxacin hydrochloride)
500 mg Ciprofloxacin 500mg tablets | 10 tablet PoM £15.00 DT = £3.85 | 20 tablet PoM £1.62–£20.00
Ciprofloxacin (as Ciprofloxacin hydrochloride)
750 mg Ciprofloxacin 750mg tablets | 10 tablet PoM £8.00 DT = £1.65

Oral suspension
CAUTIONARY AND ADVISORY LABELS 7, 9
▸ **Ciproxin** (Bayer Plc)
Ciprofloxacin 50 mg per 1 ml Ciproxin 250mg/5ml oral suspension | 100 ml PoM £21.29 DT = £21.29

Solution for infusion

ELECTROLYTES: May contain Sodium

▸ Ciprofloxacin (Non-proprietary)

Ciprofloxacin 2 mg per 1 ml Ciprofloxacin 400mg/200ml solution for infusion bottles | 10 bottle PoM £260.10 (Hospital only)
Ciprofloxacin 200mg/100ml solution for infusion bottles | 10 bottle PoM £171.10 (Hospital only)

Infusion

▸ Ciprofloxacin (Non-proprietary)

Ciprofloxacin 2 mg per 1 ml Ciprofloxacin 200mg/100ml infusion KabiPac polyethylene bottles | 10 bottle PoM £171.10 (Hospital only)
Ciprofloxacin 400mg/200ml infusion bags | 10 bag PoM £228.46 (Hospital only)
Ciprofloxacin 400mg/200ml infusion KabiPac polyethylene bottles | 10 bottle PoM £260.10 (Hospital only)

ANTIBACTERIALS > SULFONAMIDES

Co-trimoxazole

06-Feb-2023

● **DRUG ACTION** Sulfamethoxazole and trimethoprim are used in combination (as co-trimoxazole) because of their synergistic activity (the importance of the sulfonamides has decreased as a result of increasing bacterial resistance and their replacement by antibacterials which are generally more active and less toxic).

● **INDICATIONS AND DOSE**

Treatment of susceptible infections

▶ BY MOUTH

▸ Child 6 weeks–5 months: 120 mg twice daily, alternatively 24 mg/kg twice daily
▸ Child 6 months–5 years: 240 mg twice daily, alternatively 24 mg/kg twice daily
▸ Child 6–11 years: 480 mg twice daily, alternatively 24 mg/kg twice daily (max. per dose 960 mg)
▸ Child 12–17 years: 960 mg twice daily

▶ BY INTRAVENOUS INFUSION

▸ Child 6 weeks–5 years: 18 mg/kg every 12 hours; increased to 27 mg/kg every 12 hours, increased dose used in severe infection
▸ Child 6–17 years: 18 mg/kg every 12 hours (max. per dose 960 mg); increased to 27 mg/kg every 12 hours (max. per dose 1.44 g), increased dose used in severe infection

Prophylaxis of infection from human bites | Prophylaxis of infection from animal bites

▶ BY MOUTH

▸ Child 6 weeks–5 months: 120 mg twice daily for 3 days, alternatively 24 mg/kg twice daily for 3 days
▸ Child 6 months–5 years: 240 mg twice daily for 3 days, alternatively 24 mg/kg twice daily for 3 days
▸ Child 6–11 years: 480 mg twice daily for 3 days, alternatively 24 mg/kg twice daily (max. per dose 960 mg) for 3 days

Treatment of infection from human bites | Treatment of infection from animal bites

▶ BY MOUTH

▸ Child 6 weeks–5 months: 120 mg twice daily for 5–7 days, alternatively 24 mg/kg twice daily for 5–7 days
▸ Child 6 months–5 years: 240 mg twice daily for 5–7 days, alternatively 24 mg/kg twice daily for 5–7 days
▸ Child 6–11 years: 480 mg twice daily for 5–7 days, alternatively 24 mg/kg twice daily (max. per dose 960 mg) for 5–7 days

Treatment of *Pneumocystis jirovecii* (*Pneumocystis carinii*) infections (undertaken where facilities for appropriate monitoring available—consult microbiologist and product literature)

▶ BY MOUTH, OR BY INTRAVENOUS INFUSION

▸ Child: 120 mg/kg daily in 2–4 divided doses for 14–21 days, oral route preferred for children

Prophylaxis of *Pneumocystis jirovecii* (*Pneumocystis carinii*) infections

▶ BY MOUTH

▸ Child: 450 mg/m^2 twice daily (max. per dose 960 mg) for 3 days of the week (either consecutively or on alternate days), dose regimens may vary, consult local guidelines

DOSE EQUIVALENCE AND CONVERSION

▸ Doses are expressed as co-trimoxazole: the total of sulfamethoxazole (sulphamethoxazole) and trimethoprim components in a ratio of 5:1.
▸ Co-trimoxazole 480 mg consists of sulfamethoxazole 400 mg and trimethoprim 80 mg.

● **UNLICENSED USE** Co-trimoxazole may be used as detailed below, although these situations are considered unlicensed:

- treatment of *Burkholderia cepacia* infections in cystic fibrosis
- treatment of *Stenotrophomonas maltophilia* infections
- EvGr prophylaxis and treatment of infection due to human bites
- prophylaxis and treatment of infection due to animal bites ⟨A⟩

Not licensed for use in children under 6 weeks.

IMPORTANT SAFETY INFORMATION

RESTRICTIONS ON THE USE OF CO-TRIMOXAZOLE

Co-trimoxazole is licensed for the prophylaxis and treatment of *Pneumocystis jirovecii* (*Pneumocystis carinii*) pneumonia and toxoplasmosis; it is also licensed for the treatment of nocardiosis. *Stenotrophomonas maltophilia* has demonstrated susceptibility to co-trimoxazole. It should only be considered for use in acute exacerbations of chronic bronchitis and infections of the urinary tract when there is bacteriological evidence of sensitivity to co-trimoxazole and good reason to prefer this combination to a single antibacterial; similarly it should only be used in acute otitis media in children when there is good reason to prefer it.

● **CONTRA-INDICATIONS** Acute porphyrias p. 745

● **CAUTIONS** Asthma · avoid in blood disorders (unless under specialist supervision) · avoid in infants under 6 weeks (except for treatment or prophylaxis of pneumocystis pneumonia) because of the risk of kernicterus · G6PD deficiency (risk of haemolytic anaemia) · maintain adequate fluid intake · predisposition to folate deficiency · predisposition to hyperkalaemia

● **INTERACTIONS** → Appendix 1: sulfonamides · trimethoprim

● **SIDE-EFFECTS**

▶ **Common or very common** Diarrhoea · electrolyte imbalance · fungal overgrowth · headache · nausea · skin reactions
▶ **Uncommon** Vomiting
▶ **Rare or very rare** Agranulocytosis · angioedema · aplastic anaemia · appetite decreased · arthralgia · ataxia · cough · depression · dizziness · dyspnoea · eosinophilia · fever · haemolysis · haemolytic anaemia · hallucination · hepatic disorders · hypoglycaemia · leucopenia · megaloblastic anaemia · meningitis aseptic · metabolic acidosis · methaemoglobinaemia · myalgia · myocarditis allergic · nephritis tubulointerstitial · neutropenia · oral disorders · pancreatitis · peripheral neuropathy · photosensitivity reaction · pseudomembranous enterocolitis · renal impairment · renal tubular acidosis · respiratory disorders · rhabdomyolysis · seizure · serum sickness · severe cutaneous adverse reactions (SCARs) · systemic lupus erythematosus (SLE) · thrombocytopenia · tinnitus · uveitis · vasculitis · vertigo

- **Frequency not known** Haemophagocytic lymphohistiocytosis · psychotic disorder

SIDE-EFFECTS, FURTHER INFORMATION Co-trimoxazole is associated with rare but serious side effects. Discontinue immediately if blood disorders (including leucopenia, thrombocytopenia, megaloblastic anaemia, eosinophilia, haemophagocytic lymphohistiocytosis) or rash/skin reactions (including Stevens-Johnson syndrome, toxic epidermal necrolysis, acute generalised exanthematous pustulosis, drug reaction with eosinophilia and systemic symptoms) develop.

- **ALLERGY AND CROSS-SENSITIVITY** EvGr Contra-indicated if previous hypersensitivity to trimethoprim, sulfonamides or co-trimoxazole. Contra-indicated if previous Stevens-Johnson syndrome (SJS), toxic epidermal necrolysis (TEN) or drug reaction with eosinophilia and systemic symptoms (DRESS) with the use of co-trimoxazole. Contra-indicated if previous drug-induced thrombocytopenia with trimethoprim, sulfonamides or co-trimoxazole. (M)
- **PREGNANCY** Teratogenic risk in first trimester (trimethoprim is a folate antagonist). Neonatal haemolysis and methaemoglobinaemia in third trimester; fear of increased risk of kernicterus in neonates appears to be unfounded.
- **BREAST FEEDING** Small risk of kernicterus in jaundiced infants and of haemolysis in G6PD-deficient infants (due to sulfamethoxazole).
- **HEPATIC IMPAIRMENT** Manufacturer advises avoid in severe liver disease.
- **RENAL IMPAIRMENT** EvGr Avoid if creatinine clearance less than 15 mL/minute or in severe insufficiency where plasma-sulfamethoxazole concentration cannot be monitored. Monitor plasma-sulfamethoxazole concentrations (consult product literature). (M)

  Dose adjustments See p. 16.

  EvGr Use half normal dose if creatinine clearance 15–30 mL/minute (consult product literature). (M)
- **MONITORING REQUIREMENTS**
  - EvGr Monitor serum potassium and sodium in patients at risk of hyperkalaemia or hyponatraemia.
  - Monitor blood counts on prolonged treatment. (M)
  - Plasma concentration monitoring may be required with high doses; seek expert advice
- **DIRECTIONS FOR ADMINISTRATION** For intermittent *intravenous infusion*, manufacturer advises may be further diluted in Glucose 5% and 10% *or* Sodium Chloride 0.9%. Dilute contents of 1 ampoule (5 mL) to 125 mL, 2 ampoules (10 mL) to 250 mL or 3 ampoules (15 mL) to 500 mL; suggested duration of infusion 60–90 minutes (but may be adjusted according to fluid requirements); if fluid restriction necessary, 1 ampoule (5 mL) may be diluted with 75 mL Glucose 5% and the required dose infused over max. 60 minutes; check container for haze or precipitant during administration. Expert sources advise in severe fluid restriction may be given undiluted via a central venous line.
- **PRESCRIBING AND DISPENSING INFORMATION** For choice of antibacterial therapy, see Pneumocystis pneumonia p. 470, Skin infections, antibacterial therapy p. 373.

- **MEDICINAL FORMS** There can be variation in the licensing of different medicines containing the same drug.

Solution for infusion

EXCIPIENTS: May contain Alcohol, propylene glycol, sulfites

ELECTROLYTES: May contain Sodium

- Co-trimoxazole (Non-proprietary)

  Trimethoprim 16 mg per 1 ml, Sulfamethoxazole 80 mg per 1 ml Co-trimoxazole 80mg/400mg/5ml solution for infusion ampoules | 10 ampoule PoM £47.15 DT = £47.15

Oral tablet

CAUTIONARY AND ADVISORY LABELS 9

- Co-trimoxazole (Non-proprietary)

  Trimethoprim 80 mg, Sulfamethoxazole 400 mg Co-trimoxazole 80mg/400mg tablets | 28 tablet PoM £3.95 DT = £1.24 | 100 tablet PoM £4.43–£10.91

  Trimethoprim 160 mg, Sulfamethoxazole 800 mg Co-trimoxazole 160mg/800mg tablets | 10 tablet PoM £4.35 | 14 tablet PoM £4.35 | 50 tablet PoM £11.73 | 100 tablet PoM £30.52 DT = £10.78

Oral suspension

CAUTIONARY AND ADVISORY LABELS 9

- Co-trimoxazole (Non-proprietary)

  Trimethoprim 8 mg per 1 ml, Sulfamethoxazole 40 mg per 1 ml Co-trimoxazole 40mg/200mg/5ml oral suspension sugar free | 100 ml PoM £15.65 DT = £16.78 SF

  Trimethoprim 16 mg per 1 ml, Sulfamethoxazole 80 mg per 1 ml Co-trimoxazole 80mg/400mg/5ml oral suspension | 100 ml PoM £10.95–£18.36 DT = £26.00

Sulfadiazine
03-Nov-2021

(Sulphadiazine)

- **DRUG ACTION** Sulfadiazine is a short-acting sulphonamide with bacteriostatic activity against a broad spectrum of organisms. The importance of the sulfonamides has decreased as a result of increasing bacterial resistance and their replacement by antibacterials which are generally more active and less toxic.

- **INDICATIONS AND DOSE**

Toxoplasmosis in pregnancy (in combination with pyrimethamine and folinic acid)

- BY MOUTH
  - Child 12–17 years: 1 g 3 times a day until delivery

Congenital toxoplasmosis (in combination with pyrimethamine and folinic acid)

- BY MOUTH
  - Neonate: 50 mg/kg twice daily for 12 months.

- **UNLICENSED USE** Not licensed for use in toxoplasmosis.

IMPORTANT SAFETY INFORMATION

SAFE PRACTICE

Sulfadiazine has been confused with sulfasalazine; care must be taken to ensure the correct drug is prescribed and dispensed.

- **CONTRA-INDICATIONS** Acute porphyrias p. 745
- **CAUTIONS** Asthma · avoid in blood disorders · G6PD deficiency (risk of haemolytic anaemia) · maintain adequate fluid intake · neonates (risk of kernicterus) · predisposition to folate deficiency
- **INTERACTIONS** → Appendix 1: sulfonamides
- **SIDE-EFFECTS**
  - **Rare or very rare** Haemolytic anaemia
  - **Frequency not known** Agranulocytosis · aplastic anaemia · appetite decreased · ataxia · back pain · blood disorders · cough · crystalluria · cyanosis · depression · diarrhoea · dizziness · drowsiness · dyspnoea · eosinophilia · erythema nodosum · fatigue · fever · haematuria · hallucination · headache · hepatic disorders · hypoglycaemia · hypoprothrombinaemia · hypothyroidism · idiopathic intracranial hypertension · idiopathic pulmonary fibrosis · insomnia · kernicterus (in neonates) · leucopenia · meningitis aseptic · myocarditis · nausea · nephritis tubulointerstitial · nephrotoxicity · nerve disorders · neurological effects · neutropenia · oral disorders · pancreatitis · photosensitivity reaction · pseudomembranous enterocolitis · psychosis · pulmonary eosinophilia · renal impairment · renal tubular necrosis · seizure · serum sickness-like reaction · severe cutaneous

adverse reactions (SCARs) · skin reactions · systemic lupus erythematosus (SLE) · thrombocytopenia · tinnitus · vasculitis · vertigo · vomiting

SIDE-EFFECTS, FURTHER INFORMATION Discontinue immediately if blood disorders (including leucopenia, thrombocytopenia, megaloblastic anaemia, eosinophilia) or rash (including Stevens-Johnson syndrome, toxic epidermal necrolysis) develop.

- **PREGNANCY** Risk of neonatal haemolysis and methaemoglobinaemia in third trimester; fear of increased risk of kernicterus in neonates appears to be unfounded.
- **BREAST FEEDING** Small risk of kernicterus in jaundiced infants and of haemolysis in G6PD-deficient infants.
- **HEPATIC IMPAIRMENT** Manufacturer advises caution in mild to moderate impairment; avoid in severe impairment or jaundice.
- **RENAL IMPAIRMENT** EvGr Caution in mild to moderate impairment; avoid in severe impairment (risk of crystalluria). (M)

  Dose adjustments EvGr Dose reduction may be necessary. (M)
- **MONITORING REQUIREMENTS** Monitor blood counts on prolonged treatment.

- **MEDICINAL FORMS** There can be variation in the licensing of different medicines containing the same drug. Forms available from special-order manufacturers include: oral suspension

Oral tablet

CAUTIONARY AND ADVISORY LABELS 9, 27

▸ Sulfadiazine (Non-proprietary)

Sulfadiazine 500 mg Sulfadiazine 500mg tablets | 56 tablet PoM £395.42–£636.30 DT = £395.42

ANTIBACTERIALS › TETRACYCLINES AND RELATED DRUGS

Tetracyclines

Overview

The tetracyclines are broad-spectrum antibiotics whose value has decreased owing to increasing bacterial resistance. In children over 12 years of age they are useful for infections caused by chlamydia (trachoma, psittacosis, salpingitis, urethritis, and lymphogranuloma venereum), rickettsia (including Q-fever), brucella (doxycycline p. 434 with either streptomycin p. 380 or rifampicin p. 449), and the spirochaete, *Borrelia burgdorferi* (See Lyme disease). They are also used in respiratory and genital mycoplasma infections, in acne, in destructive (refractory) periodontal disease, in exacerbations of chronic respiratory diseases (because of their activity against *Haemophilus influenzae*), and for leptospirosis in penicillin hypersensitivity (as an alternative to erythromycin p. 406).

Microbiologically, there is little to choose between the various tetracyclines, the only exception being minocycline p. 436 which has a broader spectrum; it is active against *Neisseria meningitidis* and has been used for meningococcal prophylaxis but is no longer recommended because of side-effects including dizziness and vertigo. Compared to other tetracyclines, minocycline is associated with a greater risk of lupus-erythematosus-like syndrome. Minocycline sometimes causes irreversible pigmentation.

Tetracyclines have a role in the management of meticillin-resistant *Staphylococcus aureus* (MRSA) infections.

Tetracyclines

- **CAUTIONS** Myasthenia gravis (muscle weakness may be increased) · systemic lupus erythematosus (may be exacerbated)
- **SIDE-EFFECTS**
  - ▸ **Common or very common** Angioedema · diarrhoea · headache · Henoch-Schönlein purpura · hypersensitivity · nausea · pericarditis · photosensitivity reaction · skin reactions · systemic lupus erythematosus exacerbated · vomiting
  - ▸ **Uncommon** Dizziness · pancreatitis
  - ▸ **Rare or very rare** Appetite decreased · discolouration of thyroid gland · dysphagia · eosinophilia · fontanelle bulging (in infants) · gastrointestinal disorders · glossitis · haemolytic anaemia · hepatic disorders · idiopathic intracranial hypertension · increased risk of infection · neutropenia · pseudomembranous enterocolitis · Stevens-Johnson syndrome · thrombocytopenia
  - ▸ **Frequency not known** Tooth discolouration

  SIDE-EFFECTS, FURTHER INFORMATION Headache and visual disturbances may indicate benign intracranial hypertension (discontinue treatment if raised intracranial pressure develops).
- **PREGNANCY** Should **not** be given to pregnant women; effects on skeletal development have been documented in the first trimester in *animal* studies. Administration during the second or third trimester may cause discoloration of the child's teeth, and maternal hepatotoxicity has been reported with large parenteral doses.
- **BREAST FEEDING** Should **not** be given to women who are breast-feeding (although absorption and therefore discoloration of teeth in the infant is probably usually prevented by chelation with calcium in milk).
- **HEPATIC IMPAIRMENT** In general, manufacturers advise caution.

above

Demeclocycline hydrochloride 20-Jan-2022

- **INDICATIONS AND DOSE**

Susceptible infections (e.g. chlamydia, rickettsia and mycoplasma)

▸ BY MOUTH

▸ Child 12–17 years: 150 mg 4 times a day, alternatively 300 mg twice daily

- **CONTRA-INDICATIONS** Children under 12 years (deposition in growing bone and teeth, by binding to calcium, causes staining and occasionally dental hypoplasia)
- **CAUTIONS** Photosensitivity more common than with other tetracyclines
- **INTERACTIONS** → Appendix 1: tetracyclines
- **SIDE-EFFECTS**
  - ▸ **Rare or very rare** Agranulocytosis · aplastic anaemia · hearing impairment · nephritis · severe cutaneous adverse reactions (SCARs)
  - ▸ **Frequency not known** Intracranial pressure increased · muscle weakness · nephrogenic diabetes insipidus · stomatitis · vision disorders
- **HEPATIC IMPAIRMENT**

  Dose adjustments Manufacturer advises maximum 1 g daily in divided doses.
- **RENAL IMPAIRMENT** EvGr Avoid unless potential benefit outweighs risk (risk of accumulation). (M)

  Dose adjustments EvGr Reduce dose if use is essential. (M)
- **PATIENT AND CARER ADVICE** Patients should be advised to avoid exposure to sunlight or sun lamps.

● **MEDICINAL FORMS** There can be variation in the licensing of different medicines containing the same drug. Forms available from special-order manufacturers include: oral tablet, oral suspension, oral solution

Oral tablet

▸ **Demeclocycline hydrochloride (Non-proprietary)**

Demeclocycline hydrochloride 150 mg Demeclocycline 150mg tablets | 100 tablet PoM ⊠

Oral capsule

CAUTIONARY AND ADVISORY LABELS 7, 9, 11, 23

▸ **Demeclocycline hydrochloride (Non-proprietary)**

Demeclocycline hydrochloride 150 mg Demeclocycline 150mg capsules | 28 capsule PoM £238.41–£381.46 DT = £238.41

Demeclocycline hydrochloride 300 mg Ledermycin 300mg capsules | 16 capsule PoM ⊠

Demeclocycline 300mg capsules | 28 capsule PoM £452.98 DT = £452.98

⚑ 433

Doxycycline

18-Apr-2025

● **INDICATIONS AND DOSE**

Susceptible infections (e.g. chlamydia, rickettsia and mycoplasma)

▶ BY MOUTH USING IMMEDIATE-RELEASE MEDICINES

▸ Child 8–11 years (administered on expert advice) (body-weight up to 45 kg): Initially 4.4 mg/kg daily in 1–2 divided doses for 1 day, then 2.2 mg/kg daily in 1–2 divided doses

▸ Child 8–11 years (administered on expert advice) (body-weight 45 kg and above): Initially 200 mg daily in 1–2 divided doses for 1 day, then 100 mg daily

▸ Child 12–17 years: Initially 200 mg daily in 1–2 divided doses for 1 day, then 100 mg daily

Severe infections (including refractory urinary-tract infections)

▶ BY MOUTH USING IMMEDIATE-RELEASE MEDICINES

▸ Child 8–11 years (administered on expert advice) (body-weight up to 45 kg): Initially 4.4 mg/kg daily in 1–2 divided doses for 1 day, then 2.2–4.4 mg/kg daily in 1–2 divided doses

▸ Child 8–11 years (administered on expert advice) (body-weight 45 kg and above): 200 mg daily

▸ Child 12–17 years: 200 mg daily

Acute sinusitis | Acute cough [if systemically very unwell or at higher risk of complications] | Community-acquired pneumonia

▶ BY MOUTH USING IMMEDIATE-RELEASE MEDICINES

▸ Child 12–17 years: Initially 200 mg for 1 dose on first day, then 100 mg once daily for 5 days in total

Acute exacerbation of bronchiectasis

▶ BY MOUTH USING IMMEDIATE-RELEASE MEDICINES

▸ Child 12–17 years: Initially 200 mg for 1 dose on first day, then 100 mg once daily for 7–14 days in total

Prophylaxis of infection from human bites [in combination with other drugs] | Prophylaxis of infection from animal bites [in combination with other drugs]

▶ BY MOUTH USING IMMEDIATE-RELEASE MEDICINES

▸ Child 12–17 years: Initially 200 mg daily on first day, then 100–200 mg daily for 3 days in total

Treatment of infection from human bites [in combination with other drugs] | Treatment of infection from animal bites [in combination with other drugs]

▶ BY MOUTH USING IMMEDIATE-RELEASE MEDICINES

▸ Child 12–17 years: Initially 200 mg daily on first day, then 100–200 mg daily for 5–7 days in total

Acne vulgaris [adjunct to topical treatment]

▶ BY MOUTH USING IMMEDIATE-RELEASE MEDICINES

▸ Child 12–17 years: 100 mg once daily

Early syphilis | Asymptomatic contacts of patients with infectious syphilis

▶ BY MOUTH USING IMMEDIATE-RELEASE MEDICINES

▸ Child 12–17 years: 100 mg twice daily for 14 days

Late latent syphilis

▶ BY MOUTH USING IMMEDIATE-RELEASE MEDICINES

▸ Child 12–17 years: 100 mg twice daily for 28 days

Uncomplicated genital chlamydia | Non-gonococcal urethritis

▶ BY MOUTH USING IMMEDIATE-RELEASE MEDICINES

▸ Child 12–17 years: 100 mg twice daily for 7 days

Pelvic inflammatory disease

▶ BY MOUTH USING IMMEDIATE-RELEASE MEDICINES

▸ Child 12–17 years: 100 mg twice daily for 14 days

Lyme disease [erythema migrans and/or non-focal symptoms] | Lyme disease [affecting cranial nerves or peripheral nervous system] | Lyme carditis

▶ BY MOUTH USING IMMEDIATE-RELEASE MEDICINES

▸ Child 9–11 years (administered on expert advice) (body-weight up to 45 kg): Initially 5 mg/kg in 2 divided doses on day 1, then 2.5 mg/kg daily in 1–2 divided doses for a total of 21 days, increased if necessary up to 5 mg/kg daily for 21 days, increased dose used in severe infections; maximum 200 mg per day

▸ Child 9–11 years (administered on expert advice) (body-weight 45 kg and above): 200 mg daily in 1–2 divided doses for 21 days

▸ Child 12–17 years (administered on expert advice): 200 mg daily in 1–2 divided doses for 21 days

Lyme disease [affecting central nervous system]

▶ BY MOUTH USING IMMEDIATE-RELEASE MEDICINES

▸ Child 9–11 years (administered on expert advice) (body-weight up to 45 kg): Initially 5 mg/kg in 2 divided doses on day 1, then 2.5 mg/kg daily in 1–2 divided doses for a total of 21 days, increased if necessary up to 5 mg/kg daily, increased dose used in severe infections

▸ Child 9–11 years (administered on expert advice) (body-weight 45 kg and above): 400 mg daily in 1–2 divided doses for 21 days

▸ Child 12–17 years (administered on expert advice): 400 mg daily in 1–2 divided doses for 21 days

Lyme arthritis | Acrodermatitis chronica atrophicans

▶ BY MOUTH USING IMMEDIATE-RELEASE MEDICINES

▸ Child 9–11 years (administered on expert advice) (body-weight up to 45 kg): Initially 5 mg/kg in 2 divided doses on day 1, then 2.5 mg/kg daily in 1–2 divided doses for a total of 28 days, increased if necessary up to 5 mg/kg daily for 28 days, increased dose used in severe infections; maximum 200 mg per day

▸ Child 9–11 years (administered on expert advice) (body-weight 45 kg and above): 200 mg daily in 1–2 divided doses for 28 days

▸ Child 12–17 years (administered on expert advice): 200 mg daily in 1–2 divided doses for 28 days

Anthrax (treatment or post-exposure prophylaxis)

▶ BY MOUTH USING IMMEDIATE-RELEASE MEDICINES

▸ Child 1 month–11 years: 2.5 mg/kg twice daily (max. per dose 100 mg), only to be used in children under 12 years if alternative antibacterial cannot be given

▸ Child 12–17 years: 100 mg twice daily

Prophylaxis of malaria

▶ BY MOUTH USING IMMEDIATE-RELEASE MEDICINES

▸ Child 12–17 years (body-weight 25 kg and above): 100 mg once daily, to be started 1–2 days before entering endemic area and continued for 4 weeks after leaving

Adjunct to quinine in treatment of *Plasmodium falciparum* malaria

▶ BY MOUTH USING IMMEDIATE-RELEASE MEDICINES

▸ Child 12–17 years: 200 mg daily for 7 days

Periodontitis (as an adjunct to gingival scaling and root planing)

▶ BY MOUTH USING IMMEDIATE-RELEASE MEDICINES

▸ Child 12–17 years: 20 mg twice daily for 3 months

Rocky Mountain spotted fever

▶ BY MOUTH USING DISPERSIBLE TABLETS

▸ Child (administered on expert advice) (body-weight up to 45 kg): 2.2 mg/kg twice daily continue treatment for at least 3 days after fever subsides, minimum treatment duration is 5–7 days

▸ Child (administered on expert advice) (body-weight 45 kg and above): 100 mg twice daily continue treatment for at least 3 days after fever subsides, minimum treatment duration is 5–7 days

● **UNLICENSED USE** Doxycycline may be used as detailed below, although these situations are considered outside the scope of its licence:
- EvGr duration of treatment for acute sinusitis;
- dose for treatment of acne vulgaris;
- dose for treatment of early syphilis and late latent syphilis;
- dose for treatment of asymptomatic contacts of patients with infectious syphilis;
- Lyme disease (A);
- treatment or post-exposure prophylaxis of anthrax;
- malaria prophylaxis during pregnancy.

● **CAUTIONS** Alcohol dependence · children 8–11 years—use only in acute or severe infections when there are no adequate alternatives (deposition in growing bone and teeth, by binding to calcium, causes staining and occasionally dental hypoplasia) · children under 8 years—use only in severe or life-threatening conditions (e.g. Rocky Mountain spotted fever) when there are no adequate alternatives (deposition in growing bone and teeth, by binding to calcium, causes staining and occasionally dental hypoplasia)

● **INTERACTIONS** → Appendix 1: tetracyclines

● **SIDE-EFFECTS**

▶ **Common or very common** Dyspnoea · hypotension · peripheral oedema · tachycardia

▶ **Uncommon** Gastrointestinal discomfort

▶ **Rare or very rare** Anxiety · arthralgia · Clostridioides difficile colitis · flushing · intracranial pressure increased with papilloedema · Jarisch-Herxheimer reaction · myalgia · photoonycholysis · severe cutaneous adverse reactions (SCARs) · skin hyperpigmentation (long term use) · stomatitis · tinnitus · vision disorders

● **PREGNANCY**

▸ When used for Prophylaxis of malaria UKHSA advises avoid—when travel to malarious areas is unavoidable and other regimens are unsuitable, doxycycline can be used if the entire course can be completed before 15 weeks' gestation. See also *Pregnancy* in Malaria, prophylaxis p. 476.

● **BREAST FEEDING**

▸ When used for Prophylaxis of malaria See *Breast-feeding* in Malaria, prophylaxis p. 476.

● **MONITORING REQUIREMENTS** When used for periodontitis, monitor for superficial fungal infection, particularly if predisposition to oral candidiasis.

● **DIRECTIONS FOR ADMINISTRATION** Manufacturer advises capsules and tablets should be swallowed whole with plenty of fluid, while sitting or standing.

● **PRESCRIBING AND DISPENSING INFORMATION** For choice of antibacterial therapy, see Anthrax p. 444, Genital system infections, antibacterial therapy p. 368, Lyme disease p. 444, Malaria, prophylaxis p. 476, Malaria, treatment p. 482, Nose infections, antibacterial therapy p. 370, Respiratory system infections, antibacterial therapy p. 371, Skin infections, antibacterial therapy p. 373, Urinary-tract infections p. 454.

● **PATIENT AND CARER ADVICE** Counselling on administration advised.

Photosensitivity Patients should be advised to avoid exposure to sunlight or sun lamps.

● **PROFESSION SPECIFIC INFORMATION**

Dental practitioners' formulary Doxycycline Capsules 100 mg may be prescribed. Dispersible tablets may be prescribed as Dispersible Doxycycline Tablets. Tablets may be prescribed as Doxycycline Tablets 20 mg.

● **MEDICINAL FORMS** There can be variation in the licensing of different medicines containing the same drug. Forms available from special-order manufacturers include: oral suspension, oral solution

Oral tablet

CAUTIONARY AND ADVISORY LABELS 6, 11, 27

▸ **Periostat** (Universal Medicines Ltd)

Doxycycline (as Doxycycline hyclate) 20 mg Periostat 20mg tablets | 56 tablet PoM £17.30 DT = £17.30

Dispersible tablet

CAUTIONARY AND ADVISORY LABELS 6, 9, 11, 13

▸ **Vibramycin-D** (Pfizer Ltd)

Doxycycline (as Doxycycline monohydrate) 100 mg Vibramycin-D 100mg dispersible tablets | 8 tablet PoM £4.91 DT = £4.91 SF

Modified-release capsule

CAUTIONARY AND ADVISORY LABELS 6, 11, 27

▸ **Efracea** (Galderma (UK) Ltd)

Doxycycline (as Doxycycline monohydrate) 40 mg Efracea 40mg modified-release capsules | 14 capsule PoM £7.99 DT = £7.99

Oral capsule

CAUTIONARY AND ADVISORY LABELS 6, 9, 11, 27

▸ **Doxycycline (Non-proprietary)**

Doxycycline (as Doxycycline hyclate) 50 mg Doxycycline 50mg capsules | 28 capsule PoM £2.10 DT = £1.41

Doxycycline (as Doxycycline hyclate) 100 mg Doxycycline 100mg capsules | 6 capsule PoM £0.57–£1.00 | 8 capsule PoM £3.00 DT = £0.69 | 14 capsule PoM £5.25 | 50 capsule PoM £4.31–£19.00

433

Lymecycline

20-Jan-2022

● **INDICATIONS AND DOSE**

Susceptible infections (e.g. chlamydia, rickettsia and mycoplasma)

▶ BY MOUTH

▸ Child 12–17 years: 408 mg twice daily, dose to be increased to 1.224–1.632 g per day in severe infection

Acne vulgaris [adjunct to topical treatment]

▶ BY MOUTH

▸ Child 12–17 years: 408 mg once daily

● **CONTRA-INDICATIONS** Children under 8 years (deposition in growing bone and teeth, by binding to calcium, causes staining and occasionally dental hypoplasia)

● **INTERACTIONS** → Appendix 1: tetracyclines

● **SIDE-EFFECTS**

▶ **Common or very common** Gastrointestinal discomfort

▶ **Frequency not known** Visual impairment

● **RENAL IMPAIRMENT** EvGr Caution; avoid in overt renal insufficiency. (M)

● **MEDICINAL FORMS** There can be variation in the licensing of different medicines containing the same drug.

Oral capsule

CAUTIONARY AND ADVISORY LABELS 6, 9

▸ **Lymecycline (Non-proprietary)**

Lymecycline 408 mg Lymecycline 408mg capsules | 28 capsule PoM £5.99 DT = £3.50 | 56 capsule PoM £14.13 DT = £7.00

▸ **Tetralysal** (Galderma (UK) Ltd)

Lymecycline 408 mg Tetralysal 300 capsules | 28 capsule PoM £6.95 DT = £3.50 | 56 capsule PoM £11.53 DT = £7.00

433

Minocycline

10-Feb-2022

- **INDICATIONS AND DOSE**

Susceptible infections (e.g. chlamydia, rickettsia and mycoplasma)

▶ BY MOUTH USING IMMEDIATE-RELEASE MEDICINES
- Child 12–17 years: 100 mg twice daily

Acne

▶ BY MOUTH USING IMMEDIATE-RELEASE MEDICINES
- Child 12–17 years: 100 mg once daily, alternatively 50 mg twice daily

▶ BY MOUTH USING MODIFIED-RELEASE MEDICINES
- Child 12–17 years: 100 mg daily

- **CONTRA-INDICATIONS** Children under 12 years (deposition in growing bone and teeth, by binding to calcium, causes staining and occasionally dental hypoplasia)
- **CAUTIONS** Systemic lupus erythematosus
- **INTERACTIONS** → Appendix 1: tetracyclines
- **SIDE-EFFECTS**

▶ **Rare or very rare** Acute kidney injury · hearing impairment · respiratory disorders · tinnitus

▶ **Frequency not known** Alopecia · arthralgia · ataxia · breast secretion · conjunctival discolouration · drug reaction with eosinophilia and systemic symptoms (DRESS) · dyspepsia · hyperbilirubinaemia · hyperhidrosis · oral discolouration · polyarteritis nodosa · sensation abnormal · tear discolouration · tongue discolouration · vertigo

- **RENAL IMPAIRMENT** EvGr Caution in severe impairment (risk of accumulation). (M)

Dose adjustments EvGr Dose reduction may be required in severe impairment. (M)

- **MONITORING REQUIREMENTS** If treatment continued for longer than 6 months, monitor every 3 months for hepatotoxicity, pigmentation and for systemic lupus erythematosus—discontinue if these develop or if pre-existing systemic lupus erythematosus worsens.
- **DIRECTIONS FOR ADMINISTRATION** Manufacturer advises tablets or capsules should be swallowed whole with plenty of fluid while sitting or standing.
- **PATIENT AND CARER ADVICE** Counselling on administration advised (posture).
- **LESS SUITABLE FOR PRESCRIBING** Less suitable for prescribing (compared with other tetracyclines, minocycline is associated with a greater risk of lupus-erythematosus-like syndrome; it sometimes causes irreversible pigmentation).

- **MEDICINAL FORMS** There can be variation in the licensing of different medicines containing the same drug. Forms available from special-order manufacturers include: oral suspension, oral solution

Modified-release capsule

CAUTIONARY AND ADVISORY LABELS 6, 25

▸ Acnamino MR (Dexcel-Pharma Ltd)
Minocycline (as Minocycline hydrochloride) 100 mg Acnamino MR 100mg capsules | 56 capsule PoM £21.14 DT = £20.08

▸ Minocin MR (Viatris UK Healthcare Ltd)
Minocycline (as Minocycline hydrochloride) 100 mg Minocin MR 100mg capsules | 56 capsule PoM £20.08 DT = £20.08

433

Oxytetracycline

20-Jan-2022

- **INDICATIONS AND DOSE**

Susceptible infections (e.g. chlamydia, rickettsia and mycoplasma)

▶ BY MOUTH
- Child 12–17 years: 250–500 mg 4 times a day

Acne

▶ BY MOUTH
- Child 12–17 years: 500 mg twice daily

- **CONTRA-INDICATIONS** Children under 12 years (deposition in growing bone and teeth, by binding to calcium, causes staining and occasionally dental hypoplasia)
- **INTERACTIONS** → Appendix 1: tetracyclines
- **SIDE-EFFECTS** Gastrointestinal discomfort · renal impairment
- **HEPATIC IMPAIRMENT**

Dose adjustments Manufacturer advises avoid in high doses.

- **RENAL IMPAIRMENT** EvGr Avoid unless potential benefit outweighs risk (risk of accumulation). (M)

Dose adjustments EvGr Reduce dose and/or increase dosing interval if use is essential. (M)

- **PROFESSION SPECIFIC INFORMATION**

Dental practitioners' formulary Oxytetracycline Tablets may be prescribed.

- **MEDICINAL FORMS** There can be variation in the licensing of different medicines containing the same drug. Forms available from special-order manufacturers include: oral suspension

Oral tablet

CAUTIONARY AND ADVISORY LABELS 7, 9, 23

▸ Oxytetracycline (Non-proprietary)
Oxytetracycline (as Oxytetracycline dihydrate)
250 mg Oxytetracycline 250mg tablets | 28 tablet PoM £61.00 DT = £30.29

433

Tetracycline

26-Jul-2023

- **INDICATIONS AND DOSE**

Susceptible infections (e.g. chlamydia, rickettsia, mycoplasma)

▶ BY MOUTH
- Child 12–17 years: 250 mg 4 times a day, increased if necessary to 500 mg 3–4 times a day, increased dose used in severe infections

Acne

▶ BY MOUTH
- Child 12–17 years: 500 mg twice daily

Non-gonococcal urethritis

▶ BY MOUTH
- Child 12–17 years: 500 mg 4 times a day for 7–14 days (21 days if failure or relapse after first course)

- **CONTRA-INDICATIONS** Children under 12 years (deposition in growing bone and teeth, by binding to calcium, causes staining and occasionally dental hypoplasia)
- **INTERACTIONS** → Appendix 1: tetracyclines
- **SIDE-EFFECTS**

▶ **Rare or very rare** Agranulocytosis · aplastic anaemia · nephritis · renal impairment

▶ **Frequency not known** Gastrointestinal discomfort · stomatitis · toxic epidermal necrolysis

- **HEPATIC IMPAIRMENT**

Dose adjustments Manufacturer advises avoid in high doses.

- **RENAL IMPAIRMENT** EvGr Avoid unless potential benefit outweighs risk (risk of accumulation). (M)

Dose adjustments EvGr Reduce dose and/or increase dosing interval if use is essential. (M)

- **DIRECTIONS FOR ADMINISTRATION** Manufacturer advises tablets should be swallowed whole with plenty of fluid while sitting or standing.

- **PRESCRIBING AND DISPENSING INFORMATION** For choice of antibacterial therapy, see Genital system infections, antibacterial therapy p. 368.
- **PATIENT AND CARER ADVICE** Counselling on administration advised.
- **PROFESSION SPECIFIC INFORMATION**

Dental practitioners' formulary Tetracycline Tablets may be prescribed.

- **MEDICINAL FORMS** There can be variation in the licensing of different medicines containing the same drug. Forms available from special-order manufacturers include: oral capsule, oral solution

Oral tablet

CAUTIONARY AND ADVISORY LABELS 7, 9, 23

▸ **Tetracycline (Non-proprietary)**
Tetracycline hydrochloride 250 mg Tetracycline 250mg tablets | 28 tablet PoM £50.00 DT = £41.33

Tigecycline

02-Dec-2020

- **DRUG ACTION** Tigecycline is a glycylcycline antibacterial structurally related to the tetracyclines. Tigecycline is active against Gram-positive and Gram-negative bacteria, including tetracycline-resistant organisms, and some anaerobes. It is also active against meticillin-resistant *Staphylococcus aureus* and vancomycin-resistant enterococci, but *Pseudomonas aeruginosa* and many strains of *Proteus* spp. are resistant to tigecycline.

- **INDICATIONS AND DOSE**

Complicated skin and soft tissue infections (when other antibiotics are not suitable) | Complicated intra-abdominal infections (when other antibiotics are not suitable)

▶ BY INTRAVENOUS INFUSION
▸ Child 8–11 years (under expert supervision): 1.2 mg/kg every 12 hours (max. per dose 50 mg) for 5–14 days
▸ Child 12–17 years (under expert supervision): 50 mg every 12 hours for 5–14 days

- **CONTRA-INDICATIONS** Children under 8 years (deposition in growing bone and teeth, by binding to calcium, causes staining and occasionally dental hypoplasia) · Diabetic foot infections
- **CAUTIONS** Cholestasis
- **INTERACTIONS** → Appendix 1: tigecycline
- **SIDE-EFFECTS**

▶ **Common or very common** Abscess · appetite decreased · diarrhoea · dizziness · gastrointestinal discomfort · headache · healing impaired · hyperbilirubinaemia · hypoglycaemia · hypoproteinaemia · increased risk of infection · nausea · sepsis · skin reactions · vomiting
▶ **Uncommon** Hepatic disorders · pancreatitis · thrombocytopenia · thrombophlebitis
▶ **Frequency not known** Acidosis · azotaemia · hyperphosphataemia · hypofibrinogenaemia · idiopathic intracranial hypertension · photosensitivity reaction · pseudomembranous enterocolitis · severe cutaneous adverse reactions (SCARs) · tooth discolouration

SIDE-EFFECTS, FURTHER INFORMATION Side-effects similar to those of the tetracyclines can potentially occur.

- **ALLERGY AND CROSS-SENSITIVITY** EvGr Contra-indicated in patients hypersensitive to tetracyclines. ⟨M⟩
- **PREGNANCY** Tetracyclines should **not** be given to pregnant women; effects on skeletal development have been documented in the first trimester in *animal* studies. Administration during the second or third trimester may cause discoloration of the child's teeth, and maternal hepatotoxicity has been reported with large parenteral doses.
- **BREAST FEEDING** Manufacturer advises avoid—present in milk in *animal* studies.
- **HEPATIC IMPAIRMENT** Manufacturer advises caution in severe impairment.

Dose adjustments Manufacturer advises dose reduction of 50% in severe impairment.

- **MONITORING REQUIREMENTS** Manufacturer advises monitor liver function tests, amylase, lipase, coagulation and haematology parameters before starting treatment, and regularly during treatment.
- **DIRECTIONS FOR ADMINISTRATION** For *intravenous infusion* (*Tygacil*®), give intermittently *in* Glucose 5% *or* Sodium Chloride 0.9%. Reconstitute each vial with 5.3 mL infusion fluid to produce a 10 mg/mL solution; dilute requisite dose in 100 mL infusion fluid; give over 30–60 minutes (preferably 60 minutes).
- **PATIENT AND CARER ADVICE**

Driving and skilled tasks Manufacturer advises patients and carers should be cautioned on the effects on driving and performance of skilled tasks—increased risk of dizziness.

- **MEDICINAL FORMS** There can be variation in the licensing of different medicines containing the same drug.

Powder for solution for infusion

▸ **Tigecycline (Non-proprietary)**
Tigecycline 50 mg Tigecycline 50mg powder for solution for infusion vials | 10 vial PoM £290.79–£323.10 (Hospital only)

▸ **Tygacil** (Pfizer Ltd)
Tigecycline 50 mg Tygacil 50mg powder for solution for infusion vials | 10 vial PoM £323.10 (Hospital only)

ANTIBACTERIALS › OTHER

Chloramphenicol

24-Jul-2024

- **DRUG ACTION** Chloramphenicol is a potent broad-spectrum antibiotic.

- **INDICATIONS AND DOSE**

Life threatening infections particularly those caused by *Haemophilus influenzae* | Typhoid fever

▶ BY MOUTH, OR BY INTRAVENOUS INJECTION, OR BY INTRAVENOUS INFUSION
▸ Child: 12.5 mg/kg every 6 hours, dose may be doubled in severe infections such as septicaemia, meningitis and epiglottitis providing plasma-chloramphenicol concentrations are measured and high doses reduced as soon as indicated

▶ BY INTRAVENOUS INJECTION
▸ Neonate up to 14 days: 12.5 mg/kg twice daily, doses should be checked carefully as overdosage can be fatal.
▸ Neonate 14 days to 28 days: 12.5 mg/kg 2–4 times a day, doses should be checked carefully as overdosage can be fatal.

Cystic fibrosis for the treatment of respiratory *Burkholderia cepacia* infection resistant to other antibacterials

▶ BY MOUTH, OR BY INTRAVENOUS INFUSION, OR BY INTRAVENOUS INJECTION
▸ Child: (consult product literature)

- **CONTRA-INDICATIONS** Acute porphyrias p. 745
- **CAUTIONS** Avoid repeated courses and prolonged treatment
- **INTERACTIONS** → Appendix 1: chloramphenicol
- **SIDE-EFFECTS**

▶ **Rare or very rare**
▸ With parenteral use Aplastic anaemia (reversible or irreversible, with reports of resulting leukaemia)

5 Infection

- **Frequency not known**
  - With oral use Bone marrow disorders · circulatory collapse · diarrhoea · enterocolitis · nausea · optic neuritis · oral disorders · ototoxicity · vomiting
  - With parenteral use Agranulocytosis · bone marrow disorders · depression · diarrhoea · dry mouth · fungal superinfection · headache · nausea · nerve disorders · thrombocytopenic purpura · urticaria · vision disorders · vomiting

SIDE-EFFECTS, FURTHER INFORMATION Associated with serious haematological side-effects when given systemically and should therefore be reserved for the treatment of life-threatening infections.

Grey syndrome Grey baby syndrome (abdominal distension, pallid cyanosis, circulatory collapse) may follow excessive doses in neonates with immature hepatic metabolism.

- **PREGNANCY** Manufacturer advises avoid; neonatal 'grey-baby syndrome' if used in third trimester.
- **BREAST FEEDING** Manufacturer advises avoid; use another antibiotic; may cause bone-marrow toxicity in infant; concentration in milk usually insufficient to cause 'grey syndrome'.
- **HEPATIC IMPAIRMENT** Manufacturer advises caution (increased risk of bone-marrow depression)—monitor plasma-chloramphenicol concentration.
  Dose adjustments Manufacturer advises consider dose reduction.
- **RENAL IMPAIRMENT** EvGr Caution (increased risk of bone-marrow depression)—monitor plasma-chloramphenicol concentration. (M)
  Dose adjustments EvGr Consider dose reduction. (M)
- **MONITORING REQUIREMENTS**
  - Plasma concentration monitoring preferred in those under 4 years of age.
  - In neonates Plasma concentration monitoring required in neonates. Grey baby syndrome may follow excessive doses in neonates with immature hepatic metabolism.
  - Recommended peak plasma concentration (approx. 2 hours after administration by mouth, intravenous injection or infusion) 10–25 mg/litre; pre-dose ('trough') concentration should not exceed 15 mg/litre.
  - Blood counts required before and periodically during treatment.
- **DIRECTIONS FOR ADMINISTRATION** Displacement value may be significant for injection, consult local guidelines. EvGr For *intermittent intravenous infusion*, dilute reconstituted solution further in Glucose 5% *or* Sodium Chloride 0.9%. (M)
- **PRESCRIBING AND DISPENSING INFORMATION** For choice of antibacterial therapy, see Central nervous system infections, antibacterial therapy p. 365.

- **MEDICINAL FORMS** There can be variation in the licensing of different medicines containing the same drug.

Powder for solution for injection

ELECTROLYTES: May contain Sodium

- **Chloramphenicol (Non-proprietary)**
  Chloramphenicol (as Chloramphenicol sodium succinate)
  1 gram Chloramphenicol 1g powder for solution for injection vials | 1 vial PoM £65.00-£79.99 (Hospital only) | 1 vial PoM £92.34-£92.40

Oral capsule

- **Chloramphenicol (Non-proprietary)**
  Chloramphenicol 250 mg Chloramphenicol 250mg capsules | 60 capsule PoM £377.00

Daptomycin

18-Aug-2021

- **DRUG ACTION** Daptomycin is a lipopeptide antibacterial with a spectrum of activity similar to vancomycin but its efficacy against enterococci has not been established. It needs to be given with other antibacterials for mixed infections involving Gram-negative bacteria and some anaerobes.

- **INDICATIONS AND DOSE**

Complicated skin and soft-tissue infections caused by Gram-positive bacteria

- BY INTRAVENOUS INFUSION
  - Child 12–23 months: 10 mg/kg once daily for up to 14 days, alternatively 12 mg/kg once daily, higher dose only if associated with *Staphylococcus aureus* bacteraemia—duration of treatment in accordance with risk of complications in individual patients
  - Child 2–6 years: 9 mg/kg once daily for up to 14 days, alternatively 12 mg/kg once daily, higher dose only if associated with *Staphylococcus aureus* bacteraemia—duration of treatment in accordance with risk of complications in individual patients
  - Child 7–11 years: 7 mg/kg once daily for up to 14 days, alternatively 9 mg/kg once daily, higher dose only if associated with *Staphylococcus aureus* bacteraemia—duration of treatment in accordance with risk of complications in individual patients
  - Child 12–17 years: 5 mg/kg once daily for up to 14 days, alternatively 7 mg/kg once daily, higher dose only if associated with *Staphylococcus aureus* bacteraemia—duration of treatment in accordance with risk of complications in individual patients

- **CAUTIONS** Obesity (limited information on safety and efficacy)
- **INTERACTIONS** → Appendix 1: daptomycin
- **SIDE-EFFECTS**
  - **Common or very common** Anaemia · anxiety · asthenia · constipation · diarrhoea · dizziness · fever · flatulence · gastrointestinal discomfort · headache · hypertension · hypotension · increased risk of infection · insomnia · nausea · pain · skin reactions · vomiting
  - **Uncommon** Appetite decreased · arrhythmias · arthralgia · electrolyte imbalance · eosinophilia · flushing · glossitis · hyperglycaemia · muscle weakness · myalgia · myopathy · paraesthesia · renal impairment · taste altered · thrombocytosis · tremor · vertigo
  - **Rare or very rare** Jaundice
  - **Frequency not known** Acute generalised exanthematous pustulosis (AGEP) · chills · Clostridioides difficile colitis · cough · infusion related reaction · peripheral neuropathy · respiratory disorders · syncope

SIDE-EFFECTS, FURTHER INFORMATION If unexplained muscle pain, tenderness, weakness, or cramps develop during treatment, measure creatine kinase every 2 days; discontinue if unexplained muscular symptoms and creatine elevated markedly.

- **PREGNANCY** Manufacturer advises use only if potential benefit outweighs risk—no information available.
- **BREAST FEEDING** Present in milk in small amounts, but absorption from gastrointestinal tract negligible.
- **HEPATIC IMPAIRMENT** Manufacturer advises caution in severe impairment—no information available.
- **RENAL IMPAIRMENT** Manufacturer advises the dosage regimen has not been established—use with caution and monitor renal function regularly.
- **MONITORING REQUIREMENTS**
  - Manufacturer advises monitor plasma creatine phosphokinase (CPK) before treatment and then at least weekly during treatment; monitor CPK more frequently in

patients at higher risk of developing myopathy, including those with renal impairment, taking other drugs associated with myopathy, or if CPK elevated more than 5 times upper limit of normal before treatment.
- Manufacturer advises monitor renal function regularly during concomitant administration of potentially nephrotoxic drugs.

- **EFFECT ON LABORATORY TESTS** Interference with assay for prothrombin time and INR—take blood sample immediately before daptomycin dose.
- **DIRECTIONS FOR ADMINISTRATION** For *intravenous infusion*, manufacturer advises give intermittently in Sodium Chloride 0.9%; reconstitute with Sodium Chloride 0.9% (350 mg in 7 mL, 500 mg in 10 mL); gently rotate vial without shaking; allow to stand for at least 10 minutes then rotate gently to dissolve; dilute requisite dose in 50 mL infusion fluid and give over 60 minutes for children aged 1–6 years and over 30 minutes for children aged 7–17 years.
- **HANDLING AND STORAGE** Manufacturer advises store in a refrigerator (2–8 °C)—consult product literature for further information regarding storage after reconstitution and dilution.

- **MEDICINAL FORMS** There can be variation in the licensing of different medicines containing the same drug.

Powder for solution for infusion

- **Daptomycin (Non-proprietary)**
  - **Daptomycin 350 mg** Daptomycin 350mg powder for solution for infusion vials | 1 vial PoM £59.00–£62.00 (Hospital only) | 1 vial PoM £55.80–£60.00
  - **Daptomycin 500 mg** Daptomycin 500mg powder for solution for infusion vials | 1 vial PoM £87.00–£88.57 (Hospital only) | 1 vial PoM £79.71–£88.00
- **Cubicin** (Merck Sharp & Dohme (UK) Ltd)
  - **Daptomycin 350 mg** Cubicin 350mg powder for concentrate for solution for infusion vials | 1 vial PoM £62.00 (Hospital only)
  - **Daptomycin 500 mg** Cubicin 500mg powder for concentrate for solution for infusion vials | 1 vial PoM £88.57 (Hospital only)

Fidaxomicin

16-Aug-2023

- **DRUG ACTION** Fidaxomicin is a macrocyclic antibacterial that is poorly absorbed from the gastro-intestinal tract, and, therefore, it should not be used to treat systemic infections.

- **INDICATIONS AND DOSE**

***Clostridioides difficile* infection**

- BY MOUTH
  - Neonate (body-weight up to 4 kg): 40 mg every 12 hours for 10 days.
  - Neonate (body-weight 4–6 kg): 80 mg every 12 hours for 10 days.
  - Child (body-weight up to 4 kg): 40 mg every 12 hours for 10 days
  - Child (body-weight 4–6 kg): 80 mg every 12 hours for 10 days
  - Child (body-weight 7–8 kg): 120 mg every 12 hours for 10 days
  - Child (body-weight 9–12.4 kg): 160 mg every 12 hours for 10 days
  - Child (body-weight 12.5 kg and above): 200 mg every 12 hours for 10 days

- **INTERACTIONS** → Appendix 1: fidaxomicin
- **SIDE-EFFECTS**
  - **Common or very common** Constipation · nausea · vomiting
  - **Uncommon** Abdominal distension · appetite decreased · dizziness · dry mouth · flatulence · headache · skin reactions · taste altered
- **ALLERGY AND CROSS-SENSITIVITY** EvGr Use with caution in macrolide hypersensitivity. ⓜ
- **PREGNANCY** Manufacturer advises avoid—no information available.
- **BREAST FEEDING** Manufacturer advises avoid—no information available.
- **HEPATIC IMPAIRMENT** Manufacturer advises caution in moderate to severe impairment—limited information available.
- **RENAL IMPAIRMENT** EvGr Caution in severe impairment (limited information available). ⓜ
- **DIRECTIONS FOR ADMINISTRATION** Fidaxomicin oral suspension can be administered via an enteral feeding tube—consult product literature.
- **PATIENT AND CARER ADVICE** Patient or carer counselling is advised for fidaxomicin oral suspension.

- **MEDICINAL FORMS** There can be variation in the licensing of different medicines containing the same drug.

Oral tablet

CAUTIONARY AND ADVISORY LABELS 9, 25
EXCIPIENTS: May contain Lecithin

- **Fidaxomicin (Non-proprietary)**
  - **Fidaxomicin 200 mg** Fidaxomicin 200mg tablets | 20 tablet PoM £1,350.00 DT = £1,350.00

Oral suspension

CAUTIONARY AND ADVISORY LABELS 9

- **Fidaxomicin (Non-proprietary)**
  - **Fidaxomicin 40 mg per 1 ml** Fidaxomicin 40mg/ml oral suspension sugar free | 110 ml PoM £1,350.00 DT = £1,350.00 SF

Fosfomycin

28-Jul-2021

- **DRUG ACTION** Fosfomycin, a phosphonic acid antibacterial, is active against a range of Gram-positive and Gram-negative bacteria including *Staphylococcus aureus* and Enterobacteriaceae.

- **INDICATIONS AND DOSE**

Acute uncomplicated lower urinary-tract infections (in females)

- BY MOUTH USING GRANULES
  - Child 12–17 years (female): 3 g for 1 dose.

Osteomyelitis when first-line treatments are inappropriate or ineffective | Hospital-acquired lower respiratory-tract infections when first-line treatments are inappropriate or ineffective

- BY INTRAVENOUS INFUSION
  - Neonate up to 40 weeks corrected gestational age: 100 mg/kg daily in 2 divided doses.
  - Neonate 40 weeks to 44 weeks corrected gestational age: 200 mg/kg daily in 3 divided doses.
  - Child 1–11 months (body-weight up to 10 kg): 200–300 mg/kg daily in 3 divided doses, consider using the high-dose regimen in severe infection, particularly when suspected or known to be caused by less sensitive organisms
  - Child 1–11 years (body-weight 10–39 kg): 200–400 mg/kg daily in 3–4 divided doses, consider using the high-dose regimen in severe infection, particularly when suspected or known to be caused by less sensitive organisms
  - Child 12–17 years (body-weight 40 kg and above): 12–24 g daily in 2–3 divided doses (max. per dose 8 g), use the high-dose regimen in severe infection, particularly when suspected or known to be caused by less sensitive organisms

continued →

Complicated urinary-tract infections when first-line treatment ineffective or inappropriate

▶ BY INTRAVENOUS INFUSION

- Neonate up to 40 weeks corrected gestational age: 100 mg/kg daily in 2 divided doses.
- Neonate 40 weeks to 44 weeks corrected gestational age: 200 mg/kg daily in 3 divided doses.
- Child 1–11 months (body-weight up to 10 kg): 200–300 mg/kg daily in 3 divided doses, consider using the high-dose regimen in severe infection, particularly when suspected or known to be caused by less sensitive organisms
- Child 1–11 years (body-weight 10–39 kg): 200–400 mg/kg daily in 3–4 divided doses, consider using the high-dose regimen in severe infection, particularly when suspected or known to be caused by less sensitive organisms
- Child 12–17 years (body-weight 40 kg and above): 12–16 g daily in 2–3 divided doses (max. per dose 8 g), use the high-dose regimen in severe infection, particularly when suspected or known to be caused by less sensitive organisms

Bacterial meningitis when first-line treatment ineffective or inappropriate

▶ BY INTRAVENOUS INFUSION

- Neonate up to 40 weeks corrected gestational age: 100 mg/kg daily in 2 divided doses.
- Neonate 40 weeks to 44 weeks corrected gestational age: 200 mg/kg daily in 3 divided doses.
- Child 1–11 months (body-weight up to 10 kg): 200–300 mg/kg daily in 3 divided doses, consider using the high-dose regimen in severe infection, particularly when suspected or known to be caused by less sensitive organisms
- Child 1–11 years (body-weight 10–39 kg): 200–400 mg/kg daily in 3–4 divided doses, consider using the high-dose regimen in severe infection, particularly when suspected or known to be caused by less sensitive organisms
- Child 12–17 years (body-weight 40 kg and above): 16–24 g daily in 3–4 divided doses (max. per dose 8 g), use the high-dose regimen in severe infection suspected or known to be caused by less sensitive organisms

● **CAUTIONS**

- With intravenous use Cardiac insufficiency · hyperaldosteronism · hypernatraemia · hypertension · pulmonary oedema

● **SIDE-EFFECTS**

GENERAL SIDE-EFFECTS

- **Common or very common** Abdominal pain · diarrhoea · headache · nausea · vomiting
- **Uncommon** Skin reactions
- **Frequency not known** Antibiotic associated colitis · Clostridioides difficile colitis · pseudomembranous enterocolitis

SPECIFIC SIDE-EFFECTS

- **Common or very common**
  - With oral use Dizziness · vulvovaginal infection
- **Uncommon**
  - With parenteral use Appetite decreased · dyspnoea · electrolyte imbalance · fatigue · oedema · taste altered · vertigo
- **Rare or very rare**
  - With parenteral use Bone marrow disorders · eosinophilia · hepatic disorders · visual impairment
- **Frequency not known**
  - With parenteral use Agranulocytosis · asthmatic attack · confusion · leucopenia · neutropenia · tachycardia · thrombocytopenia

● **PREGNANCY** Manufacturer advises use only if potential benefit outweighs risk.

● **BREAST FEEDING** Manufacturer advises use only if potential benefit outweighs risk—present in milk.

● **RENAL IMPAIRMENT** See p. 16.

- With oral use EvGr Avoid if creatinine clearance less than 10 mL/minute. ⟨M⟩
- With intravenous use Child under 12 years (body-weight up to 40 kg)—no information available. EvGr Child 12–17 years (body-weight 40 kg and above)—caution if creatinine clearance 40–80 mL/minute; consult product literature if creatinine clearance less than 40 mL/minute. ⟨M⟩

● **MONITORING REQUIREMENTS**

- With intravenous use Monitor electrolytes and fluid balance.

● **DIRECTIONS FOR ADMINISTRATION**

- With intravenous use Displacement value may be significant when reconstituting injection, consult local guidelines. Manufacturer advises reconstitute each 2-g or 4-g vial with 20 mL and 8-g vial with 40 mL Glucose 5% *or* Glucose 10% *or* Water for Injections; dilute reconstituted solution to a concentration of 40 mg/mL; do not exceed infusion rate of 133 mg/minute.
- With oral use Manufacturer advises granules should be taken on an empty stomach (about 2–3 hours before or after a meal), preferably before bedtime and after emptying the bladder. The granules should be dissolved into a glass of water and taken immediately.

● **PRESCRIBING AND DISPENSING INFORMATION** Doses expressed as fosfomycin base.

● **NATIONAL FUNDING/ACCESS DECISIONS**

For full details see funding body website

Scottish Medicines Consortium (SMC) decisions

- **Fosfomycin (*Fomicyt*®) for the treatment of the following infections in adults and children including neonates: acute osteomyelitis; complicated urinary tract infections; nosocomial lower respiratory tract infections; bacterial meningitis; bacteraemia that occurs in association with, or is suspected to be associated with, any of the infections listed above (March 2015)** SMC No. 1033/15 Recommended with restrictions
- **Fosfomycin trometamol (*Monuril*®) for the treatment of acute lower uncomplicated urinary tract infections, caused by pathogens sensitive to fosfomycin in adult and adolescent female, and for prophylaxis in diagnostic and surgical transurethral procedures (September 2016)** SMC No. 1163/16 Recommended

● **MEDICINAL FORMS** There can be variation in the licensing of different medicines containing the same drug.

Granules for oral solution

CAUTIONARY AND ADVISORY LABELS 9, 13, 23

EXCIPIENTS: May contain Sucrose

- **Fosfomycin (Non-proprietary)**
  Fosfomycin (as Fosfomycin trometamol) 3 gram Fosfomycin 3g granules for oral solution sachets | 1 sachet PoM £4.86–£7.90 DT = £7.58
- **Monuril** (Zambon UK Ltd)
  Fosfomycin (as Fosfomycin trometamol) 3 gram Monuril 3g granules for oral solution sachets | 1 sachet PoM £4.86 DT = £7.58

Powder for solution for infusion

ELECTROLYTES: May contain Sodium

- **Fosfomycin (Non-proprietary)**
  Fosfomycin (as Fosfomycin sodium) 5 gram Infectofos 5g powder for solution for infusion vials | 10 vial PoM ⊠ (Hospital only)
- **Fomicyt** (InfectoPharm Ltd)
  Fosfomycin (as Fosfomycin sodium) 2 gram Fomicyt 2g powder for solution for infusion vials | 10 vial PoM £160.03 (Hospital only)

Fosfomycin (as Fosfomycin sodium) 4 gram Fomicyt 4g powder for solution for infusion vials | 10 vial [PoM] £320.06 (Hospital only)

Fusidic acid

05-Oct-2021

● **DRUG ACTION** Fusidic acid and its salts are narrow-spectrum antibiotics used for staphylococcal infections.

● **INDICATIONS AND DOSE**

Staphylococcal skin infection

▶ TO THE SKIN
- Child: Apply 3–4 times a day usually for 7 days

▶ BY MOUTH USING TABLETS
- Child 12–17 years: 250 mg every 12 hours for 5-10 days, dose expressed as sodium fusidate

Non-bullous impetigo [in patients who are not systemically unwell or at high risk of complications] | Secondary bacterial infection of eczema [for localised infections only]

▶ TO THE SKIN
- Child: Apply 3 times a day for 5–7 days

Penicillin-resistant staphylococcal infection including osteomyelitis | Staphylococcal endocarditis in combination with other antibacterials

▶ BY MOUTH USING ORAL SUSPENSION
- Neonate: 15 mg/kg 3 times a day.
- Child 1-11 months: 15 mg/kg 3 times a day
- Child 1-4 years: 250 mg 3 times a day
- Child 5-11 years: 500 mg 3 times a day
- Child 12-17 years: 750 mg 3 times a day

▶ BY MOUTH USING TABLETS
- Child 12-17 years: 500 mg every 8 hours, dose expressed as sodium fusidate, increased to 1 g every 8 hours, dose expressed as sodium fusidate, increased dose used for severe infections

Staphylococcal infections due to susceptible organisms

▶ BY INTRAVENOUS INFUSION
- Child (body-weight up to 50 kg): 6–7 mg/kg 3 times a day, dose expressed as sodium fusidate
- Child (body-weight 50 kg and above): 500 mg 3 times a day, dose expressed as sodium fusidate

DOSE EQUIVALENCE AND CONVERSION
- With oral use
- Fusidic acid is incompletely absorbed and doses recommended for suspension are proportionately higher than those for sodium fusidate tablets.

● **CAUTIONS**
- With systemic use Impaired transport and metabolism of bilirubin
- With topical use Avoid contact of cream or ointment with eyes

CAUTIONS, FURTHER INFORMATION
- Avoiding resistance
- With topical use To avoid the development of resistance, fusidic acid should not be used for longer than 10 days and local microbiology advice should be sought before using it in hospital.

● **INTERACTIONS** → Appendix 1: fusidate

● **SIDE-EFFECTS**

GENERAL SIDE-EFFECTS
- **Uncommon** Skin reactions

SPECIFIC SIDE-EFFECTS
- **Common or very common**
- With intravenous use Thrombophlebitis · vascular pain (reduced if given via central vein)
- With oral use Diarrhoea · gastrointestinal discomfort · nausea · vomiting
- With systemic use Dizziness · drowsiness · hepatic disorders · hyperbilirubinaemia
- **Uncommon**
- With oral use Rash pustular
- With systemic use Appetite decreased · asthenia · headache · malaise · rhabdomyolysis
- **Rare or very rare**
- With topical use Angioedema · conjunctivitis
- **Frequency not known**
- With systemic use Agranulocytosis · anaemia · leucopenia · neutropenia · pancytopenia · renal failure · thrombocytopenia

SIDE-EFFECTS, FURTHER INFORMATION Elevated liver enzymes, hyperbilirubinaemia and jaundice can occur with systemic use—these effects are usually reversible following withdrawal of therapy.

● **PREGNANCY**
- With systemic use Not known to be harmful; manufacturer advises use only if potential benefit outweighs risk.

● **BREAST FEEDING**
- With systemic use Present in milk—manufacturer advises caution.

● **HEPATIC IMPAIRMENT**
- With systemic use Manufacturer advises caution.

● **MONITORING REQUIREMENTS**
- With systemic use Manufacturer advises monitor liver function with high doses or on prolonged therapy; monitoring also advised for patients with biliary tract obstruction, those taking potentially hepatotoxic medication, or those taking concurrent medication with a similar excretion pathway.

● **DIRECTIONS FOR ADMINISTRATION** Manufacturer advises *for intravenous infusion*, give intermittently in Sodium Chloride 0.9% or Glucose 5%; reconstitute each vial with 10 mL buffer solution, then add contents of vial to 500 mL infusion fluid to give a solution containing approximately 1 mg/mL. Give requisite dose via a central line over 2 hours (give over at least 6 hours if administered via a large peripheral vein).

● **PRESCRIBING AND DISPENSING INFORMATION** For choice of antibacterial therapy, see Cardiovascular system infections, antibacterial therapy p. 364, Musculoskeletal system infections, antibacterial therapy p. 369, Skin infections, antibacterial therapy p. 373.

● **PROFESSION SPECIFIC INFORMATION**

Dental practitioners' formulary May be prescribed as Sodium Fusidate ointment.

● **MEDICINAL FORMS** There can be variation in the licensing of different medicines containing the same drug. Forms available from special-order manufacturers include: oral suspension

Oral tablet

CAUTIONARY AND ADVISORY LABELS 9

▶ **Fusidic acid (Non-proprietary)**
Sodium fusidate 250 mg Sodium fusidate 250mg tablets | 1 tablet [PoM] [X]

Cutaneous ointment

EXCIPIENTS: May contain Cetostearyl alcohol (including cetyl and stearyl alcohol), woolfat and related substances (including lanolin)

▶ **Fucidin** (LEO Pharma)
Sodium fusidate 20 mg per 1 gram Fucidin 20mg/g ointment | 15 gram [PoM] £2.68 DT = £2.68 | 30 gram [PoM] £4.55 DT = £4.55

Oral suspension

CAUTIONARY AND ADVISORY LABELS 9

▶ **Fucidin** (LEO Pharma)
Fusidic acid 50 mg per 1 ml Fucidin 250mg/5ml oral suspension | 90 ml [PoM] £12.11 DT = £12.11

Cutaneous cream

EXCIPIENTS: May contain Butylated hydroxyanisole, cetostearyl alcohol (including cetyl and stearyl alcohol)

▸ **Fusidic acid (Non-proprietary)**
Fusidic acid 20 mg per 1 gram Fusidic acid 2% cream | 15 gram [PoM] £3.14 DT = £1.92 | 30 gram [PoM] £6.60 DT = £3.59

▸ **Fucidin** (LEO Pharma)
Fusidic acid 20 mg per 1 gram Fucidin 20mg/g cream | 15 gram [PoM] £1.92 DT = £1.92 | 30 gram [PoM] £3.59 DT = £3.59

Powder and solvent for solution for infusion
ELECTROLYTES: May contain Sodium

▸ **Fusidic acid (Non-proprietary)**
Sodium fusidate 500 mg Sodium fusidate 500mg powder and solvent for solution for infusion vials | 1 vial [PoM] £21.95

Linezolid

21-Apr-2026

● **DRUG ACTION** Linezolid, an oxazolidinone antibacterial, is active against Gram-positive bacteria including meticillin-resistant *Staphylococcus aureus* (MRSA), and glycopeptide-resistant enterococci. Resistance to linezolid can develop with prolonged treatment or if the dose is less than that recommended. Linezolid is **not** active against common Gram-negative organisms; it must be given in combination with other antibacterials for mixed infections that also involve Gram-negative organisms.

● **INDICATIONS AND DOSE**

Pneumonia (when other antibacterials e.g. a glycopeptide, such as vancomycin, cannot be used) (initiated under specialist supervision) | Complicated skin and soft-tissue infections caused by Gram-positive bacteria, when other antibacterials cannot be used (initiated under specialist supervision)

▸ BY MOUTH, OR BY INTRAVENOUS INFUSION

▸ Neonate up to 7 days: 10 mg/kg every 12 hours, increased if necessary to 10 mg/kg every 8 hours, increased dose can be used if poor response.

▸ Neonate 7 days to 28 days: 10 mg/kg every 8 hours.

▸ Child 1 month–11 years: 10 mg/kg every 8 hours (max. per dose 600 mg)

▸ Child 12–17 years: 600 mg every 12 hours

Cellulitis (specialist use only) | Erysipelas (specialist use only)

▸ BY MOUTH, OR BY INTRAVENOUS INFUSION

▸ Child 1 month–11 years: 10 mg/kg every 8 hours (max. per dose 600 mg)

▸ Child 12–17 years: 600 mg every 12 hours

● **UNLICENSED USE** Not licensed for use in children.

IMPORTANT SAFETY INFORMATION

CHM ADVICE (OPTIC NEUROPATHY)

Severe optic neuropathy may occur rarely, particularly if linezolid is used for longer than 28 days. The CHM recommends that:

- patients should be warned to report symptoms of visual impairment (including blurred vision, visual field defect, changes in visual acuity and colour vision) immediately;
- patients experiencing new visual symptoms (regardless of treatment duration) should be evaluated promptly, and referred to an ophthalmologist if necessary;
- visual function should be monitored regularly if treatment is required for longer than 28 days.

BLOOD DISORDERS

Haematopoietic disorders (including thrombocytopenia, anaemia, leucopenia, and pancytopenia) have been reported in patients receiving linezolid. It is recommended that full blood counts are monitored weekly. Close monitoring is recommended in patients who:

- receive treatment for more than 10–14 days;
- have pre-existing myelosuppression;
- are receiving drugs that may have adverse effects on haemoglobin, blood counts, or platelet function;
- have severe renal impairment.

If significant myelosuppression occurs, treatment should be stopped unless it is considered essential, in which case intensive monitoring of blood counts and appropriate management should be implemented.

● **CAUTIONS** Acute confusional states · bipolar depression · carcinoid tumour · history of seizures · phaeochromocytoma · schizophrenia · thyrotoxicosis · uncontrolled hypertension

CAUTIONS, FURTHER INFORMATION

▸ Close observation Unless close observation and blood pressure monitoring possible, linezolid should be avoided in uncontrolled hypertension, phaeochromocytoma, carcinoid tumour, thyrotoxicosis, bipolar depression, schizophrenia, or acute confusional states.

● **INTERACTIONS** → Appendix 1: linezolid

● **SIDE-EFFECTS**

▸ **Common or very common** Anaemia · constipation · diarrhoea · dizziness · gastrointestinal discomfort · headache · hypertension · increased risk of infection · insomnia · localised pain · nausea · skin reactions · taste altered · thrombocytopenia · vomiting

▸ **Uncommon** Angioedema · antibiotic associated colitis · arrhythmias · bone marrow disorders · chills · dry mouth · eosinophilia · fatigue · gastritis · hyperhidrosis · hyponatraemia · leucopenia · nerve disorders · neutropenia · oral disorders · pancreatitis · polyuria · pseudomembranous enterocolitis · renal failure · seizure · sensation abnormal · thirst · thrombophlebitis · tinnitus · tongue discolouration · transient ischaemic attack · vision disorders · vulvovaginal disorder

▸ **Rare or very rare** Hypersensitivity vasculitis · lactic acidosis · rhabdomyolysis · severe cutaneous adverse reactions (SCARs) · tooth discolouration

▸ **Frequency not known** Alopecia · Clostridioides difficile colitis · serotonin syndrome · SIADH

● **PREGNANCY** Manufacturer advises use only if potential benefit outweighs risk—no information available.

● **BREAST FEEDING** Manufacturer advises avoid—present in milk in *animal* studies.

● **HEPATIC IMPAIRMENT** Manufacturer advises caution in severe impairment (no information available).

● **RENAL IMPAIRMENT** [EvGr] Use with caution if creatinine clearance less than 30 mL/minute (metabolites may accumulate), ⟨M⟩ see p. 16.

● **MONITORING REQUIREMENTS** Monitor full blood count (including platelet count) weekly.

● **DIRECTIONS FOR ADMINISTRATION**

▸ With intravenous use Manufacturer advises infusion to be administered over 30–120 minutes.

● **PRESCRIBING AND DISPENSING INFORMATION** For choice of antibacterial therapy, see Respiratory system infections, antibacterial therapy p. 371, Skin infections, antibacterial therapy p. 373.

There is limited information on use in children and expert advice should be sought.

● **PATIENT AND CARER ADVICE** Patients should be advised to read the patient information leaflet given with linezolid.
Driving and skilled tasks Patients and carers should be cautioned on the effects on driving and performance of skilled tasks—increased risk of dizziness.

● **MEDICINAL FORMS** There can be variation in the licensing of different medicines containing the same drug.

Infusion

EXCIPIENTS: May contain Glucose

ELECTROLYTES: May contain Sodium

▸ **Linezolid (Non-proprietary)**

Linezolid 2 mg per 1 ml Linezolid 600mg/300ml infusion KabiPac polyethylene bottles | 10 bottle PoM £706.30 (Hospital only) Linezolid 600mg/300ml infusion bags | 10 bag PoM £445.00 (Hospital only)

▸ **Zyvox** (Pfizer Ltd)

Linezolid 2 mg per 1 ml Zyvox 600mg/300ml infusion bags | 10 bag PoM £445.00 (Hospital only)

Oral tablet

CAUTIONARY AND ADVISORY LABELS 9, 10

▸ **Linezolid (Non-proprietary)**

Linezolid 600 mg Linezolid 600mg tablets | 10 tablet PoM £239.16–£392.77 (Hospital only) | 10 tablet PoM £22.02–£445.00

▸ **Zyvox** (Pfizer Ltd)

Linezolid 600 mg Zyvox 600mg tablets | 10 tablet PoM £445.00

Oral suspension

CAUTIONARY AND ADVISORY LABELS 9, 10

EXCIPIENTS: May contain Aspartame

▸ **Zyvox** (Pfizer Ltd)

Linezolid 20 mg per 1 ml Zyvox 100mg/5ml granules for oral suspension | 150 ml PoM £222.50 DT = £222.50

Trimethoprim

15-Jul-2025

● **INDICATIONS AND DOSE**

Respiratory-tract infections

▶ BY MOUTH

- Neonate: Initially 3 mg/kg for 1 dose, then 1–2 mg/kg twice daily.
- Child 4–5 weeks: 4 mg/kg twice daily (max. per dose 200 mg)
- Child 6 weeks–5 months: 4 mg/kg twice daily (max. per dose 200 mg), alternatively 25 mg twice daily
- Child 6 months–5 years: 4 mg/kg twice daily (max. per dose 200 mg), alternatively 50 mg twice daily
- Child 6–11 years: 4 mg/kg twice daily (max. per dose 200 mg), alternatively 100 mg twice daily
- Child 12–17 years: 200 mg twice daily

Treatment of mild to moderate *Pneumocystis jirovecii* (*Pneumocystis carinii*) pneumonia in patients who cannot tolerate co-trimoxazole (in combination with dapsone)

▶ BY MOUTH

- Child: 5 mg/kg every 6–8 hours

Shigellosis | Invasive salmonella infection

▶ BY MOUTH

- Child: (consult product literature)

Acute pyelonephritis

▶ BY MOUTH

- Child 16–17 years: 200 mg twice daily for 14 days

Urinary-tract infection (catheter-associated)

▶ BY MOUTH

- Child 3–5 months: 4 mg/kg twice daily (max. per dose 200 mg) for 7–10 days, alternatively 25 mg twice daily for 7–10 days
- Child 6 months–5 years: 4 mg/kg twice daily (max. per dose 200 mg) for 7–10 days, alternatively 50 mg twice daily for 7–10 days
- Child 6–11 years: 4 mg/kg twice daily (max. per dose 200 mg) for 7–10 days, alternatively 100 mg twice daily for 7–10 days
- Child 12–15 years: 200 mg twice daily for 7–10 days
- Child 16–17 years: 200 mg twice daily for 7 days (14 days if upper urinary-tract symptoms are present)

Lower urinary-tract infection

▶ BY MOUTH

- Neonate: Initially 3 mg/kg for 1 dose, then 1–2 mg/kg twice daily.
- Child 4–5 weeks: 4 mg/kg twice daily (max. per dose 200 mg)
- Child 6 weeks–2 months: 4 mg/kg twice daily (max. per dose 200 mg), alternatively 25 mg twice daily
- Child 3–5 months: 4 mg/kg twice daily (max. per dose 200 mg) for 3 days, alternatively 25 mg twice daily for 3 days
- Child 6 months–5 years: 4 mg/kg twice daily (max. per dose 200 mg) for 3 days, alternatively 50 mg twice daily for 3 days
- Child 6–11 years: 4 mg/kg twice daily (max. per dose 200 mg) for 3 days, alternatively 100 mg twice daily for 3 days
- Child 12–15 years: 200 mg twice daily for 3 days
- Child 16–17 years: 200 mg twice daily for 3 days (7 days in males)

Prophylaxis of recurrent urinary-tract infection in non-pregnant females [using single-dose antibacterial prophylaxis]

▶ BY MOUTH

- Child 16–17 years: 200 mg for 1 dose, dose to be taken following exposure to a trigger

Prophylaxis of recurrent urinary-tract infection [using daily antibacterial prophylaxis]

▶ BY MOUTH

- Child 16–17 years: 100 mg once daily, dose to be taken at night, seek specialist advice if considering use for prophylaxis in male patients, or for recurrent upper urinary-tract infection or recurrent complicated lower urinary-tract infection

Prophylaxis of recurrent urinary-tract infection [using daily antibacterial prophylaxis] (initiated under specialist supervision)

▶ BY MOUTH

- Neonate: 2 mg/kg once daily, dose to be taken at night.
- Child 4–5 weeks: 2 mg/kg once daily, dose to be taken at night
- Child 6 weeks–5 months: 2 mg/kg once daily, dose to be taken at night, alternatively 12.5 mg once daily, dose to be taken at night
- Child 6 months–5 years: 2 mg/kg once daily (max. per dose 100 mg), dose to be taken at night, alternatively 25 mg once daily, dose to be taken at night
- Child 6–11 years: 2 mg/kg once daily (max. per dose 100 mg), dose to be taken at night, alternatively 50 mg once daily, dose to be taken at night
- Child 12–15 years: 100 mg once daily, dose to be taken at night

● **UNLICENSED USE** Not licensed for treatment of pneumocystis pneumonia. EvGr Trimethoprim is used as a single-dose regimen for the prophylaxis of recurrent urinary-tract infection, (A) but this is not licensed.

Not licensed for use in children under 6 weeks.

EvGr Trimethoprim is used for the prophylaxis of recurrent urinary-tract infection in children aged under 6 months, (A) but this is not licensed.

● **CONTRA-INDICATIONS** Blood dyscrasias

● **CAUTIONS** Acute porphyrias p. 745 · neonates (specialist supervision required) · predisposition to folate deficiency

● **INTERACTIONS** → Appendix 1: trimethoprim

● **SIDE-EFFECTS**

▶ **Common or very common** Diarrhoea · electrolyte imbalance · fungal overgrowth · headache · nausea · skin reactions · vomiting

- **Rare or very rare** Agranulocytosis · angioedema · anxiety · appetite decreased · arthralgia · behaviour abnormal · bone marrow disorders · confusion · constipation · cough · depression · dizziness · dyspnoea · eosinophilia · erythema nodosum · fever · haemolysis · haemolytic anaemia · haemorrhage · hallucination · hepatic disorders · hypoglycaemia · lethargy · leucopenia · meningitis aseptic · movement disorders · myalgia · neutropenia · oral disorders · pancreatitis · paraesthesia · peripheral neuritis · photosensitivity reaction · pseudomembranous enterocolitis · renal impairment · seizure · severe cutaneous adverse reactions (SCARs) · sleep disorders · syncope · systemic lupus erythematosus (SLE) · thrombocytopenia · tinnitus · tremor · uveitis · vasculitis · vertigo · wheezing
- **Frequency not known** Gastrointestinal disorder · megaloblastic anaemia · methaemoglobinaemia

● **PREGNANCY** Teratogenic risk in first trimester (folate antagonist). Manufacturers advise avoid during pregnancy.

● **BREAST FEEDING** Present in milk—short-term use not known to be harmful.

● **RENAL IMPAIRMENT** Manufacturer advises caution in impairment.

Dose adjustments Manufacturer advises dose reduction to half normal dose after 3 days if estimated glomerular filtration rate 15–30 mL/minute/1.73 m^2.

Manufacturer advises dose reduction to half normal dose if estimated glomerular filtration rate less than 15 mL/minute/1.73 m^2.

● **MONITORING REQUIREMENTS**

- Manufacturer advises monitor blood counts with long-term use and in those with, or at risk of, folate deficiency.
- Manufacturer advises monitor serum electrolytes in patients at risk of developing hyperkalaemia, and consider monitoring in other patients, particularly with long-term use.
- Manufacturer advises consider monitoring renal function, particularly with long-term use.
- Manufacturer advises monitoring of plasma-trimethoprim concentration may be considered with long-term use and under specialist advice.

● **PRESCRIBING AND DISPENSING INFORMATION** For choice of antibacterial therapy, see Gastro-intestinal system infections, antibacterial therapy p. 367, Pneumocystis pneumonia p. 470, Respiratory system infections, antibacterial therapy p. 371, Urinary-tract infections p. 454.

● **PATIENT AND CARER ADVICE**

Blood disorders On long-term treatment, patients and their carers should be told how to recognise signs of blood disorders and advised to seek immediate medical attention if symptoms such as fever, sore throat, rash, mouth ulcers, purpura, bruising or bleeding develop.

Medicines for Children leaflet: Trimethoprim for bacterial infections
www.medicinesforchildren.org.uk/medicines/trimethoprim-for-bacterial-infections/

● **MEDICINAL FORMS** There can be variation in the licensing of different medicines containing the same drug. Forms available from special-order manufacturers include: oral suspension, oral solution

Oral tablet

CAUTIONARY AND ADVISORY LABELS 9

- **Trimethoprim (Non-proprietary)**
  Trimethoprim 100 mg Trimethoprim 100mg tablets | 28 tablet [PoM] £8.00 DT = £4.57
  Trimethoprim 200 mg Trimethoprim 200mg tablets | 6 tablet [PoM] £2.15 DT = £1.62 | 14 tablet [PoM] £6.90 DT = £3.78

Oral suspension

CAUTIONARY AND ADVISORY LABELS 9

- **Trimethoprim (Non-proprietary)**
  Trimethoprim 10 mg per 1 ml Trimethoprim 50mg/5ml oral suspension sugar free | 100 ml [PoM] £21.00 DT = £7.31 [SF]

Combinations available: ***Co-trimoxazole,*** p. 431

1.1 Anthrax

Anthrax

03-Apr-2021

Treatment and post-exposure prophylaxis

Anthrax is a notifiable disease in the UK. For further information, see *Notifiable diseases* in Antibacterials, principles of therapy p. 358. If anthrax infection is suspected, discuss with an infectious disease specialist and arrange urgent consultation. For community level outbreaks, specialist advice should be sought from Public Health England (tel. 020 8200 4400) or, in Scotland, Health Protection Scotland (tel. 0141 300 1191).

Inhalation or *gastro-intestinal anthrax* should be treated initially with either ciprofloxacin p. 429 or, in patients over 12 years, doxycycline p. 434 [unlicensed use] and combined with one or two other antibacterials (such as benzylpenicillin sodium p. 415, clindamycin, rifampicin, and vancomycin). Alternatively, the combination of amoxicillin p. 417 and imipenem with cilastatin, or meropenem and chloramphenicol may be given.

Cutaneous anthrax should be treated with either oral ciprofloxacin [unlicensed use] or, in patients over 12 years, doxycycline [unlicensed use] for 7 days; treatment should be switched to amoxicillin if the infecting strain is susceptible.

Oral ciprofloxacin, doxycycline [unlicensed use], or amoxicillin may be given for *post-exposure prophylaxis*. Antibacterial prophylaxis should continue for up to 60 days, however a shorter period may be recommended. Vaccination against anthrax may be considered in selected cases. For further information, see Anthrax vaccine p. 962.

Useful resources

Recommendations reflect Chemical, biological, radiological and nuclear incidents: clinical management and health protection. Second Edition. Public Health England. May 2018.

www.gov.uk/government/publications/chemical-biological-radiological-and-nuclear-incidents-recognise-and-respond

Chapter 13, Anthrax, in *Immunisation against infectious disease*- 'The Green Book'. Public Health England. February 2017.

www.gov.uk/government/publications/anthrax-the-green-book-chapter-13

1.2 Lyme disease

Lyme disease

14-Nov-2018

Description of condition

Lyme disease, also known as Lyme borreliosis, is an infection caused by bacteria called *Borrelia burgdorferi*. It is transmitted to humans by the bite of an infected tick. Ticks are mainly found in grassy and wooded areas including urban gardens and parks. Most tick bites do not cause Lyme disease, and the prompt and correct removal of the tick reduces the risk of infection.

Lyme disease usually presents with a characteristic erythema migrans rash. This usually becomes visible 1–4 weeks after a tick bite, but can appear from 3 days to

3 months, and last for several weeks. It may be accompanied by non-focal (non-organ related) symptoms, such as fever, swollen glands, malaise, fatigue, neck pain or stiffness, joint or muscle pain, headache, cognitive impairment, or paraesthesia.

Other signs and symptoms of Lyme disease may also appear months or years after the initial infection and are typically characterised by focal symptoms (relating to at least 1 organ system). These include neurological (affecting cranial nerves, peripheral and central nervous systems), joint (Lyme arthritis), cardiac (Lyme carditis), or skin (acrodermatitis chronica atrophicans) manifestations.

Drug treatment

EvGr The diagnosis and management of Lyme disease in children should be discussed with a specialist unless the child presents with a single erythema migrans lesion and no other symptoms. Children diagnosed with Lyme disease should be given treatment with an antibacterial drug; the choice of drug should be based on presenting symptoms. (A)

Child aged 9 years and over

EvGr In children presenting with *erythema migrans rash with or without non-focal symptoms* oral doxycycline p. 434 [unlicensed] is recommended as first-line treatment. If doxycycline p. 434 cannot be given, oral amoxicillin p. 417 should be used as an alternative. Oral azithromycin p. 402 [unlicensed] should be given if both doxycycline p. 434 and amoxicillin p. 417 are unsuitable.

In children presenting with focal symptoms of *cranial nerve or peripheral nervous system* involvement, oral doxycycline p. 434 [unlicensed] is recommended as first-line treatment. If doxycycline p. 434 cannot be given, oral amoxicillin p. 417 should be used as an alternative.

In children presenting with symptoms of *central nervous system* involvement, intravenous ceftriaxone p. 391 is recommended as first-line treatment. Oral doxycycline p. 434 [unlicensed] should be used as an alternative if ceftriaxone p. 391 cannot be given, or when switching to oral antibacterial treatment.

In children with symptoms of *Lyme arthritis or acrodermatitis chronica atrophicans*, oral doxycycline p. 434 [unlicensed] is recommended as first-line treatment. If doxycycline p. 434 cannot be given, oral amoxicillin p. 417 should be used as an alternative. Intravenous ceftriaxone p. 391 should be used if both doxycycline p. 434 and amoxicillin p. 417 are unsuitable.

In children with symptoms of *Lyme carditis* who are *haemodynamically stable*, oral doxycycline p. 434 [unlicensed] is recommended as first-line treatment. If doxycycline p. 434 cannot be given, intravenous ceftriaxone p. 391 should be used as an alternative.

In children with symptoms of *Lyme carditis who are haemodynamically unstable*, intravenous ceftriaxone p. 391 is recommended. If ceftriaxone p. 391 cannot be given, oral doxycycline p. 434 [unlicensed] should be used as an alternative. (A)

Child aged under 9 years

EvGr In children presenting with *erythema migrans rash with or without non-focal symptoms*, oral amoxicillin p. 417 is recommended as first-line treatment. If oral amoxicillin p. 417 cannot be given, oral azithromycin p. 402 [unlicensed] should be used as an alternative.

In children presenting with focal symptoms of *cranial nerve or peripheral nervous system* involvement, oral amoxicillin p. 417 is recommended.

In children presenting with symptoms of *central nervous system* involvement, intravenous ceftriaxone p. 391 is recommended.

In children with symptoms of *Lyme arthritis or acrodermatitis chronica atrophicans*, oral amoxicillin p. 417 is recommended as first-line treatment. If amoxicillin p. 417 cannot be given, intravenous ceftriaxone p. 391 should be used as an alternative.

In children with symptoms of *Lyme carditis (both haemodynamically stable and unstable)*, intravenous ceftriaxone p. 391 is recommended. (A)

Ongoing symptom management

EvGr If symptoms continue to persist or worsen after antibacterial treatment, patients should be assessed for possible alternative causes, re-infection with Lyme disease, treatment failure or non-adherence to previous antibacterial treatment, or progression to organ damage caused by Lyme disease (such as nerve palsy).

A second course of antibacterial treatment should be given to patients presenting with signs and symptoms of re-infection. In patients presenting with ongoing symptoms due to possible treatment failure, treatment with an alternative antibacterial drug should be considered. A third course of antibacterial treatment is not recommended, and further management should be discussed with a national reference laboratory or suitable specialist depending on symptoms (for example, a rheumatologist or neurologist). (A)

Useful Resources

Lyme disease. National Institute for Health and Care Excellence. NICE guideline 95. April 2018.
www.nice.org.uk/guidance/ng95

'Be tick aware'–Toolkit for raising awareness of the potential risk posed by ticks and tick-borne disease in England. Public Health England. March 2018.
www.gov.uk/government/publications/tick-bite-risks-and-prevention-of-lyme-disease

1.3 Meticillin-resistant Staphylococcus aureus

MRSA

15-Jan-2025

Management

Meticillin-resistant *Staphylococcus aureus* (MRSA) are strains of *Staphylococcus aureus* that are resistant to a number of commonly used antibacterials including beta-lactam antibacterials (e.g. meticillin [now discontinued] and flucloxacillin). As with *Staph. aureus* colonisation, MRSA may colonise the skin, gut, or nose without displaying signs or symptoms of infection. Infection with MRSA can be difficult to manage; management includes appropriate infection control measures, adherence to local policies, and treatment guided by the sensitivity of the infecting strain. Consult a microbiologist or the local infection control team where appropriate.

EvGr Oral doxycycline p. 434, trimethoprim p. 443, ciprofloxacin p. 429, or co-trimoxazole p. 431 can be considered for lower *urinary-tract infections* caused by MRSA according to susceptibility. A **glycopeptide** can be considered for complicated urinary-tract infections. (A)

For information on the management of MRSA-associated *skin and soft-tissue infections, hospital-acquired pneumonia, endocarditis, osteomyelitis,* and *septic arthritis*, see the corresponding treatment summary: Skin infections, antibacterial therapy p. 373, Respiratory system infections, antibacterial therapy p. 371, Cardiovascular system infections, antibacterial therapy p. 364, and Musculoskeletal system infections, antibacterial therapy p. 369.

For information on MRSA eradication of the nasal carriage, see Nose p. 868.

5 Infection

1.4 Tuberculosis

Tuberculosis

06-Nov-2025

Overview

Tuberculosis is a curable infectious disease caused by bacteria of the *Mycobacterium tuberculosis* complex (*M. tuberculosis*, *M. africanum*, *M. bovis* or *M. microti*) and is spread by breathing in infected respiratory droplets from a person with infectious tuberculosis. The most common form of tuberculosis infection is in the lungs (**pulmonary**) but infection can also spread and develop in other parts of the body (**extrapulmonary**).

The initial infection with tuberculosis clears in the majority of individuals. However, in some cases the bacteria may become dormant and remain in the body with no symptoms (**latent** tuberculosis) or progress to being symptomatic (**active** tuberculosis) over the following weeks or months. In individuals with latent tuberculosis only a small proportion will develop active tuberculosis.

Many cases of tuberculosis can be prevented by public health measures and when clinical disease does occur most individuals can be cured if treated properly with the correct dose, combination and duration of treatment. Drug-resistant strains of tuberculosis are much harder to treat and significantly increase an individual's risk of long-term complications or death.

Treatment phases, overview

The standard treatment of active tuberculosis is completed in two phases—an **initial phase** using four drugs and a **continuation phase** using two drugs, in fully sensitive cases. EvGr The management and investigation of tuberculosis in children should be undertaken by either a paediatrician with experience and training in tuberculosis or a general paediatrician with advice from a specialist clinician. This tuberculosis service should include specialised nurses and health visitors. Ⓐ

Within the UK there are two regimens recommended for the treatment of tuberculosis: **unsupervised** or **supervised**; with the choice of either regimen dependent on a risk assessment to identify if a child needs enhanced case management.

EvGr In all phases of treatment for tuberculosis, fixed-dose combination tablets should be used, and a daily dosing schedule should be offered in active pulmonary tuberculosis and considered as first choice in active extrapulmonary tuberculosis. Ⓐ

Initial phase

EvGr As standard treatment for children with active tuberculosis, offer rifampicin p. 449, ethambutol hydrochloride p. 452, pyrazinamide p. 454 and isoniazid p. 453 (with pyridoxine hydrochloride p. 784) in the initial phase of treatment; modified according to drug susceptibility testing; and continued for 2 months.

Treatment should be started without waiting for culture results if clinical signs and symptoms are consistent with a tuberculosis diagnosis; consider completing the standard treatment even if subsequent culture results are negative. Ⓐ

Continuation phase

EvGr After the initial phase, offer standard continuation treatment with rifampicin and isoniazid (with pyridoxine hydrochloride) for a further 4 months in children with active tuberculosis without central nervous system involvement. Longer treatment of 10 months should be offered to children with active tuberculosis of the central nervous system, with or without spinal involvement. Treatment should be modified according to drug susceptibility testing. Ⓐ

Unsupervised treatment

The unsupervised treatment regimen is for children who are likely to take antituberculosis drugs (or have treatment administered by a parent or carer) reliably and willingly without supervision by a healthcare worker.

Supervised treatment

For children or families requiring supervised treatment (directly observed therapy, DOT), this is offered as part of enhanced case management. EvGr Daily supervised treatment is the preferred option wherever feasible. A 3 times weekly dosing schedule can be considered in children with active tuberculosis if they require enhanced case management and daily directly observed therapy is not available. Antituberculosis treatment dosing regimens of fewer than 3 times a week are not recommended.

Directly observed therapy should be offered to children or to children whose carers:

- have a current risk or history of non-adherence;
- have previously been treated for tuberculosis;
- have a history of homelessness, drug or alcohol misuse;
- are in a young offender institution, or have been in the past 5 years;
- have a major psychiatric, memory or cognitive disorder;
- are in denial of the tuberculosis diagnosis;
- have multi-drug resistant tuberculosis;
- request directly observed therapy after discussion with the clinical team;
- are too ill to self-administer treatment.

Advice and support should be offered to those children and their carers to assist with treatment completion. Ⓐ

Individuals with comorbidities or coexisting conditions, including the immunocompromised

EvGr Children with comorbidities or coexisting conditions (such as HIV, severe liver disease or diabetes) should be managed by a specialist multidisciplinary team with experience in managing tuberculosis and the comorbidity or coexisting condition.

In children who are HIV-positive with active tuberculosis, treatment with the standard regimen should not routinely exceed 6 months, unless the tuberculosis has central nervous system involvement, in which case treatment should not routinely extend beyond 12 months.

Care should be taken to avoid drug interactions when co-prescribing antiretroviral and antituberculosis drugs. Ⓐ For further information on the **management of tuberculosis in HIV infection** consult the Children's HIV Association of UK and Ireland (www.chiva.org.uk/professionals/clinical-guidelines/).

Extrapulmonary tuberculosis

Central nervous system tuberculosis

EvGr Children with central nervous system tuberculosis should be offered standard treatment with **initial phase** drugs for 2 months (see *Initial phase* for specific drugs). After completion of the initial treatment phase, standard treatment with **continuation phase** drugs should then be offered (see *Continuation phase* for specific drugs); and continued for a further 10 months. Treatment for tuberculosis meningitis should be offered if clinical signs and other laboratory findings are consistent with the diagnosis, even if a rapid diagnostic test is negative.

An initial high dose of *dexamethasone* or *prednisolone* should be offered at the same time as antituberculosis treatment, then slowly withdrawn over 4–8 weeks.

Referral for surgery should only be considered in children who have raised intracranial pressure; or have spinal TB with spinal instability or evidence of spinal cord compression. Ⓐ

Recommended dosage for standard unsupervised 6-month treatment

Isoniazid	Child: 10 mg/kg once daily (max. per dose 300 mg) for 6 months (initial and continuation phases)
Rifampicin	Child: ▸ body-weight up to 50 kg 15 mg/kg once daily for 6 months (initial and continuation phases); maximum 450 mg per day ; ▸ body-weight 50 kg and above 15 mg/kg once daily for 6 months (initial and continuation phases); maximum 600 mg per day
Pyrazinamide	Child: ▸ body-weight up to 50 kg 35 mg/kg once daily for 2 months (initial phase); maximum 1.5 g per day ; ▸ body-weight 50 kg and above 35 mg/kg once daily for 2 months (initial phase); maximum 2 g per day
Ethambutol hydrochloride	Child: 20 mg/kg once daily for 2 months (initial phase)

In general, doses should be rounded up to facilitate administration of suitable volumes of liquid or an appropriate strength of tablet. The exception is ethambutol hydrochloride p. 452 due to the risk of toxicity. Doses may also need to be recalculated to allow for weight gain in younger children.
The fixed-dose combination preparations (*Rifater*®, *Rifinah*®) are unlicensed for use in children. Consideration may be given to use of these preparations in older children, provided the respective dose of each drug is appropriate for the weight of the child.

Recommended dosage for intermittent supervised 6-month treatment

Isoniazid	Child: 15 mg/kg 3 times a week (max. per dose 900 mg) for 6 months (initial and continuation phases)
Rifampicin	Child: 15 mg/kg 3 times a week (max. per dose 900 mg) for 6 months (initial and continuation phases)
Pyrazinamide	Child: ▸ body-weight up to 50 kg 50 mg/kg 3 times a week (max. per dose 2 g 3 times a week) for 2 months (initial phase) ; ▸ body-weight 50 kg and above 50 mg/kg 3 times a week (max. per dose 2.5 g 3 times a week) for 2 months (initial phase)
Ethambutol hydrochloride	Child: 30 mg/kg 3 times a week for 2 months (initial phase)

In general, doses should be rounded up to facilitate administration of suitable volumes of liquid or an appropriate strength of tablet. The exception is ethambutol hydrochloride due to the risk of toxicity. Doses may also need to be recalculated to allow for weight gain in younger children.
The fixed-dose combination preparations (*Rifater*®, *Rifinah*®) are unlicensed for use in children. Consideration may be given to use of these preparations in older children, provided the respective dose of each drug is appropriate for the weight of the child.

Pericardial tuberculosis

EvGr An initial high dose of oral *prednisolone* should be offered to children with active pericardial tuberculosis, at the same time as antituberculosis treatment, then slowly withdrawn over 2–3 weeks. ⟨A⟩

Latent tuberculosis

Some children with latent tuberculosis are at increased risk of developing active tuberculosis (such as children who are HIV-positive, diabetic or receiving treatment with an anti-tumor necrosis factor alpha inhibitor). EvGr These children and their carers should be informed of the risks and symptoms of active tuberculosis. ⟨A⟩

Close contacts

EvGr Children who are a close contact (prolonged, frequent or intense contact, for example household contacts) of a person with pulmonary or laryngeal tuberculosis should be tested for latent tuberculosis. Children aged under 2 years should be assessed by a specialist. ⟨A⟩

Immunocompromised

EvGr Children who are anticipated to be, or who are currently immunocompromised should be referred to a specialist if latent tuberculosis is suspected (for example if they are from a high incidence country or have been in close contact with people with *suspected infectious* or *confirmed* pulmonary or laryngeal tuberculosis). ⟨A⟩

Treatment of latent tuberculosis

EvGr **Neonates** who have been in close contact with a person with tuberculosis which has not yet been treated for at least two weeks, should start treatment with isoniazid p. 453 (with pyridoxine hydrochloride p. 784) followed by a Mantoux test after 6 weeks of treatment.

If the Mantoux test is positive (and active tuberculosis is not present) treatment should be continued for 6 months; if negative (and confirmed by a negative interferon-gamma release assay), the treatment should be stopped and a BCG vaccination given. If the interferon-gamma release assay result is positive (and active tuberculosis is not present) treatment should be continued for 6 months.

Children aged 4 weeks to 2 years who have been in close contact with a person with tuberculosis which has not been treated for at least two weeks, should start treatment for latent tuberculosis and have a Mantoux test. Treatment is either isoniazid (with pyridoxine hydrochloride) alone for 6 months (preferred regimen if interactions with rifamycins are a concern) or rifampicin p. 449 and isoniazid (with pyridoxine hydrochloride) for 3 months (recommended when hepatotoxicity is a concern).

If the Mantoux test is positive (and active tuberculosis is not present), the treatment course should be completed. If the test is negative, treatment should be continued and the child should be re-assessed for active tuberculosis after 6 weeks. If the results are then negative (and confirmed by a negative interferon-gamma release assay), the treatment should be stopped and a BCG vaccination given (if the child has not already had one). If the result is positive (and active tuberculosis is not present), the course of treatment should be continued.

Children aged over 2 years should be offered a Mantoux test, and if positive (and active tuberculosis is not present), then treat as above for children aged 4 weeks to 2 years. If the test is negative, then offer an interferon-gamma release assay after 6 weeks and repeat the Mantoux test. ⟨A⟩

The choice of regimen is dependent on clinical factors, including age, risk of hepatotoxicity and possible drug interactions. EvGr Testing for HIV, hepatitis B and hepatitis C should be offered before starting antituberculosis treatment as this may affect choice of therapy.

Children with severe liver disease should be treated under the care of a specialist team. Careful monitoring of liver function is necessary in children with non-severe liver disease, abnormal liver function, or who misuse alcohol or drugs. ⟨A⟩

For advice on tuberculin testing and immunisation against tuberculosis, see Bacillus Calmette-Guérin vaccine p. 963.

Treatment failure

Major causes of treatment failure include incorrect prescribing by the clinician and inadequate compliance by the child or carer. EvGr All children diagnosed with tuberculosis should have an allocated case manager to help with the development of a health and social care plan, supervision of treatment, and support with the completion of treatment. Multidisciplinary tuberculosis teams should implement strategies (such as random urine tests, pill counts, home visits, health education counselling, and language appropriate reminder services) to help with adherence to, and successful completion of treatment. Ⓐ

Treatment interruptions

A break in antituberculosis treatment of at least 2 weeks (during the initial phase) or missing more than 20% of prescribed doses is classified as treatment interruption. Re-establishing treatment appropriately following interruptions is key to ensuring treatment success without relapse, drug resistance or further adverse events. EvGr If an adverse reaction recurs upon re-introducing a particular drug, do not give that drug in future regimens and consider extending the total regimen accordingly. Ⓐ

Treatment interruptions due to drug-induced hepatotoxicity

EvGr Following treatment interruption due to drug-induced hepatotoxicty, all potential causes of hepatotoxicity should be investigated. Once aspartate or alanine transaminase levels fall below twice the upper limit of normal, bilirubin levels have returned to the normal range, and hepatotoxic symptoms have resolved, antituberculosis therapy should be sequentially re-introduced at previous full doses over a period of no more than 10 days. Start with ethambutol hydrochloride p. 452 and either isoniazid (with pyridoxine hydrochloride) or rifampicin.

In children with severe or highly infectious tuberculosis who need to interrupt the standard regimen, consider continuing treatment with at least 2 drugs with low risk of hepatotoxicity, such as ethambutol hydrochloride and streptomycin p. 380 (with or without a fluoroquinolone antibacterial, such as levofloxacin [unlicensed use] or moxifloxacin [unlicensed use]), with ongoing monitoring by a liver specialist. Ⓐ Due to the risk of disabling and potentially long-lasting or irreversible side-effects associated with fluoroquinolones, the MHRA/CHM have issued further advice on the restrictions and precautions for use of fluoroquinolone antibacterials, for further information, see *Important safety information* in levofloxacin or moxifloxacin drug monographs.

Treatment interruptions due to cutaneous reactions

EvGr If a child with severe or highly infectious tuberculosis has a cutaneous reaction, consider continuing treatment with a combination of at least 2 drugs with low risk for causing cutaneous reactions, such as ethambutol hydrochloride and streptomycin, with monitoring by a dermatologist. Ⓐ

Drug-resistant tuberculosis

EvGr Treatment of drug-resistant tuberculosis should be managed by a multidisciplinary team with experience in such cases, and where appropriate facilities for infection-control exist. Ⓐ The risk of resistance is minimised by ensuring therapy is administered in the correct dose and combination for the prescribed duration.

Single drug-resistant tuberculosis

EvGr For single drug-resistance in individuals with tuberculosis with central nervous system involvement, refer to a specialist with experience in managing drug-resistant tuberculosis. Ⓐ For those without central nervous system involvement, the following treatment regimens are recommended:

Resistance to isoniazid:

- EvGr First 2 months (initial phase): rifampicin, pyrazinamide p. 454 and ethambutol hydrochloride;
- Continue with (continuation phase): rifampicin and ethambutol hydrochloride for 7 months (up to 10 months for extensive disease). Ⓐ

Resistance to pyrazinamide:

- EvGr First 2 months (initial phase): rifampicin, ethambutol hydrochloride and isoniazid (with pyridoxine hydrochloride);
- Continue with (continuation phase): rifampicin and isoniazid (with pyridoxine hydrochloride) for 7 months. Ⓐ

Resistance to ethambutol hydrochloride:

- EvGr First 2 months (initial phase): rifampicin, pyrazinamide and isoniazid (with pyridoxine hydrochloride);
- Continue with (continuation phase): rifampicin p. 449 and isoniazid p. 453 (with pyridoxine hydrochloride p. 784) for 4 months. Ⓐ

Resistance to rifampicin:

- EvGr Rifampicin-resistant tuberculosis should be managed in the same way as multi-drug resistant tuberculosis. Ⓐ

Multi-drug resistant tuberculosis (MDR-TB)

EvGr Advice on the management of patients with MDR-TB (resistance to isoniazid and rifampicin, with or without any other resistance), should be sought from local specialist advisory services for MDR-TB and the **British Thoracic Society** MDR-TB Clinical Advice Service (see: www.brit-thoracic.org.uk/quality-improvement/bts-mdr-tb-clinical-advice-service/). Testing for resistance to second-line drugs is recommended and treatment should be modified according to susceptibility. Ⓐ Treatment regimens are comprised of different combinations of drugs such as bedaquiline, clofazimine [unlicensed use], delamanid [unlicensed], levofloxacin [unlicensed use] or moxifloxacin [unlicensed use], linezolid [unlicensed use], pretomanid [unlicensed], and pyrazinamide.

Useful Resources

Tuberculosis. National Institute for Health and Care Excellence. NICE guideline NG33. September 2019, updated February 2024.
www.nice.org.uk/guidance/ng33

ANTIMYCOBACTERIALS > RIFAMYCINS

Rifabutin

30-May-2023

● INDICATIONS AND DOSE

Prophylaxis of *Mycobacterium avium* complex infections in immunosuppressed patients with low CD4 count

▶ BY MOUTH

- Child 1 month–11 years: 5 mg/kg once daily (max. per dose 300 mg), also consult product literature
- Child 12–17 years: 300 mg once daily, also consult product literature

Treatment of non-tuberculous mycobacterial disease, in combination with other drugs

▶ BY MOUTH

- Child 1 month–11 years: 5 mg/kg once daily for up to 6 months after cultures negative
- Child 12–17 years: 450–600 mg once daily for up to 6 months after cultures negative

Treatment of pulmonary tuberculosis, in combination with other drugs

▶ BY MOUTH

- Child 12–17 years: 150–450 mg once daily for at least 6 months

- **UNLICENSED USE** Not licensed for use in children.
- **CAUTIONS** Acute porphyrias p. 745 · discolours soft contact lenses
- **INTERACTIONS** → Appendix 1: rifamycins
- **SIDE-EFFECTS** Agranulocytosis · anaemia · arthralgia · bronchospasm · chest pain · corneal deposits · decreased leucocytes · dyspnoea · eosinophilia · fever · haemolysis · hepatic disorders · influenza like illness · myalgia · nausea · neutropenia · pancytopenia · skin reactions · thrombocytopenia · urine discolouration · uveitis (more common following high doses or concomitant use with drugs that increase plasma concentration) · vomiting
- **ALLERGY AND CROSS-SENSITIVITY** EvGr Contra-indicated in patients with rifamycin hypersensitivity. (M)
- **CONCEPTION AND CONTRACEPTION**
  Important Rifabutin induces hepatic enzymes and the effectiveness of hormonal contraceptives is reduced; alternative family planning advice should be offered.
- **PREGNANCY** Manufacturer advises avoid—no information available.
- **BREAST FEEDING** Manufacturer advises avoid—no information available.
- **HEPATIC IMPAIRMENT** Manufacturer advises caution in severe impairment.
- **RENAL IMPAIRMENT**
  Dose adjustments See p. 16.
  In adults, manufacturer advises use half normal dose if creatinine clearance less than 30 mL/minute (consult product literature).
- **MONITORING REQUIREMENTS**
  - *Renal function* should be checked before treatment.
  - *Hepatic function* should be checked before treatment. If there is no evidence of liver disease (and pre-treatment liver function is normal), further checks are only necessary if the patient develops fever, malaise, vomiting, jaundice or unexplained deterioration during treatment. However, hepatic function should be monitored on prolonged therapy.
  - Blood counts should be monitored on prolonged therapy.
- **PRESCRIBING AND DISPENSING INFORMATION** If treatment interruption occurs, re-introduce with low dosage and increase gradually.
- **PATIENT AND CARER ADVICE**
  Soft contact lenses Patients or their carers should be advised that rifabutin discolours soft contact lenses.
  Hepatic disorders Patients or their carers should be told how to recognise signs of liver disorder, and advised to discontinue treatment and seek immediate medical attention if symptoms such as persistent nausea, vomiting, malaise or jaundice develop.

- **MEDICINAL FORMS** There can be variation in the licensing of different medicines containing the same drug. Forms available from special-order manufacturers include: oral suspension, oral solution

Oral capsule

CAUTIONARY AND ADVISORY LABELS 8, 14

- **Mycobutin** (Pfizer Ltd)
  Rifabutin 150 mg Mycobutin 150mg capsules | 30 capsule PoM £90.38 DT = £90.38

Rifampicin

30-May-2023

- **INDICATIONS AND DOSE**

Brucellosis in combination with other antibacterials | Legionnaires disease in combination with other antibacterials | Serious staphylococcal infections in combination with other antibacterials

- BY MOUTH, OR BY INTRAVENOUS INFUSION
  - Neonate: 5–10 mg/kg twice daily.
  - Child 1-11 months: 5–10 mg/kg twice daily
  - Child 1-17 years: 10 mg/kg twice daily (max. per dose 600 mg)

Tuberculosis, in combination with other drugs (intermittent supervised 6-month treatment) (under expert supervision)

- BY MOUTH
  - Child: 15 mg/kg 3 times a week (max. per dose 900 mg) for 6 months (initial and continuation phases)

Tuberculosis, in combination with other drugs (standard unsupervised 6-month treatment)

- BY MOUTH
  - Child (body-weight up to 50 kg): 15 mg/kg once daily for 6 months (initial and continuation phases); maximum 450 mg per day
  - Child (body-weight 50 kg and above): 15 mg/kg once daily for 6 months (initial and continuation phases); maximum 600 mg per day

Congenital tuberculosis

- BY MOUTH
  - Neonate: 15 mg/kg once daily for 6 months (initial and continuation phases).

Prevention of tuberculosis in susceptible close contacts or those who have become tuberculin positive, in combination with isoniazid

- BY MOUTH
  - Child 1 month-11 years (body-weight up to 50 kg): 15 mg/kg daily for 3 months; maximum 450 mg per day
  - Child 1 month-11 years (body-weight 50 kg and above): 15 mg/kg daily for 3 months; maximum 600 mg per day
  - Child 12-17 years (body-weight up to 50 kg): 450 mg daily for 3 months
  - Child 12-17 years (body-weight 50 kg and above): 600 mg daily for 3 months

Prevention of tuberculosis in susceptible close contacts or those who have become tuberculin positive, who are isoniazid-resistant

- BY MOUTH
  - Child 1 month-11 years (body-weight up to 50 kg): 15 mg/kg daily for 6 months; maximum 450 mg per day
  - Child 1 month-11 years (body-weight 50 kg and above): 15 mg/kg daily for 6 months; maximum 600 mg per day
  - Child 12-17 years (body-weight up to 50 kg): 450 mg daily for 6 months
  - Child 12-17 years (body-weight 50 kg and above): 600 mg daily for 6 months

Prevention of secondary case of *Haemophilus influenzae* type b disease

- BY MOUTH
  - Child 1-2 months: 10 mg/kg once daily for 4 days
  - Child 3 months-11 years: 20 mg/kg once daily (max. per dose 600 mg) for 4 days
  - Child 12-17 years: 600 mg once daily for 4 days

continued →

5 Infection

Prevention of secondary case of meningococcal meningitis
- BY MOUTH
  - Neonate: 5 mg/kg every 12 hours for 2 days.
  - Child 1-11 months: 5 mg/kg every 12 hours for 2 days
  - Child 1-11 years: 10 mg/kg every 12 hours (max. per dose 600 mg), for 2 days
  - Child 12-17 years: 600 mg every 12 hours for 2 days

Pruritus due to cholestasis
- BY MOUTH
  - Child: 5–10 mg/kg once daily (max. per dose 600 mg)

- **UNLICENSED USE** Not licensed for use in children for pruritus due to cholestasis.
- **CONTRA-INDICATIONS** Acute porphyrias p. 745 · jaundice
- **CAUTIONS** Discolours soft contact lenses
- **INTERACTIONS** → Appendix 1: rifamycins
- **SIDE-EFFECTS**

GENERAL SIDE-EFFECTS
- **Common or very common** Nausea · thrombocytopenia · vomiting
- **Uncommon** Diarrhoea · leucopenia
- **Frequency not known** Abdominal discomfort · acute kidney injury · adrenal insufficiency · agranulocytosis · appetite decreased · disseminated intravascular coagulation · dyspnoea · eosinophilia · eye disorders · flushing · gastrointestinal disorders · haemolytic anaemia · hepatitis · hypersensitivity · influenza · intracranial haemorrhage · menstrual disorder · muscle weakness · myopathy · oedema · pseudomembranous enterocolitis · red discolouration of body fluids · severe cutaneous adverse reactions (SCARs) · shock · skin reactions · sputum discolouration · sweat changes · urine discolouration · vasculitis · wheezing

SPECIFIC SIDE-EFFECTS
- With intravenous use Bone pain · hyperbilirubinaemia · psychotic disorder
- With oral use Psychosis

SIDE-EFFECTS, FURTHER INFORMATION Side-effects that mainly occur with intermittent therapy include influenza-like symptoms (with chills, fever, dizziness, bone pain), respiratory symptoms (including shortness of breath), collapse and shock, haemolytic anaemia, thrombocytopenic purpura, and acute renal failure.

Discontinue if serious side-effects develop.

- **ALLERGY AND CROSS-SENSITIVITY** [EvGr] Contra-indicated in patients with rifamycin hypersensitivity. ⟨M⟩
- **CONCEPTION AND CONTRACEPTION**

Important Effectiveness of hormonal contraceptives is reduced and alternative family planning advice should be offered.

- **PREGNANCY** Manufacturers advise very high doses teratogenic in *animal* studies in first trimester; risk of neonatal bleeding may be increased in third trimester.
- **BREAST FEEDING** Amount too small to be harmful.
- **HEPATIC IMPAIRMENT** Manufacturer advises caution—monitor liver function weekly for two weeks, then every two weeks for the next six weeks.

Dose adjustments Manufacturer advises maximum 8 mg/kg per day.

- **RENAL IMPAIRMENT** Use with caution if doses above 10 mg/kg daily.
- **MONITORING REQUIREMENTS**
  - *Renal function* should be checked before treatment.
  - *Hepatic function* should be checked before treatment. If there is no evidence of liver disease (and pre-treatment liver function is normal), further checks are only necessary if the patient develops fever, malaise, vomiting, jaundice or unexplained deterioration during treatment. However, liver function should be monitored on prolonged therapy.
  - Blood counts should be monitored in patients on prolonged therapy.
- **DIRECTIONS FOR ADMINISTRATION** Displacement value may be significant, consult local reconstitution guidelines; reconstitute with solvent provided. Expert sources advise may be further diluted with Glucose 5% *or* Sodium Chloride 0.9% to a final concentration of 1.2 mg/mL; infuse over 2–3 hours.
- **PRESCRIBING AND DISPENSING INFORMATION** If treatment interruption occurs, re-introduce with low dosage and increase gradually.

Flavours of syrup may include raspberry.

- With oral use In general, doses should be rounded up to facilitate administration of suitable volumes of liquid or an appropriate strength of tablet. Doses may also need to be recalculated to allow for weight gain in younger children.

- **PATIENT AND CARER ADVICE**

Soft contact lenses Patients or their carers should be advised that rifampicin discolours soft contact lenses.

Hepatic disorders Patients or their carers should be told how to recognise signs of liver disorder, and advised to discontinue treatment and seek immediate medical attention if symptoms such as persistent nausea, vomiting, malaise or jaundice develop.

Medicines for Children leaflet: Rifampicin for meningococcal prophylaxis www.medicinesforchildren.org.uk/medicines/rifampicin-for-meningococcal-prophylaxis/

Medicines for Children leaflet: Rifampicin for treatment of tuberculosis www.medicinesforchildren.org.uk/medicines/rifampicin-for-treatment-of-tuberculosis/

- **MEDICINAL FORMS** There can be variation in the licensing of different medicines containing the same drug. Forms available from special-order manufacturers include: oral suspension, oral solution

Powder and solvent for solution for injection
- **Rifampicin (Non-proprietary)**

Rifampicin 300 mg RIFA parenteral 300mg powder and solvent for solution for injection vials | 1 vial [PoM] [X] (Hospital only)

Oral suspension

CAUTIONARY AND ADVISORY LABELS 8, 14, 23

EXCIPIENTS: May contain Sucrose
- **Rifadin** (Sanofi)

Rifampicin 20 mg per 1 ml Rifadin 100mg/5ml syrup | 120 ml [PoM] £4.82 DT = £4.27

Oral capsule

CAUTIONARY AND ADVISORY LABELS 8, 14, 23
- **Rifampicin (Non-proprietary)**

Rifampicin 150 mg Rifampicin 150mg capsules | 100 capsule [PoM] £73.47–£105.00

Rifampicin 300 mg Rifampicin 300mg capsules | 60 capsule [PoM] £69.20 | 100 capsule [PoM] £165.18 DT = £140.20
- **Rifadin** (Sanofi)

Rifampicin 150 mg Rifadin 150mg capsules | 100 capsule [PoM] £20.66

Rifampicin 300 mg Rifadin 300mg capsules | 100 capsule [PoM] £41.31 DT = £140.20
- **Rimactane** (Sandoz Ltd)

Rifampicin 300 mg Rimactane 300mg capsules | 60 capsule [PoM] £21.98

Powder and solvent for solution for infusion

ELECTROLYTES: May contain Sodium
- **Rifampicin (Non-proprietary)**

Rifampicin 600 mg Rifampicin 600mg powder and solvent for solution for infusion vials | 1 vial [PoM] [X]
- **Rifadin** (Sanofi)

Rifampicin 600 mg Rifadin 600mg powder and solvent for solution for infusion vials | 1 vial [PoM] £9.20

Rifampicin with isoniazid
10-Mar-2020

The properties listed below are those particular to the combination only. For the properties of the components please consider, rifampicin p. 449, isoniazid p. 453.

- **INDICATIONS AND DOSE**

Treatment of tuberculosis (continuation phase)

▶ BY MOUTH

▶ Child: Although not licensed in children, consideration may be given to use of *Rifinah*® in older children, provided the respective dose of each drug is appropriate for the weight of the child (consult local protocol).

DOSE EQUIVALENCE AND CONVERSION

▶ *Rifinah*® Tablets contain rifampicin and isoniazid; the proportions are expressed in the form x/y where x and y are the strengths in milligrams of rifampicin and isoniazid respectively.

▶ Each *Rifinah*® 150/100 Tablet contains rifampicin 150 mg and isoniazid 100 mg.

▶ Each *Rifinah*® 300/150 Tablet contains rifampicin 300 mg and isoniazid 150 mg.

- **UNLICENSED USE** Not licensed for use in children.
- **INTERACTIONS** → Appendix 1: isoniazid · rifamycins
- **PATIENT AND CARER ADVICE**

Medicines for Children leaflet: Isoniazid and rifampicin combination for latent tuberculosis www.medicinesforchildren.org.uk/medicines/isoniazid-and-rifampicin-combination-for-latent-tuberculosis/

- **MEDICINAL FORMS** There can be variation in the licensing of different medicines containing the same drug.

Oral tablet

CAUTIONARY AND ADVISORY LABELS 8, 14, 23

▶ **Rifampicin with isoniazid (Non-proprietary)**
Isoniazid 150 mg, Rifampicin 300 mg Rifampicin 300mg / Isoniazid 150mg tablets | 1 tablet PoM

▶ **Rifinah** (Sanofi)
Isoniazid 100 mg, Rifampicin 150 mg Rifinah 150mg/100mg tablets | 84 tablet PoM £19.09 DT = £19.09
Isoniazid 150 mg, Rifampicin 300 mg Rifinah 300mg/150mg tablets | 56 tablet PoM £25.22 DT = £25.22

Rifampicin with isoniazid and pyrazinamide

The properties listed below are those particular to the combination only. For the properties of the components please consider, rifampicin p. 449, isoniazid p. 453, pyrazinamide p. 454.

- **INDICATIONS AND DOSE**

Initial treatment of tuberculosis (in combination with ethambutol)

▶ Child: Although not licensed in children, consideration may be given to use of *Rifater*® in older children, provided the respective dose of each drug is appropriate for the weight of the child (consult local protocol).

DOSE EQUIVALENCE AND CONVERSION

▶ Tablet quantities refer to the number of *Rifater*® Tablets which should be taken. Each *Rifater*® Tablet contains isoniazid 50 mg, pyrazinamide 300 mg and rifampicin 120 mg.

- **UNLICENSED USE** Not licensed for use in children.
- **INTERACTIONS** → Appendix 1: isoniazid · pyrazinamide · rifamycins
- **MEDICINAL FORMS** There can be variation in the licensing of different medicines containing the same drug.

Oral tablet

CAUTIONARY AND ADVISORY LABELS 8, 14, 22

▶ **Rifampicin with isoniazid and pyrazinamide (Non-proprietary)**
Isoniazid 50 mg, Rifampicin 120 mg, Pyrazinamide 300 mg Rifater tablets | 1 tablet PoM

▶ **Rifater** (Sanofi)
Isoniazid 50 mg, Rifampicin 120 mg, Pyrazinamide 300 mg Rifater tablets | 100 tablet PoM £26.34

ANTIMYCOBACTERIALS › OTHER

Bedaquiline
04-Apr-2023

- **INDICATIONS AND DOSE**

Multiple-drug resistant pulmonary tuberculosis, in combination with other drugs (under expert supervision)

▶ BY MOUTH

▶ Child 5–17 years (body-weight 15–19 kg): Initially 160 mg once daily for 2 weeks, then 80 mg 3 times a week for 22 weeks, intervals of at least 48 hours between each dose, continue appropriate combination therapy after bedaquiline

▶ Child 5–17 years (body-weight 20–29 kg): Initially 200 mg once daily for 2 weeks, then 100 mg 3 times a week for 22 weeks, intervals of at least 48 hours between each dose, continue appropriate combination therapy after bedaquiline

▶ Child 5–17 years (body-weight 30 kg and above): Initially 400 mg once daily for 2 weeks, then 200 mg 3 times a week for 22 weeks, intervals of at least 48 hours between each dose, continue appropriate combination therapy after bedaquiline

- **CONTRA-INDICATIONS** QTc interval more than 500 milliseconds (derived using Fridericia's formula) · ventricular arrhythmia
- **CAUTIONS** Hypothyroidism · QTc interval (derived using Fridericia's formula) 450–500 milliseconds · risk factors for QT interval prolongation (e.g. electrolyte disturbances, heart failure, history of symptomatic arrhythmias, bradycardia, congenital long QT syndrome)
- **INTERACTIONS** → Appendix 1: bedaquiline
- **SIDE-EFFECTS**

▶ **Common or very common** Arthralgia · diarrhoea · dizziness · headache · hepatic function abnormal · myalgia · nausea · QT interval prolongation · vomiting

SIDE-EFFECTS, FURTHER INFORMATION If syncope occurs, obtain ECG to identify if QT interval prolongation present.

- **PREGNANCY** Manufacturer advises avoid unless potential benefit outweighs risk.
- **BREAST FEEDING** Manufacturer advises avoid—present in milk in *animal* studies.
- **HEPATIC IMPAIRMENT** Manufacturer advises caution in moderate impairment; avoid in severe impairment—no information available.
- **RENAL IMPAIRMENT** EvGr Caution if creatinine clearance less than 30 mL/minute, ⟨M⟩ see p. 16.
- **MONITORING REQUIREMENTS**

▶ Determine serum potassium, calcium, and magnesium before starting treatment (correct if abnormal)—remeasure if QT prolongation occurs during treatment.

▶ Obtain ECG before starting treatment, and then at least monthly during treatment or more frequently if concomitant use with other drugs known to prolong the QT interval.

▶ Monitor liver function before starting treatment and then at least monthly during treatment—discontinue treatment if severe abnormalities in liver function tests.

5 Infection

- **PATIENT AND CARER ADVICE**
Missed doses If a dose is missed during the first two weeks of treatment, the missed dose should not be taken and the next dose should be taken at the usual time; if a dose is missed during weeks 3–24 of treatment, the missed dose should be taken as soon as possible and then the usual regimen resumed.
Driving and skilled tasks Dizziness may affect performance of skilled tasks (e.g. driving).
- **NATIONAL FUNDING/ACCESS DECISIONS**
For full details see funding body website
All Wales Medicines Strategy Group (AWMSG) decisions
 ▸ **Bedaquiline (*Sirturo*®) for use as part of an appropriate combination regimen for pulmonary multidrug-resistant tuberculosis (MDR-TB) in adult and paediatric patients (5 years to less than 18 years of age and weighing at least 15 kg) when an effective treatment regimen cannot otherwise be composed for reasons of resistance or tolerability (November 2022)** AWMSG No. 4860 Recommended
- **MEDICINAL FORMS** There can be variation in the licensing of different medicines containing the same drug.
Oral tablet
CAUTIONARY AND ADVISORY LABELS 4, 8, 21
 ▸ Sirturo (Janssen-Cilag Ltd)
Bedaquiline (as Bedaquiline fumarate) 20 mg Sirturo 20mg tablets | 60 tablet PoM £1,193.64 (Hospital only)
Bedaquiline (as Bedaquiline fumarate) 100 mg Sirturo 100mg tablets | 24 tablet PoM £2,387.28 (Hospital only)

Cycloserine

- **INDICATIONS AND DOSE**
Tuberculosis resistant to first-line drugs, in combination with other drugs
 ▸ BY MOUTH
 ▸ Child 2-11 years: Initially 5 mg/kg twice daily (max. per dose 250 mg), then increased if necessary up to 10 mg/kg twice daily (max. per dose 500 mg), dose to be increased according to blood concentration and response
 ▸ Child 12-17 years: Initially 250 mg every 12 hours for 2 weeks, then increased if necessary up to 500 mg every 12 hours, dose to be increased according to blood concentration and response
PHARMACOKINETICS
 ▸ Cycloserine penetrates the CNS.
- **UNLICENSED USE** Licensed for use in children (age range not specified by manufacturer).
- **CONTRA-INDICATIONS** Alcohol dependence · depression · epilepsy · psychotic states · severe anxiety
- **INTERACTIONS** → Appendix 1: cycloserine
- **SIDE-EFFECTS** Behaviour abnormal · coma · confusion · congestive heart failure · drowsiness · dysarthria · headache · hyperirritability · megaloblastic anaemia · memory loss · neurological effects · paraesthesia · paresis · psychosis · rash · reflexes increased · seizures · suicidal ideation · tremor · vertigo
SIDE-EFFECTS, FURTHER INFORMATION **CNS toxicity** Discontinue or reduce dose if symptoms of CNS toxicity occur.
Rashes or allergic dermatitis Discontinue or reduce dose if rashes or allergic dermatitis develop.
- **PREGNANCY** Manufacturer advises use only if potential benefit outweighs risk—crosses the placenta.
- **BREAST FEEDING** Present in milk—amount too small to be harmful.
- **RENAL IMPAIRMENT**
Dose adjustments Increase interval between doses if creatinine clearance less than 50 mL/minute/1.73 m^2.
Monitoring Monitor blood-cycloserine concentration if creatinine clearance less than 50 mL/minute/1.73 m^2.
- **MONITORING REQUIREMENTS**
 ▸ Blood concentration should not exceed a peak concentration of 30 mg/litre (measured 3–4 hours after the dose).
 ▸ Monitor haematological, renal, and hepatic function.
- **MEDICINAL FORMS** There can be variation in the licensing of different medicines containing the same drug.
Oral capsule
CAUTIONARY AND ADVISORY LABELS 2, 8
 ▸ Cycloserine (Non-proprietary)
Cycloserine 250 mg Cycloserine 250mg capsules | 100 capsule PoM £597.00

Ethambutol hydrochloride

26-Oct-2021

- **INDICATIONS AND DOSE**
Tuberculosis, in combination with other drugs (standard unsupervised 6-month treatment)
 ▸ BY MOUTH
 ▸ Child: 20 mg/kg once daily for 2 months (initial phase)
Tuberculosis, in combination with other drugs (intermittent supervised 6-month treatment) (under expert supervision)
 ▸ BY MOUTH
 ▸ Child: 30 mg/kg 3 times a week for 2 months (initial phase)
Congenital tuberculosis, in combination with other drugs
 ▸ BY MOUTH
 ▸ Neonate: 20 mg/kg once daily for 2 months (initial phase).
- **CONTRA-INDICATIONS** Optic neuritis · poor vision
- **CAUTIONS** Young children
CAUTIONS, FURTHER INFORMATION
 ▸ Understanding warnings Patients who cannot understand warnings about visual side-effects should, if possible, be given an alternative drug. In particular, ethambutol should be used with caution in children until they are at least 5 years old and capable of reporting symptomatic visual changes accurately.
- **INTERACTIONS** → Appendix 1: ethambutol
- **SIDE-EFFECTS**
 ▸ **Common or very common** Hyperuricaemia · nerve disorders · visual impairment
 ▸ **Rare or very rare** Nephritis tubulointerstitial
 ▸ **Frequency not known** Alveolitis allergic · appetite decreased · asthenia · confusion · dizziness · eosinophilia · fever · flatulence · gastrointestinal discomfort · gout · hallucination · headache · jaundice · leucopenia · nausea · nephrotoxicity · neutropenia · photosensitive lichenoid eruption · sensation abnormal · severe cutaneous adverse reactions (SCARs) · skin reactions · taste metallic · thrombocytopenia · tremor · vomiting
SIDE-EFFECTS, FURTHER INFORMATION Ocular toxicity is more common where excessive dosage is used or if the patient's renal function is impaired. Early discontinuation of the drug is almost always followed by recovery of eyesight.
- **PREGNANCY** Not known to be harmful.
- **BREAST FEEDING** Amount too small to be harmful.
- **RENAL IMPAIRMENT** Risk of optic nerve damage. EvGr Should preferably be avoided in patients with renal impairment. (M)

Dose adjustments EvGr If creatinine clearance less than 30 mL/minute, use 15–25 mg/kg (max. 2.5 g) 3 times a week—monitor plasma-ethambutol concentration. (M) See p. 16.

- **MONITORING REQUIREMENTS**
- 'Peak' concentration (2–2.5 hours after dose) should be 2–6 mg/litre (7–22 micromol/litre); 'trough' (pre-dose) concentration should be less than 1 mg/litre (4 micromol/litre).
- Renal function should be checked before treatment.
- Visual acuity should be tested by Snellen chart before treatment with ethambutol.
- In young children, routine ophthalmological monitoring recommended.
- **PRESCRIBING AND DISPENSING INFORMATION** The RCPCH and NPPG recommend that, when a liquid special of ethambutol is required, the following strength is used: 400 mg/5 mL.
- **PATIENT AND CARER ADVICE**

Ocular toxicity The earliest features of ocular toxicity are subjective and patients should be advised to discontinue therapy immediately if they develop deterioration in vision and promptly seek further advice.

Medicines for Children leaflet: Ethambutol for treatment of tuberculosis www.medicinesforchildren.org.uk/medicines/ethambutol-for-treatments-of-tuberculosis/

- **MEDICINAL FORMS** There can be variation in the licensing of different medicines containing the same drug. Forms available from special-order manufacturers include: oral suspension, oral solution

Oral tablet

CAUTIONARY AND ADVISORY LABELS 8

- Ethambutol hydrochloride (Non-proprietary)

Ethambutol hydrochloride 100 mg Ethambutol 100mg tablets | 56 tablet PoM £40.00 DT = £40.00

Ethambutol hydrochloride 400 mg Ethambutol 400mg tablets | 56 tablet PoM £70.00 DT = £50.00

Isoniazid

10-Nov-2021

- **INDICATIONS AND DOSE**

Tuberculosis, in combination with other drugs (standard unsupervised 6-month treatment)

- BY MOUTH, OR BY INTRAMUSCULAR INJECTION, OR BY INTRAVENOUS INJECTION
- Child: 10 mg/kg once daily (max. per dose 300 mg) for 6 months (initial and continuation phases)

Tuberculosis, in combination with other drugs (intermittent supervised 6-month treatment) (under expert supervision)

- BY MOUTH, OR BY INTRAMUSCULAR INJECTION, OR BY INTRAVENOUS INJECTION
- Child: 15 mg/kg 3 times a week (max. per dose 900 mg) for 6 months (initial and continuation phases)

Congenital tuberculosis, in combination with other drugs

- BY MOUTH, OR BY INTRAMUSCULAR INJECTION, OR BY INTRAVENOUS INJECTION
- Neonate: 10 mg/kg daily for 6 months (initial and continuation phases).

Prevention of tuberculosis in susceptible close contacts or those who have become tuberculin positive

- INITIALLY BY MOUTH, OR BY INTRAMUSCULAR INJECTION, OR BY INTRAVENOUS INJECTION
- Neonate: 10 mg/kg daily for 6 months.
- Child 1 month–11 years: 10 mg/kg daily (max. per dose 300 mg) for 6 months, alternatively (by mouth) 10 mg/kg daily (max. per dose 300 mg) for 3 months, to be taken in combination with rifampicin
- Child 12–17 years: 300 mg daily for 6 months, alternatively (by mouth) 300 mg daily for 3 months, to be taken in combination with rifampicin

- **CONTRA-INDICATIONS** Drug-induced liver disease
- **CAUTIONS** Acute porphyrias p. 745 · alcohol dependence · diabetes mellitus · epilepsy · history of psychosis · HIV infection · malnutrition · slow acetylator status (increased risk of side-effects)

CAUTIONS, FURTHER INFORMATION

- Peripheral neuropathy Pyridoxine hydrochloride p. 784 should be given prophylactically in all patients from the start of treatment. Peripheral neuropathy is more likely to occur where there are pre-existing risk factors such as diabetes, alcohol dependence, chronic renal failure, pregnancy, malnutrition and HIV infection.

- **INTERACTIONS** → Appendix 1: isoniazid
- **SIDE-EFFECTS**

GENERAL SIDE-EFFECTS

- **Uncommon** Hepatic disorders
- **Rare or very rare** Severe cutaneous adverse reactions (SCARs)
- **Frequency not known** Agranulocytosis · aplastic anaemia · fever · gynaecomastia · haemolytic anaemia · nerve disorders · seizure · vasculitis

SPECIFIC SIDE-EFFECTS

- With oral use Acidosis · constipation · deafness · dry mouth · dysuria · erythema multiforme · euphoric mood · gastrointestinal disorder · hypoglycaemia · interstitial lung disease · lupus erythematosus · nausea · nicotinic acid deficiency · pancreatitis acute · psychiatric disorder · psychotic disorder · tinnitus · vertigo · vomiting · withdrawal syndrome
- With parenteral use Alopecia · anaemia · eosinophilia · hyperglycaemia · lupus-like syndrome · optic atrophy · pancreatitis · pellagra · psychosis · skin reactions · thrombocytopenia

- **PREGNANCY** Not known to be harmful; prophylactic pyridoxine recommended.
- **BREAST FEEDING** Theoretical risk of convulsions and neuropathy; prophylactic pyridoxine advisable in mother.

Monitoring In breast-feeding, monitor infant for possible toxicity.

- **HEPATIC IMPAIRMENT** Manufacturer advises caution (increased risk of hepatotoxicity).

Monitoring In patients with pre-existing liver disease or hepatic impairment monitor liver function regularly and particularly frequently in the first 2 months.

- **RENAL IMPAIRMENT** EvGr Use with caution (risk of ototoxicity and peripheral neuropathy; prophylactic pyridoxine hydrochloride p. 784 recommended). (M)

Dose adjustments

- With parenteral use EvGr Dose reduction may be required in severe impairment (consult product literature). (M)

- **MONITORING REQUIREMENTS**
- *Renal function* should be checked before treatment.
- *Hepatic function* should be checked before treatment. If there is no evidence of liver disease (and pre-treatment liver function is normal), further checks are only necessary if the patient develops fever, malaise, vomiting, jaundice or unexplained deterioration during treatment.
- **PRESCRIBING AND DISPENSING INFORMATION**
- With oral use In general, doses should be rounded up to facilitate administration of suitable volumes of liquid or an appropriate strength of tablet. The RCPCH and NPPG recommend that, when a liquid special of isoniazid is required, the following strength is used: 50 mg/5 mL.

Doses may need to be recalculated to allow for weight gain in younger children.

● **PATIENT AND CARER ADVICE**
Hepatic disorders Patients or their carers should be told how to recognise signs of liver disorder, and advised to discontinue treatment and seek immediate medical attention if symptoms such as persistent nausea, vomiting, malaise or jaundice develop.
Medicines for Children leaflet: Isoniazid for latent tuberculosis www.medicinesforchildren.org.uk/medicines/isoniazid-for-latent-tuberculosis/
Medicines for Children leaflet: Isoniazid for treatment of tuberculosis www.medicinesforchildren.org.uk/medicines/isoniazid-for-treatment-of-tuberculosis/

● **MEDICINAL FORMS** There can be variation in the licensing of different medicines containing the same drug. Forms available from special-order manufacturers include: oral suspension, oral solution, solution for injection

Solution for injection

▸ Isoniazid (Non-proprietary)
Isoniazid 20 mg per 1 ml Tebesium-S 100mg/5ml solution for injection ampoules | 12 ampoule PoM (Hospital only)
Isoniazid 60 mg per 1 ml Cemidon Intravenoso 300mg/5ml solution for injection ampoules | 5 ampoule PoM (Hospital only)

Oral tablet

CAUTIONARY AND ADVISORY LABELS 8, 22

▸ Isoniazid (Non-proprietary)
Isoniazid 50 mg Isoniazid 50mg tablets | 56 tablet PoM £23.81 DT = £23.81
Isoniazid 100 mg Isoniazid 100mg tablets | 28 tablet PoM £54.34 DT = £54.34
Isoniazid 300 mg Isoniazid 300mg tablets | 30 tablet PoM (Hospital only)

Combinations available: ***Rifampicin with isoniazid***, p. 451 · ***Rifampicin with isoniazid and pyrazinamide***, p. 451

Pyrazinamide

11-Nov-2021

● **INDICATIONS AND DOSE**

Tuberculosis, in combination with other drugs (standard unsupervised 6-month treatment)

▶ BY MOUTH
▸ Child (body-weight up to 50 kg): 35 mg/kg once daily for 2 months (initial phase); maximum 1.5 g per day
▸ Child (body-weight 50 kg and above): 35 mg/kg once daily for 2 months (initial phase); maximum 2 g per day

Tuberculosis, in combination with other drugs (intermittent supervised 6-month treatment) (under expert supervision)

▶ BY MOUTH
▸ Child (body-weight up to 50 kg): 50 mg/kg 3 times a week (max. per dose 2 g 3 times a week) for 2 months (initial phase)
▸ Child (body-weight 50 kg and above): 50 mg/kg 3 times a week (max. per dose 2.5 g 3 times a week) for 2 months (initial phase)

Congenital tuberculosis, in combination with other drugs

▶ BY MOUTH
▸ Neonate: 35 mg/kg once daily for 2 months (initial phase).

● **CAUTIONS** Diabetes

● **INTERACTIONS** → Appendix 1: pyrazinamide

● **SIDE-EFFECTS** Appetite decreased · arthralgia · dysuria · flushing · gout aggravated · hepatic disorders · malaise · nausea · peptic ulcer aggravated · photosensitivity reaction · sideroblastic anaemia · skin reactions · splenomegaly · vomiting

● **PREGNANCY** Manufacturer advises use only if potential benefit outweighs risk.

● **BREAST FEEDING** Amount too small to be harmful.

● **HEPATIC IMPAIRMENT** Manufacturer advises avoid in severe impairment, acute hepatic disease and for up to 6 months after occurrence of hepatitis (risk of increased exposure).

● **RENAL IMPAIRMENT**
Dose adjustments If estimated glomerular filtration rate less than 30 mL/minute/1.73 m², use 25–30 mg/kg 3 times a week.

● **MONITORING REQUIREMENTS**
▸ *Renal function* should be checked before treatment.
▸ *Hepatic function* should be checked before treatment. If there is no evidence of liver disease (and pre-treatment liver function is normal), further checks are only necessary if the patient develops fever, malaise, vomiting, jaundice or unexplained deterioration during treatment.

● **PRESCRIBING AND DISPENSING INFORMATION** In general, doses should be rounded up to facilitate administration of suitable volumes of liquid or an appropriate strength of tablet. Doses may also need to be recalculated to allow for weight gain in younger children.

The RCPCH and NPPG recommend that, when a liquid special of pyrazinamide is required, the following strength is used: 500 mg/5 mL.

● **PATIENT AND CARER ADVICE**
Hepatic disorders Patients or their carers should be told how to recognise signs of liver disorder, and advised to discontinue treatment and seek immediate medical attention if symptoms such as persistent nausea, vomiting, malaise or jaundice develop.
Medicines for Children leaflet: Pyrazinamide for the treatment of tuberculosis www.medicinesforchildren.org.uk/medicines/pyrazinamide-for-the-treatment-of-tuberculosis/

● **MEDICINAL FORMS** There can be variation in the licensing of different medicines containing the same drug. Forms available from special-order manufacturers include: oral suspension, oral solution

Oral tablet

CAUTIONARY AND ADVISORY LABELS 8

▸ Pyrazinamide (Non-proprietary)
Pyrazinamide 500 mg Pyrazinamide 500mg tablets | 30 tablet PoM £31.35–£50.00 DT = £40.06

▸ Zinamide (Genus Pharmaceuticals Ltd)
Pyrazinamide 500 mg Zinamide 500mg tablets | 30 tablet PoM £31.35 DT = £40.06

Combinations available: ***Rifampicin with isoniazid and pyrazinamide***, p. 451

1.5 Urinary tract infections

Urinary-tract infections

02-Jan-2025

Description of condition

Urinary-tract infections (UTIs) are common infections that can affect any part of the urinary tract; the terms ‘male’ and ‘female’ refer to all patients with a male urinary tract, and female urinary tract, respectively. UTIs occur more frequently in females, and are usually independent of any risk factor. The risk of a UTI is greater in children aged under 1 year, in those with functional and structural abnormalities that may cause urinary retention, and in those who are sexually active. UTIs are predominantly caused by bacteria from the gastrointestinal tract entering the urinary tract, with *Escherichia coli* being the most common cause.

Lower UTIs are associated with inflammation of the bladder (cystitis) and urethra (urethritis). A complicated lower UTI is a lower UTI with an increased risk of a more serious outcome or treatment failure, for example in a child with a structural or functional abnormality of the urinary tract, or an underlying disease. In some children the infection can ascend the urinary tract and lead to an upper UTI. Upper UTIs affect the proximal part of the ureters (pyelitis) or the proximal part of the ureters and the kidneys (pyelonephritis). Acute pyelonephritis, especially in children with vesicoureteric reflux, may lead to renal scarring, hypertension or failure, and sepsis.

In pregnant females, asymptomatic bacteriuria is a risk factor for pyelonephritis and premature labour. UTIs in pregnant females have been associated with developmental delay and cerebral palsy in the infant, as well as fetal death.

Insertion of a catheter into the urinary tract also increases the risk of developing a UTI, and the longer the catheter is in place for, further increases the risk of bacteriuria.

UTIs are considered recurrent in children aged 16 years and over after at least two episodes within 6 months or three or more episodes within 12 months. For children aged under 16 years, UTIs are considered recurrent after at least two episodes of acute pyelonephritis, three episodes of a lower UTI, or one episode of acute pyelonephritis in addition to one or more episodes of a lower UTI.

Aims of treatment

The aims of treatment are to relieve symptoms, treat the underlying infection, prevent systemic infection, and to reduce the risk of complications.

Non-drug treatment

EvGr Parents or carers of children with a UTI should be advised to ensure their child drinks plenty of fluids to avoid dehydration, and to use self-care strategies to reduce the risk of recurrent infections. These include wiping from front to back after defaecation, not delaying urination, avoiding constipation, and not wearing occlusive underwear.

To reduce the risk of recurrent infections, some females (non-pregnant) aged 16 years and over with recurrent UTIs may wish to try cranberry products (evidence of benefit uncertain) or D-mannose. In children aged under 16 years cranberry products may be tried on the advice of a paediatric specialist. Children and their parents or carers should be advised to consider the sugar content of these products. There is no evidence to support the use of cranberry products for the treatment of UTIs. Ⓐ

Drug treatment

EvGr When prescribing antibacterial therapy the severity of symptoms, risk of developing complications, previous urine culture and susceptibility results, and previous antibacterial use should be taken into consideration.

If a urine sample is required it should be collected before antibacterials are started. However for children with a high risk of serious illness, antibacterial treatment should not be delayed if a urine sample cannot be obtained.

With the exception of pregnant females, asymptomatic bacteriuria is not routinely treated with antibacterials. Ⓐ

For other considerations such as for children receiving prophylactic antibacterial therapy, switching from *intravenous* to *oral* antibacterials, and for advice to give to children and their parents, or carers, see Antibacterials, principles of therapy p. 358.

EvGr Reassess children if symptoms worsen at any time, or do not start to improve within 48 hours of starting treatment.

Refer children to hospital if they have any symptoms or signs suggestive of a more serious illness or condition.

Review choice of antibacterial when microbiological results are available, and change treatment as appropriate if susceptibility results indicate bacterial resistance.

Advise parents or carers that paracetamol or ibuprofen can be used for pain relief as appropriate. In acute pyelonephritis, codeine may also be considered (child aged 12 years and over). Ⓐ

Child under 3 months of age

EvGr Children under 3 months of age with a suspected UTI should be referred to a paediatric specialist. A urine sample should also be sent for urgent microscopy and culture, and the child managed in line with NICE guideline: **Fever in under 5s: assessment and initial management** (available at: www.nice.org.uk/guidance/ng143). Ⓐ

Uncomplicated lower urinary-tract infection

For complicated lower UTI, see *pyelonephritis, acute* for antibacterial choices.

Non-pregnant females aged 16 years and over

EvGr Acute, uncomplicated lower UTIs in these individuals can be self-limiting and for some, delaying antibacterial treatment with a back-up prescription to see if symptoms will resolve, may be an option. Consider a back-up antibacterial prescription for use if symptoms worsen or do not improve within 48 hours **or** an immediate antibacterial prescription. Ⓐ

Choice of antibacterial therapy

- ***Oral** first line* :
  - EvGr Nitrofurantoin p. 458, or trimethoprim p. 443 (if low risk of resistance). Ⓐ
- ***Oral** second line* (if no improvement after at least 48 hours **or** first line not suitable):
  - EvGr Nitrofurantoin (if not used first line), fosfomycin p. 439, pivmecillinam hydrochloride p. 424, or amoxicillin p. 417 (high rate of resistance, so only use if culture susceptible). Ⓐ

Males aged 16 years and over

EvGr An immediate antibacterial prescription should be given and a midstream urine sample obtained before treatment is taken and sent for culture and susceptibility testing. Ⓐ

Choice of antibacterial therapy

- ***Oral** first line* :
  - EvGr Nitrofurantoin, or trimethoprim. Ⓐ
- ***Oral** second line* (if no improvement after at least 48 hours, or first line not suitable):
  - Consider pyelonephritis or prostatitis. See *pyelonephritis, acute* below, or *prostatitis, acute* in BNF for guidance.

Pregnant females aged 12 years and over

EvGr An immediate antibacterial prescription should be given and a urine sample obtained before treatment is taken and sent for culture and susceptibility testing. Ⓐ

Choice of antibacterial therapy

- ***Oral** first line* :
  - EvGr Nitrofurantoin. Ⓐ
- ***Oral** second line* (if no improvement after at least 48 hours, **or** first line not suitable):
  - EvGr Amoxicillin p. 417 (only if culture susceptible), or cefalexin p. 385. Ⓐ
- ***Alternative** second line* :
  - EvGr Consult local microbiologist. Ⓐ
- ***Asymptomatic bacteriuria***:
  - EvGr Amoxicillin, cefalexin, or nitrofurantoin p. 458. Ⓐ

Children aged 3 months to under 16 years of age

EvGr An immediate antibacterial prescription should be given. For information on urine testing, see NICE guidance: **Urinary tract infection in under 16s: diagnosis and management** (see *Useful resources*). Ⓐ

Choice of antibacterial therapy

- ***Oral** first line* :
  - EvGr Nitrofurantoin, or trimethoprim p. 443 (if low risk of resistance). Ⓐ

- ***Oral** second line* (if no improvement after at least 48 hours **or** first line not suitable):
  - EvGr Nitrofurantoin (if not used first line), or amoxicillin (if culture susceptible), or cefalexin. (A)

Pyelonephritis, acute

EvGr An immediate antibacterial prescription should be given and a urine sample obtained before treatment is taken and sent for culture and susceptibility testing.

Consider referring children aged 3 months to 16 years to a paediatric specialist, and consider referring or seeking specialist advice for children aged 16 years and over who are significantly dehydrated or are unable to take oral fluids and medicines, are pregnant, or have a higher risk of developing complications. (A)

Males and non-pregnant females aged 16 years and over

Choice of antibacterial therapy

- ***Oral** first line* :
  - EvGr Cefalexin. If sensitivity known: co-amoxiclav p. 420, or trimethoprim. If other first line antibacterials are inappropriate, ciprofloxacin p. 429 may be used. (A)
- ***Intravenous** first line* (if severely unwell or unable to take oral treatment). EvGr Antibacterials may be combined if concerned about susceptibility or sepsis.
  - Amikacin p. 377, ceftriaxone p. 391, cefuroxime p. 388, or gentamicin p. 378. Co-amoxiclav may be used if given in combination or sensitivity known. If other first line antibacterials are inappropriate, ciprofloxacin may be used. (A)
- ***Intravenous** second line* :
  - EvGr Consult local microbiologist. (A)

Pregnant females aged 12 years and over

Choice of antibacterial therapy

- ***Oral** first line* :
  - EvGr Cefalexin. (A)
- ***Intravenous** first line* (if severely unwell or unable to take oral treatment):
  - EvGr Cefuroxime. (A)
- *Second line* or combining antibacterials if concerned about susceptibility or sepsis:
  - EvGr Consult local microbiologist. (A)

Children aged 3 months to under 16 years

Choice of antibacterial therapy

- ***Oral** first line* :
  - EvGr Cefalexin, or co-amoxiclav (if sensitivity known). (A)
- ***Intravenous** first line* (if severely unwell or unable to take oral treatment). EvGr Antibacterials may be combined if concerned about susceptibility or sepsis.
  - Amikacin, ceftriaxone, cefuroxime, gentamicin, or co-amoxiclav (if given in combination or sensitivity known). (A)
- ***Intravenous** second line* :
  - EvGr Consult local microbiologist. (A)

Recurrent urinary-tract infection

EvGr Seek specialist advice for children aged under 16 years, males aged 16 years and over, those who have had gender reassignment surgery that involved structural alteration of the urethra, females aged 16 years and over who are pregnant, patients with suspected cancer, and those presenting with recurrent upper UTI, or recurrent lower UTI with an unknown cause. (A)

Non-pregnant females aged 16 years and over

When behavioural and personal hygiene measures are not effective or appropriate, consider these alternative options in the following order to prevent recurrent UTIs, if appropriate for the patient:

- EvGr Consider single-dose antibacterial prophylaxis [unlicensed indication] when there has been exposure to an identifiable trigger;
- Methenamine hippurate p. 457 may be considered for prophylaxis of recurrent uncomplicated lower UTI. Specialist advice should be sought if considering use in non-pregnant females with recurrent upper UTI or complicated lower UTI (lack of evidence to inform when methenamine hippurate may be beneficial in these patients). Treatment should be reviewed within 6 months and then annually, or earlier if required;
- Daily antibacterial prophylaxis should be considered if there is no improvement with the above measures. (A)

Children aged under 16 years, males and pregnant females aged 16 years and over

EvGr When behavioural and personal hygiene measures alone are not effective or appropriate, seek specialist advice if considering methenamine hippurate for prophylaxis of recurrent UTI (lack of evidence to inform when methenamine hippurate may be beneficial in these patients). Treatment should be reviewed within 6 months and then annually, or earlier if required. If methenamine hippurate is not effective, with specialist advice, consider daily antibacterial prophylaxis as an alternative. (A)

Choice of antibacterial therapy

- ***Oral** first line* :
  - EvGr Trimethoprim, or nitrofurantoin. (A)
- ***Oral** second line* :
  - EvGr Amoxicillin [unlicensed indication], or cefalexin.

Advise parents or carers about the risk of resistance with long-term antibacterial use, seeking medical help if the child develops symptoms of an acute UTI, and to return for review within 6 months.

Review the success, and ongoing need of prophylaxis at least every 6 months. If antibacterial prophylaxis is stopped, ensure the child has rapid access to treatment if they develop an acute UTI. (A)

Catheter-associated urinary-tract infection

EvGr For children with a catheter-associated urinary-tract infection, consider removing or changing the catheter as soon as possible if it has been in place for longer than 7 days, without delaying antibacterial treatment. An immediate antibacterial prescription should be given and a urine sample obtained before treatment is taken and sent for culture and susceptibility testing.

Consider referring or seeking specialist advice for children with a catheter-associated UTI who are significantly dehydrated or unable to take oral fluids and medicines, are pregnant, have a higher risk of developing complications, have recurrent catheter-associated UTIs, or have bacteria resistant to oral antibacterials. (A)

Males and non-pregnant females aged 16 years and over

Choice of antibacterial therapy

- ***Oral** first line* (if **no** upper UTI symptoms):
  - EvGr Amoxicillin (only if culture susceptible), nitrofurantoin, or trimethoprim (if low risk of resistance). (A)
- ***Oral** second line* (if **no** upper UTI symptoms and first line not suitable):
  - EvGr Pivmecillinam hydrochloride p. 424. (A)
- ***Oral** first line* (upper UTI symptoms):
  - EvGr Cefalexin, co-amoxiclav (only if culture susceptible), or trimethoprim (only if culture susceptible). If other first line antibacterials are inappropriate, ciprofloxacin may be used. (A)
- ***Intravenous** first line* (if severely unwell or unable to take oral treatment). EvGr Antibacterials may be combined if concerned about susceptibility or sepsis.

- Amikacin, ceftriaxone, cefuroxime, gentamicin, or co-amoxiclav (only in combination, unless culture results confirm susceptibility). If other first line antibacterials are inappropriate, ciprofloxacin may be used. (A)
- ***Intravenous** second line* :
- EvGr Consult local microbiologist. (A)

Pregnant females aged 12 years and over
Choice of antibacterial therapy

- ***Oral** first line* :
- EvGr Cefalexin. (A)
- ***Intravenous** first line* (if severely unwell or unable to take oral treatment)
- EvGr Cefuroxime. (A)
- *Second line or combining if concerned about susceptibility or sepsis*:
- EvGr Consult local microbiologist. (A)

Children aged 3 months to under 16 years
Choice of antibacterial therapy

- ***Oral** first line* :
- EvGr Cefalexin p. 385 or trimethoprim p. 443 (if low risk of resistance), amoxicillin p. 417 (if culture susceptible), or co-amoxiclav p. 420 (if culture susceptible). (A)
- ***Intravenous** first line* (if severely unwell or unable to take oral treatment). EvGr Antibacterials may be combined if concerned about susceptibility or sepsis.
- Amikacin p. 377, ceftriaxone p. 391, cefuroxime p. 388, gentamicin p. 378, or co-amoxiclav (only in combination, unless culture results confirm susceptibility). (A)
- ***Intravenous** second line* :
- EvGr Consult local microbiologist. (A)

Useful Resources

Urinary tract infection (lower): antimicrobial prescribing. National Institute for Health and Care Excellence. NICE Guideline NG109. October 2018.
www.nice.org.uk/guidance/ng109

Management of suspected bacterial lower urinary tract infection in adult women. Scottish Intercollegiate Guidelines Network. Clinical guideline 160. September 2020.
www.sign.ac.uk/our-guidelines/management-of-suspected-bacterial-lower-urinary-tract-infection-in-adult-women/

Pyelonephritis (acute): antimicrobial prescribing. National Institute for Health and Care Excellence. NICE guideline NG111. October 2018, updated September 2024.
www.nice.org.uk/guidance/ng111

Urinary tract infection (recurrent): antimicrobial prescribing. National Institute for Health and Care Excellence. NICE guideline NG112. October 2018, updated December 2024.
www.nice.org.uk/guidance/ng112

Urinary tract infection (catheter-associated): antimicrobial prescribing. National Institute for Health and Care Excellence. NICE guideline NG113. November 2018, updated September 2024.
www.nice.org.uk/guidance/ng113

Patient decision aids: Urinary tract infection (lower) National Institute for Health and Care Excellence. November 2018, updated April 2022.
www.nice.org.uk/about/what-we-do/our-programmes/nice-guidance/nice-guidelines/shared-decision-making

Urinary tract infection in under 16s: diagnosis and management. National Institute for Health and Care Excellence. NICE guideline NG224. July 2022.
www.nice.org.uk/guidance/ng224

ANTIBACTERIALS

Methenamine hippurate

29-Oct-2024

(Hexamine hippurate)

- **DRUG ACTION** Methenamine hippurate is a urinary antiseptic which requires an acidic urine for its action. It has decreased effect on urea-degrading bacteria e.g. *Pseudomonas* and some strains of *Proteus*; these organisms usually affect patients with complicated urinary tract infections.

- **INDICATIONS AND DOSE**

Prophylaxis of uncomplicated lower urinary-tract infection

▶ BY MOUTH
- Child 6–11 years (specialist use only): 500 mg twice daily
- Child 12–15 years (specialist use only): 1 g twice daily

▶ BY MOUTH
- Child 16–17 years: 1 g twice daily, seek specialist advice if considering use for prophylaxis during pregnancy, in male patients, or for recurrent upper UTI or recurrent complicated lower UTI (lack of evidence to inform when methenamine hippurate may be beneficial in these patients)

- **UNLICENSED USE** Methenamine hippurate is considered unlicensed for the situations detailed below:
  - prophylaxis of recurrent upper UTI;
  - prophylaxis of recurrent complicated lower UTI.
- **CONTRA-INDICATIONS** Gout · metabolic acidosis · renal parenchymal infection · severe dehydration
- **INTERACTIONS** → Appendix 1: methenamine
- **SIDE-EFFECTS**
  - ▶ **Uncommon** Gastrointestinal discomfort · nausea · skin reactions · vomiting
  - ▶ **Frequency not known** Diarrhoea
- **PREGNANCY** Specialist sources indicate not known to be harmful, however limited human data available.
- **BREAST FEEDING** EvGr Amount too small to be harmful (M) (recommendation also supported by tertiary sources).
- **HEPATIC IMPAIRMENT** EvGr Avoid (M) (risk of accumulation of ammonia metabolite).
- **RENAL IMPAIRMENT** Risk of hippurate crystalluria. EvGr Avoid if creatinine clearance less than 10 mL/minute. (M) see p. 16.
- **EFFECT ON LABORATORY TESTS** False results for urinary steroids, catecholamines and 5-hydroxyindole acetic acid can occur.
- **PATIENT AND CARER ADVICE** Patients and their carers should be advised to avoid using over-the-counter urinary-tract infection relief sachets containing potassium citrate or sodium citrate that make urine less acidic as this may reduce the effectiveness of methenamine. Patients and their carers should be advised to seek medical help if symptoms of acute urinary-tract infection occur.

- **MEDICINAL FORMS** There can be variation in the licensing of different medicines containing the same drug.

Oral tablet

- ▶ **Methenamine hippurate (Non-proprietary)**
  Methenamine hippurate 1 gram Methenamine hippurate 1g tablets | 60 tablet PoM £19.74–£39.38 DT = £17.20
- ▶ **Hiprex** (Viatris UK Healthcare Ltd)
  Methenamine hippurate 1 gram Hiprex 1g tablets | 60 tablet PoM £19.74 DT = £17.20

Nitrofurantoin

15-Jul-2025

- **INDICATIONS AND DOSE**

Lower urinary-tract infections

▶ BY MOUTH USING IMMEDIATE-RELEASE MEDICINES

- Child 3 months–11 years: 750 micrograms/kg 4 times a day (max. per dose 50 mg) for 3 days
- Child 12–15 years: 50 mg 4 times a day for 3 days (7 days in pregnant women)
- Child 16–17 years: 50 mg 4 times a day for 3 days (7 days in males and pregnant women)

▶ BY MOUTH USING MODIFIED-RELEASE MEDICINES

- Child 12–15 years: 100 mg twice daily for 3 days (7 days in pregnant women)
- Child 16–17 years: 100 mg twice daily for 3 days (7 days in males and pregnant women)

Urinary-tract infections (catheter-associated)

▶ BY MOUTH USING IMMEDIATE-RELEASE MEDICINES

- Child 16–17 years: 50 mg 4 times a day for 7 days, to be used if modified-release preparations are unavailable

▶ BY MOUTH USING MODIFIED-RELEASE MEDICINES

- Child 16–17 years: 100 mg twice daily for 7 days

Severe chronic recurrent urinary-tract infections

▶ BY MOUTH USING IMMEDIATE-RELEASE MEDICINES

- Child 12–17 years: 100 mg 4 times a day for 3–7 days

Prophylaxis of recurrent urinary-tract infection in non-pregnant females [using single-dose antibacterial prophylaxis]

▶ BY MOUTH USING IMMEDIATE-RELEASE MEDICINES

- Child 16–17 years: 100 mg for 1 dose, dose to be taken following exposure to a trigger

Prophylaxis of recurrent urinary-tract infection [using daily antibacterial prophylaxis]

▶ BY MOUTH USING IMMEDIATE-RELEASE MEDICINES

- Child 16–17 years: 50–100 mg once daily, dose to be taken at night, seek specialist advice if considering use for prophylaxis during pregnancy (avoid at term), in male patients, or for recurrent upper urinary-tract infection or recurrent complicated lower urinary-tract infection

Prophylaxis of recurrent urinary-tract infection [using daily antibacterial prophylaxis] (initiated under specialist supervision)

▶ BY MOUTH USING IMMEDIATE-RELEASE MEDICINES

- Child 3 months–11 years: 1 mg/kg once daily, dose to be taken at night
- Child 12–15 years: 50–100 mg once daily, dose to be taken at night

Genito-urinary surgical prophylaxis

▶ BY MOUTH USING MODIFIED-RELEASE MEDICINES

- Child 12–17 years: 100 mg twice daily on day of procedure and for 3 days after

- **UNLICENSED USE** Nitrofurantoin may be used as detailed below, although these situations are considered unlicensed:
  - EvGr shorter duration of treatment for lower urinary-tract infections;
  - single-dose regimen for the prophylaxis of recurrent urinary-tract infection. Ⓐ

  See Urinary-tract infections p. 454 for further information.

IMPORTANT SAFETY INFORMATION

MHRA/CHM ADVICE: NITROFURANTOIN: REMINDER OF THE RISKS OF PULMONARY AND HEPATIC ADVERSE DRUG REACTIONS (APRIL 2023)

Following a report of fatality in a patient who developed acute pulmonary damage and respiratory failure after a 10-day course of nitrofurantoin for the treatment of urinary-tract infection, the MHRA reminds healthcare professionals to:

- increase vigilance for acute pulmonary reactions in the first week of treatment;
- closely monitor patients on long-term therapy for new or worsening respiratory symptoms;
- discontinue treatment immediately if new or worsening symptoms of pulmonary damage occur;
- use caution when prescribing to patients with pulmonary disease which may mask the signs and symptoms of adverse reactions.

In addition, following discussion with NHS England about the risks of hepatic adverse reactions, the MHRA reminds healthcare professionals to:

- be vigilant for signs and symptoms of hepatic dysfunction, especially with long-term therapy, and periodically monitor for signs and changes in biochemical tests that would indicate hepatitis or liver injury;
- use caution when prescribing to patients with hepatic dysfunction which may mask the signs and symptoms of adverse reactions.

Patients and their carers should be counselled to seek immediate medical advice if symptoms of pulmonary or hepatic adverse reactions develop.

- **CONTRA-INDICATIONS** Acute porphyrias p. 745 · G6PD deficiency · infants less than 3 months old
- **CAUTIONS** Anaemia · diabetes mellitus · electrolyte imbalance · folate deficiency · pulmonary disease · susceptibility to peripheral neuropathy · urine may be coloured yellow or brown · vitamin B deficiency
- **INTERACTIONS** → Appendix 1: nitrofurantoin
- **SIDE-EFFECTS** Agranulocytosis · alopecia · anaemia · angioedema · aplastic anaemia · appetite decreased · arthralgia · asthenia · chest pain · chills · circulatory collapse · confusion · cough · cyanosis · depression · diarrhoea · dizziness · drowsiness · dyspnoea · eosinophilia · euphoric mood · fever · granulocytopenia · haemolytic anaemia · headache · hepatic disorders · idiopathic intracranial hypertension · increased risk of infection · interstitial pneumonitis · leucopenia · lupus-like syndrome · nausea · nerve disorders · nystagmus · pancreatitis · psychotic disorder · pulmonary fibrosis · pulmonary hypersensitivity · pulmonary reaction (possible association with lupus erythematosus-like syndrome) · respiratory disorders · skin reactions · Stevens-Johnson syndrome · thrombocytopenia · urine discolouration · vertigo · vomiting

  SIDE-EFFECTS, FURTHER INFORMATION Discontinue treatment if otherwise unexplained haematological or neurological syndromes (such as peripheral neuropathy) occur.

  Hepatic reactions Hepatic reactions, including fatal cases, have been reported. Discontinue treatment immediately if hepatitis occurs.

  Pulmonary reactions Acute pulmonary reactions usually occur within the first week of treatment and are reversible with cessation of therapy. Chronic pulmonary reactions can develop insidiously. Discontinue treatment immediately if pulmonary reactions occur.
- **PREGNANCY** Avoid at term—may produce neonatal haemolysis.
- **BREAST FEEDING** Avoid; only small amounts in milk but enough to produce haemolysis in G6PD-deficient infants.
- **HEPATIC IMPAIRMENT** Manufacturer advises caution.
- **RENAL IMPAIRMENT** Risk of peripheral neuropathy; antibacterial efficacy depends on renal secretion of the drug into urinary tract. Avoid if estimated glomerular filtration rate less than 45 mL/minute/1.73 m^2; may be used with caution if estimated glomerular filtration rate 30–44 mL/minute/1.73 m^2 as a short-course only (3 to 7 days), to treat uncomplicated lower urinary-tract

infection caused by suspected or proven multidrug resistant bacteria and only if potential benefit outweighs risk.

- **MONITORING REQUIREMENTS** On long-term therapy, monitor liver function and monitor for pulmonary symptoms (discontinue if deterioration in lung function).
- **EFFECT ON LABORATORY TESTS** False positive urinary glucose (if tested for reducing substances).
- **PATIENT AND CARER ADVICE** Patients and their carers should be advised to seek immediate medical attention if signs or symptoms of pulmonary, hepatic, haematological, or neurological adverse reactions develop.

Medicines for Children leaflet: Nitrofurantoin for urinary tract infections www.medicinesforchildren.org.uk/medicines/nitrofurantoin-for-urinary-tract-infections/

Driving and skilled tasks Patients and carers should be counselled on the effects on driving and performance of skilled tasks—increased risk of dizziness and drowsiness.

- **MEDICINAL FORMS** There can be variation in the licensing of different medicines containing the same drug. Forms available from special-order manufacturers include: oral suspension, oral solution

Oral tablet

CAUTIONARY AND ADVISORY LABELS 9, 14, 21

▸ **Nitrofurantoin (Non-proprietary)**

Nitrofurantoin 50 mg Nitrofurantoin 50mg tablets | 28 tablet PoM £31.33 DT = £3.39 | 100 tablet PoM £17.11–£111.89

Nitrofurantoin 100 mg Nitrofurantoin 100mg tablets | 28 tablet PoM £12.58 DT = £3.71 | 100 tablet PoM £17.07–£22.14

Oral suspension

CAUTIONARY AND ADVISORY LABELS 9, 14, 21

▸ **Nitrofurantoin (Non-proprietary)**

Nitrofurantoin 5 mg per 1 ml Nitrofurantoin 25mg/5ml oral suspension sugar free | 300 ml PoM £525.17 DT = £254.30 SF

Modified-release capsule

CAUTIONARY AND ADVISORY LABELS 9, 14, 21, 25

▸ **Nitrofurantoin (Non-proprietary)**

Nitrofurantoin 100 mg Nitrofurantoin 100mg modified-release capsules | 14 capsule PoM £7.70–£9.50 DT = £9.50

Oral capsule

CAUTIONARY AND ADVISORY LABELS 9, 14, 21

▸ **Nitrofurantoin (Non-proprietary)**

Nitrofurantoin 50 mg Nitrofurantoin 50mg capsules | 30 capsule PoM £15.42 DT = £1.45

Nitrofurantoin 100 mg Nitrofurantoin 100mg capsules | 30 capsule PoM £13.56 DT = £7.64

2 Fungal infection

Antifungals, systemic use

31-Jan-2025

Fungal infections

The systemic treatment of common fungal infections is outlined below; specialist treatment is required in most forms of systemic or disseminated fungal infections. Local treatment is suitable for a number of fungal infections (genital, bladder, eye, ear, oropharynx, and skin).

Aspergillosis

Aspergillosis most commonly affects the respiratory tract but in severely immunocompromised patients, invasive forms can affect the heart, brain, and skin. Voriconazole p. 468 is the treatment of choice for aspergillosis; liposomal amphotericin B p. 462 is an alternative first-line treatment when voriconazole cannot be used. Caspofungin p. 460 or itraconazole p. 465 can be used in patients who are refractory to, or intolerant of voriconazole and liposomal amphotericin B. Itraconazole is also used for the treatment of chronic pulmonary aspergillosis or as an adjunct in the treatment of allergic bronchopulmonary aspergillosis [unlicensed indication].

Candidiasis

Many superficial candidal infections, including infections of the skin, are treated locally. Systemic antifungal treatment is required in widespread or intractable infection. Vaginal candidiasis can be treated with locally acting antifungals; alternatively, fluconazole p. 463 can be given by mouth.

Oropharyngeal candidiasis generally responds to topical therapy but oral therapy may be required in some cases; see Oropharyngeal fungal infections p. 883 for further information.

For *invasive or disseminated candidiasis*, either amphotericin B by intravenous infusion or an **echinocandin** can be used. Fluconazole is an alternative for *Candida albicans* infection in clinically stable children who have not received an azole antifungal recently. Amphotericin B should be considered for the initial treatment of CNS candidiasis. Voriconazole can be used for infections caused by fluconazole-resistant *Candida* spp. when oral therapy is required, or in children intolerant of amphotericin B or an echinocandin. In refractory cases, flucytosine p. 469 can be used with intravenous amphotericin B.

Cryptococcosis

Cryptococcosis is uncommon but infection in the immunocompromised, especially in HIV-positive patients, can be life-threatening; cryptococcal meningitis is the most common form of fungal meningitis. The treatment of choice in cryptococcal meningitis is amphotericin B by intravenous infusion and flucytosine by intravenous infusion for 2 weeks, followed by fluconazole by mouth for 8 weeks or until cultures are negative. In cryptococcosis, fluconazole is sometimes given alone as an alternative in HIV-positive patients with mild, localised infections or in those who cannot tolerate amphotericin B. Following successful treatment, fluconazole can be used for prophylaxis against relapse until immunity recovers.

Histoplasmosis

Histoplasmosis is rare in temperate climates; it can be life-threatening, particularly in HIV-infected persons. Itraconazole can be used for the treatment of immunocompetent patients with indolent non-meningeal infection, including chronic pulmonary histoplasmosis. Amphotericin B by intravenous infusion is used for the initial treatment of fulminant or severe infections, followed by a course of itraconazole by mouth. Following successful treatment, itraconazole can be used for prophylaxis against relapse until immunity recovers.

Skin and nail infections

Mild localised fungal infections of the skin (including tinea corporis, tinea cruris, and tinea pedis) respond to topical therapy. Systemic therapy is appropriate if topical therapy fails, if many areas are affected, or if the site of infection is difficult to treat such as in infections of the nails (onychomycosis) and of the scalp (tinea capitis).

Oral imidazole or triazole antifungals (particularly itraconazole) and terbinafine p. 901 are used more frequently than griseofulvin p. 470 because they have a broader spectrum of activity and require a shorter duration of treatment.

Tinea capitis is treated systemically; additional topical application of an antifungal may reduce transmission. Griseofulvin is used for tinea capitis in adults and children; it is effective against infections caused by *Trichophyton tonsurans* and *Microsporum* spp. Terbinafine is used for tinea capitis caused by *T. tonsurans* [unlicensed indication]. The role of terbinafine in the management of *Microsporum* infections is uncertain. Fluconazole or itraconazole are alternatives in the treatment of tinea capitis caused by *T. tonsurans* or *Microsporum* spp. [both unlicensed indications].

5 Infection

Pityriasis versicolor may be treated with itraconazole by mouth if topical therapy is ineffective; fluconazole by mouth is an alternative. Oral terbinafine is **not** effective for pityriasis versicolor.

Antifungal treatment may not be necessary in asymptomatic patients with tinea infection of the nails. If treatment is necessary, a systemic antifungal is more effective than topical therapy. Terbinafine and itraconazole have largely replaced griseofulvin for the systemic treatment of *onychomycosis*, particularly of the toenail; they should be used under specialist advice in children. Although terbinafine is not licensed for use in children, it is considered to be the drug of choice for onychomycosis. Itraconazole can be administered as intermittent 'pulse' therapy. Topical antifungals also have a role in the treatment of onychomycosis.

Immunocompromised children

Immunocompromised children are at particular risk of fungal infections and may receive antifungal drugs prophylactically; oral triazole antifungals are the drugs of choice for prophylaxis. Fluconazole is more reliably absorbed than itraconazole, but fluconazole is not effective against *Aspergillus* spp. Itraconazole is preferred in patients at risk of invasive aspergillosis. Micafungin p. 461 can be used for prophylaxis of candidiasis in patients undergoing haematopoietic stem cell transplantation when fluconazole or itraconazole cannot be used.

Amphotericin B by intravenous infusion or caspofungin is used for the empirical *treatment* of serious fungal infections in immunocompromised children; caspofungin is not effective against fungal infections of the CNS.

Triazole antifungals

Triazole antifungal drugs have a role in the prevention and systemic treatment of fungal infections.

Fluconazole is very well absorbed after oral administration. It also achieves good penetration into the cerebrospinal fluid to treat fungal meningitis. Fluconazole is excreted largely unchanged in the urine and can be used to treat candiduria.

Itraconazole is active against a wide range of dermatophytes. There is limited information available on use in children. Itraconazole capsules require an acid environment in the stomach for optimal absorption. Itraconazole has been associated with liver damage and should be avoided or used with caution in patients with liver disease; fluconazole is less frequently associated with hepatotoxicity.

Voriconazole is a broad-spectrum antifungal drug which is licensed in adults for use in life-threatening infections.

Imidazole antifungals

The imidazole antifungals include clotrimazole p. 635, econazole nitrate p. 900, ketoconazole p. 900, and tioconazole p. 901. They are used for the local treatment of vaginal candidiasis and for dermatophyte infections. Miconazole p. 884 can be used locally for oral infections; it is also effective in intestinal infections. Systemic absorption may follow use of miconazole oral gel and may result in significant drug interactions.

Polyene antifungals

The polyene antifungals include amphotericin B and nystatin p. 885; neither drug is absorbed when given by mouth. Nystatin is used for oral, oropharyngeal, and perioral infections by local application in the mouth. Nystatin is also used for *Candida albicans* infection of the skin.

Amphotericin B p. 462 by intravenous infusion is used for the treatment of systemic fungal infections and is active against most fungi and yeasts. It is highly protein bound and penetrates poorly into body fluids and tissues. When given parenterally amphotericin B is toxic and side-effects are common. Lipid formulations of amphotericin B are significantly less toxic and are recommended when the conventional formulation of amphotericin B is contra-indicated because of toxicity, especially nephrotoxicity or when response to conventional amphotericin B is inadequate; lipid formulations are more expensive.

Echinocandin antifungals

The echinocandin antifungals include caspofungin below and micafungin p. 461. They are only active against *Aspergillus* spp. and *Candida* spp.; however, micafungin is not used for the treatment of aspergillosis. Echinocandins are not effective against fungal infections of the CNS. Echinocandin antifungals have a role in the prevention and systemic treatment of fungal infections.

Other antifungals

Flucytosine p. 469 is used with amphotericin B in a synergistic combination. Bone marrow depression can occur which limits its use, particularly in HIV-positive patients; weekly blood counts are necessary during prolonged therapy. Resistance to flucytosine can develop during therapy and sensitivity testing is essential before and during treatment. Flucytosine has a role in the treatment of systemic candidiasis and cryptococcal meningitis.

Griseofulvin p. 470 is effective for widespread or intractable dermatophyte infections but has been superseded by newer antifungals, particularly for nail infections. Griseofulvin is used in the treatment of tinea capitis. It is the drug of choice for trichophyton infections in children. Duration of therapy is dependent on the site of the infection and may extend to a number of months.

Terbinafine p. 901 is the drug of choice for fungal nail infections and is also used for ringworm infections where oral treatment is considered appropriate.

ANTIFUNGALS › ECHINOCANDIN ANTIFUNGALS

Caspofungin

07-Aug-2020

● **INDICATIONS AND DOSE**

Invasive aspergillosis | Invasive candidiasis | Empirical treatment of systemic fungal infections in patients with neutropenia

▶ BY INTRAVENOUS INFUSION

- Neonate: 25 mg/m^2 once daily.

- Child 1–2 months: 25 mg/m^2 once daily
- Child 3–11 months: 50 mg/m^2 once daily
- Child 1–17 years: Loading dose 70 mg/m^2 for 1 dose (max. per dose 70 mg), then maintenance 50 mg/m^2 once daily (max. per dose 70 mg); increased if necessary to 70 mg/m^2 once daily (max. per dose 70 mg), dose may be increased if lower dose tolerated but inadequate response

DOSE ADJUSTMENTS DUE TO INTERACTIONS

- Manufacturer advises increase dose to 70 mg/m^2 daily (max. 70 mg daily) with concurrent use of some enzyme inducers (such as carbamazepine, dexamethasone, phenytoin, and rifampicin).

● **INTERACTIONS** → Appendix 1: caspofungin

● **SIDE-EFFECTS**

▶ **Common or very common** Arrhythmias · arthralgia · diarrhoea · dyspnoea · electrolyte imbalance · fever · flushing · headache · hyperhidrosis · hypotension · nausea · skin reactions · vomiting

▶ **Uncommon** Anaemia · anxiety · appetite decreased · ascites · chest discomfort · coagulation disorder · congestive heart failure · constipation · cough · disorientation · dizziness · drowsiness · dry mouth · dysphagia · excessive tearing · eyelid oedema · fatigue · flatulence · fluid overload ·

gastrointestinal discomfort · haematuria · hepatic disorders · hyperbilirubinaemia · hyperglycaemia · hypertension · hypoxia · induration · insomnia · laryngeal pain · leucopenia · malaise · metabolic acidosis · muscle weakness · myalgia · nasal congestion · oedema · pain · palpitations · renal impairment · respiratory disorders · sensation abnormal · taste altered · thrombocytopenia · thrombophlebitis · tremor · vision blurred
- **Frequency not known** Severe cutaneous adverse reactions (SCARs)

- **PREGNANCY** Manufacturer advises avoid unless essential—toxicity in *animal* studies.
- **BREAST FEEDING** Present in milk in *animal* studies—manufacturer advises avoid.
- **HEPATIC IMPAIRMENT** No information available for severe impairment.
Dose adjustments Usual initial dose, then use 70% of normal maintenance dose in moderate impairment.
- **DIRECTIONS FOR ADMINISTRATION** For *intravenous infusion* (*Cancidas*®), manufacturer advises allow vial to reach room temperature; initially reconstitute 50 mg with 10.5 mL Water for Injections to produce a 5.2 mg/mL solution, or reconstitute 70 mg with 10.5 mL Water for Injections to produce a 7.2 mg/mL solution; mix gently to dissolve; dilute requisite dose to a final concentration not exceeding 500 micrograms/mL with Sodium Chloride 0.9%; give over 60 minutes; incompatible with glucose solutions.

- **MEDICINAL FORMS** There can be variation in the licensing of different medicines containing the same drug.

Powder for solution for infusion
- Caspofungin (Non-proprietary)
Caspofungin (as Caspofungin acetate) 50 mg Caspofungin 50mg powder for concentrate for solution for infusion vials | 1 vial PoM £265.41–£327.67 (Hospital only)
Caspofungin (as Caspofungin acetate) 70 mg Caspofungin 70mg powder for concentrate for solution for infusion vials | 1 vial PoM £337.59–£416.78 (Hospital only)

Micafungin

28-Apr-2021

- **INDICATIONS AND DOSE**

Invasive candidiasis
- BY INTRAVENOUS INFUSION
  - Neonate (administered on expert advice): 2 mg/kg once daily for at least 14 days; increased if necessary to 4 mg/kg once daily for at least 14 days (total course), increased dose to be used if response inadequate.
  - Child (body-weight up to 40 kg): 2 mg/kg once daily for at least 14 days; increased if necessary to 4 mg/kg once daily for at least 14 days (total course), increased dose to be used if response inadequate
  - Child (body-weight 40 kg and above): 100 mg once daily for at least 14 days; increased if necessary to 200 mg once daily for at least 14 days (total course), increased dose to be used if response inadequate

Oesophageal candidiasis
- BY INTRAVENOUS INFUSION
  - Child 16–17 years (body-weight up to 40 kg): 3 mg/kg once daily
  - Child 16–17 years (body-weight 40 kg and above): 150 mg once daily

Prophylaxis of candidiasis in patients undergoing bone-marrow transplantation or who are expected to become neutropenic for over 10 days
- BY INTRAVENOUS INFUSION
  - Neonate: 1 mg/kg once daily continue for at least 7 days after neutrophil count is in desirable range.
  - Child (body-weight up to 40 kg): 1 mg/kg once daily continue for at least 7 days after neutrophil count is in desirable range
  - Child (body-weight 40 kg and above): 50 mg once daily continue for at least 7 days after neutrophil count is in desirable range

- **INTERACTIONS** → Appendix 1: micafungin
- **SIDE-EFFECTS** Anaemia · anxiety · appetite decreased · arrhythmias · confusion · constipation · diarrhoea · disseminated intravascular coagulation · dizziness · drowsiness · dyspnoea · electrolyte imbalance · eosinophilia · flushing · gastrointestinal discomfort · haemolysis · haemolytic anaemia · headache · hepatic disorders · hepatic failure (potentially life-threatening) · hyperbilirubinaemia · hyperhidrosis · hypersensitivity · hypertension · hypoalbuminaemia · hypotension · insomnia · leucopenia · nausea · neutropenia · palpitations · pancytopenia · peripheral oedema · renal impairment · severe cutaneous adverse reactions (SCARs) · shock · skin reactions · taste altered · thrombocytopenia · tremor · vomiting
- **PREGNANCY** Manufacturer advises avoid unless essential—toxicity in *animal* studies.
- **BREAST FEEDING** Manufacturer advises use only if potential benefit outweighs risk—present in milk in *animal* studies.
- **HEPATIC IMPAIRMENT** Manufacturer advises caution in chronic impairment; avoid in severe impairment (limited information available).
- **RENAL IMPAIRMENT** EvGr Use with caution; renal function may deteriorate. ⟨M⟩
- **MONITORING REQUIREMENTS**
  - Monitor renal function.
  - Monitor liver function—discontinue if significant and persistent abnormalities in liver function tests develop.
- **DIRECTIONS FOR ADMINISTRATION** For *intravenous infusion*, manufacturer advises reconstitute each vial with 5 mL Glucose 5% *or* Sodium Chloride 0.9%; gently rotate vial, without shaking, to dissolve; dilute requisite dose to a concentration of 0.5–2 mg/mL with Glucose 5% *or* Sodium Chloride 0.9%; protect infusion from light; give over 60 minutes.

- **MEDICINAL FORMS** There can be variation in the licensing of different medicines containing the same drug.

Powder for solution for infusion
- Micafungin (Non-proprietary)
Micafungin (as Micafungin sodium) 50 mg Micafungin 50mg powder for concentrate for solution for infusion vials | 1 vial PoM £196.08 (Hospital only)
Micafungin (as Micafungin sodium) 100 mg Micafungin 100mg powder for concentrate for solution for infusion vials | 1 vial PoM £341.00 (Hospital only)
- Mycamine (Sandoz Ltd)
Micafungin (as Micafungin sodium) 50 mg Mycamine 50mg powder for solution for infusion vials | 1 vial PoM £196.08
Micafungin (as Micafungin sodium) 100 mg Mycamine 100mg powder for solution for infusion vials | 1 vial PoM £341.00

ANTIFUNGALS > POLYENE ANTIFUNGALS

Amphotericin B
07-Feb-2025

(Amphotericin)

● **INDICATIONS AND DOSE**

FUNGIZONE®

Systemic fungal infections

▶ BY INTRAVENOUS INFUSION

▸ Neonate: 1 mg/kg once daily, increased if necessary to 1.5 mg/kg daily for 7 days, then reduced to 1–1.5 mg/kg once daily on alternate days if required.

▸ Child: Test dose 100 micrograms/kg (max. per dose 1 mg), included as part of first dose of 250 micrograms/kg daily, then increased if tolerated to 1 mg/kg daily, dose is gradually increased over 2–4 days; in severe infection max. 1.5 mg/kg daily or on alternate days. Prolonged treatment usually necessary; if interrupted for longer than 7 days recommence at 250 micrograms/kg daily and increase gradually

DOSE EQUIVALENCE AND CONVERSION

▸ *Fungizone*® is a conventional formulation; it is not interchangeable with other formulations of amphotericin B.

LIPOSOMAL AMPHOTERICIN B

Severe systemic or deep mycoses (including disseminated candidiasis and aspergillosis)

▶ BY INTRAVENOUS INFUSION

▸ Neonate: 1 mg/kg once daily, increased if necessary to 3 mg/kg once daily, maximum 5 mg/kg per day.

▸ Child: 3–5 mg/kg once daily for a minimum of 14 days

Mucormycosis

▶ BY INTRAVENOUS INFUSION

▸ Child: 5–10 mg/kg once daily, slow escalation of doses should be avoided

Suspected or confirmed fungal infection in febrile neutropenic patients unresponsive to broad-spectrum antibacterials and where investigations have failed to define a bacterial or viral cause

▶ BY INTRAVENOUS INFUSION

▸ Neonate: 1 mg/kg once daily, increased if necessary to 3 mg/kg once daily, maximum 5 mg/kg per day.

▸ Child: 3–5 mg/kg once daily continue treatment until patient is afebrile for 3 consecutive days; treatment should not exceed 42 days

Visceral leishmaniasis (unresponsive to the antimonial alone) (under expert supervision)

▶ BY INTRAVENOUS INFUSION

▸ Child: 1–3 mg/kg once daily for 10–21 days to a cumulative dose of 21–30 mg/kg, alternatively initially 3 mg/kg once daily for 5 consecutive days, followed by 3 mg/kg for 1 dose, to be given 6 days later

HIV-associated cryptococcal meningitis (adjunct to flucytosine and fluconazole)

▶ BY INTRAVENOUS INFUSION

▸ Child: 10 mg/kg for 1 dose, to be administered on day 1 in combination with flucytosine and fluconazole—consult product literature

DOSE EQUIVALENCE AND CONVERSION

▸ Liposomal amphotericin B is **not** interchangeable with conventional formulations of amphotericin B, e.g. *Fungizone*®.

● **UNLICENSED USE**

FUNGIZONE® Intravenous conventional formulation amphotericin B (*Fungizone*®) is licensed for use in children (age range not specified by manufacturer).

LIPOSOMAL AMPHOTERICIN B Liposomal amphotericin B is not licensed for use in neonates.

IMPORTANT SAFETY INFORMATION

MHRA/CHM ADVICE: LIPOSOMAL AND LIPID-COMPLEX FORMULATIONS: NAME CHANGE TO REDUCE MEDICATION ERRORS (JULY 2020)

Serious harm and fatal overdoses have occurred following confusion between liposomal, pegylated-liposomal, lipid-complex, and conventional formulations of the same drug substance. Medicines with these formulations will explicitly include 'liposomal', 'pegylated-liposomal', or 'lipid-complex' within their name to reduce the risk of potentially fatal medication errors.

The MHRA reminds healthcare professionals that liposomal, pegylated-liposomal, lipid-complex, and conventional formulations containing the same drug substance are **not** interchangeable. Healthcare professionals are advised to make a clear distinction between formulations when prescribing, dispensing, administering, and communicating about amphotericin B. The product name and dose should be verified before administration and the maximum dose should not be exceeded.

● **CAUTIONS** Infusion-related reactions

CAUTIONS, FURTHER INFORMATION [EvGr] Infusion-related reactions can be managed by stopping the infusion and restarting at a slower rate (over at least 2 hours), or by administering antipyretics, antihistamines or hydrocortisone as premedication. (M)

FUNGIZONE® Avoid rapid infusion (risk of arrhythmia)

● **INTERACTIONS** → Appendix 1: amphotericin B

● **SIDE-EFFECTS**

▶ **Common or very common** Anaemia · appetite decreased · azotaemia · chills · diarrhoea · dyspnoea · electrolyte imbalance · fever · headache · hepatic function abnormal (discontinue) · hyposthenuria · hypotension · nausea · nephrocalcinosis · renal impairment · renal tubular acidosis · skin reactions · vomiting

▶ **Uncommon** Agranulocytosis · arrhythmias · bronchospasm · flushing · gastrointestinal discomfort · hepatic disorders · leucopenia · myalgia · peripheral neuropathy · thrombocytopenia

▶ **Rare or very rare** Alveolitis allergic · arthralgia · cardiac arrest · coagulation disorder · deafness · encephalopathy · eosinophilia · haemorrhage · heart failure · hypersensitivity · hypertension · malaise · nephrogenic diabetes insipidus · pain · pulmonary oedema non-cardiogenic · seizure · severe cutaneous adverse reactions (SCARs) · shock · tinnitus · vertigo · vision disorders · weight decreased

● **PREGNANCY** Specialist sources indicate can be used if potential benefit outweighs risk (crosses human placenta).

● **BREAST FEEDING** Specialist sources indicate no information available but probably compatible due to high molecular weight, high protein binding, and poor oral absorption.

● **RENAL IMPAIRMENT** [EvGr] Liposomal amphotericin B may be less nephrotoxic than conventional, non-liposomal amphotericin B (*Fungizone*®). (M)

● **MONITORING REQUIREMENTS** [EvGr] Monitor hepatic function, renal function, serum electrolytes (especially magnesium and potassium concentration) and full blood count at least once weekly—consider dose reduction, treatment interruption, or discontinuation if there is clinically significant worsening of renal function or other clinical parameters. ⟨M⟩

- **EFFECT ON LABORATORY TESTS** Liposomal amphotericin B may cause false elevations of serum phosphate—consult product literature.
- **DIRECTIONS FOR ADMINISTRATION** The product name and dose should be verified before administration to ensure that the correct amphotericin B preparation is administered.

FUNGIZONE ® **Amphotericin B (as sodium deoxycholate complex)** EvGr Incompatible with Sodium Chloride solutions.

For *intravenous infusion*, reconstitute each vial with 10 mL Water for Injections, and shake immediately to produce a 5 mg/mL clear colloidal solution. Dilute further in Glucose 5% to a concentration of 100 micrograms/mL (expert sources advise that concentrations up to 400 micrograms/mL may be given via a central line for fluid-restricted patients); the pH of Glucose 5% should not be below 4.2 (check each container—consult product literature if pH less than 4.2). Infuse the test dose over 20–30 minutes, and subsequent doses over 2–6 hours; an in-line filter (pore size no less than 1 micron) may be used.

When starting treatment, patient should be carefully observed throughout administration of test dose and for a minimum of 30 minutes after. ⟨M⟩

LIPOSOMAL AMPHOTERICIN B EvGr Incompatible with Sodium Chloride solutions. For *intravenous infusion*, reconstitute each vial with 12 mL Water for Injections and shake vigorously for 30 seconds to produce a 4 mg/mL dispersion. Using the 5 micron filter provided, dilute requisite dose in Glucose 5%, 10% or 20% to a final concentration of 0.2–2 mg/mL. Infuse over 30–60 minutes; for doses greater than 5 mg/kg, or to prevent infusion-related reactions—infuse over 2 hours. An in-line filter (pore size no less than 1 micron) may be used. ⟨M⟩

- **HANDLING AND STORAGE**

FUNGIZONE ® Store in a refrigerator (2–8°C) and protect from light. For storage conditions after reconstitution and dilution—consult product literature.

LIPOSOMAL AMPHOTERICIN B Store at room temperature (below 25°C). For storage conditions after reconstitution and dilution—consult product literature.

- **MEDICINAL FORMS** There can be variation in the licensing of different medicines containing the same drug.

Powder for dispersion for infusion

▸ Amphotericin b (Non-proprietary)

Amphotericin B liposomal 50 mg Amphotericin B liposomal 50mg powder for dispersion for infusion vials | 1 vial PoM £81.00 (Hospital only) | 10 vial PoM £800.00 (Hospital only)

Powder for solution for infusion

▸ Fungizone (Neon Healthcare Ltd)

Amphotericin B 50 mg Fungizone 50mg powder for concentrate for solution for infusion vials | 1 vial PoM £16.21 DT = £16.21

ANTIFUNGALS › TRIAZOLE ANTIFUNGALS

Fluconazole

15-Nov-2024

- **INDICATIONS AND DOSE**

Candidal balanitis

▶ BY MOUTH

▸ Child 16–17 years: 150 mg for 1 dose

Vaginal candidiasis

▶ BY MOUTH

▸ Child 12–17 years: 150 mg for 1 dose

Vulvovaginal candidiasis (recurrent)

▶ BY MOUTH

▸ Child 12–17 years: Initially 150 mg every 72 hours for 3 doses, then 150 mg once weekly for 6 months

Oropharyngeal candidiasis | Oesophageal candidiasis

▶ BY MOUTH, OR BY INTRAVENOUS INFUSION

▸ Neonate up to 15 days: Initially 6 mg/kg for 1 dose, to be given on first day, then 3 mg/kg every 72 hours, treatment continued according to response.

▸ Neonate 15 days to 28 days: Initially 6 mg/kg for 1 dose, to be given on first day, then 3 mg/kg every 48 hours, treatment continued according to response.

▸ Child 1 month–11 years: Initially 6 mg/kg for 1 dose (max. per dose 400 mg), to be given on first day, then 3 mg/kg once daily (max. per dose 200 mg), treatment continued according to response

Oropharyngeal candidiasis

▶ BY MOUTH, OR BY INTRAVENOUS INFUSION

▸ Child 12–17 years: Initially 6 mg/kg for 1 dose (max. per dose 400 mg), to be given on first day, then 3 mg/kg once daily (max. per dose 200 mg), treatment continued according to response, alternatively initially 200–400 mg for 1 dose, to be given on first day, then 100–200 mg once daily for 7–21 days (duration may be increased in severely immunocompromised patients)

Oesophageal candidiasis

▶ BY MOUTH, OR BY INTRAVENOUS INFUSION

▸ Child 12–17 years: Initially 6 mg/kg for 1 dose (max. per dose 400 mg), to be given on first day, then 3 mg/kg once daily (max. per dose 200 mg), treatment continued according to response, alternatively initially 200–400 mg for 1 dose, to be given on first day, then 100–200 mg once daily for 14–30 days (duration may be increased in severely immunocompromised patients)

Tinea pedis

▶ BY MOUTH

▸ Child: 3 mg/kg once daily (max. per dose 50 mg) for up to 6 weeks

Tinea corporis | Tinea cruris | Pityriasis versicolor [Tinea versicolor] | Dermal candidiasis

▶ BY MOUTH

▸ Child: 3 mg/kg once daily (max. per dose 50 mg) for 2–4 weeks; maximum duration of treatment 6 weeks

Invasive candidal infections (including candidaemia and disseminated candidiasis)

▶ BY MOUTH, OR BY INTRAVENOUS INFUSION

▸ Neonate up to 15 days: 6–12 mg/kg every 72 hours, dose dependent on the severity of the infection, treatment continued according to response.

▸ Neonate 15 days to 28 days: 6–12 mg/kg every 48 hours, dose dependent on the severity of the infection, treatment continued according to response.

▸ Child 1 month–11 years: 6–12 mg/kg once daily (max. per dose 400 mg), dose dependent on the severity of the infection, treatment continued according to response

▸ Child 12–17 years: 6–12 mg/kg once daily (max. per dose 400 mg), dose dependent on the severity of the infection, treatment continued according to response, alternatively initially 800 mg for 1 dose, to be given on first day, then 400 mg once daily, in candidaemia continue treatment for 2 weeks after first negative blood culture and resolution of signs and symptoms

continued →

Cryptococcal meningitis

▶ BY MOUTH, OR BY INTRAVENOUS INFUSION

- Neonate up to 15 days: 6–12 mg/kg every 72 hours, dose dependent on the severity of the infection, treatment continued according to response.
- Neonate 15 days to 28 days: 6–12 mg/kg every 48 hours, dose dependent on the severity of the infection, treatment continued according to response.
- Child 1 month–11 years: 6–12 mg/kg once daily (max. per dose 400 mg), dose dependent on the severity of the infection, treatment continued according to response
- Child 12–17 years: 6–12 mg/kg once daily (max. per dose 400 mg), dose dependent on the severity of the infection, treatment continued according to response, alternatively initially 400 mg for 1 dose, to be given on first day, then 200–400 mg once daily, dose can be increased to 800 mg once daily in life-threatening infections, treatment continued according to response, usually for at least 6–8 weeks

Prevention of candidal infections in immunocompromised patients

▶ BY MOUTH, OR BY INTRAVENOUS INFUSION

- Neonate up to 15 days: 3–12 mg/kg every 72 hours, start treatment before anticipated onset of neutropenia and continue for 7 days after neutrophil count in desirable range, dose according to extent and duration of neutropenia.
- Neonate 15 days to 28 days: 3–12 mg/kg every 48 hours, start treatment before anticipated onset of neutropenia and continue for 7 days after neutrophil count in desirable range, dose according to extent and duration of neutropenia.
- Child: 3–12 mg/kg once daily (max. per dose 400 mg), start treatment before anticipated onset of neutropenia and continue for 7 days after neutrophil count in desirable range, dose according to extent and duration of neutropenia

Prevention of relapse of cryptococcal meningitis in patients at high risk of recurrence

▶ BY MOUTH, OR BY INTRAVENOUS INFUSION

- Neonate up to 15 days: 6 mg/kg every 72 hours.
- Neonate 15 days to 28 days: 6 mg/kg every 48 hours.
- Child: 6 mg/kg once daily (max. per dose 200 mg)

- **UNLICENSED USE** Fluconazole may be used as detailed below, although these situations are considered unlicensed:
  - vaginal candidiasis, and vulvovaginal candidiasis (recurrent), in females aged under 16 years;
  - tinea infections;
  - dermal candidiasis.
- **CONTRA-INDICATIONS** Acute porphyrias p. 745
- **CAUTIONS** Susceptibility to QT interval prolongation
- **INTERACTIONS** → Appendix 1: antifungals, azoles
- **SIDE-EFFECTS**

GENERAL SIDE-EFFECTS

▶ **Common or very common** Diarrhoea · gastrointestinal discomfort · headache · nausea · skin reactions · vomiting

▶ **Uncommon** Dizziness · flatulence · hepatic disorders · seizure · taste altered

▶ **Rare or very rare** Agranulocytosis · alopecia · dyslipidaemia · hypokalaemia · leucopenia · neutropenia · QT interval prolongation · severe cutaneous adverse reactions (SCARs) · thrombocytopenia · torsade de pointes

SPECIFIC SIDE-EFFECTS

▶ **Uncommon**

▸ With parenteral use Anaemia · appetite decreased · asthenia · constipation · drowsiness · dry mouth · fever · hyperhidrosis · insomnia · malaise · myalgia · paraesthesia · vertigo

▶ **Rare or very rare**

▸ With parenteral use Angioedema · face oedema · tremor

▶ **Frequency not known**

▸ With oral use Cardio-respiratory distress · oedema

SIDE-EFFECTS, FURTHER INFORMATION If rash occurs, discontinue treatment (or monitor closely if infection invasive or systemic); severe cutaneous reactions are more likely in patients with AIDS.

- **CONCEPTION AND CONTRACEPTION** EvGr After single dose treatment in females of childbearing potential, a washout period of 1 week is recommended before becoming pregnant. For longer courses of treatment in females of childbearing potential, effective contraception should be considered during and for 1 week after treatment. ⟨M⟩
- **PREGNANCY** EvGr Avoid unless potential benefit outweighs risk (multiple congenital abnormalities reported with long-term high doses). ⟨M⟩
- **BREAST FEEDING** Present in milk but amount probably too small to be harmful.
- **HEPATIC IMPAIRMENT** Manufacturer advises caution—limited information available.
- **RENAL IMPAIRMENT** EvGr Use with caution. ⟨M⟩

  Dose adjustments EvGr Usual initial dose then halve subsequent doses if creatinine clearance less than 50 mL/minute (consult product literature). ⟨M⟩ See p. 16.
- **MONITORING REQUIREMENTS** Monitor liver function with high doses or extended courses—discontinue if signs or symptoms of hepatic disease (risk of hepatic necrosis).
- **DIRECTIONS FOR ADMINISTRATION** For *intravenous infusion*, give over 10–30 minutes; do not exceed an infusion rate of 5–10 mL/minute.
- **PRESCRIBING AND DISPENSING INFORMATION** Flavours of oral liquid formulations may include orange.
- **PATIENT AND CARER ADVICE**

  Medicines for Children leaflet: Fluconazole for yeast and fungal infections www.medicinesforchildren.org.uk/medicines/fluconazole-for-yeast-and-fungal-infections/
- **PROFESSION SPECIFIC INFORMATION**

  Dental practitioners' formulary Fluconazole Capsules 50 mg may be prescribed. Fluconazole Oral Suspension 50 mg/5 mL may be prescribed.
- **EXCEPTIONS TO LEGAL CATEGORY** Fluconazole capsules can be sold to the public for vaginal candidiasis and associated candidal balanitis in those aged 16–60 years, in a container or packaging containing not more than 150 mg and labelled to show a max. dose of 150 mg.

- **MEDICINAL FORMS** There can be variation in the licensing of different medicines containing the same drug.

Infusion

▸ **Fluconazole (Non-proprietary)**

Fluconazole 2 mg per 1 ml Fluconazole 200mg/100ml infusion KabiPac polyethylene bottles | 10 bottle PoM £510.90 (Hospital only)
Fluconazole 200mg/100ml infusion polyethylene bottles | 20 bottle PoM £748.00 (Hospital only)

Solution for infusion

ELECTROLYTES: May contain Sodium

▸ **Fluconazole (Non-proprietary)**

Fluconazole 2 mg per 1 ml Fluconazole 50mg/25ml solution for infusion vials | 1 vial PoM £20.00
Fluconazole 100mg/50ml solution for infusion vials | 5 vial PoM £12.60 (Hospital only)
Fluconazole 200mg/100ml solution for infusion bottles | 10 bottle PoM £427.20 (Hospital only)

Oral suspension

CAUTIONARY AND ADVISORY LABELS 9

- **Fluconazole (Non-proprietary)**
  - **Fluconazole 10 mg per 1 ml** Fluconazole 50mg/5ml oral suspension | 35 ml PoM £29.95 DT = £29.63
- **Diflucan** (Pfizer Ltd)
  - **Fluconazole 10 mg per 1 ml** Diflucan 50mg/5ml oral suspension | 35 ml PoM £16.61 DT = £29.63
  - **Fluconazole 40 mg per 1 ml** Diflucan 200mg/5ml oral suspension | 35 ml PoM £66.42 DT = £66.42

Oral capsule

CAUTIONARY AND ADVISORY LABELS 9 (50 mg and 200 mg strengths only)

- **Fluconazole (Non-proprietary)**
  - **Fluconazole 50 mg** Fluconazole 50mg capsules | 7 capsule PoM £1.43 DT = £0.73
  - **Fluconazole 150 mg** Fluconazole 150mg capsules | 1 capsule PoM £0.68 DT = £0.70
  - **Fluconazole 200 mg** Fluconazole 200mg capsules | 7 capsule PoM £6.02 DT = £2.90
- **Diflucan** (Pfizer Ltd)
  - **Fluconazole 50 mg** Diflucan 50mg capsules | 7 capsule PoM £16.61 DT = £0.73
  - **Fluconazole 150 mg** Diflucan 150mg capsules | 1 capsule PoM £7.12 DT = £0.70
  - **Fluconazole 200 mg** Diflucan 200mg capsules | 7 capsule PoM £66.42 DT = £2.90

Itraconazole

08-Dec-2025

● INDICATIONS AND DOSE

Oropharyngeal candidiasis

▶ BY MOUTH

- Child 1 month–11 years: 3–5 mg/kg once daily (max. per dose 100 mg) for 15 days
- Child 12–17 years: 100 mg once daily for 15 days

Oropharyngeal candidiasis in patients with AIDS or neutropenia

▶ BY MOUTH

- Child 1 month–11 years: 3–5 mg/kg once daily (max. per dose 200 mg) for 15 days
- Child 12–17 years: 200 mg once daily for 15 days

Systemic candidiasis where other antifungal drugs inappropriate or ineffective

▶ BY MOUTH

- Child: 5 mg/kg once daily (max. per dose 200 mg), increased to 5 mg/kg twice daily (max. per dose 200 mg), increased dose used in invasive or disseminated disease

▶ BY INTRAVENOUS INFUSION

- Child: 2.5 mg/kg every 12 hours (max. per dose 200 mg) for 2 days, then 2.5 mg/kg once daily (max. per dose 200 mg) for max. 12 days

Pityriasis versicolor

▶ BY MOUTH

- Child 1 month–11 years: 3–5 mg/kg once daily (max. per dose 200 mg) for 7 days
- Child 12–17 years: 200 mg once daily for 7 days

Tinea pedis | Tinea manuum

▶ BY MOUTH

- Child 1 month–11 years: 3–5 mg/kg once daily (max. per dose 100 mg) for 30 days
- Child 12–17 years: 100 mg once daily for 30 days, alternatively 200 mg twice daily for 7 days

Tinea corporis | Tinea cruris

▶ BY MOUTH

- Child 1 month–11 years: 3–5 mg/kg once daily (max. per dose 100 mg) for 15 days
- Child 12–17 years: 100 mg once daily for 15 days, alternatively 200 mg once daily for 7 days

Tinea capitis

▶ BY MOUTH

- Child 1–17 years: 3–5 mg/kg once daily (max. per dose 200 mg) for 2–6 weeks

Onychomycosis

▶ BY MOUTH

- Child 1–11 years: 5 mg/kg daily (max. per dose 200 mg) for 7 days, subsequent courses repeated after 21-day intervals; fingernails 2 courses, toenails 3 courses
- Child 12–17 years: 200 mg once daily for 3 months, alternatively 200 mg twice daily for 7 days, subsequent courses repeated after 21-day intervals; fingernails 2 courses, toenails 3 courses

Systemic aspergillosis where other antifungal drugs inappropriate or ineffective

▶ BY INTRAVENOUS INFUSION

- Child: 2.5 mg/kg every 12 hours (max. per dose 200 mg) for 2 days, then 2.5 mg/kg once daily (max. per dose 200 mg) for max. 12 days

▶ BY MOUTH

- Child: 5 mg/kg once daily (max. per dose 200 mg), increased to 5 mg/kg twice daily (max. per dose 200 mg), increased dose used in invasive or disseminated disease

Histoplasmosis

▶ BY MOUTH

- Child: 5 mg/kg 1–2 times a day (max. per dose 200 mg)

Systemic cryptococcosis including cryptococcal meningitis where other antifungal drugs inappropriate or ineffective

▶ BY MOUTH

- Child: 5 mg/kg once daily (max. per dose 200 mg), increased to 5 mg/kg twice daily (max. per dose 200 mg), increased dose used in invasive or disseminated disease and in cryptococcal meningitis

▶ BY INTRAVENOUS INFUSION

- Child: 2.5 mg/kg every 12 hours (max. per dose 200 mg) for 2 days, then 2.5 mg/kg once daily (max. per dose 200 mg) for max. 12 days

Maintenance in HIV-infected patients to prevent relapse of underlying fungal infection and prophylaxis in neutropenia when standard therapy inappropriate

▶ BY MOUTH

- Child: 5 mg/kg once daily (max. per dose 200 mg), increased to 5 mg/kg twice daily (max. per dose 200 mg), increased dose used only if low plasma-itraconazole concentration

Prophylaxis of deep fungal infections (when standard therapy inappropriate) in patients with haematological malignancy or undergoing bone-marrow transplantation who are expected to become neutropenic

▶ BY MOUTH USING ORAL SOLUTION

- Child: 2.5 mg/kg twice daily, to be started before transplantation or before chemotherapy (taking care to avoid interaction with cytotoxic drugs) and continued until neutrophil count recovers, safety and efficacy not established

DOSE ADJUSTMENTS DUE TO INTERACTIONS

- EvGr Max. dose 200 mg daily with concurrent use of cobicistat-boosted regimens. (M)

DOSE EQUIVALENCE AND CONVERSION

- With oral use
- Itraconazole oral solution is **not** interchangeable with capsules on a milligram-for-milligram basis due to differences in bioavailability—higher exposure with oral solution than with capsules when the same dose is given.

● UNLICENSED USE

Not licensed for use in children (age range not specified by manufacturer).

- **CONTRA-INDICATIONS** Acute porphyrias p. 745
- **CAUTIONS** Active liver disease · history of hepatotoxicity with other drugs · susceptibility to congestive heart failure

CAUTIONS, FURTHER INFORMATION
- Susceptibility to congestive heart failure There have been reports of heart failure associated with itraconazole. Those at risk may include patients receiving higher daily doses and longer courses, patients with cardiac disease, patients with chronic lung disease, and patients receiving treatment with calcium channel blockers. Manufacturer advises avoid in patients with ventricular dysfunction, such as history of congestive heart failure, unless the infection is serious.
- **INTERACTIONS** → Appendix 1: antifungals, azoles
- **SIDE-EFFECTS**

GENERAL SIDE-EFFECTS
- **Common or very common** Alopecia · constipation · diarrhoea · dyspnoea · gastrointestinal discomfort · headache · heart failure · hepatic disorders · hyperbilirubinaemia · hypotension · nausea · oedema · pulmonary oedema · skin reactions · vision disorders · vomiting
- **Uncommon** Hearing loss · taste altered
- **Rare or very rare** Angioedema · hypersensitivity vasculitis · hypertriglyceridaemia · pancreatitis · photosensitivity reaction · severe cutaneous adverse reactions (SCARs)
- **Frequency not known** Peripheral neuropathy (discontinue)

SPECIFIC SIDE-EFFECTS
- **Common or very common**
- With intravenous use Chest pain · confusion · cough · dizziness · drowsiness · electrolyte imbalance · fatigue · gastrointestinal disorder · granulocytopenia · hyperglycaemia · hyperhidrosis · hypersensitivity · hypertension · myalgia · pain · renal impairment · tachycardia · tremor · urinary incontinence
- **Uncommon**
- With intravenous use Dysphonia · numbness · thrombocytopenia
- With oral use Flatulence · increased risk of infection · menstrual disorder
- **Rare or very rare**
- With oral use Erectile dysfunction · leucopenia · sensation abnormal · serum sickness · tinnitus · urinary frequency increased

SIDE-EFFECTS, FURTHER INFORMATION Potentially life-threatening hepatotoxicity reported very rarely—discontinue if signs of hepatitis develop.
- **CONCEPTION AND CONTRACEPTION** Ensure effective contraception during treatment and until the next menstrual period following end of treatment.
- **PREGNANCY** Manufacturer advises use only in life-threatening situations (toxicity at high doses in *animal* studies).
- **BREAST FEEDING** Small amounts present in milk—may accumulate; manufacturer advises avoid.
- **HEPATIC IMPAIRMENT** Manufacturer advises use only in serious or life-saving situations where potential benefit outweighs risk of hepatotoxicity.
- **RENAL IMPAIRMENT**
- With oral use Manufacturer advises caution (risk of congestive heart failure).
- With intravenous use Manufacturer advises caution in mild to moderate impairment (risk of congestive heart failure); avoid if creatinine clearance less than 30 mL/minute. See p. 16.

Dose adjustments
- With oral use In adults, manufacturer advises dose adjustment may be considered (bioavailability possibly reduced; consult product literature).
- **MONITORING REQUIREMENTS**
- Absorption reduced in AIDS and neutropenia (monitor plasma-itraconazole concentration and increase dose if necessary).
- Monitor liver function if treatment continues for longer than one month, if receiving other hepatotoxic drugs, or if history of hepatotoxicity with other drugs.
- **DIRECTIONS FOR ADMINISTRATION** For *intravenous infusion*, manufacturer advises dilute 250 mg with 50 mL Sodium Chloride 0.9% and give requisite dose through an in-line filter (0.2 micron) over 60 minutes.

For *oral liquid*, manufacturer advises do not take with food; swish around mouth and swallow, do not rinse afterwards.
- **PRESCRIBING AND DISPENSING INFORMATION** Flavours of oral liquid formulations may include cherry.
- **PATIENT AND CARER ADVICE** Patients should be told how to recognise signs of liver disorder and advised to seek prompt medical attention if symptoms such as anorexia, nausea, vomiting, fatigue, abdominal pain or dark urine develop.

Patients or carers should be given advice on how to administer itraconazole oral liquid.

- **MEDICINAL FORMS** There can be variation in the licensing of different medicines containing the same drug. Forms available from special-order manufacturers include: oral suspension, oral solution

Solution for infusion

EXCIPIENTS: May contain Propylene glycol
- **Itraconazole (Non-proprietary)**

Itraconazole 10 mg per 1 ml Itraconazole 250mg/25ml concentrate and solvent for solution for infusion ampoules | 1 ampoule PoM £87.55 (Hospital only)

Oral solution

CAUTIONARY AND ADVISORY LABELS 9, 23
- **Itraconazole (Non-proprietary)**

Itraconazole 10 mg per 1 ml Itraconazole 50mg/5ml oral solution sugar free | 150 ml PoM £58.34 DT = £43.27 SF

Oral suspension

CAUTIONARY AND ADVISORY LABELS 9, 23

Oral capsule

CAUTIONARY AND ADVISORY LABELS 5, 9, 21, 25
- **Itraconazole (Non-proprietary)**

Itraconazole 100 mg Itraconazole 100mg capsules | 15 capsule PoM £13.77 DT = £5.12 | 28 capsule PoM £8.68 | 60 capsule PoM £28.25–£55.10

Posaconazole

15-Sep-2025

- **INDICATIONS AND DOSE**

Invasive aspergillosis either refractory to, or in patients intolerant of, itraconazole or amphotericin B | Fusariosis either refractory to, or in patients intolerant of, amphotericin B | Chromoblastomycosis and mycetoma either refractory to, or in patients intolerant of, itraconazole | Coccidioidomycosis either refractory to, or in patients intolerant of, amphotericin B, itraconazole, or fluconazole

- BY MOUTH USING TABLETS
- Child 2–17 years (body-weight 41 kg and above): Loading dose 300 mg twice daily on first day, then 300 mg once daily
- BY INTRAVENOUS INFUSION
- Child 2–17 years: Loading dose 6 mg/kg twice daily (max. per dose 300 mg) on first day, then 6 mg/kg once daily (max. per dose 300 mg), switch from intravenous to oral route when appropriate

Prophylaxis of invasive fungal infections in patients at high risk and undergoing high-dose immunosuppressive therapy for haematopoietic stem cell transplantation or receiving chemotherapy for acute myeloid leukaemia or myelodysplastic syndrome and expected to develop prolonged neutropenia

▶ BY MOUTH USING TABLETS
- Child 2–17 years (body-weight 41 kg and above): Loading dose 300 mg twice daily on first day, then 300 mg once daily, for chemotherapy patients, start several days before the expected onset of neutropenia and continue for 7 days after neutrophil count rises above 500 cells/mm^3

▶ BY INTRAVENOUS INFUSION
- Child 2–17 years: Loading dose 6 mg/kg twice daily (max. per dose 300 mg) on first day, then 6 mg/kg once daily (max. per dose 300 mg), switch from intravenous to oral route when appropriate, for chemotherapy patients, start several days before the expected onset of neutropenia and continue for 7 days after neutrophil count rises above 500 cells/mm^3

NOXAFIL® GASTRO-RESISTANT POWDER AND SOLVENT FOR ORAL SUSPENSION

Invasive aspergillosis either refractory to, or in patients intolerant of, itraconazole or amphotericin B | Fusariosis either refractory to, or in patients intolerant of, amphotericin B | Chromoblastomycosis and mycetoma either refractory to, or in patients intolerant of, itraconazole | Coccidioidomycosis either refractory to, or in patients intolerant of, amphotericin B, itraconazole, or fluconazole

▶ BY MOUTH USING ORAL SUSPENSION
- Child 2–17 years (body-weight 10–11 kg): Loading dose 90 mg twice daily on first day, then 90 mg once daily
- Child 2–17 years (body-weight 12–16 kg): Loading dose 120 mg twice daily on first day, then 120 mg once daily
- Child 2–17 years (body-weight 17–20 kg): Loading dose 150 mg twice daily on first day, then 150 mg once daily
- Child 2–17 years (body-weight 21–25 kg): Loading dose 180 mg twice daily on first day, then 180 mg once daily
- Child 2–17 years (body-weight 26–35 kg): Loading dose 210 mg twice daily on first day, then 210 mg once daily
- Child 2–17 years (body-weight 36–40 kg): Loading dose 240 mg twice daily on first day, then 240 mg once daily

Prophylaxis of invasive fungal infections in patients at high risk and undergoing high-dose immunosuppressive therapy for haematopoietic stem cell transplantation or receiving chemotherapy for acute myeloid leukaemia or myelodysplastic syndrome and expected to develop prolonged neutropenia

▶ BY MOUTH USING ORAL SUSPENSION
- Child 2–17 years (body-weight 10–11 kg): Loading dose 90 mg twice daily on first day, then 90 mg once daily, for chemotherapy patients, start several days before the expected onset of neutropenia and continue for 7 days after neutrophil count rises above 500 cells/mm^3
- Child 2–17 years (body-weight 12–16 kg): Loading dose 120 mg twice daily on first day, then 120 mg once daily, for chemotherapy patients, start several days before the expected onset of neutropenia and continue for 7 days after neutrophil count rises above 500 cells/mm^3
- Child 2–17 years (body-weight 17–20 kg): Loading dose 150 mg twice daily on first day, then 150 mg once daily, for chemotherapy patients, start several days before the expected onset of neutropenia and continue for 7 days after neutrophil count rises above 500 cells/mm^3
- Child 2–17 years (body-weight 21–25 kg): Loading dose 180 mg twice daily on first day, then 180 mg once daily, for chemotherapy patients, start several days before the expected onset of neutropenia and continue for 7 days after neutrophil count rises above 500 cells/mm^3
- Child 2–17 years (body-weight 26–35 kg): Loading dose 210 mg twice daily on first day, then 210 mg once daily, for chemotherapy patients, start several days before the expected onset of neutropenia and continue for 7 days after neutrophil count rises above 500 cells/mm^3
- Child 2–17 years (body-weight 36–40 kg): Loading dose 240 mg twice daily on first day, then 240 mg once daily, for chemotherapy patients, start several days before the expected onset of neutropenia and continue for 7 days after neutrophil count rises above 500 cells/mm^3

DOSE EQUIVALENCE AND CONVERSION
- *Noxafil®* gastro-resistant powder and solvent for oral suspension is **not** interchangeable with other oral suspensions (licensed for use in adults).

IMPORTANT SAFETY INFORMATION

Posaconazole gastro-resistant powder and solvent for oral suspension is **not** bioequivalent with other oral suspensions (licensed for use in adults) and should not be used interchangeably, due to differences in dosing frequency, administration with regards to food, and the plasma-drug concentration achieved. Directly switching between these preparations can lead to incorrect dosing which may result in a lack of efficacy if underdosed, or serious side-effects if overdosed. Prescribers should specify the dosage form for posaconazole on every prescription, and pharmacists should ensure that the correct preparation is supplied.

- **CONTRA-INDICATIONS** Acute porphyrias p. 745
- **CAUTIONS** Administration by intravenous infusion, particularly by peripheral catheter (increased risk of QTc interval prolongation) · body-weight over 120 kg (risk of treatment failure possibly increased) · body-weight under 50 kg (risk of side-effects increased) · bradycardia · cardiomyopathy · history of QTc interval prolongation · symptomatic arrhythmias
- **INTERACTIONS** → Appendix 1: antifungals, azoles
- **SIDE-EFFECTS**
  - ▶ **Common or very common** Appetite decreased · asthenia · constipation · diarrhoea · dizziness · drowsiness · dry mouth · electrolyte imbalance · fever · gastrointestinal discomfort · gastrointestinal disorders · headache · hypertension · nausea · neutropenia · sensation abnormal · skin reactions · taste altered · vomiting
  - ▶ **Uncommon** Alopecia · anaemia · aphasia · arrhythmias · burping · chest discomfort · chills · confusion · cough · embolism and thrombosis · eosinophilia · feeling jittery · haemorrhage · hepatic disorders · hiccups · hyperglycaemia · hypoglycaemia · hypotension · leucopenia · long QT syndrome · lymphadenopathy · malaise · menstrual disorder · mucositis · nasal congestion · oedema · oral disorders · pain · palpitations · pancreatitis · peripheral neuropathy · renal impairment · respiratory disorders · seizure · sleep disorders · splenic infarction · thrombocytopenia · tremor · vasculitis · vision disorders
  - ▶ **Rare or very rare** Adrenal insufficiency · breast pain · cardiac arrest · coagulation disorder · depression · encephalopathy · haemolytic uraemic syndrome · hearing impairment · heart failure · interstitial lung disease · myocardial infarction · nephritis tubulointerstitial · pancytopenia · pseudoaldosteronism · psychotic disorder · pulmonary hypertension · renal tubular acidosis · Stevens-Johnson syndrome · stroke · sudden cardiac death · syncope
  - ▶ **Frequency not known** Photosensitivity reaction
- **CONCEPTION AND CONTRACEPTION** Manufacturer recommends effective contraception during treatment.
- **PREGNANCY** Manufacturer advises avoid unless potential benefit outweighs risk; toxicity in *animal* studies.

- **BREAST FEEDING** Manufacturer advises avoid—present in milk in *animal* studies.
- **HEPATIC IMPAIRMENT** Manufacturer advises caution (risk of increased exposure, limited information available).
- **RENAL IMPAIRMENT**
  - With intravenous use EvGr Monitor efficacy in severe impairment (variable exposure expected). (M) Caution if creatinine clearance less than 50 mL/minute (intravenous vehicle may accumulate). See p. 16.
- **MONITORING REQUIREMENTS**
  - Monitor electrolytes (including potassium, magnesium, and calcium) before and during therapy.
  - Monitor liver function before and during therapy.
- **DIRECTIONS FOR ADMINISTRATION** For *intravenous infusion* (*Noxafil*®), give continuously in Glucose 5% *or* Sodium Chloride 0.9%; dilute requisite dose in infusion fluid to produce a final concentration of 1–2 mg/mL; give via a central venous catheter or peripherally inserted central catheter over approx. 90 minutes (can give a single dose via peripheral venous catheter if central access not established—dilute to a final concentration of 2 mg/mL and give over approx. 30 minutes).
  For *gastro-resistant powder and solvent for oral suspension* (*Noxafil*®), mix each sachet with 9 mL of solvent, shake well for 45 seconds, and use within 30 minutes—consult product literature.
- **HANDLING AND STORAGE**
  - With intravenous use Store in a refrigerator (2–8 °C).
- **PATIENT AND CARER ADVICE** Patients and carers should be advised on how to administer *Noxafil*® gastro-resistant powder and solvent for oral suspension.
  Driving and skilled tasks Patients and carers should be counselled on the effects on driving and performance of skilled tasks—increased risk of dizziness and somnolence.
  NOXAFIL ® GASTRO-RESISTANT POWDER AND SOLVENT FOR ORAL SUSPENSION A user manual should be provided.

- **MEDICINAL FORMS** There can be variation in the licensing of different medicines containing the same drug.

Solution for infusion

ELECTROLYTES: May contain Sodium

- **Posaconazole (Non-proprietary)**
  Posaconazole 18 mg per 1 ml Posaconazole 300mg/16.7ml concentrate for solution for infusion vials | 1 vial PoM £211.00 (Hospital only)
- **Noxafil** (Merck Sharp & Dohme (UK) Ltd)
  Posaconazole 18 mg per 1 ml Noxafil 300mg/16.7ml concentrate for solution for infusion vials | 1 vial PoM £211.00 (Hospital only)

Gastro resistant powder and solvent for oral suspension

CAUTIONARY AND ADVISORY LABELS 3, 9, 11

EXCIPIENTS: May contain Hydroxybenzoates (parabens), potassium sorbate, propylene glycol, sorbitol

- **Noxafil** (Merck Sharp & Dohme (UK) Ltd)
  Posaconazole 30 mg per 1 ml Noxafil 300mg/10ml gastro-resistant powder and solvent for oral suspension | 8 sachet PoM £596.96 (Hospital only) SF

Gastro-resistant tablet

CAUTIONARY AND ADVISORY LABELS 3, 9, 11, 25

- **Posaconazole (Non-proprietary)**
  Posaconazole 100 mg Posaconazole 100mg gastro-resistant tablets | 24 tablet PoM £596.96 DT = £596.96 | 24 tablet PoM £498.00-£596.96 DT = £596.96 (Hospital only) | 96 tablet PoM £1,150.00-£2,360.00 | 96 tablet PoM £1,050.00-£2,387.85 (Hospital only)
- **Noxafil** (Merck Sharp & Dohme (UK) Ltd)
  Posaconazole 100 mg Noxafil 100mg gastro-resistant tablets | 24 tablet PoM £596.96 DT = £596.96 | 96 tablet PoM £2,387.85

Voriconazole

02-Aug-2021

- **INDICATIONS AND DOSE**

Invasive aspergillosis | Serious infections caused by *Scedosporium* spp., *Fusarium* spp., or invasive fluconazole-resistant *Candida* spp. (including *C. krusei*)

- BY MOUTH
  - Child 2–11 years: Treatment should be initiated with intravenous regimen, and oral regimen should be considered only after there is a significant clinical improvement; maintenance 9 mg/kg every 12 hours, adjusted in steps of 1 mg/kg and increased if necessary up to 350 mg every 12 hours, then adjusted in steps of 50 mg as required
  - Child 12–14 years (body-weight up to 50 kg): Treatment should be initiated with intravenous regimen, and oral regimen should be considered only after there is a significant clinical improvement; maintenance 9 mg/kg every 12 hours, adjusted in steps of 1 mg/kg and increased if necessary up to 350 mg every 12 hours, then adjusted in steps of 50 mg as required
  - Child 12–14 years (body-weight 50 kg and above): Initially 400 mg every 12 hours for 2 doses, then 200 mg every 12 hours, increased if necessary to 300 mg every 12 hours
  - Child 15–17 years (body-weight up to 40 kg): Initially 200 mg every 12 hours for 2 doses, then 100 mg every 12 hours, increased if necessary to 150 mg every 12 hours
  - Child 15–17 years (body-weight 40 kg and above): Initially 400 mg every 12 hours for 2 doses, then 200 mg every 12 hours, increased if necessary to 300 mg every 12 hours
- BY INTRAVENOUS INFUSION
  - Child 2–11 years: Initially 9 mg/kg every 12 hours for 2 doses, then 8 mg/kg every 12 hours; adjusted in steps of 1 mg/kg as required; for max. 6 months
  - Child 12–14 years (body-weight up to 50 kg): Initially 9 mg/kg every 12 hours for 2 doses, then 8 mg/kg every 12 hours; adjusted in steps of 1 mg/kg as required; for max. 6 months
  - Child 12–14 years (body-weight 50 kg and above): Initially 6 mg/kg every 12 hours for 2 doses, then 4 mg/kg every 12 hours; reduced if not tolerated to 3 mg/kg every 12 hours; for max. 6 months
  - Child 15–17 years: Initially 6 mg/kg every 12 hours for 2 doses, then 4 mg/kg every 12 hours; reduced if not tolerated to 3 mg/kg every 12 hours; for max. 6 months

DOSE ADJUSTMENTS DUE TO INTERACTIONS

- Manufacturer advises increasing the maintenance dose with concurrent use of fosphenytoin, phenytoin, or rifabutin—no specific recommendations made for children.

- **CONTRA-INDICATIONS** Acute porphyrias p. 745
- **CAUTIONS** Avoid exposure to sunlight · bradycardia · cardiomyopathy · electrolyte disturbances · history of QT interval prolongation · patients at risk of pancreatitis · symptomatic arrhythmias
- **INTERACTIONS** → Appendix 1: antifungals, azoles
- **SIDE-EFFECTS**

GENERAL SIDE-EFFECTS

- **Common or very common** Acute kidney injury · agranulocytosis · alopecia · anaemia · anxiety · arrhythmias · asthenia · bone marrow disorders · chest pain · chills · confusion · constipation · depression · diarrhoea · dizziness · drowsiness · dyspnoea · electrolyte imbalance · eye disorders · eye inflammation · fever · gastrointestinal discomfort · haemorrhage · hallucination · headache · hepatic disorders · hypoglycaemia · hypotension · increased risk of infection · insomnia · leucopenia · muscle tone increased · nausea · neutropenia · oedema · oral disorders · pain · pulmonary oedema · respiratory disorders · seizure · sensation abnormal · skin reactions · syncope · tetany · thrombocytopenia · tremor · vision disorders · vomiting

- **Uncommon** Adrenal insufficiency · arthritis · brain oedema · duodenitis · encephalopathy · eosinophilia · gallbladder disorders · hearing impairment · hypothyroidism · influenza like illness · lymphadenopathy · lymphangitis · movement disorders · nephritis · nerve disorders · pancreatitis · parkinsonism · phototoxicity · proteinuria · pseudomembranous enterocolitis · QT interval prolongation · renal tubular necrosis · severe cutaneous adverse reactions (SCARs) · taste altered · thrombophlebitis · tinnitus · vertigo
- **Rare or very rare** Angioedema · cardiac conduction disorders · disseminated intravascular coagulation · hyperthyroidism
- **Frequency not known** Cutaneous lupus erythematosus · periostitis (more common in transplant patients) · squamous cell carcinoma (more common in presence of phototoxicity)

SPECIFIC SIDE-EFFECTS
- With intravenous use Infusion related reaction

SIDE-EFFECTS, FURTHER INFORMATION **Hepatotoxicity** Hepatitis, cholestasis, and acute hepatic failure have been reported; risk of hepatotoxicity increased in patients with haematological malignancy. Consider treatment discontinuation if severe abnormalities in liver function tests.

Phototoxicity Phototoxicity occurs uncommonly. If phototoxicity occurs, consider treatment discontinuation; if treatment is continued, monitor for pre-malignant skin lesions and squamous cell carcinoma, and discontinue treatment if they occur.

- **CONCEPTION AND CONTRACEPTION** Effective contraception required during treatment.
- **PREGNANCY** Toxicity in *animal* studies—manufacturer advises avoid unless potential benefit outweighs risk.
- **BREAST FEEDING** Manufacturer advises avoid—no information available.
- **HEPATIC IMPAIRMENT** Manufacturer advises caution, particularly in severe impairment (no information available).

Dose adjustments
- Child 12–17 years Manufacturer advises use usual initial loading dose then halve maintenance doses in mild to moderate cirrhosis.

- **RENAL IMPAIRMENT** EvGr Intravenous vehicle may accumulate if creatinine clearance less than 50 mL/minute—use intravenous infusion only if potential benefit outweighs risk, and monitor renal function; alternatively, use tablets or oral suspension (no dose adjustment required). ⟨M⟩ See p. 16.
- **MONITORING REQUIREMENTS**
  - Monitor renal function.
  - Monitor liver function before starting treatment, then at least weekly for 1 month, and then monthly during treatment.
- **DIRECTIONS FOR ADMINISTRATION** For *intravenous infusion*, manufacturer advises reconstitute each 200 mg with 19 mL Water for Injections *or* Sodium Chloride 0.9% to produce a 10 mg/mL solution; dilute dose to concentration of 0.5–5 mg/mL with Glucose 5% or Sodium Chloride 0.9% and give intermittently at a rate not exceeding 3 mg/kg/hour.
- **PRESCRIBING AND DISPENSING INFORMATION** Flavours of oral liquid formulations may include orange.
- **PATIENT AND CARER ADVICE** Patients and their carers should be told how to recognise symptoms of liver disorder, and advised to seek immediate medical attention if symptoms such as persistent nausea, vomiting, malaise or jaundice develop.

Patients and their carers should be advised that patients should avoid exposure to direct sunlight, and to avoid the use of sunbeds. In sunlight, patients should cover sun-exposed areas of skin and use a sunscreen with a high sun protection factor. Patients should seek medical attention if they experience sunburn or a severe skin reaction following exposure to light or sun.

Patients and their carers should be advised to keep the alert card with them at all times.

- **MEDICINAL FORMS** There can be variation in the licensing of different medicines containing the same drug.

Oral tablet

CAUTIONARY AND ADVISORY LABELS 9, 11, 23

- **Voriconazole (Non-proprietary)**
  Voriconazole 50 mg Voriconazole 50mg tablets | 28 tablet PoM £191.62–£275.68 DT = £275.68 | 28 tablet PoM £65.50–£275.68 DT = £275.68 (Hospital only)
  Voriconazole 100 mg Voriconazole 100mg tablets | 28 tablet PoM £275.68 DT = £275.68
  Voriconazole 200 mg Voriconazole 200mg tablets | 28 tablet PoM £758.92–£1,102.74 DT = £1,102.74 | 28 tablet PoM £218.00-£1,102.75 DT = £1,102.74 (Hospital only)
- **VFEND** (Pfizer Ltd)
  Voriconazole 50 mg VFEND 50mg tablets | 28 tablet PoM £275.68 DT = £275.68
  Voriconazole 200 mg VFEND 200mg tablets | 28 tablet PoM £1,102.74 DT = £1,102.74

Oral suspension

CAUTIONARY AND ADVISORY LABELS 9, 11, 23

- **Voriconazole (Non-proprietary)**
  Voriconazole 40 mg per 1 ml Voriconazole 200mg/5ml oral suspension | 70 ml PoM £551.37 DT = £551.37
- **VFEND** (Pfizer Ltd)
  Voriconazole 40 mg per 1 ml VFEND 40mg/ml oral suspension | 70 ml PoM £551.37 DT = £551.37

Powder for solution for infusion

EXCIPIENTS: May contain Sulfobutylether beta cyclodextrin sodium
ELECTROLYTES: May contain Sodium

- **Voriconazole (Non-proprietary)**
  Voriconazole 200 mg Voriconazole 200mg powder for solution for infusion vials | 1 vial PoM £69.43–£77.14 (Hospital only)
- **VFEND** (Pfizer Ltd)
  Voriconazole 200 mg VFEND 200mg powder for solution for infusion vials | 1 vial PoM £77.14 (Hospital only)

ANTIFUNGALS > OTHER

Flucytosine

17-Nov-2020

- **INDICATIONS AND DOSE**

Systemic yeast and fungal infections | Adjunct to amphotericin B in severe systemic candidiasis and in other severe or long-standing infections

- BY INTRAVENOUS INFUSION, OR BY MOUTH
  - Neonate: 50 mg/kg every 12 hours.
  - Child: Usual dose 50 mg/kg every 6 hours usually for not more than 7 days, alternatively 25–37.5 mg/kg every 6 hours usually for not more than 7 days, lower dose may be sufficient for sensitive organisms

Cryptococcal meningitis (adjunct to amphotericin B)

- BY INTRAVENOUS INFUSION, OR BY MOUTH
  - Neonate: 50 mg/kg every 12 hours.
  - Child: 25 mg/kg every 6 hours for 2 weeks

- **UNLICENSED USE** Tablets not licensed.

> **IMPORTANT SAFETY INFORMATION**
>
> **MHRA/CHM ADVICE: FLUCYTOSINE (*ANCOTIL*®): NEW CONTRA-INDICATION IN PATIENTS WITH DPD DEFICIENCY (OCTOBER 2020)**
>
> Patients with partial or complete dihydropyrimidine dehydrogenase (DPD) deficiency are at increased risk of severe and fatal toxicity during treatment with fluoropyrimidines. Healthcare professionals are advised that pre-treatment testing for DPD deficiency is not required in order to avoid delay in antimycotic therapy with flucytosine. However, if drug toxicity is confirmed or suspected, testing of DPD activity and withdrawal of treatment should be considered. Flucytosine is contra-indicated in patients with known complete DPD deficiency.

- **CONTRA-INDICATIONS** Complete dihydropyrimidine dehydrogenase deficiency
- **CAUTIONS** Blood disorders · partial dihydropyrimidine dehydrogenase deficiency
- **INTERACTIONS** → Appendix 1: flucytosine
- **SIDE-EFFECTS** Agranulocytosis · aplastic anaemia · blood disorder · cardiotoxicity · confusion · diarrhoea · hallucination · headache · hepatic disorders · leucopenia · nausea · rash · sedation · seizure · thrombocytopenia · toxic epidermal necrolysis · ventricular dysfunction · vertigo · vomiting
- **PREGNANCY** Teratogenic in *animal* studies; manufacturer advises use only if potential benefit outweighs risk.
- **BREAST FEEDING** Manufacturer advises avoid.
- **RENAL IMPAIRMENT**

Dose adjustments Use normal dose every 12 hours if creatinine clearance 20–40 mL/minute; use normal dose every 24 hours if creatinine clearance 10–20 mL/minute; use initial normal dose if creatinine clearance less than 10 mL/minute and then adjust dose according to plasma-flucytosine concentration.

Monitoring In renal impairment liver- and kidney-function tests and blood counts required weekly.

- **MONITORING REQUIREMENTS**
  - For plasma concentration monitoring, blood should be taken shortly before starting the next infusion; plasma concentration for optimum response 25–50 mg/litre (200–400 micromol/litre)—should not be allowed to exceed 80 mg/litre (620 micromol/litre).
  - Liver- and kidney-function tests and blood counts required (weekly in blood disorders).
- **DIRECTIONS FOR ADMINISTRATION** For *intravenous infusion*, manufacturer advises give over 20–40 minutes.

- **MEDICINAL FORMS** Forms available from special-order manufacturers include: oral solution

Griseofulvin

16-Jan-2020

- **INDICATIONS AND DOSE**

Dermatophyte infections of the skin, scalp, hair and nails where topical therapy has failed or is inappropriate

▶ BY MOUTH

- Child 1 month–11 years: Usual dose 10 mg/kg daily (max. per dose 500 mg), increased if necessary to 20 mg/kg daily (max. per dose 1 g), for severe infections; reduce dose when response occurs, daily dose may be taken once daily or in divided doses
- Child 12–17 years: 500 mg daily, increased if necessary to 1 g daily, for severe infections; reduce dose when response occurs, daily dose may be taken once daily or in divided doses

Tinea capitis caused by *Trichophyton tonsurans*

▶ BY MOUTH

- Child 1 month–11 years: 15–20 mg/kg once daily (max. per dose 1 g), alternatively 15–20 mg/kg daily in divided doses (max. per dose 1 g)
- Child 12–17 years: 1 g once daily, alternatively 1 g daily in divided doses

- **UNLICENSED USE** Licensed for use in children (age range not specified by manufacturer).
- **CONTRA-INDICATIONS** Acute porphyrias p. 745 · systemic lupus erythematosus (risk of exacerbation)
- **INTERACTIONS** → Appendix 1: griseofulvin
- **SIDE-EFFECTS**
  - **Common or very common** Diarrhoea · epigastric discomfort · headache · nausea · vomiting
  - **Uncommon** Appetite decreased · confusion · coordination abnormal · dizziness · drowsiness · insomnia · irritability · peripheral neuropathy · photosensitivity reaction · skin reactions · taste altered · toxic epidermal necrolysis
  - **Rare or very rare** Anaemia · hepatic disorders · leucopenia · neutropenia · systemic lupus erythematosus (SLE)
- **CONCEPTION AND CONTRACEPTION** Effective contraception required during and for at least 1 month after administration to women (important: effectiveness of oral contraceptives may be reduced, additional contraceptive precautions e.g. barrier method, required). Men should avoid fathering a child during and for at least 6 months after administration
- **PREGNANCY** Avoid (fetotoxicity and teratogenicity in *animals*).
- **BREAST FEEDING** Avoid—no information available.
- **HEPATIC IMPAIRMENT** Manufacturer advises caution in mild to moderate impairment (risk of deterioration); avoid in severe impairment.
- **PATIENT AND CARER ADVICE**

Medicines for Children leaflet: Griseofulvin for fungal infections www.medicinesforchildren.org.uk/medicines/griseofulvin-for-fungal-infections/

Driving and skilled tasks May impair performance of skilled tasks (e.g. driving); effects of alcohol enhanced.

- **MEDICINAL FORMS** There can be variation in the licensing of different medicines containing the same drug. Forms available from special-order manufacturers include: oral suspension

Oral tablet

CAUTIONARY AND ADVISORY LABELS 9, 21

- **Griseofulvin (Non-proprietary)**

Griseofulvin 125 mg Griseofulvin 125mg tablets | 100 tablet [PoM] £121.80 DT = £121.80

Griseofulvin 500 mg Griseofulvin 500mg tablets | 100 tablet [PoM] £113.82 DT = £113.82

2.1 Pneumocystis pneumonia

Pneumocystis pneumonia

25-Mar-2024

Overview

Pneumonia caused by *Pneumocystis jirovecii* (*Pneumocystis carinii*) occurs in immunosuppressed patients; it is a common cause of pneumonia in AIDS. Pneumocystis pneumonia should generally be treated by those experienced in its management. Blood gas measurement is used to assess disease severity.

Treatment

The recommended duration of treatment is generally 14–21 days.

Mild to moderate disease
Co-trimoxazole p. 431 in high dosage is the drug of choice for the treatment of mild to moderate pneumocystis pneumonia.

Atovaquone p. 472 or a combination of dapsone below with trimethoprim p. 443 is given by mouth for the treatment of mild to moderate disease [unlicensed indication] in children who cannot tolerate co-trimoxazole.

A combination of clindamycin p. 400 and primaquine p. 488 may be used in the treatment of mild to moderate disease [unlicensed indication].

Severe disease
Co-trimoxazole in high dosage, given by mouth or by intravenous infusion, is the drug of choice for the treatment of severe pneumocystis pneumonia. Pentamidine isetionate p. 472 given by intravenous infusion is an alternative for children who cannot tolerate co-trimoxazole, or who have not responded to it. Pentamidine isetionate is a potentially toxic drug that can cause severe hypotension during or immediately after infusion. If there is clinical improvement after 7–10 days of intravenous therapy with pentamidine isetionate, patients can be switched to oral treatment (e.g. atovaquone) to complete 21 days treatment.

Corticosteroid treatment can be lifesaving in those with severe pneumocystis pneumonia.

Adjunctive therapy
In moderate to severe pneumocystis infections associated with HIV infection, prednisolone p. 548 is given by mouth for 5 days (alternatively, hydrocortisone p. 544 may be given parenterally); the dose is then reduced over the next 16 days and then stopped. Corticosteroid treatment should ideally be started at the same time as the anti-pneumocystis therapy and certainly no later than 24–72 hours afterwards. The corticosteroid should be withdrawn before anti-pneumocystis treatment is complete.

Prophylaxis

Prophylaxis against pneumocystis pneumonia should be given to all children with a history of this infection, and to all HIV-infected infants aged 1 month–1 year. Prophylaxis against pneumocystis pneumonia should also be considered for severely immunocompromised children. Prophylaxis should continue until immunity recovers sufficiently. It should not be discontinued if the child has oral candidiasis, continues to lose weight, or is receiving cytotoxic therapy or long-term immunosuppressant therapy.

Prophylaxis should also be given to infants aged 1 month–1 year who are suspected to be HIV-positive, *or* whose mothers had a viral load greater than 1000 HIV RNA copies/mL between 36 weeks' gestation and delivery; prophylaxis should be continued until HIV infection is excluded or until immunity recovers.

Co-trimoxazole by mouth is the drug of choice for prophylaxis against pneumocystis pneumonia. Co-trimoxazole may be used in infants born to mothers with a high risk of transmission of infection.

Inhaled pentamidine isetionate is better tolerated than parenteral pentamidine isetionate. Intermittent inhalation of pentamidine isetionate is used for prophylaxis against pneumocystis pneumonia in children unable to tolerate co-trimoxazole. It is effective but children may be prone to extrapulmonary infection. Alternatively, dapsone can be used.

ANTIMYCOBACTERIALS

Dapsone

13-May-2025

● **INDICATIONS AND DOSE**

Treatment of mild to moderate *Pneumocystis jirovecii* (*Pneumocystis carinii*) pneumonia (in combination with trimethoprim)
▶ BY MOUTH
▸ Child 1 month–11 years: 2 mg/kg once daily (max. per dose 100 mg)
▸ Child 12–17 years: 100 mg once daily

Prophylaxis of *Pneumocystis jirovecii* (*Pneumocystis carinii*) pneumonia
▶ BY MOUTH
▸ Child: 2 mg/kg once daily (max. per dose 100 mg)

● **UNLICENSED USE** Not licensed for treatment of pneumocystis (*P. jirovecii*) pneumonia.
Monotherapy not licensed for children for prophylaxis of *P. jirovecii* pneumonia.

● **CAUTIONS** Anaemia (treat severe anaemia before starting) · avoid in Acute porphyrias p. 745 · cardiac disease · G6PD deficiency (avoid in severe deficiency) · pulmonary disease · susceptibility to haemolysis

CAUTIONS, FURTHER INFORMATION
▸ Susceptibility to haemolysis Patients deficient in G6PD or methaemoglobin reductase, or with haemoglobin M are more susceptible to the haemolytic effects of dapsone.

● **INTERACTIONS** → Appendix 1: dapsone

● **SIDE-EFFECTS**
▶ **Common or very common** Haemolysis · methaemoglobinaemia
▶ **Uncommon** Appetite decreased · haemolytic anaemia · headache · hepatic disorders · hypoalbuminaemia · insomnia · nausea · peripheral neuropathy · photosensitivity reaction · psychosis · skin reactions · tachycardia · vomiting
▶ **Rare or very rare** Agranulocytosis · severe cutaneous adverse reactions (SCARs)

SIDE-EFFECTS, FURTHER INFORMATION If drug reaction with eosinophilia and systemic symptoms (DRESS) occurs (rash with fever and eosinophilia)—discontinue immediately (may progress to exfoliative dermatitis, hepatitis, hypoalbuminaemia, psychosis and death).

● **PREGNANCY** Folic acid p. 710 (higher dose) should be given to mother throughout pregnancy; neonatal haemolysis and methaemoglobinaemia reported in third trimester.

● **BREAST FEEDING** Haemolytic anaemia; although significant amount in milk, risk to infant very small unless infant is G6PD deficient.

● **MONITORING REQUIREMENTS** EvGr Monitor full blood count regularly during treatment. Ⓜ

● **PATIENT AND CARER ADVICE**
Blood disorders On long-term treatment, patients and their carers should be told how to recognise signs of blood disorders and advised to seek immediate medical attention if symptoms such as fever, sore throat, rash, mouth ulcers, purpura, bruising or bleeding develop.

● **MEDICINAL FORMS** There can be variation in the licensing of different medicines containing the same drug. Forms available from special-order manufacturers include: oral suspension, oral solution

Oral tablet
CAUTIONARY AND ADVISORY LABELS 8
▸ Dapsone (Non-proprietary)
Dapsone 50 mg Dapsone 50mg tablets | 28 tablet PoM £32.00 DT = £5.20

5 Infection

Dapsone 100 mg Dapsone 100mg tablets | 28 tablet [PoM] £95.00 DT = £13.80

ANTIPROTOZOALS

Atovaquone

09-Sep-2021

● **INDICATIONS AND DOSE**

Treatment of mild to moderate *Pneumocystis jirovecii* (*Pneumocystis carinii*) pneumonia in patients intolerant of co-trimoxazole

▶ BY MOUTH

▸ Child 1-2 months: 15–20 mg/kg twice daily for 14–21 days, dose to be taken with food, particularly high fat food

▸ Child 3 months-1 year: 22.5 mg/kg twice daily for 14–21 days, dose to be taken with food, particularly high fat food

▸ Child 2-17 years: 15–20 mg/kg twice daily (max. per dose 750 mg) for 14–21 days, dose to be taken with food, particularly high fat food

● **UNLICENSED USE** Not licensed for use in children.

● **CAUTIONS** Initial diarrhoea and difficulty in taking with food may reduce absorption (and require alternative therapy) · other causes of pulmonary disease should be sought and treated

● **INTERACTIONS** → Appendix 1: antimalarials

● **SIDE-EFFECTS**

▶ **Common or very common** Anaemia · angioedema · bronchospasm · diarrhoea · headache · hypersensitivity · hyponatraemia · insomnia · nausea · neutropenia · skin reactions · throat tightness · vomiting

▶ **Frequency not known** Stevens-Johnson syndrome

● **PREGNANCY** Manufacturer advises avoid unless potential benefit outweighs risk—no information available.

● **BREAST FEEDING** Manufacturer advises avoid.

● **HEPATIC IMPAIRMENT** Manufacturer advises use with caution in significant impairment and monitor closely—no information available.

● **RENAL IMPAIRMENT** [EvGr] Caution in significant impairment (no information available). ⟨M⟩

● **PRESCRIBING AND DISPENSING INFORMATION** Flavours of oral liquid formulations may include tutti-frutti.

● **MEDICINAL FORMS** There can be variation in the licensing of different medicines containing the same drug.

Oral suspension

CAUTIONARY AND ADVISORY LABELS 21

▸ Atovaquone (Non-proprietary)

Atovaquone 150 mg per 1 ml Atovaquone 750mg/5ml oral suspension sugar free | 226 ml [PoM] £470.60–£724.00 DT = £486.37 [SF]

▸ Wellvone (GlaxoSmithKline UK Ltd)

Atovaquone 150 mg per 1 ml Wellvone 750mg/5ml oral suspension | 226 ml [PoM] £486.37 DT = £486.37 [SF]

Pentamidine isetionate

05-Oct-2021

● **INDICATIONS AND DOSE**

Treatment of *Pneumocystis jirovecii* (*Pneumocystis carinii*) pneumonia (specialist use only)

▶ BY INTRAVENOUS INFUSION

▸ Child: 4 mg/kg once daily for at least 7–10 days

Prophylaxis of *Pneumocystis jirovecii* (*Pneumocystis carinii*) pneumonia (specialist use only)

▶ BY INHALATION OF NEBULISED SOLUTION

▸ Child 5-17 years: 300 mg every 4 weeks, use suitable equipment—consult product literature, alternatively 150 mg every 2 weeks, use suitable equipment—consult product literature

Visceral leishmaniasis (specialist use only)

▶ BY DEEP INTRAMUSCULAR INJECTION

▸ Child 1-17 years: 3–4 mg/kg once daily on alternate days maximum total of 10 injections, course may be repeated if necessary

Cutaneous leishmaniasis (specialist use only)

▶ BY DEEP INTRAMUSCULAR INJECTION

▸ Child 1-17 years: 3–4 mg/kg 1–2 times a week until condition resolves

Trypanosomiasis (specialist use only)

▶ BY DEEP INTRAMUSCULAR INJECTION, OR BY INTRAVENOUS INFUSION

▸ Child 1-17 years: 4 mg/kg once daily or on alternate days for a total of 7–10 injections

● **UNLICENSED USE** Not licensed for prevention of pneumocystis pneumonia in children.

● **CAUTIONS** Anaemia · bradycardia · cardiac disease · history of ventricular arrhythmias · hyperglycaemia · hypertension · hypoglycaemia · hypokalaemia · hypomagnesaemia · hypotension · leucopenia · risk of severe hypotension following administration · thrombocytopenia

● **INTERACTIONS** → Appendix 1: pentamidine

● **SIDE-EFFECTS**

GENERAL SIDE-EFFECTS

▶ **Common or very common** Dizziness · hypoglycaemia (can be severe and sometimes fatal) · hypotension (can be severe and sometimes fatal) · local reaction · nausea · rash · taste altered

▶ **Rare or very rare** QT interval prolongation

▶ **Frequency not known** Pancreatitis acute (can be severe and sometimes fatal)

SPECIFIC SIDE-EFFECTS

▶ **Common or very common**

▸ When used by inhalation Cough · dyspnoea · respiratory disorders

▸ With parenteral use Acute kidney injury · anaemia · azotaemia · electrolyte imbalance · flushing · haematuria · hyperglycaemia · induration · leucopenia · localised pain · myopathy · syncope · thrombocytopenia · vomiting

▶ **Rare or very rare**

▸ With parenteral use Arrhythmia (can be severe and sometimes fatal) · pancreatitis (can be severe and sometimes fatal)

▶ **Frequency not known**

▸ When used by inhalation Angioedema · appetite decreased · bradycardia · fatigue · renal failure

▸ With parenteral use Arrhythmias · perioral hypoaesthesia · sensation abnormal · Stevens-Johnson syndrome

● **PREGNANCY** Manufacturer advises avoid unless essential.

● **BREAST FEEDING** Manufacturer advises avoid unless essential—no information available.

● **HEPATIC IMPAIRMENT** Manufacturer advises caution.

● **RENAL IMPAIRMENT** [EvGr] Use with caution. ⟨M⟩

Dose adjustments [EvGr] Reduce intravenous dose for pneumocystis pneumonia if creatinine clearance less than 10 mL/minute: in *life-threatening infection*, use 4 mg/kg once daily for 7–10 days, then 4 mg/kg on alternate days to complete course of at least 14 doses; in *less severe infection*, use 4 mg/kg on alternate days for at least 14 doses. ⟨M⟩ See p. 16.

● **MONITORING REQUIREMENTS**

▶ Monitor blood pressure before starting treatment, during administration, and at regular intervals, until treatment concluded.

▶ Carry out laboratory monitoring according to product literature.

- **DIRECTIONS FOR ADMINISTRATION** Manufacturer advises patient should be lying down when receiving drug parenterally. Direct intravenous injection should be avoided whenever possible and **never** given rapidly; intramuscular injections should be deep and preferably given into the buttock. For *intravenous infusion*, manufacturer advises reconstitute 300 mg with 3–5 mL Water for Injections (displacement value may be significant), then dilute required dose with 50–250 mL Glucose 5% *or* Sodium Chloride 0.9%; give over at least 60 minutes.
  Powder for injection (dissolved in water for injection) may be used for nebulisation.
- **HANDLING AND STORAGE** Pentamidine isetionate is toxic and personnel should be adequately protected during handling and administration—consult product literature.

- **MEDICINAL FORMS** There can be variation in the licensing of different medicines containing the same drug.

Powder for solution for injection

- **Pentamidine isetionate (Non-proprietary)**
  Pentamidine isetionate 300 mg Pentamidine 300mg powder for solution for injection vials | 5 vial PoM £1,710.00 DT = £158.86 (Hospital only)
- **Pentacarinat** (The Simple Pharma Company UK Ltd)
  Pentamidine isetionate 300 mg Pentacarinat 300mg powder for solution for injection vials | 5 vial PoM £158.86 DT = £158.86

3 Helminth infection

Helminth infections

11-May-2026

Specialist centres

Advice on prophylaxis and treatment of helminth infections is available from the following specialist centres:

Birmingham	(0121) 424 0357
Scotland	Contact local Infectious Diseases Unit
Liverpool	(0151) 705 3100
London	0845 155 5000 (treatment)

Threadworms

Anthelmintics are effective in threadworm (pinworms, *Enterobius vermicularis*) infections, but their use needs to be combined with hygienic measures to break the cycle of auto-infection. All members of the family require treatment.

Adult threadworms do not live for longer than 6 weeks and for development of fresh worms, ova must be swallowed and exposed to the action of digestive juices in the upper intestinal tract. Direct multiplication of worms does not take place in the large bowel. Adult female worms lay ova on the perianal skin which causes pruritus; scratching the area then leads to ova being transmitted on fingers to the mouth, often via food eaten with unwashed hands. Washing hands and scrubbing nails before each meal and after each visit to the toilet is essential. A bath taken immediately after rising will remove ova laid during the night.

Mebendazole p. 475 is the drug of choice for treating threadworm infection in patients of all ages over 6 months. It is given as a single dose; as reinfection is very common, a second dose may be given after 2 weeks.

Ascaricides (common roundworm infections)

Mebendazole is effective against *Ascaris lumbricoides* and is generally considered to be the drug of choice.

Levamisole [unlicensed] is no longer recommended due to the risk of leukoencephalopathy.

Tapeworm infections

Taenicides

Niclosamide [unlicensed] (available from 'special-order' manufacturers or specialist importing companies) is the most widely used drug for tapeworm infections and side-effects are limited to occasional gastro-intestinal upset, lightheadedness, and pruritus; it is not effective against larval worms. Fears of developing cysticercosis in *Taenia solium* infections have proved unfounded. All the same, an antiemetic can be given before treatment and a laxative can be given 2 hours after niclosamide.

Praziquantel p. 475 [unlicensed] (available from 'special-order' manufacturers or specialist importing companies) is as effective as niclosamide.

Hydatid disease

Cysts caused by *Echinococcus granulosus* grow slowly and asymptomatic patients do not always require treatment. Surgical treatment remains the method of choice in many situations. Albendazole p. 474 [unlicensed] (available from 'special-order' manufacturers or specialist importing companies) is used in conjunction with surgery to reduce the risk of recurrence or as primary treatment in inoperable cases. Alveolar echinococcosis due to *E. multilocularis* is usually fatal if untreated. Surgical removal with albendazole cover is the treatment of choice, but where effective surgery is impossible, repeated cycles of albendazole (for a year or more) may help. Careful monitoring of liver function is particularly important during drug treatment.

Hookworms

Hookworms (ancylostomiasis, necatoriasis) live in the upper small intestine and draw blood from the point of their attachment to their host. An iron-deficiency anaemia may occur and, if present, effective treatment of the infection requires not only expulsion of the worms but treatment of the anaemia.

Mebendazole has a useful broad-spectrum activity, and is effective against hookworms. Albendazole [unlicensed] (available from 'special-order' manufacturers or specialist importing companies) is an alternative. Levamisole [unlicensed] is no longer recommended due to the risk of leukoencephalopathy.

Schistosomicides (bilharziasis)

Adult *Schistosoma haematobium* worms live in the genito-urinary veins and adult *S. mansoni* in those of the colon and mesentery. *S. japonicum* is more widely distributed in veins of the alimentary tract and portal system.

Praziquantel [unlicensed] is available from Merck Serono (*Cysticide*®) and is effective against all human schistosomes. No serious adverse effects have been reported. Of all the available schistosomicides, it has the most attractive combination of effectiveness, broad-spectrum activity, and low toxicity.

Filaricides

Diethylcarbamazine [unlicensed] (available from 'special-order' manufacturers or specialist importing companies) is effective against microfilariae and adults of *Loa loa*, *Wuchereria bancrofti*, and *Brugia malayi*. To minimise reactions, treatment in adults and children over 1 month, is commenced with a dose of diethylcarbamazine citrate on the first day and increased gradually over 3 days. Length of treatment varies according to infection type, and usually gives a radical cure for these infections. Close medical supervision is necessary particularly in the early phase of treatment.

In heavy infections there may be a febrile reaction, and in heavy *Loa loa* infection there is a small risk of encephalopathy. In such cases specialist advice should be sought, and treatment must be given under careful in-patient supervision and stopped at the first sign of cerebral involvement.

Ivermectin below [unlicensed] is very effective in *onchocerciasis* and it is now the drug of choice; reactions are usually slight. Diethylcarbamazine or suramin should no longer be used for *onchocerciasis* because of their toxicity.

Cutaneous larva migrans (creeping eruption)

Dog and cat hookworm larvae may enter human skin where they produce slowly extending itching tracks usually on the foot. Single tracks can be treated with topical tiabendazole (no commercial preparation available). Multiple infections respond to ivermectin, albendazole or **tiabendazole** (thiabendazole) by mouth [all unlicensed].

Strongyloidiasis

Adult *Strongyloides stercoralis* live in the gut and produce larvae which penetrate the gut wall and invade the tissues, setting up a cycle of auto-infection. Ivermectin is the treatment of choice for chronic *Strongyloides* infection in adults and children over 5 years. Albendazole [unlicensed] (available from 'special order' manufacturers or specialist importing companies) is an alternative given to adults and children over 2 years.

ANTHELMINTICS

Albendazole

03-Jun-2024

● **INDICATIONS AND DOSE**

Chronic *Strongyloides* infection

▶ BY MOUTH

▸ Child 2–17 years: 400 mg twice daily for 3 days, dose may be repeated after 3 weeks if necessary

Hydatid disease, in conjunction with surgery to reduce the risk of recurrence or as primary treatment in inoperable cases

▶ BY MOUTH

▸ Child 2–17 years: 7.5 mg/kg twice daily (max. per dose 400 mg) for 28 days followed by 14-day break, to be repeated for up to 2–3 cycles

Hookworm infections

▶ BY MOUTH

▸ Child 2–17 years: 400 mg for 1 dose

● **UNLICENSED USE** Albendazole is an unlicensed drug.

● **CAUTIONS** Pre-existing neurocysticercosis (may trigger neurological symptoms)

● **INTERACTIONS** → Appendix 1: albendazole

● **SIDE-EFFECTS**

▶ **Common or very common** Abdominal pain · alopecia (reversible) · dizziness · gastrointestinal disorder · hair thinning · headache · nausea · vomiting

▶ **Uncommon** Diarrhoea · hepatic disorders · leucopenia · skin reactions

▶ **Rare or very rare** Agranulocytosis · bone marrow disorders · bone pain · proteinuria · Stevens-Johnson syndrome

● **PREGNANCY** Specialist sources indicate low risk due to poor oral bioavailability but consider avoiding during first trimester.

● **BREAST FEEDING** Specialist sources indicate present in milk but amount is clinically insignificant; a single oral dose is compatible with breast-feeding.

● **HEPATIC IMPAIRMENT** [EvGr] Caution in pre-existing liver disease (no information available). ⟨M⟩

● **MEDICINAL FORMS** There can be variation in the licensing of different medicines containing the same drug. Forms available from special-order manufacturers include: oral tablet, chewable tablet, oral suspension

Oral tablet

CAUTIONARY AND ADVISORY LABELS 9

▸ **Albendazole (Non-proprietary)**

Albendazole 400 mg Eskazole 400mg tablets | 60 tablet [PoM] [X]

Chewable tablet

CAUTIONARY AND ADVISORY LABELS 9

EXCIPIENTS: May contain Propylene glycol

▸ **Albendazole (Non-proprietary)**

Albendazole 200 mg Zentel 200mg chewable tablets | 6 tablet [PoM] [X] (Hospital only)

Albendazole 400 mg Zentel 400mg chewable tablets | 1 tablet [PoM] [X]

Diethylcarbamazine

● **INDICATIONS AND DOSE**

***Wuchereria bancrofti* infections | *Brugia malayi* infections**

▶ BY MOUTH

▸ Child 1 month–9 years: Initially 1 mg/kg daily in divided doses on the first day, then increased to 3 mg/kg daily in divided doses, dose to be increased gradually over 3 days

▸ Child 10–17 years: Initially 1 mg/kg daily in divided doses on the first day, then increased to 6 mg/kg daily in divided doses, dose to be increased gradually over 3 days

***Loa loa* infections**

▶ BY MOUTH

▸ Child 1 month–9 years: Initially 1 mg/kg daily in divided doses on the first day, then increased to 3 mg/kg daily in divided doses, dose to be increased gradually over 3 days

▸ Child 10–17 years: Initially 1 mg/kg daily in divided doses on the first day, then increased to 6 mg/kg daily in divided doses, dose to be increased gradually over 3 days

● **UNLICENSED USE** Diethylcarbamazine is an unlicensed drug.

● **MEDICINAL FORMS** No licensed medicines listed.

Ivermectin

07-Jul-2024

● **INDICATIONS AND DOSE**

Onchocerciasis

▶ BY MOUTH

▸ Child 5–17 years: 150 micrograms/kg for 1 dose, repeat at intervals of 6 to 12 months, depending on symptoms, must be given until adult worms die out

Scabies

▶ BY MOUTH

▸ Child (body-weight 15 kg and above): 200 micrograms/kg for 1 dose, recovery may take up to 4 weeks after treatment; only repeat the dose within 2 weeks if new specific lesions occur or if a parasitologic examination is positive at this date

Hyperkeratotic (crusted or 'Norwegian') scabies

▶ BY MOUTH

▸ Child (body-weight 15 kg and above): 200 micrograms/kg for 1 dose, a repeat dose within 8 to 15 days may be necessary for recovery

Gastrointestinal strongyloidiasis

▶ BY MOUTH

▸ Child (body-weight 15–24 kg): 3 mg for 1 dose

▸ Child (body-weight 25–35 kg): 6 mg for 1 dose

- ▸ Child (body-weight 36–50 kg): 9 mg for 1 dose
- ▸ Child (body-weight 51–65 kg): 12 mg for 1 dose
- ▸ Child (body-weight 66–79 kg): 15 mg for 1 dose
- ▸ Child (body-weight 80 kg and above): 18 mg for 1 dose

Microfilaraemia in patients with lymphatic filariasis due to *Wuchereria bancrofti* infection

▶ BY MOUTH

- ▸ Child (body-weight 15 kg and above): 150–200 micrograms/kg for 1 dose, to be repeated every 6 months. Consult product literature for more information

- **UNLICENSED USE** Ivermectin is used for the treatment of *onchocerciasis*, but is not licensed for this indication.
- **INTERACTIONS** → Appendix 1: ivermectin
- **SIDE-EFFECTS**
  - ▶ **Common or very common** Skin reactions
  - ▶ **Frequency not known** Abdominal pain · abnormal sensation in eye · anaemia · appetite decreased · arthralgia · asthenia · asthma exacerbated · coma · confusion · constipation · diarrhoea · difficulty standing · difficulty walking · dizziness · drowsiness · dyspnoea · encephalopathy · eye erythema · eye inflammation · fever · gastrointestinal disorders · haemorrhage · headache · hepatic disorders · hyperbilirubinaemia · hypereosinophilia · leucopenia · lymphatic abnormalities · Mazzotti reaction · myalgia · nausea · oedema · pain · postural hypotension · psychiatric disorder · severe cutaneous adverse reactions (SCARs) · stupor · tachycardia · tremor · urinary incontinence · vertigo · vomiting
- **PREGNANCY** EvGr Use only if potential benefit outweighs risk—no adverse effects in limited human data (recommendation also supported by specialist sources). (M)
- **BREAST FEEDING** Specialist sources indicate present in milk but amount probably too small to be harmful.
- **DIRECTIONS FOR ADMINISTRATION** EvGr Tablets can be crushed before swallowing. (M)
- **PATIENT AND CARER ADVICE** Patients and carers should be advised to take ivermectin on an empty stomach; 2 hours before or 2 hours after food (effect of food on absorption is unknown).

- **MEDICINAL FORMS** There can be variation in the licensing of different medicines containing the same drug. Forms available from special-order manufacturers include: oral tablet

Oral tablet

▸ Ivermectin (Non-proprietary)

Ivermectin 3 mg Stromectol 3mg tablets | 4 tablet PoM ⊠ DT = £105.57

Ivermectin 3mg tablets | 4 tablet PoM £57.75–£95.67 DT = £105.57 | 8 tablet PoM £191.34

Mebendazole

10-Nov-2021

- **INDICATIONS AND DOSE**

Threadworm infections

▶ BY MOUTH

- ▸ Child 6 months–17 years: 100 mg for 1 dose, if reinfection occurs, second dose may be needed after 2 weeks

Whipworm infections | Hookworm infections

▶ BY MOUTH

- ▸ Child 1–17 years: 100 mg twice daily for 3 days

Roundworm infections

▶ BY MOUTH

- ▸ Child 1 year: 100 mg twice daily for 3 days
- ▸ Child 2–17 years: 100 mg twice daily for 3 days, alternatively 500 mg for 1 dose

Threadworm infections (dose approved for use by community practitioner nurse prescribers)

▶ BY MOUTH

- ▸ Child 2–17 years: 100 mg for 1 dose, if reinfection occurs, second dose may be needed after 2 weeks

- **UNLICENSED USE** Not licensed for use as a single dose of 500 mg in roundworm infections.
  Not licensed for use in children under 2 years.
- **INTERACTIONS** → Appendix 1: mebendazole
- **SIDE-EFFECTS**
  - ▶ **Common or very common** Gastrointestinal discomfort
  - ▶ **Uncommon** Diarrhoea · flatulence
  - ▶ **Rare or very rare** Alopecia · dizziness · hepatitis · neutropenia · seizure · severe cutaneous adverse reactions (SCARs) · skin reactions
- **PREGNANCY** Manufacturer advises avoid—toxicity in *animal* studies.
- **BREAST FEEDING** Amount present in milk too small to be harmful but manufacturer advises avoid.
- **PRESCRIBING AND DISPENSING INFORMATION** Flavours of oral liquid formulations may include banana.
- **PATIENT AND CARER ADVICE**
  Medicines for Children leaflet: Mebendazole for worm infections www.medicinesforchildren.org.uk/medicines/mebendazole-for-worm-infections/
- **EXCEPTIONS TO LEGAL CATEGORY** Mebendazole tablets can be sold to the public if supplied for oral use in the treatment of enterobiasis in adults and children over 2 years provided its container or package is labelled to show a max. single dose of 100 mg and it is supplied in a container or package containing not more than 800 mg.

- **MEDICINAL FORMS** There can be variation in the licensing of different medicines containing the same drug.

Oral suspension

▸ Vermox (Janssen-Cilag Ltd)

Mebendazole 20 mg per 1 ml Vermox 100mg/5ml oral suspension | 30 ml PoM £1.55 DT = £1.55

Chewable tablet

▸ Vermox (Janssen-Cilag Ltd)

Mebendazole 100 mg Vermox 100mg chewable tablets | 6 tablet PoM £1.34 DT = £1.34 SF

Praziquantel

- **INDICATIONS AND DOSE**

Tapeworm infections (*Taenia solium*)

▶ BY MOUTH

- ▸ Child 4–17 years: 5–10 mg/kg for 1 dose, to be taken after a light breakfast

Tapeworm infections (*Hymenolepis nana*)

▶ BY MOUTH

- ▸ Child 4–17 years: 25 mg/kg for 1 dose, to be taken after a light breakfast

***Schistosoma haematobium* worm infections | *Schistosoma mansoni* worm infections**

▶ BY MOUTH

- ▸ Child 4–17 years: 20 mg/kg, followed by 20 mg/kg after 4–6 hours

***Schistosoma japonicum* worm infections**

▶ BY MOUTH

- ▸ Child 4–17 years: 20 mg/kg 3 times a day for 1 day

- **UNLICENSED USE** Praziquantel is an unlicensed drug.
- **INTERACTIONS** → Appendix 1: praziquantel

- **MEDICINAL FORMS** There can be variation in the licensing of different medicines containing the same drug. Forms available from special-order manufacturers include: oral tablet

Oral tablet

▸ Praziquantel (Non-proprietary)

Praziquantel 150 mg Cesol 150mg tablets | 6 tablet PoM ☒

Praziquantel 600 mg Biltricide 600mg tablets | 6 tablet PoM ☒

4 Protozoal infection

Antiprotozoal drugs

31-Jan-2025

Amoebicides

Metronidazole p. 409 is the drug of choice for *acute invasive amoebic dysentery* since it is very effective against vegetative forms of *Entamoeba histolytica* in ulcers. Tinidazole is also effective. Metronidazole and tinidazole are also active against amoebae which may have migrated to the liver. Treatment with metronidazole (or tinidazole) is followed by a 10-day course of diloxanide furoate.

Diloxanide furoate is the drug of choice for asymptomatic patients with *E. histolytica* cysts in the faeces; metronidazole and tinidazole are relatively ineffective. Diloxanide furoate is relatively free from toxic effects and the usual course is of 10 days, given alone for chronic infections or following metronidazole or tinidazole treatment.

For *amoebic abscesses* of the liver metronidazole is effective; tinidazole is an alternative. Aspiration of the abscess is indicated where it is suspected that it may rupture or where there is no improvement after 72 hours of metronidazole; the aspiration may need to be repeated. Aspiration aids penetration of metronidazole and, for abscesses with large volumes of pus, if carried out in conjunction with drug therapy, may reduce the period of disability.

Diloxanide furoate is not effective against hepatic amoebiasis, but a 10-day course should be given at the completion of metronidazole or tinidazole treatment to destroy any amoebae in the gut.

Trichomonacides

Metronidazole is the treatment of choice for *Trichomonas vaginalis* infection. Contact tracing is recommended and sexual contacts should be treated simultaneously. If metronidazole is ineffective, tinidazole may be tried.

Antigiardial drugs

Metronidazole is the treatment of choice for *Giardia lamblia* infections. Tinidazole may be used as an alternative to metronidazole.

Leishmaniacides

Cutaneous leishmaniasis frequently heals spontaneously but if skin lesions are extensive or unsightly, treatment is indicated, as it is in visceral leishmaniasis (kala-azar). Leishmaniasis should be treated under specialist supervision.

Sodium stibogluconate, an organic pentavalent antimony compound, is used for visceral leishmaniasis. The dosage varies with different geographical regions and expert advice should be obtained. Skin lesions can also be treated with sodium stibogluconate.

Amphotericin B p. 462 is used with or after an antimony compound for visceral leishmaniasis unresponsive to the antimonial alone; side-effects may be reduced by using liposomal amphotericin B.

Pentamidine isetionate p. 472 (pentamidine isethionate) has been used in antimony-resistant visceral leishmaniasis, but although the initial response is often good, the relapse rate is high; it is associated with serious side-effects. Other treatments include paromomycin [unlicensed] (available from 'special-order' manufacturers or specialist importing companies).

Trypanocides

The prophylaxis and treatment of trypanosomiasis is difficult and differs according to the strain of organism. Expert advice should therefore be obtained.

Toxoplasmosis

Most infections caused by *Toxoplasma gondii* are self-limiting, and treatment is not necessary. Exceptions are patients with eye involvement (toxoplasma choroidoretinitis), and those who are immunosuppressed. Toxoplasmic encephalitis is a common complication of AIDS. The treatment of choice is a combination of pyrimethamine p. 490 and sulfadiazine p. 432, given for several weeks (expert advice **essential**). Pyrimethamine is a folate antagonist, and adverse reactions to this combination are relatively common (folinic acid supplements and weekly blood counts needed). Alternative regimens use combinations of pyrimethamine with clindamycin p. 400 or clarithromycin p. 403 or azithromycin p. 402. Long-term secondary prophylaxis is required after treatment of toxoplasmosis in immunocompromised patients; prophylaxis should continue until immunity recovers.

If toxoplasmosis is acquired in pregnancy, transplacental infection may lead to severe disease in the fetus; specialist advice should be sought on management. Spiramycin [unlicensed] (available from 'special-order' manufacturers or specialist importing companies) may reduce the risk of transmission of maternal infection to the fetus. When there is evidence of placental or fetal infection, pyrimethamine may be given with sulfadiazine and folinic acid p. 683 after the first trimester.

In neonates without signs of toxoplasmosis, but born to mothers known to have become infected, spiramycin is given while awaiting laboratory results. If toxoplasmosis is confirmed in the infant, pyrimethamine and sulfadiazine are given for 12 months, together with folinic acid.

4.1 Malaria

Malaria, prophylaxis

14-Aug-2025

Prophylaxis against malaria

The recommendations on prophylaxis reflect guidelines agreed by the UK Malaria Expert Advisory Group (UKMEAG), published in the UKHSA Guidelines for malaria prevention in travellers from the UK, 2024. The advice is aimed at residents of the UK who travel to malaria-endemic areas.

For specialist centres offering advice on specific malaria-related problems, see Malaria, treatment p. 482.

The choice of drug for a particular individual should take into account:

- risk of exposure to malaria
- extent of drug resistance
- efficacy of the recommended drugs
- side-effects of the drugs
- patient-related factors (e.g. age, pregnancy, renal or hepatic impairment, compliance with prophylactic regimen)

Prophylactic doses are based on guidelines agreed by UK malaria experts and may differ from advice in the product literature. **Weight is a better guide than age**. If in doubt obtain advice from a specialist centre, see Malaria, treatment p. 482.

Key to recommended regimens for prophylaxis against malaria

Codes for regimens	Details of regimens for prophylaxis against malaria
-	No risk
1	Chemoprophylaxis not recommended, but avoid mosquito bites and consider malaria if fever presents
2	Chloroquine only
3	Chloroquine or atovaquone with proguanil hydrochloride or doxycycline or mefloquine
4	Atovaquone with proguanil hydrochloride or doxycycline or mefloquine
5	Atovaquone with proguanil hydrochloride or doxycycline

Specific recommendations

Country	Comments on risk of malaria and regional or seasonal variation	Codes for regimens
Afghanistan	Low risk below 2000 m from May–November	1
	Very low risk below 2000 m from December–April	1
Andaman and Nicobar Islands (India)	Low risk	1
Angola	High risk	4
Argentina	No risk	1
Azerbaijan	No risk	1
Bangladesh	High risk in Chittagong Hill Tract districts (but not Chittagong city)	4
	Very low risk in Chittagong city and other areas, except Chittagong Hill Tract districts	1
Belize	No risk	1
Benin	High risk	4
Bhutan	Low risk in southern belt districts, along border with India: Chukha, Geyleg-phug, Samchi, Samdrup Jonkhar, and Shemgang	1
	No risk in areas other than those above	-
Bolivia	Low risk in Amazon basin	1
	Low risk in rural areas below 2500 m (other than above)	1
	No risk above 2500 m	-
Botswana	High risk from November–June in northern half, including Okavango Delta area	4
	Low risk from July–October in northern half, including Okavango Delta area	1
	Very low risk in southern half	1
Brazil	Low risk in Amazon basin, including city of Manaus	1
	Very low risk in areas other than those above	1
	No risk in Iguaçu Falls	-
Brunei Darussalam	Very low risk	1
Burkina Faso	High risk	4
Burundi	High risk	4
Cambodia	Low risk. Mefloquine resistance widespread in western provinces bordering Thailand	1
	Very low risk in Angkor Wat and Lake Tonle Sap, including Siem Reap	1
	No risk in Phnom Penh	-
Cameroon	High risk	4
Cape Verde	No risk	1
Central African Republic	High risk	4
Chad	High risk	4
China	No risk	1
	No risk in Hong Kong	-
Colombia	Low risk in rural areas below 1600 m	1
	Very low risk above 1600 m and in Cartagena	1
Comoros	High risk	4
Congo	High risk	4
Costa Rica	Low risk in Limon province, but not city of Limon (Puerto Limon)	1
	Very low risk in areas other than those above	1

Country	Comments on risk of malaria and regional or seasonal variation	Codes for regimens
Cote d'Ivoire (Ivory Coast)	High risk	4
Democratic Republic of the Congo	High risk	4
Djibouti	High risk	4
Dominican Republic	Low risk	1
	No risk in cities of Santiago and Santo Domingo	-
East Timor (Timor-Leste)	Very low risk	1
Ecuador	Low risk in areas below 1500 m including coastal provinces and Amazon basin	1
	No risk in Galapagos islands or city of Guayaquil	-
Egypt	No risk	1
El Salvador	No risk	1
Equatorial Guinea	High risk	4
Eritrea	High risk below 2200 m	4
	No risk in Asmara or in areas above 2200 m	-
Eswatini	Risk present in the northern and eastern regions bordering Mozambique and South Africa, including all the Lubombo district and Big Bend, Mhlume, Simunye, and Tshaneni regions	4
	Very low risk in areas other than those above	1
Ethiopia	High risk below 2000 m	4
	No risk in Addis Ababa or in areas above 2000 m	-
French Guiana	Risk present (particularly in border areas)	4
	Low risk in city of Cayenne or Devil's Island (Ile du Diable)	1
Gabon	High risk	4
Gambia	High risk	4
Georgia	Very low risk from June-October in rural south east	1
	No risk from November-May in rural south east	-
Ghana	High risk	4
Guatemala	Low risk below 1500 m	1
	No risk in Guatemala City, Antigua, or Lake Atitlan, and in areas above 1500 m	-
Guinea	High risk	4
Guinea-Bissau	High risk	4
Guyana	Risk present in all interior regions	4
	Very low risk in Georgetown and coastal region	1
Haiti	Risk present	3
Honduras	Low risk below 1000 m and in Roatán and other Bay Islands	1
	No risk in San Pedro Sula and Tegucigalpa and areas above 1000 m	-
India	Risk present in states of Assam and Orissa, districts of East Godavari, Srikakulam, Vishakhapatnam, and Vizianagaram in the state of Andhra Pradesh, and districts of Balaghat, Dindori, Mandla, and Seoni in the state of Madhya Pradesh	4
	Low risk in areas other than those above or below (including Goa, Andaman and Nicobar islands)	1
	No risk in Lakshadweep islands	-
Indonesia	High risk in Irian Jaya (Papua)	4
	Low risk in Bali, Lombok, and islands of Java and Sumatra	1
	No risk in city of Jakarta	-
Indonesia (Borneo)	Low risk	1
Iran	Low risk from March-November in rural south eastern provinces and in north, along Azerbaijan border in Ardabil, and near Turkmenistan border in North Khorasan	1
	Very low risk in areas other than those above	1
Iraq	Very low risk from May-November in rural northern area below 1500 m	1
	No risk in areas other than those above	-
Kenya	High risk	4
	Very low risk in city of Nairobi and in the highlands above 2500 m	1
Lao People's Democratic Republic (Laos)	Low risk	1
	Very low risk in city of Vientiane	1

Key to recommended regimens for prophylaxis against malaria

Codes for regimens	Details of regimens for prophylaxis against malaria
-	No risk
1	Chemoprophylaxis not recommended, but avoid mosquito bites and consider malaria if fever presents
2	Chloroquine only
3	Chloroquine or atovaquone with proguanil hydrochloride or doxycycline or mefloquine
4	Atovaquone with proguanil hydrochloride or doxycycline or mefloquine
5	Atovaquone with proguanil hydrochloride or doxycycline

Specific recommendations

Country	Comments on risk of malaria and regional or seasonal variation	Codes for regimens
Liberia	High risk	4
Madagascar	High risk	4
Malawi	High risk	4
Malaysia	Low risk in mainland Malaysia	1
Malaysia (Borneo)	Low risk in inland areas of Sabah and in inland, forested areas of Sarawak	1
	Very low risk in areas other than those above, including coastal areas of Sabah and Sarawak	1
Mali	High risk	4
Mauritania	High risk all year in southern provinces, and from July-October in the northern provinces	4
	Low risk from November-June in the northern provinces	1
Mauritius	No risk	1
Mayotte	Low risk	1
Mexico	Very low risk	1
Mozambique	High risk	4
Myanmar	Risk present at altitudes below 1000 m and on the border area with Thailand	5
Namibia	High risk in regions of Caprivi Strip, Kavango, and Kunene river	4
	Very low risk in areas other than those above	1
Nepal	Low risk below 1500 m, including the Terai district	1
	No risk in city of Kathmandu and on typical Himalayan treks	-
Nicaragua	Low risk	1
	Very low risk in Managua	1
Niger	High risk	4
Nigeria	High risk	4
North Korea	Very low risk in some southern areas	1
Pakistan	Low risk below 2000 m	1
	Very low risk above 2000 m	1
Panama	Low risk east of Canal Zone	1
	Very low risk west of Canal Zone	1
	No risk in Panama City or Canal Zone itself	-
Papua New Guinea	High risk below 1800 m	4
	Very low risk above 1800 m	1
Peru	Low risk in Amazon basin along border with Brazil, particularly in Loreto province and in rural areas below 2000 m including the Amazon basin bordering Bolivia	1
	No risk in city of Lima and coastal region south of Chiclayo	-
Philippines	Low risk in rural areas below 600 m and on islands of Luzon, Mindanao, Mindoro, and Palawan	1
	No risk in cities or on islands of Boracay, Bohol, Catanduanes, Cebu, or Leyte	-
Rwanda	High risk	4
São Tomé and Principe	High risk	4

Country	Comments on risk of malaria and regional or seasonal variation	Codes for regimens
Saudi Arabia	Low risk in south-western provinces along border with Yemen, including below 2000 m in Asir province	1
	No risk in cities of Jeddah, Makkah (Mecca), Medina, Riyadh, and Ta'if, or above 2000 m in Asir province	-
Senegal	High risk	4
Sierra Leone	High risk	4
Singapore	No risk	1
Solomon Islands	High risk	4
Somalia	High risk	4
South Africa	Risk from September–May in low altitude areas of Mpumalanga and Limpopo, particularly those bordering Mozambique, Eswatini, and Zimbabwe, including Kruger National Park	4
	Low risk from September–May in north-east KwaZulu-Natal and in designated areas of Mpumalanga and Limpopo	1
	Very low risk all year in North West Province (adjacent to Molopo river) and Northern Cape Province (adjacent to Orange river); and from June–August in low altitude areas of Mpumalanga and Limpopo, particularly those bordering Mozambique, Eswatini, and Zimbabwe, including Kruger National Park	1
South Korea	Very low risk in northern areas, in Gangwon-do and Gyeonggi-do provinces, and Incheon city (towards Demilitarized Zone)	1
South Sudan	High risk	4
Sri Lanka	No risk	1
Sudan	Risk present in all areas including Khartoum	4
Suriname	Low risk	1
	No risk in city of Paramaribo	-
Syria	Very low risk in small, remote foci of El Hasakah; possibility of additional cases cannot be excluded as up-to-date data not available	1
Tajikistan	No risk	1
Tanzania	High risk below 1800 m; risk also present in Zanzibar	4
	No risk above 1800 m	-
Thailand	Mefloquine resistance present. Low risk in rural forested borders with Cambodia, Laos, and Myanmar	1
	Very low risk in areas other than those above, including Kanchanaburi (Kwai Bridge)	1
	No risk in cities of Bangkok, Chiang Mai, Chiang Rai, Koh Phangan, Koh Samui, and Pattaya	-
Togo	High risk	4
Turkey	Very low risk	1
Uganda	High risk	4
Uzbekistan	No risk	1
Vanuatu	Risk present	4
Venezuela	Risk present (particularly in the Amazonas, Bolívar, Delta Amacuro, and Sucre states)	4
	No risk in city of Caracas or on Margarita Island	1
Vietnam	Low risk in rural areas, and in southern provinces of Tay Ninh, Lam Dong, Dak Lak, Gia Lai, and Kon Tum	1
	No risk in large cities (including Ho Chi Minh City (Saigon) and Hanoi), the Red River delta, coastal areas north of Nha Trang, and Phu Quoc Island	1
Western Sahara	No risk	1
Yemen	Risk present below 2000 m	4
	Very low risk on Socrota Island	1
	No risk above 2000 m, including Sana'a city	1
Zambia	High risk	4
Zimbabwe	High risk all year in Zambezi valley, and from November–June in areas below 1200 m	4
	Low risk from July–October in areas below 1200 m	1
	Very low risk all year in Harare and Bulawayo	1

For guidance on risk assessment when advising on malaria prevention, see UKHSA: **Guidelines for malaria prevention in travellers from the UK** (see *Useful resources*).

Protection against bites

Prophylaxis is not absolute, and breakthrough infection can occur with any of the drugs recommended. Personal protection against being bitten is very important and is recommended even in malaria-free areas as a preventive measure against other insect vector-borne diseases. Mosquito bed nets impregnated with a pyrethroid insecticide (such as permethrin p. 904) improve protection and should be used unless sleeping in a well screened room with mosquito netting on windows and doors, or a room with switched on functioning air conditioning that is also sufficiently well sealed, into which mosquitoes cannot enter. The use of plug-in vaporised insecticides are also useful. Long-sleeved clothing, long trousers, and socks also provide protection against bites; clothing may be sprayed or impregnated with an insecticide such as permethrin.

Insect repellents give protection against bites, but attention to the correct application of the product is required. They should only be applied to exposed areas of skin, although some preparations can be sprayed onto clothing. A repellent should still be applied to exposed skin even if clothing has been sprayed or impregnated.

Diethyltoluamide (DEET) is available in various preparations including sprays and modified-release formulations. A 50% DEET-based insect repellent is recommended as the first choice; there is no further increase in duration of protection beyond a DEET concentration of 50%. DEET is safe and effective when applied to the skin of children over 2 months of age. It can be used during pregnancy and breast-feeding, however, ingestion should be avoided and so breast-feeding mothers should wash their hands and breast tissue before handling infants. DEET can be sprayed onto clothing, but it may damage synthetic fibres. When sunscreen is also required, DEET should be applied after the sunscreen. DEET reduces the SPF of sunscreen, so a sunscreen of SPF 30–50 should be applied. For alternative options if DEET is not tolerated or is unavailable, see UKHSA: **Guidelines for malaria prevention in travellers from the UK** (see *Useful resources*).

Length of prophylaxis

Prophylaxis should generally be started before travel into an endemic area; 1 week before travel for chloroquine p. 485; 2–3 weeks before travel for mefloquine p. 486; and 1–2 days before travel for doxycycline p. 434 (children aged 12 years and over) or atovaquone with proguanil hydrochloride p. 484. Prophylaxis should be continued for 4 weeks after leaving the area (except for atovaquone with proguanil hydrochloride prophylaxis which should be stopped 1 week after leaving). For extensive journeys across different regions, the traveller must be protected in all areas of risk.

In those requiring long-term prophylaxis, chloroquine may be used, however there is considerable concern over the protective efficacy of chloroquine in certain areas where it was previously useful. Mefloquine is licensed for use up to 1 year (although, if it is tolerated in the short term, there is no evidence of harm when it is used for up to 3 years). Doxycycline (children aged 12 years and over) can be used for up to 2 years, and atovaquone with proguanil hydrochloride for up to 1 year. Prophylaxis with mefloquine, doxycycline, or atovaquone with proguanil hydrochloride may be considered for longer durations if it is justified by the risk of exposure to malaria. Specialist advice may be sought for long-term prophylaxis.

Return from malarial region

It is important to consider that any illness that occurs within 1 year and especially within 3 months of return, might be malaria, even if all recommended precautions against malaria were taken. Children and their parents/carers should be warned of this and told that if they develop any illness after their return they should see a doctor early, and specifically mention their risk of exposure to malaria.

Malaria is a notifiable disease in England, Northern Ireland, and Wales. For further information, see *Notifiable diseases* in Antibacterials, principles of therapy p. 358.

Epilepsy

Both chloroquine and mefloquine are unsuitable for malaria prophylaxis in children with a history of epilepsy. In these patients, doxycycline (children aged 12 years and over) or atovaquone with proguanil hydrochloride may be used. However doxycycline may interact with some antiepileptics and its dose may need to be adjusted, see *interactions* information in the doxycycline drug monograph.

Asplenia

Children with asplenia (or those with severe splenic dysfunction) are at particular risk of severe malaria and should avoid travel to malarious areas where possible; if travel to malarious areas is unavoidable, rigorous precautions are required against contracting the disease.

Pregnancy

Travel to malarious areas should be avoided during pregnancy; if travel is unavoidable, pregnant individuals must be informed about the risks and benefits of effective prophylaxis. Chloroquine can be given during all trimesters of pregnancy, but is not appropriate for most areas because its effectiveness has declined due to drug resistance. If travelling to high-risk areas or there is resistance to other drugs, mefloquine may be considered during the second or third trimester of pregnancy. Mefloquine can be used in the first trimester with caution if the benefits outweigh the risks. Doxycycline is contra-indicated during pregnancy, however it can be used for malaria prophylaxis if other regimens are unsuitable and if the entire course of doxycycline can be completed before 15 weeks' gestation [unlicensed]. Atovaquone with proguanil hydrochloride should be avoided during pregnancy, however it can be considered during the second and third trimesters if there is no suitable alternative. Folic acid p. 710 (dosed as a pregnancy at 'high-risk' of neural tube defects) should be given for the length of time that atovaquone with proguanil hydrochloride is used during pregnancy, and in those planning on becoming pregnant.

Breast-feeding

Chloroquine p. 485 and mefloquine p. 486 are considered safe for use during breast-feeding. Atovaquone with proguanil hydrochloride p. 484 and doxycycline p. 434 should generally be avoided but can be used if other antimalarial options are unsuitable.

Prophylaxis is required in breast-fed infants; although antimalarials are present in breast milk, the amounts are too low to give reliable protection.

Anticoagulants

Children taking warfarin sodium should begin chemoprophylaxis 2–3 weeks before departure and the INR should be stable before departure. It should be measured before starting chemoprophylaxis, 7 days after starting, and after completing the course. For prolonged stays, the INR should be checked at regular intervals.

Some antimalarials may alter the anticoagulant effect of warfarin, see *Interactions* in individual drug monographs for information.

Other medical conditions

For additional information on malaria prophylaxis in children with other medical conditions, see UKHSA: **Guidelines for malaria prevention in travellers from the UK** (see *Useful resources*). Patients already taking hydroxychloroquine sulfate p. 798 for another indication, and for whom chloroquine would be an appropriate antimalarial, can remain on hydroxychloroquine sulfate.

Emergency standby treatment

Children and their parents/carers on prophylaxis who are visiting remote, malarious areas should carry standby emergency treatment if they are likely to be more than 24 hours away from medical care. Standby emergency treatment should also be considered in long-term travellers living in or visiting remote, malarious areas that may be far from appropriate medical attention; this does not replace the need to consider prophylaxis. Self-medication should be **avoided** if medical help is accessible.

In order to use standby treatment appropriately, children and their parents/carers should be provided with written instructions which include seeking urgent medical attention if fever (38°C or more) develops more than 7 days after arriving in a malarious area, and that self-treatment is indicated if medical help is not available within 24 hours of fever onset.

In view of the continuing emergence of resistant strains and of the different regimens required for different areas, expert advice should be sought on the best treatment course for an individual traveller. A drug used for chemoprophylaxis should not be considered for standby treatment for the same traveller due to concerns over drug resistance and to minimise drug toxicity.

Malaria prophylaxis, specific recommendations

Travellers planning journeys across continents can travel into areas that have different malaria prophylaxis recommendations. The choice of prophylaxis medication must reflect overall risk to ensure protection in all areas; it may be possible to change from one regimen to another. Those travelling to remote or little-visited areas may require expert advice. For further information, see *Recommended regimens for prophylaxis against malaria*, and UKHSA: **Guidelines for malaria prevention in travellers from the UK** (see *Useful resources*).

Some countries not listed in *Recommended regimens for prophylaxis against malaria* may experience occasional instances of malaria transmission. For further guidance, see the National Travel Health Network and Centre (nathnac.net/).

Important

Settled immigrants (or long-term visitors) in the UK may be unaware that any immunity they may have acquired while living in malarious areas is lost rapidly after migration to the UK, or that any non-malarious areas where they lived previously may now be malarious.

Useful resources

UK Health Security Agency: Guidelines for malaria prevention in travellers from the UK. July 2024.
www.gov.uk/government/publications/malaria-prevention-guidelines-for-travellers-from-the-uk

Malaria, treatment

28-Jan-2026

Advice for healthcare professionals

A number of specialist centres are able to provide advice on specific problems.

UKHSA Malaria Reference Laboratory (prophylaxis) www.gov.uk/government/collections/malaria-reference-laboratory-mrl

National Travel Health Network and Centre (NaTHNaC) www.travelhealthpro.org.uk/

Hospital for Tropical Diseases (HTD) (treatment) www.uclh.nhs.uk/our-services/find-service/tropical-and-infectious-diseases/htd-guidelines

Liverpool School of Tropical Medicine (LSTM) (treatment) 0151 705 3100 Monday to Friday: 9 a.m.–5 p.m. and via Royal Liverpool Hospital switchboard at all other times 0151 706 2000 www.lstmed.ac.uk/

Birmingham Infectious Diseases and Tropical Medicine 0121 424 2358

Advice for travellers

Hospital for Tropical Diseases travel clinic www.uclh.nhs.uk/our-services/find-service/tropical-and-infectious-diseases/travel-clinic-services

WHO advice on international travel and health www.who.int/travel-advice

National Travel Health Network and Centre (NaTHNaC) www.travelhealthpro.org.uk/

Treatment of malaria

Malaria is a notifiable disease in England, Northern Ireland, and Wales. For further information, see *Notifiable diseases* in Antibacterials, principles of therapy p. 358.

The recommendations on treatment reflect UK malaria treatment guidelines 2016, agreed by the UK Malaria Expert Advisory Group (see *Useful resources*). They are aimed for residents of the UK and for use in a non-endemic setting. Choice will depend on the age of the child.

Expert advice must be sought in all children suspected to have malaria. If malaria is diagnosed in a returned traveller, other members of the family or travelling group should be advised that they may have shared the same exposure risk and they should seek medical attention if they develop symptoms.

If the infective species is **not known**, or if the infection is **mixed** and includes falciparum parasites, initial treatment should be as for *falciparum malaria*.

Falciparum malaria

Falciparum malaria is caused by *Plasmodium falciparum*. Children with falciparum malaria should be observed in hospital initially for at least 24 hours due to the possibility of rapid progression and also to ensure that they are tolerating oral treatment.

Artemisinin combination therapy (artemether with lumefantrine p. 483, or piperaquine phosphate with artenimol p. 487 [unlicensed (available as *Eurartesim*®)]) is recommended as first-line treatment of uncomplicated *P. falciparum* malaria. Oral quinine p. 488 is an alternative if artemisinin combination therapy is not suitable. Quinine is highly effective but poorly-tolerated in prolonged treatment and should be used in combination with an additional drug, usually oral doxycycline p. 434 (or clindamycin p. 400 [unlicensed use] in pregnant females and young children). Atovaquone with proguanil hydrochloride p. 484 can also be used for the treatment of uncomplicated malaria in children.

Severe or complicated falciparum malaria in children should be managed in a high dependency unit or paediatric intensive care with advice from a specialist. Intravenous artesunate p. 484 is the preferred treatment over intravenous quinine [unlicensed]. A full course of oral treatment (such as artemisinin combination therapy) should be given following a minimum of 24 hours of intravenous artesunate treatment, and when the child has improved and is able to take oral treatment.

However, treatment should not be delayed whilst obtaining artesunate. Quinine by intravenous infusion [unlicensed] should be given if artesunate is not immediately available; it should be continued until the child can take an oral antimalarial treatment (such as an artemisinin combination therapy, oral quinine with doxycycline (or clindamycin [unlicensed use]), or atovaquone with proguanil hydrochloride).

In most parts of the world, *P. falciparum* is now resistant to chloroquine which should therefore not be used for treatment. Mefloquine is also no longer recommended for treatment because of concerns about adverse effects and non-completion of courses. Reduced sensitivity to artemisinin combination therapies has been observed in some African countries and the Greater Mekong Subregion, resulting in late treatment failure (recrudescence). Specialist advice should be sought when managing a second episode of falciparum malaria without intervening travel to a malaria-endemic country (presumed recrudescence). For further guidance, see UKHSA guidance: **Management of treatment failure (recrudescence) in falciparum malaria** (available at: www.gov.uk/government/publications/management-of-treatment-failure-recrudescence-in-falciparum-malaria).

Pregnancy

Falciparum malaria in pregnancy carries a higher risk of severe disease; it requires prompt treatment by specialists in hospital and close observation. Uncomplicated falciparum malaria in the second and third trimesters of pregnancy should be treated with artemether with lumefantrine; if unsuitable, piperaquine phosphate with artenimol [unlicensed] can be used. Quinine with clindamycin [unlicensed use] can be used in all trimesters. Quinine can increase the risk of uterine contractions and hypoglycaemia.

Severe or complicated falciparum malaria is associated with a high risk of fatality, pregnancy loss, and complications. Due to efficacy, treatment with intravenous artesunate in any trimester of pregnancy is preferred; intravenous quinine [unlicensed] (with clindamycin [unlicensed use]) can be used as an alternative.

Non-falciparum malaria

Non-falciparum malaria is usually caused by *Plasmodium vivax* and less commonly by *P. ovale*, *P. malariae*, and *P. knowlesi*. *P. knowlesi* is present in the Asia-Pacific region.

Either an artemisinin combination therapy (artemether with lumefantrine below [unlicensed use] or piperaquine phosphate with artenimol [unlicensed (available as *Eurartesim*®)]), or chloroquine p. 485 can be used for the treatment of non-falciparum malaria. Chloroquine-resistant *P. vivax* has been reported in the Indonesian archipelago, the Malay Peninsula, including Myanmar, and eastward to Southern Vietnam. Chloroquine can still be used for treatment of non-falciparum malaria from these regions with appropriate follow-up, however artemisinin combination therapy may be preferred.

Chloroquine alone is adequate for *P. malariae* and *P. knowlesi* infections but in the case of *P. vivax* and *P. ovale*, a *radical cure* (to destroy parasites in the liver and thus prevent relapses) is required. For a radical cure, primaquine p. 488 [unlicensed] is given with chloroquine treatment; the dose is dependent on the infecting organism. Patients should be screened for G6PD deficiency before primaquine treatment, as primaquine may cause haemolysis in G6PD deficient individuals.

Severe or complicated non-falciparum malaria in children should be treated with intravenous artesunate or quinine [unlicensed] as for treatment of severe or complicated falciparum malaria.

Pregnancy

Chloroquine can be given for non-falciparum malaria treatment throughout pregnancy. An artemisinin combination therapy (either artemether with lumefantrine [unlicensed use] or piperaquine phosphate with artenimol [unlicensed]) can be used in the second and third trimesters, and quinine may be used in the first trimester if there is concern about chloroquine-resistant *P. vivax*. In the case of *P. vivax* or *P. ovale* however, the radical cure with primaquine [unlicensed] should be **postponed** until the pregnancy (and breast-feeding) is over; instead weekly chloroquine prophylaxis should be continued until delivery or completion of breast-feeding.

Useful resources

UK malaria treatment guidelines. UK Malaria Expert Advisory Group (formerly known as the Advisory Committee on Malaria Prevention). February 2016.

www.gov.uk/government/collections/uk-malaria-expert-advisory-group

ANTIPROTOZOALS › ANTIMALARIALS

Artemether with lumefantrine

02-Jun-2025

● **INDICATIONS AND DOSE**

Treatment of acute uncomplicated falciparum malaria | Treatment of chloroquine-resistant non-falciparum malaria

▶ BY MOUTH

- Child (body-weight 5–14 kg): 1 tablet for 6 doses, to be given at 0, 8, 24, 36, 48, and 60 hours (total 6 tablets over 60 hours)
- Child (body-weight 15–24 kg): 2 tablets for 6 doses, to be given at 0, 8, 24, 36, 48, and 60 hours (total 12 tablets over 60 hours)
- Child (body-weight 25–34 kg): 3 tablets for 6 doses, to be given at 0, 8, 24, 36, 48, and 60 hours (total 18 tablets over 60 hours)
- Child (body-weight 35 kg and above): 4 tablets for 6 doses, to be given at 0, 8, 24, 36, 48, and 60 hours (total 24 tablets over 60 hours)

● **UNLICENSED USE** Use in treatment of non-falciparum malaria is an unlicensed indication.

● **CONTRA-INDICATIONS** Family history of congenital QT interval prolongation · family history of sudden death · history of arrhythmias · history of clinically relevant bradycardia · history of congestive heart failure accompanied by reduced left ventricular ejection fraction

● **CAUTIONS** Avoid in Acute porphyrias p. 745 · electrolyte disturbances (correct before and during treatment)

● **INTERACTIONS** → Appendix 1: antimalarials

● **SIDE-EFFECTS**

▶ **Common or very common** Abdominal pain · appetite decreased · arthralgia · asthenia · cough · diarrhoea · dizziness · headache · myalgia · nausea · palpitations · QT interval prolongation · skin reactions · sleep disorders · vomiting

▶ **Uncommon** Clonus · drowsiness

▶ **Frequency not known** Angioedema

● **PREGNANCY** Toxicity in *animal* studies with artemether. Manufacturer advises use only if potential benefit outweighs risk.

● **BREAST FEEDING** Manufacturer advises avoid breastfeeding for at least 1 week after last dose. Present in milk in *animal* studies.

● **HEPATIC IMPAIRMENT** Manufacturer advises caution in severe impairment (no information available)—monitor ECG and plasma potassium concentration.

● **RENAL IMPAIRMENT** EvGr Caution in severe impairment (limited information available)—monitor ECG and plasma potassium concentration. (M)

● **MONITORING REQUIREMENTS** Monitor patients unable to take food (greater risk of recrudescence).

● **DIRECTIONS FOR ADMINISTRATION** Manufacturer advises tablets may be crushed just before administration.

● **PATIENT AND CARER ADVICE**

Driving and skilled tasks Dizziness may affect performance of skilled tasks (e.g. driving).

● **MEDICINAL FORMS** There can be variation in the licensing of different medicines containing the same drug.

Oral tablet

CAUTIONARY AND ADVISORY LABELS 21

▶ **Riamet** (Novartis Pharmaceuticals UK Ltd)

Artemether 20 mg, Lumefantrine 120 mg Riamet tablets | 24 tablet PoM £22.50 DT = £22.50

Artesunate
16-Jan-2025

● **INDICATIONS AND DOSE**

Severe malaria (under expert supervision)

▶ BY INTRAVENOUS INJECTION

▸ Neonate: 3 mg/kg every 12 hours for 3 doses, to be given at 0, 12, and 24 hours, if patient is unable to switch to oral antimalarial treatment after initial 3 doses, continue to give every 24 hours until they are able to do so. If intravenous treatment is required for more than 7 days, consult an infectious disease specialist.

▸ Child (body-weight up to 20 kg): 3 mg/kg every 12 hours for 3 doses, to be given at 0, 12, and 24 hours, if patient is unable to switch to oral antimalarial treatment after initial 3 doses, continue to give every 24 hours until they are able to do so. If intravenous treatment is required for more than 7 days, consult an infectious disease specialist

▸ Child (body-weight 20 kg and above): 2.4 mg/kg every 12 hours for 3 doses, to be given at 0, 12, and 24 hours, if patient is unable to switch to oral antimalarial treatment after initial 3 doses, continue to give every 24 hours until they are able to do so. If intravenous treatment is required for more than 7 days, consult an infectious disease specialist

● **INTERACTIONS** → Appendix 1: antimalarials

● **SIDE-EFFECTS**

▶ **Common or very common** Abdominal pain · acute kidney injury · anaemia · bradycardia · cough · diarrhoea · dizziness · fever · haemoglobinuria · haemolysis (delayed) · headache · hyperbilirubinaemia · hypotension · jaundice · reticulocytopenia · rhinitis · taste altered · vomiting

▶ **Uncommon** Appetite decreased · constipation · fatigue · flushing · nausea · skin reactions · Stevens-Johnson syndrome

● **PREGNANCY** Specialist sources indicate benefit to the mother outweighs potential risk to the unborn child (limited information available). See also *Pregnancy* in Malaria, treatment p. 482.

● **BREAST FEEDING** Specialist sources indicate present in milk but not known to be harmful.

● **MONITORING REQUIREMENTS** EvGr Monitor for haemolytic anaemia for 4 weeks after starting treatment (risk of post-artesunate delayed haemolysis, particularly in younger children and those with hyperparasitaemia). (M)

● **MEDICINAL FORMS** There can be variation in the licensing of different medicines containing the same drug.

Powder and solvent for solution for injection

▸ Artesunate (non-proprietary) ▼

Artesunate 60 mg Artesun 60mg powder and solvent for solution for injection vials | 1 vial PoM (Hospital only)

Artesunate 110 mg Artesunate 110mg powder and solvent for solution for injection vials | 2 vial PoM £1,750.00 (Hospital only)

Atovaquone with proguanil hydrochloride
18-Apr-2025

● **INDICATIONS AND DOSE**

Prophylaxis of falciparum malaria, particularly where resistance to other antimalarial drugs suspected [using 250 mg/100 mg tablets]

▶ BY MOUTH

▸ Child (body-weight 40 kg and above): 1 tablet once daily, to be started 1–2 days before entering endemic area and continued for 1 week after leaving

Prophylaxis of falciparum malaria, particularly where resistance to other antimalarial drugs suspected [using 62.5 mg/25 mg tablets]

▶ BY MOUTH

▸ Child (body-weight 5–7 kg): 0.5 tablet once daily, to be started 1–2 days before entering endemic area and continued for 1 week after leaving

▸ Child (body-weight 8–9 kg): 0.75 tablet once daily, to be started 1–2 days before entering endemic area and continued for 1 week after leaving

▸ Child (body-weight 10–19 kg): 1 tablet once daily, to be started 1–2 days before entering endemic area and continued for 1 week after leaving

▸ Child (body-weight 20–29 kg): 2 tablets once daily, to be started 1–2 days before entering endemic area and continued for 1 week after leaving

▸ Child (body-weight 30–39 kg): 3 tablets once daily, to be started 1–2 days before entering endemic area and continued for 1 week after leaving

▸ Child (body-weight 40 kg and above): Use 250 mg/100 mg tablets

Treatment of acute uncomplicated falciparum malaria [using 250 mg/100 mg tablets] | Treatment of non-falciparum malaria [using 250 mg/100 mg tablets]

▶ BY MOUTH

▸ Child (body-weight 11–20 kg): 1 tablet once daily for 3 days

▸ Child (body-weight 21–30 kg): 2 tablets once daily for 3 days

▸ Child (body-weight 31–40 kg): 3 tablets once daily for 3 days

▸ Child (body-weight 41 kg and above): 4 tablets once daily for 3 days

Treatment of acute uncomplicated falciparum malaria [using 62.5 mg/25 mg tablets] | Treatment of non-falciparum malaria [using 62.5 mg/25 mg tablets]

▶ BY MOUTH

▸ Child (body-weight 5–8 kg): 2 tablets once daily for 3 days

▸ Child (body-weight 9–10 kg): 3 tablets once daily for 3 days

▸ Child (body-weight 11 kg and above): Use 250 mg/100 mg tablets

DOSE EQUIVALENCE AND CONVERSION

▸ Each 250 mg/100 mg tablet contains 250 mg of atovaquone and 100 mg of proguanil hydrochloride.

▸ Each 62.5 mg/25 mg tablet contains 62.5 mg of atovaquone and 25 mg of proguanil hydrochloride.

● **UNLICENSED USE** Not licensed for treatment of non-falciparum malaria. Not licensed for prophylaxis of malaria in children under 11 kg.

Dosing for prophylaxis of malaria differs from product literature and adheres to Public Health England guidelines.

● **CAUTIONS** Diarrhoea or vomiting (reduced absorption of atovaquone) · efficacy not evaluated in cerebral or complicated malaria (including hyperparasitaemia, pulmonary oedema or renal failure)

● **INTERACTIONS** → Appendix 1: antimalarials

● **SIDE-EFFECTS**

▶ **Common or very common** Abdominal pain · appetite decreased · cough · depression · diarrhoea · dizziness · fever · headache · nausea · skin reactions · sleep disorders · vomiting

▶ **Uncommon** Alopecia · anxiety · blood disorder · hyponatraemia · oral disorders · palpitations

▶ **Frequency not known** Hallucination · hepatic disorders · photosensitivity reaction · seizure · Stevens-Johnson syndrome · tachycardia · vasculitis

● **PREGNANCY**
- When used for Prophylaxis of malaria UKHSA advises avoid but may be considered during second and third trimesters if no suitable alternative available. See also *Pregnancy* in Malaria, prophylaxis p. 476.
- When used for Treatment of malaria EvGr Use only if potential benefit outweighs risk. (M)

● **BREAST FEEDING** Specialist sources indicate use only if no suitable alternative available.

● **RENAL IMPAIRMENT** EvGr Avoid for malaria prophylaxis (and if possible for malaria treatment) if creatinine clearance less than 30 mL/minute, (M) see p. 16.

● **DIRECTIONS FOR ADMINISTRATION** *Malarone paediatric®* tablets may be crushed and mixed with food or a milky drink just before administration.

● **PATIENT AND CARER ADVICE** Warn travellers about **importance** of avoiding mosquito bites, **importance** of taking prophylaxis regularly, and **importance** of immediate visit to doctor if ill within 1 year and **especially** within 3 months of return.
Medicines for Children leaflet: Malarone for prevention of malaria www.medicinesforchildren.org.uk/medicines/malarone-for-prevention-of-malaria/

● **NATIONAL FUNDING/ACCESS DECISIONS**
NHS restrictions Drugs for malaria prophylaxis are not prescribable in NHS primary care; health authorities may investigate circumstances under which antimalarials are prescribed.

● **MEDICINAL FORMS** There can be variation in the licensing of different medicines containing the same drug.

Oral tablet

CAUTIONARY AND ADVISORY LABELS 21
- **Atovaquone with proguanil hydrochloride (Non-proprietary)**
  Proguanil hydrochloride 25 mg, Atovaquone 62.5 mg Proguanil 25mg / Atovaquone 62.5mg tablets | 12 tablet PoM £6.26 DT = £6.26
  Proguanil hydrochloride 100 mg, Atovaquone 250 mg Proguanil 100mg / Atovaquone 250mg tablets | 12 tablet PoM £31.50 DT = £25.21
- **Malarone** (GlaxoSmithKline UK Ltd)
  Proguanil hydrochloride 25 mg, Atovaquone 62.5 mg Malarone Paediatric 62.5mg/25mg tablets | 12 tablet PoM £6.26 DT = £6.26
  Proguanil hydrochloride 100 mg, Atovaquone 250 mg Malarone 250mg/100mg tablets | 12 tablet PoM £25.21 DT = £25.21

Chloroquine

16-Apr-2025

● **INDICATIONS AND DOSE**

Prophylaxis of malaria

▶ BY MOUTH USING SYRUP
- Child (body-weight up to 4.5 kg): 25 mg once weekly, started 1 week before entering endemic area and continued for 4 weeks after leaving
- Child (body-weight 4.5–7 kg): 50 mg once weekly, started 1 week before entering endemic area and continued for 4 weeks after leaving
- Child (body-weight 8–10 kg): 75 mg once weekly, started 1 week before entering endemic area and continued for 4 weeks after leaving
- Child (body-weight 11–14 kg): 100 mg once weekly, started 1 week before entering endemic area and continued for 4 weeks after leaving
- Child (body-weight 15–16.4 kg): 125 mg once weekly, started 1 week before entering endemic area and continued for 4 weeks after leaving
- Child (body-weight 16.5–24 kg): 150 mg once weekly, started 1 week before entering endemic area and continued for 4 weeks after leaving
- Child (body-weight 25–44 kg): 225 mg once weekly, started 1 week before entering endemic area and continued for 4 weeks after leaving
- Child (body-weight 45 kg and above): 300 mg once weekly, started 1 week before entering endemic area and continued for 4 weeks after leaving

▶ BY MOUTH USING TABLETS
- Child (body-weight up to 6 kg): 38.75 mg once weekly, started 1 week before entering endemic area and continued for 4 weeks after leaving
- Child (body-weight 6–9 kg): 77.5 mg once weekly, started 1 week before entering endemic area and continued for 4 weeks after leaving
- Child (body-weight 10–15 kg): 116.25 mg once weekly, started 1 week before entering endemic area and continued for 4 weeks after leaving
- Child (body-weight 16–24 kg): 155 mg once weekly, started 1 week before entering endemic area and continued for 4 weeks after leaving
- Child (body-weight 25–44 kg): 232.5 mg once weekly, started 1 week before entering endemic area and continued for 4 weeks after leaving
- Child (body-weight 45 kg and above): 310 mg once weekly, started 1 week before entering endemic area and continued for 4 weeks after leaving

Treatment of non-falciparum malaria

▶ BY MOUTH
- Child: Initially 10 mg/kg (max. per dose 620 mg), then 5 mg/kg after 6–8 hours (max. per dose 310 mg), then 5 mg/kg daily (max. per dose 310 mg) for 2 days

***P. vivax* or *P. ovale* infection during pregnancy while radical cure is postponed**

▶ BY MOUTH
- Child: 10 mg/kg once weekly (max. per dose 310 mg)

DOSE EQUIVALENCE AND CONVERSION
- Doses expressed as chloroquine base.
- Each tablet contains 155 mg of chloroquine base (equivalent to 250 mg of chloroquine phosphate). Syrup contains 50 mg/5 mL of chloroquine base (equivalent to 80 mg/5 mL of chloroquine phosphate).

● **UNLICENSED USE** Chloroquine doses for the treatment and prophylaxis of malaria in BNF Publications may differ from those in product literature.

IMPORTANT SAFETY INFORMATION

MHRA/CHM ADVICE: HYDROXYCHLOROQUINE, CHLOROQUINE: INCREASED RISK OF CARDIOVASCULAR EVENTS WHEN USED WITH MACROLIDE ANTIBIOTICS; REMINDER OF PSYCHIATRIC REACTIONS (FEBRUARY 2022)

An observational study has shown that co-administration of azithromycin with hydroxychloroquine in patients with rheumatoid arthritis was associated with an increased risk of cardiovascular events (including angina or chest pain and heart failure) and mortality. Healthcare professionals are reminded to consider the benefits and risks of co-prescribing systemic macrolides with chloroquine because of its similar safety profile to hydroxychloroquine. If such use cannot be avoided, caution is recommended in patients with risk factors for cardiac events and they should be advised to seek urgent medical attention if any signs or symptoms develop.

A European safety review has reported that psychiatric reactions associated with chloroquine (including rare cases of suicidal behaviour) typically occurred within the first month of treatment; events have been reported in patients with no history of psychiatric disorders. Healthcare professionals are reminded to be vigilant for psychiatric reactions, and counsel patients and carers to seek medical advice if any new or worsening mental health symptoms develop.

● **CAUTIONS** Acute porphyrias p. 745 · diabetes (may lower blood glucose) · G6PD deficiency · long-term therapy (risk of retinopathy and cardiomyopathy) · may aggravate myasthenia gravis · may exacerbate psoriasis · neurological disorders, especially epilepsy (may lower seizure threshold)—avoid for prophylaxis of malaria if history of epilepsy · severe gastro-intestinal disorders

- **INTERACTIONS** → Appendix 1: antimalarials
- **SIDE-EFFECTS**
  - **Rare or very rare** Cardiomyopathy · hallucination · hepatitis
  - **Frequency not known** Abdominal pain · agranulocytosis · alopecia · anxiety · atrioventricular block · behaviour abnormal · bone marrow disorders · concentration impaired · confusion · corneal deposits · delusions · depression · diarrhoea · eye disorders · gastrointestinal disorder · headache · hearing impairment · hypoglycaemia · hypotension · interstitial lung disease · mania · movement disorders · myopathy · nausea · neuromyopathy · neutropenia · photosensitivity reaction · psychiatric disorder · psychosis · QT interval prolongation · seizure · severe cutaneous adverse reactions (SCARs) · skin reactions · sleep disorders · suicidal behaviour · thrombocytopenia · tinnitus · tongue protrusion · vision disorders · vomiting

SIDE-EFFECTS, FURTHER INFORMATION Side-effects which occur at doses used in the prophylaxis or treatment of malaria are generally not serious.

Overdose Chloroquine is very toxic in overdosage; overdosage is extremely hazardous and difficult to treat. Urgent advice from the National Poisons Information Service is essential. Life-threatening features include arrhythmias (which can have a very rapid onset) and convulsions (which can be intractable).

- **PREGNANCY**
  - When used for Prophylaxis of malaria or Treatment of malaria UKHSA advises can be used during all trimesters. See also *Pregnancy* in Malaria, prophylaxis p. 476 and Malaria, treatment p. 482.
- **BREAST FEEDING**
  - When used for Prophylaxis of malaria [EvGr] Present in milk but amount probably too small to be harmful. (M)
  - When used for Treatment of malaria PHE advises safe for use.
- **HEPATIC IMPAIRMENT** Manufacturer advises caution, particularly in cirrhosis.
- **RENAL IMPAIRMENT** Manufacturers advise caution.

  Dose adjustments Only partially excreted by the kidneys and reduction of the dose is not required for prophylaxis of malaria except in severe impairment.
- **MONITORING REQUIREMENTS** Expert sources advise ophthalmic examination with long-term therapy.
- **PATIENT AND CARER ADVICE** Warn travellers going to malarious areas about **importance** of avoiding mosquito bites, **importance** of taking prophylaxis regularly, and **importance** of immediate visit to doctor if ill within 1 year and **especially** within 3 months of return.
- **NATIONAL FUNDING/ACCESS DECISIONS**

  NHS restrictions Drugs for malaria prophylaxis are not prescribable in NHS primary care; health authorities may investigate circumstances under which antimalarials are prescribed.
- **EXCEPTIONS TO LEGAL CATEGORY** *Tablets* can be sold to the public provided it is licensed and labelled for the prophylaxis of malaria.

- **MEDICINAL FORMS** There can be variation in the licensing of different medicines containing the same drug. Forms available from special-order manufacturers include: oral solution

Oral solution

CAUTIONARY AND ADVISORY LABELS 5

- **Malarivon** (Wallace Manufacturing Chemists Ltd)

  Chloroquine phosphate 16 mg per 1 ml Malarivon 80mg/5ml syrup | 75 ml [PoM] £30.00

Mefloquine

18-Apr-2025

- **INDICATIONS AND DOSE**

Treatment of malaria

- BY MOUTH
  - Child: (consult product literature)

Prophylaxis of malaria

- BY MOUTH
  - Child (body-weight 5–15 kg): 62.5 mg once weekly, dose to be started 2–3 weeks before entering endemic area and continued for 4 weeks after leaving
  - Child (body-weight 16–24 kg): 125 mg once weekly, dose to be started 2–3 weeks before entering endemic area and continued for 4 weeks after leaving
  - Child (body-weight 25–44 kg): 187.5 mg once weekly, dose to be started 2–3 weeks before entering endemic area and continued for 4 weeks after leaving
  - Child (body-weight 45 kg and above): 250 mg once weekly, dose to be started 2–3 weeks before entering endemic area and continued for 4 weeks after leaving

- **UNLICENSED USE** Mefloquine doses in BNF Publications may differ from those in product literature.

  Not licensed for use in children under 5 kg body-weight and under 3 months.
- **CONTRA-INDICATIONS** Avoid for prophylaxis if history of psychiatric disorders (including depression) or convulsions · avoid for standby treatment if history of convulsions · history of blackwater fever
- **CAUTIONS** Cardiac conduction disorders · epilepsy (avoid for prophylaxis) · infants less than 3 months (limited experience) · not recommended in infants under 5 kg · traumatic brain injury

CAUTIONS, FURTHER INFORMATION

- Neuropsychiatric reactions Mefloquine is associated with potentially serious neuropsychiatric reactions. Abnormal dreams, insomnia, anxiety, and depression occur commonly. Psychosis, suicidal ideation, and suicide have also been reported. Psychiatric symptoms such as insomnia, nightmares, acute anxiety, depression, restlessness, or confusion should be regarded as potentially prodromal for a more serious event. Adverse reactions may occur and persist up to several months after discontinuation because mefloquine has a long half-life. For a prescribing checklist, and further information on side-effects, particularly neuropsychiatric side-effects, which may be associated with the use of mefloquine for malaria prophylaxis, see the *Guide for Healthcare Professionals* provided by the manufacturer.

- **INTERACTIONS** → Appendix 1: antimalarials
- **SIDE-EFFECTS**
  - **Common or very common** Anxiety · depression · diarrhoea · dizziness · gastrointestinal discomfort · headache · nausea · skin reactions · sleep disorders · vision disorders · vomiting
  - **Frequency not known** Acute kidney injury · agranulocytosis · alopecia · aplastic anaemia · appetite decreased · arrhythmias · arthralgia · asthenia · behaviour abnormal · cardiac conduction disorders · cataract · chest pain · chills · concentration impaired · confusion · cranial nerve paralysis · delusional disorder · depersonalisation · drowsiness · dyspnoea · encephalopathy · eye disorder · fever · flushing · gait abnormal · hallucination · hearing impairment · hepatic disorders · hyperacusia · hyperhidrosis · hypertension · hypotension · leucocytosis · leucopenia · malaise · memory loss · mood altered · movement disorders · muscle complaints · muscle weakness · nephritis · nerve disorders · oedema · palpitations · pancreatitis · paraesthesia · pneumonia · pneumonitis · psychosis · seizure · self-endangering behaviour · speech disorder · Stevens-Johnson syndrome ·

suicidal behaviours · syncope · thrombocytopenia · tinnitus · tremor · vertigo

- **ALLERGY AND CROSS-SENSITIVITY** EvGr Contra-indicated in patients with hypersensitivity to quinine. (M)
- **CONCEPTION AND CONTRACEPTION** Manufacturer advises adequate contraception during prophylaxis and for 3 months after stopping (teratogenicity in *animal* studies).
- **PREGNANCY**
  - When used for Treatment of malaria EvGr Not known to be harmful, (M) but see also *Pregnancy* in Malaria, treatment p. 482.
  - When used for Prophylaxis of malaria UKHSA advises that use may be considered if travelling to high-risk areas or there is resistance to other drugs. See also *Pregnancy* in Malaria, prophylaxis p. 476.
- **BREAST FEEDING** Specialist sources indicate present in milk but amount probably too small to be harmful.
- **HEPATIC IMPAIRMENT** Manufacturer advises avoid in severe impairment—elimination may be prolonged.
- **RENAL IMPAIRMENT** Manufacturer advises caution.
- **DIRECTIONS FOR ADMINISTRATION** Expert sources advise tablet may be crushed and mixed with food such as jam or honey just before administration.
- **PATIENT AND CARER ADVICE** Manufacturer advises that patients receiving mefloquine for malaria prophylaxis should be informed to discontinue its use if neuropsychiatric symptoms occur and seek immediate medical advice so that mefloquine can be replaced with an alternative antimalarial. Travellers should also be warned about **importance** of avoiding mosquito bites, **importance** of taking prophylaxis regularly, and **importance** of immediate visit to doctor if ill within 1 year and especially within 3 months of return.

  A patient alert card should be provided.

  Driving and skilled tasks Dizziness or a disturbed sense of balance may affect performance of skilled tasks (e.g. driving); effects may occur and persist up to several months after stopping mefloquine.
- **NATIONAL FUNDING/ACCESS DECISIONS**

  NHS restrictions Drugs for malaria prophylaxis are not prescribable in NHS primary care; health authorities may investigate circumstances under which antimalarials are prescribed.

- **MEDICINAL FORMS** There can be variation in the licensing of different medicines containing the same drug.

Oral tablet

CAUTIONARY AND ADVISORY LABELS 10, 21, 27

- **Mefloquine (Non-proprietary)**
  Mefloquine (as Mefloquine hydrochloride) 250 mg Mefloquine 250mg tablets | 1 tablet PoM
- **Lariam** (Neon Healthcare Ltd)
  Mefloquine (as Mefloquine hydrochloride) 250 mg Lariam 250mg tablets | 8 tablet PoM £14.53 DT = £14.53

Piperaquine phosphate with artenimol

01-Feb-2026

(Piperaquine tetraphosphate with dihydroartemisinin)

- **INDICATIONS AND DOSE**

Treatment of uncomplicated falciparum malaria [using 320 mg/40 mg tablets] | Treatment of uncomplicated non-falciparum malaria [using 320 mg/40 mg tablets]

▶ BY MOUTH

- Child 6 months–17 years (body-weight 5–7 kg): 0.5 tablet once daily for 3 days, max. 2 courses in 12 months; second course given at least 2 months after first course
- Child 6 months–17 years (body-weight 8–10 kg): 0.75 tablet once daily for 3 days, max. 2 courses in 12 months; second course given at least 2 months after first course
- Child 6 months–17 years (body-weight 11–16 kg): 1 tablet once daily for 3 days, max. 2 courses in 12 months; second course given at least 2 months after first course
- Child 6 months–17 years (body-weight 17–24 kg): 1.5 tablets once daily for 3 days, max. 2 courses in 12 months; second course given at least 2 months after first course
- Child 6 months–17 years (body-weight 25–35 kg): 2 tablets once daily for 3 days, max. 2 courses in 12 months; second course given at least 2 months after first course
- Child 6 months–17 years (body-weight 36–74 kg): 3 tablets once daily for 3 days, max. 2 courses in 12 months; second course given at least 2 months after first course
- Child 6 months–17 years (body-weight 75 kg and above): 4 tablets once daily for 3 days, max. 2 courses in 12 months; second course given at least 2 months after first course

DOSE EQUIVALENCE AND CONVERSION

- Each 320 mg/40 mg tablet contains piperaquine phosphate 320 mg and artenimol 40 mg.

- **UNLICENSED USE** Piperaquine phosphate with artenimol is not licensed in the UK. Expert sources advise that it is used as detailed below:
  - Treatment of uncomplicated falciparum malaria
  - Treatment of uncomplicated non-falciparum malaria
- **CONTRA-INDICATIONS** Bradycardia · congenital long QT syndrome · electrolyte disturbances (particularly hypokalaemia, hypocalcaemia, or hypomagnesaemia) · family history of sudden death · heart failure with reduced left ventricular ejection fraction · history of symptomatic arrhythmias · left ventricular hypertrophy · risk factors for QT_c interval prolongation · severe hypertension
- **INTERACTIONS** → Appendix 1: antimalarials
- **SIDE-EFFECTS**
  - **Common or very common** Abdominal pain · anaemia · appetite decreased · asthenia · conjunctivitis · cough · diarrhoea · fever · increased risk of infection · leucocytosis · leucopenia · neutropenia · QT interval prolongation · skin reactions · thrombocytopenia · vomiting
  - **Uncommon** Arthralgia · cardiac conduction disorder · epistaxis · headache · hepatic disorders · hypochromia · lymphadenopathy · nausea · rhinorrhoea · seizure · splenomegaly · stomatitis · thrombocytosis
  - **Frequency not known** Eosinophilia · haemolytic anaemia · sinus tachycardia

  SIDE-EFFECTS, FURTHER INFORMATION Haemolytic anaemia and autoimmune haemolytic anaemia can occur up to one month after starting treatment.
- **PREGNANCY** EvGr Avoid in first trimester (teratogenic in *animal* studies); may be used in second and third trimester when other artemisinin combination therapies are unsuitable (large amount of data indicates no fetotoxicity); (M) recommendation also supported by specialist sources.
- **BREAST FEEDING** Specialist sources indicate present in milk but not known to be harmful.
- **HEPATIC IMPAIRMENT** EvGr Caution in jaundice or in moderate to severe impairment (no information available)—monitor ECG and plasma potassium concentration. (M)
- **RENAL IMPAIRMENT** EvGr Caution in moderate to severe impairment (no information available)—monitor ECG and plasma potassium concentration. (M)
- **MONITORING REQUIREMENTS**
  - EvGr Consider obtaining ECG in all patients before third dose and 4–6 hours after third dose due to increased risk of

5 Infection

QT_C interval prolongation. If QT_C interval more than 500 milliseconds, discontinue treatment and monitor ECG for a further 24–48 hours due to risk of potentially life-threatening ventricular tachyarrhythmias.

- Obtain ECG as soon as possible after starting treatment then continue monitoring in children at a higher risk of arrhythmias due to QT_C interval prolongation, such as those taking medicines that increase plasma-piperaquine concentration, in children who are vomiting, or in females. ⟨M⟩

- **DIRECTIONS FOR ADMINISTRATION** Each dose should be taken at least 3 hours before or at least 3 hours after food intake.

For children unable to swallow tablets or where a partial dose is required, the tablets can be crushed and dispersed in water immediately before administration and the required volume administered.

For example, for a 0.75 tablet dose, crush and disperse a 320 mg/40 mg tablet in 10 mL of water and administer 7.5 mL; discard the remaining mixture.

- **PRESCRIBING AND DISPENSING INFORMATION** Available as *Eurartesim*® from the wholesaler Mawdsleys or specialist tropical disease centres.

- **PATIENT AND CARER ADVICE** Patients and carers should be given advice on how to administer tablets containing piperaquine phosphate with artenimol.

Delayed haemolytic anaemia Patients and carers should be advised of the signs and symptoms of post-treatment haemolysis, such as pallor, jaundice, dark-coloured urine, fever, fatigue, shortness of breath, dizziness, and confusion, and to seek medical advice if they occur.

Vomiting [EvGr] If vomiting occurs within 30 minutes of taking a dose, a full replacement dose should be taken; if vomiting occurs within 30–60 minutes of taking a dose, half the dose should be taken. Re-dosing should not be attempted more than once—if vomiting occurs following the second dose, alternative antimalarial treatment should be given. ⟨M⟩

- **MEDICINAL FORMS** No licensed medicines listed.

Primaquine

02-Sep-2024

- **INDICATIONS AND DOSE**

Adjunct in the treatment of non-falciparum malaria caused by *Plasmodium vivax* infection

- BY MOUTH
  - Child 6 months–17 years: 500 micrograms/kg daily (max. per dose 30 mg) for 14 days

Adjunct in the treatment of non-falciparum malaria caused by *Plasmodium ovale* infection

- BY MOUTH
  - Child 6 months–17 years: 250 micrograms/kg daily (max. per dose 15 mg) for 14 days

Adjunct in the treatment of non-falciparum malaria caused by *Plasmodium vivax* infection in patients with mild G6PD deficiency (administered on expert advice) | Adjunct in the treatment of non-falciparum malaria caused by *Plasmodium ovale* infection in patients with mild G6PD deficiency (administered on expert advice)

- BY MOUTH
  - Child: 750 micrograms/kg once weekly for 8 weeks; maximum 45 mg per week

Treatment of mild to moderate pneumocystis infection (in combination with clindamycin)

- BY MOUTH
  - Child: (consult product literature)

- **UNLICENSED USE** Not licensed.

- **CAUTIONS** G6PD deficiency · systemic diseases associated with granulocytopenia (e.g. rheumatoid arthritis, lupus erythematosus)

- **INTERACTIONS** → Appendix 1: antimalarials

- **SIDE-EFFECTS** Arrhythmia · dizziness · gastrointestinal discomfort · haemolytic anaemia (in G6PD deficiency) · leucopenia · methaemoglobinaemia (in NADH methaemoglobin reductase deficiency) · nausea · QT interval prolongation · skin reactions · vomiting

- **PREGNANCY** Risk of neonatal haemolysis and methaemoglobinaemia in third trimester.

- **BREAST FEEDING** No information available; theoretical risk of haemolysis in G6PD-deficient infants.

- **PRE-TREATMENT SCREENING** Before starting primaquine, blood should be tested for glucose-6-phosphate dehydrogenase (G6PD) activity since the drug can cause haemolysis in G6PD-deficient patients. Specialist advice should be obtained in G6PD deficiency.

- **MEDICINAL FORMS** There can be variation in the licensing of different medicines containing the same drug. Forms available from special-order manufacturers include: oral tablet, oral suspension

Oral tablet

- **Primaquine (Non-proprietary)**

Primaquine (as Primaquine phosphate) 15 mg Primaquine 15mg tablets | 100 tablet [PoM] (Hospital only)

Quinine

27-Jul-2020

- **INDICATIONS AND DOSE**

Non-falciparum malaria

- BY INTRAVENOUS INFUSION
  - Child: 10 mg/kg every 8 hours (max. per dose 700 mg), infused over 4 hours, given if patient is unable to take oral therapy. Change to oral chloroquine as soon as the patient's condition permits, reduce dose to 5–7 mg/kg if parenteral treatment is required for more than 48 hours

Falciparum malaria

- BY MOUTH
  - Child: 10 mg/kg every 8 hours (max. per dose 600 mg) for 7 days, to be given together with or followed by either doxycycline (in children over 12 years), or clindamycin
- BY INTRAVENOUS INFUSION
  - Neonate: Loading dose 20 mg/kg, infused over 4 hours, the loading dose of 20 mg/kg should **not** be used if the patient has received quinine or mefloquine during the previous 12 hours, then maintenance 10 mg/kg every 8 hours until patient can swallow oral medication to complete the 7-day course, maintenance dose to be given 8 hours after the start of the loading dose and infused over 4 hours, to be given together with or followed by clindamycin, reduce maintenance dose to 5–7 mg/kg if parenteral treatment is required for more than 48 hours.
  - Child: Loading dose 20 mg/kg (max. per dose 1.4 g), infused over 4 hours, the loading dose of 20 mg/kg should **not** be used if the patient has received quinine or mefloquine during the previous 12 hours, then maintenance 10 mg/kg every 8 hours (max. per dose 700 mg) until patient can swallow tablets to complete the 7-day course, maintenance dose to be given 8 hours after the start of the loading dose and infused over 4 hours, to be given together with or followed by either doxycycline (in children over 12 years), or clindamycin, reduce maintenance dose to 5–7 mg/kg if

parenteral treatment is required for more than 48 hours

Falciparum malaria (in intensive care unit)

▶ BY INTRAVENOUS INFUSION

▶ Neonate: Loading dose 7 mg/kg, infused over 30 minutes, followed immediately by 10 mg/kg, infused over 4 hours, then maintenance 10 mg/kg every 8 hours until patient can swallow oral medication to complete the 7-day course, maintenance dose to be given 8 hours after the start of the loading dose and infused over 4 hours, to be given together with or followed by clindamycin, reduce maintenance dose to 5–7 mg/kg if parenteral treatment is required for more than 48 hours.

▶ Child: Loading dose 7 mg/kg, infused over 30 minutes, followed immediately by 10 mg/kg, infused over 4 hours, then maintenance 10 mg/kg every 8 hours (max. per dose 700 mg) until patient can swallow tablets to complete the 7-day course, maintenance dose to be given 8 hours after the start of the loading dose and infused over 4 hours, to be given together with or followed by either doxycycline (in children over 12 years), or clindamycin, reduce maintenance dose to 5–7 mg/kg if parenteral treatment is required for more than 48 hours

DOSE EQUIVALENCE AND CONVERSION

▶ When using quinine for malaria, doses are valid for quinine hydrochloride, dihydrochloride, and sulfate; they are **not valid** for quinine bisulfate which contains a correspondingly smaller amount of quinine.

▶ Quinine (anhydrous base) 100 mg = quinine bisulfate 169 mg; quinine dihydrochloride 122 mg; quinine hydrochloride 122 mg; and quinine sulfate 121 mg. Quinine bisulfate 300 mg tablets are available but provide less quinine than 300 mg of the dihydrochloride, hydrochloride, or sulfate.

● **UNLICENSED USE** Injection not licensed.

IMPORTANT SAFETY INFORMATION

MHRA/CHM ADVICE: REMINDER OF DOSE-DEPENDENT QT-PROLONGING EFFECTS (NOVEMBER 2017)

Quinine has been associated with dose-dependent QT-interval-prolonging effects and should be used with caution in patients with risk factors for QT prolongation or in those with atrioventricular block—see Cautions for further information.

● **CONTRA-INDICATIONS** Haemoglobinuria · myasthenia gravis · optic neuritis · tinnitus

● **CAUTIONS** Atrial fibrillation (monitor ECG during parenteral treatment) · cardiac disease (monitor ECG during parenteral treatment) · conduction defects (monitor ECG during parenteral treatment) · electrolyte disturbance · G6PD deficiency · heart block (monitor ECG during parenteral treatment)

● **INTERACTIONS** → Appendix 1: antimalarials

● **SIDE-EFFECTS** Abdominal pain · agitation · agranulocytosis · angioedema · asthma · atrioventricular conduction changes · bronchospasm · cardiotoxicity · cerebral impairment · coagulation disorders · coma · confusion · death · diarrhoea · dyspnoea · fever · flushing · gastrointestinal disorder · haemoglobinuria · haemolysis · haemolytic uraemic syndrome · headache · hearing impairment · hypersensitivity · loss of consciousness · muscle weakness · myasthenia gravis aggravated · nausea · ocular toxicity · oedema · pancytopenia · photosensitivity reaction · QT interval prolongation · renal impairment · skin reactions · thrombocytopenia · tinnitus · vertigo · vision disorders · vomiting

Overdose Quinine is very toxic in overdosage; life-threatening features include arrhythmias (which can have a very rapid onset) and convulsions (which can be intractable).

For details on the management of poisoning, see Emergency treatment of poisoning p. 1036.

● **PREGNANCY** High doses are teratogenic in *first trimester*, but in malaria benefit of treatment outweighs risk.

● **BREAST FEEDING** Present in milk but not known to be harmful.

● **HEPATIC IMPAIRMENT**

▶ With oral use Manufacturer advises caution (risk of prolonged half-life).

Dose adjustments

▶ With intravenous use For treatment of malaria in severe impairment, reduce parenteral maintenance dose to 5–7 mg/kg of quinine salt.

▶ With oral use Manufacturer advises dose reduction or increased dose interval.

● **RENAL IMPAIRMENT**

Dose adjustments

▶ With intravenous use For treatment of malaria in severe impairment, reduce parenteral maintenance dose to 5–7 mg/kg of quinine salt.

● **MONITORING REQUIREMENTS**

▶ With intravenous use Monitor blood glucose and electrolyte concentration during parenteral treatment.

● **DIRECTIONS FOR ADMINISTRATION** For *intravenous infusion*, expert sources advise dilute to a concentration of 2 mg/mL (max. 30 mg/mL in fluid restriction) with Glucose 5% *or* Sodium Chloride 0.9% and give over 4 hours.

● **PRESCRIBING AND DISPENSING INFORMATION** Intravenous injection of quinine is so hazardous that it has been superseded by infusion.

● **MEDICINAL FORMS** There can be variation in the licensing of different medicines containing the same drug. Forms available from special-order manufacturers include: oral capsule, oral suspension, oral solution, solution for infusion

Oral tablet

▶ Quinine (Non-proprietary)

Quinine sulfate 200 mg Quinine sulfate 200mg tablets | 28 tablet [PoM] £7.61 DT = £2.21

Quinine bisulfate 300 mg Quinine bisulfate 300mg tablets | 28 tablet [PoM] £50.00 DT = £3.51

Quinine sulfate 300 mg Quinine sulfate 300mg tablets | 28 tablet [PoM] £3.60 DT = £1.88

4.2 Toxoplasmosis

ANTIBACTERIALS › MACROLIDES

Spiramycin

03-Dec-2020

● **INDICATIONS AND DOSE**

Toxoplasmosis in pregnancy

▶ BY MOUTH

▶ Child 12–17 years: 1.5 g twice daily until delivery

Chemoprophylaxis of congenital toxoplasmosis

▶ BY MOUTH

▶ Neonate: 50 mg/kg twice daily.

DOSE EQUIVALENCE AND CONVERSION

▶ 3000 units ≡ 1 mg spiramycin.

● **UNLICENSED USE** Spiramycin is not licensed in the UK. Expert sources advise that it is used as detailed below:

- Toxoplasmosis in pregnancy
- Chemoprophylaxis of congenital toxoplasmosis

- **CAUTIONS** Arrhythmias · cardiac disease · G6PD deficiency · predisposition to QT interval prolongation
- **SIDE-EFFECTS**
  - ▶ **Rare or very rare** Vasculitis
  - ▶ **Frequency not known** Angioedema · diarrhoea · haemolysis · nausea · paraesthesia · pseudomembranous enterocolitis · skin reactions · vomiting
- **ALLERGY AND CROSS-SENSITIVITY** EvGr Contra-indicated if hypersensitivity to other macrolides. ⟨M⟩
- **BREAST FEEDING** Present in breast milk.
- **HEPATIC IMPAIRMENT** Manufacturer advises caution.

- **MEDICINAL FORMS** There can be variation in the licensing of different medicines containing the same drug.

Oral tablet

▸ **Spiramycin (Non-proprietary)**

Spiramycin 1.5 mega unit Rovamycine 1.5million unit tablets | 16 tablet PoM ✗ (Hospital only)

Spiramycin 3 mega unit Rovamycine 3million unit tablets | 10 tablet PoM ✗ (Hospital only)

Powder for solution for infusion

▸ **Spiramycin (Non-proprietary)**

Spiramycin (as Spiramycin adipate) 1.5 mega unit Rovamycine 1.5million unit powder for solution for infusion vials | 1 vial PoM ✗ (Hospital only)

ANTIPROTOZOALS

Pyrimethamine

13-Jan-2022

- **INDICATIONS AND DOSE**

Toxoplasmosis in pregnancy (in combination with sulfadiazine and folinic acid)

▶ BY MOUTH

▸ Child 12–17 years: 50 mg once daily until delivery

Congenital toxoplasmosis (in combination with sulfadiazine and folinic acid)

▶ BY MOUTH

▸ Neonate: 1 mg/kg twice daily for 2 days, then 1 mg/kg once daily for 6 months, then 1 mg/kg 3 times a week for 6 months.

- **UNLICENSED USE** Not licensed for use in children under 5 years.
- **CAUTIONS** History of seizures—avoid large loading doses · predisposition to folate deficiency
- **INTERACTIONS** → Appendix 1: antimalarials
- **SIDE-EFFECTS**
  - ▶ **Common or very common** Anaemia · diarrhoea · dizziness · headache · leucopenia · nausea · skin reactions · thrombocytopenia · vomiting
  - ▶ **Uncommon** Fever
  - ▶ **Rare or very rare** Abdominal pain · oral ulceration · pancytopenia · pneumonia eosinophilic · seizure
- **PREGNANCY** Theoretical teratogenic risk in *first trimester* (folate antagonist). Adequate folate supplements should be given to the mother.
- **BREAST FEEDING** Significant amount in milk—avoid administration of other folate antagonists to infant. Avoid breast-feeding during toxoplasmosis treatment.
- **HEPATIC IMPAIRMENT** Manufacturer advises caution (limited information available).

  Dose adjustments Manufacturer advises consider dose reduction.
- **RENAL IMPAIRMENT** Manufacturer advises caution.
- **MONITORING REQUIREMENTS** Blood counts required with prolonged treatment.

- **MEDICINAL FORMS** There can be variation in the licensing of different medicines containing the same drug. Forms available from special-order manufacturers include: oral suspension

Oral tablet

▸ **Daraprim** (GlaxoSmithKline UK Ltd)

Pyrimethamine 25 mg Daraprim 25mg tablets | 30 tablet PoM £13.00 DT = £13.00

5 Viral infection

5.1 Coronavirus

COVID-19

08-Apr-2026

Description of condition

COVID-19 is the syndrome caused by a novel coronavirus, SARS-CoV-2, which was originally detected late 2019 in Wuhan, Hubei Province, China. SARS-CoV-2 is primarily transmitted between people through respiratory particles, direct human contact, and contact with contaminated surfaces. A child can be infected when respiratory particles are inhaled, or come into contact with the eyes, nose or mouth.

COVID-19 is predominantly a respiratory illness and in general, children are at very low risk of severe disease or death from COVID-19 compared to adults, and generally exhibit milder symptoms. Common symptoms in children include fever, a new continuous cough, shortness of breath, loss or change in sense of smell or taste, loss of appetite, abdominal pain, nausea or vomiting, diarrhoea, fatigue, muscle aches, headache, sore throat, and nasal congestion or rhinorrhoea. In children, additional symptoms to those found in adults may include grunting, nasal flare, and conjunctivitis. COVID-19 infection varies in severity from no symptoms in some children to severe pneumonia in others. Rarely, some children may develop a multisystem inflammatory response (known as paediatric multisystem inflammatory syndrome (PIMS)). For further information on PIMS, see Royal College of Paediatrics and Child Health (RCPCH): **Paediatric multisystem inflammatory syndrome temporally associated with COVID-19 (PIMS)** (available at: www.rcpch.ac.uk/resources/paediatric-multisystem-inflammatory-syndrome-temporally-associated-covid-19-pims-guidance).

Children with pre-existing health conditions are at a greater risk of severe disease from COVID-19, although there is limited evidence to associate severe COVID-19 disease with specific health conditions. Children may be at higher risk if they are medically complex; have long-term dependence on technological support (e.g. tracheostomy); have developmental delay, genetic abnormalities, or respiratory or cardiac co-morbidities. The risk also increases in pregnancy and in those with obesity. Children with cystic fibrosis may also be at greater risk of deterioration if they become infected.

After acute infection with COVID-19, children may experience prolonged symptoms that persist for more than 4 weeks (known as 'long COVID'). For guidance on the management of 'long COVID', see NICE, SIGN and the Royal College of General Practitioners (RCGP) COVID-19 rapid guideline: **Managing the long-term effects of COVID-19** (available at: www.nice.org.uk/guidance/ng188).

COVID-19 vaccination significantly reduces the risk of infection, hospitalisation, and death. However, fully vaccinated children can still become infected with SARS-CoV-2 and transmit the infection to other individuals. For information on vaccination against COVID-19, see COVID-19 vaccines p. 964.

Management

COVID-19 is a notifiable disease in the UK. For further information, see *Notifiable diseases* in Antibacterials, principles of therapy p. 358.

For guidance on infection prevention and control, and sampling and diagnostics, see the UKHSA collection: **Coronavirus (COVID-19): guidance** (available at: www.gov.uk/government/collections/coronavirus-covid-19-list-of-guidance).

For guidance on the management of COVID-19, see NICE rapid guideline: **Managing COVID-19** (see *Useful resources*).

Drug treatment

Children with COVID-19 have an increased risk of venous thromboembolism (VTE), but for children aged under 16 years the risk of VTE is uncertain in the context of COVID-19. For guidance on the prophylaxis and management of VTE, see NICE rapid guideline: **Managing COVID-19** (see *Useful resources*) and SIGN rapid guideline: **Prevention and management of venous thromboembolism in patients with COVID-19** (available at: www.sign.ac.uk/our-guidelines/prevention-and-management-of-venous-thromboembolism-in-covid-19/).

Dexamethasone p. 543 should be offered to children with COVID-19 who need supplemental oxygen, or who have a level of hypoxia that requires supplemental oxygen but are unable to have or tolerate it. If dexamethasone is unsuitable or unavailable, an alternative corticosteroid such as prednisolone p. 548 can be used.

Specialist advice should be sought on the use of other treatments for children hospitalised due to COVID-19, and for symptomatic children who are at high risk of progression to severe disease. Treatment options include antivirals (such as remdesivir below) or a Janus kinase inhibitor (such as baricitinib [unlicensed use]). For further guidance on drug treatments for COVID-19, see NICE rapid guideline: **Managing COVID-19** (see *Useful resources*).

Antibacterials are not recommended for preventing or treating pneumonia if it is likely to be caused by SARS-CoV-2, another virus, or a fungal infection. Empirical antibacterials should be started if a secondary bacterial infection is suspected in children with COVID-19. For guidance on the management of suspected or confirmed bacterial pneumonia, see Respiratory system infections, antibacterial therapy p. 371.

Antifungals should only be offered for treatment of COVID-19-associated pulmonary aspergillosis (CAPA) if diagnosis is confirmed, or CAPA is suspected and a multidisciplinary team or local protocols support starting treatment.

For guidance on the management of COVID-19 infection in pregnancy, including therapies that should be offered to pregnant or postpartum females with COVID-19, see Royal College of Obstetricians and Gynaecologists, Royal College of Midwives, Royal College of Paediatrics and Child Health, PHE and Public Health Scotland guidance: **Coronavirus (COVID-19) infection in pregnancy** (available at: www.rcog.org.uk/guidance/coronavirus-covid-19-pregnancy-and-women-s-health/). Exposure to COVID-19 antivirals in pregnant females should be reported to the UK COVID-19 antivirals in pregnancy registry. For further information, see uktis.org/covid-19-antivirals-pregnancy-registry/.

For information on the fetal and neonatal risks of exposure to COVID-19 treatments, see UK Teratology Information Service (UKTIS): **Medications used to treat COVID-19 in pregnancy** (available at: uktis.org/monographs/medications-used-to-treat-covid-19-in-pregnancy/).

For breastfeeding advice on drugs that may be used for COVID-19, see UK Drugs in Lactation Advisory Service (UKDILAS) guidance on the Specialist Pharmacy Service website (available at: www.sps.nhs.uk/articles/managing-covid-19-and-breastfeeding/).

Management of COVID-19 symptoms

Children with a cough should be encouraged to avoid lying on their backs, if possible, because this may make coughing less effective. Cough should be initially managed using simple non-drug measures (such as honey). Seek specialist advice for suppressing coughing that is distressing in a child with COVID-19. For further information on the management of acute cough, see *Cough, acute* in Respiratory system infections, antibacterial therapy p. 371.

Children with fever should be advised to drink fluids regularly to avoid dehydration, and to take an antipyretic (such as paracetamol or ibuprofen) as appropriate (whilst both fever and other symptoms that antipyretics would help treat are present). For guidance on the management of children presenting with a feverish illness, see Fever p. 348.

Reversible causes of breathlessness (such as pulmonary oedema, pulmonary embolism, and asthma) should be identified and treated accordingly. When other significant medical pathology has been excluded or further investigation is inappropriate, non-drug management (such as relaxation and breathing techniques, and changing body positioning) may help to manage breathlessness as part of supportive care. If hypoxia is the likely cause of breathlessness, consider a trial of oxygen therapy if appropriate.

Seek specialist advice for management of anxiety or agitation, and end of life care.

Useful Resources

COVID-19 rapid guideline: managing COVID-19. National Institute for Health and Care Excellence. NICE guideline 191. March 2021, updated May 2025.
www.nice.org.uk/guidance/ng191

ANTIVIRALS

Remdesivir

16-Apr-2026

- **DRUG ACTION** Remdesivir is an RNA polymerase inhibitor that disrupts the production of viral RNA, preventing multiplication of SARS-CoV-2.

- **INDICATIONS AND DOSE**

COVID-19 in patients hospitalised with pneumonia and requiring low-flow supplemental oxygen (under close medical supervision)

▶ BY INTRAVENOUS INFUSION

▶ Child (body-weight 3–39 kg): Loading dose 5 mg/kg for 1 dose, then maintenance 2.5 mg/kg once daily for up to 5 days in total, treatment should be initiated within 10 days of initial COVID-19 symptoms, consider stopping treatment if continuous deterioration despite 48 hours of mechanical ventilation, course may be repeated if readmitted with COVID-19—consult interim clinical commissioning policy for further details (see *Prescribing and dispensing information*)

▶ Child (body-weight 40 kg and above): Loading dose 200 mg for 1 dose, then maintenance 100 mg once daily for up to 5 days in total, treatment should be initiated within 10 days of initial COVID-19 symptoms, consider stopping treatment if continuous deterioration despite 48 hours of mechanical ventilation, course may be repeated if readmitted with COVID-19—consult interim clinical commissioning policy for further details (see *Prescribing and dispensing information*)

COVID-19 in immunocompromised patients hospitalised with pneumonia (under close medical supervision)

▶ BY INTRAVENOUS INFUSION

▶ Child (body-weight 3–39 kg): Loading dose 5 mg/kg for 1 dose, then maintenance 2.5 mg/kg once daily for up to 10 days in total following a multidisciplinary assessment, consider stopping treatment

continued →

if continuous deterioration despite 48 hours of mechanical ventilation, course may be repeated if readmitted with COVID-19—consult interim clinical commissioning policy for further details (see *Prescribing and dispensing information*)

- Child (body-weight 40 kg and above): Loading dose 200 mg for 1 dose, then maintenance 100 mg once daily for up to 10 days in total following a multidisciplinary assessment, consider stopping treatment if continuous deterioration despite 48 hours of mechanical ventilation, course may be repeated if readmitted with COVID-19—consult interim clinical commissioning policy for further details (see *Prescribing and dispensing information*)

COVID-19 in patients who do not require oxygen supplementation and are at an increased risk of progression to severe COVID-19 infection (under close medical supervision)

- BY INTRAVENOUS INFUSION
- Child (body-weight 40 kg and above): Loading dose 200 mg for 1 dose, then maintenance 100 mg once daily for 3 days in total, treatment should be initiated within 7 days of initial COVID-19 symptoms

- **UNLICENSED USE** EvGr Remdesivir is used in the doses provided for the treatment of COVID-19, (A) but these may differ from those licensed.

IMPORTANT SAFETY INFORMATION

MHRA/CHM ADVICE: COVID-19 ANTIVIRALS: REPORTING TO THE UK COVID-19 ANTIVIRALS PREGNANCY REGISTRY (FEBRUARY 2022)

The safety of COVID-19 antiviral treatment, such as remdesivir, during pregnancy has not been established. The MHRA, in collaboration with the UK Teratology Information Service (UKTIS), is operating the UK COVID-19 Antivirals Pregnancy Registry to collect information about and enable follow-up of reported exposures to COVID-19 antivirals in pregnancy; it is also collecting information on the outcomes of pregnancies, where conception occurred during or shortly after paternal exposure to antiviral treatment.

Healthcare professionals in England, Scotland, and Wales (as well as patients and their partners) are advised to report exposure to remdesivir during pregnancy or around the time of conception, or of partners on remdesivir around the time of conception. Healthcare professionals in Northern Ireland cannot currently report on behalf of a pregnant female or their partner but should encourage them to self-report. Since exposure can occur in very early pregnancy before pregnancy is recognised, healthcare professionals are advised to report (or to encourage patients to self-report), even if some time has passed since the end of remdesivir treatment.

An exposed pregnancy should be reported by telephone to UKTIS–for more information, see the UKTIS Registry website (available at: www.medicinesinpregnancy.org/bumps/COVID-19-Antivirals-Pregnancy-Registry/).

- **INTERACTIONS** → Appendix 1: remdesivir
- **SIDE-EFFECTS**
  - **Common or very common** Headache · nausea · rash
  - **Rare or very rare** Hypersensitivity · infusion related reaction
  - **Frequency not known** Sinus bradycardia

SIDE-EFFECTS, FURTHER INFORMATION Manufacturer advises slower infusion rates, with a maximum infusion time of up to 120 minutes, to prevent signs and symptoms of hypersensitivity. If significant hypersensitivity occurs, discontinue immediately.

- **CONCEPTION AND CONTRACEPTION** Manufacturer advises females of childbearing potential should use effective contraception during treatment.
- **PREGNANCY** EvGr Avoid unless potential benefit outweighs risk—no information available. (M) See also *Important safety information*.
- **BREAST FEEDING** Specialist sources indicate use with caution—limited information. Minimal oral absorption expected, but monitor breast-fed infants for adverse reactions such as diarrhoea, rash, hypotension, liver and renal impairment (increased risk of accumulation due to long half-life).
- **HEPATIC IMPAIRMENT** Manufacturer advises caution (no information available)—treatment should not be started if ALT is ≥ 5 times the upper limit of normal. If ALT increases during treatment, remdesivir may need to be withheld, consult product literature for further information.
- **RENAL IMPAIRMENT** Manufacturer advises avoid if eGFR less than 30 mL/minute/1.73 m^2— *Veklury*® formulation excipient (sulfobutylether beta cyclodextrin sodium) may accumulate. See p. 16.
- **MONITORING REQUIREMENTS**
  - Manufacturer advises monitor liver function at baseline and periodically during treatment as indicated.
  - Manufacturer advises monitor eGFR at baseline and periodically during treatment as indicated—severe renal toxicity in *animal* studies.
- **DIRECTIONS FOR ADMINISTRATION** EvGr For *intravenous infusion*, reconstitute each vial with 19 mL Water for Injections, then dilute in Sodium Chloride 0.9%; give over 30–120 minutes. (M) For further information on dilution and infusion rates—consult product literature.
- **PRESCRIBING AND DISPENSING INFORMATION** NHS England Interim Clinical Commissioning Policy: Remdesivir for patients hospitalised due to COVID-19 (adults and children 12 years and older) (available at: www.england.nhs.uk/coronavirus/documents/interim-clinical-commissioning-policy-remdesivir-for-patients-hospitalised-due-to-covid-19-adults-and-adolescents-12-years-and-older/).
- **NATIONAL FUNDING/ACCESS DECISIONS** For full details see funding body website

NICE decisions

- **Remdesivir and tixagevimab plus cilgavimab for treating COVID-19 (May 2024)** NICE TA971 Recommended with restrictions

Scottish Medicines Consortium (SMC) decisions

- **Remdesivir (*Veklury*®) for the treatment of COVID-19 in adults and paediatric patients (updated February 2026)** SMC No. SMC2550 Recommended with restrictions

- **MEDICINAL FORMS** There can be variation in the licensing of different medicines containing the same drug.

Powder for solution for infusion

EXCIPIENTS: May contain Sulfobutylether beta cyclodextrin sodium

- **Veklury** (Gilead Sciences Ltd)
  Remdesivir 100 mg Veklury 100mg powder for concentrate for solution for infusion vials | 1 vial PoM £340.00 (Hospital only)

5.2 Hepatitis

Hepatitis

15-Mar-2023

Overview

Acute infectious hepatitis is a notifiable disease in the UK. For further information, see *Notifiable diseases* in Antibacterials, principles of therapy p. 358.

Treatment for viral hepatitis should be initiated by a specialist. The management of uncomplicated acute viral hepatitis is largely symptomatic. Hepatitis B and hepatitis C viruses are major causes of chronic hepatitis. Active or passive immunisation against hepatitis A and B infections is available, see Hepatitis A vaccine p. 967 and Hepatitis B vaccine p. 968.

Chronic hepatitis B

Treatment of chronic hepatitis B infection should be initiated by a specialist.

EvGr Entecavir, peginterferon alfa, tenofovir alafenamide below, and tenofovir disoproxil p. 519 are options for the treatment of chronic hepatitis B infection in children, if treatment is deemed necessary. (A)

For information on the treatment of HIV and chronic hepatitis B co-infection, see HIV infection p. 505.

Chronic hepatitis C

Treatment of chronic hepatitis C infection should be initiated by a specialist. Before starting treatment, the genotype of the infecting hepatitis C virus should be determined and the viral load measured as this may affect the choice and duration of treatment.

Direct-acting antiviral agents (e.g. sofosbuvir p. 496 in combination with ribavirin, sofosbuvir with velpatasvir p. 496, ledipasvir with sofosbuvir p. 495 (with or without ribavirin), glecaprevir with pibrentasvir p. 497, elbasvir with grazoprevir below (with or without ribavirin)) and ribavirin p. 494 in combination with peginterferon alfa p. 498 are licensed for the treatment of chronic hepatitis C infection in children.

5.3 Hepatitis infections

5.3a Chronic hepatitis B

Other drugs used for Chronic hepatitis B Lamivudine, p. 518

ANTIVIRALS › NUCLEOSIDE REVERSE TRANSCRIPTASE INHIBITORS

513

Tenofovir alafenamide

01-Dec-2020

● **INDICATIONS AND DOSE**

Chronic hepatitis B (initiated by a specialist)

▶ BY MOUTH

▸ Child 12–17 years (body-weight 35 kg and above): 25 mg once daily, for duration of treatment—consult product literature

● **CAUTIONS** Decompensated liver disease · HIV co-infection

● **INTERACTIONS** → Appendix 1: tenofovir alafenamide

● **SIDE-EFFECTS**

▶ **Common or very common** Abdominal distension · arthralgia

▶ **Frequency not known** Hepatitis aggravated (during or following treatment) · nephrotoxicity

● **BREAST FEEDING** Manufacturer advises avoid—present in milk in *animal* studies.

● **HEPATIC IMPAIRMENT** Manufacturer advises caution in decompensated hepatic disease (no information available).

● **PRE-TREATMENT SCREENING** Manufacturer advises HIV antibody testing should be offered to those with unknown HIV-1 status before initiation of treatment.

● **MONITORING REQUIREMENTS** Manufacturer advises monitor liver function tests at repeated intervals during treatment and for at least 6 months after last dose—recurrent hepatitis may occur on discontinuation.

● **PATIENT AND CARER ADVICE**

Missed doses Manufacturer advises if a dose is more than 18 hours late, the missed dose should not be taken and the next dose should be taken at the normal time.

● **MEDICINAL FORMS** There can be variation in the licensing of different medicines containing the same drug.

Oral tablet

CAUTIONARY AND ADVISORY LABELS 21

▸ **Vemlidy** (Gilead Sciences Ltd)

Tenofovir alafenamide (as Tenofovir alafenamide fumarate) 25 mg Vemlidy 25mg tablets | 30 tablet PoM £325.73 (Hospital only)

5.3b Chronic hepatitis C

ANTIVIRALS › HCV INHIBITORS

Elbasvir with grazoprevir

16-Aug-2022

● **DRUG ACTION** Elbasvir is an HCV NS5A inhibitor and grazoprevir is an HCV NS3/4A protease inhibitor; they reduce viral load by inhibiting hepatitis C virus RNA replication.

● **INDICATIONS AND DOSE**

Chronic hepatitis C infection of genotypes 1 or 4 [with or without ribavirin] (initiated by a specialist)

▶ BY MOUTH

▸ Child 12–17 years (body-weight 30 kg and above): 50/100 mg once daily for 12 weeks (may extend to 16 weeks in some circumstances—consult product literature)

DOSE EQUIVALENCE AND CONVERSION

▸ Dose expressed as *x*/*y* mg of elbasvir/grazoprevir.

IMPORTANT SAFETY INFORMATION

MHRA/CHM ADVICE: DIRECT-ACTING ANTIVIRALS TO TREAT CHRONIC HEPATITIS C: RISK OF INTERACTION WITH VITAMIN K ANTAGONISTS AND CHANGES IN INR (JANUARY 2017)

An EU-wide review has identified that changes in liver function, secondary to hepatitis C treatment with direct-acting antivirals, may affect the efficacy of vitamin K antagonists; the MHRA has advised that INR should be monitored closely in patients receiving concomitant treatment.

MHRA/CHM ADVICE: DIRECT-ACTING ANTIVIRAL INTERFERON-FREE REGIMENS TO TREAT CHRONIC HEPATITIS C: RISK OF HEPATITIS B REACTIVATION (JANUARY 2017)

An EU-wide review has concluded that direct-acting antiviral interferon-free regimens for chronic hepatitis C can cause hepatitis B reactivation in patients co-infected with hepatitis B and C viruses; the MHRA recommends to screen patients for hepatitis B before starting treatment—patients infected with both hepatitis B and C viruses must be monitored and managed according to current clinical guidelines.

MHRA/CHM ADVICE: DIRECT-ACTING ANTIVIRALS FOR CHRONIC HEPATITIS C: RISK OF HYPOGLYCAEMIA IN PATIENTS WITH DIABETES (DECEMBER 2018)

Rapid reduction in hepatitis C viral load during direct-acting antiviral therapy for hepatitis C may improve glucose metabolism in patients with diabetes and result in symptomatic hypoglycaemia if diabetic treatment is continued at the same dose.

The MHRA advises healthcare professionals:

- to monitor glucose levels closely in patients with diabetes during direct-acting antiviral therapy for hepatitis C, especially within the first 3 months of treatment and modify diabetic medication or doses when necessary;

- to be vigilant for changes in glucose tolerance and advise patients of the risk of hypoglycaemia;
- to inform the healthcare professional in charge of the diabetic care of the patient when direct-acting antiviral therapy is initiated.

● **CAUTIONS** Hepatitis B co-infection · re-treatment following previous exposure to elbasvir with grazoprevir, or to drugs of the same classes (NS5A inhibitors or NS3/4A inhibitors other than telaprevir, simeprevir, boceprevir)—efficacy not demonstrated

● **INTERACTIONS** → Appendix 1: elbasvir · grazoprevir

● **SIDE-EFFECTS**
- **Common or very common** Alopecia · anxiety · appetite decreased · arthralgia · asthenia · constipation · depression · diarrhoea · dizziness · dry mouth · gastrointestinal discomfort · headache · insomnia · irritability · myalgia · nausea · pruritus · vomiting
- **Frequency not known** Anaemia · hepatitis B reactivation · transient ischaemic attack

● **PREGNANCY** Manufacturer advises use only if potential benefit outweighs risk.

● **BREAST FEEDING** Manufacturer advises avoid—present in milk in *animal* studies.

● **HEPATIC IMPAIRMENT** Manufacturer advises avoid in moderate to severe impairment.

● **MONITORING REQUIREMENTS** Manufacturer advises monitor liver function before treatment, at week 8 in all patients, at week 12 in patients receiving 16 weeks of treatment, and then as clinically indicated—consider discontinuing treatment if alanine aminotransferase (ALT) is greater than 10 times the upper limit of normal; discontinue treatment if ALT elevation is accompanied by signs or symptoms of hepatic impairment or inflammation.

● **PATIENT AND CARER ADVICE**
Hepatic effects Patients and their carers should consult a healthcare professional if signs and symptoms of hepatic dysfunction occur (including fatigue, weakness, lack of appetite, nausea and vomiting, jaundice or discoloured faeces).
Vomiting If vomiting occurs within 4 hours of a dose, an additional dose should be taken.
Missed doses If a dose is more than 16 hours late, the missed dose should not be taken and the next dose should be taken at the normal time.

● **NATIONAL FUNDING/ACCESS DECISIONS**
For full details see funding body website

All Wales Medicines Strategy Group (AWMSG) decisions
- **Elbasvir with grazoprevir (*Zepatier*®) for the treatment of chronic hepatitis C of genotypes 1 or 4 in paediatric patients 12 years of age and older who weigh at least 30 kg (July 2022)** AWMSG No. 4980 Recommended

● **MEDICINAL FORMS** There can be variation in the licensing of different medicines containing the same drug.

Oral tablet
CAUTIONARY AND ADVISORY LABELS 3
ELECTROLYTES: May contain Sodium
- **Zepatier** (Merck Sharp & Dohme (UK) Ltd)
  Elbasvir 50 mg, Grazoprevir 100 mg Zepatier 50mg/100mg tablets | 28 tablet PoM £12,166.67

ANTIVIRALS > NUCLEOSIDE ANALOGUES

Ribavirin
30-Dec-2024

(Tribavirin)

● **INDICATIONS AND DOSE**

Bronchiolitis
- BY INHALATION OF AEROSOL, OR BY INHALATION OF NEBULISED SOLUTION
  - Child 1–23 months: Inhale a solution containing 20 mg/mL for 12–18 hours for at least 3 days, maximum of 7 days, to be administered via small particle aerosol generator

Life-threatening RSV, parainfluenza virus, and adenovirus infection in immunocompromised children (administered on expert advice)
- BY INTRAVENOUS INFUSION
  - Child: 33 mg/kg for 1 dose, to be administered over 15 minutes, then 16 mg/kg every 6 hours for 4 days, then 8 mg/kg every 8 hours for 3 days

REBETOL ® CAPSULES

Chronic hepatitis C (in combination with interferon alfa or peginterferon alfa) in previously untreated children without liver decompensation
- BY MOUTH
  - Child 3-17 years (body-weight up to 47 kg): 15 mg/kg daily in 2 divided doses
  - Child 3-17 years (body-weight 47-49 kg): 200 mg, dose to be given in the morning and 400 mg, dose to be given in the evening
  - Child 3-17 years (body-weight 50-64 kg): 400 mg twice daily
  - Child 3-17 years (body-weight 65-80 kg): 400 mg, dose to be given in the morning and 600 mg, dose to be given in the evening
  - Child 3-17 years (body-weight 81-104 kg): 600 mg twice daily
  - Child 3-17 years (body-weight 105 kg and above): 600 mg, dose to be given in the morning and 800 mg, dose to be given in the evening

● **UNLICENSED USE**
- When used by inhalation Inhalation preparation not licensed.
- With intravenous use Intravenous preparation not licensed.

● **CONTRA-INDICATIONS**
- With systemic use Consult product literature for specific contra-indications when ribavirin used in combination with other medicinal products · haemoglobinopathies · severe, uncontrolled cardiac disease in children with chronic hepatitis C

● **CAUTIONS**
- When used by inhalation Maintain standard supportive respiratory and fluid management therapy
- With systemic use Cardiac disease (assessment including ECG recommended before and during treatment—discontinue if deterioration) · consult product literature for specific cautions when ribavirin used in combination with other medicinal products · patients with a transplant—risk of rejection · risk of growth retardation in children, the reversibility of which is uncertain—if possible, consider starting treatment after pubertal growth spurt

● **INTERACTIONS** → Appendix 1: ribavirin

● **SIDE-EFFECTS**
- **Common or very common** Alopecia · anaemia · anxiety · appetite decreased · arrhythmias · arthralgia · arthritis · asthenia · behaviour abnormal · chest pain · chills · concentration impaired · constipation · cough · depression · diarrhoea · dizziness · drowsiness · dry mouth · dysphagia · dyspnoea · ear pain · eye disorders · eye inflammation · eye

pain · fever · gastrointestinal discomfort · gastrointestinal disorders · haemorrhage · headaches · hyperthyroidism · hypotension · hypothyroidism · increased risk of infection · influenza like illness · lymphadenopathy · malaise · memory loss · mood altered · muscle complaints · muscle weakness · nasal congestion · nausea · neutropenia · oral disorders · pain · palpitations · peripheral oedema · photosensitivity reaction · respiratory disorders · sensation abnormal · sexual dysfunction · skin reactions · sleep disorders · sweat changes · syncope · taste altered · thirst · throat pain · thrombocytopenia · tinnitus · tremor · vasodilation · vertigo · vision disorders · vomiting · weight decreased

- **Uncommon** Dehydration · diabetes mellitus · hallucination · hearing loss · hepatic disorders · hypertension · nerve disorders · sarcoidosis · suicidal behaviours · thyroiditis
- **Rare or very rare** Angina pectoris · angioedema · bone marrow disorders · cardiac inflammation · cerebral ischaemia · cholangitis · coma · congestive heart failure · facial paralysis · hepatic failure (discontinue) · hypersensitivity · interstitial pneumonitis · intracranial haemorrhage · myocardial infarction · myopathy · pancreatitis · psychotic disorder · pulmonary embolism · retinopathy · seizure · severe cutaneous adverse reactions (SCARs) · systemic lupus erythematosus (SLE) · vasculitis
- **Frequency not known** Haemolytic anaemia · homicidal ideation · nephrotic syndrome · pure red cell aplasia · renal failure · solid organ transplant rejection · tongue discolouration · ulcerative colitis

SIDE-EFFECTS, FURTHER INFORMATION Side effects listed are reported when oral ribavirin is used in combination with peginterferon alfa or interferon alfa, consult product literature for details.

- **CONCEPTION AND CONTRACEPTION**
- With systemic use Exclude pregnancy before treatment in females of childbearing age. Effective contraception essential during treatment and for 4 months after treatment in females and for 7 months after treatment in males of childbearing age. Routine monthly pregnancy tests recommended. Condoms must be used if partner of male patient is pregnant (ribavirin excreted in semen).
- When used by inhalation Women planning pregnancy should avoid exposure to aerosol.
- **PREGNANCY** Avoid; teratogenicity in *animal* studies.
- When used by inhalation Pregnant women should avoid exposure to aerosol.
- **BREAST FEEDING** Avoid—no information available.
- **RENAL IMPAIRMENT** Plasma-ribavirin concentration increased. Manufacturer advises avoid oral ribavirin if estimated glomerular filtration rate less than 50 mL/minute/1.73 m^2—monitor haemoglobin concentration closely.

  Manufacturer advises use intravenous preparation with caution if estimated glomerular filtration rate less than 30 mL/minute/1.73 m^2.
- **MONITORING REQUIREMENTS**
- When used by inhalation Monitor electrolytes closely. Monitor equipment for precipitation.
- With systemic use Determine full blood count, platelets, electrolytes, serum creatinine, liver function tests and uric acid before starting treatment and then on weeks 2 and 4 of treatment, then as indicated clinically—adjust dose if adverse reactions or laboratory abnormalities develop (consult product literature). Test thyroid function before treatment and then every 3 months.
- With oral use Eye examination recommended before treatment. Eye examination also recommended during treatment if pre-existing ophthalmological disorder or if decrease in vision reported—discontinue treatment if ophthalmological disorder deteriorates or if new ophthalmological disorder develops.
- **PRESCRIBING AND DISPENSING INFORMATION** Flavours of oral liquid formulations may include bubble-gum.
- **NATIONAL FUNDING/ACCESS DECISIONS**
  For full details see funding body website

NICE decisions

- **Peginterferon alfa and ribavirin for treating chronic hepatitis C in children and young people (November 2013) NICE TA300** Recommended
- **LESS SUITABLE FOR PRESCRIBING** Ribavirin inhalation is less suitable for prescribing.

- **MEDICINAL FORMS** There can be variation in the licensing of different medicines containing the same drug.

Oral capsule

CAUTIONARY AND ADVISORY LABELS 21

- Ribavirin (Non-proprietary)

Ribavirin 200 mg Ribavirin 200mg capsules | 84 capsule PoM £160.69 | 140 capsule PoM £267.81 | 168 capsule PoM £321.38

ANTIVIRALS > NUCLEOTIDE ANALOGUES

Ledipasvir with sofosbuvir 08-Mar-2023

The properties listed below are those particular to the combination only. For the properties of the components please consider, sofosbuvir p. 496.

- **DRUG ACTION** Sofosbuvir is a nucleotide analogue inhibitor and ledipasvir is an HCV inhibitor; they reduce viral load by inhibiting hepatitis C virus RNA replication.

- **INDICATIONS AND DOSE**

Chronic hepatitis C infection (under expert supervision)

- BY MOUTH USING GRANULES
- Child 3–17 years (body-weight up to 17 kg): 33.75/150 mg once daily, for treatment duration—consult product literature
- BY MOUTH
- Child 3–17 years (body-weight 17–34 kg): 45/200 mg once daily, for treatment duration—consult product literature
- Child 3–17 years (body-weight 35 kg and above): 90/400 mg once daily, for treatment duration—consult product literature

DOSE ADJUSTMENTS DUE TO INTERACTIONS

- Manufacturer advises reduce dose of concurrent H_2-receptor antagonist if above a dose comparable to famotidine 40 mg twice daily.
- Manufacturer advises reduce dose of concurrent proton pump inhibitor if above a dose comparable to omeprazole 20 mg; take at the same time as sofosbuvir with ledipasvir.

DOSE EQUIVALENCE AND CONVERSION

- Dose expressed as *x/y* mg ledipasvir/sofosbuvir.

- **CAUTIONS** Retreatment following treatment failure—efficacy not established
- **INTERACTIONS** → Appendix 1: ledipasvir · sofosbuvir
- **SIDE-EFFECTS**
- **Common or very common** Fatigue · headache · rash
- **Frequency not known** Angioedema · hepatitis B reactivation · Stevens-Johnson syndrome
- **DIRECTIONS FOR ADMINISTRATION** Granules may be swallowed or mixed with non-acidic soft food that is at or below room temperature, and swallowed within 30 minutes without chewing.
- **PRESCRIBING AND DISPENSING INFORMATION** Dispense tablets in original container (contains desiccant).
- **PATIENT AND CARER ADVICE** Patients or carers should be given advice on how to administer granules.
  Vomiting If vomiting occurs within 5 hours of

administration, an additional dose should be taken.
Missed doses If a dose is more than 18 hours late, the missed dose should not be taken and the next dose should be taken at the normal time.

- **NATIONAL FUNDING/ACCESS DECISIONS**

For full details see funding body website

Scottish Medicines Consortium (SMC) decisions

- **Ledipasvir with sofosbuvir (*Harvoni*®) for the treatment of chronic hepatitis C infection in adolescents aged 12 up to 18 years (June 2018)** SMC No. 1343/18 Recommended with restrictions

- **MEDICINAL FORMS** There can be variation in the licensing of different medicines containing the same drug.

Oral tablet

CAUTIONARY AND ADVISORY LABELS 25

- Harvoni (Gilead Sciences Ltd)

Ledipasvir 90 mg, Sofosbuvir 400 mg Harvoni 90mg/400mg tablets | 28 tablet PoM £12,993.33 (Hospital only)

Sofosbuvir

22-Mar-2023

- **INDICATIONS AND DOSE**

Chronic hepatitis C infection (under expert supervision)

- BY MOUTH USING GRANULES
  - Child 3–17 years (body-weight up to 17 kg): 150 mg once daily, for duration of treatment—consult product literature
- BY MOUTH
  - Child 3–17 years (body-weight 17–34 kg): 200 mg once daily, for duration of treatment—consult product literature
  - Child 3–17 years (body-weight 35 kg and above): 400 mg once daily, for duration of treatment—consult product literature

IMPORTANT SAFETY INFORMATION

MHRA/CHM ADVICE: DIRECT-ACTING ANTIVIRALS TO TREAT CHRONIC HEPATITIS C: RISK OF INTERACTION WITH VITAMIN K ANTAGONISTS AND CHANGES IN INR (JANUARY 2017)

An EU-wide review has identified that changes in liver function, secondary to hepatitis C treatment with direct-acting antivirals, may affect the efficacy of vitamin K antagonists; the MHRA has advised that INR should be monitored closely in patients receiving concomitant treatment.

MHRA/CHM ADVICE: DIRECT-ACTING ANTIVIRAL INTERFERON-FREE REGIMENS TO TREAT CHRONIC HEPATITIS C: RISK OF HEPATITIS B REACTIVATION (JANUARY 2017)

An EU-wide review has concluded that direct-acting antiviral interferon-free regimens for chronic hepatitis C can cause hepatitis B reactivation in patients co-infected with hepatitis B and C viruses; the MHRA recommends to screen patients for hepatitis B before starting treatment—patients infected with both hepatitis B and C viruses must be monitored and managed according to current clinical guidelines.

MHRA/CHM ADVICE: DIRECT-ACTING ANTIVIRALS FOR CHRONIC HEPATITIS C: RISK OF HYPOGLYCAEMIA IN PATIENTS WITH DIABETES (DECEMBER 2018)

Rapid reduction in hepatitis C viral load during direct-acting antiviral therapy for hepatitis C may improve glucose metabolism in patients with diabetes and result in symptomatic hypoglycaemia if diabetic treatment is continued at the same dose.

The MHRA advises healthcare professionals:

- to monitor glucose levels closely in patients with diabetes during direct-acting antiviral therapy for hepatitis C, especially within the first 3 months of treatment and modify diabetic medication or doses when necessary;
- to be vigilant for changes in glucose tolerance and advise patients of the risk of hypoglycaemia;
- to inform the healthcare professional in charge of the diabetic care of the patient when direct-acting antiviral therapy is initiated.

- **INTERACTIONS** → Appendix 1: sofosbuvir
- **SIDE-EFFECTS**
  - **Common or very common** Alopecia · anaemia · anxiety · appetite decreased · arthralgia · asthenia · chest pain · chills · concentration impaired · constipation · cough · depression · diarrhoea · dizziness · dry mouth · dyspnoea · fever · gastrointestinal discomfort · gastroesophageal reflux disease · headaches · influenza like illness · insomnia · irritability · memory loss · muscle complaints · nasopharyngitis · nausea · neutropenia · pain · skin reactions · vision blurred · vomiting · weight decreased
  - **Frequency not known** Hepatitis B reactivation · Stevens-Johnson syndrome

SIDE-EFFECTS, FURTHER INFORMATION Side-effects listed are reported when sofosbuvir is used in combination with ribavirin or with ribavirin and peginterferon alfa.

- **PREGNANCY** Manufacturer advises avoid—limited information available.
- **BREAST FEEDING** Manufacturer advises avoid—present in milk in *animal* studies.
- **RENAL IMPAIRMENT** See p. 16. EvGr Caution if estimated glomerular filtration rate is less than 30 mL/minute/1.73 m^2 (accumulation may occur; limited information available). ⟨M⟩
- **DIRECTIONS FOR ADMINISTRATION** Granules may be swallowed or mixed with non-acidic soft food that is at or below room temperature, and swallowed within 30 minutes without chewing.
- **PATIENT AND CARER ADVICE** Patients or carers should be given advice on how to administer granules.

Vomiting If vomiting occurs within 2 hours of administration, an additional dose should be taken.
Missed doses If a dose is more than 18 hours late, the missed dose should not be taken and the next dose should be taken at the normal time.
Driving and skilled tasks Patients and carers should be cautioned on the effects on driving and performance of skilled tasks—increased risk of dizziness, impaired concentration, and blurred vision.

- **MEDICINAL FORMS** There can be variation in the licensing of different medicines containing the same drug.

Oral tablet

CAUTIONARY AND ADVISORY LABELS 21, 25

- Sovaldi (Gilead Sciences Ltd)

Sofosbuvir 400 mg Sovaldi 400mg tablets | 28 tablet PoM £11,660.98 (Hospital only)

Sofosbuvir with velpatasvir

22-Mar-2023

The properties listed below are those particular to the combination only. For the properties of the components please consider, sofosbuvir above.

- **DRUG ACTION** Sofosbuvir is a nucleotide analogue inhibitor and velpatasvir is an HCV inhibitor; they reduce viral load by inhibiting hepatitis C virus RNA replication.

- **INDICATIONS AND DOSE**

Chronic hepatitis C infection (under expert supervision)

- BY MOUTH USING GRANULES
  - Child 3–17 years (body-weight up to 17 kg): 150/37.5 mg once daily for 12 weeks

▸ BY MOUTH
▸ Child 3–17 years (body-weight 17–29 kg): 200/50 mg once daily for 12 weeks
▸ Child 3–17 years (body-weight 30 kg and above): 400/100 mg once daily for 12 weeks

DOSE ADJUSTMENTS DUE TO INTERACTIONS
▸ Manufacturer advises reduce dose of concurrent H_2-receptor antagonist if above a dose comparable to famotidine 40 mg twice daily.
▸ Manufacturer advises reduce dose of concurrent proton pump inhibitor if above a dose comparable to omeprazole 20 mg; take 4 hours after sofosbuvir with velpatasvir.

DOSE EQUIVALENCE AND CONVERSION
▸ Dose expressed as *x*/*y* mg sofosbuvir/velpatasvir.

● **INTERACTIONS** → Appendix 1: sofosbuvir · velpatasvir
● **SIDE-EFFECTS**
▸ **Common or very common** Rash · vomiting
▸ **Uncommon** Angioedema
▸ **Frequency not known** Fatigue · headache · hepatitis B reactivation · nausea · Stevens-Johnson syndrome

● **DIRECTIONS FOR ADMINISTRATION** Granules may be swallowed or mixed with non-acidic soft food that is at or below room temperature, and swallowed within 15 minutes without chewing.

● **PATIENT AND CARER ADVICE** Patients or carers should be given advice on how to administer granules.
Vomiting If vomiting occurs within 3 hours of administration, an additional dose should be taken.
Missed doses If a dose is more than 18 hours late, the missed dose should not be taken and the next dose should be taken at the normal time.

● **NATIONAL FUNDING/ACCESS DECISIONS**
For full details see funding body website

All Wales Medicines Strategy Group (AWMSG) decisions
▸ **Sofosbuvir with velpatasvir (*Epclusa*®) for the treatment of chronic hepatitis C virus (HCV) infection in patients from 3 years of age to less than 18 years of age (February 2023)** AWMSG No. 4573 Recommended

● **MEDICINAL FORMS** There can be variation in the licensing of different medicines containing the same drug.

Oral tablet
CAUTIONARY AND ADVISORY LABELS 25
▸ **Epclusa** (Gilead Sciences Ltd)
Velpatasvir 50 mg, Sofosbuvir 200 mg Epclusa 200mg/50mg tablets | 28 tablet [PoM] £12,993.33 (Hospital only)
Velpatasvir 100 mg, Sofosbuvir 400 mg Epclusa 400mg/100mg tablets | 28 tablet [PoM] £12,993.33 (Hospital only)

Oral granules
CAUTIONARY AND ADVISORY LABELS 25
▸ **Epclusa** (Gilead Sciences Ltd)
Velpatasvir 37.5 mg, Sofosbuvir 150 mg Epclusa 150mg/37.5mg granules sachets | 28 sachet [PoM] £12,993.33 (Hospital only) [SF]
Velpatasvir 50 mg, Sofosbuvir 200 mg Epclusa 200mg/50mg granules sachets | 28 sachet [PoM] £12,993.33 (Hospital only) [SF]

ANTIVIRALS > PROTEASE INHIBITORS, HEPATITIS

Glecaprevir with pibrentasvir
08-Dec-2021

● **INDICATIONS AND DOSE**

Chronic hepatitis C (specialist use only)
▸ BY MOUTH
▸ Child 12–17 years: 300/120 mg once daily, for duration of treatment, consult product literature

DOSE EQUIVALENCE AND CONVERSION
▸ Dose expressed as x/y mg glecaprevir/pibrentasvir.

IMPORTANT SAFETY INFORMATION

HEPATITIS B INFECTION
Cases of hepatitis B reactivation, sometimes fatal, have been reported in patients co-infected with hepatitis B and C viruses; manufacturer advises to assess patients for hepatitis B prior to initiation of therapy and manage according to current clinical guidelines.

MHRA/CHM ADVICE: DIRECT-ACTING ANTIVIRALS TO TREAT CHRONIC HEPATITIS C: RISK OF INTERACTION WITH VITAMIN K ANTAGONISTS AND CHANGES IN INR (JANUARY 2017)
An EU-wide review has identified that changes in liver function, secondary to hepatitis C treatment with direct-acting antivirals, may affect the efficacy of vitamin K antagonists; the MHRA has advised that INR should be monitored closely in patients receiving concomitant treatment.

MHRA/CHM ADVICE: DIRECT-ACTING ANTIVIRALS FOR CHRONIC HEPATITIS C: RISK OF HYPOGLYCAEMIA IN PATIENTS WITH DIABETES (DECEMBER 2018)
Rapid reduction in hepatitis C viral load during direct-acting antiviral therapy for hepatitis C may improve glucose metabolism in patients with diabetes and result in symptomatic hypoglycaemia if diabetic treatment is continued at the same dose.

The MHRA advises healthcare professionals:
- to monitor glucose levels closely in patients with diabetes during direct-acting antiviral therapy for hepatitis C, especially within the first 3 months of treatment and modify diabetic medication or doses when necessary;
- to be vigilant for changes in glucose tolerance and advise patients of the risk of hypoglycaemia;
- to inform the healthcare professional in charge of the diabetic care of the patient when direct-acting antiviral therapy is initiated.

● **CAUTIONS** Hepatitis B infection · post-liver transplant patients · re-treatment of patients with prior exposure to NS3/4A- or NS5A-inhibitors—efficacy not established
● **INTERACTIONS** → Appendix 1: glecaprevir · pibrentasvir
● **SIDE-EFFECTS**
▸ **Common or very common** Asthenia · diarrhoea · headache · nausea
▸ **Uncommon** Angioedema
▸ **Frequency not known** Hepatitis B reactivation · pruritus · transient ischaemic attack
● **PREGNANCY** Manufacturer advises avoid—limited information available.
● **BREAST FEEDING** Manufacturer advises avoid—present in milk in *animal* studies.
● **HEPATIC IMPAIRMENT** Manufacturer advises avoid in moderate to severe impairment (risk of increased exposure).
● **PATIENT AND CARER ADVICE**
Missed doses Manufacturer advises if a dose is more than 18 hours late, the missed dose should not be taken and the next dose should be taken at the normal time.
● **NATIONAL FUNDING/ACCESS DECISIONS**
For full details see funding body website

Scottish Medicines Consortium (SMC) decisions
▸ **Glecaprevir with pibrentasvir (*Mavire*t®) for the treatment of chronic hepatitis C virus (HCV) infection in adolescents aged 12 years up to 18 years (November 2019)** SMC No. SMC2214 Recommended

All Wales Medicines Strategy Group (AWMSG) decisions
▸ **Glecaprevir with pibrentasvir (*Maviret*®) granules for the treatment of chronic hepatitis C virus (HCV) infection in**

5 Infection

children aged 3 years up to 12 years (November 2021) AWMSG No. 4917 Recommended
- **Glecaprevir with pibrentasvir (*Maviret*®) tablets for the treatment of chronic hepatitis C virus (HCV) infection in adolescents aged 12 years up to 18 years (November 2021)** AWMSG No. 4917 Recommended

- **MEDICINAL FORMS** There can be variation in the licensing of different medicines containing the same drug.

Oral tablet

CAUTIONARY AND ADVISORY LABELS 21, 25
- Glecaprevir with pibrentasvir (Non-proprietary)
  Pibrentasvir 40 mg, Glecaprevir 100 mg Glecaprevir 100mg / Pibrentasvir 40mg tablets | 84 tablet PoM £12,993.66 (Hospital only)

IMMUNOSTIMULANTS > INTERFERONS

Peginterferon alfa

15-Dec-2021

- **DRUG ACTION** Polyethylene glycol-conjugated ('pegylated') derivatives of interferon alfa (**peginterferon alfa-2a** and **peginterferon alfa-2b**) are available; pegylation increases the persistence of the interferon in the blood.

- **INDICATIONS AND DOSE**

PEGASYS®

Chronic hepatitis C (in combination with ribavirin) in previously untreated children without liver decompensation
- BY SUBCUTANEOUS INJECTION
- Child 5-17 years: (consult product literature)

- **CONTRA-INDICATIONS** Severe psychiatric illness

CONTRA-INDICATIONS, FURTHER INFORMATION For contra-indications consult product literature.
- **CAUTIONS** For cautions consult product literature.
- **INTERACTIONS** → Appendix 1: interferons
- **SIDE-EFFECTS**
- **Common or very common** Alopecia · anaemia · anxiety · appetite decreased · arthralgia · asthenia · behaviour abnormal · chills · concentration impaired · cough · depression · diabetes mellitus · diarrhoea · dizziness · drowsiness · dyspnoea · ear pain · eye discomfort · face oedema · feeling cold · fever · flushing · gastrointestinal discomfort · growth retardation · haemorrhage · headaches · hypotension · hypothyroidism · increased risk of infection · influenza like illness · laryngeal pain · leucopenia · lymphadenopathy · malaise · mood altered · muscle complaints · nausea · neutropenia · oral disorders · pain · palpitations · skin reactions · sleep disorders · syncope · tachycardia · taste altered · thrombocytopenia · urinary disorders · urinary tract disorder · vertigo · vision disorders · vomiting
- **Uncommon** Akathisia · chest discomfort · dysmenorrhoea · hallucination · hypersensitivity · keratitis · muscle contractions involuntary · nasal complaints · pallor · photosensitivity reaction · proteinuria · retinal exudate · sensation abnormal · tremor · vaginal discharge · wheezing

SIDE-EFFECTS, FURTHER INFORMATION Respiratory symptoms should be investigated and if pulmonary infiltrates are suspected or lung function is impaired the discontinuation of peginterferon alfa should be considered.
- **CONCEPTION AND CONTRACEPTION** Effective contraception required during treatment—consult product literature.
- **PREGNANCY** Manufacturers recommend avoid unless potential benefit outweighs risk (toxicity in *animal* studies).
- **BREAST FEEDING** Manufacturers advise avoid—no information available.
- **HEPATIC IMPAIRMENT** Manufacturer advises avoid in severe impairment and decompensated cirrhosis.
- **RENAL IMPAIRMENT**

Dose adjustments See p. 16.

In adults, manufacturer advises reduce dose if creatinine clearance less than 30 mL/minute (consult product literature).
- **MONITORING REQUIREMENTS**
- Monitoring of lipid concentration is recommended.
- Monitoring of hepatic function is recommended.
- **NATIONAL FUNDING/ACCESS DECISIONS**

For full details see funding body website

NICE decisions
- **Peginterferon alfa and ribavirin for treating chronic hepatitis C in children and young people (November 2013) NICE TA300** Recommended

- **MEDICINAL FORMS** There can be variation in the licensing of different medicines containing the same drug.

Solution for injection

EXCIPIENTS: May contain Benzyl alcohol
- Pegasys (pharmaand GmbH)
  Interferon alfa-2a (as Peginterferon alfa-2a) 180 microgram per 1 ml Pegasys 90micrograms/0.5ml solution for injection pre-filled syringes | 1 pre-filled disposable injection PoM £76.51 (Hospital only)
  Interferon alfa-2a (as Peginterferon alfa-2a) 270 microgram per 1 ml Pegasys 135micrograms/0.5ml solution for injection pre-filled syringes | 1 pre-filled disposable injection PoM £107.76 (Hospital only)
  Interferon alfa-2a (as Peginterferon alfa-2a) 360 microgram per 1 ml Pegasys 180micrograms/0.5ml solution for injection pre-filled syringes | 4 pre-filled disposable injection PoM £497.60 (Hospital only)

5.4 Herpesvirus infections

Herpesvirus infections

13-Oct-2025

Herpes simplex infections

Herpes infection of the mouth and lips and in the eye is generally associated with herpes simplex virus serotype 1 (HSV-1); other areas of the skin may also be infected, especially in immunodeficiency. Genital infection is most often associated with HSV-2 and also HSV-1.

EvGr Topical antiviral treatment is not routinely recommended in immunocompetent children with uncomplicated infection of the lips (herpes labialis or cold sores) or herpetic gingivostomatitis. However, some children may find application of a topical antiviral drug helpful when used from the onset of the prodromal phase. Oral paracetamol p. 325 and/or ibuprofen p. 821 may be given to relieve pain and fever. Other preparations that may be considered for symptom relief include topical anaesthetics or analgesics, and mouthwashes. Oral antiviral treatment may be considered in children with severe, frequent or persistent oral infection.

Primary or recurrent genital herpes simplex infection is treated with an antiviral drug given by mouth.

Children suspected of having ocular herpes simplex infection should be referred for urgent, same-day specialist referral; treatment should not be initiated whilst awaiting review. If same-day review is not possible, specialist advice should be sought which may include topical antiviral treatment in primary care. Some optometrists with appropriate expertise and training can initiate topical antiviral treatment in certain suspected cases.

Refer or seek specialist advice for treatment of herpes simplex infection in pregnancy. Ⓐ

Neonatal herpes is a notifiable disease in England. For further information, see *Notifiable diseases* in Antibacterials, principles of therapy p. 358.

Varicella-zoster infections

Varicella (chickenpox) is an acute disease caused by the varicella-zoster virus. EvGr Specialist advice should be sought on the management of chickenpox in neonates due to the higher risk of severe disease and complications. Chickenpox in otherwise healthy children is usually self-limiting and complications are rare; antiviral treatment is not routinely recommended.

Chickenpox is more severe in adolescents (aged 14 years and over) and adults than in children; antiviral treatment started within 24 hours of the onset of rash may be considered, particularly for those with severe infection or at risk of complications. Specialist advice should be sought on the diagnosis and management of chickenpox in immunocompromised children. Ⓐ

Pregnant females who develop severe chickenpox may be at risk of complications, especially varicella pneumonia. EvGr Immediate specialist advice should be sought for the treatment of chickenpox during pregnancy. Ⓐ

Chickenpox is a notifiable disease in England and Northern Ireland. For further information, see *Notifiable diseases* in Antibacterials, principles of therapy p. 358.

Herpes zoster (shingles) is a viral infection of an individual nerve and the skin surface affected by the nerve. The infection is caused by the reactivation of the varicella-zoster virus, the same virus that causes chickenpox. EvGr Immunocompetent children do not usually require treatment. Oral antiviral treatment should be offered to children with shingles who have non-truncal involvement (e.g. neck, limbs, perineum), or those with moderate to severe pain or rash. Treatment with the antiviral should be started within 72 hours of the onset of rash. All immunocompromised children or those with shingles in the ophthalmic distribution of the trigeminal nerve, should be admitted to hospital or specialist advice should be sought. Ⓐ

Chronic pain which persists after the rash has healed (post-herpetic neuralgia) requires specific management. For further information, see Neuropathic pain p. 348.

The risk and incidence of varicella-zoster infections can be reduced through vaccination of selected individuals. For further information, see Varicella-zoster vaccines p. 983.

Post-exposure prophylaxis

UKHSA recommends post-exposure prophylaxis to attenuate disease and reduce the risk of complications (such as pneumonitis) in individuals at increased risk of severe chickenpox, such as neonates (especially in the first 7 days of life), certain children aged under 1 year, pregnant females, and immunosuppressed children, who have had a significant exposure to varicella-zoster virus during the infectious period and who are susceptible to the virus.

Neonates whose mothers develop chickenpox (but not shingles) 7 days before, or 7 days after delivery, should be given intravenous varicella-zoster immunoglobulin p. 958 (VZIG) [unlicensed] as soon as possible following exposure. If VZIG cannot be commenced within 96 hours of exposure, intravenous normal immunoglobulin p. 955 (IVIG) [unlicensed use] should be given instead. Intravenous aciclovir p. 500 [unlicensed use] should also be commenced as soon as possible after exposure, and continued until day 21 post-delivery; after a minimum of 48 hours, treatment can be switched to oral aciclovir [unlicensed use].

For all other susceptible patient groups who are non-immune, post-exposure prophylaxis with oral aciclovir [unlicensed use] is recommended. This includes pregnant females, immunosuppressed children, neonates exposed to chickenpox or shingles other than in the mother in the first 7 days of life, children aged under 1 year who have remained in hospital since birth who were either born before 28 weeks gestation or weighed less than 1000 g at birth, or children who have a severe congenital or other underlying condition that requires prolonged intensive or special care during the first year of life. Valaciclovir p. 502 [unlicensed use] can be used as an alternative to aciclovir as appropriate for children over the age of 3 months, but should only be used on specialist advice in children under the age of 2 years. Children on long term aciclovir or valaciclovir prophylaxis may require their dose to be temporarily increased. Oral antivirals may also be considered for other groups who have increased risk of severe disease, such as those with neurodisabilities. In susceptible children where antivirals are contra-indicated or otherwise unsuitable (e.g. if there are significant concerns about renal impairment or intestinal malabsorption), intravenous normal immunoglobulin (IVIG) [unlicensed use] may be considered instead.

For further information on risk assessment and post-exposure guidance for specific risk groups, including guidance on subsequent exposures, see UKHSA guidance: **Guidelines on post exposure prophylaxis (PEP) for varicella or shingles** (available at: www.gov.uk/government/publications/post-exposure-prophylaxis-for-chickenpox-and-shingles).

At-risk children who develop chickenpox despite post-exposure prophylaxis require treatment with an antiviral.

During outbreaks in nurseries and pre-school settings where chickenpox is co-circulating with group A streptococcus infections (such as scarlet fever), post-exposure prophylaxis with the chickenpox varicella-zoster vaccine p. 1004 may be given to certain non-immune individuals in these settings. For further guidance, see *Post-exposure management of varicella (chickenpox)* in Varicella-zoster vaccines p. 983.

Drug choice for treatment

Aciclovir is active against herpesviruses but does not eradicate them. EvGr Uses of aciclovir include systemic treatment of varicella-zoster and the systemic and topical treatment of herpes simplex infections of the skin and mucous membranes. Ⓐ Aciclovir eye ointment p. 847 is licensed for herpes simplex infections of the eye.

Valaciclovir p. 502 is an ester of aciclovir, licensed for herpes simplex infections of the skin and mucous membranes (including genital herpes), and for preventing cytomegalovirus disease following solid organ transplantation.

Cytomegalovirus infection

Cytomegalovirus (CMV) is a member of the herpesvirus group. In immunocompetent children, CMV infection is often asymptomatic and self-limiting therefore treatment is not always required. In immunocompromised children, the infection manifests more severely causing diseases associated with greater morbidity and mortality.

Drugs licensed for use in the management of CMV disease include ganciclovir p. 503 (related to aciclovir), valaciclovir, and valganciclovir p. 504 (an ester of ganciclovir). There is a possibility of ganciclovir resistance in those who repeatedly have a poor treatment response or when viral excretion continues despite treatment.

Foscarnet sodium p. 504 [unlicensed] is deposited in teeth, bone and cartilage, and *animal* studies have shown that deposition is greater in young animals. Its effect on skeletal development in children is not known.

ANTIVIRALS > NUCLEOSIDE ANALOGUES

Aciclovir
13-Oct-2025

(Acyclovir)

● **INDICATIONS AND DOSE**

Herpes simplex, treatment

▶ BY MOUTH

- Child 1–23 months: 100 mg 5 times a day usually for 5 days (longer if new lesions appear during treatment or if healing incomplete)
- Child 2–17 years: 200 mg 5 times a day usually for 5 days (longer if new lesions appear during treatment or if healing incomplete)

▶ BY INTRAVENOUS INFUSION

- Neonate: 20 mg/kg every 8 hours for 14 days (for at least 21 days if CNS involvement—confirm cerebrospinal fluid negative for herpes simplex virus before stopping treatment).

- Child 1–2 months: 20 mg/kg every 8 hours for 14 days (for at least 21 days if CNS involvement—confirm cerebrospinal fluid negative for herpes simplex virus before stopping treatment)
- Child 3 months–11 years: 250 mg/m^2 every 8 hours usually for 5 days
- Child 12–17 years: 5 mg/kg every 8 hours usually for 5 days

Herpes simplex, treatment, in immunocompromised or if absorption impaired

▶ BY MOUTH

- Child 1–23 months: 200 mg 5 times a day usually for 5 days (longer if new lesions appear during treatment or if healing incomplete)
- Child 2–17 years: 400 mg 5 times a day usually for 5 days (longer if new lesions appear during treatment or if healing incomplete)

Herpes simplex, treatment, in immunocompromised or in simplex encephalitis

▶ BY INTRAVENOUS INFUSION

- Child 3 months–11 years: 500 mg/m^2 every 8 hours usually for 5 days (given for at least 21 days in encephalitis—confirm cerebrospinal fluid negative for herpes simplex virus before stopping treatment)
- Child 12–17 years: 10 mg/kg every 8 hours usually for 5 days (given for at least 14 days in encephalitis and for at least 21 days if also immunocompromised—confirm cerebrospinal fluid negative for herpes simplex virus before stopping treatment)

Herpes simplex, suppression

▶ BY MOUTH

- Child 12–17 years: 400 mg twice daily, alternatively 200 mg 4 times a day; increased to 400 mg 3 times a day, dose may be increased if recurrences occur on standard suppressive therapy or for suppression of genital herpes during late pregnancy (from 36 weeks gestation)

Herpes simplex, prophylaxis in the immunocompromised

▶ BY MOUTH

- Child 1–23 months: 100–200 mg 4 times a day
- Child 2–17 years: 200–400 mg 4 times a day

Post-exposure prophylaxis of varicella zoster infection [neonates exposed to maternal chickenpox 7 days before or after delivery]

▶ BY INTRAVENOUS INFUSION

- Neonate: 20 mg/kg every 8 hours for 21 days post-delivery, after a minimum of 48 hours, treatment can be converted to oral if preferred.

Post-exposure prophylaxis of varicella zoster infection [neonates exposed to chickenpox or shingles other than in the mother in first 7 days of life]

▶ BY MOUTH

- Neonate: 20 mg/kg 4 times a day for 14 days, start course on day 7 after exposure.

Post-exposure prophylaxis of varicella zoster infection [infants who have remained in hospital since birth, or who require intensive or special care]

▶ BY MOUTH

- Neonate: 20 mg/kg 4 times a day for 14 days, start course on day 7 after exposure.

- Child 1–11 months: 10 mg/kg 4 times a day for 14 days, start course on day 7 after exposure

Post-exposure prophylaxis of varicella zoster infection

▶ BY MOUTH

- Child 1–23 months: 10 mg/kg 4 times a day for 7 days, start course on day 7 after exposure; if the patient presents after this, the course may be started up to day 14 after exposure
- Child 2–11 years: 10 mg/kg 4 times a day for 7 days, start course on day 7 after exposure; if the patient presents after this, the course may be started up to day 14 after exposure
- Child 12–17 years: 10 mg/kg 4 times a day (max. per dose 800 mg) for 7 days, start course on day 7 after exposure; if the patient presents after this, the course may be started up to day 14 after exposure

Varicella zoster (chickenpox), treatment | Herpes zoster (shingles), treatment

▶ BY MOUTH

- Child 1–23 months: 200 mg 4 times a day for 5 days
- Child 2–5 years: 400 mg 4 times a day for 5 days
- Child 6–11 years: 800 mg 4 times a day for 5 days
- Child 12–17 years: 800 mg 5 times a day for 7 days

▶ BY INTRAVENOUS INFUSION

- Neonate: 10–20 mg/kg every 8 hours for at least 7 days, higher end of dose range to be used if chickenpox develops despite prophylaxis with varicella-zoster immunoglobulin.

- Child 1–2 months: 10–20 mg/kg every 8 hours for at least 7 days
- Child 3 months–11 years: 250 mg/m^2 every 8 hours usually for 5 days
- Child 12–17 years: 5 mg/kg every 8 hours usually for 5 days

Varicella zoster (chickenpox), treatment in encephalitis | Herpes zoster (shingles), treatment in encephalitis

▶ BY INTRAVENOUS INFUSION

- Neonate: 10–20 mg/kg every 8 hours given for 10–14 days, possibly longer if also immunocompromised.

- Child 1–2 months: 10–20 mg/kg every 8 hours given for 10–14 days, possibly longer if also immunocompromised
- Child 3 months–11 years: 500 mg/m^2 every 8 hours given for 10–14 days, possibly longer if also immunocompromised
- Child 12–17 years: 10 mg/kg every 8 hours given for 10–14 days, possibly longer if also immunocompromised

Varicella zoster (chickenpox), treatment in immunocompromised

▶ BY INTRAVENOUS INFUSION

- Child 3 months–11 years: 500 mg/m^2 every 8 hours usually for 5 days

- Child 12–17 years: 10 mg/kg every 8 hours usually for 5 days

Herpes zoster (shingles), treatment in immunocompromised

- BY MOUTH
- Child 1–23 months: 200 mg 4 times a day continued for 2 days after crusting of lesions
- Child 2–5 years: 400 mg 4 times a day continued for 2 days after crusting of lesions
- Child 6–11 years: 800 mg 4 times a day continued for 2 days after crusting of lesions
- Child 12–17 years: 800 mg 5 times a day continued for 2 days after crusting of lesions
- BY INTRAVENOUS INFUSION
- Child 3 months–11 years: 500 mg/m^2 every 8 hours usually for 5 days
- Child 12–17 years: 10 mg/kg every 8 hours usually for 5 days

DOSES AT EXTREMES OF BODY-WEIGHT
- With intravenous use To avoid excessive dosage in obese patients, dose should be calculated on the basis of ideal body-weight for height.

● **UNLICENSED USE**
- With oral use UKHSA advises aciclovir is used for post-exposure prophylaxis of varicella zoster infection, but it is not licensed for this indication. Tablets and suspension not licensed for suppression of herpes simplex or for treatment of herpes zoster in children (age range not specified by manufacturer).
- With intravenous use Intravenous infusion not licensed for herpes zoster.
- With systemic use Aciclovir doses in BNF Publications may differ from those in product literature.

IMPORTANT SAFETY INFORMATION
- With intravenous use

Be aware that some doses are calculated either using mg/kg or mg/m^2, depending on the age of the child.

● **CAUTIONS** Maintain adequate hydration (especially with infusion or high doses)

● **INTERACTIONS** → Appendix 1: aciclovir

● **SIDE-EFFECTS**

GENERAL SIDE-EFFECTS
- **Common or very common** Abdominal pain · diarrhoea · dizziness · fatigue · fever · headache · nausea · photosensitivity reaction · skin reactions · vomiting
- **Uncommon** Anaemia · leucopenia · thrombocytopenia
- **Rare or very rare** Agitation · angioedema · ataxia · coma · confusion · drowsiness · dysarthria · dyspnoea · encephalopathy · hallucination · hepatic disorders · psychosis · renal impairment · renal pain · seizure · tremor
- **Frequency not known** Crystalluria

SPECIFIC SIDE-EFFECTS
- **Rare or very rare**
  - With intravenous use Inflammation localised
- **Frequency not known**
  - With oral use Alopecia

● **PREGNANCY** Not known to be harmful—manufacturers advise use only when potential benefit outweighs risk.

● **BREAST FEEDING** Significant amount in milk after systemic administration—not known to be harmful but manufacturer advises caution.

● **RENAL IMPAIRMENT** See p. 16.

Risk of neurological reactions increased. Maintain adequate hydration (especially during renal impairment).

Dose adjustments Consider dose reduction.
- With intravenous use Use *normal intravenous dose* every 12 hours if estimated glomerular filtration rate 25–50 mL/minute/1.73 m^2 (every 24 hours if estimated glomerular filtration rate 10–25 mL/minute/1.73 m^2). Consult product literature for intravenous dose if estimated glomerular filtration rate less than 10 mL/minute/1.73 m^2.
- With oral use For *herpes zoster*, use normal oral dose every 8 hours if estimated glomerular filtration rate 10–25 mL/minute/1.73 m^2 (every 12 hours if estimated glomerular filtration rate less than 10 mL/minute/1.73 m^2). For *herpes simplex*, use normal dose every 12 hours if estimated glomerular filtration rate less than 10 mL/minute/1.73 m^2.

● **DIRECTIONS FOR ADMINISTRATION** For *intravenous infusion*, reconstitute to 25 mg/mL with Water for Injections or Sodium Chloride 0.9% then dilute to concentration of 5 mg/mL with Sodium Chloride 0.9% or Sodium Chloride and Glucose and give over 1 hour; alternatively, may be administered in a concentration of 25 mg/mL using a suitable infusion pump and central venous access and given over 1 hour.

● **PRESCRIBING AND DISPENSING INFORMATION** For further information on *herpes simplex*, *varicella zoster*, and *herpes zoster*, see Herpesvirus infections p. 498.

Flavours of oral liquid preparations may include banana, or orange.
- With oral use for Herpes simplex, suppression Interrupt therapy every 6–12 months to reassess recurrence frequency—consider restarting after two or more recurrences.

● **PATIENT AND CARER ADVICE**
Medicines for Children leaflet: Aciclovir (oral) for viral infections www.medicinesforchildren.org.uk/medicines/aciclovir-oral-for-viral-infections/

● **PROFESSION SPECIFIC INFORMATION**
Dental practitioners' formulary Aciclovir Tablets 200 mg or 800 mg may be prescribed. Aciclovir Oral Suspension 200 mg/5mL may be prescribed.

● **MEDICINAL FORMS** There can be variation in the licensing of different medicines containing the same drug.

Oral tablet

CAUTIONARY AND ADVISORY LABELS 9
- **Aciclovir (Non-proprietary)**
  - **Aciclovir 200 mg** Aciclovir 200mg tablets | 25 tablet PoM £2.28 DT = £0.98
  - **Aciclovir 400 mg** Aciclovir 400mg tablets | 56 tablet PoM £6.00 DT = £2.18
  - **Aciclovir 800 mg** Aciclovir 800mg tablets | 35 tablet PoM £8.40 DT = £2.37

Dispersible tablet

CAUTIONARY AND ADVISORY LABELS 9
- **Aciclovir (Non-proprietary)**
  - **Aciclovir 200 mg** Aciclovir 200mg dispersible tablets | 25 tablet PoM £1.32 DT = £1.15
  - **Aciclovir 400 mg** Aciclovir 400mg dispersible tablets | 56 tablet PoM £4.55 DT = £4.08
  - **Aciclovir 800 mg** Aciclovir 800mg dispersible tablets | 35 tablet PoM £5.68 DT = £4.80
- **Zovirax** (GlaxoSmithKline UK Ltd)
  - **Aciclovir 200 mg** Zovirax 200mg dispersible tablets | 25 tablet PoM £2.85 DT = £1.15

Oral suspension

CAUTIONARY AND ADVISORY LABELS 9
- **Aciclovir (Non-proprietary)**
  - **Aciclovir 40 mg per 1 ml** Aciclovir 200mg/5ml oral suspension sugar free | 125 ml PoM £32.00 DT = £27.97 SF
  - **Aciclovir 80 mg per 1 ml** Aciclovir 400mg/5ml oral suspension sugar free | 100 ml PoM £38.80 DT = £31.00 SF
- **Zovirax** (GlaxoSmithKline UK Ltd)
  - **Aciclovir 40 mg per 1 ml** Zovirax 200mg/5ml oral suspension | 125 ml PoM £29.56 DT = £27.97 SF
  - **Aciclovir 80 mg per 1 ml** Zovirax Double Strength 400mg/5ml oral suspension | 100 ml PoM £33.02 DT = £31.00 SF

Solution for infusion

ELECTROLYTES: May contain Sodium

▸ **Aciclovir (Non-proprietary)**

Aciclovir (as Aciclovir sodium) 25 mg per 1 ml Aciclovir 250mg/10ml concentrate for solution for infusion vials | 5 vial PoM £50.00–£55.00 (Hospital only)

Aciclovir 1g/40ml concentrate for solution for infusion vials | 1 vial PoM £40.00 (Hospital only)

Aciclovir 500mg/20ml concentrate for solution for infusion vials | 5 vial PoM £100.00–£110.00 (Hospital only)

Powder for solution for infusion

ELECTROLYTES: May contain Sodium

▸ **Aciclovir (Non-proprietary)**

Aciclovir (as Aciclovir sodium) 250 mg Aciclovir 250mg powder for solution for Infusion vials | 5 vial PoM £16.50 (Hospital only)

Aciclovir 250mg powder for solution for infusion vials | 5 vial PoM £49.30 (Hospital only) | 10 vial PoM £91.30–£98.60 (Hospital only)

Aciclovir (as Aciclovir sodium) 500 mg Aciclovir 500mg powder for solution for infusion vials | 10 vial PoM £182.00 (Hospital only)

▸ **Zovirax I.V.** (GlaxoSmithKline UK Ltd)

Aciclovir (as Aciclovir sodium) 250 mg Zovirax I.V. 250mg powder for solution for infusion vials | 5 vial PoM £16.70 (Hospital only)

Aciclovir (as Aciclovir sodium) 500 mg Zovirax I.V. 500mg powder for solution for infusion vials | 5 vial PoM £17.00 (Hospital only)

Valaciclovir

23-Sep-2022

● **INDICATIONS AND DOSE**

Post-exposure prophylaxis of varicella zoster infection

▸ BY MOUTH

▸ Child 2–17 years: 20 mg/kg 3 times a day (max. per dose 1000 mg) for 7 days, start course on day 7 after exposure; if the patient presents after this, the course may be started up to day 14 after exposure

Herpes zoster infection, treatment in immunocompromised patients

▸ BY MOUTH

▸ Child 12–17 years: 1 g 3 times a day for at least 7 days and continued for 2 days after crusting of lesions

Herpes simplex, treatment of first infective episode

▸ BY MOUTH

▸ Child 12–17 years: 500 mg twice daily for 5 days (longer if new lesions appear during treatment or healing is incomplete)

Herpes simplex infections treatment of first episode in immunocompromised or HIV-positive patients

▸ BY MOUTH

▸ Child 12–17 years: 1 g twice daily for 10 days

Herpes simplex, treatment of recurrent infections

▸ BY MOUTH

▸ Child 12–17 years: 500 mg twice daily for 3–5 days

Treatment of recurrent herpes simplex infections in immunocompromised or HIV-positive patients

▸ BY MOUTH

▸ Child 12–17 years: 1 g twice daily for 5–10 days

Herpes labialis treatment

▸ BY MOUTH

▸ Child 12–17 years: Initially 2 g, then 2 g after 12 hours

Herpes simplex, suppression of infections

▸ BY MOUTH

▸ Child 12–17 years: 500 mg daily in 1–2 divided doses, therapy to be interrupted every 6–12 months to reassess recurrence frequency—consider restarting after two or more recurrences

Herpes simplex, suppression of infections in immunocompromised or HIV-positive patients

▸ BY MOUTH

▸ Child 12–17 years: 500 mg twice daily, therapy to be interrupted every 6–12 months to reassess recurrence frequency—consider restarting after two or more recurrences

Prevention of cytomegalovirus disease following solid organ transplantation when valganciclovir or ganciclovir cannot be used

▸ BY MOUTH

▸ Child 12–17 years: 2 g 4 times a day usually for 90 days, preferably starting within 72 hours of transplantation

● **UNLICENSED USE** UKHSA advises valaciclovir is used for post-exposure prophylaxis of varicella zoster infection, but it is not licensed for this indication.

Not licensed for treatment of herpes zoster in children.

Not licensed for treatment or suppression of herpes simplex infection in immunocompromised or HIV-positive children.

● **CAUTIONS** Maintain adequate hydration (especially with high doses)

● **INTERACTIONS** → Appendix 1: valaciclovir

● **SIDE-EFFECTS**

▸ **Common or very common** Diarrhoea · dizziness · headache · nausea · photosensitivity reaction · skin reactions · vomiting

▸ **Uncommon** Abdominal discomfort · agitation · confusion · dyspnoea · haematuria · hallucination · leucopenia · level of consciousness decreased · renal pain · thrombocytopenia · tremor

▸ **Rare or very rare** Angioedema · ataxia · coma · delirium · dysarthria · encephalopathy · nephrolithiasis · psychosis · renal impairment · seizure

▸ **Frequency not known** Microangiopathic haemolytic anaemia

SIDE-EFFECTS, FURTHER INFORMATION Neurological reactions more frequent with higher doses.

● **PREGNANCY** Not known to be harmful—manufacturers advise use only when potential benefit outweighs risk.

● **BREAST FEEDING** Significant amount in milk after systemic administration—not known to be harmful but manufacturer advises caution.

● **HEPATIC IMPAIRMENT** Manufacturer advises caution with doses of 4 g or more per day (no information available).

● **RENAL IMPAIRMENT** See p. 16. Maintain adequate hydration.

Dose adjustments Consider dose reduction.

For *herpes zoster*, 1 g every 12 hours if estimated glomerular filtration rate 30–50 mL/minute/1.73 m^2 (1 g every 24 hours if estimated glomerular filtration rate 10–30 mL/minute/1.73 m^2; 500 mg every 24 hours if estimated glomerular filtration rate less than 10 mL/minute/1.73 m^2).

For *treatment of herpes simplex*, 500 mg (1 g in immunocompromised or HIV-positive children) every 24 hours if estimated glomerular filtration rate less than 30 mL/minute/1.73 m^2.

For *treatment of herpes labialis*, if estimated glomerular filtration rate 30–50 mL/minute/1.73 m^2, initially 1 g, then 1 g 12 hours after initial dose (if estimated glomerular filtration rate 10–30 mL/minute/1.73 m^2, initially 500 mg, then 500 mg 12 hours after initial dose; if estimated glomerular filtration rate less than 10 mL/minute/1.73 m^2, 500 mg as a single dose).

For *suppression of herpes simplex*, 250 mg (500 mg in immunocompromised or HIV-positive children) every 24 hours if estimated glomerular filtration rate less than 30 mL/minute/1.73 m^2.

Reduce dose according to estimated glomerular filtration rate for *cytomegalovirus prophylaxis* following solid organ transplantation (consult product literature).

● **PRESCRIBING AND DISPENSING INFORMATION** Valaciclovir is a pro-drug of aciclovir.

- **MEDICINAL FORMS** There can be variation in the licensing of different medicines containing the same drug. Forms available from special-order manufacturers include: oral suspension

Oral tablet

CAUTIONARY AND ADVISORY LABELS 9

- Valaciclovir (Non-proprietary)
  - **Valaciclovir (as Valaciclovir hydrochloride) 250 mg** Valaciclovir 250mg tablets | 60 tablet PoM £123.28 DT = £123.28
  - **Valaciclovir (as Valaciclovir hydrochloride) 500 mg** Valaciclovir 500mg tablets | 10 tablet PoM £25.00 DT = £12.20 | 42 tablet PoM £16.46–£86.30
  - **Valaciclovir (as Valaciclovir hydrochloride) 1 gram** Valaciclovir 1g tablets | 10 tablet PoM £33.98 DT = £33.98 | 21 tablet PoM £71.36–£73.47
- Valtrex (GlaxoSmithKline UK Ltd)
  - **Valaciclovir (as Valaciclovir hydrochloride) 250 mg** Valtrex 250mg tablets | 60 tablet PoM £123.28 DT = £123.28
  - **Valaciclovir (as Valaciclovir hydrochloride) 500 mg** Valtrex 500mg tablets | 10 tablet PoM £20.59 DT = £12.20 | 42 tablet PoM £86.30

5.4a Cytomegalovirus infections

ANTIVIRALS > NUCLEOSIDE ANALOGUES

Ganciclovir

15-Dec-2020

- **INDICATIONS AND DOSE**

Prevention of cytomegalovirus disease [pre-emptive therapy in patients with drug-induced immunosuppression]

▶ BY INTRAVENOUS INFUSION

- Child 12–17 years: Initially 5 mg/kg every 12 hours for 7–14 days, then maintenance 5 mg/kg once daily, alternatively maintenance 6 mg/kg 5 times a week

Prevention of cytomegalovirus disease [universal prophylaxis in patients with drug-induced immunosuppression]

▶ BY INTRAVENOUS INFUSION

- Neonate: (consult product literature).
- Child 1 month–16 years: (consult product literature)
- Child 17 years: 5 mg/kg once daily, alternatively 6 mg/kg 5 times a week

Treatment of cytomegalovirus disease [in immunocompromised patients]

▶ BY INTRAVENOUS INFUSION

- Child: Initially 5 mg/kg every 12 hours for 14–21 days, then maintenance 5 mg/kg once daily, alternatively maintenance 6 mg/kg 5 times weekly, maintenance only for patients at risk of relapse; if disease progresses initial induction treatment may be repeated

Congenital cytomegalovirus infection of the CNS

▶ BY INTRAVENOUS INFUSION

- Neonate: 6 mg/kg every 12 hours for 6 weeks.

- **UNLICENSED USE** Not licensed for use in children under 12 years for the treatment of cytomegalovirus disease in immunocompromised patients.

  Not licensed for congenital cytomegalovirus infection of the CNS.

- **CONTRA-INDICATIONS** Abnormally low haemoglobin count (consult product literature) · abnormally low neutrophil count (consult product literature) · abnormally low platelet count (consult product literature)
- **CAUTIONS** History of cytopenia · potential carcinogen (including long-term carcinogenicity) · potential teratogen (including long-term teratogenicity) · radiotherapy
- **INTERACTIONS** → Appendix 1: ganciclovir
- **SIDE-EFFECTS**
  - **Common or very common** Anaemia · anxiety · appetite decreased · arthralgia · asthenia · bone marrow disorders · chest pain · chills · confusion · constipation · cough · depression · diarrhoea · dizziness · dysphagia · dyspnoea · ear pain · eye disorders · eye inflammation · eye pain · fever · flatulence · gastrointestinal discomfort · headache · hepatic function abnormal · increased risk of infection · insomnia · leucopenia · malaise · muscle complaints · nausea · neutropenia · night sweats · pain · peripheral neuropathy · renal impairment · seizure · sensation abnormal · sepsis · skin reactions · taste altered · thinking abnormal · thrombocytopenia · vomiting · weight decreased
  - **Uncommon** Alopecia · arrhythmia · deafness · haematuria · hypotension · infertility male · oral ulceration · pancreatitis · psychotic disorder · tremor · visual impairment
  - **Rare or very rare** Agranulocytosis · hallucination
- **ALLERGY AND CROSS-SENSITIVITY** EvGr Contra-indicated in patients hypersensitive to valganciclovir.

  Caution in patients hypersensitive to aciclovir, valaciclovir, or famciclovir. (M)

- **CONCEPTION AND CONTRACEPTION** Manufacturer advises women of childbearing potential should use effective contraception during and for at least 30 days after treatment; men with partners of childbearing potential should be advised to use barrier contraception during and for at least 90 days after treatment. Ganciclovir may cause temporary or permanent inhibition of spermatogenesis—impaired fertility observed in *animal* studies.
- **PREGNANCY** Manufacturer advises avoid unless potential benefit outweighs risk—teratogenicity in *animal* studies.
- **BREAST FEEDING** Manufacturer advises avoid—present in milk in *animal* studies.
- **RENAL IMPAIRMENT**

  Dose adjustments Manufacturer advises reduce dose for patients receiving mg/kg dosing if creatinine clearance less than 70 mL/minute—consult product literature. See p. 16.

- **MONITORING REQUIREMENTS** Monitor full blood count closely (severe deterioration may require correction and possibly treatment interruption).
- **DIRECTIONS FOR ADMINISTRATION** Manufacturer advises, for *intravenous infusion*, give intermittently in Glucose 5% or Sodium Chloride 0.9%. Reconstitute with Water for Injections (500 mg/10 mL) then dilute requisite dose to a concentration of not more than 10 mg/mL with infusion fluid; give over 1 hour into a vein with adequate flow, preferably using a plastic cannula.
- **HANDLING AND STORAGE**

  Caution in handling Ganciclovir is a potential teratogen and carcinogen. Manufacturer advises avoid inhalation of the powder or direct contact of the powder or reconstituted solution with the skin or mucous membranes; if contact occurs, wash thoroughly with soap and water; rinse eyes thoroughly with plain water.

- **MEDICINAL FORMS** There can be variation in the licensing of different medicines containing the same drug.

Powder for solution for infusion

ELECTROLYTES: May contain Sodium

- Ganciclovir (Non-proprietary)
  - **Ganciclovir (as Ganciclovir sodium) 500 mg** Ganciclovir 500mg powder for concentrate for solution for infusion vials | 5 vial PoM £145.00–£148.82 (Hospital only)
- Cymevene (Neon Healthcare Ltd)
  - **Ganciclovir (as Ganciclovir sodium) 500 mg** Cymevene 500mg powder for concentrate for solution for infusion vials | 5 vial PoM £148.83 (Hospital only)

Valganciclovir

06-Aug-2021

- **INDICATIONS AND DOSE**

Prevention of cytomegalovirus disease [following solid organ transplantation from a cytomegalovirus positive donor]

▶ BY MOUTH

▶ Neonate: (consult product literature).

▶ Child: (consult product literature)

- **CONTRA-INDICATIONS** Abnormally low haemoglobin count (consult product literature) · abnormally low neutrophil count (consult product literature) · abnormally low platelet count (consult product literature)
- **CAUTIONS** History of cytopenia · potential carcinogen (including long-term carcinogenicity) · potential teratogen (including long-term teratogenicity) · radiotherapy
- **INTERACTIONS** → Appendix 1: valganciclovir
- **SIDE-EFFECTS**

▶ **Common or very common** Anaemia · anxiety · appetite decreased · arthralgia · asthenia · bone marrow disorders · chest pain · confusion · constipation · cough · depression · diarrhoea · dizziness · dysphagia · dyspnoea · ear pain · eye disorders · eye inflammation · eye pain · flatulence · gastrointestinal discomfort · headache · hepatic function abnormal · increased risk of infection · insomnia · leucopenia · malaise · muscle complaints · nausea · neutropenia · night sweats · pain · peripheral neuropathy · renal impairment · seizure · sensation abnormal · sepsis · skin reactions · taste altered · thinking abnormal · thrombocytopenia · vomiting · weight decreased

▶ **Uncommon** Alopecia · arrhythmia · deafness · haematuria · hallucination · hypotension · infertility male · oral ulceration · pancreatitis · psychotic disorder · tremor · visual impairment

- **ALLERGY AND CROSS-SENSITIVITY** EvGr Contra-indicated in patients hypersensitive to ganciclovir.

  Caution in patients hypersensitive to aciclovir, valaciclovir, or famciclovir. ⟨M⟩
- **CONCEPTION AND CONTRACEPTION** Manufacturer advises women of childbearing potential should use effective contraception during and for at least 30 days after treatment; men with partners of childbearing potential should be advised to use barrier contraception during and for at least 90 days after treatment. *Ganciclovir* may cause temporary or permanent inhibition of spermatogenesis—impaired fertility observed in *animal* studies.
- **PREGNANCY** Manufacturer advises avoid unless potential benefit outweighs risk—teratogenicity observed with *ganciclovir* in *animal* studies.
- **BREAST FEEDING** Manufacturer advises avoid— *ganciclovir* present in milk in *animal* studies.
- **MONITORING REQUIREMENTS** Monitor full blood count closely (severe deterioration may require correction and possibly treatment interruption).
- **PRESCRIBING AND DISPENSING INFORMATION** Valganciclovir is a pro-drug of ganciclovir.

  Flavours of oral liquid formulations may include tutti-frutti.
- **HANDLING AND STORAGE** Manufacturer advises reconstituted powder for oral solution should be stored in a refrigerator (2–8°C) for up to 49 days.

  Caution in handling Valganciclovir is a potential teratogen and carcinogen. Manufacturer advises caution when handling the powder, reconstituted solution, or broken tablets and avoid inhalation of powder; if contact with skin or mucous membranes occurs, wash thoroughly with soap and water; rinse eyes thoroughly with plain water.
- **MEDICINAL FORMS** There can be variation in the licensing of different medicines containing the same drug. Forms available from special-order manufacturers include: oral solution

Oral tablet

CAUTIONARY AND ADVISORY LABELS 21

▶ Valganciclovir (Non-proprietary)

Valganciclovir (as Valganciclovir hydrochloride) 450 mg Valganciclovir 450mg tablets | 60 tablet PoM £1,081.46 DT = £1,081.46

▶ Valcyte (Neon Healthcare Ltd)

Valganciclovir (as Valganciclovir hydrochloride) 450 mg Valcyte 450mg tablets | 60 tablet PoM £1,081.46 DT = £1,081.46

Oral solution

CAUTIONARY AND ADVISORY LABELS 21

▶ Valcyte (Neon Healthcare Ltd)

Valganciclovir (as Valganciclovir hydrochloride) 50 mg per 1 ml Valcyte 50mg/ml oral solution | 88 ml PoM £230.32 DT = £230.32 SF

ANTIVIRALS › OTHER

Foscarnet sodium

27-Apr-2021

- **INDICATIONS AND DOSE**

Cytomegalovirus disease

▶ BY INTRAVENOUS INFUSION

▶ Child (under expert supervision): Initially 60 mg/kg every 8 hours 2–3 weeks, then maintenance 60 mg/kg daily, increased if tolerated to 90–120 mg/kg daily, if disease progresses on maintenance dose, repeat induction regimen

Mucocutaneous herpes simplex virus infections unresponsive to aciclovir in immunocompromised patients

▶ BY INTRAVENOUS INFUSION

▶ Child (under expert supervision): 40 mg/kg every 8 hours for 2–3 weeks or until lesions heal

- **UNLICENSED USE** Not licensed for use in children.
- **CAUTIONS** Conditions where excess sodium should be avoided · ensure adequate hydration
- **INTERACTIONS** → Appendix 1: foscarnet
- **SIDE-EFFECTS**

▶ **Common or very common** Aggression · anaemia · anxiety · appetite decreased · arrhythmias · asthenia · chest pain · chills · confusion · constipation · coordination abnormal · dehydration · depression · diarrhoea · dizziness · electrolyte imbalance · fever · gastrointestinal discomfort · genital discomfort (due to high concentrations excreted in urine) · genital ulceration (due to high concentrations excreted in urine) · haemorrhage · headache · hepatic function abnormal · hypertension · hypotension · leucopenia · malaise · muscle contractions involuntary · myalgia · nausea (reduce infusion rate) · neutropenia · numbness · oedema · palpitations · pancreatitis · paraesthesia (reduce infusion rate) · peripheral neuropathy · proteinuria · renal impairment · seizure · sepsis · skin reactions · thrombocytopenia · thrombophlebitis · tremor · urinary disorders · vomiting

▶ **Uncommon** Acidosis · angioedema · glomerulonephritis · nephropathy · pancytopenia

▶ **Frequency not known** Anaphylactoid reaction · diabetes insipidus · muscle weakness · myopathy · oesophageal ulcer · QT interval prolongation · renal pain · renal tubular acidosis · severe cutaneous adverse reactions (SCARs)

- **CONCEPTION AND CONTRACEPTION** Men should avoid fathering a child during and for 6 months after treatment.
- **PREGNANCY** Manufacturer advises avoid.
- **BREAST FEEDING** Avoid—present in milk in *animal* studies.
- **RENAL IMPAIRMENT** Manufacturer advises caution.

  Dose adjustments In adults, manufacturer advises dose reduction (consult product literature).

- **MONITORING REQUIREMENTS**
  - Monitor electrolytes, particularly calcium and magnesium.
  - Monitor serum creatinine every second day during induction and every week during maintenance.
- **DIRECTIONS FOR ADMINISTRATION** For *intravenous infusion*, manufacturer advises give undiluted solution via a central venous catheter; alternatively dilute to a concentration of 12 mg/mL with Glucose 5% *or* Sodium Chloride 0.9% for administration via a peripheral vein; give over at least 1 hour (give doses greater than 60 mg/kg over 2 hours).

- **MEDICINAL FORMS** There can be variation in the licensing of different medicines containing the same drug.

Solution for infusion

ELECTROLYTES: May contain Sodium

- **Foscarnet sodium (Non-proprietary)**
  Foscarnet sodium 24 mg per 1 ml Foscarnet sodium 6g/250ml solution for infusion bottles | 1 bottle PoM £199.00 (Hospital only)
- **Foscavir** (Clinigen Healthcare Ltd)
  Foscarnet sodium 24 mg per 1 ml Foscavir 6g/250ml solution for infusion bottles | 1 bottle PoM £75.00 (Hospital only)

5.5 HIV infection

HIV infection

03-Jul-2024

Overview

The human immunodeficiency virus (HIV) is a retrovirus that causes immunodeficiency by infecting and destroying cells of the immune system, particularly the CD4 cells. The prognosis of HIV has greatly improved due to more effective and better tolerated antiretroviral therapy (ART). The greatest risk to excess mortality and morbidity is delayed HIV diagnosis and treatment.

Drug treatment should only be prescribed by specialists within a paediatric HIV clinical network.

Further information on the management of children with HIV can be obtained from the Children's HIV Association (CHIVA) www.chiva.org.uk. For further information on antiretroviral use and toxicity in children see Paediatric European Network for Treatment of AIDS (PENTA) guidelines for treatment of paediatric HIV-1 infection available at: penta-id.org and the British HIV Association guidelines available at: bhiva.org/clinical-guidelines/.

Aims of treatment

Treatment aims to achieve an undetectable viral load, to preserve immune function, and to reduce the mortality and morbidity associated with chronic HIV infection whilst minimising drug toxicity. Treatment with a combination of ART aims to improve the physical and psychological well-being of infected children and optimise general health for a full and productive adult life.

Initiation of treatment

EvGr Antiretroviral therapy (ART) should be started in all children diagnosed with HIV irrespective of age, CD4 count and viral load. Infants born to women living with HIV require urgent diagnosis and treatment. The choice of antiviral treatment for children should take into account the method and frequency of administration, risk of side-effects, compatibility of drugs with food, palatability, and the appropriateness of the formulation. Additionally, potential transmitted resistance and resistance resulting from maternal or infant antiretroviral exposure during failed vertical transmission treatment should also be considered. Ⓐ Commitment to treatment and strict adherence over many years are required.

EvGr In children, treatment of HIV infection is initiated with a combination of two nucleoside reverse transcriptase inhibitors (NRTI) as a backbone regimen plus *one* of the following as a third drug: an integrase inhibitor (INSTI), a non-nucleoside reverse transcriptase inhibitor (NNRTI), *or* a boosted protease inhibitor (PI).

Abacavir with lamivudine p. 514 is the NRTI backbone combination of choice for initial therapy however, abacavir should not be given to children who are positive for the HLA-B*5701 allele. Alternative NRTI backbones regimens and third drug options, depending on the age of the child, can be found at: penta-id.org.

The metabolism of many antiretroviral drugs varies in young children, it may therefore be necessary to adjust the dose according to the plasma-drug concentration. Children who require treatment for both HIV and chronic hepatitis B should be treated with antivirals active against both diseases. Ⓐ

Switching therapy

EvGr Deterioration of the condition (including clinical, virological, and CD4 cell count changes) may require a change in therapy. The choice of an alternative regimen should be guided by factors such as the response to previous treatment, tolerability, drug-drug interactions, and the possibility of drug resistance. Ⓐ For further information see Paediatric European Network for Treatment of AIDS (PENTA) HIV first and second line antiretroviral treatment guidelines available at: www.chiva.org.uk.

HIV infection and pregnancy

EvGr Management of HIV infection in pregnancy should focus on the well-being of the women living with HIV, by ensuring that their ART regimen maximally suppresses viral replication as early as possible (if possible before conception) in order to minimise vertical transmission of HIV. Information on the teratogenic potential of most antiretroviral drugs is limited, however, all pregnant women living with HIV who conceive whilst on effective ART should continue this treatment throughout their pregnancy. All other women should start ART during their pregnancy. The recommended regimen is a NRTI backbone of either tenofovir disoproxil p. 519 or abacavir, with either emtricitabine p. 516 or lamivudine; the third drug should be efavirenz p. 510 or atazanavir p. 521 boosted with ritonavir p. 524. All treatment options require careful assessment by a specialist. Ⓐ For further information, including alternative ART options, see British HIV Association guidelines for the management of HIV in pregnancy and postpartum available at: bhiva.org/clinical-guidelines/.

EvGr Pregnancies in women with HIV and babies born to them should be reported prospectively to the National Study of HIV in Pregnancy and Childhood at: www.ucl.ac.uk/nshpc/ **and** to the Antiretroviral Pregnancy Registry at: www.apregistry.com. Ⓐ

HIV infection and breast-feeding

EvGr Breast-feeding by HIV-positive mothers may cause HIV infection in the infant and should be avoided. Ⓐ For further information see British HIV Association guidelines for the management of HIV in pregnancy and postpartum available at: bhiva.org/clinical-guidelines/.

HIV infection, post-exposure prophylaxis

EvGr Children exposed to HIV infection through needlestick injury or by another route should be sent immediately to an accident and emergency department for post-exposure prophylaxis [unlicensed indication]. Ⓐ For further information see recommendations produced by the Children's HIV Association available at: www.chiva.org.uk.

Drug treatment

Drugs that are licensed for the treatment of HIV/AIDS in children are listed below according to drug class.

Nucleoside reverse transcriptase inhibitors (NRTI or 'nucleoside analogue'): abacavir, emtricitabine, lamivudine, tenofovir alafenamide fumarate p. 493 (tenofovir AF), tenofovir disoproxil fumarate (tenofovir DF), and zidovudine p. 519.

Non-nucleoside reverse transcriptase inhibitors (NNRTI): efavirenz, etravirine p. 510, nevirapine p. 511, and rilpivirine p. 512.

Protease inhibitors (PI): atazanavir, darunavir p. 521, fosamprenavir p. 523, lopinavir, and ritonavir.

CCR5 antagonist: maraviroc p. 524.

Integrase inhibitors (INSTI): bictegravir, dolutegravir p. 508, elvitegravir, and raltegravir p. 509.

Fusion inhibitor: enfuvirtide below.

Pharmacokinetic enhancers: cobicistat p. 525, and low-dose ritonavir. They boost the concentrations of other antiretrovirals metabolised by CYP3A4.

HIV infection in neonates

EvGr In order to prevent transmission of infection, neonates born to HIV-positive mothers should be given post-exposure prophylaxis as soon as possible (within 4 hours) after birth and starting no later than 72 hours after birth. Zidovudine monotherapy can be given where there is a very low or low risk of HIV transmission. Risk is determined by the mother's viral load at the time of delivery and whether the mother has been on combination ART for more than 10 weeks. Combination ART should be given to neonates at high risk of infection or whose mothers are found to be HIV positive after delivery. The preferred treatment regimen is zidovudine and lamivudine as the NRTI backbone and nevirapine as the third drug. Prophylaxis is given for 2–4 weeks depending on the risk of infection. Ⓐ For further information see British HIV Association guidelines for the management of HIV in pregnancy and postpartum available at: bhiva.org/clinical-guidelines/.

ANTIVIRALS › HIV-FUSION INHIBITORS

Enfuvirtide

04-Sep-2020

- **DRUG ACTION** Enfuvirtide inhibits the fusion of HIV to the host cell.

- **INDICATIONS AND DOSE**

HIV infection in combination with other antiretroviral drugs for resistant infection or for patients intolerant to other antiretroviral regimens

▶ BY SUBCUTANEOUS INJECTION

▸ Child 6–15 years: 2 mg/kg twice daily (max. per dose 90 mg)

▸ Child 16–17 years: 90 mg twice daily

- **INTERACTIONS** → Appendix 1: enfuvirtide
- **SIDE-EFFECTS**

▶ **Common or very common** Anxiety · appetite decreased · asthenia · concentration impaired · conjunctivitis · diabetes mellitus · gastrooesophageal reflux disease · haematuria · hypertriglyceridaemia · increased risk of infection · influenza like illness · irritability · lymphadenopathy · myalgia · nasal congestion · nephrolithiasis · nightmare · numbness · pancreatitis · peripheral neuropathy · skin papilloma · skin reactions · tremor · vertigo · weight decreased

▶ **Frequency not known** Diarrhoea · hypersensitivity · immune reconstitution inflammatory syndrome · nausea · osteonecrosis

SIDE-EFFECTS, FURTHER INFORMATION **Hypersensitivity** Hypersensitivity reactions including rash, fever, nausea, vomiting, chills, rigors, low blood pressure, respiratory distress, glomerulonephritis, and raised liver enzymes reported; discontinue immediately if any signs or symptoms of systemic hypersensitivity develop and do not rechallenge.

Osteonecrosis Osteonecrosis has been reported in patients with advanced HIV disease or following long-term exposure to combination antiretroviral therapy.

- **PREGNANCY** Manufacturer advises use only if potential benefit outweighs risk.
- **HEPATIC IMPAIRMENT** Manufacturer advises caution (no information available); increased risk of hepatic side effects in patients with chronic hepatitis B or C.
- **DIRECTIONS FOR ADMINISTRATION** For *subcutaneous injection*, manufacturer advises reconstitute with 1.1 mL Water for Injections and allow to stand (for up to 45 minutes) to dissolve; do **not** shake or invert vial.
- **PATIENT AND CARER ADVICE**

Hypersensitivity reactions Patients or carers should be told how to recognise signs of hypersensitivity, and advised to discontinue treatment and seek immediate medical attention if symptoms develop.

- **MEDICINAL FORMS** No licensed medicines listed.

ANTIVIRALS › HIV-INTEGRASE INHIBITORS

Cabotegravir

21-Nov-2025

- **DRUG ACTION** Cabotegravir is an inhibitor of HIV integrase.

- **INDICATIONS AND DOSE**

APRETUDE TABLETS ®

Pre-exposure prophylaxis of HIV-1 infection [oral lead-in therapy] (specialist use only)

▶ BY MOUTH

▸ Child 12–17 years (body-weight 35 kg and above): 30 mg once daily for approximately 1 month (at least 28 days) then, if tolerated, switch to intramuscular treatment with cabotegravir at month 2, for oral dose recommendations if cabotegravir injection is missed—consult product literature

APRETUDE ® INJECTION

Pre-exposure prophylaxis of HIV-1 infection (specialist use only)

▶ BY INTRAMUSCULAR INJECTION

▸ Child 12–17 years (body-weight 35 kg and above): Initially 600 mg every month for 2 doses, to be started on the last day of oral lead-in therapy with cabotegravir or within 3 days thereafter (if used), then maintenance 600 mg every 2 months, to be given 2 months after previous injection

VOCABRIA TABLETS ®

HIV-1 infection [oral lead-in therapy, in combination with rilpivirine] (specialist use only)

▶ BY MOUTH

▸ Child 12–17 years (body-weight 35 kg and above): 30 mg once daily for approximately 1 month (at least 28 days) then, if tolerated, switch to intramuscular treatment with cabotegravir and rilpivirine at month 2, for oral dose recommendations if cabotegravir injection and rilpivirine injection are missed—consult product literature

VOCABRIA® INJECTION

HIV-1 infection [in combination with rilpivirine prolonged-release injection] (specialist use only)

▶ BY INTRAMUSCULAR INJECTION

▶ Child 12–17 years (body-weight 35 kg and above): Initially 600 mg for 1 dose, to be started on the last day of oral lead-in therapy with cabotegravir and rilpivirine (if used), or on the last day of current regimen, then maintenance 400 mg every month, to be given 1 month after initial injection, alternatively initially 600 mg every month for 2 doses, to be started on the last day of oral lead-in therapy with cabotegravir and rilpivirine (if used), or on the last day of current regimen, then maintenance 600 mg every 2 months, to be given 2 months after previous injection

DOSE EQUIVALENCE AND CONVERSION

▶ For dose recommendations if switching between maintenance injections given every month or every 2 months—consult product literature.

● **CAUTIONS**

▶ When used for HIV-1 infection [in combination with rilpivirine prolonged-release injection] Co-infection with hepatitis B or C · risk factors for virological failure

▶ When used for HIV-1 infection [oral lead-in therapy, in combination with rilpivirine] Co-infection with hepatitis B or C · risk factors for virological failure

▶ When used for Pre-exposure prophylaxis of HIV-1 infection Psychiatric illness (may exacerbate underlying illness)

▶ When used for Pre-exposure prophylaxis of HIV-1 infection [oral lead-in therapy] Psychiatric illness (may exacerbate underlying illness)

CAUTIONS, FURTHER INFORMATION

▶ Risk factors for virological failure

▶ When used for HIV-1 infection [oral lead-in therapy, in combination with rilpivirine] or HIV-1 infection [in combination with rilpivirine prolonged-release injection] EvGr Use with caution in patients with HIV-1 subtype A6/A1 or BMI of 30 kg/m^2 or more, if treatment history uncertain and pre-treatment resistance analyses absent. (M)

● **INTERACTIONS** → Appendix 1: cabotegravir

● **SIDE-EFFECTS**

GENERAL SIDE-EFFECTS

▶ **Common or very common** Anxiety · asthenia · depression · diarrhoea · dizziness · feeling hot · fever · flatulence · gastrointestinal discomfort · headache · malaise · myalgia · nausea · skin reactions · sleep disorders · vomiting · weight increased

▶ **Uncommon** Angioedema · drowsiness · hepatotoxicity · suicidal behaviours

SPECIFIC SIDE-EFFECTS

▶ With intramuscular use Pancreatitis

● **PREGNANCY**

▶ With oral use EvGr Avoid unless potential benefit outweighs risk—no information available. (M)

▶ With intramuscular use EvGr Avoid unless potential benefit outweighs risk—may remain in systemic circulation for up to 12 months or longer after last prolonged-release injection. (M)

● **BREAST FEEDING**

▶ With oral use EvGr Avoid—present in milk in *animal* studies. (M)

▶ With intramuscular use EvGr Avoid—may be present in milk for up to 12 months or longer after last prolonged-release injection. (M)

● **HEPATIC IMPAIRMENT** EvGr Caution in severe impairment (no information available). (M)

● **MONITORING REQUIREMENTS** EvGr Monitor liver function—discontinue treatment if hepatotoxicity develops. (M)

● **TREATMENT CESSATION**

▶ With intramuscular use EvGr May remain in circulation for up to 12 months or longer. (M) With *Vocabria®*, start an alternative regimen no later than 1 month after final monthly injection or 2 months after final 2-month injection. With *Apretude®*, start an alternative regimen no later than 2 months after final injection.

● **DIRECTIONS FOR ADMINISTRATION** For *intramuscular injection*, inject into the gluteal muscle. Injections may be given up to 7 days before or after the scheduled dose. If injections are missed—consult product literature. For *Vocabria®*, cabotegravir and rilpivirine injections must be administered into separate gluteal muscle sites.

● **PRESCRIBING AND DISPENSING INFORMATION** The manufacturer of *Apretude®* has provided a *Guide for Prescribers* and a *Checklist for Prescribers*.

● **PATIENT AND CARER ADVICE** Patients or carers should be given advice on how to administer cabotegravir tablets.

With *Apretude®* patients and carers should be counselled on the risks of suicidal ideation and behaviours prior to initiation and periodically throughout treatment.

Patient guide and reminder card An *Apretude®* guide, and reminder card for individuals at risk must be provided.

Missed doses If an **oral** dose is more than 12 hours late, the missed dose should not be taken and the next dose should be taken at the normal time. If vomiting occurs within 4 hours of taking an **oral** dose, a replacement dose should be taken.

Driving and skilled tasks Patients and carers should be counselled on the effects on driving and performance of skilled tasks—increased risk of fatigue, dizziness and somnolence.

● **NATIONAL FUNDING/ACCESS DECISIONS**

For full details see funding body website

NICE decisions

▶ **Cabotegravir for preventing HIV-1 in adults and young people (November 2025)** NICE TA1106 Recommended with restrictions

Scottish Medicines Consortium (SMC) decisions

▶ **Cabotegravir (*Apretude®*) in combination with safer sex practices for pre-exposure prophylaxis to reduce the risk of sexually acquired HIV-1 infection in high-risk adults and adolescents, weighing at least 35 kg (February 2025)** SMC No. SMC2718 Recommended with restrictions

● **MEDICINAL FORMS** There can be variation in the licensing of different medicines containing the same drug.

Prolonged-release suspension for injection

EXCIPIENTS: May contain Polysorbates

▶ **Apretude** (ViiV Healthcare UK Ltd) ▼

Cabotegravir 200 mg per 1 ml Apretude 600mg/3ml prolonged-release suspension for injection vials | 1 vial PoM £1,197.02 (Hospital only)

▶ **Vocabria** (ViiV Healthcare UK Ltd) ▼

Cabotegravir 200 mg per 1 ml Vocabria 600mg/3ml prolonged-release suspension for injection vials | 1 vial PoM £1,197.02 (Hospital only)

Oral tablet

▶ **Apretude** (ViiV Healthcare UK Ltd) ▼

Cabotegravir 30 mg Apretude 30mg tablets | 30 tablet PoM £638.57 (Hospital only)

▶ **Vocabria** (ViiV Healthcare UK Ltd) ▼

Cabotegravir 30 mg Vocabria 30mg tablets | 30 tablet PoM £638.57 (Hospital only)

Dolutegravir

20-Jul-2023

● **DRUG ACTION** Dolutegravir is an inhibitor of HIV integrase.

● **INDICATIONS AND DOSE**

HIV infection without resistance to other inhibitors of HIV integrase [in combination with other antiretroviral drugs] (specialist use only)

▶ BY MOUTH USING TABLETS

- Child 6–11 years (body-weight 14–19 kg): 40 mg once daily, alternatively 20 mg twice daily
- Child 6–17 years (body-weight 20 kg and above): 50 mg once daily, alternatively 25 mg twice daily

▶ BY MOUTH USING DISPERSIBLE TABLETS

- Child 1–5 months (body-weight 3–5 kg): 5 mg once daily
- Child 1–5 months (body-weight 6–9 kg): 10 mg once daily, alternatively 5 mg twice daily
- Child 6 months–17 years (body-weight 6–9 kg): 15 mg once daily, alternatively 10 mg twice daily
- Child 6 months–17 years (body-weight 10–13 kg): 20 mg once daily, alternatively 10 mg twice daily
- Child 6 months–17 years (body-weight 14–19 kg): 25 mg once daily, alternatively 15 mg twice daily
- Child 6 months–17 years (body-weight 20 kg and above): 30 mg once daily, alternatively 15 mg twice daily

HIV infection [in combination with other antiretroviral drugs (with concomitant carbamazepine, efavirenz, etravirine (without boosted protease inhibitors, but see also Interactions), fosphenytoin, phenobarbital, phenytoin, primidone, nevirapine, oxcarbazepine, St John's wort, or rifampicin)] (specialist use only)

▶ BY MOUTH USING TABLETS

- Child 6–11 years (body-weight 14–19 kg): 40 mg twice daily, avoid concomitant use with these drugs if resistance to other inhibitors of HIV integrase suspected
- Child 6–17 years (body-weight 20 kg and above): 50 mg twice daily, avoid concomitant use with these drugs if resistance to other inhibitors of HIV integrase suspected

▶ BY MOUTH USING DISPERSIBLE TABLETS

- Child 1–5 months (body-weight 3–5 kg): 5 mg twice daily, avoid concomitant use with these drugs if resistance to other inhibitors of HIV integrase suspected
- Child 1–5 months (body-weight 6–9 kg): 10 mg twice daily, avoid concomitant use with these drugs if resistance to other inhibitors of HIV integrase suspected
- Child 6 months–17 years (body-weight 6–9 kg): 15 mg twice daily, avoid concomitant use with these drugs if resistance to other inhibitors of HIV integrase suspected
- Child 6 months–17 years (body-weight 10–13 kg): 20 mg twice daily, avoid concomitant use with these drugs if resistance to other inhibitors of HIV integrase suspected
- Child 6 months–17 years (body-weight 14–19 kg): 25 mg twice daily, avoid concomitant use with these drugs if resistance to other inhibitors of HIV integrase suspected
- Child 6 months–17 years (body-weight 20 kg and above): 30 mg twice daily, avoid concomitant use with these drugs if resistance to other inhibitors of HIV integrase suspected

DOSE EQUIVALENCE AND CONVERSION

- *Tivicay*® film-coated tablets and *Tivicay*® dispersible tablets are **not** bioequivalent. Follow correct dosing recommendations for the dosage form when switching formulations.

IMPORTANT SAFETY INFORMATION

MHRA/CHM ADVICE: DOLUTEGRAVIR (*TIVICAY*®, *TRIUMEQ*®, *JULUCA*®): UPDATED ADVICE ON INCREASED RISK OF NEURAL TUBE DEFECTS (OCTOBER 2020)

The MHRA has updated its safety recommendations based on an ongoing European review evaluating cases of neural tube defects in babies born to mothers who became pregnant during dolutegravir treatment that found a smaller increased risk than previously thought, almost comparable to other HIV drugs.

Healthcare professionals are advised to counsel women of childbearing potential on the possible risk of neural tube defects with dolutegravir, including consideration of effective contraceptive measures. The benefits and risks of continuing treatment in women who are trying to become pregnant should be discussed with the patient. If pregnancy is confirmed in the first trimester during treatment, the benefits and risks of continuing dolutegravir versus switching to another antiretroviral regimen should also be discussed, considering the gestational age and the critical time period of neural tube defect development.

● **INTERACTIONS** → Appendix 1: dolutegravir

● **SIDE-EFFECTS**

▶ **Common or very common** Anxiety · depression · diarrhoea · dizziness · fatigue · flatulence · gastrointestinal discomfort · headache · nausea · skin reactions · sleep disorders · vomiting

▶ **Uncommon** Arthralgia · hepatic disorders · hypersensitivity · immune reconstitution inflammatory syndrome · myalgia · suicidal behaviours

SIDE-EFFECTS, FURTHER INFORMATION **Hypersensitivity** Hypersensitivity reactions (including severe rash, or rash accompanied by fever, malaise, arthralgia, myalgia, blistering, oral lesions, conjunctivitis, angioedema, eosinophilia, or raised liver enzymes) reported uncommonly. Discontinue immediately if any sign or symptoms of hypersensitivity reactions develop.

Osteonecrosis Osteonecrosis has been reported in patients with advanced HIV disease or following long-term exposure to combination antiretroviral therapy.

● **PREGNANCY** EvGr Specialist sources indicate dolutegravir may be considered from 6 weeks' gestation if expected benefit outweighs risk—see *Important Safety Information*. Higher dose folic acid is recommended due to increased risk of neural tube defects—see *Prevention of neural tube defects (in those in the high-risk group who wish to become pregnant or who are at risk of becoming pregnant)* in folic acid p. 710. ⟨A⟩

● **HEPATIC IMPAIRMENT** Manufacturer advises caution in severe impairment—no information available.

● **DIRECTIONS FOR ADMINISTRATION** EvGr *Tivicay*® dispersible tablets may be dispersed in water and given within 30 minutes, or swallowed whole one at a time. Do not chew, cut, or crush. ⟨M⟩

● **PATIENT AND CARER ADVICE** Patients or carers should be given advice on how to administer dolutegravir film-coated tablets and dispersible tablets.

Missed doses If a dose is more than 20 hours late on the once-daily regimen (or more than 8 hours late on the twice-daily regimen), the missed dose should not be taken and the next dose should be taken at the normal time.

Driving and skilled tasks Patients and carers should be counselled on the effects on driving and performance of skilled tasks—increased risk of dizziness.

- **NATIONAL FUNDING/ACCESS DECISIONS** For full details see funding body website

Scottish Medicines Consortium (SMC) decisions

- **Dolutegravir (*Tivicay*®) for use in combination with other antiretroviral medicinal products for the treatment of Human Immunodeficiency Virus (HIV) infected adolescents above 12 years of age (May 2014)** SMC No. 961/14 Recommended
- **Dolutegravir (*Tivicay*®) for use in combination with other anti-retroviral medicinal products for the treatment of Human Immunodeficiency Virus (HIV) infected children aged 6 to 12 years of age (July 2017)** SMC No. 1253/17 Recommended

All Wales Medicines Strategy Group (AWMSG) decisions

- **Dolutegravir (*Tivicay*®) for the treatment of Human Immunodeficiency Virus (HIV) infected adolescents and children above 6 years of age, in combination with other anti-retroviral medicinal products (October 2017)** AWMSG No. 3373 Recommended
- **Dolutegravir 5 mg dispersible tablets (*Tivicay*®) in combination with other anti-retroviral medicinal products for the treatment of Human Immunodeficiency Virus (HIV) infected adults, adolescents and children of at least 4 weeks of age or older and weighing at least 3 kg (September 2021)** AWMSG No. 4611 Recommended

- **MEDICINAL FORMS** There can be variation in the licensing of different medicines containing the same drug.

Dispersible tablet

- Tivicay (ViiV Healthcare UK Ltd)
  Dolutegravir (as Dolutegravir sodium) 5 mg Tivicay 5mg dispersible tablets | 60 tablet PoM £159.60 (Hospital only) SF

Oral tablet

- Tivicay (ViiV Healthcare UK Ltd)
  Dolutegravir (as Dolutegravir sodium) 50 mg Tivicay 50mg tablets | 30 tablet PoM £498.75 (Hospital only)

Combinations available: *Abacavir with dolutegravir and lamivudine*, p. 514 · ***Lamivudine with dolutegravir*,** p. 518

Raltegravir

10-Nov-2020

- **DRUG ACTION** Raltegravir is an inhibitor of HIV integrase.

- **INDICATIONS AND DOSE**

HIV-1 infection (initiated by a specialist)

▶ BY MOUTH USING TABLETS

- Child (body-weight 25 kg and above): 400 mg twice daily
- Child (body-weight 40 kg and above): 1200 mg once daily, once daily dosing for use in patients who are treatment naive or virologically suppressed on an initial regimen of 400 mg twice daily—use 600 mg tablets only

▶ BY MOUTH USING CHEWABLE TABLETS

- Child (body-weight 11–13 kg): 75 mg twice daily
- Child (body-weight 14–19 kg): 100 mg twice daily
- Child (body-weight 20–27 kg): 150 mg twice daily
- Child (body-weight 28–39 kg): 200 mg twice daily
- Child (body-weight 40 kg and above): 300 mg twice daily

▶ BY MOUTH USING ORAL SUSPENSION

- Neonate up to 7 days (body-weight 2 kg): 4 mg once daily.
- Neonate up to 7 days (body-weight 3 kg): 5 mg once daily.
- Neonate up to 7 days (body-weight 4 kg): 7 mg once daily.
- Neonate 7 days to 28 days (body-weight 2 kg): 8 mg twice daily.
- Neonate 7 days to 28 days (body-weight 3 kg): 10 mg twice daily.
- Neonate 7 days to 28 days (body-weight 4 kg): 15 mg twice daily.
- Child (body-weight 3 kg): 25 mg twice daily
- Child (body-weight 4–5 kg): 30 mg twice daily
- Child (body-weight 6–7 kg): 40 mg twice daily
- Child (body-weight 8–10 kg): 60 mg twice daily
- Child (body-weight 11–13 kg): 80 mg twice daily
- Child (body-weight 14–19 kg): 100 mg twice daily

DOSE EQUIVALENCE AND CONVERSION

- Raltegravir granules for oral suspension and chewable tablets are **not** bioequivalent or interchangeable with the 400 mg and 600 mg *standard* tablets.

- **CONTRA-INDICATIONS** Pre-term neonates—no information available
- **CAUTIONS** Psychiatric illness (may exacerbate underlying illness including depression) · risk factors for myopathy · risk factors for rhabdomyolysis
- **INTERACTIONS** → Appendix 1: raltegravir
- **SIDE-EFFECTS**
  - **Common or very common** Akathisia · appetite abnormal · asthenia · behaviour abnormal · depression · diarrhoea · dizziness · fever · gastrointestinal discomfort · gastrointestinal disorders · headaches · nausea · skin reactions · sleep disorders · vertigo · vomiting
  - **Uncommon** Alopecia · anaemia · anxiety · arrhythmias · arthralgia · arthritis · body fat disorder · burping · cachexia · chest discomfort · chills · cognitive disorder · concentration impaired · confusion · constipation · diabetes mellitus · drowsiness · dry mouth · dyslipidaemia · dysphonia · erectile dysfunction · feeling jittery · glossitis · gynaecomastia · haemorrhage · hepatic disorders · hot flush · hyperglycaemia · hypersensitivity · hypertension · immune reconstitution inflammatory syndrome · increased risk of infection · lipodystrophy · lymph node abscess · lymphatic abnormalities · malaise · memory loss · menopausal symptoms · mood altered · myalgia · myopathy · nasal congestion · nephritis · nephrolithiasis · nerve disorders · neutropenia · nocturia · odynophagia · oedema · osteopenia · pain · palpitations · pancreatitis acute · polydipsia · psychiatric disorder · renal cyst · renal impairment · sensation abnormal · severe cutaneous adverse reactions (SCARs) · skin papilloma · submandibular mass · suicidal behaviours · sweat changes · taste altered · tendinitis · thrombocytopenia · tinnitus · tremor · visual impairment · weight increased
  - **Frequency not known** Osteonecrosis

  SIDE-EFFECTS, FURTHER INFORMATION Rash occurs commonly. Discontinue if severe rash or rash accompanied by fever, malaise, arthralgia, myalgia, blistering, mouth ulceration, conjunctivitis, angioedema, hepatitis, or eosinophilia.
- **PREGNANCY** Manufacturer advises avoid—toxicity in *animal* studies.
- **HEPATIC IMPAIRMENT** Manufacturer advises caution in severe impairment (no information available), and in patients with chronic hepatitis B or C (consider interrupting or discontinuing treatment if impairment worsens; increased risk of hepatic side-effects).
- **DIRECTIONS FOR ADMINISTRATION** Manufacturer advises for *chewable tablets*, the 100 mg strength can be divided into equal 50 mg doses.
- **PRESCRIBING AND DISPENSING INFORMATION** Dispense raltegravir chewable tablets in original container (contains desiccant).
- **NATIONAL FUNDING/ACCESS DECISIONS** For full details see funding body website

Scottish Medicines Consortium (SMC) decisions

- **Raltegravir chewable and 400 mg film-coated tablets (*Isentress*®) in combination with other anti-retroviral medicinal products for the treatment of human immunodeficiency virus (HIV-1) infection in adolescents and** children aged 2 to 17 years (September 2013) SMC No. 902/13 Recommended with restrictions

- **Raltegravir granules for oral suspension (*Isentress*®) for the treatment of human immunodeficiency virus (HIV-1) infection (November 2015)** SMC No. 1102/15 Recommended with restrictions
- **Raltegravir chewable tablets (*Isentress*®) in combination with other anti-retroviral medicinal products for the treatment of human immunodeficiency virus (HIV-1) infection in children from the age of 4 weeks up to 2 years (November 2015)** SMC No. 1113/15 Recommended with restrictions
- **Raltegravir 600 mg film-coated tablets (*Isentress*®) in combination with other anti-retroviral medicinal products for the treatment of human immunodeficiency virus (HIV-1) infection in adults and paediatric patients weighing at least 40 kg (November 2017)** SMC No. 1280/17 Recommended with restrictions

● **MEDICINAL FORMS** There can be variation in the licensing of different medicines containing the same drug.

Oral tablet

CAUTIONARY AND ADVISORY LABELS 25

- Raltegravir (Non-proprietary)
  Raltegravir 600 mg Raltegravir 600mg tablets | 60 tablet PoM £249.85–£471.41
- Isentress (Merck Sharp & Dohme (UK) Ltd)
  Raltegravir 400 mg Isentress 400mg tablets | 60 tablet PoM £471.41 (Hospital only)
  Raltegravir 600 mg Isentress 600mg tablets | 60 tablet PoM £471.41 (Hospital only)

Granules for oral suspension

EXCIPIENTS: May contain Sorbitol

- Isentress (Merck Sharp & Dohme (UK) Ltd)
  Raltegravir 100 mg Isentress 100mg granules for oral suspension sachets | 60 sachet PoM £213.02 (Hospital only)

Chewable tablet

CAUTIONARY AND ADVISORY LABELS 24

EXCIPIENTS: May contain Aspartame

- Isentress (Merck Sharp & Dohme (UK) Ltd)
  Raltegravir 25 mg Isentress 25mg chewable tablets | 60 tablet PoM £29.46 (Hospital only)
  Raltegravir 100 mg Isentress 100mg chewable tablets | 60 tablet PoM £117.85 (Hospital only)

ANTIVIRALS > NON-NUCLEOSIDE REVERSE TRANSCRIPTASE INHIBITORS

Efavirenz

27-Apr-2021

● **INDICATIONS AND DOSE**

HIV infection in combination with other antiretroviral drugs

▶ BY MOUTH USING CAPSULES

- Child 3 months–17 years (body-weight 3.5–4 kg): 100 mg once daily
- Child 3 months–17 years (body-weight 5–7.4 kg): 150 mg once daily
- Child 3 months–17 years (body-weight 7.5–14 kg): 200 mg once daily
- Child 3 months–17 years (body-weight 15–19 kg): 250 mg once daily
- Child 3 months–17 years (body-weight 20–24 kg): 300 mg once daily
- Child 3 months–17 years (body-weight 25–32.4 kg): 350 mg once daily
- Child 3 months–17 years (body-weight 32.5–39 kg): 400 mg once daily
- Child 3 months–17 years (body-weight 40 kg and above): 600 mg once daily

▶ BY MOUTH USING TABLETS

- Child (body-weight 40 kg and above): 600 mg once daily

● **CAUTIONS** Acute porphyrias p. 745 · history of psychiatric disorders · history of seizures · risk of QT interval prolongation

● **INTERACTIONS** → Appendix 1: NNRTIs

● **SIDE-EFFECTS**

- **Common or very common** Abdominal pain · anxiety · concentration impaired · depression · diarrhoea · dizziness · drowsiness · dyslipidaemia · fatigue · headache · movement disorders · nausea · skin reactions · sleep disorders · vomiting
- **Uncommon** Behaviour abnormal · confusion · flushing · gynaecomastia · hallucination · hepatic disorders · memory loss · mood altered · pancreatitis · psychosis · seizure · Stevens-Johnson syndrome · suicidal behaviours · thinking abnormal · tinnitus · tremor · vertigo · vision blurred
- **Rare or very rare** Delusions · photosensitivity reaction
- **Frequency not known** Immune reconstitution inflammatory syndrome · osteonecrosis

SIDE-EFFECTS, FURTHER INFORMATION **Rash** Rash, usually in the first 2 weeks, is the most common side-effect; discontinue if severe rash with blistering, desquamation, mucosal involvement or fever; if rash mild or moderate, may continue without interruption—usually resolves within 1 month.

CNS effects Administration at bedtime especially in first 2–4 weeks reduces CNS effects.

Abnormal hepatic function Manufacturer advises interrupt or discontinue treatment if transaminases more than 5 times the upper limit of normal.

● **PREGNANCY** Reports of neural tube defects when used in first trimester.

● **HEPATIC IMPAIRMENT** Greater risk of hepatic side-effects in chronic hepatitis B or C. Manufacturer advises avoid in severe impairment (limited information available).

● **RENAL IMPAIRMENT** Manufacturer advises caution in severe renal failure—no information available.

● **MONITORING REQUIREMENTS** Monitor liver function if receiving other hepatotoxic drugs.

● **DIRECTIONS FOR ADMINISTRATION** Manufacturer advises for patients who cannot swallow capsules, the capsule may be opened and contents added to a small amount of food—consult product literature. No additional food should be consumed for up to 2 hours after administration of efavirenz.

● **PATIENT AND CARER ADVICE**

Psychiatric disorders Patients or their carers should be advised to seek immediate medical attention if symptoms such as severe depression, psychosis or suicidal ideation occur.

● **MEDICINAL FORMS** There can be variation in the licensing of different medicines containing the same drug.

Oral tablet

CAUTIONARY AND ADVISORY LABELS 23

- Efavirenz (Non-proprietary)
  Efavirenz 600 mg Efavirenz 600mg tablets | 30 tablet PoM £22.50–£452.94 (Hospital only)

Etravirine

15-Oct-2021

● **INDICATIONS AND DOSE**

HIV infection in combination with other antiretroviral drugs (including a boosted protease inhibitor) in patients previously treated with antiretrovirals (initiated by a specialist)

▶ BY MOUTH

- Child 2–17 years (body-weight 10–19 kg): 100 mg twice daily, to be taken after food

- Child 2-17 years (body-weight 20-24 kg): 125 mg twice daily, to be taken after food
- Child 2-17 years (body-weight 25-29 kg): 150 mg twice daily, to be taken after food
- Child 2-17 years (body-weight 30 kg and above): 200 mg twice daily, to be taken after food

- **CONTRA-INDICATIONS** Acute porphyrias p. 745
- **INTERACTIONS** → Appendix 1: NNRTIs
- **SIDE-EFFECTS**
  - **Common or very common** Anaemia · anxiety · appetite decreased · asthenia · constipation · diabetes mellitus · diarrhoea · drowsiness · dry mouth · dyslipidaemia · dyspnoea exertional · gastrointestinal discomfort · gastrointestinal disorders · headache · hyperglycaemia · hypersensitivity · hypertension · memory loss · myocardial infarction · nausea · peripheral neuropathy · renal failure · sensation abnormal · skin reactions · sleep disorders · stomatitis · sweat changes · thrombocytopenia · vision blurred · vomiting
  - **Uncommon** Angina pectoris · angioedema · atrial fibrillation · bronchospasm · concentration impaired · confusion · gynaecomastia · haematemesis · hepatic disorders · immune reconstitution inflammatory syndrome · pancreatitis · seizure · syncope · tremor · vertigo
  - **Rare or very rare** Haemorrhagic stroke · severe cutaneous adverse reactions (SCARs) · Stevens-Johnson syndrome (especially in children and adolescents)
  - **Frequency not known** Osteonecrosis

  SIDE-EFFECTS, FURTHER INFORMATION Rash, usually in the second week, is the most common side-effect and appears more frequently in females. Life-threatening hypersensitivity reactions reported usually during week 3–6 of treatment and characterised by rash, eosinophilia, and systemic symptoms (including fever, general malaise, myalgia, arthralgia, blistering, oral lesions, conjunctivitis, and hepatitis). Discontinue permanently if hypersensitivity reaction or severe rash develop. If rash mild or moderate (without signs of hypersensitivity reaction), may continue without interruption—usually resolves within 2 weeks.
- **HEPATIC IMPAIRMENT** Manufacturer advises caution in moderate impairment and in patients with hepatitis B or C (increased risk of hepatic side effects); avoid in severe impairment (no information available).
- **DIRECTIONS FOR ADMINISTRATION** Manufacturer advises patients with swallowing difficulties may disperse tablets in a glass of water just before administration.
- **PRESCRIBING AND DISPENSING INFORMATION** Dispense in original container (contains desiccant).
- **PATIENT AND CARER ADVICE**

  Hypersensitivity reactions Patients or carers should be told how to recognise hypersensitivity reactions and advised to seek immediate medical attention if hypersensitivity reaction or severe rash develop.

  Vomiting If vomiting occurs 4 hours after taking tablets, no additional dose should be taken and the next dose should be taken at the usual time.

  Missed doses If a dose is more than 6 hours late, the missed dose should not be taken and the next dose should be taken at the normal time.
- **NATIONAL FUNDING/ACCESS DECISIONS**

  For full details see funding body website

  All Wales Medicines Strategy Group (AWMSG) decisions
  - **Etravirine (*Intelence*®) in combination with a boosted protease inhibitor and other antiretroviral medicinal products, for the treatment of human immunodeficiency virus type 1 (HIV-1) infection in antiretroviral treatment-experienced adults and in antiretroviral treatment-experienced paediatric patients from 2 years of age (September 2021)** AWMSG No. 4506 Recommended
- **MEDICINAL FORMS** There can be variation in the licensing of different medicines containing the same drug.

  Oral tablet

  CAUTIONARY AND ADVISORY LABELS 21
  - **Intelence** (Janssen-Cilag Ltd)

    Etravirine 100 mg Intelence 100mg tablets | 120 tablet [PoM] £301.27 (Hospital only)

    Etravirine 200 mg Intelence 200mg tablets | 60 tablet [PoM] £301.27 (Hospital only)

Nevirapine

27-Apr-2021

- **INDICATIONS AND DOSE**

  HIV infection in combination with other antiretroviral drugs (initial dose)
  - BY MOUTH USING IMMEDIATE-RELEASE MEDICINES
    - Child: Initially 150–200 mg/m^2 once daily (max. per dose 200 mg) for first 14 days, initial dose titration using 'immediate-release' preparation should not exceed 28 days; if rash occurs and is not resolved within 28 days, alternative treatment should be sought. If treatment interrupted for more than 7 days, restart using the lower dose of the 'immediate-release' preparation for the first 14 days as for new treatment

  HIV infection in combination with other antiretroviral drugs (maintenance dose following initial dose titration if no rash present)
  - BY MOUTH USING IMMEDIATE-RELEASE MEDICINES
    - Child 1 month-2 years: 150–200 mg/m^2 twice daily (max. per dose 200 mg), alternatively 300–400 mg/m^2 once daily (max. per dose 400 mg)
    - Child 3-17 years: 150–200 mg/m^2 twice daily (max. per dose 200 mg)

  HIV infection in combination with other antiretroviral drugs (maintenance dose following initial dose titration if no rash present)
  - BY MOUTH USING IMMEDIATE-RELEASE MEDICINES
    - Child 3-17 years (body surface area 0.58-0.83 m^2): 200 mg once daily
    - Child 3-17 years (body surface area 0.84-1.17 m^2): 300 mg once daily
    - Child 3-17 years (body surface area 1.18 m^2 and above): 400 mg once daily
  - BY MOUTH USING MODIFIED-RELEASE MEDICINES
    - Child 3-17 years (body surface area 0.58-0.83 m^2): 200 mg once daily
    - Child 3-17 years (body surface area 0.84-1.17 m^2): 300 mg once daily
    - Child 3-17 years (body surface area 1.18 m^2 and above): 400 mg once daily
- **UNLICENSED USE** 'Immediate-release' tablets not licensed for use in children weighing less than 50 kg or with body surface area less than 1.25 m^2; 'immediate-release' tablets and suspension not licensed for once daily dose after the initial dose titration.
- **CONTRA-INDICATIONS** Acute porphyrias p. 745 · post-exposure prophylaxis
- **CAUTIONS** Females (at greater risk of hepatic side effects) · high CD4 cell count (at greater risk of hepatic side effects)
- **INTERACTIONS** → Appendix 1: NNRTIs
- **SIDE-EFFECTS**
  - **Common or very common** Abdominal pain · angioedema · diarrhoea · fatigue · fever · headache · hepatic disorders · hypersensitivity · hypertransaminasaemia · nausea · skin reactions · vomiting
  - **Uncommon** Anaemia · arthralgia · myalgia · severe cutaneous adverse reactions (SCARs)
  - **Frequency not known** Eosinophilia · osteonecrosis · weight increased

5 Infection

SIDE-EFFECTS, FURTHER INFORMATION **Hepatic effects** Potentially life-threatening hepatotoxicity including fatal fulminant hepatitis reported usually in first 6 weeks; discontinue permanently if abnormalities in liver function tests accompanied by hypersensitivity reaction (rash, fever, arthralgia, myalgia, lymphadenopathy, hepatitis, renal impairment, eosinophilia, granulocytopenia); suspend if severe abnormalities in liver function tests but no hypersensitivity reaction—discontinue permanently if significant liver function abnormalities recur; monitor patient closely if mild to moderate abnormalities in liver function tests with no hypersensitivity reaction.

Rash Rash, usually in first 6 weeks, is most common side-effect; incidence reduced if introduced at low dose and dose increased gradually (after 14 days); Discontinue permanently if severe rash or if rash accompanied by blistering, oral lesions, conjunctivitis, facial oedema, general malaise or hypersensitivity reactions; if rash mild or moderate may continue without interruption but dose should not be increased until rash resolves.

Osteonecrosis Osteonecrosis has been reported in patients with advanced HIV disease or following long-term exposure to combination antiretroviral therapy.

- **HEPATIC IMPAIRMENT** For *modified-release* preparations, manufacturer advises avoid (no information available). For *immediate-release* preparations, manufacturer advises caution in moderate impairment and chronic hepatitis (increased risk of hepatic side effects; consider interrupting or discontinuing treatment if hepatic function worsens); avoid in severe impairment (no information available).
- **RENAL IMPAIRMENT** Manufacturer advises avoid *modified-release* preparation—no information available.
- **MONITORING REQUIREMENTS**
  - Hepatic disease Close monitoring of liver function required during first 18 weeks; monitor liver function before treatment then every 2 weeks for 2 months then after 1 month and then regularly.
  - Rash Monitor closely for skin reactions during first 18 weeks.
- **PATIENT AND CARER ADVICE**
  Hypersensitivity reactions Patients or carers should be told how to recognise hypersensitivity reactions and advised to discontinue treatment and seek immediate medical attention if severe skin reaction, hypersensitivity reactions, or symptoms of hepatitis develop.

- **MEDICINAL FORMS** There can be variation in the licensing of different medicines containing the same drug.

Oral tablet
- Nevirapine (Non-proprietary)
  Nevirapine 200 mg Nevirapine 200mg tablets | 60 tablet PoM £170.00 (Hospital only)

Oral suspension
- Viramune (Boehringer Ingelheim Ltd)
  Nevirapine (as Nevirapine hemihydrate) 10 mg per 1 ml Viramune 50mg/5ml oral suspension | 240 ml PoM £50.40 (Hospital only)

Modified-release tablet
CAUTIONARY AND ADVISORY LABELS 25
- Nevirapine (Non-proprietary)
  Nevirapine 400 mg Nevirapine 400mg modified-release tablets | 30 tablet PoM £127.50 (Hospital only)

Rilpivirine

27-Feb-2025

- **INDICATIONS AND DOSE**

HIV-1 infection [in combination with other antiretroviral drugs] (specialist use only)
- BY MOUTH USING FILM-COATED TABLETS
  - Child 2–17 years (body-weight 25 kg and above): 25 mg once daily, dose to be taken with food

HIV-1 infection [oral lead-in therapy, in combination with cabotegravir] (specialist use only)
- BY MOUTH USING FILM-COATED TABLETS
  - Child 12–17 years (body-weight 35 kg and above): 25 mg once daily for approximately 1 month (at least 28 days) with food then, if tolerated, switch to intramuscular treatment with cabotegravir and rilpivirine at month 2, for oral dose recommendations if cabotegravir injection and rilpivirine injection are missed—consult product literature

HIV-1 infection [in combination with cabotegravir prolonged-release injection] (specialist use only)
- BY INTRAMUSCULAR INJECTION
  - Child 12–17 years (body-weight 35 kg and above): Initially 900 mg for 1 dose, to be started on the last day of oral lead-in therapy with cabotegravir and rilpivirine (if used), or on the last day of current regimen, then maintenance 600 mg every month, to be given 1 month after initial injection, alternatively initially 900 mg every month for 2 doses, to be started on the last day of oral lead-in therapy with cabotegravir and rilpivirine (if used), or on the last day of current regimen, then maintenance 900 mg every 2 months, to be given 2 months after previous injection

DOSE EQUIVALENCE AND CONVERSION
- For dose recommendations if switching between maintenance injections given every month or every 2 months—consult product literature.

- **CAUTIONS** Acute porphyrias p. 745 · co-infection with hepatitis B or C · risk factors for virological failure

CAUTIONS, FURTHER INFORMATION
- Risk factors for virological failure EvGr Use with caution in patients with HIV-1 subtype A6/A1 or BMI of 30 kg/m² or more, if treatment history uncertain and pre-treatment resistance analyses absent. (M)

- **INTERACTIONS** → Appendix 1: NNRTIs
- **SIDE-EFFECTS**
  - **Common or very common** Appetite decreased · depression · dizziness · drowsiness · dry mouth · fatigue · gastrointestinal discomfort · headache · nausea · rash · sleep disorders · vomiting
  - **Uncommon** Immune reconstitution inflammatory syndrome
- **PREGNANCY**
  - With oral use EvGr Use only if potential benefit outweighs risk—no toxicity observed in *animal* studies. If used, monitoring of viral load is recommended. (M)
  - With intramuscular use EvGr Avoid unless potential benefit outweighs risk—no information available. May remain in systemic circulation for up to 4 years after last prolonged-release injection. If used, monitoring of viral load is recommended. (M)
- **BREAST FEEDING**
  - With oral use EvGr Avoid—present in milk in *animal* studies. (M)
  - With intramuscular use EvGr Avoid—may be present in milk for up to 4 years after last prolonged-release injection. (M)
- **HEPATIC IMPAIRMENT** Manufacturer advises caution in moderate impairment (limited information available); avoid in severe impairment (no information available).
- **RENAL IMPAIRMENT** Manufacturer advises caution in severe impairment.
- **MONITORING REQUIREMENTS** EvGr Monitor liver function in patients with hepatitis C—limited information available. (M)
- **TREATMENT CESSATION**
  - With intramuscular use EvGr May remain in circulation for up to 4 years; start an alternative regimen no later than

1 month after monthly regimen or 2 months after 2-monthly regimen. ⟨M⟩

- **DIRECTIONS FOR ADMINISTRATION** For *Rekambys*®, rilpivirine and cabotegravir injections must be administered into separate gluteal muscle sites. Maintenance injections may be given up to 7 days before or after the scheduled dose. If injections are missed—consult product literature.
- **HANDLING AND STORAGE** Store rilpivirine prolonged-release injection (*Rekambys*®) in a refrigerator (2°C to 8°C)—may be stored unopened at room temperature (below 25°C) for up to 6 hours before use.
- **PATIENT AND CARER ADVICE** Patients or carers should be given advice on how to administer rilpivirine tablets.
Missed doses If an **oral** dose is more than 12 hours late, the missed dose should not be taken and the next dose should be taken at the normal time. If vomiting occurs within 4 hours of taking an **oral** dose, a replacement dose should be taken.
Driving and skilled tasks Patients and carers should be counselled on the effects on driving and performance of skilled tasks—increased risk of fatigue, dizziness and somnolence.
- **NATIONAL FUNDING/ACCESS DECISIONS**
For full details see funding body website
All Wales Medicines Strategy Group (AWMSG) decisions
▶ **Rilpivirine (*Edurant*®) for treatment of human immunodeficiency virus type 1 (HIV-1) infection in antiretroviral treatment-naive patients from 12 years old to less than 18 years old with a viral load less than or equal to 100,000 HIV-1 RNA copies/ml (October 2016)** AWMSG No. 2936 Recommended

- **MEDICINAL FORMS** There can be variation in the licensing of different medicines containing the same drug.

Prolonged-release suspension for injection
▸ **Rekambys** (ViiV Healthcare UK Ltd) ▼
Rilpivirine 300 mg per 1 ml Rekambys 900mg/3ml prolonged-release suspension for injection vials | 1 vial [PoM] £440.47 (Hospital only)

Oral tablet
CAUTIONARY AND ADVISORY LABELS 3, 21, 25
▸ **Edurant** (Janssen-Cilag Ltd)
Rilpivirine (as Rilpivirine hydrochloride) 25 mg Edurant 25mg tablets | 30 tablet [PoM] £200.27 (Hospital only)

Combinations available: *Emtricitabine with rilpivirine and tenofovir alafenamide*, p. 516

ANTIVIRALS › NUCLEOSIDE REVERSE TRANSCRIPTASE INHIBITORS

Nucleoside reverse transcriptase inhibitors

- **SIDE-EFFECTS**
▶ **Common or very common** Abdominal pain · anaemia (may require transfusion) · asthenia · diarrhoea · dizziness · fever · flatulence · headache · insomnia · nausea · neutropenia · skin reactions · vomiting
▶ **Uncommon** Angioedema · pancreatitis
▶ **Rare or very rare** Lactic acidosis
▶ **Frequency not known** Immune reconstitution inflammatory syndrome · osteonecrosis · weight increased
SIDE-EFFECTS, FURTHER INFORMATION Osteonecrosis has been reported in patients with advanced HIV disease or following long-term exposure to combination antiretroviral therapy.
- **PREGNANCY**
Monitoring Mitochondrial dysfunction has been reported in infants exposed to nucleoside reverse transcriptase inhibitors in utero; the main effects include haematological, metabolic, and neurological disorders; all infants whose mothers received nucleoside reverse transcriptase inhibitors during pregnancy should be monitored for relevant signs or symptoms.
- **HEPATIC IMPAIRMENT** In general, manufacturers advise caution in patients with chronic hepatitis B or C (increased risk of hepatic side-effects).

F above

Abacavir

28-Apr-2021

- **INDICATIONS AND DOSE**

HIV infection in combination with other antiretroviral drugs
▶ BY MOUTH
▸ Child 3 months–11 years: 8 mg/kg twice daily (max. per dose 300 mg), alternatively 16 mg/kg once daily (max. per dose 600 mg)
▸ Child 3 months–11 years (body-weight 14–20 kg): 150 mg twice daily, alternatively 300 mg once daily
▸ Child 3 months–11 years (body-weight 21–29 kg): 150 mg, taken in the morning and 300 mg, taken in the evening, alternatively 450 mg once daily
▸ Child 3 months–11 years (body-weight 30 kg and above): 300 mg twice daily, alternatively 600 mg once daily
▸ Child 12–17 years: 300 mg twice daily, alternatively 600 mg once daily

- **CAUTIONS** Patients at high risk of cardiovascular disease
- **INTERACTIONS** → Appendix 1: NRTIs
- **SIDE-EFFECTS**
▶ **Common or very common** Appetite decreased · lethargy
▶ **Rare or very rare** Severe cutaneous adverse reactions (SCARs)
▶ **Frequency not known** Hypersensitivity
SIDE-EFFECTS, FURTHER INFORMATION Life-threatening hypersensitivity reactions have been reported—characterised by fever or rash and possibly nausea, vomiting, diarrhoea, abdominal pain, dyspnoea, cough, lethargy, malaise, headache, and myalgia; less frequently mouth ulceration, oedema, hypotension, sore throat, acute respiratory distress syndrome, anaphylaxis, paraesthesia, arthralgia, conjunctivitis, lymphadenopathy, lymphocytopenia and renal failure; rarely myolysis. Laboratory abnormalities may include raised liver function tests and creatine kinase; symptoms usually appear in the first 6 weeks, but may occur at any time. Discontinue immediately if any symptom of hypersensitivity develops and do not rechallenge (risk of more severe hypersensitivity reaction).
- **ALLERGY AND CROSS-SENSITIVITY** [EvGr] Caution—increased risk of hypersensitivity reaction in presence of HLA-B*5701 allele. ⟨M⟩
- **HEPATIC IMPAIRMENT** Manufacturer advises caution in mild impairment; consider avoiding in moderate to severe impairment (no information available).
- **RENAL IMPAIRMENT** Manufacturer advises avoid in end-stage renal disease.
- **PRE-TREATMENT SCREENING** Test for HLA-B*5701 allele before treatment or if restarting treatment and HLA-B*5701 status not known.
- **MONITORING REQUIREMENTS** Monitor for symptoms of hypersensitivity reaction every 2 weeks for 2 months.
- **PRESCRIBING AND DISPENSING INFORMATION** Flavours of oral liquid formulations may include banana, or strawberry.
- **PATIENT AND CARER ADVICE** Patients and their carers should be told the importance of regular dosing (intermittent therapy may increase the risk of

sensitisation), how to recognise signs of hypersensitivity, and advised to seek immediate medical attention if symptoms develop or before re-starting treatment.

Patients should be provided with an alert card and advised to keep it with them at all times.

- **MEDICINAL FORMS** There can be variation in the licensing of different medicines containing the same drug.

Oral tablet

- **Abacavir (Non-proprietary)**
 Abacavir (as Abacavir sulfate) 300 mg Abacavir 300mg tablets | 60 tablet [PoM] £177.60–£177.61 (Hospital only)
- **Ziagen** (ViiV Healthcare UK Ltd)
 Abacavir (as Abacavir sulfate) 300 mg Ziagen 300mg tablets | 60 tablet [PoM] £208.95 (Hospital only)

Oral solution

EXCIPIENTS: May contain Propylene glycol

- **Ziagen** (ViiV Healthcare UK Ltd)
 Abacavir (as Abacavir sulfate) 20 mg per 1 ml Ziagen 20mg/ml oral solution | 240 ml [PoM] £55.72 (Hospital only) [SF]

Abacavir with dolutegravir and lamivudine

28-Jul-2021

The properties listed below are those particular to the combination only. For the properties of the components please consider, abacavir p. 513, lamivudine p. 518, dolutegravir p. 508.

- **INDICATIONS AND DOSE**

HIV infection

- BY MOUTH
- Child 12–17 years (body-weight 40 kg and above): 1 tablet once daily

- **INTERACTIONS** → Appendix 1: dolutegravir · NRTIs
- **RENAL IMPAIRMENT** [EvGr] Avoid if creatinine clearance less than 50 mL/minute (consult product literature). ⟨M⟩ See p. 16.
- **PATIENT AND CARER ADVICE**
 Missed doses If a dose is more than 20 hours late, the missed dose should not be taken and the next dose should be taken at the normal time.
- **MEDICINAL FORMS** There can be variation in the licensing of different medicines containing the same drug.

Oral tablet

- **Triumeq** (ViiV Healthcare UK Ltd)
 Dolutegravir (as Dolutegravir sodium) 50 mg, Lamivudine 300 mg, Abacavir (as Abacavir sulfate) 600 mg Triumeq 50mg/600mg/300mg tablets | 30 tablet [PoM] £798.16 (Hospital only)

Abacavir with lamivudine

28-Jul-2021

The properties listed below are those particular to the combination only. For the properties of the components please consider, abacavir p. 513, lamivudine p. 518.

- **INDICATIONS AND DOSE**

HIV infection in combination with other antiretrovirals

- BY MOUTH
- Child 12–17 years (body-weight 40 kg and above): 1 tablet once daily

- **INTERACTIONS** → Appendix 1: NRTIs
- **RENAL IMPAIRMENT** [EvGr] Avoid if creatinine clearance less than 50 mL/minute (consult product literature). ⟨M⟩ See p. 16.
- **MEDICINAL FORMS** There can be variation in the licensing of different medicines containing the same drug.

Oral tablet

- **Abacavir with lamivudine (Non-proprietary)**
 Lamivudine 300 mg, Abacavir 600 mg Abacavir 600mg / Lamivudine 300mg tablets | 30 tablet [PoM] £299.41 DT = £352.25 (Hospital only)
- **Kivexa** (ViiV Healthcare UK Ltd)
 Lamivudine 300 mg, Abacavir 600 mg Kivexa 600mg/300mg tablets | 30 tablet [PoM] £352.25 DT = £352.25 (Hospital only)

Abacavir with lamivudine and zidovudine

28-Jul-2021

The properties listed below are those particular to the combination only. For the properties of the components please consider, abacavir p. 513, lamivudine p. 518, zidovudine p. 519.

- **INDICATIONS AND DOSE**

HIV infection (use only if patient is stabilised for 6–8 weeks on the individual components in the same proportions)

- BY MOUTH
- Child (body-weight 30 kg and above): 1 tablet twice daily

- **UNLICENSED USE** *Trizivir*® not licensed for use in children.
- **INTERACTIONS** → Appendix 1: NRTIs
- **RENAL IMPAIRMENT** [EvGr] Avoid if creatinine clearance less than 50 mL/minute (consult product literature). ⟨M⟩ See p. 16.
- **MEDICINAL FORMS** No licensed medicines listed.

Bictegravir with emtricitabine and tenofovir alafenamide

05-Jul-2024

The properties listed below are those particular to the combination only. For the properties of the components please consider, emtricitabine p. 516, tenofovir alafenamide p. 493.

- **INDICATIONS AND DOSE**

HIV-1 infection [doses for 30/120/15 mg tablets] (initiated by a specialist)

- BY MOUTH
- Child 2–17 years (body-weight 14–24 kg): 1 tablet once daily

HIV-1 infection [doses for 50/200/25 mg tablets] (initiated by a specialist)

- BY MOUTH
- Child 2–17 years (body-weight 25 kg and above): 1 tablet once daily

DOSE EQUIVALENCE AND CONVERSION

- Tablet strength expressed as x/y/z mg representing bictegravir/emtricitabine/tenofovir alafenamide, respectively.

- **INTERACTIONS** → Appendix 1: bictegravir · tenofovir alafenamide
- **SIDE-EFFECTS**
 - **Common or very common** Depression · diarrhoea · dizziness · fatigue · headache · nausea · sleep disorders
 - **Uncommon** Anaemia · angioedema · anxiety · arthralgia · flatulence · gastrointestinal discomfort · hyperbilirubinaemia · skin reactions · suicidal behaviours · vomiting
 - **Rare or very rare** Stevens-Johnson syndrome
 - **Frequency not known** Osteonecrosis

- **PREGNANCY** EvGr Use only if potential benefit outweighs risk (limited information on bictegravir). ⟨M⟩
- **HEPATIC IMPAIRMENT** EvGr Avoid in severe impairment (no information available). ⟨M⟩
- **RENAL IMPAIRMENT** EvGr Avoid if creatinine clearance is less than 30 mL/minute (limited information available). ⟨M⟩ See p. 16. EvGr Caution in patients weighing <35kg with any degree of renal impairment (no information available). ⟨M⟩
- **PRESCRIBING AND DISPENSING INFORMATION** Dispense in original container (contains desiccant).
- **PATIENT AND CARER ADVICE**
  Vomiting If vomiting occurs within 1 hour of taking a dose, a replacement dose should be taken.
  Missed doses If a dose is more than 18 hours late, the missed dose should not be taken and the next dose should be taken at the normal time.
  Driving and skilled tasks Patients and carers should be counselled on the effects on driving and performance of skilled tasks—increased risk of dizziness.

- **MEDICINAL FORMS** There can be variation in the licensing of different medicines containing the same drug.

Oral tablet

CAUTIONARY AND ADVISORY LABELS 25

- **Biktarvy** (Gilead Sciences Ltd)
  Tenofovir alafenamide (as Tenofovir alafenamide fumarate) 15 mg, Bictegravir (as Bictegravir sodium) 30 mg, Emtricitabine 120 mg Biktarvy 30mg/120mg/15mg tablets | 30 tablet PoM £879.51 (Hospital only)
  Tenofovir alafenamide (as Tenofovir alafenamide fumarate) 25 mg, Bictegravir (as Bictegravir sodium) 50 mg, Emtricitabine 200 mg Biktarvy 50mg/200mg/25mg tablets | 30 tablet PoM £879.51 (Hospital only)

Elvitegravir with cobicistat, emtricitabine and tenofovir alafenamide

22-Oct-2020

The properties listed below are those particular to the combination only. For the properties of the components please consider, emtricitabine p. 516, elvitegravir, cobicistat p. 525, tenofovir alafenamide p. 493.

- **INDICATIONS AND DOSE**

HIV-1 infection (specialist use only)

- BY MOUTH
- Child 6–11 years (body-weight 25 kg and above): 1 tablet once daily
- Child 12–17 years (body-weight 35 kg and above): 1 tablet once daily

IMPORTANT SAFETY INFORMATION

MHRA/CHM ADVICE: ELVITEGRAVIR BOOSTED WITH COBICISTAT: AVOID USE IN PREGNANCY DUE TO RISK OF TREATMENT FAILURE AND MATERNAL-TO-CHILD TRANSMISSION OF HIV-1 (APRIL 2019)

Pharmacokinetic data show mean exposure of elvitegravir boosted with cobicistat (available in combination in *Genvoya*® and *Stribild*®) to be lower during the second and third trimesters of pregnancy than postpartum. Low elvitegravir exposure may be associated with an increased risk of treatment failure and an increased risk of HIV-1 transmission to the unborn child. For further information, see *Pregnancy*.

- **INTERACTIONS** → Appendix 1: cobicistat · elvitegravir · tenofovir alafenamide
- **SIDE-EFFECTS**
  - **Common or very common** Abnormal dreams · diarrhoea · dizziness · fatigue · flatulence · gastrointestinal discomfort · headache · nausea · skin reactions · vomiting
  - **Uncommon** Anaemia · depression · suicidal behaviours
  - **Frequency not known** Nephrotoxicity · osteonecrosis · weight increased
- **CONCEPTION AND CONTRACEPTION** Manufacturer advises effective contraception in women of childbearing potential; if using a hormonal contraceptive, it must contain drospirenone or norgestimate as the progestogen and at least 30 micrograms ethinylestradiol.
- **PREGNANCY** Manufacturer advises not to be initiated during pregnancy due to low elvitegravir exposure; women who become pregnant during therapy should be switched to an alternative regimen.
- **HEPATIC IMPAIRMENT** Manufacturer advises caution (increased risk of hepatic side-effects); avoid in severe impairment (no information available).
- **RENAL IMPAIRMENT** Manufacturer advises avoid if creatinine clearance less than 30 mL/minute—limited information available. See p. 16. Manufacturer advises caution in children under 12 years with renal impairment—no information available.
- **PRESCRIBING AND DISPENSING INFORMATION** Dispense in original container—contains desiccant.
- **PATIENT AND CARER ADVICE**
  Missed doses Manufacturer advises if a dose is more than 18 hours late, the missed dose should not be taken and the next dose should be taken at the normal time.
  Driving and skilled tasks Manufacturer advises patients and carers should be counselled on the effects on driving and performance of skilled tasks—increased risk of dizziness.
- **NATIONAL FUNDING/ACCESS DECISIONS**
  For full details see funding body website

Scottish Medicines Consortium (SMC) decisions

- **Elvitegravir, cobicistat, emtricitabine, tenofovir alafenamide (*Genvoya*®) for the treatment of adults and adolescents (aged 12 years and older with body weight at least 35 kg) infected with human immunodeficiency virus-1 (HIV-1) without any known mutations associated with resistance to the integrase inhibitor class, emtricitabine or tenofovir (May 2016)** SMC No. 1142/16 Recommended

All Wales Medicines Strategy Group (AWMSG) decisions

- **Elvitegravir / cobicistat / emtricitabine / tenofovir alafenamide (*Genvoya*®) for the treatment of adults and adolescents (aged 12 years and older with body weight at least 35 kg) infected with human immunodeficiency virus-1 (HIV-1) without any known mutations associated with resistance to the integrase inhibitor class, emtricitabine or tenofovir (July 2016)** AWMSG No. 2248 Recommended

- **MEDICINAL FORMS** There can be variation in the licensing of different medicines containing the same drug.

Oral tablet

CAUTIONARY AND ADVISORY LABELS 21

- **Genvoya** (Gilead Sciences Ltd)
  Tenofovir alafenamide (as Tenofovir alafenamide fumarate) 6 mg, Cobicistat 90 mg, Elvitegravir 90 mg, Emtricitabine 120 mg Genvoya 90mg/90mg/120mg/6mg tablets | 30 tablet PoM £879.51 (Hospital only)
  Tenofovir alafenamide (as Tenofovir alafenamide fumarate) 10 mg, Cobicistat 150 mg, Elvitegravir 150 mg, Emtricitabine 200 mg Genvoya 150mg/150mg/200mg/10mg tablets | 30 tablet PoM £879.51 (Hospital only)

513

Emtricitabine

26-Jul-2021

(FTC)

● **INDICATIONS AND DOSE**

HIV infection in combination with other antiretroviral drugs

▶ BY MOUTH USING CAPSULES

- Child (body-weight 33 kg and above): 200 mg once daily

▶ BY MOUTH USING ORAL SOLUTION

- Child 4 months–17 years (body-weight up to 33 kg): 6 mg/kg once daily
- Child 4 months–17 years (body-weight 33 kg and above): 240 mg once daily

DOSE EQUIVALENCE AND CONVERSION

- 240 mg oral solution ≡ 200 mg capsule; where appropriate the capsule may be used instead of the oral solution.

● **SIDE-EFFECTS**

▶ **Common or very common** Abnormal dreams · dyspepsia · hyperbilirubinaemia · hyperglycaemia · hypersensitivity · hypertriglyceridaemia · pain · rash pustular

● **HEPATIC IMPAIRMENT**

Monitoring On discontinuation, monitor patients with hepatitis B (risk of exacerbation of hepatitis).

● **RENAL IMPAIRMENT**

Dose adjustments See p. 16.

In adults, manufacturer advises reduce dose or increase dosage interval if creatinine clearance less than 30 mL/minute (consult product literature).

● **PRESCRIBING AND DISPENSING INFORMATION** Flavours of oral liquid formulations may include candy.

● **PATIENT AND CARER ADVICE**

Missed doses If a dose is more than 12 hours late, the missed dose should not be taken and the next dose should be taken at the normal time.

● **MEDICINAL FORMS** There can be variation in the licensing of different medicines containing the same drug.

Oral solution

ELECTROLYTES: May contain Sodium

▸ Emtriva (Gilead Sciences Ltd)

Emtricitabine 10 mg per 1 ml Emtriva 10mg/ml oral solution | 170 ml [PoM] £39.53 (Hospital only) [SF]

Oral capsule

▸ Emtriva (Gilead Sciences Ltd)

Emtricitabine 200 mg Emtriva 200mg capsules | 30 capsule [PoM] £138.98 (Hospital only)

Combinations available: *Darunavir with cobicistat, emtricitabine and tenofovir alafenamide,* p. 522

Emtricitabine with rilpivirine and tenofovir alafenamide

21-Aug-2020

The properties listed below are those particular to the combination only. For the properties of the components please consider, emtricitabine above, rilpivirine p. 512, tenofovir alafenamide p. 493.

● **INDICATIONS AND DOSE**

HIV infection in patients with plasma HIV-1 RNA concentration of 100 000 copies/mL or less (specialist use only)

▶ BY MOUTH

- Child 12–17 years (body-weight 35 kg and above): 1 tablet once daily

● **INTERACTIONS** → Appendix 1: NNRTIs · tenofovir alafenamide

● **SIDE-EFFECTS**

▶ **Common or very common** Appetite decreased · depression · diarrhoea · dizziness · drowsiness · dry mouth · fatigue · flatulence · gastrointestinal discomfort · headache · nausea · skin reactions · sleep disorders · vomiting

▶ **Uncommon** Anaemia · angioedema · arthralgia · immune reconstitution inflammatory syndrome · severe cutaneous adverse reactions (SCARs)

▶ **Frequency not known** Conjunctivitis · eosinophilia · fever · osteonecrosis

SIDE-EFFECTS, FURTHER INFORMATION Systemic symptoms reported with severe skin reactions include fever, blisters, conjunctivitis, angioedema, elevated liver function tests, and eosinophilia.

● **HEPATIC IMPAIRMENT** Manufacturer advises caution in moderate impairment (increased risk of hepatic side-effects); avoid in severe impairment (no information available).

● **RENAL IMPAIRMENT** Manufacturer advises avoid if creatinine clearance less than 30 mL/minute—no information available. See p. 16.

● **PATIENT AND CARER ADVICE**

Vomiting Manufacturer advises if vomiting occurs within 4 hours of taking a dose, a replacement dose should be taken.

Driving and skilled tasks Manufacturer advises patients and carers should be counselled on the effects on driving and performance of skilled tasks—increased risk of dizziness.

● **NATIONAL FUNDING/ACCESS DECISIONS**

For full details see funding body website

Scottish Medicines Consortium (SMC) decisions

▶ **Emtricitabine/rilpivirine/tenofovir alafenamide (*Odefsey*®) for the treatment of HIV-1 without known mutations associated with resistance to the non nucleoside reverse transcriptase inhibitor class, tenofovir or emtricitabine, and with a viral load HIV-1 RNA of 100,000 copies/mL or less (October 2016)** SMC No. 1189/16 Recommended

All Wales Medicines Strategy Group (AWMSG) decisions

▶ **Emtricitabine/rilpivirine/tenofovir alafenamide (*Odefsey*®) for the treatment of HIV-1 without known mutations associated with resistance to the non-nucleoside reverse transcriptase inhibitor class, tenofovir or emtricitabine, and with a viral load HIV-1 RNA of 100,000 copies/mL or less (November 2016)** AWMSG No. 3031 Recommended

● **MEDICINAL FORMS** There can be variation in the licensing of different medicines containing the same drug.

Oral tablet

CAUTIONARY AND ADVISORY LABELS 3, 21

▸ Odefsey (Gilead Sciences Ltd)

Rilpivirine (as Rilpivirine hydrochloride) 25 mg, Tenofovir alafenamide (as Tenofovir alafenamide fumarate) 25 mg, Emtricitabine 200 mg Odefsey 200mg/25mg/25mg tablets | 30 tablet [PoM] £525.95 (Hospital only)

Emtricitabine with tenofovir alafenamide

10-Mar-2025

The properties listed below are those particular to the combination only. For the properties of the components please consider, emtricitabine p. 516, tenofovir alafenamide p. 493.

● **INDICATIONS AND DOSE**

HIV-1 infection in combination with other antiretroviral drugs [doses for 200/10 mg or 200/25 mg tablets] (initiated by a specialist)

▶ BY MOUTH

▸ Child 12–17 years (body-weight 35 kg and above): 1 tablet once daily, tablet strength is dependent on drug regimen—consult product literature

Pre-exposure prophylaxis of HIV-1 infection [doses for 200/25 mg tablets] (initiated by a specialist)

▶ BY MOUTH

▸ Child 12–17 years (body-weight 35 kg and above and male): 1 tablet once daily.

DOSE EQUIVALENCE AND CONVERSION

▸ Tablet strength expressed as *x/y* mg representing emtricitabine/tenofovir alafenamide, respectively.

● **INTERACTIONS** → Appendix 1: tenofovir alafenamide

● **SIDE-EFFECTS**

▶ **Common or very common** Abnormal dreams · diarrhoea · dizziness · fatigue · flatulence · gastrointestinal discomfort · headache · nausea · skin reactions · vomiting

▶ **Uncommon** Anaemia · angioedema · arthralgia

▶ **Frequency not known** Immune reconstitution inflammatory syndrome · nephrotoxicity · osteonecrosis

● **HEPATIC IMPAIRMENT** EvGr Caution (increased risk of hepatic side-effects). ⟨M⟩

● **RENAL IMPAIRMENT** EvGr Avoid if creatinine clearance less than 30 mL/minute (limited information available). ⟨M⟩ See p. 16.

● **PATIENT AND CARER ADVICE**

Missed doses If a dose is more than 18 hours late, the missed dose should not be taken and the next dose should be taken at the normal time.

Driving and skilled tasks Patients and carers should be counselled on the effects on driving and performance of skilled tasks—increased risk of dizziness.

● **NATIONAL FUNDING/ACCESS DECISIONS**

For full details see funding body website

Scottish Medicines Consortium (SMC) decisions

▶ **Emtricitabine / tenofovir alafenamide (*Descovy*®) in combination with other antiretroviral agents for the treatment of adults and adolescents (aged 12 years and older with body weight at least 35 kg) infected with human immunodeficiency virus type 1 (August 2016)** SMC No. 1169/16 Recommended

All Wales Medicines Strategy Group (AWMSG) decisions

▶ **Emtricitabine / tenofovir alafenamide (*Descovy*®) for treatment of adults and adolescents (aged 12 years and older with body weight at least 35 kg) infected with human immunodeficiency virus type 1 (HIV 1) (October 2016)** AWMSG No. 2771 Recommended

▶ **Emtricitabine / tenofovir alafenamide (*Descovy*®) for pre-exposure prophylaxis to reduce the risk of sexually acquired HIV-1 infection in at-risk men who have sex with men, including adolescents (with body weight at least 35 kg) (February 2025)** AWMSG No. 2566 Recommended with restrictions

● **MEDICINAL FORMS** There can be variation in the licensing of different medicines containing the same drug.

Oral tablet

CAUTIONARY AND ADVISORY LABELS 25

▸ **Descovy** (Gilead Sciences Ltd)

Tenofovir alafenamide (as Tenofovir alafenamide fumarate) 25 mg, Emtricitabine 200 mg Descovy 200mg/25mg tablets | 30 tablet PoM £355.73 DT = £355.73 (Hospital only)

Tenofovir alafenamide (as Tenofovir alafenamide fumarate) 10 mg, Emtricitabine 200 mg Descovy 200mg/10mg tablets | 30 tablet PoM £355.73 DT = £355.73 (Hospital only)

Emtricitabine with tenofovir disoproxil

12-Oct-2020

The properties listed below are those particular to the combination only. For the properties of the components please consider, tenofovir disoproxil p. 519, emtricitabine p. 516.

● **INDICATIONS AND DOSE**

HIV-1 infection (initiated by a specialist)

▶ BY MOUTH

▸ Child 12–17 years (body-weight 35 kg and above): 200/245 mg once daily

Pre-exposure prophylaxis of HIV-1 infection (initiated by a specialist)

▶ BY MOUTH

▸ Child 12–17 years (body-weight 35 kg and above): 200/245 mg once daily

DOSE EQUIVALENCE AND CONVERSION

▸ Dose expressed as x/y mg emtricitabine/tenofovir disoproxil.

● **INTERACTIONS** → Appendix 1: tenofovir disoproxil

● **HEPATIC IMPAIRMENT** Manufacturer advises caution (increased risk of hepatic side-effects).

● **RENAL IMPAIRMENT** Manufacturer advises avoid.

● **DIRECTIONS FOR ADMINISTRATION** Patients with swallowing difficulties may disperse tablet in half a glass of water, orange juice, or grape juice.

● **PATIENT AND CARER ADVICE** Patients or carers should be given advice on how to administer emtricitabine with tenofovir tablets.

Missed doses If a dose is more than 12 hours late, the missed dose should not be taken and the next dose should be taken at the normal time.

● **MEDICINAL FORMS** There can be variation in the licensing of different medicines containing the same drug. Forms available from special-order manufacturers include: oral tablet

Oral tablet

CAUTIONARY AND ADVISORY LABELS 21

▸ **Emtricitabine with tenofovir disoproxil (Non-proprietary)**

Emtricitabine 200 mg, Tenofovir disoproxil 245 mg Emtricitabine 200mg / Tenofovir disoproxil 245mg tablets | 30 tablet PoM £302.37 DT = £355.73 (Hospital only) | 30 tablet PoM ⊠ DT = £355.73

▸ **Truvada** (Gilead Sciences Ltd)

Emtricitabine 200 mg, Tenofovir disoproxil 245 mg Truvada 200mg/245mg tablets | 30 tablet PoM £355.73 DT = £355.73 (Hospital only)

513

Lamivudine

25-Jul-2021

(3TC)

● **INDICATIONS AND DOSE**

EPIVIR ® ORAL SOLUTION

HIV infection in combination with other antiretroviral drugs

▶ BY MOUTH

- Child 1–2 months: 4 mg/kg twice daily
- Child 3 months–11 years (body-weight up to 14 kg): 4 mg/kg twice daily (max. per dose 150 mg), alternatively 8 mg/kg once daily (max. per dose 300 mg)
- Child 3 months–11 years (body-weight 14–20 kg): 4 mg/kg twice daily (max. per dose 150 mg), alternatively 8 mg/kg once daily (max. per dose 300 mg), alternatively 75 mg twice daily, alternatively 150 mg once daily
- Child 3 months–11 years (body-weight 21–29 kg): 4 mg/kg twice daily (max. per dose 150 mg), alternatively 8 mg/kg once daily (max. per dose 300 mg), alternatively 75 mg daily, dose to be taken in the morning and 150 mg daily, dose to be taken in the evening, alternatively 225 mg once daily
- Child 3 months–11 years (body-weight 30 kg and above): 4 mg/kg twice daily (max. per dose 150 mg), alternatively 8 mg/kg once daily (max. per dose 300 mg), alternatively 150 mg twice daily, alternatively 300 mg once daily
- Child 12–17 years: 150 mg twice daily, alternatively 300 mg once daily

EPIVIR ® TABLETS

HIV infection in combination with other antiretroviral drugs

▶ BY MOUTH

- Child 1–2 months: 4 mg/kg twice daily
- Child 3 months–11 years (body-weight up to 14 kg): 4 mg/kg twice daily, alternatively 8 mg/kg once daily
- Child 3 months–11 years (body-weight 14–20 kg): 4 mg/kg twice daily (max. per dose 150 mg), alternatively 8 mg/kg once daily (max. per dose 300 mg), alternatively 75 mg twice daily, alternatively 150 mg once daily
- Child 3 months–11 years (body-weight 21–29 kg): 4 mg/kg twice daily (max. per dose 150 mg), alternatively 8 mg/kg once daily (max. per dose 300 mg), alternatively 75 mg daily, dose to be taken in the morning and 150 mg daily, dose to be taken in the evening, alternatively 225 mg once daily
- Child 3 months–11 years (body-weight 30 kg and above): 4 mg/kg twice daily (max. per dose 150 mg), alternatively 8 mg/kg once daily (max. per dose 300 mg), alternatively 150 mg twice daily, alternatively 300 mg once daily
- Child 12–17 years: 150 mg twice daily, alternatively 300 mg once daily

ZEFFIX ®

Chronic hepatitis B infection either with compensated liver disease (with evidence of viral replication and histology of active liver inflammation or fibrosis) when first-line treatments cannot be used, or (in combination with another antiviral drug without cross-resistance to lamivudine) with decompensated liver disease

▶ BY MOUTH

- Child 2–11 years: 3 mg/kg once daily (max. per dose 100 mg), children receiving lamivudine for concomitant HIV infection should continue to receive lamivudine in a dose appropriate for HIV infection
- Child 12–17 years: 100 mg once daily, patients receiving lamivudine for concomitant HIV infection should continue to receive lamivudine in a dose appropriate for HIV infection

● **UNLICENSED USE**

EPIVIR ® ORAL SOLUTION Not licensed for use in children under 3 months.

EPIVIR ® TABLETS Not licensed for use in children under 3 months.

ZEFFIX ® Not licensed for use in children.

● **CAUTIONS** Recurrent hepatitis in patients with chronic hepatitis B may occur on discontinuation of lamivudine

● **INTERACTIONS** → Appendix 1: NRTIs

● **SIDE-EFFECTS**

▶ **Common or very common** Alopecia · arthralgia · cough · gastrointestinal discomfort · hepatic disorders · malaise · muscle complaints · myopathy · nasal disorder

▶ **Uncommon** Thrombocytopenia

▶ **Rare or very rare** Paraesthesia · peripheral neuropathy · pure red cell aplasia

▶ **Frequency not known** Respiratory tract infection · throat complaints

● **BREAST FEEDING** Can be used with caution in women infected with chronic hepatitis B alone, providing that adequate measures are taken to prevent hepatitis B infection in infants.

● **RENAL IMPAIRMENT**

Dose adjustments EvGr Reduce dose if creatinine clearance less than 50 mL/minute (consult product literature). Ⓜ See p. 16.

● **MONITORING REQUIREMENTS** When treating chronic hepatitis B with lamivudine, monitor liver function tests every 3 months, and viral markers of hepatitis B every 3–6 months, more frequently in patients with advanced liver disease or following transplantation (monitoring to continue for at least 1 year after discontinuation—recurrent hepatitis may occur on discontinuation).

● **PRESCRIBING AND DISPENSING INFORMATION** Flavours of oral liquid formulations may include banana and strawberry.

● **MEDICINAL FORMS** There can be variation in the licensing of different medicines containing the same drug.

Oral tablet

▸ **Epivir** (ViiV Healthcare UK Ltd)

Lamivudine 150 mg Epivir 150mg tablets | 60 tablet PoM £143.32 DT = £143.32 (Hospital only)

Lamivudine 300 mg Epivir 300mg tablets | 30 tablet PoM £157.51 DT = £157.51 (Hospital only)

▸ **Zeffix** (GlaxoSmithKline UK Ltd)

Lamivudine 100 mg Zeffix 100mg tablets | 28 tablet PoM £78.09 DT = £78.09

Oral solution

EXCIPIENTS: May contain Sucrose

▸ **Epivir** (ViiV Healthcare UK Ltd)

Lamivudine 10 mg per 1 ml Epivir 50mg/5ml oral solution | 240 ml PoM £39.01 DT = £39.01 (Hospital only)

Lamivudine with dolutegravir

23-Oct-2020

The properties listed below are those particular to the combination only. For the properties of the components please consider, lamivudine above, dolutegravir p. 508.

● **INDICATIONS AND DOSE**

HIV-1 infection

▶ BY MOUTH

- Child 12–17 years (body-weight 40 kg and above): 300/50 mg once daily

DOSE EQUIVALENCE AND CONVERSION
- Dose expressed as x/y mg lamivudine/dolutegravir.

- **INTERACTIONS** → Appendix 1: dolutegravir · NRTIs
- **RENAL IMPAIRMENT** Manufacturer advises avoid if creatinine clearance less than 50 mL/minute. See p. 16.
- **PATIENT AND CARER ADVICE**
Missed doses Manufacturer advises if a dose is more than 20 hours late, the missed dose should not be taken and the next dose should be taken at the normal time.
- **NATIONAL FUNDING/ACCESS DECISIONS**
For full details see funding body website
Scottish Medicines Consortium (SMC) decisions
- **Dolutegravir / lamivudine (*Dovato*®) for treatment of Human Immunodeficiency Virus type 1 (HIV-1) infection in adults and adolescents above 12 years of age weighing at least 40 kg, with no known or suspected resistance to the integrase inhibitor class, or lamivudine (September 2019)** SMC No. SMC2205 Recommended

All Wales Medicines Strategy Group (AWMSG) decisions
- **Dolutegravir / lamivudine (*Dovato*®) for treatment of Human Immunodeficiency Virus type 1 (HIV-1) infection in adults and adolescents above 12 years of age weighing at least 40 kg, with no known or suspected resistance to the integrase inhibitor class, or lamivudine (February 2020)** AWMSG No. 3659 Recommended

- **MEDICINAL FORMS** There can be variation in the licensing of different medicines containing the same drug.

Oral tablet
- Dovato (ViiV Healthcare UK Ltd)
Dolutegravir (as Dolutegravir sodium) 50 mg, Lamivudine 300 mg Dovato 50mg/300mg tablets | 30 tablet PoM £656.26

513

Tenofovir disoproxil

23-Aug-2021

- **INDICATIONS AND DOSE**

HIV infection in combination with other antiretroviral drugs when first-line nucleoside reverse transcriptase inhibitors cannot be used because of resistance or contra-indications
- BY MOUTH
- Child 2–17 years: 6.5 mg/kg once daily (max. per dose 245 mg)
- Child 6–17 years (body-weight 17–21 kg): 123 mg once daily
- Child 6–17 years (body-weight 22–27 kg): 163 mg once daily
- Child 6–17 years (body-weight 28–34 kg): 204 mg once daily
- Child 6–17 years (body-weight 35 kg and above): 245 mg once daily

Chronic hepatitis B infection with compensated liver disease (with evidence of viral replication, and histology of active liver inflammation or fibrosis)
- BY MOUTH
- Child 12–17 years (body-weight 35 kg and above): 245 mg once daily

DOSE EQUIVALENCE AND CONVERSION
- 7.5 scoops of granules contains approx. 245 mg tenofovir disoproxil (as fumarate).

- **INTERACTIONS** → Appendix 1: tenofovir disoproxil
- **SIDE-EFFECTS**
- **Common or very common** Abdominal distension
- **Uncommon** Renal tubular disorders
- **Rare or very rare** Acute tubular necrosis · hepatic disorders · nephritis · nephrogenic diabetes insipidus · renal impairment
- **HEPATIC IMPAIRMENT** Manufacturer advises caution in decompensated hepatic disease (limited information available).
- **RENAL IMPAIRMENT** EvGr Avoid (no information available). (M)
- **MONITORING REQUIREMENTS**
- Test renal function and serum phosphate before treatment, then every 4 weeks (more frequently if at increased risk of renal impairment) for 1 year and then every 3 months, interrupt treatment if renal function deteriorates or serum phosphate decreases.
- When treating chronic hepatitis B with tenofovir, monitor liver function tests every 3 months and viral markers for hepatitis B every 3–6 months during treatment (continue monitoring for at least 1 year after discontinuation—recurrent hepatitis may occur on discontinuation).
- **DIRECTIONS FOR ADMINISTRATION** *Granules*: Manufacturer advises mix 1 scoop of granules with 1 tablespoon of soft food (e.g. yoghurt, apple sauce) and take immediately without chewing. Do **not** mix granules with liquids.
- **PATIENT AND CARER ADVICE** Patients or carers should be given advice on how to administer tenofovir granules.
Missed doses If a dose is more than 12 hours late, the missed dose should not be taken and the next dose should be taken at the normal time.

- **MEDICINAL FORMS** There can be variation in the licensing of different medicines containing the same drug.

Oral tablet
CAUTIONARY AND ADVISORY LABELS 21
- Tenofovir disoproxil (Non-proprietary)
Tenofovir disoproxil 245 mg Tenofovir disoproxil 245mg tablets | 30 tablet PoM £28.39 | 30 tablet PoM £11.60–£204.39 (Hospital only)
- Viread (Gilead Sciences Ltd)
Tenofovir disoproxil 123 mg Viread 123mg tablets | 30 tablet PoM £102.60 (Hospital only)
Tenofovir disoproxil 163 mg Viread 163mg tablets | 30 tablet PoM £135.98 (Hospital only)
Tenofovir disoproxil 204 mg Viread 204mg tablets | 30 tablet PoM £170.19 (Hospital only)
Tenofovir disoproxil 245 mg Viread 245mg tablets | 30 tablet PoM £204.39 (Hospital only)

Oral granules
CAUTIONARY AND ADVISORY LABELS 21
- Viread (Gilead Sciences Ltd)
Tenofovir disoproxil 33 mg per 1 gram Viread 33mg/g granules | 60 gram PoM £54.50 (Hospital only)

513

Zidovudine

02-Sep-2021

(Azidothymidine; AZT)

- **INDICATIONS AND DOSE**

HIV infection in combination with other antiretroviral drugs
- BY MOUTH
- Child: 180 mg/m^2 twice daily (max. per dose 300 mg)
- Child (body-weight 8–13 kg): 100 mg twice daily
- Child (body-weight 14–20 kg): 100 mg, to be taken in the morning and 200 mg, to be taken in the evening
- Child (body-weight 21–27 kg): 200 mg twice daily
- Child (body-weight 28–29 kg): 200–250 mg twice daily
- Child (body-weight 30 kg and above): 250–300 mg twice daily

HIV infection in combination with other antiretroviral drugs (dose expressed in mg/kg)
- BY MOUTH
- Child (body-weight 4–8 kg): 12 mg/kg twice daily
- Child (body-weight 9–29 kg): 9 mg/kg twice daily

continued →

5 Infection

Prevention of maternal-fetal HIV transmission
- BY MOUTH, OR BY INTRAVENOUS INFUSION
  - Child: Seek specialist advice (combination therapy preferred) (consult local protocol)

HIV infection in combination with other antiretroviral drugs in patients temporarily unable to take zidovudine by mouth
- BY INTRAVENOUS INFUSION
  - Child 3 months–11 years: 60–80 mg/m^2 every 6 hours usually for not more than 2 weeks, dose approximating to 9–12 mg/kg twice daily by mouth
  - Child 12–17 years: 0.8–1 mg/kg every 4 hours usually for not more than 2 weeks, dose approximating to 1.2–1.5 mg/kg every 4 hours by mouth

- **CONTRA-INDICATIONS** Abnormally low haemoglobin concentration (consult product literature) · abnormally low neutrophil counts (consult product literature) · neonates with hyperbilirubinaemia requiring treatment other than phototherapy, or with raised transaminase (consult product literature)
- **CAUTIONS** Lactic acidosis · risk of haematological toxicity particularly with high dose and advanced disease · vitamin B_{12} deficiency (increased risk of neutropenia)

  CAUTIONS, FURTHER INFORMATION
  - Lactic acidosis Lactic acidosis associated with hepatomegaly and hepatic steatosis has been reported with zidovudine. Use with caution in patients with hepatomegaly, hepatitis, or other risk factors for liver disease and hepatic steatosis (including obesity and alcohol abuse). Manufacturer advises discontinue treatment if symptoms of hyperlactataemia, lactic acidosis, progressive hepatomegaly or rapid deterioration of liver function become apparent.
- **INTERACTIONS** → Appendix 1: NRTIs
- **SIDE-EFFECTS**
  - **Common or very common** Leucopenia · malaise · myalgia
  - **Uncommon** Bone marrow disorders · dyspnoea · generalised pain · myopathy · thrombocytopenia
  - **Rare or very rare** Alertness decreased · anxiety · appetite decreased · cardiomyopathy · chest pain · chills · cough · depression · drowsiness · dyspepsia · gynaecomastia · hepatic disorders · hyperhidrosis · influenza like illness · nail discolouration · oral discolouration · paraesthesia · pure red cell aplasia · seizure · taste altered · urinary frequency increased
  - **Frequency not known** Lipoatrophy

  SIDE-EFFECTS, FURTHER INFORMATION **Anaemia and myelosuppression** If anaemia or myelosuppression occur, reduce dose or interrupt treatment according to product literature, or consider other treatment.

  Lipodystrophy syndrome Metabolic effects may occur with zidovudine; plasma lipids and blood glucose concentrations should be measured routinely.
- **HEPATIC IMPAIRMENT** Manufacturer advises caution in moderate to severe impairment (increased risk of accumulation).

  Dose adjustments Manufacturer advises consider dose reduction in moderate to severe impairment—consult product literature.
- **RENAL IMPAIRMENT**

  Dose adjustments See p. 16.

  [EvGr] Reduce dose if creatinine clearance less than 10 mL/minute (consult product literature). ⟨M⟩
- **MONITORING REQUIREMENTS** Monitor full blood count after 4 weeks of treatment, then every 3 months.
- **DIRECTIONS FOR ADMINISTRATION** For *intermittent intravenous infusion*, manufacturer advises dilute to a concentration of 2 mg/mL or 4 mg/mL with Glucose 5% and give over 1 hour.
- **PRESCRIBING AND DISPENSING INFORMATION** The abbreviation AZT which is sometimes used for zidovudine has also been used for another drug.
- **PATIENT AND CARER ADVICE**

  Medicines for Children leaflet: Zidovudine for treatment of HIV infection www.medicinesforchildren.org.uk/medicines/zidovudine-for-the-treatment-of-hiv-infection/

- **MEDICINAL FORMS** There can be variation in the licensing of different medicines containing the same drug.

Solution for infusion
- **Retrovir** (ViiV Healthcare UK Ltd)

  Zidovudine 10 mg per 1 ml Retrovir IV 200mg/20ml concentrate for solution for infusion vials | 5 vial [PoM] £52.48 (Hospital only)

Oral solution
- **Retrovir** (ViiV Healthcare UK Ltd)

  Zidovudine 10 mg per 1 ml Retrovir 100mg/10ml oral solution | 200 ml [PoM] £20.91 (Hospital only) [SF]

Oral capsule
- **Zidovudine (Non-proprietary)**

  Zidovudine 100 mg Zidovudine 100mg capsules | 60 capsule [PoM] £53.31 (Hospital only)

  Zidovudine 250 mg Zidovudine 250mg capsules | 60 capsule [PoM] £13.32 (Hospital only)
- **Retrovir** (ViiV Healthcare UK Ltd)

  Zidovudine 100 mg Retrovir 100mg capsules | 100 capsule [PoM] £104.54 (Hospital only)

  Zidovudine 250 mg Retrovir 250mg capsules | 40 capsule [PoM] £104.54 (Hospital only)

Zidovudine with lamivudine

29-Jul-2021

The properties listed below are those particular to the combination only. For the properties of the components please consider, zidovudine p. 519, lamivudine p. 518.

- **INDICATIONS AND DOSE**

HIV infection in combination with other antiretroviral drugs
- BY MOUTH
  - Child (body-weight 14–20 kg): 0.5 tablet twice daily
  - Child (body-weight 21–29 kg): 0.5 tablet daily, to be given in the morning and 1 tablet daily, to be given in the evening
  - Child (body-weight 30 kg and above): 1 tablet twice daily

- **INTERACTIONS** → Appendix 1: NRTIs
- **RENAL IMPAIRMENT** [EvGr] Avoid if creatinine clearance less than 50 mL/minute (consult product literature). ⟨M⟩ See p. 16.
- **DIRECTIONS FOR ADMINISTRATION**

  COMBIVIR® TABLETS Manufacturer advises tablets may be crushed and mixed with semi-solid food or liquid just before administration.

- **MEDICINAL FORMS** There can be variation in the licensing of different medicines containing the same drug.

Oral tablet
- **Zidovudine with lamivudine (Non-proprietary)**

  Lamivudine 150 mg, Zidovudine 300 mg Zidovudine 300mg / Lamivudine 150mg tablets | 60 tablet [PoM] £240.10–£255.10 DT = £300.12 (Hospital only)
- **Combivir** (ViiV Healthcare UK Ltd)

  Lamivudine 150 mg, Zidovudine 300 mg Combivir 150mg/300mg tablets | 60 tablet [PoM] £300.12 DT = £300.12 (Hospital only)

ANTIVIRALS › PROTEASE INHIBITORS, HIV

Protease inhibitors

- **CONTRA-INDICATIONS** Acute porphyrias p. 745
- **CAUTIONS** Haemophilia (increased risk of bleeding)

● **SIDE-EFFECTS**
- **Common or very common** Angioedema · anxiety · appetite abnormal · arthralgia · asthenia · diabetes mellitus · diarrhoea · dizziness · dyslipidaemia · fever · gastrointestinal discomfort · gastrointestinal disorders · headache · hepatic disorders · hypersensitivity · hypertension · myalgia · nausea · oral ulceration · pancreatitis · peripheral neuropathy · seizure · skin reactions · sleep disorders · syncope · taste altered · urinary frequency increased · vomiting
- **Uncommon** Alopecia · dry mouth · immune reconstitution inflammatory syndrome · myocardial infarction · osteonecrosis · weight increased
- **Rare or very rare** Stevens-Johnson syndrome

● **HEPATIC IMPAIRMENT** In general, manufacturers advise use with caution in patients with chronic hepatitis B or C (increased risk of hepatic side-effects).

520

Atazanavir

26-Apr-2023

● **INDICATIONS AND DOSE**

HIV infection, in combination with other antiretroviral drugs—with low-dose ritonavir (initiated by a specialist)

▶ BY MOUTH
- Child 6–17 years (body-weight 15–34 kg): 200 mg once daily
- Child 6–17 years (body-weight 35 kg and above): 300 mg once daily

HIV infection, in combination with other antiretroviral drugs—with cobicistat (initiated by a specialist)

▶ BY MOUTH
- Child 12–17 years (body-weight 35 kg and above): 300 mg once daily

● **CAUTIONS** Cardiac conduction disorders · electrolyte disturbances · predisposition to QT interval prolongation

● **INTERACTIONS** → Appendix 1: HIV-protease inhibitors

● **SIDE-EFFECTS**
- **Uncommon** Chest pain · chronic kidney disease · depression · disorientation · drowsiness · drug reaction with eosinophilia and systemic symptoms (DRESS) · dyspnoea · gallbladder disorders · gynaecomastia · haematuria · malaise · memory loss · myopathy · nephritis tubulointerstitial · nephrolithiasis · proteinuria · torsade de pointes
- **Rare or very rare** Gait abnormal · oedema · palpitations · QT interval prolongation · renal pain · vasodilation

SIDE-EFFECTS, FURTHER INFORMATION Mild to moderate rash occurs commonly, usually within the first 3 weeks of therapy. Severe rash occurs less frequently and may be accompanied by systemic symptoms. Discontinue if severe rash develops.

● **PREGNANCY** [EvGr] Theoretical risk of hyperbilirubinaemia in neonate if used at term. (M)

Monitoring [EvGr] In pregnancy, monitor viral load and plasma-atazanavir concentration during second and third trimesters. Postpartum patients should be closely monitored for adverse reactions. (M)

● **HEPATIC IMPAIRMENT** Manufacturer advises caution in mild impairment; avoid in moderate to severe impairment (no information available).

● **RENAL IMPAIRMENT** [EvGr] Avoid in patients undergoing haemodialysis (limited information available). (M)

● **MEDICINAL FORMS** There can be variation in the licensing of different medicines containing the same drug.

Oral capsule

CAUTIONARY AND ADVISORY LABELS 5, 21

▶ Atazanavir (Non-proprietary)

Atazanavir (as Atazanavir sulfate) 200 mg Atazanavir 200mg capsules | 60 capsule [PoM] £303.38 (Hospital only)

Atazanavir (as Atazanavir sulfate) 300 mg Atazanavir 300mg capsules | 30 capsule [PoM] £257.87–£303.38 (Hospital only)

520

Darunavir

15-Dec-2020

● **INDICATIONS AND DOSE**

HIV infection in combination with other antiretroviral drugs in patients previously treated with antiretroviral therapy—with low-dose ritonavir

▶ BY MOUTH
- Child 3–17 years (body-weight 15–29 kg): 375 mg twice daily
- Child 3–17 years (body-weight 30–39 kg): 450 mg twice daily
- Child 3–17 years (body-weight 40 kg and above): 600 mg twice daily
- Child 12–17 years: 800 mg once daily, once daily dose only to be used if no resistance to darunavir, if plasma HIV-RNA concentration less than 100 000 copies/mL, and if CD4 cell count greater than 100 cells × 10^6/ litre

HIV infection in combination with other antiretroviral drugs in patients previously treated with antiretroviral therapy—with cobicistat

▶ BY MOUTH
- Child 12–17 years (body-weight 40 kg and above): 800 mg once daily, dose appropriate if no resistance to darunavir, if plasma HIV-RNA concentration less than 100 000 copies/mL, and if CD4 cell count greater than 100 cells × 10^6/litre

HIV infection in combination with other antiretroviral drugs in patients not previously treated with antiretroviral therapy—with low-dose ritonavir

▶ BY MOUTH
- Child 12–17 years (body-weight 40 kg and above): 800 mg once daily

HIV infection in combination with other antiretroviral drugs in patients not previously treated with antiretroviral therapy—with cobicistat

▶ BY MOUTH
- Child 12–17 years (body-weight 40 kg and above): 800 mg once daily

● **INTERACTIONS** → Appendix 1: HIV-protease inhibitors

● **SIDE-EFFECTS**
- **Uncommon** Anaemia · angina pectoris · arrhythmias · burping · chest pain · concentration impaired · confusion · constipation · cough · depression · drowsiness · dry eye · dyspnoea · eye erythema · feeling hot · flushing · gout · gynaecomastia · haemorrhage · herpes simplex · hyperglycaemia · hypothyroidism · leucopenia · malaise · memory loss · mood altered · muscle spasms · muscle weakness · nail discolouration · nephrolithiasis · neutropenia · oral disorders · osteoporosis · pain · peripheral oedema · polydipsia · QT interval prolongation · renal impairment · sensation abnormal · sexual dysfunction · sweat changes · throat irritation · thrombocytopenia · urinary disorders · urine abnormalities · vertigo
- **Rare or very rare** Arthritis · chills · feeling abnormal · joint stiffness · musculoskeletal stiffness · palpitations · rhinorrhoea · severe cutaneous adverse reactions (SCARs) · visual impairment

SIDE-EFFECTS, FURTHER INFORMATION Mild to moderate rash occurs commonly, usually within the first 4 weeks of therapy and resolves without stopping treatment. Severe skin rash (including Stevens-Johnson syndrome and toxic epidermal necrolysis) occurs less frequently and may be accompanied by fever, malaise, arthralgia, myalgia, oral lesions, conjunctivitis, hepatitis, or eosinophilia; treatment should be stopped if this develops.

- **ALLERGY AND CROSS-SENSITIVITY** EvGr Use with caution in patients with sulfonamide sensitivity. (M)
- **PREGNANCY** Manufacturer advises use only if potential benefit outweighs risk; if required, use the twice daily dose regimen.
- **HEPATIC IMPAIRMENT** Manufacturer advises caution in mild to moderate impairment; avoid in severe impairment (no information available).
- **MONITORING REQUIREMENTS** Monitor liver function before and during treatment.
- **PRESCRIBING AND DISPENSING INFORMATION** Flavours of oral liquid formulations may include strawberry.
- **PATIENT AND CARER ADVICE**
  Vomiting EvGr If vomiting occurs more than 4 hours after a dose is taken, the missed dose should not be taken and the next dose should be taken at the normal time. (M)
  Missed doses EvGr If a dose is more than 6 hours late on the twice-daily regimen (or more than 12 hours late on the once-daily regimen), the missed dose should not be taken and the next dose should be taken at the normal time. (M)

- **MEDICINAL FORMS** There can be variation in the licensing of different medicines containing the same drug.

Oral tablet

CAUTIONARY AND ADVISORY LABELS 21

▸ Darunavir (Non-proprietary)

Darunavir 400 mg Darunavir 400mg tablets | 60 tablet PoM £297.80 (Hospital only)

Darunavir 600 mg Darunavir 600mg tablets | 60 tablet PoM £400.00–£446.70 (Hospital only)

Darunavir 800 mg Darunavir 800mg tablets | 30 tablet PoM £297.80 DT = £268.00 (Hospital only)

▸ Prezista (Janssen-Cilag Ltd)

Darunavir 800 mg Prezista 800mg tablets | 30 tablet PoM £297.80 DT = £268.00 (Hospital only)

Oral suspension

CAUTIONARY AND ADVISORY LABELS 21

▸ Prezista (Janssen-Cilag Ltd)

Darunavir (as Darunavir ethanolate) 100 mg per 1 ml Prezista 100mg/ml oral suspension | 200 ml PoM £248.17 (Hospital only) SF

Darunavir with cobicistat

09-Dec-2020

The properties listed below are those particular to the combination only. For the properties of the components please consider, cobicistat p. 525, darunavir p. 521.

- **INDICATIONS AND DOSE**

HIV infection, in combination with other antiretroviral drugs (initiated by a specialist)

▸ BY MOUTH

▸ Child 12–17 years (body-weight 40 kg and above): 800/150 mg once daily

DOSE EQUIVALENCE AND CONVERSION

▸ Dose expressed as x/y mg of darunavir/cobicistat.

IMPORTANT SAFETY INFORMATION

MHRA/CHM ADVICE: DARUNAVIR BOOSTED WITH COBICISTAT: AVOID USE IN PREGNANCY DUE TO RISK OF TREATMENT FAILURE AND MATERNAL-TO-CHILD TRANSMISSION OF HIV-1 (JULY 2018)

Pharmacokinetic data show mean exposure of darunavir boosted with cobicistat (available in combination in *Rezolsta*® and *Symtuza*®) to be lower during the second and third trimesters of pregnancy than during 6–12 weeks postpartum. Low darunavir exposure may be associated with an increased risk of treatment failure and an increased risk of HIV-1 transmission to the unborn child. For further information, see *Pregnancy*.

- **CONTRA-INDICATIONS** Treatment-experienced patients with 1 or more darunavir resistance-associated mutations, plasma HIV-RNA concentration of 100 000 copies/mL or greater, or CD4 count less than 100 cells × 10^6/litre
- **INTERACTIONS** → Appendix 1: cobicistat · HIV-protease inhibitors
- **PREGNANCY** Manufacturer advises not to be initiated during pregnancy due to low darunavir exposure; women who become pregnant during therapy should be switched to an alternative regimen. Darunavir with ritonavir may be considered as an alternative.
- **NATIONAL FUNDING/ACCESS DECISIONS**
  For full details see funding body website

All Wales Medicines Strategy Group (AWMSG) decisions

▸ **Darunavir with cobicistat (*Rezolsta*®) in combination with other antiretroviral medicinal products for the treatment of human immunodeficiency virus-1 (HIV-1) infection in adults and adolescents (aged 12 years and older with body weight at least 40 kg) (November 2020)** AWMSG No. 3779 Recommended

- **MEDICINAL FORMS** There can be variation in the licensing of different medicines containing the same drug.

Oral tablet

CAUTIONARY AND ADVISORY LABELS 21

▸ Rezolsta (Janssen-Cilag Ltd)

Cobicistat 150 mg, Darunavir (as Darunavir ethanolate) 800 mg Rezolsta 800mg/150mg tablets | 30 tablet PoM £317.24 (Hospital only)

Darunavir with cobicistat, emtricitabine and tenofovir alafenamide

10-Aug-2021

The properties listed below are those particular to the combination only. For the properties of the components please consider, darunavir p. 521, cobicistat p. 525, emtricitabine p. 516, tenofovir alafenamide p. 493.

- **INDICATIONS AND DOSE**

HIV infection (initiated by a specialist)

▸ BY MOUTH

▸ Child 12–17 years (body-weight 40 kg and above): 1 tablet once daily

IMPORTANT SAFETY INFORMATION

MHRA/CHM ADVICE: DARUNAVIR BOOSTED WITH COBICISTAT: AVOID USE IN PREGNANCY DUE TO RISK OF TREATMENT FAILURE AND MATERNAL-TO-CHILD TRANSMISSION OF HIV-1 (JULY 2018)

Pharmacokinetic data show mean exposure of darunavir boosted with cobicistat (available in combination in *Rezolsta*® and *Symtuza*®) to be lower during the second and third trimesters of pregnancy than during 6–12 weeks postpartum. Low darunavir exposure may be associated with an increased risk of treatment failure and an increased risk of HIV-1 transmission to the unborn child. For further information, see *Pregnancy*.

- **INTERACTIONS** → Appendix 1: cobicistat · HIV-protease inhibitors · tenofovir alafenamide
- **PREGNANCY** Manufacturer advises not to be initiated during pregnancy due to low darunavir exposure; women who become pregnant during therapy should be switched to an alternative regimen.
- **RENAL IMPAIRMENT** EvGr Avoid if creatinine clearance less than 30 mL/minute (no information available). (M) See p. 16.

● **PATIENT AND CARER ADVICE**
Driving and skilled tasks Manufacturer advises patients and carers should be counselled on the effects on driving and performance of skilled tasks—increased risk of dizziness.

● **NATIONAL FUNDING/ACCESS DECISIONS**
For full details see funding body website

Scottish Medicines Consortium (SMC) decisions

- **Darunavir, cobicistat, emtricitabine, tenofovir alafenamide (*Symtuza*®) for the treatment of human immunodeficiency virus type 1 (HIV-1) infection in adults and adolescents (aged 12 years and older with body weight at least 40 kg) (January 2018)** SMC No. 1290/18 Recommended

All Wales Medicines Strategy Group (AWMSG) decisions

- **Darunavir / cobicistat / emtricitabine / tenofovir alafenamide (*Symtuza*®) for the treatment of human immunodeficiency virus type 1 (HIV-1) infection in adults and adolescents (aged 12 years and older with body weight at least 40 kg) (March 2018)** AWMSG No. 2418 Recommended

● **MEDICINAL FORMS** There can be variation in the licensing of different medicines containing the same drug.

Oral tablet

CAUTIONARY AND ADVISORY LABELS 21

- **Symtuza** (Janssen-Cilag Ltd)
Tenofovir alafenamide (as Tenofovir alafenamide fumarate) 10 mg, Cobicistat 150 mg, Emtricitabine 200 mg, Darunavir (as Darunavir ethanolate) 800 mg Symtuza 800mg/150mg/200mg/10mg tablets | 30 tablet PoM £672.97 (Hospital only)

F 520

Fosamprenavir

03-Aug-2020

● **DRUG ACTION** Fosamprenavir is a pro-drug of amprenavir.

● **INDICATIONS AND DOSE**

HIV infection in combination with other antiretroviral drugs—with low-dose ritonavir

- BY MOUTH
- Child 6–17 years (body-weight 25–39 kg): 18 mg/kg twice daily (max. per dose 700 mg)
- Child 6–17 years (body-weight 40 kg and above): 700 mg twice daily

DOSE EQUIVALENCE AND CONVERSION

- 700 mg fosamprenavir is equivalent to approximately 600 mg amprenavir.

● **INTERACTIONS** → Appendix 1: HIV-protease inhibitors

● **SIDE-EFFECTS**

- **Common or very common** Oral paraesthesia

SIDE-EFFECTS, FURTHER INFORMATION Rash may occur, usually in the second week of therapy; discontinue permanently if severe rash with systemic or allergic symptoms or, mucosal involvement; if rash mild or moderate, may continue without interruption—usually resolves and may respond to antihistamines.

● **PREGNANCY** Toxicity in *animal* studies; manufacturer advises use only if potential benefit outweighs risk.

● **HEPATIC IMPAIRMENT** Manufacturer advises caution.
Dose adjustments In adults, manufacturer advises dose reduction—consult product literature.

● **DIRECTIONS FOR ADMINISTRATION** Manufacturer advises in children, oral suspension should be taken with food.

● **PRESCRIBING AND DISPENSING INFORMATION** Flavours of oral liquid formulations may include grape, bubblegum, or peppermint.

● **PATIENT AND CARER ADVICE** Patients or carers should be given advice on how to administer fosamprenavir oral suspension.

● **MEDICINAL FORMS** No licensed medicines listed.

F 520

Lopinavir with ritonavir

21-Dec-2021

● **INDICATIONS AND DOSE**

HIV infection in combination with other antiretroviral drugs

- BY MOUTH USING TABLETS
- Child 2–17 years (body-weight up to 40 kg and body surface area 0.5–0.7 m^2): 200/50 mg twice daily
- Child 2–17 years (body-weight up to 40 kg and body surface area 0.8–1.1 m^2): 300/75 mg twice daily
- Child 2–17 years (body-weight 40 kg and above and body surface area 1.2 m^2 and above): 400/100 mg twice daily
- BY MOUTH USING ORAL SOLUTION
- Child 14 days–5 months: 3.75 mL/m^2 twice daily
- Child 6 months–17 years: 2.9 mL/m^2 twice daily (max. per dose 5 mL)

DOSE EQUIVALENCE AND CONVERSION

- Oral solution contains 400 mg lopinavir, 100 mg ritonavir/5 mL (or 80 mg lopinavir, 20 mg ritonavir/mL).

● **CAUTIONS** Cardiac conduction disorders · pancreatitis · patients at high risk of cardiovascular disease · structural heart disease

● **INTERACTIONS** → Appendix 1: HIV-protease inhibitors

● **SIDE-EFFECTS**

- **Common or very common** Anaemia · increased risk of infection · leucopenia · lymphadenopathy · menstrual cycle irregularities · migraine · muscle spasms · muscle weakness · myopathy · neutropenia · night sweats · pain · sexual dysfunction
- **Uncommon** Atherosclerosis · atrioventricular block · cholangitis · constipation · deep vein thrombosis · haemorrhage · hyperbilirubinaemia · hypogonadism · nephritis · stomatitis · stroke · tinnitus · tremor · tricuspid valve incompetence · vasculitis · vertigo · visual impairment

SIDE-EFFECTS, FURTHER INFORMATION Signs and symptoms suggestive of pancreatitis (including raised serum lipase) should be evaluated—discontinue if pancreatitis diagnosed.

● **PREGNANCY** For *tablets*, manufacturer advises only use if potential benefit outweighs risk—toxicity in *animal* studies (recommendation also supported by specialist sources). Avoid *oral solution* due to high alcohol and propylene glycol content.

● **HEPATIC IMPAIRMENT** For *oral solution*, manufacturer advises avoid due to propylene glycol content (risk of toxicity). For *tablets*, manufacturer advises avoid in severe impairment (no information available).

● **RENAL IMPAIRMENT** EvGr Avoid *oral solution* due to high propylene glycol content. ◈

● **MONITORING REQUIREMENTS**

- Manufacturer advises monitor liver function before and during treatment.
- For *oral solution*, manufacturer advises monitor for signs of alcohol and propylene glycol toxicity (particularly in infants).

● **PRESCRIBING AND DISPENSING INFORMATION** For *oral solution*, manufacturer advises high alcohol (42 % v/v) and propylene glycol content—consider total amounts from all medicines that are to be given to infants in order to avoid toxicity; caution in patients for which consumption may be harmful.

● **PATIENT AND CARER ADVICE** Oral solution tastes bitter.

● **NATIONAL FUNDING/ACCESS DECISIONS**
For full details see funding body website

Scottish Medicines Consortium (SMC) decisions

- **Lopinavir/ritonavir (*Kaletra*®) oral solution in combination with other antiretroviral medicinal products for the treatment**

of human immunodeficiency virus (HIV-1) infected children aged from 14 days up to 2 years (February 2018)
SMC No. 1302/18 Recommended

- **Lopinavir 200 mg, ritonavir 50 mg tablet (*Kaletra*®) for the treatment of HIV-1 infected adults and children above the age of 2 years in combination with other antiretroviral agents (November 2006)** SMC No. 326/06 Recommended

All Wales Medicines Strategy Group (AWMSG) decisions

- **Lopinavir/ritonavir (*Kaletra*®) oral solution for treatment of human immunodeficiency virus (HIV-1) infected children aged from 14 days to less than 2 years old (March 2018)** AWMSG No. 3557 Recommended

● **MEDICINAL FORMS** There can be variation in the licensing of different medicines containing the same drug.

Oral solution

CAUTIONARY AND ADVISORY LABELS 21
EXCIPIENTS: May contain Alcohol, propylene glycol

- **Kaletra** (AbbVie Ltd)
Ritonavir 20 mg per 1 ml, Lopinavir 80 mg per 1 ml Kaletra 80mg/20mg/1ml oral solution | 120 ml PoM £122.96 (Hospital only) | 300 ml PoM £307.39 (Hospital only)

520

Ritonavir

20-Jul-2023

● **INDICATIONS AND DOSE**

HIV infection in combination with other antiretroviral drugs (high-dose ritonavir)

- BY MOUTH
- Child 2–17 years: Initially 250 mg/m² twice daily, increased in steps of 50 mg/m² every 2–3 days; increased to 350 mg/m² twice daily (max. per dose 600 mg twice daily), tolerability of this regimen is poor

Low-dose ritonavir to increase the effect of atazanavir

- BY MOUTH
- Child 6–17 years (body-weight 15 kg and above): 100 mg once daily

Low-dose ritonavir to increase the effect of darunavir

- BY MOUTH
- Child 3–17 years (body-weight 15–29 kg): 50 mg twice daily
- Child 3–17 years (body-weight 30–39 kg): 60 mg twice daily
- Child 3–17 years (body-weight 40 kg and above): 100 mg twice daily
- Child 12–17 years (body-weight 40 kg and above): 100 mg once daily for use in patients taking darunavir once daily

Low-dose ritonavir to increase the effect of fosamprenavir

- BY MOUTH
- Child 6–17 years (body-weight 25–32 kg): 3 mg/kg twice daily
- Child 6–17 years (body-weight 33 kg and above): 100 mg twice daily

● **CAUTIONS** Cardiac conduction disorders · pancreatitis · structural heart disease

● **INTERACTIONS** → Appendix 1: HIV-protease inhibitors

● **SIDE-EFFECTS**

- **Common or very common** Back pain · concentration impaired · confusion · cough · dehydration · feeling hot · flushing · gastrointestinal haemorrhage · gout · hypotension · menorrhagia · myopathy · oedema · oral paraesthesia · oropharyngeal pain · paraesthesia · peripheral coldness · pharyngitis · renal impairment · thrombocytopenia · vision blurred
- **Rare or very rare** Hyperglycaemia · toxic epidermal necrolysis

SIDE-EFFECTS, FURTHER INFORMATION Signs and symptoms suggestive of pancreatitis (including raised serum lipase) should be evaluated — discontinue if pancreatitis diagnosed.

● **PREGNANCY**
Dose adjustments Only use low-dose booster to increase the effect of other protease inhibitors.

● **HEPATIC IMPAIRMENT** When used as a *low-dose booster*, manufacturer advises caution in severe impairment; avoid in decompensated liver disease. When used in *high-doses*, manufacturer advises avoid in severe impairment.
Dose adjustments Manufacturer advises consult product literature of co-administered protease inhibitor.

● **PATIENT AND CARER ADVICE**
Driving and skilled tasks Patients and carers should be counselled on the effects on driving and performance of skilled tasks— increased risk of dizziness.

● **MEDICINAL FORMS** There can be variation in the licensing of different medicines containing the same drug.

Oral tablet

CAUTIONARY AND ADVISORY LABELS 21, 25

- **Ritonavir (Non-proprietary)**
Ritonavir 100 mg Ritonavir 100mg tablets | 30 tablet PoM £16.52–£19.44 (Hospital only)
- **Norvir** (AbbVie Ltd)
Ritonavir 100 mg Norvir 100mg tablets | 30 tablet PoM £19.44 (Hospital only)

ANTIVIRALS > OTHER

Maraviroc

31-Aug-2020

● **DRUG ACTION** Maraviroc is an antagonist of the CCR5 chemokine receptor.

● **INDICATIONS AND DOSE**

CCR5-tropic HIV infection in combination with other antiretroviral drugs in patients previously treated with antiretrovirals

- BY MOUTH
- Child: (consult local protocol)

● **UNLICENSED USE** Not licensed for use in children.

● **CAUTIONS** Cardiovascular disease

● **INTERACTIONS** → Appendix 1: maraviroc

● **SIDE-EFFECTS**

- **Common or very common** Abdominal pain · anaemia · appetite decreased · asthenia · depression · diarrhoea · flatulence · headache · insomnia · nausea · rash
- **Uncommon** Hyperbilirubinaemia · increased risk of infection · myopathy · postural hypotension · proteinuria · renal failure · seizure
- **Rare or very rare** Angina pectoris · granulocytopenia · hepatic disorders · metastases · neoplasms · pancytopenia · severe cutaneous adverse reactions (SCARs)
- **Frequency not known** Fever · hypersensitivity · immune reconstitution inflammatory syndrome · organ dysfunction · osteonecrosis

SIDE-EFFECTS, FURTHER INFORMATION **Osteonecrosis** Osteonecrosis has been reported in patients with advanced HIV disease or following long-term exposure to combination antiretroviral therapy.

Hepatotoxicity Manufacturer advises consider discontinuation if signs or symptoms of acute hepatitis, or increased liver transaminases with systemic symptoms of hypersensitivity occur.

● **PREGNANCY** Manufacturer advises use only if potential benefit outweighs risk—toxicity in *animal* studies.

● **HEPATIC IMPAIRMENT** Manufacturer advises caution in impairment and in patients with chronic hepatitis (increased risk of hepatic side-effects; limited information available).

● **RENAL IMPAIRMENT** If estimated glomerular filtration rate less than 80 mL/minute/1.73 m², consult product literature.

- **MEDICINAL FORMS** There can be variation in the licensing of different medicines containing the same drug.

Oral tablet

▸ **Maraviroc (Non-proprietary)**
Maraviroc 150 mg Maraviroc 150mg tablets | 60 tablet PoM £467.23 (Hospital only)
Maraviroc 300 mg Maraviroc 300mg tablets | 60 tablet PoM £467.23 (Hospital only)

▸ **Celsentri** (ViiV Healthcare UK Ltd)
Maraviroc 150 mg Celsentri 150mg tablets | 60 tablet PoM £519.14 (Hospital only)
Maraviroc 300 mg Celsentri 300mg tablets | 60 tablet PoM £519.14 (Hospital only)

PHARMACOKINETIC ENHANCERS

Cobicistat 06-Aug-2021

- **INDICATIONS AND DOSE**

Pharmacokinetic enhancer used to increase the effect of atazanavir
▶ BY MOUTH
▸ Child 12–17 years (body-weight 35 kg and above): 150 mg once daily

Pharmacokinetic enhancer used to increase the effect of darunavir
▶ BY MOUTH
▸ Child 12–17 years (body-weight 40 kg and above): 150 mg once daily

- **INTERACTIONS** → Appendix 1: cobicistat
- **PREGNANCY** EvGr Not to be initiated during pregnancy. (M) For use with darunavir, see darunavir with cobicistat p. 522 or darunavir with cobicistat, emtricitabine and tenofovir alafenamide p. 522. For use with elvitegravir, see elvitegravir with cobicistat, emtricitabine and tenofovir alafenamide p. 515.
- **HEPATIC IMPAIRMENT** Manufacturer advises avoid in severe impairment—no information available.
- **RENAL IMPAIRMENT** EvGr No dose adjustment required; inhibits tubular secretion of creatinine; when any co-administered drug requires dose adjustment based on renal function, avoid initiating cobicistat if creatinine clearance less than 70 mL/minute. (M) See p. 16.
- **PRESCRIBING AND DISPENSING INFORMATION** Dispense in original container (contains desiccant).
- **PATIENT AND CARER ADVICE**

Missed doses If a dose is more than 12 hours late, the missed dose should not be taken and the next dose should be taken at the normal time.

- **MEDICINAL FORMS** There can be variation in the licensing of different medicines containing the same drug.

Oral tablet

CAUTIONARY AND ADVISORY LABELS 21

▸ **Tybost** (Gilead Sciences Ltd)
Cobicistat 150 mg Tybost 150mg tablets | 30 tablet PoM £21.38 (Hospital only)

Combinations available: ***Darunavir with cobicistat,*** p. 522 · ***Darunavir with cobicistat, emtricitabine and tenofovir alafenamide,*** p. 522 · ***Elvitegravir with cobicistat, emtricitabine and tenofovir alafenamide,*** p. 515

5.6 Influenza

Influenza 05-Jan-2026

Description of condition

Influenza is a highly infectious, acute respiratory infection caused by influenza viruses, of which there are three types (A, B, and C). Influenza A is more virulent and occurs more frequently; influenza B presents a milder course of disease but still has the potential to cause outbreaks; and influenza C causes mild or asymptomatic disease, similar to the common cold. Types A and B can be further categorised into subtypes depending on their principal H and N antigens. Transmission occurs via droplets, aerosols, or direct contact with respiratory secretions from an infected person, and the usual incubation period is 1–3 days.

Influenza illness is classified as severe or non-severe. The most common symptoms of non-severe influenza include sudden onset cough, sore throat, fever, rhinorrhoea, headache, myalgia, and severe malaise. Gastro-intestinal symptoms (especially in children) and, less commonly, ocular symptoms may also be associated with influenza. Symptoms usually appear suddenly and recovery usually occurs within a week without requiring medical attention. Severe influenza is characterised by clinical complications that directly result from influenza virus infection, such as pneumonia, sepsis, multi-organ failure, encephalopathy, or exacerbation of an underlying chronic condition; most cases require management in hospital.

The risk of progression to severe influenza and hospitalisation is greater for those in *at-risk groups* such as, children aged under 6 months, pregnant females (including females up to 2 weeks post-partum), patients with long-term conditions (such as respiratory, renal, hepatic, neurological, or cardiovascular disease, diabetes mellitus, or morbid obesity (BMI $\geq 40\,kg/m^2$)), or those who may be immunosuppressed. Patients with severe immunosuppression are at higher risk of developing severe illness or resistance to antivirals. For further information on at-risk groups and severe immunosuppression, see UKHSA **Guidance on use of antiviral agents for the treatment and prophylaxis of seasonal influenza** (see *Useful resources*).

Other types of influenza include pandemic influenza, avian influenza, and swine influenza. For information and guidance on their management, see www.gov.uk/guidance/pandemic-flu, www.gov.uk/government/publications/avian-influenza-managing-human-exposures-to-incidents-in-birds-or-animals, and www.gov.uk/guidance/swine-influenza.

Influenza of zoonotic origin is a notifiable disease in England. For further information, see *Notifiable diseases* in Antibacterials, principles of therapy p. 358.

Aims of treatment

The management of influenza aims to reduce the duration and severity of illness, reduce the risk of complications, and to prevent infection.

Management

Consider antiviral treatment for patients with virologically confirmed influenza and influenza-like illness when national influenza surveillance indicates that influenza is circulating above baseline levels or where there is evidence of increased local circulation. Information on the dominant circulating strain can be found in UKHSA's national influenza reports available at: www.gov.uk/government/collections/weekly-national-flu-reports.

There are two classes of direct-acting antivirals (DAAs), neuraminidase inhibitors (NAIs) (oseltamivir and zanamivir) and cap-dependent endonuclease inhibitors (CENIs) (baloxavir marboxil); they are used for both treatment and post-exposure prophylaxis of influenza. However, there is evidence that some strains of influenza are more likely to develop resistance to oseltamivir or CENIs, with the risk being higher in patients who are severely immunosuppressed. The risk of developing oseltamivir resistance is considered to be greater for N1-containing influenza viruses, such as A(H1N1)pdm09 virus, with rapid emergence as early as 48 hours after starting treatment and is far more common than resistance to zanamivir. The risk of developing resistance to CENis is considered to be greater with A(H3N2) influenza infections in children. A greater viral burden and/or prolonged duration of infection might be seen in patients with antiviral resistance, or those at greater risk of developing antiviral resistance, such as young children and infants.

The impact of DAAs on viral replication is greatest at the onset of illness, or as post-exposure prophylaxis. In patients where severe influenza is suspected (based on clinical presentation and/or influenza is currently circulating or they are part of a confirmed outbreak) treatment should be started promptly without waiting for test results. All patients with severe respiratory illness should be tested for influenza as soon as possible; however, this should not delay initiation of DAA treatment. If test results show antiviral treatment is not clinically indicated, treatment may be stopped. In patients being tested for antiviral resistance, treatment interruption should be avoided while awaiting test results, as this may be associated with the development of resistance.

Specialist advice regarding the management of influenza for individual patients can be obtained from local infection specialists where required; additional advice can be obtained from virologists at regional public health laboratories or the UKHSA national Respiratory Virus Unit (RVU Colindale).

For information on vaccination against influenza, see Influenza vaccine p. 971.

Treatment of suspected or confirmed influenza

Where treatment with oseltamivir or zanamivir is indicated, it should be started as soon as possible, ideally within 48 hours of symptom onset. There is evidence to suggest that the risk of mortality may be reduced even if treatment is started up to 5 days after symptom onset (up to 6 days for intravenous zanamivir); treatment initiation beyond 48 hours of onset is unlicensed and specialist advice should be sought. Where treatment with baloxavir marboxil is indicated, treatment initiation should not be delayed due to supply issues—an alternative option that is readily available should be used.

Inhaled zanamivir should be considered in patients with a poor clinical response to oseltamivir, a confirmed strain with potential for oseltamivir resistance, evidence of gastro-intestinal dysfunction requiring discontinuation of oseltamivir, or other reasons for which oseltamivir cannot be given. If oseltamivir has already been started, discuss with a local infection specialist before changing treatment to a second- or third-line DAA.

Non-severe influenza

Patients with non-severe influenza are usually managed in the community or accident and emergency departments. All patients should be advised about the symptoms of severe influenza and to seek medical attention if their condition worsens.

For patients who are otherwise healthy (excluding pregnant females), no antiviral treatment is usually needed. For patients in an at-risk group or those considered to be at risk of developing serious complications, offer oseltamivir p. 527 as first-line treatment for any circulating strain. If oseltamivir is unsuitable, offer inhaled zanamivir p. 528 as second-line treatment.

Where virological testing (using validated diagnostic tests for respiratory viruses) is unavailable, or if the patient has symptom onset during a virologically confirmed influenza outbreak in a closed setting, prompt treatment prior to testing is recommended. Treatment may also be considered for influenza case-patients in order to reduce transmission to severely immunosuppressed household contacts.

For further information, see UKHSA **Guidance on use of antiviral agents for the treatment and prophylaxis of seasonal influenza** (see *Useful resources*).

Severe influenza

All patients should be tested and treated, often in hospital—do not wait for laboratory test results to treat. For patients with severe influenza from any dominant circulating strain, offer oseltamivir p. 527 as first-line treatment. In patients where oseltamivir is unsuitable, offer inhaled zanamivir p. 528 as second-line treatment. If there is a poor clinical response, or concerns about the development of oseltamivir resistance, consider either adding baloxavir marboxil p. 527 or, switching to intravenous zanamivir as third-line treatment options—seek specialist advice. Intravenous zanamivir can also be considered if oral or inhaled routes are unsuitable. For further information, see UKHSA **Guidance on use of antiviral agents for the treatment and prophylaxis of seasonal influenza** (see *Useful resources*).

Post-exposure prophylaxis

Contacts in an at-risk group who are not adequately protected through vaccination (either due to infection by a different circulating strain, exposure within 14 days post-vaccination, or not vaccinated within the same influenza season) should be offered prophylaxis following exposure to a person in the same household or residential setting with influenza-like illness (when influenza is circulating). Certain populations that are susceptible to localised outbreaks (such as those in care homes, prisons, or detention centres) may be considered for antiviral prophylaxis regardless of vaccination status. For information on prophylaxis in these settings, refer to individual guidelines available at: www.gov.uk/government/collections/seasonal-influenza-guidance-data-and-analysis.

Prophylaxis should be started as soon as possible following exposure—ideally within 48 hours for oseltamivir and 36 hours for inhaled zanamivir. Initiation beyond these times is unlicensed and specialist advice should be sought.

For patients in an at-risk group, offer oseltamivir as first-line prophylaxis for any dominant strain, except if index case strain is oseltamivir resistant. If oseltamivir is unsuitable, offer inhaled zanamivir as second-line prophylaxis. For patients exposed to a strain with confirmed oseltamivir resistance, offer inhaled zanamivir as first-line prophylaxis; on specialist advice, baloxavir marboxil may be offered as second-line prophylaxis—ideally within 48 hours.

For severely immunosuppressed patients who are unable to use inhaled zanamivir (due to underlying severe respiratory disease or inability to use the device) and children aged under 5 years in an at-risk group, offer oseltamivir and advise patients or carers to seek immediate medical attention if symptoms develop subsequently. For patients exposed to suspected or confirmed oseltamivir resistant influenza who are unable to use inhaled zanamivir, including children aged under 5 years, specialist advice should be sought; monitor closely for influenza-like illness, with arrangements made for prompt treatment if symptoms develop. On specialist advice, baloxavir marboxil may be considered.

Specialist advice is available through local health protection teams and regional public health virologists.

For further information, including post-exposure prophylaxis in neonates exposed after birth, see UKHSA **Guidance on use of antiviral agents for the treatment and prophylaxis of seasonal influenza** (see *Useful resources*).

Pregnancy

For pregnant females, offer oseltamivir as first-line treatment for any circulating strain of influenza, or as first-line prophylaxis for any dominant strain (except if index case strain is oseltamivir resistant). If oseltamivir is unsuitable, offer inhaled zanamivir as a second-line option. Pregnant females who meet additional criteria for requiring zanamivir first-line should be discussed with a local infection specialist.

For further information, see UKHSA **Guidance on use of antiviral agents for the treatment and prophylaxis of seasonal influenza** (see *Useful resources*).

Useful Resources

Recommendations reflect Guidance on use of antiviral agents for the treatment and prophylaxis of seasonal influenza. UK Health Security Agency. January 2026.
www.gov.uk/government/publications/influenza-treatment-and-prophylaxis-using-anti-viral-agents

ANTIVIRALS › CAP-DEPENDENT ENDONUCLEASE INHIBITORS

Baloxavir marboxil
05-Mar-2026

- **DRUG ACTION** Baloxavir marboxil (a pro-drug of baloxavir) reduces replication of influenza A and B viruses by inhibiting viral cap-dependent endonuclease.

- **INDICATIONS AND DOSE**

Post-exposure prophylaxis of influenza | Treatment of influenza

▶ BY MOUTH

- Neonate 21 days to 28 days (body-weight up to 19 kg): 2 mg/kg for 1 dose.
- Child (body-weight up to 19 kg): 2 mg/kg for 1 dose
- Child (body-weight 20–79 kg): 40 mg for 1 dose
- Child (body-weight 80 kg and above): 80 mg for 1 dose

- **INTERACTIONS** → Appendix 1: baloxavir marboxil
- **SIDE-EFFECTS**
  - ▶ **Common or very common** Diarrhoea · skin reactions · vomiting
  - ▶ **Frequency not known** Angioedema
- **PREGNANCY** EvGr Avoid—limited information available. ⟨M⟩
- **BREAST FEEDING** EvGr Avoid—present in milk in *animal* studies. ⟨M⟩
- **HEPATIC IMPAIRMENT** EvGr Use with caution in severe impairment (no information available). ⟨M⟩
- **DIRECTIONS FOR ADMINISTRATION** Baloxavir marboxil oral suspension can be administered via an enteral feeding tube—consult product literature.

- **MEDICINAL FORMS** There can be variation in the licensing of different medicines containing the same drug.

Oral tablet

▸ **Xofluza** (Roche Products Ltd, Imported (Germany))

Baloxavir marboxil 20 mg Xofluza 20mg tablets | 2 tablet PoM (Hospital only)

Baloxavir marboxil 40 mg Xofluza 40mg tablets | 1 tablet PoM £100.00

Baloxavir marboxil 80 mg Xofluza 80mg tablets | 1 tablet PoM £100.00

Oral suspension

CAUTIONARY AND ADVISORY LABELS 13

▸ **Baloxavir marboxil (Non-proprietary)**

Baloxavir marboxil 2 mg per 1 ml Xofluza 2mg/ml oral suspension | 20 ml PoM (Hospital only) SF

ANTIVIRALS › NEURAMINIDASE INHIBITORS

Oseltamivir
05-Mar-2026

- **DRUG ACTION** Reduces replication of influenza A and B viruses by inhibiting viral neuraminidase.

- **INDICATIONS AND DOSE**

Post-exposure prophylaxis of influenza

▶ BY MOUTH

- Neonate up to 36 weeks corrected gestational age: Seek specialist advice.
- Neonate: 3 mg/kg once daily for 10 days for post-exposure prophylaxis.
- Child 1–11 months: 3 mg/kg once daily (max. per dose 30 mg) for 10 days for post-exposure prophylaxis
- Child 1–12 years (body-weight up to 16 kg): 30 mg once daily for 10 days for post-exposure prophylaxis; for up to 6 weeks (or up to 12 weeks if immunocompromised) during an epidemic
- Child 1–12 years (body-weight 16–23 kg): 45 mg once daily for 10 days for post-exposure prophylaxis; for up to 6 weeks (or up to 12 weeks if immunocompromised) during an epidemic
- Child 1–12 years (body-weight 24–40 kg): 60 mg once daily for 10 days for post-exposure prophylaxis; for up to 6 weeks (or up to 12 weeks if immunocompromised) during an epidemic
- Child 1–12 years (body-weight 41 kg and above): 75 mg once daily for 10 days for post-exposure prophylaxis; for up to 6 weeks (or up to 12 weeks if immunocompromised) during an epidemic
- Child 13–17 years (body-weight up to 41 kg): 60 mg once daily for 10 days for post-exposure prophylaxis; for up to 6 weeks (or up to 12 weeks if immunocompromised) during an epidemic
- Child 13–17 years (body-weight 41 kg and above): 75 mg once daily for 10 days for post-exposure prophylaxis; for up to 6 weeks (or up to 12 weeks if immunocompromised) during an epidemic

Treatment of influenza

▶ BY MOUTH

- Neonate up to 36 weeks corrected gestational age: 1 mg/kg twice daily for 5 days (10 days if immunocompromised).
- Neonate: 3 mg/kg twice daily for 5 days (10 days if immunocompromised).
- Child 1–11 months: 3 mg/kg twice daily (max. per dose 30 mg) for 5 days (10 days if immunocompromised)
- Child 1–12 years (body-weight 10–15 kg): 30 mg twice daily for 5 days (10 days if immunocompromised)
- Child 1–12 years (body-weight 16–23 kg): 45 mg twice daily for 5 days (10 days if immunocompromised)
- Child 1–12 years (body-weight 24–40 kg): 60 mg twice daily for 5 days (10 days if immunocompromised)
- Child 1–12 years (body-weight 41 kg and above): 75 mg twice daily for 5 days (10 days if immunocompromised)
- Child 13–17 years (body-weight up to 41 kg): 60 mg twice daily for 5 days (10 days if immunocompromised)
- Child 13–17 years (body-weight 41 kg and above): 75 mg twice daily for 5 days (10 days if immunocompromised)

- **UNLICENSED USE** UKHSA advises oseltamivir may be used in premature infants (i.e. those with a corrected gestational age of less than 36 weeks) for the post-exposure prophylaxis or treatment of influenza, but it is not licensed for this age group.

  UKHSA advises oseltamivir is used in BNFC as detailed below, although these situations are considered unlicensed:

- post-exposure prophylaxis of influenza in children aged 1–12 years weighing less than 10 kg;
- post-exposure prophylaxis or treatment of influenza in children aged 13 years and over weighing less than 40 kg.

● **INTERACTIONS** → Appendix 1: oseltamivir

● **SIDE-EFFECTS**

▸ **Common or very common** Dizziness · gastrointestinal discomfort · herpes simplex · nausea · sleep disorders · vertigo · vomiting

▸ **Uncommon** Arrhythmia · seizure · skin reactions

▸ **Rare or very rare** Angioedema · anxiety · behaviour abnormal · confusion · delirium · delusions · gastrointestinal haemorrhage · hallucination · hepatic disorders · self-injurious behaviour · severe cutaneous adverse reactions (SCARs) · thrombocytopenia · visual impairment

● **PREGNANCY** Although safety data are limited, oseltamivir can be used in women who are pregnant when the potential benefit outweighs the risk (e.g. during a pandemic).

● **BREAST FEEDING** Although safety data are limited, oseltamivir can be used in women who are breast-feeding when the potential benefit outweighs the risk (e.g. during a pandemic). Oseltamivir is the preferred drug in women who are breast-feeding.

● **RENAL IMPAIRMENT** See p. 16.

Dose adjustments For *treatment*, use 40% of normal dose twice daily if estimated glomerular filtration rate 30–60 mL/minute/1.73 m^2 (40% of normal dose once daily if estimated glomerular filtration rate 10–30 mL/minute/1.73 m^2).

For *post-exposure prophylaxis*, use 40% of normal dose once daily if estimated glomerular filtration rate 30–60 mL/minute/1.73 m^2 (40% of normal dose every 48 hours if estimated glomerular filtration rate 10–30 mL/minute/1.73 m^2).

● **DIRECTIONS FOR ADMINISTRATION** If suspension not available, manufacturer advises capsules can be opened and the contents mixed with a small amount of sweetened food, such as sugar water or chocolate syrup, just before administration.

● **PRESCRIBING AND DISPENSING INFORMATION** Flavours of oral liquid formulations may include tutti-frutti.

UKHSA advises that oseltamivir oral suspension should be reserved for children under the age of 1 year. Children over 1 year of age, adults with swallowing difficulties, and those receiving nasogastric oseltamivir, should use capsules which can be opened and mixed into an appropriate sugary liquid.

● **PATIENT AND CARER ADVICE**

Medicines for Children leaflet: Oseltamivir for influenza (flu) www.medicinesforchildren.org.uk/medicines/oseltamivir-for-influenza-flu/

● **NATIONAL FUNDING/ACCESS DECISIONS**

For full details see funding body website

NICE decisions

▸ **Oseltamivir, zanamivir, and amantadine for prophylaxis of influenza (September 2008)** NICE TA158 Recommended with restrictions

▸ **Oseltamivir, zanamivir, and amantadine for treatment of influenza (February 2009)** NICE TA168 Recommended with restrictions

NHS restrictions *Tamiflu*® is not prescribable in NHS primary care except for the treatment and prophylaxis of influenza as indicated in the NICE guidance; endorse prescription 'SLS'.

● **MEDICINAL FORMS** There can be variation in the licensing of different medicines containing the same drug. Forms available from special-order manufacturers include: oral suspension, oral solution

Oral solution

CAUTIONARY AND ADVISORY LABELS 9

Oral suspension

CAUTIONARY AND ADVISORY LABELS 9

EXCIPIENTS: May contain Sorbitol

▸ **Tamiflu** (Roche Products Ltd)

Oseltamivir (as Oseltamivir phosphate) 6 mg per 1 ml Tamiflu 6mg/ml oral suspension | 50 ml [PoM] £10.27 DT = £10.27 [SF]

Oral capsule

CAUTIONARY AND ADVISORY LABELS 9

▸ **Oseltamivir (Non-proprietary)**

Oseltamivir (as Oseltamivir phosphate) 30 mg Oseltamivir 30mg capsules | 10 capsule [PoM] £6.50 DT = £7.71

Oseltamivir (as Oseltamivir phosphate) 75 mg Oseltamivir 75mg capsules | 10 capsule [PoM] £14.64 DT = £15.41

▸ **Tamiflu** (Roche Products Ltd)

Oseltamivir (as Oseltamivir phosphate) 30 mg Tamiflu 30mg capsules | 10 capsule [PoM] £7.71 DT = £7.71

Oseltamivir (as Oseltamivir phosphate) 45 mg Tamiflu 45mg capsules | 10 capsule [PoM] £15.41 DT = £15.41

Oseltamivir (as Oseltamivir phosphate) 75 mg Tamiflu 75mg capsules | 10 capsule [PoM] £15.41 DT = £15.41

Zanamivir

05-Mar-2026

● **DRUG ACTION** Reduces replication of influenza A and B viruses by inhibiting viral neuraminidase.

● **INDICATIONS AND DOSE**

Post-exposure prophylaxis of influenza

▶ BY INHALATION OF POWDER

▸ Child 5-17 years: 10 mg once daily for 10 days

Prophylaxis of seasonal influenza during an epidemic

▶ BY INHALATION OF POWDER

▸ Child 5-17 years: 10 mg once daily for up to 28 days

Treatment of influenza

▶ BY INHALATION OF POWDER

▸ Child 5-17 years: 10 mg twice daily for 5 days

Treatment of severe influenza [resistant to other treatments and/or other treatments are unsuitable]

▶ BY INTRAVENOUS INFUSION

▸ Child 6 months-5 years: 14 mg/kg twice daily for 5 to 10 days

▸ Child 6-17 years: 12 mg/kg twice daily (max. per dose 600 mg) for 5 to 10 days

● **CAUTIONS**

▸ When used by inhalation Asthma · chronic pulmonary disease · uncontrolled chronic illness

CAUTIONS, FURTHER INFORMATION

▸ Asthma and chronic pulmonary disease

▸ When used by inhalation Risk of bronchospasm—short-acting bronchodilator should be available. Avoid in severe asthma unless close monitoring possible and appropriate facilities available to treat bronchospasm.

● **INTERACTIONS** → Appendix 1: zanamivir

● **SIDE-EFFECTS**

GENERAL SIDE-EFFECTS

▶ **Common or very common** Skin reactions

▶ **Uncommon** Oropharyngeal oedema

▶ **Rare or very rare** Face oedema · severe cutaneous adverse reactions (SCARs)

▶ **Frequency not known** Behaviour abnormal · delirium · hallucination · level of consciousness decreased · seizure

SPECIFIC SIDE-EFFECTS

▶ **Common or very common**

▸ With intravenous use Diarrhoea · hepatocellular injury

- **Uncommon**
  - When used by inhalation Bronchospasm · dehydration · dyspnoea · presyncope · throat tightness
- **Frequency not known**
  - When used by inhalation Psychiatric disorder

SIDE-EFFECTS, FURTHER INFORMATION Neurological and psychiatric disorders occur more commonly in children and adolescents.

- **PREGNANCY** Manufacturer advises avoid unless potential benefit outweighs risk (e.g. during a pandemic)—limited information available; *animal* studies do not indicate toxicity.
- **BREAST FEEDING** Manufacturer advises use only if potential benefit outweighs risk (e.g. during a pandemic)—limited information available; present in low levels in milk in *animal* studies.
- **RENAL IMPAIRMENT**

Dose adjustments

- With intravenous use Manufacturer advises reduce dose if creatinine clearance less than 80 mL/minute—consult product literature for details. See p. 16.

- **DIRECTIONS FOR ADMINISTRATION**
  - When used by inhalation Manufacturer advises other inhaled drugs should be administered before zanamivir.
  - With intravenous use Manufacturer advises for *intermittent intravenous infusion*, give undiluted or dilute to a concentration of not less than 200 micrograms/mL with Sodium Chloride 0.9%; give over 30 minutes.
- **NATIONAL FUNDING/ACCESS DECISIONS**

For full details see funding body website

NICE decisions

- **Oseltamivir, zanamivir, and amantadine for prophylaxis of influenza (September 2008)** NICE TA158 Recommended with restrictions
- **Oseltamivir, zanamivir, and amantadine for treatment of influenza (February 2009)** NICE TA168 Recommended with restrictions

Scottish Medicines Consortium (SMC) decisions

- **Zanamivir (*Dectova*®) for the treatment of complicated and potentially life-threatening influenza A or B virus infection in patients (aged 6 months and older) when the patient's influenza virus is known or suspected to be resistant to anti-influenza medicinal products other than zanamivir, and/or other anti-viral medicinal products for treatment of influenza, including inhaled zanamivir, are not suitable for the individual patient (December 2019)** SMC No. SMC2204 Recommended

All Wales Medicines Strategy Group (AWMSG) decisions

- **Zanamivir (*Dectova*®) for the treatment of complicated and potentially life-threatening influenza A or B virus infection in patients (aged 6 months and older) when the patient's influenza virus is known or suspected to be resistant to anti-influenza medicinal products other than zanamivir, and/or other anti-viral medicinal products for treatment of influenza, including inhaled zanamivir, are not suitable for the individual patient (October 2019)** AWMSG No. 4130 Recommended

NHS restrictions *Relenza*® is not prescribable in NHS primary care except for the treatment and prophylaxis of influenza as indicated in the NICE guidance; endorse prescription 'SLS'.

- **MEDICINAL FORMS** There can be variation in the licensing of different medicines containing the same drug.

Solution for infusion

ELECTROLYTES: May contain Sodium

- Dectova (GlaxoSmithKline UK Ltd) ▼

Zanamivir 10 mg per 1 ml Dectova 200mg/20ml solution for infusion vials | 1 vial PoM £27.83 (Hospital only)

Inhalation powder

- Relenza (GlaxoSmithKline UK Ltd)

Zanamivir 5 mg Relenza 5mg inhalation powder blisters with Diskhaler | 20 blister PoM £16.36 DT = £16.36

Chapter 6
Endocrine system

CONTENTS

1 Antidiuretic hormone disorders

Posterior pituitary hormones and antagonists

Posterior pituitary hormones

Diabetes insipidus

Diabetes insipidus is caused by either a deficiency of antidiuretic hormone (ADH, vasopressin p. 74) secretion (cranial, neurogenic, or pituitary diabetes insipidus) or by failure of the renal tubules to react to secreted antidiuretic hormone (nephrogenic diabetes insipidus).

Vasopressin (antidiuretic hormone, ADH) is used in the treatment of *pituitary diabetes insipidus* as is its analogue desmopressin below. Dosage is tailored to produce a regular diuresis every 24 hours to avoid water intoxication. Treatment may be required permanently or for a limited period only in diabetes insipidus following trauma or pituitary surgery.

Desmopressin is more potent and has a longer duration of action than vasopressin; unlike vasopressin it has no vasoconstrictor effect. It is given by mouth or intranasally for maintenance therapy, and by injection in the postoperative period or in unconscious patients. Desmopressin is also used in the differential diagnosis of diabetes insipidus; following an intramuscular or intranasal dose, restoration of the ability to concentrate urine after water deprivation confirms a diagnosis of pituitary diabetes insipidus. Failure to respond suggests nephrogenic diabetes insipidus. Fluid input must be managed carefully to avoid hyponatraemia; this test is not usually recommended in young children.

In *nephrogenic* and *partial pituitary diabetes insipidus* benefit may be gained from the paradoxical antidiuretic effect of thiazides.

Other uses

Desmopressin is also used to boost factor VIII concentration in mild to moderate haemophilia and in von Willebrand's disease; it is also used to test fibrinolytic response. Desmopressin also has a role in nocturnal enuresis.

Vasopressin infusion is used to control variceal bleeding in portal hypertension, before introducing more definitive treatment. Terlipressin acetate, a derivative of vasopressin with reportedly less pressor and antidiuretic activity, and octreotide are used similarly but experience in children is limited.

1.1 Diabetes insipidus

Other drugs used for Diabetes insipidus Chlorothiazide, p. 130

PITUITARY AND HYPOTHALAMIC HORMONES AND ANALOGUES › VASOPRESSIN AND ANALOGUES

Desmopressin

01-Sep-2023

- **DRUG ACTION** Desmopressin is an analogue of vasopressin.

- **INDICATIONS AND DOSE**

Diabetes insipidus, treatment

▶ BY MOUTH

- Neonate: Initially 1–4 micrograms 2–3 times a day, adjusted according to response.
- Child 1-23 months: Initially 10 micrograms 2–3 times a day, adjusted according to response; usual dose 30–150 micrograms daily
- Child 2-11 years: Initially 50 micrograms 2–3 times a day, adjusted according to response; usual dose 100–800 micrograms daily
- Child 12-17 years: Initially 100 micrograms 2–3 times a day, adjusted according to response; usual dose 0.2–1.2 mg daily

▶ BY SUBLINGUAL ADMINISTRATION
▸ Child 2–17 years: Initially 60 micrograms 3 times a day, adjusted according to response; usual dose 40–240 micrograms 3 times a day
▶ BY INTRANASAL ADMINISTRATION
▸ Neonate: Initially 100–500 nanograms, adjusted according to response; usual dose 1.25–10 micrograms daily in 1–2 divided doses.
▸ Child 1–23 months: Initially 2.5–5 micrograms 1–2 times a day, adjusted according to response
▸ Child 2–11 years: Initially 5–20 micrograms 1–2 times a day, adjusted according to response
▸ Child 12–17 years: Initially 10–20 micrograms 1–2 times a day, adjusted according to response
▶ BY INTRAMUSCULAR INJECTION
▸ Neonate: Initially 100 nanograms once daily, adjusted according to response.
▶ BY SUBCUTANEOUS INJECTION, OR BY INTRAMUSCULAR INJECTION
▸ Child 1 month–11 years: Initially 400 nanograms once daily, adjusted according to response
▸ Child 12–17 years: Initially 1–4 micrograms once daily, adjusted according to response

Primary nocturnal enuresis
▶ BY MOUTH USING TABLETS
▸ Child 5–17 years: 200 micrograms once daily, increased if necessary to 400 micrograms once daily, dose to be taken at bedtime, limit fluid intake from 1 hour before to 8 hours after administration, dose to be increased only if lower dose not effective, reassess after 3 months by withdrawing treatment for at least 1 week
▶ BY MOUTH USING ORAL SOLUTION
▸ Child 5–17 years: 180 micrograms once daily, increased if necessary to 360 micrograms once daily, dose to be taken at bedtime, limit fluid intake from 1 hour before to 8 hours after administration, dose to be increased only if lower dose not effective, reassess after 3 months by withdrawing treatment for at least 1 week
▶ BY SUBLINGUAL ADMINISTRATION
▸ Child 5–17 years: 120 micrograms once daily, increased if necessary to 240 micrograms once daily, dose to be taken at bedtime, limit fluid intake from 1 hour before to 8 hours after administration, dose to be increased only if lower dose not effective, reassess after 3 months by withdrawing treatment for at least 1 week

Diabetes insipidus, diagnosis (water deprivation test)
▶ BY INTRANASAL ADMINISTRATION
▸ Neonate: Not recommended, use trial of treatment.
▸ Child 1–23 months: 5–10 micrograms for 1 dose, manage fluid input carefully to avoid hyponatraemia, not usually recommended
▸ Child 2–11 years: 10–20 micrograms for 1 dose, manage fluid input carefully to avoid hyponatraemia
▸ Child 12–17 years: 20 micrograms for 1 dose, manage fluid input carefully to avoid hyponatraemia
▶ BY INTRAMUSCULAR INJECTION, OR BY SUBCUTANEOUS INJECTION
▸ Neonate: Not recommended, use trial of treatment.
▸ Child 1–23 months: 400 nanograms for 1 dose, manage fluid input carefully to avoid hyponatraemia, not usually recommended
▸ Child 2–11 years: 0.5–1 microgram for 1 dose, manage fluid input carefully to avoid hyponatraemia
▸ Child 12–17 years: 1–2 micrograms for 1 dose, manage fluid input carefully to avoid hyponatraemia

Renal function testing
▶ BY INTRANASAL ADMINISTRATION
▸ Child 1–11 months: 10 micrograms, empty bladder at time of administration and restrict fluid intake to 50% at next 2 feeds to avoid fluid overload
▸ Child 1–14 years: 20 micrograms, empty bladder at time of administration and restrict fluid intake to 500 mL from 1 hour before until 8 hours after administration to avoid fluid overload
▸ Child 15–17 years: 40 micrograms, empty bladder at time of administration and limit fluid intake to 500 mL from 1 hour before until 8 hours after administration to avoid fluid overload
▶ BY SUBCUTANEOUS INJECTION, OR BY INTRAMUSCULAR INJECTION
▸ Child 1–11 months: 400 nanograms, empty bladder at time of administration and restrict fluid intake to 50% at next 2 feeds to avoid fluid overload
▸ Child 1–17 years: 2 micrograms, empty bladder at time of administration and restrict fluid intake to 500 mL from 1 hour before until 8 hours after administration to avoid fluid overload

Mild to moderate haemophilia and von Willebrand's disease
▶ BY INTRANASAL ADMINISTRATION
▸ Child 1–17 years: 4 micrograms/kg for 1 dose, for pre-operative use give 2 hours before procedure
▶ BY INTRAVENOUS INFUSION, OR BY SUBCUTANEOUS INJECTION
▸ Child: 300 nanograms/kg for 1 dose, to be administered immediately before surgery or after trauma; may be repeated at intervals of 12 hours if no tachycardia

Fibrinolytic response testing
▶ BY INTRAVENOUS INFUSION, OR BY SUBCUTANEOUS INJECTION
▸ Child 2–17 years: 300 nanograms/kg for 1 dose, blood to be sampled after 20 minutes for fibrinolytic activity

Assessment of antidiuretic hormone secretion (congenital deficiency suspected) (specialist use only)
▶ BY INTRANASAL ADMINISTRATION
▸ Child 1–23 months: Initially 100–500 nanograms for 1 dose

Assessment of antidiuretic hormone secretion (congenital deficiency not suspected) (specialist use only)
▶ BY INTRANASAL ADMINISTRATION
▸ Child 1–23 months: 1–5 micrograms for 1 dose

DOSE EQUIVALENCE AND CONVERSION
▸ *Tablets*, *intranasal spray*, and *solution for injection* contain desmopressin acetate; doses are expressed as desmopressin acetate.
▸ *Sublingual tablets*, *oral lyophilisate*, and *oral solution* contain desmopressin acetate; doses are expressed as desmopressin. For example, 1 mL of *Demovo®* oral solution contains 400 micrograms of desmopressin acetate equivalent to 360 micrograms of desmopressin.

● **UNLICENSED USE** Desmopressin is used in the doses provided in BNF Publications for the treatment of diabetes insipidus, but these may differ from those licensed.
Consult product literature for individual preparations.
Not licensed for assessment of antidiuretic hormone secretion.
Oral use of *DDAVP®* intravenous injection is not licensed.

● **CONTRA-INDICATIONS** Cardiac insufficiency · conditions treated with diuretics · history of hyponatraemia · polydipsia in alcohol dependence · psychogenic polydipsia · syndrome of inappropriate ADH secretion · von Willebrand's Disease Type IIB (may result in pseudothrombocytopenia)

● **CAUTIONS** Avoid fluid overload · cardiovascular disease (not indicated for nocturia associated with multiple sclerosis) · conditions which might be aggravated by water retention · cystic fibrosis · epilepsy · hypertension (not indicated for nocturia associated with multiple sclerosis) · nocturia—limit fluid intake to minimum from 1 hour before dose until 8 hours afterwards · nocturnal enuresis—limit fluid intake to minimum from 1 hour before dose until 8 hours afterwards

- **INTERACTIONS** → Appendix 1: desmopressin
- **SIDE-EFFECTS**

GENERAL SIDE-EFFECTS
- **Common or very common** Headache · nausea
- **Rare or very rare** Allergic dermatitis · emotional disorder · hyponatraemia
- **Frequency not known** Aggression · fluid retention

SPECIFIC SIDE-EFFECTS
- **Common or very common**
- With intranasal use Asthenia · conjunctivitis
- With oral use Abdominal pain
- **Uncommon**
- With intranasal use Epistaxis · gastrointestinal discomfort · nasal congestion · rhinitis · vomiting
- **Rare or very rare**
- With intranasal use Brain oedema
- **Frequency not known**
- With intramuscular use Abdominal pain
- With intravenous use Abdominal pain · vasodilation
- With oral use Brain oedema
- With subcutaneous use Abdominal pain
- With sublingual use Abdominal pain

SIDE-EFFECTS, FURTHER INFORMATION Treatment with desmopressin without restricting fluid intake may lead to fluid retention and/or hyponatraemia.

- **PREGNANCY** Small oxytocic effect in third trimester; increased risk of pre-eclampsia.
- **BREAST FEEDING** Amount too small to be harmful.
- **RENAL IMPAIRMENT** EvGr Caution with *injection*, *nasal spray*, and *tablets* (antidiuretic effect may be reduced). ⟨M⟩ EvGr Avoid *oral lyophilisate*, *oral solution*, and *sublingual tablets* in moderate or severe impairment. ⟨M⟩
- **MONITORING REQUIREMENTS** In *nocturia*, periodic blood pressure and weight checks are needed to monitor for fluid overload.
- **DIRECTIONS FOR ADMINISTRATION** Desmopressin oral lyophilisates are for sublingual administration.

Expert sources advise *DDAVP*® and *Desmotabs*® tablets may be crushed.

Expert sources advise *DDAVP*® injection may be administered orally.

EvGr For *intravenous infusion* (*DDAVP*®, *Octim*®), give intermittently in Sodium Chloride 0.9%; dilute with 50 mL and give over 20 minutes. ⟨M⟩

Expert sources advise higher doses of *DDAVP*® by *intravenous infusion*, used in mild to moderate haemophilia and von Willebrand's disease, may be diluted with 30–50 mL Sodium Chloride 0.9% intravenous infusion.

- **PATIENT AND CARER ADVICE**

Hyponatraemic convulsions Patients being treated for primary nocturnal enuresis should be warned to avoid fluid overload (including during swimming) and to stop taking desmopressin during an episode of vomiting or diarrhoea (until fluid balance normal).

Medicines for Children leaflet: Desmopressin for bedwetting www.medicinesforchildren.org.uk/medicines/desmopressin-for-bedwetting/

- **MEDICINAL FORMS** There can be variation in the licensing of different medicines containing the same drug. Forms available from special-order manufacturers include: oral capsule, oral suspension, oral solution, nasal drops, spray

Oral tablet

- **Desmopressin (Non-proprietary)**

Desmopressin acetate 100 microgram Desmopressin 100microgram tablets | 90 tablet PoM £76.62 DT = £39.73

Desmopressin acetate 200 microgram Desmopressin 200microgram tablets | 30 tablet PoM £31.00 DT = £16.92

- **DDAVP** (Ferring Pharmaceuticals Ltd)

Desmopressin acetate 100 microgram DDAVP 0.1mg tablets | 90 tablet PoM £44.12 DT = £39.73

Desmopressin acetate 200 microgram DDAVP 0.2mg tablets | 90 tablet PoM £88.23

- **Desmotabs** (Ferring Pharmaceuticals Ltd)

Desmopressin acetate 200 microgram Desmotabs 0.2mg tablets | 30 tablet PoM £29.43 DT = £16.92

Solution for injection

- **DDAVP** (Ferring Pharmaceuticals Ltd)

Desmopressin acetate 4 microgram per 1 ml DDAVP 4micrograms/1ml solution for injection ampoules | 10 ampoule PoM £13.16 DT = £13.16

- **Octim** (Ferring Pharmaceuticals Ltd)

Desmopressin acetate 15 microgram per 1 ml Octim 15micrograms/1ml solution for injection ampoules | 10 ampoule PoM £192.20 (Hospital only)

Spray

- **Desmopressin (Non-proprietary)**

Desmopressin acetate 2.5 microgram per 1 dose Minirin 2.5micrograms/dose nasal spray | 50 dose PoM ⊠

Desmopressin acetate 10 microgram per 1 dose Desmopressin 10micrograms/dose nasal spray | 60 dose PoM £34.95–£35.25 DT = £75.59

Desmopressin acetate 150 microgram per 1 dose Desmopressin 150micrograms/dose nasal spray | 25 dose PoM ⊠

Oral solution

- **Demovo** (Alturix Ltd)

Desmopressin (as Desmopressin acetate) 360 microgram per 1 ml Demovo 360micrograms/ml oral solution | 15 ml PoM £19.95 DT = £19.95 SF

Sublingual tablet

CAUTIONARY AND ADVISORY LABELS 26

EXCIPIENTS: May contain Aspartame

- **Desmopressin (Non-proprietary)**

Desmopressin acetate 60 microgram Desmopressin 60microgram sublingual tablets sugar free | 100 tablet PoM £27.79–£51.14 DT = £27.79 SF

Desmopressin acetate 120 microgram Desmopressin 120microgram sublingual tablets sugar free | 30 tablet PoM £16.69–£30.34 DT = £16.69 SF | 100 tablet PoM £80.85 SF

Desmopressin acetate 240 microgram Desmopressin 240microgram sublingual tablets sugar free | 30 tablet PoM £33.37–£60.68 DT = £33.37 SF | 100 tablet PoM £111.14–£161.71 DT = £111.14 SF

Oral lyophilisate

CAUTIONARY AND ADVISORY LABELS 26

- **Desmopressin (Non-proprietary)**

Desmopressin (as Desmopressin acetate) 120 microgram Desmopressin 120microgram oral lyophilisates sugar free | 30 tablet PoM £23.27–£50.00 DT = £30.34 SF

Desmopressin (as Desmopressin acetate) 240 microgram Desmopressin 240microgram oral lyophilisates sugar free | 30 tablet PoM £46.53–£100.00 DT = £60.68 SF

- **DDAVP Melt** (Ferring Pharmaceuticals Ltd)

Desmopressin (as Desmopressin acetate) 60 microgram DDAVP Melt 60microgram oral lyophilisates | 100 tablet PoM £50.53 DT = £50.53 SF

Desmopressin (as Desmopressin acetate) 120 microgram DDAVP Melt 120microgram oral lyophilisates | 100 tablet PoM £101.07 DT = £101.07 SF

Desmopressin (as Desmopressin acetate) 240 microgram DDAVP Melt 240microgram oral lyophilisates | 100 tablet PoM £202.14 SF

- **DesmoMelt** (Ferring Pharmaceuticals Ltd)

Desmopressin (as Desmopressin acetate) 120 microgram DesmoMelt 120microgram oral lyophilisates | 30 tablet PoM £30.34 DT = £30.34 SF

Desmopressin (as Desmopressin acetate)
240 microgram DesmoMelt 240microgram oral lyophilisates | 30 tablet PoM £60.68 DT = £60.68 SF

▸ **Noqdirna** (Ferring Pharmaceuticals Ltd)

Desmopressin (as Desmopressin acetate) 25 microgram Noqdirna 25microgram oral lyophilisates | 30 tablet PoM £15.16 DT = £15.16 SF

Desmopressin (as Desmopressin acetate)
50 microgram Noqdirna 50microgram oral lyophilisates | 30 tablet PoM £15.16 DT = £15.16 SF

2 Bone metabolism disorders

Bone metabolism

Disorders of bone metabolism

The two main disorders of bone metabolism that occur in children are rickets and osteoporosis. The two most common forms of rickets are Vitamin D deficiency rickets and hypophosphataemic rickets. See also calcium.

Osteoporosis

Osteoporosis in children may be primary (e.g. *osteogenesis imperfecta* and *idiopathic juvenile osteoporosis*), or secondary (e.g. due to inflammatory disorders, immobilisation, or corticosteroids); specialist management is required.

Corticosteroid-induced osteoporosis

To reduce the risk of osteoporosis doses of oral corticosteroids should be as low as possible and courses of treatment as short as possible.

Calcitonin

Calcitonin is involved with parathyroid hormone in the regulation of bone turnover and hence in the maintenance of calcium balance and homoeostasis. Calcitonin (salmon) p. 536 (synthetic or recombinant salmon calcitonin) is used by specialists to lower the plasma-calcium concentration in children with hypercalcaemia associated with malignancy.

Bisphosphonates

A bisphosphonate such as pamidronate disodium p. 535 is used in the management of severe forms of *osteogenesis imperfecta* and other causes of osteoporosis in children to reduce the number of fractures; the long-term effects of bisphosphonates in children has not been established. Single doses of biphosphonates are also used to manage hypercalcaemia. Treatment should be initiated under specialist advice **only**.

Other drugs used for Bone metabolism disorders
Calcitriol, p. 788

BISPHOSPHONATES

Bisphosphonates

● **DRUG ACTION** Bisphosphonates are adsorbed onto hydroxyapatite crystals in bone, slowing both their rate of growth and dissolution, and therefore reducing the rate of bone turnover.

IMPORTANT SAFETY INFORMATION

MHRA/CHM ADVICE: BISPHOSPHONATES: ATYPICAL FEMORAL FRACTURES (JUNE 2011)

Atypical femoral fractures have been reported rarely with bisphosphonate treatment, mainly in patients receiving long-term treatment for osteoporosis.

The need to continue bisphosphonate treatment for osteoporosis should be re-evaluated periodically based on an assessment of the benefits and risks of treatment for individual patients, particularly after 5 or more years of use.

Patients should be advised to report any thigh, hip, or groin pain during treatment with a bisphosphonate.

Discontinuation of bisphosphonate treatment in patients suspected to have an atypical femoral fracture should be considered after an assessment of the benefits and risks of continued treatment.

MHRA/CHM ADVICE: BISPHOSPHONATES: OSTEONECROSIS OF THE JAW (NOVEMBER 2009) AND INTRAVENOUS BISPHOSPHONATES: OSTEONECROSIS OF THE JAW—FURTHER MEASURES TO MINIMISE RISK (JULY 2015)

The risk of osteonecrosis of the jaw is substantially greater for patients receiving intravenous bisphosphonates in the treatment of cancer than for patients receiving oral bisphosphonates for osteoporosis or Paget's disease.

Risk factors for developing osteonecrosis of the jaw that should be considered are: potency of bisphosphonate (highest for zoledronate), route of administration, cumulative dose, duration and type of malignant disease, concomitant treatment, smoking, comorbid conditions, and history of dental disease.

All patients with cancer and patients with poor dental status should have a dental check-up (and any necessary remedial work should be performed) before bisphosphonate treatment, or as soon as possible after starting treatment. Patients should also maintain good oral hygiene, receive routine dental check-ups, and report any oral symptoms such as dental mobility, pain, or swelling, non-healing sores or discharge to a doctor and dentist during treatment.

Before prescribing an intravenous bisphosphonate, patients should be given a patient reminder card and informed of the risk of osteonecrosis of the jaw. Advise patients to tell their doctor if they have any problems with their mouth or teeth before starting treatment, and if the patient wears dentures, they should make sure their dentures fit properly. Patients should tell their doctor and dentist that they are receiving an intravenous bisphosphonate if they need dental treatment or dental surgery.

Guidance for dentists in primary care is included in *Oral Health Management of Patients at Risk of Medication-related Osteonecrosis of the Jaw: Dental Clinical Guidance*, Scottish Dental Clinical Effectiveness Programme, March 2017 (available at www.sdcep.org.uk/published-guidance/medication-related-osteonecrosis-of-the-jaw/).

MHRA/CHM ADVICE: BISPHOSPHONATES: OSTEONECROSIS OF THE EXTERNAL AUDITORY CANAL (DECEMBER 2015)

Benign idiopathic osteonecrosis of the external auditory canal has been reported very rarely with bisphosphonate treatment, mainly in patients receiving long-term therapy (2 years or longer).

The possibility of osteonecrosis of the external auditory canal should be considered in patients receiving bisphosphonates who present with ear symptoms, including chronic ear infections, or suspected cholesteatoma.

Risk factors for developing osteonecrosis of the external auditory canal include: steroid use, chemotherapy, infection, an ear operation, or cotton-bud use.

Patients should be advised to report any ear pain, discharge from the ear, or an ear infection during treatment with a bisphosphonate.

● **SIDE-EFFECTS**

▸ **Common or very common** Alopecia · anaemia · appetite decreased · arthralgia · asthenia · chills · constipation · diarrhoea · dizziness · dysphagia · electrolyte imbalance ·

eye inflammation · fever · gastritis · gastrointestinal discomfort · headache · influenza like illness · malaise · myalgia · nausea · oesophageal ulcer (discontinue) · oesophagitis (discontinue) · pain · peripheral oedema · renal impairment · skin reactions · taste altered · vomiting
- **Uncommon** Anaphylactic reaction · angioedema · bronchospasm · oesophageal stenosis (discontinue) · osteonecrosis
- **Rare or very rare** Atypical femur fracture · Stevens-Johnson syndrome

- **PATIENT AND CARER ADVICE**
Atypical femoral fractures Patients should be advised to report any thigh, hip, or groin pain during treatment with a bisphosphonate.
Osteonecrosis of the jaw During bisphosphonate treatment patients should maintain good oral hygiene, receive routine dental check-ups, and report any oral symptoms.
Osteonecrosis of the external auditory canal Patients should be advised to report any ear pain, discharge from ear or an ear infection during treatment with a bisphosphonate.

533

Alendronic acid

16-Nov-2022

(Alendronate)

- **INDICATIONS AND DOSE**

Osteoporosis (due to osteogenesis imperfecta and other causes) (initiated under specialist supervision) | Hypercalcaemia (initiated under specialist supervision)
- BY MOUTH
  - Child: (consult local protocol)

- **UNLICENSED USE** Not licensed for use in children.
- **CONTRA-INDICATIONS** Abnormalities of oesophagus · hypocalcaemia · other factors which delay emptying (e.g. stricture or achalasia)
- **CAUTIONS** Active gastro-intestinal bleeding · atypical femoral fractures · duodenitis · dysphagia · exclude other causes of osteoporosis · gastritis · history (within 1 year) of ulcers · surgery of the upper gastro-intestinal tract · symptomatic oesophageal disease · ulcers · upper gastro-intestinal disorders
- **INTERACTIONS** → Appendix 1: bisphosphonates
- **SIDE-EFFECTS**
  - **Common or very common** Gastrointestinal disorders · joint swelling · vertigo
  - **Uncommon** Haemorrhage
  - **Rare or very rare** Femoral stress fracture · oropharyngeal ulceration · photosensitivity reaction · severe cutaneous adverse reactions (SCARs)

  SIDE-EFFECTS, FURTHER INFORMATION Severe oesophageal reactions (oesophagitis, oesophageal ulcers, oesophageal stricture and oesophageal erosions) have been reported; patients should be advised to stop taking the tablets and to seek medical attention if they develop symptoms of oesophageal irritation such as dysphagia, new or worsening heartburn, pain on swallowing or retrosternal pain.
- **PREGNANCY** Avoid.
- **BREAST FEEDING** Manufacturer advises avoid—no information available.
- **RENAL IMPAIRMENT** EvGr Avoid if creatinine clearance less than 35 mL/minute. (M) See p. 16.
- **MONITORING REQUIREMENTS** Correct disturbances of calcium and mineral metabolism (e.g. vitamin-D deficiency, hypocalcaemia) before starting treatment. Monitor serum-calcium concentration during treatment.
- **DIRECTIONS FOR ADMINISTRATION** Manufacturer advises tablets should be swallowed whole and oral solution should be swallowed as a single 100 mL dose. Doses should be taken with plenty of water while sitting or standing, on an empty stomach at least 30 minutes before breakfast (or another oral medicine); patient should stand or sit upright for at least 30 minutes after administration.
- **PATIENT AND CARER ADVICE** Patients or their carers should be given advice on how to administer alendronic acid tablets and oral solution.
Oesophageal reactions Patients (or their carers) should be advised to stop taking alendronic acid and to seek medical attention if they develop symptoms of oesophageal irritation such as dysphagia, new or worsening heartburn, pain on swallowing or retrosternal pain.

- **MEDICINAL FORMS** There can be variation in the licensing of different medicines containing the same drug. Forms available from special-order manufacturers include: oral solution

Oral tablet
- Alendronic acid (Non-proprietary)
  Alendronic acid (as Alendronate sodium) 70 mg Alendronic acid 70mg tablets | 4 tablet PoM £2.28 DT = £0.97
- Fosamax Once Weekly (Organon Pharma (UK) Ltd)
  Alendronic acid (as Alendronate sodium) 70 mg Fosamax Once Weekly 70mg tablets | 4 tablet PoM £22.80 DT = £0.97

Oral solution
- Alendronic acid (Non-proprietary)
  Alendronic acid 700 microgram per 1 ml Alendronic acid 70mg/100ml oral solution unit dose sugar free | 4 unit dose PoM £29.80 DT = £24.94 SF

Effervescent tablet
- Binosto (Internis Pharmaceuticals Ltd)
  Alendronic acid (as Alendronate sodium) 70 mg Binosto 70mg effervescent tablets | 4 tablet PoM £11.60 DT = £11.60 SF

533

Clodronate disodium

14-Apr-2026

(Sodium clodronate)

- **INDICATIONS AND DOSE**

Osteoporosis (due to osteogenesis imperfecta or other causes) (specialist use only) | Hypercalcaemia (specialist use only)
- BY MOUTH
  - Child: (consult local protocol)

- **UNLICENSED USE** Not licensed for use in children.
- **CONTRA-INDICATIONS** Acute severe gastro-intestinal inflammatory conditions
- **CAUTIONS** Atypical femoral fractures · maintain adequate fluid intake during treatment · upper gastro-intestinal disorders
- **INTERACTIONS** → Appendix 1: bisphosphonates
- **SIDE-EFFECTS** Proteinuria · respiratory disorder
- **PREGNANCY** Avoid.
- **BREAST FEEDING** Manufacturer advises avoid—no information available.
- **RENAL IMPAIRMENT** Manufacturer advises avoid if creatinine clearance less than 10 mL/minute.
Dose adjustments See p. 16.
In adults, manufacturer advises reduce dose if creatinine clearance 10–50 mL/minute (consult product literature).
- **MONITORING REQUIREMENTS** Monitor renal function, serum calcium and serum phosphate before and during treatment.
- **DIRECTIONS FOR ADMINISTRATION** Manufacturer advises avoid food or fluids (other than plain water) for 2 hours before and 1 hour after treatment, particularly calcium-containing products e.g. milk; also avoid iron and mineral supplements and antacids; maintain adequate fluid intake.
- **PATIENT AND CARER ADVICE** Patients or carers should be given advice on how to administer clodronate disodium capsules and tablets.

● **MEDICINAL FORMS** There can be variation in the licensing of different medicines containing the same drug.

Oral tablet

CAUTIONARY AND ADVISORY LABELS 10

▸ **Clasteon** (Kent Pharma (UK) Ltd)
Sodium clodronate 800 mg Clasteon 800mg tablets | 60 tablet PoM £146.43 DT = £146.43

▸ **Loron** (Esteve Pharmaceuticals Ltd)
Sodium clodronate 520 mg Loron 520mg tablets | 60 tablet PoM £114.44 DT = £114.44

Oral capsule

▸ **Clasteon** (Kent Pharma (UK) Ltd)
Sodium clodronate 400 mg Clasteon 400mg capsules | 30 capsule PoM £34.96 DT = £34.96 | 120 capsule PoM £139.83 DT = £139.83

533

Pamidronate disodium

11-Nov-2025

(Formerly called aminohydroxypropylidenediphosphonate disodium (APD))

● **INDICATIONS AND DOSE**

Osteoporosis (due to osteogenesis imperfecta and other causes) (specialist use only) | Hypercalcaemia (specialist use only)

▸ BY INTRAVENOUS INFUSION

▸ Child: (consult local protocols or specialist resources)

● **UNLICENSED USE** Not licensed for use in children.

● **CAUTIONS** Atypical femoral fractures · cardiac disease · ensure adequate hydration · previous thyroid surgery (risk of hypocalcaemia)

● **INTERACTIONS** → Appendix 1: bisphosphonates

● **SIDE-EFFECTS**

▸ **Common or very common** Decreased leucocytes · drowsiness · flushing · hypertension · insomnia · paraesthesia · tetany · thrombocytopenia

▸ **Uncommon** Agitation · dyspnoea · hypotension · muscle cramps · seizure

▸ **Rare or very rare** Acute respiratory distress syndrome (ARDS) · confusion · glomerulonephritis · haematuria · heart failure · interstitial lung disease · nephritis tubulointerstitial · nephrotic syndrome · oedema · pulmonary oedema · reactivation of infections · renal disorder exacerbated · renal tubular disorder · visual hallucinations · xanthopsia

▸ **Frequency not known** Atrial fibrillation

● **PREGNANCY** Avoid—toxicity in *animal* studies.

● **BREAST FEEDING** Avoid.

● **HEPATIC IMPAIRMENT** Manufacturer advises caution in severe hepatic impairment (no information available).

● **DIRECTIONS FOR ADMINISTRATION** For *slow intravenous infusion*, consult local protocols or specialist resources for information on dilution and rate of administration.

● **PATIENT AND CARER ADVICE** A patient reminder card should be provided (risk of osteonecrosis of the jaw).

Driving and skilled tasks Patients should be warned against performing skilled tasks (e.g. cycling, driving or operating machinery) immediately after treatment (somnolence or dizziness can occur).

● **MEDICINAL FORMS** There can be variation in the licensing of different medicines containing the same drug.

Solution for infusion

▸ **Pamidronate disodium (Non-proprietary)**
Pamidronate disodium 3 mg per 1 ml Pamidronate disodium 30mg/10ml solution for infusion vials | 1 vial PoM £59.66 (Hospital only)
Pamidronate disodium 9 mg per 1 ml Pamidronate disodium 90mg/10ml solution for infusion vials | 1 vial PoM £170.45 (Hospital only)

533

Risedronate sodium

21-Jul-2021

● **INDICATIONS AND DOSE**

Osteoporosis (due to osteogenesis imperfecta and other causes) (specialist use only) | Hypercalcaemia (specialist use only)

▸ BY MOUTH

▸ Child: (consult local protocol)

● **UNLICENSED USE** Not licensed for use in children.

● **CONTRA-INDICATIONS** Hypocalcaemia

● **CAUTIONS** Atypical femoral fractures · oesophageal abnormalities · other factors which delay transit or emptying (e.g. stricture or achalasia) · upper gastro-intestinal disorders

● **INTERACTIONS** → Appendix 1: bisphosphonates

● **SIDE-EFFECTS**

▸ **Uncommon** Gastrointestinal disorders

▸ **Rare or very rare** Glossitis

▸ **Frequency not known** Amblyopia · apnoea · chest pain · corneal lesion · dry eye · hypersensitivity · hypersensitivity vasculitis · increased risk of infection · leg cramps · liver disorder · muscle weakness · neoplasms · nocturia · tinnitus · toxic epidermal necrolysis · weight decreased

● **PREGNANCY** Avoid.

● **BREAST FEEDING** Avoid.

● **RENAL IMPAIRMENT** EvGr Avoid if creatinine clearance less than 30 mL/minute. Ⓜ See p. 16.

● **MONITORING REQUIREMENTS**

▸ Correct hypocalcaemia before starting.

▸ Correct other disturbances of bone and mineral metabolism (e.g. vitamin-D deficiency) at onset of treatment.

● **DIRECTIONS FOR ADMINISTRATION** Manufacturer advises swallow tablets whole with full glass of water; on rising, take on an empty stomach at least 30 minutes before first food or drink of the day **or**, if taking at any other time of the day, avoid food and drink for at least 2 hours before or after risedronate (particularly avoid calcium-containing products e.g. milk; also avoid iron and mineral supplements and antacids); stand or sit upright for at least 30 minutes; do not take tablets at bedtime or before rising.

● **PATIENT AND CARER ADVICE** Patients or carers should be given advice on how to administer risedronate sodium tablets.

Oesophageal reactions Patients should be advised to stop taking the tablets and seek medical attention if they develop symptoms of oesophageal irritation such as dysphagia, pain on swallowing, retrosternal pain, or heartburn.

Medicines for Children leaflet: Risedronate for brittle bones
www.medicinesforchildren.org.uk/medicines/risedronate-for-brittle-bones/

● **MEDICINAL FORMS** There can be variation in the licensing of different medicines containing the same drug. Forms available from special-order manufacturers include: oral suspension, oral solution

Oral tablet

▸ **Risedronate sodium (Non-proprietary)**
Risedronate sodium 5 mg Risedronate sodium 5mg tablets | 28 tablet PoM £24.78 DT = £20.52
Risedronate sodium 30 mg Risedronate sodium 30mg tablets | 28 tablet PoM £143.83 DT = £143.83
Risedronate sodium 35 mg Risedronate sodium 35mg tablets | 4 tablet PoM £17.56 DT = £0.96

▸ **Actonel** (Teva UK Ltd)
Risedronate sodium 35 mg Actonel 35mg tablets | 4 tablet PoM DT = £0.96

CALCIUM REGULATING DRUGS › BONE RESORPTION INHIBITORS

Calcitonin (salmon) (Salcatonin)

01-Jun-2021

● **INDICATIONS AND DOSE**

Hypercalcaemia (limited experience in children) (specialist use only)

▶ BY SUBCUTANEOUS INJECTION, OR BY INTRAMUSCULAR INJECTION

▶ Child: 2.5–5 units/kg every 12 hours (max. per dose 400 units every 6–8 hours), adjusted according to response, no additional benefit with doses over 8 units/kg every 6 hours

▶ BY INTRAVENOUS INFUSION

▶ Child: 5–10 units/kg, to be administered by slow intravenous infusion over at least 6 hours

Osteoporosis (specialist use only)

▶ BY INTRAMUSCULAR INJECTION, OR BY SUBCUTANEOUS INJECTION

▶ Child: Refer for specialist advice, experience very limited

● **UNLICENSED USE** Not licensed in children.

● **CONTRA-INDICATIONS** Hypocalcaemia

● **CAUTIONS** History of allergy (skin test advised) · risk of malignancy—avoid prolonged use (use lowest effective dose for shortest possible time)

● **INTERACTIONS** → Appendix 1: calcitonins

● **SIDE-EFFECTS**

▶ **Common or very common** Abdominal pain · arthralgia · diarrhoea · dizziness · fatigue · flushing · headache · musculoskeletal pain · nausea · secondary malignancy (long term use) · taste altered · vomiting

▶ **Uncommon** Hypersensitivity · hypertension · influenza like illness · oedema · polyuria · skin reactions · visual impairment

▶ **Rare or very rare** Bronchospasm · throat swelling · tongue swelling

▶ **Frequency not known** Hypocalcaemia · tremor

● **PREGNANCY** Avoid unless potential benefit outweighs risk (toxicity in *animal* studies).

● **BREAST FEEDING** Avoid; inhibits lactation in *animals*.

● **RENAL IMPAIRMENT** EvGr Use with caution in end-stage renal disease (reduced renal metabolism; limited information available). Ⓜ

● **MONITORING REQUIREMENTS** Monitor bone growth.

● **DIRECTIONS FOR ADMINISTRATION** For *intravenous infusion*, manufacturer advises dilute injection solution (e.g. 400 units in 500 mL) with Sodium Chloride 0.9% and give over at least 6 hours; glass or hard plastic containers should not be used; use diluted solution without delay.

● **MEDICINAL FORMS** There can be variation in the licensing of different medicines containing the same drug.

Solution for injection

▶ **Calcitonin (salmon) (Non-proprietary)**

Calcitonin (salmon) 100 unit per 1 ml Calcitonin (salmon) 100units/1ml solution for injection ampoules | 5 ampoule PoM £248.79

DRUGS AFFECTING BONE STRUCTURE AND MINERALISATION › MONOCLONAL ANTIBODIES

Denosumab

25-May-2022

● **DRUG ACTION** Denosumab is a human monoclonal antibody that inhibits osteoclast formation, function, and survival, thereby decreasing bone resorption.

● **INDICATIONS AND DOSE**

XGEVA®

Giant cell tumour of bone that is unresectable or where surgical resection is likely to result in severe morbidity in skeletally mature adolescents

▶ BY SUBCUTANEOUS INJECTION

▶ Child: 120 mg every 4 weeks, give additional dose on days 8 and 15 of the first month of treatment only, supplementation of at least calcium 500 mg and Vitamin D 400 units daily should also be taken unless hypercalcaemia is present, to be administered into the thigh, abdomen or upper arm

IMPORTANT SAFETY INFORMATION

MHRA/CHM ADVICE: DENOSUMAB: ATYPICAL FEMORAL FRACTURES (FEBRUARY 2013)

Atypical femoral fractures have been reported rarely in patients receiving denosumab for the long-term treatment (2.5 or more years) of postmenopausal osteoporosis.

Patients should be advised to report any new or unusual thigh, hip, or groin pain during treatment with denosumab.

Discontinuation of denosumab in patients suspected to have an atypical femoral fracture should be considered after an assessment of the benefits and risks of continued treatment.

MHRA/CHM ADVICE: DENOSUMAB: MINIMISING THE RISK OF OSTEONECROSIS OF THE JAW; MONITORING FOR HYPOCALCAEMIA—UPDATED RECOMMENDATIONS (SEPTEMBER 2014) AND DENOSUMAB: OSTEONECROSIS OF THE JAW—FURTHER MEASURES TO MINIMISE RISK (JULY 2015)

Denosumab is associated with a risk of osteonecrosis of the jaw (ONJ) and with a risk of hypocalcaemia.

Osteonecrosis of the jaw Osteonecrosis of the jaw is a well-known and common side-effect in patients receiving denosumab 120 mg for cancer. Risk factors include smoking, poor oral hygiene, invasive dental procedures (including tooth extractions, dental implants, oral surgery), comorbidity (including dental disease, anaemia, coagulopathy, infection), advanced cancer, previous treatment with bisphosphonates, and concomitant treatments (including chemotherapy, anti-angiogenic biologics, corticosteroids, and radiotherapy to head and neck). The following precautions are now recommended to reduce the risk of ONJ:

Denosumab 120 mg (cancer indication)

- A dental examination and appropriate preventative dentistry before starting treatment are now recommended for all patients
- Do not start denosumab in patients with a dental or jaw condition requiring surgery, or in patients who have unhealed lesions from dental or oral surgery

All patients should be given a patient reminder card and informed of the risk of ONJ. Advise patients to tell their doctor if they have any problems with their mouth or teeth before starting treatment, if they wear dentures they should make sure their dentures fit properly before starting treatment, to maintain good oral hygiene, receive routine dental check-ups during treatment, and immediately report any oral symptoms such as dental mobility, pain, swelling, non-healing sores or discharge to a doctor and dentist. Patients should tell their doctor and dentist that they are receiving denosumab if they need dental treatment or dental surgery.

Hypocalcaemia Denosumab is associated with a risk of hypocalcaemia. This risk increases with the degree of renal impairment. Hypocalcaemia usually occurs in the first weeks of denosumab treatment, but it can also occur later in treatment.

Plasma-calcium concentration monitoring is recommended for denosumab 120 mg (cancer indication):

- before the first dose
- within two weeks after the initial dose
- if suspected symptoms of hypocalcaemia occur
- consider monitoring more frequently in patients with risk factors for hypocalcaemia (e.g. severe renal impairment, creatinine clearance less than 30 mL/minute)

All patients should be advised to report symptoms of hypocalcaemia to their doctor (e.g. muscle spasms, twitches, cramps, numbness or tingling in the fingers, toes, or around the mouth).

MHRA/CHM ADVICE: DENOSUMAB: REPORTS OF OSTEONECROSIS OF THE EXTERNAL AUDITORY CANAL (JUNE 2017)

Osteonecrosis of the external auditory canal has been reported with denosumab and this should be considered in patients who present with ear symptoms including chronic ear infections or in those with suspected cholesteatoma. Possible risk factors include steroid use and chemotherapy, with or without local risk factors such as infection or trauma. The MHRA recommends advising patients to report any ear pain, discharge from the ear, or an ear infection during denosumab treatment.

MHRA/CHM ADVICE: DENOSUMAB (*XGEVA*®) FOR GIANT CELL TUMOUR OF BONE: RISK OF CLINICALLY SIGNIFICANT HYPERCALCAEMIA FOLLOWING DISCONTINUATION (JUNE 2018)

Cases of clinically significant hypercalcaemia (rebound hypercalcaemia) have been reported up to 9 months after discontinuation of denosumab treatment for giant cell tumour of bone. The MHRA recommends that prescribers should monitor patients for signs and symptoms of hypercalcaemia after discontinuation, consider periodic assessment of serum calcium, re-evaluate the patient's calcium and vitamin D supplementation requirements, and advise patients to report symptoms of hypercalcaemia.

Denosumab is not recommended in patients with growing skeletons.

MHRA/CHM ADVICE: DENOSUMAB 60 MG (*PROLIA*®): SHOULD NOT BE USED IN PATIENTS UNDER 18 YEARS DUE TO THE RISK OF SERIOUS HYPERCALCAEMIA (MAY 2022)

Cases of serious and life-threatening hypercalcaemia requiring hospitalisation and leading to acute kidney injury have been reported in children and adolescents aged under 18 years who were given denosumab 60 mg in clinical trials and during off-label use. Hypercalcaemia occurred during treatment or in the weeks to months after the last dose.

Healthcare professionals are reminded that:

- *Prolia*® is only licensed for the treatment of osteoporosis and other bone loss conditions in patients aged 18 years and older;
- patients younger than 18 years currently receiving *Prolia*® in clinical trials or off-label should be counselled alongside their carers to seek advice from healthcare professionals.

- **CONTRA-INDICATIONS** Hypocalcaemia

XGEVA® Unhealed lesions from dental or oral surgery

- **CAUTIONS** Risk factors for osteonecrosis of the external auditory canal · risk factors for osteonecrosis of the jaw—consider temporary interruption of denosumab if occurs during treatment
- **INTERACTIONS** → Appendix 1: denosumab
- **SIDE-EFFECTS**

▶ **Common or very common** Abdominal discomfort · alopecia · constipation · diarrhoea · dyspnoea · hyperhidrosis · hypocalcaemia (including fatal cases) · hypophosphataemia · increased risk of infection · osteonecrosis · pain · sciatica · second primary malignancy · skin reactions

▶ **Uncommon** Atypical femur fracture · cellulitis (seek prompt medical attention) · hypercalcaemia (on discontinuation)

▶ **Rare or very rare** Hypersensitivity · hypersensitivity vasculitis

▶ **Frequency not known** Facial swelling

- **CONCEPTION AND CONTRACEPTION** Ensure effective contraception in women of child-bearing potential, during treatment and for at least 5 months after stopping treatment.
- **PREGNANCY** Manufacturer advises avoid—toxicity in *animal* studies; risk of toxicity increases with each trimester.
- **BREAST FEEDING** Manufacturer advises avoid.
- **RENAL IMPAIRMENT** Increased risk of hypocalcaemia if creatinine clearance less than 30 mL/minute, see p. 16.
- **MONITORING REQUIREMENTS** Correct hypocalcaemia and vitamin D deficiency before starting. Monitor plasma-calcium concentration during therapy.
- **PATIENT AND CARER ADVICE**

Atypical femoral fractures Patients should be advised to report any new or unusual thigh, hip, or groin pain during treatment with denosumab.

Osteonecrosis of the jaw All patients should be informed to maintain good oral hygiene, receive routine dental check-ups, and immediately report any oral symptoms such as dental mobility, pain, or swelling to a doctor and dentist.

Hypocalcaemia All patients should be advised to report symptoms of hypocalcaemia to their doctor (e.g. muscle spasms, twitches, cramps, numbness or tingling in the fingers, toes, or around the mouth).

Patient reminder card A patient reminder card should be provided (risk of osteonecrosis of the jaw).

- **MEDICINAL FORMS** There can be variation in the licensing of different medicines containing the same drug.

Solution for injection

CAUTIONARY AND ADVISORY LABELS 10

EXCIPIENTS: May contain Sorbitol

▸ **Xgeva** (Amgen Ltd)

Denosumab 70 mg per 1 ml Xgeva 120mg/1.7ml solution for injection vials | 1 vial PoM £309.86 DT = £309.86

3 Corticosteroid responsive conditions

CORTICOSTEROIDS

Corticosteroids, general use 08-Jun-2021

Overview

Dosages of corticosteroids vary widely in different diseases and in different patients. If the use of a corticosteroid can save or prolong life, as in exfoliative dermatitis, pemphigus, acute leukaemia or acute transplant rejection, high doses may need to be given, because the complications of therapy are likely to be less serious than the effects of the disease itself.

When long-term corticosteroid therapy is used in some chronic diseases, the adverse effects of treatment may become greater than the disabilities caused by the disease. To minimise side-effects the maintenance dose should be kept as low as possible.

When potentially less harmful measures are ineffective, corticosteroids are used topically for the treatment of inflammatory conditions of the skin. Corticosteroids should be avoided or used only under specialist supervision in psoriasis.

Corticosteroids are used both topically (by rectum) and systemically (by mouth or intravenously) in the management of ulcerative colitis and Crohn's disease.

Use can be made of the mineralocorticoid activity of fludrocortisone acetate p. 544 to treat postural hypotension in autonomic neuropathy.

High-dose corticosteroids should be avoided for the management of septic shock. However, low-dose hydrocortisone p. 544 can be used in septic shock that is resistant to volume expansion and catecholamines, and is accompanied by suspected or proven adrenal insufficiency.

The suppressive action of glucocorticoids on the hypothalamic-pituitary-adrenal axis is greatest and most prolonged when they are given at night. In most adults a single dose of dexamethasone p. 543 at night is sufficient to inhibit corticotropin secretion for 24 hours. This is the basis of the 'overnight dexamethasone suppression test' for diagnosing Cushing's syndrome.

Betamethasone p. 542 and dexamethasone are also appropriate for conditions where water retention would be a disadvantage.

A corticosteroid may be used in the management of raised intracranial pressure or cerebral oedema that occurs as a result of malignancy (see Prescribing in palliative care p. 20). However, a corticosteroid should **not** be used for the management of head injury or stroke because it is unlikely to be of benefit and may even be harmful.

Corticosteroids are no longer recommended for the routine emergency treatment of anaphylaxis. For guidance on the management of anaphylaxis, see Antihistamines, allergen immunotherapy and allergic emergencies p. 199.

EvGr In the management of asthma, corticosteroids are preferably used by inhalation. Systemic therapy along with bronchodilators is required for the treatment of acute asthma and in some very severe cases of chronic asthma. (A)

Betamethasone is used in women at risk of preterm delivery to reduce the incidence of neonatal respiratory distress syndrome [unlicensed use].

Dexamethasone should not be used routinely for the prophylaxis and treatment of chronic lung disease in neonates because of an association with adverse neurological effects.

Corticosteroids may be useful in conditions such as autoimmune hepatitis, rheumatoid arthritis, and sarcoidosis; they may also lead to remissions of acquired haemolytic anaemia and thrombocytopenic purpura.

High doses of a corticosteroid (usually prednisolone p. 548) are used in the treatment of *glomerular kidney disease*, including *nephrotic syndrome*. The condition frequently recurs; a corticosteroid given in high doses and for prolonged periods may delay relapse but the higher incidence of adverse effects limits the overall benefit. Those who suffer frequent relapses may be treated with prednisolone given in a low dose (daily or on alternate days) for 3–6 months; the dose should be adjusted to minimise effects on growth and development. Other drugs used in the treatment of glomerular kidney disease include levamisole p. 645, cyclophosphamide p. 663, chlorambucil p. 663, and ciclosporin p. 640. *Congenital nephrotic syndrome* may be resistant to corticosteroids and immunosuppressants; indometacin p. 824 and an ACE inhibitor such as captopril p. 131 have been used.

Corticosteroids can improve the prognosis of serious conditions such as systemic lupus erythematosus and polyarteritis nodosa; the effects of the disease process may be suppressed and symptoms relieved, but the underlying condition is not cured, although it may ultimately remit. It is usual to begin therapy in these conditions at fairly high dose and then to reduce the dose to the lowest commensurate with disease control.

For other references to the use of corticosteroids see: Prescribing in palliative care, immunosuppression, rheumatic diseases, eye, otitis externa, allergic rhinitis, and aphthous ulcers.

Side-effects

MHRA/CHM advice: Corticosteroids: rare risk of central serous chorioretinopathy with local as well as systemic administration (August 2017)

Central serous chorioretinopathy is a retinal disorder that has been linked to the systemic use of corticosteroids. Recently, it has also been reported after local administration of corticosteroids via inhaled and intranasal, epidural, intra-articular, topical dermal, and periocular routes. The MHRA recommends that patients should be advised to report any blurred vision or other visual disturbances with corticosteroid treatment given by any route; consider referral to an ophthalmologist for evaluation of possible causes if a patient presents with vision problems.

Mineralocorticoid and glucocorticoid side-effects

Overdosage or prolonged use can exaggerate some of the normal physiological actions of corticosteroids leading to mineralocorticoid and glucocorticoid side-effects.

Mineralocorticoid side-effects

- hypertension
- sodium retention
- water retention
- potassium loss
- calcium loss

Mineralocorticoid side-effects are most marked with fludrocortisone, but are significant with hydrocortisone, corticotropin, and tetracosactide. Mineralocorticoid actions are negligible with the high potency glucocorticoids, betamethasone and dexamethasone, and occur only slightly with methylprednisolone, prednisolone, and triamcinolone.

Glucocorticoid side-effects

- diabetes
- osteoporosis
- in addition high doses are associated with avascular necrosis of the femoral head
- muscle wasting (proximal myopathy) can also occur
- corticosteroid therapy is also weakly linked with peptic ulceration and perforation
- psychiatric reactions may also occur

Managing side-effects

Side-effects can be minimised by using the lowest effective dose for the minimum period possible. The suppressive action of a corticosteroid on cortisol secretion is least when it is given as a single dose in the morning. In an attempt to reduce pituitary-adrenal suppression further, the total dose for two days can sometimes be taken as a single dose on alternate days; alternate-day administration has not been very successful in the management of asthma. Pituitary-adrenal suppression can also be reduced by means of intermittent therapy with short courses. In some conditions it may be possible to reduce the dose of corticosteroid by adding a small dose of an immunosuppressive drug.

For information on the cessation of oral corticosteroid treatment, see *Treatment cessation*, for systemic corticosteroids (e.g. prednisolone).

Whenever possible *local treatment* with creams, intra-articular injections, inhalations, eye-drops, or enemas should be used in preference to *systemic treatment*.

Inhaled corticosteroids have considerably fewer systemic effects than oral corticosteroids, but adverse effects including adrenal suppression have been reported. Use of other corticosteroid therapy (including topical) or concurrent use of drugs which inhibit corticosteroid metabolism should be taken into account when assessing systemic risk. In children being treated for asthma, administration of medium or high dose inhaled corticosteroids may be associated with systemic side-effects such as growth failure, reduced bone mineral density and adrenal suppression, but this risk is likely to be outweighed by their ability to reduce the need for multiple courses of oral corticosteroids for acute asthma attacks.

Adrenal insufficiency

23-Mar-2023

Description of condition

Adrenal insufficiency occurs as a result of inadequate production of steroid hormones in the adrenal cortex of the adrenal glands. Glucocorticoids (e.g. cortisol) and mineralocorticoids (e.g. aldosterone) are the two main groups of steroid hormones produced by the adrenal cortex; their production is primarily regulated by the hypothalamic-pituitary-adrenal (HPA) axis and renin-angiotensin system, respectively. These hormones affect a number of body systems such as those involved in metabolic activity, water and electrolyte balance, and the body's response to stress. Symptoms of adrenal insufficiency can be mild, non-specific, and may include fatigue, gastrointestinal upset, anorexia, weight loss, musculoskeletal symptoms, salt cravings, and dizziness or syncope due to hypotension.

Adrenal insufficiency is classified as either primary, secondary, or tertiary, and results from disorders that affect the adrenal cortex (e.g. Addison's disease, congenital adrenal hyperplasia), the anterior pituitary gland (e.g. pituitary tumour or subarachnoid haemorrhage), or the hypothalamus (e.g. HPA axis suppression), respectively.

Some drugs can also cause adrenal insufficiency, with the systemic use of glucocorticoids being the most common cause due to suppression of the HPA axis. If glucocorticoids are stopped or decreased too quickly after prolonged use, endogenous glucocorticoid production may not be sufficient to meet the body's needs. Some patients on glucocorticoid therapy (oral, inhaled, topical, intranasal, and intra-articular) are at particular risk of adrenal insufficiency (with risk likely to be influenced by factors such as the child's age and weight, the drug, dose, route of administration and duration of use).

Adrenal insufficiency can lead to adrenal crisis (acute adrenal insufficiency) if not identified and treated. Adrenal crisis can also occur in patients at risk of adrenal insufficiency when glucocorticoid levels are insufficient, such as when exogenous glucocorticoids have been omitted, delayed, or given at inadequate doses. This may occur particularly during times of increased need (e.g. surgery, infection, or trauma) as patients are unable to mount a stress response by increasing endogenous glucocorticoid production. Life-threatening symptoms such as severe dehydration, hypotension, hypovolaemic shock, altered consciousness, seizures, stroke, or cardiac arrest may develop; if left untreated, adrenal crisis may lead to death or permanent disability.

Steroid Cards

A patient-held Steroid Treatment Card and an Adrenal Insufficiency Card are available; children with adrenal insufficiency and steroid dependence who are at risk of adrenal crisis should have an Adrenal Insufficiency card. For further information, see *Important safety information* and *Patient and carer advice* in drug monographs.

Aims of treatment

Treatment aims to reduce symptoms, reduce the risk of complications such as adrenal crisis, and to improve overall quality of life.

Management of adrenal insufficiency

Recommendations on the management of adrenal insufficiency are from the *Emergency and peri-operative management of adrenal insufficiency in children and young people: BSPED consensus guidelines. British Society for Paediatric Endocrinology and Diabetes (BSPED) (November 2022).*

If adrenal crisis (acute adrenal insufficiency) is suspected, prompt treatment should be given without delay. For further information, see *Adrenal Crisis*.

Adrenal insufficiency is treated by physiological glucocorticoid replacement with hydrocortisone p. 544 (most similar to cortisol). Children with primary adrenal insufficiency usually also require mineralocorticoid replacement with fludrocortisone acetate p. 544 due to aldosterone deficiency.

Glucocorticoid replacement during stress

Children with adrenal insufficiency and those considered to be at risk of adrenal insufficiency (and their parents or carers) should be educated on the importance of 'stress' glucocorticoid doses (increased doses) for the prevention of adrenal crisis during times of stress (e.g. surgical or invasive procedures), in order to maintain cortisol levels as close to the physiological concentration as possible. Children with adrenal insufficiency who do not usually require maintenance glucocorticoids should still be advised of the likely need for glucocorticoid replacement during times of stress.

In children with adrenal insufficiency and intercurrent illness, 'sick day rules' should be followed. Children on long-acting hydrocortisone preparations should switch to short-acting, more rapidly absorbed preparations during an intercurrent illness. For severe intercurrent illness (e.g. persistent vomiting from gastrointestinal viral illnesses), intramuscular or intravenous hydrocortisone should be given. Children with adrenal insufficiency are at higher risk of glucocorticoid deficiency if they are vomiting or have diarrhoea. Children with established adrenal insufficiency, and their family/carers, should be provided with a hydrocortisone emergency injection kit, be trained in the administration of intramuscular hydrocortisone, and advised to go to hospital if vomiting or diarrhoeal illness persist. For children who are usually on fludrocortisone, high-dose hydrocortisone provides sufficient mineralocorticoid cover. Oral fludrocortisone should be re-commenced when tolerated.

For information on glucocorticoid cover during stress and sick day rules for children on exogenous steroids who are at an increased risk of adrenal insufficiency, see the British Society for Paediatric Endocrinology and Diabetes guidance: **Emergency and peri-operative management of adrenal insufficiency in children and young people: BSPED consensus guidelines** (see *Useful resources*).

Management of adrenal crisis

Recommendations on the management of adrenal crisis are from the *Emergency and peri-operative management of adrenal insufficiency in children and young people: BSPED consensus guidelines. British Society for Paediatric Endocrinology and Diabetes (BSPED) (November 2022).*

Adrenal crisis (acute adrenal insufficiency) is a medical emergency. All children who are considered to be at risk of, or suspected of having adrenal crisis should be treated immediately, especially pregnant females; investigations can be initiated once the patient is clinically stable.

Treatment involves prompt glucocorticoid replacement with parenteral hydrocortisone and rehydration using a crystalloid fluid (e.g. sodium chloride 0.9%). A safe approach is to administer emergency hydrocortisone in any unwell child with adrenal insufficiency. For children usually on fludrocortisone, high-dose hydrocortisone provides sufficient mineralocorticoid cover.

Particular care is required in children with diabetes insipidus and adrenal insufficiency related to hypothalamic-pituitary disease who are treated with desmopressin, as they are at risk of uncontrolled diabetes insipidus if doses of desmopressin are omitted, or hyponatraemia if excess fluid is given.

All children should be referred to an endocrinologist for advice on ongoing treatment and education around 'sick day rules' prior to hospital discharge.

Congenital adrenal hyperplasia

In *congenital adrenal hyperplasia*, the pituitary gland increases production of corticotropin to compensate for reduced formation of cortisol; this results in excessive adrenal androgen production. Treatment is aimed at suppressing corticotropin using hydrocortisone p. 544. Careful and continual dose titration is required to avoid growth retardation and toxicity; for this reason potent, synthetic glucocorticoids such as dexamethasone are usually reserved for use in adolescents. The dose is adjusted according to clinical response and measurement of adrenal androgens and 17-hydroxyprogesterone. Salt-losing forms of congenital adrenal hyperplasia (where there is a lack of aldosterone production) also require mineralocorticoid replacement and salt supplementation (particularly in early life). The dose of mineralocorticoid is adjusted according to electrolyte concentration and plasma-renin activity.

Useful Resources

Emergency and peri-operative management of adrenal insufficiency in children and young people: BSPED consensus guidelines. British Society for Paediatric Endocrinology and Diabetes (BSPED). November 2022. www.bsped.org.uk/clinical-resources/bsped-adrenal-insufficiency-consensus-guidelines/

Glucocorticoid therapy

Glucocorticoid and mineralocorticoid activity

In comparing the relative potencies of corticosteroids in terms of their anti-inflammatory (glucocorticoid) effects it should be borne in mind that high glucocorticoid activity in itself is of no advantage unless it is accompanied by relatively low mineralocorticoid activity (see Disadvantages of Corticosteroids). The mineralocorticoid activity of fludrocortisone acetate p. 544 is so high that its anti-inflammatory activity is of no clinical relevance.

Equivalent anti-inflammatory doses of corticosteroids

This table takes no account of mineralocorticoid effects, nor does it take account of variations in duration of action

Prednisolone 1 mg	≡	Betamethasone 150 micrograms
	≡	Deflazacort 1.2 mg
	≡	Dexamethasone 150 micrograms
	≡	Hydrocortisone 4 mg
	≡	Methylprednisolone 800 micrograms
	≡	Triamcinolone 800 micrograms

The relatively high mineralocorticoid activity of hydrocortisone p. 544, and the resulting fluid retention, makes it unsuitable for disease suppression on a long-term basis. However, hydrocortisone can be used for adrenal replacement therapy. Hydrocortisone is used on a short-term basis by intravenous injection for the emergency management of some conditions. The relatively moderate anti-inflammatory potency of hydrocortisone also makes it a useful topical corticosteroid for the management of inflammatory skin conditions because side-effects (both topical and systemic) are less marked.

Prednisolone p. 548 has predominantly glucocorticoid activity and is the corticosteroid most commonly used by mouth for long-term disease suppression.

Betamethasone p. 542 and dexamethasone p. 543 have very high glucocorticoid activity in conjunction with insignificant mineralocorticoid activity. This makes them particularly suitable for high-dose therapy in conditions where fluid retention would be a disadvantage.

Betamethasone and dexamethasone also have a long duration of action and this, coupled with their lack of mineralocorticoid action makes them particularly suitable for conditions which require suppression of corticotropin (corticotrophin) secretion.

Some esters of betamethasone and of beclometasone dipropionate (beclomethasone) exert a considerably more marked topical effect (e.g. on the skin or the lungs) than when given by mouth; use is made of this to obtain topical effects whilst minimising systemic side-effects (e.g. for skin applications and asthma inhalations).

Deflazacort p. 542 has a high glucocorticoid activity; it is derived from prednisolone.

Corticosteroids (systemic)

IMPORTANT SAFETY INFORMATION

MHRA/CHM ADVICE: CORTICOSTEROIDS: RARE RISK OF CENTRAL SEROUS CHORIORETINOPATHY WITH LOCAL AS WELL AS SYSTEMIC ADMINISTRATION (AUGUST 2017)

Central serous chorioretinopathy is a retinal disorder that has been linked to the systemic use of corticosteroids. Recently, it has also been reported after local administration of corticosteroids via inhaled and intranasal, epidural, intra-articular, topical dermal, and periocular routes. The MHRA recommends that patients should be advised to report any blurred vision or other visual disturbances with corticosteroid treatment given by any route; consider referral to an ophthalmologist for evaluation of possible causes if a patient presents with vision problems.

ADRENAL INSUFFICIENCY CARD (APRIL 2023)

The British Society for Paediatric Endocrinology and Diabetes (BSPED) has developed an Adrenal Insufficiency Card which should be issued to children with adrenal insufficiency and steroid dependence. The card includes a management summary for the emergency treatment of adrenal crisis and sick day dosing, and can be issued by any healthcare professional managing such patients. The BSPED Adrenal Insufficiency Card is available at: www.bsped.org.uk/adrenal-insufficiency.

- **CONTRA-INDICATIONS** Avoid injections containing benzyl alcohol in neonates · avoid live virus vaccines in those receiving immunosuppressive doses (serum antibody response diminished) · systemic infection (unless specific therapy given)

CONTRA-INDICATIONS, FURTHER INFORMATION

- With intra-articular use or intradermal use or intralesional use For further information on contra-indications associated with intra-articular, intradermal and intralesional preparations, consult product literature.

- **CAUTIONS** Congestive heart failure · diabetes mellitus (including a family history of) · diverticular disease (increased risk of diverticular perforation) · diverticulitis · epilepsy · glaucoma (including a family history of or susceptibility to) · history of steroid myopathy · history of tuberculosis or X-ray changes (frequent monitoring required) · hypertension · hypothyroidism · infection (particularly untreated) · long-term use · myasthenia gravis · ocular herpes simplex (risk of corneal perforation) · osteoporosis · peptic ulcer · psychiatric reactions · recent intestinal anastomoses · recent myocardial infarction (rupture reported) · severe affective disorders (particularly if history of steroid-induced psychosis) · thromboembolic disorders · ulcerative colitis

CAUTIONS, FURTHER INFORMATION

- **With intra-articular use or intradermal use or intralesional use** For further information on cautions associated with intra-articular, intradermal, and intralesional preparations, consult product literature.

- **SIDE-EFFECTS**
- **Common or very common** Anxiety · appetite increased · behaviour abnormal · cataract subcapsular · cognitive impairment · Cushing's syndrome · electrolyte imbalance · fluid retention · gastrointestinal discomfort · growth retardation · headache · healing impaired · hirsutism · hypertension · increased risk of infection · menstrual cycle irregularities · mood altered · nausea · osteoporosis · peptic ulcer · psychotic disorder · skin reactions · sleep disorder · vision blurred · weight increased
- **Uncommon** Adrenal suppression · alkalosis hypokalaemic · bone fractures · diabetic control impaired · glaucoma · haemorrhage · hyperhidrosis · myopathy · osteonecrosis · pancreatitis · papilloedema · seizure · thromboembolism · tuberculosis reactivation · vertigo
- **Rare or very rare** Tendon rupture
- **Frequency not known** Chorioretinopathy · eye disorders · intracranial pressure increased with papilloedema (usually after withdrawal) · leucocytosis

SIDE-EFFECTS, FURTHER INFORMATION **Adrenal suppression** During prolonged therapy with corticosteroids, particularly with systemic use, adrenal atrophy develops and can persist for years after stopping. Abrupt withdrawal after a prolonged period can lead to acute adrenal insufficiency, hypotension, or death. To compensate for a diminished adrenocortical response caused by prolonged corticosteroid treatment, any significant intercurrent illness, trauma, or surgical procedure requires a temporary increase in corticosteroid dose, or if already stopped, a temporary reintroduction of corticosteroid treatment. For vamorolone, there is no evidence on the effects of increasing the dose, and temporary supplementation with hydrocortisone is advised.

Infections Prolonged courses of corticosteroids increase susceptibility to infections and severity of infections; clinical presentation of infections may also be atypical. Serious infections e.g. septicaemia and tuberculosis may reach an advanced stage before being recognised, and amoebiasis or strongyloidiasis may be activated or exacerbated (exclude before initiating a corticosteroid in those at risk or with suggestive symptoms). Fungal or viral ocular infections may also be exacerbated.

Chickenpox Unless they have had chickenpox, patients receiving oral or parenteral corticosteroids for purposes other than replacement should be regarded as being at risk of severe chickenpox. Manifestations of fulminant illness include pneumonia, hepatitis and disseminated intravascular coagulation; rash is not necessarily a prominent feature. Passive immunisation with varicella–zoster immunoglobulin is needed for exposed non–immune patients receiving systemic corticosteroids or for those who have used them within the previous 3 months. Confirmed chickenpox warrants specialist care and urgent treatment. Corticosteroids should not be stopped and dosage may need to be increased.

Measles Patients taking corticosteroids should be advised to take particular care to avoid exposure to measles and to seek immediate medical advice if exposure occurs. Prophylaxis with intramuscular normal immunoglobulin may be needed.

Psychiatric reactions Systemic corticosteroids, particularly in high doses, are linked to psychiatric reactions including euphoria, insomnia, irritability, mood lability, suicidal thoughts, psychotic reactions, and behavioural disturbances. These reactions frequently subside on reducing the dose or discontinuing the corticosteroid but they may also require specific management. Patients should be advised to seek medical advice if psychiatric symptoms (especially depression and suicidal thoughts) occur and they should also be alert to the rare possibility of such reactions during withdrawal of corticosteroid treatment. Systemic corticosteroids should be prescribed with care in those predisposed to psychiatric reactions, including those who have previously suffered corticosteroid–induced psychosis, or who have a personal or family history of psychiatric disorders.

- **PREGNANCY** The benefit of treatment with corticosteroids during pregnancy outweighs the risk. Corticosteroid cover is required during labour. Following a review of the data on the safety of systemic corticosteroids used in pregnancy and breast-feeding the CSM (May 1998) concluded that corticosteroids vary in their ability to cross the placenta but there is no convincing evidence that systemic corticosteroids increase the incidence of congenital abnormalities such as cleft palate or lip. When administration is prolonged or repeated during pregnancy, systemic corticosteroids increase the risk of intra-uterine growth restriction; there is no evidence of intra-uterine growth restriction following short-term treatment (e.g. prophylactic treatment for neonatal respiratory distress syndrome). Any adrenal suppression in the neonate following prenatal exposure usually resolves spontaneously after birth and is rarely clinically important.
Monitoring Pregnant women with pre-eclampsia or fluid retention should be monitored closely when given systemic corticosteroids.
- **BREAST FEEDING** The benefit of treatment with corticosteroids during breast-feeding outweighs the risk.
- **HEPATIC IMPAIRMENT** In general, manufacturers advise caution (risk of increased exposure).
- **RENAL IMPAIRMENT** In general, manufacturers advise caution.
- **MONITORING REQUIREMENTS**
- EvGr The following baseline measurements should be taken before starting treatment and at regular intervals during the course of long-term treatment:
  - blood pressure
  - body weight
  - BMI
  - height (children and adolescents)
  - HbA_{1c}
  - triglycerides
  - potassium
  - eye examination (for glaucoma and cataract)
- In addition monitor the following during treatment, depending on clinical judgement:
  - osteoporosis risk
  - falls risk assessment
  - adrenal suppression (A)

- **EFFECT ON LABORATORY TESTS** May suppress skin test reactions.
- **TREATMENT CESSATION** The magnitude and speed of dose reduction in corticosteroid withdrawal should be determined on a case-by-case basis, taking into consideration the underlying condition that is being treated, and individual patient factors such as the likelihood of relapse and the duration of corticosteroid treatment. *Gradual* withdrawal of systemic corticosteroids should be considered in those whose disease is unlikely to relapse and have:
  - received more than 40 mg prednisolone (or equivalent) daily for more than 1 week *or* 2 mg/kg daily for 1 week *or* 1 mg/kg daily for 1 month;
  - been given repeat doses in the evening;
  - received more than 3 weeks' treatment;
  - recently received repeated courses (particularly if taken for longer than 3 weeks);
  - taken a short course within 1 year of stopping long-term therapy;
  - other possible causes of adrenal suppression.

  Systemic corticosteroids may be stopped abruptly in those whose disease is unlikely to relapse *and* who have received treatment for 3 weeks or less *and* who are not included in the patient groups described above.

  During corticosteroid withdrawal the dose may be reduced rapidly down to physiological doses (equivalent to prednisolone 2–2.5 mg/m^2 daily) and then reduced more slowly. Assessment of the disease may be needed during withdrawal to ensure that relapse does not occur.
- **PATIENT AND CARER ADVICE**

  Advice for patients A patient information leaflet should be supplied to every patient when a systemic corticosteroid is prescribed. Patients should especially be advised of potential side-effects including adrenal suppression, immunosuppression, and psychiatric reactions (for further details, see *Side-effects, further information*).

  Steroid Treatment Card Steroid Treatment Cards should be issued where appropriate to support communication of the risks associated with treatment and to record details of the prescriber, drug, dosage, and duration of treatment. Steroid treatment cards are available for purchase from the NHS Print online ordering portal cmswebshop.corp.xerox.com/NHS/Login.aspx.

  GP practices can obtain supplies through Primary Care Support England. NHS Trusts can order supplies via the online ordering portal.

  In **Scotland**, steroid treatment cards can be obtained from APS Group Scotland by emailing stockorders.dppas@apsgroup.co.uk or by fax on 0131 629 9967.

  Adrenal Insufficiency Card The British Society for Paediatric Endocrinology and Diabetes (BSPED) has developed an Adrenal Insufficiency Card which should be issued to children with adrenal insufficiency and steroid dependence. The card includes a management summary for the emergency treatment of adrenal crisis and sick day dosing, and can be issued by any healthcare professional managing such patients.

  The BSPED Adrenal Insufficiency Card is available at: www.bsped.org.uk/adrenal-insufficiency.

  In **Wales** see: www.weds-wales.co.uk/steroid-therapy/.

F 540

Betamethasone

26-Jul-2025

- **DRUG ACTION** Betamethasone has very high glucocorticoid activity and insignificant mineralocorticoid activity.

- **INDICATIONS AND DOSE**

Suppression of inflammatory and allergic disorders | Congenital adrenal hyperplasia

▶ BY SLOW INTRAVENOUS INJECTION, OR BY INTRAVENOUS INFUSION

- Child 1–11 months: 1 mg, dose may be repeated up to 4 times in 24 hours according to response
- Child 1–5 years: 2 mg, dose may be repeated up to 4 times in 24 hours according to response
- Child 6–11 years: 4 mg, dose may be repeated up to 4 times in 24 hours according to response
- Child 12–17 years: 4–20 mg, dose may be repeated up to 4 times in 24 hours according to response

- **INTERACTIONS** → Appendix 1: corticosteroids
- **SIDE-EFFECTS** Hiccups · malaise · myocardial rupture (following recent myocardial infarction) · oedema · Stevens-Johnson syndrome
- **PREGNANCY** Readily crosses the placenta. Transient effect on fetal movements and heart rate.
- **DIRECTIONS FOR ADMINISTRATION** For *intravenous infusion*, dilute with Glucose 5% or Sodium Chloride 0.9%.

- **MEDICINAL FORMS** There can be variation in the licensing of different medicines containing the same drug.

Solution for injection

CAUTIONARY AND ADVISORY LABELS 10

▶ Betamethasone (Non-proprietary)

Betamethasone (as Betamethasone sodium phosphate) 4 mg per 1 ml Betamethasone 4mg/1ml solution for injection ampoules | 5 ampoule PoM £112.36–£126.54

F 540

Deflazacort

26-Jul-2025

- **DRUG ACTION** Deflazacort is derived from prednisolone; it has predominantly glucocorticoid activity.

- **INDICATIONS AND DOSE**

Inflammatory and allergic disorders

▶ BY MOUTH

- Child 1 month–11 years: 0.25–1.5 mg/kg once daily or on alternate days; increased if necessary up to 2.4 mg/kg daily (max. per dose 120 mg), in emergency situations
- Child 12–17 years: 3–18 mg once daily or on alternate days; increased if necessary up to 2.4 mg/kg daily (max. per dose 120 mg), in emergency situations

Nephrotic syndrome

▶ BY MOUTH

- Child: Initially 1.5 mg/kg once daily (max. per dose 120 mg), reduced to the lowest effective dose for maintenance

- **INTERACTIONS** → Appendix 1: corticosteroids
- **SIDE-EFFECTS**
  - **Uncommon** Carbohydrate intolerance · depressed mood · oedema
  - **Frequency not known** Confusion · delusions · epilepsy exacerbated · hallucination · heart failure · hypertrophic cardiomyopathy (in preterm infants) · idiopathic intracranial hypertension · memory loss · peptic ulcer perforation · schizophrenia exacerbated · severe cutaneous adverse reactions (SCARs) · suicidal thoughts · telangiectasia · tendinitis · tumour lysis syndrome
- **HEPATIC IMPAIRMENT**

  Dose adjustments Manufacturer advises adjust to the minimum effective dose.

● **MEDICINAL FORMS** There can be variation in the licensing of different medicines containing the same drug. Forms available from special-order manufacturers include: oral tablet

Oral tablet

CAUTIONARY AND ADVISORY LABELS 5, 10

▸ **Calcort** (Neon Healthcare Ltd)

Deflazacort 6 mg Calcort 6mg tablets | 60 tablet PoM £15.82 DT = £15.82

F 540

Dexamethasone

26-Jul-2025

● **DRUG ACTION** Dexamethasone has very high glucocorticoid activity and insignificant mineralocorticoid activity.

● **INDICATIONS AND DOSE**

Suppression of inflammatory and allergic disorders

▶ BY MOUTH

▸ Child: 10–100 micrograms/kg daily in 1–2 divided doses, adjusted according to response; up to 300 micrograms/kg daily may be required in emergency situations

▶ BY INTRAMUSCULAR INJECTION, OR BY SLOW INTRAVENOUS INJECTION, OR BY INTRAVENOUS INFUSION

▸ Child 1 month–11 years: 83–333 micrograms/kg daily in 1–2 divided doses; maximum 20 mg per day

▸ Child 12–17 years: Initially 0.4–20 mg daily

Congenital adrenal hyperplasia (under expert supervision)

▶ BY MOUTH

▸ Child 16–17 years: 300–500 micrograms once daily

Mild croup

▶ BY MOUTH

▸ Child: 150 micrograms/kg for 1 dose

Severe croup (or mild croup that might cause complications)

▶ INITIALLY BY MOUTH

▸ Child: Initially 150 micrograms/kg for 1 dose, to be given before transfer to hospital, then (by mouth or by intravenous injection) 150 micrograms/kg for 1 dose, then (by mouth or by intravenous injection) 150 micrograms/kg for 1 dose, to be given 12 hours after previous dose if required

Adjunctive treatment of suspected bacterial meningitis

▶ BY INTRAVENOUS INJECTION

▸ Child 3 months–15 years: 150 micrograms/kg every 6 hours (max. per dose 10 mg), to be started before or up to 12 hours after the first dose of antibacterial—seek specialist advice if more than 12 hours have elapsed after starting antibacterials, continued for 4 days in patients with meningitis caused by *Streptococcus pneumoniae* (pneumococcus) or *Haemophilus influenzae* type b—discontinue treatment if another cause is suspected or confirmed

▸ Child 16–17 years: 10 mg every 6 hours, to be started before or up to 12 hours after the first dose of antibacterial—seek specialist advice if more than 12 hours have elapsed after starting antibacterials, continued for 4 days in patients with meningitis caused by *Streptococcus pneumoniae* (pneumococcus) or *Haemophilus influenzae* type b—discontinue treatment if another cause is suspected or confirmed

Life-threatening cerebral oedema

▶ BY INTRAVENOUS INJECTION

▸ Child (body-weight up to 35 kg): Initially 16.6 mg for 1 dose, then 3.3 mg every 3 hours for 3 days, then 3.3 mg every 6 hours for 1 day, then 1.7 mg every 6 hours for 4 days, dose then reduced in steps of 0.83 mg per day, continue dose reduction to discontinue over the following 7–10 days or change to oral dexamethasone maintenance if required

▸ Child (body-weight 35 kg and above): Initially 20.8 mg for 1 dose, then 3.3 mg every 2 hours for 3 days, then 3.3 mg every 4 hours for 1 day, then 3.3 mg every 6 hours for 4 days, dose then reduced in steps of 1.7 mg per day, continue dose reduction to discontinue over the following 7–10 days or change to oral dexamethasone maintenance if required

COVID-19 requiring supplemental oxygen

▶ BY MOUTH, OR BY NASOGASTRIC TUBE, OR BY INTRAVENOUS INJECTION

▸ Child: 150 micrograms/kg once daily (max. per dose 6 mg) for 10 days, or until the day of discharge if this is sooner

DOSE EQUIVALENCE AND CONVERSION

▸ With intramuscular use or intravenous use or oral use or when used by local infiltration

▸ Doses expressed as dexamethasone base. Dexamethasone base 3.3 mg is equivalent to dexamethasone phosphate 4 mg. Dexamethasone base 3.3 mg is equivalent to dexamethasone sodium phosphate 4.3 mg.

● **UNLICENSED USE** EvGr Dexamethasone is used for the treatment of suspected bacterial meningitis, ⟨A⟩ but is not licensed for this indication.

NICE and the Royal College of Paediatrics and Child Health (RCPCH) advise dexamethasone is used for the treatment of COVID-19 in children, but it is not licensed in children aged under 12 years.

● **INTERACTIONS** → Appendix 1: corticosteroids

● **SIDE-EFFECTS**

▸ With oral use Heart failure · hiccups · hyperglycaemia · hypotension · malaise · myocardial rupture (following recent myocardial infarction) · protein catabolism · telangiectasia

▸ With parenteral use Hypotension · perineal irritation (may occur following the intravenous injection of large doses of the phosphate ester) · telangiectasia

● **PREGNANCY** Dexamethasone readily crosses the placenta.

● **DIRECTIONS FOR ADMINISTRATION** For administration *by mouth* tablets may be dispersed in water or injection solution given by mouth.

For *intravenous infusion* dilute with Glucose 5% or Sodium Chloride 0.9%; give over 15–20 minutes.

● **PRESCRIBING AND DISPENSING INFORMATION**

▸ With systemic use Dexamethasone 3.8 mg/mL Injection has replaced dexamethasone 4 mg/mL Injection.

▸ When used for COVID-19 requiring supplemental oxygen Royal College of Paediatrics and Child Health (RCPCH) advises a specialist should be consulted when considering use in children under 5 years.

● **PATIENT AND CARER ADVICE**

Medicines for Children leaflet: Dexamethasone for croup www.medicinesforchildren.org.uk/medicines/dexamethasone-for-croup/

● **MEDICINAL FORMS** There can be variation in the licensing of different medicines containing the same drug. Forms available from special-order manufacturers include: oral capsule, oral suspension, oral solution

Oral tablet

CAUTIONARY AND ADVISORY LABELS 10, 21

▸ **Dexamethasone (Non-proprietary)**

Dexamethasone 500 microgram Dexamethasone 500microgram tablets | 28 tablet PoM £54.08 DT = £2.07 | 30 tablet PoM £1.82-£77.78

Dexamethasone 1 mg Dexamethasone 1mg tablets | 30 tablet PoM £4.97-£7.00 DT = £4.97

Dexamethasone 2 mg Dexamethasone 2mg tablets | 28 tablet PoM £1.64-£24.00 | 50 tablet PoM £42.85 DT = £2.99 | 100 tablet PoM £5.84-£8.50

Dexamethasone 4 mg Dexamethasone 4mg tablets | 30 tablet PoM £25.25 | 50 tablet PoM £120.00 DT = £36.15 | 100 tablet PoM £84.16

Soluble tablet

CAUTIONARY AND ADVISORY LABELS 10, 13, 21
ELECTROLYTES: May contain Sodium

▸ Dexamethasone (Non-proprietary)

Dexamethasone (as Dexamethasone sodium phosphate) 2 mg Dexamethasone 2mg soluble tablets sugar free | 50 tablet PoM £29.99–£44.80 DT = £48.86 SF

Dexamethasone (as Dexamethasone sodium phosphate) 4 mg Dexamethasone 4mg soluble tablets sugar free | 50 tablet PoM £60.00 DT = £60.00 SF

Dexamethasone (as Dexamethasone sodium phosphate) 8 mg Dexamethasone 8mg soluble tablets sugar free | 50 tablet PoM £120.00 DT = £120.00 SF

Dexamethasone (as Dexamethasone sodium phosphate) 10 mg Dexamethasone 10mg soluble tablets sugar free | 10 tablet PoM £10.00 DT = £10.00 SF

Dexamethasone (as Dexamethasone sodium phosphate) 20 mg Dexamethasone 20mg soluble tablets sugar free | 10 tablet PoM £20.00 DT = £20.00 SF

Solution for injection

CAUTIONARY AND ADVISORY LABELS 10
EXCIPIENTS: May contain Disodium edetate, propylene glycol

▸ Dexamethasone (Non-proprietary)

Dexamethasone (as Dexamethasone sodium phosphate) 3.3 mg per 1 ml Dexamethasone (base) 6.6mg/2ml solution for injection ampoules | 10 ampoule PoM £24.00–£48.00
Dexamethasone (base) 6.6mg/2ml solution for injection vials | 5 vial PoM £24.00 DT = £24.00
Dexamethasone (base) 3.3mg/1ml solution for injection ampoules | 10 ampoule PoM £23.93–£28.79 DT = £9.92 (Hospital only) | 10 ampoule PoM £9.41–£26.80 DT = £9.92

Dexamethasone (as Dexamethasone sodium phosphate) 3.8 mg per 1 ml Dexamethasone (base) 3.8mg/1ml solution for injection vials | 10 vial PoM £19.99 DT = £19.99

Oral solution

CAUTIONARY AND ADVISORY LABELS 10, 21

▸ Dexamethasone (Non-proprietary)

Dexamethasone (as Dexamethasone sodium phosphate) 400 microgram per 1 ml Dexamethasone 2mg/5ml oral solution sugar free | 150 ml PoM £42.30 DT = £23.33 SF

Dexamethasone (as Dexamethasone sodium phosphate) 2 mg per 1 ml Dexamethasone 10mg/5ml oral solution sugar free | 150 ml PoM £161.49 DT = £161.49 SF

▸ Dexsol (Rosemont Pharmaceuticals Ltd)

Dexamethasone (as Dexamethasone sodium phosphate) 400 microgram per 1 ml Dexsol 2mg/5ml oral solution | 75 ml PoM £21.15 SF | 150 ml PoM £42.30 DT = £23.33 SF

F 540

Fludrocortisone acetate

26-Jul-2025

● **DRUG ACTION** Fludrocortisone has very high mineralocorticoid activity and insignificant glucocorticoid activity.

● **INDICATIONS AND DOSE**

Primary adrenal insufficiency [if mineralocorticoid replacement needed alongside glucocorticoid replacement] | Congenital adrenal hyperplasia [if mineralocorticoid replacement needed alongside glucocorticoid replacement]

▶ BY MOUTH

▸ Neonate: Initially 50–200 micrograms once daily, adjust dose according to response, higher doses may be required, dose adjustment may be required if salt supplements are given.

▸ Child 1–11 months: Initially 50–200 micrograms once daily, adjust dose according to response, higher doses may be required, dose adjustment may be required if salt supplements are given

▸ Child 1–15 years: Initially 50–300 micrograms once daily, adjust dose according to response, higher doses may be required, dose adjustment may be required if salt supplements are given

▸ Child 16–17 years: Initially 50 micrograms once daily, increased if necessary up to 300 micrograms once daily, adjust dose according to response, consider a higher daily dose for physically active people

● **UNLICENSED USE** EvGr Fludrocortisone acetate is used in the doses provided for the treatment of primary adrenal insufficiency, and congenital adrenal hyperplasia (A), but these may differ from those licensed.

● **INTERACTIONS** → Appendix 1: corticosteroids

● **SIDE-EFFECTS**

▶ **Common or very common** Congestive heart failure · muscle weakness · oedema · swelling

▶ **Uncommon** Appetite decreased · cardiomegaly · delusions · diarrhoea · epilepsy · hallucination · illusion · loss of consciousness · syncope · taste altered

▶ **Frequency not known** Adrenocortical unresponsiveness · confusion · depression · diabetes mellitus exacerbated · drug dependence · fatigue · idiopathic intracranial hypertension · increased insulin requirement · insomnia · lupus-like rash · memory loss · neuritis · oesophagitis ulcerative · paraesthesia · pituitary unresponsiveness · posterior subcapsular cataract · psychiatric disorders · schizophrenia exacerbated · thrombophlebitis · vasculitis necrotising

● **PRESCRIBING AND DISPENSING INFORMATION** Oral solution (Aristo Pharma) is an oily liquid; it is not recommended for patients with swallowing difficulties due to risk if aspirated.

● **PATIENT AND CARER ADVICE**
Medicines for Children leaflet: Fludrocortisone for hormone replacement www.medicinesforchildren.org.uk/medicines/fludrocortisone-for-hormone-replacement/

● **MEDICINAL FORMS** There can be variation in the licensing of different medicines containing the same drug. Forms available from special-order manufacturers include: oral capsule, oral suspension

Oral tablet

CAUTIONARY AND ADVISORY LABELS 10

▸ Fludrocortisone acetate (Non-proprietary)

Fludrocortisone acetate 50 microgram Fludrocortisone 50microgram tablets | 30 tablet PoM £13.60–£24.48 DT = £13.60

Fludrocortisone acetate 100 microgram Fludrocortisone 100microgram tablets | 30 tablet PoM £17.10 DT = £2.80 | 100 tablet PoM £10.83–£17.73

Oral solution

CAUTIONARY AND ADVISORY LABELS 10

▸ Fludrocortisone acetate (Non-proprietary)

Fludrocortisone acetate 100 microgram per 1 ml Fludrocortisone 100micrograms/ml oral solution sugar free | 50 ml PoM £135.00–£236.74 DT = £135.00 SF

F 540

Hydrocortisone

26-Jul-2025

● **DRUG ACTION** Hydrocortisone has equal glucocorticoid and mineralocorticoid activity.

● **INDICATIONS AND DOSE**

Adrenal crisis [in patients with adrenal insufficiency who are steroid-dependent]

▶ INITIALLY BY INTRAMUSCULAR INJECTION, OR BY INTRAVENOUS INJECTION

▸ Child 16–17 years: Initially 100 mg for 1 dose, then (by continuous intravenous infusion) 200 mg/24 hours, dilute in Glucose 5%, alternatively (by intramuscular injection or by intravenous injection) 50 mg every 6 hours, dose increased to 100 mg every 6 hours in patients who are severely obese

Adrenal crisis in the community [in patients with adrenal insufficiency who are steroid-dependent]

▶ BY INTRAMUSCULAR INJECTION, OR BY INTRAVENOUS INJECTION

- Neonate: 25 mg for 1 dose, patients should be admitted to hospital after the first dose, steroid treatment must not be stopped.
- Child 1-11 months: 25 mg for 1 dose, patients should be admitted to hospital after the first dose, steroid treatment must not be stopped
- Child 1-5 years: 50 mg for 1 dose, patients should be admitted to hospital after the first dose, steroid treatment must not be stopped
- Child 6-15 years: 100 mg for 1 dose, patients should be admitted to hospital after the first dose, steroid treatment must not be stopped

Adrenal crisis in hospital when illness is severe [in patients with adrenal insufficiency who are steroid-dependent]

▶ BY INTRAVENOUS INJECTION, OR BY INTRAVENOUS INFUSION

- Neonate: 4 mg/kg every 4–6 hours.

▶ INITIALLY BY INTRAMUSCULAR INJECTION, OR BY INTRAVENOUS INJECTION

- Child 1-11 months: Initially 25 mg for 1 dose, alternatively (by intravenous injection or by intravenous infusion) initially 2 mg/kg for 1 dose, then (by intravenous injection or by intravenous infusion) 2 mg/kg every 4–6 hours
- Child 1-5 years: Initially 50 mg for 1 dose, alternatively (by intravenous injection or by intravenous infusion) initially 2 mg/kg for 1 dose (max. per dose 100 mg), then (by intravenous injection or by intravenous infusion) 2 mg/kg every 4–6 hours (max. per dose 100 mg)
- Child 6-15 years: Initially 100 mg for 1 dose, alternatively (by intravenous injection or by intravenous infusion) initially 2 mg/kg for 1 dose (max. per dose 100 mg), then (by intravenous injection or by intravenous infusion) 2 mg/kg every 4–6 hours (max. per dose 100 mg)

Adrenal crisis in hospital when stable and improving [in patients with adrenal insufficiency who are steroid-dependent]

▶ BY INTRAVENOUS INJECTION, OR BY INTRAVENOUS INFUSION

- Neonate: 2 mg/kg every 4–6 hours.
- Child 1 month-15 years: 1 mg/kg every 4–6 hours (max. per dose 50 mg)

Adrenal crisis in hospital when stable and tolerating drinks and diet [in patients with adrenal insufficiency who are steroid-dependent]

▶ BY MOUTH

- Neonate: 7.5 mg/m^2 4 times a day, restart fludrocortisone if indicated.
- Child 1 month-15 years: 7.5 mg/m^2 4 times a day, restart fludrocortisone if indicated

Congenital adrenal hyperplasia

▶ BY MOUTH USING IMMEDIATE-RELEASE MEDICINES

- Neonate: 9–15 mg/m^2 daily in 3 divided doses, a larger dose to be given in the morning and a smaller dose in the evening, to be adjusted according to response.
- Child: 9–15 mg/m^2 daily in 3 divided doses, a larger dose to be given in the morning and a smaller dose in the evening, to be adjusted according to response

Congenital adrenal hyperplasia [in patients who have not completed growth]

▶ BY MOUTH USING MODIFIED-RELEASE CAPSULES

- Child 12-17 years: 10–15 mg/m^2 daily in 2 divided doses, take morning dose 1 hour before food and the evening dose at least 2 hours after last meal, at initiation, give two-thirds to three-quarters of the dose in the evening, and the remainder in the morning; adjust dose thereafter based on response. A lower dose may be sufficient in patients with remaining endogenous cortisol production; maximum 25 mg per day

Congenital adrenal hyperplasia [in patients who have completed growth]

▶ BY MOUTH USING MODIFIED-RELEASE CAPSULES

- Child 12-17 years: 15–25 mg daily in 2 divided doses, take morning dose 1 hour before food and the evening dose at least 2 hours after last meal, at initiation, give two-thirds to three-quarters of the dose in the evening, and the remainder in the morning; adjust dose thereafter based on response. A lower dose may be sufficient in patients with remaining endogenous cortisol production

Adrenal hypoplasia | Addison's disease, chronic maintenance or replacement therapy

▶ BY MOUTH USING IMMEDIATE-RELEASE MEDICINES

- Neonate: 8–10 mg/m^2 daily in 3 divided doses, a larger dose to be given in the morning and a smaller dose in the evening, higher doses may be needed.
- Child: 8–10 mg/m^2 daily in 3 divided doses, a larger dose to be given in the morning and a smaller dose in the evening, higher doses may be needed

Inflammatory bowel disease—induction of remission

▶ BY INTRAVENOUS INJECTION

- Child 2-17 years: 2.5 mg/kg every 6 hours (max. per dose 100 mg)

▶ BY CONTINUOUS INTRAVENOUS INFUSION

- Child 2-17 years: 10 mg/kg/24 hours (max. per dose 400 mg/24 hours)

Acute hypersensitivity reactions | Angioedema

▶ BY INTRAMUSCULAR INJECTION, OR BY INTRAVENOUS INJECTION

- Child 1-5 months: Initially 25 mg 3 times a day, dose to be adjusted according to response
- Child 6 months-5 years: Initially 50 mg 3 times a day, dose to be adjusted according to response
- Child 6-11 years: Initially 100 mg 3 times a day, dose to be adjusted according to response
- Child 12-17 years: Initially 200 mg 3 times a day, dose to be adjusted according to response

Hypotension resistant to inotropic treatment and volume replacement [limited evidence]

▶ BY INTRAVENOUS INJECTION

- Neonate: Initially 2.5 mg/kg for 1 dose, then 2.5 mg/kg for 1 dose, to be given 4 hours after first dose if required, followed by 2.5 mg/kg every 6 hours for 48 hours or until blood pressure recovers, dose to then be reduced gradually over at least 48 hours.
- Child: 1 mg/kg every 6 hours (max. per dose 100 mg)

Severe acute asthma | Life-threatening acute asthma

▶ BY INTRAVENOUS INJECTION

- Child 1 month-1 year: 4 mg/kg every 6 hours (max. per dose 100 mg) until conversion to oral prednisolone is possible, dose given, preferably, as sodium succinate, alternatively 25 mg every 6 hours until conversion to oral prednisolone is possible, dose given, preferably, as sodium succinate
- Child 2-4 years: 4 mg/kg every 6 hours (max. per dose 100 mg) until conversion to oral

continued →

prednisolone is possible, dose given, preferably, as sodium succinate, alternatively 50 mg every 6 hours until conversion to oral prednisolone is possible, dose given, preferably, as sodium succinate

- Child 5–11 years: 4 mg/kg every 6 hours (max. per dose 100 mg) until conversion to oral prednisolone is possible, dose given, preferably, as sodium succinate, alternatively 100 mg every 6 hours until conversion to oral prednisolone is possible, dose given, preferably, as sodium succinate
- Child 12–17 years: 4 mg/kg every 6 hours (max. per dose 100 mg) until conversion to oral prednisolone is possible, dose given, preferably, as sodium succinate, alternatively 100 mg every 6 hours until conversion to oral prednisolone is possible, dose given, preferably, as sodium succinate

IMPORTANT SAFETY INFORMATION

MHRA/CHM ADVICE: HYDROCORTISONE MUCO-ADHESIVE BUCCAL TABLETS: SHOULD NOT BE USED OFF-LABEL FOR ADRENAL INSUFFICIENCY IN CHILDREN DUE TO SERIOUS RISKS (DECEMBER 2018)

The MHRA has received reports of off-label use of hydrocortisone muco-adhesive buccal tablets for adrenal insufficiency in children.

Healthcare professionals are advised that:

- hydrocortisone muco-adhesive buccal tablets are indicated only for local use in the mouth for aphthous ulceration and should not be used to treat adrenal insufficiency;
- substitution of licensed oral hydrocortisone formulations with muco-adhesive buccal tablets can result in insufficient cortisol absorption and, in stress situations, life-threatening adrenal crisis;
- only hydrocortisone products licensed for adrenal replacement therapy should be used.

MHRA/CHM ADVICE: *ALKINDI*® (HYDROCORTISONE GRANULES): RISK OF ACUTE ADRENAL INSUFFICIENCY IN CHILDREN WHEN SWITCHING FROM HYDROCORTISONE TABLET FORMULATIONS TO GRANULES (FEBRUARY 2021)

Adrenal crisis has been reported in an infant who was switched from hydrocortisone soluble tablets to hydrocortisone granules (*Alkindi*®). Acute adrenal insufficiency could also occur when switching from crushed hydrocortisone tablets to granules due to a potential risk of inaccurate dosing.

Healthcare professionals should advise parents or carers of children switching from hydrocortisone tablets to *Alkindi*® to carefully observe the child for symptoms of adrenal insufficiency during the first week. They should be counselled on what to do if symptoms of adrenal insufficiency develop, including the need to seek immediate medical advice and administer extra doses of *Alkindi*® if appropriate. A long-term increase in the daily dose of *Alkindi*® should be considered if additional doses are required during the first week after switching.

● **INTERACTIONS** → Appendix 1: corticosteroids

● **SIDE-EFFECTS**

- With oral use Dyslipidaemia · fatigue · hypotension · malaise · myocardial rupture (following recent myocardial infarction) · oedema
- With parenteral use Heart failure · hiccups · Kaposi's sarcoma · lipomatosis · malaise · myocardial rupture (following recent myocardial infarction)

● **DIRECTIONS FOR ADMINISTRATION**

- With intravenous use EvGr For *intravenous administration*, dilute with Glucose 5% or Sodium Chloride 0.9%. Ⓜ For *intermittent infusion* give over 20–30 minutes.
- With oral use EvGr For *Alkindi*®, capsules should be opened and granules either administered directly into the mouth and then followed immediately with a drink, or sprinkled onto a spoonful of soft food (such as yoghurt) and given immediately. Granules should not be chewed or added to liquid before administration due to the bitter taste, and they should not be given via an enteral tube as it may cause blockage. Ⓜ

● **PRESCRIBING AND DISPENSING INFORMATION**

- When used for Asthma For choice of therapy, see Asthma, acute p. 174 and Asthma, chronic p. 171.
- With oral use The RCPCH and NPPG recommend that, when a liquid special of hydrocortisone is required, the following strength is used: 5 mg/5 mL.

● **NATIONAL FUNDING/ACCESS DECISIONS**

For full details see funding body website

Scottish Medicines Consortium (SMC) decisions

- **Hydrocortisone (*Alkindi*®) for the replacement therapy of adrenal insufficiency in infants, children and adolescents (aged from birth to less than 18 years old) (October 2018)** SMC No. SMC2088 Recommended with restrictions
- **Hydrocortisone modified-release (*Efmody*®) for the treatment of congenital adrenal hyperplasia (CAH) in adolescents aged 12 years and over and adults (March 2022)** SMC No. SMC2414 Not recommended

All Wales Medicines Strategy Group (AWMSG) decisions

- **Hydrocortisone MR (*Efmody*®) for the treatment of congenital adrenal hyperplasia (CAH) in adolescents aged 12 years and over and adults (October 2022)** AWMSG No. 3017 Recommended with restrictions

● **LESS SUITABLE FOR PRESCRIBING**

- With intravenous use Hydrocortisone as the sodium phosphate is less suitable for prescribing as paraesthesia and pain (particularly in the perineal region) may follow intravenous injection.

● **EXCEPTIONS TO LEGAL CATEGORY**

- With intramuscular use or intravenous use Prescription only medicine restriction does not apply where administration is for saving life in emergency.

● **MEDICINAL FORMS** There can be variation in the licensing of different medicines containing the same drug. Forms available from special-order manufacturers include: oral capsule, oral suspension, oral solution

Oral tablet

CAUTIONARY AND ADVISORY LABELS 10, 21

- **Hydrocortisone (Non-proprietary)**
  - **Hydrocortisone 2.5 mg** Hydrocortisone 2.5mg tablets | 30 tablet PoM £39.53–£59.70 DT = £56.69
  - **Hydrocortisone 5 mg** Hydrocortisone 5mg tablets | 30 tablet PoM £38.12 DT = £18.36
  - **Hydrocortisone 10 mg** Hydrocortisone 10mg tablets | 30 tablet PoM £19.99 DT = £1.42
  - **Hydrocortisone 15 mg** Hydrocortisone 15mg tablets | 30 tablet PoM £33.51–£44.78 DT = £33.51
  - **Hydrocortisone 20 mg** Hydrocortisone 20mg tablets | 30 tablet PoM £4.60 DT = £3.32
- **Hydventia** (GlucoRx Ltd)
  - **Hydrocortisone 10 mg** Hydventia 10mg tablets | 30 tablet PoM £10.47 DT = £1.42
  - **Hydrocortisone 20 mg** Hydventia 20mg tablets | 30 tablet PoM £20.94 DT = £3.32
- **Sontirco** (Silicon Pharma Ltd)
  - **Hydrocortisone 10 mg** Sontirco 10mg tablets | 30 tablet PoM £1.45 DT = £1.42
  - **Hydrocortisone 20 mg** Sontirco 20mg tablets | 30 tablet PoM £3.45 DT = £3.32

Soluble tablet

CAUTIONARY AND ADVISORY LABELS 10, 13, 21

ELECTROLYTES: May contain Sodium

- **Hydrocortisone (Non-proprietary)**
  - **Hydrocortisone (as Hydrocortisone sodium phosphate) 10 mg** Hydrocortisone 10mg soluble tablets sugar free | 30 tablet PoM £37.50–£67.50 DT = £37.50 SF

Powder for solution for injection

▸ **Hydrocortisone (Non-proprietary)**
Hydrocortisone (as Hydrocortisone sodium succinate)
100 mg Hydrocortisone sodium succinate 100mg powder for solution for injection vials | 10 vial PoM £17.18 DT = £17.18

Powder and solvent for solution for injection

CAUTIONARY AND ADVISORY LABELS 10

▸ **Hydrocortisone (Non-proprietary)**
Hydrocortisone (as Hydrocortisone sodium succinate)
100 mg Solu-Cortef Act-O-Vial 100mg powder and solvent for solution for injection vials | 1 vial PoM ☒ DT = £2.61
Hydrocortisone sodium succinate 100mg powder and solvent for solution for injection vials | 1 vial PoM £2.61 DT = £2.61

Solution for injection

CAUTIONARY AND ADVISORY LABELS 10

▸ **Hydrocortisone (Non-proprietary)**
Hydrocortisone (as Hydrocortisone sodium phosphate) 100 mg per 1 ml Hydrocortisone sodium phosphate 100mg/1ml solution for injection ampoules | 5 ampoule PoM £10.60 DT = £10.60

Modified-release capsule

CAUTIONARY AND ADVISORY LABELS 10, 23, 25

▸ **Efmody** (Neurocrine UK Ltd)
Hydrocortisone 5 mg Efmody 5mg modified-release capsules | 50 capsule PoM £135.00 DT = £135.00
Hydrocortisone 10 mg Efmody 10mg modified-release capsules | 50 capsule PoM £275.00 DT = £275.00

Oral solution

▸ **Hydrocortisone (Non-proprietary)**
Hydrocortisone sodium phosphate 1 mg per 1 ml Hydrocortisone 5mg/5ml oral solution sugar free | 100 ml PoM £135.00 DT = £135.00 SF
Hydrocortisone sodium phosphate 2 mg per 1 ml Hydrocortisone 10mg/5ml oral solution sugar free | 100 ml PoM £270.00 DT = £270.00 SF

Oral granules

CAUTIONARY AND ADVISORY LABELS 10

▸ **Alkindi** (Neurocrine UK Ltd)
Hydrocortisone 500 microgram Alkindi 0.5mg granules in capsules for opening | 50 capsule PoM £33.75 DT = £33.75
Hydrocortisone 1 mg Alkindi 1mg granules in capsules for opening | 50 capsule PoM £67.50 DT = £67.50
Hydrocortisone 2 mg Alkindi 2mg granules in capsules for opening | 50 capsule PoM £135.00 DT = £135.00
Hydrocortisone 5 mg Alkindi 5mg granules in capsules for opening | 50 capsule PoM £337.50 DT = £337.50

F 540

Methylprednisolone

26-Jul-2025

● **DRUG ACTION** Methylprednisolone exerts predominantly glucocorticoid effects with minimal mineralcorticoid effects.

● **INDICATIONS AND DOSE**

Inflammatory and allergic disorders

▶ BY MOUTH, OR BY SLOW INTRAVENOUS INJECTION, OR BY INTRAVENOUS INFUSION
▸ Child: 0.5–1.7 mg/kg daily in 2–4 divided doses, divide doses depending on condition and response

Treatment of graft rejection reactions

▶ BY INTRAVENOUS INJECTION
▸ Child: 10–20 mg/kg once daily for 3 days, alternatively 400–600 mg/m² once daily (max. per dose 1 g) for 3 days

Severe erythema multiforme | Lupus nephritis | Systemic onset juvenile idiopathic arthritis

▶ BY INTRAVENOUS INJECTION
▸ Child: 10–30 mg/kg once daily or on alternate days (max. per dose 1 g) for up to 3 doses

DEPO-MEDRONE®

Suppression of inflammatory and allergic disorders

▶ BY DEEP INTRAMUSCULAR INJECTION
▸ Child: Seek specialist advice, to be injected into the gluteal muscle

IMPORTANT SAFETY INFORMATION

MHRA/CHM ADVICE: METHYLPREDNISOLONE INJECTABLE MEDICINE CONTAINING LACTOSE (*SOLU-MEDRONE®* 40 MG): DO NOT USE IN PATIENTS WITH COWS' MILK ALLERGY (OCTOBER 2017)

▸ With intramuscular use or intravenous use
An EU-wide review has concluded that *Solu-Medrone®* 40 mg may contain trace amounts of milk proteins and should not be used in patients with a known or suspected allergy to cows' milk. Serious allergic reactions, including bronchospasm and anaphylaxis, have been reported in patients allergic to cows' milk proteins. If a patient's symptoms worsen or new allergic symptoms occur, administration should be stopped and the patient treated accordingly.

MHRA/CHM ADVICE: *SOLU-MEDRONE®* 40 MG (METHYLPREDNISOLONE AS SODIUM SUCCINATE): CHANGE FROM LACTOSE-CONTAINING TO A LACTOSE-FREE FORMULATION—RISK OF SERIOUS ALLERGIC REACTIONS IF FORMULATIONS ARE CONFUSED (NOVEMBER 2020)

▸ With intramuscular use or intravenous use
Solu-Medrone® 40 mg powder and solvent for solution for injection has been reformulated to a lactose-free preparation in which the lactose is replaced with sucrose. There is a risk of serious allergic reactions if the new lactose-free preparation is confused with the lactose-containing preparation. Healthcare professionals should take extra care to ensure that patients who have been treated with the lactose-free preparation do not inadvertently receive the lactose-containing preparation. They should also be aware of the transition to the lactose-free preparation in their respective practices, and the precautionary measures taken by the manufacturer to differentiate between the packaging and labelling of the old (lactose-containing) and new (lactose-free) formulations to help avoid potential medication errors. Prescribers are advised to ensure patients who are allergic to cow's milk proteins and require the new lactose-free formulation are prescribed *Solu-Medrone®* injection 40 mg lactose free or methylprednisolone injection 40 mg lactose free.

● **CAUTIONS**

▸ With intravenous use Rapid intravenous administration of large doses associated with cardiovascular collapse
▸ With systemic use Systemic sclerosis (increased incidence of scleroderma renal crisis)

● **INTERACTIONS** → Appendix 1: corticosteroids

● **SIDE-EFFECTS**

▶ **Common or very common**
▸ With oral use Depressed mood
▶ **Frequency not known**
▸ With oral use Confusion · delusions · diarrhoea · dizziness · dyslipidaemia · fatigue · hallucination · hiccups · hypotension · insomnia · Kaposi's sarcoma · lipomatosis · malaise · myocardial rupture (following recent myocardial infarction) · oedema · schizophrenia · suicidal ideation · telangiectasia · withdrawal syndrome
▸ With parenteral use Confusion · delusions · depressed mood · diarrhoea · dizziness · dyslipidaemia · fatigue · hallucination · hiccups · hypotension · Kaposi's sarcoma · lipomatosis · malaise · oedema · schizophrenia · suicidal thoughts · telangiectasia · vomiting · withdrawal syndrome

● **MONITORING REQUIREMENTS** Manufacturer advises monitor blood pressure and renal function (s-creatinine) routinely in patients with systemic sclerosis—increased incidence of scleroderma renal crisis.

● **DIRECTIONS FOR ADMINISTRATION**

▸ With intravenous use Intravenous injection given over 30 minutes. For intravenous infusion, may be diluted with sodium chloride intravenous infusion 0.9% or 0.45%, or glucose intravenous infusion 5% or 10%.

● **PRESCRIBING AND DISPENSING INFORMATION**

▸ With intramuscular use or intravenous use For warnings about the different formulations of *Solu-Medrone*® 40 mg, see *Important safety information*.

● **MEDICINAL FORMS** There can be variation in the licensing of different medicines containing the same drug. Forms available from special-order manufacturers include: oral suspension

Oral tablet

CAUTIONARY AND ADVISORY LABELS 10, 21

▸ **Medrone** (Pfizer Ltd)

Methylprednisolone 2 mg Medrone 2mg tablets | 30 tablet PoM £3.88 DT = £3.88

Methylprednisolone 4 mg Medrone 4mg tablets | 30 tablet PoM £6.19 DT = £6.19

Methylprednisolone 16 mg Medrone 16mg tablets | 30 tablet PoM £17.17 DT = £17.17

Methylprednisolone 100 mg Medrone 100mg tablets | 20 tablet PoM £48.32 DT = £48.32

Powder and solvent for solution for injection

CAUTIONARY AND ADVISORY LABELS 10

▸ **Methylprednisolone (Non-proprietary)**

Methylprednisolone (as Methylprednisolone sodium succinate) 40 mg Methylprednisolone sodium succinate 40mg powder and solvent for solution for injection vials | 1 vial PoM £1.58 DT = £1.58

Methylprednisolone (as Methylprednisolone sodium succinate) 125 mg Methylprednisolone sodium succinate 125mg powder and solvent for solution for injection vials | 1 vial PoM £4.75

Methylprednisolone (as Methylprednisolone sodium succinate) 500 mg Methylprednisolone sodium succinate 500mg powder and solvent for solution for injection vials | 1 vial PoM £9.60

Methylprednisolone (as Methylprednisolone sodium succinate) 1 gram Methylprednisolone sodium succinate 1g powder and solvent for solution for injection vials | 1 vial PoM £17.30

▸ **Solu-Medrone** (Pfizer Ltd)

Methylprednisolone (as Methylprednisolone sodium succinate) 40 mg Solu-Medrone 40mg powder and solvent for solution for injection vials | 1 vial PoM £1.58 DT = £1.58

Methylprednisolone (as Methylprednisolone sodium succinate) 125 mg Solu-Medrone 125mg powder and solvent for solution for injection vials | 1 vial PoM £4.75

Methylprednisolone (as Methylprednisolone sodium succinate) 500 mg Solu-Medrone 500mg powder and solvent for solution for injection vials | 1 vial PoM £9.60

Methylprednisolone (as Methylprednisolone sodium succinate) 1 gram Solu-Medrone 1g powder and solvent for solution for injection vials | 1 vial PoM £17.30

Suspension for injection

CAUTIONARY AND ADVISORY LABELS 10

▸ **Depo-Medrone** (Pfizer Ltd)

Methylprednisolone acetate 40 mg per 1 ml Depo-Medrone 40mg/1ml suspension for injection vials | 1 vial PoM £3.44 DT = £3.44 | 10 vial PoM £34.04

Depo-Medrone 80mg/2ml suspension for injection vials | 1 vial PoM £6.18 DT = £6.18 | 10 vial PoM £61.39

Depo-Medrone 120mg/3ml suspension for injection vials | 1 vial PoM £8.96 DT = £8.96 | 10 vial PoM £88.81

F 540

Prednisolone

26-Jul-2025

● **DRUG ACTION** Prednisolone exerts predominantly glucocorticoid effects with minimal mineralocorticoid effects.

● **INDICATIONS AND DOSE**

Severe croup (before transfer to hospital) | Mild croup that might cause complications (before transfer to hospital)

▸ BY MOUTH

▸ Child: 1–2 mg/kg

Mild to moderate acute asthma (when oral corticosteroid taken for more than a few days) | Severe or life-threatening acute asthma (when oral corticosteroid taken for more than a few days)

▸ BY MOUTH

▸ Child 1 month–11 years: 2 mg/kg once daily (max. per dose 60 mg) for up to 3 days, longer if necessary

Mild to moderate acute asthma | Severe or life-threatening acute asthma

▸ BY MOUTH

▸ Child 1 month–11 years: 1–2 mg/kg once daily (max. per dose 40 mg) for up to 3 days, longer if necessary

▸ Child 12–17 years: 40–50 mg once daily for at least 5 days

Adrenal insufficiency [regular glucocorticoid replacement in patients who have completed growth]

▸ BY MOUTH

▸ Child 1–17 years: Initially 3–5 mg daily in 1–2 divided doses, dose to be adjusted according to response

Congenital adrenal hyperplasia [regular glucocorticoid replacement in patients who have completed growth]

▸ BY MOUTH

▸ Child 1–17 years: Initially 3–5 mg daily in 1–2 divided doses, dose to be adjusted according to response, consider higher doses with specialist advice if needed

Autoimmune inflammatory disorders (including juvenile idiopathic arthritis, connective tissue disorders and systemic lupus erythematosus)

▸ BY MOUTH

▸ Child: Initially 1–2 mg/kg once daily (max. per dose 60 mg), to be reduced after a few days if appropriate

Autoimmune hepatitis

▸ BY MOUTH

▸ Child: Initially 2 mg/kg once daily (max. per dose 40 mg), to be reduced to minimum effective dose

Infantile spasms (initial dose) [in combination with vigabatrin] (under expert supervision)

▸ BY MOUTH

▸ Child 1–23 months: Initially 10 mg 4 times a day for 14 days then gradually reduce dose, dose can be increased to 20 mg 3 times a day for 7 days if seizures not controlled after initial 7 days

Infantile spasms (dose reduction in patient taking 40 mg per day) [in combination with vigabatrin] (under expert supervision)

▸ BY MOUTH

▸ Child 1–23 months: 10 mg 3 times a day for 5 days, then reduced to 10 mg twice daily for 5 days, then reduced to 10 mg once daily for 5 days, then stop

Infantile spasms (dose reduction in patient taking 60 mg per day) [in combination with vigabatrin] (under expert supervision)

▸ BY MOUTH

▸ Child 1–23 months: 10 mg 4 times a day for 5 days, then reduced to 10 mg twice daily for 5 days, then reduced to 10 mg once daily for 5 days, then stop

Idiopathic thrombocytopenic purpura
▶ BY MOUTH
▸ Child 1–9 years: 1–2 mg/kg daily for maximum of 14 days, alternatively 4 mg/kg daily for a maximum of 4 days

Nephrotic syndrome
▶ BY MOUTH
▸ Child: Initially 60 mg/m^2 once daily for 4–6 weeks until proteinuria ceases, then reduced to 40 mg/m^2 once daily on alternate days for 4–6 weeks, then withdraw by reducing dose gradually; maximum 80 mg per day

Nephrotic syndrome (prevention of relapse)
▶ BY MOUTH
▸ Child: 0.5–1 mg/kg once daily or on alternate days for 3–6 months

Ulcerative colitis | Crohn's disease
▶ BY MOUTH
▸ Child 2–17 years: 2 mg/kg once daily (max. per dose 60 mg) until remission occurs, followed by reducing doses

Pneumocystis pneumonia in moderate to severe infections associated with HIV infection
▶ BY MOUTH
▸ Child: 2 mg/kg daily for 5 days, the dose is then reduced over the next 16 days and then stopped, corticosteroid treatment should ideally be started at the same time as the anti-pneumocystis therapy and certainly no later than 24–72 hours afterwards, the corticosteroid should be withdrawn before anti-pneumocystis treatment is complete; maximum 80 mg per day

Proctitis
▶ BY RECTUM USING RECTAL FOAM
▸ Child 12–17 years: 1 metered application 1–2 times a day for 2 weeks, continued for further 2 weeks if good response, to be inserted into the rectum, 1 metered application contains 20 mg prednisolone
▶ BY RECTUM USING SUPPOSITORIES
▸ Child 2–17 years: 5 mg twice daily, to be inserted into the rectum morning and night, after a bowel movement

Distal ulcerative colitis
▶ BY RECTUM USING RECTAL FOAM
▸ Child 12–17 years: 1 metered application 1–2 times a day for 2 weeks, continued for further 2 weeks if good response, to be inserted into the rectum, 1 metered application contains 20 mg prednisolone

Rectal complications of Crohn's disease
▶ BY RECTUM USING SUPPOSITORIES
▸ Child 2–17 years: 5 mg twice daily, to be inserted into the rectum morning and night, after a bowel movement

COVID-19 requiring supplemental oxygen [when dexamethasone cannot be used or is unavailable]
▶ BY MOUTH, OR BY NASOGASTRIC TUBE
▸ Child: 1 mg/kg once daily (max. per dose 40 mg) for 10 days, or until the day of discharge if this is sooner

● **UNLICENSED USE** EvGr Prednisolone is used in the doses provided for the treatment of adrenal insufficiency, and congenital adrenal hyperplasia ⟨A⟩, but these may differ from those licensed.
▸ With oral use EvGr Prednisolone as combination therapy with vigabatrin is used for the treatment of infantile spasms, ⟨B⟩ but such use is not licensed for this indication.
▸ With rectal use Prednisolone rectal foam not licensed for use in children (age range not specified by manufacturer).

IMPORTANT SAFETY INFORMATION
SAFE PRACTICE
▸ With systemic use
Prednisolone has been confused with propranolol; care must be taken to ensure the correct drug is prescribed and dispensed.

● **CONTRA-INDICATIONS**
▸ With rectal use Abdominal or local infection · bowel perforation · extensive fistulas · intestinal obstruction · recent intestinal anastomoses

● **CAUTIONS**
▸ With rectal use Systemic absorption may occur with rectal preparations
▸ With systemic use Duchenne's muscular dystrophy (possible transient rhabdomyolysis and myoglobinuria following strenuous physical activity) · systemic sclerosis (increased incidence of scleroderma renal crisis with a daily dose of 15 mg or more)

● **INTERACTIONS** → Appendix 1: corticosteroids

● **SIDE-EFFECTS**
▸ With oral use Diarrhoea · dizziness · dyslipidaemia · fatigue · heart failure · insomnia · lipomatosis · malaise · protein catabolism · scleroderma renal crisis · telangiectasia

SIDE-EFFECTS, FURTHER INFORMATION Since systemic absorption can follow local administration, also consider the side-effects of systemic corticosteroids.

● **PREGNANCY** As it crosses the placenta 88% of prednisolone is inactivated.
Monitoring ▸ With systemic use Pregnant women with fluid retention should be monitored closely.

● **BREAST FEEDING** Prednisolone appears in small amounts in breast milk but maternal doses of up to 40 mg daily are unlikely to cause systemic effects in the infant.
Monitoring ▸ With systemic use Infant should be monitored for adrenal suppression if mother is taking a dose higher than 40 mg.

● **MONITORING REQUIREMENTS**
▸ With systemic use Manufacturer advises monitor blood pressure and renal function (s-creatinine) routinely in patients with systemic sclerosis—increased incidence of scleroderma renal crisis.
▸ With oral use EvGr Monitor blood pressure and urinary glucose weekly. ⟨A⟩
▸ When used for Infantile spasms EvGr Monitor closely for additive side-effects when used as combination therapy with vigabatrin. ⟨E⟩

● **PRESCRIBING AND DISPENSING INFORMATION**
▸ When used for Asthma For choice of therapy, see Asthma, acute p. 174 and Asthma, chronic p. 171.
▸ When used for COVID-19 requiring supplemental oxygen Royal College of Paediatrics and Child Health (RCPCH) advises a specialist should be consulted when considering use in children under 5 years.

● **PATIENT AND CARER ADVICE**
Medicines for Children leaflet: Prednisolone for nephrotic syndrome www.medicinesforchildren.org.uk/medicines/prednisolone-for-nephrotic-syndrome/
Medicines for Children leaflet: Prednisolone for asthma www.medicinesforchildren.org.uk/medicines/prednisolone-for-asthma/

6 Endocrine system

● **MEDICINAL FORMS** There can be variation in the licensing of different medicines containing the same drug. Forms available from special-order manufacturers include: oral suspension, oral solution

Oral tablet

CAUTIONARY AND ADVISORY LABELS 10, 21

▸ Prednisolone (Non-proprietary)

Prednisolone 500 microgram Prednisolone 500microgram tablets | 28 tablet PoM £4.75–£8.08 DT = £4.75

Prednisolone 1 mg Prednisolone 1mg tablets | 28 tablet PoM DT = £0.63 (Hospital only) | 28 tablet PoM £1.31 DT = £0.63

Prednisolone 2 mg Prednisolone 2mg tablets | 28 tablet PoM £5.00–£8.50 DT = £5.00

Prednisolone 2.5 mg Prednisolone 2.5mg tablets | 28 tablet PoM £6.00 DT = £3.94

Prednisolone 3 mg Prednisolone 3mg tablets | 28 tablet PoM £5.50–£9.36 DT = £5.50

Prednisolone 4 mg Prednisolone 4mg tablets | 28 tablet PoM £5.75–£11.85

Prednisolone 5 mg Prednisolone 5mg tablets | 28 tablet PoM £9.86 DT = £0.65 | 28 tablet PoM DT = £0.65 (Hospital only)

Prednisolone 10 mg Prednisolone 10mg tablets | 28 tablet PoM £14.60 DT = £9.70

Prednisolone 20 mg Prednisolone 20mg tablets | 28 tablet PoM £29.40 DT = £19.46

Prednisolone 25 mg Prednisolone 25mg tablets | 56 tablet PoM £80.00 DT = £49.50

Prednisolone 30 mg Prednisolone 30mg tablets | 28 tablet PoM £47.00 DT = £29.12

Gastro-resistant tablet

CAUTIONARY AND ADVISORY LABELS 5, 10, 25

▸ Prednisolone (Non-proprietary)

Prednisolone 1 mg Prednisolone 1mg gastro-resistant tablets | 100 tablet PoM £32.49–£51.70 DT = £32.49

Prednisolone 2.5 mg Prednisolone 2.5mg gastro-resistant tablets | 28 tablet PoM £3.90 DT = £0.92 | 30 tablet PoM £0.87–£1.13

Prednisolone 5 mg Prednisolone 5mg gastro-resistant tablets | 28 tablet PoM £6.50 DT = £1.00 | 30 tablet PoM £0.96–£1.24

Soluble tablet

CAUTIONARY AND ADVISORY LABELS 10, 13, 21

▸ Prednisolone (Non-proprietary)

Prednisolone (as Prednisolone sodium phosphate)

5 mg Prednisolone 5mg soluble tablets sugar free | 30 tablet PoM £53.48 DT = £53.48 SF

Suppository

▸ Prednisolone (Non-proprietary)

Prednisolone (as Prednisolone sodium phosphate)

5 mg Prednisolone sodium phosphate 5mg suppositories | 10 suppository PoM £263.78 DT = £215.09

Rectal foam

▸ Prednisolone (Non-proprietary)

Prednisolone (as Prednisolone sodium metasulfobenzoate)

20 mg per 1 application Prednisolone 20mg/application foam enema | 14 dose PoM £246.48–£320.61 DT = £320.61

Oral solution

CAUTIONARY AND ADVISORY LABELS 10

▸ Prednisolone (Non-proprietary)

Prednisolone 1 mg per 1 ml Prednisolone 5mg/5ml oral solution unit dose | 10 unit dose PoM £11.41–£16.98 DT = £17.56

Prednisolone 10 mg per 1 ml Prednisolone 10mg/ml oral solution sugar free | 30 ml PoM £55.50–£105.50 DT = £55.50 SF

3.1 Cushing's syndrome and disease

Cushing's syndrome 07-Apr-2021

Management

Cushing's syndrome results from chronic exposure to excess cortisol; exogenous corticosteroid use is the most common cause. Endogenous causes include adrenocorticotrophic hormone (ACTH)-secreting pituitary tumours (Cushing's disease), cortisol-secreting adrenal tumours, and rarely, ectopic ACTH-secreting tumours. Most types of endogenous Cushing's syndrome are treated surgically.

Metyrapone p. 551 is licensed for the management of Cushing's syndrome. Expert sources advise it can be used to prepare the child for surgery.

Ketoconazole below is licensed in children aged over 12 years for the treatment of endogenous Cushing's syndrome.

ENZYME INHIBITORS

Ketoconazole 30-May-2023

● **DRUG ACTION** An imidazole derivative which acts as a potent inhibitor of cortisol and aldosterone synthesis by inhibiting the activity of 17α-hydroxylase, 11-hydroxylation steps and at higher doses the cholesterol side-chain cleavage enzyme. It also inhibits the activity of adrenal C17-20 lyase enzymes resulting in androgen synthesis inhibition, and may have a direct effect on corticotropic tumour cells in patients with Cushing's disease.

● **INDICATIONS AND DOSE**

Endogenous Cushing's syndrome (specialist use only)

▸ BY MOUTH

▸ Child 12–17 years: Initially 400–600 mg daily in 2–3 divided doses, increased to 800–1200 mg daily; maintenance 400–800 mg daily in 2–3 divided doses, for dose titrations in patients with established dose, adjustments in adrenal insufficiency, or concomitant corticosteroid replacement therapy, consult product literature; maximum 1200 mg per day

DOSE ADJUSTMENTS DUE TO INTERACTIONS

▸ EvGr Max. dose 200 mg daily with concurrent use of cobicistat-boosted regimens. Ⓜ

IMPORTANT SAFETY INFORMATION

CHMP ADVICE: KETOCONAZOLE (JULY 2013)

The CHMP has recommended that the marketing authorisation for oral ketoconazole to treat fungal infections should be suspended. The CHMP concluded that the risk of hepatotoxicity associated with oral ketoconazole is greater than the benefit in treating fungal infections. Doctors should review patients who are being treated with oral ketoconazole for fungal infections, with a view to stopping treatment or choosing an alternative treatment. Patients with a prescription of oral ketoconazole for fungal infections should be referred back to their doctors.

Oral ketoconazole for Cushing's syndrome and topical products containing ketoconazole are not affected by this advice.

● **CONTRA-INDICATIONS** Acquired QTc prolongation · Acute porphyrias p. 745 · avoid concomitant use of hepatotoxic drugs · congenital QTc prolongation

● **CAUTIONS** Pre-treatment liver enzymes should not exceed 2 times the normal upper limit · risk of adrenal insufficiency

● **INTERACTIONS** → Appendix 1: antifungals, azoles

● **SIDE-EFFECTS**

▸ **Common or very common** Adrenal insufficiency · diarrhoea · gastrointestinal discomfort · nausea · skin reactions · vomiting

▸ **Uncommon** Allergic conditions · alopecia · angioedema · asthenia · dizziness · drowsiness · headache · thrombocytopenia

▸ **Rare or very rare** Fever · hepatic disorders · taste altered

▸ **Frequency not known** Alcohol intolerance · appetite abnormal · arthralgia · azoospermia · dry mouth · epistaxis ·

flatulence · fontanelle bulging · gynaecomastia · hot flush · insomnia · intracranial pressure increased · malaise · menstrual disorder · myalgia · nervousness · papilloedema · paraesthesia · peripheral oedema · photophobia · photosensitivity reaction · tongue discolouration

SIDE-EFFECTS, FURTHER INFORMATION Potentially life-threatening hepatotoxicity reported rarely with oral use. Manufacturer advises reduce dose if hepatic enzymes increased to less than 3 times the upper limit of normal—consult product literature; discontinue permanently if hepatic enzymes at least 3 times the upper limit of normal.

- **CONCEPTION AND CONTRACEPTION** Effective contraception must be used in women of child-bearing potential.
- **PREGNANCY** Manufacturer advises avoid—teratogenic in *animal* studies.
- **BREAST FEEDING** Manufacturer advises avoid—present in breast milk.
- **HEPATIC IMPAIRMENT** Manufacturer advises avoid.
- **MONITORING REQUIREMENTS**
  - Monitor ECG before and one week after initiation, and then as clinically indicated thereafter.
  - Adrenal insufficiency Monitor adrenal function within one week of initiation, then regularly thereafter. When cortisol levels are normalised or close to target and effective dose established, monitor every 3–6 months as there is a risk of autoimmune disease development or exacerbation after normalisation of cortisol levels. If symptoms suggestive of adrenal insufficiency such as fatigue, anorexia, nausea, vomiting, hypotension, hyponatraemia, hyperkalaemia, and/or hypoglycaemia occur, measure cortisol levels and discontinue treatment temporarily (can be resumed thereafter at lower dose) or reduce dose and if necessary, initiate corticosteroid substitution.
  - Hepatotoxicity Monitor liver function before initiation of treatment, then weekly for 1 month after initiation, then monthly for 6 months—more frequently if dose adjusted or abnormal liver function detected.
- **PATIENT AND CARER ADVICE** Patients or their carers should be told how to recognise signs of liver disorder, and advised to discontinue treatment and seek prompt medical attention if symptoms such as anorexia, nausea, vomiting, fatigue, jaundice, abdominal pain, or dark urine develop. Patients or their carers should also be told how to recognise signs of adrenal insufficiency.
  Driving and skilled tasks Dizziness and somnolence may affect the performance of skilled tasks (e.g. driving).
- **MEDICINAL FORMS** There can be variation in the licensing of different medicines containing the same drug. Forms available from special-order manufacturers include: oral suspension

Oral tablet

CAUTIONARY AND ADVISORY LABELS 2, 5, 21

- Ketoconazole (non-proprietary) ▼
  Ketoconazole 200 mg Ketoconazole 200mg tablets | 60 tablet PoM £648.90 DT = £648.90

Metyrapone 14-Dec-2020

- **DRUG ACTION** Metyrapone is a competitive inhibitor of 11β-hydroxylation in the adrenal cortex; the resulting inhibition of cortisol (and to a lesser extent aldosterone) production leads to an increase in ACTH production which, in turn, leads to increased synthesis and release of cortisol precursors. Metyrapone may be used as a test of anterior pituitary function.
- **INDICATIONS AND DOSE**

Differential diagnosis of ACTH-dependent Cushing's syndrome (specialist supervision in hospital)

- BY MOUTH
  - Child: 15 mg/kg every 4 hours for 6 doses, alternatively 300 mg/m^2 every 4 hours for 6 doses; usual dose 250–750 mg every 4 hours

Management of Cushing's syndrome (specialist supervision in hospital)

- BY MOUTH
  - Child: Usual dose 0.25–6 g daily, dose to be tailored to cortisol production, dose is either low, and tailored to cortisol production, or high, in which case corticosteroid replacement therapy is also needed

- **CONTRA-INDICATIONS** Adrenocortical insufficiency
- **CAUTIONS** Avoid in Acute porphyrias p. 745 · gross hypopituitarism (risk of precipitating acute adrenal failure) · hypertension on long-term administration · hypothyroidism (delayed response)
- **INTERACTIONS** → Appendix 1: metyrapone
- **SIDE-EFFECTS**
  - **Common or very common** Dizziness · headache · hypotension · nausea · sedation · vomiting
  - **Rare or very rare** Abdominal pain · adrenal insufficiency · allergic dermatitis · hirsutism
  - **Frequency not known** Alopecia · bone marrow failure · hypertension
- **PREGNANCY** Avoid (may impair biosynthesis of fetal-placental steroids).
- **BREAST FEEDING** Avoid—no information available.
- **HEPATIC IMPAIRMENT** Manufacturer advises caution (risk of delayed response).
- **PATIENT AND CARER ADVICE**
  Driving and skilled tasks Drowsiness may affect the performance of skilled tasks (e.g. driving).
- **MEDICINAL FORMS** There can be variation in the licensing of different medicines containing the same drug.

Oral capsule

CAUTIONARY AND ADVISORY LABELS 21

- Metyrapone (Non-proprietary)
  Metyrapone 250 mg Metyrapone 250mg capsules | 100 capsule PoM £552.60 DT = £552.60

4 Diabetes mellitus and hypoglycaemia

4.1 Diabetes mellitus

Diabetes 07-Sep-2023

Description of condition

Diabetes mellitus is a group of metabolic disorders in which persistent hyperglycaemia is caused by deficient insulin secretion or by resistance to the action of insulin. This leads to the abnormalities of carbohydrate, fat and protein metabolism that are characteristic of diabetes mellitus.

Type 1 diabetes below and Type 2 diabetes p. 555 are the two most common classifications of diabetes. Other common types of diabetes are gestational diabetes (develops during pregnancy and resolves after delivery, see Diabetes, pregnancy and breast-feeding p. 559) and secondary diabetes (may be caused by pancreatic damage, hepatic cirrhosis, or endocrine disease). Treatment with endocrine, antiviral or antipsychotic drugs may also cause secondary diabetes. In children, conditions such as cystic fibrosis can lead to diabetes; monogenic diabetes (previously known as maturity onset diabetes in the young) can also occur due to a single gene defect.

Driving

Information on the requirements for driving vehicles by young people receiving treatment for diabetes is available in BNF or from the DVLA at www.gov.uk/guidance/diabetes-mellitus-assessing-fitness-to-drive.

Alcohol

Adolescents and their carers should be made aware that alcohol can make the signs of hypoglycaemia less clear, and can cause delayed hypoglycaemia; (note: specialist sources recommend that **adult** patients with diabetes should drink alcohol only in moderation, and when accompanied by food).

Oral glucose tolerance tests

The oral glucose tolerance test is used mainly for diagnosis of impaired glucose tolerance; it is **not** recommended or necessary for routine diagnostic use of diabetes when severe symptoms of hyperglycaemia are present. In children who have less severe symptoms and blood-glucose levels that do not establish or exclude diabetes (e.g. impaired fasting glycaemia), an oral glucose tolerance test may be required. It may be useful for diagnosis of monogenic diabetes or cystic fibrosis related diabetes, and is used to establish the presence of gestational diabetes.

An oral glucose tolerance test involves measuring the blood-glucose concentration after fasting, and then 2 hours after drinking a standard anhydrous glucose drink. Anhydrous glucose may alternatively be given as the appropriate amount of *Polycal*® or as *Rapilose*® OGTT oral solution.

HbA1c measurement

Glycated haemoglobin (HbA1c) forms when red blood cells are exposed to glucose in the plasma. The HbA1c test reflects average plasma glucose over the previous 2 to 3 months and provides a good indicator of glycaemic control. Unlike the oral glucose tolerance test, an HbA1c test can be performed at any time of the day and does not require any special preparation such as fasting.

HbA1c values are expressed in *mmol of glycated haemoglobin per mol of haemoglobin (mmol/mol)*, a standardised unit specific for HbA1c created by the International Federation of Clinical Chemistry and Laboratory Medicine (IFCC). HbA1c values were previously aligned to the assay used in the Diabetes Control and Complications Trial (DCCT) and expressed as a percentage.

Equivalent values

IFCC-HbA1c (mmol/mol)	DCCT-HbA1c (%)
42	6.0
48	6.5
53	7.0
59	7.5
64	8.0
69	8.5
75	9.0

The HbA1c test is used for monitoring glycaemic control in both Type 1 diabetes below and Type 2 diabetes p. 555 in children, and for diagnosis of type 2 diabetes in adults. EvGr HbA1c should not be used to diagnose diabetes in children. Ⓐ

HbA1c is also a reliable predictor of microvascular and macrovascular complications and mortality. Lower HbA1c is associated with a lower risk of long term vascular complications, and children and their carers should be supported to aim for an individualised HbA1c target (see Type 1 diabetes below and Type 2 diabetes p. 555). EvGr HbA1c should usually be measured in children with type 1 and type 2 diabetes every 3 months; and more frequently in children with type 1 diabetes if blood-glucose is poorly controlled. Ⓐ

HbA1c monitoring is invalid in children with disturbed erythrocyte turnover or in children with a lack of, or abnormal haemoglobin (for example, any anaemia, a recent blood transfusion, or an altered red cell lifespan). In these cases, quality-controlled plasma glucose profiles, total glycated haemoglobin estimation (if there is abnormal haemoglobin), or fructosamine estimation can be used.

Laboratory measurement of fructosamine concentration measures the glycated fraction of all plasma proteins over the previous 14 to 21 days but is a less accurate measure of glycaemic control than HbA1c.

Type 1 diabetes

07-Sep-2023

Description of condition

Type 1 diabetes describes an absolute insulin deficiency in which there is little or no endogenous insulin secretory capacity due to destruction of insulin-producing beta-cells in the pancreatic islets of Langerhans. This form of the disease has an auto-immune basis in most cases, and it can occur at any age, but most commonly before adulthood.

Loss of insulin secretion results in hyperglycaemia and other metabolic abnormalities. If poorly managed, the resulting tissue damage has both short-term and long-term adverse effects on health; this can result in retinopathy, nephropathy, premature cardiovascular disease, and peripheral artery disease.

Typical features in children presenting with type 1 diabetes are hyperglycaemia (random blood-glucose concentration above 11 mmol/litre), polyuria, polydipsia, weight loss, and excessive tiredness.

Aims of treatment

Treatment is aimed at using insulin regimens to achieve as optimal a level of blood-glucose control as is feasible, while avoiding or reducing the frequency of hypoglycaemic episodes, in order to minimise the risk of long-term microvascular and macrovascular complications. Disability from complications can often be prevented by early detection and active management of the disease (see Diabetic complications p. 556).

EvGr The target for glycaemic control should be individualised for each child, considering factors such as daily activities, aspirations, likelihood of complications, adherence to treatment, comorbidities, and history of hypoglycaemia. Tighter control of blood-glucose is now recommended for children with type 1 diabetes and treatment should attempt to reach near normal glycated haemoglobin (HbA1c) levels and blood-glucose concentration. Aim for a target HbA1c level of 48 mmol/mol (6.5%) or lower in children with type 1 diabetes to minimise the risk of long-term complications. Ⓐ For further information on HbA1c, including monitoring frequency, see Diabetes p. 551.

EvGr Continuous glucose monitoring (CGM) should be offered to support children to self-manage their diabetes.

Children using CGM will still need to take capillary blood-glucose measurements, but can do this less often. Children who are unwilling to or unable to use CGM should be offered capillary blood-glucose monitoring and be advised to measure their blood-glucose concentration at least five times a day. The optimal blood-glucose targets for children are:

- fasting blood-glucose concentration of 4–7 mmol/litre on waking;
- a blood-glucose concentration of 4–7 mmol/litre before meals at other times of the day;
- a blood-glucose concentration of 5–9 mmol/litre after meals;
- a blood-glucose concentration of at least 5 mmol/litre when driving, as recommended by the Driver and Vehicle Licensing Agency (DVLA). (A)

For further guidance on blood-glucose management, see NICE guideline: **Diabetes (type 1 and type 2) in children and young people: diagnosis and management** (see *Useful resources*).

Management

EvGr Type 1 diabetes requires insulin replacement, supported when necessary by active management of other associated cardiovascular risk factors such as hypertension. Tight glycaemic control may be achieved by intensive insulin management (multiple daily injections or insulin pump therapy) from diagnosis, accompanied by carbohydrate counting.

The effectiveness of metformin in combination with insulin is not yet known in children, and so should not be used; acarbose or sulfonylureas should not be used in combination with insulin as their use may increase the risk of hypoglycaemia.

Dietary control is important in both type 1 and type 2 diabetes and children (with their families) should be encouraged to develop good knowledge of nutrition and how it affects their diabetes and insulin requirements. Healthy eating, regular exercise, and control of body-weight can reduce cardiovascular risk and help improve glycaemic control.

Children with type 1 diabetes should receive immunisation against influenza and pneumococcal infection—see Influenza vaccine p. 971 and Pneumococcal vaccine p. 975. (A)

Insulin therapy in type 1 diabetes

EvGr All children with type 1 diabetes require insulin therapy (**see also Insulin p. 554**). Treatment should be initiated and managed by clinicians with relevant expertise; there are three basic types of insulin regimen, although each regimen should be individualised.

Children and their family or carers (if appropriate) should also be offered carbohydrate-counting training as part of a structured education programme if using a multiple daily insulin injection regimen or an insulin pump. (A)

Multiple daily injection basal-bolus insulin regimens

One or more separate daily injections of intermediate-acting insulin or long-acting insulin analogue as the basal insulin; alongside multiple bolus injections of short-acting insulin before meals. This regimen offers flexibility to tailor insulin therapy with the carbohydrate load of each meal.

Mixed (biphasic) regimen

One, two, or three insulin injections per day of short-acting insulin mixed with intermediate-acting insulin. The insulin preparations may be mixed by the patient at the time of injection, or a premixed product can be used.

Continuous subcutaneous insulin infusion (insulin pump)

A regular or continuous amount of insulin (usually in the form of a rapid-acting insulin analogue or soluble insulin), delivered by a programmable pump and insulin storage reservoir via a subcutaneous needle or cannula.

Recommended insulin regimens

EvGr Children should be offered a multiple daily injection basal-bolus regimen initiated at diagnosis, considering personal and family circumstances, and personal preferences. Children and their family/carers should be encouraged to adjust the insulin dose as appropriate after each blood-glucose measurement, and advised to inject rapid-acting insulin analogues before eating (rather than after eating); this reduces blood-glucose concentrations after meals and helps to optimise blood-glucose control.

If a multiple daily injection basal-bolus insulin regimen is unsuitable, or if the child does not have optimal blood-glucose control, it may be necessary to offer an alternative insulin regimen as well as additional support (such as increased contact with their specialist diabetes team). Consider a continuous subcutaneous insulin infusion (insulin pump); a once-, twice- or three-times daily mixed injection regimen may also be considered.

Continuous subcutaneous insulin infusion therapy may be considered under the care of a specialist team. It should only be offered to children over 12 years who suffer disabling hypoglycaemia while attempting to achieve their target HbA1c level, or, who have high HbA1c levels (69 mmol/mol [8.5%] or above) with multiple daily injection therapy (including, if appropriate, the use of long-acting insulin analogues) despite a high level of care. Children under 12 years may be offered insulin pump therapy if a multiple daily injection regimen is impractical or inappropriate, but they should undergo a trial of a multiple dose injection regimen between the ages of 12 and 18 years.

If the chosen regimen is a twice daily injection regimen, the insulin dose should be adjusted according to the general trend in pre-meal, bedtime and occasional night-time blood-glucose concentration. (A)

Insulin requirements

EvGr The dosage of insulin must be determined individually for each child and should be adjusted as necessary according to the results of regular monitoring of blood-glucose concentrations.

Prescribers and patients should be aware that initiation of insulin may be followed by a **temporary** partial remission phase or 'honeymoon period' when lower doses of insulin may be required than are subsequently necessary to maintain glycaemic control with an HbA1c level of less than 48 mmol/mol (6.5%). (A)

EvGr Insulin doses should be reviewed after puberty (around 1 year after menarche or after the growth spurt in boys) as insulin resistance falls after puberty, and maintenance of pubertal doses may increase the risk for excessive weight gain. (E)

Persistent poor glucose control, leading to erratic insulin requirements or episodes of hypoglycaemia, may be due to many factors, including adherence, injection technique, injection site problems, blood-glucose monitoring skills, lifestyle issues (including diet and exercise), psychological issues, and organic causes such as renal disease, thyroid disorders, coeliac disease, Addison's disease or gastroparesis. These factors should be considered before changes are made to a previously optimised regimen. EvGr A review of the child's injection sites should be offered at each clinic visit. (A)

Infection, stress, accidental or surgical trauma, and puberty may all increase the required insulin dose. Insulin requirements may be decreased (and therefore susceptibility to hypoglycaemia increased) by physical activity, intercurrent illness, reduced food intake, and in certain endocrine disorders, such as anterior pituitary or adrenocortical insufficiency and hypothyroidism.

EvGr Rapid-acting insulin analogues should be supplied for use during intercurrent illness and episodes of hyperglycaemia. (A)

Risks of hypoglycaemia with insulin

EvGr Hypoglycaemia is an inevitable adverse effect of insulin treatment, and children and their carers should be advised of the warning signs and actions to take (for guidance on management, see Hypoglycaemia p. 578). (A)

Impaired awareness of hypoglycaemia can occur, when the ability to recognise usual symptoms is lost, or when the symptoms are blunted or no longer present. EvGr Awareness of hypoglycaemia should be discussed and assessed with the child and their carer approximately every 3 months. (E)

An increase in the frequency of hypoglycaemic episodes may reduce the warning symptoms experienced by the child. Impaired awareness of symptoms below 3 mmol/litre is associated with a significantly increased risk of severe hypoglycaemia. Beta-blockers can also blunt hypoglycaemic awareness, by reducing warning signs such as tremor.

Loss of warning of hypoglycaemia among insulin-treated children can be a serious hazard, especially for adolescents who are drivers, cyclists, or in dangerous occupations. Advice should be given in line with the Driver and Vehicle Licensing Agency (DVLA) guidance (see *Driving*, under Diabetes p. 551).

EvGr To restore the warning signs, episodes of hypoglycaemia must be minimised. Insulin regimens, doses and blood-glucose targets should be reviewed and continuous subcutaneous insulin infusion therapy and real-time continuous glucose monitoring should be considered. (A)

EvGr Children and their family/carers should receive structured education to ensure they are following the principles of a flexible insulin regimen correctly, with additional education regarding avoiding and treating hypoglycaemia for those who continue to have impaired awareness. If recurrent severe episodes of hypoglycaemia continue despite appropriate interventions, the child should be referred to a specialist centre. (E)

Manufacturers advise any switch between brands or formulation of insulin (including switching from animal to human insulin) should be done under strict supervision; a change in dose may be required.

Hypodermic equipment

EvGr Children and their carers should be advised on the safe disposal of lancets, single-use syringes, and needles, and should be provided with suitable disposal containers. Arrangements should be made for the suitable disposal of these containers. (A)

Lancets, needles, syringes, and accessories are listed under Hypodermic Equipment in Part IXA of the Drug Tariff (Part III of the Northern Ireland Drug Tariff, Part 3 of the Scottish Drug Tariff). The Drug Tariffs can be accessed online at:

- National Health Service Drug Tariff for England and Wales: www.nhsbsa.nhs.uk/pharmacies-gp-practices-and-appliance-contractors/drug-tariff
- Health and Personal Social Services for Northern Ireland Drug Tariff: bso.hscni.net/directorates/operations/family-practitioner-services/pharmacy/contractor-information/drug-tariff-and-related-materials/drug-tariff-2/
- Scottish Drug Tariff: publichealthscotland.scot/resources-and-tools/medical-practice-and-pharmaceuticals/scottish-drug-tariff/

Useful Resources

Diabetes (type 1 and type 2) in children and young people: diagnosis and management. National Institute for Health and Care Excellence. NICE guideline NG18. August 2015, updated May 2023.
www.nice.org.uk/guidance/ng18

Insulin

16-Sep-2021

Overview

For recommended insulin regimens see Type 1 diabetes p. 552 and Type 2 diabetes p. 555.

Insulin is a polypeptide hormone secreted by pancreatic beta-cells. Insulin increases glucose uptake by adipose tissue and muscles, and suppresses hepatic glucose release. The role of insulin is to lower blood-glucose concentrations in order to prevent hyperglycaemia and its associated microvascular, macrovascular and metabolic complications.

The natural profile of insulin secretion in the body consists of basal insulin (a low and steady secretion of background insulin that controls the glucose continuously released from the liver) and meal-time bolus insulin (secreted in response to glucose absorbed from food and drink).

Sources of insulin

Three types of insulin are available in the UK: human insulin, human insulin analogues, and animal insulin. Animal insulins are extracted and purified from animal sources (bovine or porcine insulin). Although widely used in the past, animal insulins are no longer initiated in people with diabetes but may still be used by some adult patients who cannot, or do not wish to, change to human insulins.

Human insulins are produced by recombinant DNA technology and have the same amino acid sequence as endogenous human insulin. Human insulin analogues are produced in the same way as human insulins, but the insulin is modified to produce a desired kinetic characteristic, such as an extended duration of action or faster absorption and onset of action.

Immunological resistance to insulin is uncommon and true insulin allergy is rare. Human insulin and insulin analogues are less immunogenic than animal insulins.

Administration of insulin

Insulin is inactivated by gastro-intestinal enzymes and must therefore be given by injection; the subcutaneous route is ideal in most circumstances. Insulin should be injected into a body area with plenty of subcutaneous fat—usually the abdomen (fastest absorption rate) or outer thighs/buttocks (slower absorption compared with the abdomen or inner thighs).

Absorption from a limb site can vary considerably (by as much as 20–40%) day-to-day, particularly in children. Local tissue reactions, changes in insulin sensitivity, injection site, blood flow, depth of injection, and the amount of insulin injected can all affect the rate of absorption. Increased blood flow around the injection site due to exercise can also increase insulin absorption.

EvGr Lipohypertrophy can occur due to repeatedly injecting into the same small area, and can cause erratic absorption of insulin, and contribute to poor glycaemic control. Patients should be advised not to use affected areas for further injection until the skin has recovered. Lipohypertrophy can be minimised by using different injection sites in rotation. Injection sites should be checked for signs of infection, swelling, bruising, and lipohypertrophy before administration. (A)

Insulin preparations

Insulin preparations can be broadly categorised into three groups based on their time-action profiles: short-acting insulins (including soluble insulin and rapid-acting insulins), intermediate-acting insulins and long-acting insulins. The duration of action of each particular type of insulin varies considerably from one patient to another, and needs to be assessed individually.

Short-acting insulins

Short-acting insulins have a short duration and a relatively rapid onset of action, to replicate the insulin normally produced by the body in response to glucose absorbed from a meal. These are available as soluble Insulin p. 569 (human and, bovine or porcine—both rarely used), and the rapid-acting insulin analogues (insulin aspart p. 570, insulin glulisine p. 570 and insulin lispro p. 571).

Soluble insulin

Soluble insulin is usually given subcutaneously but some preparations can be given intravenously and intramuscularly. For maintenance regimens, it is usual to inject the insulin 15 to 30 minutes before meals, depending on the insulin preparation used.

When injected subcutaneously, soluble insulin has a rapid onset of action (30 to 60 minutes), a peak action between 1 and 4 hours, and a duration of action of up to 9 hours.

When injected intravenously, soluble insulin has a short half-life of only a few minutes and its onset of action is instantaneous.

Soluble insulin administered intravenously is the most appropriate form of insulin for use in diabetic emergencies e.g. diabetic ketoacidosis and peri-operatively.

Rapid-acting insulin

Insulin aspart, insulin glulisine, and insulin lispro have a faster onset of action (within 15 minutes) and shorter duration of action (approximately 2–5 hours) than soluble insulin, and are usually given by subcutaneous injection.

EvGr For maintenance regimens, these insulins should ideally be injected immediately before meals. Rapid-acting insulin, administered before meals, has an advantage over short-acting soluble insulin in terms of improved glucose control, reduction of HbA1c, and reduction in the incidence of severe hypoglycaemia, including nocturnal hypoglycaemia.

The routine use of *post-meal* injections of rapid-acting insulin should be avoided—when given during or after meals, they are associated with poorer glucose control, an increased risk of high postprandial-glucose concentration, and subsequent hypoglycaemia. (A)

Intermediate-acting insulin

Intermediate-acting insulins (isophane insulin p. 572) have an intermediate duration of action, designed to mimic the effect of endogenous basal insulin. When given by subcutaneous injection, they have an onset of action of approximately 1–2 hours, a maximal effect at 3–12 hours, and a duration of action of 11–24 hours.

Isophane insulin is a suspension of insulin with protamine; it may be given as one or more daily injections alongside separate meal-time short-acting insulin injections, or mixed with a short-acting (soluble or rapid-acting) insulin in the same syringe—for recommended insulin regimens see Type 1 diabetes p. 552 and Type 2 diabetes below. Isophane insulin may be mixed with a short-acting insulin by the patient, or a pre-mixed biphasic insulin can be supplied (biphasic isophane insulin p. 571, biphasic insulin aspart p. 572 and biphasic insulin lispro p. 572).

Biphasic insulins (biphasic isophane insulin, biphasic insulin aspart, biphasic insulin lispro) are pre-mixed insulin preparations containing various combinations of short-acting insulin (soluble insulin or rapid-acting analogue insulin) and an intermediate-acting insulin.

The percentage of short-acting insulin varies from 15% to 50%. These preparations should be administered by subcutaneous injection immediately before a meal.

Long-acting insulin

Like intermediate-acting insulins, the long-acting insulins (protamine zinc insulin, insulin zinc suspension, insulin detemir p. 573, insulin glargine p. 573, insulin degludec p. 573) mimic endogenous basal insulin secretion, but their duration of action may last up to 36 hours. They achieve a steady-state level after 2–4 days to produce a constant level of insulin.

Insulin glargine and insulin degludec are given once daily and insulin detemir is given once or twice daily according to individual requirements. The older long-acting insulins, (insulin zinc suspension and protamine zinc insulin) are now rarely prescribed.

Type 2 diabetes

07-Sep-2023

Description of condition

Type 2 diabetes is a chronic metabolic condition characterised by insulin resistance and insufficient pancreatic insulin production, resulting in high blood-glucose levels (hyperglycaemia).

Type 2 diabetes in children is associated with increased body-weight, increased risk of renal complications, hypertension, and dyslipidaemia; therefore it increases cardiovascular risk. It is associated with long-term microvascular and macrovascular complications, together with reduced quality of life and life expectancy.

Type 2 diabetes typically develops later in life, but despite previously being considered a disease of adulthood, it is increasingly being diagnosed in children.

Aims of treatment

Treatment is aimed at minimising the risk of long-term microvascular and macrovascular complications by effective blood-glucose control and maintenance of glycated haemoglobin (HbA1c) at or below the target value set for each individual child.

Management

EvGr Children with suspected type 2 diabetes should have their diagnosis confirmed and their care, immediate and continuing, provided by a multidisciplinary paediatric diabetes team.

Lifestyle modifications (including weight loss, smoking cessation, and regular exercise) can help to reduce both hyperglycaemia and cardiovascular risk and should be encouraged where appropriate. Children and their parents/carers should also receive advice from a paediatric dietitian to help optimise body-weight and blood-glucose control.

Lifestyle modifications alone are often unsuccessful at achieving glycaemic control in children, therefore antidiabetic drugs should be offered and initiated alongside lifestyle interventions from the time of diagnosis.

Children with type 2 diabetes should receive immunisation against influenza and pneumococcal infection—see Influenza vaccine p. 971 and Pneumococcal vaccine p. 975. (A)

For guidance on the management of diabetes in pregnancy and breastfeeding, see Diabetes, pregnancy and breast-feeding p. 559.

For guidance on the management of complications associated with diabetes, see Diabetic complications p. 556.

Antidiabetic drugs

In children, type 2 diabetes does not usually occur until adolescence and information on the use of oral antidiabetic drugs in children is limited. For recommended treatment regimens and the place in therapy of each drug, see *Treatment of type 2 diabetes*.

Metformin hydrochloride p. 559 has an anti-hyperglycaemic effect, lowering both basal and postprandial blood-glucose concentrations. Metformin hydrochloride does not stimulate insulin secretion and therefore, when given alone, does not cause hypoglycaemia.

EvGr The dose of standard-release metformin hydrochloride should be increased gradually to minimise the risk of gastro-intestinal side-effects. (A)

Glucagon-like peptide-1 (GLP-1) receptor agonists, such as dulaglutide p. 560 and liraglutide p. 562, and sodium-glucose co-transporter 2 (SGLT2) inhibitors, such as empagliflozin, in addition to lowering blood-glucose, also promote weight loss. Liraglutide and dulaglutide may be slightly more effective at managing blood glucose levels than empagliflozin.

There is little experience of the use of other non-insulin antidiabetic drugs in children, with most evidence extrapolated from adult studies.

Several **sulfonylureas** (such as gliclazide p. 566, glibenclamide p. 566 and tolbutamide p. 567) are available but experience in children is limited; they are not the recommended choice of treatment in children. The sulfonylureas may cause hypoglycaemia which may be more common in children than in adults. Hypoglycaemia is more likely with long-acting sulfonylureas such as glibenclamide, which has been associated with severe, prolonged and sometimes fatal cases—for this reason sulfonylureas are usually avoided in children.

Treatment of type 2 diabetes

EvGr A target HbA1c level of 48 mmol/mol (6.5%) or lower is ideal to minimise the risk of long-term complications, however an individualised lowest achievable target should be agreed with each child and their parent/carer taking into account factors such as daily activities, individual life goals, complications, and comorbidities. HbA1c levels should be monitored every 3 months.

Consider relaxing the target HbA1c level on a case-by-case basis, with particular consideration for children where tight blood-glucose control is not appropriate or poses a high risk of the consequences of hypoglycaemia. (A)

For further guidance on HbA1c, see Diabetes p. 551, and for guidance on self-monitoring of capillary blood-glucose and continuous glucose monitoring, see NICE guideline: **Diabetes (type 1 and type 2) in children and young people: diagnosis and management** (see *Useful resources*).

EvGr Metformin hydrochloride monotherapy is the first-line choice for initial treatment in children and should be offered from diagnosis, alongside dietary and lifestyle advice. For children with an HbA1c level of 69 mmol/mol (8.5%) or more at diagnosis, insulin should be offered in addition to metformin; a basal-bolus insulin regimen should be offered if the child has ketosis but not diabetic ketoacidosis.

4 weeks after diagnosing type 2 diabetes, data from glucose monitoring should be reviewed, and if needed, treatment changed.

Children aged 10 years or over who are on metformin monotherapy, should be offered liraglutide or dulaglutide in addition to metformin if, they have not achieved the HbA1c target level; or they have a plasma glucose level of more than 7 mmol/litre on 4 or more days a week when fasting or before meals; or they have a plasma glucose level of more than 9 mmol/litre on 4 or more days a week, 2 hours after meals. Empagliflozin [unlicensed use] in addition to metformin, may be considered as an alternative in children unable to tolerate liraglutide or dulaglutide, or who have a preference for empagliflozin. Insulin should be offered to children in whom the target HbA1c level cannot be achieved using metformin in combination with liraglutide, or dulaglutide, or empagliflozin.

For children aged 10 years or over who have been on metformin and insulin since diagnosis, insulin therapy should be gradually reduced with the aim of stopping it if, they have achieved the HbA1c target level; or they have a plasma glucose level of 4 mmol/litre to 7 mmol/litre on 4 or more days a week, when fasting or before meals; or they have a plasma glucose level of 5 mmol/litre to 9 mmol/litre on 4 or more days a week, 2 hours after meals. Children who have not met these targets should be offered liraglutide or dulaglutide in addition to metformin and insulin, rather than increasing their insulin. Empagliflozin [unlicensed use] in addition to current treatment, may be considered as an alternative in children unable to tolerate liraglutide or dulaglutide, or who have a preference for empagliflozin. Insulin should only be increased if the child's HbA1c or glucose levels are not in the target ranges despite also taking metformin with liraglutide, dulaglutide, or empagliflozin, or if liraglutide, dulaglutide, and empagliflozin are not tolerated or are contra-indicated. (A)

Weight gain may occur and can be particularly problematic in children with type 2 diabetes when insulin therapy is initiated, unless there is careful attention and adherence to dietary measures. EvGr The importance of diet and exercise should be emphasised. (A)

Useful Resources

Diabetes (type 1 and type 2) in children and young people: diagnosis and management. National Institute for Health and Care Excellence. NICE guideline 18. May 2023.
www.nice.org.uk/guidance/ng18

Diabetic complications

15-Dec-2021

See also

Diabetes p. 551
Type 1 diabetes p. 552
Type 2 diabetes p. 555
Diabetic foot infections, antibacterial therapy p. 366. For guidance on other diabetic foot problems, see NICE guideline **Diabetic foot problems** (available at: www.nice.org/guidance/ng19).

Diabetes and cardiovascular disease

Diabetes is a strong risk factor for cardiovascular disease later in life. EvGr Other risk factors for cardiovascular disease that should also be addressed are: smoking, hypertension, obesity and dyslipidaemia. (A) The use of an ACE inhibitor (or an angiotensin-II receptor antagonist) and lipid-regulating drugs can be beneficial in children with diabetes and a high cardiovascular disease risk. ACE inhibitors and angiotensin-II receptor antagonists may also have a role in the management of diabetic nephropathy. For guidance on stopping smoking, see Smoking cessation p. 353.

Diabetic nephropathy

EvGr In diabetic children with nephropathy, blood pressure should be reduced to the lowest achievable level to slow the rate of decline of glomerular filtration rate and reduce proteinuria. Microalbuminuria can occur transiently during puberty. Provided there are no contra-indications, all diabetic children with nephropathy causing proteinuria or with established microalbuminuria should be treated with an ACE inhibitor or an angiotensin-II receptor antagonist, even if the blood pressure is normal. ACE inhibitors or angiotensin-II receptor antagonists should also be given as monotherapy, or combined therapy, in children with chronic kidney disease and proteinuria, to reduce the rate of progression of chronic kidney disease. (A)

ACE inhibitors can potentiate the hypoglycaemic effect of insulin and oral antidiabetic drugs; this effect is more likely during the first weeks of combined treatment and in children with renal impairment.

See also treatment of hypertension in diabetes in Hypertension p. 116.

Diabetic neuropathy

Clinical neuropathy is rare in children whose diabetes is well controlled.

Visual impairment

EvGr Optimal diabetic control and blood pressure control (<130/80 mmHg) should be maintained to prevent onset and progression of diabetic eye disease, Ⓐ see Type 1 diabetes p. 552 and Type 2 diabetes p. 555 for diabetic target thresholds.

Diabetic hyperglycaemic emergencies

13-May-2024

Description of condition

Diabetic ketoacidosis (DKA) and the hyperosmolar hyperglycaemic state ((HHS), previously referred to as hyperosmolar non-ketotic (HONK) coma) are medical emergencies with significant morbidity and mortality. HHS has a higher mortality than DKA.

Precipitating factors for DKA include absolute insulin deficiency, insufficient insulin, infection, or stress; and for HHS, these include undiagnosed diabetes, infection, stress, trauma, or substance abuse.

DKA develops rapidly (within hours to days) and usually occurs in children with type 1 diabetes. Unlike DKA, HHS can take days or weeks to fully develop, and consequently the dehydration and electrolyte disturbances are more severe at presentation. HHS is more likely to occur in children with type 2 diabetes, especially in those with learning difficulties or other factors preventing proper hydration.

DKA is characterised by **hyperglycaemia** (blood glucose above 11 mmol/L or known diabetes mellitus), **ketonaemia** (capillary or blood ketone above 3 mmol/L or significant ketonuria of 2+ or more), and **acidosis** (bicarbonate less than 15 mmol/L and/or venous pH less than 7.3). Common signs and symptoms of DKA include dehydration due to polydipsia and polyuria, weight loss, fatigue, nausea, vomiting, abdominal pain, Kussmaul respiration (rapid and deep respiration) with acetone breath, and reduced consciousness.

Characteristic features of HHS are **hypovolaemia**, **marked hyperglycaemia** (blood glucose above 33.3 mmol/L without significant hyperketonaemia or acidosis), and **hyperosmolality** (osmolality above 320 mOsm/kg); however, a mixed picture of DKA and HHS may occur. Common signs and symptoms of HHS include dehydration due to polyuria and polydipsia, nausea, vomiting, dry mucous membranes, poor skin turgor, hypotension, and altered levels of consciousness.

Aims of treatment

The treatment of DKA aims to restore circulatory volume, correct electrolyte imbalance and hyperglycaemia, clear ketones and suppress ketogenesis, identify and treat any precipitating causes, and prevent complications.

The treatment of HHS aims to correct fluid and electrolyte losses, hyperosmolality and hyperglycaemia, identify and treat any underlying or precipitating causes, and prevent complications.

Diabetic ketoacidosis

Children with suspected DKA should be diagnosed promptly and managed intensively. They should be immediately referred to a hospital with facilities for paediatric resuscitation and discussed with the consultant paediatrician on-call (or senior clinician).

For children who are clinically dehydrated, nauseated or vomiting, or not alert, the initial drug management of DKA involves intravenous fluid replacement, followed by intravenous insulin. For children who normally take long acting insulin, consider continuing their usual dose(s) throughout treatment. Potassium replacement and glucose administration may also be required to prevent subsequent hypokalaemia and hypoglycaemia, depending on potassium levels or urine output, and blood glucose concentrations, respectively.

Children who are alert, not clinically dehydrated, and not nauseated or vomiting, can usually tolerate oral rehydration and subcutaneous insulin. They should be monitored regularly to ensure that they are improving and their ketone levels are falling.

For further information on the management of DKA, see BSPED guideline: **Guideline for the Management of Children and Young People under the age of 18 years with Diabetic Ketoacidosis**, and NICE guideline: **Diabetes (type 1 and type 2) in children and young people** (see *Useful resources*). For individuals aged 16–18 years being managed by an adult diabetes team, the JBDS guideline: **The Management of Diabetic Ketoacidosis in Adults** (see *Useful resources*) can be followed.

Hyperosmolar hyperglycaemic state

Children with suspected HHS should be diagnosed promptly and managed intensively. They should be referred to a hospital with facilities for paediatric resuscitation, reviewed by a senior paediatrician, and discussed with consultants who have expertise in paediatric diabetes and paediatric intensive care.

The initial drug management of HHS involves intravenous fluid replacement, followed by intravenous insulin only once adequate fluid resuscitation and rehydration has been achieved. For patients with significant ketosis or acidosis (a mixed DKA/HHS picture), insulin can be started earlier. Potassium, magnesium, and phosphate replacement may also be required.

For further information on the management of HHS, see ACDC and BSPED guideline: **Practical Management of Hyperglycaemic Hyperosmolar State (HHS) in children** (see *Useful resources*). For individuals aged 16–18 years being managed by an adult diabetes team, the JBDS guideline: **The Management of the Hyperosmolar Hyperglycaemic State (HHS) in Adults with Diabetes** (see *Useful resources*) can be followed.

Useful Resources

Recommendations reflect BSPED Guideline for the Management of Children and Young People under the age of 18 years with Diabetic Ketoacidosis. British Society for Paediatric Endocrinology and Diabetes. November 2021.
www.bsped.org.uk/clinical-resources/guidelines/#diabetes

The Management of the Hyperosmolar Hyperglycaemic State (HHS) in Adults with diabetes Guideline. Joint British Diabetes Societies for Inpatient Care Group. February 2022.
abcd.care/joint-british-diabetes-societies-jbds-inpatient-care-group

Diabetes (type 1 and type 2) in children and young people: diagnosis and management. National Institute for Health and Care Excellence. NICE guideline 18. August 2015 (updated May 2023).
www.nice.org.uk/guidance/ng18

The Management of Diabetic Ketoacidosis in Adults Guideline. Joint British Diabetes Societies for Inpatient Care Group. March 2023.
abcd.care/joint-british-diabetes-societies-jbds-inpatient-care-group

Practical Management of Hyperglycaemic Hyperosmolar State (HHS) in children. Association of Children's Diabetes Clinicians, British Society for Paediatric Endocrinology and Diabetes, and Children and Young People's National Diabetes Network. Clinical guideline. April 2021
www.a-c-d-c.org/endorsed-guidelines/

Diabetes, surgery and medical illness

16-Sep-2021

Management of diabetes during surgery

EvGr Children with diabetes should undergo surgery in centres with facilities and expertise for the care of children with diabetes. Detailed local protocols should be available to all healthcare professionals involved in the treatment of these children. All surgery requiring general anaesthesia in children with type 1 and type 2 diabetes requires hospital admission. (A)

Note: The following recommendations provide general guidance for the management of diabetes during surgery. **Local protocols and guidelines should be referred to where they exist.**

Use of insulin during surgery

Elective surgery—minor procedures

EvGr *Minor procedures* (procedures of less than 2 hours requiring either general anaesthesia or heavy sedation) in children who have type 1 or type 2 diabetes should not have a major impact on glycaemic control, and a slight modification of the usual regimen may be all that is necessary—adjustments should be made following local protocol; taking into consideration the type of insulin or antidiabetic drugs the child usually takes, whether fasting is required, the time of day of the operation, and requirement for intravenous fluids and glucose. All children who are usually prescribed insulin require intravenous insulin during surgery, to avoid ketoacidosis. (A)

Elective surgery—major procedures

EvGr *Major procedures* (procedures requiring general anaesthesia for more than 2 hours) in children who have type 1 or type 2 diabetes, should ideally be performed when diabetes is under optimal control. If glycaemic control is poor, the procedure should be delayed if possible; otherwise it is advisable to admit the child well in advance of surgery for stabilisation of glycaemic control.

Blood-glucose concentration should be maintained within the usual target range of 5–10 mmol/litre throughout the peri-operative period for all surgical procedures.

Children usually prescribed insulin for type 1 or type 2 diabetes require an intravenous insulin infusion p. 569 during surgery (even if fasting) to avoid ketoacidosis. Detailed local protocols should be consulted. In general, the following steps should be followed:

- on the *evening before surgery*, the usual insulin regimen should be given as normal; the usual bedtime snack should be given and hourly capillary blood-glucose monitoring should be initiated to detect hypoglycaemia or hyperglycaemia before the procedure. Ketones should also be checked if blood-glucose is above 14 mmol/litre, and an appropriate dose of short-acting insulin should be administered to restore blood-glucose to the target range;
- on the *morning of surgery* the **usual** insulin dose should be omitted;
- at least 2 *hours before the procedure*, a maintenance fluid infusion of sodium chloride 0.45 % and glucose 5 % (sodium chloride with glucose p. 730) intravenous infusion should be started. A switch to sodium chloride 0.9 % infusion p. 728 may be required if sodium concentration falls and there is risk of hyponatraemia. After surgery, potassium chloride p. 744 should be added to the intravenous fluid, according to the child's body weight and fluid requirements. Electrolytes must be measured frequently throughout, and adjustments to the infusion made as necessary;
- soluble human insulin 1 unit/mL in sodium chloride 0.9 % intravenous infusion should be started with the maintenance fluids at an infusion rate appropriate to the blood-glucose concentration, to maintain a concentration between 5 and 10 mmol/litre, adjusted according to hourly blood-glucose monitoring;
- if the blood-glucose concentration falls below 6 mmol/litre the insulin infusion should **not** be stopped as this will cause rebound hyperglycaemia; instead the rate should be reduced; however, if blood-glucose concentration drops below 4 mmol/litre the insulin infusion can be stopped temporarily for 10–15 minutes.

After surgery, continue the glucose infusion, and the intravenous insulin infusion or additional short-acting insulin as necessary, until the child can eat and drink normally and their usual treatment regimen can resume. A short-acting insulin can also be given if required to reduce hyperglycaemia. (A)

Emergency surgery

EvGr Children with diabetes (type 1 and 2) requiring emergency surgery, should always have their blood-glucose, blood or urinary ketone concentration, and serum electrolytes checked before surgery. If ketones are high, blood gases should also be checked. If ketoacidosis is present, recommendations for diabetic ketoacidosis should be followed immediately, and surgery delayed if possible. If there is no acidosis, intravenous fluids and an insulin infusion should be started and managed as for *major elective surgery* (above). (A)

Use of antidiabetic drugs during surgery

EvGr If elective *minor surgical procedures* only require a short-fasting period (just one missed meal), it may be possible to adjust antidiabetic drugs to avoid a switch to a variable rate intravenous insulin infusion; normal drug treatment can continue.

Children who usually take **sulfonylureas** should have their medication stopped on the day of surgery. (A)

EvGr **Sulfonylureas** are associated with hypoglycaemia in the fasted state and therefore should not be recommenced until the child is eating and drinking normally. (E)

EvGr Children undergoing *minor procedures* require hourly blood-glucose monitoring and, if blood-glucose concentration rises above 10 mmol/litre, should be treated with subcutaneous rapid-acting insulin no more frequently than every 3 hours.

Children undergoing a *major surgical* procedure expected to last at least 2 hours should be managed on an intravenous insulin infusion following the recommendations for *Elective surgery* (above). (A)

EvGr Insulin is almost always required in medical and surgical emergencies. (E)

EvGr **Metformin hydrochloride p. 559** is renally excreted; renal impairment may lead to accumulation and lactic acidosis during surgery. In children undergoing *major surgery* lasting more than 2 hours, metformin hydrochloride should be discontinued 24 hours before the procedure. Children having minor surgery lasting less than 2 hours may stop their metformin on the day of surgery. Metformin hydrochloride should not be restarted until at least 48 hours after surgery or after the child is eating again, and only once normal renal function has been established. (A)

The manufacturer advises that metformin should also be omitted if contrast medium is administered during surgery to reduce the risk of contrast-induced nephropathy. It should be stopped prior to, or at the time of the test, and not to be restarted until 48 hours afterwards, and only once normal renal function has been established.

Use of antidiabetic drugs during medical illness

Manufacturers of some antidiabetic drugs recommend that they may need to be replaced temporarily with insulin during intercurrent illness when the drug is unlikely to control hyperglycaemia (such as coma, severe infection, trauma and other medical emergencies). Consult individual product literature.

Diabetes, pregnancy and breast-feeding

04-Apr-2022

Description of condition

Diabetes in pregnancy is associated with increased risks to the young woman (such as pre-eclampsia and rapidly worsening retinopathy), and to the developing fetus, compared with pregnancy in non-diabetic young women. Effective blood-glucose control before conception and throughout pregnancy reduces (but does not eliminate) the risk of adverse outcomes such as miscarriage, congenital malformation, stillbirth, and neonatal death.

Management of pre-existing diabetes

EvGr Young women with pre-existing diabetes who are planning on becoming pregnant should aim to keep their HbA1c concentration below 48 mmol/mol (6.5%) if possible without causing problematic hypoglycaemia. Any reduction towards this target is likely to reduce the risk of congenital malformations in the newborn.

Young women with pre-existing diabetes who are planning to become pregnant should be advised to take folic acid at the dose for young women who are at high-risk of conceiving a child with a neural tube defect, see folic acid p. 710. (A)

Overview

Oral antidiabetic drugs

EvGr All oral antidiabetic drugs, except metformin hydrochloride below, should be discontinued before pregnancy (or as soon as an unplanned pregnancy is identified) and substituted with insulin therapy. Young women with diabetes may be treated with metformin hydrochloride below as an adjunct or alternative to insulin in the preconception period and during pregnancy when the likely benefits from improved blood-glucose control outweigh the potential for harm. Metformin hydrochloride below can be continued immediately after birth and during breast-feeding for those with pre-existing Type 2 diabetes p. 555. All other antidiabetic drugs should be avoided while breast-feeding. (A)

Insulin

Limited evidence suggests that the rapid-acting insulin analogues (insulin aspart p. 570 and insulin lispro p. 571) can be associated with fewer episodes of hypoglycaemia, a reduction in postprandial glucose excursions, and an improvement in overall glycaemic control compared with regular human insulin.

EvGr Isophane insulin p. 572 is the first-choice for long-acting insulin during pregnancy, however in young women who have good blood-glucose control before pregnancy with the long-acting insulin analogues (insulin detemir p. 573 or insulin glargine p. 573), it may be appropriate to continue their use throughout pregnancy.

Continuous subcutaneous insulin infusion p. 569 (insulin pump therapy) may be appropriate for young women who have difficulty achieving glycaemic control with multiple daily injections of insulin p. 569 without significant disabling hypoglycaemia.

All young women treated with insulin p. 569 during pregnancy should be aware of the risks of hypoglycaemia, particularly in the first trimester, and should be advised to always carry a fast-acting form of glucose, such as dextrose tablets or a glucose-containing drink. Pregnant young women with Type 1 diabetes p. 552 should also be prescribed glucagon p. 579 for use if needed.

Young women with pre-existing diabetes treated with insulin p. 569 during pregnancy are at increased risk of hypoglycaemia in the postnatal period and should reduce their insulin immediately after birth. Blood-glucose levels should be monitored carefully to establish the appropriate dose. (A)

Medication for diabetic complications

EvGr Angiotensin-converting enzyme inhibitors and angiotensin-II receptor antagonists should be discontinued and replaced with an alternative antihypertensive suitable for use in pregnancy before conception or as soon as pregnancy is confirmed. Statins should not be prescribed during pregnancy and should be discontinued before a planned pregnancy. (A)

Gestational diabetes

EvGr Young women with gestational diabetes who have a fasting plasma glucose below 7 mmol/litre at diagnosis, should first attempt a change in diet and exercise alone in order to reduce blood-glucose. If blood-glucose targets are not met within 1 to 2 weeks, metformin hydrochloride below may be prescribed. Insulin p. 569 may be prescribed if metformin is contra-indicated or not acceptable, and may also be added to treatment if metformin is not effective alone.

Young women who have a fasting plasma glucose above 7 mmol/litre at diagnosis should be treated with insulin p. 569 immediately with or without metformin hydrochloride below, in addition to a change in diet and exercise.

Young women who have a fasting plasma glucose between 6 and 6.9 mmol/litre alongside complications, such as macrosomia or hydramnios, should be considered for immediate insulin p. 569 treatment, with or without metformin hydrochloride below.

Young women with gestational diabetes should discontinue hypoglycaemic treatment immediately after giving birth. (A)

Useful Resources

Diabetes in pregnancy: management from preconception to the postnatal period. National Institute for Health and Care Excellence. NICE guideline NG3. February 2015 (updated December 2020).
www.nice.org.uk/guidance/ng3

BLOOD GLUCOSE LOWERING DRUGS ›
BIGUANIDES

Metformin hydrochloride

07-May-2024

- **DRUG ACTION** Metformin exerts its effect mainly by decreasing gluconeogenesis and by increasing peripheral utilisation of glucose; since it acts only in the presence of endogenous insulin it is effective only if there are some residual functioning pancreatic islet cells.

- **INDICATIONS AND DOSE**

Type 2 diabetes mellitus [monotherapy or in combination with other antidiabetic drugs (including insulin)]

▶ BY MOUTH USING IMMEDIATE-RELEASE MEDICINES
- Child 8–9 years (specialist use only): Initially 200–250 mg once daily; increased if necessary up to 2 g daily in 2–3 divided doses, dose to be adjusted according to response at intervals of at least 1 week
- Child 10–17 years (specialist use only): Initially 500 mg once daily; increased if necessary to 2 g daily in 2–3 divided doses, dose to be adjusted according to response at intervals of at least 1 week

- **UNLICENSED USE** EvGr Metformin is used in the doses provided in BNF publications for the treatment of type 2 diabetes mellitus, (E) but these may differ from those licensed.

EvGr Metformin may be used in children aged 8–9 years for the treatment of type 2 diabetes, Ⓔ but is not licensed for this age group.

IMPORTANT SAFETY INFORMATION

MHRA/CHM ADVICE: METFORMIN IN PREGNANCY: STUDY SHOWS NO SAFETY CONCERNS (MARCH 2022)

European and CHM reviews of data from a large cohort study of Finnish population registries did not identify any safety issues with the use of metformin during pregnancy. Product literature for single-ingredient metformin preparations was subsequently updated to permit its use as an adjunct or alternative to insulin during pregnancy and the periconception period, if clinically indicated.

MHRA/CHM ADVICE: METFORMIN AND REDUCED VITAMIN B_{12} LEVELS: NEW ADVICE FOR MONITORING PATIENTS AT RISK (JUNE 2022)

A European review, with input from the MHRA, has found vitamin B_{12} deficiency to be a common side-effect in patients treated with metformin, especially in those receiving a higher dose or longer treatment duration and in those with risk factors for vitamin B_{12} deficiency.

Healthcare professionals are advised to check serum-vitamin B_{12} levels if deficiency is suspected and consider periodic monitoring in patients with risk factors for deficiency. Vitamin B_{12} deficiency should be treated according to current guidelines and treatment with metformin continued for as long as it is tolerated. Patients and their carers should be counselled on the signs and symptoms of vitamin B_{12} deficiency and advised to seek medical advice if these occur. Patients should continue taking metformin unless they are advised to stop.

- **CONTRA-INDICATIONS** Acute metabolic acidosis (including lactic acidosis and diabetic ketoacidosis)
- **CAUTIONS** Risk factors for lactic acidosis

CAUTIONS, FURTHER INFORMATION Manufacturer advises caution in chronic stable heart failure (monitor cardiac function), and concomitant use of drugs that can acutely impair renal function; interrupt treatment if dehydration occurs, and avoid in conditions that can acutely worsen renal function, or cause tissue hypoxia.

- **INTERACTIONS** → Appendix 1: metformin
- **SIDE-EFFECTS**
  - **Common or very common** Abdominal pain · appetite decreased · diarrhoea · gastrointestinal disorder · nausea · taste altered · vitamin B12 deficiency · vomiting
  - **Rare or very rare** Hepatitis · lactic acidosis (discontinue) · skin reactions

SIDE-EFFECTS, FURTHER INFORMATION Gastrointestinal side-effects are most frequent during treatment initiation and usually resolve spontaneously. A slow increase in dose may improve tolerability.

- **PREGNANCY** EvGr Can be used in pregnancy for both pre-existing and gestational diabetes. Women with gestational diabetes should discontinue treatment after giving birth. Ⓐ See also *Important safety information.*
- **BREAST FEEDING** EvGr May be used during breast-feeding in women with pre-existing diabetes. Ⓐ
- **HEPATIC IMPAIRMENT** Withdraw if tissue hypoxia likely.
- **RENAL IMPAIRMENT** See p. 16. Manufacturer advises avoid if estimated glomerular filtration rate is less than 30 mL/minute/1.73 m^2.

Dose adjustments Manufacturer advises consider dose reduction in moderate impairment.

- **MONITORING REQUIREMENTS** Determine renal function before treatment and at least annually (at least twice a year in patients with additional risk factors for renal impairment, or if deterioration suspected).
- **PATIENT AND CARER ADVICE** Manufacturer advises that patients and their carers should be informed of the risk of lactic acidosis and told to seek immediate medical attention if symptoms such as dyspnoea, muscle cramps, abdominal pain, hypothermia, or asthenia occur.

Medicines for Children leaflet: Metformin for diabetes www.medicinesforchildren.org.uk/medicines/metformin-for-diabetes/

- **MEDICINAL FORMS** There can be variation in the licensing of different medicines containing the same drug. Forms available from special-order manufacturers include: oral capsule, oral suspension, oral solution

Oral tablet

CAUTIONARY AND ADVISORY LABELS 21

▸ **Metformin hydrochloride (Non-proprietary)**

Metformin hydrochloride 500 mg Metformin 500mg tablets | 28 tablet PoM £1.80 DT = £0.55 | 84 tablet PoM £1.62–£5.20 | 500 tablet PoM £9.64–£14.11 | 1000 tablet PoM £20.00–£25.89

Metformin hydrochloride 850 mg Metformin 850mg tablets | 56 tablet PoM £5.20 DT = £0.78 | 200 tablet PoM £2.69 | 300 tablet PoM £3.30–£10.00

Metformin hydrochloride 1 gram Metformin 1g tablets | 28 tablet PoM £44.21 DT = £3.09

▸ **Axpinet** (GlucoRx Ltd)

Metformin hydrochloride 500 mg Axpinet 500mg tablets | 28 tablet PoM £0.50 DT = £0.55

Metformin hydrochloride 850 mg Axpinet 850mg tablets | 56 tablet PoM £0.95 DT = £0.78

▸ **Glucophage** (Merck Serono Ltd)

Metformin hydrochloride 500 mg Glucophage 500mg tablets | 84 tablet PoM £2.88

Metformin hydrochloride 850 mg Glucophage 850mg tablets | 56 tablet PoM £3.20 DT = £0.78

Oral solution

CAUTIONARY AND ADVISORY LABELS 21

▸ **Metformin hydrochloride (Non-proprietary)**

Metformin hydrochloride 100 mg per 1 ml Metformin 500mg/5ml oral solution sugar free | 100 ml PoM £5.00–£30.00 SF | 150 ml PoM £31.34 DT = £4.97 SF | 300 ml PoM £45.10 SF

Metformin hydrochloride 170 mg per 1 ml Metformin 850mg/5ml oral solution sugar free | 150 ml PoM £81.60 DT = £68.00 SF

Metformin hydrochloride 200 mg per 1 ml Metformin 1g/5ml oral solution sugar free | 150 ml PoM £116.78 DT = £80.00 SF

Powder for oral solution

CAUTIONARY AND ADVISORY LABELS 13

▸ **Metformin hydrochloride (Non-proprietary)**

Metformin hydrochloride 500 mg Metformin 500mg oral powder sachets sugar free | 30 sachet PoM £12.60–£22.68 DT = £12.60 SF

Metformin hydrochloride 1 gram Metformin 1g oral powder sachets sugar free | 30 sachet PoM £12.60 DT = £12.60 SF

BLOOD GLUCOSE LOWERING DRUGS ›
GLUCAGON-LIKE PEPTIDE-1 RECEPTOR AGONISTS

Dulaglutide

26-Feb-2026

- **DRUG ACTION** Dulaglutide is a long-acting glucagon-like peptide 1 (GLP-1) receptor agonist that augments glucose-dependent insulin secretion, and slows gastric emptying.
- **INDICATIONS AND DOSE**

Type 2 diabetes mellitus as monotherapy (if metformin inappropriate), or in combination with other antidiabetic drugs (including insulin), if existing treatment fails to achieve adequate glycaemic control

▸ BY SUBCUTANEOUS INJECTION

▸ Child 10–17 years: 0.75 mg once weekly; increased if necessary to 1.5 mg once weekly, dose increased after at least 4 weeks

DOSE ADJUSTMENTS DUE TO INTERACTIONS
- Dose of concomitant insulin or drugs that stimulate insulin secretion may need to be reduced.

IMPORTANT SAFETY INFORMATION

MHRA/CHM ADVICE: GLP-1 RECEPTOR AGONISTS: REPORTS OF DIABETIC KETOACIDOSIS WHEN CONCOMITANT INSULIN WAS RAPIDLY REDUCED OR DISCONTINUED (JUNE 2019)

Serious and life-threatening cases of diabetic ketoacidosis have been reported in patients with type 2 diabetes mellitus on a combination of a glucagon-like peptide-1 (GLP-1) receptor agonist and insulin, particularly after discontinuation or rapid dose reduction of concomitant insulin. Healthcare professionals are advised that any dose reduction of insulin should be done in a stepwise manner with careful blood glucose self-monitoring, particularly when GLP-1 receptor agonist therapy is initiated. Patients should be informed of the risk factors for and signs and symptoms of diabetic ketoacidosis, and advised to seek immediate medical attention if these develop.

MHRA/CHM ADVICE: GLP-1 RECEPTOR AGONISTS: REMINDER OF THE POTENTIAL SIDE EFFECTS AND TO BE AWARE OF THE POTENTIAL FOR MISUSE (OCTOBER 2024)

The MHRA reminds healthcare professionals to ensure that patients are aware of potential side-effects associated with glucagon-like peptide-1 (GLP-1) receptor agonists following anecdotal evidence and Yellow Card reports suggesting misuse of these medicines for weight management outside of their licence. The only GLP-1 receptor agonists licensed for weight management are liraglutide p. 562 (*Saxenda*®), semaglutide p. 77 (*Wegovy*®), and tirzepatide (*Mounjaro*®; licensed in adults only), which is also a glucose-dependent insulinotropic polypeptide (GIP) receptor agonist. The benefits and risks of these medicines for weight loss in individuals who are not obese, or who are not overweight with weight-related co-morbidities, have not been studied.

Healthcare professionals should inform patients and carers upon initial prescription and at any dose increase about the common risk of gastro-intestinal side-effects (including nausea, vomiting, diarrhoea, and constipation) associated with GLP-1 receptor agonists; these are usually non-serious but can persist for several days and may lead to serious complications such as severe dehydration and kidney damage, resulting in hospitalisation. For this reason, patients should be advised to stay well hydrated by drinking plenty of fluids throughout treatment. They should also be informed of other serious but less common side-effects, including acute gallstone disease, pancreatitis, and serious allergic reactions.

Patients and carers should be advised to ensure that prescriptions are only obtained from registered healthcare professionals and that private prescriptions are dispensed from authorised sources to avoid the risk of receiving falsified pens. Patients and carers should consult the patient information leaflet for instructions on the use of GLP-1 receptor agonists, and be advised to only administer the prescribed dose.

MHRA/CHM ADVICE: GLP-1 AND DUAL GIP/GLP-1 RECEPTOR AGONISTS: POTENTIAL RISK OF PULMONARY ASPIRATION DURING GENERAL ANAESTHESIA OR DEEP SEDATION (JANUARY 2025)

An EU review has concluded that glucagon-like peptide-1 (GLP-1) and dual glucose-dependent insulinotropic polypeptide (GIP)/GLP-1 receptor agonists are associated with a potential risk of pulmonary aspiration in patients undergoing surgery or procedures requiring general anaesthesia or deep sedation. These medicines are known to slow gastric emptying, thereby increasing the risk of residual gastric contents despite preoperative fasting, which could lead to pulmonary aspiration and other severe complications, such as aspiration pneumonia.

The MHRA advises healthcare professionals to identify the increased risk of aspiration as early as possible, ideally at the pre-assessment clinic before surgery, in patients using GLP-1 or dual GIP/GLP-1 receptor agonists. Anaesthetists should complete an individualised preoperative risk assessment and consider the following:
- patients with underlying diabetic gastroparesis, as well as other co-morbidities such as obesity or gastroesophageal reflux disease, and symptoms of delayed gastric emptying (such as nausea, vomiting and abdominal pain) may have a higher risk of aspiration;
- directly asking patients or their carers about their use of GLP-1 or dual GIP/GLP-1 receptor agonists, as private prescriptions may not be included in the patient's medical notes or drug history, and patients who may have purchased these medications for use in aesthetic weight loss may not readily disclose this information (see also advice issued in October 2024, above).

There is limited evidence to support any recommendations on a time frame to withhold GLP-1 or dual GIP/GLP-1 receptor agonists prior to anaesthesia, new fasting guidelines, or an appropriate medical procedure to confirm an empty stomach. Anaesthetists should manage aspiration risk in line with usual anaesthetic practice and retain flexibility to provide individualised assessment.

Healthcare professionals should counsel patients or their carers to continue taking their prescribed medicines and not stop treatment without first discussing with their doctor. They should also be advised regarding the risk of aspiration and that there may be a need to modify pre-procedure instruction and anaesthetic technique.

MHRA/CHM ADVICE: GLP-1 RECEPTOR AGONISTS AND DUAL GLP-1/GIP RECEPTOR AGONISTS: STRENGTHENED WARNINGS ON ACUTE PANCREATITIS, INCLUDING NECROTISING AND FATAL CASES (JANUARY 2026)

Following rare reports of necrotising and fatal pancreatitis associated with glucagon-like peptide-1 (GLP-1) and dual GLP-1/glucose-dependent insulinotropic polypeptide (GIP) receptor agonists, healthcare professionals are advised to:
- remain vigilant to the risk, and signs and symptoms of acute pancreatitis;
- use these drugs with caution in patients with a history of pancreatitis;
- enquire about privately prescribed GLP-1 or dual GLP-1/GIP receptor agonists if a patient presents with suspected symptoms, as such use may not appear in their medical history;
- discontinue treatment immediately if pancreatitis is suspected, and not to restart treatment if confirmed;
- counsel patients or their carers to seek urgent medical attention if they develop persistent severe abdominal pain that may radiate to the back, and may be accompanied by nausea and vomiting.

- **CONTRA-INDICATIONS** Severe gastro-intestinal disease—no information available
- **CAUTIONS** General anaesthesia or deep sedation (risk of pulmonary aspiration due to delayed gastric emptying) · history of pancreatitis
- **INTERACTIONS** → Appendix 1: glucagon-like peptide-1 receptor agonists

- **SIDE-EFFECTS**
  - **Common or very common** Appetite decreased · atrioventricular block · burping · constipation · diarrhoea · fatigue · gastrointestinal discomfort · gastrointestinal disorders · hypoglycaemia · nausea · sinus tachycardia · vomiting
  - **Uncommon** Dehydration · gallbladder disorders
  - **Rare or very rare** Angioedema · pancreatitis acute (discontinue)
  - **Frequency not known** Necrotising pancreatitis (discontinue)

  SIDE-EFFECTS, FURTHER INFORMATION Discontinue if symptoms of acute pancreatitis occur, such as persistent, severe abdominal pain; fatal cases reported. If pancreatitis confirmed, do not restart treatment.
- **PREGNANCY** Manufacturer advises avoid—toxicity in *animal* studies.
- **BREAST FEEDING** Manufacturer advises avoid— no information available.
- **RENAL IMPAIRMENT** EvGr Avoid if estimated glomerular filtration rate less than 15 mL/minute/1.73 m^2 (limited information available), (M) see p. 16.
- **PRESCRIBING AND DISPENSING INFORMATION** Dulaglutide is a biological medicine. Biological medicines must be prescribed and dispensed by brand name, see *Biological medicines* and *Biosimilar medicines*, under Guidance on prescribing p. 1; record the brand name and batch number after each administration.

  For choice of therapy, see Type 2 diabetes p. 555.
- **HANDLING AND STORAGE** **Refrigerated storage** is usually necessary (2 °C – 8 °C). Once in use, may be stored unrefrigerated for up to 14 days at a temperature not above 30 °C.
- **PATIENT AND CARER ADVICE** Patients or carers should be given advice on how to administer dulaglutide injection.

  Acute pancreatitis Patients should be told how to recognise signs and symptoms of acute pancreatitis and advised to seek medical attention if symptoms such as persistent, severe abdominal pain develop.

  Dehydration Patients should be informed of the potential risk of dehydration in relation to gastro-intestinal side-effects and advised to take precautions to avoid fluid depletion.

  Missed doses If a dose is missed, it should be administered as soon as possible only if there are at least 3 days until the next scheduled dose; if less than 3 days remain before the next scheduled dose, the missed dose should not be taken and the next dose should be taken at the normal time.

- **MEDICINAL FORMS** There can be variation in the licensing of different medicines containing the same drug.

Solution for injection

EXCIPIENTS: May contain Polysorbates

- Trulicity (Eli Lilly and Company Ltd)

  Dulaglutide 1.5 mg per 1 ml Trulicity 0.75mg/0.5ml solution for injection pre-filled pens | 4 pre-filled disposable injection PoM £73.25 DT = £73.25

  Dulaglutide 3 mg per 1 ml Trulicity 1.5mg/0.5ml solution for injection pre-filled pens | 4 pre-filled disposable injection PoM £73.25 DT = £73.25

  Dulaglutide 6 mg per 1 ml Trulicity 3mg/0.5ml solution for injection pre-filled pens | 4 pre-filled disposable injection PoM £73.25 DT = £73.25

  Dulaglutide 9 mg per 1 ml Trulicity 4.5mg/0.5ml solution for injection pre-filled pens | 4 pre-filled disposable injection PoM £73.25 DT = £73.25

Liraglutide

26-Feb-2026

- **DRUG ACTION** Liraglutide binds to, and activates, the GLP-1 (glucagon-like peptide-1) receptor to increase insulin secretion, suppresses glucagon secretion, and slows gastric emptying.

- **INDICATIONS AND DOSE**

Type 2 diabetes mellitus as monotherapy (if metformin inappropriate), or in combination with other antidiabetic drugs (including insulin) if existing treatment fails to achieve adequate glycaemic control

- BY SUBCUTANEOUS INJECTION
  - Child 10–17 years: Initially 0.6 mg once daily for at least 1 week, then increased to 1.2 mg once daily for at least 1 week, then increased if necessary to 1.8 mg once daily

Adjunct in weight management [in conjunction with dietary measures and increased physical activity in individuals with a BMI corresponding to 30 kg/m^2 or more in adults, and body-weight above 60 kg]

- BY SUBCUTANEOUS INJECTION
  - Child 12–17 years: Initially 0.6 mg once daily, then dose to be increased in steps of 0.6 mg at intervals of at least 1 week up to a maintenance dose of 3 mg once daily or the maximum tolerated dose whichever is lower. Consider discontinuation if escalation to the next dose is not tolerated for 2 consecutive weeks. Discontinue if at least 4% of initial body-weight has not been lost after 12 weeks at maximum dose

DOSE ADJUSTMENTS DUE TO INTERACTIONS

- Dose of concomitant insulin or sulfonylurea may need to be reduced.

DOSE EQUIVALENCE AND CONVERSION

- Liraglutide preparations are indication-specific; use the appropriate preparation—consult product literature. See also *Prescribing and dispensing information*.

IMPORTANT SAFETY INFORMATION

MHRA/CHM ADVICE: GLP-1 RECEPTOR AGONISTS: REPORTS OF DIABETIC KETOACIDOSIS WHEN CONCOMITANT INSULIN WAS RAPIDLY REDUCED OR DISCONTINUED (JUNE 2019)

- When used for Type 2 diabetes mellitus

Serious and life-threatening cases of diabetic ketoacidosis have been reported in patients with type 2 diabetes mellitus on a combination of a glucagon-like peptide-1 (GLP-1) receptor agonist and insulin, particularly after discontinuation or rapid dose reduction of concomitant insulin. Healthcare professionals are advised that any dose reduction of insulin should be done in a stepwise manner with careful blood glucose self-monitoring, particularly when GLP-1 receptor agonist therapy is initiated. Patients should be informed of the risk factors for and signs and symptoms of diabetic ketoacidosis, and advised to seek immediate medical attention if these develop.

MHRA/CHM ADVICE: *SAXENDA*® (LIRAGLUTIDE): VIGILANCE REQUIRED DUE TO POTENTIALLY HARMFUL FALSIFIED PRODUCTS (NOVEMBER 2023)

Falsified *Saxenda*® preparations, some containing insulin, have been found in the UK. Healthcare professionals are advised to remind patients to always obtain prescription medicines from qualified healthcare providers, and not to use preparations they suspect are falsified as this may lead to serious harm. Healthcare professionals should remain vigilant for symptoms associated with hypoglycaemia in patients who may have obtained a falsified preparation containing insulin; patients should be advised to seek immediate medical attention if such symptoms occur. Suspected falsified preparations should be quarantined and reported to the Yellow Card scheme.

MHRA/CHM ADVICE: GLP-1 RECEPTOR AGONISTS: REMINDER OF THE POTENTIAL SIDE EFFECTS AND TO BE AWARE OF THE POTENTIAL FOR MISUSE (OCTOBER 2024)

The MHRA reminds healthcare professionals to ensure that patients are aware of potential side-effects associated with glucagon-like peptide-1 (GLP-1) receptor agonists following anecdotal evidence and Yellow Card reports suggesting misuse of these medicines for weight management outside of their licence. The only GLP-1 receptor agonists licensed for weight management are liraglutide p. 562 (*Saxenda*®), semaglutide p. 77 (*Wegovy*®), and tirzepatide (*Mounjaro*®; licensed in adults only), which is also a glucose-dependent insulinotropic polypeptide (GIP) receptor agonist. The benefits and risks of these medicines for weight loss in individuals who are not obese, or who are not overweight with weight-related co-morbidities, have not been studied.

Healthcare professionals should inform patients and carers upon initial prescription and at any dose increase about the common risk of gastro-intestinal side-effects (including nausea, vomiting, diarrhoea, and constipation) associated with GLP-1 receptor agonists; these are usually non-serious but can persist for several days and may lead to serious complications such as severe dehydration and kidney damage, resulting in hospitalisation. For this reason, patients should be advised to stay well hydrated by drinking plenty of fluids throughout treatment. They should also be informed of other serious but less common side-effects, including acute gallstone disease, pancreatitis, and serious allergic reactions. Healthcare professionals are advised that hypoglycaemia can occur in non-diabetic patients using liraglutide for weight management and therefore to ensure patients and carers know the signs and symptoms to be aware of, and to seek immediate medical attention if these occur.

Patients and carers should be advised to ensure that prescriptions are only obtained from registered healthcare professionals and that private prescriptions are dispensed from authorised sources to avoid the risk of receiving falsified pens (see also advice issued in November 2023, above). Patients and carers should consult the patient information leaflet for instructions on the use of GLP-1 receptor agonists, and be advised to only administer the prescribed dose.

MHRA/CHM ADVICE: GLP-1 AND DUAL GIP/GLP-1 RECEPTOR AGONISTS: POTENTIAL RISK OF PULMONARY ASPIRATION DURING GENERAL ANAESTHESIA OR DEEP SEDATION (JANUARY 2025)

An EU review has concluded that glucagon-like peptide-1 (GLP-1) and dual glucose-dependent insulinotropic polypeptide (GIP)/GLP-1 receptor agonists are associated with a potential risk of pulmonary aspiration in patients undergoing surgery or procedures requiring general anaesthesia or deep sedation. These medicines are known to slow gastric emptying, thereby increasing the risk of residual gastric contents despite preoperative fasting, which could lead to pulmonary aspiration and other severe complications, such as aspiration pneumonia.

The MHRA advises healthcare professionals to identify the increased risk of aspiration as early as possible, ideally at the pre-assessment clinic before surgery, in patients using GLP-1 or dual GIP/GLP-1 receptor agonists. Anaesthetists should complete an individualised preoperative risk assessment and consider the following:

- patients with underlying diabetic gastroparesis, as well as other co-morbidities such as obesity or gastroesophageal reflux disease, and symptoms of delayed gastric emptying (such as nausea, vomiting and abdominal pain) may have a higher risk of aspiration;
- directly asking patients or their carers about their use of GLP-1 or dual GIP/GLP-1 receptor agonists, as private prescriptions may not be included in the patient's medical notes or drug history, and patients who may have purchased these medications for use in aesthetic weight loss may not readily disclose this information (see also advice issued in October 2024, above).

There is limited evidence to support any recommendations on a time frame to withhold GLP-1 or dual GIP/GLP-1 receptor agonists prior to anaesthesia, new fasting guidelines, or an appropriate medical procedure to confirm an empty stomach. Anaesthetists should manage aspiration risk in line with usual anaesthetic practice and retain flexibility to provide individualised assessment.

Healthcare professionals should counsel patients or their carers to continue taking their prescribed medicines and not stop treatment without first discussing with their doctor. They should also be advised regarding the risk of aspiration and that there may be a need to modify pre-procedure instruction and anaesthetic technique.

MHRA/CHM ADVICE: GLP-1 RECEPTOR AGONISTS AND DUAL GLP-1/GIP RECEPTOR AGONISTS: STRENGTHENED WARNINGS ON ACUTE PANCREATITIS, INCLUDING NECROTISING AND FATAL CASES (JANUARY 2026)

Following rare reports of necrotising and fatal pancreatitis associated with glucagon-like peptide-1 (GLP-1) and dual GLP-1/glucose-dependent insulinotropic polypeptide (GIP) receptor agonists, healthcare professionals are advised to:

- remain vigilant to the risk, and signs and symptoms of acute pancreatitis;
- use these drugs with caution in patients with a history of pancreatitis;
- enquire about privately prescribed GLP-1 or dual GLP-1/GIP receptor agonists if a patient presents with suspected symptoms, as such use may not appear in their medical history;
- discontinue treatment immediately if pancreatitis is suspected, and not to restart treatment if confirmed;
- counsel patients or their carers to seek urgent medical attention if they develop persistent severe abdominal pain that may radiate to the back, and may be accompanied by nausea and vomiting.

● CONTRA-INDICATIONS

GENERAL CONTRA-INDICATIONS Diabetic gastroparesis · inflammatory bowel disease

SPECIFIC CONTRA-INDICATIONS

- ▸ **When used for Type 2 diabetes mellitus** Diabetic ketoacidosis
- ▸ **When used for Weight management** Obesity secondary to endocrinological or eating disorders
- ▸ **When used for Weight management** Concomitant use with other products for weight management

● CAUTIONS General anaesthesia or deep sedation (risk of pulmonary aspiration due to delayed gastric emptying) · history of pancreatitis · severe congestive heart failure (no information available) · thyroid disease

● INTERACTIONS → Appendix 1: glucagon-like peptide-1 receptor agonists

● SIDE-EFFECTS

- ▸ **Common or very common** Appetite decreased (in patients with type 2 diabetes) · asthenia · burping · constipation · diarrhoea · dizziness · dry mouth · gallbladder disorders · gastrointestinal discomfort · gastrointestinal disorders · headache · hypoglycaemia · increased risk of infection ·

insomnia · nausea · skin reactions · taste altered · toothache · vomiting
- **Uncommon** Dehydration · malaise · pancreatitis (discontinue) · renal impairment · tachycardia
- **Frequency not known** Angioedema · cutaneous amyloidosis · necrotising pancreatitis (discontinue) · pancreatitis acute (discontinue) · thyroid disorder

SIDE-EFFECTS, FURTHER INFORMATION Discontinue if symptoms of acute pancreatitis occur, such as persistent, severe abdominal pain; fatal cases reported. If pancreatitis confirmed, do not restart treatment.

- **PREGNANCY** EvGr Avoid (toxicity in *animal* studies) ⓜ (recommendation also supported by specialist sources).
- **BREAST FEEDING** Specialist sources indicate use with caution, especially if breast-feeding a neonate or preterm infant (no information available). Large molecular weight suggests limited excretion into milk and drug molecule likely to be partially destroyed in the infant's gastro-intestinal tract. Blood glucose monitoring of the infant should be considered.
- **HEPATIC IMPAIRMENT** EvGr Avoid in severe impairment (risk of decreased exposure). ⓜ
  - When used for Weight management EvGr Use with caution in mild to moderate impairment. ⓜ
- **RENAL IMPAIRMENT**
  - When used for Type 2 diabetes mellitus EvGr Avoid in end-stage renal disease (limited information available). ⓜ
  - When used for Weight management EvGr Avoid if creatinine clearance less than 30 mL/minute. ⓜ See p. 16.
- **DIRECTIONS FOR ADMINISTRATION** Inject into the abdomen, thigh, or upper arm; rotate injection site. Liraglutide pre-filled pen may be self-administered or administered by a carer after appropriate training in subcutaneous injection technique.
- **PRESCRIBING AND DISPENSING INFORMATION** Liraglutide is a biological medicine. Biological medicines must be prescribed and dispensed by brand name, see *Biological medicines* and *Biosimilar medicines*, under Guidance on prescribing p. 1; record the brand name and batch number after each administration.

  Licensed indications differ between preparations—further information can be found in the product literature for the individual preparations. *Diavic*® and *Zegluxen*® are licensed for the treatment of type 2 diabetes mellitus—for choice of therapy, see Type 2 diabetes p. 555. *Biolide*®, *Nevolat*®, and *Saxenda*® are licensed for weight management.
- **HANDLING AND STORAGE** Store in a refrigerator (2–8°C)—after first use can also be stored below 30°C and used within 1 month; keep cap on pen to protect from light.
- **PATIENT AND CARER ADVICE** Patients and their carers should be advised that glucagon-like peptide-1 (GLP-1) receptor agonists should only be used if they have been prescribed by a healthcare professional and should not be switched, including between brands containing the same GLP-1 receptor agonist, without prior consultation, in order to reduce the risk of adverse effects or loss of treatment efficacy. Patients and their carers should be given advice on how to administer liraglutide injection and when to discard it, including not attempting to extract any remaining medicine. Patients and their carers should be informed of the symptoms of cholelithiasis and cholecystitis, and of increased heart rate.

  Acute pancreatitis Patients and their carers should be told how to recognise signs and symptoms of acute pancreatitis and advised to seek immediate medical attention if symptoms such as persistent, severe abdominal pain develop.

  Dehydration Patients and their carers should be informed of the potential risk of dehydration in relation to gastro-intestinal side-effects and advised to take precautions to avoid fluid depletion.

  Information for patients The MHRA has produced guidance for patients on GLP-1 medicines for weight loss and diabetes: www.gov.uk/government/publications/glp-1-medicines-for-weight-loss-and-diabetes-what-you-need-to-know/glp-1-medicines-for-weight-loss-and-diabetes-what-you-need-to-know.

  Missed doses
  - When used for Weight management If a dose is more than 12 hours late, the missed dose should not be administered and the next dose should be administered at the normal time.

  Driving and skilled tasks
  - When used for Weight management Patients and their carers should be cautioned on the effects of driving and performance of skilled tasks—increased risk of dizziness, particularly during first 3 months of treatment.
- **MEDICINAL FORMS** There can be variation in the licensing of different medicines containing the same drug.

Solution for injection

EXCIPIENTS: May contain Propylene glycol

- **Liraglutide (Non-proprietary)**
  Liraglutide 6 mg per 1 ml Liraglutide 6mg/ml solution for injection 3ml pre-filled disposable devices | 2 pre-filled disposable injection PoM £50.49–£51.00 DT = £50.49 | 3 pre-filled disposable injection PoM £75.74–£76.50
- **Biolide** (Biocon Pharma UK Ltd)
  Liraglutide 6 mg per 1 ml Biolide 6mg/ml solution for injection 3ml pre-filled pens | 3 pre-filled disposable injection PoM £76.50 | 5 pre-filled disposable injection PoM £127.50
- **Diavic** (Sun Pharma UK Ltd)
  Liraglutide 6 mg per 1 ml Diavic 6mg/ml solution for injection 3ml pre-filled pens | 2 pre-filled disposable injection PoM £50.49 DT = £50.49 | 3 pre-filled disposable injection PoM £76.00
- **Nevolat** (Zentiva Pharma UK Ltd)
  Liraglutide 6 mg per 1 ml Nevolat 6mg/ml solution for injection 3ml pre-filled pens | 3 pre-filled disposable injection PoM £76.52 | 5 pre-filled disposable injection PoM £127.53
- **Plaobes** (Cipla EU Ltd)
  Liraglutide 6 mg per 1 ml Plaobes 6mg/ml solution for injection 3ml pre-filled pens | 3 pre-filled disposable injection PoM £76.26 | 5 pre-filled disposable injection PoM £127.10
- **Saxenda** (Novo Nordisk Ltd)
  Liraglutide 6 mg per 1 ml Saxenda 6mg/ml solution for injection 3ml pre-filled pens | 5 pre-filled disposable injection PoM £196.20
- **Zegluxen** (Zentiva Pharma UK Ltd)
  Liraglutide 6 mg per 1 ml Zegluxen 6mg/ml solution for injection 3ml pre-filled pens | 2 pre-filled disposable injection PoM £50.49 DT = £50.49 | 3 pre-filled disposable injection PoM £75.52

BLOOD GLUCOSE LOWERING DRUGS > SODIUM GLUCOSE CO-TRANSPORTER 2 INHIBITORS

Dapagliflozin

24-Jul-2025

- **DRUG ACTION** Reversibly inhibits sodium-glucose co-transporter 2 (SGLT2) in the renal proximal convoluted tubule to reduce glucose reabsorption and increase urinary glucose excretion.

- **INDICATIONS AND DOSE**

Type 2 diabetes mellitus [as monotherapy if metformin inappropriate] | Type 2 diabetes mellitus [in combination with insulin or other antidiabetic drugs]

- BY MOUTH
  - Child 10–17 years: 10 mg once daily

DOSE ADJUSTMENTS DUE TO INTERACTIONS
- Dose of concomitant insulin or drugs that stimulate insulin secretion may need to be reduced (risk of hypoglycaemia)—consult product literature.

IMPORTANT SAFETY INFORMATION

MHRA/CHM ADVICE (UPDATED APRIL 2016): RISK OF DIABETIC KETOACIDOSIS WITH SODIUM-GLUCOSE CO-TRANSPORTER 2 (SGLT2) INHIBITORS (CANAGLIFLOZIN, DAPAGLIFLOZIN OR EMPAGLIFLOZIN)

A review by the European Medicines Agency has concluded that serious, life-threatening, and fatal cases of diabetic ketoacidosis (DKA) have been reported rarely in patients taking an SGLT2 inhibitor. In several cases, the presentation of DKA was atypical with patients having only moderately elevated blood glucose levels, and some of them occurred during off-label use.

To minimise the risk of such effects when treating patients with a SGLT2 inhibitor, the European Medicines Agency has issued the following advice:

- inform patients of the signs and symptoms of DKA, (including rapid weight loss, nausea or vomiting, abdominal pain, fast and deep breathing, sleepiness, a sweet smell to the breath, a sweet or metallic taste in the mouth, or a different odour to urine or sweat), and advise them to seek immediate medical advice if they develop any of these
- test for raised ketones in patients with signs and symptoms of DKA, even if plasma glucose levels are near-normal
- use dapagliflozin with caution in patients with risk factors for DKA, (including a low beta cell reserve, conditions leading to restricted food intake or severe dehydration, sudden reduction in insulin, increased insulin requirements due to acute illness, surgery or alcohol abuse), and discuss these risk factors with patients
- discontinue treatment if DKA is suspected or diagnosed
- do not restart treatment with any SGLT2 inhibitor in patients who experienced DKA during use, unless another cause for DKA was identified and resolved
- interrupt SGLT2 inhibitor treatment in patients who are hospitalised for major surgery or acute serious illnesses; treatment may be restarted once the patient's condition has stabilised

MHRA/CHM ADVICE: SGLT2 INHIBITORS: MONITOR KETONES IN BLOOD DURING TREATMENT INTERRUPTION FOR SURGICAL PROCEDURES OR ACUTE SERIOUS MEDICAL ILLNESS (MARCH 2020)

New recommendations have been issued following a European review of peri-operative diabetic ketoacidosis in patients taking SGLT2 inhibitors. Healthcare professionals are advised to monitor ketone levels during SGLT2 inhibitor treatment interruption in patients who have been hospitalised for major surgery or acute serious illness—measurement of blood ketone levels is preferred to urine. Treatment may be restarted once ketone levels are normal and the patient's condition has stabilised.

MHRA/CHM ADVICE: SGLT2 INHIBITORS: REPORTS OF FOURNIER'S GANGRENE (NECROTISING FASCIITIS OF THE GENITALIA OR PERINEUM) (FEBRUARY 2019)

Fournier's gangrene, a rare but serious and potentially life-threatening infection, has been associated with the use of sodium-glucose co-transporter 2 (SGLT2) inhibitors. If Fournier's gangrene is suspected, stop the SGLT2 inhibitor and urgently start treatment (including antibiotics and surgical debridement).

Patients should be advised to seek urgent medical attention if they experience severe pain, tenderness, erythema, or swelling in the genital or perineal area, accompanied by fever or malaise—urogenital infection or perineal abscess may precede necrotising fasciitis.

MHRA/CHM ADVICE: *FORXIGA*® (DAPAGLIFLOZIN) 5 MG SHOULD NO LONGER BE USED FOR THE TREATMENT OF TYPE 1 DIABETES MELLITUS (NOVEMBER 2021)

Dapagliflozin 5 mg is no longer authorised for the treatment of patients with type 1 diabetes mellitus (T1DM) and should no longer be used in this population. Discontinuation of dapagliflozin in patients with T1DM must be made by or in consultation with a physician specialised in diabetes care as soon as clinically practical. After stopping dapagliflozin, frequent blood glucose monitoring is recommended, and the insulin dose should be increased carefully to minimise the risk of hypoglycaemia.

- **CONTRA-INDICATIONS** Diabetic ketoacidosis · type 1 diabetes mellitus (increased risk of diabetic ketoacidosis)
- **CAUTIONS** Hypotension · risk of volume depletion

CAUTIONS, FURTHER INFORMATION
- Volume depletion Correct hypovolaemia before starting treatment.

- **INTERACTIONS** → Appendix 1: sodium glucose co-transporter 2 inhibitors
- **SIDE-EFFECTS**
  - **Common or very common** Back pain · balanoposthitis · cystitis · dizziness · dyslipidaemia · hypoglycaemia (in combination with insulin or sulfonylurea) · increased risk of infection · prostatitis · skin reactions · urinary disorders · vulvovaginal disorders
  - **Uncommon** Constipation · dry mouth · fluid imbalance · genital pruritus · hypotension · thirst · weight decreased
  - **Rare or very rare** Angioedema · diabetic ketoacidosis (discontinue immediately) · Fournier's gangrene (discontinue and initiate treatment promptly) · nephritis tubulointerstitial

SIDE-EFFECTS, FURTHER INFORMATION **Volume depletion** Interrupt treatment if volume depletion occurs.

Urinary tract infections Urinary glucose excretion may be associated with an increased risk of urinary tract infection. Consider temporarily interrupting treatment with dapagliflozin when treating pyelonephritis or urosepsis.

Renal function changes Creatinine levels may increase during initial treatment. These increases in creatinine are generally transient with continued treatment or reversible after stopping treatment.

- **PREGNANCY** Avoid—toxicity in *animal* studies.
- **BREAST FEEDING** Avoid—present in milk in *animal* studies.
- **HEPATIC IMPAIRMENT** EvGr Caution in severe impairment (risk of increased exposure; limited information available). (M)

Dose adjustments EvGr Initially 5 mg daily in severe impairment, increased if tolerated to 10 mg daily. (M)

- **RENAL IMPAIRMENT** See p. 16. EvGr Avoid initiation if estimated glomerular filtration rate less than 15 mL/minute/1.73 m^2.

Consider additional antidiabetic drugs with dapagliflozin if estimated glomerular filtration rate less than 45 mL/minute/1.73 m^2 (reduced efficacy). (M)

- **PATIENT AND CARER ADVICE** Patients should be informed of the signs and symptoms of diabetic ketoacidosis, see MHRA advice.

- **MEDICINAL FORMS** There can be variation in the licensing of different medicines containing the same drug.

Oral tablet
- **Dapagliflozin (Non-proprietary)**

Dapagliflozin (as Dapagliflozin propanediol monohydrate)
5 mg Dapagliflozin 5mg tablets | 28 tablet PoM £36.59 DT = £5.21

Dapagliflozin (as Dapagliflozin propanediol monohydrate)
10 mg Dapagliflozin 10mg tablets | 28 tablet PoM £36.59 DT = £4.10

▸ **Forxiga** (AstraZeneca UK Ltd)
Dapagliflozin (as Dapagliflozin propanediol monohydrate)
5 mg Forxiga 5mg tablets | 28 tablet PoM £36.59 DT = £5.21
Dapagliflozin (as Dapagliflozin propanediol monohydrate)
10 mg Forxiga 10mg tablets | 28 tablet PoM £36.59 DT = £4.10

BLOOD GLUCOSE LOWERING DRUGS › SULFONYLUREAS

Sulfonylureas

- **DRUG ACTION** The sulfonylureas act mainly by augmenting insulin secretion and consequently are effective only when some residual pancreatic beta-cell activity is present; during long-term administration they also have an extrapancreatic action.
- **CONTRA-INDICATIONS** Presence of ketoacidosis
- **CAUTIONS** Can encourage weight gain · G6PD deficiency
- **SIDE-EFFECTS**
  - **Common or very common** Abdominal pain · diarrhoea · hypoglycaemia · nausea · vomiting
  - **Uncommon** Hepatic disorders
  - **Rare or very rare** Agranulocytosis · erythropenia · granulocytopenia · haemolytic anaemia · leucopenia · pancytopenia · thrombocytopenia
  - **Frequency not known** Allergic dermatitis (usually in the first 6–8 weeks of therapy) · constipation · photosensitivity reaction · skin reactions · visual impairment
- **HEPATIC IMPAIRMENT** In general, manufacturers advise avoid in severe impairment (increased risk of hypoglycaemia).
- **RENAL IMPAIRMENT** Sulfonylureas should be used with care in those with mild to moderate renal impairment, because of the hazard of hypoglycaemia. Care is required to use the lowest dose that adequately controls blood glucose. Avoid where possible in severe renal impairment.
- **PATIENT AND CARER ADVICE**
  Driving and skilled tasks Drivers need to be particularly careful to avoid hypoglycaemia and should be warned of the problems.

above

Glibenclamide

22-Apr-2021

- **INDICATIONS AND DOSE**

Neonatal diabetes mellitus (initiated by a specialist)

▸ BY MOUTH USING ORAL SUSPENSION

▸ Neonate: Initially 0.2 mg/kg daily in 2 divided doses, before feeding, increase dose according to product literature; usual maintenance 0.2–0.5 mg/kg daily in 2–4 divided doses, oral suspension is available in 2 different strengths and contains sodium benzoate—see *Prescribing and dispensing information* for information regarding the maximum volume per day.

▸ Child: Initially 0.2 mg/kg daily in 2 divided doses, before feeding, increase dose according to product literature; usual maintenance 0.2–0.5 mg/kg daily in 2–4 divided doses, oral suspension is available in 2 different strengths and contains sodium benzoate—see *Prescribing and dispensing information* for information regarding the maximum volume per day

- **CONTRA-INDICATIONS** Avoid where possible in Acute porphyrias p. 745
- **INTERACTIONS** → Appendix 1: sulfonylureas
- **SIDE-EFFECTS**
  - **Common or very common** Dyspepsia · neutropenia · tooth discolouration
  - **Frequency not known** Bone marrow depression · hypereosinophilia · vision disorders
- **HEPATIC IMPAIRMENT** EvGr Caution in mild or moderate impairment. Ⓜ
  Dose adjustments EvGr In mild or moderate impairment, use the lowest dose that adequately controls blood glucose. Ⓜ
- **PRESCRIBING AND DISPENSING INFORMATION** Care is required when prescribing and dispensing glibenclamide oral suspension as 2 different strengths are available. The prescriber must state the strength of the oral suspension to be used.
  Glibenclamide oral suspension contains sodium benzoate, and the maximum volume that can be given is 1 mL/kg per day, regardless of the strength of the suspension. If the calculated daily dose exceeds this maximum volume using the lower-strength suspension, the higher-strength suspension must be used to administer the dose—consult product literature.
- **MEDICINAL FORMS** There can be variation in the licensing of different medicines containing the same drug. Forms available from special-order manufacturers include: oral suspension

Oral suspension

ELECTROLYTES: May contain Sodium

▸ **Amglidia** (Bioprojet UK Ltd)
Glibenclamide 600 microgram per 1 ml Amglidia 0.6mg/ml oral suspension with 1ml oral syringe | 30 ml PoM £882.00 (Hospital only) SF

above

Gliclazide

17-Mar-2025

- **INDICATIONS AND DOSE**

Type 2 diabetes mellitus

▸ BY MOUTH USING IMMEDIATE-RELEASE MEDICINES

▸ Child 12–17 years: Initially 20 mg once daily, dose to be taken with breakfast, increased if necessary up to 160 mg 1–2 times a day, dose to be adjusted according to response

Maturity-onset diabetes of the young (specialist use only)

▸ BY MOUTH USING IMMEDIATE-RELEASE MEDICINES

▸ Child 12–17 years: Initially 20 mg once daily, dose to be taken with breakfast, increased if necessary up to 160 mg 1–2 times a day, dose to be adjusted according to response

- **UNLICENSED USE** Not licensed for use in children.
- **CONTRA-INDICATIONS** Avoid where possible in Acute porphyrias p. 745
- **INTERACTIONS** → Appendix 1: sulfonylureas
- **SIDE-EFFECTS** Anaemia · angioedema · dyspepsia · gastrointestinal disorder · hypersensitivity vasculitis · hyponatraemia · severe cutaneous adverse reactions (SCARs)
- **PREGNANCY** The use of sulfonylureas in pregnancy should generally be avoided because of the risk of neonatal hypoglycaemia.
- **BREAST FEEDING** Avoid—theoretical possibility of hypoglycaemia in the infant.
- **RENAL IMPAIRMENT** If necessary, gliclazide which is principally metabolised in the liver, can be used in renal impairment but careful monitoring of blood-glucose concentration is essential.

- **PATIENT AND CARER ADVICE**
Medicines for Children leaflet: Gliclazide for type 2 diabetes mellitus and maturity-onset diabetes of the young
www.medicinesforchildren.org.uk/medicines/gliclazide-for-type-2-diabetes-mellitus-and-maturity-onset-diabetes-of-the-young/

- **MEDICINAL FORMS** There can be variation in the licensing of different medicines containing the same drug. Forms available from special-order manufacturers include: oral suspension

Oral tablet

CAUTIONARY AND ADVISORY LABELS 21

▸ **Gliclazide (Non-proprietary)**
Gliclazide 40 mg Gliclazide 40mg tablets | 28 tablet PoM £3.36 DT = £0.75
Gliclazide 80 mg Gliclazide 80mg tablets | 28 tablet PoM £3.75 DT = £0.71 | 60 tablet PoM £0.81–£1.85

▸ **Glydex** (Medreich Plc)
Gliclazide 160 mg Glydex 160mg tablets | 28 tablet PoM £15.00 DT = £15.00

▸ **Zicron** (Bristol Laboratories Ltd)
Gliclazide 40 mg Zicron 40mg tablets | 28 tablet PoM £3.36 DT = £0.75

F 566

Tolbutamide

- **INDICATIONS AND DOSE**

Type 2 diabetes mellitus

▶ BY MOUTH
▸ Child 12–17 years (specialist use only): 0.5–1.5 g daily in divided doses, dose to be taken with or immediately after meals, alternatively 0.5–1.5 g once daily, dose to be taken with or immediately after breakfast; maximum 2 g per day

- **UNLICENSED USE** Not licensed for use in children.
- **CONTRA-INDICATIONS** Avoid where possible in Acute porphyrias p. 745
- **INTERACTIONS** → Appendix 1: sulfonylureas
- **SIDE-EFFECTS**
▶ **Rare or very rare** Aplastic anaemia · blood disorder
▶ **Frequency not known** Alcohol intolerance · appetite abnormal · erythema multiforme (usually in the first 6–8 weeks of therapy) · exfoliative dermatitis (usually in the first 6–8 weeks of therapy) · fever (usually in the first 6–8 weeks of therapy) · headache · hypersensitivity (usually in the first 6–8 weeks of therapy) · paraesthesia · tinnitus · weight increased
- **PREGNANCY** The use of sulfonylureas in pregnancy should generally be avoided because of the risk of neonatal hypoglycaemia.
- **BREAST FEEDING** The use of sulfonylureas in breast-feeding should be avoided because there is a theoretical possibility of hypoglycaemia in the infant.
- **RENAL IMPAIRMENT** If necessary, the short-acting drug tolbutamide can be used in renal impairment but careful monitoring of blood-glucose concentration is essential.

- **MEDICINAL FORMS** There can be variation in the licensing of different medicines containing the same drug. Forms available from special-order manufacturers include: oral suspension

Oral tablet

▸ **Tolbutamide (Non-proprietary)**
Tolbutamide 500 mg Tolbutamide 500mg tablets | 28 tablet PoM £120.00 DT = £84.00

DISEASE-MODIFYING ANTIDIABETIC DRUGS

Teplizumab

07-Oct-2025

- **DRUG ACTION** Teplizumab is a humanised monoclonal antibody that binds to CD3 antigens on T-lymphocytes, thereby limiting the autoimmune destruction and preserving the function of pancreatic islet insulin-producing beta cells.

- **INDICATIONS AND DOSE**

Type 1 diabetes mellitus [to delay onset of stage 3 in those with stage 2 disease]

▶ BY INTRAVENOUS INFUSION
▸ Child 8–17 years: 65 micrograms/m^2 once daily on day 1, then 125 micrograms/m^2 once daily on day 2, then 250 micrograms/m^2 once daily on day 3, then 500 micrograms/m^2 once daily on day 4, then 1030 micrograms/m^2 once daily on days 5–14

- **CONTRA-INDICATIONS** Absolute neutrophil count less than 1×10^9 cells/litre in patients of African descent or less than 1.5×10^9 cells/litre in all other groups (do not initiate) · active serious infection except localised skin infections (do not initiate) · chronic active infection except localised skin infections (do not initiate) · elevated alanine aminotransferase (ALT) exceeding 2 times the upper limit of normal (do not initiate) · elevated aspartate aminotransferase (AST) exceeding 2 times the upper limit of normal (do not initiate) · elevated bilirubin exceeding 1.5 times the upper limit of normal (do not initiate) · evidence of acute cytomegalovirus infection (do not initiate) · evidence of acute Epstein-Barr virus infection (do not initiate) · haemoglobin less than 10 g/dL (do not initiate) · lymphocyte count less than 1×10^9 cells/litre (do not initiate) · platelet count less than 150×10^9 cells/litre (do not initiate)

CONTRA-INDICATIONS, FURTHER INFORMATION
▸ Vaccination against infection EvGr To reduce the risk of infection, patients should receive all recommended vaccinations prior to initiation; teplizumab treatment may also interfere with the immune response and decrease vaccine efficacy. Live attenuated vaccines are not recommended within the 8 weeks before starting, during, or up to 52 weeks after, treatment (safety of immunisation during treatment unknown). Inactivated or mRNA vaccines are not recommended within the 2 weeks before starting, during, or 6 weeks after, treatment. (M)

- **CAUTIONS** Risk of cytokine release syndrome

CAUTIONS, FURTHER INFORMATION
▸ Cytokine release syndrome (CRS) EvGr To mitigate CRS, patients should be premedicated with an NSAID or paracetamol, an antihistamine, and, if needed, an antiemetic for the first 5 days of treatment; additional doses of premedication may be given as required. If severe CRS develops, consider temporarily interrupting treatment for 1–2 days or discontinuing treatment—consult product literature. (M)

- **INTERACTIONS** → Appendix 1: monoclonal antibodies
- **SIDE-EFFECTS**
▶ **Common or very common** Chills · cytokine release syndrome · diarrhoea · fever · headache · increased risk of infection · leucopenia · lymphopenia (discontinue if severe and prolonged) · nausea · neutropenia · skin reactions · thrombocytopenia
▶ **Frequency not known** Abscess · fatigue · hypersensitivity · illness · pain · sepsis · vomiting

SIDE-EFFECTS, FURTHER INFORMATION Manufacturer advises discontinue treatment if transaminase levels more than 5 times the upper limit of normal or blood bilirubin more than 3 times the upper limit of normal—consult product literature.

- **PREGNANCY** EvGr Avoid use during, and for at least 30 days before planned, pregnancy (limited information available). (M)
- **BREAST FEEDING** Specialist sources indicate use with caution (no information available). Large molecular weight suggests limited excretion into milk and drug molecule likely to be partially destroyed in the infant's gastro-intestinal tract; waiting for at least 2 weeks postpartum to resume treatment may minimise transfer to infant.
- **MONITORING REQUIREMENTS**
  - EvGr Monitor for signs and symptoms of infection during and after treatment—discontinue treatment if serious infection develops.
  - A full blood count should be performed prior to initiation; monitor white blood cell count during treatment—discontinue treatment if lymphocyte count is less than 0.5×10^9 cells/litre for 1 week or longer.
  - Liver enzyme tests should be performed prior to initiation and monitored during treatment—discontinue treatment if alanine aminotransferase (ALT) or aspartate aminotransferase (AST) exceeds 5 times the upper limit of normal (ULN) or bilirubin exceeds 3 times the ULN. (M)
- **DIRECTIONS FOR ADMINISTRATION** For *intermittent intravenous infusion* (*Tzield®*), dilute to an initial concentration of 100 micrograms/mL with Sodium Chloride 0.9% then dilute requisite dose with 25 mL of Sodium Chloride 0.9%; give over 30 minutes—consult product literature.

  Missed doses If a dose is missed, resume dosing by administering all remaining doses on consecutive days to complete the 14-day treatment course.
- **PRESCRIBING AND DISPENSING INFORMATION** The manufacturer of *Tzield®* has provided a *Guide for Healthcare Professionals*.
- **HANDLING AND STORAGE** Store in a refrigerator (2–8°C) and protect from light—consult product literature for storage conditions after dilution.
- **PATIENT AND CARER ADVICE**

  Risk minimisation materials A patient guide should be provided.

  Driving and skilled tasks Patients and carers should be cautioned on the effects on driving and performance of skilled tasks—increased risk of fatigue.

- **MEDICINAL FORMS** There can be variation in the licensing of different medicines containing the same drug.

Solution for infusion

EXCIPIENTS: May contain Polysorbates

- **Tzield** (Sanofi) ▼

  Teplizumab 1 mg per 1 ml Tzield 2mg/2ml concentrate for solution for infusion vials | 1 vial PoM £10,939.12 (Hospital only)

INSULINS

Insulins

IMPORTANT SAFETY INFORMATION

NHS ENGLAND PATIENT SAFETY ALERT: RISK OF SEVERE HARM AND DEATH DUE TO WITHDRAWING INSULIN FROM PEN DEVICES (NOVEMBER 2016)

Insulin should not be extracted from insulin pen devices.

The strength of insulin in pen devices can vary by multiples of 100 units/mL. Insulin syringes have graduations only suitable for calculating doses of standard 100 units/mL. If insulin extracted from a pen or cartridge is of a higher strength, and that is not considered in determining the volume required, it can lead to a significant and potentially fatal overdose.

NHS NEVER EVENT: OVERDOSE OF INSULIN DUE TO ABBREVIATIONS OR INCORRECT DEVICE (JANUARY 2018)

The words 'unit' or 'international units' should **not** be abbreviated.

Specific insulin administration devices should always be used to measure insulin i.e. insulin syringes and pens.

Insulin should **not** be withdrawn from an insulin pen or pen refill and then administered using a syringe and needle.

HEALTH SERVICES SAFETY INVESTIGATIONS BODY (HSSIB) PATIENT SAFETY INVESTIGATIONS: ADMINISTERING HIGH-STRENGTH INSULIN FROM A PEN DEVICE IN HOSPITAL (JULY 2022)

A review of an accidental overdose of high-strength insulin, leading to hypoglycaemia, identified that high-strength insulin was extracted from an insulin pen device using an insulin syringe. To reduce the risk of similar incidents occurring, the HSSIB has issued advice: www.hssib.org.uk/patient-safety-investigations/administering-high-strength-insulin-from-a-pen-device-in-hospital/.

MHRA/CHM ADVICE: INSULINS (ALL TYPES): RISK OF CUTANEOUS AMYLOIDOSIS AT INJECTION SITE (SEPTEMBER 2020)

A European review concluded that injection of insulin (all types) can lead to deposits of amyloid protein under the skin (cutaneous amyloidosis) at the injection site. Insulin-derived cutaneous amyloidosis interferes with insulin absorption, and administration of insulin at an affected site may affect glycaemic control. The MHRA advises healthcare professionals should consider cutaneous amyloidosis as a differential diagnosis to lipodystrophy when patients present with subcutaneous lumps at an insulin injection site. Patients should be reminded to rotate injection sites within the same body region to reduce or prevent the risk of cutaneous amyloidosis and other skin reactions. Patients should also be advised that injecting into an affected 'lumpy' area may reduce the effectiveness of insulin. Those currently injecting into a 'lumpy' area should contact their doctor before changing injection site due to the risk of hypoglycaemia; blood glucose should be closely monitored after changing injection site, and dose adjustment of insulin or other antidiabetic medication may be required.

- **SIDE-EFFECTS**
  - **Common or very common** Oedema
  - **Uncommon** Lipodystrophy
  - **Frequency not known** Cutaneous amyloidosis

  Overdose Overdose causes hypoglycaemia.
- **PREGNANCY**

  Dose adjustments During pregnancy, insulin requirements may alter and doses should be assessed frequently by an experienced diabetes physician.

  The dose of insulin generally needs to be increased in the second and third trimesters of pregnancy.
- **BREAST FEEDING**

  Dose adjustments During breast-feeding, insulin requirements may alter and doses should be assessed frequently by an experienced diabetes physician.
- **HEPATIC IMPAIRMENT** Insulin requirements may be decreased.
- **RENAL IMPAIRMENT** The compensatory response to hypoglycaemia is impaired in renal impairment.

  Dose adjustments EvGr Insulin requirements may decrease in patients with renal impairment and therefore dose reduction may be necessary. (M)
- **MONITORING REQUIREMENTS**
  - Many patients now monitor their own blood-glucose concentrations; all carers and children need to be trained to do this.

- Since blood-glucose concentration varies substantially throughout the day, 'normoglycaemia' cannot always be achieved throughout a 24-hour period without causing damaging hypoglycaemia.
- It is therefore best to recommend that patients should maintain a blood-glucose concentration of between 4 and 9 mmol/litre for most of the time (4–7 mmol/litre before meals and less than 9 mmol/litre after meals).
- While accepting that on occasions, for brief periods, the blood-glucose concentration will be above these values; strenuous efforts should be made to prevent it from falling below 4 mmol/litre. Patients using multiple injection regimens should understand how to adjust their insulin dose according to their carbohydrate intake. With fixed-dose insulin regimens, the carbohydrate intake needs to be regulated, and should be distributed throughout the day to match the insulin regimen. The intake of energy and of simple and complex carbohydrates should be adequate to allow normal growth and development but obesity must be avoided.

● **DIRECTIONS FOR ADMINISTRATION** Insulin is generally given by *subcutaneous injection*; the injection site should be rotated to prevent lipodystrophy and cutaneous amyloidosis. Injection devices ('pens'), which hold the insulin in a cartridge and meter the required dose, are convenient to use. Insulin syringes (for use with needles) are required for insulins not available in cartridge form, but are less popular with children and carers.

● **PRESCRIBING AND DISPENSING INFORMATION** Insulins must be prescribed and dispensed by brand name.

Show container to patient or carer and confirm the expected version is dispensed.

Units The word 'unit' should **not** be abbreviated.

● **PATIENT AND CARER ADVICE**

Hypoglycaemia Hypoglycaemia is a potential problem with insulin therapy. All patients must be carefully instructed on how to avoid it; this involves appropriate adjustment of insulin type, dose and frequency together with suitable timing and quantity of meals and snacks.

Insulin Passport Insulin Passports and patient information booklets should be offered to patients receiving insulin. The Insulin Passport provides a record of the patient's current insulin preparations and contains a section for emergency information. The patient information booklet provides advice on the safe use of insulin. They are available for purchase from:

3M Security Print and Systems Limited
Gorse Street, Chadderton
Oldham
OL9 9QH
Tel: 0845 610 1112

GP practices can obtain supplies through their Local Area Team stores.

NHS Trusts can order supplies from cmswebshop.corp.xerox.com/NHS/Login.aspx. Further information is available at www.england.nhs.uk/improvement-hub/wp-content/uploads/sites/44/2017/11/Safe-use-of-insulin-and-you-patient-info-booklet.pdf.

Driving and skilled tasks Drivers need to be particularly careful to avoid hypoglycaemia and should be warned of the problems.

INSULINS › RAPID-ACTING

568

Insulin

26-Feb-2025

(Neutral Insulin; Soluble Insulin)

● **DRUG ACTION** Soluble insulin is a natural or recombinant insulin with a short duration of action.

● **INDICATIONS AND DOSE**

Diabetes mellitus
- BY SUBCUTANEOUS INJECTION
  - Child: According to requirements

Hyperglycaemia during illness
- BY INTRAVENOUS INFUSION
  - Neonate: 0.02–0.125 unit/kg/hour, dose to be adjusted according to blood-glucose concentration.
  - Child: 0.025–0.1 unit/kg/hour, dose to be adjusted according to blood-glucose concentration

Neonatal hyperglycaemia | Neonatal diabetes
- BY INTRAVENOUS INFUSION
  - Neonate: 0.02–0.125 unit/kg/hour, dose to be adjusted according to blood-glucose concentration.

Diabetic ketoacidosis | Diabetes during surgery
- BY INTRAVENOUS INFUSION
  - Child: (consult local protocol)

● **INTERACTIONS** → Appendix 1: insulin

● **SIDE-EFFECTS**
- **Uncommon** Skin reactions
- **Rare or very rare** Refraction disorder

● **DIRECTIONS FOR ADMINISTRATION** Short-acting injectable insulins can be given by continuous subcutaneous infusion using a portable infusion pump. This device delivers a continuous basal insulin infusion and patient-activated bolus doses at meal times. This technique can be useful for patients who suffer recurrent hypoglycaemia or marked morning rise in blood-glucose concentration despite optimised multiple-injection regimens. Patients on subcutaneous insulin infusion must be highly motivated, able to monitor their blood-glucose concentration, and have expert training, advice and supervision from an experienced healthcare team. Some insulin preparations are not recommended for use in subcutaneous insulin infusion pumps—may precipitate in catheter or needle—consult product literature.
- With intravenous use For *intravenous infusion*, dilute to a concentration of 1 unit/mL with Sodium Chloride 0.9% and mix thoroughly; insulin may be adsorbed by plastics, flush giving set with 5 mL of infusion fluid containing insulin. *For intravenous infusion in neonatal intensive care*, dilute 5 units to a final volume of 50 mL with Sodium Chloride 0.9% and mix thoroughly; an intravenous infusion rate of 0.1 mL/kg/hour provides a dose of 0.01 units/kg/hour.

● **PRESCRIBING AND DISPENSING INFORMATION** A sterile solution of insulin (i.e. bovine or porcine) or of human insulin; pH 6.6–8.0.

● **NATIONAL FUNDING/ACCESS DECISIONS**
For full details see funding body website

NICE decisions
- **Continuous subcutaneous insulin infusion for the treatment of diabetes mellitus (type 1) (July 2008)** NICE TA151
  Recommended
- **Hybrid closed loop systems for managing blood glucose levels in type 1 diabetes (December 2023)** NICE TA943
  Recommended

● **MEDICINAL FORMS** There can be variation in the licensing of different medicines containing the same drug. Forms available from special-order manufacturers include: solution for injection, solution for infusion

Solution for injection

▸ **Insulin (Non-proprietary)**

Insulin human 500 unit per 1 ml Humulin R 500units/ml solution for injection 20ml vials | 1 vial PoM

Humulin R KwikPen 500units/ml solution for injection 3ml pre-filled pens | 2 pre-filled disposable injection PoM

▸ **Actrapid** (Novo Nordisk Ltd)

Insulin human (as Insulin soluble human) 100 unit per 1 ml Actrapid 100units/ml solution for injection 10ml vials | 1 vial PoM £7.48 DT = £15.68

▸ **Humulin S** (Eli Lilly and Company Ltd)

Insulin human (as Insulin soluble human) 100 unit per 1 ml Humulin S 100units/ml solution for injection 10ml vials | 1 vial PoM £15.68 DT = £15.68

Humulin S 100units/ml solution for injection 3ml cartridges | 5 cartridge PoM £19.08 DT = £19.08

▸ **Hypurin Porcine Neutral** (C P Pharmaceuticals Ltd)

Insulin porcine (as Insulin soluble porcine) 100 unit per 1 ml Hypurin Porcine Neutral 100units/ml solution for injection 3ml cartridges | 5 cartridge PoM £59.08 DT = £59.08

Combinations available: ***Biphasic insulin aspart***, p. 572 · ***Biphasic insulin lispro***, p. 572 · ***Biphasic isophane insulin***, p. 571 · ***Insulin degludec***, p. 573 · ***Insulin detemir***, p. 573 · ***Insulin glargine***, p. 573 · ***Isophane insulin***, p. 572

F 568

Insulin aspart

26-Feb-2025

● **DRUG ACTION** Insulin aspart is a recombinant human insulin analogue with a rapid onset and short duration of action.

● **INDICATIONS AND DOSE**

FIASP®

Diabetes mellitus

▸ BY SUBCUTANEOUS INJECTION

▸ Child 1–17 years: Administer immediately before meals or when necessary shortly after meals, according to requirements

▸ BY SUBCUTANEOUS INFUSION, OR BY INTRAVENOUS INFUSION

▸ Child 1–17 years: According to requirements

NOVORAPID®

Diabetes mellitus

▸ BY SUBCUTANEOUS INJECTION

▸ Child: Administer immediately before meals or when necessary shortly after meals, according to requirements

▸ BY SUBCUTANEOUS INFUSION, OR BY INTRAVENOUS INFUSION

▸ Child: According to requirements

PHARMACOKINETICS

▸ *Fiasp*® and *NovoRapid*® are **not** interchangeable due to differences in bioavailability; *Fiasp*® has a quicker onset of action and shorter duration.

● **UNLICENSED USE** Not licensed for use in children under 1 year.

● **INTERACTIONS** → Appendix 1: insulin

● **SIDE-EFFECTS**

▸ **Common or very common** Skin reactions

▸ **Uncommon** Refraction disorder

● **PREGNANCY** Not known to be harmful—may be used during pregnancy.

● **BREAST FEEDING** Not known to be harmful—may be used during lactation.

● **DIRECTIONS FOR ADMINISTRATION** Short-acting injectable insulins can be given by continuous subcutaneous infusion using a portable infusion pump. This device delivers a continuous basal insulin infusion and patient-activated bolus doses at meal times. This technique can be useful for patients who suffer recurrent hypoglycaemia or marked morning rise in blood-glucose concentration despite optimised multiple-injection regimens. Patients on subcutaneous insulin infusion must be highly motivated, able to monitor their blood-glucose concentration, and have expert training, advice and supervision from an experienced healthcare team.

Manufacturer advises for *intravenous infusion* of *Fiasp*®, give continuously in Glucose 5% or Sodium Chloride 0.9%; dilute to 0.5–1 unit/mL with infusion fluid.

Manufacturer advises for *intravenous infusion* of *NovoRapid*®, give continuously in Glucose 5% or Sodium Chloride 0.9%; dilute to 0.05–1 unit/mL with infusion fluid; adsorbed to some extent by plastics of infusion set.

● **PRESCRIBING AND DISPENSING INFORMATION** Insulin aspart is a biological medicine. Biological medicines must be prescribed and dispensed by brand name, see *Biological medicines* and *Biosimilar medicines*, under Guidance on prescribing p. 1. Dose adjustments and close metabolic monitoring is recommended if switching between insulin aspart preparations.

● **NATIONAL FUNDING/ACCESS DECISIONS**

For full details see funding body website

NICE decisions

▸ **Continuous subcutaneous insulin infusion for the treatment of diabetes mellitus (type 1) (July 2008)** NICE TA151 Recommended

● **MEDICINAL FORMS** There can be variation in the licensing of different medicines containing the same drug.

Solution for injection

▸ **Fiasp** (Novo Nordisk Ltd)

Insulin aspart 100 unit per 1 ml Fiasp 100units/ml solution for injection 10ml vials | 1 vial PoM £14.08 DT = £14.08

▸ **Fiasp Penfill** (Novo Nordisk Ltd)

Insulin aspart 100 unit per 1 ml Fiasp Penfill 100units/ml solution for injection 3ml cartridges | 5 cartridge PoM £28.31 DT = £28.31

▸ **NovoRapid** (Novo Nordisk Ltd)

Insulin aspart 100 unit per 1 ml NovoRapid 100units/ml solution for injection 10ml vials | 1 vial PoM £14.08 DT = £14.08

▸ **NovoRapid FlexPen** (Novo Nordisk Ltd)

Insulin aspart 100 unit per 1 ml NovoRapid FlexPen 100units/ml solution for injection 3ml pre-filled pens | 5 pre-filled disposable injection PoM £30.60 DT = £30.60

▸ **NovoRapid Penfill** (Novo Nordisk Ltd)

Insulin aspart 100 unit per 1 ml NovoRapid Penfill 100units/ml solution for injection 3ml cartridges | 5 cartridge PoM £28.31 DT = £28.31

▸ **NovoRapid PumpCart** (Novo Nordisk Ltd)

Insulin aspart 100 unit per 1 ml NovoRapid PumpCart 100units/ml solution for injection 1.6ml cartridges | 5 cartridge PoM £15.10 DT = £15.10

F 568

Insulin glulisine

26-Feb-2025

● **DRUG ACTION** Insulin glulisine is a recombinant human insulin analogue with a rapid onset and short duration of action.

● **INDICATIONS AND DOSE**

Diabetes mellitus

▸ BY SUBCUTANEOUS INJECTION

▸ Child: Administer immediately before meals or when necessary shortly after meals, according to requirements

▸ BY SUBCUTANEOUS INFUSION, OR BY INTRAVENOUS INFUSION

▸ Child: According to requirements

● **UNLICENSED USE** Not licensed for children under 6 years.

● **INTERACTIONS** → Appendix 1: insulin

● **DIRECTIONS FOR ADMINISTRATION** Short-acting injectable insulins can be given by continuous subcutaneous infusion using a portable infusion pump. This device delivers a continuous basal insulin infusion and patient-activated bolus doses at meal times. This technique can be useful for patients who suffer recurrent hypoglycaemia or marked morning rise in blood-glucose concentration despite optimised multiple-injection regimens. Patients on subcutaneous insulin infusion must be highly motivated, able to monitor their blood-glucose concentration, and have expert training, advice and supervision from an experienced healthcare team.

- **NATIONAL FUNDING/ACCESS DECISIONS** For full details see funding body website

NICE decisions

- **Continuous subcutaneous insulin infusion for the treatment of diabetes mellitus (type 1) (July 2008)** NICE TA151
Recommended

Scottish Medicines Consortium (SMC) decisions

- **Insulin glulisine (*Apidra*®) for adolescents and children with diabetes mellitus (November 2008)** SMC No. 512/08
Recommended with restrictions

- **MEDICINAL FORMS** There can be variation in the licensing of different medicines containing the same drug.

Solution for injection

- **Apidra** (Sanofi)
Insulin glulisine 100 unit per 1 ml Apidra 100units/ml solution for injection 10ml vials | 1 vial PoM £16.00 DT = £16.00
Apidra 100units/ml solution for injection 3ml cartridges | 5 cartridge PoM £28.30 DT = £28.30
- **Apidra SoloStar** (Sanofi)
Insulin glulisine 100 unit per 1 ml Apidra 100units/ml solution for injection 3ml pre-filled SoloStar pens | 5 pre-filled disposable injection PoM £28.30 DT = £28.30

568

Insulin lispro

26-Feb-2025

- **DRUG ACTION** Insulin lispro is a recombinant human insulin analogue with a rapid onset and short duration of action.

- **INDICATIONS AND DOSE**

Diabetes mellitus

- BY SUBCUTANEOUS INJECTION
  - Child 1 month–1 year: Administer shortly before meals or when necessary shortly after meals, according to requirements
  - Child 2–17 years: Administer shortly before meals or when necessary shortly after meals, according to requirements
- BY SUBCUTANEOUS INFUSION, OR BY INTRAVENOUS INFUSION, OR BY INTRAVENOUS INJECTION
  - Child 1 month–1 year: According to requirements
  - Child 2–17 years: According to requirements

- **UNLICENSED USE** Not licensed for use in children under 2 years.
- **INTERACTIONS** → Appendix 1: insulin
- **PREGNANCY** Not known to be harmful—may be used during pregnancy.
- **BREAST FEEDING** Not known to be harmful—may be used during lactation.
- **DIRECTIONS FOR ADMINISTRATION** Short-acting injectable insulins can be given by continuous subcutaneous infusion using a portable infusion pump. This device delivers a continuous basal insulin infusion and patient-activated bolus doses at meal times. This technique can be useful for patients who suffer recurrent hypoglycaemia or marked morning rise in blood-glucose concentration despite optimised multiple-injection regimens (see also NICE guidance, below). Patients on subcutaneous insulin infusion must be highly motivated, able to monitor their blood-glucose concentration, and have expert training, advice and supervision from an experienced healthcare team.
  - With intravenous use For *intravenous infusion*, dilute to a concentration of 0.1–1 unit/mL with Glucose 5% or Sodium Chloride 0.9% and mix thoroughly; insulin may be adsorbed by plastics, flush giving set with 5 mL of infusion fluid containing insulin.
- **PRESCRIBING AND DISPENSING INFORMATION** Insulin lispro is a biological medicine. Biological medicines must be prescribed and dispensed by brand name, see *Biological medicines* and *Biosimilar medicines*, under Guidance on prescribing p. 1.
- **NATIONAL FUNDING/ACCESS DECISIONS** For full details see funding body website

NICE decisions

- **Continuous subcutaneous insulin infusion for the treatment of diabetes mellitus (type 1) (July 2008)** NICE TA151
Recommended

- **MEDICINAL FORMS** There can be variation in the licensing of different medicines containing the same drug.

Solution for injection

- **Admelog** (Sanofi)
Insulin lispro 100 unit per 1 ml Admelog 100units/ml solution for injection 10ml vials | 1 vial PoM £14.12 DT = £16.61
Admelog 100units/ml solution for injection 3ml cartridges | 5 cartridge PoM £21.23 DT = £28.31
Admelog 100units/ml solution for injection 3ml pre-filled pens | 5 pre-filled disposable injection PoM £22.10 DT = £29.46
- **Humalog (Insulin lispro)** (Eli Lilly and Company Ltd)
Insulin lispro 100 unit per 1 ml Humalog 100units/ml solution for injection 10ml vials | 1 vial PoM £16.61 DT = £16.61
Humalog 100units/ml solution for injection 3ml cartridges | 5 cartridge PoM £28.31 DT = £28.31
- **Humalog Junior KwikPen** (Eli Lilly and Company Ltd)
Insulin lispro 100 unit per 1 ml Humalog Junior KwikPen 100units/ml solution for injection 3ml pre-filled pens | 5 pre-filled disposable injection PoM £29.46 DT = £29.46
- **Humalog KwikPen** (Eli Lilly and Company Ltd)
Insulin lispro 100 unit per 1 ml Humalog KwikPen 100units/ml solution for injection 3ml pre-filled pens | 5 pre-filled disposable injection PoM £29.46 DT = £29.46
Insulin lispro 200 unit per 1 ml Humalog KwikPen 200units/ml solution for injection 3ml pre-filled pens | 5 pre-filled disposable injection PoM £58.92 DT = £58.92
- **Lyumjev** (Eli Lilly and Company Ltd)
Insulin lispro 100 unit per 1 ml Lyumjev 100units/ml solution for injection 3ml cartridges | 5 cartridge PoM £28.31 DT = £28.31
Lyumjev 100units/ml solution for injection 10ml vials | 1 vial PoM £16.61 DT = £16.61
- **Lyumjev Junior KwikPen** (Eli Lilly and Company Ltd)
Insulin lispro 100 unit per 1 ml Lyumjev Junior KwikPen 100units/ml solution for injection 3ml pre-filled pens | 5 pre-filled disposable injection PoM £29.46 DT = £29.46
- **Lyumjev KwikPen** (Eli Lilly and Company Ltd)
Insulin lispro 100 unit per 1 ml Lyumjev KwikPen 100units/ml solution for injection 3ml pre-filled pens | 5 pre-filled disposable injection PoM £29.46 DT = £29.46
Insulin lispro 200 unit per 1 ml Lyumjev KwikPen 200units/ml solution for injection 3ml pre-filled pens | 5 pre-filled disposable injection PoM £58.92 DT = £58.92

INSULINS › INTERMEDIATE-ACTING

568

Biphasic isophane insulin

26-Feb-2025

- **DRUG ACTION** Biphasic isophane insulin is a mixture of natural or recombinant insulins with a short onset and intermediate duration of action.

- **INDICATIONS AND DOSE**

Diabetes mellitus

- BY SUBCUTANEOUS INJECTION
  - Child: Dose according to requirements

- **INTERACTIONS** → Appendix 1: insulin

- **SIDE-EFFECTS**
  - **Rare or very rare** Angioedema
  - **Frequency not known** Hypokalaemia · weight increased
- **PRESCRIBING AND DISPENSING INFORMATION** A sterile buffered suspension of either porcine or human insulin complexed with protamine sulfate (or another suitable protamine) in a solution of insulin of the same species.

  Check product container—the proportions of the two components should be checked carefully (the order in which the proportions are stated may not be the same in other countries).

- **MEDICINAL FORMS** There can be variation in the licensing of different medicines containing the same drug.

Suspension for injection

- **Humulin M3** (Eli Lilly and Company Ltd)
  Insulin human (as Insulin soluble human) 30 unit per 1 ml, Insulin human (as Insulin isophane human) 70 unit per 1 ml Humulin M3 100units/ml suspension for injection 3ml cartridges | 5 cartridge [PoM] £19.08 DT = £19.08
  Humulin M3 100units/ml suspension for injection 10ml vials | 1 vial [PoM] £15.68 DT = £15.68
- **Humulin M3 KwikPen** (Eli Lilly and Company Ltd)
  Insulin human (as Insulin soluble human) 30 unit per 1 ml, Insulin human (as Insulin isophane human) 70 unit per 1 ml Humulin M3 KwikPen 100units/ml suspension for injection 3ml pre-filled pens | 5 pre-filled disposable injection [PoM] £21.70 DT = £21.70
- **Hypurin Porcine 30/70 Mix** (C P Pharmaceuticals Ltd)
  Insulin porcine (as Insulin soluble porcine) 30 unit per 1 ml, Insulin porcine (as Insulin isophane porcine) 70 unit per 1 ml Hypurin Porcine 30/70 Mix 100units/ml suspension for injection 3ml cartridges | 5 cartridge [PoM] £59.08 DT = £59.08

F 568

Isophane insulin

26-Feb-2025

(Isophane Protamine Insulin; NPH Insulin)

- **DRUG ACTION** Isophane insulin is a natural or recombinant insulin with an intermediate duration of action.

- **INDICATIONS AND DOSE**

  Diabetes mellitus
  - BY SUBCUTANEOUS INJECTION
  - Child: According to requirements

- **INTERACTIONS** → Appendix 1: insulin
- **PREGNANCY** Recommended where longer-acting insulins are needed.
- **PRESCRIBING AND DISPENSING INFORMATION** A sterile suspension of bovine or porcine insulin or of human insulin in the form of a complex obtained by the addition of protamine sulfate or another suitable protamine.

- **MEDICINAL FORMS** There can be variation in the licensing of different medicines containing the same drug.

Suspension for injection

- **Humulin I** (Eli Lilly and Company Ltd)
  Insulin human (as Insulin isophane human) 100 unit per 1 ml Humulin I 100units/ml suspension for injection 10ml vials | 1 vial [PoM] £15.68 DT = £15.68
  Humulin I 100units/ml suspension for injection 3ml cartridges | 5 cartridge [PoM] £19.08 DT = £19.08
- **Humulin I KwikPen** (Eli Lilly and Company Ltd)
  Insulin human (as Insulin isophane human) 100 unit per 1 ml Humulin I KwikPen 100units/ml suspension for injection 3ml pre-filled pens | 5 pre-filled disposable injection [PoM] £21.70 DT = £21.70
- **Hypurin Porcine Isophane** (C P Pharmaceuticals Ltd)
  Insulin porcine (as Insulin isophane porcine) 100 unit per 1 ml Hypurin Porcine Isophane 100units/ml suspension for injection 3ml cartridges | 5 cartridge [PoM] £59.08 DT = £59.08
- **Insulatard** (Novo Nordisk Ltd)
  Insulin human (as Insulin isophane human) 100 unit per 1 ml Insulatard 100units/ml suspension for injection 10ml vials | 1 vial [PoM] £7.48 DT = £15.68

INSULINS > INTERMEDIATE-ACTING COMBINED WITH RAPID-ACTING

F 568

Biphasic insulin aspart

26-Feb-2025

- **DRUG ACTION** Biphasic insulin aspart is a mixture of recombinant human insulin analogues with a rapid onset and intermediate duration of action.

- **INDICATIONS AND DOSE**

  Diabetes mellitus
  - BY SUBCUTANEOUS INJECTION
  - Child: Administer up to 10 minutes before or soon after a meal, according to requirements

- **INTERACTIONS** → Appendix 1: insulin
- **SIDE-EFFECTS**
  - **Uncommon** Skin reactions
- **PRESCRIBING AND DISPENSING INFORMATION** Check product container—the proportions of the two components should be checked carefully (the order in which the proportions are stated may not be the same in other countries).

- **MEDICINAL FORMS** There can be variation in the licensing of different medicines containing the same drug.

Suspension for injection

- **NovoMix 30 FlexPen** (Novo Nordisk Ltd)
  Insulin aspart 30 unit per 1 ml, Insulin aspart (as Insulin aspart protamine) 70 unit per 1 ml NovoMix 30 FlexPen 100units/ml suspension for injection 3ml pre-filled pens | 5 pre-filled disposable injection [PoM] £29.89 DT = £29.89
- **NovoMix 30 Penfill** (Novo Nordisk Ltd)
  Insulin aspart 30 unit per 1 ml, Insulin aspart (as Insulin aspart protamine) 70 unit per 1 ml NovoMix 30 Penfill 100units/ml suspension for injection 3ml cartridges | 5 cartridge [PoM] £28.79 DT = £28.79

F 568

Biphasic insulin lispro

26-Feb-2025

- **DRUG ACTION** Biphasic insulin lispro is a mixture of recombinant human insulin analogues with a rapid onset and intermediate duration of action.

- **INDICATIONS AND DOSE**

  Diabetes mellitus
  - BY SUBCUTANEOUS INJECTION
  - Child: Administer up to 15 minutes before or soon after a meal, according to requirements

- **CAUTIONS** Children under 12 years (use only if benefit likely compared to soluble insulin)
- **INTERACTIONS** → Appendix 1: insulin
- **PRESCRIBING AND DISPENSING INFORMATION** Check product container—the proportions of the two components should be checked carefully (the order in which the proportions are stated may not be the same in other countries).

- **MEDICINAL FORMS** There can be variation in the licensing of different medicines containing the same drug.

Suspension for injection

- **Humalog Mix25** (Eli Lilly and Company Ltd)
  Insulin lispro 25 unit per 1 ml, Insulin lispro (as Insulin lispro protamine) 75 unit per 1 ml Humalog Mix25 100units/ml suspension for injection 10ml vials | 1 vial [PoM] £16.61 DT = £16.61
  Humalog Mix25 100units/ml suspension for injection 3ml cartridges | 5 cartridge [PoM] £29.46 DT = £29.46
- **Humalog Mix25 KwikPen** (Eli Lilly and Company Ltd)
  Insulin lispro 25 unit per 1 ml, Insulin lispro (as Insulin lispro protamine) 75 unit per 1 ml Humalog Mix25 KwikPen 100units/ml suspension for injection 3ml pre-filled pens | 5 pre-filled disposable injection [PoM] £30.98 DT = £30.98

▸ **Humalog Mix50** (Eli Lilly and Company Ltd)
Insulin lispro 50 unit per 1 ml, Insulin lispro (as Insulin lispro protamine) 50 unit per 1 ml Humalog Mix50 100units/ml suspension for injection 3ml cartridges | 5 cartridge PoM £29.46 DT = £29.46

▸ **Humalog Mix50 KwikPen** (Eli Lilly and Company Ltd)
Insulin lispro 50 unit per 1 ml, Insulin lispro (as Insulin lispro protamine) 50 unit per 1 ml Humalog Mix50 KwikPen 100units/ml suspension for injection 3ml pre-filled pens | 5 pre-filled disposable injection PoM £30.98 DT = £30.98

INSULINS > LONG-ACTING

568

Insulin degludec

26-Feb-2025

● **DRUG ACTION** Insulin degludec is a recombinant human insulin analogue with a long duration of action.

● **INDICATIONS AND DOSE**

Diabetes mellitus

▸ BY SUBCUTANEOUS INJECTION

▸ Child 1–17 years: Dose to be given according to requirements

IMPORTANT SAFETY INFORMATION

NATIONAL PATIENT SAFETY ALERT: POTENTIAL FOR INAPPROPRIATE DOSING OF INSULIN WHEN SWITCHING *TRESIBA*® (INSULIN DEGLUDEC) PRODUCTS (DECEMBER 2023)

In response to a shortage of *Tresiba*® FlexTouch® 100 units/mL pre-filled pens, some patients may have been switched to *Tresiba*® FlexTouch® 200 units/mL pre-filled pens. However, there have been reports of patients being incorrectly advised to reduce the number of units of insulin, resulting in one patient requiring hospitalisation for diabetic ketoacidosis.

Healthcare professionals are reminded that *Tresiba*® FlexTouch® pen delivery devices show the number of **units** that will be injected rather than the volume of solution, therefore no dose conversion is necessary when switching patients from one strength to another. Patients who have been switched to a different *Tresiba*® FlexTouch® pen must be made aware of this.

When prescribing *Tresiba*® 100 units/mL Penfill® **cartridges**, patients should also be given a compatible Novo Nordisk insulin delivery system and appropriate needles.

All patients initiated on a new device should be counselled on the change and given training on use, including signposting to training videos, and the potential need for closer monitoring of blood glucose concentration.

● **INTERACTIONS** → Appendix 1: insulin

● **SIDE-EFFECTS**

▸ **Rare or very rare** Urticaria

● **PREGNANCY** Evidence of the safety of long-acting insulin analogues in pregnancy is limited, therefore isophane insulin is recommended where longer-acting insulins are needed; insulin detemir may also be considered.

● **PRESCRIBING AND DISPENSING INFORMATION** Insulin degludec (*Tresiba*®) is available in strengths of 100 units/mL (allows 1-unit dose adjustment) and 200 units/mL (allows 2-unit dose adjustment)—ensure correct strength prescribed.

● **NATIONAL FUNDING/ACCESS DECISIONS**
For full details see funding body website

All Wales Medicines Strategy Group (AWMSG) decisions

▸ **Insulin degludec (*Tresiba*®) for the treatment of diabetes mellitus in adults, adolescents and children from the age of 1 year (October 2022)** AWMSG No. 5196 Recommended

● **MEDICINAL FORMS** There can be variation in the licensing of different medicines containing the same drug.

Solution for injection

▸ **Tresiba FlexTouch** (Novo Nordisk Ltd)
Insulin degludec 200 unit per 1 ml Tresiba FlexTouch 200units/ml solution for injection 3ml pre-filled pens | 3 pre-filled disposable injection PoM £55.92 DT = £55.92

▸ **Tresiba Penfill** (Novo Nordisk Ltd)
Insulin degludec 100 unit per 1 ml Tresiba Penfill 100units/ml solution for injection 3ml cartridges | 5 cartridge PoM £46.60 DT = £46.60

568

Insulin detemir

26-Feb-2025

● **DRUG ACTION** Insulin detemir is a recombinant human insulin analogue with a long duration of action.

● **INDICATIONS AND DOSE**

Diabetes mellitus

▸ BY SUBCUTANEOUS INJECTION

▸ Child 1–17 years: According to requirements

● **INTERACTIONS** → Appendix 1: insulin

● **SIDE-EFFECTS**

▸ **Uncommon** Refraction disorder

● **PREGNANCY** Evidence of the safety of long-acting insulin analogues in pregnancy is limited, therefore isophane insulin p. 572 is recommended where longer-acting insulins are needed; insulin detemir may also be considered where longer-acting insulins are needed.

● **NATIONAL FUNDING/ACCESS DECISIONS**
For full details see funding body website

Scottish Medicines Consortium (SMC) decisions

▸ **Insulin detemir (*Levemir*®) for the treatment of diabetes mellitus (March 2016)** SMC No. 1126/16 Recommended with restrictions

● **MEDICINAL FORMS** There can be variation in the licensing of different medicines containing the same drug.

Solution for injection

▸ **Levemir FlexPen** (Novo Nordisk Ltd)
Insulin detemir 100 unit per 1 ml Levemir FlexPen 100units/ml solution for injection 3ml pre-filled pens | 5 pre-filled disposable injection PoM £42.00 DT = £42.00

▸ **Levemir Penfill** (Novo Nordisk Ltd)
Insulin detemir 100 unit per 1 ml Levemir Penfill 100units/ml solution for injection 3ml cartridges | 5 cartridge PoM £42.00 DT = £42.00

568

Insulin glargine

26-Feb-2025

● **DRUG ACTION** Insulin glargine is a recombinant human insulin analogue with a long duration of action.

● **INDICATIONS AND DOSE**

Diabetes mellitus

▸ BY SUBCUTANEOUS INJECTION

▸ Child 2–17 years: According to requirements

● **INTERACTIONS** → Appendix 1: insulin

● **SIDE-EFFECTS**

▸ **Rare or very rare** Myalgia · taste altered

▸ **Frequency not known** Sodium retention

● **PREGNANCY** Evidence of the safety of long-acting insulin analogues in pregnancy is limited, therefore isophane insulin is recommended where longer-acting insulins are needed; insulin detemir may also be considered.

● **PRESCRIBING AND DISPENSING INFORMATION** Insulin glargine is a biological medicine. Biological medicines must be prescribed and dispensed by brand name, see *Biological medicines* and *Biosimilar medicines*, under Guidance on prescribing p. 1. Dose adjustments and close metabolic monitoring is recommended if switching between insulin glargine preparations.

● **NATIONAL FUNDING/ACCESS DECISIONS**
For full details see funding body website

Scottish Medicines Consortium (SMC) decisions

▸ **Insulin glargine (*Lantus*®) for the treatment of diabetes mellitus in adults, adolescents and children aged 2 years and above (April 2013)** SMC No. 860/13 Recommended with restrictions

● **MEDICINAL FORMS** There can be variation in the licensing of different medicines containing the same drug.

Solution for injection

▸ **Abasaglar** (Eli Lilly and Company Ltd)
Insulin glargine 100 unit per 1 ml Abasaglar 100units/ml solution for injection 3ml cartridges | 5 cartridge PoM £35.28 DT = £34.75

▸ **Abasaglar KwikPen** (Eli Lilly and Company Ltd)
Insulin glargine 100 unit per 1 ml Abasaglar KwikPen 100units/ml solution for injection 3ml pre-filled pens | 5 pre-filled disposable injection PoM £35.28 DT = £34.75

▸ **Lantus** (Sanofi)
Insulin glargine 100 unit per 1 ml Lantus 100units/ml solution for injection 3ml cartridges | 5 cartridge PoM £34.75 DT = £34.75
Lantus 100units/ml solution for injection 3ml pre-filled SoloStar pens | 5 pre-filled disposable injection PoM £34.75 DT = £34.75
Lantus 100units/ml solution for injection 10ml vials | 1 vial PoM £25.69 DT = £25.69

▸ **Semglee** (Biocon Biologics Ireland Ltd)
Insulin glargine 100 unit per 1 ml Semglee 100units/ml solution for injection 3ml pre-filled pens | 5 pre-filled disposable injection PoM £29.99 DT = £34.75

▸ **Toujeo** (Sanofi)
Insulin glargine 300 unit per 1 ml Toujeo 300units/ml solution for injection 1.5ml pre-filled SoloStar pens | 3 pre-filled disposable injection PoM £32.14 DT = £32.14

▸ **Toujeo DoubleStar** (Sanofi)
Insulin glargine 300 unit per 1 ml Toujeo 300units/ml solution for injection 3ml pre-filled DoubleStar pens | 3 pre-filled disposable injection PoM £64.27 DT = £64.27

4.1a Diabetes, diagnosis and monitoring

Diabetes mellitus, diagnostic and monitoring devices

24-May-2022

Urinalysis: urinary glucose

Reagent strips are available for measuring for glucose in the urine. Tests for ketones by patients are rarely required unless they become unwell—see Blood Monitoring.

Microalbuminuria can be detected with *Micral-Test II*® but this should be followed by confirmation in the laboratory, since false positive results are common.

Blood glucose monitoring

In the UK blood-glucose concentration is expressed in mmol/litre and Diabetes UK advises that these units should be used for self-monitoring of blood-glucose. In other European countries units of mg/100 mL (or mg/dL) are commonly used.

It is advisable to check that the meter is pre-set in the correct units.

Capillary blood-glucose monitoring using a meter gives a direct measure of the glucose concentration at the time of the test and can detect hypoglycaemia as well as hyperglycaemia. Carers and children should be properly

Meters and test strips

Meter (all NHS)	Type of monitoring	Compatible test strips	Test strip net price	Sensitivity range (mmol/litre)	Manufacturer
Accu-Chek® Active	Blood glucose	Active®	50 strip= £0.00	0.6- 33.3 mmol/litre	Roche Diabetes Care Ltd
Accu-Chek® Aviva	Blood glucose	Aviva®	50 strip= £12.99	0.6- 33.3 mmol/litre	Roche Diabetes Care Ltd
Accu-Chek® Aviva Expert	Blood glucose	Aviva®	50 strip= £12.99	0.6- 33.3 mmol/litre	Roche Diabetes Care Ltd
Accu-Chek® Mobile	Blood glucose	Mobile®	50 device= £10.24	0.3- 33.3 mmol/litre	Roche Diabetes Care Ltd
Accu-Chek® Aviva Nano	Blood glucose	Aviva®	50 strip= £12.99	0.6- 33.3 mmol/litre	Roche Diabetes Care Ltd
BGStar® Free of charge from diabetes healthcare professionals	Blood glucose	BGStar®	50 strip= £0.00	1.1- 33.3 mmol/litre	Sanofi
Breeze 2®	Blood glucose	Breeze 2®	50 strip= £15.00	0.6- 33.3 mmol/litre	Bayer Plc
CareSens N® Free of charge from diabetes healthcare professionals	Blood glucose	CareSens N®	50 strip= £12.75	1.1- 33.3 mmol/litre	Spirit Healthcare Ltd
Contour®	Blood glucose	Contour®	50 strip= £10.15	0.6- 33.3 mmol/litre	Ascensia Diabetes Care UK Ltd
Contour® XT	Blood glucose	Contour® Next	50 strip= £16.21	0.6- 33.3 mmol/litre	Ascensia Diabetes Care UK Ltd
Element®	Blood glucose	Element®	50 strip= £9.89	0.55- 33.3 mmol/litre	Neon Diagnostics Ltd
FreeStyle® Meter no longer available	Blood glucose	FreeStyle®	50 strip= £0.00	1.1- 27.8 mmol/litre	Abbott Laboratories Ltd

Meter (all NHS)	Type of monitoring	Compatible test strips	Test strip net price	Sensitivity range (mmol/litre)	Manufacturer
FreeStyle Freedom® Meter no longer available	Blood glucose	FreeStyle®	50 strip= £0.00	1.1- 27.8 mmol/litre	Abbott Laboratories Ltd
FreeStyle Freedom Lite®	Blood glucose	FreeStyle Lite®	50 strip= £16.41	1.1- 27.8 mmol/litre	Abbott Laboratories Ltd
FreeStyle InsuLinx®	Blood glucose	FreeStyle Lite®	50 strip= £16.41	1.1- 27.8 mmol/litre	Abbott Laboratories Ltd
FreeStyle Lite®	Blood glucose	FreeStyle Lite®	50 strip= £16.41	1.1- 27.8 mmol/litre	Abbott Laboratories Ltd
FreeStyle Mini® Meter no longer available	Blood glucose	FreeStyle®	50 strip= £0.00	1.1- 27.8 mmol/litre	Abbott Laboratories Ltd
FreeStyle Optium®	Blood glucose	FreeStyle Optium®	50 strip= £16.30	1.1- 27.8 mmol/litre	Abbott Laboratories Ltd
FreeStyle Optium®	Blood ketones	FreeStyle Optium® β-ketone	10 strip= £21.94	0- 8.0 mmol/litre	Abbott Laboratories Ltd
FreeStyle Optium Neo®	Blood glucose	FreeStyle Optium®	50 strip= £16.30	1.1- 27.8 mmol/litre	Abbott Laboratories Ltd
FreeStyle Optium Neo®	Blood ketones	FreeStyle Optium® β-ketone	10 strip= £21.94	0- 8.0 mmol/litre	Abbott Laboratories Ltd
GlucoDock® module For use with iPhone®, iPod touch®, and iPad®	Blood glucose	GlucoDock®	50 strip= £14.90	1.1- 33.3 mmol/litre	Medisana Healthcare (UK) Ltd
GlucoLab®	Blood glucose	GlucoLab®	50 strip= £9.89	0.55- 33.3 mmol/litre	Neon Diagnostics Ltd
GlucoRx® Free of charge from diabetes healthcare professionals	Blood glucose	GlucoRx®	50 strip= £5.45	1.1- 33.3 mmol/litre	GlucoRx Ltd
GlucoRx Nexus® Free of charge from diabetes healthcare professionals	Blood glucose	GlucoRx Nexus®	50 strip= £8.95	1.1- 33.3 mmol/litre	GlucoRx Ltd
Glucotrend® Meter no longer available	Blood glucose	Active®	50 strip= £0.00	0.6- 33.3 mmol/litre	Roche Diabetes Care Ltd
iBGStar®	Blood glucose	BGStar®	50 strip= £0.00	1.1- 33.3 mmol/litre	Sanofi
Mendor Discreet®	Blood glucose	Mendor Discreet®	50 strip= £14.75	1.1- 33.3 mmol/litre	SpringMed Solutions Ltd
Microdot®+ Free of charge from diabetes healthcare professionals	Blood glucose	Microdot®+	50 strip= £0.00	1.1- 29.2 mmol/litre	Cambridge Sensors Ltd
MyGlucoHealth®	Blood glucose	MyGlucoHealth®	50 strip= £15.50	0.6- 33.3 mmol/litre	Entra Health Systems Ltd
One Touch® VerioPro Free of charge from diabetes healthcare professionals	Blood glucose	One Touch® Verio	50 strip= £15.12	1.1- 33.3 mmol/litre	LifeScan
SD CodeFree®	Blood glucose	SD CodeFree®	50 strip= £7.40	0.6- 33.3 mmol/litre	Home Health (UK) Ltd
Sensocard Plus® Meter no longer available	Blood glucose	Sensocard®	50 strip= £16.30	1.1- 33.3 mmol/litre	BBI Healthcare Ltd
TRUEyou mini®	Blood glucose	TRUEyou®	50 strip= £0.00	1.1- 33.3 mmol/litre	Trividia Health UK Ltd
WaveSense JAZZ® Free of charge from diabetes healthcare professionals	Blood glucose	WaveSense JAZZ®	50 strip= £8.74	1.1- 33.3 mmol/litre	AgaMatrix Europe Ltd

trained in the use of blood-glucose monitoring systems and the appropriate action to take on the results obtained. Inadequate understanding of the normal fluctuations in blood-glucose can lead to confusion and inappropriate action.

Continuous glucose monitoring may be appropriate in certain children with diabetes. A continuous glucose monitor is a device that measures interstitial fluid glucose levels and sends the readings to a display device or smartphone.

For further information on self-monitoring of capillary blood-glucose, and continuous glucose monitoring, see NICE guideline: **Diabetes (type 1 and type 2) in children and young people: diagnosis and management** (available at: www.nice.org.uk/guidance/ng18).

Children using multiple injection regimens should understand how to adjust their insulin dose according to their carbohydrate intake. With fixed-dose insulin regimens, the carbohydrate intake needs to be regulated, and should be distributed throughout the day to match the insulin regimen.

If the blood-glucose level is high or if the child is unwell, blood **ketones** should be measured according to local guidelines in order to detect diabetic ketoacidosis. Children and their carers should be trained in the use of blood ketone monitoring systems and to take appropriate action on the results obtained, including when to seek medical attention.

Other drugs used for Diabetes, diagnosis and monitoring
Glucose, p. 730

Blood glucose testing strips

● **BLOOD GLUCOSE TESTING STRIPS**

4SURE testing strips (Nipro Medical UK Ltd)
50 strip • NHS indicative price = £7.99 • Drug Tariff (Part IXr)

Accu-Chek Inform II testing strips (Roche Diagnostics Ltd)
50 strip • No NHS indicative price available • Drug Tariff (Part IXr)

Advocate Redi-Code+ testing strips (Diabetes Care Technology Ltd)
50 strip • NHS indicative price = £9.95 • Drug Tariff (Part IXr)

AgaMatrix Agile testing strips (AgaMatrix Europe Ltd)
50 strip • NHS indicative price = £5.43 • Drug Tariff (Part IXr)

AutoSense testing strips (Advance Diagnostic Products (NI) Ltd)
25 strip • NHS indicative price = £4.50 • Drug Tariff (Part IXr)

Aviva testing strips (Roche Diabetes Care Ltd)
50 strip • NHS indicative price = £12.99 • Drug Tariff (Part IXr)

Betachek C50 cassette (National Diagnostic Products)
50 device • NHS indicative price = £9.95 • Drug Tariff (Part IXr) | 100 device • NHS indicative price = £19.90 • Drug Tariff (Part IXr)

Betachek G5 testing strips (National Diagnostic Products)
50 strip • NHS indicative price = £5.50 • Drug Tariff (Part IXr)

Betachek Visual testing strips (National Diagnostic Products)
50 strip • NHS indicative price = £5.50 • Drug Tariff (Part IXr)

Breeze 2 testing discs (Bayer Plc)
50 strip • NHS indicative price = £15.00 • Drug Tariff (Part IXr)

CareSens N testing strips (Spirit Healthcare Ltd)
50 strip • NHS indicative price = £12.75 • Drug Tariff (Part IXr)

CareSens PRO testing strips (Spirit Healthcare Ltd)
50 strip • NHS indicative price = £9.95 • Drug Tariff (Part IXr)

CareSens S testing strips (Spirit Healthcare Ltd)
50 strip • NHS indicative price = £5.45 • Drug Tariff (Part IXr)

Contour Next testing strips (Ascensia Diabetes Care UK Ltd)
50 strip • NHS indicative price = £16.21 • Drug Tariff (Part IXr)

Contour Plus testing strips (Ascensia Diabetes Care UK Ltd)
50 strip • NHS indicative price = £5.95 • Drug Tariff (Part IXr)

Contour testing strips (Ascensia Diabetes Care UK Ltd)
50 strip • NHS indicative price = £10.15 • Drug Tariff (Part IXr)

Dario Lite testing strips (LabStyle Innovations Ltd)
50 strip • NHS indicative price = £9.95 • Drug Tariff (Part IXr)

Dario testing strips (LabStyle Innovations Ltd)
50 strip • NHS indicative price = £14.95 • Drug Tariff (Part IXr)

Element testing strips (Neon Diagnostics Ltd)
50 strip • NHS indicative price = £9.89 • Drug Tariff (Part IXr)

Finetest Lite testing strips (Neon Diagnostics Ltd)
50 strip • NHS indicative price = £5.15 • Drug Tariff (Part IXr)

Fora Advanced pro GD40 testing strips (Miller Medical Supplies Ltd)
50 strip • NHS indicative price = £7.95 • Drug Tariff (Part IXr)

FreeStyle Lite testing strips (Abbott Laboratories Ltd)
50 strip • NHS indicative price = £16.41 • Drug Tariff (Part IXr)

FreeStyle Optium H testing strips (Abbott Laboratories Ltd)
100 strip • No NHS indicative price available • Drug Tariff (Part IXr)

FreeStyle Optium Neo H testing strips (Abbott Laboratories Ltd)
100 strip • No NHS indicative price available • Drug Tariff (Part IXr)

FreeStyle Optium testing strips (Abbott Laboratories Ltd)
50 strip • NHS indicative price = £16.30 • Drug Tariff (Part IXr)

FreeStyle Precision Pro testing strips (Abbott Laboratories Ltd)
100 strip • No NHS indicative price available • Drug Tariff (Part IXr)

GluNEO testing strips (Neon Diagnostics Ltd)
50 strip • NHS indicative price = £9.89 • Drug Tariff (Part IXr)

GlucoDock testing strips (Medisana Healthcare (UK) Ltd)
50 strip • NHS indicative price = £14.90 • Drug Tariff (Part IXr)

GlucoLab testing strips (Neon Diagnostics Ltd)
50 strip • NHS indicative price = £9.89 • Drug Tariff (Part IXr)

GlucoMen areo Sensor testing strips (A. Menarini Diagnostics Ltd)
50 strip • NHS indicative price = £7.25 • Drug Tariff (Part IXr)

GlucoRx GO Professional testing strips (GlucoRx Ltd)
50 strip • NHS indicative price = £9.95 • Drug Tariff (Part IXr)

GlucoRx GO testing strips (GlucoRx Ltd)
50 strip • NHS indicative price = £9.95 • Drug Tariff (Part IXr)

GlucoRx HCT Glucose testing strips (GlucoRx Ltd)
50 strip • NHS indicative price = £8.95 • Drug Tariff (Part IXr)

GlucoRx Nexus testing strips (GlucoRx Ltd)
50 strip • NHS indicative price = £8.95 • Drug Tariff (Part IXr)

GlucoRx Q testing strips (GlucoRx Ltd)
50 strip • NHS indicative price = £5.45 • Drug Tariff (Part IXr)

GlucoRx Smart Glucose testing strips (GlucoRx Ltd)
50 strip • NHS indicative price = £5.45 • Drug Tariff (Part IXr)

GlucoRx Vivid testing strips (GlucoRx Ltd)
50 strip • NHS indicative price = £5.45 • Drug Tariff (Part IXr)

GlucoRx X6 Glucose testing strips (GlucoRx Ltd)
50 strip • NHS indicative price = £15.95 • Drug Tariff (Part IXr)

Glucofix Tech Sensor testing strips (A. Menarini Diagnostics Ltd)
50 strip • NHS indicative price = £5.95 • Drug Tariff (Part IXr)

Glucoflex-R testing strips (National Diagnostic Products)
50 strip • NHS indicative price = £5.50 • Drug Tariff (Part IXr)

Guide testing strips (Roche Diabetes Care Ltd)
50 strip • NHS indicative price = £16.21 • Drug Tariff (Part IXr)

Instant testing strips (Roche Diabetes Care Ltd)
50 strip • NHS indicative price = £5.95 • Drug Tariff (Part IXr)

Kinetik Wellbeing AG-607 testing strips (Kinetik Medical Devices Ltd)
50 strip • NHS indicative price = £8.49 • Drug Tariff (Part IXr) | 100 strip • NHS indicative price = £13.98 • Drug Tariff (Part IXr)

Kinetik Wellbeing BG-710/BG-710b testing strips (Kinetik Medical Devices Ltd)
50 strip • NHS indicative price = £7.50 • Drug Tariff (Part IXr) | 100 strip • NHS indicative price = £13.00 • Drug Tariff (Part IXr)

MODZ testing strips (Modz Oy)
50 strip • NHS indicative price = £14.00 • Drug Tariff (Part IXr)

MediTouch 2 testing strips (Medisana Healthcare (UK) Ltd)
50 strip • NHS indicative price = £12.49 • Drug Tariff (Part IXr)

MediTouch testing strips (Medisana Healthcare (UK) Ltd)
50 strip • NHS indicative price = £14.90 • Drug Tariff (Part IXr)

Mendor Discreet testing strips (SpringMed Solutions Ltd)
50 strip • NHS indicative price = £14.75 • Drug Tariff (Part IXr)

Mobile cassette (Roche Diabetes Care Ltd)
50 device • NHS indicative price = £10.24 • Drug Tariff (Part IXr)

Myglucohealth testing strips (Entra Health Systems Ltd)
50 strip • NHS indicative price = £15.50 • Drug Tariff (Part IXr)

Mylife Aveo testing strips (Pikdare S.p.A.)
50 strip • NHS indicative price = £6.95 • Drug Tariff (Part IXr)

Mylife Pura testing strips (Pikdare S.p.A.)
50 strip • NHS indicative price = £9.50 • Drug Tariff (Part IXr)

Mylife Unio testing strips (Pikdare S.p.A.)
50 strip • NHS indicative price = £9.50 • Drug Tariff (Part IXr)

Neon GK+ Glucose testing strips (Neon Diagnostics Ltd)
50 strip • NHS indicative price = £5.39 • Drug Tariff (Part IXr)

OKmeter Core testing strips (Syringa UK Ltd)
50 strip • NHS indicative price = £9.90 • Drug Tariff (Part IXr)

Oh'Care Lite testing strips (Neon Diagnostics Ltd)
50 strip • NHS indicative price = £8.88 • Drug Tariff (Part IXr)

On Call Extra testing strips (Connect2Pharma Ltd)
50 strip • NHS indicative price = £5.20 • Drug Tariff (Part IXr)

On Call Sure testing strips (Connect2Pharma Ltd)
50 strip • NHS indicative price = £8.50 • Drug Tariff (Part IXr)

On-Call Advanced testing strips (Point Of Care Testing Ltd)
50 strip • NHS indicative price = £13.65 • Drug Tariff (Part IXr)

OneTouch Select Plus testing strips (LifeScan)
50 strip • NHS indicative price = £9.99 • Drug Tariff (Part IXr)

OneTouch Verio testing strips (LifeScan)
50 strip • NHS indicative price = £15.12 • Drug Tariff (Part IXr)

Performa testing strips (Roche Diabetes Care Ltd)
50 strip • NHS indicative price = £5.99 • Drug Tariff (Part IXr)

SD CodeFree testing strips (Home Health (UK) Ltd)
50 strip • NHS indicative price = £7.40 • Drug Tariff (Part IXr)

SURESIGN Resure testing strips (Ciga Healthcare Ltd)
50 strip • NHS indicative price = £8.49 • Drug Tariff (Part IXr)

Sensocard testing strips (BBI Healthcare Ltd)
50 strip • NHS indicative price = £16.30 • Drug Tariff (Part IXr)

StatStrip testing strips (Nova Biomedical)
50 strip • No NHS indicative price available • Drug Tariff (Part IXr)

TEE2 testing strips (Spirit Healthcare Ltd)
50 strip • NHS indicative price = £7.75 • Drug Tariff (Part IXr)

True Metrix testing strips (Trividia Health UK Ltd)
50 strip • NHS indicative price = £4.95 • Drug Tariff (Part IXr) | 100 strip • NHS indicative price = £9.90 • Drug Tariff (Part IXr)

VivaChek Ino testing strips (JR Biomedical Ltd)
50 strip • NHS indicative price = £8.99 • Drug Tariff (Part IXr)

WaveSense JAZZ testing strips (AgaMatrix Europe Ltd)
50 strip • NHS indicative price = £8.74 • Drug Tariff (Part IXr)

Xceed Precision Pro testing strips (Abbott Laboratories Ltd)
10 strip • No NHS indicative price available | 50 strip • No NHS indicative price available • Drug Tariff (Part IXr) | 100 strip • No NHS indicative price available • Drug Tariff (Part IXr)

palmdoc iCare Advanced Solo testing strips (Palmdoc Ltd)
50 strip • NHS indicative price = £13.50 • Drug Tariff (Part IXr)

palmdoc iCare Advanced testing strips (Palmdoc Ltd)
50 strip • NHS indicative price = £9.70 • Drug Tariff (Part IXr)

palmdoc testing strips (Palmdoc Ltd)
50 strip • NHS indicative price = £5.90 • Drug Tariff (Part IXr)

Blood ketones testing strips

● BLOOD KETONES TESTING STRIPS

4SURE beta-ketone testing strips (Nipro Medical UK Ltd) | 10 strip • NHS indicative price = £9.92 • Drug Tariff (Part IXr)

Fora Advanced pro GD40 Ketone testing strips (Miller Medical Supplies Ltd) | 10 strip • NHS indicative price = £8.95 • Drug Tariff (Part IXr)

FreeStyle Optium H beta-ketone testing strips (Abbott Laboratories Ltd) | 10 strip • No NHS indicative price available • Drug Tariff (Part IXr)

FreeStyle Optium beta-ketone testing strips (Abbott Laboratories Ltd) | 10 strip • NHS indicative price = £21.94 • Drug Tariff (Part IXr)

FreeStyle Precision Pro beta-ketone testing strips (Abbott Laboratories Ltd) | 50 strip • No NHS indicative price available

GlucoMen areo Ketone Sensor testing strips (A. Menarini Diagnostics Ltd) | 10 strip • NHS indicative price = £9.95 • Drug Tariff (Part IXr)

GlucoRx HCT Ketone testing strips (GlucoRx Ltd) | 10 strip • NHS indicative price = £9.95 • Drug Tariff (Part IXr)

GlucoRx Smart Ketone testing strips (GlucoRx Ltd) | 10 strip • NHS indicative price = £8.95 • Drug Tariff (Part IXr)

GlucoRx X6 Ketone testing strips (GlucoRx Ltd) | 10 strip • NHS indicative price = £15.95 • Drug Tariff (Part IXr)

Glucofix Tech beta-ketone Sensor testing strips (A. Menarini Diagnostics Ltd) | 10 strip • NHS indicative price = £9.95 • Drug Tariff (Part IXr)

KetoSens testing strips (Spirit Healthcare Ltd) | 10 strip • NHS indicative price = £9.95 • Drug Tariff (Part IXr)

Neon GK+ Ketone testing strips (Neon Diagnostics Ltd) | 10 strip • NHS indicative price = £7.95 • Drug Tariff (Part IXr)

StatStrip beta-ketone testing strips (Nova Biomedical) | 50 strip • No NHS indicative price available

Xceed Precision Pro beta-ketone testing strips (Abbott Laboratories Ltd) | 10 strip • No NHS indicative price available • Drug Tariff (Part IXr) | 50 strip • No NHS indicative price available | 100 strip • No NHS indicative price available

Glucose interstitial fluid detection sensors

● GLUCOSE INTERSTITIAL FLUID DETECTION SENSORS

A8 TouchCare Nano Sensor (Medtrum Ltd)
2 kit • No NHS indicative price available • Drug Tariff (Part IXa)

A8 TouchCare Nano Transmitter (Medtrum Ltd)
1 device • No NHS indicative price available • Drug Tariff (Part IXa)

ALLYcgm Sensor (AgaMatrix Europe Ltd)
1 kit • NHS indicative price = £31.87 • Drug Tariff (Part IXa)

Accu-Chek SmartGuide Sensor (Roche Diagnostics Ltd)
1 kit • NHS indicative price = £35.00 • Drug Tariff (Part IXa)

CareSens Air Sensor (Spirit Healthcare Ltd)
1 kit • NHS indicative price = £31.87 • Drug Tariff (Part IXa)

Dexcom G6 Receiver (Dexcom International Ltd)
1 device • No NHS indicative price available • Drug Tariff (Part IXa)

Dexcom G6 Sensor (Dexcom International Ltd)
1 kit • No NHS indicative price available • Drug Tariff (Part IXa) | 3 kit • No NHS indicative price available • Drug Tariff (Part IXa)

Dexcom G6 Transmitter (Dexcom International Ltd)
1 device • No NHS indicative price available • Drug Tariff (Part IXa)

Dexcom G7 Receiver (Dexcom International Ltd)
1 device • No NHS indicative price available • Drug Tariff (Part IXa)

Dexcom G7 Sensor (Dexcom International Ltd)
1 kit • No NHS indicative price available • Drug Tariff (Part IXa)

Dexcom One+ Sensor (Dexcom International Ltd)
1 kit • NHS indicative price = £24.97 • Drug Tariff (Part IXa)

FreeStyle Libre 2 Plus Sensor (Abbott Laboratories Ltd)
1 kit • NHS indicative price = £37.50 • Drug Tariff (Part IXa)

FreeStyle Libre 3 Plus Sensor (Abbott Laboratories Ltd)
1 kit • NHS indicative price = £45.00 • Drug Tariff (Part IXa)

GlucoMen iCan Sensor (A. Menarini Diagnostics Ltd)
1 kit • NHS indicative price = £37.25 • Drug Tariff (Part IXa)

GlucoRx AiDEX Sensor (GlucoRx Ltd)
1 kit • NHS indicative price = £29.76 • Drug Tariff (Part IXa)

GlucoRx AiDEX Transmitter (GlucoRx Ltd)
1 device • NHS indicative price = £19.95 • Drug Tariff (Part IXa)

Guardian 4 Link Transmitter Replacement (Medtronic Ltd)
1 device • No NHS indicative price available • Drug Tariff (Part IXa)

Guardian 4 Sensor (Medtronic Ltd)
1 device • No NHS indicative price available • Drug Tariff (Part IXa) | 5 device • No NHS indicative price available | 10 device • No NHS indicative price available | 15 device • No NHS indicative price available

Sibionics GS3-R Sensor (Shenzhen Sisensing Co., Ltd)
1 kit • NHS indicative price = £35.00 • Drug Tariff (Part IXa)

Hypodermic insulin injection pens

● HYPODERMIC INSULIN INJECTION PENS

AUTOPEN® 24

Autopen® 24 (for use with Sanofi- Aventis 3-mL insulin cartridges), allowing 1-unit dosage adjustment, max. 21 units (single-unit version) or 2-unit dosage adjustment, max. 42 units (2- unit version).

AUTOPEN® CLASSIC

Autopen® Classic (for use with Lilly and Wockhardt 3-mL insulin cartridges), allowing 1-unit dosage adjustment, max. 21 units (single-unit version) or 2-unit dosage adjustment, max. 42 units (2-unit version).

HUMAPEN® LUXURA HD

For use with *Humulin®* and *Humalog®* 3-mL cartridges; allowing 0.5-unit dosage adjustment, max. 30 units.

NOVOPEN ECHO® PLUS

For use with *Penfill®* 3-mL insulin cartridges; allowing 0.5-unit dosage adjustment, max. 30 units.

NovoPen Echo Plus hypodermic insulin injection pen reusable for 3ml cartridge 0.5 unit dial up / range 0.5-30 units (Novo Nordisk Ltd)
1 device • NHS indicative price = £26.86 • Drug Tariff (Part IXa)

NovoPen Echo Plus hypodermic insulin injection pen reusable for 3ml cartridge 0.5 unit dial up / range 0.5-30 units (Novo Nordisk Ltd)
1 device • NHS indicative price = £26.86 • Drug Tariff (Part IXa)

NOVOPEN® 6

For use with *Penfill®* 3-mL insulin cartridges; allowing 1-unit dosage adjustment, max. 60 units.

NovoPen 6 hypodermic insulin injection pen reusable for 3ml cartridge 1 unit dial up / range 1-60 units (Novo Nordisk Ltd)
1 device • NHS indicative price = £26.86 • Drug Tariff (Part IXa)

NovoPen 6 hypodermic insulin injection pen reusable for 3ml cartridge 1 unit dial up / range 1-60 units (Novo Nordisk Ltd)
1 device • NHS indicative price = £26.86 • Drug Tariff (Part IXa)

Needle free insulin delivery systems

● **NEEDLE FREE INSULIN DELIVERY SYSTEMS**

INSUJET®

For use with any 10-mL vial or 3-mL cartridge of insulin, allowing 1-unit dosage adjustment, max 40 units. Available as *starter set* (*InsuJet®* device, nozzle cap, nozzle and piston, 1 × 10-mL adaptor, 1 × 3-mL adaptor, 1 cartridge cap removal key), *nozzle pack* (15 nozzles), *cartridge adaptor pack* (15 adaptors), or *vial adaptor pack* (15 adaptors).

Urine glucose testing strips

● **URINE GLUCOSE TESTING STRIPS**

Diastix testing strips (Ascensia Diabetes Care UK Ltd)
50 strip • NHS indicative price = £2.96 • Drug Tariff (Part IXr)

Medi-Test Glucose testing strips (BHR Pharmaceuticals Ltd)
50 strip • NHS indicative price = £2.36 • Drug Tariff (Part IXr)

Urine ketone testing strips

● **URINE KETONES TESTING STRIPS**

GlucoRx KetoRx Sticks 2GK testing strips (GlucoRx Ltd)
50 strip • NHS indicative price = £2.25 • Drug Tariff (Part IXr)

Ketostix testing strips (Ascensia Diabetes Care UK Ltd)
50 strip • NHS indicative price = £3.13 • Drug Tariff (Part IXr)

Urine protein testing strips

● **URINE PROTEIN TESTING STRIPS**

Albustix testing strips (Siemens Medical Solutions Diagnostics Ltd)
50 strip • NHS indicative price = £4.42 • Drug Tariff (Part IXr)

Medi-Test Protein 2 testing strips (BHR Pharmaceuticals Ltd)
50 strip • NHS indicative price = £3.31 • Drug Tariff (Part IXr)

4.2 Hypoglycaemia

Hypoglycaemia

07-Apr-2021

Description of condition

Hypoglycaemia results from an imbalance between glucose supply, glucose utilisation, and existing insulin concentration. Clinical hypoglycaemia is defined as a blood-glucose concentration low enough to cause symptoms or signs of impaired brain function. In clinical practice, a glucose value of ≤ 3.9 mmol/litre is used as the threshold value to initiate treatment for hypoglycaemia in children with diabetes.

Symptoms of hypoglycaemia in the young include shakiness, pounding heart, sweatiness, headache, drowsiness, and difficulty concentrating. In young children, behavioural changes such as irritability, agitation, quietness, and tantrums, may be prominent.

Short-term complications of severe hypoglycaemia include transient neurological symptoms such as paresis, convulsions, encephalopathy, loss of consciousness, and rarely, subsequent neurological damage and mild intellectual impairment.

Diabetes mellitus, idiopathic ketotic hypoglycaemia, adrenal insufficiency, hyperinsulinism, fatty acid oxidation disorders, and glycogen storage disease (amongst others), may cause acute hypoglycaemia in children. Common clinical precipitants for hypoglycaemia in children with diabetes may include insufficient food consumption (i.e. missed meals, nocturnal hypoglycaemia), excessive insulin dosing, exercise, alcohol ingestion (in adolescents), and sulfonylureas [unlicensed].

Treatment of acute hypoglycaemia

For a quick reference resource with doses for the treatment of hypoglycaemia, see *Hypoglycaemia* in Medical emergencies in the community p. 1480.

Prompt treatment of hypoglycaemia in children is essential whatever the cause. Hypoglycaemia caused by a sulfonylurea (although rarely used in children) or a long acting insulin, may persist for up to 24–36 hours following the last dose, especially if there is concurrent renal impairment (rare in children). EvGr Close monitoring is required and hospital care should be considered. Ⓔ

Severe hypoglycaemia

Intravenous management

Hypoglycaemia which causes unconsciousness or seizures is an emergency. EvGr If the child is in hospital and rapid intravenous access is possible, severe hypoglycaemia should be treated with glucose 10% intravenous infusion p. 730. Ⓐ EvGr A bolus dose using glucose 10% can be given before the glucose infusion to rapidly increase the plasma-glucose concentration, in order to allow glucose to cross the blood brain barrier and alleviate neuroglycopaenia. Ⓔ

Pain and phlebitis may occur during administration, particularly if infused too quickly. Glucose 50% intravenous infusion is not recommended as it is hypertonic, thus increases the risk of extravasation injury, and is viscous, making administration difficult.

Oral and intramuscular management

EvGr Severe hypoglycaemia outside of hospital or when rapid intravenous access is not available, may be treated with concentrated oral glucose solution, as long as the child is **conscious and able to swallow.** Ⓐ Proprietary products of fast-acting carbohydrate, as glucose 40% gel (e.g. *Glucogel®*, *Dextrogel®*, or *Rapilose®*, see glucose) are available for the patient to keep at hand in case of severe hypoglycaemia.

EvGr If the child is **unconscious or unable to swallow,** intramuscular glucagon p. 579 should be given and blood-glucose concentration monitored. (A) Glucagon increases blood glucose by mobilising glycogen stored in the liver. The manufacturer advises that it is ineffective in patients whose liver glycogen is depleted, therefore should not be used in anyone who has fasted for a prolonged period, has adrenal insufficiency, chronic hypoglycaemia, or alcohol-induced hypoglycaemia. EvGr Glucagon may also be less effective in children taking a sulfonylurea; in these cases, intravenous glucose will be required. (E)

EvGr As symptoms improve or normoglycaemia is restored, and the child is sufficiently awake, an oral long-acting carbohydrate snack (e.g. two biscuits, one banana) or a meal should be given to maintain normal blood-glucose concentration. The blood-glucose concentration should be checked repeatedly in children and young people who have persistently reduced consciousness after a severe hypoglycaemic episode, to determine whether further glucose is needed. (A)

Advice for parents or carers

EvGr Parents or carers of insulin-treated children should be trained and equipped to give intramuscular glucagon for emergency use in severe hypoglycaemic attacks.

Parents or carers should be advised to seek medical assistance if glucagon is not effective within 10 minutes as intravenous glucose is required. (A)

Non-severe hypoglycaemia

EvGr In children who are **conscious and able to swallow**, non-severe hypoglycaemia is treated with a fast-acting carbohydrate by mouth, preferably in liquid form. (A)

EvGr Fast-acting carbohydrates include *Lift*® glucose liquid (previously *Glucojuice*®), glucose tablets, glucose 40% gels (e.g. *Glucogel*®, *Dextrogel*®, or *Rapilose*®), and sugar (sucrose) dissolved in an appropriate volume of water. Oral glucose formulations are preferred as absorption occurs more quickly. Glucose 40% gel may be given buccally in children who are uncooperative, but who are conscious and able to swallow. (E)

EvGr Chocolates and biscuits should be avoided if possible, because they have a lower sugar content and their high fat content may delay stomach emptying.

Administration of fast-acting carbohydrates may need to be in frequent small amounts, because hypoglycaemia can cause vomiting. (A) Blood-glucose concentrations should rise within 5–15 minutes; EvGr if hypoglycaemia persists after 15 minutes, repeat the fast-acting glucose. As symptoms improve or normoglycaemia is restored, a long-acting carbohydrate snack (e.g. two biscuits, one banana) or a meal, can be given to prevent blood-glucose concentration from falling again. (A)

Neonatal hypoglycaemia in term babies

Infants at risk of impaired metabolic adaptation and hypoglycaemia include infants of mothers with diabetes (including gestational diabetes), those whose mothers have taken beta-blockers, and those with intra-uterine growth restriction. EvGr Severe or persistent hypoglycaemia may be a presenting feature of an underlying inborn error of metabolism and requires urgent medical review.

Asymptomatic neonatal hypoglycaemia may be treated by increasing breast-feeding frequency, supplementing with a breast milk substitute (i.e. formula), or intravenous glucose therapy. Buccal glucose gel may be used in conjunction with a feeding plan. When feeding interventions are offered, blood-glucose concentrations should be re-checked in 1 hour to ensure there has been a response. If feeding interventions are not effective, glucose 10% intravenous infusion should be given, and blood-glucose re-tested within 15 minutes.

Symptomatic hypoglycaemic neonates should be treated immediately with a glucose intravenous infusion. If there is a delay in obtaining intravenous access, consider either buccal glucose gel or intramuscular glucagon. If blood glucose is <1 mmol/litre, buccal glucose gel should only be used as an interim measure while arranging treatment with intravenous glucose infusion. Neonates requiring 12 mg/kg/minute or more of glucose to maintain normoglycaemia, should be investigated for congenital hyperinsulinism. (E)

GLYCOGENOLYTIC HORMONES

Glucagon

10-Nov-2021

● **INDICATIONS AND DOSE**

Diabetic hypoglycaemia

▶ BY SUBCUTANEOUS INJECTION, OR BY INTRAMUSCULAR INJECTION

- Neonate: 20 micrograms/kg.
- Child 1 month–8 years (body-weight up to 25 kg): 500 micrograms, if no response within 10 minutes intravenous glucose must be given
- Child 9–17 years (body-weight 25 kg and above): 1 mg, if no response within 10 minutes intravenous glucose must be given

Endogenous hyperinsulinism

▶ BY INTRAMUSCULAR INJECTION, OR BY INTRAVENOUS INJECTION

- Neonate: 200 micrograms/kg (max. per dose 1 mg) for 1 dose.
- Child 1 month–1 year: 1 mg for 1 dose

▶ BY CONTINUOUS INTRAVENOUS INFUSION

- Neonate: 1–18 micrograms/kg/hour (max. per dose 50 micrograms/kg/hour), adjusted according to response.
- Child 1 month–1 year: 1–10 micrograms/kg/hour, dose to be adjusted as necessary

Diagnosis of growth hormone secretion (specialist use only)

▶ BY INTRAMUSCULAR INJECTION

- Child: 100 micrograms/kg (max. per dose 1 mg) for 1 dose, dose may vary, consult local guidelines

Severe hypotension, heart failure or cardiogenic shock due to acute overdosage of beta-blockers

▶ INITIALLY BY INTRAVENOUS INJECTION

- Child: 50–150 micrograms/kg (max. per dose 10 mg), administered over 1–2 minutes, followed by (by intravenous infusion) 50 micrograms/kg/hour, titrated according to response

DOSE EQUIVALENCE AND CONVERSION

- 1 unit of glucagon = 1 mg of glucagon.

● **UNLICENSED USE** TOXBASE advises glucagon is used for the treatment of severe hypotension, heart failure or cardiogenic shock due to acute overdosage of beta-blockers, but it is not licensed for this indication.

Not licensed for growth hormone test and hyperinsulinism.

● **CONTRA-INDICATIONS** Phaeochromocytoma

● **CAUTIONS** Glucagonoma · ineffective in chronic hypoglycaemia, starvation, and adrenal insufficiency · insulinoma · when used in the diagnosis of growth hormone secretion, delayed hypoglycaemia may result—deaths reported (ensure a meal is eaten before discharge)

● **INTERACTIONS** → Appendix 1: glucagon

● **SIDE-EFFECTS**

▶ **Common or very common** Nausea

▶ **Uncommon** Vomiting

▶ **Rare or very rare** Abdominal pain · hypertension · hypotension · tachycardia

- **DIRECTIONS FOR ADMINISTRATION** For *intravenous infusion*, TOXBASE advises reconstituted solution may be used undiluted or diluted in Glucose 5%.
  Incompatibility For *intravenous infusion*, expert sources advise do not add to infusion fluids containing calcium—precipitation may occur.
- **PATIENT AND CARER ADVICE**
  Medicines for Children leaflet: Glucagon for hypoglycaemia www.medicinesforchildren.org.uk/medicines/glucagon-for-hypoglycaemia/
- **EXCEPTIONS TO LEGAL CATEGORY** Prescription-only medicine restriction does not apply where administration is for saving life in emergency.

- **MEDICINAL FORMS** There can be variation in the licensing of different medicines containing the same drug.
  Powder and solvent for solution for injection
  ▸ **GlucaGen Hypokit** (Novo Nordisk Ltd)
  Glucagon hydrochloride 1 mg GlucaGen Hypokit 1mg powder and solvent for solution for injection | 1 vial PoM £11.52 DT = £11.52

4.2a Chronic hypoglycaemia

Other drugs used for Chronic hypoglycaemia
Chlorothiazide, p. 130

GLYCOGENOLYTIC HORMONES

Diazoxide

17-May-2021

- **INDICATIONS AND DOSE**
  Resistant hypertension
  ▸ BY MOUTH
  ▸ Neonate: Initially 1.7 mg/kg 3 times a day, adjusted according to response; maximum 15 mg/kg per day.
  ▸ Child: Initially 1.7 mg/kg 3 times a day, adjusted according to response; maximum 15 mg/kg per day
  Chronic intractable hypoglycaemia
  ▸ BY MOUTH
  ▸ Neonate: Initially 5 mg/kg twice daily, adjusted according to response, initial dose used to establish response; maintenance 1.5–3 mg/kg 2–3 times a day; increased if necessary up to 7 mg/kg 3 times a day, higher doses are unlikely to be beneficial, but may be required in some cases.
  ▸ Child: Initially 1.7 mg/kg 3 times a day, adjusted according to response; maintenance 1.5–3 mg/kg 2–3 times a day, increased if necessary up to 5 mg/kg 3 times a day, doses up to 5 mg/kg may be required in some cases, but higher doses are unlikely to be beneficial
- **UNLICENSED USE** Not licensed for resistant hypertension.
- **CAUTIONS** Aortic coarctation · aortic stenosis · arteriovenous shunt · heart failure · hyperuricaemia · impaired cardiac circulation · impaired cerebral circulation
- **INTERACTIONS** → Appendix 1: diazoxide
- **SIDE-EFFECTS** Abdominal pain · albuminuria · appetite decreased (long term use) · arrhythmia · azotaemia · cardiomegaly · cataract · constipation · diabetic hyperosmolar coma · diarrhoea · dizziness · dyspnoea · eosinophilia · extrapyramidal symptoms · face abnormal · fever · fluid retention · galactorrhoea · haemorrhage · headache · heart failure · hirsutism · hyperglycaemia · hyperuricaemia (long term use) · hypogammaglobulinaemia · hypotension · ileus · ketoacidosis · leucopenia · libido decreased · musculoskeletal pain · nausea · nephritic syndrome · oculogyric crisis · pancreatitis · parkinsonism · pulmonary hypertension · skin reactions · sodium retention · taste altered · thrombocytopenia · tinnitus · vision disorders · voice alteration (long term use) · vomiting
- **PREGNANCY** Use only if essential; alopecia and hypertrichosis reported in neonates with prolonged use; may inhibit uterine activity during labour.
- **BREAST FEEDING** Manufacturer advises avoid—no information available.
- **RENAL IMPAIRMENT**
  Dose adjustments EvGr Dose reduction may be required. Ⓜ
- **MONITORING REQUIREMENTS**
  ▸ Monitor blood pressure.
  ▸ Monitor white cell and platelet count during prolonged use.
  ▸ Regularly assess growth, bone, and psychological development during prolonged use.

- **MEDICINAL FORMS** There can be variation in the licensing of different medicines containing the same drug. Forms available from special-order manufacturers include: oral capsule, oral suspension, oral solution
  Oral tablet
  ▸ **Eudemine** (RPH Pharmaceuticals AB)
  Diazoxide 50 mg Eudemine 50mg tablets | 100 tablet PoM £108.61 DT = £108.61
  Oral capsule
  ▸ **Diazoxide (Non-proprietary)**
  Diazoxide 25 mg Proglycem 25 capsules | 100 capsule PoM

PITUITARY AND HYPOTHALAMIC HORMONES AND ANALOGUES › SOMATOSTATIN ANALOGUES

Somatostatin analogues

- **CAUTIONS** Diabetes mellitus (antidiabetic requirements may be altered) · insulinoma (increased depth and duration of hypoglycaemia may occur—observe patients and monitor blood glucose levels when initiating treatment and changing doses)
- **SIDE-EFFECTS**
  ▸ **Common or very common** Alopecia · appetite decreased · asthenia · cholecystitis · cholelithiasis (following long term use) · cholestasis · constipation · diabetes mellitus · diarrhoea · dizziness · gastrointestinal discomfort · gastrointestinal disorders · glucose tolerance impaired (following long term use) · headache · hyperglycaemia (long term use) · hypoglycaemia · myalgia · nausea · pruritus · sinus bradycardia · vomiting
- **DIRECTIONS FOR ADMINISTRATION** Injection sites should be rotated.

above

Octreotide

14-Sep-2020

- **INDICATIONS AND DOSE**
  Persistent hyperinsulinaemic hypoglycaemia unresponsive to diazoxide and glucose
  ▸ BY SUBCUTANEOUS INJECTION
  ▸ Neonate: Initially 2–5 micrograms/kg every 6–8 hours, adjusted according to response; increased if necessary up to 7 micrograms/kg every 4 hours, dosing up to 7 micrograms/kg may rarely be required.
  ▸ Child: Initially 1–2 micrograms/kg every 4–6 hours, adjusted according to response; increased if necessary up to 7 micrograms/kg every 4 hours, dosing up to 7 micrograms/kg may rarely be required

Bleeding from oesophageal or gastric varices
- ▶ BY CONTINUOUS INTRAVENOUS INFUSION
- ▶ Child: 1 microgram/kg/hour, higher doses may be required initially, when no active bleeding reduce dose over 24 hours; Usual maximum 50 micrograms/hour

- **UNLICENSED USE** Not licensed in children.
- **INTERACTIONS** → Appendix 1: octreotide
- **SIDE-EFFECTS**
- ▶ **Common or very common** Arrhythmias · biliary sludge · dyspnoea · hyperbilirubinaemia · hypothyroidism · skin reactions · thyroid disorder
- ▶ **Uncommon** Dehydration
- ▶ **Frequency not known** Hepatic disorders · pancreatitis acute (after administration) · thrombocytopenia

SIDE-EFFECTS, FURTHER INFORMATION Administering non-depot injections of octreotide between meals and at bedtime may reduce gastrointestinal side-effects.

- **CONCEPTION AND CONTRACEPTION** Effective contraception required during treatment.
- **PREGNANCY** Possible effect on fetal growth; manufacturer advises use only if potential benefit outweighs risk.
- **BREAST FEEDING** Manufacturer advises avoid—present in milk in *animal* studies.
- **HEPATIC IMPAIRMENT** Manufacturer advises caution (risk of increased half-life in cirrhosis).

Dose adjustments In adults, manufacturer advises consider dose reduction—consult product literature.

- **MONITORING REQUIREMENTS**
- ▶ Monitor thyroid function on long-term therapy.
- ▶ Monitor liver function.
- **TREATMENT CESSATION** Avoid abrupt withdrawal of short-acting subcutaneous octreotide (associated with biliary colic and pancreatitis).
- **DIRECTIONS FOR ADMINISTRATION** For *intravenous injection or intravenous infusion*, manufacturer advises dilute requisite dose to a ratio of at least 1:1 and up to a maximum of 1:9 by volume with Sodium Chloride 0.9%.

- **MEDICINAL FORMS** There can be variation in the licensing of different medicines containing the same drug.

Solution for injection

▶ **Octreotide (Non-proprietary)**

Octreotide (as Octreotide acetate) 50 microgram per 1 ml Octreotide 50micrograms/1ml solution for injection pre-filled syringes | 5 pre-filled disposable injection [PoM] £35.00–£64.00 DT = £35.00

Octreotide 50micrograms/1ml solution for injection ampoules | 5 ampoule [PoM] £12.64–£18.60 DT = £14.87

Octreotide (as Octreotide acetate) 100 microgram per 1 ml Octreotide 100micrograms/1ml solution for injection ampoules | 5 ampoule [PoM] £27.75–£32.65 DT = £27.97

Octreotide 100micrograms/1ml solution for injection pre-filled syringes | 5 pre-filled disposable injection [PoM] £55.00–£100.00 DT = £55.00

Octreotide 100micrograms/1ml solution for injection vials | 5 vial [PoM] £32.65 DT = £32.65 (Hospital only) | 5 vial [PoM] £32.65 DT = £32.65

Octreotide (as Octreotide acetate) 200 microgram per 1 ml Octreotide 1mg/5ml solution for injection vials | 1 vial [PoM] £65.00 DT = £65.00

Octreotide (as Octreotide acetate) 500 microgram per 1 ml Octreotide 500micrograms/1ml solution for injection vials | 5 vial [PoM] £158.25 DT = £158.25

Octreotide 500micrograms/1ml solution for injection pre-filled syringes | 5 pre-filled disposable injection [PoM] £250.00–£460.00 DT = £250.00

Octreotide 500micrograms/1ml solution for injection ampoules | 5 ampoule [PoM] £115.15–£169.35 DT = £135.47

▶ **Sandostatin** (Novartis Pharmaceuticals UK Ltd)

Octreotide (as Octreotide acetate) 50 microgram per 1 ml Sandostatin 50micrograms/1ml solution for injection ampoules | 5 ampoule [PoM] £14.87 DT = £14.87

Octreotide (as Octreotide acetate) 100 microgram per 1 ml Sandostatin 100micrograms/1ml solution for injection ampoules | 5 ampoule [PoM] £27.97 DT = £27.97

Octreotide (as Octreotide acetate) 500 microgram per 1 ml Sandostatin 500micrograms/1ml solution for injection ampoules | 5 ampoule [PoM] £135.47 DT = £135.47

Powder and solvent for suspension for injection

▶ **Olatuton** (Teva UK Ltd)

Octreotide (as Octreotide acetate) 10 mg Olatuton 10mg powder and solvent for prolonged-release suspension for injection vials | 1 vial [PoM] £494.74 DT = £549.71

Octreotide (as Octreotide acetate) 20 mg Olatuton 20mg powder and solvent for prolonged-release suspension for injection vials | 1 vial [PoM] £719.40 DT = £799.33

Octreotide (as Octreotide acetate) 30 mg Olatuton 30mg powder and solvent for prolonged-release suspension for injection vials | 1 vial [PoM] £898.57 DT = £998.41

▶ **Sandostatin LAR** (Novartis Pharmaceuticals UK Ltd)

Octreotide (as Octreotide acetate) 10 mg Sandostatin LAR 10mg powder and solvent for suspension for injection vials | 1 vial [PoM] £549.71 DT = £549.71

Octreotide (as Octreotide acetate) 20 mg Sandostatin LAR 20mg powder and solvent for suspension for injection vials | 1 vial [PoM] £799.33 DT = £799.33

Octreotide (as Octreotide acetate) 30 mg Sandostatin LAR 30mg powder and solvent for suspension for injection vials | 1 vial [PoM] £998.41 DT = £998.41

5 Gonadotrophin responsive conditions

PITUITARY AND HYPOTHALAMIC HORMONES AND ANALOGUES > GONADOTROPHIN-RELEASING HORMONES

Goserelin

16-Jul-2024

- **DRUG ACTION** Administration of gonadorelin analogues produces an initial phase of stimulation; continued administration is followed by down-regulation of gonadotrophin-releasing hormone receptors, thereby reducing the release of gonadotrophins (follicle stimulating hormone and luteinising hormone) which in turn leads to inhibition of androgen and oestrogen production.

- **INDICATIONS AND DOSE**

ZOLADEX LA ®

Gonadotrophin-dependent precocious puberty
- ▶ BY SUBCUTANEOUS INJECTION
- ▶ Child: 10.8 mg every 12 weeks, to be administered into the anterior abdominal wall, injections may be required more frequently in some cases

ZOLADEX ®

Gonadotrophin-dependent precocious puberty
- ▶ BY SUBCUTANEOUS INJECTION
- ▶ Child: 3.6 mg every 28 days, to be administered into the anterior abdominal wall, injections may be required more frequently in some cases

- **UNLICENSED USE** Not licensed for use in children.
- **CONTRA-INDICATIONS** Undiagnosed vaginal bleeding
- **CAUTIONS** Depression · patients with metabolic bone disease (decrease in bone mineral density can occur)
- **SIDE-EFFECTS** Asthma · body hair change · breast abnormalities · depression · headache · hypersensitivity · mood altered · ovarian cyst · paraesthesia · skin reactions · vaginal haemorrhage · visual impairment · weight change · withdrawal bleed
- **CONCEPTION AND CONTRACEPTION** Non-hormonal, barrier methods of contraception should be used during entire

treatment period. Pregnancy should be excluded before treatment, the first injection should be given during menstruation or shortly afterwards or use barrier contraception for 1 month beforehand.

- **PREGNANCY** Avoid.
- **BREAST FEEDING** Avoid.
- **MONITORING REQUIREMENTS** Monitor bone mineral density.
- **DIRECTIONS FOR ADMINISTRATION** Rotate injection site to prevent atrophy and nodule formation.
- **NATIONAL FUNDING/ACCESS DECISIONS**

NHS restrictions Goserelin is not prescribable in NHS primary care for puberty suppression [unlicensed use] except in children who meet the criteria listed in part XVIIIB of the Drug Tariff. The prescription must be endorsed 'SLS'.

- **MEDICINAL FORMS** There can be variation in the licensing of different medicines containing the same drug.

Prolonged-release subcutaneous implant

- Zoladex (AstraZeneca UK Ltd)
  Goserelin (as Goserelin acetate) 3.6 mg Zoladex 3.6mg implant SafeSystem pre-filled syringes | 1 pre-filled disposable injection PoM £70.00 DT = £70.00
- Zoladex LA (AstraZeneca UK Ltd)
  Goserelin (as Goserelin acetate) 10.8 mg Zoladex LA 10.8mg implant SafeSystem pre-filled syringes | 1 pre-filled disposable injection PoM £235.00 DT = £235.00

Leuprorelin acetate

14-Jan-2025

- **DRUG ACTION** Administration of gonadorelin analogues produces an initial phase of stimulation; continued administration is followed by down-regulation of gonadotrophin-releasing hormone receptors, thereby reducing the release of gonadotrophins (follicle stimulating hormone and luteinising hormone) which in turn leads to inhibition of androgen and oestrogen production.

- **INDICATIONS AND DOSE**

PROSTAP 3 DCS®

Gonadotrophin-dependent precocious puberty (specialist use only)

- BY SUBCUTANEOUS INJECTION
- Child (body-weight up to 19 kg): 5.625 mg every 3 months, dose may be increased if necessary. Discontinue when bone maturation consistent with age of 12 years in girls or 13 years in boys
- Child (body-weight 20 kg and above): 11.25 mg every 3 months, dose may be increased if necessary. Discontinue when bone maturation consistent with age of 12 years in girls or 13 years in boys

PROSTAP PD DCS®

Gonadotrophin-dependent precocious puberty (specialist use only)

- BY SUBCUTANEOUS INJECTION
- Child (body-weight up to 19 kg): 1.88 mg every month, dose may be increased if necessary. Discontinue when bone maturation consistent with age of 12 years in girls or 13 years in boys

PROSTAP SR DCS®

Gonadotrophin-dependent precocious puberty (specialist use only)

- BY SUBCUTANEOUS INJECTION
- Child (body-weight up to 19 kg): 1.88 mg every month, dose may be increased if necessary. Discontinue when bone maturation consistent with age of 12 years in girls or 13 years in boys
- Child (body-weight 20 kg and above): 3.75 mg every month, dose may be increased if necessary. Discontinue when bone maturation consistent with age of 12 years in girls or 13 years in boys

- **CONTRA-INDICATIONS**

PROSTAP 3 DCS® Undiagnosed vaginal bleeding

PROSTAP PD DCS® Undiagnosed vaginal bleeding

PROSTAP SR DCS® Undiagnosed vaginal bleeding

- **CAUTIONS** Patients with metabolic bone disease (decrease in bone mineral density can occur)
- **SIDE-EFFECTS**
  - **Common or very common** Depression · emotional lability · gastrointestinal discomfort · haemorrhage · headache · metrorrhagia · nausea · skin reactions · vaginal discharge · vomiting
  - **Uncommon** Myalgia
  - **Frequency not known** Idiopathic intracranial hypertension · interstitial lung disease · seizure · severe cutaneous adverse reactions (SCARs)
- **PREGNANCY** Avoid—teratogenic in *animal* studies.
- **BREAST FEEDING** Avoid.
- **MONITORING REQUIREMENTS**
  - Monitor bone maturation every 6–12 months during treatment.
  - Monitor weight gain regularly during treatment.
- **DIRECTIONS FOR ADMINISTRATION** Rotate injection site to prevent atrophy and nodule formation.

STALADEX® 11.25MG To be administered under the skin of the abdomen.

- **PATIENT AND CARER ADVICE** Patients and carers should be counselled on the signs and symptoms of idiopathic intracranial hypertension (such as severe or recurrent headache, vision disturbances and tinnitus)—consider discontinuing treatment if these occur. Patients and carers should be informed of the increased risk of depression during treatment.

PROSTAP 3 DCS® Patients and carers should be counselled on the signs and symptoms of severe cutaneous adverse reactions (SCARs) when starting treatment—treatment should be immediately discontinued if these occur.

PROSTAP PD DCS® Patients and carers should be counselled on the signs and symptoms of severe cutaneous adverse reactions (SCARs) when starting treatment—treatment should be immediately discontinued if these occur.

PROSTAP SR DCS® Patients and carers should be counselled on the signs and symptoms of severe cutaneous adverse reactions (SCARs) when starting treatment—treatment should be immediately discontinued if these occur.

- **NATIONAL FUNDING/ACCESS DECISIONS**

NHS restrictions Leuprorelin acetate is not prescribable in NHS primary care for puberty suppression [unlicensed use] except in children who meet the criteria listed in part XVIIIB of the Drug Tariff. The prescription must be endorsed 'SLS'.

- **MEDICINAL FORMS** There can be variation in the licensing of different medicines containing the same drug.

Powder and solvent for prolonged-release suspension for inj

EXCIPIENTS: May contain Polysorbates

- Prostap 3 DCS (Takeda UK Ltd)
  Leuprorelin acetate 11.25 mg Prostap 3 DCS 11.25mg powder and solvent for prolonged-release suspension for injection pre-filled syringes | 1 pre-filled disposable injection PoM £225.72 DT = £225.72

- ▸ **Prostap PD DCS** (Takeda UK Ltd)
  Leuprorelin acetate 1.88 mg Prostap PD DCS 1.88mg powder and solvent for prolonged-release suspension for injection pre-filled syringes | 1 pre-filled disposable injection [PoM] £60.00 DT = £60.00
- ▸ **Prostap SR DCS** (Takeda UK Ltd)
  Leuprorelin acetate 3.75 mg Prostap SR DCS 3.75mg powder and solvent for prolonged-release suspension for injection pre-filled syringes | 1 pre-filled disposable injection [PoM] £75.24 DT = £75.24

Triptorelin

23-Jan-2025

- **DRUG ACTION** Administration of gonadorelin analogues produces an initial phase of stimulation; continued administration is followed by down-regulation of gonadotrophin-releasing hormone receptors, thereby reducing the release of gonadotrophins (follicle stimulating hormone and luteinising hormone) which in turn leads to inhibition of androgen and oestrogen production.

- **INDICATIONS AND DOSE**

DECAPEPTYL ® SR 11.25MG

Gonadotrophin-dependent precocious puberty (specialist use only)

▶ BY INTRAMUSCULAR INJECTION
- ▸ Child: 11.25 mg every 3 months, discontinue when bone maturation consistent with age of 12 years in girls or 13–14 years in boys

DECAPEPTYL ® SR 22.5MG

Gonadotrophin-dependent precocious puberty (specialist use only)

▶ BY INTRAMUSCULAR INJECTION
- ▸ Child: 22.5 mg every 6 months, discontinue when bone maturation consistent with age of 12–13 years in girls or 13–14 years in boys

GONAPEPTYL DEPOT ®

Gonadotrophin-dependent precocious puberty

▶ BY SUBCUTANEOUS INJECTION, OR BY DEEP INTRAMUSCULAR INJECTION
- ▸ Child (body-weight up to 20 kg): Initially 1.875 mg every 2 weeks for 3 doses, to be administered on days 0, 14, and 28 of treatment, then 1.875 mg every 3–4 weeks, discontinue when bone maturation consistent with age over 12 years in girls and over 13 years in boys
- ▸ Child (body-weight 20-30 kg): Initially 2.5 mg every 2 weeks for 3 doses, to be administered on days 0, 14, and 28 of treatment, then 2.5 mg every 3–4 weeks, discontinue when bone maturation consistent with age over 12 years in girls and over 13 years in boys
- ▸ Child (body-weight 31 kg and above): Initially 3.75 mg every 2 weeks for 3 doses, to be administered on days 0, 14, and 28 of treatment, then 3.75 mg every 3–4 weeks, discontinue when bone maturation consistent with age over 12 years in girls and over 13 years in boys

- **CONTRA-INDICATIONS** Undiagnosed vaginal bleeding
- **SIDE-EFFECTS**
  - ▶ **Common or very common** Depression · mood altered
  - ▶ **Uncommon** Anaphylactic reaction · haemorrhage · nausea · vaginal discharge · vomiting
  - ▶ **Frequency not known** Alopecia · angioedema · epiphysiolysis · gastrointestinal discomfort · headache · hot flush · malaise · myalgia · nervousness · pain · skin reactions · vision disorders · weight increased
- **CONCEPTION AND CONTRACEPTION** Non-hormonal, barrier methods of contraception should be used during entire treatment period. Pregnancy should be excluded before treatment, the first injection should be given during menstruation or shortly afterwards or use barrier contraception for 1 month beforehand.
- **PREGNANCY** Avoid.
- **BREAST FEEDING** Avoid.
- **MONITORING REQUIREMENTS** Monitor bone mineral density.
- **DIRECTIONS FOR ADMINISTRATION** Rotate injection site to prevent atrophy and nodule formation.
- **PRESCRIBING AND DISPENSING INFORMATION**
  DECAPEPTYL ® SR 11.25MG Each vial includes an overage to allow accurate administration of an 11.25 mg dose.
  DECAPEPTYL ® SR 22.5MG Each vial includes an overage to allow accurate administration of a 22.5 mg dose.
- **NATIONAL FUNDING/ACCESS DECISIONS**
  NHS restrictions Triptorelin is not prescribable in NHS primary care for puberty suppression [unlicensed use] except in children who meet the criteria listed in part XVIIIB of the Drug Tariff. The prescription must be endorsed 'SLS'.

- **MEDICINAL FORMS** There can be variation in the licensing of different medicines containing the same drug.

Powder and solvent for prolonged-release suspension for inj

- ▸ **Decapeptyl SR** (Ipsen Ltd)
  Triptorelin 11.25 mg Decapeptyl SR 11.25mg powder and solvent for suspension for injection vials | 1 vial [PoM] £207.00 DT = £207.00
  Triptorelin (as Triptorelin embonate) 22.5 mg Decapeptyl SR 22.5mg powder and solvent for suspension for injection vials | 1 vial [PoM] £414.00 DT = £414.00
- ▸ **Gonapeptyl Depot** (Ferring Pharmaceuticals Ltd)
  Triptorelin (as Triptorelin acetate) 3.75 mg Gonapeptyl Depot 3.75mg powder and solvent for suspension for injection pre-filled syringes | 1 pre-filled disposable injection [PoM] £81.69 DT = £81.69

6 Hypothalamic and anterior pituitary hormone related disorders

Hypothalamic and anterior pituitary hormones

10-Jul-2025

Anterior pituitary hormones

Corticotrophins

Tetracosactide p. 584 (tetracosactrin), an analogue of corticotropin (adrenocorticotrophic hormone, ACTH), is used to test adrenocortical function; failure of plasma-cortisol concentration to rise after administration of tetracosactide indicates adrenocortical insufficiency. A low-dose test is considered by some clinicians to be more sensitive when used to confirm established, partial adrenal suppression.

Tetracosactide should be given only if no other ACTH preparations have been given previously. Tetracosactide depot injection (*Synacthen Depot*®) is also used in the treatment of infantile spasms but it is contra-indicated in neonates because of the presence of benzyl alcohol in the injection. Corticotropin-releasing factor, corticorelin p. 585, (also known as corticotropin-releasing hormone, CRH) is used to test anterior pituitary function and secretion of corticotropin.

Gonadotrophins

Gonadotrophins are occasionally used in the treatment of hypogonadotrophic hypogonadism and associated oligospermia. There is no justification for their use in primary gonadal failure.

Growth hormone

Growth hormone is used to treat proven deficiency of the hormone, Prader-Willi syndrome, Turner's syndrome, growth disturbance in children born small for corrected gestational age, chronic renal insufficiency, and short stature homeobox-containing gene (SHOX) deficiency. Growth hormone is also used in idiopathic short stature [unlicensed use] and Noonan syndrome under specialist management. Treatment should be initiated and monitored by a paediatrician with expertise in managing growth-hormone disorders; treatment can be continued under a shared-care protocol by a general practitioner.

Growth hormone of human origin (HGH; somatotrophin) has been replaced by recombinant growth hormone of human sequence; somatropin p. 586, and the long-acting forms somapacitan p. 585 and somatrogon p. 586, may be used.

Mecasermin p. 588, a human insulin-like growth factor-I (rhIGF-I), is licensed to treat growth failure in children with severe primary insulin-like growth factor-I deficiency.

Hypothalamic hormones

Gonadorelin p. 585 when injected intravenously in post-pubertal girls leads to a rapid rise in plasma concentrations of both luteinising hormone (LH) and follicle-stimulating hormone (FSH). It has not proved to be very helpful, however, in distinguishing hypothalamic from pituitary lesions. It is used in the assessment of delayed or precocious puberty.

Other growth hormone stimulation tests involve the use of insulin, glucagon p. 579, arginine p. 763, and clonidine hydrochloride p. 120 [all unlicensed uses]. The tests should be carried out in specialist centres.

6.1 Adrenocortical function testing

PITUITARY AND HYPOTHALAMIC HORMONES AND ANALOGUES > CORTICOTROPHINS

Tetracosactide

30-Sep-2022

(Tetracosactrin)

● **INDICATIONS AND DOSE**

Diagnosis of adrenocortical insufficiency (diagnostic 30-minute test), standard-dose test

▶ BY INTRAMUSCULAR INJECTION, OR BY INTRAVENOUS INJECTION

▸ Child: 145 micrograms/m^2 (max. per dose 250 micrograms) for 1 dose

Diagnosis of adrenocortical insufficiency (diagnostic 30-minute test), low-dose test

▶ BY INTRAMUSCULAR INJECTION, OR BY INTRAVENOUS INJECTION

▸ Child: 0.3 microgram/m^2 for 1 dose

Infantile spasms (under expert supervision)

▶ BY INTRAMUSCULAR INJECTION USING DEPOT INJECTION

▸ Child 1–23 months: 500 micrograms once daily on alternate days for 2 weeks; increased if necessary up to 750 micrograms once daily on alternate days, increased dose to be used if spasms continue or recur after the first 7 days

● **UNLICENSED USE** Not licensed for low-dose test for adrenocortical insufficiency. EvGr Tetracosactide is used for the treatment of infantile spasms, (B) but is not licensed for this indication.

● **CONTRA-INDICATIONS** Acute psychosis · adrenogenital syndrome · allergic disorders · asthma · avoid injections containing benzyl alcohol in neonates · Cushing's syndrome · infectious diseases · peptic ulcer · primary adrenocortical insufficiency · refractory heart failure

● **CAUTIONS** Active infectious diseases (should not be used unless adequate disease-specific therapy is being given) · active systemic diseases (should not be used unless adequate disease-specific therapy is being given) · diabetes mellitus · diverticulitis · history of asthma · history of atopic allergy · history of eczema · history of hayfever · history of hypersensitivity · hypertension · latent amoebiasis (may become activated) · latent tuberculosis (may become activated) · myasthenia gravis · ocular herpes simplex · osteoporosis · predisposition to thromboembolism · psychological disturbances may be triggered · recent intestinal anastomosis · reduced immune response (should not be used unless adequate disease-specific therapy is being given) · ulcerative colitis

CAUTIONS, FURTHER INFORMATION

▸ Risk of anaphylaxis Should only be administered under medical supervision—consult product literature.

▸ Hypertension Patients already receiving medication for moderate to severe hypertension must have their dosage adjusted if treatment started.

▸ Diabetes mellitus Patients already receiving medication for diabetes mellitus must have their dosage adjusted if treatment started.

● **SIDE-EFFECTS** Abdominal distension · abscess · adrenocortical unresponsiveness · angioedema · appetite increased · bone fractures · congestive heart failure · Cushing's syndrome · diabetes mellitus exacerbated · dizziness · dyspnoea · electrolyte imbalance · exophthalmos · fluid retention · flushing · gastrointestinal disorders · glaucoma · growth retardation · haemorrhage · headache · healing impaired · hirsutism · hyperglycaemia · hyperhidrosis · hypersensitivity (may be more severe in patients susceptible to allergies, especially asthma) · hypertension · idiopathic intracranial hypertension exacerbated · increased risk of infection · leucocytosis · malaise · menstruation irregular · muscle weakness · myopathy · nausea · osteonecrosis · osteoporosis · pancreatitis · papilloedema · pituitary unresponsiveness · posterior subcapsular cataract · protein catabolism · psychiatric disorder · seizure · skin reactions · tendon rupture · thromboembolism · vasculitis necrotising · ventricular hypertrophy · vertigo · vomiting · weight increased

● **ALLERGY AND CROSS-SENSITIVITY** EvGr Contra-indicated in patients with history of hypersensitivity to tetracosactide/corticotrophins or excipients. (M)

● **PREGNANCY** Avoid (but may be used diagnostically if essential).

● **BREAST FEEDING** Avoid (but may be used diagnostically if essential).

● **HEPATIC IMPAIRMENT** For *depot injection*, manufacturer advises caution in cirrhosis (may enhance effect of tetracosactide therapy).

● **RENAL IMPAIRMENT** EvGr Use with caution in renal failure. (M)

● **EFFECT ON LABORATORY TESTS** May suppress skin test reactions.

Post administration total plasma cortisol levels during 30-minute test for diagnosis of adrenocotical insufficiency might be misleading due to altered cortisol binding globulin levels in some special clinical situations including, patients on oral contraceptives, post-operative patients, critical illness, severe liver disease and nephrotic syndrome.

● **DIRECTIONS FOR ADMINISTRATION** For *intravenous injection*, expert sources advise may be diluted in sodium chloride 0.9% to 250 nanograms/mL.

- **MEDICINAL FORMS** There can be variation in the licensing of different medicines containing the same drug.

Solution for injection

▸ **Synacthen** (Atnahs Pharma UK Ltd)
Tetracosactide acetate 250 microgram per 1 ml Synacthen 250micrograms/1ml solution for injection ampoules | 1 ampoule [PoM] £38.00 DT = £38.00

Suspension for injection

EXCIPIENTS: May contain Benzyl alcohol

▸ **Tetracosactide (Non-proprietary)**
Tetracosactide acetate 1 mg per 1 ml Tetracosactide 1mg/1ml suspension for injection ampoules | 1 ampoule [PoM] [X]

▸ **Synacthen Depot** (Atnahs Pharma UK Ltd)
Tetracosactide acetate 1 mg per 1 ml Synacthen Depot 1mg/1ml suspension for injection ampoules | 1 ampoule [PoM] £346.28

6.2 Assessment of pituitary function

DIAGNOSTIC AGENTS

Corticorelin

(Corticotrophin-releasing hormone; CRH)

- **INDICATIONS AND DOSE**

Test of anterior pituitary function

▸ BY INTRAVENOUS INJECTION

▸ Child: 1 microgram/kg for 1 dose (max. per dose 100 micrograms), to be administered over 30 seconds

- **UNLICENSED USE** Not licensed.
- **SIDE-EFFECTS** Angioedema · cardiac arrest · chest tightness · dyspnoea · flushing · hypersensitivity · hypotension · loss of consciousness · tachycardia · urticaria · wheezing
- **PREGNANCY** Avoid.
- **BREAST FEEDING** Avoid.
- **MEDICINAL FORMS** No licensed medicines listed.

PITUITARY AND HYPOTHALAMIC HORMONES AND ANALOGUES › GONADOTROPHIN-RELEASING HORMONES

Gonadorelin

16-Jul-2024

(Gonadotrophin-releasing hormone; GnRH; LH-RH)

- **INDICATIONS AND DOSE**

Assessment of anterior pituitary function | Assessment of delayed puberty

▸ BY INTRAVENOUS INJECTION, OR BY SUBCUTANEOUS INJECTION

▸ Child 1–17 years: 2.5 micrograms/kg for 1 dose (max. per dose 100 micrograms)

- **CAUTIONS** Pituitary adenoma
- **SIDE-EFFECTS**

▸ **Uncommon** Pain · skin reactions · swelling

▸ **Rare or very rare** Abdominal discomfort · bronchospasm · dizziness · eye erythema · flushing · headache · nausea · tachycardia

▸ **Frequency not known** Menorrhagia · sepsis · thrombophlebitis

- **PREGNANCY** Avoid.
- **BREAST FEEDING** Avoid.
- **NATIONAL FUNDING/ACCESS DECISIONS**

NHS restrictions Gonadorelin is not prescribable in NHS primary care for puberty suppression [unlicensed use] except in children who meet the criteria listed in part XVIIIB of the Drug Tariff. The prescription must be endorsed 'SLS'.

- **MEDICINAL FORMS** There can be variation in the licensing of different medicines containing the same drug.

Powder for solution for injection

▸ **Gonadorelin (Non-proprietary)**
Gonadorelin (as Gonadorelin hydrochloride)
100 microgram Gonadorelin 100microgram powder for solution for injection vials | 1 vial [PoM] £75.00 (Hospital only)

6.3 Growth hormone disorders

PITUITARY AND HYPOTHALAMIC HORMONES AND ANALOGUES › HUMAN GROWTH HORMONES

Somapacitan

08-Jul-2025

- **DRUG ACTION** Somapacitan is a long-acting recombinant human growth hormone derivative.
- **INDICATIONS AND DOSE**

Deficiency of growth hormone (under expert supervision)

▸ BY SUBCUTANEOUS INJECTION

▸ Child 3–17 years: 160 micrograms/kg once weekly, for advice on dose adjustments and treatment evaluation or discontinuation—consult product literature

DOSE EQUIVALENCE AND CONVERSION

▸ For patients switching from another growth hormone therapy, the initial dose of somapacitan should be administered at least 8 hours after the last dose of daily growth hormone or 1 week after the last dose of weekly growth hormone.

- **CONTRA-INDICATIONS** Complications in acute critical illness (consult product literature) · evidence of tumour activity (complete antitumour therapy and ensure intracranial lesions are inactive before starting) · not to be used for growth promotion in children with closed epiphyses
- **CAUTIONS** Diabetes mellitus (adjustment of antidiabetic therapy may be necessary) · glucose intolerance or risk factors for diabetes (additional monitoring may be necessary) · history of malignant disease or benign tumour · hypoadrenalism (initiation or adjustment of glucocorticoid replacement therapy may be necessary) · hypothyroidism (periodic thyroid function tests recommended) · resolved intracranial hypertension (monitor closely)
- **INTERACTIONS** → Appendix 1: somapacitan
- **SIDE-EFFECTS**

▸ **Common or very common** Adrenal insufficiency · arthralgia · fatigue · headache · hyperglycaemia · hypothyroidism · pain · peripheral oedema

- **PREGNANCY** [EvGr] Avoid (toxicity in *animal* studies). ⟨M⟩
- **BREAST FEEDING** [EvGr] Avoid (present in milk in *animal* studies). ⟨M⟩
- **MONITORING REQUIREMENTS** Monitor serum insulin-like growth factor-1 concentrations during treatment—consult product literature.
- **DIRECTIONS FOR ADMINISTRATION** Inject into the abdomen, thighs, buttocks, or upper arms; rotate injection site weekly to prevent lipoatrophy. *Sogroya*® may be self-administered or administered by a carer after appropriate training in subcutaneous injection technique.
- **PRESCRIBING AND DISPENSING INFORMATION** Somapacitan is a biological medicine. Biological medicines must be prescribed and dispensed by brand name, see *Biological medicines* and *Biosimilar medicines*, under

6 Endocrine system

Guidance on prescribing p. 1; record the brand name and batch number after each administration.

- **HANDLING AND STORAGE** Store in a refrigerator (2–8°C) and protect from light—consult product literature for further information regarding storage outside the refrigerator.
- **PATIENT AND CARER ADVICE**
Self-administration Patients and their carers should be given training in subcutaneous injection technique, if appropriate.
Missed doses If a dose is more than 3 days late, the missed dose should not be administered and the next dose should be administered on the usual scheduled day.
If two or more doses are missed, the next dose should be administered on the usual scheduled day.
- **NATIONAL FUNDING/ACCESS DECISIONS**
For full details see funding body website
NICE decisions
  - **Somapacitan for treating growth hormone deficiency in people 3 to 17 years (June 2025)** NICE TA1066 Recommended

Scottish Medicines Consortium (SMC) decisions
  - **Somapacitan (*Sogroya*®) for the replacement of endogenous growth hormone in children aged 3 years and above, and adolescents with growth failure due to growth hormone deficiency, and in adults with growth hormone deficiency (November 2024)** SMC No. SMC2629 Recommended with restrictions

- **MEDICINAL FORMS** There can be variation in the licensing of different medicines containing the same drug.
Solution for injection
  - **Sogroya** (Novo Nordisk Ltd) ▼
Somapacitan 6.7 mg per 1 ml Sogroya 10mg/1.5ml solution for injection pre-filled pens | 1 pre-filled disposable injection PoM £285.45
Somapacitan 10 mg per 1 ml Sogroya 15mg/1.5ml solution for injection pre-filled pens | 1 pre-filled disposable injection PoM £428.18

Somatrogon

30-May-2025

- **DRUG ACTION** Somatrogon is a long-acting recombinant human growth hormone analogue.

- **INDICATIONS AND DOSE**

Deficiency of growth hormone
  - BY SUBCUTANEOUS INJECTION
  - Child 3–17 years: 660 micrograms/kg once weekly, to be given on the same day each week, dose to be adjusted according to response, for advice on dose titration and treatment evaluation or discontinuation—consult product literature

- **CONTRA-INDICATIONS** Complications in acute critical illness (consult product literature) · evidence of tumour activity (complete antitumour therapy and ensure intracranial lesions inactive before starting) · not to be used for growth promotion in children with closed epiphyses
- **CAUTIONS** Diabetes mellitus (adjustment of antidiabetic therapy may be necessary) · disorders of the epiphysis (monitor for limping and hip or knee pain) · glucose intolerance or risk factors for diabetes (additional monitoring may be necessary) · history of malignant disease · hypoadrenalism (initiation or adjustment of glucocorticoid replacement therapy may be necessary) · hypothyroidism (periodic thyroid function tests recommended) · Prader-Willi syndrome (consult product literature) · resolved intracranial hypertension (monitor closely)
- **INTERACTIONS** → Appendix 1: somatrogon
- **SIDE-EFFECTS**
  - **Common or very common** Anaemia · arthralgia · conjunctivitis allergic · eosinophilia · fever · headache · hypothyroidism · pain in extremity
  - **Uncommon** Adrenal insufficiency · rash generalised
- **PREGNANCY** EvGr Avoid—limited information available. ⟨M⟩
- **BREAST FEEDING** EvGr Avoid—no information available. ⟨M⟩
- **MONITORING REQUIREMENTS**
  - EvGr Monitor serum insulin-like growth factor 1 concentrations during treatment.
  - Funduscopic examination should be carried out before starting treatment and as clinically indicated. ⟨M⟩
- **DIRECTIONS FOR ADMINISTRATION** EvGr Inject into the thigh or abdomen, or upper arm or buttocks (if not self-administered); rotate injection site. ⟨M⟩ Patients may self-administer *Ngenla*® after appropriate training in administration.
- **PRESCRIBING AND DISPENSING INFORMATION** Somatrogon is a biological medicine. Biological medicines must be prescribed and dispensed by brand name, see *Biological medicines* and *Biosimilar medicines*, under Guidance on prescribing p. 1; record the brand name and batch number after each administration.
- **HANDLING AND STORAGE** Store in a refrigerator (2–8°C) and protect from light—consult product literature for further information regarding storage outside refrigerator.
- **PATIENT AND CARER ADVICE**
Self-administration If appropriate, patients and their carers should be given training in subcutaneous injection technique.
Missed doses If a dose is more than 3 days late, the missed dose should not be administered and the next dose should be administered on the usual scheduled day.
- **NATIONAL FUNDING/ACCESS DECISIONS**
For full details see funding body website
NICE decisions
  - **Somatrogon for treating growth disturbance in children and young people aged 3 years and over (February 2023)** NICE TA863 Recommended

Scottish Medicines Consortium (SMC) decisions
  - **Somatrogon (*Ngenla*®) for the treatment of children and adolescents from 3 years of age with growth disturbance due to insufficient secretion of growth hormone (August 2022)** SMC No. SMC2493 Recommended

- **MEDICINAL FORMS** There can be variation in the licensing of different medicines containing the same drug.
Solution for injection
  - **Ngenla** (Pfizer Ltd) ▼
Somatrogon 20 mg per 1 ml Ngenla 24mg/1.2ml solution for injection pre-filled pens | 1 pre-filled disposable injection PoM £166.08 CD4-2
Somatrogon 50 mg per 1 ml Ngenla 60mg/1.2ml solution for injection pre-filled pens | 1 pre-filled disposable injection PoM £415.20 DT = £415.20 CD4-2

Somatropin

30-May-2025

- **DRUG ACTION** Somatropin is a recombinant human growth hormone.

- **INDICATIONS AND DOSE**

Gonadal dysgenesis (Turner syndrome)
  - BY SUBCUTANEOUS INJECTION
  - Child: 1.4 mg/m^2 daily, alternatively 45–50 micrograms/kg daily

Deficiency of growth hormone
- ▶ BY SUBCUTANEOUS INJECTION, OR BY INTRAMUSCULAR INJECTION
  - ▸ Child: 23–39 micrograms/kg daily, alternatively 0.7–1 mg/m^2 daily

Growth disturbance in children born small for gestational age whose growth has not caught up by 4 years or later
- ▶ BY SUBCUTANEOUS INJECTION
  - ▸ Child 4-17 years: 35 micrograms/kg daily, alternatively 1 mg/m^2 daily

Noonan syndrome
- ▶ BY SUBCUTANEOUS INJECTION
  - ▸ Child: 66 micrograms/kg daily, alternatively 33 micrograms/kg daily, lower dose may be sufficient for some patients

Prader-Willi syndrome, in children with growth velocity greater than 1 cm/year, in combination with energy-restricted diet
- ▶ BY SUBCUTANEOUS INJECTION
  - ▸ Child: 1 mg/m^2 daily, alternatively 35 micrograms/kg daily; maximum 2.7 mg per day

Chronic renal insufficiency (renal function decreased to less than 50%)
- ▶ BY SUBCUTANEOUS INJECTION
  - ▸ Child: 45–50 micrograms/kg daily, alternatively 1.4 mg/m^2 daily, higher doses may be needed, adjust if necessary after 6 months

SHOX deficiency
- ▶ BY SUBCUTANEOUS INJECTION
  - ▸ Child: 45–50 micrograms/kg daily

DOSE EQUIVALENCE AND CONVERSION
- ▸ Dose formerly expressed in units; somatropin 1 mg ≡ 3 units.

- **CONTRA-INDICATIONS** Avoid injections containing benzyl alcohol in neonates · discontinue at the time of renal transplantation · evidence of tumour activity (complete antitumour therapy and ensure intracranial lesions inactive before starting) · not to be used for growth promotion in children with closed epiphyses (or near closure in Prader-Willi syndrome) · severe obesity in Prader-Willi syndrome · severe respiratory impairment in Prader-Willi syndrome
- **CAUTIONS** Diabetes mellitus (adjustment of antidiabetic therapy may be necessary) · disorders of the epiphysis of the hip (monitor for limping) · history of malignant disease · hypoadrenalism (initiation or adjustment of glucocorticoid replacement therapy may be necessary) · initiation of treatment close to puberty not recommended in child born small for corrected gestational age · papilloedema · resolved intracranial hypertension (monitor closely) · risk of hypothyroidism—manufacturers recommend periodic thyroid function tests · Silver-Russell syndrome
- **INTERACTIONS** → Appendix 1: somatropin
- **SIDE-EFFECTS**
  - ▶ **Common or very common** Headache · lipoatrophy
  - ▶ **Uncommon** Arthralgia · carpal tunnel syndrome · fluid retention · gynaecomastia · idiopathic intracranial hypertension · musculoskeletal stiffness · myalgia · oedema · paraesthesia
  - ▶ **Rare or very rare** Hyperglycaemia · hyperinsulinism · hypothyroidism · osteonecrosis of femur · pancreatitis · slipped capital femoral epiphysis
  - ▶ **Frequency not known** Leukaemia

SIDE-EFFECTS, FURTHER INFORMATION Funduscopy for papilloedema recommended if severe or recurrent headache, visual problems, nausea and vomiting occur—if papilloedema confirmed consider benign intracranial hypertension (rare cases reported).

- **PREGNANCY** Discontinue if pregnancy occurs—no information available.
- **BREAST FEEDING** No information available. Absorption from milk unlikely.
- **DIRECTIONS FOR ADMINISTRATION** Rotate subcutaneous injection sites to prevent lipoatrophy.
- **PRESCRIBING AND DISPENSING INFORMATION** Somatropin is a biological medicine. Biological medicines must be prescribed and dispensed by brand name, see *Biological medicines* and *Biosimilar medicines*, under Guidance on prescribing p. 1.

GENOTROPIN® PREPARATIONS Cartridges are for use with *Genotropin®* Pen device (non-NHS but available free of charge from clinics).

NORDITROPIN® PREPARATIONS Cartridges are for use with appropriate *NordiPen®* device (non-NHS but available free of charge from clinics).

Multidose disposable prefilled pens for use with *NovoFine®* or *NovoTwist®* needles.

NUTROPINAQ® For use with *NutropinAq®* Pen device (non-NHS but available free of charge from clinics).

OMNITROPE® For use with *Omnitrope Pen* 5® and *Omnitrope Pen* 10® devices (non-NHS but available free of charge from clinics).

SAIZEN® POWDER AND SOLVENT FOR SOLUTION FOR INJECTION For use with *one. click®* autoinjector device or *cool.click®* needle-free autoinjector device or *easypod®* autoinjector device (non-NHS but available free of charge from clinics).

SAIZEN® SOLUTION FOR INJECTION For use with *cool.click®* needle-free autoinjector device or *easypod®* autoinjector device (non-NHS but available free of charge from clinics).

ZOMACTON® 4 mg vial for use with *ZomaJet* 2® *Vision* needle-free device (non-NHS but available free of charge from clinics) or with needles and syringes.

10 mg vial for use with *ZomaJet Vision X®* needle-free device (non-NHS but available free of charge from clinics) or with needles and syringes.

- **NATIONAL FUNDING/ACCESS DECISIONS**
For full details see funding body website

NICE decisions
- ▶ **Somatropin for the treatment of growth failure in children (May 2010)** NICE TA188 Recommended

---

- **MEDICINAL FORMS** There can be variation in the licensing of different medicines containing the same drug.

Solution for injection

EXCIPIENTS: May contain Benzyl alcohol

- ▸ **Norditropin FlexPro** (Novo Nordisk Ltd)
  - **Somatropin (epr) 3.3 mg per 1 ml** Norditropin FlexPro 5mg/1.5ml solution for injection pre-filled pens | 1 pre-filled disposable injection PoM £106.35 CD4-2
  - **Somatropin (epr) 6.7 mg per 1 ml** Norditropin FlexPro 10mg/1.5ml solution for injection pre-filled pens | 1 pre-filled disposable injection PoM £212.70 DT = £212.70 CD4-2
  - **Somatropin (epr) 10 mg per 1 ml** Norditropin FlexPro 15mg/1.5ml solution for injection pre-filled pens | 1 pre-filled disposable injection PoM £319.05 DT = £319.05 CD4-2
- ▸ **Omnitrope SurePal** (Sandoz Ltd)
  - **Somatropin (rbe) 3.333 mg per 1 ml** Omnitrope SurePal 5 5mg/1.5ml solution for injection cartridges | 5 cartridge PoM £368.74 DT = £368.74 CD4-2
  - **Somatropin (rbe) 6.667 mg per 1 ml** Omnitrope SurePal 10 10mg/1.5ml solution for injection cartridges | 5 cartridge PoM £737.49 DT = £737.49 CD4-2
  - **Somatropin (rbe) 10 mg per 1 ml** Omnitrope SurePal 15 15mg/1.5ml solution for injection cartridges | 5 cartridge PoM £1,106.22 DT = £1,106.22 CD4-2
- ▸ **Saizen** (Merck Serono Ltd)
  - **Somatropin (rmc) 5.825 mg per 1 ml** Saizen 6mg/1.03ml solution for injection cartridges | 1 cartridge PoM £139.08 DT = £139.08 CD4-2

Somatropin (rmc) 8 mg per 1 ml Saizen 12mg/1.5ml solution for injection cartridges | 1 cartridge PoM £278.16 DT = £278.16 CD4-2
Saizen 20mg/2.5ml solution for injection cartridges | 1 cartridge PoM £463.60 DT = £463.60 CD4-2

Powder and solvent for solution for injection

EXCIPIENTS: May contain Benzyl alcohol

▸ Genotropin (Pfizer Ltd)

Somatropin (rbe) 5.3 mg Genotropin 5.3mg powder and solvent for solution for injection cartridges | 1 cartridge PoM £92.15 DT = £92.15 CD4-2

Somatropin (rbe) 12 mg Genotropin 12mg powder and solvent for solution for injection cartridges | 1 cartridge PoM £208.65 DT = £208.65 CD4-2

▸ Genotropin GoQuick (Pfizer Ltd)

Somatropin (rbe) 5.3 mg Genotropin GoQuick 5.3mg powder and solvent for solution for injection pre-filled pens | 1 pre-filled disposable injection PoM £92.15 DT = £92.15 CD4-2

Somatropin (rbe) 12 mg Genotropin GoQuick 12mg powder and solvent for solution for injection pre-filled pens | 1 pre-filled disposable injection PoM £208.65 DT = £208.65 CD4-2

▸ Genotropin MiniQuick (Pfizer Ltd)

Somatropin (rbe) 200 microgram Genotropin MiniQuick 200microgram powder and solvent for solution for injection pre-filled disposable devices | 7 pre-filled disposable injection PoM £24.35 DT = £24.35 CD4-2

Somatropin (rbe) 400 microgram Genotropin MiniQuick 400microgram powder and solvent for solution for injection pre-filled disposable devices | 7 pre-filled disposable injection PoM £48.68 DT = £48.68 CD4-2

Somatropin (rbe) 600 microgram Genotropin MiniQuick 600microgram powder and solvent for solution for injection pre-filled disposable devices | 7 pre-filled disposable injection PoM £73.03 DT = £73.03 CD4-2

Somatropin (rbe) 800 microgram Genotropin MiniQuick 800microgram powder and solvent for solution for injection pre-filled disposable devices | 7 pre-filled disposable injection PoM £97.37 DT = £97.37 CD4-2

Somatropin (rbe) 1 mg Genotropin MiniQuick 1mg powder and solvent for solution for injection pre-filled disposable devices | 7 pre-filled disposable injection PoM £121.71 DT = £121.71 CD4-2

Somatropin (rbe) 1.2 mg Genotropin MiniQuick 1.2mg powder and solvent for solution for injection pre-filled disposable devices | 7 pre-filled disposable injection PoM £146.06 DT = £146.06 CD4-2

Somatropin (rbe) 1.4 mg Genotropin MiniQuick 1.4mg powder and solvent for solution for injection pre-filled disposable devices | 7 pre-filled disposable injection PoM £170.39 DT = £170.39 CD4-2

Somatropin (rbe) 1.6 mg Genotropin MiniQuick 1.6mg powder and solvent for solution for injection pre-filled disposable devices | 7 pre-filled disposable injection PoM £194.74 DT = £194.74 CD4-2

Somatropin (rbe) 1.8 mg Genotropin MiniQuick 1.8mg powder and solvent for solution for injection pre-filled disposable devices | 7 pre-filled disposable injection PoM £219.08 DT = £219.08 CD4-2

Somatropin (rbe) 2 mg Genotropin MiniQuick 2mg powder and solvent for solution for injection pre-filled disposable devices | 7 pre-filled disposable injection PoM £243.42 DT = £243.42 CD4-2

▸ Zomacton (Ferring Pharmaceuticals Ltd)

Somatropin (rbe) 4 mg Zomacton 4mg powder and solvent for solution for injection vials | 1 vial PoM £68.28 CD4-2

6.3a Insulin-like growth factor-I deficiency

PITUITARY AND HYPOTHALAMIC HORMONES AND ANALOGUES › SOMATOMEDINS

Mecasermin

30-May-2025

(rhIGF-1)

● **DRUG ACTION** Mecasermin, a recombinant human insulin-like growth factor-1 (rhIGF-1), is the principal mediator of the somatotropic effects of human growth hormone.

● **INDICATIONS AND DOSE**

Treatment of growth failure in children with severe primary insulin-like growth factor-I deficiency

▸ BY SUBCUTANEOUS INJECTION

▸ Child 2–17 years: Initially 40 micrograms/kg twice daily for 1 week, increased, if tolerated, in steps of 40 micrograms/kg (max. per dose 120 micrograms/kg twice daily), discontinue if no response within 1 year, reduce dose if hypoglycaemia occurs despite adequate food intake; withhold injection if patient unable to eat

IMPORTANT SAFETY INFORMATION

MHRA/CHM ADVICE: MECASERMIN (*INCRELEX*®): RISK OF BENIGN AND MALIGNANT NEOPLASIA (JANUARY 2020)

Cases of benign and malignant tumours have been observed in children and adolescents treated with mecasermin; the risk of neoplasia is higher when used outside the licensed indication or dose. If a physician determines that there is a clinical need for such use, the patient and their carers should be consulted and fully informed of the potential benefits and risks, and the final decision made jointly. Physicians should be vigilant for the development of potential malignancies in such patients.

Healthcare professionals are advised that mecasermin is contra-indicated in children and adolescents with active or suspected neoplasia and in any condition or medical history that increases the risk of benign or malignant neoplasia. If benign or malignant neoplasm develops during treatment, mecasermin should be permanently discontinued.

● **CONTRA-INDICATIONS** Evidence of tumour activity (discontinue treatment)

● **CAUTIONS** Correct hypothyroidism before initiating treatment · diabetes mellitus (adjustment of antidiabetic therapy may be necessary) · papilloedema

● **SIDE-EFFECTS**

▸ **Common or very common** Adenoidal hypertrophy · arthralgia · dizziness · ear discomfort · gastrointestinal discomfort · gynaecomastia · hair texture abnormal · headache · hearing impairment · hyperglycaemia · hypoglycaemia · melanocytic naevus · myalgia · otitis media · pain in extremity · papilloedema · scoliosis · seizures · skin hypertrophy · sleep apnoea · snoring · tachycardia · thymus enlargement · tonsillar hypertrophy · tremor · vomiting

▸ **Uncommon** Cardiac hypertrophy · cardiac valve disorders · depression · idiopathic intracranial hypertension · lipohypertrophy · nervousness · weight increased

▸ **Frequency not known** Alopecia · benign neoplasm (discontinue permanently) · neoplasm malignant (discontinue permanently)

SIDE-EFFECTS, FURTHER INFORMATION Funduscopy for papilloedema recommended regularly during treatment and if severe or recurrent headache, visual problems, nausea and vomiting occur—if papilloedema confirmed consider benign intracranial hypertension.

- **CONCEPTION AND CONTRACEPTION** Contraception advised in women of child-bearing potential.
- **PREGNANCY** Avoid unless essential.
- **BREAST FEEDING** Avoid.
- **MONITORING REQUIREMENTS**
  - Monitor ECG before and on termination of treatment (and during treatment if ECG abnormal).
  - Monitor for disorders of the epiphysis of the hip (monitor for limping).
  - Monitor for signs of tonsillar hypertrophy (snoring, sleep apnoea, and chronic middle ear effusions).
- **DIRECTIONS FOR ADMINISTRATION** Manufacturer advises dose should be administered just before or after food.
- **PATIENT AND CARER ADVICE** Patients or carers should be given advice on how to administer mecasermin injection. **Missed doses** Patients or carers should be advised not to increase dose if a dose is missed.

- **MEDICINAL FORMS** There can be variation in the licensing of different medicines containing the same drug.

Solution for injection

EXCIPIENTS: May contain Benzyl alcohol

- **Increlex** (Esteve Pharmaceuticals Ltd) ▼
  Mecasermin 10 mg per 1 ml Increlex 40mg/4ml solution for injection vials | 1 vial PoM £605.00

7 Sex hormone responsive conditions

Sex hormones

Hormone replacement therapy

Sex hormone replacement therapy is indicated in children for the treatment of gonadotrophin deficiency, gonadal disorders, or delayed puberty that interferes with quality of life. Indications include constitutional delay in puberty, congenital or acquired hypogonadotrophic hypogonadism, hypergonadotrophic hypogonadism (Turner's syndrome, Klinefelter's syndrome), endocrine disorders (Cushing's syndrome or hyperprolactinaemia), and chronic illnesses, such as cystic fibrosis or sickle-cell disease, that may affect the onset of puberty.

Replacement therapy is generally started at the appropriate age for the development of puberty and should be managed by a paediatric endocrinologist. Patients with constitutional delay, chronic illness, or eating disorders may need only small doses of hormone supplements for 4 to 6 months to induce puberty and endogenous sex hormone production, which is then sustained. Patients with organic causes of hormone deficiency will require life-long replacement, adjusted to allow normal development.

Inadequate treatment may lead to poor bone mineralisation, resulting in fractures and osteoporosis.

Female sex hormones

Oestrogens

Oestrogens are necessary for the development of female secondary sexual characteristics. If onset of puberty is delayed because of organic pathology, puberty can be induced with ethinylestradiol p. 590 in increasing doses, guided by breast staging and uterine scans. Cyclical progestogen replacement is added after 12–18 months of oestrogen treatment. Once the adult dosage of oestrogen has been reached, it may be more convenient to provide replacement either as a low-dose oestrogen containing oral contraceptive formulation [unlicensed indication] or as a combined oestrogen and progestogen hormone replacement therapy preparation [unlicensed indication]. There is limited experience in the use of transdermal patches or gels in children; compliance and skin irritation are sometimes a problem.

Ethinylestradiol is occasionally used, under **specialist supervision**, for the management of hereditary haemorrhagic telangiectasia (but evidence of benefit is limited), for the prevention of tall stature, and in tests of growth hormone secretion.

Topical oestrogen creams are used in the treatment of labial adhesions.

Progestogens

There are two main groups of progestogen, *progesterone and its analogues* (dydrogesterone and medroxyprogesterone acetate p. 632) and *testosterone analogues* (norethisterone p. 591 and norgestrel). The newer progestogens (desogestrel p. 626, norgestimate, and gestodene) are all derivatives of norgestrel; levonorgestrel p. 628 is the active isomer of norgestrel and has twice its potency. Progesterone and its analogues are less androgenic than the testosterone derivatives and neither progesterone nor dydrogesterone causes virilisation.

In delayed puberty cyclical progestogen is added after 12–18 months of oestrogen therapy to establish a menstrual cycle.

Norethisterone is also used to postpone menstruation during a cycle; treatment is started 3 days before the expected onset of menstruation.

Heavy menstrual bleeding

11-Jun-2021

Description of condition

Heavy menstrual bleeding, also known as menorrhagia, is excessive menstrual blood loss of 80 mL or more, and/or for a duration of more than 7 days, which results in the need to change menstrual products every 1–2 hours. Heavy menstrual bleeding occurs regularly, every 24–35 days.

Drug treatment

EvGr The choice of treatment should be guided by the presence or absence of fibroids (including size, number and location), polyps, endometrial pathology or adenomyosis, other symptoms (such as pressure or pain), co-morbidities, and patient preference.

In females with heavy menstrual bleeding and unidentified pathology, fibroids less than 3 cm in diameter causing no distortion of the uterine cavity, or suspected or diagnosed adenomyosis, a levonorgestrel-releasing intra-uterine system p. 628 is the first-line treatment option. Patients should be advised that irregular menstrual bleeding can occur particularly during the first months of use and that the full benefit of treatment may take at least 6 months.

If a levonorgestrel-releasing intra-uterine system p. 628 is unsuitable, either tranexamic acid p. 92, an NSAID, a combined hormonal contraceptive, or a cyclical oral progestogen should be considered. Progestogen-only contraceptives may suppress menstruation and be beneficial to females with heavy menstrual bleeding. A non-hormonal treatment is recommended in patients actively trying to conceive.

If drug treatment is unsuccessful or declined by the patient, or if symptoms are severe, referral to a specialist for alternative drug treatment or surgery should be considered.

In females with fibroids of 3 cm or more in diameter, referral to a specialist should be considered. Treatment options include tranexamic acid, an NSAID, a levonorgestrel-releasing intra-uterine system p. 628, a combined hormonal contraceptive, a cyclical oral progestogen, uterine artery embolisation, or surgery. Treatment choice depends on the size, number and location of the fibroids, and severity of symptoms. If drug treatment is required while investigations and definitive treatment is being organised, either tranexamic acid, or an NSAID, or both, can be given.

The effectiveness of drug treatment for heavy menstrual bleeding may be limited in females with fibroids that are substantially greater than 3 cm in diameter. Treatment with a gonadotrophin-releasing hormone analogue before hysterectomy and myomectomy should be considered if uterine fibroids are causing an enlarged or distorted uterus. Ⓐ

Useful Resources

Heavy menstrual bleeding: assessment and management. National Institute for Health and Care Excellence. NICE guideline 88. March 2018 (updated May 2021). www.nice.org.uk/guidance/ng88

7.1 Female sex hormone responsive conditions

Other drugs used for Female sex hormone responsive conditions Medroxyprogesterone acetate, p. 632

OESTROGENS

Ethinylestradiol
22-May-2020

(Ethinyloestradiol)

● **INDICATIONS AND DOSE**

Induction of sexual maturation in girls

▶ BY MOUTH

▶ Child (female): Initially 2 micrograms daily for 6 months, then increased to 5 micrograms daily for 6 months, then increased to 10 micrograms daily for 6 months, then increased to 20 micrograms daily, after 12–18 months of treatment give progestogen for 7 days of each 28-day cycle.

Maintenance of sexual maturation in girls

▶ BY MOUTH

▶ Child (female): 20 micrograms daily, to be given with cyclical progestogen for 7 days of each 28-day cycle.

Prevention of tall stature in girls

▶ BY MOUTH

▶ Child 2-11 years (female): 20–50 micrograms daily.

● **UNLICENSED USE** Unlicensed for use in children.

● **CONTRA-INDICATIONS** Active or recent arterial thromboembolic disease (e.g. angina or myocardial infarction) · Acute porphyrias p. 745 · cardiovascular disease (risk of fluid retention) · family history of thromboembolism · history of breast cancer · history of venous thromboembolism · liver disease (where liver function tests have failed to return to normal) · oestrogen-dependent cancer · thrombophilic disorder · undiagnosed vaginal bleeding · untreated endometrial hyperplasia

CONTRA-INDICATIONS, FURTHER INFORMATION

▶ Combined hormonal contraception For more information on contra-indications for ethinylestradiol in *contraception* see combined hormonal contraceptive preparations containing ethinylestradiol.

● **CAUTIONS** Diabetes (increased risk of heart disease) · history of breast nodules or fibrocystic disease—closely monitor breast status (risk of breast cancer) · history of endometrial hyperplasia · history of hypertriglyceridaemia (increased risk of pancreatitis) · hypophyseal tumours · increased risk of gall-bladder disease · migraine (migraine-like headaches) · presence of antiphospholipid antibodies (increased risk of thrombotic events) · prolonged exposure to unopposed oestrogens may increase risk of developing endometrial cancer · risk factors for oestrogen-dependent tumours (e.g. breast cancer in first-degree relative) · risk factors for venous thromboembolism · symptoms of endometriosis may be exacerbated · uterine fibroids may increase in size

CAUTIONS, FURTHER INFORMATION

▶ Combined hormonal contraception For more information on cautions for ethinylestradiol in *contraception* see combined hormonal contraceptive preparations containing ethinylestradiol.

● **INTERACTIONS** → Appendix 1: hormone replacement therapy

● **SIDE-EFFECTS** Breast abnormalities · cervical mucus increased · cholelithiasis · contact lens intolerance · depression · electrolyte imbalance · embolism and thrombosis · erythema nodosum · feminisation · fluid retention · headaches · hypertension · jaundice cholestatic · metrorrhagia · mood altered · myocardial infarction · nausea · neoplasms · skin reactions · stroke · uterine disorders · vomiting · weight change

● **PREGNANCY** Avoid.

● **BREAST FEEDING** Avoid until weaning or for 6 months after birth (adverse effects on lactation).

● **HEPATIC IMPAIRMENT** Manufacturer advises caution; avoid in acute or active disease.

● **MEDICINAL FORMS** Forms available from special-order manufacturers include: oral tablet, oral capsule, oral suspension

PROGESTOGENS

Dienogest
17-Feb-2020

● **DRUG ACTION** Dienogest is a nortestosterone derivative that has a progestogenic effect in the uterus, reducing the production of estradiol and thereby suppressing endometriotic lesions.

● **INDICATIONS AND DOSE**

Endometriosis

▶ BY MOUTH

▶ Females of childbearing potential: 2 mg once daily, can be started on any day of cycle, dose should be taken continuously at the same time each day

● **CONTRA-INDICATIONS** Arterial disease (past or present) · cardiovascular disease (past or present) · diabetes with vascular involvement · liver tumours (past or present) · sex hormone-dependent malignancies (confirmed or suspected) · undiagnosed vaginal bleeding · venous thromboembolism (active)

● **CAUTIONS** Diabetes (progestogens can decrease glucose tolerance—monitor patient closely) · history of depression · history of ectopic pregnancy · history of gestational diabetes · patients at risk of osteoporosis · patients at risk of venous thromboembolism

CAUTIONS, FURTHER INFORMATION

▶ Immobilisation Manufacturer advises to discontinue treatment during prolonged immobilisation. For elective surgery, treatment should be discontinued at least 4 weeks before surgery; treatment may be restarted 2 weeks after complete remobilisation.

● **INTERACTIONS** → Appendix 1: dienogest

● **SIDE-EFFECTS**

▶ **Common or very common** Alopecia · anxiety · asthenic conditions · breast abnormalities · depression ·

gastrointestinal discomfort · gastrointestinal disorders · haemorrhage · headaches · hot flush · libido loss · mood altered · nausea · ovarian cyst · pain · skin reactions · sleep disorder · vomiting · vulvovaginal disorders · weight changes
- **Uncommon** Anaemia · appetite increased · autonomic dysfunction · broken nails · circulatory system disorder · concentration impaired · constipation · dandruff · diarrhoea · dry eye · dyspnoea · genital discharge · hair changes · hyperhidrosis · hypotension · increased risk of infection · limb discomfort · muscle spasms · oedema · palpitations · pelvic pain · photosensitivity reaction · tinnitus
- **Frequency not known** Glucose tolerance impaired · insulin resistance · menstrual cycle irregularities

● **CONCEPTION AND CONTRACEPTION** Manufacturer advises that, if contraception is required, females of childbearing potential should use non-hormonal contraception during treatment. The menstrual cycle usually returns to normal within 2 months after stopping treatment.

● **BREAST FEEDING** Manufacturer advises avoid—present in milk in *animal* studies.

● **HEPATIC IMPAIRMENT** Manufacturer advises avoid in severe impairment (no information available).

● **PATIENT AND CARER ADVICE** Manufacturer advises patients with a history of chloasma gravidarum to avoid sunlight or UV radiation exposure during treatment.
Missed doses Manufacturer advises if one or more tablets are missed, or if vomiting and/or diarrhoea occurs within 3–4 hours of taking a tablet, another tablet should be taken as soon as possible and the next dose taken at the normal time.

● **MEDICINAL FORMS** There can be variation in the licensing of different medicines containing the same drug.

Oral tablet

- **Dienogest (Non-proprietary)**
  Dienogest 2 mg Dienogest 2mg tablets | 28 tablet PoM £20.50-£22.00 DT = £20.50 | 84 tablet PoM £61.50 DT = £61.50
- **Dimetrum** (Besins Healthcare (UK) Ltd)
  Dienogest 2 mg Dimetrum 2mg tablets | 28 tablet PoM £16.40 DT = £20.50
- **Sawis** (Gedeon Richter (UK) Ltd)
  Dienogest 2 mg Sawis 2mg tablets | 28 tablet PoM £20.50 DT = £20.50

Norethisterone

19-Dec-2023

● **INDICATIONS AND DOSE**

Postponement of menstruation
- BY MOUTH
- Females of childbearing potential: 5 mg 3 times a day, to be started 3 days before expected onset (menstruation occurs 2–3 days after stopping)

Induction and maintenance of sexual maturation in females (combined with an oestrogen after 12–18 months oestrogen therapy)
- BY MOUTH
- Child: 5 mg once daily for the last 7 days of 28-day cycle

Short-term contraception
- BY DEEP INTRAMUSCULAR INJECTION
- Females of childbearing potential: 200 mg, to be administered within first 5 days of cycle or immediately after parturition (duration 8 weeks). To be injected into the gluteal muscle, then 200 mg after 8 weeks if required

Contraception
- BY MOUTH
- Females of childbearing potential: 350 micrograms daily, dose to be taken at same time each day, starting on day 1 of cycle then continuously, if administration delayed for 3 hours or more it should be regarded as a 'missed pill'

● **UNLICENSED USE**
- When used for Induction and maintenance of sexual maturation in females or Postponement of menstruation Not licensed for use in children.
- When used for Contraception Consult product literature for the licensing status of individual preparations.

● **CONTRA-INDICATIONS**

GENERAL CONTRA-INDICATIONS Acute porphyrias p. 745 · current breast cancer (unless progestogens are being used in the management of this condition) · history during pregnancy of idiopathic jaundice (non-contraceptive indications) · history during pregnancy of pemphigoid gestationis (non-contraceptive indications) · history during pregnancy of severe pruritus (non-contraceptive indications)

SPECIFIC CONTRA-INDICATIONS
- With oral use History of thromboembolism (non-contraceptive indications) · undiagnosed vaginal bleeding (non-contraceptive indications)

● **CAUTIONS**

GENERAL CAUTIONS Cardiac dysfunction · conditions that may worsen with fluid retention · diabetes (progestogens can decrease glucose tolerance—monitor patient closely) · history of breast cancer—seek specialist advice before use · hypertension · liver tumours—seek specialist advice before use · migraine · multiple risk factors for cardiovascular disease—seek specialist advice before intramuscular use · positive antiphospholipid antibodies · rheumatoid arthritis · risk factors for venous thromboembolism · systemic lupus erythematosus

SPECIFIC CAUTIONS
- With intramuscular use Cervical cancer
- When used for Contraception History of stroke (including transient ischaemic attack)—seek specialist advice before intramuscular use · ischaemic heart disease—seek specialist advice before intramuscular use · undiagnosed vaginal bleeding—seek specialist advice before intramuscular use
- With oral use for Contraception Malabsorption syndromes

● **INTERACTIONS** → Appendix 1: norethisterone

● **SIDE-EFFECTS**

GENERAL SIDE-EFFECTS
- **Common or very common** Menstrual cycle irregularities
- **Uncommon** Breast tenderness
- **Frequency not known** Hepatic cancer · thromboembolism

SPECIFIC SIDE-EFFECTS
- **Common or very common**
  - With intramuscular use Dizziness · haemorrhage · headache · hypersensitivity · nausea · skin reactions · weight increased
- **Uncommon**
  - With intramuscular use Abdominal distension · depressed mood
- **Frequency not known**
  - With oral use Appetite change · depression · fatigue · gastrointestinal disorder · headaches · hypertension · libido disorder · nervousness · rash · weight change

SIDE-EFFECTS, FURTHER INFORMATION **Breast cancer risk with contraceptive use** The benefits of using progestogen-only contraceptives (POCs), such as norethisterone, should be weighed against the possible risks for each individual woman.

There is a possible small increase in the risk of breast cancer in women using, or who have recently used, progestogen-only contraception. Causal association is not clearly established, and absolute risk remains very small, and is like that of current or recent use of combined hormonal contraception.

The most important risk factor for breast cancer appears to be the age the contraceptive is stopped rather than the duration of use; the risk gradually disappears during the 10 years after stopping.

- **PREGNANCY** Not known to be harmful in contraceptive doses. Avoid in other indications.
- **BREAST FEEDING** Progestogen-only contraceptives do not affect lactation.
  - With intramuscular use Withhold breast-feeding for neonates with severe or persistent jaundice requiring medical treatment.
- **HEPATIC IMPAIRMENT** Manufacturers advise caution; avoid in severe or active disease.
- **RENAL IMPAIRMENT**
  - With oral use EvGr Use with caution. (M)
- **PATIENT AND CARER ADVICE**

Diarrhoea and vomiting with oral contraceptives Vomiting and persistent, severe diarrhoea can interfere with the absorption of oral progestogen-only contraceptives. If vomiting occurs within 2 hours of taking an oral progestogen-only contraceptive, another pill should be taken as soon as possible. If a replacement pill is not taken within 3 hours of the normal time for taking the progestogen-only pill, or in cases of persistent vomiting or very severe diarrhoea, additional precautions should be used during illness and for 2 days after recovery.

Starting routine for oral contraceptives One tablet daily, on a continuous basis, starting on day 1 of cycle and taken at the same time each day (if delayed by longer than 3 hours contraceptive protection may be lost). Additional contraceptive precautions are not required if norethisterone is started up to and including day 5 of the menstrual cycle; if started after this time, additional contraceptive precautions are required for 2 days.

Changing from a combined oral contraceptive Start on the day following completion of the combined oral contraceptive course without a break (or in the case of *everyday* (ED) tablets, omitting the inactive tablets).

After childbirth (not breast-feeding) Oral progestogen-only contraceptives can be started before 21 days postpartum without the need for additional contraceptive precautions. If started 21 days or more postpartum, additional contraceptive precautions are required for 2 days.

Contraceptives by injection Full counselling backed by *patient information leaflet* required before administration—likelihood of menstrual disturbance and the potential for a delay in return to full fertility. Delayed return of fertility and irregular cycles may occur after discontinuation of treatment but there is no evidence of permanent infertility.

Missed oral contraceptive pill The following advice is recommended: 'If you forget a pill, take it as soon as you remember and carry on with the next pill at the right time (this may mean taking 2 pills at the same time). If the pill was more than 3 hours overdue you are not protected. Continue normal pill-taking but you must also use another method, such as the condom, for the next 2 days'.

The CoSRH recommends emergency contraception if one or more progestogen-only contraceptive tablets are missed or taken more than 3 hours late and unprotected intercourse has occurred before 2 further tablets have been correctly taken.

- **MEDICINAL FORMS** There can be variation in the licensing of different medicines containing the same drug. Forms available from special-order manufacturers include: oral suspension

Solution for injection

- **Noristerat** (Bayer Plc)
  Norethisterone enantate 200 mg per 1 ml Noristerat 200mg/1ml solution for injection ampoules | 1 ampoule PoM £4.05 DT = £4.05

Oral tablet

- **Norethisterone (Non-proprietary)**
  Norethisterone 5 mg Norethisterone 5mg tablets | 30 tablet PoM £10.00 DT = £5.57
- **Noriday** (Pfizer Ltd)
  Norethisterone 350 microgram Noriday 350microgram tablets | 84 tablet PoM £2.10 DT = £2.10
- **Primolut N** (Bayer Plc)
  Norethisterone 5 mg Primolut N 5mg tablets | 30 tablet PoM £2.26 DT = £5.57
- **Utovlan** (Pfizer Ltd)
  Norethisterone 5 mg Utovlan 5mg tablets | 30 tablet PoM £1.40 DT = £5.57 | 90 tablet PoM £4.21

7.2 Male sex hormone responsive conditions

Androgens, anti-androgens and anabolic steroids

14-Aug-2020

Androgens

Androgens cause masculinisation; they are used as replacement therapy in androgen deficiency, in delayed puberty, and in those who are hypogonadal due to either pituitary or testicular disease.

When given to patients with hypopituitarism androgens can lead to normal sexual development and potency but not to fertility. If fertility is desired, the usual treatment is with gonadotrophins or pulsatile gonadotrophin-releasing hormone which stimulates spermatogenesis as well as androgen production.

Intramuscular depot preparations of **testosterone esters** are preferred for replacement therapy. Testosterone enantate or propionate or alternatively *Sustanon*®, which consists of a mixture of testosterone esters and has a longer duration of action, can be used. For induction of puberty, depot testosterone injections are given monthly and the doses increased every 6 to 12 months according to response. Single ester testosterone injections may need to be given more frequently.

Oral **testosterone undecanoate** is used for induction of puberty. An alternative approach that promotes growth rather than sexual maturation uses oral oxandrolone p. 593.

Testosterone topical gel is also available but experience of use in children under 15 years is limited. Topical testosterone is applied to the penis in the treatment of microphallus; an extemporaneously prepared cream should be used because the alcohol in proprietary gel formulations causes irritation.

Anti-androgens and precocious puberty

The gonadorelin stimulation test is used to distinguish between *gonadotrophin-dependent (central) precocious puberty* and *gonadotrophin-independent precocious puberty*. Treatment requires specialist management.

Gonadorelin analogues, used in the management of gonadotrophin-dependent precocious puberty, delay development of secondary sexual characteristics and growth velocity.

Testolactone p. 595 and cyproterone acetate p. 594 are used in the management of gonadotrophin-independent precocious puberty, resulting from McCune-Albright syndrome, familial male precocious puberty (testotoxicosis), hormone-secreting tumours, and ovarian and testicular disorders. Testolactone inhibits the aromatisation of testosterone, the rate limiting step in oestrogen synthesis. Cyproterone acetate is a progestogen with anti-androgen properties. The MHRA/CHM have released important safety information on the use of cyproterone acetate and risk of meningioma. For further information, see *Important safety information* for cyproterone acetate.

Spironolactone p. 147 is sometimes used in combination with testolactone because it has some androgen receptor blocking properties.

High blood concentration of sex hormones may activate release of gonadotrophin releasing hormone, leading to development of secondary, central gonadotrophin-dependent precocious puberty. This may require the addition of gonadorelin analogues to prevent progression of pubertal development and skeletal maturation.

Anabolic steroids

Anabolic steroids have some androgenic activity but they cause less virilisation than androgens in girls. They are used in the treatment of some *aplastic anaemias*.

Oxandrolone is used to stimulate late pre-pubertal growth prior to induction of sexual maturation in boys with short stature and in girls with Turner's syndrome; specialist management is required.

ANABOLIC STEROIDS

Oxandrolone

19-Oct-2023

- **INDICATIONS AND DOSE**

Stimulation of late pre-pubertal growth in boys (of appropriate age) with short stature

▸ BY MOUTH

▸ Child 10–17 years (male): 1.25–2.5 mg daily for 3–6 months.

Stimulation of late pre-pubertal growth in girls with Turner's syndrome

▸ BY MOUTH

▸ Child (female): 0.625–2.5 mg daily, to be taken in combination with growth hormone.

- **CONTRA-INDICATIONS** History of primary liver tumours · hypercalcaemia · nephrosis
- **CAUTIONS** Cardiac impairment · diabetes mellitus · epilepsy · hypertension · migraine · skeletal metastases (risk of hypercalcaemia)
- **INTERACTIONS** → Appendix 1: oxandrolone
- **SIDE-EFFECTS**
  - ▸ **Common or very common** Androgenetic alopecia · androgenic effects · anxiety · asthenia · bone formation increased · depression · electrolyte imbalance · epiphyses premature fusion (in pre-pubertal males) · gastrointestinal haemorrhage · gynaecomastia · headache · hirsutism · hypertension · jaundice cholestatic · nausea · oedema · paraesthesia · polycythaemia · precocious puberty (in pre-pubertal males) · seborrhoea · sexual dysfunction · skin reactions · spermatogenesis reduced · virilism · weight increased
  - ▸ **Rare or very rare** Hepatic neoplasm
  - ▸ **Frequency not known** Sleep apnoea
- **PREGNANCY** Avoid—causes masculinisation of female fetus.
- **BREAST FEEDING** Avoid; may cause masculinisation in the female infant or precocious development in the male infant. High doses suppress lactation.
- **HEPATIC IMPAIRMENT** Avoid if possible—fluid retention and dose-related toxicity.
- **RENAL IMPAIRMENT** [EvGr] Use with caution (risk of oedema with or without congestive heart failure). ⟨M⟩
- **MEDICINAL FORMS** There can be variation in the licensing of different medicines containing the same drug. Forms available from special-order manufacturers include: oral tablet

Oral tablet

▸ **Oxandrolone (Non-proprietary)**

Oxandrolone 2.5 mg Oxandrin 2.5mg tablets | 100 tablet [PoM] [CD4-2]

ANDROGENS

Androgens

- **CONTRA-INDICATIONS** Breast cancer in males · history of liver tumours · hypercalcaemia · prostate cancer
- **CAUTIONS** Cardiac impairment · diabetes mellitus · epilepsy · hypertension · ischaemic heart disease · migraine · pre-pubertal boys (fusion of epiphyses is hastened and may result in short stature)—statural growth and sexual development should be monitored · risk factors for venous thromboembolism · skeletal metastases—risk of hypercalcaemia or hypercalciuria (if this occurs, treat appropriately and restart treatment once normal serum calcium concentration restored) · sleep apnoea · stop treatment or reduce dose if severe polycythaemia occurs · thrombophilia—increased risk of thrombosis · tumours—risk of hypercalcaemia or hypercalciuria (if this occurs, treat appropriately and restart treatment once normal serum calcium concentration restored)
- **SIDE-EFFECTS**
  - ▸ **Common or very common** Hypertension
  - ▸ **Uncommon** Headache
  - ▸ **Rare or very rare** Pulmonary oil microembolism
  - ▸ **Frequency not known** Alopecia · anxiety · asthenia · behaviour abnormal · depression · dizziness · dyspnoea · dysuria · epiphyses premature fusion · fluid retention · gynaecomastia · hot flush · hyperhidrosis · insomnia · jaundice · nausea · oedema · oligozoospermia · paraesthesia · polycythaemia · precocious puberty · prostate abnormalities · prostate cancer · seborrhoea · sexual dysfunction · skin reactions · sleep apnoea · urinary tract obstruction · weight increased

  SIDE-EFFECTS, FURTHER INFORMATION Stop treatment or reduce dose if severe polycythaemia occurs.
- **PREGNANCY** Avoid—causes masculinisation of female fetus.
- **BREAST FEEDING** Avoid.
- **HEPATIC IMPAIRMENT** In general, manufacturers advise caution (increased risk of fluid retention and heart failure).
- **RENAL IMPAIRMENT** In general, manufacturers advise caution (increased risk of fluid retention and heart failure).
- **MONITORING REQUIREMENTS** Monitor haematocrit and haemoglobulin before treatment, every three months for the first year, and yearly thereafter.

above

Testosterone enantate

13-May-2020

- **INDICATIONS AND DOSE**

Induction and maintenance of sexual maturation in males (specialist use only)

▸ BY DEEP INTRAMUSCULAR INJECTION

▸ Child 12–17 years: 25–50 mg/m^2 every month, dose to be increased every 6–12 months according to response

- **UNLICENSED USE** Not licensed for use in children.
- **INTERACTIONS** → Appendix 1: testosterone
- **SIDE-EFFECTS** Bone formation increased · circulatory system disorder · gastrointestinal disorder · gastrointestinal haemorrhage · hepatomegaly · hypercalcaemia · neoplasms · spermatogenesis abnormal

● **MEDICINAL FORMS** There can be variation in the licensing of different medicines containing the same drug.

Solution for injection

▸ Testosterone enantate (Non-proprietary)

Testosterone enantate 250 mg per 1 ml Testosterone enantate 250mg/1ml solution for injection ampoules | 3 ampoule PoM £101.33 DT = £101.33 CD4-2

593

Testosterone propionate

13-May-2020

● **INDICATIONS AND DOSE**

Delayed puberty in males

▸ BY INTRAMUSCULAR INJECTION

▸ Child: 50 mg once weekly

Treatment of microphallus (specialist use only)

▸ TO THE SKIN USING CREAM

▸ Child: Apply 3 times a day for 3 weeks

● **INTERACTIONS** → Appendix 1: testosterone

● **MEDICINAL FORMS** Forms available from special-order manufacturers include: solution for injection, cutaneous cream

593

Testosterone undecanoate

13-May-2020

● **INDICATIONS AND DOSE**

Induction and maintenance of sexual maturation in males (specialist use only)

▸ BY MOUTH

▸ Child 12–17 years: 40 mg once daily on alternate days, adjusted according to response to 120 mg daily

● **INTERACTIONS** → Appendix 1: testosterone

● **SIDE-EFFECTS** Azoospermia · diarrhoea · fluid imbalance · gastrointestinal discomfort · hepatic function abnormal · lipid metabolism change · mood altered · myalgia · penis enlarged

● **MEDICINAL FORMS** No licensed medicines listed.

7.2a Male sex hormone antagonism

ANTI-ANDROGENS

Cyproterone acetate

01-Dec-2020

● **INDICATIONS AND DOSE**

Gonadotrophin-independent precocious puberty (specialist use only)

▸ BY MOUTH

▸ Child: Initially 25 mg twice daily, adjusted according to response

● **UNLICENSED USE** Unlicensed for use in children.

IMPORTANT SAFETY INFORMATION

MHRA/CHM ADVICE: CYPROTERONE ACETATE: NEW ADVICE TO MINIMISE RISK OF MENINGIOMA (JUNE 2020)

Cyproterone acetate has been associated with an overall rare, but cumulative dose-dependent, increased risk of meningioma (single and multiple), mainly at doses of 25 mg/day and higher. Healthcare professionals are advised to monitor patients for meningiomas, and to permanently discontinue treatment if diagnosed. Use of cyproterone acetate, including co-cyprindiol, for all indications is contra-indicated in those with meningioma or a history of meningioma. Treatment with high doses of cyproterone acetate for any indication, except prostate cancer, should be restricted to when alternative treatments or interventions are unavailable or considered inappropriate.

● **CONTRA-INDICATIONS** Dubin-Johnson syndrome · existing or history of thromboembolic disorders · malignant diseases · meningioma or history of meningioma · previous or existing liver tumours · Rotor syndrome · severe depression · severe diabetes (with vascular changes) · sickle-cell anaemia · wasting diseases · youths under 18 years (may arrest bone maturation and testicular development)

● **CAUTIONS** Diabetes mellitus

● **INTERACTIONS** → Appendix 1: anti-androgens

● **SIDE-EFFECTS**

▸ **Common or very common** Depressed mood · dyspnoea · fatigue · gynaecomastia · hepatic disorders · hot flush · hyperhidrosis · nipple pain · restlessness · weight change

▸ **Uncommon** Skin reactions

▸ **Rare or very rare** Galactorrhoea · meningioma (increased risk with increasing cumulative dose) · neoplasms

▸ **Frequency not known** Adrenocortical suppression · anaemia · azoospermia · hair changes · hypotrichosis · osteoporosis · sebaceous gland underactivity (may clear acne) · thromboembolism

SIDE-EFFECTS, FURTHER INFORMATION Direct hepatic toxicity including jaundice, hepatitis and hepatic failure have been reported (fatalities reported, usually after several months, at dosages of 100 mg and above). If hepatotoxicity is confirmed, cyproterone should normally be withdrawn unless the hepatotoxicity can be explained by another cause such as metastatic disease (in which case cyproterone should be continued only if the perceived benefit exceeds the risk).

● **HEPATIC IMPAIRMENT** Manufacturer advises avoid.

● **MONITORING REQUIREMENTS**

▸ Monitor blood counts initially and throughout treatment.

▸ Monitor adrenocortical function regularly.

▸ Monitor hepatic function regularly—liver function tests should be performed before and regularly during treatment and whenever symptoms suggestive of hepatotoxicity occur.

● **PATIENT AND CARER ADVICE**

Driving and skilled tasks Fatigue and lassitude may impair performance of skilled tasks (e.g. driving).

● **MEDICINAL FORMS** There can be variation in the licensing of different medicines containing the same drug. Forms available from special-order manufacturers include: oral tablet, oral capsule, oral suspension, oral solution

Oral tablet

CAUTIONARY AND ADVISORY LABELS 21

▸ Cyproterone acetate (Non-proprietary)

Cyproterone acetate 50 mg Cyproterone 50mg tablets | 56 tablet PoM £98.85 DT = £101.76

Cyproterone acetate 100 mg Cyproterone 100mg tablets | 84 tablet PoM £260.00 DT = £132.57

▸ Androcur (Advanz Pharma)

Cyproterone acetate 50 mg Androcur 50mg tablets | 60 tablet PoM £31.34

▸ Cyprostat (Advanz Pharma)

Cyproterone acetate 50 mg Cyprostat 50mg tablets | 160 tablet PoM £82.86

HORMONE ANTAGONISTS AND RELATED AGENTS › AROMATASE INHIBITORS

Testolactone

● **INDICATIONS AND DOSE**

Gonadotrophin-independent precocious puberty (specialist use only)

▶ BY MOUTH

▶ Child: 5 mg/kg 3–4 times a day; increased if necessary up to 10 mg/kg 4 times a day

● **SIDE-EFFECTS**

▶ **Common or very common** Appetite decreased · diarrhoea · hair growth abnormal · hypertension · nausea · peripheral neuropathy · vomiting · weight change

▶ **Rare or very rare** Hypersensitivity · rash

● **PREGNANCY** Avoid.

● **BREAST FEEDING** No information available.

● **MEDICINAL FORMS** There can be variation in the licensing of different medicines containing the same drug.

Oral tablet

▶ Testolactone (Non-proprietary)

Testolactone 50 mg Teslac 50mg tablets | 100 tablet PoM

8 Thyroid disorders

8.1 Hyperthyroidism

Hyperthyroidism

09-Dec-2019

Description of condition

Hyperthyroidism results from the excessive production and secretion of thyroid hormones leading to thyrotoxicosis (an excess of circulating thyroid hormones). Signs and symptoms of hyperthyroidism include a goitre, hyperactivity, fatigue, palpitations, nervousness, heat intolerance, weight loss, rapid growth in height, and diarrhoea. Complications include Graves' orbitopathy, or thyroid storm (thyrotoxic crisis) which is a life-threatening medical emergency. Risk factors include smoking, a family history of thyroid disease, or autoimmune disorders.

Primary hyperthyroidism refers to when the condition arises from the thyroid gland rather than due to a pituitary or hypothalamic disorder. It is mainly caused by Graves' disease (an autoimmune disorder mediated by antibodies that stimulate the thyroid-stimulating hormone (TSH) receptor), or rarely due to toxic nodular goitre (autonomously functioning thyroid nodules that secrete excess thyroid hormone).

Primary hyperthyroidism is more common in females than males and can be classified as either overt or subclinical; both of which may or may not be symptomatic. Overt hyperthyroidism is characterised by TSH levels below the reference range and free thyroxine (FT4) and/or free tri-iodothyronine (FT3) levels above the reference range. In subclinical hyperthyroidism, TSH is suppressed but FT4 and FT3 levels are within the reference range.

Thyrotoxicosis can also occur without hyperthyroidism; this is usually transient, and can occur because of excess intake of levothyroxine or thyroiditis.

Aims of treatment

Treatment aims to alleviate symptoms, align thyroid function tests within or close to the reference range, and to reduce the risk of long-term complications.

Non-drug treatment

EvGr Radioactive iodine or surgery (such as total thyroidectomy or hemithyroidectomy) may be considered by specialists in the management of Graves' disease or toxic nodular goitre. Whilst awaiting these treatments, antithyroid drugs should be offered to control hyperthyroidism, see *Graves' disease* and *Toxic nodular goitre* in *Primary hyperthyroidism*. (A)

Primary Hyperthyroidism

EvGr Explain to children, and their family or carers if appropriate, that:

- Some children may feel well even when their thyroid function tests are outside the reference range;
- Even when they have no symptoms, treatment may be advised to reduce the risk of long-term complications;
- Symptoms may lag behind treatment changes for several weeks to months.

For children aged 16 years and over, consider antithyroid drugs alongside supportive treatment (for example, beta-blockers) whilst awaiting specialist assessment and further treatment. Carbimazole p. 596 is the recommended choice of antithyroid drug, with propylthiouracil p. 597 considered for those in whom carbimazole is unsuitable. For further information, see *Graves' disease* and *Toxic nodular goitre*.

Before starting antithyroid drugs in children, check full blood count and liver function tests. (A)

The MHRA/CHM have released important safety information regarding the use of carbimazole p. 596 and the risk of acute pancreatitis. For further information, see *Important safety information* for carbimazole p. 596.

For guidance on follow up and monitoring of hyperthyroidism, see NICE guideline: **Thyroid disease** (see *Useful resources*).

Graves' disease

Children aged under 16 years

EvGr Under specialist care, carbimazole p. 596 [unlicensed in children under 2 years] is recommended as first-line definitive treatment using a titration regimen (dose based on thyroid function tests), for at least 2 years (and possibly longer). Review the need for treatment every 2 years and consider continuing or restarting antithyroid drugs, or discussing other non-drug treatment options if the child relapses.

If agranulocytosis develops during antithyroid treatment, stop and do not restart treatment. (A)

Children aged 16 years and over

EvGr Under specialist care, radioactive iodine is recommended as first-line definitive treatment unless it is unsuitable or remission is likely to be achieved with antithyroid drugs. For children in whom an antithyroid drug is likely to achieve remission (such as in mild and uncomplicated cases), a choice of either carbimazole p. 596 or radioactive iodine should be offered. Carbimazole p. 596 should be offered as first-line definitive treatment if radioactive iodine and surgery are unsuitable treatment options.

Offer carbimazole p. 596 as a 12–18 month course using either a block and replace regimen (combination of fixed high-dose carbimazole with levothyroxine sodium p. 599), or a titration regimen (dose based on thyroid function tests), and review the need for further treatment. If children have persistent or relapsed hyperthyroidism despite antithyroid drug treatment, consider radioactive iodine or surgery.

Consider propylthiouracil for children who experience side-effects to carbimazole p. 596, are pregnant or trying to conceive within the following 6 months, or have a history of pancreatitis.

If agranulocytosis develops during antithyroid treatment, stop and do not restart treatment. (A)

Toxic nodular goitre

Children aged under 16 years

EvGr Under specialist care, offer carbimazole below [unlicensed in children under 2 years] using a titration regimen to children with hyperthyroidism secondary to a single or multiple nodules, and discuss the role of surgery and radioactive iodine.

If agranulocytosis develops during antithyroid treatment, stop and do not restart treatment. (A)

Children aged 16 years and over

EvGr Under specialist care, radioactive iodine is recommended as first-line definitive treatment for children with hyperthyroidism secondary to multiple nodules; offer total thyroidectomy or life-long antithyroid drugs if radioactive iodine is unsuitable. For children with hyperthyroidism secondary to a single nodule, offer radioactive iodine or surgery (hemithyroidectomy) as first-line definitive treatment; if these options are unsuitable, offer life-long antithyroid drugs. Consider treatment with a titration regimen of carbimazole below when offering life-long antithyroid drugs.

Consider propylthiouracil for children who experience side-effects to carbimazole, are pregnant or are trying to conceive within the following 6 months, or have a history of pancreatitis.

If agranulocytosis develops during antithyroid treatment, stop and do not restart treatment. (A)

Subclinical hyperthyroidism

EvGr For children aged under 16 years, consider seeking specialist advice on managing subclinical hyperthyroidism. Consider measuring TSH, FT4 and FT3 every 3 months for untreated subclinical hyperthyroidism.

For children aged 16 years and over, consider seeking specialist advice if they have 2 TSH readings lower than 0.1 mIU/litre at least 3 months apart and evidence of thyroid disease or symptoms of thyrotoxicosis. Consider measuring TSH every 6 months for untreated subclinical hyperthyroidism. (A)

For further information on monitoring in subclinical hyperthyroidism, see NICE guideline: **Thyroid disease** (see *Useful resources*).

Thyrotoxicosis without hyperthyroidism

EvGr Transient thyrotoxicosis without hyperthyroidism usually only needs supportive treatment (for example, beta-blockers). (A)

Useful Resources

Thyroid disease: assessment and management. National Institute for Health and Care Excellence. NICE guideline 145. November 2019, updated February 2020.
www.nice.org.uk/guidance/ng145

Other drugs used for Hyperthyroidism Propranolol hydrochloride, p. 123

ANTITHYROID DRUGS › SULFUR-CONTAINING IMIDAZOLES

Carbimazole

02-Sep-2020

● **INDICATIONS AND DOSE**

Hyperthyroidism (blocking-replacement regimen) in combination with levothyroxine

▶ BY MOUTH

▶ Child: Therapy usually given for 12 to 24 months (consult product literature or local protocols)

Hyperthyroidism (including Graves' disease)

▶ BY MOUTH

▶ Neonate: Initially 750 micrograms/kg daily until patient is euthyroid, usually after 8 to 12 weeks, then gradually reduce to a maintenance dose of 30–60% of the initial dose; higher initial doses (up to 1 mg/kg daily) are occasionally required, particularly in thyrotoxic crisis, dose may be given in single or divided doses.

▶ Child 1 month-11 years: Initially 750 micrograms/kg daily until patient is euthyroid, usually after 4–8 weeks, then gradually reduce to a maintenance dose of 30–60% of the initial dose; higher initial doses are occasionally required, particularly in thyrotoxic crisis, dose may be given in single or divided doses; maximum 30 mg per day

▶ Child 12-17 years: Initially 30 mg daily until euthyroid, usually after 4–8 weeks, then gradually reduce to a maintenance dose of 30–60% of the initial dose; higher initial doses are occasionally required, particularly in thyrotoxic crisis, dose may be given in single or divided doses

DOSE EQUIVALENCE AND CONVERSION

▶ When substituting, carbimazole 1 mg is considered equivalent to propylthiouracil 10 mg but the dose may need adjusting according to response.

IMPORTANT SAFETY INFORMATION

NEUTROPENIA AND AGRANULOCYTOSIS

Manufacturer advises of the importance of recognising bone marrow suppression induced by carbimazole and the need to stop treatment promptly.

- Patient should be asked to report symptoms and signs suggestive of infection, especially sore throat.
- A white blood cell count should be performed if there is any clinical evidence of infection.
- Carbimazole should be stopped promptly if there is clinical or laboratory evidence of neutropenia.

MHRA/CHM ADVICE: CARBIMAZOLE: INCREASED RISK OF CONGENITAL MALFORMATIONS; STRENGTHENED ADVICE ON CONTRACEPTION (FEBRUARY 2019)

Carbimazole is associated with an increased risk of congenital malformations when used during pregnancy, especially in the first trimester and at high doses (daily dose of 15 mg or more).

Women of childbearing potential should use effective contraception during treatment with carbimazole. It should only be considered in pregnancy after a thorough benefit-risk assessment, and at the lowest effective dose without additional administration of thyroid hormones—close maternal, fetal, and neonatal monitoring is recommended.

MHRA/CHM ADVICE: CARBIMAZOLE: RISK OF ACUTE PANCREATITIS (FEBRUARY 2019)

Cases of acute pancreatitis have been reported during treatment with carbimazole. It should be stopped immediately and permanently if acute pancreatitis occurs.

Carbimazole should not be used in patients with a history of acute pancreatitis associated with previous treatment—re-exposure may result in life-threatening acute pancreatitis with a decreased time to onset.

● **CONTRA-INDICATIONS** Severe blood disorders

● **INTERACTIONS** → Appendix 1: carbimazole

● **SIDE-EFFECTS**

▶ **Rare or very rare** Bone marrow disorders · haemolytic anaemia · severe cutaneous adverse reactions (SCARs) · thrombocytopenia

▶ **Frequency not known** Agranulocytosis · alopecia · angioedema · dyspepsia · eosinophilia · fever ·

gastrointestinal disorder · generalised lymphadenopathy · haemorrhage · headache · hepatic disorders · insulin autoimmune syndrome · leucopenia · malaise · myopathy · nausea · nerve disorders · neutropenia · pancreatitis acute (discontinue permanently) · salivary gland enlargement · skin reactions · taste loss

- **CONCEPTION AND CONTRACEPTION** The MHRA advises that females of childbearing potential should use effective contraception during treatment.
- **PREGNANCY** The MHRA advises consider use only after a thorough benefit-risk assessment. See *Important Safety Information* for further information.
- **BREAST FEEDING** Present in breast milk but this does not preclude breast-feeding as long as neonatal development is closely monitored and the lowest effective dose is used. Amount in milk may be sufficient to affect neonatal thyroid function therefore lowest effective dose should be used.
- **HEPATIC IMPAIRMENT** Manufacturer advises use with caution in mild to moderate insufficiency—half-life may be prolonged; avoid in severe insufficiency.
- **PATIENT AND CARER ADVICE** Warn patient or carers to tell doctor **immediately** if sore throat, mouth ulcers, bruising, fever, malaise, or non-specific illness develops.

Medicines for Children leaflet: Carbimazole for overactive thyroid www.medicinesforchildren.org.uk/medicines/carbimazole-for-overactive-thyroid/

- **MEDICINAL FORMS** There can be variation in the licensing of different medicines containing the same drug. Forms available from special-order manufacturers include: oral capsule, oral suspension, oral solution

Oral tablet

- Carbimazole (Non-proprietary)
  - **Carbimazole 5 mg** Carbimazole 5mg tablets | 100 tablet [PoM] £87.20 DT = £1.57
  - **Carbimazole 10 mg** Carbimazole 10mg tablets | 100 tablet [PoM] £96.00 DT = £65.81
  - **Carbimazole 15 mg** Carbimazole 15mg tablets | 100 tablet [PoM] £420.00 DT = £281.42
  - **Carbimazole 20 mg** Carbimazole 20mg tablets | 100 tablet [PoM] £208.17 DT = £1.81

ANTITHYROID DRUGS › THIOURACILS

Propylthiouracil

18-Aug-2021

- **INDICATIONS AND DOSE**

Hyperthyroidism (including Graves' disease)

▶ BY MOUTH

- Neonate: Initially 2.5–5 mg/kg twice daily until euthyroid, usually after 8 to 12 weeks, then gradually reduce to a maintenance dose of 30–60% of the initial dose; higher initial doses are occasionally required, particularly in thyrotoxic crisis.
- Child 1–11 months: Initially 2.5 mg/kg 3 times a day until euthyroid, usually after 4 to 8 weeks, then gradually reduce to a maintenance dose of 30–60% of the initial dose; higher initial doses are occasionally required, particularly in thyrotoxic crisis
- Child 1–4 years: Initially 25 mg 3 times a day until euthyroid, usually after 4 to 8 weeks, then gradually reduce to a maintenance dose of 30–60% of the initial dose; higher initial doses are occasionally required, particularly in thyrotoxic crisis
- Child 5–11 years: Initially 50 mg 3 times a day until euthyroid, usually after 4 to 8 weeks, then gradually reduce to a maintenance dose of 30–60% of the initial dose; higher initial doses are occasionally required, particularly in thyrotoxic crisis
- Child 12–17 years: Initially 100 mg 3 times a day until euthyroid, usually after 4 to 8 weeks, then gradually reduce to a maintenance dose of 30–60% of the initial dose; higher initial doses are occasionally required, particularly in thyrotoxic crisis

DOSE EQUIVALENCE AND CONVERSION

- When substituting, carbimazole 1 mg is considered equivalent to propylthiouracil 10 mg but the dose may need adjusting according to response.

- **UNLICENSED USE** Not licensed for use in children under 6 years of age.
- **INTERACTIONS** → Appendix 1: propylthiouracil
- **SIDE-EFFECTS**
  - **Rare or very rare** Agranulocytosis · bone marrow disorders · glomerulonephritis acute · hearing impairment · leucopenia · thrombocytopenia · vomiting
  - **Frequency not known** Alopecia · arthralgia · arthritis · encephalopathy · fever · gastrointestinal disorder · haemorrhage · headache · hepatic disorders · hypoprothrombinaemia · interstitial pneumonitis · lupus-like syndrome · lymphadenopathy · myopathy · nausea · nephritis · skin reactions · taste altered · vasculitis

SIDE-EFFECTS, FURTHER INFORMATION Severe hepatic reactions have been reported, including fatal cases and cases requiring liver transplant—discontinue if significant liver-enzyme abnormalities develop.

- **PREGNANCY** Propylthiouracil can be given but the blocking-replacement regimen is **not** suitable. Propylthiouracil crosses the placenta and in high doses may cause fetal goitre and hypothyroidism—the lowest dose that will control the hyperthyroid state should be used (requirements in Graves' disease tend to fall during pregnancy).
- **BREAST FEEDING** Present in breast milk but this does not preclude breast-feeding as long as neonatal development is closely monitored and the lowest effective dose is used. Amount in milk probably too small to affect infant; high doses may affect neonatal thyroid function.
  Monitoring Monitor infant's thyroid status.
- **HEPATIC IMPAIRMENT** Manufacturer advises caution (risk of increased half life).
  Dose adjustments Manufacturer advises consider dose reduction.
- **RENAL IMPAIRMENT**
  Dose adjustments See p. 16.
  [EvGr] Use 75% of normal dose if estimated glomerular filtration rate 10–50 mL/minute/1.73 m^2.
  Use 50% of normal dose if estimated glomerular filtration rate less than 10 mL/minute/1.73 m^2. [M]
- **MONITORING REQUIREMENTS** Monitor for hepatotoxicity.
- **PATIENT AND CARER ADVICE** Patients should be told how to recognise signs of liver disorder and advised to seek prompt medical attention if symptoms such as anorexia, nausea, vomiting, fatigue, abdominal pain, jaundice, dark urine, or pruritus develop.

- **MEDICINAL FORMS** There can be variation in the licensing of different medicines containing the same drug. Forms available from special-order manufacturers include: oral suspension, oral solution

Oral tablet

- Propylthiouracil (Non-proprietary)
  - **Propylthiouracil 25 mg** Propylthiouracil 25mg tablets | 28 tablet [PoM] £27.65–£44.00 DT = £37.65
  - **Propylthiouracil 50 mg** Propylthiouracil 50mg tablets | 56 tablet [PoM] £58.19 DT = £7.95 | 100 tablet [PoM] £12.00–£59.20
  - **Propylthiouracil 100 mg** Propylthiouracil 100mg tablets | 56 tablet [PoM] £44.48–£56.05 DT = £44.48

VITAMINS AND TRACE ELEMENTS

Iodide with iodine

(Lugol's Solution; Aqueous Iodine Oral Solution)

● **INDICATIONS AND DOSE**

Thyrotoxicosis (pre-operative)

▶ BY MOUTH USING ORAL SOLUTION

▶ Neonate: 0.1–0.3 mL 3 times a day.

▶ Child: 0.1–0.3 mL 3 times a day

Neonatal thyrotoxicosis

▶ BY MOUTH USING ORAL SOLUTION

▶ Neonate: 0.05–0.1 mL 3 times a day.

Thyrotoxic crisis

▶ BY MOUTH USING ORAL SOLUTION

▶ Child 1 month–1 year: 0.2–0.3 mL 3 times a day

DOSE EQUIVALENCE AND CONVERSION

▶ Doses based on the use of an aqueous oral solution containing iodine 50 mg/mL and potassium iodide 100 mg/mL.

● **CAUTIONS** Children · not for long-term treatment

● **SIDE-EFFECTS** Conjunctivitis · depression (long term use) · erectile dysfunction (long term use) · excessive tearing · headache · hypersensitivity · increased risk of infection · influenza like illness · insomnia (long term use) · rash · salivary gland pain

● **PREGNANCY** Neonatal goitre and hypothyroidism.

● **BREAST FEEDING** Stop breast-feeding. Danger of neonatal hypothyroidism or goitre. Appears to be concentrated in milk.

● **DIRECTIONS FOR ADMINISTRATION** For oral solution, dilute well with milk or water.

● **MEDICINAL FORMS** There can be variation in the licensing of different medicines containing the same drug. Forms available from special-order manufacturers include: oral solution

Oral solution

CAUTIONARY AND ADVISORY LABELS 27

8.2 Hypothyroidism

Hypothyroidism

18-Jun-2024

Description of condition

Hypothyroidism results from the underproduction and secretion of thyroid hormones. Signs and symptoms of hypothyroidism include fatigue, weight gain, constipation, slow growth, depression, intolerance to the cold, and reduced body and scalp hair. Complications include cardiovascular disease and an increase in cardiovascular risk factors (such as hypercholesterolaemia), and myxoedema coma (which is a life-threatening medical emergency).

Primary hypothyroidism refers to when the condition arises from the thyroid gland and can be congenital or due to an autoimmune disease (such as Hashimoto's thyroiditis), rather than due to a pituitary or hypothalamic disorder (secondary hypothyroidism). Primary hypothyroidism is more common in females than males and can be classified as either overt or subclinical. Overt hypothyroidism is characterised by thyroid stimulating hormone (TSH) levels above the reference range and free thyroxine (FT4) levels below the reference range. In subclinical hypothyroidism, TSH levels are above the reference range but FT4 and free tri-iodothyronine (FT3) levels are within the reference range.

Aims of treatment

The aims of treatment are to alleviate symptoms, align thyroid function tests within or close to the reference range, and to reduce the risk of long-term complications.

Management of primary hypothyroidism

EvGr Explain to children, and their family or carers if appropriate, that:

- Some children may feel well even when their thyroid function tests are outside the reference range;
- Even when they have no symptoms, treatment may be advised to reduce the risk of long-term complications;
- Symptoms may lag behind treatment changes for several weeks to months. (A)

Overt hypothyroidism

EvGr Offer levothyroxine sodium p. 599 as first-line treatment and aim to maintain thyroid stimulating hormone (TSH) levels within the reference range. If symptoms persist, even after achieving normal TSH levels, consider adjusting the dose to achieve optimal well-being whilst avoiding doses that cause TSH suppression or thyrotoxicosis.

For children whose TSH level was very high before starting treatment or who have had a prolonged period of untreated disease, the TSH level can take up to 6 months to return to the reference range.

For children aged 28 days to under 2 years, consider measuring free thyroxine (FT4) and TSH every 4–8 weeks until the TSH level is stable, then every 2–3 months until 1 year of age, then every 3–4 months until 2 years of age.

For children aged 2 years to under 16 years, consider measuring FT4 and TSH every 6–12 weeks until the TSH is stable, then every 4–6 months until puberty, then yearly thereafter.

For children aged 16 years and over, consider measuring TSH levels every 3 months until a stable level has been achieved, then yearly thereafter. Monitoring free thyroxine (FT4) should also be considered in those who continue to be symptomatic.

Due to the uncertainty around the long-term adverse effects and the insufficient evidence of benefit over levothyroxine monotherapy, the use of natural thyroid extract is not recommended in children. Liothyronine (either alone or in combination with levothyroxine) is not routinely recommended in children for the same reasons. NHS England have produced guidance on the prescribing of liothyronine, for further information see: www.england.nhs.uk/long-read/liothyronine-advice-for-prescribers/. (A)

Subclinical hypothyroidism

EvGr When considering whether to start treatment for subclinical hypothyroidism, take into account features suggesting underlying thyroid disease.

In children aged 28 days to under 2 years, consider levothyroxine sodium p. 599 for those who have a TSH level of 10 mIU/L or higher.

In children aged 2 years to under 16 years, consider levothyroxine sodium p. 599 for those who have a TSH level:

- of 20 mIU/litre or higher, or
- between 10–20 mIU/litre on 2 separate occasions 3 months apart, or
- between 5–10 mIU/litre on 2 separate occasions 3 months apart and have
  - ▶ thyroid dysgenesis (underdeveloped thyroid gland), or
  - ▶ signs or symptoms of thyroid dysfunction.

For children aged 16 years and over, consider levothyroxine sodium p. 599 in those who have a TSH level of 10 mIU/L or higher on 2 separate occasions 3 months apart.

For all children, if symptoms persist, even after achieving normal TSH levels, consider adjusting the dose to achieve optimal well-being whilst avoiding doses that cause TSH suppression or thyrotoxicosis.

For children whose TSH level was very high before starting treatment or who have had a prolonged period of untreated disease, the TSH level can take up to 6 months to return to the reference range.

For children in whom treatment with levothyroxine is started, monitor TSH and FT4 levels according to their age as outlined in *Overt hypothyroidism*.

For symptomatic children aged 16 years and over with a TSH level above the reference range, but lower than 10 mIU/L on 2 separate occasions 3 months apart, consider a 6-month trial of levothyroxine sodium treatment below. If symptoms do not improve after starting levothyroxine, re-measure TSH and if the level remains elevated, adjust the dose. If symptoms persist when the serum TSH is within the reference range, consider stopping levothyroxine and follow the recommendations on *Monitoring untreated subclinical hypothyroidism and monitoring after stopping treatment* in the NICE guideline: **Thyroid disease** (see *Useful resources*). Ⓐ

Useful Resources

Thyroid disease: assessment and management. National Institute for Health and Care Excellence. NICE guideline 145. November 2019, updated February 2020
www.nice.org.uk/guidance/ng145

THYROID HORMONES

Levothyroxine sodium

18-Aug-2025

(Thyroxine sodium)

● **INDICATIONS AND DOSE**

Hypothyroidism

▶ BY MOUTH

▶ Neonate: Initially 10–15 micrograms/kg once daily (max. per dose 50 micrograms); adjusted in steps of 5 micrograms/kg every 2 weeks, alternatively adjusted in steps of 5 micrograms/kg as required; maintenance 20–50 micrograms daily, levothyroxine should be taken at the same time each day, preferably 30–60 minutes before meals, caffeine-containing drinks, or other medicines; this could be before breakfast or another more convenient time.

▶ Child 1 month–1 year: Initially 5 micrograms/kg once daily (max. per dose 50 micrograms); adjusted in steps of 10–25 micrograms every 2–4 weeks until metabolism normalised; maintenance 25–75 micrograms daily, levothyroxine should be taken at the same time each day, preferably 30–60 minutes before meals, caffeine-containing drinks, or other medicines; this could be before breakfast or another more convenient time

▶ Child 2–11 years: Initially 50 micrograms once daily; adjusted in steps of 25 micrograms every 2–4 weeks until metabolism normalised; maintenance 75–100 micrograms daily, levothyroxine should be taken at the same time each day, preferably 30–60 minutes before meals, caffeine-containing drinks, or other medicines; this could be before breakfast or another more convenient time

▶ Child 12–17 years: Initially 50 micrograms once daily; adjusted in steps of 25–50 micrograms every 3–4 weeks until metabolism normalised; maintenance 100–200 micrograms daily, levothyroxine should be taken at the same time each day, preferably 30–60 minutes before meals, caffeine-containing drinks, or other medicines; this could be before breakfast or another more convenient time

Hyperthyroidism (blocking-replacement regimen) in combination with carbimazole

▶ BY MOUTH

▶ Child: Therapy usually given for 12 to 24 months (consult product literature or local protocols)

IMPORTANT SAFETY INFORMATION

MHRA/CHM ADVICE: LEVOTHYROXINE: NEW PRESCRIBING ADVICE FOR PATIENTS WHO EXPERIENCE SYMPTOMS ON SWITCHING BETWEEN DIFFERENT LEVOTHYROXINE PRODUCTS (MAY 2021)

A small proportion of patients treated with levothyroxine report symptoms, often consistent with thyroid dysfunction, when switching between different tablet formulations of levothyroxine. Healthcare professionals are advised that if a patient reports symptoms after changing to a different tablet of levothyroxine, a thyroid function test should be considered; if a patient is persistently symptomatic, whether they are biochemically euthyroid or have evidence of abnormal thyroid function, consistently prescribing a specific levothyroxine tablet known to be well tolerated by the patient should be considered. If symptoms or poor control of thyroid function persist despite adhering to a specific tablet, consider prescribing levothyroxine in an oral solution formulation.

● **CONTRA-INDICATIONS** Thyrotoxicosis

● **CAUTIONS** Cardiac disorders (monitor ECG; start at low dose and carefully titrate) · diabetes insipidus · diabetes mellitus (dose of antidiabetic drugs including insulin may need to be increased) · long-standing hypothyroidism · panhypopituitarism (initiate corticosteroid therapy before starting levothyroxine) · predisposition to adrenal insufficiency (initiate corticosteroid therapy before starting levothyroxine)

● **INTERACTIONS** → Appendix 1: thyroid hormones

● **SIDE-EFFECTS**

▶ **Common or very common** Anxiety · arrhythmias · headache · hyperthyroidism · insomnia · palpitations

▶ **Rare or very rare** Idiopathic intracranial hypertension (particularly in children)

▶ **Frequency not known** Alopecia · angina pectoris · angioedema · arthralgia · circulatory collapse (in low birth weight pre-term neonates) · diarrhoea · dyspnoea · epiphyses premature fusion · fever · flushing · heat intolerance · hyperhidrosis · malaise · menstruation irregular · muscle cramps · muscle spasms · muscle weakness · nausea · oedema · skin reactions · thyrotoxic crisis · tremor · vomiting · weight decreased

SIDE-EFFECTS, FURTHER INFORMATION If metabolism increases too rapidly following initial dosage (causing diarrhoea, nervousness, rapid pulse, insomnia, tremors and sometimes anginal pain where there is latent myocardial ischaemia), reduce dose or withhold for 1–2 days and start again at a lower dose.

● **PREGNANCY** Levothyroxine may cross the placenta. Excessive or insufficient maternal thyroid hormones can be detrimental to fetus.

Dose adjustments Levothyroxine requirement may increase during pregnancy.

Monitoring Assess maternal thyroid function before conception (if possible), at diagnosis of pregnancy, at antenatal booking, during both the second and third trimesters, and after delivery (more frequent monitoring required on initiation or adjustment of levothyroxine).

● **BREAST FEEDING** Amount too small to affect tests for neonatal hypothyroidism.

● **MONITORING REQUIREMENTS**

▶ When used for Primary hypothyroidism EvGr In those *aged between 28 days and 2 years*, consider measuring free thyroxine (FT4) and thyroid stimulating hormone (TSH) levels every 4–8 weeks until TSH level stabilised (two similar measurements within the reference range, 2 months apart), then every 2–3 months during the first year of life, and every 3–4 months during the second year of life. In those *aged 2 years and older*, consider measuring FT4 and TSH levels every 6–12 weeks until TSH level stabilised (two similar measurements within the reference range, 3 months apart), then every 4–6 months until after puberty, then yearly thereafter. (A)

- **EFFECT ON LABORATORY TESTS** EvGr Biotin may interfere with thyroid immunoassays that are based on biotin/streptavidin interaction, and the risk of interference increases with higher doses of biotin. Possible biotin interference should be considered when interpreting test results as these may be falsely high or low, leading to misdiagnosis, or inappropriate management or dose adjustment of levothyroxine. If the patient is taking biotin-containing products, laboratory personnel should be informed before tests are ordered as alternative assays may be available. (M)
- **PRESCRIBING AND DISPENSING INFORMATION** Levothyroxine equivalent to 100 micrograms/m^2/day can be used as a guide to the requirements in children.
- **PATIENT AND CARER ADVICE** Patients or their carers should be routinely asked about use of biotin-containing products (see *Effect on laboratory tests*).

Medicines for Children leaflet: Levothyroxine for hypothyroidism www.medicinesforchildren.org.uk/medicines/levothyroxine-for-hypothyroidism/

- **MEDICINAL FORMS** There can be variation in the licensing of different medicines containing the same drug. Forms available from special-order manufacturers include: oral capsule, oral suspension, oral solution

Oral tablet

- Levothyroxine sodium (Non-proprietary)

Levothyroxine sodium anhydrous 12.5 microgram Levothyroxine sodium 12.5microgram tablets | 28 tablet PoM £21.24 DT = £9.01 | 56 tablet PoM £20.10–£30.38

Levothyroxine sodium anhydrous 25 microgram Levothyroxine sodium 25microgram tablets | 28 tablet PoM £3.05 DT = £0.67 | 500 tablet PoM £41.61–£54.46

Levothyroxine sodium 25microgram tablets lactose free | 100 tablet PoM ☒

Levothyroxine sodium anhydrous 50 microgram Levothyroxine sodium 50microgram tablets lactose free | 100 tablet PoM ☒

Levothyroxine sodium 50microgram tablets | 28 tablet PoM £1.28 DT = £0.65 | 1000 tablet PoM £21.78–£47.85

Levothyroxine sodium anhydrous 75 microgram Levothyroxine sodium 75microgram tablets | 28 tablet PoM £4.20 DT = £1.92 | 56 tablet PoM £4.70–£5.68

Levothyroxine sodium anhydrous 100 microgram Levothyroxine sodium 100microgram tablets lactose free | 100 tablet PoM ☒

Levothyroxine sodium 100microgram tablets | 28 tablet PoM £1.24 DT = £0.65 | 1000 tablet PoM £22.13–£43.57

- Eltroxin (Advanz Pharma)

Levothyroxine sodium anhydrous 25 microgram Eltroxin 25microgram tablets | 28 tablet PoM £2.54 DT = £0.67

Levothyroxine sodium anhydrous 50 microgram Eltroxin 50microgram tablets | 28 tablet PoM £1.77 DT = £0.65

Levothyroxine sodium anhydrous 100 microgram Eltroxin 100microgram tablets | 28 tablet PoM £1.78 DT = £0.65

- Vencamil (Aristo Pharma Ltd)

Levothyroxine sodium anhydrous 25 microgram Vencamil 25microgram tablets | 28 tablet PoM £2.53 DT = £0.67

Levothyroxine sodium anhydrous 50 microgram Vencamil 50microgram tablets | 28 tablet PoM £1.76 DT = £0.65

Levothyroxine sodium anhydrous 75 microgram Vencamil 75microgram tablets | 28 tablet PoM £2.53 DT = £1.92

Oral capsule

- Levothyroxine sodium (Non-proprietary)

Levothyroxine sodium anhydrous 25 microgram Tirosint 25microgram capsules | 28 capsule PoM ☒ DT = £67.49

Levothyroxine sodium anhydrous 50 microgram Tirosint 50microgram capsules | 28 capsule PoM ☒ DT = £40.02

Levothyroxine sodium anhydrous 100 microgram Tirosint 100microgram capsules | 28 capsule PoM ☒

Oral solution

- Levothyroxine sodium (Non-proprietary)

Levothyroxine sodium anhydrous 5 microgram per 1 ml Levothyroxine sodium 25micrograms/5ml oral solution sugar free | 100 ml PoM £95.00 DT = £29.10 SF

Levothyroxine sodium anhydrous 10 microgram per 1 ml Levothyroxine sodium 50micrograms/5ml oral solution sugar free | 100 ml PoM £91.27 DT = £28.12 SF

Levothyroxine sodium anhydrous 15 microgram per 1 ml Levothyroxine sodium 75micrograms/5ml oral solution sugar free | 100 ml PoM £163.50 DT = £163.50 SF

Levothyroxine sodium anhydrous 20 microgram per 1 ml Levothyroxine sodium 100micrograms/5ml oral solution sugar free | 100 ml PoM £165.00 DT = £61.33 SF

Levothyroxine sodium anhydrous 25 microgram per 1 ml Levothyroxine sodium 125micrograms/5ml oral solution sugar free | 100 ml PoM £185.00–£333.00 DT = £185.00 SF

Liothyronine sodium

18-Aug-2025

(L-Tri-iodothyronine sodium)

- **INDICATIONS AND DOSE**

Hypothyroidism

▶ BY MOUTH

- Child 12–17 years: Initially 10–20 micrograms daily; increased to 60 micrograms daily in 2–3 divided doses

Hypothyroid coma

▶ BY SLOW INTRAVENOUS INJECTION

- Child 12–17 years: 5–20 micrograms every 12 hours, increased to 5–20 micrograms every 4 hours if required, alternatively initially 50 micrograms for 1 dose, then 25 micrograms every 8 hours, reduced to 25 micrograms twice daily

Hypothyroidism (replacement for oral levothyroxine)

▶ BY SLOW INTRAVENOUS INJECTION

- Child: Convert daily levothyroxine dose to liothyronine and give in 2–3 divided doses, adjusted according to response

DOSE EQUIVALENCE AND CONVERSION

- 20–25 micrograms of liothyronine sodium is equivalent to approximately 100 micrograms of levothyroxine sodium.
- Brands without a UK licence may not be bioequivalent and dose adjustment may be necessary.

- **CONTRA-INDICATIONS** Thyrotoxicosis
- **CAUTIONS** Cardiac disorders (monitor ECG; start at low dose and carefully titrate) · diabetes insipidus · diabetes mellitus (dose of antidiabetic drugs including insulin may need to be increased) · prolonged hypothyroidism (initiate corticosteroid therapy in adrenal insufficiency) · severe hypothyroidism (initiate corticosteroid therapy in adrenal insufficiency)
- **INTERACTIONS** → Appendix 1: thyroid hormones
- **SIDE-EFFECTS**

GENERAL SIDE-EFFECTS Alopecia · angina pectoris · anxiety · arrhythmias · diarrhoea · fever · flushing · headache · heat intolerance · hyperhidrosis · insomnia · muscle cramps · muscle weakness · palpitations · tremor · vomiting · weight decreased

SPECIFIC SIDE-EFFECTS

▶ **Rare or very rare**
- With intravenous use Idiopathic intracranial hypertension

▶ **Frequency not known**
- With intravenous use Epiphyses premature fusion · menstruation irregular

- **PREGNANCY** Does not cross the placenta in significant amounts. Excessive or insufficient maternal thyroid hormones can be detrimental to fetus.

Dose adjustments Liothyronine requirement may increase during pregnancy.

Monitoring Assess maternal thyroid function before conception (if possible), at diagnosis of pregnancy, at antenatal booking, during both the second and third trimesters, and after delivery (more frequent monitoring required on initiation or adjustment of liothyronine).

- **BREAST FEEDING** Amount too small to affect tests for neonatal hypothyroidism.
- **EFFECT ON LABORATORY TESTS** EvGr Biotin may interfere with thyroid immunoassays that are based on biotin/streptavidin interaction, and the risk of interference increases with higher doses of biotin. Possible biotin interference should be considered when interpreting test results as these may be falsely high or low, leading to misdiagnosis, or inappropriate management or dose adjustment of liothyronine. If the patient is taking biotin-containing products, laboratory personnel should be informed before tests are ordered as alternative assays may be available. ⟨M⟩
- **PRESCRIBING AND DISPENSING INFORMATION**
Switching to a different brand Patients switched to a different brand should be monitored (particularly if pregnant or if heart disease present) as brands without a UK licence may not be bioequivalent. Pregnant women or those with heart disease should undergo an early review of thyroid status, and other patients should have thyroid function assessed if experiencing a significant change in symptoms. If liothyronine is continued long-term, thyroid function tests should be repeated 1–2 months after any change in brand.
- **PATIENT AND CARER ADVICE** Patients or their carers should be routinely asked about use of biotin-containing products (see *Effect on laboratory tests*).
- **MEDICINAL FORMS** There can be variation in the licensing of different medicines containing the same drug. Forms available from special-order manufacturers include: oral tablet, oral capsule, oral suspension, oral solution, solution for injection

Oral tablet

▸ Liothyronine sodium (Non-proprietary)

Liothyronine sodium 5 microgram Liothyronine 5microgram tablets | 28 tablet PoM £123.38 DT = £51.25

Liothyronine sodium 10 microgram Liothyronine 10microgram tablets | 28 tablet PoM £280.00 DT = £152.44

Liothyronine sodium 15 microgram Liothyronine 15microgram tablets | 28 tablet PoM £152.44

Liothyronine sodium 20 microgram Liothyronine 20microgram tablets | 28 tablet PoM £147.14 DT = £28.30

Liothyronine sodium 25 microgram Cytomel 25microgram tablets | 100 tablet PoM ⊠

Liothyronine 25microgram tablets | 28 tablet PoM £152.44

Powder for solution for injection

▸ Liothyronine sodium (Non-proprietary)

Liothyronine sodium 20 microgram Liothyronine 20microgram powder for solution for injection vials | 5 vial PoM £1,567.50

Oral capsule

▸ Liothyronine sodium (Non-proprietary)

Liothyronine sodium 5 microgram Liothyronine 5microgram capsules | 28 capsule PoM £55.00 DT = £55.00

Liothyronine sodium 10 microgram Liothyronine 10microgram capsules | 28 capsule PoM £65.00 DT = £65.00

Liothyronine sodium 20 microgram Liothyronine 20microgram capsules | 28 capsule PoM £55.00 DT = £55.00

Oral solution

▸ Enolio (Eclosix Ltd)

Liothyronine sodium 10 microgram per 1 ml Enolio 10micrograms/ml oral solution | 50 ml PoM £32.23 SF

Chapter 7
Genito-urinary system

CONTENTS

1 Bladder and urinary disorders

1.1 Urinary frequency, enuresis, and incontinence

Urinary frequency, enuresis and incontinence

Urinary incontinence

Antimuscarinic drugs reduce symptoms of urgency and urge incontinence and increase bladder capacity; oxybutynin hydrochloride p. 603 also has a direct relaxant effect on urinary smooth muscle. Oxybutynin hydrochloride can be considered first for children under 12 years. Side-effects limit the use of oxybutynin hydrochloride, but they may be reduced by starting at a lower dose and then slowly titrating upwards; alternatively oxybutynin hydrochloride can be given by intravesicular instillation. Tolterodine tartrate p. 604 is also effective for urinary incontinence; it can be considered for children over 12 years, or for younger children who have failed to respond to oxybutynin hydrochloride. Modified-release preparations of oxybutynin hydrochloride and tolterodine tartrate are available; they may have fewer side-effects. Antimuscarinic treatment should be reviewed soon after it is commenced, and then at regular intervals; a response generally occurs within 6 months but occasionally may take longer. Children with nocturnal enuresis may require specific additional measures if night-time symptoms also need to be controlled.

See also Nocturnal enuresis in children below.

Nocturnal enuresis in children

23-May-2017

Description of condition

Nocturnal enuresis is the involuntary discharge of urine during sleep, which is common in young children. Children are generally expected to be dry by a developmental age of 5 years, and historically it has been common practice to consider children for treatment only when they reach 7 years; however, symptoms may still persist in a small proportion by the age of 10 years.

Treatment

Children under 5 years

EvGr For children under 5 years, treatment is usually unnecessary as the condition is likely to resolve spontaneously. Reassurance and advice can be useful for some families. (A)

Non Drug Treatment

EvGr Initially, advice should be given on fluid intake, diet, toileting behaviour, and use of reward systems. For children who do not respond to this advice (more than 1–2 wet beds per week), an enuresis alarm should be the recommended treatment for motivated, well-supported children. Alarms in children under 7 years should be considered depending on the child's maturity, motivation and understanding of the alarm. Alarms have a lower relapse rate than drug treatment when discontinued.

Treatment using an alarm should be reviewed after 4 weeks and continued until a minimum of 2 weeks' uninterrupted dry nights have been achieved. If complete dryness is not achieved after 3 months but the condition is still improving and the child remains motivated to use the alarm, it is recommended to continue the treatment. Combined treatment with desmopressin p. 530, or the use of desmopressin alone, is recommended if the initial alarm treatment is unsuccessful or it is no longer appropriate or desirable. (A)

Drug Treatment

EvGr Treatment with oral or sublingual desmopressin is recommended for children over 5 years of age when alarm use is inappropriate or undesirable, or when rapid or short-term results are the priority (for example, to cover periods away from home). Desmopressin alone can also be used if there has been a partial response to a combination of desmopressin and an alarm following initial treatment with an alarm alone. Treatment should be assessed after 4 weeks and continued for 3 months if there are signs of response. Repeated courses of desmopressin can be used in responsive children who experience repeated recurrences of bedwetting, but should be withdrawn **gradually** at regular intervals (for 1 week every 3 months) for full reassessment.

Under specialist supervision, nocturnal enuresis associated with daytime symptoms (overactive bladder) can be managed with desmopressin alone or in combination with an antimuscarinic drug (such as oxybutynin hydrochloride below or tolterodine tartrate p. 604 [unlicensed indication]). Treatment should be continued for 3 months; the course can be repeated if necessary.

The tricyclic antidepressant imipramine hydrochloride p. 291 can be considered for children who have not responded to all other treatments and have undergone specialist assessment, however relapse is common after withdrawal and children and their carers should be aware of the dangers of overdose. Initial treatment should continue for 3 months; further courses can be considered following a medical review every 3 months. Tricyclic antidepressants should be withdrawn gradually. Ⓐ

Useful Resources

Bedwetting in under 19s. National Institute for Health and Care Excellence. Clinical guideline CG111. October 2010.
www.nice.org.uk/guidance/cg111

ANTIMUSCARINICS

Antimuscarinics (systemic)

- **CONTRA-INDICATIONS** Angle-closure glaucoma · gastro-intestinal obstruction · intestinal atony · myasthenia gravis (but some antimuscarinics may be used to decrease muscarinic side-effects of anticholinesterases) · paralytic ileus · pyloric stenosis · severe ulcerative colitis · significant bladder outflow obstruction · toxic megacolon · urinary retention
- **CAUTIONS** Arrhythmias (may be worsened) · autonomic neuropathy · cardiac insufficiency (due to association with tachycardia) · cardiac surgery (due to association with tachycardia) · children (increased risk of side-effects) · conditions characterised by tachycardia · congestive heart failure (may be worsened) · coronary artery disease (may be worsened) · diarrhoea · gastro-oesophageal reflux disease · hiatus hernia with reflux oesophagitis · hypertension · hyperthyroidism (due to association with tachycardia) · individuals susceptible to angle-closure glaucoma · pyrexia · ulcerative colitis
- **SIDE-EFFECTS**
  - ▶ **Common or very common** Confusion · constipation · dizziness · drowsiness · dry mouth · dyspepsia · flushing · headache · nausea · palpitations · skin reactions · tachycardia · urinary disorders · vision disorders · vomiting
  - ▶ **Rare or very rare** Angioedema
- **PATIENT AND CARER ADVICE**
  Driving and skilled tasks Antimuscarinics can affect the performance of skilled tasks (e.g. driving).

ANTIMUSCARINICS › URINARY

F above

Oxybutynin hydrochloride

16-Oct-2024

- **INDICATIONS AND DOSE**

Urinary frequency | Urinary urgency | Urinary incontinence | Neurogenic bladder instability

▶ BY MOUTH USING IMMEDIATE-RELEASE MEDICINES
- ▶ Child 2–4 years: 1.25–2.5 mg 2–3 times a day
- ▶ Child 5–11 years: Initially 2.5–3 mg twice daily, increased to 5 mg 2–3 times a day
- ▶ Child 12–17 years: Initially 5 mg 2–3 times a day, increased if necessary up to 5 mg 4 times a day

▶ BY MOUTH USING MODIFIED-RELEASE TABLETS
- ▶ Child 5–17 years: Initially 5 mg once daily, dose can be adjusted in steps of 5 mg every week according to response up to a maximum of 15 mg per day

Neurogenic detrusor overactivity (under expert supervision)

▶ BY INTRAVESICAL INSTILLATION
- ▶ Child 6–11 years: Initially 2 mg once daily, higher starting doses may be necessary—consult product literature, increased if necessary up to 10 mg 3 times a day, dose to be adjusted according to response
- ▶ Child 12–17 years: Initially 5 mg twice daily, higher starting doses may be necessary—consult product literature, increased if necessary up to 10 mg 4 times a day, dose to be adjusted according to response

Nocturnal enuresis associated with overactive bladder

▶ BY MOUTH USING IMMEDIATE-RELEASE MEDICINES
- ▶ Child 5–17 years: 2.5–3 mg twice daily, last dose to be taken before bedtime, increased to 5 mg 2–3 times a day, last dose to be taken before bedtime

▶ BY MOUTH USING MODIFIED-RELEASE TABLETS
- ▶ Child 5–17 years: Initially 5 mg once daily, dose can be adjusted in steps of 5 mg every week according to response up to a maximum of 15 mg per day

- **UNLICENSED USE** Not licensed for use in children under 5 years.
- **CAUTIONS** Acute porphyrias p. 745
- **INTERACTIONS** → Appendix 1: oxybutynin
- **SIDE-EFFECTS**

GENERAL SIDE-EFFECTS
- ▶ **Common or very common** Diarrhoea · dry eye
- ▶ **Frequency not known** Cognitive disorder · hallucination · seizure

SPECIFIC SIDE-EFFECTS
- ▶ **Uncommon**
  - ▶ With oral use Abdominal discomfort · appetite decreased · dysphagia
- ▶ **Frequency not known**
  - ▶ With intravesical use Abnormal sensation in eye · agoraphobia · akathisia · anticholinergic syndrome · apathy · chest discomfort · concentration impaired · consciousness impaired · fatigue · feeling cold · gastrointestinal discomfort · haematuria · hyperprolactinaemia · hypotension · increased risk of infection · insomnia · proteinuria · supraventricular tachycardia · sweat changes · taste altered · thirst · vertigo
  - ▶ With oral use Anxiety · arrhythmia · depressive symptom · drug dependence · gastrointestinal disorders · glaucoma · heat stroke · hypohidrosis · mydriasis · nightmare · paranoia · photosensitivity reaction · urinary tract infection
- **PREGNANCY** Manufacturers advise avoid unless essential—toxicity in *animal* studies.
- **BREAST FEEDING** Specialist sources indicate probably compatible (limited information available). High plasma-protein binding suggests limited excretion into milk and poor oral bioavailability suggests limited absorption by the infant; monitor breast-fed infants for adverse reactions.
- **HEPATIC IMPAIRMENT** Manufacturer advises caution.
- **RENAL IMPAIRMENT** Manufacturer advises caution.
- **PRESCRIBING AND DISPENSING INFORMATION** The need for therapy for urinary indications should be reviewed soon after it has been commenced and then at regular intervals; a response usually occurs within 6 months but may take longer.
- **PATIENT AND CARER ADVICE** Patients or carers should be trained on administration of *intravesical* solution.
  Medicines for Children leaflet: Oxybutynin for daytime urinary symptoms www.medicinesforchildren.org.uk/medicines/oxybutynin-for-daytime-urinary-symptoms/

- **MEDICINAL FORMS** There can be variation in the licensing of different medicines containing the same drug. Forms available from special-order manufacturers include: oral suspension, oral solution

Oral tablet

CAUTIONARY AND ADVISORY LABELS 3

▸ Oxybutynin hydrochloride (Non-proprietary)

Oxybutynin hydrochloride 2.5 mg Oxybutynin 2.5mg tablets | 56 tablet PoM £6.58 DT = £2.66 | 84 tablet PoM £1.50–£7.00

Oxybutynin hydrochloride 5 mg Oxybutynin 5mg tablets | 56 tablet PoM £7.40 DT = £3.10 | 84 tablet PoM £1.80–£7.80

Modified-release tablet

CAUTIONARY AND ADVISORY LABELS 3, 25

▸ Oxybutynin hydrochloride (Non-proprietary)

Oxybutynin hydrochloride 5 mg Oxybutynin 5mg modified-release tablets | 28 tablet PoM £7.21–£15.50 DT = £4.28

Oxybutynin hydrochloride 10 mg Oxybutynin 10mg modified-release tablets | 28 tablet PoM £23.61–£52.36 DT = £18.40

Oral solution

CAUTIONARY AND ADVISORY LABELS 3

▸ Oxybutynin hydrochloride (Non-proprietary)

Oxybutynin hydrochloride 500 microgram per 1 ml Oxybutynin 2.5mg/5ml oral solution sugar free | 150 ml PoM £214.84 DT = £127.54 SF

Oxybutynin hydrochloride 1 mg per 1 ml Oxybutynin 5mg/5ml oral solution sugar free | 150 ml PoM £235.53 DT = £131.60 SF

Intravesical solution

CAUTIONARY AND ADVISORY LABELS 3

▸ Velariq (Medice UK Ltd)

Oxybutynin hydrochloride 1 mg per 1 ml Velariq 10mg/10ml intravesical solution pre-filled syringes | 12 pre-filled disposable injection PoM £204.00 | 96 pre-filled disposable injection PoM £1,632.00

603

Solifenacin succinate

23-Jul-2020

- **INDICATIONS AND DOSE**

Neurogenic detrusor overactivity

▸ BY MOUTH

▸ Child 2–17 years (body-weight 9–15 kg): Initially 2 mg once daily, increased if necessary up to 4 mg once daily

▸ Child 2–17 years (body-weight 16–30 kg): Initially 3 mg once daily, increased if necessary up to 5 mg once daily

▸ Child 2–17 years (body-weight 31–45 kg): Initially 3 mg once daily, increased if necessary up to 6 mg once daily

▸ Child 2–17 years (body-weight 46–60 kg): Initially 4 mg once daily, increased if necessary up to 8 mg once daily

▸ Child 2–17 years (body-weight 61 kg and above): Initially 5 mg once daily, increased if necessary up to 10 mg once daily

DOSE ADJUSTMENTS DUE TO INTERACTIONS

▸ Manufacturer advises no more than the initial daily dose, according to body-weight, with concurrent use of potent inhibitors of CYP3A4; avoid concurrent use in patients who also have moderate hepatic impairment or severe renal impairment.

- **CAUTIONS** Susceptibility to QT-interval prolongation
- **INTERACTIONS** → Appendix 1: solifenacin
- **SIDE-EFFECTS**

▸ **Common or very common** Gastrointestinal discomfort

▸ **Uncommon** Cystitis · dry eye · dry throat · fatigue · gastrointestinal disorders · nasal dryness · peripheral oedema · taste altered · urinary tract infection

▸ **Rare or very rare** Hallucination

▸ **Frequency not known** Anaphylactic reaction · appetite decreased · arrhythmias · delirium · dysphonia · glaucoma · hyperkalaemia · liver disorder · muscle weakness · QT interval prolongation · renal impairment

- **PREGNANCY** Manufacturer advises caution—no information available.
- **BREAST FEEDING** Manufacturer advises avoid—present in milk in *animal* studies.
- **HEPATIC IMPAIRMENT** Manufacturer advises caution in moderate impairment (risk of increased half-life); avoid in severe impairment (no information available).

Dose adjustments Manufacturer advises no more than the initial daily dose, according to body-weight, in moderate impairment.

- **RENAL IMPAIRMENT** Manufacturer advises caution in severe impairment.

Dose adjustments See p. 16.

Manufacturer advises no more than the initial daily dose, according to body-weight, if creatinine clearance 30 mL/minute or less.

- **DIRECTIONS FOR ADMINISTRATION** Manufacturer advises for *oral suspension*, doses should be followed by a glass of water—ingestion with food or other drinks may lead to the release of solifenacin in the mouth, causing a bitter taste and numbness in the mouth.
- **PRESCRIBING AND DISPENSING INFORMATION** Manufacturer advises the need for continuing therapy for neurogenic detrusor overactivity should be reviewed at least every 12 months.
- **MEDICINAL FORMS** There can be variation in the licensing of different medicines containing the same drug. Forms available from special-order manufacturers include: oral suspension

Oral suspension

CAUTIONARY AND ADVISORY LABELS 3

EXCIPIENTS: May contain Ethanol, hydroxybenzoates (parabens), propylene glycol

▸ Vesicare (Astellas Pharma Ltd)

Solifenacin succinate 1 mg per 1 ml Vesicare 1mg/ml oral suspension | 150 ml PoM £27.62 DT = £27.62 SF

603

Tolterodine tartrate

25-Feb-2022

- **INDICATIONS AND DOSE**

Urinary frequency | Urinary urgency | Urinary incontinence

▸ BY MOUTH USING IMMEDIATE-RELEASE MEDICINES

▸ Child 2–17 years: 1 mg once daily, then increased if necessary up to 2 mg twice daily, adjusted according to response

▸ BY MOUTH USING MODIFIED-RELEASE CAPSULES

▸ Child 2–17 years: 4 mg once daily

Nocturnal enuresis associated with overactive bladder

▸ BY MOUTH USING IMMEDIATE-RELEASE MEDICINES

▸ Child 5–17 years: 1 mg once daily, dose to be taken at bedtime, then increased if necessary up to 2 mg twice daily, adjusted according to response

DOSE EQUIVALENCE AND CONVERSION

▸ Children stabilised on immediate-release tolterodine tartrate 2 mg twice daily may be transferred to modified-release tolterodine tartrate 4 mg once daily.

- **UNLICENSED USE** Not licensed for use in children.
- **CAUTIONS** History of QT-interval prolongation
- **INTERACTIONS** → Appendix 1: tolterodine
- **SIDE-EFFECTS**

▸ **Common or very common** Abdominal pain · bronchitis · chest pain · diarrhoea · dry eye · fatigue · gastrointestinal disorders · paraesthesia · peripheral oedema · vertigo · weight increased

▸ **Uncommon** Arrhythmia · heart failure · memory loss · nervousness

▸ **Frequency not known** Hallucination

- **PREGNANCY** Manufacturer advises avoid—toxicity in *animal* studies.
- **BREAST FEEDING** Manufacturer advises avoid—no information available.
- **HEPATIC IMPAIRMENT** Manufacturer advises caution (risk of increased exposure).

Dose adjustments In adults, manufacturers advise dose reduction—consult product literature.

- **RENAL IMPAIRMENT** Manufacturer advises caution (risk of increased exposure).
  Dose adjustments See p. 16.
  In adults, manufacturer advises reduce dose if eGFR less than or equal to 30 mL/minute/1.73 m^2 (consult product literature).
- **PRESCRIBING AND DISPENSING INFORMATION** The need for therapy for urinary indications should be reviewed soon after it has been commenced and then at regular intervals; a response usually occurs within 6 months but may take longer.

- **MEDICINAL FORMS** There can be variation in the licensing of different medicines containing the same drug. Forms available from special-order manufacturers include: oral suspension, oral solution, oral powder

Oral tablet

CAUTIONARY AND ADVISORY LABELS 3

- **Tolterodine tartrate (Non-proprietary)**
  Tolterodine tartrate 1 mg Tolterodine 1mg tablets | 56 tablet PoM £29.03 DT = £6.53
  Tolterodine tartrate 2 mg Tolterodine 2mg tablets | 56 tablet PoM £30.56 DT = £3.72
- **Detrusitol** (Viatris UK Healthcare Ltd)
  Tolterodine tartrate 1 mg Detrusitol 1mg tablets | 56 tablet PoM £29.03 DT = £6.53
  Tolterodine tartrate 2 mg Detrusitol 2mg tablets | 56 tablet PoM £30.56 DT = £3.72

Oral suspension

- **Tolterodine tartrate (Non-proprietary)**
  Tolterodine tartrate 400 microgram per 1 ml Tolterodine 2mg/5ml oral suspension sugar free | 150 ml PoM £140.00 SF

Modified-release capsule

CAUTIONARY AND ADVISORY LABELS 3, 25

- **Tolterodine tartrate (Non-proprietary)**
  Tolterodine tartrate 2 mg Tolterodine 2mg modified-release capsules | 1 capsule PoM 🅇
  Tolterodine tartrate 4 mg Tolterodine 4mg modified-release capsules | 1 capsule PoM 🅇
- **Detrusitol XL** (Viatris UK Healthcare Ltd)
  Tolterodine tartrate 4 mg Detrusitol XL 4mg capsules | 28 capsule PoM £25.78 DT = £12.89
- **Mariosea XL** (Teva UK Ltd)
  Tolterodine tartrate 2 mg Mariosea XL 2mg capsules | 28 capsule PoM £11.59 DT = £11.60
  Tolterodine tartrate 4 mg Mariosea XL 4mg capsules | 28 capsule PoM £12.79 DT = £12.89
- **Neditol XL** (Aspire Pharma Ltd)
  Tolterodine tartrate 2 mg Neditol XL 2mg capsules | 28 capsule PoM £11.60 DT = £11.60
  Tolterodine tartrate 4 mg Neditol XL 4mg capsules | 28 capsule PoM £12.89 DT = £12.89
- **Tolterma XL** (Macleods Pharma UK Ltd)
  Tolterodine tartrate 2 mg Tolterma XL 2mg capsules | 28 capsule PoM £12.74 DT = £11.60
  Tolterodine tartrate 4 mg Tolterma XL 4mg capsules | 28 capsule PoM £14.89 DT = £12.89
- **Tolthen XL** (Northumbria Pharma Ltd)
  Tolterodine tartrate 2 mg Tolthen XL 2mg capsules | 28 capsule PoM £6.99 DT = £11.60
  Tolterodine tartrate 4 mg Tolthen XL 4mg capsules | 28 capsule PoM £6.99 DT = £12.89

F 603

Trospium chloride

11-Dec-2018

- **INDICATIONS AND DOSE**

Urinary frequency | Urinary urgency | Urge incontinence

- BY MOUTH USING IMMEDIATE-RELEASE MEDICINES
- Child 12–17 years: 20 mg twice daily, to be taken before food

- **INTERACTIONS** → Appendix 1: trospium
- **SIDE-EFFECTS**
  - **Common or very common** Abdominal pain
  - **Uncommon** Chest pain · diarrhoea · flatulence
  - **Rare or very rare** Arthralgia · asthenia · dyspnoea · myalgia
  - **Frequency not known** Agitation · anaphylactic reaction · hallucination · severe cutaneous adverse reactions (SCARs)
- **PREGNANCY** Manufacturer advises caution.
- **BREAST FEEDING** Manufacturer advises caution.
- **HEPATIC IMPAIRMENT** Manufacturer advises caution in mild to moderate impairment; avoid in severe impairment (no information available).
- **RENAL IMPAIRMENT** Use with caution. Avoid *Regurin® XL*.
  Dose adjustments Reduce dose to 20 mg once daily or 20 mg on alternate days if eGFR 10–30 mL/minute/1.73m^2.
- **PRESCRIBING AND DISPENSING INFORMATION** The need for continuing therapy for urinary incontinence should be reviewed every 4–6 weeks until symptoms stabilise, and then every 6–12 months.

- **MEDICINAL FORMS** There can be variation in the licensing of different medicines containing the same drug.

Oral tablet

CAUTIONARY AND ADVISORY LABELS 23

- **Trospium chloride (Non-proprietary)**
  Trospium chloride 20 mg Trospium chloride 20mg tablets | 60 tablet PoM £13.00–£30.70 DT = £22.62
- **Regurin** (Viatris UK Healthcare Ltd)
  Trospium chloride 20 mg Regurin 20mg tablets | 60 tablet PoM £26.00 DT = £22.62

1.2 Urinary retention

Urinary retention

31-May-2017

Description of condition

Urinary retention is the inability to voluntarily urinate. Causes in children can include severe voiding dysfunction, urethral blockage, drug treatment (such as opioids and antimuscarinic drugs), conditions that reduce detrusor contractions or interfere with relaxation of the urethra, and neurogenic causes.

Acute urinary retention is a medical emergency characterised by the abrupt (over a period of hours) development of the inability to pass urine, associated with increasing pain and the presence of a distended bladder, which can be palpated on examination.

Chronic urinary retention is the gradual (over months or years) development of the inability to empty the bladder completely, characterised by difficulties with initiating and maintaining urinary stream, urinary overflow, no sensation for needing to void and a post-void residual.

Treatment

EvGr Treatment of urinary retention depends on the underlying condition. Catheterisation is used as an effective initial management strategy, which should be followed by diagnostic evaluation and appropriate treatment of the underlying cause. Clean intermittent catheterisation on a long-term basis is effective for children with idiopathic or neurogenic bladder dysfunction.

The selective alpha-adrenoceptor blockers, doxazosin p. 606 and tamsulosin hydrochloride p. 606, have been shown to be of use in primary bladder neck dysfunction and dysfunctional voiding; they reduce urethral sphincteric pressure, thereby improving bladder emptying in children. Treatment should be under specialist advice only. Ⓔ

ALPHA-ADRENOCEPTOR BLOCKERS

Doxazosin

19-Jan-2024

● **INDICATIONS AND DOSE**

Hypertension

▶ BY MOUTH USING IMMEDIATE-RELEASE MEDICINES

▸ Child 6–11 years: Initially 0.5 mg once daily, then increased to 2–4 mg once daily, dose should be increased at intervals of 1 week

▸ Child 12–17 years: Initially 1 mg once daily for 1–2 weeks, then increased to 2 mg once daily, then increased if necessary to 4 mg once daily, rarely doses of up to 16 mg per day may be required

Dysfunctional voiding (initiated under specialist supervision)

▶ BY MOUTH USING IMMEDIATE-RELEASE MEDICINES

▸ Child 4–11 years: Initially 0.5 mg daily, adjusted according to response, dose should be increased at monthly intervals; maximum 2 mg per day

▸ Child 12–17 years: Initially 1 mg daily, adjusted according to response, dose may be doubled at intervals of 1 month; usual maintenance 2–4 mg daily; maximum 8 mg per day

● **UNLICENSED USE** Not licensed for use in children.

● **CONTRA-INDICATIONS** History of postural hypotension

● **CAUTIONS** Care with initial dose (postural hypotension) · cataract surgery (risk of intra-operative floppy iris syndrome) · heart failure · pulmonary oedema due to aortic or mitral stenosis

● **INTERACTIONS** → Appendix 1: alpha blockers

● **SIDE-EFFECTS**

▶ **Common or very common** Arrhythmias · asthenia · chest pain · cough · cystitis · dizziness · drowsiness · dry mouth · dyspnoea · gastrointestinal discomfort · headache · hypotension · increased risk of infection · influenza like illness · muscle complaints · nausea · oedema · pain · palpitations · skin reactions · urinary disorders · vertigo

▶ **Uncommon** Angina pectoris · anxiety · appetite abnormal · arthralgia · constipation · depression · diarrhoea · gastrointestinal disorders · gout · haemorrhage · insomnia · myocardial infarction · sensation abnormal · sexual dysfunction · stroke · syncope · tinnitus · tremor · vomiting · weight increased

▶ **Rare or very rare** Alopecia · bronchospasm · flushing · gynaecomastia · hepatic disorders · leucopenia · malaise · muscle weakness · thrombocytopenia · vision blurred

▶ **Frequency not known** Floppy iris syndrome

● **PREGNANCY** No evidence of teratogenicity; manufacturers advise use only when potential benefit outweighs risk.

● **BREAST FEEDING** Accumulates in milk in *animal* studies—manufacturer advises avoid.

● **HEPATIC IMPAIRMENT** Manufacturer advises caution in mild to moderate impairment (limited information available); avoid in severe impairment (no information available).

● **PATIENT AND CARER ADVICE** Patient counselling is advised for doxazosin tablets (initial dose).

Driving and skilled tasks May affect performance of skilled tasks e.g. driving.

● **MEDICINAL FORMS** There can be variation in the licensing of different medicines containing the same drug. Forms available from special-order manufacturers include: oral capsule, oral suspension, oral solution

Oral tablet

▸ **Doxazosin (Non-proprietary)**

Doxazosin (as Doxazosin mesilate) 1 mg Doxazosin 1mg tablets | 28 tablet PoM £10.56 DT = £0.68

Doxazosin (as Doxazosin mesilate) 2 mg Doxazosin 2mg tablets | 28 tablet PoM £14.08 DT = £0.70

Doxazosin (as Doxazosin mesilate) 4 mg Doxazosin 4mg tablets | 28 tablet PoM £14.08 DT = £0.78

Doxazosin (as Doxazosin mesilate) 8 mg Doxazosin 8mg tablets | 28 tablet PoM £34.77 DT = £41.51

▸ **Cardura** (Viatris UK Healthcare Ltd)

Doxazosin (as Doxazosin mesilate) 1 mg Cardura 1mg tablets | 28 tablet PoM £10.56 DT = £0.68

Doxazosin (as Doxazosin mesilate) 2 mg Cardura 2mg tablets | 28 tablet PoM £14.08 DT = £0.70

▸ **Doxadura** (Dexcel-Pharma Ltd)

Doxazosin (as Doxazosin mesilate) 4 mg Doxadura 4mg tablets | 28 tablet PoM £1.11 DT = £0.78

Modified-release tablet

CAUTIONARY AND ADVISORY LABELS 25

▸ **Doxazosin (Non-proprietary)**

Doxazosin (as Doxazosin mesilate) 4 mg Doxazosin 4mg modified-release tablets | 28 tablet PoM £6.08 DT = £5.24

▸ **Cardura XL** (Viatris UK Healthcare Ltd)

Doxazosin (as Doxazosin mesilate) 4 mg Cardura XL 4mg tablets | 28 tablet PoM £5.00 DT = £5.24

Doxazosin (as Doxazosin mesilate) 8 mg Cardura XL 8mg tablets | 28 tablet PoM £9.98 DT = £9.98

▸ **Doxadura XL** (Dexcel-Pharma Ltd)

Doxazosin (as Doxazosin mesilate) 4 mg Doxadura XL 4mg tablets | 28 tablet PoM £4.75 DT = £5.24

▸ **Raporsin XL** (Accord-UK Ltd)

Doxazosin (as Doxazosin mesilate) 4 mg Raporsin XL 4mg tablets | 28 tablet PoM £5.70 DT = £5.24

Tamsulosin hydrochloride

14-Jan-2025

● **INDICATIONS AND DOSE**

Dysfunctional voiding (administered on expert advice)

▶ BY MOUTH USING MODIFIED-RELEASE MEDICINES

▸ Child 12–17 years: 400 micrograms once daily

● **UNLICENSED USE** Not licensed for use in children.

● **CONTRA-INDICATIONS** History of postural hypotension

● **CAUTIONS** Care with initial dose (postural hypotension) · cataract surgery (risk of intra-operative floppy iris syndrome)

● **INTERACTIONS** → Appendix 1: alpha blockers

● **SIDE-EFFECTS**

▶ **Common or very common** Dizziness · sexual dysfunction

▶ **Uncommon** Asthenia · constipation · diarrhoea · headache · nausea · palpitations · postural hypotension · rhinitis · skin reactions · vomiting

▶ **Rare or very rare** Angioedema · Stevens-Johnson syndrome · syncope

▶ **Frequency not known** Dry mouth · epistaxis · vision disorders

● **HEPATIC IMPAIRMENT** Manufacturer advises avoid in severe impairment.

● **RENAL IMPAIRMENT** EvGr Use with caution if creatinine clearance less than 10 mL/minute. (M) See p. 16.

● **PATIENT AND CARER ADVICE**

Driving and skilled tasks May affect performance of skilled tasks e.g. driving.

● **MEDICINAL FORMS** There can be variation in the licensing of different medicines containing the same drug.

Modified-release tablet

CAUTIONARY AND ADVISORY LABELS 25

▸ **Faramsil** (Sandoz Ltd)

Tamsulosin hydrochloride 400 microgram Faramsil 400microgram modified-release tablets | 30 tablet PoM £8.89 DT = £10.47

▸ **Flomaxtra XL** (Astellas Pharma Ltd)

Tamsulosin hydrochloride 400 microgram Flomaxtra XL 400microgram tablets | 30 tablet PoM £10.47 DT = £10.47

Modified-release capsule

CAUTIONARY AND ADVISORY LABELS 25

- **Tamsulosin hydrochloride (Non-proprietary)**
  Tamsulosin hydrochloride 400 microgram Tamsulosin 400microgram modified-release capsules | 30 capsule PoM £3.80 DT = £0.92 | 200 capsule PoM £22.20–£67.60
- **Contiflo XL** (Sun Pharma UK Ltd)
  Tamsulosin hydrochloride 400 microgram Contiflo XL 400microgram capsules | 30 capsule PoM £7.44 DT = £0.92
- **Pamsvax XL** (Accord-UK Ltd)
  Tamsulosin hydrochloride 400 microgram Pamsvax XL 400microgram capsules | 30 capsule PoM £1.27 DT = £0.92
- **Tabphyn MR** (Genus Pharmaceuticals Ltd)
  Tamsulosin hydrochloride 400 microgram Tabphyn MR 400microgram capsules | 30 capsule PoM £4.45 DT = £0.92
- **Tamfrex XL** (Milpharm Ltd)
  Tamsulosin hydrochloride 400 microgram Tamfrex XL 400microgram capsules | 30 capsule PoM £28.51 DT = £0.92
- **Tamsumac** (Macleods Pharma UK Ltd)
  Tamsulosin hydrochloride 400 microgram Tamsumac 0.4mg modified-release capsules | 30 capsule PoM £3.87 DT = £0.92
- **Tamurex** (Somex Pharma)
  Tamsulosin hydrochloride 400 microgram Tamurex 400microgram modified-release capsules | 30 capsule PoM £3.87 DT = £0.92

1.3 Urolithiasis

Renal and ureteric stones 03-Apr-2019

Description of condition

Renal and ureteric stones are crystalline calculi that may form anywhere in the upper urinary tract. They are often asymptomatic but may cause pain when they move or obstruct the flow of urine. Most stones are composed of calcium salts (calcium oxalate, calcium phosphate or both). The rest are composed of struvite, uric acid, cystine and other substances. Patients are susceptible to stone formation when there is a decrease in urine volume and/or an excess of stone forming substances in the urine.

The following are risk factors that have been associated with stone formation: dehydration, change in urine pH, positive family history, obesity, urinary anatomical abnormalities, and excessive dietary intake of oxalate, urate, sodium, and animal protein. Certain diseases which alter urinary volume, pH, and concentrations of certain ions (such as calcium, phosphate, oxalate, sodium, and uric acid) may also increase the risk of stone formation. Certain drugs such as calcium or vitamin D supplements, protease inhibitors, or diuretics may also increase the risk of stone formation.

Symptoms of acute renal or ureteric stones can include an abrupt onset of severe unilateral abdominal pain radiating to the groin (known as renal colic) that may be accompanied with nausea, vomiting, haematuria, increased urinary frequency, dysuria and fever (if concomitant urinary infection is present).

Stones can pass spontaneously and will depend on a number of factors, including the size of the stone (stones greater than 6 mm have a very low chance of spontaneous passage), the location (distal ureteral stones are more likely to pass than proximal ureteral stones), and the degree of obstruction.

Aims of treatment

EvGr The aim of treatment is to improve the detection, clearance and prevention of renal and ureteric stones thereby reducing pain and improving quality of life. Ⓐ

Non-drug treatment

EvGr Consider watchful waiting for asymptomatic renal stones if they are less than 5mm in diameter. If they are larger than this then the specialist will discuss the risk and benefit of this option with the patient or parents.

Options for surgical stone removal should be discussed by the specialist team in hospital depending on severity of obstruction, patient factors, size and site of stone. Options include shockwave lithotripsy, percutaneous nephrolithotomy and ureteroscopy.

For patients with recurrent calcium stones avoid excessive intake of oxalate-rich products, such as rhubarb, spinach, cocoa, tea, nuts, soy products, strawberries, and wheat bran. For patients with recurrent uric acid stones, avoid excessive dietary intake of urate rich products, such as liver, kidney, calf thymus, poultry skin, and certain fish (herring with skin, sardines and anchovies). Ⓐ

Child aged under 16 years

EvGr Consider referring children and young patients with renal or ureteric stones to a paediatric nephrologist or urologist with expertise in this area for assessment and metabolic investigations.

Advise children to drink or carers to give their children 1–2 litres of water a day (depending on age) with the addition of fresh lemon juice and to avoid carbonated drinks. Advise children or carers to maintain a normal daily calcium intake of 350–1000mg and daily salt intake of 2–6g (depending on age). Ⓐ

Child aged 16 years and over

EvGr Consider stone analysis and measure serum calcium for children with recurring renal or ureteric stones.

Along with maintaining a healthy lifestyle, advise children to drink 2.5–3 litres of water a day with the addition of fresh lemon juice and to avoid carbonated drinks. Maintain a normal daily calcium intake of 700–1,200mg and salt intake of no more than 6g a day. Ⓐ

Pain Management

EvGr Offer NSAIDs as first line treatment for the management of pain associated with suspected renal colic or renal and ureteric stones. If NSAIDs are contra-indicated or not sufficiently controlling the pain, consider intravenous paracetamol. Subsequently, opioids can be used if both paracetamol and NSAIDs are contra-indicated or not sufficiently controlling the pain. Do not offer antispasmodics to patients with suspected renal colic. Ⓐ

Medical Expulsive Therapy

EvGr Consider alpha-adrenoceptor blockers for children with distal ureteric stones less than 10mm in diameter. Ⓐ

Child aged 16 years and over

EvGr Alpha-adrenoceptor blockers may also be considered as adjunctive therapy for children having shockwave lithotripsy for ureteric stones less than 10mm. Ⓐ

Prevention of recurrence of stones

Child aged under 16 years

EvGr Alongside lifestyle advice, consider potassium citrate [unlicensed] in children with recurrent stones composed of at least 50% calcium oxalate, and those with hypercalciuria and hypocitraturia. Ⓐ

Child aged 16 years and over

EvGr Alongside lifestyle advice, consider potassium citrate [unlicensed] in children with recurrent stones composed of at least 50% calcium oxalate. Thiazides [unlicensed] may be given if children also have hypercalciuria after restricting their sodium intake to no more than 6g a day. Ⓐ

1.4 Urological pain

Urological pain

03-Apr-2019

Treatment

Lidocaine hydrochloride gel is a useful topical application in *urethral pain* or to relieve the discomfort of catheterisation.

For information on the management of pain in renal and ureteric stones, see Renal and ureteric stones p. 607.

Alkalinisation of urine

Alkalinisation of urine can be undertaken with potassium citrate. The alkalinising action may relieve the discomfort of *cystitis* caused by lower urinary tract infections.

ALKALISING DRUGS

Citric acid with potassium citrate

25-Apr-2022

● **INDICATIONS AND DOSE**

Relief of discomfort in mild urinary-tract infections | Alkalinisation of urine

▶ BY MOUTH USING ORAL SOLUTION

▸ Child 1–5 years: 5 mL 3 times a day, to be diluted well with water

▸ Child 6–17 years: 10 mL 3 times a day, to be diluted well with water

● **CONTRA-INDICATIONS** Addison's disease · dehydration · hyperkalaemia · ventricular arrhythmia

● **CAUTIONS** Cardiac disease

● **INTERACTIONS** → Appendix 1: potassium citrate

● **SIDE-EFFECTS** Hyperkalaemia · nausea · vomiting

● **RENAL IMPAIRMENT** EvGr Consider avoiding (risk of hyperkalaemia). (M)

● **PRESCRIBING AND DISPENSING INFORMATION** When prepared extemporaneously, the BP states Potassium Citrate Mixture BP consists of potassium citrate 30%, citric acid monohydrate 5% in a suitable vehicle with a lemon flavour. Extemporaneous preparations should be recently prepared according to the following formula: potassium citrate 3 g, citric acid monohydrate 500 mg, syrup 2.5 mL, quillaia tincture 0.1 mL, lemon spirit 0.05 mL, double-strength chloroform water 3 mL, water to 10 mL. Contains about 28 mmol K^+/10 mL.

● **EXCEPTIONS TO LEGAL CATEGORY** Proprietary brands of potassium citrate are on sale to the public for the relief of discomfort in mild urinary-tract infections.

● **MEDICINAL FORMS** There can be variation in the licensing of different medicines containing the same drug.

Oral solution

CAUTIONARY AND ADVISORY LABELS 27

▸ **Citric acid with potassium citrate (Non-proprietary)**

Citric acid monohydrate 50 mg per 1 ml, Potassium citrate 300 mg per 1 ml Potassium citrate mixture | 200 ml P £2.45 DT = £3.96

Effervescent tablet

▸ **Effercitrate** (Cambridge Healthcare Supplies Ltd)

Citric acid 250 mg, Potassium citrate 1.5 gram Effercitrate tablets | 12 tablet GSL £6.29 DT = £6.29 SF

2 Bladder instillations and urological surgery

ANTISEPTICS AND DISINFECTANTS

Chlorhexidine

23-Feb-2022

● **INDICATIONS AND DOSE**

Bladder irrigation and catheter patency solutions

▶ BY INTRAVESICAL INSTILLATION

▸ Child: (consult product literature)

● **MEDICINAL FORMS** There can be variation in the licensing of different medicines containing the same drug. Forms available from special-order manufacturers include: irrigation solution

Cutaneous or intravesical irrigation solution

▸ **Chlorhexidine (Non-proprietary)**

Chlorhexidine acetate 200 microgram per 1 ml Chlorhexidine acetate 0.02% irrigation solution 1litre bottles | 1 bottle P ⊠

Chlorhexidine acetate 500 microgram per 1 ml Chlorhexidine acetate 0.05% irrigation solution 1litre bottles | 1 bottle P ⊠

Catheter maintenance solutions

● **CATHETER MAINTENANCE SOLUTIONS**

Curion CuriFlush Solutio G citric acid 3.23% catheter maintenance solution (Mediq Healthcare UK Ltd)
50 ml • NHS indicative price = £3.49 • Drug Tariff (Part IXa) | 100 ml • NHS indicative price = £3.49 • Drug Tariff (Part IXa)

Curion CuriFlush Solutio R citric acid 6% catheter maintenance solution (Mediq Healthcare UK Ltd)
50 ml • NHS indicative price = £3.49 • Drug Tariff (Part IXa) | 100 ml • NHS indicative price = £3.49 • Drug Tariff (Part IXa)

OptiFlo G citric acid 3.23% catheter maintenance solution (Bard Ltd)
50 ml • NHS indicative price = £4.05 • Drug Tariff (Part IXa) | 100 ml • NHS indicative price = £4.05 • Drug Tariff (Part IXa)

OptiFlo R citric acid 6% catheter maintenance solution (Bard Ltd)
50 ml • NHS indicative price = £4.05 • Drug Tariff (Part IXa) | 100 ml • NHS indicative price = £4.05 • Drug Tariff (Part IXa)

Uro-Tainer PHMB polihexanide 0.02% catheter maintenance solution (B.Braun Medical Ltd)
100 ml • NHS indicative price = £3.90 • Drug Tariff (Part IXa)

Uro-Tainer Twin Solutio R citric acid 6% catheter maintenance solution (B.Braun Medical Ltd)
60 ml • NHS indicative price = £5.50 • Drug Tariff (Part IXa)

Uro-Tainer Twin Suby G citric acid 3.23% catheter maintenance solution (B.Braun Medical Ltd)
60 ml • NHS indicative price = £5.50 • Drug Tariff (Part IXa)

UroFlush G citric acid 3.23% catheter maintenance solution (TriOn Pharma Ltd)
50 ml • NHS indicative price = £3.15 • Drug Tariff (Part IXa) | 100 ml • NHS indicative price = £3.15 • Drug Tariff (Part IXa)

UroFlush R citric acid 6% catheter maintenance solution (TriOn Pharma Ltd)
100 ml • NHS indicative price = £3.15 • Drug Tariff (Part IXa)

Curion CuriFlush sodium chloride 0.9% catheter maintenance solution (Mediq Healthcare UK Ltd) **Sodium chloride 9 mg per 1 ml**
50 ml • NHS indicative price = £3.49 • Drug Tariff (Part IXa) | 100 ml • NHS indicative price = £3.49 • Drug Tariff (Part IXa)

OptiFlo S saline 0.9% catheter maintenance solution (Bard Ltd)
Sodium chloride 9 mg per 1 ml 50 ml • NHS indicative price = £3.82 • Drug Tariff (Part IXa) | 100 ml • NHS indicative price = £3.82 • Drug Tariff (Part IXa)

Uro-Tainer M sodium chloride 0.9% catheter maintenance solution (B.Braun Medical Ltd) **Sodium chloride 9 mg per 1 ml** 50 ml • No NHS indicative price available • Drug Tariff (Part IXa) | 100 ml • No NHS indicative price available • Drug Tariff (Part IXa)

Uro-Tainer sodium chloride 0.9% catheter maintenance solution (B.Braun Medical Ltd) **Sodium chloride 9 mg per 1 ml** 50 ml • NHS indicative price = £3.85 • Drug Tariff (Part IXa) | 100 ml • NHS indicative price = £3.85 • Drug Tariff (Part IXa)

UroFlush Saline 0.9% catheter maintenance solution (TriOn Pharma Ltd) **Sodium chloride 9 mg per 1 ml** 50 ml • NHS indicative price = £3.15 • Drug Tariff (Part IXa) | 100 ml • NHS indicative price = £3.15 • Drug Tariff (Part IXa)

3 Contraception

Contraceptives, hormonal

14-Oct-2025

Overview

Hormonal contraception includes combined hormonal contraception (containing an oestrogen and a progestogen) and progestogen-only contraception.

EvGr When prescribing contraception, information should be given on all available methods taking into consideration medical eligibility. This should include contraceptive effectiveness (including factors that alter efficacy), non-contraceptive benefits, health risks, and side-effects to allow an informed decision to be made on the most suitable choice. (A)

In adolescents, hormonal contraception is used after menarche. When prescribing contraception for females aged under 16 years, it is considered good practice for health professionals to follow the criteria commonly known as the Fraser Guidelines, available at: cosrh.org/Public/Documents/fsrh-ceu-guidance-young-people-mar-2010.aspx.

For information on contraceptive use in specific populations such as young people, overweight or obese individuals, individuals with eating disorders, those with inflammatory bowel disease, and after pregnancy, see FSRH guidance available at: www.cosrh.org/Public/Public/Standards-and-Guidance/Contraception-for-Specific-Populations.aspx.

For the UK Medical Eligibility Criteria for Contraceptive Use, which includes information on risk categorisation for patients with pre-existing medical conditions, see FSRH guidance available at: www.cosrh.org/Public/Public/Standards-and-Guidance/uk-medical-eligibility-criteria-for-contraceptive-use-ukmec.aspx.

Contraception in patients taking medication with teratogenic potential: FSRH (February 2018) and MHRA (March 2019) guidance

Females of childbearing potential should be advised to use highly effective contraception if they or their male partners are taking known teratogenic drugs or drugs with potential teratogenic effects. Highly effective contraception should be used both during treatment and for the recommended duration after discontinuation to avoid unintended pregnancy. Pregnancy testing should be performed before treatment initiation to exclude pregnancy and repeat testing may be required.

Methods of contraception considered to be 'highly effective' include male and female sterilisation, and the long-acting reversible contraceptives (LARC)—copper intra-uterine device (Cu-IUD), levonorgestrel intra-uterine device (LNG-IUD) and progestogen-only implant (IMP). Females using the IMP must not take any interacting drugs that could reduce contraceptive effectiveness; for further information see Contraceptives, interactions p. 614.

For further guidance, see the FSRH CEU statement (cosrh.org/Public/Documents/fsrh-ceu-statement-contraception-for-women-using-known-teratogenic-drugs.aspx), MHRA drug safety update (www.gov.uk/drug-safety-update/medicines-with-teratogenic-potential-what-is-effective-contraception-and-how-often-is-pregnancy-testing-needed), and the UK teratogenic information service (www.uktis.org).

Combined hormonal contraceptives

Combined hormonal contraceptives (CHC) are available as tablets (COC), transdermal patches (CTP), and vaginal rings (CVR). They are highly user-dependant methods where the failure rate if used perfectly (i.e. correctly and consistently) is less than 1%. Certain factors such as the person's weight, malabsorption (COC only), and drug interactions may contribute to contraceptive failure. Prescriptions of up to 12 months' supply for CHC initiation or continuation may be appropriate to avoid unwanted discontinuation and increased risk of pregnancy.

CHC use may be associated with some health benefits such as:

- Reduced risk of ovarian, endometrial and colorectal cancer;
- Predictable bleeding patterns;
- Reduced dysmenorrhoea and menorrhagia;
- Management of symptoms of polycystic ovary syndrome (PCOS), endometriosis and premenstrual syndrome;
- Improvement of acne;
- Reduced menopausal symptoms;
- Maintaining bone mineral density in peri-menopausal females under the age of 50 years.

However, the use of CHC is also associated with health risks. For information on these risks, and further information on the benefits, see FSRH clinical guideline: **Combined Hormonal Contraception** (see *Useful resources*).

For information on advice to give to patients on the management of incorrect CHC use, see FSRH clinical guidance: **Incorrect use of Combined Hormonal Contraception** (see *Useful resources*).

Preparation choice

COCs containing a fixed amount of an oestrogen and a progestogen in each active tablet are termed 'monophasic'; those with varying amounts of the two hormones are termed 'multiphasic'.

COCs usually contain ethinylestradiol as the oestrogen component; mestranol, estetrol and estradiol are also used. The ethinylestradiol content of COCs range from 20–40 micrograms. EvGr A monophasic preparation containing 30 micrograms or less of ethinylestradiol in combination with levonorgestrel or norethisterone (to minimise cardiovascular risk), is generally used as the first line option. However, choice should be made taking into account the patients medical history, personal preference, previous contraceptive experience, and any age related considerations.

Due to potential reduced efficacy, non-oral CHC should be considered if there are concerns over absorption. In females who weigh 90 kg or more, consider non-topical options or use additional precautions with CTP. (A)

Combined Oral Contraceptives Monophasic 21-day preparations

Oestrogen content	Progestogen content	Brand
Ethinylestradiol 20 micrograms	Desogestrel 150 micrograms	Bimizza®
Ethinylestradiol 20 micrograms	Desogestrel 150 micrograms	Gedarel® 20/150
Ethinylestradiol 20 micrograms	Desogestrel 150 micrograms	Mercilon®
Ethinylestradiol 20 micrograms	Gestodene 75 micrograms	Akizza® 20/75
Ethinylestradiol 20 micrograms	Gestodene 75 micrograms	Femodette®
Ethinylestradiol 20 micrograms	Gestodene 75 micrograms	Millinette® 20/75

7 Genito-urinary system

Oestrogen content	Progestogen content	Brand
Ethinylestradiol 20 micrograms	Gestodene 75 micrograms	Sunya® 20/75
Ethinylestradiol 30 micrograms	Desogestrel 150 micrograms	Cimizt®
Ethinylestradiol 30 micrograms	Desogestrel 150 micrograms	Gedarel® 30/150
Ethinylestradiol 30 micrograms	Desogestrel 150 micrograms	Marvelon®
Ethinylestradiol 30 micrograms	Drospirenone 3 mg	Dretine®
Ethinylestradiol 30 micrograms	Drospirenone 3 mg	Lucette®
Ethinylestradiol 30 micrograms	Drospirenone 3 mg	Yacella®
Ethinylestradiol 30 micrograms	Drospirenone 3 mg	Yasmin®
Ethinylestradiol 30 micrograms	Drospirenone 3 mg	Yiznell®
Ethinylestradiol 30 micrograms	Gestodene 75 micrograms	Akizza® 30/75
Ethinylestradiol 30 micrograms	Gestodene 75 micrograms	Femodene®
Ethinylestradiol 30 micrograms	Gestodene 75 micrograms	Katya® 30/75
Ethinylestradiol 30 micrograms	Gestodene 75 micrograms	Millinette® 30/75
Ethinylestradiol 30 micrograms	Levonorgestrel 150 micrograms	Ambelina®
Ethinylestradiol 30 micrograms	Levonorgestrel 150 micrograms	Elevin®
Ethinylestradiol 30 micrograms	Levonorgestrel 150 micrograms	Levest®
Ethinylestradiol 30 micrograms	Levonorgestrel 150 micrograms	Maexeni®
Ethinylestradiol 30 micrograms	Levonorgestrel 150 micrograms	Microgynon® 30
Ethinylestradiol 30 micrograms	Levonorgestrel 150 micrograms	Ovranette®
Ethinylestradiol 30 micrograms	Levonorgestrel 150 micrograms	Rigevidon®
Ethinylestradiol 35 micrograms	Norethisterone 500 micrograms	Brevinor®
Ethinylestradiol 35 micrograms	Norethisterone 1 mg	Norimin®
Ethinylestradiol 35 micrograms	Norgestimate 250 micrograms	Cilique®
Ethinylestradiol 35 micrograms	Norgestimate 250 micrograms	Lizinna®
Mestranol 50 micrograms	Norethisterone 1 mg	Norinyl-1®

Combined Oral Contraceptives Monophasic 28-day preparations

Oestrogen content	Progestogen content	Brand
Estetrol 14.2 mg	Drospirenone 3 mg	Drovelis®
Estradiol (as hemihydrate) 1.5 mg	Nomegestrol acetate 2.5 mg	Zoely®
Ethinylestradiol 20 micrograms	Drospirenone 3 mg	Eloine®
Ethinylestradiol 30 micrograms	Gestodene 75 micrograms	Femodene® ED
Ethinylestradiol 30 micrograms	Levonorgestrel 150 micrograms	Microgynon® 30 ED

Combined Oral Contraceptives Multiphasic 21-day preparations

Oestrogen content	Progestogen content	Brand
Ethinylestradiol 30 micrograms	Levonorgestrel 50 micrograms	
Ethinylestradiol 40 micrograms	Levonorgestrel 75 micrograms	Logynon®
Ethinylestradiol 30 micrograms	Levonorgestrel 125 micrograms	
Ethinylestradiol 30 micrograms	Levonorgestrel 50 micrograms	
Ethinylestradiol 40 micrograms	Levonorgestrel 75 micrograms	TriRegol®
Ethinylestradiol 30 micrograms	Levonorgestrel 125 micrograms	
Ethinylestradiol 35 micrograms	Norethisterone 500 micrograms	
Ethinylestradiol 35 micrograms	Norethisterone 1 mg	Synphase®
Ethinylestradiol 35 micrograms	Norethisterone 500 micrograms	

Combined Oral Contraceptives Multiphasic 28-day preparations

Oestrogen content	Progestogen content	Brand
Estradiol valerate 3 mg		
Estradiol valerate 2 mg	Dienogest 2 mg	
Estradiol valerate 2 mg	Dienogest 3 mg	Qlaira®
Estradiol valerate 1 mg		
Ethinylestradiol 30 micrograms	Levonorgestrel 50 micrograms	
Ethinylestradiol 40 micrograms	Levonorgestrel 75 micrograms	Logynon® ED
Ethinylestradiol 30 micrograms	Levonorgestrel 125 micrograms	

Regimen choice

EvGr Information should be given to females on both the traditional 21 day CHC regimen with a monthly withdrawal bleed during the 7 day hormone free interval (HFI), and 'tailored' CHC regimens [unlicensed use]. Tailored CHC regimens can only be used with monophasic CHC containing ethinylestradiol [unlicensed use]; they offer the choice of either a shortened, or less frequent, or no hormone free interval based on the person's preference.

The following tailored regimens may be used [unlicensed use]:

- Shortened HFI: 21 days of continuous use followed by a 4 day HFI;
- Extended use (tricycling): 9 weeks of continuous use followed by a 4 or 7 day HFI;
- Flexible extended use: continuous use for 21 days or more followed by a 4 day HFI when breakthrough bleeding occurs;
- Continuous use: continuous CHC use with no HFI. Ⓐ

Withdrawal bleeds do not represent physiological menstruation and there is no difference in efficacy or safety of using the traditional 21 day regimen, which mimics the natural menstrual cycle, over using extended or continuous regimens. Use of the traditional regimen may be associated with disadvantages such as heavy or painful withdrawal bleeds, headaches, mood changes, and increased risk of incorrect use with subsequent unplanned pregnancy. EvGr Withdrawal bleeds during traditional CHC use has been reported in females who are pregnant and should therefore not be relied on as reassurance of a person's pregnancy status. Ⓐ

Follow up

EvGr A review of continued medical eligibility, satisfaction and adherence, drug interactions, and consideration of alternative contraception should be undertaken annually. Body mass index and blood pressure should also be checked annually. Ⓐ

Surgery

EvGr CHC use should be discontinued at least 4 weeks prior to major elective surgery, any surgery to the legs or pelvis, or surgery that involves prolonged immobilisation of a lower limb. An alternative method of contraception should be used to prevent unintentional pregnancy, and CHC may be recommenced 2 weeks after full remobilisation. When discontinuation is not possible, e.g. after trauma or if a patient admitted for an elective procedure is still on CHC, thromboprophylaxis should be considered. Ⓜ

When to seek further advice

EvGr All females should be advised to seek advice from a healthcare professional if they experience any troublesome side-effects, have a significant health event, start any new medication, would like to discontinue CHC, or to discuss alternative methods at any time. For further information, see FSRH guidance: **Combined Hormonal Contraception** (see *Useful resources*). Ⓐ

Progestogen-only contraceptives

Progestogen-only contraceptive options are available in oral, injectable, subdermal, and intra-uterine form. Some forms are highly user-dependent (e.g. oral tablet) whilst others rely on timely re-administration (e.g. depot injection); the failure rate if used perfectly (i.e. correctly and consistently) is less than 1%. The primary mechanism of action differs between contraceptive options, however progestogenic effects leading to contraceptive action include changes to the cervical mucus affecting sperm penetration, endometrial changes affecting implantation, effects on tubal motility, and ovulation suppression.

Oral progestogen-only contraceptives

Oral progestogen-only preparations contain either levonorgestrel p. 628, norethisterone p. 591, desogestrel p. 626, or drospirenone p. 627. EvGr Desogestrel and drospirenone suppress ovulation more consistently and may improve symptoms of dysmenorrhoea, however there is insufficient evidence to compare the contraceptive effectiveness of oral progestogen-only contraceptives with each other. Incorrect use, vomiting or severe diarrhoea, and drug interactions may contribute to contraceptive failure. Prescriptions of up to 12 months' supply at initial and subsequent visits may be appropriate. Follow-up in the form of an annual review is recommended, with the advice to return at any time if any problems arise. Ⓐ

For further information on progestogen-only pills, see FSRH guidance: **Progestogen-only Pills** (see *Useful resources*).

Parenteral progestogen-only contraceptives

Parenteral long-acting progestogens include the injections medroxyprogesterone acetate p. 632 and norethisterone enantate, and the implant etonogestrel p. 631. These are long-acting reversible contraceptive options that work primarily by suppressing ovulation along with other progestogenic effects. EvGr As they often lead to amenorrhoea or reduced bleeding, they may benefit those with menstrual problems (such as heavy bleeding or dysmenorrhoea). Ⓐ

Injections

The failure rate for injectable progestogen-only contraception during the first year is approximately only 0.2% with perfect use (used consistently and correctly), the failure rate with typical use (includes incorrect/inconsistent use) is approximately 6%. The typical failure rates are higher compared to other long-acting methods and may be due to the relative frequency of repeat injections.

EvGr Depot medroxyprogesterone acetate is administered every 13 weeks. Its use is associated with a small loss of bone mineral density, which largely recovers after discontinuation. However, due to the concerns and uncertainties around bone-loss the following is advised regarding its use:

- Females aged under 18 years may use depot medroxyprogesterone acetate after all options have been discussed and are considered unsuitable or unacceptable.
- In all females, although there is no definitive upper duration limit, use should be reviewed every 2 years and continuation benefits and risks discussed.
- In females with significant risk factors for osteoporosis, other methods of contraception should be considered.

Patients should be informed that there can be a delayed return of fertility of up to 1 year after discontinuation of depot medroxyprogesterone acetate. However, patients who discontinue use and do not wish to conceive, should be advised to start an alternative contraceptive method before or at the time of their next scheduled injection. Ⓐ

Norethisterone enantate is less commonly used in the UK. EvGr It is used for short-term contraception (duration of 8 weeks) for females whose partners undergo a vasectomy until the vasectomy is effective, and after rubella immunisation. Ⓐ

For further information on progestogen-only injections including dosing interval of repeat injections and management of side-effects, see FSRH guidance: **Progestogen-only Injectable Contraception** (see *Useful resources*).

Implant

EvGr The etonogestrel implant is inserted subdermally and provides highly effective contraception for up to 3 years. The contraceptive failure rate for both perfect and typical use is approximately 0.05% in the first year of use. Routine follow-up during implant use, removal or replacement is not generally required, however patients should be advised to see their healthcare professional if the implant cannot be felt or problematic bleeding occurs. Ⓐ

For further information on progestogen-only implant, see FSRH guidance: **Progestogen-only Implant** (see *Useful resources*).

Intra-uterine progestogen-only devices

Intra-uterine devices (IUDs) containing levonorgestrel are long-acting reversible contraceptive options that have a duration of use that ranges from 3–10 years depending on the device used, and the age of the female at insertion. A foreign-body effect may be a contributing factor to the contraceptive action, in addition to progestogenic effects. Ovulation is not suppressed in the majority of females (over 75%) who use an IUD. An IUD releasing 20mcg/24hour of levonorgestrel may also have health benefits such as improving pain associated with dysmenorrhoea, endometriosis or adenomyosis.

FSRH CEU have issued recommendations on the management of pain and anxiety associated with insertion of intra-uterine contraception, available at: www.cosrh.org/Public/Documents/fsrh-statement-pain-associated-with-insertion-of-intrauterine.aspx.

EvGr Patients should be advised to seek medical advice if they develop symptoms of pelvic infection, pain, abnormal bleeding, non-palpable threads or they can feel the stem of the IUD. (A)

For further information on progestogen-only IUDs, see FSRH guidance: **Intra-uterine Contraception** (see *Useful resources*).

Surgery

In accordance with the UK Medical Eligibility Criteria for Contraceptive Use, progestogen-only pills, injections, implants, and intra-uterine devices are suitable for use as contraceptives in females undergoing surgery. For further information, see FSRH guidance: **UK Medical Eligibility Criteria for Contraceptive Use** (available at: www.cosrh.org/Public/Public/Standards-and-Guidance/uk-medical-eligibility-criteria-for-contraceptive-use-ukmec.aspx).

Useful Resources

Combined Hormonal Contraception. The Faculty of Sexual & Reproductive Healthcare. Clinical guideline. January 2019, updated October 2023.
www.cosrh.org/Public/Documents/fsrh-guideline-combined-hormonal-contraception.aspx

Recommended actions after incorrect use of combined hormonal contraception (e.g. late or missed pills, ring and patch). The Faculty of Sexual & Reproductive Healthcare Clinical Effectiveness Unit. Guidance. March 2020.
www.cosrh.org/Public/Documents/fsrh-ceu-guidance-recommended-actions-after-incorrect-use.aspx

Progestogen-only Pills. The Faculty of Sexual & Reproductive Healthcare. Clinical guidance. August 2022, updated July 2023.
www.cosrh.org/Public/Documents/ceu-guideline-progestogen-only-pills.aspx

Progestogen-only Injectable Contraception. The Faculty of Sexual & Reproductive Healthcare. Clinical guidance. December 2014, updated July 2023.
www.cosrh.org/Public/Documents/fsrh-ceu-guidance-progestogen-only-injectables.aspx

Progestogen-only Implant. The Faculty of Sexual & Reproductive Healthcare. Clinical guidance. February 2021, updated July 2023.
www.cosrh.org/Public/Documents/clinical-guidance-progestogen-only-implants.aspx

Intra-uterine Contraception. The Faculty of Sexual & Reproductive Healthcare. Clinical guidance. March 2023, updated July 2023.
www.cosrh.org/Public/Documents/ceu-guidance-intrauterine-contraception.aspx

Contraceptives, non-hormonal

14-Oct-2025

Contraception in patients taking medication with teratogenic potential: FSRH (February 2018) and MHRA (March 2019) guidance

Females of childbearing potential should be advised to use highly effective contraception if they or their male partners are taking known teratogenic drugs or drugs with potential teratogenic effects. Highly effective contraception should be used both during treatment and for the recommended duration after discontinuation to avoid unintended pregnancy. Pregnancy testing should be performed before treatment initiation to exclude pregnancy and repeat testing may be required.

Methods of contraception considered to be 'highly effective' include male and female sterilisation, and the long-acting reversible contraceptives (LARC)—copper intra-uterine device (Cu-IUD), levonorgestrel intra-uterine device (LNG-IUD) and progestogen-only implant (IMP). Females using the IMP must not take any interacting drugs that could reduce contraceptive effectiveness; for further information, see Contraceptives, interactions p. 614.

For further guidance, see the FSRH Clinical Effectiveness Unit (CEU) statement (cosrh.org/Public/Documents/fsrh-ceu-statement-contraception-for-women-using-known-teratogenic-drugs.aspx), MHRA drug safety update (www.gov.uk/drug-safety-update/medicines-with-teratogenic-potential-what-is-effective-contraception-and-how-often-is-pregnancy-testing-needed), and the UK teratogenic information service (www.uktis.org).

Barrier methods

Barrier methods include condoms (male and female), diaphragms and cervical caps. Male condoms are less effective than some other contraception methods but are effective when used consistently and correctly, and provide significant protection against some sexually transmitted infections (STIs). Female condoms are also available; they are pre-lubricated with a non-spermicidal lubricant.

There is no evidence that condoms lubricated with spermicide provide additional protection against pregnancy or STIs. EvGr Diaphragms and caps must be used in conjunction with a **spermicide** and should not be removed until at least 6 hours after the last episode of intercourse. (A)

Spermicidal contraceptives

Spermicidal contraceptives are useful additional safeguards but do **not** give adequate protection if used alone. They have two components: a spermicide and a vehicle for its delivery (e.g. vaginal gel). EvGr They are suitable for use with barrier methods, such as diaphragms or caps; however, spermicidal contraceptives are not recommended for use with condoms, as there is no evidence of any additional protection compared with non-spermicidal lubricants.

Spermicidal contraceptives are not suitable for use in those with or at high risk of sexually transmitted infections (including HIV); (A) high frequency use of the spermicide nonoxinol '9' p. 633 has been associated with genital lesions, which may increase the risk of acquiring these infections.

Contraceptive devices

Intra-uterine devices

EvGr The intra-uterine device (IUD) is a suitable contraceptive for young women irrespective of parity; (A) however they may be unsuitable in women with certain conditions such as those with pelvic inflammatory disease or unexplained vaginal bleeding. The UK Medical Eligibility Criteria for Contraceptive Use (published by FSRH) provides guidance on safe use of contraceptive methods including restrictions for intra-uterine devices; full guidance is available at: www.cosrh.org/Public/Public/Standards-and-Guidance/uk-medical-eligibility-criteria-for-contraceptive-use-ukmec.aspx.

EvGr Copper intra-uterine devices (Cu-IUDs) are effective immediately after insertion and can be used for contraception for 5 or 10 years depending on the device. (A) Framed Cu-IUDs in the UK have a copper surface area of 300 mm^2 or more, with either banded copper arms, a copper stem only, or copper arms with a silver-containing stem. A frameless, copper-bearing intra-uterine device (*GyneFix*®) is also available.

EvGr Cu-IUDs are also highly effective emergency contraception that can be retained to provide ongoing contraception. (A) For further information, see Emergency contraception below.

For guidance on the management of pain and anxiety associated with insertion of intra-uterine contraception, see FSRH Clinical Effectiveness Unit (CEU) statement: **Pain associated with insertion of intra-uterine contraception**, available at: www.cosrh.org/Public/Documents/fsrh-statement-pain-associated-with-insertion-of-intrauterine.aspx.

Caution with oil-based lubricants

Products such as petroleum jelly (*Vaseline*®), baby oil and oil-based vaginal and rectal preparations are likely to damage condoms, contraceptive diaphragms, and caps made from latex rubber, and may render them less effective as a barrier method of contraception and as a protection from sexually transmitted infections (including HIV).

Useful resources

Barrier Methods for Contraception and STI Prevention. The Faculty of Sexual & Reproductive Healthcare. Clinical guidance. August 2012, updated October 2015.
www.cosrh.org/Public/Documents/ceu-guidance-barrier-methods-for-contraception.aspx

Intra-uterine Contraception. The Faculty of Sexual & Reproductive Healthcare. Clinical guidance. March 2023, updated July 2023.
www.cosrh.org/Public/Documents/ceu-guidance-intrauterine-contraception.aspx

Emergency contraception

14-Oct-2025

Overview

EvGr Emergency contraception is intended for occasional use, to reduce the risk of pregnancy after unprotected sexual intercourse (UPSI). It does not replace effective regular contraception.

Females of childbearing potential who do not wish to conceive should be offered emergency contraception after UPSI that has taken place on any day of a natural menstrual cycle. Emergency contraception should also be offered after UPSI from day 21 after childbirth (unless the criteria for lactational amenorrhoea are met), and from day 5 after abortion, miscarriage, ectopic pregnancy or uterine evacuation for gestational trophoblastic disease.

Emergency contraception should also be offered to females whose regular contraception has been compromised or has been used incorrectly. (A)

Emergency contraceptive methods

Copper intra-uterine devices

EvGr Insertion of a copper intra-uterine device (see intra-uterine contraceptive devices (copper) p. 624) is the most effective form of emergency contraception and should be offered (if appropriate) to all females who have had UPSI and do not wish to conceive. A copper intra-uterine contraceptive device can be inserted up to 120 hours (5 days) after the first UPSI in a natural menstrual cycle, or up to 5 days after the earliest estimated date of ovulation (i.e. within the minimum period before implantation), whichever is later. (A) For information on the use of copper intra-uterine devices as emergency contraception in females using hormonal contraception, see FSRH guideline: **Emergency Contraception** (see *Useful resources*).

EvGr Antibacterial cover may be considered for copper intra-uterine contraceptive device insertion if there is a significant risk of sexually transmitted infection that could be associated with ascending pelvic infection.

A copper intra-uterine device is not known to be affected by BMI, body-weight, or by other drugs. (A)

For further guidance on the use of copper intra-uterine devices as emergency contraception, see FSRH guideline: **Emergency Contraception** (see *Useful resources*).

For guidance on the management of pain and anxiety associated with insertion of intra-uterine contraception, see FSRH Clinical Effectiveness Unit (CEU) statement: **Pain associated with insertion of intra-uterine contraception**, available at: www.cosrh.org/Public/Documents/fsrh-statement-pain-associated-with-insertion-of-intrauterine.aspx.

Due to the current shortage of banded copper intra-uterine devices, which is thought to be due to a shortfall in global copper supply, the FSRH CEU have issued guidance to support clinical practice during this time, available at: www.cosrh.org/Public/Documents/fsrh-statement-copper-intrauterine-device-shortage.aspx.

Hormonal methods

EvGr Oral emergency hormonal contraceptives (includes levonorgestrel p. 628 and ulipristal acetate p. 626) should be offered as soon as possible if a copper intra-uterine device is not appropriate or is not acceptable to the patient and there has been UPSI within the last 5 days; either drug should be taken as soon as possible to increase efficacy. Oral emergency contraception administered after ovulation is ineffective.

Levonorgestrel is effective if taken within 72 hours (3 days) of UPSI and may also be used between 72 and 96 hours after UPSI [unlicensed use], but efficacy decreases with time. Ulipristal acetate is effective if taken within 120 hours (5 days) of UPSI. Ulipristal acetate has been demonstrated to be more effective than levonorgestrel for emergency contraception.

There is the possibility that a higher body-weight or BMI could reduce the effectiveness of oral emergency contraception, particularly levonorgestrel. If the patient's BMI is greater than 26 kg/m^2 or their body-weight is greater than 70 kg, it is recommended that either ulipristal acetate or a double dose of levonorgestrel [unlicensed indication] is given (see *Emergency contraception* under levonorgestrel). It is unknown which is more effective.

Ulipristal acetate should be considered as the first-line oral emergency contraceptive for females who have had UPSI within the last 96–120 hours (even if they have also had additional instances of UPSI within the last 96 hours). It should also be considered first line for females who have had UPSI within the last 5 days if it is likely to have taken place during the 5 days before the estimated day of ovulation.

Levonorgestrel may be considered for oral emergency contraception in females on a regular combined hormonal contraceptive who have missed contraception within the first week of restarting their contraceptive. (A) See FSRH guideline: **Emergency Contraception** (see *Useful resources*) for further information.

EvGr Ulipristal acetate and levonorgestrel can be used as oral emergency contraception more than once in the same cycle. (A) Note that the manufacturer of levonorgestrel advises that there may be an increased risk of side-effects (such as menstrual irregularities) with repeated administration of levonorgestrel as emergency contraception more than once in the same cycle.

For further information on the use of oral hormonal methods as emergency contraception, see FSRH guideline: **Emergency Contraception** (see *Useful resources*).

Emergency hormonal contraception interactions

See Contraceptives, interactions below.

Starting hormonal contraception after emergency hormonal contraception

The copper intra-uterine device immediately provides effective ongoing contraception, whereas oral emergency hormonal contraception methods do **not**.

EvGr After taking levonorgestrel, females should start suitable hormonal contraception immediately. They must use condoms reliably or abstain from intercourse until contraception becomes effective.

Females should wait 5 days after taking ulipristal acetate before starting suitable hormonal contraception; they must use condoms reliably or abstain from intercourse during the 5 day waiting period and also until their contraceptive method is effective. However, hormonal contraception can be started immediately in females who are on a regular combined hormonal contraceptive who have missed contraception within the first week of restarting after a scheduled hormone-free interval, and have taken ulipristal acetate as emergency contraception; they must use condoms reliably or abstain from intercourse for 7 days until contraception becomes effective. (A) For further information on delaying versus immediately restarting combined hormonal contraception after taking ulipristal acetate, see FSRH CEU statement: **Response to recent publication** (available at: www.cosrh.org/Public/Documents/fsrh-ceu-statement-response-to-recent-publication-regarding.aspx).

Useful Resources

Emergency Contraception. The Faculty of Sexual and Reproductive Healthcare. FSRH guideline. March 2017, updated July 2023.
www.cosrh.org/Public/Documents/ceu-clinical-guidance-emergency-contraception-march-2017.aspx

Contraceptives, interactions

01-Dec-2024

Overview

Contraceptive providers should take a drug history (including any herbal products) and check for drug interactions prior to provision of hormonal contraception. The effectiveness of *combined* oral contraceptives, *progestogen-only* oral contraceptives, contraceptive patches, vaginal rings, subdermal implants, and emergency hormonal contraception can be considerably reduced by interaction with drugs that induce hepatic enzyme activity (e.g. carbamazepine p. 234, eslicarbazepine acetate p. 236, efavirenz p. 510, nevirapine p. 511, oxcarbazepine p. 246, phenytoin p. 249, phenobarbital p. 264, primidone p. 265, rifabutin p. 448, rifampicin p. 449, ritonavir p. 524, St John's wort, and topiramate p. 257), requiring additional or alternative methods of contraception to be used (see below). A condom together with a long-acting method (such as an injectable contraceptive) may be more suitable for patients with HIV infection or at risk of HIV infection; advice on the possibility of interaction with antiretroviral drugs should be sought from HIV specialists. Note that the MHRA recommends that concurrent use of St John's wort with any form of hormonal contraception should be avoided; for further guidance, see MHRA drug safety update: **St John's wort: interaction with hormonal contraceptives, including implants** (available at: www.gov.uk/drug-safety-update/st-john-s-wort-interaction-with-hormonal-contraceptives-including-implants).

For further information on other drug interactions with hormonal contraceptives, see the *Interactions* section of the relevant drug monograph.

Hormonal contraception with concurrent use of enzyme-inducing and teratogenic drugs

In females taking a teratogenic or potentially teratogenic drug that is an enzyme inducer, or if an enzyme-inducing drug is also being taken with a teratogen or potential teratogen, the preferred method of contraception is a copper intra-uterine device (IUD) or a progestogen-only IUD (levonorgestrel p. 628). If a progestogen-only injectable contraceptive (such as medroxyprogesterone acetate p. 632) is used, this should be in combination with reliable use of condoms. Use of combined hormonal contraception, progestogen-only pills, and the etonogestrel implant is not recommended; for further guidance, see FSRH Clinical Effectiveness Unit (CEU) statement (cosrh.org/Public/Documents/fsrh-ceu-statement-contraception-for-women-using-known-teratogenic-drugs.aspx), MHRA drug safety update (www.gov.uk/drug-safety-update/medicines-with-teratogenic-potential-what-is-effective-contraception-and-how-often-is-pregnancy-testing-needed), and the UK teratogenic information service (www.uktis.org).

Combined hormonal contraceptive interactions

Interactions with enzyme-inducing drugs

Females using combined hormonal contraceptive patches, vaginal rings, or oral tablets who require enzyme-inducing drugs should always be advised to change to a reliable contraceptive method that is unaffected by enzyme-inducers, such as a copper IUD, a progestogen-only IUD (levonorgestrel), or a progestogen-only injectable contraceptive (such as medroxyprogesterone acetate). This should be continued for the duration of treatment and for 4 weeks after stopping.

If a change in contraceptive method is undesirable or inappropriate, the following options should be discussed:

Short-term use (2 months or less) of an enzyme-inducing drug (except rifampicin or rifabutin)

Continuing the combined hormonal contraceptive method may be considered if used in combination with consistent and careful use of condoms for the duration of treatment and for 4 weeks after stopping the enzyme-inducing drug.

Continued use (over 2 months) of an enzyme-inducing drug (except rifampicin or rifabutin)

In exceptional circumstances, the use of a monophasic combined oral contraceptive containing ethinylestradiol p. 590 at a higher daily dose [unlicensed use] may be considered and used either continuously or 'tricycled' (i.e. taking three packets of monophasic tablets without a break followed by a shortened tablet-free interval of 4 days [unlicensed use]); continue for the duration of treatment with the interacting drug and for 4 weeks after stopping. However, contraceptive effectiveness is not guaranteed. For further guidance, see FSRH guidance: **Drug Interactions with Hormonal Contraception** (see *Useful resources*).

If breakthrough bleeding occurs (and all other causes are ruled out) additional precautions should be used, or contraception should be changed to a method unaffected by the interacting drugs.

Use of contraceptive patches and vaginal rings (including concurrent use of two patches or two vaginal rings) is not recommended for females taking enzyme-inducing drugs over a long period.

Females taking rifampicin or rifabutin

An alternative method of contraception that is unaffected by enzyme-inducers is **always** recommended because they are such potent enzyme-inducing drugs; the alternative method of contraception should be continued for 4 weeks after stopping the enzyme-inducing drug.

Interactions with HIV-protease inhibitors
Note that despite ritonavir being an enzyme inducer, the CoSRH (formerly FSRH) suggests that concurrent use of HIV-protease inhibitors boosted with ritonavir are not expected to affect the efficacy of the combined hormonal contraceptives, but some caution is required if they are given with combined hormonal contraceptives because the increased risk of side-effects might impact adherence.

For HIV-protease inhibitors boosted with cobicistat, CoSRH recommends caution or an alternative effective method of contraception.

Interactions with lamotrigine
It is possible that lamotrigine p. 243 could reduce the efficacy of combined hormonal contraceptives, therefore the additional reliable use of condoms is recommended. However, combined hormonal contraceptives can decrease lamotrigine concentrations, which might result in reduced efficacy (e.g. seizure control). If combined hormonal contraceptive use is unavoidable, consider increasing the lamotrigine dose and monitoring lamotrigine concentrations. A continuous combined hormonal contraceptive regimen (with no hormone-free interval) could be used to avoid cyclical changes in lamotrigine concentrations [unlicensed use].

Oral progestogen-only contraceptives interactions

Interactions with enzyme-inducing drugs
The efficacy of oral progestogen-only preparations is reduced by enzyme-inducing drugs and an alternative contraceptive method, unaffected by the interacting drug, such as a copper IUD, a progestogen-only IUD (levonorgestrel), or a progestogen-only injectable contraceptive (such as medroxyprogesterone acetate) is recommended during treatment with an interacting drug and for at least 4 weeks afterwards.

For short-term use of an enzyme-inducing drug (less than 2 months), continuing the progestogen-only oral method may be appropriate if used in combination with consistent and careful use of condoms for the duration of treatment and for 4 weeks after stopping the enzyme-inducing drug.

Note that despite ritonavir being an enzyme inducer, the CoSRH suggests that concurrent use of HIV-protease inhibitors boosted with ritonavir are not expected to affect the efficacy of the oral progestogen-only contraceptives but might increase their concentrations. They therefore state that no extra precautions are needed in those taking HIV-protease inhibitors boosted with ritonavir.

Interactions with lamotrigine
It is possible that lamotrigine could reduce the efficacy of progestogen-only oral contraceptives, therefore the additional reliable use of condoms is recommended. Desogestrel p. 626 might increase lamotrigine concentrations, but evidence for other oral progestogen-only contraceptives is lacking. Patients should be advised to be vigilant for signs of lamotrigine toxicity if starting progestogen-only contraceptives and consideration given to monitoring lamotrigine concentrations on stopping the contraceptive.

Parenteral (including *subdermal*) progestogen-only contraceptives interactions

Interactions with enzyme-inducing drugs
The effectiveness of intramuscular norethisterone injection p. 591 and intramuscular and subcutaneous medroxyprogesterone acetate injections p. 632 is not affected by enzyme-inducing drugs and they may be continued as normal during courses of these drugs. FSRH guidance on drug interactions between HIV antiretroviral therapy and contraception (see *Useful resources*) suggests that for patients with a high BMI or those taking efavirenz and rifampicin, the use of intra-uterine contraception, or additional use of condoms, or shortening the dosing interval of medroxyprogesterone acetate injection might be considered.

Effectiveness of the etonogestrel-releasing subdermal implant p. 631 may be reduced by enzyme-inducing drugs and an alternative contraceptive method, unaffected by the interacting drug, such as a copper IUD, a progestogen-only IUD (levonorgestrel p. 628), or a progestogen-only injectable contraceptive (such as medroxyprogesterone acetate), is recommended during treatment with the interacting drug and for at least 4 weeks after stopping. For a short course of an enzyme-inducing drug, if a change in contraceptive method is undesirable or inappropriate, continued contraception with the implant may be appropriate if used in combination with consistent and careful use of condoms for the duration of treatment and for 4 weeks after stopping the enzyme-inducing drug. Note that despite ritonavir being an enzyme inducer, the CoSRH suggests that concurrent use of HIV-protease inhibitors boosted with ritonavir are not expected to affect the efficacy of the etonogestrel implant but might increase etonogestrel concentrations. They therefore state that no extra precautions are needed in those taking HIV-protease inhibitors boosted with ritonavir.

Interactions with lamotrigine
It is possible that lamotrigine could reduce the efficacy of the progestogen-only subdermal implant, therefore the additional reliable use of condoms is recommended. Contraceptive effectiveness of progestogen-only injectable contraceptives is not expected to be affected by lamotrigine, however progestogen-only contraceptives might increase lamotrigine concentrations. Patients should be advised to be vigilant for signs of lamotrigine toxicity if starting progestogen-only contraceptives and consideration given to monitoring lamotrigine concentrations on stopping the contraceptive.

Emergency hormonal contraception interactions

The effectiveness of levonorgestrel and ulipristal acetate p. 626 could be reduced in females taking enzyme-inducing drugs (and for at least 4 weeks after stopping). EvGr A copper IUD can be offered instead. If the copper IUD is declined or unsuitable, the dose of levonorgestrel should be increased (See *Dose adjustments due to interactions* under levonorgestrel). ⟨A⟩ If levonorgestrel is also unsuitable, a standard dose of ulipristal acetate may be considered. Females should be advised that the effectiveness of emergency hormonal contraception when enzyme-inducing drugs are being taken is unknown. Note that despite ritonavir being an enzyme inducer, the CoSRH suggests that concurrent use of HIV-protease inhibitors boosted with ritonavir do not affect the efficacy of levonorgestrel emergency hormonal contraception but might increase levonorgestrel concentrations. They therefore do not extend the advice for enzyme inducers to HIV-protease inhibitors boosted with ritonavir.

The effectiveness of ulipristal acetate for emergency contraception in females using drugs that increase gastric pH is unknown. A copper IUD or levonorgestrel can be offered instead. If these are unsuitable, ulipristal acetate can be offered, but it is possible that effectiveness could be reduced.

EvGr Hormonal contraception should not be newly initiated in a patient until 5 days after administration of ulipristal acetate as emergency hormonal contraception—the contraceptive effect of ulipristal acetate will be reduced. Consistent and careful use of condoms is recommended. Females on a regular combined oral contraceptive may in certain circumstances be able to restart regular contraception immediately after administration of ulipristal acetate as emergency hormonal contraception. ⟨A⟩ For further information, see *Starting hormonal contraception after emergency hormonal contraception* under *Emergency contraceptive methods* in Emergency contraception p. 613.

When a progestogen (including levonorgestrel for emergency contraception) is given 7 days before, or 5 days after administration of ulipristal acetate as emergency hormonal contraception, the contraceptive effect of ulipristal acetate may be reduced.

Antibacterials that do not induce liver enzymes

Due to anecdotal reports of contraceptive failures, there had been concerns that some antibacterials that do not induce liver enzymes (e.g. ampicillin p. 419, doxycycline p. 434) reduce the efficacy of *combined* oral contraceptives by impairing the bacterial flora responsible for recycling ethinylestradiol p. 590 from the large bowel. However, there is a lack of evidence to support this interaction. It is recommended by the CoSRH that no additional contraceptive precautions are required when hormonal contraceptives, including emergency hormonal contraceptives, are used with antibacterials that do not induce liver enzymes, unless diarrhoea or vomiting occur when using oral contraceptives. These recommendations should be discussed with the female, who should also be advised that guidance in patient information leaflets may differ.

Useful Resources

Drug Interactions with Hormonal Contraception. The Faculty of Sexual and Reproductive Healthcare Clinical Effectiveness Unit. Clinical guidance. May 2022.
www.cosrh.org/Public/Documents/ceu-clinical-guidance-drug-interactions-with-hormonal.aspx

Emergency Contraception. The Faculty of Sexual and Reproductive Healthcare. FSRH guideline. March 2017, updated December 2020.
www.cosrh.org/Public/Documents/ceu-clinical-guidance-emergency-contraception-march-2017.aspx

Drug Interactions Between HIV Antiretroviral Therapy (ART) and Contraception. The Faculty of Sexual and Reproductive Healthcare Clinical Effectiveness Unit. Clinical guidance. February 2023.
www.cosrh.org/Public/Documents/fsrh-ceu-guidance-drug-interactions-between-hiv-art-and-contraception.aspx

3.1 Contraception, combined

OESTROGENS COMBINED WITH PROGESTOGENS

Combined hormonal contraceptives

- **CONTRA-INDICATIONS** Acute porphyrias p. 745 · atrial fibrillation · benign hepatocellular adenoma · Budd-Chiari syndrome · cardiomyopathy with impaired cardiac function · complicated congenital heart disease · complicated valvular heart disease · current breast cancer · hepatocellular carcinoma · hypertension (blood pressure systolic 160 mmHg or diastolic 100 mmHg or higher) · hypertensive retinopathy · ischaemic heart disease · known thrombogenic mutations (e.g. factor V Leiden, prothrombin mutation, protein S, protein C and antithrombin deficiencies) · less than 3 weeks postpartum in non-breastfeeding women with other risk factors for venous thromboembolism · less than 6 weeks postpartum in breastfeeding women · major surgery with prolonged immobilisation · migraine with aura · peripheral vascular disease with intermittent claudication · positive antiphospholipid antibodies · previous or current venous thrombosis · stroke · systemic lupus erythematosus with antiphospholipid antibodies · transient ischaemic attack
- **CAUTIONS**

GENERAL CAUTIONS Carrier of breast cancer gene mutations e.g. BRCA1, BRCA2—seek specialist advice before use · cervical intraepithelial neoplasia or cancer · cholestasis during pregnancy · cholestasis with previous use of combined hormonal contraception—seek specialist advice before use · focal nodular hyperplasia · gallbladder disease—if medically treated or current, seek specialist advice before use · history of breast cancer—seek specialist advice before use · history of negative mood changes induced by hormonal contraceptive (a product containing an alternative progestogen may be tried) · inflammatory bowel disease · organ transplantation—when complicated, seek specialist advice before use · personal or family history of hypertriglyceridaemia (increased risk of pancreatitis) · prolactinoma—seek specialist advice before use · risk factors for cardiovascular disease · risk factors for venous thromboembolism · sickle-cell disease · undiagnosed mass or breast symptoms during combined hormonal contraception treatment—if symptoms exist prior to initiation, seek specialist advice before use · undiagnosed vaginal bleeding · viral hepatitis during combined hormonal contraception treatment—if condition exists prior to initiation, seek specialist advice before use

SPECIFIC CAUTIONS

▶ With oral use Bariatric surgery with body mass index 30 kg/m^2 to 34 kg/m^2 (possible reduction in contraceptive efficacy)—if body mass index $\geq$ 35 kg/m^2, seek specialist advice before use · severe diarrhoea (possible reduction in contraceptive efficacy) · vomiting (possible reduction in contraceptive efficacy)

CAUTIONS, FURTHER INFORMATION

▶ Risk of venous thromboembolism There is an increased risk of venous thromboembolic disease in users of combined hormonal contraceptives particularly during the first year and possibly after restarting combined hormonal contraceptives following a break of four weeks or more. This risk is smaller than that associated with pregnancy and the postpartum period. In all cases the risk of venous thromboembolism increases with age and in the presence of other risk factors, such as obesity. The risk also varies depending on the type of progestogen and oestrogen dose.

▶ Risk factors for venous thromboembolism Use with **caution** if any of following factors present. If multiple risk factors are present, clinical judgement must be applied to decide whether the risk of using the combined hormonal contraceptive outweighs the benefit; referral to a specialist contraceptive provider may be required (for risk factors where treatment with combined hormonal contraceptives should be avoided, see *Contra-indications*).

- 6 weeks to 6 months *postpartum in breastfeeding women*;
- 3 to 6 weeks *postpartum in non-breastfeeding women* in the absence of additional risk factors for venous thromboembolism—if 3 to 6 weeks postpartum with risk factors, or if less than 3 weeks postpartum without risk factors, seek specialist advice before use;
- *Smoking*;
- *Obesity* with body mass index 30 kg/m^2 to 34 kg/m^2—if body mass index $\geq$ 35 kg/m^2, seek specialist advice before use;
- *History of hypertension during pregnancy* in currently normotensive women;
- *Family history of venous thromboembolism* in a first-degree relative aged 45 years and older—if first-degree relative is under 45 years, seek specialist advice before use;
- *Major surgery* without prolonged immobilisation;
- *Long-term immobility* (e.g. wheelchair use, debilitating illness)—seek specialist advice before use;

- *Superficial venous thrombosis*;
- *Uncomplicated valvular heart disease*;
- *Uncomplicated congenital heart disease*;
- *Cardiomyopathy* with normal cardiac function;
- *Long QT syndrome*;
- *Systemic lupus erythematosus* with no antiphospholipid antibodies;
- *High altitudes*: women travelling above 4500 m or 14500 feet for more than 1 week should consider alternative contraceptive methods (risk of thrombosis).

Combined Hormonal Contraception and Risk of Venous Thromboembolism

Progestogen in Combined Hormonal Contraceptive	Estimated incidence per 10 000 women per year of use
Non-pregnant, not using combined hormonal contraception	2
Levonorgestrel[1]	5-7
Norgestimate[1]	5-7
Norethisterone[1]	5-7
Etonogestrel[1]	6-12
Norelgestromin[1]	6-12
Gestodene[1]	9-12
Desogestrel[1]	9-12
Drospirenone[1]	9-12
Dienogest[2]	Not known—insufficient data
Nomegestrol[2]	Not known—insufficient data

[1] Combined with ethinylestradiol [2] Combined with estradiol

- ▸ Risk of cardiovascular disease Combined hormonal contraceptives also slightly increase the risk of *cardiovascular disease* such as myocardial infarction and ischaemic stroke; risk appears to be greater with higher oestrogen doses.
- ▸ Risk factors for cardiovascular disease Use with **caution** if any one of following factors present. If multiple risk factors are present, clinical judgement must be applied to decide whether the risk of using the combined hormonal contraceptive outweighs the benefit; referral to a specialist contraceptive provider may be required (for risk factors where treatment with combined hormonal contraceptives should be avoided, see *Contra-indications*).
  - *Smoking*;
  - *Hypertension* if adequately controlled or if blood pressure *systolic* 140–159 *mmHg* or *diastolic* 90–99 *mmHg*, seek specialist advice before use;
  - *History of hypertension during pregnancy* in currently normotensive women;
  - *Dyslipidaemias*;
  - *Non-migrainous headache (mild or severe)* during combined hormonal contraceptive use;
  - *Migraine without aura* prior to initiation of combined hormonal contraceptives—if *migraine without aura* occurs during combined hormonal contraceptive use or when history of *migraine with aura* is 5 or more years ago, seek specialist advice;
  - *Idiopathic intracranial hypertension*;
  - *Uncomplicated valvular heart disease*;
  - *Uncomplicated congenital heart disease*;
  - *Cardiomyopathy* with normal cardiac function;
  - *Long QT syndrome*;
  - *Diabetes mellitus*—if vascular disease present, seek specialist advice before use;
  - *Rheumatoid arthritis*;
  - *Systemic lupus erythematosus* without antiphospholipid antibodies.

● **SIDE-EFFECTS**

- ▸ **Common or very common** Abdominal pain · breast abnormalities · diarrhoea · fluid retention · headaches · metrorrhagia · mood altered · nausea · sexual dysfunction · skin reactions · vaginal discharge · vomiting · weight increased
- ▸ **Uncommon** Alopecia
- ▸ **Rare or very rare** Embolism and thrombosis

SIDE-EFFECTS, FURTHER INFORMATION **Breast cancer** There is a small increase in the risk of having breast cancer diagnosed in women taking the combined oral contraceptive pill; this relative risk may be due to an earlier diagnosis. In users of combined oral contraceptive pills the cancers are more likely to be localised to the breast. The most important factor for diagnosing breast cancer appears to be the age at which the contraceptive is stopped rather than the duration of use; any increase in the rate of diagnosis diminishes gradually during the 10 years after stopping and disappears by 10 years.

Cervical cancer Use of combined oral contraceptives for 5 years or longer is associated with a small increased risk of cervical cancer; the risk diminishes after stopping and disappears by about 10 years. The possible small increase in the risk of breast cancer and cervical cancer should be weighed against the protective effect against cancers of the ovary and endometrium.

● **PREGNANCY** Not known to be harmful.

● **BREAST FEEDING** CoSRH advises usually suitable for use from 6 weeks postpartum (benefits generally outweigh risks); safe for use 6 months or more postpartum.

● **HEPATIC IMPAIRMENT** In general, manufacturer advises caution; avoid in acute disease, severe chronic disease, or liver tumour.

● **DIRECTIONS FOR ADMINISTRATION**

- ▸ With oral use Each tablet should be taken at approximately same time each day; if delayed, contraceptive protection may be lost. CoSRH advises if reasonably certain woman is not pregnant, first course can be started on any day of cycle—if starting on day 6 of cycle or later, additional precautions (barrier methods) necessary during first 7 days; for estradiol-containing preparations, additional precautions (barrier methods) necessary for 7 days (9 days for *Qlaira*®) if started after day 1 of cycle.

Changing to combined preparation containing different progestogen

- ▸ With oral use CoSRH advises if previous contraceptive used correctly, or pregnancy can reasonably be excluded, start the first active tablet of new brand immediately. Consult product literature for requirements of specific preparations.

Changing from progestogen-only tablet

- ▸ With oral use CoSRH advises if previous contraceptive used correctly, or pregnancy can reasonably be excluded, start new brand immediately, additional precautions (barrier methods) necessary for first 7 days (9 days for *Qlaira*®).

Secondary amenorrhoea (exclude pregnancy)

- ▸ With oral use CoSRH advises start any day, additional precautions (barrier methods) necessary during first 7 days (9 days for *Qlaira*®).

After childbirth (not breast-feeding)

- ▸ With oral use CoSRH advises start 3 weeks after childbirth except on specialist advice in the absence of additional risk factors for thromboembolism, or 6 weeks after childbirth in the presence of additional risk factors for thromboembolism (increased risk of thrombosis if started earlier); additional precautions (barrier methods) necessary for first 7 days (9 days for *Qlaira*®).

After abortion, miscarriage, ectopic pregnancy or gestational trophoblastic disease

- ▸ With oral use CoSRH advises additional contraceptive precautions (barrier methods) required for 7 days if started after day 5 following treatment; for estradiol-containing preparations, additional contraceptive precautions (barrier methods) required for 7 days (9 days for *Qlaira*®) if started after day 1 following treatment.

● **PATIENT AND CARER ADVICE**

Travel Women taking oral contraceptives or using the patch or vaginal ring are at an increased risk of deep vein thrombosis during travel involving long periods of immobility (over 3 hours). The risk may be reduced by appropriate exercise during the journey and possibly by wearing graduated compression hosiery.

Diarrhoea and vomiting Vomiting and severe diarrhoea can interfere with the absorption of combined oral contraceptives. The CoSRH advises following the instructions for missed pills if vomiting occurs within 3 hours of taking a combined oral contraceptive or severe diarrhoea occurs for more than 24 hours. Use of non-oral contraception should be considered if diarrhoea or vomiting persist.

Missed doses The critical time for loss of contraceptive protection is when a pill is omitted at the *beginning* or *end* of a cycle (which lengthens the pill-free interval). If a woman forgets to take a pill, it should be taken as soon as she remembers, and the next one taken at the normal time (even if this means taking 2 pills together). A missed pill is one that is 24 or more hours late. If a woman misses only one pill, she should take an active pill as soon as she remembers and then resume normal pill-taking. No additional precautions are necessary. If a woman misses 2 or more pills (especially from the first 7 in a packet), she may not be protected. She should take an active pill as soon as she remembers and then resume normal pill-taking. In addition, she must either abstain from sex or use an additional method of contraception such as a condom for the next 7 days. If these 7 days run beyond the end of the packet, the next packet should be started at once, omitting the pill-free interval (or, in the case of *everyday* (ED) pills, omitting the 7 inactive tablets). Emergency contraception is recommended if 2 or more combined oral contraceptive tablets are missed from the first 7 tablets in a packet and unprotected intercourse has occurred since finishing the last packet.

616

Dienogest with estradiol valerate

17-Feb-2021

● **INDICATIONS AND DOSE**

Contraception with 28-day combined preparations | Menstrual symptoms with 28-day combined preparations

▶ BY MOUTH

▸ Females of childbearing potential: 1 active tablet daily for 26 days, followed by 1 inactive tablet daily for 2 days, to be started on day 1 of cycle with first active tablet (withdrawal bleeding may occur during the 2-day interval of inactive tablets); subsequent courses repeated without interval

● **UNLICENSED USE** Consult product literature for the licensing status.

● **INTERACTIONS** → Appendix 1: combined hormonal contraceptives

● **SIDE-EFFECTS**

▶ **Common or very common** Gastrointestinal discomfort · increased risk of infection · menstrual cycle irregularities

▶ **Uncommon** Appetite increased · cervical abnormalities · crying · depression · dizziness · fatigue · haemorrhage · hot flush · hyperhidrosis · hypertension · muscle spasms · neoplasms · oedema · ovarian and fallopian tube disorders · painful sexual intercourse · pelvic disorders · sleep disorders · uterine cramps · vulvovaginal disorders · weight decreased

▶ **Rare or very rare** Aggression · anxiety · asthma · chest pain · cholecystitis chronic · concentration impaired · constipation · contact lens intolerance · dry eye · dry mouth · dyspnoea · eye swelling · fever · galactorrhoea · gastrooesophageal reflux disease · genital discharge · hair changes · hypertriglyceridaemia · hypotension · lymphadenopathy · malaise · myocardial infarction · pain · palpitations · paraesthesia · seborrhoea · sensation of pressure · urinary tract pain · vascular disorders · vertigo

● **DIRECTIONS FOR ADMINISTRATION**

Changing to *Qlaira*® Start the first active *Qlaira*® tablet on the day after taking the last active tablet of the previous brand.

● **PATIENT AND CARER ADVICE**

Diarrhoea and vomiting In cases of persistent vomiting or severe diarrhoea lasting more than 12 hours in women taking *Qlaira*®, refer to product literature.

Missed doses A missed pill for a patient taking *Qlaira*® is one that is 12 hours or more late; for information on how to manage missed pills in women taking *Qlaira*®, refer to product literature.

● **MEDICINAL FORMS** There can be variation in the licensing of different medicines containing the same drug.

Form unstated

▸ **Qlaira** (Bayer Plc)

Qlaira tablets | 84 tablet PoM £25.18

616

Drospirenone with estetrol

19-Dec-2023

● **INDICATIONS AND DOSE**

Contraception

▶ BY MOUTH

▸ Females of childbearing potential: 1 active tablet once daily for 24 days, followed by 1 inactive tablet once daily for 4 days, to be started on day 1 of cycle with first active tablet (withdrawal bleeding may occur during the 4-day interval of inactive tablets) —if starting on day 2 to 5 of cycle, additional precautions (barrier methods) necessary during first 7 days; subsequent courses repeated without interval, see Contraceptives, hormonal p. 609 for recommendations from the CoSRH on 'tailored' regimens in which there is a shortened, less frequent, or no interval where *inactive* tablets are taken.

● **INTERACTIONS** → Appendix 1: combined hormonal contraceptives · drospirenone

● **SIDE-EFFECTS**

▶ **Common or very common** Anger · haemorrhage · menstrual cycle irregularities · weight change

▶ **Uncommon** Anxiety · appetite disorder · chest pain · crying · depression · dizziness · drowsiness · dry mouth · fatigue · feeling abnormal · gastrointestinal discomfort · hot flush · increased risk of infection · insomnia · oedema · pain · painful sexual intercourse · paraesthesia · sweat changes · uterine disorders · vulvovaginal disorders

▶ **Rare or very rare** Bladder spasm · breast fibroadenoma · constipation · dry eye · facial swelling · gastrointestinal disorders · hirsutism · hyperkalaemia · hypertension · hyperthermia · hypotension · joint swelling · lactation disorder · limb discomfort · lip swelling · malaise · memory loss · muscle spasms · ovarian cyst · pelvic pain · performance status decreased · seborrhoea · urine odour abnormal · varicose veins · vertigo · vision disorders

● **MEDICINAL FORMS** There can be variation in the licensing of different medicines containing the same drug.

Oral tablet

▸ **Drovelis** (Gedeon Richter (UK) Ltd) ▼
Drospirenone 3 mg, Estetrol (as Estetrol monohydrate) 14.2 mg Drovelis 3mg/14.2mg tablets | 28 tablet PoM £8.60 DT = £8.60

616

Estradiol with nomegestrol

13-Sep-2020

● **INDICATIONS AND DOSE**

Contraception

▸ BY MOUTH

▸ Females of childbearing potential: 1 active tablet daily for 24 days, followed by 1 inactive tablet daily for 4 days, to be started on day 1 of cycle with first active tablet (withdrawal bleeding occurs when inactive tablets being taken); subsequent courses repeated without interval

● **INTERACTIONS** → Appendix 1: combined hormonal contraceptives · estradiol

● **SIDE-EFFECTS**

▸ **Common or very common** Depression · menstrual cycle irregularities · pelvic pain

▸ **Uncommon** Abdominal distension · appetite abnormal · galactorrhoea · hot flush · hyperhidrosis · oedema · painful sexual intercourse · seborrhoea · sensation of pressure · uterine cramps · vulvovaginal disorders

▸ **Rare or very rare** Cerebrovascular insufficiency · concentration impaired · contact lens intolerance · dry eye · dry mouth · gallbladder disorders · hypertrichosis

▸ **Frequency not known** Meningioma

● **PREGNANCY** Toxicity in *animal* studies.

● **DIRECTIONS FOR ADMINISTRATION** *Zoely® (every day (ED) combined (monophasic) preparation)*, 1 *active* tablet daily for 24 days, followed by 1 *inactive* tablet daily for 4 days, starting on day 1 of cycle with first *active* tablet; subsequent courses repeated without interval (withdrawal bleeding occurs when *inactive* tablets being taken).
Changing to *Zoely®* Start the first active *Zoely®* tablet on the day after taking the last active tablet of the previous brand or, at the latest, the day after the tablet-free or inactive tablet interval of the previous brand.

● **PATIENT AND CARER ADVICE**
Diarrhoea and vomiting In cases of persistent vomiting or severe diarrhoea lasting more than 12 hours in women taking *Zoely®*, refer to product literature.
Missed doses A missed pill for a patient taking *Zoely®* is one that is 12 hours or more late; for information on how to manage missed pills in women taking *Zoely®*, refer to product literature.

● **MEDICINAL FORMS** There can be variation in the licensing of different medicines containing the same drug.

Oral tablet

▸ **Zoely** (Theramex HQ UK Ltd)
Estradiol (as Estradiol hemihydrate) 1.5 mg, Nomegestrol acetate 2.5 mg Zoely 2.5mg/1.5mg tablets | 84 tablet PoM £19.80 DT = £19.80

616

Ethinylestradiol with desogestrel

14-Mar-2021

● **INDICATIONS AND DOSE**

Menstrual symptoms with 21-day combined preparations

▸ BY MOUTH

▸ Females of childbearing potential: 1 tablet once daily for 21 days; subsequent courses repeated after 7-day interval, withdrawal bleeding occurs during the 7-day interval, if reasonably certain woman is not pregnant, first course can be started on any day of cycle—if starting on day 6 of cycle or later, additional precautions (barrier methods) necessary during first 7 days, tablets should be taken at approximately the same time each day

Contraception with 21-day combined preparations

▸ BY MOUTH

▸ Females of childbearing potential: 1 tablet once daily for 21 days; subsequent courses repeated after hormone-free interval, withdrawal bleeding occurs during the hormone-free interval, if reasonably certain woman is not pregnant, first course can be started on any day of cycle—if starting on day 6 of cycle or later, additional precautions (barrier methods) necessary during first 7 days, tablets should be taken at approximately the same time each day, see Contraceptives, hormonal p. 609 for recommendations from the CoSRH on 'traditional' and 'tailored' regimens in which there is a shortened, less frequent, or no hormone-free interval.

● **UNLICENSED USE** Consult product literature for the licensing status.

● **INTERACTIONS** → Appendix 1: combined hormonal contraceptives · desogestrel · ethinylestradiol

● **SIDE-EFFECTS**

▸ **Common or very common** Depressed mood

▸ **Rare or very rare** Contact lens intolerance · erythema nodosum · weight decreased

▸ **Frequency not known** Angioedema aggravated

● **MEDICINAL FORMS** There can be variation in the licensing of different medicines containing the same drug.

Oral tablet

▸ **Bimizza** (Morningside Healthcare Ltd)
Ethinylestradiol 20 microgram, Desogestrel 150 microgram Bimizza 150microgram/20microgram tablets | 63 tablet PoM £5.04 DT = £5.98

▸ **Cimizt** (Morningside Healthcare Ltd)
Ethinylestradiol 30 microgram, Desogestrel 150 microgram Cimizt 30microgram/150microgram tablets | 63 tablet PoM £3.80 DT = £4.93

▸ **Gedarel** (Gedeon Richter (UK) Ltd)
Ethinylestradiol 20 microgram, Desogestrel 150 microgram Gedarel 20microgram/150microgram tablets | 63 tablet PoM £5.98 DT = £5.98
Ethinylestradiol 30 microgram, Desogestrel 150 microgram Gedarel 30microgram/150microgram tablets | 63 tablet PoM £4.93 DT = £4.93

▸ **Marvelon** (Organon Pharma (UK) Ltd)
Ethinylestradiol 30 microgram, Desogestrel 150 microgram Marvelon tablets | 63 tablet PoM £7.10 DT = £4.93

▸ **Mercilon** (Organon Pharma (UK) Ltd)
Ethinylestradiol 20 microgram, Desogestrel 150 microgram Mercilon 150microgram/20microgram tablets | 63 tablet PoM £8.44 DT = £5.98

616

Ethinylestradiol with drospirenone

19-Dec-2023

● **INDICATIONS AND DOSE**

Menstrual symptoms with 21-day combined preparations

▸ BY MOUTH

▸ Females of childbearing potential: 1 tablet once daily for 21 days; subsequent courses repeated after 7-day interval, withdrawal bleeding occurs during the 7-day interval

Contraception with 21-day combined preparations

▸ BY MOUTH

▸ Females of childbearing potential: 1 tablet once daily for 21 days; subsequent courses repeated after hormone-free interval, withdrawal bleeding occurs continued →

during the hormone-free interval, see Contraceptives, hormonal p. 609 for recommendations from the CoSRH on 'traditional' and 'tailored' regimens in which there is a shortened, less frequent, or no hormone-free interval.

Menstrual symptoms with 28-day combined preparations

▶ BY MOUTH

▸ Females of childbearing potential: 1 active tablet once daily for 24 days, followed by 1 inactive tablet once daily for 4 days, to be started on day 1 of cycle with first active tablet (withdrawal bleeding may occur during the 4-day interval of inactive tablets); subsequent courses repeated without interval

Contraception with 28-day combined preparations

▶ BY MOUTH

▸ Females of childbearing potential: 1 active tablet once daily for 24 days, followed by 1 inactive tablet once daily for 4 days, to be started on day 1 of cycle with first active tablet (withdrawal bleeding may occur during the 4-day interval of inactive tablets); subsequent courses repeated without interval, see Contraceptives, hormonal p. 609 for recommendations from the CoSRH on 'tailored' regimens in which there is a shortened, less frequent, or no interval where *inactive* tablets are taken.

● **UNLICENSED USE** Consult product literature for the licensing status.

● **INTERACTIONS** → Appendix 1: combined hormonal contraceptives · drospirenone · ethinylestradiol

● **SIDE-EFFECTS**

▶ **Common or very common** Depressed mood · increased risk of infection · menstrual disorder

▶ **Uncommon** Hypertension · hypotension · weight decreased

▶ **Rare or very rare** Asthma · erythema nodosum · hearing impairment

● **PATIENT AND CARER ADVICE**

Pill-free interval Withdrawal bleeding can occur during the 7-day tablet-free interval.

● **MEDICINAL FORMS** There can be variation in the licensing of different medicines containing the same drug.

Oral tablet

▸ **Dretine** (Theramex HQ UK Ltd)
Ethinylestradiol 30 microgram, Drospirenone 3 mg Dretine 0.03mg/3mg tablets | 63 tablet PoM £8.34 DT = £14.70

▸ **ELOINE** (Bayer Plc)
Ethinylestradiol 20 microgram, Drospirenone 3 mg Eloine 0.02mg/3mg tablets | 84 tablet PoM £14.70 DT = £14.70

▸ **Lucette** (Gedeon Richter (UK) Ltd)
Ethinylestradiol 30 microgram, Drospirenone 3 mg Lucette 0.03mg/3mg tablets | 63 tablet PoM £11.00 DT = £14.70

▸ **Yacella** (Morningside Healthcare Ltd)
Ethinylestradiol 30 microgram, Drospirenone 3 mg Yacella 0.03mg/3mg tablets | 63 tablet PoM £8.30 DT = £14.70

▸ **Yasmin** (Bayer Plc)
Ethinylestradiol 30 microgram, Drospirenone 3 mg Yasmin tablets | 63 tablet PoM £14.70 DT = £14.70

F 616

Ethinylestradiol with etonogestrel

14-Mar-2021

● **INDICATIONS AND DOSE**

Menstrual symptoms

▶ BY VAGINA

▸ Females of childbearing potential: 1 unit, insert the ring into the vagina on day 1 of cycle and leave in for 3 weeks; remove ring on day 22; subsequent courses repeated after 7-day ring free interval (during which withdrawal bleeding occurs)

Contraception

▶ BY VAGINA

▸ Females of childbearing potential: 1 unit, insert the ring into the vagina on day 1 of cycle and leave in for 3 weeks; remove ring on day 22; subsequent courses repeated after 7-day ring free interval (during which withdrawal bleeding occurs), see Contraceptives, hormonal p. 609 for recommendations from the CoSRH on 'tailored' regimens in which there is a shortened, less frequent, or no ring-free interval.

● **INTERACTIONS** → Appendix 1: combined hormonal contraceptives · ethinylestradiol · etonogestrel

● **SIDE-EFFECTS**

▶ **Common or very common** Depression · device complications · genital pruritus · increased risk of infection · menstrual cycle irregularities · pelvic disorders

▶ **Uncommon** Abdominal distension · appetite increased · cervical abnormalities · constipation · cystitis · dizziness · fatigue · hot flush · malaise · muscle spasms · oedema · pain · painful sexual intercourse · sensation abnormal · urinary disorders · uterine cramps · visual impairment · vulvovaginal disorders

▶ **Rare or very rare** Galactorrhoea

▶ **Frequency not known** Angioedema aggravated · penis disorder

● **DIRECTIONS FOR ADMINISTRATION**

Changing from combined hormonal contraception to vaginal ring Manufacturer advises insert ring at the latest on the day after the usual tablet-free, patch-free, or inactive-tablet interval. If previous contraceptive used correctly, or pregnancy can reasonably be excluded, can switch to ring on any day of cycle.

Changing from progestogen-only method to vaginal ring From an implant or intra-uterine progestogen-only device, manufacturer advises insert ring on the day implant or intra-uterine progestogen-only device removed; from an injection, insert ring when next injection due; from oral preparation, first ring may be inserted on any day after stopping pill. For all methods additional precautions (barrier methods) should be used concurrently for first 7 days.

● **PATIENT AND CARER ADVICE** Patients or carers should be given advice on how to administer vaginal ring.

Counselling The presence of the ring should be checked regularly.

Missed doses

Expulsion, delayed insertion or removal, or broken vaginal ring If the vaginal ring is expelled for *less than* 3 *hours*, rinse the ring with cool water and reinsert immediately; no additional contraception is needed.

If the ring remains outside the vagina for *more than* 3 *hours* or if the user does not know when the ring was expelled, contraceptive protection may be reduced:

- If ring expelled during week 1 or 2 of cycle, rinse ring with cool water and reinsert; use additional precautions (barrier methods) for next 7 days;
- If ring expelled during week 3 of cycle, either insert a new ring to start a new cycle *or* allow a withdrawal bleed and insert a new ring no later than 7 days after ring was expelled; latter option only available if ring was used continuously for at least 7 days before expulsion.

If insertion of a new ring at the start of a new cycle is delayed, contraceptive protection is lost. A new ring should be inserted as soon as possible; additional precautions (barrier methods) should be used for the first 7 days of the new cycle. If intercourse occurred during the extended ring-free interval, pregnancy should be considered.

No additional contraception is required if removal of the ring is delayed by up to 1 week (4 weeks of continuous use). The 7-day ring-free interval should be observed and subsequently a new ring should be inserted. Contraceptive protection may be reduced with continuous use of the ring for more than 4 weeks—pregnancy should be ruled out before inserting a new ring.

If the ring breaks during use, remove it and insert a new ring immediately; additional precautions (barrier methods) should be used for the first 7 days of the new cycle.

● **MEDICINAL FORMS** There can be variation in the licensing of different medicines containing the same drug.

Vaginal delivery system

▸ NuvaRing (Organon Pharma (UK) Ltd)
Ethinylestradiol 2.7 mg, Etonogestrel 11.7 mg NuvaRing 0.12mg/0.015mg per day vaginal delivery system | 3 system PoM £29.70 DT = £29.70

616

Ethinylestradiol with gestodene

14-Mar-2021

● **INDICATIONS AND DOSE**

Menstrual symptoms with 21-day combined preparations

▶ BY MOUTH

▸ Females of childbearing potential: 1 tablet once daily for 21 days; subsequent courses repeated after 7-day interval, withdrawal bleeding occurs during the 7-day interval, if reasonably certain woman is not pregnant, first course can be started on any day of cycle—if starting on day 6 of cycle or later, additional precautions (barrier methods) necessary during first 7 days, tablets should be taken at approximately the same time each day

Contraception with 21-day combined preparations

▶ BY MOUTH

▸ Females of childbearing potential: 1 tablet once daily for 21 days; subsequent courses repeated after hormone-free interval, withdrawal bleeding occurs during the hormone-free interval, if reasonably certain woman is not pregnant, first course can be started on any day of cycle—if starting on day 6 of cycle or later, additional precautions (barrier methods) necessary during first 7 days, tablets should be taken at approximately the same time each day, see Contraceptives, hormonal p. 609 for recommendations from the CoSRH on 'traditional' and 'tailored' regimens in which there is a shortened, less frequent, or no hormone-free interval.

Menstrual symptoms with 28-day combined preparations

▶ BY MOUTH

▸ Females of childbearing potential: 1 active tablet once daily for 21 days, followed by 1 inactive tablet daily for 7 days; subsequent courses repeated without interval, withdrawal bleeding occurs during the 7-day interval of *inactive* tablets being taken, if reasonably certain woman is not pregnant, first course can be started on any day of cycle—if starting on day 6 of cycle or later, additional precautions (barrier methods) necessary during first 7 days, tablets should be taken at approximately the same time each day

Contraception with 28-day combined preparations

▶ BY MOUTH

▸ Females of childbearing potential: 1 active tablet once daily for 21 days, followed by 1 inactive tablet daily for 7 days; subsequent courses repeated without interval, withdrawal bleeding occurs during the interval of *inactive* tablets being taken, if reasonably certain woman is not pregnant, first course can be started on any day of cycle—if starting on day 6 of cycle or later, additional precautions (barrier methods) necessary during first 7 days, tablets should be taken at approximately the same time each day, see Contraceptives, hormonal p. 609 for recommendations from the CoSRH on 'tailored' regimens in which *inactive* tablets are taken for a shortened, less frequent, or absent interval.

● **UNLICENSED USE** Consult product literature for the licensing status.

● **INTERACTIONS** → Appendix 1: combined hormonal contraceptives · ethinylestradiol

● **SIDE-EFFECTS**

▶ **Common or very common** Depression · dizziness · increased risk of infection · menstrual cycle irregularities · nervousness

▶ **Uncommon** Appetite abnormal · hirsutism · hypertension · hypertriglyceridaemia

▶ **Rare or very rare** Angioedema · chorea exacerbated · ear disorders · erythema nodosum · eye irritation · gallbladder disorders · gastrointestinal disorders · haemolytic uraemic syndrome · hepatic disorders · hypersensitivity · inflammatory bowel disease · neoplasms · optic neuritis · pancreatitis · systemic lupus erythematosus exacerbated · varicose veins exacerbated · weight decreased

● **MEDICINAL FORMS** There can be variation in the licensing of different medicines containing the same drug.

Oral tablet

▸ Ethinylestradiol with gestodene (Non-proprietary)
Ethinylestradiol 30 microgram, Gestodene 50 microgram Ethinylestradiol 30microgram / Gestodene 50microgram tablets | 18 tablet PoM Ⓧ
Ethinylestradiol 40 microgram, Gestodene 70 microgram Ethinylestradiol 40microgram / Gestodene 70microgram tablets | 15 tablet PoM Ⓧ
Ethinylestradiol 30 microgram, Gestodene 100 microgram Ethinylestradiol 30microgram / Gestodene 100microgram tablets | 30 tablet PoM Ⓧ

▸ Akizza (Morningside Healthcare Ltd)
Ethinylestradiol 30 microgram, Gestodene 75 microgram Akizza 75microgram/30microgram tablets | 63 tablet PoM £8.85 DT = £6.73
Ethinylestradiol 20 microgram, Gestodene 75 microgram Akizza 75microgram/20microgram tablets | 63 tablet PoM £6.73 DT = £8.85

▸ Femodene (Bayer Plc)
Ethinylestradiol 30 microgram, Gestodene 75 microgram Femodene tablets | 63 tablet PoM £6.73 DT = £6.73

▸ Femodette (Bayer Plc)
Ethinylestradiol 20 microgram, Gestodene 75 microgram Femodette tablets | 63 tablet PoM £8.85 DT = £8.85

▸ Millinette (Gedeon Richter (UK) Ltd)
Ethinylestradiol 30 microgram, Gestodene 75 microgram Millinette 30microgram/75microgram tablets | 63 tablet PoM £4.85 DT = £6.73
Ethinylestradiol 20 microgram, Gestodene 75 microgram Millinette 20microgram/75microgram tablets | 63 tablet PoM £6.37 DT = £8.85

616

Ethinylestradiol with levonorgestrel

14-Mar-2021

● **INDICATIONS AND DOSE**

Menstrual symptoms with 21-day combined preparations

▶ BY MOUTH

▸ Females of childbearing potential: 1 tablet once daily for 21 days; subsequent courses repeated after 7-day interval, withdrawal bleeding occurs during the 7-day interval, if reasonably certain woman is not pregnant, first course can be started on any day of cycle—if starting on day 6 of cycle or later, additional precautions (barrier methods) necessary during first 7 days, tablets should be taken at approximately the same time each day

continued →

Contraception with 21-day combined preparations
- ▶ BY MOUTH
- ▸ Females of childbearing potential: 1 tablet once daily for 21 days; subsequent courses repeated after hormone-free interval, withdrawal bleeding occurs during the hormone-free interval, if reasonably certain woman is not pregnant, first course can be started on any day of cycle—if starting on day 6 of cycle or later, additional precautions (barrier methods) necessary during first 7 days, tablets should be taken at approximately the same time each day, see Contraceptives, hormonal p. 609 for recommendations from the CoSRH on 'traditional' and 'tailored' regimens in which there is a shortened, less frequent, or no hormone-free interval.

Menstrual symptoms with 28-day combined preparations
- ▶ BY MOUTH
- ▸ Females of childbearing potential: 1 active tablet once daily for 21 days, followed by 1 inactive tablet once daily for 7 days, withdrawal bleeding occurs during the 7-day interval of *inactive* tablets being taken, if reasonably certain woman is not pregnant, first course can be started on any day of cycle—if starting on day 6 of cycle or later, additional precautions (barrier methods) necessary during first 7 days, tablets should be taken at approximately the same time each day. Subsequent courses repeated without interval

Contraception with 28-day combined preparations
- ▶ BY MOUTH
- ▸ Females of childbearing potential: 1 active tablet once daily for 21 days, followed by 1 inactive tablet once daily for 7 days, withdrawal bleeding occurs during the interval of *inactive* tablets being taken, if reasonably certain woman is not pregnant, first course can be started on any day of cycle—if starting on day 6 of cycle or later, additional precautions (barrier methods) necessary during first 7 days, tablets should be taken at approximately the same time each day. Subsequent courses repeated without interval, see Contraceptives, hormonal p. 609 for recommendations from the CoSRH on 'tailored' regimens in which there is a shortened, less frequent, or no interval where *inactive* tablets are taken.

● **UNLICENSED USE** Consult product literature for the licensing status of individual preparations.

● **INTERACTIONS** → Appendix 1: combined hormonal contraceptives · ethinylestradiol · levonorgestrel

● **SIDE-EFFECTS**
- ▶ **Common or very common** Depressed mood
- ▶ **Rare or very rare** Contact lens intolerance · erythema nodosum · weight decreased
- ▶ **Frequency not known** Angioedema aggravated · chorea exacerbated · hepatic function abnormal · hypertriglyceridaemia · inflammatory bowel disease · menstrual cycle irregularities

● **MEDICINAL FORMS** There can be variation in the licensing of different medicines containing the same drug.

Oral tablet
- ▸ Ethinylestradiol with levonorgestrel (Non-proprietary)
  Ethinylestradiol 30 microgram, Levonorgestrel 50 microgram Ethinylestradiol 30microgram / Levonorgestrel 50microgram tablets | 6 tablet PoM
  Ethinylestradiol 40 microgram, Levonorgestrel 75 microgram Ethinylestradiol 40microgram / Levonorgestrel 75microgram tablets | 5 tablet PoM
  Ethinylestradiol 30 microgram, Levonorgestrel 125 microgram Ethinylestradiol 30microgram / Levonorgestrel 125microgram tablets | 10 tablet PoM
- ▸ Ambelina (Crescent Pharma Ltd)
  Ethinylestradiol 30 microgram, Levonorgestrel 150 microgram Ambelina 150microgram/30microgram tablets | 63 tablet PoM £2.60 DT = £2.82
- ▸ Elevin (Genesis Pharmaceuticals Ltd)
  Ethinylestradiol 30 microgram, Levonorgestrel 150 microgram Elevin 150microgram/30microgram tablets | 63 tablet PoM £29.25 DT = £2.82
- ▸ Levest (Morningside Healthcare Ltd)
  Ethinylestradiol 30 microgram, Levonorgestrel 150 microgram Levest 150/30 tablets | 63 tablet PoM £1.80 DT = £2.82
- ▸ Maexeni (Lupin Healthcare (UK) Ltd)
  Ethinylestradiol 30 microgram, Levonorgestrel 150 microgram Maexeni 150microgram/30microgram tablets | 63 tablet PoM £1.88 DT = £2.82
- ▸ Microgynon 30 (Bayer Plc)
  Ethinylestradiol 30 microgram, Levonorgestrel 150 microgram Microgynon 30 tablets | 63 tablet PoM £2.82 DT = £2.82
- ▸ Ovranette (Pfizer Ltd)
  Ethinylestradiol 30 microgram, Levonorgestrel 150 microgram Ovranette 150microgram/30microgram tablets | 63 tablet PoM £2.20 DT = £2.82
- ▸ Rigevidon (Gedeon Richter (UK) Ltd)
  Ethinylestradiol 30 microgram, Levonorgestrel 150 microgram Rigevidon tablets | 63 tablet PoM £1.89 DT = £2.82

616

Ethinylestradiol with norelgestromin

14-Mar-2021

● **INDICATIONS AND DOSE**

Menstrual symptoms
- ▶ BY TRANSDERMAL APPLICATION
- ▸ Females of childbearing potential: Apply 1 patch once weekly for 3 weeks, apply first patch on day 1 of cycle, change patch on days 8 and 15; remove third patch on day 22 and apply new patch after 7-day patch-free interval to start subsequent contraceptive cycle, subsequent courses repeated after a 7-day patch free interval (during which withdrawal bleeding occurs)

Contraception
- ▶ BY TRANSDERMAL APPLICATION
- ▸ Females of childbearing potential: Apply 1 patch once weekly for 3 weeks, apply first patch on day 1 of cycle, change patch on days 8 and 15; remove third patch on day 22 and apply new patch after a patch-free interval to start subsequent contraceptive cycle, subsequent courses repeated after a patch-free interval (during which withdrawal bleeding occurs), see Contraceptives, hormonal p. 609 for recommendations from the CoSRH on 'traditional' and 'tailored' regimens in which there is a shortened, less frequent, or no patch-free interval.

● **UNLICENSED USE** Consult product literature for the licensing status of individual preparations.

● **CAUTIONS** Body-weight 90 kg and above (possible reduction in contraceptive efficacy)

● **INTERACTIONS** → Appendix 1: combined hormonal contraceptives · ethinylestradiol

● **SIDE-EFFECTS**
- ▶ **Common or very common** Abdominal distension · anxiety · dizziness · fatigue · increased risk of infection · malaise · menstrual cycle irregularities · muscle spasms · uterine cramps · vaginal haemorrhage
- ▶ **Uncommon** Appetite increased · dyslipidaemia · hypertension · insomnia · lactation disorders · oedema · photosensitivity reaction · vulvovaginal dryness
- ▶ **Rare or very rare** Gallbladder disorders · genital discharge · myocardial infarction · neoplasms · stroke · swelling
- ▶ **Frequency not known** Anger · angioedema · cervical dysplasia · colitis · contact lens intolerance · erythema nodosum · hepatic disorders · hyperglycaemia · intracranial haemorrhage · pulmonary artery thrombosis · taste altered

● **DIRECTIONS FOR ADMINISTRATION** Manufacturer advises adhesives or bandages should not be used to hold patch in place. If no longer sticky do not reapply but use a new patch.

Changing to a transdermal combined hormonal contraceptive

Changing from combined oral contraception Manufacturer advises apply patch on the first day of withdrawal bleeding; if no withdrawal bleeding within 5 days of taking last *active* tablet, rule out pregnancy before applying first patch. Unless patch is applied on first day of withdrawal bleeding, additional precautions (barrier methods) should be used concurrently for first 7 days.

Changing from progestogen-only method Manufacturer advises

- from an implant, apply first patch on the day implant removed
- from an injection, apply first patch when next injection due
- from oral progestogen, first patch may be applied on any day after stopping pill

For all methods additional precautions (barrier methods) should be used concurrently for first 7 days.

After childbirth (not breast-feeding) Manufacturer advises start 4 weeks after birth; if started later than 4 weeks after birth additional precautions (barrier methods) should be used for first 7 days.

After abortion or miscarriage Manufacturer advises before 20 weeks' gestation start immediately; no additional contraception required if started immediately. After 20 weeks' gestation start on day 21 after abortion or on the first day of first spontaneous menstruation; additional precautions (barrier methods) should be used for first 7 days after applying the patch.

- **PATIENT AND CARER ADVICE** Patients and carers should be given advice on how to administer patches.

Travel Women using patches are at an increased risk of deep vein thrombosis during travel involving long periods of immobility (over 3 hours). The risk may be reduced by appropriate exercise during the journey and possibly by wearing graduated compression hosiery.

Missed doses

Delayed application or detached patch If a patch is partly detached for less than 24 hours, reapply to the same site or replace with a new patch immediately; no additional contraception is needed and the next patch should be applied on the usual 'change day'. If a patch remains detached for more than 24 hours or if the user is not aware when the patch became detached, then stop the current contraceptive cycle and start a new cycle by applying a new patch, giving a new 'Day 1'; an additional non-hormonal contraceptive must be used concurrently for the first 7 days of the new cycle.

If application of a new patch at the start of a new cycle is delayed, contraceptive protection is lost. A new patch should be applied as soon as remembered giving a new 'Day 1'; additional non-hormonal methods of contraception should be used for the first 7 days of the new cycle. If application of a patch in the middle of the cycle is delayed (i.e. the patch is not changed on day 8 or day 15):

- for up to 48 hours, apply a new patch immediately; next patch 'change day' remains the same and no additional contraception is required;
- for more than 48 hours, contraceptive protection may have been lost. Stop the current cycle and start a new 4-week cycle immediately by applying a new patch giving a new 'Day 1'; additional non-hormonal contraception should be used for the first 7 days of the new cycle.

If the patch is not removed at the end of the cycle (day 22), remove it as soon as possible and start the next cycle on the usual 'change day', the day after day 28; no additional contraception is required.

- **NATIONAL FUNDING/ACCESS DECISIONS**

For full details see funding body website

Scottish Medicines Consortium (SMC) decisions

- **Ethinylestradiol with norelgestromin (*Evra*®) for use as female contraception (September 2003)** SMC No. 48/03 Recommended with restrictions

- **MEDICINAL FORMS** There can be variation in the licensing of different medicines containing the same drug.

Transdermal patch

- **Evra** (Gedeon Richter (UK) Ltd)
  Ethinylestradiol 33.9 microgram per 24 hour, Norelgestromin 203 microgram per 24 hour Evra transdermal patches | 9 patch PoM £19.51 DT = £19.51

616

Ethinylestradiol with norethisterone

14-Mar-2021

- **INDICATIONS AND DOSE**

Menstrual symptoms with 21-day combined preparations

▶ BY MOUTH

▶ Females of childbearing potential: 1 tablet once daily for 21 days; subsequent courses repeated after 7-day interval, withdrawal bleeding occurs during the 7-day interval, if reasonably certain woman is not pregnant, first course can be started on any day of cycle—if starting on day 6 of cycle or later, additional precautions (barrier methods) necessary during first 7 days, tablets should be taken at approximately the same time each day

Contraception with 21-day combined preparations

▶ BY MOUTH

▶ Females of childbearing potential: 1 tablet once daily for 21 days; subsequent courses repeated after hormone-free interval, withdrawal bleeding occurs during the hormone-free interval, if reasonably certain woman is not pregnant, first course can be started on any day of cycle—if starting on day 6 of cycle or later, additional precautions (barrier methods) necessary during first 7 days, tablets should be taken at approximately the same time each day, see Contraceptives, hormonal p. 609 for recommendations from the CoSRH on 'traditional' and 'tailored' regimens in which there is a shortened, less frequent, or no hormone-free interval.

- **UNLICENSED USE** Consult product literature for the licensing status.
- **INTERACTIONS** → Appendix 1: combined hormonal contraceptives · ethinylestradiol · norethisterone
- **SIDE-EFFECTS** Angioedema aggravated

- **MEDICINAL FORMS** There can be variation in the licensing of different medicines containing the same drug.

Oral tablet

- **Ethinylestradiol with norethisterone (Non-proprietary)**
  Ethinylestradiol 35 microgram, Norethisterone 500 microgram Ethinylestradiol 35microgram / Norethisterone 500microgram tablets | 5 tablet PoM ⊠
  Ethinylestradiol 35 microgram, Norethisterone 750 microgram Ethinylestradiol 35microgram / Norethisterone 750microgram tablets | 21 tablet PoM ⊠
  Ethinylestradiol 35 microgram, Norethisterone 1 mg Ethinylestradiol 35microgram / Norethisterone 1mg tablets | 9 tablet PoM ⊠
- **Brevinor** (Pfizer Ltd)
  Ethinylestradiol 35 microgram, Norethisterone 500 microgram Brevinor 500microgram/35microgram tablets | 63 tablet PoM £1.99 DT = £1.99
- **Norimin** (Pfizer Ltd)
  Ethinylestradiol 35 microgram, Norethisterone 1 mg Norimin 1mg/35microgram tablets | 63 tablet PoM £2.28 DT = £2.28

616

Ethinylestradiol with norgestimate

15-Mar-2021

● **INDICATIONS AND DOSE**

Menstrual symptoms with 21-day combined preparations

▶ BY MOUTH

▶ Females of childbearing potential: 1 tablet once daily for 21 days; subsequent courses repeated after 7-day interval, withdrawal bleeding occurs during the 7-day interval, if reasonably certain woman is not pregnant, first course can be started on any day of cycle—if starting on day 6 of cycle or later, additional precautions (barrier methods) necessary during first 7 days, tablets should be taken at approximately the same time each day

Contraception with 21-day combined preparations

▶ BY MOUTH

▶ Females of childbearing potential: 1 tablet once daily for 21 days; subsequent courses repeated after hormone-free interval, withdrawal bleeding occurs during the hormone-free interval, if reasonably certain woman is not pregnant, first course can be started on any day of cycle—if starting on day 6 of cycle or later, additional precautions (barrier methods) necessary during first 7 days, tablets should be taken at approximately the same time each day, see Contraceptives, hormonal p. 609 for recommendations from the CoSRH on 'traditional' and 'tailored' regimens in which there is a shortened, less frequent, or no hormone-free interval.

● **UNLICENSED USE** Consult product literature for the licensing status.

● **INTERACTIONS** → Appendix 1: combined hormonal contraceptives · ethinylestradiol

● **SIDE-EFFECTS**

▶ **Common or very common** Anxiety · asthenic conditions · chest pain · constipation · depression · dizziness · gastrointestinal discomfort · gastrointestinal disorders · genital discharge · hypersensitivity · increased risk of infection · insomnia · menstrual cycle irregularities · muscle complaints · oedema · pain

▶ **Uncommon** Appetite abnormal · cervical dysplasia · dry eye · dyspnoea · hirsutism · hot flush · hypertension · ovarian cyst · palpitations · paraesthesia · syncope · visual impairment · vulvovaginal dryness · weight changes

▶ **Rare or very rare** Hepatic disorders · pancreatitis · photosensitivity reaction · sweat changes · tachycardia · vertigo

▶ **Frequency not known** Angioedema · contact lens intolerance · dyslipidaemia · erythema nodosum · neoplasms · seizure · suppressed lactation

● **MEDICINAL FORMS** There can be variation in the licensing of different medicines containing the same drug.

Oral tablet

▶ **Cilique** (Gedeon Richter (UK) Ltd)
Ethinylestradiol 35 microgram, Norgestimate 250 microgram Cilique 250microgram/35microgram tablets | 63 tablet [PoM] £4.65 DT = £4.65

▶ **Lizinna** (Morningside Healthcare Ltd)
Ethinylestradiol 35 microgram, Norgestimate 250 microgram Lizinna 250microgram/35microgram tablets | 63 tablet [PoM] £4.64 DT = £4.65

616

Norethisterone with mestranol

● **INDICATIONS AND DOSE**

Contraception | Menstrual symptoms

▶ BY MOUTH

▶ Females of childbearing potential: 1 tablet once daily for 21 days; subsequent courses repeated after 7-day interval, withdrawal bleeding can occur during the 7-day interval, if reasonably certain woman is not pregnant, first course can be started on any day of cycle—if starting on day 6 of cycle or later, additional precautions (barrier methods) necessary during first 7 days, tablets should be taken at the same time each day

● **UNLICENSED USE** Consult product literature for the licensing status of individual preparations.

● **INTERACTIONS** → Appendix 1: combined hormonal contraceptives · norethisterone

● **MEDICINAL FORMS** No licensed medicines listed.

3.2 Contraception, devices

Other drugs used for Contraception, devices
Levonorgestrel, p. 628

CONTRACEPTIVE DEVICES

Intra-uterine contraceptive devices (copper)

06-Mar-2024

● **INDICATIONS AND DOSE**

Contraception

▶ BY INTRA-UTERINE ADMINISTRATION

▶ Females of childbearing potential: (consult product literature)

IMPORTANT SAFETY INFORMATION

MHRA/CHM ADVICE (JUNE 2015) INTRA-UTERINE CONTRACEPTION: UTERINE PERFORATION—UPDATED INFORMATION ON RISK FACTORS

Uterine perforation most often occurs during insertion, but might not be detected until sometime later. The risk of uterine perforation is increased when the device is inserted up to 36 weeks postpartum or in patients who are breastfeeding. Before inserting an intra-uterine contraceptive device, inform patients that perforation occurs in approximately 1 in every 1000 insertions and signs and symptoms include:

- severe pelvic pain after insertion (worse than period cramps);
- pain or increased bleeding after insertion which continues for more than a few weeks;
- sudden changes in periods;
- pain during intercourse;
- unable to feel the threads.

Patients should be informed on how to check their threads and to arrange a check-up if threads cannot be felt, especially if they also have significant pain. Partial perforation may occur even if the threads can be seen; consider this if there is severe pain following insertion and perform an ultrasound.

● **CONTRA-INDICATIONS** Active trophoblastic disease (until return to normal of urine and plasma-gonadotrophin concentration) · genital malignancy · medical diathermy · pelvic inflammatory disease · post-abortion sepsis ·

postpartum sepsis · recent sexually transmitted infection (if not fully investigated and treated) · severe anaemia · unexplained uterine bleeding · Wilson's disease

- **CAUTIONS** Anaemia · anatomical abnormalities—seek specialist advice · anticoagulant therapy · cardiac disease—seek specialist advice · endometriosis · epilepsy (risk of seizure at time of insertion) · immunosuppression (risk of infection)—seek specialist advice · menorrhagia (progestogen intra-uterine device might be preferable) · postpartum—seek specialist advice · risk of sexually transmitted infections · severe primary dysmenorrhoea · young age

CAUTIONS, FURTHER INFORMATION EvGr If removal is after day 7 of the menstrual cycle, intercourse should be avoided or another method of contraception used for at least 7 days before removal of intra-uterine device. (M)

▸ Sexually transmitted infections and pelvic inflammatory disease The main excess risk of pelvic infection occurs in the first 3 weeks after insertion and is believed to be related to existing carriage of a sexually transmitted infection.

The CoSRH advises pre-insertion screening (for chlamydia and, depending on sexual history and local prevalence of disease, *Neisseria gonorrhoeae*) be performed in women at risk of sexually transmitted infections. If results are unavailable at the time of fitting an intra-uterine device for emergency contraception, consider appropriate prophylactic antibacterial cover.

- **SIDE-EFFECTS** Abdominal pain lower · anaemia · back pain · device complications · menstrual cycle irregularities · pelvic inflammatory disease · uterine injuries
- **ALLERGY AND CROSS-SENSITIVITY** EvGr Contra-indicated if patient has a copper allergy. (M)
- **PREGNANCY** If an intra-uterine device fails and the woman wishes to continue to full-term the device should be removed in the first trimester if possible. Remove device; if pregnancy occurs, increased likelihood that it may be ectopic.
- **BREAST FEEDING** Not known to be harmful.
- **MONITORING REQUIREMENTS** Gynaecological examination before insertion, 6–8 weeks after insertion, then annually.
- **DIRECTIONS FOR ADMINISTRATION** The healthcare professional inserting (or removing) the device should be fully trained in the technique and should provide full counselling backed, where available, by the patient information leaflet.
- **PRESCRIBING AND DISPENSING INFORMATION**

ANCORA® 375 CU For uterine length over 6.5 cm; replacement every 5 years.

COPPER T380 A® For uterine length 6.5–9 cm; replacement every 10 years.

EUROGINE T 380® AG '*Mini*' size for minimum uterine length 5 cm; '*Normal*' size for uterine length 6.5–9 cm; replacement every 5 years.

EUROGINE T 380® CU '*Mini*' size for minimum uterine length 5 cm; '*Normal*' size for uterine length 6.5–9 cm; replacement every 5 years.

FLEXI-T® 300 For uterine length over 5 cm; replacement every 5 years.

FLEXI-T® + 380 For uterine length over 6 cm; replacement every 5 years.

GYNEFIX® Suitable for all uterine sizes; replacement every 5 years.

IUB BALLERINE MIDI® For uterine length over 6 cm; replacement every 5 years.

LOAD® 375 For uterine length over 7 cm; replacement every 5 years.

MINI TT380® SLIMLINE For minimum uterine length 5 cm; replacement every 5 years.

MULTI-SAFE® 375 For uterine length 6–9 cm; replacement every 5 years.

MULTILOAD® CU375 For uterine length 6–9 cm; replacement every 5 years.

NEO-SAFE® T380 For uterine length 6.5–9 cm; replacement every 5 years.

NOVA-T® 380 For uterine length 6.5–9 cm; replacement every 5 years.

T-SAFE® 380A QL For uterine length 6.5–9 cm; replacement every 10 years.

TT380® SLIMLINE For uterine length 6.5–9 cm; replacement every 10 years.

UT380 SHORT® For uterine length 5–7 cm; replacement every 5 years.

UT380 STANDARD® For uterine length 6.5–9 cm; replacement every 5 years.

- **MEDICINAL FORMS** There can be variation in the licensing of different medicines containing the same drug.

Products without form

▸ **Intra-uterine contraceptive devices** (R.F. Medical Supplies Ltd, Durbin Plc, Williams Medical Supplies Ltd, Bayer Plc)
Copper T380 A intra-uterine contraceptive device | 1 device £9.08
Load 375 intra-uterine contraceptive device | 1 device £8.52
T-Safe 380A QL intra-uterine contraceptive device | 1 device £11.38
UT380 Standard intra-uterine contraceptive device | 1 device £11.22
Nova-T 380 intra-uterine contraceptive device | 1 device £15.20
Flexi-T+ 380 intra-uterine contraceptive device | 1 device £10.06
Eurogine T 380 Cu intra-uterine contraceptive device normal | 1 device £10.95
Mini TT380 Slimline intra-uterine contraceptive device | 1 device £12.46
Eurogine T 380 Ag intra-uterine contraceptive device mini | 1 device £12.69
Eurogine T 380 Ag intra-uterine contraceptive device normal | 1 device £12.69
Flexi-T 300 intra-uterine contraceptive device | 1 device £9.47
Eurogine T 380 Cu intra-uterine contraceptive device mini | 1 device £10.95
Multi-Safe 375 intra-uterine contraceptive device | 1 device £8.96
GyneFix intra-uterine contraceptive device | 1 device £27.11
TT380 Slimline intra-uterine contraceptive device | 1 device £12.46
Neo-Safe T380 intra-uterine contraceptive device | 1 device £13.40
UT380 Short intra-uterine contraceptive device | 1 device £11.22

Silicone contraceptive pessaries

- **SILICONE CONTRACEPTIVE PESSARIES**

FemCap 22mm (Durbin Plc)
| 1 device · NHS indicative price = £15.29 · Drug Tariff (Part IXa)

FemCap 26mm (Durbin Plc)
| 1 device · NHS indicative price = £15.29 · Drug Tariff (Part IXa)

FemCap 30mm (Durbin Plc)
| 1 device · NHS indicative price = £15.29 · Drug Tariff (Part IXa)

3.3 Contraception, emergency

Other drugs used for Contraception, emergency Intra-uterine contraceptive devices (copper), p. 624 · Levonorgestrel, p. 628

PROGESTERONE RECEPTOR MODULATORS

Ulipristal acetate 03-Sep-2025

- **DRUG ACTION** Ulipristal acetate is a synthetic, selective progesterone receptor modulator with a partial progesterone antagonist effect.

- **INDICATIONS AND DOSE**

Emergency contraception

▶ BY MOUTH

▶ Females of childbearing potential: 30 mg for 1 dose, to be taken as soon as possible after coitus, but no later than after 120 hours

- **CONTRA-INDICATIONS** Breast cancer · cervical cancer · ovarian cancer · severe asthma controlled by oral glucocorticoids · undiagnosed vaginal bleeding · uterine cancer
- **INTERACTIONS** → Appendix 1: ulipristal
- **SIDE-EFFECTS**
- ▶ **Common or very common** Asthenia · breast abnormalities · dizziness · endometrial thickening · gastrointestinal discomfort · headaches · hot flush · menstrual cycle irregularities · mood altered · myalgia · nausea · ovarian and fallopian tube disorders · pain · pelvic pain · skin reactions · vertigo · vomiting · weight increased
- ▶ **Uncommon** Alopecia · anxiety · appetite disorder · chills · concentration impaired · constipation · diarrhoea · drowsiness · dry mouth · fever · flatulence · genital abnormalities · hyperhidrosis · increased risk of infection · insomnia · libido disorder · malaise · oedema · urinary incontinence · vision disorders · vulvovaginal disorders
- ▶ **Rare or very rare** Abnormal sensation in eye · disorientation · dry throat · epistaxis · eye erythema · painful sexual intercourse · syncope · taste altered · thirst · tremor
- ▶ **Frequency not known** Angioedema
- **PREGNANCY** EvGr Limited information available—if pregnancy occurs, report to the *ellaOne*® pregnancy registry. Ⓜ
- **BREAST FEEDING** Specialist sources indicate use with caution (very limited information available). Negligible levels present in milk. No interruption to breast-feeding is considered necessary after taking a single dose. Although adverse effects are unlikely, monitor infant for drowsiness, irritability, vomiting, diarrhoea, and poor feeding.
- **HEPATIC IMPAIRMENT** EvGr Avoid in severe impairment—no information available. Ⓜ
- **PATIENT AND CARER ADVICE** When prescribing or supplying hormonal emergency contraception, women should be told:
  - if vomiting occurs within 3 hours of taking a dose, a replacement dose should be taken;
  - that their next period may be early or late;
  - to seek medical attention promptly if any lower abdominal pain occurs because this could signify an ectopic pregnancy.

  The CoSRH also advises women should be told:
  - that a barrier method of contraception needs to be used—see Emergency contraception p. 613 for further information;
  - that a pregnancy test should be performed if the next menstrual period is delayed by more than 7 days, is lighter than usual, or is associated with abdominal pain that is not typical of the woman's usual dysmenorrhoea;
  - that a pregnancy test should be performed if hormonal contraception is started soon after use of emergency contraception even if they have bleeding; bleeding associated with the contraceptive method may not represent menstruation.

  Driving and skilled tasks Patients and carers should be counselled on the effects on driving and performance of skilled tasks—increased risk of dizziness.

- **MEDICINAL FORMS** There can be variation in the licensing of different medicines containing the same drug.

Oral tablet

▶ **Ulipristal acetate (Non-proprietary)**

Ulipristal acetate 30 mg Ulipristal 30mg tablets | 1 tablet Ⓟ £11.50–£19.60 DT = £14.05

▶ **Ellaone** (Omega Pharma Ltd)

Ulipristal acetate 30 mg EllaOne 30mg tablets | 1 tablet Ⓟ £14.05 DT = £14.05

3.4 Contraception, oral progestogen-only

Other drugs used for Contraception, oral progestogen-only Norethisterone, p. 591

PROGESTOGENS

Desogestrel 02-May-2024

- **INDICATIONS AND DOSE**

Contraception

▶ BY MOUTH

▶ Females of childbearing potential: 75 micrograms once daily, dose to be taken at same time each day, if administration delayed for 12 hours or more it should be regarded as a 'missed pill', to be started on day 1 of cycle

- **UNLICENSED USE** Consult product literature for the licensing status of individual preparations.
- **CONTRA-INDICATIONS** Acute porphyrias p. 745 · current breast cancer
- **CAUTIONS** Cardiac dysfunction · diabetes (progestogens can decrease glucose tolerance—monitor patient closely) · history of breast cancer—seek specialist advice before use · history of stroke (including transient ischaemic attack) · history of venous thromboembolism · ischaemic heart disease · liver tumours—seek specialist advice before use · malabsorption states · migraine with aura · multiple risk factors for cardiovascular disease · positive antiphospholipid antibodies · rheumatoid arthritis · systemic lupus erythematosus · undiagnosed vaginal bleeding
- **INTERACTIONS** → Appendix 1: desogestrel
- **SIDE-EFFECTS**
- ▶ **Common or very common** Breast abnormalities · depressed mood · headache · libido decreased · menstrual cycle irregularities · mood altered · nausea · skin reactions · weight increased
- ▶ **Uncommon** Alopecia · contact lens intolerance · fatigue · ovarian cyst · vomiting · vulvovaginal infection
- ▶ **Rare or very rare** Erythema nodosum
- ▶ **Frequency not known** Angioedema · arterial thromboembolism · neoplasms

SIDE-EFFECTS, FURTHER INFORMATION The benefits of using progestogen-only contraceptives (POCs), such as desogestrel, should be weighed against the possible risks for each individual woman.

There is a possible small increase in the risk of breast cancer in women using, or who have recently used, progestogen-only contraception. Causal association is not clearly established, and absolute risk remains very small, and is like that of current or recent use of combined hormonal contraception.

The most important risk factor for breast cancer appears to be the age the contraceptive is stopped rather than the duration of use; the risk gradually disappears during the 10 years after stopping.

- **ALLERGY AND CROSS-SENSITIVITY** EvGr *Lovima*® tablets contra-indicated in patients with hypersensitivity or allergy to peanuts or soya. ⟨M⟩
- **PREGNANCY** Not known to be harmful.
- **BREAST FEEDING** EvGr Suitable for use, however, a small amount of its active metabolite etonogestrel is present in milk ⟨M⟩ (recommendation also supported by primary literature). EvGr A decrease in milk production has been reported infrequently. ⟨M⟩
- **HEPATIC IMPAIRMENT** Manufacturer advises caution; avoid in severe or active disease.
- **PATIENT AND CARER ADVICE**

Surgery All progestogen-only contraceptives are suitable for use as an alternative to combined hormonal contraceptives before major elective surgery, before all surgery to the legs, or before surgery which involves prolonged immobilisation of a lower limb.

Starting routine One tablet daily, on a continuous basis, starting on day 1 of cycle and taken at the same time each day (if delayed by longer than 12 hours contraceptive protection may be lost). Additional contraceptive precautions are not required if desogestrel is started up to and including day 5 of the menstrual cycle; if started after this time, additional contraceptive precautions are required for 2 days.

Changing from a combined oral contraceptive Start on the day following completion of the combined oral contraceptive course without a break (or in the case of *everyday* (ED) tablets, omitting the inactive tablets).

After childbirth (not breast-feeding) Oral progestogen-only contraceptives can be started before 21 days postpartum without the need for additional contraceptive precautions. If started 21 days or more postpartum, additional contraceptive precautions are required for 2 days.

Diarrhoea and vomiting Vomiting and persistent, severe diarrhoea can interfere with the absorption of oral progestogen-only contraceptives. If vomiting occurs within 2 hours of taking desogestrel, another pill should be taken as soon as possible. If a replacement pill is not taken within 12 hours of the normal time for taking desogestrel, or in cases of persistent vomiting or very severe diarrhoea, additional precautions should be used during illness and for 2 days after recovery.

Missed doses The following advice is recommended: 'If you forget a pill, take it as soon as you remember and carry on with the next pill at the right time (this may mean taking 2 pills at the same time). If the pill was more than 12 hours overdue you are not protected. Continue normal pill-taking but you must also use another method, such as the condom, for the next 2 days'.

The CoSRH recommends emergency contraception if one or more tablets are missed or taken more than 12 hours late and unprotected intercourse has occurred before 2 further tablets have been correctly taken.

- **NATIONAL FUNDING/ACCESS DECISIONS**

For full details see funding body website

Scottish Medicines Consortium (SMC) decisions

- **Desogestrel (*Cerazette*®) for use as contraception (September 2003)** SMC No. 36/03 Recommended with restrictions

- **EXCEPTIONS TO LEGAL CATEGORY** *Lovima*® 75 microgram tablets can be sold to the public for use as oral contraception in females of childbearing potential, following a clinical assessment.

- **MEDICINAL FORMS** There can be variation in the licensing of different medicines containing the same drug.

Oral tablet

- **Desogestrel (Non-proprietary)**
  Desogestrel 75 microgram Desogestrel 75microgram tablets | 84 tablet PoM £9.55 DT = £2.31
- **Cerazette** (Organon Pharma (UK) Ltd)
  Desogestrel 75 microgram Cerazette 75microgram tablets | 84 tablet PoM £9.55 DT = £2.31
- **Cerelle** (Gedeon Richter (UK) Ltd)
  Desogestrel 75 microgram Cerelle 75microgram tablets | 84 tablet PoM £4.30 DT = £2.31
- **Desorex** (Somex Pharma)
  Desogestrel 75 microgram Desorex 75microgram tablets | 84 tablet PoM £2.45 DT = £2.31
- **Zelleta** (Morningside Healthcare Ltd)
  Desogestrel 75 microgram Zelleta 75microgram tablets | 84 tablet PoM £3.51 DT = £2.31

Drospirenone

19-Dec-2023

- **INDICATIONS AND DOSE**

Contraception

- BY MOUTH
- Females of childbearing potential: 1 active tablet once daily for 24 days, followed by 1 inactive tablet once daily for 4 days, to be started on day 1 of cycle with first active tablet (withdrawal bleeding may occur during the 4-day interval of inactive tablets); subsequent courses repeated without interval, if administration delayed for 24 hours or more it should be regarded as a 'missed pill'

- **CONTRA-INDICATIONS** Acute porphyrias p. 745 · current breast cancer
- **CAUTIONS** Diabetes (progestogens can decrease glucose tolerance—monitor patient closely) · history of breast cancer—seek specialist advice before use · history of stroke (including transient ischaemic attack) · history of venous thromboembolism · hyperkalaemia · hypoaldosteronism—consider assessing urea and electrolytes, and blood pressure · ischaemic heart disease · liver tumours—seek specialist advice before use · multiple risk factors for cardiovascular disease · undiagnosed vaginal bleeding
- **INTERACTIONS** → Appendix 1: drospirenone
- **SIDE-EFFECTS**
  - **Common or very common** Abdominal pain · breast abnormalities · headache · libido disorder · menstrual cycle irregularities · mood altered · nausea · skin reactions · vaginal haemorrhage · weight changes
  - **Uncommon** Alopecia · anaemia · anxiety · appetite disorder · constipation · depression · diarrhoea · dizziness · fatigue · hot flush · hyperhidrosis · hyperkalaemia · hypertension · ovarian cyst · pelvic pain · peripheral oedema · seborrhoea · uterine leiomyoma · vomiting · vulvovaginal disorders · vulvovaginal infection
  - **Rare or very rare** Cervical dysplasia · contact lens intolerance · galactorrhoea · polyuria
- **PREGNANCY** EvGr Not known to be harmful. ⟨M⟩
- **BREAST FEEDING** EvGr Progestogen-only contraceptives do not affect lactation. ⟨M⟩
- **HEPATIC IMPAIRMENT** EvGr Avoid in severe disease. ⟨M⟩
- **RENAL IMPAIRMENT** EvGr Avoid in severe renal insufficiency or acute renal failure (potential risk of hyperkalaemia). ⟨M⟩ The CoSRH advises caution in mild to moderate impairment, or significant risk factors for chronic kidney disease particularly if aged over 50 years—consider assessing urea and electrolytes, and blood pressure.

● **PATIENT AND CARER ADVICE**
Surgery All progestogen-only contraceptives are suitable for use as an alternative to combined hormonal contraceptives before major elective surgery, before all surgery to the legs, or before surgery which involves prolonged immobilisation of a lower limb.
Starting routine One tablet daily, on a continuous basis, starting on day 1 of cycle and taken at the same time each day (if delayed by longer than 24 hours contraceptive protection may be lost). If started at any other time, additional contraceptive precautions are required for 7 days.
Changing from a combined oral contraceptive Start on the day following completion of the combined oral contraceptive course without a break (or in the case of *everyday* (ED) tablets, omitting the inactive tablets).
After childbirth (not breast-feeding) Oral progestogen-only contraceptives can be started before 21 days postpartum without the need for additional contraceptive precautions. If started 21 days or more postpartum, additional contraceptive precautions are required for 7 days.
Diarrhoea and vomiting Vomiting and persistent, severe diarrhoea can interfere with the absorption of oral progestogen-only contraceptives. If vomiting occurs within 3–4 hours of taking drospirenone, another pill should be taken as soon as possible. If a replacement pill is not taken within 24 hours of the normal time for taking drospirenone, or in cases of persistent vomiting or very severe diarrhoea, additional precautions should be used during illness and for 7 days after recovery.
Missed doses The following advice is recommended: 'If you forget any active pill, take it as soon as you remember and carry on with the next pill at the right time (this may mean taking 2 pills at the same time). If the active pill was more than 24 hours overdue you are not protected. Continue normal pill-taking but you must also use another method, such as the condom, for the next 7 days. If these 7 days run into or beyond the end of the packet, the next packet should be started at once, omitting the 4 inactive pills'.
The CoSRH recommends emergency contraception if:
- any active tablets are missed or taken more than 24 hours late and unprotected intercourse has occurred before 7 further tablets have been correctly taken *or*
- active tablets are missed or taken more than 24 hours late on days 1–7 and unprotected intercourse has occurred during the preceding 4-day interval of inactive tablets or during week 1.

● **MEDICINAL FORMS** There can be variation in the licensing of different medicines containing the same drug.
Oral tablet
▸ Slynd (Exeltis UK Ltd)
Drospirenone 4 mg Slynd 4mg tablets | 84 tablet PoM £14.70 DT = £14.70

Levonorgestrel

24-Mar-2026

● **INDICATIONS AND DOSE**
Emergency contraception
▶ BY MOUTH
▸ Females of childbearing potential: 1.5 mg for 1 dose, taken as soon as possible after coitus, preferably within 12 hours and no later than after 72 hours (may also be used between 72–96 hours after coitus but efficacy decreases with time), alternatively 3 mg for 1 dose, taken as soon as possible after coitus, preferably within 12 hours and no later than after 72 hours (may also be used between 72–96 hours after coitus but efficacy decreases with time). Higher dose should be considered for patients with body-weight over 70 kg or BMI over 26 kg/m^2

Contraception
▶ BY MOUTH
▸ Females of childbearing potential: 30 micrograms daily starting on day 1 of the cycle then continuously, dose is to be taken at the same time each day, if administration delayed for 3 hours or more it should be regarded as a "missed pill"

DOSE ADJUSTMENTS DUE TO INTERACTIONS
▸ When used orally as an emergency contraceptive, the effectiveness of levonorgestrel could be reduced in women taking enzyme-inducing drugs (and for up to 4 weeks after stopping); a copper intra-uterine device should preferably be used instead. If the copper intra-uterine device is undesirable or inappropriate, the dose of levonorgestrel should be increased to a total of 3 mg taken as a single dose; pregnancy should be excluded following use, and medical advice sought if pregnancy occurs.

BENILEXA ® ONE HANDED 20MICROGRAMS/24HOURS INTRA-UTERINE DELIVERY SYSTEM
Contraception | Menorrhagia
▶ BY INTRA-UTERINE ADMINISTRATION
▸ Females of childbearing potential: Insert within 5 days of onset of menstruation, post-abortion or miscarriage, or at any time if replacement within licensed duration of use or if reasonably certain female is not pregnant and there is no risk of conception; postpartum insertions should be performed ≤48 hours after delivery, or delayed until ≥4 weeks and, either inserted within 5 days of onset of menstruation, or at any time if criteria for lactational amenorrhoea method are met. If the above criteria are not met, additional contraceptive precautions, e.g. barrier methods, should be used for at least 7 days before replacement or following insertion. Effective for 8 years when used for contraception if age <45, or until age 55 if age ≥45 at time of insertion; effective for 3 years when used for menorrhagia

Prevention of endometrial hyperplasia during oestrogen replacement therapy
▶ BY INTRA-UTERINE ADMINISTRATION
▸ Females of childbearing potential: Insert during last days of menstruation or withdrawal bleeding or at any time if amenorrhoeic; effective for 5 years

JAYDESS ® 13.5MG INTRA-UTERINE DEVICE
Contraception
▶ BY INTRA-UTERINE ADMINISTRATION
▸ Females of childbearing potential: Insert within 5 days of onset of menstruation, post-abortion or miscarriage, or at any time if replacement within licensed duration of use or if reasonably certain female is not pregnant and there is no risk of conception; postpartum insertions should be performed ≤48 hours after delivery, or delayed until ≥4 weeks and, either inserted within 5 days of onset of menstruation, or at any time if criteria for lactational amenorrhoea method are met. If the above criteria are not met, additional contraceptive precautions, e.g. barrier methods, should be used for at least 7 days before replacement or following insertion. Effective for 3 years

KYLEENA ® 19.5MG INTRA-UTERINE DEVICE
Contraception
▶ BY INTRA-UTERINE ADMINISTRATION
▸ Females of childbearing potential: Insert within 5 days of onset of menstruation, post-abortion or miscarriage, or at any time if replacement within licensed duration of use or if reasonably certain female is not pregnant and there is no risk of conception; postpartum insertions

should be performed ≤48 hours after delivery, or delayed until ≥4 weeks and, either inserted within 5 days of onset of menstruation, or at any time if criteria for lactational amenorrhoea method are met. If the above criteria are not met, additional contraceptive precautions, e.g. barrier methods, should be used for at least 7 days before replacement or following insertion. Effective for 5 years

LEVOSERT® 20MICROGRAMS/24HOURS INTRA-UTERINE DEVICE

Contraception | Menorrhagia

▶ BY INTRA-UTERINE ADMINISTRATION

▸ Females of childbearing potential: Insert within 5 days of onset of menstruation, post-abortion or miscarriage, or at any time if replacement within licensed duration of use or if reasonably certain female is not pregnant and there is no risk of conception; postpartum insertions should be performed ≤48 hours after delivery, or delayed until ≥4 weeks and, either inserted within 5 days of onset of menstruation, or at any time if criteria for lactational amenorrhoea method are met. If the above criteria are not met, additional contraceptive precautions, e.g. barrier methods, should be used for at least 7 days before replacement or following insertion. Effective for 8 years when used for contraception if age <45, or until age 55 if age ≥45 at time of insertion; effective for 3 years when used for menorrhagia

Prevention of endometrial hyperplasia during oestrogen replacement therapy

▶ BY INTRA-UTERINE ADMINISTRATION

▸ Females of childbearing potential: Insert during last days of menstruation or withdrawal bleeding or at any time if amenorrhoeic; effective for 5 years

MIRENA® 20MICROGRAMS/24HOURS INTRA-UTERINE DEVICE

Contraception | Menorrhagia

▶ BY INTRA-UTERINE ADMINISTRATION

▸ Females of childbearing potential: Insert within 5 days of onset of menstruation, post-abortion or miscarriage, or at any time if replacement within licensed duration of use or if reasonably certain female is not pregnant and there is no risk of conception; postpartum insertions should be performed ≤48 hours after delivery, or delayed until ≥4 weeks and, either inserted within 5 days of onset of menstruation, or at any time if criteria for lactational amenorrhoea method are met. If the above criteria are not met, additional contraceptive precautions, e.g. barrier methods, should be used for at least 7 days before replacement or following insertion. Effective for 8 years when used for contraception if age <45, or until age 55 if age ≥45 at time of insertion; effective for 5 years when used for menorrhagia

Prevention of endometrial hyperplasia during oestrogen replacement therapy

▶ BY INTRA-UTERINE ADMINISTRATION

▸ Females of childbearing potential: Insert during last days of menstruation or withdrawal bleeding or at any time if amenorrhoeic; effective for 5 years

● UNLICENSED USE

▸ With intra-uterine use The CoSRH advises levonorgestrel is used as detailed below, although these situations are considered unlicensed:

- Insertion at any time if reasonably certain the woman is not pregnant or at risk of pregnancy;
- Additional precautions (e.g. barrier methods) for at least 7 days before replacement even if immediate replacement is intended;
- Insertion immediately following termination of pregnancy if successful expulsion is confirmed;
- Postpartum insertions within 48 hours or 4 weeks after delivery;
- Duration of use for 52 mg levonorgestrel intra-uterine devices for contraception and prevention of endometrial hyperplasia during oestrogen replacement therapy.

▸ With oral use The CoSRH advises levonorgestrel is used as detailed below, although these situations are considered unlicensed:

- Higher dose option for emergency contraception in patients with body-weight over 70 kg or BMI over 26 kg/m^2;
- Use for emergency contraception between 72–96 hours after coitus.

▸ With intra-uterine use or oral use Consult product literature for licensing status of individual preparations.

BENILEXA® ONE HANDED 20MICROGRAMS/24HOURS INTRA-UTERINE DELIVERY SYSTEM The CoSRH advises *Benilexa®* is used for the prevention of endometrial hyperplasia, although this is considered unlicensed.

LEVOSERT® 20MICROGRAMS/24HOURS INTRA-UTERINE DEVICE The CoSRH advises *Levosert®* is used for the prevention of endometrial hyperplasia, although this is considered unlicensed.

IMPORTANT SAFETY INFORMATION

MHRA/CHM ADVICE (JUNE 2015) INTRA-UTERINE CONTRACEPTION: UTERINE PERFORATION—UPDATED INFORMATION ON RISK FACTORS

Uterine perforation most often occurs during insertion, but might not be detected until sometime later. The risk of uterine perforation is increased when the device is inserted up to 36 weeks postpartum or in patients who are breastfeeding. Before inserting an intra-uterine contraceptive device, inform patients that perforation occurs in approximately 1 in every 1000 insertions and signs and symptoms include:

- severe pelvic pain after insertion (worse than period cramps);
- pain or increased bleeding after insertion which continues for more than a few weeks;
- sudden changes in periods;
- pain during intercourse;
- unable to feel the threads.

Patients should be informed on how to check their threads and to arrange a check-up if threads cannot be felt, especially if they also have significant pain. Partial perforation may occur even if the threads can be seen; consider this if there is severe pain following insertion and perform an ultrasound.

● CONTRA-INDICATIONS

GENERAL CONTRA-INDICATIONS Current breast cancer (use with caution for emergency contraception)

SPECIFIC CONTRA-INDICATIONS

▸ With intra-uterine use Active trophoblastic disease (until return to normal of urine- and plasma-gonadotrophin concentration) · acute malignancies affecting the blood (use with caution in remission) · not suitable for emergency contraception · pelvic inflammatory disease · post-abortion sepsis · postpartum sepsis · recent sexually transmitted infection (if not fully investigated and treated) · unexplained uterine bleeding · uterine or cervical malignancy

▸ With oral use Acute porphyrias p. 745

● CAUTIONS

GENERAL CAUTIONS Cardiac disease—seek specialist advice for intra-uterine insertion · diabetes · history of breast cancer—seek specialist advice before use · history of stroke (including transient ischaemic attack) · history of venous thromboembolism · ischaemic heart disease · migraine · multiple risk factors for cardiovascular disease · positive antiphospholipid antibodies · rheumatoid arthritis · systemic lupus erythematosus

SPECIFIC CAUTIONS

▸ With intra-uterine use Anatomical abnormalities—seek specialist advice before use · cervical intraepithelial neoplasia · epilepsy (risk of seizure at time of insertion) · immunosuppression (risk of infection)—seek specialist advice before use · postpartum—seek specialist advice before use · risk of sexually transmitted infections · young age

▸ With oral use Malabsorption states

▸ With oral use for Contraception Undiagnosed vaginal bleeding

CAUTIONS, FURTHER INFORMATION

▸ With intra-uterine use EvGr If removal is after day 7 of the menstrual cycle, intercourse should be avoided or another method of contraception used for at least 7 days before removal of intra-uterine device. (M)

▸ Sexually transmitted infections and pelvic inflammatory disease

▸ With intra-uterine use The main excess risk of pelvic infection occurs in the first 3 weeks after insertion and is believed to be related to existing carriage of a sexually transmitted infection. The CoSRH advises pre-insertion screening (for chlamydia and, depending on sexual history and local prevalence of disease, *Neisseria gonorrhoeae*) be performed in women at risk of sexually transmitted infections.

MIRENA ® 20MICROGRAMS/24HOURS INTRA-UTERINE DEVICE Advanced uterine atrophy

- **INTERACTIONS** → Appendix 1: levonorgestrel
- **SIDE-EFFECTS**

GENERAL SIDE-EFFECTS

▸ **Common or very common** Dizziness · gastrointestinal discomfort · haemorrhage · headaches · menstrual cycle irregularities · nausea · skin reactions

SPECIFIC SIDE-EFFECTS

▸ **Common or very common**

▸ With intra-uterine use Back pain · breast abnormalities · depression · device expulsion · hirsutism · increased risk of infection · libido decreased · nervousness · ovarian cyst · pelvic disorders · vulvovaginal disorders · weight increased

▸ With oral use Breast tenderness · diarrhoea · fatigue · vomiting

▸ **Uncommon**

▸ With intra-uterine use Alopecia · endometritis · oedema · uterine rupture

▸ **Rare or very rare**

▸ With oral use Face oedema · pelvic pain

▸ **Frequency not known**

▸ With intra-uterine use Breast cancer

▸ With oral use Arterial thromboembolism · cerebrovascular insufficiency · depressed mood · diabetes mellitus · neoplasms · sexual dysfunction · weight changes

SIDE-EFFECTS, FURTHER INFORMATION **Breast cancer risk with contraceptive use** The benefits of using progestogen-only contraceptives (POCs), such as levonorgestrel, should be weighed against the possible risks for each individual woman.

There is a possible small increase in the risk of breast cancer in women using, or who have recently used, progestogen-only contraception. Causal association is not clearly established, and absolute risk remains very small, and is like that of current or recent use of combined hormonal contraception.

The most important risk factor for breast cancer appears to be the age the contraceptive is stopped rather than the duration of use; the risk gradually disappears during the 10 years after stopping.

With intra-uterine use Patients should be informed about the device that has been inserted and when it should be removed or replaced (including referring them to a patient information leaflet and other sources of information).

Patients may experience irregular, prolonged or infrequent menstrual bleeding in the 3–6 months following insertion; bleeding pattern improves with time but persists in some patients.

Progestogenic side-effects resolve with time (after the first few months).

- **PREGNANCY**

▸ With oral use Not known to be harmful.

▸ With intra-uterine use If an intra-uterine device fails and the woman wishes to continue to full-term, the device should be removed in the first trimester if possible. Avoid—if pregnancy occurs remove intra-uterine device.

- **BREAST FEEDING** Progestogen-only contraceptives do not affect lactation.
- **HEPATIC IMPAIRMENT**

▸ With intra-uterine use or oral use for Contraception Manufacturer advises avoid in liver tumour.

▸ With oral use for Contraception or Emergency contraception Manufacturer advises avoid in severe impairment.

▸ With intra-uterine use Manufacturer advises avoid in acute hepatic disease or in severe impairment (no information available)—consult product literature.

- **MONITORING REQUIREMENTS**

▸ With intra-uterine use Gynaecological examination before insertion, 4–6 weeks after insertion, then annually.

- **DIRECTIONS FOR ADMINISTRATION**

▸ With intra-uterine use The doctor or nurse inserting (or removing) the device should be fully trained in the technique and should provide full counselling reinforced by the patient information leaflet.

- **PRESCRIBING AND DISPENSING INFORMATION** Levonorgestrel-releasing intra-uterine devices vary in licensed indication, duration of use and insertion technique—the MHRA recommends to prescribe and dispense by brand name to avoid inadvertent switching.
- **PATIENT AND CARER ADVICE**

Diarrhoea and vomiting with use as an oral contraceptive Vomiting and persistent, severe diarrhoea can interfere with the absorption of oral progestogen-only contraceptives. If vomiting occurs within 2 hours of taking an oral progestogen-only contraceptive, another pill should be taken as soon as possible. If a replacement pill is not taken within 3 hours of the normal time for taking the progestogen-only pill, or in cases of persistent vomiting or very severe diarrhoea, additional precautions should be used during illness and for 2 days after recovery.

Starting routine

▸ With oral use for Contraception One tablet daily, on a continuous basis, starting on day 1 of cycle and taken at the same time each day (if delayed by longer than 3 hours contraceptive protection may be lost). Additional contraceptive precautions are not required if levonorgestrel is started up to and including day 5 of the menstrual cycle; if started after this time, additional contraceptive precautions are required for 2 days.

Changing from a combined oral contraceptive Start on the day following completion of the combined oral contraceptive course without a break (or in the case of *everyday* (ED) tablets, omitting the inactive tablets).

After childbirth (not breast-feeding) Oral progestogen-only contraceptives can be started before 21 days postpartum without the need for additional contraceptive precautions. If started 21 days or more postpartum, additional contraceptive precautions are required for 2 days.

▸ With oral use for Emergency contraception When prescribing or supplying hormonal emergency contraception, manufacturer advises women should be told:

- if vomiting occurs within 3 hours, a replacement dose should be taken;
- that their next period may be early or late;

- to seek medical attention promptly if any lower abdominal pain occurs because this could signify an ectopic pregnancy.

The CoSRH also advises women should be told:
- that a barrier method of contraception needs to be used—see Emergency contraception p. 613 for further information;
- that a pregnancy test should be performed if the next menstrual period is delayed by more than 7 days, is lighter than usual, or is associated with abdominal pain that is not typical of the woman's usual dysmenorrhoea;
- that a pregnancy test should be performed if hormonal contraception is started soon after use of emergency contraception even if they have bleeding; bleeding associated with the contraceptive method may not represent menstruation.

▸ With intra-uterine use Counsel women on the signs, symptoms and risks of perforation and ectopic pregnancy.

Missed doses When used as an oral contraceptive, the following advice is recommended 'If you forget a pill, take it as soon as you remember and carry on with the next pill at the right time (this may mean taking 2 pills at the same time). If the pill was more than 3 hours overdue you are not protected. Continue normal pill-taking but you must also use another method, such as the condom, for the next 2 days'.

The CoSRH recommends emergency contraception if one or more progestogen-only contraceptive tablets are missed or taken more than 3 hours late and unprotected intercourse has occurred before 2 further tablets have been correctly taken.

● **NATIONAL FUNDING/ACCESS DECISIONS**
For full details see funding body website

Scottish Medicines Consortium (SMC) decisions
▶ **Levonorgestrel (*Kyleena*®) for contraception for up to 5 years (February 2018)** SMC No. 1299/18 Recommended

All Wales Medicines Strategy Group (AWMSG) decisions
▶ **Levonorgestrel (*Kyleena*®) for contraception for up to 5 years (September 2018)** AWMSG No. 3582 Recommended

● **EXCEPTIONS TO LEGAL CATEGORY** *Levonelle® One Step* can be sold to women over 16 years; when supplying emergency contraception to the public, pharmacists should refer to guidance issued by the Royal College of Pharmacy.

● **MEDICINAL FORMS** There can be variation in the licensing of different medicines containing the same drug.

Oral tablet

▸ **Levonorgestrel (Non-proprietary)**
Levonorgestrel 1.5 mg Levonorgestrel 1.5mg tablets | 1 tablet [PoM] £1.67–£3.74 DT = £1.67

▸ **Emerres** (Morningside Healthcare Ltd)
Levonorgestrel 1.5 mg Emerres 1.5mg tablets | 1 tablet [PoM] £3.65 DT = £1.67

▸ **Levonelle** (Bayer Plc)
Levonorgestrel 1.5 mg Levonelle 1500microgram tablets | 1 tablet [PoM] £5.20 DT = £1.67

▸ **Norgeston** (Bayer Plc)
Levonorgestrel 30 microgram Norgeston 30microgram tablets | 35 tablet [PoM] £0.92 DT = £0.92

▸ **Upostelle** (Gedeon Richter (UK) Ltd)
Levonorgestrel 1.5 mg Upostelle 1500microgram tablets | 1 tablet [PoM] £3.75 DT = £1.67

Intra-uterine device

▸ **Benilexa One Handed** (Gedeon Richter (UK) Ltd)
Levonorgestrel 20 microgram per 24 hour Benilexa One Handed 20micrograms/24hours intra-uterine delivery system | 1 device [PoM] £71.00 DT = £88.00

▸ **Jaydess** (Bayer Plc) ▼
Levonorgestrel 13.5 mg Jaydess 13.5mg intra-uterine device | 1 device [PoM] £69.22 DT = £69.22

▸ **Kyleena** (Bayer Plc)
Levonorgestrel 19.5 mg Kyleena 19.5mg intra-uterine device | 1 device [PoM] £76.00 DT = £76.00

▸ **Levosert** (Gedeon Richter (UK) Ltd)
Levonorgestrel 20 microgram per 24 hour Levosert 20micrograms/24hours intra-uterine device | 1 device [PoM] £66.00 DT = £88.00

▸ **Mirena** (Bayer Plc)
Levonorgestrel 20 microgram per 24 hour Mirena 20micrograms/24hours intra-uterine device | 1 device [PoM] £88.00 DT = £88.00

3.5 Contraception, parenteral progestogen-only

Other drugs used for Contraception, parenteral progestogen-only Norethisterone, p. 591

PROGESTOGENS

Etonogestrel

11-Mar-2021

● **INDICATIONS AND DOSE**

Contraception [no hormonal contraceptive use in previous month]

▶ BY SUBDERMAL IMPLANTATION
▸ Females of childbearing potential: 1 implant, which can be left in place for up to 3 years, when inserted during the first 5 days of cycle, no additional contraceptive precautions are needed, when inserted at any other time, additional precautions (e.g. barrier methods) advised for next 7 days

Contraception [postpartum]

▶ BY SUBDERMAL IMPLANTATION
▸ Females of childbearing potential: 1 implant, which can be left in place for up to 3 years, when inserted within 20 days after delivery (or up to 6 months postpartum if fully breast-feeding and amenorrhoeic), no additional contraceptive precautions are needed, when inserted at any other time, additional precautions (e.g. barrier methods) advised for next 7 days

Contraception [following abortion or miscarriage]

▶ BY SUBDERMAL IMPLANTATION
▸ Females of childbearing potential: 1 implant, which can be left in place for up to 3 years, when inserted within 5 days after abortion or miscarriage, no additional contraceptive precautions are needed, when inserted at any other time, additional precautions (e.g. barrier methods) advised for next 7 days

Contraception [changing from other hormonal contraceptive]

▶ BY SUBDERMAL IMPLANTATION
▸ Females of childbearing potential: 1 implant, which can be left in place for up to 3 years, consult product literature for advice on when to insert and additional contraceptive precautions

● **UNLICENSED USE** The CoSRH advises that the etonogestrel implant is used as detailed below, although these situations are considered unlicensed:
- females outside the age range of 18–40 years;
- postpartum insertions within 20 days after delivery (or up to 6 months postpartum if fully breast-feeding and amenorrhoeic);

- insertion within 5 days after abortion or miscarriage in the second trimester.

IMPORTANT SAFETY INFORMATION

MHRA/CHM ADVICE (UPDATED FEBRUARY 2020): *NEXPLANON®* (ETONOGESTREL) CONTRACEPTIVE IMPLANTS: NEW INSERTION SITE TO REDUCE RARE RISK OF NEUROVASCULAR INJURY AND IMPLANT MIGRATION

There have been reports of neurovascular injury and migration of *Nexplanon®* implants from the insertion site to the vasculature, including the pulmonary artery in rare cases. Correct subdermal insertion by an appropriately trained and accredited healthcare professional is recommended to reduce the risk of these events. Healthcare professionals are advised to review the updated guidance from the manufacturer and the statement from the CoSRH on how to correctly insert the implant. Patients should be advised on how to locate the implant, informed to check this occasionally and report any concerns. An implant that cannot be palpated at its insertion site should be located and removed as soon as possible; if unable to locate implant within the arm, the MHRA recommends using chest imaging. Implants inserted at a previous site that can be palpated should not pose a risk and should only be replaced if there are issues with its location or if a routine replacement is due.

- **CONTRA-INDICATIONS** Acute porphyrias p. 745 · current breast cancer
- **CAUTIONS** Cardiac dysfunction · cervical cancer · diabetes (progestogens can decrease glucose tolerance—monitor patient closely) · history of breast cancer—seek specialist advice before use · history of stroke (including transient ischaemic attack) · history of venous thromboembolism · ischaemic heart disease · liver tumours—seek specialist advice before use · migraine · multiple risk factors for cardiovascular disease · positive antiphospholipid antibodies · rheumatoid arthritis · systemic lupus erythematosus · undiagnosed vaginal bleeding—seek specialist advice before use
- **INTERACTIONS** → Appendix 1: etonogestrel
- **SIDE-EFFECTS**
  - **Common or very common** Abdominal pain · alopecia · anxiety · appetite increased · breast abnormalities · depressed mood · dizziness · emotional lability · fatigue · flatulence · headaches · hot flush · increased risk of infection · influenza like illness · libido decreased · menstrual cycle irregularities · nausea · ovarian cyst · pain · skin reactions · weight changes
  - **Uncommon** Arthralgia · constipation · diarrhoea · drowsiness · dysuria · fever · galactorrhoea · genital abnormalities · hypertrichosis · insomnia · myalgia · oedema · vomiting · vulvovaginal discomfort
  - **Frequency not known** Abscess · angioedema · embolism and thrombosis · haemorrhage · insulin resistance · neoplasms · paraesthesia · seborrhoea

  SIDE-EFFECTS, FURTHER INFORMATION The benefits of using progestogen-only contraceptives (POCs), such as etonogestrel, should be weighed against the possible risks for each individual woman.

  There is a possible small increase in the risk of breast cancer in women using, or who have recently used, progestogen-only contraception. Causal association is not clearly established, and absolute risk remains very small, and is like that of current or recent use of combined hormonal contraception.

  The most important risk factor for breast cancer appears to be the age the contraceptive is stopped rather than the duration of use; the risk gradually disappears during the 10 years after stopping.
- **PREGNANCY** Not known to be harmful, remove implant if pregnancy occurs.
- **BREAST FEEDING** Progestogen-only contraceptives do not affect lactation.
- **DIRECTIONS FOR ADMINISTRATION** The doctor or nurse administering (or removing) the system should be fully trained in the technique and should provide full counselling reinforced by the patient information leaflet.
- **PATIENT AND CARER ADVICE** Full counselling backed by patient information leaflet required before administration.
- **MEDICINAL FORMS** There can be variation in the licensing of different medicines containing the same drug.

Prolonged-release subcutaneous implant

- **Nexplanon** (Organon Pharma (UK) Ltd)
  Etonogestrel 68 mg Nexplanon 68mg implant | 1 device PoM £83.43 DT = £83.43

Medroxyprogesterone acetate 05-Dec-2024

- **INDICATIONS AND DOSE**

Contraception

- BY DEEP INTRAMUSCULAR INJECTION
  - Females of childbearing potential: 150 mg, to be administered within the first 5 days of cycle or within first 5 days after parturition (delay until 6 weeks after parturition if breast-feeding)
- BY SUBCUTANEOUS INJECTION
  - Females of childbearing potential: 104 mg, to be administered within first 5 days of cycle or within 5 days postpartum (delay until 6 weeks postpartum if breast-feeding), injected into anterior thigh or abdomen, dose only suitable if no hormonal contraceptive use in previous month

Long-term contraception

- BY DEEP INTRAMUSCULAR INJECTION
  - Females of childbearing potential: 150 mg every 12 weeks, first dose to be administered within the first 5 days of cycle or within first 5 days after parturition (delay until 6 weeks after parturition if breast-feeding)
- BY SUBCUTANEOUS INJECTION
  - Females of childbearing potential: 104 mg every 13 weeks, first dose to be administered within first 5 days of cycle or within 5 days postpartum (delay until 6 weeks postpartum if breast-feeding), injected into anterior thigh or abdomen, dose only suitable if no hormonal contraceptive use in previous month

Contraception (when patient changing from other hormonal contraceptive)

- BY SUBCUTANEOUS INJECTION
  - Females of childbearing potential: (consult product literature)

IMPORTANT SAFETY INFORMATION

MHRA/CHM ADVICE: MEDROXYPROGESTERONE ACETATE: RISK OF MENINGIOMA AND MEASURES TO MINIMISE THIS RISK (OCTOBER 2024)

A French epidemiological study has identified a small increased risk of developing meningioma with high-dose medroxyprogesterone acetate (all parenteral preparations and oral preparations containing 100 mg or more), mainly after prolonged use of several years. When used for contraception, high-dose medroxyprogesterone acetate is contra-indicated in patients with meningioma or a history of meningioma—if meningioma is diagnosed, it must be stopped.

This advice does not apply to lower doses (less than 100 mg) or combination preparations.

- **CONTRA-INDICATIONS** Acute porphyrias p. 745 · current breast cancer (unless progestogens are being used in the management of this condition) · current or history of meningioma

- **CAUTIONS** Cardiac dysfunction · cervical cancer · conditions that may worsen with fluid retention · diabetes (progestogens can decrease glucose tolerance—monitor patient closely) · history of breast cancer—seek specialist advice before use · history of stroke (including transient ischaemic attack)—seek specialist advice before use · history of venous thromboembolism · hypertension · ischaemic heart disease—seek specialist advice before use · liver tumours—seek specialist advice before use · migraine · multiple risk factors for cardiovascular disease—seek specialist advice before use · positive antiphospholipid antibodies · rheumatoid arthritis · risk factors for thromboembolism · systemic lupus erythematosus · undiagnosed vaginal bleeding—seek specialist advice before use
- **INTERACTIONS** → Appendix 1: medroxyprogesterone
- **SIDE-EFFECTS**
  - **Common or very common** Anxiety · asthenia · breast abnormalities · depression · dizziness · gastrointestinal discomfort · headaches · insomnia · menstrual cycle irregularities · mood altered · nausea · pain · sexual dysfunction · skin reactions · vulvovaginal infection · weight changes
  - **Uncommon** Alopecia · appetite abnormal · arthralgia · drowsiness · fever · fluid retention · galactorrhoea · hirsutism · hot flush · hypertension · muscle spasms · ovarian cyst · painful sexual intercourse · tachycardia · uterine haemorrhage · varicose veins · vertigo · vulvovaginal disorders
  - **Rare or very rare** Breast cancer · embolism and thrombosis · lipodystrophy
  - **Frequency not known** Hepatic disorders · meningioma (with high doses, particularly in long term use) · osteoporosis · osteoporotic fractures · seizure

  SIDE-EFFECTS, FURTHER INFORMATION Reduction in bone mineral density is greater with increasing duration of use. The loss is mostly recovered on discontinuation.

  Breast cancer risk with contraceptive use The benefits of using progestogen-only contraceptives (POCs), such as medroxyprogesterone acetate, should be weighed against the possible risks for each individual woman.

  There is a possible small increase in the risk of breast cancer in women using, or who have recently used, progestogen-only contraception. Causal association is not clearly established, and absolute risk remains very small, and is like that of current or recent use of combined hormonal contraception.

  The most important risk factor for breast cancer appears to be the age the contraceptive is stopped rather than the duration of use; the risk gradually disappears during the 10 years after stopping.
- **CONCEPTION AND CONTRACEPTION**
  - With intramuscular use If interval between dose is greater than 12 weeks and 5 days (in long-term contraception), rule out pregnancy before next injection and advise patient to use additional contraceptive measures (e.g. barrier) for 14 days after the injection.
  - With subcutaneous use If interval between dose is greater than 13 weeks and 7 days (in long-term contraception), rule out pregnancy before next injection.
- **PREGNANCY** Not known to be harmful.
- **BREAST FEEDING** Present in milk—no adverse effects reported. Progestogen-only contraceptives do not affect lactation. The manufacturers advise that in women who are breast-feeding, the first dose should be delayed until 6 weeks after birth; however, evidence suggests no harmful effect to infant if given earlier. The benefits of using medroxyprogesterone acetate in breast-feeding women outweigh any risks.
- **HEPATIC IMPAIRMENT**
  - With oral use Manufacturer advises caution; avoid in acute or active disease.
  - With intramuscular use or subcutaneous use Manufacturer advises caution; avoid in severe or active disease.
- **PATIENT AND CARER ADVICE** Full counselling backed by *patient information leaflet* required before administration—likelihood of menstrual disturbance and the potential for a delay in return to full fertility. Delayed return of fertility and irregular cycles may occur after discontinuation of treatment but there is no evidence of permanent infertility.

- **MEDICINAL FORMS** There can be variation in the licensing of different medicines containing the same drug.

Suspension for injection

- **Depo-Provera** (Pfizer Ltd)
  Medroxyprogesterone acetate 150 mg per 1 ml Depo-Provera 150mg/1ml suspension for injection pre-filled syringes | 1 pre-filled disposable injection PoM £6.01 DT = £6.01
- **Sayana Press** (Pfizer Ltd)
  Medroxyprogesterone acetate 160 mg per 1 ml Sayana Press 104mg/0.65 ml suspension for injection pre-filled disposable devices | 1 pre-filled disposable injection PoM £6.90 DT = £6.90

3.6 Contraception, spermicidal

SPERMICIDALS

Nonoxinol

- **INDICATIONS AND DOSE**

Spermicidal contraceptive in conjunction with barrier methods of contraception such as diaphragms or caps

- BY VAGINA
  - Females of childbearing potential: (consult product literature)

- **SIDE-EFFECTS** Genital erosion · increased risk of HIV infection · pain · paraesthesia · skin reactions · vaginal redness

  SIDE-EFFECTS, FURTHER INFORMATION High frequency use of the spermicide nonoxinol-9 has been associated with genital lesions, which may increase the risk of acquiring sexually transmitted infections.
- **CONCEPTION AND CONTRACEPTION** No evidence of harm to diaphragms.
- **PREGNANCY** Toxicity in *animal* studies.
- **BREAST FEEDING** Present in milk in *animal* studies.

- **MEDICINAL FORMS** No licensed medicines listed.

4 Vaginal and vulval conditions

Vaginal and vulval conditions 06-Aug-2021

Management

Pre-pubertal girls may be particularly susceptible to vulvovaginitis. EvGr Barrier preparations applied after cleansing can be useful when the symptoms are due to non-specific irritation. Systemic drugs may be considered if there is clinical infection rather than colonisation. Intravaginal preparations, particularly those that require the use of an applicator, are not generally suitable for young girls; topical preparations may be useful in some adolescent girls.

Genito-urinary system 7

In post-pubertal girls, symptoms are often restricted to the vulva, but infections almost invariably involve the vagina, which should also be treated; treatment should be as for adults. (E)

Vaginal and vulval changes

EvGr Topical oestrogen creams are used in the treatment of labial adhesions; treatment is usually restricted to symptomatic cases. Estriol cream [unlicensed use] should be applied to the adhesions once or twice daily for 2–6 weeks; adhesions may recur following treatment. (E)

Vaginal and vulval infections

Vulvovaginal candidiasis

Vulvovaginal candidiasis (genital thrush) is symptomatic inflammation of the vagina and/or vulva caused by a superficial fungal infection; most cases are caused by *Candida albicans*. It is not normally a problem in younger girls (pre-puberty) but can occur in adolescents. EvGr Candidal vulvitis can be treated locally with cream, but is almost invariably associated with vaginal infection which should also be treated.

Acute vulvovaginal candidiasis can be treated with an intravaginal imidazole pessary or cream inserted high into the vagina; however, these are not recommended for pre-pubertal girls and treatment with an external cream may be more appropriate. (E) Local irritation may occur on application of intravaginal imidazole drug preparations and may be mistaken for treatment failure.

EvGr Intravaginal imidazole drugs (e.g. clotrimazole p. 635, econazole nitrate) are effective against candida in short courses of 1 to 3 days according to the preparation used. Treatment can be repeated if the initial course fails to control symptoms or if symptoms recur; vaginal applications may be supplemented with a topical antifungal cream for vulvitis and to treat other superficial sites of infection.

Oral treatment of vaginal infection with fluconazole p. 463 may be considered for girls post-puberty. (E)

Vulvovaginal candidiasis in pregnancy

EvGr Symptomatic vulvovaginal candidiasis is common during pregnancy and can be treated with intravaginal application of an imidazole. Pregnant females need a longer duration of treatment, usually about 7 days, to clear the infection. (E) There is limited systemic absorption of imidazoles from the vagina. EvGr Treatment with an oral azole drug should be avoided during pregnancy. (E)

Recurrent vulvovaginal candidiasis

Recurrent vulvovaginal candidiasis is very rare in children, but can occur if there are predisposing factors such as recent antibacterial therapy, poorly controlled diabetes mellitus, pregnancy, immunosuppression, or possibly oral contraceptive use.

EvGr Treatment of recurrent vulvovaginal candidiasis may need to be extended for 6 months. (E)

Other infections

Systemic drugs are required in the treatment of infections such as gonorrhoea and syphilis. See Genital system infections, antibacterial therapy p. 368.

EvGr Trichomonal infections commonly involve the lower urinary tract as well as the genital system and need systemic treatment with metronidazole p. 409. (A)

EvGr Treatment with oral metronidazole is indicated for bacterial vaginosis; intravaginal clindamycin cream below [unlicensed use] and metronidazole gel [unlicensed use] can also be used. In pre-pubertal girls, intravaginal treatment is not recommended and oral treatment may be more appropriate. (E)

EvGr The antiviral drugs aciclovir p. 500 and valaciclovir p. 502 can be used in the treatment of genital infection due to herpes simplex virus; they have a beneficial effect on virus shedding, and reducing the severity and duration of episodes. (A) For further information, see Herpesvirus infections p. 498.

For information on the human papillomavirus vaccine, see Human papillomavirus vaccine p. 970.

4.1 Vaginal and vulval infections

4.1a Vaginal and vulval bacterial infections

ANTIBACTERIALS > LINCOSAMIDES

Clindamycin 22-Mar-2024

- **INDICATIONS AND DOSE**

DALACIN ® CREAM

Bacterial vaginosis

▶ BY VAGINA

▶ Child: 1 applicatorful once daily for 3–7 nights, dose to be administered at night

DOSE EQUIVALENCE AND CONVERSION

▶ 1 applicatorful delivers a 5 g dose of clindamycin 2%.

- **UNLICENSED USE** Not licensed for use in children.
- **CAUTIONS** Avoid intravaginal preparations (particularly those that require the use of an applicator) in young girls who are not sexually active, unless there is no alternative
- **INTERACTIONS** → Appendix 1: clindamycin
- **SIDE-EFFECTS**

▶ **Common or very common** Diarrhoea (discontinue) · skin reactions

▶ **Frequency not known** Constipation · dizziness · gastrointestinal discomfort · headache · increased risk of infection · nausea · vertigo · vomiting · vulvovaginal irritation

SIDE-EFFECTS, FURTHER INFORMATION Clindamycin 2% cream is poorly absorbed into the blood—low risk of systemic effects.

- **CONCEPTION AND CONTRACEPTION** Damages latex condoms and diaphragms.
- **PRESCRIBING AND DISPENSING INFORMATION** For choice of antibacterial therapy, see Genital system infections, antibacterial therapy p. 368.
- **PATIENT AND CARER ADVICE** Patients and their carers should be advised to discontinue and contact a doctor immediately if severe, prolonged or bloody diarrhoea develops.
- **MEDICINAL FORMS** There can be variation in the licensing of different medicines containing the same drug.

Vaginal cream

EXCIPIENTS: May contain Benzyl alcohol, cetostearyl alcohol (including cetyl and stearyl alcohol), polysorbates, propylene glycol

▶ **Dalacin** (Pfizer Ltd)

Clindamycin (as Clindamycin phosphate) 20 mg per 1 gram Dalacin 2% cream | 40 gram PoM £10.86 DT = £10.86

CARBOXYLIC ACIDS

Lactic acid 24-Nov-2020

- **INDICATIONS AND DOSE**

BALANCE ACTIV RX ® GEL

Prevention of bacterial vaginosis

▶ BY VAGINA

▶ Child: 5 mL 1–2 times a week, insert the content of 1 tube (5 mL)

- **ALLERGY AND CROSS-SENSITIVITY** EvGr Contra-indicated in shellfish allergy. (M)

- **MEDICINAL FORMS** There can be variation in the licensing of different medicines containing the same drug.

Products without form

EXCIPIENTS: May contain Propylene glycol

▸ **Balance Activ** (BBI Healthcare Ltd)
Balance Activ BV vaginal pH correction gel | 7 device £5.30

4.1b Vaginal and vulval fungal infections

Other drugs used for Vaginal and vulval fungal infections
Fluconazole, p. 463

ANTIFUNGALS > IMIDAZOLE ANTIFUNGALS

Clotrimazole

10-Nov-2021

- **INDICATIONS AND DOSE**

Superficial sites of infection in vaginal and vulval candidiasis (dose for 1% or 2% cream)

▸ BY VAGINA USING CREAM

▸ Child: Apply 2–3 times a day, to be applied to anogenital area

Vaginal candidiasis (dose for 10% intravaginal cream)

▸ BY VAGINA USING VAGINAL CREAM

▸ Child: 5 g for 1 dose, one applicatorful to be inserted into the vagina at night, dose can be repeated once if necessary

Vaginal candidiasis

▸ BY VAGINA USING PESSARIES

▸ Child: 200 mg once daily for 3 nights, course can be repeated once if necessary, alternatively 500 mg once daily for 1 night, dose can be repeated once if necessary

Recurrent vulvovaginal candidiasis

▸ BY VAGINA USING PESSARIES

▸ Child: 500 mg every week for 6 months, dose to be administered following topical imidazole for 10–14 days

- **UNLICENSED USE** Consult product literature for individual preparations.

- **CAUTIONS** Avoid intravaginal preparations (particularly those that require use of an applicator) in young girls who are not sexually active, unless there is no alternative
- **INTERACTIONS** → Appendix 1: antifungals, azoles
- **SIDE-EFFECTS** Abdominal pain · discomfort · genital peeling · oedema · paraesthesia · pelvic pain · skin reactions · vaginal haemorrhage
- **CONCEPTION AND CONTRACEPTION** Cream and pessaries may damage latex condoms and diaphragms.
- **PREGNANCY**

Dose adjustments Pregnant women need a longer duration of treatment, usually about 7 days, to clear the infection. Oral antifungal treatment should be avoided during pregnancy.

- **PATIENT AND CARER ADVICE**

Medicines for Children leaflet: Clotrimazole for fungal infections www.medicinesforchildren.org.uk/medicines/clotrimazole-for-fungal-infections/

- **EXCEPTIONS TO LEGAL CATEGORY** Brands for sale to the public include *Canesten*® Internal Cream.

- **MEDICINAL FORMS** There can be variation in the licensing of different medicines containing the same drug.

Pessary

EXCIPIENTS: May contain Benzyl alcohol, cetostearyl alcohol (including cetyl and stearyl alcohol), polysorbates

▸ **Canesten (clotrimazole)** (Bayer Plc)
Clotrimazole 100 mg Canesten 100mg pessaries | 6 pessary P £3.85 DT = £3.85
Clotrimazole 200 mg Canesten 200mg pessaries | 3 pessary P £3.41 DT = £3.41
Clotrimazole 500 mg Canesten 500mg pessaries | 1 pessary PoM £2.00 DT = £4.64

Cutaneous cream

EXCIPIENTS: May contain Benzyl alcohol, cetostearyl alcohol (including cetyl and stearyl alcohol), polysorbates

▸ **Clotrimazole (Non-proprietary)**
Clotrimazole 10 mg per 1 gram Clotrimazole 1% cream | 20 gram P £2.33 DT = £1.42 | 50 gram P £3.67 DT = £3.55

▸ **Canesten (clotrimazole)** (Bayer Plc)
Clotrimazole 10 mg per 1 gram Canesten 1% cream | 20 gram P £2.89 DT = £1.42 | 50 gram P £4.71 DT = £3.55
Clotrimazole 20 mg per 1 gram Canesten Thrush External 2% cream | 20 gram P £6.41 DT = £6.41

Vaginal cream

EXCIPIENTS: May contain Benzyl alcohol, cetostearyl alcohol (including cetyl and stearyl alcohol), polysorbates

▸ **Canesten (clotrimazole)** (Bayer Plc)
Clotrimazole 100 mg per 1 gram Canesten 10% vaginal cream | 5 gram PoM £4.50 DT = £8.36

Chapter 8 Immune system and malignant disease

CONTENTS

Immune system

1 Immune system disorders and transplantation

Immune response

13-Oct-2025

Inflammatory bowel disease

Azathioprine p. 638, mercaptopurine p. 671, or once weekly methotrexate p. 672 are used to induce remission in unresponsive or chronically active Crohn's disease. Azathioprine or mercaptopurine may also be helpful for retaining remission in frequently relapsing inflammatory bowel disease; once weekly methotrexate is used in Crohn's disease when azathioprine or mercaptopurine are ineffective or not tolerated. Response to azathioprine or mercaptopurine may not become apparent for several months. Folic acid p. 710 should be given to reduce the possibility of methotrexate toxicity. Folic acid is usually given weekly on a different day to the methotrexate; alternative regimens may be used in some settings.

Ciclosporin p. 640 (cyclosporin) is a potent immunosuppressant and is markedly nephrotoxic. In children with severe ulcerative colitis unresponsive to other treatment, ciclosporin may reduce the need for urgent colorectal surgery.

Immunosuppressant therapy

Immunosuppressants are used to suppress rejection in organ transplant recipients and to treat a variety of chronic inflammatory and autoimmune diseases. Solid organ transplant patients are maintained on drug regimens, which may include antiproliferative drugs (azathioprine or mycophenolate mofetil p. 648), calcineurin inhibitors (ciclosporin or tacrolimus p. 642), corticosteroids, or sirolimus p. 641. Choice is dependent on the type of organ, time after transplant, and clinical condition of the patient. Specialist management is required and other immunomodulators may be used to initiate treatment or to treat rejection.

Impaired immune responsiveness

Infections in the immunocompromised child can be severe and show atypical features. Specific local protocols should be followed for the management of infection. Corticosteroids may suppress clinical signs of infection and allow diseases such as septicaemia or tuberculosis to reach an advanced stage before being recognised— **important**: normal immunoglobulin administration should be considered as soon as possible after measles exposure in a non-immune child, and an antiviral [unlicensed use] and/or varicella-zoster immunoglobulin [unlicensed], or normal immunoglobulin [unlicensed use], may be required for non-immune neonates and children exposed to varicella (chickenpox) or herpes zoster (shingles); for further information, see Immunoglobulins p. 951 and Herpesvirus infections p. 498. Wherever possible, immunisation or additional booster doses for children with immunosuppression should be carried out either before immunosuppression occurs or deferred until an improvement in immunity has been seen. Specialist advice should be sought on the use of live vaccines for those being treated with immunosuppressive drugs.

Antiproliferative immunosuppressants

Azathioprine is widely used for transplant recipients and it is also used to treat a number of auto-immune conditions, usually when corticosteroid therapy alone provides inadequate control. It is metabolised to mercaptopurine, and doses should be reduced (to one quarter of the original dose in children) when allopurinol p. 685 is given concurrently.

Mycophenolate mofetil is metabolised to mycophenolic acid which has a more selective mode of action than azathioprine.

There is evidence that compared with similar regimens incorporating azathioprine, mycophenolate mofetil may reduce the risk of acute rejection episodes; the risk of opportunistic infections (particularly due to tissue-invasive cytomegalovirus) and the occurrence of blood disorders such as leucopenia may be higher. Children may suffer a high incidence of side-effects, particularly gastrointestinal effects, calling for temporary reduction in dose or interruption of treatment.

Cyclophosphamide p. 663 is less commonly prescribed as an immunosuppressant.

Corticosteroids and other immunosuppressants

The corticosteroids prednisolone p. 548 and dexamethasone p. 543 are widely used in paediatric oncology; they have a marked antitumour effect. Dexamethasone is preferred for acute lymphoblastic leukaemia whilst prednisolone may be used for Hodgkin's disease, non-Hodgkin's lymphoma, and B-cell lymphoma and leukaemia.

Dexamethasone is the corticosteroid of choice in paediatric supportive and palliative care. For children who are not receiving a corticosteroid as a component of their chemotherapy, dexamethasone may be used to reduce raised intracranial pressure, or to help control emesis when combined with an appropriate anti-emetic.

The corticosteroids are also powerful immunosuppressants. They are used to prevent organ transplant rejection, and in high dose to treat rejection episodes.

Ciclosporin (cyclosporin), a calcineurin inhibitor, is a potent immunosuppressant which is virtually non-myelotoxic but markedly nephrotoxic. It may be used in organ and tissue transplantation, for prevention of graft rejection following bone marrow, kidney, liver, pancreas, heart, lung, and heart-lung transplantation, and for prophylaxis and treatment of graft-versus-host disease. Ciclosporin also has a role in steroid-sensitive and steroid-resistant nephrotic syndrome; in corticosteroid-sensitive nephrotic syndrome it may be given with prednisolone.

Tacrolimus is also a calcineurin inhibitor. Although not chemically related to ciclosporin it has a similar mode of action and side-effects.

Other drugs used for Immune system disorders and transplantation Anakinra, p. 799 · Eculizumab, p. 702 · Hydroxychloroquine sulfate, p. 798 · Rituximab, p. 659 · Ruxolitinib, p. 692 · Tocilizumab, p. 800

ALKALOIDS › PLANT ALKALOIDS

Colchicine

04-Apr-2025

● **INDICATIONS AND DOSE**

Prophylaxis of familial Mediterranean fever (recurrent polyserositis) (under expert supervision)

▶ BY MOUTH

▸ Child 1 month–4 years: Initially 500 micrograms once daily, increased if necessary up to 2 mg daily in 1–2 divided doses, dose increased in increments, such as 250 micrograms, in patients who do not respond or those with amyloid nephropathy; monitor closely for side-effects

▸ Child 5–10 years: Initially 1 mg once daily, increased if necessary up to 2 mg daily in 1–2 divided doses, dose increased in increments, such as 250 micrograms, in patients who do not respond or those with amyloid nephropathy; monitor closely for side-effects

▸ Child 11–17 years: Initially 1.5 mg daily in 1–2 divided doses, increased if necessary up to 2 mg daily in 1–2 divided doses, dose increased in increments, such as 250 micrograms, in patients who do not respond or those with amyloid nephropathy; monitor closely for side-effects

DOSE ADJUSTMENTS DUE TO INTERACTIONS

▶ Manufacturer advises reduce dose by half with concurrent use of moderate inhibitors of CYP3A4.

▶ Manufacturer advises reduce dose by 75% (to one quarter of usual dose) with concurrent use of potent inhibitors of CYP3A4 or P-glycoprotein inhibitors; avoid concurrent use in patients with hepatic or renal impairment.

IMPORTANT SAFETY INFORMATION

MHRA/CHM ADVICE: COLCHICINE: REMINDER ON RISK OF SERIOUS AND FATAL TOXICITY IN OVERDOSE (NOVEMBER 2009)

Colchicine has a narrow therapeutic window and a risk of serious and fatal toxicity in overdose. Patients at particular risk are those with renal or hepatic impairment, gastro-intestinal or cardiac disease, and patients at extremes of age. Colchicine overdose is complex and specialist advice should be promptly obtained. There is often a delay of up to 6 hours before toxicity is apparent, and some features of toxicity may be delayed by 1 week or longer. Healthcare professionals are advised to refer all patients, even in the absence of early symptoms, for immediate medical assessment. Further information on the presentation and management of colchicine overdose is available from TOXBASE.

● **CONTRA-INDICATIONS** Blood disorders

● **CAUTIONS** Cardiac disease · gastro-intestinal disease

● **INTERACTIONS** → Appendix 1: colchicine

● **SIDE-EFFECTS**

▶ **Common or very common** Abdominal pain · diarrhoea · nausea · vomiting

▶ **Frequency not known** Agranulocytosis · alopecia · bone marrow disorders · gastrointestinal haemorrhage · kidney injury · liver injury · menstrual cycle irregularities · myopathy · nerve disorders · rash · sperm abnormalities · thrombocytopenia

Overdose Early signs of toxicity include abdominal pain, diarrhoea, nausea, and vomiting. Features after 1 to 7 days include arrhythmias, bone marrow depression, confusion, decreased cardiac output, hepatic impairment, hyperpyrexia, renal impairment, and respiratory distress.

● **PREGNANCY** Specialist sources indicate that, although teratogenicity was noted in *animal* studies, human data suggested risk to the fetus is low.

● **BREAST FEEDING** EvGr Present in milk. ⟨M⟩ Specialist sources indicate use with caution and note that no adverse effects have been reported in the breast-fed infant. Breast feeding can be delayed for 6–8 hours after a maternal dose to avoid peak milk concentrations.

● **HEPATIC IMPAIRMENT** EvGr Caution in mild to moderate impairment; avoid in severe impairment. ⟨M⟩

Dose adjustments EvGr Reduce initial dose by 50% in mild to moderate impairment. ⟨M⟩

● **RENAL IMPAIRMENT** EvGr Caution in mild to moderate impairment; avoid in severe impairment. ⟨M⟩

Dose adjustments EvGr Reduce initial dose by 50% in mild to moderate impairment. ⟨M⟩

● **MONITORING REQUIREMENTS** EvGr Monitor full blood count periodically in patients on long-term therapy. ⟨M⟩

● **DIRECTIONS FOR ADMINISTRATION** EvGr Some tablet formulations may be dispersed in water and taken orally immediately, or administered via a nasogastric tube—consult product literature. ⟨M⟩

● **PATIENT AND CARER ADVICE** Patients and their carers should be instructed to stop treatment and seek urgent medical attention if signs or symptoms of toxicity or blood disorders occur.

● **MEDICINAL FORMS** There can be variation in the licensing of different medicines containing the same drug.

Oral tablet

▸ Colchicine (Non-proprietary)

Colchicine 500 microgram Colchicine 500microgram tablets | 28 tablet PoM £2.54 | 100 tablet PoM £21.95 DT = £1.71

IMMUNE SERA AND IMMUNOGLOBULINS › IMMUNOGLOBULINS

Antithymocyte immunoglobulin (rabbit)

29-Sep-2025

● **INDICATIONS AND DOSE**

Prophylaxis of organ rejection in heart allograft recipients

▶ BY INTRAVENOUS INFUSION

▸ Child: 1–2.5 mg/kg daily for 3–5 days, start treatment on day of transplantation, to be given over at least 6 hours

continued →

Prophylaxis of organ rejection in renal allograft recipients
- BY INTRAVENOUS INFUSION
  - Child 1–17 years: 1–1.5 mg/kg daily for 3–9 days, start treatment on day of transplantation, to be given over at least 6 hours

Treatment of corticosteroid-resistant allograft rejection in renal transplantation
- BY INTRAVENOUS INFUSION
  - Child 1–17 years: 1.5 mg/kg daily for 7–14 days, to be given over at least 6 hours

DOSES AT EXTREMES OF BODY-WEIGHT
- To avoid excessive dosage in obese patients, calculate dose on the basis of ideal body weight.

- **CONTRA-INDICATIONS** Infection
- **INTERACTIONS** → Appendix 1: immunoglobulins
- **SIDE-EFFECTS**
  - **Common or very common** Chills · diarrhoea · dysphagia · dyspnoea · fever · hypotension · infection · lymphopenia · myalgia · nausea · neoplasm malignant · neoplasms · neutropenia · reactivation of infection · secondary malignancy · sepsis · skin reactions · thrombocytopenia · vomiting
  - **Uncommon** Cytokine release syndrome · hepatic disorders · hypersensitivity · infusion related reaction

  SIDE-EFFECTS, FURTHER INFORMATION Tolerability is increased by pretreatment with an intravenous corticosteroid and antihistamine; an antipyretic drug such as paracetamol may also be beneficial.
- **PREGNANCY** Manufacturer advises use only if potential benefit outweighs risk—no information available.
- **BREAST FEEDING** Manufacturer advises avoid—no information available.
- **MONITORING REQUIREMENTS** Monitor blood count.
- **DIRECTIONS FOR ADMINISTRATION** For *continuous intravenous infusion*, manufacturer advises reconstitute each vial with 5 mL Water for Injections to produce a solution of 5 mg/mL; gently rotate to dissolve. Dilute requisite dose with Glucose 5% *or* Sodium Chloride 0.9% to an approx. concentration of 0.5 mg/mL; begin infusion immediately after dilution; give through an in-line filter (pore size 0.22 micron); incompatible with heparin and hydrocortisone in glucose infusion—precipitation reported.
- **NATIONAL FUNDING/ACCESS DECISIONS**
  For full details see funding body website

  NICE decisions
  - **Immunosuppressive therapy for kidney transplant in children and young people (October 2017)** NICE TA482 Not recommended

- **MEDICINAL FORMS** There can be variation in the licensing of different medicines containing the same drug.

  Solution for infusion
  - **Antithymocyte immunoglobulin (rabbit) (Non-proprietary)**
    Antithymocyte immunoglobulin (rabbit) 20 mg per 1 ml Grafalon 100mg/5ml concentrate for solution for infusion vials | 1 vial PoM (Hospital only)

  Powder and solvent for solution for infusion
  - **Thymoglobulin** (Sanofi)
    Antithymocyte immunoglobulin (rabbit) 25 mg Thymoglobuline 25mg powder and solvent for solution for infusion vials | 1 vial PoM £158.77 (Hospital only)

IMMUNOSTIMULANTS › PROTEIN KINASE INHIBITORS

Leniolisib

29-Apr-2025

- **DRUG ACTION** Leniolisib is an inhibitor of the delta isoform of phosphoinositide-3 kinase (PI3Kδ) that restores normal development and proliferation of B- and T-lymphocytes, thereby normalising the hyperactive PI3Kδ pathway.

- **INDICATIONS AND DOSE**

  Activated phosphoinositide 3-kinase delta (PI3Kδ) syndrome (APDS)
  - BY MOUTH
    - Child 12–17 years (body-weight 45 kg and above): 70 mg twice daily, dose to be given approx. 12 hours apart

- **INTERACTIONS** → Appendix 1: leniolisib
- **SIDE-EFFECTS**
  - **Common or very common** Alopecia · arrhythmias · diarrhoea · fatigue · fever · headache · pain · sinusitis · skin reactions
- **CONCEPTION AND CONTRACEPTION** EvGr Females of childbearing potential should use effective contraception during treatment and for at least 1 week after last treatment. ⟨M⟩
- **PREGNANCY** EvGr Avoid (embryotoxic in *animal* studies). ⟨M⟩
- **BREAST FEEDING** EvGr Avoid during treatment and for 1 week after last treatment (present in milk in *animal* studies). ⟨M⟩
- **HEPATIC IMPAIRMENT** EvGr Avoid in moderate to severe impairment (no information available but leniolisib is extensively metabolised in the liver). ⟨M⟩
- **PATIENT AND CARER ADVICE**
  Missed doses If a dose is more than 6 hours late, the missed dose should not be taken and the next dose should be taken at the normal time.
- **NATIONAL FUNDING/ACCESS DECISIONS**
  For full details see funding body website

  NICE decisions
  - **Leniolisib for treating activated phosphoinositide 3-kinase delta syndrome in people 12 years and over (April 2025)** NICE HST33 Recommended

- **MEDICINAL FORMS** There can be variation in the licensing of different medicines containing the same drug.

  Oral tablet
  - **Joenja** (Pharming Technologies B.V.) ▼
    Leniolisib (as Leniolisib phosphate) 70 mg Joenja 70mg tablets | 60 tablet PoM £36,670.00 (Hospital only)

IMMUNOSUPPRESSANTS › ANTIMETABOLITES

Azathioprine

03-Jun-2025

- **DRUG ACTION** Azathioprine is metabolised to mercaptopurine.

- **INDICATIONS AND DOSE**

  Severe ulcerative colitis | Severe Crohn's disease
  - BY MOUTH
    - Child 2–17 years: Initially 2 mg/kg once daily, then increased if necessary up to 2.5 mg/kg once daily

  Systemic lupus erythematosus | Vasculitis | Autoimmune conditions usually when corticosteroid therapy alone has proved inadequate
  - BY MOUTH
    - Child: Initially 1 mg/kg daily, then adjusted according to response to 3 mg/kg daily, consider withdrawal if no

improvement within 3 months; maximum 3 mg/kg per day

Suppression of transplant rejection

▶ BY MOUTH, OR BY INTRAVENOUS INFUSION

▶ Child: Maintenance 1–3 mg/kg daily, adjusted according to response, consult local treatment protocol for details, oral route preferred, but if oral route is not possible then can be given by intravenous infusion, the total daily dose may alternatively be given in 2 divided doses

DOSE ADJUSTMENTS DUE TO INTERACTIONS

▶ Manufacturer advises reduce dose to one-quarter of the usual dose with concurrent use of allopurinol.

IMPORTANT SAFETY INFORMATION

MHRA/CHM ADVICE: THIOPURINES AND INTRAHEPATIC CHOLESTASIS OF PREGNANCY (MAY 2025)

Intrahepatic cholestasis of pregnancy (ICP) has been reported in a small number of patients taking azathioprine or mercaptopurine. Due to similar metabolic pathways, the risk of ICP is considered applicable to all drugs in the thiopurine class, including tioguanine. Thiopurine-induced ICP usually occurs earlier in pregnancy than non-drug-induced ICP and may not respond to ursodeoxycholic acid, however, stopping or reducing the dose of the thiopurine may improve liver-function tests. Some case reports resulted in fetal death, therefore early diagnosis and discontinuation or dose reduction of the thiopurine may minimise adverse effects in the fetus.

Healthcare professionals are advised to undertake a case-by-case assessment if ICP occurs and consider the risks versus benefits of stopping or continuing thiopurine treatment. Non-fasting serum-bile acids should be measured in patients with ICP to identify pregnancies at particular risk of spontaneous preterm birth (≥ 40 micromol/litre) or stillbirth (≥ 100 micromol/litre).

Patients and carers should be advised to seek immediate medical attention if signs or symptoms of ICP occur.

● **CAUTIONS** Reduced thiopurine methyltransferase activity

● **INTERACTIONS** → Appendix 1: azathioprine

● **SIDE-EFFECTS**

GENERAL SIDE-EFFECTS

▶ **Common or very common** Bone marrow depression (dose-related) · increased risk of infection · leucopenia · pancreatitis · thrombocytopenia

▶ **Uncommon** Anaemia · hepatic disorders · hypersensitivity

▶ **Rare or very rare** Agranulocytosis · alopecia · bone marrow disorders · diarrhoea · gastrointestinal disorders · neoplasms · photosensitivity reaction · pneumonitis · severe cutaneous adverse reactions (SCARs)

▶ **Frequency not known** Nodular regenerative hyperplasia · sinusoidal obstruction syndrome

SPECIFIC SIDE-EFFECTS

▶ With oral use Nausea

SIDE-EFFECTS, FURTHER INFORMATION Side-effects may require drug withdrawal.

Hypersensitivity reactions Hypersensitivity reactions (including malaise, dizziness, vomiting, diarrhoea, fever, rigors, myalgia, arthralgia, rash, hypotension and renal dysfunction) call for immediate withdrawal.

Neutropenia and thrombocytopenia Neutropenia is dose-dependent. Management of neutropenia and thrombocytopenia requires careful monitoring and dose adjustment.

● **ALLERGY AND CROSS-SENSITIVITY** EvGr Contra-indicated in hypersensitivity to mercaptopurine. (M)

● **PREGNANCY** Transplant patients immunosuppressed with azathioprine should not discontinue it on becoming pregnant. However, there have been reports of premature birth and low birth-weight following exposure to azathioprine, particularly in combination with corticosteroids. Spontaneous abortion has been reported following maternal or paternal exposure. Azathioprine is teratogenic in *animal* studies. The use of azathioprine during pregnancy needs to be supervised in specialist units. Treatment should not generally be initiated during pregnancy.

● **BREAST FEEDING** Present in milk in low concentration. No evidence of harm in small studies—use if potential benefit outweighs risk.

● **HEPATIC IMPAIRMENT** Manufacturer advises caution (impaired metabolism)—monitor liver function and complete blood count more frequently in those with severe impairment.

Dose adjustments Manufacturer advises use doses at lower end of the dose range in hepatic failure; reduce dose if hepatic or haematological toxicity occur.

● **RENAL IMPAIRMENT** EvGr Caution (may result in slower elimination)—monitor complete blood count more frequently in those with severe impairment. (M)

Dose adjustments EvGr Consider reducing starting dose (limited information available). (M)

● **PRE-TREATMENT SCREENING**

Thiopurine methyltransferase The enzyme thiopurine methyltransferase (TPMT) metabolises thiopurine drugs (azathioprine, mercaptopurine, tioguanine); the risk of myelosuppression is increased in patients with reduced activity of the enzyme, particularly for the few individuals in whom TPMT activity is undetectable. Manufacturer advises consider measuring TPMT activity before starting azathioprine, mercaptopurine, or tioguanine therapy. Seek specialist advice for those with reduced or absent TPMT activity.

● **MONITORING REQUIREMENTS**

▶ Monitor for toxicity throughout treatment.

▶ Monitor full blood count weekly (more frequently with higher doses or if severe renal impairment) for first 4 weeks (manufacturer advises weekly monitoring for 8 weeks but evidence of practical value unsatisfactory), thereafter reduce frequency of monitoring to at least every 3 months.

▶ Blood tests and monitoring for signs of myelosuppression are essential in long-term treatment.

● **DIRECTIONS FOR ADMINISTRATION**

▶ With intravenous use Consult local treatment protocol for details. For *intravenous infusion*, manufacturer advises reconstitute 50 mg with 5–15 mL Water for Injections; dilute requisite dose to a concentration of 0.25–2.5 mg/mL with infusion fluid. Expert sources advise give in Glucose 5% *or* Sodium Chloride 0.9%. Intravenous injection is alkaline and very irritant. Manufacturer advises intravenous route should therefore be used **only** if oral route not feasible and discontinued as soon as oral route can be tolerated.

● **PRESCRIBING AND DISPENSING INFORMATION** The RCPCH and NPPG recommend that, when a liquid special of azathioprine is required, the following strength is used: 50 mg/5 mL.

● **PATIENT AND CARER ADVICE**

Bone marrow suppression Patients and their carers should be warned to report immediately any signs or symptoms of bone marrow suppression e.g. inexplicable bruising or bleeding, infection.

Medicines for Children leaflet: Azathioprine for inflammatory bowel disease www.medicinesforchildren.org.uk/medicines/azathioprine-for-inflammatory-bowel-disease/

Medicines for Children leaflet: Azathioprine for renal transplant www.medicinesforchildren.org.uk/medicines/azathioprine-for-renal-transplant/
Medicines for Children leaflet: Azathioprine for severe atopic eczema www.medicinesforchildren.org.uk/medicines/azathioprine-for-severe-atopic-eczema/

- **MEDICINAL FORMS** There can be variation in the licensing of different medicines containing the same drug. Forms available from special-order manufacturers include: oral capsule, oral suspension, oral solution

Oral tablet

CAUTIONARY AND ADVISORY LABELS 21

- Azathioprine (Non-proprietary)
  Azathioprine 25 mg Azathioprine 25mg tablets | 28 tablet PoM £2.67 DT = £1.00 | 100 tablet PoM £3.18–£9.52
  Azathioprine 50 mg Azathioprine 50mg tablets | 56 tablet PoM £5.50 DT = £1.25 | 100 tablet PoM £3.25–£12.77
  Azathioprine 75 mg Azathioprine 75mg tablets | 100 tablet PoM £32.97
  Azathioprine 100 mg Azathioprine 100mg tablets | 100 tablet PoM £43.96

Oral suspension

- Jayempi (Nova Laboratories Ltd)
  Azathioprine 10 mg per 1 ml Jayempi 10mg/ml oral suspension | 200 ml PoM £250.00 DT = £250.00 SF

IMMUNOSUPPRESSANTS > CALCINEURIN INHIBITORS AND RELATED DRUGS

Ciclosporin

06-Feb-2026

(Cyclosporin)

- **DRUG ACTION** Ciclosporin inhibits production and release of lymphokines, thereby suppressing cell-mediated immune response.

- **INDICATIONS AND DOSE**

Refractory ulcerative colitis

▶ BY MOUTH

- Child 2–17 years: Initially 2 mg/kg twice daily (max. per dose 5 mg/kg twice daily), dose adjusted according to blood-ciclosporin concentration and response

▶ BY INTRAVENOUS INFUSION

- Child 3–17 years: Initially 0.5–1 mg/kg twice daily, dose adjusted according to blood-ciclosporin concentration and response

Short-term treatment of severe atopic dermatitis where conventional therapy ineffective or inappropriate (administered on expert advice)

▶ BY MOUTH

- Child: Initially 1.25 mg/kg twice daily (max. per dose 2.5 mg/kg twice daily) usual maximum duration of 8 weeks but may be used for longer under specialist supervision, if good initial response not achieved within 2 weeks, increase dose rapidly up to maximum

Short-term treatment of very severe atopic dermatitis where conventional therapy ineffective or inappropriate (administered on expert advice)

▶ BY MOUTH

- Child: 2.5 mg/kg twice daily usual maximum duration of 8 weeks but may be used for longer under specialist supervision

Severe psoriasis where conventional therapy ineffective or inappropriate (administered on expert advice)

▶ BY MOUTH

- Child: Initially 1.25 mg/kg twice daily (max. per dose 2.5 mg/kg twice daily), increased gradually to maximum if no improvement within 1 month, initial dose of 2.5 mg/kg twice daily justified if condition requires rapid improvement; discontinue if inadequate response after 3 months at the optimum dose; max. duration of treatment usually 1 year unless other treatments cannot be used

Prevention of graft rejection following bone-marrow, kidney, liver, pancreas, heart, lung, and heart-lung transplantation | Prevention and treatment of graft-versus-host disease

▶ BY MOUTH, OR BY INTRAVENOUS INFUSION

- Child: (consult local protocol)

Nephrotic syndrome

▶ BY MOUTH

- Child: 3 mg/kg twice daily, dose can be increased if necessary in corticosteroid-resistant disease; for maintenance reduce to lowest effective dose according to whole blood-ciclosporin concentrations, proteinuria, and renal function

DOSE ADJUSTMENTS DUE TO INTERACTIONS

- With oral use Manufacturer advises increase dose by 50% or switch to intravenous administration with concurrent use of octreotide.

- **UNLICENSED USE** Not licensed for use in children under 3 months. Not licensed for use in children under 16 years for atopic eczema (dermatitis) or psoriasis. Not licensed for use in ulcerative colitis.

IMPORTANT SAFETY INFORMATION

MHRA/CHM ADVICE: CICLOSPORIN MUST BE PRESCRIBED AND DISPENSED BY BRAND NAME (DECEMBER 2009)

Patients should be stabilised on a particular brand of oral ciclosporin because switching between formulations without close monitoring may lead to clinically important changes in blood-ciclosporin concentration.

- **CONTRA-INDICATIONS** Malignancy (in non-transplant indications) · uncontrolled hypertension (in non-transplant indications) · uncontrolled infections (in non-transplant indications)
- **CAUTIONS** Hyperuricaemia · in atopic dermatitis, active herpes simplex infections—allow infection to clear before starting (if they occur during treatment withdraw if severe) · in atopic dermatitis, *Staphylococcus aureus* skin infections—not absolute contra-indication providing controlled (but avoid erythromycin unless no other alternative) · in psoriasis treat, patients with malignant or pre-malignant conditions of skin only after appropriate treatment (and if no other option) · in uveitis, Behcet's syndrome (monitor neurological status) · lymphoproliferative disorders (discontinue treatment) · malignancy

CAUTIONS, FURTHER INFORMATION

- Malignancy In psoriasis, exclude malignancies (including those of skin and cervix) before starting (biopsy any lesions not typical of psoriasis) and treat patients with malignant or pre-malignant conditions of skin only after appropriate treatment (and if no other option); discontinue if lymphoproliferative disorder develops.

- **INTERACTIONS** → Appendix 1: ciclosporin
- **SIDE-EFFECTS**
  - **Common or very common** Appetite decreased · diarrhoea · electrolyte imbalance · eye inflammation · fatigue · fever · flushing · gastrointestinal discomfort · gingival hyperplasia · hair changes · headaches · hepatic disorders · hyperglycaemia · hyperlipidaemia · hypertension · hyperuricaemia · leucopenia · muscle complaints · nausea · paraesthesia · peptic ulcer · renal impairment (renal structural changes on long-term administration) · seizure · skin reactions · tremor · vomiting
  - **Uncommon** Anaemia · encephalopathy · oedema · thrombocytopenia · weight increased
  - **Rare or very rare** Gynaecomastia · haemolytic anaemia · idiopathic intracranial hypertension · menstrual disorder ·

Immune system and malignant disease 8

multifocal motor neuropathy · muscle weakness · myopathy · pancreatitis

- **Frequency not known** Pain in extremity · thrombotic microangiopathy

- **PREGNANCY** Crosses placenta; manufacturer advises avoid unless potential benefit outweighs risk—toxicity in *animal* studies.
- **BREAST FEEDING** Manufacturer advises avoid—present in milk.
- **HEPATIC IMPAIRMENT** Manufacturer advises caution in severe impairment (risk of increased exposure).
  Dose adjustments Manufacturer advises consider dose reduction in severe impairment to maintain blood-ciclosporin concentration in target range—monitor until concentration stable.
- **RENAL IMPAIRMENT** In non-transplant indications, manufacturer advises establishing baseline renal function before initiation of treatment; if baseline function is impaired in non-transplant indications, except nephrotic syndrome—avoid.
  Dose adjustments See p. 16. In nephrotic syndrome, manufacturer advises initial dose should not exceed 2.5 mg/kg daily in patients with baseline renal impairment. *During treatment* for non-transplant indications, manufacturer recommends if the estimated glomerular filtration rate decreases by more than 25% below baseline on more than one measurement, reduce dose by 25–50%. If the estimated glomerular filtration rate decrease from baseline exceeds 35%, further dose reduction should be considered (even if within normal range); discontinue if reduction not successful within 1 month.
- **MONITORING REQUIREMENTS**
  - Monitor whole blood ciclosporin concentration (trough level dependent on indication—consult local treatment protocol for details).
  - In long-term management of nephrotic syndrome, perform renal biopsies every 1–2 years.
- **DIRECTIONS FOR ADMINISTRATION**
  - With oral use Manufacturer advises mix solution with orange or apple juice, or other soft drink (to improve taste) immediately before taking (and rinse with more to ensure total dose). Do not mix with grapefruit juice. Total daily dose should be taken in 2 divided doses.
  - With intravenous use For intermittent *intravenous infusion*, manufacturer advises dilute to a concentration of 0.5–2.5 mg/mL with Glucose 5% *or* Sodium Chloride 0.9%; give over 2–6 hours; not to be used with PVC equipment. Observe patient for signs of anaphylaxis for at least 30 minutes after starting infusion and at frequent intervals thereafter.
- **PRESCRIBING AND DISPENSING INFORMATION**
  Brand name prescribing Prescribing and dispensing of ciclosporin should be by brand name to avoid inadvertent switching. If it is necessary to switch a patient to a different brand of ciclosporin, the patient should be monitored closely for changes in blood-ciclosporin concentration, serum creatinine, blood pressure, and transplant function (for transplant indications).
  Sandimmun® capsules and oral solution are available direct from Novartis for patients who cannot be transferred to a different oral preparation.
- **PATIENT AND CARER ADVICE** Patients and carers should be counselled on the administration of different formulations of ciclosporin. Manufacturer advises avoid excessive exposure to UV light, including sunlight. In psoriasis and atopic dermatitis, avoid use of UVB or PUVA.
  Medicines for Children leaflet: Ciclosporin for nephrotic syndrome www.medicinesforchildren.org.uk/medicines/ciclosporin-for-nephrotic-syndrome/
- **MEDICINAL FORMS** There can be variation in the licensing of different medicines containing the same drug.

Oral capsule

CAUTIONARY AND ADVISORY LABELS 11
EXCIPIENTS: May contain Ethanol, ethyl lactate, propylene glycol

- **Capimune** (Viatris UK Healthcare Ltd)
  Ciclosporin 25 mg Capimune 25mg capsules | 30 capsule PoM £13.05 DT = £18.37
  Ciclosporin 50 mg Capimune 50mg capsules | 30 capsule PoM £25.50 DT = £35.97
  Ciclosporin 100 mg Capimune 100mg capsules | 30 capsule PoM £48.50 DT = £68.28
- **Capsorin** (Morningside Healthcare Ltd)
  Ciclosporin 25 mg Capsorin 25mg capsules | 30 capsule PoM £11.14 DT = £18.37
  Ciclosporin 50 mg Capsorin 50mg capsules | 30 capsule PoM £21.80 DT = £35.97
  Ciclosporin 100 mg Capsorin 100mg capsules | 30 capsule PoM £41.59 DT = £68.28
- **Deximune** (Dexcel-Pharma Ltd)
  Ciclosporin 25 mg Deximune 25mg capsules | 30 capsule PoM £13.06 DT = £18.37
  Ciclosporin 50 mg Deximune 50mg capsules | 30 capsule PoM £25.60 DT = £35.97
  Ciclosporin 100 mg Deximune 100mg capsules | 30 capsule PoM £48.90 DT = £68.28
- **Neoral** (Novartis Pharmaceuticals UK Ltd)
  Ciclosporin 10 mg Neoral 10mg capsules | 60 capsule PoM £18.25 DT = £18.25
  Ciclosporin 25 mg Neoral 25mg capsules | 30 capsule PoM £18.37 DT = £18.37
  Ciclosporin 50 mg Neoral 50mg capsules | 30 capsule PoM £35.97 DT = £35.97
  Ciclosporin 100 mg Neoral 100mg capsules | 30 capsule PoM £68.28 DT = £68.28
- **Vanquoral** (Teva UK Ltd)
  Ciclosporin 25 mg Vanquoral 25mg capsules | 30 capsule PoM £13.05 DT = £18.37
  Ciclosporin 50 mg Vanquoral 50mg capsules | 30 capsule PoM £25.59 DT = £35.97
  Ciclosporin 100 mg Vanquoral 100mg capsules | 30 capsule PoM £48.89 DT = £68.28

Solution for infusion

CAUTIONARY AND ADVISORY LABELS 11
EXCIPIENTS: May contain Alcohol, polyoxyl castor oils

- **Sandimmun** (Novartis Pharmaceuticals UK Ltd)
  Ciclosporin 50 mg per 1 ml Sandimmun 250mg/5ml concentrate for solution for infusion ampoules | 10 ampoule PoM £110.05
  Sandimmun 50mg/1ml concentrate for solution for infusion ampoules | 10 ampoule PoM £23.23

Oral solution

CAUTIONARY AND ADVISORY LABELS 11
EXCIPIENTS: May contain Alcohol, propylene glycol

- **Neoral** (Novartis Pharmaceuticals UK Ltd)
  Ciclosporin 100 mg per 1 ml Neoral 100mg/ml oral solution | 50 ml PoM £102.30 DT = £102.30 SF

Sirolimus

19-Mar-2025

- **DRUG ACTION** Sirolimus is a non-calcineurin inhibiting immunosuppressant.

- **INDICATIONS AND DOSE**

As a component of immunosuppressive therapy for renal transplantation in children and adolescents only if intolerance necessitates the withdrawal of a calcineurin inhibitor

- BY MOUTH
  - Child: (consult local protocol)

DOSE EQUIVALENCE AND CONVERSION

- For *tablets*, the 500 microgram strength tablet is not bioequivalent to the 1 mg and 2 mg strength tablets. Multiples of 500 microgram tablets should **not** be used as a substitute for other tablet strengths.

- **UNLICENSED USE** Not licensed for use in children.

- **CAUTIONS** Hyperlipidaemia · increased susceptibility to infection (especially urinary-tract infection) · increased susceptibility to lymphoma and other malignancies, particularly of the skin (limit exposure to UV light)
- **INTERACTIONS** → Appendix 1: sirolimus
- **SIDE-EFFECTS**
  - **Common or very common** Abdominal pain · anaemia · arthralgia · ascites · constipation · diabetes mellitus · diarrhoea · dyslipidaemia · electrolyte imbalance · embolism and thrombosis · fever · haemolytic uraemic syndrome · haemorrhage · headache · healing impaired · hyperglycaemia · hypertension · increased risk of infection · interstitial lung disease · leucopenia · lymphatic vessel disorders · menstrual cycle irregularities · nausea · neoplasms · neutropenia · oedema · osteonecrosis · ovarian cyst · pain · pancreatitis · pericardial effusion · pleural effusion · proteinuria · sepsis · skin reactions · stomatitis · tachycardia · thrombocytopenia
  - **Uncommon** Clostridioides difficile colitis · focal segmental glomerulosclerosis · hepatic failure · nephrotic syndrome · pancytopenia · post transplant lymphoproliferative disorder
  - **Frequency not known** Posterior reversible encephalopathy syndrome (PRES)
- **CONCEPTION AND CONTRACEPTION** EvGr Ensure effective contraception during and for 12 weeks after treatment. (M)
- **PREGNANCY** EvGr Avoid unless essential (toxicity in *animal* studies). (M)
- **BREAST FEEDING** EvGr Discontinue breast-feeding (no information available). (M) Specialist sources also note a lack of data and that safer alternatives are preferable, especially with regards to premature infants, or in the neonatal period. However, the large molecular weight and high plasma-protein binding mean excretion into milk is unlikely, and poor oral bioavailability would suggest limited absorption by an infant, and so it may be compatible in some circumstances.
- **HEPATIC IMPAIRMENT** EvGr Caution (risk of increased exposure) (M).

  Dose adjustments In adults, manufacturer advises maintenance dose reduction in severe impairment—consult product literature.
- **MONITORING REQUIREMENTS** Monitor kidney function when given with ciclosporin; monitor lipids; monitor urine proteins.
- **DIRECTIONS FOR ADMINISTRATION** EvGr Food may affect absorption (take at the same time with respect to food). Sirolimus oral solution should be mixed with at least 60 mL water or orange juice in a glass or plastic container immediately before taking; refill container with at least 120 mL of water or orange juice and drink immediately (to ensure total dose). Do not mix with any other liquids. (M)
- **HANDLING AND STORAGE** Protect from light. Oral solution and topical gel: store in a refrigerator (2-8°C).
- **PATIENT AND CARER ADVICE** Advise patients to avoid excessive exposure to UV light including sunlight.
- **NATIONAL FUNDING/ACCESS DECISIONS**

  For full details see funding body website

  NICE decisions
  - **Immunosuppressive therapy for kidney transplant in children and young people (October 2017)** NICE TA482 Not recommended

  Scottish Medicines Consortium (SMC) decisions
  - **Sirolimus (*Hyftor*®) for the treatment of adult and paediatric patients aged 6 and above with facial angiofibroma associated with tuberous sclerosis complex (January 2025)** SMC No. SMC2710 Recommended

- **MEDICINAL FORMS** There can be variation in the licensing of different medicines containing the same drug.

Oral tablet

- **Sirolimus (Non-proprietary)**
  - **Sirolimus 500 microgram** Sirolimus 500microgram tablets | 30 tablet PoM £69.00 DT = £69.00
  - **Sirolimus 1 mg** Sirolimus 1mg tablets | 30 tablet PoM £86.49 DT = £86.49
  - **Sirolimus 2 mg** Sirolimus 2mg tablets | 30 tablet PoM £172.98 DT = £172.98
- **Rapamune** (Pfizer Ltd)
  - **Sirolimus 500 microgram** Rapamune 0.5mg tablets | 30 tablet PoM £69.00 DT = £69.00
  - **Sirolimus 1 mg** Rapamune 1mg tablets | 30 tablet PoM £86.49 DT = £86.49
  - **Sirolimus 2 mg** Rapamune 2mg tablets | 30 tablet PoM £172.98 DT = £172.98

Oral solution

EXCIPIENTS: May contain Ethanol

- **Rapamune** (Pfizer Ltd)
  - **Sirolimus 1 mg per 1 ml** Rapamune 1mg/ml oral solution | 60 ml PoM £162.41 DT = £162.41 SF

Tacrolimus

27-Sep-2024

- **DRUG ACTION** Tacrolimus is a calcineurin inhibitor.
- **INDICATIONS AND DOSE**

ADOPORT®

Prophylaxis of graft rejection following liver transplantation, starting 12 hours after transplantation

▶ BY MOUTH

- Neonate: Initially 150 micrograms/kg twice daily, then maintenance, dose to be adjusted according to response and whole blood-tacrolimus trough concentrations—doses are usually reduced in the post-transplant period.
- Child: Initially 150 micrograms/kg twice daily, then maintenance, dose to be adjusted according to response and whole blood-tacrolimus trough concentrations—doses are usually reduced in the post-transplant period

Prophylaxis of graft rejection following kidney transplantation, starting within 24 hours of transplantation

▶ BY MOUTH

- Neonate: Initially 150 micrograms/kg twice daily, then maintenance, dose to be adjusted according to response and whole blood-tacrolimus trough concentrations—doses are usually reduced in the post-transplant period.
- Child: Initially 150 micrograms/kg twice daily, a lower initial dose of 100 micrograms/kg twice daily has been used in adolescents to prevent very high 'trough' concentrations, then maintenance, dose to be adjusted according to response and whole blood-tacrolimus trough concentrations—doses are usually reduced in the post-transplant period

Prophylaxis of graft rejection following heart transplantation following antibody induction, starting within 5 days of transplantation

▶ BY MOUTH

- Neonate: Initially 50–150 micrograms/kg twice daily, then maintenance, dose to be adjusted according to response and whole blood-tacrolimus trough concentrations—doses are usually reduced in the post-transplant period.
- Child: Initially 50–150 micrograms/kg twice daily, then maintenance, dose to be adjusted according to response and whole blood-tacrolimus trough

concentrations—doses are usually reduced in the post-transplant period

Prophylaxis of graft rejection following heart transplantation without antibody induction, starting within 12 hours of transplantation

▶ BY MOUTH

- Neonate: Initially 150 micrograms/kg twice daily, dose to be given as soon as clinically possible (8–12 hours after discontinuation of intravenous infusion), then maintenance, dose to be adjusted according to response and whole blood-tacrolimus trough concentrations—doses are usually reduced in the post-transplant period.
- Child: Initially 150 micrograms/kg twice daily, dose to be given as soon as clinically possible (8–12 hours after discontinuation of intravenous infusion), then maintenance, dose to be adjusted according to response and whole blood-tacrolimus trough concentrations—doses are usually reduced in the post-transplant period

Allograft rejection resistant to conventional immunosuppressive therapy

▶ BY MOUTH

- Child: Seek specialist advice

MODIGRAF®

Prophylaxis of graft rejection following liver transplantation, starting 12 hours after transplantation

▶ BY MOUTH

- Neonate: Initially 150 micrograms/kg twice daily, then maintenance, dose to be adjusted according to response and whole blood-tacrolimus trough concentrations—doses are usually reduced in the post-transplant period.
- Child: Initially 150 micrograms/kg twice daily, then maintenance, dose to be adjusted according to response and whole blood-tacrolimus trough concentrations—doses are usually reduced in the post-transplant period

Prophylaxis of graft rejection following kidney transplantation, starting within 24 hours of transplantation

▶ BY MOUTH

- Neonate: Initially 150 micrograms/kg twice daily, then maintenance, dose to be adjusted according to response and whole blood-tacrolimus trough concentrations—doses are usually reduced in the post-transplant period.
- Child: Initially 150 micrograms/kg twice daily, a lower initial dose of 100 micrograms/kg twice daily has been used in adolescents to prevent very high 'trough' concentrations, then maintenance, dose to be adjusted according to response and whole blood-tacrolimus trough concentrations—doses are usually reduced in the post-transplant period

Prophylaxis of graft rejection following heart transplantation following antibody induction, starting within 5 days of transplantation

▶ BY MOUTH

- Neonate: Initially 50–150 micrograms/kg twice daily, then maintenance, dose to be adjusted according to response and whole blood-tacrolimus trough concentrations—doses are usually reduced in the post-transplant period.
- Child: Initially 50–150 micrograms/kg twice daily, then maintenance, dose to be adjusted according to response and whole blood-tacrolimus trough concentrations—doses are usually reduced in the post-transplant period

Prophylaxis of graft rejection following heart transplantation without antibody induction, starting within 12 hours of transplantation

▶ BY MOUTH

- Neonate: Initially 150 micrograms/kg twice daily, dose to be given as soon as clinically possible (8–12 hours after discontinuation of intravenous infusion), then maintenance, dose to be adjusted according to response and whole blood-tacrolimus trough concentrations—doses are usually reduced in the post-transplant period.
- Child: Initially 150 micrograms/kg twice daily, dose to be given as soon as clinically possible (8–12 hours after discontinuation of intravenous infusion), then maintenance, dose to be adjusted according to response and whole blood-tacrolimus trough concentrations—doses are usually reduced in the post-transplant period

Allograft rejection resistant to conventional immunosuppressive therapy

▶ BY MOUTH

- Child: Seek specialist advice

PROGRAF® CAPSULES

Prophylaxis of graft rejection following liver transplantation, starting 12 hours after transplantation

▶ BY MOUTH

- Neonate: Initially 150 micrograms/kg twice daily, then maintenance, dose to be adjusted according to response and whole blood-tacrolimus trough concentrations—doses are usually reduced in the post-transplant period.
- Child: Initially 150 micrograms/kg twice daily, then maintenance, dose to be adjusted according to response and whole blood-tacrolimus trough concentrations—doses are usually reduced in the post-transplant period

Prophylaxis of graft rejection following kidney transplantation, starting within 24 hours of transplantation

▶ BY MOUTH

- Neonate: Initially 150 micrograms/kg twice daily, then maintenance, dose to be adjusted according to response and whole blood-tacrolimus trough concentrations—doses are usually reduced in the post-transplant period.
- Child: Initially 150 micrograms/kg twice daily, a lower initial dose of 100 micrograms/kg twice daily has been used in adolescents to prevent very high 'trough' concentrations, then maintenance, dose to be adjusted according to response and whole blood-tacrolimus trough concentrations—doses are usually reduced in the post-transplant period

Prophylaxis of graft rejection following heart transplantation following antibody induction, starting within 5 days of transplantation

▶ BY MOUTH

- Neonate: Initially 50–150 micrograms/kg twice daily, then maintenance, dose to be adjusted according to response and whole blood-tacrolimus trough concentrations—doses are usually reduced in the post-transplant period.
- Child: Initially 50–150 micrograms/kg twice daily, then maintenance, dose to be adjusted according to response and whole blood-tacrolimus trough concentrations—doses are usually reduced in the post-transplant period

continued →

Prophylaxis of graft rejection following heart transplantation without antibody induction, starting within 12 hours of transplantation

▸ BY MOUTH

▸ Neonate: Initially 150 micrograms/kg twice daily, dose to be given as soon as clinically possible (8–12 hours after discontinuation of intravenous infusion), then maintenance, dose to be adjusted according to response and whole blood-tacrolimus trough concentrations—doses are usually reduced in the post-transplant period.

▸ Child: Initially 150 micrograms/kg twice daily, dose to be given as soon as clinically possible (8–12 hours after discontinuation of intravenous infusion), then maintenance, dose to be adjusted according to response and whole blood-tacrolimus trough concentrations—doses are usually reduced in the post-transplant period

Allograft rejection resistant to conventional immunosuppressive therapy

▸ BY MOUTH

▸ Child: Seek specialist advice

PROGRAF® INFUSION

Prophylaxis of graft rejection following liver transplantation, starting 12 hours after transplantation when oral route not appropriate

▸ BY CONTINUOUS INTRAVENOUS INFUSION

▸ Neonate: Initially 50 micrograms/kg/24 hours for up to 7 days (then transfer to oral therapy).

▸ Child: Initially 50 micrograms/kg/24 hours for up to 7 days (then transfer to oral therapy)

Prophylaxis of graft rejection following kidney transplantation, starting within 24 hours of transplantation when oral route not appropriate

▸ BY CONTINUOUS INTRAVENOUS INFUSION

▸ Neonate: Initially 75–100 micrograms/kg/24 hours for up to 7 days (then transfer to oral therapy).

▸ Child: Initially 75–100 micrograms/kg/24 hours for up to 7 days (then transfer to oral therapy)

Prophylaxis of graft rejection following heart transplantation without antibody induction, starting within 12 hours of transplantation

▸ BY CONTINUOUS INTRAVENOUS INFUSION

▸ Neonate: Initially 30–50 micrograms/kg/24 hours for up to 7 days (then transfer to oral therapy).

▸ Child: Initially 30–50 micrograms/kg/24 hours for up to 7 days (then transfer to oral therapy)

Allograft rejection resistant to conventional immunosuppressive therapy

▸ BY CONTINUOUS INTRAVENOUS INFUSION

▸ Child: Seek specialist advice (consult local protocol)

DOSE EQUIVALENCE AND CONVERSION

▸ For *Prograf*®: intravenous and oral doses are **not** interchangeable due to differences in bioavailability. Follow correct dosing recommendations for the dosage form when switching formulations.

IMPORTANT SAFETY INFORMATION

MHRA/CHM ADVICE: ORAL TACROLIMUS PRODUCTS: PRESCRIBE AND DISPENSE BY BRAND NAME ONLY, TO MINIMISE THE RISK OF INADVERTENT SWITCHING BETWEEN PRODUCTS, WHICH HAS BEEN ASSOCIATED WITH REPORTS OF TOXICITY AND GRAFT REJECTION (JUNE 2012; NOVEMBER 2017)

Inadvertent switching between oral tacrolimus products has been associated with reports of toxicity and graft rejection. To ensure maintenance of therapeutic response when a patient is stabilised on a particular brand, oral tacrolimus products should be prescribed and dispensed by brand name only.

- *Adoport*® and *Prograf*® are immediate-release capsules that are taken twice daily, once in the morning and once in the evening;
- *Modigraf*® granules are used to prepare an immediate-release oral suspension which is taken twice daily, once in the morning and once in the evening.

Switching between tacrolimus brands requires careful supervision and therapeutic monitoring by an appropriate specialist.

● **CAUTIONS** Increased risk of infections · increased susceptibility to lymphoproliferative disorders · malignancies · neurotoxicity · risk factors for cardiomyopathies · risk factors for QT-interval prolongation · UV light (avoid excessive exposure to sunlight and sunlamps)

● **INTERACTIONS** → Appendix 1: tacrolimus

● **SIDE-EFFECTS**

GENERAL SIDE-EFFECTS

▸ **Common or very common** Alopecia · anaemia · anxiety · appetite decreased · arrhythmias · ascites · asthenic conditions · bile duct disorders · confusion · consciousness impaired · constipation · coronary artery disease · cough · depression · diabetes mellitus · diarrhoea · dizziness · dysgraphia · dyslipidaemia · dyspnoea · electrolyte imbalance · embolism and thrombosis · eye disorder · febrile disorders · fluid imbalance · gastrointestinal discomfort · gastrointestinal disorders · gastrointestinal inflammatory disorders · haemorrhage · hallucination · headache · hepatic disorders · hyperglycaemia · hyperhidrosis · hypertension · hyperuricaemia · hypotension · increased risk of infection · interstitial lung disease · ischaemia · joint disorders · leucocytosis · leucopenia · metabolic acidosis · mood altered · muscle spasms · nasal complaints · nausea · nephropathy · nerve disorders · nervous system disorder · oedema · oral disorders · pain · peripheral vascular disease · primary transplant dysfunction · psychiatric disorder · renal impairment · renal tubular necrosis · respiratory disorders · seizure · sensation abnormal · skin reactions · sleep disorders · temperature sensation altered · thrombocytopenia · tinnitus · tremor · urinary tract disorder · urine abnormal · vision disorders · vomiting · weight changes

▸ **Uncommon** Asthma · cardiac arrest · cardiomyopathy · cataract · central nervous system haemorrhage · chest discomfort · coagulation disorders · coma · dysmenorrhoea · encephalopathy · feeling abnormal · haemolytic anaemia · hearing impairment · heart failure · hypoglycaemia · hypoproteinaemia · influenza like illness · memory loss · multi organ failure · neutropenia · palpitations · pancreatitis · pancytopenia · paralysis · paresis · photosensitivity reaction · psychotic disorder · shock · speech disorder · stroke · ventricular hypertrophy

▸ **Rare or very rare** Fall · hirsutism · mobility decreased · muscle tone increased · muscle weakness · pancreatic pseudocyst · pericardial effusion · QT interval prolongation · severe cutaneous adverse reactions (SCARs) · sinusoidal obstruction syndrome · thirst · ulcer

▸ **Frequency not known** Agranulocytosis · anaphylactoid reaction (due to excipient) · neoplasm malignant · neoplasms · polyomavirus-associated nephropathy · progressive multifocal leukoencephalopathy (PML) · pure red cell aplasia

SIDE-EFFECTS, FURTHER INFORMATION Cardiomyopathy has been reported to occur primarily in children with tacrolimus blood trough concentrations much higher than the recommended maximum levels. Patients should be monitored by echocardiography for hypertrophic changes—consider dose reduction or discontinuation if these occur.

- **ALLERGY AND CROSS-SENSITIVITY** EvGr Contra-indicated if history of hypersensitivity to macrolides. For *Prograf*® capsules, use only if benefit outweighs potential risk in patients with hypersensitivity to peanuts or soya (printing ink on the capsules contains soya lecithin). ⟨M⟩
- **CONCEPTION AND CONTRACEPTION** Exclude pregnancy before treatment.
- **PREGNANCY** Specialist sources indicate avoid unless benefit outweighs potential risk—crosses the placenta and risk of premature delivery, intra-uterine growth restriction, hyperkalaemia and renal toxicity. Maternal risk of hyperglycaemia, hypertension, pre-eclampsia and renal impairment.
- **BREAST FEEDING** Specialist sources indicate present in milk (following systemic administration) but amount probably too small to be harmful—monitor exclusively breastfed infants, including blood concentrations, if there are concerns regarding toxicity.
- **HEPATIC IMPAIRMENT** Manufacturer advises caution in severe impairment.
  Dose adjustments Manufacturer advises consider dose reduction in severe impairment.
- **MONITORING REQUIREMENTS**
  - EvGr After initial dosing, and for maintenance treatment, tacrolimus doses should be adjusted according to response and whole blood-tacrolimus trough concentrations (especially during episodes of diarrhoea). Patients of black African or African–Caribbean family origin may require higher doses. Consult local treatment protocols for further details of therapeutic drug monitoring.
  - Monitor blood pressure, ECG (for hypertrophic changes—risk of cardiomyopathy), fasting blood-glucose concentration, haematological and coagulation parameters, plasma protein, electrolytes, neurological (including visual) status, hepatic and renal function. Monitor for posterior reversible encephalopathy syndrome (PRES). ⟨M⟩
- **DIRECTIONS FOR ADMINISTRATION** For *continuous intravenous infusion* manufacturer advises give over 24 hours, dilute to a concentration of 4–100 micrograms/mL with Glucose 5% *or* Sodium Chloride 0.9%, to a total volume between 20–500mL. Tacrolimus is incompatible with PVC.
- **PRESCRIBING AND DISPENSING INFORMATION** The RCPCH and NPPG recommend that, when a liquid special of tacrolimus is required, the following strength is used: 5 mg/5 mL.
  PROGRAF® INFUSION Intravenous route should only be used if oral route is inappropriate.
- **PATIENT AND CARER ADVICE** Advise patients to avoid excessive exposure to UV light including sunlight and to report symptoms of eye disorders for prompt evaluation by an ophthalmologist.
  Medicines for Children leaflet: Tacrolimus for prevention of transplant rejection www.medicinesforchildren.org.uk/medicines/tacrolimus-for-prevention-of-transplant-rejection/
  Driving and skilled tasks May affect performance of skilled tasks (e.g. driving).
- **NATIONAL FUNDING/ACCESS DECISIONS**
  For full details see funding body website

NICE decisions

- **Immunosuppressive therapy for kidney transplant in children and young people [for immediate-release tacrolimus] (October 2017)** NICE TA482 Recommended with restrictions
- **Immunosuppressive therapy for kidney transplant in children and young people [for prolonged-release tacrolimus] (October 2017)** NICE TA482 Not recommended

Scottish Medicines Consortium (SMC) decisions

- **Tacrolimus granules for suspension (*Modigraf*®) for prophylaxis of transplant rejection in adult and paediatric, kidney, liver or heart allograft recipients or for treatment of allograft rejection resistant to treatment with other immunosuppressive medicinal products in adult and paediatric patients (December 2010)** SMC No. 657/10 Recommended with restrictions

- **MEDICINAL FORMS** There can be variation in the licensing of different medicines containing the same drug.

Oral capsule

CAUTIONARY AND ADVISORY LABELS 23
EXCIPIENTS: May contain Gelatin, lecithin, propylene glycol

- **Adoport** (Sandoz Ltd)
  Tacrolimus 500 microgram Adoport 0.5mg capsules | 50 capsule PoM £42.92 DT = £61.88
  Tacrolimus 1 mg Adoport 1mg capsules | 50 capsule PoM £55.69 DT = £80.28 | 100 capsule PoM £111.36
  Tacrolimus 5 mg Adoport 5mg capsules | 50 capsule PoM £205.74 DT = £296.58
- **Prograf** (Astellas Pharma Ltd)
  Tacrolimus 500 microgram Prograf 500microgram capsules | 50 capsule PoM £61.88 DT = £61.88
  Tacrolimus 1 mg Prograf 1mg capsules | 50 capsule PoM £80.28 DT = £80.28 | 100 capsule PoM £160.54
  Tacrolimus 5 mg Prograf 5mg capsules | 50 capsule PoM £296.58 DT = £296.58

Solution for infusion

EXCIPIENTS: May contain Polyoxyl castor oils

- **Prograf** (Astellas Pharma Ltd)
  Tacrolimus 5 mg per 1 ml Prograf 5mg/1ml solution for infusion ampoules | 10 ampoule PoM £584.51

Granules for oral suspension

CAUTIONARY AND ADVISORY LABELS 13, 23

- **Modigraf** (Astellas Pharma Ltd)
  Tacrolimus (as Tacrolimus monohydrate) 200 microgram Modigraf 0.2mg granules for oral suspension sachets | 50 sachet PoM £71.30 DT = £71.30 SF
  Tacrolimus (as Tacrolimus monohydrate) 1 mg Modigraf 1mg granules for oral suspension sachets | 50 sachet PoM £356.65 DT = £356.65 SF

IMMUNOSUPPRESSANTS › IMMUNOMODULATING DRUGS

Levamisole

01-May-2026

- **INDICATIONS AND DOSE**

Nephrotic syndrome (initiated under specialist supervision)

- BY MOUTH
- Child: 2.5 mg/kg once daily on alternate days (max. per dose 150 mg)

- **UNLICENSED USE** Not licensed.

IMPORTANT SAFETY INFORMATION

LEUKOENCEPHALOPATHY

An EU-wide safety review (February 2026) has confimed leukoencephalopathy as a rare but serious side-effect of levamisole, and therefore the EU marketing authorisation for the treatment of helminth infections has been withdrawn as the benefits do not outweigh the risks. Cases of leukoencephalopathy and CNS demyelination have been reported when levamisole is used for any indication, or in the context of misuse or accidental exposure. Leukoencephalopathy may occur even after a single dose, and symptoms may occur in a period of one day to several months after treatment. No risk factors or risk minimisation measures were identified.

- **CONTRA-INDICATIONS** Blood disorders

- **CAUTIONS** Epilepsy · juvenile idiopathic arthritis · Sjögren's syndrome
- **INTERACTIONS** → Appendix 1: levamisole
- **SIDE-EFFECTS** Arthralgia (long term use) · blood disorder (long term use) · diarrhoea · dizziness · headache · influenza like illness (long term use) · insomnia (long term use) · myalgia (long term use) · nausea · rash (long term use) · seizure (long term use) · taste altered (long term use) · vasculitis (long term use) · vomiting
- **PREGNANCY** Embryotoxic in *animal* studies, avoid if possible.
- **BREAST FEEDING** No information available.
- **HEPATIC IMPAIRMENT**
  Dose adjustments Use with caution—dose adjustment may be necessary.
- **PATIENT AND CARER ADVICE**
  Medicines for Children leaflet: Levamisole for nephrotic syndrome www.medicinesforchildren.org.uk/medicines/levamisole-for-nephrotic-syndrome/

- **MEDICINAL FORMS** There can be variation in the licensing of different medicines containing the same drug. Forms available from special-order manufacturers include: oral tablet

Oral tablet

CAUTIONARY AND ADVISORY LABELS 4

▸ **Ergamisol** (Imported (Belgium))
Levamisole (as Levamisole hydrochloride) 50 mg Ergamisol 50mg tablets | 20 tablet [PoM] [Ⓧ]

IMMUNOSUPPRESSANTS › INTERLEUKIN INHIBITORS

Satralizumab

11-Mar-2024

- **DRUG ACTION** Satralizumab is a recombinant humanised monoclonal antibody that inhibits interleukin-6 signalling.

- **INDICATIONS AND DOSE**

Neuromyelitis optica spectrum disorder (initiated under specialist supervision)

▸ BY SUBCUTANEOUS INJECTION

▸ Child 12–17 years (body-weight 40 kg and above): Initially 120 mg every 2 weeks for the first 3 doses, followed by maintenance 120 mg every 4 weeks

- **CAUTIONS** Active infection (delay treatment until infection is controlled) · immunisation
  CAUTIONS, FURTHER INFORMATION
  ▸ Immunisation [EvGr] Patients should receive all recommended vaccinations before starting treatment—immunisation during treatment has not been studied. Live or live attenuated vaccines should be avoided during treatment—safety is unknown. ⟨M⟩
- **INTERACTIONS** → Appendix 1: monoclonal antibodies
- **SIDE-EFFECTS**
  ▸ **Common or very common** Allergic rhinitis · arthralgia · bradycardia · gastritis · headaches · hyperlipidaemia · hypertension · hypofibrinogenaemia · injection related reaction · insomnia · musculoskeletal stiffness · peripheral oedema · skin reactions · weight increased
  SIDE-EFFECTS, FURTHER INFORMATION If increased liver transaminase, low platelet count, or low neutrophil count occurs treatment should be interrupted or discontinued—consult product literature.
- **PREGNANCY** [EvGr] Avoid (limited information available). ⟨M⟩
- **BREAST FEEDING** Specialist sources indicate use with caution, especially if breast-feeding a newborn or premature infant (limited information available). Risk of transfer to infant may be minimised by resuming treatment at least 2 weeks postpartum.
- **MONITORING REQUIREMENTS**
  ▸ [EvGr] Monitor liver transaminases every 4 weeks for the first 3 months of treatment, then every 3 months for 1 year, and as clinically indicated thereafter ⟨M⟩—consult product literature for further information.
  ▸ [EvGr] Monitor neutrophil count 4 to 8 weeks after starting treatment and as clinically indicated thereafter ⟨M⟩—consult product literature for further information.
- **DIRECTIONS FOR ADMINISTRATION** Inject into the thigh or abdomen (except for the 5 cm around the navel); rotate injection site and avoid moles, scars, or skin that is tender, bruised, red, hardened, or broken.
  Adult carers may administer *Enspryng*® after appropriate training in subcutaneous injection technique.
- **PRESCRIBING AND DISPENSING INFORMATION** Satralizumab is a biological medicine. Biological medicines must be prescribed and dispensed by brand name, see *Biological medicines* and *Biosimilar medicines*, under Guidance on prescribing p. 1; record the brand name and batch number after each administration.
- **HANDLING AND STORAGE** Store in a refrigerator (2–8°C) and protect from light and moisture—consult product literature for further information regarding storage outside refrigerator.
- **PATIENT AND CARER ADVICE** Patients and their carers should be instructed to seek early medical attention if signs and symptoms of infection develop during treatment.
  Self-administration Patients and their carers should be given training in subcutaneous injection technique if appropriate.
  A patient card should be provided.
  Missed doses For information on delayed or missed doses—consult product literature.

- **MEDICINAL FORMS** There can be variation in the licensing of different medicines containing the same drug.

Solution for injection

▸ **Enspryng** (Roche Products Ltd) ▼
Satralizumab 120 mg per 1 ml Enspryng 120mg/1ml solution for injection pre-filled syringes | 1 pre-filled disposable injection [PoM] £7,030.00 (Hospital only)

IMMUNOSUPPRESSANTS › MONOCLONAL ANTIBODIES

Canakinumab

17-May-2021

- **DRUG ACTION** Canakinumab is a recombinant human monoclonal antibody that selectively inhibits interleukin-1 beta receptor binding.

- **INDICATIONS AND DOSE**

Cryopyrin-associated periodic syndromes (specialist use only)

▸ BY SUBCUTANEOUS INJECTION

▸ Child 2–3 years (body-weight 7.5–14 kg): 4 mg/kg every 8 weeks, to be administered to the upper thigh, abdomen, upper arm or buttocks, additional doses may be considered if clinical response not achieved within 7 days—consult product literature

▸ Child 4–17 years (body-weight 7.5–14 kg): 4 mg/kg every 8 weeks, to be administered to the upper thigh, abdomen, upper arm or buttocks, additional doses may be considered if clinical response not achieved within 7 days—consult product literature

▸ Child 4–17 years (body-weight 15–40 kg): 2 mg/kg every 8 weeks, to be administered to the upper thigh, abdomen, upper arm or buttocks, additional doses may

be considered if clinical response not achieved within 7 days—consult product literature
- Child 4–17 years (body-weight 41 kg and above): 150 mg every 8 weeks, to be administered to the upper thigh, abdomen, upper arm or buttocks, additional doses may be considered if clinical response not achieved within 7 days—consult product literature

Tumour necrosis factor receptor associated periodic syndrome (specialist use only) | Hyperimmunoglobulin D syndrome (specialist use only) | Familial Mediterranean fever (specialist use only)

▶ BY SUBCUTANEOUS INJECTION
- Child 2–17 years (body-weight 7.5–40 kg): 2 mg/kg every 4 weeks, to be administered to the upper thigh, abdomen, upper arm or buttocks, a second dose may be considered if clinical response not achieved within 7 days—consult product literature
- Child 2–17 years (body-weight 41 kg and above): 150 mg every 4 weeks, to be administered to the upper thigh, abdomen, upper arm or buttocks, a second dose may be considered if clinical response not achieved within 7 days—consult product literature

Still's disease (specialist use only)

▶ BY SUBCUTANEOUS INJECTION
- Child 2–17 years (body-weight 7.5 kg and above): 4 mg/kg every 4 weeks (max. per dose 300 mg), to be administered to the upper thigh, abdomen, upper arm or buttocks

● **CONTRA-INDICATIONS** Active severe infection · leucopenia · neutropenia

● **CAUTIONS** History of recurrent infection · latent and active tuberculosis · predisposition to infection

CAUTIONS, FURTHER INFORMATION
- Vaccinations EvGr Patients should receive all recommended vaccinations (including pneumococcal and inactivated influenza vaccine) before starting treatment; avoid live vaccines unless potential benefit outweighs risk—consult product literature for further information. ⟨M⟩

● **INTERACTIONS** → Appendix 1: monoclonal antibodies

● **SIDE-EFFECTS**
- **Common or very common** Abdominal pain upper · arthralgia · asthenia · dizziness · increased risk of infection · leucopenia · neutropenia · pain · proteinuria · vertigo
- **Uncommon** Gastrooesophageal reflux disease

● **CONCEPTION AND CONTRACEPTION** Effective contraception required during treatment and for up to 3 months after last dose.

● **PREGNANCY** Manufacturer advises avoid unless potential benefit outweighs risk.

● **BREAST FEEDING** Consider if benefit outweighs risk—not known if present in human milk.

● **PRE-TREATMENT SCREENING** Patients should be evaluated for latent and active tuberculosis before starting treatment.

● **MONITORING REQUIREMENTS**
- Manufacturer advises monitor full blood count including neutrophil count before starting treatment, 1–2 months after starting treatment, and periodically thereafter.
- Manufacturer advises monitor for signs and symptoms of infection (including tuberculosis) during and after treatment.

● **HANDLING AND STORAGE** Manufacturer advises store in a refrigerator (2–8 °C).

● **PATIENT AND CARER ADVICE** Manufacturer advises patients and carers should be instructed to seek medical advice if signs or symptoms suggestive of tuberculosis (including persistent cough, weight loss and subfebrile temperature) occur.

Driving and skilled tasks Manufacturer advises patients and carers should be counselled on the effects on driving and performance of skilled tasks—increased risk of dizziness and drowsiness.

● **MEDICINAL FORMS** There can be variation in the licensing of different medicines containing the same drug.

Solution for injection
- **Ilaris** (Novartis Pharmaceuticals UK Ltd)
  Canakinumab 150 mg per 1 ml Ilaris 150mg/1ml solution for injection vials | 1 vial PoM £9,927.80
  Ilaris 150mg/1ml solution for injection pre-filled pens | 1 pre-filled disposable injection PoM £9,927.80 (Hospital only)

IMMUNOSUPPRESSANTS › MONOCLONAL ANTIBODIES › ANTI-LYMPHOCYTE

Basiliximab

23-Mar-2021

● **DRUG ACTION** Basiliximab is a monoclonal antibody that acts as an interleukin-2 receptor antagonist and prevents T-lymphocyte proliferation.

● **INDICATIONS AND DOSE**

Prophylaxis of acute rejection in allogeneic renal transplantation used in combination with ciclosporin and corticosteroid-containing immunosuppression regimens (specialist use only)

▶ BY INTRAVENOUS INJECTION, OR BY INTRAVENOUS INFUSION
- Child 1–17 years (body-weight up to 35 kg): Initially 10 mg, dose to be administered within 2 hours before transplant surgery, followed by 10 mg after 4 days, dose administered after transplant surgery, withhold second dose if severe hypersensitivity or graft loss occurs
- Child 1–17 years (body-weight 35 kg and above): Initially 20 mg, administered within 2 hours before transplant surgery, followed by 20 mg after 4 days, dose to be administered after surgery, withhold second dose if severe hypersensitivity or graft loss occurs

● **CAUTIONS** Off-label use in cardiac transplantation—increased risk of serious cardiac side-effects

● **INTERACTIONS** → Appendix 1: monoclonal antibodies

● **SIDE-EFFECTS** Capillary leak syndrome · constipation · cytokine release syndrome · dyspnoea · fever · heart failure · hypersensitivity · hypertension · hypertrichosis · hypotension · increased risk of infection · myocardial infarction · pulmonary oedema · respiratory disorders · sepsis · skin reactions · sneezing · tachycardia

● **CONCEPTION AND CONTRACEPTION** Adequate contraception must be used during treatment and for 16 weeks after last dose.

● **PREGNANCY** Manufacturer advises avoid—no information available.

● **BREAST FEEDING** Manufacturer advises avoid—no information available.

● **DIRECTIONS FOR ADMINISTRATION** For *intravenous infusion*, manufacturer advises dilute reconstituted solution to a concentration not exceeding 400 micrograms/mL, with Glucose 5% *or* Sodium Chloride 0.9%; give over 20–30 minutes.

● **NATIONAL FUNDING/ACCESS DECISIONS** For full details see funding body website

NICE decisions
- **Immunosuppressive therapy for kidney transplant in children and young people (October 2017)** NICE TA482 Recommended

- **MEDICINAL FORMS** There can be variation in the licensing of different medicines containing the same drug.

Powder and solvent for solution for injection

- Simulect (Novartis Pharmaceuticals UK Ltd)
  Basiliximab 10 mg Simulect 10mg powder and solvent for solution for injection vials | 1 vial PoM £758.69 (Hospital only)

Belimumab

28-Nov-2022

- **INDICATIONS AND DOSE**

Systemic lupus erythematosus (under expert supervision)

▶ BY INTRAVENOUS INFUSION

- Child 5–17 years: 10 mg/kg every 2 weeks for 3 doses, then 10 mg/kg every 4 weeks, review treatment if no response within 6 months

IMPORTANT SAFETY INFORMATION

MHRA/CHM ADVICE: BELIMUMAB (*BENLYSTA*®): INCREASED RISK OF SERIOUS PSYCHIATRIC EVENTS SEEN IN CLINICAL TRIALS (APRIL 2019)

Clinical trials show an increased risk of depression, suicidal ideation or behaviour, or self-injury in patients with systemic lupus erythematosus on belimumab. Healthcare professionals should assess patients for these risks before starting treatment, monitor for new or worsening signs of these risks during treatment, and advise patients to seek immediate medical attention if new or worsening symptoms occur.

- **CAUTIONS** Do not initiate until active infections controlled · history or development of malignancy · predisposition to infection
- **INTERACTIONS** → Appendix 1: monoclonal antibodies
- **SIDE-EFFECTS**

▶ **Common or very common** Depression · diarrhoea · fever · hypersensitivity · increased risk of infection · infusion related reaction · leucopenia · migraine · nausea · pain in extremity · skin reactions

▶ **Uncommon** Angioedema · suicidal behaviours

▶ **Frequency not known** Progressive multifocal leukoencephalopathy (PML) · psychiatric disorder · self-injurious behaviour · severe cutaneous adverse reactions (SCARs)

SIDE-EFFECTS, FURTHER INFORMATION Hypersensitivity reactions and infusion reactions can occur, and can be severe or life-threatening. Hypersensitivity reactions are possible several days after administration. Before infusion, premedication with an antihistamine, with or without an antipyretic may be considered.

- **CONCEPTION AND CONTRACEPTION** Manufacturer advises adequate contraception during treatment and for at least 4 months after last dose.
- **PREGNANCY** Avoid unless essential.
- **BREAST FEEDING** Avoid—present in milk in *animal* studies.
- **RENAL IMPAIRMENT** EvGr Caution in severe impairment (limited information available). ⓜ
- **MONITORING REQUIREMENTS** Delay in the onset of acute hypersensitivity reactions has been observed; patients should remain under clinical supervision for several hours following at least the first 2 infusions.
- **DIRECTIONS FOR ADMINISTRATION** EvGr For *intravenous infusion*, give intermittently in Sodium Chloride 0.9%; reconstitute with Water for Injections (120 mg in 1.5 mL, 400 mg in 4.8 mL) to produce a solution containing 80 mg/mL; gently swirl vial for 60 seconds, then allow to stand; swirl vial (without shaking) for 60 seconds every 5 minutes until dissolved; dilute requisite dose with infusion fluid to a final volume of 250 mL and give over 1 hour. ⓜ
- **PRESCRIBING AND DISPENSING INFORMATION** Belimumab is a biological medicine. Biological medicines must be prescribed and dispensed by brand name, see *Biological medicines* and *Biosimilar medicines*, under Guidance on prescribing p. 1; record the brand name and batch number after each administration.
- **HANDLING AND STORAGE** Store in a refrigerator (2–8°C) and protect from light.
- **PATIENT AND CARER ADVICE** Patients and their carers should be advised to seek immediate medical attention if signs or symptoms of infection or hypersensitivity reaction occur.
- **NATIONAL FUNDING/ACCESS DECISIONS**

For full details see funding body website

NICE decisions

▶ **Belimumab for treating active autoantibody-positive systemic lupus erythematosus (December 2021)** NICE TA752
Recommended with restrictions

Scottish Medicines Consortium (SMC) decisions

▶ **Belimumab powder for concentrate for solution for infusion (*Benlysta*®) as add-on therapy in patients aged 5 years and older with active, autoantibody-positive systemic lupus erythematosus (SLE) with a high degree of disease activity (e.g., positive anti-dsDNA and low complement) despite standard therapy (November 2022)** SMC No. SMC2477
Recommended with restrictions

All Wales Medicines Strategy Group (AWMSG) decisions

▶ **Belimumab powder for concentrate for solution for infusion (*Benlysta*®) for the treatment of systemic lupus erythematosus in children (August 2020)** AWMSG No. 3778
Recommended with restrictions

- **MEDICINAL FORMS** There can be variation in the licensing of different medicines containing the same drug.

Powder for solution for infusion

EXCIPIENTS: May contain Polysorbates

- Benlysta (GlaxoSmithKline UK Ltd) ▼
  Belimumab 120 mg Benlysta 120mg powder for concentrate for solution for infusion vials | 1 vial PoM £121.50 (Hospital only)
  Belimumab 400 mg Benlysta 400mg powder for concentrate for solution for infusion vials | 1 vial PoM £405.00 (Hospital only)

IMMUNOSUPPRESSANTS › PURINE SYNTHESIS INHIBITORS

Mycophenolate mofetil

05-Oct-2021

- **INDICATIONS AND DOSE**

Prophylaxis of acute rejection in renal transplantation (in combination with a corticosteroid and ciclosporin) (under expert supervision)

▶ BY MOUTH

- Child: 600 mg/m^2 twice daily (max. per dose 1000 mg), consult local protocol for details

Prophylaxis of acute rejection in renal transplantation (in combination with a corticosteroid and tacrolimus) (under expert supervision)

▶ BY MOUTH

- Child: 300 mg/m^2 twice daily (max. per dose 1000 mg), consult local protocol for details

Prophylaxis of acute rejection in hepatic transplantation (in combination with a corticosteroid and ciclosporin or tacrolimus) (under expert supervision)

▶ BY MOUTH

- Child: 10 mg/kg twice daily (max. per dose 1000 mg), dose can be increased to 20 mg/kg twice daily, consult local protocol for details

- **UNLICENSED USE** Not licensed for use in children under 2 years for the prophylaxis of acute rejection in renal transplantation. Not licensed for use in children for the prophylaxis of acute rejection in hepatic transplantation.

> **IMPORTANT SAFETY INFORMATION**
>
> **MHRA/CHM ADVICE: MYCOPHENOLATE MOFETIL, MYCOPHENOLIC ACID: UPDATED CONTRACEPTION ADVICE FOR MALE PATIENTS (FEBRUARY 2018)**
>
> Available clinical evidence does not indicate an increased risk of malformations or miscarriage in pregnancies where the father was taking mycophenolate medicines, however mycophenolate mofetil and mycophenolic acid are genotoxic and a risk cannot be fully excluded; for further information, see *Conception and contraception* and *Patient and carer advice*.

- **CAUTIONS** Active serious gastro-intestinal disease (risk of haemorrhage, ulceration and perforation) · children (higher incidence of side-effects may call for temporary reduction of dose or interruption) · delayed graft function · increased susceptibility to skin cancer (avoid exposure to strong sunlight) · risk of hypogammaglobulinaemia or bronchiectasis when used in combination with other immunosuppressants

CAUTIONS, FURTHER INFORMATION

- Hypogammaglobulinaemia or bronchiectasis Measure serum immunoglobulin levels if recurrent infections develop, and consider bronchiectasis or pulmonary fibrosis if persistent respiratory symptoms such as cough and dyspnoea develop.

- **INTERACTIONS** → Appendix 1: mycophenolate
- **SIDE-EFFECTS**
  - **Common or very common** Acidosis · alopecia · anaemia · anxiety · appetite decreased · arthralgia · asthenia · bone marrow disorders · burping · chills · confusion · constipation · cough · depression · diarrhoea · dizziness · drowsiness · dyslipidaemia · dyspnoea · electrolyte imbalance · fever · gastrointestinal discomfort · gastrointestinal disorders · gastrointestinal haemorrhage · gout · headache · hepatic disorders · hyperbilirubinaemia · hyperglycaemia · hypertension · hyperuricaemia · hypotension · increased risk of infection · insomnia · leucocytosis · leucopenia · malaise · nausea · neoplasms · neuromuscular dysfunction · oedema · oral disorders · pain · pancreatitis · paraesthesia · renal impairment · respiratory disorders · seizure · sepsis · skin reactions · tachycardia · taste altered · thinking abnormal · thrombocytopenia · tremor · vasodilation · vomiting · weight decreased
  - **Uncommon** Agranulocytosis
  - **Frequency not known** Endocarditis · hypogammaglobulinaemia · interstitial lung disease · malignancy · meningitis · neutropenia · polyomavirus-associated nephropathy · progressive multifocal leukoencephalopathy (PML) · pulmonary fibrosis · pure red cell aplasia

SIDE-EFFECTS, FURTHER INFORMATION Cases of pure red cell aplasia have been reported with mycophenolate mofetil; dose reduction or discontinuation should be considered under specialist supervision.

- **CONCEPTION AND CONTRACEPTION**

Pregnancy prevention The MHRA advises to exclude pregnancy in females of child-bearing potential before treatment—2 pregnancy tests 8–10 days apart are recommended. Women should use at least 1 method of effective contraception before and during treatment, and for 6 weeks after discontinuation—2 methods of effective contraception are preferred. Male patients or their female partner should use effective contraception during treatment and for 90 days after discontinuation.

- **PREGNANCY** Avoid unless no suitable alternative—congenital malformations and spontaneous abortions reported.
- **BREAST FEEDING** Manufacturer advises avoid—present in milk in *animal* studies.
- **RENAL IMPAIRMENT**

Dose adjustments Manufacturer advises consider dose reduction if estimated glomerular filtration rate less than 25 mL/minute/1.73 m^2.

- **MONITORING REQUIREMENTS** Monitor full blood count every week for 4 weeks then twice a month for 2 months then every month in the first year (consider interrupting treatment if neutropenia develops).
- **PRESCRIBING AND DISPENSING INFORMATION** Tablets and capsules not appropriate for dose titration in children with body surface are less than 1.25 m^2.
- **PATIENT AND CARER ADVICE**

Pregnancy prevention advice The MHRA advises that prescribers should ensure that female patients understand the need to comply with the pregnancy prevention advice, and they should be informed to seek immediate medical attention if there is a possibility of pregnancy; male patients planning to conceive children should be informed of the implications of both immunosuppression and the effect of the prescribed medications on the pregnancy.

Bone marrow suppression Patients should be warned to report immediately any signs or symptoms of bone marrow suppression e.g. infection or inexplicable bruising or bleeding.

Medicines for Children leaflet: Mycophenolate mofetil for nephrotic syndrome www.medicinesforchildren.org.uk/medicines/mycophenolate-mofetil-for-nephrotic-syndrome/

- **NATIONAL FUNDING/ACCESS DECISIONS**

For full details see funding body website

NICE decisions

- **Immunosuppressive therapy for kidney transplant in children and young people (October 2017)** NICE TA482 Recommended

---

- **MEDICINAL FORMS** There can be variation in the licensing of different medicines containing the same drug. Forms available from special-order manufacturers include: oral suspension

Oral tablet

- **Mycophenolate mofetil (Non-proprietary)**
  Mycophenolate mofetil 500 mg Mycophenolate mofetil 500mg tablets | 50 tablet [PoM] £74.03 DT = £5.52
- **CellCept** (Roche Products Ltd)
  Mycophenolate mofetil 500 mg CellCept 500mg tablets | 50 tablet [PoM] £82.26 DT = £5.52
- **Myfenax** (Teva UK Ltd)
  Mycophenolate mofetil 500 mg Myfenax 500mg tablets | 50 tablet [PoM] £78.15 DT = £5.52

Oral suspension

EXCIPIENTS: May contain Aspartame

- **Mycophenolate mofetil (Non-proprietary)**
  Mycophenolate mofetil 200 mg per 1 ml Mycophenolate mofetil 1g/5ml oral suspension sugar free | 175 ml [PoM] £115.16-£180.00 [SF]
- **CellCept** (Roche Products Ltd)
  Mycophenolate mofetil 200 mg per 1 ml CellCept 1g/5ml oral suspension | 160 ml [PoM] £115.16 DT = £115.16 [SF]

Oral capsule

- **Mycophenolate mofetil (Non-proprietary)**
  Mycophenolate mofetil 250 mg Mycophenolate mofetil 250mg capsules | 100 capsule [PoM] £82.26 DT = £14.71
- **CellCept** (Roche Products Ltd)
  Mycophenolate mofetil 250 mg CellCept 250mg capsules | 100 capsule [PoM] £82.26 DT = £14.71
- **Myfenax** (Teva UK Ltd)
  Mycophenolate mofetil 250 mg Myfenax 250mg capsules | 100 capsule [PoM] £78.15 DT = £14.71

RHO KINASE INHIBITORS

Belumosudil
05-Mar-2024

● **INDICATIONS AND DOSE**

Chronic graft-versus-host disease (under expert supervision)

▶ BY MOUTH

▸ Child 12–17 years: 200 mg once daily

DOSE ADJUSTMENTS DUE TO INTERACTIONS

▸ EvGr Increase dose to 200 mg twice daily with concurrent use of potent CYP3A4 inducers or proton pump inhibitors. (M)

● **INTERACTIONS** → Appendix 1: belumosudil

● **SIDE-EFFECTS**

▶ **Common or very common** Anaemia · appetite decreased · arthralgia · asthenia · constipation · cough · diarrhoea · dizziness · dyspnoea · fever · gastrointestinal discomfort · headache · hyperglycaemia · hypertension · increased risk of infection · leucopenia · malaise · muscle spasms · nausea · neutropenia · oedema · pain · peripheral neuropathy · pruritus · swelling · vomiting · weight decreased

▶ **Frequency not known** Microangiopathic haemolytic anaemia · multi organ failure

● **CONCEPTION AND CONTRACEPTION** EvGr Females of childbearing potential and male patients, if their female partner is of childbearing potential, should use highly effective contraception during treatment and for at least 1 week after the last treatment. (M)

● **PREGNANCY** EvGr Avoid—toxicity in *animal* studies. (M)

● **BREAST FEEDING** EvGr Avoid during treatment and for at least 1 week after the last treatment—no information available. (M)

● **HEPATIC IMPAIRMENT** EvGr Caution in severe impairment (no information available); increased exposure in mild or moderate impairment—no dose adjustment required. (M)

● **MONITORING REQUIREMENTS**

▶ EvGr A complete blood count should be performed before starting treatment.

▶ Monitor liver function tests before starting treatment and at least monthly during treatment. Treatment should be withheld or permanently discontinued in patients who develop hepatotoxicity—consult product literature. (M)

● **PATIENT AND CARER ADVICE**

Vomiting If vomiting occurs after taking tablets, no additional dose should be taken on that day and the next dose should be taken at the usual time.

Missed doses If a dose is more than 12 hours late, the missed dose should not be taken and the next dose should be taken at the normal time.

Driving and skilled tasks Patients and carers should be cautioned on the effects on driving and performance of skilled tasks—increased risk of fatigue and dizziness.

● **NATIONAL FUNDING/ACCESS DECISIONS**

For full details see funding body website

NICE decisions

▶ **Belumosudil for treating chronic graft-versus-host disease after 2 or more systemic treatments in people 12 years and over (February 2024)** NICE TA949 Recommended

● **MEDICINAL FORMS** There can be variation in the licensing of different medicines containing the same drug.

Oral tablet

CAUTIONARY AND ADVISORY LABELS 21

▸ Rezurock (Sanofi) ▼

Belumosudil (as Belumosudil mesilate) 200 mg Rezurock 200mg tablets | 30 tablet PoM £6,708.00

1.1 Multiple sclerosis

IMMUNOSUPPRESSANTS › IMMUNOMODULATING DRUGS

Fingolimod
18-Jan-2023

● **DRUG ACTION** Fingolimod is a sphingosine-1-phosphate receptor modulator, which prevents movement of lymphocytes out of lymph nodes, thereby limiting inflammation in the central nervous system.

● **INDICATIONS AND DOSE**

Multiple sclerosis (initiated by a specialist)

▶ BY MOUTH

▸ Child 10–17 years (body-weight up to 40 kg): 250 micrograms once daily

▸ Child 10–17 years (body-weight 40 kg and above): 500 micrograms once daily

IMPORTANT SAFETY INFORMATION

MHRA/CHM ADVICE: FINGOLIMOD—NOT RECOMMENDED FOR PATIENTS AT KNOWN RISK OF CARDIOVASCULAR EVENTS. ADVICE FOR EXTENDED MONITORING FOR THOSE WITH SIGNIFICANT BRADYCARDIA OR HEART BLOCK AFTER THE FIRST DOSE AND FOLLOWING TREATMENT INTERRUPTION (JANUARY 2013)

Fingolimod is known to cause transient bradycardias and heart block after the first dose—see *Cautions*, *Contra-indications*, and *Monitoring* for further information.

MHRA/CHM ADVICE: FINGOLIMOD: NEW CONTRA-INDICATIONS IN RELATION TO CARDIAC RISK (DECEMBER 2017)

Fingolimod can cause persistent bradycardia, which can increase the risk of serious cardiac arrhythmias. New contra-indications have been introduced for patients with pre-existing cardiac disorders—see *Contra-indications* for further information.

MHRA/CHM ADVICE: MULTIPLE SCLEROSIS THERAPIES: SIGNAL OF REBOUND EFFECT AFTER STOPPING OR SWITCHING THERAPY (APRIL 2017)

A signal of rebound syndrome in multiple sclerosis patients whose treatment with fingolimod was stopped or switched to other treatments has been reported in two recently published articles. The MHRA advise to be vigilant for such events and report any suspected adverse effects relating to fingolimod, or other treatments for multiple sclerosis, via the Yellow Card Scheme, while this report is under investigation.

MHRA/CHM ADVICE: FINGOLIMOD: UPDATED ADVICE ABOUT RISK OF CANCERS AND SERIOUS INFECTIONS (DECEMBER 2017)

Fingolimod has an immunosuppressive effect and can increase the risk of skin cancers and lymphoma. Following a recent EU review, the MHRA has recommended the following strengthened warnings:

- re-assess the benefit-risk balance of fingolimod therapy in individual patients, particularly those with additional risk factors for malignancy—either closely monitor for skin cancers or consider discontinuation on a case-by-case basis
- examine all patients for skin lesions before they start fingolimod and then re-examine at least every 6 to 12 months
- advise patients to protect themselves against UV radiation exposure and seek urgent medical advice if they notice any skin lesions
- refer patients with suspicious lesions to a dermatologist

Fingolimod has also been associated with risk of fatal fungal infections and reports of progressive multifocal leukoencephalopathy (PML)—see *Monitoring* and *Side effects* for further information.

MHRA/CHM ADVICE: FINGOLIMOD (*GILENYA*®): INCREASED RISK OF CONGENITAL MALFORMATIONS; NEW CONTRA-INDICATION DURING PREGNANCY AND IN WOMEN OF CHILDBEARING POTENTIAL NOT USING EFFECTIVE CONTRACEPTION (SEPTEMBER 2019)

An increased risk of major congenital malformations, including cardiac, renal, and musculoskeletal defects, has been associated with the use of fingolimod in pregnancy. Females of childbearing potential must use effective contraception during, and for 2 months after stopping, treatment. Healthcare professionals are advised that fingolimod is contra-indicated in pregnancy and that female patients should be informed of the risk of congenital malformations and given a pregnancy-specific patient reminder card. Pregnancy should be excluded before starting treatment, and pregnancy testing repeated at suitable intervals during treatment. Fingolimod should be stopped 2 months before planning a pregnancy. If a female taking fingolimod becomes pregnant, treatment should be stopped immediately, and the patient referred to an obstetrician for close monitoring. Exposed pregnancies should be enrolled on the pregnancy registry.

MHRA/CHM ADVICE: FINGOLIMOD (*GILENYA*®): UPDATED ADVICE ABOUT THE RISKS OF SERIOUS LIVER INJURY AND HERPES MENINGOENCEPHALITIS (JANUARY 2021)

A European review of safety data identified 7 cases of clinically significant liver injury that developed between 10 days and 5 years of starting fingolimod, including 3 reports of acute hepatic failure requiring liver transplantation. The guidance for monitoring liver function and criteria for discontinuation have been strengthened to minimise the risks of liver injury.

Liver function tests including serum bilirubin should be performed before starting and during treatment at months 1, 3, 6, 9, and 12, then periodically thereafter until 2 months after discontinuation.

In the absence of clinical symptoms, if liver transaminases (AST or ALT) exceed:

- 3 times the upper limit of normal (ULN) but less than 5 times the ULN without increase in serum bilirubin, liver function tests should be monitored more frequently;
- 5 times the ULN or at least 3 times the ULN with any increase in serum bilirubin, fingolimod should be discontinued; treatment may be restarted when serum levels have returned to normal, after careful benefit-risk assessment of the underlying cause.

In the presence of clinical symptoms suggestive of hepatic dysfunction, liver function tests should be checked promptly and fingolimod discontinued if significant liver injury is confirmed; further treatment may be restarted after recovery, only if an alternative cause of hepatic dysfunction is established.

The review also considered reported cases of herpes zoster/herpes simplex infections with visceral or CNS dissemination (e.g. herpes meningoencephalitis), some of which were fatal. Healthcare professionals are reminded to continue to be vigilant for infections with fingolimod.

Patients should be advised to seek urgent medical attention if they develop any signs or symptoms of liver injury or brain infection (during fingolimod treatment and for 8 weeks after the last dose in the case of the latter).

- **CONTRA-INDICATIONS** Active malignancies · baseline QTc interval 500 milliseconds or greater · cerebrovascular disease (including transient ischaemic attack) in the previous 6 months · decompensated heart failure (requiring inpatient treatment) in the previous 6 months · heart failure in the previous 6 months (New York Heart Association class III/IV) · increased risk for opportunistic infections (including immunosuppression) · myocardial infarction in the previous 6 months · second-degree Mobitz type II atrioventricular block or third-degree AV block, or sick-sinus syndrome, if the patient does not have a pacemaker · severe active infection · severe cardiac arrhythmias requiring treatment with class Ia or class III anti-arrhythmic drugs · unstable angina in the previous 6 months
- **CAUTIONS** Body-weight less than 40 kg (limited information available) · check varicella zoster virus status—consult product literature for further information · children should be brought up-to-date with current immunisation schedule before starting treatment · children under 12 years (limited information available) · chronic obstructive pulmonary disease · history of myocardial infarction · history of symptomatic bradycardia or recurrent syncope · patients receiving anti-arrhythmic or heart-rate lowering drugs, including beta-blockers and heart rate-lowering calcium-channel blockers (seek advice from cardiologist regarding switching to alternative drugs, or appropriate monitoring if unable to switch) · pulmonary fibrosis · severe respiratory disease · severe sleep apnoea · significant QT prolongation (QTc greater than 460 milliseconds in females, or QTc greater than 450 milliseconds in males); if QTc 500 milliseconds or greater—see *Contra-indications* · susceptibility to QT-interval prolongation (including electrolyte disturbances) · Tanner stage I (limited information available) · uncontrolled hypertension

CAUTIONS, FURTHER INFORMATION

- Washout period A washout period is recommended when switching treatment from some disease modifying therapies—consult product literature for further information.
- Bradycardia and cardiac rhythm disturbance Fingolimod may cause transient bradycardia, atrioventricular conduction delays and heart block after the first dose. Fingolimod is not recommended in patients with the cardiovascular risks listed above unless the anticipated benefits outweigh the potential risks, and advice from a cardiologist (including monitoring advice) is sought before initiation.

- **INTERACTIONS** → Appendix 1: fingolimod
- **SIDE-EFFECTS**
  - **Common or very common** Alopecia · arthralgia · asthenia · atrioventricular block · back pain · bradycardia · cough · decreased leucocytes · depression · diarrhoea · dizziness · dyspnoea · headaches · hypertension · increased risk of infection · myalgia · neoplasms · skin reactions · vision blurred · weight decreased
  - **Uncommon** Macular oedema · nausea · seizures · thrombocytopenia
  - **Rare or very rare** Posterior reversible encephalopathy syndrome (PRES)
  - **Frequency not known** Anxiety · autoimmune haemolytic anaemia · haemophagocytic lymphohistiocytosis · hepatic disorders · peripheral oedema · progressive multifocal leukoencephalopathy (PML)

SIDE-EFFECTS, FURTHER INFORMATION **Basal-cell carcinoma** Patients should be advised to seek medical advice if they have any signs of basal-cell carcinoma including skin nodules, patches or open sores that do not heal within weeks.

Progressive multifocal leukoencephalopathy (PML) and other opportunistic infections Patients should be advised to seek medical attention if they have any signs of PML or any other infections. Suspension of treatment should be considered if a patient develops a severe infection, taking into consideration the risk-benefit.

- **CONCEPTION AND CONTRACEPTION** Manufacturer advises females of childbearing potential should use effective contraception during treatment and for 2 months after last treatment—see *Important safety information* for further information.

- **PREGNANCY** Manufacturer advises avoid—teratogenic.
- **BREAST FEEDING** Avoid.
- **HEPATIC IMPAIRMENT** Manufacturer advises caution when initiating treatment in mild to moderate impairment; avoid in severe impairment.
- **MONITORING REQUIREMENTS**
  - **All** patients receiving fingolimod should be monitored at treatment initiation, (first dose monitoring—before, during and after dose), and after treatment interruption (see note below); monitoring should include:
  - **Pre-treatment**
    - an ECG and blood pressure measurement before starting
  - **During the first 6 hours of treatment**
    - continuous ECG monitoring for 6 hours
    - blood pressure and heart rate measurement every hour
  - **After 6 hours of treatment**
    - a further ECG and blood pressure measurement
  - If heart rate at the end of the 6 hour period is at its lowest since fingolimod was first administered, monitoring should be extended by at least 2 hours and until heart rate increases.
  - If post-dose bradyarrhythmia-related symptoms occur, appropriate clinical management should be initiated and monitoring should be continued until the symptoms have resolved. If pharmacological intervention is required during the first-dose monitoring, overnight monitoring should follow, and the first-dose monitoring should then be repeated after the second dose.
  - If after 6 hours, the heart rate is less than 55 beats per minute in children aged 12 years and above, or less than 60 beats per minute in children under 12 years, or the ECG shows new onset second degree or higher grade AV block, or a QTc interval of 500 milliseconds or greater, monitoring should be extended (at least overnight, until side-effect resolution).
  - The occurrence at any time of third degree AV block requires extended monitoring (at least overnight, until side-effect resolution).
  - In case of T-wave inversion, ensure there are no associated signs or symptoms of myocardial ischaemia—if suspected seek advice from a cardiologist.
  - **Note**
  - First dose monitoring as above **should be repeated** in all patients whose treatment is interrupted for:
    - 1 day or more during the first 2 weeks of treatment
    - more than 7 days during weeks 3 and 4 of treatment
    - more than 2 weeks after one month of treatment
  - If the treatment interruption is of shorter duration than the above, treatment should be continued with the next dose as planned.
  - Manufacturer advises eye examination recommended 3–4 months after initiation of treatment (and before initiation of treatment in patients with diabetes or history of uveitis).
  - Manufacturer advises skin examination for skin lesions before starting treatment and then every 6 to 12 months thereafter or as clinically indicated.
  - The MHRA advises to monitor liver function—see *Important Safety Information.*
  - Monitor full blood count before treatment, at 3 months, then at least yearly thereafter and if signs of infection (interrupt treatment if lymphocyte count reduced)—consult product literature.
  - Monitor for signs and symptoms of haemophagocytic syndrome (including pyrexia, asthenia, hepato-splenomegaly and adenopathy—may be associated with hepatic failure and respiratory distress; also progressive cytopenia, elevated serum-ferritin concentrations, hypertriglyceridaemia, hypofibrinogenaemia, coagulopathy, hepatic cytolysis, hyponatraemia)—initiate treatment immediately.
  - Manufacturer advises to monitor routine MRI for lesions suggestive of progressive multifocal leukoencephalopathy (PML), particularly in patients considered at increased risk; monitor for signs and symptoms of new neurological dysfunction.
- **PRESCRIBING AND DISPENSING INFORMATION** The manufacturer of *Gilenya*® has provided a *Prescriber's checklist*.
- **PATIENT AND CARER ADVICE**

Patient reminder card Patients should be given a patient reminder card.

Female patients of childbearing potential should also be given a pregnancy-specific patient reminder card.

- **NATIONAL FUNDING/ACCESS DECISIONS**

For full details see funding body website

Scottish Medicines Consortium (SMC) decisions

- **Fingolimod (*Gilenya*®) as a single disease modifying therapy in highly active relapsing remitting multiple sclerosis for patients aged 10 to less than 18 years: with highly active disease despite a full course of treatment with at least one disease modifying therapy or with rapidly evolving severe relapsing remitting multiple sclerosis (June 2019)** SMC No. SMC2154 Recommended

All Wales Medicines Strategy Group (AWMSG) decisions

- **Fingolimod (*Gilenya*®) as a single disease modifying therapy in highly active relapsing remitting multiple sclerosis for patients aged 10 to 17 years: with highly active disease despite a full course of treatment with at least one disease modifying therapy or with rapidly evolving severe relapsing remitting multiple sclerosis (June 2019)** AWMSG No. 2777 Recommended

NHS restrictions

NHS England Clinical Commissioning Policy NHS England (May 2014) has provided guidance on the use of fingolimod for the treatment of multiple sclerosis in England. An NHS England Clinical Commissioning Policy outlines the funding arrangements and the criteria for initiating and discontinuing this treatment option, see www.england.nhs.uk/commissioning/spec-services/npc-crg/group-d/neurology/.

- **MEDICINAL FORMS** There can be variation in the licensing of different medicines containing the same drug.

Oral capsule

- **Fingolimod (non-proprietary)** ▼

Fingolimod (as Fingolimod hydrochloride)

500 microgram Fingolimod 500microgram capsules | 7 capsule PoM £312.00–£367.50 | 7 capsule PoM £312.38–£330.75 (Hospital only) | 28 capsule PoM £1,470.00 DT = £1,470.00 (Hospital only) | 28 capsule PoM £1,250.00–£1,470.00 DT = £1,470.00

- **Gilenya** (Novartis Pharmaceuticals UK Ltd)

Fingolimod (as Fingolimod hydrochloride)

250 microgram Gilenya 0.25mg capsules | 28 capsule PoM £1,470.00

Fingolimod (as Fingolimod hydrochloride)

500 microgram Gilenya 0.5mg capsules | 7 capsule PoM £367.50 | 28 capsule PoM £1,470.00 DT = £1,470.00

IMMUNOSUPPRESSANTS › PYRIMIDINE SYNTHESIS INHIBITORS

Teriflunomide

23-Jun-2022

- **DRUG ACTION** Teriflunomide is a metabolite of leflunomide which has immunomodulating and anti-inflammatory properties.

- **INDICATIONS AND DOSE**

Multiple sclerosis (initiated by a specialist)

- BY MOUTH
  - Child 10–17 years (body-weight up to 40 kg): 7 mg once daily

▸ Child 10–17 years (body-weight 40 kg and above): 14 mg once daily

- **CONTRA-INDICATIONS** Anaemia · leucopenia · neutropenia · serious infection · severe hypoproteinaemia · severe immunodeficiency · significantly impaired bone-marrow function · thrombocytopenia
- **CAUTIONS** Anaemia · dyspnoea—assess for interstitial lung disease and consider suspending treatment · hypoproteinaemia (avoid if severe) · impaired bone-marrow function (avoid if severe) · latent tuberculosis · leucopenia · persistent cough—assess for interstitial lung disease and consider suspending treatment · severe infection—delay or suspend treatment until resolved · significant alcohol consumption · signs or symptoms of serious skin reactions (including ulcerative stomatitis, Stevens-Johnson syndrome, and toxic epidermal necrolysis)—discontinue treatment · switching between other immunomodulating drugs · thrombocytopenia
- **INTERACTIONS** → Appendix 1: teriflunomide
- **SIDE-EFFECTS**

▸ **Common or very common** Alopecia · anaemia · anxiety · arthralgia · cystitis · diarrhoea · gastrointestinal discomfort · headache · hypersensitivity · hypertension · increased risk of infection · menorrhagia · myalgia · nausea · nerve disorders · neutropenia · oral disorders · pain · palpitations · pancreatitis · sensation abnormal · skin reactions · urinary frequency increased · vomiting · weight decreased

▸ **Uncommon** Colitis · dyslipidaemia · interstitial lung disease · nail disorder · sepsis · severe cutaneous adverse reactions (SCARs) · thrombocytopenia

▸ **Rare or very rare** Hepatic disorders

▸ **Frequency not known** Pulmonary hypertension

SIDE-EFFECTS, FURTHER INFORMATION **Hepatic injury** Discontinue treatment if signs or symptoms of hepatic injury, or if liver enzymes exceed 3 times the upper limit of reference range.

Important: accelerated elimination procedure recommended following discontinuation due to serious adverse effects (consult product literature).

- **CONCEPTION AND CONTRACEPTION** Effective contraception essential for women of child-bearing potential during treatment and for up to 2 years after treatment. In patients undergoing treatment with teriflunomide that are planning to conceive, the accelerated elimination procedure should be used prior to conception. Use of non-oral contraception is recommended during the accelerated elimination procedure—consult product literature.
- **PREGNANCY** Avoid—toxicity in animal studies.
- **BREAST FEEDING** Present in milk in *animal* studies—manufacturer advises avoid.
- **HEPATIC IMPAIRMENT** EvGr Avoid in severe impairment. (M)

Monitoring EvGr In patients with pre-existing liver disease, monitor liver function every 2 weeks for the first 6 months during treatment, then every 8 weeks thereafter for at least 2 years. Increase to weekly monitoring if alanine aminotransferase (ALT) is 2–3 times the upper limit of normal; discontinue treatment if signs or symptoms of hepatic injury occur, or if liver enzymes exceed 3 times the upper limit of normal. (M)

- **MONITORING REQUIREMENTS**

▸ EvGr Monitor full blood count (including differential white cell count and platelet count) before treatment and as clinically indicated during treatment.

▸ Monitor blood pressure before treatment and periodically thereafter.

▸ Monitor liver function before treatment and every 4 weeks for the first 6 months during treatment, then as clinically indicated. (M) Additional monitoring required in pre-existing liver disease or if alanine aminotransferase (ALT) increases during treatment, see *Hepatic impairment*.

- **TREATMENT CESSATION**

Accelerated elimination procedures To aid drug elimination in case of serious adverse effect or before conception, stop treatment and give *either* colestyramine p. 151 *or* activated charcoal p. 1043. After the accelerated elimination procedure a plasma concentration of less than 20 micrograms/litre (measured on 2 occasions at least 14 days apart) and a waiting period of one and a half months are necessary before conception.

- **PRESCRIBING AND DISPENSING INFORMATION** The manufacturer of *Aubagio*® has provided a guide for healthcare professionals.
- **PATIENT AND CARER ADVICE** Patients and their carers should be advised to report symptoms of infections to a doctor.

Patients and their carers should be counselled on the symptoms of pancreatitis.

Patients or their carers should be given a patient card.

- **NATIONAL FUNDING/ACCESS DECISIONS**

For full details see funding body website

All Wales Medicines Strategy Group (AWMSG) decisions

▸ **Teriflunomide (*Aubagio*®) for the treatment of relapsing-remitting multiple sclerosis in children aged 10 to 17 years (May 2022)** AWMSG No. 4033 Recommended with restrictions

- **MEDICINAL FORMS** There can be variation in the licensing of different medicines containing the same drug.

Oral tablet

▸ **Teriflunomide (Non-proprietary)**

Teriflunomide 14 mg Teriflunomide 14mg tablets | 28 tablet PoM £870.00–£1,037.84 (Hospital only) | 28 tablet PoM £705.00–£1,037.84

Malignant disease

1 Antibody responsive malignancy

ANTINEOPLASTIC DRUGS › MONOCLONAL ANTIBODIES

Blinatumomab [Specialist drug] 18-Sep-2025

- **INDICATIONS AND DOSE**

Acute lymphoblastic leukaemia

▸ BY CONTINUOUS INTRAVENOUS INFUSION

▸ Child 1–17 years: Specialist drug – access specialist resources for dosing information

- **INTERACTIONS** → Appendix 1: monoclonal antibodies
- **SIDE-EFFECTS**

▸ **Common or very common** Abdominal pain · anaemia · arrhythmias · ataxia · chest discomfort · chills · cognitive disorder · confusion · constipation · cough · cranial nerve disorder · cytokine release syndrome · decreased leucocytes · diarrhoea · dizziness · drowsiness · dyspnoea · encephalopathy · facial swelling · fever · flushing · headache · hyperbilirubinaemia · hypersensitivity · hypertension · hypogammaglobulinaemia · hypoglobulinaemia · hypotension · increased risk of infection · infusion related reaction · insomnia · leucocytosis · memory loss · nausea · neutropenia · oedema · pain · respiratory disorders · seizure · sensation abnormal · sepsis · skin reactions · speech impairment · thrombocytopenia · tremor · tumour lysis syndrome · vomiting · weight increased

- **Uncommon** Capillary leak syndrome · cytokine storm · haemophagocytic lymphohistiocytosis · lymphadenopathy · pancreatitis
- **Frequency not known** Consciousness impaired · device related infection · hypoxia · multi organ failure · psychiatric disorder · viral infection reactivation

SIDE-EFFECTS, FURTHER INFORMATION **Cytokine release syndrome, infusion-reactions, and tumour lysis syndrome** Life-threatening (including fatal) cases of cytokine release syndrome and tumour lysis syndrome have been reported in patients taking blinatumomab; temporary interruption or discontinuation might be required.

Neurological events There is potentially a higher risk of neurological events in patients with clinically relevant CNS pathology.

Pancreatitis Life-threatening or fatal cases of pancreatitis have been reported; temporary interruption or discontinuation might be required.

- **CONCEPTION AND CONTRACEPTION** Manufacturer advises effective contraception during treatment and for at least 48 hours after treatment in women of child-bearing potential.
- **PATIENT AND CARER ADVICE** A patient alert card should be provided. Educational materials should be provided to patients and carers to ensure blinatumomab is used in a safe and effective way, and to prevent the risk of medication errors and neurological events—consult product information.
  Driving and skilled tasks Manufacturer advises patients and carers should be counselled about the effects on driving and performance of skilled tasks—increased risk of confusion, disorientation, co-ordination and balance disorders, seizures and disturbances in consciousness.
- **NATIONAL FUNDING/ACCESS DECISIONS**
  For full details see funding body website

Scottish Medicines Consortium (SMC) decisions

- **Blinatumomab (*Blincyto*®) as monotherapy for the treatment of paediatric patients aged 1 year or older with Philadelphia chromosome-negative CD19-positive B-cell precursor acute lymphoblastic leukaemia which is refractory or in relapse after receiving at least two prior therapies or in relapse after receiving prior allogeneic hematopoietic stem cell transplantation (April 2019)** SMC No. SMC2148 Recommended

All Wales Medicines Strategy Group (AWMSG) decisions

- **Blinatumomab (*Blincyto*®) as monotherapy for the treatment of paediatric patients aged 1 year or older with Philadelphia chromosome-negative CD19-positive B-cell precursor acute lymphoblastic leukaemia (ALL) which is refractory or in relapse after receiving at least two prior therapies or in relapse after receiving prior allogeneic haematopoietic stem cell transplantation (April 2019)** AWMSG No. 3769 Recommended

---

- **MEDICINAL FORMS** There can be variation in the licensing of different medicines containing the same drug.

Powder and solution for solution for infusion

EXCIPIENTS: May contain Polysorbates

- **Blincyto** (Amgen Ltd) ▼
  Blinatumomab 38.5 microgram Blincyto 38.5micrograms powder for concentrate and solution for infusion vials | 1 vial [PoM] £2,017.00 (Hospital only)

Dinutuximab beta [Specialist drug]

04-Nov-2020

- **INDICATIONS AND DOSE**

Neuroblastoma

- BY INTRAVENOUS INFUSION
  - Child 1–17 years: Specialist drug – access specialist resources for dosing information

IMPORTANT SAFETY INFORMATION

Resuscitation facilities should be available during administration.

- **CONTRA-INDICATIONS** Acute grade 3 or 4, or extensive chronic graft-versus-host disease
- **INTERACTIONS** → Appendix 1: monoclonal antibodies
- **SIDE-EFFECTS**
  - **Common or very common** Anaemia · anxiety · appetite decreased · arthralgia · ascites · capillary leak syndrome · chest pain · chills · constipation · cough · cytokine release syndrome · decreased leucocytes · device related infection · diarrhoea · dizziness · dyspnoea · electrolyte imbalance · eye disorders · eye inflammation · fever · fluid imbalance · gastrointestinal discomfort · gastrointestinal disorders · haematuria · headache · heart failure · hyperhidrosis · hypersensitivity · hypertension · hypertriglyceridaemia · hypoalbuminaemia · hypotension · hypoxia · increased risk of infection · left ventricular dysfunction · muscle spasms · nausea · neutropenia · oedema · oral disorders · pain · paraesthesia · pericardial effusion · peripheral neuropathy · photosensitivity reaction · pulmonary oedema · renal impairment · respiratory disorders · seizure · sepsis · skin reactions · tachycardia · thrombocytopenia · tremor · urinary retention · urine abnormalities · vision disorders · vomiting · weight changes
  - **Uncommon** Disseminated intravascular coagulation · eosinophilia · hepatocellular injury · hypovolaemic shock · intracranial pressure increased · peripheral vascular disease · posterior reversible encephalopathy syndrome (PRES)
  - **Frequency not known** Erythropenia
- **CONCEPTION AND CONTRACEPTION** Manufacturer advises women of childbearing potential should use contraception during and for 6 months after stopping treatment.
- **PATIENT AND CARER ADVICE**
  Driving and skilled tasks Manufacturer advises patients should not use or drive machines during treatment.
- **NATIONAL FUNDING/ACCESS DECISIONS**
  For full details see funding body website

NICE decisions

- **Dinutuximab beta for treating neuroblastoma (August 2018)** NICE TA538 Recommended with restrictions

Scottish Medicines Consortium (SMC) decisions

- **Dinutuximab beta (*Qarziba*®) for the treatment of high-risk neuroblastoma in patients aged 12 months and above, who have previously received induction chemotherapy and achieved at least a partial response, followed by myeloablative therapy and stem cell transplantation, as well as patients with history of relapsed or refractory neuroblastoma, with or without residual disease (November 2018)** SMC No. SMC2105 Recommended

---

- **MEDICINAL FORMS** There can be variation in the licensing of different medicines containing the same drug.

Solution for infusion

- **Qarziba** (Recordati UK Ltd) ▼
  Dinutuximab beta 4.5 mg per 1 ml Qarziba 20mg/4.5ml concentrate for solution for infusion vials | 1 vial [PoM] £7,610.00 (Hospital only)

Gemtuzumab ozogamicin [Specialist drug]

06-Nov-2020

● **INDICATIONS AND DOSE**

Acute myeloid leukaemia

▸ BY INTRAVENOUS INFUSION

▸ Child 15–17 years: Specialist drug – access specialist resources for dosing information

IMPORTANT SAFETY INFORMATION

Resuscitation facilities should be available during administration.

● **INTERACTIONS** → Appendix 1: gemtuzumab ozogamicin

● **SIDE-EFFECTS**

▸ **Common or very common** Anaemia · appetite decreased · arrhythmias · ascites · asthenia · bone marrow disorders · bronchospasm · central nervous system haemorrhage · chills · constipation · decreased leucocytes · diarrhoea · dyspnoea · facial swelling · fever · gastrointestinal discomfort · gastrointestinal disorders · haemorrhage · headache · hepatic disorders · hyperbilirubinaemia · hyperglycaemia · hypersensitivity · hypertension · hyperthermia · hypotension · increased risk of infection · infusion related reaction (including fatal cases) · lethargy · malaise · mucositis · multi organ failure · nausea · neutropenia · oedema · oral disorders · oropharyngeal complaints · periorbital oedema · sepsis · sinusoidal obstruction syndrome · skin reactions · thrombocytopenia · tumour lysis syndrome (including fatal cases) · vomiting

▸ **Frequency not known** Interstitial pneumonia

SIDE-EFFECTS, FURTHER INFORMATION Infusion-related reactions (including fatal cases) can occur during the first 24 hours after administration. Manufacturer advises interrupt treatment immediately and treat as clinically indicated; permanent discontinuation should be strongly considered in patients who develop signs and symptoms of anaphylaxis.

● **CONCEPTION AND CONTRACEPTION** Manufacturer advises women of childbearing potential should use 2 methods of effective contraception during treatment and for at least 7 months after the last dose; male patients should use 2 methods of effective contraception during treatment and for at least 4 months after the last dose if their partner is of childbearing potential.

● **PATIENT AND CARER ADVICE**

Driving and skilled tasks Manufacturer advises patients and carers should be counselled on the effects on driving and performance of skilled tasks—increased risk of fatigue and headache.

● **NATIONAL FUNDING/ACCESS DECISIONS**

For full details see funding body website

NICE decisions

▸ **Gemtuzumab ozogamicin for untreated acute myeloid leukaemia (November 2018)** NICE TA545 Recommended with restrictions

Scottish Medicines Consortium (SMC) decisions

▸ **Gemtuzumab ozogamicin (*Mylotarg*®) as combination therapy with daunorubicin and cytarabine for the treatment of patients age 15 years and above with previously untreated, *de novo* CD33-positive acute myeloid leukaemia, except acute promyelocytic leukaemia (October 2018)** SMC No. SMC2089 Recommended with restrictions

● **MEDICINAL FORMS** There can be variation in the licensing of different medicines containing the same drug.

Powder for solution for infusion

▸ **Mylotarg** (Pfizer Ltd)

Gemtuzumab ozogamicin 5 mg Mylotarg 5mg powder for concentrate for solution for infusion vials | 1 vial PoM £6,300.00 (Hospital only)

Ipilimumab [Specialist drug]

06-Jun-2025

● **INDICATIONS AND DOSE**

Melanoma

▸ BY INTRAVENOUS INFUSION

▸ Child 12–17 years: Specialist drug – access specialist resources for dosing information

IMPORTANT SAFETY INFORMATION

MHRA/CHM ADVICE: IPILIMUMAB (*YERVOY*®): REPORTS OF CYTOMEGALOVIRUS (CMV) GASTROINTESTINAL INFECTION OR REACTIVATION (JANUARY 2019)

There have been post-marketing cases of gastrointestinal CMV infection or reactivation in ipilimumab-treated patients reported to have corticosteroid-refractory immune-related colitis, including fatal cases.

Patients should be advised to contact their healthcare professional immediately at the onset of symptoms of colitis. Possible causes, including infections, should be investigated; a stool infection work-up should be performed and patients screened for CMV. For patients with corticosteroid-refractory immune-related colitis, use of an additional immunosuppressive agent should only be considered if other causes are excluded using viral PCR on biopsy, and eliminating other viral, bacterial, and parasitic causes.

MHRA/CHM ADVICE: ATEZOLIZUMAB (*TECENTRIQ*®) AND OTHER IMMUNE-STIMULATORY ANTI-CANCER DRUGS: RISK OF SEVERE CUTANEOUS ADVERSE REACTIONS (SCARS) (JUNE 2021)

Severe cutaneous adverse reactions (SCARs), including cases of Stevens-Johnson syndrome (SJS) and toxic epidermal necrolysis (TEN), have been reported in patients treated with immunostimulant antineoplastic drugs, such as ipilimumab. Healthcare professionals are advised to monitor patients for suspected severe skin reactions and exclude other causes. Patients should be advised to seek urgent medical attention if severe skin reactions occur. If a SCAR is suspected, ipilimumab therapy should be withheld and the patient referred to a specialist for diagnosis and treatment. Ipilimumab should be permanently discontinued for any grade confirmed SJS or TEN, and for any grade 4 SCAR. Caution is recommended when considering the use of ipilimumab in patients with a history of severe or life-threatening SCAR associated with other immunostimulant antineoplastic drugs.

● **INTERACTIONS** → Appendix 1: monoclonal antibodies

● **SIDE-EFFECTS**

▸ **Common or very common** Allergic rhinitis · alopecia · anaemia · appetite decreased · arrhythmias · arthralgia · arthritis · asthenia · brain oedema · cancer pain · chills · confusion · constipation · cough · decreased leucocytes · dehydration · depression · diarrhoea · dizziness · dyspnoea · electrolyte imbalance · eye discomfort · fever · gastrointestinal discomfort · gastrointestinal disorders · haemorrhage · headache · hepatic disorders · hypophysitis · hypopituitarism · hypotension · hypothyroidism · increased risk of infection · influenza like illness · lethargy · mucositis · muscle complaints · musculoskeletal discomfort · nausea · nerve disorders · neutropenia · night sweats · oedema · pain · renal failure · sepsis · skin reactions · stomatitis ·

thrombocytopenia · vasodilation · vision disorders · vomiting · weight decreased
- **Uncommon** Adrenal hypofunction · alkalosis · amenorrhoea · cystitis · dysarthria · eosinophilia · eye inflammation · glomerulonephritis · haemolytic anaemia · hair colour changes · hypersensitivity · hyperthyroidism · hypogonadism · infusion related reaction · libido decreased · meningitis aseptic · movement disorders · multi organ failure · muscle weakness · myopathy · nephritis autoimmune · pancreatitis · paraneoplastic syndrome · peripheral vascular disease · pneumonitis · polymyalgia rheumatica · proteinuria · psychiatric disorder · pulmonary oedema · renal tubular acidosis · respiratory disorders · severe cutaneous adverse reactions (SCARs) · syncope · systemic inflammatory response syndrome · tremor · tumour lysis syndrome · vascular disorders · vasculitis
- **Rare or very rare** Diabetic ketoacidosis · myasthenia gravis · serous retinal detachment · thyroiditis · type 1 diabetes mellitus
- **Frequency not known** Cardiomyopathy · cytokine release syndrome · cytomegalovirus infection reactivation · erythema nodosum · haemophagocytic lymphohistiocytosis · hyperglycaemia · hyperpituitarism · hypoparathyroidism · lymphocytosis · meningism · myocarditis · neurosensory hypoacusis · pericardial effusion · polycythaemia · sarcoidosis · solid organ transplant rejection

SIDE-EFFECTS, FURTHER INFORMATION A corticosteroid can be used after starting ipilimumab, to treat immune-related reactions.

- **CONCEPTION AND CONTRACEPTION** Use effective contraception.
- **PATIENT AND CARER ADVICE** A patient information guide and alert card should be provided.

Driving and skilled tasks Patients and carers should be counselled on the effects on driving and performance of skilled tasks—increased risk of fatigue.

- **NATIONAL FUNDING/ACCESS DECISIONS**

For full details see funding body website

Scottish Medicines Consortium (SMC) decisions
- **Ipilimumab (*Yervoy*®) for the treatment of advanced (unresectable or metastatic) melanoma in adolescents 12 years of age and older (October 2018)** SMC No. SMC2094 Recommended

All Wales Medicines Strategy Group (AWMSG) decisions
- **Ipilimumab (*Yervoy*®) as monotherapy for the treatment of advanced (unresectable or metastatic) melanoma in adolescents 12 years of age to less than 18 years of age (November 2018)** AWMSG No. 3604 Recommended

- **MEDICINAL FORMS** There can be variation in the licensing of different medicines containing the same drug.

Solution for infusion

ELECTROLYTES: May contain Sodium
- **Yervoy** (Bristol-Myers Squibb Pharmaceuticals Ltd)

Ipilimumab 5 mg per 1 ml Yervoy 50mg/10ml concentrate for solution for infusion vials | 1 vial PoM £3,750.00 (Hospital only)
Yervoy 200mg/40ml concentrate for solution for infusion vials | 1 vial PoM £15,000.00 (Hospital only)

Nivolumab [Specialist drug] 26-Feb-2026

- **INDICATIONS AND DOSE**

Melanoma
- BY INTRAVENOUS INFUSION
- Child 12-17 years: Specialist drug – access specialist resources for dosing information

IMPORTANT SAFETY INFORMATION

MHRA/CHM ADVICE: NIVOLUMAB (*OPDIVO*®): REPORTS OF ORGAN TRANSPLANT REJECTION (JULY 2017)

A European review of worldwide data concluded that nivolumab may increase the risk of rejection in organ transplant recipients. The MHRA recommends considering the benefit of treatment with nivolumab versus the risk of possible organ transplant rejection for each patient.

MHRA/CHM ADVICE: NIVOLUMAB (*OPDIVO*®): REPORTS OF CYTOMEGALOVIRUS (CMV) GASTROINTESTINAL INFECTION OR REACTIVATION (OCTOBER 2019)

A European review of worldwide data identified cases suggestive of gastrointestinal CMV infection or reactivation in nivolumab-treated patients, including fatal cases.

Patients should be advised to contact their healthcare professional immediately at the onset of symptoms of colitis. Possible causes, including infections, should be investigated; a stool infection work-up should be performed and patients screened for CMV. For patients with corticosteroid-refractory immune-related colitis, use of an additional immunosuppressive agent should only be considered if other causes are excluded using viral PCR on biopsy, and eliminating other viral, bacterial, and parasitic causes.

MHRA/CHM ADVICE: ATEZOLIZUMAB (*TECENTRIQ*®) AND OTHER IMMUNE-STIMULATORY ANTI-CANCER DRUGS: RISK OF SEVERE CUTANEOUS ADVERSE REACTIONS (SCARS) (JUNE 2021)

Severe cutaneous adverse reactions (SCARs), including cases of Stevens-Johnson syndrome (SJS) and toxic epidermal necrolysis (TEN), have been reported in patients treated with immunostimulant antineoplastic drugs, such as nivolumab. Healthcare professionals are advised to monitor patients for suspected severe skin reactions and exclude other causes. Patients should be advised to seek urgent medical attention if severe skin reactions occur. If a SCAR is suspected, nivolumab therapy should be withheld and the patient referred to a specialist for diagnosis and treatment. Nivolumab should be permanently discontinued for any grade confirmed SJS or TEN, and for any grade 4 SCAR. Caution is recommended when considering the use of nivolumab in patients with a history of severe or life-threatening SCAR associated with other immunostimulant antineoplastic drugs.

- **INTERACTIONS** → Appendix 1: monoclonal antibodies
- **SIDE-EFFECTS**
- **Common or very common** Abdominal pain · alopecia · anaemia · appetite decreased · arrhythmias · arthralgia · arthritis · chest pain · constipation · cough · cytokine release syndrome · decreased leucocytes · dehydration · diarrhoea · dizziness · dry eye · dry mouth · dyspnoea · electrolyte imbalance · fatigue · fever · gastrointestinal disorders · haemolytic anaemia · headache · hyperglycaemia · hypersensitivity · hypertension · hyperthyroidism · hypoalbuminaemia · hypoglycaemia · hypothyroidism · increased risk of infection · inflammation · infusion related reaction · interstitial lung disease · muscle complaints · musculoskeletal discomfort · nausea · nerve disorders · neutropenia · oedema · pain · renal impairment · respiratory disorders · skin reactions ·

stomatitis · thrombocytopenia · thyroiditis · vision blurred · vomiting · weight decreased
- **Uncommon** Adrenal hypofunction · cardiac inflammation · connective tissue disorders · diabetes mellitus · eosinophilia · eye inflammation · hepatic disorders · hypophysitis · hypopituitarism · metabolic acidosis · pancreatitis · paresis · pericardial disorders · sarcoidosis
- **Rare or very rare** Cystitis · demyelination · diabetic ketoacidosis · histiocytic necrotising lymphadenitis · hypoparathyroidism · meningitis aseptic · myopathy · nephritis · neuromuscular dysfunction · severe cutaneous adverse reactions (SCARs) · vasculitis
- **Frequency not known** Cytomegalovirus infection reactivation · haemophagocytic lymphohistiocytosis · solid organ transplant rejection · thyroid disorder · tumour lysis syndrome

SIDE-EFFECTS, FURTHER INFORMATION **Immune-related reactions** Manufacturer advises that most immune-related adverse reactions improved or resolved with appropriate management, including initiation of corticosteroids and treatment modifications.

Infusion-related reactions Manufacturer advises that patients with mild or moderate infusion reactions can continue treatment with close monitoring and use of pre-medication according to local guidelines; discontinue treatment if severe infusion reactions occur.

- **CONCEPTION AND CONTRACEPTION** EvGr Ensure effective contraception during and for at least 5 months after treatment in females of childbearing potential. (M)
- **PATIENT AND CARER ADVICE** Patients should be provided with a patient alert card with each prescription.

Driving and skilled tasks Patients and carers should be counselled on the effects on driving and performance of skilled tasks—increased risk of fatigue.

- **MEDICINAL FORMS** There can be variation in the licensing of different medicines containing the same drug.

Solution for infusion

EXCIPIENTS: May contain Polysorbates
ELECTROLYTES: May contain Sodium

- **Opdivo** (Bristol-Myers Squibb Pharmaceuticals Ltd)

Nivolumab 10 mg per 1 ml Opdivo 40mg/4ml concentrate for solution for infusion vials | 1 vial PoM £439.00 (Hospital only)
Opdivo 120mg/12ml concentrate for solution for infusion vials | 1 vial PoM £1,317.00 (Hospital only)
Opdivo 100mg/10ml concentrate for solution for infusion vials | 1 vial PoM £1,097.00 (Hospital only)
Opdivo 240mg/24ml concentrate for solution for infusion vials | 1 vial PoM £2,633.00 (Hospital only)

Nivolumab with relatlimab [Specialist drug]

01-Aug-2024

The properties listed below are those particular to the combination only. For the properties of the components please consider, nivolumab p. 656.

- **INDICATIONS AND DOSE**

Melanoma
- BY INTRAVENOUS INFUSION
- Child 12-17 years: Specialist drug – access specialist resources for dosing information

- **INTERACTIONS** → Appendix 1: monoclonal antibodies
- **SIDE-EFFECTS**
- **Common or very common** Abdominal pain · adrenal hypofunction · alopecia · anaemia · appetite decreased · arthralgia · arthritis · chills · confusion · constipation · cough · decreased leucocytes · dehydration · diabetes mellitus · diarrhoea · dizziness · dry eye · dry mouth · dysphagia · dyspnoea · electrolyte imbalance · eosinophilia · eye disorders · eye inflammation · fatigue · fever · gastrointestinal disorders · headache · hepatitis · hyperthyroidism · hyperuricaemia · hypoalbuminaemia · hypoglycaemia · hypophysitis · hypothyroidism · increased risk of infection · influenza like illness · infusion related reaction · interstitial lung disease · muscle spasms · muscle weakness · myocarditis · nasal congestion · nausea · nerve disorders · neutropenia · oedema · pain · pancreatitis · photosensitivity reaction · proteinuria · renal impairment · skin reactions · stomatitis · taste altered · thrombocytopenia · thyroiditis · visual impairment · vomiting · weight decreased
- **Uncommon** Asthma · azoospermia · cholangitis · connective tissue disorders · haemolytic anaemia · hypogonadism · hypopituitarism · myopathy · nephritis · pericardial effusion · systemic lupus erythematosus (SLE)
- **Frequency not known** Endocrine disorders · haemophagocytic lymphohistiocytosis · hypersensitivity · lung infiltration

- **PATIENT AND CARER ADVICE** A patient card should be provided.
- **NATIONAL FUNDING/ACCESS DECISIONS**

For full details see funding body website

NICE decisions
- **Nivolumab-relatlimab for untreated unresectable or metastatic melanoma in people 12 years and over (February 2024)** NICE TA950 Recommended with restrictions

Scottish Medicines Consortium (SMC) decisions
- **Nivolumab with relatlimab (*Opdualag*®) for first-line treatment of advanced (unresectable or metastatic) melanoma in adults and adolescents 12 years of age and over (July 2024)** SMC No. SMC2645 Recommended

- **MEDICINAL FORMS** There can be variation in the licensing of different medicines containing the same drug.

Solution for infusion

EXCIPIENTS: May contain Polysorbates

- **Opdualag** (Bristol-Myers Squibb Pharmaceuticals Ltd) ▼

Relatlimab 4 mg per 1 ml, Nivolumab 12 mg per 1 ml Opdualag 240mg/20ml / 80mg/20ml concentrate for solution for infusion vials | 1 vial PoM £6,134.75 (Hospital only)

Pembrolizumab [Specialist drug]

21-Apr-2026

- **INDICATIONS AND DOSE**

Classical Hodgkin lymphoma
- BY INTRAVENOUS INFUSION
- Child 3-17 years: Specialist drug – access specialist resources for dosing information

Melanoma
- BY INTRAVENOUS INFUSION
- Child 12-17 years: Specialist drug – access specialist resources for dosing information

IMPORTANT SAFETY INFORMATION

MHRA/CHM ADVICE: PEMBROLIZUMAB (*KEYTRUDA*®): REPORTS OF ORGAN TRANSPLANT REJECTION (JULY 2017)

A European review of worldwide data concluded that pembrolizumab may increase the risk of rejection in organ transplant recipients. The MHRA recommends considering the benefit of treatment with pembrolizumab versus the risk of possible organ transplant rejection for each patient.

MHRA/CHM ADVICE: ATEZOLIZUMAB (*TECENTRIQ*®) AND OTHER IMMUNE-STIMULATORY ANTI-CANCER DRUGS: RISK OF SEVERE CUTANEOUS ADVERSE REACTIONS (SCARS) (JUNE 2021)

Severe cutaneous adverse reactions (SCARs), including cases of Stevens-Johnson syndrome (SJS) and toxic epidermal necrolysis (TEN), have been reported in patients treated with immunostimulant antineoplastic drugs, such as pembrolizumab. Healthcare professionals are advised to monitor patients for suspected severe skin reactions and exclude other causes. Patients should be advised to seek urgent medical attention if severe skin reactions occur. If a SCAR is suspected, pembrolizumab therapy should be withheld and the patient referred to a specialist for diagnosis and treatment. Pembrolizumab should be permanently discontinued for any grade confirmed SJS or TEN, and for any grade 4 SCAR. Caution is recommended when considering the use of pembrolizumab in patients with a history of severe or life-threatening SCAR associated with other immunostimulant antineoplastic drugs.

- **INTERACTIONS** → Appendix 1: monoclonal antibodies
- **SIDE-EFFECTS**
  - **Common or very common** Alopecia · anaemia · appetite decreased · arrhythmias · arthritis · asthenia · chills · connective tissue disorders · constipation · cough · cytokine release syndrome · decreased leucocytes · diarrhoea · dizziness · dry eye · dry mouth · dyspnoea · electrolyte imbalance · enterocolitis haemorrhagic · eye inflammation · eyelid hypopigmentation · fever · fluid imbalance · gastrointestinal discomfort · gastrointestinal disorders · genital abnormalities · headache · hepatic disorders · hypersensitivity · hypertension · hyperthyroidism · hypothyroidism · immune-mediated lung disease · increased risk of infection · influenza like illness · infusion related reaction · insomnia · interstitial lung disease · joint disorders · lethargy · lip swelling · musculoskeletal discomfort · myalgia · myopathy · myxoedema · nausea · nerve disorders · neutropenia · oedema · pain · severe cutaneous adverse reactions (SCARs) · skin reactions · taste altered · thrombocytopenia · torticollis · vomiting
  - **Uncommon** Adrenal hypofunction · cardiac inflammation · diabetic ketoacidosis · eosinophilia · epilepsy · glomerulonephritis · hair colour changes · hypophysitis · hypopituitarism · immune-mediated pancreatitis · lymphocytic hypophysitis · nephritis · nephrotic syndrome · neuromuscular dysfunction · pancreatitis · pericardial effusion · renal impairment · sarcoidosis · tendon disorders · thyroid disorder · thyroiditis · type 1 diabetes mellitus
  - **Rare or very rare** Aortitis · cholangitis sclerosing · cystitis · encephalitis non-infective · erythema nodosum · haemolytic anaemia · haemophagocytic lymphohistiocytosis · hypoparathyroidism · meningitis · meningitis non-infective · pure red cell aplasia · transverse myelitis · vasculitis
  - **Frequency not known** Solid organ transplant rejection

SIDE-EFFECTS, FURTHER INFORMATION **Immune-related reactions** Most immune-related adverse reactions are reversible and managed by temporarily stopping treatment and administration of a corticosteroid.

Infusion-related reactions Manufacturer advises to permanently discontinue treatment in patients with severe infusion reactions.

- **CONCEPTION AND CONTRACEPTION** Manufacturer recommends effective contraception during treatment and for at least 4 months after treatment in women of childbearing potential.
- **PATIENT AND CARER ADVICE** Patients should be provided with an alert card and advised to keep it with them at all times. A patient information brochure highlighting important safety information to minimise the risk of immune-related side-effects is also available.

Driving and skilled tasks Patients should be counselled on the effects on driving and performance of skilled tasks—increased risk of dizziness and fatigue.

- **NATIONAL FUNDING/ACCESS DECISIONS**

For full details see funding body website

NICE decisions

- **Pembrolizumab for adjuvant treatment of resected stage 2B or 2C melanoma (October 2022)** NICE TA837 Recommended
- **Pembrolizumab for treating relapsed or refractory classical Hodgkin lymphoma after stem cell transplant or at least 2 previous therapies (February 2022)** NICE TA772 Recommended with restrictions
- **Pembrolizumab for treating relapsed or refractory classical Hodgkin lymphoma in people 3 years and over (May 2024)** NICE TA967 Recommended with restrictions

Scottish Medicines Consortium (SMC) decisions

- **Pembrolizumab (*Keytruda*®) as monotherapy for the adjuvant treatment of adults and adolescents aged 12 years and older with stage 2B or 2C melanoma and who have undergone complete resection (April 2023)** SMC No. SMC2526 Recommended
- **Pembrolizumab (*Keytruda*®) as monotherapy for the treatment of adult and paediatric patients aged 3 years and older with relapsed or refractory classical Hodgkin lymphoma who have failed autologous stem cell transplant (ASCT), or following at least two prior therapies when ASCT is not a treatment option (November 2021)** SMC No. SMC2380 Recommended with restrictions

- **MEDICINAL FORMS** There can be variation in the licensing of different medicines containing the same drug.

Solution for infusion

EXCIPIENTS: May contain Polysorbates

- **Keytruda** (Merck Sharp & Dohme (UK) Ltd)
  Pembrolizumab 25 mg per 1 ml Keytruda 100mg/4ml concentrate for solution for infusion vials | 2 vial PoM £5,260.00 (Hospital only)

IMMUNOSUPPRESSANTS › MONOCLONAL ANTIBODIES › ANTI-LYMPHOCYTE

Anti-lymphocyte monoclonal antibodies

- **DRUG ACTION** The anti-lymphocyte monoclonal antibodies cause lysis of B lymphocytes.

IMPORTANT SAFETY INFORMATION

All anti-lymphocyte monoclonal antibodies should be given under the supervision of an experienced specialist, in an environment where full resuscitation facilities are immediately available.

- **SIDE-EFFECTS**
  - **Common or very common** Alopecia · anaemia · anaphylactic reaction · anxiety · arthralgia · asthenia · conjunctivitis · constipation · cough · cytokine release syndrome · depression · diarrhoea · fever · headache · hypersensitivity (discontinue permanently) · increased risk of infection · infusion related reaction · leucopenia · myocardial infarction · neutropenia · pain · pruritus · thrombocytopenia · vomiting
  - **Uncommon** Haemolytic anaemia · progressive multifocal leukoencephalopathy (PML)

SIDE-EFFECTS, FURTHER INFORMATION **Infusion-related side-effects** In rare cases infusion reactions may be fatal. Infusion-related side-effects occur predominantly during the first infusion. Patients should receive premedication before administration of anti-lymphocyte monoclonal antibodies to reduce these effects—consult product literature for details of individual regimens. The infusion may have to be stopped temporarily and the infusion-related effects treated—consult product literature for appropriate management.

Cytokine release syndrome Fatalities following severe cytokine release syndrome (characterised by severe dyspnoea) and associated with features of tumour lysis syndrome have occurred after infusions of anti-lymphocyte monoclonal antibodies. Patients with a high tumour burden as well as those with pulmonary insufficiency or infiltration are at increased risk and should be monitored very closely (and a slower rate of infusion considered).

Progressive Multifocal Leukoencephalopathy (PML) If suspected, treatment should be suspended until PML has been excluded. If a patient develops an opportunistic infection or PML, anti-lymphocyte monoclonal antibodies should be permanently discontinued.

- **PRE-TREATMENT SCREENING** All patients should be screened for hepatitis B before treatment.

658

Rituximab

11-Nov-2022

- **INDICATIONS AND DOSE**

Severe cases of resistant immune modulated disease [including idiopathic thrombocytopenia purpura, haemolytic anaemia, and systemic lupus erythematosus] (under expert supervision)

▶ BY INTRAVENOUS INFUSION

▶ Child: Patients should receive premedication before each dose (consult product literature for details) (consult local protocol)

Post-transplantation lymphoproliferative disease (specialist use only) | Non-Hodgkin's lymphoma (specialist use only) | Hodgkin's lymphoma (specialist use only)

▶ BY INTRAVENOUS INFUSION

▶ Child: Specialist indication – access specialist resources for dosing information

- **UNLICENSED USE** Not licensed for use in children.
- **CAUTIONS** History of cardiovascular disease (in adults exacerbation of angina, arrhythmia, and heart failure have been reported) · patients receiving cardiotoxic chemotherapy (in adults exacerbation of angina, arrhythmia, and heart failure have been reported) · predisposition to infection · transient hypotension occurs frequently during infusion (anti-hypertensives may need to be withheld for 12 hours before infusion)

CAUTIONS, FURTHER INFORMATION For full details on cautions, consult product literature or local treatment protocol.

▶ Hepatitis B infection and reactivation Hepatitis B infection and reactivation (including fatal cases) have been reported in patients taking **rituximab**. Manufacturer advises patients with positive hepatitis B serology should be referred to a liver specialist for monitoring and initiation of antiviral therapy before treatment initiation; treatment should not be initiated in patients with evidence of current hepatitis B infection until the infection has been adequately treated. Manufacturer also advises patients should be closely monitored for clinical and laboratory signs of active hepatitis B infection (consult product literature).

- **INTERACTIONS** → Appendix 1: monoclonal antibodies
- **SIDE-EFFECTS**

▶ **Common or very common** Angioedema · appetite decreased · arrhythmias · bone marrow disorders · bursitis · cancer pain · cardiac disorder · chest pain · chills · dizziness · dysphagia · dyspnoea · ear pain · electrolyte imbalance · gastrointestinal discomfort · gastrointestinal disorders · hepatitis B · hypercholesterolaemia · hyperglycaemia · hypertension · hypotension · insomnia · lacrimation disorder · malaise · migraine · multi organ failure · muscle complaints · muscle tone increased · nausea · nerve disorders · oedema · oral disorders · osteoarthritis · respiratory disorders · sensation abnormal · sepsis · skin reactions · sweat changes · throat irritation · tinnitus · vasodilation · weight decreased

▶ **Uncommon** Asthma · coagulation disorder · heart failure · hypoxia · ischaemic heart disease · lymphadenopathy · taste altered

▶ **Rare or very rare** Facial paralysis · hepatitis B reactivation · interstitial lung disease · renal failure · Stevens-Johnson syndrome (discontinue) · toxic epidermal necrolysis · tumour lysis syndrome · vasculitis · vision disorders

▶ **Frequency not known** Epistaxis · hearing loss · hypogammaglobulinaemia · infective thrombosis · influenza like illness · irritability · muscle weakness · nasal congestion · posterior reversible encephalopathy syndrome (PRES) · psychiatric disorder · seizure · skin papilloma · tremor

SIDE-EFFECTS, FURTHER INFORMATION Associated with infections, sometimes severe, including tuberculosis, septicaemia, and hepatitis B reactivation.

Progressive multifocal leucoencephalopathy has been reported in association with rituximab; patients should be monitored for cognitive, neurological, or psychiatric signs and symptoms. If progressive multifocal leucoencephalopathy is suspected, suspend treatment until it has been excluded.

- **CONCEPTION AND CONTRACEPTION** Effective contraception in females of childbearing potential required during and for 12 months after treatment.
- **PREGNANCY** Avoid unless potential benefit to mother outweighs risk of B-lymphocyte depletion in fetus.
- **BREAST FEEDING** Avoid breast-feeding during and for 12 months after treatment.
- **MONITORING REQUIREMENTS** For full details on monitoring requirements consult product literature.
- **PRESCRIBING AND DISPENSING INFORMATION** Rituximab is a biological medicine. Biological medicines must be prescribed and dispensed by brand name, see *Biological medicines* and *Biosimilar medicines*, under Guidance on prescribing p. 1.

- **MEDICINAL FORMS** There can be variation in the licensing of different medicines containing the same drug.

Solution for infusion

EXCIPIENTS: May contain Polysorbates

ELECTROLYTES: May contain Sodium

▶ **Ituxredi** (Dr Reddy's Laboratories (UK) Ltd) ▼

Rituximab 10 mg per 1 ml Ituxredi 500mg/50ml concentrate for solution for infusion vials | 1 vial PoM £873.15 (Hospital only)
Ituxredi 100mg/10ml concentrate for solution for infusion vials | 2 vial PoM £349.25 (Hospital only)

▶ **MabThera** (Roche Products Ltd)

Rituximab 10 mg per 1 ml MabThera 100mg/10ml concentrate for solution for infusion vials | 2 vial PoM £349.25 (Hospital only)
MabThera 500mg/50ml concentrate for solution for infusion vials | 1 vial PoM £873.15 (Hospital only)

▶ **Rixathon** (Sandoz Ltd)

Rituximab 10 mg per 1 ml Rixathon 100mg/10ml concentrate for solution for infusion vials | 3 vial PoM £471.50 (Hospital only)
Rixathon 500mg/50ml concentrate for solution for infusion vials | 2 vial PoM £1,571.67 (Hospital only)

▶ **Ruxience** (Pfizer Ltd)

Rituximab 10 mg per 1 ml Ruxience 100mg/10ml concentrate for solution for infusion vials | 1 vial PoM £157.17 (Hospital only)
Ruxience 500mg/50ml concentrate for solution for infusion vials | 1 vial PoM £785.84 (Hospital only)

▶ **Truxima** (Celltrion Healthcare UK Ltd)

Rituximab 10 mg per 1 ml Truxima 100mg/10ml concentrate for solution for infusion vials | 2 vial PoM £314.33 (Hospital only)
Truxima 500mg/50ml concentrate for solution for infusion vials | 1 vial PoM £785.84 (Hospital only)

2 Cytotoxic responsive malignancy

Cytotoxic drugs

13-Oct-2025

Overview

The management of childhood cancer is complex and is generally confined to specialist regional centres and some associated shared-care units.

Cytotoxic drugs have both anti-cancer activity and the potential for damage to normal tissue. In children, chemotherapy is almost always started with curative intent, but may be continued as palliation if the disease is refractory.

Chemotherapy with a combination of two or more cytotoxic drugs aims to reduce the development of resistance and to improve cytotoxic effect. Treatment protocols generally incorporate a series of treatment courses at defined intervals with clear criteria for starting each course, such as adequate bone-marrow recovery and renal or cardiac function. The principal component of treatment for leukaemias in children is cytotoxic therapy, whereas solid tumours may be managed with surgery or radiotherapy in addition to chemotherapy.

Only medical or nursing staff who have received appropriate training should administer parenteral cytotoxics. In most instances central venous access will be required for the intravenous administration of cytotoxics to children; care is required to avoid the risk of extravasation (see Side-effects of Cytotoxic Drugs and their Management).

Cytotoxic drug handling guidelines

- Trained personnel should reconstitute cytotoxics
- Reconstitution should be carried out in designated pharmacy areas
- Protective clothing (including gloves, gowns, and masks) should be worn
- The eyes should be protected and means of first aid should be specified
- Pregnant staff should avoid exposure to cytotoxic drugs (all females of child-bearing age should be informed of the reproductive hazard)
- Use local procedures for dealing with spillages and safe disposal of waste material, including syringes, containers, and absorbent material
- Staff exposure to cytotoxic drugs should be monitored

Intrathecal chemotherapy

A Health Service Circular (HSC 2008/001) provides guidance on the introduction of safe practice in NHS Trusts where intrathecal chemotherapy is administered; written local guidance covering all aspects of national guidance should be available. Support for training programmes is also available. Copies, and further information may be obtained from the Department of Health and Social Care website (www.gov.uk/government/organisations/department-of-health-and-social-care).

Safe systems for cytotoxic medicines

Safe system requirements for cytotoxic medicines:

- Cytotoxic drugs for the treatment of cancer should be given as part of a wider pathway of care that is co-ordinated by a multi-disciplinary team
- Cytotoxic drugs should be prescribed, dispensed and administered only in the context of a written protocol or treatment plan
- Injectable cytotoxic drugs should only be dispensed if they are prepared for administration
- Oral cytotoxic medicines should be dispensed with clear directions for use

Cytotoxic drugs: important safety information

Risks of incorrect dosing of oral anti-cancer medicines

The National Patient Safety Agency has advised (January 2008) that the prescribing and use of oral cytotoxic medicines should be carried out to the same standard as parenteral cytotoxic therapy. Standards to be followed to achieve this include:

- non-specialists who prescribe or administer on-going oral cytotoxic medication should have access to written protocols and treatment plans, including guidance on the monitoring and treatment of toxicity;
- staff dispensing oral cytotoxic medicines should confirm that the prescribed dose is appropriate for the patient. Patients should have written information that includes details of the intended oral anti-cancer regimen, the treatment plan, and arrangements for monitoring, taken from the original protocol from the initiating hospital. Staff dispensing oral cytotoxic medicines should also have access to this information, and to advice from an experienced cancer pharmacist in the initiating hospital.

Cytotoxic drug doses

Doses of cytotoxic drugs are determined using a variety of different methods including age, body-surface area, or body-weight. Alternatively, doses may be fixed. Doses may be further adjusted following consideration of a patient's neutrophil count, renal and hepatic function, and history of previous adverse effects to the cytotoxic drug. Doses may also differ depending on whether a drug is used alone or in combination.

Because of the complexity of dosage regimens in the treatment of malignant disease, dose statements have been omitted from many of the drug entries in this chapter.

Cytotoxic drugs: effect on pregnancy and reproductive function

Most cytotoxic drugs are teratogenic and should not be administered during pregnancy, especially during the first trimester. Exclude pregnancy before treatment with cytotoxic drugs. Considerable caution is necessary if a pregnant female presents with cancer requiring chemotherapy, and specialist advice should always be sought.

Contraceptive advice should be given to males and females before cytotoxic therapy begins (and should cover the duration of contraception required after therapy has ended).

Alkylating drugs can have an adverse effect on gametogenesis, which may be reversible particularly in females. Regimens that do not contain an alkylating drug or procarbazine may have less effect on fertility, but those with an alkylating drug or procarbazine carry the risk of causing permanent male sterility (there is no effect on potency). Pretreatment counselling and consideration of sperm storage may be appropriate. Females are less severely affected, though the span of reproductive life may be shortened by the onset of a premature menopause. No increase in fetal abnormalities or abortion rate has been recorded in patients who remain fertile after cytotoxic chemotherapy. Amenorrhoea may occur, which also may be reversible.

Management of cytotoxic drug side-effects

Gastro-intestinal effects

Management of gastrointestinal effects of cytotoxic drugs includes the use of antacids, H_2-receptor antagonists, and proton pump inhibitors to protect the gastric mucosa, laxatives to treat constipation, and enteral and parenteral nutritional support.

Oral mucositis

Good oral hygiene keeps the mouth clean and moist and helps to prevent mucositis; prevention is more effective than treatment of the complication. Good oral hygiene measures for children over 6 months include brushing teeth with a soft small brush with fluoride toothpaste 2–3 times daily, and rinsing the mouth frequently. Daily fluoride supplements can be used on the advice of the child's dental team. For children under 6 months or when it is not possible to brush teeth, carers should be instructed how to clean the mouth using an oral sponge moistened with water or with an antimicrobial solution such as diluted chlorhexidine. Mucositis related to chemotherapy can be extremely painful and may, in some circumstances, require opioid analgesia. Secondary infection with candida is frequent; treatment with a systemically absorbed antifungal, such as fluconazole p. 463, is effective.

Nausea and vomiting

Nausea and vomiting cause considerable distress to many children who receive chemotherapy, and to a lesser extent abdominal radiotherapy, and may lead to refusal of further treatment; prophylaxis of nausea and vomiting is therefore extremely important. Symptoms may be acute (occurring within 24 hours of treatment), delayed (first occurring more than 24 hours after treatment), or anticipatory (occurring prior to subsequent doses). Delayed and anticipatory symptoms are more difficult to control than acute symptoms and require different management.

Susceptibility to nausea and vomiting may increase with repeated exposure to the cytotoxic drug.

Drugs may be divided according to their emetogenic potential and some examples are given below, but the symptoms vary according to the dose, to other drugs administered, and to the individual's susceptibility to emetogenic stimuli.

Mildly emetogenic treatment—fluorouracil, etoposide p. 677, low doses of methotrexate p. 672, the vinca alkaloids, and abdominal radiotherapy.

Moderately emetogenic treatment— carboplatin p. 676, doxorubicin hydrochloride p. 668, intermediate and low doses of cyclophosphamide p. 663, mitoxantrone p. 669, and high doses of methotrexate.

Highly emetogenic treatment— cisplatin p. 677, dacarbazine p. 664, and high doses of alkylating drugs.

Anti-emetic drugs, when given regularly, help prevent or ameliorate emesis associated with chemotherapy in children.

Prevention of acute symptoms: For patients at low risk of emesis, pretreatment with a $5HT_3$-receptor antagonist may be of benefit.

For patients at high risk of *emesis* or when other treatment is inadequate, a $5HT_3$-receptor antagonist is often highly effective. The addition of dexamethasone p. 543 and other anti-emetics may also be required.

Prevention of delayed symptoms: dexamethasone, given by mouth, is the drug of choice for preventing delayed symptoms; it is used alone or with metoclopramide hydrochloride p. 315. Due to the risks of neurological side-effects, metoclopramide hydrochloride should only be used in children as a second-line option. The $5HT_3$-receptor antagonists may have a role in preventing uncontrolled symptoms. Aprepitant p. 316 given in combination with a $5HT_3$-receptor antagonist (with or without dexamethasone) is licensed for prevention of nausea and vomiting associated with highly and moderately emetogenic cancer chemotherapy.

Prevention of anticipatory symptoms: Good symptom control is the best way to prevent anticipatory symptoms. Lorazepam p. 272 can be helpful for its amnesiac, sedative, and anxiolytic effects.

For information on the treatment of nausea and vomiting, see Nausea and labyrinth disorders p. 311.

Bone-marrow suppression

All cytotoxic drugs except vincristine sulfate p. 678 and bleomycin p. 675 cause bone-marrow suppression. This commonly occurs 7 to 10 days after administration, but is delayed for certain drugs, such as melphalan p. 665. Peripheral blood counts must be checked before each treatment. The duration and severity of neutropenia can be reduced by the use of granulocyte-colony stimulating factors; their use should be reserved for children who have previously experienced severe neutropenia.

Cytotoxic drugs may be contra-indicated in children with acute infection; any infection should be treated before, or when starting, cytotoxic drugs.

Infection in a child with neutropenia requires immediate broad-spectrum antibacterial treatment that covers all likely pathogens. Appropriate bacteriological investigations should be conducted as soon as possible. Children taking cytotoxic drugs who have signs or symptoms of infection (or their carers) should be advised to seek prompt medical attention. All children should be investigated and treated under the supervision of an appropriate oncology or haematology specialist. Antifungal treatment may be required in a child with prolonged neutropenia or fever lasting longer than 4–5 days. Chickenpox and measles can be particularly hazardous in immunocompromised children. If a non-immune child has had close contact with varicella (chickenpox) or herpes zoster (shingles), post-exposure prophylaxis with an antiviral [unlicensed use] or normal immunoglobulin [unlicensed use], may be required. If a non-immune child has come into close contact with an infectious individual with measles, normal immunoglobulin p. 955 should be given. For further information on post-exposure prophylaxis in immunocompromised children following exposure to chickenpox or shingles, see Herpesvirus infections p. 498, and for measles, see Immunoglobulins p. 951.

Alopecia

Reversible hair loss is a common complication, although it varies in degree between drugs and individual patients.

Long-term and delayed toxicity

Cytotoxic drugs may produce specific organ-related toxicity in children (e.g. cardiotoxicity with doxorubicin hydrochloride or nephrotoxicity with cisplatin and ifosfamide p. 665). Manifestations of such toxicity may not appear for several months or even years after cancer treatment. Careful follow-up of survivors of childhood cancer is therefore vital; national and local guidelines have been developed to facilitate this.

Thromboembolism

Venous thromboembolism can be a complication of cancer itself, but chemotherapy increases the risk.

Tumour lysis syndrome

Tumour lysis syndrome occurs secondary to spontaneous or treatment related rapid destruction of malignant cells. Patients at risk of tumour lysis syndrome include those with non-Hodgkin's lymphoma (especially if high grade and bulky disease), Burkitt's lymphoma, acute lymphoblastic leukaemia and acute myeloid leukaemia (particularly if high white blood cell counts or bulky disease), and occasionally those with solid tumours. Pre-existing hyperuricaemia, dehydration and renal impairment are also predisposing factors. Features, include hyperkalaemia, hyperuricaemia, and hyperphosphataemia with hypocalcaemia; renal damage and arrhythmias can follow. Early recognition of patients at risk, and initiation of prophylaxis or therapy for tumour lysis syndrome, is essential.

Treatment of cytotoxic drug side-effects

Hyperuricaemia

Hyperuricaemia, which may be present in high-grade lymphoma and leukaemia, can be markedly worsened by chemotherapy and is associated with acute renal failure.

Allopurinol p. 685 is used routinely in children at low to moderate risk of hyperuricaemia. It should be started 24 hours before treatment; patients should be adequately hydrated (consideration should be given to omitting phosphate and potassium from hydration fluids). The dose of mercaptopurine p. 671 or azathioprine p. 638 should be reduced if allopurinol is given concomitantly.

Rasburicase p. 684 is a recombinant urate oxidase used in children who are at high-risk of developing hyperuricaemia. It rapidly reduces plasma-uric acid concentration and may be of particular value in preventing complications following treatment of leukaemias or bulky lymphomas.

Methotrexate-induced mucositis and myelosuppression

Folinic acid p. 683 (given as calcium folinate) is used to counteract the folate-antagonist action of methotrexate and thus speed recovery from methotrexate-induced mucositis or myelosuppression ('folinic acid rescue').

The calcium salt of levofolinic acid p. 683, a single isomer of folinic acid, is also used following methotrexate administration. The dose of calcium levofolinate is generally half that of calcium folinate.

The disodium salts of folinic acid and levofolinic acid are also used for rescue therapy following methotrexate administration.

The efficacy of high dose methotrexate is enhanced by delaying initiation of folinic acid p. 683 for at least 24 hours, local protocols define the correct time. Folinic acid is normally continued until the plasma-methotrexate concentration falls to 45–90 nanograms/mL (100–200 nanomol/litre).

In the treatment of methotrexate overdose, folinate should be administered immediately; other measures to enhance the elimination of methotrexate are also necessary.

Urothelial toxicity

Haemorrhagic cystitis is a common manifestation of urothelial toxicity which occurs with the oxazaphosphorines, cyclophosphamide p. 663 and ifosfamide p. 665; it is caused by the metabolite acrolein. Adequate hydration is essential to reduce the risk of urothelial toxicity. Mesna reacts specifically with acrolein in the urinary tract, preventing toxicity. Mesna p. 682 is given for the same duration as cyclophosphamide or ifosfamide. It is generally given intravenously; the dose of mesna is equal to or greater than that of the oxazaphosphorine.

Cytotoxic antibiotics

Cytotoxic antibiotics are widely used. Many act as radiomimetics and simultaneous use of radiotherapy should be **avoided** because it may markedly increase toxicity.

Daunorubicin p. 667, doxorubicin hydrochloride p. 668, and epirubicin hydrochloride p. 668 are anthracycline antibiotics. Mitoxantrone p. 669 (mitozantrone) is an anthracycline derivative.

Epirubicin hydrochloride and mitoxantrone are considered less toxic than the other anthracycline antibiotics, and may be suitable for children who have received high cumulative doses of other anthracyclines.

Vinca alkaloids

The vinca alkaloids, vinblastine sulfate p. 678 and vincristine sulfate p. 678 are used to treat a variety of cancers including leukaemias, lymphomas, and some solid tumours.

Antimetabolites

Antimetabolites are incorporated into new nuclear material or they combine irreversibly with cellular enzymes and prevent normal cellular division. Cytarabine p. 670, fludarabine phosphate p. 670, mercaptopurine p. 671, methotrexate p. 672, and tioguanine p. 675 are commonly used in paediatric chemotherapy.

Other antineoplastic drugs

Asparaginase

Asparaginase is used almost exclusively in the treatment of acute lymphoblastic leukaemia. Hypersensitivity reactions may occur and facilities for the management of anaphylaxis should be available. A number of different preparations of asparaginase exist and only the product specified in the treatment protocol should be used.

ANTINEOPLASTIC DRUGS > ALKYLATING AGENTS

Busulfan [Specialist drug] 08-Jul-2020

(Busulphan)

● INDICATIONS AND DOSE

Conditioning treatment before haematopoietic progenitor cell transplantation

▶ BY MOUTH, OR BY INTRAVENOUS INFUSION

▶ Child: Specialist drug – access specialist resources for dosing information

IMPORTANT SAFETY INFORMATION

RISKS OF INCORRECT DOSING OF ORAL ANTI-CANCER MEDICINES

See Cytotoxic drugs p. 660.

● **CONTRA-INDICATIONS** Acute porphyrias p. 745

● **INTERACTIONS** → Appendix 1: alkylating agents

● **SIDE-EFFECTS**

GENERAL SIDE-EFFECTS

▶ **Common or very common** Alopecia · diarrhoea · hepatic disorders · interstitial lung disease · nausea · sinusoidal obstruction syndrome · skin reactions · thrombocytopenia · vomiting

▶ **Uncommon** Seizure

▶ **Rare or very rare** Cataract · eye disorders

SPECIFIC SIDE-EFFECTS

▶ **Common or very common**

▶ With intravenous use Anaemia · anxiety · appetite decreased · arrhythmias · arthralgia · ascites · asthenia · asthma · cardiomegaly · chest pain · chills · confusion · constipation · cough · depression · dizziness · dyspnoea · dysuria · electrolyte imbalance · embolism and thrombosis · fever · gastrointestinal discomfort · gastrointestinal disorders · haemorrhage · headache · hiccups · hyperglycaemia · hypersensitivity · hypertension · hypoalbuminaemia · hypotension · increased risk of infection · insomnia · mucositis · myalgia · nervous system disorder · neutropenia · oedema · pain · pancytopenia · pericardial effusion · pericarditis · reactivation of infections · renal disorder · renal impairment · respiratory disorders · stomatitis · vasodilation · weight increased

▶ With oral use Amenorrhoea (may be reversible) · azoospermia · bone marrow disorders · cardiac tamponade · delayed puberty · hyperbilirubinaemia · infertility male · leucopenia · leukaemia · menopausal symptoms · oral disorders · ovarian and fallopian tube disorders · testicular atrophy

▶ **Uncommon**

▶ With intravenous use Capillary leak syndrome · delirium · encephalopathy · hallucination · hypoxia · intracranial haemorrhage

▶ **Rare or very rare**

▶ With oral use Dry mouth · erythema nodosum · gynaecomastia · myasthenia gravis · radiation injury · Sjögren's syndrome

- ▶ **Frequency not known**
- ▸ With intravenous use Hypogonadism · ovarian failure · premature menopause · sepsis

SIDE-EFFECTS, FURTHER INFORMATION **Lung toxicity** Discontinue if lung toxicity develops.

Secondary malignancy Use of busulfan is associated with an increased incidence of secondary malignancy.

Fluid retention Alkylating drugs can cause fluid retention with oedema and dilutional hyponatraemia in younger children; the risk of this complication is higher in the first 2 days and also when given with concomitant vinca alkaloids.

- **CONCEPTION AND CONTRACEPTION** Manufacturers advise effective contraception during and for 6 months after treatment in men or women.

- **MEDICINAL FORMS** There can be variation in the licensing of different medicines containing the same drug. Forms available from special-order manufacturers include: oral capsule, oral suspension, oral solution

Oral tablet

▸ Busulfan (Non-proprietary)

Busulfan 2 mg Busulfan 2mg tablets | 25 tablet PoM £14.43

Solution for infusion

▸ Busulfan (Non-proprietary)

Busulfan 6 mg per 1 ml Busulfan 60mg/10ml concentrate for solution for infusion vials | 8 vial PoM £1,529.50–£2,816.40 (Hospital only)

Chlorambucil

13-Jul-2020

- **INDICATIONS AND DOSE**

Hodgkin's disease (specialist use only) | Non-Hodgkin's lymphoma (specialist use only)

▶ BY MOUTH

▸ Child: Specialist indication – access specialist resources for dosing information

Relapsing steroid-sensitive nephrotic syndrome (initiated in specialist centres)

▶ BY MOUTH

▸ Child 3 months–17 years: 200 micrograms/kg daily for 8 weeks

- **UNLICENSED USE** Not licensed for use in nephrotic syndrome.

IMPORTANT SAFETY INFORMATION

RISKS OF INCORRECT DOSING OF ORAL ANTI-CANCER MEDICINES

See Cytotoxic drugs p. 660.

- **CAUTIONS** History of epilepsy (increased seizure risk) · nephrotic syndrome (increased seizure risk)
- **INTERACTIONS** → Appendix 1: alkylating agents
- **SIDE-EFFECTS**
- ▶ **Common or very common** Anaemia · bone marrow disorders · diarrhoea · gastrointestinal disorder · leucopenia · nausea · neoplasms · neutropenia · oral ulceration · seizures · thrombocytopenia · vomiting
- ▶ **Uncommon** Skin reactions
- ▶ **Rare or very rare** Cystitis · fever · hepatic disorders · interstitial pneumonia · movement disorders · muscle twitching · peripheral neuropathy · pulmonary fibrosis · severe cutaneous adverse reactions (SCARs) · tremor
- ▶ **Frequency not known** Amenorrhoea · azoospermia

SIDE-EFFECTS, FURTHER INFORMATION **Secondary malignancy** Use of chlorambucil is associated with an increased incidence of acute leukaemia, particularly with prolonged use.

Skin reactions Manufacturer advises assessing continued use if rash occurs—has been reported to progress to Stevens-Johnson syndrome and toxic epidermal necrolysis.

Fluid retention Alkylating drugs can cause fluid retention with oedema and dilutional hyponatraemia in younger children; the risk of this complication is higher in the first 2 days and also when given with concomitant vinca alkaloids.

- **CONCEPTION AND CONTRACEPTION** Contraceptive advice required.
- **PREGNANCY** Avoid. See also *Pregnancy and reproductive function* in Cytotoxic drugs p. 660.
- **BREAST FEEDING** Discontinue breast-feeding.
- **HEPATIC IMPAIRMENT** Manufacturer advises caution—monitor for signs and symptoms of toxicity.

Dose adjustments Manufacturer advises consider dose reduction in severe impairment—limited information available.

- **MONITORING REQUIREMENTS** Monitor full blood count regularly throughout treatment.
- **PATIENT AND CARER ADVICE**

Medicines for Children leaflet: Chlorambucil for nephrotic syndrome www.medicinesforchildren.org.uk/medicines/chlorambucil-for-nephrotic-syndrome/

- **MEDICINAL FORMS** There can be variation in the licensing of different medicines containing the same drug.

Oral tablet

▸ Chlorambucil (Non-proprietary)

Chlorambucil 2 mg Chlorambucil 2mg tablets | 25 tablet PoM £11.15

Cyclophosphamide

04-Aug-2023

- **INDICATIONS AND DOSE**

Acute lymphoblastic leukaemia, non-Hodgkin's lymphoma, retinoblastoma, neuroblastoma, rhabdomyosarcoma, soft-tissue sarcomas, Ewing tumour, neuroectodermal tumours (including medulloblastoma), infant brain tumours, ependymona, high-dose conditioning for bone marrow transplantation, lupus nephritis (specialist use only)

▶ BY MOUTH, OR BY INTRAVENOUS INFUSION

▸ Child: Specialist indication – access specialist resources for dosing information

Steroid-sensitive nephrotic syndrome (under expert supervision)

▶ BY MOUTH

▸ Child 3 months–17 years: 2–3 mg/kg daily for 8 weeks

▶ BY INTRAVENOUS INFUSION

▸ Child 3 months–17 years: 500 mg/m^2 once a month for 6 months

- **UNLICENSED USE** Not licensed for use in children.

IMPORTANT SAFETY INFORMATION

RISKS OF INCORRECT DOSING OF ORAL ANTI-CANCER MEDICINES

See Cytotoxic drugs p. 660.

- **CAUTIONS** Avoid in Acute porphyrias p. 745 · diabetes mellitus · haemorrhagic cystitis · previous or concurrent mediastinal irradiation—risk of cardiotoxicity
- **INTERACTIONS** → Appendix 1: alkylating agents
- **SIDE-EFFECTS**

GENERAL SIDE-EFFECTS

- ▶ **Common or very common** Agranulocytosis · alopecia · anaemia · asthenia · bone marrow disorders · cystitis · decreased leucocytes · fever · haemolytic uraemic syndrome · haemorrhage · hepatic disorders · immunosuppression · increased risk of infection · mucosal abnormalities · neutropenia · progressive multifocal

leukoencephalopathy (PML) · reactivation of infections · sperm abnormalities · thrombocytopenia
- **Uncommon** Appetite decreased · flushing · hypersensitivity · ovarian and fallopian tube disorders · sepsis
- **Rare or very rare** Bladder disorders · chest pain · confusion · constipation · diarrhoea · disseminated intravascular coagulation · dizziness · eye inflammation · fluid imbalance · headache · hyponatraemia · menstrual cycle irregularities · myocardial infarction · nail discolouration · nausea · neoplasms · oral disorders · pancreatitis acute · renal failure · rhabdomyolysis · secondary neoplasm · seizure · severe cutaneous adverse reactions (SCARs) · SIADH · skin reactions · visual impairment · vomiting
- **Frequency not known** Abdominal pain · altered smell sensation · arrhythmias · arthralgia · ascites · cardiac inflammation · cardiogenic shock · cardiomyopathy · cough · deafness · dyspnoea · embolism and thrombosis · encephalopathy · excessive tearing · facial swelling · gastrointestinal disorders · heart failure · hyperhidrosis · hypoxia · infertility · influenza like illness · interstitial lung disease · multi organ failure · muscle complaints · myelopathy · nasal complaints · nephrogenic diabetes insipidus · nephrotoxicity · nerve disorders · neuralgia · neurotoxicity · oedema · oropharyngeal pain · palpitations · pericardial effusion · peripheral ischaemia · pulmonary fibrosis · pulmonary hypertension · pulmonary oedema · QT interval prolongation · radiation injuries · renal tubular disorder · renal tubular necrosis · respiratory disorders · scleroderma · sensation abnormal · sinusoidal obstruction syndrome · taste altered · testicular atrophy · tinnitus · tremor · tumour lysis syndrome · vasculitis

SPECIFIC SIDE-EFFECTS
- With intravenous use Infusion site necrosis · injection site necrosis

SIDE-EFFECTS, FURTHER INFORMATION **Haemorrhagic cystitis** A urinary metabolite of cyclophosphamide, acrolein, can cause haemorrhagic cystitis; this is a rare but serious complication that may be prevented by increasing fluid intake for 24–48 hours after intravenous injection. Mesna can also help prevent cystitis.

Secondary malignancy As with all cytotoxic therapy, treatment with cyclophosphamide is associated with an increased incidence of secondary malignancies.

Fluid retention Alkylating drugs can cause fluid retention with oedema and dilutional hyponatraemia in younger children; the risk of this complication is higher in the first 2 days and also when given with concomitant vinca alkaloids.

- **CONCEPTION AND CONTRACEPTION** EvGr Females of childbearing potential should use effective contraception during treatment and for at least 12 months after last treatment; male patients should use effective contraception during treatment and for at least 6 months after last treatment if their partner is of childbearing potential. ⟨M⟩ See also *Pregnancy and reproductive function* in Cytotoxic drugs p. 660.
- **PREGNANCY** Avoid. See also *Pregnancy and reproductive function* in Cytotoxic drugs p. 660.
- **BREAST FEEDING** Discontinue breast-feeding during and for 36 hours after stopping treatment.
- **HEPATIC IMPAIRMENT** Manufacturer advises caution (risk of decreased cyclophosphamide activation and increased risk of veno-occlusive liver disease).
 Dose adjustments Manufacturer advises consider dose adjustment in severe impairment—consult product literature.
- **RENAL IMPAIRMENT**
 Dose adjustments EvGr Consider dose reduction (consult product literature). ⟨M⟩
- **DIRECTIONS FOR ADMINISTRATION** Consult local treatment protocol for details.
- **PATIENT AND CARER ADVICE**
 Medicines for Children leaflet: Cyclophosphamide for nephrotic syndrome www.medicinesforchildren.org.uk/medicines/cyclophosphamide-for-nephrotic-syndrome/
- **MEDICINAL FORMS** There can be variation in the licensing of different medicines containing the same drug. Forms available from special-order manufacturers include: oral tablet, oral suspension, oral solution, solution for injection, solution for infusion

Oral tablet

CAUTIONARY AND ADVISORY LABELS 25, 27
- Cyclophosphamide (Non-proprietary)
 Cyclophosphamide (as Cyclophosphamide monohydrate) 50 mg Cyclophosphamide 50mg tablets | 100 tablet PoM £153.00
- Cytoxan (Imported (United States))
 Cyclophosphamide 25 mg Cytoxan 25mg tablets | 100 tablet PoM ⊠

Powder for solution for injection
- Cyclophosphamide (Non-proprietary)
 Cyclophosphamide (as Cyclophosphamide monohydrate) 500 mg Cyclophosphamide 500mg powder for solution for injection vials | 1 vial PoM £8.21–£10.63 (Hospital only)
 Cyclophosphamide (as Cyclophosphamide monohydrate) 1 gram Cyclophosphamide 1g powder for solution for injection vials | 1 vial PoM £15.22–£19.70 (Hospital only)
 Cyclophosphamide (as Cyclophosphamide monohydrate) 2 gram Cyclophosphamide 2g powder for solution for injection vials | 1 vial PoM £28.22 (Hospital only)

Dacarbazine [Specialist drug] 24-Jun-2021

- **INDICATIONS AND DOSE**

Hodgkin's disease | Paediatric solid tumours
- BY INTRAVENOUS INJECTION, OR BY INTRAVENOUS INFUSION
- Child: Specialist drug – access specialist resources for dosing information

- **INTERACTIONS** → Appendix 1: alkylating agents
- **SIDE-EFFECTS**
 - **Common or very common** Anaemia · appetite decreased · leucopenia · nausea · thrombocytopenia · vomiting
 - **Uncommon** Alopecia · infection · influenza like illness · photosensitivity reaction · skin reactions
 - **Rare or very rare** Agranulocytosis · confusion · diarrhoea · flushing · headache · hepatic disorders · lethargy · pancytopenia · paraesthesia · renal impairment · seizure · visual impairment
- **CONCEPTION AND CONTRACEPTION** Ensure effective contraception during and for at least 6 months after treatment in men or women.
- **MEDICINAL FORMS** There can be variation in the licensing of different medicines containing the same drug.

Powder for solution for infusion
- Dacarbazine (Non-proprietary)
 Dacarbazine (as Dacarbazine citrate) 500 mg Dacarbazine 500mg powder for solution for infusion vials | 1 vial PoM £37.50
 Dacarbazine (as Dacarbazine citrate) 1 gram Dacarbazine 1g powder for solution for infusion vials | 1 vial PoM £70.00

Powder for solution for injection
- Dacarbazine (Non-proprietary)
 Dacarbazine (as Dacarbazine citrate) 100 mg Dacarbazine 100mg powder for solution for injection vials | 10 vial PoM £90.00
 Dacarbazine (as Dacarbazine citrate) 200 mg Dacarbazine 200mg powder for solution for injection vials | 10 vial PoM £160.00

Ifosfamide [Specialist drug] 30-Jan-2022

● **INDICATIONS AND DOSE**

Rhabdomyosarcoma | Soft-tissue sarcomas | Ewing tumour | Germ cell tumour | Osteogenic sarcoma

▶ BY INTRAVENOUS INFUSION

▶ Child: Specialist drug – access specialist resources for dosing information

● **CONTRA-INDICATIONS** Acute infection · Acute porphyrias p. 745 · cystitis · urinary-tract obstruction · urothelial damage

● **INTERACTIONS** → Appendix 1: alkylating agents

● **SIDE-EFFECTS**

▶ **Common or very common** Alopecia · appetite decreased · bone marrow disorders · haemorrhage · hepatic disorders · infection · leucopenia · nausea · reactivation of infection · renal impairment · thrombocytopenia · vomiting

▶ **Uncommon** Cardiotoxicity · diarrhoea · hypotension · oral disorders

▶ **Rare or very rare** Skin reactions

▶ **Frequency not known** Abdominal pain · agranulocytosis · amenorrhoea · anaemia · angina pectoris · angioedema · arrhythmias · arthralgia · asterixis · behaviour abnormal · blood disorders · bone disorders · cancer progression · capillary leak syndrome · cardiac arrest · cardiomyopathy · chills · conjunctivitis · constipation · cough · deafness · delirium · delusions · disseminated intravascular coagulation · dysarthria · dyspnoea · electrolyte imbalance · embolism and thrombosis · encephalopathy · eye irritation · Fanconi syndrome acquired · fatigue · fever · flushing · gait abnormal · gastrointestinal disorders · growth retardation · haemolytic anaemia · heart failure · hyperglycaemia · hyperhidrosis · hyperphosphaturia · hypertension · hypoxia · immunosuppression · infertility · interstitial lung disease · malaise · mania · memory loss · metabolic acidosis · movement disorders · mucosal ulceration · multi organ failure · muscle complaints · myocardial infarction · nail disorder · neoplasms · nephritis tubulointerstitial · nephrogenic diabetes insipidus · neurotoxicity · oedema · ovarian and fallopian tube disorders · pain · pancreatitis · panic attack · peripheral neuropathy · polydipsia · premature menopause · psychiatric disorders · pulmonary fibrosis · pulmonary hypertension · pulmonary oedema · radiation recall reaction · respiratory disorders · rhabdomyolysis · secondary malignancy · sensation abnormal · sepsis · severe cutaneous adverse reactions (SCARs) · SIADH · sinusoidal obstruction syndrome · sperm abnormalities · status epilepticus · tinnitus · tumour lysis syndrome · urinary disorders · vasculitis · vertigo · visual impairment

SIDE-EFFECTS, FURTHER INFORMATION **Urothelial toxicity** Mesna is routinely given with ifosfamide to reduce urothelial toxicity.

Secondary malignancy Use of ifosfamide is associated with an increased incidence of acute leukaemia.

Fluid retention Alkylating drugs can cause fluid retention with oedema and dilutional hyponatraemia in younger children; the risk of this complication is higher in the first 2 days and also when given with concomitant vinca alkaloids.

● **CONCEPTION AND CONTRACEPTION** Manufacturer advises adequate contraception during and for at least 6 months after treatment in men or women.

● **MEDICINAL FORMS** There can be variation in the licensing of different medicines containing the same drug.

Powder for solution for injection

▶ **Ifosfamide (Non-proprietary)**

Ifosfamide 1 gram Ifosfamide 1g powder for concentrate for solution for injection vials | 1 vial [PoM] £151.49

Ifosfamide 2 gram Ifosfamide 2g powder for concentrate for solution for injection vials | 1 vial [PoM] £298.41

Melphalan [Specialist drug] 21-Mar-2023

● **INDICATIONS AND DOSE**

High intravenous dose with haematopoietic stem cell transplantation in the treatment of childhood neuroblastoma and some other advanced embryonal tumours

▶ BY INTRAVENOUS INFUSION

▶ Child: Specialist drug – access specialist resources for dosing information

● **UNLICENSED USE** Not licensed for use in embryonal tumours.

● **INTERACTIONS** → Appendix 1: alkylating agents

● **SIDE-EFFECTS**

▶ **Common or very common** Alopecia · anaemia · bone marrow depression (delayed) · diarrhoea · feeling hot · myalgia · myopathy · nausea · paraesthesia · stomatitis · thrombocytopenia · vomiting

▶ **Rare or very rare** Haemolytic anaemia · hepatic disorders · interstitial pneumonitis · peripheral vascular disease · pulmonary fibrosis · skin reactions

SIDE-EFFECTS, FURTHER INFORMATION **Secondary malignancy** Use of melphalan is associated with an increased incidence of acute leukaemias.

Fluid retention Alkylating drugs can cause fluid retention with oedema and dilutional hyponatraemia in younger children; the risk of this complication is higher in the first 2 days and also when given with concomitant vinca alkaloids.

● **CONCEPTION AND CONTRACEPTION** Manufacturer advises adequate contraception during treatment in men or women.

● **MEDICINAL FORMS** There can be variation in the licensing of different medicines containing the same drug.

Powder and solvent for solution for injection

▶ **Melphalan (Non-proprietary)**

Melphalan (as Melphalan hydrochloride) 50 mg Melphalan 50mg powder and solvent for solution for injection vials | 1 vial [PoM] £26.64–£105.00 (Hospital only)

▶ **Phelinun** (Adienne Pharma & Biotech)

Melphalan (as Melphalan hydrochloride) 50 mg Phelinun 50mg powder and solvent for concentrate for solution for infusion vials | 1 vial [PoM] £129.81 (Hospital only)

Temozolomide [Specialist drug] 10-May-2021

● **INDICATIONS AND DOSE**

Malignant glioma

▶ BY MOUTH

▶ Child 3–17 years: Specialist drug – access specialist resources for dosing information

IMPORTANT SAFETY INFORMATION

RISKS OF INCORRECT DOSING OF ORAL ANTI-CANCER MEDICINES

See Cytotoxic drugs p. 660.

● **INTERACTIONS** → Appendix 1: alkylating agents

● **SIDE-EFFECTS**

▶ **Common or very common** Alopecia · anaemia · anxiety · appetite decreased · arthralgia · asthenia · cognitive impairment · concentration impaired · confusion · constipation · cough · Cushing's syndrome · decreased leucocytes · depression · diarrhoea · dizziness · drowsiness · dysphagia · dyspnoea · ear pain · embolism and thrombosis · eye pain · fever · gastrointestinal discomfort ·

haemorrhage · headache · hearing impairment · hemiparesis · hyperglycaemia · hypersensitivity · hypertension · increased risk of infection · influenza like illness · insomnia · level of consciousness decreased · malaise · memory loss · movement disorders · muscle weakness · myalgia · myopathy · nausea · nerve disorders · neutropenia · oedema · oral disorders · pain · peripheral swelling · radiation injuries · seizures · sensation abnormal · skin reactions · speech impairment · taste altered · thrombocytopenia · tinnitus · tremor · urinary disorders · vertigo · vision disorders · vomiting · weight changes

- **Uncommon** Altered smell sensation · angioedema · aplastic anaemia (sometimes fatal) · behaviour disorder · breast pain · chills · condition aggravated · diabetes insipidus · dry eye · dry mouth · emotional lability · erectile dysfunction · gait abnormal · gastrointestinal disorders · hallucination · hemiplegia · hepatic disorders · hepatic failure (sometimes fatal) · hepatitis B reactivation (sometimes fatal) · hyperacusia · hyperbilirubinaemia · hyperhidrosis · hypokalaemia · interstitial lung disease · intracranial haemorrhage · meningoencephalitis herpetic (sometimes fatal) · menstrual cycle irregularities · nasal congestion · neoplasms · nervous system disorder · palpitations · pancytopenia (sometimes prolonged) · photosensitivity reaction · pulmonary fibrosis · reactivation of infections · respiratory failure (sometimes fatal) · secondary malignancy · sepsis (sometimes fatal) · severe cutaneous adverse reactions (SCARs) · thirst · tongue discolouration · vasodilation

● **CONCEPTION AND CONTRACEPTION** Manufacturer advises adequate contraception during treatment. Men should avoid fathering a child during and for at least 6 months after treatment.

● **MEDICINAL FORMS** There can be variation in the licensing of different medicines containing the same drug. Forms available from special-order manufacturers include: oral suspension

Oral capsule

CAUTIONARY AND ADVISORY LABELS 23, 25

- **Temozolomide (Non-proprietary)**
  - **Temozolomide 5 mg** Temozolomide 5mg capsules | 5 capsule PoM £10.06 | 5 capsule PoM £10.06–£16.00 (Hospital only)
  - **Temozolomide 20 mg** Temozolomide 20mg capsules | 5 capsule PoM £40.23–£65.00 (Hospital only)
  - **Temozolomide 100 mg** Temozolomide 100mg capsules | 5 capsule PoM £211.00 | 5 capsule PoM £201.18–£325.00 (Hospital only)
  - **Temozolomide 140 mg** Temozolomide 140mg capsules | 5 capsule PoM £296.47–£465.00 (Hospital only)
  - **Temozolomide 180 mg** Temozolomide 180mg capsules | 5 capsule PoM £381.18–£586.00 (Hospital only)
  - **Temozolomide 250 mg** Temozolomide 250mg capsules | 5 capsule PoM £529.00 | 5 capsule PoM £529.42–£814.00 (Hospital only)
- **Temodal** (Merck Sharp & Dohme (UK) Ltd)
  - **Temozolomide 5 mg** Temodal 5mg capsules | 5 capsule PoM £10.59 (Hospital only)
  - **Temozolomide 20 mg** Temodal 20mg capsules | 5 capsule PoM £42.35 (Hospital only)
  - **Temozolomide 100 mg** Temodal 100mg capsules | 5 capsule PoM £211.77 (Hospital only)
  - **Temozolomide 140 mg** Temodal 140mg capsules | 5 capsule PoM £296.48 (Hospital only)
  - **Temozolomide 180 mg** Temodal 180mg capsules | 5 capsule PoM £381.19 (Hospital only)
  - **Temozolomide 250 mg** Temodal 250mg capsules | 5 capsule PoM £529.43 (Hospital only)

Thiotepa [Specialist drug] 16-Nov-2020

● **INDICATIONS AND DOSE**

Conditioning treatment before haematopoietic stem cell transplantation in the treatment of haematological disease or solid tumours

- BY INTRAVENOUS INFUSION
  - Child: Specialist drug – access specialist resources for dosing information

● **CONTRA-INDICATIONS** Acute porphyrias p. 745

● **INTERACTIONS** → Appendix 1: alkylating agents

● **SIDE-EFFECTS**

- **Common or very common** Abdominal pain · anaemia · appetite decreased · ataxia · bladder disorder · cardiac arrest · cardiovascular insufficiency · diarrhoea · encephalopathy · fever · gastrointestinal disorders · graft versus host disease · growth retardation · haemorrhage · headache · hearing impairment · heart failure · hepatic failure · hyperglycaemia · hypertension · hypogonadism · hypopituitarism · hypothyroidism · hypoxia · increased risk of infection · interstitial lung disease · intracranial haemorrhage · memory loss · mucositis · multi organ failure · nausea · neutropenia · pain · pancytopenia · paresis · psychiatric disorder · pulmonary oedema · renal failure · respiratory arrest · secondary malignancy · seizure · sepsis · sinusoidal obstruction syndrome · skin reactions · stomatitis · thrombocytopenia · vomiting
- **Frequency not known** Pulmonary arterial hypertension · severe cutaneous adverse reactions (SCARs)

SIDE-EFFECTS, FURTHER INFORMATION Alkylating drugs can cause fluid retention with oedema and dilutional hyponatraemia in younger children; the risk of this complication is higher in the first 2 days and also when given with concomitant vinca alkaloids.

● **CONCEPTION AND CONTRACEPTION** Contraceptive advice required.

● **NATIONAL FUNDING/ACCESS DECISIONS**

For full details see funding body website

Scottish Medicines Consortium (SMC) decisions

- **Thiotepa (*Tepadina*®) in combination with other chemotherapy as conditioning treatment in adults or children with haematological diseases, or solid tumours prior to haematopoietic stem cell transplantation (July 2012)** SMC No. 790/12 Not recommended

● **MEDICINAL FORMS** There can be variation in the licensing of different medicines containing the same drug.

Powder for solution for infusion

- **Thiotepa (Non-proprietary)**
  - **Thiotepa 15 mg** Thiotepa 15mg powder for concentrate for solution for infusion vials | 1 vial PoM £123.00–£250.00 (Hospital only)
  - **Thiotepa 100 mg** Thiotepa 100mg powder for concentrate for solution for infusion vials | 1 vial PoM £736.00–£850.00 (Hospital only)
- **Tepadina** (Adienne Pharma & Biotech)
  - **Thiotepa 15 mg** Tepadina 15mg powder for concentrate for solution for infusion vials | 1 vial PoM £123.00 (Hospital only)
  - **Thiotepa 100 mg** Tepadina 100mg powder for concentrate for solution for infusion vials | 1 vial PoM £736.00 (Hospital only)

Treosulfan [Specialist drug] 05-Jul-2023

● **INDICATIONS AND DOSE**

TRECONDI®

Conditioning treatment before allogeneic haematopoietic stem cell transplantation in patients with malignant disease

- BY INTRAVENOUS INFUSION
  - Child: Specialist drug – access specialist resources for dosing information

- **CONTRA-INDICATIONS** Active uncontrolled infection · acute porphyrias p. 745 · concomitant use of live vaccines · Fanconi anaemia and other DNA repair disorders · severe concomitant cardiac, lung, liver and renal impairment
- **INTERACTIONS** → Appendix 1: alkylating agents
- **SIDE-EFFECTS**
  - ▶ **Common or very common** Alopecia · anaemia · bone marrow disorders · diarrhoea · dysphagia · fever · gastrointestinal discomfort · haemorrhage · leucopenia · nausea · oral disorders · oropharyngeal pain · skin reactions · thrombocytopenia · vomiting
  - ▶ **Uncommon** Neoplasms
  - ▶ **Rare or very rare** Addison's disease · alveolitis · cardiomyopathy · hypoglycaemia · inflammation localised · influenza like illness · pneumonia · pulmonary fibrosis · scleroderma
  - ▶ **Frequency not known** Alkalosis · amenorrhoea · capillary leak syndrome · chills · colitis neutropenic · constipation · cystitis · dry eye · electrolyte imbalance · fatigue · febrile neutropenia · headache · hepatic disorders · hypertension · hypotension · hypoxia · ovarian suppression · pain · paraesthesia · pulmonary toxicity · renal impairment · scrotal erythema · seizure · sinusoidal obstruction syndrome · skin ulcer · treatment related secondary malignancy

  SIDE-EFFECTS, FURTHER INFORMATION Prolonged use of treosulfan is associated with an increased incidence of acute non-lymphocytic leukaemia.
- **CONCEPTION AND CONTRACEPTION** Manufacturer advises females of childbearing potential and male patients with partners of childbearing potential should use effective contraception during and for 6 months after treatment.
- **PATIENT AND CARER ADVICE**

  Driving and skilled tasks Patients and carers should be counselled on the effects on driving and performance of skilled tasks—increased risk of nausea, vomiting or dizziness.
- **NATIONAL FUNDING/ACCESS DECISIONS**

  For full details see funding body website

  NICE decisions
  - ▶ **Treosulfan with fludarabine for malignant disease before allogeneic stem cell transplant (August 2020)** NICE TA640 Recommended

  Scottish Medicines Consortium (SMC) decisions
  - ▶ **Treosulfan (*Trecondi*®) in combination with fludarabine as part of conditioning treatment prior to allogeneic haematopoietic stem cell transplantation in adult patients with malignant and non-malignant diseases, and in paediatric patients older than one month with malignant diseases (June 2023)** SMC No. SMC2527 Recommended with restrictions

- **MEDICINAL FORMS** There can be variation in the licensing of different medicines containing the same drug.

  Powder for solution for injection
  - ▶ **Trecondi** (medac UK)

    Treosulfan 1 gram Trecondi 1g powder for solution for infusion | 5 vial [PoM] £494.40 (Hospital only)

    Treosulfan 5 gram Trecondi 5g powder for solution for infusion | 5 vial [PoM] £2,434.25 (Hospital only)

ANTINEOPLASTIC DRUGS > ANTHRACYCLINES AND RELATED DRUGS

Daunorubicin [Specialist drug]

19-Dec-2021

- **INDICATIONS AND DOSE**

  Acute myelogenous leukaemia | Acute lymphocytic leukaemia
  - ▶ BY INTRAVENOUS INFUSION
  - ▶ Child: Specialist drug – access specialist resources for dosing information

  DOSE EQUIVALENCE AND CONVERSION
  - ▶ Daunorubicin is available as *conventional* and *liposomal* formulations; these formulations are **not** interchangeable.
- **UNLICENSED USE** *DaunoXome*® is not licensed for use in children.

> **IMPORTANT SAFETY INFORMATION**
>
> **MHRA/CHM ADVICE: LIPOSOMAL AND LIPID-COMPLEX FORMULATIONS: NAME CHANGE TO REDUCE MEDICATION ERRORS (JULY 2020)**
>
> Serious harm and fatal overdoses have occurred following confusion between liposomal, pegylated-liposomal, lipid-complex, and conventional formulations of the same drug substance. Medicines with these formulations will explicitly include 'liposomal', 'pegylated-liposomal', or 'lipid-complex' within their name to reduce the risk of potentially fatal medication errors.
>
> The MHRA reminds healthcare professionals that liposomal, pegylated-liposomal, lipid-complex, and conventional formulations containing the same drug substance are **not** interchangeable. Healthcare professionals are advised to make a clear distinction between formulations when prescribing, dispensing, administering, and communicating about daunorubicin. The product name and dose should be verified before administration and the maximum dose should not be exceeded.

- **CONTRA-INDICATIONS** Myocardial insufficiency · previous treatment with maximum cumulative doses of daunorubicin or other anthracycline · recent myocardial infarction · severe arrhythmia
- **INTERACTIONS** → Appendix 1: anthracyclines
- **SIDE-EFFECTS** Abdominal pain · alopecia · amenorrhoea · anaemia · arrhythmias · ascites · atrioventricular block · azoospermia · bone marrow disorders · cardiac inflammation · cardiomyopathy · chills · congestive heart failure · cyanosis · death · dehydration · diarrhoea · dyspnoea · extravasation necrosis · fever · flushing · gastrointestinal disorders · haemorrhage · hepatomegaly · hyperpyrexia · hyperuricaemia · hypoxia · infection · ischaemic heart disease · leucopenia · mucositis · myocardial infarction · nail discolouration · nausea · nephropathy · neutropenia · oedema · pain · paraesthesia · pleural effusion · posterior reversible encephalopathy syndrome (PRES) · radiation injuries · shock · skin reactions · stomatitis · thrombocytopenia · thrombophlebitis · urine discolouration · venous sclerosis · vomiting

  SIDE-EFFECTS, FURTHER INFORMATION Cardiotoxicity is cumulative and may be irreversible, however responds to treatment if detected early.
- **CONCEPTION AND CONTRACEPTION** Contraceptive advice required.

● **MEDICINAL FORMS** There can be variation in the licensing of different medicines containing the same drug.

Powder for solution for infusion

▸ Daunorubicin (Non-proprietary)

Daunorubicin (as Daunorubicin hydrochloride)

20 mg Daunorubicin 20mg powder for solution for infusion vials | 10 vial PoM £715.00 (Hospital only)

Doxorubicin hydrochloride [Specialist drug]

05-Oct-2021

● **INDICATIONS AND DOSE**

Paediatric malignancies including Ewing's sarcoma, osteogenic sarcoma, Wilm's tumour, neuroblastoma, retinoblastoma, some liver tumours, acute lymphoblastic leukaemia, Hodgkin's lymphoma, non-Hodgkin's lymphoma (conventional formulation only)

▸ BY INTRAVENOUS INFUSION

▸ Child: Specialist drug – access specialist resources for dosing information

IMPORTANT SAFETY INFORMATION

MHRA/CHM ADVICE: LIPOSOMAL AND LIPID-COMPLEX FORMULATIONS: NAME CHANGE TO REDUCE MEDICATION ERRORS (JULY 2020)

Serious harm and fatal overdoses have occurred following confusion between liposomal, pegylated-liposomal, lipid-complex, and conventional formulations of the same drug substance. Medicines with these formulations will explicitly include 'liposomal', 'pegylated-liposomal', or 'lipid-complex' within their name to reduce the risk of potentially fatal medication errors.

The MHRA reminds healthcare professionals that liposomal, pegylated-liposomal, lipid-complex, and conventional formulations containing the same drug substance are **not** interchangeable. Healthcare professionals are advised to make a clear distinction between formulations when prescribing, dispensing, administering, and communicating about doxorubicin. The product name and dose should be verified before administration and the maximum dose should not be exceeded.

● **CONTRA-INDICATIONS** Acute inflammatory heart disease · increased haemorrhagic tendency · marked persisting myelosuppression induced by previous treatment · marked persisting stomatitis induced by previous treatment · previous myocardial infarction · previous treatment with maximum cumulative doses of doxorubicin · previous treatment with maximum cumulative doses of other anthracycline · severe arrhythmia · severe myocardial insufficiency

● **INTERACTIONS** → Appendix 1: anthracyclines

● **SIDE-EFFECTS**

▸ **Common or very common** Alopecia · anaemia · anxiety · appetite decreased · arrhythmias · arthralgia · asthenia · bone marrow depression · breast pain · cachexia · cardiovascular disorder · chest discomfort · chills · constipation · cough · decreased leucocytes · dehydration · depression · diarrhoea · dizziness · drowsiness · dry mouth · dysphagia · dyspnoea · dysuria · electrolyte imbalance · epistaxis · eye inflammation · fever · gastrointestinal discomfort · gastrointestinal disorders · headache · hyperhidrosis · hypersensitivity · hypertension · hyperthermia · hypotension · increased risk of infection · influenza like illness · infusion related reaction · insomnia · malaise · mucosal abnormalities · muscle complaints · muscle tone increased · muscle weakness · nail disorder · nausea · nerve disorders · neutropenia · oedema · oral disorders · pain · scrotal erythema · sensation abnormal · sepsis · skin reactions · skin ulcer · syncope · taste altered · thrombocytopenia · vasodilation · vision blurred · vomiting · weight decreased

▸ **Uncommon** Confusion · embolism and thrombosis

▸ **Rare or very rare** Secondary oral neoplasms · severe cutaneous adverse reactions (SCARs)

▸ **Frequency not known** Asthma · congestive heart failure · secondary malignancy · throat tightness

SIDE-EFFECTS, FURTHER INFORMATION Extravasation can cause tissue necrosis.

Cardiotoxicity All anthracycline antibiotics have been associated with varying degrees of cardiac toxicity—this may be idiosyncratic and reversible, but is commonly related to total cumulative dose and is irreversible.

● **CONCEPTION AND CONTRACEPTION** Manufacturer advises effective contraception during and for at least 6 months after treatment in men or women.

● **MEDICINAL FORMS** There can be variation in the licensing of different medicines containing the same drug. Forms available from special-order manufacturers include: solution for injection, solution for infusion

Solution for injection

▸ Doxorubicin hydrochloride (Non-proprietary)

Doxorubicin hydrochloride 2 mg per 1 ml Doxorubicin 50mg/25ml solution for injection Cytosafe vials | 1 vial PoM £103.00 (Hospital only)

Doxorubicin 50mg/25ml solution for infusion vials | 1 vial PoM £103.00 (Hospital only)

Doxorubicin 10mg/5ml solution for injection Cytosafe vials | 1 vial PoM £20.60 (Hospital only)

Doxorubicin 10mg/5ml concentrate for solution for infusion vials | 1 vial PoM £19.57–£20.60 (Hospital only)

Doxorubicin 10mg/5ml solution for infusion vials | 1 vial PoM £20.60 (Hospital only)

Doxorubicin 50mg/25ml concentrate for solution for infusion vials | 1 vial PoM £96.00–£97.85 (Hospital only)

Solution for infusion

▸ Doxorubicin hydrochloride (Non-proprietary)

Doxorubicin hydrochloride 2 mg per 1 ml Doxorubicin 200mg/100ml solution for infusion vials | 1 vial PoM £412.00 (Hospital only)

Doxorubicin 20mg/10ml concentrate for solution for infusion vials | 1 vial PoM £22.00 (Hospital only)

Doxorubicin 100mg/50ml concentrate for solution for infusion vials | 1 vial PoM £235.00 (Hospital only)

Doxorubicin 200mg/100ml solution for injection Cytosafe vials | 1 vial PoM £412.00 (Hospital only)

Doxorubicin 200mg/100ml concentrate for solution for infusion vials | 1 vial PoM £389.00–£391.40 (Hospital only)

Doxorubicin hydrochloride (as Doxorubicin hydrochloride pegylated liposomal) 2 mg per 1 ml Doxorubicin pegylated liposomal 50mg/25ml concentrate for solution for infusion vials | 1 vial PoM £712.00–£712.49 (Hospital only) | 1 vial PoM £712.48

Doxorubicin pegylated liposomal 20mg/10ml concentrate for solution for infusion vials | 1 vial PoM £360.00–£360.23 (Hospital only) | 1 vial PoM £360.22

Epirubicin hydrochloride [Specialist drug]

21-May-2021

● **INDICATIONS AND DOSE**

Recurrent acute lymphoblastic leukaemia | Rhabdomyosarcoma | Other soft-tissue tumours of childhood

▸ BY INTRAVENOUS INFUSION

▸ Child: Specialist drug – access specialist resources for dosing information

● **UNLICENSED USE** Not licensed for use in children.

● **CONTRA-INDICATIONS** Myocardiopathy · previous treatment with maximum cumulative doses of epirubicin or other anthracycline · recent myocardial infarction · severe arrhythmia · severe myocardial insufficiency · unstable angina

- **INTERACTIONS** → Appendix 1: anthracyclines
- **SIDE-EFFECTS**
  - **Common or very common** Alopecia · amenorrhoea · anaemia · appetite decreased · arrhythmias · cardiac conduction disorders · chills · congestive heart failure · dehydration · diarrhoea · eye inflammation · fever · gastrointestinal discomfort · gastrointestinal disorders · haemorrhage · increased risk of infection · leucopenia · malaise · mucositis · nail discolouration · nausea · neutropenia · oral disorders · skin reactions · thrombocytopenia · urine discolouration · vasodilation · vomiting
  - **Uncommon** Asthenia · embolism and thrombosis · sepsis
  - **Rare or very rare** Hyperuricaemia
  - **Frequency not known** Bone marrow depression · cardiomyopathy · cardiotoxicity · photosensitivity reaction · radiation injuries · shock

  SIDE-EFFECTS, FURTHER INFORMATION **Cardiotoxicity** All anthracycline antibiotics have been associated with varying degrees of cardiac toxicity—this may be idiosyncratic and reversible, but is commonly related to total cumulative dose and is irreversible.

  Cumulative doses of other anthracycline Epirubicin is considered less toxic than other anthracyline antibiotics, and may be suitable for children who have received high cumulative doses of other anthracyclines.
- **CONCEPTION AND CONTRACEPTION** Females of childbearing potential should use effective contraception during treatment and for at least 6.5 months after last dose; male patients should use effective contraception during treatment and for at least 3.5 months after last dose.

- **MEDICINAL FORMS** There can be variation in the licensing of different medicines containing the same drug. Forms available from special-order manufacturers include: solution for injection, solution for infusion

Solution for injection

- **Epirubicin hydrochloride (Non-proprietary)**
  Epirubicin hydrochloride 2 mg per 1 ml Epirubicin 50mg/25ml solution for injection vials | 1 vial [PoM] £86.89–£106.19 (Hospital only)
  Epirubicin 10mg/5ml solution for injection vials | 1 vial [PoM] £17.38–£21.24 (Hospital only)
- **Pharmorubicin** (Pfizer Ltd)
  Epirubicin hydrochloride 2 mg per 1 ml Pharmorubicin 50mg/25ml solution for injection Cytosafe vials | 1 vial [PoM] £106.19 (Hospital only)
  Pharmorubicin 10mg/5ml solution for injection Cytosafe vials | 1 vial [PoM] £21.24 (Hospital only)

Solution for infusion

- **Epirubicin hydrochloride (Non-proprietary)**
  Epirubicin hydrochloride 2 mg per 1 ml Epirubicin 100mg/50ml solution for infusion vials | 1 vial [PoM] £201.76 (Hospital only)
  Epirubicin 200mg/100ml solution for infusion vials | 1 vial [PoM] £347.55–£366.85 (Hospital only)

Mitoxantrone [Specialist drug] (Mitozantrone)

25-Jun-2020

- **INDICATIONS AND DOSE**

Acute myeloid leukaemia | Recurrent acute lymphoblastic leukaemia

- BY INTRAVENOUS INFUSION
  - Child: Specialist drug – access specialist resources for dosing information

- **UNLICENSED USE** Not licensed for use in children.
- **INTERACTIONS** → Appendix 1: anthracyclines
- **SIDE-EFFECTS**
  - **Uncommon** Urine discolouration
  - **Frequency not known** Abdominal pain · acute leukaemia · alopecia · amenorrhoea · anxiety · appetite decreased · arrhythmia · asthenia · bone marrow depression · confusion · constipation · diarrhoea · drowsiness · dyspnoea · fever · gastrointestinal haemorrhage · heart failure · mucositis · nail discolouration · nail dystrophy · nausea · neurological effects · paraesthesia · scleral discolouration · skin discolouration · stomatitis · thrombocytopenia · vomiting

  SIDE-EFFECTS, FURTHER INFORMATION Cardiac toxicity, including irreversible and fatal congestive heart failure, may occur either during treatment with mitoxantrone or months to years after discontinuation; the risk increases with cumulative dose.
- **CONCEPTION AND CONTRACEPTION** Manufacturer advises effective contraception during and for at least 6 months after treatment in men or women.

- **MEDICINAL FORMS** There can be variation in the licensing of different medicines containing the same drug.

Solution for infusion

- **Onkotrone** (Baxter Healthcare Ltd)
  Mitoxantrone (as Mitoxantrone hydrochloride) 2 mg per 1 ml Onkotrone 20mg/10ml solution for infusion vials | 1 vial [PoM] £121.85 (Hospital only)
  Onkotrone 25mg/12.5ml solution for infusion vials | 1 vial [PoM] £152.33 (Hospital only)

ANTINEOPLASTIC DRUGS > ANTIMETABOLITES

Clofarabine [Specialist drug]

13-Dec-2021

- **INDICATIONS AND DOSE**

Acute lymphoblastic leukaemia

- BY INTRAVENOUS INFUSION
  - Child 1–17 years: Specialist drug – access specialist resources for dosing information

- **UNLICENSED USE** Not licensed for use in children under 1 year.
- **INTERACTIONS** → Appendix 1: clofarabine
- **SIDE-EFFECTS**
  - **Common or very common** Alopecia · anxiety · appetite decreased · arthralgia · capillary leak syndrome · chills · cough · dehydration · diarrhoea · dizziness · drowsiness · dyspnoea · fatigue · feeling abnormal · feeling hot · fever · flushing · gastrointestinal discomfort · haemorrhage · headache · hearing impairment · hepatic disorders · hyperbilirubinaemia · hyperhidrosis · hypersensitivity · hypotension · increased risk of infection · irritability · mucositis · multi organ failure · myalgia · nausea · neutropenia · oedema · oral disorders · pain · paraesthesia · pericardial effusion · peripheral neuropathy · psychiatric disorder · renal impairment · respiratory disorders · sepsis · sinusoidal obstruction syndrome · skin reactions · systemic inflammatory response syndrome · tachycardia · tremor · tumour lysis syndrome · vomiting · weight decreased
  - **Frequency not known** Clostridioides difficile colitis · gastrointestinal disorders · hyponatraemia · pancreatitis · severe cutaneous adverse reactions (SCARs)
- **CONCEPTION AND CONTRACEPTION** Contraceptive advice required.

- **MEDICINAL FORMS** There can be variation in the licensing of different medicines containing the same drug.

Solution for infusion

ELECTROLYTES: May contain Sodium

- **Clofarabine (Non-proprietary)**
  Clofarabine 1 mg per 1 ml Clofarabine 20mg/20ml concentrate for solution for infusion vials | 1 vial [PoM] £1,300.00 (Hospital only)

Cytarabine [Specialist drug]

05-Oct-2021

● **INDICATIONS AND DOSE**

Acute lymphoblastic leukaemia | Acute myeloid leukaemia | Non-Hodgkin's lymphoma

▶ BY INTRAVENOUS INJECTION, OR BY INTRAVENOUS INFUSION, OR BY SUBCUTANEOUS INJECTION

▶ Child: Specialist drug – access specialist resources for dosing information

Meningeal leukaemia | Meningeal neoplasms

▶ BY INTRATHECAL INJECTION

▶ Child: Specialist drug – access specialist resources for dosing information

IMPORTANT SAFETY INFORMATION

Not all cytarabine preparations can be given by intrathecal injection—consult product literature.

● **INTERACTIONS** → Appendix 1: cytarabine

● **SIDE-EFFECTS**

▶ **Common or very common** Alopecia · anaemia · appetite decreased · consciousness impaired · diarrhoea · dysarthria · dysphagia · eye disorders · eye inflammation · eye stinging · fever · gastrointestinal discomfort · gastrointestinal disorders · haemorrhagic conjunctivitis (consider prophylactic corticosteroid eye drops) · hyperuricaemia · leucopenia · nausea · oral disorders · renal impairment · skin reactions · thrombocytopenia · urinary retention · vasculitis · vision disorders · vomiting

▶ **Uncommon** Arthralgia · dyspnoea · headache · increased risk of infection · myalgia · nerve disorders · pain · paralysis · pericarditis · sepsis · skin ulcer · throat pain

▶ **Rare or very rare** Arrhythmias

▶ **Frequency not known** Acute respiratory distress syndrome (ARDS) · amenorrhoea · ataxia · azoospermia · bone marrow disorders · cardiomyopathy · cerebellar dysfunction · chest pain · coma · confusion · cytarabine syndrome · dizziness · drowsiness · haemorrhage · hand and foot syndrome (palmar-plantar erythrodysaesthesia syndrome) · hepatic disorders · hyperbilirubinaemia · neurotoxicity · neurotoxicity rash · neutropenia · pancreatitis · personality change · pulmonary oedema · reticulocytopenia · rhabdomyolysis · seizure · tremor

● **CONCEPTION AND CONTRACEPTION** Contraceptive advice required.

● **MEDICINAL FORMS** There can be variation in the licensing of different medicines containing the same drug. Forms available from special-order manufacturers include: solution for injection

Solution for injection

▶ **Cytarabine (Non-proprietary)**

Cytarabine 20 mg per 1 ml Cytarabine 100mg/5ml solution for injection vials | 5 vial [PoM] £20.48–£30.00 (Hospital only)

Cytarabine 100 mg per 1 ml Cytarabine 500mg/5ml solution for injection vials | 5 vial [PoM] £89.78 (Hospital only)

Cytarabine 100mg/1ml solution for injection vials | 5 vial [PoM] £26.93 (Hospital only)

Cytarabine 2g/20ml solution for injection vials | 1 vial [PoM] £73.63–£79.00 (Hospital only)

Cytarabine 1g/10ml solution for injection vials | 1 vial [PoM] £37.05–£40.00 (Hospital only)

Fludarabine phosphate [Specialist drug]

13-Aug-2021

● **INDICATIONS AND DOSE**

Poor prognosis or relapsed acute myeloid leukaemia | Relapsed acute lymphoblastic leukaemia | Conditioning before bone marrow transplantation

▶ BY MOUTH, OR BY INTRAVENOUS INJECTION, OR BY INTRAVENOUS INFUSION

▶ Child: Specialist drug – access specialist resources for dosing information

● **UNLICENSED USE** Not licensed for use in children.

IMPORTANT SAFETY INFORMATION

RISKS OF INCORRECT DOSING OF ORAL ANTI-CANCER MEDICINES

See Cytotoxic drugs p. 660.

● **CONTRA-INDICATIONS** Haemolytic anaemia

● **INTERACTIONS** → Appendix 1: fludarabine

● **SIDE-EFFECTS**

GENERAL SIDE-EFFECTS

▶ **Common or very common** Anaemia · appetite decreased · asthenia · bone marrow depression (may be cumulative) · chills · cough · diarrhoea · fever · increased risk of infection · malaise · mucositis · nausea · neoplasms · nerve disorders · neutropenia · oedema · stomatitis · thrombocytopenia · vision disorders · vomiting

▶ **Uncommon** Autoimmune disorder · confusion · dyspnoea · haemorrhage · pneumonitis · pulmonary fibrosis · pulmonary toxicity · tumour lysis syndrome

▶ **Rare or very rare** Agitation · arrhythmia · coma · heart failure · seizure · severe cutaneous adverse reactions (SCARs)

SPECIFIC SIDE-EFFECTS

▶ **Common or very common**

▶ With oral use Progressive multifocal leukoencephalopathy (PML) · skin reactions · viral infection reactivation

▶ With parenteral use Rash

▶ **Uncommon**

▶ With oral use Acquired haemophilia · crystalluria · electrolyte imbalance · haemolytic anaemia · hyperuricaemia · metabolic acidosis · renal failure

▶ **Frequency not known**

▶ With oral use Posterior reversible encephalopathy syndrome (PRES)

▶ With parenteral use Encephalopathy · intracranial haemorrhage

● **CONCEPTION AND CONTRACEPTION** Manufacturer advises effective contraception during and for at least 6 months after treatment in men or women.

● **MEDICINAL FORMS** There can be variation in the licensing of different medicines containing the same drug.

Solution for injection

▶ **Fludarabine phosphate (Non-proprietary)**

Fludarabine phosphate 25 mg per 1 ml Fludarabine phosphate 50mg/2ml concentrate for solution for injection vials | 1 vial [PoM] £155.00–£156.00 (Hospital only)

Oral tablet

▶ **Fludara** (Sanofi)

Fludarabine phosphate 10 mg Fludara 10mg tablets | 20 tablet [PoM] £403.31 (Hospital only)

Mercaptopurine
03-Jun-2025
(6-Mercaptopurine)

● **INDICATIONS AND DOSE**

Severe ulcerative colitis (under expert supervision) | Severe Crohn's disease (under expert supervision)

▶ BY MOUTH
- Child 2–17 years: 1–1.5 mg/kg once daily, initial max. dose 50 mg once daily; may be increased if necessary up to max. 75 mg once daily

Acute lymphoblastic leukaemia (specialist use only) | Lymphoblastic lymphomas (specialist use only)

▶ BY MOUTH
- Child: Specialist indication – access specialist resources for dosing information

DOSE ADJUSTMENTS DUE TO INTERACTIONS
- Manufacturer advises reduce dose to one-quarter of the usual dose with concurrent use of allopurinol.

DOSE EQUIVALENCE AND CONVERSION
- Mercaptopurine tablets and *Xaluprine*® oral suspension are **not** bioequivalent.

● **UNLICENSED USE** Not licensed for use in ulcerative colitis and Crohn's disease.

Not licensed for use in children for acute lymphoblastic lymphoma or T-cell non-Hodgkins lymphoma.

IMPORTANT SAFETY INFORMATION

SAFE PRACTICE

Mercaptopurine has been confused with mercaptamine; care must be taken to ensure the correct drug is prescribed and dispensed.

RISKS OF INCORRECT DOSING OF ORAL ANTI-CANCER MEDICINES

See Cytotoxic drugs p. 660.

MHRA/CHM ADVICE: THIOPURINES AND INTRAHEPATIC CHOLESTASIS OF PREGNANCY (MAY 2025)

Intrahepatic cholestasis of pregnancy (ICP) has been reported in a small number of patients taking azathioprine or mercaptopurine. Due to similar metabolic pathways, the risk of ICP is considered applicable to all drugs in the thiopurine class, including tioguanine. Thiopurine-induced ICP usually occurs earlier in pregnancy than non-drug-induced ICP and may not respond to ursodeoxycholic acid, however, stopping or reducing the dose of the thiopurine may improve liver-function tests. Some case reports resulted in fetal death, therefore early diagnosis and discontinuation or dose reduction of the thiopurine may minimise adverse effects in the fetus.

Healthcare professionals are advised to undertake a case-by-case assessment if ICP occurs and consider the risks versus benefits of stopping or continuing thiopurine treatment. Non-fasting serum-bile acids should be measured in patients with ICP to identify pregnancies at particular risk of spontaneous preterm birth (≥ 40 micromol/litre) or stillbirth (≥ 100 micromol/litre).

Patients and carers should be advised to seek immediate medical attention if signs or symptoms of ICP occur.

● **CONTRA-INDICATIONS**
- When used for Non-cancer indications Absent thiopurine methyltransferase activity

● **CAUTIONS** Reduced thiopurine methyltransferase activity

CAUTIONS, FURTHER INFORMATION
- Thiopurine methyltransferase The enzyme thiopurine methyltransferase (TPMT) metabolises thiopurine drugs (azathioprine, mercaptopurine, tioguanine); the risk of myelosuppression is increased in patients with reduced activity of the enzyme, particularly for the few individuals in whom TPMT activity is undetectable. Those with reduced TPMT activity may be treated under specialist supervision.

● **INTERACTIONS** → Appendix 1: mercaptopurine

● **SIDE-EFFECTS**
- **Common or very common** Anaemia · appetite decreased · bone marrow depression · diarrhoea · hepatic disorders · hepatotoxicity (more common at high doses) · leucopenia · nausea · oral disorders · pancreatitis · thrombocytopenia · vomiting
- **Uncommon** Arthralgia · fever · increased risk of infection · neutropenia · rash
- **Rare or very rare** Alopecia · face oedema · intestinal ulcer · neoplasms · oligozoospermia
- **Frequency not known** Hypoglycaemia · photosensitivity reaction

● **CONCEPTION AND CONTRACEPTION** Contraceptive advice required, see *Pregnancy and reproductive function* in Cytotoxic drugs p. 660.

● **PREGNANCY** EvGr Use only if potential benefit outweighs risk. ⟨M⟩ See also *Pregnancy and reproductive function* in Cytotoxic drugs p. 660.

● **BREAST FEEDING** Discontinue breast-feeding.

● **HEPATIC IMPAIRMENT** Manufacturer advises caution (risk of increased exposure).

Dose adjustments Manufacturer advises consider dose reduction.

● **RENAL IMPAIRMENT** EvGr Use with caution. ⟨M⟩

Dose adjustments EvGr Consider dose reduction. ⟨M⟩

● **PRE-TREATMENT SCREENING** Manufacturer advises consider measuring thiopurine methyltransferase (TPMT) activity before starting mercaptopurine therapy.

● **MONITORING REQUIREMENTS**
- Monitor liver function—discontinue if jaundice develops.
- When used for Severe ulcerative colitis or Severe Crohn's disease Monitor for toxicity throughout treatment. Monitor full blood count weekly (more frequently with higher doses or if severe hepatic or renal impairment) for first 4 weeks (manufacturer advises weekly monitoring for 8 weeks but evidence of practical value unsatisfactory), thereafter reduce frequency of monitoring to at least every 3 months.

● **PRESCRIBING AND DISPENSING INFORMATION** Flavours of oral liquid formulations may include raspberry.

● **MEDICINAL FORMS** There can be variation in the licensing of different medicines containing the same drug. Forms available from special-order manufacturers include: oral tablet, oral capsule, oral suspension

Oral tablet

- **Mercaptopurine (Non-proprietary)**

Mercaptopurine 10 mg Mercaptopurine 10mg tablets | 100 tablet PoM ☒ DT = £152.68

Mercaptopurine 50 mg Mercaptopurine 50mg tablets | 25 tablet PoM £15.30 DT = £16.87

- **Hanixol** (Fontus Health Ltd)

Mercaptopurine 50 mg Hanixol 50mg tablets | 25 tablet PoM £34.39 DT = £16.87

Oral suspension

EXCIPIENTS: May contain Aspartame

- **Xaluprine** (Nova Laboratories Ltd)

Mercaptopurine 20 mg per 1 ml Xaluprine 20mg/ml oral suspension | 100 ml PoM £170.00 DT = £170.00

Methotrexate

15-Apr-2025

● **DRUG ACTION** Methotrexate inhibits the enzyme dihydrofolate reductase, essential for the synthesis of purines and pyrimidines.

● **INDICATIONS AND DOSE**

Severe Crohn's disease (under expert supervision)

▶ BY SUBCUTANEOUS INJECTION, OR BY INTRAMUSCULAR INJECTION

▸ Child 7–17 years: 15 mg/m^2 once weekly (max. per dose 25 mg)

Maintenance of remission of severe Crohn's disease (under expert supervision)

▶ BY MOUTH, OR BY SUBCUTANEOUS INJECTION, OR BY INTRAMUSCULAR INJECTION

▸ Child 7–17 years: 15 mg/m^2 once weekly (max. per dose 25 mg), dose reduced according to response to lowest effective dose

Juvenile idiopathic arthritis (under expert supervision) | Juvenile dermatomyositis (under expert supervision) | Vasculitis (under expert supervision) | Uveitis (under expert supervision) | Systemic lupus erythematosus (under expert supervision) | Localised scleroderma (under expert supervision) | Sarcoidosis (under expert supervision)

▶ BY MOUTH, OR BY SUBCUTANEOUS INJECTION, OR BY INTRAMUSCULAR INJECTION

▸ Child: Initially 10–15 mg/m^2 once weekly, then increased if necessary up to 25 mg/m^2 once weekly

Maintenance and remission of acute lymphoblastic leukaemia, lymphoblastic lymphoma (specialist use only)

▶ BY MOUTH

▸ Child: Specialist indication – access specialist resources for dosing information

Treatment of early stage Burkitt's lymphoma, non-Hodgkin's lymphoma, osteogenic sarcoma, some CNS tumours including infant brain tumours, acute lymphoblastic leukaemia (specialist use only)

▶ BY INTRAVENOUS INJECTION, OR BY INTRAVENOUS INFUSION

▸ Child: Specialist indication – access specialist resources for dosing information

Meningeal leukaemia, treatment and prevention of CNS involvement of leukaemia (specialist use only)

▶ BY INTRATHECAL INJECTION

▸ Child: Specialist indication – access specialist resources for dosing information

Severe psoriasis unresponsive to conventional therapy (under expert supervision)

▶ BY MOUTH

▸ Child 2–17 years: Initially 200 micrograms/kg once weekly (max. per dose 10 mg), then increased if necessary to 400 micrograms/kg once weekly (max. per dose 25 mg), dose to be adjusted according to response, stop treatment if inadequate response after 3 months at the optimum dose

● **UNLICENSED USE** *Metoject*® is licensed for use in children over 3 years for polyarticular forms of juvenile idiopathic arthritis; other preparations not licensed for use in children for non-malignant conditions.

IMPORTANT SAFETY INFORMATION

NHS NEVER EVENT: OVERDOSE OF METHOTREXATE FOR NON-CANCER TREATMENT (JANUARY 2018)

Patients given methotrexate, by any route, for non-cancer treatment should not be given more than their intended weekly dose.

WEEKLY DOSING

Note that the dose is a **weekly** dose. To avoid error with low-dose methotrexate, it is recommended that:

- the patient or their carer is carefully advised of the **dose** and **frequency** and the reason for taking methotrexate and any other prescribed medication (e.g. folic acid);
- only one strength of methotrexate tablet (usually 2.5 mg) is prescribed and dispensed;
- the prescription and the dispensing label clearly show the dose and frequency of methotrexate administration;
- the patient or their carer is warned to report immediately the onset of any feature of blood disorders (e.g. sore throat, bruising, and mouth ulcers), liver toxicity (e.g. nausea, vomiting, abdominal discomfort, and dark urine), and respiratory effects (e.g. shortness of breath).

MHRA/CHM ADVICE: METHOTREXATE ONCE-WEEKLY FOR AUTOIMMUNE DISEASES: NEW MEASURES TO REDUCE RISK OF FATAL OVERDOSE DUE TO INADVERTENT DAILY INSTEAD OF WEEKLY DOSING (SEPTEMBER 2020)

▸ With oral use

Methotrexate should be taken **once a week** in autoimmune conditions and, less commonly, in some cancer therapy regimens. A European review highlighted continued reports of inadvertent overdose due to more frequent dosing (including daily administration), which has resulted in some fatalities. Subsequently, new measures have been implemented by the MHRA. Prescribers are advised to:

- ensure patients can understand and comply with once-weekly dosing before prescribing methotrexate, decide with the patient which day of the week they will take their dose, and note this down in full on the prescription;
- consider the patient's overall polypharmacy burden when deciding which formulation to prescribe, especially in those with a high pill burden;
- inform patients and carers of the potentially fatal risk of accidental overdose if methotrexate is taken more frequently than once a week, and reaffirm that it should not be taken daily;
- advise patients and carers to seek immediate medical attention if overdose is suspected.

The MHRA further advises dispensers to remind patients of the once-weekly dosing and the risks of potentially fatal overdose if they take more than directed. Where possible, the day of the week for dosing should be written in full in the space provided on the outer packaging. Patients should be encouraged to write the day of the week for dosing in their patient alert card and carry it with them.

MHRA/CHM ADVICE: METHOTREXATE: ADVISE PATIENTS TO TAKE PRECAUTIONS IN THE SUN TO AVOID PHOTOSENSITIVITY REACTIONS (AUGUST 2023)

Photosensitivity reactions, including phototoxicity, are known side-effects of methotrexate that may occur with low- and high-dose treatment. These reactions are distinct from radiation recall reactions, and can appear as severe sunburn (e.g. rashes with papules or blistering, and sometimes swelling); rarely, photosensitivity reactions have contributed to deaths from secondary infections.

Healthcare professionals are reminded to inform patients and their carers of the risk and signs of photosensitivity reactions during methotrexate treatment, and advise them to:

- avoid exposure to UV light (including intense sunlight, especially between 11 a.m. and 3 p.m., sunlamps, and sunbeds);

- use a sunscreen with a high sun protection factor (SPF) and wear protective clothing during sun exposure;
- speak to a healthcare professional if they have concerns about a skin reaction.

- **CONTRA-INDICATIONS** Active infection · ascites · immunodeficiency syndromes · significant pleural effusion
- **CAUTIONS** Dehydration (increased risk of toxicity) · diarrhoea · extreme caution in blood disorders (avoid if severe) · peptic ulceration (avoid in active disease) · photosensitivity · risk of accumulation in pleural effusion or ascites—drain before treatment · ulcerative colitis · ulcerative stomatitis

CAUTIONS, FURTHER INFORMATION
- Blood count Bone marrow suppression can occur abruptly; factors likely to increase toxicity include advanced age, renal impairment, and concomitant use with another anti-folate drug (e.g. trimethoprim). Manufacturer advises a clinically significant drop in white cell count or platelet count calls for immediate withdrawal of methotrexate and introduction of supportive therapy.
- Gastro-intestinal toxicity Manufacturer advises withdraw treatment if stomatitis or diarrhoea develops—may be first sign of gastro-intestinal toxicity.
- Photosensitivity Psoriasis lesions may be aggravated by UV radiation—skin ulceration has been reported.
  Radiation recall reaction has been reported in both radiation- and sun-damaged skin.
- Liver toxicity Liver cirrhosis reported. Manufacturer advises treatment should not be started or should be discontinued if any abnormality of liver function or liver biopsy is present or develops during therapy. Abnormalities can return to normal within 2 weeks after which treatment may be recommenced if judged appropriate. Persistent increases in liver transaminases may necessitate dose reduction or discontinuation; abrupt withdrawal can lead to disease flare in juvenile idiopathic arthritis.
- Pulmonary toxicity Manufacturer advises children and carers to seek medical attention if dyspnoea, cough or fever develops; monitor for symptoms at each visit—discontinue if pneumonitis suspected.

- **INTERACTIONS** → Appendix 1: methotrexate
- **SIDE-EFFECTS**

GENERAL SIDE-EFFECTS
- **Uncommon** Seizure

SPECIFIC SIDE-EFFECTS
- **Common or very common**
- With systemic use Anaemia · appetite decreased · diarrhoea · drowsiness · fatigue · gastrointestinal discomfort · headache · increased risk of infection · interstitial lung disease · leucopenia · nausea · oral disorders · respiratory disorders · skin reactions · throat ulcer · thrombocytopenia · vomiting
- **Uncommon**
- With parenteral use Drug toxicity · local reaction
- With systemic use Agranulocytosis · alopecia · arthralgia · bone marrow disorders · chills · confusion · cystitis · depression · diabetes mellitus · dysuria · fever · gastrointestinal disorders · haemorrhage · healing impaired · hepatic disorders · myalgia · neoplasms · nephropathy · osteoporosis · photosensitivity reaction · pulmonary fibrosis · rheumatoid arthritis aggravated · severe cutaneous adverse reactions (SCARs) · vasculitis · vertigo · vulvovaginal disorders
- **Rare or very rare**
- With oral use Asthma · brain oedema · cognitive impairment · paresis · psychosis · speech impairment
- With parenteral use Apnoea · asthma-like conditions
- With systemic use Azotaemia · conjunctivitis · cough · dyspnoea · embolism and thrombosis · eosinophilia · gynaecomastia · hypotension · immune deficiency · infertility · insomnia · lymphadenopathy · meningism · meningitis aseptic · menstrual cycle irregularities · mood altered · muscle weakness · nail discolouration · neutropenia · pain · pancreatitis · pericardial disorders · pericarditis · proteinuria · radiation injuries · reactivation of infection · renal impairment · retinopathy · sensation abnormal · sepsis · sexual dysfunction · sperm abnormalities · stress fracture · taste altered · telangiectasia · tinnitus · vision disorders
- **Frequency not known**
- With intrathecal use Arachnoiditis · cerebrospinal fluid pressure increased · Guillain-Barre syndrome · leukoencephalopathy · paresis · pulmonary oedema
- With oral use Chest pain · death · electrolyte imbalance · encephalopathy · neurotoxicity · pulmonary oedema ·
- With parenteral use Aphasia · cognitive disorder · hemiparesis · injection site necrosis · leukoencephalopathy · metabolic change · necrosis · sudden death
- With systemic use Defective oogenesis · dizziness · mucositis · oedema · progressive multifocal leukoencephalopathy (PML) · skin ulcer

SIDE-EFFECTS, FURTHER INFORMATION Give folic acid to reduce side-effects. Folic acid decreases mucosal and gastrointestinal side-effects of methotrexate and may prevent hepatotoxicity; there is no evidence of a reduction in haematological side-effects.

Withdraw treatment if ulcerative stomatitis develops—may be first sign of gastro-intestinal toxicity.

Treatment with folinic acid (as calcium folinate) may be required in acute toxicity.

- **CONCEPTION AND CONTRACEPTION** EvGr Females of childbearing potential should use effective contraception during treatment and for at least 6 months after last treatment; male patients should use effective contraception during treatment and for at least 3 months after last treatment if their partner is of childbearing potential. (M)
- **PREGNANCY** Avoid (teratogenic; fertility may be reduced during therapy but this may be reversible).
- **BREAST FEEDING** Discontinue breast-feeding—present in milk.
- **HEPATIC IMPAIRMENT** When used for malignancy, avoid in severe hepatic impairment—consult local treatment protocol for details. Avoid with hepatic impairment in non-malignant conditions—dose-related toxicity.
- **RENAL IMPAIRMENT** Risk of nephrotoxicity at high doses. EvGr Use with caution; avoid in severe impairment. (M)
  Dose adjustments EvGr Reduce dose (consult product literature). (M)
- **PRE-TREATMENT SCREENING** Exclude pregnancy before treatment.
  Patients should have full blood count and renal and liver function tests before starting treatment.
  Check immunity to varicella-zoster and consider vaccination before initiating therapy.
- **MONITORING REQUIREMENTS** Full blood count and liver function tests repeated fortnightly for at least the first 4 weeks of treatment and at this frequency after any change in dose until therapy stabilised, thereafter monthly; renal function tests should be performed regularly during treatment.
- **PRESCRIBING AND DISPENSING INFORMATION** Folinic acid following methotrexate administration helps to prevent methotrexate-induced mucositis and myelosuppression.
  The licensed routes of administration for parenteral preparations vary—further information can be found in the product literature for the individual preparations.
  Risk minimisation materials documents are available for healthcare professionals.

● **PATIENT AND CARER ADVICE** Patients and their carers should be warned to report immediately the onset of any feature of blood disorders (e.g. sore throat, bruising, and mouth ulcers), liver toxicity (e.g. nausea, vomiting, abdominal discomfort and dark urine), and respiratory effects (e.g. shortness of breath). Patients and their carers should be advised to avoid exposure to UV light (including intense sunlight, sunlamps, and sunbeds)—see *Important safety information*.

Children and carers should be advised to avoid self-medication with over-the-counter ibuprofen.

Children and their carers should be counselled on the dose and use of NSAIDs.

▸ With oral use A patient alert card should be provided to patients on once-weekly dosing—see also *Important safety information*.

Medicines for Children leaflet: Methotrexate for skin conditions www.medicinesforchildren.org.uk/medicines/methotrexate-for-skin-conditions/

● **MEDICINAL FORMS** There can be variation in the licensing of different medicines containing the same drug. Forms available from special-order manufacturers include: oral suspension, oral solution, solution for injection

Oral tablet

CAUTIONARY AND ADVISORY LABELS 10, 11

▸ **Methotrexate (Non-proprietary)**
Methotrexate 2.5 mg Methotrexate 2.5mg tablets | 24 tablet PoM £1.28–£3.27 | 28 tablet PoM DT = £1.54 | 100 tablet PoM £4.61–£14.01
Methotrexate 10 mg Methotrexate 10mg tablets | 100 tablet PoM £55.74 DT = £53.77

Solution for injection

▸ **Methotrexate (Non-proprietary)**
Methotrexate (as Methotrexate sodium) 2.5 mg per 1 ml Methotrexate 5mg/2ml solution for injection vials | 5 vial PoM £36.00 (Hospital only)
Methotrexate (as Methotrexate sodium) 25 mg per 1 ml Methotrexate 1g/40ml solution for injection vials | 1 vial PoM £1,452.55 (Hospital only)
Methotrexate 500mg/20ml solution for injection vials | 1 vial PoM £48.00 (Hospital only)
Methotrexate 50mg/2ml solution for injection vials | 1 vial PoM £72.63 (Hospital only) | 5 vial PoM £35.00 (Hospital only)
Methotrexate (as Methotrexate sodium) 100 mg per 1 ml Methotrexate 1g/10ml solution for injection vials | 1 vial PoM £80.75–£85.00 (Hospital only)

▸ **Methofill** (Accord-UK Ltd)
Methotrexate 50 mg per 1 ml Methofill 12.5mg/0.25ml solution for injection pre-filled injector | 1 pre-filled disposable injection PoM £14.34 DT = £14.35
Methofill 30mg/0.6ml solution for injection pre-filled syringes | 1 pre-filled disposable injection PoM £14.55 DT = £14.55
Methofill 22.5mg/0.45ml solution for injection pre-filled injector | 1 pre-filled disposable injection PoM £16.10 DT = £16.11
Methofill 30mg/0.6ml solution for injection pre-filled injector | 1 pre-filled disposable injection PoM £16.55 DT = £16.56
Methofill 27.5mg/0.55ml solution for injection pre-filled injector | 1 pre-filled disposable injection PoM £16.49 DT = £16.50
Methofill 7.5mg/0.15ml solution for injection pre-filled injector | 1 pre-filled disposable injection PoM £12.86 DT = £12.87
Methofill 20mg/0.4ml solution for injection pre-filled injector | 1 pre-filled disposable injection PoM £15.55 DT = £15.56
Methofill 10mg/0.2ml solution for injection pre-filled injector | 1 pre-filled disposable injection PoM £13.25 DT = £13.26
Methofill 15mg/0.3ml solution for injection pre-filled injector | 1 pre-filled disposable injection PoM £14.40 DT = £14.41
Methofill 17.5mg/0.35ml solution for injection pre-filled injector | 1 pre-filled disposable injection PoM £15.24 DT = £15.25
Methofill 25mg/0.5ml solution for injection pre-filled injector | 1 pre-filled disposable injection PoM £16.12 DT = £16.13
Methotrexate (as Methotrexate sodium) 50 mg per 1 ml Methofill 15mg/0.3ml solution for injection pre-filled syringes | 1 pre-filled disposable injection PoM £12.40 DT = £12.40
Methofill 25mg/0.5ml solution for injection pre-filled syringes | 1 pre-filled disposable injection PoM £14.24 DT = £14.24
Methofill 10mg/0.2ml solution for injection pre-filled syringes | 1 pre-filled disposable injection PoM £11.25 DT = £11.25
Methofill 7.5mg/0.15ml solution for injection pre-filled syringes | 1 pre-filled disposable injection PoM £10.86 DT = £10.86
Methofill 17.5mg/0.35ml solution for injection pre-filled syringes | 1 pre-filled disposable injection PoM £13.24 DT = £13.24
Methofill 27.5mg/0.55ml solution for injection pre-filled syringes | 1 pre-filled disposable injection PoM £14.49
Methofill 22.5mg/0.45ml solution for injection pre-filled syringes | 1 pre-filled disposable injection PoM £14.10 DT = £14.10
Methofill 12.5mg/0.25ml solution for injection pre-filled syringes | 1 pre-filled disposable injection PoM £12.34 DT = £12.34
Methofill 20mg/0.4ml solution for injection pre-filled syringes | 1 pre-filled disposable injection PoM £13.55 DT = £13.55

▸ **Metoject PEN** (medac UK)
Methotrexate 50 mg per 1 ml Metoject PEN 27.5mg/0.55ml solution for injection pre-filled pens | 1 pre-filled disposable injection PoM £16.50 DT = £16.50
Metoject PEN 17.5mg/0.35ml solution for injection pre-filled pens | 1 pre-filled disposable injection PoM £15.25 DT = £15.25
Metoject PEN 30mg/0.6ml solution for injection pre-filled pens | 1 pre-filled disposable injection PoM £16.56 DT = £16.56
Metoject PEN 12.5mg/0.25ml solution for injection pre-filled pens | 1 pre-filled disposable injection PoM £14.35 DT = £14.35
Metoject PEN 10mg/0.2ml solution for injection pre-filled pens | 1 pre-filled disposable injection PoM £13.26 DT = £13.26
Metoject PEN 15mg/0.3ml solution for injection pre-filled pens | 1 pre-filled disposable injection PoM £14.41 DT = £14.41
Metoject PEN 22.5mg/0.45ml solution for injection pre-filled pens | 1 pre-filled disposable injection PoM £16.11 DT = £16.11
Metoject PEN 7.5mg/0.15ml solution for injection pre-filled pens | 1 pre-filled disposable injection PoM £12.87 DT = £12.87
Metoject PEN 25mg/0.5ml solution for injection pre-filled pens | 1 pre-filled disposable injection PoM £16.13 DT = £16.13
Metoject PEN 20mg/0.4ml solution for injection pre-filled pens | 1 pre-filled disposable injection PoM £15.56 DT = £15.56

▸ **Nordimet** (Nordic Pharma Ltd)
Methotrexate 25 mg per 1 ml Nordimet 15mg/0.6ml solution for injection pre-filled pens | 1 pre-filled disposable injection PoM £14.92 DT = £14.92
Nordimet 20mg/0.8ml solution for injection pre-filled pens | 1 pre-filled disposable injection PoM £16.06 DT = £16.06
Nordimet 22.5mg/0.9ml solution for injection pre-filled pens | 1 pre-filled disposable injection PoM £16.61 DT = £16.61
Nordimet 12.5mg/0.5ml solution for injection pre-filled pens | 1 pre-filled disposable injection PoM £14.85 DT = £14.85
Nordimet 10mg/0.4ml solution for injection pre-filled pens | 1 pre-filled disposable injection PoM £13.77 DT = £13.77
Nordimet 17.5mg/0.7ml solution for injection pre-filled pens | 1 pre-filled disposable injection PoM £15.75 DT = £15.75
Nordimet 25mg/1ml solution for injection pre-filled pens | 1 pre-filled disposable injection PoM £16.64 DT = £16.64
Nordimet 7.5mg/0.3ml solution for injection pre-filled pens | 1 pre-filled disposable injection PoM £13.37 DT = £13.37

▸ **Zlatal** (Nordic Pharma Ltd)
Methotrexate (as Methotrexate sodium) 25 mg per 1 ml Zlatal 17.5mg/0.7ml solution for injection pre-filled syringes | 1 pre-filled disposable injection PoM £15.75 DT = £15.75
Zlatal 10mg/0.4ml solution for injection pre-filled syringes | 1 pre-filled disposable injection PoM £13.77 DT = £13.77
Zlatal 25mg/1ml solution for injection pre-filled syringes | 1 pre-filled disposable injection PoM £16.64 DT = £16.64
Zlatal 20mg/0.8ml solution for injection pre-filled syringes | 1 pre-filled disposable injection PoM £16.06 DT = £16.06
Zlatal 12.5mg/0.5ml solution for injection pre-filled syringes | 1 pre-filled disposable injection PoM £14.85 DT = £14.85
Zlatal 7.5mg/0.3ml solution for injection pre-filled syringes | 1 pre-filled disposable injection PoM £13.37 DT = £13.37
Zlatal 22.5mg/0.9ml solution for injection pre-filled syringes | 1 pre-filled disposable injection PoM £16.61 DT = £16.61
Zlatal 15mg/0.6ml solution for injection pre-filled syringes | 1 pre-filled disposable injection PoM £14.92 DT = £14.92

Oral suspension

CAUTIONARY AND ADVISORY LABELS 10, 11

Solution for infusion

▸ **Methotrexate (Non-proprietary)**
Methotrexate (as Methotrexate sodium) 100 mg per 1 ml Methotrexate 5g/50ml solution for infusion vials | 1 vial PoM £380.00–£400.00 (Hospital only)

Oral solution

CAUTIONARY AND ADVISORY LABELS 10, 11

▸ **Methotrexate (Non-proprietary)**
Methotrexate (as Methotrexate sodium) 2 mg per 1 ml Methotrexate 2mg/ml oral solution sugar free | 35 ml PoM

£95.00–£152.00 DT = £95.00 SF | 65 ml PoM £125.00 DT = £125.00 SF

▸ **Jylamvo** (Esteve Pharmaceuticals Ltd)
Methotrexate (as Methotrexate sodium) 2 mg per 1 ml Jylamvo 2mg/ml oral solution | 60 ml PoM £112.50 SF

Nelarabine [Specialist drug]

10-Nov-2020

● **INDICATIONS AND DOSE**

T-cell acute lymphoblastic leukaemia | T-cell lymphoblastic lymphoma

▸ BY INTRAVENOUS INFUSION

▸ Child: Specialist drug – access specialist resources for dosing information

● **INTERACTIONS** → Appendix 1: nelarabine

● **SIDE-EFFECTS**

▸ **Common or very common** Anaemia · arthralgia · asthenia · ataxia · confusion · constipation · diarrhoea · drowsiness · electrolyte imbalance · fever · headache · hyperbilirubinaemia · hypoglycaemia · increased risk of infection · leucopenia · nausea · neutropenia · pain in extremity · peripheral neuropathy · seizures · sensation abnormal · sepsis · stomatitis · thrombocytopenia · tremor · vomiting

▸ **Rare or very rare** Rhabdomyolysis

SIDE-EFFECTS, FURTHER INFORMATION If signs or symptoms of neurotoxicity occur, treatment should be discontinued immediately.

● **CONCEPTION AND CONTRACEPTION** Manufacturer advises effective contraception during and for at least 3 months after treatment in men and women.

● **PATIENT AND CARER ADVICE**

Driving and skilled tasks Drowsiness may affect performance of skilled tasks (e.g. cycling or driving).

● **NATIONAL FUNDING/ACCESS DECISIONS**

For full details see funding body website

Scottish Medicines Consortium (SMC) decisions

▸ **Nelarabine (*Atriance*®) for the treatment of patients with T-cell acute lymphoblastic leukaemia (T-ALL) and T-cell lymphoblastic lymphoma (T-LBL) (April 2008)** SMC No. 454/08 Recommended with restrictions

● **MEDICINAL FORMS** There can be variation in the licensing of different medicines containing the same drug.

Solution for infusion

ELECTROLYTES: May contain Sodium

▸ **Atriance** (Sandoz Ltd) ▼
Nelarabine 5 mg per 1 ml Atriance 250mg/50ml solution for infusion vials | 1 vial PoM £222.00 (Hospital only)

Tioguanine [Specialist drug] (Thioguanine)

03-Jun-2025

● **INDICATIONS AND DOSE**

Infant acute lymphoblastic leukaemia

▸ BY MOUTH

▸ Child: Specialist drug – access specialist resources for dosing information

IMPORTANT SAFETY INFORMATION

RISKS OF INCORRECT DOSING OF ORAL ANTI-CANCER MEDICINES
See Cytotoxic drugs p. 660.

MHRA/CHM ADVICE: THIOPURINES AND INTRAHEPATIC CHOLESTASIS OF PREGNANCY (MAY 2025)
Intrahepatic cholestasis of pregnancy (ICP) has been reported in a small number of patients taking azathioprine or mercaptopurine. Due to similar metabolic pathways, the risk of ICP is considered applicable to all drugs in the thiopurine class, including tioguanine. Thiopurine-induced ICP usually occurs earlier in pregnancy than non-drug-induced ICP and may not respond to ursodeoxycholic acid, however, stopping or reducing the dose of the thiopurine may improve liver-function tests. Some case reports resulted in fetal death, therefore early diagnosis and discontinuation or dose reduction of the thiopurine may minimise adverse effects in the fetus.

Healthcare professionals are advised to undertake a case-by-case assessment if ICP occurs and consider the risks versus benefits of stopping or continuing thiopurine treatment. Non-fasting serum-bile acids should be measured in patients with ICP to identify pregnancies at particular risk of spontaneous preterm birth (≥ 40 micromol/litre) or stillbirth (≥ 100 micromol/litre).

Patients and carers should be advised to seek immediate medical attention if signs or symptoms of ICP occur.

● **INTERACTIONS** → Appendix 1: tioguanine

● **SIDE-EFFECTS**

▸ **Common or very common** Bone marrow failure · gastrointestinal disorders · hepatic disorders · hyperbilirubinaemia · hyperuricaemia · hyperuricosuria · nodular regenerative hyperplasia · oesophageal varices · sinusoidal obstruction syndrome · splenomegaly · stomatitis · thrombocytopenia · uric acid nephropathy · weight increased

▸ **Frequency not known** Photosensitivity reaction

SIDE-EFFECTS, FURTHER INFORMATION Manufacturer advises tioguanine is not recommended for maintenance or long-term continuous therapy because of the high risk of hepatic toxicity. If hepatic toxicity develops, discontinue treatment.

● **CONCEPTION AND CONTRACEPTION** Ensure effective contraception during treatment in men or women.

● **MEDICINAL FORMS** There can be variation in the licensing of different medicines containing the same drug. Forms available from special-order manufacturers include: oral capsule

Oral tablet

▸ **Tioguanine (Non-proprietary)**
Tioguanine 40 mg Tioguanine 40mg tablets | 25 tablet PoM £76.35 DT = £76.35

ANTINEOPLASTIC DRUGS › CYTOTOXIC ANTIBIOTICS AND RELATED SUBSTANCES

Bleomycin [Specialist drug]

19-Sep-2023

● **INDICATIONS AND DOSE**

Some germ cell tumours | Hodgkin's lymphoma

▸ BY INTRAVENOUS INFUSION

▸ Child: Specialist drug – access specialist resources for dosing information

● **UNLICENSED USE** Not licensed for use in children.

● **CONTRA-INDICATIONS** Ataxia telangiectasia · pulmonary infection · significantly reduced lung function

● **INTERACTIONS** → Appendix 1: bleomycin

● **SIDE-EFFECTS**

▸ **Common or very common** Alopecia · appetite decreased · chills · dyspnoea · embolism and thrombosis · fever (after administration) · fingertip swelling · fingertip tenderness · headache · hypersensitivity · idiosyncratic drug reaction · induration · interstitial lung disease · malaise · mucositis · nausea · oedema · pulmonary fibrosis · respiratory disorders · skin reactions · stomatitis · vomiting · weight decreased

- **Uncommon** Angular cheilitis · arthralgia · bone marrow disorders · cancer pain · confusion · diarrhoea · dizziness · haemorrhage · hypotension · leucopenia · myalgia · nail discolouration · nail disorder · neutropenia · oliguria · thrombocytopenia · urinary disorders · vein wall hypertrophy
- **Rare or very rare** Cerebrovascular insufficiency · chest pain · haemolytic uraemic syndrome · hepatic impairment · myocardial infarction · pericarditis · peripheral vascular disease · scleroderma · thrombotic microangiopathy · tumour lysis syndrome
- **Frequency not known** Anaemia · sepsis

SIDE-EFFECTS, FURTHER INFORMATION Pulmonary reactions, including interstitial pneumonitis, pulmonary fibrosis, and pulmonary toxicity have been reported. Pulmonary toxicity occurs more frequently in those who have received total doses greater than 400 units. Pulmonary toxicity has also been reported in young patients receiving low doses. If pulmonary changes occur, discontinue treatment and investigate.

- **CONCEPTION AND CONTRACEPTION** EvGr Ensure effective contraception during and for 6 months after treatment in male and female patients. ⟨M⟩

- **MEDICINAL FORMS** There can be variation in the licensing of different medicines containing the same drug.

Powder for solution for injection

- **Bleomycin (Non-proprietary)**
  Bleomycin (as Bleomycin sulfate) 15000 unit Bleomycin 15,000unit powder for solution for injection vials | 1 vial PoM £19.06–£62.00 (Hospital only)

Dactinomycin [Specialist drug] 28-Jul-2020
(Actinomycin D)

- **INDICATIONS AND DOSE**

Wilms' tumour | Childhood rhabdomyosarcoma and other soft-tissue sarcomas | Ewing's sarcoma

- BY INTRAVENOUS INJECTION
- Child: Specialist drug – access specialist resources for dosing information

- **UNLICENSED USE** Not licensed for use in children under 12 years.
- **INTERACTIONS** → Appendix 1: dactinomycin
- **SIDE-EFFECTS** Agranulocytosis · alopecia · anaemia · appetite decreased · ascites · bone marrow disorders · diarrhoea · dysphagia · fatigue · fever · gastrointestinal discomfort · gastrointestinal disorders · growth retardation · healing impaired · hepatic disorders · hypocalcaemia · increased risk of infection · lethargy · leucopenia · leukaemia secondary · malaise · myalgia · nausea · neutropenia · oedema · oral disorders · pneumonitis · renal impairment · reticulocytopenia · secondary neoplasm · sepsis · severe cutaneous adverse reactions (SCARs) · sinusoidal obstruction syndrome · skin reactions · soft tissue damage · thrombocytopenia · tumour lysis syndrome · venous thrombosis · vomiting
- **CONCEPTION AND CONTRACEPTION** Exclude pregnancy before treatment with cytotoxic drugs. Contraceptive advice should be given to men and women before cytotoxic therapy begins (and should cover the duration of contraception required after therapy has ended). Regimens that do not contain an alkylating drug or procarbazine may have less effect on fertility, but those with an alkylating drug or procarbazine carry the risk of causing permanent male sterility (there is no effect on potency). Pretreatment counselling and consideration of sperm storage may be appropriate. Women are less severely affected, though the span of reproductive life may be shortened by the onset of a premature menopause. No increase in fetal abnormalities or abortion rate has been recorded in patients who remain fertile after cytotoxic chemotherapy.

- **MEDICINAL FORMS** There can be variation in the licensing of different medicines containing the same drug.

Powder for solution for injection

- **Cosmegen** (Recordati Rare Diseases UK Ltd)
  Dactinomycin 500 microgram Cosmegen Lyovac 500microgram powder for solution for injection vials | 1 vial PoM £52.58

ANTINEOPLASTIC DRUGS › PLATINUM COMPOUNDS

Carboplatin [Specialist drug] 16-Aug-2021

- **INDICATIONS AND DOSE**

Stage 4 neuroblastoma | Germ cell tumours | Low-grade gliomas (including astrocytomas) | Neuroectodermal tumours (including medulloblastoma) | Rhabdomyosarcoma (metastatic and non-metastatic disease) | Soft-tissue sarcomas | Retinoblastoma | High risk Wilms' tumour | Some liver tumours

- BY INTRAVENOUS INFUSION
- Child: Specialist drug – access specialist resources for dosing information

- **UNLICENSED USE** Not licensed for use in children.
- **INTERACTIONS** → Appendix 1: platinum compounds
- **SIDE-EFFECTS**
  - **Common or very common** Alopecia · anaemia · asthenia · cardiovascular disorder · constipation · diarrhoea · gastrointestinal discomfort · haemorrhage · hypersensitivity · increased risk of infection · interstitial lung disease · leucopenia · mucosal abnormalities · musculoskeletal disorder · nausea · neutropenia · ototoxicity · peripheral neuropathy · reflexes decreased · respiratory disorders · sensation abnormal · skin reactions · taste altered · thrombocytopenia · urogenital disorder · vision disorders · vomiting
  - **Rare or very rare** Angioedema
  - **Frequency not known** Appetite decreased · bone marrow failure · chills · dehydration · embolism · encephalopathy · extravasation necrosis · fever · haemolytic uraemic syndrome · heart failure · hypertension · hyponatraemia · hypotension · injection site necrosis · malaise · pancreatitis · pulmonary fibrosis · stomatitis · stroke · treatment related secondary malignancy · tumour lysis syndrome
- **CONCEPTION AND CONTRACEPTION** Contraceptive advice required.
- **NATIONAL FUNDING/ACCESS DECISIONS**
  For full details see funding body website

NICE decisions

- **Bevacizumab in combination with paclitaxel and carboplatin for the first-line treatment of advanced ovarian cancer (May 2013)** NICE TA284 Not recommended
- **Bevacizumab in combination with gemcitabine and carboplatin for treating the first recurrence of platinum-sensitive advanced ovarian cancer (May 2013)** NICE TA285 Not recommended

- **MEDICINAL FORMS** There can be variation in the licensing of different medicines containing the same drug.

Solution for infusion

- **Carboplatin (Non-proprietary)**
  Carboplatin 10 mg per 1 ml Carboplatin 50mg/5ml concentrate for solution for infusion vials | 1 vial PoM £20.20–£28.33 (Hospital only)
  Carboplatin 150mg/15ml concentrate for solution for infusion vials | 1 vial PoM £56.92–£73.17 (Hospital only)
  Carboplatin 600mg/60ml concentrate for solution for infusion vials | 1 vial PoM £232.64–£334.29 (Hospital only)
  Carboplatin 600mg/60ml solution for infusion vials | 1 vial PoM £260.00 (Hospital only)

Carboplatin 450mg/45ml concentrate for solution for infusion vials | 1 vial [PoM] £168.85–£217.13 (Hospital only)
Carboplatin 450mg/45ml solution for infusion vials | 1 vial [PoM] £197.48 (Hospital only)
Carboplatin 150mg/15ml solution for infusion vials | 1 vial [PoM] £65.83 (Hospital only)
Carboplatin 50mg/5ml solution for infusion vials | 1 vial [PoM] £22.86 (Hospital only)

Cisplatin [Specialist drug] 07-Feb-2022

● **INDICATIONS AND DOSE**

Osteogenic sarcoma | Stage 4 neuroblastoma | Some liver tumours | Infant brain tumours | Intra-cranial germ-cell tumours

▶ BY INTRAVENOUS INFUSION

▸ Child: Specialist drug – access specialist resources for dosing information

● **UNLICENSED USE** Not licensed for use in children.

● **INTERACTIONS** → Appendix 1: platinum compounds

● **SIDE-EFFECTS**

▶ **Common or very common** Anaemia · arrhythmias · bone marrow failure · electrolyte imbalance · extravasation necrosis · fever · leucopenia · nephrotoxicity (dose-related and potentially cumulative) · sepsis · thrombocytopenia

▶ **Uncommon** Anaphylactoid reaction · ototoxicity (dose-related and potentially cumulative) · spermatogenesis abnormal

▶ **Rare or very rare** Acute leukaemia · cardiac arrest · encephalopathy · myocardial infarction · nerve disorders · seizure · stomatitis

▶ **Frequency not known** Alopecia · appetite decreased · asthenia · autonomic dysfunction · cardiac disorder · cerebrovascular insufficiency · deafness · dehydration · diarrhoea · haemolytic anaemia · hiccups · hyperuricaemia · infection · Lhermitte's sign · malaise · muscle spasms · myelopathy · nausea · papilloedema · pulmonary embolism · rash · Raynaud's phenomenon · renal impairment · renal tubular disorder · retinal discolouration · SIADH · taste loss · tetany · thrombotic microangiopathy · tinnitus · vision disorders · vomiting

● **CONCEPTION AND CONTRACEPTION** Manufacturer advises effective contraception during and for at least 6 months after treatment in men or women.

● **MEDICINAL FORMS** There can be variation in the licensing of different medicines containing the same drug.

Solution for infusion

▸ **Cisplatin (Non-proprietary)**

Cisplatin 1 mg per 1 ml Cisplatin 50mg/50ml concentrate for solution for infusion vials | 1 vial [PoM] £26.70–£28.11 (Hospital only)
Cisplatin 100mg/100ml solution for infusion vials | 1 vial [PoM] £50.22 (Hospital only)
Cisplatin 50mg/50ml solution for infusion vials | 1 vial [PoM] £25.37 (Hospital only)
Cisplatin 10mg/10ml concentrate for solution for infusion vials | 1 vial [PoM] £5.36 (Hospital only)
Cisplatin 100mg/100ml concentrate for solution for infusion vials | 1 vial [PoM] £52.86–£55.64 (Hospital only)

ANTINEOPLASTIC DRUGS › PODOPHYLLOTOXIN DERIVATIVES

Etoposide [Specialist drug] 21-Jun-2021

● **INDICATIONS AND DOSE**

Stage 4 neuroblastoma | Germ-cell tumours | Intracranial germ-cell tumours | Rhabdomyosarcoma | Soft-tissue sarcomas | Neuroectodermal tumours (including medulloblastoma) | Relapsed Hodgkin's disease | Non-Hodgkin's lymphoma | Ewing tumour | Acute lymphoblastic leukaemia | Acute myeloid leukaemia

▶ BY MOUTH, OR BY INTRAVENOUS INFUSION

▸ Child: Specialist drug – access specialist resources for dosing information

● **UNLICENSED USE** Not licensed for use in children.

IMPORTANT SAFETY INFORMATION

RISKS OF INCORRECT DOSING OF ORAL ANTI-CANCER MEDICINES

See Cytotoxic drugs p. 660.

● **INTERACTIONS** → Appendix 1: etoposide

● **SIDE-EFFECTS**

GENERAL SIDE-EFFECTS

▶ **Common or very common** Abdominal pain · acute leukaemia · alopecia · anaemia · appetite decreased · arrhythmia · asthenia · bone marrow depression · constipation · diarrhoea · dizziness · hepatotoxicity · hypertension · leucopenia · malaise · mucositis · myocardial infarction · nausea · neutropenia · skin reactions · thrombocytopenia · vomiting

▶ **Uncommon** Nerve disorders

▶ **Rare or very rare** Dysphagia · interstitial pneumonitis · neurotoxicity · pulmonary fibrosis · radiation recall reaction · seizure · severe cutaneous adverse reactions (SCARs) · taste altered · vision loss

SPECIFIC SIDE-EFFECTS

▶ **Common or very common**

▸ With intravenous use Anaphylactic reaction · hypotension · infection

▸ With oral use Oesophagitis · stomatitis · transient systolic hypotension

▶ **Uncommon**

▸ With intravenous use Haemorrhage

▶ **Rare or very rare**

▸ With intravenous use Fever

▸ With oral use Drowsiness

▶ **Frequency not known**

▸ With intravenous use Angioedema · bronchospasm · extravasation necrosis · infertility · tumour lysis syndrome

● **CONCEPTION AND CONTRACEPTION** Contraceptive advice required.

● **MEDICINAL FORMS** There can be variation in the licensing of different medicines containing the same drug.

Solution for infusion

▸ **Etoposide (Non-proprietary)**

Etoposide 20 mg per 1 ml Etoposide 100mg/5ml concentrate for solution for infusion vials | 1 vial [PoM] £16.25–£21.25 (Hospital only)
Etoposide 500mg/25ml concentrate for solution for infusion vials | 1 vial [PoM] £81.42–£106.29 (Hospital only)

Oral capsule

CAUTIONARY AND ADVISORY LABELS 23

▸ **Etoposide (Non-proprietary)**

Etoposide 50 mg Etoposide 50mg capsules | 20 capsule [PoM] £199.64 DT = £194.65

Etoposide 100 mg Etoposide 100mg capsules | 10 capsule [PoM] £174.46 DT = £170.11

Powder for solution for injection

▸ **Etoposide (Non-proprietary)**

Etoposide (as Etoposide phosphate) 100 mg Etoposide 100mg powder for solution for injection vials | 1 vial [PoM] [H]

▸ **Etopophos** (Neon Healthcare Ltd)
Etoposide (as Etoposide phosphate) 100 mg Etopophos 100mg powder for solution for injection vials | 10 vial PoM £261.68

ANTINEOPLASTIC DRUGS › VINCA ALKALOIDS

Vinblastine sulfate [Specialist drug]

02-Jul-2020

● **INDICATIONS AND DOSE**

Hodgkin's disease and other lymphomas

▸ BY INTRAVENOUS INJECTION

▸ Child: Specialist drug – access specialist resources for dosing information

● **UNLICENSED USE** Licensed for use in children (age range not specified by manufacturer).

IMPORTANT SAFETY INFORMATION
Vinblastine is for **intravenous administration only**. Inadvertent intrathecal administration can cause severe neurotoxicity, which is usually fatal.

The National Patient Safety Agency has advised (August 2008) that adult and teenage patients treated in an adult or adolescent unit should receive their vinca alkaloid dose in a 50 mL minibag. Teenagers and children treated in a child unit may receive their vinca alkaloid dose in a syringe.

● **CONTRA-INDICATIONS** Intrathecal injection **contra-indicated.**

● **INTERACTIONS** → Appendix 1: vinca alkaloids

● **SIDE-EFFECTS**

▸ **Rare or very rare** Hearing impairment · nerve disorders · vestibular damage

▸ **Frequency not known** Abdominal pain · alopecia (reversible) · anaemia · appetite decreased · asthenia · balance impaired · cancer pain · constipation · depression · diarrhoea · dizziness · dyspnoea · haemorrhage · headache · hypertension · ileus · increased risk of infection · leucopenia (dose-limiting) · malaise · myalgia · nausea · nystagmus · oral blistering · pain · Raynaud's phenomenon · reflexes absent · respiratory disorders · seizure · sensation abnormal · SIADH · skin reactions · thrombocytopenia · vertigo · vomiting

SIDE-EFFECTS, FURTHER INFORMATION **Constipation** Prophylactic use of laxatives may be considered.

● **CONCEPTION AND CONTRACEPTION** Contraceptive advice required.

● **MEDICINAL FORMS** There can be variation in the licensing of different medicines containing the same drug.

Solution for injection

▸ **Vinblastine sulfate (Non-proprietary)**
Vinblastine sulfate 1 mg per 1 ml Vinblastine 10mg/10ml solution for injection vials | 5 vial PoM £85.00 (Hospital only)

Vincristine sulfate [Specialist drug]

03-Jul-2020

● **INDICATIONS AND DOSE**

Acute leukaemias | Lymphomas | Paediatric solid tumours

▸ BY INTRAVENOUS INJECTION

▸ Child: Specialist drug – access specialist resources for dosing information

● **UNLICENSED USE** Licensed for use in children (age range not specified by manufacturer).

IMPORTANT SAFETY INFORMATION
Vincristine injections are for **intravenous administration only.** Inadvertent intrathecal administration can cause severe neurotoxicity, which is usually fatal.

The National Patient Safety Agency has advised (August 2008) that adult and teenage patients treated in an adult or adolescent unit should receive their vinca alkaloid dose in a 50 mL minibag. Teenagers and children treated in a child unit may receive their vinca alkaloid dose in a syringe.

● **CONTRA-INDICATIONS** Avoid injections containing benzyl alcohol in neonates

CONTRA-INDICATIONS, FURTHER INFORMATION Intrathecal injection **contra-indicated.**

● **INTERACTIONS** → Appendix 1: vinca alkaloids

● **SIDE-EFFECTS**

▸ **Rare or very rare** Hypersensitivity · rash · SIADH

▸ **Frequency not known** Abdominal cramps · adrenal disorder · alopecia · anaemia · appetite decreased · azotaemia · bladder atony · bronchospasm · connective tissue disorders · constipation · coronary artery disease · dehydration · diarrhoea · dizziness · dyspnoea · eighth cranial nerve damage · eye disorders · fever · gait abnormalities · gastrointestinal disorders · haemolytic anaemia · headache · hearing impairment · hypertension · hyponatraemia · hypotension · infection · leucopenia · movement disorders · muscle atrophy · myalgia · myocardial infarction · nausea · neuromuscular effects (dose-limiting) · neutropenia · oedema · oral disorders · pain · paralysis · paresis · reflexes absent · renal disorder · secondary malignancy · seizure · sensation abnormal · sepsis · throat pain · thrombocytopenia · urinary disorders · vertigo · vestibular damage · vision loss · vomiting · weight decreased

SIDE-EFFECTS, FURTHER INFORMATION **Bronchospasm** Severe bronchospasm following administration is more common when used in combination with mitomycin-C.

Neurotoxicity Sensory and motor neuropathies are common and are cumulative. Manufacturer advises monitoring patients for symptoms of neuropathy, such as hypoesthesia, hyperesthesia, paresthesia, hyporeflexia, areflexia, neuralgia, jaw pain, decreased vibratory sense, cranial neuropathy, ileus, burning sensation, arthralgia, myalgia, muscle spasm, or weakness, both before and during treatment—requires dose reduction, treatment interruption or treatment discontinuation, depending on severity.

Motor weakness can also occur and dose reduction or discontinuation of therapy may be appropriate if motor weakness increases. Recovery from neurotoxic effects is usually slow but complete.

Constipation Prophylactic use of laxatives may be considered.

● **CONCEPTION AND CONTRACEPTION** Contraceptive advice required.

● **MEDICINAL FORMS** There can be variation in the licensing of different medicines containing the same drug.

Solution for injection

▸ **Vincristine sulfate (Non-proprietary)**
Vincristine sulfate 1 mg per 1 ml Vincristine 1mg/1ml solution for injection vials | 1 vial PoM £13.47 (Hospital only) | 5 vial PoM £67.35 (Hospital only)
Vincristine 2mg/2ml solution for injection vials | 1 vial PoM £26.66 (Hospital only) | 5 vial PoM £133.30 (Hospital only)

ANTINEOPLASTIC DRUGS > OTHER

Asparaginase [Specialist drug] 03-Nov-2020

- **INDICATIONS AND DOSE**

Acute lymphoblastic leukaemia

▸ BY INTRAVENOUS INFUSION

▸ Neonate: Specialist drug – access specialist resources for dosing information.

▸ Child: Specialist drug – access specialist resources for dosing information

IMPORTANT SAFETY INFORMATION
Resuscitation facilities should be available during administration.

- **CONTRA-INDICATIONS** History of pancreatitis related to asparaginase therapy · history of serious haemorrhage related to asparaginase therapy · history of serious thrombosis related to asparaginase therapy · pancreatitis · pre-existing known coagulopathy
- **INTERACTIONS** → Appendix 1: asparaginase
- **SIDE-EFFECTS**

▸ **Common or very common** Agitation · anaemia · angioedema · appetite decreased · arthralgia · bronchospasm · coagulation disorders · confusion · depression · diarrhoea · dizziness · drowsiness · dyspnoea · embolism and thrombosis · fatigue · flushing · gastrointestinal discomfort · haemorrhage · hallucination · hyperglycaemia · hypersensitivity · hypoalbuminaemia · hypoglycaemia · hypotension · increased risk of infection · leucopenia · nausea · neurological effects · oedema · pain · pancreatitis acute · skin reactions · thrombocytopenia · vomiting · weight decreased

▸ **Uncommon** Headache · hyperammonaemia · hyperuricaemia

▸ **Rare or very rare** Coma · consciousness impaired · diabetic ketoacidosis · hepatic disorders · hyperparathyroidism · hypoparathyroidism · ischaemic stroke · necrotising pancreatitis · pancreatic pseudocyst · pancreatitis (sometimes fatal) · posterior reversible encephalopathy syndrome (PRES) · secondary hypothyroidism · seizure · tremor

SIDE-EFFECTS, FURTHER INFORMATION There have been rare reports of cholestasis, icterus, hepatic cell necrosis and hepatic failure with fatal outcome; manufacturer advises interrupt treatment if these symptoms develop.

- **CONCEPTION AND CONTRACEPTION** Manufacturer advises effective contraception in men and women of child-bearing potential during treatment and for at least 3 months after last dose; asparaginase may reduce effectiveness of oral contraceptives—additional precautions (e.g. barrier method) are required.
- **PATIENT AND CARER ADVICE**

Driving and skilled tasks Manufacturer advises asparaginase has moderate influence on driving and performance of skilled tasks—increased risk of dizziness and somnolence.

- **NATIONAL FUNDING/ACCESS DECISIONS**

For full details see funding body website

Scottish Medicines Consortium (SMC) decisions

▸ **Asparaginase (*Spectrila*®) as a component of antineoplastic combination therapy for the treatment of acute lymphoblastic leukaemia in paediatric patients from birth to 18 years and adult patients (April 2018)** SMC No. 1319/18 Recommended

- **MEDICINAL FORMS** There can be variation in the licensing of different medicines containing the same drug.

Powder for solution for infusion

▸ Spectrila (medac UK)

Asparaginase 10000 unit Spectrila 10,000unit powder for concentrate for solution for infusion vials | 1 vial PoM £450.00 (Hospital only)

Crisantaspase [Specialist drug] 07-Aug-2020

- **INDICATIONS AND DOSE**

Acute lymphoblastic leukaemia

▸ BY INTRAVENOUS INFUSION, OR BY INTRAMUSCULAR INJECTION

▸ Child 4 months–17 years: Specialist drug – access specialist resources for dosing information

IMPORTANT SAFETY INFORMATION
Resuscitation facilities should be available during administration.

- **CONTRA-INDICATIONS** History of pancreatitis related to asparaginase therapy
- **INTERACTIONS** → Appendix 1: crisantaspase
- **SIDE-EFFECTS**

▸ **Common or very common** Anaemia · anxiety · appetite decreased · arthralgia · diarrhoea · dizziness · dyslipidaemia · dyspnoea · embolism and thrombosis · encephalopathy · fatigue · febrile disorders · fever · gastrointestinal discomfort · haemorrhage · headache · hepatic disorders · hyperammonaemia · hyperglycaemia · hypersensitivity · hypoalbuminaemia · hypoglycaemia · hypotension · increased risk of infection · infusion related reaction · irritability · ischaemia · leucopenia · level of consciousness decreased · mucositis · myalgia · nausea · necrotising pancreatitis · neurotoxicity · neutropenia · pain · pancreatitis · pseudocyst · sepsis · skin reactions · thrombocytopenia · vomiting · weight decreased

▸ **Uncommon** Diabetic ketoacidosis · renal impairment · seizures

▸ **Frequency not known** Arthritis reactive · bone marrow depression · coagulation disorders · glucose tolerance impaired · hypertension · toxic epidermal necrolysis

- **ALLERGY AND CROSS-SENSITIVITY** Children who are hypersensitive to asparaginase derived from one organism may tolerate asparaginase derived from another organism but cross-sensitivity occurs in about 20–30% of individuals.
- **CONCEPTION AND CONTRACEPTION** Contraceptive advice required.
- **MEDICINAL FORMS** There can be variation in the licensing of different medicines containing the same drug.

Powder for solution for injection

▸ Erwinase (Porton Biopharma Ltd)

Crisantaspase 10000 unit Erwinase 10,000unit powder for solution for injection vials | 5 vial PoM £3,822.50 (Hospital only)

Hydroxycarbamide 04-Sep-2020
(Hydroxyurea)

- **INDICATIONS AND DOSE**

SIKLOS®

Sickle-cell disease [prevention of recurrent vaso-occlusive crises] (initiated by a specialist)

▸ BY MOUTH

▸ Child 2–17 years: Initially 10–15 mg/kg once daily, increased in steps of 2.5–5 mg/kg daily, dose to be

continued →

increased every 12 weeks according to response; usual dose 15–30 mg/kg daily; maximum 35 mg/kg per day

XROMI®

Sickle-cell disease [prevention of vaso-occlusive complications] (under expert supervision)

- BY MOUTH
- Child 2-17 years: Initially 15 mg/kg daily, increased in steps of 5 mg/kg daily, dose to be increased every 8 weeks according to response; usual maintenance 20–25 mg/kg daily; maximum 35 mg/kg per day

> IMPORTANT SAFETY INFORMATION
> RISKS OF INCORRECT DOSING OF ORAL ANTI-CANCER MEDICINES
> See Cytotoxic drugs p. 660.

- **CAUTIONS** Leg ulcers (review treatment if cutaneous vasculitic ulcerations develop)
- **INTERACTIONS** → Appendix 1: hydroxycarbamide
- **SIDE-EFFECTS**
- **Common or very common** Alopecia · anaemia · appetite decreased · asthenia · bone marrow disorders · chills · constipation · cutaneous vasculitis · dermatomyositis · diarrhoea · disorientation · dizziness · drowsiness · dyspnoea · dysuria · fever · gastrointestinal discomfort · haemorrhage · hallucination · headache · hepatic disorders · leucopenia · lung infiltration · malaise · mucositis · nail discolouration · nail disorder · nausea · neoplasms · neutropenia · oral disorders · pancreatitis · peripheral neuropathy · pulmonary fibrosis · pulmonary oedema · red blood cell abnormalities · seizure · skin reactions · skin ulcers · sperm abnormalities · thrombocytopenia · vomiting
- **Rare or very rare** Cutaneous lupus erythematosus · gangrene · systemic lupus erythematosus (SLE)
- **Frequency not known** Amenorrhoea · gastrointestinal disorders · hypomagnesaemia · Parvovirus B19 infection · vitamin D deficiency · weight increased
- **CONCEPTION AND CONTRACEPTION** Manufacturer advises effective contraception before and during treatment. See also *Pregnancy and reproductive function* in Cytotoxic drugs p. 660.
- **PREGNANCY** Avoid (teratogenic in *animal* studies). See also *Pregnancy and reproductive function* in Cytotoxic drugs p. 660.
- **BREAST FEEDING** Discontinue breast-feeding.
- **HEPATIC IMPAIRMENT** Manufacturer advises caution in mild to moderate impairment; avoid in severe impairment (unless used for malignant conditions).
- **RENAL IMPAIRMENT** In sickle-cell disease, avoid if estimated glomerular filtration rate less than 30 mL/minute/1.73 m^2.

Dose adjustments In sickle-cell disease, reduce initial dose by 50% if estimated glomerular filtration rate less than 60 mL/minute/1.73 m^2.

- **MONITORING REQUIREMENTS**
- Monitor renal and hepatic function before and during treatment.
- Monitor full blood count before treatment, and repeatedly throughout use; in sickle-cell disease monitor every 2 weeks for the first 2 months and then every 2 to 3 months thereafter (or every 2 weeks if on maximum dose).
- Patients receiving long-term therapy for malignant disease should be monitored for secondary malignancies.
- **PATIENT AND CARER ADVICE** Patients receiving long-term therapy with hydroxycarbamide should be advised to protect skin from sun exposure.

Medicines for Children leaflet: Hydroxycarbamide for sickle cell disease www.medicinesforchildren.org.uk/medicines/hydroxycarbamide-for-sickle-cell-disease/

- **NATIONAL FUNDING/ACCESS DECISIONS**

For full details see funding body website

Scottish Medicines Consortium (SMC) decisions

- Hydroxycarbamide oral solution (*Xromi®*) for the prevention of vaso-occlusive complications of sickle-cell disease in patients over 2 years of age (August 2020) SMC No. SMC2271 Recommended with restrictions

All Wales Medicines Strategy Group (AWMSG) decisions

- Hydroxycarbamide oral solution (*Xromi®*) for the prevention of vaso-occlusive complications of sickle-cell disease in patients over 2 years of age (August 2020) AWMSG No. 4264 Recommended with restrictions

- **MEDICINAL FORMS** There can be variation in the licensing of different medicines containing the same drug.

Oral tablet

- **Siklos** (Masters Pharmaceuticals Ltd)

Hydroxycarbamide 100 mg Siklos 100mg tablets | 60 tablet PoM £100.00 DT = £100.00

Hydroxycarbamide 1 gram Siklos 1000mg tablets | 30 tablet PoM £500.00 DT = £500.00

Oral solution

CAUTIONARY AND ADVISORY LABELS 27

EXCIPIENTS: May contain Hydroxybenzoates (parabens)

- **Xromi** (Nova Laboratories Ltd)

Hydroxycarbamide 100 mg per 1 ml Xromi 100mg/ml oral solution | 150 ml PoM £250.00 DT = £250.00 SF

Mitotane [Specialist drug]

09-Sep-2021

- **INDICATIONS AND DOSE**

Adrenocortical carcinoma

- BY MOUTH
- Child: Specialist drug – access specialist resources for dosing information

- **UNLICENSED USE** Not licensed for use in children.

> IMPORTANT SAFETY INFORMATION
> RISKS OF INCORRECT DOSING OF ORAL ANTI-CANCER MEDICINES
> See Cytotoxic drugs p. 660.

- **CONTRA-INDICATIONS** Acute porphyrias p. 745
- **INTERACTIONS** → Appendix 1: mitotane
- **SIDE-EFFECTS**
- **Common or very common** Adrenal insufficiency · anaemia · appetite decreased · asthenia · cognitive impairment · confusion · diarrhoea · dizziness · drowsiness · dyslipidaemia · gastrointestinal discomfort · gynaecomastia · headache · hepatic disorders · leucopenia · movement disorders · mucositis · muscle weakness · nausea · paraesthesia · polyneuropathy · rash · thrombocytopenia · vertigo · vomiting
- **Frequency not known** Encephalopathy · eye disorders · flushing · fungal infection · generalised pain · growth retardation · haemorrhage · hyperpyrexia · hypersalivation · hypertension · hypothyroidism · hypouricaemia · lens opacity · neuro-psychological retardation · ovarian cyst · postural hypotension · proteinuria · taste altered · thyroid disorder · vision disorders
- **CONCEPTION AND CONTRACEPTION** Contraceptive advice required.
- **PATIENT AND CARER ADVICE** Patients should be warned to contact doctor immediately if injury, infection, or illness occurs (because of risk of acute adrenal insufficiency—treatment may need to be temporarily discontinued and exogenous steroids administered).

Patient card A patient card should be provided.

Driving and skilled tasks Central nervous system toxicity may affect performance of skilled tasks (e.g. driving).

● **MEDICINAL FORMS** There can be variation in the licensing of different medicines containing the same drug.

Oral tablet

CAUTIONARY AND ADVISORY LABELS 2, 10, 21

▸ **Mitotane (Non-proprietary)**

Mitotane 500 mg Mitotane 500mg tablets | 100 tablet PoM £780.08 DT = £780.08

Pegaspargase [Specialist drug] 25-Aug-2020

● **INDICATIONS AND DOSE**

Acute lymphoblastic leukaemia

▶ BY INTRAMUSCULAR INJECTION, OR BY INTRAVENOUS INFUSION

▸ Neonate: Specialist drug – access specialist resources for dosing information.

▸ Child: Specialist drug – access specialist resources for dosing information

IMPORTANT SAFETY INFORMATION

Resuscitation facilities should be available during administration.

● **CONTRA-INDICATIONS** History of pancreatitis · history of serious haemorrhagic event with previous L-asparaginase therapy · history of serious thrombosis with previous L-asparaginase therapy

● **INTERACTIONS** → Appendix 1: pegaspargase

● **SIDE-EFFECTS**

▶ **Common or very common** Abdominal pain · anaemia · appetite decreased · ascites · coagulation disorders · diarrhoea · dyslipidaemia · embolism and thrombosis · febrile neutropenia · hepatic disorders · hyperglycaemia · hypersensitivity · hypoalbuminaemia · hypokalaemia · hypoxia · increased risk of infection · nausea · pain in extremity · pancreatitis (discontinue if suspected and do not restart if confirmed) · peripheral neuropathy · seizure · sepsis · skin reactions · stomatitis · syncope · vomiting · weight decreased

▶ **Rare or very rare** Encephalopathy · haemorrhage · necrotising pancreatitis

▶ **Frequency not known** Acute kidney injury · bone marrow disorders · confusion · diabetic ketoacidosis · drowsiness · fever · hyperammonaemia (monitor if symptoms present) · hyperglycaemic hyperosmolar nonketotic syndrome · hypoglycaemia · pancreatic pseudocyst · stroke · toxic epidermal necrolysis · tremor

SIDE-EFFECTS, FURTHER INFORMATION There have been rare reports of cholestasis, icterus, hepatic cell necrosis and hepatic failure with fatal outcome in patients receiving pegaspargase.

● **CONCEPTION AND CONTRACEPTION** Manufacturer advises effective contraception in men and women of child-bearing potential during treatment and for at least 6 months after discontinuing treatment; pegaspargase may reduce effectiveness of oral contraceptives—additional precautions (e.g. barrier method) are required.

● **PATIENT AND CARER ADVICE**

Pancreatitis Manufacturer advises patients and carers should be told how to recognise signs and symptoms of pancreatitis and advised to seek medical attention if symptoms such as persistent, severe abdominal pain develop.

Driving and skilled tasks Manufacturer advises patients and carers should be counselled on the effects on driving and performance of skilled tasks—increased risk of confusion and somnolence.

● **NATIONAL FUNDING/ACCESS DECISIONS**

For full details see funding body website

NICE decisions

▶ **Pegaspargase for treating acute lymphoblastic leukaemia (September 2016)** NICE TA408 Recommended

Scottish Medicines Consortium (SMC) decisions

▶ **Pegaspargase (*Oncaspar*®) as a component of antineoplastic combination therapy in acute lymphoblastic leukaemia (ALL) in paediatric patients from birth to 18 years, and adult patients (November 2016)** SMC No. 1197/16 Recommended

● **MEDICINAL FORMS** There can be variation in the licensing of different medicines containing the same drug.

Powder for solution for injection

▸ **Oncaspar** (Servier Laboratories Ltd)

Pegaspargase 3750 unit Oncaspar 3,750unit powder for solution for injection vials | 1 vial PoM £1,296.19 (Hospital only)

Procarbazine [Specialist drug] 16-Nov-2021

● **INDICATIONS AND DOSE**

Hodgkin's lymphoma

▶ BY MOUTH

▸ Child: Specialist drug – access specialist resources for dosing information

IMPORTANT SAFETY INFORMATION

RISKS OF INCORRECT DOSING OF ORAL ANTI-CANCER MEDICINES

See Cytotoxic drugs p. 660.

● **CONTRA-INDICATIONS** Pre-existing severe leucopenia · pre-existing severe thrombocytopenia

● **INTERACTIONS** → Appendix 1: procarbazine

● **SIDE-EFFECTS**

▶ **Common or very common** Appetite decreased

▶ **Frequency not known** Azoospermia · hepatic disorders · infection · lethargy · leucopenia · nausea · neutropenia · ovarian failure · pneumonitis · skin reactions · thrombocytopenia · vomiting

● **CONCEPTION AND CONTRACEPTION** Contraceptive advice required.

● **MEDICINAL FORMS** There can be variation in the licensing of different medicines containing the same drug.

Oral capsule

CAUTIONARY AND ADVISORY LABELS 4

▸ **Procarbazine (Non-proprietary)**

Procarbazine (as Procarbazine hydrochloride)

50 mg Procarbazine 50mg capsules | 50 capsule PoM £503.61–£555.23 DT = £555.23

RETINOID AND RELATED DRUGS

Tretinoin [Specialist drug] 06-Nov-2023

(Retinoic acid; Vitamin A acid)

● **INDICATIONS AND DOSE**

Acute promyelocytic leukaemia

▶ BY MOUTH

▸ Child: Specialist drug – access specialist resources for dosing information

IMPORTANT SAFETY INFORMATION

MHRA/CHM ADVICE: ORAL RETINOID MEDICINES: REVISED AND SIMPLIFIED PREGNANCY PREVENTION EDUCATIONAL MATERIALS FOR HEALTHCARE PROFESSIONALS AND WOMEN (JUNE 2019)

Materials to support the Pregnancy Prevention Programme in women and girls of childbearing potential taking oral acitretin, alitretinoin, or isotretinoin have been updated. Oral tretinoin and bexarotene do not have a Pregnancy Prevention Programme in light of their oncology indication and specialist care setting. However, healthcare professionals are advised that these medicines are extremely teratogenic and product information should be consulted for contraceptive and pregnancy testing requirements when used in females of childbearing potential.

Neuropsychiatric reactions have been reported in patients taking oral retinoids. Healthcare professionals are advised to monitor patients for signs of depression or suicidal ideation and refer for appropriate treatment, if necessary; particular care is needed in those with a history of depression. Patients should be advised to speak to their doctor if they experience any changes in mood or behaviour, and encouraged to ask family and friends to look out for any change in mood.

- **INTERACTIONS** → Appendix 1: retinoids
- **SIDE-EFFECTS**
  - **Common or very common** Abdominal pain · alopecia · anxiety · appetite decreased · arrhythmia · asthma · bone pain · cheilitis · chest pain · chills · confusion · conjunctival disorder · constipation · depression · diarrhoea · dizziness · dry mouth · flushing · headache · hearing impairment · hyperhidrosis · idiopathic intracranial hypertension (children particularly susceptible - consider dose reduction if intractable headache in children) · insomnia · intracranial pressure increased · malaise · nasal dryness · nausea · pancreatitis · paraesthesia · respiratory disorders · skin reactions · visual impairment · vomiting
  - **Frequency not known** Embolism and thrombosis · erythema nodosum · genital ulceration · hypercalcaemia · increased leucocytes · mood altered · myocardial infarction · myositis · necrotising fasciitis · stroke · thrombocytopenia · vasculitis

  SIDE-EFFECTS, FURTHER INFORMATION Children are particularly susceptible to nervous system effects.

  Retinoic acid syndrome Fever, dyspnoea, acute respiratory distress, pulmonary infiltrates, pleural effusion, hyperleucocytosis, hypotension, oedema, weight gain, hepatic, renal and multi-organ failure requires immediate treatment—consult product literature.
- **ALLERGY AND CROSS-SENSITIVITY** [EvGr] Contra-indicated in patients with hypersensitivity to peanuts or soya (capsule filling contains soya-bean oil). ⟨M⟩
- **CONCEPTION AND CONTRACEPTION** [EvGr] Ensure effective contraception during and for at least 1 month after treatment. ⟨M⟩
- **PATIENT AND CARER ADVICE**

  Risk of neuropsychiatric reactions The MHRA advises patients and carers to seek medical attention if changes in mood or behaviour occur.

- **MEDICINAL FORMS** There can be variation in the licensing of different medicines containing the same drug.

Oral capsule

CAUTIONARY AND ADVISORY LABELS 21, 25

- **Tretinoin (Non-proprietary)**

  Tretinoin 10 mg Tretinoin 10mg capsules | 100 capsule [PoM] £400.00 DT = £400.00

2.1 Cytotoxic drug-induced side effects

Other drugs used for Cytotoxic drug-induced side effects
Sodium thiosulfate, p. 1044

ANTIDOTES AND CHELATORS

Glucarpidase

16-Nov-2023

- **DRUG ACTION** Glucarpidase is a recombinant bacterial enzyme that converts methotrexate to its inactive metabolites.
- **INDICATIONS AND DOSE**

  Reduction of toxic plasma-methotrexate concentration
  - BY INTRAVENOUS INJECTION
    - Child: 50 units/kg for 1 dose, dose to be given without delay; the optimal administration timeframe for patients with delayed methotrexate elimination is within 48–60 hours from the start of high-dose methotrexate infusion, folinic acid rescue should continue to be given at least 2 hours after glucarpidase administration—see also *Interactions*
- **INTERACTIONS** → Appendix 1: glucarpidase
- **SIDE-EFFECTS**
  - **Uncommon** Feeling hot · flushing · headache · sensation abnormal
  - **Rare or very rare** Abdominal pain upper · crystalluria · diarrhoea · drowsiness · fever · hypersensitivity · hypotension · nausea · pleural effusion · skin reactions · tachycardia · throat tightness · tremor · vomiting
- **PREGNANCY** Specialist sources indicate probably compatible (no information available).
- **BREAST FEEDING** Specialist sources indicate probably compatible (no information available).
- **EFFECT ON LABORATORY TESTS** May interfere with measurement of methotrexate concentration by immunoassay if carried out within 48 hours of administration—consult product literature.
- **DIRECTIONS FOR ADMINISTRATION** For *intravenous injection*, reconstitute each vial with 1 mL Sodium Chloride 0.9% and give over 5 minutes.
- **PRESCRIBING AND DISPENSING INFORMATION** Glucarpidase is a biological medicine. Biological medicines must be prescribed and dispensed by brand name, see *Biological medicines* and *Biosimilar medicines*, under Guidance on prescribing p. 1; record the brand name and batch number after each administration.
- **HANDLING AND STORAGE** Store in a refrigerator (2–8°C)—consult product literature for storage conditions after reconstitution.

- **MEDICINAL FORMS** There can be variation in the licensing of different medicines containing the same drug.

Powder for solution for injection

- **Voraxaze** (Protherics Medicines Development Ltd) ▼

  Glucarpidase 1000 unit Voraxaze 1,000unit powder for solution for injection vials | 1 vial [PoM] £25,385.00 (Hospital only)

DETOXIFYING DRUGS › UROPROTECTIVE DRUGS

Mesna

16-Dec-2020

- **INDICATIONS AND DOSE**

  Urothelial toxicity following oxazaphosphorine therapy
  - BY INTRAVENOUS INJECTION, OR BY CONTINUOUS INTRAVENOUS INFUSION
    - Child: (consult local protocol)

  Mucolytic in cystic fibrosis
  - BY INHALATION OF NEBULISED SOLUTION
    - Child: 3–6 mL twice daily, use a 20% solution
- **UNLICENSED USE** Not licensed for use in children.

- **SIDE-EFFECTS**
  - **Common or very common** Appetite decreased · arthralgia · asthenia · chest pain · chills · concentration impaired · conjunctivitis · constipation · cough · dehydration · diarrhoea · dizziness · drowsiness · dry mouth · dyspnoea · dysuria · fever · flatulence · flushing · gastrointestinal discomfort · haemorrhage · headache · hyperhidrosis · influenza like illness · laryngeal discomfort · lymphadenopathy · malaise · mucosal irritation · myalgia · nasal congestion · nausea · oral irritation · pain · palpitations · respiratory disorders · sensation abnormal · skin reactions · sleep disorders · syncope · vision disorders · vomiting
  - **Frequency not known** Acute kidney injury · angioedema · drug reaction with eosinophilia and systemic symptoms (DRESS) · hypotension · hypoxia · oedema · tachycardia · ulcer
- **ALLERGY AND CROSS-SENSITIVITY** EvGr Caution if history of hypersensitivity to thiol-containing compounds. ⟨M⟩
- **PREGNANCY** Not known to be harmful. See also *Pregnancy and reproductive function* in Cytotoxic drugs p. 660.
- **MEDICINAL FORMS** There can be variation in the licensing of different medicines containing the same drug.

Solution for injection

- **Mesna (Non-proprietary)**
  Mesna 100 mg per 1 ml Mesna 1g/10ml solution for injection ampoules | 15 ampoule PoM £527.10 (Hospital only)
  Mesna 400mg/4ml solution for injection ampoules | 15 ampoule PoM £240.30 (Hospital only)

VITAMINS AND TRACE ELEMENTS › FOLATES

Folinic acid

04-Mar-2026

- **INDICATIONS AND DOSE**

Reduction of methotrexate-induced toxicity

- BY MOUTH, OR BY INTRAVENOUS INFUSION, OR BY INTRAVENOUS INJECTION
  - Child: (consult local protocol)

Methotrexate overdose

- BY INTRAVENOUS INFUSION, OR BY INTRAVENOUS INJECTION
  - Child: (consult local protocol)

Megaloblastic anaemia due to folate deficiency

- BY MOUTH
  - Child 1 month–11 years: 250 micrograms/kg once daily
  - Child 12–17 years: 15 mg once daily

Metabolic disorders leading to folate deficiency

- BY MOUTH, OR BY INTRAVENOUS INFUSION
  - Child: 15 mg once daily, larger doses may be required in older children

Prevention of megaloblastic anaemia associated with pyrimethamine and sulfadiazine treatment of congenital toxoplasmosis

- BY MOUTH
  - Neonate: 5 mg 3 times a week; increased if necessary up to 20 mg 3 times a week, if the patient is neutropenic.
  - Child 1–11 months: 10 mg 3 times a week

SODIOFOLIN®

As an antidote to methotrexate

- BY INTRAVENOUS INFUSION, OR BY INTRAVENOUS INJECTION
  - Child: (consult product literature)

- **UNLICENSED USE** Consult product literature for licensing status of individual preparations.
- **CONTRA-INDICATIONS** Intrathecal injection
- **CAUTIONS** Avoid simultaneous administration of methotrexate · **not** indicated for pernicious anaemia or other megaloblastic anaemias caused by vitamin B_{12} deficiency
- **INTERACTIONS** → Appendix 1: folates
- **SIDE-EFFECTS**

GENERAL SIDE-EFFECTS
  - **Common or very common** Diarrhoea
  - **Uncommon** Fever
  - **Rare or very rare** Agitation (with high doses) · depression (with high doses) · epilepsy exacerbated · gastrointestinal disorder (with high doses) · insomnia (with high doses)

SPECIFIC SIDE-EFFECTS
  - **Common or very common**
    - With intravenous use Bone marrow failure · dehydration · mucositis · nausea · oral disorders · skin reactions · vomiting
  - **Rare or very rare**
    - With intravenous use Sensitisation
  - **Frequency not known**
    - With intravenous use Hyperammonaemia
    - With oral use Leucopenia · stomatitis · thrombocytopenia
- **PREGNANCY** Not known to be harmful; benefit outweighs risk.
- **BREAST FEEDING** Presence in milk unknown but benefit outweighs risk.
- **MEDICINAL FORMS** There can be variation in the licensing of different medicines containing the same drug. Forms available from special-order manufacturers include: oral suspension, oral solution

Oral tablet

- **Folinic acid (Non-proprietary)**
  Folinic acid (as Calcium folinate) 15 mg Calcium folinate 15mg tablets | 10 tablet PoM £66.80 DT = £37.85
- **Refolinon** (Pfizer Ltd)
  Folinic acid (as Calcium folinate) 15 mg Refolinon 15mg tablets | 30 tablet PoM £85.74 DT = £85.74

Solution for injection

- **Folinic acid (Non-proprietary)**
  Folinic acid (as Calcium folinate) 10 mg per 1 ml Calcium folinate 200mg/20ml solution for injection vials | 10 vial PoM ⊠ (Hospital only)
  Calcium folinate 300mg/30ml solution for injection vials | 1 vial PoM £100.00 (Hospital only)
  Calcium folinate 350mg/35ml solution for injection vials | 1 vial PoM £166.79 (Hospital only) | 10 vial PoM £1,667.90 (Hospital only)
  Calcium folinate 100mg/10ml solution for injection vials | 1 vial PoM £37.50–£54.31 (Hospital only) | 10 vial PoM £375.00–£543.10 (Hospital only)
  Calcium folinate 50mg/5ml solution for injection vials | 1 vial PoM £20.00–£29.53 (Hospital only) | 1 vial PoM £30.56 | 10 vial PoM £305.60 | 10 vial PoM £200.00 (Hospital only)
- **Sodiofolin** (medac UK)
  Folinic acid (as Disodium folinate) 50 mg per 1 ml Sodiofolin 400mg/8ml solution for injection vials | 1 vial PoM £126.25 (Hospital only)
  Sodiofolin 100mg/2ml solution for injection vials | 1 vial PoM £35.09 (Hospital only)

Levofolinic acid

17-Feb-2021

- **DRUG ACTION** Levofolinic acid is an isomer of folinic acid.
- **INDICATIONS AND DOSE**

Reduction of methotrexate-induced toxicity

- BY INTRAMUSCULAR INJECTION, OR BY INTRAVENOUS INJECTION, OR BY INTRAVENOUS INFUSION
  - Child: (consult local protocol)

Methotrexate overdose

- BY INTRAMUSCULAR INJECTION, OR BY INTRAVENOUS INJECTION, OR BY INTRAVENOUS INFUSION
  - Child: (consult local protocol)

- **CONTRA-INDICATIONS** Intrathecal injection
- **CAUTIONS** Avoid simultaneous administration of methotrexate · **not** indicated for pernicious anaemia or

other megaloblastic anaemias caused by vitamin B_{12} deficiency

- **INTERACTIONS** → Appendix 1: folates
- **SIDE-EFFECTS**
  - **Common or very common** Dehydration · diarrhoea · mucosal toxicity · nausea · vomiting
  - **Uncommon** Fever
  - **Rare or very rare** Agitation (with high doses) · depression (with high doses) · epilepsy exacerbated · gastrointestinal disorder · insomnia (with high doses) · urticaria
- **PREGNANCY** Not known to be harmful; benefit outweighs risk.
- **BREAST FEEDING** Presence in milk unknown but benefit outweighs risk.

- **MEDICINAL FORMS** There can be variation in the licensing of different medicines containing the same drug.

Solution for injection

- Levofolinic acid (Non-proprietary)
  Levofolinic acid (as Disodium levofolinate) 50 mg per 1 ml Levofolinic acid 50mg/1ml solution for injection vials | 1 vial PoM £24.70 (Hospital only)
  Levofolinic acid 200mg/4ml solution for injection vials | 1 vial PoM £80.40 (Hospital only)
- Isovorin (Pfizer Ltd)
  Levofolinic acid (as Calcium levofolinate) 10 mg per 1 ml Isovorin 175mg/17.5ml solution for injection vials | 1 vial PoM £81.33 (Hospital only)

2.1a Hyperuricaemia associated with cytotoxic drugs

DETOXIFYING DRUGS > URATE OXIDASES

Rasburicase 06-Oct-2025

- **DRUG ACTION** Rasburicase is a recombinant urate oxidase enzyme which catalyses oxidation of uric acid into allantoin, which is then renally excreted.

- **INDICATIONS AND DOSE**

Prophylaxis and treatment of acute hyperuricaemia, before and during initiation of chemotherapy, in patients with haematological malignancy and high tumour burden at risk of rapid tumour lysis (under expert supervision)

- BY INTRAVENOUS INFUSION
  - Neonate: 200 micrograms/kg once daily for up to 7 days according to plasma-uric acid concentration.
  - Child: 200 micrograms/kg once daily for up to 7 days according to plasma-uric acid concentration

IMPORTANT SAFETY INFORMATION

NATIONAL PATIENT SAFETY ALERT: HARM FROM DELAYED ADMINISTRATION OF RASBURICASE FOR TUMOUR LYSIS SYNDROME (SEPTEMBER 2025)

Reviews of reported incidents have identified cases of delayed or omitted doses of rasburicase which have led to fatalities, development of tumour lysis syndrome (TLS) leading to intensive care admission, and significant deterioration. To minimise the risk of harm from TLS, the British Society for Haematology (BSH) has updated guidelines for diagnosis and management of TLS in patients with haematological malignancies, available at: onlinelibrary.wiley.com/doi/10.1111/bjh.70092.

The overall use of rasburicase should be reviewed locally and protocols should be aligned with BSH recommendations, including:

- documented personalised risk assessments for TLS and prescription of appropriate prophylaxis prior to initiating new treatment for patients with a haematological malignancy;
- clear documentation of indication, dose and monitoring requirements for rasburicase, to negate the need for further validation outside of the immediate specialist clinical team;
- limiting routine use of rasburicase to clinical areas with sufficient expertise;
- if, by exception, rasburicase is used in a clinical area without sufficient expertise, specialist staff should ensure it is prescribed on a chart accessible to the clinical area, any relevant information is documented, and that there are sufficient stocks available for the full treatment course;
- sufficient quantities of both strengths of rasburicase (1.5 mg and 7.5 mg) should be available in relevant clinical areas for administration within 1 hour of prescribing.

- **CONTRA-INDICATIONS** G6PD deficiency
- **CAUTIONS** Atopic allergies
- **SIDE-EFFECTS**
  - **Common or very common** Diarrhoea · fever · headache · hypersensitivity · nausea · skin reactions · vomiting
  - **Uncommon** Bronchospasm · haemolysis (discontinue immediately) · haemolytic anaemia · hypotension · methaemoglobinaemia (discontinue immediately) · seizure
  - **Rare or very rare** Rhinitis
  - **Frequency not known** Muscle contractions involuntary
- **PREGNANCY** EvGr Avoid unless essential; (M) (recommendation also supported by specialist sources—limited information available).
- **BREAST FEEDING** EvGr Use only if potential benefit outweighs risk (no information available). (M) Specialist sources indicate that large molecular weight suggests limited excretion into milk and drug molecule likely to be partially destroyed in the infant's gastro-intestinal tract.
- **MONITORING REQUIREMENTS** Monitor closely for hypersensitivity.
- **EFFECT ON LABORATORY TESTS** Interferes with plasma-uric acid concentrations—consult product literature.
- **DIRECTIONS FOR ADMINISTRATION** For *intravenous infusion* (*Fasturtec*®), give intermittently in Sodium Chloride 0.9%; reconstitute with solvent provided; gently swirl vial without shaking to dissolve; dilute requisite dose to 50 mL with infusion fluid and give over 30 minutes.
- **PRESCRIBING AND DISPENSING INFORMATION** Rasburicase is a biological medicine. Biological medicines must be prescribed and dispensed by brand name, see *Biological medicines* and *Biosimilar medicines*, under Guidance on prescribing p. 1; record the brand name and batch number after each administration.
- **HANDLING AND STORAGE** Store in a refrigerator (2–8°C) and protect from light.

- **MEDICINAL FORMS** There can be variation in the licensing of different medicines containing the same drug.

Powder and solvent for solution for infusion

- Fasturtec (Sanofi)
  Rasburicase 1.5 mg Fasturtec 1.5mg powder and solvent for solution for infusion vials | 3 vial PoM £208.39 (Hospital only)
  Rasburicase 7.5 mg Fasturtec 7.5mg powder and solvent for solution for infusion vials | 1 vial PoM £347.32 (Hospital only)

XANTHINE OXIDASE INHIBITORS

Allopurinol

12-Mar-2025

● **INDICATIONS AND DOSE**

Prophylaxis of hyperuricaemia associated with cancer chemotherapy | Prophylaxis of hyperuricaemic nephropathy | Enzyme disorders causing increased serum urate e.g Lesch-Nyhan syndrome

▶ BY MOUTH

▸ Child 1 month–14 years: 10–20 mg/kg once daily (max. per dose 400 mg), to be taken preferably after food, if once-daily dose exceeds 300 mg consider dividing the dose to reduce gastro-intestinal intolerance

▸ Child 15–17 years: Initially 100 mg once daily, to be taken preferably after food, increased if necessary up to 300 mg 3 times a day, to be taken preferably after food, dose to be adjusted according to response

● **CAUTIONS** Ensure adequate fluid intake · for hyperuricaemia associated with cancer therapy, allopurinol treatment should be started before cancer therapy · thyroid disorders

● **INTERACTIONS** → Appendix 1: allopurinol

● **SIDE-EFFECTS**

▶ **Common or very common** Rash (discontinue therapy; if rash mild re-introduce cautiously but discontinue immediately if recurrence)

▶ **Uncommon** Hypersensitivity · nausea · vomiting

▶ **Rare or very rare** Agranulocytosis · alopecia · angina pectoris · angioedema · angioimmunoblastic T-cell lymphoma · aplastic anaemia · asthenia · ataxia · boil · bradycardia · cataract · coma · depression · diabetes mellitus · drowsiness · erectile dysfunction · fever · gastrointestinal disorders · gynaecomastia · haemorrhage · hair colour changes · headache · hepatic disorders · hyperlipidaemia · hypertension · infertility male · maculopathy · malaise · oedema · paraesthesia · paralysis · peripheral neuropathy · severe cutaneous adverse reactions (SCARs) · skin reactions · stomatitis · taste altered · thrombocytopenia · vertigo · visual impairment

● **PREGNANCY** Toxicity not reported. Manufacturer advises use only if no safer alternative and disease carries risk for mother or child.

● **BREAST FEEDING** Present in milk—not known to be harmful.

● **HEPATIC IMPAIRMENT** Manufacturer advises monitor liver function periodically during early stages of therapy.

Dose adjustments Manufacturer advises reduce dose.

● **RENAL IMPAIRMENT** [EvGr] Use with caution (risk of accumulation). ⟨M⟩ Increased risk of hypersensitivity skin reactions.

Dose adjustments [EvGr] Reduce dose or increase dose interval in severe impairment; adjust dose to maintain plasma-oxipurinol concentration below 100 micromol/litre. ⟨M⟩

● **PATIENT AND CARER ADVICE**

Medicines for Children leaflet: Allopurinol for hyperuricaemia www.medicinesforchildren.org.uk/medicines/allopurinol-for-hyperuricaemia/

● **MEDICINAL FORMS** There can be variation in the licensing of different medicines containing the same drug. Forms available from special-order manufacturers include: oral suspension, oral solution

Oral tablet

CAUTIONARY AND ADVISORY LABELS 8, 21, 27

▸ **Allopurinol (Non-proprietary)**

Allopurinol 100 mg Allopurinol 100mg tablets | 28 tablet [PoM] £2.28 DT = £0.59 | 100 tablet [PoM] £5.50–£10.89

Allopurinol 200 mg Allopurinol 200mg tablets | 28 tablet [PoM] £14.24 | 30 tablet [PoM] £14.24–£25.62 DT = £14.24

Allopurinol 300 mg Allopurinol 300mg tablets | 28 tablet [PoM] £5.85 DT = £0.73 | 100 tablet [PoM] £6.10–£13.03

▸ **Zyloric** (Aspen Pharma Trading Ltd)

Allopurinol 100 mg Zyloric 100mg tablets | 100 tablet [PoM] £10.19

Allopurinol 300 mg Zyloric 300mg tablets | 28 tablet [PoM] £7.31 DT = £0.73

Oral suspension

▸ **Allopurinol (Non-proprietary)**

Allopurinol 60 mg per 1 ml Allopurinol 300mg/5ml oral suspension sugar free | 150 ml [PoM] £265.00 [SF]

3 Immunotherapy responsive malignancy

IMMUNOSTIMULANTS › INTERFERONS

Interferon gamma-1b (Immune interferon)

25-May-2021

● **INDICATIONS AND DOSE**

To reduce the frequency of serious infection in chronic granulomatous disease

▶ BY SUBCUTANEOUS INJECTION

▸ Child 6 months–17 years (body surface area up to 0.6 m^2): 1.5 micrograms/kg 3 times a week

▸ Child 6 months–17 years (body surface area 0.6 m^2 and above): 50 micrograms/m^2 3 times a week

To reduce the frequency of serious infection in severe malignant osteopetrosis

▶ BY SUBCUTANEOUS INJECTION

▸ Child (body surface area up to 0.6 m^2): 1.5 micrograms/kg 3 times a week

▸ Child (body surface area 0.6 m^2 and above): 50 micrograms/m^2 3 times a week

● **CONTRA-INDICATIONS** Simultaneous administration of foreign proteins including immunological products (such as vaccines)—risk of exaggerated immune response

● **CAUTIONS** Arrhythmias · cardiac disease · congestive heart failure · ischaemia · seizure disorders (including seizures associated with fever)

● **SIDE-EFFECTS**

▶ **Common or very common** Abdominal pain · arthralgia · back pain · chills · depression · diarrhoea · fatigue · fever · headache · nausea · rash · vomiting

▶ **Frequency not known** Atrioventricular block · chest discomfort · confusion · connective tissue disorders · embolism and thrombosis · gait abnormal · gastrointestinal haemorrhage · hallucination · heart failure · hepatic failure · hypertriglyceridaemia · hypoglycaemia · hyponatraemia · hypotension · influenza like illness · interstitial lung disease · myocardial infarction · neutropenia · pancreatitis · parkinsonism · proteinuria · renal failure · respiratory disorders · seizure · syncope · systemic lupus erythematosus (SLE) · tachycardia · thrombocytopenia · transient ischaemic attack

● **CONCEPTION AND CONTRACEPTION** Effective contraception required during treatment—consult product literature.

● **PREGNANCY** Manufacturers recommend avoid unless potential benefit outweighs risk (toxicity in *animal* studies).

● **BREAST FEEDING** Manufacturers advise avoid—no information available.

● **HEPATIC IMPAIRMENT** Manufacturer advises caution in severe impairment (increased risk of accumulation).

● **RENAL IMPAIRMENT** Manufacturer advises caution in severe impairment—risk of accumulation.

- **MONITORING REQUIREMENTS** Monitor before and during treatment: haematological tests (including full blood count, differential white cell count, and platelet count), blood chemistry tests (including renal and liver function tests) and urinalysis.

- **MEDICINAL FORMS** There can be variation in the licensing of different medicines containing the same drug.

Solution for injection

▸ **Immukin** (Clinigen Healthcare Ltd)

Interferon gamma-1b (recombinant human) 200 microgram per 1 ml Immukin 100micrograms/0.5ml solution for injection vials | 6 vial PoM £930.00

IMMUNOSTIMULANTS › OTHER

Mifamurtide [Specialist drug] 20-Sep-2024

- **INDICATIONS AND DOSE**

Osteosarcoma

▸ BY INTRAVENOUS INFUSION

▸ Child 2–17 years: Specialist drug – access specialist resources for dosing information

- **INTERACTIONS** → Appendix 1: mifamurtide
- **SIDE-EFFECTS**

▸ **Common or very common** Alopecia · anaemia · anxiety · appetite decreased · arthralgia · asthenia · cancer pain · chest discomfort · chills · confusion · constipation · cough · cyanosis · dehydration · depression · diarrhoea · dizziness · drowsiness · dysmenorrhoea · dyspnoea · feeling cold · fever · flushing · gastrointestinal discomfort · haemorrhage · headache · hearing loss · hepatic pain · hyperhidrosis · hypertension · hypokalaemia · hypotension · hypothermia · increased risk of infection · insomnia · laryngeal pain · leucopenia · malaise · mucositis · muscle complaints · musculoskeletal stiffness · nasal congestion · nausea · neutropenia · oedema · pain · pallor · palpitations · respiratory disorders · sensation abnormal · sepsis · skin reactions · tachycardia · thrombocytopenia · tinnitus · tremor · urinary disorders · vertigo · vision blurred · vomiting · weight decreased

▸ **Frequency not known** Pericardial effusion

- **CONCEPTION AND CONTRACEPTION** EvGr Females of childbearing potential should use effective contraception. ⟨M⟩
- **PATIENT AND CARER ADVICE**

Driving and skilled tasks Patients and carers should be counselled on the effects on driving and performance of skilled tasks—increased risk of dizziness, vertigo, fatigue, and blurred vision.

- **NATIONAL FUNDING/ACCESS DECISIONS** For full details see funding body website

NICE decisions

▸ **Mifamurtide for the treatment of osteosarcoma (October 2011)** NICE TA235 Recommended

- **MEDICINAL FORMS** There can be variation in the licensing of different medicines containing the same drug.

Powder for dispersion for infusion

▸ **Mifamurtide (Non-proprietary)**

Mifamurtide 4 mg Mifamurtide 4mg powder for concentrate for dispersion for infusion vials | 1 vial PoM £2,375.00 (Hospital only)

4 Targeted therapy responsive malignancy

ANTINEOPLASTIC DRUGS › PROTEIN KINASE INHIBITORS

Crizotinib [Specialist drug] 07-Jan-2025

- **INDICATIONS AND DOSE**

Inflammatory myofibroblastic tumour | Systemic anaplastic large cell lymphoma

▸ BY MOUTH

▸ Child 6–17 years: Specialist drug – access specialist resources for dosing information

IMPORTANT SAFETY INFORMATION

RISKS OF INCORRECT DOSING OF ORAL ANTI-CANCER MEDICINES

See Cytotoxic drugs p. 660.

MHRA/CHM ADVICE (NOVEMBER 2015): RISK OF CARDIAC FAILURE

Severe, sometimes fatal cases of cardiac failure have been reported in adult patients treated with crizotinib. The MHRA has issued the following advice:

- monitor all patients for signs and symptoms of heart failure (including dyspnoea, oedema, or rapid weight gain from fluid retention)
- consider reducing the dose, or interrupting or stopping treatment if symptoms of heart failure occur

VISION DISORDERS

Vision disorders, including risk of severe visual loss, have been reported as a very common side-effect in patients treated with crizotinib. As vision disorders are harder to identify in children, patients and carers should be counselled on the symptoms of vision disorders and the potential risk of visual loss, and advised to seek immediate medical attention if symptoms develop. Ophthalmological monitoring should be carried out before starting treatment, within the first month and every 3 months thereafter. Dose reduction or treatment discontinuation may be required if vision disorders occur.

- **INTERACTIONS** → Appendix 1: crizotinib
- **SIDE-EFFECTS**

▸ **Common or very common** Anaemia · appetite decreased · arrhythmias · constipation · decreased leucocytes · diarrhoea · dizziness · fatigue · gait abnormal · gastrointestinal discomfort · hypophosphataemia · muscle weakness · nausea · neutropenia · oedema · oesophagitis · paraesthesia · periorbital oedema · peripheral neuropathy · QT interval prolongation · rash · taste altered · thrombocytopenia · vision disorders · vitreous floater · vomiting

▸ **Frequency not known** Drug-induced liver injury · pneumonitis

SIDE-EFFECTS, FURTHER INFORMATION **Interstitial lung disease** Interstitial lung disease and pneumonitis, including fatal events, have been reported; withdraw treatment if suspected, and permanently discontinue treatment if diagnosed.

- **CONCEPTION AND CONTRACEPTION** EvGr Ensure effective contraception during and for at least 90 days after treatment. ⟨M⟩
- **PATIENT AND CARER ADVICE**

Gastrointestinal perforation Patients and carers should be counselled on the signs and symptoms of gastrointestinal perforation and advised to seek immediate medical attention if symptoms develop.

Vision disorders Patients and carers should be counselled on the signs and symptoms of vision disorders and advised to seek immediate medical attention if symptoms develop—risk of severe visual loss.
Photosensitivity Patients and carers should be advised to minimise exposure to sunlight, and protect skin by wearing sun-protective clothing and/or using sunscreen.
Patient Information Booklet A patient information booklet, including a patient alert card, should be provided.
Missed doses If a dose is more than 6 hours late, the missed dose should not be taken and the next dose should be taken at the normal time.
Driving and skilled tasks Patients and carers should be cautioned on the effects on driving and performance of skilled tasks—increased risk of symptomatic bradycardia (including syncope, dizziness, and hypotension), vision disorder and fatigue.

- **MEDICINAL FORMS** There can be variation in the licensing of different medicines containing the same drug.

Oral capsule

CAUTIONARY AND ADVISORY LABELS 11, 25

- **Xalkori** (Pfizer Ltd)
  Crizotinib 200 mg Xalkori 200mg capsules | 60 capsule PoM £4,689.00 (Hospital only)
  Crizotinib 250 mg Xalkori 250mg capsules | 60 capsule PoM £4,689.00 (Hospital only)

Dabrafenib [Specialist drug]

18-Sep-2024

- **INDICATIONS AND DOSE**

Low-grade glioma | High-grade glioma

▶ BY MOUTH USING DISPERSIBLE TABLETS
- Child 1–17 years: Specialist drug – access specialist resources for dosing information

IMPORTANT SAFETY INFORMATION

RISKS OF INCORRECT DOSING OF ORAL ANTI-CANCER MEDICINES

See Cytotoxic drugs p. 660.

- **CONTRA-INDICATIONS** BRAF wild-type glioma
- **INTERACTIONS** → Appendix 1: dabrafenib
- **SIDE-EFFECTS**

▶ **Common or very common** Abdominal pain · alopecia · anaemia · appetite decreased · arthralgia · asthenia · bradycardia · chills · CNS haemorrhage · constipation · cough · dehydration · diarrhoea · dizziness · dyspnoea · electrolyte imbalance · eye inflammation · fever · haemorrhage · headache · hyperglycaemia · hypersensitivity · hypertension · hypotension · increased risk of infection · influenza like illness · leucopenia · malaise · mucositis · muscle complaints · musculoskeletal stiffness · nausea · neutropenia · oedema · pain in extremity · pancreatitis · panniculitis · skin papilloma · skin reactions · stomatitis · thrombocytopenia · vertigo · vision disorders · vomiting · weight increased
▶ **Uncommon** Gastrointestinal disorders · retinal detachment · sweat changes

- **CONCEPTION AND CONTRACEPTION** EvGr Females of childbearing potential should use effective non-hormonal contraception during treatment and for 2 weeks after last treatment. Ⓜ
- **PATIENT AND CARER ADVICE** Patients and carers should be informed to immediately report new skin lesions—risk of cutaneous squamous cell carcinoma and new primary melanoma. Patients and carers should be counselled on the administration of dabrafenib.

Breast milk or formula may be given on demand if a child is unable to tolerate the fasting conditions.

If vomiting occurs after taking dabrafenib, no additional dose should be taken and the next dose should be taken at the normal time.
Missed doses If a dose is more than 6 hours late, the missed dose should not be taken and the next dose should be taken at the normal time.
Driving and skilled tasks Patients and carers should be counselled on the effects on driving and performance of skilled tasks—increased risk of fatigue, dizziness, and visual disturbances.

- **NATIONAL FUNDING/ACCESS DECISIONS**

For full details see funding body website

NICE decisions

▶ **Dabrafenib with trametinib for treating BRAF V600E mutation-positive glioma in children and young people aged 1 year and over (May 2024)** NICE TA977 Recommended

Scottish Medicines Consortium (SMC) decisions

▶ **Dabrafenib (*Finlee*®) in combination with trametinib for the treatment of paediatric patients aged 1 year and older with: low-grade glioma with a BRAF V600 mutation who require systemic therapy; or high-grade glioma with a BRAF V600 mutation who have received at least one prior radiation and/or chemotherapy treatment (September 2024)** SMC No. SMC2667 Recommended

- **MEDICINAL FORMS** There can be variation in the licensing of different medicines containing the same drug.

Dispersible tablet

CAUTIONARY AND ADVISORY LABELS 13, 23

EXCIPIENTS: May contain Benzyl alcohol, propylene glycol

- **Finlee** (Novartis Pharmaceuticals UK Ltd)
  Dabrafenib (as Dabrafenib mesilate) 10 mg Finlee 10mg dispersible tablets | 420 tablet PoM £2,800.00 (Hospital only) SF

Dasatinib [Specialist drug]

03-Jun-2025

- **INDICATIONS AND DOSE**

Chronic myeloid leukaemia | Acute lymphoblastic leukaemia

▶ BY MOUTH
- Child 1–17 years: Specialist drug – access specialist resources for dosing information

DOSE EQUIVALENCE AND CONVERSION
- *Sprycel*® film-coated tablets and *Sprycel*® powder for oral suspension are **not** bioequivalent.

UXIL®

Acute lymphoblastic leukaemia

▶ BY MOUTH
- Child 1–17 years: Specialist drug – access specialist resources for dosing information

DOSE EQUIVALENCE AND CONVERSION
- *Uxil*® film-coated tablets and other dasatinib preparations are **not** bioequivalent.

IMPORTANT SAFETY INFORMATION

Sprycel® formulations are **not** bioequivalent and should not be used interchangeably.

Uxil® film-coated tablets and other dasatinib preparations are **not** bioequivalent and should not be used interchangeably.

RISKS OF INCORRECT DOSING OF ORAL ANTI-CANCER MEDICINES

See Cytotoxic drugs p. 660.

MHRA/CHM ADVICE (MAY 2016): RISK OF HEPATITIS B VIRUS REACTIVATION WITH BCR-ABL TYROSINE KINASE INHIBITORS

An EU wide review has concluded that dasatinib can cause hepatitis B reactivation; the MHRA recommends establishing hepatitis B virus status in all patients before initiation of treatment. Patients who are carriers of hepatitis B virus should be closely monitored for signs and symptoms of active infection throughout treatment and for several months after stopping treatment; expert advice should be sought for patients who test positive for hepatitis B virus and in those with active infection.

- **INTERACTIONS** → Appendix 1: dasatinib
- **SIDE-EFFECTS**
  - **Common or very common** Alopecia · anaemia · appetite abnormal · arrhythmias · arthralgia · asthenia · bone disorders · bone marrow depression · cardiac disorder · cardiomyopathy · chest pain · chills · constipation · cough · depression · diarrhoea · dizziness · drowsiness · dry eye · dyspnoea · eye inflammation · facial swelling · fever · fluid imbalance · flushing · gastrointestinal discomfort · gastrointestinal disorders · genital abnormalities · growth retardation · haemorrhage · headache · heart failure · hypertension · hyperuricaemia · increased risk of infection · insomnia · interstitial lung disease · milia · mucositis · muscle complaints · muscle weakness · musculoskeletal stiffness · myocardial dysfunction · nausea · nerve disorders · neutropenia · oedema · oral disorders · pain · palpitations · pericardial effusion · perinephric effusion · peripheral swelling · pulmonary hypertension · pulmonary oedema · respiratory disorders · sepsis · skin reactions · sweat changes · taste altered · thrombocytopenia · tinnitus · vision disorders · vomiting · weight changes
  - **Uncommon** Acute coronary syndrome · anxiety · arthritis · ascites · asthma · cardiac inflammation · cardiomegaly · cerebrovascular insufficiency · cholecystitis · CNS haemorrhage · confusion · dysphagia · embolism and thrombosis · emotional lability · excessive tearing · gynaecomastia · hair disorder · hearing loss · hepatic disorders · hypercholesterolaemia · hypoalbuminaemia · hypotension · hypothyroidism · ischaemic heart disease · libido decreased · lymphadenopathy · lymphopenia · malaise · memory loss · menstrual disorder · movement disorders · myopathy · nail disorder · osteonecrosis · pancreatitis · panniculitis · penile disorders · photosensitivity reaction · proteinuria · QT interval prolongation · renal impairment · scrotal oedema · skin ulcer · syncope · tendinitis · testicular swelling · tremor · tumour lysis syndrome · urinary frequency increased · vertigo · vulvovaginal swelling
  - **Rare or very rare** Cardiac arrest · dementia · diabetes mellitus · facial paralysis · gait abnormal · hypersensitivity vasculitis · hyperthyroidism · pure red cell aplasia · seizure · thyroiditis
  - **Frequency not known** Electrolyte imbalance · hepatitis B reactivation · nephrotic syndrome · Stevens-Johnson syndrome · thrombotic microangiopathy
- **CONCEPTION AND CONTRACEPTION** Effective contraception required during treatment.
- **PATIENT AND CARER ADVICE**
  Interstitial lung disease Patients and carers should be advised to report acute or unexplained worsening of respiratory symptoms, such as cough, difficulty breathing, or painful breathing.
- **NATIONAL FUNDING/ACCESS DECISIONS**
  For full details see funding body website

Scottish Medicines Consortium (SMC) decisions

- **Dasatinib (*Sprycel*®) tablets for the treatment of paediatric patients with newly diagnosed Philadelphia chromosome positive chronic myelogenous leukaemia in chronic phase (Ph+ CML-CP) or Ph+ CML-CP resistant or intolerant to prior therapy including imatinib (April 2019)** SMC No. SMC2142 Recommended

All Wales Medicines Strategy Group (AWMSG) decisions

- **Dasatinib (*Sprycel*®) tablets for the treatment of paediatric patients weighing 10 kg and above with newly diagnosed Philadelphia chromosome positive (Ph+) chronic myelogenous leukaemia (CML) in chronic phase (Ph+CML-CP) or Ph+CML-CP resistant or intolerant to prior therapy including imatinib (March 2019)** AWMSG No. 1514 Recommended

- **MEDICINAL FORMS** There can be variation in the licensing of different medicines containing the same drug.

Oral tablet

CAUTIONARY AND ADVISORY LABELS 5, 25

- **Dasatinib (Non-proprietary)**
  - **Dasatinib (as Dasatinib monohydrate) 20 mg** Dasatinib 20mg tablets | 60 tablet PoM £626.24–£1,064.61 (Hospital only) | 60 tablet PoM £650.00
  - **Dasatinib (as Dasatinib monohydrate) 50 mg** Dasatinib 50mg tablets | 60 tablet PoM £1,150.00–£2,129.22 (Hospital only) | 60 tablet PoM £1,200.00
  - **Dasatinib (as Dasatinib monohydrate) 80 mg** Dasatinib 80mg tablets | 30 tablet PoM £1,200.00 | 30 tablet PoM £1,252.48–£2,129.22 (Hospital only)
  - **Dasatinib (as Dasatinib monohydrate) 100 mg** Dasatinib 100mg tablets | 30 tablet PoM £1,200.00 | 30 tablet PoM £1,175.00–£2,129.22 (Hospital only)
  - **Dasatinib (as Dasatinib monohydrate) 140 mg** Dasatinib 140mg tablets | 30 tablet PoM £1,200.00 | 30 tablet PoM £2,129.22 (Hospital only)
- **Sprycel** (Bristol-Myers Squibb Pharmaceuticals Ltd)
  - **Dasatinib (as Dasatinib monohydrate) 20 mg** Sprycel 20mg tablets | 60 tablet PoM £1,252.48
  - **Dasatinib (as Dasatinib monohydrate) 50 mg** Sprycel 50mg tablets | 60 tablet PoM £2,504.96
  - **Dasatinib (as Dasatinib monohydrate) 80 mg** Sprycel 80mg tablets | 30 tablet PoM £2,504.96
  - **Dasatinib (as Dasatinib monohydrate) 100 mg** Sprycel 100mg tablets | 30 tablet PoM £2,504.96
  - **Dasatinib (as Dasatinib monohydrate) 140 mg** Sprycel 140mg tablets | 30 tablet PoM £2,504.96

Oral suspension

CAUTIONARY AND ADVISORY LABELS 5

EXCIPIENTS: May contain Benzyl alcohol, sucrose

- **Sprycel** (Imported (Germany))
  - **Dasatinib (as Dasatinib monohydrate) 10 mg per 1 ml** Sprycel 10mg/ml oral suspension | 90 ml PoM

Entrectinib [Specialist drug]

22-Mar-2023

- **INDICATIONS AND DOSE**

Solid tumours

- BY MOUTH
  - Child 12–17 years: Specialist drug – access specialist resources for dosing information

IMPORTANT SAFETY INFORMATION

RISKS OF INCORRECT DOSING OF ORAL ANTI-CANCER MEDICINES

See Cytotoxic drugs p. 660.

- **CONTRA-INDICATIONS** Congenital long QT syndrome
- **INTERACTIONS** → Appendix 1: entrectinib
- **SIDE-EFFECTS**
  - **Common or very common** Abdominal pain · anaemia · anxiety · appetite decreased · arthralgia · asthenia · bone fractures · cognitive disorder · concentration impaired · confusion · constipation · cough · delirium · depression · diarrhoea · dizziness · drowsiness · dysphagia · dyspnoea · fever · fluid imbalance · gait abnormal · hallucinations · headache · heart failure · hyperuricaemia · hypotension · increased risk of infection · memory impairment · mood altered · movement disorders · muscle weakness · myalgia · nausea · neutropenia · oedema · pain · peripheral neuropathy · peripheral swelling · photosensitivity reaction · pleural effusion · psychiatric disorders · pulmonary oedema · QT interval prolongation · sensation abnormal · skin reactions · sleep disorders · syncope · taste altered · urinary disorders · vertigo · vision disorders · vomiting · weight increased
  - **Uncommon** Tumour lysis syndrome

- **CONCEPTION AND CONTRACEPTION** Manufacturer advises females of childbearing potential should use effective contraception during treatment and for 5 weeks after last treatment; male patients should use effective contraception during treatment and for 3 months after last treatment if their partner is of childbearing potential. Additional barrier method recommended in females using hormonal contraceptives.
- **PATIENT AND CARER ADVICE**
Missed doses Manufacturer advises if a dose is more than 12 hours late, the missed dose should not be taken and the next dose should be taken at the normal time. If vomiting occurs immediately after a dose is taken, patients may repeat the dose.
Driving and skilled tasks Manufacturer advises patients and carers should be counselled on the effects on driving and performance of skilled tasks—increased risk of cognitive disorders, syncope, blurred vision, or dizziness.
- **NATIONAL FUNDING/ACCESS DECISIONS**
For full details see funding body website
NICE decisions
▸ **Entrectinib for treating NTRK fusion-positive solid tumours (August 2020)** NICE TA644 Recommended
Scottish Medicines Consortium (SMC) decisions
▸ **Entrectinib (*Rozlytrek*®) for the treatment of adult and paediatric patients 12 years of age and older, with solid tumours that have a neurotrophic tyrosine receptor kinase (NTRK) gene fusion (March 2021)** SMC No. SMC2295 Recommended

- **MEDICINAL FORMS** There can be variation in the licensing of different medicines containing the same drug.
Oral capsule
CAUTIONARY AND ADVISORY LABELS 25
▸ **Rozlytrek** (Roche Products Ltd) ▼
Entrectinib 100 mg Rozlytrek 100mg capsules | 30 capsule PoM £860.00 (Hospital only)
Entrectinib 200 mg Rozlytrek 200mg capsules | 90 capsule PoM £5,160.00 (Hospital only)

Everolimus

19-Dec-2022

- **DRUG ACTION** Everolimus is a protein kinase inhibitor.

- **INDICATIONS AND DOSE**

VOTUBIA® DISPERSIBLE TABLETS

Subependymal giant cell astrocytoma associated with tuberous sclerosis complex (initiated by a specialist)
▸ BY MOUTH USING DISPERSIBLE TABLETS
▸ Child 1–17 years: (consult product literature)

Adjunctive treatment of refractory partial-onset seizures, with or without secondary generalisation, associated with tuberous sclerosis complex (initiated by a specialist)
▸ BY MOUTH USING DISPERSIBLE TABLETS
▸ Child 2–17 years: (consult product literature)

VOTUBIA® TABLETS

Subependymal giant cell astrocytoma associated with tuberous sclerosis complex (initiated by a specialist)
▸ BY MOUTH USING TABLETS
▸ Child 1–17 years: (consult product literature)

IMPORTANT SAFETY INFORMATION

RISKS OF INCORRECT DOSING OF ORAL ANTI-CANCER MEDICINES
See Cytotoxic drugs p. 660.

MHRA/CHM ADVICE: ANTIEPILEPTICS: RISK OF SUICIDAL THOUGHTS AND BEHAVIOUR (AUGUST 2008)
See Epilepsy p. 227.

MHRA/CHM ADVICE: ANTIEPILEPTIC DRUGS: UPDATED ADVICE ON SWITCHING BETWEEN DIFFERENT MANUFACTURERS' PRODUCTS (NOVEMBER 2017)
See Epilepsy p. 227 and see also *Prescribing and dispensing information*.

MHRA/CHM ADVICE: ANTIEPILEPTIC DRUGS IN PREGNANCY: UPDATED ADVICE FOLLOWING COMPREHENSIVE SAFETY REVIEW (JANUARY 2021)
See Epilepsy p. 227.

- **CAUTIONS** History of bleeding disorders · peri-surgical period (impaired wound healing)
- **INTERACTIONS** → Appendix 1: everolimus
- **SIDE-EFFECTS**
▸ **Common or very common** Alopecia · anaemia · appetite decreased · arthralgia · asthenia · cough · decreased leucocytes · dehydration · diabetes mellitus · diarrhoea · dry mouth · dyslipidaemia · dysphagia · dyspnoea · electrolyte imbalance · eye inflammation · fever · gastrointestinal discomfort · haemorrhage · headache · hyperglycaemia · hypertension · increased risk of infection · insomnia · interstitial lung disease · menstrual cycle irregularities · mucositis · nail disorders · nausea · neutropenia · oral disorders · peripheral oedema · proteinuria · renal impairment · respiratory disorders · skin reactions · taste altered · thrombocytopenia · vomiting · weight decreased
▸ **Uncommon** Congestive heart failure · embolism and thrombosis · flushing · healing impaired · hepatitis B · musculoskeletal chest pain · pancytopenia · rhabdomyolysis · sepsis · urinary frequency increased
▸ **Rare or very rare** Pure red cell aplasia
▸ **Frequency not known** Hepatitis B reactivation · suicidal behaviours
SIDE-EFFECTS, FURTHER INFORMATION Reduce dose or discontinue if severe side-effects occur—consult product literature.
- **CONCEPTION AND CONTRACEPTION** Effective contraception must be used during and for up to 8 weeks after treatment. See also *Pregnancy and reproductive function* in Cytotoxic drugs p. 660.
- **PREGNANCY** Manufacturer advises avoid (toxicity in *animal* studies). See also *Pregnancy and reproductive function* in Cytotoxic drugs p. 660. See also *Pregnancy* in Epilepsy p. 227.
- **BREAST FEEDING** Manufacturer advises avoid.
- **HEPATIC IMPAIRMENT** Consult product literature.
- **MONITORING REQUIREMENTS**
▸ For *Votubia*® preparations: manufacturer advises everolimus blood concentration monitoring is required—consult product literature.
▸ Manufacturer advises monitor blood-glucose concentration, complete blood count, serum-triglycerides and serum-cholesterol before treatment and periodically thereafter.
▸ Manufacturer advises monitor renal function before treatment and periodically thereafter.
▸ Manufacturer advises monitor for signs and symptoms of infection before and during treatment.
- **DIRECTIONS FOR ADMINISTRATION**
VOTUBIA® DISPERSIBLE TABLETS Manufacturer advises tablets must be dispersed in water before administration—consult product literature for details.
VOTUBIA® TABLETS Manufacturer advises tablets may be dispersed in approximately 30 mL of water by gently stirring, immediately before drinking. After solution has been swallowed, any residue must be re-dispersed in the same volume of water and swallowed.
- **PRESCRIBING AND DISPENSING INFORMATION** *Votubia*® is available as both *tablets* and *dispersible tablets*. These formulations vary in their licensed indications and are not

interchangeable—consult product literature for information on switching between formulations.

- **PATIENT AND CARER ADVICE**
Pneumonitis Non-infectious pneumonitis reported. Manufacturer advises patients and their carers should be informed to seek urgent medical advice if new or worsening respiratory symptoms occur.
Infections Manufacturer advises patients and their carers should be informed of the risk of infection.

- **NATIONAL FUNDING/ACCESS DECISIONS**
For full details see funding body website

Scottish Medicines Consortium (SMC) decisions

- **Everolimus dispersible tablets (*Votubia*®) for the adjunctive treatment of patients aged 2 years and older whose refractory partial-onset seizures, with or without secondary generalisation, are associated with tuberous sclerosis complex (June 2018)** SMC No. 1331/18 Recommended

All Wales Medicines Strategy Group (AWMSG) decisions

- **Everolimus dispersible tablets (*Votubia*®) for the adjunctive treatment of patients aged 2 years and older whose refractory partial-onset seizures, with or without secondary generalisation, are associated with tuberous sclerosis complex (TSC) (September 2021)** AWMSG No. 2142 Recommended
- **Everolimus tablets and dispersible tablets (*Votubia*®) for the treatment of adult and paediatric patients with subependymal giant cell astrocytoma (SEGA) associated with tuberous sclerosis complex (TSC) who require therapeutic intervention but are not amenable to surgery (December 2022)** AWMSG No. 1156 Recommended

- **MEDICINAL FORMS** There can be variation in the licensing of different medicines containing the same drug.

Dispersible tablet

CAUTIONARY AND ADVISORY LABELS 13

- **Votubia** (Novartis Pharmaceuticals UK Ltd)
  - **Everolimus 2 mg** Votubia 2mg dispersible tablets | 30 tablet PoM £960.00 SF
  - **Everolimus 3 mg** Votubia 3mg dispersible tablets | 30 tablet PoM £1,440.00 SF
  - **Everolimus 5 mg** Votubia 5mg dispersible tablets | 30 tablet PoM £2,250.00 SF

Oral tablet

CAUTIONARY AND ADVISORY LABELS 25

- **Votubia** (Novartis Pharmaceuticals UK Ltd)
  - **Everolimus 2.5 mg** Votubia 2.5mg tablets | 30 tablet PoM £1,200.00
  - **Everolimus 5 mg** Votubia 5mg tablets | 30 tablet PoM £2,250.00
  - **Everolimus 10 mg** Votubia 10mg tablets | 30 tablet PoM £2,970.00

Imatinib [Specialist drug]

03-Jun-2025

- **INDICATIONS AND DOSE**

Chronic myeloid leukaemia | Acute lymphoblastic leukaemia

- BY MOUTH
- Child: Specialist drug – access specialist resources for dosing information

IMPORTANT SAFETY INFORMATION

RISKS OF INCORRECT DOSING OF ORAL ANTI-CANCER MEDICINES
See Cytotoxic drugs p. 660.

MHRA/CHM ADVICE (MAY 2016): RISK OF HEPATITIS B VIRUS REACTIVATION WITH BCR-ABL TYROSINE KINASE INHIBITORS
An EU wide review has concluded that imatinib can cause hepatitis B reactivation; the MHRA recommends establishing hepatitis B virus status in all patients before initiation of treatment. Patients who are carriers of hepatitis B virus should be closely monitored for signs and symptoms of active infection throughout treatment and for several months after stopping treatment; expert advice should be sought for patients who test positive for hepatitis B virus and in those with active infection.

- **INTERACTIONS** → Appendix 1: imatinib

- **SIDE-EFFECTS**
  - **Common or very common** Alopecia · anaemia · appetite abnormal · asthenia · bone marrow disorders · chills · constipation · cough · diarrhoea · dizziness · dry eye · dry mouth · dyspnoea · excessive tearing · eye inflammation · fever · fluid imbalance · flushing · gastrointestinal discomfort · gastrointestinal disorders · haemorrhage · headaches · insomnia · joint disorders · muscle complaints · nausea · neutropenia · oedema · pain · photosensitivity reaction · sensation abnormal · skin reactions · sweat changes · taste altered · thrombocytopenia · vision blurred · vomiting · weight changes
  - **Uncommon** Anxiety · arrhythmias · ascites · breast abnormalities · broken nails · burping · chest pain · CNS haemorrhage · congestive heart failure · depression · drowsiness · dysphagia · electrolyte imbalance · eosinophilia · eye discomfort · gout · gynaecomastia · hearing loss · hepatic disorders · hyperbilirubinaemia · hyperglycaemia · hypertension · hyperuricaemia · hypotension · increased risk of infection · laryngeal pain · lymphadenopathy · lymphopenia · malaise · memory loss · menstrual cycle irregularities · nerve disorders · oral disorders · palpitations · pancreatitis · peripheral coldness · pulmonary oedema · Raynaud's phenomenon · renal impairment · renal pain · respiratory disorders · restless legs · scrotal oedema · sepsis · sexual dysfunction · syncope · thrombocytosis · tinnitus · tremor · urinary frequency increased · vertigo
  - **Rare or very rare** Angina pectoris · angioedema · arthritis · cardiac arrest · cataract · confusion · glaucoma · haemolytic anaemia · haemorrhagic ovarian cyst · hepatic failure (including fatal cases) · hypersensitivity vasculitis · inflammatory bowel disease · intracranial pressure increased · muscle weakness · myocardial infarction · myopathy · nail discolouration · pericardial disorders · pulmonary fibrosis · pulmonary hypertension · seizure · severe cutaneous adverse reactions (SCARs) · thrombotic microangiopathy · tumour lysis syndrome
  - **Frequency not known** Embolism and thrombosis · growth retardation · hepatitis B reactivation · interstitial lung disease · neoplasm complications · osteonecrosis · pericarditis

- **CONCEPTION AND CONTRACEPTION** EvGr Females of childbearing potential should use effective contraception during treatment and for at least 15 days after last treatment. (M)

- **PATIENT AND CARER ADVICE** Patients and carers should be given advice on how to administer imatinib tablets.
Interstitial lung disease Patients and carers should be advised to report acute or unexplained worsening of respiratory symptoms, such as cough, difficulty breathing, or painful breathing.

- **MEDICINAL FORMS** There can be variation in the licensing of different medicines containing the same drug.

Oral tablet

CAUTIONARY AND ADVISORY LABELS 21, 27

- **Imatinib (Non-proprietary)**
  - **Imatinib (as Imatinib mesilate) 100 mg** Imatinib 100mg tablets | 30 tablet PoM £388.80 | 60 tablet PoM £104.49–£333.41 (Hospital only) | 60 tablet PoM £104.49–£924.65
  - **Imatinib (as Imatinib mesilate) 400 mg** Imatinib 400mg tablets | 30 tablet PoM £254.49–£1,849.34 | 30 tablet PoM £208.98–£664.58 (Hospital only)
  - **Imatinib (as Imatinib mesilate) 600 mg** Imatinib 600mg tablets | 30 tablet PoM (Hospital only)

▸ **Glivec** (Novartis Pharmaceuticals UK Ltd)
Imatinib (as Imatinib mesilate) 100 mg Glivec 100mg tablets | 60 tablet [PoM] £973.32
Imatinib (as Imatinib mesilate) 400 mg Glivec 400mg tablets | 30 tablet [PoM] £1,946.67

Larotrectinib [Specialist drug] 03-Jun-2020

● **INDICATIONS AND DOSE**

Solid tumours

▸ BY MOUTH

▸ Child: Specialist drug – access specialist resources for dosing information

IMPORTANT SAFETY INFORMATION

RISKS OF INCORRECT DOSING OF ORAL ANTI-CANCER MEDICINES

See Cytotoxic drugs p. 660.

● **INTERACTIONS** → Appendix 1: larotrectinib

● **SIDE-EFFECTS**

▸ **Common or very common** Anaemia · constipation · dizziness · fatigue · gait abnormal · leucopenia · muscle weakness · myalgia · nausea · neutropenia · paraesthesia · taste altered · vomiting · weight increased

SIDE-EFFECTS, FURTHER INFORMATION Increases in ALT and AST have been reported in patients receiving larotrectinib; withhold treatment or permanently discontinue depending on severity. The majority of ALT and AST increases occurred in the first 3 months of treatment.

● **CONCEPTION AND CONTRACEPTION** Manufacturer advises effective contraception in females of childbearing potential and in men with a partner of childbearing potential, during treatment and for 1 month after last treatment; additional barrier method recommended in women using hormonal contraceptives.

● **PATIENT AND CARER ADVICE**

Driving and skilled tasks Manufacturer advises patients and carers should be counselled on the effects on driving and performance of skilled tasks—increased risk of dizziness and fatigue.

● **NATIONAL FUNDING/ACCESS DECISIONS**

For full details see funding body website

NICE decisions

▸ **Larotrectinib for treating NTRK fusion-positive solid tumours (May 2020)** NICE TA630 Recommended with restrictions

● **MEDICINAL FORMS** There can be variation in the licensing of different medicines containing the same drug.

Oral solution

EXCIPIENTS: May contain Hydroxybenzoates (parabens), potassium sorbate, propylene glycol, sorbitol, sucrose

▸ **Vitrakvi** (Bayer Plc) ▼
Larotrectinib (as Larotrectinib sulfate) 20 mg per 1 ml Vitrakvi 20mg/ml oral solution sugar free | 100 ml [PoM] £5,000.00 (Hospital only) [SF]

Oral capsule

CAUTIONARY AND ADVISORY LABELS 25

EXCIPIENTS: May contain Gelatin, propylene glycol

▸ **Vitrakvi** (Bayer Plc) ▼
Larotrectinib (as Larotrectinib sulfate) 25 mg Vitrakvi 25mg capsules | 56 capsule [PoM] £3,500.00 (Hospital only)
Larotrectinib (as Larotrectinib sulfate) 100 mg Vitrakvi 100mg capsules | 56 capsule [PoM] £14,000.00 (Hospital only)

Nilotinib [Specialist drug] 03-Jun-2025

● **INDICATIONS AND DOSE**

Chronic myeloid leukaemia

▸ BY MOUTH

▸ Child 6–17 years: Specialist drug – access specialist resources for dosing information

IMPORTANT SAFETY INFORMATION

RISKS OF INCORRECT DOSING OF ORAL ANTI-CANCER MEDICINES

See Cytotoxic drugs p. 660.

MHRA/CHM ADVICE (MAY 2016): RISK OF HEPATITIS B VIRUS REACTIVATION WITH TYROSINE KINASE INHIBITORS

An EU wide review has concluded that nilotinib can cause hepatitis B virus reactivation; the MHRA recommends establishing hepatitis B virus status in all patients before initiation of treatment. Patients who are carriers of hepatitis B virus should be closely monitored for signs and symptoms of active infection throughout treatment and for several months after stopping treatment; expert advice should be sought for patients who test positive for hepatitis B virus and in those with active infection.

● **INTERACTIONS** → Appendix 1: nilotinib

● **SIDE-EFFECTS**

▸ **Common or very common** Alopecia · anaemia · anxiety · appetite abnormal · arrhythmias · asthenia · cardiac conduction disorders · chest discomfort · chills · constipation · cough · decreased leucocytes · depression · diabetes mellitus · diarrhoea · dizziness · dry eye · dyslipidaemia · dyspnoea · ear pain · electrolyte imbalance · erectile dysfunction · eye discomfort · eye disorders · eye inflammation · fever · flushing · gastrointestinal discomfort · gastrointestinal disorders · gout · growth retardation · haemorrhage · headaches · hepatic disorders · hyperaemia · hyperbilirubinaemia · hyperglycaemia · hypertension · hyperuricaemia · hypothyroidism · increased risk of infection · influenza like illness · insomnia · ischaemic heart disease · joint disorders · leucocytosis · malaise · menorrhagia · muscle complaints · muscle weakness · nausea · neutropenia · oedema · oral disorders · oropharyngeal pain · pain · palpitations · pancreatitis · peripheral vascular disease · QT interval prolongation · sensation abnormal · skin reactions · sweat changes · thrombocytopenia · thrombocytosis · tinnitus · urinary disorders · vertigo · vision disorders · vomiting · weight changes

▸ **Uncommon** Arthritis · atherosclerosis · breast abnormalities · cerebrovascular insufficiency · concentration impaired · confusion · dry mouth · dysphonia · eosinophilia · erythema nodosum · facial paralysis · facial swelling · fluid imbalance · gynaecomastia · hearing impairment · heart failure · hyperthyroidism · hypoglycaemia · hypotension · interstitial lung disease · intracranial haemorrhage · lethargy · loss of consciousness · memory loss · musculoskeletal stiffness · myocardial dysfunction · myocardial infarction · neoplasms · nerve disorders · oesophageal pain · pancytopenia · pericardial effusion · pericarditis · photosensitivity reaction · pulmonary hypertension · pulmonary oedema · renal failure · respiratory disorders · restless legs · sepsis · skin ulcer · syncope · taste altered · temperature sensation altered · throat complaints · thrombosis · tremor · urine discolouration

▸ **Rare or very rare** Brain oedema · chorioretinopathy · cyanosis · haemorrhagic shock · hepatitis B reactivation · hyperparathyroidism · sebaceous hyperplasia · sudden death · thyroiditis · tumour lysis syndrome

● **CONCEPTION AND CONTRACEPTION** Manufacturer advises highly effective contraception in women of childbearing potential during treatment and for up to two weeks after stopping treatment.

- **PATIENT AND CARER ADVICE**

Cardiovascular events Patients and carers should seek immediate medical attention if signs or symptoms of cardiovascular events occur.
Interstitial lung disease Patients and carers should be advised to report acute or unexplained worsening of respiratory symptoms, such as cough, difficulty breathing, or painful breathing.
All patients should be provided with the *Important Information About How to Take Your Medication* leaflet provided by the manufacturer.

- **MEDICINAL FORMS** There can be variation in the licensing of different medicines containing the same drug.

Oral capsule

CAUTIONARY AND ADVISORY LABELS 25, 27

▸ **Nilotinib (Non-proprietary)**
Nilotinib 150 mg Nilotinib 150mg capsules | 28 capsule [PoM] £547.39 (Hospital only) | 112 capsule [PoM] £2,165.24–£2,432.85 (Hospital only)
Nilotinib 200 mg Nilotinib 200mg capsules | 28 capsule [PoM] £547.39 (Hospital only) | 112 capsule [PoM] £2,165.24–£2,432.85 (Hospital only)

▸ **Tasigna** (Novartis Pharmaceuticals UK Ltd)
Nilotinib (as Nilotinib hydrochloride monohydrate)
50 mg Tasigna 50mg capsules | 120 capsule [PoM] £2,432.85
Nilotinib 150 mg Tasigna 150mg capsules | 112 capsule [PoM] £2,432.85
Nilotinib 200 mg Tasigna 200mg capsules | 112 capsule [PoM] £2,432.85

Ruxolitinib

16-Jul-2025

- **DRUG ACTION** Ruxolitinib is a selective inhibitor of the Janus-associated tyrosine kinases JAK1 and JAK2.

- **INDICATIONS AND DOSE**

Graft-versus-host disease [with inadequate response to corticosteroids] (under expert supervision)

▸ BY MOUTH

- Child 6–11 years: 5 mg twice daily, for dose adjustments or interruption due to side-effects, or for tapering after response seen—consult product literature
- Child 12–17 years: 10 mg twice daily, for dose adjustments or interruption due to side-effects, or for tapering after response seen—consult product literature

- **CONTRA-INDICATIONS** Active serious infection (delay treatment until infection resolved)
- **CAUTIONS** Major adverse cardiovascular events · thromboembolic events (history of, or risk factors for)

CAUTIONS, FURTHER INFORMATION

▸ **Major adverse cardiovascular events** [EvGr] The benefits versus risks of treatment should be considered prior to starting or continuing treatment for patients with risk factors for major adverse cardiovascular events, such as those who are current or past long-time smokers, those with a history of atherosclerotic cardiovascular disease, or those with other cardiovascular risk factors. ⟨M⟩

- **INTERACTIONS** → Appendix 1: ruxolitinib
- **SIDE-EFFECTS**

▸ **Common or very common** Anaemia · BK virus infection · bruising · constipation · dizziness · dyslipidaemia · flatulence · haemorrhage · headache · hypertension · increased risk of infection · intracranial haemorrhage · nausea · neutropenia · pancytopenia · sepsis · thrombocytopenia · weight increased
▸ **Uncommon** Hepatitis B reactivation
▸ **Frequency not known** Cardiac death · embolism and thrombosis · malignancy · myocardial infarction · neoplasms · progressive multifocal leukoencephalopathy (PML) (withhold treatment) · stroke

- **PREGNANCY** [EvGr] Avoid (toxicity in *animal* studies); ⟨M⟩ recommendation also supported by specialist sources.
- **BREAST FEEDING** Specialist sources indicate avoid breast-feeding during and for at least 2 weeks after treatment (no human data available).
- **HEPATIC IMPAIRMENT** [EvGr] Caution (risk of reduced elimination). ⟨M⟩

Dose adjustments [EvGr] In hepatic impairment not caused by Graft-versus-host disease, reduce starting dose by 50%.
In Graft-versus-host disease with hepatic involvement and raised total bilirubin exceeding 3 times the upper limit of normal, monitor blood counts more frequently for toxicity and consider dose reduction ⟨M⟩—consult product literature.

- **RENAL IMPAIRMENT**

Dose adjustments [EvGr] Reduce starting dose by 50% and administer twice daily if creatinine clearance less than 30 mL/minute. ⟨M⟩ See p. 16.

- **PRE-TREATMENT SCREENING** Patients should be evaluated for tuberculosis and hepatitis B before treatment.
- **MONITORING REQUIREMENTS**

▸ [EvGr] Monitor complete blood count (including differential white cell count) prior to initiation of treatment and every 2–4 weeks until dose stabilised, and as clinically indicated thereafter.
▸ Monitor for signs and symptoms of serious infections during treatment.
▸ Monitor for new or worsening signs and symptoms of progressive multifocal leukoencephalopathy (withhold treatment if suspected and refer to a neurologist).
▸ Periodic skin examination is recommended in patients at increased risk of skin cancer.
▸ Monitor lipid profile routinely. ⟨M⟩

- **PATIENT AND CARER ADVICE** Patients and their carers should be told how to recognise early signs and symptoms of herpes zoster and advised to seek prompt medical attention if these occur.

Driving and skilled tasks Patients and their carers should be cautioned on the effects on driving and performance of skilled tasks—increased risk of dizziness.

- **NATIONAL FUNDING/ACCESS DECISIONS**

For full details see funding body website

NICE decisions

▸ **Ruxolitinib for treating acute graft versus host disease that responds inadequately to corticosteroids in people 12 years and over (April 2025)** NICE TA1054 Recommended

Scottish Medicines Consortium (SMC) decisions

▸ **Ruxolitinib (*Jakavi*®) for the treatment of patients aged 12 years and older with acute graft versus host disease who have inadequate response to corticosteroids (June 2025)** SMC No. SMC2750 Recommended

- **MEDICINAL FORMS** There can be variation in the licensing of different medicines containing the same drug.

Oral tablet

▸ **Jakavi** (Novartis Pharmaceuticals UK Ltd)
Ruxolitinib (as Ruxolitinib phosphate) 5 mg Jakavi 5mg tablets | 56 tablet [PoM] £1,428.00
Ruxolitinib (as Ruxolitinib phosphate) 10 mg Jakavi 10mg tablets | 56 tablet [PoM] £2,856.00
Ruxolitinib (as Ruxolitinib phosphate) 15 mg Jakavi 15mg tablets | 56 tablet [PoM] £2,856.00
Ruxolitinib (as Ruxolitinib phosphate) 20 mg Jakavi 20mg tablets | 56 tablet [PoM] £2,856.00

Selpercatinib [Specialist drug] 31-Jul-2025

● **INDICATIONS AND DOSE**

Thyroid cancer

▶ BY MOUTH

▶ Child 12–17 years: Specialist drug – access specialist resources for dosing information

IMPORTANT SAFETY INFORMATION

RISKS OF INCORRECT DOSING OF ORAL ANTI-CANCER MEDICINES

See Cytotoxic drugs p. 660.

● **CONTRA-INDICATIONS** Uncontrolled hypertension

● **INTERACTIONS** → Appendix 1: selpercatinib

● **SIDE-EFFECTS**

▶ **Common or very common** Angioedema · appetite decreased · ascites · asthenia · CNS haemorrhage · constipation · cystitis · diarrhoea · disseminated intravascular coagulation · dizziness · dry mouth · empyema · epiphysiolysis of the femoral head · erectile dysfunction · eye inflammation · fever · gastrointestinal discomfort · gastrointestinal disorders · genital oedema · haemorrhage · haemorrhagic stroke · headaches · hepatic haematoma · hypersensitivity · hypertension · hypothyroidism · increased risk of infection · inflammation · interstitial lung disease · langerhans' cell histiocytosis · lymphoedema · malaise · menorrhagia · mucosal abnormalities · nausea · oedema · oral disorders · pelvic haematoma · penile oedema · postmenopausal haemorrhage · QT interval prolongation · radiation injuries · respiratory disorders · scrotal disorders · skin reactions · testicular swelling · traumatic haematoma · tumour haemorrhage · urogenital infection fungal · urosepsis · vertigo · vomiting · vulvovaginal swelling

▶ **Frequency not known** Severe cutaneous adverse reactions (SCARs) · thrombocytopenia · tumour lysis syndrome

● **CONCEPTION AND CONTRACEPTION** EvGr Females of childbearing potential and men with a partner of childbearing potential should use effective contraception during treatment and for one week after the last dose. Ⓜ The effect on human fertility is not known—impairment of fertility has been observed in *animal* studies.

● **PATIENT AND CARER ADVICE** EvGr If vomiting occurs after administration, no additional dose should be taken and the next dose should be taken at the normal time. Ⓜ

Missed doses EvGr If a dose is missed, the missed dose should not be taken and the next dose should be taken at the normal time. Ⓜ

Driving and skilled tasks EvGr Patients and their carers should be counselled on the effects on driving and skilled tasks—increased risk of fatigue and dizziness. Ⓜ

● **NATIONAL FUNDING/ACCESS DECISIONS**

For full details see funding body website

NICE decisions

▶ **Selpercatinib for advanced thyroid cancer with RET alterations after treatment with a targeted cancer drug in people 12 years and over (February 2025)** NICE TA1038 Recommended with restrictions

▶ **Selpercatinib for advanced thyroid cancer with RET alterations untreated with a targeted cancer drug in people 12 years and over (February 2025)** NICE TA1039 Recommended with restrictions

Scottish Medicines Consortium (SMC) decisions

▶ **Selpercatinib (*Retsevmo*®) as monotherapy for the treatment of adults and adolescents 12 years and older with advanced RET-mutant medullary thyroid cancer (MTC) who require systemic therapy following prior treatment with cabozantinib and/or vandetanib (September 2021)** SMC No. SMC2370 Recommended

▶ **Selpercatinib (*Retsevmo*®) as monotherapy for the treatment of adults and adolescents 12 years and older with advanced rearranged during transfection (RET)-mutant medullary thyroid cancer (June 2025)** SMC No. SMC2732 Recommended with restrictions

▶ **Selpercatinib (*Retsevmo*®) as monotherapy for the treatment of adults and adolescents 12 years and older with advanced RET fusion-positive thyroid cancer who are radioactive iodine-refractory (if radioactive iodine is appropriate) (July 2025)** SMC No. SMC2733 Recommended with restrictions

● **MEDICINAL FORMS** No licensed medicines listed.

Selumetinib 21-Aug-2023

● **DRUG ACTION** Selumetinib selectively inhibits the mitogen-activated protein kinase (MAPK) pathway, specifically mitogen-activated extracellular kinases MEK 1 and 2, thereby inhibiting the proliferation and survival of tumour cells.

● **INDICATIONS AND DOSE**

Inoperable plexiform neurofibromas in patients with neurofibromatosis type 1 (initiated by a specialist)

▶ BY MOUTH

▶ Child 3–17 years: 25 mg/m^2 twice daily (max. per dose 50 mg), each dose should be rounded to the nearest 5 or 10 mg and given about 12 hours apart, for further dosing advice based on body surface area—consult product literature, for dose adjustments, treatment interruption, or discontinuation due to side-effects—consult product literature

IMPORTANT SAFETY INFORMATION

RISKS OF INCORRECT DOSING OF ORAL ANTI-CANCER MEDICINES

See Cytotoxic drugs p. 660.

● **CAUTIONS** Patients of Asian origin (increased risk of side-effects)

● **INTERACTIONS** → Appendix 1: selumetinib

● **SIDE-EFFECTS**

▶ **Common or very common** Alopecia · anaemia · asthenia · diarrhoea · dry mouth · dyspnoea · fever · hair colour changes · hypertension · hypoalbuminaemia · increased risk of infection · nausea · oedema · periorbital oedema · skin reactions · stomatitis · vision blurred · vomiting

▶ **Uncommon** Chorioretinopathy · eye disorders · retinal occlusion (permanently discontinue) · retinal vascular thrombosis

● **CONCEPTION AND CONTRACEPTION** EvGr Effective contraception required during and for at least 1 week after treatment in male and female patients of reproductive potential; additional barrier method recommended in females using hormonal contraceptives. Ⓜ See also *Pregnancy and reproductive function* in Cytotoxic drugs p. 660.

● **PREGNANCY** EvGr Avoid—toxicity in *animal* studies. Ⓜ See also *Pregnancy and reproductive function* in Cytotoxic drugs p. 660.

● **BREAST FEEDING** EvGr Avoid—present in milk in *animal* studies. Ⓜ

● **HEPATIC IMPAIRMENT** EvGr Avoid in severe impairment; caution in moderate impairment. Ⓜ

Dose adjustments EvGr Reduce initial dose to 20 mg/m^2 twice daily in moderate impairment—consult product literature. Ⓜ

● **MONITORING REQUIREMENTS**

▶ EvGr Monitor liver function before treatment, at least

monthly during the first 6 months, and thereafter as clinically indicated.
- Assess left ventricular ejection fraction before treatment, then every 3 months or more frequently as clinically indicated.
- An ophthalmological evaluation is recommended before treatment, and whenever new visual disturbances are reported. ⟨M⟩

- **DIRECTIONS FOR ADMINISTRATION** EvGr *Koselugo*® capsules should be swallowed whole on an empty stomach; avoid food or drink, apart from water, 2 hours before and 1 hour after administration. Do not chew, dissolve, or open the capsules. ⟨M⟩
- **PRESCRIBING AND DISPENSING INFORMATION** EvGr Patients should be assessed for their ability to swallow capsules before starting treatment—children under 6 years of age, in particular, may be at risk of choking. *Koselugo*® capsules should not be given to patients unable or unwilling to swallow the capsule whole. ⟨M⟩
- **PATIENT AND CARER ADVICE** Patients and carers should be given advice on how to administer *Koselugo*® capsules. Patients and carers should be advised to report any new visual disturbances. Patients and carers should be advised that supplements containing vitamin E should not be taken while on *Koselugo*®.

Vomiting If vomiting occurs after taking a dose, no additional dose should be taken on that day and the next dose should be taken at the usual time.

Missed doses If a dose is more than 18 hours late, the missed dose should not be taken and the next dose should be taken at the normal time.

Driving and skilled tasks Patients and carers should be counselled on the effects on driving and performance of skilled tasks—increased risk of asthenia, fatigue, and visual disturbances.

- **NATIONAL FUNDING/ACCESS DECISIONS**

For full details see funding body website

NICE decisions
- **Selumetinib for treating symptomatic and inoperable plexiform neurofibromas associated with type 1 neurofibromatosis in children aged 3 and over (May 2022)** NICE HST20 Recommended

Scottish Medicines Consortium (SMC) decisions
- **Selumetinib (*Koselugo*®) as monotherapy for the treatment of symptomatic, inoperable plexiform neurofibromas in paediatric patients with neurofibromatosis type 1 aged 3 years and above (August 2023)** SMC No. SMC2540 Not recommended

- **MEDICINAL FORMS** There can be variation in the licensing of different medicines containing the same drug.

Oral capsule

CAUTIONARY AND ADVISORY LABELS 25

EXCIPIENTS: May contain Vitamin e

- **Koselugo** (AstraZeneca UK Ltd) ▼

Selumetinib (as Selumetinib hydrogen sulfate) 10 mg Koselugo 10mg capsules | 60 capsule PoM £4,223.59 (Hospital only)

Selumetinib (as Selumetinib hydrogen sulfate) 25 mg Koselugo 25mg capsules | 60 capsule PoM £10,560.00 (Hospital only)

Trametinib [Specialist drug]

20-Jun-2024

- **INDICATIONS AND DOSE**

Low-grade glioma | High-grade glioma

▶ BY MOUTH USING ORAL SOLUTION
- Child 1-17 years: Specialist drug – access specialist resources for dosing information

IMPORTANT SAFETY INFORMATION

MHRA/CHM ADVICE (MARCH 2016): TRAMETINIB: RISK OF GASTROINTESTINAL PERFORATION AND COLITIS

A review by EU medicines regulators has concluded that trametinib can cause gastrointestinal perforation or colitis.

Trametinib should be used with caution in patients with risk factors for gastrointestinal perforation, such as gastrointestinal metastases, diverticulitis, or use of concomitant medicines that can cause gastrointestinal perforation. Prescribers should be vigilant for signs and symptoms of gastrointestinal perforation and should advise patients to seek urgent medical attention if they develop severe abdominal pain.

RISKS OF INCORRECT DOSING OF ORAL ANTI-CANCER MEDICINES

See Cytotoxic drugs p. 660.

- **CONTRA-INDICATIONS** History of retinal vein occlusion
- **INTERACTIONS** → Appendix 1: trametinib
- **SIDE-EFFECTS**
  - **Common or very common** Abdominal pain · alopecia · anaemia · appetite decreased · arthralgia · asthenia · bradycardia · chills · CNS haemorrhage · constipation · cough · dehydration · diarrhoea · dizziness · dyspnoea · electrolyte imbalance · eye inflammation · fever · haemorrhage · headache · hyperglycaemia · hypersensitivity · hypertension · hypotension · increased risk of infection · influenza like illness · leucopenia · malaise · mucositis · muscle complaints · musculoskeletal stiffness · nausea · neutropenia · oedema · pain in extremity · pancreatitis · panniculitis · skin papilloma · skin reactions · stomatitis · thrombocytopenia · vertigo · vision disorders · vomiting · weight increased
  - **Uncommon** Eye disorders · gastrointestinal disorders · sweat changes
- **CONCEPTION AND CONTRACEPTION** EvGr Females of childbearing potential should use effective contraception during treatment and for 16 weeks after last treatment. ⟨M⟩
- **PATIENT AND CARER ADVICE** Patients and their carers should be told to seek immediate medical attention if symptoms of pulmonary embolism or deep vein thrombosis occur; patients and their carers should also be advised to report new visual disturbances. Patients and carers should be counselled on the administration of trametinib.

Breast milk or formula may be given on demand if a child is unable to tolerate the fasting conditions.

If vomiting occurs after taking trametinib, no additional dose should be taken and the next dose should be taken at the normal time.

Missed doses If a dose is more than 12 hours late, the missed dose should not be taken and the next dose should be taken at the normal time.

Driving and skilled tasks Patients and carers should be counselled on the effects on driving and performance of skilled tasks—increased risk of fatigue, dizziness, and visual disturbances.

- **NATIONAL FUNDING/ACCESS DECISIONS**

For full details see funding body website

NICE decisions
- **Dabrafenib with trametinib for treating BRAF V600E mutation-positive glioma in children and young people aged 1 year and over (May 2024)** NICE TA977 Recommended

- **MEDICINAL FORMS** There can be variation in the licensing of different medicines containing the same drug.

Oral solution

CAUTIONARY AND ADVISORY LABELS 23

EXCIPIENTS: May contain Potassium sorbate, sulfobutylether beta cyclodextrin sodium

ELECTROLYTES: May contain Sodium

- **Spexotras** (Novartis Pharmaceuticals UK Ltd)

Trametinib (as Trametinib dimethyl sulfoxide) 50 microgram per 1 ml Spexotras 50micrograms/ml oral solution | 90 ml PoM £376.00 (Hospital only) SF

ANTINEOPLASTIC DRUGS > OTHER

Vorasidenib [Specialist drug]

25-Mar-2026

● **INDICATIONS AND DOSE**

Astrocytoma | Oligodendroglioma

▸ BY MOUTH

▸ Child 12–17 years: Specialist drug – access specialist resources for dosing information

IMPORTANT SAFETY INFORMATION

RISKS OF INCORRECT DOSING OF ORAL ANTI-CANCER MEDICINES

See Cytotoxic drugs p. 660.

● **INTERACTIONS** → Appendix 1: vorasidenib

● **SIDE-EFFECTS**

▸ **Common or very common** Appetite decreased · asthenia · diarrhoea · gastrointestinal discomfort · gastrointestinal disorders · hyperglycaemia · hypophosphataemia

▸ **Frequency not known** Hepatic disorders

● **CONCEPTION AND CONTRACEPTION** EvGr Females of childbearing potential and male patients with a partner who is of childbearing potential should use effective contraception during treatment and for at least 3 months after last treatment; an additional barrier method of contraception should be used in female patients using hormonal contraceptives. ⟨M⟩

● **PATIENT AND CARER ADVICE**

Vomiting If vomiting occurs after taking tablets, no additional dose should be taken on that day and the next dose should be taken at the usual time.

Missed doses If a dose is more than 6 hours late, the missed dose should not be taken and the next dose should be taken at the normal time.

● **NATIONAL FUNDING/ACCESS DECISIONS**

For full details see funding body website

Scottish Medicines Consortium (SMC) decisions

▸ **Vorasidenib (*Voranigo*®) for the treatment of grade 2 astrocytoma or oligodendroglioma with a susceptible isocitrate dehydrogenase-1 mutation or isocitrate dehydrogenase-2 mutation in adults and paediatric patients 12 years and older, who are not in need of immediate chemotherapy or radiotherapy following surgical intervention (March 2026)** SMC No. SMC2844 Recommended

● **MEDICINAL FORMS** There can be variation in the licensing of different medicines containing the same drug.

Oral tablet

CAUTIONARY AND ADVISORY LABELS 23, 25

▸ **Voranigo** (Servier Laboratories Ltd) ▼

Vorasidenib (as Vorasidenib hemicitric acid hemihydrate)
10 mg Voranigo 10mg tablets | 30 tablet PoM £7,500.00 (Hospital only)

Vorasidenib (as Vorasidenib hemicitric acid hemihydrate)
40 mg Voranigo 40mg tablets | 30 tablet PoM £15,000.00 (Hospital only)

Chapter 9
Blood and nutrition

CONTENTS

Blood and blood-forming organs

1 Anaemias

Anaemias

27-Nov-2024

Anaemia treatment considerations

Before initiating treatment for anaemia, it is essential to determine which type is present. Iron salts may be harmful if given to children with anaemias other than those due to iron deficiency.

Sickle-cell anaemia

Sickle-cell disease is caused by a structural abnormality of haemoglobin resulting in deformed, less flexible red blood cells. Acute complications in the more severe forms include sickle-cell crisis, where infarction of the microvasculature and restricted blood supply to organs results in severe pain. EvGr Sickle-cell crisis usually requires hospitalisation, fluid replacement, analgesia, and treatment of any concurrent infection. Children who can be managed at home are often provided with a management plan from their secondary care team that should be followed, including when to seek medical advice. ⟨A⟩ Complications include anaemia, leg ulcers, renal failure, and increased susceptibility to infection. EvGr Pneumococcal vaccine, haemophilus influenzae type b vaccine, an annual influenza vaccine, and lifelong prophylactic penicillin reduce the risk of infection. Hepatitis B vaccine should also be given if the child is not immune.

In most forms of sickle-cell disease, varying degrees of haemolytic anaemia are present which is accompanied by increased erythropoiesis; this may increase folate requirements and supplementation with folic acid is recommended. The optimum dose should be discussed with a specialist. ⟨A⟩

Hydroxycarbamide p. 679 can prevent acute chest syndrome, reduce the frequency of painful crises, and reduce transfusion requirements in sickle-cell disease. The beneficial effects of hydroxycarbamide may not become evident for several months.

G6PD deficiency

Glucose 6-phosphate dehydrogenase (G6PD) deficiency is common in individuals originating from Africa, Asia, the Mediterranean region, and the Middle East; it can also occur less frequently in all other individuals. G6PD deficiency is more common in males than it is in females.

Individuals with G6PD deficiency are susceptible to developing acute haemolytic anaemia when they take a number of common drugs or when they have an infection. They are also susceptible to developing acute haemolytic anaemia when they eat fava beans (broad beans); this is termed *favism*.

When prescribing drugs for patients with G6PD deficiency, the following three points should be kept in mind:

- G6PD deficiency is genetically heterogeneous; susceptibility to the haemolytic risk from drugs varies; thus, a drug found to be safe in some G6PD-deficient individuals may not be equally safe in others;
- manufacturers do not routinely test drugs for their effects in G6PD-deficient individuals;
- the risk and severity of haemolysis is almost always dose-related.

The lists below should be read with these points in mind. Ideally, information about G6PD deficiency should be available before prescribing drugs that are associated with a risk of haemolysis in G6PD-deficient patients, including those listed below. However, in the absence of this information, the possibility of haemolysis should be considered, especially if the patient belongs to a group in which G6PD deficiency is common.

Very few G6PD-deficient individuals with chronic non-spherocytic haemolytic anaemia have haemolysis even in the absence of an exogenous trigger. In these children, exacerbation of haemolysis following oxidative stress, such as the administration of any of the drugs listed below, will occur.

Drugs with definite risk of haemolysis in most G6PD-deficient individuals

- Dapsone and other sulfones
- Fluoroquinolones (including ciprofloxacin, moxifloxacin, norfloxacin, and ofloxacin)
- Methylthioninium chloride
- Niridazole [not on UK market]
- Nitrofurantoin
- Pamaquin [not on UK market]
- Primaquine
- Quinolones
- Rasburicase
- Sulfonamides (including co-trimoxazole)

Drugs with possible risk of haemolysis in some G6PD-deficient individuals

- Aspirin
- Chloroquine
- Menadione, water-soluble derivatives (e.g. menadiol sodium phosphate)
- Quinine (may be acceptable in acute malaria)
- Sulfonylureas

Naphthalene in mothballs also causes haemolysis in individuals with G6PD deficiency.

Aplastic and renal anaemias

Treatment choice for aplastic anaemia is dependent on several factors including disease severity. Treatment options in children include haematopoietic stem cell transplantation or immunosuppressive therapy such as intravenous horse antithymocyte globulin in combination with ciclosporin. Prednisolone is used for the prevention of adverse effects associated with antithymocyte globulin treatment. Early reactions that may occur include fever, rash, fluid retention, rigors, acute respiratory distress syndrome, and anaphylaxis; serum sickness may occur 7–14 days later. Treatment should be given under specialist supervision in an appropriate facility. Androgens, such as oxymetholone, are also a treatment option for aplastic anaemia.

Corticosteroids have an important place in the management of haematological disorders. For further information, see Corticosteroids, general use p. 537.

Erythropoietins

Epoetins (recombinant human erythropoietins) are used to treat anaemia associated with erythropoietin deficiency in chronic renal failure.

Epoetin beta p. 700 is also licensed for the prevention of anaemia in preterm neonates of low birth-weight; a therapeutic response may take several weeks.

Darbepoetin alfa p. 698 is a glycosylated derivative of epoetin; it persists longer in the body and can be administered less frequently than epoetin.

For further guidance on the use of erythropoietins in children with chronic kidney disease and anaemia, see NICE guideline: **Chronic kidney disease: assessment and management** (available at: www.nice.org.uk/guidance/ng203).

1.1 Hypoplastic, haemolytic, and renal anaemias

ANABOLIC STEROIDS

Oxymetholone

19-Oct-2023

- **INDICATIONS AND DOSE**

Aplastic anaemia

▸ BY MOUTH

▸ Child: 1–5 mg/kg daily for 3 to 6 months

- **INTERACTIONS** → Appendix 1: oxymetholone
- **MEDICINAL FORMS** Forms available from special-order manufacturers include: oral capsule, oral suspension

EPOETINS

Epoetins

IMPORTANT SAFETY INFORMATION

MHRA/CHM ADVICE: RECOMBINANT HUMAN ERYTHROPOIETINS: VERY RARE RISK OF SEVERE CUTANEOUS ADVERSE REACTIONS (UPDATED JANUARY 2018)

The MHRA is aware of very rare cases of severe cutaneous adverse reactions, including Stevens-Johnson syndrome and toxic epidermal necrolysis, in patients treated with erythropoietins; some cases were fatal. More severe cases were recorded with long-acting agents (darbepoetin alfa and methoxy polyethylene glycol-epoetin beta).

Patients and their carers should be advised of the signs and symptoms of severe skin reactions when starting treatment and instructed to stop treatment and seek immediate medical attention if they develop widespread rash and blistering; these rashes often follow fever or flu-like symptoms—discontinue treatment permanently if such reactions occur.

ERYTHROPOIETINS—HAEMOGLOBIN CONCENTRATION

In chronic kidney disease, the use of erythropoietins can be considered in a child with anaemia. The aim of treatment is to relieve symptoms of anaemia and to avoid the need for blood transfusion. Manufacturer advises haemoglobin concentration should not be increased beyond that which provides adequate control of symptoms of anaemia. In *adults*, overcorrection of haemoglobin concentration with erythropoietins in those with chronic kidney disease may increase the risk of serious cardiovascular events and death; haemoglobin concentrations higher than 12 g/100 mL should be avoided in children.

- **CONTRA-INDICATIONS** Pure red cell aplasia following erythropoietin therapy · uncontrolled hypertension
- **CAUTIONS** Aluminium toxicity (can impair the response to erythropoietin) · concurrent infection (can impair the response to erythropoietin) · correct factors that contribute to the anaemia of chronic renal failure, such as iron or folate deficiency, before treatment · during dialysis (increase in heparin or low molecular weight heparin dose may be needed) · epilepsy · inadequately treated or poorly controlled blood pressure—interrupt treatment if blood pressure uncontrolled · ischaemic vascular disease · malignant disease · other inflammatory disease (can impair the response to erythropoietin) · risk factors for thromboembolism · sickle-cell disease (lower target haemoglobin concentration may be appropriate) · sudden stabbing migraine-like pain (warning of a hypertensive crisis) · thrombocytosis (monitor platelet count for first 8 weeks)
- **SIDE-EFFECTS**
  - **Common or very common** Arthralgia · embolism and thrombosis · headache · hypertension (dose-dependent) · influenza like illness · peripheral oedema · skin reactions · stroke
  - **Uncommon** Hypertensive crisis (in isolated patients with normal or low blood pressure) · respiratory tract congestion · seizure
  - **Rare or very rare** Angioedema · thrombocytosis
  - **Frequency not known** Hypertensive encephalopathy · pure red cell aplasia (more common following subcutaneous administration in patients with chronic renal failure) · severe cutaneous adverse reactions (SCARs)

SIDE-EFFECTS, FURTHER INFORMATION **Hypertensive crisis** In isolated patients with normal or low blood pressure, hypertensive crisis with encephalopathy-like symptoms and generalised tonic-clonic seizures requiring immediate medical attention has occurred with epoetin.

Pure red cell aplasia There have been very rare reports of pure red cell aplasia in patients treated with erythropoietins. In patients who develop a lack of efficacy with erythropoietin therapy and with a diagnosis of pure red cell aplasia, treatment with erythropoietins must be discontinued and testing for erythropoietin antibodies considered. Patients who develop pure red cell aplasia should not be switched to another form of erythropoietin.

- **MONITORING REQUIREMENTS**
  - Monitor closely blood pressure, reticulocyte counts, haemoglobin, and electrolytes—interrupt treatment if blood pressure uncontrolled.
  - Other factors, such as iron or folate deficiency, that contribute to the anaemia of chronic renal failure should be corrected before treatment and monitored during therapy. Supplemental iron may improve the response in resistant patients and in preterm neonates.

697

Darbepoetin alfa

30-Apr-2019

- **INDICATIONS AND DOSE**

Symptomatic anaemia associated with chronic renal failure in patients on dialysis

▶ BY SUBCUTANEOUS INJECTION, OR BY INTRAVENOUS INJECTION

▶ Child 11–17 years: Initially 450 nanograms/kg once weekly, dose to be adjusted according to response by approximately 25% at intervals of at least 4 weeks, maintenance dose to be given once weekly or once every 2 weeks, reduce dose by approximately 25% if rise in haemoglobin concentration exceeds 2 g/100 mL over 4 weeks or if haemoglobin concentration exceeds 12 g/100 mL; if haemoglobin concentration continues to rise, despite dose reduction, suspend treatment until haemoglobin concentration decreases and then restart at a dose approximately 25% lower than the previous dose, when changing route give same dose then adjust according to weekly or fortnightly haemoglobin measurements, adjust doses not more frequently than every 2 weeks during maintenance treatment

Symptomatic anaemia associated with chronic renal failure in patients not on dialysis

▶ BY SUBCUTANEOUS INJECTION

▶ Child 11–17 years: Initially 450 nanograms/kg once weekly, alternatively initially 750 nanograms/kg every 2 weeks, dose to be adjusted according to response by approximately 25% at intervals of at least 4 weeks, maintenance dose can be given once weekly, every 2 weeks, or once a month, subcutaneous route preferred in patients not on haemodialysis, reduce dose by approximately 25% if rise in haemoglobin concentration exceeds 2 g/100 mL over 4 weeks or if haemoglobin concentration exceeds 12 g/100 mL; if haemoglobin concentration continues to rise, despite dose reduction, suspend treatment until haemoglobin concentration decreases and then restart at a dose approximately 25% lower than the previous dose, when changing route give same dose then adjust according to weekly or fortnightly haemoglobin measurements, adjust doses not more frequently than every 2 weeks during maintenance treatment

Symptomatic anaemia associated with chronic renal failure in patients not on dialysis

▶ BY INTRAVENOUS INJECTION

▶ Child 11–17 years: Initially 450 nanograms/kg once weekly, dose to be adjusted according to response by approximately 25% at intervals of at least 4 weeks, maintenance dose given once weekly, subcutaneous route preferred in patients not on haemodialysis, reduce dose by approximately 25% if rise in haemoglobin concentration exceeds 2 g/100 mL over 4 weeks or if haemoglobin concentration exceeds 12 g/100 mL; if haemoglobin concentration continues to rise, despite dose reduction, suspend treatment until haemoglobin concentration decreases and then restart at a dose approximately 25% lower than the previous dose, when changing route give same dose then adjust according to weekly or fortnightly haemoglobin measurements, adjust doses not more frequently than every 2 weeks during maintenance treatment

- **SIDE-EFFECTS**
  - **Common or very common** Cerebrovascular insufficiency · device thrombosis · hypersensitivity · oedema · rash pustular
  - **Frequency not known** Bronchospasm
- **PREGNANCY** No evidence of harm in *animal* studies—manufacturer advises caution.
- **BREAST FEEDING** Manufacturer advises avoid—no information available.
- **HEPATIC IMPAIRMENT** Manufacturer advises caution (no information available).

- **MEDICINAL FORMS** There can be variation in the licensing of different medicines containing the same drug.

Solution for injection

- **Aranesp** (Amgen Ltd)
  - **Darbepoetin alfa 25 microgram per 1 ml** Aranesp 10micrograms/0.4ml solution for injection pre-filled syringes | 4 pre-filled disposable injection [PoM] £58.72 DT = £58.72
  - **Darbepoetin alfa 40 microgram per 1 ml** Aranesp 20micrograms/0.5ml solution for injection pre-filled syringes | 4 pre-filled disposable injection [PoM] £117.45 DT = £117.45
  - **Darbepoetin alfa 100 microgram per 1 ml** Aranesp 50micrograms/0.5ml solution for injection pre-filled syringes | 4 pre-filled disposable injection [PoM] £293.62 DT = £293.62
  - Aranesp 40micrograms/0.4ml solution for injection pre-filled syringes | 4 pre-filled disposable injection [PoM] £234.90 DT = £234.90
  - Aranesp 30micrograms/0.3ml solution for injection pre-filled syringes | 4 pre-filled disposable injection [PoM] £176.17 DT = £176.17
  - **Darbepoetin alfa 200 microgram per 1 ml** Aranesp 130micrograms/0.65ml solution for injection pre-filled syringes | 4 pre-filled disposable injection [PoM] £763.42
  - Aranesp 100micrograms/0.5ml solution for injection pre-filled syringes | 4 pre-filled disposable injection [PoM] £587.24 DT = £587.24
  - Aranesp 60micrograms/0.3ml solution for injection pre-filled syringes | 4 pre-filled disposable injection [PoM] £352.35 DT = £352.35
  - Aranesp 80micrograms/0.4ml solution for injection pre-filled syringes | 4 pre-filled disposable injection [PoM] £469.79 DT = £469.79
  - **Darbepoetin alfa 500 microgram per 1 ml** Aranesp 300micrograms/0.6ml solution for injection pre-filled syringes | 1 pre-filled disposable injection [PoM] £440.43 DT = £440.43
  - Aranesp 500micrograms/1ml solution for injection pre-filled syringes | 1 pre-filled disposable injection [PoM] £734.05 DT = £734.05
  - Aranesp 150micrograms/0.3ml solution for injection pre-filled syringes | 4 pre-filled disposable injection [PoM] £880.86 DT = £880.86
- **Aranesp SureClick** (Amgen Ltd)
  - **Darbepoetin alfa 40 microgram per 1 ml** Aranesp SureClick 20micrograms/0.5ml solution for injection pre-filled pens | 1 pre-filled disposable injection [PoM] £29.36 DT = £29.36
  - **Darbepoetin alfa 100 microgram per 1 ml** Aranesp SureClick 40micrograms/0.4ml solution for injection pre-filled pens | 1 pre-filled disposable injection [PoM] £58.72 DT = £58.72
  - Aranesp SureClick 80micrograms/0.4ml solution for injection pre-filled pens | 1 pre-filled disposable injection [PoM] £117.45 DT = £117.45
  - **Darbepoetin alfa 200 microgram per 1 ml** Aranesp SureClick 100micrograms/0.5ml solution for injection pre-filled pens | 1 pre-filled disposable injection [PoM] £146.81 DT = £146.81
  - Aranesp SureClick 60micrograms/0.3ml solution for injection pre-filled pens | 1 pre-filled disposable injection [PoM] £88.09 DT = £88.09
  - **Darbepoetin alfa 500 microgram per 1 ml** Aranesp SureClick 300micrograms/0.6ml solution for injection pre-filled pens | 1 pre-filled disposable injection [PoM] £440.43 DT = £440.43
  - Aranesp SureClick 150micrograms/0.3ml solution for injection pre-filled pens | 1 pre-filled disposable injection [PoM] £220.22 DT = £220.22
  - Aranesp SureClick 500micrograms/1ml solution for injection pre-filled pens | 1 pre-filled disposable injection [PoM] £734.05

F 697

Epoetin alfa

11-Oct-2023

- **INDICATIONS AND DOSE**

EPREX ® PRE-FILLED SYRINGES

Symptomatic anaemia associated with chronic renal failure in patients on haemodialysis

- BY INTRAVENOUS INJECTION
- Child (body-weight up to 10 kg): Initially 50 units/kg 3 times a week, adjusted in steps of 25 units/kg 3 times a week, dose adjusted according to response at intervals of at least 4 weeks; maintenance 75–150 units/kg 3 times a week, intravenous injection to be given over 1–5 minutes, reduce dose by approximately 25% if rise in haemoglobin concentration exceeds 2 g/100 mL over 4 weeks or if haemoglobin concentration exceeds 12 g/100 mL; if haemoglobin concentration continues to rise, despite dose reduction, suspend treatment until haemoglobin concentration decreases and then restart at a dose approximately 25% lower than the previous dose
- Child (body-weight 10-30 kg): Initially 50 units/kg 3 times a week, adjusted in steps of 25 units/kg 3 times a week, dose adjusted according to response at intervals of at least 4 weeks; maintenance 60–150 units/kg 3 times a week, intravenous injection to be given over 1–5 minutes, reduce dose by approximately 25% if rise in haemoglobin concentration exceeds 2 g/100 mL over 4 weeks or if haemoglobin concentration exceeds 12 g/100 mL; if haemoglobin concentration continues to rise, despite dose reduction, suspend treatment until haemoglobin concentration decreases and then restart at a dose approximately 25% lower than the previous dose
- Child (body-weight 31-60 kg): Initially 50 units/kg 3 times a week, adjusted in steps of 25 units/kg 3 times a week, dose adjusted according to response at intervals of at least 4 weeks; maintenance 30–100 units/kg 3 times a week, intravenous injection to be given over 1–5 minutes, reduce dose by approximately 25% if rise in haemoglobin concentration exceeds 2 g/100 mL over 4 weeks or if haemoglobin concentration exceeds 12 g/100 mL; if haemoglobin concentration continues to rise, despite dose reduction, suspend treatment until haemoglobin concentration decreases and then restart at a dose approximately 25% lower than the previous dose
- Child (body-weight 61 kg and above): Initially 50 units/kg 3 times a week, adjusted in steps of 25 units/kg 3 times a week, dose adjusted according to response at intervals of at least 4 weeks; maintenance 75–300 units/kg once weekly, maintenance dose can be given as a single dose or in divided doses, intravenous injection to be given over 1–5 minutes, reduce dose by approximately 25% if rise in haemoglobin concentration exceeds 2 g/100 mL over 4 weeks or if haemoglobin concentration exceeds 12 g/100 mL; if haemoglobin concentration continues to rise, despite dose reduction, suspend treatment until haemoglobin concentration decreases and then restart at a dose approximately 25% lower than the previous dose

- **SIDE-EFFECTS**
  - **Common or very common** Chills · cough · diarrhoea · fever · myalgia · nausea · pain · vomiting
  - **Uncommon** Hyperkalaemia
- **PREGNANCY** No evidence of harm. Benefits probably outweigh risk of anaemia and of blood transfusion in pregnancy.
- **BREAST FEEDING** Unlikely to be present in milk. Minimal effect on infant.
- **HEPATIC IMPAIRMENT** Manufacturer advises caution in chronic hepatic failure.
- **PRESCRIBING AND DISPENSING INFORMATION** Epoetin alfa is a biological medicine. Biological medicines must be prescribed and dispensed by brand name, see *Biological medicines* and *Biosimilar medicines*, under Guidance on prescribing p. 1.

- **MEDICINAL FORMS** There can be variation in the licensing of different medicines containing the same drug.

Solution for injection

- **Eprex** (Janssen-Cilag Ltd)
  - **Epoetin alfa 4000 unit per 1 ml** Eprex 2,000units/0.5ml solution for injection pre-filled syringes | 6 pre-filled disposable injection [PoM] £66.37 DT = £66.37
  - **Epoetin alfa 10000 unit per 1 ml** Eprex 6,000units/0.6ml solution for injection pre-filled syringes | 6 pre-filled disposable injection [PoM] £199.11 DT = £199.11
  - Eprex 4,000units/0.4ml solution for injection pre-filled syringes | 6 pre-filled disposable injection [PoM] £132.74 DT = £132.74

Eprex 5,000units/0.5ml solution for injection pre-filled syringes | 6 pre-filled disposable injection PoM £165.92
Eprex 3,000units/0.3ml solution for injection pre-filled syringes | 6 pre-filled disposable injection PoM £99.55
Eprex 10,000units/1ml solution for injection pre-filled syringes | 6 pre-filled disposable injection PoM £331.85 DT = £331.85
Eprex 8,000units/0.8ml solution for injection pre-filled syringes | 6 pre-filled disposable injection PoM £265.48
Epoetin alfa 40000 unit per 1 ml Eprex 20,000units/0.5ml solution for injection pre-filled syringes | 1 pre-filled disposable injection PoM £110.62 DT = £110.62
Eprex 30,000units/0.75ml solution for injection pre-filled syringes | 1 pre-filled disposable injection PoM £199.11
Eprex 40,000units/1ml solution for injection pre-filled syringes | 1 pre-filled disposable injection PoM £265.48 DT = £265.48

697

Epoetin beta

06-Dec-2019

● **INDICATIONS AND DOSE**

Symptomatic anaemia associated with chronic renal failure

▶ BY SUBCUTANEOUS INJECTION

▸ Neonate: Initially 20 units/kg 3 times a week for 4 weeks, increased in steps of 20 units/kg 3 times a week, according to response at intervals of 4 weeks, total weekly dose may be divided into daily doses; maintenance dose, initially reduce dose by half then adjust according to response at intervals of 1–2 weeks, total weekly maintenance dose may be given as a single dose or in 3 or 7 divided doses. Subcutaneous route preferred in patients not on haemodialysis. Reduce dose by approximately 25% if rise in haemoglobin concentration exceeds 2 g/100 mL over 4 weeks or if haemoglobin concentration approaches or exceeds 12 g/100 mL; if haemoglobin concentration continues to rise, despite dose reduction, suspend treatment until haemoglobin concentration decreases and then restart at a dose approximately 25% lower than the previous dose; maximum 720 units/kg per week.

▸ Child: Initially 20 units/kg 3 times a week for 4 weeks, increased in steps of 20 units/kg 3 times a week, according to response at intervals of 4 weeks, total weekly dose may be divided into daily doses; maintenance dose, initially reduce dose by half then adjust according to response at intervals of 1–2 weeks, total weekly maintenance dose may be given as a single dose or in 3 or 7 divided doses. Subcutaneous route preferred in patients not on haemodialysis. Reduce dose by approximately 25% if rise in haemoglobin concentration exceeds 2 g/100 mL over 4 weeks or if haemoglobin concentration approaches or exceeds 12 g/100 mL; if haemoglobin concentration continues to rise, despite dose reduction, suspend treatment until haemoglobin concentration decreases and then restart at a dose approximately 25% lower than the previous dose; maximum 720 units/kg per week

▶ BY INTRAVENOUS INJECTION

▸ Neonate: Initially 40 units/kg 3 times a week for 4 weeks, then increased to 80 units/kg 3 times a week, then increased in steps of 20 units/kg 3 times a week if required, at intervals of 4 weeks; maintenance dose, initially reduce dose by half then adjust according to response at intervals of 1–2 weeks. Intravenous injection to be administered over 2 minutes. Subcutaneous route preferred in patients not on haemodialysis. Reduce dose by approximately 25% if rise in haemoglobin concentration exceeds 2 g/100 mL over 4 weeks or if haemoglobin concentration approaches or exceeds 12 g/100 mL; if haemoglobin concentration continues to rise, despite dose reduction, suspend treatment until haemoglobin concentration decreases and then restart at a dose approximately 25% lower than the previous dose; maximum 720 units/kg per week.

▸ Child: Initially 40 units/kg 3 times a week for 4 weeks, then increased to 80 units/kg 3 times a week, then increased in steps of 20 units/kg 3 times a week if required, at intervals of 4 weeks; maintenance dose, initially reduce dose by half then adjust according to response at intervals of 1–2 weeks. Intravenous injection to be administered over 2 minutes. Subcutaneous route preferred in patients not on haemodialysis. Reduce dose by approximately 25% if rise in haemoglobin concentration exceeds 2 g/100 mL over 4 weeks or if haemoglobin concentration approaches or exceeds 12 g/100 mL; if haemoglobin concentration continues to rise, despite dose reduction, suspend treatment until haemoglobin concentration decreases and then restart at a dose approximately 25% lower than the previous dose; maximum 720 units/kg per week

Prevention of anaemias of prematurity in neonates

▶ BY SUBCUTANEOUS INJECTION

▸ Neonate up to 33 weeks corrected gestational age (body-weight 0.75-1.5 kg): 250 units/kg 3 times a week preferably started within 3 days of birth and continued for 6 weeks, using single-dose unpreserved injection.

IMPORTANT SAFETY INFORMATION

MHRA/CHM ADVICE (MAY 2015) EPOETIN BETA (NEORECORMON): INCREASED RISK OF RETINOPATHY IN PRETERM INFANTS CANNOT BE EXCLUDED

There is a possible increased risk of retinopathy in premature infants, when epoetin beta is used for preventing anaemia of prematurity. When using epoetin beta in preterm infants:
- consider the benefits and risks of treatment, including the possible risk of retinopathy,
- monitor the infant for features of retinopathy, and
- advise parents or carers that their baby's eyes will be carefully monitored for any ill effects.

● **PREGNANCY** No evidence of harm. Benefits probably outweigh risk of anaemia and of blood transfusion in pregnancy.

● **BREAST FEEDING** Unlikely to be present in milk. Minimal effect on infant.

● **HEPATIC IMPAIRMENT** Manufacturer advises caution in chronic hepatic failure.

● **MEDICINAL FORMS** There can be variation in the licensing of different medicines containing the same drug.

Solution for injection

EXCIPIENTS: May contain Phenylalanine

▸ NeoRecormon (Roche Products Ltd)

Epoetin beta 1667 unit per 1 ml NeoRecormon 500units/0.3ml solution for injection pre-filled syringes | 6 pre-filled disposable injection PoM £21.05 DT = £21.05
Epoetin beta 6667 unit per 1 ml NeoRecormon 2,000units/0.3ml solution for injection pre-filled syringes | 6 pre-filled disposable injection PoM £84.17 DT = £84.17
Epoetin beta 10000 unit per 1 ml NeoRecormon 3,000units/0.3ml solution for injection pre-filled syringes | 6 pre-filled disposable injection PoM £126.25 DT = £126.25
Epoetin beta 13333 unit per 1 ml NeoRecormon 4,000units/0.3ml solution for injection pre-filled syringes | 6 pre-filled disposable injection PoM £168.34 DT = £168.34
Epoetin beta 16667 unit per 1 ml NeoRecormon 10,000units/0.6ml solution for injection pre-filled syringes | 6 pre-filled disposable injection PoM £420.85 DT = £420.85
NeoRecormon 5,000units/0.3ml solution for injection pre-filled syringes | 6 pre-filled disposable injection PoM £210.42 DT = £210.42

Epoetin beta 20000 unit per 1 ml NeoRecormon 6,000units/0.3ml solution for injection pre-filled syringes | 6 pre-filled disposable injection PoM £252.50 DT = £252.50

Epoetin beta 50000 unit per 1 ml NeoRecormon 30,000units/0.6ml solution for injection pre-filled syringes | 4 pre-filled disposable injection PoM £841.71 DT = £841.71

697

Epoetin zeta

11-Oct-2023

● **INDICATIONS AND DOSE**

Symptomatic anaemia associated with chronic renal failure in patients on haemodialysis

▶ BY INTRAVENOUS INJECTION

▶ Child (body-weight up to 10 kg): Initially 50 units/kg 3 times a week, adjusted according to response, adjusted in steps of 25 units/kg 3 times a week, dose to be adjusted at intervals of at least 4 weeks; maintenance 75–150 units/kg 3 times a week, to be administered over 1–5 minutes, avoid increasing haemoglobin concentration at a rate exceeding 2 g/100 mL over 4 weeks

▶ Child (body-weight 10–30 kg): Initially 50 units/kg 3 times a week, adjusted according to response, adjusted in steps of 25 units/kg 3 times a week, dose to be adjusted at intervals of at least 4 weeks; maintenance 60–150 units/kg 3 times a week, to be administered over 1–5 minutes, avoid increasing haemoglobin concentration at a rate exceeding 2 g/100 mL over 4 weeks

▶ Child (body-weight 31 kg and above): Initially 50 units/kg 3 times a week, adjusted according to response, adjusted in steps of 25 units/kg 3 times a week, dose to be adjusted at intervals of at least 4 weeks; maintenance 30–100 units/kg 3 times a week, to be administered over 1–5 minutes, avoid increasing haemoglobin concentration at a rate exceeding 2 g/100 mL over 4 weeks

● **SIDE-EFFECTS**

▶ **Common or very common** Asthenia · dizziness · myocardial infarction

▶ **Uncommon** Intracranial haemorrhage

▶ **Frequency not known** Aneurysm · cerebrovascular insufficiency · myocardial ischaemia

● **PREGNANCY** No evidence of harm. Benefits probably outweigh risk of anaemia and of blood transfusion in pregnancy.

● **BREAST FEEDING** Unlikely to be present in milk. Minimal effect on infant.

● **HEPATIC IMPAIRMENT** Manufacturer advises caution in chronic hepatic failure.

● **PRESCRIBING AND DISPENSING INFORMATION** Epoetin zeta is a biological medicine. Biological medicines must be prescribed and dispensed by brand name, see *Biological medicines* and *Biosimilar medicines*, under Guidance on prescribing p. 1.

● **MEDICINAL FORMS** There can be variation in the licensing of different medicines containing the same drug.

Solution for injection

EXCIPIENTS: May contain Phenylalanine

▶ Retacrit (Pfizer Ltd)

Epoetin zeta 3333 unit per 1 ml Retacrit 2,000units/0.6ml solution for injection pre-filled syringes | 6 pre-filled disposable injection PoM £57.70

Retacrit 3,000units/0.9ml solution for injection pre-filled syringes | 6 pre-filled disposable injection PoM £86.55

Retacrit 1,000units/0.3ml solution for injection pre-filled syringes | 6 pre-filled disposable injection PoM £28.85

Epoetin zeta 10000 unit per 1 ml Retacrit 6,000units/0.6ml solution for injection pre-filled syringes | 6 pre-filled disposable injection PoM £173.09

Retacrit 10,000units/1ml solution for injection pre-filled syringes | 6 pre-filled disposable injection PoM £288.48 DT = £288.48

Retacrit 8,000units/0.8ml solution for injection pre-filled syringes | 6 pre-filled disposable injection PoM £230.79 DT = £230.79

Retacrit 4,000units/0.4ml solution for injection pre-filled syringes | 6 pre-filled disposable injection PoM £115.40

Retacrit 5,000units/0.5ml solution for injection pre-filled syringes | 6 pre-filled disposable injection PoM £144.25

Epoetin zeta 40000 unit per 1 ml Retacrit 20,000units/0.5ml solution for injection pre-filled syringes | 1 pre-filled disposable injection PoM £96.16

Retacrit 40,000units/1ml solution for injection pre-filled syringes | 1 pre-filled disposable injection PoM £193.32

Retacrit 30,000units/0.75ml solution for injection pre-filled syringes | 1 pre-filled disposable injection PoM £144.25 DT = £144.25

1.1a Atypical haemolytic uraemic syndrome and paroxysmal nocturnal haemoglobinuria

IMMUNOSUPPRESSANTS > COMPLEMENT INHIBITORS

Crovalimab

14-Jan-2025

● **DRUG ACTION** Crovalimab is a recombinant monoclonal antibody that inhibits terminal complement activation at the C5 protein, thereby reducing haemolysis.

● **INDICATIONS AND DOSE**

Paroxysmal nocturnal haemoglobinuria (initiated under specialist supervision)

▶ INITIALLY BY INTRAVENOUS INFUSION

▶ Child 12–17 years (body-weight 40–99 kg): Loading dose 1000 mg for 1 dose, to be given on day 1, then (by subcutaneous injection) 340 mg for 4 doses, to be given on days 2, 8, 15, and 22, followed by (by subcutaneous injection) maintenance 680 mg every 4 weeks, to be given from day 29 onwards

▶ Child 12–17 years (body-weight 100 kg and above): Loading dose 1500 mg for 1 dose, to be given on day 1, then (by subcutaneous injection) 340 mg for 4 doses, to be given on days 2, 8, 15, and 22, followed by (by subcutaneous injection) maintenance 1020 mg every 4 weeks, to be given from day 29 onwards

DOSE EQUIVALENCE AND CONVERSION

▶ For patients switching from another complement inhibitor, the first loading dose of crovalimab should be administered at the time of the next scheduled complement inhibitor dose.

● **CONTRA-INDICATIONS** Patients unvaccinated against *Neisseria meningitidis* · unresolved infection caused by *Neisseria meningitidis*

● **CAUTIONS** Active systemic infections (monitor for signs and symptoms of worsening infection)

CAUTIONS, FURTHER INFORMATION

▶ Vaccination against serious infection EvGr To reduce the risk of serious infection, it is advised that patients are vaccinated against *Neisseria meningitidis* (vaccines against serotypes A, C, Y, W135, and B, where available, are recommended), *Streptococcus pneumoniae*, and *Haemophilus influenzae* type b according to local guidelines, at least 2 weeks before starting treatment. If immediate treatment is needed, administer the required vaccines as soon as possible; treat with prophylactic antibiotics until 2 weeks after vaccination. (M)

● **INTERACTIONS** → Appendix 1: crovalimab

- **SIDE-EFFECTS**
- ▶ **Common or very common** Abdominal pain · arthralgia · asthenia · diarrhoea · fever · headache · hypersensitivity · increased risk of infection · infusion related reaction · injection related reaction · rash · type III hypersensitivity reaction (complex-mediated) (when switching from another C5 inhibitor)
- ▶ **Uncommon** Sepsis

SIDE-EFFECTS, FURTHER INFORMATION Monitor patients for symptoms of type III hypersensitivity reactions (such as arthralgia, rash, fever, fatigue, abdominal distress, headache and axonal neuropathy) for the first 30 days after switching between C5 inhibitors.

- **PREGNANCY** EvGr Use only if potential benefit outweighs risk (limited information available). (M) Crovalimab is an immunoglobulin G (IgG) monoclonal antibody; human IgG antibodies are known to cross the placenta.
- **BREAST FEEDING** EvGr Avoid (limited information available). (M)
- **MONITORING REQUIREMENTS**
- ▶ EvGr Monitor for early signs of meningococcal infection caused by *Neisseria meningitidis*.
- ▶ Monitor for intravascular haemolysis (including serum-lactate dehydrogenase concentration) following treatment discontinuation; consider restarting appropriate treatment if haemolysis occurs. (M)
- **DIRECTIONS FOR ADMINISTRATION** For *intermittent intravenous infusion*, dilute requisite dose to a final concentration of 4–15 mg/mL with Sodium Chloride 0.9%; give over 60–90 minutes through a 0.2 micron in-line filter.

For *subcutaneous injection*, administer into the abdomen (except for the 5 cm around the navel); rotate injection site and avoid moles, scars, and skin that is tender, bruised, red, hardened, or not intact.

Piasky® may be self-administered or administered by a carer after appropriate training in subcutaneous injection technique.

- **PRESCRIBING AND DISPENSING INFORMATION** Crovalimab is a biological medicine. Biological medicines must be prescribed and dispensed by brand name, see *Biological medicines* and *Biosimilar medicines*, under Guidance on prescribing p. 1; record the brand name and batch number after each administration.

The manufacturer of *Piasky®* has provided a *Healthcare Professional Guide*.

- **HANDLING AND STORAGE** Store in a refrigerator (2–8°C) and protect from light—consult product literature for further information regarding storage outside the refrigerator.
- **PATIENT AND CARER ADVICE** Patients and carers should be informed of the signs and symptoms of serious infections, especially meningococcal infection, and advised to seek immediate medical care if they occur.

Self administration Patients or their carers should be given training in subcutaneous injection technique if appropriate.

Patient card and guide A patient card and guide for patients and caregivers should be provided.

- **NATIONAL FUNDING/ACCESS DECISIONS** For full details see funding body website

NICE decisions

- ▶ **Crovalimab for treating paroxysmal nocturnal haemoglobinuria in people 12 years and over (November 2024)** NICE TA1019 Recommended

Scottish Medicines Consortium (SMC) decisions

- ▶ **Crovalimab (*Piasky®*) as monotherapy for the treatment of adult and paediatric patients 12 years of age or older with a weight of 40 kg and above with paroxysmal nocturnal haemoglobinuria: in patients with haemolysis with clinical symptom(s) indicative of high disease activity; or who are clinically stable after having been treated with a complement component 5 inhibitor for at least the past 6 months (January 2025)** SMC No. SMC2728 Recommended with restrictions

- **MEDICINAL FORMS** There can be variation in the licensing of different medicines containing the same drug.

Solution for injection

- ▶ **Piasky** (Roche Products Ltd) ▼

Crovalimab 170 mg per 1 ml PiaSky 340mg/2ml solution for injection vials | 1 vial PoM £9,500.00 (Hospital only)

Eculizumab

28-Mar-2024

- **DRUG ACTION** Eculizumab is a recombinant monoclonal antibody that inhibits terminal complement activation at the C5 protein and thereby reduces complement-mediated cell damage.

- **INDICATIONS AND DOSE**

Paroxysmal nocturnal haemoglobinuria (under expert supervision)

▶ BY INTRAVENOUS INFUSION

- ▶ **Child (body-weight 5–9 kg):** Initially 300 mg once weekly for 2 weeks, followed by maintenance 300 mg every 3 weeks
- ▶ **Child (body-weight 10–19 kg):** Initially 600 mg once weekly for 1 week, then reduced to 300 mg once weekly for 1 week, followed by maintenance 300 mg every 2 weeks
- ▶ **Child (body-weight 20–29 kg):** Initially 600 mg once weekly for 3 weeks, followed by maintenance 600 mg every 2 weeks
- ▶ **Child (body-weight 30–39 kg):** Initially 600 mg once weekly for 2 weeks, then increased to 900 mg once weekly for 1 week, followed by maintenance 900 mg every 2 weeks
- ▶ **Child (body-weight 40 kg and above):** Initially 600 mg once weekly for 4 weeks, then increased to 900 mg once weekly for 1 week, followed by maintenance 900 mg every 12–16 days

Atypical haemolytic uraemic syndrome (under expert supervision)

▶ BY INTRAVENOUS INFUSION

- ▶ **Child (body-weight 5–9 kg):** Initially 300 mg once weekly for 2 weeks, followed by maintenance 300 mg every 3 weeks
- ▶ **Child (body-weight 10–19 kg):** Initially 600 mg once weekly for 1 week, then reduced to 300 mg once weekly for 1 week, followed by maintenance 300 mg every 2 weeks
- ▶ **Child (body-weight 20–29 kg):** Initially 600 mg once weekly for 3 weeks, followed by maintenance 600 mg every 2 weeks
- ▶ **Child (body-weight 30–39 kg):** Initially 600 mg once weekly for 2 weeks, then increased to 900 mg once weekly for 1 week, followed by maintenance 900 mg every 2 weeks
- ▶ **Child (body-weight 40 kg and above):** Initially 900 mg once weekly for 4 weeks, then increased to 1.2 g once weekly for 1 week, followed by maintenance 1.2 g every 12–16 days

- **UNLICENSED USE** Not licensed for use in children for paroxysmal nocturnal haemoglobinuria.
- **CONTRA-INDICATIONS** Patients unvaccinated against *Neisseria meningitidis* · unresolved *Neisseria meningitidis* infection
- **CAUTIONS** Active systemic infection

CAUTIONS, FURTHER INFORMATION

- ▶ Meningococcal infection Manufacturer advises vaccinate against *Neisseria meningitidis* at least 2 weeks before treatment (vaccines against serotypes A, C, Y, W135 and B where available, are recommended); revaccinate according to current medical guidelines. Patients receiving eculizumab less than 2 weeks after receiving meningococcal vaccine must be given prophylactic antibiotics until 2 weeks after vaccination. Advise patient to report promptly any signs of meningococcal infection. Other immunisations should also be up to date.

- **INTERACTIONS** → Appendix 1: monoclonal antibodies
- **SIDE-EFFECTS**
  - **Common or very common** Alopecia · asthenia · cough · decreased leucocytes · diarrhoea · dizziness · fever · gastrointestinal discomfort · headache · hypertension · increased risk of infection · influenza like illness · joint disorders · muscle complaints · nausea · oropharyngeal pain · skin reactions · sleep disorders · taste altered · vomiting
  - **Uncommon** Abscess · anxiety · appetite decreased · chest discomfort · chills · constipation · cystitis · depression · dysuria · haemorrhage · hepatosplenic abscess · hot flush · hyperhidrosis · hypersensitivity · hypotension · infusion related reaction · limb abscess · meningitis meningococcal · mood swings · nasal complaints · oedema · pain · palpitations · paraesthesia · renal abscess · sepsis · spontaneous penile erection · throat irritation · tinnitus · tremor · vascular disorders · vertigo · vision blurred
  - **Rare or very rare** Abnormal clotting factor · conjunctival irritation · feeling hot · gastrooesophageal reflux disease · gingival discomfort · Grave's disease · jaundice · malignant melanoma · menstrual disorder · syncope · urogenital tract gonococcal infection
- **CONCEPTION AND CONTRACEPTION** Manufacturer advises effective contraception during and for 5 months after treatment.
- **PREGNANCY** Manufacturer advises use only if potential benefit outweighs risk—limited information available. Eculizumab is an immunoglobulin G (IgG) monoclonal antibody; human IgG antibodies are known to cross the placenta.
- **BREAST FEEDING** Manufacturer advises use with caution—limited information available; unlikely to be present in milk.
- **MONITORING REQUIREMENTS**
  - Monitor for 1 hour after infusion.
  - For *paroxysmal nocturnal haemoglobinuria*, monitor for intravascular haemolysis (including serum-lactate dehydrogenase concentration) during treatment and for at least 8 weeks after discontinuation.
  - For *atypical haemolytic uraemic syndrome*, monitor for thrombotic microangiopathy (measure platelet count, serum-lactate dehydrogenase concentration, and serum creatinine) during treatment and for at least 12 weeks after discontinuation.
- **DIRECTIONS FOR ADMINISTRATION** For *intravenous infusion*, manufacturer advises dilute requisite dose to a concentration of 5 mg/mL with Glucose 5% or Sodium Chloride 0.9% and mix gently; give over 1–4 hours (infusion time may be increased to 4 hours if infusion-related reactions occur).
- **PRESCRIBING AND DISPENSING INFORMATION** Eculizumab is a biological medicine. Biological medicines must be prescribed and dispensed by brand name, see *Biological medicines* and *Biosimilar medicines*, under Guidance on prescribing p. 1.

  Consult product literature for details of supplemental doses with concomitant plasmapheresis, plasma exchange, or plasma infusion.

  The manufacturer of *Soliris*® has provided a *Physician's guide* and user manual for healthcare professionals.
- **HANDLING AND STORAGE** Store in a refrigerator (2–8°C) and protect from light—consult product literature for further information regarding storage outside refrigerator.
- **PATIENT AND CARER ADVICE** Patients or carers should be advised to report promptly any signs of meningococcal infection. Advice about prevention of gonorrhoea should also be given.

  A patient information card and a patient safety card should be provided.
- **NATIONAL FUNDING/ACCESS DECISIONS** For full details see funding body website

  NICE decisions
  - **Eculizumab for treating atypical haemolytic uraemic syndrome (January 2015)** NICE HST1 Recommended
- **MEDICINAL FORMS** There can be variation in the licensing of different medicines containing the same drug.

Solution for infusion

EXCIPIENTS: May contain Polysorbates

ELECTROLYTES: May contain Sodium

- **Bekemv** (Amgen Ltd) ▼
  Eculizumab 10 mg per 1 ml Bekemv 300mg/30ml concentrate for solution for infusion vials | 1 vial PoM £3,150.00 (Hospital only)
- **Epysqli** (Samsung Bioepis NL B.V. Ltd) ▼
  Eculizumab 10 mg per 1 ml Epysqli 300mg/30ml concentrate for solution for infusion vials | 1 vial PoM £3,150.00 (Hospital only)
- **Soliris** (Alexion Pharma UK Ltd)
  Eculizumab 10 mg per 1 ml Soliris 300mg/30ml concentrate for solution for infusion vials | 1 vial PoM £3,150.00 (Hospital only)

Ravulizumab

28-Mar-2024

- **DRUG ACTION** Ravulizumab is a recombinant monoclonal antibody that inhibits terminal complement activation at the C5 protein, thereby reducing haemolysis and thrombotic microangiopathy.

- **INDICATIONS AND DOSE**

Atypical haemolytic uraemic syndrome (under expert supervision) | Paroxysmal nocturnal haemoglobinuria (under expert supervision)

▶ BY INTRAVENOUS INFUSION

- Child (body-weight 10–19 kg): Loading dose 0.6 g for 1 dose, then maintenance 0.6 g every 4 weeks, start maintenance dosing 2 weeks after the loading dose, a maintenance dose (except for the first maintenance dose) may be given up to 7 days before or after the scheduled date; the subsequent dose should be given according to the original schedule, for duration of infusion—consult product literature
- Child (body-weight 20–29 kg): Loading dose 0.9 g for 1 dose, then maintenance 2.1 g every 8 weeks, start maintenance dosing 2 weeks after the loading dose, a maintenance dose (except for the first maintenance dose) may be given up to 7 days before or after the scheduled date; the subsequent dose should be given according to the original schedule, for duration of infusion—consult product literature
- Child (body-weight 30–39 kg): Loading dose 1.2 g for 1 dose, then maintenance 2.7 g every 8 weeks, start maintenance dosing 2 weeks after the loading dose, a maintenance dose (except for the first maintenance dose) may be given up to 7 days before or after the scheduled date; the subsequent dose should be given according to the original schedule, for duration of infusion—consult product literature
- Child (body-weight 40–59 kg): Loading dose 2.4 g for 1 dose, then maintenance 3 g every 8 weeks, start maintenance dosing 2 weeks after the loading dose, a maintenance dose (except for the first maintenance dose) may be given up to 7 days before or after the scheduled date; the subsequent dose should continued →

be given according to the original schedule, for duration of infusion—consult product literature
- Child (body-weight 60-99 kg): Loading dose 2.7 g for 1 dose, then maintenance 3.3 g every 8 weeks, start maintenance dosing 2 weeks after the loading dose, a maintenance dose (except for the first maintenance dose) may be given up to 7 days before or after the scheduled date; the subsequent dose should be given according to the original schedule, for duration of infusion—consult product literature
- Child (body-weight 100 kg and above): Loading dose 3 g for 1 dose, then maintenance 3.6 g every 8 weeks, start maintenance dosing 2 weeks after the loading dose, a maintenance dose (except for the first maintenance dose) may be given up to 7 days before or after the scheduled date; the subsequent dose should be given according to the original schedule, for duration of infusion—consult product literature

DOSE EQUIVALENCE AND CONVERSION
- For patients switching from eculizumab to ravulizumab, the initial loading dose of ravulizumab should be administered 2 weeks after the last eculizumab infusion.

- **CONTRA-INDICATIONS** Patients unvaccinated against *Neisseria meningitidis* · unresolved *Neisseria meningitidis* infection
- **CAUTIONS** Active systemic infection

CAUTIONS, FURTHER INFORMATION
- Meningococcal infection EvGr Vaccinate against *Neisseria meningitidis* at least 2 weeks before treatment (vaccines against serotypes A, C, Y, W135 and B where available, are recommended); revaccinate according to current medical guidelines. Patients receiving ravulizumab less than 2 weeks after receiving meningococcal vaccine must be given prophylactic antibiotics until 2 weeks after vaccination. Other immunisations should also be up to date for all age groups. ⟨M⟩
- Vaccination EvGr Patients under 18 years should also be vaccinated against *Haemophilus influenzae* type b and pneumococcal infections. ⟨M⟩

- **INTERACTIONS** → Appendix 1: ravulizumab
- **SIDE-EFFECTS**
  - **Common or very common** Arthralgia · asthenia · back pain · diarrhoea · dizziness · fever · gastrointestinal discomfort · headache · increased risk of infection · influenza like illness · infusion related reaction · muscle complaints · nausea · skin reactions · vomiting
  - **Uncommon** Chills · hypersensitivity · meningococcal sepsis
- **CONCEPTION AND CONTRACEPTION** Manufacturer advises effective contraception during and for up to 8 months after treatment.
- **PREGNANCY** Manufacturer advises use only if potential benefit outweighs risk—no information available. Ravulizumab is an immunoglobulin G (IgG) monoclonal antibody; human IgG antibodies are known to cross the placenta.
- **BREAST FEEDING** Manufacturer advises avoid breast-feeding during and for up to 8 months after treatment—no information available.
- **MONITORING REQUIREMENTS**
  - When used for Paroxysmal nocturnal haemoglobinuria EvGr Monitor for intravascular haemolysis (including serum-lactate dehydrogenase concentration) for at least 16 weeks after stopping treatment; consider restarting ravulizumab if haemolysis occurs. ⟨M⟩
  - When used for Atypical haemolytic uraemic syndrome EvGr Monitor for thrombotic microangiopathy (measure platelet count, serum-lactate dehydrogenase concentration, and serum creatinine) after stopping treatment; consider restarting ravulizumab if thrombotic microangiopathy occurs. ⟨M⟩
- **DIRECTIONS FOR ADMINISTRATION** EvGr For *intravenous infusion* using *Ultomiris*® *300 mg/3 mL, 1100 mg/11 mL concentrate for infusion*, give intermittently in Sodium Chloride 0.9%. Dilute requisite dose with infusion fluid to a final concentration of 50 mg/mL and administer through an in-line filter (0.2 micron). For *intravenous infusion* using *Ultomiris*® *300 mg/30 mL concentrate for infusion*, give intermittently in Sodium Chloride 0.9%. Dilute requisite dose with infusion fluid to a final concentration of 5 mg/mL and administer through an in-line filter (0.2 micron). ⟨M⟩
- **PRESCRIBING AND DISPENSING INFORMATION** Ravulizumab is a biological medicine. Biological medicines must be prescribed and dispensed by brand name, see *Biological medicines* and *Biosimilar medicines*, under Guidance on prescribing p. 1; record the brand name and batch number after each administration.

  The manufacturer of *Ultomiris*® has provided a *Physician's guide* for healthcare professionals.
- **HANDLING AND STORAGE** Store in a refrigerator (2-8°C) and protect from light—consult product literature for further information regarding storage outside refrigerator.
- **PATIENT AND CARER ADVICE** Patients or carers should be advised to report promptly any signs of meningococcal infection. Advice about prevention of gonorrhoea should also be given.

  A patient information card and a patient safety card should be provided.
- **NATIONAL FUNDING/ACCESS DECISIONS**

  For full details see funding body website

  NICE decisions
  - **Ravulizumab for treating atypical haemolytic uraemic syndrome (June 2021)** NICE TA710 Recommended

  Scottish Medicines Consortium (SMC) decisions
  - **Ravulizumab (*Ultomiris*®) for the treatment of patients with a body weight of 10 kg or above with atypical haemolytic uremic syndrome who are complement inhibitor treatment-naive or have received eculizumab for at least 3 months and have evidence of response to eculizumab (May 2021)** SMC No. SMC2330 Recommended with restrictions

  All Wales Medicines Strategy Group (AWMSG) decisions
  - **Ravulizumab (*Ultomiris*®) for the treatment of paediatric patients with a body weight of 10 kg or above with paroxysmal nocturnal haemoglobinuria, who have haemolysis with clinical symptoms indicative of high disease activity or who are clinically stable after receiving eculizumab for at least 6 months (February 2022)** AWMSG No. 4869 Recommended

- **MEDICINAL FORMS** There can be variation in the licensing of different medicines containing the same drug.

Solution for infusion

EXCIPIENTS: May contain Polysorbates

ELECTROLYTES: May contain Sodium
- **Ultomiris** (Alexion Pharma UK Ltd)

  Ravulizumab 100 mg per 1 ml Ultomiris 1,100mg/11ml concentrate for solution for infusion vials | 1 vial PoM £16,621.00

  Ultomiris 300mg/3ml concentrate for solution for infusion vials | 1 vial PoM £4,533.00

1.2 Iron deficiency anaemia

Anaemia, iron deficiency
12-Feb-2025

Iron deficiency, treatment and prophylaxis

Iron deficiency anaemia is the reduction of red blood cell production due to low iron stores in the body.

Treatment with an iron preparation should be initiated for confirmed iron-deficiency anaemia. It is important to exclude any underlying causes of the anaemia (e.g. gastro-intestinal bleeding, coeliac disease, inflammatory bowel disease, or heavy menstrual bleeding), but iron treatment should not be delayed whilst awaiting investigations. The possibility of thalassaemia should be considered in children of Mediterranean or Indian subcontinent descent.

Prophylaxis with an iron preparation may be appropriate in those with a poor diet, malabsorption, menorrhagia, pregnancy, in haemodialysis patients, and in the management of low birth-weight infants such as preterm neonates.

For information on the management of anaemia in peri-operative patients, see Centre for Perioperative Care guidance: **Guideline for the Management of Anaemia in the Perioperative Pathway** (available at: cpoc.org.uk/guidelines-resources-guidelines/anaemia-perioperative-pathway).

Oral iron

Iron salts should be given by mouth unless there are good reasons for using another route.

Ferrous salts show only marginal differences between one another in efficiency of absorption of iron. Haemoglobin regeneration rate is little affected by the type of salt used provided sufficient iron is given, and in most patients the speed of response is not critical. Choice of preparation is thus usually decided by formulation, palatability, incidence of side-effects, and cost.

Treatment of iron-deficiency anaemia

Iron supplementation may also be required to produce an optimum response to erythropoietins in iron-deficient children with chronic renal failure or in preterm neonates.

When prescribing, express the dose in terms of elemental iron and iron salt and select the most appropriate preparation; specify both the iron salt and formulation on the prescription. The iron content of artificial formula feeds should also be considered.

EvGr An initial once-daily or alternate-day dose regimen of oral iron salts (depending on preparation used) is recommended, as these may be just as effective as multiple daily dose regimens (such as two or three times a day dosing), with a lower incidence of side-effects and better compliance. Haemoglobin and ferritin concentrations should be monitored within the first 6 weeks to 3 months of starting treatment to assess response and to ensure concentrations are increasing. Once haemoglobin is within the normal range, treatment should be continued for around a further 3 months to replenish iron stores. An increased dose of oral iron salts may be considered if the therapeutic response is slow and treatment is tolerated. For guidance on iron dosing, see ferrous fumarate p. 707, ferrous gluconate p. 708, ferrous sulfate p. 708, and sodium feredetate p. 709. Ⓔ

Iron content of different iron salts

Iron salt/amount	Content of ferrous iron
ferrous fumarate 210 mg	69 mg
ferrous gluconate 300 mg	35 mg
ferrous sulfate, dried 200 mg	65 mg
sodium feredetate 190 mg/5 mL	27.5 mg/5 mL

Prophylaxis of iron deficiency

In neonates, haemoglobin and haematocrit concentrations change rapidly. These changes are not due to iron deficiency and cannot be corrected by iron supplementation. Similarly, neonatal anaemia resulting from repeated blood sampling does not respond to iron therapy.

All babies, including preterm neonates, are born with substantial iron stores but these stores can become depleted unless dietary intake is adequate. All babies require an iron intake of 400–700 nanograms daily to maintain body stores. Iron in breast milk is well absorbed but that in artificial feeds or in cow's milk is less so. Most artificial formula feeds are sufficiently fortified with iron to prevent deficiency and their iron content should be taken into account when considering further iron supplementation.

EvGr Prophylactic iron supplementation is given to preterm or low birth-weight infants who are partially or solely breast-fed; supplementation is usually started 2–6 weeks after birth and continued for 6–12 months or until the infant is receiving iron-rich formula or food. For further guidance on iron supplementation in preterm or low birth-weight infants, see British Dietetic Association Neonatal Dieticians guideline: **The routine supplementation of vitamins and iron and the management of zinc deficiency in preterm and small for gestational age infants** (available at: www.bda.uk.com/specialist-groups-and-branches/paediatric-specialist-group/paediatric-sub-groups-home/neonatal-dietitians-sub-group/clinical-guidelines.html). Ⓔ

Infants with a poor diet may become anaemic in the second year of life, particularly if cow's milk, rather than fortified formula feed, is a major part of the diet.

Compound preparations

Some oral preparations contain ascorbic acid p. 786 to aid absorption of the iron, but the therapeutic advantage of such preparations is minimal and cost may be increased.

There is no justification for the inclusion of other ingredients, such as the **B group of vitamins**, except folic acid p. 710 for pregnant women.

Modified-release preparations

EvGr Modified-release preparations of iron do not enhance iron absorption and are **not** recommended. Ⓔ

Parenteral iron

Iron can be administered parenterally as iron dextran p. 707, iron sucrose p. 707 or ferric carboxymaltose p. 706. Parenteral iron is generally reserved for use when oral therapy is unsuccessful because the child cannot tolerate oral iron, or does not take it reliably, or if there is continuing blood loss, or in malabsorption.

Many children with chronic renal failure who are receiving haemodialysis (and some who are receiving peritoneal dialysis) also require iron by the intravenous route on a regular basis.

With the exception of children with severe renal failure receiving haemodialysis, parenteral iron does not produce a faster haemoglobin response than oral iron provided that the oral iron preparation is taken reliably and is absorbed adequately. If parenteral iron is necessary, the dose should be calculated according to the child's body-weight and total iron deficit. Depending on the preparation used, parenteral iron is given as a total dose or in divided doses. Further treatment should be guided by monitoring haemoglobin and serum iron concentrations.

MINERALS AND TRACE ELEMENTS > IRON, INJECTABLE

Iron (injectable)

IMPORTANT SAFETY INFORMATION

MHRA/CHM ADVICE: SERIOUS HYPERSENSITIVITY REACTIONS WITH INTRAVENOUS IRON (AUGUST 2013)

Serious hypersensitivity reactions, including life-threatening and fatal anaphylactic reactions, have been reported in patients receiving intravenous iron. These reactions can occur even when a previous administration has been tolerated (including a negative test dose). Test doses are no longer recommended and caution is needed with every dose of intravenous iron.

Intravenous iron products should only be administered when appropriately trained staff and resuscitation facilities are immediately available; patients should be closely monitored for signs of hypersensitivity during and for at least 30 minutes after every administration. In the event of a hypersensitivity reaction, treatment should be stopped immediately and appropriate management initiated.

The risk of hypersensitivity is increased in patients with known allergies, immune or inflammatory conditions, or those with a history of severe asthma, eczema, or other atopic allergy; in these patients, intravenous iron should only be used if the benefits outweigh the risks.

Intravenous iron should be avoided in the first trimester of pregnancy and used in the second or third trimesters only if the benefit outweighs the potential risks for both mother and fetus.

- **CONTRA-INDICATIONS** Disturbances in utilisation of iron · iron overload
- **CAUTIONS** Allergic disorders · eczema · hepatic dysfunction · immune conditions · infection (discontinue if ongoing bacteraemia) · inflammatory conditions · oral iron should not be given until 5 days after the last injection · severe asthma
- **SIDE-EFFECTS**
  - **Common or very common** Dizziness · flushing · headache · hypertension · hypophosphataemia · hypotension · nausea · skin reactions · taste altered
  - **Uncommon** Arrhythmias · arthralgia · bronchospasm · chest pain · chills · constipation · diarrhoea · dyspnoea · fatigue · fever · gastrointestinal discomfort · hyperhidrosis · hypersensitivity · loss of consciousness · malaise · muscle complaints · pain · peripheral oedema · sensation abnormal · vision blurred · vomiting
  - **Rare or very rare** Angioedema · anxiety · circulatory collapse · influenza like illness · pallor · palpitations · psychiatric disorder · seizure · syncope · tremor
  - **Frequency not known** Kounis syndrome

SIDE-EFFECTS, FURTHER INFORMATION **Hypersensitivity reactions** Anaphylactic reactions can occur with parenteral administration of iron complexes and facilities for cardiopulmonary resuscitation must be available. If children complain of acute symptoms particularly nausea, back pain, breathlessness, or develop hypotension, the infusion should be stopped.

Skin reactions Skin discolouration (sometimes permanent) can occur with parenteral iron administration. This can occur both at the site of administration and on other areas of the body.

Overdose For details on the management of poisoning, see Iron salts, under Emergency treatment of poisoning p. 1036.

- **PREGNANCY** EvGr Avoid in first trimester. (M)

Monitoring in pregnancy EvGr Fetal monitoring is recommended during administration due to the risk of fetal bradycardia. (M)

F 705

Ferric carboxymaltose

14-Apr-2025

- **INDICATIONS AND DOSE**

Iron-deficiency anaemia

- BY SLOW INTRAVENOUS INJECTION, OR BY INTRAVENOUS INFUSION
  - Child 1–17 years: Dose calculated according to body-weight and iron deficit (consult product literature)

IMPORTANT SAFETY INFORMATION

MHRA/CHM ADVICE: FERRIC CARBOXYMALTOSE (*FERINJECT*®): RISK OF SYMPTOMATIC HYPOPHOSPHATAEMIA LEADING TO OSTEOMALACIA AND FRACTURES (NOVEMBER 2020)

A European review of worldwide data concluded that ferric carboxymaltose is associated with hypophosphataemia, resulting in hypophosphataemic osteomalacia and fractures, particularly in patients with existing risk factors and following prolonged exposure to high doses—some cases required clinical intervention, including surgery. The risk of persistent hypophosphataemia and osteomalacia may be higher with ferric carboxymaltose than with other intravenous iron formulations.

Healthcare professionals are advised to monitor serum phosphate levels in patients requiring multiple high-dose administrations, on long-term treatment, or with pre-existing risk factors for hypophosphataemia. Patients experiencing symptoms of hypophosphataemia (including new musculoskeletal symptoms or worsening tiredness) should seek medical advice—be aware that these symptoms may be confused with those of iron deficiency anaemia. If hypophosphataemia persists, ferric carboxymaltose treatment should be re-evaluated.

- **INTERACTIONS** → Appendix 1: iron
- **SIDE-EFFECTS**
  - **Rare or very rare** Gastrointestinal disorders
  - **Frequency not known** Face oedema · thirst
- **PREGNANCY** EvGr *Animal* studies indicate may influence skeletal development. (M)
- **HEPATIC IMPAIRMENT** Manufacturer advises caution—monitor iron status to avoid iron overload; avoid where iron overload increases risk of impairment (particularly porphyria cutanea tarda).
- **DIRECTIONS FOR ADMINISTRATION** For *intravenous infusion* (*Ferinject*®), give intermittently in Sodium Chloride 0.9%. Dilute 200–500 mg in up to 100 mL infusion fluid and give over at least 6 minutes; dilute 0.5–1 g in up to 250 mL infusion fluid and give over at least 15 minutes.
- **PRESCRIBING AND DISPENSING INFORMATION** A ferric carboxymaltose complex containing 5% (50 mg/mL) of iron.

- **MEDICINAL FORMS** There can be variation in the licensing of different medicines containing the same drug.

Dispersion for injection

ELECTROLYTES: May contain Sodium

- **Ferric carboxymaltose (Non-proprietary)**

Iron (as Ferric carboxymaltose) 50 mg per 1 ml Feristark 1000mg/20ml dispersion for injection vials | 1 vial PoM £138.81 (Hospital only)

Feristark 100mg/2ml dispersion for injection vials | 5 vial PoM £85.95 (Hospital only)

Feristark 500mg/10ml dispersion for injection vials | 5 vial PoM £429.75 (Hospital only)

- **Ferinject** (Vifor Pharma UK Ltd)

Iron (as Ferric carboxymaltose) 50 mg per 1 ml Ferinject 1000mg/20ml dispersion for injection vials | 1 vial PoM £154.23 (Hospital only)

Ferinject 500mg/10ml dispersion for injection vials | 5 vial PoM £477.50 (Hospital only)

705

Iron dextran
14-Apr-2025

- **INDICATIONS AND DOSE**

Iron-deficiency anaemia

▶ BY DEEP INTRAMUSCULAR INJECTION

▶ Child 14–17 years: Intramuscular injection to be administered into the gluteal muscle, doses calculated according to body-weight and iron deficit (consult product literature)

▶ BY SLOW INTRAVENOUS INJECTION, OR BY INTRAVENOUS INFUSION

▶ Child: Doses calculated according to body-weight and iron deficit (consult product literature)

- **UNLICENSED USE** Not licensed for use in children under 14 years.

IMPORTANT SAFETY INFORMATION
CosmoFer® should only be administered when appropriately trained staff and resuscitation facilities are immediately available; patients should be closely monitored during and for at least 30 minutes following each injection.

- **INTERACTIONS** → Appendix 1: iron
- **SIDE-EFFECTS**
▶ **Uncommon** Feeling hot
▶ **Rare or very rare** Deafness (transient) · haemolysis
▶ **Frequency not known** Injection site necrosis · rheumatoid arthritis aggravated
- **HEPATIC IMPAIRMENT** Manufacturer advises avoid in decompensated cirrhosis and hepatitis.
- **RENAL IMPAIRMENT** EvGr Avoid in acute renal failure. (M)
- **PRESCRIBING AND DISPENSING INFORMATION** A complex of ferric hydroxide with dextran containing 5% (50 mg/mL) of iron.
- **MEDICINAL FORMS** There can be variation in the licensing of different medicines containing the same drug.

Solution for injection

▶ **CosmoFer** (Pharmacosmos UK Ltd)
Iron (as iron dextran) 50 mg per 1 ml CosmoFer 500mg/10ml solution for injection ampoules | 2 ampoule PoM £79.70 DT = £79.70
CosmoFer 100mg/2ml solution for injection ampoules | 5 ampoule PoM £39.85 DT = £39.85

705

Iron sucrose
14-Apr-2025

- **INDICATIONS AND DOSE**

Iron-deficiency anaemia

▶ BY SLOW INTRAVENOUS INJECTION, OR BY INTRAVENOUS INFUSION

▶ Child (body-weight up to 67 kg): Dose calculated according to body-weight and iron deficit, each divided dose should not exceed 3 mg/kg/dose (consult product literature)

▶ Child (body-weight 67 kg and above): Dose calculated according to body-weight and iron deficit, each divided dose should not exceed max. 200 mg/dose (consult product literature)

- **UNLICENSED USE** Not licensed for use in children.
- **INTERACTIONS** → Appendix 1: iron
- **SIDE-EFFECTS**
▶ **Uncommon** Asthenia
▶ **Rare or very rare** Drowsiness · urine discolouration
▶ **Frequency not known** Cold sweat · confusion · level of consciousness decreased · thrombophlebitis
- **HEPATIC IMPAIRMENT** Manufacturer advises caution—monitor iron status to avoid iron overload; avoid where iron overload is a precipitating factor (particularly porphyria cutanea tarda).
- **PRESCRIBING AND DISPENSING INFORMATION** A complex of ferric hydroxide with sucrose containing 2% (20 mg/mL) of iron.
- **MEDICINAL FORMS** There can be variation in the licensing of different medicines containing the same drug.

Solution for injection

▶ **Venofer** (Imported (United States), Vifor Pharma UK Ltd)
Iron (as iron sucrose) 20 mg per 1 ml Venofer 50mg/2.5ml solution for injection vials | 5 vial PoM
Venofer 100mg/5ml solution for injection vials | 5 vial PoM £51.20 DT = £51.20

MINERALS AND TRACE ELEMENTS › IRON, ORAL

Iron (oral)

- **SIDE-EFFECTS**
▶ **Common or very common** Constipation · diarrhoea · gastrointestinal discomfort · nausea
▶ **Uncommon** Vomiting
▶ **Frequency not known** Appetite decreased · gastrointestinal disorders

SIDE-EFFECTS, FURTHER INFORMATION Iron can be constipating and occasionally lead to faecal impaction. Oral iron can exacerbate diarrhoea in patients with inflammatory bowel disease; care is also needed in patients with intestinal strictures and diverticular disease.

Overdose Iron preparations are an important cause of accidental overdose in children and as little as 20 mg/kg of elemental iron can lead to symptoms of toxicity.

For details on the management of poisoning, see Iron salts, under Emergency treatment of poisoning p. 1036.

- **MONITORING REQUIREMENTS** EvGr Monitor haemoglobin and ferritin concentrations within the first 6 weeks to 3 months of treatment to assess response and ensure concentrations are increasing. Further monitoring thereafter as needed if the child remains symptomatic. Once haemoglobin is within the normal range, treatment should be continued for around a further 3 months to replenish iron stores. (E)
- **PRESCRIBING AND DISPENSING INFORMATION** Express the dose in terms of elemental iron and iron salt and select the most appropriate preparation; specify both the iron salt and formulation on the prescription.

The iron content of artificial formula feeds should also be considered.

The most common reason for lack of response in children is poor compliance; poor absorption is rare in children.

- **PATIENT AND CARER ADVICE** It is recommended to take iron on an empty stomach to allow for better absorption, although it can be taken after food to reduce gastro-intestinal side-effects if necessary. Certain food and drinks, such as milk or dairy products, unprocessed bran, tea, and coffee can reduce the absorption of oral iron. May discolour stools. EvGr When used in neonates and infants, iron supplements may be given just before a milk feed or diluted in a small volume of the milk feed. (E)

above

Ferrous fumarate
27-Jan-2025

- **INDICATIONS AND DOSE**

Iron-deficiency anaemia [treatment and prophylaxis]

▶ BY MOUTH USING TABLETS

▶ Child 6–11 years: 210 mg once daily on alternate days

▶ Child 12–17 years: Initially 210 mg once daily, reduced if not tolerated to 210 mg once daily on

continued →

9 Blood and nutrition

alternate days, alternatively initially 322 mg once daily, reduced if not tolerated to 322 mg once daily on alternate days

- ▶ BY MOUTH USING CAPSULES
- ▸ Child 12–17 years: 305 mg once daily, reduced if not tolerated to 305 mg once daily on alternate days
- ▶ BY MOUTH USING ORAL SOLUTION
- ▸ Neonate: 1 mL once daily, reduced if not tolerated to 1 mL once daily on alternate days.
- ▸ Child 1–11 months: 1.2 mL once daily, reduced if not tolerated to 1.2 mL once daily on alternate days
- ▸ Child 1–4 years: 2.5 mL once daily, reduced if not tolerated to 2.5 mL once daily on alternate days
- ▸ Child 5–11 years: 5 mL once daily, reduced if not tolerated to 5 mL once daily on alternate days
- ▸ Child 12–17 years: 5–10 mL once daily, reduced if not tolerated to 5–10 mL once daily on alternate days

Iron-deficiency anaemia [prophylaxis in preterm or low birth-weight babies who are solely or partially breast-fed]

- ▶ BY MOUTH USING ORAL SOLUTION
- ▸ Neonate: 0.3–0.6 mL once daily, supplementation is usually started 2–6 weeks after birth.
- ▸ Child 1–11 months: 0.3–0.6 mL once daily, supplementation is usually started 2–6 weeks after birth and continued for 6–12 months or until receiving sufficient iron-rich formula, dose can be increased if necessary to 1.2 mL once daily

DOSE EQUIVALENCE AND CONVERSION

- ▸ Tablets contain ferrous fumarate 210 mg (equivalent to 69 mg elemental iron) or ferrous fumarate 322 mg (equivalent to 106 mg elemental iron).
- ▸ Capsules contain ferrous fumarate 305 mg equivalent to 100 mg elemental iron.
- ▸ Oral solutions contain ferrous fumarate 28 mg/mL equivalent to 9 mg/mL elemental iron.

● **UNLICENSED USE** Ferrous fumarate may be used as detailed below, although doses may differ from those licensed:

- EvGr treatment and prophylaxis of iron-deficiency anaemia in neonates and children aged under 12 years; ⟨E⟩
- EvGr treatment and prophylaxis of iron-deficiency anaemia in children aged 12–17 years; ⟨A⟩
- EvGr prophylaxis of iron-deficiency anaemia in preterm or low birth-weight babies. ⟨E⟩

● **INTERACTIONS** → Appendix 1: iron

● **SIDE-EFFECTS** Haemosiderosis

● **PATIENT AND CARER ADVICE**
Medicines for Children leaflet: Ferrous fumarate for iron-deficiency anaemia www.medicinesforchildren.org.uk/medicines/ferrous-fumarate-for-iron-deficiency-anaemia/

● **MEDICINAL FORMS** There can be variation in the licensing of different medicines containing the same drug.

Oral tablet

- ▸ Ferrous fumarate (Non-proprietary)
Ferrous fumarate 210 mg Ferrous fumarate 210mg tablets | 84 tablet P £4.00 DT = £2.38
Ferrous fumarate 322 mg Ferrous fumarate 322mg tablets | 28 tablet P £1.00 DT = £1.00

Oral solution

- ▸ Ferrous fumarate (Non-proprietary)
Ferrous fumarate 28 mg per 1 ml Ferrous fumarate 140mg/5ml oral solution | 200 ml P £3.92 DT = £3.92
- ▸ Galfer (Thornton & Ross Ltd)
Ferrous fumarate 28 mg per 1 ml Galfer 140mg/5ml syrup | 300 ml P £5.33 DT = £5.33 SF

Oral capsule

- ▸ Galfer (Thornton & Ross Ltd)
Ferrous fumarate 305 mg Galfer 305mg capsules | 100 capsule P £5.00 DT = £5.00 | 250 capsule P £12.50

707

Ferrous gluconate

27-Jan-2025

● **INDICATIONS AND DOSE**

Iron-deficiency anaemia [treatment and prophylaxis]

- ▶ BY MOUTH USING TABLETS
- ▸ Child 6–11 years: 300 mg once daily, reduced if not tolerated to 300 mg once daily on alternate days
- ▸ Child 12–17 years: 600 mg once daily, reduced if not tolerated to 600 mg once daily on alternate days

DOSE EQUIVALENCE AND CONVERSION

- ▸ Tablets contain ferrous gluconate 300 mg equivalent to 35 mg elemental iron.

● **UNLICENSED USE** Ferrous gluconate may be used as detailed below, although doses may differ from those licensed:

- EvGr treatment and prophylaxis of iron-deficiency anaemia in children aged 6–11 years; ⟨E⟩
- EvGr treatment and prophylaxis of iron-deficiency anaemia in children aged 12–17 years. ⟨A⟩

● **INTERACTIONS** → Appendix 1: iron

● **PATIENT AND CARER ADVICE**
Medicines for Children leaflet: Ferrous gluconate for iron-deficiency anaemia www.medicinesforchildren.org.uk/medicines/ferrous-gluconate-for-iron-deficiency-anaemia/

● **MEDICINAL FORMS** There can be variation in the licensing of different medicines containing the same drug.

Oral tablet

- ▸ Ferrous gluconate (Non-proprietary)
Ferrous gluconate 300 mg Ferrous gluconate 300mg tablets | 28 tablet P £5.49 DT = £5.84 | 1000 tablet P £47.86–£119.64

707

Ferrous sulfate

27-Jan-2025

● **INDICATIONS AND DOSE**

Iron-deficiency anaemia [treatment and prophylaxis]

- ▶ BY MOUTH USING TABLETS
- ▸ Child 6–11 years: 200 mg once daily on alternate days
- ▸ Child 12–17 years: 200 mg once daily, reduced if not tolerated to 200 mg once daily on alternate days
- ▶ BY MOUTH USING ORAL DROPS
- ▸ Neonate: 0.3 mL once daily, reduced if not tolerated to 0.3 mL once daily on alternate days.
- ▸ Child 1–11 months: 0.4 mL once daily, reduced if not tolerated to 0.4 mL once daily on alternate days
- ▸ Child 1–4 years: 0.8 mL once daily, reduced if not tolerated to 0.8 mL once daily on alternate days
- ▸ Child 5–11 years: 1.6 mL once daily, reduced if not tolerated to 1.6 mL once daily on alternate days
- ▸ Child 12–17 years: 2–4 mL once daily, reduced if not tolerated to 2–4 mL once daily on alternate days

Iron-deficiency anaemia [prophylaxis in preterm or low birth-weight babies who are solely or partially breast-fed]

- ▶ BY MOUTH USING ORAL DROPS
- ▸ Neonate: 0.1–0.2 mL once daily, supplementation is usually started 2–6 weeks after birth.
- ▸ Child 1–11 months: 0.1–0.2 mL once daily, supplementation is usually started 2–6 weeks after birth and continued for 6–12 months or until receiving sufficient iron-rich formula, dose can be increased if necessary to 0.4 mL once daily

DOSE EQUIVALENCE AND CONVERSION
- Tablets contain ferrous sulfate 200 mg (equivalent to 65 mg elemental iron) or ferrous sulfate 325 mg (equivalent to 105 mg elemental iron).
- Oral drops contain ferrous sulfate 125 mg/mL equivalent to 25 mg/mL elemental iron.

- **UNLICENSED USE** Ferrous sulfate may be used as detailed below, although doses may differ from those licensed:
  - EvGr treatment and prophylaxis of iron-deficiency anaemia in neonates and children aged under 12 years; (E)
  - EvGr treatment and prophylaxis of iron-deficiency anaemia in children aged 12–17 years; (A)
  - EvGr prophylaxis of iron-deficiency anaemia in preterm or low birth-weight babies. (E)
- **INTERACTIONS** → Appendix 1: iron
- **SIDE-EFFECTS** Tooth discolouration
- **PATIENT AND CARER ADVICE**
Medicines for Children leaflet: Ferrous sulfate for iron-deficiency anaemia www.medicinesforchildren.org.uk/medicines/ferrous-sulfate-for-iron-deficiency-anaemia/
- **MEDICINAL FORMS** There can be variation in the licensing of different medicines containing the same drug.

Oral tablet
- Ferrous sulfate (Non-proprietary)
Ferrous sulfate dried 200 mg Ferrous sulfate 200mg tablets | 28 tablet P £1.41 DT = £0.91 | 60 tablet P £2.28–£3.05 | 100 tablet P £3.00–£5.00 | 1000 tablet P £38.21–£47.66

Oral drops
- Ironorm (Wallace Manufacturing Chemists Ltd)
Ferrous sulfate 125 mg per 1 ml Ironorm 125mg/ml oral drops | 15 ml P £30.00 DT = £30.00 SF

707

Sodium feredetate
27-Jan-2025

(Sodium ironedetate)

- **INDICATIONS AND DOSE**

Iron-deficiency anaemia [treatment and prophylaxis]

▶ BY MOUTH USING ORAL SOLUTION
- Neonate: 1.5 mL once daily, reduced if not tolerated to 1.5 mL once daily on alternate days.
- Child 1-11 months: 2 mL once daily, reduced if not tolerated to 2 mL once daily on alternate days
- Child 1-4 years: 4 mL once daily, reduced if not tolerated to 4 mL once daily on alternate days
- Child 5-11 years: 8 mL once daily, reduced if not tolerated to 8 mL once daily on alternate days
- Child 12-17 years: 10–15 mL once daily, reduced if not tolerated to 10–15 mL once daily on alternate days

Iron-deficiency anaemia [prophylaxis in preterm or low birth-weight babies who are solely or partially breast-fed]

▶ BY MOUTH USING ORAL SOLUTION
- Neonate: 0.5–1 mL once daily, supplementation is usually started 2–6 weeks after birth.
- Child 1-11 months: 0.5–1 mL once daily, supplementation is usually started 2–6 weeks after birth and continued for 6–12 months or until receiving sufficient iron-rich formula, dose can be increased if necessary to 2 mL once daily

DOSE EQUIVALENCE AND CONVERSION
- *Feredet*® and *Sodifer*® oral solutions contain sodium feredetate 38 mg/mL equivalent to 5.5 mg/mL elemental iron.
- *Sytron*® oral solution contains sodium feredetate trihydrate 41.5 mg/mL equivalent to 5.5 mg/mL elemental iron.

- **UNLICENSED USE** Sodium feredetate may be used as detailed below, although doses may differ from those licensed:
  - EvGr treatment and prophylaxis of iron-deficiency anaemia in neonates and children aged under 12 years; (E)
  - EvGr treatment and prophylaxis of iron-deficiency anaemia in children aged 12–17 years; (A)
  - EvGr prophylaxis of iron-deficiency anaemia in preterm or low birth-weight babies. (E)
- **INTERACTIONS** → Appendix 1: iron
- **PATIENT AND CARER ADVICE**
Medicines for Children leaflet: Sodium feredetate for the prevention of anaemia www.medicinesforchildren.org.uk/medicines/sodium-feredetate-for-the-prevention-of-anaemia/
Medicines for Children leaflet: Sodium feredetate for the treatment of anaemia www.medicinesforchildren.org.uk/medicines/sodium-feredetate-for-the-treatment-of-anaemia/
- **MEDICINAL FORMS** There can be variation in the licensing of different medicines containing the same drug.

Oral solution
EXCIPIENTS: May contain Ethanol, hydroxybenzoates (parabens), sorbitol
- Sytron (Grunenthal Ltd)
Iron (as Sodium feredetate) 5.5 mg per 1 ml Sytron oral solution | 500 ml P £14.95 DT = £14.95 SF

1.3 Megaloblastic anaemia

Anaemia, megaloblastic
12-Jul-2022

Overview

Megaloblastic anaemias are rare in children; they may result from a lack of either vitamin B_{12} or folate and it is essential to establish in every case which deficiency is present and the underlying cause. In emergencies, when delay might be dangerous, it is sometimes necessary to administer both substances after the bone marrow test while plasma assay results are awaited. Normally, however, appropriate treatment should not be instituted until the results of tests are available.

Vitamin B_{12} is used in the treatment of megaloblastosis caused by *prolonged nitrous oxide anaesthesia*, which inactivates the vitamin, and in the rare disorders of *congenital transcobalamin II deficiency* and *homocystinuria*.

Vitamin B_{12} should be given prophylactically after *total ileal resection*.

Apart from dietary deficiency, all other causes of vitamin B_{12} deficiency are attributable to malabsorption. There is little place for the use of low-dose vitamin B_{12} orally and none for vitamin B_{12} intrinsic factor complexes given by mouth. Vitamin B_{12} in larger oral doses may be effective.

Hydroxocobalamin p. 711 is retained in the body longer than cyanocobalamin p. 711 and thus for maintenance therapy can be given at intervals of up to 3 months. Treatment is generally initiated with frequent administration of intramuscular injections to replenish the depleted body stores. Thereafter, maintenance treatment, which is usually for life, can be instituted. There is no evidence that doses larger than those recommended provide any additional benefit in vitamin B_{12} neuropathy.

Folic acid p. 710 has few indications for long-term therapy since most causes of folate deficiency are self-limiting or will yield to a short course of treatment. It should not be used in undiagnosed megaloblastic anaemia unless vitamin B_{12} is administered concurrently otherwise neuropathy may be precipitated.

In *folate-deficient megaloblastic anaemia* (e.g. because of poor nutrition, pregnancy, or antiepileptic drugs), daily folic acid supplementation for 4 months brings about haematological remission and replenishes body stores; higher doses may be necessary in malabsorption states. In pregnancy, folic acid daily is continued to term.

For prophylaxis in *chronic haemolytic states*, *malabsorption*, or *in renal dialysis*, folic acid is given daily or sometimes weekly, depending on the diet and the rate of haemolysis.

Folic acid is also used for the prevention of methotrexate-induced side-effects in juvenile idiopathic arthritis, severe Crohn's disease and severe psoriasis.

Folic acid is actively excreted in breast milk and is well absorbed by the infant. It is also present in cow's milk and artificial formula feeds but is heat labile. Serum and red cell folate concentrations fall after delivery and urinary losses are high, particularly in low birth-weight neonates. Although symptomatic deficiency is rare in the absence of malabsorption or prolonged diarrhoea, it is common for neonatal units to give supplements of folic acid to all preterm neonates from 2 weeks of age until full-term corrected age is reached, particularly if heated breast milk is used without an artificial formula fortifier.

Folinic acid p. 683 is also effective in the treatment of folate deficient megaloblastic anaemia but it is normally only used in association with cytotoxic drugs; it is given as calcium folinate.

There is **no** justification for prescribing multiple ingredient vitamin preparations containing vitamin B_{12} or folic acid.

For the use of folic acid before and during pregnancy, see Neural tube defects (prevention in pregnancy) p. 796.

VITAMINS AND TRACE ELEMENTS › FOLATES

Folic acid

10-Nov-2021

● **INDICATIONS AND DOSE**

Folate-deficient megaloblastic anaemia

▶ BY MOUTH

- Neonate: Initially 500 micrograms/kg once daily for up to 4 months.
- Child 1–11 months: Initially 500 micrograms/kg once daily (max. per dose 5 mg) for up to 4 months, doses up to 10 mg per day may be required in malabsorption states
- Child 1–17 years: 5 mg once daily for 4 months (until term in pregnant women), doses up to 15 mg per day may be required in malabsorption states

Folate supplementation in neonates

▶ BY MOUTH

- Neonate: 50 micrograms once daily.

Prevention of neural tube defects [in those at a low risk of conceiving a child with a neural tube defect]

▶ BY MOUTH

- Females of childbearing potential: 400 micrograms once daily to be taken before conception and until week 12 of pregnancy

Prevention of neural tube defects [in those in the high-risk group who wish to become pregnant or who are at risk of becoming pregnant]

▶ BY MOUTH

- Females of childbearing potential: 5 mg once daily to be taken before conception and until week 12 of pregnancy

Prevention of neural tube defects [in those with sickle-cell disease]

▶ BY MOUTH

- Females of childbearing potential: 5 mg once daily, patient should continue taking their normal dose of folic acid 5 mg once daily (or increase the dose to 5 mg once daily) before conception and continue this throughout pregnancy

Prevention of methotrexate side-effects in severe Crohn's disease | Prevention of methotrexate side-effects in severe psoriasis

▶ BY MOUTH

- Child: 5 mg once weekly, dose to be taken on a different day to methotrexate dose

Prophylaxis of folate deficiency in dialysis

▶ BY MOUTH

- Child 1 month–11 years: 250 micrograms/kg once daily (max. per dose 10 mg)
- Child 12–17 years: 5–10 mg once daily

Haemolytic anaemia | Metabolic disorders

▶ BY MOUTH

- Child 1 month–11 years: 2.5–5 mg once daily
- Child 12–17 years: 5–10 mg once daily

Prevention of methotrexate side-effects in juvenile idiopathic arthritis

▶ BY MOUTH

- Child: 1 mg once daily, dose to be adjusted according to local guidelines, alternatively 5 mg once weekly, weekly dose to be taken on a different day to methotrexate dose, dose to be adjusted according to local guidelines

● **UNLICENSED USE** Unlicensed for limiting methotrexate toxicity.

● **CAUTIONS** Should never be given alone for pernicious anaemia or other megaloblastic anaemias caused by vitamin B_{12} deficiency (may precipitate subacute combined degeneration of the spinal cord)

● **INTERACTIONS** → Appendix 1: folates

● **SIDE-EFFECTS** Abdominal distension · appetite decreased · flatulence · nausea · vitamin B12 deficiency exacerbated

● **PATIENT AND CARER ADVICE**

Medicines for Children leaflet: Folic acid for megaloblastic anaemia caused by folate deficiency and haemolytic anaemia www.medicinesforchildren.org.uk/medicines/folic-acid-for-megaloblastic-anaemia-caused-by-folate-deficiency-and-haemolytic-anaemia/

● **EXCEPTIONS TO LEGAL CATEGORY** Can be sold to the public provided daily doses do not exceed 500 micrograms.

● **MEDICINAL FORMS** There can be variation in the licensing of different medicines containing the same drug. Forms available from special-order manufacturers include: oral capsule, oral suspension, oral solution

Oral tablet

- **Folic acid (Non-proprietary)**
  Folic acid 400 microgram Folic acid 400microgram tablets | 90 tablet [P] £9.95–£17.12 DT = £5.54
  Folic acid 5 mg Folic acid 5mg tablets | 28 tablet [PoM] £0.95 DT = £0.66

Oral solution

- **Folic acid (Non-proprietary)**
  Folic acid 500 microgram per 1 ml Folic acid 2.5mg/5ml oral solution sugar free | 150 ml [PoM] £9.16 DT = £9.16 [SF]
  Folic acid 1 mg per 1 ml Folic acid 5mg/5ml oral solution sugar free | 150 ml [PoM] £48.02–£83.07 DT = £77.26 [SF]
- **Lexpec** (Rosemont Pharmaceuticals Ltd)
  Folic acid 500 microgram per 1 ml Lexpec Folic Acid 2.5mg/5ml oral solution | 150 ml [PoM] £9.16 DT = £9.16 [SF]

VITAMINS AND TRACE ELEMENTS › VITAMIN B GROUP

Cyanocobalamin

28-Mar-2024

● **INDICATIONS AND DOSE**

Prophylaxis of macrocytic anaemias associated with vitamin B_{12} deficiency

▶ BY INTRAMUSCULAR INJECTION
- Child: 0.25–1 mg once a month

Pernicious anaemia and other macrocytic anaemias without neurological involvement

▶ BY INTRAMUSCULAR INJECTION
- Child: Initially 0.25–1 mg once daily on alternate days for 1 to 2 weeks, then 0.25 mg once weekly until blood count normal; maintenance 1 mg once a month

Pernicious anaemia and other macrocytic anaemias with neurological involvement

▶ BY INTRAMUSCULAR INJECTION
- Child: 1 mg once daily on alternate days as long as improvement occurs; maintenance 1 mg once a month

Dietary vitamin B_{12} deficiency

▶ BY MOUTH
- Child: 50 micrograms once daily, dose to be taken between meals, dose may be adjusted as clinically indicated

Dietary vitamin B_{12} deficiency during pregnancy or breast feeding

▶ BY MOUTH
- Child 16–17 years: 1 mg once daily, dose to be taken between meals, dose may be increased as clinically indicated

Vitamin B_{12} deficiency due to malabsorption

▶ BY MOUTH
- Child 16–17 years: 1 mg once daily, dose to be taken between meals, dose may be increased as clinically indicated

● **UNLICENSED USE** Cyanocobalamin is used in the doses provided in BNFC from the age of 16 years in the situations detailed below, although these may differ from those licensed:
- EvGr dietary vitamin B_{12} deficiency during pregnancy or breast feeding
- vitamin B_{12} deficiency due to malabsorption ⟨A⟩

IMPORTANT SAFETY INFORMATION

MHRA/CHM ADVICE: VITAMIN B_{12} (CYANOCOBALAMIN): ADVISE PATIENTS WITH KNOWN COBALT ALLERGY TO BE VIGILANT FOR SENSITIVITY REACTIONS (DECEMBER 2023)

Following a report via the Yellow Card Scheme, the MHRA conducted a review and found evidence in the literature of cobalt sensitivity-type reactions in patients being treated for vitamin B_{12} deficiency; other similar reports have also been received. Such reactions typically present with cutaneous symptoms of chronic or subacute allergic contact dermatitis (an erythema multiforme-like eruption may infrequently be triggered); onset may be immediate or delayed up to 72 hours after vitamin B_{12} administration. Vitamin B_{12} (i.e. cyanocobalamin or hydroxocobalamin) contains cobalt and 1 to 3% of the general population is estimated to have cobalt allergy.

Healthcare professionals are recommended to assess the benefits and risks of continuing treatment in patients who develop cobalt sensitivity-type reactions and, if necessary to continue, advise such patients on appropriate symptom management. Patients with known cobalt allergy should be advised to speak to a healthcare professional if they are prescribed vitamin B_{12} and be alert for symptoms of cobalt sensitivity-type reactions. All patients should be counselled to seek medical advice if they develop allergic skin reactions whilst on vitamin B_{12} therapy; urgent medical attention must be sought if symptoms of a serious allergic reaction, such as extensive or blistering rash, wheeze, difficulty breathing, or feeling faint, occur.

● **PRESCRIBING AND DISPENSING INFORMATION** Currently available brands of the tablet may not be suitable for vegans.

● **NATIONAL FUNDING/ACCESS DECISIONS**
NHS restrictions *Cytamen*® injection is not prescribable in NHS primary care.

● **LESS SUITABLE FOR PRESCRIBING** Cyanocobalamin injection is less suitable for prescribing.

● **MEDICINAL FORMS** There can be variation in the licensing of different medicines containing the same drug.

Oral tablet

▶ **Cyanocobalamin (Non-proprietary)**
Cyanocobalamin 50 microgram Cyanocobalamin 50microgram tablets | 50 tablet P £30.00 DT = £2.42
Cyanocobalamin 500 microgram Acyanocomin 500microgram tablets | 50 tablet £6.89
Cyanocobalamin 1 mg Behepan 1mg tablets | 100 tablet PoM ⊠

▶ **ActivB12** (MaN Pharma Ltd)
Cyanocobalamin 100 microgram ActivB12 100microgram tablets | 28 tablet £1.95 | 50 tablet £3.22

▶ **CyanocoB12** (TriOn Pharma Ltd)
Cyanocobalamin 100 microgram CyanocoB12 100microgram tablets | 28 tablet £1.94 | 50 tablet £3.19
Cyanocobalamin 500 microgram CyanocoB12 500microgram tablets | 50 tablet £6.89

▶ **CyanocoMinn** (Essential-Healthcare Ltd)
Cyanocobalamin 100 microgram CyanocoMinn 100microgram tablets | 28 tablet £1.87 | 50 tablet £3.21

▶ **Orobalin** (Northumbria Pharma Ltd)
Cyanocobalamin 1 mg Orobalin 1mg tablets | 30 tablet PoM £9.99 DT = £9.99

▶ **SunVit-Pro (Cyanocobalamin)** (SunVit-D3 Ltd)
Cyanocobalamin 100 microgram SunVit-Pro Vitamin B12 100microgram tablets | 50 tablet £3.79

Hydroxocobalamin

29-Jan-2024

● **INDICATIONS AND DOSE**

Macrocytic anaemia without neurological involvement

▶ BY INTRAMUSCULAR INJECTION
- Child: Initially 0.25–1 mg once daily on alternate days for 1–2 weeks, then 0.25 mg once weekly until blood count normal, then 1 mg every 2–3 months

Macrocytic anaemia with neurological involvement

▶ BY INTRAMUSCULAR INJECTION
- Child: Initially 1 mg once daily on alternate days until no further improvement, then 1 mg every 2 months

Prophylaxis of macrocytic anaemias associated with vitamin B_{12} deficiency

▶ BY INTRAMUSCULAR INJECTION
- Child: 1 mg every 2–3 months

Leber's optic atrophy

▶ BY INTRAMUSCULAR INJECTION
- Child: Initially 1 mg daily for 2 weeks, then 1 mg twice weekly until no further improvement, then 1 mg every 1–3 months

Congenital transcobalamin II deficiency

▶ BY INTRAMUSCULAR INJECTION
- Neonate: 1 mg 3 times a week for 1 year, then reduced to 1 mg once weekly, adjusted as appropriate.
- Child: 1 mg 3 times a week for 1 year, then reduced to 1 mg once weekly, adjusted as appropriate

continued →

Methylmalonic acidaemia and homocystinuria
- ▶ BY INTRAMUSCULAR INJECTION
- ▸ Child: Initially 1 mg daily for 5–7 days, then adjusted according to response to up to 1 mg 1–2 times a week, this is the maintenance dose

Methylmalonic acidaemia, maintenance once intramuscular response established
- ▶ BY MOUTH
- ▸ Child: 5–10 mg 1–2 times a week, some children do not respond to oral route

CYANOKIT®

Poisoning with cyanides
- ▶ BY INTRAVENOUS INFUSION
- ▸ Child (body-weight 5 kg and above): Initially 70 mg/kg (max. per dose 5 g), to be given over 15 minutes, then 70 mg/kg (max. per dose 5 g) if required, this second dose can be given over 15 minutes–2 hours depending on severity of poisoning and patient stability

● **UNLICENSED USE**
- ▸ With intramuscular use or oral use Licensed for use in children (age not specified by manufacturers). Not licensed for use in inborn errors of metabolism.

IMPORTANT SAFETY INFORMATION

MHRA/CHM ADVICE: VITAMIN B_{12} (HYDROXOCOBALAMIN): ADVISE PATIENTS WITH KNOWN COBALT ALLERGY TO BE VIGILANT FOR SENSITIVITY REACTIONS (DECEMBER 2023)

Following a report via the Yellow Card Scheme, the MHRA conducted a review and found evidence in the literature of cobalt sensitivity-type reactions in patients being treated for vitamin B_{12} deficiency; other similar reports have also been received. Such reactions typically present with cutaneous symptoms of chronic or subacute allergic contact dermatitis (an erythema multiforme-like eruption may infrequently be triggered); onset may be immediate or delayed up to 72 hours after vitamin B_{12} administration. Vitamin B_{12} (i.e. cyanocobalamin or hydroxocobalamin) contains cobalt and 1 to 3% of the general population is estimated to have cobalt allergy.

Healthcare professionals are recommended to assess the benefits and risks of continuing treatment in patients who develop cobalt sensitivity-type reactions and, if necessary to continue, advise such patients on appropriate symptom management. Patients with known cobalt allergy should be advised to speak to a healthcare professional if they are prescribed vitamin B_{12} and be alert for symptoms of cobalt sensitivity-type reactions. All patients should be counselled to seek medical advice if they develop allergic skin reactions whilst on vitamin B_{12} therapy; urgent medical attention must be sought if symptoms of a serious allergic reaction, such as extensive or blistering rash, wheeze, difficulty breathing, or feeling faint, occur.

Hydroxocobalamin preparations used for the treatment of known or suspected cyanide poisoning are excluded from these precautions because the potentially life-saving benefit of treatment in a medical emergency outweighs the risk of an allergic reaction.

● **CAUTIONS** Diagnosis of vitamin B_{12} deficiency should be confirmed before giving hydroxocobalamin

● **SIDE-EFFECTS**

GENERAL SIDE-EFFECTS Diarrhoea · dizziness · headache · hot flush · nausea · skin reactions · urine discolouration

SPECIFIC SIDE-EFFECTS
- ▸ With intramuscular use Arrhythmia · chills · drug fever · hypokalaemia · malaise · pain · thrombocytosis · tremor · vomiting
- ▸ With intravenous use Angioedema · dysphagia · extrasystole · gastrointestinal discomfort · memory loss · mucosal discolouration red · peripheral oedema · pleural effusion · rash pustular · red discolouration of plasma · restlessness · swelling · throat complaints

● **BREAST FEEDING** Present in milk but not known to be harmful.

● **EFFECT ON LABORATORY TESTS**
- ▸ With intravenous use Deep red colour of hydroxocobalamin may interfere with laboratory tests.

● **DIRECTIONS FOR ADMINISTRATION** For *intravenous infusion (Cyanokit®)*, give intermittently *in* Sodium Chloride 0.9%, reconstitute 5 g vial with 200 mL Sodium Chloride 0.9%; gently invert vial for at least 1 minute to mix (do not shake).

For administration by *mouth*, expert sources advise injection solution may be given orally.

● **PRESCRIBING AND DISPENSING INFORMATION**
- ▸ With intramuscular use The BP directs that when vitamin B_{12} injection is prescribed or demanded, hydroxocobalamin injection shall be dispensed or supplied.

Poisoning by cyanides
- ▸ With intravenous use *Cyanokit®* is the only preparation of hydroxocobalamin that is suitable for use in victims of smoke inhalation who show signs of significant cyanide poisoning.

● **NATIONAL FUNDING/ACCESS DECISIONS**

NHS restrictions *Cobalin-H®* is not prescribable in NHS primary care.

Neo-Cytamen® is not prescribable in NHS primary care.

● **MEDICINAL FORMS** There can be variation in the licensing of different medicines containing the same drug. Forms available from special-order manufacturers include: oral suspension, oral solution

Solution for injection
- ▸ **Hydroxocobalamin (Non-proprietary)**
  Hydroxocobalamin 1 mg per 1 ml Hydroxocobalamin 1mg/1ml solution for injection ampoules | 5 ampoule PoM £20.60 DT = £11.06
  Hydroxocobalamin 2.5 mg per 1 ml Hepavit 5mg/2ml solution for injection ampoules | 2 ampoule PoM (Hospital only)
  Hydroxocobalamin 5 mg per 1 ml Megamilbedoce 10mg/2ml solution for injection ampoules | 10 ampoule PoM
- ▸ **Neo-Cytamen** (RPH Pharmaceuticals AB)
  Hydroxocobalamin 1 mg per 1 ml Neo-Cytamen 1000micrograms/1ml solution for injection ampoules | 5 ampoule PoM £12.49 DT = £11.06

Powder for solution for infusion
- ▸ **Cyanokit** (SERB)
  Hydroxocobalamin 5 gram Cyanokit 5g powder for solution for infusion vials | 1 vial PoM £772.00 (Hospital only)

2 Iron overload

Iron overload

Overview

Severe tissue iron overload can occur in aplastic and other refractory anaemias, mainly as the result of repeated blood transfusions. It is a particular problem in refractory anaemias with hyperplastic bone marrow, especially *thalassaemia major*, where excessive iron absorption from the gut and inappropriate iron therapy can add to the tissue siderosis.

Iron overload associated with haemochromatosis can be treated with repeated venesection. Venesection may also be used for patients who have received multiple transfusions and whose bone marrow has recovered. Where venesection is contra-indicated, and in thalassaemia, the long-term administration of the iron chelating compound desferrioxamine mesilate p. 714 is useful. Desferrioxamine mesilate (up to 2 g per unit of blood) may also be given at the time of blood transfusion, provided that the desferrioxamine mesilate is **not** added to the blood and is **not** given through the same line as the blood (but the two may be given through the same cannula).

Iron excretion induced by desferrioxamine mesilate is enhanced by ascorbic acid p. 786 (vitamin C) daily by mouth; it should be given separately from food since it also enhances iron absorption. Ascorbic acid should not be given to children with cardiac dysfunction; in children with normal cardiac function ascorbic acid should be introduced 1 month after starting desferrioxamine mesilate.

Desferrioxamine mesilate infusion can be used to treat *aluminium overload* in dialysis patients; theoretically 100 mg of desferrioxamine binds with 4.1 mg of aluminium.

ANTIDOTES AND CHELATORS > IRON CHELATORS

Deferasirox

23-Nov-2020

● **DRUG ACTION** Deferasirox is an oral iron chelator.

● **INDICATIONS AND DOSE**

Transfusion-related chronic iron overload when desferrioxamine is contra-indicated or inadequate in patients with beta thalassaemia major who receive frequent blood transfusions (7 mL/kg/month or more of packed red blood cells) (specialist use only)

▶ BY MOUTH

▸ Child 2–5 years: Initially 7–21 mg/kg once daily, dose adjusted according to serum-ferritin concentration and amount of transfused blood—consult product literature, then adjusted in steps of 3.5–7 mg/kg every 3–6 months, maintenance dose adjusted according to serum-ferritin concentration; maximum 28 mg/kg per day; Usual maximum 21 mg/kg

Transfusion-related chronic iron overload in patients with beta thalassaemia major who receive frequent blood transfusions (7 mL/kg/month or more of packed red blood cells) (specialist use only)

▶ BY MOUTH

▸ Child 6–17 years: Initially 7–21 mg/kg once daily, dose adjusted according to serum-ferritin concentration and amount of transfused blood—consult product literature, then adjusted in steps of 3.5–7 mg/kg every 3–6 months, maintenance dose adjusted according to serum-ferritin concentration; maximum 28 mg/kg per day; Usual maximum 21 mg/kg

Transfusion-related chronic iron overload when desferrioxamine is contra-indicated or inadequate in patients with beta thalassaemia major who receive infrequent blood transfusions (less than 7 mL/kg/month of packed red blood cells) (specialist use only) | Transfusion-related chronic iron overload when desferrioxamine is contra-indicated or inadequate in patients with other anaemias (specialist use only)

▶ BY MOUTH

▸ Child 2–17 years: Initially 7–21 mg/kg once daily, dose adjusted according to serum-ferritin concentration and amount of transfused blood—consult product literature, then adjusted in steps of 3.5–7 mg/kg every 3–6 months, maintenance dose adjusted according to serum-ferritin concentration; maximum 28 mg/kg per day; Usual maximum 21 mg/kg

Chronic iron overload when desferrioxamine is contra-indicated or inadequate in non-transfusion-dependent thalassaemia syndromes (specialist use only)

▶ BY MOUTH

▸ Child 10–17 years: Initially 7 mg/kg once daily, maintenance dose adjusted according to serum-ferritin concentration and liver-iron concentration (consult product literature); maximum 7 mg/kg per day

● **CAUTIONS** History of liver cirrhosis · not recommended in conditions which may reduce life expectancy (e.g. high-risk myelodysplastic syndromes) · platelet count less than $50x10^9$/litre · risk of gastro-intestinal ulceration and haemorrhage · unexplained cytopenia—consider treatment interruption

● **INTERACTIONS** → Appendix 1: iron chelators

● **SIDE-EFFECTS**

▶ **Common or very common** Constipation · diarrhoea · gastrointestinal discomfort · headache · nausea · skin reactions · urine abnormalities · vomiting

▶ **Uncommon** Anxiety · cataract · cholelithiasis · dizziness · fatigue · fever · gastrointestinal disorders · gastrointestinal haemorrhage (including fatal cases) · hearing impairment · hepatic disorders · laryngeal pain · maculopathy · oedema · renal tubular disorders · sleep disorder

▶ **Rare or very rare** Optic neuritis · severe cutaneous adverse reactions (SCARs)

▶ **Frequency not known** Acute kidney injury · alopecia · anaemia aggravated · hyperammonaemic encephalopathy · hypersensitivity vasculitis · lens opacity · leucopenia · metabolic acidosis · nephritis tubulointerstitial · nephrolithiasis · neutropenia · pancreatitis acute · pancytopenia · renal tubular necrosis · thrombocytopenia

● **PREGNANCY** Manufacturer advises avoid unless essential— toxicity in *animal* studies.

● **BREAST FEEDING** Manufacturer advises avoid—present in milk in *animal* studies.

● **HEPATIC IMPAIRMENT** Manufacturer advises caution in moderate impairment; avoid in severe impairment.
Dose adjustments Manufacturer advises reduce initial dose considerably then gradually increase to max. 50% of normal dose in moderate impairment.

● **RENAL IMPAIRMENT** Manufacturer advises avoid if estimated creatinine clearance less than 60 mL/minute.
Dose adjustments See p. 16.

Manufacturer advises reduce dose if serum-creatinine increased above age-appropriate limits or creatinine clearance less than 90 mL/minute on 2 consecutive occasions—consult product literature.

● **MONITORING REQUIREMENTS**

▶ Manufacturer advises monitoring of the following patient parameters: baseline serum creatinine twice and creatinine clearance once before initiation of treatment, weekly in the first month after treatment initiation or modification, then monthly thereafter; proteinuria before treatment initiation then monthly thereafter, and other markers of renal tubular function as needed; liver function before treatment initiation, every 2 weeks during the first month of treatment, then monthly thereafter; eye and ear examinations before treatment and annually during treatment; serum-ferritin concentration monthly.

▶ Manufacturer advises monitor liver-iron concentration every three months in children with non-transfusion-dependent thalassaemia syndromes when serum ferritin is ≤800 micrograms/litre.

▶ Manufacturer advises monitor body-weight, height, and sexual development before treatment and then annually thereafter.

● **DIRECTIONS FOR ADMINISTRATION** For *film-coated tablets*, manufacturer advises tablets may be crushed and sprinkled on to soft food (yoghurt or apple sauce), then administered immediately.

● **PATIENT AND CARER ADVICE** Patient or carers should be given advice on how to administer deferasirox tablets.
Medicines for Children leaflet: Deferasirox for removing excess iron
www.medicinesforchildren.org.uk/medicines/deferasirox-for-removing-excess-iron/

● **NATIONAL FUNDING/ACCESS DECISIONS**
For full details see funding body website

Scottish Medicines Consortium (SMC) decisions

▸ **Deferasirox (*Exjade*®) for the treatment of chronic iron overload due to blood transfusions when deferoxamine therapy is contra-indicated or inadequate, in adult and paediatric patients aged 2 years and older with rare acquired or inherited anaemias (January 2017)** SMC No. 347/07 Recommended with restrictions

▸ **Deferasirox (*Exjade*®) for the treatment of chronic iron overload: due to frequent blood transfusions in patients with beta thalassaemia major aged 6 years and over; due to blood transfusions when deferoxamine therapy is contra-indicated or inadequate in other patient groups (June 2017)** SMC No. 1246/17 Recommended with restrictions

● **MEDICINAL FORMS** There can be variation in the licensing of different medicines containing the same drug.

Oral tablet

CAUTIONARY AND ADVISORY LABELS 25

▸ **Deferasirox (Non-proprietary)**

Deferasirox 90 mg Deferasirox 90mg tablets | 30 tablet [PoM] £126.00 DT = £126.00 | 30 tablet [PoM] £105.00–£126.00 DT = £126.00 (Hospital only)

Deferasirox 180 mg Deferasirox 180mg tablets | 30 tablet [PoM] £252.00 DT = £252.00 | 30 tablet [PoM] £210.00–£252.00 DT = £252.00 (Hospital only)

Deferasirox 360 mg Deferasirox 360mg tablets | 30 tablet [PoM] £504.00 DT = £504.00 | 30 tablet [PoM] £424.00–£507.00 DT = £504.00 (Hospital only)

▸ **Exjade** (Novartis Pharmaceuticals UK Ltd) ▼

Deferasirox 90 mg Exjade 90mg tablets | 30 tablet [PoM] £126.00 DT = £126.00

Deferasirox 180 mg Exjade 180mg tablets | 30 tablet [PoM] £252.00 DT = £252.00

Deferasirox 360 mg Exjade 360mg tablets | 30 tablet [PoM] £504.00 DT = £504.00

Deferiprone

28-Jun-2021

● **DRUG ACTION** Deferiprone is an oral iron chelator.

● **INDICATIONS AND DOSE**

Treatment of iron overload in patients with thalassaemia major in whom desferrioxamine is contra-indicated or is inadequate

▸ BY MOUTH

▸ Child 6–17 years: 25 mg/kg 3 times a day; maximum 100 mg/kg per day

● **CONTRA-INDICATIONS** History of agranulocytosis or recurrent neutropenia

● **INTERACTIONS** → Appendix 1: iron chelators

● **SIDE-EFFECTS**

▸ **Common or very common** Abdominal pain (reducing dose and increasing gradually may improve tolerance) · agranulocytosis · appetite increased · arthralgia · diarrhoea (reducing dose and increasing gradually may improve tolerance) · fatigue · headache · nausea (reducing dose and increasing gradually may improve tolerance) · neutropenia · urine discolouration · vomiting (reducing dose and increasing gradually may improve tolerance)

▸ **Frequency not known** Skin reactions · zinc deficiency

● **CONCEPTION AND CONTRACEPTION** Manufacturer advises avoid before intended conception—teratogenic and embryotoxic in *animal* studies. Contraception advised in females of child-bearing potential.

● **PREGNANCY** Manufacturer advises avoid during pregnancy—teratogenic and embryotoxic in *animal* studies.

● **BREAST FEEDING** Manufacturer advises avoid—no information available.

● **HEPATIC IMPAIRMENT** Manufacturer advises caution (no information available)—monitor hepatic function and consider interrupting treatment if persistent elevation in serum alanine aminotransferase. Manufacturer advises caution in patients with hepatitis C (ensure iron chelation is optimal)—monitor liver histology.

● **RENAL IMPAIRMENT** [EvGr] Caution in end-stage renal disease (no information available). ⟨M⟩

● **MONITORING REQUIREMENTS** Monitor neutrophil count weekly and discontinue treatment if neutropenia develops.

● **PATIENT AND CARER ADVICE**
Blood disorders Patients or their carers should be told how to recognise signs of neutropenia and advised to seek immediate medical attention if symptoms such as fever or sore throat develop.

● **MEDICINAL FORMS** There can be variation in the licensing of different medicines containing the same drug. Forms available from special-order manufacturers include: oral capsule, oral suspension, oral solution

Oral tablet

CAUTIONARY AND ADVISORY LABELS 14

▸ **Deferiprone (Non-proprietary)**

Deferiprone 500 mg Deferiprone 500mg tablets | 100 tablet [PoM] £78.00–£130.00

▸ **Ferriprox** (Chiesi Ltd)

Deferiprone 500 mg Ferriprox 500mg tablets | 100 tablet [PoM] £130.00

Deferiprone 1 gram Ferriprox 1000mg tablets | 50 tablet [PoM] £130.00

Oral solution

CAUTIONARY AND ADVISORY LABELS 14

▸ **Ferriprox** (Chiesi Ltd)

Deferiprone 100 mg per 1 ml Ferriprox 100mg/ml oral solution | 500 ml [PoM] £152.39 [SF]

Desferrioxamine mesilate

09-Jun-2021

(Deferoxamine Mesilate)

● **INDICATIONS AND DOSE**

Iron poisoning

▸ BY CONTINUOUS INTRAVENOUS INFUSION

▸ Neonate: Initially up to 15 mg/kg/hour, max. 80 mg/kg in 24 hours, dose to be reduced after 4–6 hours, in severe cases, higher doses may be given on advice from the National Poisons Information Service.

▸ Child: Initially up to 15 mg/kg/hour, max. 80 mg/kg in 24 hours, dose to be reduced after 4–6 hours, in severe cases, higher doses may be given on advice from the National Poisons Information Service

Aluminium overload in dialysis patients

▸ BY INTRAVENOUS INFUSION

▸ Child: 5 mg/kg once weekly

Chronic iron overload (low iron overload)

▸ BY SUBCUTANEOUS INFUSION

▸ Child: Initially up to 30 mg/kg 3–7 times a week, to be given over 8–12 hours, the dose should reflect the degree of iron overload

Chronic iron overload (established overload)

▸ BY SUBCUTANEOUS INFUSION

▸ Child: 20–50 mg/kg daily

● **UNLICENSED USE**

▸ When used for Iron poisoning Licensed for use in children (age range not specified by manufacturer).

● **CAUTIONS** Aluminium-related encephalopathy (may exacerbate neurological dysfunction)

● **INTERACTIONS** → Appendix 1: iron chelators

● **SIDE-EFFECTS**
▸ **Common or very common** Arthralgia · bone disorder · fever · growth retardation · headache · muscle complaints · nausea · skin reactions
▸ **Uncommon** Abdominal pain · asthma · deafness neurosensory · tinnitus · vomiting
▸ **Rare or very rare** Angioedema · blood disorder · cataract · diarrhoea · dizziness · encephalopathy · eye disorders · hypersensitivity · hypotension (more common when given too rapidly by intravenous injection) · increased risk of infection · nerve disorders · nervous system disorder · paraesthesia · respiratory disorders · shock · tachycardia · thrombocytopenia · vision disorders
▸ **Frequency not known** Acute kidney injury · hypocalcaemia · leucopenia · renal tubular disorder · seizure · urine discolouration

● **PREGNANCY** Teratogenic in *animal* studies. Manufacturer advises use only if potential benefit outweighs risk.

● **BREAST FEEDING** Manufacturer advises use only if potential benefit outweighs risk—no information available.

● **RENAL IMPAIRMENT** EvGr Use with caution. Ⓜ

● **MONITORING REQUIREMENTS**
▸ Eye and ear examinations before treatment and at 3-month intervals during treatment.
▸ Monitor body-weight and height in children at 3-month intervals—risk of growth retardation with excessive doses.

● **DIRECTIONS FOR ADMINISTRATION** For full details and warnings relating to administration, consult product literature.

EvGr For *intravenous* or *subcutaneous infusion*, reconstitute powder with Water for Injection to a concentration of 100 mg/mL; dilute with Glucose 5% or Sodium Chloride 0.9%.

In *haemodialysis* or *haemo-filtration*, administer over the last hour of dialysis or 5 hours prior to dialysis depending on post-desferrioxamine test serum aluminium levels (consult product literature). Ⓜ Expert sources advise may be given via the dialysis fistula.

EvGr For *intraperitoneal* use, may be added to dialysis fluid. Give prior to the last exchange of the day. Ⓜ

● **MEDICINAL FORMS** There can be variation in the licensing of different medicines containing the same drug.

Powder for solution for injection

▸ **Desferrioxamine mesilate (Non-proprietary)**
Desferrioxamine mesilate 500 mg Desferrioxamine 500mg powder for solution for injection vials | 10 vial PoM £51.29 (Hospital only)
Desferrioxamine mesilate 2 gram Desferrioxamine 2g powder for solution for injection vials | 10 vial PoM £205.26

▸ **Desferal** (Novartis Pharmaceuticals UK Ltd)
Desferrioxamine mesilate 500 mg Desferal 500mg powder for solution for injection vials | 10 vial PoM £46.63

3 Neutropenia and stem cell mobilisation

3.1 Neutropenia

Neutropenia

05-Mar-2021

Management

Neutropenia is characterised by a low neutrophil count (absolute neutrophil count less than 1.5×10^9/litre). Neutropenia is a risk factor for the development of infection and sepsis, especially in patients receiving high-intensity chemotherapy regimens. Recombinant human granulocyte-colony stimulating factor (rhG-CSF) stimulates the production of neutrophils and may reduce the duration of chemotherapy-induced neutropenia and thereby reduce the incidence of associated febrile neutropenia; there is as yet no evidence that it improves overall survival. Granulocyte-colony stimulating factors include filgrastim p. 716 and lenograstim p. 717.

Filgrastim (unglycosylated rhG-CSF) and lenograstim (glycosylated rhG-CSF) have similar effects; both have been used in a variety of clinical settings for neutropenia.

Granulocyte-colony stimulating factors should only be prescribed by those experienced in their use.

Neonatal neutropenia

Expert sources advise filgrastim [unlicensed use] has been used to treat sepsis-induced neutropenia in preterm neonates. There is no clear evidence that granulocyte-colony stimulating factors improve survival or long-term outcomes.

IMMUNOSTIMULANTS › GRANULOCYTE-COLONY STIMULATING FACTORS

Granulocyte-colony stimulating factors

● **DRUG ACTION** Recombinant human granulocyte-colony stimulating factor (rhG-CSF) stimulates the production of neutrophils.

● **CAUTIONS** Malignant myeloid conditions · pre-malignant myeloid conditions · risk of splenomegaly and rupture—spleen size should be monitored · sickle-cell disease

CAUTIONS, FURTHER INFORMATION
▸ **Acute respiratory distress syndrome** There have been reports of pulmonary infiltrates leading to acute respiratory distress syndrome—patients with a recent history of pulmonary infiltrates or pneumonia may be at higher risk.

● **SIDE-EFFECTS**
▸ **Common or very common** Arthralgia · cutaneous vasculitis · dyspnoea · haemoptysis · headache · hypersensitivity · leucocytosis · pain · spleen abnormalities · thrombocytopenia
▸ **Uncommon** Acute febrile neutrophilic dermatosis · capillary leak syndrome · hypoxia · interstitial pneumonia · pulmonary fibrosis · pulmonary oedema · respiratory disorders · sickle cell anaemia with crisis

SIDE-EFFECTS, FURTHER INFORMATION Treatment should be withdrawn in patients who develop signs of pulmonary infiltration.

● **PREGNANCY** Manufacturers advise avoid—toxicity in *animal* studies.

● **BREAST FEEDING** There is no evidence for the use of granulocyte-colony stimulating factors during breast-feeding and manufacturers advise avoiding their use.

● **MONITORING REQUIREMENTS**
▸ Full blood counts including differential white cell and platelet counts should be monitored.
▸ Spleen size should be monitored during treatment—risk of splenomegaly and rupture.

F 715

Filgrastim

24-Jul-2020

(Recombinant human granulocyte-colony stimulating factor; G-CSF)

● **INDICATIONS AND DOSE**

Reduction in duration of neutropenia and incidence of febrile neutropenia in cytotoxic chemotherapy for malignancy (except chronic myeloid leukaemia and myelodysplastic syndromes) (specialist use only)

▶ BY SUBCUTANEOUS INJECTION, OR BY INTRAVENOUS INFUSION

▸ Child: 5 micrograms/kg daily until neutrophil count in normal range, usually for up to 14 days (up to 38 days in acute myeloid leukaemia), to be started at least 24 hours after cytotoxic chemotherapy. Preferably given by subcutaneous injection; if given by intravenous infusion, administer over 30 minutes

Reduction in duration of neutropenia (and associated sequelae) in myeloablative therapy followed by bone-marrow transplantation (specialist use only)

▶ BY SUBCUTANEOUS INFUSION, OR BY INTRAVENOUS INFUSION

▸ Child: 10 micrograms/kg daily, to be started at least 24 hours following cytotoxic chemotherapy and within 24 hours of bone-marrow infusion, then adjusted according to neutrophil count— consult product literature, doses administered over 30 minutes or 24 hours via intravenous route and over 24 hours via subcutaneous route

Mobilisation of peripheral blood progenitor cells for autologous infusion, used alone (specialist use only)

▶ BY SUBCUTANEOUS INFUSION, OR BY SUBCUTANEOUS INJECTION

▸ Child: 10 micrograms/kg daily for 5–7 days, to be administered over 24 hours if given by subcutaneous infusion

Mobilisation of peripheral blood progenitor cells for autologous infusion, used following adjunctive myelosuppressive chemotherapy—to improve yield (specialist use only)

▶ BY SUBCUTANEOUS INJECTION

▸ Child: 5 micrograms/kg daily until neutrophil count in normal range, to be started the day after completing chemotherapy, for timing of leucopheresis, consult product literature

Mobilisation of peripheral blood progenitor cells in normal donors for allogeneic infusion (specialist use only)

▶ BY SUBCUTANEOUS INJECTION

▸ Child 16-17 years: 10 micrograms/kg daily for 4–5 days, for timing of leucopheresis, consult product literature

Severe congenital neutropenia and history of severe or recurrent infections (distinguish carefully from other haematological disorders) (specialist use only)

▶ BY SUBCUTANEOUS INJECTION

▸ Child: Initially 12 micrograms/kg daily, adjusted according to response, can be given in single or divided doses, consult product literature and local protocol

Severe cyclic neutropenia, or idiopathic neutropenia and history of severe or recurrent infections (distinguish carefully from other haematological disorders) (specialist use only)

▶ BY SUBCUTANEOUS INJECTION

▸ Child: Initially 5 micrograms/kg daily, adjusted according to response, can be given in single or divided doses, consult product literature and local protocol

Persistent neutropenia in HIV infection (specialist use only)

▶ BY SUBCUTANEOUS INJECTION

▸ Child: Initially 1 microgram/kg daily, subsequent doses increased as necessary until neutrophil count in normal range, then adjusted to maintain neutrophil count in normal range—consult product literature; maximum 4 micrograms/kg per day

Neonatal neutropenia (specialist use only)

▶ BY SUBCUTANEOUS INJECTION

▸ Neonate: 10 micrograms/kg daily, to be discontinued if white cell count exceeds 50×10^9/litre.

Glycogen storage disease type 1b (specialist use only)

▶ BY SUBCUTANEOUS INJECTION

▸ Child: Initially 5 micrograms/kg daily, dose to be adjusted as necessary

● **UNLICENSED USE** Not licensed for treatment of glycogen storage disease or neonatal neutropenia.

● **CONTRA-INDICATIONS** Severe congenital neutropenia who develop leukaemia or have evidence of leukaemic evolution

● **CAUTIONS** Osteoporotic bone disease (monitor bone density if given for more than 6 months) · secondary acute myeloid leukaemia

● **INTERACTIONS** → Appendix 1: filgrastim

● **SIDE-EFFECTS**

▶ **Common or very common** Anaemia · diarrhoea · dysuria · haemorrhage · hepatomegaly · hyperuricaemia · hypotension · osteoporosis · rash

▶ **Uncommon** Fluid imbalance · graft versus host disease · interstitial lung disease · peripheral vascular disease · pseudogout · rheumatoid arthritis aggravated · urine abnormalities

● **MONITORING REQUIREMENTS** Regular morphological and cytogenetic bone-marrow examinations recommended in severe congenital neutropenia (possible risk of myelodysplastic syndromes or leukaemia).

● **DIRECTIONS FOR ADMINISTRATION** For *subcutaneous* or *intravenous infusion*, manufacturer advises give continuously *or* intermittently *in* Glucose 5%; for a filgrastim concentration of less than 1 500 000 units/mL (15 micrograms/mL), albumin (human albumin solution) is added to produce a final albumin concentration of 2 mg/mL; should not be diluted to a filgrastim concentration of less than 200 000 units/mL (2 micrograms/mL) and should not be diluted with sodium chloride solution.

● **PRESCRIBING AND DISPENSING INFORMATION** Filgrastim is a biological medicine. Biological medicines must be prescribed and dispensed by brand name, see *Biological medicines* and *Biosimilar medicines*, under Guidance on prescribing p. 1.

1 million units of filgrastim solution for injection contains 10 micrograms filgrastim.

● **MEDICINAL FORMS** There can be variation in the licensing of different medicines containing the same drug.

Solution for injection

▸ **Accofil** (Accord-UK Ltd)

Filgrastim 60 mega unit per 1 ml Accofil 30million units/0.5ml solution for injection pre-filled syringes | 5 pre-filled disposable injection PoM £284.20 DT = £250.75 (Hospital only) | 7 pre-filled disposable injection PoM £397.60 (Hospital only)

Accofil 12million units/0.2ml solution for injection pre-filled syringes | 5 pre-filled disposable injection PoM £113.60 (Hospital only)

Filgrastim 96 mega unit per 1 ml Accofil 48million units/0.5ml solution for injection pre-filled syringes | 5 pre-filled disposable injection PoM £455.70 (Hospital only) | 7 pre-filled disposable injection PoM £637.98 (Hospital only)

Accofil 70million units/0.73ml solution for injection pre-filled syringes | 5 pre-filled disposable injection [PoM] £662.67 (Hospital only)

▸ **Neupogen** (Amgen Ltd)

Filgrastim 30 mega unit per 1 ml Neupogen 30million units/1ml solution for injection vials | 5 vial [PoM] £263.52 DT = £263.52

▸ **Neupogen Singleject** (Amgen Ltd)

Filgrastim 60 mega unit per 1 ml Neupogen Singleject 30million units/0.5ml solution for injection pre-filled syringes | 1 pre-filled disposable injection [PoM] £52.70

Filgrastim 96 mega unit per 1 ml Neupogen Singleject 48million units/0.5ml solution for injection pre-filled syringes | 1 pre-filled disposable injection [PoM] £84.06

▸ **Nivestim** (Pfizer Ltd)

Filgrastim 60 mega unit per 1 ml Nivestim 30million units/0.5ml solution for injection pre-filled syringes | 5 pre-filled disposable injection [PoM] £246.50 DT = £250.75

Nivestim 12million units/0.2ml solution for injection pre-filled syringes | 5 pre-filled disposable injection [PoM] £153.00

Filgrastim 96 mega unit per 1 ml Nivestim 48million units/0.5ml solution for injection pre-filled syringes | 5 pre-filled disposable injection [PoM] £395.25

▸ **Zarzio** (Sandoz Ltd)

Filgrastim 60 mega unit per 1 ml Zarzio 30million units/0.5ml solution for injection pre-filled syringes | 5 pre-filled disposable injection [PoM] £250.75 DT = £250.75

Filgrastim 96 mega unit per 1 ml Zarzio 48million units/0.5ml solution for injection pre-filled syringes | 5 pre-filled disposable injection [PoM] £399.50

715

Lenograstim

20-Jul-2020

(Recombinant human granulocyte-colony stimulating factor; rHuG-CSF)

● **INDICATIONS AND DOSE**

Reduction in the duration of neutropenia and associated complications following bone-marrow transplantation for non-myeloid malignancy (specialist use only) | Reduction in the duration of neutropenia and associated complications following peripheral stem cells transplantation for non-myeloid malignancy (specialist use only)

▸ BY INTRAVENOUS INFUSION, OR BY SUBCUTANEOUS INJECTION

▸ Child 2–17 years: 150 micrograms/m^2 daily until neutrophil count stable in acceptable range (max. 28 days), to be started the day after transplantation. Intravenous infusion to be given over 30 minutes

Reduction in the duration of neutropenia and associated complications following treatment with cytotoxic chemotherapy associated with a significant incidence of febrile neutropenia (specialist use only)

▸ BY SUBCUTANEOUS INJECTION

▸ Child 2–17 years: 150 micrograms/m^2 daily until neutrophil count stable in acceptable range (max. 28 days), to be started on the day after completion of chemotherapy

Mobilisation of peripheral blood progenitor cells for harvesting and subsequent infusion, used alone (specialist use only)

▸ BY SUBCUTANEOUS INJECTION

▸ Child 2–17 years: 10 micrograms/kg daily for 4–6 days (5–6 days in healthy donors)

Mobilisation of peripheral blood progenitor cells, used following adjunctive myelosuppressive chemotherapy (to improve yield) (specialist use only)

▸ BY SUBCUTANEOUS INJECTION

▸ Child 2–17 years: 150 micrograms/m^2 daily until neutrophil count stable in acceptable range, to be started 1–5 days after completion of chemotherapy, for timing of leucopheresis, consult product literature

● **UNLICENSED USE** Not licensed for use in children for cytotoxic-induced neutropenia, mobilisation of peripheral blood progenitor cells (monotherapy or adjunctive therapy), or following peripheral stem cells transplantation.

● **INTERACTIONS** → Appendix 1: lenograstim

● **SIDE-EFFECTS**

▸ **Common or very common** Abdominal pain · asthenia

▸ **Rare or very rare** Erythema nodosum · pyoderma gangrenosum · toxic epidermal necrolysis

● **DIRECTIONS FOR ADMINISTRATION** For *intravenous infusion*, manufacturer advises dilute reconstituted solution to a concentration of not less than 2 micrograms/mL (*Granocyte*®-13) or 2.5 micrograms/mL (*Granocyte*®-34) with Glucose 5% *or* Sodium Chloride 0.9%.

● **PRESCRIBING AND DISPENSING INFORMATION** *Granocyte*® solution for injection contains 105 micrograms of lenograstim per 13.4 mega unit vial and 263 micrograms lenograstim per 33.6 mega unit vial.

● **MEDICINAL FORMS** There can be variation in the licensing of different medicines containing the same drug.

Powder and solvent for solution for injection

EXCIPIENTS: May contain Phenylalanine

▸ **Granocyte** (Chugai Pharma UK Ltd)

Lenograstim 13.4 mega unit Granocyte 13million unit powder and solvent for solution for injection pre-filled syringes | 1 pre-filled disposable injection [PoM] £40.11 | 5 pre-filled disposable injection [PoM] £200.55

Lenograstim 33.6 mega unit Granocyte 34million unit powder and solvent for solution for injection pre-filled syringes | 1 pre-filled disposable injection [PoM] £62.54 | 5 pre-filled disposable injection [PoM] £312.69

3.2 Stem cell mobilisation

IMMUNOSTIMULANTS › CHEMOKINE RECEPTOR ANTAGONISTS

Plerixafor

22-Oct-2020

● **DRUG ACTION** Plerixafor is a chemokine receptor antagonist.

● **INDICATIONS AND DOSE**

Mobilise haematopoietic stem cells to peripheral blood for collection and subsequent autologous transplantation in patients with lymphoma or solid malignant tumours (specialist use only)

▸ BY SUBCUTANEOUS INJECTION

▸ Child 1–17 years: 240 micrograms/kg daily usually for 2–4 days (and up to 7 days), to be administered 6–11 hours before initiation of apheresis, dose to be given following 4 days treatment with a granulocyte-colony stimulating factor; maximum 40 mg per day

● **SIDE-EFFECTS**

▸ **Common or very common** Arthralgia · constipation · diarrhoea · dizziness · dry mouth · erythema · fatigue · flatulence · gastrointestinal discomfort · headache · hyperhidrosis · malaise · musculoskeletal pain · nausea · oral hypoaesthesia · sleep disorders · vomiting

▸ **Frequency not known** Postural hypotension · splenomegaly · syncope

● **CONCEPTION AND CONTRACEPTION** Use effective contraception during treatment— teratogenic in *animal* studies.

● **PREGNANCY** Manufacturer advises avoid unless essential— teratogenic in *animal* studies.

● **BREAST FEEDING** Manufacturer advises avoid—no information available.

- **RENAL IMPAIRMENT** No information available if creatinine clearance less than 20 mL/minute.
  Dose adjustments Manufacturer advises reduce dose to 160 micrograms/kg (maximum 27 mg) daily if creatinine clearance 20–50 mL/minute. See p. 16.
- **MONITORING REQUIREMENTS** Monitor platelets and white blood cell count.
- **PATIENT AND CARER ADVICE**
  Driving and skilled tasks Manufacturer advises patients and carers should be cautioned on the effects on driving and performance of skilled tasks—increased risk of dizziness, fatigue, or vasovagal reactions.
- **NATIONAL FUNDING/ACCESS DECISIONS**
  For full details see funding body website
  Scottish Medicines Consortium (SMC) decisions
  ▸ **Plerixafor (*Mozobil*®) in combination with granulocyte-colony stimulating factor (G-CSF) to enhance mobilisation of haematopoietic stem cells to the peripheral blood for collection and subsequent autologous transplantation in children aged 1 year to less than 18 years with lymphoma or solid malignant tumours (February 2020)** SMC No. SMC2249 Recommended
  All Wales Medicines Strategy Group (AWMSG) decisions
  ▸ **Plerixafor (*Mozobil*®) in combination with granulocyte-colony stimulating factor (G-CSF) to enhance mobilisation of haematopoietic stem cells to the peripheral blood for collection and subsequent autologous transplantation in children aged 1 to less than 18 years with lymphoma or solid malignant tumours (February 2020)** AWMSG No. 3297 Recommended

- **MEDICINAL FORMS** There can be variation in the licensing of different medicines containing the same drug.
  Solution for injection
  ▸ Plerixafor (Non-proprietary)
  Plerixafor 20 mg per 1 ml Plerixafor 24mg/1.2ml solution for injection vials | 1 vial PoM £3,800.00–£4,882.77 (Hospital only)

4 Platelet disorders

4.1 Essential thrombocythaemia

ANTITHROMBOTIC DRUGS › CYCLIC AMP PHOSPHODIESTERASE III INHIBITORS

Anagrelide [Specialist drug]

27-May-2022

- **INDICATIONS AND DOSE**
  Essential thrombocythaemia [in patients at risk of thrombo-haemorrhagic events who have not responded adequately to other drugs or who cannot tolerate other drugs]
  ▸ BY MOUTH
  ▸ Child 7–17 years: Specialist drug – access specialist resources for dosing information
- **UNLICENSED USE** Not licensed for use in children.

IMPORTANT SAFETY INFORMATION

MHRA/CHM ADVICE: *XAGRID*® (ANAGRELIDE HYDROCHLORIDE): RISK OF THROMBOSIS, INCLUDING CEREBRAL INFARCTION, IF TREATMENT DISCONTINUED ABRUPTLY [ALSO APPLICABLE TO GENERIC FORMS] (APRIL 2022)

There is an increased risk of potentially fatal thrombosis, including cerebral infarction, due to the rebound in platelet count when anagrelide treatment is discontinued abruptly. The platelet count will typically start to increase within 4 days after discontinuation and return to baseline levels within 1 to 2 weeks, but may rebound above these values.

Healthcare professionals are advised to:
- avoid abrupt treatment discontinuation;
- monitor platelet counts frequently during dosage interruption or treatment withdrawal;
- counsel patients or their carers on how to recognise early signs and symptoms of thrombosis, including cerebral infarction, and to seek urgent medical advice if they occur.

- **INTERACTIONS** → Appendix 1: anagrelide
- **SIDE-EFFECTS**
  ▸ **Common or very common** Anaemia · arrhythmias · asthenia · diarrhoea · dizziness · fluid retention · gastrointestinal discomfort · gastrointestinal disorders · headaches · nausea · palpitations · skin reactions · vomiting
  ▸ **Uncommon** Alopecia · appetite decreased · arthralgia · chest pain · chills · confusion · congestive heart failure · constipation · depression · dry mouth · dyspnoea · erectile dysfunction · fever · haemorrhage · hypertension · insomnia · malaise · memory loss · myalgia · nervousness · oedema · pain · pancreatitis · pancytopenia · pneumonia · pulmonary hypertension · respiratory disorders · sensation abnormal · syncope · thrombocytopenia · weight changes
  ▸ **Rare or very rare** Angina pectoris · cardiomegaly · cardiomyopathy · coordination abnormal · drowsiness · dysarthria · influenza like illness · myocardial infarction · nocturia · pericardial effusion · postural hypotension · renal failure · tinnitus · vasodilation · vision disorders
  ▸ **Frequency not known** Hepatitis · interstitial lung disease · nephritis tubulointerstitial · thrombosis (on abrupt discontinuation)
- **CONCEPTION AND CONTRACEPTION** Effective contraception required during treatment.
- **PATIENT AND CARER ADVICE**
  Driving and skilled tasks Dizziness may affect performance of skilled tasks (e.g. cycling, driving).

- **MEDICINAL FORMS** There can be variation in the licensing of different medicines containing the same drug.
  Oral capsule
  ▸ Anagrelide (Non-proprietary)
  Anagrelide (as Anagrelide hydrochloride) 500 microgram Anagrelide 500microgram capsules | 100 capsule PoM ⊠ DT = £249.99 (Hospital only) | 100 capsule PoM £404.57 DT = £249.99
  ▸ Xagrid (Takeda UK Ltd)
  Anagrelide (as Anagrelide hydrochloride) 500 microgram Xagrid 500microgram capsules | 100 capsule PoM £404.57 DT = £249.99

4.2 Thrombocytopenias

4.2a Acquired thrombotic thrombocytopenic purpura

ANTITHROMBOTIC DRUGS

Caplacizumab

12-Jan-2021

- **DRUG ACTION** Caplacizumab is a monoclonal antibody fragment (nanobody) that binds to von Willebrand factor, thereby inhibiting platelet adhesion.

- **INDICATIONS AND DOSE**
  Acquired thrombotic thrombocytopenic purpura (specialist use only)
  ▸ INITIALLY BY INTRAVENOUS INJECTION
  ▸ Child 12–17 years (body-weight 40 kg and above): Initially 10 mg for 1 dose, given before plasma exchange, followed by (by subcutaneous injection) 10 mg once daily given after each plasma exchange during, and for

30 days after finishing, daily plasma exchange therapy, treatment may be continued after this if there is evidence of unresolved immunological disease

- **CONTRA-INDICATIONS** Active bleeding (interrupt treatment)
- **CAUTIONS** Increased risk of bleeding
- **INTERACTIONS** → Appendix 1: caplacizumab
- **SIDE-EFFECTS**
  - **Common or very common** Cerebral infarction · dyspnoea · fatigue · fever · haemorrhage · headache · menorrhagia · myalgia · subarachnoid haemorrhage · urticaria
- **PREGNANCY** Manufacturer advises avoid—no information available.
- **BREAST FEEDING** Manufacturer advises avoid—no information available.
- **HEPATIC IMPAIRMENT** Manufacturer advises caution in severe impairment (no information available).
- **DIRECTIONS FOR ADMINISTRATION** Manufacturer advises injection into the abdomen. Patients may self-administer *Cablivi*® after appropriate training in subcutaneous injection technique.
- **PRESCRIBING AND DISPENSING INFORMATION** Caplacizumab is a biological medicine. Biological medicines must be prescribed and dispensed by brand name, see *Biological medicines* and *Biosimilar medicines*, under Guidance on prescribing p. 1.
- **HANDLING AND STORAGE** Manufacturer advises store in a refrigerator (2-8°C) and protect from light—consult product literature for further information regarding storage outside refrigerator.
- **PATIENT AND CARER ADVICE**
  Missed doses Manufacturer advises if a dose is more than 12 hours late, the missed dose should not be given and the next dose should be given at the normal time.
- **NATIONAL FUNDING/ACCESS DECISIONS**
  For full details see funding body website

NICE decisions

- **Caplacizumab with plasma exchange and immunosuppression for treating acute acquired thrombotic thrombocytopenic purpura (December 2020)** NICE TA667 Recommended

---

- **MEDICINAL FORMS** There can be variation in the licensing of different medicines containing the same drug.

Powder and solvent for solution for injection

EXCIPIENTS: May contain Polysorbates

- **Cablivi** (Sanofi)
  Caplacizumab 10 mg Cablivi 10mg powder and solvent for solution for injection vials | 1 vial [PoM] £4,143.00 (Hospital only)

4.2b Immune thrombocytopenia

Immune thrombocytopenic purpura

12-Apr-2021

Overview

Acute immune (idiopathic) thrombocytopenic purpura is usually self-limiting in children, with spontaneous remission more likely in younger children. [EvGr] Most children with newly diagnosed immune thrombocytopenic purpura can be managed with watchful waiting under the supervision of a haematologist.

Treatment to increase platelet counts consists of corticosteroids, intravenous normal immunoglobulin p. 955, or less commonly, intravenous anti-D immunoglobulins [unlicensed use]. In general, corticosteroids are used for minor or mild bleeding, or in children who are unresponsive to normal immunoglobulin. If there is moderate or severe bleeding, immunoglobulin preparations may be used to give a temporary rapid rise in platelets.

In children with *persistent or chronic* immune thrombocytopenic purpura, treatment primarily consists of thrombopoietin receptor agonists (eltrombopag below and romiplostim p. 720), rituximab p. 659 [unlicensed use], or mycophenolate mofetil [unlicensed use]. ⟨A⟩

Splenectomy is very rarely indicated in childhood immune thrombocytopenic purpura.

ANTIHAEMORRHAGICS › THROMBOPOIETIN RECEPTOR AGONISTS

Eltrombopag

29-Mar-2022

- **DRUG ACTION** Eltrombopag is a thrombopoietin receptor agonist that binds to and activates the thrombopoietin (TPO) receptor, thereby increasing platelet production.

- **INDICATIONS AND DOSE**

Chronic immune (idiopathic) thrombocytopenic purpura in patients of East or Southeast Asian origin refractory to other treatments (such as corticosteroids or immunoglobulins) (under expert supervision)

▶ BY MOUTH

- Child 1–17 years: Initially 25 mg once daily, dose to be adjusted to achieve a platelet count of $50x10^9$/litre or more—consult product literature for dose adjustments, dose can be increased if necessary up to maximum 75 mg per day, discontinue if inadequate response after 4 weeks treatment at maximum dose

Chronic immune (idiopathic) thrombocytopenic purpura in patients refractory to other treatments (such as corticosteroids or immunoglobulins) (under expert supervision)

▶ BY MOUTH

- Child 1–5 years: Initially 25 mg once daily, dose to be adjusted to achieve a platelet count of $50x10^9$/litre or more—consult product literature for dose adjustments, dose can be increased if necessary up to maximum 75 mg per day, discontinue if inadequate response after 4 weeks treatment at maximum dose
- Child 6–17 years: Initially 50 mg once daily, dose to be adjusted to achieve a platelet count of $50x10^9$/litre or more—consult product literature for dose adjustments, dose can be increased if necessary up to maximum 75 mg per day, discontinue if inadequate response after 4 weeks treatment at maximum dose

DOSE EQUIVALENCE AND CONVERSION

- Powder for oral suspension may lead to higher eltrombopag exposure than oral tablet; platelet counts should be monitored weekly for 2 weeks when switching between preparations.

IMPORTANT SAFETY INFORMATION

MHRA/CHM ADVICE: ELTROMBOPAG (*REVOLADE*®): REPORTS OF INTERFERENCE WITH BILIRUBIN AND CREATININE TEST RESULTS (JULY 2018)

See *Effect on laboratory tests*.

- **CAUTIONS** Patients of East or Southeast Asian origin · risk factors for thromboembolism
- **INTERACTIONS** → Appendix 1: eltrombopag
- **SIDE-EFFECTS**
  - **Common or very common** Alopecia · anaemia · appetite decreased · asthenia · chest pain · cough · depression · diarrhoea · drowsiness · dry eye · dry mouth · ear pain · electrolyte imbalance · embolism and thrombosis · eosinophilia · eye pain · fever · gastrointestinal discomfort · gastrointestinal disorders · haemorrhage · headaches · hepatic disorders · hyperbilirubinaemia · increased

9 Blood and nutrition

leucocytes · increased risk of infection · malaise · menorrhagia · muscle complaints · nasal complaints · nausea · oral disorders · oropharyngeal complaints · pain · renal impairment · renal thrombotic microangiopathy · sensation abnormal · skin reactions · sleep disorder · sweat changes · urine abnormalities · vasodilation · vertigo · vision disorders · vomiting

- **Uncommon** Anisocytosis · arrhythmias · balance impaired · cardiovascular disorder · cataract cortical · cyanosis · excessive tearing · eye inflammation · feeling hot · feeling jittery · food poisoning · gout · haemolytic anaemia · hemiparesis · lens opacity · mood altered · muscle weakness · myocardial infarction · nephritis lupus · nerve disorders · nocturia · QT interval prolongation · rectosigmoid cancer · retinal pigment epitheliopathy · sinus disorder · sleep apnoea · speech disorder · sunburn · tremor · wound inflammation
- **Frequency not known** Cerebral infarction

- **CONCEPTION AND CONTRACEPTION** Ensure effective contraception during treatment.
- **PREGNANCY** Avoid—toxicity in *animal* studies.
- **BREAST FEEDING** Manufacturer advises avoid.
- **HEPATIC IMPAIRMENT** Manufacturer advises consider avoiding.

  Dose adjustments Manufacturer advises initial dose reduction to 25 mg once daily and wait at least 3 weeks before upwards titration of dose.
- **RENAL IMPAIRMENT** EvGr Use with caution. (M)
- **MONITORING REQUIREMENTS**
  - Manufacturer advises monitor liver function before treatment, every two weeks when adjusting the dose, and monthly thereafter.
  - Manufacturer advises regular ophthalmological examinations for cataract formation.
  - Manufacturer advises peripheral blood smear prior to initiation to establish baseline level of cellular morphologic abnormalities; once stabilised, full blood count with white blood cell count differential should be performed monthly.
  - Manufacturer advises monitor full blood count including platelet count and peripheral blood smears every week during treatment until a stable platelet count is reached ($50x10^9$/litre or more for at least 4 weeks), then monthly thereafter; monitor platelet count weekly for 4 weeks following treatment discontinuation.
- **EFFECT ON LABORATORY TESTS** Eltrombopag is highly coloured and can cause serum discolouration and interference with total bilirubin and creatinine testing. If laboratory results are inconsistent with clinical observations, manufacturer advises re-testing using another method to help determine the validity of the result.
- **DIRECTIONS FOR ADMINISTRATION** EvGr Each dose should be taken at least 2 hours before or 4 hours after any dairy products (or foods containing calcium), indigestion remedies, or medicines containing aluminium, calcium, iron, magnesium, zinc, or selenium to reduce possible interference with absorption. For *powder for oral suspension*, disperse dose in 20 mL of water and administer using an oral syringe. Discard suspension if not administered within 30 minutes of preparation. (M)
- **PATIENT AND CARER ADVICE** Patients or carers should be given advice on how to administer eltrombopag tablets and powder for oral suspension.
- **NATIONAL FUNDING/ACCESS DECISIONS**

  For full details see funding body website

  Scottish Medicines Consortium (SMC) decisions
  - **Eltrombopag (*Revolade*®) for chronic immune (idiopathic) thrombocytopenic purpura (ITP) patients aged 1 year to 17 years who are refractory to other treatments (e.g. corticosteroids, immunoglobulins) (January 2017)** SMC No. 1206/17 Recommended with restrictions

  All Wales Medicines Strategy Group (AWMSG) decisions
  - **Eltrombopag (*Revolade*®) for treatment of chronic immune (idiopathic) thrombocytopenic purpura (ITP) patients aged 1 year to 17 years who are refractory to other treatments (e.g. corticosteroids, immunoglobulins) (October 2016)** AWMSG No. 2692 Recommended

- **MEDICINAL FORMS** There can be variation in the licensing of different medicines containing the same drug.

Oral tablet

- **Eltrombopag (Non-proprietary)**

  Eltrombopag (as Eltrombopag olamine) 12.5 mg Promacta 12.5mg tablets | 30 tablet PoM (Hospital only)

  Eltrombopag (as Eltrombopag olamine) 25 mg Eltrombopag 25mg tablets | 28 tablet PoM £693.00 DT = £770.00 | 28 tablet PoM £770.00 DT = £770.00 (Hospital only)

  Eltrombopag (as Eltrombopag olamine) 50 mg Eltrombopag 50mg tablets | 28 tablet PoM £1,540.00 DT = £1,540.00 (Hospital only) | 28 tablet PoM £1,386.00 DT = £1,540.00

  Eltrombopag (as Eltrombopag olamine) 75 mg Eltrombopag 75mg tablets | 28 tablet PoM £2,079.00 DT = £2,310.00 | 28 tablet PoM £2,310.00 DT = £2,310.00 (Hospital only)
- **Revolade** (Novartis Pharmaceuticals UK Ltd)

  Eltrombopag (as Eltrombopag olamine) 25 mg Revolade 25mg tablets | 28 tablet PoM £770.00 DT = £770.00

  Eltrombopag (as Eltrombopag olamine) 50 mg Revolade 50mg tablets | 28 tablet PoM £1,540.00 DT = £1,540.00

  Eltrombopag (as Eltrombopag olamine) 75 mg Revolade 75mg tablets | 28 tablet PoM £2,310.00 DT = £2,310.00

Powder for oral suspension

CAUTIONARY AND ADVISORY LABELS 13

- **Revolade** (Novartis Pharmaceuticals UK Ltd)

  Eltrombopag (as Eltrombopag olamine) 25 mg Revolade 25mg oral powder sachets | 30 sachet PoM £825.00 (Hospital only) SF

Romiplostim

22-Oct-2020

- **DRUG ACTION** Romiplostim is an Fc–peptide fusion protein that binds to and activates the thrombopoietin (TPO) receptor, thereby increasing platelet production.

- **INDICATIONS AND DOSE**

Chronic immune (idiopathic) thrombocytopenic purpura in patients refractory to other treatments (such as corticosteroids or immunoglobulins) (under expert supervision)

- BY SUBCUTANEOUS INJECTION
  - Child 1–17 years: Initially 1 microgram/kg once weekly, adjusted in steps of 1 microgram/kg once weekly (max. per dose 10 micrograms/kg once weekly) until a stable platelet count of $50x10^9$/litre or more is reached, consult product literature for further details of dose adjustments; reassess bodyweight every 12 weeks, discontinue treatment if inadequate response after 4 weeks at maximum dose

- **CAUTIONS** Risk factors for thromboembolism
- **INTERACTIONS** → Appendix 1: romiplostim
- **SIDE-EFFECTS**
  - **Common or very common** Anaemia · angioedema · arthralgia · asthenia · bone marrow disorders · chills · constipation · cough · diarrhoea · dizziness · embolism and thrombosis · eye inflammation · fever · flushing · gastrointestinal discomfort · headaches · hypersensitivity · increased risk of infection · influenza like illness · muscle complaints · nausea · oropharyngeal pain · pain · palpitations · peripheral oedema · peripheral swelling · sensation abnormal · skin reactions · sleep disorders
  - **Uncommon** Alopecia · appetite decreased · chest pain · clonus · dehydration · depression · dry throat · dysphagia · dyspnoea · erythromelalgia · eye disorders · eye pruritus · feeling hot · feeling jittery · gastrooesophageal reflux

disease · gout · haemorrhage · hair growth abnormal · hypotension · irritability · leucocytosis · malaise · muscle weakness · myocardial infarction · nasal complaints · neoplasms · oral disorders · peripheral ischaemia · peripheral neuropathy · photosensitivity reaction · pleuritic pain · portal vein thrombosis · skin nodule · splenomegaly · taste altered · thrombocytosis · tooth discolouration · vertigo · vision disorders · vomiting · weight changes

- **PREGNANCY** Manufacturer advises avoid—toxicity in *animal* studies.
- **BREAST FEEDING** Manufacturer advises avoid—no information available.
- **HEPATIC IMPAIRMENT** Manufacturer advises caution; consider avoiding in moderate to severe impairment (risk of thromboembolic complications).
- **RENAL IMPAIRMENT** Manufacturer advises caution—no information available.
- **MONITORING REQUIREMENTS**
  - Manufacturer advises monitor full blood count and peripheral blood smears for morphological abnormalities before and during treatment.
  - Manufacturer advises monitor platelet count weekly until platelet count reaches 50×10^9/litre or more for at least 4 weeks without dose adjustment, then monthly thereafter.
  - Manufacturer advises monitor platelet count following treatment discontinuation—risk of bleeding.
- **PATIENT AND CARER ADVICE**
  Driving and skilled tasks Manufacturer advises that patients and their carers should be counselled on the effects on driving and the performance of skilled tasks—increased risk of dizziness.
- **NATIONAL FUNDING/ACCESS DECISIONS**
  For full details see funding body website

  Scottish Medicines Consortium (SMC) decisions
  - **Romiplostim (*Nplate*®) for chronic immune (idiopathic) thrombocytopenic purpura patients one year of age and older who are refractory to other treatments (e.g. corticosteroids, immunoglobulins) (February 2019)** SMC No. SMC2126 Recommended with restrictions

  All Wales Medicines Strategy Group (AWMSG) decisions
  - **Romiplostim (*Nplate*®) for the treatment of chronic immune (idiopathic) thrombocytopenic purpura (ITP) patients aged 1 year to less than 18 years who are refractory to other treatments (for example, corticosteroids, immunoglobulins) (March 2019)** AWMSG No. 3103 Recommended

---

- **MEDICINAL FORMS** There can be variation in the licensing of different medicines containing the same drug.

  Powder for solution for injection
  - **Nplate** (Amgen Ltd)
    Romiplostim 125 microgram Nplate 125microgram powder for solution for injection vials | 1 vial PoM £241.00 (Hospital only)

Nutrition and metabolic disorders

1 Acid-base imbalance

1.1 Metabolic acidosis

ALKALISING DRUGS

Potassium citrate with potassium bicarbonate

13-Oct-2022

- **INDICATIONS AND DOSE**

  Distal renal tubular acidosis
  - BY MOUTH
    - Child 1-3 years: Initially 4 mEq/kg daily in 2 divided doses, adjusted in steps of 1.5 mEq/kg daily if required, to be adjusted until optimal response is achieved, use the lowest maximum daily dose; maximum 10 mEq/kg per day; maximum 336 mEq per day
    - Child 4-11 years: Initially 2 mEq/kg daily in 2 divided doses, adjusted in steps of 1.5 mEq/kg daily if required, to be adjusted until optimal response is achieved, use the lowest maximum daily dose; maximum 10 mEq/kg per day; maximum 336 mEq per day
    - Child 12-17 years: Initially 1 mEq/kg daily in 2 divided doses, adjusted in steps of 1 mEq/kg daily if required, to be adjusted until optimal response is achieved, use the lowest maximum daily dose; maximum 10 mEq/kg per day; maximum 336 mEq per day

  DOSE EQUIVALENCE AND CONVERSION
  - When switching from other alkalising therapy, treatment should be initiated at the target dose used with the previous therapy, in mEq/kg per day, and adjusted as necessary.

- **CONTRA-INDICATIONS** Hyperkalaemia
- **CAUTIONS** Conditions predisposing to hyperkalaemia · gastrointestinal disorders

  CAUTIONS, FURTHER INFORMATION
  - Gastrointestinal disorders EvGr Gastrointestinal disorders such as malabsorption, delayed gastric emptying, diarrhoea, nausea and vomiting could affect efficacy and safety. Monitor plasma bicarbonate levels regularly and adjust dose as clinically indicated. (M)
- **SIDE-EFFECTS**
  - **Common or very common** Diarrhoea · gastrointestinal discomfort · gastrointestinal disorder · nausea · vomiting
- **PREGNANCY** EvGr Use only if potential benefit outweighs risk—increased risk of developing hyperkalaemia. (M)
- **BREAST FEEDING** EvGr Present in milk but not known to be harmful. (M)
- **RENAL IMPAIRMENT** See p. 16. EvGr Avoid if estimated GFR is less than 45 mL/min/1.73m².

  Avoid if estimated GFR is between 45 and 59 mL/min/1.73m² and plasma potassium levels are elevated.

  Caution if estimated GFR is between 45 and 59 mL/min/1.73m²—monitor renal function and plasma potassium levels prior to and after initiation of treatment or dose increase, then at least twice yearly thereafter. (M)
- **DIRECTIONS FOR ADMINISTRATION** Granules should be swallowed whole with a large glass of water, preferably during meals. Alternatively, granules can be mixed (without crushing) with small amounts of soft food (e.g.

9 Blood and nutrition

yoghurt, fruit puree) and taken immediately without chewing. Do **not** mix granules with hot liquids, hot foods or alcohol. Granules should not be given via an enteral feeding tube as they may cause blockage.

- **PATIENT AND CARER ADVICE** Patients or carers should be given advice on how to administer *Sibnayal®* granules.
Missed doses If vomiting occurs within 2 hours of taking a dose, a replacement dose should be taken.
- **NATIONAL FUNDING/ACCESS DECISIONS**
For full details see funding body website
Scottish Medicines Consortium (SMC) decisions
▶ **Potassium citrate and potassium hydrogen carbonate (*Sibnayal®*) for the treatment of distal renal tubular acidosis in adults, adolescents and children aged one year and older (August 2022)** SMC No. SMC2409 Recommended

- **MEDICINAL FORMS** There can be variation in the licensing of different medicines containing the same drug.

Modified-release granules

CAUTIONARY AND ADVISORY LABELS 25, 27
ELECTROLYTES: May contain Potassium

▸ Sibnayal (Advicenne S.A.)
Potassium citrate 282 mg, Potassium bicarbonate 527 mg Sibnayal 8mEq prolonged-release granules sachets | 60 sachet PoM £120.00 (Hospital only) SF
Potassium citrate 847 mg, Potassium bicarbonate 1.582 gram Sibnayal 24mEq prolonged-release granules sachets | 60 sachet PoM £360.00 (Hospital only) SF

Trometamol

(THAM; Tris(hydroxymethyl)aminomethane)

- **INDICATIONS AND DOSE**

Metabolic acidosis

▶ BY INTRAVENOUS INFUSION
▸ Child: To be administered at an amount appropriate to the body base deficit

- **UNLICENSED USE** Unlicensed preparation.
- **CONTRA-INDICATIONS** Anuria · chronic respiratory acidosis
- **CAUTIONS** Extravasation can cause severe tissue damage
- **SIDE-EFFECTS** Hepatic necrosis (following administration via umbilical vein) (in neonates) · hyperkalaemia (in renal impairment) · hypoglycaemia · respiratory depression
SIDE-EFFECTS, FURTHER INFORMATION Respiratory support may be required because trometamol induces respiratory depression.
- **PREGNANCY** Limited information available, hypoglycaemia may harm fetus.
- **BREAST FEEDING** No information available.
- **RENAL IMPAIRMENT** Use with caution, may cause hyperkalaemia.
- **MEDICINAL FORMS** There can be variation in the licensing of different medicines containing the same drug. Forms available from special-order manufacturers include: solution for infusion

Solution for infusion

▸ Trometamol (Non-proprietary)
Trometamol 363.4 mg per 1 ml Tris 36.34% solution for infusion 20ml ampoules | 10 ampoule PoM (Hospital only)

2 Fluid and electrolyte imbalances

Fluids and electrolytes

15-Jan-2025

Electrolyte replacement therapy

The electrolyte concentrations (intravenous fluid) table and the electrolyte content (gastro-intestinal secretions) table may be helpful in planning replacement electrolyte therapy; faeces, vomit, or aspiration should be saved and analysed where possible if abnormal losses are suspected.

Oral preparations for fluid and electrolyte imbalance

Sodium and potassium salts, may be given by mouth to prevent deficiencies or to treat established deficiencies of mild or moderate degree.

Oral potassium

Compensation for potassium loss is especially necessary:

- in children in whom secondary hyperaldosteronism occurs, e.g. renal artery stenosis, renal tubule disorder, the nephrotic syndrome, and severe heart failure;
- in children with excessive losses of potassium in the faeces, e.g. chronic diarrhoea associated with intestinal malabsorption or laxative abuse;
- in those taking digoxin or anti-arrhythmic drugs, where potassium depletion may induce arrhythmias.

Measures to compensate for potassium loss may be required during long-term administration of drugs known to induce potassium loss (e.g. corticosteroids). Potassium supplements are **seldom required** with the small doses of diuretics given to treat hypertension; **potassium-sparing diuretics** (rather than potassium supplements) are recommended for prevention of hypokalaemia due to diuretics such as furosemide p. 163 or the thiazides when these are given to eliminate oedema.

If potassium salts are used for the *prevention of hypokalaemia*, then doses of potassium chloride p. 744 daily by mouth are suitable in patients taking a normal diet. Smaller doses must be used if there is renal insufficiency to reduce the risk of **hyperkalaemia**.

Potassium salts cause nausea and vomiting and poor compliance is a major limitation to their effectiveness (small divided doses may minimise gastric irritation); when appropriate, potassium-sparing diuretics are preferable. When there is *established potassium depletion* larger doses may be necessary, the quantity depending on the severity of any continuing potassium loss (monitoring of plasma-potassium concentration and specialist advice would be required). Potassium depletion is frequently associated with chloride depletion and with metabolic alkalosis, and these disorders require correction.

Management of hyperkalaemia

Acute severe hyperkalaemia calls for urgent treatment with intravenous infusion of **soluble insulin** (0.3–0.6 units/kg/hour in neonates and 0.05–0.2 units/kg/hour in children over 1 month) with glucose 0.5–1 g/kg/hour (5–10 mL/kg of glucose 10%; 2.5–5 mL/kg of glucose 20% via a central venous catheter may also be considered). If insulin cannot be used, salbutamol p. 181 can be given by intravenous injection, but it has a slower onset of action and may be less effective for reducing plasma-potassium concentration.

Calcium gluconate p. 735 is given by slow intravenous injection to manage cardiac excitability caused by hyperkalaemia.

The correction of causal or compounding acidosis with sodium bicarbonate infusion p. 725 should be considered (**important**: preparations of sodium bicarbonate and calcium salts should not be administered in the same line—risk of precipitation). Intravenous furosemide can also be given but is less effective in children with renal impairment. Drugs exacerbating hyperkalaemia should be reviewed and stopped as appropriate; dialysis may occasionally be required.

Ion-exchange resins may be used to remove excess potassium in *mild hyperkalaemia* or in *moderate hyperkalaemia* when there are no ECG changes. Calcium polystyrene sulfonate is preferred unless plasma-calcium concentrations are high.

Oral sodium and water

Sodium chloride p. 728 is indicated in states of sodium depletion. In preterm neonates in the first few weeks of life and in chronic conditions associated with mild or moderate degrees of sodium depletion, e.g. in salt-losing bowel or renal disease, oral supplements of sodium chloride may be sufficient. Sodium chloride solutions suitable for use by mouth in neonates are available from 'special-order' manufacturers or specialist importing companies, they should be used with care because they are hypertonic. Supplementation with sodium chloride may be required to replace losses in children with cystic fibrosis particularly in warm weather.

Oral rehydration therapy (ORT)

Diarrhoea in children is usually self-limiting, however, in children under 6 months of age, and more particularly in those under 3 months, symptoms of dehydration may be less obvious and there is a risk of rapid and severe deterioration. Intestinal absorption of sodium and water is enhanced by glucose (and other carbohydrates). Replacement of fluid and electrolytes lost through diarrhoea can therefore be achieved by giving solutions containing sodium, potassium, and glucose or another carbohydrate such as rice starch.

Oral rehydration solutions should:

- enhance the absorption of water and electrolytes;
- replace the electrolyte deficit adequately and safely;
- contain an alkalinising agent to counter acidosis;
- be slightly hypo-osmolar (about 250 mmol/litre) to prevent the possible induction of osmotic diarrhoea;
- be simple to use in hospital and at home;
- be palatable and acceptable, especially to children;
- be readily available.

It is the policy of the World Health Organization (WHO) to promote a single oral rehydration solution but to use it flexibly (e.g. by giving extra water between drinks of oral rehydration solution to moderately dehydrated infants).

The WHO oral rehydration salts formulation contains sodium chloride 2.6 g, potassium chloride 1.5 g, sodium citrate 2.9 g, anhydrous glucose 13.5 g. It is dissolved in sufficient water to produce 1 litre (providing Na^+ 75 mmol, K^+ 20 mmol, Cl^- 65 mmol, citrate 10 mmol, glucose 75 mmol/litre). This formulation is recommended by the WHO and the United Nations Children's fund, but it is not commonly used in the UK.

Oral rehydration solutions used in the UK are lower in sodium (50–60 mmol/litre) than the WHO formulation since, in general, patients suffer less severe sodium loss.

Rehydration should be rapid over 3 to 4 hours (except in hypernatraemic dehydration in which case rehydration should occur more slowly over 12 hours). The patient should be reassessed after initial rehydration and if still dehydrated rapid fluid replacement should continue.

Once rehydration is complete further dehydration is prevented by encouraging the patient to drink normal volumes of an appropriate fluid and by replacing continuing losses with an oral rehydration solution; in infants, breast-feeding or formula feeds should be offered between oral rehydration drinks.

Oral bicarbonate

Sodium bicarbonate is given by mouth for *chronic acidotic states* such as uraemic acidosis or renal tubular acidosis. The dose for correction of metabolic acidosis is not predictable and the response must be assessed. For severe *metabolic acidosis*, sodium bicarbonate can be given intravenously.

Sodium supplements may increase blood pressure or cause fluid retention and pulmonary oedema in those at risk; hypokalaemia may be exacerbated.

Sodium bicarbonate p. 725 may affect the stability or absorption of other drugs if administered at the same time. If possible, allow 1–2 hours before administering other drugs orally.

Where *hyperchloraemic acidosis* is associated with potassium deficiency, as in some renal tubular and gastrointestinal disorders it may be appropriate to give oral **potassium bicarbonate**, although acute or severe deficiency should be managed by intravenous therapy.

Parenteral preparations for fluid and electrolyte imbalance

For guidance on intravenous fluids in the management of suspected sepsis, see Sepsis p. 362.

Electrolytes and water

Solutions of electrolytes are given intravenously, to meet normal fluid and electrolyte requirements or to replenish substantial deficits or continuing losses when it is not possible or desirable to use the oral route. When intravenous administration is not possible, fluid (as sodium chloride 0.9% p. 728 or glucose 5% p. 730) can also be given subcutaneously by hypodermoclysis.

In an individual patient the nature and severity of the electrolyte imbalance must be assessed from the history and clinical and biochemical examination. Sodium, potassium, chloride, magnesium, phosphate, and water depletion can occur singly and in combination with or without disturbances of acid-base balance.

Isotonic solutions may be infused safely into a peripheral vein. Solutions more concentrated than plasma, for example 15% glucose, are best given through an indwelling catheter positioned in a large vein.

Maintenance fluid requirements in children are usually derived from the relationship that exists between body-weight and metabolic rate; the figures in the table below may be used as a guide outside the neonatal period. The glucose requirement is that needed to minimise gluconeogenesis from amino acids obtained as substrate from muscle breakdown. Maintenance fluids are intended only to provide hydration for a short period until enteral or parenteral nutrition can be established.

It is usual to meet these requirements by using a standard solution of sodium chloride with glucose p. 730. Solutions containing 20 mmol/litre of potassium chloride p. 744 meet usual potassium requirements when given in the suggested volumes; adjustments may be needed if there is an inability to excrete fluids or electrolytes, excessive renal loss or continuing extra-renal losses. The exact requirements depend upon the nature of the clinical situation and types of losses incurred.

Fluid requirements for children over 1 month:	
Body-weight	24-hour fluid requirement
Under 10 kg	100 mL/kg
10-20 kg	100 mL/kg for the first 10 kg + 50 mL/kg for each 1 kg body-weight over 10 kg
Over 20 kg	100 mL/kg for the first 10 kg + 50 mL/kg for each 1 kg body-weight between 10-20 kg + 20 mL/kg for each 1 kg body-weight over 20 kg (max. 2 litres in females, 2.5 litres in males)

Important The baseline fluid requirements shown in the table should be adjusted to take account of factors that reduce water loss (e.g. increased antidiuretic hormone, renal failure, hypothermia, and high ambient humidity) or increase water loss (e.g. pyrexia or burns).

Replacement therapy: initial intravenous replacement fluid is generally required if the child is over 10% dehydrated, or if 5–10% dehydrated and oral or enteral rehydration is not tolerated or possible. Oral rehydration is adequate, if tolerated, in the majority of those less than 10% dehydrated. Subsequent fluid and electrolyte requirements are determined by clinical assessment of fluid balance.

Intravenous sodium

Intravenous sodium chloride in isotonic (0.9%) solution provides the most important extracellular ions in near physiological concentrations and is indicated in *sodium depletion*. It may be given for initial treatment of acute fluid loss and to replace ongoing gastro-intestinal losses from the upper gastro-intestinal tract. Intravenous sodium chloride is commonly given as a component of maintenance and replacement therapy, usually in combination with other electrolytes and glucose.

Chronic hyponatraemia should ideally be corrected by fluid restriction. However, if sodium chloride is required, the deficit should be corrected slowly to avoid the risk of osmotic demyelination syndrome; the rise in plasma sodium concentration should be no more than 10 mmol/litre in 24 hours.

Sodium chloride with glucose solutions are indicated when there is combined *water and sodium depletion*. A 1:1 mixture of isotonic sodium chloride and glucose 5% allows some of the water (free of sodium) to enter body cells which suffer most from dehydration while the sodium salt with a volume of water determined by the normal plasma Na^+ remains extracellular.

Combined sodium, potassium, chloride, and water depletion may occur, for example, with severe diarrhoea or persistent vomiting; replacement is carried out with sodium chloride 0.9% intravenous infusion and glucose 5% intravenous infusion with potassium as appropriate.

Compound sodium lactate (Hartmann's solution) can be used instead of isotonic sodium chloride solution during or after surgery, or in the initial management of the injured or wounded.

Intravenous glucose

Glucose solutions are used mainly to replace water deficit. Water depletion (dehydration) tends to occur when losses are not matched by a comparable intake, as may occur in coma or dysphagia.

Electrolyte concentrations—intravenous fluids

	Millimoles per litre				
Intravenous infusion	Na^+	K^+	HCO_3^-	Cl^-	Ca^{2+}
Normal plasma values	142	4.5	26	103	2.5
Sodium Chloride 0.9%	150	–	–	150	–
Compound Sodium Lactate (Hartmann's)	131	5	29	111	2
Sodium Chloride 0.18% and Glucose 4% (Adults only)	30	–	–	30	–
Sodium Chloride 0.45% and Glucose 5% (Children only)	75	–	–	75	–
Potassium Chloride 0.15% and Glucose 5% (Children only)	–	20	–	20	–
Potassium Chloride 0.15% and Sodium Chloride 0.9% (Children only)	150	20	–	170	–
Potassium Chloride 0.3% and Glucose 5%	–	40	–	40	–
Potassium Chloride 0.3% and Sodium Chloride 0.9%	150	40	–	190	–
To correct metabolic acidosis					
Sodium Bicarbonate 1.26%	150	–	150	–	–
Sodium Bicarbonate 8.4% for cardiac arrest	1000	–	1000	–	–
Sodium Lactate (m/6)	167	–	167	–	–

Electrolyte content—gastro-intestinal secretions

	Millimoles per litre				
Type of fluid	H^+	Na^+	K^+	HCO_3^-	Cl^-
Gastric	40-60	20-80	5-20	–	100-150
Biliary	–	120-140	5-15	30-50	80-120
Pancreatic	–	120-140	5-15	70-110	40-80
Small bowel	–	120-140	5-15	20-40	90-130

Water loss rarely exceeds electrolyte losses but this can occur in fevers, hyperthyroidism, and in uncommon water-losing renal states such as diabetes insipidus or hypercalcaemia. The volume of glucose solution needed to replace deficits varies with the severity of the disorder; the rate of infusion should be adjusted to return the plasma-sodium concentration to normal over 48 hours.

Glucose solutions are also used to correct and prevent hypoglycaemia and to provide a source of energy in those too ill to be fed adequately by mouth; glucose solutions are a key component of parenteral nutrition.

Glucose solutions are given with insulin for the emergency management of *hyperkalaemia*. They are also given, after correction of hyperglycaemia, during treatment of diabetic ketoacidosis, when they must be accompanied by continuous insulin infusion.

Intravenous potassium

Potassium chloride with sodium chloride intravenous infusion p. 728 is the initial treatment for the correction of *severe hypokalaemia* and when sufficient potassium cannot be taken by mouth.

Repeated measurements of plasma-potassium concentration are necessary to determine whether further infusions are required and to avoid the development of hyperkalaemia, which is especially likely in renal impairment.

Initial potassium replacement therapy should **not** involve glucose infusions, because glucose may cause a further decrease in the plasma-potassium concentration.

Bicarbonate and trometamol

Sodium bicarbonate is used to control severe *metabolic acidosis* (pH < 7.1) particularly that caused by loss of bicarbonate (as in renal tubular acidosis or from excessive gastro-intestinal losses). Mild metabolic acidosis associated with volume depletion should first be managed by appropriate fluid replacement because acidosis usually resolves as tissue and renal perfusion are restored. In more severe metabolic acidosis or when the acidosis remains unresponsive to correction of anoxia or hypovolaemia, sodium bicarbonate (1.26%) below can be infused over 3–4 hours with plasma-pH and electrolyte monitoring. In severe shock, metabolic acidosis can develop without sodium depletion; in these circumstances sodium bicarbonate is best given intravenously as a small volume of hypertonic solution, such as 8.4%; plasma pH and electrolytes should be monitored. For *chronic acidotic states*, sodium bicarbonate can be given by mouth.

Trometamol p. 722 (tris(hydroxymethyl)aminomethane, THAM), an organic buffer, corrects metabolic acidosis by causing an increase in urinary pH and an osmotic diuresis. It is indicated when sodium bicarbonate is unsuitable as in carbon dioxide retention, hypernatraemia, or renal impairment. It is also used during cardiac bypass surgery and, very rarely, in cardiac arrest.

Plasma and plasma substitutes

Albumin p. 736, prepared from whole blood, contain soluble proteins and electrolytes but no clotting factors, blood group antibodies, or plasma cholinesterases; they may be given without regard to the recipient's blood group.

Albumin is usually used after the acute phase of illness to correct a plasma-volume deficit; hypoalbuminaemia itself is not an appropriate indication. The use of albumin in acute plasma or blood loss may be wasteful; plasma substitutes are more appropriate. Concentrated albumin may also be used to obtain a diuresis in hypoalbuminaemic patients (e.g. in nephrotic syndrome).

Recent evidence does not support the previous view that the use of albumin increases mortality.

Plasma substitutes

Gelatin p. 737 is a macromolecular substance that is metabolised slowly. Gelatin may be used at the outset to expand and maintain blood volume in shock arising from conditions such as burns; it may also be used as an immediate short-term measure to treat haemorrhage until blood is available. Gelatin is rarely needed when shock is due to sodium and water depletion because, in these circumstances, the shock responds to water and electrolyte repletion; see also the management of shock.

Plasma substitutes should **not** be used to maintain plasma volume in conditions such as burns or peritonitis where there is loss of plasma protein, water, and electrolytes over periods of several days or weeks. In these situations, plasma or plasma protein fractions containing large amounts of albumin should be given.

Large volumes of *some* plasma substitutes can increase the risk of bleeding through depletion of coagulation factors.

Parenteral preparations for fluid and electrolyte imbalance in neonates

Electrolytes and water

Neonates lose water through the skin and nose, particularly if preterm or if the skin is damaged. The basic fluid requirement for a term baby in average ambient humidity is 40–60 mL/kg/day plus urinary losses. Preterm babies have very high transepidermal losses particularly in the first few days of life; they may need more fluid replacement than full term babies and up to 180 mL/kg/day may be required. Local guidelines for fluid management in the neonatal period should be consulted.

Intravenous sodium

The sodium requirement for most healthy neonates is 3 mmol/kg daily. Preterm neonates, particularly below 30 weeks gestation, may require up to 6 mmol/kg daily. *Hyponatraemia* may be caused by excessive renal loss of sodium; it may also be dilutional and restriction of fluid intake may be appropriate. Sodium supplementation is likely to be required if the serum sodium concentration is significantly reduced.

Hypernatraemia may also occur, most often due to dehydration (e.g. breast milk insufficiency). Severe hypernatraemia and hyponatraemia can cause fits and rarely brain damage. Sodium in drug preparations, delivered via continuous infusions, or in infusions to maintain the patency of intravascular or umbilical lines, can result in significant amounts of sodium being delivered, (e.g. 1 mL/hour of sodium chloride 0.9% infused over 24 hours is equivalent to 3.6 mmol/day of sodium).

BICARBONATE

Sodium bicarbonate

19-Apr-2022

● **INDICATIONS AND DOSE**

Chronic acidotic states such as uraemic acidosis or renal tubular acidosis

▶ BY MOUTH

- Neonate: Initially 1–2 mmol/kg daily in divided doses, adjusted according to response.
- Child: Initially 1–2 mmol/kg daily in divided doses, adjusted according to response

Severe metabolic acidosis

▶ BY SLOW INTRAVENOUS INJECTION

- Child: Administer an amount appropriate to the body base deficit, to be given using a strong solution (up to 8.4%)

▶ BY CONTINUOUS INTRAVENOUS INFUSION

- Child: Administer an amount appropriate to the body base deficit, to be given using a weak solution (usually 1.26%)

continued →

Renal hyperkalaemia

▶ BY SLOW INTRAVENOUS INJECTION

▶ Neonate: 1 mmol/kg daily.

▶ Child: 1 mmol/kg daily

Persistent cyanotic spell in a child with congenital heart disease despite optimal use of 100% oxygen and propranolol

▶ BY INTRAVENOUS INFUSION

▶ Child: 1 mmol/kg, dose given to correct acidosis (or dose calculated according to arterial blood gas results), sodium bicarbonate 4.2% intravenous infusion is appropriate for a child under 1 year and sodium bicarbonate 8.4% intravenous infusion in children over 1 year

● **CONTRA-INDICATIONS**

▶ With systemic use Hypokalaemia · salt restricted diet

▶ With intravenous use for metabolic acidosis Conditions associated with sodium retention · history of urinary calculi

With systemic use for metabolic acidosis Hypernatraemia · hypocalcaemia · hypochlorhydria · metabolic or respiratory alkalosis

● **CAUTIONS**

▶ With intravenous use Respiratory acidosis

▶ With oral use for metabolic acidosis Conditions associated with sodium retention

With systemic use for metabolic acidosis Hypoventilation

● **INTERACTIONS** → Appendix 1: sodium bicarbonate

● **SIDE-EFFECTS**

▶ With intravenous use Skin exfoliation · soft tissue necrosis · ulcer

▶ With oral use Anxiety · appetite decreased · asthenia · dizziness · dyspnoea · flatulence · fluid retention · gastrointestinal discomfort · headache · hypertension · hypokalaemia · inflammation · metabolic alkalosis · mood altered · muscle complaints · nausea · nephrolithiasis (long term use) · pulmonary oedema · taste unpleasant · urinary frequency increased · vomiting

● **PREGNANCY** EvGr Use with caution. Ⓜ

● **HEPATIC IMPAIRMENT**

▶ With oral use Manufacturer advises caution in cirrhosis.

● **RENAL IMPAIRMENT**

▶ With oral use EvGr Caution (risk of metabolic alkalosis, hypokalaemia and sodium retention). Ⓜ

● **MONITORING REQUIREMENTS**

▶ With systemic use EvGr Monitor plasma-pH and electrolytes regularly during treatment. Ⓜ

● **DIRECTIONS FOR ADMINISTRATION**

▶ With intravenous use For *peripheral infusion* dilute 8.4% solution at least 1 in 10. For *central line infusion* dilute 1 in 5 with Glucose 5% or 10% *or* Sodium Chloride 0.9%. Extravasation can cause severe tissue damage.

▶ With oral use Sodium bicarbonate may affect the stability or absorption of other drugs if administered at the same time. If possible, allow 1–2 hours before administering other drugs orally.

● **PRESCRIBING AND DISPENSING INFORMATION**

▶ With oral use *Sodium bicarbonate* 500*mg* capsules contain approximately 6 mmol each of Na^+ and HCO_3^-; *Sodium bicarbonate* 600*mg* capsules contain approximately 7 mmol each of Na^+ and HCO_3^-. Oral solutions of sodium bicarbonate are required occasionally; these are available from 'special-order' manufacturers or specialist importing companies; the strength of sodium bicarbonate should be stated on the prescription.

▶ With intravenous use Usual strength Sodium bicarbonate 1.26% (12.6 g, 150 mmol each of Na^+ and HCO_3^-/litre), various other strengths available.

● **PATIENT AND CARER ADVICE** Patients or carers should be given advice on the administration of sodium bicarbonate oral medicines.

Medicines for Children leaflet: Sodium bicarbonate for acidosis www.medicinesforchildren.org.uk/medicines/sodium-bicarbonate-for-acidosis/

● **MEDICINAL FORMS** There can be variation in the licensing of different medicines containing the same drug. Forms available from special-order manufacturers include: oral capsule, oral suspension, oral solution, solution for injection

Oral tablet

▶ Sodium bicarbonate (Non-proprietary)

Sodium bicarbonate 600 mg Sodium bicarbonate 600mg tablets | 100 tablet GSL ⊠

Solution for injection

▶ Sodium bicarbonate (Non-proprietary)

Sodium bicarbonate 84 mg per 1 ml Sodium bicarbonate 8.4% (1mmol/ml) solution for infusion 100ml bottles | 10 bottle PoM £127.00 DT = £127.00 (Hospital only)

Sodium bicarbonate 8.4% (1mmol/ml) solution for injection 100ml bottles | 10 bottle PoM £127.00 DT = £127.00

Sodium bicarbonate 8.4% (1mmol/ml) solution for infusion 250ml bottles | 10 bottle PoM £127.00 DT = £127.00 (Hospital only)

Sodium bicarbonate 8.4% (1mmol/ml) solution for injection 10ml ampoules | 10 ampoule PoM £131.20–£208.44 DT = £208.44

Sodium bicarbonate 8.4% (1mmol/ml) solution for injection 250ml bottles | 10 bottle PoM £127.00 DT = £127.00

Oral capsule

▶ Sodium bicarbonate (Non-proprietary)

Sodium bicarbonate 500 mg Sodium bicarbonate 500mg capsules | 56 capsule PoM £9.00–£11.56 DT = £5.08

Oral solution

▶ Sodium bicarbonate (Non-proprietary)

Sodium bicarbonate 84 mg per 1 ml S-Bicarb 420mg/5ml (1mmol/ml) oral solution | 100 ml ⊠

Sodium bicarbonate 420mg/5ml (1mmol/ml) oral solution sugar free | 100 ml PoM £39.80 DT = £35.82 SF

▶ Thamicarb (SyriMed)

Sodium bicarbonate 84 mg per 1 ml Thamicarb 84mg/1ml oral solution | 100 ml PoM £35.82 DT = £35.82 SF | 500 ml PoM £179.28 DT = £179.28 SF

Infusion

▶ Sodium bicarbonate (Non-proprietary)

Sodium bicarbonate 12.6 mg per 1 ml Polyfusor sodium bicarbonate 1.26% infusion 500ml bottles | 12 bottle PoM £376.56

Sodium bicarbonate 14 mg per 1 ml Polyfusor sodium bicarbonate 1.4% infusion 500ml bottles | 12 bottle PoM £376.56

Sodium bicarbonate 27.4 mg per 1 ml Polyfusor sodium bicarbonate 2.74% infusion 500ml bottles | 12 bottle PoM £376.56

Sodium bicarbonate 42 mg per 1 ml Polyfusor sodium bicarbonate 4.2% infusion 500ml bottles | 12 bottle PoM £376.56

Sodium bicarbonate 84 mg per 1 ml Polyfusor sodium bicarbonate 8.4% infusion 200ml bottles | 12 bottle PoM £376.56

ELECTROLYTES AND MINERALS › POTASSIUM

Potassium chloride with calcium chloride dihydrate and sodium chloride

(Ringer's solution)

The properties listed below are those particular to the combination only. For the properties of the components please consider, potassium chloride p. 744, sodium chloride p. 728.

● **INDICATIONS AND DOSE**

Electrolyte imbalance

▶ BY INTRAVENOUS INFUSION

▶ Child: Dosed according to the deficit or daily maintenance requirements (consult product literature)

● **INTERACTIONS** → Appendix 1: potassium chloride

● **PRESCRIBING AND DISPENSING INFORMATION** Ringer's solution for injection provides the following ions (in mmol/litre), Ca^{2+} 2.2, K^{+} 4, Na^{+} 147, Cl^{-} 156.

● **MEDICINAL FORMS** No licensed medicines listed.

Potassium chloride with calcium chloride, sodium chloride and sodium lactate

26-Feb-2026

(Sodium Lactate Intravenous Infusion, Compound; Compound, Hartmann's Solution for Injection; Ringer-Lactate Solution for Injection)

The properties listed below are those particular to the combination only. For the properties of the components please consider, potassium chloride p. 744, sodium chloride p. 728, calcium chloride p. 734.

● **INDICATIONS AND DOSE**

For prophylaxis, and replacement therapy, requiring the use of sodium chloride and lactate, with minimal amounts of calcium and potassium

▶ BY INTRAVENOUS INFUSION

▸ Child: (consult product literature)

● **INTERACTIONS** → Appendix 1: calcium compounds · potassium chloride

● **PRESCRIBING AND DISPENSING INFORMATION** Compound sodium lactate intravenous infusion contains Na^{+} 131 mmol, K^{+} 5 mmol, Ca^{2+} 2 mmol, HCO_3^{-} (as lactate) 29 mmol, Cl^{-} 111 mmol/litre.

For information on the use of compound sodium lactate intravenous infusion (Hartmann's solution) in sepsis, see Sepsis p. 362.

● **MEDICINAL FORMS** There can be variation in the licensing of different medicines containing the same drug.

Infusion

▸ Potassium chloride with calcium chloride, sodium chloride and sodium lactate (Non-proprietary)

Calcium chloride 270 microgram per 1 ml, Potassium chloride 400 microgram per 1 ml, Sodium lactate 3.17 mg per 1 ml, Sodium chloride 6 mg per 1 ml Sodium lactate compound (Hartmann's Solution) infusion 1litre bags | 10 bag [PoM] £30.00 (Hospital only)

Sodium lactate compound (Hartmann's Solution) infusion 1litre Viaflo bags | 10 bag [PoM] £46.60

Sodium lactate compound (Hartmann's Solution) infusion 1litre Cosinus bags | 10 bag [PoM] £49.50

Sodium lactate compound (Hartmann's Solution) infusion 1litre Freeflex bags | 10 bag [PoM] £22.10

Potassium chloride with glucose

The properties listed below are those particular to the combination only. For the properties of the components please consider, potassium chloride p. 744, glucose p. 730.

● **INDICATIONS AND DOSE**

Electrolyte imbalance

▶ BY INTRAVENOUS INFUSION

▸ Child: Dosed according to the deficit or daily maintenance requirements

● **INTERACTIONS** → Appendix 1: potassium chloride

● **PRESCRIBING AND DISPENSING INFORMATION** Potassium chloride 0.3% contains 40 mmol each of K^{+} and Cl^{-}/litre or 0.15% contains 20 mmol each of K^{+} and Cl^{-}/litre with 5% of anhydrous glucose.

● **MEDICINAL FORMS** There can be variation in the licensing of different medicines containing the same drug. Forms available from special-order manufacturers include: infusion, solution for infusion

Infusion

▸ Potassium chloride with glucose (Non-proprietary)

Presentations available from various suppliers include

Potassium chloride 1.5 mg per 1 ml, Glucose anhydrous 50 mg per 1 ml Potassium chloride 0.15% (potassium 20mmol/1litre) / Glucose 5% infusion | 1litre bags [PoM]

Potassium chloride 1.5 mg per 1 ml, Glucose (as Glucose monohydrate) 50 mg per 1 ml Potassium chloride 0.15% (potassium 10mmol/500ml) / Glucose 5% infusion | 500ml bottles [PoM] (Hospital only)

Potassium chloride 0.15% (potassium 20mmol/1litre) / Glucose 5% infusion | 1litre bottles [PoM] (Hospital only)

Potassium chloride 1.5 mg per 1 ml, Glucose anhydrous 100 mg per 1 ml Potassium chloride 0.15% (potassium 10mmol/500ml) / Glucose 10% infusion | 500ml bags [PoM] (Hospital only)

Potassium chloride 3 mg per 1 ml, Glucose anhydrous 50 mg per 1 ml Potassium chloride 0.3% (potassium 20mmol/500ml) / Glucose 5% infusion | 500ml bags [PoM]

Potassium chloride 0.3% (potassium 40mmol/1litre) / Glucose 5% infusion | 1litre bags [PoM]

Potassium chloride 3 mg per 1 ml, Glucose (as Glucose monohydrate) 50 mg per 1 ml Potassium chloride 0.3% (potassium 20mmol/500ml) / Glucose 5% infusion | 500ml bottles [PoM] (Hospital only)

Potassium chloride 0.3% (potassium 40mmol/1litre) / Glucose 5% infusion | 1litre bottles [PoM] (Hospital only)

Potassium chloride with glucose and sodium chloride

The properties listed below are those particular to the combination only. For the properties of the components please consider, potassium chloride p. 744, glucose p. 730, sodium chloride p. 728.

● **INDICATIONS AND DOSE**

Electrolyte imbalance

▶ BY INTRAVENOUS INFUSION

▸ Child: Dosed according to the deficit or daily maintenance requirements

● **INTERACTIONS** → Appendix 1: potassium chloride

● **PRESCRIBING AND DISPENSING INFORMATION** Concentration of potassium chloride to be specified by the prescriber (usually K^{+} 10–40 mmol/litre).

● **MEDICINAL FORMS** There can be variation in the licensing of different medicines containing the same drug. Forms available from special-order manufacturers include: infusion, solution for infusion

Infusion

▸ Potassium chloride with glucose and sodium chloride (Non-proprietary)

Presentations available from various suppliers include

Potassium chloride 1.5 mg per 1 ml, Sodium chloride 1.8 mg per 1 ml, Glucose anhydrous 40 mg per 1 ml Potassium chloride 0.15% (potassium 20mmol/1litre) / Glucose 4% / Sodium chloride 0.18% infusion | 1litre bags [PoM]

Potassium chloride 1.5 mg per 1 ml, Sodium chloride 1.8 mg per 1 ml, Glucose (as Glucose monohydrate) 40 mg per 1 ml Potassium chloride 0.15% (potassium 10mmol/500ml) / Glucose 4% / Sodium chloride 0.18% infusion | 500ml bottles [PoM] (Hospital only)

Potassium chloride 0.15% (potassium 20mmol/1litre) / Glucose 4% / Sodium chloride 0.18% infusion | 1litre bottles [PoM] (Hospital only)

Potassium chloride 1.5 mg per 1 ml, Sodium chloride 4.5 mg per 1 ml, Glucose anhydrous 50 mg per 1 ml Potassium chloride 0.15% (potassium 10mmol/500ml) / Glucose 5% / Sodium chloride 0.45% infusion | 500ml bags [PoM]

Sodium chloride 1.8 mg per 1 ml, Potassium chloride 3 mg per 1 ml, Glucose anhydrous 40 mg per 1 ml Potassium chloride 0.3% (potassium 40mmol/1litre) / Glucose 4% / Sodium chloride 0.18% infusion | 1litre bags [PoM]

Sodium chloride 1.8 mg per 1 ml, Potassium chloride 3 mg per 1 ml, Glucose (as Glucose monohydrate) 40 mg per 1 ml Potassium chloride 0.3% (potassium 20mmol/500ml) / Glucose 4% / Sodium chloride 0.18% infusion | 500ml bottles [PoM] (Hospital only)
Potassium chloride 0.3% (potassium 40mmol/1litre) / Glucose 4% / Sodium chloride 0.18% infusion | 1litre bottles [PoM] (Hospital only)

Potassium chloride with potassium bicarbonate

09-May-2025

The properties listed below are those particular to the combination only. For the properties of the components please consider, potassium chloride p. 744.

● **INDICATIONS AND DOSE**

Potassium depletion

▶ BY MOUTH

▶ Child: Dosed according to the deficit or daily maintenance requirements (consult product literature)

● **INTERACTIONS** → Appendix 1: potassium chloride

● **DIRECTIONS FOR ADMINISTRATION** The RCPCH and NPPG recommend that, for part doses using *Sando-K®* effervescent tablets, one 12 mmol tablet should be dissolved in 11 mL of water to give a final concentration of approximately 1 mmol/mL. Once the tablet has fully dispersed and fizzing has stopped, the required dose should be withdrawn using an oral syringe and any remaining solution discarded.

● **PRESCRIBING AND DISPENSING INFORMATION** Each *Sando-K®* tablet contains potassium 470 mg (12 mmol of K^+) and chloride 285 mg (8 mmol of Cl^-).
Administration of 'part doses' using effervescent tablets The RCPCH and NPPG recommend that doses should be rounded to enable measurement, and clear instructions provided on the dispensing label and when counselling patients or their carer. Appropriate equipment for administration should also be provided, such as:
- a 20 mL oral syringe to measure the initial volume of water required for tablet dispersion;
- a reusable plastic medicine pot in which the tablet can be dispersed in water;
- another smaller oral syringe to measure and administer the required dose (a 1 mL syringe is required for dose volume less than 1 mL).

For further details, see the position statement from the RCPCH and NPPG, available at: nppg.org.uk/wp-content/uploads/2025/04/Position-Statement-CalciumPhosphate-and-PotassiumV3.pdf.

● **PATIENT AND CARER ADVICE**
Medicines for Children leaflet: Potassium chloride for potassium depletion www.medicinesforchildren.org.uk/medicines/potassium-chloride-for-potassium-depletion/
Medicines for Children leaflet: How to give calcium, phosphate or potassium using effervescent tablets www.medicinesforchildren.org.uk/advice-guides/giving-medicines/how-to-give-phosphate-or-calcium-from-effervescent-tablets/

● **MEDICINAL FORMS** There can be variation in the licensing of different medicines containing the same drug.

Effervescent tablet

CAUTIONARY AND ADVISORY LABELS 13, 21

▶ **AabKCL** (TriOn Pharma Ltd)
Potassium bicarbonate 400 mg, Potassium chloride 600 mg AabKCL effervescent tablets | 100 tablet £7.97 [SF]

▶ **Aace K** (Essential-Healthcare Ltd)
Potassium bicarbonate 400 mg, Potassium chloride 600 mg Aace K effervescent tablets | 100 tablet £7.91 [SF]

▶ **Sando-K** (Stirling Anglian Pharmaceuticals Ltd)
Potassium bicarbonate 400 mg, Potassium chloride 600 mg Sando-K effervescent tablets | 100 tablet [P] £24.95 DT = £24.95

Potassium chloride with sodium chloride

The properties listed below are those particular to the combination only. For the properties of the components please consider, potassium chloride p. 744, sodium chloride below.

● **INDICATIONS AND DOSE**

Electrolyte imbalance

▶ BY INTRAVENOUS INFUSION

▶ Child: Depending on the deficit or the daily maintenance requirements (consult product literature)

● **INTERACTIONS** → Appendix 1: potassium chloride

● **PRESCRIBING AND DISPENSING INFORMATION** Potassium chloride 0.15% with sodium chloride 0.9% contains K^+ 20 mmol, Na^+ 150 mmol, and Cl^- 170 mmol/litre or potassium chloride 0.3% with sodium chloride 0.9% contains K^+ 40 mmol, Na^+ 150 mmol, and Cl^- 190 mmol/litre.

● **MEDICINAL FORMS** There can be variation in the licensing of different medicines containing the same drug. Forms available from special-order manufacturers include: infusion, solution for infusion

Infusion

▶ **Potassium chloride with sodium chloride (Non-proprietary)**
Presentations available from various suppliers include
Potassium chloride 1.5 mg per 1 ml, Sodium chloride 9 mg per 1 ml Potassium chloride 0.15% (potassium 10mmol/500ml) / Sodium chloride 0.9% infusion | 500ml bags [PoM] | 500ml bottles [PoM] (Hospital only)
Potassium chloride 0.15% (potassium 20mmol/1litre) / Sodium chloride 0.9% infusion | 1litre bags [PoM] | 1litre bottles [PoM] (Hospital only)
Potassium chloride 3 mg per 1 ml, Sodium chloride 9 mg per 1 ml Potassium chloride 0.3% (potassium 20mmol/500ml) / Sodium chloride 0.9% infusion | 500ml bags [PoM] | 500ml bottles [PoM] (Hospital only)
Potassium chloride 0.3% (potassium 40mmol/1litre) / Sodium chloride 0.9% infusion | 1litre bags [PoM] | 1litre bottles [PoM] (Hospital only)

ELECTROLYTES AND MINERALS > SODIUM CHLORIDE

Sodium chloride

26-Feb-2026

● **INDICATIONS AND DOSE**

Sodium deficiency

▶ BY MOUTH USING ORAL SOLUTION

▶ Neonate: Initially 3–5 mmol/kg daily in divided doses, adjusted according to requirements.

▶ BY MOUTH

▶ Child: Initially 1–2 mmol/kg daily in divided doses, adjusted according to requirements

Chronic renal salt wasting

▶ BY MOUTH

▶ Child: 1–2 mmol/kg daily in divided doses, adjusted according to requirements

Sodium supplementation [preterm neonates 30 weeks' gestation or less]

▶ BY MOUTH USING ORAL SOLUTION

▶ Neonate: 2 mmol daily in divided doses, dose to be administered for each 100 mL of formula feed consumed (consult dietician). Additional sodium replacement may be needed for deficiency, alternatively 3–4 mmol daily in divided doses, dose to be administered for each 100 mL of breast milk consumed (consult dietician). Additional sodium replacement may be needed for deficiency.

Fluid and electrolyte replacement

- BY INTRAVENOUS INFUSION
- Child: The volume of sodium chloride solution needed to replace deficits may vary (consult product literature)

Diabetic ketoacidosis (when systolic blood pressure below 90 mmHg)

- BY INTRAVENOUS INFUSION
- Child: (consult local protocol)

DOSE EQUIVALENCE AND CONVERSION

- With oral use
- Each *Slow Sodium*® modified-release tablet contains approx. 10 mmol each of Na^+ and Cl^-. Oral solution doses are expressed as mmol of sodium.

● **CAUTIONS**

- With intravenous use Avoid excessive administration · cardiac failure · cardio-respiratory diseases · children receiving glucocorticoids · dilutional hyponatraemia · hepatic cirrhosis · hypertension · peripheral oedema · pulmonary oedema · reduced fluid loss · renal insufficiency · restrict intake in impaired renal function · toxaemia of pregnancy

CAUTIONS, FURTHER INFORMATION

- Reduced fluid loss
- With intravenous use The volume of fluid infused should take into account the possibility of reduced fluid loss owing to increased antidiuretic hormone and factors such as renal failure, hypothermia, and high humidity.
- Dilutional hyponatraemia
- With intravenous use Dilutional hyponatraemia is a rare but potentially fatal risk of parenteral hydration. It may be caused by inappropriate use of hypotonic fluids such as sodium chloride 0.18% and glucose 4% intravenous infusion, especially in the postoperative period when antidiuretic hormone secretion is increased. Dilutional hyponatraemia is characterized by a rapid fall in plasma-sodium concentration leading to cerebral oedema and seizures; any child with severe hyponatraemia or rapidly changing plasma-sodium concentration should be referred urgently to a paediatric high dependency facility.

● **SIDE-EFFECTS**

- With intravenous use Chills · fever · hypervolaemia · hyponatraemia · hyponatraemic encephalopathy · hypotension · local reaction · localised pain · paraesthesia · skin reactions · tremor · vascular irritation · venous thrombosis
- With oral use Abdominal cramps · acidosis hyperchloraemic · diarrhoea · generalised oedema · hyperhidrosis · hypertension · hypotension · irritability · muscle complaints · nausea · vomiting

● **MONITORING REQUIREMENTS**

- With intravenous use During parenteral hydration, fluids and electrolytes should be monitored closely and any disturbance corrected by slow infusion of an appropriate solution.

● **DIRECTIONS FOR ADMINISTRATION**

- With oral use For neonates and infants, *oral solution* should be diluted and thoroughly mixed into breast milk, formula feed, or water immediately before administration. Example dilutions are 2 mmol sodium diluted in 100 mL formula feed, or 3–4 mmol sodium diluted in 100 mL breast milk. For older children, *oral solution* may be diluted and thoroughly mixed into water.
  Slow Sodium® *modified-release tablets* should be swallowed whole with water (approx. 70 mL per tablet in patients with normal kidney function).

● **PRESCRIBING AND DISPENSING INFORMATION**

- With intravenous use Sodium chloride 0.9% intravenous infusion contains Na^+ and Cl^- each 150 mmol/litre. The term 'normal saline' should not be used to describe sodium chloride intravenous infusion 0.9%; the term 'physiological saline' is acceptable but it is preferable to give the composition (i.e. sodium chloride intravenous infusion 0.9%). For information on the use of sodium chloride 0.9% intravenous infusion in sepsis, see Sepsis p. 362.
- With oral use The RCPCH and NPPG recommend that, when a liquid formulation of sodium chloride is required, the following strength is used: 5 mmol/mL.

● **PATIENT AND CARER ADVICE** Patients or their carers should be advised on how to administer oral solutions and modified-release tablets.

Medicines for Children leaflet: Sodium chloride for hyponatraemia www.medicinesforchildren.org.uk/medicines/sodium-chloride-for-hyponatraemia/

● **PROFESSION SPECIFIC INFORMATION**

Dental practitioners' formulary Compound Sodium Chloride Mouthwash may be prescribed—see sodium bicarbonate with sodium chloride p. 878.

● **MEDICINAL FORMS** There can be variation in the licensing of different medicines containing the same drug. Forms available from special-order manufacturers include: oral capsule, oral solution, solution for injection, infusion, solution for infusion

Modified-release tablet

CAUTIONARY AND ADVISORY LABELS 25

- **Slow Sodium** (Stirling Anglian Pharmaceuticals Ltd)
  Sodium chloride 600 mg Slow Sodium 600mg tablets | 100 tablet GSL £21.95 DT = £21.95

Solution for injection

- **Sodium chloride (Non-proprietary)**
  Presentations available from various suppliers include
  Sodium chloride 9 mg per 1 ml Sodium chloride 0.9% solution for injection | 2ml, 5ml, 10ml, 20ml ampoules PoM | 50ml vials PoM
  Sodium chloride 300 mg per 1 ml Sodium chloride 30% solution for injection | 10ml ampoules PoM

Infusion

- **Sodium chloride (Non-proprietary)**
  Presentations available from various suppliers include
  Sodium chloride 1.8 mg per 1 ml Sodium chloride 0.18% infusion | 500ml bottles PoM
  Sodium chloride 4.5 mg per 1 ml Sodium chloride 0.45% infusion | 500ml bags PoM
  Sodium chloride 9 mg per 1 ml Sodium chloride 0.9% infusion | 50ml, 100ml, 250ml, 500ml, 1litre bags PoM | 50ml, 100ml, 250ml, 500ml, 1litre bottles PoM (Hospital only)
  Sodium chloride 18 mg per 1 ml Sodium chloride 1.8% infusion | 500ml bottles PoM
  Sodium chloride 27 mg per 1 ml Sodium chloride 2.7% infusion | 500ml bottles PoM
  Sodium chloride 50 mg per 1 ml Sodium chloride 5% infusion | 500ml bottles PoM

Oral solution

EXCIPIENTS: May contain Potassium sorbate

- **Sodium chloride (Non-proprietary)**
  Sodium chloride 58.5 mg per 1 ml Sodium chloride 292.5mg/5ml (1mmol/ml) oral solution | 100 ml PoM £33.16 DT = £33.16
  Sodium chloride 292 mg per 1 ml Sodium chloride 1.46g/5ml (5mmol/ml) oral solution | 100 ml PoM £22.00–£22.46 DT = £22.46
- **AcuSal** (Essential-Healthcare Ltd)
  Sodium chloride 234 mg per 1 ml AcuSal 1.17g/5ml (4mmol/ml) oral solution | 100 ml £6.87 DT = £11.77
- **Syrisal** (SyriMed)
  Sodium chloride 58.5 mg per 1 ml Syrisal 292.5mg/5ml (1mmol/ml) oral solution | 100 ml PoM £30.20 DT = £33.16

Solution for infusion

- **Sodium chloride (Non-proprietary)**
  Presentations available from various suppliers include
  Sodium chloride 300 mg per 1 ml Sodium chloride 30% concentrate for solution for infusion | 10ml ampoules PoM (Hospital only) | 50ml vials PoM | 100ml vials PoM (Hospital only)

Combinations available: ***Potassium chloride with calcium chloride dihydrate and sodium chloride,*** p. 726 · ***Potassium chloride with calcium chloride, sodium chloride and sodium lactate,*** p. 727 · ***Potassium chloride with glucose and sodium***

9 Blood and nutrition

chloride, p. 727 · ***Potassium chloride with sodium chloride***, p. 728

Sodium chloride with glucose

The properties listed below are those particular to the combination only. For the properties of the components please consider, sodium chloride p. 728, glucose below.

● **INDICATIONS AND DOSE**

Combined water and sodium depletion

▶ BY INTRAVENOUS INFUSION

▸ Child: (consult product literature)

● **CAUTIONS** Sodium chloride 0.18% and glucose 4% intravenous infusion fluid should not be used for fluid replacement in children aged 16 years or less because of the risk of hyponatraemia; availability of this infusion should be restricted to high dependency and intensive care units, and specialist wards, such as renal, liver, and cardiac units. Local guidelines on intravenous fluids should be consulted.

● **MONITORING REQUIREMENTS**

▶ Maintenance fluid should accurately reflect daily requirements and close monitoring is required to avoid fluid and electrolyte imbalance.

▶ During parenteral hydration, fluids and electrolytes should be monitored closely and any disturbance corrected by slow infusion of an appropriate solution.

● **MEDICINAL FORMS** There can be variation in the licensing of different medicines containing the same drug. Forms available from special-order manufacturers include: infusion, solution for infusion

Infusion

▸ Sodium chloride with glucose (Non-proprietary)

Presentations available from various suppliers include

Sodium chloride 1.8 mg per 1 ml, Glucose anhydrous 40 mg per 1 ml Sodium chloride 0.18% / Glucose 4% infusion | 500ml, 1litre bags PoM

Sodium chloride 1.8 mg per 1 ml, Glucose anhydrous 100 mg per 1 ml Sodium chloride 0.18% / Glucose 10% infusion | 500ml bags PoM

Sodium chloride 4.5 mg per 1 ml, Glucose anhydrous 25 mg per 1 ml Sodium chloride 0.45% / Glucose 2.5% infusion | 500ml bags PoM

Sodium chloride 4.5 mg per 1 ml, Glucose (as Glucose monohydrate) 50 mg per 1 ml Sodium chloride 0.45% / Glucose 5% infusion | 500ml bottles PoM (Hospital only)

Sodium chloride 9 mg per 1 ml, Glucose (as Glucose monohydrate) 50 mg per 1 ml Sodium chloride 0.9% / Glucose 5% infusion | 500ml bottles PoM (Hospital only)

NUTRIENTS > SUGARS

Glucose

04-Dec-2025

(Dextrose Monohydrate)

● **INDICATIONS AND DOSE**

Establish presence of gestational diabetes

▶ BY MOUTH

▸ Child: Test dose 75 g, anhydrous glucose to be given to the fasting patient and blood-glucose concentrations measured at intervals, to be given with 200–300 mL fluid

Oral glucose tolerance test

▶ BY MOUTH

▸ Child: Test dose 1.75 g/kg (max. per dose 75 g), anhydrous glucose to be given to the fasting patient and blood-glucose concentrations measured at intervals. To be given with 200–300 mL fluid

Neonatal hypoglycaemia

▶ BY INTRAVENOUS INFUSION

▸ Neonate: 500 mg/kg/hour, to be administered as Glucose 10% intravenous infusion, an initial dose of 250 mg/kg over 5 minutes may be required if hypoglycaemia is severe enough to cause loss of consciousness or seizures.

Hypoglycaemia

▶ BY MOUTH

▸ Child up to 5 years: 5 g, repeated after 15 minutes if necessary, 5 g is available from 20 mL oral glucose liquid, 1.5 glucose tablets, or half a tube of glucose 40% oral gel. If oral glucose formulations are not available, the dose may be given using another fast-acting carbohydrate; 5 g is available from approximately 1 teaspoonful of sugar dissolved in an appropriate volume of water

▸ Child 5–11 years: 10 g, repeated after 15 minutes if necessary, 10 g is available from 40 mL oral glucose liquid, 3 glucose tablets, or 1 tube of glucose 40% oral gel. If oral glucose formulations are not available, the dose may be given using another fast-acting carbohydrate; 10 g is available from approximately 2 teaspoonfuls of sugar dissolved in an appropriate volume of water

▸ Child 12–17 years: 15 g, repeated after 15 minutes if necessary, 15 g is available from 60 mL oral glucose liquid, 4 glucose tablets, or 1.5 tubes of glucose 40% oral gel. If oral glucose formulations are not available, the dose may be given using another fast-acting carbohydrate; 15 g is available from approximately 3 teaspoonfuls of sugar dissolved in an appropriate volume of water

▶ BY INTRAVENOUS INFUSION

▸ Child: 500 mg/kg, to be administered as Glucose 10% intravenous infusion into a large vein through a large-gauge needle; care is required since this concentration is irritant

Hypoglycaemia [in conscious but uncooperative patients]

▶ BY BUCCAL ADMINISTRATION

▸ Child up to 5 years: 5 g, repeated after 15 minutes if necessary, to be given as half a tube of glucose 40% oral gel

▸ Child 5–11 years: 10 g, repeated after 15 minutes if necessary, to be given as 1 tube of glucose 40% oral gel

▸ Child 12–17 years: 15 g, repeated after 15 minutes if necessary, to be given as 1.5 tubes of glucose 40% oral gel

Energy source

▶ BY INTRAVENOUS INFUSION

▸ Child: (consult product literature)

Fluid and carbohydrate replacement

▶ BY INTRAVENOUS INFUSION

▸ Child: The volume of glucose solution needed to replace deficits may vary (consult product literature)

Persistent cyanosis (in combination with propranolol) when blood glucose less than 3 mmol/litre (followed by morphine)

▶ BY INTRAVENOUS INFUSION

▸ Child: 200 mg/kg, to be administered as Glucose 10% intravenous infusion over 10 minutes

Diabetic ketoacidosis

▶ BY INTRAVENOUS INFUSION

▸ Child: (consult local protocol)

DOSE EQUIVALENCE AND CONVERSION

▸ 75 g anhydrous glucose is equivalent to Glucose BP 82.5 g.

▸ For hypoglycaemia, examples of glucose preparations which can be used to give oral doses are based on the use of oral liquid containing glucose 250 mg/mL and tablets containing glucose 4 g per tablet. Buccal dosing is based on tubes of 40% oral gel containing glucose 10 g per tube.

- **CAUTIONS** Do not give alone except when there is no significant loss of electrolytes · prolonged administration of glucose solutions without electrolytes can lead to hyponatraemia and other electrolyte disturbances
- **SIDE-EFFECTS** Chills · electrolyte imbalance · fever · fluid imbalance · hypersensitivity · local reaction · localised pain · polyuria · rash · venous thrombosis
- **DIRECTIONS FOR ADMINISTRATION**
  - With intravenous use EvGr Injections containing more than 10% glucose can be irritant and should generally be given into a central venous line except in emergencies. (M)
- **PRESCRIBING AND DISPENSING INFORMATION** Glucose BP is the monohydrate but Glucose Intravenous Infusion BP is a sterile solution of anhydrous glucose or glucose monohydrate, potency being expressed in terms of anhydrous glucose.
- **EXCEPTIONS TO LEGAL CATEGORY**
  - With intravenous use Prescription only medicine restriction does not apply where administration is for saving life in emergency.

- **MEDICINAL FORMS** There can be variation in the licensing of different medicines containing the same drug. Forms available from special-order manufacturers include: oral solution, solution for injection, solution for infusion

Solution for infusion

- Glucose (Non-proprietary)
  Glucose anhydrous 200 mg per 1 ml Glucose 20% solution for infusion 100ml vials | 1 vial PoM £10.80
  Glucose anhydrous 500 mg per 1 ml Glucose 50% solution for infusion 20ml ampoules | 10 ampoule PoM £18.94–£22.73
  Glucose 50% solution for infusion 50ml vials | 25 vial PoM £85.00–£102.00

Oral solution

- Rapilose OGTT (Penlan Healthcare Ltd)
  Glucose 250 mg per 1 ml Rapilose OGTT solution | 300 ml £3.98

Oral liquid

- Glucojuice (BBI Healthcare Ltd, Flavour Not Specified)
  Lift Fast Acting Glucose Shot liquid zesty lemon & lime | 60 ml £0.99
  Lift Fast Acting Glucose Shot liquid strawberry & lime | 60 ml £0.99
  Lift Fast Acting Glucose Shot liquid very berry | 60 ml £0.99
  Lift Fast Acting Glucose Shot liquid | 60 ml ⊠
  Lift Fast Acting Glucose Shot liquid fruity tropical | 60 ml £0.99

Oral gel

- AACE Gluco (Essential-Healthcare Ltd)
  Glucose 400 mg per 1 gram AACE Gluco 40% gel | 75 gram £4.80 DT = £7.16
- AddGluco (TriOn Pharma Ltd)
  Glucose 400 mg per 1 gram AddGluco 40% gel | 75 gram £4.75 DT = £7.16
- Dextrogel (Neoceuticals Ltd)
  Glucose 400 mg per 1 gram Dextrogel 40% gel | 75 gram £5.38 DT = £7.16 | 80 gram £5.38
- GlucoBoost (Ennogen Healthcare International Ltd)
  Glucose 400 mg per 1 gram GlucoBoost 40% gel | 75 gram £7.16 DT = £7.16 | 80 gram £6.11
- GlucoGel (BBI Healthcare Ltd)
  Glucose 400 mg per 1 gram GlucoGel 40% gel original | 75 gram £7.16 DT = £7.16 | 80 gram £6.84
- PlusGluco (MaN Pharma Ltd)
  Glucose 400 mg per 1 gram PlusGluco 40% gel | 75 gram £4.77 DT = £7.16
- Rapilose (Penlan Healthcare Ltd)
  Glucose 400 mg per 1 gram Rapilose 40% gel | 75 gram £5.49 DT = £7.16

Infusion

- Glucose (Non-proprietary)
  Presentations available from various suppliers include
  Glucose anhydrous 50 mg per 1 ml Glucose 5% infusion | 50ml, 100ml, 250ml, 500ml, 1litre bags PoM | 500ml, 1litre bottles PoM
  Glucose (as Glucose monohydrate) 50 mg per 1 ml Glucose 5% infusion | 50ml, 100ml, 250ml bottles PoM (Hospital only)
  Glucose anhydrous 100 mg per 1 ml Glucose 10% infusion | 500ml, 1litre bags PoM
  Glucose anhydrous 200 mg per 1 ml Glucose 20% infusion | 500ml bags PoM
  Glucose (as Glucose monohydrate) 300 mg per 1 ml Glucose 30% infusion | 500ml bottles PoM (Hospital only)
  Glucose anhydrous 400 mg per 1 ml Glucose 40% infusion | 500ml bags PoM
  Glucose anhydrous 500 mg per 1 ml Glucose 50% infusion | 500ml bags PoM
  Glucose anhydrous 700 mg per 1 ml Glucose 70% concentrate for solution for infusion | 500ml bags PoM (Hospital only)

Combinations available: ***Potassium chloride with glucose***, p. 727 · ***Potassium chloride with glucose and sodium chloride***, p. 727 · ***Sodium chloride with glucose***, p. 730

ORAL REHYDRATION SALTS

Disodium hydrogen citrate with glucose, potassium chloride and sodium chloride

09-May-2024

- **DRUG ACTION** Formulated as oral rehydration salts
- **INDICATIONS AND DOSE**

Fluid and electrolyte loss in diarrhoea

- BY MOUTH
  - Child 1–11 months: 1–1½ times usual feed volume to be given
  - Child 1–11 years: 200 mL, to be given after every loose motion
  - Child 12–17 years: 200–400 mL, to be given after every loose motion, dose according to fluid loss

- **DIRECTIONS FOR ADMINISTRATION** Manufacturer advises reconstitute 1 sachet with 200mL of water (freshly boiled and cooled for infants); 5 sachets reconstituted with 1 litre of water provide Na^+ 60 mmol, K^+ 20 mmol, Cl^- 60 mmol, citrate 10 mmol, and glucose 90 mmol.
- **PRESCRIBING AND DISPENSING INFORMATION** Flavours of oral powder formulations may include black currant, citrus, or natural.
- **PATIENT AND CARER ADVICE** After reconstitution any unused solution should be discarded no later than 1 hour after preparation unless stored in a refrigerator when it may be kept for up to 24 hours.
  Medicines for Children leaflet: Oral rehydration salts
  www.medicinesforchildren.org.uk/medicines/oral-rehydration-salts/

- **MEDICINAL FORMS** There can be variation in the licensing of different medicines containing the same drug.

Powder for oral solution

CAUTIONARY AND ADVISORY LABELS 13

- Dioralyte (Dendron Brands Ltd)
  Potassium chloride 300 mg, Sodium chloride 470 mg, Disodium hydrogen citrate 530 mg, Glucose 3.56 gram Dioralyte oral powder sachets blackcurrant | 20 sachet P £9.37
  Dioralyte oral powder sachets plain | 20 sachet P £9.37

Potassium chloride with rice powder, sodium chloride and sodium citrate

09-May-2024

- **DRUG ACTION** Formulated as oral rehydration salts

- **INDICATIONS AND DOSE**

Fluid and electrolyte loss in diarrhoea
▶ BY MOUTH
▸ Child 1–11 months: 1–1½ times usual feed volume to be given
▸ Child 1–11 years: 200 mL, to be given after every loose motion
▸ Child 12–17 years: 200–400 mL, to be given after every loose motion, dose according to fluid loss

- **UNLICENSED USE** *Dioralyte Relief®* not licensed for use in children under 3 months.
- **DIRECTIONS FOR ADMINISTRATION** Manufacturer advises reconstitute 1 sachet with 200 mL of water (freshly boiled and cooled for infants); 5 sachets when reconstituted with 1 litre of water provide Na^{+} 60 mmol, K^{+} 20 mmol, Cl^{-} 50 mmol and citrate 10 mmol.
- **PRESCRIBING AND DISPENSING INFORMATION** Flavours of oral powder formulations may include apricot, black currant, or raspberry.
- **PATIENT AND CARER ADVICE** Patients and carers should be advised how to reconstitute *Dioralyte®* Relief oral powder. After reconstitution any unused solution should be discarded no later than 1 hour after preparation unless stored in a refrigerator when it may be kept for up to 24 hours.
Medicines for Children leaflet: Oral rehydration salts www.medicinesforchildren.org.uk/medicines/oral-rehydration-salts/

- **MEDICINAL FORMS** There can be variation in the licensing of different medicines containing the same drug.

Powder for oral solution
CAUTIONARY AND ADVISORY LABELS 13
EXCIPIENTS: May contain Aspartame
▸ Dioralyte Relief (Dendron Brands Ltd)
Potassium chloride 300 mg, Sodium chloride 350 mg, Sodium citrate 580 mg, Rice powder pre-cooked 6 gram Dioralyte Relief oral powder sachets blackcurrant | 20 sachet [P] £10.00 [SF]

2.1 Calcium imbalance

Calcium imbalance

Calcium supplements

Calcium supplements are usually only required where dietary calcium intake is deficient. This dietary requirement varies with age and is relatively greater in childhood, pregnancy, and lactation, due to an increased demand. Hypocalcaemia may be caused by vitamin D deficiency (see Vitamin D under Vitamins p. 780), impaired metabolism, a failure of secretion (hypoparathyroidism), or resistance to parathyroid hormone (pseudohypoparathyroidism).

Mild asymptomatic hypocalcaemia may be managed with oral calcium supplements. *Severe symptomatic hypocalcaemia* requires an intravenous infusion of calcium gluconate 10% p. 735 over 5 to 10 minutes, repeating the dose if symptoms persist; in exceptional cases it may be necessary to maintain a continuous calcium infusion over a day or more. Calcium chloride injection p. 734 is also available, but is more irritant; care should be taken to prevent extravasation.

See the role of calcium gluconate in temporarily reducing the toxic effects of *hyperkalaemia*.

Persistent hypocalcaemia requires oral calcium supplements and either a vitamin D analogue (alfacalcidol p. 787 or calcitriol p. 788) for hypoparathyroidism and pseudohypoparathyroidism or natural vitamin D (calciferol) if due to vitamin D deficiency. It is important to monitor plasma and urinary calcium during long-term maintenance therapy.

Severe hypercalcaemia

Severe hypercalcaemia calls for urgent treatment before detailed investigation of the cause. Dehydration should be corrected first with intravenous infusion of sodium chloride **0.9%** p. 728. Drugs (such as thiazides and vitamin D compounds) which promote hypercalcaemia, should be discontinued and dietary calcium should be restricted.

If *severe hypercalcaemia persists* drugs which inhibit mobilisation of calcium from the skeleton may be required. The **bisphosphonates** are useful and pamidronate disodium p. 535 is probably the most effective.

Corticosteroids are widely given, but may only be useful where hypercalcaemia is due to sarcoidosis or vitamin D intoxication; they often take several days to achieve the desired effect.

Calcitonin (salmon) p. 536 can be used by specialists for the treatment of hypercalcaemia associated with malignancy; it is rarely effective where bisphosphonates have failed to reduce serum calcium adequately.

After treatment of severe hypercalcaemia the underlying cause must be established. *Further treatment* is governed by the same principles as for initial therapy. Salt and water depletion and drugs promoting hypercalcaemia should be avoided; oral administration of a bisphosphonate may be useful. Parathyroidectomy may be indicated for hyperparathyroidism.

Hypercalciuria

Hypercalciuria should be investigated for an underlying cause, which should be treated. Reducing dietary calcium intake may be beneficial but severe restriction of calcium intake has not proved beneficial and may even be harmful.

Calcium supplements in neonates

Hypocalcaemia is common in the first few days of life, particularly following birth asphyxia or respiratory distress. Late onset at 4–10 days after birth may be secondary to vitamin D deficiency, hypoparathyroidism or hypomagnesaemia and may be associated with seizures.

2.1a Hypercalcaemia and hypercalciuria

CALCIUM REGULATING DRUGS > BONE RESORPTION INHIBITORS

Cinacalcet

25-Apr-2025

- **DRUG ACTION** Cinacalcet reduces parathyroid hormone which leads to a decrease in serum calcium concentrations.

- **INDICATIONS AND DOSE**

Secondary hyperparathyroidism [in patients with end-stage renal disease on dialysis] (under expert supervision)
▶ BY MOUTH
▸ Child 3–17 years: (consult product literature)

- **CONTRA-INDICATIONS** Hypocalcaemia
- **CAUTIONS** Conditions that may worsen with a decrease in serum-calcium concentrations

CAUTIONS, FURTHER INFORMATION Manufacturer advises caution with use in patients with conditions that may worsen with a decrease in serum-calcium concentrations, including predisposition to QT-interval prolongation, history of seizures, and history of impaired cardiac function—serum-calcium concentration should be closely monitored.

- **INTERACTIONS** → Appendix 1: cinacalcet
- **SIDE-EFFECTS**
  - **Common or very common** Appetite decreased · asthenia · back pain · constipation · cough · diarrhoea · dizziness · dyspnoea · electrolyte imbalance · gastrointestinal discomfort · headache · hypersensitivity · hypotension · muscle complaints · nausea · paraesthesia · rash · seizure · upper respiratory tract infection · vomiting
  - **Frequency not known** Heart failure aggravated · QT interval prolongation · ventricular arrhythmia
- **PREGNANCY** Manufacturer advises use only if potential benefit outweighs risk—no information available.
- **BREAST FEEDING** Manufacturer advises avoid—present in milk in *animal* studies.
- **HEPATIC IMPAIRMENT** Manufacturer advises caution in moderate to severe impairment.
- **MONITORING REQUIREMENTS** Manufacturer advises measure serum-calcium concentration before initiation of treatment and within 1 week after starting treatment or adjusting dose, then weekly thereafter. Measure parathyroid hormone concentration 1–4 weeks after starting treatment or adjusting dose.
- **DIRECTIONS FOR ADMINISTRATION** Manufacturer advises capsules containing granules should be opened and the granules sprinkled on to a small amount of soft food (apple sauce or yogurt) or liquid, then administered immediately. Capsules should not be swallowed whole. For administration advice via nasogastric or gastrostomy tube—consult product literature.
- **PATIENT AND CARER ADVICE** Manufacturer advises patients and their carers should be counselled on the symptoms of hypocalcaemia and importance of serum-calcium monitoring.
  Driving and skilled tasks Manufacturer advises patients and carers should be counselled on the effects on driving and performance of skilled tasks—increased risk of dizziness and seizures.

- **MEDICINAL FORMS** There can be variation in the licensing of different medicines containing the same drug.

Oral tablet

CAUTIONARY AND ADVISORY LABELS 21

- **Cinacalcet (Non-proprietary)**
  - **Cinacalcet (as Cinacalcet hydrochloride) 30 mg** Cinacalcet 30mg tablets | 28 tablet [PoM] £113.18 DT = £4.06
  - **Cinacalcet (as Cinacalcet hydrochloride) 60 mg** Cinacalcet 60mg tablets | 28 tablet [PoM] £208.77 DT = £11.93
  - **Cinacalcet (as Cinacalcet hydrochloride) 90 mg** Cinacalcet 90mg tablets | 28 tablet [PoM] £295.77 DT = £295.77

2.1b Hypocalcaemia

ELECTROLYTES AND MINERALS > CALCIUM

Calcium salts

- **CONTRA-INDICATIONS** Conditions associated with hypercalcaemia (e.g. some forms of malignant disease) · conditions associated with hypercalciuria (e.g. some forms of malignant disease)
- **CAUTIONS** History of nephrolithiasis · sarcoidosis
- **SIDE-EFFECTS**
  - **Uncommon** Constipation · diarrhoea · hypercalcaemia · nausea
  - **Rare or very rare** Gastrointestinal disorder
- **RENAL IMPAIRMENT** [EvGr] Use with caution. ⟨M⟩

above

Calcium carbonate

09-May-2025

- **INDICATIONS AND DOSE**

Phosphate binding in renal failure and hyperphosphataemia

▶ BY MOUTH

- Child 1-11 months: 120 mg 3–4 times a day, to be taken with feeds, dose to be adjusted as necessary
- Child 1-5 years: 300 mg 3–4 times a day, to be taken prior to or with meals, dose to be adjusted as necessary
- Child 6-11 years: 600 mg 3–4 times a day, to be taken prior to or with meals, dose to be adjusted as necessary
- Child 12-17 years: 1.25 g 3–4 times a day, to be taken prior to or with meals, dose to be adjusted as necessary

Calcium deficiency

▶ BY MOUTH

- Neonate: 0.25 mmol/kg 4 times a day, dose adjusted according to response.
- Child 1 month-4 years: 0.25 mmol/kg 4 times a day, dose adjusted according to response
- Child 5-11 years: 0.2 mmol/kg 4 times a day, dose adjusted according to response
- Child 12-17 years: 10 mmol 4 times a day, dose adjusted according to response

- **INTERACTIONS** → Appendix 1: calcium compounds
- **SIDE-EFFECTS**
  - **Uncommon** Hypercalciuria
  - **Rare or very rare** Flatulence · gastrointestinal discomfort · milk-alkali syndrome · skin reactions
- **DIRECTIONS FOR ADMINISTRATION** The RCPCH and NPPG recommend that, for part doses using Calcium 500 mg effervescent tablets, one 12.5 mmol tablet should be dissolved in 12 mL of water to give a final concentration of approximately 1 mmol/mL. Once the tablet has fully dispersed and fizzing has stopped, the required dose should be withdrawn using an oral syringe and any remaining solution discarded.
- **PRESCRIBING AND DISPENSING INFORMATION** *Adcal*® contains calcium carbonate 1.5 g (calcium 600 mg or Ca^{2+} 15 mmol); *Calcichew*® contains calcium carbonate 1.25 g (calcium 500 mg or Ca^{2+} 12.5 mmol); *Calcichew Forte*® contains calcium carbonate 2.5 g (calcium 1 g or Ca^{2+} 25 mmol); *Cacit*® contains calcium carbonate 1.25 g, providing calcium citrate when dispersed in water (calcium 500 mg or Ca^{2+} 12.5 mmol); consult product literature for details of other available products.

  Flavours of chewable tablet formulations may include orange or fruit flavour.

  ▸ When used for Phosphate binding in renal failure and hyperphosphataemia The RCPCH and NPPG recommend that, when a liquid special of calcium carbonate is required, the following strength is used: 500 mg/5 mL.

  Administration of 'part doses' using effervescent tablets The RCPCH and NPPG recommend that doses should be rounded to enable measurement, and clear instructions provided on the dispensing label and when counselling patients or their carer. Appropriate equipment for administration should also be provided, such as:

  - a 20 mL oral syringe to measure the initial volume of water required for tablet dispersion;
  - a reusable plastic medicine pot in which the tablet can be dispersed in water;

- another smaller oral syringe to measure and administer the required dose (a 1 mL syringe is required for dose volume less than 1 mL).

For further details, see the position statement from the RCPCH and NPPG, available at: nppg.org.uk/wp-content/uploads/2025/04/Position-Statement-CalciumPhosphate-and-PotassiumV3.pdf.

- **PATIENT AND CARER ADVICE** Patients or carers should be counselled on how to administer part doses of effervescent tablets.

Medicines for Children leaflet: Calcium salts for kidney disease www.medicinesforchildren.org.uk/medicines/calcium-salts-for-kidney-disease/

Medicines for Children leaflet: How to give calcium, phosphate or potassium using effervescent tablets www.medicinesforchildren.org.uk/advice-guides/giving-medicines/how-to-give-phosphate-or-calcium-from-effervescent-tablets/

- **MEDICINAL FORMS** There can be variation in the licensing of different medicines containing the same drug. Forms available from special-order manufacturers include: oral tablet, oral capsule, oral suspension

Oral tablet

CAUTIONARY AND ADVISORY LABELS 25

Effervescent tablet

CAUTIONARY AND ADVISORY LABELS 13

▸ **A1-Cal** (TriOn Pharma Ltd)
Calcium carbonate 625 mg A1-Cal 250mg effervescent tablets | 10 tablet £13.87 SF
Calcium carbonate 1.25 gram A1-Cal 500mg effervescent tablets | 20 tablet £2.99 SF

▸ **AaceCa** (Essential-Healthcare Ltd)
Calcium carbonate 1.25 gram AaceCa 500mg effervescent tablets | 19 tablet £2.79 SF | 76 tablet £11.15 SF

Chewable tablet

CAUTIONARY AND ADVISORY LABELS 24
EXCIPIENTS: May contain Aspartame

▸ **Adcal** (Grunenthal Ltd)
Calcium carbonate 1.5 gram Adcal 1500mg chewable tablets | 100 tablet P £8.70 DT = £8.70 SF

▸ **Calcichew** (Forum Health Products Ltd)
Calcium carbonate 1.25 gram Calcichew 500mg chewable tablets | 100 tablet P £9.33 DT = £9.33 SF
Calcium carbonate 2.5 gram Calcichew Forte chewable tablets | 60 tablet P £14.21 DT = £14.21 SF

▸ **Rennie** (Bayer Plc)
Calcium carbonate 500 mg Rennie Orange 500mg chewable tablets | 24 tablet GSL £2.55 | 36 tablet GSL £3.19 | 72 tablet GSL £5.22

▸ **Setlers Antacid** (Thornton & Ross Ltd)
Calcium carbonate 500 mg Setlers Antacid spearmint chewable tablets | 24 tablet GSL £2.04 | 36 tablet GSL £2.04
Setlers Antacid peppermint chewable tablets | 24 tablet GSL £2.04 | 36 tablet GSL £2.04

Calcium carbonate with calcium lactate gluconate

09-May-2025

The properties listed below are those particular to the combination only. For the properties of the components please consider, calcium carbonate p. 733.

- **INDICATIONS AND DOSE**

Calcium deficiency

▸ BY MOUTH

▸ Neonate: 0.25 mmol/kg 4 times a day, adjusted according to response.

▸ Child 1 month–4 years: 0.25 mmol/kg 4 times a day, adjusted according to response

▸ Child 5–11 years: 0.2 mmol/kg 4 times a day, adjusted according to response

▸ Child 12–17 years: 10 mmol 4 times a day, adjusted according to response

- **INTERACTIONS** → Appendix 1: calcium compounds
- **DIRECTIONS FOR ADMINISTRATION** The RCPCH and NPPG recommend that, for part doses using *Calvive*® 1000 effervescent tablets, one 25 mmol tablet should be dissolved in 20 mL of water to give a final concentration of approximately 1 mmol/mL. Once the tablet has fully dispersed and fizzing has stopped, the required dose should be withdrawn using an oral syringe and any remaining solution discarded.
- **PRESCRIBING AND DISPENSING INFORMATION** Each *Calvive*® tablet contains 1 g calcium (Ca^{2+} 25 mmol); flavours of effervescent tablet formulations may include orange.

Administration of 'part doses' using effervescent tablets The RCPCH and NPPG recommend that doses should be rounded to enable measurement, and clear instructions provided on the dispensing label and when counselling patients or their carer. Appropriate equipment for administration should also be provided, such as:

- a 20 mL oral syringe to measure the initial volume of water required for tablet dispersion;
- a reusable plastic medicine pot in which the tablet can be dispersed in water;
- another smaller oral syringe to measure and administer the required dose (a 1 mL syringe is required for dose volume less than 1 mL).

For further details, see the position statement from the RCPCH and NPPG, available at: nppg.org.uk/wp-content/uploads/2025/04/Position-Statement-CalciumPhosphate-and-PotassiumV3.pdf.

- **PATIENT AND CARER ADVICE** Patients or carers should be counselled on how to administer part doses of effervescent tablets.

Medicines for Children leaflet: How to give calcium, phosphate or potassium using effervescent tablets www.medicinesforchildren.org.uk/advice-guides/giving-medicines/how-to-give-phosphate-or-calcium-from-effervescent-tablets/

- **MEDICINAL FORMS** There can be variation in the licensing of different medicines containing the same drug.

Effervescent tablet

CAUTIONARY AND ADVISORY LABELS 13
EXCIPIENTS: May contain Aspartame

▸ **Calvive** (Haleon UK Trading Ltd)
Calcium carbonate 1.75 gram, Calcium lactate gluconate 2.263 gram Calvive 1000 effervescent tablets | 30 tablet P £14.11 DT = £14.11 SF

733

Calcium chloride

10-Nov-2023

- **INDICATIONS AND DOSE**

Acute hypocalcaemia

▸ BY INTRAVENOUS INFUSION

▸ Child: (consult product literature)

- **CAUTIONS** Avoid in respiratory acidosis · avoid in respiratory failure
- **INTERACTIONS** → Appendix 1: calcium compounds
- **SIDE-EFFECTS** Soft tissue calcification · taste unpleasant · vasodilation
- **DIRECTIONS FOR ADMINISTRATION** Care should be taken to avoid extravasation. Incompatible with bicarbonates, phosphates, or sulfates.
- **PRESCRIBING AND DISPENSING INFORMATION** Non-proprietary *Calcium chloride dihydrate* 7.35% (calcium 20 mg or Ca^{2+} 500 micromol/mL); *Calcium chloride dihydrate* 10% (calcium 27.3 mg or Ca^{2+} 680 micromol/mL); *Calcium chloride dihydrate* 14.7% (calcium 40.1 mg or Ca^{2+} 1000 micromol/mL).

● **MEDICINAL FORMS** There can be variation in the licensing of different medicines containing the same drug. Forms available from special-order manufacturers include: solution for injection, solution for infusion

Solution for injection

▸ Calcium chloride (Non-proprietary)

Calcium chloride dihydrate 100 mg per 1 ml Calcium chloride 10% solution for injection 10ml pre-filled syringes | 1 pre-filled disposable injection PoM £9.89–£13.18

Calcium chloride dihydrate 147 mg per 1 ml Calcium chloride 14.7% solution for injection 5ml ampoules | 10 ampoule PoM £249.41

Calcium chloride 14.7% solution for injection 10ml ampoules | 10 ampoule PoM £107.06–£169.55

733

Calcium gluconate

09-May-2025

● **INDICATIONS AND DOSE**

Calcium deficiency | Mild asymptomatic hypocalcaemia

▶ BY MOUTH

▸ Neonate: 0.25 mmol/kg 4 times a day, dose adjusted according to response.

▸ Child 1 month–4 years: 0.25 mmol/kg 4 times a day, dose adjusted according to response

▸ Child 5–11 years: 0.2 mmol/kg 4 times a day, dose adjusted according to response

▸ Child 12–17 years: 10 mmol 4 times a day, dose adjusted according to response

Acute hypocalcaemia [urgent correction]

▶ BY SLOW INTRAVENOUS INJECTION

▸ Neonate: 0.11 mmol/kg for 1 dose, to be given over 5–10 minutes, some units use a dose of 0.46 mmol/kg (2 mL/kg calcium gluconate 10%) for hypocalcaemia in line with US practice.

▸ Child: 0.11 mmol/kg for 1 dose (max. per dose 4.5 mmol), to be given over 5–10 minutes (10 mL calcium gluconate 10% is equivalent to approximately 2.25 mmol of calcium)

Acute hypocalcaemia [maintenance]

▶ BY CONTINUOUS INTRAVENOUS INFUSION

▸ Neonate: 0.5 mmol/kg daily, adjusted according to response, dose to be given over 24 hours, use oral route as soon as possible due to risk of extravasation.

▸ Child 1 month–1 year: 1 mmol/kg daily, adjusted according to response, dose to be given over 24 hours, use oral route as soon as possible due to risk of extravasation; Usual maximum 8.8 mmol

▸ Child 2–17 years: 8.8 mmol daily, adjusted according to response, dose to be given over 24 hours, use oral route as soon as possible due to risk of extravasation

Acute severe hyperkalaemia [prevention of arrhythmias]

▶ BY SLOW INTRAVENOUS INJECTION

▸ Neonate: 0.11 mmol/kg for 1 dose, to be given over 5–10 minutes, repeat dose if ECG changes persist after 5–10 minutes.

▸ Child: 0.11 mmol/kg for 1 dose (max. per dose 6.75 mmol), to be given over 5–10 minutes (10 mL calcium gluconate 10% is equivalent to approximately 2.25 mmol of calcium), repeat dose if ECG changes persist after 5–10 minutes

DOSE EQUIVALENCE AND CONVERSION

▸ With intravenous use

▸ 0.11 mmol/kg is equivalent to 0.5 mL/kg of calcium gluconate 10%.

● **UNLICENSED USE** Calcium gluconate is used in the doses provided in BNFC for the urgent correction of acute hypocalcaemia and treatment of acute severe hyperkalaemia in neonates and children, but these may differ from those licensed. Calcium gluconate is used for the maintenance treatment of acute hypocalcaemia in neonates and children, but is not licensed for this indication.

IMPORTANT SAFETY INFORMATION

MHRA/CHM ADVICE: CALCIUM GLUCONATE INJECTION IN SMALL-VOLUME GLASS CONTAINERS: NEW CONTRA-INDICATIONS DUE TO ALUMINIUM EXPOSURE RISK (AUGUST 2010)

The MHRA has advised that repeated or prolonged administration of calcium gluconate injection packaged in 10 mL glass containers is contra-indicated in children under 18 years and in patients with renal impairment owing to the risk of aluminium accumulation; in these patients the use of calcium gluconate injection packaged in plastic containers is recommended.

● **INTERACTIONS** → Appendix 1: calcium compounds

● **SIDE-EFFECTS**

GENERAL SIDE-EFFECTS Arrhythmias

SPECIFIC SIDE-EFFECTS

▸ With intravenous use Circulatory collapse · feeling hot · hyperhidrosis · hypotension · vasodilation · vomiting

● **MONITORING REQUIREMENTS**

▸ With intravenous use for Acute hypocalcaemia [urgent correction] EvGr Plasma-calcium and ECG monitoring required for administration by slow intravenous injection (risk of arrhythmias if given too rapidly). Ⓜ

● **DIRECTIONS FOR ADMINISTRATION**

▸ With intravenous use For *intravenous infusion* dilute to at least 45 micromol/mL with Glucose 5% *or* Sodium Chloride 0.9%. Maximum administration rate 45 micromol/kg/hour (or in neonates max. 22 micromol/kg/hour). May be given more concentrated via a central venous catheter. May be used undiluted (calcium gluconate 10%) in emergencies. Avoid extravasation; should not be given by intramuscular injection. Incompatible with sodium bicarbonate and phosphate solutions.

▸ With oral use The RCPCH and NPPG recommend that, for part doses using Calcium gluconate 1 g effervescent tablets, one 2.23 mmol tablet should be dissolved in 20 mL of water to give a final concentration of approximately 0.1 mmol/mL. Once the tablet has fully dispersed and fizzing has stopped, the required dose should be withdrawn using an oral syringe and any remaining solution discarded.

● **PRESCRIBING AND DISPENSING INFORMATION** Calcium gluconate 1 g contains calcium 89 mg or Ca^{2+} 2.23 mmol.

Administration of 'part doses' using effervescent tablets The RCPCH and NPPG recommend that doses should be rounded to enable measurement, and clear instructions provided on the dispensing label and when counselling patients or their carer. Appropriate equipment for administration should also be provided, such as:

- a 20 mL oral syringe to measure the initial volume of water required for tablet dispersion;
- a reusable plastic medicine pot in which the tablet can be dispersed in water;
- another smaller oral syringe to measure and administer the required dose (a 1 mL syringe is required for dose volume less than 1 mL).

For further details, see the position statement from the RCPCH and NPPG, available at: nppg.org.uk/wp-content/uploads/2025/04/Position-Statement-CalciumPhosphate-and-PotassiumV3.pdf.

- **PATIENT AND CARER ADVICE** Patients or carers should be counselled on how to administer part doses of effervescent tablets.
Medicines for Children leaflet: How to give calcium, phosphate or potassium using effervescent tablets www.medicinesforchildren.org.uk/advice-guides/giving-medicines/how-to-give-phosphate-or-calcium-from-effervescent-tablets/

- **MEDICINAL FORMS** There can be variation in the licensing of different medicines containing the same drug. Forms available from special-order manufacturers include: oral tablet, oral capsule, oral suspension, oral solution, solution for injection, solution for infusion

Solution for injection

▸ Calcium gluconate (Non-proprietary)
Calcium gluconate 100 mg per 1 ml Calcium gluconate 10% solution for injection 10ml ampoules | 10 ampoule PoM £24.17-£28.21 | 20 ampoule PoM £30.00-£163.86 | 20 ampoule PoM £39.00 (Hospital only)

Effervescent tablet

CAUTIONARY AND ADVISORY LABELS 13
ELECTROLYTES: May contain Sodium

▸ Calcium gluconate (Non-proprietary)
Calcium gluconate 1 gram Calcium gluconate 1g effervescent tablets | 28 tablet GSL £18.35-£23.60 DT = £18.35

733

Calcium lactate

- **INDICATIONS AND DOSE**

Calcium deficiency

▸ BY MOUTH
▸ Neonate: 0.25 mmol/kg 4 times a day, adjusted according to response.
▸ Child 1 month–4 years: 0.25 mmol/kg 4 times a day, adjusted according to response
▸ Child 5–11 years: 0.2 mmol/kg 4 times a day, adjusted according to response
▸ Child 12–17 years: 10 mmol 4 times a day, adjusted according to response

- **INTERACTIONS** → Appendix 1: calcium compounds
- **MEDICINAL FORMS** No licensed medicines listed.

733

Calcium phosphate

- **INDICATIONS AND DOSE**

Indications listed in combination monographs (available in the UK only in combination with other drugs)

▸ BY MOUTH
▸ Child: Doses listed in combination monographs

- **INTERACTIONS** → Appendix 1: calcium compounds
- **SIDE-EFFECTS** Epigastric pain · hypercalciuria
- **MEDICINAL FORMS** No licensed medicines listed.

2.2 Low blood volume

BLOOD AND RELATED PRODUCTS › PLASMA PRODUCTS

Albumin

10-Apr-2026

(Human Albumin Solution)

- **INDICATIONS AND DOSE**

Acute or sub-acute loss of plasma volume e.g. in burns, pancreatitis, trauma, and complications of surgery (with isotonic solutions) | Plasma exchange (with isotonic solutions) | Severe hypoalbuminaemia associated with low plasma volume and generalised oedema where salt and water restriction with plasma volume expansion are required (with concentrated solutions 20%) | Paracentesis of large volume ascites associated with portal hypertension (with concentrated solutions 20%)

▸ BY INTRAVENOUS INFUSION
▸ Child: (consult product literature)

Adjunct in the treatment of hyperbilirubinaemia by exchange transfusion in the newborn (with concentrated solutions 20%)

▸ BY INTRAVENOUS INFUSION
▸ Child: (consult product literature)

- **CAUTIONS** Correct dehydration when administering concentrated solution · history of cardiovascular disease · increased capillary permeability · risk of haemodilution (e.g. severe anaemia or haemorrhagic disorders) · risk of hypervolaemia (e.g. oesophageal varices or pulmonary oedema) · vaccination against hepatitis A and hepatitis B may be required

CAUTIONS, FURTHER INFORMATION

▸ Volume status Manufacturer advises adjust dose and rate of infusion to avoid fluid overload.

- **SIDE-EFFECTS**

▸ **Rare or very rare** Fever · flushing · nausea · shock · urticaria

- **MONITORING REQUIREMENTS** Plasma and plasma substitutes are often used in very ill patients whose condition is unstable. Therefore, close monitoring is required and fluid and electrolyte therapy should be adjusted according to the patient's condition at all times.
- **PRESCRIBING AND DISPENSING INFORMATION** A solution containing protein derived from plasma, serum, or normal placentas; at least 95% of the protein is albumin. The solution may be isotonic (containing 3.5–5% protein) or concentrated (containing 15–25% protein).

- **MEDICINAL FORMS** There can be variation in the licensing of different medicines containing the same drug.

Solution for infusion

▸ Albumin (Non-proprietary)
Albumin solution human 200 mg per 1 ml Human Albumin Grifols 20% solution for infusion 50ml vials | 1 vial PoM £27.00 (Hospital only)
Human Albumin Grifols 20% solution for infusion 100ml vials | 1 vial PoM £54.00 (Hospital only)

▸ Albunorm (Octapharma Ltd)
Albumin solution human 50 mg per 1 ml Albunorm 5% solution for infusion 250ml bottles | 1 bottle PoM £33.75 (Hospital only)
Albunorm 5% solution for infusion 100ml bottles | 1 bottle PoM £13.50 (Hospital only)
Albunorm 5% solution for infusion 500ml bottles | 1 bottle PoM £67.50 (Hospital only)
Albumin solution human 200 mg per 1 ml Albunorm 20% solution for infusion 100ml bottles | 1 bottle PoM £54.00 (Hospital only)
Albunorm 20% solution for infusion 50ml bottles | 1 bottle PoM £27.00 (Hospital only)

- ▸ **Alburex** (CSL Behring UK Ltd)
  Albumin solution human 50 mg per 1 ml Alburex 5% solution for infusion 500ml vials | 1 vial [PoM] £67.50 (Hospital only)
  Albumin solution human 200 mg per 1 ml Alburex 20% solution for infusion 100ml vials | 1 vial [PoM] £54.00 (Hospital only)
- ▸ **Biotest** (Grifols UK Ltd)
  Albumin solution human 50 mg per 1 ml Human Albumin Biotest 5% solution for infusion 250ml vials | 1 vial [PoM] £33.75 (Hospital only)
  Albumin solution human 200 mg per 1 ml Human Albumin Biotest 20% solution for infusion 50ml vials | 1 vial [PoM] £27.00 (Hospital only)
  Human Albumin Biotest 20% solution for infusion 100ml vials | 1 vial [PoM] £54.00 (Hospital only)
- ▸ **Grifols** (Grifols UK Ltd)
  Albumin solution human 50 mg per 1 ml Human Albumin Grifols 5% solution for infusion 250ml bottles | 1 bottle [PoM] £33.75
  Human Albumin Grifols 5% solution for infusion 500ml bottles | 1 bottle [PoM] £67.50
- ▸ **Octalbin** (Octapharma Ltd)
  Albumin solution human 50 mg per 1 ml Octalbin 5% solution for infusion 250ml bottles | 1 bottle [PoM] £33.75 (Hospital only)
  Octalbin 5% solution for infusion 500ml bottles | 1 bottle [PoM] £67.50 (Hospital only)
  Albumin solution human 200 mg per 1 ml Octalbin 20% solution for infusion 100ml bottles | 1 bottle [PoM] £54.00 (Hospital only)
- ▸ **Zenalb** (Bio Products Laboratory Ltd)
  Albumin solution human 45 mg per 1 ml Zenalb 4.5% solution for infusion 250ml bottles | 1 bottle [PoM] £30.38
  Zenalb 4.5% solution for infusion 500ml bottles | 1 bottle [PoM] £60.75
  Albumin solution human 200 mg per 1 ml Zenalb 20% solution for infusion 100ml bottles | 1 bottle [PoM] £54.00
  Zenalb 20% solution for infusion 50ml bottles | 1 bottle [PoM] £27.00

PLASMA SUBSTITUTES

Gelatin

03-Mar-2026

● **INDICATIONS AND DOSE**

Low blood volume in hypovolaemic shock, burns and cardiopulmonary bypass

▸ BY INTRAVENOUS INFUSION

▸ Child: Initially 10–20 mL/kilogram

● **CAUTIONS** Cardiac disease · severe liver disease

CAUTIONS, FURTHER INFORMATION The use of plasma substitutes in children requires specialist supervision due to the risk of fluid overload; use is best restricted to an intensive care setting.

● **SIDE-EFFECTS**

▸ **Rare or very rare** Chills · dyspnoea · fever · hyperhidrosis · hypersensitivity · hypertension · hypotension · hypoxia · tachycardia · tremor · urticaria · wheezing

● **PREGNANCY** Manufacturer of *Geloplasma*® advises avoid at the end of pregnancy.

● **HEPATIC IMPAIRMENT** Manufacturers advise avoid preparations that contain lactate (risk of impaired lactate metabolism).

● **RENAL IMPAIRMENT** [EvGr] Use with caution. ⟨M⟩

● **MONITORING REQUIREMENTS**

▸ Urine output should be monitored. Care should be taken to avoid haematocrit concentration from falling below 25–30% and the patient should be monitored for hypersensitivity reactions.

▸ Plasma and plasma substitutes are often used in very ill patients whose condition is unstable. Therefore, close monitoring is required and fluid and electrolyte therapy should be adjusted according to the patient's condition at all times.

● **PRESCRIBING AND DISPENSING INFORMATION** The available preparations may not be licensed for use in all age-groups—further information can be found in the product literature for the individual preparations.

Gelaspan® contains succinylated gelatin (modified fluid gelatin, average molecular weight 26 500) 40 g (4%), Na^+ 151 mmol/litre, K^+ 4 mmol/litre, Mg^{2+} 1 mmol/litre, Cl^- 103 mmol/litre, Ca^{2+} 1 mmol/litre and acetate 24 mmol/litre.

Gelofusine® contains succinylated gelatin (modified fluid gelatin, average molecular weight 26 500) 40 g (4%), Na^+ 154 mmol/litre and Cl^- 120 mmol/litre.

Geloplasma® contains partially hydrolysed and succinylated gelatin (modified liquid gelatin) (as anhydrous gelatin) 30 g (3%), Na^+ 150 mmol/litre, K^+ 5 mmol/litre, Mg^{2+} 1.5mmol/litre, Cl^- 100 mmol/litre and lactate 30 mmol/litre.

● **MEDICINAL FORMS** There can be variation in the licensing of different medicines containing the same drug.

Infusion

- ▸ **Gelaspan** (B.Braun Medical Ltd)
  Calcium chloride dihydrate 150 mg per 1 litre, Magnesium chloride hexahydrate 200 mg per 1 litre, Potassium chloride 300 mg per 1 litre, Sodium acetate trihydrate 3.27 gram per 1 litre, Sodium chloride 5.55 gram per 1 litre, Gelatin succinylated 40 gram per 1 litre Gelaspan 4% infusion 500ml Ecobags | 20 bag [PoM] £136.00 (Hospital only)
- ▸ **Gelofusine** (B.Braun Medical Ltd)
  Gelatin succinylated 40 gram per 1 litre, Chloride 120 mmol per 1 litre, Sodium 154 mmol per 1 litre Gelofusine 4% infusion 1litre Ecobags | 10 bag [PoM] £87.90 (Hospital only)
  Gelofusine 4% infusion 500ml Ecobags | 20 bag [PoM] £94.00 (Hospital only)
- ▸ **Geloplasma** (Fresenius Kabi Ltd)
  Magnesium chloride hexahydrate 305 mg per 1 litre, Potassium chloride 373 mg per 1 litre, Sodium lactate 3.36 gram per 1 litre, Sodium chloride 5.382 gram per 1 litre, Gelatin succinylated 30 gram per 1 litre Geloplasma 3% infusion 500ml Freeflex bags | 20 bag [PoM] £85.50 (Hospital only)

2.3 Magnesium imbalance

Magnesium imbalance

08-Aug-2022

Overview

Magnesium is an essential constituent of many enzyme systems, particularly those involved in energy generation; the largest stores are in the skeleton.

Magnesium salts are not well absorbed from the gastro-intestinal tract, which explains the use of magnesium sulfate as an osmotic laxative.

[EvGr] Magnesium is excreted mainly by the kidneys and is therefore retained in renal failure, which can result in *hypermagnesaemia* (causing muscle weakness and arrhythmias). Calcium gluconate injection is used for the management of magnesium toxicity. ⟨M⟩

Hypomagnesaemia

Since magnesium is secreted in large amounts in the gastro-intestinal fluid, excessive losses in diarrhoea, stoma or fistula can cause *hypomagnesaemia*; deficiency may also occur as a result of treatment with certain drugs. Hypomagnesaemia often causes secondary hypocalcaemia, particularly in neonates, and also hypokalaemia.

Symptomatic hypomagnesaemia is usually associated with severe magnesium depletion. Magnesium can be given by intravenous infusion or by intramuscular injection of magnesium sulfate p. 739; the intramuscular injection is painful.

Patients with mild magnesium depletion are usually asymptomatic. Oral magnesium glycerophosphate p. 738 is licensed for hypomagnesaemia. Oral magnesium aspartate p. 738 and magnesium citrate p. 738 are licensed for the treatment and prevention of magnesium deficiency.

2.3a Hypomagnesaemia

ELECTROLYTES AND MINERALS › MAGNESIUM

Magnesium aspartate 24-Sep-2024

● **INDICATIONS AND DOSE**

MAGNASPARTATE®

Treatment and prevention of magnesium deficiency

▶ BY MOUTH

- Child 2–3 years: 5 mmol once daily
- Child 4–9 years: 5 mmol once daily, alternatively 10 mmol once daily
- Child 10–17 years: 10 mmol once daily

DOSE EQUIVALENCE AND CONVERSION

- Each *Magnaspartate®* sachet contains magnesium aspartate equivalent to magnesium 243 mg *or* Mg^{2+} 10 mmol; dose expressed as Mg^{2+}.
- Magnesium preparations may not be interchangeable due to differences in bioavailability, therefore caution should be exercised when switching preparations to ensure tolerability and to maintain therapeutic effect.

● **CONTRA-INDICATIONS** Disorders of cardiac conduction

● **INTERACTIONS** → Appendix 1: magnesium

● **SIDE-EFFECTS**

▶ **Uncommon** Diarrhoea · faeces soft

▶ **Rare or very rare** Fatigue · hypermagnesaemia

▶ **Frequency not known** Gastrointestinal irritation

SIDE-EFFECTS, FURTHER INFORMATION Side-effects generally occur at higher doses; if side-effects (such as diarrhoea) occur, consider interrupting treatment and restarting at a reduced dose.

Overdose Symptoms of hypermagnesaemia may include nausea, vomiting, flushing, thirst, hypotension, drowsiness, confusion, reflexes absent (due to neuromuscular blockade), respiratory depression, speech slurred, diplopia, muscle weakness, arrhythmias, coma, and cardiac arrest.

● **RENAL IMPAIRMENT** See p. 16. EvGr Avoid if estimated glomerular filtration rate less than 30 mL/minute/1.73 m^2. ⟨M⟩

● **MONITORING REQUIREMENTS** EvGr Monitor serum magnesium levels every 3–6 months. ⟨M⟩

● **DIRECTIONS FOR ADMINISTRATION** EvGr Dissolve contents of one *Magnaspartate®* sachet in 50–200 mL of water, tea, or orange juice and take immediately (or within 24 hours when dissolved in bottled water and stored below 25°C).

Dissolve half the volume of one sachet in 50–200 mL of water for a 5-mmol dose.

Magnaspartate® may be dissolved in 200 mL of water and administered immediately (or within 24 hours when dissolved in bottled water and stored below 25°C) via a gastric, duodenal, or nasal feeding tube. ⟨M⟩

● **PATIENT AND CARER ADVICE** Patients and carers should be given advice on how to administer magnesium aspartate powder.

● **MEDICINAL FORMS** There can be variation in the licensing of different medicines containing the same drug.

Powder for oral solution

EXCIPIENTS: May contain Sucrose

▸ Magnaspartate (Kora Healthcare)

Magnesium (as Magnesium aspartate) 243 mg Magnaspartate 243mg (magnesium 10mmol) oral powder sachets | 10 sachet PoM £9.45 DT = £9.45 | 20 sachet PoM £18.89

Magnesium citrate 01-Aug-2022

● **INDICATIONS AND DOSE**

Treatment and prevention of magnesium deficiency

▶ BY MOUTH

- Child 12–17 years: 4 mmol 3 times a day

DOSE EQUIVALENCE AND CONVERSION

- Each tablet contains magnesium citrate equivalent to magnesium 97.2 mg *or* Mg^{2+} 4 mmol; dose expressed as Mg^{2+}.
- Magnesium preparations may not be interchangeable due to differences in bioavailability, therefore caution should be exercised when switching preparations to ensure tolerability and to maintain therapeutic effect.

● **CAUTIONS** Disorders of cardiac conduction

● **INTERACTIONS** → Appendix 1: magnesium

● **SIDE-EFFECTS**

▶ **Common or very common** Diarrhoea (with high doses) · faeces soft (with high doses)

▶ **Rare or very rare** Fatigue (long term use)

▶ **Frequency not known** Gastrointestinal irritation (with high doses)

● **RENAL IMPAIRMENT** EvGr Avoid in severe impairment. ⟨M⟩

● **MONITORING REQUIREMENTS** EvGr Monitor serum magnesium levels every 3–6 months. ⟨M⟩

● **MEDICINAL FORMS** There can be variation in the licensing of different medicines containing the same drug.

Oral tablet

▸ Magnesium citrate (Non-proprietary)

Magnesium (as Magnesium citrate) 97.2 mg Magnesium citrate (magnesium 97.2mg (4mmol)) tablets | 60 tablet PoM £24.00 DT = £24.00

Magnesium glycerophosphate 24-Sep-2024

● **INDICATIONS AND DOSE**

Hypomagnesaemia

▶ BY MOUTH

- Child 1 month–11 years: Initially 0.2 mmol/kg 3 times a day, dose to be adjusted as necessary
- Child 12–17 years: Initially 4–8 mmol 3 times a day, dose to be adjusted as necessary

DOSE EQUIVALENCE AND CONVERSION

- Magnesium glycerophosphate 1 g is approximately equivalent to magnesium 97.2 mg *or* Mg^{2+} 4 mmol; dose expressed as Mg^{2+}.
- Magnesium preparations may not be interchangeable due to differences in bioavailability, therefore caution should be exercised when switching preparations to ensure tolerability and to maintain therapeutic effect.

NEOMAG® CHEWABLE TABLETS

Hypomagnesaemia

▶ BY MOUTH

- Child 4–11 years: Initially 4 mmol twice daily, dose to be adjusted as necessary
- Child 12–17 years: Initially 4 mmol 3 times a day, dose to be adjusted as necessary

DOSE EQUIVALENCE AND CONVERSION

- Each *Neomag®* chewable tablet contains magnesium glycerophosphate equivalent to magnesium 97.2 mg *or* Mg^{2+} 4 mmol; dose expressed as Mg^{2+}.
- Magnesium preparations may not be interchangeable due to differences in bioavailability, therefore caution should be exercised when switching preparations to ensure tolerability and to maintain therapeutic effect.

● **INTERACTIONS** → Appendix 1: magnesium

● **SIDE-EFFECTS** Diarrhoea · hypermagnesaemia

Overdose Symptoms of hypermagnesaemia may include nausea, vomiting, flushing, thirst, hypotension, drowsiness, confusion, reflexes absent (due to neuromuscular blockade), respiratory depression, speech slurred, diplopia, muscle weakness, arrhythmias, coma, and cardiac arrest.

- **RENAL IMPAIRMENT** EvGr Caution (risk of hypermagnesaemia); avoid if creatinine clearance less than 30 mL/minute. ⟨M⟩ See p. 16.
- **MONITORING REQUIREMENTS** Manufacturer advises to monitor serum magnesium levels every 3–6 months.
- **DIRECTIONS FOR ADMINISTRATION** EvGr *Neomag®* chewable tablets may be broken into quarters and chewed or swallowed with water. ⟨M⟩
- **NATIONAL FUNDING/ACCESS DECISIONS** For full details see funding body website

Scottish Medicines Consortium (SMC) decisions

▸ **Magnesium glycerophosphate (*Neomag®*) for use as an oral magnesium supplement for the treatment of patients with chronic magnesium loss or hypomagnesaemia (September 2017)** SMC No. 1267/17 Recommended

- **MEDICINAL FORMS** There can be variation in the licensing of different medicines containing the same drug. Forms available from special-order manufacturers include: oral tablet, oral capsule, oral suspension, oral solution, oral powder

Oral tablet

▸ **Magnesium glycerophosphate (Non-proprietary)**
Magnesium (as Magnesium glycerophosphate) 97.2 mg Mag-4 (magnesium 97.2mg (4mmol)) tablets | 30 tablet £84.50

Oral capsule

▸ **Magnesium glycerophosphate (Non-proprietary)**
Magnesium (as Magnesium glycerophosphate) 48.6 mg Mag-4 (magnesium 48.6mg (2mmol)) capsules | 30 capsule £85.70
Magnesium (as Magnesium glycerophosphate) 97.2 mg Mag-4 (magnesium 97.2mg (4mmol)) capsules | 30 capsule £89.30

▸ **MagnEss Gly** (Essential-Healthcare Ltd)
Magnesium (as Magnesium glycerophosphate) 39.5 mg MagnEss Gly 39.5mg (1.6mmol) capsules | 50 capsule £28.17
Magnesium (as Magnesium glycerophosphate) 48.6 mg MagnEss Gly 48.6mg (2mmol) capsules | 50 capsule £35.67
Magnesium (as Magnesium glycerophosphate) 97.2 mg MagnEss Gly 97.2mg (4mmol) capsules | 50 capsule £37.47

▸ **MagnaPhos** (TriOn Pharma Ltd)
Magnesium (as Magnesium glycerophosphate) 39.5 mg MagnaPhos 39.5mg (1.6mmol) capsules | 50 capsule £28.32
Magnesium (as Magnesium glycerophosphate) 48.6 mg MagnaPhos 48.6mg (2mmol) capsules | 50 capsule £35.87
Magnesium (as Magnesium glycerophosphate) 97.2 mg MagnaPhos 97.2mg (4mmol) capsules | 50 capsule £37.75

Oral solution

▸ **LiquaMag GP** (Fontus Health Ltd)
Magnesium (as Magnesium glycerophosphate) 24.25 mg per 1 ml LiquaMag GP (magnesium 121.25mg/5ml (5mmol/5ml)) oral solution | 200 ml £29.99 SF

▸ **MagnEss Gly** (Essential-Healthcare Ltd)
Magnesium (as Magnesium glycerophosphate) 19.44 mg per 1 ml MagnEss Gly 97.2mg/5ml (4mmol/5ml) oral solution | 200 ml £29.97 SF
Magnesium (as Magnesium glycerophosphate) 24.25 mg per 1 ml MagnEss Gly 121.25mg/5ml (5mmol/5ml) oral solution | 200 ml £31.97 SF

▸ **MagnaPhos** (TriOn Pharma Ltd)
Magnesium (as Magnesium glycerophosphate) 19.44 mg per 1 ml MagnaPhos 97.2mg/5ml (4mmol/5ml) oral solution | 200 ml £25.57 DT = £11.46
Magnesium (as Magnesium glycerophosphate) 24.25 mg per 1 ml MagnaPhos 121.25mg/5ml (5mmol/5ml) oral solution | 200 ml £37.87 DT = £37.87

Chewable tablet

EXCIPIENTS: May contain Aspartame

▸ **Magnesium glycerophosphate (Non-proprietary)**
Magnesium (as Magnesium glycerophosphate) 97.2 mg Mag-4 (magnesium 97.2mg (4mmol)) chewable tablets | 30 tablet £84.50 SF
Neomag (magnesium 97mg (4mmol)) chewable tablets | 50 tablet PoM £22.77 DT = £22.77 SF

▸ **MagnEss Gly** (Essential-Healthcare Ltd)
Magnesium (as Magnesium glycerophosphate) 97.2 mg MagnEss Gly 97.2mg (4mmol) chewable tablets | 50 tablet £15.44 DT = £22.77 SF

▸ **MagnaPhate** (Arjun Products Ltd)
Magnesium (as Magnesium glycerophosphate) 97.2 mg MagnaPhate (magnesium 97.2mg (4mmol)) chewable tablets | 50 tablet £22.64 DT = £22.77 SF

▸ **MagnaPhos** (TriOn Pharma Ltd)
Magnesium (as Magnesium glycerophosphate) 97.2 mg MagnaPhos 97.2mg (4mmol) chewable tablets | 50 tablet £15.44 DT = £22.77 SF

Magnesium sulfate

09-Jul-2025

- **INDICATIONS AND DOSE**

Severe acute asthma | Continuing respiratory deterioration in anaphylaxis

▸ BY INTRAVENOUS INFUSION

▸ Child 2–17 years: 40 mg/kg (max. per dose 2 g), to be given over 20 minutes

Persistent pulmonary hypertension of the newborn

▸ INITIALLY BY INTRAVENOUS INFUSION

▸ Neonate: Initially 200 mg/kg for 1 dose, to be given over 20–30 minutes, then (by continuous intravenous infusion) 20–75 mg/kg/hour for up to 5 days if response occurs after initial dose, dose adjusted to maintain plasma magnesium concentration between 3.5–5.5 mmol/ litre.

Hypomagnesaemia

▸ BY INTRAVENOUS INJECTION

▸ Neonate: 100 mg/kg every 6–12 hours as required, to be given over at least 10 minutes.

▸ Child 1 month–11 years: 50 mg/kg every 12 hours as required, to be given over at least 10 minutes

▸ Child 12–17 years: 1 g every 12 hours as required, to be given over at least 10 minutes

Hypomagnesaemia maintenance (e.g. in intravenous nutrition)

▸ BY INTRAVENOUS INFUSION, OR BY INTRAMUSCULAR INJECTION

▸ Child: 50–100 mg/kg daily; maximum 5 g per day

Neonatal hypocalcaemia

▸ BY DEEP INTRAMUSCULAR INJECTION, OR BY INTRAVENOUS INFUSION

▸ Neonate: 100 mg/kg every 12 hours for 2–3 doses.

Torsade de pointes

▸ BY INTRAVENOUS INJECTION

▸ Child: 25–50 mg/kg (max. per dose 2 g), to be given over 10–15 minutes, dose may be repeated once if necessary (consult local protocol)

DOSE EQUIVALENCE AND CONVERSION

▸ Magnesium sulfate heptahydrate 1 g equivalent to Mg^{2+} approx. 4 mmol.

- **UNLICENSED USE** Magnesium sulfate may be used as detailed below, although these situations are considered unlicensed:
  - severe acute asthma
  - continuing respiratory deterioration in anaphylaxis

IMPORTANT SAFETY INFORMATION

MHRA/CHM ADVICE: MAGNESIUM SULFATE: RISK OF SKELETAL ADVERSE EFFECTS IN THE NEONATE FOLLOWING PROLONGED OR REPEATED USE IN PREGNANCY (MAY 2019)

Maternal administration of magnesium sulfate for longer than 5–7 days in pregnancy has been associated with hypocalcaemia, hypermagnesaemia, and skeletal side-effects in neonates. Healthcare professionals are advised to consider monitoring neonates for abnormal calcium and magnesium levels, and skeletal side-effects if maternal treatment with magnesium sulfate during pregnancy is prolonged or repeated beyond current recommendations.

- **INTERACTIONS** → Appendix 1: magnesium
- **SIDE-EFFECTS** Bone demineralisation (reported in neonates following prolonged or repeated use in pregnancy) · electrolyte imbalance · osteopenia (reported in neonates following prolonged or repeated use in pregnancy)

  Overdose Symptoms of hypermagnesaemia may include nausea, vomiting, flushing, thirst, hypotension, drowsiness, confusion, reflexes absent (due to neuromuscular blockade), respiratory depression, speech slurred, diplopia, muscle weakness, arrhythmias, coma, and cardiac arrest.
- **PREGNANCY** For information on the risk of side-effects in neonates following prolonged or repeated maternal use of magnesium sulfate during pregnancy, see *Important Safety Information*.
  - When used for Neonatal hypocalcaemia or Hypomagnesaemia or Torsade de pointes or Severe acute asthma or Continuing respiratory deterioration in anaphylaxis Sufficient amount may cross the placenta in mothers treated with high doses e.g. in pre-eclampsia, causing hypotonia and respiratory depression in newborns.
- **HEPATIC IMPAIRMENT** Avoid in hepatic coma if risk of renal failure.
- **RENAL IMPAIRMENT** EvGr Caution in mild to moderate impairment; avoid in severe impairment (increased risk of toxicity). (M)

  Dose adjustments EvGr Reduce dose (consult product literature). (M)
- **MONITORING REQUIREMENTS** Monitor blood pressure, respiratory rate, urinary output and for signs of overdosage (loss of patellar reflexes, weakness, nausea, sensation of warmth, flushing, drowsiness, double vision, and slurred speech).
- **DIRECTIONS FOR ADMINISTRATION**
  - With intravenous use In severe hypomagnesaemia administer initially via controlled infusion device (preferably syringe pump). For *intravenous infusion*, in persistent pulmonary hypertension of the newborn, dilute to a max. concentration of 100 mg/mL (10%) (0.4 mmol/mL Mg^{2+}) magnesium sulfate heptahydrate (200 mg/mL (0.8 mmol/mL Mg^{2+}) if fluid restricted) with Glucose 5% *or* Sodium Chloride 0.9%. For neonatal hypocalcaemia, hypomagnaesemia, and torsade de pointes, dilute to 10% (100 mg magnesium sulfate heptahydrate (0.4 mmol Mg^{2+}) in 1 mL) with Glucose 5% *or* 10%, Sodium Chloride 0.45% *or* 0.9% *or* Glucose and Sodium Chloride combinations. Up to 20% solution may be given in fluid restriction. Rate of administration should not exceed 10 mg/kg/minute (0.04 mmol/kg/minute Mg^{2+}) of magnesium sulfate heptahydrate.
- **PRESCRIBING AND DISPENSING INFORMATION** The BP directs that the label states the strength as the % w/v of magnesium sulfate heptahydrate and as the approximate concentration of magnesium ions (Mg^{2+}) in mmol/mL. Magnesium Sulfate Injection BP is a sterile solution of Magnesium Sulfate Heptahydrate.
  - When used for Asthma For choice of therapy, see Asthma, acute p. 174 and Asthma, chronic p. 171.
- **MEDICINAL FORMS** There can be variation in the licensing of different medicines containing the same drug. Forms available from special-order manufacturers include: solution for injection, infusion, solution for infusion

Solution for injection

- Magnesium sulfate (Non-proprietary)

  Magnesium sulfate heptahydrate 200 mg per 1 ml Magnesium sulfate 20% (magnesium 0.8mmol/ml) solution for injection 20ml vials | 10 vial PoM £40.90 (Hospital only)

  Magnesium sulfate heptahydrate 500 mg per 1 ml Magnesium sulfate 50% (magnesium 2mmol/ml) solution for injection 10ml ampoules | 10 ampoule PoM £21.71–£100.70 | 10 ampoule PoM £56.70 (Hospital only)

  Magnesium sulfate 50% (magnesium 2mmol/ml) solution for injection 20ml vials | 10 vial PoM £122.20

  Magnesium sulfate 50% (magnesium 2mmol/ml) solution for injection 5ml ampoules | 10 ampoule PoM £67.39–£89.30

  Magnesium sulfate 50% (magnesium 2mmol/ml) solution for injection 2ml ampoules | 10 ampoule PoM £17.35–£44.10

Solution for infusion

- Magnesium sulfate (Non-proprietary)

  Magnesium sulfate heptahydrate 100 mg per 1 ml Magnesium sulfate 10% (magnesium 0.4mmol/ml) solution for injection 10ml ampoules | 10 ampoule PoM £84.18–£97.23

  Magnesium sulfate 10% (magnesium 0.4mmol/ml) solution for infusion 10ml ampoules | 10 ampoule PoM £54.00

  Magnesium sulfate heptahydrate 200 mg per 1 ml Magnesium sulfate 20% (magnesium 0.8mmol/ml) solution for infusion 10ml ampoules | 10 ampoule PoM £165.00 (Hospital only)

  Magnesium sulfate 20% (magnesium 0.8mmol/ml) solution for infusion 50ml vials | 1 vial PoM £7.63 (Hospital only)

  Magnesium sulfate heptahydrate 500 mg per 1 ml Magnesium sulfate 50% (magnesium 2mmol/ml) solution for infusion 100ml vials | 10 vial PoM £160.90

  Magnesium sulfate 50% (magnesium 2mmol/ml) solution for infusion 50ml vials | 10 vial PoM £172.50

2.4 Phosphate imbalance

Phosphate imbalance

15-Dec-2021

Phosphate supplements

Oral phosphate supplements p. 742 are licensed for the treatment of hypophosphataemia associated with vitamin D-resistant rickets in children. See also Vitamin D, under Vitamins p. 780.

For phosphate requirements in total parenteral nutrition regimens, see Intravenous nutrition p. 770.

Phosphate-binding agents

EvGr For the management of hyperphosphataemia in children with stage 4 or 5 chronic kidney disease (CKD), dietary management and dialysis (for children who are having this) should be optimised prior to starting phosphate-binding agents.

Children with stage 4 or 5 CKD should be offered a calcium-based phosphate binder. If there is an increasing trend in the serum-calcium concentration towards the upper age-adjusted limit, consider combination treatment with a calcium-based phosphate binder and sevelamer p. 741 (a non-calcium-based phosphate binder), or switching to sevelamer alone.

In children who remain hyperphosphataemic despite adherence to a calcium-based phosphate binder and serum-calcium concentration increases to the upper age-adjusted limit, consider combination treatment with, or switching to, a non-calcium-based phosphate binder such as sevelamer. (A)

For further guidance on the management of hyperphosphataemia in children with CKD, see NICE guideline: **Chronic kidney disease: assessment and management** (available at: www.nice.org.uk/guidance/ng203).

2.4a Hyperphosphataemia

ELECTROLYTES AND MINERALS › CALCIUM

733

Calcium acetate
01-Sep-2025

● **INDICATIONS AND DOSE**

PHOSEX® TABLETS

Hyperphosphataemia in patients with chronic renal failure on dialysis

▶ BY MOUTH

▸ Child: (consult product literature)

● **INTERACTIONS** → Appendix 1: calcium compounds

● **SIDE-EFFECTS**

▶ **Uncommon** Soft tissue calcification · vomiting

● **PATIENT AND CARER ADVICE**

Medicines for Children leaflet: Calcium salts for kidney disease www.medicinesforchildren.org.uk/medicines/calcium-salts-for-kidney-disease/

● **MEDICINAL FORMS** There can be variation in the licensing of different medicines containing the same drug.

Oral tablet

CAUTIONARY AND ADVISORY LABELS 25

EXCIPIENTS: May contain Gelatin, sucrose

▸ Calcium acetate (Non-proprietary)

Calcium acetate 500 mg Phosex 500mg tablets | 200 tablet PoM

▸ Renacet (Stanningley Pharma Ltd)

Calcium acetate 475 mg Renacet 475mg tablets | 200 tablet P £16.95 DT = £16.95

Calcium acetate 950 mg Renacet 950mg tablets | 200 tablet P £23.75 DT = £23.75

PHOSPHATE BINDERS

Sevelamer
23-Apr-2024

● **INDICATIONS AND DOSE**

RENAGEL®

Hyperphosphataemia in patients on haemodialysis or peritoneal dialysis

▶ BY MOUTH

▸ Child 12–17 years: Initially 0.8–1.6 g 3 times a day, dose to be given with meals and adjusted according to serum-phosphate concentration

RENVELA® 2.4G ORAL POWDER SACHETS

Hyperphosphataemia in chronic kidney disease

▶ BY MOUTH

▸ Child 6–17 years (body surface area 0.75–1.1 m^2): Initially 2.4 g daily in 3 divided doses, dose to be taken with meals and adjusted according to serum-phosphate concentration every 2–4 weeks—consult product literature

▸ Child 6–17 years (body surface area 1.2 m^2 and above): Initially 4.8 g daily in 3 divided doses, dose to be taken with meals and adjusted according to serum-phosphate concentration every 2–4 weeks—consult product literature

● **UNLICENSED USE**

RENAGEL® Not licensed for use in children under 18 years.

● **CONTRA-INDICATIONS** Bowel obstruction

● **CAUTIONS** Gastro-intestinal disorders

● **INTERACTIONS** → Appendix 1: sevelamer

● **SIDE-EFFECTS**

▶ **Common or very common** Constipation · diarrhoea · gastrointestinal discomfort · gastrointestinal disorders · nausea · vomiting

▶ **Frequency not known** Skin reactions

● **PREGNANCY** Manufacturer advises use only if potential benefit outweighs risk.

● **BREAST FEEDING**

RENAGEL® Manufacturer advises use only if potential benefit outweighs risk.

RENVELA® 2.4G ORAL POWDER SACHETS Unlikely to be present in milk (however, manufacturer advises avoid).

● **DIRECTIONS FOR ADMINISTRATION**

RENVELA® 2.4G ORAL POWDER SACHETS Manufacturer advises each sachet should be dispersed in 60 mL water, or mixed with a small amount of cool food (100 g), prior to administration and discarded if unused after 30 minutes.

● **PATIENT AND CARER ADVICE**

Medicines for Children leaflet: Sevelamer in dialysis www.medicinesforchildren.org.uk/medicines/sevelamer-in-dialysis/

RENVELA® 2.4G ORAL POWDER SACHETS Patients and carers should be advised on how to administer powder for oral suspension.

● **NATIONAL FUNDING/ACCESS DECISIONS**

RENVELA® 2.4G ORAL POWDER SACHETS For full details see funding body website

Scottish Medicines Consortium (SMC) decisions

▶ **Sevelamer carbonate (*Renvela*®) for the control of hyperphosphataemia in paediatric patients (older than 6 years of age and a Body Surface Area greater than 0.75m^2) with chronic kidney disease (February 2018)** SMC No. 1304/18 Recommended with restrictions

● **MEDICINAL FORMS** There can be variation in the licensing of different medicines containing the same drug.

Oral tablet

CAUTIONARY AND ADVISORY LABELS 25

EXCIPIENTS: May contain Propylene glycol

▸ Renagel (Sanofi)

Sevelamer 800 mg Renagel 800mg tablets | 180 tablet PoM £167.04 DT = £26.46

Powder for oral suspension

CAUTIONARY AND ADVISORY LABELS 13

▸ Renvela (Sanofi)

Sevelamer carbonate 2.4 gram Renvela 2.4g oral powder sachets | 60 sachet PoM £167.04 DT = £167.04 SF

2.4b Hypophosphataemia

DRUGS AFFECTING BONE STRUCTURE AND MINERALISATION › MONOCLONAL ANTIBODIES

Burosumab
25-Apr-2025

● **DRUG ACTION** Burosumab is a human monoclonal antibody that inhibits the activity of fibroblast growth factor 23, thereby increasing renal tubular reabsorption of phosphate and increasing serum concentration of vitamin D.

● **INDICATIONS AND DOSE**

X-linked hypophosphataemia (initiated by a specialist)

▶ BY SUBCUTANEOUS INJECTION

▸ Child 1–17 years: 0.8 mg/kg every 2 weeks (max. per dose 90 mg), dose may be administered 3 days either side of scheduled date if required, each dose should be rounded to the nearest 10 mg, dosing adjusted based on fasting serum-phosphate

continued →

concentration—consult product literature. Dose may be increased in steps of 0.4 mg/kg at intervals of at least 4 weeks up to a maximum of 2 mg/kg (max. per dose 90 mg)

- **CONTRA-INDICATIONS** Concurrent use of oral phosphate or vitamin D analogues—discontinue 1 week before initiation of burosumab
- **SIDE-EFFECTS**
  - **Common or very common** Constipation · cough · diarrhoea · dizziness · fever · headache · increased risk of infection · myalgia · nausea · oral disorders · pain in extremity · skin reactions · vomiting
  - **Frequency not known** Hypersensitivity
- **PREGNANCY** Manufacturer advises avoid— toxicity in *animal* studies.
- **BREAST FEEDING** Manufacturer advises avoid—no information available.
- **RENAL IMPAIRMENT** Manufacturer advises avoid in severe impairment— no information available.
- **MONITORING REQUIREMENTS**
  - EvGr Monitor fasting serum-phosphate concentration before treatment initiation, every 2 weeks for the first month, every 4 weeks for the following 2 months, 4 weeks after dose adjustment, and as appropriate thereafter—target the lower end of the normal reference range for age to decrease the risk of ectopic mineralisation. Periodic measurement of post-prandial serum-phosphate concentration is also advised.
  - Monitor for signs and symptoms of nephrocalcinosis at treatment initiation, every 6 months for the first 12 months, and annually thereafter. Also monitor plasma alkaline phosphatase, calcium, parathyroid hormone, and creatinine every 6 months (every 3 months for children aged 1–2 years) or as indicated, and urine calcium and phosphate every 3 months. ⟨M⟩
- **DIRECTIONS FOR ADMINISTRATION** EvGr Allow the vial to reach room temperature prior to administration. Inject into the upper arm, abdomen, buttock, or thigh. Maximum volume per injection site is 1.5 mL. If a volume over 1.5 mL is required on a given dosing day, the total volume should be split and given at 2 different injection sites. ⟨M⟩ Patients or their carers may self-administer *Crysvita*® after appropriate training in subcutaneous injection technique.
- **PRESCRIBING AND DISPENSING INFORMATION** Burosumab is a biological medicine. Biological medicines must be prescribed and dispensed by brand name, see *Biological medicines* and *Biosimilar medicines*, under Guidance on prescribing p. 1; record the brand name and batch number after each administration.
- **HANDLING AND STORAGE** Store in a refrigerator (2-8°C) and protect from light.
- **PATIENT AND CARER ADVICE**
  Self-administration Patients or their carers should be given training in subcutaneous injection technique if appropriate.
  Driving and skilled tasks Patients and carers should be counselled on the effects on driving and performance of skilled tasks—increased risk of dizziness.
- **NATIONAL FUNDING/ACCESS DECISIONS**
  For full details see funding body website

NICE decisions

- **Burosumab for treating X-linked hypophosphataemia in children and young people (updated April 2025)** NICE HST8 Recommended

Scottish Medicines Consortium (SMC) decisions

- **Burosumab (*Crysvita*®) for the treatment of X-linked hypophosphataemia in children and adolescents aged 1 to 17 years with radiographic evidence of bone disease (January 2024)** SMC No. SMC2588 Recommended

- **MEDICINAL FORMS** There can be variation in the licensing of different medicines containing the same drug.

Solution for injection

EXCIPIENTS: May contain Polysorbates, sorbitol

- **Crysvita** (Kyowa Kirin Ltd)
  Burosumab 10 mg per 1 ml Crysvita 10mg/1ml solution for injection vials | 1 vial PoM £2,992.00 (Hospital only)
  Burosumab 20 mg per 1 ml Crysvita 20mg/1ml solution for injection vials | 1 vial PoM £5,984.00 (Hospital only)
  Burosumab 30 mg per 1 ml Crysvita 30mg/1ml solution for injection vials | 1 vial PoM £8,976.00 (Hospital only)
  Crysvita 10mg/0.33ml solution for injection pre-filled syringes | 1 pre-filled disposable injection PoM £2,992.00 (Hospital only)
  Crysvita 20mg/0.67ml solution for injection pre-filled syringes | 1 pre-filled disposable injection PoM £5,984.00 (Hospital only)
  Crysvita 30mg/1ml solution for injection pre-filled syringes | 1 pre-filled disposable injection PoM £8,976.00 (Hospital only)

ELECTROLYTES AND MINERALS › PHOSPHATE

Phosphate

09-May-2025

- **INDICATIONS AND DOSE**

Hypophosphataemia | Hypophosphataemic rickets | Osteomalacia

- BY MOUTH USING EFFERVESCENT TABLETS
  - Neonate: 1 mmol/kg daily in 1–2 divided doses, dose can be taken as a supplement in breast milk—caution advised as solubility in breast milk is limited to 1.2 mmol in 100 mL if calcium also added, contact pharmacy department for details.
  - Child 1 month–4 years: 2–3 mmol/kg daily in 2–4 divided doses, dose to be adjusted as necessary, dose can be taken as a supplement in breast milk—caution advised as solubility in breast milk is limited to 1.2 mmol in 100 mL if calcium also added, contact pharmacy department for details; maximum 48 mmol per day
  - Child 5-17 years: 2–3 mmol/kg daily in 2–4 divided doses, dose to be adjusted as necessary; maximum 97 mmol per day
- BY INTRAVENOUS INFUSION
  - Neonate: 1 mmol/kg daily, dose to be adjusted as necessary.
  - Child 1 month–1 year: 0.7 mmol/kg daily, dose to be adjusted as necessary
  - Child 2-17 years: 0.4 mmol/kg daily, dose to be adjusted as necessary

IMPORTANT SAFETY INFORMATION

Some phosphate injection preparations also contain potassium. Expert sources advise for peripheral intravenous administration the *concentration* of potassium should not usually exceed 40 mmol/litre; the infusion solution should be **thoroughly mixed**. Local policies on avoiding inadvertent use of potassium concentrate should be followed. The potassium content of some phosphate preparations may also limit the *rate* at which they may be administered.

- **CAUTIONS**
  GENERAL CAUTIONS Cardiac disease · dehydration · diabetes mellitus · sodium and potassium concentrations of preparations
  SPECIFIC CAUTIONS
  - With intravenous use Avoid extravasation · severe tissue necrosis
- **INTERACTIONS** → Appendix 1: phosphate
- **SIDE-EFFECTS**
  - With intravenous use Electrolyte imbalance
  - With oral use Abdominal distress · diarrhoea · nausea

SIDE-EFFECTS, FURTHER INFORMATION Diarrhoea is a common side-effect and should prompt a reduction in dosage.

- **RENAL IMPAIRMENT**

Dose adjustments Reduce dose.

Monitoring Monitor closely in renal impairment.

- **MONITORING REQUIREMENTS** It is essential to monitor closely plasma concentrations of calcium, phosphate, potassium, and other electrolytes—excessive doses of phosphates may cause hypocalcaemia and metastatic calcification.
- **DIRECTIONS FOR ADMINISTRATION**

▸ With intravenous use Expert sources advise dilute injection with Sodium Chloride 0.9% or Glucose 5%; administration rate of phosphate should not exceed 0.05 mmol/kg/hour. In emergencies in intensive care seek specialist advice on rates of administration.

▸ With oral use The RCPCH and NPPG recommend that, for part doses using *Phosphate Sandoz®* effervescent tablets, one 16.1 mmol tablet should be dissolved in 15 mL of water to give a final concentration of approximately 1 mmol/mL. Once the tablet has fully dispersed and fizzing has stopped, the required dose should be withdrawn using an oral syringe and any remaining solution discarded.

- **PRESCRIBING AND DISPENSING INFORMATION** *Phosphate Sandoz®* contains sodium dihydrogen phosphate anhydrous (anhydrous sodium acid phosphate) 1.936 g, sodium bicarbonate 350 mg, potassium bicarbonate 315 mg, equivalent to phosphorus 500 mg (phosphate 16.1 mmol), sodium 468.8 mg (Na^+ 20.4 mmol), potassium 123 mg (K^+ 3.1 mmol); *Polyfusor NA®* contains Na^+ 162 mmol/litre, K^+ 19 mmol/litre, PO_4^{3-} 100 mmol/litre; non-proprietary *potassium dihydrogen phosphate injection* (potassium acid phosphate) 13.6% may contain 1 mmol/mL phosphate, 1 mmol/mL potassium.

Administration of 'part doses' using effervescent tablets The RCPCH and NPPG recommend that doses should be rounded to enable measurement, and clear instructions provided on the dispensing label and when counselling patients or their carer. Appropriate equipment for administration should also be provided, such as:

- a 20 mL oral syringe to measure the initial volume of water required for tablet dispersion;
- a reusable plastic medicine pot in which the tablet can be dispersed in water;
- another smaller oral syringe to measure and administer the required dose (a 1 mL syringe is required for dose volume less than 1 mL).

For further details, see the position statement from the RCPCH and NPPG, available at: nppg.org.uk/wp-content/uploads/2025/04/Position-Statement-CalciumPhosphate-and-PotassiumV3.pdf.

- **PATIENT AND CARER ADVICE** Patients or carers should be counselled on how to administer part doses of effervescent tablets.

Medicines for Children leaflet: Phosphate supplements for hypophosphataemia www.medicinesforchildren.org.uk/medicines/phosphate-supplements-for-hypophosphataemia/

Medicines for Children leaflet: How to give calcium, phosphate or potassium using effervescent tablets www.medicinesforchildren.org.uk/advice-guides/giving-medicines/how-to-give-phosphate-or-calcium-from-effervescent-tablets/

- **MEDICINAL FORMS** There can be variation in the licensing of different medicines containing the same drug. Forms available from special-order manufacturers include: infusion, solution for infusion

Effervescent tablet

CAUTIONARY AND ADVISORY LABELS 13

▸ Phosphate Sandoz (Stirling Anglian Pharmaceuticals Ltd)

Sodium dihydrogen phosphate anhydrous 1.936 gram Phosphate Sandoz effervescent tablets | 100 tablet GSL £32.50 DT = £32.50

Solution for infusion

▸ Phosphate (Non-proprietary)

Potassium dihydrogen phosphate 136 mg per 1 ml Potassium dihydrogen phosphate 13.6% (potassium 10mmol/10ml) solution for infusion 10ml ampoules | 10 ampoule PoM £164.58

Infusion

▸ Phosphate (Non-proprietary)

Potassium dihydrogen phosphate 1.295 gram per 1 litre, Disodium hydrogen phosphate anhydrous 5.75 gram per 1 litre Polyfusor phosphates infusion 500ml bottles | 12 bottle PoM £223.32 (Hospital only)

2.5 Potassium imbalance

2.5a Hyperkalaemia

Other drugs used for Hyperkalaemia Calcium gluconate, p. 735

ANTIDOTES AND CHELATORS › CATION EXCHANGE COMPOUNDS

Calcium polystyrene sulfonate

05-Oct-2021

- **INDICATIONS AND DOSE**

Hyperkalaemia associated with anuria or severe oliguria, and in dialysis patients

▸ BY MOUTH

▸ Child: 0.5–1 g/kg daily in divided doses; maximum 60 g per day

▸ BY RECTUM

▸ Neonate: 0.5–1 g/kg daily, irrigate colon to remove resin after 8–12 hours.

▸ Child: 0.5–1 g/kg daily, irrigate colon to remove resin after 8–12 hours; maximum 30 g per day

- **CONTRA-INDICATIONS** Hyperparathyroidism · metastatic carcinoma · multiple myeloma · obstructive bowel disease · reduced gut motility (in neonates) · sarcoidosis
- **CAUTIONS** Impaction of resin with excessive dosage or inadequate dilution
- **INTERACTIONS** → Appendix 1: polystyrene sulfonate
- **SIDE-EFFECTS** Appetite decreased · constipation (discontinue—avoid magnesium-containing laxatives) · diarrhoea · electrolyte imbalance · epigastric discomfort · gastrointestinal disorders · gastrointestinal necrosis (in combination with sorbitol) · hypercalcaemia (in dialysed patients and occasionally in those with renal impairment) · increased risk of infection · nausea · vomiting
- **PREGNANCY** Manufacturers advise use only if potential benefit outweighs risk—no information available.
- **BREAST FEEDING** Manufacturers advise use only if potential benefit outweighs risk—no information available.
- **MONITORING REQUIREMENTS** Monitor for electrolyte disturbances (stop if plasma-potassium concentration below 5 mmol/litre).
- **DIRECTIONS FOR ADMINISTRATION**

▸ With rectal use Manufacturer advises mix each 1 g of resin with 5 mL of water or 10% glucose.

- **MEDICINAL FORMS** There can be variation in the licensing of different medicines containing the same drug. Forms available from special-order manufacturers include: enema

Powder for oral or rectal suspension

CAUTIONARY AND ADVISORY LABELS 13

- Calcium polystyrene sulfonate (Non-proprietary)
  Calcium polystyrene sulfonate 999 mg per 1 gram Calcium polystyrene sulfonate powder sugar free | 300 gram [PoM] £82.16 DT = £82.16 [SF]

Sodium polystyrene sulfonate 05-Oct-2021

- **INDICATIONS AND DOSE**

Hyperkalaemia associated with anuria or severe oliguria, and in dialysis patients

- BY MOUTH
- Child: 0.5–1 g/kg daily in divided doses; maximum 60 g per day
- BY RECTUM
- Neonate: 0.5–1 g/kg daily, irrigate colon to remove resin after 8–12 hours.
- Child: 0.5–1 g/kg daily, irrigate colon to remove resin after 8–12 hours; maximum 30 g per day

- **CONTRA-INDICATIONS** Obstructive bowel disease · reduced gut motility (in neonates)
- **CAUTIONS** Congestive heart failure · hypertension · impaction of resin with excessive dosage or inadequate dilution · oedema
- **INTERACTIONS** → Appendix 1: polystyrene sulfonate
- **SIDE-EFFECTS** Appetite decreased · bezoar · constipation (discontinue—avoid magnesium-containing laxatives) · diarrhoea · electrolyte imbalance · epigastric discomfort · gastrointestinal disorders · increased risk of infection · nausea · necrosis (in combination with sorbitol) · vomiting
- **PREGNANCY** Manufacturers advise use only if potential benefit outweighs risk—no information available.
- **BREAST FEEDING** Manufacturers advise use only if potential benefit outweighs risk—no information available.
- **RENAL IMPAIRMENT** [EvGr] Use with caution. ⟨M⟩
- **MONITORING REQUIREMENTS** Monitor for electrolyte disturbances (stop if plasma-potassium concentration below 5 mmol/litre).
- **DIRECTIONS FOR ADMINISTRATION**
  - With rectal use Manufacturer advises mix each 1 g of resin with 5 mL of water or 10% glucose.
  - With oral use Manufacturer advises administer dose (powder) in a small amount of water or honey—do not give with fruit juice or squash, which have a high potassium content.

- **MEDICINAL FORMS** There can be variation in the licensing of different medicines containing the same drug. Forms available from special-order manufacturers include: oral suspension

Powder for oral or rectal suspension

CAUTIONARY AND ADVISORY LABELS 13

- Resonium A (Sanofi)
  Sodium polystyrene sulfonate 999.34 mg per 1 gram Resonium A powder | 454 gram [P] £81.11 DT = £81.11 [SF]

2.5b Hypokalaemia

ELECTROLYTES AND MINERALS › POTASSIUM

Potassium chloride 29-Mar-2021

- **INDICATIONS AND DOSE**

Prevention of hypokalaemia (patients with normal diet)

- BY MOUTH
- Child: 1–2 mmol/kg daily; Usual maximum 50 mmol

Electrolyte imbalance

- BY INTRAVENOUS INFUSION
- Neonate: 1–2 mmol/kg daily, dose dependent on deficit or the daily maintenance requirements.
- Child: 1–2 mmol/kg daily, dose dependent on deficit or the daily maintenance requirements

Potassium depletion

- BY MOUTH
- Neonate: 0.5–1 mmol/kg twice daily, total daily dose may alternatively be given in 3 divided doses, dose to be adjusted according to plasma-potassium concentration.
- Child: 0.5–1 mmol/kg twice daily, total daily dose may alternatively be given in 3 divided doses, dose to be adjusted according to plasma-potassium concentration

IMPORTANT SAFETY INFORMATION

SAFE PRACTICE

Potassium overdose can be fatal. Ready-mixed infusion solutions containing potassium should be used. Exceptionally, if potassium chloride concentrate is used for preparing an infusion, the infusion solution should be **thoroughly mixed**. Local policies on avoiding inadvertent use of potassium chloride concentrate should be followed.

NHS NEVER EVENT: MIS-SELECTION OF A STRONG POTASSIUM SOLUTION (JANUARY 2018)

Patients should not be inadvertently given a strong potassium solution (≥10% potassium w/v) intravenously, rather than the intended medication.

- **CONTRA-INDICATIONS** Plasma-potassium concentration above 5 mmol/litre
- **CAUTIONS**
  - With intravenous use Seek specialist advice in very severe potassium depletion or difficult cases
  - With oral use Cardiac disease · hiatus hernia (*with modified-release preparations*) · history of peptic ulcer (*with modified-release preparations*) · intestinal stricture (*with modified-release preparations*)
- **INTERACTIONS** → Appendix 1: potassium chloride
- **SIDE-EFFECTS**
  GENERAL SIDE-EFFECTS Hyperkalaemia
  SPECIFIC SIDE-EFFECTS
  - With oral use Abdominal cramps · diarrhoea · gastrointestinal disorders · nausea · vomiting
- **RENAL IMPAIRMENT** Avoid in severe impairment.
  Dose adjustments Smaller doses must be used in the prevention of hypokalaemia, to reduce the risk of hyperkalaemia.
  Monitoring Close monitoring required in renal impairment—high risk of hyperkalaemia.
- **MONITORING REQUIREMENTS**
  - Regular monitoring of plasma-potassium concentration is essential in those taking potassium supplements.
  - With intravenous use ECG monitoring should be performed in difficult cases.

- **DIRECTIONS FOR ADMINISTRATION**
  - With oral use in neonates Potassium chloride solutions suitable for use by mouth in neonates are available from 'special order' manufacturers; expert sources advise give with feeds to minimise gastric irritation.
  - With intravenous use Ready-mixed infusion solutions should be used when possible. EvGr If potassium chloride concentrate is used, it must be diluted and **thoroughly mixed** with Sodium Chloride 0.9% intravenous infusion. (M) For *peripheral intravenous infusion*, EvGr the concentration of potassium should not usually exceed 40 mmol/L. (M) Expert sources advise potassium infusions should be given slowly and at a rate not exceeding 0.2 mmol/kg/hour EvGr (max. 20 mmol/hour). (M) Expert sources advise higher concentrations of potassium chloride or faster infusion rates may be given in very severe depletion, but require specialist advice.
- **PRESCRIBING AND DISPENSING INFORMATION** *Kay-Cee-L®* contains 1 mmol/mL each of K^+ and Cl^-.
  Potassium Tablets Do not confuse Effervescent Potassium Tablets BPC 1968 with effervescent potassium chloride tablets. Effervescent Potassium Tablets BPC 1968 do not contain chloride ions and their use should be restricted to hyperchloraemic states.
- **PATIENT AND CARER ADVICE** Patient or carers should be given advice on how to administer potassium chloride modified-release tablets.
  Salt substitutes A number of salt substitutes which contain significant amounts of potassium chloride are readily available as health food products (e.g. *LoSalt®* and *Ruthmol®*). These should not be used by patients with renal failure as potassium intoxication may result.
- **LESS SUITABLE FOR PRESCRIBING** Modified-release tablets are less suitable for prescribing. Modified-release preparations should be avoided unless effervescent tablets or liquid preparations inappropriate.

- **MEDICINAL FORMS** There can be variation in the licensing of different medicines containing the same drug. Forms available from special-order manufacturers include: modified-release tablet, oral solution, infusion, solution for infusion

Modified-release tablet

CAUTIONARY AND ADVISORY LABELS 25, 27

- **Potassium chloride (Non-proprietary)**
  Potassium chloride 600 mg Kaleorid LP 600mg tablets | 30 tablet PoM (X)
  Duro-K 600mg tablets | 100 tablet PoM (X)

Solution for infusion

- **Potassium chloride (Non-proprietary)**
  Potassium chloride 150 mg per 1 ml Potassium chloride 15% (potassium 20mmol/10ml) solution for infusion 10ml ampoules | 10 ampoule PoM £7.00 | 20 ampoule PoM £29.24 | 20 ampoule PoM £14.00 (Hospital only)
  Potassium chloride 15% (potassium 20mmol/10ml) concentrate for solution for infusion 10ml ampoules | 20 ampoule PoM £16.80
  Potassium chloride 200 mg per 1 ml Potassium chloride 20% (potassium 13.3mmol/5ml) solution for infusion 5ml ampoules | 10 ampoule PoM £14.00

Oral solution

CAUTIONARY AND ADVISORY LABELS 21

- **Potassium chloride (Non-proprietary)**
  Potassium chloride 75 mg per 1 ml Potassium chloride 375mg/5ml (potassium 5mmol/5ml) oral solution sugar free | 500 ml P £55.00 SF

Infusion

- **Potassium chloride (Non-proprietary)**
  Potassium chloride 30 mg per 1 ml Potassium chloride 3% (potassium 40mmol/100ml) infusion 100ml bags | 1 bag PoM (X) (Hospital only)
  Potassium chloride 3% (potassium 20mmol/50ml) infusion 50ml bags | 1 bag PoM (X) (Hospital only)

3 Metabolic disorders

Metabolic disorders

10-May-2021

Use of medicines in metabolic disorders

Metabolic disorders should be managed under the guidance of a specialist. As many preparations are unlicensed and may be difficult to obtain, arrangements for continued prescribing and supply should be coordinated between the specialist centre, and local secondary and primary care.

General advice on the use of medicines in metabolic disorders can be obtained from:

Alder Hey Children's Hospital, Medicines Information Centre
(0151) 252 5837

and

Great Ormond Street Hospital for Children, pharmacy
(020) 7405 9200

Urea cycle disorders

EvGr Sodium benzoate p. 764 [unlicensed use] and sodium phenylbutyrate p. 766 are used in the management of urea cycle disorders. (A) Sodium phenylbutyrate is licensed as adjunctive therapy in all patients with neonatal-onset disease and in those with late-onset disease who have a history of hyperammonaemic encephalopathy. Expert sources advise sodium benzoate [unlicensed use] is also used in non-ketotic hyperglycinaemia.

EvGr The long-term management of urea cycle disorders includes oral maintenance treatment with sodium benzoate [unlicensed use] and sodium phenylbutyrate combined with a low protein diet and other drugs such as arginine p. 763 or citrulline p. 764, depending on the specific disorder. (A)

Emergency management

For further information on the emergency management of urea cycle disorders, consult the British Inherited Metabolic Disease Group (BIMDG) website at: www.bimdg.org.uk.

3.1 Acute porphyrias

Acute porphyrias

05-May-2022

Overview

The acute porphyrias (acute intermittent porphyria, variegate porphyria, hereditary coproporphyria, and 5-aminolaevulinic acid dehydratase deficiency porphyria) are hereditary disorders of haem biosynthesis; they have a prevalence of about 1 in 75 000 of the population.

Great care must be taken when prescribing for patients with acute porphyria, since certain drugs can induce acute porphyric crises. Since acute porphyrias are hereditary, relatives of affected individuals should be screened and advised about the potential danger of certain drugs.

EvGr Where there is no safe alternative, drug treatment for serious or life-threatening conditions should not be withheld from patients with acute porphyria. Where possible, the clinical situation should be discussed with a porphyria specialist for advice on how to proceed and monitor the patient. In the UK clinical advice can be obtained from the National Acute Porphyria Service or from the UK Porphyria Medicines Information Service (UKPMIS) (see *Useful resources*). (E)

Haem arginate p. 747 is administered by short intravenous

infusion as haem replacement in moderate, severe, or unremitting acute porphyria crises.

In the United Kingdom the National Acute Porphyria Service (NAPS) provides clinical support and treatment with haem arginate from two centres (Cardiff and Vale University Health Board and King's College Hospital) (see *Useful resources*).

Drugs unsafe for use in acute porphyrias

EvGr The following list contains drugs that have been classified as 'unsafe' in porphyria because they have been shown to be porphyrinogenic in animals or in vitro, or have been associated with acute attacks in patients. Absence of a drug from the following lists does not necessarily imply that the drug is safe. For many drugs no information about porphyria is available. (E)

An up-to-date list of drugs considered safe in acute porphyrias is available from the UKPMIS (see *Useful resources*).

Further information may be obtained from the European Porphyria Network (available at: porphyria.eu/) and UKPMIS (see *Useful resources*).

Quite modest changes in chemical structure can lead to changes in porphyrinogenicity but where possible general statements have been made about groups of drugs; these should be checked first.

Unsafe Drug Groups (check first)

- Anabolic steroids
- Antidepressants, MAOIs (contact UKPMIS for advice)
- Antidepressants, Tricyclic and related (contact UKPMIS for advice)
- Barbiturates (includes primidone and thiopental)
- Contraceptives, hormonal (for detailed advice contact UKPMIS or a porphyria specialist)
- Hormone replacement therapy (for detailed advice contact UKPMIS or a porphyria specialist)
- Imidazole antifungals (applies to oral and intravenous use; topical antifungals are thought to be safe due to low systemic exposure)
- Non-nucleoside reverse transcriptase inhibitors (contact UKPMIS for advice)
- Progestogens (for detailed advice contact UKPMIS or a porphyria specialist)
- Protease inhibitors (contact UKPMIS for advice)
- Sulfonamides (includes co-trimoxazole and sulfasalazine)
- Sulfonylureas (glipizide and glimepiride are thought to be safe)
- Taxanes (contact UKPMIS for advice)
- Triazole antifungals (applies to oral and intravenous use; topical antifungals are thought to be safe due to low systemic exposure)

Unsafe Drugs (check groups above first)

- Aceclofenac
- Alcohol
- Amiodarone
- Aprepitant
- Artemether with lumefantrine
- Bexarotene
- Bosentan
- Busulfan
- Carbamazepine
- Chloral hydrate (although evidence of hazard is uncertain, manufacturer advises avoid)
- Chloramphenicol
- Chloroform (small amounts in medicines probably safe)
- Clemastine
- Clindamycin
- Cocaine
- Danazol
- Dapsone
- Diltiazem
- Disopyramide
- Disulfiram
- Ergometrine
- Ergotamine
- Erythromycin
- Etamsylate
- Ethosuximide
- Etomidate
- Flutamide
- Fosaprepitant
- Fosphenytoin
- Griseofulvin
- Hydralazine
- Ifosfamide
- Indapamide
- Isometheptene mucate
- Isoniazid (safety uncertain, contact UKPMIS for advice)
- Ketamine
- Mefenamic acid (safety uncertain, contact UKPMIS for advice)
- Meprobamate
- Methyldopa
- Metolazone
- Metyrapone
- Mifepristone
- Minoxidil (safety uncertain, contact UKPMIS for advice)
- Mitotane
- Nalidixic acid
- Nitrazepam
- Nitrofurantoin
- Orphenadrine
- Oxcarbazepine
- Oxybutynin
- Pentazocine
- Pentoxifylline
- Pergolide
- Phenoxybenzamine
- Phenytoin
- Pivmecillinam
- Pizotifen
- Porfimer
- Raloxifene
- Rifabutin (safety uncertain, contact UKPMIS for advice)
- Rifampicin
- Riluzole
- Risperidone
- Spironolactone
- Sulfinpyrazone
- Tamoxifen
- Temoporfin
- Thiotepa
- Tiagabine
- Tibolone
- Topiramate
- Toremifene
- Trimethoprim
- Valproate
- Verapamil
- Xipamide

Useful Resources

Cardiff and Vale University Health Board National Acute Porphyria Service.
cavuhb.nhs.wales/our-services/laboratory-medicine/medical-biochemistry-and-immunology/porphyria-service-cardiff/national-acute-porphyria-service-naps/

King's College Hospital National Acute Porphyria Service.
www.kch.nhs.uk/service/a-z/porphyria

UK Porphyria Medicines Information Service. Drugs in porphyrias.
www.wmic.wales.nhs.uk/specialist-services/drugs-in-porphyria

9 Blood and nutrition

BLOOD AND RELATED PRODUCTS > HAEM DERIVATIVES

Haem arginate
05-Oct-2021

(Human hemin)

● **INDICATIONS AND DOSE**

Acute porphyrias | Acute intermittent porphyria | Porphyria variegata | Hereditary coproporphyria

▶ BY INTRAVENOUS INFUSION

▶ Child: Initially 3 mg/kg once daily for 4 days, if response inadequate, repeat 4-day course with close biochemical monitoring; maximum 250 mg per day

● **SIDE-EFFECTS**

▶ **Common or very common** Poor venous access

▶ **Rare or very rare** Fever

▶ **Frequency not known** Headache · injection site necrosis · skin discolouration · venous thrombosis

● **PREGNANCY** Manufacturer advises avoid unless essential.

● **BREAST FEEDING** Manufacturer advises avoid unless essential—no information available.

● **DIRECTIONS FOR ADMINISTRATION** Manufacturer advises administer over at least 30 minutes through a filter via large antebrachial or central vein; dilute requisite dose in 100 mL Sodium Chloride 0.9% in glass bottle; administer within 1 hour after dilution; max. concentration 2.5 mg/mL.

● **MEDICINAL FORMS** There can be variation in the licensing of different medicines containing the same drug.

Solution for infusion

▶ **Normosang** (Recordati Rare Diseases UK Ltd)

Haem arginate 25 mg per 1 ml Normosang 250mg/10ml solution for infusion ampoules | 4 ampoule PoM £1,737.00 (Hospital only)

DRUGS FOR METABOLIC DISORDERS > SMALL INTERFERING RIBONUCLEIC ACID

Givosiran
13-May-2022

● **DRUG ACTION** Givosiran is a small interfering RNA, which reduces production of the enzyme ALAS1 involved in haem synthesis in the liver, thereby reducing accumulation of neurotoxic intermediates that cause acute porphyria attacks and symptoms.

● **INDICATIONS AND DOSE**

Acute hepatic porphyria (initiated under specialist supervision)

▶ BY SUBCUTANEOUS INJECTION

▶ Child 12-17 years: 2.5 mg/kg once a month

● **INTERACTIONS** → Appendix 1: givosiran

● **SIDE-EFFECTS**

▶ **Common or very common** Fatigue · hypersensitivity · nausea · renal impairment · skin reactions

● **PREGNANCY** EvGr Use only if potential benefit outweighs risk—toxicity in *animal* studies. (M)

● **BREAST FEEDING** EvGr Avoid—present in milk in *animal* studies. (M)

● **RENAL IMPAIRMENT** EvGr Monitor renal function during treatment—progression of impairment reported. (M)

● **MONITORING REQUIREMENTS** EvGr Monitor liver function before treatment, every 4 weeks for the first 6 months of treatment, then as clinically indicated thereafter. For transaminase elevations consider discontinuing or interrupting treatment; restarting treatment at a reduced dose may be considered—consult product literature. (M)

● **DIRECTIONS FOR ADMINISTRATION** EvGr Maximum 1.5 mL per injection site; inject into the abdomen, thigh or upper arm and rotate injection site. Avoid injecting into scar tissue or skin that is reddened, inflamed or swollen. (M)

● **PRESCRIBING AND DISPENSING INFORMATION** EvGr The efficacy and safety data in acute hepatic porphyria (AHP) subtypes other than acute intermittent porphyria (hereditary coproporphyria, variegate porphyria and 5-aminolaevulinic acid dehydratase-deficient porphyria) are limited; this should be taken into consideration when assessing the individual benefit-risk in these rare AHP subtypes. (M)

● **NATIONAL FUNDING/ACCESS DECISIONS**
For full details see funding body website

NICE decisions

▶ **Givosiran for treating acute hepatic porphyria (November 2021)** NICE HST16 Recommended with restrictions

● **MEDICINAL FORMS** There can be variation in the licensing of different medicines containing the same drug.

Solution for injection

▶ **Givlaari** (Alnylam UK Ltd) ▼

Givosiran (as Givosiran sodium) 189 mg per 1 ml Givlaari 189mg/1ml solution for injection vials | 1 vial PoM £41,884.43 (Hospital only)

3.2 Alpha-mannosidosis

ENZYMES

Velmanase alfa
19-Dec-2023

● **DRUG ACTION** Velmanase alfa is an enzyme produced by recombinant DNA technology that provides replacement therapy for the treatment of alpha-mannosidosis, a lysosomal storage disorder caused by deficiency of alpha-mannosidase.

● **INDICATIONS AND DOSE**

Non-neurological manifestations of alpha-mannosidosis (under expert supervision)

▶ BY INTRAVENOUS INFUSION

▶ Neonate: 1 mg/kg once weekly.

▶ Child: 1 mg/kg once weekly

● **CAUTIONS** Infusion-related reactions

CAUTIONS, FURTHER INFORMATION EvGr Infusion-related reactions can occur and velmanase alfa should only be administered when appropriately trained staff are available; pre-medication with an antihistamine and/or corticosteroid may prevent subsequent reactions in those who required symptomatic treatment. Patients should be closely monitored for signs of infusion-related reactions during and for at least 1 hour after administration, and managed appropriately—consult product literature. (M)

● **SIDE-EFFECTS**

▶ **Common or very common** Acute kidney injury · appetite increased · bradycardia · chills · confusion · cyanosis · diarrhoea · dizziness · epistaxis · eye erythema · eye irritation · eyelid oedema · fatigue · feeling hot · fever · gastrointestinal discomfort · headache · hyperhidrosis · hypersensitivity · insomnia · joint disorders · loss of consciousness · malaise · myalgia · nausea · pain · procedural headache · psychotic disorder · reflux gastritis · syncope · tremor · urticaria · vomiting · weight increased

▶ **Frequency not known** Hyperthermia · infusion related reaction

● **PREGNANCY** EvGr Avoid unless essential—limited information available. (M)

- **BREAST FEEDING** EvGr Suitable for use in breast-feeding—no information available but absorption by the infant is considered to be minimal. (M)
- **DIRECTIONS FOR ADMINISTRATION** EvGr For *intermittent intravenous infusion* (*Lamzede*®), reconstitute each 10-mg vial with 5 mL Water for Injections to produce a 2 mg/mL solution; give requisite dose through a low-protein binding 0.22 micron in-line filter via an infusion pump, according to the recommended rate (max. 25 mL/hour) and duration (min. 50 minutes)—consult product literature. Patients tolerating their infusions well may be considered for home infusion—consult product literature. (M)
- **PRESCRIBING AND DISPENSING INFORMATION** Velmanase alfa is a biological medicine. Biological medicines must be prescribed and dispensed by brand name, see *Biological medicines* and *Biosimilar medicines*, under Guidance on prescribing p. 1; record the brand name and batch number after each administration.
- **HANDLING AND STORAGE** Store in a refrigerator (2–8°C) and protect from light—consult product literature for storage conditions after reconstitution.
- **PATIENT AND CARER ADVICE** EvGr Patients or their carers should be given training in infusion technique, and be counselled on the signs and management of infusion-related reactions, if appropriate. (M)
- **NATIONAL FUNDING/ACCESS DECISIONS**
For full details see funding body website

NICE decisions
- **Velmanase alfa for treating alpha-mannosidosis (December 2023)** NICE HST29 Recommended with restrictions

---

- **MEDICINAL FORMS** There can be variation in the licensing of different medicines containing the same drug.

Powder for solution for infusion
- Lamzede (Chiesi Ltd) ▼
Velmanase alfa 10 mg Lamzede 10mg powder for solution for infusion vials | 1 vial PoM £886.61 (Hospital only)

3.3 Carnitine deficiency

AMINO ACIDS AND DERIVATIVES

Levocarnitine

29-Jun-2021

(Carnitine)

- **INDICATIONS AND DOSE**

Primary carnitine deficiency due to inborn errors of metabolism
- BY MOUTH
  - Neonate: Up to 200 mg/kg daily in 2–4 divided doses.
  - Child: Up to 200 mg/kg daily in 2–4 divided doses; maximum 3 g per day
- INITIALLY BY INTRAVENOUS INFUSION
  - Neonate: Initially 100 mg/kg, to be administered over 30 minutes, followed by (by continuous intravenous infusion) 4 mg/kg/hour.
  - Child: Initially 100 mg/kg, to be administered over 30 minutes, followed by (by continuous intravenous infusion) 4 mg/kg/hour
- BY SLOW INTRAVENOUS INJECTION
  - Neonate: Up to 100 mg/kg daily in 2–4 divided doses, to be administered over 2–3 minutes.
  - Child: Up to 100 mg/kg daily in 2–4 divided doses, to be administered over 2–3 minutes

Secondary carnitine deficiency in haemodialysis patients
- INITIALLY BY SLOW INTRAVENOUS INJECTION
  - Child: 20 mg/kg, to be administered over 2–3 minutes, after each dialysis session, dosage adjusted according to plasma-carnitine concentration, then (by mouth) maintenance 1 g daily, administered if benefit is gained from first intravenous course

Organic acidaemias
- BY MOUTH
  - Neonate: Up to 200 mg/kg daily in 2–4 divided doses.
  - Child: Up to 200 mg/kg daily in 2–4 divided doses; maximum 3 g per day
- INITIALLY BY INTRAVENOUS INFUSION
  - Neonate: Initially 100 mg/kg, to be administered over 30 minutes, followed by (by continuous intravenous infusion) 4 mg/kg/hour.
  - Child: Initially 100 mg/kg, to be administered over 30 minutes, followed by (by continuous intravenous infusion) 4 mg/kg/hour
- BY SLOW INTRAVENOUS INJECTION
  - Neonate: Up to 100 mg/kg daily in 2–4 divided doses, to be administered over 2–3 minutes.
  - Child: Up to 100 mg/kg daily in 2–4 divided doses, to be administered over 2–3 minutes

- **UNLICENSED USE** Not licensed for use in organic acidaemias.
Not licensed for use by intravenous infusion.
Tablets, chewable tablets, and oral liquid (10%) not licensed in children under 12 years. Paediatric oral solution (30%) not licensed in children over 12 years.
- **CAUTIONS** Diabetes mellitus
- **SIDE-EFFECTS**
  - **Rare or very rare** Abdominal cramps · diarrhoea · nausea · skin odour abnormal · vomiting

SIDE-EFFECTS, FURTHER INFORMATION Side-effects may be dose-related—monitor tolerance during first week and after any dose increase.
- **PREGNANCY** Appropriate to use; no evidence of teratogenicity in *animal* studies.
- **RENAL IMPAIRMENT** Accumulation of metabolites may occur with chronic oral administration of high doses in severe impairment.
- **MONITORING REQUIREMENTS**
  - Monitoring of free and acyl carnitine in blood and urine recommended.
- **DIRECTIONS FOR ADMINISTRATION** For *intravenous infusion*, expert sources advise dilute injection with Sodium Chloride 0.9% or Glucose 5% or 10%.
- **PRESCRIBING AND DISPENSING INFORMATION**
  - When used for Organic acidaemias Levocarnitine is used in the treatment of some organic acidaemias; however, use in fatty acid oxidation is controversial.
- **PATIENT AND CARER ADVICE**
Medicines for Children leaflet: Carnitine for metabolic disorders www.medicinesforchildren.org.uk/medicines/carnitine-for-metabolic-disorders/

- **MEDICINAL FORMS** There can be variation in the licensing of different medicines containing the same drug. Forms available from special-order manufacturers include: oral capsule

Oral solution
- Levocarnitine (Non-proprietary)
L-Carnitine 300 mg per 1 ml Levocarnitine 1.5g/5ml (30%) oral solution paediatric sugar free | 20 ml PoM £46.99–£71.40 DT = £71.40 SF | 40 ml PoM £142.00 SF | 50 ml PoM £178.50 DT = £178.50 SF | 100 ml PoM £234.95 SF

Oral capsule

▸ Levocarnitine (Non-proprietary)

L-Carnitine 250 mg Bio-Carnitine 250mg capsules | 125 capsule £17.04

3.4 Cystinosis

3.4a Nephropathic cystinosis

AMINO ACIDS AND DERIVATIVES

Mercaptamine (Cysteamine)

27-Nov-2025

● **INDICATIONS AND DOSE**

Corneal cystine crystal deposits in patients with cystinosis (specialist use only)

▶ TO THE EYE

▸ Child 2–17 years: Apply 1 drop 4 times a day, to be applied to both eyes (minimum 4 hours between doses); dose may be reduced according to response (minimum daily dose 1 drop in each eye)

CYSTAGON®

Nephropathic cystinosis (specialist use only)

▶ BY MOUTH

▸ Neonate: Initially one-sixth to one-quarter of the expected maintenance dose, increased gradually over 4–6 weeks to avoid intolerance, dose increased if there is adequate tolerance and the leucocyte-cystine concentration remains above 1 nanomol hemicystine/mg protein, maintenance 325 mg/m^2 4 times a day; maximum 1.95 g/m^2 per day.

▸ Child 1 month–11 years (body-weight up to 50 kg): Initially one-sixth to one-quarter of the expected maintenance dose, increased gradually over 4–6 weeks to avoid intolerance, dose increased if there is adequate tolerance and the leucocyte-cystine concentration remains above 1 nanomol hemicystine/mg protein, maintenance 325 mg/m^2 4 times a day; maximum 1.95 g/m^2 per day

▸ Child 12–17 years (body-weight up to 50 kg): Initially one-sixth to one-quarter of the expected maintenance dose, increased gradually over 4–6 weeks to avoid intolerance, dose increased if there is adequate tolerance and the leucocyte-cystine concentration remains above 1 nanomol hemicystine/mg protein, maintenance 325 mg/m^2 4 times a day; maximum 1.95 g/m^2 per day

▸ Child 12–17 years (body-weight 50 kg and above): Initially one-sixth to one-quarter of the expected maintenance dose, increased gradually over 4–6 weeks to avoid intolerance, dose increased if there is adequate tolerance and the leucocyte-cystine concentration remains above 1 nanomol hemicystine/mg protein, maintenance 500 mg 4 times a day; maximum 1.95 g/m^2 per day

PROCYSBI®

Nephropathic cystinosis (specialist use only)

▶ BY MOUTH

▸ Neonate: Initially one-sixth to one-quarter of the expected maintenance dose, increased if there is adequate tolerance and the leucocyte-cystine concentration remains above 1 nanomol hemicystine/mg protein (measured using the mixed leucocyte assay), maintenance 650 mg/m^2 twice daily, administered every 12 hours; for approximations of maintenance dose—consult product literature; maximum 1.95 g/m^2 per day.

▸ Child: Initially one-sixth to one-quarter of the expected maintenance dose, increased if there is adequate tolerance and the leucocyte-cystine concentration remains above 1 nanomol hemicystine/mg protein (measured using the mixed leucocyte assay), maintenance 650 mg/m^2 twice daily, administered every 12 hours; for approximations of maintenance dose—consult product literature; maximum 1.95 g/m^2 per day

IMPORTANT SAFETY INFORMATION

SAFE PRACTICE

Mercaptamine has been confused with mercaptopurine; care must be taken to ensure the correct drug is prescribed and dispensed.

● **CAUTIONS**

▸ When used by eye Contact lens wearers

▸ With oral use Dose of phosphate supplement may need to be adjusted if transferring from phosphocysteamine to mercaptamine

● **SIDE-EFFECTS**

▶ **Common or very common**

▸ When used by eye Dry eye · eye discomfort · eye disorders · vision blurred

▸ With oral use Appetite decreased · asthenia · breath odour · diarrhoea · drowsiness · encephalopathy · fever · gastroenteritis · gastrointestinal discomfort · headache · nausea · skin reactions · vomiting

▶ **Uncommon**

▸ With oral use Compression fracture · gastrointestinal ulcer · hair colour changes · hallucination · joint hyperextension · leg pain · leucopenia · musculoskeletal disorders · nephrotic syndrome · nervousness · osteopenia · seizure

▶ **Frequency not known**

▸ With oral use Depression · intracranial pressure increased · papilloedema

● **ALLERGY AND CROSS-SENSITIVITY** EvGr Contra-indicated if history of hypersensitivity to penicillamine. Ⓜ

● **PREGNANCY**

▸ With oral use Manufacturer advises avoid—teratogenic and toxic in *animal* studies.

● **BREAST FEEDING**

▸ With oral use Manufacturer advises avoid—no information available.

● **MONITORING REQUIREMENTS**

▸ With oral use Manufacturer advises leucocyte-cystine concentration, liver function, and haematological monitoring required—consult product literature. Manufacturer advises monitor for skin and bone abnormalities; dose reduction or treatment discontinuation may be required—consult product literature.

▸ All patients receiving mercaptamine should be registered (contact local specialist centre for details).

● **DIRECTIONS FOR ADMINISTRATION**

CYSTAGON® Manufacturer advises for children aged 6 years and under at risk of aspiration, capsules can be opened and contents sprinkled on food (at a temperature suitable for eating); avoid adding to acidic drinks (e.g. orange juice).

PROCYSBI® Manufacturer advises for children aged 6 years and under at risk of aspiration, capsules can be opened and contents sprinkled on food or liquid—consult product literature.

Manufacturer advises capsules can be opened and contents sprinkled on food, water, acidic fruit juice or administered via an enteral feeding tube—consult product

9 Blood and nutrition

literature. Avoid dairy products and meals (rich in fats and protein) at least 1 hour before and after taking a dose.

- **PRESCRIBING AND DISPENSING INFORMATION** Mercaptamine has a very unpleasant taste and smell, which can affect compliance.
- **HANDLING AND STORAGE**
  - When used by eye Manufacturer advises store in a refrigerator (2–8°C)—after opening store at room temperature up to 25°C for up to 7 days; protect from light.

  PROCYSBI® Manufacturer advises store in a refrigerator (2–8°C).
- **PATIENT AND CARER ADVICE** Medicines for Children leaflet: Mercaptamine eye drops for ocular symptoms of cystinosis www.medicinesforchildren.org.uk/medicines/mercaptamine-eye-drops-for-ocular-symptoms-of-cystinosis/

  Driving and skilled tasks
  - With oral use Manufacturer advises patients and carers should be counselled on the effects on driving and performance of skilled tasks—increased risk of drowsiness.
  - When used by eye Manufacturer advises patients and carers should be counselled on the effects on driving and performance of skilled tasks—increased risk of blurred vision and visual disturbances.

  PROCYSBI® **Missed doses** Manufacturer advises if a dose is within 4 hours of the next dose, the missed dose should not be taken and the next dose should be taken at the normal time.
- **NATIONAL FUNDING/ACCESS DECISIONS** For full details see funding body website

  Scottish Medicines Consortium (SMC) decisions
  - **Mercaptamine (*Procysbi*®) for the treatment of proven nephropathic cystinosis (November 2025)** SMC No. SMC2824 Recommended

  All Wales Medicines Strategy Group (AWMSG) decisions
  - **Mercaptamine bitartrate (*Procysbi*®) for the treatment of proven nephropathic cystinosis (May 2022)** AWMSG No. 4804 Recommended

- **MEDICINAL FORMS** There can be variation in the licensing of different medicines containing the same drug. Forms available from special-order manufacturers include: eye drops

Gastro-resistant capsule

CAUTIONARY AND ADVISORY LABELS 25

- **Procysbi** (Chiesi Ltd)

  Mercaptamine (as Mercaptamine bitartrate) 25 mg Procysbi 25mg gastro-resistant capsules | 60 capsule PoM £335.97 DT = £335.97

  Mercaptamine (as Mercaptamine bitartrate) 75 mg Procysbi 75mg gastro-resistant capsules | 250 capsule PoM £4,199.65 DT = £4,199.65

Eye drops

EXCIPIENTS: May contain Benzalkonium chloride, disodium edetate

- **Mercaptamine (Non-proprietary)**

  Mercaptamine (as Mercaptamine hydrochloride) 4.4 mg per 1 ml Cystaran 0.44% eye drops | 15 ml PoM (Hospital only)
- **Cystadrops** (Recordati Rare Diseases UK Ltd)

  Mercaptamine (as Mercaptamine hydrochloride) 3.8 mg per 1 ml Cystadrops 3.8mg/ml eye drops | 5 ml PoM £865.00 DT = £865.00

Oral capsule

CAUTIONARY AND ADVISORY LABELS 21

- **Cystagon** (Recordati Rare Diseases UK Ltd)

  Mercaptamine (as Mercaptamine bitartrate) 50 mg Cystagon 50mg capsules | 100 capsule PoM £70.00 DT = £70.00

  Mercaptamine (as Mercaptamine bitartrate) 150 mg Cystagon 150mg capsules | 100 capsule PoM £190.00 DT = £190.00

3.5 Fabry's disease

ENZYMES

Agalsidase alfa

21-Aug-2024

- **DRUG ACTION** Agalsidase alfa is a form of recombinant human alpha-galactosidase A used for long-term enzyme replacement therapy in Fabry's disease.

- **INDICATIONS AND DOSE**

  Fabry's disease (under expert supervision)
  - BY INTRAVENOUS INFUSION
    - Child 7–17 years: 200 micrograms/kg every 2 weeks

- **INTERACTIONS** → Appendix 1: agalsidase alfa
- **SIDE-EFFECTS**
  - **Common or very common** Arrhythmias · asthenia · chest discomfort · chills · cough · diarrhoea · dizziness · dyspnoea · excessive tearing · fever · flushing · gastrointestinal discomfort · headache · hoarseness · hypersomnia · hypertension · increased risk of infection · influenza like illness · joint disorders · malaise · musculoskeletal discomfort · myalgia · nausea · ototoxicity · pain · palpitations · peripheral oedema · peripheral swelling · rhinorrhoea · sensation abnormal · skin reactions · taste altered · temperature sensation altered · throat complaints · tremor · vomiting
  - **Uncommon** Altered smell sensation · angioedema · hypersensitivity · sensation of pressure
  - **Frequency not known** Heart failure · hyperhidrosis · hypotension · myocardial ischaemia

  SIDE-EFFECTS, FURTHER INFORMATION Infusion-related reactions; manage by interrupting the infusion, or minimise by pre-treatment with an antihistamine or corticosteroid — consult product literature.
- **PREGNANCY** Use with caution.
- **BREAST FEEDING** Use with caution—no information available.
- **DIRECTIONS FOR ADMINISTRATION** Administration for *intravenous infusion*, manufacturer advises dilute requisite dose with 100 mL Sodium Chloride 0.9% and give over 40 minutes using an in-line filter.

- **MEDICINAL FORMS** There can be variation in the licensing of different medicines containing the same drug.

Solution for infusion

- **Replagal** (Takeda UK Ltd)

  Agalsidase alfa 1 mg per 1 ml Replagal 3.5mg/3.5ml solution for infusion vials | 1 vial PoM £1,049.94 (Hospital only)

Agalsidase beta

21-Aug-2024

- **DRUG ACTION** Agalsidase beta is a form of recombinant human alpha-galactosidase A used for long-term enzyme replacement therapy in Fabry's disease.

- **INDICATIONS AND DOSE**

  Fabry's disease (under expert supervision)
  - BY INTRAVENOUS INFUSION
    - Child 8–17 years: 1 mg/kg every 2 weeks

- **INTERACTIONS** → Appendix 1: agalsidase beta
- **SIDE-EFFECTS**
  - **Common or very common** Angioedema · arrhythmias · arthralgia · asthenia · chest discomfort · chills · cough · diarrhoea · dizziness · drowsiness · dyspnoea · eye disorders · fever · gastrointestinal discomfort · headache · hypertension · hyperthermia · hypotension · increased risk of infection · muscle complaints · musculoskeletal stiffness · nasal complaints · nausea · oedema · oral hypoaesthesia ·

pain · pallor · palpitations · respiratory disorders · sensation abnormal · skin reactions · syncope · temperature sensation altered · throat complaints · tinnitus · vasodilation · vertigo · vomiting

- **Uncommon** Dysphagia · ear discomfort · eye pruritus · influenza like illness · malaise · peripheral coldness · tremor
- **Frequency not known** Anaphylactoid reaction · hypersensitivity vasculitis · hypoxia

SIDE-EFFECTS, FURTHER INFORMATION Infusion-related reactions; manage by slowing the infusion rate, or minimise by pre-treatment with an antihistamine, antipyretic, or corticosteroid — consult product literature.

- **PREGNANCY** Use with caution.
- **BREAST FEEDING** Use with caution—no information available.
- **DIRECTIONS FOR ADMINISTRATION** For *intravenous infusion*, manufacturer advises give intermittently *in* Sodium Chloride 0.9%, reconstitute initially with Water for Injections (5 mg in 1.1 mL, 35 mg in 7.2 mL) to produce a solution containing 5 mg/mL. Dilute with Sodium Chloride 0.9% (for doses less than 35 mg dilute with at least 50 mL; doses 35–70 mg dilute with at least 100 mL; doses 70–100 mg dilute with at least 250 mL; doses greater than 100 mg dilute with 500 mL) and give through an in-line low protein-binding 0.2 micron filter at an initial rate of no more than 15 mg/hour; for subsequent infusions, infusion rate may be increased gradually once tolerance has been established.

- **MEDICINAL FORMS** There can be variation in the licensing of different medicines containing the same drug.

Powder for solution for infusion

- **Fabrazyme** (Sanofi)
  - **Agalsidase beta 5 mg** Fabrazyme 5mg powder for concentrate for solution for infusion vials | 1 vial PoM £315.08
  - **Agalsidase beta 35 mg** Fabrazyme 35mg powder for concentrate for solution for infusion vials | 1 vial PoM £2,196.59

ENZYME STABILISER

Migalastat

04-Oct-2023

- **DRUG ACTION** Migalastat is a pharmacological chaperone that binds to the active sites of certain mutant forms of alpha-galactosidase A, thereby stabilising these mutant forms in the endoplasmic reticulum, and facilitating normal trafficking to lysosomes.

- **INDICATIONS AND DOSE**

Fabry's disease (under expert supervision)

- BY MOUTH
  - Child 12–17 years (body-weight 45 kg and above): 123 mg once daily on alternate days, to be taken at the same time of day

IMPORTANT SAFETY INFORMATION

SAFE PRACTICE

Migalastat could be confused with miglustat; care must be taken to ensure the correct drug is prescribed and dispensed.

- **SIDE-EFFECTS**
- **Common or very common** Constipation · defaecation urgency · depression · diarrhoea · dizziness · dry mouth · dyspnoea · epistaxis · fatigue · gastrointestinal discomfort · headache · muscle complaints · nausea · pain · palpitations · proteinuria · sensation abnormal · skin reactions · torticollis · vertigo · weight increased
- **PREGNANCY** Manufacturer advises avoid—toxicity in *animal* studies.
- **BREAST FEEDING** Manufacturer advises avoid—present in milk in *animal* studies.
- **RENAL IMPAIRMENT** See p. 16. Manufacturer advises avoid if estimated glomerular filtration rate less than 30 mL/minute/1.73 m^2.
- **MONITORING REQUIREMENTS** Manufacturer advises monitor renal function, echocardiographic parameters and biochemical markers every 6 months.
- **DIRECTIONS FOR ADMINISTRATION** Food should not be consumed at least 2 hours before and 2 hours after taking *Galafold*® capsules (minimum 4 hours fast).
- **PATIENT AND CARER ADVICE** Patients or carers should be given advice on how to administer *Galafold*® capsules.
Missed doses If a dose is more than 12 hours late, the missed dose should not be taken and the next dose should be taken on the normal day and at the normal time (not to be taken on 2 consecutive days).
- **NATIONAL FUNDING/ACCESS DECISIONS** For full details see funding body website

NICE decisions

- **Migalastat for treating Fabry disease (February 2017)**
NICE HST4 Recommended with restrictions

Scottish Medicines Consortium (SMC) decisions

- **Migalastat (*Galafold*®) for long-term treatment of adults and adolescents aged 16 years and older with a confirmed diagnosis of Fabry disease (α-galactosidase A deficiency) and who have an amenable mutation (November 2016)**
SMC No. 1196/16 Recommended with restrictions

All Wales Medicines Strategy Group (AWMSG) decisions

- **Migalastat (*Galafold*®) for the long-term treatment of adolescents aged 12 years to 16 years with a confirmed diagnosis of Fabry disease (alpha-galactosidase A deficiency) and who have an amenable mutation (November 2022)**
AWMSG No. 4268 Recommended with restrictions

- **MEDICINAL FORMS** There can be variation in the licensing of different medicines containing the same drug.

Oral capsule

CAUTIONARY AND ADVISORY LABELS 25

- **Galafold** (Amicus Therapeutics UK Operations Ltd)
  - **Migalastat (as Migalastat hydrochloride) 123 mg** Galafold 123mg capsules | 14 capsule PoM £16,153.85 (Hospital only)

3.6 Gaucher's disease

ENZYMES

Imiglucerase

21-Jul-2020

- **DRUG ACTION** Imiglucerase is an enzyme produced by recombinant DNA technology that is administered as enzyme replacement therapy for non-neurological manifestations of type I or type III Gaucher's disease, a familial disorder affecting principally the liver, spleen, bone marrow, and lymph nodes.

- **INDICATIONS AND DOSE**

Gaucher's disease type I (specialist use only)

- BY INTRAVENOUS INFUSION
  - Neonate: Initially 60 units/kg every 2 weeks, adjusted according to response, doses as low as 30 units/kg once every 2 weeks may be appropriate.
  - Child: Initially 60 units/kg every 2 weeks, adjusted according to response, doses as low as 30 units/kg once every 2 weeks may be appropriate

continued →

Gaucher's disease type III (specialist use only)

▶ BY INTRAVENOUS INFUSION

- Neonate: Initially 60–120 units/kg every 2 weeks, adjusted according to response.
- Child: Initially 60–120 units/kg every 2 weeks, adjusted according to response

- **UNLICENSED USE** Expert sources advise that imiglucerase is used in the doses provided in BNFC for the treatment of Gaucher's disease, but these may differ from those licensed.
- **SIDE-EFFECTS**
  - **Common or very common** Angioedema · cough · dyspnoea · hypersensitivity · skin reactions
  - **Uncommon** Abdominal cramps · arthralgia · back pain · chest discomfort · chills · cyanosis · diarrhoea · dizziness · fatigue · fever · flushing · headache · hypotension · nausea · paraesthesia · tachycardia · vomiting
- **PREGNANCY** Manufacturer advises use with caution—limited information available.
- **BREAST FEEDING** No information available.
- **MONITORING REQUIREMENTS**
  - Monitor for immunoglobulin G (IgG) antibodies to imiglucerase.
  - When stabilised, monitor all parameters and response to treatment at intervals of 6–12 months.
- **DIRECTIONS FOR ADMINISTRATION** For *intravenous infusion* (*Cerezyme*®), manufacturer advises give intermittently in Sodium Chloride 0.9%; initially reconstitute with Water for Injections (400 units in 10.2 mL) to give 40 units/mL solution; dilute requisite dose with infusion fluid to a final volume of 100–200 mL and give initial dose at a rate not exceeding 0.5 units/kg/minute, subsequent doses to be given at a rate not exceeding 1 unit/kg/minute; administer within 3 hours after reconstitution.

- **MEDICINAL FORMS** There can be variation in the licensing of different medicines containing the same drug.

Powder for solution for infusion

ELECTROLYTES: May contain Sodium

▶ Cerezyme (Sanofi)

Imiglucerase 400 unit Cerezyme 400unit powder for concentrate for solution for infusion vials | 1 vial PoM £1,071.29 (Hospital only)

Velaglucerase alfa

29-Jul-2020

- **DRUG ACTION** Velaglucerase alfa is an enzyme produced by recombinant DNA technology that is administered as enzyme replacement therapy for the treatment of type I Gaucher's disease.

- **INDICATIONS AND DOSE**

Type I Gaucher's disease (specialist use only)

▶ BY INTRAVENOUS INFUSION

- Child 4–17 years: Initially 60 units/kg every 2 weeks; adjusted according to response to 15–60 units/kg every 2 weeks

- **SIDE-EFFECTS**
  - **Common or very common** Arthralgia · asthenia · chest discomfort · dizziness · dyspnoea · fever · flushing · gastrointestinal discomfort · headache · hypersensitivity · hypertension · hypotension · infusion related reaction · nausea · pain · skin reactions · tachycardia

  SIDE-EFFECTS, FURTHER INFORMATION Infusion-related reactions are very common; manage by slowing the infusion rate, or interrupting the infusion, or minimise by pre-treatment with an antihistamine, antipyretic, or corticosteroid—consult product literature.
- **PREGNANCY** Manufacturer advises use with caution—limited information available.
- **BREAST FEEDING** Manufacturer advises use with caution—no information available.
- **MONITORING REQUIREMENTS** Monitor immunoglobulin G (IgG) antibody concentration in severe infusion-related reactions or if there is a lack or loss of effect with velaglucerase alfa.
- **DIRECTIONS FOR ADMINISTRATION** For *intravenous infusion*, manufacturer advises reconstitute each 400-unit vial with 4.3 mL Water for Injections; dilute requisite dose in 100 mL Sodium Chloride 0.9% and give over 60 minutes through a 0.22 micron filter; start infusion within 24 hours of reconstitution.

- **MEDICINAL FORMS** There can be variation in the licensing of different medicines containing the same drug.

Powder for solution for infusion

ELECTROLYTES: May contain Sodium

▶ VPRIV (Takeda UK Ltd)

Velaglucerase alfa 400 unit VPRIV 400units powder for solution for infusion vials | 1 vial PoM £1,410.20 (Hospital only)

3.7 Homocystinuria

METHYL DONORS

Betaine

03-Nov-2020

- **INDICATIONS AND DOSE**

Adjunctive treatment of homocystinuria involving deficiencies or defects in cystathionine beta-synthase, 5,10-methylene-tetrahydrofolate reductase, or cobalamin cofactor metabolism (specialist use only)

▶ BY MOUTH

- Neonate: Initially 50 mg/kg twice daily (max. per dose 75 mg/kg), adjusted according to response; maximum 150 mg/kg per day.
- Child 1 month–9 years: Initially 50 mg/kg twice daily (max. per dose 75 mg/kg), adjusted according to response; maximum 150 mg/kg per day
- Child 10–17 years: 3 g twice daily (max. per dose 10 g), adjusted according to response; maximum 20 g per day

- **SIDE-EFFECTS**
  - **Uncommon** Abdominal discomfort · agitation · alopecia · appetite decreased · brain oedema · diarrhoea · glossitis · irritability · nausea · skin reactions · urinary incontinence · vomiting
- **PREGNANCY** Manufacturer advises avoid unless essential—limited information available.
- **BREAST FEEDING** Manufacturer advises caution—no information available.
- **MONITORING REQUIREMENTS** Monitor plasma-methionine concentration before and during treatment—interrupt treatment if symptoms of cerebral oedema occur.
- **DIRECTIONS FOR ADMINISTRATION** Manufacturer advises powder should be mixed with water, juice, milk, formula, or food until completely dissolved and taken immediately; measuring spoons are provided to measure 1 g, 150 mg, and 100 mg of *Cystadane*® powder.
- **PRESCRIBING AND DISPENSING INFORMATION** Betaine should be used in conjunction with dietary restrictions and may be given with supplements of vitamin B_{12}, pyridoxine, and folate under specialist advice.

● **NATIONAL FUNDING/ACCESS DECISIONS**
For full details see funding body website

Scottish Medicines Consortium (SMC) decisions

▶ **Betaine anhydrous (*Cystadane*®) for the adjunctive treatment of homocystinuria involving deficiencies or defects in cystathionine beta-synthase (CBS), 5,10-methylene-tetrahydrofolate reductase (MTHFR) or cobalamin cofactor metabolism (cbl) (August 2010)** SMC No. 407/07 Recommended with restrictions

● **MEDICINAL FORMS** There can be variation in the licensing of different medicines containing the same drug. Forms available from special-order manufacturers include: oral tablet, oral solution

Oral powder

▸ Amversio (SERB)
Betaine 1 gram per 1 gram Amversio oral powder | 180 gram PoM £305.00 DT = £347.00

▸ Cystadane (Recordati Rare Diseases UK Ltd)
Betaine 1 gram per 1 gram Cystadane oral powder | 180 gram PoM £347.00 DT = £347.00

3.8 Hypophosphatasia

ENZYMES

Asfotase alfa

21-Mar-2023

● **DRUG ACTION** Asfotase alfa is a human recombinant tissue-nonspecific alkaline phosphatase that promotes mineralisation of the skeleton.

● **INDICATIONS AND DOSE**

Paediatric-onset hypophosphatasia (initiated by a specialist)

▶ BY SUBCUTANEOUS INJECTION

▸ Neonate: 2 mg/kg 3 times a week, alternatively 1 mg/kg 6 times a week, dosing frequency depends on body-weight—consult product literature for further information.

▸ Child: 2 mg/kg 3 times a week, alternatively 1 mg/kg 6 times a week, dosing frequency depends on body-weight—consult product literature for further information

● **CAUTIONS** Hypersensitivity reactions

CAUTIONS, FURTHER INFORMATION Reactions, including signs and symptoms consistent with anaphylaxis, have occurred within minutes of administration and can occur in patients on treatment for more than one year; if these reactions occur, manufacturer advises immediate discontinuation of treatment and initiation of appropriate medical treatment. For information on re-administration, consult product literature.

● **SIDE-EFFECTS**

▶ **Common or very common** Bruising tendency · chills · cough · cutis laxa · fever · headache · hypersensitivity · hypocalcaemia · irritability · myalgia · nausea · nephrolithiasis · oral hypoaesthesia · pain · skin reactions · tachycardia · vasodilation · vomiting

SIDE-EFFECTS, FURTHER INFORMATION Injection-site reactions including hypertrophy, induration, skin discolouration, and cellulitis may occur, particularly in patients receiving treatment 6 times a week. Manufacturer advises rotation of injection sites to manage these reactions; interrupt treatment if severe reactions occur and administer appropriate medical therapy.

● **PREGNANCY** Manufacturer advises avoid—no information available.

● **BREAST FEEDING** Manufacturer advises avoid—no information available.

● **MONITORING REQUIREMENTS**

▶ Manufacturer advises monitor serum parathyroid hormone and calcium concentrations—supplements of calcium and oral vitamin D may be required.

▶ Manufacturer advises periodic ophthalmological examination and renal ultrasounds.

▶ Manufacturer advises monitor for increased intracranial pressure (including fundoscopy for signs of papilloedema) periodically in patients below 5 years of age—prompt intervention required if increased intracranial pressure develops.

● **DIRECTIONS FOR ADMINISTRATION** Manufacturer advises max. 1 mL per injection site; administer multiple injections if more than 1 mL is required—consult product literature.

● **HANDLING AND STORAGE** Manufacturer advises store in a refrigerator (2–8 °C).

● **PATIENT AND CARER ADVICE**

Injection guides The manufacturer has produced injection guides for patients and carers to support training given by health care professionals.

● **NATIONAL FUNDING/ACCESS DECISIONS**
For full details see funding body website

NICE decisions

▶ **Asfotase alfa for treating paediatric-onset hypophosphatasia (March 2023)** NICE HST23 Recommended with restrictions

● **MEDICINAL FORMS** There can be variation in the licensing of different medicines containing the same drug.

Solution for injection

▸ Strensiq (Alexion Pharma UK Ltd) ▼
Asfotase alfa 40 mg per 1 ml Strensiq 18mg/0.45ml solution for injection vials | 12 vial PoM £12,700.80 (Hospital only)
Strensiq 28mg/0.7ml solution for injection vials | 12 vial PoM £19,756.80 (Hospital only)
Strensiq 40mg/1ml solution for injection vials | 12 vial PoM £28,224.00 (Hospital only)
Asfotase alfa 100 mg per 1 ml Strensiq 80mg/0.8ml solution for injection vials | 12 vial PoM £56,448.00 (Hospital only)

3.9 Leptin deficiency

DRUGS FOR METABOLIC DISORDERS › LEPTIN ANALOGUES

Metreleptin

16-Mar-2021

● **DRUG ACTION** Metreleptin is a recombinant human leptin analogue which binds to, and activates the leptin receptor to increase fat breakdown in the blood, muscles and liver, thereby correcting some abnormalities in patients with lipodystrophy.

● **INDICATIONS AND DOSE**

Leptin deficiency in lipodystrophy (specialist use only)

▶ BY SUBCUTANEOUS INJECTION

▸ Child 2–17 years: (consult product literature)

● **CAUTIONS** Autoimmune disease · haematological abnormalities · severe infection

● **INTERACTIONS** → Appendix 1: metreleptin

● **SIDE-EFFECTS**

▶ **Common or very common** Alopecia · appetite abnormal · fatigue · gastrointestinal discomfort · headache · hypoglycaemia · menorrhagia · nausea · weight changes

▶ **Frequency not known** Anaplastic large cell lymphoma · arthralgia · cough · deep vein thrombosis · diabetes mellitus · diarrhoea · dyspnoea · hypertension exacerbated · increased risk of infection · insulin resistance · malaise ·

9 Blood and nutrition

myalgia · pancreatitis · peripheral swelling · pleural effusion · skin reactions · tachycardia · vomiting

- **CONCEPTION AND CONTRACEPTION** EvGr May increase fertility due to restoration of luteinising hormone release. Females of childbearing potential should use additional, effective non-hormonal contraception during treatment. ⟨M⟩
- **PREGNANCY** EvGr Avoid—toxicity in *animal* studies. ⟨M⟩
- **BREAST FEEDING** Specialist sources indicate use with caution—no information available. Large molecular weight and short half-life suggest limited excretion into milk, but monitor breast-fed infants for adverse reactions such as hypoglycaemia, decreased weight and abdominal pain.
- **TREATMENT CESSATION** EvGr Treatment should be withdrawn gradually over 2 weeks in conjunction with a low fat diet, to reduce the risk of increased hypertriglyceridaemia and pancreatitis—monitor triglyceride levels and consider the initiation or adjustment of lipid-lowering therapies as needed. ⟨M⟩
- **DIRECTIONS FOR ADMINISTRATION** EvGr Inject into the thigh, abdomen, or upper arm; rotate injection site—max. 1 mL per injection site. ⟨M⟩ Patients may self-administer *Myalepta*® after appropriate training in reconstitution and subcutaneous injection technique.
- **PRESCRIBING AND DISPENSING INFORMATION** The manufacturer of *Myalepta*® has provided a *Healthcare Professional Guide* and a *Specialist Prescriber Guide*.
  EvGr Prescribe the appropriate dose in milligrams and in millilitres—dosage should be based on actual body-weight. ⟨M⟩
- **HANDLING AND STORAGE** Store in a refrigerator (2-8°C) and protect from light—consult product literature about storage after reconstitution.
- **PATIENT AND CARER ADVICE**
  Self-administration Patients and their carers should be given training on reconstitution and subcutaneous injection technique if appropriate—a review of technique is recommended every 6 months.
  Information for patients The manufacturer of *Myalepta*® has provided a *Patient Care Guide* and a *Patient Dose Information Card*.
  Missed doses If a dose is missed, it should be injected when remembered and the next dose should be injected at the normal time.
  Driving and skilled tasks Patients and their carers should be counselled on the effects on driving and performance of skilled tasks—increased risk of fatigue and dizziness.
- **NATIONAL FUNDING/ACCESS DECISIONS**
  For full details see funding body website
  NICE decisions
  - **Metreleptin for treating lipodystrophy [in patients aged 2 years and over with generalised lipodystrophy] (February 2021)** NICE HST14 Recommended
  - **Metreleptin for treating lipodystrophy [in patients aged 12 years and over with partial lipodystrophy] (February 2021)** NICE HST14 Recommended with restrictions

---

- **MEDICINAL FORMS** There can be variation in the licensing of different medicines containing the same drug.

Powder for solution for injection

CAUTIONARY AND ADVISORY LABELS 10

EXCIPIENTS: May contain Polysorbates

- Myalepta (Chiesi Ltd) ▼
  Metreleptin 3 mg Myalepta 3mg powder for solution for injection vials | 30 vial PoM £17,512.50 (Hospital only)
  Metreleptin 5.8 mg Myalepta 5.8mg powder for solution for injection vials | 30 vial PoM £35,025.00 (Hospital only)
  Metreleptin 11.3 mg Myalepta 11.3mg powder for solution for injection vials | 30 vial PoM £70,050.00 (Hospital only)

3.10 Lysosomal acid lipase deficiency

ENZYMES

Sebelipase alfa

09-Jul-2024

- **DRUG ACTION** Sebelipase alfa is a recombinant human lysosomal acid lipase used as enzyme replacement therapy in lysosomal acid lipase deficiency (such as Wolman disease).

- **INDICATIONS AND DOSE**

Lysosomal acid lipase deficiency [rapidly progressive; Wolman disease] (under expert supervision)

▶ BY INTRAVENOUS INFUSION

- Neonate: Initially 1 mg/kg every week for at least 4 doses, then increased if necessary to 3 mg/kg every week, then increased if necessary to 5 mg/kg every week, further dose adjustments can be made according to response; doses higher than 7.5 mg/kg once weekly have not been studied, alternatively initially 3 mg/kg every week, then increased if necessary to 5 mg/kg every week, further dose adjustments can be made according to response; doses higher than 7.5 mg/kg once weekly have not been studied.
- Child 1-5 months: Initially 1 mg/kg every week for at least 4 doses, then increased if necessary to 3 mg/kg every week, then increased if necessary to 5 mg/kg every week, further dose adjustments can be made according to response; doses higher than 7.5 mg/kg once weekly have not been studied, alternatively initially 3 mg/kg every week, then increased if necessary to 5 mg/kg every week, further dose adjustments can be made according to response; doses higher than 7.5 mg/kg once weekly have not been studied

Lysosomal acid lipase deficiency (under expert supervision)

▶ BY INTRAVENOUS INFUSION

- Child 6 months–17 years: 1 mg/kg every 2 weeks, then increased if necessary to 3 mg/kg every 2 weeks

- **CAUTIONS** Hypersensitivity reactions
  CAUTIONS, FURTHER INFORMATION Hypersensitivity reactions, including anaphylaxis, have been reported, usually during or within 4 hours of an infusion; anaphylaxis has occurred during infusion as long as 1 year after treatment initiation. EvGr *Kanuma*® should only be administered by appropriately trained staff, and patients should be observed for 1 hour after the initial infusion or after any dose increase; manage hypersensitivity reactions by temporarily interrupting the infusion, reducing the rate of infusion and/or treatment with antihistamines, antipyretics, and/or corticosteroids. If a severe reaction occurs, stop infusion immediately and start appropriate medical treatment; caution is advised on re-administration. Pre-treatment with antipyretics and/or antihistamines may prevent subsequent reactions. ⟨M⟩
- **SIDE-EFFECTS**
  - **Common or very common** Chest discomfort · diarrhoea · dizziness · dyspnoea · eyelid oedema · fatigue · fever · gastrointestinal discomfort · hyperaemia · hypersensitivity · hyperthermia · hypotension · respiratory distress · skin reactions · tachycardia · vomiting
- **ALLERGY AND CROSS-SENSITIVITY** EvGr *Kanuma*® is contra-indicated in patients with egg allergy (may contain traces of egg proteins). ⟨M⟩

- **PREGNANCY** EvGr Avoid as a precaution (no information available). (M)
- **BREAST FEEDING** EvGr Avoid (no information available). (M)
- **DIRECTIONS FOR ADMINISTRATION** For *intravenous infusion* (*Kanuma*®), dilute requisite dose in Sodium Chloride 0.9% to a final concentration of 0.1–1.5 mg/mL and infuse over approximately 2 hours using a low protein-binding 0.2 micron in-line filter. For changes to duration of infusion—consult product literature.
- **PRESCRIBING AND DISPENSING INFORMATION** Sebelipase alfa is a biological medicine. Biological medicines must be prescribed and dispensed by brand name, see *Biological medicines* and *Biosimilar medicines*, under Guidance on prescribing p. 1; record the brand name and batch number after each administration.

  The manufacturer of *Kanuma*® has provided a User Manual and a Guide for Healthcare Professionals.
- **HANDLING AND STORAGE** Store in a refrigerator (2–8°C) and protect from light—consult product literature for storage conditions after dilution.
- **PATIENT AND CARER ADVICE**

  Driving and skilled tasks Patients and carers should be cautioned on the effects on driving and performance of skilled tasks—increased risk of dizziness.
- **NATIONAL FUNDING/ACCESS DECISIONS**

  For full details see funding body website

  NICE decisions
  - **Sebelipase alfa for treating Wolman disease (January 2024)** NICE HST30 Recommended with restrictions

- **MEDICINAL FORMS** There can be variation in the licensing of different medicines containing the same drug.

  Solution for infusion

  ELECTROLYTES: May contain Sodium
  - **Kanuma** (Alexion Pharma UK Ltd) ▼

    Sebelipase alfa 2 mg per 1 ml Kanuma 20mg/10ml concentrate for solution for infusion vials | 1 vial PoM £6,286.00 (Hospital only)

3.11 Mitochondrial disorders

NEUROPROTECTIVE DRUGS

Omaveloxolone

20-Mar-2026

- **DRUG ACTION** Omaveloxolone activates the nuclear factor (erythroid-derived 2)-like 2 (Nrf2) pathway, although it's exact mechanism of action is unknown.

- **INDICATIONS AND DOSE**

  Friedreich's ataxia (under expert supervision)
  - BY MOUTH
  - Child 16–17 years: 150 mg once daily

  DOSE ADJUSTMENTS DUE TO INTERACTIONS
  - EvGr Reduce dose to 50 mg once daily if concurrent use of potent CYP3A4 inhibitors is unavoidable; stop concurrent use if side-effects occur.
  - Reduce dose to 100 mg once daily if concurrent use of moderate CYP3A4 inhibitors, ciclosporin, ciprofloxacin, or fluvoxamine is unavoidable; further reduce dose to 50 mg once daily if side-effects occur. (M)

- **INTERACTIONS** → Appendix 1: omaveloxolone
- **SIDE-EFFECTS**
  - **Common or very common** Appetite decreased · back pain · diarrhoea · dyslipidaemia · dysmenorrhoea · fatigue · gastrointestinal discomfort · headache · increased risk of infection · muscle spasms · nausea · oropharyngeal pain · vomiting · weight decreased
- **CONCEPTION AND CONTRACEPTION** EvGr Females of childbearing potential should use effective contraception during treatment and for 28 days after last treatment; an additional barrier method of contraception or an alternative non-hormonal method of contraception (e.g. intra-uterine device) should be used in females using hormonal contraceptives. (M)
- **PREGNANCY** EvGr Avoid (toxicity in *animal* studies). (M)
- **BREAST FEEDING** Specialist sources indicate use with caution, especially if breast-feeding a neonate or preterm infant (no information available). High plasma-protein binding suggests limited excretion into milk.
- **HEPATIC IMPAIRMENT**

  EvGr Caution in moderate impairment (risk of increased exposure); avoid in severe impairment (limited information available). (M)

  Dose adjustments EvGr Reduce dose to 100 mg once daily in moderate impairment; consider further dose reduction to 50 mg once daily if side-effects occur. (M)
- **MONITORING REQUIREMENTS**
  - EvGr Monitor liver function prior to initiation, monthly for the first 3 months, then as clinically indicated thereafter—interrupt treatment if alanine aminotransferase (ALT) or aspartate aminotransferase (AST) exceeds 5 times the upper limit of normal (ULN), or if ALT or AST exceeds 3 times the ULN and bilirubin exceeds 2 times the ULN. Treatment may be resumed once liver abnormalities resolve.
  - Monitor lipid profile prior to initiation and periodically during treatment.
  - Monitor B-type natriuretic peptide (BNP) prior to initiation and periodically during treatment—consult product literature. (M)
- **DIRECTIONS FOR ADMINISTRATION** EvGr Capsules may be swallowed whole with water. Alternatively, capsules may be opened and the contents sprinkled onto 2 tablespoons of apple sauce and administered immediately. (M)
- **PATIENT AND CARER ADVICE** Patients and carers should be informed of the signs and symptoms of congestive heart failure and advised to seek immediate medical attention if they occur. Patients and carers should be advised to monitor for weight loss. Patients and carers should be given advice on how to administer *Skyclarys*® capsules.

  Missed doses If a dose is missed, it should not be taken and the next dose should be taken at the normal time.

  Driving and skilled tasks Patients and carers should be counselled on the effects on driving and performance of skilled tasks—increased risk of fatigue.
- **NATIONAL FUNDING/ACCESS DECISIONS**

  For full details see funding body website

  Scottish Medicines Consortium (SMC) decisions
  - **Omaveloxolone (*Skyclarys*®) for the treatment of Friedreich's ataxia in adults and adolescents aged 16 years and older (March 2026)** SMC No. SMC2845 Not recommended

- **MEDICINAL FORMS** There can be variation in the licensing of different medicines containing the same drug.

  Oral capsule

  CAUTIONARY AND ADVISORY LABELS 23
  - **Skyclarys** (Biogen Idec Ltd) ▼

    Omaveloxolone 50 mg Skyclarys 50mg capsules | 90 capsule PoM £20,235.04 (Hospital only)

VITAMINS AND TRACE ELEMENTS

Ubidecarenone 16-Feb-2021

(Ubiquinone; Co-enzyme Q10)

● **INDICATIONS AND DOSE**

Mitochondrial disorders

▶ BY MOUTH

▸ Neonate: Initially 5 mg 1–2 times a day, adjusted according to response, dose too be taken with food, increased if necessary up to 200 mg daily.

▸ Child: Initially 5 mg 1–2 times a day, adjusted according to response, dose to be taken with food, increased if necessary up to 300 mg daily

● **UNLICENSED USE** Not licensed.

● **CAUTIONS** May reduce insulin requirement in diabetes mellitus

● **SIDE-EFFECTS**

▶ **Common or very common** Diarrhoea · dyspepsia · nausea

▶ **Rare or very rare** Agitation · dizziness · headache · irritability

● **HEPATIC IMPAIRMENT**

Dose adjustments Reduce dose in moderate and severe impairment.

● **PATIENT AND CARER ADVICE**

Medicines for Children leaflet: Ubidecarenone for mitochondrial disease www.medicinesforchildren.org.uk/medicines/ubidecarenone-for-mitochondrial-disease/

● **MEDICINAL FORMS** There can be variation in the licensing of different medicines containing the same drug. Forms available from special-order manufacturers include: oral solution, oral drops

Oral tablet

▸ Ubidecarenone (Non-proprietary)

Ubidecarenone 30 mg Higher Nature Co-enzyme Q10 30mg tablets | 90 tablet £18.40

Oral capsule

▸ Ubidecarenone (Non-proprietary)

Ubidecarenone 30 mg Vega Co-Enzyme Q10 30mg capsules | 60 capsule £12.47

Ubidecarenone 100 mg Bio-Quinone Q10 GOLD 100mg capsules | 60 capsule £23.58 | 150 capsule £47.31

Myoquinone 100mg capsules | 60 capsule [X]

▸ ACo Q10 (Essential-Healthcare Ltd)

Ubidecarenone 30 mg ACo Q10 30mg capsules | 60 capsule £7.95

Ubidecarenone 100 mg ACo Q10 100mg capsules | 60 capsule £13.87

Ubidecarenone 200 mg ACo Q10 200mg capsules | 60 capsule £17.59

▸ BioActive Q10 Uniquinol (Pharma Nord (UK) Ltd)

Ubidecarenone 30 mg Bio-Ubiquinol Active QH 30mg capsules | 60 capsule £12.05 | 150 capsule £23.96

Ubidecarenone 100 mg Bio-Ubiquinol Active QH 100mg capsules | 60 capsule £31.86 | 150 capsule £57.91

▸ Super Bio-Quinone (Pharma Nord (UK) Ltd)

Ubidecarenone 30 mg Bio-Quinone Q10 Super 30mg capsules | 30 capsule £5.26 | 60 capsule £10.72 | 150 capsule £19.37

Oral drops

▸ Ubidecarenone (Non-proprietary)

Ubidecarenone 5 mg per 1 ml Ubicor 5mg/ml oral drops | 10 ml PoM [X]

Oral solution

▸ Ubidecarenone (Non-proprietary)

Ubidecarenone 5 mg per 1 ml 10-Q Ubidecarenone 25mg/5ml oral solution | 100 ml £54.83 SF

Ubidecarenone 10 mg per 1 ml 10-Q Ubidecarenone 50mg/5ml oral solution | 100 ml £64.78 SF

Chewable tablet

▸ Ubidecarenone (Non-proprietary)

Ubidecarenone 25 mg Kirkman Coenzyme Q10 25mg chewable tablets | 250 tablet PoM [X] SF

3.12 Molybdenum cofactor deficiency

DRUGS FOR METABOLIC DISORDERS

Fosdenopterin 21-Apr-2026

(Cyclic pyranopterin monophosphate; cPMP)

● **DRUG ACTION** Fosdenopterin is a synthetic form of cyclic pyranopterin monophosphate (cPMP) used as substrate replacement therapy in molybdenum cofactor deficiency (MoCD) type A.

● **INDICATIONS AND DOSE**

Molybdenum cofactor deficiency (MoCD) type A [gestational age less than 37 weeks] (under expert supervision)

▶ BY INTRAVENOUS INFUSION

▸ Neonate: Initially 400 micrograms/kg once daily for 1 month, then increased to 700 micrograms/kg once daily for 2 months; maintenance 900 micrograms/kg once daily.

▸ Child 1-11 months: Initially 400 micrograms/kg once daily for 1 month, then increased to 700 micrograms/kg once daily for 2 months; maintenance 900 micrograms/kg once daily

Molybdenum cofactor deficiency (MoCD) type A [gestational age 37 weeks and above] (under expert supervision)

▶ BY INTRAVENOUS INFUSION

▸ Neonate: Initially 550 micrograms/kg once daily for 1 month, then increased to 750 micrograms/kg once daily for 2 months; maintenance 900 micrograms/kg once daily.

▸ Child 1-11 months: Initially 550 micrograms/kg once daily for 1 month, then increased to 750 micrograms/kg once daily for 2 months; maintenance 900 micrograms/kg once daily

Molybdenum cofactor deficiency (MoCD) type A (under expert supervision)

▶ BY INTRAVENOUS INFUSION

▸ Child 1-17 years: 900 micrograms/kg once daily

● **PREGNANCY** EvGr Avoid (limited information available). (M)

● **BREAST FEEDING** EvGr Avoid (no information available). (M)

● **DIRECTIONS FOR ADMINISTRATION** For *intravenous infusion* (*Nulibry*®), reconstitute each vial with 5 mL Water for Injections to produce a 1.9 mg/mL solution; give requisite dose through di-2-ethylhexylphthalate (DEHP)-free tubing with a 0.2 micron in-line filter, via a syringe pump, at a rate of 1.5 mL/minute if dose volume is 2 mL or more—consult product literature for further details, including if dose volume is less than 2 mL. Patients stabilised on their infusions may be considered for home infusion—consult product literature.

● **HANDLING AND STORAGE** Store in a freezer (-25 to -10°C) and protect from light—consult product literature for storage conditions after reconstitution.

● **PATIENT AND CARER ADVICE**

Photosensitivity Photosensitivity is a theoretical risk, based on *animal* studies, and patients should be advised to follow sun protection strategies—consult product literature.

Self-administration Patients and carers should be given training in intravenous administration technique, if appropriate; the *Home Infusion Guide* and *Infusion Diary* should be provided.

Missed doses If a dose is missed, the next dose should be administered as soon as possible and the next scheduled dose administered at least 6 hours later.

● **MEDICINAL FORMS** There can be variation in the licensing of different medicines containing the same drug.

Powder for solution for injection

EXCIPIENTS: May contain Sucrose

▸ **Nulibry** (Sentynl Therapeutics, Inc.) ▼

Fosdenopterin (as Fosdenopterin hydrobromide dihydrate)
9.5 mg Nulibry 9.5mg powder for solution for injection vials | 1 vial PoM £1,205.51 (Hospital only)

3.13 Mucopolysaccharidosis

ENZYMES

Elosulfase alfa

04-May-2022

● **DRUG ACTION** Elosulfase alfa is an enzyme produced by recombinant DNA technology that provides replacement therapy in conditions caused by N-acetylgalactosamine-6-sulfatase (GALNS) deficiency.

● **INDICATIONS AND DOSE**

Mucopolysaccharidosis IVA (specialist use only)

▸ BY INTRAVENOUS INFUSION

▸ Neonate: 2 mg/kg once weekly.

▸ Child: 2 mg/kg once weekly

● **CAUTIONS** Infusion-related reactions

CAUTIONS, FURTHER INFORMATION Infusion-related reactions can occur; manufacturer advises these may be minimised by pre-treatment with an antihistamine and antipyretic, given 30-60 minutes before treatment. If reaction is severe, stop infusion and start appropriate treatment. Caution and close monitoring is advised during re-administration following a severe reaction.

● **SIDE-EFFECTS**

▸ **Common or very common** Chills · diarrhoea · dizziness · dyspnoea · fever · gastrointestinal discomfort · headache · hypersensitivity · myalgia · nausea · oropharyngeal pain · vomiting

▸ **Frequency not known** Infusion related reaction

● **PREGNANCY** Manufacturer advises avoid unless essential—limited information available.

● **BREAST FEEDING** Manufacturer advises use only if potential benefit outweighs risk—present in milk in *animal* studies.

● **DIRECTIONS FOR ADMINISTRATION** For *intravenous infusion* (*Vimizim*®), manufacturer advises give intermittently *in* Sodium Chloride 0.9%; body-weight under 25 kg, dilute requisite dose to final volume of 100 mL infusion fluid and mix gently, give over 4 hours through in-line filter (0.2 micron) initially at a rate of 3 mL/hour, then increase to a rate of 6 mL/hour after 15 minutes, then increase gradually if tolerated every 15 minutes by 6 mL/hour to max. 36 mL/hour; body-weight 25 kg or over, dilute requisite dose to final volume of 250 mL and mix gently, give over 4 hours through in-line filter (0.2 micron) initially at a rate of 6 mL/hour, then increase to a rate of 12 mL/hour after 15 minutes, then increase gradually if tolerated every 15 minutes by 12 mL/hour to max. 72 mL/hour.

● **HANDLING AND STORAGE** Manufacturer advises store in a refrigerator at 2–8°C. After dilution use immediately or, if necessary, store at 2-8°C for max. 24 hours, followed by up to 24 hours at 23–27°C.

● **PATIENT AND CARER ADVICE**

Driving and skilled tasks Manufacturer advises patients and carers should be counselled about the effects on driving and performance of skilled tasks—increased risk of dizziness.

● **NATIONAL FUNDING/ACCESS DECISIONS**

For full details see funding body website

NICE decisions

▸ **Elosulfase alfa for treating mucopolysaccharidosis type 4A (April 2022)** NICE HST19 Recommended

● **MEDICINAL FORMS** There can be variation in the licensing of different medicines containing the same drug.

Solution for infusion

EXCIPIENTS: May contain Polysorbates, sorbitol

ELECTROLYTES: May contain Sodium

▸ **Vimizim** (BioMarin (U.K.) Ltd) ▼

Elosulfase alfa 1 mg per 1 ml Vimizim 5mg/5ml concentrate for solution for infusion vials | 1 vial PoM £750.00 (Hospital only)

Galsulfase

21-Oct-2024

● **DRUG ACTION** Galsulfase is a recombinant form of human N-acetylgalactosamine-4-sulfatase.

● **INDICATIONS AND DOSE**

Mucopolysaccharidosis VI (specialist use only)

▸ BY INTRAVENOUS INFUSION

▸ Child 5–17 years: 1 mg/kg once weekly

● **CAUTIONS** Acute febrile illness (consider delaying treatment) · acute respiratory illness (consider delaying treatment) · infusion-related reactions can occur · respiratory disease

● **SIDE-EFFECTS**

▸ **Common or very common** Abdominal pain · angioedema · apnoea · arthralgia · asthma · chest pain · chills · conjunctivitis · corneal opacity · cough · dyspnoea · ear pain · fever · headache · hearing impairment · hypertension · hypotension · increased risk of infection · malaise · nasal congestion · nausea · pain · reflexes absent · respiratory disorders · skin reactions · tremor · umbilical hernia · vomiting

▸ **Frequency not known** Arrhythmias · cyanosis · hypoxia · infusion related reaction · nerve disorders · pallor · paraesthesia · shock

SIDE-EFFECTS, FURTHER INFORMATION Infusion-related reactions often occur, they can be managed by slowing the infusion rate or interrupting the infusion, and can be minimised by pre-treatment with an antihistamine and an antipyretic. Recurrent infusion-related reactions may require pre-treatment with a corticosteroid — consult product literature for details.

● **PREGNANCY** Manufacturer advises avoid unless essential.

● **BREAST FEEDING** Manufacturer advises avoid—no information available.

● **DIRECTIONS FOR ADMINISTRATION** For *intravenous infusion*, manufacturer advises dilute requisite dose with Sodium Chloride 0.9% to a final volume of 250 mL and mix gently; infuse through a 0.2 micron in-line filter; give approx. 2.5% of the total volume over 1 hour, then infuse remaining volume over next 3 hours; if body-weight under 20 kg and at risk of fluid overload, dilute requisite dose in 100 mL Sodium Chloride 0.9% and give over at least 4 hours.

- **NATIONAL FUNDING/ACCESS DECISIONS** For full details see funding body website

All Wales Medicines Strategy Group (AWMSG) decisions

▶ **Galsulfase (*Naglazyme*®) for long-term enzyme replacement therapy in patients with a confirmed diagnosis of mucopolysaccharidosis VI (October 2024)** AWMSG No. 155 Recommended

- **MEDICINAL FORMS** There can be variation in the licensing of different medicines containing the same drug.

Solution for infusion

▸ **Naglazyme** (BioMarin (U.K.) Ltd)

Galsulfase 1 mg per 1 ml Naglazyme 5mg/5ml solution for infusion vials | 1 vial PoM £982.00 (Hospital only)

Idursulfase

16-Jul-2020

- **DRUG ACTION** Idursulfase is an enzyme produced by recombinant DNA technology licensed for long-term replacement therapy in mucopolysaccharidosis II (Hunter syndrome), a lysosomal storage disorder caused by deficiency of iduronate-2-sulfatase.

- **INDICATIONS AND DOSE**

Mucopolysaccharidosis II (specialist use only)

▶ BY INTRAVENOUS INFUSION

▸ Child 16 months–17 years: 500 micrograms/kg once weekly

- **CAUTIONS** Acute febrile respiratory illness (consider delaying treatment) · infusion-related reactions can occur · severe respiratory disease
- **SIDE-EFFECTS**

▶ **Common or very common** Arrhythmias · arthralgia · chest pain · cough · cyanosis · diarrhoea · dizziness · dyspnoea · fever · flushing · gastrointestinal discomfort · headache · hypertension · hypotension · hypoxia · infusion related reaction · nausea · oedema · respiratory disorders · skin reactions · tongue swelling · tremor · vomiting

▶ **Frequency not known** Hypersensitivity

SIDE-EFFECTS, FURTHER INFORMATION Infusion-related reactions often occur, they can be managed by slowing the infusion rate or interrupting the infusion, and can be minimised by pre-treatment with an antihistamine and an antipyretic. Recurrent infusion-related reactions may require pre-treatment with a corticosteroid—consult product literature for details.

- **CONCEPTION AND CONTRACEPTION** Contra-indicated in women of child-bearing potential.
- **PREGNANCY** Manufacturer advises avoid.
- **BREAST FEEDING** Manufacturer advises avoid—present in milk in *animal* studies.
- **DIRECTIONS FOR ADMINISTRATION** For *intravenous infusion*, manufacturer advises dilute requisite dose in 100 mL Sodium Chloride 0.9% and mix gently (do not shake); give over 3 hours (gradually reduced to 1 hour if no infusion-related reactions).

- **MEDICINAL FORMS** There can be variation in the licensing of different medicines containing the same drug.

Solution for infusion

▸ **Elaprase** (Takeda UK Ltd) ▼

Idursulfase 2 mg per 1 ml Elaprase 6mg/3ml concentrate for solution for infusion vials | 1 vial PoM £1,985.00 (Hospital only)

Laronidase

09-Dec-2024

- **DRUG ACTION** Laronidase is an enzyme produced by recombinant DNA technology licensed for long-term replacement therapy in the treatment of non-neurological manifestations of mucopolysaccharidosis I, a lysosomal storage disorder caused by deficiency of alpha-L-iduronidase.

- **INDICATIONS AND DOSE**

Non-neurological manifestations of mucopolysaccharidosis I (specialist use only)

▶ BY INTRAVENOUS INFUSION

▸ Child: 100 units/kg once weekly

- **CAUTIONS** Infusion-related reactions can occur
- **INTERACTIONS** → Appendix 1: laronidase
- **SIDE-EFFECTS**

▶ **Common or very common** Abdominal pain · alopecia · anaphylactic reaction · angioedema · chills · cough · diarrhoea · dizziness · dyspnoea · fatigue · fever · flushing · headache · hypotension · influenza like illness · joint disorders · nausea · pain · pallor · paraesthesia · peripheral coldness · respiratory disorders · restlessness · skin reactions · sweat changes · tachycardia · temperature sensation altered · vomiting

▶ **Frequency not known** Cyanosis · hypoxia · oedema

SIDE-EFFECTS, FURTHER INFORMATION Infusion-related reactions often occur, they can be managed by slowing the infusion rate or interrupting the infusion, and can be minimised by pre-treatment with an antihistamine and an antipyretic. Recurrent infusion-related reactions may require pre-treatment with a corticosteroid—consult product literature for details.

- **PREGNANCY** Manufacturer advises avoid unless essential—no information available.
- **BREAST FEEDING** Manufacturer advises avoid—no information available.
- **MONITORING REQUIREMENTS** Monitor immunoglobulin G (IgG) antibody concentration.
- **DIRECTIONS FOR ADMINISTRATION** For *intravenous infusion*, manufacturer advises dilute with Sodium Chloride 0.9%; body-weight under 20 kg, dilute to 100 mL, body-weight over 20 kg dilute to 250 mL; give through in-line filter (0.2 micron) initially at a rate of 2 units/kg/hour then increase gradually every 15 minutes to max. 43 units/kg/hour.

- **MEDICINAL FORMS** There can be variation in the licensing of different medicines containing the same drug.

Solution for infusion

ELECTROLYTES: May contain Sodium

▸ **Aldurazyme** (Sanofi)

Laronidase 100 unit per 1 ml Aldurazyme 500units/5ml concentrate for solution for infusion vials | 1 vial PoM £444.70

Vestronidase alfa

23-Sep-2024

- **DRUG ACTION** Vestronidase alfa is an enzyme produced by recombinant DNA technology used for long-term replacement therapy of non-neurological manifestations of mucopolysaccharidosis VII (Sly syndrome), a lysosomal storage disorder caused by deficiency of beta-glucuronidase.

- **INDICATIONS AND DOSE**

Non-neurological manifestations of mucopolysaccharidosis VII (under expert supervision)

▶ BY INTRAVENOUS INFUSION

▸ Neonate: 4 mg/kg every 2 weeks.

▸ Child: 4 mg/kg every 2 weeks

- **CAUTIONS** Acute febrile illness (delay treatment) · acute respiratory illness (delay treatment) · hypersensitivity reactions

CAUTIONS, FURTHER INFORMATION
- Hypersensitivity reactions [EvGr] Serious hypersensitivity reactions, including anaphylaxis, have been reported; these may be minimised by pre-treatment with a non-sedating antihistamine with or without an antipyretic, given 30–60 minutes before the start of the infusion. *Mepsevii*® should only be administered by appropriately trained staff, and patients should be observed for at least 1 hour after the infusion; manage hypersensitivity reactions by temporarily interrupting the infusion, reducing the rate of infusion and/or treatment with antihistamines, antipyretics, and/or corticosteroids. If a severe reaction occurs, stop infusion immediately and start appropriate medical treatment; caution is advised on re-administration. ⟨M⟩

- **SIDE-EFFECTS**
  - **Common or very common** Diarrhoea · febrile seizure · hypersensitivity · skin reactions
- **PREGNANCY** [EvGr] Avoid unless potential benefit outweighs risk (no information available). ⟨M⟩
- **BREAST FEEDING** Specialist sources indicate use with caution (no information available). Large molecular weight suggests limited excretion into milk and drug molecule likely to be destroyed in the infant's gastro-intestinal tract; monitor breast-fed infants carefully.
- **DIRECTIONS FOR ADMINISTRATION** [EvGr] For *intravenous infusion* (*Mepsevii*®), dilute with Sodium Chloride 0.9%; give through a low-protein binding 0.2 micron in-line filter. Initially infuse 2.5% of the total volume in the first hour, then infuse remaining volume over the next 3 hours according to the recommended rate—consult product literature. ⟨M⟩
- **PRESCRIBING AND DISPENSING INFORMATION** Vestronidase alfa is a biological medicine. Biological medicines must be prescribed and dispensed by brand name, see *Biological medicines* and *Biosimilar medicines*, under Guidance on prescribing p. 1; record the brand name and batch number after each administration.
- **HANDLING AND STORAGE** Store in a refrigerator at 2–8°C and protect from light—consult product literature for storage conditions after dilution.

- **MEDICINAL FORMS** There can be variation in the licensing of different medicines containing the same drug.

Solution for infusion

EXCIPIENTS: May contain Polysorbates
ELECTROLYTES: May contain Sodium

- **Mepsevii** (Ultragenyx UK Ltd) ▼
  Vestronidase alfa 2 mg per 1 ml Mepsevii 10mg/5ml concentrate for solution for infusion vials | 1 vial [PoM] £1,713.00 (Hospital only)

3.14 Niemann-Pick disease

ENZYME INHIBITORS › GLUCOSYLCERAMIDE SYNTHASE INHIBITORS

Miglustat

21-Oct-2024

- **DRUG ACTION** Miglustat is an inhibitor of glucosylceramide synthase.

- **INDICATIONS AND DOSE**

Treatment of progressive neurological manifestations of Niemann-Pick type C disease (under expert supervision)

▶ BY MOUTH
- Child 4–11 years (body surface area up to 0.48 m^2): 100 mg once daily
- Child 4–11 years (body surface area 0.48–0.73 m^2): 100 mg twice daily
- Child 4–11 years (body surface area 0.74–0.88 m^2): 100 mg 3 times a day
- Child 4–11 years (body surface area 0.89–1.25 m^2): 200 mg twice daily
- Child 4–11 years (body surface area 1.26 m^2 and above): 200 mg 3 times a day
- Child 12–17 years: 200 mg 3 times a day

IMPORTANT SAFETY INFORMATION

SAFE PRACTICE

Miglustat could be confused with migalastat; care must be taken to ensure the correct drug is prescribed and dispensed.

- **SIDE-EFFECTS**
  - **Common or very common** Appetite decreased · asthenia · chills · constipation · depression · diarrhoea · dizziness · flatulence · gastrointestinal discomfort · headache · insomnia · libido decreased · malaise · muscle spasms · muscle weakness · nausea · peripheral neuropathy · sensation abnormal · thrombocytopenia · tremor · vomiting · weight decreased
  - **Uncommon** Feeling jittery
  - **Frequency not known** Growth retardation
- **CONCEPTION AND CONTRACEPTION** [EvGr] Effective contraception must be used during treatment. Male patients should avoid fathering a child during and for 3 months after treatment. ⟨M⟩
- **PREGNANCY** [EvGr] Avoid (toxicity in *animal* studies). ⟨M⟩
- **BREAST FEEDING** [EvGr] Avoid (no information available). ⟨M⟩
- **HEPATIC IMPAIRMENT** Manufacturer advises caution (no information available).
- **RENAL IMPAIRMENT** Avoid if estimated glomerular filtration less than 30 mL/minute/1.73 m^2. Child under 12 years—consult product literature.
  Dose adjustments Child 12–17 years, initially 200 mg twice daily if estimated glomerular filtration rate 50–70 mL/minute/1.73 m^2. Initially 100 mg twice daily if estimated glomerular filtration rate 30–50 mL/minute/1.73 m^2.
- **MONITORING REQUIREMENTS**
  - Monitor cognitive and neurological function.
  - Monitor growth and platelet count in Niemann-Pick type C disease.
- **NATIONAL FUNDING/ACCESS DECISIONS**
  For full details see funding body website

  All Wales Medicines Strategy Group (AWMSG) decisions
  - **Miglustat for the treatment of progressive neurological manifestations in adult patients and paediatric patients with Niemann-Pick type C disease (October 2024)** AWMSG No. 371 Recommended

- **MEDICINAL FORMS** There can be variation in the licensing of different medicines containing the same drug.

Oral capsule

- **Miglustat (Non-proprietary)**
  Miglustat 100 mg Miglustat 100mg capsules | 84 capsule [PoM] £2,850.00–£3,934.00 (Hospital only) | 84 capsule [PoM] £3,442.00
- **Opfolda** (Amicus Therapeutics UK Operations Ltd)
  Miglustat 65 mg Opfolda 65mg capsules | 4 capsule [PoM] £116.69 (Hospital only) | 24 capsule [PoM] £700.14 (Hospital only)
- **Yargesa** (Piramal Critical Care Ltd)
  Miglustat 100 mg Yargesa 100mg capsules | 84 capsule [PoM] £3,500.00 (Hospital only)
- **Zavesca** (Janssen-Cilag Ltd)
  Miglustat 100 mg Zavesca 100mg capsules | 84 capsule [PoM] £3,934.17 (Hospital only)

ENZYMES

Olipudase alfa
25-Apr-2025

- **DRUG ACTION** Olipudase alfa is an enzyme produced by recombinant DNA technology that is administered as enzyme replacement therapy for the treatment of acid sphingomyelinase deficiency (Niemann-Pick disease) type A/B or B, a lysosomal storage disorder affecting the normal function of tissues and organs such as the liver, spleen, lungs, heart, and brain.

- **INDICATIONS AND DOSE**

Non-neurological manifestations of acid sphingomyelinase deficiency (Niemann-Pick disease) type A/B or B (under expert supervision)

▶ BY INTRAVENOUS INFUSION

▶ Neonate: Initially 30 micrograms/kg for 1 dose, subsequent doses to be administered every 2 weeks according to dose escalation regimen until maintenance phase is reached after 16 weeks—consult product literature; usual maintenance 3 mg/kg every 2 weeks.

▶ Child: Initially 30 micrograms/kg for 1 dose, subsequent doses to be administered every 2 weeks according to dose escalation regimen until maintenance phase is reached after 16 weeks—consult product literature; usual maintenance 3 mg/kg every 2 weeks

DOSES AT EXTREMES OF BODY-WEIGHT

▶ Doses should be calculated on the basis of optimal body-weight in patients with BMI > 30 kg/m^2—consult product literature.

- **CAUTIONS** Infusion-related reactions

CAUTIONS, FURTHER INFORMATION EvGr Serious infusion-related reactions can occur and olipudase alfa should only be administered when appropriately trained staff and resuscitation facilities are available; these reactions may be minimised by pre-medication with an antihistamine, antipyretic, and corticosteroid. Patients should be closely monitored for signs of infusion-related reactions during and after administration, and managed appropriately—consult product literature. (M)

- **SIDE-EFFECTS**

▶ **Common or very common** Angioedema · arthralgia · asthenia · chills · diarrhoea · dyspnoea · eye discomfort · eye erythema · fever · gastrointestinal discomfort · headache · hepatic pain · hypersensitivity · hypotension · myalgia · nausea · pain · palpitations · respiratory disorders · skin reactions · tachycardia · throat complaints · vasodilation · vomiting

- **PREGNANCY** EvGr Avoid unless potential benefit outweighs risk—toxicity in *animal* studies. (M)

- **BREAST FEEDING** Specialist sources indicate use with caution—no information available. Large molecular weight suggests limited excretion into milk and drug molecule likely to be partially destroyed in the infant's gastro-intestinal tract.

- **MONITORING REQUIREMENTS** EvGr Monitor hepatic transaminases (ALT and AST) within 1 month before treatment initiation, then within 72 hours before the next scheduled infusion during dose escalation or when resuming treatment, and as clinically indicated during maintenance phase—consult product literature. (M)

- **DIRECTIONS FOR ADMINISTRATION** EvGr For *intermittent intravenous infusion* (*Xenpozyme*®), reconstitute initially with Water for Injections then dilute requisite dose with Sodium Chloride 0.9%; give through a low-protein binding 0.2 micron in-line filter, preferably via an infusion pump, according to the recommended rate and duration—consult product literature. Patients stabilised on a maintenance dose may be considered for home infusion under the supervision of a healthcare professional—consult product literature. (M)

- **PRESCRIBING AND DISPENSING INFORMATION** Olipudase alfa is a biological medicine. Biological medicines must be prescribed and dispensed by brand name, see *Biological medicines* and *Biosimilar medicines*, under Guidance on prescribing p. 1; record the brand name and batch number after each administration.

- **HANDLING AND STORAGE** Store in a refrigerator (2–8°C)—consult product literature for storage conditions after reconstitution and dilution.

- **PATIENT AND CARER ADVICE**

Driving and skilled tasks Patients and carers should be cautioned on the effects on driving and performance of skilled tasks—increased risk of hypotension.

- **NATIONAL FUNDING/ACCESS DECISIONS**

For full details see funding body website

NICE decisions

▶ **Olipudase alfa for treating acid sphingomyelinase deficiency (Niemann-Pick disease) type AB and type B (April 2025)**
NICE HST32 Not recommended

- **MEDICINAL FORMS** There can be variation in the licensing of different medicines containing the same drug.

Powder for solution for infusion

EXCIPIENTS: May contain Sucrose
ELECTROLYTES: May contain Sodium

▶ Xenpozyme (Sanofi) ▼
Olipudase alfa 20 mg Xenpozyme 20mg powder for concentrate for solution for infusion vials | 1 vial PoM £3,612.00 (Hospital only)

3.15 Pompe disease

ENZYMES

Alglucosidase alfa
28-May-2024

- **DRUG ACTION** Alglucosidase alfa is an enzyme produced by recombinant DNA technology licensed for long-term replacement therapy in Pompe disease, a lysosomal storage disorder caused by deficiency of acid alpha-glucosidase.

- **INDICATIONS AND DOSE**

Pompe disease (specialist use only)

▶ BY INTRAVENOUS INFUSION

▶ Neonate: 20 mg/kg every 2 weeks.

▶ Child: 20 mg/kg every 2 weeks

- **CAUTIONS** Cardiac dysfunction · infusion-related reactions—consult product literature · respiratory dysfunction

- **SIDE-EFFECTS**

▶ **Common or very common** Anxiety · arrhythmias · chest discomfort · chills · cough · cyanosis · diarrhoea · dizziness · fever · flushing · hyperhidrosis · hypersensitivity · hypertension · irritability · local swelling · muscle complaints · nausea · oedema · pallor · paraesthesia · respiratory disorders · skin reactions · temperature sensation altered · throat complaints · tremor · vomiting

▶ **Frequency not known** Angioedema · apnoea · arthralgia · asthenia · cardiac arrest · drowsiness · dysphagia · dyspnoea · excessive tearing · eye inflammation · gastrointestinal discomfort · headache · hypotension · hypoxia · influenza like illness · infusion related reaction · malaise · musculoskeletal chest pain · nephrotic syndrome · palpitations · peripheral coldness · proteinuria · skin ulcer · vasoconstriction

SIDE-EFFECTS, FURTHER INFORMATION Infusion-related reactions are very common, calling for use of antihistamine, antipyretic, or corticosteroid; consult product literature for details.

- **PREGNANCY** Toxicity in *animal* studies, but treatment should not be withheld.
- **BREAST FEEDING** Manufacturer advises avoid—no information available.
- **MONITORING REQUIREMENTS**
  - Monitor closely if cardiac dysfunction.
  - Monitor closely if respiratory dysfunction.
  - Monitor immunoglobulin G (IgG) antibody concentration.
- **DIRECTIONS FOR ADMINISTRATION** For *intravenous infusion*, manufacturer advises reconstitute 50 mg with 10.3 mL Water for Injections to produce 5 mg/mL solution; gently rotate vial without shaking; dilute requisite dose with Sodium Chloride 0.9% to give a final concentration of 0.5–4 mg/mL; give through a low protein-binding in-line filter (0.2 micron) at an initial rate of 1 mg/kg/hour increased by 2 mg/kg/hour every 30 minutes to max. 7mg/kg/hour.
- **NATIONAL FUNDING/ACCESS DECISIONS**
  For full details see funding body website

  All Wales Medicines Strategy Group (AWMSG) decisions
  - **Alglucosidase alfa (*Myozyme*®) for long-term enzyme replacement therapy in patients with a confirmed diagnosis of Pompe disease (acid alpha-glucosidase deficiency) (May 2024)**
    AWMSG No. 17 Recommended

- **MEDICINAL FORMS** There can be variation in the licensing of different medicines containing the same drug.

  Powder for solution for infusion
  - **Myozyme** (Sanofi)
    Alglucosidase alfa 50 mg Myozyme 50mg powder for concentrate for solution for infusion vials | 1 vial PoM £356.06 (Hospital only)

Avalglucosidase alfa

25-Jul-2023

- **DRUG ACTION** Avalglucosidase alfa, a modification of alglucosidase alfa, is an enzyme produced by recombinant DNA technology that is administered as enzyme replacement therapy in Pompe disease, a lysosomal storage disorder caused by deficiency of acid alpha-glucosidase.

- **INDICATIONS AND DOSE**

  Pompe disease (under expert supervision)
  - BY INTRAVENOUS INFUSION
  - Child 7 months–17 years: 20 mg/kg every 2 weeks; increased if necessary to 40 mg/kg every 2 weeks, dose may only be increased in patients with infantile-onset disease who do not respond adequately to standard dosing, and in the absence of safety concerns

- **CAUTIONS** Cardiac dysfunction · infusion-related reactions · respiratory dysfunction · susceptibility to fluid volume overload

  CAUTIONS, FURTHER INFORMATION
  - Infusion-related reactions EvGr Infusion-related reactions can occur and avalglucosidase alfa should only be administered when appropriately trained staff are available; these reactions may be minimised by premedication with an antihistamine, antipyretic, and/or corticosteroid. Patients should be monitored for signs of infusion-related reactions during and after administration, and managed appropriately—consult product literature. (M)
- **SIDE-EFFECTS**
  - **Common or very common** Asthenia · chest discomfort · chills · cough · diarrhoea · dizziness · dyspnoea · eye disorders · headache · hypersensitivity · hypertension · influenza like illness · muscle complaints · nausea · oral disorders · pain · skin reactions · tremor · vomiting
  - **Uncommon** Angioedema · arrhythmias · conjunctivitis · drowsiness · dysphagia · eye pruritus · fever · flushing · gastrointestinal discomfort · hyperhidrosis · hyperthermia · hypotension · localised oedema · paraesthesia · peripheral swelling · respiratory disorders · throat irritation
  - **Frequency not known** Infusion related reaction
- **PREGNANCY** EvGr Use only if potential benefit outweighs risk—no information available. (M)
- **BREAST FEEDING** EvGr Use only if potential benefit outweighs risk—no information available. (M)
- **DIRECTIONS FOR ADMINISTRATION** EvGr For *intermittent intravenous infusion* (*Nexviadyme*®), reconstitute each 100-mg vial with 10 mL Water for Injections then dilute requisite dose to a concentration of 0.5–4 mg/mL with Glucose 5%; give through a low protein-binding 0.2 micron in-line filter, according to the recommended rate (initially 1 mg/kg/hour) and duration—consult product literature. Patients tolerating their infusions well may be considered for home infusion under the supervision of a healthcare professional—consult product literature. (M)
- **PRESCRIBING AND DISPENSING INFORMATION** Avalglucosidase alfa is a biological medicine. Biological medicines must be prescribed and dispensed by brand name, see *Biological medicines* and *Biosimilar medicines*, under Guidance on prescribing p. 1; record the brand name and batch number after each administration.

  The manufacturer of *Nexviadyme*® has provided *Risk minimisation materials* documents for healthcare professionals.
- **HANDLING AND STORAGE** Store in refrigerator (2–8°C)—consult product literature for storage conditions after reconstitution and dilution.
- **PATIENT AND CARER ADVICE**
  Driving and skilled tasks Patients and carers should be counselled on the effects on driving and performance of skilled tasks—increased risk of dizziness.
- **NATIONAL FUNDING/ACCESS DECISIONS**
  For full details see funding body website

  NICE decisions
  - **Avalglucosidase alfa for treating Pompe disease (August 2022)**
    NICE TA821 Recommended

  Scottish Medicines Consortium (SMC) decisions
  - **Avalglucosidase alfa (*Nexviadyme*®) as a long-term enzyme replacement therapy for the treatment of patients with Pompe disease (acid alpha-glucosidase deficiency) (July 2023)**
    SMC No. SMC2546 Recommended

- **MEDICINAL FORMS** There can be variation in the licensing of different medicines containing the same drug.

  Powder for solution for infusion
  EXCIPIENTS: May contain Polysorbates
  - **Nexviadyme** (Sanofi) ▼
    Avalglucosidase alfa 100 mg Nexviadyme 100mg powder for concentrate for solution for infusion vials | 1 vial PoM £783.33 (Hospital only)

9 Blood and nutrition

3.16 Primary hyperoxaluria

DRUGS FOR METABOLIC DISORDERS › SMALL INTERFERING RIBONUCLEIC ACID

Lumasiran

04-Jul-2023

- **DRUG ACTION** Lumasiran is a double-stranded small interfering RNA, which reduces production of the enzyme glycolate oxidase involved in the synthesis of glyoxylate and oxalate, thereby reducing urinary and plasma oxalate levels.

- **INDICATIONS AND DOSE**

Primary hyperoxaluria type 1 (under expert supervision)

▶ BY SUBCUTANEOUS INJECTION

- Neonate (body-weight up to 10 kg): Loading dose 6 mg/kg once a month for 3 doses, then maintenance 3 mg/kg once a month, to be started 1 month after the last loading dose.
- Child (body-weight up to 10 kg): Loading dose 6 mg/kg once a month for 3 doses, then maintenance 3 mg/kg once a month, to be started 1 month after the last loading dose
- Child (body-weight 10-19 kg): Loading dose 6 mg/kg once a month for 3 doses, then maintenance 6 mg/kg every 3 months, to be started 1 month after the last loading dose
- Child (body-weight 20 kg and above): Loading dose 3 mg/kg once a month for 3 doses, then maintenance 3 mg/kg every 3 months, to be started 1 month after the last loading dose

- **CAUTIONS** Children under 1 year of age (limited information available)
- **SIDE-EFFECTS**
  - ▶ **Common or very common** Gastrointestinal discomfort
- **PREGNANCY** EvGr Use only if potential benefit outweighs risk (limited information available). (M)
- **BREAST FEEDING** EvGr Avoid (no information available). (M)
- **HEPATIC IMPAIRMENT** EvGr Caution in moderate or severe impairment (potential for decreased efficacy). (M)
- **RENAL IMPAIRMENT** Monitor for signs and symptoms of metabolic acidosis in severe impairment (increased plasma-glycolate levels caused by lumasiran therapy may increase the risk of, or worsen pre-existing, metabolic acidosis).
- **DIRECTIONS FOR ADMINISTRATION** Maximum 1.5 mL per injection site; inject into the abdomen, thigh, or upper arm and rotate injection site. Avoid injecting into scar tissue or skin that is reddened, inflamed, or swollen.
- **HANDLING AND STORAGE** Protect from light.
- **NATIONAL FUNDING/ACCESS DECISIONS** For full details see funding body website

NICE decisions

- ▶ **Lumasiran for treating primary hyperoxaluria type 1 (April 2023)** NICE HST25 Recommended

- **MEDICINAL FORMS** There can be variation in the licensing of different medicines containing the same drug.

Solution for injection

- ▶ **Oxlumo** (Alnylam UK Ltd)
  Lumasiran (as Lumasiran sodium) 189 mg per 1 ml Oxlumo 94.5mg/0.5ml solution for injection vials | 1 vial PoM £61,068.98 (Hospital only)

3.17 Tyrosinaemia type I

ENZYME INHIBITORS › 4-HYDROXYPHENYLPYRUVATE DIOXYGENASE INHIBITORS

Nitisinone

19-Jul-2022

(NTBC)

- **DRUG ACTION** Nitisinone is a competitive inhibitor of 4-hydroxyphenylpyruvate dioxygenase which inhibits catabolism of tyrosine and thereby prevents accumulation of harmful metabolites.

- **INDICATIONS AND DOSE**

Hereditary tyrosinaemia type I (in combination with dietary restriction of tyrosine and phenylalanine) (specialist use only)

▶ BY MOUTH

- Neonate: Initially 1 mg/kg daily in 1–2 divided doses, adjusted according to response; maximum 2 mg/kg per day.
- Child: Initially 1 mg/kg daily in 1–2 divided doses, adjusted according to response; maximum 2 mg/kg per day

ORFADIN® CAPSULES

Hereditary tyrosinaemia type I (in combination with dietary restriction of tyrosine and phenylalanine) (specialist use only)

▶ BY MOUTH USING CAPSULES

- Neonate: Initially 1 mg/kg daily in 1–2 divided doses, adjusted according to response; maximum 2 mg/kg per day.
- Child: Initially 1 mg/kg daily in 1–2 divided doses, adjusted according to response; maximum 2 mg/kg per day

ORFADIN® ORAL SUSPENSION

Hereditary tyrosinaemia type I (in combination with dietary restriction of tyrosine and phenylalanine) (specialist use only)

▶ BY MOUTH USING ORAL SUSPENSION

- Neonate: Initially 1 mg/kg daily in 1–2 divided doses, adjusted according to response; maximum 2 mg/kg per day.
- Child: Initially 1 mg/kg daily in 1–2 divided doses, adjusted according to response; maximum 2 mg/kg per day

- **INTERACTIONS** → Appendix 1: nitisinone
- **SIDE-EFFECTS**
  - ▶ **Common or very common** Corneal opacity · eye inflammation · eye pain · granulocytopenia · increased risk of infection · leucopenia · photophobia · skin reactions · thrombocytopenia
  - ▶ **Uncommon** Leucocytosis
- **PREGNANCY** Manufacturer advises avoid unless potential benefit outweighs risk—toxicity in *animal* studies.
- **BREAST FEEDING** Manufacturer advises avoid—adverse effects in *animal* studies.
- **MONITORING REQUIREMENTS** EvGr Slit-lamp examination of eyes is recommended before treatment and at least once a year thereafter. Monitor plasma tyrosine levels—consult product literature. Monitor platelet and white blood cell count every 6 months. Monitor liver function regularly. (M)

- **DIRECTIONS FOR ADMINISTRATION** Manufacturer advises capsules can be opened and the contents suspended in a small amount of water or formula diet and taken immediately.
- **HANDLING AND STORAGE** Store in a refrigerator (2–8°C).
- **PATIENT AND CARER ADVICE** Patients and carers should be advised to seek immediate medical attention if symptoms of visual disorders develop during treatment.

Driving and skilled tasks Patients and carers should be cautioned on the effects on driving and performance of skilled tasks—increased risk of visual disorders.

ORFADIN® ORAL SUSPENSION Patients or carers should be given advice on how to administer *Orfadin®* oral suspension.

- **MEDICINAL FORMS** There can be variation in the licensing of different medicines containing the same drug.

Oral suspension

CAUTIONARY AND ADVISORY LABELS 21
EXCIPIENTS: May contain Polysorbates
ELECTROLYTES: May contain Sodium

- **Orfadin** (Swedish Orphan Biovitrum Ltd)
  Nitisinone 4 mg per 1 ml Orfadin 4mg/1ml oral suspension | 90 ml PoM £1,692.00 (Hospital only) SF

Oral capsule

- **Nitisinone (Non-proprietary)**
  Nitisinone 2 mg Nitisinone 2mg capsules | 60 capsule PoM £423.00
  Nitisinone 5 mg Nitisinone 5mg capsules | 60 capsule PoM £845.25
  Nitisinone 10 mg Nitisinone 10mg capsules | 60 capsule PoM £1,546.50
  Nitisinone 20 mg Nitisinone 20mg capsules | 60 capsule PoM £3,384.00
- **Orfadin** (Swedish Orphan Biovitrum Ltd)
  Nitisinone 2 mg Orfadin 2mg capsules | 60 capsule PoM £423.00 (Hospital only)
  Nitisinone 5 mg Orfadin 5mg capsules | 60 capsule PoM £845.25 (Hospital only)
  Nitisinone 10 mg Orfadin 10mg capsules | 60 capsule PoM £1,546.50 (Hospital only)
  Nitisinone 20 mg Orfadin 20mg capsules | 60 capsule PoM £3,384.00 (Hospital only)

3.18 Urea cycle disorders

AMINO ACIDS AND DERIVATIVES

Arginine

03-Mar-2020

- **INDICATIONS AND DOSE**

Acute hyperammonaemia in carbamylphosphate synthetase deficiency (specialist use only) | Acute hyperammonaemia in ornithine transcarbamylase deficiency (specialist use only)

▶ BY INTRAVENOUS INFUSION

- Neonate: 6 mg/kg/hour.
- Child (body-weight up to 40 kg): 6 mg/kg/hour
- Child (body-weight 40 kg and above): 4 mg/kg/hour

Maintenance treatment of hyperammonaemia in carbamylphosphate synthetase deficiency (specialist use only) | Maintenance treatment of hyperammonaemia in ornithine transcarbamylase deficiency (specialist use only)

▶ BY MOUTH

- Neonate: 100–200 mg/kg daily in 3–4 divided doses, dose to be taken with feeds.
- Child (body-weight up to 20 kg): 100–200 mg/kg daily in 3–4 divided doses, dose to be given with feeds or meals
- Child (body-weight 20 kg and above): 2.5–6 g/m^2 daily in 3–4 divided doses, dose to be taken with meals; maximum 6 g per day

Acute hyperammonaemia in citrullinaemia (specialist use only) | Acute hyperammonaemia in arginosuccinic aciduria (specialist use only)

▶ BY INTRAVENOUS INFUSION

- Neonate: Initially 300 mg/kg, to be administered over 90 minutes, followed by 12.5 mg/kg/hour, to be administered over 24 hours (maximum 25 mg/kg/hour thereafter).
- Child (body-weight up to 40 kg): Initially 300 mg/kg, to be administered over 90 minutes, followed by 12.5 mg/kg/hour, to be administered over 24 hours (maximum 25 mg/kg/hour thereafter)
- Child (body-weight 40 kg and above): 21 mg/kg/hour

Maintenance treatment of hyperammonaemia in citrullinaemia (specialist use only) | Maintenance treatment of hyperammonaemia in arginosuccinic aciduria (specialist use only)

▶ BY MOUTH

- Neonate: 100–300 mg/kg daily in 3–4 divided doses, dose to be taken with feeds.
- Child (body-weight up to 20 kg): 100–300 mg/kg daily in 3–4 divided doses, dose to be taken with feed or meals
- Child (body-weight 20 kg and above): 2.5–6 g/m^2 daily in 3–4 divided doses, doses to be taken with meals; maximum 6 g per day

- **UNLICENSED USE**
  - With intravenous use Injection not licensed in children.
  - With oral use Tablets not licensed in children. Powder licensed for urea cycle disorders in children.
- **CONTRA-INDICATIONS** Not to be used in the treatment of arginase deficiency
- **SIDE-EFFECTS** Acidosis hyperchloraemic · flushing · headache · hypotension · nausea · numbness · vomiting
- **PREGNANCY** No information available.
- **BREAST FEEDING** No information available.
- **MONITORING REQUIREMENTS** Monitor plasma pH and chloride.
- **DIRECTIONS FOR ADMINISTRATION** For *intravenous infusion*, dilute to a max. concentration of 50 mg/mL with glucose 10%.
- **PRESCRIBING AND DISPENSING INFORMATION**
  - With oral use Powder to be prescribed as a borderline substance (ACBS). For use as a supplement in urea cycle disorders other than arginase deficiency, such as hyperammonaemia types I and II, citrullinaemia, arginosuccinic aciduria, and deficiency of N-acetyl glutamate synthetase.
- **PATIENT AND CARER ADVICE**
  Medicines for Children leaflet: Arginine for urea cycle disorders www.medicinesforchildren.org.uk/medicines/arginine-for-urea-cycle-disorders/
- **MEDICINAL FORMS** There can be variation in the licensing of different medicines containing the same drug. Forms available from special-order manufacturers include: oral tablet, oral capsule, oral solution, solution for infusion

Oral tablet

- **Arginine (Non-proprietary)**
  L-Arginine 500 mg HealthAid L-Arginine 500mg tablets | 60 tablet £7.25
  L-Arginine 1 gram Arginine 1g tablets | 90 tablet £12.26

Oral capsule

- **Arginine (Non-proprietary)**
  L-Arginine 500 mg SynBio L-Arginine 500mg capsules | 60 capsule £4.75

9 Blood and nutrition

Solution for infusion

▸ Arginine (Non-proprietary)

L-Arginine monohydrochloride 210.7 mg per 1 ml L-Arginin-Hydrochlorid 21% concentrate for solution for infusion 20ml ampoules | 5 ampoule PoM (Hospital only)

Oral solution

▸ Aactigin (TriOn Pharma Ltd)

L-Arginine 100 mg per 1 ml Aactigin 500mg/5ml oral solution | 200 ml £37.09 SF

▸ Aargin (Essential-Healthcare Ltd)

L-Arginine 100 mg per 1 ml Aargin 500mg/5ml oral solution | 200 ml £37.89 DT = £46.99

Carglumic acid

24-Jul-2020

● **INDICATIONS AND DOSE**

Hyperammonaemia due to N-acetylglutamate synthase deficiency (under expert supervision)

▸ BY MOUTH

▸ Neonate: Initially 50–125 mg/kg twice daily, to be taken immediately before feeds, dose adjusted according to plasma–ammonia concentration; maintenance 5–50 mg/kg twice daily, the total daily dose may alternatively be given in 3–4 divided doses.

▸ Child: Initially 50–125 mg/kg twice daily, to be taken immediately before food, dose adjusted according to plasma–ammonia concentration; maintenance 5–50 mg/kg twice daily, the total daily dose may alternatively be given in 3–4 divided doses

Hyperammonaemia due to organic acidaemia (under expert supervision)

▸ BY MOUTH

▸ Neonate: Initially 50–125 mg/kg twice daily, to be taken immediately before feeds, dose adjusted according to plasma-ammonia concentration, the total daily dose may alternatively be given in 3–4 divided doses.

▸ Child: Initially 50–125 mg/kg twice daily, to be taken immediately before food, dose adjusted according to plasma-ammonia concentration, the total daily dose may alternatively be given in 3–4 divided doses

IMPORTANT SAFETY INFORMATION

EMERGENCY MANAGEMENT OF UREA CYCLE DISORDERS

For further information on the emergency management of urea cycle disorders consult the British Inherited Metabolic Disease Group (BIMDG) website at www.bimdg.org.uk

● **SIDE-EFFECTS**

▸ **Common or very common** Hyperhidrosis

▸ **Uncommon** Bradycardia · diarrhoea · fever · vomiting

▸ **Frequency not known** Rash

● **PREGNANCY** Manufacturer advises avoid unless essential—no information available.

● **BREAST FEEDING** Manufacturer advises avoid—present in milk in *animal* studies.

● **DIRECTIONS FOR ADMINISTRATION** Manufacturer advises dispersible tablets must be dispersed in at least 5–10 mL of water and taken orally immediately, or administered via a nasogastric tube.

● **MEDICINAL FORMS** There can be variation in the licensing of different medicines containing the same drug.

Dispersible tablet

CAUTIONARY AND ADVISORY LABELS 13

▸ Carglumic acid (Non-proprietary)

Carglumic acid 200 mg Carglumic acid 200mg dispersible tablets sugar free | 5 tablet PoM £218.69 SF | 15 tablet PoM £625.37 SF | 60 tablet PoM £2,624.30 SF

▸ Carbaglu (Recordati Rare Diseases UK Ltd)

Carglumic acid 200 mg Carbaglu 200mg dispersible tablets | 5 tablet PoM £299.00 SF | 60 tablet PoM £3,499.00 SF

▸ Ucedane (Eurocept International bv)

Carglumic acid 200 mg Ucedane 200mg dispersible tablets | 12 tablet PoM £660.00 SF | 60 tablet PoM £3,300.00 SF

Citrulline

23-Oct-2020

● **INDICATIONS AND DOSE**

Carbamyl phosphate synthase deficiency | Ornithine carbamyl transferase deficiency

▸ BY MOUTH

▸ Neonate: 150 mg/kg daily in 3–4 divided doses, adjusted according to response.

▸ Child: 150 mg/kg daily in 3–4 divided doses, adjusted according to response

● **PREGNANCY** No information available.

● **BREAST FEEDING** No information available.

● **DIRECTIONS FOR ADMINISTRATION** Manufacturer advises powder may be mixed with drinks or taken as a paste.

● **MEDICINAL FORMS** There can be variation in the licensing of different medicines containing the same drug. Forms available from special-order manufacturers include: oral tablet, oral solution, oral powder

Oral solution

▸ Citrulline (Non-proprietary)

L-Citrulline 100 mg per 1 ml Stimol oral solution 10ml sachets | 36 sachet PoM (Hospital only) SF

BENZOATES

Sodium benzoate

16-Aug-2023

● **INDICATIONS AND DOSE**

Acute hyperammonaemia due to urea cycle disorder (specialist use only)

▸ BY INTRAVENOUS INFUSION

▸ Neonate: Initially 250 mg/kg, to be administered over 90 minutes, followed by 10 mg/kg/hour, adjusted according to response.

▸ Child: Initially 250 mg/kg, to be administered over 90 minutes, followed by 10 mg/kg/hour, adjusted according to response

Maintenance treatment of hyperammonaemia due to urea cycle disorders (specialist use only) | Non-ketotic hyperglycinaemia (specialist use only)

▸ BY MOUTH

▸ Neonate: Up to 250 mg/kg daily in 3–4 divided doses, dose to be taken with feeds.

▸ Child: Up to 250 mg/kg daily in 3–4 divided doses, dose to be taken with feeds or meals; maximum 12 g per day

● **UNLICENSED USE** Sodium benzoate is not licensed in the UK. It is used as detailed below:

- Acute hyperammonaemia due to urea cycle disorders;
- Maintenance treatment of hyperammonaemia due to urea cycle disorders;
- Non-ketotic hyperglycinaemia.

IMPORTANT SAFETY INFORMATION

EMERGENCY MANAGEMENT OF UREA CYCLE DISORDERS

For further information on the emergency management of urea cycle disorders, consult the British Inherited Metabolic Disease Group (BIMDG) website at: www.bimdg.org.uk

- **CAUTIONS** Conditions involving sodium retention with oedema (preparations contain significant amounts of sodium) · congestive heart failure (preparations contain significant amounts of sodium) · neonates (risk of kernicterus and increased side-effects)
- **SIDE-EFFECTS** Appetite decreased · coma · irritability · lethargy · nausea · vomiting

  SIDE-EFFECTS, FURTHER INFORMATION Gastro-intestinal side-effects may be reduced by giving smaller doses more frequently.
- **PREGNANCY** No information available.
- **BREAST FEEDING** No information available.
- **RENAL IMPAIRMENT** Use with caution (preparations contain significant amounts of sodium).
- **DIRECTIONS FOR ADMINISTRATION** For administration *by mouth*, expert sources advise oral solution or powder may be administered in fruit drinks.

  For *intravenous infusion*, expert sources advise dilute to a max. concentration of 50 mg/mL with Glucose 10%.
- **PATIENT AND CARER ADVICE**

  Medicines for Children leaflet: Sodium benzoate for urea cycle disorders www.medicinesforchildren.org.uk/medicines/sodium-benzoate-for-urea-cycle-disorders/
- **MEDICINAL FORMS** There can be variation in the licensing of different medicines containing the same drug. Forms available from special-order manufacturers include: oral tablet, oral capsule, oral solution, solution for infusion

  Solution for infusion

  ELECTROLYTES: May contain Sodium

DRUGS FOR METABOLIC DISORDERS › ACETIC ACIDS

Sodium dichloroacetate

- **INDICATIONS AND DOSE**

  Pyruvate dehydrogenase defects

  ▶ BY MOUTH

  ▸ Neonate: Initially 12.5 mg/kg 4 times a day, adjusted according to response, increased if necessary up to 200 mg/kg daily.

  ▸ Child: Initially 12.5 mg/kg 4 times a day, adjusted according to response, increased if necessary up to 200 mg/kg daily
- **SIDE-EFFECTS** Metabolic acidosis · oxalate metabolism abnormal · polyneuropathy (long term use)
- **PREGNANCY** No information available.
- **BREAST FEEDING** No information available.
- **MEDICINAL FORMS** No licensed medicines listed.

DRUGS FOR METABOLIC DISORDERS › AMMONIA LOWERING DRUGS

Glycerol phenylbutyrate

18-Nov-2020

- **DRUG ACTION** Glycerol phenylbutyrate is a nitrogen-binding agent that provides an alternative vehicle for waste nitrogen excretion.
- **INDICATIONS AND DOSE**

  Urea cycle disorders (specialist use only)

  ▶ BY MOUTH, OR BY GASTROSTOMY TUBE, OR BY NASOGASTRIC TUBE

  ▸ Neonate (body surface area up to 1.3 m^2): Initially 9.4 g/m^2 daily in divided doses, usual maintenance 5.3–12.4 g/m^2 daily in divided doses, each dose should be rounded up to the nearest 0.1 mL and given with each feed. For dose adjustments based on individual requirements—consult product literature.

  ▸ Child 1–23 months (body surface area up to 1.3 m^2): Initially 9.4 g/m^2 daily in divided doses, usual maintenance 5.3–12.4 g/m^2 daily in divided doses, each dose should be rounded up to the nearest 0.1 mL and given with each meal or feed. For dose adjustments based on individual requirements—consult product literature

  ▸ Child 2–17 years (body surface area up to 1.3 m^2): Initially 9.4 g/m^2 daily in divided doses, usual maintenance 5.3–12.4 g/m^2 daily in divided doses, each dose should be rounded up to the nearest 0.5 mL and given with each meal. For dose adjustments based on individual requirements—consult product literature

  ▸ Child 2–17 years (body surface area 1.3 m^2 and above): Initially 8 g/m^2 daily in divided doses, usual maintenance 5.3–12.4 g/m^2 daily in divided doses, each dose should be rounded up to the nearest 0.5 mL and given with each meal. For dose adjustments based on individual requirements—consult product literature

  DOSE EQUIVALENCE AND CONVERSION

  ▶ 1 mL of liquid contains 1.1 g of glycerol phenylbutyrate.

  ▶ For patients switching from sodium phenylbutyrate or sodium benzoate—consult product literature.

> **IMPORTANT SAFETY INFORMATION**
>
> **EMERGENCY MANAGEMENT OF UREA CYCLE DISORDERS**
>
> For further information on the emergency management of urea cycle disorders consult the British Inherited Metabolic Disease Group (BIMDG) website at www.bimdg.org.uk.

- **CONTRA-INDICATIONS** Treatment of acute hyperammonaemia
- **CAUTIONS** Intestinal malabsorption · pancreatic insufficiency
- **INTERACTIONS** → Appendix 1: glycerol phenylbutyrate
- **SIDE-EFFECTS**

  ▶ **Common or very common** Appetite abnormal · constipation · diarrhoea · dizziness · fatigue · food aversion · gastrointestinal discomfort · gastrointestinal disorders · headache · menstrual cycle irregularities · nausea · oral disorders · peripheral oedema · skin reactions · tremor · vomiting

  ▶ **Uncommon** Akathisia · alopecia · biliary colic · bladder pain · burping · confusion · depressed mood · drowsiness · dry mouth · dysphonia · epistaxis · fever · gastrointestinal infection viral · hot flush · hyperhidrosis · hypoalbuminaemia · hypokalaemia · hypothyroidism · joint swelling · muscle spasms · nasal congestion · oropharyngeal pain · pain · paraesthesia · plantar fasciitis · speech disorder · taste altered · throat irritation · ventricular arrhythmia · weight changes

  ▶ **Frequency not known** Anaemia · nail ridging · thrombocytosis
- **PREGNANCY** Manufacturer advises avoid unless essential—toxicity in *animal* studies.
- **BREAST FEEDING** Manufacturer advises avoid—no information available.
- **HEPATIC IMPAIRMENT** Manufacturer advises caution (risk of increased exposure).

  Dose adjustments Manufacturer advises use lowest possible dose—consult product literature.
- **RENAL IMPAIRMENT** Manufacturer advises use with caution in severe impairment—no information available.
- **DIRECTIONS FOR ADMINISTRATION** Manufacturer advises may be added to a small amount of apple sauce, ketchup,

or squash puree and used within 2 hours. For administration advice via nasogastric or gastrostomy tube—consult product literature.

- **HANDLING AND STORAGE** Manufacturer advises discard contents of bottle 14 days after opening.
- **PATIENT AND CARER ADVICE**
Driving and skilled tasks Manufacturer advises patients and carers should be counselled on the effects on driving and performance of skilled tasks—increased risk of dizziness.
- **NATIONAL FUNDING/ACCESS DECISIONS**
For full details see funding body website

Scottish Medicines Consortium (SMC) decisions
- **Glycerol phenylbutyrate (*Ravicti*®) as adjunctive therapy for chronic management of adult and paediatric patients aged 2 months and older with urea cycle disorders who cannot be managed by dietary protein restriction and/or amino acid supplementation alone (August 2018)** SMC No. 1342/18 Recommended

All Wales Medicines Strategy Group (AWMSG) decisions
- **Glycerol phenylbutyrate (*Ravicti*®) as adjunctive therapy for chronic management of patients with urea cycle disorders who cannot be managed by dietary protein restriction and/or amino acid supplementation alone (December 2019)** AWMSG No. 2127 Recommended

- **MEDICINAL FORMS** There can be variation in the licensing of different medicines containing the same drug.

Gastroenteral or oral liquid
- **Ravicti** (Immedica Pharma AB)
Glycerol phenylbutyrate 1.1 gram per 1 ml Ravicti 1.1g/ml oral liquid | 25 ml [PoM] £161.00

Sodium phenylbutyrate 05-Oct-2021

- **INDICATIONS AND DOSE**

Acute hyperammonaemia due to urea cycle disorders (specialist use only)
- BY INTRAVENOUS INFUSION
  - Neonate: Initially 250 mg/kg, to be administered over 90 minutes, followed by 10 mg/kg/hour, adjusted according to response.
  - Child: Initially 250 mg/kg, to be administered over 90 minutes, followed by 10 mg/kg/hour, adjusted according to response

Maintenance treatment of hyperammonaemia due to urea cycle disorders (specialist use only)
- BY MOUTH
  - Neonate: Up to 250 mg/kg daily in 3–4 divided doses, with feeds.
  - Child (body-weight up to 20 kg): Up to 250 mg/kg daily in 3–4 divided doses, with feeds or meals
  - Child (body-weight 20 kg and above): 5 g/m^2 daily in 3–4 divided doses, with meals; maximum 12 g per day

- **UNLICENSED USE**
  - With intravenous use Injection not licensed for use in children.

IMPORTANT SAFETY INFORMATION

EMERGENCY MANAGEMENT OF UREA CYCLE DISORDERS

For further information on the emergency management of urea cycle disorders consult the British Inherited Metabolic Disease Group (BIMDG) website at www.bimdg.org.uk.

- **CAUTIONS** Conditions involving sodium retention with oedema (preparations contain significant amounts of sodium) · congestive heart failure (preparations contain significant amounts of sodium)
- **INTERACTIONS** → Appendix 1: sodium phenylbutyrate
- **SIDE-EFFECTS**
  - **Common or very common** Abdominal pain · anaemia · appetite decreased · constipation · depression · headache · irritability · leucocytosis · leucopenia · menstrual cycle irregularities · metabolic acidosis · metabolic alkalosis · nausea · oedema · renal tubular acidosis · skin reactions · syncope · taste altered · thrombocytopenia · thrombocytosis · vomiting · weight increased
  - **Uncommon** Anorectal haemorrhage · aplastic anaemia · arrhythmia · gastrointestinal disorders · pancreatitis
- **CONCEPTION AND CONTRACEPTION** Manufacturer advises adequate contraception during administration in women of child-bearing potential.
- **PREGNANCY** Avoid—toxicity in *animal* studies.
- **BREAST FEEDING** Manufacturer advises avoid—no information available.
- **HEPATIC IMPAIRMENT** Manufacturer advises caution.
- **RENAL IMPAIRMENT** Manufacturer advises use with caution (preparations contain significant amounts of sodium).
- **DIRECTIONS FOR ADMINISTRATION**
  - With oral use Expert sources advise oral dose may be mixed with fruit drinks, milk, or feeds. [EvGr] *Pheburane*® granules may be directly swallowed with a drink or sprinkled on a spoonful of food, during feeds or mealtimes. Granules must not be administered by nasogastric or gastrostomy tubes. ⟨M⟩
  - With intravenous use For *intravenous infusion*, expert sources advise dilute to a maximum concentration of 50 mg/mL with Glucose 10%.
- **PATIENT AND CARER ADVICE**
Medicines for Children leaflet: Sodium phenylbutyrate for urea cycle disorders www.medicinesforchildren.org.uk/medicines/sodium-phenylbutyrate-for-urea-cycle-disorders/

- **MEDICINAL FORMS** There can be variation in the licensing of different medicines containing the same drug. Forms available from special-order manufacturers include: oral capsule, oral suspension, oral solution, solution for infusion

Oral tablet
- **Ammonaps** (Immedica Pharma AB)
Sodium phenylbutyrate 500 mg Ammonaps 500mg tablets | 250 tablet [PoM] £493.00 DT = £493.00

Solution for infusion

ELECTROLYTES: May contain Sodium

Oral solution
- **Pheburane** (Eurocept International bv)
Sodium phenylbutyrate 350 mg per 1 ml Pheburane 350mg/ml oral solution | 100 ml [PoM] £190.12 (Hospital only) [SF]

Oral granules
- **Pheburane** (Eurocept International bv)
Sodium phenylbutyrate 483 mg per 1 gram Pheburane 483mg/g granules | 174 gram [PoM] £331.00

ENZYMES

Pegzilarginase 20-Mar-2026

- **DRUG ACTION** Pegzilarginase is an enzyme produced by recombinant DNA technology that is administered as enzyme replacement therapy for the treatment of arginase-1 deficiency (hyperargininaemia).

- **INDICATIONS AND DOSE**

Arginase-1 deficiency [hyperargininaemia] (under expert supervision)
- BY INTRAVENOUS INFUSION, OR BY SUBCUTANEOUS INJECTION
  - Child 2–17 years: Initially 0.1 mg/kg once weekly, dose should then be adjusted in steps of 0.05 mg/kg according to plasma-arginine concentrations—consult

product literature, doses exceeding 0.2 mg/kg once weekly have not been studied

IMPORTANT SAFETY INFORMATION

EMERGENCY MANAGEMENT OF UREA CYCLE DISORDERS

For further information on the emergency management of urea cycle disorders consult the British Inherited Metabolic Disease Group (BIMDG) website at www.bimdg.org.uk.

- **CAUTIONS** Hypersensitivity reactions

CAUTIONS, FURTHER INFORMATION

- With intravenous use EvGr Reactions, including facial swelling, rash, and flushing, have occurred usually with the first few doses; initial doses of pegzilarginase should be administered, under medical observation, by appropriately trained staff. These reactions may be managed by temporarily interrupting or reducing the rate of the infusion, and/or treatment with antihistamines and/or corticosteroids. Pre-medication with an antihistamine and/or corticosteroid should be considered on re-administration. (M)
- **SIDE-EFFECTS**
  - **Common or very common** Hypersensitivity
- **PREGNANCY** EvGr Avoid (toxicity in *animal* studies). (M)
- **BREAST FEEDING** EvGr Avoid (no information available). (M)
- **DIRECTIONS FOR ADMINISTRATION** For *intermittent intravenous infusion*, dilute requisite dose with Sodium Chloride 0.9% (up to a maximum concentration of 0.5 mg/mL) and give over at least 30 minutes.

  For *subcutaneous injection*, inject into the abdomen (except for area directly surrounding the navel), lateral part of the thigh, or side or back of the upper arm; if more than one injection is needed for a single dose, injection sites should be at least 3 cm apart. Rotate injection site and avoid skin that is scarred, red, inflamed, or swollen.

  After at least 8 weeks of treatment, *Loargys*® may be self-administered or administered by a carer if appropriate training in subcutaneous injection technique has been given.
- **PRESCRIBING AND DISPENSING INFORMATION** Pegzilarginase is a biological medicine. Biological medicines must be prescribed and dispensed by brand name, see *Biological medicines* and *Biosimilar medicines*, under Guidance on prescribing p. 1; record the brand name and batch number after each administration.
- **HANDLING AND STORAGE** Store in a refrigerator (2–8°C) and protect from light; may be stored at room temperature (below 25°C) for up to 2 hours—consult product literature for further information regarding storage after preparation.
- **PATIENT AND CARER ADVICE**
  - With subcutaneous use Patients and their carers should be advised to stop administration and seek immediate medical attention if early signs of severe hypersensitivity reactions occur—consider prescribing medication for treatment of a potential severe hypersensitivity reaction.

  Self-administration Patients or their carers should be given training in subcutaneous injection technique if appropriate. A patient guide on self-administration at home should be provided.

  Missed doses If a dose is missed, it should be administered as soon as possible; there should be a minimum of 4 days between doses.
- **NATIONAL FUNDING/ACCESS DECISIONS** For full details see funding body website

NICE decisions

- **Pegzilarginase for treating arginase-1 deficiency in people 2 years and over (March 2026)** NICE HST35 Recommended

- **MEDICINAL FORMS** There can be variation in the licensing of different medicines containing the same drug.

Solution for injection

- Loargys (Immedica Pharma AB) ▼

  Pegzilarginase 5 mg per 1 ml Loargys 2mg/0.4ml solution for injection vials | 1 vial PoM £4,690.00 (Hospital only)

3.19 Wilson's disease

ANTIDOTES AND CHELATORS › COPPER ABSORPTION INHIBITORS

Zinc acetate

23-Jul-2020

- **DRUG ACTION** Zinc prevents the absorption of copper in Wilson's disease.
- **INDICATIONS AND DOSE**

Wilson's disease (initiated under specialist supervision)

- BY MOUTH
  - Child 1–5 years: 25 mg twice daily
  - Child 6–15 years (body-weight up to 57 kg): 25 mg 3 times a day
  - Child 6–15 years (body-weight 57 kg and above): 50 mg 3 times a day
  - Child 16–17 years: 50 mg 3 times a day

DOSE EQUIVALENCE AND CONVERSION

- Doses expressed as elemental zinc.

PHARMACOKINETICS

- Symptomatic Wilson's disease patients should be treated initially with a chelating agent because zinc has a slow onset of action. When transferring from chelating treatment to zinc maintenance therapy, chelating treatment should be co-administered for 2–3 weeks until zinc produces its maximal effect.

- **CAUTIONS** Portal hypertension (risk of hepatic decompensation when switching from chelating agent)
- **INTERACTIONS** → Appendix 1: zinc
- **SIDE-EFFECTS**
  - **Common or very common** Epigastric discomfort (usually transient)
  - **Uncommon** Leucopenia · sideroblastic anaemia
  - **Frequency not known** Condition aggravated

  SIDE-EFFECTS, FURTHER INFORMATION Transient gastric irritation may be reduced if first dose is taken mid-morning or with a little protein.
- **PREGNANCY**

  Dose adjustments Usual dose 25 mg 3 times daily adjusted according to plasma-copper concentration and urinary copper excretion.
- **BREAST FEEDING** Manufacturer advises avoid; present in milk—may cause zinc-induced copper deficiency in infant.
- **MONITORING REQUIREMENTS** Monitor full blood count and serum cholesterol.
- **DIRECTIONS FOR ADMINISTRATION** Manufacturer advises capsules may be opened and the contents mixed with water.

- **MEDICINAL FORMS** There can be variation in the licensing of different medicines containing the same drug.

Oral capsule

CAUTIONARY AND ADVISORY LABELS 23

- Wilzin (Recordati Rare Diseases UK Ltd)

  Zinc (as Zinc acetate) 25 mg Wilzin 25mg capsules | 250 capsule PoM £132.00 DT = £132.00

  Zinc (as Zinc acetate) 50 mg Wilzin 50mg capsules | 250 capsule PoM £242.00 DT = £242.00

ANTIDOTES AND CHELATORS › COPPER CHELATORS

Penicillamine 22-Dec-2025

● **DRUG ACTION** Penicillamine aids the elimination of copper ions in Wilson's disease (hepatolenticular degeneration).

● **INDICATIONS AND DOSE**

Wilson's disease

▶ BY MOUTH

▸ Child 1 month–11 years: 20 mg/kg daily in 2–3 divided doses, to be taken 1 hour before food; maximum 2 g per day

▸ Child 12–17 years: Initially 20 mg/kg daily in 2–3 divided doses. maintenance 0.75–1 g daily, to be taken 1 hour before food; maximum 2 g per day

Cystinuria

▶ BY MOUTH

▸ Child: 20–30 mg/kg daily in 2–3 divided doses, lower doses may be used initially and increased gradually, doses to be adjusted to maintain 24-hour urinary cystine below 1 mmol/litre, maintain adequate fluid intake, to be taken 1 hour before food; maximum 3 g per day

IMPORTANT SAFETY INFORMATION

NHS ENGLAND NATIONAL PATIENT SAFETY ALERT: HARM FROM INCORRECT RECORDING OF A PENICILLIN ALLERGY AS A PENICILLAMINE ALLERGY (NOVEMBER 2025)

A review of national incident data has identified cases of penicillin allergy being recorded as penicillamine allergy in electronic prescribing systems by healthcare staff. The review identified one patient death as a result of an anaphylactic reaction to a penicillin-based antibiotic, which was inadvertently prescribed due to their penicillin allergy being documented as a penicillamine allergy on their GP record. All other relevant incidents were recorded as low or no harm due to healthcare staff identifying issues before it became clinically significant. To help resolve this issue and prevent reoccurrence, the following actions should be completed as soon as possible but no later than 20 November 2026:

- primary and secondary care organisations must form working groups to identify affected patients records, clinically review the accuracy of the allergy status, and update allergy records accordingly;
- in secondary care, allergy guidance and training must cover safe recording of allergy status in electronic prescribing systems and related digital healthcare systems, including checking and correcting allergy status on admission and discharge;
- in primary care, additional checks should be implemented when inputting allergy status into GP systems, particularly if this is completed by non-clinical staff;
- all organisations should work with digital system suppliers and user groups to develop technical mitigations and safety features (e.g. adding alerts and modifying search terms) to reduce the likelihood of inadvertent recording of the wrong allergy, and prioritise safe deployment of these upgrades once developed;
- the working group should strongly consider producing regular reports on allergy status until the issue is resolved.

● **CONTRA-INDICATIONS** Lupus erythematosus

● **CAUTIONS** Neurological involvement in Wilson's disease

● **INTERACTIONS** → Appendix 1: penicillamine

● **SIDE-EFFECTS**

▶ **Common or very common** Proteinuria · thrombocytopenia

▶ **Rare or very rare** Alopecia · breast enlargement (males and females) · connective tissue disorders · haematuria (discontinue immediately if cause unknown) · hypersensitivity · oral disorders · skin reactions

▶ **Frequency not known** Agranulocytosis · aplastic anaemia · appetite decreased · fever · glomerulonephritis · Goodpasture's syndrome · haemolytic anaemia · increased risk of infection · jaundice cholestatic · leucopenia · lupus-like syndrome · myasthenia gravis · nausea · nephrotic syndrome · neurological deterioration in Wilson's Disease · neutropenia · pancreatitis · pneumonitis · polymyositis · pulmonary haemorrhage · rash (consider dose reduction) · respiratory tract inflammation · Stevens-Johnson syndrome · taste loss (mineral supplements not recommended) · vomiting · yellow nail syndrome

● **ALLERGY AND CROSS-SENSITIVITY** Patients who are hypersensitive to penicillin may react rarely to penicillamine.

● **PREGNANCY** Fetal abnormalities reported rarely; avoid if possible.

● **BREAST FEEDING** Manufacturer advises avoid unless potential benefit outweighs risk—no information available.

● **RENAL IMPAIRMENT** EvGr Caution in mild impairment; avoid in moderate to severe impairment. ⟨M⟩

Dose adjustments EvGr Dose reduction may be required in mild impairment depending on indication (consult product literature). ⟨M⟩

● **MONITORING REQUIREMENTS**

▶ Consider withdrawal if platelet count falls below 120 000/mm^3 or white blood cells below 2500/mm^3 or if 3 successive falls within reference range (can restart at reduced dose when counts return to within reference range but permanent withdrawal necessary if recurrence of leucopenia or thrombocytopenia).

▶ Monitor urine for proteinuria.

▶ Monitor blood and platelet count regularly.

● **PATIENT AND CARER ADVICE** Counselling on the symptoms of blood disorders is advised. Warn patient and carers to tell doctor immediately if sore throat, fever, infection, non-specific illness, unexplained bleeding and bruising, purpura, mouth ulcers, or rashes develop.

● **MEDICINAL FORMS** There can be variation in the licensing of different medicines containing the same drug. Forms available from special-order manufacturers include: oral solution

Oral tablet

CAUTIONARY AND ADVISORY LABELS 6, 22

▸ **Penicillamine (Non-proprietary)**

Penicillamine 125 mg Penicillamine 125mg tablets | 56 tablet PoM £139.66 DT = £93.11

Penicillamine 250 mg Penicillamine 250mg tablets | 56 tablet PoM £173.00 DT = £140.00

Trientine 14-Jun-2023

● **DRUG ACTION** Trientine is a chelating agent that binds to copper, forming a complex that is readily excreted by the kidneys; it may also inhibit the absorption of copper from the gastro-intestinal tract.

● **INDICATIONS AND DOSE**

Wilson's disease in patients intolerant of penicillamine [using Tillomed generic capsules] (initiated by a specialist)

▶ BY MOUTH

▸ Child 5–17 years: Initially 20 mg/kg daily in 2–3 divided doses, each dose should be rounded to the nearest 250 mg; usual initial dose 500–1250 mg daily. Dose should then be adjusted according to response and serum-copper concentrations

DOSE EQUIVALENCE AND CONVERSION
- For Tillomed generic: each capsule contains trientine base equivalent to 250 mg trientine dihydrochloride; doses expressed as trientine dihydrochloride.
- Preparations are not interchangeable on a milligram-for-milligram basis due to differences in bioavailability.

CUFENCE®

Wilson's disease in patients intolerant of penicillamine (initiated by a specialist)
- BY MOUTH
- Child 5–17 years: Initially 400–1000 mg daily in 2–4 divided doses, dose should then be adjusted according to response and serum-copper concentrations

DOSE EQUIVALENCE AND CONVERSION
- For *Cufence*®: each capsule contains trientine dihydrochloride equivalent to 200 mg trientine base; doses expressed as trientine base.
- Preparations are not interchangeable on a milligram-for-milligram basis due to differences in bioavailability.

CUPRIOR®

Wilson's disease in patients intolerant of penicillamine (initiated by a specialist)
- BY MOUTH
- Child 5–17 years: Initially 225–600 mg daily in 2–4 divided doses, dose should then be adjusted according to response and serum-copper concentrations

DOSE EQUIVALENCE AND CONVERSION
- For *Cuprior*®: each tablet contains trientine tetrahydrochloride equivalent to 150 mg of trientine base; doses expressed as trientine base.
- Preparations are not interchangeable on a milligram-for-milligram basis due to differences in bioavailability.

- **INTERACTIONS** → Appendix 1: trientine
- **SIDE-EFFECTS**
- **Common or very common** Nausea
- **Uncommon** Anaemia · aplastic anaemia · dystonia · skin reactions · tremor
- **Frequency not known** Dysarthria · gastrointestinal disorders · lupus-like syndrome · muscle rigidity · nephritis lupus · neurological decompensation
- **PREGNANCY** EvGr Teratogenic in *animal* studies—use only if benefit outweighs risk. Monitor maternal and neonatal serum-copper concentrations. (M)
- **BREAST FEEDING** EvGr Specialist sources indicate caution—limited information available; effect on copper levels in milk conflicting and impact on infant unknown. (D)
- **DIRECTIONS FOR ADMINISTRATION**
CUPRIOR® Tablets can be divided into 2 equal halves.
- **PRESCRIBING AND DISPENSING INFORMATION** Trientine is **not** an alternative to penicillamine for rheumatoid arthritis or cystinuria. Penicillamine-induced systemic lupus erythematosus may not resolve on transfer to trientine.
- **NATIONAL FUNDING/ACCESS DECISIONS**
For full details see funding body website

Scottish Medicines Consortium (SMC) decisions
- **Trientine tetrahydrochloride (*Cuprior*®) for the treatment of Wilson's disease in adults, adolescents and children aged 5 years and older, intolerant to D-penicillamine therapy (November 2019)** SMC No. SMC2222 Recommended

- **MEDICINAL FORMS** There can be variation in the licensing of different medicines containing the same drug.

Oral tablet

CAUTIONARY AND ADVISORY LABELS 7, 23
- **Cuprior** (Orphalan UK Ltd)
Trientine (as Trientine tetrahydrochloride) 150 mg Cuprior 150mg tablets | 72 tablet PoM £2,725.00 (Hospital only)

Oral capsule

CAUTIONARY AND ADVISORY LABELS 7, 23, 25
- **Trientine (Non-proprietary)**
Trientine (as Trientine dihydrochloride) 200 mg Trientine 200mg capsules | 100 capsule PoM £2,998.46–£3,075.13
Trientine dihydrochloride 250 mg Metalite 250mg capsules | 100 capsule PoM ⊠
Trientine dihydrochloride 250mg capsules | 100 capsule PoM £1,498.00 (Hospital only)
- **Cufence** (Univar Solutions B.V.)
Trientine (as Trientine dihydrochloride) 100 mg Cufence 100mg capsules | 200 capsule PoM £3,075.13
Trientine (as Trientine dihydrochloride) 200 mg Cufence 200mg capsules | 100 capsule PoM £3,075.13

4 Mineral and trace elements deficiencies

4.1 Zinc deficiency

Zinc deficiency

22-Mar-2021

Overview

Zinc is an essential trace element, involved in a number of body enzyme systems, and is found in a variety of foods. Patients with malnutrition, inflammatory bowel disease, and malabsorption syndromes are at an increased risk of zinc deficiency.

Zinc supplements can be given for zinc deficiency or in zinc-losing conditions. Continuous zinc supplementation is generally safe, however higher doses should be limited to short-term use due to an increased risk of gastro-intestinal adverse effects, copper deficiency, reduced immunity, anaemia, and genitourinary complications with long-term use.

Zinc is used in the treatment of Wilson's disease, and in acrodermatitis enteropathica, a rare inherited disorder characterised by impaired zinc absorption.

Parenteral nutrition regimens usually include trace amounts of zinc, see also Intravenous nutrition p. 770. Further zinc can be added to intravenous feeding regimens if required.

ELECTROLYTES AND MINERALS › ZINC

Zinc sulfate

09-May-2025

- **INDICATIONS AND DOSE**

Zinc deficiency or supplementation in zinc-losing conditions
- BY MOUTH USING EFFERVESCENT TABLETS
- Neonate: 1 mg/kg daily, dose expressed as elemental zinc, to be dissolved in water and taken after food.
- Child (body-weight up to 10 kg): 22.5 mg daily, dose to be adjusted as necessary, to be dissolved in water and taken after food, dose expressed as elemental zinc
- Child (body-weight 10-30 kg): 22.5 mg 1–3 times a day, dose to be adjusted as necessary, to be dissolved in water and taken after food, dose expressed as elemental zinc

continued →

▸ Child (body-weight 31 kg and above): 45 mg 1–3 times a day, dose to be adjusted as necessary, to be dissolved in water and taken after food, dose expressed as elemental zinc

Acrodermatitis enteropathica

▶ BY MOUTH USING EFFERVESCENT TABLETS

▸ Neonate: 0.5–1 mg/kg twice daily, dose to be adjusted as necessary, total daily dose may alternatively be given in 3 divided doses, dose expressed as elemental zinc.

▸ Child: 0.5–1 mg/kg twice daily, dose to be adjusted as necessary, total daily dose may alternatively be given in 3 divided doses, dose expressed as elemental zinc

- **UNLICENSED USE** *Solvazinc*® is not licensed for use in acrodermatitis enteropathica.

IMPORTANT SAFETY INFORMATION

ZINC-INDUCED COPPER DEFICIENCY

Zinc inhibits the absorption of copper, thereby reducing copper levels and potentially causing copper deficiency. The risk of copper deficiency is greater with higher doses of zinc and with long-term treatment, particularly if zinc deficiency is no longer present. Signs of copper deficiency include neurological and haematological symptoms.

- **CONTRA-INDICATIONS** Copper deficiency
- **INTERACTIONS** → Appendix 1: zinc
- **SIDE-EFFECTS** Copper deficiency · diarrhoea · gastritis · gastrointestinal discomfort · nausea · vomiting
- **PREGNANCY** Crosses placenta; risk theoretically minimal, but no information available.
- **BREAST FEEDING** Present in milk; risk theoretically minimal, but no information available.
- **RENAL IMPAIRMENT** EvGr Use with caution (accumulation may occur in renal failure). (M)
- **DIRECTIONS FOR ADMINISTRATION** The RCPCH and NPPG recommend that, for part doses using *Solvazinc*® effervescent tablets, one 45 mg tablet should be dissolved in 8.5 mL of water to give a final concentration of approximately 5 mg/mL. Once the tablet has fully dispersed and fizzing has stopped, the required dose should be withdrawn using an oral syringe and any remaining solution discarded.
- **PRESCRIBING AND DISPENSING INFORMATION** Each *Solvazinc*® tablet contains zinc sulfate monohydrate 125 mg (45 mg elemental zinc).

Administration of 'part doses' using effervescent tablets The RCPCH and NPPG recommend that doses should be rounded to enable measurement, and clear instructions provided on the dispensing label and when counselling patients or their carer. Appropriate equipment for administration should also be provided, such as:

- a 20 mL oral syringe to measure the initial volume of water required for tablet dispersion;
- a reusable plastic medicine pot in which the tablet can be dispersed in water;
- another smaller oral syringe to measure and administer the required dose (a 1 mL syringe is required for dose volume less than 1 mL).

For further details, see the position statement from the RCPCH and NPPG, available at: nppg.org.uk/wp-content/uploads/2025/04/Position-Statement-CalciumPhosphate-and-PotassiumV3.pdf.

- **MEDICINAL FORMS** There can be variation in the licensing of different medicines containing the same drug.

Effervescent tablet

CAUTIONARY AND ADVISORY LABELS 13, 21

EXCIPIENTS: May contain Sorbitol

ELECTROLYTES: May contain Sodium

▸ **Solvazinc** (Galen Ltd)

Zinc sulfate monohydrate 125 mg Solvazinc 125mg effervescent tablets | 90 tablet P £17.72 DT = £17.72 SF

5 Nutrition (intravenous)

Intravenous nutrition

Overview

When adequate feeding through the alimentary tract is not possible, nutrients may be given by intravenous infusion. This may be in addition to oral or enteral tube feeding—**supplemental parenteral nutrition**, or may be the sole source of nutrition— **total parenteral nutrition** (TPN). Complete enteral starvation is undesirable and total parenteral nutrition is a last resort.

Indications for parenteral nutrition include prematurity; severe or prolonged disorders of the gastro-intestinal tract; preparation of undernourished patients for surgery, chemotherapy, or radiation therapy; major surgery, trauma, or burns; prolonged coma or inability to eat; and some patients with renal or hepatic failure. The composition of proprietary preparations used in children is given under Proprietary Infusion Fluids for Parenteral Feeding p. 771.

Parenteral nutrition requires the use of a solution containing amino acids, glucose, lipids, electrolytes, trace elements, and vitamins. This is now commonly provided by the pharmacy in the form of an amino-acid, glucose, electrolyte bag, and a separate lipid infusion or, in older children a single 'all-in-one' bag. If the patient is able to take small amounts by mouth, vitamins may be given orally.

The nutrition solution is infused through a central venous catheter inserted under full surgical precautions. Alternatively, infusion through a peripheral vein may be used for supplementary as well as total parenteral nutrition, depending on the availability of peripheral veins; factors prolonging cannula life and preventing thrombophlebitis include the use of soft polyurethane paediatric cannulas and use of nutritional solutions of low osmolality and neutral pH. Nutritional fluids should be given by a dedicated intravenous line; if not possible, compatibility with any drugs or fluids should be checked as precipitation of components may occur. Extravasation of parenteral nutrition solution can cause severe tissue damage and injury; the infusion site should be regularly monitored.

Before starting intravenous nutrition the patient should be clinically stable and renal function and acid-base status should be assessed. Appropriate biochemical tests should have been carried out beforehand and serious deficits corrected. Nutritional and electrolyte status must be monitored throughout treatment. The nutritional components of parenteral nutrition regimens are usually increased gradually over a number of days to prevent metabolic complications and to allow metabolic adaptation to the infused nutrients. The solutions are usually infused over 24 hours but this may be gradually reduced if long-term nutrition is required. Home parenteral nutrition is usually infused over 12 hours overnight.

Complications of long-term parenteral nutrition include gall bladder sludging, gall stones, cholestasis and abnormal liver function tests. For details of the prevention and management of parenteral nutrition complications, specialist literature should be consulted.

Proprietary Infusion Fluids for Parenteral Feeding

Preparation	Nitrogen g/litre	[1,2]Energy kJ/litre	Electrolytes					Other components/litre
			K^+	Mg^{2+}	Na^+	$Acet^-$	Cl^-	
Aminoplasmal 10% (B.Braun Medical Ltd) Net price (10-bottle pack) 500 ml = £230.00; Net price (6-bottle pack) 1 litre = £320.00	15.8	-	-	-	-	28.0	-	citrate 1-2 mmol
Aminoplasmal 15% (B.Braun Medical Ltd) Net price (10-bottle pack) 500 ml = £230.00; Net price (6-bottle pack) 1 litre = £324.00	24.0	-	-	-	5.3	-	-	
Clinimix N14G30E (Baxter Healthcare Ltd) Net price (dual compartment bag of amino acids with electrolytes 1000 mL and glucose 30% with calcium 1000 mL) 2 litre = £31.52	7.0	2520	30.0	2.5	35.0	70.0	40.0	Ca^{2+} 2.3 mmol, phosphate 15 mmol, anhydrous glucose 150 g
ClinOleic 20% (Baxter Healthcare Ltd) Net price 100 ml = £6.28; Net price 250 ml = £10.08; Net price 500 ml = £13.88	-	8360	-	-	-	-	-	purified olive and soya oil 200 g, glycerol 22.5 g, egg phospholipids 12 g
Intralipid 10% (Fresenius Kabi Ltd) Net price (10-bag pack) 100 ml = £48.50; Net price (12-bag pack) 500 ml = £127.20	-	4600	-	-	-	-	-	soya oil 100 g, glycerol 22 g, purified egg phospholipids 12 g, phosphate 15 mmol
Intralipid 20% (Fresenius Kabi Ltd) Net price (10-bag pack) 100 ml = £73.00; Net price (10-bag pack) 250 ml = £119.50; Net price (12-bag pack) 500 ml = £190.80	-	8400	-	-	-	-	-	soya oil 200 g, glycerol 22 g, purified egg phospholipids 12 g, phosphate 15 mmol
Kabiven (Fresenius Kabi Ltd) Net price (triple compartment bag of amino acids and electrolytes 450 mL, glucose 790 mL, lipid emulsion 300 mL; 4-bag pack) 1.54 litre = £207.48; Net price (triple compartment bag of amino acids and electrolytes 600 mL, glucose 1053 mL, lipid emulsion 400 mL; 4-bag pack) 2.053 litre = £270.20; Net price (triple compartment bag of amino acids and electrolytes 750 mL, glucose 1316 mL, lipid emulsion 500 mL; 3-bag pack) 2.566 litre = £211.47	5.3	3275	23.0	4.0	31.0	38.0	45.0	Ca^{2+} 2 mmol, phosphate 9.7 mmol, anhydrous glucose 97 g, soya oil 39 g
Kabiven peripheral (Fresenius Kabi Ltd) Net price (triple compartment bag of amino acids and electrolytes 300 mL, glucose 885 mL, lipid emulsion 255 mL; 4-bag pack) 1.44 litre = £144.80; Net price (triple compartment bag of amino acids and electrolytes 400 mL, glucose 1180 mL, lipid emulsion 340 mL; 4-bag pack) 1.92 litre = £207.48; Net price (triple compartment bag of amino acids and electrolytes 500 mL, glucose 1475 mL, lipid emulsion 425 mL; 3-bag pack) 2.4 litre = £196.65	3.75	2625	17.0	2.8	22.0	27.0	33.0	Ca^{2+} 1.4 mmol, phosphate 7.5 mmol, anhydrous glucose 67.5 g, soya oil 35.4 g
Lipidem (B.Braun Medical Ltd) Net price 500 ml: no price available; Net price (6-bottle pack) 1 litre = £500.00	-	7900	-	-	-	-	-	omega-3-acid triglycerides 20 g, soya oil 80 g, medium chain triglycerides 100 g

1 1000 kcal = 4200kJ; 1000 kJ = 238.8 kcal. All entries are Prescription-only medicines.

2 Excludes protein- or amino acid-derived energy

Preparation	Nitrogen g/litre	[1,2]Energy kJ/litre	Electrolytes K^{+}	Mg^{2+}	Na^{+}	Acet^{-}	Cl^{-}	Other components/litre
Lipoflex peri (B.Braun Medical Ltd) Net price (triple compartment bag of amino acids 500 mL, glucose 500 mL, lipid emulsion 250 mL) 1.25 litre: no price available; Net price (triple compartment bag of amino acids 750 mL, glucose 750 mL, lipid emulsion 375 mL) 1.875 litre: no price available; Net price (triple compartment bag of amino acids 1000 mL, glucose 1000 mL, lipid emulsion 500 mL) 2.5 litre: no price available	4.6	2665	24.0	2.4	40.0	32.0	38.0	Ca^{2+} 2.4 mmol, Zn^{2+} 24 micromol, phosphate 6 mmol, anhydrous glucose 64 g, soya oil 20 g, medium-chain triglycerides 20 g
Lipoflex plus (B.Braun Medical Ltd) Net price (triple compartment bag of amino acids 500 mL, glucose 500 mL, lipid emulsion 250 mL) 1.25 litre: no price available; Net price (triple compartment bag of amino acids 750 mL, glucose 750 mL, lipid emulsion 375 mL) 1.875 litre: no price available; Net price (triple compartment bag of amino acids 1000 mL, glucose 1000 mL, lipid emulsion 500 mL) 2.5 litre: no price available	5.4	3600	28.0	3.2	40.0	36.0	36.0	Ca^{2+} 3.2 mmol, Zn^{2+} 24 micromol, phosphate 12 mmol, anhydrous glucose 120 g, soya oil 20 g, medium-chain triglycerides 20 g
Lipoflex special (B.Braun Medical Ltd) Net price (triple compartment bag of amino acids 500 mL, glucose 500 mL, lipid emulsion 250 mL) 1.25 litre: no price available; Net price (triple compartment bag of amino acids 750 mL, glucose 750 mL, lipid emulsion 375 mL) 1.875 litre: no price available	8.0	4005	37.6	4.2	53.6	48.0	48.0	Ca^{2+} 4.2 mmol, Zn^{2+} 30 micromol, phosphate 16 mmol, anhydrous glucose 144 g, soya oil 20 g, medium-chain triglycerides 20 g
Lipoflex special without electrolytes (B.Braun Medical Ltd) Net price (triple compartment bag of amino acids 750 mL, glucose 750 mL, lipid emulsion 375 mL) 1.875 litre: no price available	8.0	4005	-	-	-	-	-	anhydrous glucose 144 g, soya oil 20 g, medium-chain triglycerides 20 g
Lipofundin MCT/LCT 20% (B.Braun Medical Ltd) Net price 500 ml: no price available	-	8095	-	-	-	-	-	soya oil 100 g, medium-chain triglycerides 100 g
Nutriflex basal (B.Braun Medical Ltd) Net price (dual compartment bag of amino acids 800 mL, glucose 1200 mL) 2 litre: no price available	4.6	2093	30.0	5.7	49.9	35.0	50.0	Ca^{2+} 3.6 mmol, phosphate 12.8 mmol, anhydrous glucose 125 g
Nutriflex peri (B.Braun Medical Ltd) Net price (dual compartment bag of amino acids 800 mL, glucose 1200 mL) 2 litre: no price available	5.7	1340	15.0	4.0	27.0	19.5	31.6	Ca^{2+} 2.5 mmol, phosphate 5.7 mmol, anhydrous glucose 80 g
Nutriflex plus (B.Braun Medical Ltd) Net price (dual compartment bag of amino acids 800 mL, glucose 1200 mL) 2 litre: no price available	6.8	2512	25.0	5.7	37.2	22.9	35.5	Ca^{2+} 3.6 mmol, phosphate 20 mmol, anhydrous glucose 150 g
Nutriflex special (B.Braun Medical Ltd) Net price (dual compartment bag of amino acids 750 mL, glucose 750 mL) 1.5 litre: no price available	10.0	4019	25.7	5.0	40.5	22.0	49.5	Ca^{2+} 4.1 mmol, phosphate 14.7 mmol, anhydrous glucose 240 g

1 1000 kcal = 4200kJ; 1000 kJ = 238.8 kcal. All entries are Prescription-only medicines.
2 Excludes protein- or amino acid-derived energy

Preparation	Nitrogen g/litre	[1,2]Energy kJ/litre	Electrolytes K$^+$	Mg^{2+}	Na$^+$	Acet$^-$	Cl$^-$	Other components/litre
Omeflex peri (B.Braun Medical Ltd) Net price (triple compartment bag of amino acids 500 mL, glucose 500 mL, lipid emulsion 250 mL) 1.25 litre: no price available; Net price (triple compartment bag of amino acids 750 mL, glucose 750 mL, lipid emulsion 375 mL) 1.875 litre: no price available; Net price (triple compartment bag of amino acids 1000 mL, glucose 1000 mL, lipid emulsion 500 mL) 2.5 litre: no price available	4.6	2665	24.0	2.4	40.0	32.0	38.0	Ca^{2+} 2.4 mmol, Zn^{2+} 24 micromol, phosphate 6 mmol, anhydrous glucose 64 g, soya oil 16 g, medium-chain triglycerides 20 g, omega-3-acid triglycerides 4 g
Omeflex plus (B.Braun Medical Ltd) Net price (triple compartment bag of amino acids 500 mL, glucose 500 mL, lipid emulsion 250 mL) 1.25 litre: no price available; Net price (triple compartment bag of amino acids 750 mL, glucose 750 mL, lipid emulsion 375 mL) 1.875 litre: no price available; Net price (triple compartment bag of amino acids 1000 mL, glucose 1000 mL, lipid emulsion 500 mL) 2.5 litre: no price available	5.4	3600	28.0	3.2	40.0	36.0	36.0	Ca^{2+} 3.2 mmol, Zn^{2+} 24 micromol, phosphate 12 mmol, anhydrous glucose 120 g, soya oil 16 g, medium-chain triglycerides 20 g, omega-3-acid triglycerides 4 g
Omeflex special (B.Braun Medical Ltd) Net price (triple compartment bag of amino acids 250 mL, glucose 250 mL, lipid emulsion 125 mL) 625 ml: no price available; Net price (triple compartment bag of amino acids 500 mL, glucose 500 mL, lipid emulsion 250 mL) 1.25 litre: no price available; Net price (triple compartment bag of amino acids 750 mL, glucose 750 mL, lipid emulsion 375 mL) 1.875 litre: no price available	8.0	4005	37.6	4.2	53.6	48.0	48.0	Ca^{2+} 4.2 mmol, Zn^{2+} 30 micromol, phosphate 16 mmol, anhydrous glucose 144 g, soya oil 16 g, medium-chain triglycerides 20 g, omega-3-acid triglycerides 4 g
Omeflex special without electrolytes (B.Braun Medical Ltd) Net price (triple compartment bag of amino acids 500 mL, glucose 500 mL, lipid emulsion 250 mL) 1.25 litre: no price available; Net price (triple compartment bag of amino acids 750 mL, glucose 750 mL, lipid emulsion 375 mL) 1.875 litre: no price available	8.0	4005	-	-	-	-	-	anhydrous glucose 144 g, soya oil 16 g, medium-chain triglycerides 20 g
Plasma-Lyte 148 (water) (Baxter Healthcare Ltd) Net price 500 ml = £1.46; Net price 1 litre = £1.83	-	-	5.0	1.5	140.0	27.0	98.0	gluconate 23 mmol
Plasma-Lyte 148 (dextrose 5%) (Baxter Healthcare Ltd) Net price 500 ml = £1.46; Net price 1 litre = £1.83	-	840	5.0	1.5	140.0	27.0	98.0	gluconate 23 mmol, glucose monohydrate 55 g
Primene 10% (Baxter Healthcare Ltd) Net price 100 ml = £5.78; Net price 250 ml = £7.92	15.0	-	-	-	-	-	19.0	

1 1000 kcal = 4200kJ; 1000 kJ = 238.8 kcal. All entries are Prescription-only medicines.
2 Excludes protein- or amino acid-derived energy

Preparation	Nitrogen g/litre	[1,2]Energy kJ/litre	Electrolytes K^+	Mg^{2+}	Na^+	$Acet^-$	Cl^-	Other components/litre
SmofKabiven (Fresenius Kabi Ltd) Net price (triple compartment bag of amino acids and electrolytes 250 mL, glucose 149 mL, lipid emulsion 94 mL; 6-bag pack) 493 ml = £348.00; Net price (triple compartment bag of amino acids and electrolytes 500 mL, glucose 298 mL, lipid emulsion 188 mL; 4-bag pack) 986 ml = £299.20; Net price (triple compartment bag of amino acids and electrolytes 750 mL, glucose 446 mL, lipid emulsion 281 mL; 4-bag pack) 1.477 litre = £301.40; Net price (triple compartment bag of amino acids and electrolytes 1000 mL, glucose 595 mL, lipid emulsion 375 mL; 4-bag pack) 1.97 litre = £318.72	8.0	3780	30.0	5.1	41.0	106.0	36.0	Ca^{2+} 2.5 mmol, phosphate 13 mmol, anhydrous glucose 127 g, fish oil 5.7 g, olive oil 9.5 g, soya oil 11.4 g, medium-chain triglycerides 11.4 g
SmofKabiven Electrolyte Free (Fresenius Kabi Ltd) Net price (triple compartment bag of amino acids 500 mL, glucose 298 mL, lipid emulsion 188 mL; 4-bag pack) 986 ml = £299.20; Net price (triple compartment bag of amino acids 750 mL, glucose 446 mL, lipid emulsion 281 mL; 4-bag pack) 1.477 litre = £301.40; Net price (triple compartment bag of amino acids 1000 mL, glucose 595 mL, lipid emulsion 375 mL; 4-bag pack) 1.97 litre = £318.72	8.0	3780	-	-	-	74.5	-	phosphate 2.8 mmol, anhydrous glucose 127 g, fish oil 5.7 g, olive oil 9.5 g, soya oil 11.4 g, medium-chain triglycerides 11.4 g
SmofKabiven extra Nitrogen (Fresenius Kabi Ltd) Net price (triple compartment bag of amino acids and electrolytes 662 mL, glucose 204 mL, lipid emulsion 146 mL; 4-bag pack) 1.012 litre = £300.00; Net price (triple compartment bag of amino acids and electrolytes 993 mL, glucose 306 mL, lipid emulsion 219 mL; 4-bag pack) 1.518 litre = £320.00; Net price (triple compartment bag of amino acids and electrolytes 1325 mL, glucose 408 mL, lipid emulsion 292 mL; 4-bag pack) 2.025 litre = £356.00	10.5	2633	30.5	5.1	40.8	125.0	35.6	Ca^{2+} 2.6 mmol, phosphate 12.7 mmol, anhydrous glucose 84.7 g, fish oil 4.3 g, olive oil 7.2 g, soya oil 8.7 g, medium-chain triglycerides 8.7 g
SmofKabiven extra Nitrogen Electrolyte free (Fresenius Kabi Ltd) Net price (triple compartment bag of amino acids 993 mL, glucose 306 mL, lipid emulsion 219 mL; 4-bag pack) 1.518 litre = £320.00; Net price (triple compartment bag of amino acids 1325 mL, glucose 408 mL, lipid emulsion 292 mL; 4-bag pack) 2.025 litre = £356.00	10.5	2633	-	-	-	96.0	-	phosphate 2.2 mmol, anhydrous glucose 84.7 g, fish oil 4.3 g, olive oil 7.2 g, soya oil 8.7 g, medium-chain triglycerides 8.7 g

1 1000 kcal = 4200kJ; 1000 kJ = 238.8 kcal. All entries are Prescription-only medicines.

2 Excludes protein- or amino acid-derived energy

Preparation	Nitrogen g/litre	1,2 Energy kJ/litre	Electrolytes					Other components/litre
			K^+	Mg^{2+}	Na^+	$Acet^-$	Cl^-	
SmofKabiven Low Osmo Peripheral (Fresenius Kabi Ltd) Net price (triple compartment bag of amino acids and electrolytes 350 mL, glucose 805 mL, lipid emulsion 245 mL; 4-bag pack) 1.4 litre = £232.00; Net price (triple compartment bag of amino acids and electrolytes 488 mL, glucose 1121 mL, lipid emulsion 341 mL; 4-bag pack) 1.95 litre = £244.00; Net price (triple compartment bag of amino acids and electrolytes 625 mL, glucose 1438 mL, lipid emulsion 438 mL; 3-bag pack) 2.5 litre = £204.00	4.0	2617	15.0	2.5	20.0	52.0	18.0	Ca^{2+} 1.3 mmol, phosphate 7.5 mmol, anhydrous glucose 68 g, fish oil 5.3 g, olive oil 8.8 g, soya oil 11 g, medium-chain triglycerides 11 g
SmofKabiven Peripheral (Fresenius Kabi Ltd) Net price (triple compartment bag of amino acids and electrolytes 600 mL, glucose 1036 mL, lipid emulsion 268 mL; 4-bag pack) 1.904 litre = £255.36	5.1	2520	19.0	3.2	25.0	66.0	22.0	Ca^{2+} 1.6 mmol, phosphate 8.2 mmol, anhydrous glucose 71 g, fish oil 4.2 g, olive oil 7 g, soya oil 8.5 g, medium-chain triglycerides 8.5 g
SMOFlipid (Fresenius Kabi Ltd) Net price (10-bottle pack) 100 ml = £87.50; Net price (10-bottle pack) 250 ml = £140.00; Net price (10-bottle pack) 500 ml = £205.00	-	8400	-	-	-	-	-	fish oil 30 g, olive oil 50 g, soya oil 60 g, medium-chain triglycerides 60 g
Synthamin 9 EF (electrolyte-free) (Baxter Healthcare Ltd) Net price 500 ml = £6.97; Net price 1 litre = £12.92	9.1	-	-	-	-	44.0	22.0	
Synthamin 14 EF (electrolyte-free) (Baxter Healthcare Ltd) Net price 500 ml = £9.87; Net price 1 litre = £17.51	14.0	-	-	-	-	68.0	34.0	
Synthamin 17 EF (electrolyte-free) (Baxter Healthcare Ltd) Net price 500 ml = £12.66; Net price 3 litre = £55.00	16.5	-	-	-	-	82.0	40.0	
Vamin 14 (electrolyte-free) (Fresenius Kabi Ltd) Net price (10-bottle pack) 500 ml = £111.50; Net price (6-bottle pack) 1 litre = £113.10	13.5	-	-	-	-	90.0	-	
Vamin 18 (electrolyte-free) (Fresenius Kabi Ltd) Net price (10-bottle pack) 500 ml = £141.00; Net price (6-bottle pack) 1 litre = £165.00	18.0	-	-	-	-	110.0	-	
Vaminolact (Fresenius Kabi Ltd) Net price (10-bottle pack) 100 ml: no price available; Net price (10-bottle pack) 500 ml: no price available	9.3	-	-	-	-	-	-	

1 1000 kcal = 4200kJ; 1000 kJ = 238.8 kcal. All entries are Prescription-only medicines.

2 Excludes protein- or amino acid-derived energy

Protein (nitrogen) is given as mixtures of essential and non-essential synthetic L-amino acids. Ideally, all essential amino acids should be included with a wide variety of non-essential ones to provide sufficient nitrogen together with electrolytes. Solutions vary in their composition of amino acids; they often contain an energy source (usually glucose) and electrolytes. Solutions for use in neonates and children under 1 year of age are based on the amino acid profile of umbilical cord blood (*Primene*®) or breast milk (*Vaminolact*®) and contain amino acids that are essential in this age group; these amino acids may not be present in sufficient quantities in preparations designed for older children and adults.

Energy requirements must be met if amino acids are to be utilised for tissue maintenance. An appropriate energy to protein ratio is essential and requirements will vary depending on the child's age and condition. A mixture of carbohydrate and fat energy sources (usually 30–50% as fat) gives better utilisation of amino acids than glucose alone.

Glucose p. 730 is the preferred source of carbohydrate, but frequent monitoring of blood glucose is required particularly during initiation and build-up of the regimen; insulin may be necessary. Glucose above a concentration of 12.5% must be infused through a central venous catheter to avoid thrombosis; the maximum concentration of glucose that should normally be infused in fluid restricted children is 20–25%.

In parenteral nutrition regimens, it is necessary to provide adequate **phosphate** in order to allow phosphorylation of glucose and to prevent hypophosphataemia. Neonates, particularly preterm neonates, and young children also require phosphorus and calcium to ensure adequate bone mineralisation. The compatibility and solubility of calcium and phosphorus salts is complex and unpredictable; precipitation is a risk and specialist pharmacy advice should be sought.

Fat (lipid) emulsions have the advantages of a high energy to fluid volume ratio, neutral pH, and iso-osmolarity with plasma, and provide essential fatty acids. Several days of adaptation may be required to attain maximal utilisation. Reactions include occasional febrile episodes (usually only with 20% emulsions) and rare anaphylactic responses. Interference with biochemical measurements such as those for blood gases and calcium may occur if samples are taken before fat has been cleared. Regular monitoring of plasma cholesterol and triglyceride is necessary to ensure clearance from the plasma, particularly in conditions where fat metabolism may be disturbed e.g. infection. Emulsions containing 20% or 30% fat should be used in neonates as they are cleared more efficiently. **Additives should not be mixed with fat emulsions unless compatibility is known.**

Electrolytes are usually provided as the chloride salts of potassium and sodium. Acetate salts can be used to reduce the amount of chloride infused; hyperchloraemic acidosis or hypochloraemic alkalosis can occur in preterm neonates or children with renal impairment.

Adminstration

Because of the complex requirements relating to parenteral nutrition full details relating to administration have been omitted. In all cases *specialist pharmacy advice, product literature and other specialist literature should be consulted.*

NUTRIENTS › PARENTERAL NUTRITION

Parenteral nutrition supplements

18-Aug-2025

- **INDICATIONS AND DOSE**

Supplement in intravenous nutrition

▶ BY INTRAVENOUS INFUSION, OR BY SLOW INTRAVENOUS INJECTION

▸ Child: (consult product literature)

DIPEPTIVEN 20G/100ML CONCENTRATE FOR SOLUTION FOR INFUSION BOTTLES

Amino acid supplement for hypercatabolic or hypermetabolic states

▶ BY INTRAVENOUS INFUSION

▸ Child: 300–400 mg/kg daily, dose not to exceed 20% of total amino acid intake

IMPORTANT SAFETY INFORMATION

MHRA/CHM ADVICE: PARENTERAL NUTRITION PRODUCTS: LIGHT PROTECTION REQUIRED TO REDUCE THE RISK OF SERIOUS ADVERSE EFFECTS IN PREMATURE NEONATES (SEPTEMBER 2019)

Containers and administration sets of parenteral nutrition products containing amino acids and/or lipids should be protected from light during administration to neonates and children under 2 years of age. Studies found that light exposure caused formation of peroxides and other degradation products that may lead to adverse effects when given to premature neonates (who are considered to be at high risk of oxidative stress); this advice was extended to all neonates and children aged under 2 years as a precautionary measure.

- **CAUTIONS**

PEDITRACE SOLUTION FOR INFUSION 10ML VIALS Reduced biliary excretion · reduced biliary excretion in cholestatic liver disease · reduced biliary excretion in markedly reduced urinary excretion (careful biochemical monitoring required) · total parenteral nutrition exceeding one month

CAUTIONS, FURTHER INFORMATION

▸ Total parenteral nutrition exceeding one month Measure serum manganese concentration and check liver function before commencing treatment and regularly during treatment—discontinue if manganese concentration raised or if cholestasis develops.

- **EFFECT ON LABORATORY TESTS** EvGr Biotin may interfere with laboratory tests that are based on biotin/streptavidin interaction, such as thyroid immunoassays, and the risk of interference increases with higher doses of biotin. Possible biotin interference should be considered when interpreting test results as these may be falsely high or low, leading to misdiagnosis or inappropriate management. If the patient is taking biotin-containing products, laboratory personnel should be informed before tests are ordered as alternative assays may be available. ⟨M⟩

- **DIRECTIONS FOR ADMINISTRATION** Because of the complex requirements relating to parenteral nutrition, full details relating to administration have been omitted. In all cases *specialist pharmacy advice, product literature, and other specialist literature should be consulted.* Compatibility with the infusion solution must be ascertained before adding supplementary preparations. **Additives should not be mixed with fat emulsions unless compatibility is known.**

ADDIPHOS® VIALS For addition to *Vamin*® solutions and glucose intravenous infusions.

ADDITRACE SOLUTION FOR INFUSION 10ML AMPOULES For addition to *Vamin*® solutions and glucose intravenous infusions.

CERNEVIT® POWDER FOR SOLUTION FOR INJECTION VIALS Dissolve in 5 mL water for injections or Glucose 5% or Sodium Chloride 0.9% for adding to infusion solutions.

DECAN CONCENTRATE FOR SOLUTION FOR INFUSION 40ML BOTTLES For addition to infusion solutions.

DIPEPTIVEN 20G/100ML CONCENTRATE FOR SOLUTION FOR INFUSION BOTTLES For addition to infusion solutions containing amino acids.

PEDITRACE SOLUTION FOR INFUSION 10ML VIALS For addition to *Vaminolact*®, *Vamin*® 14 *Electrolyte-Free* solutions, and glucose intravenous infusions.

SOLIVITO N POWDER FOR SOLUTION FOR INFUSION VIALS Dissolve in water for injections or glucose intravenous infusion for adding to glucose intravenous infusion or *Intralipid*®; dissolve in *Vitlipid N*® or *Intralipid*® for adding to *Intralipid*® only.

- **PRESCRIBING AND DISPENSING INFORMATION**

ADDIPHOS® VIALS *Addiphos*® sterile solution contains phosphate 40 mmol, K^+ 30 mmol, Na^+ 30 mmol/20 mL.

ADDITRACE SOLUTION FOR INFUSION 10ML AMPOULES For patients over 40 kg.

Additrace® solution contains traces of Fe^{3+}, Zn^{2+}, Mn^{2+}, Cu^{2+}, Cr^{3+}, Se^{4+}, Mo^{6+}, F^-, I^-.

CERNEVIT® POWDER FOR SOLUTION FOR INJECTION VIALS *Cernevit*® powder for reconstitution contains *dl*-alpha tocopherol 10.2 mg, ascorbic acid 125 mg, biotin 69 micrograms, colecalciferol 220 units, cyanocobalamin 6 micrograms, folic acid 414 micrograms, nicotinamide 46 mg, pantothenic acid (as dexpanthenol) 17.25 mg, pyridoxine hydrochloride 5.5 mg, retinol (as palmitate) 3500 units, riboflavin (as dihydrated sodium phosphate) 4.14 mg, thiamine (as cocarboxylase tetrahydrate) 3.51 mg.

For adults and children over 11 years.

DECAN CONCENTRATE FOR SOLUTION FOR INFUSION 40ML BOTTLES For patients over 40 kg.
Decan® solution contains trace elements Fe^{2+}, Zn^{2+}, Cu^{2+}, Mn^{2+}, F^-, Co^{2+}, I^-, Se^{4+}, Mo^{6+}, Cr^{3+}.

DIPEPTIVEN 20G/100ML CONCENTRATE FOR SOLUTION FOR INFUSION BOTTLES *Dipeptiven*® solution contains N(2)-L-alanyl-L-glutamine 200 mg/mL (providing L-alanine 82 mg, L-glutamine 134.6 mg).

PEDITRACE SOLUTION FOR INFUSION 10ML VIALS For use in neonates (when kidney function established, usually second day of life), infants, and children.
Peditrace® solution contains traces of Zn^{2+}, Cu^{2+}, Mn^{2+}, Se^{4+}, F^-, I^-.

SOLIVITO N POWDER FOR SOLUTION FOR INFUSION VIALS *Solivito N*® powder for reconstitution contains biotin 60 micrograms, cyanocobalamin 5 micrograms, folic acid 400 micrograms, glycine 300 mg, nicotinamide 40 mg, pyridoxine hydrochloride 4.9 mg, riboflavin sodium phosphate 4.9 mg, sodium ascorbate 113 mg, sodium pantothenate 16.5 mg, thiamine mononitrate 3.1 mg.

- **MEDICINAL FORMS** There can be variation in the licensing of different medicines containing the same drug. Forms available from special-order manufacturers include: solution for infusion

Solution for infusion

- **Parenteral nutrition supplements (Non-proprietary)**
  Sodium glycerophosphate (as Sodium glycerophosphate pentahydrate) 216 mg per 1 ml Sodium glycerophosphate 4.32g/20ml concentrate for solution for infusion ampoules | 20 ampoule PoM £175.80
- **Dipeptiven** (Fresenius Kabi Ltd)
  N(2)-L-alanyl-L-glutamine 200 mg per 1 ml Dipeptiven 20g/100ml concentrate for solution for infusion bottles | 10 bottle PoM £305.00
- **Peditrace** (Fresenius Kabi Ltd)
  Manganese (as Manganese chloride) 1 microgram per 1 ml, Iodine (as Potassium iodide) 1 microgram per 1 ml, Selenium (as Sodium selenite) 2 microgram per 1 ml, Copper (as Copper chloride) 20 microgram per 1 ml, Fluoride (as Sodium fluoride) 57 microgram per 1 ml, Zinc (as Zinc chloride) 250 microgram per 1 ml Peditrace solution for infusion 10ml vials | 10 vial PoM £35.50
- **Tracutil** (B.Braun Medical Ltd)
  Sodium molybdate dihydrate 2.42 microgram per 1 ml, Chromic chloride 5.3 microgram per 1 ml, Sodium selenite pentahydrate 7.89 microgram per 1 ml, Potassium iodide 16.6 microgram per 1 ml, Sodium fluoride 126 microgram per 1 ml, Manganese chloride 197.9 microgram per 1 ml, Copper chloride 204.6 microgram per 1 ml, Zinc chloride 681.5 microgram per 1 ml, Ferrous chloride 695.8 microgram per 1 ml Tracutil concentrate for solution for infusion 10ml ampoules | 5 ampoule PoM £9.50 (Hospital only)

Powder for solution for infusion

- **Solivito N** (Fresenius Kabi Ltd)
  Cyanocobalamin 5 microgram, Biotin 60 microgram, Folic acid 400 microgram, Thiamine nitrate 3.1 mg, Pyridoxine hydrochloride 4.9 mg, Riboflavin sodium phosphate 4.9 mg, Sodium pantothenate 16.5 mg, Nicotinamide 40 mg, Sodium ascorbate 113 mg Solivito N powder for concentrate for solution for infusion vials | 10 vial PoM £23.20

Powder for solution for injection

EXCIPIENTS: May contain Glycocholic acid

- **Cernevit** (Baxter Healthcare Ltd)
  Cyanocobalamin 6 microgram, Biotin 69 microgram, Folic acid 414 microgram, Thiamine 3.51 mg, Riboflavin (as Riboflavin sodium phosphate) 4.14 mg, Pyridoxine (as Pyridoxine hydrochloride) 4.53 mg, Pantothenic acid (as Dexpanthenol) 17.25 mg, Nicotinamide 46 mg, Ascorbic acid 125 mg, Alpha tocopherol 11.2 unit, Colecalciferol 220 unit, Retinol 3500 unit Cernevit powder for solution for injection vials | 10 vial PoM £50.50

6 Nutrition (oral)

Enteral nutrition

Overview

Children have higher nutrient requirements per kg bodyweight, different metabolic rates, and physiological responses compared to adults. They have low nutritional stores and are particularly vulnerable to growth and nutritional problems during critical periods of development. Major illness, operations, or trauma impose increased metabolic demands and can rapidly exhaust nutritional reserves.

Every effort should be made to optimise oral food intake before beginning enteral tube feeding; this may include change of posture, special seating, feeding equipment, oral desensitisation, food texture changes, thickening of liquids, increasing energy density of food, treatment of reflux or oesophagitis, as well as using age-specific nutritional supplements.

Enteral tube feeding has a role in both short-term rehabilitation and long-term nutritional management in paediatrics. It can be used as supportive therapy, in which the enteral feed supplies a proportion of the required nutrients, or as primary therapy, in which the enteral feed delivers all the necessary nutrients. Most children receiving tube feeds should also be encouraged to take oral food and drink. Tube feeding should be considered in the following situations:

- unsafe swallowing and risk of aspiration
- inability to consume at least 60% of energy needs by mouth
- total feeding time of more than 4 hours per day
- weight loss or no weight gain for a period of 3 months (less for younger children and infants)
- weight for height (or length) less than 2nd percentile for age and sex

Most feeds for enteral use contain protein derived from cows' milk or soya. Elemental feeds containing protein hydrolysates or free amino acids can be used for children who have diminished ability to break down protein, for example in inflammatory bowel disease or pancreatic insufficiency.

Even when nutritionally complete feeds are given, water and electrolyte balance should be monitored. Haematological and biochemical parameters should also be monitored, particularly in the clinically unstable child. Extra minerals (e.g. magnesium and zinc) may be needed in patients where gastro-intestinal secretions are being lost. Additional vitamins may also be needed.

Choosing the best formula for children depends on several factors including: nutritional requirements, gastro-intestinal function, underlying disease, nutrient restrictions, age, and feed characteristics (nutritional composition, viscosity, osmolality, availability and cost). Children have specific dietary requirements and in many situations liquid feeds prepared for adults are totally unsuitable and should not be given. Expert advice from a dietician should be sought before prescribing enteral feeds for a child.

Infant formula feeds

Child 0–12 months. Term infants with normal gastro-intestinal function are given either breast milk or normal infant formula during the first year of life. The average intake is between 150 mL and 200 mL/kg/day. Infant milk formulas are based on whey- or casein-dominant protein, lactose with or without maltodextrin, amylose, vegetable oil and milk fat. The composition of all normal and soya infant formulas have to meet The Infant Formula and Follow-on Formula Regulations (England and Wales) 2007, which enact the European Community Regulations 2006/141/EC; the composition of other enteral and specialist feeds has to meet the Commission Directive (1999/21/EC) on Dietary Foods for Special Medical Purposes.

A high-energy feed, which contains 9–11% of energy derived from protein can be used for infants who fail to grow adequately. Alternatively, energy supplements may be added to normal infant formula to achieve a higher energy content (but this will reduce the protein to energy ratio) or the normal infant formula concentration may be increased slightly. Care should be taken not to present an osmotic load of more than 500 milliosmols/kg water to the normal functioning gut, otherwise osmotic diarrhoea will result. Concentrating or supplementing feeds should not be attempted without the advice of a paediatric dietician.

Enteral feeds

Child 1–6 years (body-weight 8–20 kg). Ready-to-use feeds based on caseinates, maltodextrin and vegetable oils (with or without added medium chain triglyceride (MCT) oil or fibre) are well tolerated and effective in improving nutritional status in this age group. Although originally designed for children 1–6 years (body-weight 8–20 kg), some products have ACBS approval for use in children weighing up to 30 kg (approx. 10 years of age). Enteral feeds formulated for children 1–6 years are low in sodium and potassium; electrolyte intake and biochemical status should be monitored. Older children in this age range taking small feed volumes may need to be given additional micronutrients. Fibre-enriched feeds may be helpful for children with chronic constipation or diarrhoea.

Child 7–12 years (body-weight 21–45 kg). Depending on age, weight, clinical condition and nutritional requirements, ready-to-use feeds formulated for 7–12 year olds may be given at appropriate rates.

Child over 12 years (body-weight over 45 kg). As there are no standard enteral feeds formulated for this age group, adult formulations are used. The intake of protein, electrolytes, vitamins, and trace minerals should be carefully assessed and monitored. Note: Adult feeds containing more than 6 g/100 mL protein or 2 g/100 mL fibre should be used with caution and expert advice.

Specialised formula

It is essential that any infant who is intolerant of breast milk or normal infant formula, or whose condition requires nutrient-specific adaptation, is prescribed an adequate volume of a nutritionally complete replacement formula. In the first 4 months of life, a volume of 150–200 mL/kg/day is recommended. After 6 months, should the formula still be required, a volume of 600 mL/day should be maintained, in addition to solid food.

Products for cow's milk protein intolerance or lactose intolerance. There are a number of infant formulas formulated for cow's milk protein intolerance or lactose intolerance; these feeds may contain a residual amount of lactose (less than 1 g/100 mL formula)—sometimes described as clinically lactose-free or 'lactose-free' by manufacturers. If the total daily intake of these formulas is low, it may be necessary to supplement with calcium, and a vitamin and mineral supplement.

Soya-based infant formulas have a high phytoestrogen content and this may be a long-term reproductive health risk. The Chief Medical Officer has advised that soya-based infant formulas should not be used as the first choice for the management of infants with proven cow's milk sensitivity, lactose intolerance, galactokinase deficiency and galactosaemia. Most UK paediatricians with expertise in inherited metabolic disease still advocate soya-based formulations for infants with galactosaemia as there are concerns about the residual lactose content of low lactose formulas and protein hydrolysates based on cow's milk protein.

Low lactose infant formulations, based on whole cow's milk protein, are unsuitable for children with cow's milk protein intolerance. Liquid soya milks purchased from supermarkets and health food stores are not nutritionally complete and should never be used for infants under 1 year of age.

Protein hydrolysate formulas. Non-milk, peptide-based feeds containing hydrolysates of casein, whey, meat and soya protein, are suitable for infants with disaccharide or whole protein intolerance. The total daily intake of electrolytes, vitamins and minerals should be carefully assessed and modified to meet the child's nutritional requirements; these feeds have a high osmolality when given at recommended dilution and need gradual and careful introduction.

Elemental (amino acid based formula). Specially formulated elemental feeds containing essential and nonessential amino acids are available for use in infants and children under 6 years with proven whole protein intolerance. Adult elemental formula may be used for children over 6 years; the intake of electrolytes, vitamins and minerals should be carefully assessed and modified to meet nutritional requirements. These feeds have a high osmolality when given at the recommended concentration and therefore need gradual and careful introduction.

Modular feeds. Modular feeds (see Specialised Formulas for Specific Clinical Conditions) are based on individual protein, fat, carbohydrate, vitamin and mineral components or modules which can be combined to meet the specific needs of a child. Modular feeds are used when nutritionally complete specialised formula are not tolerated, or if the fluid and nutrient requirements change e.g. in gastro-intestinal, renal or liver disease. The main advantage of modular feeds is their flexibility; disadvantages include their complexity and preparation difficulties. Modular feeds should not be used without the supervision of a paediatric dietician.

Specialised formula. Highly specialised formulas are designed to meet the specific requirements in various clinical conditions such as renal and liver diseases. When using these formulas, both the biochemical status of the child and their growth parameters need to be monitored.

Feed thickeners

Carob based thickeners may be used to thicken feeds for infants under 1 year with significant gastro-oesophageal reflux. Breast-fed infants can be given the thickener mixed to a paste with water or breast-milk prior to feeds.

Pre-thickened formula Milk-protein- or casein-dominant infant formula, which contains small quantities of pre-gelatinized starch, is recommended primarily for infants with mild gastro-oesophageal reflux. Pre-thickened formula is prepared in the same way as normal infant formula and flows through a standard teat. The feeds do not thicken on standing but thicken in the stomach when exposed to acid pH.

Starched based thickeners can be used to thicken liquids and feeds for children over 1 year of age with dysphagia.

Dietary supplements for oral use

Three types of prescribable fortified dietary supplements are available: fortified milk and non-milk tasting (juice-style) drinks, and fortified milk-based semi-solid preparations. The recommended daily quantity is age-dependent. The following is a useful guide: 1–2 years, 200 kcal (840 kJ); 3–5 years, 400 kcal (1680 kJ); 6–11 years, 600 kcal (2520 kJ); and over 12 years, 800 kcal (3360 kJ). Supplements containing 1.5 kcal/mL are high in protein and should not be used for children under 3 years of age. Many supplements are high in sugar or maltodextrin; care should be taken to prevent prolonged contact with teeth. Ideally supplements should be administered after meals or at bedtime so as not to affect appetite.

Products for metabolic diseases

There is a large range of disease-specific infant formulas and amino acid-based supplements available for use in children with metabolic diseases (see under specific metabolic diseases). Some of these formulas are nutritionally incomplete and supplementation with vitamins and other nutrients may be necessary. Many of the product names are similar; to prevent metabolic complications in children who cannot tolerate specific amino acids it is important to ensure the correct supplement is supplied.

Enteral feeding tubes

Care is required in choosing an appropriate formulation of a drug for administration through a nasogastric narrow-bore feeding tube or through a percutaneous endoscopic gastrostomy (PEG) or jejunostomy tube. Liquid preparations (or soluble tablets) are preferred; injection solutions may also be suitable for administration through an enteral tube.

If a solid formulation of a medicine needs to be given, it should be given as a suspension of particles fine enough to pass through the tube. It is possible to crush many immediate-release tablets but enteric-coated or modified-release preparations should **not** be crushed.

Enteral feeds may affect the absorption of drugs and it is therefore important to consider the timing of drug administration in relation to feeds. If more than one drug needs to be given, they should be given separately and the tube should be flushed with water after each drug has been given.

Clearing blockages

Carbonated (sugar-free) drinks may be marginally more effective than water in unblocking feeding tubes, but mildly acidic liquids (such as pineapple juice or cola-based drinks) can coagulate protein in feeds, causing further blockage. If these measures fail to clear the enteral feeding tube, an alkaline solution containing pancreatic enzymes may be introduced into the tube (followed after at least 5 minutes by water). Specific products designed to break up blockages caused by formula feeds are also available.

6.1 Special diets

Nutrition in special diets 06-Apr-2021

Overview

In certain clinical conditions, some food preparations are regarded as drugs and can be prescribed within the NHS if they have been approved by the Advisory Committee on Borderline Substances (ACBS). There is also a large range of disease-specific infant formulas and amino acid-based supplements available for use in children with metabolic diseases (see *Borderline Substances*).

Coeliac disease

Coeliac disease is caused by an abnormal immune response to gluten. For further information, see Coeliac disease p. 29.

Phenylketonuria

Phenylketonuria results from the inability to metabolise phenylalanine. EvGr The treatment of phenylketonuria usually involves restricting dietary intake of phenylalanine to a small amount sufficient for tissue building and repair, in addition to phenylalanine-free L-amino acid supplementation.

A subset of children with phenylketonuria may be responsive to sapropterin dihydrochloride below (A), a synthetic form of tetrahydrobiopterin. It is licensed as an adjunct to dietary restriction of phenylalanine in the management of children with phenylketonuria and tetrahydrobiopterin deficiency.

Aspartame (used as a sweetener in some foods and medicines) contributes to phenylalanine intake and may affect control of phenylketonuria. EvGr If aspartame-free alternatives are unavailable, children with phenylketonuria should not be denied access to appropriate medication. (A) Where the presence of aspartame in a preparation is specified in the product literature, it is listed as an excipient against the preparation in individual drug monographs. The child or carer should be informed the preparation contains aspartame.

6.1a Phenylketonuria

DRUGS FOR METABOLIC DISORDERS ›
TETRAHYDROBIOPTERIN AND DERIVATIVES

Sapropterin dihydrochloride 18-Oct-2021

- **DRUG ACTION** Sapropterin is synthetic 6R-tetrahydrobiopterin (6R-BH4), a cofactor for phenylalanine hydroxylase, and therefore restores the activity of phenylalanine hydroxylase and reduces phenylalanine concentration in the blood.

- **INDICATIONS AND DOSE**

Phenylketonuria (adjunct to dietary restriction of phenylalanine) (specialist use only)

▶ BY MOUTH

▶ Neonate: Initially 10 mg/kg once daily, adjusted according to response; usual dose 5–20 mg/kg once daily, dose to be taken preferably in the morning.

▶ Child: Initially 10 mg/kg once daily, adjusted according to response; usual dose 5–20 mg/kg once daily, dose to be taken preferably in the morning

Tetrahydrobiopterin deficiency (adjunct to dietary restriction of phenylalanine) (specialist use only)

▶ BY MOUTH

▶ Neonate: Initially 2–5 mg/kg daily in 2–3 divided doses, adjusted according to response; maximum 20 mg/kg per day.

▶ Child: Initially 2–5 mg/kg daily in 2–3 divided doses, adjusted according to response; maximum 20 mg/kg per day

- **CAUTIONS** History of convulsions
- **INTERACTIONS** → Appendix 1: sapropterin
- **SIDE-EFFECTS**

▶ **Common or very common** Cough · diarrhoea · gastrointestinal discomfort · headache · laryngeal pain · nasal complaints · nausea · vomiting

▶ **Frequency not known** Gastrointestinal disorders · rash

- **PREGNANCY** Manufacturer advises caution—consider only if strict dietary management inadequate.
- **BREAST FEEDING** Manufacturer advises avoid—no information available.
- **HEPATIC IMPAIRMENT** Manufacturer advises caution (no information available).
- **RENAL IMPAIRMENT** Manufacturer advises caution—no information available.
- **MONITORING REQUIREMENTS**

▶ Monitor blood-phenylalanine concentration before and after first week of treatment—if unsatisfactory response increase dose at weekly intervals to max. dose and monitor blood-phenylalanine concentration weekly; discontinue treatment if unsatisfactory response after 1 month.

▶ Monitor blood-phenylalanine and tyrosine concentrations 1–2 weeks after dose adjustment and during treatment.

- **DIRECTIONS FOR ADMINISTRATION** Manufacturer advises tablets should be dissolved in water and taken within 20 minutes.
- **PATIENT AND CARER ADVICE** Patient or carers should be given advice on how to administer sapropterin dihydrochloride dispersible tablets.
- **NATIONAL FUNDING/ACCESS DECISIONS** For full details see funding body website

NICE decisions

- ▶ **Sapropterin for treating hyperphenylalaninaemia in phenylketonuria (September 2021)** NICE TA729 Recommended with restrictions

Scottish Medicines Consortium (SMC) decisions

- ▶ **Sapropterin (*Kuvan*®) for the treatment of hyperphenylalaninaemia (HPA) in adults and paediatric patients of all ages with phenylketonuria (PKU) who have been shown to be responsive to such treatment (August 2018)** SMC No. 558/09 Not recommended

- **MEDICINAL FORMS** There can be variation in the licensing of different medicines containing the same drug.

Soluble tablet

CAUTIONARY AND ADVISORY LABELS 13, 21

▶ **Sapropterin dihydrochloride (Non-proprietary)**

Sapropterin dihydrochloride 100 mg Sapropterin 100mg soluble tablets sugar free | 30 tablet PoM £537.50 (Hospital only) SF | 120 tablet PoM £2,150.00 (Hospital only) SF

7 Vitamin deficiency

Vitamins

09-Dec-2025

Overview

Vitamins are used for the prevention and treatment of specific deficiency states or where the diet is known to be inadequate; they may be prescribed in the NHS to prevent or treat deficiency but not as dietary supplements. Except for iron-deficiency anaemia, a primary vitamin or mineral deficiency due to simple dietary inadequacy is rare in the developed world. Some children may be at risk of developing deficiencies because of an inadequate intake, impaired vitamin synthesis or malabsorption in disease states such as cystic fibrosis and Crohn's disease.

The use of vitamins as general 'pick-me-ups' is of unproven value and, the 'fad' for mega-vitamin therapy with water-soluble vitamins, such as ascorbic acid p. 786 and pyridoxine hydrochloride p. 784, is unscientific and can be harmful. Many vitamin supplements are described as 'multivitamin' but few contain the whole range of essential vitamins and many contain relatively high amounts of vitamins A and D. Care should be taken to ensure the correct dose is not exceeded.

Dietary reference values for vitamins are available in the Department of Health publication:

Dietary Reference Values for Food Energy and Nutrients for the United Kingdom: Report of the Panel on Dietary Reference Values of the Committee on Medical Aspects of Food Policy. *Report on Health and Social Subjects* 41. London: HMSO, 1991.

Dental patients

It is unjustifiable to treat stomatitis or glossitis with mixtures of vitamin preparations; this delays diagnosis and correct treatment.

Most patients who develop a nutritional deficiency despite an adequate intake of vitamins have malabsorption and if this is suspected the patient should be referred to a medical practitioner.

Vitamin A

Deficiency of vitamin A p. 783 (retinol) is associated with ocular defects (particularly xerophthalmia) and an increased susceptibility to infections, but deficiency is rare in the UK (even in disorders of fat absorption).

Vitamin A supplementation may be required in children with liver disease, particularly cholestatic liver disease, due to the malabsorption of fat soluble vitamins. In those with complete biliary obstruction an intramuscular dose once a month may be appropriate.

Preterm neonates have low plasma concentrations of vitamin A and are usually given vitamin A supplements, often as part of an oral multivitamin preparation once enteral feeding has been established.

Vitamin B group

Deficiency of the B vitamins, other than vitamin B_{12}, is rare in the UK and is usually treated by preparations containing thiamine p. 785 (B_1), and riboflavin (B_2). Other members (or substances traditionally classified as members) of the vitamin B complex such as aminobenzoic acid, biotin, choline, inositol nicotinate, and pantothenic acid or panthenol may be included in vitamin B preparations, but there is no evidence of their value as supplements; however, they can be used in the management of certain metabolic disorders. Anaphylaxis has been reported with parenteral B vitamins.

As with other vitamins of the B group, pyridoxine hydrochloride (B_6) deficiency is rare, but it may occur during isoniazid p. 453 therapy or penicillamine p. 768 treatment in Wilson's disease and is characterised by peripheral neuritis. High doses of pyridoxine hydrochloride are given in some metabolic disorders, such as hyperoxaluria, cystathioninuria and homocystinuria; folic acid p. 710 supplementation may also be beneficial in these disorders. Pyridoxine hydrochloride is also used in sideroblastic anaemia. Rarely, seizures in the neonatal period or during infancy respond to pyridoxine hydrochloride treatment; pyridoxine hydrochloride should be tried in all cases of early-onset intractable seizures and status epilepticus. Pyridoxine hydrochloride has been tried for a wide variety of other disorders, but there is little sound evidence to support the claims of efficacy.

A number of mitochondrial disorders may respond to treatment with certain B vitamins but these disorders require specialist management. Thiamine is used in the treatment of maple syrup urine disease, mitochondrial respiratory chain defects and, together with riboflavin, in the treatment of congenital lactic acidosis; riboflavin is also used in glutaric acidaemias and cytochrome oxidase deficiencies; biotin is used in carboxylase defects.

Folic acid and vitamin B_{12} are used in the treatment of megaloblastic anaemia. Folinic acid p. 683 (available as calcium folinate) is used in association with cytotoxic therapy.

Vitamin C

Vitamin C (ascorbic acid) therapy is essential in scurvy, but less florid manifestations of vitamin C deficiency have been reported. Vitamin C is used to enhance the excretion of iron one month after starting desferrioxamine mesilate p. 714 therapy; it is given separately from food as it also enhances iron absorption. Vitamin C is also used in the treatment of some inherited metabolic disorders, particularly mitochondrial disorders; specialist management of these conditions is required.

Severe scurvy causes gingival swelling and bleeding margins as well as petechiae on the skin. This is, however, exceedingly rare and a child with these signs is more likely to have leukaemia. Investigation should not be delayed by a trial period of vitamin treatment.

Claims that vitamin C ameliorates colds or promotes wound healing have not been proved.

Vitamin D

The term Vitamin D is used for a range of compounds including ergocalciferol p. 792 (calciferol, vitamin D_2), colecalciferol p. 788 (vitamin D_3), dihydrotachysterol, alfacalcidol p. 787 (1α-hydroxycholecalciferol), and calcitriol p. 788 (1,25-dihydroxycholecalciferol).

Asymptomatic vitamin D deficiency is common in the United Kingdom; symptomatic deficiency may occur in certain ethnic groups, particularly as rickets or hypocalcaemia, and rarely in association with malabsorption. Deficiency can occur in children whose exposure to sunlight is limited and in those whose diet is deficient in vitamin D. Specific populations at risk of deficiency may include children with dark skin (such as those of African, African-Caribbean and South Asian origin) as their skin is less efficient at synthesising vitamin D, children who have low or no exposure to the sun (such as those who are housebound or confined indoors, or who cover their skin for cultural reasons), pregnant and breastfeeding females, and all children aged under 4 years. EvGr Supplements containing vitamin D (e.g. *Healthy Start*) should be considered for all pregnant and breastfeeding females, and children aged under 4 years, to prevent vitamin D deficiency (if clinically appropriate); Ⓐ information on the Healthy Start scheme can be found at: www.healthystart.nhs.uk/. The amount of vitamin D required in infancy is related to the stores built up *in-utero* and subsequent exposure to sunlight. The amount of vitamin D in breast milk varies and some breast-fed babies, particularly if preterm or born to vitamin D deficient mothers, may become deficient. Most formula milk and supplement feeds contain adequate vitamin D to prevent deficiency; EvGr infants fed with vitamin D fortified formula will only require additional supplementation if they consume less than 500 mL of formula daily. Ⓐ

Simple, nutritional vitamin D deficiency can be prevented by oral supplementation of ergocalciferol p. 792 (calciferol, vitamin D_2) or colecalciferol p. 788 (vitamin D_3) daily, using multi-vitamin drops, preparations of vitamins A and D, manufactured 'special' solutions, or as calcium and ergocalciferol tablets (although the calcium and other vitamins in supplements are unnecessary); excessive supplementation may cause hypercalcaemia.

Inadequate bone mineralisation can be caused by a deficiency, or a lack of action of vitamin D or its active metabolite. In childhood this causes bowing and distortion of bones (rickets). In nutritional vitamin D deficiency rickets, initial high doses of ergocalciferol or colecalciferol should be reduced to supplemental doses after 8–12 weeks, as there is a significant risk of hypercalcaemia. However, calcium supplements are recommended if there is hypocalcaemia or evidence of a poor dietary calcium intake. A single large dose of ergocalciferol or colecalciferol can also be effective for the treatment of nutritional vitamin D deficiency rickets.

Poor bone mineralisation in neonates and young children may also be due to inadequate intake of phosphate or calcium particularly during long-term parenteral nutrition—supplementation with phosphate or calcium may be required.

Hypophosphataemic rickets occurs due to abnormal phosphate excretion; treatment with high doses of oral phosphate, and hydroxylated (activated) forms of vitamin D allow bone mineralisation and optimise growth.

EvGr Nutritional deficiency of vitamin D is treated with oral colecalciferol, or ergocalciferol if the patient cannot take colecalciferol. Ⓐ Preparations containing calcium and colecalciferol are also occasionally used in children where there is evidence of combined calcium and vitamin D deficiency. Vitamin D deficiency caused by *intestinal malabsorption* may require vitamin D in pharmacological doses under specialist supervision. Hypocalcaemia of *hypoparathyroidism* often requires higher doses in order to achieve normocalcaemia and alfacalcidol p. 787 is generally preferred.

Vitamin D supplementation is often given in combination with calcium supplements for persistent hypocalcaemia in neonates, and in chronic renal disease.

EvGr Specialist advice should be obtained for children with vitamin D deficiency and severe liver disease, and for children with end-stage chronic kidney disease who may require activated forms such as alfacalcidol or calcitriol p. 788 [unlicensed use]. Ⓐ

Paricalcitol p. 793, a synthetic vitamin D analogue, is licensed for the prevention and treatment of secondary hyperparathyroidism associated with chronic kidney disease.

Vitamin E

The daily requirement of vitamin E (tocopherol) has not been well defined. Vitamin E supplements are given to children with fat malabsorption such as in cystic fibrosis and cholestatic liver disease. In children with abetalipoproteinaemia abnormally low vitamin E concentrations may occur in association with neuromuscular problems; this usually responds to high doses of vitamin E. Some neonatal units still administer a single intramuscular dose of vitamin E at birth to preterm neonates to reduce the risk of complications; no trials of long-term outcome have been carried out. The intramuscular route should also be considered in children with severe liver disease when response to oral therapy is inadequate.

Vitamin E has been tried for various other conditions but there is little scientific evidence of its value.

Vitamin K

Vitamin K is necessary for the production of blood clotting factors and proteins necessary for the normal calcification of bone.

Because vitamin K is fat soluble, children with fat malabsorption, especially in biliary obstruction or hepatic disease, may become deficient. For oral administration to prevent vitamin K deficiency in malabsorption syndromes, a water-soluble synthetic vitamin K derivative, menadiol sodium phosphate p. 794 can be used if supplementation with phytomenadione p. 795 by mouth has been insufficient.

Oral coumarin anticoagulants act by interfering with vitamin K metabolism in the hepatic cells and their effects can be antagonised by giving vitamin K; see advice on the use of vitamin K in haemorrhage.

Vitamin K deficiency bleeding

Neonates are relatively deficient in vitamin K and those who do not receive supplements of vitamin K are at risk of serious bleeding including intracranial bleeding. The Chief Medical Officer and the Chief Nursing Officer have recommended that all newborn babies should receive vitamin K to prevent vitamin K deficiency bleeding (previously termed haemorrhagic disease of the newborn). An appropriate regimen should be selected after discussion with parents in the antenatal period.

Vitamin K (as phytomenadione) may be given by a single intramuscular injection at birth; this prevents vitamin K deficiency bleeding in virtually all babies.

Alternatively, in healthy babies who are not at particular risk of bleeding disorders, vitamin K may be given by mouth, and arrangements must be in place to ensure the appropriate regimen is followed. Two doses of a colloidal (mixed micelle) preparation of phytomenadione should be given by mouth in the first week, the first dose being given at birth and the second dose at 4–7 days. For exclusively breast-fed babies, a third dose of colloidal phytomenadione is given by mouth at 1 month of age; the third dose is omitted in formula-fed babies because formula feeds contain adequate vitamin K. An alternative regimen is to give one dose of phytomenadione by mouth at birth (using the contents of a phytomenadione capsule) to protect from the risk of vitamin K deficiency bleeding in the first week; for exclusively breast-fed babies, further doses of phytomenadione are given by mouth (using the contents of a phytomenadione capsule) at weekly intervals for 12 weeks.

Multivitamins

Multivitamin supplements are used in children with vitamin deficiencies and also in malabsorption conditions such as cystic fibrosis or liver disease. Supplementation is not required if nutrient enriched feeds are used; consult a dietician for further advice.

VITAMINS AND TRACE ELEMENTS › MULTIVITAMINS

Vitamins A and D

07-Sep-2021

The properties listed below are those particular to the combination only. For the properties of the components please consider, vitamin A p. 783, colecalciferol p. 788.

● **INDICATIONS AND DOSE**

Prevention of vitamin A and D deficiency (using 4500 units vitamin A/450 units vitamin D_3 capsules)

▶ BY MOUTH

▸ Child 7–17 years: 1 capsule daily, increased if necessary to 2 capsules daily, dose increase to be guided by serum values

Prevention of vitamin A and D deficiency (using 4000 units vitamin A/400 units vitamin D capsules)

▶ BY MOUTH

▸ Child 1–17 years: 1 capsule daily

DOSE EQUIVALENCE AND CONVERSION

▸ Each 4500 units vitamin A/450 units vitamin D_3 capsule contains the equivalent of 11 micrograms vitamin D_3.

▸ Each 4000 units vitamin A/400 units vitamin D capsule (vitamins A and D capsules BPC 1973) contains the equivalent of 10 micrograms vitamin D.

● **INTERACTIONS** → Appendix 1: vitamin A · vitamin D substances

● **SIDE-EFFECTS**

Overdose Prolonged excessive ingestion of vitamins A and D can lead to hypervitaminosis.

● **BREAST FEEDING** Manufacturer advises avoid—present in milk.

● **PRESCRIBING AND DISPENSING INFORMATION** This drug contains vitamin D; consult individual vitamin D monographs.

● **MEDICINAL FORMS** There can be variation in the licensing of different medicines containing the same drug.

Oral capsule

EXCIPIENTS: May contain Gelatin

▸ **Vitamins a and d (Non-proprietary)**
Vitamin D 400 unit, Vitamin A 4000 unit Vitamins A and D capsules BPC 1973 | 28 capsule GSL ⊠
Colecalciferol 450 unit, Retinol palmitate 4500 unit Retinol 4,500unit / Colecalciferol 450unit capsules | 84 capsule P £25.95

Vitamins A, B group, C and D

● **INDICATIONS AND DOSE**

Prevention of deficiency

▶ BY MOUTH USING CAPSULES

▸ Child 1–11 years: 1 capsule daily

▸ Child 12–17 years: 2 capsules daily

Cystic Fibrosis: prevention of deficiency

▶ BY MOUTH USING CAPSULES

▸ Child 1–17 years: 2–3 capsules daily

ABIDEC MULTIVITAMIN DROPS®

Prevention of deficiency

▶ BY MOUTH USING ORAL DROPS

▸ Preterm neonate: 0.6 mL daily.

▸ Neonate: 0.3 mL daily.

▸ Child 1–11 months: 0.3 mL daily

▸ Child 1–17 years: 0.6 mL daily

Cystic Fibrosis: prevention of deficiency

▶ BY MOUTH USING ORAL DROPS

▸ Child 1–11 months: 0.6 mL daily

▸ Child 1–17 years: 1.2 mL daily

DALIVIT ORAL DROPS®

Prevention of deficiency

▶ BY MOUTH USING ORAL DROPS

▸ Preterm neonate: 0.3 mL daily.

▸ Neonate: 0.3 mL daily.

▸ Child 1–11 months: 0.3 mL daily

▸ Child 1–17 years: 0.6 mL daily

Cystic Fibrosis: prevention of deficiency

▶ BY MOUTH USING ORAL DROPS

▸ Child 1–11 months: 0.6 mL daily

▸ Child 1–17 years: 1 mL daily

● **UNLICENSED USE** *Dalivit*® not licensed for use in children under 6 weeks.

● **PRESCRIBING AND DISPENSING INFORMATION** This drug contains vitamin D; consult individual vitamin D monographs.

To avoid potential toxicity, the content of all vitamin preparations, particularly vitamin A, should be considered when used together with other supplements.

Vitamin A concentration of preparations varies.

ABIDEC MULTIVITAMIN DROPS® *Abidec*® contains 1333 units of vitamin A (as palmitate) per 0.6 mL dose.

DALIVIT ORAL DROPS® *Dalivit*® contains 5000 units of vitamin A (as palmitate) per 0.6 mL dose.

● **MEDICINAL FORMS** There can be variation in the licensing of different medicines containing the same drug.

Oral capsule

▸ **Vitamins a, b group, c and d (Non-proprietary)**
Riboflavin 500 microgram, Thiamine hydrochloride 1 mg, Nicotinamide 7.5 mg, Ascorbic acid 15 mg, Vitamin D 300 unit, Vitamin A 2500 unit Vitamins capsules | 84 capsule ⊠ DT = £1.43 | 1000 capsule £23.52
Aa BPC Vitamin capsules | 84 capsule £1.43 DT = £1.43 | 1000 capsule £11.73

▸ **AVITA BPC** (TriOn Pharma Ltd)
Riboflavin 500 microgram, Thiamine hydrochloride 1 mg, Nicotinamide 7.5 mg, Ascorbic acid 15 mg, Vitamin D 300 unit, Vitamin A 2500 unit AVITA BPC Vitamin capsules | 28 capsule £0.49 | 84 capsule £1.19 DT = £1.43 | 1000 capsule £10.09

Oral drops

EXCIPIENTS: May contain Arachis (peanut) oil, sucrose

▸ **Abidec Multivitamin** (Omega Pharma Ltd)
Nicotinamide 1333 microgram per 1 ml, Pyridoxine hydrochloride 1333 microgram per 1 ml, Riboflavin 1333 microgram per 1 ml, Thiamine hydrochloride 1.67 mg per 1 ml, Ascorbic acid 66.7 mg per 1 ml, Ergocalciferol 667 unit per 1 ml, Retinol (as Vitamin A palmitate) 2222 unit per 1 ml Abidec Multivitamin drops | 25 ml GSL £4.32

▸ **Dalivit** (Dendron Brands Ltd)
Riboflavin 667 microgram per 1 ml, Pyridoxine 833 microgram per 1 ml, Thiamine 1667 microgram per 1 ml, Nicotinamide 8.3 mg per 1 ml, Ascorbic acid 83 mg per 1 ml, Ergocalciferol 667 unit per

1 ml, Vitamin A 8333 unit per 1 ml Dalivit oral drops | 25 ml GSL £8.12 | 50 ml GSL £13.74

Vitamins A, C and D

05-May-2020

The properties listed below are those particular to the combination only. For the properties of the components please consider, vitamin A below, ascorbic acid p. 786.

- **INDICATIONS AND DOSE**

Prevention of vitamin deficiency

▶ BY MOUTH

- Child 1 month–4 years: 5 drops daily, 5 drops contain vitamin A approx. 700 units, vitamin D approx. 300 units (7.5 micrograms), ascorbic acid approx. 20 mg

- **INTERACTIONS** → Appendix 1: ascorbic acid · vitamin A
- **PRESCRIBING AND DISPENSING INFORMATION** This drug contains vitamin D; consult individual vitamin D monographs.

Available free of charge to children under 4 years in families on the Healthy Start Scheme, or alternatively may be available direct to the public—further information for healthcare professionals can be accessed at www.healthystart.nhs.uk. Beneficiaries can contact their midwife or health visitor for further information on where to obtain supplies.

Healthy Start Vitamins for women (containing ascorbic acid, vitamin D, and folic acid) are also available free of charge to women on the Healthy Start Scheme during pregnancy and until their baby is one year old, or alternatively may be available direct to the public—further information for healthcare professionals can be accessed at www.healthystart.nhs.uk. Beneficiaries can contact their midwife or health visitor for further information on where to obtain supplies.

- **MEDICINAL FORMS** There can be variation in the licensing of different medicines containing the same drug.

Oral drops

▶ Healthy Start Children's Vitamin (Secretary of State for Health)

Vitamin A and D3 concentrate.55 mg per 1 ml, Sodium ascorbate 18.58 mg per 1 ml, Ascorbic acid 150 mg per 1 ml, Vitamin D 2000 unit per 1 ml, Vitamin A 5000 unit per 1 ml Healthy Start Children's Vitamin drops | 10 ml

VITAMINS AND TRACE ELEMENTS > VITAMIN A

Vitamin A

(Retinol)

- **INDICATIONS AND DOSE**

Vitamin A deficiency

▶ BY MOUTH

- Neonate: 5000 units daily, higher doses may be used initially for treatment of severe deficiency.
- Child 1–11 months: 5000 units daily, to be taken with or after food, higher doses may be used initially for treatment of severe deficiency
- Child 1–17 years: 10 000 units daily, to be taken with or after food, higher doses may be used initially for treatment of severe deficiency

Prevention of deficiency in complete biliary obstruction

▶ BY INTRAMUSCULAR INJECTION

- Neonate: 50 000 units once a month.
- Child 1–11 months: 50 000 units once a month

- **UNLICENSED USE** Preparations containing only vitamin A are not licensed.
- **INTERACTIONS** → Appendix 1: vitamin A
- **SIDE-EFFECTS**

Overdose Massive overdose can cause rough skin, dry hair, an enlarged liver, and increases in erythrocyte sedimentation rate, serum calcium and serum alkaline phosphatase concentration.

- **PREGNANCY** Excessive doses may be teratogenic. In view of evidence suggesting that high levels of vitamin A may cause birth defects, women who are (or may become) pregnant are advised not to take vitamin A supplements (including tablets and fish liver oil drops), except on the advice of a doctor or an antenatal clinic; nor should they eat liver or products such as liver paté or liver sausage.
- **BREAST FEEDING** Theoretical risk of toxicity in infants of mothers taking large doses.
- **MONITORING REQUIREMENTS** Treatment is sometimes initiated with very high doses of vitamin A and the child should be monitored closely; very high doses are associated with acute toxicity.
- **MEDICINAL FORMS** There can be variation in the licensing of different medicines containing the same drug. Forms available from special-order manufacturers include: oral drops, solution for injection

Solution for injection

▶ Vitamin a (Non-proprietary)

Retinol (as Vitamin A palmitate) 50000 unit per 1 ml Aquasol A Parenteral 100,000units/2ml solution for injection vials | 1 vial PoM
Nepalm Vitamin A 100,000units/2ml solution for injection ampoules | 6 ampoule PoM

Oral drops

▶ Vitamin a (Non-proprietary)

Vitamin A 150000 unit per 1 ml Arovit 150,000units/ml drops | 7.5 ml PoM

Combinations available: ***Vitamins A and D***, p. 782 · ***Vitamins A, C and D***, above

VITAMINS AND TRACE ELEMENTS > VITAMIN B GROUP

Biotin

18-Aug-2025

(Vitamin H)

- **INDICATIONS AND DOSE**

Isolated carboxylase defects

▶ BY MOUTH, OR BY SLOW INTRAVENOUS INJECTION

- Neonate: 5 mg once daily, adjusted according to response, maintenance 10–50 mg daily, higher doses may be required.
- Child: 10 mg once daily, adjusted according to response; maintenance 10–50 mg daily, increased if necessary up to 100 mg daily

Defects of biotin metabolism

▶ BY MOUTH, OR BY SLOW INTRAVENOUS INJECTION

- Neonate: Initially 10 mg once daily, adjusted according to response; maintenance 5–20 mg daily, higher doses may be required.
- Child: Initially 10 mg once daily, adjusted according to response; maintenance 5–20 mg daily, higher doses may be required

- **PREGNANCY** No information available.
- **BREAST FEEDING** No information available.
- **EFFECT ON LABORATORY TESTS** EvGr Biotin may interfere with laboratory tests that are based on biotin/streptavidin interaction, such as thyroid immunoassays, and the risk of interference increases with higher doses of biotin. Possible biotin interference should be considered when interpreting test results as these may be falsely high or

9 Blood and nutrition

low, leading to misdiagnosis or inappropriate management. If the patient is taking biotin-containing products, laboratory personnel should be informed before tests are ordered as alternative assays may be available. (M)

- **DIRECTIONS FOR ADMINISTRATION** For administration *by mouth*, expert sources advise tablets may be crushed and mixed with food or drink.
- **PATIENT AND CARER ADVICE**
  Medicines for Children leaflet: Biotin for metabolic disorders www.medicinesforchildren.org.uk/medicines/biotin-for-metabolic-disorders/

- **MEDICINAL FORMS** There can be variation in the licensing of different medicines containing the same drug. Forms available from special-order manufacturers include: oral tablet, oral suspension, oral solution

Oral tablet

- **Biotin (Non-proprietary)**
  Biotin 5 mg Biotin-ratiopharm 5 tablets | 30 tablet PoM ⊠ DT = £28.70
  Biotin 10 mg Biotisan Biotin S 10mg FORTE tablets | 30 tablet ⊠
- **AactiBio** (TriOn Pharma Ltd)
  Biotin 10 mg AactiBio 10mg tablets | 28 tablet £36.98

Solution for injection

- **Biotin (Non-proprietary)**
  Biotin 5 mg per 1 ml Biodermatin 5mg/1ml solution for injection vials | 10 vial PoM ⊠ (Hospital only)

Pyridoxine hydrochloride

05-Oct-2021

(Vitamin B$_6$)

- **INDICATIONS AND DOSE**

Isoniazid-induced neuropathy (prophylaxis)

▶ BY MOUTH

- Neonate: 5 mg daily.
- Child 1 month–11 years: 5–10 mg daily
- Child 12–17 years: 10 mg daily

Isoniazid-induced neuropathy (treatment)

▶ BY MOUTH

- Neonate: 5–10 mg daily.
- Child 1 month–11 years: 10–20 mg 2–3 times a day
- Child 12–17 years: 30–50 mg 2–3 times a day

Prevention of penicillamine-induced neuropathy in Wilson's disease

▶ BY MOUTH

- Child 1–11 years: 5–10 mg daily
- Child 12–17 years: 10 mg daily

Metabolic diseases | Cystathioninuria | Homocystinuria

▶ BY MOUTH

- Neonate: 50–100 mg 1–2 times a day.
- Child: 50–250 mg 1–2 times a day

Pyridoxine-dependent seizures

▶ INITIALLY BY INTRAVENOUS INJECTION

- Neonate: Test dose 50–100 mg, repeated if necessary, if responsive, followed by an oral maintenance dose; (by mouth) maintenance 50–100 mg once daily, dose to be adjusted as necessary.
- Child 1 month–11 years: Test dose 50–100 mg daily, if responsive, followed by an oral maintenance dose, (by mouth) maintenance 20–50 mg 1–2 times a day, dose to be adjusted as necessary, (by mouth) increased if necessary up to 30 mg/kg daily, alternatively (by mouth) increased if necessary up to 1 g daily

- **UNLICENSED USE** Not licensed for prophylaxis of penicillamine-induced neuropathy in Wilson's disease. Not licensed for use in children.
- **CAUTIONS**
  ▶ With intravenous use Risk of cardiovascular collapse (with intravenous injection—resuscitation facilities must be available and monitor closely)
- **SIDE-EFFECTS** Peripheral neuritis
  Overdose Overdosage induces toxic effects.

- **MEDICINAL FORMS** There can be variation in the licensing of different medicines containing the same drug. Forms available from special-order manufacturers include: oral capsule, oral suspension, oral solution, solution for injection

Oral tablet

- **Pyridoxine hydrochloride (Non-proprietary)**
  Pyridoxine hydrochloride 10 mg Pyridoxine 10mg tablets | 28 tablet PoM £18.00–£31.90 DT = £14.00
  Pyridoxine hydrochloride 50 mg Pyridoxine 50mg tablets | 28 tablet PoM £5.56–£31.02 DT = £4.74
- **ActiPyrid** (Northumbria Pharma Ltd)
  Pyridoxine hydrochloride 20 mg ActiPyrid 20mg tablets | 28 tablet £18.87
- **PyriDose** (TriOn Pharma Ltd)
  Pyridoxine hydrochloride 20 mg PyriDose 20mg tablets | 28 tablet £18.87
- **Pyrid** (Ennogen Healthcare International Ltd)
  Pyridoxine hydrochloride 20 mg Pyrid-20 tablets | 30 tablet £89.80
- **PyridoxEss** (Essential-Healthcare Ltd)
  Pyridoxine hydrochloride 20 mg PyridoxEss 20mg tablets | 28 tablet £18.93

Solution for injection

- **Pyridoxine hydrochloride (Non-proprietary)**
  Pyridoxine hydrochloride 25 mg per 1 ml Sicovit B6 50mg/2ml solution for injection vials | 5 vial PoM ⊠ (Hospital only)
  Pyridoxine hydrochloride 50 mg per 1 ml Vitamin B6 Streuli 100mg/2ml solution for injection ampoules | 10 ampoule PoM ⊠ (Hospital only)

Oral capsule

- **Pyridoxine hydrochloride (Non-proprietary)**
  Pyridoxine hydrochloride 100 mg Solgar Vitamin B6 100mg capsules | 100 capsule ⊠
  G & G Vitamin B6 100mg capsules | 120 capsule £5.00

Oral solution

- **Apyrid** (Essential-Healthcare Ltd)
  Pyridoxine hydrochloride 20 mg per 1 ml Apyrid 100mg/5ml oral solution | 100 ml £23.97 DT = £22.92
- **PyriDose** (TriOn Pharma Ltd)
  Pyridoxine hydrochloride 20 mg per 1 ml PyriDose 100mg/5ml oral solution | 100 ml £23.88 DT = £22.92

Riboflavin

(Riboflavine; Vitamin B$_2$)

- **INDICATIONS AND DOSE**

Metabolic diseases

▶ BY MOUTH

- Neonate: 50 mg 1–2 times a day, to be adjusted according to response.
- Child: 50–100 mg 1–2 times a day, to be adjusted according to response up to 400 mg per day

- **UNLICENSED USE** Not licensed in children.
- **SIDE-EFFECTS** Urine discolouration
- **PREGNANCY** Crosses the placenta but no adverse effects reported, information at high doses limited.
- **BREAST FEEDING** Present in breast milk but no adverse effects reported, information at high doses limited.

- **MEDICINAL FORMS** There can be variation in the licensing of different medicines containing the same drug. Forms available from special-order manufacturers include: oral tablet, modified-release tablet, oral capsule, oral suspension, oral solution

Oral tablet

- Riboflavin (Non-proprietary)
  Riboflavin 10 mg Beflavine 10mg tablets | 20 tablet [NHS]
  Riboflavin 100 mg Freeda Pure Vitamin B2 100mg tablets | 100 tablet [NHS]

Modified-release tablet

- RiboEss (Essential-Healthcare Ltd)
  Riboflavin 100 mg RiboEss 100mg sustained release tablets | 50 tablet £47.22

Oral capsule

- Riboflavin (Non-proprietary)
  Riboflavin 50 mg Riboflavin 50mg capsules | 30 capsule £3.96
- B-2-50 (Bio-Tech Pharmacal Inc)
  Riboflavin 50 mg B-2-50 capsules | 100 capsule [NHS]
- E-B2 (Ennogen Healthcare International Ltd)
  Riboflavin 100 mg E-B2 100mg capsules | 30 capsule £89.20
- RiboEss (Essential-Healthcare Ltd)
  Riboflavin 50 mg RiboEss 50mg capsules | 30 capsule £41.37
  Riboflavin 100 mg RiboEss 100mg capsules | 30 capsule £58.78

Oral solution

- AabRibof (TriOn Pharma Ltd)
  Riboflavin 20 mg per 1 ml AabRibof 100mg/5ml oral solution | 100 ml £49.86 [SF]

Thiamine
(Vitamin B_1)

04-Feb-2021

- **INDICATIONS AND DOSE**

Maple syrup urine disease

▶ BY MOUTH

- Neonate: 5 mg/kg daily, dose to be adjusted as necessary.
- Child: 5 mg/kg daily, dose to be adjusted as necessary

Metabolic disorders | Congenital lactic acidosis

▶ INITIALLY BY MOUTH, OR BY INTRAVENOUS INFUSION

- Neonate: 50–200 mg once daily, dose to be adjusted as necessary, the total dose may alternatively be given in 2–3 divided doses, administer intravenous infusion over 30 minutes.
- Child: 100–300 mg once daily, dose to be adjusted as necessary, the total dose may alternatively be given in 2–3 divided doses, administer intravenous infusion over 30 minutes, (by mouth) increased if necessary up to 2 g daily

- **UNLICENSED USE** Not licensed in children.

IMPORTANT SAFETY INFORMATION

MHRA/CHM ADVICE (SEPTEMBER 2007)

Although potentially serious allergic adverse reactions may rarely occur during, or shortly after, parenteral administration, the CHM has recommended that:

- This should not preclude the use of parenteral thiamine in patients where this route of administration is required, particularly in patients at risk of Wernicke-Korsakoff syndrome where treatment with thiamine is essential;
- Intravenous administration should be by infusion over 30 minutes;
- Facilities for treating anaphylaxis (including resuscitation facilities) should be available when parenteral thiamine is administered.

- **CAUTIONS** Anaphylaxis may occasionally follow injection, see *Important safety information*
- **BREAST FEEDING** Severely thiamine-deficient mothers should avoid breast-feeding as toxic methyl-glyoxal present in milk.
- **PRESCRIBING AND DISPENSING INFORMATION**
  ▶ With intravenous use Some preparations may contain phenol as a preservative.
- **MEDICINAL FORMS** There can be variation in the licensing of different medicines containing the same drug. Forms available from special-order manufacturers include: oral suspension, oral solution

Oral tablet

- Thiamine (Non-proprietary)
  Thiamine hydrochloride 50 mg Thiamine 50mg tablets | 28 tablet [P] £1.10–£3.00 | 100 tablet [P] £6.72 DT = £3.00
  Thiamine hydrochloride 100 mg Thiamine 100mg tablets | 28 tablet [P] £1.35–£6.72 | 100 tablet [P] £11.55 DT = £3.50

Modified-release tablet

- Athiam (Essential-Healthcare Ltd)
  Thiamine hydrochloride 100 mg Athiam 100mg sustained release tablets | 30 tablet £3.19
- ThiaDose (TriOn Pharma Ltd)
  Thiamine hydrochloride 100 mg ThiaDose 100mg modified-release tablets | 30 tablet £3.19

Solution for injection

- Thiamine (Non-proprietary)
  Thiamine hydrochloride 50 mg per 1 ml Thiamine 100mg/2ml solution for injection ampoules | 5 ampoule [PoM] [NHS] (Hospital only)
  Vitamin B1 - Injektopas 100mg/2ml solution for injection ampoules | 10 ampoule [PoM] [NHS] (Hospital only)
  Thiamine 250mg/5ml solution for injection ampoules | 6 ampoule [PoM] £16.23 DT = £16.23
  Bevitine 100mg/2ml solution for injection ampoules | 5 ampoule [PoM] [NHS] (Hospital only)
  Thiamine hydrochloride 100 mg per 1 ml Vitamin B1 Streuli 100mg/1ml solution for injection ampoules | 10 ampoule [PoM] [NHS] (Hospital only)
  Thiamine 200mg/2ml solution for injection vials | 25 vial [PoM] [NHS] (Hospital only)
  Thiamine hydrochloride 125 mg per 1 ml Thiamine 250mg/2ml solution for injection ampoules | 10 ampoule [PoM] £27.00

Oral solution

- Athiam (Essential-Healthcare Ltd)
  Thiamine hydrochloride 20 mg per 1 ml Athiam 100mg/5ml oral solution | 100 ml £21.73 [SF]
- ThiaDose (TriOn Pharma Ltd)
  Thiamine hydrochloride 20 mg per 1 ml ThiaDose 100mg/5ml oral solution | 100 ml £22.90 [SF]

Vitamin B complex

21-May-2021

- **INDICATIONS AND DOSE**

Treatment of deficiency

▶ BY MOUTH USING SYRUP

- Child 1–11 months: 5 mL 3 times a day, this dose is for *Vigranon B®* syrup.
- Child 1–11 years: 10 mL 3 times a day, this dose is for *Vigranon B®* syrup.
- Child 12–17 years: 10–15 mL 3 times a day, this dose is for *Vigranon B®* syrup.

Prophylaxis of deficiency

▶ BY MOUTH USING SYRUP

- Child 1–11 months: 5 mL once daily, this dose is for *Vigranon B®* syrup.
- Child 1–11 years: 5 mL twice daily, this dose is for *Vigranon B®* syrup.
- Child 12–17 years: 5 mL 3 times a day, this dose is for *Vigranon B®* syrup.

- **NATIONAL FUNDING/ACCESS DECISIONS**
  NHS restrictions *Vigranon B®* syrup is not prescribable in NHS primary care.
- **LESS SUITABLE FOR PRESCRIBING** *Vigranon B®* syrup is less suitable for prescribing.

● **MEDICINAL FORMS** There can be variation in the licensing of different medicines containing the same drug.

Oral solution

▸ Vigranon-B (Wallace Manufacturing Chemists Ltd)
Pyridoxine hydrochloride 400 microgram per 1 ml, Riboflavin sodium phosphate 548 microgram per 1 ml, Dexpanthenol 600 microgram per 1 ml, Thiamine hydrochloride 1 mg per 1 ml, Nicotinamide 4 mg per 1 ml Vigranon-B syrup | 150 ml [P] £26.00 [SF]

Vitamins with minerals and trace elements

18-Aug-2025

● **INDICATIONS AND DOSE**

FORCEVAL® CAPSULES

Vitamin and mineral deficiency and as adjunct in synthetic diets

▶ BY MOUTH

▸ Child 12–17 years: 1 capsule daily, one hour after a meal

KETOVITE® LIQUID

Prevention of vitamin deficiency in disorders of carbohydrate or amino-acid metabolism | Adjunct in restricted, specialised, or synthetic diets

▶ BY MOUTH

▸ Child: 5 mL daily, use with *Ketovite® Tablets* for complete vitamin supplementation.

KETOVITE® TABLETS

Prevention of vitamin deficiency in disorders of carbohydrate or amino-acid metabolism | Adjunct in restricted, specialised, or synthetic diets

▶ BY MOUTH

▸ Child: 1 tablet 3 times a day, use with *Ketovite® Liquid* for complete vitamin supplementation.

● **EFFECT ON LABORATORY TESTS** [EvGr] Biotin may interfere with laboratory tests that are based on biotin/streptavidin interaction, such as thyroid immunoassays, and the risk of interference increases with higher doses of biotin. Possible biotin interference should be considered when interpreting test results as these may be falsely high or low, leading to misdiagnosis or inappropriate management. If the patient is taking biotin-containing products, laboratory personnel should be informed before tests are ordered as alternative assays may be available. (M)

● **PRESCRIBING AND DISPENSING INFORMATION** To avoid potential toxicity, the content of all vitamin preparations, particularly vitamin A, should be considered when used together with other supplements.

● **PATIENT AND CARER ADVICE**

KETOVITE® LIQUID *Ketovite®* liquid may be mixed with milk, cereal, or fruit juice.

KETOVITE® TABLETS Tablets may be crushed immediately before use.

● **MEDICINAL FORMS** There can be variation in the licensing of different medicines containing the same drug.

Oral emulsion

▸ Vitamins with minerals and trace elements (Non-proprietary)
Cyanocobalamin 2.5 microgram per 1 ml, Choline chloride 30 mg per 1 ml, Ergocalciferol 80 unit per 1 ml, Vitamin A 500 unit per 1 ml Ketovite liquid | 150 ml [P] £119.10 [SF]

Oral tablet

▸ Ketovite (Essential Pharmaceuticals Ltd)
Biotin 170 microgram, Folic acid 250 microgram, Pyridoxine hydrochloride 330 microgram, Acetomenaphthone 500 microgram, Riboflavin 1 mg, Thiamine hydrochloride 1 mg, Calcium pantothenate 1.16 mg, Nicotinamide 3.3 mg, Alpha tocopheryl acetate 5 mg, Ascorbic acid 16.6 mg, Inositol 50 mg Ketovite tablets | 100 tablet £28.19

Oral capsule

▸ Forceval (Alliance Pharmaceuticals Ltd)
Cyanocobalamin 3 microgram, Selenium 50 microgram, Biotin 100 microgram, Iodine 140 microgram, Chromium 200 microgram, Molybdenum 250 microgram, Folic acid 400 microgram, Thiamine 1.2 mg, Riboflavin 1.6 mg, Copper 2 mg, Pyridoxine 2 mg, Manganese 3 mg, Pantothenic acid 4 mg, Potassium 4 mg, Tocopheryl acetate 10 mg, Iron 12 mg, Zinc 15 mg, Nicotinamide 18 mg, Magnesium 30 mg, Ascorbic acid 60 mg, Phosphorus 77 mg, Calcium 100 mg, Ergocalciferol 400 unit, Vitamin A 2500 unit Forceval capsules | 15 capsule [P] £6.28 | 30 capsule [P] £11.41 | 90 capsule [P] £33.09

VITAMINS AND TRACE ELEMENTS › VITAMIN C

Ascorbic acid (Vitamin C)

19-Feb-2021

● **INDICATIONS AND DOSE**

Treatment of scurvy

▶ BY MOUTH

▸ Child 1 month–3 years: 125–250 mg daily in 1–2 divided doses

▸ Child 4–11 years: 250–500 mg daily in 1–2 divided doses

▸ Child 12–17 years: 0.5–1 g daily in 1–2 divided doses

Adjunct to desferrioxamine (to enhance the excretion of iron 1 month after treatment)

▶ BY MOUTH

▸ Child: 100–200 mg daily, to be taken 1 hour before food

Metabolic disorders | Tyrosinaemia type III | Transient tyrosinaemia of the newborn | Glutathione synthase deficiency | Hawkinsinuria

▶ BY MOUTH

▸ Neonate: 50–200 mg daily, dose to be adjusted as necessary.

▸ Child: 200–400 mg daily in 1–2 divided doses, dose to be adjusted as necessary, increased if necessary up to 1 g daily

● **UNLICENSED USE** Not licensed for metabolic disorders.

● **CONTRA-INDICATIONS** Hyperoxaluria

● **INTERACTIONS** → Appendix 1: ascorbic acid

● **SIDE-EFFECTS** Diarrhoea · gastrointestinal disorder · hyperoxaluria · oxalate nephrolithiasis · polyuria

● **PRESCRIBING AND DISPENSING INFORMATION** It is rarely necessary to prescribe more than 100 mg daily except early in the treatment of scurvy.

● **MEDICINAL FORMS** There can be variation in the licensing of different medicines containing the same drug. Forms available from special-order manufacturers include: oral tablet, oral suspension, oral solution

Oral tablet

EXCIPIENTS: May contain Aspartame

▸ Ascorbic acid (Non-proprietary)
Ascorbic acid 50 mg Ascorbic acid 50mg tablets | 28 tablet [GSL] £189.54 DT = £72.70
Ascorbic acid 100 mg Ascorbic acid 100mg tablets | 28 tablet [GSL] £198.46 DT = £48.06
Ascorbic acid 200 mg Ascorbic acid 200mg tablets | 28 tablet [GSL] £197.20 DT = £40.15
Ascorbic acid 250 mg Ascorbic acid 250mg tablets | 1000 tablet [PoM] [X]
Ascorbic acid 500 mg Ascorbic acid 500mg tablets | 28 tablet [GSL] £66.00 DT = £36.12

Oral capsule

▸ Ascorbic acid (Non-proprietary)
Ascorbic acid 500 mg BioCare Vitamin C 500mg capsules | 60 capsule £9.54 | 180 capsule £24.73

▸ Liposil (Ascorbic acid) (Silicon Pharma Ltd)
Ascorbic acid 500 mg LipoSil Liposomal Vitamin C 500mg capsules | 30 capsule £9.88

Chewable tablet

CAUTIONARY AND ADVISORY LABELS 24

EXCIPIENTS: May contain Aspartame

▸ Ascorbic acid (Non-proprietary)

Ascorbic acid 60 mg Tesco Vitamin C One A Day 60mg chewable tablets | 60 tablet ⊠

Ascorbic acid 500 mg Premier Vitamin C 500mg chewable tablets | 30 tablet £2.30 | 60 tablet £4.13

Numark Vitamin C 500mg chewable tablets | 30 tablet £1.44

HealthAid Vitamin C 500mg chewable tablets | 60 tablet £5.58 | 100 tablet £7.25

Tesco Vitamin C One A Day 500mg chewable tablets | 60 tablet ⊠

Ascorbic acid 1 gram HealthAid Vitamin C 1000mg chewable tablets | 30 tablet £5.58 | 60 tablet £8.37 | 100 tablet £11.16

Combinations available: ***Vitamins A, C and D***, p. 783

VITAMINS AND TRACE ELEMENTS › VITAMIN D AND ANALOGUES

Vitamin D and analogues (systemic)

- **CONTRA-INDICATIONS** Hypercalcaemia · metastatic calcification
- **SIDE-EFFECTS**
  - ▸ **Common or very common** Abdominal pain · headache · hypercalcaemia · hypercalciuria · nausea · skin reactions
  - ▸ **Uncommon** Appetite decreased · asthenia · constipation · diarrhoea · dry mouth · myalgia · vomiting
  - ▸ **Frequency not known** Arrhythmia · weight decreased

  Overdose Symptoms of overdosage include anorexia, lassitude, nausea and vomiting, diarrhoea, constipation, weight loss, polyuria, sweating, headache, thirst, vertigo, and raised concentrations of calcium and phosphate in plasma and urine.
- **PREGNANCY** High doses teratogenic in *animals* but therapeutic doses unlikely to be harmful.
- **BREAST FEEDING** Caution with high doses; may cause hypercalcaemia in infant—monitor serum-calcium concentration.
- **MONITORING REQUIREMENTS** **Important**: all patients receiving pharmacological doses of vitamin D should have their plasma-calcium concentration checked at intervals as clinically indicated and whenever nausea or vomiting occur.

above

Alfacalcidol

10-Apr-2026

(1α-Hydroxycholecalciferol)

- **INDICATIONS AND DOSE**

Hypophosphataemic rickets (under expert supervision) | Persistent hypocalcaemia due to hypoparathyroidism or pseudohypoparathyroidism (under expert supervision)

▸ BY MOUTH, OR BY INTRAVENOUS INJECTION

- ▸ Child 1 month–11 years: 25–50 nanograms/kg once daily (max. per dose 1000 nanograms), dose to be adjusted as necessary
- ▸ Child 12–17 years: 1 microgram once daily, dose to be adjusted as necessary

Persistent neonatal hypocalcaemia (under expert supervision)

▸ BY MOUTH, OR BY INTRAVENOUS INJECTION

- ▸ Neonate: 50–100 nanograms/kg once daily, dose to be adjusted according to response, in resistant cases higher doses may be needed and can be increased if necessary up to 2 micrograms/kg per day.

Prevention of vitamin D deficiency in renal or cholestatic liver disease (under expert supervision)

▸ BY MOUTH, OR BY INTRAVENOUS INJECTION

- ▸ Neonate: 20 nanograms/kg once daily, dose to be adjusted as necessary.
- ▸ Child 1 month–11 years (body-weight up to 20 kg): 15–30 nanograms/kg once daily (max. per dose 500 nanograms)
- ▸ Child 1 month–11 years (body-weight 20 kg and above): 250–500 nanograms once daily, dose to be adjusted as necessary
- ▸ Child 12–17 years: 250–500 nanograms once daily, dose to be adjusted as necessary

DOSE EQUIVALENCE AND CONVERSION

- ▸ One drop of alfacalcidol 2 microgram/mL oral drops contains approximately 100 nanograms alfacalcidol.

- **CAUTIONS** Granulomatous diseases (risk of increased sensitivity to vitamin D) · nephrolithiasis · take care to ensure correct dose in infants
- **INTERACTIONS** → Appendix 1: vitamin D substances
- **SIDE-EFFECTS**
  - ▸ **Common or very common** Abdominal discomfort · hyperphosphataemia · rash pustular
  - ▸ **Uncommon** Malaise · urolithiases
  - ▸ **Rare or very rare** Dizziness
  - ▸ **Frequency not known** Confusion · renal impairment
- **RENAL IMPAIRMENT** EvGr Monitor plasma-calcium and phosphate concentration closely in renal impairment. ⟨M⟩
- **MONITORING REQUIREMENTS** EvGr Monitor plasma-calcium concentration (ideally corrected for protein binding), especially in patients receiving high doses—if hypercalcaemia occurs, withhold treatment until calcium returns to normal, then restart at half the previous dose. Also monitor plasma-phosphate, parathyroid hormone, alkaline phosphatase and calcium phosphate. Measure parameters every week initially, then every 2–4 weeks when the dose is stabilised. ⟨M⟩
- **DIRECTIONS FOR ADMINISTRATION** For *injection*, manufacturer advises shake ampoule for at least 5 seconds before use, and give over 30 seconds.
- **HANDLING AND STORAGE**
  - ▸ With intravenous use Store in a refrigerator (2–8°C) and protect from light.

- **MEDICINAL FORMS** There can be variation in the licensing of different medicines containing the same drug. Forms available from special-order manufacturers include: oral suspension, oral solution

Solution for injection

EXCIPIENTS: May contain Alcohol, propylene glycol

▸ One-Alpha (Neon Healthcare Ltd)

Alfacalcidol 2 microgram per 1 ml One-Alpha 2micrograms/1ml solution for injection ampoules | 10 ampoule PoM £41.13 DT = £41.13

One-Alpha 1micrograms/0.5ml solution for injection ampoules | 10 ampoule PoM £21.57

Oral capsule

EXCIPIENTS: May contain Potassium sorbate, sesame oil, vitamin e

▸ Alfacalcidol (Non-proprietary)

Alfacalcidol 250 nanogram Alfacalcidol 250nanogram capsules | 30 capsule PoM £4.94 DT = £1.90

Alfacalcidol 500 nanogram Alfacalcidol 500nanogram capsules | 30 capsule PoM £9.90 DT = £3.42

Alfacalcidol 1 microgram Alfacalcidol 1microgram capsules | 30 capsule PoM £8.75 DT = £8.75

▸ AlfaD (Theramex HQ UK Ltd)

Alfacalcidol 250 nanogram AlfaD 0.25microgram capsules | 30 capsule PoM £5.00 DT = £1.90

Alfacalcidol 500 nanogram AlfaD 0.5microgram capsules | 30 capsule PoM £10.00 DT = £3.42

Alfacalcidol 1 microgram AlfaD 1microgram capsules | 30 capsule PoM £14.00 DT = £8.75

▸ **One-Alpha** (Neon Healthcare Ltd)
Alfacalcidol 250 nanogram One-Alpha 250nanogram capsules | 30 capsule PoM £3.37 DT = £1.90
Alfacalcidol 500 nanogram One-Alpha 0.5microgram capsules | 30 capsule PoM £6.27 DT = £3.42
Alfacalcidol 1 microgram One-Alpha 1microgram capsules | 30 capsule PoM £8.75 DT = £8.75

Oral drops

EXCIPIENTS: May contain Alcohol, hydroxybenzoates (parabens), polyoxyl castor oils, sorbitol, vitamin e

▸ **One-Alpha** (Neon Healthcare Ltd)
Alfacalcidol 2 microgram per 1 ml One-Alpha 2micrograms/ml oral drops | 10 ml PoM £21.30 DT = £21.30 SF

F 787

Calcitriol

12-Mar-2026

(1,25-Dihydroxycholecalciferol)

● **INDICATIONS AND DOSE**

Vitamin D dependent rickets (under expert supervision) | Hypophosphataemic rickets (under expert supervision) | Persistent hypocalcaemia due to hypoparathyroidism (under expert supervision) | Pseudo-hypoparathyroidism (limited experience) (under expert supervision)

▶ BY MOUTH

▸ Child 1 month–11 years: Initially 15 nanograms/kg once daily (max. per dose 250 nanograms), increased in steps of 5 nanograms/kg daily (max. per dose 250 nanograms) if required, dose to be increased every 2–4 weeks

▸ Child 12–17 years: Initially 250 nanograms once daily, increased in steps of 5 nanograms/kg daily (max. per dose 250 nanograms) if required, dose to be increased every 2–4 weeks; usual dose 0.5–1 microgram daily

● **UNLICENSED USE** Not licensed for use in children.

● **CAUTIONS** Take care to ensure correct dose in infants

● **INTERACTIONS** → Appendix 1: vitamin D substances

● **SIDE-EFFECTS**

▶ **Common or very common** Urinary tract infection

▶ **Frequency not known** Abdominal pain upper · apathy · dehydration · drowsiness · fever · growth retardation · muscle weakness · paralytic ileus · polydipsia · psychiatric disorder · sensory disorder · thirst · urinary disorders

● **RENAL IMPAIRMENT** Manufacturer advises avoid—no information available.

● **MONITORING REQUIREMENTS** EvGr Monitor plasma-calcium, phosphate, and creatinine concentrations regularly, particularly during dose titration. (M)

● **MEDICINAL FORMS** There can be variation in the licensing of different medicines containing the same drug. Forms available from special-order manufacturers include: oral suspension, oral solution

Oral solution

▸ **Calcitriol (Non-proprietary)**
Calcitriol 1 microgram per 1 ml Rocaltrol 1micrograms/ml oral solution | 10 ml PoM (X) SF

Oral capsule

EXCIPIENTS: May contain Butylated hydroxyanisole, butylated hydroxytoluene, sorbitol

▸ **Calcitriol (Non-proprietary)**
Calcitriol 250 nanogram Calcitriol 250nanogram capsules | 30 capsule PoM £18.04 (Hospital only) | 30 capsule PoM £5.41–£8.92
Calcitriol 500 nanogram Calcitriol 500nanogram capsules | 30 capsule PoM £32.25 (Hospital only) | 30 capsule PoM £9.68–£15.96

▸ **Rocaltrol** (Atnahs Pharma UK Ltd)
Calcitriol 250 nanogram Rocaltrol 250nanogram capsules | 100 capsule PoM £18.04 DT = £18.04
Calcitriol 500 nanogram Rocaltrol 500nanogram capsules | 100 capsule PoM £32.25 DT = £32.25

F 787

Colecalciferol

20-Oct-2022

(Cholecalciferol; Vitamin D_3)

● **INDICATIONS AND DOSE**

Primary prevention of vitamin D deficiency (if breastfed or formula-fed and consume less than 500mL formula per day)

▶ BY MOUTH

▸ Child up to 11 months: 340–400 units daily

Primary prevention of vitamin D deficiency

▶ BY MOUTH

▸ Child 1–17 years: 400 units daily

Treatment of vitamin D deficiency [Loading dose]

▶ BY MOUTH

▸ Child 1–5 months: 3000 units daily for 8 to 12 weeks, loading dosing may be given daily or the equivalent dose given intermittently e.g. weekly or fortnightly

▸ Child 6 months–11 years: 6000 units daily for 8 to 12 weeks, loading dosing may be given daily or the equivalent dose given intermittently e.g. weekly or fortnightly

▸ Child 12–17 years: 10 000 units daily for 8 to 12 weeks, loading dosing may be given daily or the equivalent dose given intermittently e.g. weekly or fortnightly. A single or divided loading dose totalling 300 000 units can be considered if there are concerns about compliance

Treatment of vitamin D deficiency [Maintenance dose]

▶ BY MOUTH

▸ Child 1 month–11 years: 400–600 units daily, maintenance to be started one month after loading dose completed, or if correction of vitamin D deficiency is less urgent, maintenance may be started without the use of loading doses

▸ Child 12–17 years: 400–600 units daily, maintenance dosing may be given daily or the equivalent dose given intermittently. Maintenance to be started one month after loading dose completed, or if correction of vitamin D deficiency is less urgent, maintenance may be started without the use of loading doses. Higher maintenance doses may be necessary in those at high risk of vitamin D deficiency; maximum 4000 units per day

DOSE EQUIVALENCE AND CONVERSION

▸ Colecalciferol 400 units is equivalent to 10 micrograms; dose expressed as units.

● **UNLICENSED USE** EvGr Colecalciferol is used in the doses provided in BNF publications, for the primary prevention and treatment of vitamin D deficiency, (A) but these may differ from those licensed.

● **CAUTIONS** Sarcoidosis · take care to ensure correct dose in infants

● **INTERACTIONS** → Appendix 1: vitamin D substances

● **MONITORING REQUIREMENTS**

▸ When used for Treatment of vitamin D deficiency EvGr Monitor plasma-25-hydroxyvitamin D concentration and bone profile after last loading dose. (A)

● **DIRECTIONS FOR ADMINISTRATION**

INVITA D3® ORAL SOLUTION Manufacturer advises may be mixed with a small amount of milk or cold or lukewarm food immediately before administration.

● **MEDICINAL FORMS** There can be variation in the licensing of different medicines containing the same drug. Forms available from special-order manufacturers include: oral tablet, oral capsule, oral suspension, oral solution, oral drops

Oral tablet

▸ **Colecalciferol (Non-proprietary)**
Colecalciferol 400 unit FSC Vitamin D3 400unit tablets | 60 tablet £1.35
Prohealth Vitamin D3 10micrograms (400units) tablets | 120 tablet ⊠
Dekristol 400unit tablets | 100 tablet ⊠
Colecalciferol 800 unit Colecalciferol 800unit tablets | 30 tablet PoM £6.00 DT = £5.80
Colecalciferol 1000 unit Colecalciferol 1,000unit tablets | 30 tablet PoM £3.16–£5.30
Colecalciferol 2000 unit Colecalciferol 2,000unit tablets | 30 tablet PoM £13.50–£22.26
Colecalciferol 5000 unit Vitamin D3 High Strength 5,000unit tablets | 60 tablet £8.37

▸ **Aace D3** (Essential-Healthcare Ltd)
Colecalciferol 2200 unit Aace D3 2,200unit tablets | 28 tablet £7.03

▸ **Aactive D3** (TriOn Pharma Ltd)
Colecalciferol 2200 unit Aactive D3 2,200unit tablets | 30 tablet £7.49
Colecalciferol 3000 unit Aactive D3 3,000unit tablets | 30 tablet £3.89
Colecalciferol 10000 unit Aactive D3 10,000unit tablets | 30 tablet £5.24
Colecalciferol 50000 unit Aactive D3 50,000unit tablets | 10 tablet £11.96

▸ **AceCal D3** (Essential-Healthcare Ltd)
Colecalciferol 3000 unit AceCal D3 3,000unit tablets | 28 tablet £3.87
Colecalciferol 5000 unit AceCal D3 5,000unit tablets | 28 tablet £4.19
Colecalciferol 10000 unit AceCal D3 10,000unit tablets | 28 tablet £5.29
Colecalciferol 20000 unit AceCal D3 20,000unit tablets | 28 tablet £7.89

▸ **Aciferol D3** (Fontus Health Ltd)
Colecalciferol 400 unit Aciferol D3 400unit tablets | 90 tablet £12.95
Colecalciferol 2200 unit Aciferol D3 2,200unit tablets | 90 tablet £29.95
Colecalciferol 3000 unit Aciferol D3 3,000unit tablets | 60 tablet £16.99
Colecalciferol 5000 unit Aciferol D3 5,000unit tablets | 60 tablet £21.95
Colecalciferol 10000 unit Aciferol D3 10,000unit tablets | 30 tablet £15.99
Colecalciferol 20000 unit Aciferol D3 20,000unit tablets | 30 tablet £21.95

▸ **Actium D3** (MaN Pharma Ltd)
Colecalciferol 400 unit Actium D3 400unit tablets | 30 tablet £2.25
Colecalciferol 5000 unit Actium D3 5,000unit tablets | 28 tablet £4.19
Colecalciferol 20000 unit Actium D3 20,000unit tablets | 28 tablet £7.46
Colecalciferol 50000 unit Actium D3 50,000unit tablets | 10 tablet £11.97

▸ **ColeDose D3** (TriOn Pharma Ltd)
Colecalciferol 5000 unit ColeDose D3 5,000unit tablets | 30 tablet £4.49
Colecalciferol 20000 unit ColeDose D3 20,000unit tablets | 30 tablet £7.45

▸ **ColeKal-D3** (Essential-Healthcare Ltd)
Colecalciferol 400 unit ColeKal-D3 400unit tablets | 30 tablet £2.23

▸ **Colextra-D3** (Synergy Biologics Ltd)
Colecalciferol 25000 unit Colextra-D3 25,000unit tablets | 12 tablet PoM £12.40 DT = £17.00

▸ **Cubicole D3** (Cubic Pharmaceuticals Ltd)
Colecalciferol 400 unit Cubicole D3 400unit tablets | 30 tablet £3.55

▸ **Desunin** (Viatris UK Healthcare Ltd)
Colecalciferol 800 unit Desunin 800unit tablets | 30 tablet PoM £3.60 DT = £5.80 | 90 tablet PoM £10.17
Colecalciferol 4000 unit Desunin 4,000unit tablets | 70 tablet PoM £15.90 DT = £15.90

▸ **E-D3** (Ennogen Healthcare International Ltd)
Colecalciferol 400 unit E-D3 400unit tablets | 30 tablet £78.50
Colecalciferol 10000 unit E-D3 10,000unit tablets | 30 tablet £95.00
Colecalciferol 20000 unit E-D3 20,000unit tablets | 30 tablet £95.90

▸ **Healthmarque** (Kinerva Ltd)
Colecalciferol 20000 unit Healthmarque D3 20,000unit tablets | 15 tablet £3.33

▸ **Pro D3** (Synergy Biologics Ltd)
Colecalciferol 400 unit Pro D3 400unit tablets | 30 tablet £1.90

▸ **Stexerol-D3** (Grunenthal Ltd)
Colecalciferol 1000 unit Stexerol-D3 1,000unit tablets | 28 tablet PoM £2.95 DT = £2.95
Colecalciferol 25000 unit Stexerol-D3 25,000unit tablets | 12 tablet PoM £17.00 DT = £17.00

▸ **SunVit D3** (SunVit-D3 Ltd)
Colecalciferol 400 unit SunVit-D3 400unit Vegan tablets | 60 tablet £5.00
SunVit-D3 400unit tablets | 28 tablet £3.07
Colecalciferol 3000 unit SunVit-D3 3,000unit tablets | 28 tablet £6.60
Colecalciferol 5000 unit SunVit-D3 5,000unit tablets | 28 tablet £6.00
Colecalciferol 10000 unit SunVit-D3 10,000unit tablets | 28 tablet £8.40
Colecalciferol 20000 unit SunVit-D3 20,000unit tablets | 28 tablet £5.29
Colecalciferol 50000 unit SunVit-D3 50,000unit tablets | 15 tablet £24.03

▸ **YPV Vitamin D3** (GlucoRx Ltd)
Colecalciferol 400 unit YPV Vitamin D3 400unit tablets | 180 tablet £4.95
Colecalciferol 20000 unit YPV Vitamin D3 20,000unit tablets | 14 tablet £4.95

Oral capsule

CAUTIONARY AND ADVISORY LABELS 25

▸ **Colecalciferol (Non-proprietary)**
Colecalciferol 400 unit Colecalciferol 400unit capsules | 30 capsule PoM ⊠
Colecalciferol 800 unit Colecalciferol 800unit capsules | 30 capsule PoM £3.60 DT = £3.60
Colecalciferol 1000 unit Colecalciferol 1,000unit capsules | 30 capsule PoM £10.00 DT = £5.34
Colecalciferol 3000 unit FSC High Strength Vitamin D3 3,000unit capsules | 60 capsule £1.65
Colecalciferol 3200 unit Colecalciferol 3,200unit capsules | 30 capsule PoM £13.32 DT = £13.32
Colecalciferol 5000 unit Colecalciferol 5,000unit capsules | 100 capsule PoM ⊠
Colecalciferol 10000 unit Colecalciferol 10,000unit capsules | 20 capsule PoM £14.32 DT = £13.68
Colecalciferol 20000 unit Colecalciferol 20,000unit capsules | 10 capsule PoM £9.67 | 20 capsule PoM £13.15–£20.95 | 30 capsule PoM £29.00 DT = £29.00

▸ **Aace D3** (Essential-Healthcare Ltd)
Colecalciferol 600 unit Aace D3 600unit capsules | 28 capsule £4.17
Colecalciferol 2200 unit Aace D3 2,200unit capsules | 28 capsule £4.67
Colecalciferol 2500 unit Aace D3 2,500unit capsules | 28 capsule £4.59
Colecalciferol 3000 unit Aace D3 3,000unit capsules | 28 capsule £3.59
Colecalciferol 30000 unit Aace D3 30,000unit capsules | 10 capsule £7.43

▸ **Aactive D3** (TriOn Pharma Ltd)
Colecalciferol 600 unit Aactive D3 600unit capsules | 30 capsule £4.49
Colecalciferol 2200 unit Aactive D3 2,200unit capsules | 30 capsule £4.99
Colecalciferol 2500 unit Aactive D3 2,500unit capsules | 30 capsule £4.59
Colecalciferol 3000 unit Aactive D3 3,000unit capsules | 28 capsule £3.85
Colecalciferol 30000 unit Aactive D3 30,000unit capsules | 10 capsule £14.49
Colecalciferol 40000 unit Aactive D3 40,000unit capsules | 10 capsule £7.64

▸ **Aciferol D3** (Fontus Health Ltd)
Colecalciferol 30000 unit Aciferol D3 30,000unit capsules | 10 capsule £24.95

- ▸ **Actium D3** (MaN Pharma Ltd)
  - **Colecalciferol 600 unit** Actium D3 600unit capsules | 28 capsule £11.97
  - **Colecalciferol 2500 unit** Actium D3 2,500unit capsules | 30 capsule £5.00
- ▸ **ColeKal-D3** (Essential-Healthcare Ltd)
  - **Colecalciferol 40000 unit** ColeKal-D3 40,000unit capsules | 10 capsule £7.59
- ▸ **Colextra-D3** (Synergy Biologics Ltd)
  - **Colecalciferol 800 unit** Colextra-D3 800unit capsules | 30 capsule PoM £2.40 DT = £3.60
  - **Colecalciferol 20000 unit** Colextra-D3 20,000unit capsules | 10 capsule PoM £5.90 | 30 capsule PoM £15.90 DT = £29.00
- ▸ **Cubicole D3** (Cubic Pharmaceuticals Ltd)
  - **Colecalciferol 600 unit** Cubicole D3 600unit capsules | 30 capsule £4.95
  - **Colecalciferol 2200 unit** Cubicole D3 2,200unit capsules | 30 capsule £5.55
  - **Colecalciferol 3000 unit** Cubicole D3 3,000unit capsules | 30 capsule £5.95
- ▸ **E-D3** (Ennogen Healthcare International Ltd)
  - **Colecalciferol 600 unit** E-D3 600unit capsules | 30 capsule £82.10
  - **Colecalciferol 2200 unit** E-D3 2,200unit capsules | 30 capsule £86.20
  - **Colecalciferol 2500 unit** E-D3 2,500unit capsules | 30 capsule £86.20
  - **Colecalciferol 3000 unit** E-D3 3,000unit capsules | 30 capsule £88.60
  - **Colecalciferol 30000 unit** E-D3 30,000unit capsules | 10 capsule £94.40
- ▸ **Fultium-D3** (Internis Pharmaceuticals Ltd)
  - **Colecalciferol 800 unit** Fultium-D3 800unit capsules | 90 capsule PoM £8.85 DT = £8.85
  - **Colecalciferol 3200 unit** Fultium-D3 3,200unit capsules | 30 capsule PoM £13.32 DT = £13.32 | 90 capsule PoM £39.96
  - **Colecalciferol 20000 unit** Fultium-D3 20,000unit capsules | 15 capsule PoM £17.04 DT = £17.04 | 30 capsule PoM £29.00 DT = £29.00
- ▸ **InVita D3** (Consilient Health Ltd)
  - **Colecalciferol 5600 unit** InVita D3 5,600unit capsules | 4 capsule PoM £2.50 DT = £2.50
  - **Colecalciferol 25000 unit** InVita D3 25,000unit capsules | 3 capsule PoM £3.95 DT = £3.95
  - **Colecalciferol 50000 unit** InVita D3 50,000unit capsules | 3 capsule PoM £4.95 DT = £4.95
- ▸ **LipoSil (Colecalciferol)** (Silicon Pharma Ltd)
  - **Colecalciferol 2000 unit** LipoSil Liposomal D3 2,000unit capsules | 30 capsule £9.67
- ▸ **Plenachol** (Accord-UK Ltd)
  - **Colecalciferol 20000 unit** Plenachol D3 20,000unit capsules | 10 capsule PoM £9.00
- ▸ **Pro D3** (Synergy Biologics Ltd)
  - **Colecalciferol 2500 unit** Pro D3 2,500unit capsules | 30 capsule £9.99
  - **Colecalciferol 30000 unit** Pro D3 30,000unit capsules | 10 capsule £12.00
- ▸ **RestorD3** (TriOn Pharma Ltd)
  - **Colecalciferol 40000 unit** RestorD3 40,000unit capsules | 10 capsule £7.59
- ▸ **Strivit-D3** (Strides Pharma UK Ltd)
  - **Colecalciferol 800 unit** Strivit-D3 800unit capsules | 30 capsule PoM £2.50 DT = £3.60
  - **Colecalciferol 1000 unit** Strivit-D3 1,000unit capsules | 30 capsule PoM £2.50 DT = £5.34
  - **Colecalciferol 3200 unit** Strivit-D3 3,200unit capsules | 30 capsule PoM £9.32 DT = £13.32
  - **Colecalciferol 20000 unit** Strivit-D3 20,000unit capsules | 10 capsule PoM £9.60 | 20 capsule PoM £13.15
- ▸ **SunVit D3** (SunVit-D3 Ltd)
  - **Colecalciferol 600 unit** SunVit-D3 600unit capsules | 60 capsule £8.00
  - **Colecalciferol 2200 unit** SunVit-D3 2,200unit capsules | 28 capsule £6.00
  - **Colecalciferol 2500 unit** SunVit-D3 2,500unit capsules | 28 capsule £6.60
  - **Colecalciferol 40000 unit** SunVit-D3 40,000unit capsules | 10 capsule £12.01

Oral drops

- ▸ **Colecalciferol (Non-proprietary)**
  - **Colecalciferol 400 unit per 1 ml** Life On Vitokid-D3 400unit oral drops sugar free | 30 ml £2.78 SF
  - **Colecalciferol 20000 unit per 1 ml** Vigantol 20,000units/ml oral drops | 10 ml
  - **Colecalciferol 400 unit per 1 drop** Prohealth Vitamin D3 10micrograms/drop (400units/drop) oral drops | 2.4 ml £2.49 SF
  - **Colecalciferol 1000 unit per 1 drop** Vitamin D3 1,000unit oral drops | 30 ml £9.49 SF
- ▸ **Aactive D3** (TriOn Pharma Ltd)
  - **Colecalciferol 400 unit per 1 ml** Aactive D3 400units/ml oral drops | 50 ml £3.99 SF
  - **Colecalciferol 2000 unit per 1 ml** Aactive D3 2,000units/ml oral drops | 20 ml £5.82 SF
  - **Colecalciferol 200 unit per 1 drop** Aactive D3 200units/drop oral drops | 15 ml £5.19 SF
- ▸ **ColeKal-D3** (Essential-Healthcare Ltd)
  - **Colecalciferol 400 unit per 1 ml** ColeKal-D3 400units/ml oral drops | 30 ml £3.97 SF
- ▸ **E-D3** (Ennogen Healthcare International Ltd)
  - **Colecalciferol 2000 unit per 1 ml** E-D3 2,000units/ml oral drops | 20 ml SF
- ▸ **Fultium-D3** (Internis Pharmaceuticals Ltd)
  - **Colecalciferol 2740 unit per 1 ml** Fultium-D3 2,740units/ml oral drops | 25 ml PoM £10.70 DT = £10.70 SF
- ▸ **Healthmarque** (Kinerva Ltd)
  - **Colecalciferol 400 unit per 1 drop** Healthmarque D3 400units/drop oral drops | 7.5 ml £5.83 SF
  - **Colecalciferol 1000 unit per 1 drop** Healthmarque D3 1,000unit oral drops | 20 ml £7.49 SF
- ▸ **InVita D3** (Consilient Health Ltd)
  - **Colecalciferol 2400 unit per 1 ml** InVita D3 2,400units/ml oral drops | 10 ml PoM £3.60 DT = £3.60 SF
- ▸ **Pro D3** (Synergy Biologics Ltd)
  - **Colecalciferol 2000 unit per 1 ml** Pro D3 2,000units/ml liquid drops | 20 ml £9.80 SF
    Pro D3 2,000units/ml Vegan liquid drops | 20 ml £11.00 SF
- ▸ **Provitavit Vitamin D** (Cuttlefish Ltd)
  - **Colecalciferol 200 unit per 1 drop** Provitavit Vitamin D 200units/drop oral drops | 7 ml £4.95 SF
- ▸ **SunVit D3** (SunVit-D3 Ltd)
  - **Colecalciferol 2000 unit per 1 ml** SunVit-D3 2,000units/ml oral drops | 20 ml £7.45 SF
- ▸ **Thorens** (Galen Ltd)
  - **Colecalciferol 10000 unit per 1 ml** Thorens 10,000units/ml oral drops | 10 ml PoM £5.85 DT = £5.85 SF

Oral solution

CAUTIONARY AND ADVISORY LABELS 21

- ▸ **Colecalciferol (Non-proprietary)**
  - **Colecalciferol 3000 unit per 1 ml** Colecalciferol 3,000units/ml oral solution sugar free | 100 ml PoM £89.23–£144.00 DT = £89.23 SF
    E-D3 15,000units/5ml oral solution | 50 ml
  - **Colecalciferol 10000 unit per 1 ml** ZymaD 10,000units/ml oral solution | 10 ml PoM
- ▸ **Aactive D3** (TriOn Pharma Ltd)
  - **Colecalciferol 2000 unit per 1 ml** Aactive D3 2,000units/ml oral solution | 50 ml £8.96 SF
- ▸ **Aciferol D3** (Fontus Health Ltd)
  - **Colecalciferol 2000 unit per 1 ml** Aciferol D3 2,000units/ml liquid | 100 ml £24.95
  - **Colecalciferol 3000 unit per 1 ml** Aciferol D3 3,000units/ml liquid | 100 ml £65.99
- ▸ **Baby D** (Arok Healthcare)
  - **Colecalciferol 1000 unit per 1 ml** BabyD 1,000units/ml oral solution | 30 ml £4.50
  - **Colecalciferol 1440 unit per 1 ml** BabyD 1,440units/ml oral solution | 10 ml £2.77 SF
- ▸ **E-D3** (Ennogen Healthcare International Ltd)
  - **Colecalciferol 1000 unit per 1 ml** E-D3 1,000units/ml oral solution | 15 ml
  - **Colecalciferol 3000 unit per 1 ml** E-D3 3,000units/ml oral solution | 50 ml
- ▸ **InVita D3** (Consilient Health Ltd)
  - **Colecalciferol 25000 unit per 1 ml** InVita D3 25,000units/1ml oral solution | 3 ampoule PoM £4.45 DT = £4.45 SF
  - **Colecalciferol 50000 unit per 1 ml** InVita D3 50,000units/1ml oral solution | 3 ampoule PoM £6.25 DT = £6.25 SF

▸ **Pro D3** (Synergy Biologics Ltd)
Colecalciferol 2000 unit per 1 ml Pro D3 2,000units/ml liquid | 50 ml £15.80 | 100 ml £22.50
Pro D3 2,000units/ml Vegan liquid | 50 ml £17.80
Colecalciferol 3000 unit per 1 ml Pro D3 forte 3,000units/ml liquid | 50 ml £18.90

▸ **SunVit D3** (SunVit-D3 Ltd)
Colecalciferol 2000 unit per 1 ml SunVit-D3 10,000units/5ml oral solution | 50 ml £10.70 [SF]
SunVit-D3 2,000units/ml oral solution | 50 ml £10.70 [SF]

▸ **Thorens** (Galen Ltd)
Colecalciferol 10000 unit per 1 ml Thorens 25,000units/2.5ml oral solution | 2.5 ml [PoM] £1.55 DT = £1.55 [SF] | 10 ml [PoM] £5.85 DT = £5.85 [SF]

Chewable tablet

▸ **Urgent-D** (Vega Nutritionals Ltd)
Colecalciferol 2000 unit Urgent-D 2,000unit chewable tablets | 60 tablet £4.42

Form unstated

▸ **Colecalciferol (Non-proprietary)**
Colecalciferol 400 unit per 1 dose BetterYou D400 Junior Vitamin D 400units Daily oral spray | 15 ml £4.16 [SF]
BetterYou Infant Vitamin D 400units Daily oral spray | 15 ml £4.16 [SF]
Colecalciferol 1000 unit per 1 dose BetterYou D1000 Vitamin D 1,000units Daily oral spray | 15 ml £4.44 [SF]
BetterYou Vitamin D High Strength Daily oral spray | 15 ml £3.15 [SF]
Colecalciferol 2900 unit per 1 dose BetterYou Vitamin D 40,000units Weekly oral spray | 15 ml £7.23 [SF]
Colecalciferol 3000 unit per 1 dose BetterYou Vitamin D 3,000units Daily oral spray | 15 ml £5.28 [SF]
Colecalciferol 4000 unit per 1 dose BetterYou D4000 Vitamin D 4,000units Daily oral spray | 15 ml £5.56 [SF]

▸ **DailyD** (Arok Healthcare)
Colecalciferol 400 unit per 1 dose DailyD Vitamin D3 400units oral spray | 30 ml £4.99 [SF]
Colecalciferol 1000 unit per 1 dose DailyD Vitamin D3 1,000units oral spray | 30 ml £8.88 [SF]

▸ **ToddlerD** (Arok Healthcare)
Colecalciferol 200 unit per 1 dose ToddlerD Vitamin D3 200units oral spray | 30 ml £4.99 [SF]

Orodispersible tablet

▸ **Colecalciferol (Non-proprietary)**
Colecalciferol 2000 unit Vitamin D3 Lemon Melts 2,000unit tablets | 120 tablet £7.81 [SF]

Combinations available: ***Vitamins A and D***, p. 782

Colecalciferol with calcium carbonate

The properties listed below are those particular to the combination only. For the properties of the components please consider, colecalciferol p. 788, calcium carbonate p. 733.

● **INDICATIONS AND DOSE**

Prevention and treatment of vitamin D and calcium deficiency

▶ BY MOUTH

▸ Child: Dosed according to the deficit or daily maintenance requirements (consult product literature)

● **UNLICENSED USE** *Adcal-D3*® and *Calceos*® are not licensed for use in children under 12 years. *Cacit*® D3, *Calcichew-D*$_3$® *Forte*, *Calcichew- D*$_3$® and *Kalcipos- D*® not licensed for use in children (age range not specified by manufacturers). *Accrete D3*® and *Natecal D3*® not licensed for use in children under 18 years.

● **INTERACTIONS** → Appendix 1: calcium compounds · vitamin D substances

● **PRESCRIBING AND DISPENSING INFORMATION** *Accrete D3*® contains calcium carbonate 1.5 g (calcium 600 mg or Ca^{2+} 15 mmol), colecalciferol 10 micrograms (400 units); *Adcal-D3*® tablets contain calcium carbonate 1.5 g (calcium 600 mg or Ca^{2+} 15 mmol), colecalciferol 10 micrograms (400 units); *Cacit*® *D3* contains calcium carbonate 1.25 g (calcium 500 mg or Ca^{2+} 12.5 mmol), colecalciferol 11 micrograms (440 units)/sachet; *Calceos*® contains calcium carbonate 1.25 g (calcium 500 mg or Ca^{2+} 12.5 mmol), colecalciferol 10 micrograms (400 units); *Calcichew-D3*® tablets contain calcium carbonate 1.25 g (calcium 500 mg or Ca^{2+} 12.5 mmol), colecalciferol 5 micrograms (200 units); *Calcichew-D3*® *Forte* tablets contain calcium carbonate 1.25 g (calcium 500 mg or Ca^{2+} 12.5 mmol), colecalciferol 10 micrograms (400 units); *Calcichew-D3*® 500 mg/400 unit caplets contain calcium carbonate (calcium 500 mg or Ca^{2+} 12.5 mmol), colecalciferol 10 micrograms (400 units); *Kalcipos-D*® contains calcium carbonate (calcium 500 mg or Ca^{2+} 12.5 mmol), colecalciferol 20 micrograms (800 units); *Natecal D3*® contains calcium carbonate 1.5 g (calcium 600 mg or Ca^{2+} 15 mmol), colecalciferol 10 micrograms (400 units); consult product literature for details of other available products.

Flavours of chewable and soluble forms may include orange, lemon, aniseed, peppermint, molasses, or tutti-frutti.

● **MEDICINAL FORMS** There can be variation in the licensing of different medicines containing the same drug.

Oral tablet

EXCIPIENTS: May contain Propylene glycol

▸ **Accrete D3** (Thornton & Ross Ltd)
Calcium carbonate 1.5 gram, Colecalciferol 400 unit Accrete D3 tablets | 60 tablet [P] £3.58 DT = £3.58

▸ **Adcal-D3** (Grunenthal Ltd)
Calcium carbonate 750 mg, Colecalciferol 200 unit Adcal-D3 750mg/200unit caplets | 112 tablet [P] £4.25 DT = £4.25

Effervescent granules

CAUTIONARY AND ADVISORY LABELS 13

▸ **Colecalciferol with calcium carbonate (Non-proprietary)**
Calcium carbonate 2.5 gram, Colecalciferol 880 unit Colecalciferol 880unit / Calcium carbonate 2.5g effervescent granules sachets | 24 sachet [PoM] [X]

▸ **Cacit D3** (Theramex HQ UK Ltd)
Calcium carbonate 1.25 gram, Colecalciferol 440 unit Cacit D3 effervescent granules sachets | 30 sachet [PoM] £4.06 DT = £4.06

Effervescent tablet

CAUTIONARY AND ADVISORY LABELS 13

▸ **AaCa D3** (TriOn Pharma Ltd)
Calcium carbonate 1.5 gram, Colecalciferol 400 unit AaCa D3 1.5g/400unit effervescent tablets sugar free | 56 tablet £4.97 [SF]

▸ **Adcal-D3** (Grunenthal Ltd)
Calcium carbonate 1.5 gram, Colecalciferol 400 unit Adcal-D3 Dissolve 1500mg/400unit effervescent tablets | 56 tablet [P] £6.74 DT = £6.74

▸ **SunVit-D3 (Colecalciferol + Calcium carbonate)** (SunVit-D3 Ltd)
Calcium carbonate 1.5 gram, Colecalciferol 400 unit SunVit-D3 400unit/1500mg effervescent tablets | 56 tablet £6.99 [SF]

Chewable tablet

CAUTIONARY AND ADVISORY LABELS 24

EXCIPIENTS: May contain Aspartame

▸ **Colecalciferol with calcium carbonate (Non-proprietary)**
Calcium carbonate 1.5 gram, Colecalciferol 400 unit Colecalciferol 400unit / Calcium carbonate 1.5g chewable tablets | 56 tablet [P] £5.12 DT = £5.12

▸ **A1-Cal D3** (TriOn Pharma Ltd)
Calcium carbonate 1.25 gram, Colecalciferol 400 unit A1-Cal D3 500mg/400unit chewable tablets sugar free | 60 tablet £3.49 [SF] | 100 tablet £4.98 [SF]

▸ **A1-Cal D3 Max** (TriOn Pharma Ltd)
Calcium carbonate 1.5 gram, Colecalciferol 400 unit A1-Cal D3 Max 600mg/400unit chewable tablets sugar free | 56 tablet £2.49 [SF] | 112 tablet £4.89 [SF]

▸ **AaCa D3** (TriOn Pharma Ltd)
Calcium carbonate 1.25 gram, Colecalciferol 200 unit AaCa D3 1.25g/200unit chewable tablets sugar free | 100 tablet £6.99 [SF]
Calcium carbonate 2.5 gram, Colecalciferol 800 unit AaCa D3 Plus 2.5g/800unit chewable tablets | 28 tablet £4.68 [SF]
Calcium carbonate 2.5 gram, Colecalciferol 1000 unit AaCa D3 Max 2.5g/1,000unit chewable tablets | 28 tablet £3.18 [SF]

- **AaceCa D3** (Essential-Healthcare Ltd)
  Calcium carbonate 1.25 gram, Colecalciferol 400 unit AaceCa D3 1250mg/400unit chewable tablets | 56 tablet £2.76 SF | 100 tablet £4.93 SF
  Calcium carbonate 1.5 gram, Colecalciferol 400 unit AaceCa D3 1500mg/400unit chewable tablets | 56 tablet £2.49 SF
- **Accrete D3 One a Day** (Thornton & Ross Ltd)
  Calcium carbonate 2.5 gram, Colecalciferol 880 unit Accrete D3 One a Day 1000mg/880unit chewable tablets | 30 tablet P £3.58 DT = £3.95
- **Adcal-D3** (Grunenthal Ltd)
  Calcium carbonate 1.5 gram, Colecalciferol 400 unit Adcal-D3 Lemon chewable tablets | 56 tablet P £5.12 DT = £5.12 | 112 tablet P £10.52
  Adcal-D3 chewable tablets tutti frutti | 56 tablet P £5.12 DT = £5.12 | 112 tablet P £10.52
- **Calceos** (Galen Ltd)
  Calcium carbonate 1.25 gram, Colecalciferol 400 unit Calceos 500mg/400unit chewable tablets | 60 tablet P £4.05 DT = £4.24
- **Calci-D** (Forum Health Products Ltd)
  Calcium carbonate 2.5 gram, Colecalciferol 1000 unit Calci-D 1000mg/1,000unit chewable tablets | 28 tablet P £3.48 DT = £3.48
- **Calcichew D3** (Forum Health Products Ltd)
  Calcium carbonate 1.25 gram, Colecalciferol 200 unit Calcichew D3 chewable tablets | 100 tablet P £7.68 DT = £7.68
  Calcium carbonate 2.5 gram, Colecalciferol 800 unit Calcichew D3 1000mg/800unit Once Daily chewable tablets | 30 tablet P £7.29 DT = £7.29
- **Calcichew D3 Forte** (Forum Health Products Ltd)
  Calcium carbonate 1.25 gram, Colecalciferol 400 unit Calcichew D3 Forte chewable tablets | 60 tablet P £4.24 DT = £4.24 | 100 tablet P £7.08
- **Evacal D3** (Teva UK Ltd)
  Calcium carbonate 1.5 gram, Colecalciferol 400 unit Evacal D3 1500mg/400unit chewable tablets | 56 tablet P £4.12 DT = £5.12 | 112 tablet P £8.25
- **Natecal** (Chiesi Ltd)
  Calcium carbonate 1.5 gram, Colecalciferol 400 unit Natecal D3 600mg/400unit chewable tablets | 60 tablet P £3.63
- **TheiCal-D3** (Stirling Anglian Pharmaceuticals Ltd)
  Calcium carbonate 2.5 gram, Colecalciferol 880 unit TheiCal-D3 1000mg/880unit chewable tablets | 30 tablet P £3.95 DT = £3.95

F 787

Ergocalciferol

20-Oct-2022

(Calciferol; Vitamin D_2)

● **INDICATIONS AND DOSE**

Primary prevention of vitamin D deficiency (if breastfed or formula-fed and consume less than 500mL formula per day)

▶ BY MOUTH
- Child up to 11 months: 340–400 units daily

Primary prevention of vitamin D deficiency

▶ BY MOUTH
- Child 1–17 years: 400 units daily

Treatment of vitamin D deficiency [Loading dose]

▶ BY MOUTH
- Child 1–5 months: 3000 units daily for 8 to 12 weeks, loading dosing may be given daily or the equivalent dose given intermittently e.g. weekly or fortnightly
- Child 6 months–11 years: 6000 units daily for 8 to 12 weeks, loading dosing may be given daily or the equivalent dose given intermittently e.g. weekly or fortnightly
- Child 12–17 years: 10 000 units daily for 8 to 12 weeks, loading dosing may be given daily or the equivalent dose given intermittently e.g. weekly or fortnightly. A single or divided loading dose totalling 300 000 units can be considered if there are concerns about compliance

Treatment of vitamin D deficiency [Maintenance dose]

▶ BY MOUTH
- Child 1 month–11 years: 400–600 units daily, maintenance to be started one month after loading dose completed, or if correction of vitamin D deficiency is less urgent, maintenance may be started without the use of loading doses
- Child 12–17 years: 400–600 units daily, maintenance dosing may be given daily or the equivalent dose given intermittently. Maintenance to be started one month after loading dose completed, or if correction of vitamin D deficiency is less urgent, maintenance may be started without the use of loading doses. Higher maintenance doses may be necessary in those at high risk of vitamin D deficiency; maximum 4000 units per day

Vitamin D deficiency caused by intestinal malabsorption or chronic liver disease (under expert supervision)

▶ BY INTRAMUSCULAR INJECTION
- Child 1–17 years: 300 000 units, to be given as a bolus dose in 2 divided doses, dose to be adjusted as necessary

DOSE EQUIVALENCE AND CONVERSION
- Ergocalciferol 400 units is equivalent to 10 micrograms; dose expressed as units.

● **UNLICENSED USE** EvGr Ergocalciferol is used in the doses provided in BNF publications, for the primary prevention and treatment of vitamin D deficiency, Ⓐ but these may differ from those licensed.

● **CAUTIONS** Take care to ensure correct dose in infants

● **INTERACTIONS** → Appendix 1: vitamin D substances

● **SIDE-EFFECTS**

▶ **Common or very common**
- With intramuscular use Hypoparathyroidism · pseudohypoparathyroidism

▶ **Rare or very rare**
- With intramuscular use Psychosis

▶ **Frequency not known**
- With intramuscular use Acidosis · albuminuria · azotaemia · bone pain · conjunctival deposit · drowsiness · hypercholesterolaemia · hypertension · hyperthermia · irritability · libido decreased · muscle weakness · nephrocalcinosis · pancreatitis · photophobia · polydipsia · rhinorrhoea · soft tissue calcification · taste metallic · urinary disorders · vascular calcification

● **MONITORING REQUIREMENTS**
- When used for Treatment of vitamin D deficiency EvGr Monitor plasma-25-hydroxyvitamin D concentration and bone profile after last loading dose. Ⓐ

● **PRESCRIBING AND DISPENSING INFORMATION** The BP directs that when calciferol is prescribed or demanded, colecalciferol or ergocalciferol should be dispensed or supplied.

When the strength of the tablets ordered or prescribed is not clear, the intention of the prescriber with respect to the strength (expressed in micrograms or milligrams per tablet) should be ascertained.

● **MEDICINAL FORMS** There can be variation in the licensing of different medicines containing the same drug. Forms available from special-order manufacturers include: oral tablet, oral capsule, oral suspension, oral solution, solution for injection

Oral tablet

- **Ergocalciferol (Non-proprietary)**
  Ergocalciferol 12.5 microgram Ergo-D2 12.5microgram tablets | 30 tablet ☒
- **AacErgo** (Essential-Healthcare Ltd)
  Ergocalciferol 12.5 microgram AacErgo 500unit tablets | 30 tablet £19.43
  Ergocalciferol 250 microgram AacErgo 10,000unit tablets | 30 tablet £29.83
- **Ergoral** (Cubic Pharmaceuticals Ltd)
  Ergocalciferol 250 microgram Ergoral D2 10,000unit tablets | 30 tablet £10.95

Solution for injection

▸ **Ergocalciferol (Non-proprietary)**

Ergocalciferol 300000 unit per 1 ml Ergocalciferol 300,000units/1ml solution for injection ampoules | 5 ampoule PoM £70.15 DT = £70.15

Ergocalciferol 400000 unit per 1 ml Sterogyl 15H 600,000units/1.5ml solution for injection ampoules | 1 ampoule PoM ⊠

Oral capsule

▸ **Ergocalciferol (Non-proprietary)**

Ergocalciferol 1.25 mg Ergo-D2 1.25mg capsules | 30 capsule £96.80

▸ **AacErgo** (Essential-Healthcare Ltd)

Ergocalciferol 1.25 mg AacErgo 50,000unit capsules | 10 capsule £23.41

▸ **Eciferol** (Fontus Health Ltd)

Ergocalciferol 1.25 mg Eciferol D2 50,000unit capsules | 10 capsule £39.99

Oral solution

▸ **Ergocalciferol (Non-proprietary)**

Ergocalciferol 1500 unit per 1 ml Uvesterol D 1,500units/ml oral solution | 20 ml PoM ⊠ SF

▸ **Eciferol** (Fontus Health Ltd)

Ergocalciferol 3000 unit per 1 ml Eciferol D2 3,000units/ml liquid | 60 ml £95.00 DT = £36.70

Ergocalciferol with calcium lactate and calcium phosphate

28-Jun-2023

(Calcium and vitamin D)

The properties listed below are those particular to the combination only. For the properties of the components please consider, ergocalciferol p. 792, calcium lactate p. 736, calcium phosphate p. 736.

● **INDICATIONS AND DOSE**

Prevention of calcium and vitamin D deficiency | Treatment of calcium and vitamin D deficiency

▸ BY MOUTH

▸ Child: (consult product literature)

● **UNLICENSED USE** Calcium and Ergocalciferol tablets not licensed for use in children under 6 years.

● **INTERACTIONS** → Appendix 1: calcium compounds · vitamin D substances

● **DIRECTIONS FOR ADMINISTRATION** Manufacturer advises tablets may be crushed before administration, or may be chewed.

● **PRESCRIBING AND DISPENSING INFORMATION** Each tablet contains calcium lactate 300 mg, calcium phosphate 150 mg (calcium 97 mg or Ca^{2+} 2.4 mmol), ergocalciferol 10 micrograms (400 units).

● **PATIENT AND CARER ADVICE** Patient or carers should be given advice on how to administer calcium and ergocalciferol tablets.

● **MEDICINAL FORMS** There can be variation in the licensing of different medicines containing the same drug.

Oral tablet

▸ **A1 Cal-E** (TriOn Pharma Ltd)

Ergocalciferol 10 microgram, Calcium phosphate 150 mg, Calcium lactate 300 mg A1 Cal-E tablets | 28 tablet £7.41 DT = £4.26

▸ **Acteos** (MaN Pharma Ltd)

Ergocalciferol 10 microgram, Calcium phosphate 150 mg, Calcium lactate 300 mg Acteos tablets | 28 tablet £7.43 DT = £4.26

▸ **CalciErgo** (Essential-Healthcare Ltd)

Ergocalciferol 10 microgram, Calcium phosphate 150 mg, Calcium lactate 300 mg CalciErgo tablets | 28 tablet £7.41 DT = £4.26

F 787

Paricalcitol

27-Oct-2022

● **INDICATIONS AND DOSE**

Prevention and treatment of secondary hyperparathyroidism associated with chronic kidney disease

▸ BY MOUTH

▸ Child 10–17 years: (consult product literature)

● **INTERACTIONS** → Appendix 1: vitamin D substances

● **SIDE-EFFECTS**

▸ **Common or very common** Electrolyte imbalance

▸ **Uncommon** Breast tenderness · dizziness · gastrointestinal discomfort · gastrooesophageal reflux disease · hypoparathyroidism · malaise · muscle spasms · pain · palpitations · peripheral oedema · pneumonia · taste altered

▸ **Frequency not known** Angioedema · laryngeal oedema

● **PREGNANCY** Manufacturer advises avoid—toxicity in *animal* studies.

● **BREAST FEEDING** Manufacturer advises avoid—no information available.

● **MONITORING REQUIREMENTS** EvGr Monitor plasma-calcium, phosphate and parathyroid hormone concentration regularly, particularly at initiation of treatment and during dose titration. ⟨M⟩

● **MEDICINAL FORMS** There can be variation in the licensing of different medicines containing the same drug.

Oral capsule

EXCIPIENTS: May contain Ethanol

▸ **Zemplar** (AbbVie Ltd)

Paricalcitol 1 microgram Zemplar 1microgram capsules | 28 capsule PoM £69.44 DT = £69.44

Paricalcitol 2 microgram Zemplar 2microgram capsules | 28 capsule PoM £138.88 DT = £138.88

VITAMINS AND TRACE ELEMENTS > VITAMIN E

Alpha tocopherol

04-Feb-2021

(Tocopherol)

● **INDICATIONS AND DOSE**

Vitamin E deficiency because of malabsorption in congenital or hereditary chronic cholestasis

▸ BY MOUTH USING ORAL SOLUTION

▸ Neonate: 17 mg/kg daily, dose to be adjusted as necessary.

▸ Child: 17 mg/kg daily, dose to be adjusted as necessary

● **CONTRA-INDICATIONS** Preterm neonates

● **CAUTIONS** Predisposition to thrombosis

● **INTERACTIONS** → Appendix 1: vitamin E substances

● **SIDE-EFFECTS**

▸ **Common or very common** Diarrhoea

▸ **Uncommon** Alopecia · asthenia · headache · skin reactions

▸ **Frequency not known** Abdominal pain

● **PREGNANCY** Manufacturer advises caution, no evidence of harm in *animal* studies.

● **BREAST FEEDING** Manufacturer advises use only if potential benefit outweighs risk—no information available.

● **HEPATIC IMPAIRMENT** Manufacturer advises caution.

● **RENAL IMPAIRMENT** Manufacturer advises caution. Risk of renal toxicity due to polyethylene glycol content.
Monitoring Manufacturer advises monitor closely in renal impairment.

- **PRESCRIBING AND DISPENSING INFORMATION** Tocofersolan is a water-soluble form of D-alpha tocopherol.

- **MEDICINAL FORMS** There can be variation in the licensing of different medicines containing the same drug.

Oral solution

- **Vedrop** (Recordati Rare Diseases UK Ltd) ▼
  D-alpha tocopherol (as Tocofersolan) 50 mg per 1 ml Vedrop 50mg/ml oral solution | 60 ml PoM £163.65 SF

9 Blood and nutrition

Alpha tocopheryl acetate

04-Feb-2021

(Tocopherol)

- **INDICATIONS AND DOSE**

Vitamin E deficiency

▶ BY MOUTH

- Neonate: 10 mg/kg once daily.
- Child: 2–10 mg/kg daily, increased if necessary up to 20 mg/kg daily

Malabsorption in cystic fibrosis

▶ BY MOUTH

- Child 1-11 months: 50 mg once daily, dose to be adjusted as necessary, to be taken with food and pancreatic enzymes
- Child 1-11 years: 100 mg once daily, dose to be adjusted as necessary, to be taken with food and pancreatic enzymes
- Child 12-17 years: 100–200 mg once daily, dose to be adjusted as necessary, to be taken with food and pancreatic enzymes

Vitamin E deficiency in cholestasis and severe liver disease

▶ BY MOUTH

- Neonate: 10 mg/kg daily.
- Child 1 month-11 years: Initially 100 mg daily, adjusted according to response, increased if necessary up to 200 mg/kg daily
- Child 12-17 years: Initially 200 mg daily, adjusted according to response, increased if necessary up to 200 mg/kg daily

▶ BY INTRAMUSCULAR INJECTION

- Neonate: 10 mg/kg once a month.
- Child: 10 mg/kg once a month (max. per dose 100 mg)

Malabsorption in abetalipoproteinaemia

▶ BY MOUTH

- Neonate: 100 mg/kg once daily.
- Child: 50–100 mg/kg once daily

- **CAUTIONS** Increased risk of necrotising enterocolitis in neonate weighing less than 1.5 kg or in a preterm neonate · predisposition to thrombosis
- **INTERACTIONS** → Appendix 1: vitamin E substances
- **SIDE-EFFECTS** Abdominal pain (more common at high doses) · bleeding tendency · diarrhoea (more common at high doses) · increased risk of thrombosis
- **PREGNANCY** No evidence of safety of high doses.
- **BREAST FEEDING** Excreted in milk; minimal risk, although caution with large doses.
- **MONITORING REQUIREMENTS** Increased bleeding tendency in vitamin-K deficient patients or those taking anticoagulants (prothrombin time and INR should be monitored).
- **DIRECTIONS FOR ADMINISTRATION** Consider dilution of oral suspension for use in neonates due to high osmolality.
- **MEDICINAL FORMS** There can be variation in the licensing of different medicines containing the same drug. Forms available from special-order manufacturers include: chewable tablet, solution for injection

Solution for injection

- **Alpha tocopheryl acetate (Non-proprietary)**
  Alpha tocopheryl acetate 50 mg per 1 ml E-Vicotrat 100mg/2ml solution for injection ampoules | 10 ampoule PoM ⊠

Oral suspension

EXCIPIENTS: May contain Sucrose

- **Alpha tocopheryl acetate (Non-proprietary)**
  Alpha tocopheryl acetate 100 mg per 1 ml AlphaToc-E 500mg/5ml oral suspension | 100 ml £47.19 SF
  Alpha tocopheryl acetate 500mg/5ml oral suspension | 100 ml GSL £76.81–£84.49 DT = £84.49

Oral capsule

- **Alpha tocopheryl acetate (Non-proprietary)**
  Alpha tocopherol 400 unit Vitamin E 400unit capsules | 30 capsule £2.68
- **AlphaToc-E** (Essential-Healthcare Ltd)
  Alpha tocopherol 75 unit AlphaToc-E 75unit capsules | 100 capsule £5.83
  Alpha tocopherol 200 unit AlphaToc-E 200unit capsules | 100 capsule £12.93
  Alpha tocopherol 400 unit AlphaToc-E 400unit capsules | 100 capsule £19.82
- **E-Caps** (Ennogen Healthcare International Ltd)
  Alpha tocopherol 75 unit E-Caps 75unit capsules | 100 capsule £109.50
  Alpha tocopherol 100 unit E-Caps 100unit capsules | 30 capsule £84.40
  Alpha tocopherol 200 unit E-Caps 200unit capsules | 30 capsule £89.50
  Alpha tocopherol 400 unit E-Caps 400unit capsules | 30 capsule £128.50
  Alpha tocopherol 1000 unit E-Caps 1,000unit capsules | 30 capsule £130.20
- **Nutra-E** (TriOn Pharma Ltd)
  Alpha tocopherol 75 unit Nutra-E 75unit capsules | 100 capsule £5.86
  Alpha tocopherol 200 unit Nutra-E 200unit capsules | 100 capsule £12.88
  Alpha tocopherol 400 unit Nutra-E 400unit capsules | 100 capsule £19.82
- **Vita-E** (Typharm Ltd)
  Alpha tocopherol 75 unit Vita-E 75unit capsules | 100 capsule £9.65
  Alpha tocopherol 200 unit Vita-E 200unit capsules | 30 capsule £7.38 | 100 capsule £20.69
  Alpha tocopherol 400 unit Vita-E 400unit capsules | 30 capsule £11.03 | 100 capsule £30.16

Chewable tablet

- **Alpha-E** (TriOn Pharma Ltd)
  Alpha tocopheryl acetate 100 mg Alpha-E 100mg chewable tablets | 30 tablet £37.25
- **AlphaToc-E** (Essential-Healthcare Ltd)
  Alpha tocopheryl acetate 100 mg AlphaToc-E 100mg chewable tablets | 30 tablet £29.67
- **E-Tabs** (Ennogen Healthcare International Ltd)
  Alpha tocopheryl acetate 100 mg E-Tabs 100mg chewable tablets | 30 tablet £87.30
- **Ephynal** (Imported (Italy))
  Alpha tocopheryl acetate 100 mg Ephynal 100mg chewable tablets | 30 tablet ⊠

VITAMINS AND TRACE ELEMENTS › VITAMIN K

Menadiol sodium phosphate

24-May-2021

- **INDICATIONS AND DOSE**

Supplementation in vitamin K malabsorption

▶ BY MOUTH

- Child 1-11 years: 5–10 mg daily, dose to be adjusted as necessary
- Child 12-17 years: 10–20 mg daily, dose to be adjusted as necessary

- **CONTRA-INDICATIONS** Infants · neonates

- **CAUTIONS** G6PD deficiency (risk of haemolysis) · vitamin E deficiency (risk of haemolysis)
- **PREGNANCY** Avoid in late pregnancy and labour unless benefit outweighs risk of neonatal haemolytic anaemia, hyperbilirubinaemia, and kernicterus in neonate.

- **MEDICINAL FORMS** There can be variation in the licensing of different medicines containing the same drug.

Oral tablet

▸ Menadiol sodium phosphate (Non-proprietary)
Menadiol phosphate (as Menadiol sodium phosphate)
10 mg Menadiol 10mg tablets | 100 tablet [P] £273.42 DT = £273.42

Phytomenadione 15-Apr-2026
(Vitamin K_1)

- **INDICATIONS AND DOSE**

Neonatal prophylaxis of vitamin-K deficiency bleeding
▶ BY INTRAMUSCULAR INJECTION
▸ Preterm neonate: 400 micrograms/kg for 1 dose (max. per dose 1 mg), to be given at birth, the intravenous route may be used in preterm neonates with very low birth-weight if intramuscular injection is not possible, however, it may not provide the prolonged protection of the intramuscular injection, any neonate receiving intravenous vitamin-K should be given subsequent oral doses.
▸ Neonate: 1 mg for 1 dose, to be given at birth.

Neonatal hypoprothrombinaemia | Vitamin-K deficiency bleeding
▶ BY INTRAVENOUS INJECTION
▸ Neonate: 1 mg every 8 hours as required.

Neonatal biliary atresia and liver disease
▶ BY MOUTH
▸ Neonate: 1 mg daily.

Reversal of coumarin anticoagulation when continued anticoagulation required or if no significant bleeding—seek specialist advice
▶ BY INTRAVENOUS INJECTION
▸ Child: 15–30 micrograms/kg for 1 dose (max. per dose 1 mg), dose may be repeated as necessary

Reversal of coumarin anticoagulation when anticoagulation not required or if significant bleeding—seek specialist advice | Treatment of haemorrhage associated with vitamin-K deficiency—seek specialist advice
▶ BY INTRAVENOUS INJECTION
▸ Child: 250–300 micrograms/kg for 1 dose (max. per dose 10 mg)

KONAKION® MM PAEDIATRIC

Neonatal prophylaxis of vitamin-K deficiency bleeding in healthy babies who are not at risk of bleeding disorders
▶ BY MOUTH
▸ Neonate: Initially 2 mg for 1 dose, to be given at birth, then 2 mg for 1 dose, to be given at 4–7 days of age.

Neonatal prophylaxis of vitamin-K deficiency bleeding in healthy babies who are not at risk of bleeding disorders (exclusively breast fed babies)
▶ BY MOUTH
▸ Neonate: Initially 2 mg for 1 dose, to be given at birth, then 2 mg for 1 dose, to be given at 4–7 days of age, then 2 mg for 1 dose, to be given at 1 month of age.

NEOKAY®

Neonatal prophylaxis of vitamin-K deficiency bleeding in healthy babies who are not at particular risk of bleeding disorders
▶ BY MOUTH
▸ Neonate: 1 mg for 1 dose, to be given at birth (to protect from the risk of vitamin-K deficiency bleeding in the first week).

Neonatal prophylaxis of vitamin-K deficiency bleeding in healthy babies who are not at particular risk of bleeding disorders (exclusively breast-fed babies)
▶ BY MOUTH
▸ Neonate: Initially 1 mg for 1 dose, to be given at birth, then 1 mg every week for 12 weeks.

- **CAUTIONS** Intravenous injections should be given very slowly—reports of anaphylactoid reactions

KONAKION® MM PAEDIATRIC
▸ With intravenous use Parenteral administration in premature infant or neonate of less than 2.5 kg (increased risk of kernicterus)

- **PREGNANCY** Use if potential benefit outweighs risk.
- **BREAST FEEDING** Present in milk.
- **HEPATIC IMPAIRMENT**

KONAKION® MM Manufacturer advises caution—monitor INR in patients with severe impairment (contains glycocholic acid which may displace bilirubin).

- **DIRECTIONS FOR ADMINISTRATION**

▸ With oral use in neonates Manufacturer advises contents of one capsule should be administered by cutting the narrow tubular tip off and squeezing the liquid contents into the mouth; if the baby spits out the dose or is sick within three hours of administration a replacement dose should be given.

KONAKION® MM *Konakion® MM* may be administered by slow intravenous injection or by intravenous infusion in glucose 5%; **not** for intramuscular injection.

KONAKION® MM PAEDIATRIC *Konakion® MM Paediatric* may be administered *by mouth* or *by intramuscular injection* or *by intravenous injection*. For *intravenous injection*, expert sources advise may be diluted with Glucose 5% if necessary.

- **MEDICINAL FORMS** There can be variation in the licensing of different medicines containing the same drug. Forms available from special-order manufacturers include: oral capsule, oral suspension, oral solution

Solution for injection

EXCIPIENTS: May contain Glycocholic acid, lecithin

▸ Phytomenadione (Non-proprietary)
Phytomenadione 10 mg per 1 ml Phytomenadione 2mg/0.2ml solution for injection ampoules | 5 ampoule [PoM] £11.49 DT = £11.01
Phytomenadione 10mg/1ml solution for injection ampoules | 10 ampoule [PoM] £11.49 DT = £11.01

7.1 Neural tube defects (prevention in pregnancy)

Neural tube defects (prevention in pregnancy)

01-Oct-2021

Description of condition

Neural tube defects represent a group of congenital defects, caused by incomplete closure of the neural tube within 28 days of conception. The most common forms are anencephaly, spina bifida and encephalocele.

The main risk factors are maternal folate deficiency, maternal vitamin B_{12} deficiency, previous history of having an infant with a neural tube defect, smoking, diabetes, obesity, and use of antiepileptic drugs. For information on smoking cessation see Smoking cessation p. 353.

Prevention in pregnancy

EvGr Pregnant women or women who wish to become pregnant should be advised to take supplementation with folic acid p. 710 before conception and until week 12 of pregnancy.

A higher daily dose (see folic acid) is recommended for women at a high risk of conceiving a child with a neural tube defect, including women who have previously had an infant with a neural tube defect, who are receiving antiepileptic medication (see Epilepsy p. 227), or who have diabetes or sickle-cell disease. (A)

Healthy Start vitamins for women (containing folic acid, ascorbic acid, and vitamin D) are available for pregnant women through the Healthy Start scheme. For further information, see www.healthystart.nhs.uk/. Vitamins for children are also available through the scheme.

Useful Resources

Fertility problems: assessment and treatment. National Institute for Health and Care Excellence. Clinical guideline 156. February 2013.
www.nice.org.uk/guidance/cg156

Chapter 10
Musculoskeletal system

CONTENTS

1 Arthritis

Juvenile idiopathic arthritis 16-Apr-2021

Overview

Management of juvenile idiopathic arthritis requires symptomatic treatment to relieve pain, swelling, and stiffness, together with treatment to control and suppress disease activity. Treatment options include Non-steroidal anti-inflammatory drugs p. 816 (NSAIDs), a disease modifying anti-rheumatic drug (DMARD) such as methotrexate p. 672 or a cytokine modulator, and intra-articular, intravenous, or oral corticosteroids. For further information, see Rheumatic disease, suppressing drugs below and Corticosteroids, inflammatory disorders p. 829.

Rheumatic disease, suppressing drugs 14-Oct-2022

Overview

Certain drugs, such as methotrexate p. 672, cytokine modulators, and sulfasalazine p. 35 [unlicensed], are used to suppress the disease process in *juvenile idiopathic arthritis* (juvenile chronic arthritis); these drugs are known as disease-modifying antirheumatic drugs (DMARDs). In children, DMARDs should be used under specialist supervision.

Some children with juvenile idiopathic arthritis do not require DMARDs. Methotrexate is effective in juvenile idiopathic arthritis; sulfasalazine [unlicensed] is an alternative but should be avoided in *systemic-onset juvenile idiopathic arthritis*. Gold and penicillamine are no longer used. Cytokine modulators have a role in some forms of *juvenile idiopathic arthritis*.

Unlike NSAIDs, DMARDs can affect the progression of disease but they may require 3–6 months of treatment for a full therapeutic response. Response to a DMARD may allow the dose of the NSAID to be reduced.

DMARDs can improve not only the symptoms of inflammatory joint disease but also extra-articular manifestations. They reduce the erythrocyte sedimentation rate and C-reactive protein.

Antimalarials

The antimalarial hydroxychloroquine sulfate p. 798 is rarely used to treat juvenile idiopathic arthritis.
Hydroxychloroquine sulfate can also be useful for systemic or discoid lupus erythematosus, particularly involving the skin and joints, and in sarcoidosis.

Retinopathy rarely occurs provided that the recommended doses are not exceeded.

Mepacrine hydrochloride is used on rare occasions to treat discoid lupus erythematosus [unlicensed].

Drugs affecting the immune response

Methotrexate, given as a once weekly dose, is the DMARD of choice in the treatment of juvenile idiopathic arthritis and also has a role in juvenile dermatomyositis, vasculitis, uveitis, systemic lupus erythematosus, localised scleroderma, and sarcoidosis; for these indications it is given by the subcutaneous, oral, or rarely, the intramuscular route. Absorption from intramuscular or subcutaneous routes may be more predictable than from the oral route; if the oral route is ineffective subcutaneous administration is generally preferred. Folic acid may reduce mucosal or gastro-intestinal side-effects of methotrexate. The dosage regimen for folic acid p. 710 has not been established—in children over 2 years a weekly dose [unlicensed], may be given on a different day from the methotrexate.

Azathioprine p. 638 may be used in children for vasculitis which has failed to respond to other treatments, for the management of severe cases of *systemic lupus erythematosus* and other connective tissue disorders, in conjunction with corticosteroids for patients with severe or progressive renal disease, and in cases of *polymyositis* which are resistant to corticosteroids. Azathioprine has a corticosteroid-sparing effect in patients whose corticosteroid requirements are excessive.

Ciclosporin p. 640 is rarely used in juvenile idiopathic arthritis, connective tissue diseases, vasculitis, and uveitis; it may be considered if the condition has failed to respond to other treatments.

Cytokine modulators

Cytokine modulators should be used under specialist supervision.

Adalimumab p. 806, etanercept p. 808, and infliximab p. 39 inhibit the activity of tumour necrosis factor alpha (TNF-α). Adalimumab can be used for the management of active polyarticular juvenile idiopathic arthritis and enthesitis-related arthritis. Etanercept is licensed for the treatment of the following subtypes of juvenile idiopathic arthritis: polyarticular juvenile idiopathic arthritis in children who have had an inadequate response to methotrexate or who cannot tolerate it, oligoarthritis in children who have had an inadequate response to methotrexate or who cannot tolerate it, psoriatic arthritis in children over 12 years who have had an inadequate response to methotrexate or cannot tolerate it, and enthesitis-related arthritis in children over 12 years who have had an inadequate response to conventional therapy or cannot tolerate it. Infliximab has been used in refractory polyarticular juvenile idiopathic arthritis [unlicensed] when other treatments, such as etanercept, have failed.

Abatacept p. 805 prevents the full activation of T-lymphocytes; it can be used for the management of active polyarticular juvenile idiopathic arthritis. Abatacept is not recommended for use in combination with TNF inhibitors.

Canakinumab p. 646 inhibits the activity of interleukin-1 beta (IL-1β) and is licensed for the treatment of active systemic juvenile idiopathic arthritis in children over 2 years, when there has been an inadequate response to NSAIDs and systemic corticosteroids.

Tocilizumab p. 800 antagonises the actions of interleukin-6; it can be used for the management of active systemic juvenile idiopathic arthritis when there has been an inadequate response to NSAIDs and systemic corticosteroids and polyarticular juvenile idiopathic arthritis when there has been an inadequate response to methotrexate. Tocilizumab can be used in combination with methotrexate, or as monotherapy if methotrexate is not tolerated or is contra-indicated. Tocilizumab is not recommended for use with other cytokine modulators.

Tofacitinib p. 803 inhibits the Janus-associated tyrosine kinases JAK1 and JAK3 and may be used for the treatment of active polyarticular juvenile idiopathic arthritis and juvenile psoriatic arthritis in certain children.

Anakinra p. 799 inhibits the activity of interleukin-1 and may be used for the treatment of systemic juvenile idiopathic arthritis in certain children.

Sulfasalazine

Sulfasalazine [unlicensed] has a beneficial effect in suppressing the inflammatory activity associated with some forms of juvenile idiopathic arthritis; it is generally not used in systemic-onset disease.

Other drugs used for Arthritis Diclofenac potassium, p. 817 · Diclofenac sodium, p. 818 · Etoricoxib, p. 820 · Flurbiprofen, p. 820 · Ibuprofen, p. 821 · Indometacin, p. 824 · Meloxicam, p. 826 · Naproxen, p. 826 · Piroxicam, p. 828

DISEASE-MODIFYING ANTI-RHEUMATIC DRUGS

Hydroxychloroquine sulfate

16-Apr-2025

● **INDICATIONS AND DOSE**

Active rheumatoid arthritis (including juvenile idiopathic arthritis) (administered on expert advice) | Systemic and discoid lupus erythematosus (administered on expert advice) | Dermatological conditions caused or aggravated by sunlight (administered on expert advice)

▶ BY MOUTH

▶ Child: 5–6.5 mg/kg once daily (max. per dose 400 mg), dose given based on ideal body-weight

IMPORTANT SAFETY INFORMATION

MHRA/CHM ADVICE: HYDROXYCHLOROQUINE, CHLOROQUINE: INCREASED RISK OF CARDIOVASCULAR EVENTS WHEN USED WITH MACROLIDE ANTIBIOTICS; REMINDER OF PSYCHIATRIC REACTIONS (FEBRUARY 2022)

An observational study has shown that co-administration of azithromycin with hydroxychloroquine in patients with rheumatoid arthritis was associated with an increased risk of cardiovascular events (including angina or chest pain and heart failure) and mortality. Healthcare professionals are reminded to consider the benefits and risks of co-prescribing systemic azithromycin, or other systemic macrolides, with hydroxychloroquine. If such use cannot be avoided, caution is recommended in patients with risk factors for cardiac events and they should be advised to seek urgent medical attention if any signs or symptoms develop.

A European safety review has reported that psychiatric reactions associated with hydroxychloroquine (including rare cases of suicidal behaviour) typically occurred within the first month of treatment; events have been reported in patients with no history of psychiatric disorders. Healthcare professionals are reminded to be vigilant for psychiatric reactions, and counsel patients and carers to seek medical advice if any new or worsening mental health symptoms develop.

● **CAUTIONS** Acute porphyrias p. 745 · diabetes (may lower blood glucose) · G6PD deficiency · maculopathy · may aggravate myasthenia gravis · may exacerbate psoriasis · neurological disorders (especially in those with a history of epilepsy—may lower seizure threshold) · severe gastro-intestinal disorders

● **INTERACTIONS** → Appendix 1: hydroxychloroquine

● **SIDE-EFFECTS**

▶ **Common or very common** Abdominal pain · appetite decreased · diarrhoea · headache · mood altered · nausea · skin reactions · vision disorders · vomiting

▶ **Uncommon** Alopecia · anxiety · corneal oedema · dizziness · eye disorders · hair colour changes · neuromuscular dysfunction · retinopathy · seizure · tinnitus · vertigo

▶ **Frequency not known** Acute hepatic failure · agranulocytosis · anaemia · angioedema · bone marrow disorders · bronchospasm · cardiac conduction disorders · cardiomyopathy · confusion · delusions · depression · hallucination · hearing loss · hypoglycaemia · leucopenia · movement disorders · muscle weakness · myopathy · photosensitivity reaction · psychiatric disorder · psychosis · QT interval prolongation · reflexes absent · severe cutaneous adverse reactions (SCARs) · sleep disorder · suicidal behaviour · thrombocytopenia · tremor · ventricular hypertrophy

Overdose Hydroxychloroquine is very toxic in overdosage; overdosage is extremely hazardous and difficult to treat. Urgent advice from the National Poisons Information Service is essential. Life-threatening features include arrhythmias (which can have a very rapid onset) and convulsions (which can be intractable).

● **PREGNANCY** EvGr Hydroxychloroquine is the antimalarial drug of choice in females with rheumatic disease planning a pregnancy, and may be continued during pregnancy. (A)

● **BREAST FEEDING** EvGr May be used during breast-feeding. (A) EvGr Present in milk in very small amounts—very long plasma half-life increases risk of accumulation in the infant, however no adverse effects reported with longer term use. Although adverse effects are unlikely, monitor infant for irritability, insomnia, skin reactions, vomiting, diarrhoea, poor feeding, and adequate weight gain. Avoid in infants with G6PD deficiency, hyperbilirubinaemia, or jaundice (risk of haemolytic anaemia and kernicterus). (E)

● **HEPATIC IMPAIRMENT** Manufacturer advises caution.

Dose adjustments Manufacturer advises consider dose adjustment in severe impairment.

● **RENAL IMPAIRMENT** EvGr Caution—monitor plasma-hydroxychloroquine concentration in severe impairment. (M)

Dose adjustments EvGr Consider dose adjustment in severe impairment. (M)

● **MONITORING REQUIREMENTS** A review group convened by the Royal College of Ophthalmologists has updated guidelines on monitoring for chloroquine and hydroxychloroquine retinopathy (*Hydroxychloroquine and Chloroquine Retinopathy: Recommendations on Monitoring*

2020). There are no reports of hydroxychloroquine retinopathy in patients under the age of 18 years, or evidence for monitoring paediatric patients for drug toxicity. However, the guideline recommends long-term users of hydroxychloroquine under the age of 18 years who otherwise satisfy the monitoring criteria should be referred for monitoring.

- **PRESCRIBING AND DISPENSING INFORMATION** To avoid excessive dosage in obese patients, the dose of hydroxychloroquine should be calculated on the basis of ideal body-weight.

- **MEDICINAL FORMS** There can be variation in the licensing of different medicines containing the same drug. Forms available from special-order manufacturers include: oral suspension, oral solution

Oral tablet

CAUTIONARY AND ADVISORY LABELS 21

- Hydroxychloroquine sulfate (Non-proprietary)
  - **Hydroxychloroquine sulfate 200 mg** Hydroxychloroquine 200mg tablets 60 tablet PoM £8.64 DT = £1.87
  - **Hydroxychloroquine sulfate 300 mg** Hydroxychloroquine 300mg tablets 30 tablet PoM £18.69 DT = £18.69
- Quinoric (Bristol Laboratories Ltd)
  - **Hydroxychloroquine sulfate 200 mg** Quinoric 200mg tablets | 60 tablet PoM DT = £1.87

IMMUNOSUPPRESSANTS › INTERLEUKIN INHIBITORS

Anakinra

04-May-2021

- **INDICATIONS AND DOSE**

Cryopyrin-associated periodic syndromes (specialist use only)

▶ BY SUBCUTANEOUS INJECTION

- Child 3 months–17 years (body-weight 10 kg and above): 1–2 mg/kg daily, for severe cryopyrin-associated periodic syndromes, usual maintenance is 3–4 mg/kg daily, up to a maximum of 8 mg/kg daily

Still's disease (specialist use only)

▶ BY SUBCUTANEOUS INJECTION

- Child 8 months–17 years (body-weight 10–49 kg): 1–2 mg/kg daily, increased if necessary up to 4 mg/kg daily
- Child 8 months–17 years (body-weight 50 kg and above): 100 mg daily, increased if necessary up to 4 mg/kg daily

- **CONTRA-INDICATIONS** Active infection · neutropenia (absolute neutrophil count less than 1.5×10^9/litre)—do not initiate · pre-existing malignancy
- **CAUTIONS** History of asthma (increased risk of serious infection) · history of recurrent infection · predisposition to infection
- **INTERACTIONS** → Appendix 1: anakinra
- **SIDE-EFFECTS**
  - **Common or very common** Headache · infection · neutropenia · thrombocytopenia
  - **Uncommon** Skin reactions
  - **Frequency not known** Hepatitis

  SIDE-EFFECTS, FURTHER INFORMATION Neutropenia reported commonly—discontinue if neutropenia develops.
- **PREGNANCY** Manufacturer advises avoid.
- **BREAST FEEDING** Manufacturer advises avoid—no information available.
- **HEPATIC IMPAIRMENT** Manufacturer advises caution in severe impairment.
- **RENAL IMPAIRMENT** Manufacturer advises caution in moderate impairment.

  Dose adjustments Manufacturer advises consider alternate day dosing in severe impairment.
- **PRE-TREATMENT SCREENING** Manufacturer advises patients should be screened for latent tuberculosis and viral hepatitis prior to initiation of treatment.
- **MONITORING REQUIREMENTS**
  - Manufacturer advises monitor neutrophil count before treatment, then every month for 6 months, then every 3 months thereafter.
  - When used for Cryopyrin-associated periodic syndromes Manufacturer advises monitor for CNS inflammation (including ear and eye tests) 3 months after starting treatment, then every 6 months until effective treatment doses have been identified, then yearly thereafter.
  - When used for Still's disease Manufacturer advises consider routine monitoring of hepatic enzymes during the first month of treatment.
- **PRESCRIBING AND DISPENSING INFORMATION** The manufacturer of *Kineret*® has provided a *Guide for Healthcare Professionals*.
- **PATIENT AND CARER ADVICE**

  Blood disorders Patients should be instructed to seek medical advice if symptoms suggestive of neutropenia (such as fever, sore throat, bruising or, bleeding) develop.
  - When used for Still's disease A patient card and patient booklet should be provided.
  - When used for Cryopyrin-associated periodic syndromes A patient booklet should be provided.
- **NATIONAL FUNDING/ACCESS DECISIONS**

  For full details see funding body website

  NICE decisions
  - **Anakinra for treating Still's disease (March 2021)** NICE TA685 Recommended with restrictions

  Scottish Medicines Consortium (SMC) decisions
  - **Anakinra (*Kineret*®) for the treatment of Still's disease, as monotherapy or in combination with other anti-inflammatory drugs and disease-modifying antirheumatic drugs (October 2018)** SMC No. SMC2104 Recommended

- **MEDICINAL FORMS** There can be variation in the licensing of different medicines containing the same drug.

Solution for injection

- Kineret (Swedish Orphan Biovitrum Ltd)
  - **Anakinra 150 mg per 1 ml** Kineret 100mg/0.67ml solution for injection pre-filled syringes | 7 pre-filled disposable injection PoM £183.61

Secukinumab

05-Mar-2024

- **DRUG ACTION** Secukinumab is a recombinant human monoclonal antibody that selectively binds to cytokine interleukin-17A (IL-17A) and inhibits the release of proinflammatory cytokines and chemokines.

- **INDICATIONS AND DOSE**

Plaque psoriasis (under expert supervision)

▶ BY SUBCUTANEOUS INJECTION

- Child 6–17 years (body-weight up to 50 kg): 75 mg every week for 5 doses, then maintenance 75 mg every month, review treatment if no response within 16 weeks of initial dose
- Child 6–17 years (body-weight 50 kg and above): 150 mg every week for 5 doses, then maintenance 150 mg every month, dose may be increased to 300 mg according to clinical response. Review treatment if no response within 16 weeks of initial dose

Enthesitis-related arthritis (under expert supervision) | Juvenile psoriatic arthritis (under expert supervision)

▶ BY SUBCUTANEOUS INJECTION

- Child 6–17 years (body-weight up to 50 kg): 75 mg every week for 5 doses, then maintenance 75 mg every month, review treatment if no response within 16 weeks of initial dose

continued →

- Child 6-17 years (body-weight 50 kg and above): 150 mg every week for 5 doses, then maintenance 150 mg every month, review treatment if no response within 16 weeks of initial dose

- **CONTRA-INDICATIONS** Severe active infection
- **CAUTIONS** Chronic infection · history of recurrent infection · inflammatory bowel disease (discontinue if signs or symptoms develop, or an exacerbation occurs) · predisposition to infection (discontinue if new serious infection develops)

CAUTIONS, FURTHER INFORMATION
- Tuberculosis EvGr Anti-tuberculosis therapy should be considered before starting secukinumab in patients with latent tuberculosis. ⟨M⟩
- Immunisation EvGr Children should receive all appropriate immunisations before starting treatment. ⟨M⟩

- **INTERACTIONS** → Appendix 1: monoclonal antibodies
- **SIDE-EFFECTS**
  - **Common or very common** Diarrhoea · fatigue · headache · increased risk of infection · nausea · rhinorrhoea
  - **Uncommon** Conjunctivitis · inflammatory bowel disease · neutropenia (usually mild and reversible) · skin reactions
  - **Rare or very rare** Anaphylactic reaction · hypersensitivity vasculitis
  - **Frequency not known** Pyoderma gangrenosum
- **CONCEPTION AND CONTRACEPTION** Manufacturer advises that women of childbearing potential should use effective contraception during treatment and for at least 20 weeks after stopping treatment.
- **PREGNANCY** Manufacturer advises avoid—no information available.
- **BREAST FEEDING** Manufacturer advises avoid during treatment and for up to 20 weeks after discontinuing treatment—no information available.
- **DIRECTIONS FOR ADMINISTRATION** Take syringe or pen out of the refrigerator and allow to reach room temperature before administration—consult product literature. Avoid injecting into areas of the skin that show psoriasis. Patients may self-administer *Cosentyx*® after appropriate training in subcutaneous injection technique.
- **PRESCRIBING AND DISPENSING INFORMATION** Secukinumab is a biological medicine. Biological medicines must be prescribed and dispensed by brand name, see *Biological medicines* and *Biosimilar medicines*, under Guidance on prescribing p. 1; EvGr record the brand name and batch number after each administration. ⟨M⟩
- **HANDLING AND STORAGE** Store in a refrigerator (2–8°C) and protect from light. Once removed from refrigerator, may be stored at room temperature (below 30°C) for up to 4 days.
- **PATIENT AND CARER ADVICE**
  Self-administration Patients and their carers should be given training in subcutaneous injection technique.
  Infection Patients and their carers should be advised to seek immediate medical attention if symptoms of infection develop during treatment with secukinumab.
- **NATIONAL FUNDING/ACCESS DECISIONS**
  For full details see funding body website

NICE decisions
- **Secukinumab for treating moderate to severe plaque psoriasis in children and young people (October 2021)** NICE TA734 Recommended with restrictions

- **MEDICINAL FORMS** There can be variation in the licensing of different medicines containing the same drug.

Solution for injection

EXCIPIENTS: May contain Polysorbates
- **Cosentyx** (Novartis Pharmaceuticals UK Ltd)
  Secukinumab 150 mg per 1 ml Cosentyx 150mg/1ml solution for injection pre-filled pens | 2 pre-filled disposable injection PoM £1,218.78 (Hospital only)
  Cosentyx 150mg/1ml solution for injection pre-filled syringes | 2 pre-filled disposable injection PoM £1,218.78 (Hospital only)
  Cosentyx 300mg/2ml solution for injection pre-filled pens | 1 pre-filled disposable injection PoM £1,218.78 (Hospital only)
  Cosentyx 75mg/0.5ml solution for injection pre-filled syringes | 1 pre-filled disposable injection PoM £304.70 (Hospital only)

Tocilizumab

04-Mar-2026

- **DRUG ACTION** Tocilizumab is a recombinant humanised monoclonal antibody that binds to interleukin-6 receptors thereby blocking the activity of pro-inflammatory cytokines.

- **INDICATIONS AND DOSE**

Systemic juvenile idiopathic arthritis (initiated by a specialist)

▶ BY INTRAVENOUS INFUSION
- Child 2-17 years (body-weight up to 30 kg): 12 mg/kg every 2 weeks, for dose adjustments in patients with liver enzyme abnormalities, or low absolute neutrophil or platelet count—consult product literature, review treatment if no improvement within 6 weeks
- Child 2-17 years (body-weight 30 kg and above): 8 mg/kg every 2 weeks, for dose adjustments in patients with liver enzyme abnormalities, or low absolute neutrophil or platelet count— consult product literature, review treatment if no improvement within 6 weeks

▶ BY SUBCUTANEOUS INJECTION
- Child 1-17 years (body-weight 10-30 kg): 162 mg every 2 weeks, administer to abdomen, thigh or upper arm, for dose adjustments in patients with liver enzyme abnormalities, or low absolute neutrophil or platelet count—consult product literature, review treatment if no improvement within 12 weeks
- Child 1-17 years (body-weight 30 kg and above): 162 mg once weekly, administer to abdomen, thigh or upper arm, for dose adjustments in patients with liver enzyme abnormalities, or low absolute neutrophil or platelet count—consult product literature, review treatment if no improvement within 12 weeks

Polyarticular juvenile idiopathic arthritis (initiated by a specialist)

▶ BY INTRAVENOUS INFUSION
- Child 2-17 years (body-weight up to 30 kg): 10 mg/kg every 4 weeks, for dose adjustments in patients with liver enzyme abnormalities, or low absolute neutrophil or platelet count— consult product literature, review treatment if no improvement within 12 weeks
- Child 2-17 years (body-weight 30 kg and above): 8 mg/kg every 4 weeks, for dose adjustments in patients with liver enzyme abnormalities, or low absolute neutrophil or platelet count—consult product literature, review treatment if no improvement within 12 weeks

▶ BY SUBCUTANEOUS INJECTION
- Child 2-17 years (body-weight up to 30 kg): 162 mg every 3 weeks, administer to abdomen, thigh or upper arm, for dose adjustments in patients with liver enzyme abnormalities, or low absolute neutrophil or platelet count—consult product literature, review treatment if no improvement within 12 weeks
- Child 2-17 years (body-weight 30 kg and above): 162 mg every 2 weeks, administer to abdomen, thigh or upper arm, for dose adjustments in patients with liver

enzyme abnormalities, or low absolute neutrophil or platelet count—consult product literature, review treatment if no improvement within 12 weeks

Cytokine release syndrome (initiated by a specialist)

▶ BY INTRAVENOUS INFUSION

▸ Child 2–17 years (body-weight up to 30 kg): 12 mg/kg (max. per dose 800 mg), if no improvement in symptoms after the first dose, up to 3 additional doses may be administered. The interval between the infusions should be at least 8 hours

▸ Child 2–17 years (body-weight 30 kg and above): 8 mg/kg (max. per dose 800 mg), if no improvement in symptoms after the first dose, up to 3 additional doses may be administered. The interval between the infusions should be at least 8 hours

IMPORTANT SAFETY INFORMATION

MHRA/CHM ADVICE: TOCILIZUMAB (*ROACTEMRA®*): RARE RISK OF SERIOUS LIVER INJURY INCLUDING CASES REQUIRING TRANSPLANTATION (JULY 2019)

There have been reports of rare but serious cases of drug-induced liver injury, including acute liver failure and hepatitis, in patients treated with tocilizumab; some cases required liver transplantation. Serious liver injury was reported from 2 weeks to more than 5 years after initiation of tocilizumab. Healthcare professionals are advised to initiate tocilizumab treatment with caution in patients with active hepatic disease or hepatic impairment. Patients and their carers should be advised to seek immediate medical attention if signs and symptoms of liver injury, such as tiredness, abdominal pain, and jaundice, occur. For further information see *Cautions*, *Contra-indications* and *Monitoring requirements*.

● **CONTRA-INDICATIONS**

GENERAL CONTRA-INDICATIONS Severe active infection

SPECIFIC CONTRA-INDICATIONS

▸ When used for Systemic juvenile idiopathic arthritis or Polyarticular juvenile idiopathic arthritis Do not initiate if hepatic enzymes more than 5 times the upper limit of normal · do not initiate in patients not previously treated with *RoActemra®* if absolute neutrophil count less than 2×10^9/litre

● **CAUTIONS**

▸ When used for Systemic juvenile idiopathic arthritis or Polyarticular juvenile idiopathic arthritis Hepatic enzymes more than 1.5 times the upper limit of normal · history of diverticulitis · history of intestinal ulceration · history of recurrent or chronic infection (interrupt treatment if serious infection occurs) · low absolute neutrophil count (discontinue treatment if neutrophil count less than 0.5×10^9/litre) · platelet count less than 100×10^3/microlitre (discontinue treatment if platelet count less than 50×10^3/microlitre) · predisposition to infection (interrupt treatment if serious infection occurs)

CAUTIONS, FURTHER INFORMATION

▸ Tuberculosis

▸ When used for Systemic juvenile idiopathic arthritis or Polyarticular juvenile idiopathic arthritis EvGr Patients with latent tuberculosis should be treated with standard therapy before starting tocilizumab. ⓜ

● **INTERACTIONS** → Appendix 1: monoclonal antibodies

● **SIDE-EFFECTS**

▶ **Common or very common** Abdominal pain · conjunctivitis · cough · diarrhoea · dizziness · dyslipidaemia · dyspnoea · gastrointestinal disorders · headache · hypersensitivity · hypertension · hypofibrinogenaemia · increased risk of infection · infusion related reaction · leucopenia · nausea · neutropenia · oral disorders · peripheral oedema · skin reactions · weight increased

▶ **Uncommon** Hypothyroidism · nephrolithiasis

▶ **Rare or very rare** Hepatic disorders · Stevens-Johnson syndrome

▶ **Frequency not known** Sepsis

● **CONCEPTION AND CONTRACEPTION** Effective contraception required during and for 3 months after treatment.

● **PREGNANCY** Manufacturer advises avoid unless essential—toxicity in *animal* studies.

● **BREAST FEEDING** Specialist sources indicate use with caution. Monitor breast-fed infants for adequate feeding, fever, frequent infections, diarrhoea, or unusual behaviour.

● **HEPATIC IMPAIRMENT** Manufacturer advises caution—consult product literature.

● **RENAL IMPAIRMENT**

▸ With intravenous use Manufacturer advises monitor renal function closely in moderate-to-severe impairment—no information available.

▸ With subcutaneous use Manufacturer advises monitor renal function closely in severe impairment—no information available.

● **PRE-TREATMENT SCREENING**

Tuberculosis

▸ When used for Systemic juvenile idiopathic arthritis or Polyarticular juvenile idiopathic arthritis Patients should be evaluated for tuberculosis before treatment.

● **MONITORING REQUIREMENTS**

▸ When used for Systemic juvenile idiopathic arthritis or Polyarticular juvenile idiopathic arthritis EvGr Monitor lipid profile 4–8 weeks after starting treatment and then as indicated. Monitor for demyelinating disorders. Monitor hepatic transaminases before starting treatment, every 4–8 weeks for first 6 months of treatment, then every 12 weeks thereafter. Monitor neutrophil and platelet count before starting treatment, at the time of the second dose, and then as indicated. ⓜ

● **DIRECTIONS FOR ADMINISTRATION** For *intravenous infusion*, manufacturer advises for body-weight less than 30 kg, give intermittently in Sodium chloride 0.9%, dilute requisite dose to a volume of 50 mL with infusion fluid and give over 1 hour; body-weight 30 kg or greater, give intermittently in Sodium chloride 0.9%, dilute requisite dose to a volume of 100 mL with infusion fluid and give over 1 hour.

For *subcutaneous injection*, manufacturer advises rotate injection site and avoid skin that is tender, damaged or scarred. Patients may self-administer *RoActemra®*, after appropriate training in subcutaneous injection technique.

● **PRESCRIBING AND DISPENSING INFORMATION** Tocilizumab is a biological medicine. Biological medicines must be prescribed and dispensed by brand name, see *Biological medicines* and *Biosimilar medicines*, under Guidance on prescribing p. 1; record the brand name and batch number after each administration.

RoActemra® solution for injection pre-filled pen is not suitable for children under 12 years of age—consult product literature for further information.

● **HANDLING AND STORAGE** Manufacturer advises protect from light and store in a refrigerator (2–8 °C)—consult product literature for further information regarding storage conditions outside refrigerator and after preparation of the infusion.

● **PATIENT AND CARER ADVICE** Patients and carers should be advised to seek immediate medical attention if symptoms of infection occur, or if symptoms of diverticular perforation such as abdominal pain, haemorrhage, or fever accompanying change in bowel habits occur.

An alert card and patient information brochure highlighting important safety information should be provided.

Missed doses

▸ With subcutaneous use If an injection administered once every 2 weeks or once every 3 weeks is missed and it is within 7 days of the scheduled dose, it should be administered as soon as possible and the next dose taken at the normal time.

Driving and skilled tasks Patients and carers should be counselled on the effects on driving and performance of skilled tasks—increased risk of dizziness.

● **NATIONAL FUNDING/ACCESS DECISIONS**
For full details see funding body website

NICE decisions

▸ **Tocilizumab for the treatment of systemic juvenile idiopathic arthritis (December 2011)** NICE TA238 Recommended with restrictions

▸ **Abatacept, adalimumab, etanercept and tocilizumab for treating juvenile idiopathic arthritis (December 2015)** NICE TA373 Recommended with restrictions

● **MEDICINAL FORMS** There can be variation in the licensing of different medicines containing the same drug.

Solution for injection

EXCIPIENTS: May contain Polysorbates

▸ **Avtozma** (Celltrion Healthcare UK Ltd) ▼
Tocilizumab 180 mg per 1 ml Avtozma 162mg/0.9ml solution for injection pre-filled syringes | 4 pre-filled disposable injection PoM £821.00 (Hospital only)
Avtozma 162mg/0.9ml solution for injection pre-filled pens | 4 pre-filled disposable injection PoM £821.00 (Hospital only)

▸ **RoActemra** (Roche Products Ltd)
Tocilizumab 180 mg per 1 ml RoActemra 162mg/0.9ml solution for injection pre-filled syringes | 4 pre-filled disposable injection PoM £913.12 (Hospital only)
RoActemra 162mg/0.9ml solution for injection pre-filled pens | 4 pre-filled disposable injection PoM £913.12

▸ **Tyenne** (Fresenius Kabi Ltd) ▼
Tocilizumab 180 mg per 1 ml Tyenne 162mg/0.9ml solution for injection pre-filled pens | 4 pre-filled disposable injection PoM £821.81 (Hospital only)
Tyenne 162mg/0.9ml solution for injection pre-filled syringes | 4 pre-filled disposable injection PoM £821.81 (Hospital only)

Solution for infusion

EXCIPIENTS: May contain Polysorbates
ELECTROLYTES: May contain Sodium

▸ **Avtozma** (Celltrion Healthcare UK Ltd) ▼
Tocilizumab 20 mg per 1 ml Avtozma 200mg/10ml concentrate for solution for infusion vials | 1 vial PoM £230.00 (Hospital only)
Avtozma 400mg/20ml concentrate for solution for infusion vials | 1 vial PoM £460.00 (Hospital only)
Avtozma 80mg/4ml concentrate for solution for infusion vials | 1 vial PoM £92.00 (Hospital only)

▸ **RoActemra** (Roche Products Ltd)
Tocilizumab 20 mg per 1 ml RoActemra 400mg/20ml concentrate for solution for infusion vials | 1 vial PoM £512.00 (Hospital only)
RoActemra 200mg/10ml concentrate for solution for infusion vials | 1 vial PoM £256.00 (Hospital only)
RoActemra 80mg/4ml concentrate for solution for infusion vials | 1 vial PoM £102.40 (Hospital only)

▸ **Tyenne** (Fresenius Kabi Ltd) ▼
Tocilizumab 20 mg per 1 ml Tyenne 400mg/20ml concentrate for solution for infusion vials | 1 vial PoM £460.80 (Hospital only)
Tyenne 200mg/10ml concentrate for solution for infusion vials | 1 vial PoM £230.40 (Hospital only)
Tyenne 80mg/4ml concentrate for solution for infusion vials | 1 vial PoM £92.16 (Hospital only)

IMMUNOSUPPRESSANTS › JAK INHIBITORS

Baricitinib

16-Apr-2025

● **DRUG ACTION** Baricitinib selectively and reversibly inhibits the Janus-associated tyrosine kinases JAK1 and JAK2.

● **INDICATIONS AND DOSE**

Atopic eczema (initiated by a specialist)

▸ BY MOUTH

▸ Child 2–17 years (body-weight 10–29 kg): 2 mg once daily, consider discontinuation of treatment if no response after 8 weeks, for dose adjustments due to clinical response or treatment interruption due to side-effects—consult product literature

▸ Child 2–17 years (body-weight 30 kg and above): 4 mg once daily, consider discontinuation of treatment if no response after 8 weeks, for dose adjustments due to clinical response or treatment interruption due to side-effects—consult product literature

Enthesitis-related arthritis (initiated by a specialist) | Polyarticular juvenile idiopathic arthritis (initiated by a specialist) | Juvenile psoriatic arthritis (initiated by a specialist)

▸ BY MOUTH

▸ Child 2–17 years (body-weight 10–29 kg): 2 mg once daily, consider discontinuation of treatment if no response after 12 weeks

▸ Child 2–17 years (body-weight 30 kg and above): 4 mg once daily, consider discontinuation of treatment if no response after 12 weeks

IMPORTANT SAFETY INFORMATION

MHRA/CHM ADVICE: BARICITINIB (*OLUMIANT*®): RISK OF VENOUS THROMBOEMBOLISM (MARCH 2020)

Clinical trial data have shown that baricitinib is associated with an increased frequency of venous thromboembolism (VTE) compared with placebo. Healthcare professionals are advised to use baricitinib with caution in patients with additional risk factors for VTE. Patients should be informed of the signs and symptoms of VTE before starting treatment and advised to seek urgent medical attention if these develop. Baricitinib should be permanently discontinued if clinical features of VTE occur.

MHRA/CHM ADVICE: BARICITINIB (*OLUMIANT*®): INCREASED RISK OF DIVERTICULITIS, PARTICULARLY IN PATIENTS WITH RISK FACTORS (AUGUST 2020)

A European review of worldwide data concluded that baricitinib is associated with an increased risk of diverticulitis. The MHRA recommends healthcare professionals use baricitinib with caution in patients with pre-existing diverticular disease, and in patients on long-term concomitant medicines associated with an increased risk of diverticulitis (including NSAIDs, corticosteroids, and opioids). Patients should be advised to seek immediate medical attention if they experience severe abdominal pain especially accompanied with fever, nausea and vomiting, or other symptoms of diverticulitis. Prompt evaluation is needed of any patients treated with baricitinib who present with new-onset abdominal signs and symptoms to identify early diverticulitis or gastro-intestinal perforation.

MHRA/CHM ADVICE: JANUS KINASE (JAK) INHIBITORS: NEW MEASURES TO REDUCE RISKS OF MAJOR CARDIOVASCULAR EVENTS, MALIGNANCY, VENOUS THROMBOEMBOLISM, SERIOUS INFECTIONS AND INCREASED MORTALITY (APRIL 2023)

In 2022, the EMA conducted a review of all JAK inhibitors indicated for chronic inflammatory diseases and concluded that the risks associated with the use of tofacitinib could be considered a class effect (see

Important safety information in tofacitinib below). Following a further review by the MHRA, some existing warnings for tofacitinib have been updated and implemented for all JAK inhibitors included in the review, such as baricitinib.

Healthcare professionals are advised to:
- avoid use in patients who are current or past long-time smokers, and in patients with other cardiovascular disease or malignancy risk factors, unless there are no suitable alternatives;
- use with caution in patients with risk factors for VTE;
- use lower doses in patients with risk factors, where applicable;
- periodically examine all patients' skin for malignancy;
- inform patients and their carers of these risks, and the signs and symptoms that warrant urgent medical attention.

● **CONTRA-INDICATIONS** Absolute lymphocyte count less than 0.5 × 10^9 cells/litre (do not initiate) · absolute neutrophil count less than 1 × 10^9 cells/litre (do not initiate) · haemoglobin less than 8 g/dL (do not initiate) · tuberculosis (active)

● **CAUTIONS** Active, chronic, or recurrent infection (interrupt treatment if no response to standard therapy) · history of atherosclerotic cardiovascular disease or other cardiovascular risk factors · risk factors for deep-vein thrombosis or pulmonary embolism · risk factors for malignancy · risk of diverticulitis · risk of viral reactivation (consult product literature)

CAUTIONS, FURTHER INFORMATION
- Tuberculosis EvGr Consider anti-tuberculosis therapy prior to initiation of baricitinib in patients with previously untreated latent tuberculosis. ⓜ
- Immunisation EvGr Patients should receive all recommended vaccinations before starting treatment; live vaccines are not recommended immediately before, or during, treatment. ⓜ

● **INTERACTIONS** → Appendix 1: baricitinib

● **SIDE-EFFECTS**
- **Common or very common** Abdominal pain · dyslipidaemia · embolism and thrombosis · headache · herpes zoster (interrupt treatment) · increased risk of infection · nausea · neutropenia · skin reactions · thrombocytosis
- **Uncommon** Facial swelling · weight increased
- **Frequency not known** Cardiovascular event · gastrointestinal perforation · hypersensitivity (discontinue) · malignancy · neoplasms · reactivation of infections

● **CONCEPTION AND CONTRACEPTION** Manufacturer advises effective contraception during and for at least 1 week after treatment in women of child-bearing potential.

● **PREGNANCY** EvGr Avoid (toxicity in *animal* studies). ⓜ

● **BREAST FEEDING** EvGr Avoid (present in milk in *animal* studies). ⓜ

● **HEPATIC IMPAIRMENT** Manufacturer advises avoid in severe impairment (no information available).

● **RENAL IMPAIRMENT** EvGr Avoid if creatinine clearance less than 30 mL/minute. ⓜ

Dose adjustments EvGr Use 50% of normal dose if creatinine clearance 30–60 mL/minute. ⓜ See p. 16.

● **PRE-TREATMENT SCREENING** Manufacturer advises patients should be evaluated for tuberculosis and viral hepatitis before treatment.

● **MONITORING REQUIREMENTS**
- EvGr Monitor patients with hepatitis B surface antibody and hepatitis B core antibody, without hepatitis B surface antigen, for expression of hepatitis B virus (HBV) DNA—if HBV DNA detected, consult liver specialist for advice.
- Monitor lipid profile 12 weeks after treatment initiation—hyperlipidaemia should be managed according to international clinical guidelines; monitor hepatic transaminases routinely—interrupt treatment if drug-induced liver injury suspected.
- Monitor for haematological abnormalities; interrupt treatment if absolute neutrophil count less than 1 × 10^9 cells/litre, absolute lymphocyte count less than 0.5 × 10^9 cells/litre, or haemoglobin less than 8 g/dL—treatment may be restarted when levels return above these values.
- Periodic skin examination is recommended in all patients, particularly those at increased risk of skin cancer. ⓜ

● **DIRECTIONS FOR ADMINISTRATION** EvGr In patients unable to swallow tablets whole, Eli Lilly tablets may be dispersed in 5-10 mL of water by gently swirling—consult product literature for details. ⓜ

● **PRESCRIBING AND DISPENSING INFORMATION** The manufacturer has provided guides for healthcare professionals.

● **PATIENT AND CARER ADVICE** Patients or their carers should be given advice on how to administer Eli Lilly tablets if they are unable to swallow tablets whole.

Alert card A patient alert card should be provided.

● **MEDICINAL FORMS** There can be variation in the licensing of different medicines containing the same drug.

Oral tablet

EXCIPIENTS: May contain Lecithin

▸ **Baricitinib (Non-proprietary)**

Baricitinib 2 mg Baricitinib 2mg tablets | 28 tablet PoM £805.56 DT = £805.56

Baricitinib 4 mg Baricitinib 4mg tablets | 28 tablet PoM £805.56 DT = £805.56

Tofacitinib

10-Nov-2023

● **DRUG ACTION** Tofacitinib selectively inhibits the Janus-associated tyrosine kinases JAK1 and JAK3.

● **INDICATIONS AND DOSE**

Polyarticular juvenile idiopathic arthritis (specialist use only) | Juvenile psoriatic arthritis (specialist use only)

▸ BY MOUTH USING ORAL SOLUTION
- Child 2–17 years (body-weight 10–19 kg): 3.2 mg twice daily, consider treatment discontinuation if no response 18 weeks after initial dose, for dose interruption or treatment discontinuation due to side-effects—consult product literature

▸ BY MOUTH USING ORAL SOLUTION
- Child 2–17 years (body-weight 20–39 kg): 4 mg twice daily, consider treatment discontinuation if no response 18 weeks after initial dose, for dose interruption or treatment discontinuation due to side-effects—consult product literature

▸ BY MOUTH USING FILM-COATED TABLETS, OR BY MOUTH USING ORAL SOLUTION
- Child 2–17 years (body-weight 40 kg and above): 5 mg twice daily, consider treatment discontinuation if no response 18 weeks after initial dose, for dose interruption or treatment discontinuation due to side-effects—consult product literature

DOSE ADJUSTMENTS DUE TO INTERACTIONS
- EvGr Reduce total daily dose by half with concurrent use of potent CYP3A4 inhibitors, or concurrent use of a moderate CYP3A4 inhibitor and a potent CYP2C19

continued →

10 Musculoskeletal system

inhibitor, or concurrent use of drugs which are both moderate CYP3A4 and potent CYP2C19 inhibitors. (M)

IMPORTANT SAFETY INFORMATION

MHRA/CHM ADVICE: TOFACITINIB (*XELJANZ*®): NEW MEASURES TO MINIMISE RISK OF VENOUS THROMBOEMBOLISM AND OF SERIOUS AND FATAL INFECTIONS (MARCH 2020)

New recommendations have been issued following a European safety review that found a dose-dependent increased risk of serious venous thromboembolism (VTE) associated with tofacitinib. Healthcare professionals are advised to use tofacitinib with caution in any patients with known risk factors for VTE, in addition to the underlying disease. The recommended daily dose of tofacitinib should not be exceeded— *see Indications and dose*. Patients and carers should be informed of the signs and symptoms of VTE before starting treatment and advised to seek urgent medical attention if these develop. Tofacitinib should be permanently discontinued if signs of VTE occur.

Tofacitinib was also found to increase the risk of serious and fatal infections.

MHRA/CHM ADVICE: TOFACITINIB (*XELJANZ*®): NEW MEASURES TO MINIMISE RISK OF MAJOR ADVERSE CARDIOVASCULAR EVENTS AND MALIGNANCIES (OCTOBER 2021)

Data from a clinical trial of patients with rheumatoid arthritis and at least one cardiovascular risk factor showed an increased incidence of major adverse cardiovascular events and malignancies, particularly lung cancer and lymphoma (excluding non-melanoma skin cancer), when comparing tofacitinib with tumour necrosis factor alpha inhibitors. Healthcare professionals are advised to inform patients and carers of the risks associated with tofacitinib treatment and should only use tofacitinib in patients who are current or past smokers, patients with other cardiovascular risk factors (such as diabetes or coronary artery disease), and patients with other malignancy risk factors if no suitable alternatives are available.

MHRA/CHM ADVICE: JANUS KINASE (JAK) INHIBITORS: NEW MEASURES TO REDUCE RISKS OF MAJOR CARDIOVASCULAR EVENTS, MALIGNANCY, VENOUS THROMBOEMBOLISM, SERIOUS INFECTIONS AND INCREASED MORTALITY (APRIL 2023)

In 2022, the EMA conducted a review of all JAK inhibitors indicated for chronic inflammatory diseases and concluded that the risks associated with the use of tofacitinib could be considered a class effect. Following a further review by the MHRA, some existing warnings for tofacitinib have been updated and implemented for all JAK inhibitors included in the review.

Healthcare professionals are advised to:

- avoid use in patients who are current or past long-time smokers, and in patients with other cardiovascular disease or malignancy risk factors, unless there are no suitable alternatives;
- use with caution in patients with risk factors for VTE;
- use lower doses in patients with risk factors, where applicable;
- periodically examine all patients' skin for malignancy;
- inform patients and their carers of these risks, and the signs and symptoms that warrant urgent medical attention.

10

Musculoskeletal system

- **CONTRA-INDICATIONS** Absolute lymphocyte count less than 750 cells/mm³ (do not initiate) · absolute neutrophil count less than 1200 cells/mm³ (do not initiate) · active infection including localised infection · active tuberculosis · haemoglobin less than 10 g/dL (do not initiate)
- **CAUTIONS** History of atherosclerotic cardiovascular disease or other cardiovascular risk factors · known risk factors for fractures · patients at risk of gastro-intestinal perforation (new onset abdominal signs and symptoms should be evaluated promptly) · predisposition to infection · raised serum transaminases (particularly in combination with potentially hepatotoxic drugs) · recurrent infection or history of serious infection · risk factors for malignancy · risk factors for venous thromboembolism (VTE) · risk of diverticulitis · risk of viral reactivation (consult product literature) · tuberculosis exposure

CAUTIONS, FURTHER INFORMATION

- ▸ **Immunisation** EvGr Patients should receive all recommended vaccinations before starting treatment (consider prophylactic varicella zoster vaccination); live vaccines should be given at least 2 weeks, but preferably 4 weeks, before treatment initiation—consult product literature. (M)
- ▸ **Tuberculosis** EvGr Anti-tuberculosis therapy should be initiated in patients with latent tuberculosis before starting tofacitinib. Consider anti-tuberculosis therapy prior to initiation of tofacitinib in patients with a history of previously untreated latent or active tuberculosis or in patients at risk of tuberculosis infection. Use tofacitinib with caution in patients who have travelled or resided in areas of endemic mycoses, or who have had previous exposure to tuberculosis. (M)

- **INTERACTIONS** → Appendix 1: tofacitinib
- **SIDE-EFFECTS**
- ▸ **Common or very common** Abdominal pain (more common in patients with juvenile idiopathic arthritis) · anaemia · cough (more common in patients with juvenile idiopathic arthritis) · diarrhoea · dyspepsia · fatigue · fever (more common in patients with juvenile idiopathic arthritis) · gastrointestinal disorders · headache (more common in patients with juvenile idiopathic arthritis) · hypertension · increased risk of infection · influenza (more common in patients with juvenile idiopathic arthritis) · joint disorders · nausea (more common in patients with juvenile idiopathic arthritis) · peripheral oedema · pharyngitis (more common in patients with juvenile idiopathic arthritis) · sinusitis (more common in patients with juvenile idiopathic arthritis) · skin reactions · vomiting (more common in patients with juvenile idiopathic arthritis)
- ▸ **Uncommon** Decreased leucocytes · dehydration · dyslipidaemia · dyspnoea · embolism and thrombosis · hepatic steatosis · insomnia · ligament sprain · muscle strain · musculoskeletal pain · myocardial infarction · neoplasms · neutropenia · paraesthesia · sinus congestion · tendinitis · viral infection (more common in patients with juvenile idiopathic arthritis) · weight increased
- ▸ **Rare or very rare** Meningitis · sepsis
- ▸ **Frequency not known** Angioedema · BK virus infection · cardiovascular event · epidural empyema · interstitial lung disease (including fatal cases) · limb abscess · malignancy · reactivation of infections · ulcerative colitis aggravated
- **CONCEPTION AND CONTRACEPTION** Manufacturer advises effective contraception during and for at least 4 weeks after treatment in women of child-bearing potential.
- **PREGNANCY** Manufacturer advises avoid—toxicity in *animal* studies.
- **BREAST FEEDING** Manufacturer advises avoid—present in milk in *animal* studies.
- **HEPATIC IMPAIRMENT** Manufacturer advises caution in moderate impairment; avoid in severe impairment.
  Dose adjustments Manufacturer advises dose reduction in moderate impairment—consult product literature.
- **RENAL IMPAIRMENT**
  Dose adjustments Manufacturer advises reduce dose in severe impairment—consult product literature.
- **PRE-TREATMENT SCREENING** Manufacturer advises patients should be evaluated for tuberculosis and viral hepatitis before treatment.

- **MONITORING REQUIREMENTS**
- EvGr Monitor for signs and symptoms of infection during and after treatment.
- Monitor liver function routinely; monitor lipid profile 8 weeks after treatment initiation.
- Monitor lymphocytes at baseline and every 3 months thereafter; neutrophils and haemoglobin should be monitored at baseline, after 4 to 8 weeks of treatment and every 3 months thereafter.
- Periodic skin examination is recommended in all patients, particularly those at increased risk of skin cancer. ⟨M⟩
- **DIRECTIONS FOR ADMINISTRATION** EvGr *Xeljanz® film-coated tablets* may be crushed and taken with water. *Xeljanz® oral solution* should be administered with the reusable oral syringe provided. ⟨M⟩
- **PRESCRIBING AND DISPENSING INFORMATION** The manufacturer of *Xeljanz®* has provided a *Prescriber Brochure*, *Initiation Checklist*, and *Maintenance Checklist*.
- **PATIENT AND CARER ADVICE** Patients or their carers should be given advice on how to administer *Xeljanz® oral solution*. Any unused portion must be discarded 60 days after opening.
Alert card A patient alert card should be provided.
- **NATIONAL FUNDING/ACCESS DECISIONS**
For full details see funding body website

NICE decisions
- **Tofacitinib for treating juvenile idiopathic arthritis [and juvenile psoriatic arthritis] (October 2021) NICE TA735** Recommended with restrictions

- **MEDICINAL FORMS** There can be variation in the licensing of different medicines containing the same drug.

Oral tablet
- **Xeljanz** (Pfizer Ltd)
Tofacitinib (as Tofacitinib citrate) 5 mg Xeljanz 5mg tablets | 56 tablet PoM £690.03 (Hospital only)
Tofacitinib (as Tofacitinib citrate) 10 mg Xeljanz 10mg tablets | 56 tablet PoM £1,380.06 (Hospital only)

Oral solution
EXCIPIENTS: May contain Propylene glycol
- **Xeljanz** (Pfizer Ltd)
Tofacitinib (as Tofacitinib citrate) 1 mg per 1 ml Xeljanz 1mg/ml oral solution | 240 ml PoM £591.40 (Hospital only) SF

IMMUNOSUPPRESSANTS › T-CELL ACTIVATION INHIBITORS

Abatacept
10-Aug-2021

- **INDICATIONS AND DOSE**

Moderate-to-severe active polyarticular juvenile idiopathic arthritis (specialist use only)
- BY INTRAVENOUS INFUSION
- Child 6–17 years (body-weight up to 75 kg): 10 mg/kg every 2 weeks for 3 doses, then 10 mg/kg every 4 weeks, review treatment if no response within 6 months
- Child 6–17 years (body-weight 75–100 kg): 750 mg every 2 weeks for 3 doses, then 750 mg every 4 weeks, review treatment if no response within 6 months
- Child 6–17 years (body-weight 101 kg and above): 1 g every 2 weeks for 3 doses, then 1 g every 4 weeks, review treatment if no response within 6 months

Moderate-to-severe active polyarticular juvenile idiopathic arthritis (specialist use only)
- BY SUBCUTANEOUS INJECTION
- Child 2–17 years (body-weight 10–24 kg): 50 mg once weekly, review treatment if no response within 6 months
- Child 2–17 years (body-weight 25–49 kg): 87.5 mg once weekly, review treatment if no response within 6 months
- Child 2–17 years (body-weight 50 kg and above): 125 mg once weekly, review treatment if no response within 6 months

- **CONTRA-INDICATIONS** Severe infection
- **CAUTIONS** Children should be brought up to date with current immunisation schedule before initiating therapy · do not initiate until active infections are controlled · predisposition to infection (screen for latent tuberculosis and viral hepatitis) · progressive multifocal leucoencephalopathy (discontinue treatment if neurological symptoms present)
- **INTERACTIONS** → Appendix 1: abatacept
- **SIDE-EFFECTS**
- **Common or very common** Asthenia · cough · diarrhoea · dizziness · gastrointestinal discomfort · headaches · hypertension · increased risk of infection · nausea · oral ulceration · skin reactions · vomiting
- **Uncommon** Alopecia · anxiety · arrhythmias · arthralgia · bruising tendency · conjunctivitis · depression · dry eye · dyspnoea · gastritis · hyperhidrosis · hypotension · influenza like illness · leucopenia · menstrual cycle irregularities · neoplasms · pain in extremity · palpitations · paraesthesia · respiratory disorders · sepsis · sleep disorders · throat tightness · thrombocytopenia · vasculitis · vasodilation · vertigo · visual acuity decreased · weight increased
- **Rare or very rare** Pelvic inflammatory disease
- **CONCEPTION AND CONTRACEPTION** Effective contraception required during treatment and for 14 weeks after last dose.
- **PREGNANCY** Manufacturer advises avoid unless essential.
- **BREAST FEEDING** Present in milk in *animal* studies—manufacturer advises avoid breast-feeding during treatment and for 14 weeks after last dose.
- **DIRECTIONS FOR ADMINISTRATION** For *intravenous infusion*, manufacturer advises give intermittently *in* Sodium chloride 0.9%; reconstitute each vial with 10 mL water for injections using the silicone-free syringe provided; dilute requisite dose in Sodium Chloride 0.9% to 100 mL (using the same silicone-free syringe); give over 30 minutes through a low protein-binding filter (pore size 0.2–1.2 micron).
- **NATIONAL FUNDING/ACCESS DECISIONS**
For full details see funding body website

NICE decisions
- **Abatacept, adalimumab, etanercept and tocilizumab for treating juvenile idiopathic arthritis (December 2015)** NICE TA373 Recommended

- **MEDICINAL FORMS** There can be variation in the licensing of different medicines containing the same drug.

Solution for injection
- **Orencia** (Imported (Germany), Bristol-Myers Squibb Pharmaceuticals Ltd)
Abatacept 125 mg per 1 ml Orencia 50mg/0.4ml solution for injection pre-filled syringes | 4 pre-filled disposable injection PoM ⊠ (Hospital only)
Orencia 125mg/1ml solution for injection pre-filled syringes | 4 pre-filled disposable injection PoM £1,209.60 (Hospital only)
Orencia 87.5mg/0.7ml solution for injection pre-filled syringes | 4 pre-filled disposable injection PoM ⊠ (Hospital only)
- **Orencia ClickJect** (Bristol-Myers Squibb Pharmaceuticals Ltd)
Abatacept 125 mg per 1 ml Orencia ClickJect 125mg/1ml solution for injection pre-filled pens | 4 pre-filled disposable injection PoM £1,209.60 DT = £1,209.60

Powder for solution for infusion
ELECTROLYTES: May contain Sodium
- **Orencia** (Bristol-Myers Squibb Pharmaceuticals Ltd)
Abatacept 250 mg Orencia 250mg powder for concentrate for solution for infusion vials | 1 vial PoM £302.40 (Hospital only)

10 Musculoskeletal system

IMMUNOSUPPRESSANTS › TUMOR NECROSIS FACTOR ALPHA (TNF-α) INHIBITORS

Adalimumab

15-Jan-2024

● **INDICATIONS AND DOSE**

Plaque psoriasis (initiated by a specialist)

▶ BY SUBCUTANEOUS INJECTION

▶ Child 4–17 years (body-weight 15–29 kg): Initially 20 mg once weekly for 2 doses, then 20 mg every 2 weeks, review treatment if no response within 16 weeks

▶ Child 4–17 years (body-weight 30 kg and above): Initially 40 mg once weekly for 2 doses, then 40 mg every 2 weeks, review treatment if no response within 16 weeks

Polyarticular juvenile idiopathic arthritis (initiated by a specialist)

▶ BY SUBCUTANEOUS INJECTION

▶ Child 2–17 years (body-weight 10–29 kg): 20 mg every 2 weeks, review treatment if no response within 12 weeks

▶ Child 2–17 years (body-weight 30 kg and above): 40 mg every 2 weeks, review treatment if no response within 12 weeks

Enthesitis-related arthritis (initiated by a specialist)

▶ BY SUBCUTANEOUS INJECTION

▶ Child 6–17 years (body-weight 15–29 kg): 20 mg every 2 weeks

▶ Child 6–17 years (body-weight 30 kg and above): 40 mg every 2 weeks

Crohn's disease (initiated by a specialist)

▶ BY SUBCUTANEOUS INJECTION

▶ Child 6–17 years (body-weight up to 40 kg): Initially 40 mg, then 20 mg after 2 weeks; maintenance 20 mg every 2 weeks, increased if necessary to 20 mg once weekly, review treatment if no response within 12 weeks

▶ Child 6–17 years (body-weight 40 kg and above): Initially 80 mg, then 40 mg after 2 weeks; maintenance 40 mg every 2 weeks, increased if necessary to 40 mg once weekly, alternatively 80 mg every 2 weeks, review treatment if no response within 12 weeks

Crohn's disease (accelerated regimen) (initiated by a specialist)

▶ BY SUBCUTANEOUS INJECTION

▶ Child 6–17 years (body-weight up to 40 kg): Initially 80 mg, then 40 mg after 2 weeks; maintenance 20 mg every 2 weeks, increased if necessary to 20 mg once weekly, review treatment if no response within 12 weeks

▶ Child 6–17 years (body-weight 40 kg and above): Initially 160 mg, dose can alternatively be given as divided injections over 2 days, then 80 mg after 2 weeks; maintenance 40 mg every 2 weeks, then increased if necessary to 40 mg once weekly, alternatively 80 mg every 2 weeks, review treatment if no response within 12 weeks

Ulcerative colitis (initiated by a specialist)

▶ BY SUBCUTANEOUS INJECTION

▶ Child 6–17 years (body-weight up to 40 kg): Initially 80 mg, followed by 40 mg after 2 weeks, then maintenance 40 mg every 2 weeks, review treatment if no response within 8 weeks

▶ Child 6–17 years (body-weight 40 kg and above): Initially 160 mg, dose can alternatively be given as divided injections over 2 days, followed by 80 mg after 2 weeks, then maintenance 80 mg every 2 weeks, review treatment if no response within 8 weeks

Hidradenitis suppurativa (initiated by a specialist)

▶ BY SUBCUTANEOUS INJECTION

▶ Child 12–17 years (body-weight 30 kg and above): Initially 80 mg, followed by 40 mg after 1 week, then maintenance 40 mg every 2 weeks; increased if necessary to 40 mg once weekly, alternatively 80 mg every 2 weeks, review treatment if no response within 12 weeks; if treatment interrupted—consult product literature

Uveitis (initiated by a specialist)

▶ BY SUBCUTANEOUS INJECTION

▶ Child 2–17 years (body-weight up to 30 kg): Initially 40 mg, then 20 mg after 1 week; maintenance 20 mg every 2 weeks

▶ Child 2–17 years (body-weight 30 kg and above): Initially 80 mg, then 40 mg after 1 week; maintenance 40 mg every 2 weeks

● **CONTRA-INDICATIONS** Moderate or severe heart failure · severe infections

● **CAUTIONS** Children should be brought up to date with current immunisation schedule before initiating therapy · demyelinating disorders (risk of exacerbation) · development of malignancy · do not initiate until active infections are controlled (discontinue if new serious infection develops) · hepatitis B virus—monitor for active infection · history of malignancy · mild heart failure (discontinue if symptoms develop or worsen) · predisposition to infection

CAUTIONS, FURTHER INFORMATION

▶ **Tuberculosis** Active tuberculosis should be treated with standard treatment for at least 2 months before starting adalimumab. Patients who have previously received adequate treatment for tuberculosis can start adalimumab but should be monitored every 3 months for possible recurrence. In patients without active tuberculosis but who were previously not treated adequately, chemoprophylaxis should ideally be completed before starting adalimumab. In patients at high risk of tuberculosis who cannot be assessed by tuberculin skin test, chemoprophylaxis can be given concurrently with adalimumab.

● **INTERACTIONS** → Appendix 1: monoclonal antibodies

● **SIDE-EFFECTS**

▶ **Common or very common** Agranulocytosis · alopecia · anaemia · anxiety · arrhythmias · asthma · broken nails · chest pain · coagulation disorder · connective tissue disorders · cough · dehydration · depression · dyspnoea · electrolyte imbalance · eye inflammation · fever · flushing · gastrointestinal discomfort · gastrointestinal disorders · haemorrhage · headaches · healing impaired · hyperglycaemia · hypersensitivity · hypertension · increased risk of infection · insomnia · leucocytosis · leucopenia · mood altered · muscle spasms · musculoskeletal pain · nausea · neoplasms · nerve disorders · neutropenia · oedema · renal impairment · seasonal allergy · sensation abnormal · sepsis · skin reactions · sweat changes · thrombocytopenia · vertigo · vision disorders · vomiting

▶ **Uncommon** Aortic aneurysm · arterial occlusion · congestive heart failure · deafness · dysphagia · embolism and thrombosis · erectile dysfunction · gallbladder disorders · hepatic disorders · inflammation · interstitial lung disease · lupus erythematosus · meningitis viral · myocardial infarction · nocturia · pancreatitis · respiratory disorders · rhabdomyolysis · sarcoidosis · solid organ neoplasm · stroke · tinnitus · tremor · vasculitis

▶ **Rare or very rare** Bone marrow disorders · cardiac arrest · demyelinating disorders · pulmonary fibrosis · reactivation of infections · Stevens-Johnson syndrome

▶ **Frequency not known** Weight increased

SIDE-EFFECTS, FURTHER INFORMATION Associated with infections sometimes severe, including tuberculosis, septicaemia, and hepatitis B reactivation.

- **CONCEPTION AND CONTRACEPTION** Manufacturer advises effective contraception required during treatment and for at least 5 months after last dose.
- **PREGNANCY** Manufacturer advises use only if potential benefit outweighs risk.
- **BREAST FEEDING** Manufacturer advises can be used—excreted in breast milk at very low concentrations (limited information available).
- **PRE-TREATMENT SCREENING**

Tuberculosis Manufacturer advises patients should be evaluated for active and latent tuberculosis before treatment.

- **MONITORING REQUIREMENTS**

▸ Manufacturer advises monitor for infection before, during, and for 4 months after treatment.
▸ Manufacturer advises monitor for non-melanoma skin cancer before and during treatment, especially in patients with a history of PUVA treatment for psoriasis or extensive immunosuppressant therapy.
▸ *For uveitis*, manufacturer advises patients should be assessed for pre-existing or developing central demyelinating disorders before and at regular intervals during treatment.

- **PRESCRIBING AND DISPENSING INFORMATION** Adalimumab is a biological medicine. Biological medicines must be prescribed and dispensed by brand name, see *Biological medicines* and *Biosimilar medicines*, under Guidance on prescribing p. 1.
- **PATIENT AND CARER ADVICE** When used to treat *hidradenitis suppurativa*, patients and their carers should be advised to use a daily topical antiseptic wash on lesions during treatment with adalimumab.

Tuberculosis Patients and their carers should be advised to seek medical attention if symptoms suggestive of tuberculosis (e.g. persistent cough, weight loss, and fever) develop.

Blood disorders Patients and their carers should be advised to seek medical attention if symptoms suggestive of blood disorders (such as fever, sore throat, bruising, or bleeding) develop.

Alert card An alert card should be provided.

- **NATIONAL FUNDING/ACCESS DECISIONS**

For full details see funding body website

NICE decisions

▸ **Abatacept, adalimumab, etanercept and tocilizumab for treating juvenile idiopathic arthritis (December 2015)** NICE TA373 Recommended
▸ **Adalimumab, etanercept and ustekinumab for treating plaque psoriasis in children and young people (July 2017)** NICE TA455 Recommended with restrictions

Scottish Medicines Consortium (SMC) decisions

▸ **Adalimumab (*Humira*®) for the treatment of active enthesitis-related arthritis in patients, 6 years of age and older, who have had an inadequate response to, or who are intolerant of, conventional therapy (May 2015)** SMC No. 1050/15 Recommended with restrictions
▸ **Adalimumab (*Humira*®) for the treatment of active moderate to severe hidradenitis suppurativa (HS) (acne inversa) in adolescents from 12 years of age with an inadequate response to conventional systemic HS therapy (June 2017)** SMC No. 1243/17 Recommended

All Wales Medicines Strategy Group (AWMSG) decisions

▸ **Adalimumab (*Humira*®) for the treatment of moderately to severely active Crohn's disease in paediatric patients (from 6 years of age) who have had an inadequate response to conventional therapy including primary nutrition therapy and a corticosteroid and/or an immunomodulator, or who are intolerant to or have contra-indications for such therapies (January 2017)** AWMSG No. 3118 Recommended
▸ **Adalimumab (*Humira*®) for the treatment of active moderate to severe hidradenitis suppurativa (acne inversa) in adolescents from 12 years of age with an inadequate response to conventional systemic hidradenitis suppurativa (HS) therapy (August 2017)** AWMSG No. 3371 Recommended
▸ **Adalimumab (*Humira*®) for the treatment of paediatric chronic non-infectious anterior uveitis in patients from two years of age who have had an inadequate response to or are intolerant to conventional therapy, or in whom conventional therapy is inappropriate (December 2017)** AWMSG No. 3035 Recommended
▸ **Adalimumab 40 mg and 80 mg solution for injection (*Humira*®) for the treatment of moderately to severely active ulcerative colitis in paediatric patients (from 6 years of age) who have had an inadequate response to conventional therapy including corticosteroids and/or 6-mercaptopurine or azathioprine, or who are intolerant to or have medical contra-indications for such therapies (March 2022)** AWMSG No. 4526 Recommended

- **MEDICINAL FORMS** There can be variation in the licensing of different medicines containing the same drug.

Solution for injection

CAUTIONARY AND ADVISORY LABELS 10

▸ **Amgevita** (Amgen Ltd)
Adalimumab 100 mg per 1 ml Amgevita HCF 40mg/0.4ml solution for injection pre-filled pens | 2 pre-filled disposable injection PoM £633.60 (Hospital only)
Amgevita HCF 40mg/0.4ml solution for injection pre-filled syringes | 2 pre-filled disposable injection PoM £633.60 (Hospital only)
Amgevita HCF 20mg/0.2ml solution for injection pre-filled syringes | 1 pre-filled disposable injection PoM £158.40 (Hospital only)
Amgevita HCF 80mg/0.8ml solution for injection pre-filled syringes | 1 pre-filled disposable injection PoM £633.60 (Hospital only)
Amgevita HCF 80mg/0.8ml solution for injection pre-filled pens | 1 pre-filled disposable injection PoM £633.60 (Hospital only) | 2 pre-filled disposable injection PoM £1,267.20 (Hospital only)

▸ **Humira** (AbbVie Ltd)
Adalimumab 100 mg per 1 ml Humira 40mg/0.4ml solution for injection pre-filled pens | 2 pre-filled disposable injection PoM £704.28
Humira 80mg/0.8ml solution for injection pre-filled pens | 1 pre-filled disposable injection PoM £704.28
Humira 20mg/0.2ml solution for injection pre-filled syringes | 2 pre-filled disposable injection PoM £352.14
Humira 40mg/0.4ml solution for injection pre-filled syringes | 2 pre-filled disposable injection PoM £704.28

▸ **Hyrimoz** (Sandoz Ltd)
Adalimumab 50 mg per 1 ml Hyrimoz 40mg/0.8ml solution for injection pre-filled syringes | 2 pre-filled disposable injection PoM £646.18
Adalimumab 100 mg per 1 ml Hyrimoz 40mg/0.4ml solution for injection pre-filled syringes | 2 pre-filled disposable injection PoM £646.18
Hyrimoz 40mg/0.4ml solution for injection pre-filled pens | 2 pre-filled disposable injection PoM £646.18 (Hospital only)

▸ **Idacio** (Fresenius Kabi Ltd)
Adalimumab 50 mg per 1 ml Idacio 40mg/0.8ml solution for injection vials | 1 vial PoM £316.93 (Hospital only)
Idacio 40mg/0.8ml solution for injection pre-filled syringes | 2 pre-filled disposable injection PoM £633.86
Idacio 40mg/0.8ml solution for injection pre-filled pens | 2 pre-filled disposable injection PoM £633.86 (Hospital only)

▸ **Imraldi** (Biogen Idec Ltd)
Adalimumab 50 mg per 1 ml Imraldi 40mg/0.8ml solution for injection pre-filled pens | 2 pre-filled disposable injection PoM £633.85
Imraldi 40mg/0.8ml solution for injection pre-filled syringes | 2 pre-filled disposable injection PoM £633.85
Adalimumab 100 mg per 1 ml Imraldi 40mg/0.4ml solution for injection pre-filled syringes | 2 pre-filled disposable injection PoM £633.85 (Hospital only)
Imraldi 40mg/0.4ml solution for injection pre-filled pens | 2 pre-filled disposable injection PoM £633.85 (Hospital only)

▶ **Yuflyma** (Celltrion Healthcare UK Ltd) ▼
Adalimumab 100 mg per 1 ml Yuflyma 40mg/0.4ml solution for injection pre-filled pens | 2 pre-filled disposable injection PoM £633.70
Yuflyma 80mg/0.8ml solution for injection pre-filled pens | 1 pre-filled disposable injection PoM £633.70 (Hospital only)
Yuflyma 20mg/0.2ml solution for injection pre-filled syringes | 2 pre-filled disposable injection PoM £316.93

Etanercept

14-Mar-2022

● **INDICATIONS AND DOSE**

Plaque psoriasis (initiated by a specialist)

▶ BY SUBCUTANEOUS INJECTION

▶ Child 6–17 years: 800 micrograms/kg once weekly (max. per dose 50 mg) for up to 24 weeks, discontinue if no response after 12 weeks

Polyarthritis (initiated by a specialist) | Oligoarthritis (initiated by a specialist)

▶ BY SUBCUTANEOUS INJECTION

▶ Child 2–17 years: 400 micrograms/kg twice weekly (max. per dose 25 mg), to be given at an interval of 3–4 days between doses, alternatively 800 micrograms/kg once weekly (max. per dose 50 mg), consider discontinuation if no response after 4 months

Psoriatic arthritis (initiated by a specialist) | Enthesitis-related arthritis (initiated by a specialist)

▶ BY SUBCUTANEOUS INJECTION

▶ Child 12–17 years: 400 micrograms/kg twice weekly (max. per dose 25 mg), to be given at an interval of 3–4 days between doses, alternatively 800 micrograms/kg once weekly (max. per dose 50 mg), consider discontinuation if no response after 4 months

● **CONTRA-INDICATIONS** Active infection

● **CAUTIONS** Children should be brought up to date with current immunisation schedule before initiating therapy · development of malignancy · diabetes mellitus · heart failure (risk of exacerbation) · hepatitis B virus—monitor for active infection · hepatitis C infection (monitor for worsening infection) · history of blood disorders · history of malignancy · history or increased risk of demyelinating disorders · predisposition to infection (avoid if predisposition to septicaemia) · significant exposure to herpes zoster virus—interrupt treatment and consider varicella–zoster immunoglobulin

CAUTIONS, FURTHER INFORMATION

▶ Tuberculosis Active tuberculosis should be treated with standard treatment for at least 2 months before starting etanercept. Patients who have previously received adequate treatment for tuberculosis can start etanercept but should be monitored every 3 months for possible recurrence. In patients without active tuberculosis but who were previously not treated adequately, chemoprophylaxis should ideally be completed before starting etanercept. In patients at high risk of tuberculosis who cannot be assessed by tuberculin skin test, chemoprophylaxis can be given concurrently with etanercept.

● **INTERACTIONS** → Appendix 1: etanercept

● **SIDE-EFFECTS**

▶ **Common or very common** Cystitis · fever · headache · hypersensitivity · increased risk of infection · skin reactions

▶ **Uncommon** Abscess · anaemia · angioedema · bursitis · cholecystitis · diarrhoea · endocarditis · eye inflammation · gastrointestinal disorders · heart failure · hepatic disorders · inflammatory bowel disease · leucopenia · myositis · neoplasms · neutropenia · sepsis · skin ulcers · thrombocytopenia · vasculitis

▶ **Rare or very rare** Bone marrow disorders · cutaneous lupus erythematosus · demyelination · interstitial lung disease · lupus-like syndrome · nerve disorders · pulmonary fibrosis · sarcoidosis · seizure · severe cutaneous adverse reactions (SCARs) · transverse myelitis

▶ **Frequency not known** Abdominal pain · depression · dermatomyositis exacerbated · hepatitis B reactivation · macrophage activation syndrome · nausea · personality disorder · post procedural infection · type 1 diabetes mellitus · vomiting

SIDE-EFFECTS, FURTHER INFORMATION Associated with infections, sometimes severe, including tuberculosis, septicaemia, and hepatitis B reactivation.

● **CONCEPTION AND CONTRACEPTION** Manufacturer advises effective contraception required during treatment and for 3 weeks after last dose.

● **PREGNANCY** EvGr Use only if essential. ⟨M⟩

● **BREAST FEEDING** Manufacturer advises avoid—present in milk in *animal* studies.

● **HEPATIC IMPAIRMENT** Manufacturer advises caution in moderate to severe alcoholic hepatitis.

● **PRE-TREATMENT SCREENING**

Tuberculosis Patients should be evaluated for tuberculosis before treatment.

● **MONITORING REQUIREMENTS** EvGr Monitor for skin cancer during treatment, particularly in patients with risk factors or psoriasis. ⟨M⟩

● **PRESCRIBING AND DISPENSING INFORMATION** Etanercept is a biological medicine. Biological medicines must be prescribed and dispensed by brand name, see *Biological medicines* and *Biosimilar medicines*, under Guidance on prescribing p. 1.

● **HANDLING AND STORAGE** Store in a refrigerator (2–8°C)—consult product literature for further information regarding storage conditions outside refrigerator.

● **PATIENT AND CARER ADVICE**

Blood disorders Patients and their carers should be advised to seek medical attention if symptoms suggestive of blood disorders (such as fever, sore throat, bruising, or bleeding) develop.

Tuberculosis Patients and their carers should be advised to seek medical attention if symptoms suggestive of tuberculosis (e.g. persistent cough, weight loss, and fever) develop.

Patient card A patient card should be provided.

Medicines for Children leaflet: Etanercept for juvenile idiopathic arthritis www.medicinesforchildren.org.uk/medicines/etanercept-for-juvenile-idiopathic-arthritis/

● **NATIONAL FUNDING/ACCESS DECISIONS**

For full details see funding body website

NICE decisions

▶ **Adalimumab, etanercept and ustekinumab for treating plaque psoriasis in children and young people (July 2017)** NICE TA455 Recommended with restrictions

▶ **Abatacept, adalimumab, etanercept and tocilizumab for treating juvenile idiopathic arthritis (December 2015)** NICE TA373 Recommended

Scottish Medicines Consortium (SMC) decisions

▶ **Etanercept (*Enbrel*®) for the treatment of polyarthritis (rheumatoid factor positive or negative) and extended oligoarthritis in children and adolescents (February 2013)** SMC No. 842/13 Recommended with restrictions

● **MEDICINAL FORMS** There can be variation in the licensing of different medicines containing the same drug.

Solution for injection

CAUTIONARY AND ADVISORY LABELS 10

▸ **Benepali** (Biogen Idec Ltd)

Etanercept 50 mg per 1 ml Benepali 25mg/0.5ml solution for injection pre-filled syringes | 4 pre-filled disposable injection PoM £328.00 (Hospital only)

Benepali 50mg/1ml solution for injection pre-filled pens | 4 pre-filled disposable injection PoM £656.00 (Hospital only)

Benepali 50mg/1ml solution for injection pre-filled syringes | 4 pre-filled disposable injection PoM £656.00 (Hospital only)

▸ **Enbrel** (Pfizer Ltd)

Etanercept 50 mg per 1 ml Enbrel 50mg/1ml solution for injection pre-filled syringes | 4 pre-filled disposable injection PoM £715.00 (Hospital only)

Enbrel 25mg/0.5ml solution for injection pre-filled syringes | 4 pre-filled disposable injection PoM £357.50 (Hospital only)

▸ **Enbrel MyClic** (Pfizer Ltd)

Etanercept 50 mg per 1 ml Enbrel 25mg/0.5ml solution for injection pre-filled MyClic pens | 4 pre-filled disposable injection PoM £357.50 (Hospital only)

Enbrel 50mg/1ml solution for injection pre-filled MyClic pens | 4 pre-filled disposable injection PoM £715.00 (Hospital only)

▸ **Erelzi** (Sandoz Ltd) ▼

Etanercept 50 mg per 1 ml Erelzi 50mg/1ml solution for injection pre-filled pens | 4 pre-filled disposable injection PoM £643.50 (Hospital only)

Erelzi 50mg/1ml solution for injection pre-filled syringes | 4 pre-filled disposable injection PoM £643.50 (Hospital only)

Erelzi 25mg/0.5ml solution for injection pre-filled syringes | 4 pre-filled disposable injection PoM £321.75 (Hospital only)

Powder and solvent for solution for injection

CAUTIONARY AND ADVISORY LABELS 10

▸ **Enbrel** (Pfizer Ltd)

Etanercept 10 mg Enbrel Paediatric 10mg powder and solvent for solution for injection vials | 4 vial PoM £143.00 (Hospital only)

Etanercept 25 mg Enbrel 25mg powder and solvent for solution for injection vials | 4 vial PoM £357.50 (Hospital only)

Golimumab

06-Nov-2020

● **INDICATIONS AND DOSE**

Polyarticular juvenile idiopathic arthritis (initiated by a specialist)

▶ BY SUBCUTANEOUS INJECTION

▸ Child (body-weight 40 kg and above): 50 mg once a month, on the same date each month, review treatment if no response after 3–4 doses

● **CONTRA-INDICATIONS** Moderate or severe heart failure · severe active infection

● **CAUTIONS** Active infection (do not initiate until active infections are controlled; discontinue if new serious infection develops until infection controlled) · children should be brought up to date with current immunisation schedule before initiating therapy · demyelinating disorders (risk of exacerbation) · hepatitis B virus—monitor for active infection · history or development of malignancy · mild heart failure (discontinue if symptoms develop or worsen) · predisposition to infection · risk factors for dysplasia or carcinoma of the colon—screen for dysplasia regularly

CAUTIONS, FURTHER INFORMATION

▸ Tuberculosis Active tuberculosis should be treated with standard treatment for at least 2 months before starting golimumab. Patients who have previously received adequate treatment for tuberculosis can start golimumab but should be monitored every 3 months for possible recurrence. In patients without active tuberculosis but who were previously not treated adequately, chemoprophylaxis should ideally be completed before starting golimumab. In patients at high risk of tuberculosis who cannot be assessed by tuberculin skin test, chemoprophylaxis can be given concurrently with golimumab. Patients who have tested negative for latent tuberculosis, and those who are receiving or who have completed treatment for latent tuberculosis, should be monitored closely for symptoms of active infection.

● **INTERACTIONS** → Appendix 1: monoclonal antibodies

● **SIDE-EFFECTS**

▶ **Common or very common** Abscess · alopecia · anaemia · asthenia · asthma · bone fracture · chest discomfort · depression · dizziness · fever · gastrointestinal discomfort · gastrointestinal disorders · gastrointestinal inflammatory disorders · headache · hypersensitivity · hypertension · increased risk of infection · insomnia · nausea · paraesthesia · respiratory disorders · skin reactions · stomatitis

▶ **Uncommon** Arrhythmia · balance impaired · bone marrow disorders · breast disorder · cholelithiasis · constipation · eye inflammation · eye irritation · flushing · goitre · hyperthyroidism · hypothyroidism · interstitial lung disease · leucopenia · liver disorder · menstrual disorder · myocardial ischaemia · neoplasms · sepsis · thrombocytopenia · thrombosis · thyroid disorder · vision disorders

▶ **Rare or very rare** Bladder disorder · congestive heart failure · demyelination · healing impaired · hepatitis B reactivation · lupus-like syndrome · Raynaud's phenomenon · renal disorder · sarcoidosis · taste altered · vasculitis

SIDE-EFFECTS, FURTHER INFORMATION Associated with infections, sometimes severe, including tuberculosis, septicaemia, and hepatitis B reactivation.

● **CONCEPTION AND CONTRACEPTION** Manufacturer advises adequate contraception during treatment and for at least 6 months after last dose.

● **PREGNANCY** Use only if essential.

● **BREAST FEEDING** Manufacturer advises avoid during and for at least 6 months after treatment—present in milk in *animal* studies.

● **HEPATIC IMPAIRMENT** Manufacturer advises caution (no information available).

● **PRE-TREATMENT SCREENING**

Tuberculosis Patients should be evaluated for tuberculosis before treatment.

● **MONITORING REQUIREMENTS** Monitor for infection before, during, and for 5 months after treatment.

● **DIRECTIONS FOR ADMINISTRATION**

Missed doses If dose administered more than 2 weeks late, manufacturer advises subsequent doses should be administered on the new monthly due date.

● **PATIENT AND CARER ADVICE**

Tuberculosis All patients and their carers should be advised to seek medical attention if symptoms suggestive of tuberculosis (e.g. persistent cough, weight loss, and fever) develop.

Blood disorders Patients and their carers should be advised to seek medical attention if symptoms suggestive of blood disorders (such as fever, sore throat, bruising, or bleeding) develop.

Alert card An alert card should be provided.

● **MEDICINAL FORMS** There can be variation in the licensing of different medicines containing the same drug.

Solution for injection

CAUTIONARY AND ADVISORY LABELS 10

▸ **Gobivaz** (Advanz Pharma) ▼

Golimumab 100 mg per 1 ml Gobivaz 50mg/0.5ml solution for injection pre-filled syringes | 1 pre-filled disposable injection PoM £686.67

Gobivaz 100mg/1ml solution for injection pre-filled pens | 1 pre-filled disposable injection PoM £1,373.35

Gobivaz 50mg/0.5ml solution for injection pre-filled pens | 1 pre-filled disposable injection PoM £686.67

▸ **Simponi** (Janssen-Cilag Ltd)
Golimumab 100 mg per 1 ml Simponi 100mg/1ml solution for injection pre-filled pens | 1 pre-filled disposable injection PoM £1,525.94 (Hospital only)
Simponi 50mg/0.5ml solution for injection pre-filled syringes | 1 pre-filled disposable injection PoM £762.97 (Hospital only)
Simponi 50mg/0.5ml solution for injection pre-filled pens | 1 pre-filled disposable injection PoM £762.97 (Hospital only)

2 Neuromuscular disorders

Neuromuscular disorders

Drugs that enhance neuromuscular transmission

Anticholinesterases are used as first-line treatment in *ocular myasthenia gravis* and as an adjunct to immunosuppressant therapy for *generalised myasthenia gravis*.

Corticosteroids are used when anticholinesterases do not control symptoms completely. A second-line immunosuppressant such as azathioprine p. 638 is frequently used to reduce the dose of corticosteroid.

Plasmapheresis or infusion of intravenous immunoglobulin [unlicensed indication] may induce temporary remission in severe relapses, particularly where bulbar or respiratory function is compromised or before thymectomy.

Anticholinesterases

Anticholinesterase drugs enhance neuromuscular transmission in voluntary and involuntary muscle in myasthenia gravis. Excessive dosage of these drugs can impair neuromuscular transmission and precipitate cholinergic crises by causing a depolarising block. This may be difficult to distinguish from a worsening myasthenic state.

Muscarinic side-effects of anticholinesterases include increased sweating, increased salivary and gastric secretions, increased gastro-intestinal and uterine motility, and bradycardia. These parasympathomimetic effects are antagonised by atropine sulfate p. 1013.

Neostigmine p. 814 produces a therapeutic effect for up to 4 hours. Its pronounced muscarinic action is a disadvantage, and simultaneous administration of an antimuscarinic drug such as atropine sulfate or propantheline bromide p. 69 may be required to prevent colic, excessive salivation, or diarrhoea. In severe disease neostigmine can be given every 2 hours. In infants, neostigmine by either subcutaneous or intramuscular injection is preferred for the short-term management of myasthenia.

Pyridostigmine bromide p. 814 is less powerful and slower in action than neostigmine but it has a longer duration of action. It is preferable to neostigmine because of its smoother action and the need for less frequent dosage. It is particularly preferred in patients whose muscles are weak on waking. It has a comparatively mild gastrointestinal effect but an antimuscarinic drug may still be required. It is inadvisable to use excessive doses because acetylcholine receptor down regulation may occur. Immunosuppressant therapy may be considered if high doses of pyridostigmine bromide are needed.

Neostigmine and pyridostigmine bromide should be given to neonates 30 minutes before feeds to improve suckling.

Neostigmine is also used to reverse the actions of the non-depolarising neuromuscular blocking drugs.

Immunosuppressant therapy

A course of **corticosteroids** is an established treatment in severe cases of myasthenia gravis and may be particularly useful when antibodies to the acetylcholine receptor are present in high titre. Short courses of high-dose ('pulsed') methylprednisolone p. 547 followed by maintenance therapy with oral corticosteroids may also be useful.

Corticosteroid treatment is usually initiated under specialist supervision. Transient but very serious worsening of symptoms can occur in the first 2–3 weeks, especially if the corticosteroid is started at a high dose. Once remission has occurred (usually after 2– 6 months), the dose of prednisolone p. 548 should be reduced slowly to the minimum effective dose.

Skeletal muscle relaxants

The drugs described are used for the relief of chronic muscle spasm or spasticity associated with neurological damage; they are not indicated for spasm associated with minor injuries. They act principally on the central nervous system with the exception of dantrolene, which has a peripheral site of action. They differ in action from the muscle relaxants used in anaesthesia, which block transmission at the neuromuscular junction.

The underlying cause of spasticity should be treated and any aggravating factors (e.g. pressure sores, infection) remedied. Skeletal muscle relaxants are effective in most forms of spasticity except the rare alpha variety. The major disadvantage of treatment with these drugs is that reduction in muscle tone can cause a loss of splinting action of the spastic leg and trunk muscles and sometimes lead to an increase in disability.

Dantrolene sodium p. 1025 acts directly on skeletal muscle and produces fewer central adverse effects. It is generally used in resistant cases. The dose should be increased slowly.

Baclofen p. 814 inhibits transmission at spinal level and also depresses the central nervous system. The dose should be increased slowly to avoid the major side-effects of sedation and muscular hypotonia (other adverse events are uncommon).

Diazepam p. 270 has undoubted efficacy in some children. Sedation and occasionally extensor hypotonus are disadvantages. Other benzodiazepines also have muscle-relaxant properties.

2.1 Muscular dystrophy

CORTICOSTEROIDS F 540

Vamorolone

28-Aug-2025

- **DRUG ACTION** Vamorolone is a dissociative corticosteroid that selectively binds to the glucocorticoid receptor and reduces inflammation by inhibiting cytokine production.

- **INDICATIONS AND DOSE**

Duchenne muscular dystrophy (initiated by a specialist)

▸ BY MOUTH

▸ Child 4-17 years (body-weight up to 40 kg): 6 mg/kg once daily; reduced if not tolerated to 4 mg/kg once daily, reduced if not tolerated to 2 mg/kg once daily

▸ Child 4-17 years (body-weight 40 kg and above): 240 mg once daily; reduced if not tolerated to 160 mg once daily, reduced if not tolerated to 80 mg once daily

- **INTERACTIONS** → Appendix 1: corticosteroids
- **SIDE-EFFECTS**
  ▸ **Common or very common** Diarrhoea · vomiting
  ▸ **Frequency not known** Suppression of the hypothalamic-pituitary-adrenal axis
- **PREGNANCY** EvGr Avoid unless potential benefit outweighs risk (no information available). ⟨M⟩
- **BREAST FEEDING** EvGr Discontinue breast-feeding (no information available). ⟨M⟩

- **HEPATIC IMPAIRMENT** EvGr Avoid in severe impairment; caution in moderate impairment. ⟨M⟩
  Dose adjustments EvGr Body-weight up to 40 kg, reduce dose to 2 mg/kg once daily in moderate impairment.
  Body-weight 40 kg and above, reduce dose to 80 mg once daily in moderate impairment. ⟨M⟩
- **TREATMENT CESSATION** EvGr Avoid abrupt withdrawal if treatment duration more than 1 week—reduce dose by decrements of approx. 20% over weeks, according to tolerance. ⟨M⟩
- **HANDLING AND STORAGE** Store in a refrigerator (2–8°C) after opening; discard any remaining suspension 3 months after opening.
- **PATIENT AND CARER ADVICE**
  Alert card A patient alert card should be provided.
- **NATIONAL FUNDING/ACCESS DECISIONS**
  For full details see funding body website
  NICE decisions
  - **Vamorolone for treating Duchenne muscular dystrophy in people 4 years and over (January 2025)** NICE TA1031 Recommended

  Scottish Medicines Consortium (SMC) decisions
  - **Vamorolone (*Agamree*®) for the treatment of Duchenne muscular dystrophy (DMD) in patients aged 4 years and older (January 2025)** SMC No. SMC2721 Recommended
- **MEDICINAL FORMS** There can be variation in the licensing of different medicines containing the same drug.
  Oral suspension
  - Agamree (Santhera (UK) Ltd) ▼
    Vamorolone 40 mg per 1 ml Agamree 40mg/ml oral suspension | 100 ml PoM £4,585.87 (Hospital only) SF

DRUGS FOR NEUROMUSCULAR DISORDERS

Ataluren 28-Feb-2023

- **DRUG ACTION** Ataluren restores the synthesis of dystrophin by allowing ribosomes to read through premature stop codons that cause incomplete dystrophin synthesis in nonsense mutation Duchenne muscular dystrophy.
- **INDICATIONS AND DOSE**
  Duchenne muscular dystrophy resulting from a nonsense mutation in the dystrophin gene, in ambulatory patients (initiated by a specialist)
  - BY MOUTH
    - Child 2–17 years (body-weight 12 kg and above): (consult product literature)
- **INTERACTIONS** → Appendix 1: ataluren
- **SIDE-EFFECTS**
  - **Common or very common** Appetite decreased · constipation · cough · enuresis · fever · flatulence · gastrointestinal discomfort · haemorrhage · headache · hypertension · hypertriglyceridaemia · nausea · pain · skin reactions · vomiting · weight decreased
  - **Frequency not known** Ear infection · malaise
- **PREGNANCY** Manufacturer advises avoid—toxicity in *animal* studies.
- **BREAST FEEDING** Manufacturer advises discontinue breastfeeding—present in milk in *animal* studies.
- **RENAL IMPAIRMENT** Manufacturer advises close monitoring—safety and efficacy not established.
- **MONITORING REQUIREMENTS** Manufacturer advises monitor renal function at least every 6–12 months, and cholesterol and triglyceride concentrations at least annually.
- **DIRECTIONS FOR ADMINISTRATION** Manufacturer advises the contents of each sachet should be mixed with at least 30 mL of liquid (water, milk, fruit juice), or 3 tablespoons of semi-solid food (yoghurt or apple sauce).
- **PATIENT AND CARER ADVICE** Manufacturer advises patients should maintain adequate hydration during treatment.
  Missed doses Manufacturer advises if a morning or midday dose is more than 3 hours late, or an evening dose is more than 6 hours late, the missed dose should not be taken and the next dose should be taken at the normal time.
- **NATIONAL FUNDING/ACCESS DECISIONS**
  For full details see funding body website
  NICE decisions
  - **Ataluren for treating Duchenne muscular dystrophy with a nonsense mutation in the dystrophin gene (February 2023)** NICE HST22 Recommended

  Scottish Medicines Consortium (SMC) decisions
  - **Ataluren (*Translarna*®) for the treatment of Duchenne muscular dystrophy resulting from a nonsense mutation in the dystrophin gene, in ambulatory patients aged 2 years and older (April 2021)** SMC No. SMC2327 Recommended with restrictions
- **MEDICINAL FORMS** There can be variation in the licensing of different medicines containing the same drug.
  Granules for oral suspension
  - Translarna (PTC Therapeutics Ltd) ▼
    Ataluren 125 mg Translarna 125mg granules for oral suspension sachets | 30 sachet PoM £2,532.00 (Hospital only)
    Ataluren 250 mg Translarna 250mg granules for oral suspension sachets | 30 sachet PoM £5,064.00 (Hospital only)
    Ataluren 1 gram Translarna 1,000mg granules for oral suspension sachets | 30 sachet PoM £20,256.00 (Hospital only)

Givinostat 16-Dec-2025

- **DRUG ACTION** Givinostat is a histone deacetylase inhibitor that reduces muscle loss and inflammation in dystrophic muscles, although its exact mechanism of action is unknown.
- **INDICATIONS AND DOSE**
  Duchenne muscular dystrophy
  - BY MOUTH
    - Child 6–17 years (body-weight 10–19 kg): 22.2 mg twice daily, for dose adjustments, treatment interruption, or discontinuation due to side-effects—consult product literature
    - Child 6–17 years (body-weight 20–39 kg): 31 mg twice daily, for dose adjustments, treatment interruption, or discontinuation due to side-effects—consult product literature
    - Child 6–17 years (body-weight 40–59 kg): 44.3 mg twice daily, for dose adjustments, treatment interruption, or discontinuation due to side-effects—consult product literature
    - Child 6–17 years (body-weight 60 kg and above): 53.2 mg twice daily, for dose adjustments, treatment interruption, or discontinuation due to side-effects—consult product literature

IMPORTANT SAFETY INFORMATION

INFORMATION ON REPORTED CASES OF PATIENT DEATHS AMONG DUCHENNE MUSCULAR DYSTROPHY PATIENTS RECEIVING *DUVYZAT*® (GIVINOSTAT) (NOVEMBER 2025)

Following international reports of death, including sudden death, in patients being treated with givinostat for Duchenne muscular dystrophy (DMD), the MHRA is reviewing these cases to determine if the risk-benefit ratio has changed. In the meantime, healthcare professionals are reminded of existing cautions and to follow monitoring requirements.

- **CONTRA-INDICATIONS** Platelet count less than 150 × 10^9 cells/litre (do not initiate)
- **CAUTIONS** Risk factors for ventricular arrhythmias including torsade de pointes (e.g. congenital long QT syndrome, coronary artery disease, electrolyte disturbances, concomitant use with other drugs known to prolong the QT interval)

CAUTIONS, FURTHER INFORMATION

- ECG monitoring EvGr In patients with underlying cardiac disease or using other drugs known to prolong the QT interval, an ECG should be obtained before starting treatment, during concomitant use, and as clinically indicated—withhold treatment if QTc interval exceeds 500 milliseconds or the change from baseline exceeds 60 milliseconds. (M)

- **INTERACTIONS** → Appendix 1: givinostat
- **SIDE-EFFECTS**
  - **Common or very common** Appetite decreased · arthralgia · constipation · diarrhoea · fatigue · fever · gastrointestinal discomfort · gastrointestinal disorders · hypertriglyceridaemia · myalgia · nausea · rash · thrombocytopenia · vomiting
  - **Frequency not known** Hypothyroidism
- **PREGNANCY** EvGr Avoid (toxicity in *animal* studies). (M)
- **BREAST FEEDING** Specialist sources indicate use with caution, especially if breast-feeding a newborn or pre-term infant (no information available). High plasma-protein binding suggests limited excretion into milk. Monitor breast-fed infant for side-effects.
- **MONITORING REQUIREMENTS**
  - EvGr Obtain platelet count at baseline before starting treatment and monitor blood counts every 2 weeks for the first 2 months, then at month 3, and every 3 months thereafter during treatment. Reduce dose, withhold treatment, or permanently discontinue if thrombocytopenia occurs—consult product literature.
  - Obtain triglycerides level at baseline before starting treatment and monitor at months 1, 3, and 6, then every 6 months thereafter during treatment. Reduce dose or permanently discontinue if triglycerides are elevated—consult product literature. (M)
- **NATIONAL FUNDING/ACCESS DECISIONS**
  For full details see funding body website

Scottish Medicines Consortium (SMC) decisions

- **Givinostat (*Duvyzat*®) for the treatment of Duchenne muscular dystrophy in patients 6 years of age and older (December 2025)** SMC No. SMC2856 Recommended with restrictions

- **MEDICINAL FORMS** There can be variation in the licensing of different medicines containing the same drug.

Oral suspension

CAUTIONARY AND ADVISORY LABELS 21

EXCIPIENTS: May contain Polysorbates, sorbitol

- **Duvyzat** (ITF Pharma Ltd) ▼
  Givinostat (as Givinostat hydrochloride monohydrate) 8.86 mg per 1 ml Duvyzat 8.86mg/ml oral suspension | 140 ml PoM £13,846.00 (Hospital only) SF

Nusinersen

06-Nov-2025

- **DRUG ACTION** Nusinersen is an antisense oligonucleotide that increases the production of survival motor neurone (SMN) protein, thereby helping to compensate for the defect in the SMN1 gene found in 5q spinal muscular atrophy.

- **INDICATIONS AND DOSE**

5q spinal muscular atrophy (initiated by a specialist)

▶ BY INTRATHECAL INJECTION

- Neonate: Initially 12 mg for 4 doses on days 0, 14, 28 and 63, then 12 mg every 4 months, for advice on missed doses—consult product literature.
- Child: Initially 12 mg for 4 doses on days 0, 14, 28 and 63, then 12 mg every 4 months, for advice on missed doses—consult product literature

- **UNLICENSED USE** Licensed for use in children (age range not specified by manufacturer).

IMPORTANT SAFETY INFORMATION

MHRA/CHM ADVICE: NUSINERSEN (*SPINRAZA*®): REPORTS OF COMMUNICATING HYDROCEPHALUS NOT RELATED TO MENINGITIS OR BLEEDING (JULY 2018)

Communicating hydrocephalus not related to meningitis or bleeding has been reported in patients treated with *Spinraza*®. Patients and caregivers should be informed about the signs and symptoms of hydrocephalus before *Spinraza*® is started and should be instructed to seek medical attention in case of: persistent vomiting or headache, unexplained decrease in consciousness, and in children increase in head circumference. Patients with signs and symptoms suggestive of hydrocephalus should be further investigated by a physician with expertise in its management.

- **CAUTIONS** Risk factors for renal toxicity—monitor urine protein (preferably using a first morning urine specimen) · risk factors for thrombocytopenia and coagulation disorders—monitor platelet and coagulation profile before treatment
- **SIDE-EFFECTS** Arachnoiditis · hydrocephalus · meningitis
- **PREGNANCY** Manufacturer advises avoid—no information available.
- **BREAST FEEDING** Manufacturer advises avoid—no information available.
- **RENAL IMPAIRMENT** Manufacturer advises close monitoring—safety and efficacy not established.
- **HANDLING AND STORAGE** Manufacturer advises store in a refrigerator (2–8 °C); may be stored (in the original carton, protected from light) at or below 30 °C, for up to 14 days.
- **NATIONAL FUNDING/ACCESS DECISIONS**
  For full details see funding body website

NICE decisions

- **Nusinersen for treating spinal muscular atrophy (July 2019)** NICE TA588 Recommended with restrictions

Scottish Medicines Consortium (SMC) decisions

- **Nusinersen (*Spinraza*®) for the treatment of 5q spinal muscular atrophy [type 1] (May 2018)** SMC No. 1318/18 Recommended with restrictions
- **Nusinersen (*Spinraza*®) for the treatment of 5q spinal muscular atrophy [type 2 or type 3] (October 2025)** SMC No. SMC2805 Recommended with restrictions

- **MEDICINAL FORMS** There can be variation in the licensing of different medicines containing the same drug.

Solution for injection

- Spinraza (Biogen Idec Ltd)
  Nusinersen (as Nusinersen sodium) 2.4 mg per 1 ml Spinraza 12mg/5ml solution for injection vials | 1 vial PoM £75,000.00 (Hospital only)

Risdiplam

08-Oct-2024

- **DRUG ACTION** Risdiplam is a survival motor neurone 2 (SMN2) pre-mRNA splicing modifier that increases the production of SMN protein, thereby helping to compensate for the defect in the SMN1 gene found in 5q spinal muscular atrophy.

- **INDICATIONS AND DOSE**

5q spinal muscular atrophy (initiated by a specialist)

- BY MOUTH
  - Neonate: 150 micrograms/kg once daily, to be taken after a feed at the same time each day, dose based on corrected age for preterm infants.
  - Child 1 month: 150 micrograms/kg once daily, to be taken after a feed at the same time each day, dose based on corrected age for preterm infants
  - Child 2–23 months: 200 micrograms/kg once daily, to be taken after a meal at the same time each day, dose based on corrected age for preterm infants
  - Child 2–17 years (body-weight up to 20 kg): 250 micrograms/kg once daily, to be taken after a meal at the same time each day
  - Child 2–17 years (body-weight 20 kg and above): 5 mg once daily, to be taken after a meal at the same time each day

- **INTERACTIONS** → Appendix 1: risdiplam
- **SIDE-EFFECTS**
  - **Common or very common** Arthralgia · cystitis · diarrhoea · fever · headache · hyperpyrexia · increased risk of infection · nausea · oral ulceration · skin reactions
  - **Frequency not known** Cutaneous vasculitis
- **CONCEPTION AND CONTRACEPTION** EvGr Females of childbearing potential should use highly effective contraception during treatment and for at least 1 month after last treatment; male patients should use highly effective contraception during treatment and for at least 4 months after last treatment if their partner is of childbearing potential. Male fertility may be impaired during treatment; sperm degeneration and reduced sperm numbers in *animal* studies. Ⓜ
- **PREGNANCY** EvGr Avoid—toxicity in *animal* studies. Ⓜ
- **BREAST FEEDING** EvGr Avoid—present in milk in *animal* studies. Ⓜ
- **DIRECTIONS FOR ADMINISTRATION** *Evrysdi*® must be reconstituted by a healthcare professional before dispensing. It should be administered orally with the reusable oral syringe provided; the patient should drink water after a dose to ensure that it has been completely swallowed. It should be administered after breast feeding in breast-fed infants, and not mixed with milk or formula milk. If a dose is not taken within 5 minutes of being drawn, it should be discarded and a new dose prepared. The solution can also be administered via nasogastric or gastrostomy tube.
- **PRESCRIBING AND DISPENSING INFORMATION** Patients or their carers should be counselled on the administration of the oral solution.
- **PATIENT AND CARER ADVICE** If *Evrysdi*® oral solution spills or gets on the skin, the area should be washed with soap and water. Store in a refrigerator (2–8°C); any unused portion must be discarded 64 days after reconstitution.
  Vomiting If a dose is not fully swallowed or vomiting occurs after taking a dose, no additional dose should be taken on that day and the next dose should be taken at the usual time.
  Missed doses If a dose is more than 6 hours late, the missed dose should not be taken and the next dose should be taken at the usual time.
- **NATIONAL FUNDING/ACCESS DECISIONS**
  For full details see funding body website

NICE decisions

- **Risdiplam for treating spinal muscular atrophy (updated December 2023)** NICE TA755 Recommended with restrictions

Scottish Medicines Consortium (SMC) decisions

- **Risdiplam (*Evrysdi*®) for the treatment of 5q spinal muscular atrophy (SMA) in patients two months of age and older, with a clinical diagnosis of SMA type 1, type 2 or type 3 or with one to four survival of motor neuron 2 copies (February 2022)** SMC No. SMC2401 Recommended

- **MEDICINAL FORMS** There can be variation in the licensing of different medicines containing the same drug.

Oral solution

CAUTIONARY AND ADVISORY LABELS 8
EXCIPIENTS: May contain Disodium edetate

- Evrysdi (Roche Products Ltd) ▼
  Risdiplam 750 microgram per 1 ml Evrysdi 0.75mg/ml oral solution | 80 ml PoM £7,900.00 (Hospital only) SF

2.2 Myasthenia gravis and Lambert-Eaton myasthenic syndrome

ANTICHOLINESTERASES

Anticholinesterases

- **DRUG ACTION** They prolong the action of acetylcholine by inhibiting the action of the enzyme acetylcholinesterase.
- **CONTRA-INDICATIONS** Intestinal obstruction · urinary obstruction
- **CAUTIONS** Arrhythmias · asthma (extreme caution) · atropine or other antidote to muscarinic effects may be necessary (particularly when neostigmine is given by injection) but not given routinely because it may mask signs of overdosage · bradycardia · epilepsy · hyperthyroidism · hypotension · parkinsonism · peptic ulceration · recent myocardial infarction · vagotonia
- **SIDE-EFFECTS** Abdominal cramps · diarrhoea · excessive tearing · hypersalivation · nausea · vomiting
  Overdose Signs of overdosage include bronchoconstriction, increased bronchial secretions, lacrimation, excessive sweating, involuntary defaecation, involuntary micturition, miosis, nystagmus, bradycardia, heart block, arrhythmias, hypotension, agitation, excessive dreaming, and weakness eventually leading to fasciculation and paralysis.
- **PREGNANCY** Manufacturer advises use only if potential benefit outweighs risk.
- **BREAST FEEDING** Amount probably too small to be harmful.

F 813

Neostigmine
(Neostigmine methylsulfate)

● **INDICATIONS AND DOSE**

Treatment of myasthenia gravis

▶ BY MOUTH

- Neonate: Initially 1–2 mg, then 1–5 mg every 4 hours, given 30 minutes before feeds.
- Child 1 month–5 years: Initially 7.5 mg, dose repeated at suitable intervals throughout the day, total daily dose 15–90 mg
- Child 6–11 years: Initially 15 mg, dose repeated at suitable intervals throughout the day, total daily dose 15–90 mg
- Child 12–17 years: Initially 15–30 mg, dose repeated at suitable intervals throughout the day, total daily dose 75–300 mg, the maximum that most patients can tolerate is 180 mg daily

▶ BY SUBCUTANEOUS INJECTION, OR BY INTRAMUSCULAR INJECTION

- Neonate: 150 micrograms/kg every 6–8 hours, to be given 30 minutes before feeds, then increased if necessary up to 300 micrograms/kg every 4 hours.
- Child 1 month–11 years: 200–500 micrograms, dose repeated at suitable intervals throughout the day
- Child 12–17 years: 1–2.5 mg, dose repeated at suitable intervals throughout the day

Reversal of non-depolarising (competitive) neuromuscular blockade

▶ BY INTRAVENOUS INJECTION

- Neonate: 50 micrograms/kg, to be given over 1 minute after or with glycopyrronium or atropine, followed by 25 micrograms/kg if required.
- Child 1 month–11 years: 50 micrograms/kg (max. per dose 2.5 mg), to be given over 1 minute after or with glycopyrronium or atropine, then 25 micrograms/kg if required
- Child 12–17 years: 50 micrograms/kg (max. per dose 2.5 mg), to be given over 1 minute after or with glycopyrronium or atropine, then 25 micrograms/kg (max. per dose 2.5 mg) if required

● **UNLICENSED USE**
- In neonates Dose for treatment of myasthenia gravis by subcutaneous or intramuscular injection is unlicensed.

● **CAUTIONS**
- With intravenous use Glycopyrronium or atropine should also be given when reversing neuromuscular blockade

● **INTERACTIONS** → Appendix 1: neostigmine

● **SIDE-EFFECTS**
- With parenteral use Intestinal hypermotility · muscle spasms

● **RENAL IMPAIRMENT**

Dose adjustments May need dose reduction.

● **DIRECTIONS FOR ADMINISTRATION** For *intravenous injection*, give undiluted *or* dilute with Glucose 5% *or* Sodium Chloride 0.9%.

● **MEDICINAL FORMS** There can be variation in the licensing of different medicines containing the same drug. Forms available from special-order manufacturers include: oral solution

Solution for injection

- **Neostigmine (Non-proprietary)**
  Neostigmine metilsulfate 2.5 mg per 1 ml Neostigmine 2.5mg/1ml solution for injection ampoules | 10 ampoule [PoM] £14.98–£19.50

F 813

Pyridostigmine bromide
05-Nov-2021

● **DRUG ACTION** Pyridostigmine bromide has weaker muscarinic action than neostigmine.

● **INDICATIONS AND DOSE**

Myasthenia gravis

▶ BY MOUTH

- Neonate: Initially 0.5–1 mg/kg every 4–6 hours, then increased if necessary up to 1.2 mg/kg every 4 hours, dose can be increased every 3 to 4 days, or more often during inpatient treatment with monitoring for side-effects; give 30-60 minutes before feeds.
- Child 1 month–11 years: Initially 0.5–1 mg/kg every 4–6 hours, then increased if necessary up to 1.2 mg/kg every 4 hours, dose can be increased every 3 to 4 days, or more often during inpatient treatment with monitoring for side-effects; usual maximum dose 60 mg every 4 hours
- Child 12-17 years: 30–90 mg every 4–6 hours, consider immunosuppressant therapy if total daily dose exceeds 360 mg, down-regulation of acetylcholine receptors possible if total daily dose exceeds 450 mg

● **UNLICENSED USE** [EvGr] Pyridostigmine bromide is used in the doses provided in BNFC for the treatment of myasthenia gravis, ⟨E⟩ but these are not licensed.

● **INTERACTIONS** → Appendix 1: pyridostigmine

● **SIDE-EFFECTS** Gastrointestinal hypermotility · muscle cramps · rash

● **RENAL IMPAIRMENT**

Dose adjustments [EvGr] Consider dose reduction (excreted renally). ⟨M⟩

● **MEDICINAL FORMS** There can be variation in the licensing of different medicines containing the same drug. Forms available from special-order manufacturers include: oral tablet, oral suspension, oral solution

Oral tablet

- **Pyridostigmine bromide (Non-proprietary)**
  Pyridostigmine bromide 60 mg Pyridostigmine bromide 60mg tablets | 200 tablet [PoM] £32.00 DT = £13.79
- **Mestinon** (Viatris UK Healthcare Ltd)
  Pyridostigmine bromide 60 mg Mestinon 60mg tablets | 200 tablet [PoM] £45.57 DT = £13.79

Oral solution

EXCIPIENTS: May contain Propylene glycol, sorbitol
ELECTROLYTES: May contain Sodium

- **Pyridostigmine bromide (Non-proprietary)**
  Pyridostigmine bromide 12 mg per 1 ml Pyridostigmine bromide 12mg/1ml oral solution sugar free | 150 ml [PoM] £90.00–£157.50 DT = £90.00 [SF]

2.3 Spasticity

MUSCLE RELAXANTS › CENTRALLY ACTING

Baclofen
08-Jan-2024

● **INDICATIONS AND DOSE**

Chronic severe spasticity of voluntary muscle

▶ BY MOUTH

- Child 1 month–7 years: Initially 75 micrograms/kg 4 times a day, usual maintenance up to 0.5 mg/kg 4 times a day, dose to be increased gradually at weekly intervals until satisfactory response, review treatment if no benefit within 6 weeks of achieving maximum dose; maximum 40 mg per day

- Child 8–17 years: Initially 75 micrograms/kg 4 times a day, usual maintenance up to 0.5 mg/kg 4 times a day, dose to be increased gradually at weekly intervals until satisfactory response, review treatment if no benefit within 6 weeks of achieving maximum dose; maximum 60 mg per day

Severe chronic spasticity of cerebral or spinal origin unresponsive to oral antispastic drugs (or oral therapy not tolerated) (specialist use only)

- BY INTRATHECAL INJECTION
- Child 4–17 years: Test dose 25–50 micrograms, to be given over at least 1 minute via catheter or lumbar puncture, then increased in steps of 25 micrograms (max. per dose 100 micrograms), not more often than every 24 hours to determine initial maintenance dose, then *dose-titration phase*, most often using infusion pump (implanted into chest wall or abdominal wall tissues) to establish maintenance dose retaining some spasticity to avoid sensation of paralysis; maintenance 25–200 micrograms daily, adjusted according to response

IMPORTANT SAFETY INFORMATION
Consult product literature for details on test dose and titration—important to monitor patients closely in appropriately equipped and staffed environment during screening and immediately after pump implantation. Resuscitation equipment must be available for immediate use. Treatment with continuous pump-administered intrathecal baclofen should be initiated within 3 months of a satisfactory response to intrathecal baclofen testing.

- **CONTRA-INDICATIONS**
  - With intrathecal use Local infection · systemic infection
  - With oral use Active peptic ulceration
- **CAUTIONS**
  GENERAL CAUTIONS Diabetes · epilepsy · history of peptic ulcer · history of substance abuse · hypertonic bladder sphincter · psychiatric illness · respiratory impairment
  SPECIFIC CAUTIONS
  - With intrathecal use Coagulation disorders · malnutrition (increased risk of post-surgical complications) · previous spinal fusion procedure
- **INTERACTIONS** → Appendix 1: baclofen
- **SIDE-EFFECTS**
  GENERAL SIDE-EFFECTS
  - **Common or very common** Confusion · constipation · depression · diarrhoea · dizziness · drowsiness · dry mouth · euphoric mood · hallucination · headache · hyperhidrosis · hypotension · nausea · paraesthesia · skin reactions · urinary disorders · vision disorders · vomiting
  - **Uncommon** Bradycardia · hypothermia · suicidal behaviours
  - **Rare or very rare** Withdrawal syndrome

  SPECIFIC SIDE-EFFECTS
  - **Common or very common**
  - With intrathecal use Anxiety · appetite decreased · asthenia · chills · dyspnoea · fever · hypersalivation · insomnia · neuromuscular dysfunction · oedema · pain · pneumonia · respiratory disorders · seizure · sexual dysfunction
  - With oral use Fatigue · gastrointestinal disorder · muscle weakness · myalgia · respiratory depression · sleep disorders
  - **Uncommon**
  - With intrathecal use Alopecia · deep vein thrombosis · dehydration · flushing · hypertension · hypogeusia · ileus · memory loss · pallor · paranoia
  - **Rare or very rare**
  - With oral use Abdominal pain · erectile dysfunction · hepatic function abnormal · taste altered
  - **Frequency not known**
  - With intrathecal use Scoliosis
- **PREGNANCY** Manufacturer advises use only if potential benefit outweighs risk (toxicity in *animal* studies).
- **BREAST FEEDING** Present in milk—amount probably too small to be harmful.
- **HEPATIC IMPAIRMENT**
  - With oral use Manufacturer advises use with caution—no information available.
- **RENAL IMPAIRMENT** See p. 16. [EvGr] Use with caution. ⟨M⟩
  - With oral use [EvGr] Only use if potential benefit outweighs risk if estimated glomerular filtration rate less than 15 mL/minute/1.73 m^2. ⟨M⟩

  Dose adjustments
  - With oral use [EvGr] Use smaller doses and if necessary increase dosage interval—monitor for signs and symptoms of toxicity. ⟨M⟩
- **TREATMENT CESSATION** Avoid abrupt withdrawal (risk of hyperactive state, may exacerbate spasticity, and precipitate autonomic dysfunction including hyperthermia, psychiatric reactions and convulsions; to minimise risk, discontinue by gradual dose reduction over at least 1–2 weeks (longer if symptoms occur)).
- **PRESCRIBING AND DISPENSING INFORMATION** Flavours of oral liquid formulations may include raspberry.
- **PATIENT AND CARER ADVICE**
  Medicines for Children leaflet: Baclofen for muscle spasm www.medicinesforchildren.org.uk/medicines/baclofen-for-muscle-spasm/
  Driving and skilled tasks Drowsiness may affect performance of skilled tasks (e.g. driving); effects of alcohol enhanced.

- **MEDICINAL FORMS** There can be variation in the licensing of different medicines containing the same drug. Forms available from special-order manufacturers include: oral suspension, oral solution, solution for injection

Oral tablet

CAUTIONARY AND ADVISORY LABELS 2, 8, 21
EXCIPIENTS: May contain Gluten

- **Baclofen (Non-proprietary)**
  Baclofen 5 mg Baclofen 5mg tablets | 84 tablet [PoM] £10.80
  Baclofen 10 mg Baclofen 10mg tablets | 84 tablet [PoM] £7.89 DT = £1.27
  Baclofen 20 mg Baclofen 20mg tablets | 84 tablet [PoM] £2.77
- **Lioresal** (Novartis Pharmaceuticals UK Ltd)
  Baclofen 10 mg Lioresal 10mg tablets | 100 tablet [PoM] £14.86

Solution for injection

- **Baclofen (Non-proprietary)**
  Baclofen 50 microgram per 1 ml Baclofen 50micrograms/1ml solution for injection ampoules | 10 ampoule [PoM] £40.00
  Baclofen 1 mg per 1 ml Gablofen 20mg/20ml solution for injection pre-filled syringes | 1 pre-filled disposable injection [PoM] [Ⓧ] (Hospital only)
  Gablofen 20mg/20ml solution for injection vials | 1 vial [PoM] [Ⓧ] (Hospital only)
- **Lioresal** (Novartis Pharmaceuticals UK Ltd)
  Baclofen 50 microgram per 1 ml Lioresal Intrathecal 50micrograms/1ml solution for injection ampoules | 1 ampoule [PoM] £3.16

Solution for infusion

- **Baclofen (Non-proprietary)**
  Baclofen 500 microgram per 1 ml Baclofen 10mg/20ml solution for infusion ampoules | 1 ampoule [PoM] £80.00
  Baclofen 2 mg per 1 ml Baclofen 40mg/20ml solution for infusion ampoules | 1 ampoule [PoM] £600.00
  Baclofen 10mg/5ml solution for infusion ampoules | 10 ampoule [PoM] £650.00
- **Lioresal** (Novartis Pharmaceuticals UK Ltd)
  Baclofen 500 microgram per 1 ml Lioresal Intrathecal 10mg/20ml solution for infusion ampoules | 1 ampoule [PoM] £70.01

Baclofen 2 mg per 1 ml Lioresal Intrathecal 10mg/5ml solution for infusion ampoules | 1 ampoule [PoM] £70.01

Oral solution

CAUTIONARY AND ADVISORY LABELS 2, 8, 21

▸ **Baclofen (Non-proprietary)**

Baclofen 1 mg per 1 ml Baclofen 5mg/5ml oral solution sugar free | 300 ml [PoM] £8.95 DT = £3.03 [SF]

Baclofen 2 mg per 1 ml Baclofen 10mg/5ml oral solution sugar free | 150 ml [PoM] £9.10–£14.95 DT = £14.95 [SF]

▸ **Lyflex** (Rosemont Pharmaceuticals Ltd)

Baclofen 1 mg per 1 ml Lyflex 5mg/5ml oral solution | 300 ml [PoM] £7.95 DT = £3.03 [SF]

3 Pain and inflammation in musculoskeletal disorders

Non-steroidal anti-inflammatory drugs

01-Aug-2023

Therapeutic effects

In *single doses* non-steroidal anti-inflammatory drugs (NSAIDs) have analgesic activity comparable to that of paracetamol p. 325 but paracetamol is preferred.

In regular *full dosage* NSAIDs have both a lasting analgesic and an anti-inflammatory effect which makes them particularly useful for the treatment of continuous or regular pain associated with inflammation.

Choice

Differences in anti-inflammatory activity between NSAIDs are small, but there is considerable variation in individual response and tolerance of these drugs. A large proportion of children will respond to any NSAID; of the others, those who do not respond to one may well respond to another. Pain relief starts soon after taking the first dose and a full analgesic effect should normally be obtained within a week, whereas an anti-inflammatory effect may not be achieved (or may not be clinically assessable) for up to 3 weeks. However, in juvenile idiopathic arthritis NSAIDs may take 4–12 weeks to be effective. If appropriate responses are not obtained within these times, another NSAID should be tried. The availability of appropriate formulations needs to be considered when prescribing NSAIDs for children.

NSAIDs reduce the production of prostaglandins by inhibiting the enzyme cyclo-oxygenase. They vary in their selectivity for inhibiting different types of cyclo-oxygenase; selective inhibition of cyclo-oxygenase-2 is associated with less gastro-intestinal intolerance. However, in children gastro-intestinal symptoms are rare in those taking NSAIDs for short periods. The role of selective inhibitors of cyclo-oxygenase-2 is undetermined in children.

Ibuprofen p. 821 and naproxen p. 826 are propionic acid derivatives used in children.

Ibuprofen combines anti-inflammatory, analgesic, and antipyretic properties. It has fewer side-effects than other NSAIDs but its anti-inflammatory properties are weaker.

Naproxen combines good efficacy with a low incidence of side-effects.

Diclofenac sodium p. 818, diclofenac potassium p. 817, indometacin p. 824, mefenamic acid p. 825, and piroxicam p. 828 have properties similar to those of propionic acid derivatives:

Diclofenac sodium and diclofenac potassium are similar in efficacy to naproxen.

Indometacin has an action equal to or superior to that of naproxen, but with a high incidence of side-effects including headache, dizziness, and gastro-intestinal disturbances. It is rarely used in children and should be reserved for when other NSAIDs have been unsuccessful.

Mefenamic acid has minor anti-inflammatory properties. It has occasionally been associated with diarrhoea and haemolytic anaemia which require discontinuation of treatment.

Piroxicam is as effective as naproxen and has a long duration of action which permits once-daily administration. However, it has more gastro-intestinal side-effects than most other NSAIDs, and is associated with more frequent serious skin reactions.

Meloxicam p. 826 is a selective inhibitor of cyclo-oxygenase-2. Its use may be considered in adolescents intolerant to other NSAIDs.

Ketorolac trometamol p. 1021 can be used for the short-term management of postoperative pain.

Etoricoxib p. 820, a selective inhibitor of cyclo-oxygenase-2, is licensed for the relief of pain in osteoarthritis, rheumatoid arthritis, ankylosing spondylitis, and acute gout in children aged 16 years and over.

Dental and orofacial pain

Most mild to moderate dental pain and inflammation is effectively relieved by ibuprofen, diclofenac potassium or diclofenac sodium.

NSAIDs in pregnancy

MHRA/CHM advice: NSAIDs: potential risks following prolonged use after 20 weeks of pregnancy (June 2023)

A European review of data from a 2022 study identified that prolonged (more than a few days) use of systemic NSAIDs from week 20 of pregnancy onwards may be associated with an increased risk of:

- oligohydramnios resulting from fetal renal dysfunction—this may occur shortly after treatment initiation, although usually reversible upon discontinuation;
- constriction of the ductus arteriosus—most reported cases resolved after treatment cessation.

These risks are potentially serious as they can cause restriction of fetal growth and cardiac dysfunction.

Healthcare professionals are advised to:

- avoid prescribing systemic NSAIDs from week 20 of pregnancy (the EMA review advises to avoid during the first and second trimesters) unless clinically required, in which case the lowest dose should be prescribed for the shortest time;
- consider antenatal monitoring for oligohydramnios if the mother has been exposed to systemic NSAIDs for several days after week 20 of pregnancy—the NSAID should be discontinued if oligohydramnios is detected, or if the NSAID is no longer necessary;
- continue to follow clinical guidelines about recording current and recent medicines, including over-the-counter medicines, at each antenatal appointment.

Healthcare professionals are also reminded that systemic NSAIDs are contra-indicated during the third trimester (after 28 weeks) of pregnancy due to the risk of premature closure of the ductus arteriosus, fetal renal dysfunction, prolongation of maternal bleeding time, and inhibition of uterine contractions during labour.

In addition, patients or their carers should be advised that:

- systemic NSAIDs should be avoided altogether during the third trimester of pregnancy;
- systemic NSAIDs should also be avoided from week 20 of pregnancy onwards unless otherwise advised by a doctor;
- if a systemic NSAID is used for more than a few days during later pregnancy, additional monitoring such as ultrasound scans may be required;
- some non-prescription pain relief preparations contain more than one active drug and advice should be sought from a healthcare professional if there is any uncertainty—such preparations should be used at the lowest dose for the shortest possible time;

- it is vitally important to seek medical advice if pain persists for longer than 3 days, or if there is repeated pain during pregnancy.

This advice does not apply to aspirin, COX-2 selective inhibitors, and topical NSAIDs—separate advice on the use of these during pregnancy should be followed.

NSAIDs in asthma

All NSAIDs have the potential to worsen asthma, either acutely or as a gradual worsening of symptoms; consider both prescribed NSAIDs and those that are purchased over the counter.

NSAIDs and cardiovascular events

The risk of cardiovascular events secondary to NSAID use is undetermined in children. In adults, all NSAID use (including cyclo-oxygenase-2 selective inhibitors) can, to varying degrees, be associated with a small increased risk of thrombotic events (e.g. myocardial infarction and stroke) independent of baseline cardiovascular risk factors or duration of NSAID use; however, the greatest risk may be in those patients receiving high doses long term. A small increased thrombotic risk cannot be excluded in children.

In adults, cyclo-oxygenase-2 selective inhibitors, diclofenac (150 mg daily) and ibuprofen (2.4 g daily) are associated with an increased risk of thrombotic events. The increased risk for diclofenac is similar to that of etoricoxib. Naproxen (in adults, 1 g daily) is associated with a lower thrombotic risk, and lower doses of ibuprofen p. 821 (in adults, 1.2 g daily or less) have not been associated with an increased risk of myocardial infarction.

The lowest effective dose of NSAID should be prescribed for the shortest period of time to control symptoms, and the need for long-term treatment should be reviewed periodically.

NSAIDs and gastro-intestinal events

All NSAIDs are associated with gastro-intestinal toxicity. In adults, evidence on the relative safety of NSAIDs indicates differences in the risks of serious upper gastro-intestinal side-effects— piroxicam p. 828 and ketorolac trometamol p. 1021 are associated with the highest risk; indometacin p. 824, diclofenac, and naproxen p. 826 are associated with intermediate risk, and ibuprofen with the lowest risk (although high doses of ibuprofen have been associated with intermediate risk). Selective inhibitors of cyclo-oxygenase-2 are associated with a *lower risk* of serious upper gastro-intestinal side-effects than non-selective NSAIDs.

Children appear to tolerate NSAIDs better than adults and gastro-intestinal side-effects are less common although they do still occur and can be significant; use of gastro-protective drugs may be necessary.

ANALGESICS › NON-STEROIDAL ANTI-INFLAMMATORY DRUGS

Diclofenac potassium

01-Aug-2023

- **INDICATIONS AND DOSE**

Pain and inflammation in rheumatic disease and other musculoskeletal disorders

▶ BY MOUTH

▸ Child 14–17 years: 75–100 mg daily in 2–3 divided doses

Postoperative pain

▶ BY MOUTH

▸ Child 9–13 years (body-weight 35 kg and above): Up to 2 mg/kg daily in 3 divided doses; maximum 100 mg per day

▸ Child 14–17 years: 75–100 mg daily in 2–3 divided doses

Fever in ear, nose, or throat infection

▶ BY MOUTH

▸ Child 9–17 years (body-weight 35 kg and above): Up to 2 mg/kg daily in 3 divided doses; maximum 100 mg per day

- **UNLICENSED USE** *Voltarol® Rapid* not licensed for use in children under 14 years or in fever.

> **IMPORTANT SAFETY INFORMATION**
> MHRA/CHM ADVICE: NSAIDS: POTENTIAL RISKS FOLLOWING PROLONGED USE AFTER 20 WEEKS OF PREGNANCY (JUNE 2023)
> See Non-steroidal anti-inflammatory drugs p. 816.

- **CONTRA-INDICATIONS** Active gastro-intestinal bleeding · active gastro-intestinal ulceration · cerebrovascular disease · history of gastro-intestinal bleeding related to previous NSAID therapy · history of gastro-intestinal perforation related to previous NSAID therapy · history of recurrent gastro-intestinal haemorrhage (two or more distinct episodes) · history of recurrent gastro-intestinal ulceration (two or more distinct episodes) · ischaemic heart disease · mild to severe heart failure · peripheral arterial disease
- **CAUTIONS** Allergic disorders · cardiac impairment (NSAIDs may impair renal function) · coagulation defects · connective-tissue disorders · dehydration (risk of renal impairment) · history of cardiac failure · history of gastro-intestinal disorders (e.g. ulcerative colitis, Crohn's disease) · hypertension · may mask symptoms of infection · oedema · risk factors for cardiovascular events
- **INTERACTIONS** → Appendix 1: NSAIDs
- **SIDE-EFFECTS**

▶ **Common or very common** Appetite decreased · diarrhoea · dizziness · gastrointestinal discomfort · gastrointestinal disorders · headache · nausea · skin reactions · vertigo · vomiting

▶ **Uncommon** Chest pain · heart failure · myocardial infarction · palpitations

▶ **Rare or very rare** Acute kidney injury · agranulocytosis · alopecia · anaemia · angioedema · anxiety · aplastic anaemia · asthma · confusion · constipation · depression · drowsiness · dyspnoea · erectile dysfunction · fatigue · haemolytic anaemia · haemorrhage · hearing impairment · hepatic disorders · hypersensitivity · hypertension · hypotension · inflammatory bowel disease · irritability · leucopenia · memory loss · meningitis aseptic (patients with connective-tissue disorders such as systemic lupus erythematosus may be especially susceptible) · nephritis tubulointerstitial · nephrotic syndrome · oedema · oesophageal disorder · oral disorders · pancreatitis · photosensitivity reaction · pneumonitis · proteinuria · psychotic disorder · renal papillary necrosis · seizure · sensation abnormal · severe cutaneous adverse reactions (SCARs) · shock · sleep disorders · stroke · taste altered · thrombocytopenia · tinnitus · tremor · vasculitis · vision disorders

▶ **Frequency not known** Hallucination · malaise · optic neuritis

SIDE-EFFECTS, FURTHER INFORMATION For information about cardiovascular and gastrointestinal side-effects, and a possible exacerbation of symptoms in asthma, see Non-steroidal anti-inflammatory drugs p. 816

- **ALLERGY AND CROSS-SENSITIVITY** [EvGr] Contra-indicated in patients with a history of hypersensitivity to aspirin or any other NSAID—which includes those in whom attacks of asthma, angioedema, urticaria or rhinitis have been precipitated by aspirin or any other NSAID. ⟨M⟩
- **CONCEPTION AND CONTRACEPTION** [EvGr] Caution—long-term use of some NSAIDs is associated with reduced

10 Musculoskeletal system

female fertility, which is reversible on stopping treatment. ⟨M⟩

- **PREGNANCY** Avoid use in first and second trimesters unless essential; the MHRA advises additional antenatal monitoring may be required if treatment is considered necessary by a doctor from week 20 of pregnancy onwards. Avoid use in third trimester. See *NSAIDs in Pregnancy* in Non-steroidal anti-inflammatory drugs p. 816 for further details.
- **BREAST FEEDING** Use with caution during breast-feeding. Amount in milk too small to be harmful.
- **HEPATIC IMPAIRMENT** Manufacturer advises caution in mild to moderate impairment; avoid in severe impairment.
- **RENAL IMPAIRMENT** In general, for *NSAIDs* the MHRA advises to avoid where possible; if necessary, use with caution (risk of fluid retention and further renal impairment, including renal failure). EvGr For *diclofenac potassium*, avoid in severe impairment. ⟨M⟩
- **PATIENT AND CARER ADVICE** Medicines for Children leaflet: Diclofenac for pain and inflammation www.medicinesforchildren.org.uk/medicines/diclofenac-for-pain-and-inflammation/
- **MEDICINAL FORMS** There can be variation in the licensing of different medicines containing the same drug.

Oral tablet

CAUTIONARY AND ADVISORY LABELS 21

- Voltarol Rapid (Novartis Pharmaceuticals UK Ltd)
  Diclofenac potassium 50 mg Voltarol Rapid 50mg tablets | 30 tablet PoM £7.94 DT = £7.94

Diclofenac sodium

19-Mar-2025

- **INDICATIONS AND DOSE**

Pain and inflammation in rheumatic disease including juvenile idiopathic arthritis

- BY MOUTH USING IMMEDIATE-RELEASE MEDICINES
  - Child 6 months–17 years: 1.5–2.5 mg/kg twice daily (max. per dose 75 mg), total daily dose may alternatively be given in 3 divided doses; maximum 150 mg per day

Postoperative pain

- BY RECTUM
  - Child 6 months–17 years (body-weight 8–11 kg): 12.5 mg twice daily for maximum 4 days
  - Child 6 months–17 years (body-weight 12 kg and above): 1 mg/kg 3 times a day (max. per dose 50 mg) for maximum 4 days

Inflammation | Mild to moderate pain

- BY MOUTH USING IMMEDIATE-RELEASE MEDICINES, OR BY RECTUM
  - Child 6 months–17 years: 0.3–1 mg/kg 3 times a day (max. per dose 50 mg)
- BY MOUTH USING MODIFIED-RELEASE CAPSULES
  - Child 12–17 years: 75 mg 1–2 times a day, alternatively 100 mg once daily

Pain and inflammation in rheumatic disease and other musculoskeletal disorders [using gel containing diclofenac sodium 1%] | Osteoarthritis of the knee or hand [using gel containing diclofenac sodium 1%]

- TO THE SKIN
  - Child 14–17 years: Apply 3–4 times a day review after 7 days

DOSE EQUIVALENCE AND CONVERSION

- *Voltarol® 1.16% Emulgel* contains 1.16% diclofenac diethylammonium equivalent to diclofenac sodium 1%.

VOLTAROL® SOLUTION FOR INJECTION

Postoperative pain

- BY INTRAVENOUS INFUSION, OR BY DEEP INTRAMUSCULAR INJECTION
  - Child 2–17 years: 0.3–1 mg/kg 1–2 times a day for maximum 2 days, for intramuscular injection, to be injected into the gluteal muscle; maximum 150 mg per day

- **UNLICENSED USE**
  - With systemic use Not licensed for use in children under 1 year. *Suppositories* not licensed for use in children under 6 years except for use in children over 1 year for juvenile idiopathic arthritis. Solid dose forms containing more than 25 mg not licensed for use in children. *Injection* not licensed for use in children.

> **IMPORTANT SAFETY INFORMATION**
>
> MHRA/CHM ADVICE: NSAIDS: POTENTIAL RISKS FOLLOWING PROLONGED USE AFTER 20 WEEKS OF PREGNANCY (JUNE 2023)
>
> - With systemic use
>
> See Non-steroidal anti-inflammatory drugs p. 816.

- **CONTRA-INDICATIONS**
  - With intravenous use Avoid injections containing benzyl alcohol in neonates · dehydration · history of asthma · history of confirmed or suspected cerebrovascular bleeding · history of haemorrhagic diathesis · hypovolaemia · operations with high risk of haemorrhage
  - With systemic use Active gastro-intestinal bleeding · active gastro-intestinal ulceration · avoid suppositories in proctitis · cerebrovascular disease · history of gastro-intestinal bleeding related to previous NSAID therapy · history of gastro-intestinal perforation related to previous NSAID therapy · history of recurrent gastro-intestinal haemorrhage (two or more distinct episodes) · history of recurrent gastro-intestinal ulceration (two or more distinct episodes) · ischaemic heart disease · mild to severe heart failure · peripheral arterial disease
- **CAUTIONS**
  - With systemic use Allergic disorders · cardiac impairment (NSAIDs may impair renal function) · coagulation defects · connective-tissue disorders · dehydration (risk of renal impairment) · history of cardiac failure · history of gastro-intestinal disorders (e.g. ulcerative colitis, Crohn's disease) · hypertension · may mask symptoms of infection · oedema · risk factors for cardiovascular events
  - With topical use Avoid contact with eyes · avoid contact with inflamed or broken skin · avoid contact with mucous membranes · not for use with occlusive dressings · topical application of large amounts can result in systemic effects, including hypersensitivity and asthma (renal disease has also been reported)
- **INTERACTIONS** → Appendix 1: NSAIDs
- **SIDE-EFFECTS**

GENERAL SIDE-EFFECTS

- **Common or very common** Rash (discontinue) · skin reactions
- **Rare or very rare** Angioedema · asthma · hypersensitivity · photosensitivity reaction

SPECIFIC SIDE-EFFECTS

- **Common or very common**
  - With systemic use Appetite decreased · diarrhoea · dizziness · gastrointestinal discomfort · gastrointestinal disorders · headache · nausea · vertigo · vomiting
- **Uncommon**
  - With systemic use Chest pain · heart failure · myocardial infarction · palpitations
- **Rare or very rare**
  - With parenteral use Fatigue
  - With rectal use Fatigue · ulcerative colitis aggravated

- With systemic use Acute kidney injury · agranulocytosis · alopecia · anaemia · anxiety · aplastic anaemia · confusion · constipation · depression · drowsiness · dyspnoea · erectile dysfunction · haemolytic anaemia · haemorrhage · hearing impairment · hepatic disorders · hypertension · hypotension · irritability · leucopenia · memory loss · meningitis aseptic (patients with connective-tissue disorders such as systemic lupus erythematosus may be especially susceptible) · nephritis tubulointerstitial · nephrotic syndrome · oedema · oesophageal disorder · oral disorders · pancreatitis · pneumonitis · proteinuria · psychotic disorder · renal papillary necrosis · seizure · sensation abnormal · severe cutaneous adverse reactions (SCARs) · shock · sleep disorders · stroke · taste altered · thrombocytopenia · tinnitus · tremor · vasculitis · vision disorders
- With topical use Rash pustular
- **Frequency not known**
- With oral use Fluid retention
- With parenteral use Fluid retention · injection site necrosis
- With systemic use Fertility decreased female · hallucination · malaise · optic neuritis · platelet aggregation inhibition

SIDE-EFFECTS, FURTHER INFORMATION Topical application of large amounts of diclofenac to the skin can result in systemic effects.

For information about cardiovascular and gastrointestinal side-effects, and a possible exacerbation of symptoms in asthma, see Non-steroidal anti-inflammatory drugs p. 816

- **ALLERGY AND CROSS-SENSITIVITY** [EvGr] Contra-indicated in patients with a history of hypersensitivity to aspirin or any other NSAID—which includes those in whom attacks of asthma, angioedema, urticaria or rhinitis have been precipitated by aspirin or any other NSAID. (M)
- **CONCEPTION AND CONTRACEPTION**
- With systemic use [EvGr] Caution—long-term use of some NSAIDs is associated with reduced female fertility, which is reversible on stopping treatment. (M)
- **PREGNANCY**
- With systemic use Avoid use in first and second trimesters unless essential; the MHRA advises additional antenatal monitoring may be required if treatment is considered necessary by a doctor from week 20 of pregnancy onwards. Avoid use in third trimester. See *NSAIDs in Pregnancy* in Non-steroidal anti-inflammatory drugs p. 816 for further details.
- With topical use Patient packs for topical preparations carry a warning to avoid during pregnancy.
- **BREAST FEEDING**
- With systemic use Use with caution during breast-feeding. Amount in milk too small to be harmful.
- With topical use Patient packs for topical preparations carry a warning to avoid during breast-feeding.
- **HEPATIC IMPAIRMENT**
- With systemic use Manufacturer advises caution in mild to moderate impairment; avoid in severe impairment.
- **RENAL IMPAIRMENT**
- With systemic use In general, for *NSAIDs* the MHRA advises to avoid where possible; if necessary, use with caution (risk of fluid retention and further renal impairment, including renal failure). For *diclofenac sodium*, manufacturers advise avoid in severe impairment.
- With intravenous use Manufacturers advise avoid in moderate to severe impairment.
- **DIRECTIONS FOR ADMINISTRATION** For *intravenous infusion*, dilute 75 mg with 100–500 mL Glucose 5% *or* Sodium Chloride 0.9% (previously buffered with 0.5 mL Sodium Bicarbonate 8.4% solution *or* with 1 mL Sodium Bicarbonate 4.2% solution); give over 30–120 minutes.
- **PATIENT AND CARER ADVICE** For topical preparations, patients and their carers should be advised to wash hands immediately after use. Patients and their carers using topical gels such as *Voltarol Emulgel*® should be instructed not to smoke or go near naked flames as clothing, bedding, dressings, and other fabrics that have been in contact with skin treated with these gels burn more easily and can rapidly ignite. Washing these materials may reduce build-up of these gels but not totally remove it.

Photosensitivity Patients should be advised against excessive exposure to sunlight of area treated in order to avoid possibility of photosensitivity.

Medicines for Children leaflet: Diclofenac for pain and inflammation www.medicinesforchildren.org.uk/medicines/diclofenac-for-pain-and-inflammation/

- **EXCEPTIONS TO LEGAL CATEGORY**
- With topical use for Pain and inflammation in rheumatic disease and other musculoskeletal disorders or Osteoarthritis of the knee or hand Various pack sizes of gel preparations may be available on sale to the public.

- **MEDICINAL FORMS** There can be variation in the licensing of different medicines containing the same drug. Forms available from special-order manufacturers include: dispersible tablet, oral suspension, oral solution

Gastro-resistant tablet

CAUTIONARY AND ADVISORY LABELS 5, 25

- **Diclofenac sodium (Non-proprietary)**
  Diclofenac sodium 25 mg Diclofenac sodium 25mg gastro-resistant tablets | 28 tablet [PoM] £4.13 DT = £4.13 | 84 tablet [PoM] £10.49–£14.00
  Diclofenac sodium 50 mg Diclofenac sodium 50mg gastro-resistant tablets | 28 tablet [PoM] £7.49 DT = £1.44 | 84 tablet [PoM] £14.99–£20.00

Suppository

- **Diclofenac sodium (Non-proprietary)**
  Diclofenac sodium 100 mg Diclofenac 100mg suppositories | 10 suppository [PoM] £3.04 DT = £3.64
- **Voltarol** (Novartis Pharmaceuticals UK Ltd)
  Diclofenac sodium 12.5 mg Voltarol 12.5mg suppositories | 10 suppository [PoM] £0.70 DT = £0.70
  Diclofenac sodium 25 mg Voltarol 25mg suppositories | 10 suppository [PoM] £1.24 DT = £1.24
  Diclofenac sodium 50 mg Voltarol 50mg suppositories | 10 suppository [PoM] £2.04 DT = £2.04
  Diclofenac sodium 100 mg Voltarol 100mg suppositories | 10 suppository [PoM] £3.64 DT = £3.64

Dispersible tablet

CAUTIONARY AND ADVISORY LABELS 13, 21

Solution for injection

EXCIPIENTS: May contain Benzyl alcohol, propylene glycol

- **Voltarol** (Novartis Pharmaceuticals UK Ltd)
  Diclofenac sodium 25 mg per 1 ml Voltarol 75mg/3ml solution for injection ampoules | 10 ampoule [PoM] £9.91 DT = £9.91

Modified-release capsule

CAUTIONARY AND ADVISORY LABELS 21(does not apply to Motifene® 75 mg), 25

EXCIPIENTS: May contain Propylene glycol

- **Diclomax Retard** (Galen Ltd)
  Diclofenac sodium 100 mg Diclomax Retard 100mg capsules | 28 capsule [PoM] £8.20 DT = £8.20
- **Diclomax SR** (Galen Ltd)
  Diclofenac sodium 75 mg Diclomax SR 75mg capsules | 56 capsule [PoM] £11.40 DT = £11.40
- **Motifene** (Glenwood GmbH)
  Diclofenac sodium 75 mg Motifene 75mg modified-release capsules | 56 capsule [PoM] £8.00 DT = £8.00

Cutaneous gel

CAUTIONARY AND ADVISORY LABELS 11, 15

EXCIPIENTS: May contain Benzyl alcohol, fragrances, propylene glycol

- **Diclofenac sodium (Non-proprietary)**
  Diclofenac sodium 10 mg per 1 gram Diclofenac 1% gel | 100 gram [PoM] £7.50 DT = £7.18
  Diclofenac diethylammonium 11.6 mg per 1 gram Diclofenac 1.16% gel | 30 gram [PoM] £3.29–£3.50 | 50 gram [PoM] £4.60–£4.85 | 100 gram [PoM] £4.63–£7.82 DT = £4.63
- **Voltarol Emulgel** (Haleon UK Trading Ltd)
  Diclofenac diethylammonium 11.6 mg per 1 gram Voltarol 1.16% Emulgel | 100 gram [PoM] £4.63 DT = £4.63

Etoricoxib

22-Nov-2021

- **INDICATIONS AND DOSE**

Pain and inflammation in osteoarthritis

▶ BY MOUTH

▶ Child 16–17 years: 30 mg once daily, increased if necessary to 60 mg once daily

Pain and inflammation in rheumatoid arthritis | Ankylosing spondylitis

▶ BY MOUTH

▶ Child 16–17 years: 60 mg once daily, increased if necessary to 90 mg once daily

Acute gout

▶ BY MOUTH

▶ Child 16–17 years: 120 mg once daily for maximum 8 days

- **CONTRA-INDICATIONS** Active gastro-intestinal bleeding · active gastro-intestinal ulceration · cerebrovascular disease · inflammatory bowel disease · ischaemic heart disease · mild to severe heart failure · peripheral arterial disease · uncontrolled hypertension (persistently above 140/90 mmHg)
- **CAUTIONS** Allergic disorders · cardiac impairment (NSAIDs may impair renal function) · coagulation defects · connective-tissue disorders · dehydration (risk of renal impairment) · history of cardiac failure · history of gastro-intestinal disorders · hypertension · left ventricular dysfunction · may mask symptoms of infection · oedema · risk factors for cardiovascular events
- **INTERACTIONS** → Appendix 1: NSAIDs
- **SIDE-EFFECTS**

▶ **Common or very common** Arrhythmias · asthenia · bronchospasm · constipation · diarrhoea · dizziness · fluid retention · gastrointestinal discomfort · gastrointestinal disorders · headache · hypertension · increased risk of infection · influenza like illness · nausea · oedema · oral ulceration · palpitations · skin reactions · vomiting

▶ **Uncommon** Alertness decreased · anaemia · angina pectoris · anxiety · appetite abnormal · cerebrovascular insufficiency · chest pain · congestive heart failure · conjunctivitis · cough · depression · drowsiness · dry mouth · dyspnoea · flushing · haemorrhage · hallucination · hyperkalaemia · hypersensitivity · insomnia · irritable bowel syndrome · leucopenia · myocardial infarction · pancreatitis · proteinuria · renal failure (more common in patients with pre-existing renal impairment) · sensation abnormal · taste altered · thrombocytopenia · tinnitus · vasculitis · vertigo · vision blurred · weight increased

▶ **Rare or very rare** Angioedema · confusion · hepatic disorders · muscle complaints · severe cutaneous adverse reactions (SCARs) · shock

▶ **Frequency not known** Nephritis tubulointerstitial · nephropathy

SIDE-EFFECTS, FURTHER INFORMATION For information about cardiovascular and gastrointestinal side-effects, and a possible exacerbation of symptoms in asthma, see Non-steroidal anti-inflammatory drugs p. 816

- **ALLERGY AND CROSS-SENSITIVITY** [EvGr] Contra-indicated in patients with a history of hypersensitivity to aspirin or any other NSAID—which includes those in whom attacks of asthma, angioedema, urticaria or rhinitis have been precipitated by aspirin or any other NSAID. ⟨M⟩
- **CONCEPTION AND CONTRACEPTION** Caution—long-term use of some NSAIDs is associated with reduced female fertility, which is reversible on stopping treatment.
- **PREGNANCY** Manufacturer advises avoid (teratogenic in *animal* studies). Avoid during the third trimester (risk of closure of fetal ductus arteriosus *in utero* and possibly persistent pulmonary hypertension of the newborn); onset of labour may be delayed and duration may be increased.
- **BREAST FEEDING** Use with caution during breast-feeding. Manufacturer advises avoid—present in milk in *animal* studies.
- **HEPATIC IMPAIRMENT** Manufacturer advises caution in mild to moderate impairment; avoid in severe impairment (no information available).

Dose adjustments Manufacturer advises max. 60 mg once daily in mild impairment; max. 30 mg once daily in moderate impairment.

- **RENAL IMPAIRMENT** In general, for *NSAIDs* the MHRA advises to avoid where possible; if necessary, use with caution (risk of fluid retention and further renal impairment, including renal failure). [EvGr] For *etoricoxib*, avoid if creatinine clearance less than 30 mL/minute. ⟨M⟩ See p. 16.
- **MONITORING REQUIREMENTS** Monitor blood pressure before treatment, 2 weeks after initiation and periodically during treatment.

- **MEDICINAL FORMS** There can be variation in the licensing of different medicines containing the same drug.

Oral tablet

▶ **Etoricoxib (Non-proprietary)**

Etoricoxib 30 mg Etoricoxib 30mg tablets | 28 tablet [PoM] £13.99 DT = £1.37

Etoricoxib 60 mg Etoricoxib 60mg tablets | 28 tablet [PoM] £20.11 DT = £1.73

Etoricoxib 90 mg Etoricoxib 90mg tablets | 28 tablet [PoM] £22.96 DT = £2.00

Etoricoxib 120 mg Etoricoxib 120mg tablets | 28 tablet [PoM] £24.11 DT = £4.51

▶ **Arcoxia** (Organon Pharma (UK) Ltd)

Etoricoxib 30 mg Arcoxia 30mg tablets | 28 tablet [PoM] £13.99 DT = £1.37

Etoricoxib 60 mg Arcoxia 60mg tablets | 28 tablet [PoM] £20.11 DT = £1.73

Etoricoxib 90 mg Arcoxia 90mg tablets | 28 tablet [PoM] £22.96 DT = £2.00

Etoricoxib 120 mg Arcoxia 120mg tablets | 7 tablet [PoM] £6.03 | 28 tablet [PoM] £24.11 DT = £4.51

Flurbiprofen

19-Mar-2025

- **INDICATIONS AND DOSE**

Pain and inflammation in rheumatic disease and other musculoskeletal disorders | Migraine | Postoperative analgesia | Mild to moderate pain

▶ BY MOUTH

▶ Child 12–17 years: 150–200 mg daily in 2–4 divided doses, then increased to 300 mg daily, dose to be increased only in acute conditions

Dysmenorrhoea

▶ BY MOUTH

▶ Child 12–17 years: Initially 100 mg, then 50–100 mg every 4–6 hours; maximum 300 mg per day

IMPORTANT SAFETY INFORMATION

MHRA/CHM ADVICE: NSAIDS: POTENTIAL RISKS FOLLOWING PROLONGED USE AFTER 20 WEEKS OF PREGNANCY (JUNE 2023)

See Non-steroidal anti-inflammatory drugs p. 816.

- **CONTRA-INDICATIONS** Active gastro-intestinal bleeding · active gastro-intestinal ulceration · Crohn's disease (may be exacerbated) · history of gastro-intestinal bleeding related to previous NSAID therapy · history of gastro-intestinal perforation related to previous NSAID therapy · history of recurrent gastro-intestinal haemorrhage (two or more distinct episodes) · history of recurrent gastro-intestinal ulceration (two or more distinct episodes) ·

severe heart failure · ulcerative colitis (may be exacerbated)

- **CAUTIONS** Allergic disorders · cardiac impairment (NSAIDs may impair renal function) · cerebrovascular disease · coagulation defects · connective-tissue disorders · dehydration (risk of renal impairment) · heart failure · history of gastro-intestinal disorders · ischaemic heart disease · may mask symptoms of infection · peripheral arterial disease · risk factors for cardiovascular events · uncontrolled hypertension
- **INTERACTIONS** → Appendix 1: NSAIDs
- **SIDE-EFFECTS** Agranulocytosis · angioedema · aplastic anaemia · asthma · bronchospasm · confusion · constipation · Crohn's disease · depression · diarrhoea · dizziness · drowsiness · dyspnoea · fatigue · fertility decreased female · gastrointestinal discomfort · gastrointestinal disorders · haemolytic anaemia · haemorrhage · hallucination · headache · heart failure · hepatic disorders · hypersensitivity · hypertension · malaise · meningitis aseptic (patients with connective-tissue disorders such as systemic lupus erythematosus may be especially susceptible) · nausea · nephritis tubulointerstitial · nephropathy · neutropenia · oedema · optic neuritis · oral ulceration (move lozenge around mouth) · pancreatitis · paraesthesia · photosensitivity reaction · platelet aggregation inhibition · renal failure (more common in patients with pre-existing renal impairment) · respiratory tract reaction · severe cutaneous adverse reactions (SCARs) · skin reactions · stroke · thrombocytopenia · tinnitus · vertigo · visual impairment · vomiting

  SIDE-EFFECTS, FURTHER INFORMATION For information about cardiovascular and gastrointestinal side-effects, and a possible exacerbation of symptoms in asthma, see Non-steroidal anti-inflammatory drugs p. 816
- **ALLERGY AND CROSS-SENSITIVITY** EvGr Contra-indicated in patients with a history of hypersensitivity to aspirin or any other NSAID—which includes those in whom attacks of asthma, angioedema, urticaria or rhinitis have been precipitated by aspirin or any other NSAID. ⟨M⟩
- **CONCEPTION AND CONTRACEPTION** EvGr Caution—long-term use of some NSAIDs is associated with reduced female fertility, which is reversible on stopping treatment. ⟨M⟩
- **PREGNANCY** Avoid use in first and second trimesters unless essential; the MHRA advises additional antenatal monitoring may be required if treatment is considered necessary by a doctor from week 20 of pregnancy onwards. Avoid use in third trimester. See *NSAIDs in Pregnancy* in Non-steroidal anti-inflammatory drugs p. 816 for further details.
- **BREAST FEEDING** Use with caution during breast-feeding. Small amount present in milk—manufacturer advises avoid.
- **HEPATIC IMPAIRMENT** Manufacturer advises caution in mild to moderate impairment; avoid in severe impairment.
- **RENAL IMPAIRMENT** In general, for *NSAIDs* the MHRA advises to avoid where possible; if necessary, use with caution (risk of fluid retention and further renal impairment, including renal failure). EvGr For *flurbiprofen*, avoid in severe impairment. ⟨M⟩

- **MEDICINAL FORMS** There can be variation in the licensing of different medicines containing the same drug.

Oral tablet

CAUTIONARY AND ADVISORY LABELS 21

- **Flurbiprofen (Non-proprietary)**
  - **Flurbiprofen 50 mg** Flurbiprofen 50mg tablets | 100 tablet PoM £60.54–£96.86 DT = £60.54
  - **Flurbiprofen 100 mg** Flurbiprofen 100mg tablets | 100 tablet PoM £171.20 DT = £107.00

Ibuprofen

18-Mar-2024

- **INDICATIONS AND DOSE**

Mild to moderate pain | Pain and inflammation of soft-tissue injuries | Pyrexia with discomfort

- BY MOUTH USING IMMEDIATE-RELEASE MEDICINES
  - Child 1-2 months: 5 mg/kg 3–4 times a day
  - Child 3-5 months: 50 mg 3 times a day, maximum daily dose to be given in 3–4 divided doses; maximum 30 mg/kg per day
  - Child 6-11 months: 50 mg 3–4 times a day, maximum daily dose to be given in 3–4 divided doses; maximum 30 mg/kg per day
  - Child 1-3 years: 100 mg 3 times a day, maximum daily dose to be given in 3–4 divided doses; maximum 30 mg/kg per day
  - Child 4-6 years: 150 mg 3 times a day, maximum daily dose to be given in 3–4 divided doses; maximum 30 mg/kg per day
  - Child 7-9 years: 200 mg 3 times a day, maximum daily dose to be given in 3–4 divided doses; maximum 30 mg/kg per day; maximum 2.4 g per day
  - Child 10-11 years: 300 mg 3 times a day, maximum daily dose to be given in 3–4 divided doses; maximum 30 mg/kg per day; maximum 2.4 g per day
  - Child 12-17 years: Initially 300–400 mg 3–4 times a day; maintenance 200–400 mg 3 times a day, increased if necessary up to 600 mg 4 times a day

Pain and inflammation

- BY MOUTH USING MODIFIED-RELEASE MEDICINES
  - Child 12-17 years: 1.6 g once daily, dose preferably taken in the early evening, increased to 2.4 g daily in 2 divided doses, dose to be increased only in severe cases

Pain and inflammation in rheumatic disease including juvenile idiopathic arthritis

- BY MOUTH USING IMMEDIATE-RELEASE MEDICINES
  - Child 3 months-17 years: 30–40 mg/kg daily in 3 divided doses (max. per dose 800 mg), alternatively 30–40 mg/kg daily in 4 divided doses (max. per dose 600 mg)

Pain and inflammation in systemic juvenile idiopathic arthritis

- BY MOUTH USING IMMEDIATE-RELEASE MEDICINES
  - Child 3 months-17 years (body-weight up to 40 kg): Up to 60 mg/kg daily in 4–6 divided doses
  - Child 3 months-17 years (body-weight 40 kg and above): Up to 2.4 g daily in 4–6 divided doses

Post-immunisation pyrexia in infants (on doctor's advice only)

- BY MOUTH USING IMMEDIATE-RELEASE MEDICINES
  - Child 2-3 months: 50 mg for 1 dose, followed by 50 mg for 1 dose, to be given 6 hours after first dose if required

continued →

Pain and inflammation in rheumatic disease and other musculoskeletal disorders (dose approved for use by community practitioner nurse prescribers) | Mild to moderate pain including dysmenorrhoea (dose approved for use by community practitioner nurse prescribers) | Migraine (dose approved for use by community practitioner nurse prescribers) | Dental pain (dose approved for use by community practitioner nurse prescribers) | Headache (dose approved for use by community practitioner nurse prescribers) | Fever (dose approved for use by community practitioner nurse prescribers) | Symptoms of colds and influenza (dose approved for use by community practitioner nurse prescribers) | Neuralgia (dose approved for use by community practitioner nurse prescribers)

▶ BY MOUTH USING IMMEDIATE-RELEASE MEDICINES
- Child 12–17 years: 200–400 mg 3 times a day, if symptoms worsen or persist for more than 3 days refer to doctor

Mild to moderate pain (dose approved for use by community practitioner nurse prescribers) | Pain and inflammation of soft-tissue injuries (dose approved for use by community practitioner nurse prescribers) | Pyrexia with discomfort (dose approved for use by community practitioner nurse prescribers)

▶ BY MOUTH USING IMMEDIATE-RELEASE MEDICINES
- Child 3–5 months (body-weight 5 kg and above): 20–30 mg/kg daily in divided doses, alternatively 50 mg 3 times a day for maximum of 24 hours, refer to doctor if symptoms persist for more than 24 hours
- Child 6–11 months: 50 mg 3–4 times a day, refer to doctor if symptoms persist for more than 3 days
- Child 1–3 years: 100 mg 3 times a day, refer to doctor if symptoms persist for more than 3 days
- Child 4–6 years: 150 mg 3 times a day, refer to doctor if symptoms persist for more than 3 days
- Child 7–9 years: 200 mg 3 times a day, refer to doctor if symptoms persist for more than 3 days
- Child 10–11 years: 300 mg 3 times a day, refer to doctor if symptoms persist for more than 3 days

Post-immunisation pyrexia in infants (dose approved for use by community practitioner nurse prescribers) (on doctor's advice only)

▶ BY MOUTH USING IMMEDIATE-RELEASE MEDICINES
- Child 3 months: 50 mg for 1 dose, followed by 50 mg for 1 dose, to be given 6 hours after first dose if required, if pyrexia persists refer to doctor

Acute moderate pain | Pyrexia

▶ BY INTRAVENOUS INFUSION
- Child 6–17 years (body-weight 20–29 kg): 200 mg 3 times a day as required for maximum 3 days, doses to be given at intervals of at least 6 hours; maximum 600 mg per day
- Child 6–17 years (body-weight 30–39 kg): 200 mg 4 times a day as required for maximum 3 days, doses to be given at intervals of at least 6 hours; maximum 800 mg per day
- Child 6–17 years (body-weight 40 kg and above): 200–400 mg 3 times a day as required for maximum 3 days, doses to be given at intervals of at least 6 hours; maximum 1.2 g per day

PEDEA®

Closure of ductus arteriosus (under expert supervision)

▶ BY SLOW INTRAVENOUS INJECTION
- Neonate up to 34 weeks corrected gestational age: Initially 10 mg/kg for 1 dose, to be given after the first 6 hours of life, then 5 mg/kg every 24 hours for 2 doses but see also *Monitoring requirements*, the course may be repeated after 48 hours if necessary.

● **UNLICENSED USE**
- With oral use Not licensed for use in children aged under 3 months or with body-weight under 5 kg. Maximum dose for systemic juvenile idiopathic arthritis is unlicensed.

IMPORTANT SAFETY INFORMATION

MHRA/CHM ADVICE: NSAIDS: POTENTIAL RISKS FOLLOWING PROLONGED USE AFTER 20 WEEKS OF PREGNANCY (JUNE 2023)

See Non-steroidal anti-inflammatory drugs p. 816.

● **CONTRA-INDICATIONS**

GENERAL CONTRA-INDICATIONS Active gastro-intestinal bleeding · active gastro-intestinal ulceration · history of gastro-intestinal bleeding related to previous NSAID therapy · history of gastro-intestinal perforation related to previous NSAID therapy · history of recurrent gastro-intestinal haemorrhage (two or more distinct episodes) · history of recurrent gastro-intestinal ulceration (two or more distinct episodes) · severe heart failure · varicella infection

SPECIFIC CONTRA-INDICATIONS
- With intravenous use Active bleeding (especially intracranial or gastro-intestinal) · coagulation defects (in neonates) · ductal-dependent congenital heart disease (in neonates) · known or suspected necrotising enterocolitis (in neonates) · life-threatening infection (in neonates) · marked unconjugated hyperbilirubinaemia (in neonates) · pulmonary hypertension (in neonates) · thrombocytopenia

● **CAUTIONS** Allergic disorders · cardiac impairment (NSAIDs may impair renal function) · cerebrovascular disease · coagulation defects · connective-tissue disorders · dehydration (risk of renal impairment) · heart failure · history of gastro-intestinal disorders (e.g. ulcerative colitis, Crohn's disease) · ischaemic heart disease · may mask symptoms of infection · peripheral arterial disease · risk factors for cardiovascular events · uncontrolled hypertension

CAUTIONS, FURTHER INFORMATION
- High-dose ibuprofen
- With oral use A small increase in cardiovascular risk, similar to the risk associated with cyclo-oxygenase-2 inhibitors and diclofenac, has been reported with high-dose ibuprofen (≥ 2.4 g daily); use should be avoided in patients with established ischaemic heart disease, peripheral arterial disease, cerebrovascular disease, congestive heart failure (New York Heart Association classification II-III), and uncontrolled hypertension.
- Masking of symptoms of underlying infections Ibuprofen can mask symptoms of infection, which may lead to delayed initiation of appropriate treatment and thereby worsen infection outcome. This has been observed in bacterial community-acquired pneumonia and bacterial complications to varicella. When administered for fever or pain relief in relation to infection, monitoring of infection is advised.

● **INTERACTIONS** → Appendix 1: NSAIDs

● **SIDE-EFFECTS**

GENERAL SIDE-EFFECTS
- **Common or very common** Constipation · diarrhoea · gastrointestinal discomfort · gastrointestinal disorders · haemorrhage · headache · nausea · skin reactions · vomiting
- **Uncommon** Asthma · hypersensitivity · oedema
- **Rare or very rare** Agranulocytosis · anaemia · dyspnoea · heart failure · hypertension · leucopenia · meningitis aseptic (patients with connective-tissue disorders such as systemic lupus erythematosus may be especially susceptible) · pancytopenia · renal papillary necrosis · respiratory disorders · severe cutaneous adverse reactions (SCARs) · shock · thrombocytopenia (very common in neonates)

- ▶ **Frequency not known** Fluid retention (very common in neonates) · increased risk of arterial thromboembolism

SPECIFIC SIDE-EFFECTS
- ▶ **Common or very common**
- ▶ With intravenous use Dizziness · fatigue · inflammatory bowel disease · insomnia · intraventricular haemorrhage (in neonates) · neutropenia (in neonates) · oral disorders · periventricular leukomalacia (in neonates) · vertigo
- ▶ **Uncommon**
- ▶ With intravenous use Anxiety · irritability · nephritis tubulointerstitial · nephrotic syndrome · renal impairment (very common in neonates) · tinnitus · vasculitis · vision disorders
- ▶ With oral use Rash (discontinue)
- ▶ **Rare or very rare**
- ▶ With intravenous use Alopecia · auditory disorder · confusion · depression · hepatic disorders · hypotension · infection exacerbated · myocardial infarction · neck stiffness · palpitations · pancreatitis · photosensitivity reaction · psychotic disorder · systemic lupus erythematosus (SLE)
- ▶ With oral use Acute kidney injury · angioedema · liver disorder · oral ulceration
- ▶ **Frequency not known**
- ▶ With oral use Crohn's disease · fertility decreased female · renal failure (more common in patients with pre-existing renal impairment) · respiratory tract reaction

SIDE-EFFECTS, FURTHER INFORMATION For information about cardiovascular and gastrointestinal side-effects, and a possible exacerbation of symptoms in asthma, see Non-steroidal anti-inflammatory drugs p. 816

Overdose Overdosage with ibuprofen may cause nausea, vomiting, epigastric pain, and tinnitus, but more serious toxicity is very uncommon. Activated charcoal followed by symptomatic measures are indicated if more than 100 mg/kg has been ingested within the preceding hour.

For details on the management of poisoning, see Emergency treatment of poisoning p. 1036.

● **ALLERGY AND CROSS-SENSITIVITY** EvGr Contra-indicated in patients with a history of hypersensitivity to aspirin or any other NSAID—which includes those in whom attacks of asthma, angioedema, urticaria or rhinitis have been precipitated by aspirin or any other NSAID. Ⓜ

● **CONCEPTION AND CONTRACEPTION** EvGr Caution—long-term use of some NSAIDs is associated with reduced female fertility, which is reversible on stopping treatment. Ⓜ

● **PREGNANCY** Avoid use in first and second trimesters unless essential; the MHRA advises additional antenatal monitoring may be required if treatment is considered necessary by a doctor from week 20 of pregnancy onwards. Avoid use in third trimester. See *NSAIDs in Pregnancy* in Non-steroidal anti-inflammatory drugs p. 816 for further details.

● **BREAST FEEDING** Specialist sources indicate suitable for use in breast-feeding—negligible amounts present in milk.

● **HEPATIC IMPAIRMENT**
- ▶ When used for indications relating to Pain or Pyrexia EvGr Caution in mild to moderate impairment; avoid in severe impairment. Ⓜ

Dose adjustments
- ▶ When used for indications relating to Pain or Pyrexia EvGr The lowest effective dose should be used for the shortest possible duration. Ⓜ

● **RENAL IMPAIRMENT**
- ▶ When used for indications relating to Pain or Pyrexia In general, for *NSAIDs* the MHRA advises to avoid where possible; if necessary, use with caution (risk of fluid retention and further renal impairment, including renal failure). EvGr For *ibuprofen*, avoid in severe impairment. Ⓜ
- ▶ With intravenous use in neonates EvGr Caution in mild to moderate impairment; avoid if possible in severe impairment. Ⓜ

Dose adjustments
- ▶ When used for indications relating to Pain or Pyrexia EvGr The lowest effective dose should be used for the shortest possible duration. Ⓜ

● **MONITORING REQUIREMENTS**
- ▶ With intravenous use in neonates Monitor for bleeding. Monitor gastro-intestinal function. Monitor renal function—withhold next dose until urine output returns to normal if anuria or manifest oliguria occurs after the first or second dose.

● **DIRECTIONS FOR ADMINISTRATION** For *intravenous infusion*, give over 30 minutes.

PEDEA® For *slow intravenous injection*, give over 15 minutes, preferably undiluted. May be diluted with Glucose 5% *or* Sodium Chloride 0.9%.

● **PRESCRIBING AND DISPENSING INFORMATION**
- ▶ With oral use Flavours of syrup may include orange.

● **PATIENT AND CARER ADVICE**
Medicines for Children leaflet: Ibuprofen for pain and inflammation www.medicinesforchildren.org.uk/medicines/ibuprofen-for-pain-and-inflammation/

● **PROFESSION SPECIFIC INFORMATION**
Dental practitioners' formulary Ibuprofen Oral Suspension Sugar-free may be prescribed. Ibuprofen Tablets may be prescribed.

● **EXCEPTIONS TO LEGAL CATEGORY** Oral preparations can be sold to the public in certain circumstances.

● **MEDICINAL FORMS** There can be variation in the licensing of different medicines containing the same drug. Forms available from special-order manufacturers include: oral suspension

Oral tablet

CAUTIONARY AND ADVISORY LABELS 21

- ▶ **Ibuprofen (Non-proprietary)**
  Ibuprofen 200 mg Ibuprofen 200mg tablets | 84 tablet PoM DT = £2.42 | 250 tablet PoM £9.30
  Ibuprofen sodium dihydrate 256 mg Ibuprofen sodium dihydrate 256mg tablets | 16 tablet GSL £4.19
  Ibuprofen 400 mg Ibuprofen 400mg tablets | 84 tablet PoM DT = £2.45 | 250 tablet PoM £11.20
  Ibuprofen 600 mg Ibuprofen 600mg tablets | 84 tablet PoM £9.97 DT = £7.83
  Ibuprofen 600mg tablets film coated | 84 tablet PoM £7.83 DT = £7.83
- ▶ **Brufen** (Viatris UK Healthcare Ltd)
  Ibuprofen 400 mg Brufen 400mg tablets | 60 tablet PoM £4.90
- ▶ **Feminax Express** (Bayer Plc)
  Ibuprofen lysine 342 mg Feminax Express 342mg tablets | 8 tablet GSL £2.30 DT = £2.30 | 16 tablet GSL £3.62 DT = £3.62
- ▶ **Nurofen Express (Ibuprofen sodium dihydrate)** (Reckitt Benckiser Healthcare (UK) Ltd)
  Ibuprofen sodium dihydrate 256 mg Nurofen Express 256mg tablets | 16 tablet GSL £2.46
  Nurofen Express 256mg caplets | 16 tablet GSL £2.58
- ▶ **Nurofen Maximum Strength Migraine Pain** (Reckitt Benckiser Healthcare (UK) Ltd)
  Ibuprofen lysine 684 mg Nurofen Maximum Strength Migraine Pain 684mg caplets | 12 tablet P £4.04 DT = £4.04
- ▶ **Nurofen Migraine Pain** (Reckitt Benckiser Healthcare (UK) Ltd)
  Ibuprofen lysine 342 mg Nurofen Migraine Pain 342mg caplets | 12 tablet GSL £2.26
- ▶ **Nurofen Pain Relief (Ibuprofen)** (Reckitt Benckiser Healthcare (UK) Ltd)
  Ibuprofen sodium dihydrate 256 mg Nurofen Pain Relief 256mg tablets | 16 tablet GSL £2.46
  Nurofen Pain Relief 256mg caplets | 16 tablet GSL £2.58
  Ibuprofen sodium dihydrate 512 mg Nurofen Pain Relief Max Strength 512mg tablets | 24 tablet P £6.97

Effervescent granules

CAUTIONARY AND ADVISORY LABELS 13, 21

ELECTROLYTES: May contain Sodium

▸ **Brufen** (Viatris UK Healthcare Ltd)

Ibuprofen 600 mg Brufen 600mg effervescent granules sachets | 20 sachet [PoM] £6.80 DT = £6.80

Modified-release tablet

CAUTIONARY AND ADVISORY LABELS 25, 27

▸ **Brufen Retard** (Viatris UK Healthcare Ltd)

Ibuprofen 800 mg Brufen Retard 800mg tablets | 56 tablet [PoM] £7.74 DT = £7.74

Oral suspension

CAUTIONARY AND ADVISORY LABELS 21

▸ **Ibuprofen (Non-proprietary)**

Ibuprofen 20 mg per 1 ml Ibuprofen 100mg/5ml oral suspension sugar free | 500 ml [PoM] [X] [SF]

Ibuprofen 40 mg per 1 ml Ibuprofen Twelve Plus Pain Relief 200mg/5ml oral suspension | 100 ml [P] £3.49 DT = £3.49 [SF]
Ibuprofen Seven Plus Pain Relief 200mg/5ml oral suspension | 100 ml [P] £3.49 DT = £3.49 [SF]

▸ **Nurofen** (Reckitt Benckiser Healthcare (UK) Ltd)

Ibuprofen 40 mg per 1 ml Nurofen for Children 200mg/5ml oral suspension orange | 100 ml [P] £4.85 DT = £3.49 [SF]
Nurofen for Children 200mg/5ml oral suspension strawberry | 100 ml [P] £4.85 DT = £3.49 [SF]

Modified-release capsule

▸ **Galprofen Long Lasting** (Galpharm International Ltd)

Ibuprofen 200 mg Galprofen Long Lasting 200mg capsules | 8 capsule [GSL] £0.96

▸ **Nurofen Long Lasting** (Reckitt Benckiser Healthcare (UK) Ltd)

Ibuprofen 300 mg Nurofen Long Lasting Pain Relief PR 300mg capsules | 24 capsule [P] £5.37 DT = £5.37

Oral capsule

▸ **Ibuprofen (Non-proprietary)**

Ibuprofen 400 mg Ibuprofen 400mg capsules | 100 capsule [PoM] £26.00–£47.00

▸ **Flarin** (infirst Ltd)

Ibuprofen 200 mg Flarin 200mg capsules | 12 capsule [P] £3.57 | 30 capsule [P] £7.38 DT = £5.22

▸ **Nurofen Express** (Reckitt Benckiser Healthcare (UK) Ltd)

Ibuprofen 200 mg Nurofen Express 200mg liquid capsules | 30 capsule [P] £5.22 DT = £5.22

Solution for infusion

ELECTROLYTES: May contain Sodium

▸ **Ibuprofen (Non-proprietary)**

Ibuprofen 4 mg per 1 ml Ibuprofen 400mg/100ml infusion polyethylene bottles | 10 bottle [PoM] £69.00 (Hospital only)
Ibuprofen 200mg/50ml infusion polyethylene bottles | 10 bottle [PoM] £92.00 (Hospital only)

Ibuprofen (as Ibuprofen lysine) 10 mg per 1 ml NeoProfen 20mg/2ml solution for infusion vials | 3 vial [PoM] [X] (Hospital only)

▸ **Pedea** (Recordati Rare Diseases UK Ltd)

Ibuprofen 5 mg per 1 ml Pedea 10mg/2ml solution for infusion ampoules | 4 ampoule [PoM] £288.00 (Hospital only)

Chewable capsule

▸ **Nurofen** (Reckitt Benckiser Healthcare (UK) Ltd)

Ibuprofen 100 mg Nurofen for Children 100mg chewable capsules | 12 capsule [P] £3.85 DT = £3.85

Orodispersible tablet

▸ **Nurofen Meltlets** (Reckitt Benckiser Healthcare (UK) Ltd)

Ibuprofen 200 mg Nurofen Meltlets 200mg tablets | 12 tablet [GSL] £2.58 DT = £2.58 [SF]

10

Musculoskeletal system

Indometacin

16-Apr-2026

(Indomethacin)

● **INDICATIONS AND DOSE**

Relief of pain and inflammation in rheumatic diseases including juvenile idiopathic arthritis

▸ BY MOUTH USING IMMEDIATE-RELEASE MEDICINES

▸ Child: 0.5–1 mg/kg twice daily

● **UNLICENSED USE** Expert sources advise that indometacin may be used in children for the relief of pain and inflammation in rheumatic diseases, but it is not licensed for this age group.

IMPORTANT SAFETY INFORMATION

MHRA/CHM ADVICE: NSAIDS: POTENTIAL RISKS FOLLOWING PROLONGED USE AFTER 20 WEEKS OF PREGNANCY (JUNE 2023)

See Non-steroidal anti-inflammatory drugs p. 816.

● **CONTRA-INDICATIONS** Active gastro-intestinal bleeding · active gastro-intestinal ulceration · history of gastro-intestinal bleeding related to previous NSAID therapy · history of gastro-intestinal perforation related to previous NSAID therapy · history of recurrent gastro-intestinal haemorrhage (two or more distinct episodes) · history of recurrent gastro-intestinal ulceration (two or more distinct episodes) · severe heart failure

● **CAUTIONS** Allergic disorders · cardiac impairment (NSAIDs may impair renal function) · cerebrovascular disease · coagulation defects · connective-tissue disorders · dehydration (risk of renal impairment) · epilepsy · heart failure · history of gastro-intestinal disorders (e.g. ulcerative colitis, Crohn's disease) · ischaemic heart disease · may mask symptoms of infection · peripheral arterial disease · psychiatric disturbances · risk factors for cardiovascular events · uncontrolled hypertension

● **INTERACTIONS** → Appendix 1: NSAIDs

● **SIDE-EFFECTS** Agranulocytosis · alopecia · anaphylactic reaction · angioedema · anxiety · appetite decreased · arrhythmias · asthma · blood disorder · bone marrow disorders · breast abnormalities · chest pain · coma · confusion · congestive heart failure · constipation · corneal deposits · depression · diarrhoea · disseminated intravascular coagulation · dizziness · drowsiness · dysarthria · dyspnoea · erythema nodosum · eye disorder · eye pain · fatigue · fluid retention · flushing · gastrointestinal discomfort · gastrointestinal disorders · gynaecomastia · haemolytic anaemia · haemorrhage · hallucination · headache · hearing impairment · hepatic disorders · hyperglycaemia · hyperhidrosis · hyperkalaemia · hypotension · inflammatory bowel disease · insomnia · leucopenia · malaise · movement disorders · muscle weakness · nausea · nephritis tubulointerstitial · nephrotic syndrome · oedema · oral disorders · palpitations · pancreatitis · paraesthesia · peripheral neuropathy · photosensitivity reaction · platelet aggregation inhibition · psychiatric disorders · pulmonary oedema · renal failure (more common in patients with pre-existing renal impairment) · respiratory disorders · seizures · severe cutaneous adverse reactions (SCARs) · sigmoid lesion perforation · skin reactions · syncope · thrombocytopenia · tinnitus · urine abnormalities · vasculitis · vertigo · vision disorders · vomiting

SIDE-EFFECTS, FURTHER INFORMATION For information about cardiovascular and gastrointestinal side-effects, and a possible exacerbation of symptoms in asthma, see Non-steroidal anti-inflammatory drugs p. 816

● **ALLERGY AND CROSS-SENSITIVITY** [EvGr] Contra-indicated in patients with a history of hypersensitivity to aspirin or any other NSAID—which includes those in whom attacks of asthma, angioedema, urticaria or rhinitis have been precipitated by aspirin or any other NSAID. [M]

● **CONCEPTION AND CONTRACEPTION** [EvGr] Caution—long-term use of some NSAIDs is associated with reduced female fertility, which is reversible on stopping treatment. [M]

● **PREGNANCY** Avoid use in first and second trimesters unless essential; the MHRA advises additional antenatal monitoring may be required if treatment is considered necessary by a doctor from week 20 of pregnancy onwards. Avoid use in third trimester. See *NSAIDs in Pregnancy* in

Non-steroidal anti-inflammatory drugs p. 816 for further details.

- **BREAST FEEDING** Amount probably too small to be harmful—manufacturers advise avoid. Use with caution during breast-feeding.
- **HEPATIC IMPAIRMENT** Manufacturer advises caution in mild to moderate impairment; avoid in severe impairment (increased risk of gastro-intestinal bleeding and fluid retention).
- **RENAL IMPAIRMENT** In general, for *NSAIDs* the MHRA advises to avoid where possible; if necessary, use with caution (risk of fluid retention and further renal impairment, including renal failure). EvGr For *indometacin*, avoid in severe impairment. ⟨M⟩
- **MONITORING REQUIREMENTS** During prolonged therapy ophthalmic and blood examinations particularly advisable.
- **PATIENT AND CARER ADVICE**

Driving and skilled tasks Dizziness may affect performance of skilled tasks (e.g. driving).

- **MEDICINAL FORMS** There can be variation in the licensing of different medicines containing the same drug. Forms available from special-order manufacturers include: oral suspension, oral solution

Oral capsule

CAUTIONARY AND ADVISORY LABELS 21

- **Indometacin (Non-proprietary)**
  - **Indometacin 25 mg** Indometacin 25mg capsules | 28 capsule PoM £25.30 DT = £1.24
  - **Indometacin 50 mg** Indometacin 50mg capsules | 28 capsule PoM £49.10 DT = £1.69

Suppository

- **Indometacin (Non-proprietary)**
  - **Indometacin 100 mg** Indometacin 100mg suppositories | 10 suppository PoM £17.61 DT = £17.61

Mefenamic acid

01-Aug-2023

- **INDICATIONS AND DOSE**

Acute pain including dysmenorrhoea | Menorrhagia

▶ BY MOUTH

▶ Child 12–17 years: 500 mg 3 times a day

IMPORTANT SAFETY INFORMATION

MHRA/CHM ADVICE: NSAIDS: POTENTIAL RISKS FOLLOWING PROLONGED USE AFTER 20 WEEKS OF PREGNANCY (JUNE 2023)

See Non-steroidal anti-inflammatory drugs p. 816.

- **CONTRA-INDICATIONS** Active gastro-intestinal bleeding · active gastro-intestinal ulceration · following coronary artery bypass graft (CABG) surgery · history of gastro-intestinal bleeding related to previous NSAID therapy · history of gastro-intestinal perforation related to previous NSAID therapy · history of recurrent gastro-intestinal haemorrhage (two or more distinct episodes) · history of recurrent gastro-intestinal ulceration (two or more distinct episodes) · inflammatory bowel disease · severe heart failure
- **CAUTIONS** Acute porphyrias p. 745 · allergic disorders · cardiac impairment (NSAIDs may impair renal function) · cerebrovascular disease · coagulation defects · connective-tissue disorders · dehydration (risk of renal impairment) · epilepsy · heart failure · history of gastro-intestinal disorders (e.g. ulcerative colitis, Crohn's disease) · ischaemic heart disease · may mask symptoms of infection · peripheral arterial disease · risk factors for cardiovascular events · uncontrolled hypertension
- **INTERACTIONS** → Appendix 1: NSAIDs
- **SIDE-EFFECTS** Agranulocytosis · anaemia · angioedema · appetite decreased · asthma · bone marrow disorders · confusion · constipation · Crohn's disease · depression · diarrhoea (discontinue) · disseminated intravascular coagulation · dizziness · drowsiness · dyspnoea · dysuria · ear pain · eosinophilia · eye irritation · fatigue · fertility decreased female · gastrointestinal discomfort · gastrointestinal disorders · glomerulonephritis · glucose tolerance impaired · haemolytic anaemia · haemorrhage · hallucination · headache · heart failure · hepatic disorders · hyperhidrosis · hypersensitivity · hypertension · hyponatraemia · hypotension · insomnia · leucopenia · malaise · meningitis aseptic (patients with connective-tissue disorders such as systemic lupus erythematosus may be especially susceptible) · multi organ failure · nausea · nephritis acute interstitial · nephrotic syndrome · nervousness · neutropenia · oedema · optic neuritis · oral ulceration · palpitations · pancreatitis · paraesthesia · photosensitivity reaction · proteinuria · rash (discontinue) · renal failure (more common in patients with pre-existing renal impairment) · renal failure non-oliguric · renal papillary necrosis · respiratory disorders · seizure · sepsis · severe cutaneous adverse reactions (SCARs) · skin reactions · thrombocytopenia · tinnitus · vertigo · vision disorders · vomiting

SIDE-EFFECTS, FURTHER INFORMATION For information about cardiovascular and gastrointestinal side-effects, and a possible exacerbation of symptoms in asthma, see Non-steroidal anti-inflammatory drugs p. 816

Overdose Mefenamic acid has important consequences in overdosage because it can cause convulsions, which if prolonged or recurrent, require treatment.

For details on the management of poisoning, see Emergency treatment of poisoning p. 1036, in particular, Convulsions.

- **ALLERGY AND CROSS-SENSITIVITY** EvGr Contra-indicated in patients with a history of hypersensitivity to aspirin or any other NSAID—which includes those in whom attacks of asthma, angioedema, urticaria or rhinitis have been precipitated by aspirin or any other NSAID. ⟨M⟩
- **CONCEPTION AND CONTRACEPTION** EvGr Caution—long-term use of some NSAIDs is associated with reduced female fertility, which is reversible on stopping treatment. ⟨M⟩
- **PREGNANCY** Avoid use in first and second trimesters unless essential; the MHRA advises additional antenatal monitoring may be required if treatment is considered necessary by a doctor from week 20 of pregnancy onwards. Avoid use in third trimester. See *NSAIDs in Pregnancy* in Non-steroidal anti-inflammatory drugs p. 816 for further details.
- **BREAST FEEDING** Use with caution during breast-feeding. Amount too small to be harmful but manufacturer advises avoid.
- **HEPATIC IMPAIRMENT** Manufacturer advises caution in mild to moderate impairment; avoid in severe impairment.
- **RENAL IMPAIRMENT** In general, for *NSAIDs* the MHRA advises to avoid where possible; if necessary, use with caution (risk of fluid retention and further renal impairment, including renal failure). EvGr For *mefenamic acid*, avoid in severe impairment. ⟨M⟩
- **MEDICINAL FORMS** There can be variation in the licensing of different medicines containing the same drug. Forms available from special-order manufacturers include: oral suspension

Oral tablet

CAUTIONARY AND ADVISORY LABELS 21

- **Mefenamic acid (Non-proprietary)**
  - **Mefenamic acid 250 mg** Mefenamic acid 250mg tablets | 28 tablet PoM £7.22 DT = £7.22
  - **Mefenamic acid 500 mg** Mefenamic acid 500mg tablets | 28 tablet PoM £70.00 DT = £11.03 | 84 tablet PoM £24.32–£154.38

Oral suspension

CAUTIONARY AND ADVISORY LABELS 21

EXCIPIENTS: May contain Ethanol

Oral capsule

CAUTIONARY AND ADVISORY LABELS 21

▸ Mefenamic acid (Non-proprietary)

Mefenamic acid 250 mg Mefenamic acid 250mg capsules | 100 capsule PoM £60.10 DT = £13.69

Meloxicam 01-Aug-2023

● **INDICATIONS AND DOSE**

Exacerbation of osteoarthritis (short-term)

▶ BY MOUTH

▸ Child 16–17 years: 7.5 mg once daily, then increased if necessary up to 15 mg once daily

Pain and inflammation in rheumatic disease | Ankylosing spondylitis

▶ BY MOUTH

▸ Child 16–17 years: 15 mg once daily, then reduced to 7.5 mg once daily if required

Relief of pain and inflammation in juvenile idiopathic arthritis and other musculoskeletal disorders in children intolerant to other NSAIDs

▶ BY MOUTH

▸ Child 12–17 years (body-weight up to 50 kg): 7.5 mg once daily

▸ Child 12–17 years (body-weight 50 kg and above): 15 mg once daily

● **UNLICENSED USE** Expert sources advise that meloxicam may be used from the age of 12 years for the treatment of pain and inflammation in juvenile idiopathic arthritis and other musculoskeletal disorders in children intolerant to other NSAIDS, but it is not licensed for this age group.

IMPORTANT SAFETY INFORMATION

MHRA/CHM ADVICE: NSAIDS: POTENTIAL RISKS FOLLOWING PROLONGED USE AFTER 20 WEEKS OF PREGNANCY (JUNE 2023)

See Non-steroidal anti-inflammatory drugs p. 816.

● **CONTRA-INDICATIONS** Active gastro-intestinal bleeding · active gastro-intestinal ulceration · following coronary artery bypass graft surgery · history of gastro-intestinal bleeding related to previous NSAID therapy · history of gastro-intestinal perforation related to previous NSAID therapy · history of recurrent gastro-intestinal haemorrhage (two or more distinct episodes) · history of recurrent gastro-intestinal ulceration (two or more distinct episodes) · severe heart failure

● **CAUTIONS** Allergic disorders · cardiac impairment (NSAIDs may impair renal function) · cerebrovascular disease · coagulation defects · connective-tissue disorders · dehydration (risk of renal impairment) · heart failure · history of gastro-intestinal disorders (e.g. ulcerative colitis, Crohn's disease) · ischaemic heart disease · may mask symptoms of infection · peripheral arterial disease · risk factors for cardiovascular events · uncontrolled hypertension

● **INTERACTIONS** → Appendix 1: NSAIDs

● **SIDE-EFFECTS**

▶ **Common or very common** Constipation · diarrhoea · gastrointestinal discomfort · gastrointestinal disorders · headache · nausea · vomiting

▶ **Uncommon** Anaemia · angioedema · burping · dizziness · drowsiness · electrolyte imbalance · fluid retention · flushing · haemorrhage · hepatic disorders · hypersensitivity · oedema · skin reactions · stomatitis · vertigo

▶ **Rare or very rare** Acute kidney injury · asthma · conjunctivitis · leucopenia · mood altered · nightmare · palpitations · severe cutaneous adverse reactions (SCARs) · thrombocytopenia · tinnitus · vision disorders

▶ **Frequency not known** Agranulocytosis · confusion · fertility decreased female · heart failure · increased risk of arterial thromboembolism · nephritis tubulointerstitial · nephrotic syndrome · photosensitivity reaction · renal necrosis

SIDE-EFFECTS, FURTHER INFORMATION For information about cardiovascular and gastrointestinal side-effects, and a possible exacerbation of symptoms in asthma, see Non-steroidal anti-inflammatory drugs p. 816

● **ALLERGY AND CROSS-SENSITIVITY** EvGr Contra-indicated in patients with a history of hypersensitivity to aspirin or any other NSAID—which includes those in whom attacks of asthma, angioedema, urticaria or rhinitis have been precipitated by aspirin or any other NSAID. Ⓜ

● **CONCEPTION AND CONTRACEPTION** EvGr Caution—long-term use of some NSAIDs is associated with reduced female fertility, which is reversible on stopping treatment. Ⓜ

● **PREGNANCY** Avoid use in first and second trimesters unless essential; the MHRA advises additional antenatal monitoring may be required if treatment is considered necessary by a doctor from week 20 of pregnancy onwards. Avoid use in third trimester. See *NSAIDs in Pregnancy* in Non-steroidal anti-inflammatory drugs p. 816 for further details.

● **BREAST FEEDING** Use with caution during breast-feeding. Present in milk in *animal* studies—manufacturer advises avoid.

● **HEPATIC IMPAIRMENT** Manufacturer advises caution in mild to moderate impairment; avoid in severe impairment.

● **RENAL IMPAIRMENT** In general, for *NSAIDs* the MHRA advises to avoid where possible; if necessary, use with caution (risk of fluid retention and further renal impairment, including renal failure). EvGr For *meloxicam*, avoid if creatinine clearance less than 25 mL/minute; Ⓜ see p. 16.

● **MEDICINAL FORMS** There can be variation in the licensing of different medicines containing the same drug. Forms available from special-order manufacturers include: oral suspension

Oral tablet

CAUTIONARY AND ADVISORY LABELS 21

▸ Meloxicam (Non-proprietary)

Meloxicam 7.5 mg Meloxicam 7.5mg tablets | 30 tablet PoM £3.00 DT = £0.68

Meloxicam 15 mg Meloxicam 15mg tablets | 30 tablet PoM £5.50 DT = £0.81

Orodispersible tablet

▸ Meloxicam (Non-proprietary)

Meloxicam 7.5 mg Meloxicam 7.5mg orodispersible tablets sugar free | 30 tablet PoM £49.99 DT = £49.99 SF

Meloxicam 15 mg Meloxicam 15mg orodispersible tablets sugar free | 30 tablet PoM £49.99 DT = £49.99 SF

Naproxen 01-Aug-2023

● **INDICATIONS AND DOSE**

Pain and inflammation in musculoskeletal disorders | Dysmenorrhoea

▶ BY MOUTH

▸ Child: 5 mg/kg twice daily (max. per dose 500 mg)

Pain and inflammation in juvenile idiopathic arthritis

▶ BY MOUTH

▸ Child 2–17 years: 5–7.5 mg/kg twice daily (max. per dose 500 mg)

● **UNLICENSED USE** Not licensed for use in children under 5 years for juvenile idiopathic arthritis. Not licensed for use in children under 16 years for musculoskeletal disorders or dysmenorrhoea.

IMPORTANT SAFETY INFORMATION

MHRA/CHM ADVICE: NSAIDS: POTENTIAL RISKS FOLLOWING PROLONGED USE AFTER 20 WEEKS OF PREGNANCY (JUNE 2023)

See Non-steroidal anti-inflammatory drugs p. 816.

- **CONTRA-INDICATIONS** Active gastro-intestinal bleeding · active gastro-intestinal ulceration · history of gastro-intestinal bleeding related to previous NSAID therapy · history of gastro-intestinal perforation related to previous NSAID therapy · history of recurrent gastro-intestinal haemorrhage (two or more distinct episodes) · history of recurrent gastro-intestinal ulceration (two or more distinct episodes) · severe heart failure
- **CAUTIONS** Allergic disorders · cardiac impairment (NSAIDs may impair renal function) · cerebrovascular disease · coagulation defects · connective-tissue disorders · dehydration (risk of renal impairment) · heart failure · history of gastro-intestinal disorders (e.g. ulcerative colitis, Crohn's disease) · ischaemic heart disease · may mask symptoms of infection · peripheral arterial disease · risk factors for cardiovascular events · uncontrolled hypertension
- **INTERACTIONS** → Appendix 1: NSAIDs
- **SIDE-EFFECTS**
  - **Common or very common** Constipation · diarrhoea · dizziness · fatigue · gastrointestinal discomfort · headache · hearing impairment · heart failure · hyperhidrosis · nausea · skin reactions · stomatitis · tinnitus · visual impairment · vomiting
  - **Uncommon** Cognitive impairment · concentration impaired · depression · fluid retention · gastrointestinal disorders · haemorrhage · hepatic disorders · hyperkalaemia · inflammatory bowel disease · menstrual disorder · mood altered · palpitations · seizure · sleep disorders · thirst
  - **Rare or very rare** Agranulocytosis · alopecia · angioedema · asthma · bone marrow disorders · eosinophilia · erythema nodosum · glomerulonephritis · haemolytic anaemia · hypersensitivity · increased risk of infection · leucopenia · lupus erythematosus · meningitis aseptic (patients with connective-tissue disorders such as systemic lupus erythematosus may be especially susceptible) · muscle weakness · myalgia · nephritis tubulointerstitial · nephropathy · pancreatitis · Parkinson's disease exacerbated · photosensitivity reaction · pneumonia eosinophilic · pulmonary oedema · renal failure (more common in patients with pre-existing renal impairment) · renal papillary necrosis · severe cutaneous adverse reactions (SCARs) · thrombocytopenia · vasculitis
  - **Frequency not known** Confusion · corneal opacity · drowsiness · dyspnoea · hallucination · hypertension · infertility female · malaise · neutropenia · oedema · optic neuritis · papillitis · papilloedema · paraesthesia · proteinuria · renal impairment · vertigo

  SIDE-EFFECTS, FURTHER INFORMATION For information about cardiovascular and gastrointestinal side-effects, and a possible exacerbation of symptoms in asthma, see Non-steroidal anti-inflammatory drugs p. 816
- **ALLERGY AND CROSS-SENSITIVITY** [EvGr] Contra-indicated in patients with a history of hypersensitivity to aspirin or any other NSAID—which includes those in whom attacks of asthma, angioedema, urticaria or rhinitis have been precipitated by aspirin or any other NSAID. ⟨M⟩
- **CONCEPTION AND CONTRACEPTION** [EvGr] Caution—long-term use of some NSAIDs is associated with reduced female fertility, which is reversible on stopping treatment. ⟨M⟩
- **PREGNANCY** Avoid use in first and second trimesters unless essential; the MHRA advises additional antenatal monitoring may be required if treatment is considered necessary by a doctor from week 20 of pregnancy onwards. Avoid use in third trimester. See *NSAIDs in Pregnancy* in Non-steroidal anti-inflammatory drugs p. 816 for further details.
- **BREAST FEEDING** Use with caution during breast-feeding. Amount too small to be harmful but manufacturer advises avoid.
- **HEPATIC IMPAIRMENT** Manufacturer advises caution in mild to moderate impairment; avoid in severe impairment.

  Dose adjustments Manufacturer advises consider dose reduction in mild to moderate impairment.
- **RENAL IMPAIRMENT** In general, for *NSAIDs* the MHRA advises to avoid where possible; if necessary, use with caution (risk of fluid retention and further renal impairment, including renal failure). [EvGr] For *naproxen*, avoid if creatinine clearance less than 30 mL/minute (risk of accumulation). ⟨M⟩

  Dose adjustments [EvGr] Consider dose reduction if creatinine clearance 30 mL/minute or more. ⟨M⟩ See p. 16.
- **EXCEPTIONS TO LEGAL CATEGORY** Can be sold to the public for the treatment of primary dysmenorrhoea in women aged 15–50 years subject to max. single dose of 500 mg, max. daily dose of 750 mg for max. 3 days, and a max. pack size of 9 × 250 mg tablets.

- **MEDICINAL FORMS** There can be variation in the licensing of different medicines containing the same drug. Forms available from special-order manufacturers include: oral suspension

Oral tablet

CAUTIONARY AND ADVISORY LABELS 21

- **Naproxen (Non-proprietary)**

  Naproxen 250 mg Naproxen 250mg tablets | 28 tablet [PoM] £10.94 DT = £0.83

  Naproxen 500 mg Naproxen 500mg tablets | 28 tablet [PoM] £22.99 DT = £1.30 | 250 tablet [PoM] £12.22–£12.80 | 500 tablet [PoM] £20.54–£21.00
- **Naprosyn** (Atnahs Pharma UK Ltd)

  Naproxen 250 mg Naprosyn 250mg tablets | 56 tablet [PoM] £4.29

  Naproxen 500 mg Naprosyn 500mg tablets | 56 tablet [PoM] £8.56

Gastro-resistant tablet

CAUTIONARY AND ADVISORY LABELS 5, 25

- **Naproxen (Non-proprietary)**

  Naproxen 250 mg Naproxen 250mg gastro-resistant tablets | 56 tablet [PoM] £9.98 DT = £5.15

  Naproxen 375 mg Naproxen 375mg gastro-resistant tablets | 56 tablet [PoM] £19.98 DT = £7.47

  Naproxen 500 mg Naproxen 500mg gastro-resistant tablets | 56 tablet [PoM] £25.00 DT = £14.97
- **Naprosyn EC** (Atnahs Pharma UK Ltd)

  Naproxen 250 mg Naprosyn EC 250mg tablets | 56 tablet [PoM] £4.29 DT = £5.15

  Naproxen 375 mg Naprosyn EC 375mg tablets | 56 tablet [PoM] £6.42 DT = £7.47

  Naproxen 500 mg Naprosyn EC 500mg tablets | 56 tablet [PoM] £8.56 DT = £14.97
- **Nexocin EC** (Noumed Life Sciences Ltd)

  Naproxen 250 mg Nexocin EC 250mg gastro-resistant tablets | 56 tablet [PoM] [X] DT = £5.15

  Naproxen 375 mg Nexocin EC 375mg gastro-resistant tablets | 56 tablet [PoM] [X] DT = £7.47

  Naproxen 500 mg Nexocin EC 500mg gastro-resistant tablets | 56 tablet [PoM] [X] DT = £14.97

Oral suspension

- **Naproxen (Non-proprietary)**

  Naproxen 25 mg per 1 ml Naproxen 25mg/ml oral suspension sugar free | 100 ml [PoM] £110.00 DT = £110.00 [SF]

  Naproxen 125mg/5ml oral suspension sugar free | 100 ml [PoM] £110.00 DT = £110.00 [SF]

  Naproxen 50 mg per 1 ml Naproxen 50mg/ml oral suspension | 100 ml [PoM] £45.00 DT = £45.00

Effervescent tablet
▸ **Stirlescent**(Stirling Anglian Pharmaceuticals Ltd)
Naproxen 250 mg Stirlescent 250mg effervescent tablets | 20 tablet PoM £52.72 DT = £52.72 SF

Piroxicam

01-Aug-2023

● **INDICATIONS AND DOSE**

Relief of pain and inflammation in juvenile idiopathic arthritis

▸ BY MOUTH
▸ Child 6–17 years (body-weight up to 15 kg): 5 mg daily
▸ Child 6–17 years (body-weight 15–25 kg): 10 mg daily
▸ Child 6–17 years (body-weight 26–45 kg): 15 mg daily
▸ Child 6–17 years (body-weight 46 kg and above): 20 mg daily

● **UNLICENSED USE** Expert sources advise piroxicam may be used in children from the age of 6 years for the treatment of pain and inflammation in juvenile idiopathic arthritis, but it is not licensed for this age group.

IMPORTANT SAFETY INFORMATION

CHMP ADVICE—PIROXICAM (JUNE 2007)

The CHMP has recommended restrictions on the use of piroxicam because of the increased risk of gastro-intestinal side-effects and serious skin reactions. The CHMP has advised that:

- piroxicam should be initiated only by physicians experienced in treating inflammatory or degenerative rheumatic diseases
- piroxicam should not be used as first-line treatment
- piroxicam dose should not exceed 20 mg daily
- piroxicam should no longer be used for the treatment of acute painful and inflammatory conditions
- treatment should be reviewed 2 weeks after initiating piroxicam, and periodically thereafter
- concomitant administration of a gastro-protective agent should be considered.

Topical preparations containing piroxicam are not affected by these restrictions.

MHRA/CHM ADVICE: NSAIDS: POTENTIAL RISKS FOLLOWING PROLONGED USE AFTER 20 WEEKS OF PREGNANCY (JUNE 2023)

See Non-steroidal anti-inflammatory drugs p. 816.

● **CONTRA-INDICATIONS** Active gastro-intestinal bleeding · active gastro-intestinal ulceration · history of gastro-intestinal bleeding · history of gastro-intestinal perforation · history of gastro-intestinal ulceration · inflammatory bowel disease · severe heart failure

● **CAUTIONS** Allergic disorders · cardiac impairment (NSAIDs may impair renal function) · cerebrovascular disease · coagulation defects · connective-tissue disorders · dehydration (risk of renal impairment) · heart failure · history of gastro-intestinal disorders · ischaemic heart disease · may mask symptoms of infection · peripheral arterial disease · risk factors for cardiovascular events · uncontrolled hypertension

● **INTERACTIONS** → Appendix 1: NSAIDs

● **SIDE-EFFECTS**

▸ **Common or very common** Anaemia · appetite decreased · constipation · diarrhoea · dizziness · drowsiness · eosinophilia · gastrointestinal discomfort · gastrointestinal disorders · headache · hyperglycaemia · leucopenia · nausea · oedema · rash (discontinue) · skin reactions · thrombocytopenia · tinnitus · vertigo · vomiting · weight changes

▸ **Uncommon** Hypoglycaemia · palpitations · stomatitis · vision blurred

▸ **Rare or very rare** Nephritis tubulointerstitial · nephrotic syndrome · renal failure · renal papillary necrosis · severe cutaneous adverse reactions (SCARs)

▸ **Frequency not known** Alopecia · angioedema · aplastic anaemia · bronchospasm · confusion · depression · dyspnoea · embolism and thrombosis · eye irritation · eye swelling · fertility decreased female · fluid retention · haemolytic anaemia · haemorrhage · hallucination · hearing impairment · heart failure · hepatic disorders · hypersensitivity · hypertension · malaise · mood altered · nervousness · onycholysis · pancreatitis · paraesthesia · photosensitivity reaction · sleep disorders · vasculitis

SIDE-EFFECTS, FURTHER INFORMATION For information about cardiovascular and gastrointestinal side-effects, and a possible exacerbation of symptoms in asthma, see Non-steroidal anti-inflammatory drugs p. 816

● **ALLERGY AND CROSS-SENSITIVITY** EvGr Contra-indicated in patients with a history of hypersensitivity to aspirin or any other NSAID—which includes those in whom attacks of asthma, angioedema, urticaria or rhinitis have been precipitated by aspirin or any other NSAID. ⟨M⟩

● **CONCEPTION AND CONTRACEPTION** EvGr Caution—long-term use of some NSAIDs is associated with reduced female fertility, which is reversible on stopping treatment. ⟨M⟩

● **PREGNANCY** Avoid use in first and second trimesters unless essential; the MHRA advises additional antenatal monitoring may be required if treatment is considered necessary by a doctor from week 20 of pregnancy onwards. Avoid use in third trimester. See *NSAIDs in Pregnancy* in Non-steroidal anti-inflammatory drugs p. 816 for further details.

● **BREAST FEEDING** Use with caution during breast-feeding. Amount too small to be harmful.

● **HEPATIC IMPAIRMENT** Manufacturer advises caution.

● **RENAL IMPAIRMENT** In general, for *NSAIDs* the MHRA advises to avoid where possible; if necessary, use with caution (risk of fluid retention and further renal impairment, including renal failure).

● **DIRECTIONS FOR ADMINISTRATION** Piroxicam orodispersible tablets can be taken by placing on the tongue and allowing to dissolve or by swallowing.

● **LESS SUITABLE FOR PRESCRIBING** Piroxicam is less suitable for prescribing.

● **MEDICINAL FORMS** There can be variation in the licensing of different medicines containing the same drug.

Orodispersible tablet

CAUTIONARY AND ADVISORY LABELS 10, 21
EXCIPIENTS: May contain Aspartame

▸ **Feldene Melt**(Pfizer Ltd)
Piroxicam 20 mg Feldene Melt 20mg tablets | 30 tablet PoM £10.53 DT = £10.53 SF

Oral capsule

CAUTIONARY AND ADVISORY LABELS 21

▸ **Piroxicam (Non-proprietary)**
Piroxicam 10 mg Piroxicam 10mg capsules | 56 capsule PoM £16.00 DT = £16.00
Piroxicam 20 mg Piroxicam 20mg capsules | 28 capsule PoM £24.00 DT = £24.00

▸ **Feldene**(Pfizer Ltd)
Piroxicam 10 mg Feldene 10mg capsules | 30 capsule PoM £3.86
Piroxicam 20 mg Feldene 20 capsules | 30 capsule PoM £7.71

4 Soft tissue and joint disorders

4.1 Local inflammation of joints and soft tissue

Other drugs used for Local inflammation of joints and soft tissue Dexamethasone, p. 543 · Prednisolone, p. 548

CORTICOSTEROIDS

Corticosteroids, inflammatory disorders

Systemic corticosteroids

In children with rheumatic diseases corticosteroids should be reserved for specific indications (e.g. when other therapies are unsuccessful or while waiting for DMARDs to take effect) and should be used only under the supervision of a specialist.

Systemic corticosteroids may be considered for the management of juvenile idiopathic arthritis in systemic disease or when several joints are affected. Systemic corticosteroids may also be considered in severe, possibly life-threatening conditions such as systemic lupus erythematosus, systemic vasculitis, juvenile dermatomyositis, Behçet's disease, and polyarticular joint disease.

In severe conditions, short courses ('pulses') of high dose intravenous methylprednisolone p. 547 or a pulsed oral corticosteroid may be particularly effective for providing rapid relief, and has fewer long-term adverse effects than continuous treatment.

Corticosteroid doses should be reduced with care because of the possibility of relapse if the reduction is too rapid. If complete discontinuation of corticosteroids is not possible, consideration should be given to alternate-day (or alternate high-dose, low-dose) administration; on days when no corticosteroid is given, or a lower dose is given, an additional dose of a NSAID may be helpful. In some conditions, alternative treatment using an antimalarial or concomitant use of an immunosuppressant drug, such as azathioprine p. 638, methotrexate p. 672 or cyclophosphamide p. 663 may prove useful; in less severe conditions treatment with a NSAID alone may be adequate.

Administration of corticosteroids may result in suppression of growth and may affect the development of puberty. The risk of corticosteroid-induced osteoporosis should be considered for those on long-term corticosteroid treatment; corticosteroids may also increase the risk of osteopenia in those unable to exercise. See the disadvantages of corticosteroid treatment.

For further information on corticosteroid use, see Corticosteroids, general use p. 537.

Local corticosteroid injections

Corticosteroids are injected locally for an anti-inflammatory effect. In inflammatory conditions of the joints, including juvenile idiopathic arthritis, they are given by intra-articular injection as monotherapy, or as an adjunct to long-term therapy to reduce swelling and deformity in one or a few joints. Aseptic precautions (e.g. a no-touch technique) are essential, as is a clinician skilled in the technique; infected areas should be avoided and general anaesthesia, or local anaesthesia, or conscious sedation should be used. Occasionally an acute inflammatory reaction develops after an intra-articular or soft-tissue injection of a corticosteroid. This may be a reaction to the microcrystalline suspension of the corticosteroid used, but must be distinguished from sepsis introduced into the injection site.

Triamcinolone hexacetonide p. 830 [unlicensed] is preferred for intra-articular injection because it is almost insoluble and has a long-acting (depot) effect. Triamcinolone acetonide p. 830 and methylprednisolone may also be considered for intra-articular injection into larger joints, whilst hydrocortisone acetate should be reserved for smaller joints or for soft-tissue injections. Intra-articular corticosteroid injections can cause flushing and, in adults, may affect the hyaline cartilage. Each joint should usually be treated no more than 3–4 times in one year.

A smaller amount of corticosteroid may also be injected directly into soft tissues for the relief of inflammation in conditions such as *tennis* or *golfer's elbow* or *compression neuropathies*, which occur rarely in children. In *tendinitis*, injections should be made into the tendon sheath and not directly into the tendon (due to the absence of a true tendon sheath and a high risk of rupture, the Achilles tendon should not be injected).

Corticosteroid injections are also injected into soft tissues for the treatment of skin lesions.

For further information on corticosteroid use, see Corticosteroids, general use p. 537.

540

Methylprednisolone

26-Jul-2025

- **DRUG ACTION** Methylprednisolone exerts predominantly glucocorticoid effects with minimal mineralcorticoid effects.

- **INDICATIONS AND DOSE**

DEPO-MEDRONE®

Local inflammation of joints and soft tissues

▶ BY INTRA-ARTICULAR INJECTION

▸ Child: (consult product literature)

- **CAUTIONS** Systemic sclerosis (increased incidence of scleroderma renal crisis)
- **INTERACTIONS** → Appendix 1: corticosteroids
- **SIDE-EFFECTS** Angioedema · cataract · confusion · delusions · depressed mood · diarrhoea · dizziness · drug dependence · dyslipidaemia · embolism and thrombosis · epidural lipomatosis · fatigue · gastrointestinal disorders · glucose tolerance impaired · hallucination · hepatitis · hiccups · hypopituitarism · hypotension · increased insulin requirement · insomnia · intracranial pressure increased · malaise · memory loss · metabolic acidosis · muscle weakness · myalgia · neuropathic arthropathy · peripheral oedema · psychiatric disorder · schizophrenia exacerbated · sterile abscess · suicidal ideation · vision loss · withdrawal syndrome

  SIDE-EFFECTS, FURTHER INFORMATION Since systemic absorption can follow local administration, also consider the side-effects of systemic corticosteroids.
- **MONITORING REQUIREMENTS** Manufacturer advises monitor blood pressure and renal function (s-creatinine) routinely in patients with systemic sclerosis—increased incidence of scleroderma renal crisis.

- **MEDICINAL FORMS** There can be variation in the licensing of different medicines containing the same drug.

Suspension for injection

CAUTIONARY AND ADVISORY LABELS 10

▸ **Depo-Medrone** (Pfizer Ltd)

Methylprednisolone acetate 40 mg per 1 ml Depo-Medrone 40mg/1ml suspension for injection vials | 1 vial PoM £3.44 DT = £3.44 | 10 vial PoM £34.04

Depo-Medrone 80mg/2ml suspension for injection vials | 1 vial PoM £6.18 DT = £6.18 | 10 vial PoM £61.39

Depo-Medrone 120mg/3ml suspension for injection vials | 1 vial PoM £8.96 DT = £8.96 | 10 vial PoM £88.81

F 540

Triamcinolone acetonide

26-Jul-2025

- **DRUG ACTION** Triamcinolone exerts predominantly glucocorticoid effects with minimal mineralcorticoid effect.

- **INDICATIONS AND DOSE**

ADCORTYL® INTRA-ARTICULAR/INTRADERMAL

Local inflammation of joints and soft tissues

▶ BY INTRA-ARTICULAR INJECTION

▶ Child 1–17 years: 2 mg/kg (max. per dose 15 mg), for details consult product literature, dose applies for larger joints. For doses above 15 mg use *Kenalog® Intra-articular/Intramuscular*. If appropriate repeat treatment for relapse.

KENALOG® VIALS

Local inflammation of joints and soft tissues

▶ BY INTRA-ARTICULAR INJECTION

▶ Child 1–17 years: 2 mg/kg, for details consult product literature, if appropriate repeat treatment for relapse, higher doses than usual maximum have been used; Usual maximum 40 mg

- **UNLICENSED USE** Not licensed for use in children under 6 years.
- **INTERACTIONS** → Appendix 1: corticosteroids
- **SIDE-EFFECTS** Since systemic absorption can follow local administration, also consider the side-effects of systemic corticosteroids.

- **MEDICINAL FORMS** There can be variation in the licensing of different medicines containing the same drug.

Suspension for injection

CAUTIONARY AND ADVISORY LABELS 10

EXCIPIENTS: May contain Benzyl alcohol

▶ Triamcinolone acetonide (Non-proprietary)

Triamcinolone acetonide 10 mg per 1 ml Triamcinolone acetonide 10mg/1ml suspension for injection ampoules | 1 ampoule PoM Ⓢ

Triamcinolone acetonide 40 mg per 1 ml Triamcinolone acetonide 40mg/1ml suspension for injection vials | 1 vial PoM Ⓢ

F 540

Triamcinolone hexacetonide

26-Jul-2025

- **DRUG ACTION** Triamcinolone exerts predominantly glucocorticoid effects with minimal mineralcorticoid effects.

- **INDICATIONS AND DOSE**

Symptomatic treatment of subacute and chronic inflammatory joint diseases (for details, consult product literature)

▶ BY INTRA-ARTICULAR INJECTION

▶ Child 12–17 years: 2–20 mg, according to size of the joint; if appropriate repeat treatment at intervals of 3–4 weeks, no more than 2 joints should be treated on any one day

▶ BY PERI-ARTICULAR INJECTION

▶ Child 12–17 years: 10–20 mg, according to size of the joint, no more than 2 joints should be treated on any one day

Juvenile idiopathic arthritis

▶ BY INTRA-ARTICULAR INJECTION

▶ Child 3–11 years: (consult product literature)

- **CONTRA-INDICATIONS** Avoid injections containing benzyl alcohol in neonates · consult product literature
- **CAUTIONS** Consult product literature
- **INTERACTIONS** → Appendix 1: corticosteroids
- **SIDE-EFFECTS** Heart failure · insomnia · protein catabolism

SIDE-EFFECTS, FURTHER INFORMATION Since systemic absorption can follow local administration, also consider the side-effects of systemic corticosteroids.

- **PRESCRIBING AND DISPENSING INFORMATION** Various strengths available from 'special order' manufacturers or specialist importing companies.

- **NATIONAL FUNDING/ACCESS DECISIONS**

For full details see funding body website

All Wales Medicines Strategy Group (AWMSG) decisions

▶ **Triamcinolone hexacetonide 20 mg/mL suspension for injection for the treatment of juvenile idiopathic arthritis (August 2017)** AWMSG No. 2527 Recommended

- **MEDICINAL FORMS** There can be variation in the licensing of different medicines containing the same drug.

Suspension for injection

EXCIPIENTS: May contain Benzyl alcohol

▶ Triamcinolone hexacetonide (Non-proprietary)

Triamcinolone hexacetonide 20 mg per 1 ml Triamcinolone hexacetonide 20mg/1ml suspension for injection ampoules | 10 ampoule PoM £120.00

4.2 Soft tissue disorders

Soft-tissue disorders

Soft-tissue and musculoskeletal disorders

The management of children with soft-tissue injuries and strains, and musculoskeletal disorders, may include temporary rest together with the local application of heat or cold, local massage and physiotherapy. For pain relief, paracetamol p. 325 is often adequate and should be used first. Alternatively, the lowest effective dose of a **NSAID** (e.g. ibuprofen p. 821) can be used. If pain relief with either drug is inadequate, both paracetamol (in a full dose appropriate for the child) and a low dose of a NSAID may be required.

Extravasation

Local guidelines for the management of extravasation should be followed where they exist or specialist advice sought.

Extravasation injury follows leakage of drugs or intravenous fluids from the veins or inadvertent administration into the subcutaneous or subdermal tissue. It must be dealt with **promptly** to prevent tissue necrosis.

Acidic or alkaline preparations and those with an osmolarity greater than that of plasma can cause extravasation injury; excipients including alcohol and polyethylene glycol have also been implicated. Cytotoxic drugs commonly cause extravasation injury. Very young children are at increased risk. Those receiving anticoagulants are more likely to lose blood into surrounding tissues if extravasation occurs, while those receiving sedatives or analgesics may not notice the early signs or symptoms of extravasation.

Extravasation prevention

Precautions should be taken to avoid extravasation; ideally, drugs likely to cause extravasation injury should be given through a central line and children receiving repeated doses of hazardous drugs peripherally should have the cannula resited at regular intervals. Attention should be paid to the manufacturers' recommendations for administration. Placing a glyceryl trinitrate patch p. 158 or using glyceryl trinitrate ointment distal to the cannula may improve the patency of the vessel in children with small veins or in those whose veins are prone to collapse. Children or their carers should be asked to report any pain or burning at the site of injection immediately.

Extravasation management
If extravasation is suspected the infusion should be stopped immediately but the cannula should not be removed until after an attempt has been made to aspirate the area (through the cannula) in order to remove as much of the drug as possible. Aspiration is sometimes possible if the extravasation presents with a raised bleb or blister at the injection site and is surrounded by hardened tissue, but it is often unsuccessful if the tissue is soft or soggy. **Corticosteroids** are usually given to treat inflammation, although there is little evidence to support their use in extravasation. Hydrocortisone p. 544 or dexamethasone p. 543 can be given either locally by subcutaneous injection or intravenously at a site distant from the injury. Antihistamines and analgesics may be required for symptom relief.

The management of extravasation beyond these measures is not well standardised and calls for specialist advice. Treatment depends on the nature of the offending substance; one approach is to localise and neutralise the substance whereas another is to spread and dilute it. The first method may be appropriate following extravasation of vesicant drugs and involves administration of an antidote (if available) and the application of cold compresses 3–4 times a day (consult specialist literature for details of specific antidotes). Spreading and diluting the offending substance involves infiltrating the area with physiological saline, applying warm compresses, elevating the affected limb, and administering hyaluronidase below. A saline flush-out technique (involving flushing the subcutaneous tissue with physiological saline) may be effective but requires specialist advice. Hyaluronidase should **not** be administered following extravasation of vesicant drugs (unless it is either specifically indicated or used in the saline flush-out technique).

Enzymes used in soft-tissue disorders
Hyaluronidase is used for the management of extravasation.

ENZYMES

Hyaluronidase

24-Feb-2020

● **INDICATIONS AND DOSE**

Extravasation

▸ BY LOCAL INFILTRATION

▸ Child: (consult product literature)

● **UNLICENSED USE** Licensed for use in children, but age range not specified by the manufacturer.

● **CONTRA-INDICATIONS** Avoid sites where infection is present · avoid sites where malignancy is present · do not apply direct to cornea · not for anaesthesia in unexplained premature labour · not for intravenous administration · not to be used to enhance the absorption and dispersion of dopamine and/or alpha-adrenoceptor agonists · not to be used to reduce swelling of bites · not to be used to reduce swelling of stings

● **SIDE-EFFECTS** Oedema · periorbital oedema

● **MEDICINAL FORMS** There can be variation in the licensing of different medicines containing the same drug.

Powder for solution for injection

▸ **Hyaluronidase (Non-proprietary)**

Hyaluronidase 1500 unit Hyaluronidase 1,500unit powder for solution for injection ampoules | 10 ampoule [PoM] £218.51 (Hospital only)

Chapter 11
Eye

CONTENTS

Eye

30-Nov-2020

Eye treatment: drug administration

The structure of the eye is divided into two main parts: the anterior segment and the posterior segment. Drugs are most commonly administered to the anterior segment of the eye by topical application in the form of eye drops or ointments. When a higher drug concentration is required, and when wanting to achieve therapeutic drug concentrations to the posterior segment of the eye, administration by intravitreal injection, periocular injection, or by the systemic route may be necessary.

Eye drops and eye ointments

Eye drops are generally instilled into the pocket formed by gently pulling down the lower eyelid, blinking a few times to ensure even spread, and then closing the eye; in neonates and infants it may be more appropriate to administer the drop in the inner angle of the open eye. A small amount of eye ointment is applied similarly; blinking helps to spread it. EvGr Eye drops and ointments may cause temporary blurring of vision. If affected, patients should be warned not to drive or perform other skilled tasks until vision is clear.

When two different eye preparations are used at the same time of day, the patient should leave an interval of at least 5 minutes between the two, to allow the first to be fully absorbed; eye ointment should be applied after drops. ⟨M⟩

Systemic effects may arise from absorption of drugs into the general circulation either directly from the conjunctival sac or after the excess preparation has drained down through the tear ducts into the nasal cavity. The extent of systemic absorption following ocular administration is highly variable due to a number of factors (e.g. drainage, blink rate, tear turnover). Nasal drainage of drugs is associated with eye drops much more often than with eye ointments. Applying pressure on the lacrimal punctum for at least a minute after administering eye drops reduces nasolacrimal drainage and therefore decreases systemic absorption from the nasal mucosa.

Eye-drop dispenser devices are available to aid the instillation of eye drops from plastic bottles and some are prescribable on the NHS (consult Drug Tariff—see Part IXA - Appliances). Product-specific devices may be supplied by manufacturers—consult individual manufacturers for information. They are particularly useful in patients with poor manual dexterity (e.g. due to arthritis) or reduced vision.

Eye irrigation solutions

These are solutions for the irrigation of the conjunctival sac. They act mechanically to flush out irritants or foreign bodies as a first-aid treatment. Sterile sodium chloride 0.9% solution p. 842 is usually used. Clean water will suffice in an emergency.

Other preparations administered to the eye

The intravitreal route is used to administer drug into the posterior segment of the eye for conditions such as macular oedema and age-related macular degeneration. The intracameral route can be used to deliver certain drugs to the anterior chamber, for example antibacterials after cataract surgery. These injections should only be used under specialist supervision.

Ophthalmic Specials

The Royal College of Ophthalmologists and the UK Ophthalmic Pharmacy Group have produced the Ophthalmic Special Order Products guidance to help prescribers and pharmacists manage and restrict the use of unlicensed eye preparations. 'Specials' should only be prescribed in situations where a licensed product is not suitable for a patient's needs. The Ophthalmic Special Order Products guidance can be accessed on the Royal College of Ophthalmologists website (www.rcophth.ac.uk).

Preservatives and sensitisers

Information on preservatives and substances identified as skin sensitisers is provided under Excipients statements in Medicinal form entries—see individual drug monographs. Very rarely, cases of corneal calcification have been reported with the use of phosphate-containing eye drops in patients with significantly damaged corneas—consult product literature for further information.

Eye preparations: control of microbial contamination

Preparations for the eye should be sterile when issued. Care should be taken to avoid contamination of the contents during use.

Eye preparations in multiple-application containers for use by the patient *at home* are normally discarded 4 weeks after first opening (unless otherwise stated by the manufacturer).

Multiple application eye preparations for use in *hospital general wards* are also normally discarded 4 weeks after first opening (unless otherwise stated by the manufacturer)—local practice may vary. Individual containers should be provided for each patient. A separate container should be supplied for each eye only if there are special concerns about contamination. Patients admitted with an eye infection should be supplied with a fresh container on admission. On discharge from hospital, eye preparations used during the hospital stay should be assessed for suitability (e.g. period of use, risk of contamination); if unsuitable, a fresh supply should be provided.

During formal *eye examinations* and in *eye surgery*, single-application containers should be used if possible to reduce the risk of contamination. There is a high-risk of cross-contamination in areas such as operating theatres, eye disease clinics, and ophthalmic accident and emergency departments, therefore all containers should be discarded after single patient use whether they are single- or multiple-application containers.

Compared to eye preparations containing a preservative, unpreserved eye preparations may have a shorter period of safe use; consult packaging and see Guidance on the in-use shelf life for eye drops and ointments for more information (www.sps.nhs.uk/articles/guidance-on-in-use-shelf-life-for-eye-drops-and-ointments/).

Contact lenses

Contact lenses are usually worn for their visual corrective function (e.g. myopia, astigmatism). There are two main types of lenses; hard (rigid or gas-permeable rigid) lenses or soft (hydrogel or hydrophilic) lenses. Soft lenses are the most popular type because they tend to be more comfortable, but they may not give the best vision.

Lenses are usually worn for a specified number of hours each day and removed for sleeping unless specifically designed for overnight wear. The risk of infectious and non-infectious keratitis is increased by extended continuous contact lens wear, and poor compliance with directions for use, daily cleaning, and disinfection.

Acanthamoeba keratitis, a painful and severe sight-threatening infection of the cornea, can be associated with ineffective lens cleaning and disinfection, the use of contaminated lens cases, or tap water coming into contact with the lenses. The condition, which is treated promptly by specialists, is especially associated with the use of soft lenses (particularly reusable or extended wear lenses).

Contact lenses and drug treatment

Unless medically indicated, soft lenses should be removed before instillation of the eye preparation. Alternatively, unpreserved drops can be used, as preservatives accumulate in soft lenses and can cause irritation. Eye drops, however, may be instilled while patients are wearing hard contact lenses but removal prior to instillation is still generally advised. Ointment preparations should never be used in conjunction with contact lens wear; oily eye drops can cause lens deposits and should also be avoided.

Many drugs given systemically can also have adverse effects on contact lens wear. These include drugs which can cause corneal oedema (e.g. oral contraceptives–particularly those with a higher oestrogen content), drugs which reduce eye movement and blink reflex (e.g. anxiolytics, sedative hypnotics, antihistamines, and muscle relaxants), drugs which reduce lacrimation (e.g. older generation antihistamines, phenothiazines and related drugs, some beta-blockers, diuretics, and tricyclic antidepressants), and drugs which increase lacrimation (including ephedrine hydrochloride p. 144 and hydralazine hydrochloride p. 136). Other drugs that may affect contact lens wear include isotretinoin p. 937 (can decrease tolerance to contact lens), aspirin p. 104 (can cause irritation), and rifampicin p. 449 and sulfasalazine p. 35 (can discolour lenses).

1 Allergic and inflammatory eye conditions

Eye, allergy and inflammation 05-Jun-2020

Corticosteroids

Corticosteroids administered locally to the eye or given by mouth are effective for treating anterior segment inflammation, including that which results from surgery.

Topical corticosteroids should normally only be used under expert supervision; three main dangers are associated with their use:

- a 'red eye', when the diagnosis is unconfirmed, may be due to herpes simplex virus, and a corticosteroid may aggravate the condition, leading to corneal ulceration, with possible damage to vision and even loss of the eye. Bacterial, fungal, and amoebic infections pose a similar hazard;
- 'steroid glaucoma' can follow the use of corticosteroid eye preparations in susceptible individuals;
- a 'steroid cataract' can follow prolonged use.

Products combining a corticosteroid with an antimicrobial are used after ocular surgery to reduce inflammation and prevent infection; use of combination products is otherwise rarely justified.

Systemic corticosteroids may be useful for ocular conditions. The risk of producing a 'steroid cataract' increases with the dose and duration of corticosteroid use.

Eye care, other anti-inflammatory preparations

Eye drops containing antihistamines, such as antazoline with xylometazoline below, azelastine hydrochloride p. 834, epinastine hydrochloride p. 834, ketotifen p. 834, and olopatadine p. 834, can be used for allergic conjunctivitis.

Sodium cromoglicate p. 835 and nedocromil sodium eye drops may be useful for vernal keratoconjunctivitis and other allergic forms of conjunctivitis.

Lodoxamide eye drops p. 834 are used for allergic conjunctival conditions including seasonal allergic conjunctivitis.

1.1 Allergic conjunctivitis

ANTIHISTAMINES

Antazoline with xylometazoline

06-Apr-2020

● **INDICATIONS AND DOSE**

Allergic conjunctivitis

▸ TO THE EYE
- ▸ Child 12–17 years: Apply 2–3 times a day for maximum 7 days

● **CAUTIONS** Angle-closure glaucoma · cardiovascular disease · diabetes mellitus · hypertension · hyperthyroidism · phaeochromocytoma · urinary retention

● **INTERACTIONS** → Appendix 1: antihistamines, sedating · sympathomimetics, vasoconstrictor

● **SIDE-EFFECTS** Drowsiness · eye irritation · headache · hyperhidrosis · hypertension · mydriasis · nausea · palpitations · vascular disorders · vision blurred

SIDE-EFFECTS, FURTHER INFORMATION Absorption of antazoline and xylometazoline may result in systemic side-effects.

● **MEDICINAL FORMS** No licensed medicines listed.

Azelastine hydrochloride
03-Aug-2023

● **INDICATIONS AND DOSE**

Seasonal allergic conjunctivitis

▶ TO THE EYE

▸ Child 4–17 years: Apply twice daily, increased if necessary to 4 times a day

Perennial conjunctivitis

▶ TO THE EYE

▸ Child 12–17 years: Apply twice daily for a maximum duration of 6 weeks, dose can be increased if necessary to 4 times a day

● **INTERACTIONS** → Appendix 1: antihistamines, non-sedating

● **SIDE-EFFECTS**

▶ **Common or very common** Eye irritation

▶ **Uncommon** Taste bitter

SIDE-EFFECTS, FURTHER INFORMATION Altered taste may occur after administration, often due to incorrect application.

● **MEDICINAL FORMS** There can be variation in the licensing of different medicines containing the same drug.

Eye drops

EXCIPIENTS: May contain Benzalkonium chloride, disodium edetate

▸ Azelastine hydrochloride (Non-proprietary)

Azelastine hydrochloride 500 microgram per 1 ml Azelastine 0.05% eye drops | 8 ml PoM £7.31 DT = £6.89

▸ Optilast (Ceuta Healthcare Ltd)

Azelastine hydrochloride 500 microgram per 1 ml Optilast 0.05% eye drops | 8 ml PoM £6.40 DT = £6.89

Epinastine hydrochloride
26-Mar-2020

● **INDICATIONS AND DOSE**

Seasonal allergic conjunctivitis

▶ TO THE EYE

▸ Child 12–17 years: Apply twice daily for maximum 8 weeks

● **SIDE-EFFECTS**

▶ **Common or very common** Eye discomfort

▶ **Uncommon** Dry eye · eye disorders · headache · nasal irritation · rhinitis · taste altered · visual impairment

● **MEDICINAL FORMS** There can be variation in the licensing of different medicines containing the same drug.

Eye drops

EXCIPIENTS: May contain Benzalkonium chloride, disodium edetate

▸ Relestat (AbbVie Ltd)

Epinastine hydrochloride 500 microgram per 1 ml Relestat 500micrograms/ml eye drops | 5 ml PoM £9.90 DT = £9.90

Ketotifen
14-Dec-2020

● **INDICATIONS AND DOSE**

Seasonal allergic conjunctivitis

▶ TO THE EYE

▸ Child 3–17 years: Apply twice daily

● **INTERACTIONS** → Appendix 1: antihistamines, sedating

● **SIDE-EFFECTS**

▶ **Common or very common** Eye discomfort · eye disorders · eye inflammation

▶ **Uncommon** Conjunctival haemorrhage · drowsiness · dry eye · dry mouth · headache · skin reactions · vision disorders

▶ **Frequency not known** Asthma exacerbated · facial swelling · oedema

● **NATIONAL FUNDING/ACCESS DECISIONS**
For full details see funding body website

All Wales Medicines Strategy Group (AWMSG) decisions

▶ **Ketotifen (*Ketofall*®) for symptomatic treatment of seasonal allergic conjunctivitis (June 2020)** AWMSG No. 3930 Recommended with restrictions

● **MEDICINAL FORMS** There can be variation in the licensing of different medicines containing the same drug.

Eye drops

EXCIPIENTS: May contain Benzalkonium chloride

▸ Ketofall (Scope Ophthalmics Ltd)

Ketotifen (as Ketotifen hydrogen fumarate) 250 microgram per 1 ml Ketofall 0.25mg/ml eye drops 0.4ml unit dose | 30 unit dose PoM £6.95 DT = £6.95

▸ Zaditen (Thea Pharmaceuticals Ltd)

Ketotifen (as Ketotifen fumarate) 250 microgram per 1 ml Zaditen 250micrograms/ml eye drops | 5 ml PoM £7.80 DT = £7.80

Olopatadine
25-Mar-2020

● **INDICATIONS AND DOSE**

Seasonal allergic conjunctivitis

▶ TO THE EYE

▸ Child 3–17 years: Apply twice daily for maximum 4 months

● **SIDE-EFFECTS**

▶ **Common or very common** Asthenia · dry eye · eye discomfort · headache · nasal dryness · taste altered

▶ **Uncommon** Dizziness · eye disorders · eye inflammation · increased risk of infection · numbness · skin reactions · vision disorders

▶ **Frequency not known** Drowsiness · dyspnoea · malaise · nausea · vomiting

● **MEDICINAL FORMS** There can be variation in the licensing of different medicines containing the same drug.

Eye drops

EXCIPIENTS: May contain Benzalkonium chloride

▸ Olopatadine (Non-proprietary)

Olopatadine (as Olopatadine hydrochloride) 1 mg per 1 ml Olopatadine 1mg/ml eye drops | 5 ml PoM £4.68 DT = £2.68

▸ Opatanol (Novartis Pharmaceuticals UK Ltd)

Olopatadine (as Olopatadine hydrochloride) 1 mg per 1 ml Opatanol 1mg/ml eye drops | 5 ml PoM £4.68 DT = £2.68

MAST-CELL STABILISERS

Lodoxamide
06-Apr-2020

● **INDICATIONS AND DOSE**

Allergic conjunctivitis

▶ TO THE EYE

▸ Child 4–17 years: Apply 4 times a day, improvement of symptoms may sometimes require treatment for up to 4 weeks

● **SIDE-EFFECTS**

▶ **Common or very common** Dry eye · eye discomfort · eye disorders · vision disorders

▶ **Uncommon** Corneal deposits · dizziness · eye inflammation · headache · nausea

▶ **Rare or very rare** Nasal complaints · rash · taste altered

● **EXCEPTIONS TO LEGAL CATEGORY** Lodoxamide 0.1% eye drops can be sold to the public for treatment of allergic conjunctivitis in adults and children over 4 years.

- **MEDICINAL FORMS** There can be variation in the licensing of different medicines containing the same drug.

Eye drops

EXCIPIENTS: May contain Benzalkonium chloride, disodium edetate

- **Alomide** (Novartis Pharmaceuticals UK Ltd)
  Lodoxamide (as Lodoxamide trometamol) 1 mg per 1 ml Alomide 0.1% eye drops | 10 ml [PoM] £5.21 DT = £5.21

Sodium cromoglicate

03-Aug-2023

(Sodium cromoglycate)

- **INDICATIONS AND DOSE**

Allergic conjunctivitis | Seasonal keratoconjunctivitis

▶ TO THE EYE

▶ Child: Apply 4 times a day

- **SIDE-EFFECTS** Eye stinging
- **EXCEPTIONS TO LEGAL CATEGORY** Sodium cromoglicate 2% eye drops can be sold to the public (in max. pack size of 10 mL) for treatment of acute seasonal and perennial allergic conjunctivitis.
- **MEDICINAL FORMS** There can be variation in the licensing of different medicines containing the same drug.

Eye drops

- **Sodium cromoglicate (Non-proprietary)**
  Sodium cromoglicate 20 mg per 1 ml Sodium cromoglicate 2% eye drops | 13.5 ml [PoM] £8.03 DT = £2.11
  Vividrin 2% eye drops 0.5ml unit dose preservative free | 20 unit dose [PoM] [X]
- **Catacrom** (Rayner Pharmaceuticals Ltd)
  Sodium cromoglicate 20 mg per 1 ml Catacrom 2% eye drops 0.3ml unit dose | 30 unit dose [P] £11.99 DT = £11.99
- **Eycrom** (Aspire Pharma Ltd)
  Sodium cromoglicate 20 mg per 1 ml Eycrom 2% eye drops | 13.5 ml [PoM] £8.03 DT = £8.03
- **Opticrom** (Thornton & Ross Ltd)
  Sodium cromoglicate 20 mg per 1 ml Opticrom Aqueous 2% eye drops | 13.5 ml [PoM] £8.03 DT = £2.11

1.2 Inflammatory eye conditions

Other drugs used for Inflammatory eye conditions
Adalimumab, p. 806

CORTICOSTEROIDS

F 540

Betamethasone

26-Jul-2025

- **DRUG ACTION** Betamethasone has very high glucocorticoid activity and insignificant mineralocorticoid activity.
- **INDICATIONS AND DOSE**

Local treatment of inflammation (short-term)

▶ TO THE EYE USING EYE DROP

▶ Child: Apply every 1–2 hours until controlled then reduce frequency

- **CAUTIONS** Concomitant use of ocular NSAIDs

CAUTIONS, FURTHER INFORMATION [EvGr] Concomitant use of ocular formulations containing corticosteroids with ocular formulations containing NSAIDs may increase the risk of corneal healing problems, leading to corneal melt or scarring and loss of vision. ⟨M⟩

- **INTERACTIONS** → Appendix 1: corticosteroids
- **SIDE-EFFECTS** Vision disorders

SIDE-EFFECTS, FURTHER INFORMATION Since systemic absorption can follow local administration, also consider the side-effects of systemic corticosteroids.

Vision disorders can occur with use of topical (eye) corticosteroids. Consider seeking specialist advice to evaluate cause if vision blurred or other vision disorder occurs.

- **MEDICINAL FORMS** There can be variation in the licensing of different medicines containing the same drug.

Ear/eye/nose drops solution

EXCIPIENTS: May contain Benzalkonium chloride, disodium edetate

- **Betamethasone (Non-proprietary)**
  Betamethasone sodium phosphate 1 mg per 1 ml Betamethasone 0.1% ear/eye/nose drops | 5 ml [PoM] £2.07–£3.90 | 10 ml [PoM] £2.07–£7.00 DT = £2.32
- **Betnesol** (RPH Pharmaceuticals AB)
  Betamethasone sodium phosphate 1 mg per 1 ml Betnesol 0.1% eye/ear/nose drops | 10 ml [PoM] £2.32 DT = £2.32

Combinations available: ***Betamethasone with neomycin***, p. 837

F 540

Dexamethasone

26-Jul-2025

- **DRUG ACTION** Dexamethasone has very high glucocorticoid activity and insignificant mineralocorticoid activity.
- **INDICATIONS AND DOSE**

Local treatment of inflammation (short-term)

▶ TO THE EYE USING EYE DROP

▶ Child: Apply 4–6 times a day

Short term local treatment of inflammation (severe conditions)

▶ TO THE EYE USING EYE DROP

▶ Child: Apply every 30–60 minutes until controlled, reduce frequency when control achieved

ETACORTILEN®

Local treatment of inflammation [short-term]

▶ TO THE EYE USING EYE DROP

▶ Child 13–17 years: Apply 1 drop 3–4 times a day, dose to be adjusted according to response

DOSE EQUIVALENCE AND CONVERSION

▶ *Etacortilen®* eye drops contain dexamethasone sodium phosphate 1.5 mg/mL.

- **UNLICENSED USE** *Maxidex®* not licensed for use in children under 2 years. *Dropodex®* not licensed for use in children.
- **CAUTIONS** Concomitant use of ocular NSAIDs

CAUTIONS, FURTHER INFORMATION [EvGr] Concomitant use of ocular formulations containing corticosteroids with ocular formulations containing NSAIDs may increase the risk of corneal healing problems, leading to corneal melt or scarring and loss of vision. ⟨M⟩

- **INTERACTIONS** → Appendix 1: corticosteroids
- **SIDE-EFFECTS**

▶ **Common or very common** Eye discomfort

▶ **Uncommon** Dry eye · posterior subcapsular cataract · taste altered · vision disorders

▶ **Rare or very rare** Eye inflammation · face oedema

▶ **Frequency not known** Dizziness

SIDE-EFFECTS, FURTHER INFORMATION Since systemic absorption can follow local administration, also consider the side-effects of systemic corticosteroids.

Vision disorders can occur with use of topical (eye) corticosteroids. Consider seeking specialist advice to evaluate cause if vision blurred or other vision disorder occurs.

- **PREGNANCY** Dexamethasone readily crosses the placenta.
- **PRESCRIBING AND DISPENSING INFORMATION** Although multi-dose dexamethasone eye drops commonly contain preservatives, preservative-free unit dose vials may be available.

● **MEDICINAL FORMS** There can be variation in the licensing of different medicines containing the same drug. Forms available from special-order manufacturers include: eye drops

Eye drops

EXCIPIENTS: May contain Benzalkonium chloride, disodium edetate, polysorbates

▸ **Dexamethasone (Non-proprietary)**
Dexamethasone sodium phosphate 1 mg per 1 ml Minims dexamethasone 0.1% eye drops 0.5ml unit dose | 20 unit dose [PoM] £11.92 DT = £11.92
Dexamethasone 0.1% eye drops 0.3ml unit dose preservative free | 20 unit dose [PoM] £5.53–£8.06 DT = £5.53 | 30 unit dose [PoM] £8.30 (Hospital only)

▸ **Dexafree** (Thea Pharmaceuticals Ltd)
Dexamethasone sodium phosphate 1 mg per 1 ml Dexafree 1mg/1ml eye drops 0.4ml unit dose | 30 unit dose [PoM] £9.70

▸ **Dropodex** (Rayner Pharmaceuticals Ltd)
Dexamethasone sodium phosphate 1 mg per 1 ml Dropodex 0.1% eye drops 0.4ml unit dose | 20 unit dose [PoM] £11.53 DT = £11.53

▸ **Etacortilen** (Nordic Pharma Ltd)
Dexamethasone sodium phosphate 1.5 mg per 1 ml Etacortilen 1.5mg/ml eye drops 0.3ml unit dose | 20 unit dose [PoM] £11.53

▸ **Eythalm** (Aspire Pharma Ltd)
Dexamethasone phosphate (as Dexamethasone sodium phosphate) 1 mg per 1 ml Eythalm 1mg/ml eye drops | 6 ml [PoM] £9.75 DT = £9.75

▸ **Maxidex** (Novartis Pharmaceuticals UK Ltd)
Dexamethasone 1 mg per 1 ml Maxidex 0.1% eye drops | 5 ml [PoM] £1.42 DT = £1.42

▸ **Puradex** (Aspire Pharma Ltd)
Dexamethasone phosphate (as Dexamethasone sodium phosphate) 1 mg per 1 ml Puradex 1mg/ml eye drops | 6 ml [PoM] £9.75 DT = £9.75

Combinations available: *Dexamethasone with framycetin sulfate and gramicidin,* p. 837 · *Dexamethasone with hypromellose, neomycin and polymyxin B sulfate,* p. 837

Fluorometholone

26-Jul-2025

● **INDICATIONS AND DOSE**

Local treatment of inflammation (short-term)

▶ TO THE EYE

▸ Child 2–17 years: Apply every 1 hour for 24–48 hours, then reduced to 2–4 times a day

IMPORTANT SAFETY INFORMATION

MHRA/CHM ADVICE: CORTICOSTEROIDS: RARE RISK OF CENTRAL SEROUS CHORIORETINOPATHY WITH LOCAL AS WELL AS SYSTEMIC ADMINISTRATION (AUGUST 2017)

See Corticosteroids, general use p. 537.

ADRENAL INSUFFICIENCY CARD (APRIL 2023)

The British Society for Paediatric Endocrinology and Diabetes (BSPED) has developed an Adrenal Insufficiency Card which should be issued to children with adrenal insufficiency and steroid dependence. The card includes a management summary for the emergency treatment of adrenal crisis and sick day dosing, and can be issued by any healthcare professional managing such patients. The BSPED Adrenal Insufficiency Card is available at: www.bsped.org.uk/adrenal-insufficiency.

● **CAUTIONS** Concomitant use of ocular NSAIDs

CAUTIONS, FURTHER INFORMATION [EvGr] Concomitant use of ocular formulations containing corticosteroids with ocular formulations containing NSAIDs may increase the risk of corneal healing problems, leading to corneal melt or scarring and loss of vision. ⟨M⟩

● **SIDE-EFFECTS** Cataract · eye discomfort · eye disorders · eye infection · eye inflammation · rash · taste altered · vision disorders

SIDE-EFFECTS, FURTHER INFORMATION Since systemic absorption can follow local administration, also consider the side-effects of systemic corticosteroids.

Vision disorders can occur with use of topical (eye) corticosteroids. Consider seeking specialist advice to evaluate cause if vision blurred or other vision disorder occurs.

● **PATIENT AND CARER ADVICE** If systemic absorption occurs following topical and local use, side-effects applicable to systemic corticosteroids may apply; a patient information leaflet should be supplied and the need for a Steroid Treatment Card considered, see Corticosteroids, general use p. 537.

● **MEDICINAL FORMS** There can be variation in the licensing of different medicines containing the same drug.

Eye drops

EXCIPIENTS: May contain Benzalkonium chloride, disodium edetate, polysorbates

▸ **FML Liquifilm** (AbbVie Ltd)
Fluorometholone 1 mg per 1 ml FML Liquifilm 0.1% ophthalmic suspension | 5 ml [PoM] £1.71 DT = £1.71 | 10 ml [PoM] £2.95 DT = £2.95

F 540

Prednisolone

26-Jul-2025

● **DRUG ACTION** Prednisolone exerts predominantly glucocorticoid effects with minimal mineralocorticoid effects.

● **INDICATIONS AND DOSE**

Local treatment of inflammation (short-term)

▶ TO THE EYE

▸ Child: Apply every 1–2 hours until controlled then reduce frequency

● **UNLICENSED USE** *Pred Forte*® not licensed for use in children (age range not specified by manufacturer).

● **CAUTIONS** Concomitant use of ocular NSAIDs

CAUTIONS, FURTHER INFORMATION [EvGr] Concomitant use of ocular formulations containing corticosteroids with ocular formulations containing NSAIDs may increase the risk of corneal healing problems, leading to corneal melt or scarring and loss of vision. ⟨M⟩

● **INTERACTIONS** → Appendix 1: corticosteroids

● **SIDE-EFFECTS** Eye discomfort · taste altered · visual impairment

SIDE-EFFECTS, FURTHER INFORMATION Since systemic absorption can follow local administration, also consider the side-effects of systemic corticosteroids.

Vision disorders can occur with use of topical (eye) corticosteroids. Consider seeking specialist advice to evaluate cause if vision blurred or other vision disorder occurs.

● **PRESCRIBING AND DISPENSING INFORMATION** Although multi-dose prednisolone eye drops commonly contain preservatives, preservative-free unit dose vials may be available.

● **MEDICINAL FORMS** There can be variation in the licensing of different medicines containing the same drug. Forms available from special-order manufacturers include: eye drops

Eye drops

EXCIPIENTS: May contain Benzalkonium chloride, disodium edetate, polysorbates

▸ **Prednisolone (Non-proprietary)**
Prednisolone sodium phosphate 5 mg per 1 ml Minims prednisolone sodium phosphate 0.5% eye drops 0.5ml unit dose | 20 unit dose [PoM] £14.04 DT = £14.04

▸ **Pred Forte** (AbbVie Ltd)
Prednisolone acetate 10 mg per 1 ml Pred Forte 1% eye drops | 5 ml [PoM] £1.82 DT = £1.82 | 10 ml [PoM] £3.66 DT = £3.66

Ear/eye drops solution
EXCIPIENTS May contain Benzalkonium chloride, disodium edetate

▸ **Prednisolone (Non-proprietary)**
Prednisolone sodium phosphate 5 mg per 1 ml Prednisolone sodium phosphate 0.5% ear/eye drops | 10 ml PoM £2.57 DT = £2.57

CORTICOSTEROIDS > CORTICOSTEROID COMBINATIONS WITH ANTI-INFECTIVES

Betamethasone with neomycin

20-Jun-2025

The properties listed below are those particular to the combination only. For the properties of the components please consider, betamethasone p. 835.

- **INDICATIONS AND DOSE**

Local treatment of eye inflammation and bacterial infection (short-term)

▸ TO THE EYE USING EYE DROP
▸ Child: (consult product literature)

IMPORTANT SAFETY INFORMATION

MHRA/CHM ADVICE: AMINOGLYCOSIDES (GENTAMICIN, AMIKACIN, TOBRAMYCIN, AND NEOMYCIN): INCREASED RISK OF DEAFNESS IN PATIENTS WITH MITOCHONDRIAL MUTATIONS (JANUARY 2021)

The use of aminoglycosides is associated with rare cases of ototoxicity. A safety review found an increased risk of deafness in patients with mitochondrial mutations (particularly the m.1555A>G mutation), including cases where the patient's aminoglycoside serum levels were within the recommended range. Nevertheless, these mitochondrial mutations are considered rare and penetrance is uncertain. No cases were identified with topical preparations but, based on a shared mechanism of effect, there is a potential risk with neomycin and other aminoglycosides administered at the site of toxicity i.e. the ear.

Healthcare professionals are advised to consider the need for aminoglycoside treatment versus alternative options in patients with susceptible mutations. The need for genetic testing especially in those requiring recurrent or long-term treatment with aminoglycosides should also be considered, however, urgent treatment should not be delayed. To minimise the risks of adverse effects, continuous monitoring of renal and auditory function, as well as hepatic and laboratory parameters, is recommended for all patients. Those with known mitochondrial mutations or a family history of ototoxicity are advised to inform their doctor or pharmacist before using an aminoglycoside.

- **INTERACTIONS** → Appendix 1: corticosteroids · neomycin
- **SIDE-EFFECTS** Eye disorders · glaucoma · posterior subcapsular cataract · punctate keratitis · vision blurred
- **PRE-TREATMENT SCREENING** NHS England commissions genetic testing under the *National genomic test directory* indication: R65 - Aminoglycoside exposure posing risk to hearing. The testing criteria is significant exposure to aminoglycosides posing risk of ototoxicity. This testing is relevant to individuals with a predisposition to gram-negative infections or with hearing loss who have been exposed to aminoglycosides. For further information, see www.england.nhs.uk/publication/national-genomic-test-directories/.
- **LESS SUITABLE FOR PRESCRIBING** Betamethasone with neomycin eye-drops are less suitable for prescribing.
- **MEDICINAL FORMS** There can be variation in the licensing of different medicines containing the same drug.

Ear/eye/nose drops solution
EXCIPIENTS: May contain Benzalkonium chloride, disodium edetate

▸ **Betnesol-N** (RPH Pharmaceuticals AB)
Betamethasone (as Betamethasone sodium phosphate) 1 mg per 1 ml, Neomycin sulfate 5 mg per 1 ml Betnesol-N ear/eye/nose drops | 10 ml PoM £2.39 DT = £2.39

Dexamethasone with framycetin sulfate and gramicidin

02-Mar-2021

The properties listed below are those particular to the combination only. For the properties of the components please consider, dexamethasone p. 835, framycetin sulfate p. 860.

- **INDICATIONS AND DOSE**

Local treatment of inflammation (short-term)

▸ TO THE EYE
▸ Child: Apply 4–6 times a day, may be administered every 30–60 minutes in severe conditions until controlled, then reduce frequency

- **CAUTIONS** Avoid prolonged use
- **INTERACTIONS** → Appendix 1: corticosteroids
- **LESS SUITABLE FOR PRESCRIBING** *Sofradex®* is less suitable for prescribing.
- **MEDICINAL FORMS** There can be variation in the licensing of different medicines containing the same drug.

Ear/eye drops solution
EXCIPIENTS: May contain Polysorbates

▸ **Sofradex** (Neon Healthcare Ltd)
Gramicidin 50 microgram per 1 ml, Dexamethasone (as Dexamethasone sodium metasulfobenzoate) 500 microgram per 1 ml, Framycetin sulfate 5 mg per 1 ml Sofradex ear/eye drops | 8 ml PoM £7.50

Dexamethasone with hypromellose, neomycin and polymyxin B sulfate

20-Jun-2025

The properties listed below are those particular to the combination only. For the properties of the components please consider, dexamethasone p. 835.

- **INDICATIONS AND DOSE**

Local treatment of inflammation (short-term)

▸ TO THE EYE USING EYE DROP
▸ Child: Apply every 30–60 minutes until controlled, then reduced to 4–6 times a day

▸ TO THE EYE USING EYE OINTMENT
▸ Child: Apply 3–4 times a day, alternatively apply once daily, to be applied at night, when used with eye drops

IMPORTANT SAFETY INFORMATION

MHRA/CHM ADVICE: AMINOGLYCOSIDES (GENTAMICIN, AMIKACIN, TOBRAMYCIN, AND NEOMYCIN): INCREASED RISK OF DEAFNESS IN PATIENTS WITH MITOCHONDRIAL MUTATIONS (JANUARY 2021)

The use of aminoglycosides is associated with rare cases of ototoxicity. A safety review found an increased risk of deafness in patients with mitochondrial mutations (particularly the m.1555A>G mutation), including cases where the patient's aminoglycoside serum levels were within the recommended range. Nevertheless, these mitochondrial mutations are considered rare and penetrance is uncertain. No cases were identified with topical preparations but, based on a shared mechanism of effect, there is a potential risk with neomycin and

11 Eye

other aminoglycosides administered at the site of toxicity i.e. the ear.

Healthcare professionals are advised to consider the need for aminoglycoside treatment versus alternative options in patients with susceptible mutations. The need for genetic testing especially in those requiring recurrent or long-term treatment with aminoglycosides should also be considered, however, urgent treatment should not be delayed. To minimise the risks of adverse effects, continuous monitoring of renal and auditory function, as well as hepatic and laboratory parameters, is recommended for all patients. Those with known mitochondrial mutations or a family history of ototoxicity are advised to inform their doctor or pharmacist before using an aminoglycoside.

- **INTERACTIONS** → Appendix 1: corticosteroids · neomycin · polymyxin b
- **SIDE-EFFECTS**
  - **Uncommon** Eye discomfort · eye inflammation
  - **Frequency not known** Adrenal suppression · Cushing's syndrome · eye disorders · headache · Stevens-Johnson syndrome · vision disorders
- **PRE-TREATMENT SCREENING** NHS England commissions genetic testing under the *National genomic test directory* indication: R65 - Aminoglycoside exposure posing risk to hearing. The testing criteria is significant exposure to aminoglycosides posing risk of ototoxicity. This testing is relevant to individuals with a predisposition to gram-negative infections or with hearing loss who have been exposed to aminoglycosides. For further information, see www.england.nhs.uk/publication/national-genomic-test-directories/.
- **LESS SUITABLE FOR PRESCRIBING** Dexamethasone with neomycin and polymixin B sulfate is less suitable for prescribing.

- **MEDICINAL FORMS** There can be variation in the licensing of different medicines containing the same drug.

Eye ointment

EXCIPIENTS: May contain Hydroxybenzoates (parabens), woolfat and related substances (including lanolin)

- **Maxitrol** (Novartis Pharmaceuticals UK Ltd)
  Dexamethasone 1 mg per 1 gram, Neomycin (as Neomycin sulfate) 3500 unit per 1 gram, Polymyxin B sulfate 6000 unit per 1 gram Maxitrol eye ointment | 3.5 gram PoM £1.44

Eye drops

EXCIPIENTS: May contain Benzalkonium chloride, polysorbates

- **Maxitrol** (Novartis Pharmaceuticals UK Ltd)
  Dexamethasone 1 mg per 1 ml, Neomycin (as Neomycin sulfate) 3500 unit per 1 ml, Polymyxin B sulfate 6000 unit per 1 ml Maxitrol eye drops | 5 ml PoM £1.68

IMMUNOSUPPRESSANTS › CALCINEURIN INHIBITORS AND RELATED DRUGS

Ciclosporin

06-Feb-2026

(Cyclosporin)

- **DRUG ACTION** Ciclosporin inhibits production and release of lymphokines, thereby suppressing cell-mediated immune response.

- **INDICATIONS AND DOSE**

VERKAZIA®

Severe vernal keratoconjunctivitis (initiated by a specialist)

- TO THE EYE
- Child 4–17 years: Apply 1 drop 4 times a day, to be applied to the affected eye(s) during the vernal keratoconjunctivitis season, if signs and symptoms persist after the end of the season, treatment may be continued at the recommended dose or decreased to 1 drop twice daily once adequate control is achieved. Once resolved, treatment should be discontinued, and re-initiated upon recurrence

- **CONTRA-INDICATIONS** Active or suspected ocular or peri-ocular infection · ocular or peri-ocular malignancies or premalignant conditions
- **CAUTIONS** Contact lens wearers—consult product literature · history of ocular herpes—no information available
- **INTERACTIONS** → Appendix 1: ciclosporin
- **SIDE-EFFECTS**
  - **Common or very common** Cough · eye discomfort · eye disorders · eye inflammation · headache · increased risk of infection · vision blurred
- **PREGNANCY** Manufacturer advises avoid unless potential benefit outweighs risk—no information available.
- **BREAST FEEDING** Manufacturer advises avoid—limited information.
- **MONITORING REQUIREMENTS** EvGr Regular eye examinations recommended—consult product literature. ⟨M⟩
- **DIRECTIONS FOR ADMINISTRATION** Keep eyes closed for 2 minutes after using eye drops to increase local drug action and reduce systemic absorption. If using other eye drops concomitantly, ciclosporin eye drops should be used at least 15 minutes after the other eye drops.
- **PATIENT AND CARER ADVICE**
  Driving and skilled tasks Manufacturer advises patients and carers should be counselled on the effects on driving and performance of skilled tasks—increased risk of blurred vision.
- **NATIONAL FUNDING/ACCESS DECISIONS**
  For full details see funding body website

Scottish Medicines Consortium (SMC) decisions

- **Ciclosporin (*Verkazia*®) for the treatment of severe vernal keratoconjunctivitis (VKC) in children from 4 years of age and adolescents (until the age of 18) (December 2018)** SMC No. SMC2111 Recommended

All Wales Medicines Strategy Group (AWMSG) decisions

- **Ciclosporin (*Verkazia*®) for the treatment of severe vernal keratoconjunctivitis in children and adolescents from 4 to 18 years old (March 2019)** AWMSG No. 2908 Recommended

- **MEDICINAL FORMS** There can be variation in the licensing of different medicines containing the same drug.

Eye drops

- **Verkazia** (Santen UK Ltd)
  Ciclosporin 1 mg per 1 ml Verkazia 1mg/ml eye drops emulsion 0.3ml unit dose | 120 unit dose PoM £288.00

1.2a Anterior uveitis

ANTIMUSCARINICS

Antimuscarinics (eye)

- **CAUTIONS** Children under 3 months owing to the possible association between cycloplegia and the development of amblyopia · darkly pigmented iris is more resistant to pupillary dilatation and caution should be exercised to avoid overdosage · mydriasis can precipitate acute angle-closure glaucoma (usually in those who are predisposed to the condition because of a shallow anterior chamber) · neonates at increased risk of systemic toxicity
- **SIDE-EFFECTS** Dizziness · photophobia · skin reactions · tachycardia

- **PATIENT AND CARER ADVICE** Patients may not be able to undertake skilled tasks until vision clears after mydriasis.

838

Atropine sulfate

22-Feb-2023

- **INDICATIONS AND DOSE**

Cycloplegia
- TO THE EYE USING EYE DROP
- Child 3 months–17 years: Apply twice daily for 3 days, before procedure

Anterior uveitis
- TO THE EYE USING EYE DROP
- Child 2–17 years: Apply 1 drop up to 4 times a day

- **UNLICENSED USE** Not licensed for use in children for uveitis.
- **INTERACTIONS** → Appendix 1: atropine
- **SIDE-EFFECTS** Systemic side-effects can occur.
- **PRESCRIBING AND DISPENSING INFORMATION** Although multi-dose atropine sulfate eye drops commonly contain preservatives, preservative-free unit dose vials may be available.
- **MEDICINAL FORMS** There can be variation in the licensing of different medicines containing the same drug. Forms available from special-order manufacturers include: eye drops

Eye drops
- Atropine sulfate (Non-proprietary)
  Atropine sulfate 10 mg per 1 ml Atropine 1% eye drops 0.5ml unit dose preservative free | 20 unit dose PoM £17.82–£28.52 DT = £17.82
  Atropine 1% eye drops | 5 ml PoM £80.00–£130.00 | 10 ml PoM £240.99 DT = £10.95
- Atropine sulfate (Bausch & Lomb UK Ltd)
  Atropine sulfate 10 mg per 1 ml Minims atropine sulfate 1% eye drops 0.5ml unit dose | 20 unit dose PoM £17.82 DT = £17.82
- Ocutrop (Blumont Pharma Ltd)
  Atropine sulfate 10 mg per 1 ml Ocutrop 1% eye drops | 10 ml PoM £50.00 DT = £10.95

838

Cyclopentolate hydrochloride

- **INDICATIONS AND DOSE**

Cycloplegia
- TO THE EYE
- Child 3 months–11 years: Apply 1 drop, 30–60 minutes before examination, using 1% eye drops
- Child 12–17 years: Apply 1 drop, 30–60 minutes before examination, using 0.5% eye drops

Uveitis
- TO THE EYE
- Child 3 months–17 years: Apply 1 drop 2–4 times a day, using 0.5% eye drops (1% for deeply pigmented eyes)

- **INTERACTIONS** → Appendix 1: cyclopentolate
- **SIDE-EFFECTS** Abdominal distension · arrhythmias · behaviour abnormal · cardio-respiratory distress · conjunctivitis (on prolonged administration) · constipation · dry mouth · eye oedema (on prolonged administration) · flushing · gastrointestinal disorders · hyperaemia (on prolonged administration) · mydriasis · palpitations · psychotic disorder · staggering · urinary disorders · vomiting

  SIDE-EFFECTS, FURTHER INFORMATION Systemic side-effects can occur.
- **PRESCRIBING AND DISPENSING INFORMATION** Although multi-dose cyclopentolate eye drops commonly contain preservatives, preservative-free unit dose vials may be available.
- **MEDICINAL FORMS** There can be variation in the licensing of different medicines containing the same drug.

Eye drops

EXCIPIENTS: May contain Benzalkonium chloride
- Cyclopentolate hydrochloride (Bausch & Lomb UK Ltd)
  Cyclopentolate hydrochloride 5 mg per 1 ml Minims cyclopentolate hydrochloride 0.5% eye drops 0.5ml unit dose | 20 unit dose PoM £13.08 DT = £13.08
  Cyclopentolate hydrochloride 10 mg per 1 ml Minims cyclopentolate hydrochloride 1% eye drops 0.5ml unit dose | 20 unit dose PoM £13.38 DT = £13.38
- Mydrilate (Esteve Pharmaceuticals Ltd)
  Cyclopentolate hydrochloride 5 mg per 1 ml Mydrilate 0.5% solution | 5 ml PoM £8.08 DT = £8.08
  Cyclopentolate hydrochloride 10 mg per 1 ml Mydrilate 1% solution | 5 ml PoM £8.08 DT = £8.08

838

Homatropine hydrobromide

- **INDICATIONS AND DOSE**

Anterior uveitis
- TO THE EYE
- Child 3 months–1 year: Apply 1 drop daily, alternatively apply 1 drop once daily on alternate days, adjusted according to response, only 0.5% eye drops to be used
- Child 2–17 years: Apply 1 drop twice daily, adjusted according to response

- **INTERACTIONS** → Appendix 1: homatropine
- **MEDICINAL FORMS** Forms available from special-order manufacturers include: eye drops

2 Dry eye conditions

Dry eye

08-Feb-2020

Description of condition

Dry eye presents as chronic soreness and inflammation of ocular surface associated with reduced or abnormal tear secretion (e.g. in Sjögren's syndrome). It often responds to tear replacement therapy in the form of eye drops (preferably preservative-free), eye ointment (used at night), or gels. Choice of preparation is based on the type of dry eye (e.g. aqueous-deficient or evaporative), symptoms, and patient preference.

Drug treatment

EvGr Young children presenting with symptoms of dry eye should be referred to an optometrist for specialist assessment. Urgent referral to an ophthalmologist is required for children with any corneal change (e.g. staining or vascularisation).

Hypromellose p. 841 is the most frequently used treatment for tear deficiency in patients with mild dry eye. (A) Initially, it may need to be instilled frequently (e.g. hourly) for adequate symptom relief, then at a reduced frequency. EvGr Carbomers p. 840 and polyvinyl alcohol p. 841 are suitable alternatives. (A) The ability of carbomers p. 840 and polyvinyl alcohol to cling to the eye surface and their higher viscosity may help reduce frequency of application to 4 times daily. Carbomers p. 840 can be less tolerated than hypromellose due to their impact on vision. EvGr Preservative-free tear replacement is preferred in cases of frequent and chronic application.

Ocular lubricants containing sodium hyaluronate p. 842, hydroxypropyl guar, or carmellose sodium p. 840 can be used for moderate to severe dry eye following a suitable trial (6–8 weeks) of treatment options for mild dry eye.

Eye ointments containing a paraffin (e.g. liquid paraffin with white soft paraffin and wool alcohols p. 841) can be used in addition to other options to lubricate the eye surface, especially in cases of recurrent corneal epithelial erosion. They may cause temporary visual disturbance and are best suited for application before sleep. Ointments should not be used during contact lens wear. (A)

OCULAR LUBRICANTS

Acetylcysteine 01-Aug-2024

- **INDICATIONS AND DOSE**

Tear deficiency | Impaired or abnormal mucus production

▶ TO THE EYE
- Child: Apply 3–4 times a day

- **INTERACTIONS** → Appendix 1: acetylcysteine
- **SIDE-EFFECTS** Eye discomfort · eye redness
- **MEDICINAL FORMS** There can be variation in the licensing of different medicines containing the same drug. Forms available from special-order manufacturers include: eye drops

Eye drops

EXCIPIENTS: May contain Benzalkonium chloride, disodium edetate

- Ilube (Rayner Pharmaceuticals Ltd)
  Acetylcysteine 50 mg per 1 ml Ilube 5% eye drops | 10 ml [PoM] £80.95 DT = £80.95

Carbomers 09-Feb-2021

(Polyacrylic acid)

- **INDICATIONS AND DOSE**

Dry eyes including keratoconjunctivitis sicca, unstable tear film (using 0.2% preparation)

▶ TO THE EYE
- Child: Apply 3–4 times a day, alternatively apply as required

LIQUIVISC® 0.25% EYE GEL

Dry eye conditions

▶ TO THE EYE
- Child: Apply 1–4 times a day

- **PRESCRIBING AND DISPENSING INFORMATION** Synthetic high molecular weight polymers of acrylic acid cross-linked with either allyl ethers of sucrose or allyl ethers of pentaerithrityl.
- **MEDICINAL FORMS** There can be variation in the licensing of different medicines containing the same drug.

Eye gel

EXCIPIENTS: May contain Benzalkonium chloride, cetrimide, disodium edetate

- Liquivisc (Thea Pharmaceuticals Ltd)
  Carbomer 974P 2.5 mg per 1 gram Liquivisc 0.25% eye gel | 10 gram [P] £4.50 DT = £4.50

Eye drops

- GelTears (Bausch & Lomb UK Ltd)
  Carbomer 980 2 mg per 1 gram GelTears 0.2% gel | 10 gram [P] £2.80 DT = £2.80
- Viscotears (Bausch & Lomb UK Ltd)
  Carbomer 980 2 mg per 1 gram Viscotears 2mg/g liquid gel | 10 gram [P] £1.59 DT = £2.80
  Viscotears 2mg/g eye gel 0.6ml unit dose | 30 unit dose [P] £5.42 DT = £5.42

Carmellose sodium 04-Dec-2020

- **INDICATIONS AND DOSE**

Dry eye conditions

▶ TO THE EYE
- Child: Apply as required

- **PRESCRIBING AND DISPENSING INFORMATION** Some preparations are contained units which are resealable and may be used for up to 12 hours.
- **MEDICINAL FORMS** There can be variation in the licensing of different medicines containing the same drug.

Eye drops

- Carmellose sodium (Non-proprietary)
  Carmellose 0.5% eye drops | 10 ml £7.49
  Evolve Carmellose 0.5% eye drops preservative free | 10 ml £5.25
  VIZcellose 1% eye drops preservative free | 10 ml £1.85
  VIZcellose 0.5% eye drops preservative free | 10 ml £2.88
- AaqEye Carmellose (Essential-Healthcare Ltd)
  AaqEye Carmellose 0.5% eye drops | 10 ml £1.73
- Aqualube (TriOn Pharma Ltd)
  Aqualube 0.5% eye drops | 10 ml £1.68
  AquaLube PF 0.5% eye drops preservative free | 10 ml £2.79
  Aqualube Forte 1% eye drops | 10 ml £1.58
- Carmellose (Warneford Healthcare Ltd)
  PF Drops Carmellose 0.5% eye drops preservative free | 10 ml £7.49
  PF Drops Carmellose 1% eye drops preservative free | 10 ml £7.49
- Carmize (Aspire Pharma Ltd)
  Carmize 1% eye drops | 10 ml £8.49
  Carmize 0.5% eye drops | 10 ml £7.49
- Cellusan (Farmigea S.p.A.)
  Cellusan 1% eye drops preservative free | 10 ml £4.92
  Cellusan Light 0.5% eye drops preservative free | 10 ml £4.92
- Celluvisc (AbbVie Ltd)
  Celluvisc 1% eye drops 0.4ml unit dose | 30 unit dose [P] £3.00 DT = £3.00 | 60 unit dose [P] £10.99
  Carmellose sodium 5 mg per 1 ml Celluvisc 0.5% eye drops 0.4ml unit dose | 30 unit dose [P] £4.80 DT = £4.80 | 90 unit dose [P] £15.53
- Eyeaze (Ridge Pharma Ltd)
  Eyeaze Carmellose 1% eye drops preservative free | 10 ml £1.81
  Eyeaze Carmellose 0.5% eye drops preservative free | 10 ml £2.87
- Ocu-Lube Carmellose (Sai-Meds Ltd)
  Ocu-Lube Carmellose 0.5% eye drops preservative free | 10 ml £7.49
  Ocu-Lube Carmellose 1% eye drops preservative free | 10 ml £7.49
- Ocufresh Comfort (Blumont Healthcare Ltd)
  Ocufresh Comfort Carmellose 0.5% eye drops preservative free | 10 ml £2.29
- Ocufresh Comfort Plus (Blumont Healthcare Ltd)
  Ocufresh Comfort Plus 1% eye drops preservative free | 10 ml £1.70
- Optho-Lique (Essential-Healthcare Ltd)
  Optho-Lique 0.5% eye drops | 10 ml £3.73
  Optho-Lique Forte 1% eye drops | 10 ml £2.83
- Optive (Allergan Ltd)
  Optive 0.5% eye drops | 10 ml £7.49
- Optive Plus (Allergan Ltd)
  Optive Plus 0.5% eye drops | 10 ml £7.49
- Tearvis (Sai-Meds Ltd)
  Tearvis 1% eye drops | 10 ml £8.49
  Tearvis 0.5% eye drops | 10 ml £7.49
- VisuXL (Visufarma UK Ltd)
  VisuXL Gel eye drops preservative free | 10 ml £7.49

Hydroxypropyl guar with polyethylene glycol and propylene glycol 09-May-2024

- **DRUG ACTION** Formulated as an ocular lubricant
- **INDICATIONS AND DOSE**

Dry eye conditions

▶ TO THE EYE
- Child: Apply as required

- **MEDICINAL FORMS** No licensed medicines listed.

Hyetellose (Hydroxyethylcellulose) 10-Oct-2025

● **INDICATIONS AND DOSE**

Tear deficiency

▶ TO THE EYE

▸ Child: Apply as required

● **PRESCRIBING AND DISPENSING INFORMATION** Although multi-dose hyetellose eye drops commonly contain preservatives, preservative-free unit dose vials may be available.

● **MEDICINAL FORMS** There can be variation in the licensing of different medicines containing the same drug.

Eye drops

▸ **Artificial tears** (Bausch & Lomb UK Ltd)
Hydroxyethylcellulose 4.4 mg per 1 ml Minims artificial tears 0.44% eye drops 0.5ml unit dose | 20 unit dose [P] £9.33 DT = £9.33

Hypromellose 23-Mar-2020

● **INDICATIONS AND DOSE**

Tear deficiency

▶ TO THE EYE

▸ Child: Apply as required

● **PRESCRIBING AND DISPENSING INFORMATION** Although multi-dose hypromellose eye drops commonly contain preservatives, preservative-free unit dose vials may be available.

● **MEDICINAL FORMS** There can be variation in the licensing of different medicines containing the same drug. Forms available from special-order manufacturers include: eye drops

Eye drops

EXCIPIENTS: May contain Benzalkonium chloride, cetrimide, disodium edetate

▸ **Hypromellose (Non-proprietary)**
Hypromellose 3 mg per 1 ml Hypromellose 0.3% eye drops preservative free | 10 ml £5.75
Hypromellose 0.3% eye drops | 10 ml [P] £4.99

▸ **AacuLose** (TriOn Pharma Ltd)
Hypromellose 5 mg per 1 ml AacuLose Hypromellose 0.5% eye drops | 10 ml £0.92 DT = £0.00

▸ **AaproMel** (Essential-Healthcare Ltd)
Hypromellose 5 mg per 1 ml AaproMel 0.5% eye drops | 10 ml £0.90 DT = £0.00

▸ **AddTear** (TriOn Pharma Ltd)
Hypromellose 3 mg per 1 ml AddTear Hypromellose 0.3% eye drops preservative free | 10 ml £2.99
Hypromellose 5 mg per 1 ml AddTear Hypromellose 0.5% eye drops preservative free | 10 ml £3.69

▸ **Hydromoor** (Rayner Pharmaceuticals Ltd)
Hydromoor 0.3% eye drops 0.4ml unit dose preservative free | 30 unit dose £5.99

▸ **Hypromellose** (Warneford Healthcare Ltd)
Hypromellose 3 mg per 1 ml PF Drops Hypromellose 0.3% eye drops preservative free | 10 ml £5.75

▸ **Hypromol** (Ennogen Healthcare Ltd)
Hypromellose 3 mg per 1 ml Hypromol 0.3% eye drops preservative free | 10 ml £4.55

▸ **Ocu-Lube** (Sai-Meds Ltd)
Hypromellose 3 mg per 1 ml Ocu-Lube 0.3% eye drops preservative free | 10 ml £5.75

▸ **Ocufresh (Hypromellose)** (Blumont Healthcare Ltd)
Hypromellose 3 mg per 1 ml Ocufresh Hypromellose 0.3% eye drops preservative free | 10 ml £2.99

▸ **Puroptics** (Biovantic Pharma Ltd)
Hypromellose 5 mg per 1 ml Puroptics Hypromellose 0.5% eye drops | 10 ml £0.95 DT = £0.00

▸ **Tear-Lac** (Scope Ophthalmics Ltd)
Hypromellose 3 mg per 1 ml Tear-Lac Hypromellose 0.3% eye drops preservative free | 10 ml £5.80

▸ **Teardew** (Sai-Meds Ltd)
Hypromellose 5 mg per 1 ml Teardew 0.5% eye drops | 10 ml £1.17 DT = £0.00

Hypromellose with dextran 70 07-Apr-2020

The properties listed below are those particular to the combination only. For the properties of the components please consider, hypromellose above.

● **INDICATIONS AND DOSE**

Tear deficiency

▶ TO THE EYE

▸ Child: Apply as required

● **MEDICINAL FORMS** There can be variation in the licensing of different medicines containing the same drug.

Eye drops

EXCIPIENTS: May contain Benzalkonium chloride, disodium edetate

▸ **Tears Naturale II** (Alcon Eye Care UK Ltd)
Dextran 70 1 mg per 1 ml, Hypromellose 3 mg per 1 ml Tears Naturale II eye drops | 15 ml £2.81 DT = £0.00

Liquid paraffin with white soft paraffin and wool alcohols 26-Nov-2020

● **INDICATIONS AND DOSE**

Dry eye conditions

▶ TO THE EYE

▸ Child: Apply as required, best suited for application before sleep

● **PATIENT AND CARER ADVICE** May cause temporary visual disturbance. Should not be used during contact lens wear.

● **MEDICINAL FORMS** There can be variation in the licensing of different medicines containing the same drug.

Eye ointment

▸ **Liquid paraffin with white soft paraffin and wool alcohols (Non-proprietary)**
Xailin Night eye ointment preservative free | 5 gram £2.74

▸ **Lacrilube** (AbbVie Ltd)
Wool alcohols 2 mg per 1 gram, Liquid paraffin 425 mg per 1 gram, White soft paraffin 573 mg per 1 gram Lacrilube eye ointment preservative free | 3.5 gram £2.05

Polyvinyl alcohol 17-Apr-2020

● **INDICATIONS AND DOSE**

Tear deficiency

▶ TO THE EYE

▸ Child: Apply as required

● **PRESCRIBING AND DISPENSING INFORMATION** Although multi-dose polyvinyl alcohol eye drops commonly contain preservatives, preservative-free unit dose vials may be available.

● **MEDICINAL FORMS** There can be variation in the licensing of different medicines containing the same drug. Forms available from special-order manufacturers include: eye drops

Eye drops

EXCIPIENTS: May contain Benzalkonium chloride, disodium edetate

▸ **Liquifilm Tears** (Allergan Ltd)
Polyvinyl alcohol 14 mg per 1 ml Liquifilm Tears 1.4% eye drops | 15 ml £1.93
Liquifilm Tears 1.4% eye drops 0.4ml unit dose preservative free | 30 unit dose £5.35

Retinol palmitate with white soft paraffin, light liquid paraffin, liquid paraffin and wool fat

09-May-2024

● **DRUG ACTION** Formulated as an ocular lubricant

● **INDICATIONS AND DOSE**

Dry eye conditions

▶ TO THE EYE

▶ Child: Apply as required

● **MEDICINAL FORMS** There can be variation in the licensing of different medicines containing the same drug.

Eye ointment

▶ **Hylo Night** (Scope Ophthalmics Ltd)
Hylo Night eye ointment preservative free | 5 gram £2.75

Sodium chloride

26-Feb-2026

● **INDICATIONS AND DOSE**

Tear deficiency | Ocular lubricants and astringents | Irrigation, including first-aid removal of harmful substances | Intra-ocular or topical irrigation during surgical procedures

▶ TO THE EYE

▶ Child: Apply as required, use 0.9% eye preparations

● **PRESCRIBING AND DISPENSING INFORMATION** Although multi-dose sodium chloride eye drops commonly contain preservatives, preservative-free unit dose vials may be available.

● **MEDICINAL FORMS** There can be variation in the licensing of different medicines containing the same drug. Forms available from special-order manufacturers include: eye drops, eye ointment

Eye drops

▶ **Sodium chloride (Non-proprietary)**
Sodium chloride 50 mg per 1 ml Sodium chloride 5% eye drops | 10 ml £25.25

▶ **AabChlor** (TriOn Pharma Ltd)
Sodium chloride 50 mg per 1 ml AabChlor Sodium Chloride 5% eye drops | 10 ml £7.93

▶ **AacEdem** (Essential-Healthcare Ltd)
Sodium chloride 50 mg per 1 ml AacEdem Sodium Chloride 5% eye drops | 10 ml £7.89

▶ **AcuSal** (Essential-Healthcare Ltd)
Sodium chloride 50 mg per 1 ml AcuSal 5% eye drops preservative free | 10 ml £7.29 DT = £0.00

▶ **Aeon Sodium Chloride** (Rayner Pharmaceuticals Ltd)
Sodium chloride 50 mg per 1 ml Aeon 5% eye drops preservative free | 10 ml £23.00 DT = £0.00

▶ **DROPtonic** (Kestrel Ophthalmics Ltd)
Sodium chloride 50 mg per 1 ml DROPtonic 5% eye drops preservative free | 10 ml £9.90 DT = £0.00

▶ **Hypersal** (Ennogen Healthcare Ltd)
Sodium chloride 50 mg per 1 ml Hypersal 5% eye drops | 10 ml £25.25

▶ **Natklor** (Blumont Healthcare Ltd)
Sodium chloride 50 mg per 1 ml Natklor 5% eye drops preservative free | 10 ml £7.99 DT = £0.00

▶ **ODM5** (Kestrel Ophthalmics Ltd)
Sodium chloride 50 mg per 1 ml ODM5 5% eye drops preservative free | 10 ml £24.00 DT = £0.00

▶ **Saline** (Bausch & Lomb UK Ltd)
Sodium chloride 9 mg per 1 ml Minims saline 0.9% eye drops 0.5ml unit dose | 20 unit dose Ⓟ £7.73 DT = £7.73

▶ **SodiEye** (TriOn Pharma Ltd)
SodiEye 5% eye drops 0.5ml unit dose preservative free | 20 unit dose £14.95
Sodium chloride 50 mg per 1 ml SodiEye 5% eye drops preservative free | 10 ml £15.98 DT = £0.00

▶ **Sodium chloride** (Essential Pharmaceuticals Ltd, Warneford Healthcare Ltd)
Sodium chloride 50 mg per 1 ml NaCl 5% eye drops 0.45ml unit dose preservative free | 20 unit dose £14.95
PF Drops Sodium Chloride 5% eye drops preservative free | 10 ml £25.20 DT = £0.00

Eye ointment

▶ **Sodium chloride (Non-proprietary)**
Sodium chloride 50 mg per 1 ml Sodium chloride 5% eye ointment preservative free | 5 gram £22.50

▶ **SodiEye** (TriOn Pharma Ltd)
SodiEye 6% eye ointment preservative free | 5 gram £18.92

Sodium hyaluronate

04-Dec-2020

● **INDICATIONS AND DOSE**

Dry eye conditions

▶ TO THE EYE

▶ Child: Apply as required

● **PRESCRIBING AND DISPENSING INFORMATION** Some preparations are contained in units which are resealable and may be used for up to 12 hours.

Although multi-dose sodium hyaluronate eye drops commonly contain preservatives, preservative-free unit dose vials may be available.

● **MEDICINAL FORMS** There can be variation in the licensing of different medicines containing the same drug.

Eye drops

▶ **Sodium hyaluronate (Non-proprietary)**
VIZhyal 0.4% eye drops preservative free | 10 ml £4.10
PF Drops Sodium Hyaluronate 0.4% eye drops preservative free | 10 ml £6.99
Kent Pharma Sodium Hyaluronate 0.2% eye drops preservative free | 10 ml £3.40
VIZhyal 0.1% eye drops preservative free | 10 ml £4.10
iGel 0.2% eye drops preservative free | 10 ml £4.80
PF Drops Sodium Hyaluronate 0.15% eye drops preservative free | 10 ml £6.99

▶ **Aactive HA** (TriOn Pharma Ltd)
Aactive HA 0.2% eye drops | 10 ml £3.36
Aactive HA PF 0.1% eye drops 0.4ml unit dose preservative free | 20 unit dose £3.99
Aactive HA PF 0.1% eye drops preservative free | 10 ml £3.99
Aactive HA 0.1% eye drops | 10 ml £3.93
Aactive HA PF 0.2% eye drops preservative free | 10 ml £3.46

▶ **AaqEye HA** (Essential-Healthcare Ltd)
AaqEye HA 0.2% eye drops | 10 ml £3.43
AaqEye HA 0.1% eye drops | 10 ml £3.91

▶ **Aeon Protect Plus** (Rayner Pharmaceuticals Ltd)
Aeon Protect Plus 0.3% eye drops preservative free | 10 ml £7.80

▶ **Aeon Repair** (Rayner Pharmaceuticals Ltd)
Aeon Repair 0.15% eye drops preservative free | 10 ml £4.00

▶ **Artelac Rebalance** (Bausch & Lomb UK Ltd)
Artelac Rebalance 0.15% eye drops | 10 ml £4.00

▶ **Blink Intensive** (AMO UK Ltd)
Blink Intensive Tears 0.2% eye drops 0.4ml unit dose | 20 unit dose £2.97
Blink Intensive Tears 0.2% eye drops | 10 ml £2.97

▶ **ClinOptic HA** (Warneford Healthcare Ltd)
ClinOptic HA 0.4% eye drops preservative free | 10 ml £4.15
ClinOptic HA 0.21% eye drops preservative free | 10 ml £4.15
ClinOptic HA 0.1% eye drops preservative free | 10 ml £4.15

▶ **Clinitas** (Altacor Ltd)
Clinitas Multi 0.4% eye drops preservative free | 10 ml £6.99
Clinitas 0.2% eye drops 0.5ml unit dose preservative free | 30 unit dose £5.59
Clinitas Multi 0.2% eye drops preservative free | 10 ml £5.99
Clinitas 0.4% eye drops 0.5ml unit dose preservative free | 30 unit dose £5.70

▶ **Evolve HA** (Medicom Healthcare Ltd)
Evolve HA 0.2% eye drops preservative free | 10 ml £6.05

▶ **Eyeaze** (Ridge Pharma Ltd)
Eyeaze 0.1% eye drops preservative free | 10 ml £4.05
Eyeaze 0.2% eye drops preservative free | 10 ml £4.05
Eyeaze 0.4% eye drops preservative free | 10 ml £4.05

▶ **Eyeaze Lyte** (Ridge Pharma Ltd)
Eyeaze Lyte 0.3% eye drops preservative free | 10 ml £3.89

Eyeaze Lyte 0.2% eye drops preservative free | 10 ml £3.89
Eyeaze Lyte 0.1% eye drops preservative free | 10 ml £3.89

- **Eyezin (sodium hyaluronate)** (Warneford Healthcare Ltd)
  Eyezin XL 0.4% eye drops preservative free | 10 ml £6.99
- **Hy-Opti** (Alissa Healthcare Research Ltd)
  Hy-Opti 0.1% eye drops preservative free | 12 ml £4.78
  Hy-Opti 0.2% eye drops preservative free | 12 ml £4.78
- **Hyabak** (Thea Pharmaceuticals Ltd)
  Hyabak 0.15% eye drops preservative free | 10 ml £7.99
- **Hycosan** (Scope Ophthalmics Ltd)
  Hycosan Extra 0.2% eye drops | 7.5 ml [X]
  Hycosan 0.1% eye drops | 7.5 ml [X]
- **HydraMed** (Farmigea S.p.A.)
  HydraMed Forte 0.4% eye drops 0.5ml unit dose preservative free | 30 unit dose £5.74
  HydraMed 0.2% eye drops preservative free | 10 ml £5.74
  HydraMed Forte 0.4% eye drops preservative free | 10 ml £5.74
  HydraMed 0.2% eye drops 0.5ml unit dose preservative free | 30 unit dose £5.74
- **Hylo Comod** (Ursapharm Arzneimittel GmbH)
  Hylo Comod 0.1% eye drops | 10 ml [X]
- **Hylo-Comod** (Scope Ophthalmics Ltd)
  Hylo-Tear 0.1% eye drops preservative free | 10 ml £8.50
  Hylo-Forte 0.2% eye drops preservative free | 10 ml £9.50
- **Hylo-fresh** (Scope Ophthalmics Ltd)
  Hylo-Fresh 0.03% eye drops preservative free | 10 ml £4.95
- **Ocu-Lube HA** (Sai-Meds Ltd)
  Ocu-Lube HA 0.1% eye drops preservative free | 10 ml £8.00
  Ocu-Lube HA 0.2% eye drops preservative free | 10 ml £7.90
- **Ocufresh Everyday** (Blumont Healthcare Ltd)
  Ocufresh Everyday 0.2% eye drops 0.5ml unit dose preservative free | 30 unit dose £4.70
  Ocufresh Everyday 0.2% eye drops preservative free | 10 ml £3.49
- **Ocufresh Intense Relief** (Blumont Healthcare Ltd)
  Ocufresh Intense Relief 0.4% eye drops preservative free | 10 ml £3.80
  Ocufresh Intense Relief 0.4% eye drops 0.5ml unit dose preservative free | 30 unit dose £4.80
- **Ocusan** (Agepha Pharma s.r.o.)
  Ocusan 0.2% eye drops 0.5ml unit dose | 20 unit dose £5.77
- **Oftaox** (Kestrel Ophthalmics Ltd)
  Oftaox 0.25% eye drops | 8 ml £5.50
- **Optive Fusion** (Allergan Ltd)
  Optive Fusion 0.1% eye drops | 10 ml £7.49
- **Oxya** (Bausch & Lomb UK Ltd)
  Oxya 0.15% eye drops | 10 ml £4.15
- **VIZhyal** (East Midlands Pharma Ltd)
  VIZhyal 0.2% eye drops preservative free | 10 ml £4.10
- **Viscotears HA** (Bausch & Lomb UK Ltd)
  Viscotears HA 0.1% eye drops preservative free | 10 ml £5.10
- **Vismed** (TRB Chemidica (UK) Ltd)
  Vismed Gel Multi 0.3% eye drops preservative free | 10 ml £8.44
  Vismed Multi 0.18% eye drops preservative free | 10 ml £7.23
  Vismed 0.18% eye drops 0.3ml unit dose preservative free | 20 unit dose £5.42
- **VisuXL** (Visufarma UK Ltd)
  VisuXL eye drops preservative free | 10 ml £10.30
- **Xailin HA** (Visufarma UK Ltd)
  Xailin HA 0.2% eye drops | 10 ml £7.85
- **Xailin Intense** (Visufarma UK Ltd)
  Xailin Intense HA 0.3% eye drops preservative free | 10 ml £6.10
- **Xai in Plus** (Visufarma UK Ltd)
  Xai in Plus HA 0.2% eye drops preservative free | 10 ml £4.15
- **Xailin Tears** (Visufarma UK Ltd)
  Xailin Tears HA 0.1% eye drops preservative free | 10 ml £4.15

Eye gel

- **Vismed** (TRB Chemidica (UK) Ltd)
  Vismed Gel 0.3% eye gel 0.45ml unit dose preservative free | 20 unit dose £6.35

Sodium hyaluronate with trehalose

28-Feb-2025

● **INDICATIONS AND DOSE**

Dry eye conditions

▶ TO THE EYE
- Child: Apply as required

● **PRESCRIBING AND DISPENSING INFORMATION** Sodium hyaluronate and trehalose preparations do not contain preservatives; multi-dose preparation can be used for up to 3–6 months—consult product literature.

Preparations may contain additional active ingredients—consult product literature.

● **MEDICINAL FORMS** There can be variation in the licensing of different medicines containing the same drug.

Eye drops

- **Eyeaze Pro** (Ridge Pharma Ltd)
  Eyeaze Pro eye drops preservative free | 10 ml £5.99
- **Thealoz Duo** (Thea Pharmaceuticals Ltd)
  Thealoz Duo eye drops preservative free | 10 ml £8.99
- **Trehapan** (Visufarma UK Ltd)
  Trehapan eye drops preservative free | 10 ml £5.99
- **Viscotears Tri Action** (Bausch & Lomb UK Ltd)
  Viscotears Tri Action eye drops preservative free | 10 ml £8.99

11 Eye

Yellow soft paraffin

10-Oct-2025

● **INDICATIONS AND DOSE**

Eye surface lubrication

▶ TO THE EYE
- Child: Apply as required

● **PATIENT AND CARER ADVICE** Ophthalmic preparations may cause temporary visual disturbance. Should not be used during contact lens wear.

● **MEDICINAL FORMS** There can be variation in the licensing of different medicines containing the same drug.

Eye ointment

- **Yellow soft paraffin (Non-proprietary)**
  Liquid paraffin 100 mg per 1 gram, Wool fat 100 mg per 1 gram, Yellow soft paraffin 800 mg per 1 gram Simple eye ointment | 4 gram [P] £99.84 DT = £99.84

3 Eye infections

Eye, infections

07-Jun-2020

Overview

Most acute superficial eye infections can be treated topically with eye drops or ointment. Blepharitis is often caused by staphylococci. Bacterial conjunctivitis is commonly caused by *Streptococcus pneumoniae*, *Staphylococcus aureus*, or *Haemophilus influenzae*. Keratitis may be bacterial, viral, or fungal; it can also be caused by Acanthamoeba (parasite). Endophthalmitis is usually either bacterial or fungal; it can also be non-infective (retention of foreign material).

[EvGr] Anterior bacterial blepharitis is treated by application of an antibacterial eye ointment (such as chloramphenicol p. 846) to the conjunctival sac or rubbed into the lid margins, if blepharitis is not controlled by eyelid hygiene alone. Systemic treatment (e.g. tetracyclines in patients over 12 years of age) may be required in patients with posterior blepharitis. Treatments can be intermittently stopped and restarted, based on the severity of the blepharitis and drug tolerance. (A)

Most cases of acute bacterial conjunctivitis are self-limiting and resolve within 5–7 days without treatment. [EvGr] In severe infection or where rapid resolution is required, treatment with antibacterial eye drops or ointments are used. Ongoing symptoms despite treatment may indicate viral conjunctivitis or the need for a different antibacterial; cultures or referral to a specialist may be required.

Corneal ulcer and keratitis require specialist treatment and may call for hospital admission for intensive therapy.

Endophthalmitis is a medical emergency which also calls for specialist management and may require treatment with antibacterial drugs and steroids. Surgical intervention, such as vitrectomy, is sometimes indicated. Ⓐ

Trachoma which results from chronic infection with *Chlamydia trachomatis* can be treated with azithromycin p. 845 by mouth [unlicensed indication] as recommended by the World Health Organisation.

For information on the management of ocular herpes, see Herpesvirus infections p. 498.

Fungal infections of the cornea (e.g. fungal keratitis) are rare but can occur particularly in agricultural areas and tropical climates. Antifungal preparations for the eye are not generally available. For information about supply of preparations not commercially available, contact the local Clinical Commissioning Group (CCG), or equivalent in Scotland, Wales, or Northern Ireland, or the nearest hospital ophthalmology unit, or Moorfields Eye Hospital, 162 City Road, London EC1V 2PD (tel. (020) 7253 3411) or www.moorfields.nhs.uk

Eye infections in neonates

EvGr All cases of acute bacterial conjunctivitis in neonates (ophthalmia neonatorum) must be urgently referred (same day) to an ophthalmologist to prevent serious systemic and local complications; the ongoing management usually involves input from a paediatric specialist. Where possible, the causative micro-organism should be identified. Ⓐ

Chlamydial infection is one of the most frequent causes of ophthalmia neonatorum. Azithromycin eye drops are licensed for the treatment of trachomatous conjunctivitis caused by *Chlamydia trachomatis* and purulent bacterial conjunctivitis in neonates. EvGr However, as there is a risk of simultaneous infection, such as pneumonia, in neonates and children aged under 3 months presenting with conjunctivitis caused by *Chlamydia trachomatis*, systemic treatment with oral erythromycin p. 406 is required. Ⓐ Ophthalmia neonatorum can also be caused by gonococcal, viral and other bacterial infections.

3.1 Bacterial eye infection

ANTIBACTERIALS › AMINOGLYCOSIDES

Gentamicin

▸377 20-Jun-2025

● **INDICATIONS AND DOSE**

Bacterial eye infections

▶ TO THE EYE

▸ Child: Apply 1 drop at least every 2 hours in severe infection, reduce frequency as infection is controlled and continue for 48 hours after healing, frequency of eye drops depends on the severity of the infection and the potential for irreversible ocular damage; for less severe infection 3–4 times daily is generally sufficient

● **UNLICENSED USE** Gentamicin doses in BNF Publications may differ from those in product literature.

IMPORTANT SAFETY INFORMATION

MHRA/CHM ADVICE: AMINOGLYCOSIDES (GENTAMICIN, AMIKACIN, TOBRAMYCIN, AND NEOMYCIN): INCREASED RISK OF DEAFNESS IN PATIENTS WITH MITOCHONDRIAL MUTATIONS (JANUARY 2021)

The use of aminoglycosides is associated with rare cases of ototoxicity. A safety review found an increased risk of deafness in patients with mitochondrial mutations (particularly the m.1555A>G mutation), including cases where the patient's aminoglycoside serum levels were within the recommended range. Nevertheless, these mitochondrial mutations are considered rare and penetrance is uncertain. No cases were identified with topical preparations but, based on a shared mechanism of effect, there is a potential risk with gentamicin and other aminoglycosides administered at the site of toxicity i.e. the ear.

Healthcare professionals are advised to consider the need for aminoglycoside treatment versus alternative options in patients with susceptible mutations. The need for genetic testing especially in those requiring recurrent or long-term treatment with aminoglycosides should also be considered, however, urgent treatment should not be delayed. To minimise the risks of adverse effects, continuous monitoring of renal and auditory function, as well as hepatic and laboratory parameters, is recommended for all patients. Those with known mitochondrial mutations or a family history of ototoxicity are advised to inform their doctor or pharmacist before using an aminoglycoside.

● **INTERACTIONS** → Appendix 1: aminoglycosides

● **SIDE-EFFECTS** Since systemic absorption can follow topical administration to the eye and ear, also consider the side-effects of systemic aminoglycosides.

● **PRE-TREATMENT SCREENING** NHS England commissions genetic testing under the *National genomic test directory* indication: R65 - Aminoglycoside exposure posing risk to hearing. The testing criteria is significant exposure to aminoglycosides posing risk of ototoxicity. This testing is relevant to individuals with a predisposition to gram-negative infections or with hearing loss who have been exposed to aminoglycosides. For further information, see www.england.nhs.uk/publication/national-genomic-test-directories/.

● **PRESCRIBING AND DISPENSING INFORMATION** Eye drops may be sourced as a manufactured special or from specialist importing companies.

● **MEDICINAL FORMS** There can be variation in the licensing of different medicines containing the same drug. Forms available from special-order manufacturers include: eye drops

Eye drops

EXCIPIENTS: May contain Benzalkonium chloride

Ear/eye drops solution

EXCIPIENTS: May contain Benzalkonium chloride

▸ **Gentamicin (Non-proprietary)**

Gentamicin (as Gentamicin sulfate) 3 mg per 1 ml Gentamicin 0.3% ear/eye drops | 10 ml PoM £21.92 DT = £23.84

Tobramycin

▸377 20-Jun-2025

● **INDICATIONS AND DOSE**

Local treatment of infections

▶ TO THE EYE

▸ Child 1–17 years: Apply twice daily for 6–8 days

Local treatment of infections (severe infection)

▶ TO THE EYE

▸ Child 1–17 years: Apply 4 times a day for first day, then apply twice daily for 5–7 days

IMPORTANT SAFETY INFORMATION

MHRA/CHM ADVICE: AMINOGLYCOSIDES (GENTAMICIN, AMIKACIN, TOBRAMYCIN, AND NEOMYCIN): INCREASED RISK OF DEAFNESS IN PATIENTS WITH MITOCHONDRIAL MUTATIONS (JANUARY 2021)

The use of aminoglycosides is associated with rare cases of ototoxicity. A safety review found an increased risk of deafness in patients with mitochondrial mutations (particularly the m.1555A>G mutation), including cases where the patient's aminoglycoside serum levels were within the recommended range. Nevertheless, these mitochondrial mutations are considered rare and penetrance is uncertain. No cases were identified with topical preparations but, based on a shared mechanism of effect, there is a potential risk with aminoglycosides administered at the site of toxicity i.e. the ear.

Healthcare professionals are advised to consider the need for aminoglycoside treatment versus alternative options in patients with susceptible mutations. The need for genetic testing especially in those requiring recurrent or long-term treatment with aminoglycosides should also be considered, however, urgent treatment should not be delayed. To minimise the risks of adverse effects, continuous monitoring of renal and auditory function, as well as hepatic and laboratory parameters, is recommended for all patients. Those with known mitochondrial mutations or a family history of ototoxicity are advised to inform their doctor or pharmacist before using an aminoglycoside.

- **INTERACTIONS** → Appendix 1: aminoglycosides
- **PRE-TREATMENT SCREENING** NHS England commissions genetic testing under the *National genomic test directory* indication: R65 - Aminoglycoside exposure posing risk to hearing. The testing criteria is significant exposure to aminoglycosides posing risk of ototoxicity. This testing is relevant to individuals with a predisposition to gram-negative infections or with hearing loss who have been exposed to aminoglycosides. For further information, see www.england.nhs.uk/publication/national-genomic-test-directories/.

- **MEDICINAL FORMS** No licensed medicines listed.

ANTIBACTERIALS > CEPHALOSPORINS, SECOND-GENERATION

F 384

Cefuroxime

26-Nov-2025

- **INDICATIONS AND DOSE**

Gonococcal conjunctivitis [adjunctive treatment, using 5% eye drops]

▶ TO THE EYE

▸ Child 12–17 years (body-weight 45 kg and above): Apply every 1 hour day and night for 48 hours, then apply every 1 hour daytime only for 5 days, then apply 4 times a day until complete resolution

- **UNLICENSED USE** EvGr Cefuroxime is used for the treatment of gonococcal conjunctivitis, ⟨A⟩ but is not licensed for this indication.
- **INTERACTIONS** → Appendix 1: cephalosporins
- **SIDE-EFFECTS**

▶ **Common or very common** Increased risk of infection

▶ **Frequency not known** Drug fever

- **MEDICINAL FORMS** There can be variation in the licensing of different medicines containing the same drug. Forms available from special-order manufacturers include: eye drops

ANTIBACTERIALS > MACROLIDES

F 402

Azithromycin

26-Nov-2025

- **INDICATIONS AND DOSE**

Gonococcal conjunctivitis [adjunctive treatment]

▶ TO THE EYE

▸ Child 12–17 years (body-weight 45 kg and above): Apply every 1 hour day and night for 48 hours, then apply every 1 hour daytime only for 5 days, then apply 4 times a day until complete resolution

Trachomatous conjunctivitis caused by *Chlamydia trachomatis* | Purulent bacterial conjunctivitis

▶ TO THE EYE

▸ Child: Apply twice daily for 3 days, review if no improvement after 3 days of treatment

- **UNLICENSED USE** EvGr Azithromycin is used for the treatment of gonococcal conjunctivitis, ⟨A⟩ but is not licensed for this indication.
- **INTERACTIONS** → Appendix 1: macrolides
- **SIDE-EFFECTS**

▶ **Common or very common** Eye discomfort

▶ **Uncommon** Eye allergy

- **MEDICINAL FORMS** There can be variation in the licensing of different medicines containing the same drug.

Eye drops

▸ **Azyter** (Thea Pharmaceuticals Ltd)

Azithromycin dihydrate 15 mg per 1 gram Azyter 15mg/g eye drops 0.25g unit dose | 6 unit dose PoM £6.99 DT = £6.99

ANTIBACTERIALS > QUINOLONES

F 428

Ciprofloxacin

26-Nov-2025

- **INDICATIONS AND DOSE**

Superficial bacterial eye infection

▶ TO THE EYE USING EYE DROP

▸ Child: Apply 4 times a day for maximum duration of treatment 21 days

▶ TO THE EYE USING EYE OINTMENT

▸ Child 1–17 years: Apply 1.25 centimetres 3 times a day for 2 days, then apply 1.25 centimetres twice daily for 5 days

Superficial bacterial eye infection (severe infection)

▶ TO THE EYE USING EYE DROP

▸ Child: Apply every 2 hours during waking hours for 2 days, then apply 4 times a day for maximum duration of treatment 21 days

Corneal ulcer

▶ TO THE EYE USING EYE DROP

▸ Child: Apply every 15 minutes for 6 hours, then apply every 30 minutes for the remainder of day 1, then apply every 1 hour on day 2, then apply every 4 hours on days 3–14, maximum duration of treatment 21 days, to be administered throughout the day and night

▶ TO THE EYE USING EYE OINTMENT

▸ Child 1–17 years: Apply 1.25 centimetres every 1–2 hours for 2 days, then apply 1.25 centimetres every 4 hours for the next 12 days, to be administered throughout the day and night

- **INTERACTIONS** → Appendix 1: quinolones
- **SIDE-EFFECTS**

▶ **Common or very common** Corneal deposits (reversible after completion of treatment)

▶ **Rare or very rare** Ear pain · increased risk of infection · paranasal sinus hypersecretion

- **PREGNANCY** Manufacturer advises use only if potential benefit outweighs risk.
- **BREAST FEEDING** Manufacturer advises caution.

- **MEDICINAL FORMS** There can be variation in the licensing of different medicines containing the same drug. Forms available from special-order manufacturers include: eye drops, eye ointment

Eye drops

EXCIPIENTS: May contain Benzalkonium chloride

▸ **Ciloxan** (Novartis Pharmaceuticals UK Ltd)

Ciprofloxacin (as Ciprofloxacin hydrochloride) 3 mg per 1 ml Ciloxan 0.3% eye drops | 5 ml PoM £4.70 DT = £4.70

428

Levofloxacin
15-Jul-2021

● **INDICATIONS AND DOSE**

Local treatment of eye infections

▶ TO THE EYE

▸ Child 1–17 years: Apply every 2 hours for first 2 days, to be applied maximum 8 times a day, then apply 4 times a day for 3 days

● **INTERACTIONS** → Appendix 1: quinolones

● **SIDE-EFFECTS**

▶ **Uncommon** Rhinitis

▶ **Rare or very rare** Laryngeal oedema

● **PREGNANCY** Manufacturer advises use only if potential benefit outweighs risk.

● **BREAST FEEDING** Manufacturer advises use only if potential benefit outweighs risk.

● **PRESCRIBING AND DISPENSING INFORMATION** Although multi-dose levofloxacin eye drops commonly contain preservatives, preservative-free unit dose vials may be available.

● **MEDICINAL FORMS** There can be variation in the licensing of different medicines containing the same drug.

Eye drops

EXCIPIENTS: May contain Benzalkonium chloride

▸ Levofloxacin (Non-proprietary)

Levofloxacin (as Levofloxacin hemihydrate) 5 mg per 1 ml Levofloxacin 5mg/ml eye drops | 5 ml PoM £9.28 DT = £9.76 | 5 ml PoM £10.66 DT = £9.76 (Hospital only)

▸ Eyflox (Aspire Pharma Ltd)

Levofloxacin (as Levofloxacin hemihydrate) 5 mg per 1 ml Eyflox 5mg/ml eye drops | 5 ml PoM £13.46 DT = £13.46

▸ Oftaquix (Santen UK Ltd)

Levofloxacin (as Levofloxacin hemihydrate) 5 mg per 1 ml Oftaquix 5mg/ml eye drops 0.3ml unit dose | 30 unit dose PoM £17.95 DT = £17.95

Oftaquix 5mg/ml eye drops | 5 ml PoM £6.95 DT = £9.76

▸ Oxalux (Kestrel Ophthalmics Ltd)

Levofloxacin (as Levofloxacin hemihydrate) 5 mg per 1 ml Oxalux 5mg/ml eye drops 0.5ml unit dose | 20 unit dose PoM £15.25 DT = £15.25

428

Moxifloxacin
17-Apr-2020

● **INDICATIONS AND DOSE**

Local treatment of infections

▶ TO THE EYE

▸ Child: Apply 3 times a day continue treatment for 2–3 days after infection improves; review if no improvement within 5 days

● **CAUTIONS** Not recommended for neonates

● **INTERACTIONS** → Appendix 1: quinolones

● **SIDE-EFFECTS**

▶ **Uncommon** Conjunctival haemorrhage

▶ **Rare or very rare** Laryngeal pain · nasal discomfort

▶ **Frequency not known** Corneal deposits

● **MEDICINAL FORMS** There can be variation in the licensing of different medicines containing the same drug.

Eye drops

▸ Moxifloxacin (Non-proprietary)

Moxifloxacin (as Moxifloxacin hydrochloride) 5 mg per 1 ml Moxifloxacin 0.5% eye drops | 5 ml PoM £8.99–£9.80 DT = £9.80

▸ Moxivig (Novartis Pharmaceuticals UK Ltd)

Moxifloxacin (as Moxifloxacin hydrochloride) 5 mg per 1 ml Moxivig 0.5% eye drops | 5 ml PoM £9.80 DT = £9.80

428

Ofloxacin
26-Nov-2025

● **INDICATIONS AND DOSE**

Local treatment of infections

▶ TO THE EYE

▸ Child 1–17 years: Apply every 2–4 hours for the first 2 days, then reduced to 4 times a day for maximum 10 days treatment

● **CAUTIONS** Corneal ulcer (risk of corneal perforation) · epithelial defect (risk of corneal perforation)

● **INTERACTIONS** → Appendix 1: quinolones

● **SIDE-EFFECTS** Face oedema · oropharyngeal swelling · tongue swelling

● **PREGNANCY** Manufacturer advises use only if benefit outweighs risk (systemic quinolones have caused arthropathy in *animal* studies).

● **BREAST FEEDING** Manufacturer advises avoid.

● **MEDICINAL FORMS** There can be variation in the licensing of different medicines containing the same drug.

Eye drops

EXCIPIENTS: May contain Benzalkonium chloride

▸ Exocin (AbbVie Ltd)

Ofloxacin 3 mg per 1 ml Exocin 0.3% eye drops | 5 ml PoM £2.17 DT = £2.17

ANTIBACTERIALS › OTHER

Chloramphenicol
24-Jul-2024

● **DRUG ACTION** Chloramphenicol is a potent broad-spectrum antibiotic.

● **INDICATIONS AND DOSE**

Superficial eye infections

▶ TO THE EYE USING EYE DROP

▸ Child: Apply 1 drop every 2 hours, reduce frequency as infection is controlled and continue for 48 hours after healing, frequency is dependent on the severity of the infection. For less severe infection 3–4 times daily is generally sufficient

▶ TO THE EYE USING EYE OINTMENT

▸ Child: Apply once daily, to be applied at night, once daily dosing to be used if eye drops are used during the day, alternatively apply 3–4 times a day, multiple daily dosing to be used if ointment is used alone

IMPORTANT SAFETY INFORMATION

MHRA/CHM ADVICE: CHLORAMPHENICOL EYE DROPS CONTAINING BORAX OR BORIC ACID BUFFERS: USE IN CHILDREN YOUNGER THAN 2 YEARS (JULY 2021)

Some licences for chloramphenicol eye drops containing borax or boric acid buffers were updated to restrict use in children younger than 2 years of age to reflect warnings on maximum daily limits for boron exposure. The MHRA has reviewed the available evidence and consulted independent expert advice and has concluded that the benefits of chloramphenicol eye drops containing borax or boric acid outweigh the potential risks, as the potential exposure from topical application to both eyes, in children aged 0 to 2 years old, was well below the safety limit. Healthcare professionals should advise parents and carers that these products can be safely used in children younger than 2 years as advised by a doctor or other prescriber.

● **INTERACTIONS** → Appendix 1: chloramphenicol

● **SIDE-EFFECTS** Angioedema · bone marrow disorders · eye stinging · fever · paraesthesia · skin reactions

- **PREGNANCY** Avoid unless essential—no information on *topical* use but risk of 'neonatal grey-baby syndrome' with *oral* use in third trimester.
- **BREAST FEEDING** Avoid unless essential— *theoretical* risk of bone-marrow toxicity.
- **PRESCRIBING AND DISPENSING INFORMATION** Although multi-dose chloramphenicol eye drops commonly contain preservatives, preservative-free unit dose vials may be available.
- **PATIENT AND CARER ADVICE**
Medicines for Children leaflet: Chloramphenicol for eye infections www.medicinesforchildren.org.uk/medicines/chloramphenicol-for-eye-infections/
- **EXCEPTIONS TO LEGAL CATEGORY** Chloramphenicol 0.5% eye drops (in max. pack size 10 mL) and 1% eye ointment (in max. pack size 4 g) can be sold to the public for treatment of acute bacterial conjunctivitis in adults and children over 2 years; max. duration of treatment 5 days.

- **MEDICINAL FORMS** There can be variation in the licensing of different medicines containing the same drug.

Eye drops
EXCIPIENTS: May contain Phenylmercuric acetate
- Chloramphenicol (Non-proprietary)
Chloramphenicol 5 mg per 1 ml Minims chloramphenicol 0.5% eye drops 0.5ml unit dose | 20 unit dose [PoM] £11.89 DT = £11.89
Chloramphenicol 0.5% eye drops | 10 ml [PoM] £4.00 DT = £1.48
- Eykappo (Aspire Pharma Ltd)
Chloramphenicol 5 mg per 1 ml Eykappo 5mg/ml eye drops | 10 ml [PoM] £10.12 DT = £10.12

Eye ointment
- Chloramphenicol (Non-proprietary)
Chloramphenicol 10 mg per 1 gram Chloramphenicol 1% eye ointment | 4 gram [PoM] £5.00 DT = £2.49

Fusidic acid
05-Oct-2021

- **DRUG ACTION** Fusidic acid and its salts are narrow-spectrum antibiotics used for staphylococcal infections.

- **INDICATIONS AND DOSE**

Staphylococcal eye infections
- TO THE EYE
- Child: Apply twice daily

- **INTERACTIONS** → Appendix 1: fusidate
- **SIDE-EFFECTS**
- **Common or very common** Dry eye · eye discomfort · vision blurred
- **Uncommon** Crying on application · skin reactions · watering eye
- **Frequency not known** Angioedema · eye inflammation

- **MEDICINAL FORMS** There can be variation in the licensing of different medicines containing the same drug.

Modified-release drops
EXCIPIENTS: May contain Benzalkonium chloride, disodium edetate
- Fusidic acid (Non-proprietary)
Fusidic acid 10 mg per 1 gram Fusidic acid 1% modified-release eye drops | 5 gram [PoM] £67.80 DT = £36.08

ANTIPROTOZOALS

Propamidine isetionate

- **INDICATIONS AND DOSE**

***Acanthamoeba keratitis* infections (specialist use only) | Local treatment of eye infections**
- TO THE EYE USING EYE OINTMENT
- Child: Apply 1–2 times a day
- TO THE EYE USING EYE DROP
- Child: Apply up to 4 times a day

- **UNLICENSED USE** Not licensed for *acanthamoeba keratitis* infections.
- **SIDE-EFFECTS** Eye discomfort · vision blurred
- **PREGNANCY** Manufacturer advises avoid unless essential—no information available.
- **BREAST FEEDING** Manufacturer advises avoid unless essential—no information available.

- **MEDICINAL FORMS** There can be variation in the licensing of different medicines containing the same drug.

Eye drops
EXCIPIENTS: May contain Benzalkonium chloride
- Brolene (Propamidine) (Thornton & Ross Ltd)
Propamidine isetionate 1 mg per 1 ml Brolene 0.1% eye drops | 10 ml [P] £4.35 DT = £4.35
- Golden Eye (propamidine) (Cambridge Healthcare Supplies Ltd)
Propamidine isetionate 1 mg per 1 ml Golden Eye 0.1% drops | 10 ml [P] £5.25 DT = £4.35

3.2 Viral eye infection

3.2a Ophthalmic herpes simplex

ANTIVIRALS › NUCLEOSIDE ANALOGUES

Aciclovir
13-Oct-2025

(Acyclovir)

- **INDICATIONS AND DOSE**

Herpes simplex infection (local treatment)
- TO THE EYE USING EYE OINTMENT
- Child: Apply 1 centimetre 5 times a day continue for at least 3 days after complete healing

- **INTERACTIONS** → Appendix 1: aciclovir
- **SIDE-EFFECTS**
- **Common or very common** Eye inflammation · eye pain
- **PRESCRIBING AND DISPENSING INFORMATION** For further information on *herpes simplex*, see Herpesvirus infections p. 498.
- **PATIENT AND CARER ADVICE**
Medicines for Children leaflet: Aciclovir eye ointment for herpes simplex infection www.medicinesforchildren.org.uk/medicines/aciclovir-eye-ointment-for-herpes-simplex-infection/

- **MEDICINAL FORMS** There can be variation in the licensing of different medicines containing the same drug.

Eye ointment
- Aciclovir (Non-proprietary)
Aciclovir 30 mg per 1 gram Aciclovir 30mg/g eye ointment | 4.5 gram [PoM] £45.00 DT = £45.00

4 Eye procedures

Mydriatics and cycloplegics
25-Apr-2020

Overview

Antimuscarinics dilate the pupil and paralyse the ciliary muscle; they vary in potency and duration of action.

Short-acting, relatively weak mydriatics, such as tropicamide p. 848 (action lasts for up to 6 hours), facilitate the examination of the fundus of the eye. Cyclopentolate hydrochloride p. 839 (complete recovery can take up to 24 hours) or atropine sulfate p. 839 (action up to 7 days) are also licensed for producing cycloplegia for refraction in young children. Expert sources advise tropicamide may be preferred in neonates.

Phenylephrine hydrochloride p. 849 is licensed for mydriasis in diagnostic or therapeutic procedures; mydriasis occurs within 60–90 minutes and lasts up to 5–7 hours.

EvGr Mydriatics and cycloplegics are used in the treatment of anterior uveitis, usually as an adjunct to corticosteroids. Atropine sulfate or cyclopentolate hydrochloride can prevent posterior synechiae and relieve ciliary spasm when used for anterior uveitis. (A)

Other drugs used for Eye procedures Apraclonidine, p. 856

ANTIMUSCARINICS

F 838

Tropicamide

● **INDICATIONS AND DOSE**

Funduscopy

▶ TO THE EYE

▶ Neonate: 0.5% eye drops to be applied 20 minutes before examination.

▶ Child: 0.5% eye drops to be applied 20 minutes before examination

● **INTERACTIONS** → Appendix 1: tropicamide

● **SIDE-EFFECTS** Eye erythema · eye irritation (on prolonged administration) · eye pain · headache · hypotension · nausea · syncope · vision blurred

● **PRESCRIBING AND DISPENSING INFORMATION** Although multi-dose tropicamide eye drops commonly contain preservatives, preservative-free unit dose vials may be available.

● **MEDICINAL FORMS** There can be variation in the licensing of different medicines containing the same drug.

Eye drops

EXCIPIENTS: May contain Benzalkonium chloride, edetic acid (edta)

▶ Tropicamide (Non-proprietary)

Tropicamide 10 mg per 1 ml Tropicamide 1% eye drops 0.5ml unit dose preservative free | 20 unit dose PoM £12.47 DT = £12.97

▶ Mydriacyl (Alcon Eye Care UK Ltd)

Tropicamide 10 mg per 1 ml Mydriacyl 1% eye drops | 5 ml PoM £1.60 DT = £1.60

▶ Tropicamide (Bausch & Lomb UK Ltd)

Tropicamide 5 mg per 1 ml Minims tropicamide 0.5% eye drops 0.5ml unit dose | 20 unit dose PoM £12.82 DT = £12.82

Tropicamide 10 mg per 1 ml Minims tropicamide 1% eye drops 0.5ml unit dose | 20 unit dose PoM £12.97 DT = £12.97

ANTISEPTICS AND DISINFECTANTS › IODINE PRODUCTS

Povidone-iodine

08-Feb-2022

● **INDICATIONS AND DOSE**

Cutaneous peri-ocular and conjunctival antisepsis before ocular surgery

▶ TO THE EYE

▶ Neonate: Apply, leave for 2 minutes, then irrigate thoroughly with sodium chloride 0.9%.

▶ Child: Apply, leave for 2 minutes, then irrigate thoroughly with sodium chloride 0.9%

● **CONTRA-INDICATIONS** Concomitant use of ocular antimicrobial drugs · concomitant use of ocular formulations containing mercury-based preservatives · preterm neonates

● **SIDE-EFFECTS**

▶ **Rare or very rare** Eye erythema · punctate keratitis

▶ **Frequency not known** Cytotoxicity · eye discolouration · hypothyroidism

● **BREAST FEEDING** Avoid regular or excessive use.

● **PRESCRIBING AND DISPENSING INFORMATION** Although multi-dose povidone iodine eye drops commonly contain preservatives, preservative-free unit dose vials may be available.

● **MEDICINAL FORMS** There can be variation in the licensing of different medicines containing the same drug. Forms available from special-order manufacturers include: eye lotion

Eye drops

▶ Povidone-iodine (Non-proprietary)

Povidone-Iodine 50 mg per 1 ml Povidone-Iodine 5% eye drops preservative free | 4 ml PoM £7.49 (Hospital only)

▶ Povidone iodine (Bausch & Lomb UK Ltd)

Povidone-Iodine 50 mg per 1 ml Minims povidone iodine 5% eye drops 0.4ml unit dose | 20 unit dose PoM £17.47 DT = £17.47

DIAGNOSTIC AGENTS › DYES

Fluorescein sodium

● **INDICATIONS AND DOSE**

Detection of lesions and foreign bodies

▶ TO THE EYE

▶ Child: Use sufficient amount to stain damaged areas

● **PRESCRIBING AND DISPENSING INFORMATION** Although multi-dose fluorescein eye drops commonly contain preservatives, preservative-free unit dose vials may be available.

● **MEDICINAL FORMS** There can be variation in the licensing of different medicines containing the same drug.

Eye drops

▶ Fluorescein sodium (Bausch & Lomb UK Ltd)

Fluorescein sodium 10 mg per 1 ml Minims fluorescein sodium 1% eye drops 0.5ml unit dose | 20 unit dose P £10.61 DT = £10.61

Fluorescein sodium 20 mg per 1 ml Minims fluorescein sodium 2% eye drops 0.5ml unit dose | 20 unit dose P £10.81 DT = £10.81

MIOTICS › PARASYMPATHOMIMETICS

Acetylcholine chloride

22-Feb-2021

● **INDICATIONS AND DOSE**

Cataract surgery | Penetrating keratoplasty | Iridectomy | Anterior segment surgery requiring rapid complete miosis

▶ TO THE EYE

▶ Child: (consult product literature)

● **UNLICENSED USE** Not licensed for use in children.

● **SIDE-EFFECTS** Bradycardia · corneal decompensation · corneal oedema · dyspnoea · flushing · hyperhidrosis · hypotension

● **PREGNANCY** Avoid unless potential benefit outweighs risk—no information available.

● **BREAST FEEDING** Avoid unless potential benefit outweighs risk—no information available.

● **MEDICINAL FORMS** There can be variation in the licensing of different medicines containing the same drug.

Powder and solvent for solution for intraocular irrigation

▶ Miphtel (Nordic Pharma Ltd)

Acetylcholine chloride 20 mg Miphtel 20mg powder and solvent for solution for intraocular irrigation ampoules | 6 ampoule PoM £67.08 (Hospital only)

SYMPATHOMIMETICS › VASOCONSTRICTOR

Phenylephrine hydrochloride

- **INDICATIONS AND DOSE**

Mydriasis

▶ TO THE EYE

▶ Child: Apply 1 drop, to be administered before procedure, a drop of proxymetacaine topical anaesthetic may be applied to the eye a few minutes before using phenylephrine to prevent stinging

- **CONTRA-INDICATIONS** 10% strength eye drops in children · 10% strength eye drops in neonates · aneurysms · cardiovascular disease · hypertension · thyrotoxicosis
- **CAUTIONS** Asthma · corneal epithelial damage · darkly pigmented iris is more resistant to pupillary dilatation and caution should be exercised to avoid overdosage · diabetes (avoid eye drops in long standing diabetes) · mydriasis can precipitate acute angle-closure glaucoma in the very few children who are predisposed to the condition because of a shallow anterior chamber · neonates are at an increased risk of systemic toxicity · ocular hyperaemia · susceptibility to angle-closure glaucoma
- **INTERACTIONS** → Appendix 1: sympathomimetics, vasoconstrictor
- **SIDE-EFFECTS** Arrhythmias · conjunctivitis allergic · eye discomfort · hypertension · myocardial infarction (usually after use of 10% strength in patients with pre-existing cardiovascular disease) · palpitations · periorbital pallor · vision disorders
- **PREGNANCY** Use only if potential benefit outweighs risk.
- **BREAST FEEDING** Use only if potential benefit outweighs risk—no information available.
- **PRESCRIBING AND DISPENSING INFORMATION** Although multi-dose phenylephrine eye drops commonly contain preservatives, preservative-free unit dose vials may be available.
- **PATIENT AND CARER ADVICE**

Driving and skilled tasks Patients should be warned not to undertake skilled tasks (e.g. driving) until vision clears after mydriasis.

- **MEDICINAL FORMS** There can be variation in the licensing of different medicines containing the same drug. Forms available from special-order manufacturers include: eye drops

Eye drops

EXCIPIENTS: May contain Disodium edetate, sodium metabisulfite

▶ Phenylephrine hydrochloride (Bausch & Lomb UK Ltd)

Phenylephrine hydrochloride 25 mg per 1 ml Minims phenylephrine hydrochloride 2.5% eye drops 0.5ml unit dose | 20 unit dose [P] £13.60 DT = £13.60

Phenylephrine hydrochloride 100 mg per 1 ml Minims phenylephrine hydrochloride 10% eye drops 0.5ml unit dose | 20 unit dose [P] £14.00

4.1 Post-operative pain and inflammation

ANAESTHETICS, LOCAL

Fluorescein with lidocaine

- **INDICATIONS AND DOSE**

Local anaesthesia

▶ TO THE EYE

▶ Child: Apply as required

- **CONTRA-INDICATIONS** Avoid in pre-term neonate (immature metabolising enzyme system)
- **PRESCRIBING AND DISPENSING INFORMATION** Although multi-dose lidocaine and fluorescein eye drops commonly contain preservatives, preservative-free unit dose vials may be available.
- **MEDICINAL FORMS** There can be variation in the licensing of different medicines containing the same drug.

Eye drops

▶ Lidocaine and Fluorescein (Bausch & Lomb UK Ltd)

Fluorescein sodium 2.5 mg per 1 ml, Lidocaine hydrochloride 40 mg per 1 ml Minims lidocaine and fluorescein eye drops 0.5ml unit dose | 20 unit dose [PoM] £13.40 DT = £13.40

Oxybuprocaine hydrochloride

(Benoxinate hydrochloride)

- **INDICATIONS AND DOSE**

Local anaesthetic

▶ TO THE EYE

▶ Child: Apply as required

- **CONTRA-INDICATIONS** Avoid in preterm neonates
- **INTERACTIONS** → Appendix 1: anaesthetics, local
- **PRESCRIBING AND DISPENSING INFORMATION** Although multi-dose oxybuprocaine eye drops commonly contain preservatives, preservative-free unit dose vials may be available.
- **MEDICINAL FORMS** There can be variation in the licensing of different medicines containing the same drug.

Eye drops

▶ Oxybuprocaine hydrochloride (Bausch & Lomb UK Ltd)

Oxybuprocaine hydrochloride 4 mg per 1 ml Minims oxybuprocaine hydrochloride 0.4% eye drops 0.5ml unit dose | 20 unit dose [PoM] £12.45 DT = £12.45

Proxymetacaine hydrochloride

- **INDICATIONS AND DOSE**

Local anaesthetic

▶ TO THE EYE

▶ Child: Apply as required

- **CONTRA-INDICATIONS** Avoid in preterm neonates
- **INTERACTIONS** → Appendix 1: anaesthetics, local
- **PRESCRIBING AND DISPENSING INFORMATION** Although multi-dose proxymetacaine eye drops commonly contain preservatives, preservative-free unit dose vials may be available.
- **MEDICINAL FORMS** There can be variation in the licensing of different medicines containing the same drug.

Eye drops

▶ Proxymetacaine (Bausch & Lomb UK Ltd)

Proxymetacaine hydrochloride 5 mg per 1 ml Minims proxymetacaine 0.5% eye drops 0.5ml unit dose | 20 unit dose [PoM] £14.29 DT = £14.29

Tetracaine

11-Nov-2021

(Amethocaine)

- **INDICATIONS AND DOSE**

Local anaesthetic

▶ TO THE EYE

▶ Child: Apply as required

- **UNLICENSED USE** Not licensed for use in neonates.
- **CONTRA-INDICATIONS** Avoid in preterm neonates
- **INTERACTIONS** → Appendix 1: anaesthetics, local

- **SIDE-EFFECTS** Dermatitis · eye disorders · eye inflammation · paraesthesia
- **PRESCRIBING AND DISPENSING INFORMATION** Although multi-dose tetracaine eye drops commonly contain preservatives, preservative-free unit dose vials may be available.

- **MEDICINAL FORMS** There can be variation in the licensing of different medicines containing the same drug.

Eye drops

▸ Tetracaine (Non-proprietary)
Tetracaine hydrochloride 5 mg per 1 ml Minims tetracaine hydrochloride 0.5% eye drops 0.5ml unit dose | 20 unit dose PoM £12.13 DT = £12.13
Tetracaine hydrochloride 10 mg per 1 ml Minims tetracaine hydrochloride 1% eye drops 0.5ml unit dose | 20 unit dose PoM £12.13 DT = £12.13

ANALGESICS › NON-STEROIDAL ANTI-INFLAMMATORY DRUGS

Diclofenac sodium

19-Mar-2025

- **INDICATIONS AND DOSE**

Inhibition of intra-operative miosis during cataract surgery (but does not possess intrinsic mydriatic properties) | Postoperative inflammation in cataract surgery, strabismus surgery, argon laser trabeculoplasty

▸ TO THE EYE
▸ Child: (consult product literature)

- **UNLICENSED USE** Not licensed for use in children.
- **CAUTIONS** Bleeding tendency (increased risk of ocular tissue bleeding, including hyphaema) · concomitant use of ocular corticosteroids · corneal epithelial breakdown (if evidence of, then discontinue immediately) · may mask symptoms of infection · may slow or delay wound healing · patients at increased risk of corneal side-effects

CAUTIONS, FURTHER INFORMATION

▸ Concomitant use of ocular corticosteroids EvGr Concomitant use of ocular formulations containing NSAIDs with ocular formulations containing corticosteroids may increase the risk of corneal healing problems, leading to corneal melt or scarring and loss of vision. ⟨M⟩
▸ Patients at increased risk of corneal side-effects EvGr Patients with complicated ocular surgeries, corneal denervation, corneal epithelial defects, diabetes mellitus, ocular surface diseases, rheumatoid arthritis, or repeat ocular surgeries within a short period of time may be at increased risk of corneal side-effects which may become sight threatening. ⟨M⟩

- **INTERACTIONS** → Appendix 1: NSAIDs
- **SIDE-EFFECTS**
  - ▸ **Common or very common** Skin reactions
  - ▸ **Rare or very rare** Asthma exacerbated · hypersensitivity
  - ▸ **Frequency not known** Dyspnoea · eye discomfort · eye disorders · eye inflammation · oedema · rhinitis · vision blurred

SIDE-EFFECTS, FURTHER INFORMATION Prolonged use can cause epithelial breakdown, corneal thinning, corneal erosion, corneal ulceration and corneal perforation which might be sight-threatening. Discontinue if corneal epithelial breakdown occurs and monitor closely.

- **ALLERGY AND CROSS-SENSITIVITY** EvGr Contra-indicated in patients with a history of hypersensitivity to aspirin or any other NSAID—which includes those in whom attacks of asthma, angioedema, urticaria or rhinitis have been precipitated by aspirin or any other NSAID. ⟨M⟩
- **PRESCRIBING AND DISPENSING INFORMATION** Although multi-dose diclofenac sodium eye drops commonly contain preservatives, preservative-free unit dose vials may be available.

- **MEDICINAL FORMS** There can be variation in the licensing of different medicines containing the same drug.

Eye drops

EXCIPIENTS: May contain Benzalkonium chloride, disodium edetate, propylene glycol

▸ Voltarol Ophtha (Thea Pharmaceuticals Ltd)
Diclofenac sodium 1 mg per 1 ml Voltarol Ophtha 0.1% eye drops 0.3ml unit dose | 40 unit dose PoM £32.00 DT = £32.00
▸ Voltarol Ophtha Multidose (Thea Pharmaceuticals Ltd)
Diclofenac sodium 1 mg per 1 ml Voltarol Ophtha Multidose 0.1% eye drops | 5 ml PoM £6.68 DT = £6.68

Ketorolac trometamol

19-Mar-2025

- **INDICATIONS AND DOSE**

Prophylaxis and reduction of inflammation and associated symptoms following ocular surgery

▸ TO THE EYE
▸ Child: (consult product literature)

- **UNLICENSED USE** Not licensed for use in children.
- **CAUTIONS** Bleeding tendency (increased risk of ocular tissue bleeding, including hyphaema) · concomitant use of ocular corticosteroids · corneal epithelial breakdown (if evidence of, then discontinue immediately) · may mask symptoms of infection · may slow or delay wound healing · patients at increased risk of corneal side-effects

CAUTIONS, FURTHER INFORMATION

▸ Concomitant use of ocular corticosteroids EvGr Concomitant use of ocular formulations containing NSAIDs with ocular formulations containing corticosteroids may increase the risk of corneal healing problems, leading to corneal melt or scarring and loss of vision. ⟨M⟩
▸ Patients at increased risk of corneal side-effects EvGr Patients with complicated ocular surgeries, corneal denervation, corneal epithelial defects, diabetes mellitus, ocular surface diseases, rheumatoid arthritis, or repeat ocular surgeries within a short period of time may be at increased risk of corneal side-effects which may become sight threatening. ⟨M⟩

- **INTERACTIONS** → Appendix 1: NSAIDs
- **SIDE-EFFECTS**
  - ▸ **Common or very common** Eye discomfort · eye disorders · eye infection · eye inflammation · headache · hypersensitivity · keratic deposits · retinal haemorrhage · vision disorders
  - ▸ **Uncommon** Dry eye
  - ▸ **Frequency not known** Asthma exacerbated · bronchospasm

SIDE-EFFECTS, FURTHER INFORMATION Prolonged use can cause epithelial breakdown, corneal thinning, corneal erosion, corneal ulceration and corneal perforation which might be sight-threatening. Discontinue if corneal epithelial breakdown occurs and monitor closely.

- **ALLERGY AND CROSS-SENSITIVITY** EvGr Contra-indicated in patients with a history of hypersensitivity to aspirin or any other NSAID—which includes those in whom attacks of asthma, angioedema, urticaria or rhinitis have been precipitated by aspirin or any other NSAID. ⟨M⟩

- **MEDICINAL FORMS** There can be variation in the licensing of different medicines containing the same drug.

Eye drops

EXCIPIENTS: May contain Benzalkonium chloride, disodium edetate

▸ Ketorolac trometamol (Non-proprietary)
Ketorolac trometamol 5 mg per 1 ml Ketorolac 0.5% eye drops | 5 ml PoM £9.99 DT = £4.84
▸ Acular (AbbVie Ltd)
Ketorolac trometamol 5 mg per 1 ml Acular 0.5% eye drops | 5 ml PoM £3.00 DT = £4.84

5 Glaucoma and ocular hypertension

Glaucoma

14-Sep-2020

Overview

Glaucoma describes a group of disorders characterised by a loss of visual field associated with cupping of the optic disc and optic nerve damage and is generally associated with raised intra-ocular pressure.

Glaucoma is rare in children and should always be managed by a specialist. *Primary congenital glaucoma* is the most common form of glaucoma in children, followed by *secondary glaucomas*, such as following hereditary anterior segment malformations; *juvenile open-angle glaucoma* is less common and usually occurs in older children.

Treatment of glaucoma is determined by the pathophysiology and usually involves controlling raised intra-ocular pressure with surgery. Drug therapy is generally supportive, and can be used temporarily, pre- or post-operatively, or both, to reduce intra-ocular pressure. In secondary glaucomas, drug therapy is often used first-line, and long-term treatment may be required. Drugs that reduce intra-ocular pressure by different mechanisms are available for managing glaucoma. A topical beta-blocker or a prostaglandin analogue can be used. It may be necessary to combine these drugs or add others, such as carbonic anhydrase inhibitors, or miotics to control intra-ocular pressure.

Children with an acute form of glaucoma (usually presenting with pain in older children, a cloudy cornea, and may be associated with a previous history of controlled glaucoma or recent intra-ocular surgery) need immediate referral for specialist ophthalmology assessment and treatment.

Beta-blockers for glaucoma

Topical application of a beta-blocker to the eye reduces intra-ocular pressure effectively in primary and secondary glaucomas, probably by reducing the rate of production of aqueous humour.

Prostaglandin analogues for glaucoma

The prostaglandin analogues latanoprost p. 855, and travoprost, and the synthetic prostamide, bimatoprost, increase uveoscleral outflow and subsequently reduce intra-ocular pressure. They are used to reduce intra-ocular pressure. Only latanoprost (*Xalatan*® and certain non-proprietary preparations of latanoprost) is licensed for use in children. Children receiving prostaglandin analogues should be managed by a specialist.

Sympathomimetics for glaucoma

Apraclonidine p. 856 is an alpha$_2$-adrenoceptor agonist that lowers intra-ocular pressure by reducing aqueous humour formation. Eye drops containing apraclonidine 0.5% are used for a short period to delay laser treatment or surgery for glaucoma in patients not adequately controlled by another drug; eye drops containing 1% are used for control of intra-ocular pressure after anterior segment laser surgery.

Brimonidine tartrate, an alpha$_2$-adrenoceptor agonist, is thought to lower intra-ocular pressure by reducing aqueous humour formation and increasing uveoscleral outflow.

Carbonic anhydrase inhibitors and systemic drugs for glaucoma

The **carbonic anhydrase inhibitors**, acetazolamide p. 852, brinzolamide p. 853, and dorzolamide p. 854, reduce intra-ocular pressure by reducing aqueous humour production. Systemic use of acetazolamide also produces weak diuresis.

Acetazolamide is given by mouth or, rarely in children, by intravenous injection (intramuscular injections are painful because of the alkaline pH of the solution). It is used as an adjunct to other treatment for reducing intra-ocular pressure. Acetazolamide is not generally recommended for long-term use. The MHRA/CHM have released important safety information on the use of antiepileptic drugs and the risk of suicidal thoughts and behaviour. For further information, see Epilepsy p. 227.

Dorzolamide and brinzolamide are topical carbonic anhydrase inhibitors. They are unlicensed in children but are used in those resistant to beta-blockers or those in whom beta-blockers are contra-indicated. They are used alone or as an adjunct to a topical beta-blocker. Brinzolamide can also be used as an adjunct to a prostaglandin analogue. Systemic absorption can rarely cause sulfonamide-like side-effects and may require discontinuation if severe.

Metabolic acidosis can occur in children using topical carbonic anhydrase inhibitors; symptoms may include poor feeding and lack of weight gain.

Miotics for glaucoma

Miotics act by opening up the inefficient drainage channels in the trabecular meshwork. Pilocarpine p. 855 is a miotic used pre- and post-operatively in goniotomy and trabeculotomy; it is used occasionally for aphakic glaucoma.

BETA-ADRENOCEPTOR BLOCKERS

Betaxolol

03-Apr-2020

- **INDICATIONS AND DOSE**

Primary and secondary glaucomas

▶ TO THE EYE

▶ Child: Apply twice daily

- **UNLICENSED USE** Not licensed for use in children.
- **CONTRA-INDICATIONS** Also consider contra-indications listed for systemically administered beta blockers · bradycardia · heart block
- **CAUTIONS** Patients with corneal disease

  CAUTIONS, FURTHER INFORMATION Systemic absorption can follow topical application to the eyes; consider cautions listed for systemically administered beta blockers.
- **INTERACTIONS** → Appendix 1: beta blockers, selective
- **SIDE-EFFECTS**

▶ **Common or very common** Eye discomfort · eye disorders · vision disorders

▶ **Uncommon** Dry eye · eye inflammation · rhinitis

▶ **Rare or very rare** Cataract · rhinorrhoea · skin reactions

▶ **Frequency not known** Angioedema · hypersensitivity

  SIDE-EFFECTS, FURTHER INFORMATION Systemic absorption can follow topical application to the eyes; consider side effects listed for systemically administered beta blockers.
- **PRESCRIBING AND DISPENSING INFORMATION** Although multi-dose betaxolol eye drops commonly contain preservatives, preservative-free unit dose vials may be available.

- **MEDICINAL FORMS** There can be variation in the licensing of different medicines containing the same drug.

Eye drops

EXCIPIENTS: May contain Benzalkonium chloride, disodium edetate

▸ **Betaxolol (Non-proprietary)**

Betaxolol (as Betaxolol hydrochloride) 5 mg per 1 ml Betaxolol 0.5% eye drops | 5 ml PoM ⊠ DT = £1.90

▸ **Betoptic** (Immedica Pharma AB)

Betaxolol (as Betaxolol hydrochloride) 2.5 mg per 1 ml Betoptic 0.25% suspension eye drops | 5 ml PoM £2.66 DT = £2.66

Betoptic 0.25% eye drops suspension 0.25ml unit dose | 50 unit dose [PoM] £13.77 DT = £13.77

Betaxolol (as Betaxolol hydrochloride) 5 mg per 1 ml Betoptic 0.5% eye drops | 5 ml [PoM] £1.90 DT = £1.90

Levobunolol hydrochloride

03-Apr-2020

- **INDICATIONS AND DOSE**

Primary and secondary glaucomas

▶ TO THE EYE

▶ Child: Apply 1–2 times a day

- **UNLICENSED USE** Not licensed for use in children.
- **CONTRA-INDICATIONS** Also consider contra-indications listed for systemically administered beta blockers · bradycardia · heart block
- **CAUTIONS** Patients with corneal disease

CAUTIONS, FURTHER INFORMATION Systemic absorption can follow topical application to the eyes; consider cautions listed for systemically administered beta blockers.

- **INTERACTIONS** → Appendix 1: beta blockers, non-selective
- **SIDE-EFFECTS**

▶ **Common or very common** Eye discomfort · eye inflammation

▶ **Frequency not known** Dry eye · eye disorders · eyelid eczema · vision blurred

SIDE-EFFECTS, FURTHER INFORMATION Systemic absorption can follow topical application to the eyes; consider side effects listed for systemically administered beta blockers.

- **PRESCRIBING AND DISPENSING INFORMATION** Although multi-dose levobunolol eye drops commonly contain preservatives, preservative-free unit dose vials may be available.

- **MEDICINAL FORMS** No licensed medicines listed.

F 121

Timolol maleate

05-May-2021

- **INDICATIONS AND DOSE**

Primary congenital and primary juvenile glaucoma [for a transitional period, before surgery or following failed surgery]

▶ TO THE EYE

▶ Child: Apply once daily; increased if necessary up to 2 drops daily, max. two drops daily into each affected eye. If applied twice daily, to be applied 12 hours apart. The lowest concentration solution that controls symptoms should be used

TIMOPTOL-LA ®

Reduction of intra-ocular pressure in primary and secondary glaucoma

▶ TO THE EYE

▶ Child: Apply once daily

TIOPEX ®

Reduction of intra-ocular pressure primary and secondary glaucomas

▶ TO THE EYE

▶ Child: Apply once daily, to be applied in the morning

- **UNLICENSED USE** Long-acting eye preparations are not licensed for use in children.
- **CONTRA-INDICATIONS** Also consider contra-indications listed for systemically administered beta blockers · bradycardia · heart block
- **CAUTIONS** Consider also cautions listed for systemically administered beta blockers · patients with corneal disease
- **INTERACTIONS** → Appendix 1: beta blockers, non-selective
- **SIDE-EFFECTS**

▶ **Common or very common** Eye discomfort · eye disorders · eye inflammation · vision disorders

SIDE-EFFECTS, FURTHER INFORMATION Systemic absorption can follow topical application to the eyes; consider side-effects listed for systemically administered beta blockers.

- **BREAST FEEDING** Manufacturer advises avoidance.
- **NATIONAL FUNDING/ACCESS DECISIONS**

TIOPEX ® For full details see funding body website

Scottish Medicines Consortium (SMC) decisions

▶ **Timolol eye gel (*Tiopex*®) for the reduction of the elevated intra-ocular pressure in patients with ocular hypertension or chronic open angle glaucoma.(February 2014)** SMC No. 941/14 Recommended with restrictions

- **MEDICINAL FORMS** There can be variation in the licensing of different medicines containing the same drug.

Eye gel

EXCIPIENTS: May contain Benzododecinium bromide

▶ **Timoptol-LA** (Santen UK Ltd)

Timolol (as Timolol maleate) 2.5 mg per 1 ml Timoptol-LA 0.25% ophthalmic gel-forming solution | 2.5 ml [PoM] £3.12 DT = £3.12

Timolol (as Timolol maleate) 5 mg per 1 ml Timoptol-LA 0.5% ophthalmic gel-forming solution | 2.5 ml [PoM] £3.12 DT = £3.12

Eye drops

EXCIPIENTS: May contain Benzalkonium chloride

▶ **Timolol maleate (Non-proprietary)**

Timolol (as Timolol maleate) 2.5 mg per 1 ml Timolol 0.25% eye drops | 5 ml [PoM] £5.30 DT = £2.83

Timolol (as Timolol maleate) 5 mg per 1 ml Timolol 0.5% eye drops | 5 ml [PoM] £5.00 DT = £1.52

▶ **Eysano** (Aspire Pharma Ltd)

Timolol (as Timolol maleate) 2.5 mg per 1 ml Eysano 2.5mg/ml eye drops | 5 ml [PoM] £8.45 DT = £8.45

Timolol (as Timolol maleate) 5 mg per 1 ml Eysano 5mg/ml eye drops | 5 ml [PoM] £9.65 DT = £9.65

▶ **Tiopex** (Thea Pharmaceuticals Ltd)

Timolol (as Timolol maleate) 1 mg per 1 gram Tiopex 1mg/g eye gel 0.4g unit dose | 30 unit dose [PoM] £7.49 DT = £7.49

Combinations available: ***Dorzolamide with timolol***, p. 854

CARBONIC ANHYDRASE INHIBITORS

Acetazolamide

05-Feb-2021

- **INDICATIONS AND DOSE**

Glaucoma

▶ BY MOUTH USING MODIFIED-RELEASE MEDICINES

▶ Child 12–17 years: 250–500 mg daily

Epilepsy

▶ BY MOUTH USING IMMEDIATE-RELEASE MEDICINES, OR BY SLOW INTRAVENOUS INJECTION

▶ Neonate: Initially 2.5 mg/kg 2–3 times a day, followed by maintenance 5–7 mg/kg 2–3 times a day.

▶ Child 1 month–11 years: Initially 2.5 mg/kg 2–3 times a day, followed by maintenance 5–7 mg/kg 2–3 times a day; maximum 750 mg per day

▶ Child 12–17 years: 250 mg 2–4 times a day

Reduction of intra-ocular pressure in primary and secondary glaucoma (specialist use only)

▶ BY MOUTH USING IMMEDIATE-RELEASE MEDICINES, OR BY INTRAVENOUS INJECTION

▶ Child 1 month–11 years: 5 mg/kg 2–4 times a day, adjusted according to response; maximum 750 mg per day

▶ Child 12–17 years: 250 mg 2–4 times a day

Raised intracranial pressure

▶ BY MOUTH USING IMMEDIATE-RELEASE MEDICINES, OR BY SLOW INTRAVENOUS INJECTION

▸ Child 1 month–11 years: Initially 8 mg/kg 3 times a day, then increased if necessary up to 100 mg/kg daily

- **UNLICENSED USE** Not licensed for the treatment of glaucoma.

IMPORTANT SAFETY INFORMATION

MHRA/CHM ADVICE: ANTIEPILEPTICS: RISK OF SUICIDAL THOUGHTS AND BEHAVIOUR (AUGUST 2008)

See Epilepsy p. 227.

MHRA/CHM ADVICE: ANTIEPILEPTIC DRUGS: UPDATED ADVICE ON SWITCHING BETWEEN DIFFERENT MANUFACTURERS' PRODUCTS (NOVEMBER 2017)

See Epilepsy p. 227.

MHRA/CHM ADVICE: ANTIEPILEPTIC DRUGS IN PREGNANCY: UPDATED ADVICE FOLLOWING COMPREHENSIVE SAFETY REVIEW (JANUARY 2021)

See Epilepsy p. 227.

- **CONTRA-INDICATIONS** Adrenocortical insufficiency · hyperchloraemic acidosis · hypokalaemia · hyponatraemia · long-term administration in chronic angle-closure glaucoma
- **CAUTIONS** Avoid extravasation at injection site (risk of necrosis) · diabetes mellitus · impaired alveolar ventilation (risk of acidosis) · long-term use · pulmonary obstruction (risk of acidosis) · renal calculi
- **INTERACTIONS** → Appendix 1: acetazolamide
- **SIDE-EFFECTS**

GENERAL SIDE-EFFECTS

▶ **Common or very common** Haemorrhage · metabolic acidosis · nephrolithiasis · sensation abnormal

▶ **Uncommon** Bone marrow disorders · depression · dizziness · electrolyte imbalance · hearing impairment · hepatic disorders · leucopenia · nausea · renal colic · renal impairment · renal lesions · severe cutaneous adverse reactions (SCARs) · skin reactions · thrombocytopenia · tinnitus · urinary tract discomfort · urine abnormalities · vomiting

▶ **Rare or very rare** Anaphylactic reaction · appetite disorder · confusion · diarrhoea · fatigue · fever · flushing · headache · irritability · libido decreased · paralysis · photosensitivity reaction · seizure

▶ **Frequency not known** Agranulocytosis · drowsiness · myopia · polyuria · suicidal behaviours · taste altered · thirst

SPECIFIC SIDE-EFFECTS

▶ **Uncommon**

▸ With oral use Osteomalacia

▶ **Rare or very rare**

▸ With oral use Ataxia · hyperglycaemia · hypoglycaemia · renal tubular necrosis

▶ **Frequency not known**

▸ With oral use Agitation

SIDE-EFFECTS, FURTHER INFORMATION Acetazolamide is a sulfonamide derivative; blood disorders, rashes, and other sulfonamide-related side-effects occur occasionally—patients should be told to report any unusual skin rash.

If electrolyte disturbances and metabolic acidosis occur, these can be corrected by administering bicarbonate.

- **ALLERGY AND CROSS-SENSITIVITY** EvGr Contra-indicated if history of sulfonamide hypersensitivity. Ⓜ
- **PREGNANCY** Manufacturer advises avoid, especially in first trimester (toxicity in *animal* studies). See also *Pregnancy* in Epilepsy p. 227.
- **BREAST FEEDING** Amount too small to be harmful.
- **HEPATIC IMPAIRMENT** Manufacturer advises avoid.
- **RENAL IMPAIRMENT** Avoid—risk of metabolic acidosis.
- **MONITORING REQUIREMENTS** Monitor blood count and plasma electrolyte concentrations with prolonged use.

- **MEDICINAL FORMS** There can be variation in the licensing of different medicines containing the same drug. Forms available from special-order manufacturers include: oral suspension, oral solution

Oral tablet

CAUTIONARY AND ADVISORY LABELS 3

▸ **Acetazolamide (Non-proprietary)**

Acetazolamide 250 mg Acetazolamide 250mg tablets | 112 tablet PoM £75.36 DT = £13.11

Powder for solution for injection

▸ **Acetazolamide (Non-proprietary)**

Acetazolamide 500 mg Acetazolamide 500mg powder for solution for injection vials | 1 vial PoM £14.76

▸ **Diamox** (Advanz Pharma)

Acetazolamide 500 mg Diamox Sodium Parenteral 500mg powder for solution for injection vials | 1 vial PoM £14.76

Brinzolamide

23-Jul-2021

- **INDICATIONS AND DOSE**

Reduction of intra-ocular pressure in primary and secondary glaucoma either as adjunct to beta-blockers or prostaglandin analogues or used alone if unresponsive to beta-blockers or if beta-blockers contra-indicated

▶ TO THE EYE

▸ Child: Apply twice daily, then increased if necessary up to 3 times a day

- **UNLICENSED USE** Not licensed for use in children.
- **CONTRA-INDICATIONS** Hyperchloraemic acidosis
- **CAUTIONS** Renal tubular immaturity or abnormality—risk of metabolic acidosis · systemic absorption follows topical application
- **INTERACTIONS** → Appendix 1: brinzolamide
- **SIDE-EFFECTS**

▶ **Common or very common** Eye discomfort · eye disorders · taste altered · vision disorders

▶ **Uncommon** Arrhythmias · asthenia · cardio-respiratory distress · chest discomfort · cough · depression · diarrhoea · dizziness · dry eye · dry mouth · dyspnoea · epistaxis · eye deposit · eye inflammation · feeling abnormal · foreign body in eye · gastrointestinal discomfort · gastrointestinal disorders · headache · increased risk of infection · memory impairment · motor dysfunction · muscle complaints · nasal complaints · nausea · nervousness · oral disorders · oropharyngeal pain · pain · palpitations · renal pain · scleral discolouration · sensation abnormal · sexual dysfunction · skin reactions · sleep disorders · throat complaints · vomiting

▶ **Rare or very rare** Alopecia · angina pectoris · drowsiness · irritability · respiratory disorders · tinnitus

▶ **Frequency not known** Appetite decreased · arthralgia · asthma · hypertension · malaise · peripheral oedema · severe cutaneous adverse reactions (SCARs) · tremor · urinary frequency increased · vertigo

SIDE-EFFECTS, FURTHER INFORMATION Systemic absorption can rarely cause sulfonamide-like side-effects and may require discontinuation if severe.

- **ALLERGY AND CROSS-SENSITIVITY** EvGr Contra-indicated if history of sulfonamide hypersensitivity. Ⓜ
- **PREGNANCY** Avoid—toxicity in *animal* studies.
- **BREAST FEEDING** Use only if benefit outweighs risk.
- **HEPATIC IMPAIRMENT** Manufacturer advises avoid—no information available.

- **RENAL IMPAIRMENT** EvGr Avoid if creatinine clearance less than 30 mL/minute (no information available). (M) See p. 16.

- **MEDICINAL FORMS** There can be variation in the licensing of different medicines containing the same drug.

Eye drops

EXCIPIENTS: May contain Benzalkonium chloride, disodium edetate

▸ **Brinzolamide (Non-proprietary)**
Brinzolamide 10 mg per 1 ml Brinzolamide 10mg/ml eye drops | 5 ml PoM £9.70 DT = £2.14

▸ **Azopt** (Novartis Pharmaceuticals UK Ltd)
Brinzolamide 10 mg per 1 ml Azopt 10mg/ml eye drops | 5 ml PoM £6.92 DT = £2.14

Dorzolamide

29-Jul-2021

- **INDICATIONS AND DOSE**

Raised intra-ocular pressure in primary and secondary glaucoma used alone in patients unresponsive to beta-blockers or if beta-blockers contra-indicated

▶ TO THE EYE
▸ Child: Apply 3 times a day

Raised intra-ocular pressure in primary and secondary glaucoma as adjunct to a beta-blocker

▶ TO THE EYE
▸ Child: Apply twice daily

- **UNLICENSED USE** Not licensed for use in children.
- **CONTRA-INDICATIONS** Hyperchloraemic acidosis
- **CAUTIONS** Chronic corneal defects · history of intra-ocular surgery · history of renal calculi · immature renal tubules (neonates and infants)—risk of metabolic acidosis · low endothelial cell count · systemic absorption follows topical application
- **INTERACTIONS** → Appendix 1: dorzolamide
- **SIDE-EFFECTS**

▶ **Common or very common** Asthenia · eye discomfort · eye disorders · eye inflammation · headache · nausea · taste bitter · vision disorders

▶ **Rare or very rare** Angioedema · bronchospasm · dizziness · dry mouth · dyspnoea · epistaxis · local reaction · paraesthesia · severe cutaneous adverse reactions (SCARs) · skin reactions · throat irritation · urolithiasis

▶ **Frequency not known** Hypertension · palpitations · tachycardia

SIDE-EFFECTS, FURTHER INFORMATION Systemic absorption can cause sulfonamide-like side-effects and may require discontinuation if severe.

- **ALLERGY AND CROSS-SENSITIVITY** EvGr Caution in patients with hypersensitivity to sulfonamides (systemic absorption occurs). (M)
- **PREGNANCY** Manufacturer advises avoid—toxicity in *animal* studies.
- **BREAST FEEDING** Manufacturer advises avoid—no information available.
- **HEPATIC IMPAIRMENT** Manufacturer advises caution—no information available.
- **RENAL IMPAIRMENT** EvGr Avoid if creatinine clearance less than 30 mL/minute. (M) See p. 16.
- **PRESCRIBING AND DISPENSING INFORMATION** Although multi-dose dorzolamide eye drops commonly contain preservatives, preservative-free unit dose vials may be available.

- **MEDICINAL FORMS** There can be variation in the licensing of different medicines containing the same drug.

Eye drops

EXCIPIENTS: May contain Benzalkonium chloride

▸ **Dorzolamide (Non-proprietary)**
Dorzolamide (as Dorzolamide hydrochloride) 20 mg per 1 ml Dorzolamide 20mg/ml eye drops | 5 ml PoM £6.30 DT = £2.45

▸ **Dimaz** (Scope Ophthalmics Ltd)
Dorzolamide (as Dorzolamide hydrochloride) 20 mg per 1 ml Dimaz 20mg/ml eye drops | 5 ml PoM £6.98 DT = £7.08

▸ **Eydelto** (Aspire Pharma Ltd)
Dorzolamide (as Dorzolamide hydrochloride) 20 mg per 1 ml Eydelto 20mg/ml eye drops | 5 ml PoM £7.08 DT = £7.08

▸ **Trusopt** (Santen UK Ltd)
Dorzolamide (as Dorzolamide hydrochloride) 20 mg per 1 ml Trusopt 20mg/ml eye drops | 5 ml PoM £6.33 DT = £2.45
Trusopt 20mg/ml eye drops 0.2ml unit dose preservative free | 60 unit dose PoM £24.18 DT = £24.18

▸ **Vizidor** (Bausch & Lomb UK Ltd)
Dorzolamide (as Dorzolamide hydrochloride) 20 mg per 1 ml Vizidor 20mg/ml eye drops | 5 ml PoM £7.09 DT = £7.08

Dorzolamide with timolol

The properties listed below are those particular to the combination only. For the properties of the components please consider, dorzolamide above, timolol maleate p. 852.

- **INDICATIONS AND DOSE**

Raised intra-ocular pressure in open-angle glaucoma when beta-blockers alone not adequate | Raised intra-ocular pressure in pseudo-exfoliative glaucoma when beta-blockers alone not adequate

▶ TO THE EYE
▸ Child: Apply twice daily

- **INTERACTIONS** → Appendix 1: beta blockers, non-selective · dorzolamide
- **PRESCRIBING AND DISPENSING INFORMATION** Although multi-dose dorzolamide with timolol eye drops commonly contain preservatives, preservative-free unit dose vials may be available.

- **MEDICINAL FORMS** There can be variation in the licensing of different medicines containing the same drug.

Eye drops

EXCIPIENTS: May contain Benzalkonium chloride

▸ **Dorzolamide with timolol (Non-proprietary)**
Timolol (as Timolol maleate) 5 mg per 1 ml, Dorzolamide (as Dorzolamide hydrochloride) 20 mg per 1 ml Dorzolamide 20mg/ml / Timolol 5mg/ml eye drops 0.2ml unit dose preservative free | 60 unit dose PoM £28.59 DT = £28.59
Dorzolamide 20mg/ml / Timolol 5mg/ml eye drops 0.166ml unit dose preservative free | 60 unit dose PoM £21.44–£35.54 DT = £21.44
Dorzolamide 20mg/ml / Timolol 5mg/ml eye drops | 5 ml PoM £27.16 DT = £3.08

▸ **Codimaz** (Scope Ophthalmics Ltd)
Timolol (as Timolol maleate) 5 mg per 1 ml, Dorzolamide (as Dorzolamide hydrochloride) 20 mg per 1 ml Codimaz 20mg/ml / 5mg/ml eye drops | 5 ml PoM £8.03 DT = £8.13

▸ **Cosopt** (Santen UK Ltd)
Timolol (as Timolol maleate) 5 mg per 1 ml, Dorzolamide (as Dorzolamide hydrochloride) 20 mg per 1 ml Cosopt 20mg/ml / 5mg/ml eye drops 0.2ml unit dose preservative free | 60 unit dose PoM £28.59 DT = £28.59
Cosopt 20mg/ml / 5mg/ml eye drops | 5 ml PoM £10.05 DT = £3.08

▸ **Cosopt iMulti** (Santen UK Ltd)
Timolol (as Timolol maleate) 5 mg per 1 ml, Dorzolamide (as Dorzolamide hydrochloride) 20 mg per 1 ml Cosopt iMulti 20mg/ml / 5mg/ml eye drops preservative free | 10 ml PoM £28.00

▸ **Eylamdo** (Aspire Pharma Ltd)
Timolol (as Timolol maleate) 5 mg per 1 ml, Dorzolamide (as Dorzolamide hydrochloride) 20 mg per 1 ml Eylamdo 20mg/ml / 5mg/ml eye drops | 5 ml PoM £8.13 DT = £8.13

▸ **Glaucopt** (Visufarma UK Ltd)
Timolol (as Timolol maleate) 5 mg per 1 ml, Dorzolamide (as Dorzolamide hydrochloride) 20 mg per 1 ml Glaucopt 20mg/ml /

5mg/ml eye drops 0.166ml unit dose preservative free | 60 unit dose PoM £21.44 DT = £21.44

▸ **Tidomat** (Kent Pharma (UK) Ltd)

Timolol (as Timolol maleate) 5 mg per 1 ml, Dorzolamide (as Dorzolamide hydrochloride) 20 mg per 1 ml Tidomat 20mg/ml / 5mg/ml eye drops | 5 ml PoM £10.00 DT = £3.08

▸ **Vizidor Duo** (Bausch & Lomb UK Ltd)

Timolol (as Timolol maleate) 5 mg per 1 ml, Dorzolamide (as Dorzolamide hydrochloride) 20 mg per 1 ml Vizidor Duo 20mg/ml / 5mg/ml eye drops | 5 ml PoM £8.14 DT = £8.13

MIOTICS › PARASYMPATHOMIMETICS

Pilocarpine

11-May-2021

● **DRUG ACTION** Pilocarpine acts by opening the inefficient drainage channels in the trabecular meshwork.

● **INDICATIONS AND DOSE**

Raised intra-ocular pressure

▶ TO THE EYE

▸ Child 1 month–1 year: Apply 1 drop 3 times a day, doses are for 0.5% or 1% solution

▸ Child 2-17 years: Apply 1 drop 4 times a day

Pre- and postoperatively in goniotomy and trabeculotomy

▶ TO THE EYE

▸ Child: Apply once daily, 1% or 2% solution to be applied

● **UNLICENSED USE** Not licensed for use in children.

● **CONTRA-INDICATIONS** Acute iritis · anterior uveitis · conditions where pupillary constriction is undesirable · some forms of secondary glaucoma (where pupillary constriction is undesirable)

● **CAUTIONS** A darkly pigmented iris may require a higher concentration of the miotic or more frequent administration and care should be taken to avoid overdosage · asthma · cardiac disease · care in conjunctival damage · care in corneal damage · epilepsy · gastro-intestinal spasm · hypertension · hyperthyroidism · hypotension · peptic ulceration · retinal detachment has occurred in susceptible individuals and those with retinal disease · urinary-tract obstruction

● **INTERACTIONS** → Appendix 1: pilocarpine

● **SIDE-EFFECTS**

▶ **Common or very common** Diarrhoea · headache · hyperhidrosis · hypersalivation · nausea · skin reactions · vision disorders · vomiting

▶ **Frequency not known** Bradycardia · bronchospasm · conjunctival vascular congestion · eye disorder (long term use) · eye disorders · hypotension · lens changes (long term use) · pain · paraesthesia · pulmonary oedema · sensitisation · vitreous haemorrhage

● **PREGNANCY** Avoid unless the potential benefit outweighs risk—limited information available.

● **BREAST FEEDING** Avoid unless the potential benefit outweighs risk—no information available.

● **PRE-TREATMENT SCREENING** Fundus examination is advised before starting treatment with a miotic (retinal detachment has occurred).

● **MONITORING REQUIREMENTS** Intra-ocular pressure and visual fields should be monitored in those with chronic simple glaucoma and those receiving long-term treatment with a miotic.

● **PRESCRIBING AND DISPENSING INFORMATION** Although multi-dose pilocarpine eye drops commonly contain preservatives, preservative-free unit dose vials may be available.

● **PATIENT AND CARER ADVICE**

Driving and skilled tasks Blurred vision may affect performance of skilled tasks (e.g. driving) particularly at night or in reduced lighting.

● **MEDICINAL FORMS** There can be variation in the licensing of different medicines containing the same drug. Forms available from special-order manufacturers include: eye drops

Eye drops

EXCIPIENTS: May contain Benzalkonium chloride

▸ **Pilocarpine (Non-proprietary)**

Pilocarpine hydrochloride 10 mg per 1 ml Pilocarpine hydrochloride 1% eye drops | 10 ml PoM £32.10 DT = £32.10

Pilocarpine hydrochloride 20 mg per 1 ml Pilocarpine hydrochloride 2% eye drops | 10 ml PoM £99.11 DT = £64.37

Pilocarpine hydrochloride 40 mg per 1 ml Pilocarpine hydrochloride 4% eye drops | 10 ml PoM £69.10 DT = £69.10

▸ **Pilocarpine nitrate** (Bausch & Lomb UK Ltd)

Pilocarpine nitrate 20 mg per 1 ml Minims pilocarpine nitrate 2% eye drops 0.5ml unit dose | 20 unit dose PoM £14.29 DT = £14.29

PROSTAGLANDINS AND RELATED SUBSTANCES

Latanoprost

16-Nov-2020

● **INDICATIONS AND DOSE**

Reduction of intra-ocular pressure in raised intra-ocular pressure and glaucoma

▶ TO THE EYE

▸ Child: Apply once daily, to be administered preferably in the evening

IMPORTANT SAFETY INFORMATION

MHRA/CHM ADVICE: LATANOPROST (*XALATAN®*): INCREASED REPORTING OF EYE IRRITATION SINCE REFORMULATION (JULY 2015)

Following reformulation of *Xalatan®*, to allow for long-term storage at room temperature, there has been an increase in the number of reports of eye irritation from across the EU. Patients should be advised to tell their health professional promptly (within a week) if they experience eye irritation (e.g. excessive watering) severe enough to make them consider stopping treatment. Review treatment and prescribe a different formulation if necessary.

● **CONTRA-INDICATIONS** Active herpes simplex keratitis · history of recurrent herpetic keratitis associated with prostaglandin analogues

● **CAUTIONS** Aphakia · asthma · children less than 1 year—limited information available · contact lens wearers · do not use within 5 minutes of thiomersal-containing preparations · history of significant ocular viral infections · peri-operative period of cataract surgery · preterm neonates less than 36 weeks gestational age—no information available · pseudophakia with torn posterior lens capsule or anterior chamber lenses · risk factors for cystoid macular oedema · risk factors for iritis · risk factors for uveitis

● **SIDE-EFFECTS**

▶ **Common or very common** Eye discolouration · eye discomfort · eye disorders · eye inflammation · vision disorders

▶ **Uncommon** Dry eye · rash

▶ **Rare or very rare** Asthma · chest pain · dyspnoea · unstable angina

▶ **Frequency not known** Arthralgia · dizziness · headache · myalgia · ophthalmic herpes simplex · palpitations

● **PREGNANCY** Manufacturer advises avoid.

● **BREAST FEEDING** May be present in milk—manufacturer advises avoid.

- **MONITORING REQUIREMENTS** Monitor for changes to eye coloration.
- **PRESCRIBING AND DISPENSING INFORMATION** Although multi-dose latanoprost eye drops commonly contain preservatives, preservative-free unit dose vials may be available.
- **PATIENT AND CARER ADVICE**
Changes in eye colour Before initiating treatment, patients should be warned of a possible change in eye colour as an increase in the brown pigment in the iris can occur, which may be permanent; particular care is required in those with mixed coloured irides and those receiving treatment to one eye only. Changes in eyelashes and vellus hair can also occur, and patients should also be advised to avoid repeated contact of the eye drop solution with skin as this can lead to hair growth or skin pigmentation.
- **NATIONAL FUNDING/ACCESS DECISIONS**
MONOPOST® For full details see funding body website

Scottish Medicines Consortium (SMC) decisions
- **Latanoprost (*Monopost*®) for the reduction of elevated intraocular pressure in patients with open-angle glaucoma and ocular hypertension (July 2013)** SMC No. 879/13 Recommended with restrictions

- **MEDICINAL FORMS** There can be variation in the licensing of different medicines containing the same drug.

Eye drops
EXCIPIENTS: May contain Benzalkonium chloride
- **Latanoprost (Non-proprietary)**
Latanoprost 50 microgram per 1 ml Latanoprost 50micrograms/ml eye drops | 2.5 ml PoM £12.48 DT = £1.81
- **Catiolanze** (Santen UK Ltd)
Latanoprost 50 microgram per 1 ml Catiolanze 50micrograms/ml eye drops emulsion 0.3ml unit dose | 30 unit dose PoM £7.99
- **Lotacryn** (Scope Ophthalmics Ltd)
Latanoprost 50 microgram per 1 ml Lotacryn 50micrograms/ml eye drops | 2.5 ml PoM £7.99 DT = £7.99
- **Monopost** (Thea Pharmaceuticals Ltd)
Latanoprost 50 microgram per 1 ml Monopost 50micrograms/ml eye drops 0.2ml unit dose | 30 unit dose PoM £8.49 DT = £8.49 | 90 unit dose PoM £25.47 DT = £25.47
- **Xalatan** (Viatris UK Healthcare Ltd)
Latanoprost 50 microgram per 1 ml Xalatan 50micrograms/ml eye drops | 2.5 ml PoM £12.48 DT = £1.81

SYMPATHOMIMETICS › ALPHA$_2$-ADRENOCEPTOR AGONISTS

Apraclonidine

11-May-2021

- **DRUG ACTION** Apraclonidine is an alpha$_2$-adrenoceptor agonist that lowers intra-ocular pressure by reducing aqueous humour formation. It is a derivative of clonidine.

- **INDICATIONS AND DOSE**

Control or prevention of postoperative elevation of intra-ocular pressure after anterior segment laser surgery
- TO THE EYE
- Child: Apply 1 drop, 1 hour before laser procedure, then 1 drop, immediately after completion of procedure, 1% eye drops to be administered

Short-term adjunctive treatment of chronic glaucoma in patients not adequately controlled by another drug
- TO THE EYE
- Child 12–17 years: Apply 1 drop 3 times a day usually for maximum 1 month, 0.5% eye drops to be administered, may not provide additional benefit if patient already using two drugs that suppress the production of aqueous humour

- **UNLICENSED USE** 1% drops are not licensed for use in children.
- **CONTRA-INDICATIONS** History of severe or unstable and uncontrolled cardiovascular disease
- **CAUTIONS** Cerebrovascular disease · depression · heart failure · history of angina · hypertension · loss of effect may occur over time · Raynaud's syndrome · recent myocardial infarction · reduction in vision in end-stage glaucoma (suspend treatment) · severe coronary insufficiency · thromboangiitis obliterans · vasovagal attack
- **INTERACTIONS** → Appendix 1: apraclonidine
- **SIDE-EFFECTS**
- **Common or very common** Eye disorders
- **Uncommon** Bradycardia · conjunctival haemorrhage · diarrhoea · dry eye · eye discomfort · eye inflammation · gastrointestinal discomfort · irritability · libido decreased · nasal dryness · palpitations · postural hypotension · sensation abnormal · sleep disorders · syncope · vision disorders · vomiting
- **Rare or very rare** Chest pain · dry mouth · fatigue · headache · hyperhidrosis · pain in extremity · pruritus · taste altered · temperature sensation altered

SIDE-EFFECTS, FURTHER INFORMATION Since absorption may follow topical application, systemic effects may occur– see clonidine hydrochloride p. 120.

Ocular intolerance Manufacturer advises withdrawal if eye pruritus, ocular hyperaemia, increased lacrimation, or oedema of the eyelids and conjunctiva occur.
- **PREGNANCY** Manufacturer advises avoid—no information available.
- **BREAST FEEDING** Manufacturer advises avoid—no information available.
- **HEPATIC IMPAIRMENT** Manufacturer advises use with caution and monitor, including close monitoring of cardiovascular parameters—no information available.
- **RENAL IMPAIRMENT** EvGr Use with caution in chronic renal failure. (M)
- **MONITORING REQUIREMENTS**
- Monitor intra-ocular pressure and visual fields.
- Monitor for excessive reduction in intra-ocular pressure following peri-operative use.
- **PATIENT AND CARER ADVICE**
Driving and skilled tasks Drowsiness may affect performance of skilled tasks (e.g. driving).

- **MEDICINAL FORMS** There can be variation in the licensing of different medicines containing the same drug.

Eye drops
EXCIPIENTS: May contain Benzalkonium chloride
- **Apraclonidine (Non-proprietary)**
Apraclonidine (as Apraclonidine hydrochloride) 10 mg per 1 ml Apraclonidine 1% eye drops 0.25ml unit dose preservative free | 24 unit dose PoM £110.69 DT = £110.69
- **Iopidine** (Essential Pharma Ltd)
Apraclonidine (as Apraclonidine hydrochloride) 10 mg per 1 ml Iopidine 1% eye drops 0.25ml unit dose | 24 unit dose PoM £110.69 DT = £110.69

6 Retinal disorders

6.1 Optic neuropathy

DRUGS FOR METABOLIC DISORDERS › ANTIOXIDANTS

Idebenone

11-Sep-2025

- **DRUG ACTION** Idebenone is a nootropic and antioxidant that is thought to act by restoring cellular ATP generation, thereby reactivating retinal ganglion cells.

- **INDICATIONS AND DOSE**

Leber's hereditary optic neuropathy (initiated by a specialist)

▶ BY MOUTH

▸ Child 12–17 years: 300 mg 3 times a day

- **SIDE-EFFECTS**
  - ▶ **Common or very common** Cough · diarrhoea · increased risk of infection · pain
  - ▶ **Frequency not known** Agranulocytosis · anaemia · anxiety · appetite decreased · azotaemia · delirium · dizziness · dyspepsia · hallucination · headache · hepatitis · leucopenia · malaise · movement disorders · nausea · neutropenia · poriomania · seizure · skin reactions · stupor · thrombocytopenia · urine discolouration · vomiting

  SIDE-EFFECTS, FURTHER INFORMATION The metabolites of idebenone may cause red-brown discolouration of the urine. This effect is harmless, but the manufacturer advises caution as this may mask colour changes due to other causes (e.g. renal or blood disorders).

- **PREGNANCY** Manufacturer advises avoid unless potential benefit outweighs risk—no information available.
- **BREAST FEEDING** Manufacturer advises avoid—present in milk in *animal* studies.
- **HEPATIC IMPAIRMENT** Manufacturer advises caution (no information available).
- **RENAL IMPAIRMENT** Manufacturer advises use with caution—no information available.
- **NATIONAL FUNDING/ACCESS DECISIONS**

For full details see funding body website

NICE decisions

▶ **Idebenone for treating visual impairment in Leber's hereditary optic neuropathy in people 12 years and over (August 2025)** NICE TA1093 Recommended

Scottish Medicines Consortium (SMC) decisions

▶ **Idebenone (*Raxone*®) for the treatment of visual impairment in adolescent and adult patients with Leber's Hereditary Optic Neuropathy (LHON) (May 2017)** SMC No. 1226/17 Recommended with restrictions

All Wales Medicines Strategy Group (AWMSG) decisions

▶ **Idebenone (*Raxone*®) for the treatment of visual impairment in adolescent and adult patients with Leber's hereditary optic neuropathy (March 2021)** AWMSG No. 807 Recommended

- **MEDICINAL FORMS** There can be variation in the licensing of different medicines containing the same drug. Forms available from special-order manufacturers include: oral tablet

Oral tablet

CAUTIONARY AND ADVISORY LABELS 14, 21

▸ **Raxone** (Chiesi Ltd) ▼

Idebenone 150 mg Raxone 150mg tablets | 180 tablet PoM £6,364.00 DT = £6,364.00

6.2 Retinopathy of prematurity

ANTINEOVASCULARISATION DRUGS › VASCULAR ENDOTHELIAL GROWTH FACTOR INHIBITORS

Aflibercept [Specialist drug]

12-Mar-2024

- **INDICATIONS AND DOSE**

Retinopathy of prematurity

▶ BY INTRAVITREAL INJECTION

▸ Preterm neonate: Specialist drug – access specialist resources for dosing information.

IMPORTANT SAFETY INFORMATION

MHRA/CHM ADVICE: *EYLEA*® 40 MG/ML (AFLIBERCEPT SOLUTION FOR INTRAVITREAL INJECTION): HIGHER RISK OF INTRAOCULAR PRESSURE INCREASE WITH THE PRE-FILLED SYRINGE (APRIL 2021)

Cases of increased intra-ocular pressure in adults have been reported more frequently when using the *Eylea*® prefilled syringe compared with a luer-lock syringe used with *Eylea*® solution for injection in a vial. Incorrect handling in the preparation and injection is suspected as the cause of the observed cases of increased intra-ocular pressure with the *Eylea*® prefilled syringe. Injections should be performed by healthcare professionals familiar with the handling of this presentation; the manufacturer has provided educational materials which include a *Prescriber Guide* and a training video on how to prepare and administer the intravitreal injection. The patient's vision and intra-ocular pressure should be evaluated and monitored immediately after the intravitreal injection.

ADMINISTRATION

EvGr *Eylea*® prefilled syringes contain more than the recommended dose for preterm infants, and therefore must be used in combination with the PICLEO paediatric dosing device to avoid administering a larger than recommended volume that may increase intra-ocular pressure. Ⓜ

- **CONTRA-INDICATIONS** Clinical signs of irreversible ischaemic visual function loss · ocular or periocular infection · severe intra-ocular inflammation
- **INTERACTIONS** → Appendix 1: aflibercept
- **SIDE-EFFECTS**
  - ▶ **Common or very common** Cataract · eye discomfort · eye disorders · eye inflammation · haemorrhage · retinal pigment epithelial tear · vision disorders
  - ▶ **Uncommon** Lens opacity

  SIDE-EFFECTS, FURTHER INFORMATION Discontinue treatment in the event of retinal break, rhegmatogenous retinal detachment, or if stage 3 or 4 macular holes develop.

- **MEDICINAL FORMS** There can be variation in the licensing of different medicines containing the same drug. Forms available from special-order manufacturers include: solution for injection

Solution for injection

EXCIPIENTS: May contain Polysorbates

▸ **Afqlir** (Sandoz Ltd) ▼

Aflibercept 40 mg per 1 ml Afqlir 6.6mg/165microlitres solution for injection pre-filled syringes | 1 pre-filled disposable injection PoM £734.40

▸ **Eydenzelt** (Celltrion Healthcare UK Ltd) ▼

Aflibercept 40 mg per 1 ml Eydenzelt 3.6mg/90microlitres solution for injection pre-filled syringes | 1 pre-filled disposable injection PoM £734.00 (Hospital only)

11 Eye

- **Eylea** (Bayer Plc)
  Aflibercept 40 mg per 1 ml Eylea 3.6mg/90microlitres solution for injection pre-filled syringes | 1 pre-filled disposable injection PoM £816.00 (Hospital only)
  Eylea 4mg/100microlitres solution for injection vials | 1 vial PoM £816.00 (Hospital only)
  Aflibercept 114.3 mg per 1 ml Eylea 21mg/184microlitres solution for injection pre-filled syringes | 1 pre-filled disposable injection PoM £998.00 (Hospital only)
  Eylea 30.1mg/263microlitres solution for injection vials | 1 vial PoM £998.00 (Hospital only)
- **Mynzepli** (Advanz Pharma) ▼
  Aflibercept 40 mg per 1 ml Mynzepli 3.6mg/90microlitres solution for injection pre-filled syringes | 1 pre-filled disposable injection PoM £734.40 (Hospital only)
- **Vgenfli** (MDBiologics Ltd) ▼
  Aflibercept 40 mg per 1 ml Vgenfli 6.6mg/165microlitres solution for injection pre-filled syringes | 1 pre-filled disposable injection PoM £799.00 (Hospital only)
- **Yesafili** (Biocon Biologics Ireland Ltd) ▼
  Aflibercept 40 mg per 1 ml Yesafili 3.6mg/90microlitres solution for injection pre-filled syringes | 1 pre-filled disposable injection PoM £734.40 (Hospital only)

11 Eye

Ranibizumab [Specialist drug]

28-May-2024

● INDICATIONS AND DOSE

Retinopathy of prematurity

▶ BY INTRAVITREAL INJECTION

- Preterm neonate: Specialist drug – access specialist resources for dosing information.

● CONTRA-INDICATIONS Ocular or periocular infection · severe intra-ocular inflammation

● INTERACTIONS → Appendix 1: ranibizumab

● SIDE-EFFECTS

▶ **Common or very common** Anaemia · anxiety · arthralgia · cataract · cough · dry eye · eye discomfort · eye disorders · eye inflammation · haemorrhage · headache · hypersensitivity · increased risk of infection · lens opacity · nausea · retinal pigment epithelial tear · vision disorders

▶ **Uncommon** Corneal deposits

▶ **Frequency not known** Arterial thromboembolism

SIDE-EFFECTS, FURTHER INFORMATION Discontinue treatment if rhegmatogenous retinal detachment, or stage 3 or 4 macular holes develop.

● MEDICINAL FORMS There can be variation in the licensing of different medicines containing the same drug. Forms available from special-order manufacturers include: solution for injection

Solution for injection

EXCIPIENTS: May contain Polysorbates

- **Byooviz** (Samsung Bioepis NL B.V. Ltd) ▼
  Ranibizumab 10 mg per 1 ml Byooviz 2.3mg/0.23ml solution for injection vials | 1 vial PoM £523.45 (Hospital only)
- **Lucentis** (Novartis Pharmaceuticals UK Ltd)
  Ranibizumab 10 mg per 1 ml Lucentis 2.3mg/0.23ml solution for injection vials | 1 vial PoM £551.00 (Hospital only)
  Lucentis 1.65mg/0.165ml solution for injection pre-filled syringes | 1 pre-filled disposable injection PoM £551.00
- **Ongavia** (Teva UK Ltd) ▼
  Ranibizumab 10 mg per 1 ml Ongavia 2.3mg/0.23ml solution for injection vials | 1 vial PoM £523.45 (Hospital only)
- **Rimmyrah** (Orion Pharma (UK) Ltd) ▼
  Ranibizumab 10 mg per 1 ml Rimmyrah 2.3mg/0.23ml solution for injection vials | 1 vial PoM £523.45 (Hospital only)
- **Ximluci** (Genus Pharmaceuticals Ltd) ▼
  Ranibizumab 10 mg per 1 ml Ximluci 2.3mg/0.23ml solution for injection vials | 1 vial PoM £495.90 (Hospital only)

Chapter 12
Ear, nose and oropharynx

CONTENTS

Ear

Ear

17-May-2024

Otitis externa

Otitis externa refers to inflammation of the external ear canal which in some cases may involve oedema. It is primarily caused by bacterial infection. EvGr It is important to consider underlying otitis media as otitis externa may be secondary to otorrhoea from otitis media.

Any precipitating factors should be managed and cleaning the external ear canal should be considered (using dry swabbing, microsuction, or irrigation techniques) if ear wax or debris are blocking passage of topical medicine (may require specialist referral).

A solution of **acetic acid** 2% acts as an astringent in the external ear canal by reducing the pH and reducing bacterial and fungal cell growth. It may be used to treat mild otitis externa and is comparable to an anti-infective combined with a corticosteroid; efficacy is reduced if treatment extends beyond 1 week.

If infection is present, a topical anti-infective with or without a corticosteroid may be considered. These are used for a minimum of one week but if symptoms persist they can be used until they resolve, up to a maximum of 2 weeks. Prolonged and extensive use of topical anti-infective or corticosteroid treatment may affect the flora in the ear canal, increasing the risk of fungal infections. If a mild to moderate, uncomplicated fungal infection is suspected in the context of chronic otitis externa, a topical antifungal such as clotrimazole 1% solution p. 862, acetic acid 2% spray [unlicensed indication], or clioquinol and a corticosteroid such as flumetasone pivalate with clioquinol p. 863 can be offered. Sensitivity to topical ear preparations may also occur, especially with prolonged or recurrent use. Astringent agents such as aluminium acetate ear drops p. 866 are also available. (A)

In view of reports of ototoxicity, treatment with topical **aminoglycosides** is contra-indicated in patients with a perforated tympanic membrane (eardrum). EvGr However, some specialists do use these drops cautiously in the presence of a perforation or patent grommet in patients with chronic suppurative otitis media and when other measures have failed for otitis externa; treatment should be considered only **by specialists** in the following circumstances:

- drops should only be used in the presence of obvious infection;
- treatment should be for no longer than 2 weeks;
- patients should be counselled on the risk of ototoxicity and given justification for the use of these topical antibiotics;
- baseline audiometry should be performed, if possible, before treatment is commenced.

Clinical expertise and judgement should be used to assess the risk of treatment versus the benefit to the patient in such circumstances. (E)

EvGr For severe pain associated with otitis externa, a simple analgesic, such as paracetamol p. 325 or ibuprofen p. 821, is usually sufficient; codeine phosphate p. 331 may be used for severe pain. Oral antibacterials are rarely indicated but if they are required, consider seeking specialist advice. A systemic antibacterial may be considered if the infection is spreading outside the ear canal, the patient is systemically unwell, or in a high risk group (e.g. diabetics, immunocompromised patients, patients with severe infection or at high-risk of severe infection such as pseudomonal infections). Referral should be considered if there is extensive swelling of the auditory canal. (A) For further information, see *Otitis externa* in Ear infections, antibacterial therapy p. 366.

Otitis media

Acute otitis media

Acute otitis media is a self-limiting condition that mainly affects children. It is characterised by inflammation in the middle ear associated with effusion and accompanied by the rapid onset of signs and symptoms of an ear infection. The infection can be caused by viruses or bacteria; often both are present simultaneously.

Children with acute otitis media usually present with symptoms such as ear pain, rubbing of the ear, fever, irritability, crying, poor feeding, restlessness at night, cough, or rhinorrhoea. Symptoms usually resolve within 3 to 7 days without antibacterial drugs and they make little difference to the development of complications such as short-term hearing loss, perforated eardrum or recurrent infection. Acute complications such as mastoiditis, meningitis, intracranial abscess, sinus thrombosis, and facial nerve paralysis, are rare.

EvGr Children and their carers should be given advice about the usual duration of acute otitis media, self-care of symptoms such as pain and fever with paracetamol or ibuprofen p. 821, and when to seek medical help. In addition to oral analgesics for pain relief, consider offering an ear drop containing an anaesthetic and an analgesic such as phenazone with lidocaine p. 866, if immediate antibacterial treatment is not given and there is no eardrum perforation or otorrhoea. Children and their carers should be reassured that antibacterial drugs are usually not required.

An immediate antibacterial drug should be given if the child is systemically very unwell, has signs or symptoms of a more serious illness, or is at high risk of complications such as significant heart, lung, renal, liver or neuromuscular disease, immunosuppression, cystic fibrosis, or young children who were born prematurely. An immediate antibacterial drug can also be considered if otorrhoea (discharge following perforation of the eardrum) is present, or in children under 2 years of age with bilateral otitis media. Ⓐ For further information, see *Otitis media* in Ear infections, antibacterial therapy p. 366.

EvGr Children with acute otitis media associated with a severe systemic infection or acute complications should be referred to hospital. Ⓐ

Otitis media with effusion

Otitis media with effusion (OME), also known as glue ear, is characterised by the collection of fluid within the middle ear without any signs of inflammation or infection. It occurs most frequently in children, particularly in those aged between 6 months and 4 years, and is the most common cause of hearing impairment in children. It is more prevalent in children with cleft palate, Down's syndrome, primary ciliary dyskinesia, cystic fibrosis, and allergic rhinitis.

EvGr For children with OME without hearing loss, reassurance should be provided that it will often resolve on its own over time without treatment.

For children with suspected OME with hearing loss, referral to a specialist for a formal assessment should be made. If after 3 months, hearing loss is bilateral, or is impacting on daily living or communication, non-surgical or surgical interventions such as hearing aids or grommets, respectively, may be considered.

During grommet insertion, administration of a single dose of ciprofloxacin ear drops [unlicensed use] should be considered for prevention of otorrhoea and tube blockage. If there is otorrhoea after insertion, consider treatment with non-ototoxic antibacterial ear drops, such as ciprofloxacin [unlicensed use], for 5–7 days. For otorrhoea that persists and does not respond to antibacterial ear drops, consider grommet removal.

Oral or topical antibacterials, oral or nasal corticosteroids, antihistamines, leukotriene receptor antagonists, mucolytics, and decongestants are not recommended to treat OME due to a lack of evidence supporting their use. Ⓐ

For further guidance on the management of OME, see NICE guideline: **Otitis media with effusion in under 12s** (see *Useful resources*).

Chronic suppurative otitis media

Chronic suppurative otitis media is a chronic inflammation of the middle ear and mastoid cavity, and is thought to be a complication of acute otitis media. The usual presentation is otorrhoea through a tympanic perforation and can involve infection due to a number of different bacteria or fungi. EvGr Referral to an ear, nose and throat specialist is required and treatment is likely to involve antibacterials, corticosteroids (usually topical), and intensive aural cleaning. Ⓐ

Removal of ear wax

Ear wax (cerumen) is a normal bodily secretion which provides a protective film on the lining of the ear canal and need only be removed if it causes hearing loss or other symptoms (such as discomfort or tinnitus), or interferes with a proper view of the ear canal and/or ear drum, or in order to take an impression of the ear canal.

EvGr To soften ear wax and aid removal, ear drops can be used, such as olive oil ear drops p. 867, almond oil ear drops p. 867, sodium bicarbonate ear drops p. 867, or sodium chloride 0.9% nasal drops p. 728 [unlicensed use as ear drops]. Ⓐ The drops can be used three to four times daily for several days. Lying down with the affected ear uppermost, ear drops are instilled before waiting for 5 minutes. Ear drops are not recommended for patients suspected of having a perforated tympanic membrane, active dermatitis, or active infection of the ear canal.

EvGr If necessary, ear wax may be removed by irrigation, microsuction, or another method of removal (such as removal using a probe). Pre-treatment wax softeners should be used, either immediately before ear irrigation or for up to 5 days beforehand. Pre-treatment and irrigation may need to be repeated once if unsuccessful after the first attempt; if unsuccessful after the second attempt, referral to a specialist ear care service or an ear, nose, and throat specialist is required. Ⓐ Ear irrigation is not recommended in young children, in patients unable to co-operate with the procedure, in patients with acute otitis externa with an oedematous ear canal and painful pinna, or in those with a history of otitis media in the last six weeks, any ear surgery, or any previous problem with irrigation. It should also be avoided in patients with mucus discharge from the ear within the past 12 months, a foreign body in the ear, grommets in place, cleft palate, or factors that increase the risk of trauma, infection or haemorrhage (such as dermatitis, infection/abnormalities of the ear canal, or perforated tympanic membrane or history of perforated tympanic membrane). A person who has hearing in one ear only should not have that ear irrigated because even a very slight risk of damage may lead to permanent deafness. Irrigation should be used with caution and carried out on a low setting in patients with: tinnitus, vertigo, recurrent otitis externa, recurrent otitis media, a history of radiotherapy of the head or neck, and in patients who are immunocompromised or taking anticoagulants or high-dose steroids.

Useful resources

Otitis media with effusion in under 12s. National Institute for Health and Care Excellence. NICE guideline 233. August 2023.
www.nice.org.uk/guidance/ng233

1 Otitis externa

ANTIBACTERIALS > AMINOGLYCOSIDES

Framycetin sulfate

29-Mar-2023

● INDICATIONS AND DOSE

Bacterial infection in otitis externa

▶ TO THE EAR

▶ Child: (consult product literature)

IMPORTANT SAFETY INFORMATION

MHRA/CHM ADVICE: AMINOGLYCOSIDES (GENTAMICIN, AMIKACIN, TOBRAMYCIN, AND NEOMYCIN): INCREASED RISK OF DEAFNESS IN PATIENTS WITH MITOCHONDRIAL MUTATIONS (JANUARY 2021)

The use of aminoglycosides is associated with rare cases of ototoxicity. A safety review found an increased risk of deafness in patients with mitochondrial mutations (particularly the m.1555A>G mutation), including cases where the patient's aminoglycoside serum levels were within the recommended range. Nevertheless, these mitochondrial mutations are considered rare and penetrance is uncertain. No cases were identified with topical preparations but, based on a shared mechanism of effect, there is a potential risk with aminoglycosides administered at the site of toxicity i.e. the ear.

Healthcare professionals are advised to consider the need for aminoglycoside treatment versus alternative options in patients with susceptible mutations. The need for genetic testing especially in those requiring recurrent or long-term treatment with aminoglycosides should also be considered, however, urgent treatment should not be delayed. To minimise the risks of adverse effects, continuous monitoring of renal and auditory function, as well as hepatic and laboratory parameters, is recommended for all patients. Those with known mitochondrial mutations or a family history of ototoxicity are advised to inform their doctor or pharmacist before using an aminoglycoside.

- **CONTRA-INDICATIONS** Perforated tympanic membrane
- **CAUTIONS** Avoid prolonged use
- **PRE-TREATMENT SCREENING** NHS England commissions genetic testing under the *National genomic test directory* indication: R65 - Aminoglycoside exposure posing risk to hearing. The testing criteria is significant exposure to aminoglycosides posing risk of ototoxicity. This testing is relevant to individuals with a predisposition to gram-negative infections or with hearing loss who have been exposed to aminoglycosides. For further information, see www.england.nhs.uk/publication/national-genomic-test-directories/.
- **MEDICINAL FORMS** No licensed medicines listed.

Combinations available: *Dexamethasone with framycetin sulfate and gramicidin*, p. 865

F 377

Gentamicin

20-Jun-2025

- **INDICATIONS AND DOSE**

Bacterial infection in otitis externa

▶ TO THE EAR

▸ Child: Apply 2–3 drops 4–5 times a day, (including a dose at bedtime)

- **UNLICENSED USE** Gentamicin doses in BNF Publications may differ from those in product literature.

IMPORTANT SAFETY INFORMATION

MHRA/CHM ADVICE: AMINOGLYCOSIDES (GENTAMICIN, AMIKACIN, TOBRAMYCIN, AND NEOMYCIN): INCREASED RISK OF DEAFNESS IN PATIENTS WITH MITOCHONDRIAL MUTATIONS (JANUARY 2021)

The use of aminoglycosides is associated with rare cases of ototoxicity. A safety review found an increased risk of deafness in patients with mitochondrial mutations (particularly the m.1555A>G mutation), including cases where the patient's aminoglycoside serum levels were within the recommended range. Nevertheless, these mitochondrial mutations are considered rare and penetrance is uncertain. No cases were identified with topical preparations but, based on a shared mechanism of effect, there is a potential risk with gentamicin and other aminoglycosides administered at the site of toxicity i.e. the ear.

Healthcare professionals are advised to consider the need for aminoglycoside treatment versus alternative options in patients with susceptible mutations. The need for genetic testing especially in those requiring recurrent or long-term treatment with aminoglycosides should also be considered, however, urgent treatment should not be delayed. To minimise the risks of adverse effects, continuous monitoring of renal and auditory function, as well as hepatic and laboratory parameters, is recommended for all patients. Those with known mitochondrial mutations or a family history of ototoxicity are advised to inform their doctor or pharmacist before using an aminoglycoside.

- **CONTRA-INDICATIONS** Patent grommet (although may be used by specialists, see Ear p. 859) · perforated tympanic membrane (although may be used by specialists, see Ear p. 859)
- **CAUTIONS** Avoid prolonged use
- **INTERACTIONS** → Appendix 1: aminoglycosides
- **SIDE-EFFECTS** Since systemic absorption can follow topical administration to the eye and ear, also consider the side-effects of systemic aminoglycosides.
- **PRE-TREATMENT SCREENING** NHS England commissions genetic testing under the *National genomic test directory* indication: R65 - Aminoglycoside exposure posing risk to hearing. The testing criteria is significant exposure to aminoglycosides posing risk of ototoxicity. This testing is relevant to individuals with a predisposition to gram-negative infections or with hearing loss who have been exposed to aminoglycosides. For further information, see www.england.nhs.uk/publication/national-genomic-test-directories/.
- **MEDICINAL FORMS** There can be variation in the licensing of different medicines containing the same drug.

Ear/eye drops solution

EXCIPIENTS: May contain Benzalkonium chloride

▸ Gentamicin (Non-proprietary)

Gentamicin (as Gentamicin sulfate) 3 mg per 1 ml Gentamicin 0.3% ear/eye drops | 10 ml [PoM] £21.92 DT = £23.84

Gentamicin with hydrocortisone

26-Jul-2025

- **INDICATIONS AND DOSE**

Eczematous inflammation in otitis externa

▶ TO THE EAR

▸ Child: Apply 2–4 drops 4–5 times a day, (including a dose at bedtime)

IMPORTANT SAFETY INFORMATION

MHRA/CHM ADVICE: CORTICOSTEROIDS: RARE RISK OF CENTRAL SEROUS CHORIORETINOPATHY WITH LOCAL AS WELL AS SYSTEMIC ADMINISTRATION (AUGUST 2017)

See Corticosteroids, general use p. 537.

MHRA/CHM ADVICE: AMINOGLYCOSIDES (GENTAMICIN, AMIKACIN, TOBRAMYCIN, AND NEOMYCIN): INCREASED RISK OF DEAFNESS IN PATIENTS WITH MITOCHONDRIAL MUTATIONS (JANUARY 2021)

The use of aminoglycosides is associated with rare cases of ototoxicity. A safety review found an increased risk of deafness in patients with mitochondrial mutations (particularly the m.1555A>G mutation), including cases where the patient's aminoglycoside serum levels were within the recommended range. Nevertheless, these mitochondrial mutations are considered rare and penetrance is uncertain. No cases were identified with topical preparations but, based on a shared mechanism of effect, there is a potential risk with gentamicin and other aminoglycosides administered at the site of toxicity i.e. the ear.

Healthcare professionals are advised to consider the need for aminoglycoside treatment versus alternative options in patients with susceptible mutations. The need for genetic testing especially in those requiring recurrent or long-term treatment with aminoglycosides should also be considered, however, urgent treatment should not be delayed. To minimise the risks of adverse effects, continuous monitoring of renal and auditory function, as well as hepatic and laboratory parameters, is recommended for all patients. Those with known mitochondrial mutations or a family history of ototoxicity are advised to inform their doctor or pharmacist before using an aminoglycoside.

ADRENAL INSUFFICIENCY CARD (APRIL 2023)
The British Society for Paediatric Endocrinology and Diabetes (BSPED) has developed an Adrenal Insufficiency Card which should be issued to children with adrenal insufficiency and steroid dependence. The card includes a management summary for the emergency treatment of adrenal crisis and sick day dosing, and can be issued by any healthcare professional managing such patients. The BSPED Adrenal Insufficiency Card is available at: www.bsped.org.uk/adrenal-insufficiency.

- **CONTRA-INDICATIONS** Patent grommet (although may be used by specialists, see Ear p. 859) · perforated tympanic membrane (although may be used by specialists, see Ear p. 859)
- **CAUTIONS** Avoid prolonged use
- **SIDE-EFFECTS** Local reaction
- **PRE-TREATMENT SCREENING** NHS England commissions genetic testing under the *National genomic test directory* indication: R65 - Aminoglycoside exposure posing risk to hearing. The testing criteria is significant exposure to aminoglycosides posing risk of ototoxicity. This testing is relevant to individuals with a predisposition to gram-negative infections or with hearing loss who have been exposed to aminoglycosides. For further information, see www.england.nhs.uk/publication/national-genomic-test-directories/.
- **PATIENT AND CARER ADVICE** If systemic absorption occurs following topical and local use, side-effects applicable to systemic corticosteroids may apply; a patient information leaflet should be supplied and the need for a Steroid Treatment Card considered, see Corticosteroids, general use p. 537.
  Medicines for Children leaflet: Gentamicin and hydrocortisone ear drops for inflammatory ear infections www.medicinesforchildren.org.uk/medicines/gentamicin-and-hydrocortisone-ear-drops-for-inflammatory-ear-infections/
- **MEDICINAL FORMS** There can be variation in the licensing of different medicines containing the same drug.

Ear drops

EXCIPIENTS: May contain Benzalkonium chloride, disodium edetate

▸ Gentamicin with hydrocortisone (Non-proprietary)
Gentamicin (as Gentamicin sulfate) 3 mg per 1 ml, Hydrocortisone acetate 10 mg per 1 ml Gentamicin 0.3% / Hydrocortisone acetate 1% ear drops | 10 ml PoM £48.25 DT = £33.26

ANTIBACTERIALS › QUINOLONES

428

Ciprofloxacin 26-Nov-2025

- **INDICATIONS AND DOSE**

Acute otitis externa

▶ TO THE EAR USING EAR DROPS
▸ Child 1–17 years: Apply 0.25 mL twice daily for 7 days, each 0.25 mL dose contains 0.5 mg ciprofloxacin

- **CAUTIONS** Known (or at risk of) perforated tympanic membrane
- **INTERACTIONS** → Appendix 1: quinolones
- **SIDE-EFFECTS**
  ▶ **Uncommon** Ear pruritus
- **PRESCRIBING AND DISPENSING INFORMATION** For choice of antibacterial therapy, see Ear infections, antibacterial therapy p. 366.
- **HANDLING AND STORAGE** Manufacturer advises discard any ampoules remaining 8 days after opening the pouch.
- **PATIENT AND CARER ADVICE**
  Medicines for Children leaflet: Ciprofloxacin drops for infection www.medicinesforchildren.org.uk/medicines/ciprofloxacin-drops-for-infection/
- **NATIONAL FUNDING/ACCESS DECISIONS**
  For full details see funding body website

Scottish Medicines Consortium (SMC) decisions

▶ **Ciprofloxacin (*Cetraxal*®) for the treatment of acute otitis externa in adults and children older than 1 year with an intact tympanic membrane, caused by ciprofloxacin susceptible microorganisms (April 2018)** SMC No. 1320/18 Recommended with restrictions

All Wales Medicines Strategy Group (AWMSG) decisions

▶ **Ciprofloxacin (*Cetraxal*®) for the treatment of acute otitis externa in adults and children older than 1 year with an intact tympanic membrane, caused by ciprofloxacin susceptible microorganisms (July 2018)** AWMSG No. 1343 Recommended

- **MEDICINAL FORMS** There can be variation in the licensing of different medicines containing the same drug. Forms available from special-order manufacturers include: ear drops

Ear drops

▸ Cetraxal (Aspire Pharma Ltd)
Ciprofloxacin (as Ciprofloxacin hydrochloride) 2 mg per 1 ml Cetraxal 2mg/ml ear drops 0.25ml unit dose | 15 unit dose PoM £6.01 DT = £6.01

Combinations available: *Ciprofloxacin with dexamethasone*, p. 864 · ***Ciprofloxacin with fluocinolone acetonide*,** p. 864

ANTIBACTERIALS › OTHER

Chloramphenicol 24-Jul-2024

- **DRUG ACTION** Chloramphenicol is a potent broad-spectrum antibiotic.

- **INDICATIONS AND DOSE**

Bacterial infection in otitis externa

▶ TO THE EAR
▸ Child: Apply 2–3 drops 2–3 times a day

- **CAUTIONS** Avoid prolonged use
- **INTERACTIONS** → Appendix 1: chloramphenicol
- **SIDE-EFFECTS** Blood disorder · bone marrow depression
- **PATIENT AND CARER ADVICE**
  Medicines for Children leaflet: Chloramphenicol ear drops for ear infections (otitis externa) www.medicinesforchildren.org.uk/medicines/chloramphenicol-ear-drops-for-ear-infections-otitis-externa/
- **LESS SUITABLE FOR PRESCRIBING** Chloramphenicol ear drops are less suitable for prescribing.
- **MEDICINAL FORMS** There can be variation in the licensing of different medicines containing the same drug.

Ear drops

EXCIPIENTS: May contain Propylene glycol

▸ Chloramphenicol (Non-proprietary)
Chloramphenicol 50 mg per 1 ml Chloramphenicol 5% ear drops | 10 ml PoM £154.95–£264.96 DT = £154.95
Chloramphenicol 100 mg per 1 ml Chloramphenicol 10% ear drops | 10 ml PoM £144.23–£265.38 DT = £144.23

ANTIFUNGALS › IMIDAZOLE ANTIFUNGALS

Clotrimazole 10-Nov-2021

- **INDICATIONS AND DOSE**

Fungal infection in otitis externa

▶ TO THE EAR
▸ Child: Apply 2–3 times a day continue for at least 14 days after disappearance of infection

- **INTERACTIONS** → Appendix 1: antifungals, azoles
- **SIDE-EFFECTS** Hypersensitivity · oedema · pain · paraesthesia · skin reactions
- **PATIENT AND CARER ADVICE**
Medicines for Children leaflet: Clotrimazole for fungal infections www.medicinesforchildren.org.uk/medicines/clotrimazole-for-fungal-infections/

- **MEDICINAL FORMS** There can be variation in the licensing of different medicines containing the same drug.

Cutaneous or ear solution

▸ Canesten (clotrimazole) (Bayer Plc)
Clotrimazole 10 mg per 1 ml Canesten 1% solution | 20 ml P £2.54 DT = £2.54

CORTICOSTEROIDS

908

Betamethasone

26-Jul-2025

- **DRUG ACTION** Betamethasone has very high glucocorticoid activity and insignificant mineralocorticoid activity.

- **INDICATIONS AND DOSE**

BETNESOL®

Eczematous inflammation in otitis externa
▶ TO THE EAR
▸ Child: Apply 2–3 drops every 2–3 hours, reduce frequency when relief obtained

VISTAMETHASONE®

Eczematous inflammation in otitis externa
▶ TO THE EAR
▸ Child: Apply 2–3 drops every 3–4 hours, reduce frequency when relief obtained

- **CONTRA-INDICATIONS** Avoid alone in the presence of untreated infection (combine with suitable anti-infective)
- **CAUTIONS** Avoid prolonged use
- **INTERACTIONS** → Appendix 1: corticosteroids
- **SIDE-EFFECTS** Since systemic absorption can follow local administration, also consider the side-effects of systemic corticosteroids.

- **MEDICINAL FORMS** There can be variation in the licensing of different medicines containing the same drug.

Ear/eye/nose drops solution

EXCIPIENTS: May contain Benzalkonium chloride, disodium edetate

▸ Betnesol (RPH Pharmaceuticals AB)
Betamethasone sodium phosphate 1 mg per 1 ml Betnesol 0.1% eye/ear/nose drops | 10 ml PoM £2.32 DT = £2.32

Combinations available: *Betamethasone with neomycin*, p. 864

Flumetasone pivalate with clioquinol

26-Jul-2025

- **INDICATIONS AND DOSE**

Eczematous inflammation in otitis externa | Mild bacterial or fungal infections in otitis externa
▶ TO THE EAR
▸ Child 2–17 years: 2–3 drops twice daily for 7–10 days

IMPORTANT SAFETY INFORMATION

MHRA/CHM ADVICE: CORTICOSTEROIDS: RARE RISK OF CENTRAL SEROUS CHORIORETINOPATHY WITH LOCAL AS WELL AS SYSTEMIC ADMINISTRATION (AUGUST 2017)

See Corticosteroids, general use p. 537.

ADRENAL INSUFFICIENCY CARD (APRIL 2023)

The British Society for Paediatric Endocrinology and Diabetes (BSPED) has developed an Adrenal Insufficiency Card which should be issued to children with adrenal insufficiency and steroid dependence. The card includes a management summary for the emergency treatment of adrenal crisis and sick day dosing, and can be issued by any healthcare professional managing such patients. The BSPED Adrenal Insufficiency Card is available at: www.bsped.org.uk/adrenal-insufficiency.

- **CONTRA-INDICATIONS** Iodine sensitivity
- **CAUTIONS** Avoid prolonged use · manufacturer advises avoid in perforated tympanic membrane (but used by specialists for short periods)
- **SIDE-EFFECTS** Paraesthesia · skin reactions
- **PATIENT AND CARER ADVICE** Clioquinol stains skin and clothing.
If systemic absorption occurs following topical and local use, side-effects applicable to systemic corticosteroids may apply; a patient information leaflet should be supplied and the need for a Steroid Treatment Card considered, see Corticosteroids, general use p. 537.

- **MEDICINAL FORMS** There can be variation in the licensing of different medicines containing the same drug.

Ear drops

▸ Flumetasone pivalate with clioquinol (Non-proprietary)
Flumetasone pivalate 200 microgram per 1 ml, Clioquinol 10 mg per 1 ml Flumetasone 0.02% / Clioquinol 1% ear drops | 7.5 ml PoM £11.34 DT = £11.34

908

Prednisolone

26-Jul-2025

- **DRUG ACTION** Prednisolone exerts predominantly glucocorticoid effects with minimal mineralocorticoid effects.

- **INDICATIONS AND DOSE**

Eczematous inflammation in otitis externa
▶ TO THE EAR
▸ Child: Apply 2–3 drops every 2–3 hours, frequency to be reduced when relief obtained

- **CONTRA-INDICATIONS** Avoid alone in the presence of untreated infection (combine with suitable anti-infective)
- **CAUTIONS** Avoid prolonged use
- **INTERACTIONS** → Appendix 1: corticosteroids
- **SIDE-EFFECTS** Local reaction
SIDE-EFFECTS, FURTHER INFORMATION Since systemic absorption can follow local administration, also consider the side-effects of systemic corticosteroids.

- **MEDICINAL FORMS** There can be variation in the licensing of different medicines containing the same drug. Forms available from special-order manufacturers include: ear drops

Ear drops

EXCIPIENTS: May contain Benzalkonium chloride, disodium edetate

Ear/eye drops solution

EXCIPIENTS: May contain Benzalkonium chloride, disodium edetate

▸ Prednisolone (Non-proprietary)
Prednisolone sodium phosphate 5 mg per 1 ml Prednisolone sodium phosphate 0.5% ear/eye drops | 10 ml PoM £2.57 DT = £2.57

CORTICOSTEROIDS > CORTICOSTEROID COMBINATIONS WITH ANTI-INFECTIVES

Betamethasone with neomycin

20-Jun-2025

The properties listed below are those particular to the combination only. For the properties of the components please consider, betamethasone p. 863.

● **INDICATIONS AND DOSE**

Eczematous inflammation in otitis externa

▶ TO THE EAR USING EAR DROPS

▸ Child: Apply 2–3 drops 3–4 times a day

IMPORTANT SAFETY INFORMATION

MHRA/CHM ADVICE: AMINOGLYCOSIDES (GENTAMICIN, AMIKACIN, TOBRAMYCIN, AND NEOMYCIN): INCREASED RISK OF DEAFNESS IN PATIENTS WITH MITOCHONDRIAL MUTATIONS (JANUARY 2021)

The use of aminoglycosides is associated with rare cases of ototoxicity. A safety review found an increased risk of deafness in patients with mitochondrial mutations (particularly the m.1555A>G mutation), including cases where the patient's aminoglycoside serum levels were within the recommended range. Nevertheless, these mitochondrial mutations are considered rare and penetrance is uncertain. No cases were identified with topical preparations but, based on a shared mechanism of effect, there is a potential risk with neomycin and other aminoglycosides administered at the site of toxicity i.e. the ear.

Healthcare professionals are advised to consider the need for aminoglycoside treatment versus alternative options in patients with susceptible mutations. The need for genetic testing especially in those requiring recurrent or long-term treatment with aminoglycosides should also be considered, however, urgent treatment should not be delayed. To minimise the risks of adverse effects, continuous monitoring of renal and auditory function, as well as hepatic and laboratory parameters, is recommended for all patients. Those with known mitochondrial mutations or a family history of ototoxicity are advised to inform their doctor or pharmacist before using an aminoglycoside.

● **CONTRA-INDICATIONS** Patent grommet (although may be used by specialists, see Ear p. 859) · perforated tympanic membrane (although may be used by specialists, see Ear p. 859)

● **CAUTIONS** Avoid prolonged use

● **INTERACTIONS** → Appendix 1: corticosteroids · neomycin

● **PRE-TREATMENT SCREENING** NHS England commissions genetic testing under the *National genomic test directory* indication: R65 - Aminoglycoside exposure posing risk to hearing. The testing criteria is significant exposure to aminoglycosides posing risk of ototoxicity. This testing is relevant to individuals with a predisposition to gram-negative infections or with hearing loss who have been exposed to aminoglycosides. For further information, see www.england.nhs.uk/publication/national-genomic-test-directories/.

● **MEDICINAL FORMS** There can be variation in the licensing of different medicines containing the same drug.

Ear/eye/nose drops solution

EXCIPIENTS: May contain Benzalkonium chloride, disodium edetate

▸ Betnesol-N (RPH Pharmaceuticals AB)

Betamethasone (as Betamethasone sodium phosphate) 1 mg per 1 ml, Neomycin sulfate 5 mg per 1 ml Betnesol-N ear/eye/nose drops | 10 ml PoM £2.39 DT = £2.39

Ciprofloxacin with dexamethasone

04-Nov-2020

The properties listed below are those particular to the combination only. For the properties of the components please consider, dexamethasone p. 543, ciprofloxacin p. 862.

● **INDICATIONS AND DOSE**

Acute otitis media in patients with tympanostomy tubes

▶ TO THE EAR

▸ Child 6 months–17 years: Apply 4 drops twice daily for 7 days

Acute otitis externa

▶ TO THE EAR

▸ Child 1–17 years: Apply 4 drops twice daily for 7 days

● **CONTRA-INDICATIONS** Fungal ear infections · viral ear infections

● **CAUTIONS** Avoid prolonged use

● **INTERACTIONS** → Appendix 1: corticosteroids · quinolones

● **SIDE-EFFECTS**

▶ **Common or very common** Ear discomfort

▶ **Uncommon** Ear infection fungal · flushing · irritability · malaise · otorrhoea · paraesthesia · skin reactions · taste altered · vomiting

▶ **Rare or very rare** Dizziness · headache · hearing loss · tinnitus

SIDE-EFFECTS, FURTHER INFORMATION Manufacturer advises further evaluation of underlying conditions if otorrhoea persists after a full course, or if at least two episodes of otorrhoea occur within 6 months.

● **PREGNANCY** Manufacturer advises use only if potential benefit outweighs risk—no information available.

● **BREAST FEEDING** Manufacturer advises caution—no information available.

● **PATIENT AND CARER ADVICE** Manufacturer advises counselling on administration.

● **NATIONAL FUNDING/ACCESS DECISIONS**

For full details see funding body website

Scottish Medicines Consortium (SMC) decisions

▸ **Ciprofloxacin with dexamethasone (*Cilodex*®) for treatment of the following infections in adults and children: Acute otitis media in patients with tympanostomy tubes (AOMT) (July 2017)** SMC No. 1256/17 Recommended with restrictions

● **MEDICINAL FORMS** There can be variation in the licensing of different medicines containing the same drug.

Ear drops

EXCIPIENTS: May contain Benzalkonium chloride, disodium edetate

▸ Ciprofloxacin with dexamethasone (Non-proprietary)

Dexamethasone 1 mg per 1 ml, Ciprofloxacin (as Ciprofloxacin hydrochloride) 3 mg per 1 ml Ciprofloxacin 0.3% / Dexamethasone 0.1% ear drops | 5 ml PoM £6.12–£11.50 DT = £6.12

Ciprofloxacin with fluocinolone acetonide

26-Jul-2025

The properties listed below are those particular to the combination only. For the properties of the components please consider, ciprofloxacin p. 862.

● **INDICATIONS AND DOSE**

Acute otitis externa | Acute otitis media in patients with tympanostomy tubes

▶ TO THE EAR

▸ Child 6 months–17 years: Apply 0.25 mL twice daily for 7 days

DOSE EQUIVALENCE AND CONVERSION
- Each 0.25 mL dose contains 0.75 mg ciprofloxacin and 0.0625 mg of fluocinolone acetonide.

IMPORTANT SAFETY INFORMATION

MHRA/CHM ADVICE: CORTICOSTEROIDS: RARE RISK OF CENTRAL SEROUS CHORIORETINOPATHY WITH LOCAL AS WELL AS SYSTEMIC ADMINISTRATION (AUGUST 2017)

See Corticosteroids, general use p. 537.

ADRENAL INSUFFICIENCY CARD (APRIL 2023)

The British Society for Paediatric Endocrinology and Diabetes (BSPED) has developed an Adrenal Insufficiency Card which should be issued to children with adrenal insufficiency and steroid dependence. The card includes a management summary for the emergency treatment of adrenal crisis and sick day dosing, and can be issued by any healthcare professional managing such patients. The BSPED Adrenal Insufficiency Card is available at: www.bsped.org.uk/adrenal-insufficiency.

- **CONTRA-INDICATIONS** Fungal ear infections · viral ear infections
- **INTERACTIONS** → Appendix 1: fluocinolone · quinolones
- **SIDE-EFFECTS**
  - **Common or very common** Ear discomfort · taste altered
  - **Uncommon** Crying · dizziness · fatigue · flushing · headache · hearing impairment · increased risk of infection · irritability · otorrhoea · paraesthesia · skin reactions · tinnitus · tympanic membrane disorder · vomiting

  SIDE-EFFECTS, FURTHER INFORMATION Manufacturer advises further evaluation of underlying conditions if otorrhoea persists after a full course, or if at least two episodes of otorrhoea occur within 6 months.
- **PREGNANCY** Manufacturer advises use only if potential benefit outweighs risk—limited information available.
- **BREAST FEEDING** Manufacturer advises caution.
- **PATIENT AND CARER ADVICE** Manufacturer advises counselling on administration.

  If systemic absorption occurs following topical and local use, side-effects applicable to systemic corticosteroids may apply; a patient information leaflet should be supplied and the need for a Steroid Treatment Card considered, see Corticosteroids, general use p. 537.
- **MEDICINAL FORMS** There can be variation in the licensing of different medicines containing the same drug.

Ear drops

EXCIPIENTS: May contain Polysorbates
- Cetraxal Plus (Aspire Pharma Ltd)

  Fluocinolone acetonide 250 microgram per 1 ml, Ciprofloxacin (as ciprofloxacin hydrochloride) 3 mg per 1 ml Cetraxal Plus 3mg/ml + 0.25mg/ml ear drops 0.25ml unit dose | 15 unit dose PoM £6.01 DT = £6.01

Dexamethasone with framycetin sulfate and gramicidin

02-Mar-2021

The properties listed below are those particular to the combination only. For the properties of the components please consider, dexamethasone p. 543, framycetin sulfate p. 860.

- **INDICATIONS AND DOSE**

Eczematous inflammation in otitis externa
- TO THE EAR
- Child: 2–3 drops 3–4 times a day

- **CAUTIONS** Avoid prolonged use
- **INTERACTIONS** → Appendix 1: corticosteroids
- **LESS SUITABLE FOR PRESCRIBING** *Sofradex*® is less suitable for prescribing.
- **MEDICINAL FORMS** There can be variation in the licensing of different medicines containing the same drug.

Ear/eye drops solution

EXCIPIENTS: May contain Polysorbates
- Sofradex (Neon Healthcare Ltd)

  Gramicidin 50 microgram per 1 ml, Dexamethasone (as Dexamethasone sodium metasulfobenzoate) 500 microgram per 1 ml, Framycetin sulfate 5 mg per 1 ml Sofradex ear/eye drops | 8 ml PoM £7.50

Dexamethasone with glacial acetic acid and neomycin sulfate

29-Mar-2023

The properties listed below are those particular to the combination only. For the properties of the components please consider, dexamethasone p. 543.

- **INDICATIONS AND DOSE**

Eczematous inflammation in otitis externa
- TO THE EAR
- Child 2–17 years: Apply 1 spray 3 times a day

IMPORTANT SAFETY INFORMATION

MHRA/CHM ADVICE: AMINOGLYCOSIDES (GENTAMICIN, AMIKACIN, TOBRAMYCIN, AND NEOMYCIN): INCREASED RISK OF DEAFNESS IN PATIENTS WITH MITOCHONDRIAL MUTATIONS (JANUARY 2021)

The use of aminoglycosides is associated with rare cases of ototoxicity. A safety review found an increased risk of deafness in patients with mitochondrial mutations (particularly the m.1555A>G mutation), including cases where the patient's aminoglycoside serum levels were within the recommended range. Nevertheless, these mitochondrial mutations are considered rare and penetrance is uncertain. No cases were identified with topical preparations but, based on a shared mechanism of effect, there is a potential risk with neomycin and other aminoglycosides administered at the site of toxicity i.e. the ear.

Healthcare professionals are advised to consider the need for aminoglycoside treatment versus alternative options in patients with susceptible mutations. The need for genetic testing especially in those requiring recurrent or long-term treatment with aminoglycosides should also be considered, however, urgent treatment should not be delayed. To minimise the risks of adverse effects, continuous monitoring of renal and auditory function, as well as hepatic and laboratory parameters, is recommended for all patients. Those with known mitochondrial mutations or a family history of ototoxicity are advised to inform their doctor or pharmacist before using an aminoglycoside.

- **CONTRA-INDICATIONS** Patent grommet (although may be used by specialists, see Ear p. 859) · perforated tympanic membrane (although may be used by specialists, see Ear p. 859)
- **CAUTIONS** Avoid prolonged use
- **INTERACTIONS** → Appendix 1: corticosteroids · neomycin
- **SIDE-EFFECTS** Paraesthesia · skin reactions · vision blurred
- **PRE-TREATMENT SCREENING** NHS England commissions genetic testing under the *National genomic test directory* indication: R65 - Aminoglycoside exposure posing risk to hearing. The testing criteria is significant exposure to aminoglycosides posing risk of ototoxicity. This testing is relevant to individuals with a predisposition to gram-negative infections or with hearing loss who have been

exposed to aminoglycosides. For further information, see www.england.nhs.uk/publication/national-genomic-test-directories/.

- **MEDICINAL FORMS** There can be variation in the licensing of different medicines containing the same drug.

Spray

EXCIPIENTS: May contain Hydroxybenzoates (parabens)

▸ **Dexamethasone with glacial acetic acid and neomycin sulfate (Non-proprietary)**

Dexamethasone 1 mg per 1 gram, Neomycin sulfate 5 mg per 1 gram, Acetic acid glacial 20 mg per 1 gram Dexamethasone 0.1% / Neomycin 0.5% / Acetic acid (glacial) 2% ear spray | 5 ml PoM £8.58–£16.30 DT = £8.58

Hydrocortisone with neomycin and polymyxin B sulfate

29-Mar-2023

The properties listed below are those particular to the combination only. For the properties of the components please consider, hydrocortisone p. 882.

- **INDICATIONS AND DOSE**

Bacterial infection in otitis externa

▸ TO THE EAR

▸ Child 3–17 years: Apply 3 drops 3–4 times a day for 7 days, review treatment if there is no clinical improvement

IMPORTANT SAFETY INFORMATION

MHRA/CHM ADVICE: AMINOGLYCOSIDES (GENTAMICIN, AMIKACIN, TOBRAMYCIN, AND NEOMYCIN): INCREASED RISK OF DEAFNESS IN PATIENTS WITH MITOCHONDRIAL MUTATIONS (JANUARY 2021)

The use of aminoglycosides is associated with rare cases of ototoxicity. A safety review found an increased risk of deafness in patients with mitochondrial mutations (particularly the m.1555A>G mutation), including cases where the patient's aminoglycoside serum levels were within the recommended range. Nevertheless, these mitochondrial mutations are considered rare and penetrance is uncertain. No cases were identified with topical preparations but, based on a shared mechanism of effect, there is a potential risk with neomycin and other aminoglycosides administered at the site of toxicity i.e. the ear.

Healthcare professionals are advised to consider the need for aminoglycoside treatment versus alternative options in patients with susceptible mutations. The need for genetic testing especially in those requiring recurrent or long-term treatment with aminoglycosides should also be considered, however, urgent treatment should not be delayed. To minimise the risks of adverse effects, continuous monitoring of renal and auditory function, as well as hepatic and laboratory parameters, is recommended for all patients. Those with known mitochondrial mutations or a family history of ototoxicity are advised to inform their doctor or pharmacist before using an aminoglycoside.

- **CONTRA-INDICATIONS** Patent grommet (although may be used by specialists, see Ear p. 859) · perforated tympanic membrane (although may be used by specialists, see Ear p. 859)
- **CAUTIONS** Avoid prolonged use
- **INTERACTIONS** → Appendix 1: corticosteroids · neomycin · polymyxin b
- **SIDE-EFFECTS**
  - ▸ **Rare or very rare** Headache · paraesthesia · skin reactions · telangiectasia
- **RENAL IMPAIRMENT** Manufacturer advises avoid prolonged, unsupervised use.

Dose adjustments Manufacturer advises reduce dose.

- **PRE-TREATMENT SCREENING** NHS England commissions genetic testing under the *National genomic test directory* indication: R65 - Aminoglycoside exposure posing risk to hearing. The testing criteria is significant exposure to aminoglycosides posing risk of ototoxicity. This testing is relevant to individuals with a predisposition to gram-negative infections or with hearing loss who have been exposed to aminoglycosides. For further information, see www.england.nhs.uk/publication/national-genomic-test-directories/.
- **MEDICINAL FORMS** There can be variation in the licensing of different medicines containing the same drug.

Ear drops

EXCIPIENTS: May contain Cetostearyl alcohol (including cetyl and stearyl alcohol), hydroxybenzoates (parabens), polysorbates

▸ **Otosporin** (Phenix Labs Ltd)

Hydrocortisone 10 mg per 1 ml, Neomycin sulfate 3400 unit per 1 ml, Polymyxin B sulfate 10000 unit per 1 ml Otosporin ear drops | 10 ml PoM £7.45

DERMATOLOGICAL DRUGS › ASTRINGENTS

Aluminium acetate

23-Nov-2023

- **INDICATIONS AND DOSE**

OTINOVA ®

Inflammation in otitis externa

▸ TO THE EAR

▸ Child 5–17 years: Apply 1–2 sprays twice daily for max. 7 days, to be administered in the morning and evening

DOSE EQUIVALENCE AND CONVERSION

▸ *Otinova* ® contains aluminium acetate and aluminium acetotartrate equivalent to aluminium 1.8%, and acetic acid (Burow's solution BP).

- **MEDICINAL FORMS** There can be variation in the licensing of different medicines containing the same drug.

Ear drops

▸ **Otinova** (Kestrel Medical Ltd)

Aluminium acetate 130 mg per 1 ml Otinova ear spray | 15 ml £9.04

2 Otitis media

Other drugs used for Otitis media Ciprofloxacin with dexamethasone, p. 864 · Ciprofloxacin with fluocinolone acetonide, p. 864

ANALGESICS › NON-STEROIDAL ANTI-INFLAMMATORY DRUGS

Phenazone with lidocaine

26-Nov-2020

The properties listed below are those particular to the combination only. For the properties of the components please consider, lidocaine hydrochloride p. 880.

- **INDICATIONS AND DOSE**

Acute otitis media | Barotraumatic otitis

▸ TO THE EAR

▸ Neonate: Apply 4 drops 2–3 times a day, re-evaluate therapy if symptoms do not improve within 7 days or worsen at any time.

▸ Child: Apply 4 drops 2–3 times a day, re-evaluate therapy if symptoms do not improve within 7 days or worsen at any time

- **CONTRA-INDICATIONS** Perforated tympanic membrane (risk of ototoxicity)
- **INTERACTIONS** → Appendix 1: antiarrhythmics · NSAIDs
- **SIDE-EFFECTS**
  - ▶ Rare or very rare Skin reactions · tympanic membrane hyperaemia
- **PREGNANCY** EvGr Use with caution—no information available but systemic absorption unlikely with intact tympanic membrane. ⟨M⟩
- **BREAST FEEDING** EvGr Use with caution—no information available but systemic absorption unlikely with intact tympanic membrane. ⟨M⟩
- **MEDICINAL FORMS** There can be variation in the licensing of different medicines containing the same drug.

Ear drops

EXCIPIENTS: May contain Ethanol

▸ **Otigo** (Renascience Pharma Ltd)
Lidocaine hydrochloride 10 mg per 1 gram, Phenazone 40 mg per 1 gram Otigo 40mg/g / 10mg/g ear drops | 15 ml PoM £8.92 DT = £8.92

3 Removal of earwax

BICARBONATE

Sodium bicarbonate

19-Apr-2022

- **INDICATIONS AND DOSE**

Removal of earwax (with 5% ear drop solution)

▶ TO THE EAR
▸ Child: (consult product literature)

- **INTERACTIONS** → Appendix 1: sodium bicarbonate
- **SIDE-EFFECTS** Dry ear
- **MEDICINAL FORMS** There can be variation in the licensing of different medicines containing the same drug.

Ear drops

▸ **Sodium bicarbonate (Non-proprietary)**
Sodium bicarbonate 50 mg per 1 ml Sodium bicarbonate 5% ear drops | 10 ml £1.23–£1.25

▸ **KliarVax Sodium Bicarbonate** (Essential-Healthcare Ltd)
Sodium bicarbonate 50 mg per 1 ml KliarVax Sodium Bicarbonate ear drops | 10 ml £0.94

▸ **Knoxzy** (Biovantic Pharma Ltd)
Sodium bicarbonate 50 mg per 1 ml Knoxzy Sodium Bicarbonate 5% ear drops | 10 ml £0.95

SOFTENING DRUGS

Almond oil

04-Aug-2020

- **INDICATIONS AND DOSE**

Removal of earwax

▶ TO THE EAR
▸ Child: Allow drops to warm to room temperature before use (consult product literature)

- **DIRECTIONS FOR ADMINISTRATION** Expert sources advise the patient should lie with the affected ear uppermost for 5 to 10 minutes after a generous amount of the softening remedy has been introduced into the ear.
- **MEDICINAL FORMS** There can be variation in the licensing of different medicines containing the same drug.

Form unstated

▸ **Almond oil (Non-proprietary)**
Almond oil 1 ml per 1 ml Almond oil liquid | 70 ml £1.27 | 200 ml £2.52

Docusate sodium

12-Apr-2023

(Dioctyl sodium sulphosuccinate)

- **INDICATIONS AND DOSE**

Removal of ear wax

▶ TO THE EAR
▸ Child 1–17 years: (consult product literature)

- **INTERACTIONS** → Appendix 1: docusates
- **SIDE-EFFECTS** Skin reactions
- **LESS SUITABLE FOR PRESCRIBING** Ear drops less suitable for prescribing.
- **MEDICINAL FORMS** There can be variation in the licensing of different medicines containing the same drug.

Ear drops

EXCIPIENTS: May contain Propylene glycol

▸ **Molcer** (Wallace Manufacturing Chemists Ltd)
Docusate sodium 50 mg per 1 ml Molcer ear drops | 15 ml P £5.60 DT = £5.60

▸ **Waxsol** (Ceuta Healthcare Ltd)
Docusate sodium 5 mg per 1 ml Waxsol ear drops | 10 ml P £2.93 DT = £1.95

Olive oil

04-Aug-2020

- **INDICATIONS AND DOSE**

Removal of earwax

▶ TO THE EAR
▸ Child: Apply twice daily for several days (if wax is hard and impacted)

Removal of earwax (dose approved for use by community practitioner nurse prescribers)

▶ TO THE EAR
▸ Child: (consult product literature)

- **DIRECTIONS FOR ADMINISTRATION** Expert sources advise the patient should lie with the affected ear uppermost for 5 to 10 minutes after a generous amount of the softening remedy has been introduced into the ear. Allow ear drops to warm to room temperature before use.
- **MEDICINAL FORMS** There can be variation in the licensing of different medicines containing the same drug.

Ear drops

▸ **Olive oil (Non-proprietary)**
Olive oil ear drops | 10 ml £1.35–£1.42

▸ **Cerumol (olive oil)** (Thornton & Ross Ltd)
Cerumol olive oil ear drops | 10 ml ⊠

▸ **KliarVax** (Essential-Healthcare Ltd)
KliarVax Olive Oil ear drops | 10 ml £0.81

▸ **Knoxzy** (Biovantic Pharma Ltd)
Knoxzy Olive Oil ear drops | 10 ml £0.90

▸ **Olive oil** (Thornton & Ross Ltd)
Care olive oil ear drops | 10 ml £1.42

▸ **Otadrop** (JFA Medical Ltd)
Otadrop olive oil ear drops | 10 ml £0.80

▸ **St George's** (St Georges Medical Ltd)
Olive oil ear drops | 10 ml £1.40 | 20 ml £2.70

Spray

▸ **AactiWax** (TriOn Pharma Ltd)
AactiWax Olive Oil ear spray | 10 ml £1.42

▸ **Earol** (HL Healthcare Ltd)
Earol olive oil ear spray | 10 ml ⊠

Urea hydrogen peroxide

02-Sep-2020

- **INDICATIONS AND DOSE**

Softening and removal of earwax

▶ TO THE EAR
▸ Child: (consult product literature)

- **PATIENT AND CARER ADVICE** The patient should lie with the affected ear uppermost for 5 to 10 minutes after a generous amount of the softening remedy has been introduced into the ear.
- **LESS SUITABLE FOR PRESCRIBING** Urea-hydrogen peroxide ear drops are less suitable for prescribing.

- **MEDICINAL FORMS** There can be variation in the licensing of different medicines containing the same drug.

Ear drops

▸ Otex (Diomed Developments Ltd)
Urea hydrogen peroxide 50 mg per 1 gram Otex 5% ear drops | 8 ml [P] £3.59 DT = £3.59

Nose

Nose

04-Nov-2021

Rhinitis

Rhinitis may be acute or chronic, allergic or non-allergic. Nasal spray and drop preparations often carry indications for the management of allergic rhinitis and perennial rhinitis. Many nasal preparations contain sympathomimetic drugs which may irritate the nasal mucosa.

Children with nasal congestion and obstructive sleep apnoea/hypopnoea syndrome or obesity hypoventilation syndrome may have underlying allergic or vasomotor rhinitis. For guidance on the management of rhinitis in children aged over 16 years with these syndromes, see NICE guideline: **Obstructive sleep apnoea/hypopnoea syndrome and obesity hypoventilation syndrome in over 16s** (available at: www.nice.org.uk/guidance/ng202).

Drugs used in nasal allergy

EvGr Sodium chloride 0.9% solution p. 728 may be used as nasal irrigation in allergic rhinitis for modest symptom reduction, and to reduce the need for other drug treatment.

Mild allergic rhinitis is controlled by **antihistamines** (see under Antihistamines, allergen immunotherapy and allergic emergencies p. 199) or topical **nasal corticosteroids**. Topical antihistamines (e.g. azelastine hydrochloride p. 872) are faster acting than oral antihistamines and therefore useful for controlling breakthrough symptoms in allergic rhinitis; they are less effective than topical nasal corticosteroids. Topical nasal decongestants can be used for a short period to provide quick relief from congestion and allow penetration of a topical nasal corticosteroid. Systemic nasal decongestants are weakly effective in reducing nasal obstruction but have considerable potential for side-effects, and therefore are not recommended. Sodium cromoglicate is a weakly effective alternative in children with mild symptoms, sporadic seasonal problems, or limited allergen exposure.

Moderate to severe allergic rhinitis can be relieved by topical **nasal corticosteroids** during periods of allergen exposure. Severe allergic rhinitis causing very disabling symptoms despite conventional treatment may justify the use of **oral corticosteroids** for short periods. In severe cases, oral corticosteroids may also be used in combination with nasal corticosteroids during treatment initiation to relieve severe mucosal oedema and allow the spray to penetrate the nasal cavity.

Nasal ipratropium bromide p. 872 may be added to allergic rhinitis treatment when watery rhinorrhoea persists despite treatment with topical nasal steroids and antihistamines; it has no effect on other nasal symptoms.

In seasonal allergic rhinitis (e.g. hay fever), treatment should begin 2 to 3 weeks before the season commences and/or exposure to the allergen.

Montelukast p. 194 is less effective than topical nasal corticosteroids but can be used in children with seasonal allergic rhinitis and concomitant asthma. (A)

Corticosteroids

EvGr Topical nasal corticosteroid preparations should be avoided in the presence of untreated nasal infections, after nasal surgery (until healing has occurred), and in pulmonary tuberculosis. Systemic absorption may follow nasal administration particularly if high doses are used or if treatment is prolonged. The extent of absorption varies between steroids; mometasone furoate p. 875 and fluticasone p. 874 have negligible systemic absorption, others have modest absorption, whilst betamethasone p. 873 has high systemic absorption and should only be used short-term. The growth of children receiving treatment with corticosteroids should be monitored; especially in those receiving corticosteroids via multiple routes. (A)

Nasal polyps

EvGr All children presenting with nasal polyps must be screened for cystic fibrosis and referred to an ear, nose and throat specialist for initial review. Nasal polyps may be treated with topical nasal corticosteroids (drops or spray). There may be a higher risk of side-effects with use of nasal drops compared to nasal spray due to greater systemic absorption and incorrect administration of drops. To reduce the risk, the drops must be administered with the child in the 'head down' position. A short course of a systemic corticosteroid can provide symptomatic relief but effects may be temporary and its use is rare due to concerns of systemic side-effects. If systemic corticosteroids are given, they should be used in combination with topical nasal corticosteroids. (A)

Pregnancy

EvGr If a pregnant female cannot tolerate the symptoms of allergic rhinitis, treatment may be given. (A) Although the safety of nasal corticosteroids in pregnancy has not been established through clinical trials, only minimal amounts of nasal corticosteroids are systemically absorbed. Beclometasone dipropionate p. 873, budesonide p. 873, and fluticasone are widely used in asthmatic pregnant females; fluticasone has the lowest systemic absorption when used intra-nasally. EvGr Decongestants are not recommended however, some antihistamines and sodium cromoglicate may be used. (A)

Topical nasal decongestants

The nasal mucosa is sensitive to changes in atmospheric temperature and humidity and these alone may cause slight nasal congestion. EvGr Sodium chloride 0.9% given as nasal drops, spray, or irrigation may relieve nasal congestion.

Symptoms of nasal congestion associated with allergic rhinitis, the common cold, and sinusitis may be relieved by the short-term use (usually not longer than 7 days) of decongestant nasal drops and sprays. (A) These all contain sympathomimetic drugs which exert their effect by vasoconstriction of the mucosal blood vessels which in turn reduces oedema of the nasal mucosa. Their use, especially with longer durations, can give rise to rebound congestion (rhinitis medicamentosa) on withdrawal, due to a secondary vasodilatation with a subsequent temporary increase in nasal congestion. This in turn tempts the further use of the decongestant, leading to a vicious cycle of events; tolerance with reduced effect may also be seen with excessive use.

EvGr Non-allergic watery rhinorrhoea often responds to treatment with nasal antimuscarinic ipratropium bromide. (A)

Nasal preparations for infection

Nasal staphylococci

EvGr Elimination of organisms such as staphylococci from the nasal vestibule can be achieved by the use of antimicrobial preparations such as chlorhexidine with neomycin cream p. 871 (*Naseptin*®). A nasal ointment containing mupirocin p. 871 is available if *Naseptin*® is unsuitable or ineffective.

In hospitals or in care establishments, mupirocin nasal ointment can be used for eradication of nasal carriage of meticillin-resistant *Staphylococcus aureus* (MRSA). ⟨A⟩

For information on eradication of MRSA, consult local infection control policy. See also management of MRSA p. 445.

1 Nasal congestion

SYMPATHOMIMETICS › VASOCONSTRICTOR

Ephedrine hydrochloride

29-Mar-2022

- **INDICATIONS AND DOSE**

Nasal congestion | Sinusitis affecting the maxillary antrum

▶ BY INTRANASAL ADMINISTRATION

▸ Child 12–17 years: Apply 1–2 drops up to 4 times a day as required for a maximum of 7 days, to be instilled into each nostril, administer ephedrine 0.5% nasal drops

IMPORTANT SAFETY INFORMATION

CHM/MHRA ADVICE

The CHM/MHRA has stated that non-prescription cough and cold medicines containing ephedrine can be considered for up to 5 days' treatment in children aged 6–12 years after basic principles of best care have been tried; these medicines should not be used in children under 6 years of age.

- **CAUTIONS** Avoid excessive or prolonged use · cardiovascular disease · diabetes mellitus · hypertension · hyperthyroidism
- **INTERACTIONS** → Appendix 1: sympathomimetics, vasoconstrictor
- **SIDE-EFFECTS**

▶ **Common or very common** Anxiety · headache · insomnia · nausea

▶ **Frequency not known** Appetite decreased · arrhythmia · circulation impaired · dermatitis · dizziness · drug dependence · dry mouth · dyspnoea · hallucination · hyperglycaemia · hyperhidrosis · hypersalivation · hypertension · hypokalaemia · hypotension · irritability · muscle weakness · mydriasis · pain · palpitations · paranoia · piloerection · rebound congestion · syncope · thirst · tremor · urinary disorders · vasoconstriction · vasodilation · vomiting

- **PREGNANCY** Manufacturer advises avoid.
- **BREAST FEEDING** Present in milk; manufacturer advises avoid—irritability and disturbed sleep reported.
- **PRESCRIBING AND DISPENSING INFORMATION** For nasal drops, the BP directs that if no strength is specified 0.5% drops should be supplied.
- **PROFESSION SPECIFIC INFORMATION**

Dental practitioners' formulary Ephedrine nasal drops may be prescribed.

- **EXCEPTIONS TO LEGAL CATEGORY** Ephedrine nasal drops can be sold to the public provided no more than 180 mg of ephedrine base (or salts) are supplied at one time, and pseudoephedrine salts are not supplied at the same time; for conditions that apply to supplies made at the request of a patient, see *Medicines, Ethics and Practice*, London, Pharmaceutical Press (always consult latest edition).
- **MEDICINAL FORMS** Forms available from special-order manufacturers include: nasal drops

Pseudoephedrine hydrochloride

28-Mar-2024

- **INDICATIONS AND DOSE**

Congestion of mucous membranes of upper respiratory tract

▶ BY MOUTH

▸ Child 6–11 years: 30 mg 3–4 times a day

▸ Child 12–17 years: 60 mg 3–4 times a day

IMPORTANT SAFETY INFORMATION

MHRA/CHM ADVICE: OVER-THE-COUNTER COUGH AND COLD MEDICINES FOR CHILDREN (APRIL 2009)

Children under 6 years should not be given over-the-counter cough and cold medicines containing pseudoephedrine.

MHRA/CHM ADVICE: PSEUDOEPHEDRINE: VERY RARE RISK OF POSTERIOR REVERSIBLE ENCEPHALOPATHY SYNDROME (PRES) AND REVERSIBLE CEREBRAL VASOCONSTRICTION SYNDROME (RCVS) (FEBRUARY 2024)

Healthcare professionals are reminded that PRES and RCVS are very rare side-effects of pseudoephedrine; affected patients typically recover fully within 3 months with early recognition and treatment. Pseudoephedrine-containing medicines are for short-term, symptomatic use only and are contra-indicated in patients with severe or uncontrolled hypertension, or severe renal disease. Patients and their carers should be advised on the symptoms of PRES and RCVS, and to stop taking pseudoephedrine-containing medicines and seek urgent medical attention if they develop a sudden severe headache or thunderclap headache, sudden onset of nausea or vomiting, confusion, seizures, and/or visual disturbances. Healthcare professionals should ask about the patient's medication history when presented with these symptoms.

- **CONTRA-INDICATIONS** Severe or uncontrolled hypertension
- **CAUTIONS** Diabetes · heart disease · hyperthyroidism · mild to moderate hypertension · raised intra-ocular pressure
- **INTERACTIONS** → Appendix 1: sympathomimetics, vasoconstrictor
- **SIDE-EFFECTS**

▶ **Common or very common** Anxiety · dizziness · dry mouth · headache · nausea · sleep disorders

▶ **Frequency not known** Akathisia · angioedema · angle closure glaucoma · arrhythmias · cerebrovascular insufficiency · circulation impaired · colitis ischaemic · drowsiness · hallucination · hypertension · mood altered · myocardial infarction · myocardial ischaemia · optic neuropathy · palpitations · paraesthesia · paranoid delusions · posterior reversible encephalopathy syndrome (PRES) · severe cutaneous adverse reactions (SCARs) · skin reactions · tremor · urinary disorders · vomiting

- **PREGNANCY** Defective closure of the abdominal wall (gastroschisis) reported very rarely in newborns after first trimester exposure.
- **BREAST FEEDING** May suppress lactation; avoid if lactation not well established or if milk production insufficient.
- **HEPATIC IMPAIRMENT** Manufacturer advises caution in severe impairment.
- **RENAL IMPAIRMENT** EvGr Use with caution in mild to moderate impairment; avoid in severe impairment. ⟨M⟩
- **LESS SUITABLE FOR PRESCRIBING** Pseudoephedrine hydrochloride is less suitable for prescribing.

● **EXCEPTIONS TO LEGAL CATEGORY** *Galpseud®* and *Sudafed®* can be sold to the public provided no more than 720 mg of pseudoephedrine salts are supplied, and ephedrine base (or salts) are not supplied at the same time; for details see *Medicines, Ethics and Practice*, London, Pharmaceutical Press (always consult latest edition).

● **MEDICINAL FORMS** There can be variation in the licensing of different medicines containing the same drug.

Oral tablet

▸ Pseudoephedrine hydrochloride (Non-proprietary)
Pseudoephedrine hydrochloride 60 mg Care Decongestant 60mg tablets | 12 tablet Ⓟ £2.37 DT = £3.02

▸ Sudafed Non-Drowsy Decongestant (pseudoephedrine) (McNeil Products Ltd)
Pseudoephedrine hydrochloride 60 mg Sudafed Decongestant 60mg tablets | 12 tablet Ⓟ £3.15 DT = £3.02

Oral solution

EXCIPIENTS: May contain Alcohol

▸ Sudafed Non-Drowsy Decongestant (pseudoephedrine) (McNeil Products Ltd)
Pseudoephedrine hydrochloride 6 mg per 1 ml Sudafed Decongestant 30mg/5ml liquid | 100 ml Ⓟ £2.87 DT = £2.87

Xylometazoline hydrochloride 13-Feb-2020

● **DRUG ACTION** Xylometazoline is a sympathomimetic.

● **INDICATIONS AND DOSE**

Nasal congestion

▶ BY INTRANASAL ADMINISTRATION USING NASAL DROPS

▸ Child 6–11 years: 1–2 drops 1–2 times a day as required for maximum duration of 5 days, 0.05% solution to be administered into each nostril

▸ Child 12–17 years: 2–3 drops 2–3 times a day as required for maximum duration of 7 days, 0.1% solution to be administered into each nostril

▶ BY INTRANASAL ADMINISTRATION USING NASAL SPRAY

▸ Child 12–17 years: 1 spray 1–3 times a day as required for maximum duration of 7 days, to be administered into each nostril

IMPORTANT SAFETY INFORMATION

The CHM/MHRA has stated that non-prescription cough and cold medicines containing oxymetazoline or xylometazoline can be considered for up to 5 days' treatment in children aged 6–12 years after basic principles of best care have been tried; these medicines should not be used in children under 6 years of age.

● **CAUTIONS** Angle-closure glaucoma · avoid excessive or prolonged use · cardiovascular disease · diabetes mellitus · hypertension · hyperthyroidism · rebound congestion

CAUTIONS, FURTHER INFORMATION

▸ Rebound congestion Sympathomimetic drugs are of limited value in the treatment of nasal congestion because they can, following prolonged use (more than 7 days), give rise to a rebound congestion (rhinitis medicamentosa) on withdrawal, due to a secondary vasodilatation with a subsequent temporary increase in nasal congestion. This in turn tempts the further use of the decongestant, leading to a vicious cycle of events.

● **INTERACTIONS** → Appendix 1: sympathomimetics, vasoconstrictor

● **SIDE-EFFECTS** Cardiovascular effects · headache · hypersensitivity · nasal dryness · nausea · paraesthesia · visual impairment

SIDE-EFFECTS, FURTHER INFORMATION Use of decongestants in infants and children under 6 years has been associated with agitated psychosis, ataxia, hallucinations, and even death—avoid.

● **PREGNANCY** Manufacturer advises avoid.

● **BREAST FEEDING** Manufacturer advises caution—no information available.

● **MEDICINAL FORMS** There can be variation in the licensing of different medicines containing the same drug.

Spray

▸ Xylometazoline hydrochloride (Non-proprietary)
Xylometazoline hydrochloride 1 mg per 1 ml Xylometazoline 0.1% nasal spray | 10 ml GSL £20.00 DT = £2.97

Nasal drops

▸ Otrivine (Haleon UK Trading Ltd)
Xylometazoline hydrochloride 500 microgram per 1 ml Otrivine Child nasal drops | 10 ml Ⓟ £2.80 DT = £2.80
Xylometazoline hydrochloride 1 mg per 1 ml Otrivine Adult 0.1% nasal drops | 10 ml GSL £2.50 DT = £2.50

2 Nasal infection

Sinusitis (acute) 31-Oct-2017

Description of condition

Sinusitis is an inflammation of the mucosal lining of the paranasal sinuses. Acute sinusitis (rhinosinusitis) is a self-limiting condition usually triggered by a viral upper-respiratory tract infection such as the 'common cold'. Occasionally, acute sinusitis may become complicated by a bacterial infection (*see Antibacterial therapy for acute sinusitis* in Nose infections, antibacterial therapy p. 370).

Children with acute sinusitis, particularly young children, often present with non-specific symptoms in the upper respiratory tract, including nasal blockage or congestion, discoloured nasal discharge, or cough during the day or night.

Symptoms usually improve within 2 to 3 weeks without requiring treatment.

Rarely, acute sinusitis may lead to orbital, intracranial or skeletal complications (e.g. periorbital cellulitis, symptoms or signs of meningitis).

Aims of treatment

Treatment is aimed at managing symptoms including pain, fever, and nasal congestion as well as treatment of bacterial infection if present.

Treatment

EvGr Children presenting with symptoms for around 10 *days or less*, should be given advice about the usual duration of acute sinusitis, self-care of pain or fever with paracetamol p. 325 or ibuprofen p. 821, and when to seek medical help. Children and their carers should be reassured that antibiotics are usually not required.

Children (over the age of 12) presenting with symptoms for around 10 *days or more* with no improvement could be considered for treatment with a high-dose nasal corticosteroid, such as mometasone furoate p. 875 [unlicensed use] or fluticasone p. 874 [unlicensed use] for 14 days.

If the child is systemically very unwell, has signs and symptoms of a more serious illness or condition, or is at high-risk of complications, an immediate antibiotic could be offered if deemed appropriate Ⓐ (*see Antibacterial therapy for acute sinusitis* in Nose infections, antibacterial therapy p. 370).

EvGr Children presenting with symptoms of acute sinusitis associated with a severe systemic infection or with orbital or intracranial complications should be referred to hospital. Ⓐ

Useful Resources

Sinusitis (acute): antimicrobial prescribing. National Institute for Health and Care Excellence. NICE guideline 79. October 2017.
www.nice.org.uk/guidance/ng79

ANTIBACTERIALS > AMINOGLYCOSIDES

Chlorhexidine with neomycin

20-Jun-2025

● **INDICATIONS AND DOSE**

Eradication of nasal carriage of staphylococci

▶ BY INTRANASAL ADMINISTRATION

▸ Child: Apply 4 times a day for 10 days

Preventing nasal carriage of staphylococci

▶ BY INTRANASAL ADMINISTRATION

▸ Child: Apply twice daily

IMPORTANT SAFETY INFORMATION

MHRA/CHM ADVICE: AMINOGLYCOSIDES (GENTAMICIN, AMIKACIN, TOBRAMYCIN, AND NEOMYCIN): INCREASED RISK OF DEAFNESS IN PATIENTS WITH MITOCHONDRIAL MUTATIONS (JANUARY 2021)

The use of aminoglycosides is associated with rare cases of ototoxicity. A safety review found an increased risk of deafness in patients with mitochondrial mutations (particularly the m.1555A>G mutation), including cases where the patient's aminoglycoside serum levels were within the recommended range. Nevertheless, these mitochondrial mutations are considered rare and penetrance is uncertain. No cases were identified with topical preparations but, based on a shared mechanism of effect, there is a potential risk with neomycin and other aminoglycosides administered at the site of toxicity i.e. the ear.

Healthcare professionals are advised to consider the need for aminoglycoside treatment versus alternative options in patients with susceptible mutations. The need for genetic testing especially in those requiring recurrent or long-term treatment with aminoglycosides should also be considered, however, urgent treatment should not be delayed. To minimise the risks of adverse effects, continuous monitoring of renal and auditory function, as well as hepatic and laboratory parameters, is recommended for all patients. Those with known mitochondrial mutations or a family history of ototoxicity are advised to inform their doctor or pharmacist before using an aminoglycoside.

● **PRE-TREATMENT SCREENING** NHS England commissions genetic testing under the *National genomic test directory* indication: R65 - Aminoglycoside exposure posing risk to hearing. The testing criteria is significant exposure to aminoglycosides posing risk of ototoxicity. This testing is relevant to individuals with a predisposition to gram-negative infections or with hearing loss who have been exposed to aminoglycosides. For further information, see www.england.nhs.uk/publication/national-genomic-test-directories/.

● **MEDICINAL FORMS** There can be variation in the licensing of different medicines containing the same drug.

Nasal cream

EXCIPIENTS: May contain Arachis (peanut) oil, cetostearyl alcohol (including cetyl and stearyl alcohol)

▸ Naseptin (Alliance Pharmaceuticals Ltd)
Chlorhexidine hydrochloride 1 mg per 1 gram, Neomycin sulfate 5 mg per 1 gram Naseptin nasal cream | 15 gram PoM £1.99 DT = £1.99

ANTIBACTERIALS > OTHER

Mupirocin

07-May-2021

● **INDICATIONS AND DOSE**

BACTROBAN NASAL®

For eradication of nasal carriage of staphylococci, including meticillin-resistant *Staphylococcus aureus* (MRSA)

▶ BY INTRANASAL ADMINISTRATION

▸ Child: Apply 2–3 times a day for 5 days, dose to be applied to the inner surface of each nostril, a sample should be taken 2 days after treatment to confirm eradication. Course may be repeated once if sample positive (and throat not colonised)

● **SIDE-EFFECTS**

▶ **Common or very common** Skin reactions

▶ **Uncommon** Nasal mucosal disorder

● **PREGNANCY** Manufacturer advises avoid unless potential benefit outweighs risk—no information available.

● **BREAST FEEDING** No information available.

● **MEDICINAL FORMS** There can be variation in the licensing of different medicines containing the same drug.

Nasal ointment

▸ Bactroban (GlaxoSmithKline UK Ltd)
Mupirocin (as Mupirocin calcium) 20 mg per 1 gram Bactroban 2% nasal ointment | 3 gram PoM £4.24 DT = £4.24

CORTICOSTEROIDS > CORTICOSTEROID COMBINATIONS WITH ANTI-INFECTIVES

Betamethasone with neomycin

20-Jun-2025

The properties listed below are those particular to the combination only. For the properties of the components please consider, betamethasone p. 873, neomycin sulfate p. 898.

● **INDICATIONS AND DOSE**

Nasal infection

▶ BY INTRANASAL ADMINISTRATION USING NASAL DROPS

▸ Child: Apply 2–3 drops 2–3 times a day, to be applied into each nostril

IMPORTANT SAFETY INFORMATION

MHRA/CHM ADVICE: AMINOGLYCOSIDES (GENTAMICIN, AMIKACIN, TOBRAMYCIN, AND NEOMYCIN): INCREASED RISK OF DEAFNESS IN PATIENTS WITH MITOCHONDRIAL MUTATIONS (JANUARY 2021)

The use of aminoglycosides is associated with rare cases of ototoxicity. A safety review found an increased risk of deafness in patients with mitochondrial mutations (particularly the m.1555A>G mutation), including cases where the patient's aminoglycoside serum levels were within the recommended range. Nevertheless, these mitochondrial mutations are considered rare and penetrance is uncertain. No cases were identified with topical preparations but, based on a shared mechanism of effect, there is a potential risk with neomycin and other aminoglycosides administered at the site of toxicity i.e. the ear.

Healthcare professionals are advised to consider the need for aminoglycoside treatment versus alternative options in patients with susceptible mutations. The need for genetic testing especially in those requiring recurrent or long-term treatment with aminoglycosides should also be considered, however, urgent treatment should not be delayed. To minimise the risks of adverse effects, continuous monitoring of renal and auditory function, as well as hepatic and laboratory parameters, is recommended for all patients. Those with known mitochondrial mutations or a family history of ototoxicity are advised to inform their doctor or pharmacist before using an aminoglycoside.

- **INTERACTIONS** → Appendix 1: corticosteroids · neomycin
- **SIDE-EFFECTS** Asthma · dizziness · epistaxis · growth retardation · headache · nasal complaints · nausea · smell altered · taste altered · urticaria
- **PRE-TREATMENT SCREENING** NHS England commissions genetic testing under the *National genomic test directory* indication: R65 - Aminoglycoside exposure posing risk to hearing. The testing criteria is significant exposure to aminoglycosides posing risk of ototoxicity. This testing is relevant to individuals with a predisposition to gram-negative infections or with hearing loss who have been exposed to aminoglycosides. For further information, see www.england.nhs.uk/publication/national-genomic-test-directories/.
- **LESS SUITABLE FOR PRESCRIBING** Betamethasone with neomycin nasal-drops are less suitable for prescribing; there is no evidence that topical anti-infective nasal preparations have any therapeutic value in rhinitis or sinusitis.

- **MEDICINAL FORMS** There can be variation in the licensing of different medicines containing the same drug.

Ear/eye/nose drops solution

EXCIPIENTS: May contain Benzalkonium chloride, disodium edetate

- **Betnesol-N** (RPH Pharmaceuticals AB)
  Betamethasone (as Betamethasone sodium phosphate) 1 mg per 1 ml, Neomycin sulfate 5 mg per 1 ml Betnesol-N ear/eye/nose drops | 10 ml PoM £2.39 DT = £2.39

3 Nasal inflammation, nasal polyps and rhinitis

Other drugs used for Nasal inflammation, nasal polyps and rhinitis Desloratadine, p. 202 · Fexofenadine hydrochloride, p. 203 · Ketotifen, p. 207 · Rupatadine, p. 204

ANTIHISTAMINES

Azelastine hydrochloride

03-Aug-2023

- **INDICATIONS AND DOSE**

AZELAIR®

Allergic rhinitis

- BY INTRANASAL ADMINISTRATION
- Child 6–11 years: 1 spray twice daily for a maximum duration of 4 weeks, to be administered into each nostril
- Child 12–17 years: 2 sprays once daily, to be administered into each nostril, increased if necessary up to 2 sprays twice daily, to be administered into each nostril

DOSE EQUIVALENCE AND CONVERSION

- For *Azelair*®: 1 spray equivalent to 210 micrograms.

RHINOLAST®

Allergic rhinitis

- BY INTRANASAL ADMINISTRATION
- Child 6–17 years: 1 spray twice daily, to be administered into each nostril

DOSE EQUIVALENCE AND CONVERSION

- For *Rhinolast*®: 1 spray equivalent to 140 micrograms.

- **INTERACTIONS** → Appendix 1: antihistamines, non-sedating
- **SIDE-EFFECTS**
  - **Common or very common** Taste altered
  - **Uncommon** Epistaxis · nasal complaints
  - **Rare or very rare** Asthenia · dizziness · drowsiness · skin reactions

  SIDE-EFFECTS, FURTHER INFORMATION Altered taste may occur after administration, often due to incorrect application.

- **MEDICINAL FORMS** There can be variation in the licensing of different medicines containing the same drug.

Spray

- **Azelair** (Ceuta Healthcare Ltd)
  Azelastine hydrochloride 210 microgram per 1 actuation Azelair 0.15% nasal spray | 20 ml PoM £9.90 DT = £9.90
- **Rhinolast** (Ceuta Healthcare Ltd)
  Azelastine hydrochloride 140 microgram per 1 actuation Rhinolast 140micrograms/dose nasal spray | 22 ml PoM £10.50 DT = £10.50

Combinations available: ***Fluticasone with azelastine***, p. 874

ANTIMUSCARINICS

177

Ipratropium bromide

13-Mar-2025

- **INDICATIONS AND DOSE**

Rhinorrhoea associated with allergic and non-allergic rhinitis

- BY INTRANASAL ADMINISTRATION
- Child 12–17 years: 2 sprays 2–3 times a day, dose to be sprayed into each nostril

DOSE EQUIVALENCE AND CONVERSION

- 1 metered spray of nasal spray = 21 micrograms.

- **CAUTIONS** Avoid spraying near eyes · bladder outflow obstruction · cystic fibrosis · susceptibility to angle-closure glaucoma
- **INTERACTIONS** → Appendix 1: ipratropium
- **SIDE-EFFECTS**
  - **Common or very common** Epistaxis · gastrointestinal motility disorder · headache · nasal complaints · throat complaints
  - **Uncommon** Corneal oedema · eye disorders · eye pain · nausea · respiratory disorders · stomatitis · vision disorders
  - **Rare or very rare** Palpitations

  SIDE-EFFECTS, FURTHER INFORMATION For intranasal use, also consider the side-effects of inhaled antimuscarinics.
- **ALLERGY AND CROSS-SENSITIVITY** Contra-indicated in patients with hypersensitivity to atropine or its derivatives.
- **PREGNANCY** EvGr Use only if potential benefit outweighs the risk. ⟨M⟩
- **BREAST FEEDING** No information available—manufacturer advises only use if potential benefit outweighs risk.
- **PATIENT AND CARER ADVICE** Patients or carers should be counselled on appropriate administration technique and warned against accidental contact with the eye (due to risk of ocular complications).

Driving and skilled tasks Manufacturer advises patients and carers should be counselled on the effects on driving and performance of skilled tasks—increased risk of dizziness and vision disorders.

● **MEDICINAL FORMS** There can be variation in the licensing of different medicines containing the same drug.

Spray

EXCIPIENTS: May contain Benzalkonium chloride, disodium edetate

▸ Ipratropium bromide (Non-proprietary)

Ipratropium bromide 21 microgram per 1 dose Ipratropium bromide 21micrograms/dose nasal spray | 240 dose PoM £8.72–£14.82 DT = £8.72

CORTICOSTEROIDS

Corticosteroids (intranasal)

IMPORTANT SAFETY INFORMATION

MHRA/CHM ADVICE: CORTICOSTEROIDS: RARE RISK OF CENTRAL SEROUS CHORIORETINOPATHY WITH LOCAL AS WELL AS SYSTEMIC ADMINISTRATION (AUGUST 2017)

Central serous chorioretinopathy is a retinal disorder that has been linked to the systemic use of corticosteroids. Recently, it has also been reported after local administration of corticosteroids via inhaled and intranasal, epidural, intra-articular, topical dermal, and periocular routes. The MHRA recommends that patients should be advised to report any blurred vision or other visual disturbances with corticosteroid treatment given by any route; consider referral to an ophthalmologist for evaluation of possible causes if a patient presents with vision problems.

ADRENAL INSUFFICIENCY CARD (APRIL 2023)

The British Society for Paediatric Endocrinology and Diabetes (BSPED) has developed an Adrenal Insufficiency Card which should be issued to children with adrenal insufficiency and steroid dependence. The card includes a management summary for the emergency treatment of adrenal crisis and sick day dosing, and can be issued by any healthcare professional managing such patients. The BSPED Adrenal Insufficiency Card is available at: www.bsped.org.uk/adrenal-insufficiency.

● **CAUTIONS** Avoid after nasal surgery (until healing has occurred) · avoid in pulmonary tuberculosis · avoid in the presence of untreated nasal infections · patients transferred from systemic corticosteroids may experience exacerbation of some symptoms

CAUTIONS, FURTHER INFORMATION

▸ Systemic absorption Systemic absorption may follow nasal administration particularly if high doses are used or if treatment is prolonged; therefore also consider the cautions and side-effects of systemic corticosteroids. The risk of systemic effects may be greater with nasal drops than with nasal sprays; drops are administered incorrectly more often than sprays.

● **SIDE-EFFECTS**

▸ **Common or very common** Altered smell sensation · epistaxis · headache · nasal complaints · taste altered · throat irritation

▸ **Rare or very rare** Glaucoma · nasal septum perforation (more common following nasal surgery) · vision blurred

SIDE-EFFECTS, FURTHER INFORMATION Systemic absorption may follow nasal administration particularly if high doses are used or if treatment is prolonged. Therefore also consider the side-effects of systemic corticosteroids.

● **MONITORING REQUIREMENTS** The height of children receiving prolonged treatment with nasal corticosteroids should be monitored; if growth is slowed, referral to a paediatrician should be considered.

● **PATIENT AND CARER ADVICE** If systemic absorption occurs following intranasal use, side-effects applicable to systemic corticosteroids may apply.

F above

Beclometasone dipropionate

26-Jul-2025

(Beclomethasone dipropionate)

● **INDICATIONS AND DOSE**

Prophylaxis and treatment of allergic and vasomotor rhinitis

▸ BY INTRANASAL ADMINISTRATION

▸ Child 6–17 years: 100 micrograms twice daily, dose to be administered into each nostril, reduced to 50 micrograms twice daily, dose to be administered into each nostril, dose to be reduced when symptoms controlled

● **INTERACTIONS** → Appendix 1: corticosteroids

● **MEDICINAL FORMS** There can be variation in the licensing of different medicines containing the same drug.

Spray

EXCIPIENTS: May contain Benzalkonium chloride, polysorbates

▸ Beclometasone dipropionate (Non-proprietary)

Beclometasone dipropionate 50 microgram per 1 dose Beclometasone 50micrograms/dose nasal spray | 200 dose PoM ⊠ DT = £2.63

▸ Beconase (GlaxoSmithKline UK Ltd)

Beclometasone dipropionate 50 microgram per 1 dose Beconase Aqueous 50micrograms/dose nasal spray | 200 dose PoM £2.63 DT = £2.63

▸ Nasobec (Teva UK Ltd)

Beclometasone dipropionate 50 microgram per 1 dose Nasobec Aqueous 50micrograms/dose nasal spray | 200 dose PoM £3.06 DT = £2.63

F above

Betamethasone

26-Jul-2025

● **DRUG ACTION** Betamethasone has very high glucocorticoid activity and insignificant mineralocorticoid activity.

● **INDICATIONS AND DOSE**

BETNESOL®

Non-infected inflammatory conditions of nose

▸ BY INTRANASAL ADMINISTRATION

▸ Child: Apply 2–3 drops 2–3 times a day, dose to be applied into each nostril

VISTAMETHASONE®

Non-infected inflammatory conditions of nose

▸ BY INTRANASAL ADMINISTRATION

▸ Child: Apply 2–3 drops twice daily, dose to be applied into each nostril

● **INTERACTIONS** → Appendix 1: corticosteroids

● **MEDICINAL FORMS** There can be variation in the licensing of different medicines containing the same drug.

Ear/eye/nose drops solution

EXCIPIENTS: May contain Benzalkonium chloride, disodium edetate

▸ Betnesol (RPH Pharmaceuticals AB)

Betamethasone sodium phosphate 1 mg per 1 ml Betnesol 0.1% eye/ear/nose drops | 10 ml PoM £2.32 DT = £2.32

F above

Budesonide

26-Feb-2026

● **DRUG ACTION** Budesonide is a glucocorticoid, which exerts significant local anti-inflammatory effects.

● **INDICATIONS AND DOSE**

Prophylaxis and treatment of allergic rhinitis | Nasal polyps

▸ BY INTRANASAL ADMINISTRATION

▸ Child 6–17 years: 256 micrograms once daily, to be administered as 2 sprays into each nostril in the morning, reduce dose when control

continued →

achieved, alternatively 128 micrograms twice daily, to be administered as 1 spray into each nostril in the morning and in the evening, reduce dose when control achieved

- **INTERACTIONS** → Appendix 1: corticosteroids
- **SIDE-EFFECTS**
  - **Rare or very rare** Adrenal suppression
- **MEDICINAL FORMS** There can be variation in the licensing of different medicines containing the same drug.

Spray

EXCIPIENTS: May contain Disodium edetate, polysorbates, potassium sorbate

- **Budesonide (Non-proprietary)**
  Budesonide 64 microgram per 1 dose Budesonide 64micrograms/dose nasal spray | 120 dose PoM £15.90 DT = £15.71
  Budesonide 100 microgram per 1 dose Budeflam Aquanase 100micrograms/dose nasal spray | 150 dose PoM
  Aircort 100micrograms/dose nasal spray | 200 dose PoM

873

Fluticasone

26-Jul-2025

- **INDICATIONS AND DOSE**

Prophylaxis and treatment of allergic rhinitis and perennial rhinitis

- BY INTRANASAL ADMINISTRATION USING NASAL SPRAY
  - Child 4–11 years: 50 micrograms once daily, dose to be administered into each nostril preferably in the morning, increased if necessary to 50 micrograms twice daily, dose to be administered into each nostril
  - Child 12–17 years: 100 micrograms once daily, dose to be administered into each nostril preferably in the morning, increased if necessary to 100 micrograms twice daily, dose to be administered into each nostril; reduced to 50 micrograms once daily, dose to be administered into each nostril, dose to be reduced when control achieved

Nasal polyps

- BY INTRANASAL ADMINISTRATION USING NASAL DROPS
  - Child 16–17 years: 200 micrograms 1–2 times a day, dose to be administered into each nostril (200 micrograms is equivalent to approximately 6 drops), alternative treatment should be considered if no improvement after 4–6 weeks

AVAMYS® SPRAY

Prophylaxis and treatment of allergic rhinitis

- BY INTRANASAL ADMINISTRATION
  - Child 6–11 years: 27.5 micrograms once daily, dose to be sprayed into each nostril, then increased if necessary to 55 micrograms once daily, dose to be sprayed into each nostril, reduced to 27.5 micrograms once daily, dose to be sprayed into each nostril, dose to be reduced once control achieved; use minimum effective dose
  - Child 12–17 years: 55 micrograms once daily, dose to be sprayed into each nostril, reduced to 27.5 micrograms once daily, dose to be sprayed into each nostril, dose to be reduced once control achieved; use minimum effective dose

DOSE EQUIVALENCE AND CONVERSION

- For *Avamys®* spray: 1 spray equivalent to 27.5 micrograms.

- **INTERACTIONS** → Appendix 1: corticosteroids
- **SIDE-EFFECTS** Adrenal suppression

SIDE-EFFECTS, FURTHER INFORMATION Nasal ulceration occurs commonly with nasal preparations containing fluticasone furoate.

- **MEDICINAL FORMS** There can be variation in the licensing of different medicines containing the same drug.

Spray

EXCIPIENTS: May contain Benzalkonium chloride, disodium edetate, polysorbates

- **Fluticasone (Non-proprietary)**
  Fluticasone propionate 50 microgram per 1 dose Fluticasone propionate 50micrograms/dose nasal spray | 150 dose PoM £11.01 DT = £11.01
- **Avamys** (GlaxoSmithKline UK Ltd)
  Fluticasone furoate 27.5 microgram per 1 dose Avamys 27.5micrograms/dose nasal spray | 120 dose PoM £6.44 DT = £6.44
- **Coryen** (Alissa Healthcare Research Ltd)
  Fluticasone furoate 27.5 microgram per 1 dose Coryen 27.5micrograms/dose nasal spray | 120 dose PoM £6.44 DT = £6.44
- **Flixonase** (GlaxoSmithKline UK Ltd)
  Fluticasone propionate 50 microgram per 1 dose Flixonase 50micrograms/dose aqueous nasal spray | 150 dose PoM £11.01 DT = £11.01
- **Flutikaz** (Teva UK Ltd)
  Fluticasone furoate 27.5 microgram per 1 dose Flutikaz 27.5micrograms/dose nasal spray | 120 dose PoM £6.44 DT = £6.44
- **Nasofan** (Teva UK Ltd)
  Fluticasone propionate 50 microgram per 1 dose Nasofan 50micrograms/dose aqueous nasal spray | 150 dose PoM £8.04 DT = £11.01
- **Relioz** (Zydus Pharmaceuticals UK Ltd)
  Fluticasone furoate 27.5 microgram per 1 dose Relioz 27.5micrograms/dose nasal spray | 120 dose PoM £6.44 DT = £6.44

Nasal drops

EXCIPIENTS: May contain Polysorbates

- **Fluticasone (Non-proprietary)**
  Fluticasone propionate 400 microgram Fluticasone 400microgram/unit dose nasal drops | 30 unit dose PoM £21.99–£40.46 DT = £21.99

Fluticasone with azelastine

The properties listed below are those particular to the combination only. For the properties of the components please consider, fluticasone above, azelastine hydrochloride p. 872.

- **INDICATIONS AND DOSE**

Moderate to severe seasonal and perennial allergic rhinitis, if monotherapy with antihistamine or corticosteroid is inadequate

- BY INTRANASAL ADMINISTRATION
  - Child 12–17 years: 1 spray twice daily, dose to be administered into each nostril

- **INTERACTIONS** → Appendix 1: antihistamines, non-sedating · corticosteroids
- **MEDICINAL FORMS** There can be variation in the licensing of different medicines containing the same drug.

Spray

EXCIPIENTS: May contain Benzalkonium chloride, polysorbates

- **Fluticasone with azelastine (Non-proprietary)**
  Fluticasone propionate 50 microgram per 1 dose, Azelastine hydrochloride 137 microgram per 1 dose Fluticasone propionate 50micrograms/dose / Azelastine 137micrograms/dose nasal spray | 120 dose PoM £14.80 DT = £5.60
- **Dymista** (Viatris UK Healthcare Ltd)
  Fluticasone propionate 50 microgram per 1 dose, Azelastine hydrochloride 137 microgram per 1 dose Dymista 137micrograms/dose / 50micrograms/dose nasal spray | 120 dose PoM £14.80 DT = £5.60
- **Flomister** (Strides Pharma UK Ltd)
  Fluticasone propionate 50 microgram per 1 dose, Azelastine hydrochloride 137 microgram per 1 dose Flomister 137micrograms/dose / 50micrograms/dose nasal spray | 120 dose PoM £11.10 DT = £5.60

▸ **Lutonaze** (Zentiva Pharma UK Ltd)
Fluticasone propionate 50 microgram per 1 dose, Azelastine hydrochloride 137 microgram per 1 dose Lutonaze 137micrograms/dose / 50micrograms/dose nasal spray | 120 dose PoM £11.10 DT = £5.60

F 873

Mometasone furoate

26-Jul-2025

● **INDICATIONS AND DOSE**

Prophylaxis and treatment of seasonal allergic or perennial rhinitis

▶ BY INTRANASAL ADMINISTRATION

▸ Child 3–11 years: 50 micrograms once daily, dose to be sprayed into each nostril

▸ Child 12–17 years: 100 micrograms once daily, dose to be sprayed into each nostril, increased if necessary up to 200 micrograms once daily, dose to be sprayed into each nostril; reduced to 50 micrograms once daily, dose to be sprayed into each nostril, dose to be reduced when control achieved

● **INTERACTIONS** → Appendix 1: corticosteroids

● **SIDE-EFFECTS** Nasal ulceration occurs commonly with preparations containing mometasone furoate.

● **MEDICINAL FORMS** There can be variation in the licensing of different medicines containing the same drug.

Spray

EXCIPIENTS: May contain Benzalkonium chloride, polysorbates

▸ **Mometasone furoate (Non-proprietary)**
Mometasone furoate 50 microgram per 1 dose Mometasone 50micrograms/dose nasal spray | 140 dose PoM £9.48 DT = £3.30

▸ **Nasonex** (Organon Pharma (UK) Ltd)
Mometasone furoate 50 microgram per 1 dose Nasonex 50micrograms/dose nasal spray | 140 dose PoM £7.68 DT = £3.30

Mometasone furoate with olopatadine

21-Jan-2022

The properties listed below are those particular to the combination only. For the properties of the components please consider, mometasone furoate above, olopatadine p. 834.

● **INDICATIONS AND DOSE**

Moderate to severe allergic rhinitis

▶ BY INTRANASAL ADMINISTRATION

▸ Child 12–17 years: 2 sprays twice daily into each nostril in the morning and evening

● **INTERACTIONS** → Appendix 1: corticosteroids

● **SIDE-EFFECTS**

▶ **Common or very common** Epistaxis · nasal complaints · taste altered

▶ **Uncommon** Abdominal pain · dizziness · drowsiness · dry mouth · fatigue · headaches · nausea

▶ **Rare or very rare** Anxiety · constipation · depression · dry eye · ear pain · eye discomfort · increased risk of infection · insomnia · laceration · oropharyngeal pain · throat irritation · tongue pain · vision blurred

▶ **Frequency not known** Cataract · glaucoma

SIDE-EFFECTS, FURTHER INFORMATION Systemic absorption can follow nasal administration particularly if high doses are used or if treatment is prolonged; therefore, also consider the side-effects of systemic corticosteroids.

● **PATIENT AND CARER ADVICE**

Driving and skilled tasks Patients and carers should be cautioned on the effects on driving and performance of skilled tasks—increased risk of dizziness, lethargy, fatigue, and somnolence.

● **NATIONAL FUNDING/ACCESS DECISIONS**

For full details see funding body website

Scottish Medicines Consortium (SMC) decisions

▶ **Olopatadine hydrochloride and mometasone furoate monohydrate (*Ryaltris*®) for the treatment of moderate to severe nasal symptoms associated with allergic rhinitis in adults and adolescents 12 years of age and older (December 2021)** SMC No. SMC2418 Recommended with restrictions

● **MEDICINAL FORMS** There can be variation in the licensing of different medicines containing the same drug.

Spray

EXCIPIENTS: May contain Benzalkonium chloride, disodium edetate, polysorbates

▸ **Ryaltris** (Glenmark Pharmaceuticals Europe Ltd)
Mometasone furoate 25 microgram per 1 dose, Olopatadine (as Olopatadine hydrochloride) 600 microgram per 1 dose Ryaltris 25micrograms/dose / 600micrograms/dose nasal spray | 240 dose PoM £13.32 DT = £13.32

F 873

Triamcinolone acetonide

26-Jul-2025

● **DRUG ACTION** Triamcinolone exerts predominantly glucocorticoid effects with minimal mineralcorticoid effect.

● **INDICATIONS AND DOSE**

Prophylaxis and treatment of allergic rhinitis

▶ BY INTRANASAL ADMINISTRATION

▸ Child 2–5 years: 55 micrograms once daily for maximum 3 months, dose to be sprayed into each nostril

▸ Child 6–11 years: 55 micrograms once daily, dose to be sprayed into each nostril, increased if necessary to 110 micrograms once daily, dose to be sprayed into each nostril; reduced to 55 micrograms once daily, dose to be sprayed into each nostril, reduce dose when control achieved; maximum duration of treatment 3 months

▸ Child 12–17 years: 110 micrograms once daily, dose to be sprayed into each nostril, reduced to 55 micrograms once daily, dose to be sprayed into each nostril, reduce dose when control achieved

● **UNLICENSED USE** Not licensed for use in children under 6 years.

● **INTERACTIONS** → Appendix 1: corticosteroids

● **MEDICINAL FORMS** There can be variation in the licensing of different medicines containing the same drug.

Spray

EXCIPIENTS: May contain Benzalkonium chloride, disodium edetate, polysorbates

▸ **Nasacort** (Opella POM UK Ltd)
Triamcinolone acetonide 55 microgram per 1 dose Nasacort 55micrograms/dose nasal spray | 120 dose PoM £7.39 DT = £7.39

Oropharynx

1 Dry mouth

Dry mouth

14-Dec-2020

Overview

Dry mouth (xerostomia) resulting from reduced saliva secretion may be caused by drugs such as antimuscarinics, antihistamines, tricyclic antidepressants, and some diuretics. It can also be caused by irradiation of the head and neck region, dehydration, anxiety, or Sjögren's syndrome. Children with dry mouth may be at greater risk of developing dental caries, periodontal disease, and oral infections (particularly candidiasis).

EvGr Underlying causes of dry mouth such as dehydration, anxiety, infection, or drugs causing dry mouth should be managed if appropriate. Dry mouth may be relieved by simple measures that stimulate salivation such as frequent sips of cold unsweetened drinks, or sucking pieces of ice or sugar-free fruit pastilles, or chewing sugar-free gum.

An artificial saliva substitute can be considered if simple stimulatory measures are inadequate. ⟨A⟩ The acidic pH of some artificial saliva products may be inappropriate for some children and may damage the enamel of natural teeth. Artificial saliva products below are available in oral lozenges, oral gel, oral spray, and pastille forms.

LUBRICANTS

Artificial saliva products

● **ARTIFICIAL SALIVA PRODUCTS**

AS SALIVA ORTHANA® LOZENGES

Mucin 65 mg, xylitol 59 mg, in a sorbitol basis, pH neutral

● **INDICATIONS AND DOSE**

Dry mouth as a result of having (or having undergone) radiotherapy (ACBS) | Dry mouth as a result of sicca syndrome (ACBS)

▶ BY MOUTH

▸ Child: 1 lozenge as required, allow to dissolve slowly in the mouth

● **PRESCRIBING AND DISPENSING INFORMATION** *AS Saliva Orthana®* lozenges do not contain fluoride.

AS SALIVA ORTHANA® SPRAY

Gastric mucin (porcine) 3.5%, xylitol 2%, sodium fluoride 4.2 mg/litre, with preservatives and flavouring agents, pH neutral.

● **INDICATIONS AND DOSE**

Symptomatic treatment of dry mouth

▶ BY MOUTH

▸ Child: Apply 2–3 sprays as required, spray onto oral and pharyngeal mucosa

● **PROFESSION SPECIFIC INFORMATION**

Dental practitioners' formulary *AS Saliva Orthana®* Oral Spray may be prescribed.

AS Saliva Orthana spray (CCMed Ltd)
50 ml • NHS indicative price = £4.92 • Drug Tariff (Part IXa)

BIOXTRA® DRY MOUTH GEL MOUTHSPRAY

Aqua, xylitol, hydrogenated starch hydrolysate, sorbitol, hyetellose, sodium monofluorophosphate, sodium saccharin, potassium chloride, sodium chloride, magnesium chloride, dipotassium phosphate, calcium chloride, colostrum whey, lactoperoxidase, citric acid, sodium benzoate, sodium methylparaben, sodium propylparaben, and potassium sorbate.

● **INDICATIONS AND DOSE**

Symptomatic treatment of dry mouth

▶ BY MOUTH

▸ Child: Apply as required, spray onto gums, tongue, and lips

● **PATIENT AND CARER ADVICE** Use in children aged under 7 years should be supervised to minimise swallowing.

BioXtra Dry Mouth Gel Mouthspray (R.I.S. Products Ltd)
50 ml • NHS indicative price = £4.78 • Drug Tariff (Part IXa)

BIOXTRA® DRY MOUTH ORAL GEL

Aqua, glycerin, sorbitol, hydrogenated starch hydrolysate, xylitol, hyetellose, glucose, butylene glycol, sodium polyacrylate, polyacrylic acid, colostrum whey, glucose oxidase, lactoperoxidase, lactoferrin, lysozyme, aloe barbadensis leaf juice, potassium thiocyanate and benzoic acid.

● **INDICATIONS AND DOSE**

Symptomatic treatment of dry mouth

▶ BY MOUTH

▸ Child: Apply as required, particularly at night, to oral mucosa

● **PROFESSION SPECIFIC INFORMATION**

Dental practitioners' formulary *BioXtra®* Dry Mouth Oral Gel may be prescribed as Artificial Saliva Gel.

BioXtra Dry Mouth oral gel (R.I.S. Products Ltd)
40 ml • NHS indicative price = £4.78 • Drug Tariff (Part IXa)

BIOTENE ORALBALANCE®

Lactoperoxidase, lactoferrin, lysozyme, glucose oxidase, xylitol in a gel basis

● **INDICATIONS AND DOSE**

Symptomatic treatment of dry mouth

▶ BY MOUTH

▸ Child: Apply as required, apply to gums and tongue

● **PATIENT AND CARER ADVICE** Avoid use with toothpastes containing detergents (including foaming agents).

● **PROFESSION SPECIFIC INFORMATION**

Dental practitioners' formulary *Biotene Oralbalance®* Saliva Replacement Gel may be prescribed as Artificial Saliva Gel.

Biotene Oralbalance dry mouth saliva replacement gel (Haleon UK Trading Ltd) **Glucose oxidase 12000 unit, Lactoferrin 12 mg, Lactoperoxidase 12000 unit, Muramidase 12 mg** 50 gram • NHS indicative price = £5.30 • Drug Tariff (Part IXa)

GLANDOSANE®

Carmellose sodium 500 mg, sorbitol 1.5 g, potassium chloride 60 mg, sodium chloride 42.2 mg, magnesium chloride 2.6 mg, calcium chloride 7.3 mg, and dipotassium hydrogen phosphate 17.1 mg/50 g, pH 5.75.

● **INDICATIONS AND DOSE**

Dry mouth as a result of having (or having undergone) radiotherapy (ACBS) | Dry mouth as a result of sicca syndrome (ACBS)

▶ BY MOUTH

▸ Child: Apply as required, spray onto oral and pharyngeal mucosa

● **PROFESSION SPECIFIC INFORMATION**

Dental practitioners' formulary *Glandosane®* Aerosol Spray may be prescribed.

ORALIEVE® MOISTURISING MOUTH GEL

Sorbitol, glycerin, aqua, xylitol, carbomer, sorbic acid, hyetellose, whey protein, sodium hydroxide, benzoic acid, glucose, lactoferrin, lactoperoxidase, glucose oxidase, potassium thiocyanate, disodium phosphate and aloe vera.

● **INDICATIONS AND DOSE**

Symptomatic treatment of dry mouth

▶ BY MOUTH

▸ Child 12–17 years: Apply as required, particularly at night, to oral mucosa

● **PROFESSION SPECIFIC INFORMATION**

Dental practitioners' formulary *Oralieve®* Moisturising Mouth Gel may be prescribed as Artificial Saliva Gel.

Oralieve moisturising mouth gel (Oralieve UK)
50 ml • NHS indicative price = £4.85 • Drug Tariff (Part IXa)

ORALIEVE® MOISTURISING MOUTH SPRAY
Aqua, glycerin, xylitol, poloxamer 407, sodium benzoate, sodium phosphate, xanthan gum, aroma, disodium phosphate, benzoic acid, whey protein, lactoferrin, lactoperoxidase, potassium thiocyanate, glucose oxidase, limonene, alcohol-free, detergent-free.

● **INDICATIONS AND DOSE**

Symptomatic treatment of dry mouth
▶ BY MOUTH
▸ Child 12–17 years: 1 spray as required, on the inside of each cheek, gums and tongue

Oralieve moisturising mouth spray (Oralieve UK)
50 ml • NHS indicative price = £4.95 • Drug Tariff (Part IXa)

SST®
Sugar-free, citric acid, malic acid and other ingredients in a sorbitol base.

● **INDICATIONS AND DOSE**

Symptomatic treatment of dry mouth in patients with impaired salivary gland function and patent salivary ducts
▶ BY MOUTH
▸ Child: 1 tablet as required, allow tablet to dissolve slowly in the mouth

● **PROFESSION SPECIFIC INFORMATION**
Dental practitioners' formulary May be prescribed as Saliva Stimulating Tablets.

SST saliva stimulating tablets (Sinclair IS Pharma Plc)
100 tablet • NHS indicative price = £4.86 • Drug Tariff (Part IXa)

SALIVEZE®
Carmellose sodium (sodium carboxymethylcellulose), calcium chloride, magnesium chloride, potassium chloride, sodium chloride, and dibasic sodium phosphate, pH neutral

● **INDICATIONS AND DOSE**

Dry mouth as a result of having (or having undergone) radiotherapy (ACBS) | Dry mouth as a result of sicca syndrome (ACBS)
▶ BY MOUTH
▸ Child: Apply 1 spray as required, spray onto oral mucosa

● **PROFESSION SPECIFIC INFORMATION**
Dental practitioners' formulary *Saliveze®* Oral Spray may be prescribed.

Saliveze mouth spray (Wyvern Medical Ltd)
50 ml • NHS indicative price = £3.70 • Drug Tariff (Part IXa)

SALIVIX®
Sugar-free, reddish-amber, acacia, malic acid and other ingredients.

● **INDICATIONS AND DOSE**

Symptomatic treatment of dry mouth
▶ BY MOUTH USING PASTILLES
▸ Child: 1 unit as required, suck pastille

● **PROFESSION SPECIFIC INFORMATION**
Dental practitioners' formulary *Salivix®* Pastilles may be prescribed as Artificial Saliva Pastilles.

Salivix pastilles (Galen Ltd)
50 pastille • NHS indicative price = £3.79 • Drug Tariff (Part IXa)

XEROTIN®
Sugar-free, water, sorbitol, carmellose (carboxymethylcellulose), potassium chloride, sodium chloride, potassium phosphate, magnesium chloride, calcium chloride and other ingredients, pH neutral.

● **INDICATIONS AND DOSE**

Symptomatic treatment of dry mouth
▶ BY MOUTH
▸ Child: 1 spray as required

● **PROFESSION SPECIFIC INFORMATION**
Dental practitioners' formulary *Xerotin®* Oral Spray may be prescribed as Artificial Saliva Oral Spray.

Xerotin spray (SpePharm UK Ltd)
100 ml • NHS indicative price = £6.86 • Drug Tariff (Part IXa)

2 Oral hygiene

Mouthwashes and other preparations for oropharyngeal use

01-Sep-2020

Lozenges and sprays

EvGr Lozenges containing either a local anaesthetic, an antiseptic, or a non-steroidal anti-inflammatory drug may be trialled but may only lead to a small reduction in pain. However, there is no evidence that non-medicated lozenges and local anaesthetic sprays have a beneficial action on their own in treating sore throat. Ⓐ

Mouthwashes and gargles

Expert sources advise that a saline mouthwash may be used for cleaning or freshening the mouth and can be prepared by dissolving half a teaspoonful of salt in a glassful of warm water.

Mouthwashes are generally not suitable for young children due to risk of swallowing; for further information, see individual drug monographs or manufacturers advice.

EvGr Mouthwashes containing an oxidising agent, such as hydrogen peroxide p. 878, may be useful in the treatment of acute ulcerative gingivitis whilst awaiting to be seen by a dentist. Ⓐ

Chlorhexidine below is available as a mouthwash, spray, or gel and is licensed for the management of gingivitis and maintenance of oral hygiene, particularly where there is a painful periodontal condition or if the child is unable to adequately brush their teeth (e.g. following dental procedures or due to disability). It is also licensed for the management of aphthous ulcers, oral candidiasis, and following post-periodontal treatment to promote healing. Chlorhexidine mouthwash should not be used for the prevention of endocarditis in children undergoing dental procedures.

Chlorhexidine is an effective antiseptic which has the advantage of inhibiting plaque formation on the teeth but there is limited evidence of preventing dental caries. Public Health England advise to use other treatments for preventing dental caries, such as fluoride-based products.

Chlorhexidine is incompatible with anionic agents present in some toothpastes; it has therefore been suggested to wait 30 minutes between using these two preparations.

ANTISEPTICS AND DISINFECTANTS

Chlorhexidine

23-Feb-2022

● **INDICATIONS AND DOSE**

Oral hygiene and plaque inhibition | Oral candidiasis | Gingivitis | Management of aphthous ulcers
▶ BY OROMUCOSAL ADMINISTRATION USING MOUTHWASH
▸ Child: Rinse or gargle 10 mL twice daily, rinse or gargle for about 1 minute

continued →

▶ BY OROMUCOSAL ADMINISTRATION USING OROMUCOSAL SPRAY
- Child: Apply up to 12 sprays twice daily as required, to be applied on tooth, gingival, or ulcer surfaces

Oral hygiene and plaque inhibition | Gingivitis

▶ BY OROMUCOSAL ADMINISTRATION USING DENTAL GEL
- Child: Apply 1–2 times a day, to be brushed on the teeth

Oral candidiasis | Management of aphthous ulcers

▶ BY OROMUCOSAL ADMINISTRATION USING DENTAL GEL
- Child: Apply 1–2 times a day, to affected areas

DOSE EQUIVALENCE AND CONVERSION
- Mouthwashes and oromucosal sprays contain chlorhexidine gluconate 0.2% w/v.

● **UNLICENSED USE** *Corsodyl®* not licensed for use in children under 12 years (unless on the advice of a healthcare professional).

● **SIDE-EFFECTS**
▶ **Common or very common** Dry mouth · hypersensitivity · oral disorders · taste altered · tongue discolouration · tooth discolouration

SIDE-EFFECTS, FURTHER INFORMATION If desquamation occurs with mucosal irritation, discontinue treatment.

● **PRESCRIBING AND DISPENSING INFORMATION** Chlorhexidine digluconate is a synonym for chlorhexidine gluconate.

● **PATIENT AND CARER ADVICE** Chlorhexidine gluconate may be incompatible with some ingredients in toothpaste; rinse the mouth thoroughly with water between using toothpaste and chlorhexidine-containing product.

● **PROFESSION SPECIFIC INFORMATION**

Dental practitioners' formulary *Corsodyl®* dental gel may be prescribed as Chlorhexidine Gluconate Gel; *Corsodyl®* mouthwash may be prescribed as Chlorhexidine Mouthwash; *Corsodyl®* oral spray may be prescribed as Chlorhexidine Oral Spray.

● **MEDICINAL FORMS** There can be variation in the licensing of different medicines containing the same drug.

Dental gel
- Chlorhexidine (Non-proprietary)
  Chlorhexidine gluconate 2 mg per 1 gram Perio-kin 0.2% gel | 30 ml [no NHS]
- Corsodyl (Haleon UK Trading Ltd)
  Chlorhexidine gluconate 10 mg per 1 gram Corsodyl 1% dental gel | 50 gram P £3.24 DT = £3.24 SF

Mouthwash
- Chlorhexidine (Non-proprietary)
  Chlorhexidine gluconate 2 mg per 1 ml Chlorhexidine gluconate 0.2% mouthwash original | 300 ml GSL [no NHS] DT = £3.03
  Chlorhexidine gluconate 0.2% mouthwash aniseed | 300 ml GSL £2.64 DT = £3.03
  Chlorhexidine gluconate 0.2% mouthwash peppermint | 300 ml GSL £2.64 DT = £3.03
  Chlorhexidine gluconate 0.2% mouthwash plain | 300 ml GSL £2.55 DT = £3.03

Hexetidine
06-Aug-2018

● **INDICATIONS AND DOSE**

Oral hygiene

▶ BY OROMUCOSAL ADMINISTRATION USING MOUTHWASH
- Child 12–17 years: Rinse or gargle 15 mL 2–3 times a day, to be used undiluted

● **SIDE-EFFECTS**
▶ **Rare or very rare** Anaesthesia · taste altered
▶ **Frequency not known** Cough · dry mouth · dysphagia · dyspnoea · nausea · salivary gland enlargement · vomiting

● **MEDICINAL FORMS** There can be variation in the licensing of different medicines containing the same drug.

Mouthwash
- Oraldene (McNeil Products Ltd)
  Hexetidine 1 mg per 1 ml Oraldene 0.1% mouthwash peppermint | 200 ml GSL £3.24 DT = £3.24 SF

Hydrogen peroxide
14-May-2024

● **DRUG ACTION** Hydrogen peroxide is an oxidising agent.

● **INDICATIONS AND DOSE**

Oral hygiene (with hydrogen peroxide 6%)

▶ BY MOUTH USING MOUTHWASH
- Child: Rinse or gargle 15 mL 2–3 times a day for 2–3 minutes, to be diluted in half a tumblerful of warm water

PEROXYL ®

Oral hygiene

▶ BY MOUTH USING MOUTHWASH
- Child 6–17 years: Rinse or gargle 10 mL 3 times a day for about 1 minute, for maximum 7 days, to be used after meals and at bedtime

● **PRESCRIBING AND DISPENSING INFORMATION** When prepared extemporaneously, the BP states Hydrogen Peroxide Mouthwash, BP consists of hydrogen peroxide 6% solution (= approx. 20 volume) BP.

● **HANDLING AND STORAGE** Hydrogen peroxide bleaches fabric.

● **PROFESSION SPECIFIC INFORMATION**

Dental practitioners' formulary Hydrogen Peroxide Mouthwash may be prescribed.

● **MEDICINAL FORMS** There can be variation in the licensing of different medicines containing the same drug.

Cutaneous or oromucosal liquid
- Hydrogen peroxide (Non-proprietary)
  Hydrogen peroxide 30 ml per 1 litre Hydrogen peroxide 3% solution | 100 ml PoM [no NHS]

Mouthwash
- Peroxyl (Colgate-Palmolive (UK) Ltd)
  Hydrogen peroxide 15 mg per 1 ml Peroxyl 1.5% mouthwash | 300 ml GSL £2.94 DT = £2.94 SF

Sodium bicarbonate with sodium chloride
28-Nov-2022

● **INDICATIONS AND DOSE**

Oral hygiene

▶ BY OROMUCOSAL ADMINISTRATION USING MOUTHWASH
- Child: Rinse or gargle as required

● **DIRECTIONS FOR ADMINISTRATION** To be diluted with an equal volume of warm water prior to use.

● **PRESCRIBING AND DISPENSING INFORMATION** Compound Sodium Chloride Mouthwash BP consists of sodium bicarbonate 1 % and sodium chloride 1.5 % in a suitable vehicle with peppermint flavour.

Extemporaneous mouthwash preparations should be prepared according to the following formula: sodium chloride 1.5 g, sodium bicarbonate 1 g, concentrated peppermint emulsion 2.5 mL, double-strength chloroform water 50 mL, water to 100 mL.

● **PROFESSION SPECIFIC INFORMATION**

Dental practitioners' formulary Compound sodium chloride mouthwash may be prescribed.

● **MEDICINAL FORMS** Forms available from special-order manufacturers include: mouthwash

2.1 Dental caries

Fluoride

24-Apr-2020

Overview

Fluoride is a naturally occurring mineral found in water supplies in varying amounts and in some foods; it has beneficial topical effects on teeth. Public Health England advise that all adults and children brush their teeth with fluoridated toothpaste at least twice daily to help prevent tooth decay.

Individuals who are either particularly caries prone or medically compromised may be given additional protection. Public Health England recommends the daily use of a fluoride mouthwash in adults and children aged 7 years and over who are causing concern to their dentist (e.g. those with active caries, dry mouth, or special needs). They should be used at a different time to brushing to avoid removal of the beneficial effects of fluoride in toothpaste.

Fluoride varnish is also available and can be applied topically to both primary or permanent teeth. Public Health England recommends that all children aged 3 years and over have fluoride varnish applied (usually twice a year) regardless of their risk of caries. Application of fluoride varnish at least twice a year may also be considered in adults and children aged under 3 years who are causing concern to their dentist.

Useful resources

Delivering better oral health: an evidence-based toolkit for prevention. Public Health England. March 2017.
www.gov.uk/government/publications/delivering-better-oral-health-an-evidence-based-toolkit-for-prevention

VITAMINS AND TRACE ELEMENTS

Sodium fluoride

25-Nov-2020

● **INDICATIONS AND DOSE**

Prophylaxis of dental caries for water content less than 300micrograms/litre (0.3 parts per million) of fluoride ion

▶ BY MOUTH USING TABLETS
- Child 6 months–2 years: 250 micrograms daily, doses expressed as fluoride ion (F^-)
- Child 3–5 years: 500 micrograms daily, doses expressed as fluoride ion (F^-)
- Child 6–17 years: 1 mg daily, doses expressed as fluoride ion (F^-)

Prophylaxis of dental caries for water content between 300 and 700micrograms/litre (0.3–0.7 parts per million) of fluoride ion

▶ BY MOUTH USING TABLETS
- Child 3–5 years: 250 micrograms daily, doses expressed as fluoride ion (F^-)
- Child 6–17 years: 500 micrograms daily, doses expressed as fluoride ion (F^-)

Prophylaxis of dental caries

▶ BY MOUTH USING MOUTHWASH
- Child 6–17 years: Rinse or gargle 5–10 mL daily

DOSE EQUIVALENCE AND CONVERSION
- Sodium fluoride 2.2 mg provides approx. 1 mg fluoride ion.

COLGATE DURAPHAT ® 2800PPM FLUORIDE TOOTHPASTE

Prophylaxis of dental caries

▶ BY MOUTH USING PASTE
- Child 10–17 years: Apply 1 centimetre twice daily, to be applied using a toothbrush

COLGATE DURAPHAT ® 5000PPM FLUORIDE TOOTHPASTE

Prophylaxis of dental caries

▶ BY MOUTH USING PASTE
- Child 16–17 years: Apply 2 centimetres 3 times a day, to be applied after meals using a toothbrush

EN-DE-KAY ® FLUORINSE

Prophylaxis of dental caries

▶ BY MOUTH USING MOUTHWASH
- Child 8–17 years: 5 drops daily, dilute 5 drops to 10 mL of water, alternatively 20 drops once weekly, dilute 20 drops to 10 mL

● **SIDE-EFFECTS** Dental fluorosis

● **DIRECTIONS FOR ADMINISTRATION** Manufacturer advises tablets should be sucked or dissolved in the mouth at a different time of day to tooth brushing.

Manufacturer advises for mouthwash, rinse mouth for 1 minute and then spit out.

COLGATE DURAPHAT ® 2800PPM FLUORIDE TOOTHPASTE Manufacturer advises brush teeth for 1 minute before spitting out.

COLGATE DURAPHAT ® 5000PPM FLUORIDE TOOTHPASTE Manufacturer advises brush teeth for 3 minutes before spitting out.

● **PRESCRIBING AND DISPENSING INFORMATION** Flavours of oral tablet formulations may include orange.

● **PATIENT AND CARER ADVICE**

Mouthwash Avoid eating, drinking, or rinsing mouth for 15 minutes after use.

COLGATE DURAPHAT ® 2800PPM FLUORIDE TOOTHPASTE Patients or carers should be given advice on how to administer sodium fluoride toothpaste.

Avoid drinking or rinsing mouth for 30 minutes after use.

COLGATE DURAPHAT ® 5000PPM FLUORIDE TOOTHPASTE Patients or carers should be given advice on how to administer sodium fluoride toothpaste.

● **PROFESSION SPECIFIC INFORMATION**

Dental practitioners' formulary Tablets may be prescribed as Sodium Fluoride Tablets.

Oral drops may be prescribed as Sodium Fluoride Oral Drops.

Mouthwashes may be prescribed as Sodium Fluoride Mouthwash 0.05% or Sodium Fluoride Mouthwash 2%.

COLGATE DURAPHAT ® 2800PPM FLUORIDE TOOTHPASTE May be prescribed as Sodium Fluoride Toothpaste 0.619%.

COLGATE DURAPHAT ® 5000PPM FLUORIDE TOOTHPASTE May be prescribed as Sodium Fluoride Toothpaste 1.1%.

Dental information Fluoride mouthwash, oral drops, tablets and toothpaste are prescribable on form FP10D (GP14 in Scotland, WP10D in Wales).
There are also arrangements for health authorities to supply fluoride tablets in the course of pre-school dental schemes, and they may also be supplied in school dental schemes.
Fluoride gels are not prescribable on form FP10D (GP14 in Scotland, WP10D in Wales).

● **MEDICINAL FORMS** There can be variation in the licensing of different medicines containing the same drug.

Dental paste

▸ **Colgate Duraphat** (Colgate-Palmolive (UK) Ltd)
Fluoride (as Sodium fluoride) 2.8 mg per 1 gram Colgate Duraphat 2800ppm fluoride toothpaste | 75 ml PoM £3.26 DT = £2.09 SF
Fluoride (as Sodium fluoride) 5 mg per 1 gram Colgate Duraphat 5000ppm fluoride toothpaste | 51 gram PoM £6.50 DT = £8.30 SF

3 Oral ulceration and inflammation

Oral ulceration and inflammation

09-Dec-2020

Ulceration and inflammation

Ulceration of the oral mucosa is common and usually transient but may require treatment in some cases. Causes include mechanical trauma, infections, malignant lesions, inflammatory conditions, nutritional deficiencies (e.g. iron, folic acid, vitamin B_{12}), immunodeficiency states, gastro-intestinal disease and drug therapy (see also *Chemotherapy induced mucositis and myelosuppression* under Cytotoxic drugs p. 660).

Aphthous ulcers are often recurrent and are not associated with an underlying systemic disease; they are small, round or ovoid mouth ulcers with defined margins. Aphthous ulcers may be precipitated by triggers such as certain food and drinks, allergies, anxiety, or hormonal changes. It is important to consider and exclude any possible systemic disease; treatment may include correcting the underlying cause. Treatment aims to relieve pain, reduce ulcer duration, and reduce the frequency of recurrent episodes. Secondary bacterial infections may occur with mucosal ulceration; it can increase discomfort and delay healing.

EvGr Children with an unexplained mouth ulcer of more than 3 weeks' duration should be referred urgently to a specialist to exclude oral cancer. (A)

Treatment of aphthous ulcers

EvGr Advise children and their carers to avoid known triggers for ulceration, such as oral trauma (e.g. biting during chewing, orthodontic appliances) or certain food and drinks (e.g. chocolate, gluten-containing products). If the ulcers are mild, infrequent, and do not interfere with daily activities (such as eating), treatment may not be required. (A)

Corticosteroids

EvGr Topical corticosteroids are usually considered to be first-line treatment. (A) Hydrocortisone oromucosal tablets p. 882 are licensed for use in aphthous ulceration; expert sources advise that a beclometasone dipropionate inhaler p. 185 [unlicensed indication] sprayed onto the oral mucosa, and betamethasone soluble tablets p. 881 [unlicensed indication] used as a mouthwash may also be used.

EvGr A short course of systemic corticosteroids may be prescribed for children with severe recurrent aphthous ulcers. (A)

Other therapies

EvGr Other therapies that may be used alone or in combination with topical corticosteroids include topical anaesthetics, topical analgesics/anti-inflammatory agents (e.g. benzydamine hydrochloride p. 881), and topical antimicrobial agents (e.g. chlorhexidine mouthwash p. 877). (A) EvGr Doxycycline p. 883 [unlicensed indication] rinsed in the mouth and expelled, may be considered for recurrent aphthous ulceration when other treatments are unsuccessful or unsuitable; ensure the child is able to rinse and spit prior to initiation. (E)

Expert sources advise that a saline (with or without sodium bicarbonate) mouthwash may soothe ulcers, help to maintain oral hygiene, and prevent secondary infection. Tepid water appears to be more soothing than cold or warm water.

Benzydamine hydrochloride and flurbiprofen p. 881 are non-steroidal anti-inflammatory drugs (NSAIDs). Benzydamine hydrochloride mouthwash and spray are licensed for the relief of painful inflammatory conditions associated with a variety of ulcerative conditions, as well as for discomfort of tonsillectomy and post-irradiation mucositis. Benzydamine hydrochloride mouthwash should generally be used undiluted; it can be diluted with an equal volume of water if a stinging sensation occurs. Flurbiprofen lozenges are licensed for the relief of sore throat.

When local anaesthetics are used in the mouth, care must be taken to avoid causing anaesthesia of the pharynx before meals, as this might lead to choking.

Choline salicylate p. 882 is a derivative of salicylic acid and has some analgesic properties. The dental gel is licensed for pain relief in mouth ulcers including ulcers due to dentures and orthodontic devices. EvGr Due to a potential association with Reye's syndrome, choline salicylate should be avoided in children aged under 16 years. (M)

EvGr Consider offering or advising the use of a vitamin B_{12} supplement regardless of serum vitamin B_{12} levels. (A)

ANAESTHETICS, LOCAL

Lidocaine hydrochloride

20-Nov-2025

(Lignocaine hydrochloride)

● **INDICATIONS AND DOSE**

Dental practice

▶ BY BUCCAL ADMINISTRATION USING OINTMENT
▸ Child: Rub gently into dry gum

XYLOCAINE®

Bronchoscopy | Laryngoscopy | Oesophagoscopy | Endotracheal intubation

▶ TO MUCOUS MEMBRANES
▸ Child: Up to 3 mg/kg

● **CAUTIONS** Can damage plastic cuffs of endotracheal tubes

● **INTERACTIONS** → Appendix 1: antiarrhythmics

● **ALLERGY AND CROSS-SENSITIVITY**

▸ Hypersensitivity and cross-sensitivity Hypersensitivity reactions occur mainly with the ester-type local anaesthetics, such as tetracaine; reactions are less frequent with the amide types, such as articaine, bupivacaine, levobupivacaine, lidocaine, mepivacaine, prilocaine, and ropivacaine. Cross-sensitivity reactions may be avoided by using the alternative chemical type.

● **PREGNANCY** Crosses the placenta but not known to be harmful in *animal* studies—use if benefit outweighs risk. When used as a local anaesthetic, large doses can cause fetal bradycardia; if given during delivery can also cause neonatal respiratory depression, hypotonia, or bradycardia after paracervical or epidural block.

● **BREAST FEEDING** Present in milk but amount too small to be harmful.

● **HEPATIC IMPAIRMENT** Manufacturer advises caution (risk of increased exposure).

● **RENAL IMPAIRMENT** Possible accumulation of lidocaine and active metabolite; caution in severe impairment.

● **PROFESSION SPECIFIC INFORMATION**

Dental practitioners' formulary Lidocaine ointment 5% may be prescribed.

Spray may be prescribed as Lidocaine Spray 10%

XYLOCAINE® May be prescribed as lidocaine spray 10%.

- **MEDICINAL FORMS** There can be variation in the licensing of different medicines containing the same drug. Forms available from special-order manufacturers include: ointment

Spray

- **Lidocaine hydrochloride (Non-proprietary)**
  Lidocaine 10 mg per 1 actuation Lidocaine 10mg/dose spray sugar free | 50 ml [PoM] [CD] DT = £7.41 [SF]
- **Xylocaine** (Aspen Pharma Trading Ltd)
  Lidocaine 10 mg per 1 actuation Xylocaine 10mg/dose spray | 50 ml [P] £7.41 DT = £7.41 [SF]

Ointment

- **Lidocaine hydrochloride (Non-proprietary)**
  Lidocaine hydrochloride 50 mg per 1 gram Lidocaine 5% ointment | 15 gram [P] £18.75 DT = £17.65

ANALGESICS > NON-STEROIDAL ANTI-INFLAMMATORY DRUGS

Benzydamine hydrochloride

13-Jul-2023

- **INDICATIONS AND DOSE**

Painful inflammatory conditions of oropharynx [using 0.15% preparations]

- BY OROMUCOSAL ADMINISTRATION USING MOUTHWASH
  - Child 13–17 years: Rinse or gargle 15 mL every 1.5–3 hours as required usually for not more than 7 days, dilute with an equal volume of water if stinging occurs
- BY OROMUCOSAL ADMINISTRATION USING OROMUCOSAL SPRAY
  - Child 1 month–5 years (body-weight 4–7 kg): 1 spray every 1.5–3 hours, to be administered onto affected area
  - Child 1 month–5 years (body-weight 8–11 kg): 2 sprays every 1.5–3 hours, to be administered onto affected area
  - Child 1 month–5 years (body-weight 12–15 kg): 3 sprays every 1.5–3 hours, to be administered onto affected area
  - Child 1 month–5 years (body-weight 16 kg and above): 4 sprays every 1.5–3 hours, to be administered onto affected area
  - Child 6–11 years: 4 sprays every 1.5–3 hours, to be administered onto affected area
  - Child 12–17 years: 4–8 sprays every 1.5–3 hours, to be administered onto affected area

Painful inflammatory conditions of oropharynx [using 0.3% preparations]

- BY OROMUCOSAL ADMINISTRATION USING OROMUCOSAL SPRAY
  - Child 2–5 years (body-weight 8–15 kg): 1 spray every 1.5–3 hours, to be administered onto affected area
  - Child 2–5 years (body-weight 16 kg and above): 2 sprays every 1.5–3 hours, to be administered onto affected area
  - Child 6–11 years: 2 sprays every 1.5–3 hours, to be administered onto affected area
  - Child 12–17 years: 2–4 sprays every 1.5–3 hours, to be administered onto affected area

- **CAUTIONS** Asthma
- **INTERACTIONS** → Appendix 1: NSAIDs
- **SIDE-EFFECTS**
  - **Uncommon** Oral disorders · photosensitivity reaction
  - **Rare or very rare** Angioedema · dry mouth · respiratory disorders · skin reactions
  - **Frequency not known** Nausea · vomiting
- **PREGNANCY** [EvGr] Avoid unless essential (limited information available). ⟨M⟩
- **BREAST FEEDING** [EvGr] Avoid unless essential (no information available). ⟨M⟩
- **PROFESSION SPECIFIC INFORMATION**
  Dental practitioners' formulary Benzydamine Oromucosal Spray 0.15% may be prescribed.
  Benzydamine mouthwash may be prescribed as Benzydamine Mouthwash 0.15%.
- **MEDICINAL FORMS** There can be variation in the licensing of different medicines containing the same drug.

Spray

EXCIPIENTS: May contain Benzyl alcohol, ethanol, hydroxybenzoates (parabens), polysorbates, propylene glycol

- **Benzydamine hydrochloride (Non-proprietary)**
  Benzydamine hydrochloride 1.5 mg per 1 ml Benzydamine 0.15% oromucosal spray sugar free | 30 ml [P] £4.73 DT = £1.52 [SF]
  Benzydamine hydrochloride 3 mg per 1 ml Benzydamine 0.30% oromucosal spray sugar free | 15 ml [PoM] £4.60–£7.82 DT = £4.60 [SF]
- **Difflam** (Ceuta Healthcare Ltd)
  Benzydamine hydrochloride 1.5 mg per 1 ml Difflam 0.15% spray | 30 ml [P] £4.74 DT = £1.52 [SF]

Mouthwash

- **Benzydamine hydrochloride (Non-proprietary)**
  Benzydamine hydrochloride 1.5 mg per 1 ml Benzydamine 0.15% mouthwash sugar free | 300 ml [P] £6.50 DT = £2.39 [SF]
- **Difflam** (Ceuta Healthcare Ltd)
  Benzydamine hydrochloride 1.5 mg per 1 ml Difflam Oral Rinse 0.15% solution | 300 ml [P] £6.50 DT = £2.39 [SF]
  Difflam 0.15% Sore Throat Rinse | 200 ml [P] £5.03 [SF]

Flurbiprofen

19-Mar-2025

- **INDICATIONS AND DOSE**

Relief of sore throat

- BY MOUTH USING LOZENGES
  - Child 12–17 years: 1 lozenge every 3–6 hours for maximum 3 days, allow lozenge to dissolve slowly in the mouth; maximum 5 lozenges per day

- **INTERACTIONS** → Appendix 1: NSAIDs
- **SIDE-EFFECTS** Oral ulceration (move lozenge around mouth) · taste altered
- **ALLERGY AND CROSS-SENSITIVITY** [EvGr] Contra-indicated in patients with a history of hypersensitivity to aspirin or any other NSAID—which includes those in whom attacks of asthma, angioedema, urticaria or rhinitis have been precipitated by aspirin or any other NSAID. ⟨M⟩
- **MEDICINAL FORMS** There can be variation in the licensing of different medicines containing the same drug.

Lozenge

- **Strefen** (Reckitt Benckiser Healthcare (UK) Ltd)
  Flurbiprofen 8.75 mg Strefen Orange 8.75mg lozenges sugar free | 16 lozenge [P] £4.52 [SF]
  Strefen Eucalyptus and Manuka Honey 8.75mg lozenges | 16 lozenge [P] £4.52 [SF]
  Strefen Honey and Lemon 8.75mg lozenges | 16 lozenge [P] £4.52 DT = £4.52

CORTICOSTEROIDS

F 540

Betamethasone

26-Jul-2025

- **DRUG ACTION** Betamethasone has very high glucocorticoid activity and insignificant mineralocorticoid activity.

- **INDICATIONS AND DOSE**

Oral ulceration

- BY OROMUCOSAL ADMINISTRATION USING SOLUBLE TABLETS
  - Child 12–17 years: 500 micrograms 4 times a day, to be dissolved in 20 mL water and rinsed around the mouth; not to be swallowed

- **UNLICENSED USE** Betamethasone soluble tablets not licensed for use as mouthwash or in oral ulceration.

- **CONTRA-INDICATIONS** Untreated local infection
- **INTERACTIONS** → Appendix 1: corticosteroids
- **SIDE-EFFECTS** Since systemic absorption can follow local administration, also consider the side-effects of systemic corticosteroids.
- **PATIENT AND CARER ADVICE** Patient counselling is advised for betamethasone soluble tablets (administration).
- **PROFESSION SPECIFIC INFORMATION**

Dental practitioners' formulary Betamethasone Soluble Tablets 500 micrograms may be prescribed.

- **MEDICINAL FORMS** There can be variation in the licensing of different medicines containing the same drug.

Soluble tablet

CAUTIONARY AND ADVISORY LABELS 10, 13, 21 (not for use as mouthwash for oral ulceration)

▸ Betamethasone (Non-proprietary)
Betamethasone (as Betamethasone sodium phosphate) 500 microgram Betamethasone 500microgram soluble tablets sugar free | 100 tablet [PoM] £86.90 DT = £65.82 [SF]

F 540

Hydrocortisone

26-Jul-2025

- **DRUG ACTION** Hydrocortisone has equal glucocorticoid and mineralocorticoid activity.
- **INDICATIONS AND DOSE**

Aphthous ulcers

▸ BY OROMUCOSAL ADMINISTRATION USING BUCCAL TABLET
▸ Child 1 month–11 years: Only on medical advice
▸ Child 12–17 years: 2.5 mg 4 times a day, allow buccal tablet to dissolve slowly in the mouth in contact with the ulcer

- **UNLICENSED USE** *Hydrocortisone mucoadhesive buccal tablets* licensed for use in children (under 12 years—on medical advice only).

IMPORTANT SAFETY INFORMATION

MHRA/CHM ADVICE: HYDROCORTISONE MUCO-ADHESIVE BUCCAL TABLETS: SHOULD NOT BE USED OFF-LABEL FOR ADRENAL INSUFFICIENCY IN CHILDREN DUE TO SERIOUS RISKS (DECEMBER 2018)

The MHRA has received reports of off-label use of hydrocortisone muco-adhesive buccal tablets for adrenal insufficiency in children.

Healthcare professionals are advised that:

- hydrocortisone muco-adhesive buccal tablets are indicated only for local use in the mouth for aphthous ulceration and should not be used to treat adrenal insufficiency;
- substitution of licensed oral hydrocortisone formulations with muco-adhesive buccal tablets can result in insufficient cortisol absorption and, in stress situations, life-threatening adrenal crisis;
- only hydrocortisone products licensed for adrenal replacement therapy should be used.

- **CONTRA-INDICATIONS** Untreated local infection
- **INTERACTIONS** → Appendix 1: corticosteroids
- **SIDE-EFFECTS** Since systemic absorption can follow local administration, also consider the side-effects of systemic corticosteroids.
- **PROFESSION SPECIFIC INFORMATION**

Dental practitioners' formulary Mucoadhesive buccal tablets may be prescribed as Hydrocortisone Oromucosal Tablets.

- **MEDICINAL FORMS** No licensed medicines listed.

SALICYLIC ACID AND DERIVATIVES

Choline salicylate

23-Nov-2020

- **INDICATIONS AND DOSE**

Mild oral and perioral lesions

▸ BY OROMUCOSAL ADMINISTRATION
▸ Child 16–17 years: Apply 0.5 inch, apply to the lesion with gentle massage, not more often than every 3 hours

- **CONTRA-INDICATIONS** Children under 16 years

CONTRA-INDICATIONS, FURTHER INFORMATION

▸ Reye's syndrome The CHM has advised that topical oral pain relief products containing salicylate salts should not be used in children under 16 years, as a cautionary measure due to the theoretical risk of Reye's syndrome.

- **CAUTIONS** Frequent application, especially in children, may give rise to salicylate poisoning
- **INTERACTIONS** → Appendix 1: choline salicylate
- **SIDE-EFFECTS** Bronchospasm
- **PRESCRIBING AND DISPENSING INFORMATION** When prepared extemporaneously, the BP states Choline Salicylate Dental Gel, BP consists of choline salicylate 8.7% in a flavoured gel basis.
- **PROFESSION SPECIFIC INFORMATION**

Dental practitioners' formulary Choline Salicylate Dental Gel may be prescribed.

- **MEDICINAL FORMS** There can be variation in the licensing of different medicines containing the same drug.

Oromucosal gel

▸ Bonjela (Reckitt Benckiser Healthcare (UK) Ltd)
Choline salicylate 87 mg per 1 gram Bonjela Cool Mint gel | 15 gram [GSL] £3.82 DT = £3.82 [SF]
Bonjela Original gel | 15 gram [GSL] £3.82 DT = £3.82 [SF]

Salicylic acid with rhubarb extract

17-Feb-2023

- **INDICATIONS AND DOSE**

Mild oral and perioral lesions

▸ TO THE LESION
▸ Child 16–17 years: Apply 3–4 times a day maximum duration 7 days

- **CONTRA-INDICATIONS** Children under 16 years

CONTRA-INDICATIONS, FURTHER INFORMATION

▸ Reye's syndrome The CHM has advised that topical oral pain relief products containing salicylate salts should not be used in children under 16 years, as a cautionary measure due to the theoretical risk of Reye's syndrome.

- **CAUTIONS** Frequent application, especially in children, may give rise to salicylate poisoning
- **SIDE-EFFECTS**

▸ **Common or very common** Oral discolouration · tooth discolouration

- **DIRECTIONS FOR ADMINISTRATION** [EvGr] Apply using the brush provided and avoid rinsing the mouth or eating for 15 minutes after application. ⟨M⟩
- **PATIENT AND CARER ADVICE** Patients or carers should be given advice on how to administer salicylic acid with rhubarb extract oromucosal solution. May cause temporary discolouration of teeth and oral mucosa.
- **MEDICINAL FORMS** No licensed medicines listed.

4 Oropharyngeal bacterial infections

Oropharyngeal infections, antibacterial therapy

24-Feb-2023

Pericoronitis

Public Health England advises antibacterial use only in the presence of systemic features of infection, or persistent swelling.

- Metronidazole p. 409, or *alternatively*, amoxicillin p. 417
  - ▸ *Suggested duration of treatment* 3 days or until pain reduction allows for oral hygiene.

Gingivitis (acute necrotising ulcerative)

Public Health England advises antibacterial use only in the presence of systemic features of infection.

- Metronidazole
  - ▸ *Suggested duration of treatment* 3 days.

EvGr If metronidazole is contra-indicated, use *alternative*, amoxicillin. ⟨A⟩

Abscess (periapical or periodontal)

Public Health England advises antibacterial use only if there are signs of severe infection, systemic symptoms, or a high risk of complications.

- Phenoxymethylpenicillin p. 416, or *alternatively*, amoxicillin
  - ▸ Alternative in penicillin allergy: clarithromycin p. 403
  - ▸ If signs of spreading infection (e.g. lymph node involvement, systemic signs), add metronidazole
  - ▸ *Suggested duration of treatment* up to 5 days; review at 3 days.

Periodontitis

EvGr Antibacterials may be used as an adjunct to effective mechanical debridement in severe disease or disease unresponsive to local treatment alone on the advice of a specialist. ⟨A⟩

Sore throat (acute)

Acute sore throat is usually triggered by a viral infection and is self-limiting. Symptoms can last for around 1 week, and most people will improve within this time without treatment with antibacterials, regardless of the cause. EvGr A clinical scoring system should be used in combination with clinical judgement to identify individuals most likely to benefit from an antibacterial.

Patients who are systemically very unwell, or have signs and symptoms of a more serious illness or condition, or are at high risk of complications should be offered immediate antibacterial therapy. Patients with severe systemic infection or severe suppurative complications (such as peritonsillar abscess (quinsy) or cellulitis) should be referred to hospital.

- Phenoxymethylpenicillin p. 416
  - ▸ *Suggested duration of treatment* 5 to 10 days.
- Alternative in penicillin allergy: clarithromycin p. 403 *or* erythromycin p. 406 (in pregnancy)
  - ▸ *Suggested duration of treatment* 5 days. ⟨A⟩

For further guidance on the management of acute sore throat, see NICE guideline: **Sore throat (acute): antimicrobial prescribing** (see *Useful resources*).

Other infections

For further information on antibacterial treatment used in oropharyngeal infections, see Oral bacterial infections p. 370.

Useful resources

Sore throat (acute): antimicrobial prescribing. National Institute for Health and Care Excellence. NICE guideline 84. January 2018.
www.nice.org.uk/guidance/ng84

ANTIBACTERIALS › TETRACYCLINES AND RELATED DRUGS

F 433

Doxycycline

18-Apr-2025

● **INDICATIONS AND DOSE**

Treatment of recurrent aphthous ulceration

▸ BY OROMUCOSAL ADMINISTRATION USING DISPERSIBLE TABLETS

▸ Child 12–17 years: 100 mg 4 times a day usually for 3 days, dispersible tablet can be stirred into a small amount of water then rinsed around the mouth for 2–3 minutes, it should preferably not be swallowed

● **UNLICENSED USE** Doxycycline may be used as detailed below, although considered outside the scope of its licence:
- recurrent aphthous ulceration.

● **CAUTIONS** Alcohol dependence

● **INTERACTIONS** → Appendix 1: tetracyclines

● **SIDE-EFFECTS**

▸ **Common or very common** Dyspnoea · hypotension · peripheral oedema · tachycardia

▸ **Uncommon** Gastrointestinal discomfort

▸ **Rare or very rare** Anxiety · arthralgia · Clostridioides difficile colitis · flushing · intracranial pressure increased with papilloedema · Jarisch-Herxheimer reaction · myalgia · photoonycholysis · severe cutaneous adverse reactions (SCARs) · skin hyperpigmentation (long term use) · stomatitis · tinnitus · vision disorders

● **PATIENT AND CARER ADVICE** Counselling on administration advised.

Photosensitivity Patients should be advised to avoid exposure to sunlight or sun lamps.

● **PROFESSION SPECIFIC INFORMATION**

Dental practitioners' formulary Dispersible tablets may be prescribed as Dispersible Doxycycline Tablets.

● **MEDICINAL FORMS** There can be variation in the licensing of different medicines containing the same drug.

Dispersible tablet

CAUTIONARY AND ADVISORY LABELS 6, 9, 11, 13

▸ **Vibramycin-D** (Pfizer Ltd)

Doxycycline (as Doxycycline monohydrate) 100 mg Vibramycin-D 100mg dispersible tablets | 8 tablet PoM £4.91 DT = £4.91 SF

5 Oropharyngeal fungal infections

Oropharyngeal fungal infections

19-May-2022

Overview

Fungal infections of the mouth are usually caused by *Candida* spp. (candidiasis or candidosis). Different types of oropharyngeal candidiasis are managed as follows:

12 Ear, nose and oropharynx

Thrush

Pseudomembranous candidiasis (thrush) is usually an acute infection but it may persist in chronic forms. Those at greater risk of candidal infections include children receiving inhaled corticosteroids, chemotherapy, or broad-spectrum antibacterials, and in patients with serious systemic disease associated with reduced immunity such as leukaemia, other malignancies, and HIV infection. EvGr Any predisposing condition should be managed appropriately. (A) The risk of oral candidiasis associated with corticosteroid inhaler use can be reduced by rinsing the mouth with water (or cleaning teeth) immediately after using the inhaler, use of a spacer, or using an inhaler at its lowest effective dose.

EvGr For mild and localised infections, treatment with miconazole oral gel below is recommended; if this is unsuitable, oral nystatin p. 885 may be given.

In children aged under 16 years, if the infection fails to respond to 1 week of miconazole treatment, consider extending the course if some response was seen, or switching to nystatin if no effects were seen. Refer the child to a paediatrician or specialist if there is inadequate response after 2 weeks of treatment, or the child has recurrent episodes, or the infection is severe or extensive, or if there is suspicion the child may be immunocompromised.

In children aged 16 years and over with severe or extensive infection, either refer to a specialist or considered for antifungal treatment with oral fluconazole p. 463. If the infection fails to respond to treatment after 1 week, consider extending the course for another week, swabbing to identify the causative organism, or referring to a specialist as appropriate. For immunocompromised children receiving treatment with ciclosporin, oral tacrolimus, or chemotherapy, seek specialist advice before starting antifungal treatment.

All children with evidence of systemic disease or widespread infection should be admitted to hospital. (A)

Acute erythematous candidiasis

Acute erythematous (atrophic) candidiasis is usually associated with a burning sensation of the mouth or tongue and may be caused by corticosteroid or broad-spectrum antibacterial use. EvGr Treatment of acute erythematous candidiasis is the same as for pseudomembranous candidiasis (E)—for further information, see *Thrush*.

Angular cheilitis

Angular cheilitis (angular stomatitis) is characterised by soreness, erythema, and fissuring at the angles of the mouth. It may be associated with nutritional deficiency or immunosuppression. Both yeasts (*Candida* spp.) and bacteria (*Staphylococcus aureus* and streptococci) are commonly involved as interacting, infective factors. EvGr Angular cheilitis is normally self-limiting. While the underlying cause is being identified and treated, it may be helpful to apply topical emollients, miconazole cream or ointment for mild candida infection, or fusidic acid ointment p. 441 if there is evidence of bacterial infection. If the angular cheilitis is unresponsive to treatment, hydrocortisone with miconazole cream or ointment can be used. (E)

Drugs used in oropharyngeal candidiasis

Nystatin is not absorbed from the gastro-intestinal tract and is applied locally (as a suspension) to the mouth for treating local fungal infections. Miconazole is applied locally (as an oral gel) in the mouth but it is absorbed systemically so potential interactions need to be considered. Miconazole also has some activity against Gram-positive bacteria including streptococci and staphylococci. EvGr In neonates, nystatin [unlicensed] oral suspension or miconazole [unlicensed] oral gel is used for the treatment of oropharyngeal candidiasis. (A)

For further information on systemic antifungal treatment, see Antifungals, systemic use p. 459.

12 Ear, nose and oropharynx

ANTIFUNGALS > IMIDAZOLE ANTIFUNGALS

Miconazole

23-Jun-2023

● **INDICATIONS AND DOSE**

Oral candidiasis

▶ BY OROMUCOSAL ADMINISTRATION USING ORAL GEL

- Neonate: 1 mL 2–4 times a day treatment should be continued for at least 7 days after lesions have healed or symptoms have cleared, to be smeared around the inside of the mouth after feeds.
- Child 1–23 months: 1.25 mL 4 times a day treatment should be continued for at least 7 days after lesions have healed or symptoms have cleared, to be smeared around the inside of the mouth after feeds
- Child 2–17 years: 2.5 mL 4 times a day treatment should be continued for at least 7 days after lesions have healed or symptoms have cleared, to be administered after meals, retain near oral lesions before swallowing (dental prostheses and orthodontic appliances should be removed at night and brushed with gel)

Prevention and treatment of oral candidiasis (dose approved for use by community practitioner nurse prescribers)

▶ BY OROMUCOSAL ADMINISTRATION USING ORAL GEL

- Child 4–23 months: 1.25 mL 4 times a day treatment should be continued for at least 7 days after lesions have healed or symptoms have cleared, to be smeared around the inside of the mouth after feeds
- Child 2–17 years: 2.5 mL 4 times a day treatment should be continued for at least 7 days after lesions have healed or symptoms have cleared, to be administered after meals, retain near oral lesions before swallowing (dental prostheses and orthodontic appliances should be removed at night and brushed with gel)

DOSE EQUIVALENCE AND CONVERSION

- One 5-mL spoonful of oral gel equivalent to 124 mg miconazole.

● **UNLICENSED USE** Not licensed for use in children under 4 months of age or during first 5–6 months of life of an infant born pre-term.

● **CONTRA-INDICATIONS** Infants with impaired swallowing reflex

● **CAUTIONS** Avoid in Acute porphyrias p. 745

● **INTERACTIONS** → Appendix 1: antifungals, azoles

● **SIDE-EFFECTS**

▶ **Common or very common** Dry mouth · nausea · oral disorders · vomiting

▶ **Uncommon** Skin reactions · taste altered

▶ **Frequency not known** Angioedema · choking · diarrhoea · hepatitis · severe cutaneous adverse reactions (SCARs) · tongue discolouration

● **PREGNANCY** Manufacturer advises avoid if possible—toxicity at high doses in *animal* studies.

● **BREAST FEEDING** Manufacturer advises caution—no information available.

● **HEPATIC IMPAIRMENT** Manufacturer advises avoid.

● **DIRECTIONS FOR ADMINISTRATION** Manufacturer advises oral gel should be held in mouth, after food.

● **PRESCRIBING AND DISPENSING INFORMATION** Flavours of oral gel may include orange.

● **PATIENT AND CARER ADVICE** Patients or carers should be given advice on how to administer miconazole oromucosal gel.

● **PROFESSION SPECIFIC INFORMATION**

Dental practitioners' formulary Miconazole Oromucosal Gel may be prescribed.

- **EXCEPTIONS TO LEGAL CATEGORY** 15-g tube of oral gel can be sold to the public.

- **MEDICINAL FORMS** There can be variation in the licensing of different medicines containing the same drug.

Oromucosal gel

CAUTIONARY AND ADVISORY LABELS 9

▸ **Daktarin** (McNeil Products Ltd)

Miconazole 20 mg per 1 gram Daktarin 20mg/g oromucosal gel | 80 gram PoM £4.95 DT = £4.95 SF

ANTIFUNGALS › POLYENE ANTIFUNGALS

Nystatin

10-Nov-2021

- **INDICATIONS AND DOSE**

Oral candidiasis

▸ BY OROMUCOSAL ADMINISTRATION

▸ Neonate: 100 000 units 4 times a day usually for 7 days, and continued for 48 hours after lesions have resolved, to be given after feeds.

▸ Child: 100 000 units 4 times a day usually for 7 days, and continued for 48 hours after lesions have resolved

Oral and perioral fungal infections (dose approved for use by community practitioner nurse prescribers)

▸ BY OROMUCOSAL ADMINISTRATION

▸ Neonate: 100 000 units 4 times a day usually for 7 days, and continued for 48 hours after lesions have resolved, to be given after feeds.

▸ Child: 100 000 units 4 times a day usually for 7 days, and continued for 48 hours after lesions have resolved

- **UNLICENSED USE** EvGr Nystatin may be used in neonates, ⟨E⟩ but it is not licensed for use in this patient group.

Suspension not licensed for use in neonates for the treatment of candidiasis but the Department of Health has advised that a Community Practitioner Nurse Prescriber may prescribe nystatin oral suspension for a neonate, in the doses provided in BNF Publications, provided that there is a clear diagnosis of oral thrush. The nurse prescriber must only prescribe within their own competence and must accept clinical and medicolegal responsibility for prescribing.

- **SIDE-EFFECTS** Abdominal distress · angioedema · diarrhoea · face oedema · nausea · sensitisation · skin reactions · Stevens-Johnson syndrome · vomiting

- **PATIENT AND CARER ADVICE** Counselling advised with oral suspension (use of pipette, hold in mouth, after food).

Medicines for Children leaflet: Nystatin for Candida infections www.medicinesforchildren.org.uk/medicines/nystatin-for-candida-infections/

- **PROFESSION SPECIFIC INFORMATION**

Dental practitioners' formulary Nystatin Oral Suspension may be prescribed.

- **MEDICINAL FORMS** There can be variation in the licensing of different medicines containing the same drug. Forms available from special-order manufacturers include: oral suspension

Oral suspension

CAUTIONARY AND ADVISORY LABELS 9

EXCIPIENTS: May contain Ethanol

▸ **Nystatin (Non-proprietary)**

Nystatin 100000 unit per 1 ml Nystatin 100,000units/ml oral suspension | 30 ml PoM £17.50 DT = £9.75

6 Oropharyngeal viral infections

Oropharyngeal viral infections

Management

Viral infections are the most common cause of a sore throat. It is usually a self-limiting condition which does not benefit from anti-infective treatment. Adequate analgesia may be all that is required.

Children with varicella–zoster infection often develop painful lesions in the mouth and throat. Benzydamine hydrochloride p. 881 may be used to provide local analgesia. Chlorhexidine mouthwash or gel p. 877 will control plaque accumulation if toothbrushing is painful and will also help to control secondary infection in general.

In severe herpetic stomatitis systemic aciclovir p. 500 or valaciclovir p. 502 may be used for oral lesions associated with herpes zoster. Aciclovir and valaciclovir are also used to prevent frequently recurring herpes simplex lesions of the mouth particularly when associated with the initiation of erythema multiforme. See the treatment of labial herpes simplex infections.

Chapter 13
Skin

CONTENTS

Skin conditions, management 21-Jul-2022

Topical preparations

When prescribing topical preparations for the treatment of skin conditions in children, the site of application, the condition being treated, and the child's (and carer's) preference for a particular vehicle all need to be taken into consideration.

Vehicles

The British Association of Dermatologists list of preferred unlicensed dermatological preparations (specials) is available at www.bad.org.uk/guidelines-and-standards/access-to-medicines/.

The vehicle in topical preparations for the skin affects the degree of hydration, has a mild anti-inflammatory effect, and aids the penetration of the active drug. Therefore, the vehicle, as well as the active drug, should be chosen on the basis of their suitability for the child's skin condition.

Applications are usually viscous solutions, emulsions, or suspensions for application to the skin (including the scalp) or nails.

Collodions are painted on the skin and allowed to dry to leave a flexible film over the site of application.

Creams are emulsions of oil and water and are generally well absorbed into the skin. They may contain an antimicrobial preservative unless the active ingredient or basis is intrinsically bactericidal and fungicidal. Generally, creams are cosmetically more acceptable than ointments because they are less greasy and easier to apply.

Gels consist of active ingredients in suitable hydrophilic or hydrophobic bases; they generally have a high water content. Gels are particularly suitable for application to the face and scalp.

Lotions have a cooling effect and may be preferred to ointments or creams for application over a hairy area. Lotions in alcoholic basis can sting if used on broken skin. *Shake lotions* (such as calamine lotion) contain insoluble powders which leave a deposit on the skin surface.

Ointments are greasy preparations which are normally anhydrous and insoluble in water, and are more occlusive than creams. They are particularly suitable for chronic, dry lesions. The most commonly used ointment bases consist of soft paraffin or a combination of soft, liquid, and hard paraffin. Some ointment bases have both *hydrophilic and lipophilic* properties; they may have occlusive properties on the skin surface, encourage hydration, and also be miscible with water; they often have a mild anti-inflammatory effect. *Water-soluble ointments* contain macrogols which are freely soluble in water and are therefore readily washed off; they have a limited but useful role where ready removal is desirable.

Pastes are stiff preparations containing a high proportion of finely powdered solids such as zinc oxide and starch suspended in an ointment. They are used for circumscribed lesions such as those which occur in lichen simplex, chronic eczema, or psoriasis. They are less occlusive than ointments and can be used to protect inflamed, lichenified, or excoriated skin.

Dusting powders are used only rarely. They reduce friction between opposing skin surfaces. Dusting powders should not be applied to moist areas because they can cake and abrade the skin. Talc is a lubricant but it does not absorb moisture; it can cause respiratory irritation. Starch is less lubricant but absorbs water.

Dilution

The BP directs that creams and ointments should **not** normally be diluted but that should dilution be necessary care should be taken, in particular, to prevent microbial contamination. The appropriate diluent should be used and heating should be avoided during mixing; excessive dilution may affect the stability of some creams. Diluted creams should normally be used within 2 weeks of preparation.

Suitable quantities for prescribing

Suitable quantities of dermatological preparations to be prescribed for specific areas of the body

Area of body	Creams and Ointments	Lotions
Face	15–30 g	100 mL
Both hands	25–50 g	200 mL
Scalp	50–100 g	200 mL
Both arms or both legs	100–200 g	200 mL
Trunk	400 g	500 mL
Groins and genitalia	15–25 g	100 mL

These amounts are usually suitable for children 12–18 years for twice daily application for 1 week; smaller quantities will be required for children under 12 years. These recommendations do not apply to corticosteroid preparations.

Excipients and sensitisation

Excipients in topical products rarely cause problems. If a patch test indicates allergy to an excipient, products containing the substance should be avoided (see also Anaphylaxis). The following excipients in topical preparations are associated, rarely, with sensitisation; the presence of these excipients is indicated in the entries for topical products. See also Excipients, under General Guidance.

- Beeswax
- Benzyl alcohol
- Butylated hydroxyanisole
- Butylated hydroxytoluene
- Cetostearyl alcohol (including cetyl and stearyl alcohol)
- Chlorocresol
- Edetic acid (EDTA)
- Ethylenediamine
- Fragrances
- Hydroxybenzoates (parabens)
- Imidurea
- Isopropyl palmitate
- N-(3-Chloroallyl)hexaminium chloride (quaternium 15)
- Polysorbates
- Propylene glycol
- Sodium metabisulfite
- Sorbic acid
- Wool fat and related substances including lanolin (purified versions of wool fat have reduced the problem)

Neonates

Caution is required when prescribing topical preparations for neonates—their large body surface area in relation to body mass increases susceptibility to toxicity from systemic absorption of substances applied to the skin. Topical preparations containing potentially sensitising substances such as corticosteroids, aminoglycosides, iodine, and parasiticidal drugs should be avoided. Preparations containing alcohol should be avoided because they can dehydrate the skin, cause pain if applied to raw areas, and the alcohol can cause necrosis.

In *preterm neonates*, the skin is more fragile and offers a poor barrier, especially in the first fortnight after birth. Preterm infants, especially if below 32 weeks corrected gestational age, may also require special measures to maintain skin hydration.

1 Benign neoplasms of skin

ANTINEOPLASTIC DRUGS > PROTEIN KINASE INHIBITORS

Sirolimus

19-Mar-2025

- **INDICATIONS AND DOSE**

Facial angiofibroma associated with tuberous sclerosis complex

▶ TO THE SKIN

- ▶ Child 6–11 years: Apply a thin layer of gel twice daily to the affected areas, in the morning and at bedtime. A dose of sirolimus 0.25 mg (equivalent to 125 mg of gel or approximately 0.5 cm gel strand) should be administered per 50 cm^2 lesion, and applied twice daily; maximum total daily dose sirolimus 1.2 mg (equivalent to 600 mg of gel or approximately 2 cm gel strand), discontinue treatment if no response after 12 weeks
- ▶ Child 12–17 years: Apply a thin layer of gel twice daily to the affected areas, in the morning and at bedtime. A dose of sirolimus 0.25 mg (equivalent to 125 mg of gel or approximately 0.5 cm gel strand) should be administered per 50 cm^2 lesion, and applied twice daily; maximum total daily dose sirolimus 1.6 mg (equivalent to 800 mg of gel or approximately 2.5 cm gel strand), discontinue treatment if no response after 12 weeks

- **CAUTIONS** Hyperlipidaemia · immunosuppression · increased susceptibility to lymphoma and other malignancies, particularly of the skin (limit exposure to UV light)
- **INTERACTIONS** → Appendix 1: sirolimus
- **SIDE-EFFECTS**

▶ **Common or very common** Asteatosis · conjunctivitis · eye erythema · eye irritation · increased risk of infection · nasal discomfort · photosensitivity · skin haemorrhage · skin reactions · stomatitis

- **PREGNANCY** EvGr Avoid unless essential (toxicity in *animal* studies). M
- **BREAST FEEDING** Specialist sources suggest limited systemic absorption so unlikely to affect nursing infant.
- **HEPATIC IMPAIRMENT** EvGr Avoid in severe impairment (no information available, though in general blood concentrations are low following topical administration). M
- **DIRECTIONS FOR ADMINISTRATION** EvGr Apply a thin layer of gel to the affected area and rub in gently. Do not apply on wounds, irritated, broken, or infected skin. Avoid contact with eyes and mucous membranes. M
- **HANDLING AND STORAGE** Protect from light. Topical gel: store in a refrigerator (2–8°C).
- **PATIENT AND CARER ADVICE** Advise patients to avoid excessive exposure to UV light including sunlight.

Patients and carers should be advised on the application of *Hyftor*® gel.

Missed doses If a morning dose is missed, it should be applied as soon as possible, provided it's before the evening dose. If the evening dose is missed, it should not be applied and the next dose should be applied at the normal time.

- **NATIONAL FUNDING/ACCESS DECISIONS**

For full details see funding body website

Scottish Medicines Consortium (SMC) decisions

▶ **Sirolimus (*Hyftor*®) for the treatment of adult and paediatric patients aged 6 and above with facial angiofibroma associated**

13 Skin

with tuberous sclerosis complex (January 2025)
SMC No. SMC2710 Recommended

● **MEDICINAL FORMS** There can be variation in the licensing of different medicines containing the same drug.

Cutaneous gel

CAUTIONARY AND ADVISORY LABELS 11
EXCIPIENTS: May contain Alcohol

▸ **Hyftor** (Plusultra Pharma UK Ltd)
Sirolimus 2 mg per 1 gram Hyftor 2mg/g gel | 10 gram PoM
£340.00 DT = £340.00

2 Dry and scaling skin disorders

Emollient and barrier preparations

04-Sep-2020

Borderline substances

The preparations marked 'ACBS' are regarded as drugs when prescribed in accordance with the advice of the Advisory Committee on Borderline Substances for the clinical conditions listed. Prescriptions issued in accordance with this advice and endorsed 'ACBS' will normally not be investigated (see *About Borderline Substances*).

Emollients

Emollients hydrate the skin, soften the skin, act as barrier to water and external irritants, and are indicated for all dry or scaling disorders. Their effects are short-lived and they should be applied frequently even after improvement occurs. They are useful in dry and eczematous disorders, and to a lesser extent in psoriasis; they should be applied immediately after washing or bathing to maximise the effect of skin hydration. The choice of an appropriate emollient will depend on the severity of the condition, the child's (or carer's) preference, and the site of application. Ointments may exacerbate acne and folliculitis. Some ingredients rarely cause sensitisation and this should be suspected if an eczematous reaction occurs. The use of aqueous cream as a leave-on emollient may increase the risk of skin reactions, particularly in eczema.

Preparations such as **aqueous cream** and **emulsifying ointment** can be used as soap substitutes for handwashing and in the bath; the preparation is rubbed on the skin before rinsing off completely. The addition of a bath oil may also be helpful.

Urea is occasionally used with other topical agents such as corticosteroids to enhance penetration of the skin.

Emollient bath and shower preparations

In dry skin conditions soap should be avoided.

The quantities of bath additives recommended for older children are suitable for an adult-size bath. Proportionately less should be used for a child-size bath or a washbasin; recommended bath additive quantities for younger children reflect this.

MHRA/CHM advice (updated December 2018): Emollients: new information about risk of severe and fatal burns with paraffin-containing and paraffin-free emollients

Emollients are an important and effective treatment for chronic dry skin disorders and people should continue to use these products. However, healthcare professionals must ensure that patients and their carers understand the fire risk associated with the build-up of residue on clothing and bedding and can take action to minimise the risk. There is a fire risk with all paraffin-containing emollients, regardless of paraffin concentration, and it cannot be excluded with paraffin-free emollients. A similar risk may apply to products that are applied to the skin over large body areas, or in large volumes for repeated use for more than a few days.

Healthcare professionals should advise patients not to smoke or go near naked flames because clothing, bedding, dressings, and other fabrics that have been in contact with an emollient or emollient-treated skin can rapidly ignite. Washing these materials at high temperature may reduce emollient build-up but not totally remove it.

The MHRA/CHM (August 2020) have released a toolkit of resources for health and social care professionals to support the safe use of emollients, available at: www.gov.uk/drug-safety-update/emollients-and-risk-of-severe-and-fatal-burns-new-resources-available.

Barrier preparations

Barrier preparations often contain water-repellent substances such as dimeticone (see barrier creams and ointments below), natural oils, and paraffins, to help protect the skin from abrasion and irritation; they are used to protect intact skin around stomas and pressure sores, and as a barrier against nappy rash. In neonates, barrier preparations which do not contain potentially sensitising excipients are preferred. Where the skin has broken down, barrier preparations have a limited role in protecting adjacent skin. Barrier preparations with zinc oxide or titanium salts are used to aid healing of uninfected, excoriated skin.

Nappy rash (Dermatitis)

The first line of treatment is to ensure that nappies are changed frequently and that tightly fitting water-proof pants are avoided. The rash may clear when left exposed to the air and a barrier preparation, applied with each nappy change, can be helpful. A mild corticosteroid such as hydrocortisone 0.5% or 1% p. 912 can be used if inflammation is causing discomfort, but it should be avoided in neonates. The barrier preparation should be applied after the corticosteroid preparation to prevent further damage. Preparations containing hydrocortisone should be applied for no more than a week; the hydrocortisone should be discontinued as soon as the inflammation subsides. The occlusive effect of nappies and waterproof pants may increase absorption of corticosteroids (see cautions). If the rash is associated with candidal infection, a topical antifungal such as clotrimazole cream p. 900 can be used. Topical antibacterial preparations can be used if bacterial infection is present; treatment with an oral antibacterial may occasionally be required in severe or recurrent infection. Hydrocortisone may be used in combination with antimicrobial preparations if there is considerable inflammation, erosion, and infection.

Emollients for neonates

In the *neonate*, a preservative-free paraffin-based emollient hydrates the skin without affecting the normal skin flora; substances such as olive oil are also used. The development of blisters (epidermolysis bullosa) or ichthyosis may be alleviated by applying liquid and white soft paraffin ointment while awaiting dermatological investigation.

DERMATOLOGICAL DRUGS > BARRIER PREPARATIONS

Barrier creams and ointments

13-Feb-2020

● **INDICATIONS AND DOSE**

For use as a barrier preparation

▸ TO THE SKIN
▸ Child: (consult product literature)

● **MEDICINAL FORMS** There can be variation in the licensing of different medicines containing the same drug.

Cutaneous ointment

EXCIPIENTS: May contain Woolfat and related substances (including lanolin)

▸ **Barrier creams and ointments (Non-proprietary)**
Cetostearyl alcohol 20 mg per 1 gram, Zinc oxide 75 mg per 1 gram, Beeswax white 100 mg per 1 gram, Arachis oil 305 mg per 1 gram, Castor oil 500 mg per 1 gram Ovelle zinc and castor oil ointment | 100 gram £4.41

Cutaneous cream

EXCIPIENTS: May contain Beeswax, butylated hydroxyanisole, butylated hydroxytoluene, cetostearyl alcohol (including cetyl and stearyl alcohol), chlorocresol, fragrances, hydroxybenzoates (parabens), propylene glycol, woolfat and related substances (including lanolin)

▸ **Conotrane** (Evolan Pharma AB)
Benzalkonium chloride 1 mg per 1 gram, Dimeticone 220 mg per 1 gram Conotrane cream | 500 gram GSL £9.19

▸ **Drapolene** (Supra Enterprises Ltd)
Benzalkonium chloride 100 microgram per 1 gram, Cetrimide 2 mg per 1 gram Drapolene cream | 100 gram GSL £4.06 DT = £4.06 200 gram GSL £5.93 DT = £5.93 | 350 gram GSL £9.37 DT = £9.37

▸ **Siopel** (Derma UK Ltd)
Cetrimide 3 mg per 1 gram, Dimeticone 1000 100 mg per 1 gram Siopel cream | 50 gram GSL £4.73 DT = £4.73

▸ **Sudocrem** (Teva UK Ltd)
Benzyl cinnamate 1.5 mg per 1 gram, Benzyl alcohol 3.9 mg per 1 gram, Benzyl benzoate 10.1 mg per 1 gram, Wool fat hydrous 40 mg per 1 gram, Zinc oxide 152.5 mg per 1 gram Sudocrem antiseptic healing cream | 60 gram GSL £3.53 | 125 gram GSL £5.12 | 250 gram GSL £9.06 | 400 gram GSL £12.09

DERMATOLOGICAL DRUGS › EMOLLIENTS

Emollient bath and shower products, antimicrobial-containing

15-Feb-2024

● **INDICATIONS AND DOSE**

DERMOL® 200 SHOWER EMOLLIENT

Dry and pruritic skin conditions including eczema and dermatitis

▶ TO THE SKIN
▸ Child: To be applied to the skin or used as a soap substitute

DERMOL® 600 BATH EMOLLIENT

Dry and pruritic skin conditions including eczema and dermatitis

▶ TO THE SKIN
▸ Child 1–23 months: 5–15 mL/bath, not to be used undiluted
▸ Child 2–17 years: 15–30 mL/bath, not to be used undiluted

DERMOL® WASH EMULSION

Dry and pruritic skin conditions including eczema and dermatitis

▶ TO THE SKIN
▸ Child: To be applied to the skin or used as a soap substitute

EMULSIDERM®

Dry skin conditions including eczema and ichthyosis

▶ TO THE SKIN
▸ Child 1–23 months: 5–10 mL/bath, alternatively, to be rubbed into dry skin until absorbed
▸ Child 2–17 years: 7–30 mL/bath, alternatively, to be rubbed into dry skin until absorbed

OILATUM® PLUS

Topical treatment of eczema, including eczema at risk from infection

▶ TO THE SKIN
▸ Child 6–11 months: 1 mL/bath, not to be used undiluted
▸ Child 1–17 years: 1–2 capfuls/bath, not to be used undiluted

IMPORTANT SAFETY INFORMATION

These preparations make skin and surfaces slippery—particular care is needed when bathing.

MHRA/CHM ADVICE (UPDATED DECEMBER 2018): EMOLLIENTS: NEW INFORMATION ABOUT RISK OF SEVERE AND FATAL BURNS WITH PARAFFIN-CONTAINING AND PARAFFIN-FREE EMOLLIENTS

See Emollient and barrier preparations p. 888.

● **DIRECTIONS FOR ADMINISTRATION** Emollient bath additives should be added to bath water; EvGr hydration can be improved by soaking in the bath for 5–20 minutes (consult product literature). Some bath emollients can be applied to wet skin undiluted and rinsed off. ⟨M⟩ Emollient preparations contained in tubs should be removed with a clean spoon or spatula to reduce bacterial contamination of the emollient. Emollients should be applied in the direction of hair growth to reduce the risk of folliculitis.

● **PRESCRIBING AND DISPENSING INFORMATION** Preparations containing an antibacterial should be avoided unless infection is present or is a frequent complication.

● **MEDICINAL FORMS** There can be variation in the licensing of different medicines containing the same drug.

Bath additive

CAUTIONARY AND ADVISORY LABELS 15

EXCIPIENTS: May contain Acetylated lanolin alcohols, isopropyl palmitate, polysorbates

▸ **Dermol 600** (Dermal Laboratories Ltd)
Benzalkonium chloride 5 mg per 1 gram, Isopropyl myristate 250 mg per 1 gram, Liquid paraffin 250 mg per 1 gram Dermol 600 bath emollient | 600 ml P £7.99

▸ **Emulsiderm** (Dermal Laboratories Ltd)
Benzalkonium chloride 5 mg per 1 gram, Isopropyl myristate 250 mg per 1 gram, Liquid paraffin 250 mg per 1 gram Emulsiderm emollient | 300 ml P £4.04

▸ **Oilatum Plus** (Thornton & Ross Ltd)
Triclosan 20 mg per 1 gram, Benzalkonium chloride 60 mg per 1 gram, Liquid paraffin light 525 mg per 1 gram Oilatum Plus bath additive | 500 ml GSL £8.81

Cutaneous emulsion

CAUTIONARY AND ADVISORY LABELS 15

EXCIPIENTS: May contain Cetostearyl alcohol (including cetyl and stearyl alcohol)

▸ **Dermol 200** (Dermal Laboratories Ltd)
Benzalkonium chloride 1 mg per 1 gram, Chlorhexidine hydrochloride 1 mg per 1 gram, Isopropyl myristate 25 mg per 1 gram, Liquid paraffin 25 mg per 1 gram Dermol 200 shower emollient | 200 ml P £3.76

▸ **Dermol Wash** (Dermal Laboratories Ltd)
Benzalkonium chloride 1 mg per 1 gram, Chlorhexidine hydrochloride 1 mg per 1 gram, Isopropyl myristate 25 mg per 1 gram, Liquid paraffin 25 mg per 1 gram Dermol Wash cutaneous emulsion | 200 ml P £3.76

Emollient bath and shower products, paraffin-containing

15-Aug-2024

● **INDICATIONS AND DOSE**

Dry skin conditions (using Aqueous Cream BP)

▶ TO THE SKIN
▸ Child: To be used as a soap substitute

AQUAMAX® WASH

Dry skin conditions

▶ TO THE SKIN
▸ Child: To be applied to wet or dry skin and rinse

continued →

CETRABEN® BATH

Dry skin conditions, including eczema

▶ TO THE SKIN

- Neonate: 0.5 capful/bath, alternatively, to be applied to wet skin and rinse.
- Child 1 month–11 years: 0.5–1 capful/bath, alternatively, to be applied to wet skin and rinse
- Child 12–17 years: 1–2 capfuls/bath, alternatively, to be applied to wet skin and rinse

DERMALO®

Dermatitis | Dry skin conditions, including ichthyosis

▶ TO THE SKIN

- Neonate: 5 mL/bath, alternatively, to be applied to wet skin and rinse.
- Child 1 month–11 years: 5–10 mL/bath, alternatively, to be applied to wet skin and rinse
- Child 12–17 years: 15–20 mL/bath, alternatively, to be applied to wet skin and rinse

DOUBLEBASE® EMOLLIENT BATH ADDITIVE

Dry skin conditions including dermatitis and ichthyosis

▶ TO THE SKIN

- Neonate: 5–10 mL/bath.
- Child 1 month–11 years: 5–10 mL/bath
- Child 12–17 years: 15–20 mL/bath

DOUBLEBASE® EMOLLIENT SHOWER GEL

Dry, chapped, or itchy skin conditions

▶ TO THE SKIN

- Child: To be applied to wet or dry skin and rinse, or apply to dry skin after showering

DOUBLEBASE® EMOLLIENT WASH GEL

Dry, chapped, or itchy skin conditions

▶ TO THE SKIN

- Child: To be used as a soap substitute

E45® BATH OIL

Endogenous and exogenous eczema, xeroderma, and ichthyosis

▶ TO THE SKIN

- Neonate: 5 mL/bath, alternatively, to be applied to wet skin and rinse.
- Child 1 month–11 years: 5–10 mL/bath, alternatively, to be applied to wet skin and rinse
- Child 12–17 years: 15 mL/bath, alternatively, to be applied to wet skin and rinse

E45® WASH CREAM

Endogenous and exogenous eczema, xeroderma, and ichthyosis

▶ TO THE SKIN

- Child: To be used as a soap substitute

HYDROMOL® BATH AND SHOWER EMOLLIENT

Dry skin conditions | Eczema | Ichthyosis

▶ TO THE SKIN

- Neonate: 0.5 capful/bath, alternatively apply to wet skin and rinse.
- Child 1 month–11 years: 0.5–2 capfuls/bath, alternatively apply to wet skin and rinse
- Child 12–17 years: 1–3 capfuls/bath, alternatively apply to wet skin and rinse

LPL 63.4®

Dry skin conditions

▶ TO THE SKIN

- Neonate: 0.5 capful/bath, alternatively, to be applied to wet skin and rinse.
- Child 1 month–11 years: 0.5–2 capfuls/bath, alternatively, to be applied to wet skin and rinse
- Child 12–17 years: 1–3 capfuls/bath, alternatively, to be applied to wet skin and rinse

OILATUM® EMOLLIENT BATH ADDITIVE

Dry skin conditions including dermatitis and ichthyosis

▶ TO THE SKIN

- Neonate: 0.5 capful/bath, alternatively, to be applied to wet skin and rinse.
- Child 1 month–11 years: 0.5–2 capfuls/bath, alternatively, to be applied to wet skin and rinse
- Child 12–17 years: 1–3 capfuls/bath, alternatively, to be applied to wet skin and rinse

OILATUM® JUNIOR BATH ADDITIVE

Dry skin conditions including dermatitis and ichthyosis

▶ TO THE SKIN

- Neonate: 0.5 capful/bath, alternatively, apply to wet skin and rinse.
- Child 1 month–11 years: 0.5–2 capfuls/bath, alternatively, apply to wet skin and rinse
- Child 12–17 years: 1–3 capfuls/bath, alternatively, apply to wet skin and rinse

QV® BATH OIL

Dry skin conditions including eczema, psoriasis, ichthyosis, and pruritus

▶ TO THE SKIN

- Neonate: 5 mL/bath, alternatively, to be applied to wet skin and rinse.
- Child 1–11 months: 5 mL/bath, alternatively, to be applied to wet skin and rinse
- Child 1–17 years: 10 mL/bath, alternatively, to be applied to wet skin and rinse

QV® GENTLE WASH

Dry skin conditions including eczema, psoriasis, ichthyosis, and pruritus

▶ TO THE SKIN

- Child: To be used as a soap substitute

ZEROLATUM®

Dry skin conditions | Dermatitis | Ichthyosis

▶ TO THE SKIN

- Child 1 month–11 years: 5–10 mL/bath
- Child 12–17 years: 15–20 mL/bath

IMPORTANT SAFETY INFORMATION

These preparations make the skin and surfaces slippery—particular care is needed when bathing.

MHRA/CHM ADVICE (UPDATED DECEMBER 2018): EMOLLIENTS: NEW INFORMATION ABOUT RISK OF SEVERE AND FATAL BURNS WITH PARAFFIN-CONTAINING AND PARAFFIN-FREE EMOLLIENTS

See Emollient and barrier preparations p. 888.

● **DIRECTIONS FOR ADMINISTRATION** Emollient bath additives should be added to bath water; EvGr hydration can be improved by soaking in the bath for 5–20 minutes (consult product literature). Some bath emollients can be applied to wet skin undiluted and rinsed off. ⟨M⟩ Emollient preparations contained in tubs should be removed with a clean spoon or spatula to reduce bacterial contamination of the emollient. Emollients should be applied in the direction of hair growth to reduce the risk of folliculitis.

13 Skin

● **MEDICINAL FORMS** There can be variation in the licensing of different medicines containing the same drug.

Bath additive

CAUTIONARY AND ADVISORY LABELS 15

EXCIPIENTS: May contain Acetylated lanolin alcohols, cetostearyl alcohol (including cetyl and stearyl alcohol), fragrances, isopropyl palmitate

- **Doublebase** (Dermal Laboratories Ltd)
  Liquid paraffin 650 mg per 1 gram Doublebase emollient bath additive | 500 ml GSL £5.96 DT = £5.96
- **Hydromol** (Alliance Pharmaceuticals Ltd)
  Isopropyl myristate 130 mg per 1 ml, Liquid paraffin light 378 mg per 1 ml Hydromol Bath & Shower emollient | 350 ml £4.25 | 500 ml £4.84 | 1000 ml £9.63
- **LPL** (Huxley Europe Ltd)
  Liquid paraffin light 634 mg per 1 ml LPL 63.4 bath additive and emollient | 500 ml £3.17 DT = £9.93
- **Oilatum** (Thornton & Ross Ltd)
  Liquid paraffin light 634 mg per 1 ml Oilatum Bath Formula | 150 ml GSL £3.89 DT = £3.89 | 300 ml GSL £6.42 DT = £6.42
  Oilatum Emollient | 500 ml GSL £9.93 DT = £9.93
- **Oilatum junior** (Thornton & Ross Ltd)
  Liquid paraffin light 634 mg per 1 ml Oilatum Junior bath additive | 150 ml GSL £3.89 DT = £3.89 | 300 ml GSL £6.70 DT = £6.42 | 600 ml GSL £9.54 DT = £9.54
- **Zerolatum** (Thornton & Ross Ltd)
  Acetylated wool alcohols 50 mg per 1 gram, Liquid paraffin 650 mg per 1 gram Zerolatum Emollient bath additive | 500 ml £5.05

Cutaneous wash

CAUTIONARY AND ADVISORY LABELS 15

EXCIPIENTS: May contain Cetostearyl alcohol (including cetyl and stearyl alcohol), polysorbates

- **Aquamax** (Esteve Pharmaceuticals Ltd)
  Aquamax wash | 250 gram £2.99
- **E45 emollient wash** (Karo Healthcare UK Ltd)
  E45 emollient wash cream | 250 ml £4.46

Cutaneous cream

CAUTIONARY AND ADVISORY LABELS 15

EXCIPIENTS: May contain Cetostearyl alcohol (including cetyl and stearyl alcohol)

- **Emollient bath and shower products, paraffin-containing (Non-proprietary)**
  Phenoxyethanol 10 mg per 1 gram, Liquid paraffin 60 mg per 1 gram, Emulsifying wax 90 mg per 1 gram, White soft paraffin 150 mg per 1 gram, Purified water 690 mg per 1 gram Aqueous cream | 100 gram GSL £1.15 DT = £1.19 | 500 gram GSL £10.88 DT = £5.95

Cutaneous gel

CAUTIONARY AND ADVISORY LABELS 15

EXCIPIENTS: May contain Cetostearyl alcohol (including cetyl and stearyl alcohol), polysorbates

- **Doublebase** (Dermal Laboratories Ltd)
  Isopropyl myristate 150 mg per 1 gram, Liquid paraffin 150 mg per 1 gram Doublebase Dayleve gel | 100 gram P £2.65 DT = £2.65 | 500 gram P £6.79 DT = £5.99
  Doublebase gel | 100 gram P £2.65 DT = £2.65 | 500 gram P £5.99 DT = £5.99 | 1000 gram P £10.98
  Doublebase emollient wash gel | 200 gram P £5.21
  Doublebase emollient shower gel | 200 gram P £5.21
- **Oilatum** (Thornton & Ross Ltd)
  Liquid paraffin light 700 mg per 1 gram Oilatum shower gel fragrance free | 150 gram GSL £6.62 DT = £6.62

Form unstated

CAUTIONARY AND ADVISORY LABELS 15

- **E45 emollient bath** (Karo Healthcare UK Ltd)
  E45 emollient bath oil | 500 ml £6.74

Products without form

CAUTIONARY AND ADVISORY LABELS 15

EXCIPIENTS: May contain Hydroxybenzoates (parabens)

- **QV Gentle** (Ego Pharmaceuticals)
  QV Gentle wash | 500 ml £5.60

Emollient bath and shower products, soya-bean oil-containing

19-Nov-2020

● **INDICATIONS AND DOSE**

BALNEUM® BATH OIL

Dry skin conditions including those associated with dermatitis and eczema

▶ TO THE SKIN

- Neonate: 5–15 mL/bath, not to be used undiluted.
- Child 1–23 months: 5–15 mL/bath, not to be used undiluted
- Child 2–17 years: 20–60 mL/bath, not to be used undiluted

BALNEUM® PLUS BATH OIL

Dry skin conditions including those associated with dermatitis and eczema where pruritus also experienced

▶ TO THE SKIN

- Neonate: 5 mL/bath, alternatively, to be applied to wet skin and rinse.
- Child 1–23 months: 5 mL/bath, alternatively, to be applied to wet skin and rinse
- Child 2–17 years: 10–20 mL/bath, alternatively, to be applied to wet skin and rinse

ZERONEUM®

Dry skin conditions, including eczema

▶ TO THE SKIN

- Child 1 month–11 years: 5 mL/bath
- Child 12–17 years: 20 mL/bath

IMPORTANT SAFETY INFORMATION

These preparations make skin and surfaces slippery—particular care is needed when bathing.

MHRA/CHM ADVICE (UPDATED DECEMBER 2018): EMOLLIENTS: NEW INFORMATION ABOUT RISK OF SEVERE AND FATAL BURNS WITH PARAFFIN-CONTAINING AND PARAFFIN-FREE EMOLLIENTS

See Emollient and barrier preparations p. 888.

● **DIRECTIONS FOR ADMINISTRATION** Emollient bath additives should be added to bath water; EvGr hydration can be improved by soaking in the bath for 5–20 minutes (consult product literature). Some bath emollients can be applied to wet skin undiluted and rinsed off. ⟨M⟩ Emollient preparations contained in tubs should be removed with a clean spoon or spatula to reduce bacterial contamination of the emollient. Emollients should be applied in the direction of hair growth to reduce the risk of folliculitis.

● **MEDICINAL FORMS** There can be variation in the licensing of different medicines containing the same drug.

Bath additive

CAUTIONARY AND ADVISORY LABELS 15

EXCIPIENTS: May contain Butylated hydroxytoluene, fragrances, propylene glycol

- **Balneum** (Almirall Ltd)
  Lauromacrogols 150 mg per 1 gram, Soya oil 829.5 mg per 1 gram Balneum Plus bath oil | 500 ml GSL £6.66 DT = £6.66
  Soya oil 847.5 mg per 1 gram Balneum 84.75% bath oil | 500 ml GSL £5.38 DT = £5.38
- **Zeroneum** (Thornton & Ross Ltd)
  Soya oil 833.5 mg per 1 gram Zeroneum 83.35% bath additive | 500 ml £4.72

Emollient creams and ointments, antimicrobial-containing

19-Nov-2020

● **INDICATIONS AND DOSE**

Dry and pruritic skin conditions including eczema and dermatitis

▶ TO THE SKIN

▸ Child: To be applied to the skin or used as a soap substitute

IMPORTANT SAFETY INFORMATION

These preparations make skin and surfaces slippery—particular care is needed when bathing.

MHRA/CHM ADVICE (UPDATED DECEMBER 2018): EMOLLIENTS: NEW INFORMATION ABOUT RISK OF SEVERE AND FATAL BURNS WITH PARAFFIN-CONTAINING AND PARAFFIN-FREE EMOLLIENTS

See Emollient and barrier preparations p. 888.

13 Skin

● **DIRECTIONS FOR ADMINISTRATION** Emollients should be applied immediately after washing or bathing to maximise the effect of skin hydration. Emollient preparations contained in tubs should be removed with a clean spoon or spatula to reduce bacterial contamination of the emollient. Emollients should be applied in the direction of hair growth to reduce the risk of folliculitis.

● **PRESCRIBING AND DISPENSING INFORMATION** Preparations containing an antibacterial should be avoided unless infection is present or is a frequent complication.

● **MEDICINAL FORMS** There can be variation in the licensing of different medicines containing the same drug.

Cutaneous cream

CAUTIONARY AND ADVISORY LABELS 15

EXCIPIENTS: May contain Cetostearyl alcohol (including cetyl and stearyl alcohol)

▸ **Dermol**(Dermal Laboratories Ltd)

Benzalkonium chloride 1 mg per 1 gram, Chlorhexidine hydrochloride 1 mg per 1 gram, Isopropyl myristate 100 mg per 1 gram, Liquid paraffin 100 mg per 1 gram Dermol cream | 100 gram [P] £3.08 | 500 gram [P] £7.19

Cutaneous emulsion

CAUTIONARY AND ADVISORY LABELS 15

EXCIPIENTS: May contain Cetostearyl alcohol (including cetyl and stearyl alcohol)

▸ **Dermol 500**(Dermal Laboratories Ltd)

Benzalkonium chloride 1 mg per 1 gram, Chlorhexidine hydrochloride 1 mg per 1 gram, Isopropyl myristate 25 mg per 1 gram, Liquid paraffin 25 mg per 1 gram Dermol 500 lotion | 500 ml [P] £6.52

Emollient creams and ointments, colloidal oatmeal-containing

15-Aug-2024

● **INDICATIONS AND DOSE**

Dry skin conditions | Psoriasis | Eczema | Xeroderma | Ichthyosis

▶ TO THE SKIN

▸ Child: To be applied to the skin as an emollient

IMPORTANT SAFETY INFORMATION

MHRA/CHM ADVICE (UPDATED DECEMBER 2018): EMOLLIENTS: NEW INFORMATION ABOUT RISK OF SEVERE AND FATAL BURNS WITH PARAFFIN-CONTAINING AND PARAFFIN-FREE EMOLLIENTS

See Emollient and barrier preparations p. 888.

● **DIRECTIONS FOR ADMINISTRATION** Emollients should be applied immediately after washing or bathing to maximise the effect of skin hydration. Emollient preparations contained in tubs should be removed with a clean spoon or spatula to reduce bacterial contamination of the emollient. Emollients should be applied in the direction of hair growth to reduce the risk of folliculitis.

● **MEDICINAL FORMS** There can be variation in the licensing of different medicines containing the same drug.

Form unstated

CAUTIONARY AND ADVISORY LABELS 15

EXCIPIENTS: May contain Benzyl alcohol, cetostearyl alcohol (including cetyl and stearyl alcohol), isopropyl palmitate

▸ **Aveeno**(Kenvue UK Ltd)

Aveeno cream | 100 ml(ACBS) £4.25 | 300 ml(ACBS) £8.56 | 500 ml (ACBS) £7.59

Cream

CAUTIONARY AND ADVISORY LABELS 15

EXCIPIENTS: May contain Benzyl alcohol, cetostearyl alcohol (including cetyl and stearyl alcohol), isopropyl palmitate

▸ **Emollient creams and ointments, colloidal oatmeal-containing (Non-proprietary)**

Epimax oatmeal cream | 100 gram £2.12 | 500 gram £3.19

Products without form

CAUTIONARY AND ADVISORY LABELS 15

EXCIPIENTS: May contain Benzyl alcohol, cetostearyl alcohol (including cetyl and stearyl alcohol), isopropyl palmitate

▸ **Zeroveen**(Thornton & Ross Ltd)

Zeroveen cream | 100 gram £2.86 | 500 gram £6.13

Emollient creams and ointments, hydrogenated castor oil-containing

15-Aug-2024

● **INDICATIONS AND DOSE**

Dry skin conditions | Eczema | Psoriasis

▶ TO THE SKIN

▸ Child: To be applied to the skin as an emollient or used as a soap substitute

IMPORTANT SAFETY INFORMATION

MHRA/CHM ADVICE (UPDATED DECEMBER 2018): EMOLLIENTS: NEW INFORMATION ABOUT RISK OF SEVERE AND FATAL BURNS WITH PARAFFIN-CONTAINING AND PARAFFIN-FREE EMOLLIENTS

See Emollient and barrier preparations p. 888.

MHRA/CHM ADVICE: *EPIMAX®* OINTMENT AND *EPIMAX®* PARAFFIN-FREE OINTMENT: REPORTS OF OCULAR SURFACE TOXICITY AND OCULAR CHEMICAL INJURY (JULY 2024)

Following a cluster of reports of ocular surface toxicity associated with *Epimax®* ointment and *Epimax®* paraffin-free ointment, it is advised that these preparations should not be used on the face. If contact with the eyes occurs, patients may present with pain, swelling, redness or watering, sensitivity to light, blurred vision, burning, or grittiness. Symptoms should resolve with discontinuation of the product around the eyes and can be treated with topical lubricants, antibiotics or steroids as required—see advice in manufacturer's Field Safety Notice (available from: mhra-gov.filecamp.com/s/d/icXgbJO5IVPprV2f). Patients and carers should be advised to use *Epimax®* ointment or *Epimax®* paraffin-free ointment only on the body and not on the face, to wash their hands thoroughly after use, and to avoid contact with the eyes. They should also be counselled to rinse eyes well with water and seek medical advice if these preparations accidentally get into the eyes.

● **DIRECTIONS FOR ADMINISTRATION** Emollients should be applied immediately after washing or bathing to maximise the effect of skin hydration. Emollient preparations contained in tubs should be removed with a clean spoon or spatula to reduce bacterial contamination of the emollient. Emollients should be applied in the direction of hair growth to reduce the risk of folliculitis.

● **MEDICINAL FORMS** There can be variation in the licensing of different medicines containing the same drug.

Ointment

CAUTIONARY AND ADVISORY LABELS 15

EXCIPIENTS: May contain Cetostearyl alcohol (including cetyl and stearyl alcohol)

▸ **Emollient creams and ointments, hydrogenated castor oil-containing (Non-proprietary)**
Epimax paraffin-free ointment | 500 gram £5.16

Emollient creams and ointments, paraffin-containing

15-Aug-2024

● **INDICATIONS AND DOSE**

Dry skin conditions | **Eczema** | **Psoriasis** | **Ichthyosis** | **Pruritus**

▸ TO THE SKIN

▸ Child: To be applied to the skin as an emollient

IMPORTANT SAFETY INFORMATION

MHRA/CHM ADVICE (UPDATED DECEMBER 2018): EMOLLIENTS: NEW INFORMATION ABOUT RISK OF SEVERE AND FATAL BURNS WITH PARAFFIN-CONTAINING AND PARAFFIN-FREE EMOLLIENTS

See Emollient and barrier preparations p. 888.

MHRA/CHM ADVICE: *EPIMAX*® OINTMENT AND *EPIMAX*® PARAFFIN-FREE OINTMENT: REPORTS OF OCULAR SURFACE TOXICITY AND OCULAR CHEMICAL INJURY (JULY 2024)

Following a cluster of reports of ocular surface toxicity associated with *Epimax*® ointment and *Epimax*® paraffin-free ointment, it is advised that these preparations should not be used on the face. If contact with the eyes occurs, patients may present with pain, swelling, redness or watering, sensitivity to light, blurred vision, burning, or grittiness. Symptoms should resolve with discontinuation of the product around the eyes and can be treated with topical lubricants, antibiotics or steroids as required—see advice in the manufacturer's Field Safety Notice (available from: mhra-gov.filecamp.com/s/d/icXgbJO5IVPprV2f). Patients and carers should be advised to use *Epimax*® ointment or *Epimax*® paraffin-free ointment only on the body and not on the face, to wash their hands thoroughly after use, and to avoid contact with the eyes. They should also be counselled to rinse eyes well with water and seek medical advice if these preparations accidentally get into the eyes.

● **DIRECTIONS FOR ADMINISTRATION** Emollients should be applied immediately after washing or bathing to maximise the effect of skin hydration. Emollient preparations contained in tubs should be removed with a clean spoon or spatula to reduce bacterial contamination of the emollient. Emollients should be applied in the direction of hair growth to reduce the risk of folliculitis.

● **PRESCRIBING AND DISPENSING INFORMATION** Some preparations may contain other ingredients or additives—consult product literature.

● **MEDICINAL FORMS** There can be variation in the licensing of different medicines containing the same drug.

Cutaneous ointment

CAUTIONARY AND ADVISORY LABELS 15

EXCIPIENTS: May contain Cetostearyl alcohol (including cetyl and stearyl alcohol), polysorbates

▸ **Emollient creams and ointments, paraffin-containing (Non-proprietary)**
Cetraben ointment | 125 gram £3.68 | 450 gram £5.75
Liquid paraffin 500 mg per 1 gram, White soft paraffin 500 mg per 1 gram Purosure ointment | 500 gram £3.17 DT = £0.00
Liquid paraffin 200 mg per 1 gram, Emulsifying wax 300 mg per 1 gram, White soft paraffin 500 mg per 1 gram EmulsifEss ointment | 500 gram £3.93
Emulsifying ointment | 500 gram £4.15
Magnesium sulfate dried 5 mg per 1 gram, Phenoxyethanol 10 mg per 1 gram, Wool alcohols ointment 500 mg per 1 gram Hydrous ointment | 500 gram [X]

▸ **Emelpin** (Vitame Ltd)
Emulsifying wax 300 mg per 1 gram, Yellow soft paraffin 300 mg per 1 gram Emelpin ointment | 125 gram £3.08 | 500 gram £3.97

▸ **Epaderm** (Molnlycke Health Care Ltd)
Emulsifying wax 300 mg per 1 gram, Yellow soft paraffin 300 mg per 1 gram Epaderm ointment | 125 gram £4.13 | 500 gram £7.01 | 1000 gram £13.22

▸ **Epaderm Junior** (Molnlycke Health Care Ltd)
Emulsifying wax 300 mg per 1 gram, Yellow soft paraffin 300 mg per 1 gram Epaderm Junior ointment | 125 gram £4.10

▸ **Fifty:50** (Ennogen Healthcare International Ltd)
Liquid paraffin 500 mg per 1 gram, White soft paraffin 500 mg per 1 gram Fifty:50 ointment | 250 gram £1.96 | 500 gram £3.92 DT = £0.00

▸ **Hydromol** (Alliance Pharmaceuticals Ltd)
Emulsifying wax 300 mg per 1 gram, Yellow soft paraffin 300 mg per 1 gram Hydromol ointment | 100 gram £3.36 | 125 gram £3.30 | 500 gram £5.60

▸ **KreaMoint** (Essential-Healthcare Ltd)
Liquid paraffin 500 mg per 1 gram, White soft paraffin 500 mg per 1 gram KreaMoint 50:50 ointment | 500 gram £3.11 DT = £0.00

▸ **Thirty:30** (Ennogen Healthcare International Ltd)
Emulsifying wax 300 mg per 1 gram, Yellow soft paraffin 300 mg per 1 gram Thirty:30 ointment | 125 gram £4.08 | 500 gram £6.93

▸ **Vaseline** (Unilever UK Home & Personal Care)
White soft paraffin 1 mg per 1 mg Vaseline Pure Petroleum jelly | 50 ml GSL [X]

▸ **Zeroderm** (Thornton & Ross Ltd)
Zeroderm ointment | 125 gram £2.57 | 500 gram £4.35

Cutaneous emulsion

CAUTIONARY AND ADVISORY LABELS 15

EXCIPIENTS: May contain Hydroxybenzoates (parabens), isopropyl palmitate

▸ **E45** (Karo Healthcare UK Ltd)
E45 lotion | 200 ml £3.36 | 500 ml £6.73

Spray

CAUTIONARY AND ADVISORY LABELS 15

▸ **Emollin** (C D Medical Ltd)
Emollin aerosol spray | 240 ml £7.86

Cream

CAUTIONARY AND ADVISORY LABELS 15

EXCIPIENTS: May contain Cetostearyl alcohol (including cetyl and stearyl alcohol), polysorbates

▸ **Emollient creams and ointments, paraffin-containing (Non-proprietary)**
Epimax original cream | 100 gram £0.82 | 500 gram £2.74

▸ **Aquamax** (Esteve Pharmaceuticals Ltd)
Aquamax cream | 100 gram £1.89 | 500 gram £3.99

▸ **Epaderm** (Molnlycke Health Care Ltd)
Epaderm cream | 50 gram £1.82 | 150 gram £3.81 | 500 gram £7.34

▸ **Epimax intensive cream** (Aspire Pharma Ltd)
Epimax intensive cream | 500 gram £2.84

▸ **ZeroAQS** (Thornton & Ross Ltd)
ZeroAQS emollient cream | 500 gram £3.39

Cutaneous cream

CAUTIONARY AND ADVISORY LABELS 15

EXCIPIENTS: May contain Benzyl alcohol, cetostearyl alcohol (including cetyl and stearyl alcohol), chlorocresol, disodium edetate, fragrances, hydroxybenzoates (parabens), polysorbates, propylene glycol, sorbic acid, lanolin

▸ **Cetraben** (Thornton & Ross Ltd)
Liquid paraffin light 105 mg per 1 gram, White soft paraffin 132 mg per 1 gram Cetraben cream | 50 gram £1.50 | 150 gram £4.23 | 500 gram £6.38 | 1050 gram £12.41

▸ **E45** (Karo Healthcare UK Ltd)
Wool fat 10 mg per 1 gram, Liquid paraffin light 126 mg per 1 gram, White soft paraffin 145 mg per 1 gram E45 cream | 50 gram GSL £2.77 | 125 gram GSL £4.70 | 350 gram GSL £8.40 | 500 gram GSL £7.89

▸ **Enopen** (Ennogen Healthcare International Ltd)
Liquid paraffin light 105 mg per 1 gram, White soft paraffin 132 mg per 1 gram Enopen cream | 50 gram £1.42 | 150 gram £4.03 | 500 gram £6.06 | 1050 gram £11.77

- **Epimax moisturising cream** (Aspire Pharma Ltd)
  Liquid paraffin 126 mg per 1 gram, White soft paraffin 145 mg per 1 gram Epimax moisturising cream | 100 gram £2.04 | 500 gram £3.07
- **ExCetra** (Aspire Pharma Ltd)
  Liquid paraffin light 105 mg per 1 gram, White soft paraffin 132 mg per 1 gram Epimax excetra cream | 100 gram £1.88 | 500 gram £3.18
- **Exmaben** (Ascot Laboratories Ltd)
  Liquid paraffin light 105 mg per 1 gram, White soft paraffin 132 mg per 1 gram Exmaben cream | 500 gram £4.25
- **Hydromol** (Alliance Pharmaceuticals Ltd)
  Sodium lactate 10 mg per 1 gram, Sodium pidolate 25 mg per 1 gram, Isopropyl myristate 50 mg per 1 gram, Liquid paraffin 100 mg per 1 gram Hydromol 2.5% cream | 50 gram £2.37 | 100 gram £4.42 | 500 gram £12.88
- **Lipobase** (Karo Healthcare UK Ltd)
  Lipobase cream | 50 gram [P] £1.46
- **Oilatum** (Thornton & Ross Ltd)
  Liquid paraffin light 60 mg per 1 gram, White soft paraffin 150 mg per 1 gram Oilatum cream | 150 gram [GSL] £4.18 DT = £4.18 | 500 ml [GSL] £8.57 DT = £8.57
- **Oilatum junior** (Thornton & Ross Ltd)
  Liquid paraffin light 60 mg per 1 gram, White soft paraffin 150 mg per 1 gram Oilatum Junior cream | 150 gram [GSL] £4.19 DT = £4.18 | 350 ml [GSL] £6.66 DT = £6.66 | 500 ml [GSL] £7.81 DT = £8.57
- **QV** (Ego Pharmaceuticals)
  White soft paraffin 50 mg per 1 gram, Glycerol 100 mg per 1 gram, Liquid paraffin light 100 mg per 1 gram QV cream | 100 gram £2.37 | 500 gram £6.75 | 1050 gram £12.69
- **Soffen** (Vitame Ltd)
  Liquid paraffin light 105 mg per 1 gram, White soft paraffin 132 mg per 1 gram Soffen cream | 500 gram £4.79
- **Ultrabase** (Derma UK Ltd)
  Ultrabase cream | 100 ml £2.85 | 500 ml £7.01
- **Unguentum M** (Almirall Ltd)
  Unguentum M cream | 500 gram [GSL] £8.48
- **Zerobase** (Thornton & Ross Ltd)
  Liquid paraffin 110 mg per 1 gram Zerobase 11% cream | 50 gram £1.12 | 500 gram £5.66
- **Zerocream** (Thornton & Ross Ltd)
  Liquid paraffin 126 mg per 1 gram, White soft paraffin 145 mg per 1 gram Zerocream | 50 gram £1.25 | 500 gram £4.36
- **Zeroguent** (Thornton & Ross Ltd)
  White soft paraffin 40 mg per 1 gram, Soya oil 50 mg per 1 gram, Liquid paraffin light 80 mg per 1 gram Zeroguent cream | 100 gram £2.44 | 500 gram £7.32

Cutaneous gel

CAUTIONARY AND ADVISORY LABELS 15
EXCIPIENTS: May contain Polysorbates

- **Doublebase** (Dermal Laboratories Ltd)
  Isopropyl myristate 150 mg per 1 gram, Liquid paraffin 150 mg per 1 gram Doublebase Dayleve gel | 100 gram [P] £2.65 DT = £2.65 | 500 gram [P] £6.79 DT = £5.99
  Doublebase gel | 100 gram [P] £2.65 DT = £2.65 | 500 gram [P] £5.99 DT = £5.99 | 1000 gram [P] £10.98
  Doublebase emollient wash gel | 200 gram [P] £5.21
  Doublebase emollient shower gel | 200 gram [P] £5.21

Ointment

CAUTIONARY AND ADVISORY LABELS 15
EXCIPIENTS: May contain Cetostearyl alcohol (including cetyl and stearyl alcohol)

- **Emollient creams and ointments, paraffin-containing (Non-proprietary)**
  Epimax ointment | 125 gram £2.07 | 500 gram £3.22

Products without form

CAUTIONARY AND ADVISORY LABELS 15
EXCIPIENTS: May contain Cetostearyl alcohol (including cetyl and stearyl alcohol)

- **Emollient creams and ointments, paraffin-containing (Non-proprietary)**
  Doublebase Once gel | 100 gram £2.69 | 500 gram £6.99
  Cetraben lotion | 200 ml £4.00 | 500 ml £5.92
- **Adex** (Dermal Laboratories Ltd)
  Adex gel | 100 gram £2.69 | 500 gram £5.99
- **QV intensive** (Ego Pharmaceuticals)
  QV Intensive ointment | 450 gram £6.03

13 Skin

Emollients, urea-containing

19-Nov-2020

● **DRUG ACTION** Urea is a keratin softener and hydrating agent used in the treatment of dry, scaling conditions (including ichthyosis).

● **INDICATIONS AND DOSE**

AQUADRATE ®

Dry, scaling, and itching skin
▶ TO THE SKIN
▶ Child: Apply twice daily, to be applied thinly

BALNEUM ® CREAM

Dry skin conditions
▶ TO THE SKIN
▶ Child: Apply twice daily

BALNEUM ® PLUS CREAM

Dry, scaling, and itching skin
▶ TO THE SKIN
▶ Child: Apply twice daily

CALMURID ®

Dry, scaling, and itching skin
▶ TO THE SKIN
▶ Child: Apply twice daily, apply a thick layer for 3–5 minutes, massage into area, and remove excess. Can be diluted with aqueous cream (life of diluted cream is 14 days). Half-strength cream can be used for 1 week if stinging occurs

DERMATONICS ONCE HEEL BALM ®

Dry skin on soles of feet
▶ TO THE SKIN
▶ Child 12–17 years: Apply once daily

E45 ® ITCH RELIEF CREAM

Dry, scaling, and itching skin
▶ TO THE SKIN
▶ Child: Apply twice daily

EUCERIN ® INTENSIVE CREAM

Dry skin conditions including eczema, ichthyosis, xeroderma, and hyperkeratosis
▶ TO THE SKIN
▶ Child: Apply twice daily, to be applied thinly and rubbed into area

FLEXITOL ®

Dry skin on soles of feet and heels
▶ TO THE SKIN
▶ Child 12–17 years: Apply 1–2 times a day

HYDROMOL ® INTENSIVE

Dry, scaling, and itching skin
▶ TO THE SKIN
▶ Child: Apply twice daily, to be applied thinly

IMUDERM ® EMOLLIENT

Dry skin conditions including eczema, psoriasis or dermatitis
▶ TO THE SKIN
▶ Child: Apply to skin or use as a soap substitute

NUTRAPLUS ®

Dry, scaling, and itching skin
▶ TO THE SKIN
▶ Child: Apply 2–3 times a day

IMPORTANT SAFETY INFORMATION

MHRA/CHM ADVICE (UPDATED DECEMBER 2018): EMOLLIENTS: NEW INFORMATION ABOUT RISK OF SEVERE AND FATAL BURNS WITH PARAFFIN-CONTAINING AND PARAFFIN-FREE EMOLLIENTS
See Emollient and barrier preparations p. 888.

● **DIRECTIONS FOR ADMINISTRATION** Emollients should be applied immediately after washing or bathing to maximise the effect of skin hydration. Emollient preparations contained in tubs should be removed with a clean spoon or spatula to reduce bacterial contamination of the emollient. Emollients should be applied in the direction of hair growth to reduce the risk of folliculitis.

- **MEDICINAL FORMS** There can be variation in the licensing of different medicines containing the same drug.

Cutaneous cream

CAUTIONARY AND ADVISORY LABELS 15

EXCIPIENTS: May contain Benzyl alcohol, cetostearyl alcohol (including cetyl and stearyl alcohol), hydroxybenzoates (parabens), isopropyl palmitate, polysorbates, propylene glycol, woolfat and related substances (including lanolin)

▸ **Balneum Plus** (Almirall Ltd)
Lauromacrogols 30 mg per 1 gram, Urea 50 mg per 1 gram Balneum Plus cream | 100 gram GSL £3.29 DT = £6.12 | 500 gram GSL £14.99 DT = £19.12

▸ **E45 Itch Relief** (Karo Healthcare UK Ltd)
Lauromacrogols 30 mg per 1 gram, Urea 50 mg per 1 gram E45 Itch Relief cream | 50 gram GSL £3.93 DT = £3.93 | 100 gram GSL £6.12 DT = £6.12 | 500 gram GSL £19.12 DT = £19.12

▸ **Hydromol Intensive** (Alliance Pharmaceuticals Ltd)
Urea 100 mg per 1 gram Hydromol Intensive 10% cream | 30 gram £1.78 | 100 gram £4.75

Products without form

CAUTIONARY AND ADVISORY LABELS 15

EXCIPIENTS: May contain Beeswax, benzyl alcohol, cetostearyl alcohol (including cetyl and stearyl alcohol), fragrances, lanolin

▸ **Emollients, urea-containing (Non-proprietary)**
imuDERM emollient | 500 gram £6.95

▸ **Dermatonics Once** (Dermatonics Ltd)
Dermatonics Once Heel Balm | 75 ml £3.83 | 200 ml £9.52

▸ **Flexitol** (Thornton & Ross Ltd)
Flexitol 25% Urea Heel Balm | 40 gram £2.92 | 75 gram £4.04 | 200 gram £9.99 | 500 gram £15.77

3 Epidermolysis bullosa

DERMATOLOGICAL DRUGS

Birch bark extracts

23-Jan-2026

- **DRUG ACTION** Birch bark extracts are thought to modulate inflammatory mediators and activate pathways involved in keratinocyte differentiation and migration, thereby promoting wound healing.

- **INDICATIONS AND DOSE**

Partial thickness wounds associated with dystrophic and junctional epidermolysis bullosa

▸ TO THE SKIN

▸ Child 6 months–17 years: Apply to surface of cleansed wound at a thickness of approx. 1 mm and cover with a sterile non-adhesive dressing or apply directly to the dressing—do not rub in, reapply at each wound dressing change

- **CONTRA-INDICATIONS** Avoid application to mucous membranes · avoid contact with eyes
- **CAUTIONS** Squamous cell carcinoma or other skin malignancies (discontinue treatment of affected areas) · wound infection (interrupt treatment—may be restarted once infection has resolved)
- **SIDE-EFFECTS**

▸ **Common or very common** Hypersensitivity · skin reactions · wound complications · wound infection

▸ **Uncommon** Pain

- **PREGNANCY** EvGr Not known to be harmful (limited information available but systemic exposure is negligible). ⟨M⟩
- **BREAST FEEDING** EvGr Avoid if the mother's chest area is being treated (no information available on presence in milk but systemic exposure is negligible). ⟨M⟩
- **DIRECTIONS FOR ADMINISTRATION** Each tube is for single use only and should be used immediately once opened then discarded.
- **PRESCRIBING AND DISPENSING INFORMATION** In clinical studies, the maximum total wound area treated was 5 300 cm^2 (median of 735 cm^2).
- **PATIENT AND CARER ADVICE** Patients or their carers should be counselled on the application of *Filsuvez*® gel.
- **NATIONAL FUNDING/ACCESS DECISIONS**

For full details see funding body website

NICE decisions

▸ **Birch bark extract for treating epidermolysis bullosa (September 2023)** NICE HST28 Recommended

- **MEDICINAL FORMS** There can be variation in the licensing of different medicines containing the same drug.

Cutaneous gel

▸ **Filsuvez** (Chiesi Ltd)
Filsuvez gel | 702 gram PoM £8,259.90 (Hospital only)

4 Infections of the skin

Skin infections

22-Mar-2020

Antibacterial preparations for the skin

Topical antibacterial preparations are used to treat localised bacterial skin infections caused by Gram-positive organisms (particularly by staphylococci or streptococci). Systemic antibacterial treatment is more appropriate for deep-seated skin infections.

Problems associated with the use of topical antibacterials include bacterial resistance, contact sensitisation, and superinfection. In order to minimise the development of resistance, antibacterials used systemically (e.g. fusidic acid p. 441) should not generally be chosen for topical use. *Resistant organisms* are more common in hospitals, and whenever possible swabs should be taken for bacteriological examination before beginning treatment.

Neomycin sulfate p. 898 applied topically may cause sensitisation and cross-sensitivity with other aminoglycoside antibacterials such as gentamicin p. 378 may occur. Topical antibacterials applied over large areas can cause systemic toxicity; ototoxicity with neomycin sulfate is a particular risk for neonates and children with renal impairment.

Superficial bacterial infection of the skin may be treated with a topical antiseptic such as povidone-iodine p. 944 which also softens crusts, or hydrogen peroxide 1% cream p. 945.

Bacterial infections such as *folliculitis* can be treated with a short course of topical fusidic acid; mupirocin p. 899 should be used only to treat meticillin-resistant *Staphylococcus aureus*.

Impetigo requires topical antiseptic/antibacterial or systemic antibacterial treatment, see Skin infections, antibacterial therapy p. 373.

Cellulitis and *erysipelas* require systemic antibacterial treatment, see Skin infections, antibacterial therapy p. 373.

Staphylococcal scalded-skin syndrome requires urgent treatment with a systemic antibacterial, such as flucloxacillin p. 424.

Mupirocin is not related to any other antibacterial in use; it is effective for skin infections, particularly those due to Gram-positive organisms but it is not indicated for pseudomonal infection. Although *Staphylococcus aureus* strains with low-level resistance to mupirocin are emerging, it is generally useful in infections resistant to other antibacterials. To avoid the development of resistance, mupirocin or fusidic acid should not be used for longer than 10 days and local microbiology advice should be sought before using it in hospital. In the presence of mupirocin-resistant MRSA infection, a topical antiseptic, such as povidone-iodine, chlorhexidine p. 944, or alcohol, can be used; their use should be discussed with the local microbiologist.

Mupirocin ointment contains macrogols; extensive absorption of macrogols through the mucous membranes or through application to thin or damaged skin may result in renal toxicity, especially in neonates. Mupirocin nasal ointment is formulated in a paraffin base and may be more suitable for the treatment of MRSA-infected open wound in neonates.

Metronidazole gel p. 898 is used topically in children to reduce the odour associated with anaerobic infections and for the treatment of periorificial rosacea; oral metronidazole is used to treat wounds infected with anaerobic bacteria.

Sulfadiazine silver p. 899 is licensed for the prevention and treatment of infection in burns but the use of appropriate dressings may be more effective. Systemic effects may occur following extensive application of sulfadiazine silver; its use is not recommended in neonates.

Antibacterial preparations also used systemically

Fusidic acid is a narrow-spectrum antibacterial used for staphylococcal infections.

An ointment containing fusidic acid is used in the fissures of angular cheilitis when associated with staphylococcal infection. See Oropharyngeal fungal infections p. 883 for further information on angular cheilitis.

Metronidazole is used topically to treat rosacea and to reduce the odour associated with anaerobic infections; oral metronidazole is used to treat wounds infected with anaerobic bacteria.

Antifungal preparations for the skin

Most localised fungal infections are treated with topical preparations. To prevent relapse, local antifungal treatment should be continued for 1–2 weeks after the disappearance of all signs of infection. Systemic therapy is necessary for scalp infection or if the skin infection is widespread, disseminated or intractable; although topical therapy may be used to treat some nail infections, systemic therapy is more effective. Specimens of scale, nail or hair should be sent for mycological examination before starting treatment, unless the diagnosis is certain.

Dermatophytoses

Ringworm infection can affect the scalp (tinea capitis), body (tinea corporis), groin (tinea cruris), hand (tinea manuum), foot (tinea pedis, athlete's foot), or nail (tinea unguium, onychomycosis). Tinea capitis is a common childhood infection that requires systemic treatment with an oral antifungal; additional application of a topical antifungal, during the early stages of treatment, may reduce the risk of transmission. A topical antifungal can also be used to treat asymptomatic carriers of scalp ringworm.

Tinea corporis and tinea pedis infections in children respond to treatment with a topical **imidazole** (clotrimazole p. 900, econazole nitrate p. 900, or miconazole p. 901) or terbinafine cream p. 901. Nystatin p. 885 is less effective against tinea.

Compound benzoic acid ointment (Whitfield's ointment) has been used for ringworm infections but it is cosmetically less acceptable than proprietary preparations. Antifungal dusting powders are of little therapeutic value in the treatment of fungal skin infections and may cause skin irritation; they may have some role in preventing re-infection.

Antifungal treatment may not be necessary in asymptomatic children with tinea infection of the nails. If treatment is necessary, a systemic antifungal is more effective than topical therapy. However, topical application of tioconazole p. 901 may be useful for treating early onychomycosis when involvement is limited to mild distal disease, or for superficial white onychomycosis, or where there are contra-indications to systemic therapy. Chronic paronychia on the fingers (usually due to a candidal infection) should be treated with topical clotrimazole or nystatin, but these preparations should be used with caution in children who suck their fingers. Chronic paronychia of the toes (usually due to dermatophyte infection) can be treated with topical terbinafine.

Pityriasis versicolor

Pityriasis (tinea) versicolor can be treated with ketoconazole shampoo p. 900 or **selenium sulfide** shampoo. Topical imidazole antifungals such as clotrimazole, econazole nitrate and miconazole or topical terbinafine are alternatives, but large quantities may be required.

If topical therapy fails, or if the infection is widespread, pityriasis versicolor is treated systemically with an azole antifungal. Relapse is common, especially in the immunocompromised.

Candidiasis

Candidal skin infections can be treated with topical imidazole antifungals clotrimazole, econazole nitrate, or miconazole; topical terbinafine is an alternative. Topical application of nystatin is also effective for candidiasis but it is ineffective against dermatophytosis. Refractory candidiasis requires systemic treatment generally with a triazole such as fluconazole p. 463; systemic treatment with griseofulvin p. 470 or terbinafine is **not appropriate** for refractory candidiasis. See the treatment of oral candiasis and for the management of nappy rash.

Angular cheilitis

Miconazole cream is used in the fissures of angular cheilitis when associated with *Candida*.

Compound topical preparations

Combination of an imidazole and a mild corticosteroid (such as hydrocortisone 1% p. 912) may be of value in the treatment of eczematous intertrigo and, in the first few days only, of a severely inflamed patch of ringworm. Combination of a mild corticosteroid with either an imidazole or nystatin p. 885 may be of use in the treatment of *intertriginous eczema* associated with candida.

Antiviral preparations for the skin

Aciclovir cream p. 904 is used for the treatment of initial and recurrent labial, cutaneous, and genital *herpes simplex infections* in children; treatment should begin as early as possible. Systemic treatment is necessary for buccal or vaginal infections or if cold sores recur frequently.

Herpes labialis

Aciclovir cream can be used for the treatment of initial and recurrent labial herpes simplex infections (cold sores). It is best applied at the earliest possible stage, usually when prodromal changes of sensation are felt in the lip and before vesicles appear.

Penciclovir cream is also licensed for the treatment of herpes labialis; it needs to be applied more frequently than aciclovir cream.

Parasiticidal preparations for the skin

Suitable quantities of parasiticidal preparations			
Area of body	Skin creams	Lotions	Cream rinses
Scalp (head lice)		50–100 mL	50–100 mL
Body (scabies)	30–60 g	100 mL	
Body (crab lice)	30–60 g	100 mL	
These amounts are usually suitable for a child 12–17 years for single application.			

Scabies

Permethrin p. 904 is used for the treatment of *scabies* (*Sarcoptes scabiei*); malathion p. 903 can be used if permethrin is inappropriate.

Benzyl benzoate is an irritant and should be avoided in children; it is less effective than malathion and permethrin.

Ivermectin p. 474 (available from 'special-order' manufacturers or specialist importing companies) by mouth has been used, in combination with topical drugs, for the treatment of hyperkeratotic (crusted or 'Norwegian') scabies that does not respond to topical treatment alone.

Application

Although acaricides have traditionally been applied after a hot bath, this is **not** necessary and there is even evidence that a hot bath may increase absorption into the blood, removing them from their site of action on the skin.

All members of the affected household should be treated simultaneously. Treatment should be applied to the whole body including the scalp, neck, face, and ears. Particular attention should be paid to the webs of the fingers and toes and lotion brushed under the ends of nails. It is now recommended that malathion and permethrin should be applied twice, one week apart; in the case of benzyl benzoate in adults, up to 3 applications on consecutive days may be needed. It is important to warn users to reapply treatment to the hands if they are washed. Patients with hyperkeratotic scabies may require 2 or 3 applications of acaricide on consecutive days to ensure that enough penetrates the skin crusts to kill all the mites.

Itching

The *itch* and *eczema* of scabies persists for some weeks after the infestation has been eliminated and treatment for pruritus and eczema may be required. Application of crotamiton p. 932 can be used to control itching after treatment with more effective acaricides. A topical corticosteroid may help to reduce itch and inflammation after scabies has been treated successfully; however, persistent symptoms suggest that scabies eradication was not successful. Oral administration of a **sedating antihistamine** at night may also be useful.

Head lice

Dimeticone p. 903 is effective against head lice (*Pediculus humanus capitis*) and acts on the surface of the organism. Malathion, an organophosphorus insecticide, is an alternative, but resistance has been reported. Benzyl benzoate is licensed for the treatment of head lice but it is not recommended for use in children.

Head lice infestation (pediculosis) should be treated using lotion or liquid formulations only if live lice are present. Shampoos are diluted too much in use to be effective. A contact time of 8–12 hours or overnight treatment is recommended for lotions and liquids; a 2-hour treatment is not sufficient to kill eggs.

In general, a course of treatment for head lice should be 2 applications of product 7 days apart to kill lice emerging from any eggs that survive the first application. All affected household members should be treated at the same time.

MHRA/CHM advice: Head lice eradication products: risk of serious burns if treated hair is exposed to open flames or other sources of ignition (March 2018)

Some products for the eradication of head lice infestations are combustible/flammable when on the hair and can ignite and cause serious harm in the presence of an open flame or other source of ignition such as when lighting cigarettes.

Patients and carers should be advised on the safe and correct use of head lice eradication treatments and if appropriate, should be advised that they should not smoke around treated hair and that it should be kept away from open flames or other sources of ignition, including in the morning after overnight application until hair is washed.

Wet combing methods

Head lice can be mechanically removed by combing wet hair meticulously with a plastic detection comb (probably for at least 30 minutes each time) over the whole scalp at 4-day intervals for a minimum of 2 weeks, and continued until no lice are found on 3 consecutive sessions; hair conditioner or vegetable oil can be used to facilitate the process.

Several devices for the removal of head lice such as combs and topical solutions, are available and some are prescribable on the NHS.

The Drug Tariffs can be accessed online at:

- National Health Service Drug Tariff for England and Wales: www.nhsbsa.nhs.uk/pharmacies-gp-practices-and-appliance-contractors/drug-tariff
- Health and Personal Social Services for Northern Ireland Drug Tariff: bso.hscni.net/directorates/operations/family-practitioner-services/pharmacy/contractor-information/drug-tariff-and-related-materials/drug-tariff-2/
- Scottish Drug Tariff: publichealthscotland.scot/resources-and-tools/medical-practice-and-pharmaceuticals/scottish-drug-tariff/

Crab lice

Permethrin and malathion are used to eliminate *crab lice* (*Pthirus pubis*); permethrin is not licensed for treatment of crab lice in children under 18 years. An aqueous preparation should be applied, allowed to dry naturally and washed off after 12 hours; a second treatment is needed after 7 days to kill lice emerging from surviving eggs. All surfaces of the body should be treated, including the scalp, neck, and face (paying particular attention to the eyebrows and other facial hair). A different insecticide should be used if a course of treatment fails.

Parasiticidal preparations

Dimeticone coats head lice and interferes with water balance in lice by preventing the excretion of water; it is less active against eggs and treatment should be repeated after 7 days.

Malathion is recommended for *scabies*, *head lice* and *crab lice*. The risk of systemic effects associated with 1–2 applications of malathion p. 903 is considered to be very low; however, except in the treatment of hyperkeratotic scabies in children, applications of malathion liquid repeated at intervals of less than 1 week or application for more than 3 consecutive weeks should be **avoided** since the likelihood of eradication of lice is not increased.

Permethrin p. 904 is effective for *scabies*. It is also active against *head lice* but the formulation and licensed methods of application of the current products make them unsuitable for the treatment of head lice. Permethrin is also effective against *crab lice* but it is not licensed for this purpose in children under 18 years.

4.1 Bacterial skin infections

ANTIBACTERIALS › AMINOGLYCOSIDES

Neomycin sulfate
20-Jun-2025

- **INDICATIONS AND DOSE**

Bacterial skin infections

▶ TO THE SKIN
- Child: Apply up to 3 times a day, for short-term use only

- **UNLICENSED USE** *Neomycin Cream BPC*—no information available.

IMPORTANT SAFETY INFORMATION

MHRA/CHM ADVICE: AMINOGLYCOSIDES (GENTAMICIN, AMIKACIN, TOBRAMYCIN, AND NEOMYCIN): INCREASED RISK OF DEAFNESS IN PATIENTS WITH MITOCHONDRIAL MUTATIONS (JANUARY 2021)

The use of aminoglycosides is associated with rare cases of ototoxicity. A safety review found an increased risk of deafness in patients with mitochondrial mutations (particularly the m.1555A>G mutation), including cases where the patient's aminoglycoside serum levels were within the recommended range. Nevertheless, these mitochondrial mutations are considered rare and penetrance is uncertain. No cases were identified with topical preparations but, based on a shared mechanism of effect, there is a potential risk with neomycin and other aminoglycosides administered at the site of toxicity i.e. the ear.

Healthcare professionals are advised to consider the need for aminoglycoside treatment versus alternative options in patients with susceptible mutations. The need for genetic testing especially in those requiring recurrent or long-term treatment with aminoglycosides should also be considered, however, urgent treatment should not be delayed. To minimise the risks of adverse effects, continuous monitoring of renal and auditory function, as well as hepatic and laboratory parameters, is recommended for all patients. Those with known mitochondrial mutations or a family history of ototoxicity are advised to inform their doctor or pharmacist before using an aminoglycoside.

- **CONTRA-INDICATIONS** Neonates
- **CAUTIONS**
  - Large areas If large areas of skin are being treated ototoxicity may be a hazard in children, particularly in those with renal impairment.
- **INTERACTIONS** → Appendix 1: neomycin
- **SIDE-EFFECTS** Sensitisation (cross sensitivity with other aminoglycosides may occur)
- **RENAL IMPAIRMENT** Ototoxicity may be a hazard if large areas of skin are treated.
- **PRE-TREATMENT SCREENING** NHS England commissions genetic testing under the *National genomic test directory* indication: R65 - Aminoglycoside exposure posing risk to hearing. The testing criteria is significant exposure to aminoglycosides posing risk of ototoxicity. This testing is relevant to individuals with a predisposition to gram-negative infections or with hearing loss who have been exposed to aminoglycosides. For further information, see www.england.nhs.uk/publication/national-genomic-test-directories/.
- **LESS SUITABLE FOR PRESCRIBING** Neomycin sulfate cream is less suitable for prescribing.
- **MEDICINAL FORMS** There can be variation in the licensing of different medicines containing the same drug. Forms available from special-order manufacturers include: cutaneous cream

Cutaneous cream

EXCIPIENTS: May contain Cetostearyl alcohol (including cetyl and stearyl alcohol), edetic acid (edta)

ANTIBACTERIALS › NITROIMIDAZOLE DERIVATIVES

Metronidazole
31-Oct-2025

- **DRUG ACTION** Metronidazole is an antimicrobial drug with high activity against anaerobic bacteria and protozoa.

- **INDICATIONS AND DOSE**

ACEA®

Acute inflammatory exacerbation of rosacea

▶ TO THE SKIN
- Child 1-17 years: Apply twice daily, to be applied thinly

ANABACT®

Malodorous fungating tumours and malodorous gravitational and decubitus ulcers

▶ TO THE SKIN
- Child: Apply 1–2 times a day, to be applied to clean wound and covered with non-adherent dressing

METROGEL®

Acute inflammatory exacerbation of rosacea

▶ TO THE SKIN
- Child 1-17 years: Apply twice daily, to be applied thinly

Malodorous fungating tumours

▶ TO THE SKIN
- Child: Apply 1–2 times a day, to be applied to clean wound and covered with non-adherent dressing

METROSA®

Acute exacerbation of rosacea

▶ TO THE SKIN
- Child 1-17 years: Apply twice daily, to be applied thinly

ROSICED®

Inflammatory papules and pustules of rosacea

▶ TO THE SKIN
- Child 1-17 years: Apply twice daily for 6 weeks (longer if necessary)

ROZEX® CREAM

Inflammatory papules, pustules and erythema of rosacea

▶ TO THE SKIN
- Child 1-17 years: Apply twice daily

ROZEX® GEL

Inflammatory papules, pustules and erythema of rosacea

▶ TO THE SKIN
- Child 1-17 years: Apply twice daily

ZYOMET®

Acute inflammatory exacerbation of rosacea

▶ TO THE SKIN
- Child 1-17 years: Apply twice daily, to be applied thinly

- **UNLICENSED USE**

ACEA® Not licensed for use in children under 12 years.

ANABACT® Not licensed for use in children under 12 years.

METROGEL® Not licensed for use in children.

METROSA® Not licensed for use in children.

ROSICED® Not licensed for use in children.

ROZEX® CREAM Not licensed for use in children.

ROZEX® GEL Not licensed for use in children.

ZYOMET® Not licensed for use in children.

- **CAUTIONS** Avoid exposure to strong sunlight or UV light

13 Skin

- **INTERACTIONS** → Appendix 1: metronidazole
- **SIDE-EFFECTS**
- **Common or very common** Skin reactions
- **PRESCRIBING AND DISPENSING INFORMATION** For choice of antibacterial therapy, see Skin infections, antibacterial therapy p. 373.

- **MEDICINAL FORMS** There can be variation in the licensing of different medicines containing the same drug.

Cutaneous cream

EXCIPIENTS: May contain Benzyl alcohol, isopropyl palmitate, propylene glycol

- **Rozex** (Galderma (UK) Ltd)
  Metronidazole 7.5 mg per 1 gram Rozex 0.75% cream | 50 gram PoM £12.35 DT = £12.35

Cutaneous gel

EXCIPIENTS: May contain Benzyl alcohol, disodium edetate, hydroxybenzoates (parabens), propylene glycol

- **Acea** (Ferndale Pharmaceuticals Ltd)
  Metronidazole 7.5 mg per 1 gram Acea 0.75% gel | 40 gram PoM £9.95 DT = £22.63
- **Anabact** (Cambridge Healthcare Supplies Ltd)
  Metronidazole 7.5 mg per 1 gram Anabact 0.75% gel | 15 gram PoM £5.98 DT = £5.98 | 30 gram PoM £7.89 | 40 gram PoM £15.89 DT = £22.63
- **Metrogel** (Galderma (UK) Ltd)
  Metronidazole 7.5 mg per 1 gram Metrogel 0.75% gel | 40 gram PoM £22.63 DT = £22.63
- **Metrosa** (Beaumont Pharma Ltd)
  Metronidazole 7.5 mg per 1 gram Metrosa 0.75% gel | 30 gram PoM £12.00 | 40 gram PoM £19.90 DT = £22.63
- **Rozex** (Galderma (UK) Ltd)
  Metronidazole 7.5 mg per 1 gram Rozex 0.75% gel | 50 gram PoM £12.35

ANTIBACTERIALS › SULFONAMIDES

Sulfadiazine silver

10-Oct-2025

- **INDICATIONS AND DOSE**

Prophylaxis and treatment of infection in burn wounds

- TO THE SKIN
  - Child: Apply daily, may be applied more frequently if very exudative

For conservative management of finger-tip injuries

- TO THE SKIN
  - Child: Apply every 2–3 days, consult product literature for details

Adjunct to prophylaxis of infection in skin graft donor sites and extensive abrasions

- TO THE SKIN
  - Child: (consult product literature)

Adjunct to short-term treatment of infection in pressure sores

- TO THE SKIN
  - Child: (consult product literature)

- **UNLICENSED USE** No age range specified by manufacturer.
- **CONTRA-INDICATIONS** Not recommended for neonates
- **CAUTIONS** G6PD deficiency

CAUTIONS, FURTHER INFORMATION

- Large areas Plasma-sulfadiazine concentrations may approach therapeutic levels with *side-effects* and *interactions* as for sulfonamides if large areas of skin are treated.

- **INTERACTIONS** → Appendix 1: sulfadiazine silver
- **SIDE-EFFECTS**
- **Common or very common** Leucopenia · skin reactions
- **Rare or very rare** Argyria (following treatment of large areas of skin or long term use) · renal failure

SIDE-EFFECTS, FURTHER INFORMATION Leucopenia developing 2–3 days after starting treatment of burns patients is reported usually to be self-limiting and sulfadiazine silver need not usually be discontinued provided blood counts are monitored carefully to ensure return to normality within a few days.

- **ALLERGY AND CROSS-SENSITIVITY** EvGr Caution in patients with sensitivity to sulfonamides. ⟨M⟩ See, *Cautions, further information*.
- **PREGNANCY** Risk of neonatal haemolysis and methaemoglobinaemia in third trimester.
- **BREAST FEEDING** Small risk of kernicterus in jaundiced infants and of haemolysis in G6PD-deficient infants.
- **HEPATIC IMPAIRMENT** Manufacturer advises caution in significant hepatic impairment.
- **RENAL IMPAIRMENT** Manufacturer advises caution if significant impairment.
- **MONITORING REQUIREMENTS** Monitor for leucopenia.
- **DIRECTIONS FOR ADMINISTRATION** Manufacturer advises apply with sterile applicator.

- **MEDICINAL FORMS** There can be variation in the licensing of different medicines containing the same drug.

Cutaneous cream

EXCIPIENTS: May contain Cetostearyl alcohol (including cetyl and stearyl alcohol), polysorbates, propylene glycol

- **Sulfadiazine silver (Non-proprietary)**
  Sulfadiazine silver 10 mg per 1 gram Sulfadiazine silver 1% cream | 1 gram PoM ⊠
- **Flamazine** (Smith & Nephew Healthcare Ltd)
  Sulfadiazine silver 10 mg per 1 gram Flamazine 1% cream | 20 gram PoM £2.91 | 500 gram PoM £18.27 DT = £18.27

ANTIBACTERIALS › OTHER

Mupirocin

07-May-2021

- **INDICATIONS AND DOSE**

Bacterial skin infections, particularly those caused by Gram-positive organisms (except pseudomonal infection)

- TO THE SKIN
  - Child: Apply up to 3 times a day for up to 10 days

Non-bullous impetigo [in patients who are not systemically unwell or at high risk of complications]

- TO THE SKIN
  - Child: Apply 3 times a day for 5–7 days

- **UNLICENSED USE** Mupirocin ointment licensed for use in children (age range not specified by manufacturer). *Bactroban*® cream not recommended for use in children under 1 year.
- **SIDE-EFFECTS**
- **Common or very common** Skin reactions
- **PREGNANCY** Manufacturer advises avoid unless potential benefit outweighs risk—no information available.
- **BREAST FEEDING** No information available.
- **RENAL IMPAIRMENT** EvGr Avoid using ointment in moderate to severe impairment when absorption of large quantities may occur (contains polyethylene glycol which is excreted renally). ⟨M⟩
- **PRESCRIBING AND DISPENSING INFORMATION** For choice of antibacterial therapy, see Skin infections, antibacterial therapy p. 373.

- **MEDICINAL FORMS** There can be variation in the licensing of different medicines containing the same drug.

Cutaneous ointment

- **Mupirocin (Non-proprietary)**
  Mupirocin 20 mg per 1 gram Mupirocin 2% ointment | 15 gram PoM £12.50 DT = £9.75

- Bactroban (GlaxoSmithKline UK Ltd)
  Mupirocin 20 mg per 1 gram Bactroban 2% ointment | 15 gram [PoM] £5.26 DT = £9.75

Cutaneous cream

EXCIPIENTS: May contain Benzyl alcohol, cetostearyl alcohol (including cetyl and stearyl alcohol)

- Bactroban (GlaxoSmithKline UK Ltd)
  Mupirocin (as Mupirocin calcium) 20 mg per 1 gram Bactroban 2% cream | 15 gram [PoM] £5.26 DT = £5.26

4.2 Fungal skin infections

Other drugs used for Fungal skin infections Griseofulvin, p. 470 · Hydrocortisone with clotrimazole, p. 916

ANTIFUNGALS > IMIDAZOLE ANTIFUNGALS

Clotrimazole

10-Nov-2021

- **INDICATIONS AND DOSE**

Fungal skin infections

▶ TO THE SKIN

- Child: Apply 2–3 times a day

- **CAUTIONS** Contact with eyes and mucous membranes should be avoided
- **INTERACTIONS** → Appendix 1: antifungals, azoles
- **SIDE-EFFECTS** Oedema · pain · paraesthesia · skin reactions
- **PREGNANCY** Minimal absorption from skin; not known to be harmful.
- **PRESCRIBING AND DISPENSING INFORMATION** Spray may be useful for application of clotrimazole to large or hairy areas of the skin.
- **PATIENT AND CARER ADVICE**
  Medicines for Children leaflet: Clotrimazole for fungal infections www.medicinesforchildren.org.uk/medicines/clotrimazole-for-fungal-infections/
- **MEDICINAL FORMS** There can be variation in the licensing of different medicines containing the same drug. Forms available from special-order manufacturers include: cutaneous powder

Cutaneous or ear solution

- Canesten (clotrimazole) (Bayer Plc)
  Clotrimazole 10 mg per 1 ml Canesten 1% solution | 20 ml [P] £2.54 DT = £2.54

Cutaneous cream

EXCIPIENTS: May contain Benzyl alcohol, cetostearyl alcohol (including cetyl and stearyl alcohol), polysorbates

- Clotrimazole (Non-proprietary)
  Clotrimazole 10 mg per 1 gram Clotrimazole 1% cream | 20 gram [P] £2.33 DT = £1.42 | 50 gram [P] £3.67 DT = £3.55
- Canesten (clotrimazole) (Bayer Plc)
  Clotrimazole 10 mg per 1 gram Canesten 1% cream | 20 gram [P] £2.89 DT = £1.42 | 50 gram [P] £4.71 DT = £3.55

Spray

CAUTIONARY AND ADVISORY LABELS 15

EXCIPIENTS: May contain Propylene glycol

- Canesten (clotrimazole) (Bayer Plc)
  Clotrimazole 10 mg per 1 ml Canesten Dermatological 1% spray | 40 ml [P] £4.99 DT = £4.99

Combinations available: *Hydrocortisone with clotrimazole*, p. 916

Econazole nitrate

08-May-2020

- **INDICATIONS AND DOSE**

Fungal skin infections

▶ TO THE SKIN

- Child: Apply twice daily

Fungal nail infections

▶ BY TRANSUNGUAL APPLICATION

- Child: Apply once daily, applied under occlusive dressing

- **CAUTIONS** Avoid contact with eyes and mucous membranes
- **SIDE-EFFECTS**
  ▶ **Common or very common** Pain · skin reactions
  ▶ **Uncommon** Swelling
  ▶ **Frequency not known** Angioedema

  SIDE-EFFECTS, FURTHER INFORMATION Treatment should be discontinued if side-effects are severe.
- **PREGNANCY** Minimal absorption from skin; not known to be harmful.
- **PRESCRIBING AND DISPENSING INFORMATION** *Pevaryl*® 1% cream should be used.
- **MEDICINAL FORMS** No licensed medicines listed.

Ketoconazole

30-May-2023

- **INDICATIONS AND DOSE**

Treatment of seborrhoeic dermatitis and dandruff

▶ TO THE SKIN USING SHAMPOO

- Child 12–17 years: Apply twice weekly for 2–4 weeks, leave preparation on for 3–5 minutes before rinsing

Prophylaxis of seborrhoeic dermatitis and dandruff

▶ TO THE SKIN USING SHAMPOO

- Child 12–17 years: Apply every 1–2 weeks, leave preparation on for 3–5 minutes before rinsing

Treatment of pityriasis versicolor

▶ TO THE SKIN USING SHAMPOO

- Child 12–17 years: Apply once daily for maximum 5 days, leave preparation on for 3–5 minutes before rinsing

Prophylaxis of pityriasis versicolor

▶ TO THE SKIN USING SHAMPOO

- Child 12–17 years: Apply once daily for up to 3 days before sun exposure, leave preparation on for 3–5 minutes before rinsing

- **CONTRA-INDICATIONS** Acute porphyrias p. 745
- **CAUTIONS** Avoid contact with eyes · avoid contact with mucous membranes
- **INTERACTIONS** → Appendix 1: antifungals, azoles
- **SIDE-EFFECTS**
  ▶ **Common or very common** Skin reactions
  ▶ **Uncommon** Alopecia · angioedema · excessive tearing · folliculitis · hair changes
  ▶ **Rare or very rare** Eye irritation · taste altered
- **EXCEPTIONS TO LEGAL CATEGORY** Can be sold to the public for the prevention and treatment of dandruff and seborrhoeic dermatitis of the scalp as a shampoo formulation containing ketoconazole maximum 2%, in a pack containing maximum 120 mL and labelled to show a maximum frequency of application of once every 3 days.
- **MEDICINAL FORMS** There can be variation in the licensing of different medicines containing the same drug.

Shampoo

EXCIPIENTS: May contain Imidurea

- Ketoconazole (Non-proprietary)
  Ketoconazole 20 mg per 1 gram Ketoconazole 2% shampoo | 120 ml [PoM] [S] DT = £9.38
- Dandrazol (Crescent Pharma Ltd)
  Ketoconazole 20 mg per 1 gram Dandrazol 2% shampoo | 120 ml [PoM] £5.20 DT = £9.38
- Nizoral (Thornton & Ross Ltd)
  Ketoconazole 20 mg per 1 gram Nizoral 2% shampoo | 120 ml [PoM] £3.59 DT = £9.38

Miconazole
23-Jun-2023

● **INDICATIONS AND DOSE**

Fungal skin infections

▶ TO THE SKIN

▸ Neonate: Apply twice daily continuing for 10 days after lesions have healed.

▸ Child: Apply twice daily continuing for 10 days after lesions have healed

Fungal nail infections

▶ BY TRANSUNGUAL APPLICATION

▸ Child: Apply 1–2 times a day

● **UNLICENSED USE** Licensed for use in children (age range not specified by manufacturer).

● **CAUTIONS** Avoid in Acute porphyrias p. 745 · contact with eyes and mucous membranes should be avoided

● **INTERACTIONS** → Appendix 1: antifungals, azoles

● **SIDE-EFFECTS**

▶ **Uncommon** Skin reactions

▶ **Frequency not known** Angioedema

● **PREGNANCY** Absorbed from the skin in small amounts; manufacturer advises caution.

● **BREAST FEEDING** Manufacturer advises caution—no information available.

● **PROFESSION SPECIFIC INFORMATION**

Dental practitioners' formulary Miconazole cream may be prescribed.

● **NATIONAL FUNDING/ACCESS DECISIONS**

NHS restrictions *Daktarin*® powder and *Daktarin*® cream 15 g are not prescribable in NHS primary care.

● **MEDICINAL FORMS** There can be variation in the licensing of different medicines containing the same drug.

Cutaneous powder

▸ **Daktarin** (McNeil Products Ltd)

Miconazole nitrate 20 mg per 1 gram Daktarin 2% powder | 20 gram [P] £4.46 DT = £4.46

Cutaneous cream

EXCIPIENTS: May contain Butylated hydroxyanisole

▸ **Daktarin** (McNeil Products Ltd)

Miconazole nitrate 20 mg per 1 gram Daktarin 2% cream | 15 gram [P] £3.62 | 30 gram [P] £5.30 DT = £5.30

Spray

CAUTIONARY AND ADVISORY LABELS 15

▸ **Daktarin** (McNeil Products Ltd)

Miconazole nitrate 1.6 mg per 1 gram Daktarin Aktiv 0.16% spray powder | 100 gram [GSL] £5.24 DT = £5.24

Tioconazole
03-Feb-2020

● **INDICATIONS AND DOSE**

Fungal nail infection

▶ BY TRANSUNGUAL APPLICATION

▸ Child: Apply twice daily usually for up to 6 months (may be extended to 12 months), apply to nails and surrounding skin

● **UNLICENSED USE** Licensed for use in children (age range not specified by manufacturer).

● **CAUTIONS** Contact with eyes and mucous membranes should be avoided · use with caution if child likely to suck affected digits

● **SIDE-EFFECTS**

▶ **Common or very common** Peripheral oedema

▶ **Uncommon** Skin reactions

▶ **Frequency not known** Nail disorder · pain · paraesthesia · periorbital oedema

● **PREGNANCY** Manufacturer advises avoid.

● **MEDICINAL FORMS** There can be variation in the licensing of different medicines containing the same drug.

Medicated nail lacquer

▸ **Tioconazole (Non-proprietary)**

Tioconazole 283 mg per 1 ml Tioconazole 283mg/ml medicated nail lacquer | 12 ml [PoM] £38.00 DT = £33.35

▸ **Trosyl** (Pfizer Ltd)

Tioconazole 283 mg per 1 ml Trosyl 283mg/ml nail solution | 12 ml [PoM] £27.38 DT = £33.35

ANTIFUNGALS › OTHER

Amorolfine
06-Oct-2020

● **INDICATIONS AND DOSE**

Fungal nail infections

▶ BY TRANSUNGUAL APPLICATION

▸ Child 1 month–11 years: Apply 1–2 times a week for 6 months to treat finger nails and for toe nails 9–12 months (review at intervals of 3 months), apply to infected nails after filing and cleansing, allow to dry for approximately 3 minutes

▸ Child 12–17 years: Apply 1–2 times a week for 6 months to treat finger nails and for toe nails 9–12 months (review at intervals of 3 months), apply to infected nails after filing and cleansing, allow to dry for approximately 3 minutes

● **UNLICENSED USE** Not licensed for use in children under 12 years.

● **CAUTIONS** Avoid contact with ears · avoid contact with eyes and mucous membranes · use with caution in child likely to suck affected digits

● **SIDE-EFFECTS**

▶ **Rare or very rare** Nail discolouration · skin reactions

● **PATIENT AND CARER ADVICE** Cosmetic nail varnish may be applied at least 10 minutes after amorolfine nail lacquer; the nail varnish should be removed before repeat application of amorolfine. Avoid artificial nails during treatment.

● **MEDICINAL FORMS** There can be variation in the licensing of different medicines containing the same drug.

Medicated nail lacquer

CAUTIONARY AND ADVISORY LABELS 10

▸ **Amorolfine (Non-proprietary)**

Amorolfine (as Amorolfine hydrochloride) 50 mg per 1 ml Amorolfine 5% medicated nail lacquer | 5 ml [PoM] £16.21 DT = £7.43

▸ **Loceryl** (Galderma (UK) Ltd)

Amorolfine (as Amorolfine hydrochloride) 50 mg per 1 ml Loceryl 5% medicated nail lacquer | 5 ml [PoM] £9.08 DT = £7.43

Terbinafine
16-Aug-2021

● **INDICATIONS AND DOSE**

Tinea pedis

▶ TO THE SKIN USING CREAM

▸ Child: Apply 1–2 times a day for up to 1 week, to be applied thinly

▶ BY MOUTH USING TABLETS

▸ Child 1–17 years (body-weight 10–19 kg): 62.5 mg once daily for 2–6 weeks

▸ Child 1–17 years (body-weight 20–39 kg): 125 mg once daily for 2–6 weeks

▸ Child 1–17 years (body-weight 40 kg and above): 250 mg once daily for 2–6 weeks

Tinea corporis

▶ TO THE SKIN USING CREAM

▸ Child: Apply 1–2 times a day for up to 1–2 weeks, to be applied thinly, review treatment after 2 weeks

continued →

- ▶ BY MOUTH USING TABLETS
- ▸ Child 1-17 years (body-weight 10-19 kg): 62.5 mg once daily for 4 weeks
- ▸ Child 1-17 years (body-weight 20-39 kg): 125 mg once daily for 4 weeks
- ▸ Child 1-17 years (body-weight 40 kg and above): 250 mg once daily for 4 weeks

Tinea cruris

- ▶ TO THE SKIN USING CREAM
- ▸ Child: Apply 1–2 times a day for up to 1–2 weeks, to be applied thinly, review treatment after 2 weeks
- ▶ BY MOUTH USING TABLETS
- ▸ Child 1-17 years (body-weight 10-19 kg): 62.5 mg once daily for 2–4 weeks
- ▸ Child 1-17 years (body-weight 20-39 kg): 125 mg once daily for 2–4 weeks
- ▸ Child 1-17 years (body-weight 40 kg and above): 250 mg once daily for 2–4 weeks

Tinea capitis

- ▶ BY MOUTH USING TABLETS
- ▸ Child 1-17 years (body-weight 10-19 kg): 62.5 mg once daily for 4 weeks
- ▸ Child 1-17 years (body-weight 20-39 kg): 125 mg once daily for 4 weeks
- ▸ Child 1-17 years (body-weight 40 kg and above): 250 mg once daily for 4 weeks

Dermatophyte infections of the nails

- ▶ BY MOUTH USING TABLETS
- ▸ Child 1-17 years (body-weight 10-19 kg): 62.5 mg once daily for 6 weeks–3 months (occasionally longer in toenail infections)
- ▸ Child 1-17 years (body-weight 20-39 kg): 125 mg once daily for 6 weeks–3 months (occasionally longer in toenail infections)
- ▸ Child 1-17 years (body-weight 40 kg and above): 250 mg once daily for 6 weeks–3 months (occasionally longer in toenail infections)

Cutaneous candidiasis | Pityriasis versicolor

- ▶ TO THE SKIN USING CREAM
- ▸ Child: Apply 1–2 times a day for 2 weeks, to be applied thinly, review treatment after 2 weeks

● **UNLICENSED USE** Not licensed for use in children.

● **CAUTIONS**

- ▸ With oral use Psoriasis (risk of exacerbation) · risk of lupus erythematosus
- ▸ With topical use Contact with eyes and mucous membranes should be avoided

● **INTERACTIONS** → Appendix 1: terbinafine

● **SIDE-EFFECTS**

GENERAL SIDE-EFFECTS

- ▶ **Common or very common** Skin reactions

SPECIFIC SIDE-EFFECTS

- ▶ **Common or very common**
- ▸ With oral use Appetite decreased · arthralgia · diarrhoea · gastrointestinal discomfort · gastrointestinal disorder · headache · myalgia · nausea
- ▶ **Uncommon**
- ▸ With oral use Taste altered
- ▸ With topical use Pain
- ▶ **Rare or very rare**
- ▸ With oral use Agranulocytosis · alopecia · cutaneous lupus erythematosus · dizziness · hepatic disorders · malaise · neutropenia · photosensitivity reaction · sensation abnormal · severe cutaneous adverse reactions (SCARs) · systemic lupus erythematosus (SLE) · thrombocytopenia · vertigo
- ▶ **Frequency not known**
- ▸ With oral use Anaemia · anxiety · depressive symptom · fatigue · fever · hearing impairment · influenza like illness · pancreatitis · pancytopenia · rhabdomyolysis · serum sickness-like reaction · smell altered · tinnitus · vasculitis · vision disorders
- ▸ With topical use Hypersensitivity

SIDE-EFFECTS, FURTHER INFORMATION **Liver toxicity** With oral use; discontinue treatment if liver toxicity develops (including jaundice, cholestasis and hepatitis).

Serious skin reactions With oral use; discontinue treatment in progressive skin rash (including Stevens-Johnson syndrome and toxic epidermal necrolysis).

● **PREGNANCY**

- ▸ With topical use Manufacturer advises use only if potential benefit outweighs risk— *animal* studies suggest no adverse effects.
- ▸ With oral use Manufacturer advises use only if potential benefit outweighs risk—no information available.

● **BREAST FEEDING**

- ▸ With topical use Manufacturer advises avoid—present in milk. Less than 5% of the dose is absorbed after topical application of terbinafine; avoid application to mother's chest.
- ▸ With oral use Avoid—present in milk.

● **HEPATIC IMPAIRMENT**

- ▸ With oral use Manufacturer advises avoid (risk of increased exposure).

● **RENAL IMPAIRMENT**

- ▸ With oral use EvGr Caution if creatinine clearance less than 50 mL/minute or serum creatinine concentration greater than 300 micromol/litre (limited information available). (M) See p. 16.

● **MONITORING REQUIREMENTS**

- ▸ With oral use Monitor hepatic function before treatment and then periodically after 4–6 weeks of treatment—discontinue if abnormalities in liver function tests.

● **PATIENT AND CARER ADVICE**

- ▸ With oral use Manufacturer advises that patients should immediately report any signs or symptoms suggestive of liver dysfunction such as pruritus, unexplained persistent nausea, decreased appetite, anorexia, jaundice, vomiting, fatigue, right upper abdominal pain, dark urine, or pale stools. Patients with these symptoms should discontinue taking terbinafine and the patient's liver function should be immediately evaluated.

● **EXCEPTIONS TO LEGAL CATEGORY** Preparations of terbinafine hydrochloride (maximum 1%) can be sold to the public for use in those over 16 years for external use for the treatment of tinea pedis as a cream in a pack containing maximum 15 g, or for the treatment of tinea pedis and cruris as a cream in a pack containing maximum 15 g, or for the treatment of tinea pedis, cruris, and corporis as a spray in a pack containing maximum 30 mL spray or as a gel in a pack containing maximum 30 g gel.

● **MEDICINAL FORMS** There can be variation in the licensing of different medicines containing the same drug.

Oral tablet

CAUTIONARY AND ADVISORY LABELS 9

- ▸ **Terbinafine (Non-proprietary)**
  Terbinafine (as Terbinafine hydrochloride) 250 mg Terbinafine 250mg tablets | 14 tablet PoM £18.11 DT = £1.30 | 28 tablet PoM £2.08–£36.98

Cutaneous cream

EXCIPIENTS: May contain Benzyl alcohol, cetostearyl alcohol (including cetyl and stearyl alcohol), polysorbates

- ▸ **Terbinafine (Non-proprietary)**
  Terbinafine hydrochloride 10 mg per 1 gram Terbinafine 1% cream | 15 gram PoM £3.99 DT = £1.70 | 30 gram PoM £6.52 DT = £3.40
- ▸ **Lamisil** (Karo Healthcare UK Ltd)
  Terbinafine hydrochloride 10 mg per 1 gram Lamisil 1% cream | 30 gram PoM £8.76 DT = £3.40

ANTISEPTICS AND DISINFECTANTS > UNDECENOATES

Undecenoic acid with zinc undecenoate

05-Oct-2021

● **INDICATIONS AND DOSE**

Treatment of athletes foot

▶ TO THE SKIN

▸ Child: Apply twice daily, continue use for 7 days after lesions have healed

Prevention of athletes foot

▶ TO THE SKIN

▸ Child: Apply once daily

● **UNLICENSED USE** *Mycota*® licensed for use in children (age range not specified by manufacturer).

● **CAUTIONS** Avoid broken skin · contact with eyes should be avoided · contact with mucous membranes should be avoided

● **SIDE-EFFECTS**

▶ Rare or very rare Skin irritation

SIDE-EFFECTS, FURTHER INFORMATION Treatment should be discontinued if irritation is severe.

● **MEDICINAL FORMS** There can be variation in the licensing of different medicines containing the same drug.

Cutaneous cream

EXCIPIENTS: May contain Cetostearyl alcohol (including cetyl and stearyl alcohol), fragrances

▸ Mycota (zinc undecenoate / undecenoic acid) (Thornton & Ross Ltd)

Undecenoic acid 50 mg per 1 gram, Zinc undecenoate 200 mg per 1 gram Mycota cream | 25 gram GSL £3.07 DT = £3.07

ANTISEPTICS AND DISINFECTANTS > OTHER

Chlorhexidine with nystatin

01-Mar-2021

● **INDICATIONS AND DOSE**

Skin infections due to *Candida* spp.

▶ TO THE SKIN

▸ Child: Apply 2–3 times a day continue for 7 days after lesions have healed

● **UNLICENSED USE** Licensed for use in children (age range not specified by manufacturer).

● **CAUTIONS** Avoid contact with eyes and mucous membranes

● **SIDE-EFFECTS** Hypersensitivity · skin reactions

● **MEDICINAL FORMS** There can be variation in the licensing of different medicines containing the same drug.

Cutaneous cream

EXCIPIENTS: May contain Benzyl alcohol, cetostearyl alcohol (including cetyl and stearyl alcohol), polysorbates

▸ Nystaform (Typharm Ltd)

Chlorhexidine hydrochloride 10 mg per 1 gram, Nystatin 100000 unit per 1 gram Nystaform cream | 30 gram PoM £9.50 DT = £9.50

BENZOATES

Benzoic acid with salicylic acid

22-Nov-2020

● **INDICATIONS AND DOSE**

Ringworm (tinea)

▶ TO THE SKIN

▸ Child: Apply twice daily

● **UNLICENSED USE** Licensed for use in children (age range not specified by manufacturer).

● **CAUTIONS** Avoid broken or inflamed skin · avoid contact with eyes · avoid contact with mucous membranes

CAUTIONS, FURTHER INFORMATION

▸ Salicylate toxicity Salicylate toxicity may occur particularly if applied on large areas of skin.

● **SIDE-EFFECTS** Drug toxicity · eye irritation · mucosal irritation · skin reactions

● **PRESCRIBING AND DISPENSING INFORMATION** Benzoic Acid Ointment, Compound, BP has also been referred to as Whitfield's ointment.

● **MEDICINAL FORMS** There can be variation in the licensing of different medicines containing the same drug. Forms available from special-order manufacturers include: cutaneous cream, cutaneous ointment

Cutaneous ointment

EXCIPIENTS: May contain Cetostearyl alcohol (including cetyl and stearyl alcohol)

4.3 Parasitic skin infections

Other drugs used for Parasitic skin infections Ivermectin, p. 474

PARASITICIDES

Dimeticone

04-Feb-2020

● **INDICATIONS AND DOSE**

Head lice

▶ TO THE SKIN

▸ Child: Apply once weekly for 2 doses, rub into dry hair and scalp, allow to dry naturally, shampoo after minimum 8 hours (or overnight)

● **UNLICENSED USE** Not licensed for use in children under 6 months except under medical supervision.

IMPORTANT SAFETY INFORMATION

MHRA/CHM ADVICE: HEAD LICE ERADICATION PRODUCTS: RISK OF SERIOUS BURNS IF TREATED HAIR IS EXPOSED TO OPEN FLAMES OR OTHER SOURCES OF IGNITION (MARCH 2018)

See Skin infections p. 895.

● **CAUTIONS** Avoid contact with eyes · children under 6 months, medical supervision required

● **SIDE-EFFECTS** Alopecia · dyspnoea · eye irritation · hypersensitivity · scalp changes · skin reactions

● **MEDICINAL FORMS** There can be variation in the licensing of different medicines containing the same drug.

Cutaneous solution

▸ Hedrin (Thornton & Ross Ltd)

Dimeticone 40 mg per 1 gram Hedrin 4% lotion | 150 ml P £10.00 DT = £10.00

Cutaneous spray solution

▸ Hedrin (Thornton & Ross Ltd)

Dimeticone 40 mg per 1 gram Hedrin 4% spray | 120 ml P £10.30 DT = £10.30

Malathion

04-Feb-2020

● **INDICATIONS AND DOSE**

Head lice

▶ TO THE SKIN

▸ Child: Apply once weekly for 2 doses, rub preparation into dry hair and scalp, allow to dry naturally, remove by washing after 12 hours

continued →

13 Skin

Crab lice

▶ TO THE SKIN

▸ Child: Apply once weekly for 2 doses, apply preparation over whole body, allow to dry naturally, wash off after 12 hours or overnight

Scabies

▶ TO THE SKIN

▸ Child: Apply once weekly for 2 doses, apply preparation over whole body, and wash off after 24 hours, if hands are washed with soap within 24 hours, they should be retreated

- **UNLICENSED USE** Not licensed for use in children under 6 months except under medical supervision.

IMPORTANT SAFETY INFORMATION

MHRA/CHM ADVICE: HEAD LICE ERADICATION PRODUCTS: RISK OF SERIOUS BURNS IF TREATED HAIR IS EXPOSED TO OPEN FLAMES OR OTHER SOURCES OF IGNITION (MARCH 2018)

See Skin infections p. 895.

- **CAUTIONS** Alcoholic lotions **not** recommended for head lice in children with severe eczema or asthma, or for scabies or crab lice · avoid contact with eyes · children under 6 months, medical supervision required · do not use lotion more than once a week for 3 consecutive weeks · do not use on broken or secondarily infected skin
- **SIDE-EFFECTS** Angioedema · eye swelling · hypersensitivity · skin reactions
- **PRESCRIBING AND DISPENSING INFORMATION** For scabies, manufacturer recommends application to the body but not necessarily to the head and neck. However, application should be extended to the scalp, neck, face, and ears.
- **MEDICINAL FORMS** There can be variation in the licensing of different medicines containing the same drug.

Cutaneous emulsion

EXCIPIENTS: May contain Cetostearyl alcohol (including cetyl and stearyl alcohol), fragrances, hydroxybenzoates (parabens)

▸ **Derbac-M** (G.R. Lane Health Products Ltd)

Malathion 5 mg per 1 gram Derbac-M 0.5% liquid | 150 ml [P] £15.96 DT = £15.96

Permethrin

04-Feb-2020

- **INDICATIONS AND DOSE**

Scabies

▶ TO THE SKIN

▸ Child: Apply once weekly for 2 doses, apply 5% preparation over whole body including face, neck, scalp and ears then wash off after 8–12 hours. If hands are washed with soap within 8 hours of application, they should be treated again with cream

- **UNLICENSED USE** *Dermal Cream* (scabies), not licensed for use in children under 2 months; not licensed for treatment of crab lice in children under 18 years. *Creme Rinse* (head lice) not licensed for use in children under 6 months except under medical supervision.

IMPORTANT SAFETY INFORMATION

MHRA/CHM ADVICE: HEAD LICE ERADICATION PRODUCTS: RISK OF SERIOUS BURNS IF TREATED HAIR IS EXPOSED TO OPEN FLAMES OR OTHER SOURCES OF IGNITION (MARCH 2018)

See Skin infections p. 895.

- **CAUTIONS** Avoid contact with eyes · children aged 2 months–2 years, medical supervision required for dermal cream (scabies) · children under 6 months, medical supervision required for cream rinse (head lice) · do not use on broken or secondarily infected skin
- **SIDE-EFFECTS** Scalp irritation · skin reactions
- **PRESCRIBING AND DISPENSING INFORMATION** Manufacturer recommends application to the body but to exclude head and neck. However, application should be extended to the scalp, neck, face, and ears.

  Larger patients may require up to two 30-g packs for adequate treatment.
- **LESS SUITABLE FOR PRESCRIBING** *Lyclear® Creme Rinse* is less suitable for prescribing.
- **MEDICINAL FORMS** There can be variation in the licensing of different medicines containing the same drug.

Cutaneous cream

CAUTIONARY AND ADVISORY LABELS 10 (Dermal cream only)

EXCIPIENTS: May contain Butylated hydroxytoluene, woolfat and related substances (including lanolin)

▸ **Permethrin (Non-proprietary)**

Permethrin 50 mg per 1 gram Permethrin 5% cream | 30 gram [P] £10.90 DT = £5.77

▸ **Lyclear** (Omega Pharma Ltd)

Permethrin 50 mg per 1 gram Lyclear 5% dermal cream | 30 gram [P] £7.79 DT = £5.77

Cutaneous liquid

EXCIPIENTS: May contain Cetostearyl alcohol (including cetyl and stearyl alcohol)

▸ **Lyclear** (Omega Pharma Ltd)

Permethrin 10 mg per 1 gram Lyclear 1% creme rinse | 118 ml [P] £8.08 DT = £8.08

4.4 Viral skin infections

ANTIVIRALS › NUCLEOSIDE ANALOGUES

Aciclovir

13-Oct-2025

(Acyclovir)

- **INDICATIONS AND DOSE**

Herpes simplex infection (local treatment)

▶ TO THE SKIN

▸ Child: Apply 5 times a day for 5–10 days, to be applied to lesions approximately every 4 hours, starting at first sign of attack

- **UNLICENSED USE** Cream licensed for use in children (age range not specified by manufacturer).
- **CAUTIONS** Avoid cream coming in to contact with eyes and mucous membranes
- **INTERACTIONS** → Appendix 1: aciclovir
- **SIDE-EFFECTS**

▶ **Uncommon** Skin reactions

- **PREGNANCY** Limited absorption from topical aciclovir preparations.
- **PRESCRIBING AND DISPENSING INFORMATION** For further information on *herpes simplex*, see Herpesvirus infections p. 498.
- **PATIENT AND CARER ADVICE**

Medicines for Children leaflet: Aciclovir cream for herpes (cold sore) www.medicinesforchildren.org.uk/medicines/aciclovir-cream-for-herpes-cold-sore/

- **PROFESSION SPECIFIC INFORMATION**

Dental practitioners' formulary Aciclovir Cream may be prescribed.

- **EXCEPTIONS TO LEGAL CATEGORY** A 2-g tube and a pump pack are on sale to the public for the treatment of cold sores.
- **MEDICINAL FORMS** There can be variation in the licensing of different medicines containing the same drug.

Cutaneous cream

EXCIPIENTS: May contain Cetostearyl alcohol (including cetyl and stearyl alcohol), propylene glycol

▸ **Aciclovir (Non-proprietary)**
Aciclovir 50 mg per 1 gram Aciclovir 5% cream | 2 gram PoM £2.50 DT = £2.55 | 10 gram PoM £12.21 DT = £12.18
▸ **Zovirax** (GlaxoSmithKline UK Ltd)
Aciclovir 50 mg per 1 gram Zovirax 5% cream | 2 gram PoM £4.63 DT = £2.55 | 10 gram PoM £13.96 DT = £12.18

5 Inflammatory skin conditions

5.1 Eczema and psoriasis

Eczema

06-May-2021

Types and management

Eczema (dermatitis) refers to a variety of skin conditions characterised by epidermal inflammation and itching. The main types of eczema are irritant, allergic contact, atopic, venous and discoid. *Atopic eczema* is the most common type of eczema in children and it usually involves dry skin as well as infection and lichenification caused by scratching and rubbing. Atopic eczema often has a genetic component which may cause the skin barrier to break down. This may worsen eczema as it makes the skin susceptible to trigger factors such as irritants and allergens. *Seborrhoeic dermatitis* is also common in infants.

EvGr Management of eczema involves the removal or treatment of contributory factors; known or suspected irritants and contact allergens should be avoided. Ⓐ Rarely, ingredients in topical medicinal products may sensitise the skin; the BNF for Children lists active ingredients together with excipients that have been associated with skin sensitisation.

EvGr Frequent and liberal use of emollients is advised for dry skin and itching associated with eczema. The choice of emollient is dependent on the dryness of the skin, and the child or carer preference; this can be supplemented with bath or shower emollients. Emollients can increase the efficacy of topical corticosteroids and have shown to have a steroid sparing action. The use of emollients should continue even if the eczema improves or if other treatment is being used. Aqueous cream is generally not recommended due to the high risk of developing skin reactions.

Topical corticosteroids are also often required in the management of eczema; the potency of the corticosteroid should be used in accordance to the severity and site of the condition, and the age of the child. A mild potency topical corticosteroid may be considered for short-term use on the face and neck, and a moderate to potent topical corticosteroid for severe flares or flares in vulnerable sites such as axillae and groin. Generally, moderate to potent topical corticosteroids are required for moderate or severe eczema on the scalp, limbs, and trunk. The use of very potent topical corticosteroids in children is not recommended without specialist advice. Treatment should be reviewed regularly, especially if a potent topical corticosteroid is required. In children with frequent flares (2–3 per month), a topical corticosteroid can be applied to prevent further flares using various regimens (e.g. 2 consecutive days each week). Emollient therapy should be continued during treatment with topical corticosteroids.

Under specialist supervision, bandages (including those containing ichthammol with zinc oxide p. 917) are sometimes applied over topical corticosteroids or emollients to treat eczema of the limbs. Dry-wrap dressings can be used to provide a physical barrier to help prevent scratching and improve retention of emollients. Wet elasticated viscose stockinette is used for 'wet-wrap' bandaging over topical corticosteroids or emollients to cool the skin and relieve itching, but there is an increased risk of infection and excessive absorption of the corticosteroid; 'wet-wrap' bandaging should be initiated under the supervision of a trained healthcare professional. The use of occlusive medicated dressings and dry bandages to treat infected atopic eczema is not recommended. Ⓐ

See *Wound management products and elasticated garments* in the BNF for details of elasticated viscose stockinette tubular bandages and garments, and silk clothing.

Topical pimecrolimus p. 919 is licensed for the treatment of mild to moderate atopic eczema. Tacrolimus p. 919 is licensed for topical use in the treatment of moderate to severe atopic eczema. EvGr Both are calcineurin inhibitors and should be considered as a second-line treatment option only, unless there is a specific reason to avoid or reduce the use of topical corticosteroids. Treatment of atopic eczema with topical pimecrolimus or topical tacrolimus should be initiated by a specialist.

Antihistamines are not recommended for routine use in the management of atopic eczema. However, if there is severe itching or urticaria, consider a non-sedating antihistamine. An age-appropriate sedating antihistamine may be considered in children over 6 months if itching causes sleep disturbance and has a significant impact on the child or carer. Ⓐ

Infection

EvGr Breaks in the skin caused by eczema are susceptible to bacterial infection (commonly with *Staphylococcus aureus* and occasionally with *Streptococcus pyogenes*) and may require treatment with a topical or systemic antibacterial. For further information, see *Secondary bacterial infection of common skin conditions* in Skin infections, antibacterial therapy p. 373. Episodes of infected eczema usually co-exist with a flare and will require management with treatments such as emollients and topical corticosteroids.

Widespread *herpes simplex infection* may complicate atopic eczema (eczema herpeticum) and treatment under specialist supervision with a systemic antiviral drug is indicated. If eczema herpeticum is suspected, refer the child for same-day specialist advice. Ⓐ

Severe refractory eczema

EvGr Severe refractory eczema is managed under specialist supervision; it may require phototherapy or systemic drugs that act on the immune system. Azathioprine p. 638 [unlicensed indication], mycophenolate mofetil p. 648 [unlicensed indication], and ciclosporin p. 640 are available for use in severe refractory eczema. Ⓐ

Seborrhoeic dermatitis

Seborrhoeic dermatitis (seborrhoeic eczema) is associated with species of the yeast *Malassezia*. EvGr Infantile seborrhoeic dermatitis affects particularly the body folds, nappy area and scalp; it is treated with emollients and the topical imidazoles clotrimazole p. 900 and miconazole p. 901. Topical corticosteroids are not routinely recommended however, a low potency topical corticosteroid may be beneficial for some infants with nappy rash. Infantile seborrhoeic dermatitis affecting the scalp (*cradle cap*) is treated by hydrating the scalp using natural oils, brushing the scalp and the use of a mild shampoo.

In older children, seborrhoeic dermatitis affects the scalp, paranasal areas, and eyebrows. Shampoos active against the yeast (including those containing ketoconazole p. 900) and combinations of mild topical corticosteroids with suitable antimicrobials are used to treat older children. Ⓐ

Psoriasis
11-Jan-2023

Overview

Psoriasis is an inflammatory skin disease that usually follows a relapsing and remitting course and may have nail or joint involvement. Different forms of psoriasis exist; chronic plaque psoriasis is the most common, and is characterised by epidermal thickening and scaling, commonly affecting extensor surfaces and the scalp. Guttate psoriasis is a distinctive form of psoriasis that tends to occur most often in children and young adults, often following a streptococcal throat infection or tonsillitis.

Occasionally, psoriasis is provoked or exacerbated by drugs such as lithium, chloroquine and hydroxychloroquine, beta-blockers, non-steroidal anti-inflammatory drugs, and ACE inhibitors. Psoriasis may not be seen until the drug has been taken for weeks or months.

EvGr Refer children and young people who present with any form of psoriasis to a specialist. ⟨A⟩

Treatment

EvGr Offer topical treatment first-line to all children with psoriasis. Topical treatment options include emollients, topical corticosteroids, coal tar preparations, and topical vitamin D or vitamin D analogues. When choosing topical treatment, consider the patient or carers preference, practical aspects of application, extent of psoriasis, and the variety of formulations available. ⟨A⟩

Emollients are widely used in psoriasis; they moisturise dry skin, reduce scaling, and relieve itching. They also soften cracked areas and help other topical treatment absorb through the skin to work more effectively. Some cases of mild psoriasis may settle with the use of emollients alone. EvGr Emollients may also be useful adjuncts to other more specific treatment. ⟨A⟩

Continuous long-term use of potent topical corticosteroids may cause psoriasis to become unstable, and lead to irreversible skin atrophy and striae. Widespread use (greater than 10% of body surface area affected) can also lead to systemic and local side-effects. EvGr Children and young people with psoriasis who are using topical corticosteroids of any potency should be offered a review of treatment at least annually. The use of very potent topical corticosteroids is not recommended in children and young people.

Consecutive use of potent topical corticosteroids should not be used for more than 8 weeks at any one site. Application may be restarted after a 4-week 'treatment break'; non-steroid treatments, such as topical vitamin D or vitamin D analogues, may be continued during this time. ⟨A⟩

Coal tar p. 918 has anti-inflammatory, antipruritic and anti-scaling properties and is often combined with other topical treatments for psoriasis. Several coal tar preparations are available including ointments, shampoos, and bath additives. EvGr Newer products are preferred to older products containing crude coal tar (coal tar BP), which is malodorous and usually messier to apply. ⟨A⟩

Topical vitamin D and vitamin D analogue preparations are available as ointments, gels, scalp solutions, and lotions. Tacalcitol p. 930 and calcitriol p. 930 may be less irritating than calcipotriol p. 929.

Psoriasis of the trunk and limbs

EvGr Consider treatment with either calcipotriol [unlicensed indication] (children aged over 6 years) or a once-daily potent topical corticosteroid (children aged over 1 year).

In children with treatment-resistant psoriasis of the trunk or limbs, consider treatment with short-contact dithranol p. 917. Treatment should be given in a specialist setting or the patient or carer should be provided with educational support for self-use. ⟨A⟩

Scalp psoriasis

EvGr Offer a potent topical corticosteroid applied once daily for up to 4 weeks as initial treatment. If satisfactory control is not achieved after 4 weeks, consider a different formulation of the potent topical corticosteroid (e.g. a shampoo or mousse) and/or topical agents to remove or soften adherent scale (e.g. agents containing salicylic acid, emollients, oils). These agents should be used prior to applying the potent topical corticosteroid to allow effective penetration. If response to potent corticosteroid treatment remains unsatisfactory after a further 4 weeks of treatment, offer a combination product containing calcipotriol with betamethasone p. 910 for up to 4 weeks. If treatment with calcipotriol with betamethasone for up to 4 weeks does not give a satisfactory response, offer a coal tar preparation.

In children with mild to moderate scalp psoriasis who cannot use topical corticosteroids, offer treatment with a topical vitamin D or a vitamin D analogue [unlicensed] preparation only. If treatment with a vitamin D or vitamin D analogue [unlicensed] for up to 8 weeks does not give a satisfactory response, offer a coal tar preparation. The use of coal tar-based shampoos alone for the treatment of severe scalp psoriasis is not recommended. ⟨A⟩

Facial, flexural, and genital psoriasis

EvGr Offer a mild or moderate potency topical corticosteroid applied once or twice daily. The face, flexures, and genitals are particularly vulnerable to steroid atrophy therefore topical corticosteroids should only be used short-term (e.g. 1–2 weeks per month). ⟨A⟩

Pustular or erythrodermic psoriasis

EvGr Widespread unstable psoriasis of erythrodermic or generalised pustular types requires urgent same-day specialist assessment and should be managed as a medical emergency. ⟨A⟩

Phototherapy

Phototherapy is available under the supervision of an appropriately trained healthcare professional. EvGr Narrowband ultraviolet B (UVB) phototherapy can be offered to children and young people with plaque or guttate psoriasis in whom topical treatment has failed to achieve control. ⟨A⟩

Photochemotherapy combining psoralen with ultraviolet A (PUVA) is available in specialist centres under the supervision of an appropriately trained healthcare professional. Psoralen [unlicensed] enhances the effects of UVA and is administered either by mouth or topically. EvGr PUVA irradiation can be considered with caution for the treatment of localised palmoplantar pustulosis and plaque-type psoriasis; other treatment options should be considered first. ⟨A⟩ Cumulative doses increase the risk of dysplastic and neoplastic skin lesions, especially squamous cell cancer.

Systemic treatment

Non-biological treatment

EvGr Under the supervision of a specialist, and with consideration of patient factors such as age, systemic non-biological treatment with methotrexate p. 672 [unlicensed] or ciclosporin p. 640 may be offered to some children with psoriasis that cannot be controlled with topical treatment *and* if the psoriasis has a significant impact on physical, psychological or social well-being. In addition, the psoriasis would have to be extensive, or localised with significant distress or functional impairment, or have failed phototherapy treatment.

Ciclosporin may be considered first-line in patients who need rapid or short-term disease control, have palmoplantar pustulosis, or who are considering conception (both males and females).

Only consider acitretin p. 928 in children in exceptional cases, where methotrexate [unlicensed] and ciclosporin are not appropriate, or have failed, or in children with pustular forms of psoriasis. ⟨A⟩

Biological treatment

EvGr Biological drugs for psoriasis such as interleukin inhibitors and tumor necrosis factor alpha (TNF-α) inhibitors should be initiated and supervised only by specialists experienced in the diagnosis and management of psoriasis. (A)

Other drugs used for Eczema and psoriasis Adalimumab, p. 806 · Etanercept, p. 808 · Secukinumab, p. 799 · Upadacitinib, p. 927 · Ustekinumab, p. 924

CORTICOSTEROIDS

Topical corticosteroids

08-Oct-2024

Overview

Topical corticosteroids are used for the treatment of inflammatory conditions of the skin (other than those arising from an infection), particularly eczema, contact dermatitis, insect stings, and eczema of scabies. They are generally used to relieve symptoms and suppress signs of the disorder when other measures such as emollients are ineffective. Corticosteroids suppress the inflammatory reaction during use; they are not curative and on discontinuation a withdrawal reaction (rebound or flare) may occur. Withdrawal reactions are thought to occur after long-term continuous or inappropriate use of topical corticosteroids (particularly those of moderate to high potency). Signs and symptoms are reported to happen within days to weeks of stopping long-term topical corticosteroid treatment. A flare of the underlying skin disorder is the most common withdrawal reaction. Rarely, a specific type of withdrawal reaction may occur in which skin redness extends beyond the initial area of treatment, with burning or stinging that is worse than the original condition. For further information on topical corticosteroid withdrawal reactions, see *Important safety information* in the individual drug monograph.

Children, especially infants, are particularly susceptible to side-effects. However, concern about the safety of topical corticosteroids in children should not result in the child being undertreated. The aim is to control the condition as well as possible; inadequate treatment will perpetuate the condition. Carers of young children should be advised that treatment should **not** necessarily be reserved to 'treat only the worst areas' and they may need to be advised that patient information leaflets may contain inappropriate advice for the child's condition.

In an acute flare-up of atopic eczema, it may be appropriate to use more potent formulations of topical corticosteroids for a short period to regain control of the condition.

Topical corticosteroids are not recommended in the routine treatment of urticaria; treatment should only be initiated and supervised by a specialist. Topical corticosteroids may worsen ulcerated or secondarily infected lesions. They should not be used indiscriminately in pruritus (where they will only benefit if inflammation is causing the itch) and are **not** recommended for acne vulgaris.

Systemic or very potent topical corticosteroids should be avoided or given only under specialist supervision in psoriasis because, although they may suppress the psoriasis in the short term, relapse or vigorous rebound occurs on withdrawal (sometimes precipitating severe pustular psoriasis). Topical use of potent corticosteroids on widespread psoriasis can lead to systemic as well as to local side-effects. It is reasonable, however, to prescribe a mild topical corticosteroid for a short period (2–4 weeks) for *flexural* and *facial psoriasis*, and to use a more potent corticosteroid such as betamethasone p. 909 or fluocinonide p. 912 for *psoriasis* of the *scalp*, *palms*, or *soles*.

In general, the most potent topical corticosteroids should be reserved for recalcitrant dermatoses such as *chronic discoid lupus erythematosus*, *lichen simplex chronicus*, *hypertrophic lichen planus*, and *palmoplantar pustulosis*. Potent corticosteroids should generally be avoided on the face and skin flexures, but specialists occasionally prescribe them for use on these areas in certain circumstances.

When topical treatment has failed, intralesional corticosteroid injections may be used. These are more effective than the very potent topical corticosteroid preparations and should be reserved for severe cases where there are localised lesions such as *keloid scars*, *hypertrophic lichen planus*, or *localised alopecia areata*.

Perioral lesions

Hydrocortisone cream 1% p. 912 can be used for up to 7 days to treat uninfected inflammatory lesions on the lips. Hydrocortisone with miconazole cream or ointment p. 917 is useful where infection by susceptible organisms and inflammation co-exist, particularly for initial treatment (up to 7 days) e.g. in angular cheilitis. Organisms susceptible to miconazole include *Candida* spp. and many Gram-positive bacteria including streptococci and staphylococci.

Choice

Water-miscible corticosteroid creams are suitable for moist or weeping lesions whereas ointments are generally chosen for dry, lichenified or scaly lesions or where a more occlusive effect is required. Lotions may be useful when minimal application to a large or hair-bearing area is required or for the treatment of exudative lesions. *Occlusive polythene* or *hydrocolloid dressings* increase absorption, but also increase the risk of side-effects; they are therefore used only under supervision on a short-term basis for areas of very thick skin (such as the palms and soles). Disposable nappies and tight fitting pants also increase the risk of side-effects by increasing absorption of the corticosteroid. The inclusion of urea or salicylic acid p. 950 also increases the penetration of the corticosteroid.

In BNFC, topical corticosteroids for the skin are categorised as 'mild', 'moderately potent', 'potent' or 'very potent'; the **least potent** preparation which is effective should be chosen but dilution should be avoided whenever possible.

Topical hydrocortisone is usually used in children under 1 year of age. Moderately potent and potent topical corticosteroids should be used with great care in children and for short periods (1–2 weeks) only. A very potent corticosteroid should be initiated under the supervision of a specialist.

Appropriate topical corticosteroids for specific conditions are:

- *insect bites and stings*—mild corticosteroid such as hydrocortisone 1% cream;
- *inflamed nappy rash causing discomfort* in infant over 1 month—mild corticosteroid such as hydrocortisone 0.5% or 1% for up to 7 days (combined with antimicrobial if infected);
- *mild to moderate eczema, flexural and facial eczema, or psoriasis*—mild corticosteroid such as hydrocortisone 1%;
- *severe eczema of the face and neck*—moderately potent corticosteroid for 3–5 days only, if not controlled by a mild corticosteroid;
- *severe eczema on the trunk and limbs*—moderately potent or potent corticosteroid for 1–2 weeks only, switching to a less potent preparation as the condition improves;
- *eczema affecting area with thickened skin (e.g. soles of feet)*—potent topical corticosteroid in combination with urea or salicylic acid (to increase penetration of corticosteroid).

Absorption through the skin

Mild and *moderately potent* topical corticosteroids are associated with few side-effects but particular care is required when treating neonates and infants, and in the use of *potent* and *very potent* corticosteroids. Absorption through the skin can rarely cause adrenal suppression and even Cushing's syndrome, depending on the area of the body being treated and the duration of treatment. Absorption of corticosteroid is greatest from severely inflamed skin, thin skin (especially on the face or genital area), from flexural sites (e.g. axillae, groin), and in infants where skin surface area is higher in relation to body-weight; absorption is increased by occlusion.

For further information on side-effects that may occur from absorption through the skin, see Corticosteroids, general use p. 537.

Compound preparations

The advantages of including other substances (such as antibacterials or antifungals) with corticosteroids in topical preparations are uncertain, but such combinations may have a place where inflammatory skin conditions are associated with bacterial or fungal infection, such as infected eczema. In these cases the antimicrobial drug should be chosen according to the sensitivity of the infecting organism and used regularly for a short period (typically twice daily for 1 week). Longer use increases the likelihood of resistance and of sensitisation.

The keratolytic effect of salicylic acid p. 950 facilitates the absorption of topical corticosteroids; however, excessive and prolonged use of topical preparations containing salicylic acid may cause salicylism.

Topical corticosteroid potencies

Potency of a topical corticosteroid preparation (including compound preparations) is based solely on the corticosteroid component, irrespective of the formulation and strength.

Mild
- Hydrocortisone p. 912

Moderate
- Alclometasone dipropionate p. 909
- Clobetasone butyrate p. 911
- Hydrocortisone butyrate p. 913

Potent
- Beclometasone dipropionate p. 909
- Betamethasone p. 909
- Fludroxycortide p. 911
- Fluocinolone acetonide p. 912
- Fluocinonide p. 912
- Fluticasone p. 912
- Mometasone furoate p. 913

Very potent
- Clobetasol propionate p. 911

Corticosteroids (topical)

IMPORTANT SAFETY INFORMATION

MHRA/CHM ADVICE: CORTICOSTEROIDS: RARE RISK OF CENTRAL SEROUS CHORIORETINOPATHY WITH LOCAL AS WELL AS SYSTEMIC ADMINISTRATION (AUGUST 2017)

Central serous chorioretinopathy is a retinal disorder that has been linked to the systemic use of corticosteroids. Recently, it has also been reported after local administration of corticosteroids via inhaled and intranasal, epidural, intra-articular, topical dermal, and periocular routes. The MHRA recommends that patients should be advised to report any blurred vision or other visual disturbances with corticosteroid treatment given by any route; consider referral to an ophthalmologist for evaluation of possible causes if a patient presents with vision problems.

MHRA/CHM ADVICE: TOPICAL CORTICOSTEROIDS: INFORMATION ON THE RISK OF TOPICAL STEROID WITHDRAWAL REACTIONS (SEPTEMBER 2021)

Rarely, long-term continuous or inappropriate use of topical corticosteroids, particularly those of moderate to high potency, can result in the development of rebound flares, reported as dermatitis with intense redness, stinging, and burning that can spread beyond the initial treatment area.

The MHRA advises that the lowest potency topical corticosteroid needed should be used. For patients who are currently on long-term topical corticosteroid treatment, consider reducing potency or frequency of application (or both). Healthcare professionals should also be vigilant for the signs and symptoms of topical corticosteroid withdrawal reactions.

Healthcare professionals should inform patients:
- how much should be applied, as under-use can prolong treatment duration;
- how long they should use a topical corticosteroid for, especially on sensitive areas such as the face and genitals;
- to always apply topical corticosteroids as instructed and consult the patient information leaflet provided;
- to seek medical advice before using a topical corticosteroid on a new body area, as some areas of the body are more prone to side-effects;
- to return for medical advice if their skin condition worsens while using topical corticosteroid, and advise them when it would be appropriate to re-treat without a consultation and;
- if their skin worsens within 2 weeks of stopping a topical corticosteroid, treatment should not be started again without consulting their doctor unless they have previously been advised to do so

The MHRA advises healthcare professionals to report any suspected adverse effects, via the Yellow Card Scheme, even when the adverse affects occur after stopping corticosteroid treatment.

ADRENAL INSUFFICIENCY CARD (APRIL 2023)

The British Society for Paediatric Endocrinology and Diabetes (BSPED) has developed an Adrenal Insufficiency Card which should be issued to children with adrenal insufficiency and steroid dependence. The card includes a management summary for the emergency treatment of adrenal crisis and sick day dosing, and can be issued by any healthcare professional managing such patients. The BSPED Adrenal Insufficiency Card is available at: www.bsped.org.uk/adrenal-insufficiency.

MHRA/CHM ADVICE: TOPICAL STEROIDS: INTRODUCTION OF NEW LABELLING AND A REMINDER OF THE POSSIBILITY OF SEVERE SIDE EFFECTS, INCLUDING TOPICAL STEROID WITHDRAWAL REACTIONS (MAY 2024)

The risk of serious side-effects, such as Topical Steroid Withdrawal Reactions (TSW), thinning of the skin, and systemic effects, increases with prolonged use of higher potency topical corticosteroids. Regulatory action has resulted in new labelling for topical corticosteroids with information on their potency to assist with patient counselling and correct selection. The MHRA continue to receive reports regarding TSW, particularly associated with eczema treatment; healthcare professionals are reminded to continue to follow the advice issued in 2021 (see above). In addition, healthcare professionals are advised that alternative treatments should be considered if previous discontinuation of a topical corticosteroid was associated with a reaction suspicious of TSW, and that they should support patients living with symptoms of TSW and review treatment plans alongside them.

Healthcare professionals should review the position statement from the National Eczema Society, the British

Dermatological Nursing Group, and the British Association of Dermatologists: www.bad.org.uk/topical-steroid-withdrawal-joint-statement/.

The MHRA Patient Safety Leaflet on topical corticosteroids and withdrawal reactions can be used to aid patient counselling: www.gov.uk/guidance/topical-corticosteroids-and-withdrawal-reactions.

- **CONTRA-INDICATIONS** Acne · perioral dermatitis · potent corticosteroids in widespread plaque psoriasis · rosacea · untreated bacterial, fungal or viral skin lesions
- **CAUTIONS** Avoid prolonged use (particularly on the face) · cautions applicable to systemic corticosteroids may also apply if absorption occurs following topical and local use · dermatoses of infancy, including nappy rash (extreme caution required—treatment should be limited to 5–7 days) · infection · keep away from eyes · use potent or very potent topical corticosteroids under specialist supervision
- **SIDE-EFFECTS**
  - **Common or very common** Skin reactions · telangiectasia
  - **Rare or very rare** Adrenal suppression · hypertrichosis · skin depigmentation (may be reversible)
  - **Frequency not known** Local reaction · vasodilation

  SIDE-EFFECTS, FURTHER INFORMATION Side-effects applicable to systemic corticosteroids may also apply if absorption occurs following topical and local use. In order to minimise the side-effects of a topical corticosteroid, it is important to apply it thinly to affected areas only, no more frequently than twice daily, and to use the least potent formulation which is fully effective.
- **DIRECTIONS FOR ADMINISTRATION** EvGr Topical corticosteroid preparations should be applied no more frequently than twice daily; once daily is often sufficient. (A) Topical corticosteroids should be applied in sufficient quantity to cover the affected areas. The length of cream or ointment expelled from a tube may be used to specify the quantity to be applied to a given area of skin. This length can be measured in terms of a *fingertip unit* (the distance from the tip of the adult index finger to the first crease). One fingertip unit (approximately 500 mg from a tube with a standard 5 mm diameter nozzle) is sufficient to cover an area that is twice that of the flat adult handprint (palm and fingers). EvGr Several minutes should elapse between application of topical corticosteroids and emollients. (A)

  'Wet-wrap bandaging' increases absorption into the skin, but should be initiated under the supervision of a trained healthcare professional.
- **PRESCRIBING AND DISPENSING INFORMATION** The potency of each topical corticosteroid should be included on the label with the directions for use. The label should be attached to the container (for example, the tube) rather than the outer packaging.
- **PATIENT AND CARER ADVICE** Patients and their carers should be counselled on the terms used to describe the potency of topical corticosteroid preparations. For ease of understanding, *potent* and *very potent* corticosteroids may be referred to as *strong* and *very strong* corticosteroids, respectively. If a patient is using topical corticosteroids of different potencies, the patient should be told when to use each corticosteroid. Patients and their carers should be reassured that side-effects such as skin thinning and systemic effects rarely occur when topical corticosteroids are used appropriately.

  If systemic absorption occurs following topical and local use, side-effects applicable to systemic corticosteroids may apply.

F 908

Alclometasone dipropionate

26-Jul-2025

- **INDICATIONS AND DOSE**

  Inflammatory skin disorders such as eczemas

  ▶ TO THE SKIN
  - Child: Apply 1–2 times a day, to be applied thinly

  POTENCY
  - Alclometasone dipropionate is a moderate corticosteroid.
- **UNLICENSED USE** Licensed for use in children (age range not specified by manufacturer).
- **PATIENT AND CARER ADVICE** Patients or carers should be counselled on the application of alclometasone dipropionate cream.
- **MEDICINAL FORMS** No licensed medicines listed.

F 908

Beclometasone dipropionate

26-Jul-2025

(Beclomethasone dipropionate)

- **INDICATIONS AND DOSE**

  Severe inflammatory skin disorders such as eczemas unresponsive to less potent corticosteroids | Psoriasis

  ▶ TO THE SKIN
  - Child: Apply 1–2 times a day, to be applied thinly

  POTENCY
  - Beclometasone dipropionate is a potent corticosteroid.
- **UNLICENSED USE** Not licensed for use in children under 1 year.
- **INTERACTIONS** → Appendix 1: corticosteroids
- **SIDE-EFFECTS** Vision blurred
- **MEDICINAL FORMS** There can be variation in the licensing of different medicines containing the same drug.

  Cutaneous ointment

  CAUTIONARY AND ADVISORY LABELS 28
  - Beclometasone dipropionate (Non-proprietary)

    Beclometasone dipropionate 250 microgram per 1 gram Beclometasone 0.025% ointment | 30 gram PoM £74.97 DT = £74.97

  Cutaneous cream

  CAUTIONARY AND ADVISORY LABELS 28
  - Beclometasone dipropionate (Non-proprietary)

    Beclometasone dipropionate 250 microgram per 1 gram Beclometasone 0.025% cream | 30 gram PoM £74.97 DT = £74.97

F 908

Betamethasone

26-Jul-2025

- **DRUG ACTION** Betamethasone has very high glucocorticoid activity and insignificant mineralocorticoid activity.
- **INDICATIONS AND DOSE**

  Severe inflammatory skin disorders such as eczemas unresponsive to less potent corticosteroids | Psoriasis

  ▶ TO THE SKIN
  - Child: Apply 1–2 times a day, to be applied thinly

  POTENCY
  - Betamethasone is a potent corticosteroid.
- **UNLICENSED USE** *Betacap*®, *Betnovate*® and *Betnovate-RD*® are not licensed for use in children under 1 year. *Bettamousse*® is not licensed for use in children under 6 years.
- **CAUTIONS** Use of more than 100 g per week of 0.1% preparation likely to cause adrenal suppression
- **INTERACTIONS** → Appendix 1: corticosteroids

- **SIDE-EFFECTS** Colloid milia
- **PATIENT AND CARER ADVICE** Patient counselling is advised for betamethasone cream, ointment, scalp application and foam (application).

- **MEDICINAL FORMS** There can be variation in the licensing of different medicines containing the same drug.

Cutaneous ointment

CAUTIONARY AND ADVISORY LABELS 28

- **Betamethasone (Non-proprietary)**
  Betamethasone (as Betamethasone valerate) 250 microgram per 1 gram Betamethasone valerate 0.025% ointment | 100 gram PoM £3.14–£5.30 DT = £3.15
  Betamethasone (as Betamethasone valerate) 1 mg per 1 gram Betamethasone valerate 0.1% ointment | 30 gram PoM £1.80 DT = £1.30 | 100 gram PoM £4.70 DT = £4.33
- **Betnovate** (GlaxoSmithKline UK Ltd)
  Betamethasone (as Betamethasone valerate) 250 microgram per 1 gram Betnovate RD 0.025% ointment | 100 gram PoM £3.15 DT = £3.15
  Betamethasone (as Betamethasone valerate) 1 mg per 1 gram Betnovate 0.1% ointment | 30 gram PoM £1.43 DT = £1.30 | 100 gram PoM £4.05 DT = £4.33
- **Diprosone** (Organon Pharma (UK) Ltd)
  Betamethasone (as Betamethasone dipropionate) 500 microgram per 1 gram Diprosone 0.05% ointment | 30 gram PoM £2.16 DT = £2.16

Cutaneous foam

CAUTIONARY AND ADVISORY LABELS 15, 28

EXCIPIENTS: May contain Cetostearyl alcohol (including cetyl and stearyl alcohol), polysorbates, propylene glycol

- **Bettamousse** (RPH Pharmaceuticals AB)
  Betamethasone (as Betamethasone valerate) 1 mg per 1 gram Bettamousse 0.1% cutaneous foam | 100 gram PoM £11.62 DT = £11.62

Cutaneous cream

CAUTIONARY AND ADVISORY LABELS 28

EXCIPIENTS: May contain Cetostearyl alcohol (including cetyl and stearyl alcohol), chlorocresol

- **Betamethasone (Non-proprietary)**
  Betamethasone (as Betamethasone valerate) 250 microgram per 1 gram Betamethasone valerate 0.025% cream | 100 gram PoM £3.14–£5.30 DT = £3.15
  Betamethasone (as Betamethasone valerate) 1 mg per 1 gram Betamethasone valerate 0.1% cream | 30 gram PoM £3.40 DT = £1.97 | 100 gram PoM £6.73 DT = £5.18
- **Betnovate** (GlaxoSmithKline UK Ltd)
  Betamethasone (as Betamethasone valerate) 250 microgram per 1 gram Betnovate RD 0.025% cream | 100 gram PoM £3.15 DT = £3.15
  Betamethasone (as Betamethasone valerate) 1 mg per 1 gram Betnovate 0.1% cream | 30 gram PoM £1.43 DT = £1.97 | 100 gram PoM £4.05 DT = £5.18
- **Diprosone** (Organon Pharma (UK) Ltd)
  Betamethasone (as Betamethasone dipropionate) 500 microgram per 1 gram Diprosone 0.05% cream | 100 gram PoM £6.12 DT = £6.12

Cutaneous liquid

CAUTIONARY AND ADVISORY LABELS 15(scalp lotion only), 28

EXCIPIENTS: May contain Cetostearyl alcohol (including cetyl and stearyl alcohol), hydroxybenzoates (parabens)

- **Betacap** (Dermal Laboratories Ltd)
  Betamethasone (as Betamethasone valerate) 1 mg per 1 gram Betacap 0.1% scalp application | 100 ml PoM £3.94 DT = £3.94
- **Betnovate** (GlaxoSmithKline UK Ltd)
  Betamethasone (as Betamethasone valerate) 1 mg per 1 gram Betnovate 0.1% scalp application | 100 ml PoM £4.99 DT = £3.94
  Betnovate 0.1% lotion | 100 ml PoM £4.58 DT = £4.58
- **Diprosone** (Organon Pharma (UK) Ltd)
  Betamethasone (as Betamethasone dipropionate) 500 microgram per 1 ml Diprosone 0.05% lotion | 100 ml PoM £7.80 DT = £7.80

Combinations available: ***Betamethasone with clioquinol,*** p. 914 · ***Betamethasone with clotrimazole,*** p. 914 · ***Betamethasone with fusidic acid,*** p. 914 · ***Betamethasone with neomycin,*** p. 914 · ***Betamethasone with salicylic acid,*** p. 915

Calcipotriol with betamethasone

15-Jan-2025

The properties listed below are those particular to the combination only. For the properties of the components please consider, calcipotriol p. 929, betamethasone p. 909.

- **INDICATIONS AND DOSE**

Psoriasis [using gel or ointment] (under expert supervision)

▶ TO THE SKIN

- Child 12–17 years: Apply once daily usually for up to 4 weeks, if necessary treatment may be continued for longer or repeated on the advice of a specialist, when using calcipotriol-containing preparations the maximum total dose of calcipotriol is 3.75 mg (equivalent to 75 g total amount of any formulation) in any 1 week, applied to a maximum 30% of body surface

Scalp psoriasis [using gel] (under expert supervision)

▶ TO THE SKIN

- Child 12–17 years: Apply 1–4 g once daily usually for 4 weeks, if necessary treatment may be continued for longer or repeated on the advice of a specialist, when using calcipotriol-containing preparations the maximum total dose of calcipotriol is 3.75 mg (equivalent to 75 g total amount of any formulation) in any 1 week, applied to a maximum 30% of body surface

POTENCY

- Betamethasone is a potent corticosteroid.

- **UNLICENSED USE** Not licensed for use in children.
- **CONTRA-INDICATIONS** Erythrodermic psoriasis · pustular psoriasis
- **INTERACTIONS** → Appendix 1: corticosteroids · vitamin D substances
- **PATIENT AND CARER ADVICE**
  Advice on application Patients or carers should be advised to allow calcipotriol with betamethasone preparations to remain on the scalp or skin overnight or during the day, and not to shower or bathe immediately after application.
  Hands should be washed thoroughly after application to avoid inadvertent transfer to other body areas.

- **MEDICINAL FORMS** There can be variation in the licensing of different medicines containing the same drug.

Cutaneous ointment

CAUTIONARY AND ADVISORY LABELS 28

EXCIPIENTS: May contain Butylated hydroxytoluene

- **Calcipotriol with betamethasone (Non-proprietary)**
  Calcipotriol (as Calcipotriol monohydrate) 50 microgram per 1 gram, Betamethasone (as Betamethasone dipropionate) 500 microgram per 1 gram Calcipotriol 0.005% / Betamethasone dipropionate 0.05% ointment | 30 gram PoM £26.38 DT = £19.84 | 60 gram PoM £31.74 | 120 gram PoM £59.09
- **Dovobet** (LEO Pharma)
  Calcipotriol (as Calcipotriol monohydrate) 50 microgram per 1 gram, Betamethasone (as Betamethasone dipropionate) 500 microgram per 1 gram Dovobet ointment | 30 gram PoM £19.84 DT = £19.84 | 60 gram PoM £39.68 | 120 gram PoM £73.86

Cutaneous gel

CAUTIONARY AND ADVISORY LABELS 28

EXCIPIENTS: May contain Butylated hydroxytoluene

- **Calcipotriol with betamethasone (Non-proprietary)**
  Calcipotriol (as Calcipotriol monohydrate) 50 microgram per 1 gram, Betamethasone (as Betamethasone dipropionate) 500 microgram per 1 gram Calcipotriol 0.005% / Betamethasone dipropionate 0.05% gel | 60 gram PoM £37.21 DT = £37.21 | 120 gram PoM £69.10–£74.42

▸ **Dovobet** (LEO Pharma)
Calcipotriol (as Calcipotriol monohydrate) 50 microgram per 1 gram, Betamethasone (as Betamethasone dipropionate) 500 microgram per 1 gram Dovobet gel | 60 gram PoM £37.21 DT = £37.21 | 120 gram PoM £69.11

908

Clobetasol propionate

26-Jul-2025

● **INDICATIONS AND DOSE**

Short-term treatment only of severe resistant inflammatory skin disorders such as recalcitrant eczemas unresponsive to less potent corticosteroids | Psoriasis

▸ TO THE SKIN
▸ Child 1–17 years: Apply 1–2 times a day for up to 4 weeks, to be applied thinly

POTENCY
▸ Clobetasol propionate is a very potent corticosteroid.

● **UNLICENSED USE** *Dermovate*® not licensed for use in children under 1 year.

● **PATIENT AND CARER ADVICE** Patients or carers should be given advice on how to administer clobetasol propionate foam, liquid (scalp application), cream, ointment and shampoo.
Scalp application Patients or carers should be advised to apply foam directly to scalp lesions (foam begins to subside immediately on contact with skin).

● **MEDICINAL FORMS** There can be variation in the licensing of different medicines containing the same drug. Forms available from special-order manufacturers include: cutaneous cream, cutaneous ointment, cutaneous paste

Cutaneous ointment
CAUTIONARY AND ADVISORY LABELS 28
EXCIPIENTS: May contain Propylene glycol
▸ **Clobetasol propionate (Non-proprietary)**
Clobetasol propionate 500 microgram per 1 gram Clobetasol 0.05% ointment | 30 gram PoM £2.68–£4.30 DT = £2.69 | 100 gram PoM £7.89–£12.64 DT = £7.90
▸ **Dermovate** (GlaxoSmithKline UK Ltd)
Clobetasol propionate 500 microgram per 1 gram Dermovate 0.05% ointment | 30 gram PoM £2.69 DT = £2.69 | 100 gram PoM £7.90 DT = £7.90

Cutaneous cream
CAUTIONARY AND ADVISORY LABELS 28
EXCIPIENTS: May contain Beeswax, cetostearyl alcohol (including cetyl and stearyl alcohol), chlorocresol, propylene glycol
▸ **Clobetasol propionate (Non-proprietary)**
Clobetasol propionate 500 microgram per 1 gram Clobetasol 0.05% cream | 30 gram PoM £2.68–£4.30 DT = £2.69 | 100 gram PoM £7.89–£12.64 DT = £7.90
▸ **Dermovate** (GlaxoSmithKline UK Ltd)
Clobetasol propionate 500 microgram per 1 gram Dermovate 0.05% cream | 30 gram PoM £2.69 DT = £2.69 | 100 gram PoM £7.90 DT = £7.90

Cutaneous liquid
CAUTIONARY AND ADVISORY LABELS 15, 28
▸ **Dermovate** (GlaxoSmithKline UK Ltd)
Clobetasol propionate 500 microgram per 1 gram Dermovate 0.05% scalp application | 30 ml PoM £3.07 DT = £3.07 | 100 ml PoM £10.42 DT = £10.42

Combinations available: *Clobetasol propionate with neomycin sulfate and nystatin*, p. 915

908

Clobetasone butyrate

26-Jul-2025

● **INDICATIONS AND DOSE**

Eczemas and dermatitis of all types | Maintenance between courses of more potent corticosteroids

▸ TO THE SKIN
▸ Child: Apply 1–2 times a day, to be applied thinly

POTENCY
▸ Clobetasone butyrate is a moderate corticosteroid.

● **UNLICENSED USE** Licensed for use in children (age range not specified by manufacturer).

● **PATIENT AND CARER ADVICE** Patients or carers should be advised on the application of clobetasone butyrate containing preparations.

● **EXCEPTIONS TO LEGAL CATEGORY** Cream can be sold to the public for short-term symptomatic treatment and control of patches of eczema and dermatitis (but not seborrhoeic dermatitis) in adults and children over 12 years provided pack does not contain more than 15 g.

● **MEDICINAL FORMS** There can be variation in the licensing of different medicines containing the same drug.

Cutaneous ointment
CAUTIONARY AND ADVISORY LABELS 28
▸ **Clobavate** (Teva UK Ltd)
Clobetasone butyrate 500 microgram per 1 gram Clobavate 0.05% ointment | 30 gram PoM £1.49 DT = £1.86 | 100 gram PoM £4.35 DT = £5.44
▸ **Eumovate** (GlaxoSmithKline UK Ltd)
Clobetasone butyrate 500 microgram per 1 gram Eumovate 0.05% ointment | 30 gram PoM £1.86 DT = £1.86 | 100 gram PoM £5.44 DT = £5.44

Cutaneous cream
CAUTIONARY AND ADVISORY LABELS 28
EXCIPIENTS: May contain Cetostearyl alcohol (including cetyl and stearyl alcohol), chlorocresol
▸ **Eumovate** (GlaxoSmithKline UK Ltd)
Clobetasone butyrate 500 microgram per 1 gram Eumovate 0.05% cream | 30 gram PoM £1.86 DT = £1.86 | 100 gram PoM £5.44 DT = £5.44

Combinations available: *Clobetasone butyrate with nystatin and oxytetracycline*, p. 915

908

Fludroxycortide

26-Jul-2025

(Flurandrenolone)

● **INDICATIONS AND DOSE**

Inflammatory skin disorders such as eczemas

▸ TO THE SKIN
▸ Child: Apply 1–2 times a day, to be applied thinly

POTENCY
▸ Fludroxycortide is a potent corticosteroid.

HAELAN® TAPE

Chronic localised recalcitrant dermatoses (but not acute or weeping)

▸ TO THE SKIN
▸ Child: Cut tape to fit lesion, apply to clean, dry skin shorn of hair, usually for 12 hours daily

POTENCY
▸ For *Haelan*® tape: Fludroxycortide is a potent corticosteroid.

● **UNLICENSED USE** Licensed for use in children (age range not specified by manufacturer).

● **SIDE-EFFECTS** Cushing's syndrome · increased risk of infection

● **PATIENT AND CARER ADVICE** Patients or carers should be counselled on application of fludroxycortide cream and ointment.

● **MEDICINAL FORMS** There can be variation in the licensing of different medicines containing the same drug.

Impregnated dressing
▸ **Fludroxycortide (Non-proprietary)**
Fludroxycortide 4 microgram per 1 square cm Fludroxycortide 4micrograms/square cm tape 7.5cm | 20 cm PoM £21.44–£38.24 DT = £38.45 | 50 cm PoM £37.49 DT = £68.31

908

Fluocinolone acetonide

26-Jul-2025

- **INDICATIONS AND DOSE**

Severe inflammatory skin disorders such as eczemas | Psoriasis

▶ TO THE SKIN

▶ Child 1–17 years: Apply 1–2 times a day, to be applied thinly, reduce strength as condition responds

POTENCY

▶ Fluocinolone acetonide is a potent corticosteroid.

- **UNLICENSED USE** Not licensed for use in children under 1 year.
- **INTERACTIONS** → Appendix 1: fluocinolone
- **PRESCRIBING AND DISPENSING INFORMATION** Gel is useful for application to the scalp and other hairy areas.
- **PATIENT AND CARER ADVICE** Patient counselling is advised for fluocinolone acetonide cream, gel and ointment (application).

- **MEDICINAL FORMS** There can be variation in the licensing of different medicines containing the same drug.

Cutaneous ointment

CAUTIONARY AND ADVISORY LABELS 28

EXCIPIENTS: May contain Propylene glycol, woolfat and related substances (including lanolin)

▶ Synalar (Reig Jofre UK Ltd)

Fluocinolone acetonide 62.5 microgram per 1 gram Synalar 1 in 4 Dilution 0.00625% ointment | 50 gram PoM £4.84 DT = £4.84

Fluocinolone acetonide 250 microgram per 1 gram Synalar 0.025% ointment | 30 gram PoM £4.14 DT = £4.14 | 100 gram PoM £11.75 DT = £11.75

Cutaneous cream

CAUTIONARY AND ADVISORY LABELS 28

EXCIPIENTS: May contain Benzyl alcohol, cetostearyl alcohol (including cetyl and stearyl alcohol), polysorbates, propylene glycol

▶ Synalar (Reig Jofre UK Ltd)

Fluocinolone acetonide 250 microgram per 1 gram Synalar 0.025% cream | 30 gram PoM £4.14 DT = £4.14 | 100 gram PoM £11.75 DT = £11.75

Cutaneous gel

CAUTIONARY AND ADVISORY LABELS 28

EXCIPIENTS: May contain Hydroxybenzoates (parabens), propylene glycol

▶ Synalar (Reig Jofre UK Ltd)

Fluocinolone acetonide 250 microgram per 1 gram Synalar 0.025% gel | 30 gram PoM £5.56 DT = £5.56 | 60 gram PoM £10.02 DT = £10.02

908

Fluocinonide

26-Jul-2025

- **INDICATIONS AND DOSE**

Severe inflammatory skin disorders such as eczemas unresponsive to less potent corticosteroids | Psoriasis

▶ TO THE SKIN

▶ Child: Apply 1–2 times a day, to be applied thinly

POTENCY

▶ Fluocinonide is a potent corticosteroid.

- **UNLICENSED USE** Not licensed for use in children under 1 year.
- **PATIENT AND CARER ADVICE** Patients or carers should be advised on the application of fluocinonide preparations.

- **MEDICINAL FORMS** There can be variation in the licensing of different medicines containing the same drug.

Cutaneous ointment

CAUTIONARY AND ADVISORY LABELS 28

EXCIPIENTS: May contain Propylene glycol, woolfat and related substances (including lanolin)

▶ Metosyn (Reig Jofre UK Ltd)

Fluocinonide 500 microgram per 1 gram Metosyn 0.05% ointment | 100 gram PoM £13.15 DT = £13.15

Cutaneous cream

CAUTIONARY AND ADVISORY LABELS 28

EXCIPIENTS: May contain Propylene glycol

▶ Metosyn FAPG (Reig Jofre UK Ltd)

Fluocinonide 500 microgram per 1 gram Metosyn FAPG 0.05% cream | 25 gram PoM £3.96 DT = £3.96 | 100 gram PoM £13.34 DT = £13.34

908

Fluticasone

26-Jul-2025

- **INDICATIONS AND DOSE**

Severe inflammatory skin disorders such as dermatitis and eczemas unresponsive to less potent corticosteroids | Psoriasis

▶ TO THE SKIN

▶ Child 1–2 months: Apply 1–2 times a day, to be applied thinly

▶ Child 3 months–17 years: Apply 1–2 times a day, to be applied thinly

POTENCY

▶ Fluticasone is a potent corticosteroid.

- **UNLICENSED USE** Not licensed for use in children under 3 months.
- **INTERACTIONS** → Appendix 1: corticosteroids
- **PATIENT AND CARER ADVICE** Patients or carers should be given advice on application of fluticasone creams and ointments.

- **MEDICINAL FORMS** There can be variation in the licensing of different medicines containing the same drug.

Cutaneous ointment

CAUTIONARY AND ADVISORY LABELS 28

EXCIPIENTS: May contain Propylene glycol

▶ Cutivate (GlaxoSmithKline UK Ltd)

Fluticasone propionate 50 microgram per 1 gram Cutivate 0.005% ointment | 30 gram PoM £4.24 DT = £4.24

Cutaneous cream

CAUTIONARY AND ADVISORY LABELS 28

EXCIPIENTS: May contain Cetostearyl alcohol (including cetyl and stearyl alcohol), imidurea, propylene glycol

▶ Fluticasone (Non-proprietary)

Fluticasone propionate 500 microgram per 1 gram Fluticasone 0.05% cream | 30 gram PoM £6.78 DT = £4.24

908

Hydrocortisone

26-Jul-2025

- **DRUG ACTION** Hydrocortisone has equal glucocorticoid and mineralocorticoid activity.

- **INDICATIONS AND DOSE**

Mild inflammatory skin disorders such as eczemas

▶ TO THE SKIN

▶ Child: Apply 1–2 times a day, to be applied thinly

Nappy rash

▶ TO THE SKIN

▶ Child: Apply 1–2 times a day for no longer than 1 week, to be discontinued as soon as the inflammation subsides

POTENCY

▶ Hydrocortisone is a mild corticosteroid.

- **INTERACTIONS** → Appendix 1: corticosteroids
- **PRESCRIBING AND DISPENSING INFORMATION** When hydrocortisone cream or ointment is prescribed and no strength is stated, the 1% strength should be supplied.
- **PATIENT AND CARER ADVICE** Patient counselling is advised for hydrocortisone cream and ointment (application).

- **PROFESSION SPECIFIC INFORMATION**
Dental practitioners' formulary Hydrocortisone Cream 1% 15 g may be prescribed.
- **EXCEPTIONS TO LEGAL CATEGORY** Skin creams and ointments containing hydrocortisone (alone or with other ingredients) can be sold to the public for the treatment of allergic contact dermatitis, irritant dermatitis, insect bite reactions and mild to moderate eczema in patients over 10 years, to be applied sparingly over the affected area 1–2 times daily for max. 1 week. Over-the-counter hydrocortisone preparations should not be sold without medical advice for children under 10 years or for pregnant women; they should **not** be sold for application to the face, anogenital region, broken or infected skin (including cold sores, acne, and athlete's foot).

- **MEDICINAL FORMS** There can be variation in the licensing of different medicines containing the same drug.

Cutaneous ointment
CAUTIONARY AND ADVISORY LABELS 28
- **Hydrocortisone (Non-proprietary)**
Hydrocortisone 5 mg per 1 gram Hydrocortisone 0.5% ointment | 15 gram [PoM] £55.02 DT = £102.89 | 30 gram [PoM] £101.41
Hydrocortisone 10 mg per 1 gram Hydrocortisone 1% ointment | 15 gram [PoM] £1.71 DT = £1.35 | 30 gram [PoM] £5.25 DT = £3.50 | 50 gram [PoM] £7.36 DT = £6.69
Hydrocortisone 25 mg per 1 gram Hydrocortisone 2.5% ointment | 15 gram [PoM] £52.27 DT = £52.27 | 30 gram [PoM] £95.04–£104.54

Cutaneous cream
CAUTIONARY AND ADVISORY LABELS 28
EXCIPIENTS: May contain Benzyl alcohol, cetostearyl alcohol (including cetyl and stearyl alcohol), hydroxybenzoates (parabens), propylene glycol
- **Hydrocortisone (Non-proprietary)**
Hydrocortisone 5 mg per 1 gram Hydrocortisone 0.5% cream | 30 gram [PoM] £88.00
Hydrocortisone 10 mg per 1 gram Hydrocortisone 1% cream | 15 gram [PoM] £2.50 DT = £1.75 | 30 gram [PoM] £4.44 DT = £3.28 | 50 gram [PoM] £6.96 DT = £5.00
Hydrocortisone 25 mg per 1 gram Hydrocortisone 2.5% cream | 15 gram [PoM] £56.29 DT = £100.17 | 30 gram [PoM] £95.04–£196.80
- **Hc45** (Karo Healthcare UK Ltd)
Hydrocortisone acetate 10 mg per 1 gram Hc45 Hydrocortisone 1% cream | 15 gram [P] £4.36 DT = £4.36

Combinations available: ***Hydrocortisone with benzalkonium chloride, dimeticone and nystatin***, p. 916 · ***Hydrocortisone with chlorhexidine hydrochloride and nystatin***, p. 916 · ***Hydrocortisone with clotrimazole***, p. 916 · ***Hydrocortisone with fusidic acid***, p. 916 · ***Hydrocortisone with miconazole***, p. 917 · ***Hydrocortisone with oxytetracycline***, p. 917

F 908

Hydrocortisone butyrate

26-Jul-2025

- **INDICATIONS AND DOSE**

Severe inflammatory skin disorders such as eczemas unresponsive to less potent corticosteroids | Psoriasis
- TO THE SKIN
  - Child 1–17 years: Apply 1–2 times a day, to be applied thinly

POTENCY
- Hydrocortisone butyrate is a moderate corticosteroid.

- **PATIENT AND CARER ADVICE** Patients or carers should be given advice on how to administer hydrocortisone butyrate lotion, cream, ointment and scalp lotion.
Medicines for Children leaflet: Hydrocortisone (topical) for eczema www.medicinesforchildren.org.uk/medicines/hydrocortisone-topical-for-eczema/

- **MEDICINAL FORMS** There can be variation in the licensing of different medicines containing the same drug.

Cutaneous solution
CAUTIONARY AND ADVISORY LABELS 15, 28
EXCIPIENTS: May contain Butylated hydroxytoluene, cetostearyl alcohol (including cetyl and stearyl alcohol), hydroxybenzoates (parabens), propylene glycol
- **Locoid** (Neon Healthcare Ltd)
Hydrocortisone butyrate 1 mg per 1 ml Locoid 0.1% scalp lotion | 100 ml [PoM] £6.83 DT = £6.83

Cutaneous cream
CAUTIONARY AND ADVISORY LABELS 28
EXCIPIENTS: May contain Benzyl alcohol, cetostearyl alcohol (including cetyl and stearyl alcohol), hydroxybenzoates (parabens)
- **Locoid** (Neon Healthcare Ltd)
Hydrocortisone butyrate 1 mg per 1 gram Locoid 0.1% cream | 100 gram [PoM] £4.93 DT = £4.93
- **Locoid Lipocream** (Neon Healthcare Ltd)
Hydrocortisone butyrate 1 mg per 1 gram Locoid 0.1% Lipocream | 100 gram [PoM] £5.17 DT = £4.93

Cutaneous emulsion
CAUTIONARY AND ADVISORY LABELS 15, 28
EXCIPIENTS: May contain Butylated hydroxytoluene, cetostearyl alcohol (including cetyl and stearyl alcohol), hydroxybenzoates (parabens), propylene glycol
- **Locoid Crelo** (Neon Healthcare Ltd)
Hydrocortisone butyrate 1 mg per 1 gram Locoid Crelo 0.1% topical emulsion | 100 gram [PoM] £5.91 DT = £5.91

F 908

Mometasone furoate

26-Jul-2025

- **INDICATIONS AND DOSE**

Severe inflammatory skin disorders such as eczemas unresponsive to less potent corticosteroids | Psoriasis
- TO THE SKIN
  - Child 1 month–1 year: Apply once daily, to be applied thinly (to scalp in case of lotion)
  - Child 2–17 years: Apply once daily, to be applied thinly (to scalp in case of lotion)

POTENCY
- Mometasone furoate is a potent corticosteroid.

- **UNLICENSED USE** Not licensed for use in children under 2 years.
- **INTERACTIONS** → Appendix 1: corticosteroids
- **MEDICINAL FORMS** There can be variation in the licensing of different medicines containing the same drug.

Cutaneous ointment
CAUTIONARY AND ADVISORY LABELS 28
EXCIPIENTS: May contain Beeswax, propylene glycol
- **Mometasone furoate (Non-proprietary)**
Mometasone furoate 1 mg per 1 gram Mometasone 0.1% ointment | 15 gram [PoM] £4.32 | 30 gram [PoM] £7.70 DT = £4.32 | 50 gram [PoM] £12.44 | 100 gram [PoM] £21.50 DT = £12.44
- **Elocon** (Organon Pharma (UK) Ltd)
Mometasone furoate 1 mg per 1 gram Elocon 0.1% ointment | 30 gram [PoM] £4.32 DT = £4.32 | 100 gram [PoM] £12.44 DT = £12.44

Cutaneous cream
CAUTIONARY AND ADVISORY LABELS 28
EXCIPIENTS: May contain Beeswax
- **Mometasone furoate (Non-proprietary)**
Mometasone furoate 1 mg per 1 gram Mometasone 0.1% cream | 30 gram [PoM] £8.00 DT = £3.18 | 100 gram [PoM] £24.00 DT = £10.60
- **Elocon** (Organon Pharma (UK) Ltd)
Mometasone furoate 1 mg per 1 gram Elocon 0.1% cream | 30 gram [PoM] £4.80 DT = £3.18 | 100 gram [PoM] £15.10 DT = £10.60
- **Ovixan** (Biofrontera UK Ltd)
Mometasone furoate 1 mg per 1 gram Ovixan 1mg/g cream | 30 gram [PoM] £4.40 DT = £3.18 | 100 gram [PoM] £14.10 DT = £10.60

Cutaneous liquid
CAUTIONARY AND ADVISORY LABELS 28
EXCIPIENTS: May contain Propylene glycol
- **Elocon** (Organon Pharma (UK) Ltd)
Mometasone furoate 1 mg per 1 gram Elocon 0.1% scalp lotion | 30 ml [PoM] £4.36 DT = £4.36

CORTICOSTEROIDS > CORTICOSTEROID COMBINATIONS WITH ANTI-INFECTIVES

Betamethasone with clioquinol

08-Oct-2024

The properties listed below are those particular to the combination only. For the properties of the components please consider, betamethasone p. 909.

● **INDICATIONS AND DOSE**

Severe inflammatory skin disorders such as eczemas associated with infection and unresponsive to less potent corticosteroids | Psoriasis (excluding widespread plaque psoriasis)

▶ TO THE SKIN
- Child 1–17 years: (consult product literature)

POTENCY
- Betamethasone is a potent corticosteroid.

● **INTERACTIONS** → Appendix 1: corticosteroids

● **PATIENT AND CARER ADVICE** Stains clothing. Patients or carers should be counselled on application of betamethasone with clioquinol preparations.

● **MEDICINAL FORMS** There can be variation in the licensing of different medicines containing the same drug.

Cutaneous ointment

CAUTIONARY AND ADVISORY LABELS 28

▶ **Betamethasone with clioquinol (Non-proprietary)**
Betamethasone (as Betamethasone valerate) 1 mg per 1 gram, Clioquinol 30 mg per 1 gram Betamethasone valerate 0.1% / Clioquinol 3% ointment | 30 gram PoM £49.21–£83.87

Cutaneous cream

CAUTIONARY AND ADVISORY LABELS 28

EXCIPIENTS: May contain Cetostearyl alcohol (including cetyl and stearyl alcohol), chlorocresol

▶ **Betamethasone with clioquinol (Non-proprietary)**
Betamethasone (as Betamethasone valerate) 1 mg per 1 gram, Clioquinol 30 mg per 1 gram Betamethasone valerate 0.1% / Clioquinol 3% cream | 30 gram PoM £54.08 DT = £94.44

Betamethasone with clotrimazole

08-Oct-2024

The properties listed below are those particular to the combination only. For the properties of the components please consider, betamethasone p. 909, clotrimazole p. 900.

● **INDICATIONS AND DOSE**

Short-term treatment of tinea infections and candidiasis

▶ TO THE SKIN
- Child 12–17 years: Apply twice daily for 2 weeks for tinea cruris, tinea corporis or candidiasis, or for 4 weeks for tinea pedis

POTENCY
- Betamethasone is a potent corticosteroid.

● **INTERACTIONS** → Appendix 1: antifungals, azoles · corticosteroids

● **PATIENT AND CARER ADVICE** Patients or carers should be given advice on how to administer betamethasone with clotrimazole cream.

● **MEDICINAL FORMS** There can be variation in the licensing of different medicines containing the same drug.

Cutaneous cream

CAUTIONARY AND ADVISORY LABELS 28

EXCIPIENTS: May contain Benzyl alcohol, cetostearyl alcohol (including cetyl and stearyl alcohol), propylene glycol

▶ **Lotriderm** (Organon Pharma (UK) Ltd)
Betamethasone dipropionate 640 microgram per 1 gram, Clotrimazole 10 mg per 1 gram Lotriderm cream | 30 gram PoM £6.34 DT = £6.34

Betamethasone with fusidic acid

08-Oct-2024

The properties listed below are those particular to the combination only. For the properties of the components please consider, betamethasone p. 909, fusidic acid p. 441.

● **INDICATIONS AND DOSE**

Severe inflammatory skin disorders such as eczemas associated with infection and unresponsive to less potent corticosteroids

▶ TO THE SKIN
- Child: (consult product literature)

POTENCY
- Betamethasone is a potent corticosteroid.

● **UNLICENSED USE** *Fucibet® Lipid Cream* is not licensed for use in children under 6 years.

● **INTERACTIONS** → Appendix 1: corticosteroids · fusidate

● **PATIENT AND CARER ADVICE** Patients or carers should be counselled on application of betamethasone with fusidic acid preparations.

● **MEDICINAL FORMS** There can be variation in the licensing of different medicines containing the same drug.

Cutaneous cream

CAUTIONARY AND ADVISORY LABELS 28

EXCIPIENTS: May contain Cetostearyl alcohol (including cetyl and stearyl alcohol), chlorocresol, hydroxybenzoates (parabens)

▶ **Betamethasone with fusidic acid (Non-proprietary)**
Betamethasone (as Betamethasone valerate) 1 mg per 1 gram, Fusidic acid 20 mg per 1 gram Betamethasone valerate 0.1% / Fusidic acid 2% cream | 30 gram PoM £5.80 DT = £6.38 | 60 gram PoM £12.15 DT = £12.76

▶ **Fucibet** (LEO Pharma)
Betamethasone (as Betamethasone valerate) 1 mg per 1 gram, Fusidic acid 20 mg per 1 gram Fucibet cream | 30 gram PoM £6.38 DT = £6.38 | 60 gram PoM £12.76 DT = £12.76

▶ **Xemacort** (Viatris UK Healthcare Ltd)
Betamethasone (as Betamethasone valerate) 1 mg per 1 gram, Fusidic acid 20 mg per 1 gram Xemacort 20mg/g / 1mg/g cream | 30 gram PoM £6.05 DT = £6.38 | 60 gram PoM £12.45 DT = £12.76

Betamethasone with neomycin

20-Jun-2025

The properties listed below are those particular to the combination only. For the properties of the components please consider, betamethasone p. 909, neomycin sulfate p. 898.

● **INDICATIONS AND DOSE**

Severe inflammatory skin disorders such as eczemas unresponsive to less potent corticosteroids | Psoriasis

▶ TO THE SKIN USING OINTMENT, OR TO THE SKIN USING CREAM
- Child 1–23 months: Apply 1–2 times a day, to be applied thinly
- Child 2–17 years: Apply 1–2 times a day, to be applied thinly

POTENCY
- Betamethasone is a potent corticosteroid.

● **UNLICENSED USE** Betamethasone and neomycin preparations not licensed for use in children under 2 years.

● **INTERACTIONS** → Appendix 1: corticosteroids · neomycin

● **PATIENT AND CARER ADVICE** Patient counselling is advised for betamethasone with neomycin cream and ointment (application).

● **MEDICINAL FORMS** There can be variation in the licensing of different medicines containing the same drug.

Cutaneous ointment

CAUTIONARY AND ADVISORY LABELS 28

▸ **Betamethasone with neomycin (Non-proprietary)**
Betamethasone (as Betamethasone valerate) 1 mg per 1 gram, Neomycin sulfate 5 mg per 1 gram Betamethasone valerate 0.1% / Neomycin 0.5% ointment | 30 gram PoM £42.86 DT = £42.86 | 100 gram PoM £133.22 DT = £133.22

Cutaneous cream

CAUTIONARY AND ADVISORY LABELS 28

EXCIPIENTS: May contain Cetostearyl alcohol (including cetyl and stearyl alcohol), chlorocresol

▸ **Betamethasone with neomycin (Non-proprietary)**
Betamethasone (as Betamethasone valerate) 1 mg per 1 gram, Neomycin sulfate 5 mg per 1 gram Betamethasone valerate 0.1% / Neomycin 0.5% cream | 30 gram PoM £42.86 DT = £42.86 | 100 gram PoM £133.22 DT = £133.22

Betamethasone with salicylic acid

08-Oct-2024

The properties listed below are those particular to the combination only. For the properties of the components please consider, betamethasone p. 909, salicylic acid p. 950.

● **INDICATIONS AND DOSE**

DIPROSALIC® OINTMENT

Severe inflammatory skin disorders such as eczemas unresponsive to less potent corticosteroids | Psoriasis

▸ TO THE SKIN
▸ Child: Apply 1–2 times a day, max. 60 g per week

POTENCY

▸ For *Diprosalic®* ointment: Betamethasone is a potent corticosteroid.

DIPROSALIC® SCALP APPLICATION

Severe inflammatory skin disorders such as eczemas unresponsive to less potent corticosteroids | Psoriasis

▸ TO THE SKIN
▸ Child: Apply 1–2 times a day, apply a few drops

POTENCY

▸ For *Diprosalic®* scalp application: Betamethasone is a potent corticosteroid.

● **INTERACTIONS** → Appendix 1: corticosteroids

● **PATIENT AND CARER ADVICE**

DIPROSALIC® OINTMENT Patients or carers should be counselled on application of betamethasone and salicylic acid preparations.

DIPROSALIC® SCALP APPLICATION Patients or carers should be counselled on application of betamethasone and salicylic acid scalp application.

● **MEDICINAL FORMS** There can be variation in the licensing of different medicines containing the same drug.

Cutaneous solution

CAUTIONARY AND ADVISORY LABELS 28

EXCIPIENTS: May contain Disodium edetate

▸ **Diprosalic** (Organon Pharma (UK) Ltd)
Betamethasone (as Betamethasone dipropionate) 500 microgram per 1 ml, Salicylic acid 20 mg per 1 ml Diprosalic 0.05%/2% scalp application | 100 ml PoM £10.10 DT = £10.10

Cutaneous ointment

CAUTIONARY AND ADVISORY LABELS 28

▸ **Diprosalic** (Organon Pharma (UK) Ltd)
Betamethasone (as Betamethasone dipropionate) 500 microgram per 1 gram, Salicylic acid 30 mg per 1 gram Diprosalic 0.05%/3% ointment | 30 gram PoM £3.18 DT = £3.18 | 100 gram PoM £9.14 DT = £9.14

Clobetasol propionate with neomycin sulfate and nystatin

08-Oct-2024

The properties listed below are those particular to the combination only. For the properties of the components please consider, clobetasol propionate p. 911, neomycin sulfate p. 898.

● **INDICATIONS AND DOSE**

Short-term treatment only of severe resistant inflammatory skin disorders such as recalcitrant eczemas associated with infection and unresponsive to less potent corticosteroids | Psoriasis associated with infection

▸ TO THE SKIN
▸ Child: (consult product literature)

POTENCY

▸ Clobetasol propionate is a very potent corticosteroid.

● **UNLICENSED USE** Clobetasol with neomycin and nystatin preparations not licensed for use in children under 2 years.

● **INTERACTIONS** → Appendix 1: neomycin

● **PATIENT AND CARER ADVICE** Patients or carers should be advised on application of clobetasol propionate, neomycin sulfate and nystatin containing preparations.

● **MEDICINAL FORMS** There can be variation in the licensing of different medicines containing the same drug.

Cutaneous ointment

CAUTIONARY AND ADVISORY LABELS 28

▸ **Clobetasol propionate with neomycin sulfate and nystatin (Non-proprietary)**
Clobetasol propionate 500 microgram per 1 gram, Neomycin sulfate 5 mg per 1 gram, Nystatin 100000 unit per 1 gram Clobetasol 500microgram / Neomycin 5mg / Nystatin 100,000units/g ointment | 30 gram PoM £118.61 DT = £118.61

Cutaneous cream

CAUTIONARY AND ADVISORY LABELS 28

▸ **Clobetasol propionate with neomycin sulfate and nystatin (Non-proprietary)**
Clobetasol propionate 500 microgram per 1 gram, Neomycin sulfate 5 mg per 1 gram, Nystatin 100000 unit per 1 gram Clobetasol 500microgram / Neomycin 5mg / Nystatin 100,000units/g cream | 30 gram PoM £118.61 DT = £118.61

Clobetasone butyrate with nystatin and oxytetracycline

08-Oct-2024

The properties listed below are those particular to the combination only. For the properties of the components please consider, clobetasone butyrate p. 911, oxytetracycline p. 436.

● **INDICATIONS AND DOSE**

Steroid-responsive dermatoses where candidal or bacterial infection is present

▸ TO THE SKIN
▸ Child: (consult product literature)

POTENCY

▸ Clobetasone butyrate is a moderate corticosteroid.

● **INTERACTIONS** → Appendix 1: tetracyclines

● **PATIENT AND CARER ADVICE** Stains clothing.

● **MEDICINAL FORMS** There can be variation in the licensing of different medicines containing the same drug.

Cutaneous cream

CAUTIONARY AND ADVISORY LABELS 28

EXCIPIENTS: May contain Cetostearyl alcohol (including cetyl and stearyl alcohol), chlorocresol, sodium metabisulfite

▸ **Trimovate** (Ennogen Healthcare International Ltd)
Clobetasone butyrate 500 microgram per 1 gram, Oxytetracycline (as Oxytetracycline calcium) 30 mg per 1 gram,

Nystatin 100000 unit per 1 gram Trimovate cream | 30 gram PoM £14.99 DT = £14.99

Hydrocortisone with benzalkonium chloride, dimeticone and nystatin

08-Oct-2024

The properties listed below are those particular to the combination only. For the properties of the components please consider, hydrocortisone p. 912, dimeticone p. 903.

- **INDICATIONS AND DOSE**

Mild inflammatory skin disorders such as eczemas associated with infection

▶ TO THE SKIN

▶ Child: Apply 3 times a day until lesion has healed, to be applied thinly

POTENCY

▶ Hydrocortisone is a mild corticosteroid.

- **INTERACTIONS** → Appendix 1: corticosteroids
- **PATIENT AND CARER ADVICE** Patients or carers should be advised on application of hydrocortisone with benzalkonium chloride, dimeticone and nystatin preparations.
- **MEDICINAL FORMS** There can be variation in the licensing of different medicines containing the same drug.

Cutaneous cream

CAUTIONARY AND ADVISORY LABELS 28

EXCIPIENTS: May contain Butylated hydroxyanisole, cetostearyl alcohol (including cetyl and stearyl alcohol), hydroxybenzoates (parabens), sodium metabisulfite, sorbic acid

▶ **Timodine** (Alliance Pharmaceuticals Ltd)
Benzalkonium chloride 1 mg per 1 gram, Hydrocortisone 5 mg per 1 gram, Dimeticone 350 100 mg per 1 gram, Nystatin 100000 unit per 1 gram Timodine cream | 30 gram PoM £3.37

Hydrocortisone with chlorhexidine hydrochloride and nystatin

08-Oct-2024

The properties listed below are those particular to the combination only. For the properties of the components please consider, hydrocortisone p. 912, chlorhexidine p. 944.

- **INDICATIONS AND DOSE**

Mild inflammatory skin disorders such as eczemas associated with infection

▶ TO THE SKIN

▶ Child: (consult product literature)

POTENCY

▶ Hydrocortisone is a mild corticosteroid.

- **INTERACTIONS** → Appendix 1: corticosteroids
- **PATIENT AND CARER ADVICE** Patients or carers should be given advice on application of hydrocortisone with chlorhexidine hydrochloride and nystatin preparations.
- **MEDICINAL FORMS** There can be variation in the licensing of different medicines containing the same drug.

Cutaneous ointment

CAUTIONARY AND ADVISORY LABELS 28

▶ **Nystaform HC** (Typharm Ltd)
Chlorhexidine acetate 10 mg per 1 gram, Hydrocortisone 10 mg per 1 gram, Nystatin 100000 unit per 1 gram Nystaform HC ointment | 30 gram PoM £9.66 DT = £9.66

Cutaneous cream

CAUTIONARY AND ADVISORY LABELS 28

EXCIPIENTS: May contain Benzyl alcohol, cetostearyl alcohol (including cetyl and stearyl alcohol), polysorbates

▶ **Nystaform HC** (Typharm Ltd)
Hydrocortisone 5 mg per 1 gram, Chlorhexidine hydrochloride 10 mg per 1 gram, Nystatin 100000 unit per 1 gram Nystaform HC cream | 30 gram PoM £9.66 DT = £9.66

Hydrocortisone with clotrimazole

08-Oct-2024

The properties listed below are those particular to the combination only. For the properties of the components please consider, hydrocortisone p. 912, clotrimazole p. 900.

- **INDICATIONS AND DOSE**

Mild inflammatory skin disorders such as eczemas (associated with fungal infection)

▶ TO THE SKIN

▶ Child: (consult product literature)

POTENCY

▶ Hydrocortisone is a mild corticosteroid.

- **INTERACTIONS** → Appendix 1: antifungals, azoles · corticosteroids
- **PATIENT AND CARER ADVICE** Patients or carers should be given advice on how to administer hydrocortisone with clotrimazole cream.
- **EXCEPTIONS TO LEGAL CATEGORY** A 15-g tube is on sale to the public for the treatment of athlete's foot and fungal infection of skin folds with associated inflammation in patients 10 years and over.
- **MEDICINAL FORMS** There can be variation in the licensing of different medicines containing the same drug.

Cutaneous cream

CAUTIONARY AND ADVISORY LABELS 28

EXCIPIENTS: May contain Benzyl alcohol, cetostearyl alcohol (including cetyl and stearyl alcohol)

▶ **Canesten HC** (Bayer Plc)
Clotrimazole 10 mg per 1 gram, Hydrocortisone (as Hydrocortisone acetate) 10 mg per 1 gram Canesten HC cream | 30 gram PoM £2.42 DT = £2.42

Hydrocortisone with fusidic acid

08-Oct-2024

The properties listed below are those particular to the combination only. For the properties of the components please consider, hydrocortisone p. 912, fusidic acid p. 441.

- **INDICATIONS AND DOSE**

Mild inflammatory skin disorders such as eczemas associated with infection

▶ TO THE SKIN

▶ Child: (consult product literature)

POTENCY

▶ Hydrocortisone is a mild corticosteroid.

- **INTERACTIONS** → Appendix 1: corticosteroids · fusidate
- **PATIENT AND CARER ADVICE** Patients or carers should be advised on application of hydrocortisone with fusidic acid preparations.
- **MEDICINAL FORMS** There can be variation in the licensing of different medicines containing the same drug.

Cutaneous cream

CAUTIONARY AND ADVISORY LABELS 28

EXCIPIENTS: May contain Butylated hydroxyanisole, cetostearyl alcohol (including cetyl and stearyl alcohol), polysorbates, potassium sorbate

▶ **Fucidin H (Fusidic acid / Hydrocortisone)** (LEO Pharma)
Hydrocortisone acetate 10 mg per 1 gram, Fusidic acid 20 mg per 1 gram Fucidin H cream | 30 gram PoM £6.02 DT = £6.02 | 60 gram PoM £12.05 DT = £12.05

Hydrocortisone with miconazole

08-Oct-2024

The properties listed below are those particular to the combination only. For the properties of the components please consider, hydrocortisone p. 912, miconazole p. 901.

- **INDICATIONS AND DOSE**

Mild inflammatory skin disorders such as eczemas associated with infections

▶ TO THE SKIN

▸ Child: (consult product literature)

POTENCY

▸ Hydrocortisone is a mild corticosteroid.

- **INTERACTIONS** → Appendix 1: antifungals, azoles · corticosteroids
- **PATIENT AND CARER ADVICE** Patients or carers should be advised on application of hydrocortisone with miconazole preparations.
- **PROFESSION SPECIFIC INFORMATION**

Dental practitioners' formulary May be prescribed as Miconazole and Hydrocortisone Cream or Ointment for max. 7 days.

- **EXCEPTIONS TO LEGAL CATEGORY** A 15-g tube of hydrocortisone with miconazole cream is on sale to the public for the treatment of athlete's foot and candidal intertrigo in children over 10 years.
- **MEDICINAL FORMS** There can be variation in the licensing of different medicines containing the same drug.

Cutaneous cream

CAUTIONARY AND ADVISORY LABELS 28

EXCIPIENTS: May contain Butylated hydroxyanisole, disodium edetate

▸ **Daktacort** (McNeil Products Ltd)

Hydrocortisone 10 mg per 1 gram, Miconazole nitrate 20 mg per 1 gram Daktacort Hydrocortisone cream | 15 gram [P] £5.30 DT = £5.30

Hydrocortisone with oxytetracycline

08-Oct-2024

The properties listed below are those particular to the combination only. For the properties of the components please consider, hydrocortisone p. 912, oxytetracycline p. 436.

- **INDICATIONS AND DOSE**

Mild inflammatory skin disorders such as eczemas

▶ TO THE SKIN

▸ Child 12–17 years: (consult product literature)

POTENCY

▸ Hydrocortisone is a mild corticosteroid.

- **CONTRA-INDICATIONS** Children under 12 years
- **INTERACTIONS** → Appendix 1: corticosteroids · tetracyclines
- **PREGNANCY** Tetracyclines should not be given to pregnant women. Effects on skeletal development have been documented when tetracyclines have been used in the first trimester in animal studies. Administration during the second or third trimester may cause discoloration of the child's teeth.
- **BREAST FEEDING** Tetracyclines should not be given to women who are breast-feeding (although absorption and therefore discoloration of teeth in the infant is probably usually prevented by chelation with calcium in milk).
- **PATIENT AND CARER ADVICE** Patients should be given advice on the application of hydrocortisone with oxytetracycline ointment.
- **MEDICINAL FORMS** There can be variation in the licensing of different medicines containing the same drug.

Cutaneous ointment

CAUTIONARY AND ADVISORY LABELS 28

▸ **Terra-Cortril** (Esteve Pharmaceuticals Ltd)

Hydrocortisone 10 mg per 1 gram, Oxytetracycline (as Oxytetracycline hydrochloride) 30 mg per 1 gram Terra-Cortril ointment | 30 gram [PoM] £5.01 DT = £5.01

DERMATOLOGICAL DRUGS › ANTI-INFECTIVES

Ichthammol

- **INDICATIONS AND DOSE**

Chronic lichenified eczema

▶ TO THE SKIN

▸ Child 1–17 years: Apply 1–3 times a day

- **UNLICENSED USE** No information available.
- **SIDE-EFFECTS** Skin irritation
- **MEDICINAL FORMS** Forms available from special-order manufacturers include: cutaneous ointment, cutaneous paste

Ichthammol with zinc oxide

The properties listed below are those particular to the combination only. For the properties of the components please consider, ichthammol above.

- **INDICATIONS AND DOSE**

Chronic lichenified eczema

▶ TO THE SKIN

▸ Child: (consult product literature)

- **MEDICINAL FORMS** There can be variation in the licensing of different medicines containing the same drug. Forms available from special-order manufacturers include: cutaneous cream, cutaneous ointment

Impregnated dressing

▸ **Ichthopaste** (Evolan Pharma AB)

Ichthopaste bandage 7.5cm × 6m | 1 bandage £4.07

DERMATOLOGICAL DRUGS › ANTRACEN DERIVATIVES

Dithranol

23-Nov-2020

(Anthralin)

- **INDICATIONS AND DOSE**

Subacute and chronic psoriasis

▶ TO THE SKIN

▸ Child: (consult product literature)

- **CONTRA-INDICATIONS** Acute and pustular psoriasis · hypersensitivity
- **CAUTIONS** Avoid sensitive areas of skin · avoid use near eyes
- **SIDE-EFFECTS** Skin reactions
- **PREGNANCY** No adverse effects reported.
- **BREAST FEEDING** No adverse effects reported.
- **DIRECTIONS FOR ADMINISTRATION** When applying dithranol, manufacturer advises hands should be protected by gloves or they should be washed thoroughly afterwards. Dithranol should be applied to chronic extensor plaques only, carefully avoiding normal skin.
- **PRESCRIBING AND DISPENSING INFORMATION** Treatment should be started with a low concentration such as dithranol 0.1%, and the strength increased gradually every few days up to 3%, according to tolerance.

- **PATIENT AND CARER ADVICE** Dithranol can stain the skin, hair and fabrics.
- **EXCEPTIONS TO LEGAL CATEGORY** Prescription only medicine if dithranol content more than 1%, otherwise may be sold to the public.

- **MEDICINAL FORMS** There can be variation in the licensing of different medicines containing the same drug. Forms available from special-order manufacturers include: cutaneous ointment

Cutaneous ointment

CAUTIONARY AND ADVISORY LABELS 28

Combinations available: *Coal tar with dithranol and salicylic acid*, below

Dithranol with salicylic acid and zinc oxide

The properties listed below are those particular to the combination only. For the properties of the components please consider, dithranol p. 917, salicylic acid p. 950.

- **INDICATIONS AND DOSE**

Subacute and chronic psoriasis

▶ TO THE SKIN
▶ Child: (consult local protocol)

- **MEDICINAL FORMS** There can be variation in the licensing of different medicines containing the same drug. Forms available from special-order manufacturers include: cutaneous ointment, paste

Paste

CAUTIONARY AND ADVISORY LABELS 28

DERMATOLOGICAL DRUGS › TARS

Coal tar 01-Sep-2020

- **INDICATIONS AND DOSE**

Psoriasis | Scaly scalp disorders such as psoriasis, eczema, seborrhoeic dermatitis and dandruff

▶ TO THE SKIN
▶ Child: (consult product literature)

- **CONTRA-INDICATIONS** Avoid broken or inflamed skin · avoid eye area · avoid genital area · avoid mucosal areas · avoid rectal area · infection · sore, acute, or pustular psoriasis
- **CAUTIONS**

GENERAL CAUTIONS Application to face

SPECIFIC CAUTIONS

▸ When used for Scaly scalp disorders, using shampoo Children under 12 years (consult product literature)

- **SIDE-EFFECTS** Photosensitivity reaction · skin reactions
- **PRESCRIBING AND DISPENSING INFORMATION** Coal Tar Solution BP contains coal tar 20%, Strong Coal Tar Solution BP contains coal tar 40%.
- **HANDLING AND STORAGE** Use suitable chemical protection gloves for extemporaneous preparation. May stain skin, hair and fabric.
- **PATIENT AND CARER ADVICE** May stain skin, hair and fabric.

- **MEDICINAL FORMS** There can be variation in the licensing of different medicines containing the same drug. Forms available from special-order manufacturers include: cutaneous cream, cutaneous ointment, paste

Cutaneous emulsion

EXCIPIENTS: May contain Hydroxybenzoates (parabens)

▸ **Exorex** (Teva UK Ltd)
Coal tar solution 50 mg per 1 gram Exorex lotion | 100 ml GSL £10.14 DT = £10.14 | 250 ml GSL £20.30 DT = £20.30

Shampoo

EXCIPIENTS: May contain Fragrances, hydroxybenzoates (parabens)

▸ **Polytar Scalp** (Universal Medicines Ltd)
Coal tar solution 40 mg per 1 ml Polytar Scalp shampoo | 150 ml GSL £7.57 DT = £7.57

▸ **Psoriderm** (Dermal Laboratories Ltd)
Coal tar distilled 25 mg per 1 ml Psoriderm scalp lotion | 250 ml P £5.18 DT = £5.18

Cutaneous cream

EXCIPIENTS: May contain Isopropyl palmitate, lecithin, propylene glycol

▸ **Psoriderm** (Dermal Laboratories Ltd)
Coal tar distilled 60 mg per 1 gram Psoriderm cream | 225 ml P £11.10 DT = £11.10

Coal tar with coconut oil and salicylic acid 19-Mar-2020

The properties listed below are those particular to the combination only. For the properties of the components please consider, coal tar above, salicylic acid p. 950.

- **INDICATIONS AND DOSE**

Scaly scalp disorders | Psoriasis | Seborrhoeic dermatitis | Dandruff | Cradle cap

▶ TO THE SKIN USING SHAMPOO
▶ Child: Apply daily as required

- **MEDICINAL FORMS** There can be variation in the licensing of different medicines containing the same drug.

Shampoo

▸ **Capasal** (Dermal Laboratories Ltd)
Salicylic acid 5 mg per 1 gram, Coal tar distilled 10 mg per 1 gram, Coconut oil 10 mg per 1 gram Capasal Therapeutic shampoo | 250 ml P £5.55

Coal tar with dithranol and salicylic acid

The properties listed below are those particular to the combination only. For the properties of the components please consider, coal tar above, dithranol p. 917, salicylic acid p. 950.

- **INDICATIONS AND DOSE**

Subacute and chronic psoriasis

▶ TO THE SKIN
▶ Child: Apply up to twice daily

- **UNLICENSED USE** *Psorin®* is licensed for use in children (age range not specified by manufacturer).

- **MEDICINAL FORMS** Forms available from special-order manufacturers include: cutaneous ointment

Coal tar with salicylic acid and precipitated sulfur 20-Mar-2020

The properties listed below are those particular to the combination only. For the properties of the components please consider, coal tar above, salicylic acid p. 950.

- **INDICATIONS AND DOSE**

COCOIS® OINTMENT

Scaly scalp disorders including psoriasis, eczema, seborrhoeic dermatitis and dandruff

▶ TO THE SKIN USING SCALP OINTMENT
▶ Child 6–11 years: Medical supervision required
▶ Child 12–17 years: Apply once weekly as required, alternatively apply daily for the first 3–7 days (if severe), shampoo off after 1 hour

SEBCO® OINTMENT

Scaly scalp disorders including psoriasis, eczema, seborrhoeic dermatitis and dandruff

▶ TO THE SKIN USING SCALP OINTMENT
- Child 6–11 years: Medical supervision required
- Child 12–17 years: Apply as required, alternatively apply daily for the first 3–7 days (if severe), shampoo off after 1 hour

● **MEDICINAL FORMS** There can be variation in the licensing of different medicines containing the same drug.

Cutaneous ointment

EXCIPIENTS: May contain Cetostearyl alcohol (including cetyl and stearyl alcohol)

- **Cocois** (RPH Pharmaceuticals AB)
  Salicylic acid 20 mg per 1 gram, Sulfur precipitated 40 mg per 1 gram, Coal tar solution 120 mg per 1 gram Cocois ointment | 40 gram GSL £9.35 | 100 gram GSL £14.50
- **Sebco** (Derma UK Ltd)
  Salicylic acid 20 mg per 1 gram, Sulfur precipitated 40 mg per 1 gram, Coal tar solution 120 mg per 1 gram Sebco ointment | 40 gram GSL £11.53 | 100 gram GSL £16.99

Coal tar with zinc oxide

16-Jan-2019

The properties listed below are those particular to the combination only. For the properties of the components please consider, coal tar p. 918.

● **INDICATIONS AND DOSE**

Psoriasis | Chronic atopic eczema

▶ TO THE SKIN
- Child: Apply 1–2 times a day

IMPORTANT SAFETY INFORMATION

MHRA/CHM ADVICE (UPDATED DECEMBER 2018): EMOLLIENTS: NEW INFORMATION ABOUT RISK OF SEVERE AND FATAL BURNS WITH PARAFFIN-CONTAINING AND PARAFFIN-FREE EMOLLIENTS

See Emollient and barrier preparations p. 888.

● **PRESCRIBING AND DISPENSING INFORMATION** No preparations available—when prepared extemporaneously, the BP states Zinc and Coal Tar Paste, BP consists of zinc oxide 6%, coal tar 6%, emulsifying wax 5%, starch 38%, yellow soft paraffin 45%.

● **MEDICINAL FORMS** There can be variation in the licensing of different medicines containing the same drug. Forms available from special-order manufacturers include: cutaneous ointment, cutaneous paste

Cutaneous ointment

CAUTIONARY AND ADVISORY LABELS 15

Cutaneous paste

CAUTIONARY AND ADVISORY LABELS 15

IMMUNOSUPPRESSANTS > CALCINEURIN INHIBITORS AND RELATED DRUGS

Pimecrolimus

16-May-2025

● **INDICATIONS AND DOSE**

Short-term treatment of mild to moderate atopic eczema (including flares) when topical corticosteroids cannot be used (initiated by a specialist)

▶ TO THE SKIN
- Child 3 months–17 years: Apply twice daily until symptoms resolve (stop treatment if eczema worsens or no response after 6 weeks)

● **CONTRA-INDICATIONS** Application to malignant or potentially malignant skin lesions · application under occlusion · congenital epidermal barrier defects · contact with eyes · contact with mucous membranes · generalised erythroderma · immunodeficiency · infection at treatment site

● **CAUTIONS** Alcohol consumption (risk of facial flushing and skin irritation) · avoid other topical treatments except emollients at treatment site · UV light (avoid excessive exposure to sunlight and sunlamps)

● **INTERACTIONS** → Appendix 1: pimecrolimus

● **SIDE-EFFECTS**

- ▶ **Common or very common** Increased risk of infection
- ▶ **Uncommon** Neoplasms
- ▶ **Rare or very rare** Skin discolouration
- ▶ **Frequency not known** Lymphadenopathy · malignancy

● **PREGNANCY** Specialist sources indicate low risk based on *animal* studies; systemic absorption after topical application is also minimal.

● **BREAST FEEDING** EvGr Use with caution (no information available); avoid application to the breast. (M)

● **NATIONAL FUNDING/ACCESS DECISIONS**

For full details see funding body website

NICE decisions

- ▶ **Tacrolimus and pimecrolimus for atopic eczema [for patients with mild atopic eczema or as first-line treatment for atopic eczema of any severity] (August 2004)** NICE TA82 Not recommended
- ▶ **Tacrolimus and pimecrolimus for atopic eczema [as second-line treatment for children aged 2 to 16 years with moderate atopic eczema] (August 2004)** NICE TA82 Recommended

● **MEDICINAL FORMS** There can be variation in the licensing of different medicines containing the same drug.

Cutaneous cream

CAUTIONARY AND ADVISORY LABELS 4, 11, 15, 28

EXCIPIENTS: May contain Benzyl alcohol, cetostearyl alcohol (including cetyl and stearyl alcohol), propylene glycol

- **Elidel** (Viatris UK Healthcare Ltd)
  Pimecrolimus 10 mg per 1 gram Elidel 1% cream | 30 gram PoM £19.69 DT = £19.69 | 60 gram PoM £37.41 DT = £37.41 | 100 gram PoM £59.07 DT = £59.07

Tacrolimus

27-Sep-2024

● **DRUG ACTION** Tacrolimus is a calcineurin inhibitor.

● **INDICATIONS AND DOSE**

Short-term treatment of moderate to severe atopic eczema (including flares) in patients unresponsive to, or intolerant of conventional therapy (initiated by a specialist)

▶ TO THE SKIN
- Child 2–15 years: Apply twice daily for up to 3 weeks (consider other treatment if eczema worsens or if no improvement after 2 weeks), to be applied thinly, 0.03% ointment to be used, then reduced to once daily until lesion clears, to be applied thinly, 0.03% ointment to be used
- Child 16–17 years: Apply twice daily until lesion clears (consider other treatment if eczema worsens or no improvement after 2 weeks), to be applied thinly, initially 0.1% ointment to be used; reduce frequency to once daily or strength of ointment to 0.03% if condition allows

Prevention of flares in patients with moderate to severe atopic eczema and 4 or more flares a year who have responded to initial treatment with topical tacrolimus (initiated by a specialist)

▶ TO THE SKIN
- Child 2–15 years: Apply twice weekly, to be applied thinly with an interval of 2–3 days between applications, 0.03% ointment to be used, use

continued →

13 Skin

short-term treatment regimen during an acute flare; review need for preventative therapy after 1 year
- Child 16-17 years: Apply twice weekly, to be applied thinly with an interval of 2–3 days between applications, 0.1% ointment to be used, use short-term treatment regimen during an acute flare; review need for preventative therapy after 1 year

- **CONTRA-INDICATIONS** Application to malignant or potentially malignant skin lesions · application under occlusion · avoid contact with eyes · avoid contact with mucous membranes · congenital epidermal barrier defects · generalised erythroderma · immunodeficiency · infection at treatment site
- **CAUTIONS** UV light (avoid excessive exposure to sunlight and sunlamps)
- **INTERACTIONS** → Appendix 1: tacrolimus
- **SIDE-EFFECTS**
  - **Common or very common** Alcohol intolerance · increased risk of infection · sensation abnormal · skin reactions
  - **Uncommon** Lymphadenopathy
  - **Frequency not known** Malignancy · neoplasms
- **ALLERGY AND CROSS-SENSITIVITY** EvGr Contra-indicated if history of hypersensitivity to macrolides. (M)
- **PREGNANCY** Specialist sources indicate that use can be considered if benefit outweighs potential risk—minimal systemic absorption; limited information available.
- **BREAST FEEDING** Specialist sources indicate present in milk (following systemic administration) but amount probably too small to be harmful—monitor exclusively breastfed infants, including blood concentrations, if there are concerns regarding toxicity.
- **HEPATIC IMPAIRMENT** Manufacturer advises caution in hepatic failure.
- **PATIENT AND CARER ADVICE** Advise patients to avoid excessive exposure to UV light including sunlight and to report symptoms of eye disorders for prompt evaluation by an ophthalmologist.
- **NATIONAL FUNDING/ACCESS DECISIONS**
  For full details see funding body website

NICE decisions
- **Tacrolimus and pimecrolimus for atopic eczema (August 2004)** NICE TA82 Recommended

Scottish Medicines Consortium (SMC) decisions
- **Tacrolimus 0.03 % ointment (*Protopic*®) for moderate to severe atopic dermatitis in children (March 2010)** SMC No. 608/10 Recommended with restrictions
- **Tacrolimus 0.1 % ointment (*Protopic*®) for moderate to severe atopic dermatitis in patients aged 16 years and over (April 2010)** SMC No. 609/10 Recommended with restrictions

- **MEDICINAL FORMS** There can be variation in the licensing of different medicines containing the same drug.

Cutaneous ointment

CAUTIONARY AND ADVISORY LABELS 4, 11, 28
EXCIPIENTS: May contain Beeswax

- **Tacrolimus (Non-proprietary)**
  Tacrolimus (as Tacrolimus monohydrate) 300 microgram per 1 gram Tacrolimus 0.03% ointment | 30 gram PoM £23.32–£36.00 DT = £23.33 | 60 gram PoM £42.54–£72.00 DT = £42.55
  Tacrolimus (as Tacrolimus monohydrate) 1 mg per 1 gram Tacrolimus 0.1% ointment | 30 gram PoM £25.92–£44.00 DT = £25.92 | 60 gram PoM £47.28–£84.00 DT = £47.28
- **Protopic** (LEO Pharma)
  Tacrolimus (as Tacrolimus monohydrate) 300 microgram per 1 gram Protopic 0.03% ointment | 30 gram PoM £23.33 DT = £23.33 | 60 gram PoM £42.55 DT = £42.55
  Tacrolimus (as Tacrolimus monohydrate) 1 mg per 1 gram Protopic 0.1% ointment | 30 gram PoM £25.92 DT = £25.92 | 60 gram PoM £47.28 DT = £47.28

IMMUNOSUPPRESSANTS › INTERLEUKIN INHIBITORS

Dupilumab

31-Mar-2026

- **DRUG ACTION** Dupilumab is a recombinant human monoclonal antibody that inhibits interleukin-4 and interleukin-13 signaling.

- **INDICATIONS AND DOSE**

Moderate-to-severe atopic eczema (initiated by a specialist)

▶ BY SUBCUTANEOUS INJECTION
- Child 12–17 years (body-weight 15–59 kg): Initially 400 mg, to be administered as two consecutive 200 mg injections at different injection sites, followed by 200 mg every 2 weeks, review treatment if no response after 16 weeks
- Child 12–17 years (body-weight 60 kg and above): Initially 600 mg, to be administered as two consecutive 300 mg injections at different injection sites, followed by 300 mg every 2 weeks, review treatment if no response after 16 weeks

Severe atopic eczema (initiated by a specialist)

▶ BY SUBCUTANEOUS INJECTION
- Child 6 months–5 years (body-weight 5–14 kg): Initially 200 mg, followed by 200 mg every 4 weeks, review treatment if no response after 16 weeks
- Child 6 months–5 years (body-weight 15–29 kg): Initially 300 mg, followed by 300 mg every 4 weeks, review treatment if no response after 16 weeks
- Child 6–11 years (body-weight 15–59 kg): Initially 300 mg on day 1, then 300 mg on day 15, followed by 300 mg every 4 weeks, dose may be increased to 200 mg every 2 weeks based on clinical judgement, review treatment if no response after 16 weeks
- Child 6–11 years (body-weight 60 kg and above): Initially 600 mg, to be administered as two consecutive 300 mg injections at different injection sites, followed by 300 mg every 2 weeks, review treatment if no response after 16 weeks

Severe asthma with type 2 inflammation [add-on maintenance therapy] (initiated by a specialist)

▶ BY SUBCUTANEOUS INJECTION
- Child 6–11 years (body-weight 15–29 kg): 100 mg every 2 weeks, review need for treatment yearly, alternatively 300 mg every 4 weeks, review need for treatment yearly
- Child 6–11 years (body-weight 30–59 kg): 200 mg every 2 weeks, review need for treatment yearly, alternatively 300 mg every 4 weeks, review need for treatment yearly
- Child 6–11 years (body-weight 60 kg and above): 200 mg every 2 weeks, review need for treatment yearly
- Child 12–17 years: Initially 400 mg, to be administered as two consecutive 200 mg injections at different injection sites, followed by 200 mg every 2 weeks, review need for treatment yearly

Severe asthma with type 2 inflammation [add-on maintenance therapy for patients with co-morbid severe atopic eczema] (initiated by a specialist)

▶ BY SUBCUTANEOUS INJECTION
- Child 6–11 years (body-weight 15–59 kg): Initially 300 mg on day 1, then 300 mg on day 15, followed by 300 mg every 4 weeks, dose may be increased to 200 mg every 2 weeks based on clinical judgement, review need for treatment yearly
- Child 6–11 years (body-weight 60 kg and above): Initially 600 mg, to be administered as two consecutive 300 mg injections at different injection sites, followed by 300 mg every 2 weeks, review need for treatment yearly

Severe asthma with type 2 inflammation [add-on maintenance therapy for patients currently treated with oral corticosteroids or patients with co-morbid moderate-to-severe atopic eczema] (initiated by a specialist)

▶ BY SUBCUTANEOUS INJECTION

▸ Child 12–17 years: Initially 600 mg, to be administered as two consecutive 300 mg injections at different injection sites, followed by 300 mg every 2 weeks, review need for treatment yearly

Eosinophilic oesophagitis (initiated by a specialist)

▶ BY SUBCUTANEOUS INJECTION

▸ Child 1–17 years (body-weight 15–29 kg): 200 mg every 2 weeks

▸ Child 1–17 years (body-weight 30–39 kg): 300 mg every 2 weeks

▸ Child 1–17 years (body-weight 40 kg and above): 300 mg once weekly

IMPORTANT SAFETY INFORMATION

MHRA/CHM ADVICE: DUPILUMAB (*DUPIXENT*®): RISK OF OCULAR ADVERSE REACTIONS AND NEED FOR PROMPT MANAGEMENT (NOVEMBER 2022)

The MHRA, with input from independent advisers, has reviewed the risk of dry eye and serious ocular side-effects associated with dupilumab. In patients with atopic eczema especially, common ocular side-effects include conjunctivitis, allergic conjunctivitis, eye pruritus, blepharitis, and dry eye; infrequent cases of keratitis and ulcerative keratitis have also been reported. Most ocular reactions associated with dupilumab in the UK are mild and can be managed, but it is not currently possible to predict who may experience the rarer, severe reactions; early review and intervention in ocular reactions are therefore recommended.

Healthcare professionals are advised to:

- discuss with patients or their carers the possibility of ocular side-effects and the symptoms to look out for when initiating dupilumab;
- advise patients or their carers to report new-onset or worsening eye symptoms to a healthcare professional, rather than self-managing symptoms;
- promptly review new-onset or worsening ocular symptoms, and refer patients for ophthalmological examination if necessary (for example, cases of possible keratitis, and conjunctivitis or dry eye that does not resolve after treatment);
- urgently review patients with sudden changes in vision or significant eye pain that does not settle.

● **CAUTIONS** Helminth infection

CAUTIONS, FURTHER INFORMATION

▸ Risk of infection Dupilumab may influence the immune response to helminth infections. Resolve pre-existing infection before initiating treatment; suspend treatment if resistant infection develops during therapy.

Manufacturer advises patients should be brought up-to-date with live and live attenuated vaccines before initiating treatment.

● **INTERACTIONS** → Appendix 1: monoclonal antibodies

● **SIDE-EFFECTS**

▶ **Common or very common** Arthralgia · dry eye · eosinophilia · eye inflammation · eye pruritus · increased risk of infection

▶ **Uncommon** Angioedema · facial rash

▶ **Rare or very rare** Hypersensitivity

SIDE-EFFECTS, FURTHER INFORMATION **Eosinophilic granulomatosis with polyangiitis (Churg-Strauss syndrome)** Churg-Strauss syndrome has occurred in adult patients given dupilumab; the reaction may be associated with the reduction of oral corticosteroid therapy. Churg-Strauss syndrome can present as vasculitic rash, cardiac complications, worsening pulmonary symptoms, or peripheral neuropathy in patients with eosinophilia.

Hypersensitivity Anaphylactic reactions and angioedema have occurred from minutes to up to seven days after the dupilumab injection.

● **PREGNANCY** Manufacturer advises use only if potential benefit outweighs risk—limited information available.

● **BREAST FEEDING** Manufacturer advises avoid—no information available.

● **DIRECTIONS FOR ADMINISTRATION** Manufacturer advises to inject into the thigh or abdomen (except for the 5 cm around the navel), or upper arm (if not self-administered); rotate injection site and avoid skin that is tender, damaged or scarred. Patients may self-administer *Dupixent*® after appropriate training in preparation and administration.

● **PRESCRIBING AND DISPENSING INFORMATION** Dupilumab is a biological medicine. Biological medicines must be prescribed and dispensed by brand name, see *Biological medicines* and *Biosimilar medicines*, under Guidance on prescribing p. 1; record the brand name and batch number after each administration.

EvGr *Dupixent*® pre-filled *syringe* should be used for administration to children under 12 years of age. ⟨M⟩

▸ When used for Asthma For choice of therapy, see Asthma, acute p. 174 and Asthma, chronic p. 171.

● **HANDLING AND STORAGE** Store in a refrigerator (2–8°C) and protect from light; may be kept at room temperature (max. 25°C) for max. 14 days.

● **PATIENT AND CARER ADVICE**

Missed doses If an injection administered *once weekly* is missed, it should be administered as soon as possible and a new schedule started based on this date.

If an injection administered *once every* 2 *weeks* is missed, it should be administered within 7 days of the missed dose and the next dose should be administered at the normal time. If more than 7 days has elapsed from the missed dose, it should not be administered and the next dose should be administered at the normal time.

If an injection administered *once every* 4 *weeks* is missed, it should be administered within 7 days of the missed dose and the next dose should be administered at the normal time. If more than 7 days has elapsed from the missed dose, it should be administered and a new schedule started based on this date.

● **NATIONAL FUNDING/ACCESS DECISIONS**

For full details see funding body website

NICE decisions

▶ **Dupilumab for treating severe asthma with type 2 inflammation (December 2021)** NICE TA751 Recommended with restrictions

Scottish Medicines Consortium (SMC) decisions

▶ **Dupilumab (*Dupixent*®) for the treatment of moderate-to-severe atopic dermatitis in adolescents 12 years and older who are candidates for systemic therapy (January 2020)** SMC No. SMC2232 Recommended with restrictions

▶ **Dupilumab (*Dupixent*®) as add-on maintenance treatment in adults and adolescents 12 years and older for severe asthma with type 2 inflammation, who are inadequately controlled with high dose inhaled corticosteroids plus another medicinal product for maintenance treatment (April 2021)** SMC No. SMC2317 Recommended with restrictions

All Wales Medicines Strategy Group (AWMSG) decisions

▶ **Dupilumab (*Dupixent*®) for the treatment of moderate-to-severe atopic dermatitis in adolescents 12 years and older who are candidates for systemic therapy (November 2019)** AWMSG No. 4089 Recommended with restrictions

▶ **Dupilumab (*Dupixent*®) for the treatment of severe atopic dermatitis in children 6 to 11 years old who are candidates for**

systemic therapy (March 2021) AWMSG No. 3858 Recommended with restrictions

- **Dupilumab (*Dupixent*®) as add-on maintenance treatment in children 6 to 11 years old for severe asthma with type 2 inflammation, who are inadequately controlled with medium to high dose inhaled corticosteroids plus another medicinal product for maintenance treatment (October 2022)** AWMSG No. 4017 Recommended with restrictions

- **MEDICINAL FORMS** There can be variation in the licensing of different medicines containing the same drug.

Solution for injection

EXCIPIENTS: May contain Polysorbates

- Dupixent (Sanofi)

Dupilumab 150 mg per 1 ml Dupixent 300mg/2ml solution for injection pre-filled syringes | 2 pre-filled disposable injection PoM £1,264.89 (Hospital only)

Dupixent 300mg/2ml solution for injection pre-filled pens | 2 pre-filled disposable injection PoM £1,264.89 (Hospital only)

Dupilumab 175 mg per 1 ml Dupixent 200mg/1.14ml solution for injection pre-filled syringes | 2 pre-filled disposable injection PoM £1,264.89 (Hospital only)

Dupixent 200mg/1.14ml solution for injection pre-filled pens | 2 pre-filled disposable injection PoM £1,264.89 (Hospital only)

Ixekizumab

07-Jul-2022

- **DRUG ACTION** Ixekizumab is a human monoclonal antibody that binds to interleukin-17A and inhibits the release of pro-inflammatory cytokines and chemokines.

- **INDICATIONS AND DOSE**

Moderate-to-severe plaque psoriasis (under expert supervision)

- BY SUBCUTANEOUS INJECTION
  - Child 6–17 years (body-weight 25–49 kg): Initially 80 mg for 1 dose, then maintenance 40 mg every 4 weeks, consider discontinuation of treatment if no response after 16–20 weeks
  - Child 6–17 years (body-weight 50 kg and above): Initially 160 mg for 1 dose, then maintenance 80 mg every 4 weeks, consider discontinuation of treatment if no response after 16–20 weeks

- **CONTRA-INDICATIONS** Active infections (including active tuberculosis) · inflammatory bowel disease (discontinue if signs or symptoms develop, or an exacerbation occurs)
- **CAUTIONS** Chronic or recurrent infection—monitor carefully and discontinue if serious, unresponsive infection develops

CAUTIONS, FURTHER INFORMATION

- Latent tuberculosis EvGr Patients with latent tuberculosis should complete anti-tuberculosis therapy before starting ixekizumab. ⟨M⟩

- **INTERACTIONS** → Appendix 1: monoclonal antibodies
- **SIDE-EFFECTS**
  - **Common or very common** Conjunctivitis · increased risk of infection · nausea · oropharyngeal pain · skin reactions
  - **Uncommon** Angioedema · inflammatory bowel disease · neutropenia · thrombocytopenia
  - **Rare or very rare** Anaphylactic reaction
  - **Frequency not known** Hypersensitivity (occasionally late-onset)
- **CONCEPTION AND CONTRACEPTION** Manufacturer advises effective contraception during treatment and for at least 10 weeks after treatment in women of childbearing potential.
- **PREGNANCY** Manufacturer advises avoid—limited information available.
- **BREAST FEEDING** Manufacturer advises avoid—present in milk in *animal* studies.
- **DIRECTIONS FOR ADMINISTRATION** EvGr Avoid injecting into areas of the skin that show psoriasis; injection sites may be alternated. ⟨M⟩ Patients may self-administer *Taltz*®, after appropriate training in subcutaneous injection technique; doses less than 80 mg must be prepared and administered by a healthcare professional.
- **PRESCRIBING AND DISPENSING INFORMATION** Ixekizumab is a biological medicine. Biological medicines must be prescribed and dispensed by brand name, see *Biological medicines* and *Biosimilar medicines*, under Guidance on prescribing p. 1; record the brand name and batch number after each administration.
- **HANDLING AND STORAGE** Manufacturer advises store in a refrigerator (2–8°C).
- **PATIENT AND CARER ADVICE** EvGr Patients and their carers should be advised to seek medical attention if symptoms of infection develop during treatment. ⟨M⟩

Self-administration If appropriate, patients and their carers should be given training in subcutaneous injection technique.

A Patient Leaflet and User Manual should be provided.

- **MEDICINAL FORMS** There can be variation in the licensing of different medicines containing the same drug.

Solution for injection

EXCIPIENTS: May contain Polysorbates

- Taltz (Eli Lilly and Company Ltd)

Ixekizumab 80 mg per 1 ml Taltz 80mg/1ml solution for injection pre-filled pens | 1 pre-filled disposable injection PoM £1,125.00 (Hospital only)

Taltz 80mg/1ml solution for injection pre-filled syringes | 1 pre-filled disposable injection PoM £1,125.00 (Hospital only)

Lebrikizumab

26-Nov-2024

- **DRUG ACTION** Lebrikizumab is a recombinant humanised monoclonal antibody that inhibits interleukin-13 signaling.

- **INDICATIONS AND DOSE**

Moderate-to-severe atopic eczema (initiated by a specialist)

- BY SUBCUTANEOUS INJECTION
  - Child 12–17 years (body-weight 40 kg and above): Initially 500 mg every 2 weeks for 2 doses, to be administered as two consecutive 250 mg injections at different injection sites, followed by 250 mg every 2 weeks up to week 16, review response after 16 weeks (consider discontinuing treatment if no response; if partial response consider continuing 250 mg every 2 weeks up to week 24), then maintenance 250 mg every 4 weeks

IMPORTANT SAFETY INFORMATION

MHRA/CHM ADVICE: DUPILUMAB (*DUPIXENT*®): RISK OF OCULAR ADVERSE REACTIONS AND NEED FOR PROMPT MANAGEMENT (NOVEMBER 2022)

The MHRA has reviewed the risk of dry eye and serious ocular side-effects associated with dupilumab, an inhibitor of interleukin-4 and interleukin-13 signalling. Lebrikizumab, which similarly inhibits interleukin-13, is also associated with ocular side-effects; commonly, conjunctivitis, allergic conjunctivitis, and dry eye, and less commonly, keratitis, and blepharitis. Patients who develop conjunctivitis that does not resolve following standard treatment should receive an ophthalmological examination. Healthcare professionals are advised to discuss with patients or their carers the potential for ocular side-effects and to manage any reactions promptly, especially in patients experiencing eye pain or changes to their vision.

- **CAUTIONS** Helminth infection

CAUTIONS, FURTHER INFORMATION

▸ Risk of infection EvGr Lebrikizumab may influence the immune response to helminth infections. Resolve pre-existing infection before initiating treatment; suspend treatment if resistant infection develops during therapy.

Patients should be brought up-to-date with live and live attenuated vaccines before initiating treatment. ⟨M⟩

● **INTERACTIONS** → Appendix 1: monoclonal antibodies

● **SIDE-EFFECTS**

▸ **Common or very common** Dry eye · eye inflammation

▸ **Uncommon** Eosinophilia · herpes zoster

● **PREGNANCY** EvGr Avoid as a precaution (limited information available). ⟨M⟩

● **BREAST FEEDING** EvGr Avoid—no information available. ⟨M⟩

● **DIRECTIONS FOR ADMINISTRATION** Take prefilled syringe or prefilled pen out of the refrigerator 45 minutes before administration. Inject into the thigh or abdomen (except for the 5 cm around the navel), or upper arm (if not self-administered); rotate injection site and avoid skin that is tender, damaged, bruised, or scarred. Patients may self-administer *Ebglyss*® after appropriate training in preparation and administration.

● **PRESCRIBING AND DISPENSING INFORMATION** Lebrikizumab is a biological medicine. Biological medicines must be prescribed and dispensed by brand name, see *Biological medicines* and *Biosimilar medicines*, under Guidance on prescribing p. 1; record the brand name and batch number after each administration.

● **HANDLING AND STORAGE** Store in a refrigerator (2–8°C) and protect from light; may be kept at room temperature (max. 30°C) for a maximum of 7 days.

● **PATIENT AND CARER ADVICE**

Self-administration If appropriate, patients and their carers should be given training in subcutaneous injection technique.

● **NATIONAL FUNDING/ACCESS DECISIONS**

For full details see funding body website

NICE decisions

▸ **Lebrikizumab for treating moderate to severe atopic dermatitis in people 12 years and over (July 2024)** NICE TA986 Recommended with restrictions

Scottish Medicines Consortium (SMC) decisions

▸ **Lebrikizumab (*Ebglyss*®) for the treatment of moderate-to-severe atopic dermatitis in adults and adolescents 12 years and older with a body weight of at least 40 kg who are candidates for systemic therapy (November 2024)** SMC No. SMC2707 Recommended with restrictions

● **MEDICINAL FORMS** There can be variation in the licensing of different medicines containing the same drug.

Solution for injection

EXCIPIENTS: May contain Polysorbates

▸ **Ebglyss** (Almirall Ltd) ▼

Lebrikizumab 125 mg per 1 ml Ebglyss 250mg/2ml solution for injection pre-filled pens | 2 pre-filled disposable injection PoM £2,271.26 (Hospital only)

Ebglyss 250mg/2ml solution for injection pre-filled syringes | 2 pre-filled disposable injection PoM £2,271.26 (Hospital only)

Nemolizumab

17-Apr-2026

● **DRUG ACTION** Nemolizumab is a humanised monoclonal antibody that inhibits interleukin-31 signalling.

● **INDICATIONS AND DOSE**

Moderate-to-severe atopic eczema

▸ BY SUBCUTANEOUS INJECTION

▸ Child 12–17 years (body-weight 30 kg and above): Initially 60 mg for 1 dose, to be administered as two consecutive 30 mg injections at different injection sites, followed by maintenance 30 mg every 4 weeks, patients who achieve clinical response after 16 weeks of treatment should be given maintenance dosing of 30 mg every 8 weeks, consider discontinuation of treatment if no response after 16 weeks

● **CAUTIONS** Immunisation

CAUTIONS, FURTHER INFORMATION EvGr Consider completion of immunisations according to current guidelines before initiating treatment—immunisation during treatment has not been studied. ⟨M⟩

● **INTERACTIONS** → Appendix 1: monoclonal antibodies

● **SIDE-EFFECTS**

▸ **Common or very common** Urticaria

▸ **Frequency not known** Hypersensitivity

● **PREGNANCY**

EvGr Avoid (limited information available). ⟨M⟩

● **BREAST FEEDING** Specialist sources indicate use with caution, especially if breast-feeding a neonate or pre-term infant (no information available). Large molecular weight suggests limited excretion into milk and drug molecule likely to be partially destroyed in the infant's gastro-intestinal tract; waiting for at least 2 weeks postpartum to resume treatment may minimise transfer to infant.

● **DIRECTIONS FOR ADMINISTRATION** Take carton out of the refrigerator 30 to 45 minutes before reconstitution and administration—consult product literature for further information. Inject into the abdomen (except for the 5 cm around the navel), front upper thigh, or upper arm (if not self-administered); rotate injection site and avoid skin that is tender, inflamed, swollen, damaged, bruised, or scarred. *Nemluvio*® should be used within 4 hours of reconstitution or discarded. *Nemluvio*® may be self-administered or administered by a carer after appropriate training in preparation and administration.

● **PRESCRIBING AND DISPENSING INFORMATION** Nemolizumab is a biological medicine. Biological medicines must be prescribed and dispensed by brand name, see *Biological medicines* and *Biosimilar medicines*, under Guidance on prescribing p. 1; record the brand name and batch number after each administration.

● **HANDLING AND STORAGE** Store in a refrigerator (2–8°C) and protect from light—consult product literature for further information regarding storage outside refrigerator.

● **PATIENT AND CARER ADVICE**

Self-administration If appropriate, patients and their carers should be given training in subcutaneous injection technique.

● **NATIONAL FUNDING/ACCESS DECISIONS**

For full details see funding body website

NICE decisions

▸ **Nemolizumab for treating moderate to severe atopic dermatitis in people 12 years and over (July 2025)** NICE TA1077 Recommended with restrictions

Scottish Medicines Consortium (SMC) decisions

▸ **Nemolizumab (*Nemluvio*®) for the treatment of moderate-to-severe atopic dermatitis in combination with topical corticosteroids and/or calcineurin inhibitors in adults and adolescents 12 years and older with a body weight of at least 30 kg, who are candidates for systemic therapy (April 2026)** SMC No. SMC2833 Recommended with restrictions

● **MEDICINAL FORMS** There can be variation in the licensing of different medicines containing the same drug.

Powder and solvent for solution for injection

▸ **Nemluvio** (Galderma (UK) Ltd) ▼

Nemolizumab 30 mg Nemluvio 30mg powder and solvent for solution for injection pre-filled pens | 1 pre-filled disposable injection PoM £2,257.00 (Hospital only)

Tralokinumab
02-Sep-2025

- **DRUG ACTION** Tralokinumab is a human monoclonal antibody that inhibits the interleukin-13 pathway.

- **INDICATIONS AND DOSE**

Moderate-to-severe atopic eczema (initiated by a specialist)

▶ BY SUBCUTANEOUS INJECTION

▶ Child 12–17 years: Initially 600 mg for 1 dose, followed by maintenance 300 mg every 2 weeks, patients who achieve clear or almost clear skin after 16 weeks of treatment may be considered for maintenance dosing given every 4 weeks; this may not be appropriate in patients weighing over 100 kg. Consider discontinuation of treatment if no response after 16 weeks

IMPORTANT SAFETY INFORMATION

MHRA/CHM ADVICE: DUPILUMAB (*DUPIXENT®*): RISK OF OCULAR ADVERSE REACTIONS AND NEED FOR PROMPT MANAGEMENT (NOVEMBER 2022)

The MHRA has reviewed the risk of dry eye and serious ocular side-effects associated with dupilumab, an inhibitor of interleukin-4 and interleukin-13 signalling. Tralokinumab, which similarly inhibits interleukin-13, is also associated with ocular side-effects; commonly, conjunctivitis and allergic conjunctivitis, and less commonly, keratitis. Patients who develop conjunctivitis that does not resolve following standard treatment should receive an ophthalmological examination. Healthcare professionals are advised to discuss with patients or their carers the potential for ocular side-effects and to manage any reactions promptly, especially in patients experiencing eye pain or changes to their vision.

- **CAUTIONS** Helminth infection

CAUTIONS, FURTHER INFORMATION

▶ Risk of infection EvGr Patients with pre-existing helminth infections should be treated before initiating treatment with tralokinumab. If patients become infected while receiving tralokinumab and do not respond to anthelminthic treatment, tralokinumab should be discontinued until infection resolves.

Patients should be brought up-to-date with live and live attenuated vaccines before initiating treatment. ⟨M⟩

- **INTERACTIONS** → Appendix 1: monoclonal antibodies
- **SIDE-EFFECTS**

▶ **Common or very common** Eosinophilia · eye inflammation · increased risk of infection

- **PREGNANCY** EvGr Avoid—limited information available. ⟨M⟩
- **BREAST FEEDING** Specialist sources indicate use with caution, especially if breast-feeding a neonate or preterm infant (no information available). Large molecular weight suggests limited excretion into milk and drug molecule likely to be partially destroyed in the infant's gastro-intestinal tract; waiting for at least 2 weeks postpartum to resume treatment may minimise transfer to infant.
- **DIRECTIONS FOR ADMINISTRATION** Inject into the thigh or abdomen (except for the 5 cm around the navel), or upper arm (if not self-administered); rotate injection site and avoid skin that is tender, damaged, bruised, or scarred. *Adtralza®* may be self-administered or administered by a carer after appropriate training in preparation and administration.
- **PRESCRIBING AND DISPENSING INFORMATION** Tralokinumab is a biological medicine. Biological medicines must be prescribed and dispensed by brand name, see *Biological medicines* and *Biosimilar medicines*, under Guidance on prescribing p. 1; record the brand name and batch number after each administration.
- **HANDLING AND STORAGE** Store in a refrigerator (2–8°C) and protect from light—consult product literature for further information regarding storage outside refrigerator.
- **PATIENT AND CARER ADVICE**

Self-administration If appropriate, patients and their carers should be given training in subcutaneous injection technique.

- **MEDICINAL FORMS** There can be variation in the licensing of different medicines containing the same drug.

Solution for injection

EXCIPIENTS: May contain Polysorbates

▶ Adtralza (LEO Pharma) ▼

Tralokinumab 150 mg per 1 ml Adtralza 150mg/1ml solution for injection pre-filled syringes | 4 pre-filled disposable injection PoM £1,070.00 (Hospital only)

Adtralza 300mg/2ml solution for injection pre-filled pens | 2 pre-filled disposable injection PoM £1,070.00 (Hospital only)

Ustekinumab
06-Apr-2023

- **INDICATIONS AND DOSE**

Plaque psoriasis (under expert supervision)

▶ BY SUBCUTANEOUS INJECTION

▶ Child 6–17 years (body-weight up to 60 kg): Initially 750 micrograms/kg, then 750 micrograms/kg after 4 weeks, then 750 micrograms/kg every 12 weeks, consult product literature for advice on calculating volume of injection to be given, consider discontinuation if no response within 28 weeks

▶ Child 6–17 years (body-weight 60–100 kg): Initially 45 mg, then 45 mg after 4 weeks, then 45 mg every 12 weeks, consider discontinuation if no response within 28 weeks

▶ Child 6–17 years (body-weight 101 kg and above): Initially 90 mg, then 90 mg after 4 weeks, then 90 mg every 12 weeks, consider discontinuation if no response within 28 weeks

- **CONTRA-INDICATIONS** Active infection
- **CAUTIONS** Development of malignancy · history of malignancy · predisposition to infection · start appropriate treatment if widespread erythema and skin exfoliation develop, and stop ustekinumab treatment if exfoliative dermatitis suspected

CAUTIONS, FURTHER INFORMATION

▶ Tuberculosis Active tuberculosis should be treated with standard treatment for at least 2 months before starting ustekinumab. Patients who have previously received adequate treatment for tuberculosis can start ustekinumab but should be monitored every 3 months for possible recurrence. In patients without active tuberculosis but who were previously not treated adequately, chemoprophylaxis should ideally be completed before starting ustekinumab. In patients at high risk of tuberculosis who cannot be assessed by tuberculin skin test, chemoprophylaxis can be given concurrently with ustekinumab.

- **INTERACTIONS** → Appendix 1: monoclonal antibodies
- **SIDE-EFFECTS**

▶ **Common or very common** Arthralgia · asthenia · back pain · diarrhoea · dizziness · headache · increased risk of infection · myalgia · nausea · oropharyngeal pain · skin reactions · vomiting

▶ **Uncommon** Depression · facial paralysis · hypersensitivity (may be delayed) · nasal congestion

▶ **Rare or very rare** Cutaneous lupus erythematosus · hypersensitivity vasculitis · interstitial lung disease · lupus-like syndrome · pneumonia eosinophilic

▶ **Frequency not known** Increased risk of cancer · meningitis listeria · tuberculosis reactivation

● **CONCEPTION AND CONTRACEPTION** Manufacturer advises effective contraception during treatment and for 15 weeks after stopping treatment.

● **PREGNANCY** Avoid.

● **BREAST FEEDING** Specialist sources indicate use with caution; negligible amounts present in milk which are likely to be destroyed in the infant's gastro-intestinal tract. In newborn or premature infants there may be greater intestinal absorption.

● **PRE-TREATMENT SCREENING**
Tuberculosis Patients should be evaluated for tuberculosis before treatment.

● **MONITORING REQUIREMENTS**
▶ Monitor for non-melanoma skin cancer, especially in patients with a history of PUVA treatment or prolonged immunosuppressant therapy, or those over 60 years of age.
▶ Monitor for signs and symptoms of exfoliative dermatitis or erythrodermic psoriasis.

● **DIRECTIONS FOR ADMINISTRATION** For *subcutaneous injection* (*Stelara*®), inject into the upper thigh or abdomen (except for the 5 cm around the navel), or upper arm (if not self-administered); avoid areas of the skin that show signs of psoriasis. Patients may self-administer *Stelara*®, after appropriate training in subcutaneous injection technique.

● **PRESCRIBING AND DISPENSING INFORMATION** Ustekinumab is a biological medicine. Biological medicines must be prescribed and dispensed by brand name, see *Biological medicines* and *Biosimilar medicines*, under Guidance on prescribing p. 1; record the brand name and batch number after each administration.

● **HANDLING AND STORAGE** Store in a refrigerator (2–8°C) and protect from light—consult product literature for further information regarding storage outside refrigerator.

● **PATIENT AND CARER ADVICE**
Exfoliative dermatitis Patients and carers should be advised to seek prompt medical attention if symptoms suggestive of exfoliative dermatitis or erythrodermic psoriasis (such as increased redness and shedding of skin over a larger area of the body) develop.
Infection Patients and carers should be advised to seek medical attention if symptoms of infection develop.
Tuberculosis Patients and carers should be advised to seek medical attention if symptoms suggestive of tuberculosis (e.g. persistent cough, weight loss, and fever) develop.
Lupus-related conditions Patients and carers should be advised to seek prompt medical attention if symptoms suggestive of cutaneous lupus erythematosus or lupus-like syndrome (such as skin lesions in sun exposed areas, or that are accompanied by arthralgia) develop.

● **NATIONAL FUNDING/ACCESS DECISIONS**
For full details see funding body website

NICE decisions
▶ **Adalimumab, etanercept and ustekinumab for treating plaque psoriasis in children and young people (July 2017)** NICE TA455
Recommended with restrictions

All Wales Medicines Strategy Group (AWMSG) decisions
▶ **Ustekinumab (*Stelara*®) for the treatment of moderate to severe plaque psoriasis in children and adolescent patients from the age of 6 to 11 years, who are inadequately controlled by, or are intolerant to, other systemic therapies or phototherapies (November 2021)** AWMSG No. 3687
Recommended with restrictions

● **MEDICINAL FORMS** There can be variation in the licensing of different medicines containing the same drug.

Solution for injection
CAUTIONARY AND ADVISORY LABELS 10
EXCIPIENTS: May contain Polysorbates

▶ **Imuldosa** (Accord-UK Ltd) ▼
Ustekinumab 90 mg per 1 ml Imuldosa 90mg/1ml solution for injection pre-filled syringes | 1 pre-filled disposable injection PoM £2,147.00 (Hospital only)
Imuldosa 45mg/0.5ml solution for injection pre-filled syringes | 1 pre-filled disposable injection PoM £2,147.00 (Hospital only)

▶ **Otulfi** (Fresenius Kabi Ltd) ▼
Ustekinumab 90 mg per 1 ml Otulfi 45mg/0.5ml solution for injection pre-filled syringes | 1 pre-filled disposable injection PoM £1,932.30 (Hospital only)
Otulfi 90mg/1ml solution for injection pre-filled syringes | 1 pre-filled disposable injection PoM £1,932.30 (Hospital only)

▶ **Pyzchiva** (Sandoz Ltd) ▼
Ustekinumab 90 mg per 1 ml Pyzchiva 45mg/0.5ml solution for injection pre-filled pens | 1 pre-filled disposable injection PoM £1,932.30 (Hospital only)
Pyzchiva 90mg/1ml solution for injection pre-filled syringes | 1 pre-filled disposable injection PoM £1,932.30 (Hospital only)
Pyzchiva 90mg/1ml solution for injection pre-filled pens | 1 pre-filled disposable injection PoM £1,932.30 (Hospital only)
Pyzchiva 45mg/0.5ml solution for injection pre-filled syringes | 1 pre-filled disposable injection PoM £1,932.30 (Hospital only)

▶ **Stelara** (Janssen-Cilag Ltd)
Ustekinumab 90 mg per 1 ml Stelara 90mg/1ml solution for injection pre-filled syringes | 1 pre-filled disposable injection PoM £2,147.00 (Hospital only)
Stelara 45mg/0.5ml solution for injection pre-filled pens | 1 pre-filled disposable injection PoM £2,147.00 (Hospital only)
Stelara 90mg/1ml solution for injection pre-filled pens | 1 pre-filled disposable injection PoM £2,147.00 (Hospital only)
Stelara 45mg/0.5ml solution for injection vials | 1 vial PoM £2,147.00 (Hospital only)
Stelara 45mg/0.5ml solution for injection pre-filled syringes | 1 pre-filled disposable injection PoM £2,147.00 (Hospital only)

▶ **Steqeyma** (Celltrion Healthcare UK Ltd) ▼
Ustekinumab 90 mg per 1 ml Steqeyma 90mg/1ml solution for injection pre-filled syringes | 1 pre-filled disposable injection PoM £1,932.30 (Hospital only)
Steqeyma 45mg/0.5ml solution for injection pre-filled syringes | 1 pre-filled disposable injection PoM £1,932.30 (Hospital only)

▶ **Uzpruvo** (Genus Pharmaceuticals Holdings Ltd) ▼
Ustekinumab 90 mg per 1 ml Uzpruvo 45mg/0.5ml solution for injection pre-filled syringes | 1 pre-filled disposable injection PoM £1,932.30 (Hospital only)
Uzpruvo 90mg/1ml solution for injection pre-filled syringes | 1 pre-filled disposable injection PoM £1,932.30 (Hospital only)

▶ **Wezenla** (Amgen Ltd) ▼
Ustekinumab 90 mg per 1 ml Wezenla 90mg/1ml solution for injection pre-filled pens | 1 pre-filled disposable injection PoM £2,147.00 (Hospital only)
Wezenla 45mg/0.5ml solution for injection pre-filled pens | 1 pre-filled disposable injection PoM £2,147.00 (Hospital only)
Wezenla 45mg/0.5ml solution for injection vials | 1 vial PoM £2,147.00 (Hospital only)
Wezenla 90mg/1ml solution for injection pre-filled syringes | 1 pre-filled disposable injection PoM £2,147.00 (Hospital only)
Wezenla 45mg/0.5ml solution for injection pre-filled syringes | 1 pre-filled disposable injection PoM £2,147.00 (Hospital only)

IMMUNOSUPPRESSANTS > JAK INHIBITORS

Abrocitinib

18-May-2023

- **DRUG ACTION** Abrocitinib is a selective inhibitor of the Janus-associated tyrosine kinase JAK1.

- **INDICATIONS AND DOSE**

Moderate-to-severe atopic eczema (under expert supervision)

▶ BY MOUTH

▶ Child 12–17 years: Initially 100 mg once daily, increased to 200 mg once daily if necessary and if tolerated, consider discontinuation of treatment if no response after 12 weeks, for dose adjustments, interruption or discontinuation due to clinical response or side-effects—consult product literature; maximum 200 mg per day

DOSE ADJUSTMENTS DUE TO INTERACTIONS

▶ EvGr Reduce initial dose by half with concurrent use of potent CYP2C19 inhibitors. Ⓜ

13 Skin

IMPORTANT SAFETY INFORMATION

MHRA/CHM ADVICE: JANUS KINASE (JAK) INHIBITORS: NEW MEASURES TO REDUCE RISKS OF MAJOR CARDIOVASCULAR EVENTS, MALIGNANCY, VENOUS THROMBOEMBOLISM, SERIOUS INFECTIONS AND INCREASED MORTALITY (APRIL 2023)

In 2022, the EMA conducted a review of all JAK inhibitors indicated for chronic inflammatory diseases and concluded that the risks associated with the use of tofacitinib could be considered a class effect (see *Important safety information* in tofacitinib p. 803). Following a further review by the MHRA, some existing warnings for tofacitinib have been updated and implemented for all JAK inhibitors included in the review, such as abrocitinib.

Healthcare professionals are advised to:

- avoid use in patients who are current or past long-time smokers, and in patients with other cardiovascular disease or malignancy risk factors, unless there are no suitable alternatives;
- use with caution in patients with risk factors for venous thromboembolism;
- use lower doses in patients with risk factors, where applicable;
- periodically examine all patients' skin for malignancy;
- inform patients and their carers of these risks, and the signs and symptoms that warrant urgent medical attention.

- **CONTRA-INDICATIONS** Absolute lymphocyte count less than 0.5×10^9 cells/litre (do not initiate) · absolute neutrophil count less than 1×10^9 cells/litre (do not initiate) · clinically significant active infection · haemoglobin less than 8 g/dL (do not initiate) · platelet count less than 150×10^9 cells/litre (do not initiate)

- **CAUTIONS** Chronic or recurrent infection · history of atherosclerotic cardiovascular disease or other cardiovascular risk factors · history of serious or opportunistic infection · predisposition to infection · risk factors for deep-vein thrombosis or pulmonary embolism · risk factors for malignancy · risk of viral reactivation (consult product literature) · tuberculosis exposure

CAUTIONS, FURTHER INFORMATION

▶ Tuberculosis EvGr Consider anti-tuberculosis therapy prior to initiation of abrocitinib in patients with previously untreated latent tuberculosis. Use abrocitinib with caution in patients who have travelled or resided in areas of endemic tuberculosis or endemic mycoses. Ⓜ

▶ Immunisation EvGr Patients should receive all recommended vaccinations before starting treatment; live vaccines are not recommended immediately before, or during, treatment. Ⓜ

▶ Deep-vein thrombosis or pulmonary embolism EvGr If deep-vein thrombosis or pulmonary embolism occurs during treatment, discontinuation of abrocitinib is recommended. Ⓜ

- **INTERACTIONS** → Appendix 1: abrocitinib

- **SIDE-EFFECTS**

▶ **Common or very common** Abdominal pain upper · acne · dizziness · headache · increased risk of infection · nausea · vomiting

▶ **Uncommon** Dyslipidaemia · embolism and thrombosis · lymphopenia · thrombocytopenia

▶ **Frequency not known** Cardiovascular event · malignancy · neoplasms · reactivation of infections

- **CONCEPTION AND CONTRACEPTION** EvGr Females of childbearing potential should use effective contraception during treatment and for 1 month after last treatment. Female fertility may be temporarily reduced during treatment—studies in *animals* show that the effects on fertility are reversible 1 month after stopping treatment. Ⓜ

- **PREGNANCY** EvGr Avoid—toxicity in *animal* studies. Ⓜ

- **BREAST FEEDING** EvGr Avoid—present in milk in *animal* studies. Ⓜ

- **HEPATIC IMPAIRMENT** EvGr Avoid in severe impairment (no information available). Ⓜ

- **RENAL IMPAIRMENT** EvGr Caution in moderate and severe impairment. Ⓜ

Dose adjustments EvGr Reduce dose by half in moderate impairment.

Reduce initial dose to 50 mg once daily, and increase to maximum 100 mg once daily, in severe impairment. Ⓜ

- **PRE-TREATMENT SCREENING** EvGr Patients should be evaluated for tuberculosis and viral hepatitis before treatment. Ⓜ

- **MONITORING REQUIREMENTS**

▶ EvGr Monitor lipid profile at baseline, 4 weeks after treatment initiation, and then periodically—hyperlipidaemia should be managed according to clinical guidelines.

▶ Monitor for haematological abnormalities at baseline, 4 weeks after treatment initiation, and then periodically; interrupt treatment if absolute neutrophil count less than 1×10^9 cells/litre, absolute lymphocyte count less than 0.5×10^9 cells/litre, or haemoglobin less than 8 g/dL—treatment may be restarted when levels return above these values. Discontinue treatment if platelet count less than 50×10^9 cells/litre.

▶ Monitor for viral hepatitis during treatment. Ⓜ

▶ The MHRA recommends periodic skin examination in all patients, particularly those at increased risk of skin cancer.

- **PRESCRIBING AND DISPENSING INFORMATION** The manufacturer of *Cibinqo*® has provided a *Prescriber Brochure*.

- **PATIENT AND CARER ADVICE** Patients and carers should be advised that taking *Cibinqo*® with food may improve nausea.

Risk minimisation materials A patient card should be provided.

Missed doses If a dose is more than 12 hours late, the missed dose should not be taken and the next dose should be taken at the normal time.

Driving and skilled tasks Patients and carers should be cautioned on the effects on driving and performance of skilled tasks—increased risk of dizziness.

● **NATIONAL FUNDING/ACCESS DECISIONS** For full details see funding body website

NICE decisions

▸ **Abrocitinib, tralokinumab or upadacitinib for treating moderate to severe atopic dermatitis (August 2022)** NICE TA814 Recommended with restrictions

Scottish Medicines Consortium (SMC) decisions

▸ **Abrocitinib (*Cibinqo*®) for the treatment of moderate-to-severe atopic dermatitis in adults and adolescents 12 years and older who are candidates for systemic therapy (June 2022)** SMC No. SMC2431 Recommended with restrictions

● **MEDICINAL FORMS** There can be variation in the licensing of different medicines containing the same drug.

Oral tablet

▸ Cibinqo (Pfizer Ltd) ▼
Abrocitinib 50 mg Cibinqo 50mg tablets | 28 tablet PoM £893.76
Abrocitinib 100 mg Cibinqo 100mg tablets | 28 tablet PoM £893.76
Abrocitinib 200 mg Cibinqo 200mg tablets | 28 tablet PoM £893.76 (Hospital only)

Upadacitinib

24-Apr-2025

● **DRUG ACTION** Upadacitinib is a selective and reversible inhibitor of the Janus-associated tyrosine kinase JAK1.

● **INDICATIONS AND DOSE**

Atopic eczema (under expert supervision)

▸ BY MOUTH

▸ Child 12–17 years (body-weight 30 kg and above): 15 mg once daily, consider discontinuation of treatment if no response after 12 weeks, for treatment interruption due to side-effects—consult product literature

IMPORTANT SAFETY INFORMATION

MHRA/CHM ADVICE: UPADACITINIB (*RINVOQ*®): ADVICE FOR VENOUS THROMBOEMBOLISM (MARCH 2020)

Cases of deep vein thrombosis and pulmonary embolism have been reported in patients taking upadacitinib. Healthcare professionals are advised to use upadacitinib with caution in patients with risk factors for venous thromboembolism (VTE). Patients should be informed of the signs and symptoms of VTE before starting treatment and advised to seek urgent medical attention if these develop. Upadacitinib should be discontinued if clinical features of VTE occur.

MHRA/CHM ADVICE: JANUS KINASE (JAK) INHIBITORS: NEW MEASURES TO REDUCE RISKS OF MAJOR CARDIOVASCULAR EVENTS, MALIGNANCY, VENOUS THROMBOEMBOLISM, SERIOUS INFECTIONS AND INCREASED MORTALITY (APRIL 2023)

In 2022, the EMA conducted a review of all JAK inhibitors indicated for chronic inflammatory diseases and concluded that the risks associated with the use of tofacitinib could be considered a class effect (see *Important safety information* in tofacitinib p. 803). Following a further review by the MHRA, some existing warnings for tofacitinib have been updated and implemented for all JAK inhibitors included in the review, such as upadacitinib.

Healthcare professionals are advised to:
- avoid use in patients who are current or past long-time smokers, and in patients with other cardiovascular disease or malignancy risk factors, unless there are no suitable alternatives;
- use with caution in patients with risk factors for VTE;
- use lower doses in patients with risk factors, where applicable;
- periodically examine all patients' skin for malignancy;
- inform patients and their carers of these risks, and the signs and symptoms that warrant urgent medical attention.

● **CONTRA-INDICATIONS** Absolute lymphocyte count less than 0.5 × 10^9 cells/litre · absolute neutrophil count less than 1 × 10^9 cells/litre · active serious infection including localised infection · active tuberculosis · haemoglobin less than 8 g/dL

● **CAUTIONS** Chronic or recurrent infection · history of atherosclerotic cardiovascular disease or other cardiovascular risk factors · history of serious or opportunistic infection · patients at risk of gastro-intestinal perforation (new onset abdominal signs and symptoms should be evaluated promptly) · predisposition to infection · risk factors for deep-vein thrombosis or pulmonary embolism · risk factors for malignancy · risk of viral reactivation (consult product literature) · tuberculosis exposure

CAUTIONS, FURTHER INFORMATION

▸ Immunisation EvGr Patients should receive all recommended vaccinations, including prophylactic varicella-zoster vaccination, before starting treatment; live vaccines are not recommended. ⟨M⟩

▸ Tuberculosis EvGr Consider anti-tuberculosis therapy prior to initiation of upadacitinib in patients with previously untreated latent tuberculosis or in patients at risk of tuberculosis infection. Use upadacitinib with caution in patients who have travelled or resided in areas of endemic tuberculosis or endemic mycoses. ⟨M⟩

● **INTERACTIONS** → Appendix 1: upadacitinib

● **SIDE-EFFECTS**

▸ **Common or very common** Abdominal pain · anaemia · cough · dyslipidaemia · fatigue · fever · headache · increased risk of infection · lymphopenia · nausea · neoplasms · neutropenia · skin reactions · weight increased

▸ **Uncommon** Sepsis

▸ **Frequency not known** Cardiovascular event · embolism and thrombosis · gastrointestinal perforation · malignancy · meningitis bacterial · reactivation of infections

● **CONCEPTION AND CONTRACEPTION** Manufacturer advises females of childbearing potential should use effective contraception during and for 4 weeks after treatment.

● **PREGNANCY** Manufacturer advises avoid—toxicity in *animal* studies.

● **BREAST FEEDING** Manufacturer advises avoid—present in milk in *animal* studies.

● **HEPATIC IMPAIRMENT** EvGr Avoid in severe impairment (no information available). ⟨M⟩

● **RENAL IMPAIRMENT** EvGr Caution in severe impairment (limited information available). ⟨M⟩

● **PRE-TREATMENT SCREENING** Manufacturer advises patients should be evaluated for tuberculosis and viral hepatitis before treatment.

● **MONITORING REQUIREMENTS**

▸ EvGr Monitor for signs and symptoms of infection during and after treatment.

▸ Monitor neutrophils, lymphocytes, and haemoglobin before and during treatment (no later than 12 weeks after initiation), and as clinically indicated thereafter; interrupt treatment if absolute neutrophil count less than 1 × 10^9 cells/litre, absolute lymphocyte count less than 0.5 × 10^9 cells/litre, or haemoglobin less than 8 g/dL—treatment may be restarted when levels return above these values.

▸ Monitor hepatic transaminases before starting treatment, and as clinically indicated thereafter—interrupt treatment if drug-induced liver injury suspected; monitor

lipids 12 weeks after starting treatment, and then as clinically indicated.
- Monitor for viral hepatitis reactivation during treatment; if hepatitis B virus DNA is detected, consult liver specialist for advice.
- Periodic skin examination is recommended in all patients, particularly those at increased risk of skin cancer. ◈M

- **PRESCRIBING AND DISPENSING INFORMATION** The manufacturer of *Rinvoq*® has provided a guide for healthcare professionals.
- **PATIENT AND CARER ADVICE** A patient alert card should be provided.
- **NATIONAL FUNDING/ACCESS DECISIONS**
For full details see funding body website

NICE decisions
- **Abrocitinib, tralokinumab or upadacitinib for treating moderate to severe atopic dermatitis (August 2022)** NICE TA814 Recommended with restrictions

Scottish Medicines Consortium (SMC) decisions
- **Upadacitinib (*Rinvoq*®) for the treatment of moderate to severe atopic dermatitis in adults and adolescents 12 years and older who are candidates for systemic therapy (April 2022)** SMC No. SMC2417 Recommended with restrictions

- **MEDICINAL FORMS** There can be variation in the licensing of different medicines containing the same drug.

Modified-release tablet
CAUTIONARY AND ADVISORY LABELS 25
- Rinvoq (AbbVie Ltd)
  Upadacitinib (as Upadacitinib hemihydrate) 15 mg Rinvoq 15mg modified-release tablets | 28 tablet PoM £805.56 (Hospital only)
  Upadacitinib (as Upadacitinib hemihydrate) 30 mg Rinvoq 30mg modified-release tablets | 28 tablet PoM £1,281.54 (Hospital only)
  Upadacitinib (as Upadacitinib hemihydrate) 45 mg Rinvoq 45mg modified-release tablets | 28 tablet PoM £2,087.10 (Hospital only)

RETINOID AND RELATED DRUGS

Acitretin

06-Nov-2023

- **DRUG ACTION** Acitretin is a metabolite of etretinate.

- **INDICATIONS AND DOSE**

Severe extensive psoriasis resistant to other forms of therapy (under expert supervision) | Palmoplantar pustular psoriasis (under expert supervision) | Severe congenital ichthyosis (under expert supervision)
- BY MOUTH
  - Child 1 month–11 years: 0.5 mg/kg once daily; increased if necessary to 1 mg/kg once daily, to be taken with food or milk, careful monitoring of musculoskeletal development required; maximum 35 mg per day
  - Child 12–17 years: Initially 25–30 mg daily for 2–4 weeks, then adjusted according to response to 25–50 mg daily, increased to up to 75 mg daily, dose only increased to 75 mg daily for short periods in psoriasis

Severe Darier's disease (keratosis follicularis) (under expert supervision)
- BY MOUTH
  - Child 1 month–11 years: 0.5 mg/kg once daily; increased if necessary to 1 mg/kg once daily, to be taken with food or milk, careful monitoring of musculoskeletal development required; maximum 35 mg per day
  - Child 12–17 years: Initially 10 mg daily for 2–4 weeks, then adjusted according to response to 25–50 mg daily

Harlequin ichthyosis (under expert supervision)
- BY MOUTH
  - Neonate: 0.5 mg/kg once daily; increased if necessary to 1 mg/kg once daily, to be taken with food or milk, careful monitoring of musculoskeletal development required.

IMPORTANT SAFETY INFORMATION

MHRA/CHM ADVICE: ORAL RETINOID MEDICINES: REVISED AND SIMPLIFIED PREGNANCY PREVENTION EDUCATIONAL MATERIALS FOR HEALTHCARE PROFESSIONALS AND WOMEN (JUNE 2019)

New prescriber checklists, patient reminder cards, and pharmacy checklists are available to support the Pregnancy Prevention Programme in women and girls of childbearing potential taking oral acitretin, alitretinoin, or isotretinoin. Healthcare professionals are reminded that the use of oral retinoids is contra-indicated in pregnancy due to a high risk of serious congenital malformations, and any use in females must be within the conditions of the Pregnancy Prevention Programme (see *Conception and contraception* and *Prescribing and dispensing information*).

Neuropsychiatric reactions have been reported in patients taking oral retinoids. Healthcare professionals are advised to monitor patients for signs of depression or suicidal ideation and refer for appropriate treatment, if necessary; particular care is needed in those with a history of depression. Patients should be advised to speak to their doctor if they experience any changes in mood or behaviour, and encouraged to ask family and friends to look out for any change in mood.

- **CONTRA-INDICATIONS** Hyperlipidaemia
- **CAUTIONS** Avoid excessive exposure to sunlight and unsupervised use of sunlamps · diabetes (can alter glucose tolerance—initial frequent blood glucose checks) · do not donate blood during and for 3 years after stopping therapy (teratogenic risk) · history of depression (risk of neuropsychiatric reactions) · investigate atypical musculoskeletal symptoms · use only in exceptional circumstances and monitor growth parameters and bone development (premature epiphyseal closure reported)
- **INTERACTIONS** → Appendix 1: retinoids
- **SIDE-EFFECTS**
  - **Common or very common** Abdominal pain · arthralgia · brittle nails · diarrhoea · dry mouth · eye inflammation · gastrointestinal disorder · haemorrhage · hair texture abnormal · headache · increased risk of infection · mucosal abnormalities · myalgia · nausea · oral disorders · peripheral oedema · skin reactions · thirst · vomiting · xerophthalmia
  - **Uncommon** Dizziness · hepatic disorders · photosensitivity reaction · vision disorders
  - **Rare or very rare** Bone pain · exostosis · idiopathic intracranial hypertension · peripheral neuropathy
  - **Frequency not known** Angioedema · anxiety · capillary leak syndrome · depression · drowsiness · dysphonia · flushing · glucose tolerance impaired · granuloma · hearing impairment · hyperhidrosis · malaise · mood altered · psychiatric disorder · pyogenic granuloma · retinoic acid syndrome · taste altered · tinnitus

SIDE-EFFECTS, FURTHER INFORMATION **Exostosis** Skeletal hyperostosis and extra-osseous calcification reported following long-term treatment with etretinate (of which acitretin is a metabolite) and premature epiphyseal closure in children.

Benign intracranial hypertension Discontinue if severe headache, nausea, vomiting, or visual disturbances occur.

- **CONCEPTION AND CONTRACEPTION** The MHRA advises that women and girls of childbearing potential being treated with the oral retinoids acitretin, alitretinoin, or isotretinoin must be supported on a Pregnancy Prevention Programme with regular follow-up and pregnancy testing.
Pregnancy prevention Effective contraception must be used.

In females of childbearing potential, exclude pregnancy up to 3 days before treatment, every month during treatment (unless there are compelling reasons to indicate that there is no risk of pregnancy), and every 1–3 months for 3 years after stopping treatment. Treatment should be started on day 2 or 3 of menstrual cycle. Females of childbearing age must practise effective contraception for at least 1 month before starting treatment, during treatment, and for at least 3 years after stopping treatment. Females should be advised to use at least 1 highly effective method of contraception (i.e. a user-independent form such as an intra-uterine device or implant) or 2 complementary user-dependent forms of contraception (e.g. oral contraceptives and barrier method). Females should be advised to seek medical attention immediately if they become pregnant during treatment or within 3 years of stopping treatment.

- **PREGNANCY** Manufacturer advises avoid—teratogenic.
- **BREAST FEEDING** Avoid.
- **HEPATIC IMPAIRMENT** Manufacturer advises avoid in severe impairment.
- **RENAL IMPAIRMENT** [EvGr] Avoid in severe impairment (increased risk of toxicity). (M)
- **MONITORING REQUIREMENTS**
  - Monitor serum-triglyceride and serum-cholesterol concentrations before treatment, 1 month after starting, then every 3 months.
  - Check liver function at start, at least every 4 weeks for first 2 months and then every 3 months.
- **PRESCRIBING AND DISPENSING INFORMATION**

Prescribing for females of childbearing potential The Pregnancy Prevention Programme is supported by the following materials provided by the manufacturer: *Checklists for prescribers and pharmacists*, and *Patient reminder cards*.

Each prescription for oral acitretin should be limited to a supply of up to 30 days' treatment. Pregnancy testing should ideally be carried out on the same day as prescription issuing and dispensing.

- **PATIENT AND CARER ADVICE** Females of childbearing potential should be advised to avoid alcohol during and for 2 months after stopping treatment (risk of formation of a highly teratogenic metabolite with a longer half-life).

Risk of neuropsychiatric reactions The MHRA advises patients and carers to seek medical attention if changes in mood or behaviour occur.

Pregnancy Prevention Programme Pharmacists must ensure that female patients have a patient card—see also *Important safety information*.

- **MEDICINAL FORMS** There can be variation in the licensing of different medicines containing the same drug. Forms available from special-order manufacturers include: oral suspension, oral solution

Oral capsule

CAUTIONARY AND ADVISORY LABELS 10, 11, 21

- **Acitretin (Non-proprietary)**
  - **Acitretin 10 mg** Acitretin 10mg capsules | 60 capsule [PoM] £23.80 DT = £19.49
  - **Acitretin 25 mg** Acitretin 25mg capsules | 60 capsule [PoM] £55.24 DT = £55.24
- **Neotigason** (Teva UK Ltd)
  - **Acitretin 10 mg** Neotigason 10mg capsules | 60 capsule [PoM] £17.30 DT = £19.49
  - **Acitretin 25 mg** Neotigason 25mg capsules | 60 capsule [PoM] £43.00 DT = £55.24

SALICYLIC ACID AND DERIVATIVES

Salicylic acid with zinc oxide

23-Nov-2020

- **INDICATIONS AND DOSE**

Hyperkeratotic skin disorders

▶ TO THE SKIN
- Child: Apply twice daily

- **CAUTIONS** Avoid broken skin · avoid inflamed skin

CAUTIONS, FURTHER INFORMATION
- Salicylate toxicity Salicylate toxicity may occur particularly if applied on large areas of skin or neonatal skin.

- **SIDE-EFFECTS** Skin irritation
- **PRESCRIBING AND DISPENSING INFORMATION** Zinc and Salicylic Acid Paste BP is also referred to as Lassar's Paste. When prepared extemporaneously, the BP states Zinc and Salicylic Acid Paste, BP (Lassar's Paste) consists of zinc oxide 24%, salicylic acid 2%, starch 24%, white soft paraffin 50%.
- **MEDICINAL FORMS** Forms available from special-order manufacturers include: cutaneous paste

VITAMINS AND TRACE ELEMENTS › VITAMIN D AND ANALOGUES

Calcipotriol

28-Jun-2021

- **INDICATIONS AND DOSE**

Plaque psoriasis

▶ TO THE SKIN USING OINTMENT
- Child 6–11 years: Apply twice daily, when preparations used together maximum total calcipotriol 2.5 mg in any one week (e.g. scalp solution 20 mL with ointment 30 g); maximum 50 g per week
- Child 12–17 years: Apply twice daily, when preparations used together maximum total calcipotriol 3.75 mg in any one week (e.g. scalp solution 30 mL with ointment 45 g); maximum 75 g per week

Scalp psoriasis

▶ TO THE SKIN USING SCALP LOTION
- Child 6–11 years (specialist use only): Apply twice daily, when preparations used together max. total calcipotriol 2.5 mg in any one week (e.g. scalp solution 20 mL with ointment 30 g); maximum 30 mL per week
- Child 12–17 years (specialist use only): Apply twice daily, when preparations used together maximum total calcipotriol 3.75 mg in any one week (e.g. scalp solution 30 mL with ointment 45 g); maximum 45 mL per week

- **UNLICENSED USE** Calcipotriol ointment and scalp solution not licensed for use in children.
- **CONTRA-INDICATIONS** Calcium metabolism disorders
- **CAUTIONS** Avoid excessive exposure to sunlight and sunlamps · avoid use on face · erythrodermic exfoliative psoriasis (enhanced risk of hypercalcaemia) · generalised pustular psoriasis (enhanced risk of hypercalcaemia)
- **INTERACTIONS** → Appendix 1: vitamin D substances
- **SIDE-EFFECTS**
  - **Common or very common** Skin reactions
  - **Uncommon** Hypercalcaemia · increased risk of infection
  - **Rare or very rare** Hypercalciuria · photosensitivity reaction
- **PREGNANCY** Manufacturers advise avoid unless essential.
- **BREAST FEEDING** No information available.
- **HEPATIC IMPAIRMENT** Manufacturers advise avoid in severe impairment (no information available).
- **RENAL IMPAIRMENT** [EvGr] Avoid in severe impairment (no information available). (M)

- **PATIENT AND CARER ADVICE**
Advice on application Patient information leaflet for *Dovonex*® ointment advises liberal application. However, patients should be advised of maximum recommended weekly dose.
Hands should be washed thoroughly after application to avoid inadvertent transfer to other body areas.

- **MEDICINAL FORMS** There can be variation in the licensing of different medicines containing the same drug.

Cutaneous ointment

EXCIPIENTS: May contain Disodium edetate, propylene glycol

- Calcipotriol (Non-proprietary)
  Calcipotriol 50 microgram per 1 gram Calcipotriol 50micrograms/g ointment | 30 gram PoM £9.82 DT = £8.56 | 60 gram PoM £9.83–£19.84 | 120 gram PoM £19.64–£39.28
- Dovonex (LEO Pharma)
  Calcipotriol 50 microgram per 1 gram Dovonex 50micrograms/g ointment | 30 gram PoM £5.78 DT = £8.56 | 60 gram PoM £11.56

Combinations available: *Calcipotriol with betamethasone*, p. 910

787

Calcitriol

12-Mar-2026

(1,25-Dihydroxycholecalciferol)

- **INDICATIONS AND DOSE**

Mild to moderate plaque psoriasis

- TO THE SKIN
- Child 12–17 years: Apply twice daily, not more than 35% of body surface to be treated daily; maximum 30 g per day

- **UNLICENSED USE** Not licensed for use in children.
- **CONTRA-INDICATIONS** Do not apply under occlusion · patients with calcium metabolism disorders
- **CAUTIONS** Erythrodermic exfoliative psoriasis (enhanced risk of hypercalcaemia) · generalised pustular psoriasis (enhanced risk of hypercalcaemia)
- **INTERACTIONS** → Appendix 1: vitamin D substances
- **SIDE-EFFECTS** Since systemic absorption might follow topical use, also consider the side-effects of systemic vitamin D and analogues.
- **PREGNANCY** Manufacturer advises use in restricted amounts only if clearly necessary.
Monitoring EvGr Monitor plasma-calcium concentration in pregnancy. (M)
- **BREAST FEEDING** Manufacturer advises avoid.
- **HEPATIC IMPAIRMENT** Manufacturer advises avoid.
- **RENAL IMPAIRMENT** Manufacturer advises avoid—no information available.
- **HANDLING AND STORAGE** Hands should be washed thoroughly after application to avoid inadvertent transfer to other body areas.

- **MEDICINAL FORMS** There can be variation in the licensing of different medicines containing the same drug.

Cutaneous ointment

- Silkis (Galderma (UK) Ltd)
  Calcitriol 3 microgram per 1 gram Silkis ointment | 100 gram PoM £18.06 DT = £18.06

Tacalcitol

16-Feb-2021

- **INDICATIONS AND DOSE**

Plaque psoriasis

- TO THE SKIN
- Child 12–17 years: Apply once daily, preferably at bedtime, maximum 10 g ointment or 10 mL lotion daily, when lotion and ointment used together, maximum total tacalcitol 280 micrograms in any one week (e.g. lotion 30 mL with ointment 40 g)

- **UNLICENSED USE** Expert sources advise that tacalcitol may be used in children from the age of 12 years, but it is not licensed for this age group.
- **CONTRA-INDICATIONS** Calcium metabolism disorders
- **CAUTIONS** Avoid eyes · erythrodermic exfoliative psoriasis (enhanced risk of hypercalcaemia) · generalised pustular psoriasis (enhanced risk of hypercalcaemia) · if used in conjunction with UV treatment

CAUTIONS, FURTHER INFORMATION

- UV treatment EvGr If tacalcitol is used in conjunction with UV treatment, UV radiation should be given in the morning and tacalcitol applied at bedtime. (M)

- **INTERACTIONS** → Appendix 1: vitamin D substances
- **SIDE-EFFECTS**
  - **Uncommon** Skin reactions
  - **Frequency not known** Hypercalcaemia
- **PREGNANCY** Manufacturer advises avoid unless no safer alternative—no information available.
- **BREAST FEEDING** Manufacturer advises avoid application to breast area; no information available on presence in milk.
- **RENAL IMPAIRMENT**
Monitoring Monitor serum calcium concentration.
- **MONITORING REQUIREMENTS** Monitor serum calcium if risk of hypercalcaemia.
- **PATIENT AND CARER ADVICE** Hands should be washed thoroughly after application to avoid inadvertent transfer to other body areas.

- **MEDICINAL FORMS** No licensed medicines listed.

6 Perspiration

6.1 Hyperhidrosis

Hyperhidrosis

16-Jun-2020

Overview

Hyperhidrosis is defined as sweating in excess of normal body temperature regulation. It can be localised (focal) or affect the entire skin area and can be classified by the absence (primary) or presence (secondary) of an underlying cause.

EvGr Children with primary focal hyperhidrosis affecting axillae, palmar, or plantar areas, should be offered a topical preparation containing 20% aluminium chloride hexahydrate p. 931. (A) This is a more potent antiperspirant compared to commercially available preparations and is available as a spray, roll-on, or solution. EvGr If the response to treatment is inadequate or not tolerated after 6 weeks, consider referral to a specialist.

Specialist management and treatment may also be appropriate in more severe cases of hyperhidrosis. Topical glycopyrronium bromide p. 931 as a 0.05% solution, may be used in the iontophoretic treatment of hyperhidrosis of plantar and palmar areas. *Botox*® contains botulinum toxin type A complex p. 311 and is available for intradermal use in children aged 12 years and over with severe hyperhidrosis of the axillae unresponsive to topical antiperspirant or other antihidrotic treatment. (A)

ANTIMUSCARINICS

177 603

Glycopyrronium bromide
17-Jan-2024

(Glycopyrrolate)

● **INDICATIONS AND DOSE**

Iontophoretic treatment of hyperhidrosis

▶ TO THE SKIN

▶ Child: Only 1 site to be treated at a time, maximum 2 sites treated in any 24 hours, treatment not to be repeated within 7 days (consult product literature)

● **CONTRA-INDICATIONS** Infections affecting the treatment site

CONTRA-INDICATIONS, FURTHER INFORMATION Contra-indications applicable to systemic use should be considered; however, glycopyrronium is poorly absorbed and systemic effects unlikely with topical use.

● **CAUTIONS** Cautions applicable to systemic use should be considered; however, glycopyrronium is poorly absorbed and systemic effects unlikely with topical use.

● **INTERACTIONS** → Appendix 1: glycopyrronium

● **SIDE-EFFECTS** Abdominal discomfort · eating disorder · pain · paraesthesia

SIDE-EFFECTS, FURTHER INFORMATION The possibility of systemic side-effects should be considered; however, glycopyrronium is poorly absorbed and systemic effects are unlikely with topical use.

● **MEDICINAL FORMS** No licensed medicines listed.

DERMATOLOGICAL DRUGS › ASTRINGENTS

Aluminium chloride hexahydrate
21-Nov-2020

● **INDICATIONS AND DOSE**

Hyperhidrosis affecting axillae, hands or feet

▶ TO THE SKIN

▶ Child: Apply once daily, apply liquid formulation at night to dry skin, wash off the following morning, reduce frequency as condition improves—do not bathe immediately before use

Hyperhidrosis | Bromidrosis | Intertrigo | Prevention of tinea pedis and related conditions

▶ TO THE SKIN

▶ Child: Apply powder to dry skin

● **UNLICENSED USE** Licensed for use in children (age range not specified by manufacturer).

● **CAUTIONS** Avoid contact with eyes · avoid contact with mucous membranes · avoid use on broken or irritated skin · do not shave axillae or use depilatories within 12 hours of application

● **SIDE-EFFECTS** Skin reactions

● **PATIENT AND CARER ADVICE** Avoid contact with clothing.

● **EXCEPTIONS TO LEGAL CATEGORY** A 30 mL pack of aluminium chloride hexahydrate 20% is on sale to the public.

● **MEDICINAL FORMS** There can be variation in the licensing of different medicines containing the same drug.

Cutaneous solution

CAUTIONARY AND ADVISORY LABELS 15

▶ **Anhydrol** (Dermal Laboratories Ltd)
Aluminium chloride hexahydrate 200 mg per 1 ml Anhydrol Forte 20% solution | 60 ml [P] £2.99 DT = £2.99

▶ **Driclor** (Haleon UK Trading Ltd)
Aluminium chloride hexahydrate 200 mg per 1 ml Driclor 20% solution | 75 ml [P] £7.61

7 Pruritus

Topical local antipruritics

Overview

Pruritus may be caused by systemic disease (such as obstructive jaundice, endocrine disease, chronic renal disease, iron deficiency, and certain malignant diseases), skin disease (such as eczema, psoriasis, urticaria, and scabies), drug hypersensitivity, or as a side-effect of opioid analgesics. Where possible, the underlying cause should be treated. Local antipruritics have a role in the treatment of pruritus in palliative care. Pruritus caused by cholestasis generally requires a bile acid sequestrant.

An **emollient** may be of value where the pruritus is associated with dry skin. Preparations containing calamine or crotamiton p. 932 are sometimes used but are of uncertain value.

A topical preparation containing doxepin 5% p. 932 is licensed for the relief of pruritus in eczema in children over 12 years; it can cause drowsiness and there may be a risk of sensitisation.

Topical antihistamines and local anaesthetics are only marginally effective and occasionally cause sensitisation. For *insect stings* and *insect bites*, a short course of a topical corticosteroid is appropriate. Short-term treatment with a **sedating antihistamine** may help in insect stings and in intractable pruritus where sedation is desirable. Calamine preparations are of little value for the treatment of insect stings or bites.

In *pruritus ani*, the underlying cause such as faecal soiling, eczema, psoriasis, or helminth infection should be treated.

Other drugs used for Pruritus Alimemazine tartrate, p. 205 · Cetirizine hydrochloride, p. 202 · Chlorphenamine maleate, p. 205 · Hydroxyzine hydrochloride, p. 206 · Levocetirizine hydrochloride, p. 203

ANTIPRURITICS

Calamine with zinc oxide
11-Mar-2020

● **INDICATIONS AND DOSE**

Minor skin conditions

▶ TO THE SKIN

▶ Child: (consult product literature)

IMPORTANT SAFETY INFORMATION

MHRA/CHM ADVICE (UPDATED DECEMBER 2018): EMOLLIENTS: NEW INFORMATION ABOUT RISK OF SEVERE AND FATAL BURNS WITH PARAFFIN-CONTAINING AND PARAFFIN-FREE EMOLLIENTS

See Emollient and barrier preparations p. 888.

● **CONTRA-INDICATIONS** Avoid application of preparations containing zinc oxide prior to x-ray (zinc oxide may affect outcome of x-ray)

● **LESS SUITABLE FOR PRESCRIBING** Less suitable for prescribing.

● **MEDICINAL FORMS** There can be variation in the licensing of different medicines containing the same drug.

Cutaneous cream

CAUTIONARY AND ADVISORY LABELS 15

▶ **Calamine with zinc oxide (Non-proprietary)**
Phenoxyethanol 5 mg per 1 gram, Zinc oxide 30 mg per 1 gram, Calamine 40 mg per 1 gram, Cetomacrogol emulsifying wax 50 mg per 1 gram, Self-emulsifying glyceryl monostearate 50 mg per 1 gram, Liquid paraffin 200 mg per 1 gram Aqueous calamine cream | 100 gram [GSL] £2.34 DT = £2.34

Cutaneous liquid

▸ Calamine with zinc oxide (Non-proprietary)

Phenol liquefied 5 mg per 1 ml, Sodium citrate 5 mg per 1 ml, Bentonite 30 mg per 1 ml, Glycerol 50 mg per 1 ml, Zinc oxide 50 mg per 1 ml, Calamine 150 mg per 1 ml Calamine lotion | 200 ml GSL £1.73–£4.90 DT = £2.85

Crotamiton

29-Apr-2020

● **INDICATIONS AND DOSE**

Pruritus (including pruritus after scabies)

▸ TO THE SKIN

▸ Child 1 month–2 years (on doctor's advice only): Apply once daily

▸ Child 3–17 years: Apply 2–3 times a day

● **CONTRA-INDICATIONS** Acute exudative dermatoses

● **CAUTIONS** Avoid use in buccal mucosa · avoid use near eyes · avoid use on broken skin · avoid use on very inflamed skin · use on doctor's advice for children under 3 years

● **PREGNANCY** Manufacturer advises avoid, especially during the first trimester—no information available.

● **BREAST FEEDING** No information available; avoid application to nipple area.

● **MEDICINAL FORMS** There can be variation in the licensing of different medicines containing the same drug.

Cutaneous cream

EXCIPIENTS: May contain Beeswax, cetostearyl alcohol (including cetyl and stearyl alcohol), fragrances, hydroxybenzoates (parabens)

▸ Eurax (Thornton & Ross Ltd)

Crotamiton 100 mg per 1 gram Eurax 10% cream | 30 gram GSL £3.13 DT = £3.13 | 100 gram GSL £5.91 DT = £5.91

Doxepin

20-Apr-2021

● **INDICATIONS AND DOSE**

Pruritus in eczema

▸ TO THE SKIN

▸ Child 12–17 years: Apply up to 3 g 3–4 times a day, apply thinly; coverage should be less than 10% of body surface area; maximum 12 g per day

● **CAUTIONS** Arrhythmias · avoid application to large areas · mania · severe heart disease · susceptibility to angle-closure glaucoma · urinary retention

● **INTERACTIONS** → Appendix 1: tricyclic antidepressants

● **SIDE-EFFECTS** Constipation · diarrhoea · dizziness · drowsiness · dry eye · dry mouth · dyspepsia · fever · headache · nausea · paraesthesia · skin reactions · suicidal behaviours · taste altered · urinary retention · vision blurred · vomiting

● **PREGNANCY** Manufacturer advises use only if potential benefit outweighs risk.

● **BREAST FEEDING** Manufacturer advises use only if potential benefit outweighs risk.

● **HEPATIC IMPAIRMENT** Manufacturer advises caution in severe impairment.

● **PATIENT AND CARER ADVICE** A patient information leaflet should be provided.

Driving and skilled tasks Drowsiness may affect performance of skilled tasks (e.g. driving). Effects of alcohol enhanced.

● **MEDICINAL FORMS** There can be variation in the licensing of different medicines containing the same drug.

Cutaneous cream

CAUTIONARY AND ADVISORY LABELS 2, 10

EXCIPIENTS: May contain Benzyl alcohol

▸ Xepin (Cambridge Healthcare Supplies Ltd)

Doxepin hydrochloride 50 mg per 1 gram Xepin 5% cream | 30 gram PoM £13.66 DT = £13.66

8 Rosacea and acne

Acne

18-Jun-2024

Description of condition

Acne is a common inflammatory skin condition that leads to lesions which consist of non-inflammatory comedones, and inflammatory papules, pustules, nodules and cysts. In patients with acne, lesions and/or scarring may be seen and severity can range from mild lesions to permanent disfiguration. It can also have a psychological and social impact on the patient.

Acne vulgaris is a common type of acne that primarily affects the face, back, and chest; it is most common in adolescence, but may affect those in any age group. Other types of acne include acne conglobata, a severe form of nodulo-cystic acne with interconnecting sinuses and abscesses; and acne fulminans, a very serious form of acne conglobata that is associated with systemic symptoms (such as fever and arthralgia).

The severity of acne varies along a continuum from mild to moderate to severe, that is characterised by the lesion type (s) and quantity. Patients with mild to moderate acne are those with 1 or more of the following: non-inflammatory lesions (of any number), up to 34 inflammatory lesions, up to 2 nodules. Patients with moderate to severe acne are those who have 35 or more inflammatory lesions and/or 3 or more nodules.

Aims of treatment

Treatment aims to reduce the severity of skin lesions and other complications, and to prevent recurrence and scarring.

Management of acne

Patients with acne fulminans should be urgently referred to hospital for assessment by the dermatology team within 24 hours.

Patients with acne conglobata, nodulo-cystic acne, or those with diagnostic uncertainty about their acne, should be referred to a consultant dermatologist-led team or a nationally accredited GP with an extended role (GPwER) working within a consultant dermatologist-agreed pathway.

For patients with acne vulgaris, referral to a consultant dermatologist-led team or a GPwER working within a consultant dermatologist-agreed pathway should be considered if they have scarring or persistent pigmentary changes, or if their acne or acne-related scarring is causing or contributing to persistent psychological distress or a mental health disorder.

Referral to a mental health service should also be considered for patients whose acne is contributing to psychological distress or a mental health disorder (including those who have a current or past history of suicidal ideation or self-harm, body morphic disorder, or a severe depressive or anxiety disorder).

EvGr Consider condition-specific management or specialist referral if a medication or medical disorder is contributing to the patient's acne. (A) Specialist referral should also be considered for individuals with acne and polycystic ovary syndrome (PCOS) with features of hyperandrogenism.

Non-drug treatment

EvGr Children with acne vulgaris should be advised on appropriate skin care such as using a non-alkaline, synthetic detergent cleansing product twice daily on acne-prone areas, removing make up at the end of the day, and avoiding the use of oil-based or comedogenic skincare products, sunscreens, and make-up. They should also be advised to avoid persistent picking or scratching of lesions. Ⓐ

Drug treatment

EvGr Patients with mild to moderate and moderate to severe acne vulgaris should be offered a 12-week course of a first-line treatment option, taking into account the severity and distribution of their acne, their preferences, and that the risk of scarring increases with acne severity and duration. Any potential use of oral isotretinoin in the future for severe forms of acne will be dependent on the completion of adequate courses of first-line treatments including systemic antibacterials and topical therapy, and should also be taken into consideration when deciding on initial treatment options. The use of antibacterial monotherapy or a combination of a topical and oral antibacterial are not recommended. Patients should be informed that the benefits of treatment may take between 6–8 weeks to become noticeable and hence the importance of completing the course.

Females receiving acne treatment who wish to use hormonal contraception could consider using an oral combined hormonal contraceptive, Ⓐ as combined hormonal contraceptive use may be associated with improvement of acne.

EvGr When considering treatment options that include known teratogenic drugs or drugs with teratogenic potential (such as topical or oral retinoids, or oral tetracyclines), specific contraception requirements should be taken into consideration and discussed with patients, see individual drug monographs for further information. Ⓐ

First-line treatment options for acne vulgaris

- Acne of any severity:
  - EvGr Fixed combination topical adapalene with benzoyl peroxide p. 937, or
  - Fixed combination topical tretinoin with clindamycin p. 939. Ⓐ
- Mild to moderate acne:
  - EvGr Fixed combination topical benzoyl peroxide with clindamycin p. 936. Ⓐ
- Moderate to severe acne:
  - EvGr Fixed combination topical adapalene with benzoyl peroxide **with** oral lymecycline p. 435 or doxycycline p. 434, or
  - Topical azelaic acid p. 936 **with** oral lymecycline or doxycycline. Ⓐ
  - Alternative antibacterial options if lymecycline or doxycycline unsuitable: EvGr trimethoprim p. 443 [unlicensed] **or** a macrolide (such as erythromycin p. 406). Ⓐ
- Alternative if first-line options are contra-indicated, or the patient wishes to avoid antibacterials or topical retinoids: EvGr topical benzoyl peroxide p. 936 monotherapy. Ⓐ

For further information on the management of acne vulgaris, such as the advantages and disadvantages of each treatment option, see NICE guideline: **Acne** (see *Useful resources*).

Reassessment and further treatment

EvGr Review first-line treatment after 12 weeks. For patients whose acne has cleared, maintenance options should also be considered Ⓐ (see *Maintenance*).

EvGr For patients whose treatment included an oral antibacterial and their acne has completely cleared, consider continuing their topical treatment and stopping the oral antibacterial. If their acne has improved but not cleared, consider continuing the course for up to a further 12 weeks. Treatment courses that include an antibacterial should only be continued for more than 6 months in exceptional circumstances, and should be reviewed every 3 months.

For patients with mild to moderate acne who have had an inadequate response to treatment after 12 weeks, offer another first-line option. Ⓐ For those who have mild to moderate acne unresponsive to 2 completed treatment courses, consider referral to a consultant dermatologist-led team or a GPwER working within a consultant dermatologist-agreed pathway.

EvGr For patients with moderate to severe acne who have had an inadequate response to treatment that did not include an oral antibacterial, offer another first-line option which includes an oral antibacterial. Ⓐ For those whose treatment included an oral antibacterial, consider referral to a consultant dermatologist-led team or a GPwER working within a consultant dermatologist-agreed pathway.

EvGr For females with PCOS that have not improved following treatment with a first-line option, consider adding ethinylestradiol with cyproterone (co-cyprindiol p. 934) and review at 6 months, or an alternative combined oral contraceptive pill [unlicensed]. Ⓐ

For further information on the drug treatment of acne vulgaris, including the use of intralesional corticosteroids and the management of acne-related scarring, see NICE guideline: **Acne** (see *Useful resources*).

Isotretinoin

EvGr For patients with severe acne (such as acne conglobata or fulminans, nodulo-cystic acne, or acne at risk of permanent scarring) that is resistant to adequate courses of oral antibacterial-containing first-line treatments, consider oral isotretinoin p. 937 (specialist use by a consultant dermatologist-led team or a GPwER working within a consultant dermatologist-agreed pathway). Take into account the patient's psychological wellbeing, and refer them to mental health services before starting treatment if appropriate. Ⓐ

Isotretinoin is a powerful teratogen; for females of childbearing potential isotretinoin must only be used if the conditions of the Pregnancy Prevention Programme are met. For further information, see *Important safety information*, *Conception and contraception*, and *Prescribing and dispensing information* in the isotretinoin monograph, and *Contraception in patients taking medication with teratogenic potential* in Contraceptives, hormonal p. 609.

EvGr For acne flares that occur after starting isotretinoin, a course of oral prednisolone p. 548 may be considered. Ⓐ For further information on acne flares, see NICE guideline: **Acne** (see *Useful resources*).

Relapse

EvGr For acne that responds adequately to a course of first-line treatment but then relapses, consider another 12-week course of either the same treatment or an alternative treatment option. Ⓐ For treatment options, see *First-line treatment options*.

EvGr If acne relapses after an adequate response to oral isotretinoin and is currently mild to moderate, offer an appropriate first-line treatment option. If acne relapses after an adequate response to oral isotretinoin and is currently moderate to severe, offer either a 12-week course of an appropriate first-line treatment option or re-referral if the patient is no longer under the care of a consultant dermatologist-led team or a GPwER working within a consultant dermatologist-agreed pathway. For individuals with moderate to severe acne that relapses after a second course of oral isotretinoin, further care should be provided by their dermatology team; offer re-referral if the patient is no longer under the care of the consultant dermatologist-led team or a GPwER working within a consultant dermatologist-agreed pathway. Ⓐ

Maintenance

EvGr On completion of treatment, the need for maintenance treatment is not always necessary; advise patients that appropriate skin care should be continued. In patients with a history of frequent relapse, consider maintenance treatment using a fixed combination of topical adapalene with benzoyl peroxide p. 937. If this is not tolerated or one component of the combination is contra-indicated, consider topical monotherapy with either adapalene p. 936, azelaic acid p. 936, or benzoyl peroxide p. 936. Maintenance treatments should be reviewed after 12 weeks and a decision made about continuation. (A)

Acne in neonates and infants

Lesions such as comedones, and inflammatory papules and pustules may develop at birth or within the first six weeks of life (neonatal acne); these do not usually result in scarring. Other types of self-limiting inflammatory lesions may also occur. Acne developing from 6 weeks to 1 year of age (infantile acne) may be mild to moderate in severity and usually settles within a few months. Lesions predominantly affect the cheeks and occasionally leave scarring.

EvGr Treatment options for infantile acne may include topical preparations such as benzoyl peroxide [unlicensed use] and adapalene [unlicensed use], or oral erythromycin p. 406 [unlicensed use]. In cases of severe infantile acne, oral isotretinoin [unlicensed use] may be used under expert supervision. (E)

Useful Resources

Acne vulgaris: management. National Institute for Health and Care Excellence guideline NG198. June 2021, updated December 2023.
www.nice.org.uk/guidance/ng198

Rosacea

29-Sep-2020

Rosacea

The adult form of rosacea rarely occurs in children. Persistent or repeated use of potent topical corticosteroids may cause periorificial rosacea (steroid acne). The pustules and papules of rosacea may be treated for at least 6 weeks with a topical metronidazole preparation p. 898, or a systemic antibacterial such as erythromycin p. 406, or for a child over 12 years, oxytetracycline p. 436. Tetracyclines are **contra-indicated** in children under 12 years of age.

8.1 Acne

Other drugs used for Acne Minocycline, p. 436 · Oxytetracycline, p. 436

ANTI-ANDROGENS

Clascoterone

24-Mar-2025

● **DRUG ACTION** Clascoterone is an androgen receptor inhibitor.

● **INDICATIONS AND DOSE**

Acne vulgaris

▶ TO THE SKIN

▶ Child 12–17 years: Apply twice daily, 1 g of cream to be applied thinly in the morning and evening

● **CAUTIONS** Avoid contact with broken skin · avoid contact with eczematous skin · avoid contact with eyes · avoid contact with mouth · avoid contact with mucous membranes · avoid contact with sunburned skin

● **SIDE-EFFECTS**

▶ **Common or very common** Hyperkalaemia · skin reactions · telangiectasia

▶ **Rare or very rare** Amenorrhoea · polycystic ovaries

▶ **Frequency not known** Hair colour changes · headache · suppression of the hypothalamic-pituitary-adrenal axis

● **PREGNANCY** EvGr Use with caution (limited information available). (M)

● **BREAST FEEDING** Specialist sources indicate amounts in milk are probably low and unlikely to affect breast-fed infants due to poor absorption and high plasma-protein binding (no information available); avoid application to nipple area and direct contact with treated skin.

● **MEDICINAL FORMS** There can be variation in the licensing of different medicines containing the same drug.

Cutaneous cream

EXCIPIENTS: May contain Cetostearyl alcohol (including cetyl and stearyl alcohol), disodium edetate, polysorbates, propylene glycol

▶ **Winlevi** (Glenmark Pharmaceuticals Europe Ltd) ▼
Clascoterone 10 mg per 1 gram Winlevi 10mg/g cream | 60 gram PoM £19.43 DT = £19.43

Co-cyprindiol

23-Oct-2023

● **INDICATIONS AND DOSE**

Moderate to severe acne vulgaris related to hyperandrogenism caused by polycystic ovary syndrome [adjunct in refractory acne] | Moderately severe hirsutism

▶ BY MOUTH

▶ Females of childbearing potential: 1 tablet daily for 21 days, to be started on day 1 of menstrual cycle; subsequent courses repeated after a 7-day interval (during which withdrawal bleeding occurs), time to symptom remission, at least 3 months; review need for treatment regularly

IMPORTANT SAFETY INFORMATION

MHRA/CHM ADVICE: CYPROTERONE ACETATE: NEW ADVICE TO MINIMISE RISK OF MENINGIOMA (JUNE 2020)

Cyproterone acetate has been associated with an overall rare, but cumulative dose-dependent, increased risk of meningioma (single and multiple), mainly at doses of 25 mg/day and higher. Healthcare professionals are advised to monitor patients for meningiomas, and to permanently discontinue treatment if diagnosed. Use of cyproterone acetate, including co-cyprindiol, for all indications is contra-indicated in those with meningioma or a history of meningioma.

● **CONTRA-INDICATIONS** Acute porphyrias p. 745 · atrial fibrillation · Budd-Chiari syndrome · cardiomyopathy with impaired cardiac function · complicated congenital heart disease · complicated valvular heart disease · current breast cancer · history of stroke (including transient ischaemic attack) · hypertension (blood pressure systolic 160 mmHg or diastolic 100 mmHg or higher) · hypertensive retinopathy · ischaemic heart disease · known thrombogenic mutations (e.g. factor V Leiden, prothrombin mutation, protein S, protein C and antithrombin deficiencies) · less than 3 weeks postpartum in non-breastfeeding women with other risk factors for venous thromboembolism · major surgery with prolonged immobilisation · migraine with aura · peripheral vascular disease with intermittent claudication · positive antiphospholipid antibodies · presence or history of liver tumours (benign or malignant) · previous or current venous or arterial thrombosis · severe or multiple risk factors for arterial or venous thromboembolism · systemic lupus erythematosus with antiphospholipid antibodies

- **CAUTIONS** Cervical intraepithelial neoplasia or cancer · cholestasis with previous use of combined oral contraception—seek specialist advice before use · gallbladder disease—if medically treated or current, seek specialist advice before use · gene mutations associated with breast cancer (e.g. BRCA 1)—seek specialist advice before use · history of breast cancer—seek specialist advice before use · history of cholestasis during pregnancy · history of depression · inflammatory bowel disease · migraine · organ transplantation—when complicated, seek specialist advice before use · personal or family history of hypertriglyceridaemia (increased risk of pancreatitis) · prolactinoma—seek specialist advice before use · risk factors for arterial thromboembolism · risk factors for cardiovascular disease · risk factors for venous thromboembolism · sickle-cell disease · systemic lupus erythematosus · undiagnosed breast mass—seek specialist advice before use · undiagnosed vaginal bleeding

CAUTIONS, FURTHER INFORMATION

- Venous thromboembolism There is an increased risk of venous thromboembolism in females taking co-cyprindiol, particularly during the first year of use. The incidence of venous thromboembolism is 1.5–2 times higher in females using co-cyprindiol than in females using oral combined hormonal contraceptives containing levonorgestrel, but the risk may be similar to that associated with use of oral combined hormonal contraceptives containing third generation progestogens (desogestrel and gestodene) or drospirenone.

  For more information about the risk factors for venous thromboembolism, see cautions for combined hormonal contraceptive preparations (e.g. ethinylestradiol with gestodene p. 621).
- Cardiovascular disease Co-cyprindiol also slightly increases the risk of cardiovascular disease, such as myocardial infarction and ischaemic stroke. Females requiring co-cyprindiol may have an inherently increased risk of cardiovascular disease such as that associated with polycystic ovary syndrome.

  For more information about the risk factors for cardiovascular disease, see cautions for combined hormonal contraceptive preparations (e.g. ethinylestradiol with gestodene p. 621).

- **INTERACTIONS** → Appendix 1: anti-androgens · ethinylestradiol
- **SIDE-EFFECTS**
  - **Common or very common** Abdominal pain · breast abnormalities · depression · headaches · mood altered · nausea · weight changes
  - **Uncommon** Diarrhoea · fluid retention · sexual dysfunction · skin reactions · vomiting
  - **Rare or very rare** Contact lens intolerance · erythema nodosum · thromboembolism · vaginal discharge
  - **Frequency not known** Amenorrhoea (on discontinuation) · angioedema aggravated · chorea exacerbated · hepatic function abnormal · hepatic neoplasm · hypertension · hypertriglyceridaemia · inflammatory bowel disease · menstrual cycle irregularities · suicidal behaviours
- **CONCEPTION AND CONTRACEPTION** [EvGr] Co-cyprindiol contains an anti-androgen and is an effective hormonal contraceptive. However, it should not be used solely for contraception but reserved for females who require treatment for androgen-dependent skin conditions. Patients should not take other hormonal contraceptives while being treated with co-cyprindiol. ⟨M⟩
- **PREGNANCY** Avoid—risk of feminisation of male fetus with cyproterone.
- **BREAST FEEDING** Manufacturer advises avoid; possibility of anti-androgen effects in neonate with cyproterone.
- **HEPATIC IMPAIRMENT** Manufacturer advises caution; avoid in severe or active disease
- **PRESCRIBING AND DISPENSING INFORMATION** A mixture of cyproterone acetate and ethinylestradiol in the mass proportions 2000 parts to 35 parts, respectively.
- **MEDICINAL FORMS** There can be variation in the licensing of different medicines containing the same drug.

Oral tablet

- **Co-cyprindiol (Non-proprietary)**
  Ethinylestradiol 35 microgram, Cyproterone acetate 2 mg Co-cyprindiol 2000microgram/35microgram tablets | 63 tablet [PoM] £12.45 DT = £8.87
- **Clairette** (Kent Pharma (UK) Ltd)
  Ethinylestradiol 35 microgram, Cyproterone acetate 2 mg Clairette 2000/35 tablets | 63 tablet [PoM] £5.90 DT = £8.87
- **Dianette** (Bayer Plc)
  Ethinylestradiol 35 microgram, Cyproterone acetate 2 mg Dianette tablets | 63 tablet [PoM] £7.71 DT = £8.87

ANTIBACTERIALS > LINCOSAMIDES

Clindamycin

22-Mar-2024

- **INDICATIONS AND DOSE**

DALACIN T® LOTION

Acne vulgaris

- TO THE SKIN
- Child: Apply twice daily, to be applied thinly

ZINDACLIN® GEL

Acne vulgaris

- TO THE SKIN
- Child 12–17 years: Apply once daily, to be applied thinly

- **INTERACTIONS** → Appendix 1: clindamycin
- **SIDE-EFFECTS**
  - **Common or very common** Diarrhoea (discontinue) · skin reactions
  - **Frequency not known** Abdominal pain · folliculitis gram-negative · gastrointestinal disorders · pseudomembranous enterocolitis
- **PATIENT AND CARER ADVICE** Patients and their carers should be advised to discontinue and contact a doctor immediately if severe, prolonged or bloody diarrhoea develops.
- **MEDICINAL FORMS** There can be variation in the licensing of different medicines containing the same drug.

Cutaneous gel

EXCIPIENTS: May contain Propylene glycol

- **Zindaclin** (Aspire Pharma Ltd)
  Clindamycin (as Clindamycin phosphate) 10 mg per 1 gram Zindaclin 1% gel | 30 gram [PoM] £9.95 DT = £9.95

Combinations available: *Benzoyl peroxide with clindamycin*, p. 936 · ***Tretinoin with clindamycin*,** p. 939

ANTIBACTERIALS > MACROLIDES

Erythromycin with zinc acetate

20-Apr-2020

The properties listed below are those particular to the combination only. For the properties of the components please consider, erythromycin p. 406.

- **INDICATIONS AND DOSE**

Acne vulgaris

- TO THE SKIN
- Child: Apply twice daily

- **INTERACTIONS** → Appendix 1: macrolides

● **MEDICINAL FORMS** There can be variation in the licensing of different medicines containing the same drug.

Cutaneous solution

▸ **Erythromycin with zinc acetate (Non-proprietary)**
Zinc acetate 12 mg per 1 ml, Erythromycin 40 mg per 1 ml Erythromycin 40mg/ml / Zinc acetate 12mg/ml lotion | 30 ml PoM £9.25 DT = £9.25 | 90 ml PoM £20.02 DT = £20.02

ANTISEPTICS AND DISINFECTANTS › PEROXIDES

Benzoyl peroxide
01-Nov-2021

● **INDICATIONS AND DOSE**

Acne vulgaris

▸ TO THE SKIN
▸ Child 12–17 years: Apply 1–2 times a day, preferably apply after washing with soap and water

Infantile acne

▸ TO THE SKIN
▸ Child 1–23 months: Apply 1–2 times a day

● **UNLICENSED USE** EvGr Benzoyl peroxide is used for the treatment of infantile acne, (E) but is not licensed for this indication.

● **CAUTIONS** Avoid contact with broken skin · avoid contact with eyes · avoid contact with mouth · avoid contact with mucous membranes · avoid excessive exposure to sunlight

● **SIDE-EFFECTS**
▸ **Common or very common** Skin reactions
▸ **Frequency not known** Facial swelling

● **PATIENT AND CARER ADVICE** May bleach fabrics and hair. If sun exposure is unavoidable, an appropriate sunscreen or protective clothing should be used. Patients and carers should be warned that some redness and skin peeling can occur initially but settles with time. To reduce the risk of skin irritation, treatment may be started with alternate-day or short-contact application (e.g. washing off after an hour) and progressed to standard application if tolerated. If severe irritation occurs, the frequency of application should be reduced, or treatment temporarily discontinued or stopped altogether.

● **MEDICINAL FORMS** There can be variation in the licensing of different medicines containing the same drug.

Cutaneous gel

EXCIPIENTS: May contain Fragrances, propylene glycol

▸ **Acnecide** (Galderma (UK) Ltd)
Benzoyl peroxide 50 mg per 1 gram Acnecide 5% gel | 30 gram P £6.26 DT = £6.26 | 60 gram P £12.28 DT = £12.28
Acnecide Wash 5% gel | 100 gram P £8.81

Combinations available: *Adapalene with benzoyl peroxide*, p. 937

Benzoyl peroxide with clindamycin
09-Mar-2020

The properties listed below are those particular to the combination only. For the properties of the components please consider, benzoyl peroxide above, clindamycin p. 935.

● **INDICATIONS AND DOSE**

Acne vulgaris

▸ TO THE SKIN
▸ Child 12–17 years: Apply once daily, dose to be applied in the evening

● **INTERACTIONS** → Appendix 1: clindamycin

● **MEDICINAL FORMS** There can be variation in the licensing of different medicines containing the same drug.

Cutaneous gel

EXCIPIENTS: May contain Disodium edetate

▸ **Benzoyl peroxide with clindamycin (Non-proprietary)**
Clindamycin (as Clindamycin phosphate) 10 mg per 1 gram, Benzoyl peroxide 30 mg per 1 gram Benzoyl peroxide 3% / Clindamycin 1% gel | 30 gram PoM £13.14–£21.02 DT = £13.14 | 60 gram PoM £26.28–£42.04
Clindamycin (as Clindamycin phosphate) 10 mg per 1 gram, Benzoyl peroxide 50 mg per 1 gram Benzoyl peroxide 5% / Clindamycin 1% gel | 30 gram PoM £21.02 DT = £13.14 | 60 gram PoM £42.04 DT = £26.28

▸ **Duac** (Stiefel Laboratories (UK) Ltd)
Clindamycin (as Clindamycin phosphate) 10 mg per 1 gram, Benzoyl peroxide 30 mg per 1 gram Duac Once Daily gel (3% and 1%) | 30 gram PoM £13.14 DT = £13.14 | 60 gram PoM £26.28
Clindamycin (as Clindamycin phosphate) 10 mg per 1 gram, Benzoyl peroxide 50 mg per 1 gram Duac Once Daily gel (5% and 1%) | 30 gram PoM £13.14 DT = £13.14 | 60 gram PoM £26.28 DT = £26.28

DERMATOLOGICAL DRUGS › ANTICOMEDONALS

Azelaic acid
04-Nov-2021

● **INDICATIONS AND DOSE**

FINACEA®

Acne vulgaris

▸ TO THE SKIN
▸ Child 12–17 years: Apply twice daily

SKINOREN®

Acne vulgaris

▸ TO THE SKIN
▸ Child 12–17 years: Apply twice daily

● **CAUTIONS** Avoid contact with eyes · avoid contact with mouth · avoid contact with mucous membranes

● **SIDE-EFFECTS**
▸ **Uncommon** Skin reactions
▸ **Rare or very rare** Asthma exacerbated · cheilitis
▸ **Frequency not known** Angioedema · eye swelling

● **PATIENT AND CARER ADVICE** If severe skin irritation occurs, the amount of preparation applied or frequency of application should be reduced, or treatment temporarily discontinued. In patients with sensitive skin, treatment may be started with once-daily application (in the evening) and progressed to twice-daily application if tolerated.

● **MEDICINAL FORMS** There can be variation in the licensing of different medicines containing the same drug.

Cutaneous cream

EXCIPIENTS: May contain Propylene glycol

▸ **Skinoren** (LEO Pharma)
Azelaic acid 200 mg per 1 gram Skinoren 20% cream | 50 gram PoM £7.48

Cutaneous gel

EXCIPIENTS: May contain Disodium edetate, polysorbates, propylene glycol

▸ **Finacea** (LEO Pharma)
Azelaic acid 150 mg per 1 gram Finacea 15% gel | 30 gram PoM £7.48 DT = £7.48

RETINOID AND RELATED DRUGS

Adapalene
28-Jun-2023

● **INDICATIONS AND DOSE**

Mild to moderate acne vulgaris

▸ TO THE SKIN
▸ Child 12–17 years: Apply once daily, apply thinly in the evening

13 Skin

Infantile acne
- ▶ TO THE SKIN
- ▸ Child 1–23 months: Apply once daily, apply thinly in the evening

- **UNLICENSED USE** EvGr Adapalene is used for the treatment of infantile acne, ⟨E⟩ but is not licensed for this indication.
- **CAUTIONS** Avoid accumulation in angles of the nose · avoid contact with eyes, nostrils, mouth and mucous membranes, eczematous, broken or sunburned skin · avoid exposure to UV light (including sunlight, solariums) · avoid in severe acne involving large areas · caution in sensitive areas such as the neck
- **INTERACTIONS** → Appendix 1: retinoids
- **CONCEPTION AND CONTRACEPTION** The MHRA advises females of childbearing potential should use effective contraception.
- **PREGNANCY** The MHRA advises that systemic exposure is thought to be negligible following application of topical retinoids. However, since risk cannot be excluded, use of topical retinoids is contra-indicated during pregnancy as a precaution.
- **BREAST FEEDING** Amount of drug in milk probably too small to be harmful; ensure infant does not come in contact with treated areas.
- **PATIENT AND CARER ADVICE** If sun exposure is unavoidable, an appropriate sunscreen or protective clothing should be used. To reduce the risk of skin irritation, treatment may be started with alternate-day or short-contact application (e.g. washing off after an hour) and progressed to standard application if tolerated. If severe irritation occurs, the frequency of application should be reduced, or treatment temporarily discontinued or stopped altogether.
- **MEDICINAL FORMS** There can be variation in the licensing of different medicines containing the same drug.

Cutaneous cream

CAUTIONARY AND ADVISORY LABELS 11

EXCIPIENTS: May contain Disodium edetate, hydroxybenzoates (parabens)

▸ **Differin** (Galderma (UK) Ltd)

Adapalene 1 mg per 1 gram Differin 0.1% cream | 50 gram PoM £18.26 DT = £18.26

Cutaneous gel

CAUTIONARY AND ADVISORY LABELS 11

EXCIPIENTS: May contain Disodium edetate, hydroxybenzoates (parabens), propylene glycol

▸ **Differin** (Galderma (UK) Ltd)

Adapalene 1 mg per 1 gram Differin 0.1% gel | 50 gram PoM £18.26 DT = £18.26

Adapalene with benzoyl peroxide

28-Jun-2023

The properties listed below are those particular to the combination only. For the properties of the components please consider, adapalene p. 936, benzoyl peroxide p. 936.

- **INDICATIONS AND DOSE**

Acne vulgaris
- ▶ TO THE SKIN
- ▸ Child 9–17 years: Apply once daily, to be applied thinly in the evening

- **INTERACTIONS** → Appendix 1: retinoids
- **NATIONAL FUNDING/ACCESS DECISIONS** For full details see funding body website

Scottish Medicines Consortium (SMC) decisions

▶ **Adapalene 0.1 % with benzoyl peroxide 2.5 % gel (*Epiduo*®) for the cutaneous treatment of acne vulgaris when comedones, papules and pustules are present (April 2014)** SMC No. 682/11 Recommended with restrictions

- **MEDICINAL FORMS** There can be variation in the licensing of different medicines containing the same drug.

Cutaneous gel

CAUTIONARY AND ADVISORY LABELS 11

EXCIPIENTS: May contain Disodium edetate, polysorbates, propylene glycol

▸ **Adapalene with benzoyl peroxide (Non-proprietary)**

Adapalene 3 mg per 1 gram, Benzoyl peroxide 25 mg per 1 gram Adapalene 0.3% / Benzoyl peroxide 2.5% gel | 45 gram PoM £20.75 | 60 gram PoM £27.00 DT = £27.80

Adapalene 1 mg per 1 gram, Benzoyl peroxide 25 mg per 1 gram Adapalene 0.1% / Benzoyl peroxide 2.5% gel | 30 gram PoM £13.90 | 45 gram PoM £18.26–£20.85 DT = £20.85 | 60 gram PoM £27.80 DT = £27.80

▸ **Epiduo** (Galderma (UK) Ltd)

Adapalene 3 mg per 1 gram, Benzoyl peroxide 25 mg per 1 gram Epiduo 0.3%/2.5% gel | 60 gram PoM £27.80 DT = £27.80

Adapalene 1 mg per 1 gram, Benzoyl peroxide 25 mg per 1 gram Epiduo 0.1%/2.5% gel | 60 gram PoM £27.80 DT = £27.80

Isotretinoin

30-Jan-2026

- **INDICATIONS AND DOSE**

Severe acne [(such as nodular or conglobate acne or acne at risk of permanent scarring) resistant to adequate courses of standard therapy with systemic antibacterials and topical therapy] (under expert supervision)
- ▶ BY MOUTH
- ▸ Child 12–17 years: Initially 500 micrograms/kg daily in 1–2 divided doses, increased if necessary to 1 mg/kg daily and continued until a total cumulative dose of 120–150 mg/kg is reached—treatment may be discontinued sooner if there has been an adequate response and no new lesions for 4–8 weeks, treatment course may be repeated after a period of at least 8 weeks if relapse after first course, consider dose reduction to less than 500 micrograms/kg daily for patients at increased risk of, or experiencing, side-effects; maximum 150 mg/kg per course

Severe infantile acne (specialist use only)
- ▶ BY MOUTH
- ▸ Child 1–23 months: Initially 200 micrograms/kg daily in 1–2 divided doses, increased if necessary to 1 mg/kg daily for 16–24 weeks; maximum 150 mg/kg per course

- **UNLICENSED USE** EvGr Isotretinoin is used for the treatment of severe infantile acne, ⟨E⟩ but is not licensed for this indication.

IMPORTANT SAFETY INFORMATION

MHRA/CHM ADVICE: ISOTRETINOIN (*ROACCUTANE*®): RARE REPORTS OF ERECTILE DYSFUNCTION AND DECREASED LIBIDO (OCTOBER 2017)

An EU-wide review has concluded that on rare occasions, oral isotretinoin, indicated for severe acne, may cause sexual side-effects, including erectile dysfunction and decreased libido.

MHRA/CHM ADVICE: ORAL RETINOID MEDICINES: REVISED AND SIMPLIFIED PREGNANCY PREVENTION EDUCATIONAL MATERIALS FOR HEALTHCARE PROFESSIONALS AND WOMEN (JUNE 2019)

New prescriber checklists, patient reminder cards, and pharmacy checklists are available to support the Pregnancy Prevention Programme in women and girls of childbearing potential taking oral acitretin, alitretinoin, or isotretinoin. Healthcare professionals are reminded that the use of oral retinoids is contra-indicated in pregnancy due to a high risk of serious congenital malformations, and any use in females must be within the conditions of the Pregnancy Prevention Programme (see *Conception and contraception* and *Prescribing and dispensing information*).

Neuropsychiatric reactions have been reported in patients taking oral retinoids. Healthcare professionals are advised to monitor patients for signs of depression or suicidal ideation and refer for appropriate treatment, if necessary; particular care is needed in those with a history of depression. Patients should be advised to speak to their doctor if they experience any changes in mood or behaviour, and encouraged to ask family and friends to look out for any change in mood.

MHRA/CHM ADVICE: ISOTRETINOIN (*ROACCUTANE*®): REMINDER OF IMPORTANT RISKS AND PRECAUTIONS (AUGUST 2020)

The MHRA reminds healthcare professionals that isotretinoin should only be prescribed for the treatment of severe forms of acne resistant to adequate courses of standard therapy with systemic antibacterials and topical therapy. Isotretinoin should be given under the supervision of physicians with expertise in the use of systemic retinoids, and a complete understanding of the risks of therapy and monitoring requirements (including signs of depression).

Healthcare professionals are also advised to counsel patients on the potential risks of isotretinoin, including neuropsychiatric reactions and sexual dysfunction.

The MHRA further reminds healthcare professionals that isotretinoin is a powerful teratogen associated with a high frequency of severe and life-threatening birth defects if there is exposure *in utero*; females of childbearing potential must meet the conditions of the Pregnancy Prevention Programme (see *Conception and contraception* and *Prescribing and dispensing information*).

MHRA/CHM ADVICE: ISOTRETINOIN (*ROACCUTANE*®): INTRODUCTION OF NEW SAFETY MEASURES, INCLUDING ADDITIONAL OVERSIGHT OF THE INITIATION OF TREATMENT FOR PATIENTS UNDER 18 YEARS OF AGE (OCTOBER 2023)

Based on recommendations from the CHM after a review of the potential psychiatric and sexual side-effects of isotretinoin, the MHRA has introduced new safety measures for healthcare professionals to follow. This includes new compulsory regulatory risk minimisation materials, informing patients of the benefits and risks of treatment, new roles and responsibilities such as a lead prescriber, and additional counselling and monitoring for potential mental health and sexual function side-effects.

All healthcare professionals involved in the treatment of acne, particularly those who prescribe isotretinoin, are advised to refer to the full details of the requirements in the Report of the CHM Isotretinoin Implementation Advisory Expert Working Group, available at: www.gov.uk/government/publications/report-of-the-commission-on-human-medicines-isotretinoin-implementation-advisory-expert-working-group. See also updated advice issued in January 2026, below.

MHRA/CHM ADVICE: ISOTRETINOIN: UPDATES TO PRESCRIBING GUIDANCE AND SURVEY OF SERVICES (OCTOBER 2025)

An addendum to the CHM Isotretinoin Implementation Advisory Expert Working Group's report has been published, to amend and clarify previous advice regarding follow-up consultations, pregnancy testing, and sexual function monitoring. Clinical guidance on these topics is available from the British Association of Dermatologists, see: www.bad.org.uk/guidelines-and-standards/isotretinoin-clinical-resources.

Survey data from services that prescribe isotretinoin for acne will be used to monitor adherence to risk minimisation measures, and inform the CHM's recommendations on the regulatory requirements of isotretinoin, whilst supporting patient access to treatment across all age groups. See also updated advice issued in January 2026, below.

MHRA/CHM ADVICE: ISOTRETINOIN - CHANGES TO PRESCRIBING GUIDANCE AND ADDITIONAL RISK MINIMISATION MEASURES (JANUARY 2026)

Following a review of the safety measures implemented in 2023 and the October 2025 survey of dermatology services, the CHM recommends an updated approach to the prescribing requirements for isotretinoin.

Healthcare professionals are advised that agreement from a second prescriber is no longer required when prescribing isotretinoin to patients under 18 years of age, as this has been replaced by alternative risk minimisation measures. These include an updated Acknowledgement of Risk Form for all patients, initiation of a regular clinical audit of risk minimisation measures by the British Association of Dermatologists, and a new patient information video that patients should watch before starting treatment (see *Patient and carer advice*). Patients continue to have the option to seek a second opinion from another healthcare professional if they are unsure about starting treatment.

Healthcare professionals should integrate the new measures and supporting materials into their clinical practice, and are reminded to continue to follow other existing measures:

- the lead prescriber who initiates isotretinoin must have expertise in the use of systemic retinoids for the treatment of severe acne and fully understand the monitoring requirements and risks associated with treatment;
- follow-up consultations may be carried out remotely if appropriate, however, the first appointment should be in person;
- assess patients' mental health and address any sexual function concerns before prescribing isotretinoin, and counsel patients on potential mental health and sexual function side-effects;
- monitor for mental health side-effects at each follow-up appointment;
- ask patients about sexual function at follow-up appointments, although by the third appointment, this may be brief;
- enter patients of childbearing potential into the Pregnancy Prevention Programme;
- medically supervised pregnancy testing may be performed remotely with appropriate oversight to ensure tests are performed correctly and safely;
- use the pharmacist checklist and provide a patient reminder card.

Further details of the data considered and advice given by the CHM can be found in the MHRA Review of the implementation of the recommendations of the CHM Isotretinoin Expert Working Group and Isotretinoin Implementation Advisory Expert Working Group Public Assessment Report, see: www.gov.uk/government/publications/review-of-the-impact-of-recommendations-for-the-prescribing-of-isotretinoin.

- **CONTRA-INDICATIONS** Hyperlipidaemia · hypervitaminosis A
- **CAUTIONS** Avoid blood donation during treatment and for at least 1 month after treatment · diabetes · dry eye syndrome (associated with risk of keratitis) · history of depression (risk of neuropsychiatric reactions)
- **INTERACTIONS** → Appendix 1: retinoids
- **SIDE-EFFECTS**

▶ **Common or very common** Anaemia · arthralgia · back pain · cheilitis · dry eye · eye discomfort · eye inflammation · haemorrhage · headache · increased risk of infection · myalgia · nasal dryness · neutropenia · proteinuria · skin fragility (trauma may cause blistering) · skin reactions · thrombocytopenia · thrombocytosis

- ▶ **Rare or very rare** Alopecia · anxiety · arthritis · behaviour abnormal · bronchospasm · cataract · corneal opacity · depression · diabetes mellitus · dizziness · drowsiness · dry throat · epiphyses premature fusion (following long-term use of high doses) · exostosis (following long-term use of high doses) · gastrointestinal disorders · glomerulonephritis · hair changes · hearing impairment · hepatitis · hoarseness · hyperhidrosis · hyperuricaemia · idiopathic intracranial hypertension · inflammatory bowel disease · ligament calcification (following long-term use of high doses) · lymphadenopathy · malaise · mood altered · nail dystrophy · nausea · pancreatitis · photosensitivity reaction · psychotic disorder · pyogenic granuloma · seizure · suicidal behaviours · tendinitis · tendon calcification (following long-term use of high doses) · vasculitis · vision disorders
- ▶ **Frequency not known** Psychiatric disorder · rhabdomyolysis · severe cutaneous adverse reactions (SCARs) · sexual dysfunction · vulvovaginal dryness

SIDE-EFFECTS, FURTHER INFORMATION Risk of pancreatitis if triglycerides above 9 mmol/litre—discontinue if uncontrolled hypertriglyceridaemia or pancreatitis.

Discontinue treatment if skin peeling severe or haemorrhagic diarrhoea develops.

Visual disturbances require expert referral and possible withdrawal.

Psychiatric side-effects could require expert referral.

- **ALLERGY AND CROSS-SENSITIVITY** [EvGr] Contra-indicated in patients with hypersensitivity to peanuts or soya (capsule filling contains soya-bean oil). ⟨M⟩
- **CONCEPTION AND CONTRACEPTION** The MHRA advises that women and girls of childbearing potential being treated with the oral retinoids acitretin, alitretinoin, or isotretinoin must be supported on a Pregnancy Prevention Programme with regular follow-up and pregnancy testing.

Pregnancy prevention Effective contraception must be used.

In females of childbearing potential, exclude pregnancy a few days before treatment, every month during treatment (unless there are compelling reasons to indicate that there is no risk of pregnancy), and 1 month after stopping treatment. Females of childbearing age must practise effective contraception for at least 1 month before starting treatment, during treatment, and for at least 1 month after stopping treatment. They should be advised to use at least 1 highly effective method of contraception (i.e. a user-independent form such as an intra-uterine device or implant) or 2 complementary user-dependent forms of contraception (e.g. oral contraceptives and barrier method). Females should be advised to discontinue treatment and to seek prompt medical attention if they become pregnant during treatment or within 1 month of stopping treatment.

- **PREGNANCY** Manufacturer advises avoid—teratogenic.
- **BREAST FEEDING** Avoid.
- **HEPATIC IMPAIRMENT** Manufacturer advises avoid—limited information available.
- **RENAL IMPAIRMENT**

Dose adjustments [EvGr] In severe impairment, reduce initial dose and increase gradually, if necessary, up to 1 mg/kg daily as tolerated. ⟨M⟩

- **MONITORING REQUIREMENTS** Measure hepatic function and serum lipids before treatment, 1 month after starting and then every 3 months (reduce dose or discontinue if transaminase or serum lipids persistently raised).
- **PRESCRIBING AND DISPENSING INFORMATION** Isotretinoin is an isomer of tretinoin.

The MHRA has provided an *Acknowledgement of Risk Form* and *Pharmacist Checklist*.

Applicability of the Pregnancy Prevention Programme to the patient's circumstances should be recorded on their prescription.

Prescribing for females of childbearing potential For females of childbearing potential, each prescription for oral isotretinoin should be limited to a supply of up to 30 days' treatment and dispensed within 7 days. Pregnancy testing should ideally be carried out on the same day as prescription issuing and dispensing.

For females of childbearing potential considered by the prescriber to have compelling reasons to indicate that there is no risk of pregnancy, an extended supply for longer than 30 days' treatment (up to 12 weeks if no other side-effect monitoring required) may be considered, once stable on treatment—consult *Acknowledgement of Risk Form* and *Pharmacist Checklist*.

- **PATIENT AND CARER ADVICE** Warn patient to avoid wax epilation (risk of epidermal stripping), dermabrasion, and laser skin treatments (risk of scarring) during treatment and for at least 6 months after stopping; patient should avoid exposure to UV light (including sunlight) and use sunscreen and emollient (including lip balm) preparations from the start of treatment.

Risk of neuropsychiatric reactions The MHRA advises patients and carers to seek medical attention if changes in mood or behaviour occur.

Patient Reminder Card Pharmacists must ensure that all patients have a patient reminder card—see also *Important safety information*.

Patient information video The British Association of Dermatologists, in conjunction with the MHRA and CHM, have produced a video explaining the benefits and risks of treatment, see: www.skinhealthinfo.org.uk/condition/isotretinoin-patient-video/.

- **MEDICINAL FORMS** There can be variation in the licensing of different medicines containing the same drug.

Oral capsule

CAUTIONARY AND ADVISORY LABELS 10, 11, 21

- ▶ Isotretinoin (non-proprietary) ▼
  - **Isotretinoin 5 mg** Isotretinoin 5mg capsules | 56 capsule [PoM] £29.30 DT = £14.78
  - **Isotretinoin 10 mg** Isotretinoin 10mg capsules | 30 capsule [PoM] £23.44 DT = £27.40
  - **Isotretinoin 20 mg** Isotretinoin 20mg capsules | 30 capsule [PoM] £59.98 DT = £30.31 | 56 capsule [PoM] £66.66–£104.82
- ▶ Roaccutane (Neon Healthcare Ltd) ▼
  - **Isotretinoin 10 mg** Roaccutane 10mg capsules | 30 capsule [PoM] £14.54 DT = £27.40
  - **Isotretinoin 20 mg** Roaccutane 20mg capsules | 30 capsule [PoM] £20.02 DT = £30.31

Tretinoin with clindamycin

28-Jun-2023

The properties listed below are those particular to the combination only. For the properties of the components please consider, clindamycin p. 935.

- **INDICATIONS AND DOSE**

Acne vulgaris

▶ TO THE SKIN

- ▶ Child 12–17 years: Apply once daily, to be applied thinly at bedtime

- **CONTRA-INDICATIONS** Perioral dermatitis · personal or familial history of skin cancer · rosacea
- **CAUTIONS** Allow peeling (resulting from other irritant treatments) to subside before using a topical retinoid · avoid accumulation in angles of the nose · avoid contact with eyes, nostrils, mouth and mucous membranes, eczematous, broken or sunburned skin · avoid exposure to UV light (including sunlight, solariums) · avoid use of topical retinoids with keratolytic agents, abrasive cleaners, comedogenic or astringent cosmetics · caution in sensitive areas such as the neck · severe acne
- **INTERACTIONS** → Appendix 1: clindamycin · retinoids

- **SIDE-EFFECTS** Dry skin (discontinue if severe) · eye irritation · oedema · photosensitivity reaction · skin pigmentation change (transient) · skin reactions
- **CONCEPTION AND CONTRACEPTION** The MHRA advises females of childbearing potential should use effective contraception.
- **PREGNANCY** The MHRA advises that systemic exposure is thought to be negligible following application of topical retinoids. However, since risk cannot be excluded, use of topical retinoids is contra-indicated during pregnancy as a precaution.
- **BREAST FEEDING** Amount of drug in milk after topical application probably too small to be harmful; ensure infant does not come in contact with treated areas.
- **PATIENT AND CARER ADVICE** If sun exposure is unavoidable, an appropriate sunscreen or protective clothing should be used.

  Patients and carers should be warned that some redness and skin peeling can occur initially but settles with time. To reduce the risk of skin irritation, treatment may be started with alternate-day or short-contact application (e.g. washing off after an hour) and progressed to standard application if tolerated. If severe irritation occurs, the frequency of application should be reduced or treatment suspended until the reaction subsides; if irritation persists, discontinue treatment. Several months of treatment may be needed to achieve an optimal response and the treatment should be continued until no new lesions develop.

- **MEDICINAL FORMS** There can be variation in the licensing of different medicines containing the same drug.

Cutaneous gel

CAUTIONARY AND ADVISORY LABELS 11

EXCIPIENTS: May contain Butylated hydroxytoluene, hydroxybenzoates (parabens), polysorbates

▸ Treclin (Viatris UK Healthcare Ltd)

Tretinoin 250 microgram per 1 gram, Clindamycin (as Clindamycin phosphate) 10 mg per 1 gram Treclin 1%/0.025% gel | 30 gram [PoM] £11.94 DT = £11.94

Tretinoin with erythromycin

28-Jun-2023

The properties listed below are those particular to the combination only. For the properties of the components please consider, erythromycin p. 406.

- **INDICATIONS AND DOSE**

Acne

▸ TO THE SKIN

▸ Child: Apply 1–2 times a day, to be applied thinly

- **CONTRA-INDICATIONS** Perioral dermatitis · personal or familial history of skin cancer · rosacea
- **CAUTIONS** Allow peeling (resulting from other irritant treatments) to subside before using a topical retinoid · avoid accumulation in angles of the nose · avoid contact with eyes, nostrils, mouth and mucous membranes, eczematous, broken or sunburned skin · avoid exposure to UV light (including sunlight, solariums) · avoid use of topical retinoids with keratolytic agents, abrasive cleaners, comedogenic or astringent cosmetics · caution in sensitive areas such as the neck · severe acne
- **INTERACTIONS** → Appendix 1: macrolides · retinoids
- **SIDE-EFFECTS** Dry skin (discontinue if severe) · eye irritation · oedema · photosensitivity reaction · skin eruption · skin pigmentation change (transient)
- **CONCEPTION AND CONTRACEPTION** The MHRA advises females of childbearing potential should use effective contraception.
- **PREGNANCY** The MHRA advises that systemic exposure is thought to be negligible following application of topical retinoids. However, since risk cannot be excluded, use of topical retinoids is contra-indicated during pregnancy as a precaution.
- **BREAST FEEDING** Amount of drug in milk after topical application probably too small to be harmful; ensure infant does not come in contact with treated areas.
- **PATIENT AND CARER ADVICE** If sun exposure is unavoidable, an appropriate sunscreen or protective clothing should be used.

  Patients and carers should be warned that some redness and skin peeling can occur initially but settles with time. To reduce the risk of skin irritation, treatment may be started with alternate-day or short-contact application (e.g. washing off after an hour) and progressed to standard application if tolerated. If severe irritation occurs, the frequency of application should be reduced or treatment suspended until the reaction subsides; if irritation persists, discontinue treatment. Several months of treatment may be needed to achieve an optimal response and the treatment should be continued until no new lesions develop.

- **MEDICINAL FORMS** There can be variation in the licensing of different medicines containing the same drug.

Cutaneous solution

CAUTIONARY AND ADVISORY LABELS 11

▸ Aknemycin Plus (Almirall Ltd)

Tretinoin 250 microgram per 1 gram, Erythromycin 40 mg per 1 gram Aknemycin Plus solution | 25 ml [PoM] £7.05 DT = £7.05

Trifarotene

28-May-2024

- **INDICATIONS AND DOSE**

Acne vulgaris

▸ TO THE SKIN

▸ Child 12–17 years: Apply once daily, to be applied thinly in the evening

- **CAUTIONS** Avoid contact with eyes, nostrils, mouth and mucous membranes, eczematous, broken or sunburned skin · avoid exposure to UV light (including sunlight, sunlamps)
- **SIDE-EFFECTS**
  - ▸ **Common or very common** Sunburn
  - ▸ **Uncommon** Skin reactions
  - ▸ **Rare or very rare** Cheilitis · eyelid exfoliation · eyelid oedema · flushing
- **CONCEPTION AND CONTRACEPTION** The MHRA advises females of childbearing potential should use effective contraception.
- **PREGNANCY** The MHRA advises that systemic exposure is thought to be negligible following application of topical retinoids. However, since risk cannot be excluded, use of topical retinoids is contra-indicated during pregnancy as a precaution.
- **BREAST FEEDING** Specialist sources indicate amount of drug in milk after topical application probably too small to be harmful; ensure infant does not come in contact with treated areas.
- **PATIENT AND CARER ADVICE** If sun exposure is unavoidable, an appropriate sunscreen or protective clothing should be used. To reduce the risk of skin irritation, patients should be instructed to use a moisturiser from the initiation of treatment, and if necessary the frequency of application should be reduced or treatment temporarily discontinued. If severe irritation occurs and persists despite these actions, treatment should be stopped altogether.

- **NATIONAL FUNDING/ACCESS DECISIONS** For full details see funding body website

Scottish Medicines Consortium (SMC) decisions

- **Trifarotene (*Aklief*®) for the cutaneous treatment of acne vulgaris of the face and/or the trunk in patients from 12 years of age and older, when many comedones, papules and pustules are present (September 2022) SMC No. SMC2441** Recommended

All Wales Medicines Strategy Group (AWMSG) decisions

- **Trifarotene (*Aklief*®) for the cutaneous treatment of acne vulgaris of the face and/or the trunk in patients from 12 years of age and older, when many comedones, papules and pustules are present (April 2024) AWMSG No. 3153** Recommended

- **MEDICINAL FORMS** There can be variation in the licensing of different medicines containing the same drug.

Cutaneous cream

EXCIPIENTS: May contain Ethanol, polysorbates, propylene glycol

- **Aklief** (Galderma (UK) Ltd) ▼
  Trifarotene 50 microgram per 1 gram Aklief 50micrograms/g cream | 75 gram PoM £27.75 DT = £27.75

VITAMINS AND TRACE ELEMENTS › VITAMIN B GROUP

Nicotinamide

05-Oct-2021

- **INDICATIONS AND DOSE**

Inflammatory acne vulgaris

- TO THE SKIN
  - Child: Apply twice daily, reduced to once daily or on alternate days, dose reduced if irritation occurs

- **CAUTIONS** Avoid contact with eyes · avoid contact with mucous membranes (including nose and mouth) · reduce frequency of application if excessive dryness, irritation or peeling
- **SIDE-EFFECTS** Paraesthesia · skin reactions
- **MEDICINAL FORMS** There can be variation in the licensing of different medicines containing the same drug.

Cutaneous gel

- **Freederm** (Diomed Developments Ltd)
  Nicotinamide 40 mg per 1 gram Freederm Treatment 4% gel | 25 gram P £5.56 DT = £5.56

9 Scalp and hair conditions

Scalp and hair conditions

Overview

The detergent action of shampoo removes grease (sebum) from hair. Prepubertal children produce very little grease and require shampoo less frequently than adults. Shampoos can be used as vehicles for medicinal products, but their usefulness is limited by the short time the product is in contact with the scalp and by their irritant nature.

Oils and ointments are very useful for scaly, dry scalp conditions; if a greasy appearance is cosmetically unacceptable, the preparation may be applied at night and washed out in the morning. Alcohol-based lotions are rarely used in children; alcohol causes painful stinging on broken skin and the fumes may exacerbate asthma.

Itchy, inflammatory, eczematous scalp conditions may be relieved by a simple emollient oil such as **olive oil** or **coconut oil** (arachis oil (ground nut oil, peanut oil)) is best avoided in children under 5 years). In more severe cases a topical **corticosteroid** may be required. Preparations containing **coal tar** are used for the common scaly scalp conditions of childhood including seborrhoeic dermatitis, dandruff (a mild form of seborrhoeic dermatitis), and psoriasis; salicylic acid p. 950 is used as a keratolytic in some scalp preparations.

Shampoos containing antimicrobials such as selenium below or ketoconazole p. 900 are used for seborrhoeic dermatitis and dandruff in which yeast infection has been implicated, and for tinea capitis (ringworm of the scalp). Bacterial infection affecting the scalp (usually secondary to eczema, head lice, or ringworm) may be treated with shampoos containing antimicrobials such as **pyrithione zinc**, cetrimide, or povidone-iodine p. 944.

In neonates and infants, *cradle cap* (which is also a form of seborrhoeic eczema) can be treated by massaging **coconut oil** or **olive oil** into the scalp; a bland emollient such as **emulsifying ointment** can be rubbed onto the affected area once or twice daily before bathing and a mild shampoo used.

Other drugs used for Scalp and hair conditions Coal tar, p. 918 · Coal tar with salicylic acid and precipitated sulfur, p. 918

ANTISEPTICS AND DISINFECTANTS › UNDECENOATES

Cetrimide with undecenoic acid

- **INDICATIONS AND DOSE**

Scalp psoriasis | Seborrhoeic dermatitis | Dandruff

- TO THE SKIN
  - Child: Apply 3 times a week for 1 week, then apply twice weekly

- **MEDICINAL FORMS** No licensed medicines listed.

ANTISEPTICS AND DISINFECTANTS › OTHER

Benzalkonium chloride

26-Mar-2020

- **INDICATIONS AND DOSE**

Seborrhoeic scalp conditions associated with dandruff and scaling

- TO THE SKIN
  - Child: Apply as required

- **MEDICINAL FORMS** There can be variation in the licensing of different medicines containing the same drug.

Shampoo

- **Dermax** (Dermal Laboratories Ltd)
  Benzalkonium chloride 5 mg per 1 ml Dermax Therapeutic 0.5% shampoo | 250 ml P £5.99 DT = £5.99

VITAMINS AND TRACE ELEMENTS

Selenium

- **INDICATIONS AND DOSE**

Seborrhoeic dermatitis | Dandruff

- TO THE SKIN USING SHAMPOO
  - Child 5–17 years: Apply twice weekly for 2 weeks, then apply once weekly for 2 weeks, then apply as required

Pityriasis versicolor

- TO THE SKIN USING SHAMPOO
  - Child 5–17 years: Apply once daily for 7 days, apply to the affected area and leave on for 10 minutes before rinsing off. The course may be repeated if necessary. Diluting with a small amount of water prior to application can reduce irritation

- **UNLICENSED USE** The use of selenium sulfide shampoo as a lotion for the treatment of pityriasis (tinea) versicolor is an unlicensed indication.
- **INTERACTIONS** → Appendix 1: selenium
- **PATIENT AND CARER ADVICE** Avoid using 48 hours before or after applying hair colouring, straightening or waving preparations.
- **MEDICINAL FORMS** No licensed medicines listed.

9.1 Alopecia

IMMUNOSUPPRESSANTS › JAK INHIBITORS

Ritlecitinib

03-May-2024

- **DRUG ACTION** Ritlecitinib selectively and irreversibly inhibits the Janus-associated tyrosine kinase JAK3 and the tyrosine kinase TEC.

- **INDICATIONS AND DOSE**

Alopecia areata (under expert supervision)

▸ BY MOUTH

▸ Child 12–17 years: 50 mg once daily, consider discontinuation of treatment if no response after 36 weeks

IMPORTANT SAFETY INFORMATION

MHRA/CHM ADVICE: JANUS KINASE (JAK) INHIBITORS: NEW MEASURES TO REDUCE RISKS OF MAJOR CARDIOVASCULAR EVENTS, MALIGNANCY, VENOUS THROMBOEMBOLISM, SERIOUS INFECTIONS AND INCREASED MORTALITY (APRIL 2023)

In 2022, the EMA conducted a review of all JAK inhibitors indicated for chronic inflammatory diseases and concluded that the risks associated with the use of tofacitinib could be considered a class effect (see *Important safety information* in tofacitinib p. 803). Following a further review by the MHRA, some existing warnings for tofacitinib have been updated and implemented for all JAK inhibitors included in the review.

Healthcare professionals are advised to:
- avoid use in patients who are current or past long-time smokers, and in patients with other cardiovascular disease or malignancy risk factors, unless there are no suitable alternatives;
- use with caution in patients with risk factors for venous thromboembolism;
- use lower doses in patients with risk factors, where applicable;
- periodically examine all patients' skin for malignancy;
- inform patients and their carers of these risks, and the signs and symptoms that warrant urgent medical attention.

- **CONTRA-INDICATIONS** Absolute lymphocyte count less than 0.5 × 10^9 cells/litre (do not initiate) · platelet count less than 100 × 10^9 cells/litre (do not initiate) · serious infection (active) · tuberculosis (active)
- **CAUTIONS** Chronic or recurrent infection · history of atherosclerotic cardiovascular disease or other cardiovascular risk factors · history of serious or opportunistic infection · predisposition to infection · risk factors for malignancy · risk factors for thromboembolism · risk of viral reactivation (consult product literature) · tuberculosis exposure

CAUTIONS, FURTHER INFORMATION

▸ Tuberculosis EvGr Consider anti-tuberculosis therapy prior to initiation of ritlecitinib in patients with previously untreated latent tuberculosis and those at high risk of tuberculosis infection. (M)

▸ Immunisation EvGr Patients should receive all recommended vaccinations before starting treatment; live vaccines are not recommended immediately before, or during, treatment. (M)

▸ Thromboembolism EvGr If a thromboembolic event occurs during treatment, discontinuation of ritlecitinib is recommended. (M)

- **INTERACTIONS** → Appendix 1: ritlecitinib
- **SIDE-EFFECTS**

▸ **Common or very common** Diarrhoea · dizziness · headache · increased risk of infection · skin reactions

▸ **Frequency not known** Embolism and thrombosis · malignancy · non-melanoma skin cancer · reactivation of infections · sepsis

- **CONCEPTION AND CONTRACEPTION** EvGr Females of childbearing potential should use effective contraception during treatment and for 1 month after last treatment. (M)
- **PREGNANCY** EvGr Avoid (toxicity in *animal* studies). (M)
- **BREAST FEEDING** EvGr Avoid (present in milk in *animal* studies). (M)
- **HEPATIC IMPAIRMENT** EvGr Avoid in severe impairment (no information available). (M)
- **PRE-TREATMENT SCREENING** EvGr Patients should be evaluated for tuberculosis and viral hepatitis before treatment. (M)
- **MONITORING REQUIREMENTS**

▸ EvGr Monitor for signs and symptoms of infection during and after treatment—consider treatment interruption until the infection is controlled.

▸ Monitor platelets and lymphocytes at baseline, 4 weeks after treatment initiation, and as clinically indicated thereafter. Interrupt treatment if absolute lymphocyte count less than 0.5 × 10^9 cells/litre; treatment may be restarted when levels return above this value. Discontinue treatment if platelet count less than 50 × 10^9 cells/litre.

▸ Monitor for viral reactivation (including viral hepatitis and herpes zoster) during treatment; interrupt treatment if herpes zoster infection develops and resume once resolved. If there is evidence of hepatitis reactivation, consult a liver specialist for advice.

▸ Periodic skin examination is recommended in all patients, particularly those at increased risk of skin cancer. (M)

- **PRESCRIBING AND DISPENSING INFORMATION** The manufacturer of *Litfulo*® has provided a *Prescriber Guide*, which includes a prescriber checklist.
- **HANDLING AND STORAGE** Protect from light.
- **PATIENT AND CARER ADVICE**

Patient card A patient card should be provided.

Missed doses If a dose is more than 16 hours late, the missed dose should not be taken and the next dose should be taken at the normal time.

- **NATIONAL FUNDING/ACCESS DECISIONS**

For full details see funding body website

NICE decisions

▸ **Ritlecitinib for treating severe alopecia areata in people 12 years and over (March 2024)** NICE TA958 Recommended

Scottish Medicines Consortium (SMC) decisions

▸ **Ritlecitinib (*Litfulo*®) for the treatment of severe alopecia areata in adults and adolescents aged 12 years and over (April 2024)** SMC No. SMC2610 Recommended

- **MEDICINAL FORMS** There can be variation in the licensing of different medicines containing the same drug.

Oral capsule

▸ **Litfulo** (Pfizer Ltd) ▼

Ritlecitinib (as Ritlecitinib tosylate) 50 mg Litfulo 50mg capsules | 30 capsule PoM £949.41 (Hospital only)

10 Skin cleansers, antiseptics and desloughing agents

Skin cleansers, antiseptics and desloughing agents

29-Nov-2023

Skin cleansers and antiseptics

Soap or detergent is used with water to cleanse intact skin but they can irritate infantile skin; emollient preparations such as aqueous cream or emulsifying ointment can be used in place of soap or detergent for cleansing dry or irritated skin.

An antiseptic is used for skin that is infected or that is susceptible to recurrent infection. Detergent preparations containing chlorhexidine p. 944 or povidone-iodine p. 944, which should be thoroughly rinsed off, are used. Emollients may also contain antiseptics.

Antiseptics such as chlorhexidine or povidone-iodine are used on intact skin before surgical procedures; their antiseptic effect is enhanced by an alcoholic solvent. Antiseptic solutions containing cetrimide can be used if a detergent effect is also required.

Preparations containing alcohol, and regular use of povidone-iodine, should be avoided on neonatal skin.

Hydrogen peroxide p. 945, an oxidising agent, is available as a cream and can be used for superficial bacterial skin infections.

For irrigating ulcers or wounds, lukewarm sterile sodium chloride 0.9% solution p. 728 is used but tap water is often appropriate.

Potassium permanganate solution 1 in 10 000 below, a mild antiseptic with astringent properties, can be used as a soak for exudative eczematous areas; treatment should be stopped when the skin becomes dry.

Borderline substances

Disinfectants (antiseptics) have ACBS approval (see *About Borderline Substances*) to be prescribed on an FP10 only when ordered in such quantities and with such directions as are appropriate for the treatment of patients, but not if ordered for general hygienic purposes.

Desloughing agents

Alginate, hydrogel, and hydrocolloid dressings are effective in wound debridement. Sterile larvae (maggots) (available from BioMonde) are also used for managing sloughing wounds and are prescribable on the NHS.

Desloughing solutions and creams are of little clinical value. Substances applied to an open area are easily absorbed and perilesional skin is easily sensitised.

ANTISEPTICS AND DISINFECTANTS

Potassium permanganate

26-Jul-2025

● **INDICATIONS AND DOSE**

Cleansing and deodorising suppurating eczematous reactions and wounds

▶ TO THE SKIN

▸ Child: For wet dressings or baths, use approximately 0.01% (1 in 10 000) solution

IMPORTANT SAFETY INFORMATION

NHS ENGLAND PATIENT SAFETY ALERT: RISK OF DEATH OR SERIOUS HARM FROM ACCIDENTAL INGESTION OF POTASSIUM PERMANGANATE PREPARATIONS (DECEMBER 2014)

Potassium permanganate is for external use only. Oral ingestion can cause fatality due to local inflammatory reactions that block the airways or cause perforations of the gastrointestinal tract, or through toxicity and organ failure. Potassium permanganate is subject to the requirements of Control of Substances Hazardous to Health including: separate storage, additional hazard labelling, and issue only to staff and patients who have been educated to understand its safe use. Accidental ingestion should be treated as a medical emergency.

NHS ENGLAND NATIONAL PATIENT SAFETY ALERT: INADVERTENT ORAL ADMINISTRATION OF POTASSIUM PERMANGANATE (APRIL 2022)

A review of reported incidents over a two-year period identified 35 cases of inadvertent ingestion of potassium permanganate. Of these, 15 cases were of healthcare staff administering potassium permanganate orally to patients and 9 cases, one fatal, of patients self-administering orally. To minimise the risk of harm from potassium permanganate, the British Association of Dermatologists (BAD) has issued advice on formulary management, prescribing, dispensing, storage, preparation and use, and waste: www.bad.org.uk/bad-and-nhs-england-nhs-improvement-guidance-on-the-safe-use-of-potassium-permanganate-soaks/.

The overall use of potassium permanganate should be reviewed locally and protocols for its use should be aligned with all BAD recommendations, including:

In primary care:

- patients are not on repeat prescriptions for potassium permanganate;
- prescriptions include clear instructions to dilute before use;
- dispensing label includes the warning 'harmful if swallowed'.

In secondary care:

- remove all stock supply (except for use within outpatient departments) and supply on a named patient basis only;
- potassium permanganate is prescribed as 'potassium permanganate 0.01% topical solution' and the dispensing label must include the warning 'harmful if swallowed';
- potassium permanganate is not stored with medicines for oral/internal use, including the ward drug trolley; dilution should occur away from the patient, and neither the concentrated form nor the diluted form should be left near the patient.

In all settings:

- prescriptions are only issued by an appropriate prescriber;
- if potassium permanganate is to be used in a patient's home, a risk assessment must be undertaken before prescribing;
- all patients must be supplied with a patient information leaflet, such as that produced by BAD: www.bad.org.uk/pils/potassium-permanganate-solution-soaks/.

● **CAUTIONS** Irritant to mucous membranes

● **DIRECTIONS FOR ADMINISTRATION** With potassium permanganate tablets for solution, 1 tablet dissolved in 4 litres of water provides a 0.01% (1 in 10 000) solution.

● **PATIENT AND CARER ADVICE** Can stain clothing, skin and nails (especially with prolonged use).

● **MEDICINAL FORMS** There can be variation in the licensing of different medicines containing the same drug. Forms available from special-order manufacturers include: cutaneous solution

Tablet for cutaneous solution

CAUTIONARY AND ADVISORY LABELS 10

▸ **Potassium permanganate (Non-proprietary)**

Potassium permanganate 400 mg EN-Potab 400mg tablets for cutaneous solution | 30 tablet Ⓢ DT = £30.05

- **AnateP** (Essential-Healthcare Ltd)
  Potassium permanganate 400 mg AnateP 400mg tablets for cutaneous solution | 30 tablet £17.83 DT = £30.05
- **Permitabs** (Alliance Pharmaceuticals Ltd)
  Potassium permanganate 400 mg Permitabs 400mg tablets for cutaneous solution | 30 tablet £30.05 DT = £30.05

ANTISEPTICS AND DISINFECTANTS › ALCOHOL DISINFECTANTS

Alcohol

(Industrial methylated spirit)

● **INDICATIONS AND DOSE**

Skin preparation before injection

▶ TO THE SKIN
- Child: Apply as required

● **CONTRA-INDICATIONS** Neonates

● **CAUTIONS** Avoid broken skin · flammable · patients have suffered severe burns when diathermy has been preceded by application of alcoholic skin disinfectants

● **INTERACTIONS** → Appendix 1: alcohol

● **SIDE-EFFECTS**

Overdose Features of acute alcohol intoxication include ataxia, dysarthria, nystagmus, and drowsiness, which may progress to coma, with hypotension and acidosis.

For details on the management of poisoning, see Alcohol, under Emergency treatment of poisoning p. 1036.

● **PRESCRIBING AND DISPENSING INFORMATION** Industrial methylated spirits defined by the BP as a mixture of 19 volumes of ethyl alcohol of an appropriate strength with 1 volume of approved wood naphtha.

● **MEDICINAL FORMS** No licensed medicines listed.

ANTISEPTICS AND DISINFECTANTS › IODINE PRODUCTS

Povidone-iodine

08-Feb-2022

● **INDICATIONS AND DOSE**

Skin disinfection

▶ TO THE SKIN
- Child: (consult product literature)

VIDENE ® SOLUTION

Skin disinfection

▶ TO THE SKIN
- Child: Apply undiluted in pre-operative skin disinfection and general antisepsis

VIDENE ® SURGICAL SCRUB ®

Skin disinfection

▶ TO THE SKIN
- Child: Use as a pre-operative scrub for hand and skin disinfection

VIDENE ® TINCTURE

Skin disinfection

▶ TO THE SKIN
- Child: Apply undiluted in pre-operative skin disinfection

● **CONTRA-INDICATIONS** Concomitant use of lithium · corrected gestational age under 32 weeks · infants body-weight under 1.5 kg · regular use in neonates

VIDENE ® TINCTURE Neonates

● **CAUTIONS** Broken skin · large open wounds

CAUTIONS, FURTHER INFORMATION

- Large open wounds The application of povidone–iodine to large wounds or severe burns may produce systemic adverse effects such as metabolic acidosis, hypernatraemia and impairment of renal function.

VIDENE ® TINCTURE Procedures involving hot wire cautery and diathermy

● **SIDE-EFFECTS** Acute kidney injury · goitre · hyperthyroidism · hypothyroidism · metabolic acidosis · skin burning sensation

● **PREGNANCY** Sufficient iodine may be absorbed to affect the fetal thyroid in the second and third trimester.

● **BREAST FEEDING** Avoid regular or excessive use.

● **RENAL IMPAIRMENT** EvGr Caution when applied to large wounds or severe burns (increased risk of systemic exposure). (M)

● **EFFECT ON LABORATORY TESTS** May interfere with thyroid function tests.

● **MEDICINAL FORMS** There can be variation in the licensing of different medicines containing the same drug. Forms available from special-order manufacturers include: cutaneous solution

Cutaneous solution

CAUTIONARY AND ADVISORY LABELS 15 (Only for use with alcoholic solutions)

- **Videne** (Ecolab Healthcare Division)
  Povidone-Iodine 75 mg per 1 ml Videne 7.5% surgical scrub solution | 500 ml P £8.61 DT = £8.61
  Povidone-Iodine 100 mg per 1 ml Videne 10% antiseptic solution | 200 ml P £11.78

ANTISEPTICS AND DISINFECTANTS › OTHER

Chlorhexidine

23-Feb-2022

● **INDICATIONS AND DOSE**

CEPTON ® LOTION

For skin disinfection in acne

▶ TO THE SKIN
- Child: (consult product literature)

CEPTON ® SKIN WASH

For use as skin wash in acne

▶ TO THE SKIN
- Child: (consult product literature)

HIBISCRUB ®

Pre-operative hand and skin disinfection | General hand and skin disinfection

▶ TO THE SKIN
- Child: Use as alternative to soap (consult product literature)

HIBITANE OBSTETRIC

For use in obstetrics and gynaecology as an antiseptic and lubricant

▶ TO THE SKIN
- Child: To be applied to skin around vulva and perineum and to hands of midwife or doctor

HIBI ® LIQUID HAND RUB+

Hand and skin disinfection

▶ TO THE SKIN
- Child: To be used undiluted (consult product literature)

HYDREX ® SOLUTION

For pre-operative skin disinfection

▶ TO THE SKIN
- Child: (consult product literature)

HYDREX ® SURGICAL SCRUB

For pre-operative hand and skin disinfection | General hand disinfection

▶ TO THE SKIN
- Child: (consult product literature)

UNISEPT

For cleansing and disinfecting wounds and burns and swabbing in obstetrics

▶ TO THE SKIN

▸ Child: (consult product literature)

IMPORTANT SAFETY INFORMATION

MHRA/CHM ADVICE: CHLORHEXIDINE SOLUTIONS: REMINDER OF THE RISK OF CHEMICAL BURNS IN PREMATURE INFANTS (NOVEMBER 2014)

In premature infants, use sparingly, monitor for skin reactions, and do not allow solution to pool—risk of severe chemical burns.

- **CONTRA-INDICATIONS** Alcoholic solutions not suitable for use on neonatal skin · not for use in body cavities
- **CAUTIONS** Avoid contact with brain · avoid contact with eyes · avoid contact with meninges · avoid contact with middle ear · use prior to diathermy (alcohol containing skin disinfectants)
- **SIDE-EFFECTS** Skin reactions
- **PRESCRIBING AND DISPENSING INFORMATION** Chlorhexidine digluconate is a synonym for chlorhexidine gluconate.

- **MEDICINAL FORMS** There can be variation in the licensing of different medicines containing the same drug.

Cutaneous solution

CAUTIONARY AND ADVISORY LABELS 15 (For ethanolic solutions (e.g. ChloraPrep® and Hydrex® only)

EXCIPIENTS: May contain Fragrances

▸ **Ceptor** (Dendron Brands Ltd)

Chlorhexidine gluconate 10 mg per 1 ml Cepton 1% medicated skin wash | 150 ml GSL £38.56 DT = £38.56

▸ **Hydrex** (Ecolab Healthcare Division)

Chlorhexidine gluconate 40 mg per 1 ml Hydrex 4% Surgical Scrub | 250 ml GSL £4.83 DT = £5.26 | 500 ml GSL £5.36 DT = £8.28

Cutaneous cream

▸ **Hibitane Obstetric** (Derma UK Ltd)

Chlorhexidine gluconate 10 mg per 1 gram Hibitane Obstetric 1% cream | 250 ml GSL £24.20 DT = £24.20 | 500 ml GSL £49.00 (Hospital only)

Chlorhexidine gluconate with isopropyl alcohol

The properties listed below are those particular to the combination only. For the properties of the components please consider, chlorhexidine p. 944.

- **INDICATIONS AND DOSE**

Skin disinfection before invasive procedures

▶ TO THE SKIN

▸ Child 2 months–17 years: (consult product literature)

- **MEDICINAL FORMS** There can be variation in the licensing of different medicines containing the same drug. Forms available from special-order manufacturers include: cutaneous solution

Cutaneous solution

CAUTIONARY AND ADVISORY LABELS 15

▸ **ChloraPrep** (Becton, Dickinson UK Ltd)

Chlorhexidine gluconate 20 mg per 1 ml, Isopropyl alcohol 700 ml per 1 litre ChloraPrep with Tint solution 10.5ml applicators | 25 applicator GSL £84.98 DT = £80.93

ChloraPrep solution 1ml applicators | 60 applicator GSL £21.35

ChloraPrep with Tint solution 26ml applicators | 25 applicator GSL £189.37 DT = £180.14

ChloraPrep solution 3ml applicators | 25 applicator GSL £23.58 DT = £23.58

ChloraPrep solution 1.5ml applicators | 20 applicator GSL £12.30 DT = £12.30

ChloraPrep with Tint solution 3ml applicators | 25 applicator GSL £24.86 DT = £23.58

ChloraPrep solution 10.5ml applicators | 25 applicator GSL £80.93 DT = £80.93

ChloraPrep solution 26ml applicators | 25 applicator GSL £180.14 DT = £180.14

Chlorhexidine with cetrimide

The properties listed below are those particular to the combination only. For the properties of the components please consider, chlorhexidine p. 944.

- **INDICATIONS AND DOSE**

Skin disinfection such as wound cleansing and obstetrics

▶ TO THE SKIN

▸ Child: To be used undiluted

- **MEDICINAL FORMS** There can be variation in the licensing of different medicines containing the same drug.

Cutaneous cream

▸ **Chlorhexidine with cetrimide (Non-proprietary)**

Chlorhexidine gluconate 1 mg per 1 gram, Cetrimide 5 mg per 1 gram Savlon antiseptic cream | 15 gram GSL £1.27 DT = £1.27 | 30 gram GSL £1.70 DT = £1.70 | 60 gram GSL £2.54 DT = £2.54 | 100 gram GSL £3.67 DT = £3.67

Cutaneous irrigation solution

▸ **Chlorhexidine with cetrimide (Non-proprietary)**

Chlorhexidine acetate 150 microgram per 1 ml, Cetrimide 1.5 mg per 1 ml Chlorhexidine acetate 0.015% / Cetrimide 0.15% irrigation solution 1litre bottles | 1 bottle P

Diethyl phthalate with methyl salicylate

- **INDICATIONS AND DOSE**

Skin preparation before injection

▶ TO THE SKIN

▸ Child: Apply to the area to be disinfected

- **MEDICINAL FORMS** There can be variation in the licensing of different medicines containing the same drug.

Cutaneous solution

CAUTIONARY AND ADVISORY LABELS 15

▸ **Diethyl phthalate with methyl salicylate (Non-proprietary)**

Methyl salicylate 5 ml per 1 litre, Diethyl phthalate 20 ml per 1 litre, Castor oil 25 ml per 1 litre, Industrial methylated spirit 950 ml per 1 litre Surgical spirit | 200 ml GSL £1.89 DT = £1.89

Hydrogen peroxide 14-May-2024

- **DRUG ACTION** Hydrogen peroxide is an oxidising agent.

- **INDICATIONS AND DOSE**

CRYSTACIDE®

Superficial bacterial skin infection

▶ TO THE SKIN

▸ Child: Apply 2–3 times a day for up to 3 weeks

Localised non-bullous impetigo [in patients who are not systemically unwell or at high risk of complications]

▶ TO THE SKIN

▸ Child: Apply 2–3 times a day for 5–7 days

- **CONTRA-INDICATIONS** Deep wounds · large wounds
- **CAUTIONS** Avoid on eyes · avoid on healthy skin · incompatible with products containing iodine or potassium permanganate
- **PRESCRIBING AND DISPENSING INFORMATION** The BP directs that when hydrogen peroxide is prescribed, hydrogen peroxide solution 6% (20 vols) should be dispensed.

13 Skin

Strong solutions of hydrogen peroxide which contain 27% (90 vols) and 30% (100 vols) are only for the preparation of weaker solutions.

CRYSTACIDE® For choice of therapy, see Skin infections, antibacterial therapy p. 373.

- **HANDLING AND STORAGE** Hydrogen peroxide bleaches fabric.

- **MEDICINAL FORMS** There can be variation in the licensing of different medicines containing the same drug.

Cutaneous cream

EXCIPIENTS: May contain Edetic acid (edta), propylene glycol

▸ Crystacide (Reig Jofre UK Ltd)
Hydrogen peroxide 10 mg per 1 gram Crystacide 1% cream | 25 gram [P] £8.07 DT = £8.07 | 40 gram [P] £11.62 DT = £11.62

Irrigation solutions

- **INDICATIONS AND DOSE**

Skin cleansing

▶ TO THE SKIN

▸ Child: Use for topical irrigation of wounds

- **IRRIGATION SOLUTIONS**

Flowfusor sodium chloride 0.9% irrigation solution 120ml bottles (Fresenius Kabi Ltd) **Sodium chloride 9 mg per 1 ml** 1 bottle • NHS indicative price = £2.88 • Drug Tariff (Part IXa)

Normasol sodium chloride 0.9% irrigation solution 100ml sachets (Molnlycke Health Care Ltd) **Sodium chloride 9 mg per 1 ml** 10 unit dose • NHS indicative price = £8.70 • Drug Tariff (Part IXa)

Normasol sodium chloride 0.9% irrigation solution 25ml sachets (Molnlycke Health Care Ltd) **Sodium chloride 9 mg per 1 ml** 25 unit dose • NHS indicative price = £7.05 • Drug Tariff (Part IXa)

Sodium chloride 0.9% irrigation solution 1litre bottles (Fresenius Kabi Ltd) **Sodium chloride 9 mg per 1 ml** 1 bottle • NHS indicative price = £2.57 • Drug Tariff (Part IXa)

Sodium chloride 0.9% irrigation solution 20ml AactiPod unit dose (Essential-Healthcare Ltd) **Sodium chloride 9 mg per 1 ml** 25 unit dose • NHS indicative price = £3.81 • Drug Tariff (Part IXa)

Sodium chloride 0.9% irrigation solution 20ml Clinipod unit dose (Mayors Healthcare Ltd) **Sodium chloride 9 mg per 1 ml** 25 unit dose • NHS indicative price = £4.23 • Drug Tariff (Part IXa)

Sodium chloride 0.9% irrigation solution 20ml EasyPod unit dose (TriOn Pharma Ltd) **Sodium chloride 9 mg per 1 ml** 25 unit dose • NHS indicative price = £3.81 • Drug Tariff (Part IXa)

Sodium chloride 0.9% irrigation solution 20ml ISO-POD unit dose (St Georges Medical Ltd) **Sodium chloride 9 mg per 1 ml** 25 unit dose • NHS indicative price = £4.95 • Drug Tariff (Part IXa)

Sodium chloride 0.9% irrigation solution 20ml Irripod unit dose (Crest Medical Ltd) **Sodium chloride 9 mg per 1 ml** 25 unit dose • NHS indicative price = £6.20 • Drug Tariff (Part IXa)

Sodium chloride 0.9% irrigation solution 20ml Knoxzy unit dose (Biovantic Pharma Ltd) **Sodium chloride 9 mg per 1 ml** 25 unit dose • NHS indicative price = £4.35 • Drug Tariff (Part IXa)

Sodium chloride 0.9% irrigation solution 20ml Sal-e Pods unit dose (Ennogen Healthcare International Ltd) **Sodium chloride 9 mg per 1 ml** 25 unit dose • NHS indicative price = £4.80 • Drug Tariff (Part IXa)

Sodium chloride 0.9% irrigation solution 20ml Salipod unit dose (Creed Medical Ltd) **Sodium chloride 9 mg per 1 ml** 25 unit dose • NHS indicative price = £4.99 • Drug Tariff (Part IXa)

Sodium chloride 0.9% irrigation solution 20ml Sterowash unit dose (Steroplast Healthcare Ltd) **Sodium chloride 9 mg per 1 ml** 25 unit dose • NHS indicative price = £4.29 • Drug Tariff (Part IXa)

Sodium chloride 0.9% irrigation solution 20ml unit dose (Alissa Healthcare Research Ltd) **Sodium chloride 9 mg per 1 ml** 25 unit dose • NHS indicative price = £7.36 • Drug Tariff (Part IXa)

Sodium chloride 0.9% irrigation solution 20ml unit dose (Bell, Sons & Co (Druggists) Ltd) **Sodium chloride 9 mg per 1 ml** 25 unit dose • NHS indicative price = £6.76 • Drug Tariff (Part IXa)

Sodium chloride 0.9% irrigation solution 20ml unit dose (Crest Medical Ltd) **Sodium chloride 9 mg per 1 ml** 25 unit dose • NHS indicative price = £4.99 • Drug Tariff (Part IXa)

Sodium chloride 0.9% irrigation solution 20ml unit dose (Viatris UK Healthcare Ltd) **Sodium chloride 9 mg per 1 ml** 25 unit dose • NHS indicative price = £5.50 • Drug Tariff (Part IXa)

Stericlens sodium chloride 0.9% irrigation solution aerosol spray (Crest Medical Ltd) **Sodium chloride 9 mg per 1 ml** 100 ml • No NHS indicative price available | 240 ml • NHS indicative price = £3.35 • Drug Tariff (Part IXa)

10.1 Minor cuts and abrasions

Skin adhesives

- **SKIN ADHESIVES**

Derma+Flex skin adhesive (Chemence Ltd)
0.5 ml • NHS indicative price = £5.36 • Drug Tariff (Part IXa)

Dermabond Advanced skin adhesive (Ethicon Ltd)
0.7 ml • NHS indicative price = £19.49 • Drug Tariff (Part IXa)

Dermabond Mini skin adhesive (Ethicon Ltd)
0.36 ml • NHS indicative price = £11.39 • Drug Tariff (Part IXa)

Dermabond ProPen skin adhesive (Ethicon Ltd)
0.5 ml • NHS indicative price = £19.95 • Drug Tariff (Part IXa)

Dermabond skin adhesive (Ethicon Ltd)
0.5 ml • NHS indicative price = £19.49 • Drug Tariff (Part IXa)

Histoacryl L skin adhesive (B.Braun Medical Ltd)
0.5 ml • NHS indicative price = £7.08 • Drug Tariff (Part IXa)

Histoacryl skin adhesive (B.Braun Medical Ltd)
0.5 ml • NHS indicative price = £6.85 • Drug Tariff (Part IXa)

Indermil skin adhesive (Covidien (UK) Commercial Ltd)
0.5 gram • NHS indicative price = £6.50 • Drug Tariff (Part IXa)

LiquiBand Optima skin adhesive (Advanced Medical Solutions Ltd)
0.5 gram • No NHS indicative price available • Drug Tariff (Part IXa)

LiquiBand flow control tissue adhesive (Advanced Medical Solutions Ltd)
0.5 gram • NHS indicative price = £5.50 • Drug Tariff (Part IXa)

LiquiBand tissue adhesive (Advanced Medical Solutions Ltd)
0.5 gram • NHS indicative price = £5.50 • Drug Tariff (Part IXa)

11 Skin disfigurement

Camouflages

30-Nov-2023

Overview

Disfigurement of the skin can be very distressing to patients and may have a marked psychological effect. In skilled hands, or with experience, camouflage cosmetics can be very effective in concealing scars and birthmarks. The depigmented patches in vitiligo are also very disfiguring and camouflage creams are of great cosmetic value.

Opaque cover foundation or cream is used to mask skin pigment abnormalities; careful application using a combination of dark- and light-coloured cover creams set with powder helps to minimise the appearance of skin deformities.

Borderline substances

Camouflages p. 947 marked 'ACBS' can be prescribed on the NHS (see *About Borderline Substances*) for postoperative scars and other deformities and as adjunctive therapy in the relief of emotional disturbances due to disfiguring skin disease, such as vitiligo. Cleansing creams, milks, and lotions are excluded.

Camouflages

● CAMOUFLAGES

Covermark classic foundation (Derma UK Ltd)
15 ml(ACBS) • NHS indicative price = £11.86

Covermark finishing powder (Derma UK Ltd)
25 gram(ACBS) • NHS indicative price = £11.86

Dermacolor fixing powder (Kryolan UK Ltd)
60 gram(ACBS) • NHS indicative price = £13.50

Keromask finishing powder (Bellava Ltd)
20 gram(ACBS) • NHS indicative price = £9.54

Keromask masking cream (Bellava Ltd)
15 ml(ACBS) • NHS indicative price = £9.54

Veil cover cream (Thomas Blake Cosmetic Creams Ltd)
19 gram(ACBS) • NHS indicative price = £25.40 | 44 gram(ACBS) • NHS indicative price = £37.79 | 70 gram(ACBS) • NHS indicative price = £47.70

Veil finishing powder (Thomas Blake Cosmetic Creams Ltd)
35 gram(ACBS) • NHS indicative price = £27.74

12 Sun protection and photodamage

Sunscreen 30-Nov-2023

Overview

Solar ultraviolet irradiation can be harmful to the skin. It is responsible for skin disorders such as *polymorphic light eruption*, *solar urticaria*, and it provokes the various *cutaneous porphyrias*. It may also trigger or aggravate skin lesions of *lupus erythematosus* and other *dermatoses*. Certain drugs, such as demeclocycline, phenothiazines, or amiodarone, can cause photosensitivity. Solar ultraviolet irradiation may also trigger attacks of recurrent herpes labialis.

The effects of exposure over longer periods include *ageing changes*, and more importantly the initiation of *skin cancer*.

Solar ultraviolet radiation is approximately 200–400 m in wavelength. The medium wavelengths (290–320 nm, known as UVB) are the main cause of sunburn. The long wavelengths (320–400 nm, known as UVA) are responsible for many *photosensitivity reactions* and *photodermatoses*. Both UVA and UVB contribute to long-term *photodamage* and to the changes responsible for *skin cancer* and ageing.

Sunscreen preparations contain substances that protect the skin against UVA and UVB radiation, but they are not a substitute for covering the skin and avoiding sunlight. EvGr Protective clothing and sun avoidance are recommended for children under 6 months of age. (A)

The sun protection factor (SPF, usually indicated in the preparation title) provides guidance on the degree of protection offered against UVB; it indicates the multiples of protection provided against burning, compared with unprotected skin; for example, an SPF of 8 should enable a child to remain 8 times longer in the sun without burning. However, in practice most users do not apply sufficient sunscreen product.

The EU Commission (September 2006) has recommended that the UVA protection factor for a sunscreen should be at least one-third of the sun protection factor (SPF); products that achieve this requirement will be labelled with a UVA logo alongside the SPF classification. EvGr Sunscreens should meet the minimum standards for UVA protection and the label should state that it provides good UVA protection (e.g. at least '4-star UVA protection'). They should also provide a SPF of at least 15 for UVB protection. (A) Preparations that also contain reflective substances, such as titanium dioxide, provide the most effective protection against UVA.

Sunscreen preparations may cause contact dermatitis as a result of an allergy to one of its ingredients.

For optimum photoprotection, sunscreen preparations should be applied **liberally** and **frequently** as per manufacturer instructions. As maximum protection from sunlight is desirable in patients with photodermatoses, sunscreen with the highest SPF is essential.

Borderline substances

Some sunscreen products have ACBS approval (see *About Borderline Substances*). They may be prescribed for skin protection against ultraviolet radiation and/or visible light in abnormal cutaneous photosensitivity causing severe cutaneous reactions in genetic disorders (including xeroderma pigmentosum and porphyrias), severe photodermatoses (both idiopathic and acquired) and in those with increased risk of ultraviolet radiation causing adverse effects due to chronic disease (such as haematological malignancies), medical therapies and/or procedures. Products with ACBS approval are *Anthelios*® Sunscreen Lotion SPF 50+, *Uvistat*® Lipscreen SPF 50, *Uvistat*® Suncream SPF 30, and *Uvistat*® Suncream SPF 50.

VITAMINS AND TRACE ELEMENTS › VITAMIN A

Betacarotene 06-Feb-2021

● **DRUG ACTION** Betacarotene is a precursor to vitamin A.

● **INDICATIONS AND DOSE**

Management of photosensitivity reactions in erythropoietic protoporphyria (specialist use only)

▶ BY MOUTH
- Child 1–4 years: 60–90 mg daily, to be given as a single dose or in divided doses
- Child 5–8 years: 90–120 mg daily, to be given as a single dose or in divided doses
- Child 9–11 years: 120–150 mg daily, to be given as a single dose or in divided doses
- Child 12–15 years: 150–180 mg daily, to be given as a single dose or in divided doses
- Child 16–17 years: 180–300 mg daily, to be given as a single dose or in divided doses

● **UNLICENSED USE** Not licensed.

● **CAUTIONS** Monitor vitamin A intake

CAUTIONS, FURTHER INFORMATION Protection not total—expert sources advise avoid strong sunlight and use sunscreen preparations; generally 2–6 weeks of treatment (resulting in yellow coloration of palms and soles) necessary before increasing exposure to sunlight; dose should be adjusted according to level of exposure to sunlight.

● **SIDE-EFFECTS**
▶ **Rare or very rare** Arthralgia · skin reactions
▶ **Frequency not known** Diarrhoea

● **PREGNANCY** Partially converted to vitamin A, but does not give rise to abnormally high serum concentration; manufacturer advises use only if potential benefit outweighs risk.

● **BREAST FEEDING** Use with caution—present in milk.

● **HEPATIC IMPAIRMENT** Avoid.

● **RENAL IMPAIRMENT** Use with caution.

● **MEDICINAL FORMS** There can be variation in the licensing of different medicines containing the same drug. Forms available from special-order manufacturers include: oral tablet, oral capsule

Oral capsule

CAUTIONARY AND ADVISORY LABELS 21

▸ **Betacarotene (Non-proprietary)**

Betacarotene 25 mg Carotaben 25mg capsules | 100 capsule [P] [X] (Hospital only)

Betacarotene 30 mg Lumitene 30mg capsules | 100 capsule [PoM] [X] (Hospital only)

▸ **Bio-Carotene** (Pharma Nord (UK) Ltd)

Betacarotene 9 mg Bio-Carotene 9mg capsules | 150 capsule £5.51

13 Superficial soft-tissue injuries and superficial thrombophlebitis

HEPARINOIDS

Heparinoid

● **INDICATIONS AND DOSE**

Superficial thrombophlebitis | Bruising | Haematoma

▸ TO THE SKIN

▸ Child 5–17 years: Apply up to 4 times a day

● **CONTRA-INDICATIONS** Should not be used on large areas of skin, broken or sensitive skin, or mucous membranes

● **LESS SUITABLE FOR PRESCRIBING** *Hirudoid®* is less suitable for prescribing.

● **MEDICINAL FORMS** There can be variation in the licensing of different medicines containing the same drug.

Cutaneous cream

EXCIPIENTS: May contain Cetostearyl alcohol (including cetyl and stearyl alcohol), hydroxybenzoates (parabens)

▸ **Hirudoid** (Thornton & Ross Ltd)

Heparinoid 3 mg per 1 gram Hirudoid 0.3% cream | 50 gram [P] £4.70 DT = £4.70

Cutaneous gel

EXCIPIENTS: May contain Fragrances, propylene glycol

▸ **Hirudoid** (Thornton & Ross Ltd)

Heparinoid 3 mg per 1 gram Hirudoid 0.3% gel | 50 gram [P] £4.70 DT = £4.70

14 Warts and calluses

Warts and calluses

08-Aug-2023

Cutaneous warts

Cutaneous warts are caused by infection of keratinocytes with the human papillomavirus (HPV). They can appear on any part of the body but commonly affect the feet (also known as plantar warts or verrucas) and hands. In most cases, warts resolve spontaneously usually within 2 years; sometimes within months. [EvGr] Treatment is required only if the warts are painful, unsightly, persistent, or are causing distress and the individual requests treatment. ⟨A⟩

Children with facial warts or children that are immunocompromised should be considered for specialist referral.

[EvGr] Younger children who require treatment should be offered the topical keratolytic salicylic acid p. 950.

Treatment choice in older children is dependent on patient preference and response to previous treatments. Options for non-facial warts in older children include either topical salicylic acid (or salicylic acid with lactic acid p. 950), or cryotherapy using liquid nitrogen if the child is likely to tolerate treatment, or a combination of both. A shorter cryotherapy freeze or weaker salicylic acid preparation is recommended for warts on the back of the hands, as scarring is more likely to occur. Cryotherapy is unlikely to help in the treatment of plantar warts as they can be difficult to treat. When indicated, cryotherapy should be provided by an appropriately trained healthcare professional. ⟨A⟩

Preparations of formaldehyde p. 949, and silver nitrate p. 949 are also licensed for the treatment of warts on hands and feet.

Salicylic acid with lactic acid p. 950 is also licensed for the removal of *corns and calluses*.

Anogenital warts

Anogenital warts (condylomata acuminata) in children are often asymptomatic and warts may resolve spontaneously, usually within 6 months.

[EvGr] If treatment is required, it should be given on the advice of a specialist. Options of treatment include cryotherapy with or without local topical anaesthetic, topical podophyllotoxin below [unlicensed] (the major active ingredient of podophyllum), topical imiquimod p. 949 [unlicensed], or surgical removal failing other treatment options. ⟨A⟩

ANTINEOPLASTIC DRUGS > PLANT ALKALOIDS

Podophyllotoxin

28-Jul-2020

● **INDICATIONS AND DOSE**

CONDYLINE®

Condylomata acuminata affecting the penis or the female external genitalia

▸ TO THE LESION

▸ Child 2–17 years (initiated under specialist supervision): Apply twice daily for 3 consecutive days, treatment may be repeated at weekly intervals if necessary for a total of five 3-day treatment courses, direct medical supervision for lesions in the female and for lesions greater than 4 cm^2 in the male, maximum 50 single applications ('loops') per session (consult product literature)

WARTICON® CREAM

Condylomata acuminata affecting the penis or the female external genitalia

▸ TO THE LESION

▸ Child 2–17 years (initiated under specialist supervision): Apply twice daily for 3 consecutive days, treatment may be repeated at weekly intervals if necessary for a total of four 3-day treatment courses, direct medical supervision for lesions greater than 4 cm^2

WARTICON® LIQUID

Condylomata acuminata affecting the penis or the female external genitalia

▸ TO THE LESION

▸ Child 2–17 years (initiated under specialist supervision): Apply twice daily for 3 consecutive days, treatment may be repeated at weekly intervals if necessary for a total of four 3-day treatment courses, direct medical supervision for lesions greater than 4 cm^2, maximum 50 single applications ('loops') per session (consult product literature)

● **UNLICENSED USE** Not licensed for use in children.

● **CAUTIONS** Avoid normal skin · avoid open wounds · keep away from face · very irritant to eyes

● **SIDE-EFFECTS** Balanoposthitis · skin irritation

● **PREGNANCY** Avoid.

● **BREAST FEEDING** Avoid.

● **MEDICINAL FORMS** There can be variation in the licensing of different medicines containing the same drug.

Cutaneous solution

CAUTIONARY AND ADVISORY LABELS 15

▸ **Warticon** (Phoenix Labs Ltd)

Podophyllotoxin 5 mg per 1 ml Warticon 0.5% solution | 3 ml PoM £14.86 DT = £14.86

Cutaneous cream

EXCIPIENTS: May contain Butylated hydroxyanisole, cetostearyl alcohol (including cetyl and stearyl alcohol), hydroxybenzoates (parabens), sorbic acid

▸ **Warticon** (Phoenix Labs Ltd)

Podophyllotoxin 1.5 mg per 1 gram Warticon 0.15% cream | 5 gram PoM £17.83 DT = £17.83

ANTISEPTICS AND DISINFECTANTS › ALDEHYDES AND DERIVATIVES

Formaldehyde

● **INDICATIONS AND DOSE**

Warts, particularly plantar warts

▸ TO THE LESION

▸ Child: Apply twice daily

● **UNLICENSED USE** Licensed for use in children (age range not specified by manufacturer).

● **CAUTIONS** Impaired peripheral circulation · not suitable for application to anogenital region · not suitable for application to face · not suitable for application to large areas · patients with diabetes at risk of neuropathic ulcers · protect surrounding skin and avoid broken skin · significant peripheral neuropathy

● **SIDE-EFFECTS** Asthma · cough · dysphagia · eye irritation · increased risk of infection · laryngospasm · skin reactions

● **MEDICINAL FORMS** There can be variation in the licensing of different medicines containing the same drug. Forms available from special-order manufacturers include: cutaneous solution

Cutaneous solution

▸ **Formaldehyde (Non-proprietary)**

Formaldehyde 40 mg per 1 ml Formaldehyde (Buffered) 4% solution | 1000 ml £5.88

ANTISEPTICS AND DISINFECTANTS › OTHER

Silver nitrate

● **INDICATIONS AND DOSE**

Common warts

▸ TO THE LESION

▸ Child: Apply every 24 hours for up to 3 applications, apply moistened caustic pencil tip for 1–2 minutes. Instructions in proprietary packs generally incorporate advice to remove dead skin before use by gentle filing and to cover with adhesive dressing after application

Verrucas

▸ TO THE LESION

▸ Child: Apply every 24 hours for up to 6 applications, apply moistened caustic pencil tip for 1–2 minutes. Instructions in proprietary packs generally incorporate advice to remove dead skin before use by gentle filing and to cover with adhesive dressing after application

Umbilical granulomas

▸ TO THE SKIN

▸ Child: Apply moistened caustic pencil tip (usually containing silver nitrate 40%) for 1–2 minutes, protect surrounding skin with soft paraffin

● **UNLICENSED USE** No age range specified by manufacturer.

● **CAUTIONS** Avoid broken skin · not suitable for application to ano-genital region · not suitable for application to face · not suitable for application to large areas · protect surrounding skin

● **SIDE-EFFECTS**

▸ **Rare or very rare** Argyria · methaemoglobinaemia

● **PATIENT AND CARER ADVICE** Patients should be advised that silver nitrate may stain fabric.

● **MEDICINAL FORMS** There can be variation in the licensing of different medicines containing the same drug.

Stick

▸ **Avoca** (Bray Group Ltd)

Silver nitrate 400 mg per 1 gram Avoca 40% silver nitrate pencils | 1 applicator P £1.98 DT = £1.98

Silver nitrate 750 mg per 1 gram Avoca 75% silver nitrate applicators | 100 applicator P £83.70 DT = £83.70

Avoca 75% silver nitrate applicators with thick handles | 50 applicator P £82.57

Silver nitrate 950 mg per 1 gram Avoca 95% silver nitrate applicators | 100 applicator P £89.53 DT = £89.53

Avoca 95% silver nitrate pencils | 1 applicator P £4.49 DT = £5.25

Avoca wart and verruca treatment set | 1 applicator P £5.25 DT = £5.25

ANTIVIRALS › IMMUNE RESPONSE MODIFIERS

Imiquimod

09-Nov-2020

● **INDICATIONS AND DOSE**

ALDARA ®

Warts (external genital and perianal)

▸ TO THE LESION

▸ Child (initiated under specialist supervision): Apply 3 times a week until lesions resolve (maximum 16 weeks), to be applied thinly at night

● **UNLICENSED USE** Not licensed for use in children.

● **CAUTIONS** Autoimmune disease · avoid broken skin · avoid normal skin · avoid open wounds · immunosuppressed patients · not suitable for internal genital warts · uncircumcised males (risk of phimosis or stricture of foreskin)

● **SIDE-EFFECTS**

▸ **Common or very common** Appetite decreased · arthralgia · asthenia · headaches · increased risk of infection · lymphadenopathy · myalgia · nausea · pain

▸ **Uncommon** Anorectal disorder · chills · conjunctival irritation · depression · diarrhoea · dizziness · drowsiness · dry mouth · dysuria · erectile dysfunction · eyelid oedema · face oedema · fever · flushing · gastrointestinal discomfort · genital pain · hyperhidrosis · inflammation · influenza like illness · insomnia · irritability · laryngeal pain · malaise · nasal congestion · painful sexual intercourse · paraesthesia · penis disorder · skin reactions · skin ulcer · tinnitus · uterovaginal prolapse · vomiting · vulvovaginal disorders

▸ **Rare or very rare** Autoimmune disorder exacerbated

▸ **Frequency not known** Alopecia · cutaneous lupus erythematosus · severe cutaneous adverse reactions (SCARs)

● **CONCEPTION AND CONTRACEPTION** May damage latex condoms and diaphragms.

● **PREGNANCY** No evidence of teratogenicity or toxicity in *animal* studies; manufacturer advises caution.

● **BREAST FEEDING** No information available.

● **DIRECTIONS FOR ADMINISTRATION**

▸ Important Manufacturer advises cream should be rubbed in and allowed to stay on the treated area for 6–10 hours then washed off with mild soap and water (uncircumcised males treating warts under foreskin should wash the area daily). The cream should be washed off before sexual contact.

● **PATIENT AND CARER ADVICE** A patient information leaflet should be provided.

- **MEDICINAL FORMS** There can be variation in the licensing of different medicines containing the same drug.

Cutaneous cream

CAUTIONARY AND ADVISORY LABELS 10

EXCIPIENTS: May contain Benzyl alcohol, cetostearyl alcohol (including cetyl and stearyl alcohol), hydroxybenzoates (parabens), polysorbates

▸ **Aldara** (Viatris UK Healthcare Ltd)
Imiquimod 50 mg per 1 gram Aldara 5% cream 250mg sachets | 12 sachet PoM £48.60 DT = £48.60

SALICYLIC ACID AND DERIVATIVES

Salicylic acid

24-Nov-2020

- **INDICATIONS AND DOSE**

OCCLUSAL®

Common and plantar warts

▶ TO THE LESION

▸ Child: Apply daily, treatment may need to be continued for up to 3 months

VERRUGON®

For plantar warts

▶ TO THE LESION

▸ Child: Apply daily, treatment may need to be continued for up to 3 months

- **UNLICENSED USE** Not licensed for use in children under 2 years.
- **CAUTIONS** Application to large areas · avoid broken skin · impaired peripheral circulation · not suitable for application to anogenital region · not suitable for application to face · patients with diabetes at risk of neuropathic ulcers · severe peripheral neuropathy

CAUTIONS, FURTHER INFORMATION

▸ Application to large areas and salicylate toxicity Salicylate toxicity may occur particularly if applied on large areas of skin or neonatal skin.

- **SIDE-EFFECTS** Skin irritation
- **PATIENT AND CARER ADVICE** Advise patient to apply carefully to wart and to protect surrounding skin (e.g. with soft paraffin or specially designed plaster); rub wart surface gently with file or pumice stone once weekly.
- **MEDICINAL FORMS** There can be variation in the licensing of different medicines containing the same drug.

Cutaneous solution

CAUTIONARY AND ADVISORY LABELS 15

▸ **Occlusal** (Alliance Pharmaceuticals Ltd)
Salicylic acid 260 mg per 1 ml Occlusal 26% solution | 10 ml P £3.56 DT = £3.56

Salicylic acid with lactic acid

09-Aug-2023

The properties listed below are those particular to the combination only. For the properties of the components please consider, salicylic acid above.

- **INDICATIONS AND DOSE**

DUOFILM®

Plantar and mosaic warts

▶ TO THE LESION

▸ Child: Apply daily, treatment may need to be continued for up to 3 months

SALACTOL®

Warts, particularly plantar warts | Verrucas | Corns | Calluses

▶ TO THE LESION

▸ Child: Apply daily, treatment may need to be continued for up to 3 months

SALATAC®

Warts | Verrucas | Corns | Calluses

▶ TO THE LESION

▸ Child: Apply daily, treatment may need to be continued for up to 3 months

- **PRESCRIBING AND DISPENSING INFORMATION** Preparation of salicylic acid in a collodion basis (*Salactol*®) is available but some patients may develop an allergy to colophony in the formulation.
- **MEDICINAL FORMS** There can be variation in the licensing of different medicines containing the same drug.

Cutaneous gel

CAUTIONARY AND ADVISORY LABELS 15

▸ **Salatac** (Dermal Laboratories Ltd)
Lactic acid 40 mg per 1 gram, Salicylic acid 120 mg per 1 gram Salatac gel | 8 gram P £3.26 DT = £3.26

Cutaneous paint

CAUTIONARY AND ADVISORY LABELS 15

▸ **Duofilm** (Thornton & Ross Ltd)
Lactic acid 150 mg per 1 gram, Salicylic acid 167 mg per 1 gram Duofilm paint | 15 ml P £3.40 DT = £3.40

▸ **Salactol** (Dermal Laboratories Ltd)
Lactic acid 167 mg per 1 gram, Salicylic acid 167 mg per 1 gram Salactol paint | 10 ml P £2.26 DT = £2.26

Chapter 14
Vaccines

CONTENTS

1 Immunoglobulin therapy

IMMUNE SERA AND IMMUNOGLOBULINS ›
IMMUNOGLOBULINS

Immunoglobulins

13-Oct-2025

Passive immunity

Immunity with protection against certain infective organisms can be obtained by injecting preparations made from the plasma of immune individuals with adequate levels of antibody to the disease for which protection is sought. The duration of this passive immunity varies according to the dose and the type of immunoglobulin. Passive immunity may last only a few weeks; when necessary, passive immunisation can be repeated. Antibodies of human origin are usually termed immunoglobulins. The term antiserum is applied to material prepared in animals. Because of serum sickness and other allergic-type reactions that may follow injections of antisera, this therapy has been replaced wherever possible by the use of immunoglobulins. Reactions are theoretically possible after injection of human immunoglobulins but reports of such reactions are very rare.

Two types of human immunoglobulin preparation are available, normal immunoglobulin and **disease-specific immunoglobulins**.

Human normal immunoglobulin (HNIG) is prepared from pooled plasma obtained from donors outside the UK, tested and found non-reactive for hepatitis B surface antigen and for antibodies against hepatitis C virus and human immunodeficiency virus (types 1 and 2). A global shortage of human immunoglobulin and the rapidly increasing range of clinical indications for treatment with immunoglobulins has resulted in the need for a Demand Management plan in the UK, for further information consult the Department of Health and Social Care's **Demand Management Plan for Immunoglobulin Use** and NHS England's **Clinical Commissioning Policy for the use of therapeutic immunoglobulin** (both available at: igd.mdsas.com).

For further information on the use of immunoglobulins, see UKHSA guidance: **Immunoglobulin: when to use** (www.gov.uk/government/publications/immunoglobulin-when-to-use) and **Immunisation against Infectious Disease** (www.gov.uk/government/collections/immunisation-against-infectious-disease-the-green-book).

Availability

Human normal immunoglobulin p. 955 for intramuscular administration is available from the Immunisation, Hepatitis and Blood Safety Department of PHE's Centre for Infectious Disease Surveillance and some regional PHE and NHS laboratories, for the protection of contacts and the control of outbreaks of hepatitis A, measles, and rubella only. For other indications, subcutaneous or intravenous normal immunoglobulin may be purchased from the manufacturer (see Index of manufacturers p. 1443).

Various **disease-specific immunoglobulins** for intramuscular administration are available from either the Immunisation, Hepatitis and Blood Safety Department of PHE's Centre for Infectious Disease Surveillance; some regional PHE and NHS laboratories; PHE's Rabies and Immunoglobulin Service; and/or through Bio Products Laboratory (BPL). Tetanus immunoglobulin p. 957 is available from BPL, hospital pharmacies, or blood transfusion departments. Hepatitis B immunoglobulin p. 954 required by transplant centres should be obtained commercially.

In Scotland all immunoglobulins are available from the *Scottish National Blood Transfusion Service* (SNBTS).

In Wales all immunoglobulins are available from the *Welsh Blood Service* (WBS).

In Northern Ireland all immunoglobulins are available from the *Northern Ireland Blood Transfusion Service* (NIBTS).

Normal immunoglobulin

Human normal immunoglobulin is prepared from pools of at least 1000 donations of human plasma; it contains immunoglobulin G (IgG) and antibodies to hepatitis A, measles, mumps, rubella, varicella, and other viruses that are currently prevalent in the general population.

Uses

Normal immunoglobulin (containing 10–18% protein) is administered by *intramuscular injection* for the protection of susceptible contacts against **hepatitis A** virus (infectious hepatitis), **measles** and, to a lesser extent, **rubella**. Injection of immunoglobulin produces immediate protection lasting for several weeks.

Normal immunoglobulin (containing 3–12% protein) for *intravenous administration* is used as *replacement therapy* for children with congenital agammaglobulinaemia and hypogammaglobulinaemia, and for the short-term treatment of idiopathic thrombocytopenic purpura and Kawasaki disease; it is also used for the prophylaxis of infection following bone-marrow transplantation and in children with symptomatic HIV infection who have recurrent bacterial infections. Normal immunoglobulin for replacement therapy may also be given intramuscularly or subcutaneously, but intravenous formulations are normally preferred. Intravenous immunoglobulin is also used in the treatment of Guillain-Barré syndrome as an alternative to plasma exchange, and for post-exposure prophylaxis of varicella-zoster infection in eligible children—for further information, see Herpesvirus infections p. 498.

The dose of normal immunoglobulin used as replacement therapy in patients with immunodeficiencies is **not the same** as the dose required for treatment of acute conditions. For Kawasaki disease a single dose by intravenous infusion should be given with concomitant aspirin p. 104 within 10 days of onset of symptoms (but children with a delayed diagnosis may also benefit).

14 Vaccines

For information on the use of intravenous normal immunoglobulin and alternative therapies for certain conditions, see NHS England's: **Clinical Commissioning Policy for the use of therapeutic immunoglobulin** (available at: igd.mdsas.com).

Hepatitis A
For close contacts (of the index case) who have chronic liver disease (including chronic hepatitis B or C infection), HIV infection (with a CD4 count < 200 cells per microlitre), or are immunosuppressed, normal immunoglobulin in addition to the monovalent hepatitis A vaccine p. 991 is recommended within 14 days of exposure to the index case (up to 28 days in those with chronic liver disease). Normal immunoglobulin and the monovalent hepatitis A vaccine can be given at the same time, but should be given at separate injection sites.

For further information on post-exposure prophylaxis and information on risk assessment, see Hepatitis A vaccine p. 967.

Measles
Intravenous or subcutaneous normal immunoglobulin may be given to prevent or attenuate an attack of measles in individuals who do not have adequate immunity. Children with compromised immunity who have come into contact with measles should receive intravenous or subcutaneous normal immunoglobulin as soon as possible after exposure. It is most effective if given within 72 hours but can be effective if given within 6 days.

Subcutaneous or intramuscular normal immunoglobulin should also be considered for the following individuals if they have been in contact with a confirmed case of measles or with a person associated with a local outbreak:

- non-immune pregnant women
- infants under 9 months

Further advice should be sought from the Centre for Infections, Public Health England (tel. (020) 8200 6868).

Individuals with normal immunity who are not in the above categories and who have not been fully immunised against measles, can be given measles, mumps, and rubella vaccine p. 1002 for prophylaxis following exposure to measles.

Rubella
Intramuscular immunoglobulin after exposure to rubella does **not** prevent infection in non-immune contacts and is **not** recommended for protection of pregnant women exposed to rubella. It may, however, reduce the likelihood of a clinical attack which may possibly reduce the risk to the fetus. Risk of intra-uterine transmission is greatest in the first 11 weeks of pregnancy, between 16 and 20 weeks there is minimal risk of deafness only, after 20 weeks there is no increased risk. Intramuscular normal immunoglobulin p. 955 should be used only if termination of pregnancy would be unacceptable to the pregnant woman—it should be given as soon as possible after exposure. Serological follow-up of recipients is essential to determine if the woman has become infected despite receiving immunoglobulin.

For routine prophylaxis against Rubella, see measles, mumps, and rubella vaccine p. 1002.

Tetanus
Normal immunoglobulin [unlicensed] can be used an alternative when tetanus immunoglobulin is not available (see *Tetanus immunoglobulin* in *Disease-specific immunoglobulins*).

Disease-specific immunoglobulins

Specific immunoglobulins are prepared by pooling the plasma of selected human donors with high levels of the specific antibody required. For further information, see UKHSA guidance: **Immunoglobulin: when to use** (www.gov.uk/government/publications/immunoglobulin-when-to-use).

There are no specific immunoglobulins for hepatitis A, measles, or rubella—normal immunoglobulin is used in certain circumstances. There is no specific immunoglobulin for mumps; neither normal immunoglobulin nor measles, mumps, and rubella vaccine is effective as post-exposure prophylaxis.

Hepatitis B immunoglobulin
Hepatitis B immunoglobulin p. 954 (HBIG) in addition to the hepatitis B vaccine p. 992 is recommended for post-exposure prophylaxis of children in certain high-risk groups to provide rapid protection against hepatitis B until the vaccine becomes effective. HBIG is also recommended in some known non-responders to the hepatitis B vaccine. The administration of HBIG at the same time as the vaccine will not inhibit the antibody response, but they should be given at different sites. For further information on high-risk groups and post-exposure management, see Hepatitis B vaccine p. 968.

An intravenous preparation of HBIG is licensed for the prevention of hepatitis B recurrence in HBV-DNA negative patients who have undergone liver transplantation for liver failure caused by the virus.

Rabies immunoglobulin
Post-exposure prophylaxis with rabies immunoglobulin p. 957 should be considered according to the risk assessment of rabies exposure. It provides rapid protection until rabies vaccine p. 997 (administered at a separate site) becomes effective. When indicated, rabies immunoglobulin should be infiltrated around the site of the wound if possible, as it neutralises rabies virus before the immune system can respond. There is limited benefit of intramuscular administration away from the wound site. For further guidance on risk assessment and post-exposure treatment, see Rabies vaccine p. 977, and for information about dosing and administration, see rabies immunoglobulin.

Tetanus immunoglobulin
Intravenous tetanus immunoglobulin is no longer available in the UK and the volume of intramuscular tetanus immunoglobulin required to reach a therapeutic dose would be too large in most children with tetanus. Therefore, for the management of suspected or confirmed tetanus (including localised tetanus), intravenous normal immunoglobulin [unlicensed] is recommended. For further guidance on the management of confirmed and suspected cases of tetanus (including localised tetanus), see Chapter 30, Tetanus, in *Immunisation against infectious disease*- 'The Green Book' (available at: www.gov.uk/government/publications/tetanus-the-green-book-chapter-30) and UKHSA guidance: **Tetanus** (available at: www.gov.uk/government/publications/tetanus-advice-for-health-professionals).

For the management of tetanus-prone wounds, tetanus immunoglobulin p. 957 should be considered based on a child's immunisation status and wound category. If tetanus immunoglobulin is not available, normal immunoglobulin [unlicensed] may be used. For further guidance on the management of tetanus-prone wounds, see UKHSA guidance: **Tetanus** (available at: www.gov.uk/government/publications/tetanus-advice-for-health-professionals). When indicated for post-exposure prophylaxis, tetanus immunoglobulin should be used in addition to the other preventative measures of thorough wound cleansing and administration of a tetanus-containing vaccine (depending on immunisation status). Antibacterial therapy may also be warranted depending on clinical severity. For further information, see *Post-exposure management* in Tetanus vaccine p. 981.

Varicella-zoster immunoglobulin
Varicella (chickenpox) infection can lead to severe and even life-threatening varicella disease in certain at-risk children. Post-exposure prophylaxis is recommended to attenuate disease and to reduce the risk of complications. For further

information on post-exposure prophylaxis, including risk assessment and the use of varicella-zoster immunoglobulin p. 958 in neonates exposed to maternal chickenpox within 7 days of delivery, see Herpesvirus infections p. 498.

Anti-D immunoglobulins

13-Apr-2026

(Anti-D (Rh_0) immunoglobulin)

- **DRUG ACTION** Anti-D immunoglobulins contain anti-D (Rh) antibodies which act against the Rh(D) antigen of erythrocytes, thereby suppressing sensitisation to Rh(D)-positive red cells in rhesus-negative individuals, although it's exact mechanism of action is unknown.

- **INDICATIONS AND DOSE**

To rhesus-negative woman for prevention of Rh_0(D) sensitisation, following birth of rhesus-positive infant

▶ BY DEEP INTRAMUSCULAR INJECTION

▸ Females of childbearing potential: 500 units, dose to be administered immediately or within 72 hours; for transplacental bleed of over 4 mL fetal red cells, extra 100–125 units per mL fetal red cells, subcutaneous route used for patients with bleeding disorders

To rhesus-negative woman for prevention of Rh_0(D) sensitisation, following any potentially sensitising episode (e.g. stillbirth, abortion, amniocentesis) up to 20 weeks' gestation

▶ BY DEEP INTRAMUSCULAR INJECTION

▸ Females of childbearing potential: 250 units per episode, dose to be administered immediately or within 72 hours, subcutaneous route used for patients with bleeding disorders

To rhesus-negative woman for prevention of Rh_0(D) sensitisation, following any potentially sensitising episode (e.g. stillbirth, abortion, amniocentesis) after 20 weeks' gestation

▶ BY DEEP INTRAMUSCULAR INJECTION

▸ Females of childbearing potential: 500 units per episode, dose to be administered immediately or within 72 hours, subcutaneous route used for patients with bleeding disorders

To rhesus-negative woman for prevention of Rh_0(D) sensitisation, antenatal prophylaxis

▶ BY DEEP INTRAMUSCULAR INJECTION

▸ Females of childbearing potential: 500 units, dose to be given at weeks 28 and 34 of pregnancy, if infant rhesus-positive, a further dose is still needed immediately or within 72 hours of delivery, subcutaneous route used for patients with bleeding disorders

To rhesus-negative woman for prevention of Rh_0(D) sensitisation, antenatal prophylaxis (alternative NICE recommendation)

▶ BY DEEP INTRAMUSCULAR INJECTION

▸ Females of childbearing potential: 1000–1650 units, dose to be given at weeks 28 and 34 of pregnancy, alternatively 1500 units for 1 dose, dose to be given between 28 and 30 weeks gestation

To rhesus-negative woman for prevention of Rh_0(D) sensitisation, following Rh_0(D) incompatible blood transfusion

▶ BY DEEP INTRAMUSCULAR INJECTION

▸ Females of childbearing potential: 100–125 units per mL of transfused rhesus-positive red cells, subcutaneous route used for patients with bleeding disorders

RHOPHYLAC®

To rhesus-negative woman for prevention of Rh_0(D) sensitisation, following birth of rhesus-positive infant

▶ BY INTRAMUSCULAR INJECTION, OR BY INTRAVENOUS INJECTION

▸ Females of childbearing potential: 1000–1500 units, dose to be administered immediately or within 72 hours; for large transplacental bleed, extra 100 units per mL fetal red cells (preferably by intravenous injection), intravenous route recommended for patients with bleeding disorders

To rhesus-negative woman for prevention of Rh_0(D) sensitisation, following any potentially sensitising episode (e.g. abortion, amniocentesis, chorionic villous sampling) up to 12 weeks' gestation

▶ BY INTRAMUSCULAR INJECTION, OR BY INTRAVENOUS INJECTION

▸ Females of childbearing potential: 1000 units per episode, dose to be administered immediately or within 72 hours, intravenous route recommended for patients with bleeding disorders, higher doses may be required after 12 weeks gestation

To rhesus-negative woman for prevention of Rh_0(D) sensitisation, antenatal prophylaxis

▶ BY INTRAMUSCULAR INJECTION, OR BY INTRAVENOUS INJECTION

▸ Females of childbearing potential: 1500 units, dose to be given between weeks 28–30 of pregnancy; if infant rhesus-positive, a further dose is still needed immediately or within 72 hours of delivery, intravenous route recommended for patients with bleeding disorders

To rhesus-negative woman for prevention of Rh_0(D) sensitisation, following Rh_0(D) incompatible blood transfusion

▶ BY INTRAVENOUS INJECTION

▸ Females of childbearing potential: 50 units per mL of transfused rhesus-positive blood, alternatively 100 units per of mL of erythrocyte concentrate, intravenous route recommended for patients with bleeding disorders

- **CAUTIONS** Immunoglobulin A deficiency · possible interference with live virus vaccines

CAUTIONS, FURTHER INFORMATION

▸ MMR vaccine MMR vaccine may be given in the postpartum period with anti-D immunoglobulins injection provided that separate syringes are used and the products are administered into different limbs. If blood is transfused, the antibody response to the vaccine may be inhibited—measure rubella antibodies after 6–8 weeks and revaccinate if necessary.

- **INTERACTIONS** → Appendix 1: immunoglobulins
- **SIDE-EFFECTS**

▶ **Uncommon** Chills · fever · headache · malaise · skin reactions

▶ **Rare or very rare** Arthralgia · dyspnoea · hypersensitivity · hypotension · nausea · tachycardia · vomiting

▶ **Frequency not known** Intravascular haemolysis

- **HANDLING AND STORAGE** Care must be taken to store all immunological products under the conditions recommended in the product literature, otherwise the preparation may become ineffective. **Refrigerated storage** is usually necessary; many immunoglobulins need to be stored at 2–8°C and not allowed to freeze. Immunoglobulins should be protected from light. Opened multidose vials must be used within the period recommended in the product literature.

● **NATIONAL FUNDING/ACCESS DECISIONS** For full details see funding body website

NICE decisions

▶ **Routine antenatal anti-D prophylaxis for rhesus-negative women (August 2008)** NICE TA156 Recommended

● **MEDICINAL FORMS** There can be variation in the licensing of different medicines containing the same drug.

Solution for injection

▶ **D-Gam** (Bio Products Laboratory Ltd)
Anti-D (RHO) immunoglobulin 500 unit D-Gam Anti-D immunoglobulin 500unit solution for injection vials | 1 vial PoM £54.00

▶ **Rhophylac** (CSL Behring UK Ltd)
Anti-D (RHO) immunoglobulin 750 unit per 1 ml Rhophylac 1,500units/2ml solution for injection pre-filled syringes | 1 pre-filled disposable injection PoM £76.50 (Hospital only)

Cytomegalovirus immunoglobulin

16-Apr-2020

● **INDICATIONS AND DOSE**

Prophylaxis of cytomegalovirus infection in patients taking immunosuppressants, particularly transplant recipients (specialist use only)

▶ BY INTRAVENOUS INFUSION

▶ Child: (consult product literature)

● **CONTRA-INDICATIONS** Selective IgA deficiency with IgA antibodies

● **CAUTIONS** Interference with live virus vaccines

CAUTIONS, FURTHER INFORMATION Cytomegalovirus immunoglobulin may impair the immune response to live virus vaccines; such vaccines should only be given 3 months after CMV immunoglobulin treatment. Patients receiving measles vaccines should have their antibody status checked as impairment of immune response may persist for up to 1 year.

● **INTERACTIONS** → Appendix 1: immunoglobulins

● **SIDE-EFFECTS** Arthralgia · back pain · chills · cutaneous lupus erythematosus · dizziness · embolism and thrombosis · fatigue · fever · haemolysis · haemolytic anaemia · headache · hypotension · infusion related reaction · meningitis aseptic · myocardial infarction · nausea · neutropenia · renal impairment · skin reactions · stroke · transfusion-related acute lung injury · vomiting

● **MONITORING REQUIREMENTS**

▶ Manufacturer advises monitor for signs of infusion-related reactions during and for at least one hour after each infusion in patients receiving cytomegalovirus immunoglobulin for the first time, or following a prolonged period between treatments, or when a different human immunoglobulin has been used previously; monitor all other patients for at least 20 minutes after each infusion—in case of reaction, reduce rate or stop infusion as clinically appropriate.

▶ Manufacturer advises monitor urine output and serum creatinine.

● **HANDLING AND STORAGE** Care must be taken to store all immunological products under the conditions recommended in the product literature, otherwise the preparation may become ineffective. **Refrigerated storage** is usually necessary; many immunoglobulins need to be stored at 2–8°C and not allowed to freeze. Immunoglobulins should be protected from light. Opened multidose vials must be used within the period recommended in the product literature.

● **MEDICINAL FORMS** There can be variation in the licensing of different medicines containing the same drug.

Solution for infusion

▶ **Cytotect CP Biotest** (Grifols UK Ltd)
Cytomegalovirus immunoglobulin human 100 unit per 1 ml Cytotect CP Biotest 5,000units/50ml solution for infusion vials | 1 vial PoM £917.70 (Hospital only)
Cytotect CP Biotest 1,000units/10ml solution for infusion vials | 1 vial PoM £183.54 (Hospital only)

Hepatitis B immunoglobulin

05-Feb-2024

● **INDICATIONS AND DOSE**

Post-exposure prophylaxis against hepatitis B infection

▶ BY INTRAMUSCULAR INJECTION

▶ Neonate: 250 units for 1 dose, dose to be administered as soon as possible after exposure; ideally within 24–48 hours, but no later than 7 days after exposure.

▶ Child 1 month–4 years: 250 units for 1 dose, dose to be administered as soon as possible after exposure; ideally within 24–48 hours, but no later than 7 days after exposure

▶ Child 5–9 years: 300 units for 1 dose, dose to be administered as soon as possible after exposure; ideally within 24–48 hours, but no later than 7 days after exposure

▶ Child 10–17 years: 500 units for 1 dose, dose to be administered as soon as possible after exposure; ideally within 24–48 hours, but no later than 7 days after exposure

Prevention of transmitted infection at birth

▶ BY INTRAMUSCULAR INJECTION

▶ Neonate: 250 units for 1 dose, dose to be administered as soon as possible after birth.

▶ BY INTRAVENOUS INFUSION

▶ Neonate: (consult product literature).

Post-exposure prophylaxis against hepatitis B infection [after exposure to hepatitis B virus-contaminated material]

▶ BY INTRAVENOUS INFUSION

▶ Child: Dose to be administered as soon as possible after exposure, but no later than 72 hours (consult product literature)

Prophylaxis against re-infection of transplanted liver

▶ BY INTRAVENOUS INFUSION

▶ Child: (consult product literature)

● **CAUTIONS** IgA deficiency · interference with live virus vaccines

● **INTERACTIONS** → Appendix 1: immunoglobulins

● **SIDE-EFFECTS**

▶ **Uncommon** Abdominal pain upper · headache

▶ **Rare or very rare** Cardiac discomfort · fatigue · hypersensitivity · hypertension · hypotension · muscle spasms · nasopharyngitis · oropharyngeal pain · palpitations · skin reactions

● **DIRECTIONS FOR ADMINISTRATION**

▶ With intramuscular use If more than 3 mL is to be given to young children and infants, or more than 5 mL to older children, give in divided doses at different sites.

● **PRESCRIBING AND DISPENSING INFORMATION** Vials containing 500 units (for intramuscular injection), are available from the UKHSA Rabies and Immunoglobulin Service, and are also available from Bio Products Laboratory (BPL).

● **HANDLING AND STORAGE** Care must be taken to store all immunological products under the conditions recommended in the product literature, otherwise the preparation may become ineffective. **Refrigerated storage** is usually necessary; many immunoglobulins need to be stored at 2–8°C and not allowed to freeze. Immunoglobulins should be protected from light. Opened multidose vials must be used within the period recommended in the product literature.

- **MEDICINAL FORMS** There can be variation in the licensing of different medicines containing the same drug.

Solution for injection

- **Hepatitis B immunoglobulin (Non-proprietary)**
  Hepatitis B immunoglobulin human 100 unit per 1 ml Hepatitis B immunoglobulin human 500units/5ml solution for injection vials | 1 vial PoM £600.00
- **Zutectra** (Grifols UK Ltd)
  Zutectra 500units/1ml solution for injection pre-filled syringes | 5 syringe PoM £1,500.00 (Hospital only)

Solution for infusion

- **Hepatect CP** (Grifols UK Ltd)
  Hepatitis B immunoglobulin human 50 unit per 1 ml Hepatect CP 5000units/100ml solution for infusion vials | 1 vial PoM £2,750.00 (Hospital only)
- **Omri-Hep-B** (Imported (Israel))
  Hepatitis B immunoglobulin human 50 unit per 1 ml Omri-Hep-B 5000units/100ml solution for infusion vials | 1 vial PoM (Hospital only)

Normal immunoglobulin

13-Oct-2025

- **INDICATIONS AND DOSE**

Post-exposure prophylaxis against hepatitis A infection [using Subgam®]

▶ BY DEEP INTRAMUSCULAR INJECTION

- Neonate: 500 mg for 1 dose.
- Child 1 month–9 years: 500 mg for 1 dose
- Child 10–17 years: 1000 mg for 1 dose

Rubella in pregnancy [post-exposure prophylaxis to prevent or attenuate clinical attack; only when termination of pregnancy is unacceptable]

▶ BY DEEP INTRAMUSCULAR INJECTION

- Females of childbearing potential: 750 mg for 1 dose

Post-exposure prophylaxis of varicella-zoster infection [neonates exposed to maternal chickenpox 7 days before or after delivery, if varicella-zoster immunoglobulin is unavailable]

▶ BY INTRAVENOUS INFUSION

- Neonate: 200 mg/kg for 1 dose, dose to be administered as soon as possible—preferably within 96 hours after exposure.

Post-exposure prophylaxis of varicella-zoster infection [if antivirals are contra-indicated or otherwise unsuitable]

▶ BY INTRAVENOUS INFUSION

- Neonate: 200 mg/kg for 1 dose, dose to be administered within 10 days after exposure (preferably within 7 days), but can be later if necessary.
- Child: 200 mg/kg for 1 dose, dose to be administered within 10 days after exposure (preferably within 7 days if patient is immunosuppressed), but can be later if necessary

Replacement therapy in primary immunodeficiency disorders (specialist use only) | Replacement therapy in secondary immunodeficiency disorders (specialist use only)

▶ BY SUBCUTANEOUS INFUSION, OR BY INTRAVENOUS INFUSION

- Neonate: (consult product literature).
- Child: (consult product literature)

Immune-mediated disorders (specialist use only)

▶ BY INTRAVENOUS INFUSION

- Neonate: For some indications, subcutaneous infusion may be used for maintenance treatment (consult product literature).
- Child: For some indications, subcutaneous infusion may be used for maintenance treatment (consult product literature)

Kawasaki disease [with concomitant aspirin]

▶ BY INTRAVENOUS INFUSION

- Child: 2 g/kg for 1 dose, treatment should be given within 10 days of onset of symptom (but children with a delayed diagnosis may also benefit)

- **UNLICENSED USE** The UKHSA advises normal immunoglobulin is used as detailed below, although these situations are considered unlicensed:
  - post-exposure prophylaxis against hepatitis A infection [using *Subgam*®];
  - rubella in pregnancy;
  - post-exposure prophylaxis of varicella-zoster infection.
- **CONTRA-INDICATIONS** Patients with selective IgA deficiency who have known antibodies against IgA

CONTRA-INDICATIONS, FURTHER INFORMATION For full details on contra-indications, consult product literature.

- **CAUTIONS**

GENERAL CAUTIONS Agammaglobulinaemia with or without IgA deficiency · hypogammaglobulinaemia with or without IgA deficiency

SPECIFIC CAUTIONS

- With intravenous use Ensure adequate hydration · obesity · renal insufficiency · risk factors for arterial or venous thromboembolic events · thrombophilic disorders

CAUTIONS, FURTHER INFORMATION For full details on cautions, consult product literature.

- **INTERACTIONS** → Appendix 1: immunoglobulins
- **SIDE-EFFECTS**

GENERAL SIDE-EFFECTS

- **Common or very common** Diarrhoea · dizziness · fatigue · gastrointestinal discomfort · myalgia · nausea · pain · skin reactions

SPECIFIC SIDE-EFFECTS

- **Common or very common**
- With intravenous use Arthralgia · chills · embolism and thrombosis · feeling hot · fever · haemolysis · headache · hyperaemia · hypersensitivity · hypertension · infusion related reaction · palpitations · sensory disorder · taste altered · vomiting
- With subcutaneous use Drowsiness · headaches · hypotension · local reaction
- **Uncommon**
- With intravenous use Hypothermia
- With subcutaneous use Paraesthesia
- **Frequency not known**
- With intravenous use Acute kidney injury · angina pectoris · cutaneous lupus erythematosus · dyspnoea · leucopenia · meningitis aseptic · neutropenia · shock · transfusion-related acute lung injury

SIDE-EFFECTS, FURTHER INFORMATION Adverse reactions are more likely to occur in patients receiving normal immunoglobulin for the first time, or following a prolonged period between treatments, or when a different brand of normal immunoglobulin is administered.

- **MONITORING REQUIREMENTS** Monitor for acute renal failure; consider discontinuation if renal function deteriorates. Intravenous preparations with added sucrose have been associated with cases of renal dysfunction and acute renal failure.

- **DIRECTIONS FOR ADMINISTRATION** Administration advice (including licensed route of administration, recommended rate of infusion and reconstitution requirements) varies widely between normal immunoglobulin preparations from different manufacturers—formulations are **not interchangeable**; consult product literature.
- **PRESCRIBING AND DISPENSING INFORMATION** Antibody titres can vary widely between normal immunoglobulin preparations from different manufacturers—formulations are **not interchangeable**; patients should be maintained on the same formulation throughout long-term treatment to avoid adverse effects.

  EvGr The brand name and batch number should be recorded after each administration (in case of transmission of infective agents). ⟨M⟩

  Indications, licensed age groups, and excipients differ between preparations. Some manufacturers also provide hyaluronidase to enhance the absorption of normal immunoglobulin. Further information can be found in the product literature for the individual preparations.

  ▸ With intramuscular use Available from ImmForm and from some UKHSA and NHS laboratories (for hepatitis A and rubella prophylaxis).
- **HANDLING AND STORAGE** Care must be taken to store all immunological products under the conditions recommended in the product literature, otherwise the preparation may become ineffective. **Refrigerated storage** is usually necessary; many immunoglobulins need to be stored at 2–8°C and not allowed to freeze. Immunoglobulins should be protected from light. Opened multidose vials must be used within the period recommended in the product literature.
- **MEDICINAL FORMS** There can be variation in the licensing of different medicines containing the same drug.

Solution for injection

EXCIPIENTS: May contain L-proline, polysorbates

ELECTROLYTES: May contain Sodium

▸ **Normal immunoglobulin (Non-proprietary)**

Normal immunoglobulin human 200 mg per 1 ml Hizentra 1g/5ml solution for injection pre-filled syringes | 1 pre-filled disposable injection PoM ⊠

▸ **Cutaquig** (Octapharma Ltd)

Normal immunoglobulin human 165 mg per 1 ml Cutaquig 1g/6ml solution for injection vials | 1 vial PoM £73.50 (Hospital only)
Cutaquig 2g/12ml solution for injection vials | 1 vial PoM £147.00 (Hospital only)
Cutaquig 8g/48ml solution for injection vials | 1 vial PoM £588.00 (Hospital only)
Cutaquig 4g/24ml solution for injection vials | 1 vial PoM £294.00 (Hospital only)

▸ **Hizentra** (CSL Behring UK Ltd)

Normal immunoglobulin human 200 mg per 1 ml Hizentra 4g/20ml solution for injection pre-filled syringes | 1 pre-filled disposable injection PoM £276.00 (Hospital only)
Hizentra 2g/10ml solution for injection pre-filled syringes | 1 pre-filled disposable injection PoM £138.00 (Hospital only)

▸ **Subgam** (Bio Products Laboratory Ltd)

Normal immunoglobulin human 160 mg per 1 ml Subgam 1g/6.25ml solution for injection vials | 1 vial PoM £80.00
Subgam 4g/25ml solution for injection vials | 1 vial PoM £321.00
Subgam 2g/12.5ml solution for injection vials | 1 vial PoM £161.00

▸ **Xembify** (Grifols UK Ltd) ▼

Normal immunoglobulin human 200 mg per 1 ml Xembify 4g/20ml solution for injection vials | 1 vial PoM £276.00 (Hospital only)
Xembify 2g/10ml solution for injection vials | 1 vial PoM £138.00 (Hospital only)
Xembify 1g/5ml solution for injection vials | 1 vial PoM £69.00 (Hospital only)
Xembify 10g/50ml solution for injection vials | 1 vial PoM £690.00 (Hospital only)

Solution for infusion

EXCIPIENTS: May contain Edetic acid (edta), glucose, l-proline, maltose, polysorbates, sorbitol, sucrose

ELECTROLYTES: May contain Sodium

▸ **Normal immunoglobulin (Non-proprietary)**

Normal immunoglobulin human 100 mg per 1 ml Normal immunoglobulin human 5g/50ml solution for infusion vials | 1 vial PoM ⊠
Normal immunoglobulin human 2.5g/25ml solution for infusion vials | 1 vial PoM ⊠
Normal immunoglobulin human 20g/200ml solution for infusion vials | 1 vial PoM ⊠
Normal immunoglobulin human 10g/100ml solution for infusion vials | 1 vial PoM ⊠
Normal immunoglobulin human 30g/300ml solution for infusion vials | 1 vial PoM ⊠

▸ **Cuvitru** (Takeda UK Ltd)

Normal immunoglobulin human 200 mg per 1 ml Cuvitru 4g/20ml solution for infusion vials | 1 vial PoM £276.00 (Hospital only)
Cuvitru 2g/10ml solution for infusion vials | 1 vial PoM £138.00 (Hospital only)
Cuvitru 1g/5ml solution for infusion vials | 1 vial PoM £69.00 (Hospital only)
Cuvitru 8g/40ml solution for infusion vials | 1 vial PoM £552.00 (Hospital only)
Cuvitru 10g/50ml solution for infusion vials | 1 vial PoM £690.00 (Hospital only)

▸ **Flebogammadif** (Grifols UK Ltd)

Normal immunoglobulin human 50 mg per 1 ml Flebogamma DIF 2.5g/50ml solution for infusion vials | 1 vial PoM £175.00
Flebogamma DIF 10g/200ml solution for infusion vials | 1 vial PoM £700.00
Flebogamma DIF 5g/100ml solution for infusion vials | 1 vial PoM £350.00
Flebogamma DIF 20g/400ml solution for infusion vials | 1 vial PoM £1,400.00

▸ **Gamten** (Octapharma Ltd)

Normal immunoglobulin human 100 mg per 1 ml Gamten 5g/50ml solution for infusion bottles | 1 bottle PoM £355.00 (Hospital only)
Gamten 20g/200ml solution for infusion bottles | 1 bottle PoM £1,420.00 (Hospital only)
Gamten 10g/100ml solution for infusion bottles | 1 bottle PoM £710.00 (Hospital only)

▸ **Gamunex** (Grifols UK Ltd)

Normal immunoglobulin human 100 mg per 1 ml Gamunex 10% 10g/100ml solution for infusion vials | 1 vial PoM £665.00 (Hospital only)
Gamunex 10% 20g/200ml solution for infusion vials | 1 vial PoM £1,330.00 (Hospital only)
Gamunex 10% 5g/50ml solution for infusion vials | 1 vial PoM £332.50 (Hospital only)

▸ **Hizentra** (CSL Behring UK Ltd)

Normal immunoglobulin human 200 mg per 1 ml Hizentra 2g/10ml solution for infusion vials | 1 vial PoM £138.00 (Hospital only)
Hizentra 1g/5ml solution for infusion vials | 1 vial PoM £69.00 (Hospital only)
Hizentra 4g/20ml solution for infusion vials | 1 vial PoM £276.00 (Hospital only)

▸ **Intratect** (Grifols UK Ltd)

Normal immunoglobulin human 50 mg per 1 ml Intratect 5g/100ml solution for infusion vials | 1 vial PoM £362.30 (Hospital only)
Intratect 2.5g/50ml solution for infusion vials | 1 vial PoM £181.15
Intratect 10g/200ml solution for infusion vials | 1 vial PoM £724.60 (Hospital only)

Normal immunoglobulin human 100 mg per 1 ml Intratect 10g/100ml solution for infusion vials | 1 vial PoM £724.60 (Hospital only)
Intratect 20g/200ml solution for infusion vials | 1 vial PoM £1,449.20 (Hospital only)
Intratect 5g/50ml solution for infusion vials | 1 vial PoM £362.30 (Hospital only)

▸ **Iqymune** (LFB Biopharmaceuticals Ltd)

Normal immunoglobulin human 100 mg per 1 ml Iqymune 10g/100ml solution for infusion vials | 1 vial PoM £700.00 (Hospital only)
Iqymune 2g/20ml solution for infusion vials | 1 vial PoM £140.00 (Hospital only)
Iqymune 20g/200ml solution for infusion vials | 1 vial PoM £1,400.00 (Hospital only)
Iqymune 5g/50ml solution for infusion vials | 1 vial PoM £350.00 (Hospital only)

▸ **Kiovig** (Takeda UK Ltd)
Normal immunoglobulin human 100 mg per 1 ml Kiovig 5g/50ml solution for infusion vials | 1 vial PoM £345.00 (Hospital only)
Kiovig 20g/200ml solution for infusion vials | 1 vial PoM £1,380.00 (Hospital only)
Kiovig 10g/100ml solution for infusion vials | 1 vial PoM £690.00 (Hospital only)
Kiovig 30g/300ml solution for infusion vials | 1 vial PoM £2,070.00
Kiovig 2.5g/25ml solution for infusion vials | 1 vial PoM £172.50
Kiovig 1g/10ml solution for infusion vials | 1 vial PoM £69.00

▸ **Octagam** (Octapharma Ltd)
Normal immunoglobulin human 50 mg per 1 ml Octagam 5% 10g/200ml solution for infusion bottles | 1 bottle PoM £690.00 (Hospital only)
Octagam 5% 5g/100ml solution for infusion bottles | 1 bottle PoM £345.00 (Hospital only)
Normal immunoglobulin human 100 mg per 1 ml Octagam 10% 10g/100ml solution for infusion bottles | 1 bottle PoM £710.00 (Hospital only)
Octagam 10% 5g/50ml solution for infusion bottles | 1 bottle PoM £355.00 (Hospital only)
Octagam 10% 20g/200ml solution for infusion bottles | 1 bottle PoM £1,420.00 (Hospital only)
Octagam 10% 2g/20ml solution for infusion vials | 1 vial PoM £142.00 (Hospital only)

▸ **Panzyga** (Octapharma Ltd)
Normal immunoglobulin human 100 mg per 1 ml Panzyga 20g/200ml solution for infusion bottles | 1 bottle PoM £1,380.00 (Hospital only)
Panzyga 10g/100ml solution for infusion bottles | 1 bottle PoM £690.00 (Hospital only)
Panzyga 5g/50ml solution for infusion bottles | 1 bottle PoM £345.00 (Hospital only)

▸ **Privigen** (CSL Behring UK Ltd)
Normal immunoglobulin human 100 mg per 1 ml Privigen 5g/50ml solution for infusion vials | 1 vial PoM £345.00 (Hospital only)
Privigen 10g/100ml solution for infusion vials | 1 vial PoM £690.00 (Hospital only)
Privigen 20g/200ml solution for infusion vials | 1 vial PoM £1,380.00 (Hospital only)
Privigen 2.5g/25ml solution for infusion vials | 1 vial PoM £172.50 (Hospital only)

▸ **Yimmugo** (Grifols UK Ltd) ▼
Normal immunoglobulin human 100 mg per 1 ml Yimmugo 20g/200ml solution for infusion vials | 1 vial PoM £1,444.00
Yimmugo 10g/100ml solution for infusion vials | 1 vial PoM £722.00
Yimmugo 5g/50ml solution for infusion vials | 1 vial PoM £361.00

Form unstated
EXCIPIENTS: May contain Edetic acid (edta)

▸ **HyQvia** (Takeda UK Ltd)
HyQvia 30g/300ml solution for infusion and 15ml vials | 1 pack PoM £2,070.00
HyQvia 20g/200ml solution for infusion and 10ml vials | 1 pack PoM £1,380.00
HyQvia 10g/100ml solution for infusion and 5ml vials | 1 pack PoM £690.00
HyQvia 5g/50ml solution for infusion and 2.5ml vials | 1 pack PoM £345.00
HyQvia 2.5g/25ml solution for infusion and 1.25ml vials | 1 pack PoM £172.50

Powder and solvent for solution for injection
EXCIPIENTS: May contain Glucose

▸ **Gammagard S/D** (Takeda UK Ltd)
Normal immunoglobulin human 10 gram Gammagard S/D 10g powder and solvent for solution for injection bottles | 1 bottle PoM £690.00

Rabies immunoglobulin 07-Feb-2023

● **INDICATIONS AND DOSE**

Post-exposure treatment against rabies infection

▸ BY LOCAL INFILTRATION, OR BY INTRAMUSCULAR INJECTION

▸ Child: 20 units/kg, dose administered by infiltration in and around the cleansed wound; if wound not visible or healed or if infiltration of whole volume not possible, give remainder by intramuscular injection into anterolateral thigh (remote from vaccination site). If more than 2 mL to be given by intramuscular injection then give in divided doses at different sites, to be given in combination with rabies vaccine, not required if more than 7 days have elapsed after the first dose of vaccine, or more than 1 day after the second dose of vaccine

● **CAUTIONS** IgA deficiency · interference with live virus vaccines

● **INTERACTIONS** → Appendix 1: immunoglobulins

● **SIDE-EFFECTS**

▸ **Rare or very rare** Arthralgia · chills · fatigue · fever · headache · hypersensitivity · hypotension · influenza like illness · malaise · nausea · skin reactions · tachycardia · vomiting

● **PRESCRIBING AND DISPENSING INFORMATION** The potency of individual batches of rabies immunoglobulin from the manufacturer may vary. It is therefore critical to know the potency of the batch to be used and the weight of the patient in order to calculate the specific volume required to provide the necessary dose.

Available from the Rabies and Immunoglobulin Service (RIgS) and/or Bio Products Laboratory (BPL).

● **HANDLING AND STORAGE** Care must be taken to store all immunological products under the conditions recommended in the product literature, otherwise the preparation may become ineffective. **Refrigerated storage** is usually necessary; many immunoglobulins need to be stored at 2–8°C and not allowed to freeze. Immunoglobulins should be protected from light. Opened multidose vials must be used within the period recommended in the product literature.

● **MEDICINAL FORMS** There can be variation in the licensing of different medicines containing the same drug.

Solution for injection

▸ **Rabies immunoglobulin (Non-proprietary)**
Rabies immunoglobulin human 500 unit Rabies immunoglobulin human 500unit solution for injection vials | 1 vial PoM £1,000.00

Tetanus immunoglobulin 18-Mar-2021

● **INDICATIONS AND DOSE**

Post-exposure prophylaxis

▸ BY INTRAMUSCULAR INJECTION

▸ Child: 250 units, alternatively 500 units, higher dose used if more than 24 hours have elapsed since injury, or there is risk of heavy contamination, or following burns

● **CAUTIONS** IgA deficiency · interference with live virus vaccines

● **INTERACTIONS** → Appendix 1: immunoglobulins

● **SIDE-EFFECTS**

▸ **Rare or very rare** Anaphylactic reaction · hypotension

▸ **Frequency not known** Arthralgia · chest pain · dizziness · dyspnoea · face oedema · oral disorders · tremor

● **HANDLING AND STORAGE** Care must be taken to store all immunological products under the conditions recommended in the product literature, otherwise the preparation may become ineffective. **Refrigerated storage** is usually necessary; many immunoglobulins need to be stored at 2–8°C and not allowed to freeze. Immunoglobulins should be protected from light. Opened multidose vials must be used within the period recommended in the product literature.

● **MEDICINAL FORMS** There can be variation in the licensing of different medicines containing the same drug.

Solution for injection

▸ Tetanus immunoglobulin (Non-proprietary)

Tetanus immunoglobulin human 250 unit Tetanus immunoglobulin human 250unit solution for injection vials | 1 vial PoM £300.00

Varicella-zoster immunoglobulin

15-May-2025

(Antivaricella-zoster Immunoglobulin)

● **INDICATIONS AND DOSE**

Post-exposure prophylaxis of varicella-zoster infection [neonates exposed to maternal chickenpox 7 days before or after delivery]

▸ BY INTRAVENOUS INFUSION

▸ Neonate: 50 units/kg for 1 dose (max. per dose 125 units), dose to be administered as soon as possible—preferably within 96 hours of, but no later than 10 days after, exposure.

● **UNLICENSED USE** UKHSA advises *Varitect CP*® is used for post-exposure prophylaxis of varicella-zoster infection in eligible neonates, but it is not licensed in the UK.

● **CONTRA-INDICATIONS** Selective IgA deficiency with IgA antibodies

● **CAUTIONS** Ensure adequate hydration before initiation of infusion · interference with live virus vaccines · renal insufficiency · risk factors for thromboembolic events

CAUTIONS, FURTHER INFORMATION

▸ Interference with live virus vaccines EvGr Varicella-zoster immunoglobulin may impair the immune response to live virus vaccines; such vaccines should only be given 3 months after varicella-zoster immunoglobulin treatment. Patients receiving measles vaccines should have their antibody status checked as impairment of immune response may persist for up to 1 year. Ⓜ

● **INTERACTIONS** → Appendix 1: immunoglobulins

● **SIDE-EFFECTS** Arthralgia · chills · fever · headache · hypersensitivity · hypotension · malaise · nausea · skin reactions · tachycardia · vomiting

● **MONITORING REQUIREMENTS**

▸ EvGr Monitor for signs of infusion-related reactions during and for at least one hour after each infusion in patients receiving varicella-zoster immunoglobulin for the first time, or following a prolonged period between treatments, or when a different human immunoglobulin has been used previously; monitor all other patients for at least 20 minutes after each infusion—in case of reaction, reduce rate or stop infusion as clinically appropriate.

▸ Monitor urine output and serum-creatinine levels—consider discontinuation if renal function deteriorates.

▸ Monitor for signs and symptoms of haemolysis. Ⓜ

● **EFFECT ON LABORATORY TESTS** May interfere with some serological tests, including Coombs' test, reticulocyte count, and haptoglobin, due to passive transmission of antibodies.

● **DIRECTIONS FOR ADMINISTRATION** For *intravenous infusion* (*Varitect CP*®), give at an initial rate of 0.1 mL/kg per hour for the first 10 minutes, then gradually increased to a maximum rate of 1 mL/kg per hour for the rest of the infusion.

● **PRESCRIBING AND DISPENSING INFORMATION** The brand name and batch number should be recorded after each administration (in case of transmission of infective agents).

Available from the Rabies and Immunoglobulin Service (RIgS) and selected NHS laboratories or hospital pharmacies.

● **HANDLING AND STORAGE** Care must be taken to store all immunological products under the conditions recommended in the product literature, otherwise the preparation may become ineffective. **Refrigerated storage** is usually necessary; many immunoglobulins need to be stored at 2–8°C and not allowed to freeze. Immunoglobulins should be protected from light. Opened multidose vials must be used within the period recommended in the product literature.

● **MEDICINAL FORMS** No licensed medicines listed.

2 Post-exposure prophylaxis

Botulism antitoxin

12-Jan-2021

Overview

Botulism antitoxin below (botulinum antitoxin) [unlicensed] is a polyvalent preparation that contains equine-derived immune globulins against multiple *Clostridium botulinum* serotypes. It is used for the treatment of suspected cases of botulism, such as foodborne (pre-formed toxins ingested from contaminated food) and wound botulism (associated with parenteral drug abuse). Human-derived botulism immune globulin [unlicensed] is used for the treatment of infant botulism as part of the Infant Botulism Treatment and Prevention Program. In infant botulism, neurotoxins are formed in the large intestine after ingestion of *Clostridium botulinum* spores, which are harmless to older children and adults.

Botulism is a notifiable disease in the UK, especially foodborne botulism, which is considered a public health emergency as contaminated food may be available to other individuals. For further information on reporting of suspected cases, see *Notifiable diseases* in Antibacterials, principles of therapy p. 358.

All cases of suspected botulism should be managed promptly—treatment should not be delayed while awaiting laboratory diagnosis. Supportive care (including artificial ventilation) and symptomatic treatment may also be necessary.

For individuals with wound botulism, surgical debridement and antibacterial therapy are recommended in addition to botulism antitoxin, to help reduce the organism load and toxin production.

For further information on the management of infant, foodborne and wound botulism, see Public Health England guidance: **Botulism: clinical and public health management** (see *Useful resources*).

Useful Resources

Recommendations reflect Botulism: clinical and public health management. Public Health England, December 2018.
www.gov.uk/government/publications/botulism-clinical-and-public-health-management

IMMUNE SERA AND IMMUNOGLOBULINS › ANTITOXINS

Botulism antitoxin

13-May-2021

● **INDICATIONS AND DOSE**

Treatment of botulism [suspected or confirmed]

▸ BY INTRAVENOUS INFUSION

▸ Child: (consult product literature)

14 Vaccines

- **SIDE-EFFECTS** Hypersensitivity

SIDE-EFFECTS, FURTHER INFORMATION It is essential to read the contra-indications, warnings, and details of sensitivity tests on the package insert. Prior to treatment checks should be made regarding previous administration of any antitoxin and history of any allergic condition, e.g. asthma, hay fever, etc.

- **PRE-TREATMENT SCREENING** All patients should be tested for sensitivity (diluting the antitoxin if history of allergy).
- **PRESCRIBING AND DISPENSING INFORMATION** Available from designated centres after discussion with the on-call duty doctor at Colindale, Public Health England (during and outside of working hours) for risk assessment and further advice on treatment (Tel: (020) 8200 4400).

For non-urgent queries, contact Botulism@phe.gov.uk.

- **MEDICINAL FORMS** No licensed medicines listed.

Diphtheria antitoxin

10-Nov-2023

(Dip/Ser)

- **INDICATIONS AND DOSE**

Treatment of diphtheria [confirmed or probable]

▶ BY INTRAVENOUS INFUSION

▸ Child: Dose should be given without waiting for bacteriological confirmation (consult local protocol)

- **CAUTIONS** Hypersensitivity is common after administration; resuscitation facilities should be available.

Diphtheria antitoxin is no longer used for prophylaxis because of the risk of hypersensitivity; unimmunised contacts should be promptly investigated and given antibacterial prophylaxis and vaccine.

- **SIDE-EFFECTS**

▶ **Common or very common** Hypersensitivity

- **PRE-TREATMENT SCREENING** Diphtheria antitoxin is derived from horse serum and reactions are common. Public Health England advises hypersensitivity testing should be carried out before use in certain individuals (e.g. those who have a positive history of animal allergy, or prior exposure to equine-derived immunoglobulin).
- **PRESCRIBING AND DISPENSING INFORMATION** Available from designated centres after discussion with the Duty Doctor at Colindale, Public Health England (during and outside of working hours) for risk assessment and further advice on treatment (Tel: (020) 8200 4400). In Northern Ireland, available from Public Health Laboratory, Belfast City Hospital (Tel (028) 9032 9241).
- **MEDICINAL FORMS** There can be variation in the licensing of different medicines containing the same drug.

Solution for injection

▸ Diphtheria antitoxin (Non-proprietary)

Diphtheria antitoxin 1000 unit per 1 ml Antidiphtheria serum 10,000units/10ml solution for injection ampoules | 1 ampoule PoM ⊠ (Hospital only)

3 Tuberculosis diagnostic test

DIAGNOSTIC AGENTS

Tuberculin purified protein derivative

(Tuberculin PPD)

- **INDICATIONS AND DOSE**

Mantoux test

▶ BY INTRADERMAL INJECTION

▸ Child: 2 units for one dose

Mantoux test (if first test is negative and a further test is considered appropriate)

▶ BY INTRADERMAL INJECTION

▸ Child: 10 units for 1 dose

DOSE EQUIVALENCE AND CONVERSION

▸ 2 units is equivalent to 0.1 mL of 20 units/mL strength.

▸ 10 units is equivalent to 0.1 mL of 100 units/mL strength.

- **CAUTIONS** Response to tuberculin may be suppressed by viral infection, sarcoidosis, corticosteroid therapy, or immunosuppression due to disease or treatment and the MMR vaccine. If a tuberculin skin test has already been initiated, then the MMR should be delayed until the skin test has been read unless protection against measles is required urgently. If a child has had a recent MMR, and requires a tuberculin test, then a 4 week interval should be observed. Apart from tuberculin and MMR, all other live vaccines can be administered at any time before or after tuberculin.
- **PRESCRIBING AND DISPENSING INFORMATION** Available from ImmForm (SSI brand).

The strength of tuberculin PPD in currently available products may be different to the strengths of products used previously for the Mantoux test; care is required to select the correct strength.

- **MEDICINAL FORMS** There can be variation in the licensing of different medicines containing the same drug. Forms available from special-order manufacturers include: solution for injection

Solution for injection

▸ Tuberculin purified protein derivative (Non-proprietary)

Tuberculin purified protein derivative 20 tuberculin unit per 1 ml Tuberculin PPD RT 23 SSI 20 tuberculin units/ml solution for injection 1.5ml vials | 1 vial ⊠

Tuberculin purified protein derivative 100 tuberculin unit per 1 ml Tuberculin PPD RT 23 SSI 100 tuberculin units/ml solution for injection 1.5ml vials | 1 vial ⊠

4 Vaccination

Vaccination, general principles

15-Jan-2026

Active immunity

Active immunity can be acquired by natural disease or by vaccination. Vaccines induce active immunity and provide immunological memory by stimulating the production of antibodies and cells involved in the immune response. As a result, the immune system is able to recognise and respond rapidly to natural infection at a later date. Antibodies can be detected in the patient's blood or serum, but even in the absence of detectable antibodies, immunological memory may still be present. Vaccines consist of either:

- a *live attenuated replicating* form of the virus (e.g. measles, mumps, and rubella vaccine) or bacteria (e.g. Bacillus Calmette-Guérin vaccine);
- a *live attenuated non-replicating* form of the virus (e.g. smallpox and mpox vaccine);
- *inactivated* preparations of the virus (e.g. tick-borne encephalitis vaccine) or bacteria (e.g. meningococcal vaccine);
- *inactivated toxins (toxoids)* produced by a micro-organism (e.g. tetanus and diphtheria vaccines);
- *extracts of* a micro-organism which may be derived from the organism (e.g. pneumococcal vaccine), or produced by recombinant DNA technology (e.g. hepatitis B vaccine);
- *viral vectors of* replicating (attenuated or low pathogenicity viruses) or non-replicating viruses, produced using recombinant technology; or
- *nucleic acid (DNA or RNA) of* an antigen derived from the virus (e.g. *Comirnaty*® COVID-19 vaccine) or bacteria.

Live attenuated replicating viral vaccines and replicating viral vector vaccines usually promote a full, long-lasting antibody response. In rare cases, a mild form of the disease may occur with some vaccines, such as a rash following a measles-containing vaccine.

Inactivated or non-replicating vaccines (including toxoids and non-live vaccines) produce an antibody response following a primary course, which may last for months or years. In most cases booster (reinforcing) injections are required for long-term protection. To stimulate the immune system more broadly, some polysaccharide vaccines have been enhanced by conjugation (such as the *Haemophilus influenzae* type B and meningococcal group C vaccines), while some inactivated vaccines contain an adjuvant (such as aluminium hydroxide or aluminium phosphate) to enhance the antibody response. Inactivated and non-replicating vaccines cannot cause the disease that they are designed to prevent.

For further information on how vaccines are made and what they contain, see Chapter 1, Immunity and how vaccines work, in *Immunisation against infectious disease*- 'The Green Book' (see *Useful resources*).

Passive immunity

Passive immunity is acquired through the transfer of antibodies from immune individuals either across the placenta, or from the transfusion of blood or blood products including immunoglobulins (for further information, see Immunoglobulins p. 951). Protection provided by the cross-placental transfer of antibodies provides the infant with temporary protection (commonly for a few weeks to months), and is more effective against some infections (e.g. tetanus and measles) than others (e.g. polio and pertussis).

Vaccination during pregnancy and breast-feeding

Live replicating vaccines should not be administered routinely to pregnant females due to the theoretical risk of fetal infection; these should generally be delayed until after delivery. The Immunisation and Vaccine Preventable Diseases Division at the UK Health Security Agency (UKHSA) run a UK-wide surveillance programme on the safety of certain vaccines (measles, mumps, rubella, varicella-zoster, and herpes-zoster) given inadvertently during pregnancy or shortly before conception. For advice on the reporting, risk assessment, and management of inadvertent vaccination in pregnancy, see UKHSA guidance: **Inadvertent vaccination in pregnancy (VIP)** (available at: www.gov.uk/guidance/vaccination-in-pregnancy-vip).

There is no evidence of risk from vaccinating pregnant females with inactivated viral or bacterial vaccines, or toxoids; they do not replicate so cannot harm the fetus. Some inactivated vaccines are actively recommended to prevent severe complications during pregnancy or to the new-born infant, such as the influenza vaccine, and the diphtheria, tetanus, pertussis, and poliomyelitis vaccine.

There is no evidence of risk from vaccinating females who are breast-feeding with inactivated viral or bacterial vaccines, or toxoids.

For further information on vaccination in pregnancy and breast-feeding, see individual vaccine treatment summaries.

Vaccines in immunosuppression and HIV infection

Almost all individuals can be safely vaccinated; in only a few individuals is vaccination either contra-indicated or should be deferred. Specialist advice should be sought when in doubt, if using live vaccines, or if there are queries about an individual's degree of immunosuppression. In some situations, the specialist may decide that the risk of a specific disease outweighs any potential risk from the vaccine. Antibody responses may be lower in immunosuppressed individuals, therefore additional vaccine doses may be required.

Live replicating vaccines can cause severe or fatal infections in immunosuppressed individuals due to extensive replication of the vaccine strain. Live replicating vaccines are therefore not recommended for individuals with some types of severe primary or acquired immunodeficiency, or for those who are on or have recently received high doses of certain immunosuppressive or biological therapies.

Inactivated vaccines cannot replicate so may be given to immunosuppressed individuals.

Wherever possible, immunisation or additional booster doses for individuals with immunosuppression, should be carried out either before immunosuppression occurs or deferred until an improvement in immunity has been seen. The optimal timing for any vaccination should be based upon a judgement about the relative need for rapid protection and the likely response. For infants born to females taking immunosuppressive biological therapy during pregnancy, live replicating vaccines should be delayed by 6 months; therefore, the infant will not be eligible to receive the rotavirus vaccine, and if indicated, will need to have their Bacillus Calmette-Guérin vaccine deferred.

Most live vaccines used in the UK immunisation schedule can be safely given to close contacts of an immunosuppressed individual. They carry a low risk of transmission (or the risk can be minimised with simple precautions) from a recently vaccinated close contact to an immunosuppressed individual. Close contacts of immunosuppressed individuals should be fully immunised according to the national Immunisation schedule p. 961 to reduce the risk of exposure to vaccine preventable conditions, and they should also be offered the annual Influenza vaccine p. 971.

For further information on vaccines in immunosuppression, see Chapter 6, Contra-indications and special considerations, and Chapter 7, Immunisation of individuals with underlying medical conditions in *Immunisation against infectious disease*- 'The Green Book' (see *Useful resources*).

For further information on vaccines for individuals with HIV infection, see the Children's HIV Association guidelines: **Vaccination of Children and Adolescents Living with HIV** and **Preparing children and adolescents living with HIV for travel** (available at: www.chiva.org.uk/professionals/clinical-guidelines/).

Vaccines and asplenia, splenic dysfunction, or complement disorders

The following vaccines are recommended for children with asplenia, splenic dysfunction, or complement disorders (including those taking complement inhibitors) depending on the age at which their condition is diagnosed:

- Influenza vaccine (inactivated) p. 994 or influenza vaccine (live) p. 1001;
- Meningococcal groups A, C, W135, and Y vaccine p. 996 (MenACWY) and meningococcal group B vaccine p. 995 (4CMenB);
- 13-valent or 20-valent pneumococcal polysaccharide conjugate vaccine p. 996 (PCV13 or PCV20) and/or 23-valent pneumococcal polysaccharide vaccine (PPV23); PCV20 is expected to replace PPV23 in 2025/2026. Patients on certain complement inhibitor therapy are not at increased risk of pneumococcal disease and only require routine pneumococcal vaccination.

Additional booster doses of other vaccines should be considered depending on the individual's underlying condition—specialist advice may be required. For information on specific indications for immunisation of vulnerable groups, see Chapter 7, Immunisation of individuals with underlying medical conditions, in *Immunisation against infectious disease*- 'The Green Book' (see *Useful resources*).

Children first diagnosed or presenting aged under* 1 *year should be immunised according to the Immunisation schedule below. During their first year they should also be given 2 doses of MenACWY at least 4 weeks apart, and an additional dose of PCV13 or PCV20 (in order to have received a total of 2 doses of PCV13 or PCV20 with a 4-week interval). Infants diagnosed after 16 weeks who have already received PCV13 should receive 2 doses of PCV20 (when available) with an interval of at least 4 weeks between any doses. 8 weeks following their routine 1 year booster vaccines, they should receive a booster dose of MenACWY. After their second birthday, a dose of PPV23 or PCV20 should be given at least 4 weeks after the last dose of PCV13 or PCV20. The influenza vaccine should be given annually in children aged 6 months or older.

Children first diagnosed or presenting aged* 1 *year to under* 2 *years should be immunised according to the Immunisation schedule below, including any routine vaccines due at 1 year of age if not yet administered. If the routine PCV13 booster at 1 year has already been given, a dose of PCV20 (when available) should be given at least 4 weeks later. 8 weeks following the routine 1 year booster vaccines a dose of MenACWY should be given. After their second birthday, a dose of PPV23 or PCV20 should be given at least 4 weeks after the last PCV dose. The influenza vaccine should be given annually.

Children first diagnosed or presenting aged* 2 *years to under* 10 *years should be immunised according to the Immunisation schedule below. Additionally, they should be given a dose of MenACWY, and a dose of PPV23 or PCV20. For children who have not received the full routine immunisation for 4CMenB, ensure that 2 doses, 8 weeks apart, have been given since their first birthday. The influenza vaccine should be given annually.

Children first diagnosed aged* 10 *years and over regardless of previous immunisations, should be given a dose of PPV23 or PCV20, 4CMenB, and MenACWY. After 4 weeks, an additional dose of 4CMenB should be given. The influenza vaccine should be given annually.

Vaccines and antitoxins availability

For information on availability of vaccines and antitoxins, see individual monographs.

For antivenom, see Poisoning, emergency treatment p. 1036.

Enquiries for vaccines not available commercially can also be made to:

Vaccines and Countermeasures Response Department
UK Health Security Agency
vaccinesupply@ukhsa.gov.uk

In Northern Ireland, enquiries for vaccines not available commercially should be directed to Northern Health and Social Care Trust's Pharmacy Services (www.northerntrust.hscni.net/services/pharmaceutical-services/).

In Scotland, information about availability of vaccines can be obtained from a Specialist in Pharmaceutical Public Health.

In Wales, enquiries for vaccines not available commercially should be directed to the Welsh Medicines Information Centre (www.wmic.wales.nhs.uk/about/contactus/).

Useful Resources

Recommendations reflect advice from *Immunisation against infectious disease*- 'The Green Book'. UK Health Security Agency, 2013. Chapters from the handbook (including updates since 2013) are available at: www.gov.uk/government/collections/immunisation-against-infectious-disease-the-green-book

Immunisation schedule

18-Jun-2025

Routine immunisations, sources of information

The following recommendations reflect advice from UKHSA. Recommendations specific to each vaccine can be found in *Immunisation against infectious disease*– 'The Green Book'. UKHSA, available at: www.gov.uk/government/collections/immunisation-against-infectious-disease-the-green-book.

The immunisation schedule reflects advice from the 'Complete routine immunisation schedule from 1 July 2025' produced by UKHSA. For the most up to date immunisation schedule, see: www.gov.uk/government/publications/the-complete-routine-immunisation-schedule.

The Influenza immunisation recommendations reflect advice from the 'National flu immunisation programme plan 2025/2026' produced by UKHSA, Department of Health and Social Care, and NHS England. For the most up to date letter, see: www.gov.uk/government/publications/national-flu-immunisation-programme-plan-2025-to-2026.

Vaccines for the immunisation schedule should be obtained from ImmForm at: portal.immform.ukhsa.gov.uk.

Preterm birth

Babies born preterm should receive all routine immunisations based on their actual date of birth. The risk of apnoea following vaccination is increased in preterm babies, particularly in those born at or before 28 weeks gestational age. If babies at risk of apnoea are in hospital at the time of their first immunisation, they should be monitored for respiratory complications for 48–72 hours after immunisation. If a baby develops apnoea, bradycardia, or desaturation after the first immunisation, the second immunisation should also be given in hospital with similar monitoring.

Individuals with unknown or incomplete immunisation history

For children born in the UK who present with an inadequate or unknown immunisation history, investigation into immunisations received should be carried out. Outstanding doses should be administered where the routine childhood immunisation schedule has not been completed.

For advice on dosing schedules for missed vaccinations, and the immunisation of individuals coming to the UK, consult Chapter 11, The UK immunisation schedule, in *Immunisation against infectious disease*– 'The Green Book'. UKHSA, available at: www.gov.uk/government/publications/immunisation-schedule-the-green-book-chapter-11, and UKHSA guidance: **Vaccination of individuals with uncertain or incomplete immunisation status**, available at: www.gov.uk/government/publications/vaccination-of-individuals-with-uncertain-or-incomplete-immunisation-status.

Routine immunisation schedule

When to immunise	Vaccine given and dose schedule (for details of dose, see under individual vaccines)
Neonates at risk only	▸ Bacillus Calmette-Guérin vaccine p. 1000 (around 4 weeks). Check severe combined immunodeficiency (SCID) screening outcome before giving, see Bacillus Calmette-Guérin vaccine below. ▸ Hepatitis B vaccine p. 992 (at birth and 4 weeks; **children born before** 1 July 2024 should be given an additional dose at 12 months of age, see Hepatitis B vaccine p. 968).
8 weeks	▸ Diphtheria with tetanus, pertussis, hepatitis B, poliomyelitis and haemophilus influenzae type b vaccine p. 990 (*Infanrix hexa*® or *Vaxelis*®). First dose. ▸ Meningococcal group B vaccine p. 995 (*Bexsero*®). First dose. ▸ Rotavirus vaccine p. 1003 (*Rotarix*®). Check SCID screening outcome before giving. First dose.
12 weeks	▸ Diphtheria with tetanus, pertussis, hepatitis B, poliomyelitis and haemophilus influenzae type b vaccine (*Infanrix hexa*® or *Vaxelis*®). Second dose. ▸ Meningococcal group B vaccine (*Bexsero*®). Second dose. ▸ Rotavirus vaccine (*Rotarix*®). Check SCID screening outcome before giving. Second dose.
16 weeks	▸ Diphtheria with tetanus, pertussis, hepatitis B, poliomyelitis and haemophilus influenzae type b vaccine (*Infanrix hexa*® or *Vaxelis*®). Third dose. ▸ Pneumococcal polysaccharide conjugate vaccine p. 996 (*Prevenar 13*®). Single dose.
1 year (on or after first birthday)	▸ Measles, mumps, and rubella vaccine p. 1002 (*MMR VaxPRO*® or *Priorix*®). First dose. ▸ Meningococcal group B vaccine (*Bexsero*®). Single booster dose. ▸ Pneumococcal polysaccharide conjugate vaccine (*Prevenar 13*®). Single booster dose. ▸ **For children born before** 1 July 2024, haemophilus influenzae type b and meningococcal group C vaccine p. 990 (*Menitorix*®). Single booster dose. If supplies are exhausted, give diphtheria with tetanus, pertussis, hepatitis B, poliomyelitis and haemophilus influenzae type b vaccine (*Infanrix hexa*® or *Vaxelis*®).
18 months **(for children born on or after 1 July 2024)**	▸ Diphtheria with tetanus, pertussis, hepatitis B, poliomyelitis and haemophilus influenzae type b vaccine (*Infanrix hexa*® or *Vaxelis*®). Fourth dose. ▸ Measles, mumps, and rubella vaccine (*MMR VaxPRO*® or *Priorix*®). Second dose.
2-3 years on 31 August 2025, primary school-aged children from reception to year 6, and secondary school-aged children in years 7-11	▸ Influenza vaccine (live) p. 1001. Each year from September. **Note:** live attenuated influenza nasal spray is recommended (*Fluenz*®); if contra-indicated or unsuitable, see Influenza vaccine p. 971.
3 years and 4 months, or soon after	▸ Diphtheria, tetanus, pertussis, and poliomyelitis vaccine p. 989 (*Repevax*®). Single booster dose. ▸ **For children born before** 1 July 2024, measles, mumps, and rubella vaccine (*MMR VaxPRO*® or *Priorix*®). Second dose.
11-14 years. HPV vaccine will be offered to individuals aged 12-13 years in England and Wales, those aged 12-14 years in Northern Ireland, and those aged 11-13 years in Scotland.	▸ Human papillomavirus vaccine p. 994 (*Gardasil*® *9*). 1-dose schedule. For individuals with immunosuppression or HIV infection, see Human papillomavirus vaccine p. 970.
13-15 years	▸ Meningococcal groups A, C, W135, and Y vaccine p. 996 (*MenQuadfi*®). Single dose.
13-18 years	▸ Diphtheria, tetanus, and poliomyelitis vaccine p. 989 (*Revaxis*®). Single booster dose. **Note:** Can be given at the same time as the dose of meningococcal groups A, C, W135, and Y vaccine at 13-15 years of age.
Females of child-bearing age susceptible to rubella	▸ Measles, mumps, and rubella vaccine. Females of child-bearing age who have not received 2 doses of a rubella-containing vaccine or who do not have a positive antibody test for rubella should be offered rubella immunisation (using the MMR vaccine)—exclude pregnancy before immunisation, and avoid pregnancy for one month after vaccination.
Pregnant females	▸ Acellular pertussis-containing vaccine administered as diphtheria, tetanus, and pertussis vaccine p. 988 (*Adacel*®). 1 dose from the 16th week of pregnancy, usually around the time of the fetal anomaly scan (week 20). ▸ Influenza vaccine (inactivated) p. 994. Single dose administered from September, regardless of the stage of pregnancy. For vaccine choice, see Influenza vaccine p. 971. ▸ Respiratory syncytial virus vaccine p. 998 (*Abrysvo*®). Single dose administered from the 28th week of pregnancy.

Anthrax vaccine

31-Oct-2018

Overview

Anthrax vaccine is rarely required for children.

Useful Resources

Recommendations reflect Chapter 13, Anthrax, in *Immunisation against infectious disease*– 'The Green Book'. Public Health England. February 2017.
www.gov.uk/government/publications/anthrax-the-green-book-chapter-13

Bacillus Calmette-Guérin vaccine

08-Oct-2021

Overview

The Bacillus Calmette-Guérin vaccine p. 1000 (BCG vaccine) contains a live attenuated strain derived from *Mycobacterium bovis* which is indicated for the prevention of Tuberculosis p. 446.

BCG vaccine is recommended for the following children if immunisation has not previously been carried out and they are tuberculin-negative:

- all neonates and infants (aged 0–12 months) living in areas of the UK where the annual incidence of tuberculosis is 40 cases per 100 000 or greater;
- all neonates and infants (aged 0–12 months) with a parent or grandparent born in a country where the annual incidence of tuberculosis is 40 cases per 100 000 or greater;
- previously unvaccinated children (aged 1–5 years) with a parent or grandparent born in a country where the annual incidence of tuberculosis is 40 cases per 100 000 or greater (tuberculin testing is not usually required);
- previously unvaccinated children (aged 6–15 years) with a parent or grandparent born in a country where the annual incidence of tuberculosis is 40 cases per 100 000 or greater;
- previously unvaccinated children (aged under 16 years) with close contact to cases of sputum smear-positive pulmonary or laryngeal tuberculosis;
- previously unvaccinated children (aged under 16 years) who were born in, or lived for at least 3 months in a country where the annual incidence of tuberculosis is 40 cases per 100 000 or greater.

As part of the neonatal BCG immunisation programme, immunisation is recommended for eligible neonates at 28 days of age (or soon after), to ensure that the result of the severe combined immunodeficiency (SCID) screening is available and checked prior to it being given. Vaccination may be given earlier than 28 days of age, provided that the SCID screening result is available. For further information, see UKHSA guidance: **Changing the timing of the neonatal BCG immunisation programme to a 28 day immunisation programme: effective from 1 September 2021** (see *Useful resources*).

Although protection provided by BCG vaccine may decrease with time, there is no evidence that repeat vaccination offers significant additional protection and therefore repeat BCG vaccination is not recommended.

The Bacillus Calmette-Guérin vaccine is contra-indicated in all HIV-infected children. For advice on BCG vaccination in immunosuppressed children, consult Chapter 32: Tuberculosis - 'The Green Book', Public Health England (see useful resources).

For advice on drug treatment, see Tuberculosis p. 446; for treatment of infection following vaccination, seek expert advice.

Travel

The risk of a child acquiring tuberculosis infection while travelling depends on several factors including the incidence of tuberculosis in that country, the duration of travel, the degree of contact with the local population, the reason for travel and the susceptibility and age of the child.

BCG vaccine is recommended for previously unvaccinated, tuberculin-negative children aged under 16 years who intend to travel for 3 months or more in a country where the annual incidence of tuberculosis is 40 cases per 100 000 or greater, or where the risk of multi-drug resistant tuberculosis is high. The risk of children acquiring tuberculosis infection while travelling is low and BCG vaccine is not required if no other factors are present.

A list of countries where the annual incidence of tuberculosis is 40 cases per 100 000 or greater, is available at www.gov.uk/government/publications/tuberculosis-tb-by-country-rates-per-100000-people.

Tuberculin skin testing

The tuberculin skin test (*Mantoux test*) is used to assess a child's sensitivity to tuberculin protein when BCG vaccination is being considered or as an aid to diagnosis of tuberculosis. A tuberculin skin test involves administration of tuberculin purified protein derivative p. 959 by intradermal injection. It is necessary before BCG vaccination for:

- children aged 6 years and over;
- children aged under 6 years living in a country for more than 3 months with an annual tuberculosis incidence of 40 cases per 100 000 or greater;
- those who have had close contact with a person with known tuberculosis;
- those who have a family history of tuberculosis within the last 5 years.

BCG vaccination can be given up to three months following a negative tuberculin test.

The BCG vaccine should not be administered to an individual with a positive tuberculin test—it is unnecessary and may cause a more severe local reaction. Those with a *Mantoux test* induration of 5 mm and greater should be referred to a tuberculosis clinic for assessment of the need for further investigation and treatment.

Tuberculosis is a notifiable disease in the UK. For further information, see *Notifiable diseases* in Antibacterials, principles of therapy p. 358.

Useful Resources

Recommendations reflect Chapter 32, Tuberculosis, in *Immunisation against infectious disease*– 'The Green Book'. Public Health England, August 2018.
www.gov.uk/government/publications/tuberculosis-the-green-book-chapter-32

Changing the timing of the neonatal BCG immunisation programme to a 28 day immunisation programme: effective from 1 September 2021. UK Health Security Agency. October 2021.
www.gov.uk/government/publications/bcg-vaccine-information-on-the-28-day-immunisation-programme

Cholera vaccines

08-Aug-2024

Overview

Oral cholera vaccine (inactivated) p. 987 contains inactivated Inaba (including El-Tor biotype) and Ogawa strains of *Vibrio cholerae* serotype O1, together with recombinant B-subunit of the cholera toxin produced in Inaba strains of *V. cholerae* serotype O1.

Oral cholera vaccine (live) p. 1001 contains live attenuated *V. cholerae* serotype O1 classical Inaba strain CVD 103-HgR produced by recombinant DNA technology.

Immunisation with either the inactivated or live vaccine (as appropriate) may be indicated for children from 2 years of age who are travelling to endemic or epidemic areas on the basis of current recommendations; immunisation however is not a condition for entry into any country. Following a full risk assessment, immunisation can be considered for the following children:

- children travelling with remote itineraries in areas where cholera epidemics are occurring and there is limited access to medical care;
- children travelling to potential cholera risk areas, for whom vaccination is considered potentially beneficial;
- individuals at occupational risk, such as laboratory workers who may be regularly exposed to cholera.

Immunisation with the inactivated vaccine should be completed at least one week prior to potential exposure; re-immunisation or a booster dose may be required to provide continuous protection. Immunisation with the live vaccine should be completed at least 10 days prior to potential exposure; there are no data available on re-immunisation intervals. The live vaccine should not be used in certain individuals such as those with immunosuppression, for further information, see Chapter 14, Cholera, in *Immunisation against infectious diseases*- 'The Green Book' (see *Useful resources*). Protection from immunisation with cholera vaccines may be reduced in those living with HIV infection.
For dosing schedules, see cholera vaccine (inactivated) and cholera vaccine (live).

Immunisation with either vaccine does not provide complete protection and all travellers to a country where cholera exists should be warned that scrupulous attention to food, water, and personal hygiene is essential.

Cholera is a notifiable disease in the UK. For further information, see *Notifiable diseases* in Antibacterials, principles of therapy p. 358.

Contacts

Contacts of children with cholera should maintain high standards of personal hygiene to avoid becoming infected. Cholera vaccines should not be used in the management of contacts of cases or in controlling the spread of infection.

There is a potential for transmission of the cholera vaccine (live) strain to unvaccinated close contacts caused by shedding in the stools.

Useful Resources

Recommendations reflect Chapter 14, Cholera, in *Immunisation against infectious disease*– 'The Green Book'. UK Health Security Agency. August 2024.
www.gov.uk/government/publications/cholera-the-green-book-chapter-14

COVID-19 vaccines

30-Mar-2026

Overview

Since the COVID-19 vaccination programme was initiated in December 2020, the majority of adults in the UK have been vaccinated, and most of the adult and child population have also been naturally infected. Vaccination against COVID-19 provides modest but short-term protection (lasting a few months) against infection and mild symptomatic disease, and transmission, however protection against severe disease and death appears to be greater and maintained over the medium term.

The aim of the longer-term COVID-19 vaccination programme is to reduce mortality and hospitalisation by providing ongoing protection for individuals considered to be at the highest risk of severe disease. Vaccination is therefore only offered to those at higher risk of severe COVID-19 disease through bi-annual seasonal immunisation campaigns— an autumn campaign and a spring campaign. Some individuals with severe immunosuppression may require additional vaccination doses outside of the campaigns, for further information, see *Immunosuppression and HIV*.

In individuals with confirmed COVID-19 infection, vaccination should ideally be deferred until clinical recovery. However, during care home outbreaks, residents with confirmed COVID-19 infection may receive the vaccine provided they are clinically stable. In individuals with prolonged COVID-19 symptoms, consider deferring the vaccine if they are seriously debilitated, under active investigation or have recently deteriorated, to avoid incorrect attribution of any change in symptoms to the vaccine.

COVID-19 vaccination is an area of ongoing research and recommendations may change on a seasonal basis as more data and other vaccines become available. For further information on the COVID-19 vaccination programme, see the UKHSA collection (available at: www.gov.uk/government/collections/covid-19-vaccination-programme).

Seasonal immunisation

For the Spring 2026 campaign, children aged 6 months and over who are immunosuppressed should be offered immunisation.

Eligible individuals aged 5 years and over should receive a single dose of COVID-19 vaccine p. 988 irrespective of previous vaccination history, provided that there has been an interval of at least 3 months from the previous dose.

Eligible children aged 6 months to 4 years should also receive a single dose of COVID-19 vaccine. A second dose is required for those that have not been previously vaccinated, ideally given where possible during the same seasonal campaign with an interval of 3 months from the previous dose.

For individuals who are severely immunosuppressed, additional doses may be considered; for further information, see *Immunosuppression and HIV*.

For further information on vaccination of eligible individuals, including definition of immunosuppressed and timing of additional doses, see COVID-19 - SARS-CoV-2, in *Immunisation against infectious disease*- 'The Green Book' (see *Useful resources*).

Vaccine choice

There are several COVID-19 vaccines licensed for use in the UK, however, only the messenger RNA (mRNA) monovalent vaccine, *Comirnaty*® LP.8.1, is recommended for use in children aged 6 months to 17 years in the Spring 2026 campaign. For children aged 12 years and over, if an mRNA vaccine is not suitable, the recombinant spike protein vaccine *Nuvaxovid*® JN.1 may be used on specialist advice.

For further information on vaccine choice, including when mRNA vaccines are unsuitable, see COVID-19 - SARS-CoV-2, in *Immunisation against infectious disease*- 'The Green Book' (see *Useful resources*).

Pregnancy

Females with immunosuppression who are pregnant should be offered immunisation during the seasonal campaign. The COVID-19 vaccine can be given during any stage of pregnancy and at the same time as, or at any interval before or after, other vaccines offered in pregnancy, however its administration should not be delayed so that it can be given during the same appointment as other vaccines offered during pregnancy.

Immunosuppression and HIV

Individuals with immunosuppression and HIV infection (regardless of CD4 count) are considered at higher risk and should be vaccinated against COVID-19 in accordance with JCVI recommendations (see *Seasonal immunisation*).

Eligible individuals aged 6 months and over who become, or have recently become severely immunosuppressed (such as those starting immunosuppressive therapy or those who have developed an immunosuppressive condition), should be considered for additional doses.

Unvaccinated severely immunosuppressed individuals should be considered for their first dose of vaccine regardless of the time of year, with further doses being offered based on specialist clinical judgement.

For previously vaccinated severely immunosuppressed individuals, an additional dose of COVID-19 vaccine should be considered regardless of vaccination history or time of year, and be given at least three months after any previous dose to extend protection to the next seasonal campaign.

Post-vaccination testing for individuals with severe immunosuppression may be considered by specialists managing their care; advice on whether further precautions are required to reduce their risk can then be given if appropriate.

For further information on vaccination of individuals with immunosuppression, including definition of severe immunosuppression, and timing of additional doses, see COVID-19 - SARS-CoV-2, in *Immunisation against infectious disease*- 'The Green Book' (see *Useful resources*).

Post-exposure management

COVID-19 is a notifiable disease in the UK. For further information, see *Notifiable diseases* in Antibacterials, principles of therapy p. 358.

There is limited evidence on the use of COVID-19 vaccines as post-exposure prophylaxis or to prevent transmission during outbreaks. For vulnerable individuals who require direct protection during prolonged community outbreaks, advice on post-exposure management can be sought from local health protection teams.

For the management of COVID-19 infection and links to other resources, see COVID-19 p. 490.

Useful Resources

Recommendations reflect COVID-19 - SARS-CoV-2, in *Immunisation against infectious disease*- 'The Green Book'. UK Health Security Agency. March 2026.
www.gov.uk/government/publications/covid-19-the-green-book-chapter-14a

COVID-19 vaccination programme: Information for healthcare practitioners. UK Health Security Agency. March 2026.
www.gov.uk/government/publications/covid-19-vaccination-programme-guidance-for-healthcare-practitioners

Diphtheria vaccine

18-Jun-2025

Overview

Diphtheria-containing vaccines are inactivated and prepared from a cell-free purified toxin of *Corynebacterium diphtheriae*, adsorbed on aluminium hydroxide or aluminium phosphate to improve immunogenicity. The diphtheria vaccine is only available as part of combination preparations containing other vaccines. The quantity of diphtheria toxoid in a preparation determines whether the vaccine is defined as 'high dose' (D) or 'low dose' (d), and this, as well as the need for protection against other infections, determines the choice of vaccine for each age group.

Pre-exposure prophylaxis

The objective of the immunisation programme is to provide a minimum of 5 doses of a diphtheria-containing vaccine at appropriate intervals for all individuals to provide long-term protection against diphtheria. The choice of vaccine for each age group is determined also by the need for protection against tetanus, pertussis, *Haemophilus influenzae* type b, hepatitis B, and poliomyelitis.

Laboratory and healthcare workers (including students and trainees) who may be exposed to diphtheria in the course of their work, such as in microbiology laboratories and clinical infectious disease units, are at risk and should be protected.

For additional considerations on immunisation of children with neurological conditions, see Chapter 15, Diphtheria, in *Immunisation against infectious disease*- 'The Green Book' (see *Useful resources*).

For information on immunisation in pregnancy, see *Pregnancy*.

Children with immunosuppression or HIV infection (regardless of CD4 count) should be vaccinated in accordance with the routine immunisation schedule, see *Primary immunisation* and *Boosters*. Re-immunisation after treatment completion and recovery should be considered—specialist advice may be required.

Primary immunisation

Diphtheria vaccination is given as a component of the routine childhood immunisation programme (see Immunisation schedule p. 961). If the child's routine immunisation is delayed, they should be immunised at the earliest opportunity.

Children aged under 10 years should be given a primary course consisting of 3 doses of the hexavalent diphtheria with tetanus, pertussis, hepatitis B, poliomyelitis and haemophilus influenzae type b vaccine p. 990 (DTaP/IPV/Hib/HepB vaccine) at intervals of 4 weeks—it is the only suitable vaccine containing high dose diphtheria for priming children of this age. If interrupted, the primary course should be resumed but not repeated, allowing a 4-week interval between doses. For information on circumstances where early immunisation may be considered, see UKHSA guidance: **Hexavalent DTaP/IPV/Hib/HepB combination vaccine: information for healthcare practitioners** (see *Useful resources*).

Children aged 10 years or over who are unimmunised, or have an uncertain or incomplete history, should be given a primary course consisting of 3 doses of the 'low dose' diphtheria, tetanus, and poliomyelitis vaccine p. 989 (Td/IPV vaccine) at 4-week intervals. If interrupted, the primary course should be resumed but not repeated, allowing an interval of 4 weeks between doses.

For further information, see Chapter 15, Diphtheria, in *Immunisation against infectious disease*- 'The Green Book' (see *Useful resources*).

Boosters

Following a primary course, 2 doses of a suitable diphtheria-containing booster vaccine should be given at recommended intervals. For children born on or after 1 July 2024, an additional dose of the hexavalent DTaP/IPV/Hib/HepB vaccine should be given at 18 months to provide a booster dose of a *Haemophilus influenzae* type b (Hib)-containing vaccine in the second year of life. As this hexavalent booster dose is not sufficient to provide long-term protection against diphtheria when given routinely under the age of 3 years 4 months, 2 further doses of a diphtheria-containing vaccine (termed the first and second booster) are still required before adulthood (children born before 1 July 2024 should have already received their Hib booster dose as routinely scheduled at 1 year of age).

Children aged under 10 years should receive diphtheria, tetanus, pertussis, and poliomyelitis vaccine p. 989 (dTaP/IPV vaccine) for their first booster dose. This is usually given at 3 years 4 months of age or soon after (before school entry)—see Immunisation schedule p. 961. However, when primary immunisation has been delayed, it may be given at the scheduled visit, provided it has been at least 1 year since the last dose of hexavalent DTaP/IPV/Hib/HepB vaccine.

Children aged 10 years and over should be given the Td/IPV vaccine for their first booster dose. This should be at least 5 years after the third dose of their primary course.

All children should be given the Td/IPV vaccine for their second booster dose. This is usually given 10 years after the first booster (see Immunisation schedule p. 961), but if previous doses have been delayed, it may be given at the school session or scheduled visit provided there has been at least a 5-year interval since the first booster dose.

If a child presents for their routine booster dose but has a history of being vaccinated following a tetanus-prone wound, the vaccine preparation administered at the time of injury should be determined. If this is not possible, or the vaccine administered was not the same as the vaccine due at the current visit or was not given after an appropriate interval, the routine dose should still be given to ensure long-term protection against all antigens.

For further guidance, including information on vaccination of children with uncertain or incomplete immunisation status, see Chapter 15, Diphtheria, in *Immunisation against infectious disease*- 'The Green Book' (see *Useful resources*).

Travel

All travellers to epidemic or endemic areas should ensure they are fully immunised (or are up-to-date) with their diphtheria vaccination (see *Primary immunisation* and *Boosters*). Further doses may be required in some cases, such as for those intending to live or work with local people in epidemic or endemic areas. Where protection against diphtheria is required, and more than 10 years have elapsed since the final dose of diphtheria-containing vaccine was received, Td/IPV vaccine should be given.

Post-exposure management

Advice on the management of cases, carriers, contacts, and outbreaks must be sought from local health protection teams. The immunisation history of infected individuals and their contacts should be determined.

For further information on the management of possible cases, carriers, and close contacts, see UKHSA guidance: **Public health control and management of diphtheria in England** (see *Useful resources*). For information on diphtheria control for asylum seekers, see UKHSA guidance: **Infectious diseases in asylum seekers: actions for health professionals** (available at: www.gov.uk/guidance/infectious-diseases-in-asylum-seekers-actions-for-health-professionals).

Cases

Diphtheria is a notifiable disease in the UK. For further information, see *Notifiable diseases* in Antibacterials, principles of therapy p. 358.

Diphtheria antitoxin p. 959 should only be used for the treatment of confirmed or probable cases of diphtheria in a hospital setting. Treatment should proceed as soon as possible, as the effectiveness is strongly related to time since disease onset. For further information on the use of diphtheria antitoxin, see UKHSA guidance: **Diphtheria anti-toxin** (available at: www.gov.uk/government/publications/immunoglobulin-when-to-use/diphtheria-anti-toxin-clinical-guidance-issued-may-2022). All individuals with confirmed or probable diphtheria should also receive antibacterial therapy to eliminate the organism and prevent spread. Asymptomatic carriers of toxigenic strains should be treated with the same antibacterials as cases. Individuals identified with a non-toxigenic toxin gene-bearing (NTTB) strain should be given antibacterial therapy only if clinically indicated.

Diphtheria infection may not result in adequate levels of antitoxin, and vaccination of confirmed or probable cases is recommended once the patient is clinically stable. Asymptomatic carriers of toxigenic strains should also be vaccinated. Those who are unimmunised or partially immunised against diphtheria should complete their immunisation according to the routine schedule, and fully immunised individuals should receive a reinforcing dose according to their age unless a diphtheria-containing vaccine was given within the last 12 months, see *Pre-exposure prophylaxis*.

Contacts

Close contacts of asymptomatic carriers or confirmed or probable cases should be investigated immediately, kept under surveillance, and be given antibacterial prophylaxis (see *Diphtheria: prevention of secondary cases* in Antibacterials, use for prophylaxis p. 359). Unimmunised or partially immunised close contacts should complete their immunisation according to the routine schedule, and fully immunised close contacts of asymptomatic carriers or confirmed or probable cases should receive a reinforcing dose according to their age unless a diphtheria-containing vaccine was given within the last 12 months, see *Pre-exposure prophylaxis*.

Pregnancy

Routine vaccination of pregnant females with diphtheria, tetanus, and pertussis vaccine p. 988 (Tdap vaccine) is recommended between 16 to 32 weeks of each pregnancy as part of the maternal pertussis programme, usually around the time of the fetal anomaly scan (20 weeks) for operational reasons. For further information, and for guidance for pregnant females with an uncertain or incomplete vaccination history against diphtheria, tetanus, and poliomyelitis, see UKHSA guidance: **Pertussis (whooping cough) vaccination programme for pregnant women: information for healthcare practitioners** (available at: www.gov.uk/government/publications/vaccination-against-pertussis-whooping-cough-for-pregnant-women).

Pregnant females may be given diphtheria-containing vaccines where protection is needed without delay. For information on the management of cases, see *Post-exposure management*.

Useful Resources

Recommendations reflect Chapter 15, Diphtheria, in *Immunisation against infectious disease*- 'The Green Book'. UK Health Security Agency. May 2025.
www.gov.uk/government/publications/diphtheria-the-green-book-chapter-15

Public health control and management of diphtheria in England. UK Health Security Agency. November 2023.
www.gov.uk/government/publications/diphtheria-public-health-control-and-management-in-england-and-wales

Hexavalent DTaP/IPV/Hib/HepB combination vaccine: information for healthcare practitioners. UK Health Security Agency. June 2025.
www.gov.uk/government/publications/hexavalent-combination-vaccine-programme-guidance

Haemophilus influenzae type b conjugate vaccine

18-Jun-2025

Overview

Haemophilus influenzae type b (Hib) containing vaccines are inactivated, and are made from capsular polysaccharide extracted from cultures of Hib bacteria. The polysaccharide is conjugated with a protein (such as tetanus toxoid) to increase immunogenicity, especially in young children. The Hib conjugate vaccine is only available as a combination preparation containing other vaccines.

Pre-exposure prophylaxis

For additional considerations on immunisation of individuals with neurological conditions, see Chapter 16, *Haemophilus influenzae* type b (Hib), in *Immunisation against infectious disease*- 'The Green Book' (see *Useful resources*).

Children with immunosuppression or HIV infection (regardless of CD4 count) should be vaccinated in accordance with the routine immunisation schedule (see *Primary immunisation* and *Boosters*). Re-immunisation after treatment completion and recovery should be considered—specialist advice may be required.

Primary immunisation

Hib vaccination is given as a component of the routine childhood immunisation programme to provide protection against invasive Hib disease for children aged under 10 years (see Immunisation schedule p. 961).

A primary course consists of 3 doses of the hexavalent diphtheria with tetanus, pertussis, hepatitis B, poliomyelitis and haemophilus influenzae type b vaccine p. 990 (DTaP/IPV/Hib/HepB vaccine), with an interval of 4 weeks between doses. If the child's routine immunisation is delayed, children aged under 10 years should be immunised at the earliest opportunity. Although 1 dose of a Hib-containing vaccine is effective from 1 year of age, 3 doses of the DTaP/IPV/Hib/HepB vaccine are still required to complete a primary course in all children aged under 10 years, in order to be fully protected against diphtheria, tetanus, pertussis, poliomyelitis, and hepatitis B. If interrupted, the primary course should be resumed but not repeated, allowing a 4-week interval between doses. For information on circumstances where early immunisation may be considered, see UKHSA guidance: **Hexavalent DTaP/IPV/Hib/HepB combination vaccine: information for healthcare practitioners**, and for further information on immunisation against Hib, see Chapter 16, *Haemophilus influenzae* type b (Hib), in *Immunisation against infectious disease*- 'The Green Book' (see *Useful resources*).

Boosters

For children born before 1 July 2024, the primary course should have been followed by a booster dose of haemophilus influenzae type b and meningococcal group C vaccine p. 990 (Hib/MenC vaccine) at 1 year of age (usually on or after the child's first birthday). For those aged under 10 years who did not receive their booster dose as scheduled, a single booster dose of Hib/MenC vaccine should be given (at least 4 weeks after the last dose of a Hib-containing vaccine). If Hib/MenC vaccine is unavailable (as Hib/MenC vaccine manufacturing has ceased), the hexavalent DTaP/IPV/Hib/HepB vaccine should be given instead.

For children born on or after 1 July 2024, the primary course should be followed by a booster dose of the hexavalent DTaP/IPV/Hib/HepB vaccine at 18 months of age; where there has been a delay, it can be given up until 10 years of age.

For all children (regardless of their date of birth), the booster dose of a Hib-containing vaccine is not required if the child has received at least one of their primary doses of DTaP/IPV/Hib/HepB vaccine at over 1 year of age.

For further guidance, including information on vaccination of children with uncertain or incomplete immunisation status, see Chapter 16, *Haemophilus influenzae* type b (Hib), in *Immunisation against infectious disease*- 'The Green Book' (see *Useful resources*).

Post-exposure management of invasive *Haemophilus influenzae* type b disease

Acute meningitis caused by Hib is a notifiable disease in England, Northern Ireland, and Wales. For further information, see *Notifiable diseases* in Antibacterials, principles of therapy p. 358.

Children aged under 10 years who are unimmunised or partially immunised against Hib disease and are the index case, or a household contact of the index case, or a contact of the index case in a pre-school or primary school setting, should complete their routine immunisation. Vaccination of the index case should occur after recovery from invasive Hib infection. For further information on routine immunisation, see *Pre-exposure prophylaxis*.

To reduce the risk of secondary invasive Hib disease, the index case and their household contacts should be offered antibacterial prophylaxis. Staff and children in a pre-school or primary school setting who are close contacts of the index case may be considered for antibacterial prophylaxis following an assessment of the number of cases and level of contact. For information on antibacterial prophylaxis, see *Haemophilus influenzae type b infection: prevention of secondary disease* in Antibacterials, use for prophylaxis p. 359, and for further information on prevention of secondary Hib disease, see UKHSA guidance: **Revised recommendations for the prevention of secondary *Haemophilus influenzae* type b (Hib) disease** (see *Useful resources*).

Useful Resources

Recommendations reflect Chapter 16, *Haemophilus influenzae* type b (Hib), in *Immunisation against infectious disease*- 'The Green Book'. UK Health Security Agency. May 2025.
www.gov.uk/government/publications/haemophilus-influenzae-type-hib-the-green-book-chapter-16

Revised recommendations for the prevention of secondary *Haemophilus influenzae* type b (Hib) disease. UK Health Security Agency. September 2024.
www.gov.uk/government/publications/haemophilus-influenzae-type-b-hib-revised-recommendations-for-the-prevention-of-secondary-cases

Hexavalent DTaP/IPV/Hib/HepB combination vaccine: information for healthcare practitioners. UK Health Security Agency. June 2025.
www.gov.uk/government/publications/hexavalent-combination-vaccine-programme-guidance

Hepatitis A vaccine

20-May-2022

Overview

The hepatitis A vaccine p. 991 is prepared from different strains of the virus grown in human diploid cells. The inactivated vaccine is available as a monovalent vaccine (different monovalent vaccines can be used interchangeably), or in combination with hepatitis B—vaccine choice is dependent on which infection(s) the individual requires protection from. Immunisation with normal immunoglobulin p. 955 can be used to provide immediate but temporary protection against hepatitis A.

Pre-exposure prophylaxis

Immunisation against hepatitis A is recommended for children at high risk of hepatitis A exposure, those with certain underlying medical conditions, and those at risk of complications, as listed:

- children in care homes for those with severe learning difficulties, or where personal hygiene among children may be poor;
- children with haemophilia being treated with plasma-derived clotting factors;
- children with severe liver disease regardless of the cause (consider for those with chronic hepatitis B or C infection and for patients with milder liver disease);
- children travelling to or going to reside in areas of intermediate or high prevalence, see *Travel* below;
- adolescents who are at risk due to their sexual behaviour (such as males who have sex with males);
- individuals who inject drugs.

Immunisation against hepatitis A infection requires a primary pre-exposure course. The primary immunisation regimen for monovalent hepatitis A vaccine consists of a single dose. For immunisation using the combined hepatitis A and B vaccine, the primary course depends on the product used, see hepatitis A and B vaccine p. 991 for dosing schedules (including accelerated course information).

Children with immunosuppression and HIV infection can be given hepatitis A-containing vaccines. Consider re-immunisation—specialist advice may be required. Refer to the Children's HIV Association for further information on the use of hepatitis A vaccine in HIV-positive children. See www.chiva.org.uk for further information.

Boosters
A booster dose is usually given 6–12 months after the initial dose of hepatitis A-containing vaccine, and ensures immunity beyond 10 years; however, successful boosting can occur even if the booster dose is delayed by several years. A further booster dose 25 years after full primary immunisation is only considered necessary if the risk of hepatitis A infection is still present.

Travel
Pre-exposure immunisation is recommended for individuals travelling to or going to reside in areas of high or intermediate prevalence. Immunisation should ideally be given 2 weeks prior to departure, but can be given up to the day of departure; the use of normal immunoglobulin for travel prophylaxis is no longer recommended. Care should be taken to avoid hepatitis A exposure through food and water. Further information on country-specific hepatitis A risk is available from the National Travel Health Network and Centre (travelhealthpro.org.uk/).

Post-exposure prophylaxis
Hepatitis A (acute infectious hepatitis) is a notifiable disease in the UK. For further information, see *Notifiable diseases* in Antibacterials, principles of therapy p. 358.

A risk assessment for the index case should be carried out (particularly if infection occurs in a non-household setting), and the national standard questionnaire also completed for all probable and confirmed cases. Verbal and written guidance on the importance of good hygiene practices (such as hand washing after using the toilet, changing nappies, and before preparing food) should be given to the index case, their family and other close contacts. If sexual transmission is the likely route (particularly between males who have sex with males), advice on prevention of hepatitis A spread during sex should also be given. For further information on the management of index cases and link to the national standard questionnaire, see Public Health England (PHE) guidance: **Public Health control and management of hepatitis** A (see *Useful resources*).

Close contacts of the index case(s) should have a risk assessment as soon as possible within 14 days of exposure. Prophylactic treatment choice for close contacts depends on susceptibility (determined by age and health status) and time since exposure. There should be a low threshold for considering someone a close contact.

Close contacts should be considered immune if they have a documented history of either a completed course within the past 10 years, or a single dose of monovalent vaccine within the past year, or if they have previously had laboratory-confirmed hepatitis A.

Post-exposure prophylaxis is **not** required for healthy close contacts aged under 1 year not attending childcare; immunisation should be offered to all those who assist in the child's toileting to prevent tertiary infection. For close contacts aged 2–12 months attending childcare, a dose of monovalent hepatitis A vaccine [unlicensed use] should be given within 14 days of exposure. If the child contact cannot be immunised, appropriate advice should be given on enhanced hygiene in the childcare setting; if enhanced hygiene standards cannot be met, the child should be excluded from childcare for 30 days. If exclusion of the child is not possible, all carers and children aged 2 months and above in the childcare setting should be immunised. In these cases, any child that goes on to require long-term protection against hepatitis A after their first birthday, should be given the full course of two doses.

For healthy close contacts aged 1 year and over, a single dose of monovalent hepatitis A vaccine is recommended within 14 days of exposure. A risk assessment is required to determine any continued risk of hepatitis A infection. To ensure long term protection, a second dose of the vaccine should be given after 6–12 months.

For close contacts who have chronic liver disease (including chronic hepatitis B or C infection), HIV infection (with a CD4 count < 200 cells per microlitre), or are immunosuppressed, normal immunoglobulin in addition to monovalent hepatitis A vaccine is recommended within 14 days of exposure (up to 28 days in those with chronic liver disease). To provide long term protection, a second dose of the vaccine should be given after 6–12 months.

Refer to the Children's HIV Association for further information on the use of hepatitis A vaccine in HIV-positive individuals. See www.chiva.org.uk for further information.

In households with more than one close contact, all unvaccinated household contacts seen within 8 weeks of jaundice onset in the index case should be given the monovalent hepatitis A vaccine to prevent tertiary spread within the household.

For further information on the management of susceptible close contacts and for information on outbreaks, see PHE guidance: **Public Health control and management of hepatitis A** (see *Useful resources*); and for further information on normal immunoglobulin, see Immunoglobulins p. 951.

Useful Resources
Recommendations reflect Chapter 17, Hepatitis A, in *Immunisation against infectious disease*- 'The Green Book'. UK Health Security Agency. February 2022.
www.gov.uk/government/publications/hepatitis-a-the-green-book-chapter-17

Public health control and management of hepatitis A. Public Health England. June 2017.
www.gov.uk/government/publications/hepatitis-a-infection-prevention-and-control-guidance

Hepatitis B vaccine
02-May-2026

Overview
Hepatitis B vaccines contain inactivated hepatitis B surface antigen (HBsAg) prepared from yeast cells using recombinant DNA technology, which is adsorbed onto an adjuvant. The vaccine is available as a monovalent vaccine, a bivalent vaccine in combination with hepatitis A, and a hexavalent vaccine in combination with diphtheria, tetanus, acellular pertussis, inactivated poliomyelitis, and *Haemophilus influenzae* type b (Hib).

Pre-exposure prophylaxis
The objective of the immunisation programme is to provide a complete course of hepatitis B vaccine for infants as part of the routine childhood immunisation programme, and for individuals at high risk of exposure to the virus or complications of the disease.

Routine primary immunisation in children
Hepatitis B vaccination is given as a component of the routine childhood immunisation programme to provide long-term protection against hepatitis B. Children aged under 1 year should be given a primary course consisting of 3 doses of the hexavalent diphtheria with tetanus, pertussis, hepatitis B, poliomyelitis and haemophilus influenzae type b vaccine p. 990 (DTaP/IPV/Hib/HepB vaccine), given at 4-weekly intervals (see Immunisation schedule p. 961). If interrupted, the primary course should be resumed but not repeated, allowing a 4-week interval between doses. If the child's routine immunisation is delayed, children aged under 10 years should be immunised at the earliest opportunity. For information on circumstances where early immunisation may be considered, see UKHSA guidance: **Hexavalent DTaP/IPV/Hib/HepB combination vaccine: information for healthcare practitioners** (see *Useful resources*).

Children born from 1 August 2017 who are aged under 10 years and have not received any hepatitis B-containing vaccines, should be opportunistically offered 3 doses of a hepatitis B-containing vaccine, given at least 4 weeks apart. If they are in a high-risk group or are exposed to hepatitis B, they should be proactively offered a hepatitis B vaccine course. For guidance on high-risk groups, see *Primary immunisation in high-risk children*, and for guidance on vaccination following exposure, see *Post-exposure prophylaxis*.

For further guidance on immunisation of individuals with uncertain or incomplete vaccination status, see UKHSA guidance: **Vaccination of individuals with uncertain or incomplete immunisation status** available at: www.gov.uk/government/publications/vaccination-of-individuals-with-uncertain-or-incomplete-immunisation-status

Primary immunisation in high-risk children (excluding infants who have received primary immunisation through the routine childhood schedule)
Immunisation against hepatitis B is also recommended for children in high-risk groups (those at high risk of exposure or those at risk of complications), as listed:

- people who inject drugs (PWID) and their sexual partners, other household and close family contacts;
- individuals who are likely to 'progress' to injecting drugs or who are in a close network with PWID;
- close family, household, or sexual contacts of an individual with chronic hepatitis B infection;
- individuals who change sexual partners frequently;
- gay, bisexual, and other men who have sex with men (GBMSM);
- children receiving regular blood transfusions or blood products (such as those with haemophilia), and carers responsible for the administration of such products;
- children with chronic renal failure who are on haemodialysis or a renal transplantation programme, and those predicted to require these interventions—use vaccines specifically formulated for patients with renal insufficiency;
- prospective recipients of other solid organ tranpslants (e.g. liver, heart, and lung);
- children with severe liver disease regardless of the cause, or those with milder liver disease who may share risk factors for acquiring hepatitis B infection (such as children with chronic hepatitis C);
- healthcare workers (including students and trainees) who may have direct contact with patients' blood, blood-stained body fluids, or tissues;
- laboratory staff who handle material that may contain the virus;
- other occupational risk groups;
- staff and residents of homes for those with learning difficulties (consideration may also be given for those in day care, schools, and centres for those with severe learning disability);
- staff and inmates of custodial institutions;
- individuals travelling to or going to reside in areas of high or intermediate prevalence of hepatitis B, see *Travel*;
- families adopting children from countries with a high or intermediate prevalence of hepatitis B;
- some foster carers and their families.

Immunosuppressed children with HIV infection have higher rates of developing chronic infection; HIV-positive children should be screened for evidence of hepatitis B infection or immunity and offered hepatitis B vaccination if they are non-immune. Refer to the Children's HIV Association for further information on the use of hepatitis B-containing vaccines in children with HIV infection. See www.chiva.org.uk/ for further information.

During vaccination, advice should be provided on other preventative measures (such as condom use and needle exchange), and referral to specialist services arranged if appropriate.

For immunisation of children in a high-risk group, the primary course dosing regimen depends on how rapidly protection is required, the likelihood of patient compliance, and the product used. For most children, an accelerated schedule should be given (particularly in individuals where compliance with immunisation is difficult). Alternative non-accelerated schedules are available, but should only be used when rapid protection is not required and there is a high likelihood of patient attendance for immunisation. In certain circumstances, a very rapid schedule may be given to individuals who are at immediate risk where a more rapid induction of protection is required. See hepatitis B vaccine p. 992 and hepatitis A and B vaccine p. 991 for information on dosing schedules.

Testing for response to vaccination is not routinely advised, but it is recommended for children at risk of occupational exposure, children with renal failure, and recipients and prospective recipients of solid organ transplants. For further information, see Chapter 18, Hepatitis B, in *Immunisation against infectious disease*- 'The Green Book' (see *Useful resources*).

Neonates
Neonates born to a hepatitis B-negative female who are going home to a household with another individual who has hepatitis B infection may be at immediate risk of hepatitis B infection. They should be given a dose of the monovalent hepatitis B vaccine (HepB vaccine) before being discharged from hospital. Routine childhood immunisation with the hexavalent DTaP/IPV/Hib/HepB vaccine should then be given as scheduled (see Immunisation schedule p. 961).

For post-exposure prophylaxis for neonates born to mothers who have chronic hepatitis B infection or who had acute hepatitis B during pregnancy, see *Selective neonatal immunisation programme*.

Travel
Pre-exposure immunisation is recommended for children travelling to or going to reside in areas of high or intermediate prevalence of hepatitis B and who, through their behaviour/activities may be at risk while abroad. These include sexual activity, injecting drug use, undertaking relief aid work, and/or playing contact sports. Travellers are also at risk of acquiring infection as a result of medical or dental procedures carried out in countries where unsafe therapeutic injections (e.g. the re-use of contaminated needles and syringes without sterilisation) are a risk factor for hepatitis B. Individuals at high risk of requiring medical or dental procedures in such countries should therefore be immunised, including:

- those staying for lengthy periods;
- those with chronic medical conditions that may require hospitalisation;
- those travelling for medical or dental procedures.

Further information on country-specific hepatitis B risk is available from the National Travel Health Network and Centre (travelhealthpro.org.uk/).

Boosters
Following a primary course of immunisation, most immunocompetent children do not require a reinforcing dose of a hepatitis B-containing vaccine. Children born on or after 1 July 2024 should receive an additional dose of the DTaP/IPV/Hib/HepB vaccine at 18 months of age, however, the purpose of this booster is to provide a dose of a *Haemophilus influenza* type b (Hib)-containing vaccine in the second year of life. For healthcare and laboratory workers who have not responded to the primary course of hepatitis B vaccination, children with renal failure, and individuals at the time of a subsequent significant exposure, a booster dose of a hepatitis B-containing vaccine may be required. For further information, see Chapter 18, Hepatitis B, in

Immunisation against infectious disease- 'The Green Book' (see *Useful resources*).

Post-exposure prophylaxis

Hepatitis B (acute infectious hepatitis) is a notifiable disease in the UK. For further information, see *Notifiable diseases* in Antibacterials, principles of therapy p. 358.

Post-exposure prophylaxis should be given as soon as possible to neonates born to mothers infected with hepatitis B, see *Selective neonatal immunisation programme* for further information. For females presenting in labour with unknown hepatitis B status, urgent testing should be performed; however, if HBsAg status is unknown at the time of delivery, a birth dose of vaccine can be given to the neonate.

Immediate post-exposure prophylaxis with a hepatitis B-containing vaccine should also be offered to any individual who has potentially been exposed to hepatitis B infected blood or bodily fluids, such as sexual contacts of an individual with acute hepatitis B or newly diagnosed chronic hepatitis B, or those exposed through a needle stick injury or bites from a known hepatitis B-positive individual. Advice should be sought from the nearest Emergency Department, NHS 111, occupational health services, or the local Health Protection Team. The recommended vaccine course (including use of a booster dose) is dependent on the child's vaccination history, source of exposure, and continued risk. For further information, see Chapter 18, Hepatitis B, in *Immunisation against infectious disease*- 'The Green Book' (see *Useful resources*).

Hepatitis B immunoglobulin p. 954 (HBIG) may also be given to individuals at the same time as the hepatitis B vaccine following accidental exposure to hepatitis B-infected blood or bodily fluids through percutaneous inoculation, or contamination of mucous membranes or non-intact skin. It is also recommended for use with the vaccine in sexual contacts of an individual with acute hepatitis B and may be considered in unprotected sexual contacts of an individual with newly diagnosed chronic hepatitis B, if seen within 1 week. HBIG is also recommended in some known non-responders to the hepatitis B vaccine. For further information, see UKHSA guidance: **Hepatitis B immunoglobulin** (see *Useful resources*).

Selective neonatal immunisation

Neonates born to mothers who have chronic hepatitis B infection or who had acute hepatitis B during pregnancy, should be vaccinated with a dose of the monovalent hepatitis B vaccine p. 992 (HepB vaccine) as soon as possible (ideally within 24 hours of birth), followed by a second dose at 4 weeks. Routine childhood immunisation with the hexavalent diphtheria with tetanus, pertussis, hepatitis B, poliomyelitis and haemophilus influenzae type b vaccine p. 990 (DTaP/IPV/Hib/HepB vaccine) should then be given as scheduled (see Immunisation schedule p. 961). Children born before 1 July 2024 to females who have hepatitis B infection should have been given a dose of monovalent HepB vaccine at 12 months of age (on or after their first birthday). Eligible children born on or after 1 July 2024 will no longer receive a dose at 12 months of age as they will receive an additional dose of the hexavalent DTaP/IPV/Hib/HepB vaccine at 18 months of age instead. In all eligible children, a blood test should be offered between 12 and 18 months of age, to ascertain if the child has become infected with hepatitis B virus. If this test has already been undertaken prior to the 18-month appointment and a negative result returned, the additional (fourth) dose of hexavalent vaccine will still be required at 18 months of age to provide longer term protection against Hib and hepatitis B infection. For further information on the selective neonatal immunisation programme, see UKHSA guidance: **Hexavalent DTaP/IPV/Hib/HepB combination vaccine: information for healthcare practitioners**, and **Guidance on the hepatitis B antenatal screening and selective neonatal immunisation pathway** (see *Useful resources*).

For neonates with a birth weight below 1.5 kg born to an infected mother, or neonates born to a highly infectious mother, HBIG should be given at the same time as the first dose of monovalent HepB vaccine (administered at different sites) in order to provide rapid protection until the vaccine becomes effective. For further information on the use of HBIG and which mothers are considered to be highly infectious, see UKHSA guidance: **Hepatitis B immunoglobulin** (see *Useful resources*).

Useful Resources

Recommendations reflect Chapter 18, Hepatitis B, in *Immunisation against infectious disease*– 'The Green Book'. UK Health Security Agency. February 2026.
www.gov.uk/government/publications/hepatitis-b-the-green-book-chapter-18

Hexavalent DTaP/IPV/Hib/HepB combination vaccine: information for healthcare practitioners. UK Health Security Agency. June 2025.
www.gov.uk/government/publications/hexavalent-combination-vaccine-programme-guidance

Guidance on the hepatitis B antenatal screening and selective neonatal immunisation pathway. UK Health Security Agency. June 2025.
www.gov.uk/government/publications/hepatitis-b-antenatal-screening-and-selective-neonatal-immunisation-pathway

Hepatitis B immunoglobulin. UK Health Security Agency. September 2025.
www.gov.uk/government/publications/immunoglobulin-when-to-use/hepatitis-b-immunoglobulin-issued-march-2021

Human papillomavirus vaccine 19-Jul-2024

Overview

The human papillomavirus vaccine p. 994 (HPV vaccine) consists of virus-like particles prepared from the major protein of the viral capsid that mimic the structure of the native virus, but does not contain any viral DNA. *Gardasil*® 9 is an adjuvanted nine-valent vaccine that contains HPV types 6, 11, 16, 18, 31, 33, 45, 52 and 58, and is the recommended vaccine for the national HPV vaccination programme.

It is used for the prevention of cervical and anal cancers, and pre-cancerous genital (cervical, vulvar, and vaginal) and anal lesions associated with HPV types 16 and 18. It is also effective at preventing genital warts, and may also provide some cross-protection against infection caused by other high-risk HPV types. As *Gardasil*® 9 does not protect against all strains of HPV, safe sex precautions should always be practiced; and for all females, routine cervical screening should continue at the scheduled age.

Children aged 9 to 10 years

The HPV vaccine is licensed for individuals from 9 years of age, however vaccination of children aged 9 to 10 years is not offered as part of the national vaccination programme.

Children aged 11 years and over

Immunisation is routinely recommended for children aged 11 to 14 years (the eligible age for vaccine administration varies within different countries within the UK, see Immunisation schedule p. 961 for further guidance).

Under the national programme, children in eligible cohorts (all females aged under 25 years and males born after 1st September 2006) who did not receive the HPV vaccine when scheduled can still be offered the vaccine up until their 25th birthday. Where appropriate, immunisation should also be offered to children coming into the UK if they have not been offered protection in their country of origin.

Vaccination may also be offered to children who have not already been vaccinated and who meet the eligibility criteria through the HPV vaccination programme for gay, bisexual and other men who have sex with men (GBMSM). For further guidance, see Chapter 18a, Human papillomavirus, in *Immunisation against infectious disease*- 'The Green Book' (see *Useful resources*).

A 1 dose schedule of HPV vaccine is recommended for all eligible children aged 11 years and over, except for those with immunosuppression or HIV infection. For guidance on the vaccination schedule for children with immunosuppression or HIV infection, see *Children with immunosuppression or HIV infection*.

Children with immunosuppression or HIV infection

A 3 dose schedule of HPV vaccine should be offered to eligible children who are known to be immunosuppressed at the time of immunisation. Re-immunisation may be considered after treatment is finished and/or recovery has occurred depending on the treatment received—specialist advice may be required.

A 3 dose schedule of HPV vaccine is also recommended for eligible children with HIV infection who attend HIV services, and should be given regardless of CD4 cell count, antiretroviral therapy use, or viral load.

The second dose in the 3 dose schedule should be given at least 1 month after the first dose, followed by a third dose at least 3 months after the second dose; ideally the course should be completed within a 12 month period. In cases where the second dose is given late and there is a high likelihood that the child will not return, or if it is not practical for the third dose to be given after 3 months, then the third dose can be given at least 1 month after the second dose.

Booster doses

Protection from the HPV vaccine is maintained for at least 10 years, although protection is expected to last longer. There is no recommendation for the need for booster doses.

Useful Resources

Recommendations reflect Chapter 18a, Human papillomavirus, in *Immunisation against infectious disease*- 'The Green Book'. UK Health Security Agency. June 2023. www.gov.uk/government/publications/human-papillomavirus-hpv-the-green-book-chapter-18a

HPV vaccination: guidance for healthcare practitioners. UK Health Security Agency. June 2023. www.gov.uk/government/publications/hpv-universal-vaccination-guidance-for-health-professionals

Influenza vaccine

26-Jun-2025

Overview

While most viruses are antigenically stable, the influenza viruses A and B (especially A) are constantly altering their antigenic structure as indicated by changes in the haemagglutinins (H) and neuraminidases (N) on the surface of the viruses. It is essential that influenza vaccines in use target the prevalent strain or strains recommended each year by the WHO. For the 2025/2026 influenza season, trivalent vaccines containing 2 strains of influenza A and 1 strain of influenza B are recommended.

There are several types of influenza vaccine available (see influenza vaccine (inactivated) p. 994 and influenza vaccine (live) p. 1001). The vaccines recommended in children for the 2025/2026 influenza season are the live attenuated influenza vaccine (LAIV), the inactivated cell-cultured trivalent influenza vaccine (TIVc), and the inactivated egg-cultured trivalent influenza vaccine (TIVe). The choice of vaccine is dependent on the child's age and contra-indications.

To provide optimal protection during the highest risk period (December to January), the ideal time for immunisation in children is between the beginning of September and early December.

Immunisation is recommended for children at high risk of serious complications from influenza, and to reduce transmission of infection. In the national flu immunisation programme 2025/2026, influenza vaccination is recommended for the following eligible groups:

- Children aged 6 months and over in a clinical risk group, such as those with:
  - chronic respiratory disease;
  - chronic heart disease and vascular disease;
  - chronic liver disease;
  - chronic kidney disease;
  - chronic neurological disease;
  - diabetes mellitus;
  - adrenal insufficiency;
  - splenic dysfunction or asplenia;
  - immunosuppression because of disease or treatment (including prolonged systemic corticosteroid treatment [for over 1 month at dose equivalents of prednisolone p. 548: *child under* 20 *kg*, 1 mg/kg or more daily; *child over* 20 *kg*, 20 mg or more daily], and chemotherapy);
  - HIV infection (regardless of immune status).
- All children aged 2–3 years on 31st August 2025.
- All primary school-aged children (from reception to year 6).
- Secondary school-aged children in years 7–11.
- All pregnant females (including those who become pregnant during the flu season).
- Children living in long-stay residential homes or other specific long-stay facilities, where rapid spread is likely to follow introduction of infection and cause high morbidity and mortality (this does not include, for instance, young offender institutions, or university halls of residence).
- Children who receive a carer's allowance, or who are the main carer of a disabled individual whose welfare may be at risk if the carer falls ill.
- Household contacts of immunocompromised individuals.
- Frontline health and social care workers.

Seasonal influenza vaccination should also be considered for individuals at higher risk of infection with zoonotic influenza related to their work. While this does not protect against zoonotic influenza, it may reduce the risk of co-infection with seasonal influenza viruses and, consequently, the very small theoretical risk of reassortment events that could produce a human-transmissible virus. Influenza of zoonotic origin is a notifiable disease in the UK. For further information, see *Notifiable diseases* in Antibacterials, principles of therapy p. 358.

Vaccine choice

Children aged 6 months to less than 2 years who are in a clinical risk group should be offered TIVc. If this is unavailable, TIVe may be offered.

Eligible children aged 2 to 17 years should be offered LAIV, as it has been shown to be more effective than inactivated influenza vaccines in this age group. Where parents decline LAIV for their child due to the porcine gelatine content, or if LAIV is contra-indicated or otherwise unsuitable, TIVc should be offered. If this is unavailable, TIVe may be used. For children with a household contact who is very severely immunocompromised (such as a bone marrow transplant recipient requiring isolation), TIVc (or if unavailable, TIVe) should be offered instead of LAIV.

Children aged 6 months to less than 9 years who are in a clinical risk group or who are household contacts of immunocompromised individuals should be offered 2 doses of the appropriate influenza vaccine (at least 4 weeks apart) if they have never had the influenza vaccine previously.

Pregnant females aged under 18 years should be offered TIVc. If this is unavailable, TIVe may be offered.

For further information on the annual influenza programme, see UKHSA collection: **Annual flu programme** (available at: www.gov.uk/government/collections/annual-flu-programme).

For the management of influenza, see Influenza p. 525.

Useful Resources

Recommendations reflect the National flu immunisation programme plan 2025/2026. UK Health Security Agency, Department of Health and Social Care, and NHS England. February 2025.
www.gov.uk/government/collections/annual-flu-programme#2025-to-2026-flu-season

Chapter 19, Influenza, in *Immunisation against infectious disease*- 'The Green Book'. UK Health Security Agency. May 2025.
www.gov.uk/government/publications/influenza-the-green-book-chapter-19

Flu vaccination programme 2025 to 2026: information for healthcare practitioners. UK Health Security Agency. August 2025.
www.gov.uk/government/publications/flu-vaccination-programme-information-for-healthcare-practitioners

Japanese encephalitis vaccine

14-Nov-2018

Overview

Japanese encephalitis is a mosquito-borne viral encephalitis caused by a *Flavivirus*.

Japanese encephalitis vaccine p. 995 (*IXIARO*®) is an inactivated vaccine adsorbed onto an adjuvant. It is recommended for children who are going to reside in an area where Japanese encephalitis is endemic or epidemic. Children travelling to South and South-East Asia and the Far East should be immunised if staying for a month or longer in endemic areas during the transmission season. Other children travelling with shorter exposure periods should also be immunised if the risk is considered sufficient.

The primary immunisation course of 2 doses should be completed at least one week before potential exposure to Japanese encephalitis virus.

Children (aged 2 months and over) at ongoing risk (such as long-term travellers), should receive a single booster dose 12 months after the primary immunisation course. For other children travelling, a single booster dose should be given within 12–24 months after primary immunisation, before potential re-exposure to the Japanese encephalitis virus.

Cases of Japanese encephalitis should be managed with supportive treatment.

Up-to-date information on the risk of Japanese encephalitis in specific countries can be obtained from the National Travel Health Network and Centre.

Useful Resources

Recommendations reflect Chapter 20, Japanese encephalitis, in *Immunisation against infectious disease*– 'The Green book'. Public Health England, June 2018.
www.gov.uk/government/publications/japanese-encephalitis-the-green-book-chapter-20

National Travel Health Network and Centre
nathnac.net

Measles, Mumps and Rubella vaccine

18-Jun-2025

Overview

Measles, mumps and rubella (MMR) immunisation aims to eliminate measles, mumps, and rubella (German measles) and congenital rubella syndrome. Every child should receive 2 doses of MMR vaccine by entry to primary school, unless there is a valid contra-indication. Doses given prior to 12 months of age (e.g. following exposure to a case of measles) should not be counted. MMR vaccine should be given irrespective of previous measles, mumps, or rubella infection.

The first dose of MMR vaccine is given to children at 1 year of age, on or after their first birthday. For children born on or after 1 July 2024, the second dose is given at 18 months of age. For children born before 1 July 2024, the second dose is given before starting school at 3 years 4 months of age or soon after—see Immunisation schedule p. 961.

Children aged over 12 months with an uncertain or incomplete vaccination history, should receive 2 doses in total of the MMR vaccine regardless of any history of measles, mumps, or rubella infection. A minimum interval of 4 weeks should be left between the first and second dose. For children born on or after 1 July 2024, the second dose should be given from 18 months of age. For those born before 1 July 2024, the second dose should be given from 3 years 4 months of age.

At the teenage booster session/appointment and at entry into further education, MMR immunisation should be offered to individuals who have not received 2 doses during childhood. In those who have received only a single dose in childhood, a second dose is recommended to achieve full protection. If 2 doses of MMR vaccine are required, the second dose should be given at least 4 weeks after the initial dose.

The MMR vaccine should be used to protect against rubella in unimmunised or seronegative females of childbearing age (see Immunisation schedule p. 961); unimmunised healthcare workers who might put pregnant females and other vulnerable groups at risk of rubella or measles should be vaccinated. MMR vaccine may also be offered to previously unimmunised and seronegative post-partum females—vaccination a few days after delivery is important because about 60% of congenital abnormalities from rubella infection occur in babies of females who have borne more than one child. Immigrants arriving after the age of school immunisation are particularly likely to require immunisation.

Contacts

Measles, mumps, and rubella are notifiable diseases in the UK. For further information, see *Notifiable diseases* in Antibacterials, principles of therapy p. 358.

Measles is highly infectious and can be severe, particularly in immunosuppressed individuals, young infants, and pregnant females. Post-exposure prophylaxis with MMR vaccine or normal immunoglobulin may offer some protection to exposed vulnerable contacts. The choice of prophylaxis depends on the individual's age, immune status, and vaccination history. The local Health Protection Team should be contacted for advice on contact tracing and management of contacts. For further information, see UKHSA guidance: **National measles guidelines** (see *Useful resources*).

The MMR vaccine is **not suitable** for prophylaxis following exposure to mumps or rubella since the antibody response to the mumps and rubella components is too slow for effective prophylaxis.

Travel
Unimmunised travellers, including children aged over 6 months, to areas where measles is endemic or epidemic should receive the MMR vaccine. Children immunised before 12 months of age should still receive 2 doses of MMR vaccine at the recommended ages.

Useful Resources
Advice reflects that in the handbook Immunisation against Infectious Disease (2013), which in turn reflects the guidance of the Joint Committee on Vaccination and Immunisation (JCVI). The advice also incorporates changes announced by the Chief Medical Officer and Health Department Updates. Chapters from the handbook (including updates since 2013) are available at:
www.gov.uk/government/collections/immunisation-against-infectious-disease-the-green-book

National measles guidelines. UK Health Security Agency. July 2024.
www.gov.uk/government/publications/national-measles-guidelines

Meningococcal vaccines

18-Jun-2025

Overview

Meningococcal vaccines are inactivated and are available as either conjugated vaccines or as a multicomponent protein vaccine. The conjugate vaccines are made from capsular polysaccharides of serogroups A, C, W, and Y *Neisseria meningitidis* conjugated to a carrier protein (such as tetanus toxoid) to enhance immunogenicity. The conjugate vaccines are available as a combination preparation of haemophilus influenzae type b and meningococcal group C vaccine p. 990 (Hib/MenC vaccine), or as a quadrivalent meningococcal groups A, C, W135, and Y vaccine p. 996 (MenACWY vaccine). The multicomponent protein meningococcal group B vaccine p. 995 (4CMenB vaccine) is made from 3 *N. meningitidis* proteins produced by recombinant DNA technology and a preparation of *N. meningitidis* group B outer membrane vesicles.

Pre-exposure prophylaxis

Routine childhood immunisation schedule
Meningococcal vaccinations are given as a component of the routine childhood immunisation programme (see Immunisation schedule p. 961). Immunisation against infection by serogroup B of *Neisseria meningitidis* consists of a primary course of the 4CMenB vaccine, with 2 doses given 4 weeks apart, followed by a single booster dose of the 4CMenB vaccine at 1 year of age (usually on or after the child's first birthday). Prophylactic paracetamol p. 325 is recommended in children under 1 year of age receiving 4CMenB vaccine with other routine immunisations, to prevent fever following vaccination.

Due to the very low numbers of meningitis cases caused by serogroup C *N. meningitidis*, a dose of a meningococcal group C-containing vaccine is no longer required in the second year of life. However, in order to provide continued protection against invasive Hib disease, a single booster dose of either the Hib/MenC vaccine or hexavalent diphtheria with tetanus, pertussis, hepatitis B, poliomyelitis and haemophilus influenzae type b vaccine p. 990 (DTaP/IPV/Hib/HepB vaccine) should be given in accordance with the routine immunisation schedule.

All individuals should be given a single dose of the MenACWY vaccine between the age of 13–15 years (see Immunisation schedule p. 961), including those who have already received a different meningococcal group C-containing vaccine over the age of 10 years. Individuals who have previously received the MenACWY conjugate vaccine under the age of 10 years (such as for travel reasons or because they were a close contact of a confirmed meningococcal case) will require an additional dose as scheduled. Individuals who have previously received the MenACWY vaccine at 10 years of age or over (such as for travel reasons) do not require an additional dose as part of the routine immunisation programme.

For further information on the MenACWY and 4CMenB vaccine, see UKHSA guidance: **Meningococcal ACWY vaccination programme** and **Meningococcal B vaccination programme** (see *Useful resources*).

Individuals with unknown or incomplete vaccination history
Children under 1 year of age with uncertain or incomplete vaccination histories should be given a primary course of 2 doses of the 4CMenB vaccine, given 4 weeks apart. A single booster dose of the 4CMenB vaccine should be given at 1 year of age, ensuring at least a 4-week interval between the 4CMenB primary and booster doses.

Children aged 1 year to under 2 years who have received less than 2 doses of 4CMenB vaccine within their first year of life should receive 2 doses of 4CMenB vaccine given at least 4 weeks apart.

Individuals aged under 25 years (including those who are new to the UK, and those attending further or higher education for the first time) who have missed the opportunity to receive their adolescent dose of MenACWY conjugate vaccine should be offered a dose up to their 25th birthday. No further meningococcal vaccinations are then required unless they are a close contact of a case of meningococcal infection, or for travel purposes.

For further guidance on the vaccination of individuals with uncertain or incomplete vaccination status, see Chapter 22, Meningococcal, in *Immunisation against infectious disease*-'The Green Book' (see *Useful resources*).

Immunosuppression and HIV
Individuals with asplenia, splenic dysfunction, complement disorders, or those who are taking complement inhibitors may be at increased risk of invasive meningococcal infection and require additional meningococcal vaccinations. Individuals who are taking complement inhibitors should be vaccinated at least 2 weeks prior to starting therapy. For further information on immunising individuals at increased risk of meningococcal disease, see *Vaccines and asplenia, splenic dysfunction, or complement disorders* in Vaccination, general principles p. 959.

Individuals with immunosuppression or HIV infection (regardless of CD4 count) should be given meningococcal vaccines according to the routine immunisation schedule. Re-immunisation after treatment completion and recovery should be considered—specialist advice may be required.

Travel
In some areas of the world, the risk of acquiring meningococcal infection is much higher than in the UK. For example, meningococcal infection is most common in sub-Saharan Africa, especially during the dry season (December to June). For travellers, the risk of acquiring meningococcal infection may be increased for those visiting areas prone to outbreaks or an area with a current outbreak. Travellers visiting those areas who are at greater risk include:
- long stay travellers in close contact with the local population;
- healthcare workers;
- those visiting friends and relatives;
- those who live or travel 'rough' (such as backpackers);
- individuals with asplenia, splenic dysfunction, or certain immune deficiencies.

All travellers should have a careful risk assessment prior to travel, taking into account their itinerary, duration of stay, and any planned activities. Travellers whose planned activities or medical conditions put them at an increased risk of meningococcal disease should consider vaccination with the MenACWY conjugate vaccine. Proof of vaccination against meningococcal serogroups A, C, W, and Y is required for pilgrims and seasonal workers travelling to Saudi Arabia for Hajj and Umrah (where outbreaks of serogroups A and W infections have occurred).

Further information on country-specific meningococcal risk is available from the National Travel Health Network and Centre (travelhealthpro.org.uk/).

Laboratory staff

Any laboratory staff who handle strains of or clinical samples containing *Neisseria meningitidis* must receive a primary course consisting of 1 dose of the MenACWY vaccine and 2 doses of the 4CMenB vaccine, with booster doses of both vaccines every 5 years.

Post-exposure management

Meningitis (acute) and meningococcal septicaemia are notifiable diseases in the UK. For further information, see *Notifiable diseases* in Antibacterials, principles of therapy p. 358.

Advice on the management of cases, contacts, and outbreaks must be sought from health protection teams. For further advice on management (including antibacterial prophylaxis and vaccination) to prevent secondary infection, see UKHSA: **Guidance for public health management of meningococcal disease in the UK** (see *Useful resources*), and *Meningococcal meningitis: prevention of secondary cases* in Antibacterials, use for prophylaxis p. 359.

Useful Resources

Recommendations reflect Chapter 22, Meningococcal, in *Immunisation against infectious disease*- 'The Green Book'. UK Health Security Agency. June 2025.
www.gov.uk/government/publications/meningococcal-the-green-book-chapter-22

Meningococcal ACWY vaccination programme: Information for healthcare professionals. UK Health Security Agency. June 2025.
www.gov.uk/government/publications/menacwy-programme-information-for-healthcare-professionals

Meningococcal B vaccination programme for infants: information for healthcare practitioners. UK Health Security Agency. August 2025.
www.gov.uk/government/publications/meningococcal-b-vaccine-information-for-healthcare-professionals

Guidance for public health management of meningococcal disease in the UK. UK Health Security Agency. November 2024.
www.gov.uk/government/publications/meningococcal-disease-guidance-on-public-health-management

Pertussis vaccine

18-Jun-2025

Overview

Acellular pertussis-containing vaccines are inactivated and are made from highly purified components of *Bordetella pertussis* adsorbed onto aluminium hydroxide or aluminium phosphate adjuvants to improve immunogenicity. The vaccines differ in source, number and amount of each component, and method of manufacture (resulting in differences in efficacy and frequency of side-effects), and are only available as part of combination preparations containing other vaccines.

Pre-exposure prophylaxis

For additional considerations on vaccination of individuals with neurological conditions, refer to Chapter 24, Pertussis, in *Immunisation against infectious disease*- 'The Green Book' (see *Useful resources*).

For information on immunisation in pregnancy, see *Pregnancy*.

Individuals with immunosuppression or HIV infection (regardless of CD4 count) should be vaccinated in accordance with the routine immunisation schedule, see *Primary immunisation* and *Booster dose*. Re-immunisation after treatment completion and recovery should be considered—specialist advice may be required.

Primary immunisation

Pertussis vaccination is given as a component of the routine childhood immunisation programme for all children aged under 10 years (see Immunisation schedule p. 961). If the child's routine immunisation is delayed, children aged under 10 years should be immunised at the earliest opportunity.

Immunisation consists of a primary course of 3 doses of the hexavalent diphtheria with tetanus, pertussis, hepatitis B, poliomyelitis and haemophilus influenzae type b vaccine p. 990 (DTaP/IPV/Hib/HepB vaccine), given at intervals of 4 weeks. If the course is interrupted, it should be resumed but not repeated, allowing a 4-week interval between doses. For information on circumstances where early immunisation may be considered, see UKHSA guidance: **Hexavalent DTaP/IPV/Hib/HepB combination vaccine: information for healthcare practitioners** (see *Useful resources*).

For further guidance, including information on vaccination of individuals with uncertain or incomplete vaccination status, see Chapter 24, Pertussis, in *Immunisation against infectious disease*- 'The Green Book' (see *Useful resources*).

Booster dose

For children born on or after 1 July 2024, an additional dose of the hexavalent DTaP/IPV/Hib/HepB vaccine should be given at 18 months of age to provide a booster dose of a *Haemophilus influenzae* type b (Hib)-containing vaccine in the second year of life. As this hexavalent booster dose is not sufficient to provide long-term protection against pertussis when given routinely under the age of 3 years 4 months, a further dose of a pertussis-containing vaccine (termed the pertussis booster) is still required before the age of 10 years (children born before 1 July 2024 should have already received their Hib booster dose as routinely scheduled at 1 year of age).

A single dose of the diphtheria, tetanus, pertussis, and poliomyelitis vaccine p. 989 (dTaP/IPV vaccine) should be given for the pertussis booster at 3 years 4 months of age or soon after (before school entry)—see Immunisation schedule p. 961. If the primary course was delayed, the booster dose can be given at the scheduled visit provided that it has been at least 1 year since the last dose of hexavalent DTaP/IPV/Hib/HepB vaccine.

Individuals aged 10 years or over who have only had 3 doses of a pertussis-containing vaccine do not need any further doses, except for occupational vaccination of certain healthcare workers, and during pregnancy.

If an individual presents for their routine booster dose but has a history of being vaccinated following a tetanus-prone wound, the vaccine preparation administered at the time of injury should be determined. If this is not possible, or the vaccine administered was not the same as the vaccine due at the current visit or was not given after an appropriate interval, the routine dose should still be given to ensure long-term protection against all antigens.

For further guidance, including information on vaccination of individuals with uncertain or incomplete immunisation status, see Chapter 24, Pertussis, in *Immunisation against infectious disease*- 'The Green Book' (see *Useful resources*).

Healthcare workers

Healthcare workers can be an important source of infection for vulnerable infants and pregnant females. Occupational vaccination with a single dose of dTaP/IPV vaccine or diphtheria, tetanus, and pertussis vaccine p. 988 (Tdap vaccine) should be offered to any healthcare worker who has not received a pertussis-containing vaccine in the previous 5 years and who has regular contact with pregnant females or young infants (under 3 months of age). Prioritisation of such healthcare workers for vaccination is based on their level of contact with infants and/or pregnant females. For further information on priority groups, see UKHSA guidance: **Occupational pertussis vaccination of healthcare workers** (see *Useful resources*).

Pregnancy

Routine vaccination of pregnant females with the Tdap vaccine is recommended between 16 to 32 weeks of each pregnancy as part of the maternal pertussis programme, usually around the time of the fetal anomaly scan (20 weeks) for operational reasons. Females who miss the opportunity to be vaccinated may still be immunised after week 32 of pregnancy until delivery, however, this may not offer as high a level of passive protection to the infant, particularly if they are born pre-term. Females who have not received a pertussis-containing vaccine during pregnancy can be offered it in the 8 weeks following birth; this will protect the mother and may prevent them from becoming a source of infection for the infant, but it will not provide direct protection for the infant. For further information, see UKHSA guidance: **Pertussis (whooping cough) vaccination programme for pregnant women: information for healthcare practitioners** (see *Useful resources*).

Post-exposure management

Advice on the management of cases, contacts, and outbreaks should be sought from local health protection teams. The immunisation history of infected individuals and their contacts should be determined.

For further guidance on the definition of close contacts, priority groups for public health action, and the management of cases, see UKHSA: **Guidance on the management of cases of pertussis in England during the re-emergence of pertussis in 2024** (see *Useful resources*).

Cases

Pertussis is a notifiable disease in the UK. For further information, see *Notifiable diseases* in Antibacterials, principles of therapy p. 358.

Based on clinical judgement, antibacterials may be offered to pertussis cases within 14 days from onset of cough. If the case has a household contact or other close contact who is in priority group 1 for public health action, or who is pregnant, then antibacterial treatment should be offered to the case, commencing within 21 days of onset of cough.

Unimmunised and partially immunised individuals aged up to 10 years should complete their primary and booster vaccination against pertussis once they have recovered. Routine immunisation against pertussis is not recommended for those aged 10 years and over, except for pregnant females and certain healthcare workers (see *Pregnancy* and *Healthcare workers*).

Contacts

Antibacterial prophylaxis should be offered to close contacts of the index case when coughing in the index case started within the preceding 14 days and if the close contact is in a priority group for public health action. For guidance on antibacterial prophylaxis in contacts, see *Pertussis: prevention of secondary cases* in Antibacterials, use for prophylaxis p. 359.

Unimmunised or partially immunised contacts under the age of 10 years should complete their primary and booster vaccination against pertussis. Any pregnant contacts who have reached or passed their 20th week of pregnancy and have not yet received a pertussis-containing vaccine, and females who have an infant under 8 weeks of age and who did not receive a pertussis-containing vaccine during that pregnancy should be vaccinated (see *Pregnancy*). Contacts who are healthcare workers who provide close, personal care to infants in priority group 1 or to pregnant females, should be given a booster dose of a pertussis-containing vaccine if they have not received one in the last 5 years and have not received the diphtheria, tetanus, and poliomyelitis vaccine p. 989 (Td/IPV vaccine) in the preceding month.

Useful Resources

Recommendations reflect Chapter 24, Pertussis, in *Immunisation against infectious disease*- 'The Green Book'. UK Health Security Agency. June 2025.
www.gov.uk/government/publications/pertussis-the-green-book-chapter-24

Guidance on the management of cases of pertussis in England during the re-emergence of pertussis in 2024. UK Health Security Agency. August 2024.
www.gov.uk/government/publications/pertussis-guidelines-for-public-health-management

Occupational pertussis vaccination of healthcare workers. UK Health Security Agency. August 2024.
www.gov.uk/government/publications/pertussis-occupational-vaccination-of-health-care-workers/occupational-pertussis-vaccination-of-healthcare-workers

Pertussis (whooping cough) vaccination programme for pregnant women: information for healthcare practitioners. UK Health Security Agency. August 2024
www.gov.uk/government/publications/vaccination-against-pertussis-whooping-cough-for-pregnant-women

Pneumococcal vaccine

18-Jun-2025

Overview

The pneumococcal polysaccharide conjugate vaccine p. 996 (PCV) and the pneumococcal polysaccharide vaccine (PPV) protect against infection with *Streptococcus pneumoniae* (pneumococcus). Both types of vaccines are inactivated and contain polysaccharide from capsular pneumococci. PPV contains purified polysaccharide from 23 capsular types of pneumococcus (PPV23), whereas PCV contains polysaccharide from 13 capsular types (PCV13), 15 capsular types (PCV15), or 20 capsular types (PCV20).

PCV13 is used for routine childhood immunisation, and is given as a 2-dose schedule at separate intervals (see Immunisation schedule p. 961). Children who present late for vaccination should be immunised according to *Children with unknown or incomplete vaccination history*. PCV15 is not recommended as part of the routine immunisation schedule.

PPV23 or PCV20 are recommended for children who are at high risk of serious illness from pneumococcal infection—for guidance for those in an at-risk group, including definition of risk, see *Individuals in an at-risk group*. PCV20 is expected to replace PPV23 for those at risk in 2025/2026.

Children with unknown or incomplete vaccination history

Unimmunised or partially immunised children who present late for vaccination and before the age of 1 year should receive a single dose of PCV13, followed by a booster dose on or after their first birthday, at least 4 weeks after the 1st dose.

Children aged 1 year to under 2 years who are unimmunised or partially immunised should receive a single dose of PCV13.

For further guidance, see Chapter 25, Pneumococcal, in *Immunisation against infectious disease*- 'The Green Book' (see *Useful resources*).

Individuals in an at-risk group

Immunisation against pneumococcal infection is also recommended for individuals in the following at-risk groups:

- asplenia or splenic dysfunction (including homozygous sickle cell disease and coeliac disease which could lead to splenic dysfunction);
- chronic respiratory disease (including severe asthma treated with continuous or frequent use of a systemic corticosteroid);
- chronic heart disease;
- chronic renal disease;
- chronic liver disease;
- chronic neurological or neuromuscular disease where respiratory function may be compromised (such as in cerebral palsy);
- diabetes mellitus requiring insulin or antidiabetic medication;
- immunosuppression because of disease (such as HIV infection regardless of immune status, and genetic disorders affecting the immune system) or treatment (such as prolonged systemic corticosteroid treatment for over 1 month at dose equivalents of prednisolone: *adult and child* 20 *kg and over*, 20 mg or more daily; *child under* 20 *kg*, 1 mg/kg or more daily, and chemotherapy);
- presence of cochlear implant;
- conditions where leakage of cerebrospinal fluid may occur.

Where possible, the vaccine should be given at least 2 weeks (ideally 4–6 weeks) before splenectomy, immunosuppressive treatment, chemotherapy, or radiotherapy; patients should be given advice about the increased risk of pneumococcal infection. If it is not possible to vaccinate at least 2 weeks before splenectomy, chemotherapy, or radiotherapy, the vaccine should be given at least 2 weeks after the splenectomy, and at least 3 months after completion of chemotherapy or radiotherapy. For guidance on vaccination of patients with haematological malignancies or those who have had a bone marrow transplant, and for information on patient cards and leaflets for individuals with asplenia, see Chapter 25, Pneumococcal, in *Immunisation against infectious disease*- 'The Green Book' (see *Useful resources*).

Vaccination regimens may differ depending on the individual's age, risk of pneumococcal disease, vaccination history, and immune status.

For information on revaccination with PPV23 or PCV20 for individuals in whom the antibody concentration is likely to decline rapidly, see *Revaccination*.

Children diagnosed with at-risk conditions aged under 1 year

Children in an at-risk group (excluding those with asplenia, splenic dysfunction, complement disorder, or who are severely immunocompromised) should receive PCV13 according to the Immunisation schedule p. 961. Those who present late for vaccination should be immunised according to *Children with unknown or incomplete vaccination history*. A single dose of PPV23 or PCV20 should then be given at 2 years of age, at least 4 weeks after the last dose of PCV13.

Children who are severely immunocompromised, or those with asplenia, splenic dysfunction, or complement disorders, should receive 2 doses of PCV13 or PCV20 at least 4 weeks apart (commencing no earlier than 6 weeks of age)—infants diagnosed after 16 weeks who have already received PCV13 should receive 2 doses of PCV20 (when available) with an interval of at least 4 weeks between any doses. This is followed by a booster dose of PCV13 or PCV20 given on or after their first birthday. A single dose of PPV23 or PCV20 should then be given at 2 years of age, at least 4 weeks after the last dose of PCV.

For further information on vaccination in individuals with asplenia, splenic dysfunction, or complement disorders, see Vaccination, general principles p. 959.

Children diagnosed with at-risk conditions aged 1 year to under 2 years

Children in an at-risk group (excluding those with asplenia, splenic dysfunction, complement disorder, or who are severely immunocompromised) should receive their PCV13 booster dose according to the Immunisation schedule p. 961. Those who present late for vaccination should be immunised according to *Children with unknown or incomplete vaccination history*. A single dose of PPV23 or PCV20 should then be given at 2 years of age, at least 4 weeks after the last dose of PCV13.

Children who are severely immunocompromised, or those with asplenia, splenic dysfunction, or complement disorders, should receive the routine booster dose of PCV13 or PCV20 on or after their first birthday. If a booster dose of PCV13 has already been given at 1 year of age, a booster dose of PCV20 (when available) should be given at least 4 weeks later. A single dose of PPV23 or PCV20 should then be given at 2 years of age, at least 4 weeks after the last dose of PCV.

For further information on vaccination in individuals with asplenia, splenic dysfunction, or complement disorders, see Vaccination, general principles p. 959.

Individuals diagnosed with at-risk conditions aged 2 years and over

Individuals diagnosed or first presenting with an at-risk condition (including those with asplenia, splenic dysfunction, or complement disorder, but excluding those who are severely immunocompromised) should be given a single dose of PPV23 or PCV20, regardless of immunisation status. This should be given at least 4 weeks after any previous dose of PCV.

Individuals who are severely immunocompromised should be given a single dose of PCV13 or PCV20, regardless of immunisation status. This should be followed by a further dose of PPV23 or PCV20, at least 4 weeks after the last dose of PCV.

For further information on vaccination in individuals with asplenia, splenic dysfunction, or complement disorders, see Vaccination, general principles p. 959.

Revaccination

Revaccination is not recommended for any clinical risk groups or age groups, except for individuals in whom the antibody concentration is likely to decline rapidly (e.g. asplenia, splenic dysfunction, or chronic renal disease), where revaccination is recommended every 5 years.

Management of cases

For the management of cases, contacts, and outbreaks, see Chapter 25, Pneumococcal, in *Immunisation against infectious disease*- 'The Green Book' (see *Useful resources*).

Useful Resources

Recommendations reflect Chapter 25, Pneumococcal, in *Immunisation against infectious disease*- 'The Green Book'. UK Health Security Agency. June 2025.
www.gov.uk/government/publications/pneumococcal-the-green-book-chapter-25

Poliomyelitis vaccine

18-Jun-2025

Overview

Inactivated poliomyelitis (polio) vaccine (IPV) contains 3 strains of poliovirus (serotypes 1, 2, and 3), and is only available as part of combination preparations containing other vaccines. The live oral poliomyelitis vaccine (OPV) is no longer available in the UK—for guidance on vaccination in individuals who have received some or all of their course as OPV, see Chapter 26, Polio, in *Immunisation against infectious disease*- 'The Green Book' (see *Useful resources*).

Pre-exposure prophylaxis

The objective of the immunisation programme is to provide a minimum of 5 doses of a polio-containing vaccine at appropriate intervals for all children to provide long-term protection. The choice of vaccine for each age group is determined also by the need for protection against diphtheria, tetanus, pertussis, *Haemophilus influenzae* type b, and hepatitis B.

For additional considerations on immunisation of children with neurological conditions, see Chapter 26, Polio, in *Immunisation against infectious disease*- 'The Green Book' (see *Useful resources*).

Children with immunosuppression or HIV infection (regardless of CD4 count) should be vaccinated in accordance with the routine immunisation schedule, see *Primary immunisation* and *Boosters*. Re-immunisation after treatment completion and recovery should be considered—specialist advice may be required.

Primary immunisation

Poliomyelitis vaccination is given as a component of the routine childhood immunisation programme (see Immunisation schedule p. 961). If the child's routine immunisation is delayed, they should be immunised at the earliest opportunity.

Children aged under 10 years should be given a primary course consisting of 3 doses of the hexavalent diphtheria with tetanus, pertussis, hepatitis B, poliomyelitis and haemophilus influenzae type b vaccine p. 990 (DTaP/IPV/Hib/HepB vaccine) with intervals of 4 weeks between doses. If interrupted, the primary course should be resumed but not repeated, allowing a 4-week interval between doses. For information on circumstances where early immunisation may be considered, see UKHSA guidance: **Hexavalent DTaP/IPV/Hib/HepB combination vaccine: information for healthcare practitioners** (see *Useful resources*).

Children aged 10 years and over who are unimmunised or who received a low-potency IPV, should be given a primary course consisting of 3 doses of diphtheria, tetanus, and poliomyelitis vaccine p. 989 (Td/IPV vaccine) at 4-week intervals. If interrupted, the primary course should be resumed but not repeated, allowing an interval of 4 weeks between doses.

For further guidance, including information on vaccination of children with uncertain or incomplete vaccination status, see Chapter 26, Polio, in *Immunisation against infectious disease*- 'The Green Book' (see *Useful resources*).

Boosters

Following a primary course, 2 doses of a suitable polio-containing booster vaccine should be given at recommended intervals. For children born on or after 1 July 2024, an additional dose of the hexavalent DTaP/IPV/Hib/HepB vaccine should be given at 18 months of age to provide a booster dose of a *Haemophilus influenzae* type b (Hib)-containing vaccine in the second year of life. As this hexavalent booster dose is not sufficient to provide long-term protection against poliomyelitis when given routinely under the age of 3 years 4 months, 2 further doses of a polio-containing vaccine (termed the first and second booster) are still required before adulthood (children born before 1 July 2024 should have already received their Hib booster dose as routinely scheduled at 1 year of age).

Children aged under 10 years should receive the diphtheria, tetanus, pertussis, and poliomyelitis vaccine p. 989 (dTaP/IPV vaccine) for their first booster dose. This is usually given at 3 years 4 months of age or soon after (before school entry)—see Immunisation schedule p. 961. However, when primary immunisation has been delayed, it may be given at the scheduled visit, provided it has been at least 1 year since the last dose of hexavalent DTaP/IPV/Hib/HepB vaccine.

Children aged 10 years and over should be given the Td/IPV vaccine for their first booster dose. This should be at least 5 years after the third dose of their primary course.

All children should be given the Td/IPV vaccine for their second booster dose. This is usually given 10 years after the first booster (see Immunisation schedule p. 961), but if previous doses have been delayed, it may be given at the school session or scheduled visit provided there has been at least a 5-year interval since the first booster dose.

If a child presents for their routine booster dose but has a history of being vaccinated following a tetanus-prone wound, the vaccine preparation administered at the time of injury should be determined. If this is not possible, or the vaccine administered was not the same as the vaccine due at the current visit or was not given after an appropriate interval, the routine dose should still be given to ensure long-term protection against all antigens.

Further booster doses are only necessary for individuals at special risk, such as travellers to endemic areas (see *Travel*), or laboratory staff likely to be exposed to polio, or healthcare workers in possible contact with cases; booster doses should be given to such individuals every 10 years.

For further guidance, including information on vaccination of children with uncertain or incomplete immunisation status, see Chapter 26, Polio, in *Immunisation against infectious disease*- 'The Green Book' (see *Useful resources*).

Travel

Unimmunised travellers to areas with a high incidence of poliomyelitis should receive a full 3-dose course of a preparation containing inactivated poliomyelitis vaccine. Those who have not been vaccinated in the last 10 years should receive a booster dose of Td/IPV vaccine. Information about countries with a high incidence of poliomyelitis can be obtained from the National Travel Health Network and Centre (travelhealthpro.org.uk).

Useful Resources

Recommendations reflect Chapter 26, Polio, in *Immunisation against infectious disease*- 'The Green Book'. UK Health Security Agency. June 2025.
www.gov.uk/government/publications/polio-the-green-book-chapter-26

Hexavalent DTaP/IPV/Hib/HepB combination vaccine: information for healthcare practitioners. UK Health Security Agency. June 2025.
www.gov.uk/government/publications/hexavalent-combination-vaccine-programme-guidance

Rabies vaccine

09-Jun-2023

Overview

The rabies vaccine p. 997 contains inactivated rabies virus cultured in purified chick embryo cells.

Pre-exposure prophylaxis

Immunisation with the rabies vaccine should be offered to individuals considered to be at risk of exposure to rabies within the UK, such as recreational cavers, or those who regularly handle bats, including on a voluntary basis.

Immunisation is also recommended for individuals travelling outside the UK to rabies enzootic areas, especially if:

- post-exposure medical care and rabies biologics at the destination are lacking or in short supply;
- they are undertaking higher risk activities such as cycling, running, or recreational caving;
- they are living or staying there for more than 1 month.

Immunisation against rabies requires a primary pre-exposure course of 3 doses administered over 21 or 28 days (preferred schedule if time allows), or an accelerated course of 3 doses over 7 days with an additional dose at 1 year. For dosing schedules, see rabies vaccine.

For further information on pre-exposure prophylaxis in individuals with immunosuppression and/or HIV infection, see *Immunosuppression and HIV infection*.

Boosters

The requirement for booster doses is dependent on an individual's indication for pre-exposure prophylaxis and the likely frequency of ongoing exposures.

For individuals who may have frequent unrecognised exposures to the virus (such as bat handlers) a single booster dose of rabies vaccine should be given 1 year after the primary course has been completed. Antibody levels 1 year after the last vaccine dose will determine the requirement for a further booster dose and/or further testing.

For individuals at infrequent risk of exposure but who are likely to have an unrecognised exposure (such as recreational cavers), antibody levels 1 year after the primary course will determine the requirement for a booster dose and/or further testing.

For further information on antibody testing and booster doses, see UKHSA guidance: **Guidelines on timing of rabies boosters based on antibody levels** (see *Useful resources*).

Travel

Routine booster doses are not recommended for most individuals who are travelling. A single booster dose of rabies vaccine can be considered following a risk assessment in those who have completed a primary course over 1 year ago, and who are travelling to an enzootic area again. Only 1 booster is needed in the traveller's lifetime.

Further information on country-specific rabies travel risk is available from the National Travel Health Network and Centre (travelhealthpro.org.uk/) and, in Scotland, from Health Protection Scotland (www.hps.scot.nhs.uk).

Post-exposure management

Rabies is a notifiable disease in the UK. For further information, see *Notifiable diseases* in Antibacterials, principles of therapy p. 358.

Following potential exposure to rabies, the wound or site of exposure (e.g. mucous membrane) should be cleansed under running water and washed for several minutes with soapy water as soon as possible. Disinfectant and a simple dressing can be applied, but suturing should be delayed until post-exposure treatment has begun otherwise it may increase the risk of introducing rabies virus into the nerves. Antibacterial therapy may be required for some animal bites, see *Human and animal bites* in Skin infections, antibacterial therapy p. 373 for further guidance. For puncture wounds, tetanus risk should also be assessed, see Tetanus vaccine p. 981 for information on the management of tetanus-prone wounds.

A full, rapid post-exposure risk assessment (based on detailed information about the circumstances of the potential exposure) is required so that post-exposure treatment, if indicated, can be started promptly. When post-exposure treatment is indicated, this should always be started without delay, even in the presence of other illness. If the exposure occurred many months or years previously, a full risk assessment should always be done and treatment considered as the incubation period for rabies can be prolonged.

The regimen used for post-exposure management depends on the composite rabies risk (assessed as a green, amber, or red rating using a combination of the country where the incident occurred and the type of animal involved, and the category of exposure), and the individual's past medical history (including immune status). For further information on risk assessment (including composite rabies risk) and the management of potential rabies exposure, see UKHSA guidance: **Guidelines on managing rabies post-exposure** (see *Useful resources*).

For individuals arriving in the UK who started post-exposure treatment via the intradermal route, the remaining doses should be given intramuscularly. If the regimen started was different to the UK regimen—seek specialist advice.

For post-exposure management in individuals with immunosuppression, see *Immunosuppression and HIV infection*; and for country-specific specialist contact details in England, Wales, Scotland and Northern Ireland, see Chapter 27: Rabies, in *Immunisation against infectious disease*- 'The Green Book'.

Post-exposure treatment of individuals who are fully immunised

Fully immunised individuals are those who have received at least 3 documented doses of rabies vaccine (on at least 2 separate days either as a primary pre-exposure prophylaxis course or as part of a previous post-exposure treatment course), or documented rabies virus neutralising antibody (VNA) titres of at least 0.5 IU/ml.

For *fully immunised* individuals with a *green* composite rabies risk or who have completed a rabies post-exposure treatment course in the last 3 months, no treatment is required.

For *fully immunised* individuals with an *amber* or *red* composite rabies risk, give 2 doses of rabies vaccine (first dose on day 0 and second dose between days 3–7). Rabies immunoglobulin is not needed for these individuals. If rabies immunoglobulin is inadvertently given, individuals will need to complete a 4 dose course of rabies vaccine (on days 0, 3, 7 and 21).

Post-exposure treatment of individuals who are partially immunised

Partially immunised individuals are those who have had an incomplete/inadequate primary pre-exposure prophylaxis course or documented rabies virus neutralising antibody titres consistently less than 0.5 IU/mL.

For *partially immunised* individuals with a *green* composite rabies risk, no treatment is required.

For *partially immunised* individuals with an *amber* or *red* composite rabies risk, give 4 doses in total of rabies vaccine (on days 0, 3, 7 and 21). If the fourth dose of rabies vaccine is given before day 21, a fifth dose of vaccine should be administered 2 weeks after the fourth dose. Rabies immunoglobulin is not needed for these individuals.

Post-exposure treatment of individuals who are non-immunised

Non-immunised individuals are those who have never received rabies pre- or post-exposure immunisation.

For *non-immunised* individuals with a *green* composite rabies risk, no treatment is required.

For *non-immunised* individuals with an *amber* or *red* composite rabies risk, give 4 doses in total of rabies vaccine p. 997 (on days 0, 3, 7 and 21). If the fourth dose of rabies vaccine is given before day 21, a fifth dose of vaccine should be administered 2 weeks after the fourth dose.

Individuals with a *red* composite rabies risk should also be given rabies immunoglobulin p. 957. This is not required if more than 7 days has passed since the first dose of rabies vaccine or more than 1 day since the second dose, or if the exposure was more than 12 months ago.

Immunosuppression and HIV infection

Refer to the Children's HIV Association for further information on the use of *rabies vaccine* and *rabies immunoglobulin* in children with HIV infection. See www.chiva.org.uk/ for further information.

Pre-exposure prophylaxis

Pre-exposure prophylaxis may be given to individuals with immunosuppression and/or HIV infection (regardless of CD4 count), but these individuals may not develop a full antibody response.

Individuals who are immunosuppressed or who become immunosuppressed at any point after receiving a primary course of immunisation, or after having an antibody test or booster, should be informed about the serious risks of continuing with activities that could potentially expose them to rabies as it is possible that they may not respond to post-exposure vaccine.

If vaccination is still required, antibody levels may be required 2 weeks after the last dose of vaccine to ensure an adequate immune response. For further information, see UKHSA guidance: **Guidelines on timing of rabies boosters based on antibody levels** (see *Useful resources*).

Re-immunisation should be considered upon completion of treatment and recovery has occurred, or in those with HIV when there has been immune recovery following commencement of antiretroviral treatment (such as a CD4 count >200 per mm^3).

Post-exposure management

For *immunosuppressed* individuals with a *green* composite rabies risk, no treatment is required.

For *immunosuppressed* individuals with an *amber* or *red* composite rabies risk, give 5 doses of rabies vaccine (on days 0, 3, 7, 14, and 30) and rabies immunoglobulin—specialist advice should be sought if the individual has commenced post-exposure vaccination without rabies immunoglobulin, or if the exposure was more than 12 months ago. Post-exposure treatment response should be confirmed using antibody testing at the same time as the fifth dose (day 30); further antibody tests may be required depending on the results.

Useful Resources

Recommendations reflect Chapter 27, Rabies, in *Immunisation against infectious disease*- 'The Green Book'. Public Health England, May 2023.
www.gov.uk/government/publications/rabies-the-green-book-chapter-27

Guidelines on managing rabies post-exposure. UK Health Security Agency, January 2023.
www.gov.uk/government/publications/rabies-post-exposure-prophylaxis-management-guidelines

Guidelines on timing of rabies boosters based on antibody levels. UK Health Security Agency, June 2022.
www.gov.uk/government/publications/rabies-post-exposure-treatment-timing-of-vaccine-booster

Respiratory syncytial virus immunisation

27-Feb-2026

Overview

Respiratory syncytial virus (RSV) is a common cause of respiratory tract infections in children. RSV infection can occur at any age and usually causes a mild, self-limiting infection, however infants under 1 year of age are at greatest risk of hospitalisation with more severe disease. Infection occurs year-round, but primarily between October to February, and the predominance of each subtype of RSV (A or B) changes over successive seasons.

The national RSV immunisation programme aims to reduce the incidence and severity of RSV disease in children most at risk, through maternal vaccination, and passive immunisation of very and extremely preterm infants, and high-risk infants and young children.

Maternal vaccination

All pregnant females should be offered the respiratory syncytial virus vaccine p. 998 in each pregnancy, regardless of the interval between pregnancies, to confer passive immunity against RSV to their infants. *Abrysvo*®, a bivalent, non-live recombinant vaccine containing antigens from RSV subtypes A and B, is recommended for the national maternal RSV vaccination programme.

A single dose of RSV vaccine should be given in week 28 of pregnancy, or soon after, to ensure sufficient time for high levels of maternal RSV antibodies to be produced and transferred across the placenta; this also increases the potential for infants born prematurely to benefit.

If vaccination does not occur during or soon after week 28 of pregnancy, the vaccine should still be offered up until delivery as there is evidence that transplacental antibody transfer can occur within 2 weeks of vaccination. Vaccination after week 36 of pregnancy [unlicensed use] may not confer as high a level of passive protection to the infant; however, late vaccination, including soon after delivery, may offer indirect protection by preventing maternal RSV infection and providing antibodies to the infant via breast-milk. For further information, including co-administration with other vaccines and vaccination outside of the recommended time frame, see Chapter 27a, Respiratory syncytial virus, in *Immunisation against infectious disease*- 'The Green Book' and UKHSA guidance: **Respiratory syncytial virus (RSV) programme: information for healthcare professionals** (see *Useful resources*).

Immunisation of very and extremely preterm infants

Infants born before 32 weeks gestation may have limited, if any, protection from maternal RSV vaccination. To reduce the risk of severe disease in these infants, nirsevimab p. 985 should be given immediately before or during their first RSV season.

A single dose of nirsevimab (which provides protection for at least 5 to 6 months) should be given. For infants being discharged from hospital for the first time between mid-September and the end of February, immunisation with nirsevimab should be given during their inpatient stay. Infants being discharged from hospital for the first time outside of this period should be invited for outpatient immunisation from mid-September to mid-October.

Immunisation of high-risk infants and young children

To reduce the risk of severe disease in eligible high-risk infants and young children, seasonal administration of an RSV monoclonal antibody is recommended for passive immunity, regardless of maternal vaccination. Most of these infants will already be eligible under the immunisation programme for very and extremely preterm infants (see above).

Immunisation is recommended for infants with chronic lung disease of prematurity (also known as bronchopulmonary dysplasia), infants with certain respiratory diseases who remain on oxygen or are receiving long-term ventilation at the start of the RSV season, infants with congenital heart disease, and children aged under 2 years with severe combined immunodeficiency syndrome (SCID).

A single dose of nirsevimab (which provides protection for at least 5 to 6 months) should be given. For infants being discharged from hospital for the first time between mid-September and the end of February, immunisation with nirsevimab should be given during their inpatient stay. Infants being discharged from hospital for the first time outside of this period should be invited for outpatient immunisation from mid-September to mid-October. If an infant or child is newly identified as being high-risk during the RSV season, a single dose of nirsevimab should be given up until the end of February. Certain infants, and some children aged under 2 years with SCID may be offered immunisation beyond their first RSV season.

If nirsevimab is not available, palivizumab p. 986 can be used as an alternative (for infants born after 32 weeks gestation) and should be started around calendar week 40 (the beginning of October).

For detailed eligibility criteria, including preterm infant age groups, see Chapter 27a, Respiratory syncytial virus, in *Immunisation against infectious disease*- 'The Green Book' (see *Useful resources*).

If other infants outside of these criteria are identified as being at high-risk of severe RSV infection during the RSV season, nirsevimab, or palivizumab if nirsevimab is not available, may be considered according to clinical judgement.

Useful Resources

Recommendations reflect Chapter 27a, Respiratory syncytial virus, in *Immunisation against infectious disease*- 'The Green Book'. UK Health Security Agency. February 2026.
www.gov.uk/government/publications/respiratory-syncytial-virus-the-green-book-chapter-27a

Respiratory syncytial virus (RSV) programme: information for healthcare professionals. UK Health Security Agency. March 2026.
www.gov.uk/government/publications/respiratory-syncytial-virus-rsv-programme-information-for-healthcare-professionals

Rotavirus vaccine

11-Jan-2022

Overview

Rotavirus vaccine p. 1003 is a live, oral vaccine that protects young children against gastro-enteritis caused by rotavirus infection.

Prior to vaccination with the rotavirus vaccine, the result of the severe combined immunodeficiency (SCID) screening should be checked. For further information, see PHE guidance: **The rotavirus vaccination programme: information for healthcare professionals** (see *Useful resources*).

The recommended schedule consists of 2 doses, the first at 8 weeks of age, and the second at 12 weeks of age (see Immunisation schedule p. 961). The first dose of rotavirus vaccine must be given between 6 weeks and under 15 weeks of age and the second dose should be given after an interval of at least 4 weeks; the vaccine should not be started in children 15 weeks of age or older. Ideally, the full course should be completed before 16 weeks of age to provide protection before the main burden of disease, and to avoid a temporal association between vaccination and intussusception; the course must be completed before 24 weeks of age.

Children who inadvertently receive the first dose of rotavirus vaccine at 15 weeks of age or older should still receive a second dose after at least 4 weeks, providing that they will still be under 24 weeks of age at the time.

The rotavirus vaccine virus is excreted in the stool and may be transmitted to close contacts; however, vaccination of children with *immunosuppressed* close contacts may protect the contacts from wild-type rotavirus disease and outweigh any risk from transmission of vaccine virus. Carers of a recently vaccinated child should be advised of the need to wash their hands after changing the child's nappies.

Useful Resources

Recommendations reflect Chapter 27b, Rotavirus, in *Immunisation against infectious disease*– 'The Green book'. UK Health Security Agency, August 2015.
www.gov.uk/government/publications/rotavirus-the-green-book-chapter-27b

The rotavirus vaccination programme: information for healthcare professionals. Public Health England, September 2021.
www.gov.uk/government/publications/rotavirus-qas-for-healthcare-practitioners

Smallpox and mpox vaccine

06-Feb-2023

Overview

The smallpox and mpox (monkeypox) viruses belong to the genus *orthopoxvirus*, which also includes the vaccinia virus. The smallpox and mpox vaccine (*Imvanex*®, also known as MVA-BN) is prepared from the live vaccinia virus which has been modified so that it has very limited replication capability, and should be considered as an inactivated vaccine. When supplies of the vaccine are limited, its use should be prioritised according to whether it is for pre- or post-exposure use, the risk and timing of exposure, and the ability to benefit.

Medical practitioners must notify the proper officer at their local council or local health protection team of all suspected cases of smallpox or mpox. For further information, see *Notifiable diseases* in Antibacterials, principles of therapy p. 358.

For further guidance on smallpox and mpox, see Chapter 29: Smallpox and monkeypox, in *Immunisation against infectious disease*- 'The Green Book' (see *Useful resources*) and the UKHSA collection: **Mpox (monkeypox): guidance** (available at: www.gov.uk/government/collections/monkeypox-guidance).

Pre-exposure prophylaxis

Routine immunisation against smallpox and mpox is not indicated, however staff who work in specialist roles where exposure to mpox or other orthopoxviruses is likely to be more common may be offered vaccination following a risk assessment.

During outbreaks or incidents of mpox, pre-exposure vaccination may be extended to other groups of staff, and to individuals at increased risk of exposure.

Pre-exposure vaccination regime

The primary course for individuals not previously vaccinated against smallpox or mpox consists of an initial dose of the smallpox and mpox vaccine, followed by a second dose after at least 28 days. For individuals who have previously received a single dose of the vaccine, completion of the primary course is recommended; there is no need to restart the course. Individuals who have previously been vaccinated against smallpox with a live smallpox vaccine only require a single dose of the smallpox and mpox vaccine. For information on vaccination in individuals with immunosuppression, see *Immunosuppression and HIV*.

For further guidance on pre-exposure prophylaxis, see Chapter 29: Smallpox and monkeypox, in *Immunisation against infectious disease*- 'The Green Book' and UKHSA: **Recommendations for the use of pre- and post-exposure vaccination during a monkeypox incident** (see *Useful resources*).

Post-exposure management

Post-exposure immunisation may provide protection against mpox infection, and modify disease severity in individuals with recent exposure. Individuals should be risk assessed and if appropriate, vaccination should be given within 4 days of exposure. Vaccination may be offered up to 14 days following exposure in individuals at ongoing risk of exposure or in those who are at higher risk of severe disease.

Post-exposure vaccination regime

A single dose of the smallpox and mpox vaccine should be given. For individuals who are at risk of future exposure and who have not received pre-exposure immunisation previously, a second dose should be given after at least 28 days.

For individuals who have previously received a single dose of the smallpox and mpox vaccine, completion of the primary course is recommended; there is no need to restart the course. Individuals who have previously received a

2-dose course of the vaccine, with the second dose given in the past 2 years, do not need a further dose following exposure. However, for those who are immunosuppressed and who may have had a reduced immune response, an additional dose can be considered—seek specialist advice.

For individuals with a history of receiving a single dose of a live smallpox vaccine, a single dose of the smallpox and mpox vaccine is recommended following exposure.

For individuals who have received a previous live smallpox vaccine and 1 dose of the smallpox and mpox vaccine, no further doses are recommended after exposure.

For further guidance on post-exposure vaccination, see Chapter 29: Smallpox and monkeypox, in *Immunisation against infectious disease*- 'The Green Book' and UKHSA: **Recommendations for the use of pre- and post-exposure vaccination during a monkeypox incident** (see *Useful resources*).

Antiviral treatment

Tecovirimat should be offered to patients who are hospitalised due to mpox if they meet the eligibility criteria. For further guidance, see NHS England Clinical Commissioning Rapid Policy Statement: **Tecovirimat as treatment for patients hospitalised due to monkeypox virus infection** (available at: www.england.nhs.uk/commissioning/publication/tecovirimat-as-treatment-for-patients-hospitalised-due-to-monkeypox-virus-infection/).

Booster doses

Individuals who have received a primary course of the smallpox and mpox vaccine should be offered a single booster dose 2 years after the primary course if they are considered to be at on-going risk of exposure. If the primary course included a live smallpox vaccine, seek specialist advice regarding the need for a booster dose.

Immunosuppression and HIV

The smallpox and mpox vaccine contains a replication defective virus and is considered safe to use in individuals who are immunosuppressed or living with HIV infection. The recommendations above for pre-exposure prophylaxis or post-exposure immunisation therefore apply to individuals with immunosuppression or HIV. The immune response to the vaccine could be reduced in severely immunosuppressed individuals; specialist advice on other measures may be required and additional doses should be considered for those at ongoing-risk of exposure. Refer to the British HIV Association for further information on the use of smallpox and mpox vaccine in HIV-positive individuals (available at: www.bhiva.org/rapid-guidance-on-monkeypox-virus).

Useful Resources

Recommendations reflect Chapter 29, Smallpox and monkeypox, in *Immunisation against infectious disease*- 'The Green Book'. UK Health Security Agency. September 2022.
www.gov.uk/government/publications/smallpox-and-vaccinia-the-green-book-chapter-29

Recommendations for the use of pre- and post-exposure vaccination during a monkeypox incident. UK Health Security Agency. August 2022.
www.gov.uk/government/publications/monkeypox-vaccination

Tetanus vaccine

18-Jun-2025

Overview

Tetanus-containing vaccines are inactivated and are made from a cell-free purified toxin of *Clostridium tetani* adsorbed on aluminium hydroxide or aluminium phosphate to improve immunogenicity. The tetanus vaccine is only available as part of combination preparations containing other vaccines.

Pre-exposure prophylaxis

The objective of the immunisation programme is to provide a minimum of 5 doses of a tetanus-containing vaccine at appropriate intervals for all individuals. The choice of vaccine for each age group is determined also by the need for protection against diphtheria, pertussis, *Haemophilus influenzae* type b, hepatitis B, and poliomyelitis.

Parenteral drug misusers are at a greater risk of tetanus infection—every opportunity should be taken to ensure that they are fully vaccinated against tetanus.

For additional considerations on immunisation of children with neurological conditions, see Chapter 30, Tetanus, in *Immunisation against infectious disease*- 'The Green Book' (see *Useful resources*).

For information on immunisation in pregnant females, see *Pregnancy*.

Children with immunosuppression or HIV infection (regardless of CD4 count) should be vaccinated in accordance with the routine immunisation schedule, see *Primary immunisation* and *Boosters*. Re-immunisation after treatment completion and recovery should be considered—specialist advice may be required.

Primary immunisation

Tetanus vaccination is given as a component of the routine childhood immunisation programme (see Immunisation schedule p. 961). If the child's routine immunisation is delayed, they should be immunised at the earliest opportunity.

Children aged under 10 years, should be given a primary course consisting of 3 doses of the hexavalent diphtheria with tetanus, pertussis, hepatitis B, poliomyelitis and haemophilus influenzae type b vaccine p. 990 (DTaP/IPV/Hib/HepB vaccine) at intervals of 4 weeks—it is the only suitable vaccine containing high-dose tetanus for priming children of this age. If interrupted, the primary course should be resumed but not repeated, allowing a 4-week interval between doses. For information on circumstances where early immunisation may be considered, see UKHSA guidance: **Hexavalent DTaP/IPV/Hib/HepB combination vaccine: information for healthcare practitioners** (see *Useful resources*).

Children aged 10 years and over who are unimmunised, or have an uncertain or incomplete immunisation history, should be given a primary course consisting of 3 doses of the diphtheria, tetanus, and poliomyelitis vaccine p. 989 (Td/IPV vaccine) at 4-week intervals. If interrupted, the primary course should be resumed but not repeated, allowing an interval of 4 weeks between doses.

For further information, see Chapter 30, Tetanus, in *Immunisation against infectious disease*- 'The Green Book' (see *Useful resources*).

Boosters

Following a primary course, 2 doses of a tetanus-containing booster vaccine should be given. For children born on or after 1 July 2024, an additional dose of the hexavalent DTaP/IPV/Hib/HepB vaccine should be given at 18 months of age to provide a booster dose of a *Haemophilus influenzae* type b (Hib)-containing vaccine in the second year of life. As this hexavalent booster dose is not sufficient to provide long-term protection against tetanus when given routinely under the age of 3 years 4 months, 2 further doses of a tetanus-containing vaccine (termed the first and second booster) are still required before adulthood (children born before 1 July 2024 should have already received their Hib booster dose as routinely scheduled at 1 year of age).

Children aged under 10 years should be given the diphtheria, tetanus, pertussis, and poliomyelitis vaccine p. 989 (dTaP/IPV vaccine) for their first booster dose. This is usually given at 3 years 4 months of age or soon after (before school entry)—see Immunisation schedule p. 961. However, when primary immunisation has been delayed, it may be given at the scheduled visit provided it has been at least 1 year since the last dose of hexavalent DTaP/IPV/Hib/HepB vaccine.

Children aged 10 years and over should be given the diphtheria, tetanus, and poliomyelitis vaccine (Td/IPV vaccine) for their first booster dose. This should be at least 5 years after the third dose of their primary course.

All children should be given the Td/IPV vaccine for their second booster dose. This is usually given 10 years after the first booster, but if previous doses have been delayed, it may be given at the school session or scheduled visit provided there has been at least a 5-year interval since the first booster dose.

If a child presents for their routine booster dose but has a history of being vaccinated following a tetanus-prone wound, the vaccine preparation administered at the time of injury should be determined. If this is not possible, or the vaccine administered was not the same as the vaccine due at the current visit or was not given after an appropriate interval, the routine dose should still be given to ensure long-term protection against all antigens.

Parenteral drug misusers should be given booster doses if there is any doubt about their immunisation status.

For further guidance, including information on vaccination of children with unknown or incomplete immunisation status, see Chapter 30, Tetanus, in *Immunisation against infectious disease*- 'The Green Book' (see *Useful resources*).

Travel

All travellers should ensure they are fully immunised (or are up-to-date) with their tetanus vaccination (see *Primary immunisation* and *Boosters*). Travellers who last received a tetanus booster dose more than 10 years ago and are travelling to areas where medical attention may not be accessible, should be given a booster dose of tetanus-containing vaccine prior to travel, even if they have previously received 5 doses of tetanus-containing vaccines. This is a precautionary measure in case immunoglobulin is not available to the individual in the event of a tetanus-prone injury.

Post-exposure management

Cases

Tetanus is a notifiable disease in the UK. For further information, see *Notifiable diseases* in Antibacterials, principles of therapy p. 358.

Intravenous normal immunoglobulin [unlicensed] is used for the treatment of tetanus (for further information, see Immunoglobulins p. 951). Antibacterials (such as benzylpenicillin sodium p. 415 and metronidazole p. 409) may also be required—discuss with the microbiology team. Tetanus infection may not result in immunity and vaccination is recommended following recovery (see *Pre-exposure prophylaxis*). For further guidance on the management of confirmed and suspected cases of tetanus (including localised tetanus), see Chapter 30, Tetanus, in *Immunisation against infectious disease*- 'The Green Book', and UKHSA: **Guidance on the management of suspected tetanus cases and the assessment and management of tetanus-prone wounds** (see *Useful resources*).

Prophylaxis of tetanus-prone wounds

Any wound can give rise to tetanus. *Clean wounds* (less than 6 hours old, non-penetrating and have negligible tissue damage) are considered to have a low likelihood of harbouring tetanus spores and of developing conditions that promote spore germination. *Tetanus-prone* wounds include compound fractures, certain animal bites and scratches, puncture-type injuries acquired in a contaminated environment (these are likely to contain tetanus spores), wounds or burns with systemic sepsis, and wounds containing foreign bodies—this list is not exhaustive. *High-risk tetanus-prone* wounds include any *tetanus-prone* wounds or burns that either show extensive devitalised tissue or require surgical intervention that is delayed more than 6 hours, or wounds that are heavily contaminated with material likely to contain tetanus spores (such as soil or manure).

Post-exposure management of tetanus-prone wounds depends on the child's immunisation status and wound category (*clean*, *tetanus-prone*, or *high-risk tetanus-prone*). For the risk assessment of tetanus-prone wounds, an *adequate priming course* of tetanus vaccine is considered to be at least 3 doses of tetanus-containing vaccine at appropriate intervals.

All wounds should be thoroughly cleaned, and surgical debridement of devitalised tissue in *high-risk tetanus-prone* wounds is essential for the prevention of tetanus infection.

For children aged 11 years and over who have received an adequate priming course of tetanus vaccine with the last dose given within 10 years, for children aged 5–10 years whose tetanus immunisation is up to date, and for children aged under 5 years who have received an adequate priming course, no immediate treatment is required regardless of wound category.

For children who have received an adequate priming course of tetanus vaccine but the last dose was given more than 10 years ago, and for children aged 5–10 years who have received an adequate priming course but no booster, give an immediate booster dose of a suitable tetanus-containing vaccine to children with a wound that is *tetanus-prone* or *high-risk tetanus-prone*. In addition, for a *high-risk tetanus-prone* wound, give a single dose of tetanus immunoglobulin p. 957 at a different site (or if unavailable, normal immunoglobulin [unlicensed] may be used).

For children who have not received an adequate priming course of tetanus vaccine (includes those with uncertain immunisation status), give an immediate booster dose of a suitable tetanus-containing vaccine regardless of wound category. In addition, for a *tetanus-prone* or *high-risk tetanus-prone* wound, give a single dose of tetanus immunoglobulin at a different site (or if unavailable, normal immunoglobulin [unlicensed] may be used).

Children who are severely immunosuppressed may not be adequately protected against tetanus, despite being fully immunised. An additional booster dose of a tetanus-containing vaccine and/or immunoglobulin may be required.

To ensure immunity against future exposure, all children who are not completely immunised should be given further doses of tetanus-containing vaccine as required to complete their recommended schedule (see *Pre-exposure prophylaxis*).

Antibacterial therapy may also be considered for tetanus-prone wounds depending on clinical severity, to prevent tetanus.

For further guidance on the management of tetanus-prone wounds, see Chapter 30, Tetanus, in *Immunisation against infectious disease*- 'The Green Book', and UKHSA: **Guidance on the management of suspected tetanus cases and the assessment and management of tetanus-prone wounds** (see *Useful resources*).

Pregnancy

Routine vaccination of pregnant females with diphtheria, tetanus, and pertussis vaccine p. 988 (Tdap vaccine) is recommended between 16 to 32 weeks of each pregnancy as part of the maternal pertussis programme, usually around the time of the fetal anomaly scan (20 weeks) for operational reasons. For further information, and for guidance for pregnant females with an uncertain or incomplete vaccination history against diphtheria, tetanus, and poliomyelitis, see UKHSA guidance: **Pertussis (whooping cough) vaccination programme for pregnant women: information for healthcare practitioners** (available at: www.gov.uk/government/publications/vaccination-against-pertussis-whooping-cough-for-pregnant-women).

Pregnant females may be given tetanus-containing vaccines where protection is needed without delay. For information on the management of cases and prophylaxis of tetanus-prone wounds, see *Post-exposure management*.

Useful Resources

Recommendations reflect Chapter 30, Tetanus, in *Immunisation against infectious disease*- 'The Green Book'. UK Health Security Agency. June 2025.
www.gov.uk/government/publications/tetanus-the-green-book-chapter-30

Guidance on the management of suspected tetanus cases and the assessment and management of tetanus-prone wounds. UK Health Security Agency. March 2024.
www.gov.uk/government/publications/tetanus-advice-for-health-professionals

Hexavalent DTaP/IPV/Hib/HepB combination vaccine: information for healthcare practitioners. UK Health Security Agency. June 2025.
www.gov.uk/government/publications/hexavalent-combination-vaccine-programme-guidance

Tick-borne encephalitis vaccine

04-Nov-2025

Overview

The tick-borne encephalitis (TBE) vaccine contains inactivated TBE virus (Neudörfl strain) grown in chick embryo cells. It is recommended for the protection of children at high risk of exposure to the TBE virus through work or travel.

Immunisation with tick-borne encephalitis vaccine p. 999 is therefore recommended for:

- children who travel, particularly in spring and summer, to endemic forested areas where ticks are most prevalent (including those who hike, camp, hunt, and undertake fieldwork);
- children who will be residing in an area where TBE is endemic or epidemic, especially those working in forestry, woodcutting, farming, and the military;
- laboratory workers who may be exposed to the TBE virus.

A 3 dose schedule of the tick-borne encephalitis vaccine is recommended for children aged 1 year and over. Sufficient protection can be expected for the ongoing tick season after the first 2 doses, and for at least 3 years after the 3rd dose. Booster doses are required every 3–5 years for those still at risk of TBE exposure. For dosing schedules, see tick-borne encephalitis vaccine.

Refer to the Children HIV Association for information on the use of tick-borne encephalitis vaccine in children with HIV infection. See www.chiva.org.uk/professionals/clinical-guidelines/ for further information.

Further information on preventing or reducing the risk of TBE is available from the National Travel Health Network and Centre (travelhealthpro.org.uk/).

Post-exposure prophylaxis

Unvaccinated children bitten by ticks in endemic areas should seek local medical advice. No specific therapy is available following exposure to tick-borne encephalitis; supportive treatment can significantly reduce morbidity and mortality. If tick-borne encephalitis is suspected, the referring clinician should discuss the case with a clinician at the UKHSA Rare and Imported Pathogens Laboratory (contact details are available at: www.gov.uk/guidance/tick-borne-encephalitis-epidemiology-diagnosis-and-prevention).

Acute encephalitis of any cause is a notifiable disease in the UK. For further information, see *Notifiable diseases* in Antibacterials, principles of therapy p. 358.

Useful Resources

Recommendations reflect Chapter 31, Tick-borne encephalitis, in *Immunisation against infectious disease*- 'The Green Book'. UK Health Security Agency, April 2013.
www.gov.uk/government/publications/tick-borne-encephalitis-the-green-book-chapter-31

Typhoid vaccine

20-Aug-2023

Overview

Typhoid vaccines are available as Vi capsular polysaccharide (from *Salmonella typhi*) vaccine for injection and as live, attenuated *Salmonella typhi* vaccine for oral use.

Typhoid immunisation is advised for children travelling to:

- areas where typhoid is endemic and whose planned activities put them at higher risk (country-by-country information is available from the National Travel Health Network and Centre);
- endemic areas where frequent or prolonged exposure to poor sanitation and poor food hygiene is likely.

Capsular polysaccharide typhoid vaccine (inactivated) p. 999 is given as a single dose, usually by intramuscular injection. Children under 2 years [unlicensed] may respond suboptimally to the vaccine, but children aged between 1–2 years should be immunised if the risk of typhoid fever is considered high (immunisation is not recommended for infants under 12 months). A single booster dose should be given at 3-year intervals in children over 2 years of age who remain at risk from typhoid fever.

Oral typhoid vaccine (live) p. 1003 is a live, attenuated vaccine contained in an enteric-coated capsule recommended in children aged 5 years and over. One capsule taken on alternate days for a total of 3 doses provides protection 7–10 days after the last dose. If travelling from a non-endemic area to an area where typhoid is endemic, a booster consisting of 3 doses is recommended every 3 years. The oral typhoid vaccine should be avoided in immunosuppressed and HIV-infected children.

Prevention of typhoid primarily depends on improving sanitation and water supplies in endemic areas and on scrupulous personal, food and water hygiene.

All suspected cases of typhoid fever must be notified to the local health protection unit. Where there is a community level outbreak, specialist advice should be sought from Public Health England (tel. 020 8200 4400) or, in Scotland, Health Protection Scotland (tel. 0140 300 1191).

Useful Resources

Recommendations reflect Chapter 33, Typhoid, in *Immunisation against infectious disease*–'The Green Book'. Public Health England, May 2019.
www.gov.uk/government/publications/typhoid-the-green-book-chapter-33

National Travel Health Network and Centre
nathnac.net

Varicella-zoster vaccines

13-Oct-2025

Overview

The vaccine preparations *Varilrix*® and *Varivax*® contain live, attenuated virus derived from the Oka strain of varicella-zoster virus, and provide protection against varicella (chickenpox).

Pre-exposure prophylaxis against varicella (chickenpox)

Varicella immunisation aims to protect children who are at most risk of serious illness from exposure to the varicella-zoster virus, by vaccinating specific individuals who are in regular or close contact with those at risk. Children with a definite history of chickenpox or shingles can be considered immune. However, for children born and raised overseas, a history of chickenpox is a less reliable predictor of immunity and routine testing should be considered.

Vaccination with the chickenpox varicella-zoster vaccine p. 1004 (*Varilrix*® or *Varivax*®) is recommended for:

- non-immune healthcare workers who have patient contact (including cleaners, catering staff, and receptionists);
- non-immune laboratory staff who may be exposed to varicella-zoster virus in the course of their work in virology laboratories and clinical infectious disease units;
- non-immune healthy susceptible contacts (aged 9 months and over) of immunosuppressed patients where continuing close contact is unavoidable (e.g. siblings of a leukaemic child or a child whose parent is undergoing chemotherapy).

Children aged 9–11 months should receive 2 doses of the chickenpox varicella-zoster vaccine at least 3 months apart, while those aged 1–12 years should receive 2 doses at least 4 weeks apart. Children aged 13 years and over should receive 2 doses at least 6 weeks apart.

Vaccination should be postponed in acutely unwell children until they have fully recovered, unless protection is urgently required.

A single dose of either *Varilrix*® or *Varivax*® vaccine can be given to complete the course if children have already received a single dose of varicella-zoster vaccine.

Within 1 month of vaccination, some children may develop a localised rash at the injection site or a generalised rash (papular or vesicular). Healthcare workers who develop a post-vaccine rash should consult their occupational health department for assessment before commencing work. The vaccine virus strain can also establish latent infection and reactivate to cause shingles in some individuals (the risk is substantially lower than with wild chickenpox infection)—cases of shingles should be investigated. For further information on vaccine-related cutaneous rashes, see *Cautions, further information* in varicella-zoster vaccine, and Chapter 34, Varicella, in *Immunisation against infectious disease*- 'The Green Book' (see *Useful resources*).

The chickenpox vaccines are not recommended for children with immunosuppression—seek specialist advice for those who require protection against chickenpox. Refer to the Children's HIV Association for guidance in children with HIV infection (available at: www.chiva.org.uk/professionals/clinical-guidelines/).

Post-exposure management of varicella (chickenpox)

Chickenpox is a notifiable disease in England and Northern Ireland. For further information, see *Notifiable diseases* in Antibacterials, principles of therapy p. 358.

For guidance on post-exposure prophylaxis with an antiviral [unlicensed use] and/or varicella-zoster immunoglobulin [unlicensed] or normal immunoglobulin [unlicensed use] for certain individuals who are at an increased risk of severe chickenpox, see *Post-exposure prophylaxis* in Herpesvirus infections p. 498.

During outbreaks where chickenpox is co-circulating with group A streptococcus infections (such as scarlet fever) in nurseries and pre-school settings, non-immune children aged 9 months and over and staff working in these settings can be offered 2 doses of the chickenpox varicella-zoster vaccine at least 4–8 weeks apart. The UKHSA health protection team should be contacted for advice. For further information, see UKHSA guidance: **Guidelines for the public health management of scarlet fever outbreaks in schools, nurseries and other childcare settings** (available at: www.gov.uk/government/publications/scarlet-fever-managing-outbreaks-in-schools-and-nurseries).

Pregnancy

Although there are no specific safety concerns for pregnant females or their babies if varicella-zoster vaccines are administered, the live *Varilrix*® and *Varivax*® vaccines are not recommended during pregnancy. Inadvertent exposure to these vaccines from 3 months before conception to any time during pregnancy, should be reported to the UKHSA Vaccine in Pregnancy (VIP) surveillance programme. Pregnant females should be advised to seek prompt medical advice if they develop a vesicular rash following inadvertent vaccination. For advice on the reporting, risk assessment, and management of inadvertent vaccination in pregnancy, see UKHSA guidance: **Inadvertent vaccination in pregnancy (VIP)** (available at: www.gov.uk/guidance/vaccination-in-pregnancy-vip).

Useful Resources

Recommendations reflect Chapter 34, Varicella, in *Immunisation against infectious disease*- 'The Green Book'. UK Health Security Agency, September 2024.
www.gov.uk/government/publications/varicella-the-green-book-chapter-34

Yellow fever vaccine

04-Nov-2025

MHRA/CHM advice: stronger precautions in people with weakened immunity

The MHRA and CHM have released important safety information regarding the use of the live yellow fever vaccine in those with weakened immunity. For further information, see *Important safety information* for yellow fever vaccine p. 1004.

Overview

Yellow fever vaccine is an attenuated preparation of yellow fever virus grown in chick eggs. Yellow fever vaccine is recommended for:

- children aged 9 months or older who are travelling to, or living in areas or countries with a risk of yellow fever transmission;
- children aged 9 months or older who are travelling to, or living in countries that require an International Certificate of Vaccination or Prophylaxis (ICVP) for entry (information about countries at risk of yellow fever is available from the National Health Network and Centre).

Children aged under 9 months are at higher risk of vaccine-associated encephalitis, with the risk being inversely proportional to age. Children aged under 6 months should **not** be vaccinated. Children aged 6–9 months should only be vaccinated following a detailed risk assessment, and vaccination is generally only recommended if the risk of yellow fever transmission is high (such as during epidemics/outbreaks). If travel is unavoidable, seek expert advice on whether to vaccinate.

Yellow fever vaccine should be avoided in children with primary or acquired immunodeficiency due to a congenital condition or disease process, and in children who are immunosuppressed as a result of treatment.

If the yellow fever risk is unavoidable in HIV-infected children, consult the Children's HIV Association of UK and Ireland (www.chiva.org.uk/professionals/clinical-guidelines/) or other specialist advice.

For additional guidance on the suitability of immunisation against yellow fever, the National Travel Health Network and Centre and Public Health Scotland have produced a yellow fever pre-vaccination checklist (see *Useful resources*).

A single-dose of yellow fever vaccine confers life-long immunity against yellow fever disease. Immunisation should be performed at least 10 days before travelling to an endemic area to allow protective immunity to develop and for the ICVP (if required) to become valid.

Reinforcing immunisation is not needed, except for a small subset of children at continued risk who may not have developed long-term protection from their initial yellow fever vaccine vaccination–seek expert advice.

Yellow fever is a notifiable disease in the UK. For further information, see *Notifiable diseases* in Antibacterials, principles of therapy p. 358.

Useful Resources

Recommendations reflect Chapter 35, Yellow fever, in *Immunisation against infectious disease*- 'The Green Book'. UK Health Security Agency, January 2020.
www.gov.uk/government/publications/yellow-fever-the-green-book-chapter-35

National Travel Health Network and Centre Yellow Fever Zone.
nathnacyfzone.org.uk/

Travel vaccinations and precautions

04-Nov-2025

Immunisation for travel

The National Travel Health Network and Centre have issued guidance on how to manage interrupted vaccination schedules which includes general principles for consideration, such as keeping to the recommended schedules, lengthening and shortening schedules, off-label administration and re-starting courses. For further information, see travelhealthpro.org.uk/factsheet/100/interrupted-vaccination-schedules-general-principles.

No special immunisation is required for travellers to the United States, Europe, Australia, or New Zealand, although all travellers should have immunity to tetanus and poliomyelitis (and childhood immunisations should be up to date); the tick-borne encephalitis vaccine is recommended for immunisation of those working in, or visiting, high-risk areas. Certain special precautions are required in non-European areas surrounding the Mediterranean, in Africa, the Middle East, Asia, and South America.

Travellers to areas that have a high incidence of **poliomyelitis** should be immunised with the appropriate vaccine; previously immunised travellers may be given a booster dose of a preparation containing inactivated poliomyelitis vaccine.

Immunisation against **meningococcal meningitis** is recommended for a number of areas of the world.

For guidance on immunisation against the following infectious diseases, refer to the individual treatment summaries listed:

- Cholera (see Cholera vaccines p. 963).
- Diphtheria (see Diphtheria vaccine p. 965).
- Hepatitis A (see Hepatitis A vaccine p. 967).
- Hepatitis B (see Hepatitis B vaccine p. 968).
- Japanese encephalitis (see Japanese encephalitis vaccine p. 972).
- Meningococcal meningitis (see Meningococcal vaccines p. 973).
- Rabies (see Rabies vaccine p. 977).
- Tetanus (see Tetanus vaccine p. 981).
- Tick-borne encephalitis (see Tick-borne encephalitis vaccine p. 983).
- Tuberculosis (see Bacillus Calmette-Guérin vaccine p. 963).
- Typhoid (see Typhoid vaccine p. 983).
- Yellow fever (see Yellow fever vaccine p. 984).

Immunisation requirements change from time to time, and information on the current requirements for any particular country may be obtained from the embassy or legation of the appropriate country, or the National Travel Health Network and Centre (see *Useful resources*).

Precautions for avoiding infectious disease

In areas where sanitation is poor, good food hygiene is important to help prevent hepatitis A, typhoid, cholera, and other diarrhoeal diseases (including travellers' diarrhoea). Food should be freshly prepared and hot, and uncooked vegetables (including green salads) should be avoided; only fruits which can be peeled should be eaten. Only suitable bottled water, or tap water that has been boiled or treated with sterilising tablets, should be used for drinking.

For guidance on malaria precautions, see Malaria, prophylaxis p. 476 and Malaria, treatment p. 482.

Further information on preventing or reducing the risk of infectious diseases when travelling, visiting, working, or living in high risk areas is available from the National Travel Health Network (see *Useful resources*).

Useful resources

National Travel Health Network and Centre.
nathnac.net

IMMUNE SERA AND IMMUNOGLOBULINS › MONOCLONAL ANTIBODIES

Nirsevimab

31-Jul-2025

- **DRUG ACTION** Nirsevimab is a recombinant human long-acting monoclonal antibody that binds to the prefusion conformation of the respiratory syncytial virus (RSV) F protein, thereby inhibiting viral entry into host cells and preventing RSV infection.

- **INDICATIONS AND DOSE**

Immunisation of very and extremely preterm neonates (less than 32 weeks gestational age) against respiratory syncytial virus (RSV) for first RSV season (under expert supervision)

▸ BY INTRAMUSCULAR INJECTION

▸ Neonate: 50 mg for 1 dose, to be given immediately before, or during, first RSV season.

Seasonal immunisation of high-risk children against respiratory syncytial virus (RSV) (under expert supervision)

▸ BY INTRAMUSCULAR INJECTION

▸ Neonate (body-weight up to 5 kg): 50 mg for 1 dose, to be given immediately before, or during, RSV season.

▸ Neonate (body-weight 5 kg and above): 100 mg for 1 dose, to be given immediately before, or during, RSV season.

▸ Child 1–23 months (body-weight up to 5 kg): 50 mg for 1 dose, to be given immediately before, or during, RSV season

▸ Child 1–23 months (body-weight 5 kg and above): 100 mg for 1 dose, to be given immediately before, or during, RSV season

- **UNLICENSED USE** UKHSA advises nirsevimab is used in the doses provided in BNFC for the seasonal immunisation of high-risk children against RSV, but these may differ from those licensed.

- **CAUTIONS** Acute illness · serum-nirsevimab concentration may be reduced after cardiac surgery · thrombocytopenia or any coagulation disorder (caution during administration)

CAUTIONS, FURTHER INFORMATION

▸ Acute illness UKHSA advises immunisation may be postponed if the individual is suffering from an acute illness; however, it is not necessary to postpone immunisation in patients with minor illnesses without fever or systemic upset.

- **SIDE-EFFECTS**
  - **Uncommon** Fever · skin reactions
  - **Frequency not known** Hypersensitivity
- **DIRECTIONS FOR ADMINISTRATION** For *intramuscular injection*, administration into the anterolateral aspect of the thigh is preferred.
- **PRESCRIBING AND DISPENSING INFORMATION** Nirsevimab is a biological medicine. Biological medicines must be prescribed and dispensed by brand name, see *Biological medicines* and *Biosimilar medicines*, under Guidance on prescribing p. 1; record the brand name and batch number after each administration.
  For further information on immunisation against RSV, see Respiratory syncytial virus immunisation p. 979.
- **HANDLING AND STORAGE** Store in a refrigerator (2–8°C) and protect from light; may be stored at room temperature (20–25°C) when protected from light for up to 8 hours.

- **MEDICINAL FORMS** There can be variation in the licensing of different medicines containing the same drug.

Solution for injection

EXCIPIENTS: May contain Polysorbates

- **Beyfortus** (Sanofi) ▼
  Nirsevimab 100 mg per 1 ml Beyfortus 100mg/1ml solution for injection pre-filled syringes | 1 pre-filled disposable injection PoM £1,683.00 (Hospital only)
  Beyfortus 50mg/0.5ml solution for injection pre-filled syringes | 1 pre-filled disposable injection PoM £1,683.00 (Hospital only)

Palivizumab

31-Jul-2025

- **DRUG ACTION** Palivizumab is a humanised monoclonal antibody that binds to fusion protein A on the surface of respiratory syncytial virus (RSV), which inhibits the virus from entering the host cell, thereby preventing RSV infection.

- **INDICATIONS AND DOSE**

Seasonal immunisation of high-risk children against respiratory syncytial virus (RSV) (under expert supervision)

▶ BY INTRAMUSCULAR INJECTION

- Neonate: 15 mg/kg once a month for 5 months, to start at the beginning of RSV season (calendar week 40); if treatment is started later in RSV season, give up to 5 doses until the end of calendar week 8. Where a course has been interrupted, restart and give monthly up until the end of calendar week 8.
- Child 1–23 months: 15 mg/kg once a month for 5 months, to start at the beginning of RSV season (calendar week 40); if treatment is started later in RSV season, give up to 5 doses until the end of calendar week 8. Where a course has been interrupted, restart and give monthly up until the end of calendar week 8

- **UNLICENSED USE** UKHSA advises palivizumab is used for the seasonal immunisation of high-risk children against RSV, but these recommendations may differ from those licensed.
- **CAUTIONS** Acute illness · serum-palivizumab concentration may be reduced after cardiac surgery · thrombocytopenia or any coagulation disorder (caution during administration)

CAUTIONS, FURTHER INFORMATION

- Acute illness UKHSA advises immunisation may be postponed if the individual is suffering from an acute illness; however, it is not necessary to postpone immunisation in patients with minor illnesses without fever or systemic upset.

- **SIDE-EFFECTS**
  - **Common or very common** Apnoea
  - **Uncommon** Seizure · thrombocytopenia · urticaria
  - **Frequency not known** Hypersensitivity
- **ALLERGY AND CROSS-SENSITIVITY** UKHSA advises avoid if previous anaphylactic reaction to another humanised monoclonal antibody.
- **DIRECTIONS FOR ADMINISTRATION** For *intramuscular injection*, administration into the anterolateral aspect of the thigh is preferred. EvGr Injection volume over 1 mL should be divided between more than one site. (M)
- **PRESCRIBING AND DISPENSING INFORMATION** Palivizumab is a biological medicine. Biological medicines must be prescribed and dispensed by brand name, see *Biological medicines* and *Biosimilar medicines*, under Guidance on prescribing p. 1; record the brand name and batch number after each administration.
  For further information on immunisation against RSV, see Respiratory syncytial virus immunisation p. 979.
- **HANDLING AND STORAGE** Store in a refrigerator (2–8°C) and protect from light.
- **MEDICINAL FORMS** There can be variation in the licensing of different medicines containing the same drug.

Solution for injection

- **Synagis** (AstraZeneca UK Ltd)
  Palivizumab 100 mg per 1 ml Synagis 100mg/1ml solution for injection vials | 1 vial PoM £563.64
  Synagis 50mg/0.5ml solution for injection vials | 1 vial PoM £306.34 (Hospital only)

VACCINES

Vaccines, general

12-Sep-2023

- **CAUTIONS** Acute illness · minor illnesses

CAUTIONS, FURTHER INFORMATION

- Illness UKHSA advises vaccination may be postponed if the individual is suffering from an acute illness; however, it is not necessary to postpone immunisation in patients with minor illnesses without fever or systemic upset.
- Predisposition to neurological problems UKHSA advises:
  - when there is a personal or family history of *febrile* convulsions, there is an increased risk of these occurring during fever from any cause including immunisation, but this is not a contra-indication to immunisation. In children who have had a seizure associated with fever without neurological deterioration, immunisation is *recommended*; advice on the *management of fever* should be given before immunisation. When a child has had a convulsion not associated with fever, and the neurological condition is not deteriorating, immunisation is *recommended*;
  - children with stable neurological disorders (e.g. spina bifida, congenital brain abnormality, and peri-natal hypoxic-ischaemic encephalopathy) should be immunised according to the recommended schedule;
  - when there is a *still evolving neurological problem*, including poorly controlled epilepsy, immunisation should be deferred and the child referred to a specialist. Immunisation is recommended if a cause for the neurological disorder is identified. If a cause is not identified, immunisation should be deferred until the condition is stable.
- Impaired immune response and drugs affecting immune response Immune response to vaccines may be reduced in immunosuppressed patients, UKHSA advises consider seeking specialist advice.

- **SIDE-EFFECTS**
  - **Common or very common** Abdominal pain · appetite decreased · arthralgia · diarrhoea · dizziness · fatigue · fever

- headache · lymphadenopathy · malaise · myalgia · nausea · skin reactions · vomiting
- ▶ **Uncommon** Hypersensitivity

● **ALLERGY AND CROSS-SENSITIVITY** UKHSA advises contra-indicated in patients with a confirmed anaphylactic reaction to a preceding dose of a vaccine containing the same antigens or vaccine component (such as antibacterials in viral vaccines).

● **DIRECTIONS FOR ADMINISTRATION** UKHSA advises when 2 or more injections are required (and are not available as a combined preparation), they can be administered at any time before or after each other at different sites, preferably in a different limb; if more than one injection is to be given in the same limb, they should be administered at least 2.5 cm apart. See also Cautions, further information in Bacillus Calmette-Guérin vaccine p. 1000 and in measles, mumps and rubella vaccine p. 1002.

Vaccines should not be given intravenously. Most vaccines are given by the intramuscular route, although some are given by either the intradermal, deep subcutaneous, or oral route. UKHSA advises the intramuscular route is usually avoided in patients with **bleeding disorders** such as haemophilia or thrombocytopenia; vaccines usually given by the intramuscular route can be given by deep subcutaneous injection instead.

Particular attention must be paid to instructions on the use of diluents. Vaccines which are liquid suspensions or are reconstituted before use should be adequately mixed to ensure uniformity of the material to be injected.

● **HANDLING AND STORAGE** Care must be taken to store all vaccines under the conditions recommended in the product literature, otherwise the preparation may become ineffective. **Refrigerated storage** is usually necessary; many vaccines need to be stored at 2–8°C and not allowed to freeze. Vaccines should be protected from light. Reconstituted vaccines and opened multidose vials must be used within the period recommended in the product literature. Unused vaccines should be disposed of by incineration at a registered disposal contractor.

VACCINES > INACTIVATED AND NON-REPLICATING

F 986

Chikungunya vaccine (inactivated)

06-Oct-2025

● **DRUG ACTION** The inactivated chikungunya vaccine contains adsorbed, recombinant chikungunya virus (CHIKV) virus-like particles that protect against CHIKV infection.

● **INDICATIONS AND DOSE**

Immunisation against chikungunya

▶ BY INTRAMUSCULAR INJECTION

- ▶ Child 12–17 years: 0.8 mL for 1 dose

● **SIDE-EFFECTS**
- ▶ **Common or very common** Chills
- ▶ **Uncommon** Nasal complaints
- ▶ **Rare or very rare** Gastroenteritis · lip swelling · oropharyngeal pain · pain in extremity · paraesthesia

● **PREGNANCY** EvGr Use only if potential benefit outweighs risk (limited information available). Ⓜ

● **BREAST FEEDING** EvGr Use only if potential benefit outweighs risk (no information available). Ⓜ

● **DIRECTIONS FOR ADMINISTRATION** To be administered into the deltoid region.

● **PATIENT AND CARER ADVICE** Immunisation with chikungunya vaccine (inactivated) does not provide complete protection and personal protective measures against mosquito bites are recommended.

● **MEDICINAL FORMS** There can be variation in the licensing of different medicines containing the same drug.

Suspension for injection

▶ **Vimkunya** (Bavarian Nordic UK Ltd) ▼
Vimkunya vaccine suspension for injection 0.8ml pre-filled syringes | 1 pre-filled disposable injection PoM £115.00

F 986

Cholera vaccine (inactivated)

29-Aug-2024

● **DRUG ACTION** The inactivated cholera vaccine is an oral vaccine that contains inactivated *Vibrio cholerae* and recombinant cholera toxin B-subunit. For information on the live vaccine, see cholera vaccine (live) p. 1001.

● **INDICATIONS AND DOSE**

Immunisation against cholera [primary course]

▶ BY MOUTH

- ▶ Child 2–5 years: 1 dose every 1–6 weeks for 3 doses, if more than 6 weeks have elapsed between doses, the primary course should be restarted, immunisation should be completed at least one week before potential exposure
- ▶ Child 6–17 years: 1 dose every 1–6 weeks for 2 doses, if more than 6 weeks have elapsed between doses, the primary course should be restarted, immunisation should be completed at least one week before potential exposure

Immunisation against cholera [booster dose]

▶ BY MOUTH

- ▶ Child 2–5 years: 1 dose, to be given within 6 months after primary course, if more than 6 months have elapsed since the last vaccination, the primary course should be repeated
- ▶ Child 6–17 years: 1 dose, to be given within 2 years after primary course, if more than 2 years have elapsed since the last vaccination, the primary course should be repeated

● **CONTRA-INDICATIONS** Acute gastro-intestinal illness

● **SIDE-EFFECTS**
- ▶ **Uncommon** Gastrointestinal discomfort · gastrointestinal disorders
- ▶ **Rare or very rare** Chills · cough · dehydration · drowsiness · hyperhidrosis · increased risk of infection · insomnia · pulmonary reaction · syncope · taste altered · throat pain
- ▶ **Frequency not known** Angioedema · asthenia · dyspnoea · hypertension · influenza like illness · lymphadenitis · pain · paraesthesia · sputum increased

● **DIRECTIONS FOR ADMINISTRATION** Manufacturer advises dissolve effervescent sodium bicarbonate granules in a glassful of water *or* chlorinated water (approximately 150 mL). For children over 6 years, add vaccine suspension to make one dose. For child 2–5 years, discard half (approximately 75 mL) of the solution, then add vaccine suspension to make one dose. Drink within 2 hours. Food, drink, and other oral medicines should be avoided for 1 hour before and after vaccination.

● **PATIENT AND CARER ADVICE** Counselling on administration advised. Immunisation with cholera vaccine does not provide complete protection and all travellers to a country where cholera exists should be warned that scrupulous attention to food, water, and personal hygiene is **essential**.

- **MEDICINAL FORMS** There can be variation in the licensing of different medicines containing the same drug.

Oral suspension

ELECTROLYTES: May contain Sodium

- **Dukoral** (Valneva UK Ltd)
  Dukoral cholera vaccine effervescent powder and suspension for oral suspension | 2 dose [PoM] £52.19 DT = £52.19

F 986

COVID-19 vaccine

30-Mar-2026

- **DRUG ACTION** COVID-19 vaccines are inactivated vaccines that use the spike protein of the SARS-CoV-2 virus to act as an intracellular antigen and produce an antibody response, thereby protecting against COVID-19 infection. Messenger RNA (mRNA) vaccines, such as *Comirnaty*® and *Spikevax*®, deliver viral RNA into host cells to enable expression of the spike protein. Other vaccines types include those that contain a recombinant spike protein with an adjuvant to strengthen the immune response, such as *Nuvaxovid*®.

- **INDICATIONS AND DOSE**

Immunisation against COVID-19

▸ BY INTRAMUSCULAR INJECTION

▸ Child 6 months–17 years: (consult local protocol)

- **SIDE-EFFECTS**
  - **Common or very common** Chills · crying · drowsiness · irritability · lymphatic abnormalities
  - **Uncommon** Asthenia · insomnia · pain in extremity · sweat changes
  - **Rare or very rare** Angioedema · cardiac inflammation · facial paralysis · sensation abnormal
  - **Frequency not known** Capillary leak syndrome · extensive swelling of vaccinated limb · menorrhagia
- **ALLERGY AND CROSS-SENSITIVITY** UKHSA advises individuals with a history of anaphylaxis to food, an identified drug or vaccine, or an insect sting can receive any COVID-19 vaccine, as long as they are not allergic to any of its ingredients; consider observation for 15 minutes. Individuals who had a non-allergic reaction to a first dose of COVID-19 vaccine can receive a second dose, followed by an observation period of 15 minutes. The mRNA vaccines, such as *Comirnaty*®, contain polyethylene glycol. UKHSA advises individuals with a history of immediate onset anaphylaxis to multiple classes of drugs, or unexplained anaphylaxis, (which may indicate allergy to polyethylene glycol), should only be vaccinated with *Comirnaty*® vaccine on the advice of an allergy specialist, or when at least one dose of the same vaccine has been tolerated previously. Vaccination should be administered in a setting with full resuscitation facilities, followed by an observation period of 30 minutes. Vaccination of individuals in whom mRNA vaccines are unsuitable requires an individual clinical judgement. UKHSA advises individuals with a localised allergic reaction or with systemic symptoms, but not anaphylaxis, to a previous dose of a COVID-19 vaccine can receive further doses using the same vaccine, with an observation period of at least 30 minutes, or at least 15 minutes if the reaction was delayed and self-limiting, or resolved with an oral antihistamine. Consider pre-treatment with a non-sedating antihistamine at least 30 minutes before giving further doses. Seek advice from an allergy specialist if the reaction presented with anaphylaxis or required medical attention.
- **PREGNANCY** UKHSA advises that COVID-19 vaccines are suitable.
- **BREAST FEEDING** UKHSA advises that COVID-19 vaccines are suitable.
- **MONITORING REQUIREMENTS**
  - UKHSA advises healthcare professionals to consider monitoring platelets 2 to 5 days after vaccination in patients with a history of immune thrombocytopenia.
  - UKHSA advises healthcare professionals to be alert for signs and symptoms of myocarditis and pericarditis and inform vaccinated patients to seek immediate medical attention if they experience a new onset of chest pain, shortness of breath, palpitations or arrhythmias within 10 days of vaccination.
  - For advice on further doses for those who have suspected Guillain-Barré syndrome, myocarditis, or pericarditis after vaccination, see Chapter 14a: COVID-19 - SARS-CoV-2, in *Immunisation against infectious disease*- 'The Green Book'.
- **DIRECTIONS FOR ADMINISTRATION** UKHSA advises that individuals with **bleeding disorders** may be vaccinated by the intramuscular route, on the advice of a doctor familiar with their bleeding risk. Patients treated with medicines to reduce bleeding (e.g. for haemophilia) are advised to administer their medicine shortly prior to intramuscular vaccination.
- **PRESCRIBING AND DISPENSING INFORMATION** For further information on vaccine eligibility and choice, see COVID-19 vaccines p. 964.
- **HANDLING AND STORAGE** For *Comirnaty*® LP.8.1 3 micrograms/dose and 10 micrograms/dose preparations, store in a freezer at -90°C to -60°C—consult product literature about thawing and storage after thawing.
- **PATIENT AND CARER ADVICE**
  Driving and skilled tasks Healthcare professionals are advised to inform patients not to drive for 15 minutes after vaccination—increased risk of fainting.

- **MEDICINAL FORMS** There can be variation in the licensing of different medicines containing the same drug.

Dispersion for injection

EXCIPIENTS: May contain Polysorbates

- **Comirnaty LP.8.1** (Pfizer Ltd) ▼
  Comirnaty LP.8.1 adults and adolescents from 12 years COVID-19 mRNA Vaccine 30micrograms/0.3ml dose dispersion for injection pre-filled syringes | 1 dose [PoM] £64.00 | 10 dose [PoM] £640.00
- **Comirnaty LP.8.1 Children** (Pfizer Ltd) ▼
  Comirnaty LP.8.1 Children 5-11 years COVID-19 mRNA Vaccine 10micrograms/0.3ml dose dispersion for injection single dose vials | 10 dose [PoM] £640.00
  Comirnaty LP.8.1 Children 6 months - 4 years COVID-19 mRNA Vaccine 3micrograms/0.3ml dose concentrate for dispersion for injection multidose vials | 30 dose [PoM] £1,770.00
- **Nuvaxovid JN.1** (Novavax UK Ltd) ▼
  Nuvaxovid JN.1 COVID-19 Vaccine (recombinant, adjuvanted) 5micrograms/0.5ml dose dispersion for injection pre-filled syringes | 10 dose [PoM] [X]
- **Spikevax LP.8.1** (Moderna Biotech Distributor UK Ltd) ▼
  Spikevax LP.8.1 COVID-19 mRNA Vaccine 0.1mg/1ml dispersion for injection multidose vials | 25 ml [PoM] £3,450.00

F 986

Diphtheria, tetanus, and pertussis vaccine

20-Apr-2026

- **DRUG ACTION** Diphtheria, tetanus, and pertussis vaccine is a non-live, adsorbed, combination vaccine containing diphtheria and tetanus toxoids, and pertussis antigens.

- **INDICATIONS AND DOSE**

Passive immunisation against pertussis [pregnant women in their second or third trimester]

▸ BY INTRAMUSCULAR INJECTION

▸ Females of childbearing potential: 0.5 mL for 1 dose

- **CONTRA-INDICATIONS** History of encephalopathy of unknown origin within 7 days of previous immunisation with a pertussis-containing vaccine

● **CAUTIONS** Guillain-Barre syndrome within 6 weeks of previous immunisation with a vaccine containing tetanus toxoid · progressive neurological disorders, uncontrolled epilepsy, or progressive encephalopathy (defer immunisation until condition has stabilised)

● **SIDE-EFFECTS**

▶ **Common or very common** Asthenia · axillary lymphadenopathy · chills · generalised pain · joint swelling · muscle weakness

▶ **Frequency not known** Extensive swelling of vaccinated limb · facial paralysis · myelitis · myocarditis · myositis · nerve disorders · seizure · sensation abnormal · syncope

● **PRESCRIBING AND DISPENSING INFORMATION** Details of routine immunisations are included in this monograph; for details of immunisation in other patient groups e.g. patients at high risk from infection, see Diphtheria vaccine p. 965, Tetanus vaccine p. 981, and Pertussis vaccine p. 974 respectively.

● **MEDICINAL FORMS** There can be variation in the licensing of different medicines containing the same drug.

Suspension for injection

▸ **Adacel** (Sanofi)

Adacel vaccine suspension for injection 0.5ml pre-filled syringes | 1 pre-filled disposable injection [PoM] £19.00

F 986

Diphtheria, tetanus, and poliomyelitis vaccine

20-Apr-2026

● **DRUG ACTION** Diphtheria, tetanus, and poliomyelitis vaccine is a non-live, adsorbed, combination vaccine containing diphtheria and tetanus toxoids, and inactivated poliomyelitis virus.

● **INDICATIONS AND DOSE**

Primary immunisation

▶ BY INTRAMUSCULAR INJECTION

▸ Child 10–17 years: 0.5 mL every month for 3 doses

Booster doses

▶ BY INTRAMUSCULAR INJECTION

▸ Child 10–17 years: 0.5 mL for 1 dose, first booster dose—should be given at least 5 years after primary course, then 0.5 mL for 1 dose, second booster dose—should be given 10 years after first booster dose (this interval can be reduced to a minimum of 5 years if previous doses were delayed)

● **SIDE-EFFECTS**

▶ **Common or very common** Vertigo

▶ **Frequency not known** Asthenia · chills · face oedema · influenza like illness · nerve disorders · pallor · seizure · shock · syncope · vaccination reactions

● **PRESCRIBING AND DISPENSING INFORMATION** Available as part of childhood schedule from health organisations or ImmForm.

● **MEDICINAL FORMS** There can be variation in the licensing of different medicines containing the same drug.

Suspension for injection

EXCIPIENTS: May contain Neomycin, polymyxin b, streptomycin

▸ **Revaxis** (Sanofi)

Revaxis vaccine suspension for injection 0.5ml pre-filled syringes | 1 pre-filled disposable injection [PoM] £7.80 DT = £7.80

F 986

Diphtheria, tetanus, pertussis, and poliomyelitis vaccine

20-Apr-2026

● **DRUG ACTION** Diphtheria, tetanus, pertussis, and poliomyelitis vaccine is a non-live, adsorbed, combination vaccine containing diphtheria and tetanus toxoids, pertussis antigens, and inactivated poliomyelitis virus.

● **INDICATIONS AND DOSE**

Immunisation against diphtheria, tetanus, pertussis, and poliomyelitis [booster dose]

▶ BY INTRAMUSCULAR INJECTION

▸ Child 3–9 years: 0.5 mL for 1 dose, dose to be given 3 years after primary immunisation

● **SIDE-EFFECTS**

▶ **Common or very common** Asthenia · drowsiness · irritability · joint swelling · vaccination reactions

▶ **Uncommon** Apathy · dry throat · sleep disorder

▶ **Frequency not known** Angioedema · facial paralysis · hypotonic-hyporesponsiveness episode · myelitis · nerve disorders · pallor · seizure

SIDE-EFFECTS, FURTHER INFORMATION The incidence of local and systemic reactions is lower with acellular pertussis vaccines than with whole-cell pertussis vaccines used previously.

Compared with primary vaccination, injection site reactions are more common with booster doses of vaccines containing acellular pertussis.

Public Health England has advised (2016) that the vaccine should not be withheld from children with a history to a preceding dose of: fever, irrespective of severity; hypotonic-hyporesonsive episodes; persistent crying or screaming for more than 3 hours; severe local reaction, irrespective of extent.

● **PREGNANCY** Contra-indicated in pregnant women with a history of encephalopathy of unknown origin within 7 days of previous immunisation with a pertussis-containing vaccine. Contra-indicated in pregnant women with a history of transient thrombocytopenia or neurological complications following previous immunisation against diphtheria or tetanus.

● **PRESCRIBING AND DISPENSING INFORMATION** Available as part of childhood immunisation schedule from health organisations or ImmForm.

Details of routine immunisations are included in this monograph; for details of immunisation in other patient groups e.g. patients at high risk from infection, see Diphtheria vaccine p. 965, Tetanus vaccine p. 981, Pertussis vaccine p. 974, Poliomyelitis vaccine p. 976, and Vaccination, general principles p. 959.

● **MEDICINAL FORMS** There can be variation in the licensing of different medicines containing the same drug.

Suspension for injection

EXCIPIENTS: May contain Neomycin, polymyxin b, streptomycin

▸ **Boostrix-IPV** (GlaxoSmithKline UK Ltd)

Boostrix-IPV suspension for injection 0.5ml pre-filled syringes | 1 pre-filled disposable injection [PoM] £22.74 DT = £20.00

▸ **Repevax** (Sanofi)

Repevax vaccine suspension for injection 0.5ml pre-filled syringes | 1 pre-filled disposable injection [PoM] £20.00 DT = £20.00

986

Diphtheria, tetanus, pertussis, poliomyelitis, and haemophilus influenzae type b vaccine

16-Apr-2026

- **DRUG ACTION** Diphtheria, tetanus, pertussis, poliomyelitis, and *haemophilus influenzae* type b vaccine is a non-live combination vaccine.

- **INDICATIONS AND DOSE**

Primary immunisation

▶ BY INTRAMUSCULAR INJECTION

▶ Child 2 months–9 years: 0.5 mL every month for 3 doses

- **SIDE-EFFECTS**

▶ **Common or very common** Crying abnormal · drowsiness · irritability · restlessness

▶ **Uncommon** Cough · extensive swelling of vaccinated limb · increased risk of infection · rhinorrhoea

▶ **Frequency not known** Angioedema · apnoea · hypotonic-hyporesponsiveness episode · seizure

SIDE-EFFECTS, FURTHER INFORMATION The incidence of local and systemic reactions is lower with acellular pertussis vaccines than with whole-cell pertussis vaccines used previously.

Compared with primary vaccination, injection site reactions are more common with booster doses of vaccines containing acellular pertussis.

Public Health England has advised (2016) that the vaccine should not be withheld from children with a history to a preceding dose of: fever, irrespective of severity; hypotonic-hyporesonsive episodes; persistent crying or screaming for more than 3 hours; severe local reaction, irrespective of extent.

- **PRESCRIBING AND DISPENSING INFORMATION** UKHSA advises from Autumn 2017, all babies born on or after 1 August 2017 became eligible for the hexavalent vaccine, diphtheria with tetanus, pertussis, hepatitis B, poliomyelitis and haemophilus influenzae type b vaccine below, which replaces the pentavalent vaccine in the routine childhood immunisation schedule.

- **MEDICINAL FORMS** There can be variation in the licensing of different medicines containing the same drug.

Powder and suspension for suspension for injection

▶ **Infanrix-IPV + Hib** (GlaxoSmithKline UK Ltd)
Infanrix-IPV + Hib vaccine powder and suspension for suspension for injection 0.5ml pre-filled syringes | 1 pre-filled disposable injection PoM £27.86

986

Diphtheria with tetanus, pertussis, hepatitis B, poliomyelitis and haemophilus influenzae type b vaccine

18-Aug-2025

- **DRUG ACTION** Diphtheria with tetanus, pertussis, hepatitis B, poliomyelitis and *haemophilus influenzae* type b vaccine is a non-live combination vaccine.

- **INDICATIONS AND DOSE**

Primary immunisation against diphtheria, tetanus, pertussis, hepatitis B, poliomyelitis, and *Haemophilus influenzae* type b

▶ BY INTRAMUSCULAR INJECTION

▶ Child 2 months–9 years: 0.5 mL every 4 weeks for 3 doses

Immunisation against diphtheria, tetanus, pertussis, hepatitis B, poliomyelitis, and *Haemophilus influenzae* type b [booster dose for infants born on or after 1 July 2024 who have received primary immunisation]

▶ BY INTRAMUSCULAR INJECTION

▶ Child 18 months: 0.5 mL for 1 dose

- **SIDE-EFFECTS**

▶ **Common or very common** Anxiety · crying · drowsiness · irritability

▶ **Uncommon** Appetite increased · cough · extensive swelling of vaccinated limb · hyperhidrosis · increased risk of infection · neuromuscular dysfunction · pallor · sleep disorders

▶ **Rare or very rare** Angioedema · apnoea · seizure · swelling · thrombocytopenia

- **DIRECTIONS FOR ADMINISTRATION** Anterolateral thigh is the preferred site of injection in infants under 1 year of age; deltoid muscle is preferred in older children. Administer each dose at a different injection site to that of previous dose.

- **PRESCRIBING AND DISPENSING INFORMATION** Available as part of childhood schedule from health organisations or ImmForm.

Details of routine immunisations are included in this monograph; for details of immunisation in other patient groups e.g. patients at high risk from infection, see Diphtheria vaccine p. 965, Tetanus vaccine p. 981, Pertussis vaccine p. 974, Hepatitis B vaccine p. 968, Poliomyelitis vaccine p. 976, Haemophilus influenzae type b conjugate vaccine p. 966 and Vaccination, general principles p. 959.

- **MEDICINAL FORMS** There can be variation in the licensing of different medicines containing the same drug.

Powder and suspension for suspension for injection

EXCIPIENTS: May contain Neomycin, polymyxin b

▶ **Infanrix Hexa** (GlaxoSmithKline UK Ltd)
Infanrix Hexa vaccine powder and suspension for suspension for injection 0.5ml pre-filled syringes | 1 pre-filled disposable injection PoM

Suspension for injection

EXCIPIENTS: May contain Neomycin, polymyxin b, streptomycin

▶ **Vaxelis** (Sanofi)
Vaxelis vaccine suspension for injection 0.5ml pre-filled syringes | 1 pre-filled disposable injection PoM £45.31

986

Haemophilus influenzae type b and meningococcal group C vaccine

17-Apr-2026

- **DRUG ACTION** *Haemophilus influenzae* type b and meningococcal group C vaccine is a non-live combination vaccine.

- **INDICATIONS AND DOSE**

Immunisation against *Neisseria meningitidis* group C and *Haemophilus influenzae* type b [children born before 1 July 2024 with unknown or incomplete immunisation status]

▶ BY INTRAMUSCULAR INJECTION

▶ Child 1–9 years: 0.5 mL for 1 dose

- **UNLICENSED USE** Not licensed for use in patients over 2 years.

- **SIDE-EFFECTS**

▶ **Common or very common** Drowsiness · irritability

▶ **Uncommon** Crying

▶ **Rare or very rare** Insomnia

▶ **Frequency not known** Apnoea (in neonates) · febrile seizure · meningism (but no evidence that vaccine causes meningococcal C meningitis) · muscle tone decreased

● **PRESCRIBING AND DISPENSING INFORMATION** Details on routine immunisations are included in this monograph; for details of immunisation in other patient groups e.g. patients at high risk of infection, see Haemophilus influenzae type b conjugate vaccine p. 966 and Vaccination, general principles p. 959.

Available as part of the childhood immunisation schedule from ImmForm.

● **MEDICINAL FORMS** No licensed medicines listed.

Hepatitis A and B vaccine 25-Aug-2023

The properties listed below are those particular to the combination only. For the properties of the components please consider, hepatitis A vaccine below, hepatitis B vaccine p. 992.

● **INDICATIONS AND DOSE**

AMBIRIX®

Immunisation against hepatitis A and hepatitis B infection [primary course]

▶ BY INTRAMUSCULAR INJECTION

▸ Child 1–15 years: Initially 1 mL for 1 dose, then 1 mL after 6–12 months for 1 dose, the deltoid region is the preferred site of injection in older children; anterolateral thigh may be used in infants; not to be injected into the buttock (vaccine efficacy reduced), subcutaneous route used for patients with bleeding disorders (but immune response may be reduced)

Post-exposure prophylaxis against hepatitis A infection [for rapid protection]

▶ BY INTRAMUSCULAR INJECTION

▸ Child 1–15 years: 1 mL for 1 dose, the deltoid region is the preferred site of injection in older children; anterolateral thigh may be used in infants; not to be injected into the buttock (vaccine efficacy reduced), subcutaneous route used for patients with bleeding disorders (but immune response may be reduced)

TWINRIX® ADULT

Immunisation against hepatitis A and hepatitis B infection [primary course]

▶ BY INTRAMUSCULAR INJECTION

▸ Child 16–17 years: Initially 1 mL every month for 2 doses, then 1 mL after 5 months for 1 dose, the deltoid region is the preferred site of injection; not to be injected into the buttock (vaccine efficacy reduced), subcutaneous route used for patients with bleeding disorders (but immune response may be reduced)

Immunisation against hepatitis A and hepatitis B infection [accelerated schedule for travellers departing within 1 month]

▶ BY INTRAMUSCULAR INJECTION

▸ Child 16–17 years: Initially 1 mL for 1 dose, then 1 mL after 7 days for 1 dose, then 1 mL after 14 days for 1 dose, then 1 mL for 1 dose given 12 months after the first dose, the deltoid region is the preferred site of injection; not to be injected into the buttock (vaccine efficacy reduced), subcutaneous route used for patients with bleeding disorders (but immune response may be reduced)

TWINRIX® PAEDIATRIC

Immunisation against hepatitis A and hepatitis B infection [primary course]

▶ BY INTRAMUSCULAR INJECTION

▸ Child 1–15 years: Initially 0.5 mL every month for 2 doses, then 0.5 mL after 5 months for 1 dose, the deltoid region is the preferred site of injection in older children; anterolateral thigh is the preferred site in infants; not to be injected into the buttock (vaccine efficacy reduced), subcutaneous route used for patients with bleeding disorders (but immune response may be reduced)

● **UNLICENSED USE**

AMBIRIX® Public Health England advises that *Ambirix®* may be used for post-exposure prophylaxis against hepatitis A infection where rapid protection is required, but is not licensed for this indication.

IMPORTANT SAFETY INFORMATION

Ambirix® and *Twinrix®* are not recommended for post-exposure prophylaxis following percutaneous (needle-stick), ocular, or mucous membrane exposure to hepatitis B virus.

● **PRESCRIBING AND DISPENSING INFORMATION**

AMBIRIX® Primary course should be completed with *Ambirix®* (single component vaccines given at appropriate intervals may be used for booster dose).

TWINRIX® ADULT Primary course should be completed with *Twinrix®* (single component vaccines given at appropriate intervals may be used for booster dose).

TWINRIX® PAEDIATRIC Primary course should be completed with *Twinrix®* (single component vaccines given at appropriate intervals may be used for booster dose).

● **MEDICINAL FORMS** There can be variation in the licensing of different medicines containing the same drug.

Suspension for injection

EXCIPIENTS: May contain Neomycin

▸ **Ambirix** (GlaxoSmithKline UK Ltd)
Ambirix vaccine suspension for injection 1ml pre-filled syringes | 1 pre-filled disposable injection PoM £31.18 DT = £31.18

▸ **Twinrix** (GlaxoSmithKline UK Ltd)
Twinrix Paediatric vaccine suspension for injection 0.5ml pre-filled syringes | 1 pre-filled disposable injection PoM £20.79 DT = £20.79
Twinrix Adult vaccine suspension for injection 1ml pre-filled syringes | 1 pre-filled disposable injection PoM £33.31 DT = £31.18 | 10 pre-filled disposable injection PoM £333.13

F 986

Hepatitis A vaccine 25-Aug-2023

● **DRUG ACTION** Hepatitis A vaccine is an inactivated vaccine containing adsorbed hepatitis A virus.

● **INDICATIONS AND DOSE**

AVAXIM®

Immunisation against hepatitis A infection

▶ BY INTRAMUSCULAR INJECTION

▸ Child 16–17 years: Initially 0.5 mL for 1 dose, then 0.5 mL after 6–12 months, dose given as booster; booster dose may be delayed by up to 3 years if not given after recommended interval following primary dose, the deltoid region is the preferred site of injection. The subcutaneous route may be used for patients with bleeding disorders; not to be injected into the buttock (vaccine efficacy reduced)

HAVRIX JUNIOR MONODOSE®

Immunisation against hepatitis A infection

▶ BY INTRAMUSCULAR INJECTION

▸ Child 1–15 years: Initially 0.5 mL for 1 dose, then 0.5 mL after 6–12 months, dose given as booster; booster dose may be delayed by up to 3 years if not given after recommended interval following primary dose, deltoid muscle is preferred site of injection in older children; anterolateral thigh is preferred site in infants and young children; not to be injected into the gluteal region. The subcutaneous route may be used for patients with bleeding disorders

continued →

HAVRIX MONODOSE®

Immunisation against hepatitis A infection

▶ BY INTRAMUSCULAR INJECTION

▸ Child 16–17 years: Initially 1 mL for 1 dose, then 1 mL after 6–12 months, dose given as booster; booster dose may be delayed by up to 3 years if not given after recommended interval following primary dose, the deltoid region is the preferred site of injection; not to be injected into the gluteal region. The subcutaneous route may be used for patients with bleeding disorders

VAQTA® PAEDIATRIC

Immunisation against hepatitis A infection

▶ BY INTRAMUSCULAR INJECTION

▸ Child 1–17 years: Initially 0.5 mL for 1 dose, then 0.5 mL after 6–18 months, dose given as booster, the deltoid region is the preferred site of injection. The subcutaneous route may be used for patients with bleeding disorders (but immune response may be reduced)

● **SIDE-EFFECTS**

▶ **Common or very common** Irritability

▶ **Uncommon** Anxiety · asthenia · cough · crying · drowsiness · nasal complaints · pain · sleep disorders

▶ **Rare or very rare** Allergic rhinitis · asthma · ataxia · burping · chest pain · constipation · dehydration · ear pain · eyelid crusting · feeling hot · flushing · gait abnormal · gastrointestinal discomfort · gastrointestinal disorders · infantile spitting up · influenza like illness · musculoskeletal stiffness · oropharyngeal pain · paraesthesia · respiratory tract congestion · screaming · sensation of tightness · sweat changes · synovitis

▶ **Frequency not known** Guillain-Barre syndrome · thrombocytopenia

● **MEDICINAL FORMS** There can be variation in the licensing of different medicines containing the same drug.

Suspension for injection

EXCIPIENTS: May contain Neomycin

▸ **Avaxim** (Sanofi)
Avaxim vaccine suspension for injection 0.5ml pre-filled syringes | 1 pre-filled disposable injection PoM £21.72 | 10 pre-filled disposable injection PoM £217.20

▸ **Havrix** (GlaxoSmithKline UK Ltd)
Havrix Monodose vaccine suspension for injection 1ml pre-filled syringes | 1 pre-filled disposable injection PoM £22.14 DT = £22.14 | 10 pre-filled disposable injection PoM £221.43
Havrix Junior Monodose vaccine suspension for injection 0.5ml pre-filled syringes | 1 pre-filled disposable injection PoM £16.77 | 10 pre-filled disposable injection PoM £167.68

▸ **VAQTA** (Merck Sharp & Dohme (UK) Ltd)
VAQTA Paediatric vaccine suspension for injection 0.5ml pre-filled syringes | 1 pre-filled disposable injection PoM £14.74

F 986

Hepatitis B vaccine

20-Aug-2025

● **DRUG ACTION** Hepatitis B vaccine is an inactivated vaccine containing adsorbed hepatitis B surface antigen.

● **INDICATIONS AND DOSE**

ENGERIX B®

Immunisation against hepatitis B infection

▶ BY INTRAMUSCULAR INJECTION

▸ Neonate: 10 micrograms for 1 dose, then 10 micrograms after 1 month for 1 dose, followed by 10 micrograms after 5 months for 1 dose, this dose should not be given to neonates born to hepatitis B surface antigen-positive mothers.

▸ Child 1 month–15 years: 10 micrograms for 1 dose, then 10 micrograms after 1 month for 1 dose, followed by 10 micrograms after 5 months for 1 dose

▸ Child 16–17 years: 20 micrograms for 1 dose, then 20 micrograms after 1 month for 1 dose, followed by 20 micrograms after 5 months for 1 dose

Immunisation against hepatitis B infection (accelerated schedule for pre- and post-exposure prophylaxis)

▶ BY INTRAMUSCULAR INJECTION

▸ Neonate: 10 micrograms every month for 3 doses, followed by 10 micrograms after 10 months for 1 dose, for post-exposure prophylaxis, UKHSA advises dose at 12 months not required if patient is at low risk, this dose should not be given to neonates born to hepatitis B surface antigen-positive mothers.

▸ Child 1 month–15 years: 10 micrograms every month for 3 doses, followed by 10 micrograms after 10 months for 1 dose, for post-exposure prophylaxis, UKHSA advises dose at 12 months not required if patient is at low risk

▸ Child 16–17 years: 20 micrograms every month for 3 doses, followed by 20 micrograms after 10 months for 1 dose, for post-exposure prophylaxis, UKHSA advises dose at 12 months not required if patient is at low risk

Immunisation against hepatitis B infection (alternative accelerated schedule)

▶ BY INTRAMUSCULAR INJECTION

▸ Child 11–15 years: 20 micrograms for 1 dose, followed by 20 micrograms after 6 months for 1 dose, this schedule is not suitable if high risk of infection between doses or if compliance with second dose uncertain

Immunisation against hepatitis B infection (very rapid schedule)

▶ BY INTRAMUSCULAR INJECTION

▸ Child 16–17 years: 20 micrograms for 1 dose, then 20 micrograms after 7 days for 1 dose, followed by 20 micrograms after 14 days for 1 dose, followed by 20 micrograms for 1 dose, to be given 12 months after the first dose

Immunisation against hepatitis B infection (in neonates born to hepatitis B surface antigen-positive mothers)

▶ BY INTRAMUSCULAR INJECTION

▸ Neonate: 10 micrograms every 4 weeks for 2 doses, first dose to be given ideally within 24 hours of birth, for neonates with a birth weight below 1.5 kg born to an infected mother, or neonates born to a highly infectious mother, the first dose should be given at birth with hepatitis B immunoglobulin injection (separate site).

Immunisation against hepatitis B infection (in renal insufficiency, including haemodialysis patients)

▶ BY INTRAMUSCULAR INJECTION

▸ Neonate: 10 micrograms every month for 2 doses, followed by 10 micrograms after 5 months for 1 dose, immunisation schedule and booster doses may need to be adjusted in those with low antibody concentration, this dose should not be given to neonates born to hepatitis B surface antigen-positive mothers.

▸ Child 1 month–15 years: 10 micrograms every month for 2 doses, followed by 10 micrograms after 5 months for 1 dose, immunisation schedule and booster doses may need to be adjusted in those with low antibody concentration

▸ Child 16–17 years: 40 micrograms every month for 3 doses, followed by 40 micrograms after 4 months for 1 dose, immunisation schedule and booster doses may need to be adjusted in those with low antibody concentration

Immunisation against hepatitis B infection (accelerated schedule for pre- and post-exposure prophylaxis in renal insufficiency, including haemodialysis patients)

▶ BY INTRAMUSCULAR INJECTION

- Neonate: 10 micrograms every month for 3 doses, followed by 10 micrograms after 10 months for 1 dose, for post-exposure prophylaxis, UKHSA advises dose at 12 months not required if patient is at low risk, immunisation schedule and booster doses may need to be adjusted in those with low antibody concentration, this dose should not be given to neonates born to hepatitis B surface antigen-positive mothers.
- Child 1 month–15 years: 10 micrograms every month for 3 doses, followed by 10 micrograms after 10 months for 1 dose, for post-exposure prophylaxis, UKHSA advises dose at 12 months not required if patient is at low risk, immunisation schedule and booster doses may need to be adjusted in those with low antibody concentration

FENDRIX®

Immunisation against hepatitis B infection in renal insufficiency (including pre-haemodialysis and haemodialysis patients)

▶ BY INTRAMUSCULAR INJECTION

- Child 15–17 years: 20 micrograms every month for 3 doses, followed by 20 micrograms after 4 months for 1 dose, immunisation schedule and booster doses may need to be adjusted in those with low antibody concentration

HBVAXPRO®

Immunisation against hepatitis B infection

▶ BY INTRAMUSCULAR INJECTION

- Neonate: 5 micrograms for 1 dose, followed by 5 micrograms after 1 month for 1 dose, then 5 micrograms after 5 months for 1 dose, booster doses may be required in immunocompromised patients with low antibody concentration, dose not to be used in neonates born to hepatitis B surface antigen-positive mothers.
- Child 1 month–15 years: 5 micrograms for 1 dose, followed by 5 micrograms after 1 month for 1 dose, then 5 micrograms after 5 months for 1 dose, booster doses may be required in immunocompromised patients with low antibody concentration
- Child 16–17 years: 10 micrograms for 1 dose, followed by 10 micrograms after 1 month for 1 dose, followed by 10 micrograms after 5 months for 1 dose, booster doses may be required in immunocompromised patients with low antibody concentration

Immunisation against hepatitis B infection (accelerated schedule for pre- and post-exposure prophylaxis)

▶ BY INTRAMUSCULAR INJECTION

- Neonate: 5 micrograms every month for 3 doses, followed by 5 micrograms after 10 months for 1 dose, for post-exposure prophylaxis, UKHSA advises dose at 12 months not required if patient is at low risk, booster doses may be required in immunocompromised patients with low antibody concentration, dose not to be used in neonates born to hepatitis B surface antigen-positive mothers.
- Child 1 month–15 years: 5 micrograms every month for 3 doses, followed by 5 micrograms after 10 months for 1 dose, for post-exposure prophylaxis, UKHSA advises dose at 12 months not required if patient is at low risk, booster doses may be required in immunocompromised patients with low antibody concentration
- Child 16–17 years: 10 micrograms every month for 3 doses, followed by 10 micrograms after 10 months for 1 dose, for post-exposure prophylaxis, UKHSA advises dose at 12 months not required if patient is at low risk, booster doses may be required in immunocompromised patients with low antibody concentration

Immunisation against hepatitis B infection (in neonates born to hepatitis B surface antigen-positive mothers)

▶ BY INTRAMUSCULAR INJECTION

- Neonate: 5 micrograms every 4 weeks for 2 doses, first dose to be given ideally within 24 hours of birth, for neonates with a birth weight below 1.5 kg born to an infected mother, or neonates born to a highly infectious mother, the first dose should be given at birth with hepatitis B immunoglobulin injection (separate site).

Immunisation against hepatitis B infection (in chronic haemodialysis patients)

▶ BY INTRAMUSCULAR INJECTION

- Child 16–17 years: 40 micrograms every month for 2 doses, followed by 40 micrograms after 5 months for 1 dose, booster doses may be required in those with low antibody concentration

14 Vaccines

● **UNLICENSED USE**

ENGERIX B® UKHSA advises *Engerix B®* is used in the doses provided in BNF Publications for immunisation against hepatitis B infection (very rapid schedule) in children aged 16–17 years, but these are considered unlicensed. UKHSA advises *Engerix B®* is used in the doses provided in BNFC for immunisation against hepatitis B infection in neonates born to hepatitis B surface antigen-positive mothers, but these are considered unlicensed.

HBVAXPRO® UKHSA advises *HBVAXPRO®* is used in the doses provided in BNFC for immunisation against hepatitis B infection in neonates born to hepatitis B surface antigen-positive mothers, but these are considered unlicensed.

● **SIDE-EFFECTS**

- **Common or very common** Drowsiness · gastrointestinal disorder · irritability · pain
- **Uncommon** Influenza like illness
- **Rare or very rare** Alopecia · angioedema · arthritis · asthenia · bronchospasm-like symptoms · chills · demyelinating disorders · hot flush · hypotension · increased risk of infection · nerve disorders · nervousness · paralysis · seizure · sensation abnormal · syncope · tendinitis · thirst · thrombocytopenia · transverse myelitis · uveitis · vasculitis · vertigo
- **Frequency not known** Apnoea · encephalopathy · meningitis · muscle weakness

● **DIRECTIONS FOR ADMINISTRATION** Anterolateral thigh is the preferred site of injection in infants under 1 year of age; deltoid muscle is preferred in older children. Not to be injected into the buttock (vaccine efficacy reduced).

● **PRESCRIBING AND DISPENSING INFORMATION** UKHSA advises different hepatitis B vaccine preparations can be used to complete a primary immunisation course, or to administer a booster dose. However, once the primary immunisation course has been started with *Fendrix®*, interchanging with another brand is considered unlicensed.

For details on routine immunisations and further details of immunisation in other patient groups e.g. patients at high risk of infection, see Hepatitis B vaccine p. 968 and Vaccination, general principles p. 959.

● **MEDICINAL FORMS** There can be variation in the licensing of different medicines containing the same drug.

Suspension for injection

- Engerix B (GlaxoSmithKline UK Ltd)

Hepatitis B virus surface antigen 20 microgram per 1 ml Engerix B 10micrograms/0.5ml vaccine suspension for injection pre-filled syringes | 1 pre-filled disposable injection PoM £9.67 DT = £9.67

Engerix B 20micrograms/1ml vaccine suspension for injection pre-filled syringes | 1 pre-filled disposable injection PoM £12.99 DT = £12.99 | 10 pre-filled disposable injection PoM £129.92

▸ **Fendrix** (GlaxoSmithKline UK Ltd)

Hepatitis B virus surface antigen 40 microgram per 1 ml Fendrix 20micrograms/0.5ml vaccine suspension for injection pre-filled syringes | 1 pre-filled disposable injection PoM £38.10 DT = £38.10

▸ **HBVAXPRO** (Merck Sharp & Dohme (UK) Ltd)

Hepatitis B virus surface antigen 10 microgram per 1 ml HBVAXPRO 10micrograms/1ml vaccine suspension for injection pre-filled syringes | 1 pre-filled disposable injection PoM £12.20 HBVAXPRO 5micrograms/0.5ml vaccine suspension for injection pre-filled syringes | 1 pre-filled disposable injection PoM £8.95 DT = £8.95

Hepatitis B virus surface antigen 40 microgram per 1 ml HBvaxPRO 40micrograms/1ml vaccine suspension for injection vials | 1 vial PoM £27.60 DT = £27.60

F 986

Human papillomavirus vaccine

19-Jul-2024

14 Vaccines

- **DRUG ACTION** Human papillomavirus vaccine is a non-live vaccine that contains adsorbed virus-like particles made from recombinant proteins.

- **INDICATIONS AND DOSE**

Primary immunisation against HPV-related premalignant lesions and cancer (cervical, vulvar, vaginal, and anal) and genital warts [1-dose schedule]

▸ BY INTRAMUSCULAR INJECTION

▸ Child 11–17 years: 0.5 mL for 1 dose

Immunisation against HPV-related premalignant lesions and cancer (cervical, vulvar, vaginal, and anal) and genital warts [3-dose schedule for immunocompromised or HIV-positive patients]

▸ BY INTRAMUSCULAR INJECTION

▸ Child 11–17 years: 0.5 mL for 1 dose, followed by 0.5 mL for 1 dose, second dose to be given at least 1 month after the first dose, then 0.5 mL for 1 dose, third dose to be given at least 3 months after the second dose, the 3-dose schedule should be completed within 12 months of the first dose, if the schedule is interrupted, it should be resumed but not repeated, allowing the appropriate interval between the remaining doses

- **UNLICENSED USE** UKHSA advises that *Gardasil®* 9 is used in a 1-dose immunisation schedule, but this is not licensed.

- **SIDE-EFFECTS**

▸ **Uncommon** Asthenia · chills · syncope

▸ **Frequency not known** Acute disseminated encephalomyelitis · bronchospasm · Guillain-Barre syndrome · immune thrombocytopenic purpura

- **PREGNANCY** Not known to be harmful, but vaccination should be postponed until completion of pregnancy.

- **DIRECTIONS FOR ADMINISTRATION** UKHSA advises that individuals with **bleeding disorders** may be vaccinated by the intramuscular route, on the advice of a doctor familiar with their bleeding risk. Patients treated with medicines to reduce bleeding (e.g. for haemophilia) are advised to administer their medicine shortly prior to intramuscular vaccination. Deltoid region or higher anterolateral thigh are preferred sites of injection.

- **MEDICINAL FORMS** There can be variation in the licensing of different medicines containing the same drug.

Suspension for injection

EXCIPIENTS: May contain Polysorbates

▸ **Gardasil 9** (Merck Sharp & Dohme (UK) Ltd)

Gardasil 9 vaccine suspension for injection 0.5ml pre-filled syringes | 1 pre-filled disposable injection PoM £105.00 DT = £105.00

F 986

Influenza vaccine (inactivated)

22-Aug-2025

- **DRUG ACTION** The inactivated influenza vaccines are injectable inactivated, or recombinant, vaccines that protect people at high risk from influenza and reduce transmission of infection. For information on the live vaccine, see influenza vaccine (live) p. 1001.

- **INDICATIONS AND DOSE**

Annual immunisation against seasonal influenza

▸ BY INTRAMUSCULAR INJECTION

▸ Child 6 months–17 years: 0.5 mL for 1 dose

Annual immunisation against seasonal influenza (for children in clinical risk groups, or who are household contacts of others in clinical risk groups, and who have not received seasonal influenza vaccine previously)

▸ BY INTRAMUSCULAR INJECTION

▸ Child 6 months–8 years: 0.5 mL for 1 dose, followed by 0.5 mL for 1 dose, after at least 4 weeks

- **UNLICENSED USE** The Joint Committee on Vaccination and Immunisation advises offering a second dose of vaccine for annual immunisation against seasonal influenza to children in clinical risk groups only, but this differs from licensed advice.

- **SIDE-EFFECTS**

▸ **Common or very common** Appetite change · chills · drowsiness · hyperhidrosis · irritability · local reactions · pain

▸ **Frequency not known** Angioedema · encephalomyelitis · febrile seizure · nerve disorders · nervous system disorder · paraesthesia · thrombocytopenia · vasculitis

- **ALLERGY AND CROSS-SENSITIVITY** UKHSA advises individuals with a history of egg allergy can be immunised with either an egg free influenza vaccine, if available, or an influenza vaccine with an ovalbumin content less than 120 nanograms/mL (facilities should be available to treat anaphylaxis). If an influenza vaccine containing ovalbumin is being considered in those with a history of severe anaphylaxis to egg which has previously required intensive care, these individuals should be referred to a specialist in hospital.

- **PREGNANCY** EvGr Inactivated vaccines not known to be harmful; however, the adjuvanted trivalent influenza vaccine (surface antigen, inactivated) manufactured by Seqirus is not indicated in pregnant females. ⟨M⟩

- **BREAST FEEDING** EvGr Inactivated vaccines not known to be harmful; however, the adjuvanted trivalent influenza vaccine (surface antigen, inactivated) manufactured by Seqirus is not indicated in breast-feeding females. ⟨M⟩

- **DIRECTIONS FOR ADMINISTRATION** UKHSA advises that individuals with **bleeding disorders** may be vaccinated by the intramuscular route, on the advice of a doctor familiar with their bleeding risk. Patients treated with medicines to reduce bleeding (e.g. for haemophilia) are advised to administer their medicine shortly prior to intramuscular vaccination.

- **PRESCRIBING AND DISPENSING INFORMATION** The available preparations are not licensed for use in all age-groups—further information can be found in the product literature for the individual vaccines. For choice of vaccine, see Influenza vaccine p. 971.

Ovalbumin content Preparations with a very low ovalbumin content of less than 120 nanograms/mL: the egg-cultured trivalent influenza vaccine (split virion, inactivated) manufactured by Sanofi (*Vaxigrip®*).

Preparations that are egg-free: the cell-cultured trivalent influenza vaccine (surface antigen, inactivated) manufactured by Seqirus.

● **MEDICINAL FORMS** There can be variation in the licensing of different medicines containing the same drug.

Suspension for injection

EXCIPIENTS: May contain Gentamicin, kanamycin, neomycin, polysorbates

▸ **Influenza vaccine (inactivated) (non-proprietary)** ▼
Cell-based trivalent influenza vaccine (surface antigen, inactivated) suspension for injection 0.5ml pre-filled syringes | 1 pre-filled disposable injection [PoM] £17.55 | 10 pre-filled disposable injection [PoM] £175.50
Influenza TIV MYL vaccine suspension for injection 0.5ml pre-filled syringes | 10 pre-filled disposable injection [PoM] £80.00
Adjuvanted trivalent influenza vaccine (surface antigen, inactivated) suspension for injection 0.5ml pre-filled syringes | 1 pre-filled disposable injection [PoM] £17.55 | 10 pre-filled disposable injection [PoM] £175.50

▸ **Efluelda Trivalent** (Sanofi) ▼
Efluelda Trivalent influenza vaccine (split virion, inactivated) High Dose suspension for injection 0.5ml pre-filled syringes | 10 pre-filled disposable injection [PoM] £220.00

▸ **Vaxigrip Trivalent** (Sanofi)
Vaxigrip Trivalent influenza vaccine (split virion, inactivated) suspension for injection 0.5ml pre-filled syringes | 1 pre-filled disposable injection [PoM] £8.00 | 10 pre-filled disposable injection [PoM] £80.00

986

Japanese encephalitis vaccine

25-Aug-2023

● **DRUG ACTION** Japanese encephalitis vaccine is an inactivated vaccine containing adsorbed Japanese encephalitis virus.

● **INDICATIONS AND DOSE**

Immunisation against Japanese encephalitis

▶ BY INTRAMUSCULAR INJECTION

▸ Child 2–35 months: 0.25 mL every 28 days for 2 doses, alternatively 0.25 mL every 7 days for 2 doses, anterolateral thigh may be used as the injection site in infants; deltoid muscle is preferred site in older children, immunisation should be completed at least 1 week before potential exposure

▸ Child 3–17 years: 0.5 mL every 28 days for 2 doses, alternatively 0.5 mL every 7 days for 2 doses, deltoid muscle is preferred site in older children, immunisation should be completed at least 1 week before potential exposure

First booster

▶ BY INTRAMUSCULAR INJECTION

▸ Child 14–35 months: 0.25 mL after 1–2 years, anterolateral thigh may be used as the injection site in infants; deltoid muscle is preferred site in older children, for those at continued risk, the booster dose should be given 1 year after completing the primary course

▸ Child 3–17 years: 0.5 mL after 1–2 years, deltoid muscle is preferred site in older children, for those at continued risk, the booster dose should be given 1 year after completing the primary course

● **UNLICENSED USE** The rapid schedule administered at days 0 and 7 is not licensed in children.

● **SIDE-EFFECTS** Cough · influenza like illness · irritability

● **PREGNANCY** Although manufacturer advises avoid because of limited information, miscarriage has been associated with Japanese encephalitis virus infection acquired during the first 2 trimesters of pregnancy.

● **MEDICINAL FORMS** There can be variation in the licensing of different medicines containing the same drug.

Solution for injection

▸ **Japanese encephalitis vaccine (Non-proprietary)**
Japanese encephalitis GCVC vaccine solution for injection 1ml vials | 1 vial [X]
Japanese encephalitis GCVC vaccine solution for injection 20ml vials | 1 vial [X]
Japanese encephalitis GCVC vaccine solution for injection 10ml vials | 1 vial [X]

Suspension for injection

▸ **Ixiaro** (Valneva UK Ltd)
Ixiaro vaccine suspension for injection 0.5ml pre-filled syringes | 1 pre-filled disposable injection [PoM] £62.48 DT = £62.48

986

Meningococcal group B vaccine

20-Apr-2026

● **DRUG ACTION** Meningococcal group B vaccine is a non-live vaccine that contains adsorbed recombinant *Neisseria meningitidis* serogroup B proteins.

● **INDICATIONS AND DOSE**

BEXSERO®

Primary immunisation against *Neisseria meningitidis* group B

▶ BY INTRAMUSCULAR INJECTION

▸ Child 2–3 months: 0.5 mL for 2 doses, first dose to be given at 8 weeks of age and second dose to be given at 12 weeks of age

Immunisation against *Neisseria meningitidis* group B [booster dose]

▶ BY INTRAMUSCULAR INJECTION

▸ Child 1 year: 0.5 mL for 1 dose

Immunisation against *Neisseria meningitidis* group B [patients with unknown or incomplete immunisation status presenting before 1 year of age]

▶ BY INTRAMUSCULAR INJECTION

▸ Child 3–11 months: 0.5 mL for 3 doses, first and second doses separated by an interval of at least 4 weeks, then third dose to be given between 1 and 2 years of age and at least 4 weeks after the second dose

Immunisation against *Neisseria meningitidis* group B [patients with unknown or incomplete immunisation status presenting after 1 year of age]

▶ BY INTRAMUSCULAR INJECTION

▸ Child 12–23 months: 0.5 mL for 2 doses, doses to be separated by an interval of at least 4 weeks

TRUMENBA®

Immunisation against *Neisseria meningitidis*, primary immunisation

▶ BY INTRAMUSCULAR INJECTION

▸ Child 10–17 years: 0.5 mL for 2 doses, separated by an interval of 6 months, alternatively 0.5 mL for 2 doses, separated by an interval of at least 1 month, followed by 0.5 mL as a third dose, given at least 4 months after the second dose, injected preferably into deltoid region, a booster dose should be considered for individuals at continued risk—consult product literature

● **SIDE-EFFECTS**

▶ **Common or very common** Crying abnormal · drowsiness · eating disorder · irritability

▶ **Uncommon** Seizures · vascular disorders

▶ **Frequency not known** Extensive swelling of vaccinated limb · hypotonic-hyporesponsiveness episode · meningism

● **DIRECTIONS FOR ADMINISTRATION**

BEXSERO® Anterolateral thigh is the preferred site of injection in infants under 1 year of age; deltoid muscle is preferred in older children and adults.

● **PRESCRIBING AND DISPENSING INFORMATION** Details on routine immunisations are included in this monograph; for details of immunisation in other patient groups e.g. patients at high risk of infection, see Meningococcal vaccines p. 973 and Vaccination, general principles p. 959.

BEXSERO® For information about the use of paracetamol for prophylaxis of post-immunisation pyrexia, see paracetamol p. 325.

● **MEDICINAL FORMS** There can be variation in the licensing of different medicines containing the same drug.

Suspension for injection

EXCIPIENTS: May contain Kanamycin

▸ **Bexsero** (GlaxoSmithKline UK Ltd)
Bexsero vaccine suspension for injection 0.5ml pre-filled syringes | 1 pre-filled disposable injection [PoM] £75.00 | 10 pre-filled disposable injection [PoM] £750.00

▸ **Trumenba** (Pfizer Ltd)
Trumenba vaccine suspension for injection 0.5ml pre-filled syringes | 1 pre-filled disposable injection [PoM] £75.00

986

Meningococcal groups A, C, W135, and Y vaccine

20-Apr-2026

● **DRUG ACTION** Meningococcal groups A, C, W135, and Y vaccine is a non-live conjugated vaccine.

● **INDICATIONS AND DOSE**

Primary immunisation against *Neisseria meningitidis* groups A, W135 and Y, and immunisation against *Neisseria meningitidis* group C (booster dose in those who have received primary immunisation)

▸ BY INTRAMUSCULAR INJECTION
▸ Child 13–15 years: 0.5 mL for 1 dose

Immunisation against *Neisseria meningitidis* groups A, C, W135 and Y [patients with unknown or incomplete immunisation status]

▸ BY INTRAMUSCULAR INJECTION
▸ Child 10–17 years: 0.5 mL for 1 dose

● **UNLICENSED USE** *Menveo*® is not licensed for use in children under 2 years. *MenQuadfi*® is not licensed for use in children under 1 year. *Nimenrix*® is not licensed for use in children under 6 weeks of age.

● **SIDE-EFFECTS**
▸ **Common or very common** Drowsiness · irritability
▸ **Uncommon** Crying · insomnia · numbness · pain in extremity
▸ **Frequency not known** Extensive swelling of vaccinated limb

● **DIRECTIONS FOR ADMINISTRATION** Deltoid muscle is preferred site of injection in older children and adults.

● **PRESCRIBING AND DISPENSING INFORMATION** Details on routine immunisations are included in this monograph; for details of immunisation in other patient groups e.g. patients at high risk of infection, see Meningococcal vaccines p. 973 and Vaccination, general principles p. 959.

● **MEDICINAL FORMS** There can be variation in the licensing of different medicines containing the same drug.

Solution for injection

▸ **MenQuadfi** (Sanofi)
MenQuadfi vaccine solution for injection 0.5ml vials | 1 vial [PoM] £31.50

Powder and solvent for solution for injection

EXCIPIENTS: May contain Sucrose

▸ **Menveo** (GlaxoSmithKline UK Ltd)
Menveo vaccine powder and solvent for solution for injection 0.5ml vials | 1 vial [PoM] £30.00 DT = £30.00

▸ **Nimenrix** (Pfizer Ltd)
Nimenrix vaccine powder and solvent for solution for injection 0.5ml pre-filled syringes | 1 pre-filled disposable injection [PoM] £30.00 DT = £30.00

986

Pneumococcal polysaccharide conjugate vaccine

20-Apr-2026

● **DRUG ACTION** Pneumococcal polysaccharide conjugate vaccine is an inactivated vaccine that protects against infection caused by *Streptococcus pneumoniae*. The conjugate vaccine contains adsorbed pneumococcal polysaccharide from either 13 capsular types (13-valent *Prevenar 13*®), 15 capsular types (15-valent *Vaxneuvance*®), or 20 capsular types (20-valent *Prevenar 20*®).

● **INDICATIONS AND DOSE**

Primary immunisation against pneumococcal infection

▸ BY INTRAMUSCULAR INJECTION
▸ Child 16 weeks: 0.5 mL for 1 dose

Immunisation against pneumococcal infection [booster dose]

▸ BY INTRAMUSCULAR INJECTION
▸ Child 1 year: 0.5 mL for 1 dose

Immunisation against pneumococcal infection [in patients with unknown or incomplete immunisation status]

▸ BY INTRAMUSCULAR INJECTION
▸ Child 4–11 months: 0.5 mL for 1 dose, followed by 0.5 mL for 1 dose, to be given on or after their first birthday at least 4 weeks after the first dose
▸ Child 12–23 months: 0.5 mL for 1 dose

● **SIDE-EFFECTS**
▸ **Common or very common** Drowsiness · irritability · sleep disorder
▸ **Uncommon** Crying · seizures
▸ **Rare or very rare** Hypotonic-hyporesponsiveness episode

● **DIRECTIONS FOR ADMINISTRATION** Anterolateral thigh is preferred site of injection in infants under 1 year; deltoid muscle is preferred in older children and adults.

● **PRESCRIBING AND DISPENSING INFORMATION** Details on routine immunisations are included in this monograph; for choice of vaccine and details of immunisation in other patient groups e.g. patients at high risk of infection, see Pneumococcal vaccine p. 975 and Vaccination, general principles p. 959.

Available as part of childhood immunisation schedule from ImmForm.

● **MEDICINAL FORMS** There can be variation in the licensing of different medicines containing the same drug.

Suspension for injection

▸ **Apexxnar** (Pfizer Ltd) ▼
Prevenar 20 vaccine suspension for injection 0.5ml pre-filled syringes | 1 pre-filled disposable injection [PoM] £56.50 DT = £49.10

▸ **Prevenar** (Pfizer Ltd)
Prevenar 13 vaccine suspension for injection 0.5ml pre-filled syringes | 1 pre-filled disposable injection [PoM] £49.10 DT = £49.10 | 10 pre-filled disposable injection [PoM] £491.00

▸ **Vaxneuvance** (Merck Sharp & Dohme (UK) Ltd) ▼
Vaxneuvance vaccine suspension for injection 0.5ml pre-filled syringes | 1 pre-filled disposable injection [PoM] £50.30 DT = £49.10 (Hospital only)

986

Rabies vaccine

19-Dec-2024

- **DRUG ACTION** Rabies vaccine is an inactivated vaccine containing rabies virus.

- **INDICATIONS AND DOSE**

RABIPUR®

Primary pre-exposure immunisation against rabies infection
- ▶ BY INTRAMUSCULAR INJECTION
- ▶ Child: 1 mL for 3 doses (on days 0, 7, and 28), final dose may be given from day 21 if insufficient time before travel

Primary pre-exposure immunisation against rabies infection [accelerated course]
- ▶ BY INTRAMUSCULAR INJECTION
- ▶ Child: 1 mL for 3 doses (on days 0, 3, and 7), followed by 1 mL for 1 dose, to be given at 1 year if continued travel to high-risk areas

Pre-exposure immunisation booster dose [patients at frequent risk of exposure e.g. laboratory workers who handle lyssavirus-containing material]
- ▶ BY INTRAMUSCULAR INJECTION
- ▶ Child: 1 mL for 1 dose, to be given 1 year after primary course is completed, then 1 mL, repeated if necessary, based on six-monthly antibody levels

Pre-exposure immunisation booster dose [patients who may have frequent, unrecognised exposures e.g. bat handlers]
- ▶ BY INTRAMUSCULAR INJECTION
- ▶ Child: 1 mL for 1 dose, to be given 1 year after primary course is completed, then 1 mL, repeated if necessary, based on antibody levels

Pre-exposure immunisation booster dose [patients at infrequent risk of exposure]
- ▶ BY INTRAMUSCULAR INJECTION
- ▶ Child: 1 mL for 1 dose, to be given at least 1 year after primary course is completed based on antibody levels

Post-exposure treatment [fully immunised patients with amber or red composite rabies risk] (administered on expert advice)
- ▶ BY INTRAMUSCULAR INJECTION
- ▶ Child: 1 mL for 1 dose, followed by 1 mL for 1 dose, to be given 3–7 days after the first dose, rabies immunoglobulin is not necessary

Post-exposure treatment [partially immunised patients with amber or red composite rabies risk] (administered on expert advice)
- ▶ BY INTRAMUSCULAR INJECTION
- ▶ Child: 1 mL for 4 doses (on days 0, 3, 7, and 21), rabies immunoglobulin is not necessary

Post-exposure treatment [non-immunised patients with amber or red composite rabies risk] (administered on expert advice)
- ▶ BY INTRAMUSCULAR INJECTION
- ▶ Child: 1 mL for 4 doses (on days 0, 3, 7, and 21), rabies immunoglobulin also to be given to patients with red composite rabies risk (but is not required if more than 7 days have elapsed after the first dose of vaccine, or more than 1 day after the second dose of vaccine)

Post-exposure treatment [immunosuppressed patients with amber or red composite rabies risk, regardless of immunisation status] (administered on expert advice)
- ▶ BY INTRAMUSCULAR INJECTION
- ▶ Child: 1 mL for 5 doses (on days 0, 3, 7, 14, and 30), rabies immunoglobulin also to be given

VERORAB®

Primary pre-exposure immunisation against rabies infection
- ▶ BY INTRAMUSCULAR INJECTION
- ▶ Child: 0.5 mL for 3 doses (on days 0, 7, and 28), final dose may be given from day 21 if insufficient time before travel

Primary pre-exposure immunisation against rabies infection [accelerated course]
- ▶ BY INTRAMUSCULAR INJECTION
- ▶ Child: 0.5 mL for 3 doses (on days 0, 3, and 7), followed by 0.5 mL for 1 dose, to be given at 1 year if continued travel to high-risk areas

Pre-exposure immunisation booster dose [patients at frequent risk of exposure e.g. laboratory workers who handle lyssavirus-containing material]
- ▶ BY INTRAMUSCULAR INJECTION
- ▶ Child: 0.5 mL for 1 dose, to be given 1 year after primary course is completed, then 0.5 mL, repeated if necessary, based on six-monthly antibody levels

Pre-exposure immunisation booster dose [patients who may have frequent, unrecognised exposures e.g. bat handlers]
- ▶ BY INTRAMUSCULAR INJECTION
- ▶ Child: 0.5 mL for 1 dose, to be given 1 year after primary course is completed, then 0.5 mL, repeated if necessary, based on antibody levels

Pre-exposure immunisation booster dose [patients at infrequent risk of exposure]
- ▶ BY INTRAMUSCULAR INJECTION
- ▶ Child: 0.5 mL for 1 dose, to be given at least 1 year after primary course is completed based on antibody levels

Post-exposure treatment [fully immunised patients with amber or red composite rabies risk] (administered on expert advice)
- ▶ BY INTRAMUSCULAR INJECTION
- ▶ Child: 0.5 mL for 1 dose, followed by 0.5 mL for 1 dose, to be given 3–7 days after the first dose, rabies immunoglobulin is not necessary

Post-exposure treatment [partially immunised patients with amber or red composite rabies risk] (administered on expert advice)
- ▶ BY INTRAMUSCULAR INJECTION
- ▶ Child: 0.5 mL for 4 doses (on days 0, 3, 7, and 21), rabies immunoglobulin is not necessary

Post-exposure treatment [non-immunised patients with amber or red composite rabies risk] (administered on expert advice)
- ▶ BY INTRAMUSCULAR INJECTION
- ▶ Child: 0.5 mL for 4 doses (on days 0, 3, 7, and 21), rabies immunoglobulin also to be given to patients with red composite rabies risk (but is not required if more than 7 days have elapsed after the first dose of vaccine, or more than 1 day after the second dose of vaccine)

Post-exposure treatment [immunosuppressed patients with amber or red composite rabies risk, regardless of immunisation status] (administered on expert advice)
- ▶ BY INTRAMUSCULAR INJECTION
- ▶ Child: 0.5 mL for 5 doses (on days 0, 3, 7, 14, and 30), rabies immunoglobulin also to be given

- **UNLICENSED USE** Public Health England advises rabies vaccine may be used as detailed below, although these situations are considered unlicensed:
  - dosing regimens for post-exposure treatment.
- **INTERACTIONS** → Appendix 1: rabies vaccine
- **SIDE-EFFECTS**
- ▶ **Common or very common** Abdominal discomfort · asthenia

▸ **Rare or very rare** Angioedema · chills · encephalitis · Guillain-Barre syndrome · hyperhidrosis · paraesthesia · syncope · vertigo

● **ALLERGY AND CROSS-SENSITIVITY**

RABIPUR® ▸ When used for Pre-exposure immunisation PHE advises to consider alternative rabies vaccine in individuals with a history of severe egg allergy.

▸ When used for Post-exposure treatment PHE advises it is not contra-indicated in individuals with severe egg allergies; if there is a history of hypersensitivity, specialist advice should be sought and further doses given under supervision.

● **PREGNANCY** Because of the potential consequences of untreated rabies exposure and because rabies vaccination has not been associated with fetal abnormalities, pregnancy is not considered a contra-indication to post-exposure prophylaxis. Immunisation against rabies is indicated during pregnancy if there is substantial risk of exposure to rabies and rapid access to post-exposure prophylaxis is likely to be limited.

● **DIRECTIONS FOR ADMINISTRATION** Anterolateral thigh is preferred site of injection in infants under 1 year of age; deltoid muscle is preferred in older children and adults.

● **PRESCRIBING AND DISPENSING INFORMATION**
Ovalbumin content *Rabipur*® contains residues of chicken proteins, such as ovalbumin.

● **MEDICINAL FORMS** There can be variation in the licensing of different medicines containing the same drug.

Powder and solvent for suspension for injection

EXCIPIENTS: May contain Maltose, neomycin, phenylalanine, polymyxin b, streptomycin

▸ **Verorab** (Sanofi)
Verorab powder and solvent for suspension for injection 0.5ml vials | 1 vial PoM £72.29

Powder and solvent for solution for injection

EXCIPIENTS: May contain Neomycin, sucrose

▸ **Rabipur** (Bavarian Nordic UK Ltd)
Rabipur vaccine powder and solvent for solution for injection 1ml pre-filled syringes | 1 pre-filled disposable injection PoM £48.19

F 986

Respiratory syncytial virus vaccine

21-Apr-2026

(RSV vaccine)

● **DRUG ACTION** *Abrysvo*® contains recombinant prefusion F proteins from both respiratory syncytial virus subtypes, A and B, which elicit an immune response against the virus; infants gain protection via transplacental transfer of neutralising antibodies.

● **INDICATIONS AND DOSE**

ABRYSVO®

Passive immunisation against respiratory syncytial virus [pregnant females from week 28 gestation; as part of the national immunisation programme]

▸ BY INTRAMUSCULAR INJECTION

▸ Females of childbearing potential: 0.5 mL for 1 dose

● **UNLICENSED USE**

ABRYSVO® UKHSA advises that *Abrysvo*® may be used as detailed below, although these situations are considered unlicensed:

- in pregnant females aged less than 18 years;
- in pregnant females after 36 weeks gestation.

IMPORTANT SAFETY INFORMATION

MHRA/CHM ADVICE: *ABRYSVO*® (PFIZER RSV VACCINE): BE ALERT TO A SMALL RISK OF GUILLAIN-BARRÉ SYNDROME FOLLOWING VACCINATION IN OLDER ADULTS (JULY 2025)

The MHRA has received a small number of reports of suspected Guillain-Barré syndrome in older adults after vaccination with *Abrysvo*® and further data have confirmed the risk in older adults is rare. Healthcare professionals are advised to be alert for signs and symptoms of Guillain-Barré syndrome in **all** patients receiving *Abrysvo*®. Patients or their carers should be counselled to seek urgent medical attention if symptoms such as paraesthesia in the hands and feet occur, as early intervention improves outcomes.

The CHM advises that the benefits of immunisation against RSV outweigh the small increased risk of Guillain-Barré syndrome in older adults. There is currently no evidence of this risk in pregnant females receiving *Abrysvo*®.

● **SIDE-EFFECTS**

▸ **Common or very common** Vaccination reactions

● **BREAST FEEDING** Specialist sources indicate not known to be harmful.

● **DIRECTIONS FOR ADMINISTRATION** UKHSA advises that individuals with **bleeding disorders** may be vaccinated by the intramuscular route, on the advice of a doctor familiar with their bleeding risk. Patients treated with medicines to reduce bleeding (e.g. for haemophilia) are advised to administer their medicine shortly prior to intramuscular vaccination. Deltoid muscle is preferred site of injection.

● **PRESCRIBING AND DISPENSING INFORMATION** For further information on timing of vaccination and eligibility, see Respiratory syncytial virus immunisation p. 979.

● **MEDICINAL FORMS** There can be variation in the licensing of different medicines containing the same drug.

Powder and solvent for solution for injection

EXCIPIENTS: May contain Polysorbates

▸ **Abrysvo** (Pfizer Ltd) ▼
Abrysvo vaccine powder and solvent for solution for injection 0.5ml vials | 1 vial PoM £158.00

F 986

Smallpox and mpox vaccines

30-Mar-2026

● **DRUG ACTION** Smallpox and mpox vaccines are inactivated vaccines containing live modified vaccinia virus Ankara (MVA-BN) that is replication-defective.

● **INDICATIONS AND DOSE**

Pre-exposure immunisation against smallpox and mpox [in patients previously unvaccinated against smallpox]

▸ BY DEEP SUBCUTANEOUS INJECTION, OR BY INTRAMUSCULAR INJECTION

▸ Child: 0.5 mL for 1 dose, then 0.5 mL for 1 dose, to be given at least 28 days after initial dose—a longer interval increases duration of protection

Pre-exposure immunisation against smallpox and mpox [in patients previously vaccinated against smallpox] | Post-exposure prophylaxis against smallpox and mpox

▸ BY DEEP SUBCUTANEOUS INJECTION, OR BY INTRAMUSCULAR INJECTION

▸ Child: 0.5 mL for 1 dose

● **UNLICENSED USE** UKHSA advises that *Imvanex*® is used for pre-exposure immunisation and post-exposure prophylaxis against smallpox and mpox in children, but it is not licensed for this age group—advice from UKHSA should be sought.

● **CAUTIONS** Atopic dermatitis (increased risk of injection-site reactions and generalised symptoms)

● **SIDE-EFFECTS**

▸ **Common or very common** Appetite disorder · chills · pain

▸ **Uncommon** Chest pain · cough · flushing · increased risk of infection · laryngeal pain · limb swelling · musculoskeletal stiffness · paraesthesia · sleep disorder

▸ **Rare or very rare** Angioedema · asthenia · conjunctivitis · drowsiness · dry mouth · influenza like illness · migraine ·

muscle spasms · muscle weakness · oropharyngeal pain · peripheral neuropathy · peripheral oedema · subcutaneous nodule · sweat changes · tachycardia · vertigo

▸ **Frequency not known** Facial paralysis

● **ALLERGY AND CROSS-SENSITIVITY** EvGr Contra-indicated in individuals with history of hypersensitivity to benzonase, chicken protein, ciprofloxacin, or gentamicin (*Imvanex*® contains trace residues). ⟨M⟩

● **PREGNANCY** UKHSA advises not routinely recommended during pregnancy, however, consider use if potential benefit outweighs risk (limited information available).

● **BREAST FEEDING** EvGr Use only if potential benefit outweighs risk (limited information available). ⟨M⟩ UKHSA advises suitable for use in breast-feeding females who have a significant exposure to mpox, after discussion about the risks of mpox to themselves and the breast-fed infant.

● **DIRECTIONS FOR ADMINISTRATION** Anterolateral thigh is the preferred site of injection in infants under 1 year of age; deltoid region is preferred in older children.

● **HANDLING AND STORAGE** For *Imvanex*®, store in a freezer—consult product literature about storage temperatures, thawing, and storage after thawing.

● **MEDICINAL FORMS** There can be variation in the licensing of different medicines containing the same drug.

Suspension for injection

EXCIPIENTS: May contain Gentamicin

▸ **Smallpox and mpox vaccines (non-proprietary)** ▼
Imvanex vaccine suspension for injection 0.5ml vials | 10 vial PoM (Hospital only)
Jynneos vaccine suspension for injection 0.5ml vials | 20 vial PoM (Hospital only)

▸ **Imvanex** (Bavarian Nordic UK Ltd) ▼
Imvanex vaccine suspension for injection 0.5ml vials | 10 vial PoM £1,850.00 (Hospital only) | 20 vial PoM £3,700.00 (Hospital only)

986

Tick-borne encephalitis vaccine

25-Aug-2023

● **DRUG ACTION** Tick-borne encephalitis vaccine is an inactivated vaccine containing adsorbed tick-borne encephalitis virus.

● **INDICATIONS AND DOSE**

Initial immunisation against tick-borne encephalitis

▸ BY INTRAMUSCULAR INJECTION

▸ Child 1–15 years: 0.25 mL for 1 dose, followed by 0.25 mL after 1–3 months for 1 dose, then 0.25 mL after further 5–12 months for 1 dose, to achieve more rapid protection, second dose may be given 14 days after first dose, dose to be administered in deltoid region or anterolateral thigh in infants, in immunocompromised patients (including those receiving immunosuppressants), antibody concentration may be measured 4 weeks after second dose and dose repeated if protective levels not achieved

▸ Child 16–17 years: 0.5 mL for 1 dose, followed by 0.5 mL after 1–3 months for 1 dose, then 0.5 mL after further 5–12 months for 1 dose, to achieve more rapid protection, second dose may be given 14 days after first dose, dose to be administered in deltoid region, in immunocompromised patients (including those receiving immunosuppressants), antibody concentration may be measured 4 weeks after second dose and dose repeated if protective levels not achieved

Immunisation against tick-borne encephalitis, booster doses

▸ BY INTRAMUSCULAR INJECTION

▸ Child 1–17 years: First dose to be given within 3 years after initial course completed and then every 3–5 years, dose to be administered in deltoid region or anterolateral thigh in infants (consult product literature)

● **SIDE-EFFECTS**

▸ **Common or very common** Restlessness · sleep disorder

▸ **Uncommon** Chills

▸ **Rare or very rare** Asthenia · dyspepsia · dyspnoea · encephalitis · eye pain · gait abnormal · hyperhidrosis · influenza like illness · meningism · motor dysfunction · musculoskeletal stiffness · nerve disorders · oedema · pain · seizures · sensory disorder · tinnitus · vertigo · vision disorders

● **ALLERGY AND CROSS-SENSITIVITY** PHE advises individuals with evidence of previous anaphylactic reaction to egg should not be given tick-borne encephalitis vaccine.

● **MEDICINAL FORMS** There can be variation in the licensing of different medicines containing the same drug.

Suspension for injection

EXCIPIENTS: May contain Gentamicin, neomycin

▸ **TicoVac** (Pfizer Ltd)
TicoVac Junior vaccine suspension for injection 0.25ml pre-filled syringes | 1 pre-filled disposable injection PoM £28.00
TicoVac vaccine suspension for injection 0.5ml pre-filled syringes | 1 pre-filled disposable injection PoM £32.00

986

Typhoid vaccine (inactivated)

12-Sep-2023

● **DRUG ACTION** The inactivated typhoid vaccine is an injectable polysaccharide vaccine that protects against typhoid fever caused by *Salmonella typhi* infection. For information on the live vaccine, see typhoid vaccine (live) p. 1003.

● **INDICATIONS AND DOSE**

Immunisation against typhoid fever [in children at high risk of typhoid fever]

▸ BY INTRAMUSCULAR INJECTION

▸ Child 12–23 months: 0.5 mL for 1 dose, dose should be given at least 2 weeks before potential exposure to typhoid infection, response may be suboptimal

Immunisation against typhoid fever

▸ BY INTRAMUSCULAR INJECTION

▸ Child 2–17 years: 0.5 mL for 1 dose, dose should be given at least 2 weeks before potential exposure to typhoid infection

Booster

▸ BY INTRAMUSCULAR INJECTION

▸ Child 2–17 years: 0.5 mL for 1 dose every 3 years

● **UNLICENSED USE** UKHSA advises that inactivated typhoid vaccine may be used in children aged 12–23 months at high risk of typhoid fever, but it is not licensed for this age group.

● **SIDE-EFFECTS**

▸ **Common or very common** Asthenia

▸ **Frequency not known** Asthma · shock

● **MEDICINAL FORMS** There can be variation in the licensing of different medicines containing the same drug.

Solution for injection

▸ **Typhim Vi** (Sanofi)
Salmonella typhi Vi capsular polysaccharide 50 microgram per 1 ml Typhim Vi 25micrograms/0.5ml vaccine solution for injection pre-filled syringes | 1 pre-filled disposable injection PoM £11.16 DT = £11.16 | 10 pre-filled disposable injection PoM £111.60 DT = £111.60

14 Vaccines

VACCINES > LIVE

Vaccines, live

12-Sep-2023

IMPORTANT SAFETY INFORMATION

MHRA/CHM ADVICE (UPDATED NOVEMBER 2017)

Following reports of death in neonates who received a live attenuated vaccine after exposure to a tumor necrosis factor alpha (TNF-a) inhibitor *in utero*, the MHRA has issued the following advice:

- any infant who has been exposed to immunosuppressive treatment from the mother either *in utero* during pregnancy or via breastfeeding should have any live attenuated vaccination deferred for as long as a postnatal influence on the immune status of the infant remains possible;
- in the case of infants who have been exposed to TNF-a inhibitors and other immunosuppressive biological medicines *in utero*, UKHSA advise that any live attenuated vaccination (e.g. BCG vaccine) should be deferred until the infant is age 6 months;
- UKHSA advise if there is any doubt as to whether an infant due to receive a live attenuated vaccine may be immunosuppressed due to the mother's therapy, including exposure through breast-feeding, specialist advice should be sought.

● **CONTRA-INDICATIONS**

▸ Impaired immune response UKHSA advises severely immunosuppressed patients should not be given live vaccines (including those with severe primary immunodeficiency).

● **CAUTIONS**

▸ Impaired immune response and drugs affecting immune response There is a risk of generalised infection with live vaccines.

UKHSA advises seek specialist advice for immunosuppressed patients, including those who are:

- taking high doses of corticosteroids (dose equivalents of prednisolone: **adults**, at least 40 mg daily for more than 1 week or at least 20 mg daily for more than 14 days; **children**, 2 mg/kg (or more than 40 mg) daily for more than 1 week or 1 mg/kg (or more than 20 mg) daily for more than 14 days);
- taking immunosuppressive drugs;
- receiving treatment for malignant or non-malignant conditions with chemotherapy or generalised radiotherapy.

UKHSA advises live vaccines should be postponed until at least 3 months after stopping high-dose systemic corticosteroids, or non-biological oral immune modulating drugs; and at least 6 months after stopping other immunosuppressive drugs, or generalised radiotherapy; and at least 12 months after discontinuing immunosuppressive biological therapy.

● **SIDE-EFFECTS**

▸ **Common or very common** Abdominal pain · appetite decreased · arthralgia · diarrhoea · fever · headache · malaise · myalgia · nausea · skin reactions · vomiting

▸ **Uncommon** Dizziness

● **PREGNANCY** UKHSA advises live vaccines should not be administered routinely to pregnant women because of the theoretical risk of fetal infection, but where there is a significant risk of exposure to disease the need for vaccination may outweigh any possible risk to the fetus. Termination of pregnancy following inadvertent immunisation is not recommended.

● **BREAST FEEDING** Although there is a theoretical risk of live vaccine being present in breast milk, vaccination is not contra-indicated for women who are breast-feeding when there is significant risk of exposure to disease.

● **DIRECTIONS FOR ADMINISTRATION** Manufacturer advises if alcohol or disinfectant is used for cleansing the skin it should be allowed to evaporate before vaccination to prevent possible inactivation of live vaccines.

F above F 986

Bacillus Calmette-Guérin vaccine

25-Aug-2023

(BCG vaccine)

● **DRUG ACTION** BCG (Bacillus Calmette-Guérin) vaccine is a live attenuated vaccine derived from *Mycobacterium bovis*.

● **INDICATIONS AND DOSE**

Immunisation against tuberculosis

▸ BY INTRADERMAL INJECTION

▸ Neonate: 0.05 mL, to be injected at insertion of deltoid muscle onto humerus (keloid formation more likely with sites higher on arm); tip of shoulder should be **avoided**.

▸ Child 1–11 months: 0.05 mL, to be injected at insertion of deltoid muscle onto humerus (keloid formation more likely with sites higher on arm); tip of shoulder should be **avoided**

▸ Child 1–17 years: 0.1 mL, to be injected at insertion of deltoid muscle onto humerus (keloid formation more likely with sites higher on arm); tip of shoulder should be **avoided**

● **CONTRA-INDICATIONS** Children less than 2 years of age in household contact with known or suspected case of active tuberculosis · generalised septic skin conditions · history of active or latent tuberculosis · severe combined immunodeficiency disorder

CONTRA-INDICATIONS, FURTHER INFORMATION

Manufacturer advises using a lesion-free site to administer BCG vaccine to patients with eczema.

● **CAUTIONS** When BCG is given to infants, there is no need to delay routine primary immunisations. No further vaccination should be given in the arm used for BCG vaccination for at least 3 months because of the risk of regional lymphadenitis.

● **INTERACTIONS** → Appendix 1: live vaccines

● **SIDE-EFFECTS**

▸ **Uncommon** Lymphadenitis suppurative

▸ **Rare or very rare** Osteitis · osteomyelitis

▸ **Frequency not known** Seizure · syncope

● **PRE-TREATMENT SCREENING** Apart from children under 6 years, any person being considered for BCG immunisation must first be given a skin test for hypersensitivity to tuberculoprotein (see tuberculin purified protein derivative p. 959). A skin test is not necessary for a child under 6 years provided that the child has not stayed for longer than 3 months in a country with an incidence of tuberculosis greater than 40 per 100 000, the child has not had contact with a person with tuberculosis, and there is no family history of tuberculosis within the last 5 years.

PHE advise that the results of the severe combined immunodeficiency (SCID) screening should be checked before administering BCG vaccine.

● **DIRECTIONS FOR ADMINISTRATION**

Intradermal injection technique Public Health England advises skin is stretched between thumb and forefinger and needle (size 26G) inserted (bevel upwards) for about 3 mm into superficial layers of dermis (almost parallel with surface). Needle should be short with short bevel (can usually be seen through epidermis during insertion). Tense raised blanched bleb is sign of correct injection; 7 mm bleb ≡ 0.1 mL injection, 3 mm bleb ≡ 0.05 mL injection; if considerable resistance not felt, needle too deep and should be removed and reinserted before giving more vaccine. Jet injectors and multiple puncture devices should not be used.

- **PRESCRIBING AND DISPENSING INFORMATION** Available from health organisations or direct from ImmForm.

- **MEDICINAL FORMS** There can be variation in the licensing of different medicines containing the same drug.

Powder for injection

- **Bacillus calmette-guérin vaccine (Non-proprietary)**
  BCG Vaccine AJV powder for suspension for injection 1ml vials | 10 vial PoM

F 1000 F 986

Cholera vaccine (live)

29-Aug-2024

- **DRUG ACTION** The live cholera vaccine is an oral vaccine that contains live attenuated *Vibrio cholerae*. For information on the inactivated vaccine, see cholera vaccine (inactivated) p. 987.

- **INDICATIONS AND DOSE**

Immunisation against cholera
- BY MOUTH
  - Child 2–17 years: 1 dose, immunisation should be completed at least 10 days before potential exposure

- **CONTRA-INDICATIONS** Acute gastro-intestinal illness
- **INTERACTIONS** → Appendix 1: live vaccines
- **SIDE-EFFECTS**
  - **Uncommon** Burping · constipation · dry mouth · gastrointestinal discomfort · gastrointestinal disorders
  - **Rare or very rare** Chills
- **DIRECTIONS FOR ADMINISTRATION** Administration of *Vaxchora*® and oral typhoid vaccine (live) should be separated by a 2-hour interval—transit of the capsules through the gastro-intestinal tract may be affected by the buffer administered with *Vaxchora*®.
  EvGr Mix buffer powder in 100 mL of cold or room temperature bottled water; for children aged 2–5 years, discard half (50 mL) of the buffer solution. Add active component to the buffer solution and stir for at least 30 seconds to make one dose. Drink within 15 minutes of reconstitution. Food and drink should be avoided for 1 hour before and after vaccination. ⟨M⟩
- **PATIENT AND CARER ADVICE** Counselling on administration advised. Immunisation with cholera vaccine does not provide complete protection and all travellers to a country where cholera exists should be warned that scrupulous attention to food, water, and personal hygiene is **essential**. The live cholera vaccine virus may be excreted in the stool and could be transmitted to close contacts. UKHSA advises thorough handwashing after visiting the toilet and before preparing food for at least 14 days after immunisation.

- **MEDICINAL FORMS** There can be variation in the licensing of different medicines containing the same drug.

Effervescent powder and powder for oral suspension

EXCIPIENTS: May contain Sucrose
ELECTROLYTES: May contain Sodium

- **Vaxchora** (Bavarian Nordic UK Ltd)
  Vaxchora vaccine effervescent powder and powder for oral suspension | 1 dose PoM £43.20

F 1000 F 986

Dengue vaccine

24-Aug-2023

- **DRUG ACTION** Dengue vaccine is a live, attenuated vaccine that protects against dengue virus infection.

- **INDICATIONS AND DOSE**

Immunisation against dengue
- BY SUBCUTANEOUS INJECTION
  - Child 4–17 years: 0.5 mL for 1 dose, then 0.5 mL for 1 dose, to be given 3 months after initial dose

- **INTERACTIONS** → Appendix 1: live vaccines
- **SIDE-EFFECTS**
  - **Common or very common** Asthenia · drowsiness · increased risk of infection · influenza like illness · irritability
  - **Rare or very rare** Angioedema
- **CONCEPTION AND CONTRACEPTION** EvGr Avoid pregnancy for at least 1 month after vaccination. ⟨M⟩
- **DIRECTIONS FOR ADMINISTRATION** To be administered preferably into the deltoid region.
- **PATIENT AND CARER ADVICE** Immunisation with dengue vaccine does not provide complete protection and personal protective measures against mosquito bites are recommended.

- **MEDICINAL FORMS** There can be variation in the licensing of different medicines containing the same drug.

Powder and solvent for solution for injection

- **Qdenga** (Takeda UK Ltd) ▼
  Qdenga vaccine powder and solvent for solution for injection 0.5ml pre-filled syringes | 1 pre-filled disposable injection PoM £68.75

F 1000 F 986

Influenza vaccine (live)

26-Jun-2025

- **DRUG ACTION** The live influenza vaccine is a nasal spray containing live attenuated strains; it protects people at high risk from influenza and reduces transmission of infection. For information on the inactivated vaccines, see influenza vaccine (inactivated) p. 994.

- **INDICATIONS AND DOSE**

Annual immunisation against seasonal influenza
- BY INTRANASAL ADMINISTRATION
  - Child 2–17 years: 0.2 mL for 1 dose, to be administered as 0.1 mL into each nostril

Annual immunisation against seasonal influenza (for children in clinical risk groups, or who are household contacts of others in clinical risk groups, and who have not received seasonal influenza vaccine previously)
- BY INTRANASAL ADMINISTRATION
  - Child 2–8 years: 0.2 mL for 1 dose, followed by 0.2 mL for 1 dose, after at least 4 weeks. Dose to be administered as 0.1 mL into each nostril

- **UNLICENSED USE** The Joint Committee on Vaccination and Immunisation advises offering a second dose of vaccine for annual immunisation against seasonal influenza to children in clinical risk groups only, but this differs from licensed advice.
- **CONTRA-INDICATIONS** Active wheezing · concomitant use with antiviral therapy for influenza · concomitant use with salicylates · severe asthma

CONTRA-INDICATIONS, FURTHER INFORMATION
- Concomitant use with antiviral therapy for influenza UKHSA advises avoid immunisation for at least 48 hours after stopping the influenza antiviral agent. Administration of influenza antiviral agents within two weeks of *Fluenz*® administration may reduce the effectiveness of the vaccine.

- **CAUTIONS** Nasal congestion

  CAUTIONS, FURTHER INFORMATION EvGr Vaccination should be postponed in children with heavy nasal congestion due to the potential for reduced vaccine delivery, but may proceed if there are mild symptoms of a cold without congestion. ⟨M⟩
- **INTERACTIONS** → Appendix 1: live vaccines
- **SIDE-EFFECTS**
  - **Common or very common** Nasal complaints
  - **Uncommon** Epistaxis · face oedema
  - **Frequency not known** Guillain-Barre syndrome
- **ALLERGY AND CROSS-SENSITIVITY** UKHSA advises individuals with a history of egg allergy can be immunised with either an egg free influenza vaccine, if available, or an influenza vaccine with an ovalbumin content less than 120 nanograms/mL (facilities should be available to treat anaphylaxis). If an influenza vaccine containing ovalbumin is being considered in those with a history of severe anaphylaxis to egg which has previously required intensive care, these individuals should be referred to a specialist in hospital.
- **PREGNANCY** EvGr Avoid—limited information available. ⟨M⟩
- **BREAST FEEDING** EvGr Avoid—limited information available. ⟨M⟩
- **PRESCRIBING AND DISPENSING INFORMATION** For choice of vaccine, see Influenza vaccine p. 971.

  Ovalbumin content Preparations with a very low ovalbumin content of less than 120 nanograms/mL: *Fluenz*®.
- **PATIENT AND CARER ADVICE** Avoid close contact with severely immunocompromised patients for 1–2 weeks after vaccination.

- **MEDICINAL FORMS** There can be variation in the licensing of different medicines containing the same drug.

Spray

EXCIPIENTS: May contain Gelatin, gentamicin, sucrose

- **Fluenz** (AstraZeneca UK Ltd)

  Fluenz (trivalent) vaccine nasal suspension 0.2ml unit dose | 10 unit dose PoM £180.00

F 1000 F 986

Measles, mumps, and rubella vaccine

20-Apr-2026

(MMR vaccine)

- **DRUG ACTION** Measles, mumps, and rubella vaccine is a live, attenuated combination vaccine.

- **INDICATIONS AND DOSE**

Primary immunisation against measles, mumps, and rubella [first dose]

- BY INTRAMUSCULAR INJECTION
  - Child 1 year: 0.5 mL for 1 dose

Primary immunisation against measles, mumps, and rubella [second dose for children born on or after 1 July 2024]

- BY INTRAMUSCULAR INJECTION
  - Child 18 months: 0.5 mL for 1 dose

Primary immunisation against measles, mumps, and rubella [second dose for children born before 1 July 2024]

- BY INTRAMUSCULAR INJECTION
  - Child 40 months: 0.5 mL for 1 dose

Immunisation against measles, mumps, and rubella [patients with unknown or incomplete immunisation status]

- BY INTRAMUSCULAR INJECTION
  - Child 18 months–17 years: 0.5 mL for 2 doses, doses to be separated by an interval of at least 4 weeks

IMPORTANT SAFETY INFORMATION

MMR VACCINATION AND BOWEL DISEASE OR AUTISM

Reviews undertaken on behalf of the CSM, the Medical Research Council, and the Cochrane Collaboration, have not found any evidence of a link between MMR vaccination and bowel disease or autism. Information (including fact sheets and a list of references) may be obtained from www.dh.gov.uk/immunisation.

- **CAUTIONS** Antibody response to measles component may be reduced after immunoglobulin administration or blood transfusion—leave an interval of at least 3 months before MMR immunisation

  CAUTIONS, FURTHER INFORMATION
  - Administration with other vaccines Public Health England advises MMR and yellow fever vaccines should not be administered on the same day; there should be a 4-week minimum interval between the vaccines. When protection is rapidly required, the vaccines can be given at any interval; an additional dose of MMR should be considered and re-vaccination with the yellow fever vaccine can also be considered in those at on-going risk.

    Public Health England advises MMR and varicella-zoster vaccines can be given on the same day or separated by a 4-week minimum interval. When protection is rapidly required, the vaccines can be given at any interval and an additional dose of the vaccine given second may be considered.
- **INTERACTIONS** → Appendix 1: live vaccines
- **SIDE-EFFECTS**
  - **Uncommon** Crying · increased risk of infection · rhinorrhoea
  - **Frequency not known** Angioedema · arthritis · ataxia · bronchospasm · cough · encephalopathy · eye inflammation · irritability · meningitis aseptic · nerve deafness · nerve disorders · oculomotor nerve paralysis · oedema · panniculitis · papillitis · paraesthesia · pneumonitis · regional lymphadenopathy · seizures · Stevens-Johnson syndrome · subacute sclerosing panencephalitis · syncope · throat pain · thrombocytopenia · vasculitis

  SIDE-EFFECTS, FURTHER INFORMATION Malaise, fever, or a rash can occur after the first dose of MMR vaccine—most commonly about a week after vaccination and lasting about 2 to 3 days.

  Febrile seizures occur rarely 6 to 11 days after MMR vaccination (the incidence is lower than that following measles infection).

  Idiopathic thrombocytopenic purpura Idiopathic thrombocytopenic purpura has occurred rarely following MMR vaccination, usually within 6 weeks of the first dose. The risk of idiopathic thrombocytopenic purpura after MMR vaccine is much less than the risk after infection with wild measles or rubella virus. Children who develop idiopathic thrombocytopenic purpura within 6 weeks of the first dose of MMR should undergo serological testing before the second dose is due; if the results suggest incomplete immunity against measles, mumps or rubella then a second dose of MMR is recommended. Samples should be sent to the Virus Reference Laboratory of the Health Protection Agency.

  Frequency of side effects Adverse reactions are considerably less frequent after the second dose of MMR vaccine than after the first.

- **ALLERGY AND CROSS-SENSITIVITY** PHE advises MMR vaccine can be given safely even when the child has had an anaphylactic reaction to food containing egg. Children with a confirmed anaphylactic reaction to the MMR vaccine should be assessed by a specialist. Dislike of eggs, refusal to eat egg, or confirmed anaphylactic reactions to egg-containing food is not a contra-indication to MMR vaccination.
- **CONCEPTION AND CONTRACEPTION** Exclude pregnancy before immunisation. Avoid pregnancy for at least 1 month after vaccination.
- **PRESCRIBING AND DISPENSING INFORMATION** Details on routine immunisations are included in this monograph; for details of immunisation in other patient groups e.g. patients at high risk of infection, see Measles, Mumps and Rubella vaccine p. 972 and Vaccination, general principles p. 959.

  Available as part of childhood immunisation schedule from health organisations or ImmForm.

- **MEDICINAL FORMS** There can be variation in the licensing of different medicines containing the same drug.

Powder and solvent for suspension for injection

EXCIPIENTS: May contain Gelatin, neomycin

▸ **M-M-RVAXPRO** (Merck Sharp & Dohme (UK) Ltd)
M-M-RVAXPRO vaccine powder and solvent for suspension for injection 0.5ml pre-filled syringes | 1 pre-filled disposable injection PoM £11.00 DT = £11.00

Powder and solvent for solution for injection

EXCIPIENTS: May contain Neomycin

▸ **Priorix** (GlaxoSmithKline UK Ltd)
Priorix vaccine powder and solvent for solution for injection 0.5ml pre-filled syringes | 1 pre-filled disposable injection PoM £7.64 DT = £7.64

F 1000 F 986

Rotavirus vaccine

25-Aug-2023

- **DRUG ACTION** Rotavirus vaccine is a live, oral vaccine that protects against rotavirus gastro-enteritis.

- **INDICATIONS AND DOSE**

Immunisation against gastro-enteritis caused by rotavirus

▸ BY MOUTH

▸ Child 6–23 weeks: 1.5 mL for 2 doses separated by an interval of at least 4 weeks, first dose must be given between 6–14 weeks of age; course should be completed before 24 weeks of age (preferably before 16 weeks)

IMPORTANT SAFETY INFORMATION

PUBLIC HEALTH ENGLAND: UPDATE TO GREEN BOOK (OCTOBER 2017)

Public Health England advises that immunisation with live vaccines should be delayed until 6 months of age in children born to mothers who received immunosuppressive biological therapy during pregnancy. In practice, this means that children born to mothers who were on immunosuppressive biological therapy during pregnancy will not be eligible to receive rotavirus vaccine.

- **CONTRA-INDICATIONS** History of intussusception · predisposition to intussusception · severe combined immunodeficiency disorder

  CONTRA-INDICATIONS, FURTHER INFORMATION

  ▸ Immunosuppression With the exception of severe combined immunodeficiency disorder (and children born to mothers who received immunosuppressive biological therapy during pregnancy, see *Important safety information*), rotavirus vaccine is not contra-indicated in immunosuppressed patients—benefit from vaccination is likely to outweigh the risk, if there is any doubt, Public Health England recommends seek specialist advice.
- **CAUTIONS** Diarrhoea (postpone vaccination) · immunosuppressed close contacts · vomiting (postpone vaccination)

  CAUTIONS, FURTHER INFORMATION The rotavirus vaccine virus is excreted in the stool and may be transmitted to close contacts; however, Public Health England advises vaccination of those with immunosuppressed close contacts may protect the contacts from wild-type rotavirus disease and outweigh any risk from transmission of vaccine virus.
- **INTERACTIONS** → Appendix 1: live vaccines
- **SIDE-EFFECTS**
  - ▸ **Common or very common** Irritability
  - ▸ **Uncommon** Gastrointestinal disorders
  - ▸ **Frequency not known** Apnoea · haematochezia
- **PRE-TREATMENT SCREENING** PHE advise that the results of the severe combined immunodeficiency (SCID) screening should be checked before administering rotavirus vaccine.
- **PATIENT AND CARER ADVICE** The rotavirus vaccine virus is excreted in the stool and may be transmitted to close contacts; carers of a recently vaccinated baby should be advised of the need to wash their hands after changing the baby's nappies.

- **MEDICINAL FORMS** There can be variation in the licensing of different medicines containing the same drug.

Oral suspension

▸ **Rotarix** (GlaxoSmithKline UK Ltd)
Rotarix vaccine live oral suspension 1.5ml tube | 1 tube PoM £34.76 DT = £34.76 | 10 tube PoM £347.60

F 1000 F 986

Typhoid vaccine (live)

29-Aug-2024

- **DRUG ACTION** The live typhoid vaccine is an oral attenuated vaccine that protects against typhoid fever caused by *Salmonella typhi* infection. For information on the inactivated vaccine, see typhoid vaccine (inactivated) p. 999.

- **INDICATIONS AND DOSE**

Immunisation against typhoid fever

▸ BY MOUTH

▸ Child 5–17 years: 1 capsule every 2 days for 3 doses (on days 1, 3, and 5), course should be completed at least 1 week before potential exposure to typhoid infection

Booster

▸ BY MOUTH

▸ Child 5–17 years: 1 capsule every 2 days for 3 doses (on days 1, 3, and 5) every 3 years

- **CONTRA-INDICATIONS** Acute gastro-intestinal illness
- **INTERACTIONS** → Appendix 1: live vaccines
- **SIDE-EFFECTS** Abdominal distension · asthenia · back pain · chills · flatulence · influenza like illness · paraesthesia · shock
- **DIRECTIONS FOR ADMINISTRATION** Manufacturer advises capsule should be taken one hour before a meal. Swallow as soon as possible after placing in mouth with a cold or lukewarm drink.

  Administration of capsule and oral cholera vaccine (live) (*Vaxchora*®) should be separated by a 2-hour interval—transit of the capsules through the gastro-intestinal tract may be affected by the buffer administered with *Vaxchora*®.
- **HANDLING AND STORAGE** Store capsules in a refrigerator (2–8°C).
- **PATIENT AND CARER ADVICE** Patients or carers should be given advice on how to administer and store typhoid vaccine capsules.

14 Vaccines

- **MEDICINAL FORMS** There can be variation in the licensing of different medicines containing the same drug.

Gastro-resistant capsule

CAUTIONARY AND ADVISORY LABELS 25

- **Vivotif** (Bavarian Nordic UK Ltd)
  Vivotif vaccine gastro-resistant capsules | 3 capsule PoM £14.77 DT = £14.77

F 1000 F 986

Varicella-zoster vaccine

13-Oct-2025

- **DRUG ACTION** Varicella-zoster vaccines are live attenuated vaccines that protect against varicella (chickenpox) caused by varicella-zoster virus infection.

- **INDICATIONS AND DOSE**

Immunisation against varicella infection (chickenpox)

- BY SUBCUTANEOUS INJECTION, OR BY INTRAMUSCULAR INJECTION
  - Child 9-11 months: 0.5 mL for 1 dose, then 0.5 mL for 1 dose, to be given at least 12 weeks after initial dose
  - Child 1-12 years: 0.5 mL for 1 dose, then 0.5 mL for 1 dose, to be given at least 4 weeks after initial dose
  - Child 13-17 years: 0.5 mL for 1 dose, then 0.5 mL for 1 dose, to be given at least 6 weeks after initial dose

Post-exposure prophylaxis against varicella infection (chickenpox) during co-circulating group A streptococcal infection (e.g. scarlet fever)

- BY SUBCUTANEOUS INJECTION, OR BY INTRAMUSCULAR INJECTION
  - Child 9 months–17 years: 0.5 mL for 1 dose, then 0.5 mL for 1 dose, to be given 4 to 8 weeks after initial dose

- **CAUTIONS** Post-vaccination close contact with susceptible individuals

CAUTIONS, FURTHER INFORMATION UKHSA advises that the risk of transmission of varicella-zoster vaccine virus from immunocompetent vaccinated individuals to susceptible close contacts is very low. If a localised rash develops, the lesions should be covered to reduce the risk of transmission. The risk of transmission is higher with a disseminated rash.

UKHSA advises healthcare workers who develop a generalised papular or vesicular rash on vaccination should avoid contact with patients until the lesions have crusted. Those who develop a localised rash after vaccination should cover the lesions and be allowed to continue working unless in contact with patients at high risk of severe varicella.

- Administration with MMR vaccine UKHSA advises varicella–zoster and MMR vaccines can be given on the same day or separated by a 4-week minimum interval. When protection is rapidly required, the vaccines can be given at any interval and an additional dose of the vaccine given second may be considered.

- **INTERACTIONS** → Appendix 1: live vaccines
- **SIDE-EFFECTS**
  - **Uncommon** Cough · drowsiness · increased risk of infection · irritability
  - **Rare or very rare** Conjunctivitis · Kawasaki disease · seizure · thrombocytopenia · vasculitis
  - **Frequency not known** Encephalitis (including fatal cases) · stroke
- **CONCEPTION AND CONTRACEPTION** Manufacturer advises avoid pregnancy for 1 month after vaccination.
- **DIRECTIONS FOR ADMINISTRATION** To be administered into the deltoid region or anterolateral thigh (recommended in infants aged under 1 year).
- **PRESCRIBING AND DISPENSING INFORMATION** Advice in BNF Publications may differ from that in product literature.
- **MEDICINAL FORMS** There can be variation in the licensing of different medicines containing the same drug.

Powder and solvent for suspension for injection

EXCIPIENTS: May contain Gelatin, neomycin

- **Varivax** (Merck Sharp & Dohme (UK) Ltd)
  Varivax vaccine powder and solvent for suspension for injection 0.5ml vials | 1 vial PoM £30.28 DT = £30.28

Powder and solvent for solution for injection

EXCIPIENTS: May contain Neomycin, phenylalanine

- **Varilrix** (GlaxoSmithKline UK Ltd)
  Varilrix vaccine powder and solvent for solution for injection 0.5ml vials | 1 vial PoM £27.31 DT = £27.31

F 1000 F 986

Yellow fever vaccine

25-Aug-2023

- **DRUG ACTION** Yellow fever vaccine is a live attenuated vaccine.

- **INDICATIONS AND DOSE**

Immunisation against yellow fever

- BY DEEP SUBCUTANEOUS INJECTION
  - Child 6–8 months (administered on expert advice): Infants under 9 months should be vaccinated only if the risk of yellow fever is high and unavoidable (consult product literature or local protocols)
  - Child 9 months–17 years: 0.5 mL for 1 dose

IMPORTANT SAFETY INFORMATION

MHRA/CHM ADVICE (UPDATED NOVEMBER 2019): YELLOW FEVER VACCINE: STRONGER PRECAUTIONS IN PEOPLE WITH WEAKENED IMMUNITY

The yellow fever vaccine (*Stamaril*®) has been associated with the very rare, life-threatening reactions viscerotropic disease (YEL-AVD) and neurotropic disease (YEL-AND), which both resemble yellow fever infection. It must not be given to patients who have had a thymectomy, who are taking immunosuppressive or immunomodulating biological drugs, or who have a first-degree family history of YEL-AVD or YEL-AND following vaccination that was unrelated to a known medical risk factor. It must only be administered by healthcare professionals specifically trained in the benefit-risk evaluation of yellow fever vaccine. Healthcare professionals must inform patients and carers about the early signs and symptoms of YEL-AVD and YEL-AND, and advise them to seek urgent medical attention if they occur; the manufacturer's patient information leaflet should also be provided.

Healthcare professionals administering vaccines should consult information in the YF Vaccine Centre code of practice and strengthen protocols and checklists to avoid inappropriate administration.

MHRA/CHM ADVICE: YELLOW FEVER VACCINE (*STAMARIL*®): NEW PRE-VACCINATION CHECKLIST (NOVEMBER 2021)

A standardised pre-vaccination checklist has been introduced to ensure the yellow fever vaccine is indicated for the intended travel destination and to enable vaccinators to identify existing contra-indications or precautions in individuals before vaccination. Healthcare professionals are reminded to adhere to the contra-indications (for example, in people with immunosuppression or thymus dysfunction or thymectomy) and precautions (in infants aged 6 months to 9 months, and pregnant or breast-feeding females) as this is essential to reduce the risk of very rare but potentially fatal adverse reactions.

The new checklist should be used in vaccination consultations to ensure systematic evaluation of benefits and risks for individual travellers, this however is not a replacement for the full travel health risk assessment by a qualified practitioner and additional checklists or materials that may also be used prior to vaccination, depending on clinical guidance. Patients and carers should be provided with the patient information leaflet and advised to seek emergency medical attention if they develop signs or symptoms of a severe reaction following vaccination.

- **CONTRA-INDICATIONS** Children under 6 months · history of thymus dysfunction · thymectomy
- **CAUTIONS**
  - Administration with MMR vaccine Public Health England advises yellow fever and MMR vaccines should not be administered on the same day; there should be a 4-week minimum interval between the vaccines. When protection is rapidly required, the vaccines can be given at any interval; an additional dose of MMR should be considered and re-vaccination with the yellow fever vaccine can also be considered in those at on-going risk.
- **INTERACTIONS** → Appendix 1: live vaccines
- **SIDE-EFFECTS**
  - **Common or very common** Asthenia · crying · drowsiness · irritability
  - **Rare or very rare** Rhinitis · yellow fever vaccine-associated neurotropic disease · yellow fever vaccine-associated viscerotropic disease
  - **Frequency not known** Angioedema · influenza like illness · paraesthesia

  SIDE-EFFECTS, FURTHER INFORMATION Very rare vaccine-associated adverse effects may occur, such as viscerotropic disease (yellow-fever vaccine-associated viscerotropic disease, YEL-AVD), a syndrome which may include metabolic acidosis, muscle and liver cirrhosis, and multi-organ failure. Neurological disorders (yellow fever vaccine-associated neurotropic disease, YEL-AND) such as encephalitis have also been reported. These very rare adverse effects usually occur after the first dose of yellow fever vaccine in those with no previous immunity. Increased risk of fatal reactions reported in patients aged 60 years and older and those who are immunosuppressed.
- **ALLERGY AND CROSS-SENSITIVITY** EvGr In individuals with a history of confirmed anaphylactic reaction to eggs and who are currently avoiding eggs due to ongoing hypersensitivity reactions, yellow fever vaccine should only be considered under the guidance of an allergy specialist. ⟨E⟩
- **PREGNANCY** Live yellow fever vaccine should not be given during pregnancy because there is a theoretical risk of fetal infection. Pregnant women should be advised not to travel to areas at high risk of yellow fever. If exposure cannot be avoided during pregnancy, then the vaccine should be given if the risk from disease in the mother outweighs the risk to the fetus from vaccination.
- **BREAST FEEDING** Avoid; seek specialist advice if exposure to virus cannot be avoided.

- **MEDICINAL FORMS** There can be variation in the licensing of different medicines containing the same drug.

Powder and solvent for suspension for injection

- **Stamaril** (Sanofi)

  Stamaril vaccine powder and solvent for suspension for injection 0.5ml vials | 1 vial PoM £39.72 DT = £39.72

Chapter 15
Anaesthesia

CONTENTS

General anaesthesia

Anaesthesia (general)

Overview

Several different types of drug are given together during general anaesthesia. Anaesthesia is induced with either a volatile drug given by inhalation or with an intravenously administered drug; anaesthesia is maintained with an intravenous or inhalational anaesthetic. Analgesics, usually short-acting opioids, are also used. The use of neuromuscular blocking drugs necessitates intermittent positive-pressure ventilation. Following surgery, anticholinesterases can be given to reverse the effects of neuromuscular blocking drugs; specific antagonists can be used to reverse central and respiratory depression caused by some drugs used in surgery. A local topical anaesthetic can be used to reduce pain at the injection site.

Individual requirements vary considerably and the recommended doses are only a guide. Smaller doses are indicated in ill, shocked, or debilitated children and in significant hepatic impairment, while robust individuals may require larger doses. The required dose of induction agent may be less if the patient has been premedicated with a sedative agent or if an opioid analgesic has been used.

Intravenous anaesthetics

Intravenous anaesthetics may be used either to induce anaesthesia or for maintenance of anaesthesia throughout surgery. Intravenous anaesthetics nearly all produce their effect in one arm-brain circulation time. Extreme care is required in surgery of the mouth, pharynx, or larynx where the airway may be difficult to maintain (e.g. in the presence of a tumour in the pharynx or larynx).

To facilitate tracheal intubation, induction is usually followed by a neuromuscular blocking drug or a short-acting opioid.

The doses of all intravenous anaesthetic drugs should be titrated to effect (except when using 'rapid sequence induction').

Total intravenous anaesthesia

This is a technique in which major surgery is carried out with all drugs given intravenously. Respiration can be spontaneous, or controlled with oxygen-enriched air. Neuromuscular blocking drugs can be used to provide relaxation and prevent reflex muscle movements. The main problem to be overcome is the assessment of depth of anaesthesia. Target Controlled Infusion (TCI) systems can be used to titrate intravenous anaesthetic infusions to predicted plasma-drug concentrations; specific models with paediatric pharmacokinetic data should be used for children.

Drugs used for intravenous anaesthesia

Propofol p. 1008, the most widely used intravenous anaesthetic, can be used for induction or maintenance of anaesthesia in children, but it is not commonly used in neonates. Propofol is associated with rapid recovery and less hangover effect than other intravenous anaesthetics. Propofol can also be used for sedation during diagnostic procedures.

Thiopental sodium p. 270 is a barbiturate that is used for induction of anaesthesia, but has no analgesic properties. Induction is generally smooth and rapid, but dose-related cardiovascular and respiratory depression can occur. Awakening from a moderate dose of thiopental sodium is rapid because the drug redistributes into other tissues, particularly fat. However, metabolism is slow and sedative effects can persist for 24 hours. Repeated doses have a cumulative effect particularly in neonates and recovery is much slower.

Etomidate p. 1007 is an intravenous agent associated with rapid recovery without a hangover effect. Etomidate causes less hypotension than thiopental sodium and propofol during induction. It produces a high incidence of extraneous muscle movements, which can be minimised by an opioid analgesic or a short-acting benzodiazepine given just before induction.

Ketamine p. 1023 causes less hypotension than thiopental sodium and propofol during induction. It is sometimes used in children requiring repeat anaesthesia (such as for serial burns dressings), however recovery is relatively slow and there is a high incidence of extraneous muscle movements. Ketamine can cause hallucinations, nightmares, and other transient psychotic effects; these can be reduced by a benzodiazepine such as diazepam p. 270 or midazolam p. 273.

Inhalational anaesthetics

Inhalational anaesthetics include gases and volatile liquids. *Gaseous anaesthetics* require suitable equipment for storage and administration. *Volatile liquid anaesthetics* are administered using calibrated vaporisers, using air, oxygen, or nitrous oxide-oxygen mixtures as the carrier gas. To prevent hypoxia, the inspired gas mixture should contain a minimum of 25% oxygen at all times. Higher concentrations of oxygen (greater than 30%) are usually required during inhalational anaesthesia when nitrous oxide p. 1011 is being administered.

Volatile liquid anaesthetics

Volatile liquid anaesthetics can be used for induction and maintenance of anaesthesia, and following induction with an intravenous anaesthetic.

Isoflurane p. 1010 is a volatile liquid anaesthetic. Heart rhythm is generally stable during isoflurane anaesthesia, but heart-rate can rise. Systemic arterial pressure and cardiac output can fall, owing to a decrease in systemic vascular resistance. Muscle relaxation occurs and the effects of muscle relaxant drugs are potentiated. Isoflurane is not recommended for induction of anaesthesia in infants and children of all ages because of the occurrence of cough, breath-holding, desaturation, increased secretions, and laryngospasm. Isoflurane is the preferred inhalational anaesthetic for use in obstetrics.

Desflurane p. 1010 is a rapid acting volatile liquid anaesthetic; it is reported to have about one-fifth the potency of isoflurane. Emergence and recovery from anaesthesia are particularly rapid because of its low solubility. Desflurane is not recommended for induction of anaesthesia as it is irritant to the upper respiratory tract.

Sevoflurane p. 1011 is a rapid acting volatile liquid anaesthetic and is more potent than desflurane. Emergence and recovery are particularly rapid, but slower than desflurane. Sevoflurane is non-irritant and is therefore often used for inhalational induction of anaesthesia.

Nitrous oxide

Nitrous oxide is used for maintenance of anaesthesia and, in sub-anaesthetic concentrations, for analgesia. For *anaesthesia*, it is commonly used in a concentration of 50 to 66% in oxygen as part of a balanced technique in association with other inhalational or intravenous agents. Nitrous oxide is unsatisfactory as a sole anaesthetic owing to lack of potency, but is useful as part of a combination of drugs since it allows a significant reduction in dosage.

For analgesia (without loss of consciousness), a mixture of nitrous oxide and oxygen containing 50% of each gas (*Entonox*®, *Equanox*®) is used. Self-administration using a demand valve may be used in children who are able to self-regulate their intake (usually over 5 years of age) for painful dressing changes, as an aid to postoperative physiotherapy, for wound debridement and in emergency ambulances.

Nitrous oxide may have a deleterious effect if used in children with an air-containing closed space since nitrous oxide diffuses into such a space with a resulting increase in pressure. This effect may be dangerous in conditions such as pneumothorax, which may enlarge to compromise respiration, or in the presence of intracranial air after head injury, entrapped air following recent underwater dive, or recent intra-ocular gas injection.

Malignant hyperthermia

Malignant hyperthermia is a rare but potentially lethal complication of anaesthesia. It is characterised by a rapid rise in temperature, increased muscle rigidity, tachycardia, and acidosis. The most common triggers of malignant hyperthermia are the volatile anaesthetics. Suxamethonium chloride p. 1016 has also been implicated, but malignant hyperthermia is more likely if it is given following a volatile anaesthetic. Volatile anaesthetics and suxamethonium chloride should be avoided during anaesthesia in children at high risk of malignant hyperthermia.

Dantrolene sodium p. 1025 is used in the treatment of malignant hyperthermia.

Sedation, anaesthesia, and resuscitation in dental practice

Overview

Sedation for dental procedures should be limited to conscious sedation whenever possible. Nitrous oxide p. 1011 alone and midazolam p. 273 are effective for many children.

For details of anaesthesia, sedation, and resuscitation in dental practice see *A Conscious Decision*: *A review of the use of general anaesthesia and conscious sedation in primary dental care*; report by a group chaired by the Chief Medical Officer and Chief Dental Officer, July 2000 and associated documents. Further details can also be found in *Standards for Conscious Sedation in the Provision of Dental Care*; report of an Intercollegiate Advisory Committee for Sedation in Dentistry, 2020 www.rcseng.ac.uk/dental-faculties/fds/publications-guidelines/standards-for-conscious-sedation-in-the-provision-of-dental-care-and-accreditation/.

Surgery and long-term medication

02-Mar-2021

Overview

The risk of losing disease control on stopping long-term medication before surgery is often greater than the risk posed by continuing it during surgery. It is vital that the anaesthetist knows about **all** drugs that a patient is (or has been) taking.

Patients with adrenal atrophy resulting from long-term corticosteroid use may suffer a precipitous fall in blood pressure unless corticosteroid cover is provided during anaesthesia and in the immediate postoperative period. Anaesthetists must therefore know whether a patient is, or has been, receiving corticosteroids (including high-dose inhaled corticosteroids).

Other drugs that should normally not be stopped before surgery include drugs for epilepsy, asthma, immunosuppression, and metabolic, endocrine and cardiovascular disorders (but see potassium sparing diuretics). Expert advice is required for children receiving antivirals for HIV infection. See general advice on surgery in children with diabetes in Diabetes, surgery and medical illness p. 558.

Children taking antiplatelet medication or an oral anticoagulant present an increased risk for surgery. In these circumstances, the anaesthetist and surgeon should assess the relative risks and decide jointly whether the antiplatelet or the anticoagulant drug should be stopped or replaced with heparin p. 111 or low molecular weight heparin therapy.

Drugs that should be stopped before surgery include combined hormonal contraceptives, see Contraceptives, hormonal p. 609. If antidepressants need to be stopped, they should be withdrawn gradually to avoid withdrawal symptoms. Tricyclic antidepressants need not be stopped, but there may be an increased risk of arrhythmias and hypotension (and dangerous interactions with vasopressor drugs); therefore, the anaesthetist should be informed if they are not stopped. Lithium should be stopped 24 hours before major surgery but the normal dose can be continued for minor surgery (with careful monitoring of fluids and electrolytes). Potassium-sparing diuretics may need to be withheld on the morning of surgery because hyperkalaemia may develop if renal perfusion is impaired or if there is tissue damage. Herbal medicines may be associated with adverse effects when given with anaesthetic drugs and consideration should be given to stopping them before surgery.

ANAESTHETICS, GENERAL › INTRAVENOUS

Etomidate

04-Sep-2020

● INDICATIONS AND DOSE

Induction of anaesthesia

▶ BY SLOW INTRAVENOUS INJECTION

▶ Child 1 month–14 years: 150–300 micrograms/kg (max. per dose 60 mg), to be administered over 30-60 seconds (60 seconds for children in whom hypotension might be hazardous), increased if necessary to 400 micrograms/kg

▶ Child 15–17 years: 150–300 micrograms/kg (max. per dose 60 mg), to be administered over

continued →

30–60 seconds (60 seconds for children in whom hypotension might be hazardous)

- **UNLICENSED USE** *Hypnomidate*® licensed for use in children (age range not specified by manufacturer). *Etomidate-Lipuro*® not licensed for children under 6 months except for imperative indications during inpatient treatment. Doses in BNFC may differ from those in the product literature.

> **IMPORTANT SAFETY INFORMATION**
> Etomidate should only be administered by, or under the direct supervision of, personnel experienced in its use, with adequate training in anaesthesia and airway management, and when resuscitation equipment is available.

- **CAUTIONS** Acute circulatory failure (shock) · adrenal insufficiency · avoid in Acute porphyrias p. 745 · cardiovascular disease · fixed cardiac output · hypovolaemia

CAUTIONS, FURTHER INFORMATION
- Adrenal insufficiency Etomidate suppresses adrenocortical function, particularly during continuous administration, and it should not be used for maintenance of anaesthesia. It should be used with caution in patients with underlying adrenal insufficiency, for example, those with sepsis.

- **INTERACTIONS** → Appendix 1: etomidate
- **SIDE-EFFECTS**
  - **Common or very common** Apnoea · hypotension · movement disorders · nausea · respiratory disorders · skin reactions · vascular pain · vomiting
  - **Uncommon** Arrhythmias · cough · hiccups · hypersalivation · hypertension · muscle rigidity · neuromuscular dysfunction · nystagmus · procedural complications
  - **Frequency not known** Adrenal insufficiency · atrioventricular block · cardiac arrest · embolism and thrombosis · seizures · shock · Stevens-Johnson syndrome · trismus

SIDE-EFFECTS, FURTHER INFORMATION **Pain on injection** Can be reduced by injecting into a larger vein or by giving an opioid analgesic just before induction.

Extraneous muscle movements Extraneous muscle movements can be minimised by an opioid analgesic or a short-acting benzodiazepine given just before induction.

- **PREGNANCY** May depress neonatal respiration if used during delivery.
- **BREAST FEEDING** Breast-feeding can be resumed as soon as mother has recovered sufficiently from anaesthesia.
- **HEPATIC IMPAIRMENT**
Dose adjustments Manufacturer advises reduce dose in liver cirrhosis.
- **DIRECTIONS FOR ADMINISTRATION** Manufacturer advises give over 30–60 seconds (60 seconds in patients in whom hypotension might be hazardous).
- **PATIENT AND CARER ADVICE**
Driving and skilled tasks Patients given sedatives and analgesics during minor outpatient procedures should be very carefully warned about the risk of driving or undertaking skilled tasks afterwards. For a short general anaesthetic the risk extends to **at least 24 hours** after administration. Responsible persons should be available to take patients home. The dangers of taking **alcohol** should also be emphasised.

- **MEDICINAL FORMS** There can be variation in the licensing of different medicines containing the same drug.

Solution for injection

EXCIPIENTS: May contain Propylene glycol

- **Hypnomidate** (Piramal Critical Care Ltd)
Etomidate 2 mg per 1 ml Hypnomidate 20mg/10ml solution for injection ampoules | 5 ampoule PoM £6.90 (Hospital only)

Emulsion for injection

- **Etomidate (Non-proprietary)**
Etomidate 2 mg per 1 ml Etomidate 20mg/10ml emulsion for injection ampoules | 10 ampoule PoM £21.00 (Hospital only)

Propofol

13-Aug-2020

- **INDICATIONS AND DOSE**

Induction of anaesthesia using 0.5% or 1% injection
- BY SLOW INTRAVENOUS INJECTION, OR BY INTRAVENOUS INFUSION
  - Child 1 month–16 years: Usual dose 2.5–4 mg/kg, dose adjusted according to age, body-weight and response
  - Child 17 years: Usual dose 1.5–2.5 mg/kg, to be administered at a rate of 20–40 mg every 10 seconds until response

Induction of anaesthesia using 2% injection
- BY INTRAVENOUS INFUSION
  - Child 3–16 years: Usual dose 2.5–4 mg/kg, dose adjusted according to age, body-weight and response
  - Child 17 years: Usual dose 1.5–2.5 mg/kg, to be administered at a rate of 20–40 mg every 10 seconds until response

Maintenance of anaesthesia using 1% injection
- BY CONTINUOUS INTRAVENOUS INFUSION
  - Child 1 month–16 years: Usual dose 9–15 mg/kg/hour, dose adjusted according to age, body-weight and response
  - Child 17 years: Usual dose 4–12 mg/kg/hour, adjusted according to response

Maintenance of anaesthesia using 2% injection
- BY CONTINUOUS INTRAVENOUS INFUSION
  - Child 3–16 years: Usual dose 9–15 mg/kg/hour, dose adjusted according to age, body-weight and response
  - Child 17 years: Usual dose 4–12 mg/kg/hour, adjusted according to response

Sedation of ventilated patients in intensive care using 1% or 2% injection
- BY CONTINUOUS INTRAVENOUS INFUSION
  - Child 16–17 years: Usual dose 0.3–4 mg/kg/hour, adjusted according to response

Induction of sedation for surgical and diagnostic procedures using 0.5% or 1% injection
- BY SLOW INTRAVENOUS INJECTION
  - Child 1 month–16 years: Initially 1–2 mg/kg, dose and rate of administration adjusted according to desired level of sedation and response
  - Child 17 years: Initially 0.5–1 mg/kg, to be administered over 1–5 minutes, dose and rate of administration adjusted according to desired level of sedation and response

Maintenance of sedation for surgical and diagnostic procedures using 0.5% injection
- INITIALLY BY INTRAVENOUS INFUSION
  - Child 17 years: Initially 1.5–4.5 mg/kg/hour, dose and rate of administration adjusted according to desired level of sedation and response, followed by (by slow intravenous injection) 10–20 mg, (if rapid increase in sedation required)

15 Anaesthesia

Maintenance of sedation for surgical and diagnostic procedures using 1% injection

▶ INITIALLY BY INTRAVENOUS INFUSION

▸ Child 1 month–16 years: Usual dose 1.5–9 mg/kg/hour, dose and rate of administration adjusted according to desired level of sedation and response, followed by (by slow intravenous injection) up to 1 mg/kg, (if rapid increase in sedation required)

▸ Child 17 years: Initially 1.5–4.5 mg/kg/hour, dose and rate of administration adjusted according to desired level of sedation and response, followed by (by slow intravenous injection) 10–20 mg, (if rapid increase in sedation required)

Maintenance of sedation for surgical and diagnostic procedures using 2% injection

▶ INITIALLY BY INTRAVENOUS INFUSION

▸ Child 3–16 years: Usual dose 1.5–9 mg/kg/hour, dose and rate of administration adjusted according to desired level of sedation and response

▸ Child 17 years: Initially 1.5–4.5 mg/kg/hour, dose and rate of administration adjusted according to desired level of sedation and response, followed by (by slow intravenous injection) 10–20 mg, using 0.5% or 1% injection (if rapid increase in sedation required)

IMPORTANT SAFETY INFORMATION

Propofol should only be administered by, or under the direct supervision of, personnel experienced in its use, with adequate training in anaesthesia and airway management, and when resuscitation equipment is available.

● **CONTRA-INDICATIONS** Children under 16 years receiving intensive care

CONTRA-INDICATIONS, FURTHER INFORMATION

Use in intensive care associated with a risk of propofol infusion syndrome (potentially fatal effects, including metabolic acidosis, arrhythmias, cardiac failure, rhabdomyolysis, hyperlipidaemia, hyperkalaemia, hepatomegaly, and renal failure).

● **CAUTIONS** Acute circulatory failure (shock) · cardiac impairment · cardiovascular disease · epilepsy · fixed cardiac output · hypotension · hypovolaemia · raised intracranial pressure · respiratory impairment

● **INTERACTIONS** → Appendix 1: propofol

● **SIDE-EFFECTS**

▶ **Common or very common** Apnoea · arrhythmias · headache · hypotension · localised pain · nausea · vomiting

▶ **Uncommon** Thrombosis

▶ **Rare or very rare** Epileptiform seizure (may be delayed) · movement disorders · pancreatitis · post procedural complications · pulmonary oedema · sexual dysfunction · urine discolouration

▶ **Frequency not known** Drug dependence · euphoric mood · heart failure · hepatomegaly · hyperkalaemia · hyperlipidaemia · metabolic acidosis · renal failure · respiratory depression · rhabdomyolysis

SIDE-EFFECTS, FURTHER INFORMATION **Bradycardia** Bradycardia may be profound and may be treated with intravenous administration of an antimuscarinic drug.

Pain on injection Pain on injection can be reduced by intravenous lidocaine.

Propofol infusion syndrome Prolonged infusion of propofol doses exceeding 4mg/kg/hour may result in potentially fatal effects, including metabolic acidosis, arrhythmias, cardiac failure, rhabdomyolysis, hyperlipidaemia, hyperkalaemia, hepatomegaly, and renal failure.

● **PREGNANCY** May depress neonatal respiration if used during delivery.

Dose adjustments Max. dose for maintenance of anaesthesia 6 mg/kg/hour.

● **BREAST FEEDING** Breast-feeding can be resumed as soon as mother has recovered sufficiently from anaesthesia.

● **HEPATIC IMPAIRMENT** Manufacturer advises caution.

● **RENAL IMPAIRMENT** Use with caution.

● **MONITORING REQUIREMENTS** Monitor blood-lipid concentration if risk of fat overload or if sedation longer than 3 days.

● **DIRECTIONS FOR ADMINISTRATION** Manufacturer advises shake before use; microbiological filter not recommended; may be administered via a Y-piece close to injection site co-administered with Glucose 5% *or* Sodium Chloride 0.9%. 0.5% **emulsion** for injection or intermittent infusion; manufacturer advises may be administered undiluted, or diluted with Glucose 5% *or* Sodium Chloride 0.9%; dilute to a concentration not less than 1 mg/mL. 1% **emulsion** for injection or infusion; manufacturer advises may be administered undiluted, or diluted with Glucose 5% (*Diprivan*®) or (*Propofol-Lipuro*®) *or* Sodium Chloride 0.9% (*Propofol-Lipuro*® only); dilute to a concentration not less than 2 mg/mL; use within 6 hours of preparation. 2% **emulsion** for infusion; manufacturer advises do not dilute.

● **PATIENT AND CARER ADVICE**

Driving and skilled tasks Patients given sedatives and analgesics during minor outpatient procedures should be very carefully warned about the risk of driving or undertaking skilled tasks afterwards. For a short general anaesthetic the risk extends to **at least 24 hours** after administration. Responsible persons should be available to take patients home. The dangers of taking **alcohol** should also be emphasised.

● **MEDICINAL FORMS** There can be variation in the licensing of different medicines containing the same drug.

Emulsion for infusion

▸ **Propofol (Non-proprietary)**

Propofol 10 mg per 1 ml Propofol 1% (500mg/50ml) emulsion for infusion pre-filled syringes | 1 pre-filled disposable injection PoM £13.45 (Hospital only)

Propofol 1% (1g/100ml) emulsion for infusion vials | 1 vial PoM £26.40 (Hospital only) | 10 vial PoM £225.86 (Hospital only)

Propofol 1% (500mg/50ml) emulsion for infusion vials | 1 vial PoM £13.20 (Hospital only) | 10 vial PoM £118.05 (Hospital only)

Propofol 20 mg per 1 ml Propofol 2% (1g/50ml) emulsion for infusion pre-filled syringes | 1 pre-filled disposable injection PoM £17.95 (Hospital only)

Propofol 2% (1g/50ml) emulsion for infusion vials | 1 vial PoM £26.40 (Hospital only) | 10 vial PoM £225.83 (Hospital only)

▸ **Propoven** (Fresenius Kabi Ltd)

Propofol 10 mg per 1 ml Propoven 1% emulsion for infusion 50ml vials | 10 vial PoM £132.00 (Hospital only)

Propoven 1% emulsion for infusion 100ml vials | 10 vial PoM £264.00 (Hospital only)

Propofol 20 mg per 1 ml Propoven 2% emulsion for infusion 50ml vials | 10 vial PoM £264.00 (Hospital only)

Emulsion for injection

▸ **Propofol (Non-proprietary)**

Propofol 10 mg per 1 ml Propofol 1% (200mg/20ml) emulsion for injection ampoules | 5 ampoule PoM £15.36–£20.93 (Hospital only)

Propofol 1% (200mg/20ml) emulsion for injection vials | 5 vial PoM £26.40 (Hospital only)

▸ **Propoven** (Fresenius Kabi Ltd)

Propofol 10 mg per 1 ml Propoven 1% emulsion for injection 20ml ampoules | 5 ampoule PoM £26.40 (Hospital only)

ANAESTHETICS, GENERAL › VOLATILE LIQUID

Volatile halogenated anaesthetics

IMPORTANT SAFETY INFORMATION
Should only be administered by, or under the direct supervision of, personnel experienced in their use, with adequate training in anaesthesia and airway management, and when resuscitation equipment is available.

- **CONTRA-INDICATIONS** Susceptibility to malignant hyperthermia
- **CAUTIONS** Can trigger malignant hyperthermia · neuromuscular disease (inhalational anaesthetics are very rarely associated with hyperkalaemia, resulting in cardiac arrhythmias and death) · raised intracranial pressure (can increase cerebrospinal pressure)
- **SIDE-EFFECTS**
  - **Common or very common** Agitation · apnoea · arrhythmias · chills · cough · dizziness · headache · hypersalivation · hypertension · hypotension · nausea · respiratory disorders · vomiting
  - **Uncommon** Hypoxia
  - **Frequency not known** Breath holding · cardiac arrest · haemorrhage · hepatic disorders · hyperkalaemia · malignant hyperthermia · QT interval prolongation · rhabdomyolysis · seizure
- **ALLERGY AND CROSS-SENSITIVITY** Can cause hepatotoxicity in those sensitised to halogenated anaesthetics.
- **DIRECTIONS FOR ADMINISTRATION** Volatile liquid anaesthetics are administered using calibrated vaporisers, using oxygen, oxygen-enriched air, or nitrous oxide-oxygen mixtures as the carrier gas (consult product literature).
- **PATIENT AND CARER ADVICE**
  Driving and skilled tasks Patients given sedatives and analgesics during minor outpatient procedures should be very carefully warned about the risks of driving or undertaking skilled tasks afterwards. For a short general anaesthetic, the risk extends **to at least 24 hours** after administration. Responsible persons should be available to take patients home. The dangers of taking **alcohol** should also be emphasised.

above

Desflurane

- **INDICATIONS AND DOSE**

Induction of anaesthesia (but not recommended)
▶ BY INHALATION
- Child 12–17 years: 4–11 %, to be inhaled through specifically calibrated vaporiser

Maintenance of anaesthesia (in nitrous oxide–oxygen)
▶ BY INHALATION
- Neonate: 2–6 %, to be inhaled through a specifically calibrated vaporiser.
- Child: 2–6 %, to be inhaled through a specifically calibrated vaporiser

Maintenance of anaesthesia (in oxygen or oxygen-enriched air)
▶ BY INHALATION
- Neonate: 2.5–8.5 %, to be inhaled through a specifically calibrated vaporiser.
- Child: 2.5–8.5 %, to be inhaled through a specifically calibrated vaporiser

- **INTERACTIONS** → Appendix 1: volatile halogenated anaesthetics
- **SIDE-EFFECTS**
  - **Common or very common** Coagulation disorder · conjunctivitis
  - **Uncommon** Myalgia · myocardial infarction · myocardial ischaemia · vasodilation
  - **Frequency not known** Abdominal pain · asthenia · heart failure · hypokalaemia · malaise · metabolic acidosis · pancreatitis acute · shock · skin reactions · ventricular dysfunction · visual acuity decreased
- **PREGNANCY** May depress neonatal respiration if used during delivery.
- **BREAST FEEDING** Breast-feeding can be resumed as soon as mother has recovered sufficiently from anaesthesia.
- **MEDICINAL FORMS** There can be variation in the licensing of different medicines containing the same drug.

Inhalation vapour liquid
- **Desflurane (Non-proprietary)**
  Desflurane 1 ml per 1 ml Desflurane 100% inhalation vapour liquid | 240 ml PoM £120.00 (Hospital only) | 250 ml PoM £20.00 (Hospital only)

above

Isoflurane

12-Dec-2019

- **INDICATIONS AND DOSE**

Induction of anaesthesia (in oxygen or nitrous oxide–oxygen) (but indication not recommended in infants and children of all ages)
▶ BY INHALATION
- Neonate: Initially 0.5 %, increased to 3 %, adjusted according to response, administered using specifically calibrated vaporiser.
- Child: Initially 0.5 %, increased to 3 %, adjusted according to response, administered using specifically calibrated vaporiser

Maintenance of anaesthesia (in nitrous oxide–oxygen)
▶ BY INHALATION
- Neonate: 1–2.5 %, to be administered using specifically calibrated vaporiser; an additional 0.5–1% may be required when given with oxygen alone.
- Child: 1–2.5 %, to be administered using specifically calibrated vaporiser; an additional 0.5–1% may be required when given with oxygen alone

Maintenance of anaesthesia in caesarean section (in nitrous oxide–oxygen)
▶ BY INHALATION
- Child: 0.5–0.75 %, to be administered using specifically calibrated vaporiser

IMPORTANT SAFETY INFORMATION
Isoflurane is not recommended for induction of anaesthesia in infants and children of all ages because of the occurrence of cough, breath-holding, desaturation, increased secretions, and laryngospasm.

- **CAUTIONS** Children under 2 years—limited experience
- **INTERACTIONS** → Appendix 1: volatile halogenated anaesthetics
- **SIDE-EFFECTS** Carboxyhaemoglobinaemia · chest discomfort · cognitive impairment · delirium · dyspnoea · ileus · mood altered (that can last several days) · myoglobinuria · skin reactions

15 Anaesthesia

- **PREGNANCY** May depress neonatal respiration if used during delivery.
- **BREAST FEEDING** Breast-feeding can be resumed as soon as mother has recovered sufficiently from anaesthesia.

- **MEDICINAL FORMS** There can be variation in the licensing of different medicines containing the same drug.

Inhalation vapour liquid

- Isoflurane (Non-proprietary)
  Isoflurane 1 ml per 1 ml Isoflurane 100% inhalation vapour liquid | 250 ml PoM £120.00 (Hospital only)
- AErrane (Baxter Healthcare Ltd)
  Isoflurane 1 ml per 1 ml AErrane 100% inhalation vapour liquid | 250 ml PoM £27.00 (Hospital only)

Nitrous oxide

12-Aug-2020

- **INDICATIONS AND DOSE**

Maintenance of anaesthesia in conjunction with other anaesthetic agents

▶ BY INHALATION

- Neonate: 50–66 %, to be administered using suitable anaesthetic apparatus in oxygen.
- Child: 50–66 %, to be administered using suitable anaesthetic apparatus in oxygen

Analgesia

▶ BY INHALATION

- Neonate: Up to 50 %, to be administered using suitable anaesthetic apparatus in oxygen, adjusted according to the patient's needs.
- Child: Up to 50 %, to be administered using suitable anaesthetic apparatus in oxygen, adjusted according to the patient's needs

IMPORTANT SAFETY INFORMATION

Nitrous oxide should only be administered by, or under the direct supervision of, personnel experienced in its use, with adequate training in anaesthesia and airway management, and when resuscitation equipment is available.

- **CAUTIONS** Entrapped air following recent underwater dive · pneumothorax · presence of intracranial air after head injury · recent intra-ocular gas injection
  CAUTIONS, FURTHER INFORMATION Nitrous oxide may have a deleterious effect if used in patients with an air-containing closed space since nitrous oxide diffuses into such a space with a resulting increase in pressure. This effect may be dangerous in conditions such as pneumothorax, which may enlarge to compromise respiration, or in the presence of intracranial air after head injury, entrapped air following recent underwater dive, or recent intra-ocular gas injection.
- **INTERACTIONS** → Appendix 1: nitrous oxide
- **SIDE-EFFECTS** Abdominal distension · addiction · agranulocytosis · disorientation · dizziness · euphoric mood · megaloblastic anaemia · middle ear damage · myeloneuropathy · nausea · paraesthesia · sedation · subacute combined cord degeneration · tympanic membrane perforation · vomiting
  SIDE-EFFECTS, FURTHER INFORMATION Exposure of patients to nitrous oxide for prolonged periods, either by continuous or by intermittent administration, may result in megaloblastic anaemia owing to interference with the action of vitamin B_{12}; neurological toxic effects can occur without preceding overt haematological changes. Depression of white cell formation may also occur.
- **PREGNANCY** May depress neonatal respiration if used during delivery.
- **BREAST FEEDING** Breast-feeding can be resumed as soon as mother has recovered sufficiently from anaesthesia.
- **MONITORING REQUIREMENTS**
  ▶ Assessment of plasma-vitamin B_{12} concentration should be considered in those at risk of deficiency, including the elderly, those who have a poor, vegetarian, or vegan diet, and those with a history of anaemia.
  ▶ Nitrous oxide should **not** be given continuously for longer than 24 hours or more frequently than every 4 days without close supervision and haematological monitoring.
- **DIRECTIONS FOR ADMINISTRATION** For analgesia (without loss of consciousness), manufacturer advises a mixture of nitrous oxide and oxygen containing 50% of each gas (*Entonox*®) is used.
- **HANDLING AND STORAGE** Exposure of theatre staff to nitrous oxide should be minimised (risk of serious side-effects).
- **PATIENT AND CARER ADVICE**
  Medicines for Children leaflet: Nitrous oxide for pain www.medicinesforchildren.org.uk/medicines/nitrous-oxide-for-pain/
- **MEDICINAL FORMS** There can be variation in the licensing of different medicines containing the same drug.

Inhalation gas

- Nitrous oxide (Non-proprietary)
  Nitrous oxide 1 ml per 1 ml Nitrous oxide cylinders size E | 1800 litre P ☒ CD5
  Nitrous oxide cylinders size F | 3600 litre P ☒ CD5
  Nitrous oxide cylinders size J | 18000 litre P ☒ CD5
  Nitrous oxide cylinders size G | 9000 litre P ☒ CD5
  Nitrous oxide cylinders size D | 900 litre P ☒ CD5

Sevoflurane

F 1010

- **INDICATIONS AND DOSE**

Induction of anaesthesia (in oxygen or nitrous oxide-oxygen)

▶ BY INHALATION

- Neonate: Up to 4 %, adjusted according to response, to be administered using specifically calibrated vaporiser.
- Child: Initially 0.5–1 %, then increased to up to 8 %, increased gradually, according to response, to be administered using specifically calibrated vaporiser

Maintenance of anaesthesia (in oxygen or nitrous oxide-oxygen)

▶ BY INHALATION

- Neonate: 0.5–2 %, adjusted according to response, to be administered using specifically calibrated vaporiser.
- Child: 0.5–3 %, adjusted according to response, to be administered using specifically calibrated vaporiser

- **CAUTIONS** Susceptibility to QT-interval prolongation
- **INTERACTIONS** → Appendix 1: volatile halogenated anaesthetics
- **SIDE-EFFECTS**
  ▶ **Common or very common** Drowsiness · fever · hypothermia
  ▶ **Uncommon** Asthma · atrioventricular block · confusion
  ▶ **Frequency not known** Dystonia · intracranial pressure increased · muscle rigidity · nephritis tubulointerstitial · oedema · pancreatitis
- **PREGNANCY** May depress neonatal respiration if used during delivery.
- **BREAST FEEDING** Breast-feeding can be resumed as soon as mother has recovered sufficiently from anaesthesia.
- **RENAL IMPAIRMENT** Use with caution.

- **MEDICINAL FORMS** There can be variation in the licensing of different medicines containing the same drug.

Inhalation vapour liquid

- Sevoflurane (Non-proprietary)
  Sevoflurane 1 ml per 1 ml Sevoflurane 100% inhalation vapour liquid | 250 ml [PoM] £123.00 (Hospital only)

1 Anaesthesia adjuvants

Pre-medication and peri-operative drugs

05-May-2021

Drugs that affect gastric pH

Regurgitation and aspiration of gastric contents (Mendelson's syndrome) can be a complication of general anaesthesia, particularly in obstetrics and in gastro-oesophageal reflux disease; prophylaxis against acid aspiration is not routinely used in children but may be required in high-risk cases.

An **H_2-receptor antagonist** can be used before surgery to increase the pH and reduce the volume of gastric fluid. It does not affect the pH of fluid already in the stomach and this limits its value in emergency procedures; an oral H_2-receptor antagonist can be given 1–2 hours before the procedure.

Antimuscarinic drugs

Antimuscarinic drugs are used (less commonly nowadays) as premedicants to dry bronchial and salivary secretions which are increased by intubation, upper airway surgery, or some inhalational anaesthetics. They are also used before or with neostigmine p. 814 to prevent bradycardia, excessive salivation, and other muscarinic actions of neostigmine. They also prevent bradycardia and hypotension associated with drugs such as propofol p. 1008 and suxamethonium chloride p. 1016.

Atropine sulfate p. 1013 is now rarely used for premedication but still has an emergency role in the treatment of vagotonic side-effects.

Hyoscine hydrobromide p. 320 reduces secretions and also provides a degree of amnesia, sedation, and anti-emesis. Unlike atropine sulfate it may produce bradycardia rather than tachycardia.

Glycopyrronium bromide p. 1014 reduces salivary secretions. When given intravenously it produces less tachycardia than atropine sulfate. It is widely used with neostigmine for reversal of non-depolarising muscle relaxants.

Glycopyrronium bromide or hyoscine hydrobromide are also used to control excessive secretions in upper airways or hypersalivation in palliative care and in children unable to control posture or with abnormal swallowing reflex; effective dose varies and tolerance may develop. The intramuscular route should be avoided if possible. Hyoscine hydrobromide transdermal patches may also be used.

Sedative drugs

Premedication

Fear and anxiety before a procedure (including the night before) can be minimised by using a sedative drug, usually a **benzodiazepine**. Premedication may also augment the action of anaesthetics and provide some degree of pre-operative amnesia. The choice of drug depends on the individual, the nature of the procedure, the anaesthetic to be used, and other prevailing circumstances such as outpatients, obstetrics, and availability of recovery facilities. The choice also varies between elective and emergency procedures. Oral administration is preferred if possible; the rectal route should only be used in exceptional circumstances.

Premedicants can be given the night before major surgery; a further, smaller dose may be required before surgery. Alternatively, the first dose may be given on the day of the procedure.

Oral midazolam p. 273 is the most common premedicant for children; temazepam p. 1024 may be used in older children. The antihistamine alimemazine tartrate p. 205 is occasionally used orally, but when given alone it may cause postoperative restlessness in the presence of pain.

Benzodiazepines

Benzodiazepines possess useful properties for premedication including relief of anxiety, sedation, and amnesia; short-acting benzodiazepines taken by mouth are the most common premedicants. Benzodiazepines are also used for sedation prior to clinical procedures and for sedation in intensive care.

Benzodiazepines may occasionally cause marked respiratory depression and facilities for its treatment are essential; flumazenil p. 1045 is used to antagonise the effects of benzodiazepines.

Midazolam, a water-soluble benzodiazepine, is the preferred benzodiazepine for premedication and for sedation for clinical procedures in children. It has a fast onset of action, and recovery is faster than for other benzodiazepines. Recovery may be longer in children with a low cardiac output, or after repeated dosing.

Midazolam can be given by mouth [unlicensed], but its bitter acidic taste may need to be disguised. It can also be given buccally [unlicensed indication] or intranasally [unlicensed]. Midazolam is associated with profound sedation when high doses are given or when it is used with certain other drugs. It can cause severe disinhibition and restlessness in some children. Midazolam is not recommended for prolonged sedation in neonates; drug accumulation is likely to occur.

Temazepam is given by mouth for premedication in older children and has a short duration of action. Anxiolytic and sedative effects last about 90 minutes, although there may be residual drowsiness. Temazepam is rarely used for dental procedures in children.

Lorazepam p. 272 produces more prolonged sedation than temazepam and it has marked amnesic effects.

Peri-operative use of diazepam p. 270 is not recommended in children; onset and magnitude of response are unreliable, and paradoxical effects may occur. Diazepam is not used for dental procedures in children.

Antagonists for central and respiratory depression

Respiratory depression is a major concern with opioid analgesics and it may be treated by artificial ventilation or be reversed by an opioid antagonist. Naloxone hydrochloride p. 1047 given intravenously immediately reverses opioid-induced respiratory depression but the dose may have to be repeated because of its **short duration of action**. Intramuscular injection of naloxone hydrochloride produces a more gradual and prolonged effect but absorption may be erratic. Care is required in children requiring pain relief because naloxone hydrochloride also antagonises the analgesic effect of opioids.

Flumazenil is a benzodiazepine antagonist for the reversal of the central sedative effects of benzodiazepines after anaesthetic and similar procedures. Flumazenil has a shorter half-life and duration of action than diazepam or midazolam so patients may become resedated.

Neonates

Naloxone hydrochloride is used in newborn infants to reverse respiratory depression and sedation resulting from the use of opioids by the mother, usually for pain during labour. In neonates the effects of opioids may persist for up to 48 hours and in such cases naloxone hydrochloride is often given by intramuscular injection for its prolonged effect. In severe respiratory depression after birth, breathing should first be established (using artificial means if necessary) and naloxone hydrochloride administered only if use of opioids by the mother is thought to cause the respiratory depression; the infant should be monitored closely and further doses of naloxone hydrochloride administered as necessary.

ANTIMUSCARINICS

F 603

Atropine sulfate

22-Feb-2023

● **INDICATIONS AND DOSE**

Symptomatic bradycardia due to acute overdosage of beta-blockers

▶ BY INTRAVENOUS INJECTION

▶ Child: 0.02 mg/kg (max. per dose 1.2 mg), repeat doses may be necessary

Treatment of poisoning by organophosphorus insecticide or nerve agent (in combination with pralidoxime chloride)

▶ BY INTRAVENOUS INJECTION

▶ Child: 20 micrograms/kg every 5–10 minutes (max. per dose 2 mg) until the skin becomes flushed and dry, the pupils dilate, and bradycardia is abolished, frequency of administration dependent on the severity of poisoning

Premedication

▶ BY INTRAVENOUS INJECTION

▶ Neonate: 10 micrograms/kg, to be administered immediately before induction of anaesthesia.

▶ Child 1 month–11 years: 20 micrograms/kg, to be administered immediately before induction of anaesthesia (minimum 100 micrograms, max. 600 micrograms)

▶ Child 12–17 years: 300–600 micrograms, to be administered immediately before induction of anaesthesia

▶ BY SUBCUTANEOUS INJECTION, OR BY INTRAMUSCULAR INJECTION

▶ Neonate: 10 micrograms/kg, to be administered 30–60 minutes before induction of anaesthesia.

▶ Child 1 month–11 years: 10–30 micrograms/kg, to be administered 30–60 minutes before induction of anaesthesia (minimum 100 micrograms, max. 600 micrograms)

▶ Child 12–17 years: 300–600 micrograms, to be administered 30–60 minutes before induction of anaesthesia

▶ BY MOUTH

▶ Neonate: 20–40 micrograms/kg, to be administered 1–2 hours before induction of anaesthesia.

▶ Child: 20–40 micrograms/kg (max. per dose 900 micrograms), to be administered 1–2 hours before induction of anaesthesia

Intra-operative bradycardia

▶ BY INTRAVENOUS INJECTION

▶ Neonate: 10–20 micrograms/kg.

▶ Child 1 month–11 years: 10–20 micrograms/kg

▶ Child 12–17 years: 300–600 micrograms, larger doses may be used in emergencies

Control of muscarinic side-effects of neostigmine in reversal of competitive neuromuscular block

▶ BY INTRAVENOUS INJECTION

▶ Neonate: 20 micrograms/kg.

▶ Child 1 month–11 years: 20 micrograms/kg (max. per dose 1.2 mg)

▶ Child 12–17 years: 0.6–1.2 mg

● **UNLICENSED USE** Not licensed for use in children under 12 years for intra-operative bradycardia or by intravenous route for premedication. Not licensed for use by oral route. TOXBASE advises atropine sulfate is used in the doses provided for the treatment of symptomatic bradycardia due to acute overdosage of beta-blockers, but these may vary from those licensed.

IMPORTANT SAFETY INFORMATION

▶ With systemic use for Premedication

Antimuscarinic drugs used for premedication to general anaesthesia should only be administered by, or under the direct supervision of, personnel experienced in their use.

● **INTERACTIONS** → Appendix 1: atropine

● **SIDE-EFFECTS**

▶ **Common or very common**

▶ With intramuscular or intravenous use Abdominal distension · agitation · anhidrosis · dysphagia · hyperthermia · movement disorders · speech disorder · taste loss

▶ **Uncommon**

▶ With intramuscular or intravenous use Psychotic disorder

▶ **Rare or very rare**

▶ With intramuscular or intravenous use Angina pectoris · arrhythmias · hypertensive crisis · seizure

▶ **Frequency not known**

▶ With intramuscular or intravenous use Insomnia

▶ With oral use Angle closure glaucoma · arrhythmias · bronchial secretion altered · chest pain · dysphagia · fever · gastrointestinal disorders · mydriasis · staggering · thirst

▶ With parenteral use Arrhythmias · atrioventricular block · bronchial secretion decreased · delirium · fever · gastrointestinal disorders · hallucination · mydriasis · restlessness · thirst

● **PREGNANCY** Not known to be harmful; manufacturer advises caution.

● **BREAST FEEDING** May suppress lactation; small amount present in milk—manufacturer advises caution.

● **MONITORING REQUIREMENTS**

▶ Control of muscarinic side-effects of neostigmine in reversal of competitive neuromuscular block Since atropine has a shorter duration of action than neostigmine, late unopposed bradycardia may result; close monitoring of the patient is necessary.

● **DIRECTIONS FOR ADMINISTRATION** For administration *by mouth*, expert sources advise injection solution may be given orally.

● **EXCEPTIONS TO LEGAL CATEGORY** Prescription only medicine restriction does not apply where administration is for saving life in emergency.

● **MEDICINAL FORMS** There can be variation in the licensing of different medicines containing the same drug. Forms available from special-order manufacturers include: oral suspension, oral solution, solution for injection, solution for infusion

Solution for injection

▶ **Atropine sulfate (Non-proprietary)**

Atropine sulfate 100 microgram per 1 ml Atropine 1mg/10ml solution for injection pre-filled syringes | 1 pre-filled disposable injection PoM £12.35

Atropine 500micrograms/5ml solution for injection pre-filled syringes | 1 pre-filled disposable injection PoM £13.00 | 10 pre-filled disposable injection PoM £130.00

Atropine sulfate 200 microgram per 1 ml Atropine 1mg/5ml solution for injection pre-filled syringes | 1 pre-filled disposable injection PoM £13.00 | 10 pre-filled disposable injection PoM £130.00

Atropine sulfate 300 microgram per 1 ml Atropine 3mg/10ml solution for injection pre-filled syringes | 1 pre-filled disposable injection PoM £13.00 DT = £13.00 | 10 pre-filled disposable injection PoM £130.00

Atropine sulfate 600 microgram per 1 ml Atropine 600micrograms/1ml solution for injection ampoules | 10 ampoule PoM £11.71–£14.30

Atropine sulfate 1 mg per 1 ml Atropine 1mg/1ml solution for injection ampoules | 10 ampoule PoM £183.48–£344.94

F 603

Glycopyrronium bromide

17-Jan-2024

(Glycopyrrolate)

● INDICATIONS AND DOSE

Premedication at induction

▶ BY INTRAMUSCULAR INJECTION, OR BY INTRAVENOUS INJECTION

- Neonate: 5 micrograms/kg.
- Child 1 month–11 years: 4–8 micrograms/kg (max. per dose 200 micrograms)
- Child 12–17 years: 200–400 micrograms, alternatively 4–5 micrograms/kg (max. per dose 400 micrograms)

Intra-operative bradycardia

▶ BY INTRAVENOUS INJECTION

- Neonate: 10 micrograms/kg, repeated if necessary.
- Child: 4–8 micrograms/kg (max. per dose 200 micrograms), repeated if necessary

Control of muscarinic side-effects of neostigmine in reversal of non-depolarising neuromuscular block

▶ BY INTRAVENOUS INJECTION

- Neonate: 10 micrograms/kg.
- Child 1 month–11 years: 10 micrograms/kg (max. per dose 500 micrograms)
- Child 12–17 years: 10–15 micrograms/kg, alternatively, 200 micrograms per 1 mg of neostigmine to be administered

Control of upper airways secretion | Hypersalivation

▶ BY SUBCUTANEOUS INFUSION

- Child 1 month–11 years: 12–40 micrograms/kg (max. per dose 1.2 mg) over 24 hours
- Child 12–17 years: 0.6–1.2 mg/24 hours

▶ BY SUBCUTANEOUS INJECTION, OR BY INTRAMUSCULAR INJECTION, OR BY INTRAVENOUS INJECTION

- Child 1 month–11 years: 4–10 micrograms/kg 4 times a day (max. per dose 200 micrograms) as required
- Child 12–17 years: 200 micrograms every 4 hours as required

Control of upper airways secretion (using Sialanar® 400 micrograms/mL oral solution) | Hypersalivation (using Sialanar® 400 micrograms/mL oral solution)

▶ BY MOUTH

- Child: Initially 16 micrograms/kg 3 times a day, increased in steps of 16 micrograms/kg 3 times a day, every 7 days, adjusted according to response; maximum 80 micrograms/kg 3 times a day (max. per dose 2.4 mg)

Control of upper airways secretion (using generic 1 mg/5mL oral solution) | Hypersalivation (using generic 1 mg/5mL oral solution)

▶ BY MOUTH

- Child: Initially 20 micrograms/kg 3 times a day, increased in steps of 20 micrograms/kg 3 times a day, every 7 days, adjusted according to response; maximum 100 micrograms/kg 3 times a day (max. per dose 3 mg)

Chronic pathological drooling in chronic neurological disorders (using Sialanar® 400 micrograms/mL oral solution) (under expert supervision)

▶ BY MOUTH

- Child 3–17 years: Initially 16 micrograms/kg 3 times a day, increased in steps of 16 micrograms/kg 3 times a day, every 5–7 days, adjusted according to response; maximum 80 micrograms/kg 3 times a day (max. per dose 2.4 mg)

Chronic pathological drooling in chronic neurological disorders (using generic 1 mg/5mL oral solution) (under expert supervision)

▶ BY MOUTH

- Child 3–17 years: Initially 20 micrograms/kg 3 times a day, increased in steps of 20 micrograms/kg 3 times a day, every 5–7 days, adjusted according to response; maximum 100 micrograms/kg 3 times a day (max. per dose 3 mg)

Chronic pathological drooling in chronic neurological disorders (using tablets) (under expert supervision)

▶ BY MOUTH

- Child 3–17 years: Initially 20 micrograms/kg 3 times a day, increased in steps of 20 micrograms/kg 3 times a day, every 5–7 days, adjusted according to response; maximum 100 micrograms/kg 3 times a day (max. per dose 3 mg)

DOSE EQUIVALENCE AND CONVERSION

- Glycopyrronium bromide tablets and oral solutions are not interchangeable on a microgram-for-microgram basis due to differences in bioavailability. *Sialanar*® oral solution has approximately 25% higher bioavailability and therefore equivalent doses will be lower than for tablets and generic oral solutions. *Sialanar*® oral solution contains 400 micrograms/mL of glycopyrronium bromide which is equivalent to 320 micrograms/mL of glycopyrronium. Doses in BNF Publications are expressed as glycopyrronium bromide, however *Sialanar*® oral solution doses may be expressed as glycopyrronium in other literature.

● UNLICENSED USE

- With oral use EvGr Glycopyrronium bromide is used for the control of upper airways secretion and hypersalivation, ⟨E⟩ but is not licensed for these indications.
- With intramuscular use or intravenous use or subcutaneous use Not licensed for use in control of upper airways secretion and hypersalivation.

IMPORTANT SAFETY INFORMATION

Antimuscarinic drugs used for premedication to general anaesthesia should only be administered by, or under the direct supervision of, personnel experienced in their use.

● CAUTIONS

- With oral use Compromised blood-brain barrier—monitor for behavioural changes

● INTERACTIONS → Appendix 1: glycopyrronium

● SIDE-EFFECTS

▶ **Common or very common**

- With oral use Akathisia · anxiety · behaviour abnormal · bronchial secretion decreased · concentration impaired · crying · depressed mood · diarrhoea · fever · increased risk of infection · mood altered · nasal congestion

▶ **Uncommon**

- With oral use Breath odour · dehydration · eye disorders · gastrointestinal disorders · insomnia · seizure · thirst

- ▶ **Frequency not known**
- ▶ With oral use Anhidrosis · dry eye · dysphagia · epistaxis · speech disorder
- ▶ With parenteral use Anhidrosis · bronchial secretion decreased · mydriasis

● **PREGNANCY**
- ▶ With oral use Manufacturer advises avoid—no information available.

● **BREAST FEEDING**
- ▶ With oral use Manufacturer advises avoid—no information available.

● **RENAL IMPAIRMENT** See p. 16.
- ▶ With systemic use EvGr Caution in renal impairment—duration of action may be prolonged. Repeated or large doses should be avoided in patients with uraemia due to risk of accumulation. Ⓜ
- ▶ With oral use EvGr Avoid if estimated glomerular filtration rate is less than 30 mL/minute/1.73 m^2. Ⓜ

Dose adjustments
- ▶ With oral use EvGr Reduce dose by 30% if estimated glomerular filtration rate is 30–89 mL/minute/1.73 m^2—consult product literature. Ⓜ

● **DIRECTIONS FOR ADMINISTRATION**
- ▶ With oral use Doses should be given at least 1 hour before or 2 hours after food, or at consistent times with respect to food if co-administration with food is required—high-fat food should be avoided; for administration by a nasogastric or feeding tube—consult product literature.

● **PRESCRIBING AND DISPENSING INFORMATION** Oral preparations are not interchangeable on a microgram-for-microgram basis due to differences in bioavailability. The prescriber should state the specific branded or generic oral preparation to be used; care should be taken if switching between oral preparations and dosing adjusted accordingly.
- ▶ With oral use Prescribers should consult the *Healthcare Professional Checklist* provided before initiation of treatment and at each dose adjustment.

● **PATIENT AND CARER ADVICE**
- ▶ With oral use Manufacturer advises patients and their carers should be informed to stop treatment and seek medical advice if constipation, urinary retention, pneumonia, allergic reaction, pyrexia, or changes in behaviour occur; treatment should also be stopped and medical advice sought in very hot weather.

Risk materials
- ▶ With oral use A patient alert card should be provided.

Medicines for Children leaflet: Glycopyrronium to reduce saliva production www.medicinesforchildren.org.uk/medicines/glycopyrronium-to-reduce-saliva-production/

● **NATIONAL FUNDING/ACCESS DECISIONS**
For full details see funding body website

Scottish Medicines Consortium (SMC) decisions
- ▶ **Glycopyrronium bromide (*Sialanar®*) for the symptomatic treatment of severe sialorrhoea (chronic pathological drooling) in children and adolescents aged 3 years and older with chronic neurological disorders (July 2017)** SMC No. 1254/17 Recommended

● **MEDICINAL FORMS** There can be variation in the licensing of different medicines containing the same drug. Forms available from special-order manufacturers include: oral solution

Oral tablet
- ▶ **Glycopyrronium bromide (Non-proprietary)**
  Glycopyrronium bromide 1 mg Glycopyrronium bromide 1mg tablets | 30 tablet PoM £270.18 DT = £100.36
  Glycopyrronium bromide 2 mg Glycopyrronium bromide 2mg tablets | 30 tablet PoM £290.51 DT = £198.00
- ▶ **Assicco** (Morningside Healthcare Ltd)
  Glycopyrronium bromide 1 mg Assicco 1mg tablets | 30 tablet PoM £79.00 DT = £100.36
  Glycopyrronium bromide 2 mg Assicco 2mg tablets | 30 tablet PoM £123.00 DT = £198.00

Solution for injection
- ▶ **Glycopyrronium bromide (Non-proprietary)**
  Glycopyrronium bromide 200 microgram per 1 ml Glycopyrronium bromide 200micrograms/1ml solution for injection ampoules | 10 ampoule PoM £10.50 DT = £6.77 (Hospital only) | 10 ampoule PoM £20.01 DT = £6.77
  Glycopyrronium bromide 600micrograms/3ml solution for injection ampoules | 3 ampoule PoM £8.00 | 10 ampoule PoM £21.12-£22.28 DT = £22.92 | 10 ampoule PoM £14.99 DT = £22.92 (Hospital only)

Oral solution
- ▶ **Glycopyrronium bromide (Non-proprietary)**
  Glycopyrronium bromide 200 microgram per 1 ml Glycopyrronium bromide 1mg/5ml oral solution sugar free | 150 ml PoM £111.75 DT = £49.75 SF
  Glycopyrronium bromide 400 microgram per 1 ml Glycopyrronium bromide 2mg/5ml oral solution sugar free | 60 ml PoM £76.80 DT = £76.80 SF | 250 ml PoM £320.00 DT = £320.00 SF
- ▶ **Sialanar** (Proveca Ltd)
  Glycopyrronium bromide 400 microgram per 1 ml Sialanar 320micrograms/ml oral solution | 60 ml PoM £76.80 DT = £76.80 SF | 250 ml PoM £320.00 DT = £320.00 SF

1.1 Neuromuscular blockade

Neuromuscular blockade

Neuromuscular blocking drugs

Neuromuscular blocking drugs used in anaesthesia are also known as **muscle relaxants**. By specific blockade of the neuromuscular junction they enable light anaesthesia to be used with adequate relaxation of the muscles of the abdomen and diaphragm. They also relax the vocal cords and allow the passage of a tracheal tube. Their action differs from the muscle relaxants used in musculoskeletal disorders that act on the spinal cord or brain.

Children who have received a neuromuscular blocking drug should **always** have their respiration assisted or controlled until the drug has been inactivated or antagonised. They should also receive sufficient concomitant inhalational or intravenous anaesthetic or sedative drugs to prevent awareness.

Non-depolarising neuromuscular blocking drugs
Non-depolarising neuromuscular blocking drugs (also known as competitive muscle relaxants) compete with acetylcholine for receptor sites at the neuromuscular junction and their action can be reversed with anticholinesterases such as neostigmine p. 814. Non-depolarising neuromuscular blocking drugs can be divided into the **aminosteroid** group, comprising pancuronium bromide p. 1018, rocuronium bromide p. 1019, and vecuronium bromide p. 1019, and the **benzylisoquinolinium** group, comprising atracurium besilate p. 1017, cisatracurium p. 1018, and mivacurium p. 1018.

Non-depolarising neuromuscular blocking drugs have a slower onset of action than suxamethonium chloride p. 1016. These drugs can be classified by their duration of action as short-acting (15–30 minutes), intermediate-acting (30–40 minutes), and long-acting (60–120 minutes), although duration of action is dose-dependent. Drugs with a shorter or intermediate duration of action, such as atracurium besilate and vecuronium bromide p. 1019, are more widely used than those with a longer duration of action, such as pancuronium bromide.

Non-depolarising neuromuscular blocking drugs have no sedative or analgesic effects and are not considered to trigger malignant hyperthermia.

For patients receiving intensive care and who require tracheal intubation and mechanical ventilation, a non-depolarising neuromuscular blocking drug is chosen according to its onset of effect, duration of action, and side-effects. Rocuronium bromide, with a rapid onset of effect, may facilitate intubation. Atracurium besilate or cisatracurium may be suitable for long-term neuromuscular blockade since their duration of action is not dependent on elimination by the liver or the kidneys.

Atracurium besilate, a mixture of 10 isomers, is a benzylisoquinolinium neuromuscular blocking drug with an intermediate duration of action. It undergoes non-enzymatic metabolism which is independent of liver and kidney function, thus allowing its use in children with hepatic or renal impairment. Cardiovascular effects are associated with significant histamine release; histamine release can be minimised by administering slowly or in divided doses over at least 1 minute. Neonates may be more sensitive to the effects of atracurium besilate and lower doses may be required.

Cisatracurium is a single isomer of atracurium besilate. It is more potent and has a slightly longer duration of action than atracurium besilate and provides greater cardiovascular stability because cisatracurium lacks histamine-releasing effects. In children aged 1 month to 12 years, cisatracurium has a shorter duration of action and produces faster spontaneous recovery.

Mivacurium, a benzylisoquinolinium neuromuscular blocking drug, has a short duration of action. It is metabolised by plasma cholinesterase and muscle paralysis is prolonged in individuals deficient in this enzyme. It is not associated with vagolytic activity or ganglionic blockade although histamine release can occur, particularly with rapid injection. In children under 12 years mivacurium has a faster onset, shorter duration of action, and produces more rapid spontaneous recovery.

Pancuronium bromide, an aminosteroid neuromuscular blocking drug, has a long duration of action and is often used in children receiving long-term mechanical ventilation in intensive care units. It lacks a histamine-releasing effect, but vagolytic and sympathomimetic effects can cause tachycardia and hypertension. The half-life of pancuronium bromide is prolonged in neonates; neonates should receive postoperative intermittent positive pressure ventilation.

Rocuronium bromide exerts an effect within 2 minutes and has the most rapid onset of any of the non-depolarising neuromuscular blocking drugs. It is an aminosteroid neuromuscular blocking drug with an intermediate duration of action. It is reported to have minimal cardiovascular effects; high doses produce mild vagolytic activity. In most children, the duration of action of rocuronium bromide may be shorter than in adults; however, in neonates and children under 2 years, usual doses may produce a more prolonged action.

Vecuronium bromide p. 1019, an aminosteroid neuromuscular blocking drug, has an intermediate duration of action. It does not generally produce histamine release and lacks cardiovascular effects. In most children, the duration of action of vecuronium bromide may be shorter than in adults; however, in neonates and children under 2 years, usual doses may produce a more prolonged action.

Depolarising neuromuscular blocking drugs

Suxamethonium chloride has the most rapid onset of action of any of the neuromuscular blocking drugs and is ideal if fast onset and brief duration of action are required e.g. with tracheal intubation. Neonates and young children are less sensitive to suxamethonium chloride and a higher dose may be required. Unlike the non-depolarising neuromuscular blocking drugs, its action cannot be reversed and recovery is spontaneous; anticholinesterases such as neostigmine potentiate the neuromuscular block.

Suxamethonium chloride should be given after anaesthetic induction because paralysis is usually preceded by painful muscle fasciculations. Bradycardia may occur; premedication with atropine sulfate p. 1013 reduces bradycardia as well as the excessive salivation associated with suxamethonium chloride use.

Prolonged paralysis may occur in dual block, which occurs with high or repeated doses of suxamethonium chloride and is caused by the development of a non-depolarising block following the initial depolarising block. Children with myasthenia gravis are resistant to suxamethonium chloride but can develop dual block resulting in delayed recovery. Prolonged paralysis may also occur in those with low or atypical plasma cholinesterase. Assisted ventilation should be continued until muscle function is restored.

NEUROMUSCULAR BLOCKING DRUGS › DEPOLARISING

Suxamethonium chloride

02-Dec-2020

(Succinylcholine chloride)

● **DRUG ACTION** Suxamethonium acts by mimicking acetylcholine at the neuromuscular junction but hydrolysis is much slower than for acetylcholine; depolarisation is therefore prolonged, resulting in neuromuscular blockade.

● **INDICATIONS AND DOSE**

Neuromuscular blockade (short duration) during surgery

▸ BY INTRAVENOUS INJECTION

- ▸ Neonate: 2 mg/kg, produces 5–10 minutes neuromuscular blockade.
- ▸ Child 1–11 months: 2 mg/kg
- ▸ Child 1–17 years: 1 mg/kg

▸ BY INTRAMUSCULAR INJECTION

- ▸ Neonate: Up to 4 mg/kg, produces 10–30 minutes neuromuscular blockade.
- ▸ Child 1–11 months: Up to 5 mg/kg
- ▸ Child 1–11 years: Up to 4 mg/kg (max. per dose 150 mg)

PHARMACOKINETICS

- ▸ Intramuscular injection has a duration of onset of 2–3 minutes.

IMPORTANT SAFETY INFORMATION
Should only be administered by, or under the direct supervision of, personnel experienced in its use.

● **CONTRA-INDICATIONS** Hyperkalaemia · low plasma-cholinesterase activity (including severe liver disease) · major trauma · neurological disease involving acute wasting of major muscle · personal or family history of congenital myotonic disease · personal or family history of malignant hyperthermia · prolonged immobilisation (risk of hyperkalaemia) · severe burns · skeletal muscle myopathies (e.g. Duchenne muscular dystrophy)

● **CAUTIONS** Cardiac disease · neuromuscular disease · raised intra-ocular pressure (avoid in penetrating eye injury) · respiratory disease · severe sepsis (risk of hyperkalaemia)

● **INTERACTIONS** → Appendix 1: suxamethonium

● **SIDE-EFFECTS**

▸ **Common or very common** Arrhythmias · flushing · muscle contractions involuntary · myoglobinuria · myopathy · post procedural muscle pain · rash

▸ **Rare or very rare** Apnoea · cardiac arrest · hypersensitivity · malignant hyperthermia · respiratory disorders · trismus

SIDE-EFFECTS, FURTHER INFORMATION Premedication with atropine reduces bradycardia associated with suxamethonium use.

- **ALLERGY AND CROSS-SENSITIVITY** EvGr Allergic cross-reactivity between neuromuscular blocking drugs has been reported; caution is advised in cases of hypersensitivity to these drugs. ⟨M⟩
- **PREGNANCY** Mildly prolonged maternal neuromuscular blockade may occur.
- **BREAST FEEDING** Unlikely to be present in breast milk in significant amounts (ionised at physiological pH). Breast-feeding may be resumed once the mother recovered from neuromuscular block.
- **HEPATIC IMPAIRMENT** Manufacturer advises caution, particularly in end stage hepatic failure (increased risk of prolonged apnoea due to reduced hepatic synthesis of plasma cholinesterase).
- **DIRECTIONS FOR ADMINISTRATION** For *intravenous injection*, manufacturer advises give undiluted or dilute with Glucose 5% or Sodium Chloride 0.9%.

- **MEDICINAL FORMS** There can be variation in the licensing of different medicines containing the same drug. Forms available from special-order manufacturers include: solution for injection

Solution for injection

- Suxamethonium chloride (Non-proprietary)

Suxamethonium chloride 50 mg per 1 ml Suxamethonium chloride 100mg/2ml solution for injection ampoules | 10 ampoule PoM £28.80–£50.00

NEUROMUSCULAR BLOCKING DRUGS › NON-DEPOLARISING

Non-depolarising neuromuscular blocking drugs

IMPORTANT SAFETY INFORMATION
Non-depolarising neuromuscular blocking drugs should only be administered by, or under direct supervision of, personnel experienced in their use, with adequate training in anaesthesia and airway management.

- **CAUTIONS** Burns (resistance can develop, increased doses may be required) · cardiovascular disease (reduce rate of administration) · electrolyte disturbances (response unpredictable) · fluid disturbances (response unpredictable) · hypothermia (activity prolonged, lower doses required) · myasthenia gravis (activity prolonged, lower doses required) · neuromuscular disorders (response unpredictable)
- **SIDE-EFFECTS**
  - **Common or very common** Flushing · hypotension
  - **Uncommon** Bronchospasm · hypersensitivity · skin reactions · tachycardia
  - **Rare or very rare** Circulatory collapse · muscle weakness (after prolonged use in intensive care) · myopathy (after prolonged use in intensive care) · shock
- **ALLERGY AND CROSS-SENSITIVITY** Allergic cross-reactivity between neuromuscular blocking drugs has been reported; caution is advised in cases of hypersensitivity to these drugs.
- **PREGNANCY** Non-depolarising neuromuscular blocking drugs are highly ionised at physiological pH and are therefore unlikely to cross the placenta in significant amounts.
- **BREAST FEEDING** Non-depolarising neuromuscular blocking drugs are ionised at physiological pH and are unlikely to be present in milk in significant amounts.

Breast-feeding may be resumed once the mother has recovered from neuromuscular block.

above

Atracurium besilate

(Atracurium besylate)

- **INDICATIONS AND DOSE**

Neuromuscular blockade (short to intermediate duration) for surgery

- INITIALLY BY INTRAVENOUS INJECTION
  - Neonate: Initially 300–500 micrograms/kg, followed by (by intravenous injection) 100–200 micrograms/kg, repeated if necessary, alternatively (by intravenous infusion) 300–400 micrograms/kg/hour, adjusted according to response.
  - Child: Initially 300–600 micrograms/kg, then (by intravenous injection) 100–200 micrograms/kg, repeated if necessary, alternatively (by intravenous injection) initially 300–600 micrograms/kg, followed by (by intravenous infusion) 300–600 micrograms/kg/hour, adjusted according to response

Neuromuscular blockade during intensive care

- INITIALLY BY INTRAVENOUS INJECTION
  - Neonate: Initially 300–500 micrograms/kg, followed by (by intravenous injection) 100–200 micrograms/kg, repeated if necessary, alternatively (by intravenous infusion) 300–400 micrograms/kg/hour, adjusted according to response, higher doses may be necessary.
  - Child: Initially 300–600 micrograms/kg, initial dose is optional, then (by intravenous infusion) 270–1770 micrograms/kg/hour; (by intravenous infusion) usual dose 650–780 micrograms/kg/hour

DOSES AT EXTREMES OF BODY-WEIGHT

- To avoid excessive dosage in obese patients, dose should be calculated on the basis of ideal body-weight.

- **UNLICENSED USE** Not licensed for use in neonates.
- **INTERACTIONS** → Appendix 1: neuromuscular blocking drugs, non-depolarising
- **SIDE-EFFECTS**
  - **Rare or very rare** Cardiac arrest
  - **Frequency not known** Seizure

SIDE-EFFECTS, FURTHER INFORMATION Hypotension, skin flushing, and bronchospasm is associated with histamine release. Manufacturer advises minimising effects of histamine release by administering over 1 minute in patients with cardiovascular disease or sensitivity to hypotension. Neonates may be more sensitive to the effects of atracurium and lower doses may be required.

- **DIRECTIONS FOR ADMINISTRATION** For *continuous intravenous infusion*, dilute to a concentration of 0.5–5 mg/mL with Glucose 5% or Sodium Chloride 0.9%; stability varies with diluent.
  - In neonates *Neonatal intensive care*, dilute 60 mg/kg body-weight to a final volume of 50 mL with Glucose 5% or Sodium Chloride 0.9%; minimum concentration of 500 micrograms/mL, maximum concentration of 5 mg/mL; an intravenous infusion rate of 0.1 mL/hour provides a dose of 120 micrograms/kg/hour.

- **MEDICINAL FORMS** There can be variation in the licensing of different medicines containing the same drug. Forms available from special-order manufacturers include: solution for injection

Solution for injection

- **Atracurium besilate (Non-proprietary)**
  Atracurium besilate 10 mg per 1 ml Atracurium besilate 250mg/25ml solution for injection vials | 1 vial PoM £16.50 (Hospital only) | 2 vial PoM £25.81 (Hospital only)
  Atracurium besilate 25mg/2.5ml solution for injection ampoules | 5 ampoule PoM £8.28 (Hospital only) | 10 ampoule PoM £27.50 | 10 ampoule PoM £16.56 (Hospital only)
  Atracurium besilate 50mg/5ml solution for injection ampoules | 5 ampoule PoM £15.02 (Hospital only) | 10 ampoule PoM £42.35 | 10 ampoule PoM £30.04 (Hospital only)

F 1017

Cisatracurium

24-Jul-2020

- **INDICATIONS AND DOSE**

Neuromuscular blockade (intermediate duration) during surgery

- INITIALLY BY INTRAVENOUS INJECTION
  - Child 1 month–1 year: Initially 150 micrograms/kg, then (by intravenous injection) 30 micrograms/kg every 20 minutes as required
  - Child 2–11 years: Initially 150 micrograms/kg, 80–100 micrograms/kg if not for intubation, then (by intravenous injection) 20 micrograms/kg every 10 minutes as required, alternatively (by intravenous injection) initially 150 micrograms/kg, followed by (by intravenous infusion) 180 micrograms/kg/hour, (by intravenous infusion) reduced to 60–120 micrograms/kg/hour, adjusted according to response
  - Child 12–17 years: Initially 150 micrograms/kg, then (by intravenous injection) 30 micrograms/kg every 20 minutes as required, alternatively (by intravenous injection) initially 150 micrograms/kg, followed by (by intravenous infusion) 180 micrograms/kg/hour, (by intravenous infusion) reduced to 60–120 micrograms/kg/hour, adjusted according to response

DOSES AT EXTREMES OF BODY-WEIGHT

- To avoid excessive dosage in obese patients, dose should be calculated on the basis of ideal body-weight.

- **INTERACTIONS** → Appendix 1: neuromuscular blocking drugs, non-depolarising
- **SIDE-EFFECTS**
  - **Common or very common** Bradycardia
- **DIRECTIONS FOR ADMINISTRATION** For *continuous intravenous infusion*, manufacturer advises dilute to a concentration of 0.1–2 mg/mL with Glucose 5% or Sodium Chloride 0.9%; solutions of 2 mg/mL and 5 mg/mL may be infused undiluted.
- **MEDICINAL FORMS** There can be variation in the licensing of different medicines containing the same drug.

Solution for injection

- **Cisatracurium (Non-proprietary)**
  Cisatracurium (as Cisatracurium besilate) 2 mg per 1 ml Cisatracurium besilate 10mg/5ml solution for injection ampoules | 5 ampoule PoM (Hospital only)
  Cisatracurium besilate 20mg/10ml solution for injection ampoules | 5 ampoule PoM £32.09–£37.75 (Hospital only)
  Cisatracurium besilate 10mg/5ml solution for injection vials | 1 vial PoM £30.00 (Hospital only)
  Cisatracurium (as Cisatracurium besilate) 5 mg per 1 ml Cisatracurium besilate 150mg/30ml solution for injection vials | 1 vial PoM £26.43–£31.09 (Hospital only) | 5 vial PoM £132.15 (Hospital only)

F 1017

Mivacurium

10-May-2021

- **INDICATIONS AND DOSE**

Neuromuscular blockade (short duration) during surgery

- INITIALLY BY INTRAVENOUS INJECTION
  - Child 2–5 months: Initially 150 micrograms/kg, then (by intravenous injection) 100 micrograms/kg every 6–9 minutes as required, alternatively (by intravenous infusion) 8–10 micrograms/kg/minute, (by intravenous infusion) adjusted in steps of 1 microgram/kg/minute every 3 minutes if required; (by intravenous infusion) usual dose 11–14 micrograms/kg/minute
  - Child 6 months–11 years: Initially 200 micrograms/kg, then (by intravenous injection) 100 micrograms/kg every 6–9 minutes as required, alternatively (by intravenous infusion) 8–10 micrograms/kg/minute, (by intravenous infusion) adjusted in steps of 1 microgram/kg/minute every 3 minutes if required; (by intravenous infusion) usual dose 11–14 micrograms/kg/minute
  - Child 12–17 years: Initially 70–250 micrograms/kg, then (by intravenous injection) 100 micrograms/kg every 15 minutes as required, alternatively (by intravenous infusion) 8–10 micrograms/kg/minute, (by intravenous infusion) adjusted in steps of 1 microgram/kg/minute every 3 minutes if required; (by intravenous infusion) usual dose 6–7 micrograms/kg/minute

DOSES AT EXTREMES OF BODY-WEIGHT

- To avoid excessive dosage in obese patients, dose should be calculated on the basis of ideal body-weight.

- **CAUTIONS** Burns (low plasma cholinesterase activity; dose titration required)
- **INTERACTIONS** → Appendix 1: neuromuscular blocking drugs, non-depolarising
- **HEPATIC IMPAIRMENT** Manufacturer advises caution in hepatic failure (increased duration of action).
  Dose adjustments Manufacturer advises dose reduction in hepatic failure.
- **RENAL IMPAIRMENT** EvGr Use with caution. (M)
  Dose adjustments EvGr Reduce dose according to response in end-stage renal disease (clinical effect prolonged). (M)
- **DIRECTIONS FOR ADMINISTRATION** For *intravenous injection*, give undiluted or dilute in Glucose 5% or Sodium Chloride 0.9%. Doses up to 150 micrograms/kg may be given over 5–15 seconds, higher doses should be given over 30 seconds. In asthma, cardiovascular disease or in those sensitive to reduced arterial blood pressure, give over 60 seconds.
- **MEDICINAL FORMS** There can be variation in the licensing of different medicines containing the same drug.

Solution for injection

- **Mivacurium (Non-proprietary)**
  Mivacurium (as Mivacurium chloride) 2 mg per 1 ml Mivacurium chloride 20mg/10ml solution for injection ampoules | 5 ampoule PoM £22.57 (Hospital only)
  Mivacurium chloride 10mg/5ml solution for injection ampoules | 5 ampoule PoM £13.95 (Hospital only)

F 1017

Pancuronium bromide

10-May-2021

- **INDICATIONS AND DOSE**

Neuromuscular blockade (long duration) during surgery

- BY INTRAVENOUS INJECTION
  - Neonate: Initially 100 micrograms/kg, then 50 micrograms/kg, repeated if necessary.

- Child: Initially 100 micrograms/kg, then 20 micrograms/kg, repeated if necessary

DOSES AT EXTREMES OF BODY-WEIGHT
- To avoid excessive dosage in obese patients, dose should be calculated on the basis of ideal body-weight.

- **INTERACTIONS** → Appendix 1: neuromuscular blocking drugs, non-depolarising
- **SIDE-EFFECTS** Apnoea · arrhythmia · hypersalivation · increased cardiac output · miosis

SIDE-EFFECTS, FURTHER INFORMATION Pancuronium lacks histamine-releasing effect, but vagolytic and sympathomimetic effects can cause tachycardia.
- **HEPATIC IMPAIRMENT** Manufacturer advises caution (possibly slower onset and higher dose requirements due to resistance to neuromuscular blocking action which may lead to a prolonged recovery time).
- **RENAL IMPAIRMENT** EvGr Use with caution (may prolong duration of block). (M)
- **DIRECTIONS FOR ADMINISTRATION** For *intravenous injection*, expert sources advise give undiluted or dilute in Glucose 5% or Sodium Chloride 0.9%.
- **MEDICINAL FORMS** No licensed medicines listed.

F 1017

Rocuronium bromide

10-May-2021

- **INDICATIONS AND DOSE**

Neuromuscular blockade (intermediate duration) during surgery

▶ INITIALLY BY INTRAVENOUS INJECTION
- Neonate: Initially 600 micrograms/kg, then (by intravenous injection) 150 micrograms/kg, repeated if necessary, alternatively (by intravenous infusion) 300–600 micrograms/kg/hour, adjusted according to response.
- Child: Initially 600 micrograms/kg, then (by intravenous injection) 150 micrograms/kg, repeated if necessary, alternatively (by intravenous infusion) 300–600 micrograms/kg/hour, adjusted according to response

Assisted ventilation in intensive care

▶ INITIALLY BY INTRAVENOUS INJECTION
- Child: Initially 600 micrograms/kg, initial dose is optional, then (by intravenous infusion) 300–600 micrograms/kg/hour for first hour, then (by intravenous infusion), adjusted according to response

DOSES AT EXTREMES OF BODY-WEIGHT
- To avoid excessive dosage in obese patients, dose should be calculated on the basis of ideal body-weight.

- **UNLICENSED USE** Not licensed for use in children for assisted ventilation in intensive care.
- **INTERACTIONS** → Appendix 1: neuromuscular blocking drugs, non-depolarising
- **SIDE-EFFECTS**
  - **Uncommon** Procedural complications
  - **Rare or very rare** Angioedema · face oedema · paralysis
  - **Frequency not known** Malignant hyperthermia
- **HEPATIC IMPAIRMENT** Manufacturer advises caution (may prolong duration of action).
  Dose adjustments Manufacturer advises consider dose reduction—consult product literature.
- **RENAL IMPAIRMENT** EvGr Use with caution (may prolong duration of block). (M)
  Dose adjustments EvGr Reduce maintenance dose (consult product literature). (M)
- **DIRECTIONS FOR ADMINISTRATION** EvGr For *continuous intravenous infusion* or via drip tubing, may be diluted with Glucose 5% or Sodium Chloride 0.9%. (M)
- **MEDICINAL FORMS** There can be variation in the licensing of different medicines containing the same drug.

Solution for injection

▶ **Rocuronium bromide (Non-proprietary)**

Rocuronium bromide 10 mg per 1 ml Rocuronium bromide 100mg/10ml solution for injection vials | 10 vial PoM £57.00-£102.90 (Hospital only)
Rocuronium bromide 100mg/10ml solution for injection pre-filled syringes | 1 pre-filled disposable injection PoM £56.00 (Hospital only)
Rocuronium bromide 50mg/5ml solution for injection ampoules | 10 ampoule PoM £28.00 | 10 ampoule PoM £28.00 (Hospital only) | 20 ampoule PoM £94.40 (Hospital only)
Rocuronium bromide 100mg/10ml solution for injection ampoules | 10 ampoule PoM £56.00–£57.00
Rocuronium bromide 50mg/5ml solution for injection pre-filled syringes | 1 pre-filled disposable injection PoM £28.00 (Hospital only) | 10 pre-filled disposable injection PoM £190.00 (Hospital only)
Rocuronium bromide 50mg/5ml solution for injection vials | 10 vial PoM £28.00–£50.90 (Hospital only)

F 1017

Vecuronium bromide

10-May-2021

- **INDICATIONS AND DOSE**

Neuromuscular blockade (intermediate duration) during surgery

▶ BY INTRAVENOUS INJECTION
- Neonate: (consult product literature).
- Child: (consult product literature)

DOSES AT EXTREMES OF BODY-WEIGHT
- To avoid excessive dosage in obese patients, dose should be calculated on the basis of ideal body-weight.

- **INTERACTIONS** → Appendix 1: neuromuscular blocking drugs, non-depolarising
- **SIDE-EFFECTS**
  - **Uncommon** Procedural complications
  - **Rare or very rare** Angioedema · face oedema · paralysis
- **HEPATIC IMPAIRMENT** Manufacturer advises caution in significant impairment.
- **RENAL IMPAIRMENT** EvGr Use with caution. (M)
- **MEDICINAL FORMS** There can be variation in the licensing of different medicines containing the same drug.

Powder for solution for injection

▶ **Vecuronium bromide (Non-proprietary)**

Vecuronium bromide 10 mg Vecuronium bromide 10mg powder for solution for injection vials | 10 vial PoM £75.00 (Hospital only)

1.2 Neuromuscular blockade reversal

Neuromuscular blockade reversal

Neuromuscular blockade reversal

Anticholinesterases

Anticholinesterases reverse the effects of the non-depolarising (competitive) neuromuscular blocking drugs such as pancuronium bromide p. 1018 but they prolong the action of the depolarising neuromuscular blocking drug suxamethonium chloride p. 1016.

Neostigmine p. 814 is used specifically for reversal of non-depolarising (competitive) blockade. It acts within one minute of intravenous injection and its effects last for 20 to 30 minutes; a second dose may then be necessary.

Glycopyrronium bromide p. 1014 or alternatively atropine sulfate p. 1013, given before or with neostigmine, prevent bradycardia, excessive salivation, and other muscarinic effects of neostigmine.

Other drugs for reversal of neuromuscular blockade
Sugammadex below is a modified gamma cyclodextrin that can be used in children for the routine reversal of neuromuscular blockade induced by rocuronium bromide p. 1019.

ANTICHOLINESTERASES

Neostigmine with glycopyrronium bromide

17-Jul-2020

The properties listed below are those particular to the combination only. For the properties of the components please consider, neostigmine p. 814, glycopyrronium bromide p. 1014.

- **INDICATIONS AND DOSE**

Reversal of non-depolarising neuromuscular blockade
- BY INTRAVENOUS INJECTION
- Child: 0.02 mL/kilogram, repeated if necessary, alternatively dilute to 1 in 10 solution and give 0.2 mL/kg; maximum 2 mL per course

- **INTERACTIONS** → Appendix 1: glycopyrronium · neostigmine
- **DIRECTIONS FOR ADMINISTRATION** For *intravenous injection*, manufacturer advises may be diluted with Sodium Chloride 0.9%, give over 10–30 seconds.

- **MEDICINAL FORMS** There can be variation in the licensing of different medicines containing the same drug.

Solution for injection
- Neostigmine with glycopyrronium bromide (Non-proprietary)
  Glycopyrronium bromide 500 microgram per 1 ml, Neostigmine metilsulfate 2.5 mg per 1 ml Neostigmine 2.5mg/1ml / Glycopyrronium bromide 500micrograms/1ml solution for injection ampoules | 10 ampoule PoM £11.50–£13.03

ANTIDOTES AND CHELATORS

Sugammadex

10-Aug-2021

- **INDICATIONS AND DOSE**

Routine reversal of neuromuscular blockade induced by rocuronium
- BY INTRAVENOUS INJECTION
- Child 2-17 years: 2 mg/kg (consult product literature)

IMPORTANT SAFETY INFORMATION
Should only be administered by, or under the direct supervision of, personnel experienced in its use.

- **CAUTIONS** Cardiovascular disease (recovery may be delayed) · pre-existing coagulation disorders · recurrence of neuromuscular blockade—monitor respiratory function until fully recovered · use of anticoagulants (unrelated to surgery) · wait 24 hours before re-administering rocuronium
- **INTERACTIONS** → Appendix 1: sugammadex
- **SIDE-EFFECTS**
  - **Common or very common** Abdominal pain · cough · dizziness · headache · nausea · procedural complications · skin reactions · taste altered · vomiting
  - **Frequency not known** Arrhythmias
- **PREGNANCY** Use with caution—no information available.
- **RENAL IMPAIRMENT** EvGr Avoid if creatinine clearance less than 30 mL/minute. ⟨M⟩ See p. 16.
- **DIRECTIONS FOR ADMINISTRATION** For *intravenous injection*, manufacturer advises dose may be diluted to a concentration of 10 mg/mL with Sodium Chloride 0.9%.
- **NATIONAL FUNDING/ACCESS DECISIONS**
  For full details see funding body website

Scottish Medicines Consortium (SMC) decisions
- **Sugammadex (*Bridion*®) for the routine reversal of neuromuscular blockade induced by rocuronium or vecuronium in adults and rocuronium in paediatric patients (March 2013)** SMC No. 527/09 Recommended with restrictions

- **MEDICINAL FORMS** There can be variation in the licensing of different medicines containing the same drug.

Solution for injection
ELECTROLYTES: May contain Sodium
- Sugammadex (Non-proprietary)
  Sugammadex (as Sugammadex sodium) 100 mg per 1 ml Sugammadex 500mg/5ml solution for injection vials | 10 vial PoM £1,100.00–£1,491.00 (Hospital only)
  Sugammadex 200mg/2ml solution for injection vials | 10 vial PoM £418.00–£596.40 (Hospital only)
- Bridion (Merck Sharp & Dohme (UK) Ltd)
  Sugammadex (as Sugammadex sodium) 100 mg per 1 ml Bridion 200mg/2ml solution for injection vials | 10 vial PoM £596.40 (Hospital only)

1.3 Peri-operative analgesia

Peri-operative analgesia

Non-opioid analgesics

Since non-steroidal anti-inflammatory drugs (NSAIDs) do not depress respiration, do not impair gastro-intestinal motility, and do not cause dependence, they may be useful alternatives or adjuncts to opioids for the relief of postoperative pain. NSAIDs may be inadequate for the relief of severe pain.

Diclofenac sodium p. 818, diclofenac potassium p. 817, ibuprofen p. 821, paracetamol p. 325, and ketorolac trometamol p. 1021 are used to relieve postoperative pain in children; diclofenac sodium and paracetamol can be given parenterally and rectally as well as by mouth. Ketorolac trometamol is given by intravenous injection.

Opioid analgesics

Opioid analgesics are now rarely used as premedicants; they are more likely to be administered at induction. Pre-operative use of opioid analgesics is generally limited to children who require control of existing pain. The main side-effects of opioid analgesics are respiratory depression, cardiovascular depression, nausea, and vomiting; see general notes on opioid analgesics and their use in postoperative pain.

See the management of opioid-induced respiratory depression in Pre-medication and peri-operative drugs p. 1012.

Intra-operative analgesia

Opioid analgesics given in small doses before or with induction reduce the dose requirement of some drugs used during anaesthesia.

Alfentanil p. 1022, fentanyl p. 334, and remifentanil p. 1022 are particularly useful because they act within 1–2 minutes and have short durations of action. The initial doses of alfentanil or fentanyl are followed either by successive intravenous injections or by an intravenous infusion; prolonged infusions increase the duration of effect.

In contrast to other opioids which are metabolised in the liver, remifentanil undergoes rapid metabolism by nonspecific blood and tissue esterases; its short duration of action allows prolonged administration at high dosage, without accumulation, and with little risk of residual postoperative respiratory depression. Remifentanil should not be given by intravenous injection intraoperatively, but it is well suited to continuous infusion; a supplementary analgesic is given before stopping the infusion of remifentanil.

ANALGESICS > NON-STEROIDAL ANTI-INFLAMMATORY DRUGS

Ketorolac trometamol

19-Mar-2025

● **INDICATIONS AND DOSE**

Short-term management of moderate to severe acute postoperative pain only

▶ BY INTRAMUSCULAR INJECTION, OR BY INTRAVENOUS INJECTION

▸ Child 16–17 years (body-weight up to 50 kg): Initially 10 mg, then 10–30 mg every 4–6 hours as required for maximum duration of treatment 2 days, frequency may be increased to up to every 2 hours during initial postoperative period; maximum 60 mg per day

▸ Child 16–17 years (body-weight 50 kg and above): Initially 10 mg, then 10–30 mg every 4–6 hours as required for maximum duration of treatment 2 days, frequency may be increased to up to every 2 hours during initial postoperative period; maximum 90 mg per day

▶ BY INTRAVENOUS INJECTION

▸ Child 6 months–15 years: Initially 0.5–1 mg/kg (max. per dose 15 mg), then 500 micrograms/kg every 6 hours (max. per dose 15 mg) as required for maximum duration of treatment 2 days; maximum 60 mg per day

● **UNLICENSED USE** Not licensed for use in children under 16 years.

IMPORTANT SAFETY INFORMATION

MHRA/CHM ADVICE: NSAIDS: POTENTIAL RISKS FOLLOWING PROLONGED USE AFTER 20 WEEKS OF PREGNANCY (JUNE 2023)
See Non-steroidal anti-inflammatory drugs p. 816.

● **CONTRA-INDICATIONS** Active or history of gastro-intestinal bleeding · active or history of gastro-intestinal ulceration · coagulation disorders · complete or partial syndrome of nasal polyps · confirmed or suspected cerebrovascular bleeding · dehydration · following operations with high risk of haemorrhage or incomplete haemostasis · haemorrhagic diatheses · history of gastro-intestinal bleeding related to previous NSAID therapy · history of gastro-intestinal perforation related to previous NSAID therapy · hypovolaemia · severe heart failure

● **CAUTIONS** Allergic disorders · cardiac impairment (NSAIDs may impair renal function) · cerebrovascular disease · connective-tissue disorders · heart failure · history of gastro-intestinal disorders (e.g. ulcerative colitis, Crohn's disease) · ischaemic heart disease · may mask symptoms of infection · peripheral arterial disease · risk factors for cardiovascular events · uncontrolled hypertension

● **INTERACTIONS** → Appendix 1: NSAIDs

● **SIDE-EFFECTS** Agranulocytosis · angioedema · anxiety · aplastic anaemia · appetite decreased · asthenia · asthma · azotaemia · bradycardia · burping · chest pain · concentration impaired · confusion · constipation · Crohn's disease aggravated · depression · diarrhoea · dizziness · drowsiness · dry mouth · dyspnoea · electrolyte imbalance · embolism and thrombosis · euphoric mood · fever · flank pain · fluid retention · flushing · gastrointestinal discomfort · gastrointestinal disorders · haemolytic anaemia · haemorrhage · hallucination · headache · hearing loss · heart failure · hepatic disorders · hyperhidrosis · hyperkinesia · hypersensitivity · hypertension · hypotension · infertility female · malaise · meningitis aseptic (patients with connective-tissue disorders such as systemic lupus erythematosus may be especially susceptible) · musculoskeletal disorder · myalgia · nausea · nephritis tubulointerstitial · nephropathy · neutropenia · oedema · optic neuritis · oral disorders · pallor · palpitations · pancreatitis · paraesthesia · perforation · photosensitivity reaction · platelet aggregation inhibition · psychotic disorder · pulmonary oedema · renal impairment · respiratory disorders · seizure · severe cutaneous adverse reactions (SCARs) · skin reactions · sleep disorders · taste altered · thinking abnormal · thirst · thrombocytopenia · tinnitus · ulcer · urinary disorders · vertigo · visual impairment · vomiting · weight increased · wound haemorrhage

SIDE-EFFECTS, FURTHER INFORMATION For information about cardiovascular and gastrointestinal side-effects, and a possible exacerbation of symptoms in asthma, see Non-steroidal anti-inflammatory drugs. p. 816

● **ALLERGY AND CROSS-SENSITIVITY** EvGr Contra-indicated in patients with a history of hypersensitivity to aspirin or any other NSAID—which includes those in whom attacks of asthma, angioedema, urticaria or rhinitis have been precipitated by aspirin or any other NSAID. M

● **CONCEPTION AND CONTRACEPTION** EvGr Caution—long-term use of some NSAIDs is associated with reduced female fertility, which is reversible on stopping treatment. M

● **PREGNANCY** Avoid use in first and second trimesters unless essential; the MHRA advises additional antenatal monitoring may be required if treatment is considered necessary by a doctor from week 20 of pregnancy onwards. Avoid use in third trimester. See *NSAIDs in Pregnancy* in Non-steroidal anti-inflammatory drugs p. 816 for further details.

● **BREAST FEEDING** Amount too small to be harmful.

● **HEPATIC IMPAIRMENT** Manufacturer advises caution—may increase risk of renal impairment; avoid in hepatic failure.

● **RENAL IMPAIRMENT** In general, for *NSAIDs* the MHRA advises to avoid where possible; if necessary, use with caution (risk of fluid retention and further renal impairment, including renal failure). EvGr For *ketorolac*, avoid if serum creatinine greater than 160 micromol/litre. M

Dose adjustments EvGr Max. 60 mg daily if serum creatinine 160 micromol/litre or less. M

● **DIRECTIONS FOR ADMINISTRATION** For *intravenous injection*, manufacturer advises give over at least 15 seconds.

● **MEDICINAL FORMS** There can be variation in the licensing of different medicines containing the same drug.

Solution for injection

▸ **Ketorolac trometamol (Non-proprietary)**
Ketorolac trometamol 30 mg per 1 ml Ketorolac 30mg/1ml solution for injection ampoules | 5 ampoule PoM £5.50 DT = £5.36 (Hospital only)

▸ **Toradol** (Atnahs Pharma UK Ltd)
Ketorolac trometamol 30 mg per 1 ml Toradol 30mg/1ml solution for injection ampoules | 5 ampoule PoM £5.36 DT = £5.36 (Hospital only)

15 Anaesthesia

ANALGESICS › OPIOIDS

F 327

Alfentanil

10-May-2021

● **INDICATIONS AND DOSE**

Assisted ventilation: analgesia and enhancement of anaesthesia for short procedures

▶ BY INTRAVENOUS INJECTION

▶ Neonate: Initially 5–20 micrograms/kg, dose to be administered over 30 seconds; supplemental doses up to 10 micrograms/kg.

▶ Child: Initially 10–20 micrograms/kg, dose to be administered over 30 seconds; supplemental doses up to 10 micrograms/kg

Assisted ventilation: analgesia and enhancement of anaesthesia during maintenance of anaesthesia for longer procedures

▶ BY INTRAVENOUS INFUSION

▶ Neonate: Initially 10–50 micrograms/kg, dose to be administered over 10 minutes, followed by 30–60 micrograms/kg/hour.

▶ Child: Initially 50–100 micrograms/kg, dose to be administered over 10 minutes, followed by 30–120 micrograms/kg/hour, usual dose with intravenous anaesthetic, 60 micrograms/kg/hour

DOSES AT EXTREMES OF BODY-WEIGHT

▶ To avoid excessive dosage in obese patients, dose should be calculated on the basis of ideal body-weight.

PHARMACOKINETICS

▶ Half-life is prolonged in neonates and accumulation is likely with prolonged use. Clearance may be increased in children 1 month–12 years and higher infusion doses might be needed.

● **CAUTIONS** EvGr Repeated intra-operative doses of alfentanil should be given with care since the resulting respiratory depression can persist postoperatively and occasionally it may become apparent for the first time postoperatively when monitoring of the patient might be less intensive. (M)

● **INTERACTIONS** → Appendix 1: opioids

● **SIDE-EFFECTS**

▶ **Common or very common** Apnoea · chills · fatigue · hypertension · movement disorders · muscle rigidity · procedural complications

▶ **Uncommon** Coma · hiccups · hypercapnia · pain · post procedural complications · respiratory disorders

▶ **Rare or very rare** Agitation · crying · epistaxis · vascular pain

▶ **Frequency not known** Cardiac arrest · cough · fever · loss of consciousness

SIDE-EFFECTS, FURTHER INFORMATION Alfentanil can cause muscle rigidity, particularly of the chest wall or jaw; this can be managed by the use of neuromuscular blocking drugs.

● **BREAST FEEDING** Present in milk—withhold breast-feeding for 24 hours.

● **HEPATIC IMPAIRMENT** Manufacturer advises caution.
Dose adjustments Manufacturer advises dose reduction and cautious titration.

● **RENAL IMPAIRMENT** EvGr Use with caution and titrate carefully (risk of increased and prolonged effects). (M)
Dose adjustments EvGr Dose reduction may be required in renal failure. (M)

● **DIRECTIONS FOR ADMINISTRATION** Manufacturer advises 5 mg/mL injection should be diluted in Glucose 5% *or* Sodium Chloride 0.9% before use.

● **MEDICINAL FORMS** There can be variation in the licensing of different medicines containing the same drug. Forms available from special-order manufacturers include: solution for injection

Solution for injection

▶ **Alfentanil (Non-proprietary)**

Alfentanil (as Alfentanil hydrochloride) 500 microgram per 1 ml Alfentanil 1mg/2ml solution for injection ampoules | 10 ampoule PoM £9.00 DT = £6.34 (Hospital only) CD2 | 10 ampoule PoM £9.00 DT = £6.34 CD2
Alfentanil 25mg/50ml solution for injection vials | 1 vial PoM £31.00 CD2
Alfentanil 5mg/10ml solution for injection ampoules | 5 ampoule PoM £16.50 DT = £16.00 (Hospital only) CD2 | 10 ampoule PoM £31.00 DT = £31.00 CD2

Alfentanil (as Alfentanil hydrochloride) 5 mg per 1 ml Alfentanil 5mg/1ml solution for injection ampoules | 10 ampoule PoM £25.00 DT = £23.19 CD2

▶ **Rapifen** (Piramal Critical Care Ltd)

Alfentanil (as Alfentanil hydrochloride) 500 microgram per 1 ml Rapifen 5mg/10ml solution for injection ampoules | 5 ampoule PoM £16.00 DT = £16.00 CD2
Rapifen 1mg/2ml solution for injection ampoules | 10 ampoule PoM £6.34 DT = £6.34 CD2

Alfentanil (as Alfentanil hydrochloride) 5 mg per 1 ml Rapifen Intensive Care 5mg/1ml solution for injection ampoules | 10 ampoule PoM £23.19 DT = £23.19 (Hospital only) CD2

F 327

Remifentanil

12-May-2021

● **INDICATIONS AND DOSE**

Analgesia and enhancement of anaesthesia at induction (initial bolus injection)

▶ BY INTRAVENOUS INJECTION

▶ Child 12–17 years: Initially 0.25–1 microgram/kg, dose to be administered over at least 30 seconds, if child is to be intubated more than 8 minutes after start of intravenous infusion, initial bolus intravenous injection dose is not necessary

Analgesia and enhancement of anaesthesia at induction with or without initial bolus dose

▶ BY INTRAVENOUS INFUSION

▶ Child 12–17 years: 30–60 micrograms/kg/hour, if child is to be intubated more than 8 minutes after start of intravenous infusion, initial bolus intravenous injection dose is not necessary

Assisted ventilation: analgesia and enhancement of anaesthesia during maintenance of anaesthesia (initial bolus injection)

▶ BY INTRAVENOUS INJECTION

▶ Child 1 month–11 years: Initially 0.1–1 microgram/kg, dose to be administered over at least 30 seconds (omitted if not required)

▶ Child 12–17 years: Initially 0.1–1 microgram/kg, dose to be administered over at least 30 seconds (omitted if not required)

Assisted ventilation: analgesia and enhancement of anaesthesia during maintenance of anaesthesia with or without initial bolus dose

▶ BY INTRAVENOUS INFUSION

▶ Neonate: 24–60 micrograms/kg/hour, additional doses of 1 microgram/kg can be given *by intravenous injection* during the intravenous infusion.

▶ Child 1 month–11 years: 3–78 micrograms/kg/hour, dose to be administered according to anaesthetic technique and adjusted according to response, additional doses can be given *by intravenous injection* during the intravenous infusion

▶ Child 12–17 years: 3–120 micrograms/kg/hour, dose to be administered according to anaesthetic technique and adjusted according to response, additional doses can be given *by intravenous injection* during the intravenous infusion

Spontaneous respiration: analgesia and enhancement of anaesthesia during maintenance of anaesthesia

- BY INTRAVENOUS INFUSION
- Child 12–17 years: Initially 2.4 micrograms/kg/hour, adjusted according to response; usual dose 1.5–6 micrograms/kg/hour

DOSES AT EXTREMES OF BODY-WEIGHT

- To avoid excessive dosage in obese patients, dose should be calculated on the basis of ideal body-weight.

- **UNLICENSED USE** Not licensed for use in children under 1 year.
- **CONTRA-INDICATIONS** Analgesia in conscious patients
- **INTERACTIONS** → Appendix 1: opioids
- **SIDE-EFFECTS**
- **Common or very common** Apnoea · muscle rigidity · post procedural complications
- **Uncommon** Hypoxia
- **Rare or very rare** Cardiac arrest
- **Frequency not known** Agitation · atrioventricular block · hypertension

SIDE-EFFECTS, FURTHER INFORMATION In contrast to other opioids which are metabolised in the liver, remifentanil undergoes rapid metabolism by plasma esterases; it has short duration of action which is independent of dose and duration of infusion.

Muscle rigidity Remifentanil can cause muscle rigidity that can be managed by the use of neuromuscular blocking drugs.

- **PREGNANCY** No information available.
- **BREAST FEEDING** Avoid breast-feeding for 24 hours after administration—present in milk in *animal* studies.
- **HEPATIC IMPAIRMENT** Manufacturer advises caution in severe impairment (limited information available).
- **RENAL IMPAIRMENT**

Dose adjustments EvGr No dose adjustment necessary in renal impairment. (M)

- **DIRECTIONS FOR ADMINISTRATION** For *intravenous injection*, manufacturer advises reconstitute to a concentration of 1 mg/mL; for *continuous intravenous infusion*, dilute further with Glucose 5% or Sodium Chloride 0.9% to a concentration of 20–25 micrograms/mL for child 1–12 years or 20–250 micrograms/mL (usually 50 micrograms/mL) for child 12–18 years.
- **PRESCRIBING AND DISPENSING INFORMATION** Remifentanil should not be given by intravenous injection intra-operatively, but it is well suited to continuous infusion; a supplementary analgesic is given before stopping the infusion of remifentanil.

- **MEDICINAL FORMS** There can be variation in the licensing of different medicines containing the same drug.

Powder for solution for injection

- Remifentanil (Non-proprietary)

Remifentanil (as Remifentanyl hydrochloride) 1 mg Remifentanil 1mg powder for concentrate for solution for injection vials | 5 vial PoM £25.58-£33.70 (Hospital only) CD2 | 5 vial PoM £25.50 CD2

Remifentanil (as Remifentanyl hydrochloride) 2 mg Remifentanil 2mg powder for concentrate for solution for injection vials | 5 vial PoM £51.15-£67.40 (Hospital only) CD2 | 5 vial PoM £51.00-£51.15 CD2

Remifentanil (as Remifentanyl hydrochloride) 5 mg Remifentanil 5mg powder for concentrate for solution for injection vials | 5 vial PoM £127.88-£180.00 (Hospital only) CD2 | 5 vial PoM £127.50 CD2

1.4 Peri-operative sedation

Conscious sedation for clinical procedures

Overview

Sedation of children during diagnostic and therapeutic procedures is used to reduce fear and anxiety, to control pain, and to minimise excessive movement. The choice of sedative drug will depend upon the intended procedure and whether the child is cooperative; some procedures are safer and more successful under anaesthesia.

Midazolam p. 273 and chloral hydrate p. 350 are suitable for sedating children for painless procedures, such as imaging. For painful procedures, alternative choices include nitrous oxide p. 1011, local anaesthesia, ketamine below, or concomitant use of sedation with **opioid** or **non-opioid analgesia**.

ANAESTHETICS, GENERAL > NMDA RECEPTOR ANTAGONISTS

Ketamine

04-Dec-2019

- **INDICATIONS AND DOSE**

Induction and maintenance of anaesthesia for short procedures

- BY INTRAMUSCULAR INJECTION
- Neonate: 4 mg/kg, adjusted according to response, a dose of 4 mg/kg usually produces 15 minutes of surgical anaesthesia.
- Child: 4–13 mg/kg, adjusted according to response, a dose of 4 mg/kg sufficient for some diagnostic procedures, a dose of 10 mg/kg usually produces 12–25 minutes of surgical anaesthesia
- BY INTRAVENOUS INJECTION
- Neonate: 1–2 mg/kg, adjusted according to response, to be given over at least 60 seconds, a dose of 1–2 mg/kg produces 5–10 minutes of surgical anaesthesia.
- Child 1 month–11 years: 1–2 mg/kg, adjusted according to response, to be given over at least 60 seconds, a dose of 1–2 mg/kg produces 5–10 minutes of surgical anaesthesia
- Child 12–17 years: 1–4.5 mg/kg, adjusted according to response, to be given over at least 60 seconds, a dose of 2 mg/kg usually produces 5–10 minutes of surgical anaesthesia

Induction and maintenance of anaesthesia for long procedures

- INITIALLY BY INTRAVENOUS INJECTION
- Neonate: Initially 0.5–2 mg/kg, followed by (by continuous intravenous infusion) 8 micrograms/kg/minute, adjusted according to response, doses up to 30 micrograms/kg/minute may be used to produce deep anaesthesia.
- Child: Initially 0.5–2 mg/kg, followed by (by continuous intravenous infusion) 10–45 micrograms/kg/minute, adjusted according to response

Sedation prior to invasive or painful procedures

- BY INTRAVENOUS INJECTION
- Child: 1–2 mg/kg for 1 dose

IMPORTANT SAFETY INFORMATION

Ketamine should only be administered by, or under the direct supervision of, personnel experienced in its use, with adequate training in anaesthesia and airway management, and when resuscitation equipment is available.

- **CONTRA-INDICATIONS** Acute porphyrias p. 745 · eclampsia · head trauma · hypertension · pre-eclampsia · raised intracranial pressure · severe cardiac disease · stroke
- **CAUTIONS** Acute circulatory failure (shock) · cardiovascular disease · dehydration · fixed cardiac output · hallucinations · head injury · hypertension · hypovolaemia · increased cerebrospinal fluid pressure · intracranial mass lesions · nightmares · predisposition to seizures · psychotic disorders · raised intra-ocular pressure · respiratory tract infection · thyroid dysfunction
- **INTERACTIONS** → Appendix 1: ketamine
- **SIDE-EFFECTS**
  - **Common or very common** Anxiety · behaviour abnormal · confusion · diplopia · hallucination · muscle tone increased · nausea · nystagmus · skin reactions · sleep disorders · tonic clonic movements · vomiting
  - **Uncommon** Appetite decreased · arrhythmias · hypotension · respiratory disorders
  - **Rare or very rare** Apnoea · cystitis · cystitis haemorrhagic · delirium · dysphoria · flashback · hypersalivation
  - **Frequency not known** Drug-induced liver injury

  SIDE-EFFECTS, FURTHER INFORMATION Incidence of hallucinations can be reduced by premedicaton with a benzodiazepine (such as midazolam).
- **PREGNANCY** May depress neonatal respiration if used during delivery.
- **BREAST FEEDING** Avoid for at least 12 hours after last dose.
- **HEPATIC IMPAIRMENT** Manufacturer advises caution (risk of prolonged duration of action).
  Dose adjustments Manufacturer advises consider dose reduction.
- **DIRECTIONS FOR ADMINISTRATION** For *intravenous injection*, dilute 100 mg/mL strength to a concentration of not more than 50 mg/mL with Glucose 5% *or* Sodium Chloride 0.9%. For *continuous intravenous infusion*, dilute to a concentration of 1 mg/mL with Glucose 5% *or* Sodium Chloride 0.9%; use microdrip infusion for maintenance of anaesthesia.
- **PATIENT AND CARER ADVICE**
  Driving and skilled tasks Patients given sedatives and analgesics during minor outpatient procedures should be very carefully warned about the risk of driving or undertaking skilled tasks afterwards. For a short general anaesthetic the risk extends to **at least 24 hours** after administration. Responsible persons should be available to take patients home. The dangers of taking **alcohol** should also be emphasised.
  For information on 2015 legislation regarding driving whilst taking certain controlled drugs, including ketamine, see *Drugs and driving* under Guidance on prescribing p. 1.
- **MEDICINAL FORMS** There can be variation in the licensing of different medicines containing the same drug. Forms available from special-order manufacturers include: solution for injection

Solution for injection

- Ketamine (Non-proprietary)
  Ketamine (as Ketamine hydrochloride) 10 mg per 1 ml Ketamin 10 Curamed 50mg/5ml solution for injection ampoules | 10 ampoule PoM ℞ CD2
  Ketamine 200mg/20ml solution for injection vials | 1 vial PoM £5.06–£6.04 DT = £5.06 (Hospital only) CD2
  Ketamine (as Ketamine hydrochloride) 50 mg per 1 ml Ketamine 500mg/10ml solution for injection vials | 1 vial PoM £8.77 DT = £8.77 (Hospital only) CD2 | 10 vial PoM £70.00–£87.70 CD2 | 10 vial PoM £70.00 (Hospital only) CD2
  Ketamin 100mg/2ml solution for injection ampoules | 10 ampoule PoM ℞ CD2
  Ketamine (as Ketamine hydrochloride) 100 mg per 1 ml Ketalar 200mg/2ml solution for injection vials | 5 vial PoM ℞ (Hospital only) CD2
- Ketalar (Pfizer Ltd)
  Ketamine (as Ketamine hydrochloride) 10 mg per 1 ml Ketalar 200mg/20ml solution for injection vials | 1 vial PoM £5.06 DT = £5.06 (Hospital only) CD2
  Ketamine (as Ketamine hydrochloride) 50 mg per 1 ml Ketalar 500mg/10ml solution for injection vials | 1 vial PoM £8.77 DT = £8.77 (Hospital only) CD2

HYPNOTICS, SEDATIVES AND ANXIOLYTICS > BENZODIAZEPINES

F 266

Temazepam

14-Oct-2021

- **INDICATIONS AND DOSE**
  Premedication before surgery or investigatory procedures
  - BY MOUTH
    - Child 12–17 years: 10–20 mg, to be taken 1 hour before procedure
- **UNLICENSED USE** Tablets not licensed for use in children.
- **CONTRA-INDICATIONS** Chronic psychosis · CNS depression · compromised airway · respiratory depression
- **CAUTIONS** Hypoalbuminaemia · muscle weakness · organic brain changes

  CAUTIONS, FURTHER INFORMATION
  - Paradoxical effects A paradoxical increase in hostility and aggression may be reported by patients taking benzodiazepines. The effects range from talkativeness and excitement to aggressive and antisocial acts. Adjustment of the dose (up or down) sometimes attenuates the impulses. Increased anxiety and perceptual disorders are other paradoxical effects.
- **INTERACTIONS** → Appendix 1: benzodiazepines
- **SIDE-EFFECTS** Dry mouth · gastrointestinal disorder · hypersalivation · psychosis · speech slurred · urinary incontinence
- **BREAST FEEDING** Benzodiazepines are present in milk, and should be avoided if possible during breast-feeding.
- **PATIENT AND CARER ADVICE**
  Driving and skilled tasks Patients given sedatives and analgesics during minor outpatient procedures should be very carefully warned about the risks of undertaking skilled tasks (e.g. driving) afterwards. Responsible persons should be available to take patients home afterwards. The dangers of taking **alcohol** should be emphasised.
- **PROFESSION SPECIFIC INFORMATION**
  Dental practitioners' formulary Temazepam tablets and oral solution may be prescribed.
- **MEDICINAL FORMS** There can be variation in the licensing of different medicines containing the same drug. Forms available from special-order manufacturers include: oral suspension, oral solution

Oral tablet

CAUTIONARY AND ADVISORY LABELS 19

- Temazepam (Non-proprietary)
  Temazepam 10 mg Temazepam 10mg tablets | 28 tablet PoM £43.26 DT = £24.89 CD3
  Temazepam 20 mg Temazepam 20mg tablets | 28 tablet PoM £31.25 DT = £24.79 CD3

Oral solution

CAUTIONARY AND ADVISORY LABELS 19

- Temazepam (Non-proprietary)
  Temazepam 2 mg per 1 ml Temazepam 10mg/5ml oral solution sugar free | 300 ml PoM £154.00 DT = £150.80 CD3 SF

2 Malignant hyperthermia

MUSCLE RELAXANTS > DIRECTLY ACTING

Dantrolene sodium

08-Mar-2021

- **DRUG ACTION** Acts on skeletal muscle cells by interfering with calcium efflux, thereby stopping the contractile process

- **INDICATIONS AND DOSE**

Malignant hyperthermia

▶ BY RAPID INTRAVENOUS INJECTION

▶ Child: Initially 2–3 mg/kg, then 1 mg/kg, repeated if necessary; maximum 10 mg/kg per course

Chronic severe spasticity of voluntary muscle

▶ BY MOUTH

▶ Child 5–11 years: Initially 500 micrograms/kg once daily for 7 days, then increased to 500 micrograms/kg/dose 3 times a day, then increased in steps of 500 micrograms/kg/dose every 7 days (max. per dose 2 mg/kg 3–4 times a day) until satisfactory response; maximum 400 mg per day

▶ Child 12–17 years: Initially 25 mg once daily for 7 days, then increased to 25 mg 3 times a day, then increased in steps of 500 micrograms/kg/dose every 7 days (max. per dose 2 mg/kg 3–4 times a day) until satisfactory response; maximum 400 mg per day

- **UNLICENSED USE** Not licensed for use in children.

IMPORTANT SAFETY INFORMATION

Should only be administered by, or under the direct supervision of, personnel experienced in the use of dantrolene when used for malignant hyperthermia.

- **CONTRA-INDICATIONS**

▶ With oral use Acute muscle spasm · avoid when spasticity is useful, for example, locomotion

- **CAUTIONS**

▶ With intravenous use Avoid extravasation (risk of tissue necrosis)

▶ With oral use Females (hepatotoxicity) · history of liver disorders (hepatotoxicity) · if doses greater than 400 mg daily (hepatotoxicity) · impaired cardiac function · impaired pulmonary function · therapeutic effect may take a few weeks to develop— discontinue if no response within 6–8 weeks

- **INTERACTIONS** → Appendix 1: dantrolene

- **SIDE-EFFECTS**

GENERAL SIDE-EFFECTS

▶ **Common or very common** Asthenia · diarrhoea · dizziness · drowsiness · gastrointestinal discomfort · headache · hepatic disorders · muscle weakness · nausea · respiratory disorders · seizure · skin reactions · speech disorder · vomiting

▶ **Uncommon** Arrhythmias · crystalluria · heart failure · hyperhidrosis

SPECIFIC SIDE-EFFECTS

▶ **Common or very common**

▶ With oral use Appetite decreased · cardiac inflammation · chills · confusion · depression · fever · insomnia · malaise · nervousness · vision disorders

▶ **Uncommon**

▶ With oral use Anaemia · aplastic anaemia · back pain · constipation · dysphagia · dyspnoea · excessive tearing · haemorrhage · hair growth abnormal · hallucination · hypersalivation · leucopenia · myalgia · neoplasms · photosensitivity reaction · taste altered · thrombocytopenia · urinary disorders

▶ **Rare or very rare**

▶ With oral use Erectile dysfunction

▶ **Frequency not known**

▶ With intravenous use Gastrointestinal haemorrhage · hyperkalaemia · muscle fatigue · pulmonary oedema · thrombophlebitis

▶ With oral use Dry mouth · muscle tone decreased · pericardial effusion · urine discolouration

- **PREGNANCY**

▶ With intravenous use Use only if potential benefit outweighs risk.

▶ With oral use Although teratological studies in *animals* have proved satisfactory, dantrolene sodium does cross the placenta, therefore manufacturer advises avoid.

- **BREAST FEEDING**

▶ With intravenous use Present in milk—use only if potential benefit outweighs risk.

▶ With oral use Present in milk—manufacturer advises avoid.

- **HEPATIC IMPAIRMENT**

▶ With oral use Manufacturer advises avoid in hepatic impairment.

- **MONITORING REQUIREMENTS**

▶ With oral use Test liver function before and at intervals during therapy.

- **PATIENT AND CARER ADVICE**

Hepatotoxicity

▶ With oral use Patients should be told how to recognise signs of liver disorder and advised to seek prompt medical attention if symptoms such as anorexia, nausea, vomiting, fatigue, abdominal pain, dark urine, or pruritus develop.

Driving and skilled tasks

▶ With oral use Drowsiness may affect performance of skilled tasks (e.g. driving); effects of alcohol enhanced.

- **MEDICINAL FORMS** There can be variation in the licensing of different medicines containing the same drug. Forms available from special-order manufacturers include: oral suspension, oral solution

Oral capsule

CAUTIONARY AND ADVISORY LABELS 2

▶ **Dantrium** (Forum Health Products Ltd)

Dantrolene sodium 25 mg Dantrium 25mg capsules | 100 capsule PoM £16.87 DT = £16.87

Dantrolene sodium 100 mg Dantrium 100mg capsules | 100 capsule PoM £43.07 DT = £43.07

Powder for solution for injection

▶ **Agilus** (Forum Health Products Ltd)

Dantrolene sodium 120 mg Agilus 120mg powder for solution for injection vials | 6 vial PoM £2,184.85 (Hospital only)

Local anaesthesia

Anaesthesia (local)

18-Sep-2023

Local anaesthetic drugs

The use of local anaesthetics by injection or by application to mucous membranes to produce local analgesia is discussed in this section.

Local anaesthetic drugs act by causing a reversible block to conduction along nerve fibres. They vary widely in their potency, toxicity, duration of action, stability, solubility in water, and ability to penetrate mucous membranes. These factors determine their application, e.g. topical (surface), infiltration, peripheral nerve block, intravenous regional anaesthesia (Bier's block), plexus, epidural (extradural), or spinal (intrathecal or subarachnoid) block. Local anaesthetics may also be used for postoperative pain relief, thereby reducing the need for analgesics such as opioids.

Bupivacaine hydrochloride p. 1027 has a longer duration of action than other local anaesthetics. It has a slow onset of

15 Anaesthesia

action, taking up to 30 minutes for full effect. It is often used in lumbar epidural blockade and is particularly suitable for continuous epidural analgesia in labour, or for postoperative pain relief. It is the principal drug used for spinal anaesthesia. Hyperbaric solutions containing glucose may be used for spinal block.

Levobupivacaine p. 1028, an isomer of bupivacaine hydrochloride, has anaesthetic and analgesic properties similar to bupivacaine hydrochloride, but is thought to have fewer adverse effects.

Lidocaine hydrochloride p. 1029 is effectively absorbed from mucous membranes and is a useful surface anaesthetic in concentrations up to 10%. Except for surface anaesthesia and dental anaesthesia, solutions used do not usually exceed 1% in strength. The duration of the block (with adrenaline p. 159) is about 90 minutes.

Application of a mixture of lidocaine and prilocaine (*EMLA*®) under an occlusive dressing provides surface anaesthesia for 1–2 hours. *EMLA*® does not appear to be effective in providing local anaesthesia for heel lancing in neonates.

Prilocaine hydrochloride p. 1033 is a local anaesthetic of low toxicity which is similar to lidocaine hydrochloride.

Ropivacaine hydrochloride p. 1034 is an amide-type local anaesthetic agent similar to bupivacaine hydrochloride. It is less cardiotoxic than bupivacaine hydrochloride, but also less potent.

Tetracaine p. 1034, a para-aminobenzoic acid ester, is an effective local anaesthetic for topical application; a 4% gel is indicated for anaesthesia before venepuncture or venous cannulation. Tetracaine is effective for 4–6 hours after a single application in most children. It is not recommended prior to neonatal heel lancing.

Tetracaine is rapidly absorbed from mucous membranes and should never be applied to inflamed, traumatised, or highly vascular surfaces. It should never be used to provide anaesthesia for bronchoscopy or cystoscopy because lidocaine hydrochloride is a safer alternative.

Administration by injection

The dose of local anaesthetic depends on the injection site and the procedure used. In determining the safe dosage, it is important to take account of the rate of absorption and excretion, and of the potency. The child's age, weight, physique, and clinical condition, and the vascularity of the administration site and the duration of administration, must also be considered.

Uptake of local anaesthetics into the systemic circulation determines their duration of action and produces toxicity.

NHS Improvement has advised (September 2016) that, prior to administration, all injectable medicines must be drawn directly from their original ampoule or container into a syringe and should **never** be decanted into gallipots or open containers. This is to avoid the risk of medicines being confused with other substances, e.g. skin disinfectants, and to reduce the risk of contamination.

Great care must be taken to avoid accidental intravascular injection; local anaesthetic injections should be given slowly in order to detect inadvertent intravascular administration. When prolonged analgesia is required, a long-acting local anaesthetic is preferred to minimise the likelihood of cumulative systemic toxicity. Local anaesthesia around the oral cavity may impair swallowing and therefore increases the risk of aspiration.

Epidural anaesthesia is combined with general anaesthesia for certain surgical procedures in children.

Vasoconstrictors in combination with local anaesthetics

Local anaesthetics cause dilatation of blood vessels. The addition of a vasoconstrictor such as adrenaline to the local anaesthetic preparation diminishes local blood flow, slowing the rate of absorption and thereby prolonging the anaesthetic effect. Great care should be taken to avoid inadvertent intravenous administration of a preparation containing adrenaline. The use of adrenaline with a local anaesthetic injection in digits or appendages [unlicensed use] may be associated with a risk of ischaemic necrosis though the combination is used in some circumstances (such as hand surgery that uses the Wide-awake Local Anaesthesia No Tourniquet (WALANT) technique).

Adrenaline must be used in a low concentration when administered with a local anaesthetic. Care must also be taken to calculate a safe maximum dose of local anaesthetic when using combination products.

In children with severe hypertension or unstable cardiac rhythm, the use of adrenaline with a local anaesthetic may be hazardous. For these children an anaesthetic without adrenaline should be used.

Dental anaesthesia

Lidocaine hydrochloride is widely used in dental procedures; it is most often used in combination with adrenaline. Lidocaine hydrochloride 2% combined with adrenaline 1 in 80 000 (12.5 micrograms/mL) is a safe and effective preparation; there is no justification for using higher concentrations of adrenaline. The amide-type local anaesthetics articaine and mepivacaine hydrochloride p. 1032 are also used in dentistry; they are available in cartridges suitable for dental use. Mepivacaine hydrochloride is available with or without adrenaline, and articaine is available with adrenaline. In children with severe hypertension or unstable cardiac rhythm, mepivacaine hydrochloride without adrenaline may be used. Alternatively, prilocaine hydrochloride with or without felypressin can be used but there is no evidence that it is any safer. Felypressin can cause coronary vasoconstriction when used at high doses; limit dose in children with coronary artery disease.

Toxicity induced by local anaesthesia

For management of toxicity see Severe local anaesthetic-induced cardiovascular toxicity below.

Severe local anaesthetic-induced cardiovascular toxicity

Overview

After injection of a bolus of local anaesthetic, toxicity may develop at any time in the following hour. In the event of signs of toxicity during injection, the administration of the local anaesthetic must be stopped immediately.

Cardiovascular status must be assessed and cardiopulmonary resuscitation procedures must be followed.

In the event of local anaesthetic-induced cardiac arrest, standard cardiopulmonary resuscitation should be initiated immediately. Lidocaine must not be used as anti-arrhythmic therapy.

If the patient does not respond rapidly to standard procedures, 20% lipid emulsion such as *Intralipid*® [unlicensed indication] should be given intravenously at an initial bolus dose of 1.5 mL/kg over 1 minute, followed by an infusion of 15 mL/kg/hour. After 5 minutes, if cardiovascular stability has not been restored or circulation deteriorates, give a maximum of two further bolus doses of 1.5 mL/kg over 1 minute, 5 minutes apart, and increase the infusion rate to 30 mL/kg/hour. Continue infusion until cardiovascular stability and adequate circulation are restored or maximum cumulative dose of 12 mL/kg is given.

Standard cardiopulmonary resuscitation must be maintained throughout lipid emulsion treatment.

Propofol is not a suitable alternative to lipid emulsion.

Further advice on ongoing treatment should be obtained from the National Poisons Information Service.

Detailed treatment algorithms and accompanying notes are available at www.toxbase.org *or* can be found in the Association of Anaesthetists of Great Britain and Ireland safety guideline, Management of Severe Local Anaesthetic Toxicity and Management of Severe Local Anaesthetic Toxicity – Accompanying notes.

ANAESTHETICS, LOCAL

Adrenaline with articaine hydrochloride

19-Dec-2019

(Carticaine hydrochloride with epinephrine)

- **INDICATIONS AND DOSE**

Infiltration anaesthesia in dentistry

▶ BY REGIONAL ADMINISTRATION

▶ Child 4–17 years: Consult expert dental sources

DOSES AT EXTREMES OF BODY-WEIGHT

▶ To avoid excessive dosage in obese patients, dose should be calculated on the basis of ideal body-weight.

IMPORTANT SAFETY INFORMATION

Should only be administered by, or under the direct supervision of, personnel experienced in their use, with adequate training in anaesthesia and airway management, and should not be administered parenterally unless adequate resuscitation equipment is available.

- **CONTRA-INDICATIONS** Injection into infected tissues · injection into inflamed tissues · preparations containing preservatives should not be used for caudal, epidural, or spinal block

CONTRA-INDICATIONS, FURTHER INFORMATION

▶ Injection site Manufacturer advises the local anaesthetic effect may be reduced when injected into an inflamed or infected area, due to altered local pH. Increased absorption into the blood also increases the possibility of systemic side-effects.

- **CAUTIONS** Arrhythmias · cardiovascular disease · cerebrovascular disease · children (consider dose reduction) · cor pulmonale · debilitated patients (consider dose reduction) · diabetes mellitus · epilepsy · hypercalcaemia · hyperreflexia · hypertension · hyperthyroidism · hypokalaemia · hypovolaemia · impaired cardiac conduction · impaired respiratory function · ischaemic heart disease · myasthenia gravis · obstructive cardiomyopathy · occlusive vascular disease · organic brain damage · phaeochromocytoma · prostate disorders · psychoneurosis · severe angina · shock · susceptibility to angle-closure glaucoma

CAUTIONS, FURTHER INFORMATION

▶ Use of vasoconstrictors In patients with severe hypertension or unstable cardiac rhythm, the use of adrenaline with a local anaesthetic may be hazardous. For these patients an anaesthetic without adrenaline should be used.

- **INTERACTIONS** → Appendix 1: sympathomimetics, vasoconstrictor
- **SIDE-EFFECTS** Face oedema · gingivitis · headache · nausea · sensation abnormal

SIDE-EFFECTS, FURTHER INFORMATION Toxic effects after administration of local anaesthetics are a result of excessively high plasma concentrations; severe toxicity usually results from inadvertent intravascular injection. The toxicity mainly involves the central nervous and cardiovascular systems. The onset of toxicity can be unpredictable and delayed. Monitor as per local protocol for at least 30 minutes after administration.

- **ALLERGY AND CROSS-SENSITIVITY**

▶ Hypersensitivity and cross-sensitivity Hypersensitivity reactions occur mainly with the ester-type local anaesthetics, such as tetracaine; reactions are less frequent with the amide types, such as articaine, bupivacaine, levobupivacaine, lidocaine, mepivacaine, prilocaine, and ropivacaine. Cross-sensitivity reactions may be avoided by using the alternative chemical type.

- **PREGNANCY** Use only if potential benefit outweighs risk—no information available.
- **BREAST FEEDING** Avoid breast-feeding for 48 hours after administration.
- **HEPATIC IMPAIRMENT** Manufacturer advises caution (increased risk of toxicity in severe impairment).
- **RENAL IMPAIRMENT** Manufacturers advise use with caution in severe impairment.
- **MONITORING REQUIREMENTS** Consider monitoring blood pressure and ECG (advised with systemic adrenaline).
- **MEDICINAL FORMS** There can be variation in the licensing of different medicines containing the same drug.

Solution for injection

EXCIPIENTS: May contain Sulfites

▶ **Anestadent** (Dentsply Ltd)

Adrenaline (as Adrenaline acid tartrate) 10 microgram per 1 ml, Articaine hydrochloride 40 mg per 1 ml Anestadent 4% and 1:100,000 solution for injection 2.2ml cartridges | 50 cartridge [PoM] [X] (Hospital only)

▶ **Septanest** (Septodont Ltd)

Adrenaline (as Adrenaline acid tartrate) 10 microgram per 1 ml, Articaine hydrochloride 40 mg per 1 ml Septanest 1 in 100,000 solution for injection 2.2ml cartridges | 50 cartridge [PoM] £42.45 (Hospital only)

Adrenaline (as Adrenaline acid tartrate) 5 microgram per 1 ml, Articaine hydrochloride 40 mg per 1 ml Septanest 1 in 200,000 solution for injection 2.2ml cartridges | 50 cartridge [PoM] £42.45 (Hospital only)

Bupivacaine hydrochloride

09-Dec-2019

- **INDICATIONS AND DOSE**

Surgical anaesthesia | Acute pain

▶ BY REGIONAL ADMINISTRATION

▶ Child: Doses adjusted according to child's physical status and nature of procedure, seek expert advice (consult product literature or local protocols)

DOSES AT EXTREMES OF BODY-WEIGHT

▶ To avoid excessive dosage in obese patients, dose should be calculated on the basis of ideal body-weight.

IMPORTANT SAFETY INFORMATION

The licensed doses stated may not be appropriate in some settings and expert advice should be sought.

Should only be administered by, or under the direct supervision of, personnel experienced in their use, with adequate training in anaesthesia and airway management, and should not be administered parenterally unless adequate resuscitation equipment is available.

- **CONTRA-INDICATIONS** Avoid injection into infected tissues · avoid injection into inflamed tissues · intravenous regional anaesthesia (Bier's block) · preparations containing preservatives should not be used for caudal, epidural, or spinal block

CONTRA-INDICATIONS, FURTHER INFORMATION

▶ Injection site Manufacturer advises local anaesthetics should not be injected into inflamed or infected tissues. Increased absorption into the blood increases the possibility of systemic side-effects, and the local anaesthetic effect may also be reduced by altered local pH.

- **CAUTIONS** Cardiovascular disease · cerebral atheroma · children (consider dose reduction) · complete heart block · debilitated patients (consider dose reduction) · epilepsy · hypertension · hypotension · hypovolaemia · impaired cardiac conduction · impaired respiratory function · myasthenia gravis · myocardial depression may be more severe and more resistant to treatment · shock
- **SIDE-EFFECTS**
  - **Common or very common** Arrhythmias · dizziness · hypertension · hypotension · nausea · paraesthesia · urinary retention · vomiting
  - **Uncommon** Neurotoxicity
  - **Rare or very rare** Arachnoiditis · cardiac arrest · diplopia · nerve disorders · paraplegia · paresis · respiratory depression

  SIDE-EFFECTS, FURTHER INFORMATION Toxic effects after administration of local anaesthetics are a result of excessively high plasma concentrations; severe toxicity usually results from inadvertent intravascular injection. The systemic toxicity of local anaesthetics mainly involves the central nervous and cardiovascular systems. The onset of toxicity can be unpredictable and delayed. Monitor as per local protocol for at least 30 minutes after administration.
- **ALLERGY AND CROSS-SENSITIVITY**
  - Hypersensitivity and cross-sensitivity Hypersensitivity reactions occur mainly with the ester-type local anaesthetics, such as tetracaine; reactions are less frequent with the amide types, such as articaine, bupivacaine, levobupivacaine, lidocaine, mepivacaine, prilocaine, and ropivacaine. Cross-sensitivity reactions may be avoided by using the alternative chemical type.
- **PREGNANCY** Large doses during delivery can cause neonatal respiratory depression, hypotonia, and bradycardia after epidural block.

  Dose adjustments Use lower doses for intrathecal use during late pregnancy.
- **BREAST FEEDING** Amount too small to be harmful.
- **HEPATIC IMPAIRMENT** Manufacturer advises use with caution in advanced liver dysfunction.
- **RENAL IMPAIRMENT** Use with caution in severe impairment.

- **MEDICINAL FORMS** There can be variation in the licensing of different medicines containing the same drug. Forms available from special-order manufacturers include: solution for injection, infusion, solution for infusion

Solution for injection

- Bupivacaine hydrochloride (Non-proprietary)
  - **Bupivacaine hydrochloride 2.5 mg per 1 ml** Bupivacaine 25mg/10ml (0.25%) solution for injection ampoules | 5 ampoule [PoM] £11.70 DT = £11.70 (Hospital only) | 10 ampoule [PoM] £15.84–£18.30 (Hospital only)
  - Bupivacaine 25mg/10ml (0.25%) solution for injection vials | 10 vial [PoM] [X] (Hospital only)
  - Bupivacaine 0.25% solution for injection 10ml Sure-Amp ampoules | 20 ampoule [PoM] £17.50 DT = £17.50
  - **Bupivacaine hydrochloride 5 mg per 1 ml** Bupivacaine 0.5% solution for injection 10ml Sure-Amp ampoules | 20 ampoule [PoM] £18.30 DT = £18.30 (Hospital only)
  - Bupivacaine 100mg/20ml (0.5%) solution for injection vials | 10 vial [PoM] [X] (Hospital only)
  - Bupivacaine 50mg/10ml (0.5%) solution for injection ampoules | 5 ampoule [PoM] £13.20 DT = £13.20 (Hospital only) | 10 ampoule [PoM] £7.56–£80.30 DT = £7.56 (Hospital only)
  - **Bupivacaine hydrochloride anhydrous 40 mg per 1 ml** Bupivacain Sintetica 40mg/ml (4%) solution for injection ampoules | 10 ampoule [PoM] [X] (Hospital only)

Infusion

- Bupivacaine hydrochloride (Non-proprietary)
  - **Bupivacaine hydrochloride 1 mg per 1 ml** Bupivacaine 250mg/250ml (0.1%) infusion bags | 5 bag [PoM] £60.87
  - **Bupivacaine hydrochloride 1.25 mg per 1 ml** Bupivacaine 312.5mg/250ml (0.125%) infusion bags | 5 bag [PoM] £62.12

Bupivacaine with adrenaline

19-Dec-2019

The properties listed below are those particular to the combination only. For the properties of the components please consider, bupivacaine hydrochloride p. 1027, adrenaline p. 159.

- **INDICATIONS AND DOSE**

Surgical anaesthesia

- BY LUMBAR EPIDURAL, OR BY LOCAL INFILTRATION, OR BY CAUDAL EPIDURAL
  - Child 12–17 years: (consult product literature)

Acute pain management

- BY LUMBAR EPIDURAL, OR BY LOCAL INFILTRATION
  - Child 1–17 years: (consult product literature)

- **CAUTIONS** In patients with severe hypertension or unstable cardiac rhythm, the use of adrenaline with a local anaesthetic may be hazardous. For these patients an anaesthetic without adrenaline should be used.
- **INTERACTIONS** → Appendix 1: sympathomimetics, vasoconstrictor

- **MEDICINAL FORMS** There can be variation in the licensing of different medicines containing the same drug.

Solution for injection

- Bupivacaine with adrenaline (Non-proprietary)
  - **Adrenaline (as Adrenaline acid tartrate) 5 microgram per 1 ml, Bupivacaine hydrochloride 2.5 mg per 1 ml** Bupivacaine 25mg/10ml (0.25%) / Adrenaline (base) 50micrograms/10ml (1 in 200,000) solution for injection ampoules | 10 ampoule [PoM] £46.00 DT = £46.00
  - **Adrenaline (as Adrenaline acid tartrate) 5 microgram per 1 ml, Bupivacaine hydrochloride anhydrous 2.5 mg per 1 ml** Carbostesin-adrenaline 0.25% / 100micrograms/20ml (1 in 200,000) solution for injection ampoules | 1 ampoule [PoM] [X] (Hospital only)
  - Carbostesin-adrenaline 0.25% / 25micrograms/5ml (1 in 200,000) solution for injection ampoules | 1 ampoule [PoM] [X] (Hospital only)
  - **Adrenaline (as Adrenaline acid tartrate) 5 microgram per 1 ml, Bupivacaine hydrochloride 5 mg per 1 ml** Bupivacaine 50mg/10ml (0.5%) / Adrenaline (base) 50micrograms/10ml (1 in 200,000) solution for injection ampoules | 10 ampoule [PoM] £51.75 DT = £51.75
  - **Adrenaline (as Adrenaline acid tartrate) 5 microgram per 1 ml, Bupivacaine hydrochloride anhydrous 5 mg per 1 ml** Carbostesin-adrenaline 0.5% / 25micrograms/5ml (1 in 200,000) solution for injection ampoules | 1 ampoule [PoM] [X] (Hospital only)
  - Carbostesin-adrenaline 0.5% / 100micrograms/20ml (1 in 200,000) solution for injection ampoules | 1 ampoule [PoM] [X] (Hospital only)

Levobupivacaine

08-Sep-2020

- **INDICATIONS AND DOSE**

Surgical anaesthesia | Acute pain

- BY REGIONAL ADMINISTRATION
  - Child: Doses adjusted according to child's physical status and nature of procedure, seek expert advice (consult product literature or local protocols)

DOSES AT EXTREMES OF BODY-WEIGHT

- To avoid excessive dosage in obese patients, dose should be calculated on the basis of ideal body-weight.

- **UNLICENSED USE** Not licensed for use in children except for analgesia by ilioinguinal or iliohypogastric block.

IMPORTANT SAFETY INFORMATION

The licensed doses stated may not be appropriate in some settings and expert advice should be sought.

Should only be administered by, or under the direct supervision of, personnel experienced in their use, with adequate training in anaesthesia and airway management, and should not be administered parenterally unless adequate resuscitation equipment is available.

- **CONTRA-INDICATIONS** Avoid injection into infected tissues · avoid injection into inflamed tissues · intravenous regional anaesthesia (Bier's block) · preparations containing preservatives should not be used for caudal, epidural, or spinal block

CONTRA-INDICATIONS, FURTHER INFORMATION

- Injection site Manufacturer advises local anaesthetics should not be injected into inflamed or infected tissues. Increased absorption into the blood increases the possibility of systemic side-effects, and the local anaesthetic effect may also be reduced by altered local pH.

- **CAUTIONS** Cardiovascular disease · children (consider dose reduction) · complete heart block · debilitated patients (consider dose reduction) · epilepsy · hypovolaemia · impaired cardiac conduction · impaired respiratory function · myasthenia gravis · shock

- **SIDE-EFFECTS**
  - **Common or very common** Anaemia · back pain · dizziness · fever · headache · hypotension · nausea · procedural pain · vomiting
  - **Frequency not known** Angioedema · apnoea · arrhythmias · asthenia · atrioventricular block · bladder disorder · cardiac arrest · drowsiness · eye disorders · faecal incontinence · flushing · loss of consciousness · muscle twitching · muscle weakness · nerve disorders · neurological injury · oral hypoaesthesia · paralysis · priapism · respiratory disorders · seizure · sensation abnormal · skin reactions · sneezing · sweat changes · syncope · vision blurred

SIDE-EFFECTS, FURTHER INFORMATION The systemic toxicity of local anaesthetics mainly involves the central nervous and cardiovascular systems. Systemic toxicity can occur due to inadvertent intravascular injection. The onset of toxicity can be unpredictable and delayed. Monitor as per local protocol for at least 30 minutes after administration.

- **ALLERGY AND CROSS-SENSITIVITY**
  - Hypersensitivity and cross-sensitivity Hypersensitivity reactions occur mainly with the ester-type local anaesthetics, such as tetracaine; reactions are less frequent with the amide types, such as articaine, bupivacaine, levobupivacaine, lidocaine, mepivacaine, prilocaine, and ropivacaine. Cross-sensitivity reactions may be avoided by using the alternative chemical type.

- **PREGNANCY** Large doses during delivery can cause neonatal respiratory depression, hypotonia, and bradycardia after epidural block. Avoid if possible in the first trimester—toxicity in *animal* studies. May cause fetal distress syndrome. Do not use for paracervical block in obstetrics. Do not use 7.5 mg/mL strength in obstetrics.

- **BREAST FEEDING** Amount too small to be harmful.

- **HEPATIC IMPAIRMENT** Manufacturer advises caution in impairment or patients with reduced hepatic blood flow (no information available).

- **PRESCRIBING AND DISPENSING INFORMATION** Levobupivacaine is an isomer of bupivacaine.

- **MEDICINAL FORMS** There can be variation in the licensing of different medicines containing the same drug.

Solution for injection

- Levobupivacaine (Non-proprietary)
  - **Levobupivacaine (as Levobupivacaine hydrochloride) 2.5 mg per 1 ml** Levobupivacaine 25mg/10ml (0.25%) solution for injection ampoules | 5 ampoule PoM £12.40–£13.50 (Hospital only)
  - **Levobupivacaine (as Levobupivacaine hydrochloride) 5 mg per 1 ml** Levobupivacaine 50mg/10ml (0.5%) solution for injection ampoules | 5 ampoule PoM £14.35–£22.89 (Hospital only)
  - **Levobupivacaine (as Levobupivacaine hydrochloride) 7.5 mg per 1 ml** Levobupivacaine 75mg/10ml (0.75%) solution for injection ampoules | 5 ampoule PoM £21.35–£21.78 (Hospital only)

Infusion

- Levobupivacaine (Non-proprietary)
  - **Levobupivacaine (as Levobupivacaine hydrochloride) 1.25 mg per 1 ml** Levobupivacaine 125mg/100ml (0.125%) infusion bags | 5 bag PoM £51.85–£63.30 (Hospital only)
  - Levobupivacaine 250mg/200ml (0.125%) infusion bags | 12 bag PoM £143.55 (Hospital only)

Lidocaine hydrochloride

20-Nov-2025

(Lignocaine hydrochloride)

- **INDICATIONS AND DOSE**

Infiltration anaesthesia

- BY LOCAL INFILTRATION
  - Neonate: Up to 3 mg/kg, dose to be given according to patient's weight and nature of procedure, dose may be repeated not more often than every 4 hours, 3 mg/kg equivalent to 0.3 mL/kg of 1% solution.
  - Child 1 month–11 years: Up to 3 mg/kg, dose to be given according to patient's weight and nature of procedure, dose may be repeated not more often than every 4 hours, 3 mg/kg equivalent to 0.3 mL/kg of 1% solution
  - Child 12–17 years: (max. per dose 200 mg), dose to be given according to child's weight and nature of procedure, dose may be repeated not more often than every 4 hours

DOSES AT EXTREMES OF BODY-WEIGHT

- When used by local infiltration To avoid excessive dosage in obese patients, weight-based doses for non-emergency indications may need to be calculated on the basis of ideal body-weight.

Intravenous regional anaesthesia and nerve block

- BY REGIONAL ADMINISTRATION
  - Child: Seek expert advice

Dental anaesthesia

- BY REGIONAL ADMINISTRATION
  - Child: Seek expert advice

Pain relief (in anal fissures, haemorrhoids, pruritus ani, pruritus vulvae, herpes zoster, or herpes labialis) | Lubricant in cystoscopy | Lubricant in proctoscopy

- TO THE SKIN USING OINTMENT
  - Child: Apply 1–2 mL as required, avoid long-term use

LMX 4®

Anaesthesia before venous cannulation or venepuncture

- TO THE SKIN
  - Child 1–2 months: Apply up to 1 g, apply thick layer to small area (2.5 cm × 2.5 cm) of non-irritated skin at least 30 minutes before procedure; may be applied under an occlusive dressing; max. application time 60 minutes, remove cream with gauze and perform procedure after approximately 5 minutes
  - Child 3–11 months: Apply up to 1 g, apply thick layer to small area (2.5 cm × 2.5 cm) of non-irritated skin at least 30 minutes before procedure; may be applied under an occlusive dressing; max. application time 4 hours, remove cream with gauze and perform procedure after approximately 5 minutes
  - Child 1–17 years: Apply 1–2.5 g, apply thick layer to small area (2.5 cm × 2.5 cm) of non-irritated skin at least 30 minutes before procedure; may be applied under an occlusive dressing; max. application time

continued →

15 Anaesthesia

5 hours, remove cream with gauze and perform procedure after approximately 5 minutes

IMPORTANT SAFETY INFORMATION

▸ When used by local infiltration
The licensed doses stated may not be appropriate in some settings and expert advice should be sought. Should only be administered by, or under the direct supervision of, personnel experienced in their use, with adequate training in anaesthesia and airway management, and should not be administered parenterally unless adequate resuscitation equipment is available.

- **CONTRA-INDICATIONS**
▸ When used by regional administration Avoid injection into infected tissues · avoid injection into inflamed tissues · complete heart block · preparations containing preservatives should not be used for caudal, epidural, or spinal block, or for intravenous regional anaesthesia (Bier's block)
▸ With topical use Application to the middle ear (can cause ototoxicity) · should not be applied to damaged skin
CONTRA-INDICATIONS, FURTHER INFORMATION
▸ Administration site
▸ With topical use or when used by regional administration Manufacturer advises local anaesthetics should not be injected into inflamed or infected tissues nor should they be applied to damaged skin. Increased absorption into the blood increases the possibility of systemic side-effects, and the local anaesthetic effect may also be reduced by altered local pH.
- **CAUTIONS**
▸ When used by regional administration Acute porphyrias p. 745 (consider infusion with glucose for its anti-porphyrinogenic effects) · children (consider dose reduction) · congestive cardiac failure (consider lower dose) · debilitated patients (consider dose reduction) · epilepsy · hypovolaemia · impaired cardiac conduction · impaired respiratory function · myasthenia gravis · post cardiac surgery (consider lower dose) · shock
- **INTERACTIONS** → Appendix 1: antiarrhythmics
- **SIDE-EFFECTS**
▸ With parenteral use Anxiety · arrhythmias · atrioventricular block · cardiac arrest · circulatory collapse · confusion · dizziness · drowsiness · euphoric mood · headache · hypotension (may lead to cardiac arrest) · loss of consciousness · methaemoglobinaemia · muscle twitching · myocardial contractility decreased · nausea · neurological effects · nystagmus · pain · psychosis · respiratory disorders · seizure · sensation abnormal · temperature sensation altered · tinnitus · tremor · vision blurred · vomiting
SIDE-EFFECTS, FURTHER INFORMATION **Toxic effects** The systemic toxicity of local anaesthetics mainly involves the central nervous and cardiovascular systems.
Methaemoglobinaemia Methylthioninium chloride can be used for the acute symptomatic treatment of drug-induced methaemoglobinaemia.
- **ALLERGY AND CROSS-SENSITIVITY**
▸ Hypersensitivity and cross-sensitivity Hypersensitivity reactions occur mainly with the ester-type local anaesthetics, such as tetracaine; reactions are less frequent with the amide types, such as articaine, bupivacaine, levobupivacaine, lidocaine, mepivacaine, prilocaine, and ropivacaine. Cross-sensitivity reactions may be avoided by using the alternative chemical type.
- **PREGNANCY** Crosses the placenta but not known to be harmful in *animal* studies—use if benefit outweighs risk. When used as a local anaesthetic, large doses can cause fetal bradycardia; if given during delivery can also cause neonatal respiratory depression, hypotonia, or bradycardia after paracervical or epidural block.
- **BREAST FEEDING** Present in milk but amount too small to be harmful.
- **HEPATIC IMPAIRMENT** Manufacturer advises caution (risk of increased exposure).
- **RENAL IMPAIRMENT** Possible accumulation of lidocaine and active metabolite; caution in severe impairment.
- **MONITORING REQUIREMENTS**
▸ With systemic use Monitor ECG and have resuscitation facilities available.

- **MEDICINAL FORMS** There can be variation in the licensing of different medicines containing the same drug. Forms available from special-order manufacturers include: solution for injection, ointment, cutaneous solution

Solution for injection

▸ **Lidocaine hydrochloride (Non-proprietary)**
Lidocaine hydrochloride 5 mg per 1 ml Lidocaine 50mg/10ml (0.5%) solution for injection ampoules | 10 ampoule PoM £10.00 DT = £10.00
Lidocaine hydrochloride 10 mg per 1 ml Lidocaine 100mg/10ml (1%) solution for injection Mini-Plasco ampoules | 20 ampoule PoM £13.80
Lidocaine 100mg/10ml (1%) solution for injection ampoules | 10 ampoule PoM £6.30–£7.00 DT = £8.10 | 20 ampoule PoM £14.60–£234.00 (Hospital only)
Lidocaine 200mg/20ml (1%) solution for injection vials | 10 vial PoM £26.40
Lidocaine 200mg/20ml (1%) solution for injection ampoules | 1 ampoule PoM £25.07 (Hospital only) | 10 ampoule PoM £12.60–£14.00 DT = £14.00 | 20 ampoule PoM £20.00–£501.40 (Hospital only)
Lidocaine 50mg/5ml (1%) solution for injection ampoules | 1 ampoule PoM £8.28 (Hospital only) | 10 ampoule PoM £4.00–£6.06 DT = £6.95 | 20 ampoule PoM £13.00–£165.60 (Hospital only)
Lidocaine 20mg/2ml (1%) solution for injection ampoules | 10 ampoule PoM £5.17 DT = £5.17
Lidocaine 50mg/5ml (1%) solution for injection Mini-Plasco ampoules | 20 ampoule PoM £8.05
Lidocaine hydrochloride 20 mg per 1 ml Lidocaine 100mg/5ml (2%) solution for injection ampoules | 10 ampoule PoM £5.40–£6.00 DT = £7.60 | 20 ampoule PoM £16.40–£165.00 (Hospital only)
Lidocaine 40mg/2ml (2%) solution for injection ampoules | 10 ampoule PoM £5.84 DT = £5.88
Lidocaine 100mg/5ml (2%) solution for injection Mini-Plasco ampoules | 20 ampoule PoM £12.00
Lidocaine 200mg/10ml (2%) solution for injection ampoules | 20 ampoule PoM £14.95–£382.80 (Hospital only)
Lidocaine 400mg/20ml (2%) solution for injection ampoules | 10 ampoule PoM £13.50–£15.00 DT = £15.00 | 20 ampoule PoM £32.60–£521.80 (Hospital only)

Cutaneous cream

EXCIPIENTS: May contain Benzyl alcohol, propylene glycol

▸ **LMX 4** (Ferndale Pharmaceuticals Ltd)
Lidocaine 40 mg per 1 gram LMX 4 cream | 5 gram P £2.98 DT = £2.98 | 30 gram P £14.90 DT = £14.90

Ointment

▸ **Lidocaine hydrochloride (Non-proprietary)**
Lidocaine hydrochloride 50 mg per 1 gram Lidocaine 5% ointment | 15 gram P £18.75 DT = £17.65

Lidocaine with adrenaline

19-Dec-2019

The properties listed below are those particular to the combination only. For the properties of the components please consider, lidocaine hydrochloride p. 1029, adrenaline p. 159.

- **INDICATIONS AND DOSE**

Local anaesthesia

▶ BY LOCAL INFILTRATION
▸ Child 12–17 years: Dosed according to the type of nerve block required (consult product literature)

- **INTERACTIONS** → Appendix 1: antiarrhythmics · sympathomimetics, vasoconstrictor

● **PROFESSION SPECIFIC INFORMATION**

Dental information A variety of lidocaine injections with adrenaline is available in dental cartridges.

Consult expert dental sources for specific advice in relation to dose of lidocaine for dental anaesthesia.

● **MEDICINAL FORMS** There can be variation in the licensing of different medicines containing the same drug. Forms available from special-order manufacturers include: solution for injection

Solution for injection

EXCIPIENTS: May contain Sulfites

▸ Lidocaine with adrenaline (Non-proprietary)

Adrenaline (as Adrenaline acid tartrate) 5 microgram per 1 ml, Lidocaine hydrochloride 10 mg per 1 ml Lidocaine 200mg/20ml (1%) / Adrenaline (base) 100micrograms/20ml (1 in 200,000) solution for injection vials | 5 vial PoM £11.50 (Hospital only)

Lidocaine 100mg/10ml (1%) / Adrenaline (base) 50micrograms/10ml (1 in 200,000) solution for injection ampoules | 10 ampoule PoM £90.00

Adrenaline 5 microgram per 1 ml, Lidocaine hydrochloride 20 mg per 1 ml Lidocaine 200mg/10ml (2%) / Adrenaline (base) 50micrograms/10ml (1 in 200,000) solution for injection ampoules | 10 ampoule PoM £90.00 (Hospital only)

Adrenaline (as Adrenaline acid tartrate) 5 microgram per 1 ml, Lidocaine hydrochloride 20 mg per 1 ml Lidocaine 400mg/20ml (2%) / Adrenaline (base) 100micrograms/20ml (1 in 200,000) solution for injection vials | 5 vial PoM £10.55 DT = £10.55

▸ Lignospan Special (Septodont Ltd)

Adrenaline (as Adrenaline acid tartrate) 12.5 microgram per 1 ml, Lidocaine hydrochloride 20 mg per 1 ml Lignospan Special 20mg/ml / 12.5micrograms/ml solution for injection 2.2ml cartridges | 50 cartridge PoM £35.90 DT = £35.90

Lignospan Special 20mg/ml / 12.5micrograms/ml solution for injection 1.8ml cartridges | 50 cartridge PoM £35.90 DT = £35.90

▸ Rexocaine (Henry Schein Ltd)

Adrenaline (as Adrenaline acid tartrate) 12.5 microgram per 1 ml, Lidocaine hydrochloride 20 mg per 1 ml Rexocaine 2% injection 2.2ml cartridges | 50 cartridge PoM £24.75 DT = £35.90

▸ Xylocaine with Adrenaline (Dentsply Ltd)

Adrenaline (as Adrenaline acid tartrate) 12.5 microgram per 1 ml, Lidocaine hydrochloride 20 mg per 1 ml Xylocaine 2% with Adrenaline 1 in 80,000 Dental injection 2.2ml cartridges | 50 cartridge PoM ⊠ DT = £35.90

Lidocaine with cetrimide

27-Apr-2018

The properties listed below are those particular to the combination only. For the properties of the components please consider, lidocaine hydrochloride p. 1029.

● **INDICATIONS AND DOSE**

Anaesthesia and disinfection in dental practice

▸ TO MUCOUS MEMBRANES USING OROMUCOSAL SPRAY

▸ Child 4–17 years: 10–20 mg, no more than 30 mg should be applied to the same quadrant of the buccal cavity—consult product literature, dose expressed as lidocaine

Anaesthesia in dental practice

▸ TO MUCOUS MEMBRANES USING DENTAL GEL

▸ Child 4–17 years: Apply 100–500 mg, use cotton pellet for application to dried mucosa, dose expressed as weight of gel

DOSE EQUIVALENCE AND CONVERSION

▸ 1 metered dose of *Xylonor*® spray is equivalent to 10 mg of lidocaine.

▸ 2 millimetres of *Xylonor*® gel is approximately equivalent to 100 mg of gel (approximately equivalent to 5 mg of lidocaine).

● **CAUTIONS** Sepsis (risk of rapid systemic absorption) · traumatised mucosa (risk of rapid systemic absorption)

● **INTERACTIONS** → Appendix 1: antiarrhythmics

● **MEDICINAL FORMS** There can be variation in the licensing of different medicines containing the same drug.

Oromucosal gel

▸ Xylonor (Septodont Ltd)

Cetrimide 1.5 mg per 1 gram, Lidocaine 50 mg per 1 gram Xylonor 50mg/g / 1.5mg/g gel | 15 gram P £14.90 SF

Spray

▸ Xylonor (Septodont Ltd)

Cetrimide 1.5 mg per 1 gram, Lidocaine 150 mg per 1 gram Xylonor 150mg/g / 1.5mg/g oromucosal spray | 36 gram PoM £39.00 SF

Lidocaine with phenylephrine

The properties listed below are those particular to the combination only. For the properties of the components please consider, lidocaine hydrochloride p. 1029, phenylephrine hydrochloride p. 145.

● **INDICATIONS AND DOSE**

Anaesthesia before nasal surgery, endoscopy, laryngoscopy, or removal of foreign bodies from the nose

▸ BY INTRANASAL ADMINISTRATION

▸ Child 12–17 years: Up to 8 sprays

● **INTERACTIONS** → Appendix 1: antiarrhythmics · sympathomimetics, vasoconstrictor

● **MEDICINAL FORMS** There can be variation in the licensing of different medicines containing the same drug.

Spray

▸ Lidocaine with phenylephrine (Non-proprietary)

Phenylephrine hydrochloride 5 mg per 1 ml, Lidocaine hydrochloride 50 mg per 1 ml Lidocaine 5% / Phenylephrine 0.5% nasal spray | 2.5 ml PoM £16.39–£20.01 DT = £20.01

Lidocaine with prilocaine

10-Nov-2021

The properties listed below are those particular to the combination only. For the properties of the components please consider, lidocaine hydrochloride p. 1029, prilocaine hydrochloride p. 1033.

● **INDICATIONS AND DOSE**

Anaesthesia before minor skin procedures including venepuncture

▸ TO THE SKIN

▸ Neonate: Apply up to 1 g for maximum 1 hour before procedure, to be applied under occlusive dressing, shorter application time of 15–30 minutes is recommended for children with atopic dermatitis (30 minutes before removal of mollusca); maximum 1 dose per day.

▸ Child 1–2 months: Apply up to 1 g for maximum 1 hour before procedure, to be applied under occlusive dressing, shorter application time of 15–30 minutes is recommended for children with atopic dermatitis (30 minutes before removal of mollusca); maximum 1 dose per day

▸ Child 3–11 months: Apply up to 2 g for maximum 1 hour before procedure, to be applied under occlusive dressing, shorter application time of 15–30 minutes is recommended for children with atopic dermatitis (30 minutes before removal of mollusca); maximum 2 doses per day

▸ Child 1–11 years: Apply 1–5 hours before procedure, a thick layer should be applied under occlusive dressing, shorter application time of 15–30 minutes is recommended for children with atopic dermatitis (30 minutes before removal of mollusca); maximum 2 doses per day

continued →

- Child 12–17 years: Apply 1–5 hours before procedure (2–5 hours before procedures on large areas e.g. split skin grafting), a thick layer should be applied under occlusive dressing, shorter application time of 15–30 minutes is recommended for children with atopic dermatitis (30 minutes before removal of mollusca)

Anaesthesia on genital skin before injection of local anaesthetics

- TO THE SKIN
- Child 12–17 years: Apply under occlusive dressing for 15 minutes (males) or 60 minutes (females) before procedure

Anaesthesia before surgical treatment of lesions on genital mucosa

- TO THE SKIN
- Child 12–17 years: Apply up to 10 g, to be applied 5–10 minutes before procedure, maximum dose should be proportionally reduced in adolescents with body-weight less than 20 kg

Anaesthesia before cervical curettage

- TO THE SKIN
- Child 12–17 years: Apply 10 g in lateral vaginal fornices for 10 minutes

- **CONTRA-INDICATIONS** Use in child less than 37 weeks corrected gestational age
- **CAUTIONS**

FORTACIN® Acquired methaemoglobinaemia · anaemia · congenital methaemoglobinaemia

- **INTERACTIONS** → Appendix 1: anaesthetics, local · antiarrhythmics
- **SIDE-EFFECTS**
- Rare or very rare Methaemoglobinaemia · skin reactions
- **CONCEPTION AND CONTRACEPTION**

FORTACIN® Deterioration of polyurethane-based female and male condoms has been observed. Manufacturer advises avoid in patients planning to conceive, or if it is essential to achieve penetration, then the glans penis should be washed thoroughly 5 minutes after application but before intercourse.

- **PREGNANCY**

FORTACIN® Manufacturer advises preferably avoid unless an effective male barrier contraceptive is used—limited information available.

- **HEPATIC IMPAIRMENT**

FORTACIN® Manufacturer advises caution in severe impairment (no information available).

- **DIRECTIONS FOR ADMINISTRATION**

FORTACIN® Manufacturer advises when using the spray for the first time, shake and prime the unit with 3 sprays, and before each subsequent use, shake and prime the unit with 1 spray.

- **PATIENT AND CARER ADVICE**

Medicines for Children leaflet: EMLA cream for local anaesthesia www.medicinesforchildren.org.uk/medicines/emla-cream-for-local-anaesthesia/

- **MEDICINAL FORMS** There can be variation in the licensing of different medicines containing the same drug.

Cutaneous cream

- Emla (Aspen Pharma Trading Ltd)
  Lidocaine 25 mg per 1 gram, Prilocaine 25 mg per 1 gram Emla 5% cream | 5 gram [P] £2.25-£3.74 | 25 gram [P] £12.87 | 30 gram [P] £12.30 DT = £12.30
- Nulbia (Glenmark Pharmaceuticals Europe Ltd)
  Lidocaine 25 mg per 1 gram, Prilocaine 25 mg per 1 gram Nulbia 5% cream | 5 gram [P] £1.69 | 25 gram [P] £8.44 | 30 gram [P] £9.23 DT = £12.30

Mepivacaine hydrochloride

04-Dec-2019

- **INDICATIONS AND DOSE**

Infiltration anaesthesia and nerve block in dentistry

- Child 3–17 years: Consult expert dental sources

DOSES AT EXTREMES OF BODY-WEIGHT

- To avoid excessive dosage in obese patients, dose should be calculated on the basis of ideal body-weight.

IMPORTANT SAFETY INFORMATION
Should only be administered by, or under the direct supervision of, personnel experienced in their use, with adequate training in anaesthesia and airway management, and should not be administered parenterally unless adequate resuscitation equipment is available.

- **CONTRA-INDICATIONS** Avoid injection into infected tissues · avoid injection into inflamed tissues · intravenous regional anaesthesia (Bier's block) · preparations containing preservatives should not be used for caudal, epidural, or spinal block · severe atrio-ventricular conduction disorders not controlled by a pacemaker

CONTRA-INDICATIONS, FURTHER INFORMATION

- Injection site Manufacturer advises the local anaesthetic effect may be reduced when injected into an inflamed or infected area, due to altered local pH. Increased absorption into the blood also increases the possibility of systemic side-effects.

- **CAUTIONS** Cardiovascular disease · children (consider dose reduction) · debilitated patients (consider dose reduction) · epilepsy · hypovolaemia · impaired cardiac conduction · impaired respiratory function · myasthenia gravis · shock
- **SIDE-EFFECTS**
- Common or very common Arrhythmias · dizziness · hypertension · hypotension · nausea · paraesthesia · vomiting
- Uncommon Neurotoxicity
- Rare or very rare Arachnoiditis · cardiac arrest · diplopia · nerve disorders · respiratory depression

SIDE-EFFECTS, FURTHER INFORMATION Toxic effects after administration of local anaesthetics are a result of excessively high plasma concentrations; severe toxicity usually results from inadvertent intravascular injection or too rapid injection. The systemic toxicity of local anaesthetics mainly involves the central nervous and cardiovascular systems. The onset of toxicity can be unpredictable and delayed. Monitor as per local protocol for at least 30 minutes after administration.

- **ALLERGY AND CROSS-SENSITIVITY**
- Hypersensitivity and cross-sensitivity Hypersensitivity reactions occur mainly with the ester-type local anaesthetics, such as tetracaine; reactions are less frequent with the amide types, such as articaine, bupivacaine, levobupivacaine, lidocaine, mepivacaine, prilocaine, and ropivacaine. Cross-sensitivity reactions may be avoided by using the alternative chemical type.
- **PREGNANCY** Use with caution in early pregnancy.
- **BREAST FEEDING** Use with caution.
- **HEPATIC IMPAIRMENT** Manufacturer advises caution; increased risk of toxic plasma concentrations in severe impairment.
- **RENAL IMPAIRMENT** Use with caution; increased risk of side-effects.

● **MEDICINAL FORMS** There can be variation in the licensing of different medicines containing the same drug.

Solution for injection

▸ Scandonest plain (Septodont Ltd)
Mepivacaine hydrochloride 30 mg per 1 ml Scandonest plain 3% solution for injection 2.2ml cartridges | 50 cartridge PoM £36.90

Mepivacaine with adrenaline

19-Dec-2019

The properties listed below are those particular to the combination only. For the properties of the components please consider, mepivacaine hydrochloride p. 1032, adrenaline p. 159.

● **INDICATIONS AND DOSE**

Infiltration anaesthesia and nerve block in dentistry

▶ BY LOCAL INFILTRATION

▸ Child: (consult product literature)

● **INTERACTIONS** → Appendix 1: sympathomimetics, vasoconstrictor

● **MEDICINAL FORMS** No licensed medicines listed.

Prilocaine hydrochloride

12-Nov-2020

● **INDICATIONS AND DOSE**

DOSES AT EXTREMES OF BODY-WEIGHT

To avoid excessive dosage in obese patients, dose should be calculated on the basis of ideal body-weight.

CITANEST 1%®

Infiltration anaesthesia | Nerve block

▶ BY REGIONAL ADMINISTRATION

▸ Child 6 months–11 years: Up to 5 mg/kg, dose adjusted according to site of administration and response; maximum 400 mg per course

▸ Child 12–17 years: 100–200 mg/minute, alternatively, may be given in incremental doses; dose adjusted according to site of administration and response; maximum 400 mg per course

IMPORTANT SAFETY INFORMATION

Should only be administered by, or under the direct supervision of, personnel experienced in their use, with adequate training in anaesthesia and airway management, and should not be administered parenterally unless adequate resuscitation equipment is available.

● **CONTRA-INDICATIONS** Acquired methaemoglobinaemia · anaemia · avoid injection into infected tissues · avoid injection into inflamed tissues · congenital methaemoglobinaemia · preparations containing preservatives should not be used for caudal, epidural, or spinal block

CONTRA-INDICATIONS, FURTHER INFORMATION

▸ Injection site Manufacturer advises local anaesthetics should not be injected into inflamed or infected tissues. Increased absorption into the blood increases the possibility of systemic side-effects, and the local anaesthetic effect may also be reduced by altered local pH.

● **CAUTIONS** Cardiovascular disease · children (consider dose reduction) · debilitated patients (consider dose reduction) · epilepsy · hypovolaemia · impaired cardiac conduction · impaired respiratory function · myasthenia gravis · neonates and infants under 6 months are particularly susceptible to methaemoglobinaemia · severe or untreated hypertension · shock

● **SIDE-EFFECTS**

▶ **Common or very common** Arrhythmias · dizziness · hypertension · hypotension · nausea · paraesthesia · vomiting

▶ **Uncommon** Neurotoxicity

▶ **Rare or very rare** Cardiac arrest · methaemoglobinaemia · nerve disorders

▶ **Frequency not known** Diplopia · respiratory depression

SIDE-EFFECTS, FURTHER INFORMATION **Toxic effects** Toxic effects after administration of local anaesthetics are a result of excessively high plasma concentrations; severe toxicity usually results from inadvertent intravascular injection or too rapid injection. The systemic toxicity of local anaesthetics mainly involves the central nervous and cardiovascular systems. The onset of toxicity can be unpredictable and delayed. Monitor as per local protocol for at least 30 minutes after administration.

Methaemoglobinaemia Methaemoglobinaemia can be treated with an intravenous injection of methylthioninium chloride.

● **ALLERGY AND CROSS-SENSITIVITY**

▸ Hypersensitivity and cross-sensitivity Hypersensitivity reactions occur mainly with the ester-type local anaesthetics, such as tetracaine; reactions are less frequent with the amide types, such as articaine, bupivacaine, levobupivacaine, lidocaine, mepivacaine, prilocaine, and ropivacaine. Cross-sensitivity reactions may be avoided by using the alternative chemical type.

● **PREGNANCY** Large doses during delivery can cause neonatal respiratory depression, hypotonia, and bradycardia after epidural block. Avoid paracervical or pudendal block in obstetrics (neonatal methaemoglobinaemia reported).

Dose adjustments Use lower doses for intrathecal use during late pregnancy.

● **BREAST FEEDING** Present in milk but not known to be harmful.

● **HEPATIC IMPAIRMENT** Manufacturer advises caution.

● **RENAL IMPAIRMENT** Use with caution.

Dose adjustments Lower doses may be required for intrathecal anaesthesia.

● **MEDICINAL FORMS** There can be variation in the licensing of different medicines containing the same drug.

Solution for injection

▸ Prilocaine hydrochloride (Non-proprietary)
Prilocaine hydrochloride 10 mg per 1 ml Prilocaine 500mg/50ml solution for injection vials | 1 vial PoM £7.59 (Hospital only)

▸ Prilotekal (B.Braun Medical Ltd)
Prilocaine hydrochloride 20 mg per 1 ml Prilotekal 100mg/5ml solution for injection ampoules | 10 ampoule PoM £78.75 (Hospital only)

Prilocaine with felypressin

The properties listed below are those particular to the combination only. For the properties of the components please consider, prilocaine hydrochloride above.

● **INDICATIONS AND DOSE**

Dental anaesthesia

▶ BY REGIONAL ADMINISTRATION

▸ Child: Consult expert dental sources for specific advice

● **SIDE-EFFECTS** Bradycardia · cardiac arrest · dizziness · drowsiness · hypotension · loss of consciousness · methaemoglobinaemia · myocardial contractility decreased · nervousness · respiratory arrest · seizure · tremor · vision blurred

● **MEDICINAL FORMS** There can be variation in the licensing of different medicines containing the same drug.

Solution for injection

▸ Citanest with Octapressin (Dentsply Ltd)
Felypressin 540 nanogram per 1 ml, Prilocaine hydrochloride 30 mg per 1 ml Citanest 3% with Octapressin Dental 1.19micrograms/2.2ml solution for injection cartridges | 50 cartridge PoM ⊠

Ropivacaine hydrochloride
09-Dec-2019

● **INDICATIONS AND DOSE**

Acute pain | Surgical anaesthesia

▸ BY REGIONAL ADMINISTRATION

▸ Child: Adjust according to child's physical status and nature of procedure, seek expert advice

DOSES AT EXTREMES OF BODY-WEIGHT

▸ To avoid excessive dosage in obese patients, dose may need to be calculated on the basis of ideal bodyweight.

● **UNLICENSED USE** 2 mg/mL strength not licensed for use in children under 12 years except for acute pain management by caudal epidural block and continuous epidural infusion. 7.5 mg/mL and 10 mg/mL strengths not licensed for use in children under 12 years.

IMPORTANT SAFETY INFORMATION
Should only be administered by, or under the direct supervision of, personnel experienced in their use, with adequate training in anaesthesia and airway management, and should not be administered parenterally unless adequate resuscitation equipment is available.

● **CONTRA-INDICATIONS** Avoid injection into infected tissues · avoid injection into inflamed tissues · intravenous regional anaesthesia (Bier's block) · preparations containing preservatives should not be used for caudal, epidural, or spinal block

CONTRA-INDICATIONS, FURTHER INFORMATION

▸ Injection site Manufacturer advises local anaesthetics should not be injected into inflamed or infected tissues. Increased absorption into the blood increases the possibility of systemic side-effects, and the local anaesthetic effect may also be reduced by altered local pH.

● **CAUTIONS** Acute porphyrias p. 745 · cardiovascular disease · children (consider dose reduction) · complete heart block · debilitated patients (consider dose reduction) · epilepsy · hypovolaemia · impaired cardiac conduction · impaired respiratory function · myasthenia gravis · shock

● **INTERACTIONS** → Appendix 1: anaesthetics, local

● **SIDE-EFFECTS**

▸ **Common or very common** Arrhythmias · back pain · chills · dizziness · headache · hypertension · hypotension · nausea · sensation abnormal · urinary retention · vomiting

▸ **Uncommon** Anxiety · dyspnoea · hypothermia · neurotoxicity · syncope

▸ **Rare or very rare** Cardiac arrest

▸ **Frequency not known** Dyskinesia

SIDE-EFFECTS, FURTHER INFORMATION Toxic effects after administration of local anaesthetics are a result of excessively high plasma concentrations; severe toxicity usually results from inadvertent intravascular injection. The systemic toxicity of local anaesthetics mainly involves the central nervous and cardiovascular systems. The onset of toxicity can be unpredictable and delayed. Monitor as per local protocol for at least 30 minutes after administration.

● **ALLERGY AND CROSS-SENSITIVITY**

▸ Hypersensitivity and cross-sensitivity Hypersensitivity reactions occur mainly with the ester-type local anaesthetics, such as tetracaine; reactions are less frequent with the amide types, such as articaine, bupivacaine, levobupivacaine, lidocaine, mepivacaine, prilocaine, and ropivacaine. Cross-sensitivity reactions may be avoided by using the alternative chemical type.

● **PREGNANCY** Not known to be harmful. Do not use for paracervical block in obstetrics.

● **BREAST FEEDING** Not known to be harmful.

● **HEPATIC IMPAIRMENT** Manufacturer advises caution in severe impairment.

Dose adjustments Manufacturer advises consider dose reduction for repeat doses in severe impairment.

● **RENAL IMPAIRMENT** Caution in severe impairment. Increased risk of systemic toxicity in chronic renal failure.

● **MEDICINAL FORMS** There can be variation in the licensing of different medicines containing the same drug.

Solution for injection

ELECTROLYTES: May contain Sodium

▸ Ropivacaine hydrochloride (Non-proprietary)
Ropivacaine hydrochloride 2 mg per 1 ml Ropivacaine 400mg/200ml solution for injection polyethylene bottles | 10 bottle PoM £220.00 (Hospital only)
Ropivacaine 20mg/10ml solution for injection ampoules | 5 ampoule PoM £12.79–£27.84 (Hospital only)
Ropivacaine hydrochloride 7.5 mg per 1 ml Ropivacaine 75mg/10ml solution for injection ampoules | 5 ampoule PoM £15.90–£20.40 (Hospital only)
Ropivacaine hydrochloride 10 mg per 1 ml Ropivacaine 100mg/10ml solution for injection ampoules | 5 ampoule PoM £15.87–£22.70 (Hospital only)

Infusion

ELECTROLYTES: May contain Sodium

▸ Ropivacaine hydrochloride (Non-proprietary)
Ropivacaine hydrochloride 2 mg per 1 ml Ropivacaine 400mg/200ml infusion bags | 5 bag PoM £78.50–£108.50 (Hospital only)

Tetracaine
11-Nov-2021

(Amethocaine)

● **INDICATIONS AND DOSE**

Anaesthesia before venepuncture or venous cannulation

▸ TO THE SKIN

▸ Neonate: Apply contents of tube (or appropriate proportion) to site of venepuncture or venous cannulation and cover with occlusive dressing; remove gel and dressing after 30 minutes for venepuncture and after 45 minutes for venous cannulation.

▸ Child 1 month–4 years: Apply contents of up to 1 tube (applied at separate sites at a single time or appropriate proportion) to site of venepuncture or venous cannulation and cover with occlusive dressing; remove gel and dressing after 30 minutes for venepuncture and after 45 minutes for venous cannulation

▸ Child 5–17 years: Apply contents of up to 5 tubes (applied at separate sites at a single time or appropriate proportion) to site of venepuncture or venous cannulation and cover with occlusive dressing; remove gel and dressing after 30 minutes for venepuncture and after 45 minutes for venous cannulation

● **UNLICENSED USE** Not licensed for use in neonates.

● **CONTRA-INDICATIONS** Should not be applied to damaged skin

● **INTERACTIONS** → Appendix 1: anaesthetics, local

● **SIDE-EFFECTS** Oedema · skin reactions

SIDE-EFFECTS, FURTHER INFORMATION The systemic toxicity of local anaesthetics mainly involves the central nervous system; systemic side effects unlikely as minimal absorption following topical application.

- **ALLERGY AND CROSS-SENSITIVITY**
  - Hypersensitivity and cross-sensitivity Hypersensitivity reactions occur mainly with the ester-type local anaesthetics, such as tetracaine; reactions are less frequent with the amide types, such as articaine, bupivacaine, levobupivacaine, lidocaine, mepivacaine, prilocaine, and ropivacaine. Cross-sensitivity reactions may be avoided by using the alternative chemical type.
- **BREAST FEEDING** Not known to be harmful.
- **PATIENT AND CARER ADVICE**
  Medicines for Children leaflet: Tetracaine gel for local anaesthesia www.medicinesforchildren.org.uk/medicines/tetracaine-gel-for-local-anaesthesia/
- **MEDICINAL FORMS** There can be variation in the licensing of different medicines containing the same drug.

Cutaneous gel

EXCIPIENTS: May contain Hydroxybenzoates (parabens)

- Ametop (Alliance Pharmaceuticals Ltd)
  Tetracaine 40 mg per 1 gram Ametop 4% gel | 1.5 gram [P] £1.20 DT = £1.20

Chapter 16
Emergency treatment of poisoning

CONTENTS

Poisoning, emergency treatment

01-Dec-2025

Overview

These notes provide only an overview of the treatment of poisoning, and it is strongly recommended that either **TOXBASE** or the **UK National Poisons Information Service** be consulted when there is doubt about the degree of risk or about management.

Most childhood poisoning is accidental. Other causes include intentional overdose, drug abuse, iatrogenic and deliberate poisoning. The drugs most commonly involved in childhood poisoning are paracetamol p. 325, ibuprofen p. 821, orally ingested creams, aspirin p. 104, iron preparations, cough medicines, and the contraceptive pill.

Hospital admission

Children who have features of poisoning should generally be admitted to hospital. Children who have taken poisons with delayed actions should also be admitted, even if they appear well. Delayed-action poisons include aspirin, iron, paracetamol, tricyclic antidepressants, and co-phenotrope (diphenoxylate with atropine, *Lomotil*®) p. 54; the effects of modified-release preparations are also delayed. A note of all relevant information, including what treatment has been given, should accompany the patient to hospital.

Further information

TOXBASE, the primary clinical toxicology database of the National Poisons Information Service, is available on the internet to registered users at www.toxbase.org It provides information about routine diagnosis, treatment, and management of patients exposed to drugs, household products, and industrial and agricultural chemicals.

Specialist information and advice on the treatment of poisoning is available day and night from the **UK National Poisons Information Service** on the following number: Tel: 0344 892 0111.

Advice on laboratory analytical services can be obtained from TOXBASE or from the National Poisons Information Service. Help with identifying capsules or tablets may be available from a regional medicines information centre or from the National Poisons Information Service (out of hours).

Storage of specialist antidotes

Due to the risk of unintended administration, NHS England advises emergency departments and pharmacies to ensure that 'specialist antidotes' are stored either in automatic dispensing cabinets/systems, or in a separate area specifically designated for antidotes. Those requiring refrigeration should be separated from other medicines in the medication fridge and clearly identified as antidotes. If 'specialist antidotes' are kept in the emergency/out-of-hours medicine cupboards, they should be separated from other medicines and clearly identified as antidotes.

'Specialist antidotes' are defined as those on the **Royal College of Emergency Medicine/ UK National Poisons Information Service** list (available at www.npis.org/Publications.html) and only used in emergency departments as a specific antidote.

General care

It is often impossible to establish with certainty the identity of the poison and the size of the dose. This is not usually important because only a few poisons (such as opioids, paracetamol, and iron) have specific antidotes; few patients require active removal of the poison. In most patients, treatment is directed at managing symptoms as they arise. Nevertheless, knowledge of the type and timing of poisoning can help in anticipating the course of events. All relevant information should be sought from the poisoned individual and from carers or parents. However, such information should be interpreted with care because it may not be complete or entirely reliable. Sometimes symptoms arise from other illnesses and patients should be assessed carefully. Accidents may involve domestic and industrial products (the contents of which are not generally known). The **National Poisons Information Service** should be consulted when there is doubt about any aspect of suspected poisoning.

Respiration

Respiration is often impaired in unconscious patients. An obstructed airway requires immediate attention. In the absence of trauma, the airway should be opened with simple measures such as chin lift or jaw thrust. An oropharyngeal or nasopharyngeal airway may be useful in patients with reduced consciousness to prevent obstruction, provided ventilation is adequate. Intubation and ventilation should be considered in patients whose airway cannot be protected or who have respiratory acidosis because of inadequate ventilation; such patients should be monitored in a critical care area.

Most poisons that impair consciousness also depress respiration. Assisted ventilation (either mouth-to-mouth or using a bag-valve-mask device) may be needed. Oxygen is not a substitute for adequate ventilation, although it should be given in the highest concentration possible in poisoning with carbon monoxide and irritant gases.

The potential for pulmonary aspiration of gastric contents should be considered.

Blood pressure

Hypotension is common in severe poisoning with central nervous system depressants; if severe, this may lead to irreversible brain damage or renal tubular necrosis. Hypotension should be corrected initially by raising the foot of the bed and administration of an infusion of either sodium chloride p. 728 or a colloid. Vasoconstrictor sympathomimetics are rarely required and their use may be discussed with the National Poisons Information Service or a paediatric intensive care unit.

Fluid depletion without hypotension is common after prolonged coma and after aspirin poisoning due to vomiting, sweating and hyperpnoea.

Hypertension, often transient, occurs less frequently than hypotension in poisoning; it may be associated with sympathomimetic drugs such as amfetamines, phencyclidine, and cocaine.

Heart

Cardiac conduction defects and arrhythmias can occur in acute poisoning, notably with tricyclic antidepressants, some antipsychotics, and some antihistamines. Arrhythmias often respond to correction of underlying hypoxia, acidosis, or other biochemical abnormalities, but ventricular arrhythmias that cause serious hypotension require treatment. If the QT interval is prolonged, specialist advice should be sought because the use of some anti-arrhythmic drugs may be inappropriate. Supraventricular arrhythmias are seldom life-threatening and drug treatment is best withheld until the patient reaches hospital.

Body temperature

Hypothermia may develop in patients of any age who have been deeply unconscious for some hours, particularly following overdose with barbiturates or phenothiazines. It may be missed unless core temperature is measured using a low-reading rectal thermometer or by some other means. Hypothermia should be managed by prevention of further heat loss and appropriate rewarming as clinically indicated.

Hyperthermia can develop in patients taking CNS stimulants; children and the elderly are also at risk when taking therapeutic doses of drugs with antimuscarinic properties. Hyperthermia is initially managed by removing all unnecessary clothing and using a fan. Sponging with **tepid** water will promote evaporation. Advice should be sought from the National Poisons Information Service on the management of severe hyperthermia resulting from conditions such as the serotonin syndrome.

Both hypothermia and hyperthermia require **urgent** hospitalisation for assessment and supportive treatment.

Convulsions during poisoning

Single short-lived convulsions (lasting less than 5 minutes) do not require treatment. If convulsions are protracted or recur frequently, lorazepam p. 272 or diazepam p. 270 (preferably as emulsion) should be given by slow intravenous injection into a large vein. Benzodiazepines should not be given by the intramuscular route for convulsions. If the intravenous route is not readily available, midazolam oromucosal solution p. 273 can be given by the buccal route or diazepam can be administered as a rectal solution.

Methaemoglobinaemia

Drug- or chemical-induced methaemoglobinaemia should be treated with **methylthioninium chloride p. 1049** if the methaemoglobin concentration is 30% or higher, *or* if symptoms of tissue hypoxia are present despite oxygen therapy. Methylthioninium chloride reduces the ferric iron of methaemoglobin back to the ferrous iron of haemoglobin; in high doses, methylthioninium chloride can itself cause methaemoglobinaemia.

Poison removal and elimination

Prevention of absorption

Given by mouth, **activated charcoal p. 1043** can adsorb many poisons in the gastro-intestinal system, thereby reducing their absorption. The **sooner** it is given the **more effective** it is, but it may still be effective up to 1 hour after ingestion of the poison—longer in the case of modified-release preparations or of drugs with antimuscarinic (anticholinergic) properties. It is particularly useful for the prevention of absorption of poisons that are toxic in small amounts, such as antidepressants.

A second dose may occasionally be required when blood-drug concentration continues to rise suggesting delayed drug release or delayed gastric emptying.

Active elimination techniques

Repeated doses of **activated charcoal** by mouth may *enhance the elimination* of some drugs after they have been absorbed; repeated doses are given after overdosage with:

- Carbamazepine
- Dapsone
- Phenobarbital
- Quinine
- Theophylline

If vomiting occurs after dosing, it should be treated (e.g. with an antiemetic drug) since it may reduce the efficacy of charcoal treatment. In cases of intolerance, the dose may be reduced and the frequency increased but this may compromise efficacy.

Activated charcoal should **not** be used for poisoning with petroleum distillates, corrosive substances, alcohols, malathion, cyanides and metal salts including iron and lithium salts.

Other techniques intended to enhance the elimination of poisons after absorption are only practicable in hospital and are only suitable for a small number of severely poisoned patients. Moreover, they only apply to a limited number of poisons. Examples include:

- haemodialysis for ethylene glycol, lithium, methanol, phenobarbital, salicylates, and sodium valproate;
- alkalinisation of the urine for salicylates.

Removal from the gastro-intestinal tract

Gastric lavage is rarely required as benefit rarely outweighs risk; advice should be sought from the National Poisons Information Service if a significant quantity of iron or lithium has been ingested within the previous hour.

Whole bowel irrigation (by means of a bowel cleansing preparation) has been used in poisoning with certain modified-release or enteric-coated formulations, in severe poisoning with lithium salts, and if illicit drugs are carried in the gastro-intestinal tract ('body-packing'). However, it is not clear that the procedure improves outcome and advice should be sought from the National Poisons Information Service.

The administration of **laxatives** alone has no role in the management of the poisoned child and is not a recommended method of gut decontamination. The routine use of a laxative in combination with activated charcoal has mostly been abandoned. Laxatives should not be administered to young children because of the likelihood of fluid and electrolyte imbalance.

Alcohol, acute intoxication

Acute intoxication with **alcohol** (ethanol) is common in adults but also occurs in children. The features include ataxia, dysarthria, nystagmus, and drowsiness, which may progress to coma, with hypotension and acidosis. Aspiration of vomit is a special hazard and hypoglycaemia may occur. Patients are managed supportively, with particular attention to maintaining a clear airway and measures to reduce the

Paracetamol overdose treatment graph

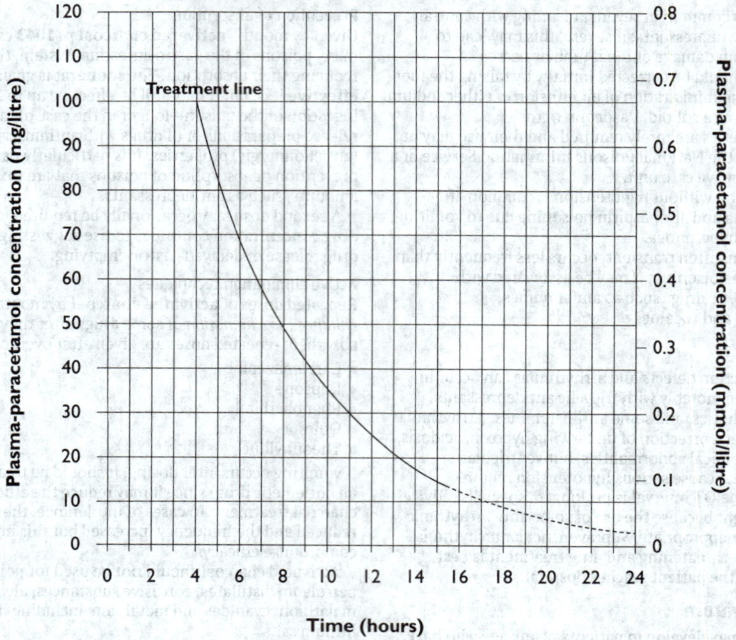

Patients whose plasma-paracetamol concentrations are on or above the **treatment line** should be treated with acetylcysteine by intravenous infusion.

The prognostic accuracy after 15 hours is uncertain, but a plasma-paracetamol concentration on or above the treatment line should be regarded as carrying a serious risk of liver damage.

Graph reproduced courtesy of Medicines and Healthcare products Regulatory Agency

risk of aspiration of gastric contents. The blood glucose is measured and glucose given if indicated.

Aspirin poisoning

The main features of salicylate poisoning are hyperventilation, tinnitus, deafness, vasodilatation, and sweating. Coma is uncommon but indicates very severe poisoning. The associated acid-base disturbances are complex.

Treatment must be in hospital, where plasma salicylate, pH, and electrolytes can be measured; absorption of aspirin may be slow and the plasma-salicylate concentration may continue to rise for several hours, requiring repeated measurement. Plasma-salicylate concentration may not correlate with clinical severity in the young, and clinical and biochemical assessment is necessary. Generally, the clinical severity of poisoning is less below a plasma-salicylate concentration of 500 mg/litre (3.6 mmol/litre), unless there is evidence of metabolic acidosis. Activated charcoal can be given within 1 hour of ingesting more than 125 mg/kg of aspirin. Fluid losses should be replaced and intravenous sodium bicarbonate may be given (ensuring plasma-potassium concentration is within the reference range) to enhance urinary salicylate excretion (optimum urinary pH 7.5–8.5).

Plasma-potassium concentration should be corrected before giving sodium bicarbonate as hypokalaemia may complicate alkalinisation of the urine.

Haemodialysis is the treatment of choice for severe salicylate poisoning and should be considered when the plasma-salicylate concentration exceeds 700 mg/litre (5.1 mmol/litre) or in the presence of severe metabolic acidosis, convulsions, respiratory failure, pulmonary oedema or persistently high plasma-salicylate concentrations unresponsive to urinary alkalinisation.

Opioid poisoning

Opioids (narcotic analgesics) cause varying degrees of coma, respiratory depression, and pinpoint pupils. The specific antidote naloxone hydrochloride p. 1047 is indicated if there is coma or bradypnoea. Since naloxone has a shorter duration of action than many opioids, close monitoring and repeated injections are necessary according to the respiratory rate and depth of coma. When repeated administration of naloxone is required, it can be given by continuous intravenous infusion instead and the rate of infusion adjusted according to vital signs. All children should be observed for at least 6 hours after the last dose of naloxone. The effects of some opioids, such as buprenorphine, are only partially reversed by naloxone. Dextropropoxyphene and methadone have very long durations of action; patients may need to be monitored for long periods following large overdoses.

Naloxone reverses the opioid effects of dextropropoxyphene. The long duration of action of dextropropoxyphene calls for prolonged monitoring and further doses of naloxone may be required. Norpropoxyphene, a metabolite of dextropropoxyphene, also has cardiotoxic effects which may require treatment with sodium bicarbonate p. 725 or magnesium sulfate p. 739, or both. Arrhythmias may occur for up to 12 hours.

Paracetamol poisoning

In all cases of **intravenous paracetamol poisoning** clinicians are encouraged to contact the National Poisons Information Service for advice on risk assessment and management.

Toxic doses of paracetamol p. 325 may cause severe hepatocellular necrosis and, much less frequently, renal tubular necrosis. Nausea and vomiting, the early features of poisoning, usually settle within 24 hours. The recurrence of nausea and vomiting after 2–3 days, often associated with the onset of right subcostal pain and tenderness, usually indicates development of hepatic necrosis. Liver damage is maximal 3–4 days after paracetamol overdose and may lead to liver failure, encephalopathy, coma, and death.

The following guidance provides only an overview of the management of paracetamol overdosage from the *National Poisons Information Service TOXBASE* database.

To avoid underestimating the potentially toxic paracetamol dose ingested by obese children who weigh more than 110 kg, use a body-weight of 110 kg (rather than their actual body-weight) when calculating the total dose of paracetamol ingested (in mg/kg).

For pregnant patients the potentially toxic paracetamol dose should be calculated using the patient's pre-pregnancy weight

Acetylcysteine p. 1048 prevents or reduces the severity of liver damage if given up to, and possibly beyond (in those at risk of severe liver disease) 24 hours of ingesting paracetamol. It is most effective if given within 8 hours of paracetamol ingestion, after which effectiveness declines. Very rarely, giving acetylcysteine by mouth [unlicensed] is an alternative if intravenous access is not possible (for further information, see **Acetylcysteine—oral doses**, available from TOXBASE).

Acute overdose

Acute overdose involves ingestion of a potentially toxic dose of paracetamol in 1 hour or less.

For **children aged under 6 years**, serious toxicity is unlikely to occur from a single ingestion of less than 150 mg/kg of paracetamol taken in less than 1 hour. Refer children to hospital for medical assessment if they meet any of the following criteria:

- are symptomatic,
- have ingested 150 mg/kg or more of paracetamol in 1 hour or less, or
- where there is uncertainty about the dose ingested or circumstance of ingestion.

For **children aged 6 years and over**, serious toxicity is unlikely to occur from a single ingestion of less than 75 mg/kg of paracetamol taken in less than 1 hour. Refer children to hospital for medical assessment if they meet any of the following criteria:

- have ingested paracetamol in the context of self-harm,
- are symptomatic,
- have ingested 75 mg/kg or more of paracetamol in 1 hour or less, or
- where the time of ingestion is uncertain but the dose ingested is 75 mg/kg or more.

Although the benefit of gastric decontamination is uncertain, activated charcoal p. 1043 should be considered if the child presents within 1 hour of ingesting paracetamol in excess of 150 mg/kg.

Children at risk of liver damage and therefore requiring acetylcysteine, can be identified from a single measurement of the plasma-paracetamol concentration related to the time from ingestion, provided this time interval is not less than 4 hours; earlier samples cannot be interpreted. The concentration is plotted on a paracetamol treatment graph, with a reference line ('treatment line') joining plots of 100 mg/litre (0.66 mmol/litre) at 4 hours and 3.13 mg/litre (0.02 mmol/litre) at 24 hours, see *Paracetamol overdose treatment graph*.

Acetylcysteine treatment should commence in children:

- whose plasma-paracetamol concentration falls on or above the *treatment line* on the paracetamol treatment graph;
- who present within 8 hours of ingestion of more than 150 mg/kg of paracetamol, if there is going to be a delay of 8 hours or more in obtaining the paracetamol concentration after the overdose;
- who present 8–24 hours of ingestion of an acute overdose of more than 150 mg/kg of paracetamol, or the amount ingested is unknown, or if the patient is symptomatic with jaundice or hepatic tenderness, even if the plasma-paracetamol concentration is not yet available;
- who present more than 24 hours of ingestion of an overdose of more than 150 mg/kg of paracetamol or the amount ingested is unknown, or if they are clearly jaundiced or have hepatic tenderness, or the paracetamol concentration is detectable.
- whose biochemical tests suggest acute liver injury, such as ALT above the upper limit of normal (children with chronically elevated ALT should be discussed with the National Poisons Information Service), or INR greater than 1.3 (in the absence of another cause), even if the plasma paracetamol concentration is below the treatment line on the paracetamol overdose treatment graph.

If the child is not at risk of liver toxicity (i.e. the paracetamol concentration is below the treatment line or undetectable; the INR and ALT are normal; and the patient is asymptomatic) no treatment with an antidote is indicated; acetylcysteine may be discontinued if it has been started.

Where the time of ingestion is unknown, patients should be managed as a *staggered overdose*.

Therapeutic excess or staggered overdose

Children who have ingested more than 150 mg/kg of paracetamol in any 24-hour period are at risk of serious toxicity. Toxicity rarely occurs with paracetamol doses between 75–150 mg/kg in any 24-hour period. Doses consistently less than 75 mg/kg in any 24-hour period are very unlikely to be toxic; however risk may be increased if this dose is repeatedly ingested over 2 or more days. Ingestion of a licensed dose of paracetamol is not considered an overdose.

Therapeutic excess is the ingestion of a potentially toxic dose of paracetamol with intent to treat pain or fever and without self-harm intent during its clinical use. All children should be referred to hospital for medical assessment if they meet any of the following criteria:

- are symptomatic,
- have ingested more than a licensed dose and more than or equal to 75 mg/kg in any 24-hour period, or
- have ingested more than the licensed dose but less than 75 mg/kg/24 hours on each day of the last 72 hours.

Children with clinical features of hepatic injury such as jaundice or hepatic tenderness should be treated urgently with acetylcysteine. For other children, management is determined by the maximum dose of paracetamol ingested in any 24-hour period (for further information, see **Paracetamol—therapeutic excess**, available from TOXBASE).

Asymptomatic children who present more than 7 days after the last dose of paracetamol was ingested, who have had no new symptoms since the time of ingestion, and who have no history of chronic kidney or liver disease, will not normally require further assessment, providing the timing of ingestion is certain.

When there is uncertainty about whether the presentation was due to therapeutic excess, the patient should be managed as a *staggered overdose*.

A **staggered overdose** involves ingestion of a potentially toxic dose of paracetamol over more than 1 hour, with the possible intention of causing self-harm. All children who have taken a staggered overdose should be referred to hospital for medical assessment. The MHRA advises that all children who have ingested a staggered overdose should be treated with acetylcysteine without delay.

Clinically significant hepatotoxicity is unlikely and the child is not considered to be at risk if, after at least 4 hours or more since the last paracetamol ingestion, the child has no symptoms suggesting liver damage, the paracetamol concentration is less than 10 mg/L, their ALT is within the normal range, and their INR is 1.3 or less. Acetylcysteine can be discontinued in children not considered to be at risk of clinically significant liver damage. If there is uncertainty about a child's risk of toxicity after paracetamol overdose, advice should be sought from the National Poisons Information Service.

Acetylcysteine dose and administration

For paracetamol overdosage, there are two intravenous acetylcysteine regimens: the standard 21-hour regimen and the modified 12-hour regimen (also known as the Scottish and Newcastle Acetylcysteine Protocol (SNAP)). The SNAP regimen [unlicensed] is not endorsed by the MHRA, but it is recommended by the Royal College of Emergency Medicine and the National Poisons Information Service. For further information, see acetylcysteine p. 1048, **Acetylcysteine SNAP Doses—Children** (for children who weigh less than 40 kg) and **Acetylcysteine SNAP Doses—Adult** (for children who weigh 40 kg or more), and **Paracetamol - Guidance for the end of the modified 12-hour IV acetylcysteine regimen (SNAP)**, available from TOXBASE.

For the standard 21-hour regimen, acetylcysteine is given in a total dose that is divided into 3 consecutive intravenous infusions over a total of 21 hours. For information on dosing/administration, see acetylcysteine, **Acetylcysteine Doses—Children** (for children who weigh less than 40 kg) and **Acetylcysteine Doses—Adults** (for children who weigh 40 kg or more), and **Paracetamol - Guidance for the end of the standard 21-hour IV acetylcysteine regimen**, available from TOXBASE.

Antidepressant poisoning

Tricyclic and related antidepressants

Tricyclic and related antidepressants cause dry mouth, coma of varying degree, hypotension, hypothermia, hyperreflexia, extensor plantar responses, convulsions, respiratory failure, cardiac conduction defects, and arrhythmias. Dilated pupils and urinary retention also occur. Metabolic acidosis may complicate severe poisoning; delirium with confusion, agitation, and visual and auditory hallucinations are common during recovery.

Assessment in hospital is strongly advised in case of poisoning by tricyclic and related antidepressants but symptomatic treatment can be given before transfer. Supportive measures to ensure a clear airway and adequate ventilation during transfer are mandatory. Intravenous lorazepam or intravenous diazepam (preferably in emulsion form) may be required to treat convulsions. Activated charcoal given within 1 hour of the overdose reduces absorption of the drug. Although arrhythmias are worrying, some will respond to correction of hypoxia and acidosis. The use of anti-arrhythmic drugs is best avoided, but intravenous infusion of sodium bicarbonate can arrest arrhythmias or prevent them in those with an extended QRS duration. Diazepam p. 270 given by mouth is usually adequate to sedate delirious patients but large doses may be required.

Selective serotonin re-uptake inhibitors (SSRIs)

Symptoms of poisoning by selective serotonin re-uptake inhibitors include nausea, vomiting, agitation, tremor, nystagmus, drowsiness, and sinus tachycardia; convulsions may occur. Rarely, severe poisoning results in the serotonin syndrome, with marked neuropsychiatric effects, neuromuscular hyperactivity, and autonomic instability; hyperthermia, rhabdomyolysis, renal failure, and coagulopathies may develop.

Management of SSRI poisoning is supportive. Activated charcoal given within 1 hour of the overdose reduces absorption of the drug. Convulsions can be treated with lorazepam p. 272, diazepam, or buccal midazolam p. 273 (see *Convulsions*). Contact the National Poisons Information Service for the management of hyperthermia or the serotonin syndrome.

Antimalarial poisoning

Overdosage with quinine, chloroquine, or hydroxychloroquine is extremely hazardous and difficult to treat. Urgent advice from the National Poisons Information Service is essential. Life-threatening features include arrhythmias (which can have a very rapid onset) and convulsions (which can be intractable).

Antipsychotic poisoning

Phenothiazines and related drugs

Phenothiazines cause less depression of consciousness and respiration than other sedatives. Hypotension, hypothermia, sinus tachycardia, and arrhythmias may complicate poisoning. Dystonic reactions can occur with therapeutic doses (particularly with prochlorperazine and trifluoperazine), and convulsions may occur in severe cases. Arrhythmias may respond to correction of hypoxia, acidosis, and other biochemical abnormalities, but specialist advice should be sought if arrhythmias result from a prolonged QT interval; the use of some anti-arrhythmic drugs can worsen such arrhythmias. Dystonic reactions are rapidly abolished by injection of drugs such as procyclidine hydrochloride p. 309 or diazepam (emulsion preferred).

Second-generation antipsychotic drugs

Features of poisoning by second-generation antipsychotic drugs include drowsiness, convulsions, extrapyramidal symptoms, hypotension, and ECG abnormalities (including prolongation of the QT interval). Management is supportive. Activated charcoal p. 1043 can be given within 1 hour of ingesting a significant quantity of a second-generation antipsychotic drug.

Benzodiazepine poisoning

Benzodiazepines taken alone cause drowsiness, ataxia, dysarthria, nystagmus, and occasionally respiratory depression, and coma. Activated charcoal can be given within 1 hour of ingesting a significant quantity of benzodiazepine, provided the patient is awake and the airway is protected. Benzodiazepines potentiate the effects of other central nervous system depressants taken concomitantly. Use of the benzodiazepine antagonist flumazenil p. 1045 [unlicensed indication] can be hazardous, particularly in mixed overdoses involving tricyclic antidepressants or in benzodiazepine-dependent patients. Flumazenil may prevent the need for ventilation, particularly in patients with severe respiratory disorders; it should be used on expert advice only and not as a diagnostic test in children with a reduced level of consciousness.

Beta-blockers poisoning

Overdosages with beta-blockers may cause cardiac effects such as bradycardia, hypotension, syncope, conduction abnormalities, and heart failure. Bradycardia is the most common arrhythmia, but some beta-blockers may induce ventricular tachyarrhythmias secondary to prolongation of QT interval (e.g. sotalol) or QRS duration (e.g. propranolol). Although the predominant effects of beta-blocker overdose are on the heart, other features may also occur, such as central nervous system effects (including drowsiness, confusion, convulsions, hallucinations, and in severe cases coma), respiratory depression, and bronchospasm. The effects of overdosage can vary from one beta-blocker to another; propranolol overdosage in particular may cause coma and convulsions.

The following guidance provides only an overview of the management of beta-blocker overdosage from the *National Poisons Information Service TOXBASE database*.

All children who have been exposed to beta-blockers as a result of self-harm should be referred for assessment. Medical assessment is recommended for all children who are symptomatic or have ingested more than a toxic dose; and in those who are treatment naive or have taken more than their therapeutic dose, and have a significant cardiac history or asthma. All children who have exceeded their prescribed daily dose of 2 or more cardiotoxic agents should also be referred for medical assessment irrespective of the dose ingested. Hospital clinicians are encouraged to discuss all serious cases with the UK National Poisons Information Service.

For children presenting with overdose, maintain a clear airway and adequate ventilation. Although the benefit of gastric decontamination is uncertain, activated charcoal p. 1043 can be considered if the child presents within 1 hour of ingestion of more than a potentially toxic dose.

For the management of hypotension, ensure adequate fluid resuscitation; in an emergency, vasopressors and inotropes can be initiated under the advice of an experienced physician. Intravenous glucagon p. 579 [unlicensed] is a treatment option for severe hypotension, heart failure, or cardiogenic shock. In severe cases, an insulin and glucose infusion can improve myocardial contractility and systemic perfusion, especially in the presence of acidosis. Consider intravenous sodium bicarbonate p. 725 for correction of metabolic acidosis that persists despite correction of hypoxia and adequate fluid resuscitation—rapid correction is particularly important if QRS duration is prolonged. For symptomatic bradycardia give intravenous atropine sulfate p. 839; dobutamine p. 143 [unlicensed] or isoprenaline [unlicensed] (available from 'special-order' manufacturers or specialist importing companies) may be considered if bradycardia is associated with hypotension. A temporary cardiac pacemaker can be used to increase the heart rate.

Treat bronchospasm with nebulised bronchodilators and corticosteroids.

If convulsions occur give oxygen, and correct acid-base and metabolic disturbances as required. Prolonged or frequent convulsions should be controlled with intravenous diazepam p. 270, lorazepam p. 272, or midazolam p. 273 [unlicensed use]. If convulsions are unresponsive to treatment, the child should be referred urgently to critical care.

Calcium-channel blockers poisoning

Features of calcium-channel blocker poisoning include nausea, vomiting, dizziness, agitation, confusion, and coma in severe poisoning. Metabolic acidosis and hyperglycaemia may occur. Verapamil and diltiazem have a profound cardiac depressant effect causing hypotension and arrhythmias, including complete heart block and asystole. The dihydropyridine calcium-channel blockers cause severe hypotension secondary to profound peripheral vasodilatation.

Activated charcoal should be considered if the patient presents within 1 hour of overdosage with a calcium-channel blocker; repeated doses of activated charcoal are considered if a modified-release preparation is involved. In patients with significant features of poisoning, calcium chloride p. 734 or calcium gluconate p. 735 is given by injection; atropine sulfate is given to correct symptomatic bradycardia. In severe cases, an insulin and glucose infusion may be required in the management of hypotension and myocardial failure. For the management of hypotension, the choice of inotropic sympathomimetic depends on whether hypotension is secondary to vasodilatation or to myocardial depression—advice should be sought from the National Poisons Information Service.

Iron salts poisoning

Iron poisoning in childhood is usually accidental. The symptoms are nausea, vomiting, abdominal pain, diarrhoea, haematemesis, and rectal bleeding. Hypotension and hepatocellular necrosis can occur later. Coma, shock, and metabolic acidosis indicate severe poisoning.

Advice should be sought from the National Poisons Information Service if a significant quantity of iron has been ingested within the previous hour.

Mortality is reduced by intensive and specific therapy with desferrioxamine mesilate p. 714, which chelates iron. The serum-iron concentration is measured as an emergency and intravenous desferrioxamine mesilate given to chelate absorbed iron in excess of the expected iron binding capacity. In severe toxicity intravenous desferrioxamine mesilate should be given immediately without waiting for the result of the serum-iron measurement.

Lithium poisoning

Most cases of lithium intoxication occur as a complication of long-term therapy and are caused by reduced excretion of the drug because of a variety of factors including dehydration, deterioration of renal function, infections, and co-administration of diuretics or NSAIDs (or other drugs that interact). Acute deliberate overdoses may also occur with delayed onset of symptoms (12 hours or more) owing to slow entry of lithium into the tissues and continuing absorption from modified-release formulations.

The early clinical features are non-specific and may include apathy and restlessness which could be confused with mental changes arising from the child's depressive illness. Vomiting, diarrhoea, ataxia, weakness, dysarthria, muscle twitching, and tremor may follow. Severe poisoning is associated with convulsions, coma, renal failure, electrolyte imbalance, dehydration, and hypotension.

Therapeutic serum-lithium concentrations are within the range of 0.4–1 mmol/litre; concentrations in excess of 2 mmol/litre are usually associated with serious toxicity and such cases may need treatment with haemodialysis if neurological symptoms or renal failure are present. In acute overdosage much higher serum-lithium concentrations may be present without features of toxicity and all that is usually necessary is to take measures to increase urine output (e.g. by increasing fluid intake but avoiding diuretics). Otherwise, treatment is supportive with special regard to electrolyte balance, renal function, and control of convulsions. Whole-bowel irrigation should be considered for significant ingestion, but advice should be sought from the National Poisons Information Service.

Stimulant-drug poisoning

Amfetamines

Amfetamines cause wakefulness, excessive activity, paranoia, hallucinations, and hypertension followed by exhaustion, convulsions, hyperthermia, and coma. The early stages can be controlled by diazepam or lorazepam; advice should be sought from the National Poisons Information Service on the management of hypertension. Later, tepid sponging, anticonvulsants, and artificial respiration may be needed.

Cocaine

Cocaine stimulates the central nervous system, causing agitation, dilated pupils, tachycardia, hypertension, hallucinations, hyperthermia, hypertonia, and hyperreflexia; cardiac effects include chest pain, myocardial infarction, and arrhythmias.

Initial treatment of cocaine poisoning involves cooling measures for hyperthermia (see Body temperature);

agitation, hypertension and cardiac effects require specific treatment and expert advice should be sought.

Ecstasy

Ecstasy (methylenedioxymethamfetamine, MDMA) may cause severe reactions, even at doses that were previously tolerated. The most serious effects are delirium, coma, convulsions, ventricular arrhythmias, hyperthermia, rhabdomyolysis, acute renal failure, acute hepatitis, disseminated intravascular coagulation, adult respiratory distress syndrome, hyperreflexia, hypotension and intracerebral haemorrhage; hyponatraemia has also been associated with ecstasy use and syndrome of inappropriate antidiuretic hormone secretion (SIADH) can occur.

Treatment of methylenedioxymethamfetamine poisoning is supportive, with diazepam p. 270 to control persistent convulsions and close monitoring including ECG. For the management of agitation, seek specialist advice. Self-induced water intoxication should be considered in patients with ecstasy poisoning.

'Liquid ecstasy' is a term used for sodium oxybate (gamma-hydroxybutyrate, GHB), which is a sedative.

Theophylline poisoning

Theophylline and related drugs are often prescribed as modified-release formulations and toxicity can therefore be delayed. They cause vomiting (which may be severe and intractable), agitation, restlessness, dilated pupils, sinus tachycardia, and hyperglycaemia. More serious effects are haematemesis, convulsions, and supraventricular and ventricular arrhythmias. Severe hypokalaemia may develop rapidly.

Repeated doses of activated charcoal p. 1043 can be used to eliminate theophylline even if more than 1 hour has elapsed after ingestion and especially if a modified-release preparation has been taken (see also under Active Elimination Techniques). Ondansetron p. 317 may be effective for severe vomiting that is resistant to other antiemetics. Hypokalaemia is corrected by intravenous infusion of potassium chloride p. 744 and may be so severe as to require high doses under ECG monitoring. Convulsions should be controlled by intravenous administration of lorazepam p. 272 or diazepam (see Convulsions). For the management of agitation associated with theophylline overdosage, seek specialist advice.

Provided the child does **not** suffer from asthma, a short-acting beta-blocker can be administered intravenously to reverse severe tachycardia, hypokalaemia, and hyperglycaemia.

Cyanide poisoning

Oxygen should be administered to children with cyanide poisoning. The choice of antidote depends on the severity of poisoning, certainty of diagnosis, and the cause. Dicobalt edetate p. 1044 is the antidote of choice when there is a strong clinical suspicion of severe cyanide poisoning, but it should **not** be used as a precautionary measure. Dicobalt edetate itself is toxic, associated with anaphylactoid reactions, and is potentially fatal if administered in the absence of cyanide poisoning. A regimen of sodium nitrite p. 1044 followed by sodium thiosulfate p. 1044 is an alternative if dicobalt edetate is not available.

Hydroxocobalamin p. 711 (*Cyanokit*®—no other preparation of hydroxocobalamin is suitable) can be considered for use in victims of smoke inhalation who show signs of significant cyanide poisoning.

Ethylene glycol and methanol poisoning

Fomepizole (available from 'special-order' manufacturers or specialist importing companies) is the treatment of choice for ethylene glycol and methanol (methyl alcohol) poisoning. If necessary, **ethanol** (by mouth or by intravenous infusion) can be used, but with caution. Advice on the treatment of ethylene glycol and methanol poisoning should be obtained from the National Poisons Information Service. It is important to start antidote treatment promptly in cases of suspected poisoning with these agents.

Heavy metal poisoning

Heavy metal antidotes include succimer (DMSA) [unlicensed], unithiol (DMPS) [unlicensed], sodium calcium edetate [unlicensed], and dimercaprol. Dimercaprol in the management of heavy metal poisoning has been superseded by other chelating agents. In all cases of heavy metal poisoning, the advice of the National Poisons Information Service should be sought.

Noxious gases poisoning

Carbon monoxide

Carbon monoxide poisoning is usually due to inhalation of smoke, car exhaust, or fumes caused by blocked flues or incomplete combustion of fuel gases in confined spaces.

Immediate treatment of carbon monoxide poisoning is essential. The patient should be moved to fresh air, the airway cleared, and high-flow **oxygen** 100% administered as soon as available. Artificial respiration should be given as necessary and continued until adequate spontaneous breathing starts, or stopped only after persistent and efficient treatment of cardiac arrest has failed. The child should be admitted to hospital because complications may arise after a delay of hours or days. Cerebral oedema may occur in severe poisoning and is treated with an intravenous infusion of mannitol p. 164. Referral for hyperbaric oxygen treatment should be discussed with the National Poisons Information Service if the patient is pregnant or in cases of severe poisoning such as if the patient is or has been unconscious, or has psychiatric or neurological features other than a headache or has myocardial ischaemia or an arrhythmia, or has a blood carboxyhaemoglobin concentration of more than 20%.

Sulfur dioxide, chlorine, phosgene, and ammonia

All of these gases can cause upper respiratory tract and conjunctival irritation. Pulmonary oedema, with severe breathlessness and cyanosis may develop suddenly up to 36 hours after exposure. Death may occur. Patients are kept under observation and those who develop pulmonary oedema are given oxygen. Assisted ventilation may be necessary in the most serious cases.

CS spray poisoning

CS spray, which is used for riot control, irritates the eyes (hence 'tear gas') and the respiratory tract; symptoms normally settle spontaneously within 15 minutes. If symptoms persist, the patient should be removed to a well-ventilated area, and the exposed skin washed with soap and water after removal of contaminated clothing. Contact lenses should be removed and rigid ones washed (soft ones should be discarded). Eye symptoms should be treated by irrigating the eyes with physiological saline (or water if saline is not available) and advice sought from an ophthalmologist. Patients with features of severe poisoning, particularly respiratory complications, should be admitted to hospital for symptomatic treatment.

Pesticide poisoning

Organophosphorus insecticides

Organophosphorus insecticides are usually supplied as powders or dissolved in organic solvents. All are absorbed through the bronchi and intact skin as well as through the gut and inhibit cholinesterase activity, thereby prolonging and intensifying the effects of acetylcholine. Toxicity between different compounds varies considerably, and onset may be delayed after skin exposure.

Anxiety, restlessness, dizziness, headache, miosis, nausea, hypersalivation, vomiting, abdominal colic, diarrhoea, bradycardia, and sweating are common features of organophosphorus poisoning. Muscle weakness and fasciculation may develop and progress to generalised flaccid paralysis, including the ocular and respiratory muscles. Convulsions, coma, pulmonary oedema with copious bronchial secretions, hypoxia, and arrhythmias occur in severe cases. Hyperglycaemia and glycosuria without ketonuria may also be present.

Further absorption of the organophosphorus insecticide should be prevented by moving the child to fresh air, removing soiled clothing, and washing contaminated skin. In severe poisoning it is vital to ensure a clear airway, frequent removal of bronchial secretions, and adequate ventilation and oxygenation; gastric lavage may be considered provided that the airway is protected. Atropine sulfate p. 839 will reverse the muscarinic effects of acetylcholine and is given by intravenous injection until the skin becomes flushed and dry, the pupils dilate, and bradycardia is abolished.

Pralidoxime chloride p. 1045, a cholinesterase reactivator, is used as an adjunct to atropine sulfate p. 839 in moderate or severe poisoning. It improves muscle tone within 30 minutes of administration. Pralidoxime chloride is continued until the patient has not required atropine sulfate for 12 hours. Pralidoxime chloride can be obtained from designated centres, the names of which are held by the National Poisons Information Service.

Snake bites and animal stings

Snake bites

Envenoming from snake bite is uncommon in the UK. Many exotic snakes are kept, some illegally, but the only indigenous venomous snake is the adder (*Vipera berus*). The bite may cause local and systemic effects. Local effects include pain, swelling, bruising, and tender enlargement of regional lymph nodes. Systemic effects include early anaphylactic symptoms (transient hypotension with syncope, angioedema, urticaria, abdominal colic, diarrhoea, and vomiting), with later persistent or recurrent hypotension, ECG abnormalities, spontaneous systemic bleeding, coagulopathy, adult respiratory distress syndrome, and acute renal failure. Fatal envenoming is rare but the potential for severe envenoming must not be underestimated.

Early anaphylactic symptoms should be treated with intramuscular adrenaline p. 159, see Antihistamines, allergen immunotherapy and allergic emergencies p. 199 for further guidance on anaphylaxis management. Indications for european viper snake venom antiserum p. 1050 treatment include *systemic envenoming*, especially hypotension, ECG abnormalities, vomiting, haemostatic abnormalities, and marked local envenoming such that after bites on the hand or foot, swelling extends beyond the wrist or ankle within 4 hours of the bite. For those children who present with clinical features of *severe envenoming* (e.g. shock, ECG abnormalities, or local swelling that has advanced from the foot to above the knee or from the hand to above the elbow within 2 hours of the bite), a higher initial dose of the european viper snake venom antiserum is recommended; if symptoms of *systemic envenoming* persist contact the National Poisons Information Service. Adrenaline injection must be immediately to hand for treatment of anaphylactic reactions to the european viper snake venom antiserum.

Antivenom is available for bites by certain foreign snakes and spiders, stings by scorpions and fish. For information on identification, management, and for supply in an emergency, telephone the National Poisons Information Service. Whenever possible the TOXBASE entry should be read, and relevant information collected, before telephoning the National Poisons Information Service.

Insect stings

Stings from ants, wasps, hornets, and bees cause local pain and swelling but seldom cause severe direct toxicity unless many stings are inflicted at the same time. If the sting is in the mouth or on the tongue local swelling may threaten the upper airway. The stings from these insects are usually treated by cleaning the area with a topical antiseptic. Bee stings should be removed as quickly as possible.
Anaphylactic reactions require immediate treatment with intramuscular **adrenaline**; self-administered (or administered by a carer) intramuscular adrenaline is the best first-aid treatment for patients with severe hypersensitivity. An inhaled bronchodilator may also be considered for patients with persisting respiratory problems, see Antihistamines, allergen immunotherapy and allergic emergencies p. 199 for further guidance on anaphylaxis management. A short course of an **oral antihistamine** or a **topical corticosteroid** may help to reduce inflammation and relieve itching. A vaccine containing extracts of bee and wasp venom can be used to reduce the risk of anaphylaxis and systemic reactions in patients with systemic hypersensitivity to bee or wasp stings.

Marine stings

The severe pain of weeverfish (*Trachinus vipera*) and Portuguese man-o'-war stings can be relieved by immersing the stung area immediately in uncomfortably hot, but not scalding, water (not more than 45° C). People stung by jellyfish and Portuguese man-o'-war around the UK coast should be removed from the sea as soon as possible. Adherent tentacles should be lifted off carefully (wearing gloves or using tweezers) or washed off with seawater. Alcoholic solutions, including suntan lotions, should **not** be applied because they can cause further discharge of stinging hairs. Ice packs can be used to reduce pain.

Other poisons

Consult either the National Poisons Information Service day and night or TOXBASE.

The **National Poisons Information Service** (Tel: 0344 892 0111) will provide specialist advice on all aspects of poisoning day and night.

1 Active elimination from the gastro-intestinal tract

ANTIDOTES AND CHELATORS › INTESTINAL ADSORBENTS

Activated charcoal

16-Sep-2025

● **INDICATIONS AND DOSE**

Reduction of absorption of poisons in the gastro-intestinal system

▶ BY MOUTH

- Neonate: 1 g/kg.
- Child 1 month–11 years: 1 g/kg (max. per dose 50 g)
- Child 12–17 years: 50 g

Active elimination of poisons

▶ BY MOUTH

- Neonate: 1 g/kg every 4 hours, dose may be reduced and the frequency increased if not tolerated, reduced dose may compromise efficacy.
- Child 1 month–11 years: 1 g/kg every 4 hours (max. per dose 50 g), dose may be reduced and the frequency increased if not tolerated, reduced dose may compromise efficacy

continued →

- Child 12–17 years: Initially 50 g, then 50 g every 4 hours, reduced if not tolerated to 25 g every 2 hours, alternatively 12.5 g every 1 hour, reduced dose may compromise efficacy

- **CAUTIONS** Comatose patient (risk of aspiration—ensure airway is protected) · drowsy patient (risk of aspiration—ensure airway protected) · reduced gastrointestinal motility (risk of obstruction)
- **SIDE-EFFECTS** Bezoar · constipation · diarrhoea · gastrointestinal disorders
- **DIRECTIONS FOR ADMINISTRATION** TOXBASE advises suspension or reconstituted powder may be mixed with soft drinks (e.g. caffeine-free diet cola) or fruit juices to mask the taste.

- **MEDICINAL FORMS** There can be variation in the licensing of different medicines containing the same drug.

Oral suspension

- Charcodote (Teva UK Ltd)
  Activated charcoal 200 mg per 1 ml Charcodote 200mg/ml oral suspension | 250 ml P £14.25 DT = £14.25 SF

Granules for gastroenteral or oral suspension

- Carbomix (Kent Pharma (UK) Ltd)
  Activated charcoal 813 mg per 1 gram Carbomix 81.3% granules for oral suspension | 50 gram P £11.90 SF

2 Chemical toxicity

2.1 Cyanide toxicity

ANTIDOTES AND CHELATORS

Dicobalt edetate

07-Oct-2021

- **INDICATIONS AND DOSE**

Severe poisoning with cyanides

- BY INTRAVENOUS INJECTION
- Child: Consult the National Poisons Information Service

- **CAUTIONS** Owing to toxicity to be used only for definite cyanide poisoning when patient tending to lose, or has lost, consciousness
- **SIDE-EFFECTS** Reflex tachycardia · vomiting
- **EXCEPTIONS TO LEGAL CATEGORY** Prescription only medicine restriction does not apply where administration is for saving life in emergency.

- **MEDICINAL FORMS** No licensed medicines listed.

Sodium nitrite

26-Jul-2025

- **INDICATIONS AND DOSE**

Poisoning with cyanides (used in conjunction with sodium thiosulfate)

- BY INTRAVENOUS INJECTION
- Child: Consult the National Poisons Information Service

IMPORTANT SAFETY INFORMATION

NHS ENGLAND NATIONAL PATIENT SAFETY ALERT: RISK OF DEATH FROM UNINTENDED ADMINISTRATION OF SODIUM NITRITE (AUGUST 2020)

Cases of unintended administration of sodium nitrite have been reported, including 2 fatalities. Sodium nitrite can cause significant side-effects such as methaemoglobinaemia and nitric oxide-induced vasodilation.

Acute trusts are advised to check all clinical areas to ensure that sodium nitrite injection has not been inadvertently supplied, and to only retain stock in emergency departments. Unlicensed sodium nitrite ampoules in emergency departments should also be destroyed appropriately and replaced with licensed vials.

For information on the storage of 'specialist antidotes', see Poisoning, emergency treatment p. 1036.

- **SIDE-EFFECTS** Arrhythmias · dizziness · headache · hypotension · methaemoglobinaemia · palpitations
- **EXCEPTIONS TO LEGAL CATEGORY** Prescription only medicine restriction does not apply where administration is for saving life in emergency.

- **MEDICINAL FORMS** There can be variation in the licensing of different medicines containing the same drug.

Solution for injection

- Sodium nitrite (Non-proprietary)
  Sodium nitrite 30 mg per 1 ml Sodium nitrite 300mg/10ml solution for injection vials | 1 vial PoM (Hospital only)

Sodium thiosulfate

06-Jun-2025

- **INDICATIONS AND DOSE**

Poisoning with cyanides

- BY INTRAVENOUS INJECTION
- Child: Consult the National Poisons Information Service

DOSE EQUIVALENCE AND CONVERSION

- 12.5 g equates to 50 mL of a 25% solution.

PEDMARQSI®

Prevention of cisplatin-induced ototoxicity

- BY INTRAVENOUS INFUSION
- Child (body-weight up to 5 kg): 6.4 g/m², for details regarding timing of administration relative to cisplatin, and premedication requirements—consult product literature
- Child (body-weight 5–10 kg): 9.6 g/m², for details regarding timing of administration relative to cisplatin, and premedication requirements—consult product literature
- Child (body-weight 11 kg and above): 12.8 g/m², for details regarding timing of administration relative to cisplatin, and premedication requirements—consult product literature

- **CONTRA-INDICATIONS**
  PEDMARQSI® Baseline serum-sodium concentration greater than 145 mmol/litre (high drug sodium content)
- **SIDE-EFFECTS**
  - **Common or very common** Electrolyte imbalance · hypersensitivity · hypertension · hypotension · metabolic acidosis · nausea · vomiting
  - **Frequency not known** Disorientation · feeling hot · headache · taste salty
- **ALLERGY AND CROSS-SENSITIVITY**
  PEDMARQSI® EvGr Caution in sulfite sensitivity (may contain traces of sodium sulfite). M
- **RENAL IMPAIRMENT**
  PEDMARQSI® EvGr Caution if estimated glomerular filtration rate falls below 60 mL/minute/1.73m². M See p. 16.
- **MONITORING REQUIREMENTS**
  - When used for Prevention of cisplatin-induced ototoxicity EvGr Monitor serum sodium, magnesium, phosphate, and potassium concentrations. Monitor blood pressure. M

● **DIRECTIONS FOR ADMINISTRATION**
PEDMARQSI® EvGr For *intravenous infusion*, give over 15 minutes via a central venous catheter. (M)

● **NATIONAL FUNDING/ACCESS DECISIONS**
For full details see funding body website

NICE decisions

▶ **Anhydrous sodium thiosulfate for preventing hearing loss caused by cisplatin chemotherapy in people 1 month to 17 years with localised solid tumours (January 2025)**
NICE TA1034 Recommended

Scottish Medicines Consortium (SMC) decisions

▶ **Sodium thiosulfate (*Pedmarqsi*®) for the prevention of ototoxicity caused by cisplatin chemotherapy in patients 1 month to less than 18 years of age with localised, non-metastatic, solid tumours (May 2025)** SMC No. SMC2730 Recommended

● **EXCEPTIONS TO LEGAL CATEGORY** Prescription only medicine restriction does not apply where administration is for saving life in emergency.

● **MEDICINAL FORMS** There can be variation in the licensing of different medicines containing the same drug.

Solution for injection

▸ **Sodium thiosulfate (Non-proprietary)**
Sodium thiosulfate 250 mg per 1 ml Sodium thiosulfate 12.5g/50ml solution for injection vials | 1 vial PoM (Hospital only)

Solution for infusion

ELECTROLYTES: May contain Sodium

▸ **Pedmarqsi** (Norgine Pharmaceuticals Ltd)
Sodium thiosulfate 80 mg per 1 ml Pedmarqsi 8g/100ml solution for infusion vials | 1 vial PoM £8,277.71 (Hospital only)

2.2 Organophosphorus toxicity

Other drugs used for Organophosphorus toxicity Atropine sulfate, p. 839

ANTIDOTES AND CHELATORS

Pralidoxime chloride

31-Jan-2022

● **INDICATIONS AND DOSE**

Adjunct to atropine in the treatment of poisoning by organophosphorus insecticide or nerve agent

▶ BY INTRAVENOUS INFUSION

- Child: Initially 30 mg/kg, to be given over 20 minutes, followed by 8 mg/kg/hour; maximum 12 g per day

● **UNLICENSED USE** Pralidoxime chloride doses may differ from those in product literature.
Licensed for use in children (age range not specified by manufacturer).

● **CONTRA-INDICATIONS** Poisoning with carbamates · poisoning with organophosphorus compounds without anticholinesterase activity

● **CAUTIONS** Myasthenia gravis

● **SIDE-EFFECTS** Dizziness · drowsiness · headache · hyperventilation · muscle weakness · nausea · tachycardia · vision disorders

● **RENAL IMPAIRMENT** EvGr Use with caution. (M)

● **DIRECTIONS FOR ADMINISTRATION** Manufacturer advises the loading dose may be administered by intravenous injection (diluted to a concentration of 50 mg/mL with water for injections) over at least 5 minutes if pulmonary oedema is present or if it is not practical to administer an intravenous infusion.
For *intravenous infusion*, manufacturer advises reconstitute each vial with 20 mL Water for Injections, then dilute to a concentration of 10–20 mg/mL with Sodium Chloride 0.9%.

● **PRESCRIBING AND DISPENSING INFORMATION** Available from designated centres for organophosphorus insecticide poisoning—see TOXBASE for list of holding centres.

● **EXCEPTIONS TO LEGAL CATEGORY** Prescription only medicine restriction does not apply where administration is for saving life in emergency.

● **MEDICINAL FORMS** There can be variation in the licensing of different medicines containing the same drug.

Powder for solution for injection

▸ **Pralidoxime chloride (Non-proprietary)**
Pralidoxime chloride 1 gram Protopam Chloride 1g powder for solution for injection vials | 6 vial PoM (Hospital only)

3 Drug toxicity

3.1 Benzodiazepine toxicity

ANTIDOTES AND CHELATORS › BENZODIAZEPINE ANTAGONISTS

Flumazenil

24-Jul-2020

● **INDICATIONS AND DOSE**

Reversal of sedative effects of benzodiazepines

▶ BY INTRAVENOUS INJECTION

▸ Neonate: 10 micrograms/kg every 1 minute if required, dose to be administered over 15 seconds.

▸ Child: 10 micrograms/kg every 1 minute (max. per dose 200 micrograms) if required, dose to be administered over 15 seconds; maximum 1 mg per course; maximum 50 micrograms/kg per course

Reversal of sedative effects of benzodiazepines (if drowsiness recurs after injection)

▶ BY INTRAVENOUS INFUSION

▸ Neonate: 2–10 micrograms/kg/hour, adjusted according to response.

▸ Child: 2–10 micrograms/kg/hour (max. per dose 400 micrograms/hour), adjusted according to response

Reversal of sedative effects of benzodiazepines in intensive care

▶ BY INTRAVENOUS INJECTION

▸ Child: 10 micrograms/kg every 1 minute (max. per dose 200 micrograms) if required, dose to be administered over 15 seconds; maximum 2 mg per course; maximum 50 micrograms/kg per course

● **UNLICENSED USE** Not licensed for use in children under 1 year. Not licensed for use by intravenous infusion in children. Not licensed for use in children in intensive care.

IMPORTANT SAFETY INFORMATION
Flumazenil should only be administered by, or under the direct supervision of, personnel experienced in its use.

● **CONTRA-INDICATIONS** Life-threatening condition (e.g. raised intracranial pressure, status epilepticus) controlled by benzodiazepines

● **CAUTIONS** Avoid rapid injection following major surgery · avoid rapid injection in high-risk or anxious patients · benzodiazepine dependence (may precipitate withdrawal symptoms) · children · ensure neuromuscular blockade cleared before giving · head injury (rapid reversal of benzodiazepine sedation may cause convulsions) · history of panic disorders (risk of recurrence) · prolonged benzodiazepine therapy for epilepsy (risk of convulsions) ·

short-acting (repeat doses may be necessary—benzodiazepine effects may persist for at least 24 hours)

- **SIDE-EFFECTS**
  - **Common or very common** Anxiety · diplopia · dry mouth · eye disorders · flushing · headache · hiccups · hyperhidrosis · hyperventilation · hypotension · insomnia · nausea · palpitations · paraesthesia · speech disorder · tremor · vertigo · vomiting
  - **Uncommon** Abnormal hearing · arrhythmias · chest pain · chills · cough · dyspnoea · nasal congestion · seizure (more common in patients with epilepsy)
  - **Frequency not known** Withdrawal syndrome
- **PREGNANCY** Not known to be harmful.
- **BREAST FEEDING** Avoid breast-feeding for 24 hours.
- **HEPATIC IMPAIRMENT** Manufacturer advises caution (risk of increased half-life).

  Dose adjustments Manufacturer advises cautious dose titration.
- **DIRECTIONS FOR ADMINISTRATION** For *continuous intravenous infusion*, manufacturer advises dilute with Glucose 5% or Sodium Chloride 0.9%.

- **MEDICINAL FORMS** There can be variation in the licensing of different medicines containing the same drug.

Solution for injection

- **Flumazenil (Non-proprietary)**

  Flumazenil 100 microgram per 1 ml Flumazenil 500micrograms/5ml solution for injection ampoules | 5 ampoule PoM £72.46 (Hospital only) | 10 ampoule PoM £150.00 | 10 ampoule PoM £150.00 (Hospital only)

3.2 Digoxin toxicity

ANTIDOTES AND CHELATORS > ANTIBODIES

Digoxin-specific antibody fragments

16-Sep-2025

- **INDICATIONS AND DOSE**

Treatment of known or strongly suspected life-threatening digoxin toxicity associated with ventricular arrhythmias or bradyarrhythmias unresponsive to atropine and when measures beyond the withdrawal of digoxin and correction of any electrolyte abnormalities are considered necessary

- BY INTRAVENOUS INFUSION
  - Child: Serious cases of digoxin toxicity should be discussed with the National Poisons Information Service (consult product literature)

- **MEDICINAL FORMS** There can be variation in the licensing of different medicines containing the same drug.

Powder for solution for infusion

- **DigiFab** (Protherics Medicines Development Ltd)

  Digoxin-specific antibody fragments 40 mg DigiFab 40mg powder for solution for infusion vials | 1 vial PoM £750.00 (Hospital only)

3.3 Heparin toxicity

ANTIDOTES AND CHELATORS

Protamine sulfate

02-Dec-2020

- **INDICATIONS AND DOSE**

Overdosage with intravenous injection or intravenous infusion of heparin (less than 30 minutes lapsed since overdose)

- BY INTRAVENOUS INJECTION
  - Child: 1 mg (max. per dose 50 mg), to be administered at a rate not exceeding 5 mg/minute, to neutralise each 100 units of heparin

Overdosage with intravenous injection or intravenous infusion of heparin (if 30–60 minutes lapsed since overdose)

- BY INTRAVENOUS INJECTION
  - Child: 500–750 micrograms (max. per dose 50 mg), to be administered at a rate not exceeding 5 mg/minute, to neutralise each 100 units of heparin

Overdosage with intravenous injection or intravenous infusion of heparin (if 60–120 minutes lapsed since overdose)

- BY INTRAVENOUS INJECTION
  - Child: 375–500 micrograms (max. per dose 50 mg), to be administered at a rate not exceeding 5 mg/minute, to neutralise each 100 units of heparin

Overdosage with intravenous injection or intravenous infusion of heparin (if over 120 minutes lapsed since overdose)

- BY INTRAVENOUS INJECTION
  - Child: 250–375 micrograms (max. per dose 50 mg), to be administered at a rate not exceeding 5 mg/minute, to neutralise each 100 units of heparin

Overdosage with subcutaneous injection of heparin

- BY INTRAVENOUS INJECTION, OR BY INTRAVENOUS INFUSION
  - Child: (max. per dose 50 mg), 50–100% of the total dose to be given by intravenous injection (rate not exceeding 5 mg/minute), then give any remainder of dose by intravenous infusion over 8–16 hours, 1 mg neutralises approx. 100 units of heparin

Overdosage with subcutaneous injection of low molecular weight heparin

- BY INTRAVENOUS INJECTION, OR BY CONTINUOUS INTRAVENOUS INFUSION
  - Child: (max. per dose 50 mg), to be administered by intermittent intravenous injection at a rate not exceeding 5 mg/minute or by continuous intravenous infusion, 1 mg neutralises approx. 100 units of low molecular weight heparin, consult product literature of low molecular weight heparin for details

- **CAUTIONS** Excessive doses can have an anticoagulant effect
- **SIDE-EFFECTS**
  - **Rare or very rare** Pulmonary oedema non-cardiogenic
  - **Frequency not known** Acute pulmonary vasoconstriction · back pain · bradycardia · circulatory collapse · dyspnoea · fatigue · feeling hot · flushing · hypertension · hypotension · nausea · pulmonary hypertension · vomiting
- **ALLERGY AND CROSS-SENSITIVITY** EvGr Caution if increased risk of allergic reaction to protamine (includes previous treatment with protamine or protamine insulin, allergy to fish, men who are infertile or who have had a vasectomy and who may have antibodies to protamine). M
- **MONITORING REQUIREMENTS** Monitor activated partial thromboplastin time or other appropriate blood clotting parameters.

● **DIRECTIONS FOR ADMINISTRATION** Manufacturer advises may be diluted if necessary with Sodium Chloride 0.9%.

● **PRESCRIBING AND DISPENSING INFORMATION** The long half-life of low molecular weight heparins should be taken into consideration when determining the dose of protamine sulfate; the effects of low molecular weight heparins can persist for up to 24 hours after administration.

● **MEDICINAL FORMS** There can be variation in the licensing of different medicines containing the same drug.

Solution for injection

▸ Protamine sulfate (Non-proprietary)

Protamine sulfate 10 mg per 1 ml Protamine sulfate 50mg/5ml solution for injection ampoules | 10 ampoule PoM £66.89

3.4 Opioid toxicity

OPIOID RECEPTOR ANTAGONISTS

Naloxone hydrochloride

03-Aug-2023

● **INDICATIONS AND DOSE**

Acute opioid overdose–high-dose regimen [when rapid titration with naloxone is necessary to reverse potentially life-threatening effects]

▶ BY INTRAVENOUS INJECTION

▸ Neonate: Initially 100 micrograms/kg, if no response, repeat at intervals of 1 minute to a total max. of 2 mg, then review diagnosis; further doses may be required if respiratory function deteriorates following initial response, intravenous administration has more rapid onset of action, doses may be given by intramuscular route but only if intravenous route is not feasible.

▸ Child 1 month–11 years: Initially 100 micrograms/kg (max. per dose 2 mg), if no response, repeat at intervals of 1 minute to a total max. of 2 mg, then review diagnosis; further doses may be required if respiratory function deteriorates following initial response, intravenous administration has more rapid onset of action, doses may be given by intramuscular route but only if intravenous route is not feasible

▸ Child 12–17 years: Initially 400 micrograms for 1 dose, then 800 micrograms for up to 2 doses at 1 minute intervals if no response to preceding dose, then increased to 2 mg for 1 dose if still no response (4 mg dose may be required in seriously poisoned patients), then review diagnosis; further doses may be required if respiratory function deteriorates following initial response, intravenous administration has more rapid onset of action, doses may be given by intramuscular route but only if intravenous route is not feasible

▶ BY CONTINUOUS INTRAVENOUS INFUSION

▸ Neonate: Using an infusion pump, adjust rate according to response, initially, rate may be set at 60% of the initial resuscitative intravenous injection dose per hour. The initial resuscitative *intravenous injection* dose is that which maintained satisfactory respiratory effort for at least 15 minutes.

▸ Child: Using an infusion pump, adjust rate according to response, initially, rate may be set at 60% of the initial resuscitative intravenous injection dose per hour. The initial resuscitative *intravenous injection* dose is that which maintained satisfactory respiratory effort for at least 15 minutes

Opioid overdose–low-dose regimen [when there is risk of acute withdrawal, or when a continued therapeutic effect is required (e.g. postoperative use, palliative care)]

▶ BY INTRAVENOUS INJECTION

▸ Neonate: Initially 1–10 micrograms/kg, if no response, repeat at intervals of 1 minute up to 5 times, if no response then give a single dose of 100 micrograms/kg then review diagnosis if still no response, further doses may be required if respiratory function deteriorates following initial response, intravenous administration has a more rapid onset of action, doses may be given by intramuscular route but only if intravenous route is not feasible.

▸ Child 1 month–11 years: Initially 1–10 micrograms/kg (max. per dose 200 micrograms), if no response, repeat at intervals of 1 minute up to 5 times, if no response then give a single dose of 100 micrograms/kg (max. dose 2 mg) then review diagnosis if still no response, further doses may be required if respiratory function deteriorates following initial response, intravenous administration has a more rapid onset of action, doses may be given by intramuscular route but only if intravenous route is not feasible

▸ Child 12–17 years: Initially 100–200 micrograms for 1 dose, then 100 micrograms for up to 2 doses at 1 minute intervals if no response to preceding dose, continue titrating up to a max. of 2 mg until adequate response achieved. If still no response, give a further 2 mg dose (4 mg dose may be required in seriously poisoned patients), then review diagnosis; further doses may be required if respiratory function deteriorates following initial response, intravenous administration has a more rapid onset of action, doses may be given by intramuscular route but only if intravenous route is not feasible

Opioid overdose in non-medical and medical settings

▶ BY INTRANASAL ADMINISTRATION

▸ Child 14–17 years: 1.8 mg, administered into one nostril, if no response, give a second dose after 2–3 minutes. If the patient responds to the first dose then relapses into respiratory depression, give the second dose immediately. Further doses should be administered into alternate nostrils

Reversal of respiratory and CNS depression resulting from opioid administration to mother during labour

▶ BY INTRAMUSCULAR INJECTION

▸ Neonate: 200 micrograms for 1 dose, to be given at birth, alternatively 60 micrograms/kg for 1 dose, to be given at birth.

▶ BY INTRAVENOUS INJECTION, OR BY SUBCUTANEOUS INJECTION

▸ Neonate: 10 micrograms/kg, repeated every 2–3 minutes if required, further doses may be required if respiratory function deteriorates following initial response, intravenous administration has a more rapid onset of action.

DOSE EQUIVALENCE AND CONVERSION

▸ With intranasal use

▸ For *Nyxoid*® nasal spray, 1 spray is equivalent to naloxone 1.8 mg. For *naloxone* 1.26 *mg nasal spray*, 1 spray is equivalent to naloxone 1.26 mg.

PHARMACOKINETICS

▸ Naloxone has a short duration of action; repeated doses or infusion may be necessary to reverse effects of opioids with longer duration of action.

- **UNLICENSED USE** TOXBASE advises naloxone is used in both high- and low-dose regimens for the management of opioid overdose, but these may differ from those licensed.

IMPORTANT SAFETY INFORMATION

SAFE PRACTICE

Doses used in acute opioid overdose may not be appropriate when there is risk of acute withdrawal (e.g. chronic opioid use), or when a continued therapeutic effect is required (e.g. postoperative use, palliative care).

- **CAUTIONS** Cardiovascular disease or those receiving cardiotoxic drugs (serious adverse cardiovascular effects reported) · chronic opioid use (risk of acute withdrawal) · maternal chronic opioid use (risk of acute withdrawal in newborn) · palliative care (risk of returning pain and acute withdrawal) · postoperative use (risk of returning pain)

CAUTIONS, FURTHER INFORMATION

- Titration of dose [EvGr] In postoperative use, the dose should be titrated for each patient in order to obtain sufficient respiratory response; however, naloxone antagonises analgesia. ⟨M⟩

- **SIDE-EFFECTS**

GENERAL SIDE-EFFECTS

- **Common or very common** Arrhythmias · dizziness · headache · hypertension · hypotension · nausea · vomiting
- **Uncommon** Diarrhoea · dry mouth · hyperhidrosis · hyperventilation · tremor
- **Rare or very rare** Cardiac arrest · erythema multiforme · pulmonary oedema

SPECIFIC SIDE-EFFECTS

- **Uncommon**
- With parenteral use Inflammation localised · pain · vascular irritation
- **Rare or very rare**
- With parenteral use Anxiety · seizure
- **Frequency not known**
- With parenteral use Analgesia reversed · asthenia · chills · death · dyspnoea · fever · irritability · nasal complaints · piloerection · yawning

- **PREGNANCY** Use only if potential benefit outweighs risk.
- **BREAST FEEDING** Not orally bioavailable.
- **MONITORING REQUIREMENTS** Specialist sources indicate that blood gases, oxygen saturation and respiratory rate should be monitored once breathing is restored. Patients should be monitored for recurrence of signs and symptoms of opioid toxicity, such as relapse in respiratory or CNS symptoms.
- **DIRECTIONS FOR ADMINISTRATION** For *continuous intravenous infusion*, dilute to a concentration of up to 200 micrograms/mL with Glucose 5% or Sodium Chloride 0.9%.
- **PRESCRIBING AND DISPENSING INFORMATION**
  - With intranasal use The manufacturer has provided a *Healthcare Professional Guidance Document*.
- **PATIENT AND CARER ADVICE**
  - With intranasal use Patients and carers should be given advice on how to administer naloxone nasal spray. Patient training and information cards should be provided.

- **MEDICINAL FORMS** There can be variation in the licensing of different medicines containing the same drug.

Solution for injection

- **Naloxone hydrochloride (Non-proprietary)**
  Naloxone hydrochloride (as Naloxone hydrochloride dihydrate) 400 microgram per 1 ml Naloxone 400micrograms/1ml solution for injection ampoules | 10 ampoule [PoM] £41.00–£49.00 | 10 ampoule [PoM] £45.00 (Hospital only)
  Naloxone hydrochloride 1 mg per 1 ml Naloxone 2mg/2ml solution for injection pre-filled syringes | 1 pre-filled disposable injection [PoM] £18.00 DT = £18.00
- **Prenoxad** (Martindale Pharmaceuticals Ltd)
  Naloxone hydrochloride 1 mg per 1 ml Prenoxad 2mg/2ml solution for injection pre-filled syringes | 1 pre-filled disposable injection [PoM] £18.00 DT = £18.00

Spray

- **Naloxone hydrochloride (Non-proprietary)**
  Naloxone (as Naloxone hydrochloride dihydrate) 12.6 mg per 1 ml Naloxone 1.26mg/0.1ml nasal spray unit dose | 2 unit dose [PoM] £25.00 DT = £25.00
- **Nyxoid** (Napp Pharmaceuticals Ltd)
  Naloxone (as Naloxone hydrochloride dihydrate) 18 mg per 1 ml Nyxoid 1.8mg/0.1ml nasal spray 0.1ml unit dose | 2 unit dose [PoM] £27.50 DT = £27.50

3.5 Paracetamol toxicity

ANTIDOTES AND CHELATORS

Acetylcysteine

01-Aug-2024

- **INDICATIONS AND DOSE**

Paracetamol overdose [12-hour SNAP regimen]

▶ BY INTRAVENOUS INFUSION

- Neonate: 100 mg/kg over 2 hours, dose to be administered as a 50 mg/mL solution in glucose 5% or sodium chloride 0.9%, then 200 mg/kg over 10 hours, dose to be administered as a 10 mg/mL solution in glucose 5% or sodium chloride 0.9%, and started immediately after completion of first infusion.
- Child (body-weight up to 40 kg): 100 mg/kg over 2 hours, dose to be administered as a 50 mg/mL solution in glucose 5% or sodium chloride 0.9%, then 200 mg/kg over 10 hours, dose to be administered as a 10 mg/mL solution in glucose 5% or sodium chloride 0.9%, and started immediately after completion of first infusion
- Child (body-weight 40 kg and above): 100 mg/kg over 2 hours, dose to be administered in 200 mL glucose 5% or sodium chloride 0.9%, then 200 mg/kg over 10 hours, dose to be administered in 1 litre glucose 5% or sodium chloride 0.9%, and started immediately after completion of first infusion

Paracetamol overdose [21-hour regimen]

▶ BY INTRAVENOUS INFUSION

- Neonate: 150 mg/kg over 1 hour, dose to be administered as a 50 mg/mL solution in glucose 5% or sodium chloride 0.9%, then 50 mg/kg over 4 hours, dose to be administered as a 6.25 mg/mL solution in glucose 5% or sodium chloride 0.9%, and started immediately after completion of first infusion, then 100 mg/kg over 16 hours, dose to be administered as a 6.25 mg/mL solution in glucose 5% or sodium chloride 0.9%, and started immediately after completion of second infusion.
- Child (body-weight up to 40 kg): 150 mg/kg over 1 hour, dose to be administered as a 50 mg/mL solution in glucose 5% or sodium chloride 0.9%, then 50 mg/kg over 4 hours, dose to be administered as a 6.25 mg/mL solution in glucose 5% or sodium chloride 0.9%, and started immediately after completion of first infusion, then 100 mg/kg over 16 hours, dose to be administered as a 6.25 mg/mL solution in glucose 5% or sodium chloride 0.9%, and started immediately after completion of second infusion
- Child (body-weight 40 kg and above): 150 mg/kg over 1 hour, dose to be administered in 200 mL glucose 5% or sodium chloride 0.9%, then 50 mg/kg over 4 hours, dose to be administered in 500 mL glucose 5% or sodium chloride 0.9%, and started immediately after completion of first infusion, then 100 mg/kg over

16 hours, dose to be administered in 1 litre glucose 5% or sodium chloride 0.9%, and started immediately after completion of second infusion

Meconium ileus

▸ BY MOUTH

- Neonate: 200–400 mg up to 3 times a day if required.

Treatment of distal intestinal obstructive syndrome

▸ BY MOUTH

- Child 1 month–1 year: 0.4–3 g as a single dose
- Child 2–6 years: 2–3 g as a single dose
- Child 7–17 years: 4–6 g as a single dose

Prevention of distal intestinal obstruction syndrome

▸ BY MOUTH

- Child 1 month–1 year: 100–200 mg 3 times a day
- Child 2–11 years: 200 mg 3 times a day
- Child 12–17 years: 200–400 mg 3 times a day

DOSES AT EXTREMES OF BODY-WEIGHT

- To avoid excessive dosage in obese patients, a ceiling weight of 110 kg should be used when calculating the dose for paracetamol overdosage.

● **UNLICENSED USE** Not licensed for use in meconium ileus or for distal intestinal obstructive syndrome in children with cystic fibrosis. TOXBASE advises acetylcysteine is used in the 12-hour SNAP regimen for paracetamol overdose, although it is considered unlicensed.

IMPORTANT SAFETY INFORMATION

PARACETAMOL OVERDOSE

There are two intravenous regimens for paracetamol overdose: the standard 21-hour regimen and the modified 12-hour regimen (also known as the Scottish and Newcastle Acetylcysteine Protocol (SNAP)).

The SNAP regimen is not endorsed by the MHRA but is recommended by the Royal College of Emergency Medicine and the National Poisons Information Service. Continued treatment after the second infusion may be necessary depending on the clinical evaluation of the individual patient—for further information, see TOXBASE.

MHRA/CHM ADVICE: INTRAVENOUS ACETYLCYSTEINE FOR PARACETAMOL OVERDOSE: REMINDER OF AUTHORISED DOSE REGIMEN; POSSIBLE NEED FOR CONTINUED TREATMENT (JANUARY 2017)

The authorised dose regimen for acetylcysteine in paracetamol overdose is 3 consecutive intravenous infusions given over a total of 21 hours.

Continued treatment (given at the dose and rate as used in the third infusion) may be necessary depending on the clinical evaluation of the individual patient.

● **CAUTIONS**

- With intravenous use Asthma · atopy · may slightly increase INR · may slightly increase prothrombin time
- With oral use Asthma · history of peptic ulceration

● **INTERACTIONS** → Appendix 1: acetylcysteine

● **SIDE-EFFECTS**

- With parenteral use Acidosis · anaphylactoid reaction · angioedema · anxiety · arrhythmias · cardiac arrest · chest discomfort · cough · cyanosis · eye pain · eye swelling · generalised seizure · hyperhidrosis · hypertension · hypotension · joint disorders · malaise · nausea · pain facial · respiratory disorders · skin reactions · syncope · thrombocytopenia · vasodilation · vision blurred · vomiting

SIDE-EFFECTS, FURTHER INFORMATION Anaphylactoid reactions (with intravenous use) can be managed by suspending treatment and initiating appropriate management. Treatment may then be restarted at lower rate.

● **PREGNANCY**

Dose adjustments TOXBASE advises that the toxic dose of *paracetamol* ingested should be calculated using the patient's pre-pregnancy body-weight and the *acetylcysteine* dose (for both regimens) should be calculated using the patient's actual pregnant body-weight.

● **DIRECTIONS FOR ADMINISTRATION** For administration *by mouth*, expert sources advise use oral granules, *or* dilute injection solution (200 mg/mL) to a concentration of 50 mg/mL; orange or blackcurrant juice or cola drink may be used as a diluent to mask the bitter taste.

EvGr For *intravenous infusion*, Glucose 5% is the preferred infusion fluid; if unsuitable then Sodium Chloride 0.9% can be used as an alternative. (M) For further information on administration, see TOXBASE.

● **MEDICINAL FORMS** There can be variation in the licensing of different medicines containing the same drug. Forms available from special-order manufacturers include: granules for oral solution, solution for infusion

Solution for infusion

ELECTROLYTES: May contain Sodium

▸ **Acetylcysteine (Non-proprietary)**

Acetylcysteine 200 mg per 1 ml Acetylcysteine 6g/30ml solution for infusion vials | 4 vial PoM ✗ (Hospital only)

Acetadote 6g/30ml solution for infusion vials | 4 vial PoM ✗ (Hospital only)

Acetylcysteine 2g/10ml solution for infusion ampoules | 10 ampoule PoM £21.26–£36.14 DT = £21.26

▸ **Parvolex** (Phoenix Labs Ltd)

Acetylcysteine 200 mg per 1 ml Parvolex 2g/10ml concentrate for solution for infusion ampoules | 10 ampoule PoM £22.50 DT = £21.26

Granules for oral solution

CAUTIONARY AND ADVISORY LABELS 13

▸ **Acetylcysteine (Non-proprietary)**

Acetylcysteine 100 mg Fluimucil N 100mg granules sachets | 20 sachet PoM ✗

Acetylcysteine 200 mg Fluimucil N 200mg granules sachets | 20 sachet PoM ✗

4 Methaemoglobinaemia

ANTIDOTES AND CHELATORS

Methylthioninium chloride

11-Feb-2022

(Methylene blue)

● **INDICATIONS AND DOSE**

Drug- or chemical-induced methaemoglobinaemia

▸ BY SLOW INTRAVENOUS INJECTION

- Neonate: Seek advice from National Poisons Information Service.
- Child 1–2 months: Seek advice from National Poisons Information Service
- Child 3 months–17 years: Initially 1–2 mg/kg, then 1–2 mg/kg after 30–60 minutes if required, to be given over 5 minutes, seek advice from National Poisons Information Service if further repeat doses are required; maximum 7 mg/kg per course

Aniline- or dapsone-induced methaemoglobinaemia

▸ BY SLOW INTRAVENOUS INJECTION

- Child 3 months–17 years: Initially 1–2 mg/kg, then 1–2 mg/kg after 30–60 minutes if required, to be given over 5 minutes, seek advice from National Poisons Information Service if further repeat doses are required; maximum 4 mg/kg per course

- **CAUTIONS** Children under 3 months (more susceptible to methaemoglobinaemia from high doses of methylthioninium) · chlorate poisoning (reduces efficacy of methylthioninium) · G6PD deficiency (seek advice from National Poisons Information Service) · methaemoglobinaemia due to treatment of cyanide poisoning with sodium nitrite (seek advice from National Poisons Information Service) · pulse oximetry may give false estimation of oxygen saturation
- **INTERACTIONS** → Appendix 1: methylthioninium chloride
- **SIDE-EFFECTS**
  - **Common or very common** Abdominal pain · anxiety · chest pain · dizziness · headache · hyperhidrosis · nausea · pain in extremity · paraesthesia · skin reactions · taste altered · urine discolouration · vomiting
  - **Frequency not known** Aphasia · arrhythmias · confusion · faeces discoloured · fever · haemolytic anaemia · hyperbilirubinaemia (in infants) · hypertension · hypotension · injection site necrosis · mydriasis · tremor
- **PREGNANCY** No information available, but risk to fetus of untreated methaemoglobinaemia likely to be significantly higher than risk of treatment.
- **BREAST FEEDING** Manufacturer advises avoid breastfeeding for up to 6 days after administration—no information available.
- **RENAL IMPAIRMENT** National Poisons Information Service advises caution in severe impairment.
  Dose adjustments Manufacturer advises lower doses may be required (consult product literature).
- **DIRECTIONS FOR ADMINISTRATION** For *intravenous injection*, manufacturer advises may be diluted with Glucose 5% to minimise injection-site pain; not compatible with Sodium Chloride 0.9%.

- **MEDICINAL FORMS** There can be variation in the licensing of different medicines containing the same drug. Forms available from special-order manufacturers include: solution for injection

Solution for injection

- **Methylthioninium chloride (Non-proprietary)**
  Methylthioninium chloride 5 mg per 1 ml Methylthioninium chloride Proveblue 50mg/10ml solution for injection ampoules | 5 ampoule PoM £196.89 (Hospital only)
  Methylthioninium chloride 10 mg per 1 ml Methylthioninium chloride (methylene blue) 50mg/5ml concentrate for solution for injection vials | 5 vial PoM £170.00 (Hospital only)

5 Snake bites

IMMUNE SERA AND IMMUNOGLOBULINS › ANTITOXINS

European viper snake venom antiserum

05-Feb-2021

- **INDICATIONS AND DOSE**

VIPERATAB®

Envenoming from *Vipera berus* bites (under expert supervision)

- BY INTRAVENOUS INFUSION
  - Child: Initially 8 mL for 1 dose, then 8 mL if required, the second and subsequent doses should only be given if signs and symptoms of envenomation persist or recur, if signs and symptoms of envenoming progress or persist contact the National Poisons Information Service

- **DIRECTIONS FOR ADMINISTRATION**
  VIPERATAB® EvGr For *intravenous infusion*, dilute with 100 mL of Sodium Chloride 0.9%; give over 30 minutes. (M)
- **PRESCRIBING AND DISPENSING INFORMATION** To order, email immform@dh.gsi.gov.uk.

- **MEDICINAL FORMS** There can be variation in the licensing of different medicines containing the same drug. Forms available from special-order manufacturers include: solution for infusion.

Emergency treatment of poisoning 16

Appendix 1
Interactions

Two or more drugs given at the same time can exert their effects independently or they can interact. Interactions may be beneficial and exploited therapeutically; this type of interaction is not within the scope of this appendix. Many interactions are harmless, and even those that are potentially harmful can often be managed, allowing the drugs to be used safely together. Nevertheless, adverse drug interactions should be reported to the Medicines and Healthcare products Regulatory Agency (MHRA), through the Yellow Card Scheme (see Adverse reactions to drugs p. 11), as for other adverse drug reactions.

Potentially harmful drug interactions may occur in only a small number of patients, but the true incidence is often hard to establish. Furthermore the severity of a harmful interaction is likely to vary from one patient to another. Patients at increased risk from drug interactions include the elderly and those with impaired renal or hepatic function.

Interactions can result in the potentiation or antagonism of one drug by another, or result in another effect, such as renal impairment. Drug interactions may develop either through pharmacokinetic or pharmacodynamic mechanisms.

Pharmacodynamic interactions

These are interactions between drugs which have similar or antagonistic pharmacological effects or side-effects. They might be due to competition at receptor sites, or occur between drugs acting on the same physiological system. They are usually predictable from a knowledge of the pharmacology of the interacting drugs; in general, those demonstrated with one drug are likely to occur with related drugs.

Pharmacokinetic interactions

These occur when one drug alters the absorption, distribution, metabolism, or excretion of another, thus increasing or decreasing the amount of drug available to produce its pharmacological effects. Pharmacokinetic interactions occurring with one drug do not necessarily occur uniformly across a group of related drugs.

Affecting absorption The rate of absorption and the total amount absorbed can both be altered by drug interactions. Delayed absorption is rarely of clinical importance unless a rapid effect is required (e.g. when giving an analgesic). Reduction in the total amount absorbed, however, can result in ineffective therapy.

Affecting distribution *Due to changes in protein binding*: To a variable extent most drugs are loosely bound to plasma proteins. Protein-binding sites are non-specific and one drug can displace another thereby increasing the proportion free to diffuse from plasma to its site of action. This only produces a detectable increase in effect if it is an extensively bound drug (more than 90%) that is not widely distributed throughout the body. Even so displacement rarely produces more than transient potentiation because this increased concentration of free drug will usually be eliminated.

Displacement from protein binding plays a part in the potentiation of warfarin by sulfonamides but these interactions become clinically relevant mainly because warfarin metabolism is also inhibited.

Induction or inhibition of drug transporter proteins: Drug transporter proteins, such as P-glycoprotein, actively transport drugs across biological membranes. Transporters can be induced or inhibited, resulting in changes in the concentrations of drugs that are substrates for the transporter. For example, rifampicin induces P-glycoprotein, particularly in the gut wall, resulting in decreased plasma concentrations of digoxin, a P-glycoprotein substrate.

Affecting metabolism Many drugs are metabolised in the liver. Drugs are either metabolised by phase I reactions (oxidation, reduction, or hydrolysis) or by phase II reactions (e.g. glucoronidation).

Phase I reactions are mainly carried out by the cytochrome P450 family of isoenzymes, of which CYP3A4 is the most important isoenzyme involved in the metabolism of drugs. Induction of cytochrome P450 isoenzymes by one drug can increase the rate of metabolism of another, resulting in lower plasma concentrations and a reduced effect. On withdrawal of the inducing drug, plasma concentrations increase and toxicity can occur.

Conversely when one drug inhibits cytochrome P450 isoenzymes, it can decrease the metabolism of another, leading to higher plasma concentrations, resulting in an increased effect with a risk of toxicity.

Isoenzymes of the hepatic cytochrome P450 system interact with a wide range of drugs. With knowledge of which isoenzymes are involved in a drug's metabolism, it is possible to predict whether certain pharmacokinetic interactions will occur. For example, carbamazepine is a potent inducer of CYP3A4, ketoconazole is potent inhibitor of CYP3A4, and midazolam is a substrate of CYP3A4. Carbamazepine reduces midazolam concentrations, and it is therefore likely that other drugs that are potent inducers of CYP3A4 will interact similarly with midazolam. Ketoconazole, however, increases midazolam concentrations, and it can be predicted that other drugs that are potent inhibitors of CYP3A4 will interact similarly.

Less is known about the enzymes involved in phase II reactions. These include UDP-glucuronyltransferases which, for example, might be induced by rifampicin, resulting in decreased metabolism of mycophenolate (a substrate for this enzyme) to its active form, mycophenolic acid.

Affecting renal excretion Drugs are eliminated through the kidney both by glomerular filtration and by active tubular secretion. Competition occurs between those which share active transport mechanisms in the proximal tubule. For example, salicylates and some other NSAIDs delay the excretion of methotrexate; serious methotrexate toxicity is possible. Changes in urinary pH can also affect the reabsorption of a small number of drugs, including methenamine.

Relative importance of interactions

Levels of severity: Most interactions have been assigned a severity; this describes the likely effect of an unmanaged interaction on the patient.

Severe—the result may be a life-threatening event or have a permanent detrimental effect.

Moderate—the result could cause considerable distress or partially incapacitate a patient; they are unlikely to be life-threatening or result in long-term effects.

Mild—the result is unlikely to cause concern or incapacitate the majority of patients.

Unknown—used for those interactions that are predicted, but there is insufficient evidence to hazard a guess at the outcome.

Levels of evidence: Most interactions have been assigned a rating to indicate the weight of evidence behind the interaction.

Study—for interactions where the information is based on formal study including those for other drugs with same mechanism (e.g. known inducers, inhibitors, or substrates of cytochrome P450 isoenzymes or P-glycoprotein).

Anecdotal—interactions based on either a single case report or a limited number of case reports.

Theoretical—interactions that are predicted based on sound theoretical considerations. The information may have been derived from *in vitro* studies or based on the way other members in the same class act.

Action messages: Each interaction describes the effect that occurs, and the action to be taken, either based on manufacturer's advice from the relevant Summary of Product Characteristics or advice from a relevant authority (e.g. MHRA). An action message is only included where the combination is to be avoided, where a dose adjustment is required, or where specific administration requirements (e.g timing of doses) are recommended. **Pharmacodynamic interactions**, with the exception of interactions with drugs that may prolong the QT interval, do not have an action message included as these will depend on individual patient circumstances.

Further information

For further information on the coverage of the interactions content, please see our *Frequently asked questions—clinical* which can be found online or in the BNF + BNFC App.

Appendix 1 structure

❶ Drugs

Drugs are listed alphabetically. If a drug is a member of a drug class, all interactions for that drug will be listed under the drug class entry; in this case the drug entry provides direction to the relevant drug class where its interactions can be found.

Within a drug or drug class entry, interactions are listed alphabetically by the interacting drug or drug class. The interactions describe the effect that occurs, and the action to be taken, either based on manufacturer's advice from the relevant Summary of Product Characteristics or advice from a relevant authority (e.g. MHRA). An action message is only included where the combination is to be avoided, where a dose adjustment is required, or where specific administration requirements (e.g. timing of doses) are recommended. If two drugs have a pharmacodynamic effect in addition to a pharmacokinetic interaction, a cross-reference to the relevant pharmacodynamic effect table is included at the end of the pharmacokinetic message.

❷ Drug classes

The drugs that are members of a drug class are listed underneath the drug class entry in a blue box. Interactions for the class are then listed alphabetically by the interacting drug or drug class. If the interaction only applies to certain drugs in the class, these drugs will be shown in brackets after the drug class name.

❸ Supplementary information

If a drug has additional important information to be considered, this is shown in a blue box underneath the drug or drug class entry. This information might be food and lifestyle advice (including smoking and alcohol consumption), relate to the pharmacology of the drug or applicability of interactions to certain routes of administration, or it might be advice about separating administration times.

❹ Pharmacodynamic effects

Tables at the beginning of Appendix 1 cover pharmacodynamic effects. If a drug is included in one or more of these tables, this will be indicated at the top of the list of interactions for the drug or drug class. In addition to the list of interactions for a drug or drug class, these tables should always be consulted.

Each table describes the relevant pharmacodynamic effect and lists those drugs that are commonly associated with the effect. Concurrent use of two or more drugs from the same table is expected to increase the risk of the pharmacodynamic effect occurring. Please note these tables are not exhaustive.

---

❶ Drug entry

- Details of interaction between **drug entry** and another **drug** or **drug class**. Action statement. Severity Evidence
- Details of interaction between **drug entry** and another **drug** or **drug class**. Action statement. Severity Evidence

→ Also see TABLE 1

Drug entry → see Drug class entry

❷ Drug class entry

Drug A · Drug B · Drug C · Drug D

- Details of interaction between **drug class entry** and another **drug** or **drug class**. Action statement. Severity Evidence

❸ Drug entry or Drug class entry

Supplementary information

❹ Drug entry or Drug class entry → see TABLE 1

TABLE 1

Name of pharmacodynamic effect

Explanation of the effect

Drug	Drug	Drug
Drug	Drug	Drug

TABLE 1

Drugs that cause hepatotoxicity

The following is a list of some drugs that cause hepatotoxicity (note that this list is not exhaustive). Concurrent use of two or more drugs from the list might increase this risk.

acitretin	dactinomycin	isotretinoin	oxandrolone	streptozocin
alectinib	decitabine	itraconazole	oxymetholone	testosterone
amiodarone	demeclocycline	lenalidomide	oxytetracycline	tetracycline
anidulafungin	doxycycline	lomitapide	paracetamol	thalidomide
asparaginase	eravacycline	lymecycline	pegaspargase	tigecycline
atorvastatin	fluconazole	mercaptopurine	pemetrexed	tioguanine
bexarotene	fludarabine	methotrexate	pomalidomide	trabectedin
capecitabine	fluorouracil	micafungin	pravastatin	valproate
carmustine	flutamide	minocycline	pyrazinamide	vitamin A
caspofungin	fluvastatin	nelarabine	ritonavir	vorasidenib
clofarabine	gemcitabine	neratinib	rosuvastatin	voriconazole
crisantaspase	heparin	nevirapine	simvastatin	zidovudine
cytarabine	isoniazid	nicotinic acid	sotorasib	

TABLE 2

Drugs that cause nephrotoxicity

The following is a list of some drugs that cause nephrotoxicity (note that this list is not exhaustive). Concurrent use of two or more drugs from the list might increase this risk.

aceclofenac	ceftazidime	foscarnet	nabumetone	sulfasalazine
aciclovir	ceftobiprole	fosinopril	naproxen	sulindac
amikacin	ceftolozane	ganciclovir	neomycin	tacrolimus
amphotericin B	ceftriaxone	gentamicin	netilmicin	tenofovir disoproxil
aspirin	cefuroxime	ibuprofen	oxaliplatin	tenoxicam
captopril	celecoxib	ifosfamide	pamidronate	tiaprofenic acid
carboplatin	ciclosporin	imidapril	parecoxib	tobramycin
cefaclor	cidofovir	indometacin	pemetrexed	tolfenamic acid
cefadroxil	cisplatin	inotersen	pentamidine	trandolapril
cefalexin	colistimethate	ketoprofen	perindopril	trimethoprim
cefazolin	deferasirox	ketorolac	phenazone	valaciclovir
cefepime	dexketoprofen	lisinopril	piroxicam	valganciclovir
cefixime	diclofenac	lithium	quinapril	vancomycin
cefotaxime	enalapril	mefenamic acid	ramipril	voclosporin
cefoxitin	etodolac	meloxicam	rifampicin	zoledronate
cefradine	etoricoxib	mesalazine	streptomycin	
ceftaroline	flurbiprofen	methotrexate	streptozocin	

TABLE 3

Drugs that cause bleeding

The following is a list of some drugs that cause bleeding (note that this list is not exhaustive). Concurrent use of two or more drugs from the list might increase this risk.

acalabrutinib	celecoxib	escitalopram	meloxicam	sertraline
aceclofenac	cilostazol	etodolac	nabumetone	sorafenib
acenocoumarol	citalopram	etoricoxib	naproxen	streptokinase
alprostadil	clopidogrel	fluoxetine	nicotinic acid	sulindac
alteplase	crisantaspase	flurbiprofen	nintedanib	sunitinib
anagrelide	dabigatran	fluvoxamine	omega-3-acid ethyl esters	tenecteplase
apixaban	dalteparin	fondaparinux	parecoxib	tenoxicam
argatroban	danaparoid	heparin	paroxetine	tiaprofenic acid
asparaginase	dapoxetine	ibrutinib	pazopanib	ticagrelor
aspirin	dasatinib	ibuprofen	pegaspargase	tinzaparin
axitinib	dexketoprofen	icosapent	pentosan	tirofiban
bemiparin	diclofenac	iloprost	phenazone	tolfenamic acid
benzydamine	dipyridamole	imatinib	phenindione	treprostinil
bismuth subsalicylate	duloxetine	indometacin	piroxicam	urokinase
bivalirudin	edoxaban	ketoprofen	ponatinib	venlafaxine
bosutinib	enoxaparin	ketorolac	prasugrel	vortioxetine
bromfenac	epoprostenol	lenvatinib	regorafenib	warfarin
cangrelor	eptifibatide	mefenamic acid	rivaroxaban	zanubrutinib

TABLE 4

Drugs that cause bradycardia

The following is a list of drugs that cause bradycardia (note that this list is not exhaustive). Concurrent use of two or more drugs from the list might increase this risk.

acebutolol
alectinib
alfentanil
amiodarone
apraclonidine
atenolol
betaxolol
bisoprolol
brigatinib
brimonidine
carvedilol
celiprolol
ceritinib
clonidine
crizotinib
digoxin
diltiazem
donepezil
dronedarone
esmolol
etrasimod
fentanyl
fingolimod
flecainide
galantamine
ivabradine
labetalol
landiolol
levobunolol
metoprolol
nadolol
nebivolol
neostigmine
ozanimod
pasireotide
pindolol
ponesimod
propafenone
propofol
propranolol
pyridostigmine
remifentanil
rivastigmine
selegiline
siponimod
sotalol
sufentanil
suxamethonium
thalidomide
ticagrelor
timolol
tizanidine
verapamil

TABLE 5

Drugs that cause first dose hypotension

The following is a list of some drugs that can cause first-dose hypotension (note that this list is not exhaustive). Concurrent use of two or more drugs from the list might increase this risk.

alfuzosin
captopril
doxazosin
enalapril
fosinopril
imidapril
indoramin
lisinopril
perindopril
prazosin
quinapril
ramipril
tamsulosin
terazosin
trandolapril

TABLE 6

Drugs that cause hypotension

The following is a list of some drugs that cause hypotension (note that this list is not exhaustive). Concurrent use of two or more drugs from the list might increase this risk.

acebutolol
alcohol
alfuzosin
aliskiren
alprostadil
amantadine
amitriptyline
amlodipine
apomorphine
apraclonidine
aripiprazole
asenapine
atenolol
avanafil
azilsartan
baclofen
bendroflumethiazide
benperidol
betaxolol
bisoprolol
bortezomib
brimonidine
bromocriptine
bumetanide
cabergoline
canagliflozin
candesartan
captopril
cariprazine
carvedilol
celiprolol
chlorothiazide
chlorpromazine
chlortalidone
clomipramine
clonidine
clozapine
dapagliflozin
desflurane
diazoxide
diltiazem
dipyridamole
dosulepin
doxazosin
doxepin
droperidol
empagliflozin
enalapril
eplerenone
epoprostenol
eprosartan
ertugliflozin
esketamine
esmolol
etomidate
felodipine
finerenone
flupentixol
fosinopril
foslevodopa
furosemide
glyceryl trinitrate
guanfacine
haloperidol
hydralazine
hydrochlorothiazide
hydroflumethiazide
iloprost
imidapril
imipramine
indapamide
indoramin
irbesartan
isocarboxazid
isoflurane
isosorbide dinitrate
isosorbide mononitrate
ketamine
labetalol
lacidipine
landiolol
lercanidipine
levobunolol
levodopa
levomepromazine
lisinopril
lofepramine
lofexidine
losartan
loxapine
lurasidone
methoxyflurane
methyldopa
metolazone
metoprolol
minoxidil
moxonidine
nadolol
nebivolol
nicardipine
nicorandil
nifedipine
nimodipine
nitroprusside
nitrous oxide
nortriptyline
olanzapine
olmesartan
paliperidone
pericyazine
perindopril
phenelzine
pimozide
pindolol
pramipexole
prazosin
prochlorperazine
promazine
propofol
propranolol
quetiapine
quinagolide
quinapril
ramipril
riociguat
risperidone
ropinirole
rotigotine
sacubitril
sapropterin
selegiline
sevoflurane
sildenafil
sodium oxybate
sotalol
sparsentan
spironolactone
sulpiride
tadalafil
tamsulosin
telmisartan
terazosin
thiopental
timolol
tizanidine
torasemide
trandolapril
tranylcypromine
treprostinil
trifluoperazine
trimipramine
valsartan
vardenafil
verapamil
vericiguat
vernakalant
xipamide
zuclopenthixol

TABLE 7
Drugs that prolong the QT interval

The following is a list of some drugs that prolong the QT-interval (note that this list is not exhaustive). In general, manufacturers advise that the use of two or more drugs that are associated with QT prolongation should be avoided. Increasing age, female sex, cardiac disease, and some metabolic disturbances (notably hypokalaemia) predispose to QT prolongation—concurrent use of drugs that reduce serum potassium might further increase this risk (see table of drugs that reduce serum potassium).

Drugs that are not known to prolong the QT interval but are predicted (by the manufacturer) to increase the risk of QT prolongation include: domperidone, etrasimod, fingolimod, granisetron, ivabradine, mefloquine, mizolastine, ozanimod, palonosetron, intravenous or intramuscular pentamidine, ponesimod, and siponimod. Most manufacturers advise avoiding concurrent use with drugs that prolong the QT interval.

amifampridine	citalopram	escitalopram	nilotinib	selpercatinib
amiodarone	clomipramine	fluconazole	ondansetron	sevoflurane
amisulpride	crizotinib	glasdegib	osilodrostat	sorafenib
anagrelide	dasatinib	haloperidol	osimertinib	sotalol
apalutamide	delamanid	hydroxychloroquine	paliperidone	sunitinib
apomorphine	desflurane	hydroxyzine	panobinostat	tetrabenazine
arsenic trioxide	disopyramide	inotuzumab ozogamicin	pasireotide	tolterodine
artemether	dronedarone	isoflurane	pazopanib	toremifene
artenimol	droperidol	ivosidenib	pimozide	vandetanib
bedaquiline	efavirenz	lapatinib	promethazine	vardenafil
bosutinib	encorafenib	lenvatinib	quinine	vemurafenib
cabozantinib	entrectinib	levomepromazine	quizartinib	vernakalant
ceritinib	eribulin	methadone	ranolazine	voclosporin
chlorpromazine	erythromycin	moxifloxacin	ribociclib	voriconazole

TABLE 8
Drugs with antimuscarinic effects

The following is a list of some drugs that have antimuscarinic effects (note that this list is not exhaustive). Concurrent use of two or more drugs from this list might increase the risk of these effects occurring.

aclidinium	cyproheptadine	haloperidol	orphenadrine	propiverine
amantadine	darifenacin	homatropine	oxybutynin	solifenacin
amitriptyline	dicycloverine	hydroxyzine	pericyazine	tiotropium
atropine	dimenhydrinate	hyoscine	pimozide	tolterodine
baclofen	disopyramide	imipramine	pridinol	trifluoperazine
chlorphenamine	dosulepin	ipratropium	prochlorperazine	trihexyphenidyl
chlorpromazine	doxepin	levomepromazine	procyclidine	trimipramine
clomipramine	fesoterodine	lofepramine	promazine	tropicamide
clozapine	flavoxate	loxapine	promethazine	trospium
cyclizine	flupentixol	nortriptyline	propafenone	umeclidinium
cyclopentolate	glycopyrronium	olanzapine	propantheline	zuclopenthixol

TABLE 9

Drugs with effects on the CNS

The following is a list of some drugs that have effects on the CNS (note that this list is not exhaustive). Concurrent use of two or more drugs from this list might increase the risk of sedation, which might affect the ability to perform skilled tasks (see 'Drugs and Driving' in Guidance on Prescribing p. 1). In some cases, concurrent use of two or more drugs from this list might also increase the risk of CNS depressant effects (which could range from sedation to unconsciousness, coma, respiratory depression, and/or cardiovascular depression).

agomelatine
alcohol
alfentanil
alimemazine
alprazolam
amisulpride
amitriptyline
apomorphine
apraclonidine
aripiprazole
asenapine
baclofen
benperidol
brimonidine
bromocriptine
buclizine
buprenorphine
cabergoline
cannabidiol
cariprazine
cenobamate
chloral hydrate
chlordiazepoxide
chlorphenamine
chlorpromazine
cinnarizine
citalopram
clobazam
clomethiazole
clomipramine
clonazepam
clonidine
clozapine
codeine
cyclizine
cyproheptadine
dapoxetine
daridorexant
desflurane
dexmedetomidine
diamorphine
diazepam
difelikefalin
dihydrocodeine
dimenhydrinate
dipipanone
dosulepin
doxepin
doxylamine
dronabinol
droperidol
duloxetine
escitalopram
esketamine
eszopiclone
etomidate
fentanyl
fluoxetine
flupentixol
flurazepam
fluvoxamine
foslevodopa
fosphenytoin
gabapentin
guanfacine
haloperidol
hydromorphone
hydroxyzine
imipramine
isoflurane
ketamine
ketotifen
lamotrigine
levetiracetam
levodopa
levomepromazine
lofepramine
lofexidine
loprazolam
lorazepam
lormetazepam
loxapine
lurasidone
melatonin
meptazinol
methadone
methocarbamol
methoxyflurane
mianserin
midazolam
mirtazapine
morphine
moxonidine
nabilone
nitrazepam
nitrous oxide
nortriptyline
olanzapine
orphenadrine
oxazepam
oxycodone
paliperidone
paroxetine
pentazocine
perampanel
pericyazine
pethidine
phenobarbital
phenytoin
pimozide
pizotifen
pramipexole
pregabalin
primidone
prochlorperazine
procyclidine
promazine
promethazine
propofol
quetiapine
quinagolide
remifentanil
remimazolam
risperidone
ropinirole
rotigotine
rufinamide
sertraline
sevoflurane
sodium oxybate
sufentanil
sulpiride
tapentadol
temazepam
tetrabenazine
thalidomide
thiopental
tizanidine
tramadol
trazodone
trifluoperazine
trihexyphenidyl
trimipramine
venlafaxine
vigabatrin
zolpidem
zopiclone
zuclopenthixol

TABLE 10

Drugs that cause peripheral neuropathy

The following is a list of some drugs that cause peripheral neuropathy (note that this list is not exhaustive). Concurrent use of two or more drugs from the list might increase this risk.

amiodarone
bortezomib
brentuximab vedotin
cabazitaxel
carboplatin
cisplatin
cytarabine
docetaxel
enfuvirtide
eribulin
isoniazid
lamivudine
leflunomide
lenalidomide
metronidazole
nitrofurantoin
oxaliplatin
paclitaxel
phenytoin
pomalidomide
teriflunomide
thalidomide
vinblastine
vincristine
vindesine
vinorelbine

TABLE 11

Drugs that cause serotonin toxicity

The following is a list of some drugs that might cause serotonin toxicity (note that this list is not exhaustive). See 'Serotonin Toxicity' and 'Monoamine-Oxidase Inhibitors' under Antidepressant drugs in BNF for more information and for specific advice on avoiding monoamine-oxidase inhibitors during and after administration of other serotonergic drugs.

citalopram
clomipramine
dapoxetine
dexamfetamine
duloxetine
escitalopram
fenfluramine
fentanyl
fluoxetine
fluvoxamine
imipramine
isocarboxazid
linezolid
lisdexamfetamine
methadone
methylthioninium chloride
moclobemide
paroxetine
pentazocine
pethidine
phenelzine
sertraline
St John's wort
tramadol
tranylcypromine
trazodone
tryptophan
venlafaxine
vortioxetine

TABLE 12

Drugs that cause myelosuppression

The following is a list of some drugs that cause myelosuppression (note that this list is not exhaustive). Concurrent use of two or more drugs from the list might increase this risk.

adalimumab
aldesleukin
alemtuzumab
amsacrine
arsenic trioxide
asparaginase
axitinib
azacitidine
azathioprine
belatacept
bendamustine
bevacizumab
bexarotene
bleomycin
blinatumomab
bortezomib
bosutinib
brentuximab vedotin
busulfan
cabazitaxel
cabozantinib
canakinumab
capecitabine
carboplatin
carfilzomib
carmustine
ceritinib
certolizumab pegol
chlorambucil
cisplatin
cladribine
clofarabine
crisantaspase
cyclophosphamide
cytarabine
dacarbazine
dactinomycin
daratumumab
dasatinib
daunorubicin
decitabine
dexrazoxane
dinutuximab
docetaxel
doxorubicin
epirubicin
eribulin
estramustine
etoposide
fludarabine
fluorouracil
ganciclovir
gemcitabine
gemtuzumab ozogamicin
golimumab
hydroxycarbamide
ibrutinib
idarubicin
ifosfamide
imatinib
infliximab
inotuzumab ozogamicin
ipilimumab
irinotecan
leflunomide
lenalidomide
lomustine
melphalan
mercaptopurine
methotrexate
mifamurtide
mitomycin
mitotane
mitoxantrone
mogamulizumab
nelarabine
nilotinib
niraparib
nivolumab
obinutuzumab
olaparib
oxaliplatin
paclitaxel
palbociclib
panobinostat
pegaspargase
peginterferon alfa
pembrolizumab
pemetrexed
pentostatin
pixantrone
pomalidomide
procarbazine
raltitrexed
ramucirumab
regorafenib
ribociclib
rituximab
ropeginterferon alfa
rucaparib
ruxolitinib
sorafenib
streptozocin
sulfasalazine
sunitinib
talazoparib
tegafur
temozolomide
temsirolimus
thalidomide
thiotepa
tioguanine
topotecan
trabectedin
trastuzumab
trastuzumab deruxtecan
trastuzumab emtansine
treosulfan
valganciclovir
vinblastine
vincristine
vindesine
vinorelbine

TABLE 13

Drugs that increase serum potassium

The following is a list of some drugs that increase serum potassium concentrations (note that this list is not exhaustive). Concurrent use of two or more drugs from this list might increase the risk of hyperkalaemia (hyperkalaemia is particularly notable when ACE inhibitors or angiotensin-II receptor antagonists are given with spironolactone or eplerenone).

aceclofenac
aliskiren
amiloride
azilsartan
bemiparin
bromfenac
candesartan
captopril
celecoxib
ciclosporin
dalteparin
dexketoprofen
diclofenac
drospirenone
enalapril
enoxaparin
eplerenone
eprosartan
etodolac
etoricoxib
finerenone
flurbiprofen
fosinopril
heparin
ibuprofen
imidapril
indometacin
irbesartan
ketoprofen
ketorolac
labetalol
lisinopril
losartan
mefenamic acid
meloxicam
nabumetone
naproxen
olmesartan
parecoxib
pentamidine
perindopril
phenazone
piroxicam
potassium aminobenzoate
potassium canrenoate
potassium chloride
quinapril
ramipril
sparsentan
spironolactone
sulindac
suxamethonium
tacrolimus
telmisartan
tenoxicam
tiaprofenic acid
tinzaparin
tolfenamic acid
tolvaptan
trandolapril
triamterene
trimethoprim
valsartan
voclosporin

TABLE 14

Drugs that reduce serum potassium

The following is a list of some drugs that reduce serum potassium concentrations (note that this list is not exhaustive and that other drugs can cause hypokalaemia in overdose). Concurrent use of two or more drugs from this list might increase the risk of hypokalaemia. Hypokalaemia can increase the risk of torsade de pointes, which might be additive with the effects of drugs that prolong the QT interval (see table of drugs that prolong the QT interval).

aminophylline
amphotericin B
beclometasone
bendroflumethiazide
betamethasone
budesonide
bumetanide
chlorothiazide
chlortalidone
deflazacort
dexamethasone
fludrocortisone
formoterol
furosemide
hydrochlorothiazide
hydrocortisone
hydroflumethiazide
indacaterol
indapamide
isoprenaline
methylprednisolone
metolazone
olodaterol
prednisolone
salbutamol
salmeterol
terbutaline
theophylline
torasemide
triamcinolone
vamorolone
vilanterol
xipamide

TABLE 15
Drugs that cause hyponatraemia

The following is a list of some drugs that reduce sodium concentrations (note that this list is not exhaustive). Concurrent use of two or more drugs from this list might increase the risk of hyponatraemia.

aceclofenac	clomipramine	furosemide	mirtazapine	sertraline
amiloride	clozapine	haloperidol	nabumetone	sulindac
amisulpride	cyclophosphamide	hydrochlorothiazide	naproxen	sulpiride
amitriptyline	desmopressin	hydroflumethiazide	nortriptyline	tenoxicam
aripiprazole	dexketoprofen	ibuprofen	olanzapine	tiaprofenic acid
asenapine	diclofenac	imipramine	oxcarbazepine	tolfenamic acid
bendroflumethiazide	dosulepin	indapamide	oxytocin	torasemide
benperidol	doxepin	indometacin	paliperidone	tramadol
bumetanide	droperidol	ketoprofen	parecoxib	trazodone
carbamazepine	duloxetine	ketorolac	paroxetine	trifluoperazine
carboplatin	escitalopram	levomepromazine	pericyazine	trimipramine
cariprazine	eslicarbazepine	lofepramine	phenazone	valproate
celecoxib	etodolac	loxapine	pimozide	venlafaxine
chlorothiazide	etoricoxib	lurasidone	piroxicam	vinblastine
chlorpromazine	fluoxetine	mannitol	prochlorperazine	vincristine
chlortalidone	flupentixol	mefenamic acid	promazine	vinorelbine
cisplatin	flurbiprofen	meloxicam	quetiapine	xipamide
citalopram	fluvoxamine	metolazone	risperidone	zuclopenthixol

TABLE 16
Drugs that cause ototoxicity

The following is a list of some drugs that cause ototoxicity (note that this list is not exhaustive). Concurrent use of two or more drugs from the list might increase this risk.

amikacin	cisplatin	mefloquine	streptomycin	vinblastine
amphotericin B	colistimethate	neomycin	teprotumumab	vincristine
bumetanide	furosemide	netilmicin	tobramycin	vindesine
carboplatin	gentamicin	oxaliplatin	torasemide	vinorelbine
chloroquine	hydroxychloroquine	quinine	vancomycin	

List of drug interactions

The following is an alphabetical list of drugs and their interactions; to avoid excessive cross-referencing each drug or group is listed twice: in the alphabetical list and also against the drug or group with which it interacts.

5-HT3-receptor antagonists → see TABLE 7 p. 1055 (QT-interval prolongation)

granisetron · ondansetron · palonosetron

- Anti-androgens **(apalutamide, enzalutamide)** are predicted to decrease the exposure to **ondansetron**. [Moderate] Study → Also see TABLE 7 p. 1055
- Antiepileptics **(carbamazepine, fosphenytoin, phenobarbital, phenytoin, primidone)** are predicted to decrease the exposure to **ondansetron**. [Moderate] Study
- Dopamine receptor agonists **(apomorphine)** increase the risk of severe hypotension when given with **ondansetron**. Avoid. [Severe] Study → Also see TABLE 7 p. 1055
- Dopamine receptor agonists **(apomorphine)** are predicted to increase the risk of severe hypotension when given with 5-HT3-receptor antagonists **(granisetron, palonosetron)**. [Severe] Theoretical
- **Encorafenib** is predicted to decrease the exposure to **ondansetron**. [Moderate] Study → Also see TABLE 7 p. 1055
- **Ivosidenib** is predicted to decrease the exposure to **ondansetron**. [Moderate] Study → Also see TABLE 7 p. 1055
- **Lumacaftor** is predicted to decrease the exposure to **ondansetron**. [Moderate] Study
- **Mitotane** is predicted to decrease the exposure to **ondansetron**. [Moderate] Study
- Rifamycins **(rifampicin)** are predicted to decrease the exposure to **ondansetron**. [Moderate] Study

Abacavir → see NRTIs

Abatacept

- **Anakinra** is predicted to increase the risk of generalised infection (possibly life-threatening) when given with **abatacept**. [Severe] Theoretical
- **Abatacept** is predicted to increase the risk of generalised infection (possibly life-threatening) when given with **etanercept**. Avoid. [Severe] Theoretical
- **Filgotinib** is predicted to increase the risk of immunosuppression when given with **abatacept**. Avoid. [Severe] Theoretical
- **Live vaccines** are predicted to increase the risk of generalised infection (possibly life-threatening) when given with **abatacept**. UKHSA advises avoid (refer to Green Book). [Severe] Theoretical
- Monoclonal antibodies **(certolizumab pegol)** are predicted to increase the risk of generalised infection (possibly life-threatening) when given with **abatacept**. Avoid. [Severe] Theoretical
- Monoclonal antibodies **(rozanolixizumab)** might decrease the concentration of **abatacept**. Avoid and for 2 weeks after stopping **rozanolixizumab**. [Moderate] Theoretical
- **Abatacept** is predicted to increase the risk of generalised infection (possibly life-threatening) when given with monoclonal antibodies **(adalimumab, golimumab, infliximab)**. Avoid. [Severe] Theoretical

Abemaciclib

- Anti-androgens **(apalutamide, enzalutamide)** are predicted to markedly decrease the exposure to **abemaciclib**. Avoid. [Severe] Study
- Antiarrhythmics **(dronedarone)** are predicted to increase the exposure to **abemaciclib**. [Moderate] Study
- Antiepileptics **(carbamazepine, fosphenytoin, phenobarbital, phenytoin, primidone)** are predicted to markedly decrease the exposure to **abemaciclib**. Avoid. [Severe] Study
- Antifungals, azoles **(fluconazole, isavuconazole)** are predicted to increase the exposure to **abemaciclib**. [Moderate] Study
- Antifungals, azoles **(itraconazole, ketoconazole, posaconazole, voriconazole)** are predicted to increase the exposure to **abemaciclib**. Avoid or adjust dose—consult product literature. [Severe] Study
- **Berotralstat** is predicted to increase the exposure to **abemaciclib**. [Moderate] Study
- Calcium-channel blockers **(diltiazem, verapamil)** are predicted to increase the exposure to **abemaciclib**. [Moderate] Study
- **Ceritinib** is predicted to increase the exposure to **abemaciclib**. Avoid or adjust dose—consult product literature. [Severe] Study
- **Cobicistat** is predicted to increase the exposure to **abemaciclib**. Avoid or adjust dose—consult product literature. [Severe] Study
- **Crizotinib** is predicted to increase the exposure to **abemaciclib**. [Moderate] Study
- **Encorafenib** is predicted to markedly decrease the exposure to **abemaciclib**. Avoid. [Severe] Study
- **Fedratinib** is predicted to increase the exposure to **abemaciclib**. [Moderate] Study
- **Grapefruit** juice is predicted to increase the exposure to **abemaciclib**. Avoid. [Moderate] Theoretical
- **HIV-protease inhibitors** are predicted to increase the exposure to **abemaciclib**. Avoid or adjust dose—consult product literature. [Severe] Study
- **Idelalisib** is predicted to increase the exposure to **abemaciclib**. Avoid or adjust dose—consult product literature. [Severe] Study
- **Imatinib** is predicted to increase the exposure to **abemaciclib**. [Moderate] Study
- **Ivosidenib** is predicted to markedly decrease the exposure to **abemaciclib**. Avoid. [Severe] Study
- **Letermovir** is predicted to increase the exposure to **abemaciclib**. [Moderate] Study
- **Lumacaftor** is predicted to markedly decrease the exposure to **abemaciclib**. Avoid. [Severe] Study
- Macrolides **(clarithromycin)** are predicted to increase the exposure to **abemaciclib**. Avoid or adjust dose—consult product literature. [Severe] Study
- Macrolides **(erythromycin)** are predicted to increase the exposure to **abemaciclib**. [Moderate] Study
- **Mitotane** is predicted to markedly decrease the exposure to **abemaciclib**. Avoid. [Severe] Study
- Neurokinin-1 receptor antagonists **(aprepitant, netupitant)** are predicted to increase the exposure to **abemaciclib**. [Moderate] Study
- **Nilotinib** is predicted to increase the exposure to **abemaciclib**. [Moderate] Study
- **Nirmatrelvir** boosted with ritonavir is predicted to increase the concentration of **abemaciclib**. Avoid or adjust dose—consult product literature. [Severe] Theoretical
- Rifamycins **(rifampicin)** are predicted to markedly decrease the exposure to **abemaciclib**. Avoid. [Severe] Study
- **St John's wort** is predicted to decrease the exposure to **abemaciclib**. Avoid. [Severe] Study
- **Tucatinib** is predicted to increase the exposure to **abemaciclib**. Avoid or adjust dose—consult product literature. [Severe] Study

Abiraterone → see anti-androgens

Abrocitinib

- Anti-androgens **(apalutamide, enzalutamide)** are predicted to decrease the exposure to **abrocitinib**. Avoid. [Moderate] Study
- Antiepileptics **(fosphenytoin, phenytoin)** are predicted to decrease the exposure to **abrocitinib**. Avoid. [Moderate] Theoretical
- Antifungals, azoles **(fluconazole)** are predicted to increase the exposure to **abrocitinib**. Adjust **abrocitinib** dose, p. 926. [Severe] Study
- **Abrocitinib** might increase the exposure to **ciclosporin**. [Moderate] Theoretical
- **Abrocitinib** might increase the exposure to **digoxin**. [Moderate] Theoretical
- **Abrocitinib** might increase the exposure to **everolimus**. [Moderate] Theoretical
- **Abrocitinib** might increase the exposure to factor XA inhibitors **(edoxaban)**. [Moderate] Theoretical
- **Live vaccines** are predicted to increase the risk of generalised infection (possibly life-threatening) when given with **abrocitinib**. Avoid. [Severe] Theoretical
- NNRTIs **(efavirenz)** are predicted to decrease the exposure to **abrocitinib**. Avoid. [Moderate] Theoretical
- Rifamycins **(rifampicin)** are predicted to decrease the exposure to **abrocitinib**. Avoid. [Moderate] Study

Abrocitinib (continued)

- **Abrocitinib** might increase the exposure to **sirolimus**. Moderate Theoretical
- SSRIs **(fluoxetine, fluvoxamine)** are predicted to increase the exposure to **abrocitinib**. Adjust **abrocitinib** dose, p. 926. Severe Study
- **Abrocitinib** slightly increases the exposure to thrombin inhibitors **(dabigatran)**. Moderate Study

Acalabrutinib → see TABLE 3 p. 1053 (bleeding)

- Anti-androgens **(apalutamide, enzalutamide)** are predicted to decrease the exposure to **acalabrutinib**. Avoid. Severe Study
- Antiarrhythmics **(dronedarone)** are predicted to increase the exposure to **acalabrutinib**. Avoid or monitor. Severe Study
- Antiepileptics **(carbamazepine, fosphenytoin, phenobarbital, phenytoin, primidone)** are predicted to decrease the exposure to **acalabrutinib**. Avoid. Severe Study
- Antifungals, azoles **(fluconazole, isavuconazole)** are predicted to increase the exposure to **acalabrutinib**. Avoid or monitor. Severe Study
- Antifungals, azoles **(itraconazole, ketoconazole, posaconazole, voriconazole)** are predicted to increase the exposure to **acalabrutinib**. Avoid. Severe Study
- **Berotralstat** is predicted to increase the exposure to **acalabrutinib**. Avoid or monitor. Severe Study
- Calcium-channel blockers **(diltiazem, verapamil)** are predicted to increase the exposure to **acalabrutinib**. Avoid or monitor. Severe Study
- **Cenobamate** is predicted to decrease the exposure to **acalabrutinib**. Adjust dose. Moderate Theoretical
- **Ceritinib** is predicted to increase the exposure to **acalabrutinib**. Avoid. Severe Study
- **Cobicistat** is predicted to increase the exposure to **acalabrutinib**. Avoid. Severe Study
- **Crizotinib** is predicted to increase the exposure to **acalabrutinib**. Avoid or monitor. Severe Study
- **Dabrafenib** is predicted to decrease the exposure to **acalabrutinib**. Severe Study
- **Encorafenib** is predicted to decrease the exposure to **acalabrutinib**. Avoid. Severe Study
- Endothelin receptor antagonists **(bosentan)** are predicted to decrease the exposure to **acalabrutinib**. Severe Study
- **Fedratinib** is predicted to increase the exposure to **acalabrutinib**. Avoid or monitor. Severe Study
- **HIV-protease inhibitors** are predicted to increase the exposure to **acalabrutinib**. Avoid. Severe Study
- **Idelalisib** is predicted to increase the exposure to **acalabrutinib**. Avoid. Severe Study
- **Imatinib** is predicted to increase the exposure to **acalabrutinib**. Avoid or monitor. Severe Study → Also see TABLE 3 p. 1053
- **Ivosidenib** is predicted to decrease the exposure to **acalabrutinib**. Avoid. Severe Study
- **Letermovir** is predicted to increase the exposure to **acalabrutinib**. Avoid or monitor. Severe Study
- **Lumacaftor** is predicted to decrease the exposure to **acalabrutinib**. Avoid. Severe Study
- Macrolides **(clarithromycin)** are predicted to increase the exposure to **acalabrutinib**. Avoid. Severe Study
- Macrolides **(erythromycin)** are predicted to increase the exposure to **acalabrutinib**. Avoid or monitor. Severe Study
- **Mitotane** is predicted to decrease the exposure to **acalabrutinib**. Avoid. Severe Study
- Neurokinin-1 receptor antagonists **(aprepitant, netupitant)** are predicted to increase the exposure to **acalabrutinib**. Avoid or monitor. Severe Study
- **Nilotinib** is predicted to increase the exposure to **acalabrutinib**. Avoid or monitor. Severe Study
- NNRTIs **(efavirenz, nevirapine)** are predicted to decrease the exposure to **acalabrutinib**. Severe Study
- Rifamycins **(rifampicin)** are predicted to decrease the exposure to **acalabrutinib**. Avoid. Severe Study
- **St John's wort** is predicted to decrease the exposure to **acalabrutinib**. Avoid. Severe Study
- **Tucatinib** is predicted to increase the exposure to **acalabrutinib**. Avoid. Severe Study

Acarbose

- **Acarbose** decreases the concentration of **digoxin**. Moderate Study
- **Fenfluramine** might decrease blood glucose concentrations when given with **acarbose**. Moderate Theoretical
- **Pancreatin** is predicted to decrease the effects of **acarbose**. Avoid. Moderate Theoretical
- **Somapacitan** might increase blood glucose concentrations, opposing the blood glucose-lowering effects of **acarbose**. Adjust dose. Moderate Theoretical
- **Somatrogon** might increase blood glucose concentrations, opposing the blood glucose-lowering effects of **acarbose**. Adjust dose. Moderate Theoretical

ACE inhibitors → see TABLE 5 p. 1054 (first-dose hypotension), TABLE 6 p. 1054 (hypotension), TABLE 2 p. 1053 (nephrotoxicity), TABLE 13 p. 1057 (increased serum potassium)

captopril · enalapril · fosinopril · imidapril · lisinopril · perindopril · quinapril · ramipril · trandolapril

- **ACE inhibitors** increase the risk of renal impairment when given with **aliskiren**. Avoid or monitor. Severe Study → Also see TABLE 6 p. 1054 → Also see TABLE 13 p. 1057
- **ACE inhibitors** are predicted to increase the risk of hypersensitivity and haematological reactions when given with **allopurinol**. Severe Anecdotal
- **ACE inhibitors** increase the risk of renal impairment when given with **angiotensin-II receptor antagonists**. Avoid or monitor. Severe Study → Also see TABLE 6 p. 1054 → Also see TABLE 13 p. 1057
- **ACE inhibitors** are predicted to increase the risk of anaemia and/or leucopenia when given with **azathioprine**. Severe Anecdotal
- **Everolimus** potentially increases the risk of angioedema when given with **ACE inhibitors**. Severe Anecdotal
- **Captopril** is predicted to increase the exposure to **gilteritinib**. Moderate Theoretical
- **ACE inhibitors** are predicted to decrease the efficacy of **icatibant** and **icatibant** is predicted to decrease the efficacy of **ACE inhibitors**. Avoid. Moderate Theoretical
- **ACE inhibitors** are predicted to increase the concentration of **lithium**. Monitor and adjust dose. Severe Anecdotal → Also see TABLE 2 p. 1053
- **ACE inhibitors** are predicted to increase the risk of angioedema when given with **temsirolimus**. Moderate Theoretical
- Oral **quinapril** (magnesium carbonate-containing forms) might decrease the absorption of oral **tetracyclines**. Avoid. Moderate Study
- **Enalapril** might enhance the antidiuretic and hypertensive effects of **vasopressin**. Moderate Theoretical

Acebutolol → see beta blockers, selective

Aceclofenac → see NSAIDs

Acenocoumarol → see coumarins

Acetazolamide

- **Acetazolamide** potentially increases the risk of toxicity when given with antiepileptics **(valproate)**. Severe Study
- **Acetazolamide** potentially increases the risk of overheating and dehydration when given with antiepileptics **(zonisamide)**. Avoid in children. Severe Theoretical
- **Acetazolamide** increases the risk of severe toxic reaction when given with **aspirin** (high-dose). Severe Study
- **Acetazolamide** alters the concentration of **lithium**. Severe Anecdotal
- **Acetazolamide** is predicted to decrease the efficacy of **methenamine**. Avoid. Moderate Theoretical
- **Acetazolamide** increases the urinary excretion of **methotrexate**. Moderate Study
- **Acetazolamide** might decrease the efficacy of **nitrofurantoin**. Unknown Theoretical

Acetylcysteine

- **Acetylcysteine** might increase the vasodilatory effects of nitrates **(glyceryl trinitrate)**. Moderate Theoretical

Aciclovir → see TABLE 2 p. 1053 (nephrotoxicity)

ROUTE-SPECIFIC INFORMATION Since systemic absorption can follow topical application, the possibility of interactions should be borne in mind.

- **Aciclovir** increases the exposure to **aminophylline**. Monitor and adjust dose. Severe Anecdotal
- **Mycophenolate** is predicted to increase the risk of haematological toxicity when given with **aciclovir**. Moderate Theoretical
- **Aciclovir** is predicted to increase the exposure to **theophylline**. Monitor and adjust dose. Severe Theoretical

Acipimox
- **Acipimox** is predicted to increase the risk of rhabdomyolysis when given with **fibrates**. Severe Theoretical
- **Acipimox** is predicted to increase the risk of rhabdomyolysis when given with **statins**. Severe Theoretical

Acitretin → see retinoids

Aclidinium → see TABLE 8 p. 1055 (antimuscarinics)
- Atypical antipsychotics **(clozapine)** can cause constipation, as can **aclidinium**; concurrent use might increase the risk of developing intestinal obstruction. Severe Theoretical → Also see TABLE 8 p. 1055

Acrivastine → see antihistamines, non-sedating

Adalimumab → see monoclonal antibodies

Adapalene → see retinoids

Adenosine → see antiarrhythmics

Adrenaline → see sympathomimetics, vasoconstrictor

Afatinib
- Antiarrhythmics **(amiodarone, dronedarone)** are predicted to increase the exposure to **afatinib**. Moderate Study
- Antiepileptics **(carbamazepine)** are predicted to decrease the exposure to **afatinib**. Moderate Study
- Antiepileptics **(phenobarbital, phenytoin)** are predicted to decrease the exposure to **afatinib**. Moderate Theoretical
- Antifungals, azoles **(itraconazole, ketoconazole)** are predicted to increase the exposure to **afatinib**. Moderate Study
- Calcium-channel blockers **(verapamil)** are predicted to increase the exposure to **afatinib**. Moderate Study
- **Ciclosporin** is predicted to increase the exposure to **afatinib**. Moderate Study
- **Cobicistat** is predicted to increase the exposure to **afatinib**. Moderate Study
- **Glecaprevir** is predicted to increase the exposure to **afatinib**. Moderate Study
- HIV-protease inhibitors **(lopinavir, ritonavir)** are predicted to increase the exposure to **afatinib**. Moderate Study
- **Lapatinib** is predicted to increase the exposure to **afatinib**. Moderate Study
- **Lorlatinib** is predicted to decrease the exposure to **afatinib**. Moderate Study
- **Macrolides** are predicted to increase the exposure to **afatinib**. Moderate Study
- **Nirmatrelvir** boosted with ritonavir is predicted to increase the concentration of **afatinib**. Moderate Theoretical
- **Pibrentasvir** is predicted to increase the exposure to **afatinib**. Moderate Study
- **Ranolazine** is predicted to increase the exposure to **afatinib**. Moderate Study
- Rifamycins **(rifampicin)** are predicted to decrease the exposure to **afatinib**. Moderate Study
- **Afatinib** is predicted to increase the exposure to the active component of **sacituzumab govitecan**. Severe Theoretical
- **St John's wort** is predicted to decrease the exposure to **afatinib**. Moderate Study
- **Tacrolimus** is predicted to increase the exposure to **afatinib**. Moderate Theoretical
- **Velpatasvir** is predicted to increase the exposure to **afatinib**. Moderate Study
- **Vemurafenib** is predicted to increase the exposure to **afatinib**. Moderate Study
- **Voxilaprevir** is predicted to increase the exposure to **afatinib**. Moderate Study

Aflibercept

ROUTE-SPECIFIC INFORMATION Interactions do not generally apply to topical use unless specified.

- Monoclonal antibodies **(rozanolixizumab)** might decrease the concentration of **aflibercept**. Avoid and for 2 weeks after stopping **rozanolixizumab**. Moderate Theoretical

Agalsidase alfa
- **Aminoglycosides** are predicted to decrease the effects of **agalsidase alfa**. Avoid. Moderate Theoretical
- Antiarrhythmics **(amiodarone)** are predicted to decrease the effects of **agalsidase alfa**. Avoid. Moderate Theoretical
- Antimalarials **(chloroquine)** are predicted to decrease the effects of **agalsidase alfa**. Avoid. Moderate Theoretical
- **Hydroxychloroquine** is predicted to decrease the effects of **agalsidase alfa**. Moderate Theoretical

Agalsidase beta
- **Aminoglycosides** are predicted to decrease the effects of **agalsidase beta**. Avoid. Moderate Theoretical
- Antiarrhythmics **(amiodarone)** are predicted to decrease the effects of **agalsidase beta**. Avoid. Moderate Theoretical
- Antimalarials **(chloroquine)** are predicted to decrease the effects of **agalsidase beta**. Avoid. Moderate Theoretical
- **Hydroxychloroquine** is predicted to decrease the exposure to **agalsidase beta**. Moderate Theoretical

Agomelatine → see TABLE 9 p. 1056 (CNS effects)

- Dose adjustment might be necessary if smoking started or stopped during treatment.
- Caution with concurrent use of drugs associated with hepatic injury.

- Antiepileptics **(fosphenytoin, phenytoin)** are predicted to decrease the exposure to **agomelatine**. Moderate Theoretical → Also see TABLE 9 p. 1056
- **Axitinib** is predicted to increase the exposure to **agomelatine**. Moderate Theoretical
- **Combined hormonal contraceptives** is predicted to increase the exposure to **agomelatine**. Moderate Study
- **Givosiran** is predicted to increase the exposure to **agomelatine**. Moderate Study
- HIV-protease inhibitors **(ritonavir)** are predicted to decrease the exposure to **agomelatine**. Moderate Theoretical
- **Leflunomide** is predicted to decrease the exposure to **agomelatine**. Moderate Theoretical
- **Mexiletine** is predicted to increase the exposure to **agomelatine**. Moderate Study
- **Osilodrostat** is predicted to increase the exposure to **agomelatine**. Moderate Study
- Quinolones **(ciprofloxacin)** are predicted to increase the exposure to **agomelatine**. Moderate Study
- Rifamycins **(rifampicin)** are predicted to decrease the exposure to **agomelatine**. Moderate Theoretical
- **Rucaparib** is predicted to increase the exposure to **agomelatine**. Moderate Study
- SSRIs **(fluvoxamine)** very markedly increase the exposure to **agomelatine**. Avoid. Severe Study → Also see TABLE 9 p. 1056
- **Teriflunomide** is predicted to decrease the exposure to **agomelatine**. Moderate Theoretical
- **Vemurafenib** is predicted to increase the exposure to **agomelatine**. Moderate Study

Albendazole
- Antiepileptics **(carbamazepine, fosphenytoin, phenobarbital, phenytoin, primidone)** decrease the concentration of **albendazole**. Moderate Study
- H_2 receptor antagonists **(cimetidine)** decrease the clearance of **albendazole**. Moderate Study
- HIV-protease inhibitors **(ritonavir)** decrease the exposure to **albendazole**. Moderate Study
- **Albendazole** slightly decreases the exposure to **levamisole** and **levamisole** moderately decreases the exposure to **albendazole**. Moderate Study

Alcohol → see TABLE 6 p. 1054 (hypotension), TABLE 9 p. 1056 (CNS effects)

ROUTE-SPECIFIC INFORMATION Interactions do not generally apply to alcohol used for topical action unless specified.

- Antiepileptics **(sultiame)** might cause a disulfiram-like reaction when given with **alcohol**. Avoid. Moderate Theoretical
- **Alcohol** potentially increases the risk of visual disturbances when given with antiepileptics **(retigabine)**. Moderate Study
- **Alcohol** potentially causes a disulfiram-like reaction when given with antifungals, azoles **(ketoconazole)**. Avoid. Moderate Anecdotal

Alcohol (continued)
- **Alcohol** causes serious, potentially fatal, CNS depression when given with **clomethiazole**. Avoid. Severe Study → Also see TABLE 9 p. 1056
- **Alcohol** (in those who drink heavily) potentially decreases the anticoagulant effect of **coumarins**. Severe Study
- **Alcohol** (excessive consumption) potentially increases the risk of gastrointestinal adverse effects when given with **dimethyl fumarate**. Avoid. Moderate Theoretical
- **Alcohol** causes an extremely unpleasant systemic reaction when given with **disulfiram**. Avoid for at least 24 hours before and up to 14 days after stopping treatment. Severe Study
- **Alcohol**-induced liver disease increases the risk of hepatotoxicity in those taking **drugs that cause hepatotoxicity** (see TABLE 1 p. 1053). Severe Theoretical
- **Alcohol** potentially causes a disulfiram-like reaction when given with **griseofulvin**. Moderate Anecdotal
- **Alcohol** potentially causes a disulfiram-like reaction when given with **levamisole**. Moderate Study
- **Alcohol** (excessive consumption) potentially increases the risk of lactic acidosis when given with **metformin**. Avoid excessive alcohol consumption. Moderate Theoretical
- **Alcohol** might increase the concentration of **methylphenidate**. Avoid. Moderate Study
- **Alcohol** potentially causes a disulfiram-like reaction when given with **metronidazole**. Avoid for at least 48 hours after stopping treatment. Moderate Study
- **Alcohol** causes rapid release of opioids **(hydromorphone, morphine)** from extended-release preparations. Avoid. Severe Study → Also see TABLE 9 p. 1056
- **Alcohol** (in those who drink heavily) causes severe liver damage when given with **paracetamol**. Severe Study
- **Alcohol** increases the risk of facial flushing and skin irritation when given with topical **pimecrolimus**. Moderate Study
- **Alcohol** potentially causes a disulfiram-like reaction when given with **procarbazine**. Moderate Anecdotal
- **Alcohol** potentially increases the concentration of retinoids **(acitretin)**. Avoid and for 2 months after stopping **acitretin**. Moderate Study
- **Alcohol** increases the risk of facial flushing and skin irritation when given with topical **tacrolimus**. Moderate Study
- **Alcohol** might decrease the antidiuretic effect of **vasopressin**. Moderate Theoretical

Aldesleukin → see TABLE 12 p. 1057 (myelosuppression)
Alectinib → see TABLE 4 p. 1054 (bradycardia), TABLE 1 p. 1053 (hepatotoxicity)
Alemtuzumab → see monoclonal antibodies
Alendronate → see bisphosphonates
Alfacalcidol → see vitamin D substances
Alfentanil → see opioids
Alfuzosin → see alpha blockers
Alimemazine → see antihistamines, sedating
Aliskiren → see TABLE 6 p. 1054 (hypotension), TABLE 13 p. 1057 (increased serum potassium)

FOOD AND LIFESTYLE Avoid apple juice and orange juice as they greatly decrease aliskiren concentrations and plasma renin activity.

- **ACE inhibitors** increase the risk of renal impairment when given with **aliskiren**. Avoid or monitor. Severe Study → Also see TABLE 6 p. 1054 → Also see TABLE 13 p. 1057
- **Angiotensin-II receptor antagonists** increase the risk of renal impairment when given with **aliskiren**. Avoid or monitor. Severe Study → Also see TABLE 6 p. 1054 → Also see TABLE 13 p. 1057
- Anti-androgens **(apalutamide)** are predicted to decrease the exposure to **aliskiren**. Monitor and adjust dose. Moderate Study
- Antiarrhythmics **(amiodarone, dronedarone)** are predicted to increase the exposure to **aliskiren**. Severe Study
- Antiepileptics **(carbamazepine)** decrease the exposure to **aliskiren**. Moderate Study
- Antifungals, azoles **(itraconazole)** markedly increase the exposure to **aliskiren**. Avoid. Severe Study
- Antifungals, azoles **(ketoconazole)** moderately increase the exposure to **aliskiren**. Moderate Study
- Calcium-channel blockers **(verapamil)** moderately increase the exposure to **aliskiren**. Moderate Study → Also see TABLE 6 p. 1054
- **Ceritinib** is predicted to increase the exposure to **aliskiren**. Moderate Theoretical
- **Ciclosporin** markedly increases the exposure to **aliskiren**. Avoid. Severe Study → Also see TABLE 13 p. 1057
- **Cobicistat** is predicted to increase the exposure to **aliskiren**. Moderate Study
- **Danicopan** is predicted to increase the exposure to **aliskiren**. Moderate Study
- **Eliglustat** is predicted to increase the exposure to **aliskiren**. Adjust dose. Moderate Study
- **Glecaprevir** is predicted to increase the exposure to **aliskiren**. Severe Theoretical
- **Grapefruit** juice moderately decreases the exposure to **aliskiren**. Avoid. Severe Study
- HIV-protease inhibitors **(ritonavir)** are predicted to increase the exposure to **aliskiren**. Moderate Theoretical
- **Ivosidenib** is predicted to alter the exposure to **aliskiren**. Moderate Theoretical
- **Lapatinib** is predicted to increase the exposure to **aliskiren**. Moderate Theoretical
- **Aliskiren** slightly decreases the exposure to loop diuretics **(furosemide)**. Moderate Study → Also see TABLE 6 p. 1054
- **Lorlatinib** decreases the exposure to **aliskiren**. Moderate Study
- Macrolides **(azithromycin)** are predicted to increase the exposure to **aliskiren**. Moderate Theoretical
- Macrolides **(clarithromycin, erythromycin)** are predicted to increase the exposure to **aliskiren**. Moderate Study
- **Mirabegron** is predicted to increase the exposure to **aliskiren**. Mild Theoretical
- **Nirmatrelvir** boosted with ritonavir is predicted to increase the concentration of **aliskiren**. Avoid. Severe Theoretical
- **Olaparib** might increase the exposure to **aliskiren**. Moderate Theoretical
- **Osimertinib** is predicted to increase the exposure to **aliskiren**. Moderate Study
- **Pibrentasvir** with glecaprevir is predicted to increase the exposure to **aliskiren**. Moderate Study
- **Pitolisant** is predicted to decrease the exposure to **aliskiren**. Mild Theoretical
- **Ranolazine** is predicted to increase the exposure to **aliskiren**. Moderate Theoretical
- Rifamycins **(rifampicin)** decrease the exposure to **aliskiren**. Moderate Study
- **Sparsentan** is predicted to increase the exposure to **aliskiren**. Avoid. Severe Theoretical → Also see TABLE 6 p. 1054 → Also see TABLE 13 p. 1057
- **St John's wort** decreases the exposure to **aliskiren**. Moderate Study
- Statins **(atorvastatin)** slightly to moderately increase the exposure to **aliskiren**. Moderate Study
- **Velpatasvir** is predicted to increase the exposure to **aliskiren**. Severe Theoretical
- **Vemurafenib** is predicted to increase the exposure to **aliskiren**. Use with caution and adjust dose. Moderate Theoretical
- **Voxilaprevir** with sofosbuvir and velpatasvir is predicted to increase the exposure to **aliskiren**. Severe Theoretical

Alitretinoin → see retinoids
Alkylating agents → see TABLE 1 p. 1053 (hepatotoxicity), TABLE 15 p. 1058 (hyponatraemia), TABLE 12 p. 1057 (myelosuppression), TABLE 2 p. 1053 (nephrotoxicity)

bendamustine · busulfan · carmustine · chlorambucil · cyclophosphamide · dacarbazine · estramustine · ifosfamide · lomustine · melphalan · temozolomide · thiotepa · treosulfan

- Oral **antacids** are predicted to decrease the absorption of oral **estramustine**. Avoid. Moderate Study
- Antifungals, azoles **(isavuconazole)** are predicted to increase the exposure to **cyclophosphamide**. Moderate Study
- Antifungals, azoles **(itraconazole)** increase the risk of busulfan toxicity when given with **busulfan**. Monitor and adjust dose. Moderate Study
- Antifungals, azoles **(miconazole)** are predicted to increase the concentration of **busulfan**. Use with caution and adjust dose. Moderate Theoretical
- Oral **calcium compounds** decrease the absorption of oral **estramustine**. Severe Study

- Iron chelators **(deferasirox)** have been reported to increase the exposure to **busulfan**. Monitor and adjust dose. Unknown Anecdotal
- **Ivosidenib** might decrease the exposure to alkylating agents **(cyclophosphamide, ifosfamide)**. Avoid or monitor efficacy. Unknown Theoretical
- **Live vaccines** are predicted to increase the risk of generalised infection (possibly life-threatening) when given with **alkylating agents**. UKHSA advises avoid (refer to Green Book). Severe Theoretical
- **Metronidazole** increases the risk of toxicity when given with **busulfan** (high-dose). Severe Study
- Neurokinin-1 receptor antagonists **(aprepitant, fosaprepitant)** are predicted to increase the exposure to **ifosfamide**. Severe Theoretical
- Neurokinin-1 receptor antagonists **(netupitant)** very slightly increase the exposure to **cyclophosphamide**. Moderate Study
- Neurokinin-1 receptor antagonists **(netupitant)** are predicted to increase the exposure to **ifosfamide**. Moderate Study
- **Paracetamol** is predicted to decrease the clearance of **busulfan**. Moderate Theoretical
- **Pemigatinib** might increase the exposure to the active metabolite of **cyclophosphamide**. Moderate Theoretical
- **Pemigatinib** might decrease the exposure to **ifosfamide**. Moderate Theoretical
- **Cyclophosphamide** (high-dose) increases the risk of toxicity when given with **pentostatin**. Avoid. Severe Anecdotal → Also see TABLE 12 p. 1057
- **Cyclophosphamide** increases the risk of prolonged neuromuscular blockade when given with **suxamethonium**. Moderate Study
- Alkylating agents **(cyclophosphamide, ifosfamide)** might enhance the antidiuretic and hypertensive effects of **vasopressin**. Moderate Theoretical
- **Vorasidenib** might decrease the concentration of **ifosfamide**. Avoid. Severe Theoretical

Allopurinol

- **ACE inhibitors** are predicted to increase the risk of hypersensitivity and haematological reactions when given with **allopurinol**. Severe Anecdotal
- **Allopurinol** potentially increases the risk of haematological toxicity when given with **azathioprine**. Adjust **azathioprine** dose, p. 638. Severe Study
- **Allopurinol** is predicted to decrease the effects of **capecitabine**. Avoid. Severe Study
- **Allopurinol** potentially increases the risk of haematological toxicity when given with **mercaptopurine**. Adjust **mercaptopurine** dose, p. 671. Severe Study
- **Allopurinol** increases the risk of skin rash when given with penicillins **(amoxicillin, ampicillin)**. Moderate Study
- **Allopurinol** is predicted to increase the risk of hyperuricaemia when given with **pyrazinamide**. Moderate Theoretical
- **Thiazide diuretics** are predicted to increase the risk of hypersensitivity reactions when given with **allopurinol**. Severe Theoretical

Almotriptan → see triptans

Alogliptin → see dipeptidylpeptidase-4 inhibitors

Alpelisib

- Anti-androgens **(apalutamide, enzalutamide)** are predicted to decrease the exposure to **alpelisib**. Avoid. Moderate Study
- Anti-androgens **(darolutamide)** are predicted to increase the exposure to **alpelisib**. Moderate Theoretical
- Antiepileptics **(carbamazepine, fosphenytoin, phenobarbital, phenytoin, primidone)** are predicted to decrease the exposure to **alpelisib**. Avoid. Moderate Study
- **Ciclosporin** is predicted to increase the exposure to **alpelisib**. Moderate Theoretical
- **Eltrombopag** is predicted to increase the exposure to **alpelisib**. Moderate Theoretical
- **Encorafenib** is predicted to decrease the exposure to **alpelisib**. Avoid. Moderate Study
- **Febuxostat** is predicted to increase the exposure to **alpelisib**. Moderate Theoretical
- **Fostamatinib** is predicted to increase the exposure to **alpelisib**. Moderate Theoretical
- **Ivosidenib** is predicted to decrease the exposure to **alpelisib**. Avoid. Moderate Study
- **Lapatinib** is predicted to increase the exposure to **alpelisib**. Moderate Theoretical
- **Leflunomide** is predicted to increase the exposure to **alpelisib**. Moderate Theoretical
- **Lumacaftor** is predicted to decrease the exposure to **alpelisib**. Avoid. Moderate Study
- **Mitotane** is predicted to decrease the exposure to **alpelisib**. Avoid. Moderate Study
- Proton pump inhibitors **(pantoprazole)** are predicted to increase the exposure to **alpelisib**. Moderate Theoretical
- Rifamycins **(rifampicin)** are predicted to decrease the exposure to **alpelisib**. Avoid. Moderate Study
- **Roxadustat** is predicted to increase the exposure to **alpelisib**. Moderate Theoretical
- **Teriflunomide** is predicted to increase the exposure to **alpelisib**. Moderate Theoretical
- **Vadadustat** is predicted to increase the exposure to **alpelisib**. Moderate Theoretical
- **Velpatasvir** is predicted to increase the exposure to **alpelisib**. Moderate Theoretical
- **Voxilaprevir** is predicted to increase the exposure to **alpelisib**. Moderate Theoretical

Alpha blockers → see TABLE 5 p. 1054 (first-dose hypotension), TABLE 6 p. 1054 (hypotension)

alfuzosin · doxazosin · indoramin · prazosin · tamsulosin · terazosin

- Antiarrhythmics **(dronedarone)** are predicted to increase the exposure to **tamsulosin**. Moderate Theoretical
- Antifungals, azoles **(fluconazole, isavuconazole)** are predicted to increase the exposure to **tamsulosin**. Moderate Theoretical
- Antifungals, azoles **(itraconazole, ketoconazole, posaconazole, voriconazole)** are predicted to increase the exposure to **doxazosin**. Moderate Study
- Antifungals, azoles **(itraconazole, ketoconazole, posaconazole, voriconazole)** are predicted to moderately increase the exposure to alpha blockers **(alfuzosin, tamsulosin)**. Use with caution or avoid. Moderate Study
- **Berotralstat** is predicted to increase the exposure to **tamsulosin**. Moderate Theoretical
- Calcium-channel blockers **(diltiazem, verapamil)** are predicted to increase the exposure to **tamsulosin**. Moderate Theoretical → Also see TABLE 6 p. 1054
- **Ceritinib** is predicted to moderately increase the exposure to alpha blockers **(alfuzosin, tamsulosin)**. Use with caution or avoid. Moderate Study
- **Ceritinib** is predicted to increase the exposure to **doxazosin**. Moderate Study
- **Cobicistat** is predicted to moderately increase the exposure to alpha blockers **(alfuzosin, tamsulosin)**. Use with caution or avoid. Moderate Study
- **Cobicistat** is predicted to increase the exposure to **doxazosin**. Moderate Study
- **Crizotinib** is predicted to increase the exposure to **tamsulosin**. Moderate Theoretical
- **Fedratinib** is predicted to increase the exposure to **tamsulosin**. Moderate Theoretical
- **HIV-protease inhibitors** are predicted to moderately increase the exposure to alpha blockers **(alfuzosin, tamsulosin)**. Use with caution or avoid. Moderate Study
- **HIV-protease inhibitors** are predicted to increase the exposure to **doxazosin**. Moderate Study
- **Idelalisib** is predicted to moderately increase the exposure to alpha blockers **(alfuzosin, tamsulosin)**. Use with caution or avoid. Moderate Study
- **Idelalisib** is predicted to increase the exposure to **doxazosin**. Moderate Study
- **Imatinib** is predicted to increase the exposure to **tamsulosin**. Moderate Theoretical
- **Letermovir** is predicted to increase the exposure to **tamsulosin**. Moderate Theoretical
- Macrolides **(clarithromycin)** are predicted to increase the exposure to **doxazosin**. Moderate Study
- Macrolides **(erythromycin)** are predicted to increase the exposure to **tamsulosin**. Moderate Theoretical

Alpha blockers (continued)

- Macrolides **(clarithromycin)** are predicted to moderately increase the exposure to alpha blockers **(alfuzosin, tamsulosin)**. Use with caution or avoid. Moderate Study
- **MAOIs, irreversible** are predicted to increase the effects of **indoramin**. Avoid. Severe Theoretical → Also see TABLE 6 p. 1054
- Neurokinin-1 receptor antagonists **(aprepitant, netupitant)** are predicted to increase the exposure to **tamsulosin**. Moderate Theoretical
- **Nilotinib** is predicted to increase the exposure to **tamsulosin**. Moderate Theoretical
- **Nirmatrelvir** boosted with ritonavir is predicted to increase the concentration of alpha blockers **(alfuzosin, tamsulosin)**. Avoid. Severe Theoretical
- **Alpha blockers** cause significant hypotensive effects when given with **phosphodiesterase type-5 inhibitors**. Patient should be stabilised on first drug then second drug should be added at the lowest recommended dose. Severe Study → Also see TABLE 6 p. 1054
- **Ribociclib** (high-dose) is predicted to increase the exposure to **alfuzosin**. Avoid. Moderate Theoretical
- **Tucatinib** is predicted to moderately increase the exposure to alpha blockers **(alfuzosin, tamsulosin)**. Use with caution or avoid. Moderate Study
- **Tucatinib** is predicted to increase the exposure to **doxazosin**. Moderate Study

Alprazolam → see benzodiazepines

Alprostadil → see TABLE 3 p. 1053 (bleeding), TABLE 6 p. 1054 (hypotension)

Alteplase → see TABLE 3 p. 1053 (bleeding)

- **Donanemab** might increase the risk of brain haemorrhage when given with **alteplase**. Avoid except in life-threatening situations. Severe Theoretical
- **Lecanemab** might increase the risk of brain haemorrhage when given with **alteplase**. Avoid except in life-threatening situations. Severe Theoretical

Aluminium hydroxide

SEPARATION OF ADMINISTRATION **Aluminium-containing antacids** should preferably not be taken at the same time as other drugs since they might impair absorption. **Aluminium-containing antacids** might damage enteric coatings designed to prevent dissolution in the stomach.

- Oral **aluminium hydroxide** might decrease the concentration of the active metabolite of oral **baloxavir marboxil**. Severe Theoretical
- Oral **aluminium hydroxide** decreases the absorption of **chenodeoxycholic acid**. Moderate Study
- **Aluminium hydroxide** increases the risk of blocked enteral or nasogastric tubes when given with **enteral feeds**. Moderate Study
- **Aluminium hydroxide** is predicted to decrease the exposure to iron chelators **(deferasirox)**. Avoid. Moderate Theoretical
- **Aluminium hydroxide** is predicted to decrease the absorption of iron chelators **(deferiprone)**. Avoid. Moderate Theoretical
- Oral **aluminium hydroxide** might decrease the exposure to oral **roxadustat**. Manufacturer advises take at least 1 hour after aluminium-containing products. Moderate Theoretical
- Oral **aluminium hydroxide** is predicted to decrease the exposure to oral **vadadustat**. Manufacturer advises take at least 1 hour before or 2 hours after aluminium-containing products. Moderate Theoretical

Amantadine → see dopamine receptor agonists

Ambrisentan → see endothelin receptor antagonists

Amfetamines → see TABLE 11 p. 1056 (serotonin toxicity)

dexamfetamine · lisdexamfetamine

- **Amfetamines** are predicted to decrease the effects of **apraclonidine**. Avoid. Severe Theoretical
- **Amfetamines** are predicted to increase the risk of adverse effects when given with **atomoxetine**. Severe Theoretical
- **Dexamfetamine** might increase the anticoagulant effect of **coumarins**. Monitor INR and adjust dose. Moderate Theoretical
- HIV-protease inhibitors **(ritonavir)** are predicted to increase the exposure to **amfetamines**. Severe Theoretical
- MAO-B inhibitors **(rasagiline, selegiline)** are predicted to increase the risk of severe hypertension when given with **amfetamines**. Avoid. Severe Theoretical
- MAO-B inhibitors **(safinamide)** are predicted to increase the risk of severe hypertension when given with **amfetamines**. Severe Theoretical
- **Amfetamines** are predicted to increase the risk of a hypertensive crisis when given with **MAOIs, irreversible**. Avoid and for 14 days after stopping the MAOI. Severe Anecdotal → Also see TABLE 11 p. 1056
- **Amfetamines** are predicted to increase the risk of a hypertensive crisis when given with **moclobemide**. Avoid. Severe Theoretical → Also see TABLE 11 p. 1056
- **Nabilone** is predicted to increase the risk of cardiovascular adverse effects when given with **amfetamines**. Severe Theoretical
- **Nirmatrelvir** boosted with ritonavir is predicted to increase the concentration of **amfetamines**. Severe Theoretical
- **Phenothiazine antipsychotics** are predicted to decrease the effects of **amfetamines** and **amfetamines** are predicted to decrease the effects of **phenothiazine antipsychotics**. Moderate Study
- SSRIs **(fluoxetine, paroxetine)** are predicted to increase the exposure to **amfetamines**. Severe Theoretical → Also see TABLE 11 p. 1056
- Volatile halogenated anaesthetics **(sevoflurane)** can cause hypertension, as can **amfetamines**. Avoid **amfetamines** for several days before surgery. Severe Theoretical

Amifampridine → see TABLE 7 p. 1055 (QT-interval prolongation)

Amikacin → see aminoglycosides

Amiloride → see potassium-sparing diuretics

Aminoglycosides → see TABLE 2 p. 1053 (nephrotoxicity), TABLE 16 p. 1058 (ototoxicity)

amikacin · gentamicin · netilmicin · streptomycin · tobramycin

ROUTE-SPECIFIC INFORMATION Since systemic absorption can follow topical application, the possibility of interactions with topical **gentamicin**, **netilmicin**, or **tobramycin** should be borne in mind.

- **Aminoglycosides** are predicted to decrease the effects of **agalsidase alfa**. Avoid. Moderate Theoretical
- **Aminoglycosides** are predicted to decrease the effects of **agalsidase beta**. Avoid. Moderate Theoretical
- Antifungals, azoles **(miconazole)** potentially decrease the exposure to **tobramycin**. Moderate Anecdotal
- **Ataluren** is predicted to increase the risk of nephrotoxicity when given with intravenous **aminoglycosides**. Avoid. Severe Study
- **Aminoglycosides** increase the risk of hypocalcaemia when given with **bisphosphonates**. Moderate Anecdotal → Also see TABLE 2 p. 1053
- **Aminoglycosides** might increase the concentration of **digoxin**. Monitor and adjust dose. Moderate Study
- **Loop diuretics** increase the risk of nephrotoxicity when given with **aminoglycosides**. Avoid. Moderate Study → Also see TABLE 16 p. 1058
- **Aminoglycosides** are predicted to decrease the effects of **neostigmine**. Moderate Theoretical
- **Aminoglycosides** might prolong the effects of **neuromuscular blocking drugs, non-depolarising**. Severe Theoretical
- **Aminoglycosides** are predicted to decrease the effects of **pyridostigmine**. Moderate Theoretical
- **Gentamicin** is predicted to increase the exposure to **relugolix**. Avoid or take relugolix first and separate administration by at least 6 hours. Moderate Theoretical
- **Aminoglycosides** might prolong the effects of **suxamethonium**. Severe Theoretical

Aminophylline → see TABLE 14 p. 1057 (reduced serum potassium)

FOOD AND LIFESTYLE Smoking can increase aminophylline clearance and increased doses of aminophylline are therefore required; dose adjustments are likely to be necessary if smoking started or stopped during treatment.

- **Aciclovir** increases the exposure to **aminophylline**. Monitor and adjust dose. Severe Anecdotal

- Aminophylline is predicted to decrease the efficacy of antiarrhythmics (adenosine). Separate administration by 24 hours. Mild Theoretical
- Antiepileptics (fosphenytoin) are predicted to decrease the exposure to aminophylline. Adjust dose. Moderate Study
- Antiepileptics (phenobarbital) are predicted to decrease the exposure to aminophylline. Adjust dose. Moderate Theoretical
- Antiepileptics (phenytoin) decrease the exposure to aminophylline. Adjust dose. Moderate Study
- Antiepileptics (primidone) are predicted to increase the clearance of aminophylline. Adjust dose. Moderate Theoretical
- Antiepileptics (stiripentol) are predicted to increase the exposure to aminophylline. Avoid. Moderate Theoretical
- Axitinib is predicted to increase the exposure to aminophylline. Moderate Theoretical
- Beta blockers, non-selective are predicted to increase the risk of bronchospasm when given with aminophylline. Avoid. Severe Theoretical
- Beta blockers, selective are predicted to increase the risk of bronchospasm when given with aminophylline. Avoid. Severe Theoretical
- Combined hormonal contraceptives is predicted to increase the exposure to aminophylline. Adjust dose. Moderate Theoretical
- Aminophylline increases the risk of agitation when given with doxapram. Moderate Study
- Esketamine is predicted to increase the risk of seizures when given with aminophylline. Avoid. Severe Theoretical
- Givosiran is predicted to increase the exposure to aminophylline. Adjust dose. Moderate Theoretical
- H_2 receptor antagonists (cimetidine) increase the concentration of aminophylline. Adjust dose. Severe Study
- HIV-protease inhibitors (ritonavir) decrease the exposure to aminophylline. Adjust dose. Moderate Study
- Interferons are predicted to slightly increase the exposure to aminophylline. Adjust dose. Moderate Theoretical
- Iron chelators (deferasirox) are predicted to increase the exposure to aminophylline. Avoid. Moderate Theoretical
- Isoniazid is predicted to affect the clearance of aminophylline. Severe Theoretical
- Leflunomide decreases the exposure to aminophylline. Adjust dose. Moderate Study
- Aminophylline is predicted to decrease the concentration of lithium. Moderate Theoretical
- Macrolides (azithromycin) are predicted to increase the exposure to aminophylline. Moderate Theoretical
- Macrolides (clarithromycin) are predicted to increase the exposure to aminophylline. Adjust dose. Moderate Theoretical
- Aminophylline is predicted to decrease the exposure to macrolides (erythromycin). Adjust dose. Severe Study
- Methotrexate is predicted to decrease the clearance of aminophylline. Moderate Theoretical
- Metreleptin might alter the exposure to aminophylline. Severe Theoretical
- Mexiletine is predicted to increase the exposure to aminophylline. Adjust dose. Moderate Theoretical
- Monoclonal antibodies (blinatumomab) are predicted to transiently increase the exposure to aminophylline. Monitor and adjust dose. Moderate Theoretical
- Monoclonal antibodies (sarilumab) potentially affect the exposure to aminophylline. Monitor and adjust dose. Moderate Theoretical
- Monoclonal antibodies (tocilizumab) are predicted to decrease the exposure to aminophylline. Monitor and adjust dose. Moderate Theoretical
- Nirmatrelvir boosted with ritonavir is predicted to decrease the concentration of aminophylline. Adjust dose. Moderate Theoretical
- Osilodrostat is predicted to increase the exposure to aminophylline. Adjust dose. Moderate Theoretical
- Pentoxifylline is predicted to increase the concentration of aminophylline. Use with caution or avoid. Severe Theoretical
- Aminophylline is predicted to slightly increase the exposure to phosphodiesterase type-4 inhibitors (roflumilast). Avoid. Moderate Theoretical
- Quinolones (ciprofloxacin) are predicted to increase the exposure to aminophylline. Adjust dose. Moderate Theoretical
- Rifamycins (rifampicin) decrease the exposure to aminophylline. Adjust dose. Moderate Study
- Rucaparib is predicted to increase the exposure to aminophylline. Adjust dose. Moderate Theoretical
- SSRIs (fluvoxamine) moderately to markedly increase the exposure to aminophylline. Avoid. Severe Study
- St John's wort is predicted to decrease the concentration of aminophylline. Severe Theoretical
- Sympathomimetics, vasoconstrictor (ephedrine) increase the risk of adverse effects when given with aminophylline. Avoid in children. Moderate Study
- Teriflunomide decreases the exposure to aminophylline. Adjust dose. Moderate Study
- Valaciclovir is predicted to increase the exposure to aminophylline. Severe Anecdotal
- Vemurafenib is predicted to increase the exposure to aminophylline. Adjust dose. Moderate Theoretical

Amiodarone → see antiarrhythmics

Amisulpride → see atypical antipsychotics

Amitriptyline → see tricyclic antidepressants

Amlodipine → see calcium-channel blockers

Amoxicillin → see penicillins

Amphotericin B → see TABLE 2 p. 1053 (nephrotoxicity), TABLE 16 p. 1058 (ototoxicity), TABLE 14 p. 1057 (reduced serum potassium)

- Amphotericin B increases the risk of toxicity when given with flucytosine. Severe Study
- Micafungin slightly increases the exposure to amphotericin B. Avoid or monitor toxicity. Moderate Study

Ampicillin → see penicillins

Amsacrine → see TABLE 12 p. 1057 (myelosuppression)

- Live vaccines are predicted to increase the risk of generalised infection (possibly life-threatening) when given with amsacrine. UKHSA advises avoid (refer to Green Book). Severe Theoretical

Anaesthetics, local

bupivacaine · levobupivacaine · mepivacaine · oxybuprocaine · prilocaine · proxymetacaine · ropivacaine · tetracaine

ROUTE-SPECIFIC INFORMATION Since systemic absorption can follow topical application, the possibility of interactions should be borne in mind.

- Antiepileptics (phenytoin) are predicted to decrease the exposure to ropivacaine. Moderate Theoretical
- Axitinib is predicted to increase the exposure to ropivacaine. Moderate Theoretical
- Combined hormonal contraceptives is predicted to increase the exposure to ropivacaine. Moderate Theoretical
- Givosiran is predicted to increase the exposure to ropivacaine. Moderate Theoretical
- HIV-protease inhibitors (ritonavir) are predicted to decrease the exposure to ropivacaine. Moderate Theoretical
- Leflunomide is predicted to decrease the exposure to ropivacaine. Moderate Theoretical
- Mexiletine is predicted to increase the exposure to ropivacaine. Moderate Theoretical
- Osilodrostat is predicted to increase the exposure to ropivacaine. Moderate Theoretical
- Quinolones (ciprofloxacin) are predicted to increase the exposure to ropivacaine. Moderate Theoretical
- Rifamycins (rifampicin) are predicted to decrease the exposure to ropivacaine. Moderate Theoretical
- Rucaparib is predicted to increase the exposure to ropivacaine. Moderate Theoretical
- SSRIs (fluvoxamine) decrease the clearance of ropivacaine. Avoid prolonged use. Moderate Study
- Teriflunomide is predicted to decrease the exposure to ropivacaine. Moderate Theoretical
- Vemurafenib is predicted to increase the exposure to ropivacaine. Moderate Theoretical

Anagrelide → see TABLE 3 p. 1053 (bleeding), TABLE 7 p. 1055 (QT-interval prolongation)

- Combined hormonal contraceptives is predicted to increase the exposure to anagrelide. Moderate Theoretical

Anagrelide (continued)

- **Givosiran** is predicted to increase the exposure to **anagrelide**. Moderate Theoretical
- **Mexiletine** is predicted to increase the exposure to **anagrelide**. Moderate Theoretical
- **Osilodrostat** is predicted to increase the exposure to **anagrelide**. Moderate Theoretical → Also see TABLE 7 p. 1055
- Quinolones **(ciprofloxacin)** are predicted to increase the exposure to **anagrelide**. Moderate Theoretical
- **Rucaparib** is predicted to increase the exposure to **anagrelide**. Moderate Theoretical
- SSRIs **(fluvoxamine)** are predicted to increase the exposure to **anagrelide**. Moderate Theoretical → Also see TABLE 3 p. 1053
- **Vemurafenib** is predicted to increase the exposure to **anagrelide**. Moderate Theoretical → Also see TABLE 7 p. 1055

Anakinra

- **Anakinra** is predicted to increase the risk of generalised infection (possibly life-threatening) when given with **abatacept**. Severe Theoretical
- **Anakinra** is predicted to increase the risk of generalised infection (possibly life-threatening) when given with **etanercept**. Avoid. Severe Theoretical
- **Filgotinib** is predicted to increase the risk of immunosuppression when given with **anakinra**. Avoid. Severe Theoretical
- **Live vaccines** are predicted to increase the risk of generalised infection (possibly life-threatening) when given with **anakinra**. UKHSA advises avoid (refer to Green Book). Severe Theoretical
- Monoclonal antibodies **(certolizumab pegol)** are predicted to increase the risk of generalised infection (possibly life-threatening) when given with **anakinra**. Avoid. Severe Theoretical
- **Anakinra** is predicted to increase the risk of generalised infection (possibly life-threatening) when given with monoclonal antibodies **(golimumab)**. Avoid. Severe Theoretical

Andexanet alfa

- **Andexanet alfa** has been reported to affect the anticoagulant effect of **heparin**. Avoid. Severe Anecdotal
- **Andexanet alfa** is predicted to affect the anticoagulant effect of **low molecular-weight heparins**. Avoid. Severe Theoretical

Angiotensin-II receptor antagonists → see TABLE 6 p. 1054 (hypotension), TABLE 13 p. 1057 (increased serum potassium)

azilsartan · candesartan · eprosartan · irbesartan · losartan · olmesartan · telmisartan · valsartan

- **ACE inhibitors** increase the risk of renal impairment when given with **angiotensin-II receptor antagonists**. Avoid or monitor. Severe Study → Also see TABLE 6 p. 1054 → Also see TABLE 13 p. 1057
- **Angiotensin-II receptor antagonists** increase the risk of renal impairment when given with **aliskiren**. Avoid or monitor. Severe Study → Also see TABLE 6 p. 1054 → Also see TABLE 13 p. 1057
- **Telmisartan** is predicted to increase the exposure to **atogepant**. Adjust **atogepant** dose. Moderate Theoretical
- **Bulevirtide** is predicted to increase the exposure to angiotensin-II receptor antagonists **(olmesartan, telmisartan, valsartan)**. Avoid or monitor. Moderate Theoretical
- **Irbesartan** is predicted to affect the efficacy of **bulevirtide**. Avoid. Severe Theoretical
- **Angiotensin-II receptor antagonists** potentially increase the concentration of **lithium**. Avoid or monitor. Severe Anecdotal
- Taxanes **(cabazitaxel)** are predicted to affect the exposure to **valsartan**. Manufacturer advises take 12 hours before or 3 hours after **cabazitaxel**. Moderate Theoretical
- **Vadadustat** is predicted to increase the exposure to **olmesartan**. Monitor and adjust dose. Moderate Study

Anidulafungin → see TABLE 1 p. 1053 (hepatotoxicity)

Antacids

SEPARATION OF ADMINISTRATION Aluminium- and magnesium-containing antacids should preferably not be taken at the same time as other drugs since they might impair absorption. Aluminium- and magnesium-containing antacids might damage enteric coatings designed to prevent dissolution in the stomach.

- Oral **antacids** are predicted to decrease the absorption of oral alkylating agents **(estramustine)**. Avoid. Moderate Study
- Oral **antacids** decrease the absorption of oral antiepileptics **(gabapentin)**. Manufacturer advises take 2 hours after antacids. Moderate Study
- Oral **antacids** decrease the absorption of oral antifungals, azoles **(itraconazole)** capsules. Manufacturer advises take 2 hours before or 1 hour after antacids. Moderate Study
- Oral **antacids** decrease the absorption of oral antifungals, azoles **(ketoconazole)**. Separate administration by at least 2 hours. Moderate Study
- Oral **antacids** decrease the absorption of oral antihistamines, non-sedating **(fexofenadine)**. Separate administration by 2 hours. Mild Study
- Oral **antacids** are predicted to decrease the absorption of oral antimalarials **(chloroquine)**. Separate administration by at least 4 hours. Moderate Theoretical
- Oral **antacids** are predicted to decrease the absorption of oral antimalarials **(proguanil)**. Separate administration by at least 2 hours. Moderate Study
- Oral **antacids** decrease the absorption of oral **aspirin** (high-dose). Moderate Study
- Oral **antacids** might decrease the concentration of the active metabolite of oral **baloxavir marboxil**. Avoid. Severe Theoretical
- **Antacids** is predicted to decrease the exposure to **belumosudil**. Separate administration by 12 hours. Moderate Theoretical
- Oral **antacids** decrease the exposure to oral **bictegravir**. Separate administration by at least 2 hours. Moderate Study
- Oral **antacids** decrease the absorption of oral bisphosphonates **(alendronate)**. Manufacturer advises take at least 30 minutes before antacids. Moderate Study
- Oral **antacids** decrease the absorption of oral bisphosphonates **(clodronate)**. Avoid antacids for 2 hours before or 1 hour after **clodronate**. Moderate Study
- Oral **antacids** are predicted to decrease the absorption of oral bisphosphonates **(ibandronate)**. Avoid antacids for at least 6 hours before or 1 hour after **ibandronate**. Moderate Theoretical
- Oral **antacids** decrease the absorption of oral bisphosphonates **(risedronate)**. Separate administration by at least 2 hours. Moderate Study
- Oral **antacids** are predicted to decrease the absorption of oral **bosutinib**. Manufacturer advises take at least 12 hours before antacids. Moderate Theoretical
- Oral **antacids** are predicted to decrease the concentration of oral **cabotegravir**. Manufacturer advises take 4 hours before or 2 hours after antacids. Moderate Theoretical
- Oral **antacids** are predicted to decrease the absorption of oral **ceritinib**. Separate administration by 2 hours. Moderate Theoretical
- Oral **antacids** are predicted to decrease the absorption of oral **cholic acid**. Separate administration by 5 hours. Mild Theoretical
- Oral **antacids** are predicted to decrease the absorption of oral corticosteroids **(deflazacort)**. Separate administration by 2 hours. Moderate Theoretical
- Oral **antacids** decrease the absorption of oral corticosteroids **(dexamethasone)**. Moderate Study
- Oral **antacids** decrease the absorption of oral **dasatinib**. Separate administration by at least 2 hours. Moderate Study
- Oral **antacids** decrease the absorption of oral **digoxin**. Separate administration by 2 hours. Mild Study
- Oral **antacids** are predicted to decrease the absorption of oral **dipyridamole** (immediate release tablets). Moderate Theoretical
- Oral **antacids** decrease the exposure to oral **dolutegravir**. Manufacturer advises take 2 hours before or 6 hours after antacids. Moderate Study
- Oral **antacids** decrease the absorption of oral **eltrombopag**. Manufacturer advises take 2 hours before or 4 hours after antacids. Severe Study
- Oral **antacids** decrease the exposure to oral **elvitegravir**. Separate administration by at least 4 hours. Moderate Study
- Oral **antacids** are predicted to decrease the absorption of oral **erlotinib**. Manufacturer advises take 2 hours before or 4 hours after antacids. Moderate Theoretical
- Oral **antacids** decrease the exposure to oral fibrates **(gemfibrozil)**. Moderate Study

- Oral **antacids** are predicted to decrease the exposure to oral **gefitinib**. Moderate Theoretical
- Oral **antacids** are predicted to decrease the absorption of oral HIV-protease inhibitors **(atazanavir)**. Manufacturer advises take 2 hours before or 1 hour after antacids. Severe Theoretical
- Oral **antacids** are predicted to decrease the absorption of oral **hydroxychloroquine**. Separate administration by at least 4 hours. Moderate Theoretical
- Oral **antacids** decrease the absorption of oral **iron**. Manufacturer advises iron should be taken 1 hour before or 2 hours after antacids. Moderate Study
- Oral **antacids** is predicted to decrease the absorption of oral **lapatinib**. Avoid. Moderate Theoretical
- Oral **antacids** are predicted to decrease the exposure to oral **ledipasvir**. Separate administration by 4 hours. Moderate Theoretical
- Oral **antacids** decrease the exposure to oral **mycophenolate**. Moderate Study
- Oral **antacids** are predicted to decrease the exposure to oral **neratinib**. Separate administration by at least 3 hours. Mild Theoretical
- Oral **antacids** might affect the absorption of oral **nilotinib**. Separate administration by at least 2 hours. Moderate Theoretical
- Oral **antacids** are predicted to decrease the exposure to oral NNRTIs **(rilpivirine)**. Manufacturer advises take 4 hours before or 2 hours after antacids. Severe Theoretical
- Oral **antacids** are predicted to decrease the absorption of oral **pazopanib**. Manufacturer advises take 1 hour before or 2 hours after antacids. Moderate Theoretical
- Oral **antacids** decrease the absorption of oral **penicillamine**. Separate administration by 2 hours. Mild Study
- Oral **antacids** decrease the absorption of oral **phenothiazine antipsychotics**. Moderate Anecdotal
- Oral **antacids** increase the risk of metabolic alkalosis when given with oral **polystyrene sulfonate**. Severe Anecdotal
- Oral **antacids** decrease the absorption of oral **quinolones**. Manufacturer advises take 2 hours before or 4 hours after antacids. Moderate Study
- Oral **antacids** decrease the exposure to oral **raltegravir**. Avoid. Moderate Study
- Oral **antacids** decrease the absorption of oral rifamycins **(rifampicin)**. Manufacturer advises take 1 hour before antacids. Moderate Study
- Oral **antacids** decrease the exposure to oral **riociguat**. Manufacturer advises take 1 hour before or 2 hours after antacids. Mild Study
- Oral **antacids** might decrease the exposure to oral **roxadustat**. Manufacturer advises take at least 1 hour after antacids. Moderate Theoretical
- **Antacids** are predicted to decrease the exposure to **selpercatinib**. Moderate Theoretical
- Oral **antacids** are predicted to decrease the exposure to oral **sotorasib**. Manufacturer advises take 4 hours before or 10 hours after antacids. Moderate Theoretical
- Oral **antacids** decrease the absorption of oral statins **(rosuvastatin)**. Separate administration by 2 hours. Moderate Study
- Oral **antacids** decrease the absorption of oral **strontium**. Separate administration by 2 hours. Moderate Study
- Oral **antacids** decrease the absorption of oral **sulpiride**. Separate administration by 2 hours. Moderate Study
- Oral **antacids** greatly decrease the absorption of oral **tetracyclines**. Separate administration by 2 to 3 hours. Moderate Study
- Oral **antacids** are predicted to decrease the absorption of oral thyroid hormones **(levothyroxine)**. Separate administration by at least 4 hours. Moderate Anecdotal
- **Antacids** might decrease the efficacy of **ulipristal** for emergency hormonal contraception. For CoSRH guidance, see Contraceptives, interactions p. 614. Unknown Theoretical
- Oral **antacids** are predicted to decrease the absorption of oral **ursodeoxycholic acid**. Separate administration by 2 hours. Moderate Theoretical
- Oral **antacids** is predicted to decrease the exposure to oral **vadadustat**. Manufacturer advises take at least 1 hour before or 2 hours after antacids. Moderate Theoretical
- Oral **antacids** are predicted to decrease the concentration of oral **velpatasvir**. Separate administration by 4 hours. Moderate Theoretical

Antazoline → see antihistamines, sedating

Anthracyclines → see TABLE 12 p. 1057 (myelosuppression)

daunorubicin · doxorubicin · epirubicin · idarubicin · mitoxantrone · pixantrone

GENERAL INFORMATION Caution is necessary with concurrent use of **anthracyclines** with cardiotoxic drugs, or drugs that reduce cardiac contractility.

- Calcium-channel blockers **(verapamil)** moderately increase the exposure to **doxorubicin**. Moderate Study
- **Ciclosporin** increases the concentration of anthracyclines **(daunorubicin, doxorubicin, epirubicin, idarubicin, mitoxantrone)**. Severe Study
- H_2 receptor antagonists **(cimetidine)** slightly increase the exposure to **epirubicin**. Avoid. Moderate Study
- **Leflunomide** is predicted to increase the exposure to anthracyclines **(daunorubicin, doxorubicin, mitoxantrone)**. Moderate Theoretical → Also see TABLE 12 p. 1057
- **Live vaccines** are predicted to increase the risk of generalised infection (possibly life-threatening) when given with **anthracyclines**. UKHSA advises avoid (refer to Green Book). Severe Theoretical
- **Anthracyclines** are predicted to increase the risk of cardiotoxicity when given with monoclonal antibodies **(trastuzumab, trastuzumab emtansine)**. Avoid. Severe Theoretical → Also see TABLE 12 p. 1057
- **Anthracyclines** are predicted to increase the risk of cardiotoxicity when given with monoclonal antibodies **(trastuzumab deruxtecan)**. Severe Theoretical → Also see TABLE 12 p. 1057
- **Pirtobrutinib** is predicted to increase the exposure to **mitoxantrone**. Moderate Theoretical
- **Teriflunomide** is predicted to increase the exposure to anthracyclines **(daunorubicin, doxorubicin, mitoxantrone)**. Moderate Theoretical

Anti-androgens → see TABLE 1 p. 1053 (hepatotoxicity), TABLE 7 p. 1055 (QT-interval prolongation)

abiraterone · apalutamide · bicalutamide · cyproterone · darolutamide · enzalutamide · flutamide

GENERAL INFORMATION Caution with concurrent chemotherapy—safety and efficacy with **abiraterone** and **enzalutamide** not established.

- Anti-androgens **(apalutamide, enzalutamide)** are predicted to decrease the exposure to 5-HT3-receptor antagonists **(ondansetron)**. Moderate Study → Also see TABLE 7 p. 1055
- Anti-androgens **(apalutamide, enzalutamide)** are predicted to markedly decrease the exposure to **abemaciclib**. Avoid. Severe Study
- Anti-androgens **(apalutamide, enzalutamide)** are predicted to decrease the exposure to **abrocitinib**. Avoid. Moderate Study
- Anti-androgens **(apalutamide, enzalutamide)** are predicted to decrease the exposure to **acalabrutinib**. Avoid. Severe Study
- **Apalutamide** is predicted to decrease the exposure to **aliskiren**. Monitor and adjust dose. Moderate Study
- Anti-androgens **(apalutamide, enzalutamide)** are predicted to decrease the exposure to **alpelisib**. Avoid. Moderate Study
- **Darolutamide** is predicted to increase the exposure to **alpelisib**. Moderate Theoretical
- Anti-androgens **(apalutamide, enzalutamide)** are predicted to decrease the exposure to anti-androgens **(abiraterone)**. Avoid. Severe Study
- Anti-androgens **(apalutamide)** are predicted to decrease the exposure to anti-androgens **(darolutamide)**. Avoid. Moderate Study
- Anti-androgens **(enzalutamide)** are predicted to decrease the exposure to anti-androgens **(darolutamide)**. Avoid. Moderate Study

A1 Interactions | Appendix 1

Anti-androgens (continued)

- Anti-androgens **(apalutamide, enzalutamide)** are predicted to decrease the exposure to antiarrhythmics **(disopyramide, dronedarone)**. Avoid. Severe Study → Also see **TABLE 7** p. 1055
- Anti-androgens **(apalutamide, enzalutamide)** are predicted to decrease the efficacy of antiarrhythmics **(propafenone)**. Moderate Study
- Anti-androgens **(apalutamide, enzalutamide)** are predicted to decrease the exposure to anticholinesterases, centrally acting **(donepezil)**. Mild Study
- Antiepileptics **(carbamazepine, eslicarbazepine, fosphenytoin, oxcarbazepine, perampanel, phenobarbital, phenytoin, primidone, rufinamide, topiramate)** are predicted to decrease the efficacy of **cyproterone** with ethinylestradiol (co-cyprindiol). Use alternative methods during treatment with, and for 28 days after, the enzyme inducing drug is stopped. Severe Study
- Antiepileptics **(carbamazepine, fosphenytoin, phenobarbital, phenytoin, primidone)** are predicted to decrease the exposure to **abiraterone**. Avoid. Severe Study
- Antiepileptics **(carbamazepine, fosphenytoin, phenobarbital, phenytoin, primidone)** are predicted to decrease the exposure to **darolutamide**. Avoid. Moderate Study
- **Enzalutamide** is predicted to slightly decrease the exposure to antiepileptics **(brivaracetam)**. Moderate Theoretical
- Anti-androgens **(apalutamide, enzalutamide)** are predicted to decrease the exposure to antiepileptics **(perampanel)**. Monitor and adjust dose. Moderate Study
- **Apalutamide** potentially decreases the exposure to antiepileptics **(valproate)**. Mild Theoretical
- **Enzalutamide** is predicted to affect the exposure to antiepileptics **(valproate)**. Use with caution or avoid. Moderate Theoretical
- Antifungals, azoles **(itraconazole)** slightly increase the exposure to **darolutamide**. Monitor and adjust dose. Moderate Study
- Antifungals, azoles **(itraconazole, ketoconazole, posaconazole, voriconazole)** are predicted to increase the exposure to **apalutamide**. Monitor and adjust dose. Mild Study → Also see **TABLE 7** p. 1055
- Antifungals, azoles **(ketoconazole)** are predicted to increase the exposure to **darolutamide**. Monitor and adjust dose. Moderate Theoretical
- Anti-androgens **(apalutamide, enzalutamide)** are predicted to decrease the exposure to antifungals, azoles **(isavuconazole)**. Avoid. Severe Study
- **Apalutamide** slightly decreases the exposure to antihistamines, non-sedating **(fexofenadine)**. Mild Study
- **Darolutamide** is predicted to increase the concentration of antihistamines, non-sedating **(fexofenadine)**. Moderate Theoretical
- Anti-androgens **(apalutamide, enzalutamide)** are predicted to decrease the exposure to antimalarials **(artemether)** with lumefantrine. Avoid. Severe Study → Also see **TABLE 7** p. 1055
- Anti-androgens **(apalutamide, enzalutamide)** are predicted to decrease the concentration of antimalarials **(piperaquine)**. Avoid. Moderate Theoretical
- **Darolutamide** is predicted to increase the exposure to **atogepant**. Adjust **atogepant** dose. Moderate Theoretical
- Anti-androgens **(apalutamide, enzalutamide)** are predicted to moderately decrease the exposure to atypical antipsychotics **(aripiprazole)**. Avoid or adjust dose—consult product literature. Moderate Study
- Anti-androgens **(apalutamide, enzalutamide)** are predicted to decrease the exposure to atypical antipsychotics **(cariprazine)**. Avoid. Severe Theoretical
- **Enzalutamide** is predicted to decrease the exposure to atypical antipsychotics **(clozapine)**. Moderate Theoretical
- Anti-androgens **(apalutamide, enzalutamide)** are predicted to decrease the exposure to atypical antipsychotics **(lurasidone)**. Avoid. Moderate Study
- Anti-androgens **(apalutamide, enzalutamide)** are predicted to decrease the exposure to atypical antipsychotics **(paliperidone)**. Monitor and adjust dose. Severe Study → Also see **TABLE 7** p. 1055
- Anti-androgens **(apalutamide, enzalutamide)** are predicted to decrease the exposure to atypical antipsychotics **(quetiapine)**. Moderate Study
- Anti-androgens **(apalutamide, enzalutamide)** are predicted to decrease the exposure to atypical antipsychotics **(risperidone)**. Adjust dose. Moderate Study
- Anti-androgens **(apalutamide, enzalutamide)** are predicted to decrease the exposure to **avacopan**. Avoid or monitor. Severe Study
- Anti-androgens **(apalutamide, enzalutamide)** are predicted to decrease the exposure to **avapritinib**. Avoid. Severe Study
- **Enzalutamide** is predicted to decrease the exposure to **avatrombopag**. Adjust **avatrombopag** dose with moderate CYP2C9 inducers in chronic immune thrombocytopenia. Moderate Study
- Anti-androgens **(apalutamide, enzalutamide)** are predicted to decrease the exposure to **axitinib**. Avoid or adjust dose. Moderate Study
- Anti-androgens **(apalutamide, enzalutamide)** decrease the exposure to **bedaquiline**. Avoid. Severe Study → Also see **TABLE 7** p. 1055
- Anti-androgens **(apalutamide, enzalutamide)** are predicted to decrease the exposure to **belumosudil**. Adjust **belumosudil** dose, p. 650. Severe Study
- Anti-androgens **(apalutamide, enzalutamide)** are predicted to decrease the exposure to benzodiazepines **(alprazolam)**. Adjust dose. Moderate Theoretical
- **Enzalutamide** is predicted to affect the exposure to benzodiazepines **(clonazepam)**. Use with caution or avoid. Moderate Theoretical
- **Apalutamide** is predicted to decrease the exposure to benzodiazepines **(diazepam)**. Avoid or monitor. Mild Study
- Anti-androgens **(apalutamide, enzalutamide)** are predicted to decrease the exposure to benzodiazepines **(midazolam)**. Monitor and adjust dose. Severe Study
- **Enzalutamide** is predicted to affect the exposure to beta blockers, non-selective **(propranolol)**. Use with caution or avoid. Moderate Theoretical
- **Enzalutamide** is predicted to affect the exposure to beta blockers, selective **(bisoprolol)**. Use with caution or avoid. Moderate Theoretical
- **Abiraterone** is predicted to increase the exposure to beta blockers, selective **(metoprolol)**. Moderate Study
- **Apalutamide** is predicted to decrease the exposure to $beta_2$ agonists **(salmeterol)**. Avoid or monitor. Moderate Study
- Anti-androgens **(apalutamide, enzalutamide)** are predicted to decrease the exposure to **bictegravir**. Avoid. Moderate Study
- Anti-androgens **(apalutamide, enzalutamide)** slightly decrease the exposure to **bortezomib**. Avoid. Severe Study
- Anti-androgens **(apalutamide, enzalutamide)** are predicted to very markedly decrease the exposure to **bosutinib**. Avoid. Severe Study → Also see **TABLE 7** p. 1055
- Anti-androgens **(apalutamide, enzalutamide)** are predicted to decrease the exposure to **brigatinib**. Avoid. Severe Study
- Anti-androgens **(apalutamide, enzalutamide)** are predicted to decrease the exposure to **buspirone**. Use with caution and adjust dose. Severe Study
- Anti-androgens **(apalutamide, enzalutamide)** moderately decrease the exposure to **cabozantinib**. Avoid. Moderate Study → Also see **TABLE 7** p. 1055
- Anti-androgens **(apalutamide, enzalutamide)** are predicted to decrease the exposure to calcium-channel blockers **(amlodipine, felodipine, lacidipine, lercanidipine, nicardipine, nifedipine, nimodipine)**. Monitor and adjust dose. Moderate Study
- **Enzalutamide** is predicted to decrease the exposure to calcium-channel blockers **(diltiazem, verapamil)**. Severe Study
- Anti-androgens **(apalutamide, enzalutamide)** are predicted to decrease the exposure to **cannabidiol**. Adjust dose. Moderate Study
- Anti-androgens **(apalutamide, enzalutamide)** are predicted to decrease the exposure to **capivasertib**. Avoid. Moderate Study
- **Cenobamate** is predicted to decrease the exposure to **darolutamide**. Avoid. Moderate Theoretical
- Anti-androgens **(apalutamide, enzalutamide)** are predicted to decrease the exposure to **ceritinib**. Avoid. Severe Study → Also see **TABLE 7** p. 1055
- **Ceritinib** is predicted to increase the exposure to **apalutamide**. Monitor and adjust dose. Mild Study → Also see **TABLE 7** p. 1055

- Anti-androgens **(apalutamide, enzalutamide)** decrease the concentration of **ciclosporin**. Severe Study
- Anti-androgens **(apalutamide, enzalutamide)** are predicted to alter the effects of **cilostazol**. Moderate Theoretical
- Anti-androgens **(apalutamide, enzalutamide)** are predicted to decrease the exposure to **cinacalcet**. Monitor and adjust dose. Moderate Study
- **Darolutamide** is predicted to increase the exposure to **cladribine**. Avoid or adjust dose. Moderate Theoretical
- Anti-androgens **(apalutamide, enzalutamide)** decrease the exposure to **clomethiazole**. Monitor and adjust dose. Moderate Study
- **Clopidogrel** is predicted to increase the exposure to **apalutamide** and **apalutamide** is predicted to increase the exposure to the active metabolite of **clopidogrel**. Avoid or monitor. Moderate Study
- **Clopidogrel** moderately increases the exposure to **enzalutamide**. Avoid or adjust **enzalutamide** dose. Severe Study
- Anti-androgens **(apalutamide, enzalutamide)** are predicted to decrease the exposure to **cobicistat**. Avoid. Severe Study
- **Cobicistat** is predicted to increase the exposure to **apalutamide**. Monitor and adjust dose. Mild Study
- Anti-androgens **(apalutamide, enzalutamide)** are predicted to decrease the exposure to **cobimetinib**. Avoid. Severe Theoretical
- **Apalutamide** is predicted to decrease the exposure to **colchicine**. Mild Study
- Anti-androgens **(apalutamide, enzalutamide)** are predicted to decrease the exposure to corticosteroids **(budesonide, deflazacort, dexamethasone, fludrocortisone, hydrocortisone, methylprednisolone, prednisolone, triamcinolone)**. Monitor and adjust dose. Moderate Study
- Anti-androgens **(apalutamide, enzalutamide)** are predicted to decrease the exposure to corticosteroids **(fluticasone)**. Unknown Theoretical
- **Apalutamide** is predicted to decrease the exposure to **coumarins**. Avoid or monitor. Mild Study
- **Enzalutamide** potentially decreases the exposure to **coumarins**. Avoid or adjust dose and monitor INR. Severe Study
- Anti-androgens **(apalutamide, enzalutamide)** are predicted to markedly decrease the exposure to **crizotinib**. Avoid. Severe Study → Also see TABLE 7 p. 1055
- Anti-androgens **(apalutamide, enzalutamide)** are predicted to decrease the exposure to **dabrafenib**. Avoid. Moderate Theoretical
- **Dabrafenib** is predicted to decrease the exposure to **darolutamide**. Avoid. Moderate Theoretical
- Anti-androgens **(apalutamide, enzalutamide)** are predicted to decrease the exposure to **daridorexant**. Severe Study
- Anti-androgens **(apalutamide, enzalutamide)** are predicted to decrease the exposure to **darifenacin**. Moderate Theoretical
- Anti-androgens **(apalutamide, enzalutamide)** are predicted to markedly decrease the exposure to **dasatinib**. Avoid. Severe Study → Also see TABLE 7 p. 1055
- Anti-androgens **(apalutamide, enzalutamide)** are predicted to slightly decrease the exposure to **delamanid**. Avoid. Moderate Study → Also see TABLE 7 p. 1055
- Anti-androgens **(apalutamide, enzalutamide)** are predicted to decrease the exposure to **deutivacaftor**. Avoid. Severe Theoretical
- Anti-androgens **(apalutamide, enzalutamide)** are predicted to markedly decrease the exposure to **dienogest**. Severe Study
- **Apalutamide** is predicted to decrease the exposure to **digoxin**. Mild Study
- **Enzalutamide** is predicted to increase the exposure to **digoxin**. Use with caution or avoid. Moderate Theoretical
- Anti-androgens **(apalutamide, enzalutamide)** are predicted to decrease the exposure to dipeptidylpeptidase-4 inhibitors **(linagliptin)**. Moderate Study
- Anti-androgens **(apalutamide, enzalutamide)** are predicted to moderately decrease the exposure to dipeptidylpeptidase-4 inhibitors **(saxagliptin)**. Moderate Study
- Anti-androgens **(apalutamide, enzalutamide)** are predicted to decrease the exposure to **dolutegravir**. Severe Study
- Anti-androgens **(apalutamide, enzalutamide)** are predicted to decrease the exposure to **dronabinol**. Avoid or adjust dose. Mild Study
- Anti-androgens **(apalutamide, enzalutamide)** are predicted to decrease the exposure to **elacestrant**. Avoid or adjust dose depending on duration—consult product literature. Severe Study
- Anti-androgens **(apalutamide, enzalutamide)** are predicted to decrease the exposure to **elbasvir**. Avoid. Severe Study
- Anti-androgens **(apalutamide, enzalutamide)** is predicted to decrease the exposure to **elexacaftor**. Avoid. Severe Theoretical
- **Abiraterone** is predicted to increase the exposure to **eliglustat**. Avoid or adjust dose—consult product literature. Severe Study
- Anti-androgens **(apalutamide, enzalutamide)** are predicted to decrease the exposure to **eliglustat**. Avoid. Severe Study
- Anti-androgens **(apalutamide, enzalutamide)** are predicted to decrease the concentration of **elvitegravir**. Avoid. Severe Study
- **Encorafenib** is predicted to decrease the exposure to **abiraterone**. Avoid. Severe Study
- Anti-androgens **(apalutamide, enzalutamide)** are predicted to decrease the exposure to **encorafenib**. Severe Theoretical → Also see TABLE 7 p. 1055
- **Encorafenib** is predicted to decrease the exposure to **darolutamide**. Avoid. Moderate Study
- Endothelin receptor antagonists **(bosentan)** are predicted to decrease the efficacy of **cyproterone** with ethinylestradiol (co-cyprindiol). Use alternative methods during treatment with, and for 28 days after, the enzyme inducing drug is stopped. Severe Study
- Endothelin receptor antagonists **(bosentan)** are predicted to decrease the exposure to **darolutamide**. Avoid. Moderate Theoretical
- Anti-androgens **(apalutamide, enzalutamide)** affect the exposure to endothelin receptor antagonists **(bosentan)**. Avoid. Severe Study
- Anti-androgens **(apalutamide, enzalutamide)** are predicted to decrease the exposure to endothelin receptor antagonists **(macitentan)**. Avoid. Severe Study
- Anti-androgens **(apalutamide, enzalutamide)** are predicted to decrease the exposure to the cytotoxic component of **enfortumab vedotin**. Moderate Theoretical
- Anti-androgens **(apalutamide, enzalutamide)** are predicted to decrease the exposure to **entrectinib**. Avoid. Severe Study → Also see TABLE 7 p. 1055
- Anti-androgens **(apalutamide, enzalutamide)** are predicted to decrease the exposure to **erdafitinib**. Avoid. Severe Study
- Anti-androgens **(apalutamide, enzalutamide)** are predicted to decrease the exposure to **erlotinib**. Avoid or adjust dose—consult product literature. Severe Study
- Anti-androgens **(apalutamide, enzalutamide)** are predicted to decrease the exposure to **esketamine**. Adjust dose. Moderate Study
- Anti-androgens **(apalutamide, enzalutamide)** are predicted to decrease the exposure to **eszopiclone**. Adjust dose. Moderate Theoretical
- **Enzalutamide** is predicted to decrease the exposure to **etrasimod**. Avoid. Severe Theoretical
- Anti-androgens **(apalutamide, enzalutamide)** are predicted to decrease the concentration of **everolimus**. Avoid or adjust dose. Severe Study
- Anti-androgens **(apalutamide, enzalutamide)** moderately decrease the exposure to **exemestane**. Moderate Study
- Anti-androgens **(apalutamide, enzalutamide)** are predicted to decrease the exposure to factor XA inhibitors **(apixaban)**. Moderate Study
- **Apalutamide** is predicted to decrease the exposure to factor XA inhibitors **(edoxaban)**. Monitor and adjust dose. Moderate Study
- Anti-androgens **(apalutamide, enzalutamide)** are predicted to decrease the exposure to factor XA inhibitors **(rivaroxaban)**. Avoid unless patient can be monitored for signs of thrombosis. Moderate Study
- Anti-androgens **(apalutamide, enzalutamide)** are predicted to decrease the exposure to **fedratinib**. Avoid. Moderate Study
- Anti-androgens **(apalutamide, enzalutamide)** are predicted to decrease the exposure to **fenfluramine**. Moderate Theoretical

Anti-androgens (continued)

- Anti-androgens **(apalutamide, enzalutamide)** are predicted to decrease the exposure to **fesoterodine**. Avoid. Moderate Study
- Fibrates **(gemfibrozil)** slightly increase the exposure to **apalutamide**. Mild Study
- Fibrates **(gemfibrozil)** moderately increase the exposure to **enzalutamide**. Avoid or adjust **enzalutamide** dose. Severe Study
- Anti-androgens **(apalutamide, enzalutamide)** are predicted to decrease the exposure to **fostamatinib**. Avoid. Severe Study
- Anti-androgens **(apalutamide, enzalutamide)** are predicted to decrease the exposure to the active metabolite of **fostemsavir**. Avoid. Severe Study
- Anti-androgens **(apalutamide, enzalutamide)** are predicted to decrease the exposure to **fruquintinib**. Avoid. Moderate Study
- Anti-androgens **(apalutamide, enzalutamide)** are predicted to decrease the exposure to **gefitinib**. Avoid. Severe Study
- **Enzalutamide** is predicted to increase the exposure to **gilteritinib**. Moderate Theoretical
- Anti-androgens **(apalutamide, enzalutamide)** are predicted to decrease the exposure to **glasdegib**. Avoid. Severe Study → Also see TABLE 7 p. 1055
- **Enzalutamide** is predicted to greatly decrease the concentration of **glecaprevir**. Avoid. Severe Study
- Anti-androgens **(apalutamide, enzalutamide)** are predicted to decrease the exposure to **grazoprevir**. Avoid. Severe Study
- **Darolutamide** is predicted to increase the exposure to **grazoprevir**. Avoid. Severe Theoretical
- Anti-androgens **(apalutamide, enzalutamide)** are predicted to decrease the concentration of **guanfacine**. Adjust **guanfacine** dose, p. 281. Moderate Study
- Anti-androgens **(apalutamide, enzalutamide)** decrease the concentration of **haloperidol**. Adjust dose. Moderate Study → Also see TABLE 7 p. 1055
- **HIV-protease inhibitors** are predicted to increase the exposure to **apalutamide**. Monitor and adjust dose. Mild Study
- HIV-protease inhibitors **(lopinavir, ritonavir)** are predicted to increase the exposure to **darolutamide**. Monitor and adjust dose. Moderate Theoretical
- HIV-protease inhibitors **(ritonavir)** are predicted to decrease the efficacy of **cyproterone** with ethinylestradiol (co-cyprindiol). Use alternative methods during treatment with, and for 28 days after, the enzyme inducing drug is stopped. Severe Study
- **Enzalutamide** is predicted to affect the exposure to HIV-protease inhibitors **(ritonavir)**. Use with caution or avoid. Moderate Theoretical
- Anti-androgens **(apalutamide, enzalutamide)** are predicted to decrease the exposure to **ibrutinib**. Avoid or monitor. Severe Study
- Anti-androgens **(apalutamide, enzalutamide)** are predicted to decrease the exposure to **idelalisib**. Avoid. Severe Study
- **Idelalisib** is predicted to increase the exposure to **apalutamide**. Monitor and adjust dose. Mild Study
- Anti-androgens **(apalutamide, enzalutamide)** are predicted to decrease the exposure to **imatinib**. Avoid. Moderate Study
- Anti-androgens **(apalutamide, enzalutamide)** are predicted to decrease the exposure to **irinotecan**. Avoid. Severe Study
- Anti-androgens **(apalutamide, enzalutamide)** are predicted to decrease the exposure to **ivabradine**. Adjust dose. Moderate Theoretical
- Anti-androgens **(apalutamide, enzalutamide)** are predicted to decrease the exposure to **ivacaftor**. Avoid. Severe Study
- **Ivosidenib** is predicted to decrease the exposure to **abiraterone**. Avoid. Severe Study
- Anti-androgens **(apalutamide, enzalutamide)** are predicted to decrease the exposure to **ivosidenib**. Avoid. Severe Theoretical → Also see TABLE 7 p. 1055
- **Ivosidenib** is predicted to decrease the exposure to **darolutamide**. Avoid. Moderate Study
- Anti-androgens **(apalutamide, enzalutamide)** are predicted to decrease the exposure to **ixazomib**. Avoid. Severe Study
- Anti-androgens **(apalutamide, enzalutamide)** are predicted to decrease the exposure to **ketamine**. Adjust dose. Moderate Theoretical
- Anti-androgens **(apalutamide, enzalutamide)** are predicted to decrease the exposure to **lapatinib**. Avoid. Severe Study → Also see TABLE 7 p. 1055
- Anti-androgens **(apalutamide, enzalutamide)** are predicted to moderately decrease the exposure to **larotrectinib**. Avoid. Moderate Study
- Anti-androgens **(apalutamide, enzalutamide)** are predicted to decrease the exposure to **lazertinib**. Avoid. Severe Study
- Anti-androgens **(apalutamide, enzalutamide)** are predicted to decrease the exposure to **lenacapavir**. Avoid. Severe Study
- Anti-androgens **(apalutamide, enzalutamide)** are predicted to decrease the exposure to **leniolisib**. Avoid. Severe Theoretical
- Anti-androgens **(apalutamide, enzalutamide)** are predicted to decrease the exposure to **lomitapide**. Monitor and adjust dose. Moderate Theoretical
- **Bicalutamide** is predicted to increase the exposure to **lomitapide**. Separate administration by 12 hours. Moderate Theoretical
- **Apalutamide** is predicted to decrease the exposure to **loperamide**. Monitor and adjust dose. Moderate Study
- Anti-androgens **(apalutamide, enzalutamide)** are predicted to decrease the exposure to **lorlatinib**. Avoid. Severe Study
- **Lorlatinib** is predicted to decrease the exposure to **darolutamide**. Avoid. Moderate Theoretical
- **Lumacaftor** is predicted to decrease the exposure to **abiraterone**. Avoid. Severe Study
- **Lumacaftor** is predicted to decrease the exposure to **darolutamide**. Avoid. Moderate Study
- Macrolides **(clarithromycin)** are predicted to increase the exposure to **apalutamide**. Monitor and adjust dose. Mild Study
- Macrolides **(clarithromycin)** are predicted to increase the exposure to **darolutamide**. Monitor and adjust dose. Moderate Theoretical
- **Enzalutamide** is predicted to affect the exposure to macrolides **(clarithromycin)**. Use with caution or avoid. Moderate Theoretical
- Anti-androgens **(apalutamide, enzalutamide)** are predicted to decrease the exposure to **maraviroc**. Adjust dose. Severe Study
- Anti-androgens **(apalutamide, enzalutamide)** are predicted to decrease the exposure to **maribavir**. Avoid or adjust **maribavir** dose. Severe Study
- Anti-androgens **(apalutamide, enzalutamide)** are predicted to decrease the exposure to **mavacamten**. Monitor and adjust dose—consult product literature. Severe Theoretical
- **Abiraterone** is predicted to increase the exposure to meglitinides **(repaglinide)**. Moderate Anecdotal
- **Darolutamide** is predicted to increase the concentration of meglitinides **(repaglinide)**. Moderate Theoretical
- Anti-androgens **(apalutamide, enzalutamide)** are predicted to decrease the exposure to meglitinides **(repaglinide)**. Monitor blood glucose and adjust dose. Moderate Study
- **Apalutamide** is predicted to decrease the exposure to **methotrexate**. Mild Study
- **Darolutamide** is predicted to increase the concentration of **methotrexate**. Moderate Theoretical
- Anti-androgens **(apalutamide, enzalutamide)** are predicted to decrease the exposure to **midostaurin**. Avoid. Severe Study
- Anti-androgens **(apalutamide, enzalutamide)** are predicted to decrease the exposure to **mifepristone**. Adjust **mifepristone** dose. Severe Study
- Mineralocorticoid receptor antagonists **(spironolactone)** might oppose the effects of **abiraterone**. Avoid. Severe Anecdotal
- Anti-androgens **(apalutamide, enzalutamide)** are predicted to decrease the exposure to mineralocorticoid receptor antagonists **(eplerenone)**. Avoid. Moderate Theoretical
- Anti-androgens **(apalutamide, enzalutamide)** are predicted to decrease the exposure to mineralocorticoid receptor antagonists **(finerenone)**. Avoid. Severe Study
- Anti-androgens **(apalutamide, enzalutamide)** are predicted to decrease the exposure to **mirtazapine**. Adjust dose. Moderate Study
- **Mitotane** is predicted to decrease the exposure to **abiraterone**. Avoid. Severe Study
- **Mitotane** is predicted to decrease the exposure to **darolutamide**. Avoid. Moderate Study

- **Apalutamide** is predicted to decrease the exposure to **moclobemide**. Avoid or monitor. Mild Study
- **Modafinil** is predicted to decrease the efficacy of **cyproterone** with ethinylestradiol (co-cyprindiol). Use alternative methods during treatment with, and for 28 days after, the enzyme inducing drug is stopped. Severe Study
- **Darolutamide** is predicted to increase the exposure to **momelotinib**. Moderate Study
- Anti-androgens **(apalutamide, enzalutamide)** are predicted to decrease the exposure to monoclonal antibodies **(polatuzumab vedotin)**. Moderate Theoretical
- Anti-androgens **(apalutamide, enzalutamide)** are predicted to decrease the exposure to the cytotoxic component of monoclonal antibodies **(trastuzumab emtansine)**. Severe Theoretical
- Anti-androgens **(apalutamide, enzalutamide)** are predicted to decrease the exposure to **montelukast**. Mild Study
- Anti-androgens **(apalutamide, enzalutamide)** are predicted to markedly decrease the exposure to **naldemedine**. Avoid. Severe Study
- Anti-androgens **(apalutamide, enzalutamide)** are predicted to markedly decrease the exposure to **naloxegol**. Avoid. Moderate Study
- Anti-androgens **(apalutamide, enzalutamide)** are predicted to decrease the exposure to **neratinib**. Avoid. Severe Study
- Neurokinin-1 receptor antagonists **(aprepitant, fosaprepitant)** are predicted to decrease the efficacy of **cyproterone** with ethinylestradiol (co-cyprindiol). Use alternative methods during treatment with, and for 28 days after, the enzyme inducing drug is stopped. Severe Study
- Anti-androgens **(apalutamide, enzalutamide)** are predicted to markedly decrease the exposure to neurokinin-1 receptor antagonists **(aprepitant)**. Avoid. Moderate Study
- Anti-androgens **(apalutamide, enzalutamide)** are predicted to decrease the exposure to neurokinin-1 receptor antagonists **(fosaprepitant)**. Avoid. Moderate Theoretical
- Anti-androgens **(apalutamide, enzalutamide)** are predicted to decrease the exposure to neurokinin-1 receptor antagonists **(netupitant)**. Avoid. Severe Study
- Anti-androgens **(apalutamide, enzalutamide)** are predicted to moderately decrease the exposure to **nilotinib**. Avoid. Severe Study → Also see TABLE 7 p. 1055
- Anti-androgens **(apalutamide, enzalutamide)** are predicted to decrease the exposure to **nirmatrelvir** boosted with ritonavir. Avoid. Severe Study
- Anti-androgens **(apalutamide, enzalutamide)** are predicted to decrease the exposure to **nitisinone**. Adjust dose. Moderate Theoretical
- NNRTIs **(efavirenz, etravirine, nevirapine)** are predicted to decrease the exposure to **darolutamide**. Avoid. Moderate Theoretical
- NNRTIs **(efavirenz, nevirapine)** are predicted to decrease the efficacy of **cyproterone** with ethinylestradiol (co-cyprindiol). Use alternative methods during treatment with, and for 28 days after, the enzyme inducing drug is stopped. Severe Study
- Anti-androgens **(apalutamide, enzalutamide)** are predicted to decrease the exposure to NNRTIs **(doravirine)**. Avoid. Severe Study
- Anti-androgens **(apalutamide, enzalutamide)** are predicted to decrease the exposure to NNRTIs **(etravirine)**. Avoid. Severe Theoretical
- Anti-androgens **(apalutamide, enzalutamide)** are predicted to decrease the exposure to NNRTIs **(nevirapine)**. Severe Study
- Anti-androgens **(apalutamide, enzalutamide)** markedly decrease the exposure to NNRTIs **(rilpivirine)**. Avoid. Severe Study
- Anti-androgens **(apalutamide, enzalutamide)** are predicted to decrease the exposure to **olaparib**. Avoid. Moderate Theoretical
- Anti-androgens **(apalutamide, enzalutamide)** are predicted to decrease the exposure to **omaveloxolone**. Avoid. Severe Study
- Anti-androgens **(apalutamide, enzalutamide)** are predicted to decrease the exposure to opioids **(alfentanil, fentanyl)**. Moderate Study
- Anti-androgens **(apalutamide, enzalutamide)** are predicted to decrease the exposure to opioids **(buprenorphine)**. Monitor and adjust dose. Moderate Theoretical
- Anti-androgens **(apalutamide, enzalutamide)** decrease the exposure to opioids **(methadone)**. Monitor and adjust dose. Severe Study → Also see TABLE 7 p. 1055
- Anti-androgens **(apalutamide, enzalutamide)** are predicted to decrease the exposure to opioids **(oxycodone)**. Monitor and adjust dose. Moderate Study
- **Enzalutamide** is predicted to affect the exposure to opioids **(tramadol)**. Use with caution or avoid. Moderate Theoretical
- Anti-androgens **(apalutamide, enzalutamide)** are predicted to decrease the exposure to **osilodrostat**. Moderate Theoretical → Also see TABLE 7 p. 1055
- Anti-androgens **(apalutamide, enzalutamide)** are predicted to moderately decrease the exposure to **osimertinib**. Avoid. Moderate Study → Also see TABLE 7 p. 1055
- Anti-androgens **(apalutamide, enzalutamide)** are predicted to moderately decrease the exposure to **ospemifene**. Moderate Study
- Anti-androgens **(apalutamide, enzalutamide)** are predicted to decrease the exposure to **palbociclib**. Avoid. Severe Study
- Anti-androgens **(apalutamide, enzalutamide)** are predicted to decrease the exposure to **panobinostat**. Avoid. Moderate Theoretical → Also see TABLE 7 p. 1055
- Anti-androgens **(apalutamide, enzalutamide)** are predicted to decrease the exposure to **pazopanib**. Avoid. Severe Theoretical → Also see TABLE 7 p. 1055
- Anti-androgens **(apalutamide, enzalutamide)** are predicted to decrease the exposure to **pemigatinib**. Avoid. Severe Study
- Anti-androgens **(apalutamide, enzalutamide)** moderately decrease the exposure to phosphodiesterase type-4 inhibitors **(apremilast)**. Avoid. Severe Study
- Anti-androgens **(apalutamide, enzalutamide)** are predicted to decrease the exposure to phosphodiesterase type-4 inhibitors **(roflumilast)**. Avoid. Moderate Study
- Anti-androgens **(apalutamide, enzalutamide)** are predicted to decrease the exposure to phosphodiesterase type-5 inhibitors **(avanafil, tadalafil)**. Avoid. Severe Study
- Anti-androgens **(apalutamide, enzalutamide)** are predicted to decrease the exposure to phosphodiesterase type-5 inhibitors **(sildenafil, vardenafil)**. Moderate Theoretical → Also see TABLE 7 p. 1055
- Anti-androgens **(apalutamide, enzalutamide)** are predicted to moderately to markedly decrease the exposure to **pibrentasvir**. Avoid. Severe Study
- **Abiraterone** slightly increases the exposure to **pioglitazone**. Moderate Study
- Anti-androgens **(apalutamide, enzalutamide)** are predicted to decrease the exposure to **pirtobrutinib**. Avoid. Moderate Study
- Anti-androgens **(apalutamide, enzalutamide)** are predicted to moderately decrease the exposure to **pitolisant**. Moderate Study
- Anti-androgens **(apalutamide, enzalutamide)** are predicted to decrease the exposure to **ponatinib**. Avoid. Moderate Theoretical
- Anti-androgens **(apalutamide, enzalutamide)** are predicted to decrease the exposure to **pralsetinib**. Avoid or adjust dose with potent CYP3A4 inducers—consult product literature. Moderate Study
- Anti-androgens **(apalutamide, enzalutamide)** are predicted to markedly decrease the exposure to **praziquantel**. Avoid. Moderate Study
- **Apalutamide** is predicted to decrease the exposure to proton pump inhibitors **(lansoprazole, rabeprazole)**. Avoid or monitor. Mild Study
- **Apalutamide** markedly decreases the exposure to proton pump inhibitors **(omeprazole)**. Avoid or monitor. Moderate Study
- Anti-androgens **(apalutamide, enzalutamide)** are predicted to decrease the exposure to **quizartinib**. Avoid. Severe Study → Also see TABLE 7 p. 1055
- Anti-androgens **(apalutamide, enzalutamide)** are predicted to decrease the exposure to **ranolazine**. Avoid. Severe Study → Also see TABLE 7 p. 1055
- Anti-androgens **(apalutamide, enzalutamide)** are predicted to decrease the exposure to **reboxetine**. Moderate Anecdotal

Anti-androgens (continued)

- Anti-androgens **(apalutamide, enzalutamide)** are predicted to decrease the exposure to **regorafenib**. Avoid. [Moderate] Study
- **Apalutamide** is predicted to decrease the exposure to **relugolix**. Avoid or adjust dose depending on indication—consult product literature. [Moderate] Study
- Anti-androgens **(apalutamide, enzalutamide)** are predicted to markedly decrease the exposure to **ribociclib**. Avoid. [Severe] Study → Also see TABLE 7 p. 1055
- Rifamycins **(rifampicin)** are predicted to decrease the exposure to **abiraterone**. Avoid. [Severe] Study
- **Rifamycins** are predicted to decrease the efficacy of **cyproterone** with ethinylestradiol (co-cyprindiol). Use alternative methods during treatment with, and for 28 days after, the enzyme inducing drug is stopped. [Severe] Study
- Rifamycins **(rifampicin)** are predicted to decrease the exposure to **darolutamide**. Avoid. [Moderate] Study
- Anti-androgens **(apalutamide, enzalutamide)** are predicted to decrease the exposure to **rimegepant**. Avoid. [Moderate] Theoretical
- Anti-androgens **(apalutamide, enzalutamide)** are predicted to decrease the exposure to **ripretinib**. Avoid or adjust dose—consult product literature. [Severe] Study
- Anti-androgens **(apalutamide, enzalutamide)** are predicted to decrease the exposure to **ruxolitinib**. Monitor and adjust dose. [Moderate] Study
- **Darolutamide** is predicted to increase the exposure to **seladelpar**. [Moderate] Study
- Anti-androgens **(apalutamide, enzalutamide)** are predicted to decrease the exposure to **selpercatinib**. Avoid. [Moderate] Study → Also see TABLE 7 p. 1055
- Anti-androgens **(apalutamide, enzalutamide)** are predicted to decrease the exposure to **selumetinib**. Avoid. [Severe] Study
- Anti-androgens **(apalutamide, enzalutamide)** are predicted to decrease the exposure to **siponimod**. Manufacturer advises caution depending on genotype—consult product literature. [Severe] Study
- Anti-androgens **(apalutamide, enzalutamide)** are predicted to decrease the concentration of **sirolimus**. Avoid or monitor and adjust dose. [Severe] Study
- Anti-androgens **(apalutamide, enzalutamide)** are predicted to decrease the exposure to **solifenacin**. [Moderate] Theoretical
- Anti-androgens **(apalutamide, enzalutamide)** are predicted to decrease the exposure to **sorafenib**. [Moderate] Theoretical → Also see TABLE 7 p. 1055
- Anti-androgens **(apalutamide, enzalutamide)** are predicted to decrease the exposure to **sotorasib**. Avoid. [Severe] Study
- **Sotorasib** is predicted to decrease the exposure to **darolutamide**. Avoid. [Moderate] Theoretical
- Anti-androgens **(apalutamide, enzalutamide)** are predicted to decrease the exposure to **sparsentan**. Avoid. [Severe] Theoretical
- **Apalutamide** is predicted to decrease the exposure to SSRIs **(citalopram)**. Avoid or monitor. [Mild] Study → Also see TABLE 7 p. 1055
- **St John's wort** is predicted to decrease the efficacy of **cyproterone** with ethinylestradiol (co-cyprindiol). Use alternative methods during treatment with, and for 28 days after, the enzyme inducing drug is stopped. [Severe] Study
- **St John's wort** is predicted to decrease the exposure to **darolutamide**. Avoid. [Moderate] Theoretical
- **Apalutamide** is predicted to decrease the exposure to statins **(atorvastatin)**. [Moderate] Study
- **Darolutamide** is predicted to increase the exposure to statins **(atorvastatin, fluvastatin)**. Avoid. [Severe] Theoretical
- **Enzalutamide** is predicted to decrease the exposure to statins **(atorvastatin, simvastatin)**. [Moderate] Study
- **Apalutamide** is predicted to decrease the exposure to statins **(fluvastatin)**. Monitor and adjust dose. [Mild] Theoretical
- **Apalutamide** is predicted to decrease the exposure to statins **(pravastatin)**. [Mild] Study
- **Darolutamide** is predicted to increase the concentration of statins **(pravastatin, simvastatin)**. [Moderate] Theoretical
- **Apalutamide** slightly decreases the exposure to statins **(rosuvastatin)**. [Mild] Study
- **Darolutamide** markedly increases the exposure to statins **(rosuvastatin)**. Avoid or adjust **rosuvastatin** dose, p. 155. [Severe] Study
- **Apalutamide** is predicted to decrease the exposure to statins **(simvastatin)**. Avoid or monitor. [Moderate] Study
- **Apalutamide** is predicted to decrease the exposure to **sulfasalazine**. [Mild] Study
- **Darolutamide** is predicted to increase the exposure to **sulfasalazine**. Avoid. [Severe] Theoretical
- **Apalutamide** is predicted to decrease the exposure to sulfonylureas **(glibenclamide)**. Monitor and adjust dose. [Mild] Theoretical
- **Darolutamide** is predicted to increase the concentration of sulfonylureas **(glibenclamide)**. [Moderate] Theoretical
- Anti-androgens **(apalutamide, enzalutamide)** are predicted to decrease the exposure to **sunitinib**. Avoid or adjust dose—consult product literature. [Moderate] Study → Also see TABLE 7 p. 1055
- Anti-androgens **(apalutamide, enzalutamide)** decrease the concentration of **tacrolimus**. Avoid or monitor and adjust dose. [Severe] Study
- **Apalutamide** is predicted to decrease the exposure to **talazoparib**. Monitor and adjust dose. [Moderate] Study
- **Enzalutamide** moderately increases the exposure to **talazoparib**. Adjust starting dose. [Moderate] Study
- Anti-androgens **(apalutamide, enzalutamide)** are predicted to decrease the exposure to taxanes **(cabazitaxel)**. Avoid. [Moderate] Study
- Anti-androgens **(apalutamide, enzalutamide)** are predicted to decrease the exposure to taxanes **(docetaxel)**. [Severe] Theoretical
- **Darolutamide** is predicted to increase the exposure to taxanes **(paclitaxel)**. [Severe] Theoretical
- Anti-androgens **(apalutamide, enzalutamide)** are predicted to decrease the exposure to taxanes **(paclitaxel)**. Avoid. [Severe] Study
- Anti-androgens **(apalutamide, enzalutamide)** are predicted to decrease the concentration of **temsirolimus**. Avoid. [Severe] Study
- **Darolutamide** is predicted to increase the exposure to **tenofovir alafenamide**. [Moderate] Theoretical
- **Darolutamide** is predicted to increase the exposure to **tenofovir disoproxil**. [Moderate] Theoretical
- **Enzalutamide** is predicted to affect the exposure to tetracyclines **(doxycycline)**. Use with caution or avoid. [Moderate] Theoretical
- Anti-androgens **(apalutamide, enzalutamide)** are predicted to decrease the exposure to tetracyclines **(eravacycline)**. Adjust **eravacycline** dose. [Moderate] Study
- Anti-androgens **(apalutamide, enzalutamide)** are predicted to decrease the exposure to **tezacaftor**. Avoid. [Severe] Theoretical
- **Apalutamide** is predicted to decrease the exposure to thrombin inhibitors **(dabigatran)**. [Mild] Study
- **Apalutamide** potentially decreases the exposure to thyroid hormones **(levothyroxine)**. [Mild] Theoretical
- **Enzalutamide** is predicted to affect the exposure to thyroid hormones **(levothyroxine)**. Use with caution or avoid. [Moderate] Theoretical
- Anti-androgens **(apalutamide, enzalutamide)** are predicted to markedly decrease the exposure to **ticagrelor**. Avoid. [Severe] Study
- Anti-androgens **(apalutamide, enzalutamide)** are predicted to decrease the exposure to the cytotoxic component of **tisotumab vedotin**. [Moderate] Theoretical
- Anti-androgens **(apalutamide, enzalutamide)** are predicted to decrease the exposure to **tivozanib**. [Severe] Study
- Anti-androgens **(apalutamide, enzalutamide)** are predicted to decrease the exposure to **tofacitinib**. Avoid. [Severe] Study
- Anti-androgens **(apalutamide, enzalutamide)** are predicted to decrease the exposure to **tolvaptan**. Use with caution or avoid depending on indication. [Severe] Study
- **Apalutamide** is predicted to decrease the exposure to **topotecan**. Monitor and adjust dose. [Moderate] Theoretical
- **Darolutamide** is predicted to increase the exposure to **topotecan**. Avoid. [Severe] Theoretical

- Anti-androgens **(apalutamide, enzalutamide)** are predicted to decrease the exposure to **toremifene**. Adjust dose. Moderate Study → Also see TABLE 7 p. 1055
- Anti-androgens **(apalutamide, enzalutamide)** are predicted to decrease the exposure to **trabectedin**. Avoid. Severe Theoretical
- **Enzalutamide** is predicted to decrease the exposure to triptans **(eletriptan)**. Severe Study
- Anti-androgens **(apalutamide, enzalutamide)** are predicted to decrease the exposure to **tucatinib**. Avoid. Severe Study
- **Tucatinib** is predicted to increase the exposure to **apalutamide**. Monitor and adjust dose. Mild Study
- **Apalutamide** is predicted to decrease the efficacy of **ulipristal**. Avoid and for 4 weeks after stopping **apalutamide**. Severe Theoretical
- **Enzalutamide** is predicted to decrease the efficacy of **ulipristal**. Avoid and for 4 weeks after stopping **enzalutamide**. Severe Theoretical
- Anti-androgens **(apalutamide, enzalutamide)** are predicted to decrease the exposure to **upadacitinib**. Moderate Study
- Anti-androgens **(apalutamide, enzalutamide)** are predicted to decrease the exposure to **vandetanib**. Avoid. Moderate Study → Also see TABLE 7 p. 1055
- Anti-androgens **(apalutamide, enzalutamide)** are predicted to decrease the exposure to **vanzacaftor**. Avoid. Severe Theoretical
- Anti-androgens **(apalutamide, enzalutamide)** are predicted to moderately decrease the exposure to **velpatasvir**. Avoid. Severe Study
- Anti-androgens **(apalutamide, enzalutamide)** are predicted to decrease the exposure to **vemurafenib**. Avoid. Severe Study → Also see TABLE 7 p. 1055
- Anti-androgens **(apalutamide, enzalutamide)** are predicted to decrease the exposure to **venetoclax**. Avoid. Severe Study
- Anti-androgens **(apalutamide, enzalutamide)** are predicted to decrease the exposure to vinca alkaloids **(vinblastine, vincristine, vindesine)**. Severe Theoretical
- Anti-androgens **(apalutamide, enzalutamide)** are predicted to decrease the exposure to vinca alkaloids **(vinorelbine)**. Use with caution or avoid. Severe Theoretical
- Anti-androgens **(apalutamide, enzalutamide)** are predicted to decrease the exposure to **vismodegib**. Avoid. Moderate Theoretical
- Anti-androgens **(apalutamide, enzalutamide)** are predicted to decrease the exposure to **voclosporin**. Avoid. Severe Study → Also see TABLE 7 p. 1055
- Anti-androgens **(apalutamide, enzalutamide)** are predicted to decrease the exposure to **vortioxetine**. Monitor and adjust dose. Moderate Study
- Anti-androgens **(apalutamide, enzalutamide)** are predicted to decrease the concentration of **voxilaprevir**. Avoid. Severe Study
- Anti-androgens **(apalutamide, enzalutamide)** are predicted to decrease the exposure to **zanubrutinib**. Avoid. Severe Study
- **Enzalutamide** is predicted to affect the exposure to **zolpidem**. Use with caution or avoid. Moderate Theoretical
- Anti-androgens **(apalutamide, enzalutamide)** are predicted to decrease the exposure to **zopiclone**. Adjust dose. Moderate Study

Anti-D immunoglobulins → see immunoglobulins

Antiarrhythmics → see TABLE 4 p. 1054 (bradycardia), TABLE 1 p. 1053 (hepatotoxicity), TABLE 6 p. 1054 (hypotension), TABLE 10 p. 1056 (peripheral neuropathy), TABLE 7 p. 1055 (QT-interval prolongation), TABLE 8 p. 1055 (antimuscarinics)

adenosine · amiodarone · disopyramide · dronedarone · flecainide · lidocaine · propafenone · vernakalant

- **Amiodarone** has a long half-life; there is potential for drug interactions to occur for several weeks (or even months) after treatment with it has been stopped.
- Since systemic absorption can follow topical application of **lidocaine**, the possibility of interactions should be borne in mind.
- Avoid intravenous class I and class III antiarrhythmics for 4 hours before and after **vernakalant**.

- **Dronedarone** is predicted to increase the exposure to **abemaciclib**. Moderate Study
- **Dronedarone** is predicted to increase the exposure to **acalabrutinib**. Avoid or monitor. Severe Study
- Antiarrhythmics **(amiodarone, dronedarone)** are predicted to increase the exposure to **afatinib**. Moderate Study
- **Amiodarone** is predicted to decrease the effects of **agalsidase alfa**. Avoid. Moderate Theoretical
- **Amiodarone** is predicted to decrease the effects of **agalsidase beta**. Avoid. Moderate Theoretical
- Antiarrhythmics **(amiodarone, dronedarone)** are predicted to increase the exposure to **aliskiren**. Severe Study
- **Dronedarone** is predicted to increase the exposure to alpha blockers **(tamsulosin)**. Moderate Theoretical
- **Aminophylline** is predicted to decrease the efficacy of **adenosine**. Separate administration by 24 hours. Mild Theoretical
- Anti-androgens **(apalutamide, enzalutamide)** are predicted to decrease the efficacy of **propafenone**. Moderate Study
- Anti-androgens **(apalutamide, enzalutamide)** are predicted to decrease the exposure to antiarrhythmics **(disopyramide, dronedarone)**. Avoid. Severe Study → Also see TABLE 7 p. 1055
- Antiarrhythmics **(propafenone)** are predicted to increase the risk of cardiodepression when given with antiarrhythmics **(amiodarone)**. Monitor and adjust dose. Severe Theoretical → Also see TABLE 4 p. 1054
- Antiarrhythmics **(amiodarone)** increase the concentration of antiarrhythmics **(flecainide)**. Adjust **flecainide** dose and monitor adverse effects. Severe Study → Also see TABLE 4 p. 1054
- Antiarrhythmics **(propafenone)** are predicted to increase the risk of cardiodepression when given with antiarrhythmics **(lidocaine)**. Moderate Study
- Antiarrhythmics **(dronedarone)** are predicted to increase the exposure to antiarrhythmics **(propafenone)**. Monitor and adjust dose. Moderate Study → Also see TABLE 4 p. 1054
- Antiepileptics **(carbamazepine, fosphenytoin, phenobarbital, phenytoin, primidone)** are predicted to decrease the efficacy of **propafenone**. Moderate Study
- Antiepileptics **(fosphenytoin, phenytoin)** are predicted to decrease the exposure to **lidocaine**. Severe Anecdotal
- Antiepileptics **(carbamazepine, fosphenytoin, phenobarbital, phenytoin, primidone)** are predicted to decrease the exposure to antiarrhythmics **(disopyramide, dronedarone)**. Avoid. Severe Study
- **Amiodarone** is predicted to slightly increase the concentration of antiepileptics **(fosphenytoin, phenytoin)**. Monitor and adjust dose. Severe Study → Also see TABLE 10 p. 1056
- Antifungals, azoles **(fluconazole)** are predicted to increase the exposure to **dronedarone**. Severe Theoretical → Also see TABLE 7 p. 1055
- Antifungals, azoles **(fluconazole, isavuconazole)** are predicted to increase the exposure to **propafenone**. Monitor and adjust dose. Moderate Study
- Antifungals, azoles **(itraconazole)** are predicted to increase the exposure to **amiodarone**. Avoid. Severe Anecdotal → Also see TABLE 1 p. 1053
- Antifungals, azoles **(itraconazole, ketoconazole, posaconazole, voriconazole)** are predicted to increase the exposure to **disopyramide**. Avoid. Severe Theoretical → Also see TABLE 7 p. 1055
- Antifungals, azoles **(itraconazole, ketoconazole, posaconazole, voriconazole)** very markedly increase the exposure to **dronedarone**. Avoid. Severe Study → Also see TABLE 7 p. 1055
- Antifungals, azoles **(itraconazole, ketoconazole, posaconazole, voriconazole)** are predicted to increase the exposure to **propafenone**. Monitor and adjust dose. Severe Study
- Antifungals, azoles **(ketoconazole, voriconazole)** are predicted to increase the exposure to **amiodarone**. Avoid. Moderate Theoretical → Also see TABLE 1 p. 1053 → Also see TABLE 7 p. 1055
- Antifungals, azoles **(miconazole)** are predicted to increase the exposure to **disopyramide**. Use with caution and adjust dose. Severe Theoretical
- **Dronedarone** is predicted to increase the exposure to antifungals, azoles **(isavuconazole)**. Moderate Theoretical
- **Amiodarone** is predicted to increase the exposure to antihistamines, non-sedating **(fexofenadine)**. Moderate Study

Antiarrhythmics (continued)

- **Dronedarone** is predicted to increase the exposure to antihistamines, non-sedating **(fexofenadine, mizolastine)**. Severe Theoretical
- **Dronedarone** is predicted to increase the exposure to antihistamines, non-sedating **(rupatadine)**. Avoid. Moderate Study
- **Dronedarone** is predicted to increase the concentration of antimalarials **(piperaquine)**. Severe Study
- **Dronedarone** is predicted to increase the exposure to atypical antipsychotics **(cariprazine)**. Monitor and adjust dose. Severe Study
- Atypical antipsychotics **(clozapine)** can cause constipation, as can antiarrhythmics **(disopyramide, propafenone)**; concurrent use might increase the risk of developing intestinal obstruction. Severe Theoretical → Also see **TABLE 8** p. 1055
- **Dronedarone** is predicted to increase the exposure to atypical antipsychotics **(lurasidone)**. Adjust **lurasidone** dose. Moderate Study
- **Dronedarone** is predicted to increase the exposure to atypical antipsychotics **(quetiapine)**. Avoid. Moderate Study
- **Dronedarone** is predicted to increase the exposure to **avapritinib**. Avoid or adjust dose—consult product literature. Moderate Study
- **Amiodarone** is predicted to increase the exposure to **avatrombopag**. Adjust **avatrombopag** dose with moderate CYP2C9 inhibitors in chronic immune thrombocytopenia. Moderate Study
- **Dronedarone** is predicted to increase the exposure to **axitinib**. Moderate Study
- **Dronedarone** might increase the exposure to **bedaquiline**. Mild Theoretical → Also see **TABLE 7** p. 1055
- **Dronedarone** is predicted to increase the exposure to benzodiazepines **(alprazolam)**. Severe Study
- **Dronedarone** is predicted to increase the exposure to benzodiazepines **(midazolam)**. Monitor adverse effects and adjust dose. Severe Study
- **Berotralstat** is predicted to increase the exposure to **propafenone**. Monitor and adjust dose. Moderate Study
- Antiarrhythmics **(amiodarone, disopyramide, dronedarone, flecainide, lidocaine)** are predicted to increase the risk of cardiovascular adverse effects when given with **beta blockers, non-selective**. Use with caution or avoid. Severe Study → Also see **TABLE 4** p. 1054 → Also see **TABLE 7** p. 1055
- **Propafenone** is predicted to increase the risk of cardiovascular adverse effects when given with beta blockers, non-selective **(labetalol, levobunolol, nadolol, pindolol, sotalol)**. Use with caution or avoid. Severe Study → Also see **TABLE 4** p. 1054
- **Propafenone** increases the risk of cardiovascular adverse effects when given with beta blockers, non-selective **(propranolol)**. Use with caution or avoid. Severe Study → Also see **TABLE 4** p. 1054
- **Propafenone** is predicted to increase the exposure to beta blockers, non-selective **(timolol)** and beta blockers, non-selective **(timolol)** are predicted to increase the risk of cardiodepression when given with **propafenone**. Severe Anecdotal → Also see **TABLE 4** p. 1054
- Antiarrhythmics **(amiodarone, disopyramide, dronedarone, flecainide, lidocaine)** are predicted to increase the risk of cardiovascular adverse effects when given with **beta blockers, selective**. Use with caution or avoid. Severe Study → Also see **TABLE 4** p. 1054
- **Propafenone** is predicted to increase the risk of cardiovascular adverse effects when given with beta blockers, selective **(acebutolol, atenolol, betaxolol, bisoprolol, celiprolol, esmolol)**. Use with caution or avoid. Severe Study → Also see **TABLE 4** p. 1054
- **Propafenone** is predicted to increase the exposure to beta blockers, selective **(metoprolol)**. Moderate Study → Also see **TABLE 4** p. 1054
- **Propafenone** is predicted to increase the exposure to beta blockers, selective **(nebivolol)** and beta blockers, selective **(nebivolol)** are predicted to increase the risk of cardiodepression when given with **propafenone**. Avoid. Severe Theoretical → Also see **TABLE 4** p. 1054
- **Dronedarone** is predicted to increase the exposure to **bosutinib**. Avoid or adjust dose. Severe Study → Also see **TABLE 7** p. 1055
- **Dronedarone** is predicted to increase the exposure to **brigatinib**. Moderate Study → Also see **TABLE 4** p. 1054
- **Dronedarone** is predicted to increase the exposure to **buspirone**. Use with caution and adjust dose. Moderate Study
- **Dronedarone** is predicted to increase the exposure to **cabozantinib**. Moderate Study → Also see **TABLE 7** p. 1055
- **Caffeine citrate** decreases the efficacy of **adenosine**. Separate administration by 24 hours. Mild Study
- Calcium-channel blockers **(diltiazem, verapamil)** increase the exposure to **dronedarone** and **dronedarone** increases the exposure to calcium-channel blockers **(diltiazem, verapamil)**. Moderate Study → Also see **TABLE 4** p. 1054
- Calcium-channel blockers **(diltiazem, verapamil)** are predicted to increase the exposure to **propafenone**. Monitor and adjust dose. Moderate Study → Also see **TABLE 4** p. 1054
- Calcium-channel blockers **(verapamil)** increase the risk of cardiodepression when given with **flecainide**. Severe Anecdotal → Also see **TABLE 4** p. 1054
- **Dronedarone** is predicted to increase the exposure to calcium-channel blockers **(amlodipine, felodipine, lacidipine, lercanidipine, nicardipine, nifedipine, nimodipine)**. Monitor and adjust dose. Moderate Study
- **Amiodarone** is predicted to increase the risk of cardiodepression when given with calcium-channel blockers **(diltiazem, verapamil)**. Avoid. Severe Theoretical → Also see **TABLE 4** p. 1054
- **Disopyramide** is predicted to increase the risk of cardiodepression when given with calcium-channel blockers **(verapamil)**. Severe Theoretical
- **Dronedarone** is predicted to increase the exposure to **capivasertib**. Adjust dose. Moderate Study
- **Ceritinib** very markedly increases the exposure to **dronedarone**. Avoid. Severe Study → Also see **TABLE 4** p. 1054 → Also see **TABLE 7** p. 1055
- **Dronedarone** is predicted to increase the exposure to **ceritinib**. Moderate Study → Also see **TABLE 4** p. 1054 → Also see **TABLE 7** p. 1055
- **Ceritinib** is predicted to increase the exposure to **propafenone**. Monitor and adjust dose. Severe Study → Also see **TABLE 4** p. 1054
- **Chloroprocaine** is predicted to increase the risk of cardiovascular adverse effects when given with antiarrhythmics **(amiodarone, dronedarone, vernakalant)**. Severe Theoretical
- **Amiodarone** increases the concentration of **ciclosporin**. Monitor concentration and adjust dose. Severe Study
- **Dronedarone** is predicted to increase the concentration of **ciclosporin**. Severe Study
- **Cobicistat** potentially increases the concentration of antiarrhythmics **(amiodarone, disopyramide, flecainide, lidocaine)**. Severe Theoretical
- **Cobicistat** very markedly increases the exposure to **dronedarone**. Avoid. Severe Study
- **Cobicistat** is predicted to increase the exposure to **propafenone**. Monitor and adjust dose. Severe Study
- **Dronedarone** is predicted to increase the exposure to **cobimetinib**. Severe Study
- **Amiodarone** is predicted to increase the exposure to **colchicine**. Avoid P-glycoprotein inhibitors or adjust **colchicine** dose, p. 637. Severe Theoretical
- **Dronedarone** is predicted to increase the exposure to **colchicine**. Adjust **colchicine** dose with moderate CYP3A4 inhibitors, p. 637. Severe Study
- **Dronedarone** is predicted to increase the exposure to corticosteroids **(methylprednisolone)**. Monitor and adjust dose. Moderate Study
- **Amiodarone** increases the anticoagulant effect of **coumarins**. Severe Study
- **Dronedarone** might increase the anticoagulant effect of **coumarins**. Moderate Anecdotal
- **Propafenone** increases the anticoagulant effect of **coumarins**. Monitor INR and adjust dose. Moderate Study

- **Dronedarone** is predicted to increase the exposure to **crizotinib**. Moderate Study → Also see **TABLE 4** p. 1054 → Also see **TABLE 7** p. 1055
- **Crizotinib** is predicted to increase the exposure to **propafenone**. Monitor and adjust dose. Moderate Study → Also see **TABLE 4** p. 1054
- **Dronedarone** is predicted to increase the exposure to **dabrafenib**. Moderate Study
- **Dronedarone** is predicted to increase the exposure to **daridorexant**. Adjust **daridorexant** dose. Severe Study
- **Dronedarone** is predicted to increase the exposure to **darifenacin**. Moderate Study
- **Darifenacin** is predicted to increase the concentration of **flecainide**. Moderate Theoretical
- **Dronedarone** is predicted to increase the exposure to **dasatinib**. Severe Study → Also see **TABLE 7** p. 1055
- **Dronedarone** is predicted to increase the exposure to **deutivacaftor**. Adjust dose, see deutivacaftor with tezacaftor and vanzacaftor p. 218. Severe Study
- **Dronedarone** is predicted to slightly increase the exposure to **dienogest**. Moderate Study
- Antiarrhythmics **(amiodarone, dronedarone)** are predicted to moderately increase the exposure to **digoxin**. Monitor and adjust **digoxin** dose, p. 91. Severe Study → Also see **TABLE 4** p. 1054
- **Propafenone** increases the concentration of **digoxin**. Monitor and adjust dose. Severe Study → Also see **TABLE 4** p. 1054
- **Dronedarone** is predicted to increase the exposure to dipeptidylpeptidase-4 inhibitors **(saxagliptin)**. Mild Study
- **Dipyridamole** increases the exposure to **adenosine**. Avoid or adjust dose. Severe Study
- **Dronedarone** is predicted to increase the exposure to **domperidone**. Avoid. Severe Study
- **Dronedarone** is predicted to increase the exposure to dopamine receptor agonists **(bromocriptine)**. Severe Theoretical
- **Dronedarone** is predicted to increase the concentration of dopamine receptor agonists **(cabergoline)**. Severe Anecdotal
- **Dronedarone** is predicted to increase the exposure to **drospirenone**. Severe Study
- **Dronedarone** is predicted to moderately increase the exposure to **dutasteride**. Mild Study
- **Dronedarone** is predicted to increase the exposure to **elacestrant**. Avoid moderate CYP3A4 inhibitors or adjust **elacestrant** dose. Severe Theoretical
- **Dronedarone** is predicted to increase the exposure to **elexacaftor**. Adjust ivacaftor with tezacaftor and elexacaftor p. 220 dose with moderate CYP3A4 inhibitors. Severe Theoretical
- Antiarrhythmics **(dronedarone, propafenone)** are predicted to increase the exposure to **eliglustat**. Avoid or adjust dose—consult product literature. Severe Study
- **Encorafenib** is predicted to decrease the exposure to antiarrhythmics **(disopyramide, dronedarone)**. Avoid. Severe Study → Also see **TABLE 7** p. 1055
- **Dronedarone** is predicted to moderately increase the exposure to **encorafenib**. Moderate Study → Also see **TABLE 7** p. 1055
- **Encorafenib** is predicted to decrease the efficacy of **propafenone**. Moderate Study
- Endothelin receptor antagonists **(bosentan)** are predicted to decrease the exposure to **dronedarone**. Severe Theoretical
- Antiarrhythmics **(amiodarone, dronedarone)** are predicted to increase the exposure to endothelin receptor antagonists **(macitentan)**. Manufacturer advises caution depending on other drugs taken—consult product literature. Moderate Theoretical
- **Dronedarone** is predicted to increase the exposure to **entrectinib**. Avoid or adjust dose with moderate CYP3A4 inhibitors—consult product literature. Severe Theoretical → Also see **TABLE 7** p. 1055
- **Amiodarone** is predicted to increase the exposure to **erdafitinib**. Adjust dose. Severe Study
- **Dronedarone** is predicted to increase the risk of ergotism when given with **ergometrine**. Severe Theoretical
- **Amiodarone** is predicted to increase the exposure to **erlotinib**. Moderate Theoretical
- **Dronedarone** is predicted to increase the exposure to **erlotinib**. Moderate Study
- **Dronedarone** is predicted to increase the exposure to **etrasimod**. Avoid in poor CYP2C9 metabolisers. Severe Theoretical → Also see **TABLE 4** p. 1054
- **Amiodarone** is predicted to increase the exposure to **everolimus**. Monitor and adjust dose. Severe Study
- **Dronedarone** is predicted to increase the concentration of **everolimus**. Avoid or adjust dose. Moderate Study
- Antiarrhythmics **(amiodarone, dronedarone)** are predicted to increase the exposure to factor XA inhibitors **(apixaban)**. Moderate Theoretical
- **Amiodarone** slightly increases the exposure to factor XA inhibitors **(edoxaban)**. Severe Study
- **Dronedarone** slightly increases the exposure to factor XA inhibitors **(edoxaban)**. Adjust **edoxaban** dose. Severe Study
- **Amiodarone** might increase the exposure to factor XA inhibitors **(rivaroxaban)**. Manufacturer advises caution in renal impairment. Moderate Study
- **Dronedarone** might increase the exposure to factor XA inhibitors **(rivaroxaban)**. Avoid. Moderate Study
- **Dronedarone** is predicted to increase the exposure to **fedratinib**. Monitor and adjust dose. Moderate Study
- **Fedratinib** is predicted to increase the exposure to **propafenone**. Monitor and adjust dose. Moderate Study
- **Dronedarone** is predicted to increase the exposure to **fesoterodine**. Adjust **fesoterodine** dose with moderate CYP3A4 inhibitors in hepatic and renal impairment. Mild Study
- Antiarrhythmics **(amiodarone, dronedarone)** are predicted to increase the exposure to **fidaxomicin**. Avoid. Moderate Study
- **Dronedarone** is predicted to increase the exposure to **gefitinib**. Moderate Study
- Antiarrhythmics **(amiodarone, dronedarone)** are predicted to increase the exposure to **gilteritinib**. Moderate Theoretical
- **Grapefruit** juice increases the exposure to **amiodarone**. Avoid. Moderate Study
- **Grapefruit** juice moderately increases the exposure to **dronedarone**. Avoid. Severe Study
- **Grapefruit** juice increases the exposure to **propafenone**. Monitor and adjust dose. Moderate Study
- Antiarrhythmics **(amiodarone, dronedarone)** are predicted to increase the exposure to **grazoprevir**. Avoid. Severe Theoretical
- **Dronedarone** is predicted to increase the concentration of **guanfacine**. Adjust **guanfacine** dose, p. 281. Moderate Theoretical
- H_2 receptor antagonists **(cimetidine)** increase the exposure to **amiodarone**. Moderate Study
- H_2 receptor antagonists **(cimetidine)** slightly increase the exposure to **flecainide**. Monitor and adjust dose. Mild Study
- H_2 receptor antagonists **(cimetidine)** increase the exposure to **lidocaine**. Monitor and adjust dose. Moderate Study
- H_2 receptor antagonists **(cimetidine)** are predicted to increase the exposure to **propafenone**. Monitor and adjust dose. Moderate Theoretical
- **HIV-protease inhibitors** are predicted to increase the exposure to **amiodarone**. Avoid. Severe Theoretical → Also see **TABLE 1** p. 1053
- **HIV-protease inhibitors** are predicted to increase the exposure to **disopyramide**. Severe Theoretical
- **HIV-protease inhibitors** very markedly increase the exposure to **dronedarone**. Avoid. Severe Study
- HIV-protease inhibitors **(ritonavir)** are predicted to increase the exposure to **flecainide**. Avoid or monitor adverse effects. Severe Theoretical
- **HIV-protease inhibitors** are predicted to increase the exposure to **lidocaine**. Avoid. Severe Study
- **HIV-protease inhibitors** are predicted to increase the exposure to **propafenone**. Monitor and adjust dose. Severe Study
- **Amiodarone** is predicted to increase the exposure to **ibrutinib**. Adjust dose—consult product literature. Severe Theoretical
- **Dronedarone** is predicted to increase the exposure to **ibrutinib**. Adjust dose with moderate CYP3A4 inhibitors—consult product literature. Severe Study
- **Idelalisib** is predicted to increase the exposure to **amiodarone**. Avoid. Moderate Theoretical
- **Idelalisib** very markedly increases the exposure to **dronedarone**. Avoid. Severe Study

Antiarrhythmics (continued)

- **Idelalisib** is predicted to increase the exposure to **propafenone**. Monitor and adjust dose. Severe Study
- **Imatinib** is predicted to increase the exposure to **dronedarone**. Severe Theoretical
- **Imatinib** is predicted to increase the exposure to **propafenone**. Monitor and adjust dose. Moderate Study
- **Dronedarone** is predicted to increase the exposure to the active metabolite of **irinotecan**. Moderate Theoretical
- **Dronedarone** is predicted to increase the exposure to **ivabradine**. Adjust **ivabradine** dose. Severe Theoretical → Also see TABLE 4 p. 1054
- **Dronedarone** is predicted to increase the exposure to **ivacaftor**. Adjust dose with moderate CYP3A4 inhibitors, see ivacaftor p. 219, tezacaftor with ivacaftor p. 223, and ivacaftor with tezacaftor and elexacaftor p. 220. Moderate Study
- **Ivosidenib** is predicted to decrease the exposure to antiarrhythmics **(disopyramide, dronedarone)**. Avoid. Severe Study → Also see TABLE 7 p. 1055
- **Dronedarone** is predicted to increase the exposure to **ivosidenib**. Monitor and adjust dose—consult product literature. Severe Study → Also see TABLE 7 p. 1055
- **Ivosidenib** is predicted to decrease the efficacy of **propafenone**. Moderate Study
- **Dronedarone** is predicted to increase the exposure to **lapatinib**. Moderate Study → Also see TABLE 7 p. 1055
- **Dronedarone** is predicted to increase the exposure to **larotrectinib**. Monitor and adjust dose. Moderate Theoretical
- **Ledipasvir** increases the risk of severe bradycardia or heart block when given with **amiodarone**. Refer to specialist literature. Severe Anecdotal
- **Dronedarone** is predicted to increase the exposure to **leniolisib**. Avoid. Moderate Study
- **Letermovir** is predicted to increase the concentration of **amiodarone**. Moderate Theoretical
- **Letermovir** is predicted to increase the exposure to **propafenone**. Monitor and adjust dose. Moderate Study
- **Amiodarone** is predicted to increase the exposure to **lomitapide**. Separate administration by 12 hours. Moderate Theoretical → Also see TABLE 1 p. 1053
- **Dronedarone** is predicted to increase the exposure to **lomitapide**. Avoid. Moderate Theoretical
- **Dronedarone** is predicted to increase the exposure to **loperamide**. Severe Theoretical
- **Lumacaftor** is predicted to decrease the exposure to antiarrhythmics **(disopyramide, dronedarone)**. Avoid. Severe Study
- **Lumacaftor** is predicted to decrease the efficacy of **propafenone**. Moderate Study
- Macrolides **(clarithromycin)** are predicted to increase the exposure to **amiodarone**. Avoid. Moderate Theoretical
- Macrolides **(clarithromycin)** very markedly increase the exposure to **dronedarone**. Avoid. Severe Study
- Macrolides **(clarithromycin)** are predicted to increase the exposure to **propafenone**. Monitor and adjust dose. Severe Study
- Macrolides **(clarithromycin, erythromycin)** are predicted to increase the exposure to **lidocaine**. Moderate Theoretical
- Macrolides **(erythromycin)** are predicted to moderately increase the exposure to **dronedarone**. Avoid. Severe Theoretical → Also see TABLE 7 p. 1055
- Macrolides **(erythromycin)** are predicted to increase the exposure to **propafenone**. Monitor and adjust dose. Moderate Study
- **Amiodarone** is predicted to increase the exposure to **mavacamten**. Monitor and adjust dose—consult product literature. Moderate Theoretical
- **Dronedarone** is predicted to increase the exposure to **mavacamten**. Adjust dose—consult product literature. Moderate Study
- **Mexiletine** is predicted to increase the risk of torsade de pointes when given with **antiarrhythmics**. Avoid. Severe Theoretical
- **Dronedarone** is predicted to increase the exposure to **midostaurin**. Moderate Theoretical
- **Amiodarone** is predicted to increase the exposure to mineralocorticoid receptor antagonists **(eplerenone)**. Adjust **eplerenone** dose. Severe Theoretical
- **Dronedarone** is predicted to increase the exposure to mineralocorticoid receptor antagonists **(eplerenone)**. Adjust **eplerenone** dose. Severe Study
- **Dronedarone** is predicted to increase the exposure to mineralocorticoid receptor antagonists **(finerenone)**. Severe Study
- **Mitotane** is predicted to decrease the exposure to antiarrhythmics **(disopyramide, dronedarone)**. Avoid. Severe Study
- **Mitotane** is predicted to decrease the efficacy of **propafenone**. Moderate Study
- **Amiodarone** is predicted to increase the risk of neutropenia when given with monoclonal antibodies **(brentuximab vedotin)**. Monitor and adjust dose. Severe Theoretical → Also see TABLE 10 p. 1056
- **Dronedarone** increases the risk of neutropenia when given with monoclonal antibodies **(brentuximab vedotin)**. Monitor and adjust dose. Severe Theoretical
- Antiarrhythmics **(amiodarone, dronedarone)** are predicted to increase the exposure to **naldemedine**. Moderate Study
- **Dronedarone** is predicted to increase the exposure to **naloxegol**. Adjust **naloxegol** dose and monitor adverse effects. Moderate Study
- **Amiodarone** is predicted to increase the exposure to **neratinib**. Avoid or adjust dose and monitor for gastrointestinal adverse effects—consult product literature. Severe Study → Also see TABLE 1 p. 1053
- **Dronedarone** is predicted to increase the exposure to **neratinib**. Avoid moderate CYP3A4 inhibitors or adjust dose and monitor for gastrointestinal adverse effects—consult product literature. Severe Study
- Neurokinin-1 receptor antagonists **(aprepitant)** increase the exposure to **dronedarone**. Severe Theoretical
- Neurokinin-1 receptor antagonists **(aprepitant, netupitant)** are predicted to increase the exposure to **propafenone**. Monitor and adjust dose. Moderate Study
- **Nilotinib** is predicted to increase the exposure to **propafenone**. Monitor and adjust dose. Moderate Study
- Antiarrhythmics **(amiodarone, dronedarone)** are predicted to increase the exposure to **nintedanib**. Moderate Study
- **Nirmatrelvir** boosted with ritonavir is predicted to increase the concentration of antiarrhythmics **(amiodarone, dronedarone, flecainide, propafenone)**. Avoid. Severe Theoretical
- **Nirmatrelvir** boosted with ritonavir is predicted to increase the concentration of antiarrhythmics **(disopyramide, lidocaine)**. Severe Theoretical
- NNRTIs **(efavirenz, etravirine, nevirapine)** are predicted to decrease the exposure to **dronedarone**. Severe Theoretical → Also see TABLE 7 p. 1055
- NSAIDs **(celecoxib)** are predicted to increase the exposure to antiarrhythmics **(flecainide, propafenone)**. Monitor and adjust dose. Moderate Theoretical
- **Dronedarone** is predicted to increase the exposure to **olaparib**. Avoid or adjust dose with moderate CYP3A4 inhibitors—consult product literature. Moderate Theoretical
- **Dronedarone** is predicted to increase the exposure to **omaveloxolone**. Avoid or adjust **omaveloxolone** dose, p. 755. Moderate Study
- **Dronedarone** is predicted to increase the exposure to opioids **(alfentanil, buprenorphine, fentanyl, oxycodone)**. Monitor and adjust dose. Moderate Study → Also see TABLE 4 p. 1054
- **Amiodarone** is predicted to increase the concentration of opioids **(fentanyl)**. Monitor and adjust dose. Moderate Theoretical → Also see TABLE 4 p. 1054
- **Dronedarone** is predicted to increase the exposure to opioids **(methadone, sufentanil)**. Moderate Theoretical → Also see TABLE 4 p. 1054 → Also see TABLE 7 p. 1055
- Antiarrhythmics **(amiodarone, dronedarone)** are predicted to increase the exposure to **panobinostat**. Adjust dose. Moderate Theoretical → Also see TABLE 7 p. 1055
- **Dronedarone** is predicted to increase the exposure to **pazopanib**. Moderate Study → Also see TABLE 7 p. 1055

- **Dronedarone** is predicted to increase the exposure to **pemigatinib**. Severe Study
- **Dronedarone** might increase the anticoagulant effect of **phenindione**. Moderate Anecdotal
- **Propafenone** is predicted to increase the anticoagulant effect of **phenindione**. Monitor and adjust dose. Moderate Theoretical
- **Dronedarone** is predicted to increase the exposure to phosphodiesterase type-5 inhibitors **(avanafil)**. Adjust **avanafil** dose. Moderate Theoretical
- **Dronedarone** is predicted to increase the exposure to phosphodiesterase type-5 inhibitors **(sildenafil)**. Monitor or adjust **sildenafil** dose with moderate CYP3A4 inhibitors, p. 139. Moderate Study
- **Dronedarone** is predicted to increase the exposure to phosphodiesterase type-5 inhibitors **(tadalafil)**. Severe Theoretical
- **Dronedarone** is predicted to increase the exposure to phosphodiesterase type-5 inhibitors **(vardenafil)**. Adjust dose. Severe Theoretical → Also see **TABLE 7** p. 1055
- **Dronedarone** is predicted to increase the exposure to **pimozide**. Avoid. Severe Theoretical → Also see **TABLE 7** p. 1055
- **Dronedarone** is predicted to increase the exposure to **ponatinib**. Moderate Study
- Antiarrhythmics **(amiodarone, dronedarone)** are predicted to increase the exposure to **pralsetinib**. Moderate Theoretical
- Quinolones **(ciprofloxacin)** slightly increase the exposure to **lidocaine**. Mild Study
- **Dronedarone** is predicted to increase the exposure to **ranolazine**. Severe Study → Also see **TABLE 7** p. 1055
- **Dronedarone** is predicted to increase the exposure to **regorafenib**. Moderate Study
- Antiarrhythmics **(amiodarone, dronedarone)** are predicted to increase the exposure to **relugolix**. Avoid or take relugolix first and separate administration by at least 6 hours. Moderate Study
- **Propafenone** is predicted to increase the exposure to **relugolix**. Avoid or take relugolix first and separate administration by at least 6 hours. Moderate Theoretical
- **Amiodarone** is predicted to increase the exposure to retinoids **(alitretinoin)**. Adjust **alitretinoin** dose. Moderate Theoretical
- **Ribociclib** (high-dose) is predicted to increase the exposure to **amiodarone**. Avoid. Moderate Theoretical → Also see **TABLE 7** p. 1055
- **Dronedarone** is predicted to increase the exposure to **ribociclib**. Moderate Study → Also see **TABLE 7** p. 1055
- Rifamycins **(rifampicin)** are predicted to decrease the efficacy of **propafenone**. Moderate Study
- Rifamycins **(rifampicin)** are predicted to decrease the exposure to antiarrhythmics **(disopyramide, dronedarone)**. Avoid. Severe Study
- **Amiodarone** is predicted to increase the exposure to **rimegepant**. Avoid another dose of rimegepant within 48 hours of concurrent use. Moderate Theoretical
- **Dronedarone** is predicted to increase the exposure to **rimegepant**. Avoid another dose of rimegepant within 48 hours of concurrent use. Moderate Study
- **Dronedarone** is predicted to increase the exposure to **ruxolitinib**. Moderate Study
- **Dronedarone** is predicted to increase the exposure to **selpercatinib**. Moderate Study → Also see **TABLE 7** p. 1055
- **Dronedarone** is predicted to increase the exposure to **selumetinib**. Avoid or adjust dose—consult product literature. Severe Study
- Antiarrhythmics **(amiodarone, dronedarone)** are predicted to increase the exposure to **siponimod**. Avoid depending on other drugs taken—consult product literature. Severe Study → Also see **TABLE 4** p. 1054
- **Amiodarone** is predicted to increase the concentration of **sirolimus**. Severe Anecdotal
- **Dronedarone** increases the concentration of **sirolimus**. Monitor and adjust dose. Moderate Study
- **Sofosbuvir** is predicted to increase the risk of severe bradycardia or heart block when given with **amiodarone**. Refer to specialist literature. Severe Anecdotal
- **Dronedarone** is predicted to increase the exposure to **sparsentan**. Moderate Study
- SSRIs **(fluvoxamine)** are predicted to increase the exposure to **propafenone**. Monitor and adjust dose. Moderate Study
- **Dronedarone** is predicted to increase the exposure to SSRIs **(citalopram, escitalopram, fluoxetine, fluvoxamine, paroxetine)**. Severe Theoretical → Also see **TABLE 7** p. 1055
- **Dronedarone** is predicted to increase the exposure to SSRIs **(dapoxetine)**. Adjust **dapoxetine** dose with moderate CYP3A4 inhibitors. Moderate Theoretical
- **Dronedarone** is predicted to increase the exposure to SSRIs **(sertraline)**. Moderate Theoretical
- **St John's wort** is predicted to decrease the exposure to **dronedarone**. Avoid. Severe Theoretical
- **Amiodarone** is predicted to increase the exposure to statins **(atorvastatin)**. Monitor and adjust dose. Moderate Theoretical → Also see **TABLE 1** p. 1053
- **Dronedarone** slightly increases the exposure to statins **(atorvastatin)**. Monitor and adjust dose. Severe Study
- **Amiodarone** is predicted to increase the exposure to statins **(fluvastatin)**. Moderate Study → Also see **TABLE 1** p. 1053
- **Dronedarone** slightly increases the exposure to statins **(rosuvastatin)**. Adjust dose. Severe Study
- **Amiodarone** increases the exposure to statins **(simvastatin)**. Adjust **simvastatin** dose, p. 156. Severe Study → Also see **TABLE 1** p. 1053
- **Dronedarone** moderately increases the exposure to statins **(simvastatin)**. Monitor and adjust dose. Severe Study
- **Amiodarone** is predicted to increase the exposure to **sulfonylureas**. Moderate Theoretical
- **Dronedarone** is predicted to increase the exposure to **sunitinib**. Moderate Study → Also see **TABLE 7** p. 1055
- **Lidocaine** is predicted to increase the effects of **suxamethonium**. Moderate Study
- **Amiodarone** is predicted to increase the concentration of **tacrolimus**. Severe Anecdotal
- **Dronedarone** is predicted to increase the concentration of **tacrolimus**. Monitor and adjust dose. Severe Theoretical
- Antiarrhythmics **(amiodarone, dronedarone)** are predicted to slightly increase the exposure to **talazoparib**. Avoid or adjust dose—consult product literature. Severe Study
- **Propafenone** is predicted to increase the exposure to **talazoparib**. Avoid or adjust dose—consult product literature. Moderate Theoretical
- **Dronedarone** is predicted to increase the exposure to taxanes **(cabazitaxel)**. Moderate Theoretical
- **Dronedarone** is predicted to increase the exposure to taxanes **(docetaxel)**. Severe Study
- **Amiodarone** is predicted to increase the exposure to taxanes **(paclitaxel)**. Severe Theoretical → Also see **TABLE 10** p. 1056
- **Dronedarone** is predicted to increase the exposure to taxanes **(paclitaxel)**. Moderate Anecdotal
- **Dronedarone** is predicted to increase the concentration of **temsirolimus**. Use with caution or avoid. Moderate Theoretical
- **Dronedarone** is predicted to increase the exposure to **tezacaftor**. Adjust dose with moderate CYP3A4 inhibitors, see tezacaftor with ivacaftor p. 223, ivacaftor with tezacaftor and elexacaftor p. 220, and deutivacaftor with tezacaftor and vanzacaftor p. 218. Severe Study
- **Theophylline** decreases the efficacy of **adenosine**. Separate administration by 24 hours. Mild Study
- **Amiodarone** increases the exposure to thrombin inhibitors **(dabigatran)**. Monitor and adjust dose. Severe Study
- **Dronedarone** moderately increases the exposure to thrombin inhibitors **(dabigatran)**. Avoid. Severe Study
- **Amiodarone** is predicted to increase the risk of thyroid dysfunction when given with **thyroid hormones**. Avoid. Moderate Study
- **Amiodarone** is predicted to increase the exposure to **ticagrelor**. Use with caution or avoid. Severe Study → Also see **TABLE 4** p. 1054
- Antiarrhythmics **(amiodarone, dronedarone)** might increase the exposure to **tigecycline**. Mild Anecdotal → Also see **TABLE 1** p. 1053
- **Dronedarone** given with a potent CYP2C19 inhibitor is predicted to increase the exposure to **tofacitinib**. Adjust **tofacitinib** dose, p. 803. Moderate Study

Antiarrhythmics (continued)

- **Dronedarone** is predicted to increase the exposure to **tolvaptan**. Manufacturer advises caution or adjust **tolvaptan** dose with moderate CYP3A4 inhibitors. Moderate Study
- Antiarrhythmics **(amiodarone, dronedarone)** are predicted to increase the exposure to **topotecan**. Severe Study
- Antiarrhythmics **(amiodarone, dronedarone)** are predicted to increase the concentration of **trametinib**. Moderate Theoretical
- **Dronedarone** is predicted to increase the exposure to **trazodone**. Moderate Theoretical
- **Dronedarone** is predicted to increase the exposure to **tricyclic antidepressants**. Avoid. Severe Theoretical → Also see TABLE 7 p. 1055
- **Propafenone** is predicted to increase the concentration of **tricyclic antidepressants**. Moderate Theoretical → Also see TABLE 8 p. 1055
- **Tucatinib** very markedly increases the exposure to **dronedarone**. Avoid. Severe Study
- **Tucatinib** is predicted to increase the exposure to **propafenone**. Monitor and adjust dose. Severe Study
- **Dronedarone** is predicted to increase the exposure to **ulipristal**. Avoid when used for uterine fibroids. Moderate Study
- **Dronedarone** is predicted to increase the exposure to **vanzacaftor**. Adjust dose, see deutivacaftor with tezacaftor and vanzacaftor p. 218. Severe Study
- **Amiodarone** is predicted to increase the concentration of **velpatasvir**. Avoid or monitor. Moderate Theoretical
- **Dronedarone** is predicted to increase the exposure to **vemurafenib**. Severe Theoretical → Also see TABLE 7 p. 1055
- **Amiodarone** is predicted to increase the exposure to **venetoclax**. Avoid or monitor for toxicity. Severe Theoretical
- **Dronedarone** is predicted to increase the exposure to **venetoclax**. Avoid or adjust dose—consult product literature. Severe Study
- **Amiodarone** might increase the exposure to **vinca alkaloids**. Severe Theoretical → Also see TABLE 10 p. 1056
- **Dronedarone** is predicted to increase the exposure to **vinca alkaloids**. Severe Theoretical
- **Dronedarone** is predicted to increase the exposure to **voclosporin**. Adjust **voclosporin** dose. Severe Study → Also see TABLE 7 p. 1055
- **Dronedarone** is predicted to increase the exposure to **zanubrutinib**. Avoid or adjust dose with moderate CYP3A4 inhibitors—consult product literature. Severe Study
- **Dronedarone** is predicted to increase the exposure to **zopiclone**. Adjust dose. Moderate Study

Anticholinesterases, centrally acting → see TABLE 4 p. 1054 (bradycardia)

donepezil · galantamine · rivastigmine

- Anti-androgens **(apalutamide, enzalutamide)** are predicted to decrease the exposure to **donepezil**. Mild Study
- Antiepileptics **(carbamazepine, fosphenytoin, phenobarbital, phenytoin, primidone)** are predicted to decrease the exposure to **donepezil**. Mild Study
- Antifungals, azoles **(itraconazole, ketoconazole, posaconazole, voriconazole)** are predicted to increase the exposure to **galantamine**. Monitor and adjust dose. Moderate Study
- **Bupropion** is predicted to increase the exposure to **galantamine**. Monitor and adjust dose. Moderate Study
- **Ceritinib** is predicted to increase the exposure to **galantamine**. Monitor and adjust dose. Moderate Study → Also see TABLE 4 p. 1054
- **Cinacalcet** is predicted to increase the exposure to **galantamine**. Monitor and adjust dose. Moderate Study
- **Cobicistat** is predicted to increase the exposure to **galantamine**. Monitor and adjust dose. Moderate Study
- **Dacomitinib** is predicted to increase the exposure to **galantamine**. Monitor and adjust dose. Moderate Study
- **Encorafenib** is predicted to decrease the exposure to **donepezil**. Mild Study
- **HIV-protease inhibitors** are predicted to increase the exposure to **galantamine**. Monitor and adjust dose. Moderate Study
- **Idelalisib** is predicted to increase the exposure to **galantamine**. Monitor and adjust dose. Moderate Study
- **Ivosidenib** is predicted to decrease the exposure to **donepezil**. Mild Study
- **Lumacaftor** is predicted to decrease the exposure to **donepezil**. Mild Study
- Macrolides **(clarithromycin)** are predicted to increase the exposure to **galantamine**. Monitor and adjust dose. Moderate Study
- **Mitotane** is predicted to decrease the exposure to **donepezil**. Mild Study
- **Anticholinesterases, centrally acting** are predicted to decrease the effects of **neuromuscular blocking drugs, non-depolarising**. Moderate Theoretical
- Rifamycins **(rifampicin)** are predicted to decrease the exposure to **donepezil**. Mild Study
- SSRIs **(fluoxetine, paroxetine)** are predicted to increase the exposure to **galantamine**. Monitor and adjust dose. Moderate Study
- **Anticholinesterases, centrally acting** increase the effects of **suxamethonium**. Moderate Theoretical → Also see TABLE 4 p. 1054
- **Terbinafine** is predicted to increase the exposure to **galantamine**. Monitor and adjust dose. Moderate Study
- **Tucatinib** is predicted to increase the exposure to **galantamine**. Monitor and adjust dose. Moderate Study

Antiepileptics → see TABLE 1 p. 1053 (hepatotoxicity), TABLE 15 p. 1058 (hyponatraemia), TABLE 10 p. 1056 (peripheral neuropathy), TABLE 9 p. 1056 (CNS effects)

brivaracetam · carbamazepine · eslicarbazepine · ethosuximide · fosphenytoin · gabapentin · lacosamide · lamotrigine · levetiracetam · oxcarbazepine · paraldehyde · perampanel · phenobarbital · phenytoin · pregabalin · primidone · retigabine · rufinamide · stiripentol · sultiame · tiagabine · topiramate · valproate · vigabatrin · zonisamide

- Manufacturer advises caution on concurrent use of **eslicarbazepine** or **lacosamide** with drugs that prolong the PR interval.
- Avoid taking milk, dairy products, carbonated drinks, fruit juices, or caffeine-containing food and drinks at the same time as **stiripentol**.

- Antiepileptics **(carbamazepine, fosphenytoin, phenobarbital, phenytoin, primidone)** are predicted to decrease the exposure to 5-HT3-receptor antagonists **(ondansetron)**. Moderate Study
- Antiepileptics **(carbamazepine, fosphenytoin, phenobarbital, phenytoin, primidone)** are predicted to markedly decrease the exposure to **abemaciclib**. Avoid. Severe Study
- Antiepileptics **(fosphenytoin, phenytoin)** are predicted to decrease the exposure to **abrocitinib**. Avoid. Moderate Theoretical
- Antiepileptics **(carbamazepine, fosphenytoin, phenobarbital, phenytoin, primidone)** are predicted to decrease the exposure to **acalabrutinib**. Avoid. Severe Study
- **Acetazolamide** potentially increases the risk of toxicity when given with **valproate**. Severe Study
- **Acetazolamide** potentially increases the risk of overheating and dehydration when given with **zonisamide**. Avoid in children. Severe Theoretical
- Antiepileptics **(phenobarbital, phenytoin)** are predicted to decrease the exposure to **afatinib**. Moderate Theoretical
- **Carbamazepine** is predicted to decrease the exposure to **afatinib**. Moderate Study
- Antiepileptics **(fosphenytoin, phenytoin)** are predicted to decrease the exposure to **agomelatine**. Moderate Theoretical → Also see TABLE 9 p. 1056
- Antiepileptics **(carbamazepine, fosphenytoin, phenobarbital, phenytoin, primidone)** decrease the concentration of **albendazole**. Moderate Study
- **Alcohol** potentially increases the risk of visual disturbances when given with **retigabine**. Moderate Study
- **Sultiame** might cause a disulfiram-like reaction when given with **alcohol**. Avoid. Moderate Theoretical
- **Carbamazepine** decreases the exposure to **aliskiren**. Moderate Study
- Antiepileptics **(carbamazepine, fosphenytoin, phenobarbital, phenytoin, primidone)** are predicted to decrease the exposure to **alpelisib**. Avoid. Moderate Study

- **Fosphenytoin** is predicted to decrease the exposure to **aminophylline**. Adjust dose. Moderate Study
- **Phenobarbital** is predicted to decrease the exposure to **aminophylline**. Adjust dose. Moderate Theoretical
- **Phenytoin** decreases the exposure to **aminophylline**. Adjust dose. Moderate Study
- **Primidone** is predicted to increase the clearance of **aminophylline**. Adjust dose. Moderate Theoretical
- **Stiripentol** is predicted to increase the exposure to **aminophylline**. Avoid. Moderate Theoretical
- **Phenytoin** is predicted to decrease the exposure to anaesthetics, local **(ropivacaine)**. Moderate Theoretical
- Oral **antacids** decrease the absorption of oral **gabapentin**. Manufacturer advises take 2 hours after antacids. Moderate Study
- Anti-androgens **(apalutamide)** potentially decrease the exposure to **valproate**. Mild Theoretical
- Anti-androgens **(apalutamide, enzalutamide)** are predicted to decrease the exposure to **perampanel**. Monitor and adjust dose. Moderate Study
- Anti-androgens **(enzalutamide)** are predicted to slightly decrease the exposure to **brivaracetam**. Moderate Theoretical
- Anti-androgens **(enzalutamide)** are predicted to affect the exposure to **valproate**. Use with caution or avoid. Moderate Theoretical
- Antiepileptics **(carbamazepine, fosphenytoin, phenobarbital, phenytoin, primidone)** are predicted to decrease the exposure to anti-androgens **(abiraterone)**. Avoid. Severe Study
- Antiepileptics **(carbamazepine, eslicarbazepine, fosphenytoin, oxcarbazepine, perampanel, phenobarbital, phenytoin, primidone, rufinamide, topiramate)** are predicted to decrease the efficacy of anti-androgens **(cyproterone)** with ethinylestradiol (co-cyprindiol). Use alternative methods during treatment with, and for 28 days after, the enzyme inducing drug is stopped. Severe Study
- Antiepileptics **(carbamazepine, fosphenytoin, phenobarbital, phenytoin, primidone)** are predicted to decrease the exposure to anti-androgens **(darolutamide)**. Avoid. Moderate Study
- Antiepileptics **(carbamazepine, fosphenytoin, phenobarbital, phenytoin, primidone)** are predicted to decrease the exposure to antiarrhythmics **(disopyramide, dronedarone)**. Avoid. Severe Study
- Antiarrhythmics **(amiodarone)** are predicted to slightly increase the concentration of antiepileptics **(fosphenytoin, phenytoin)**. Monitor and adjust dose. Severe Study → Also see **TABLE 10** p. 1056
- Antiepileptics **(fosphenytoin, phenytoin)** are predicted to decrease the exposure to antiarrhythmics **(lidocaine)**. Severe Anecdotal
- Antiepileptics **(carbamazepine, fosphenytoin, phenobarbital, phenytoin, primidone)** are predicted to decrease the efficacy of antiarrhythmics **(propafenone)**. Moderate Study
- Antiepileptics **(carbamazepine, fosphenytoin, phenobarbital, phenytoin, primidone)** are predicted to decrease the exposure to anticholinesterases, centrally acting **(donepezil)**. Mild Study
- Antiepileptics **(carbamazepine)** decrease the concentration of antiepileptics **(brivaracetam)**. Moderate Study
- Antiepileptics **(fosphenytoin, phenytoin)** decrease the concentration of antiepileptics **(brivaracetam)**. Moderate Study
- Antiepileptics **(lamotrigine)** potentially increase the concentration of antiepileptics **(carbamazepine)** and antiepileptics **(carbamazepine)** decrease the concentration of antiepileptics **(lamotrigine)**. Adjust **lamotrigine** dose and monitor **carbamazepine** concentration, p. 243, p. 234. Moderate Study
- Antiepileptics **(phenobarbital)** affect the concentration of antiepileptics **(carbamazepine)** and antiepileptics **(carbamazepine)** increase the concentration of antiepileptics **(phenobarbital)**. Adjust dose. Moderate Study
- Antiepileptics **(topiramate)** increase the risk of carbamazepine toxicity when given with antiepileptics **(carbamazepine)**. Moderate Study
- Antiepileptics **(stiripentol)** increase the concentration of antiepileptics **(carbamazepine, phenobarbital)**. Avoid in Dravet syndrome. Severe Study
- Antiepileptics **(carbamazepine)** slightly decrease the exposure to antiepileptics **(eslicarbazepine, oxcarbazepine)**. Monitor and adjust dose. Moderate Study → Also see **TABLE 15** p. 1058
- Antiepileptics **(oxcarbazepine)** are predicted to increase the concentration of antiepileptics **(fosphenytoin)**. Monitor concentration and adjust dose. Moderate Study
- Antiepileptics **(stiripentol)** are predicted to increase the concentration of antiepileptics **(fosphenytoin)**. Severe Study
- Antiepileptics **(sultiame)** might increase the concentration of antiepileptics **(fosphenytoin)**. Monitor phenytoin concentration. Severe Theoretical
- Antiepileptics **(carbamazepine)** affect the concentration of antiepileptics **(fosphenytoin, phenytoin)** and antiepileptics **(fosphenytoin, phenytoin)** decrease the concentration of antiepileptics **(carbamazepine)**. Monitor and adjust dose. Severe Study
- Antiepileptics **(eslicarbazepine)** increase the exposure to antiepileptics **(fosphenytoin, phenytoin)** and antiepileptics **(fosphenytoin, phenytoin)** decrease the exposure to antiepileptics **(eslicarbazepine)**. Monitor and adjust dose. Moderate Study
- Antiepileptics **(valproate)** affect the concentration of antiepileptics **(fosphenytoin, phenytoin)** and antiepileptics **(fosphenytoin, phenytoin)** decrease the concentration of antiepileptics **(valproate)**. Severe Study
- Antiepileptics **(vigabatrin)** decrease the concentration of antiepileptics **(fosphenytoin, phenytoin)**. Mild Study → Also see **TABLE 9** p. 1056
- Antiepileptics **(fosphenytoin)** decrease the concentration of antiepileptics **(lamotrigine)**. Monitor and adjust **lamotrigine** dose, p. 243. Moderate Study → Also see **TABLE 9** p. 1056
- Antiepileptics **(phenobarbital, phenytoin, primidone)** decrease the concentration of antiepileptics **(lamotrigine)**. Monitor and adjust **lamotrigine** dose, p. 243. Moderate Study → Also see **TABLE 9** p. 1056
- Antiepileptics **(valproate)** increase the exposure to antiepileptics **(lamotrigine)**. Adjust **lamotrigine** dose and monitor rash, p. 243. Severe Study
- Antiepileptics **(lamotrigine)** are predicted to increase the concentration of antiepileptics **(oxcarbazepine)** and antiepileptics **(oxcarbazepine)** are predicted to decrease the concentration of antiepileptics **(lamotrigine)**. Monitor adverse effects and adjust dose. Moderate Study
- Antiepileptics **(carbamazepine, fosphenytoin)** are predicted to decrease the exposure to antiepileptics **(perampanel)**. Monitor and adjust dose. Moderate Study → Also see **TABLE 9** p. 1056
- Antiepileptics **(oxcarbazepine)** decrease the concentration of antiepileptics **(perampanel)** and antiepileptics **(perampanel)** increase the concentration of antiepileptics **(oxcarbazepine)**. Monitor and adjust dose. Moderate Study
- Antiepileptics **(phenobarbital, phenytoin, primidone)** are predicted to decrease the exposure to antiepileptics **(perampanel)**. Monitor and adjust dose. Moderate Study → Also see **TABLE 9** p. 1056
- Antiepileptics **(phenytoin)** increase the concentration of antiepileptics **(phenobarbital)** and antiepileptics **(phenobarbital)** affect the concentration of antiepileptics **(phenytoin)**. Moderate Study → Also see **TABLE 9** p. 1056
- Antiepileptics **(fosphenytoin)** increase the concentration of antiepileptics **(phenobarbital, primidone)** and antiepileptics **(phenobarbital, primidone)** affect the concentration of antiepileptics **(fosphenytoin)**. Moderate Study → Also see **TABLE 9** p. 1056
- Antiepileptics **(oxcarbazepine)** are predicted to increase the concentration of antiepileptics **(phenytoin)**. Monitor concentration and adjust dose. Moderate Study
- Antiepileptics **(stiripentol)** are predicted to increase the concentration of antiepileptics **(phenytoin)**. Avoid in Dravet syndrome. Severe Study
- Antiepileptics **(sultiame)** might increase the concentration of antiepileptics **(phenytoin)**. Severe Study
- Antiepileptics **(carbamazepine)** potentially decrease the concentration of antiepileptics **(primidone)** and antiepileptics **(primidone)** potentially decrease the concentration of antiepileptics **(carbamazepine)**. Adjust dose. Moderate Anecdotal

Antiepileptics (continued)
- Antiepileptics **(phenytoin)** increase the concentration of antiepileptics **(primidone)** and antiepileptics **(primidone)** affect the concentration of antiepileptics **(phenytoin)**. [Moderate] Study → Also see TABLE 9 p. 1056
- Antiepileptics **(stiripentol)** are predicted to increase the concentration of antiepileptics **(primidone)**. [Severe] Theoretical
- Antiepileptics **(valproate)** affect the concentration of antiepileptics **(primidone)**. Monitor and adjust dose. [Severe] Study
- Antiepileptics **(carbamazepine)** slightly increase the clearance of antiepileptics **(retigabine)**. [Moderate] Study
- Antiepileptics **(fosphenytoin, phenytoin)** are predicted to slightly increase the clearance of antiepileptics **(retigabine)**. [Moderate] Study
- Antiepileptics **(valproate)** increase the exposure to antiepileptics **(rufinamide)**. Adjust **rufinamide** dose, p. 250. [Moderate] Study
- Antiepileptics **(primidone)** might increase the adverse effects of antiepileptics **(sultiame)**. [Moderate] Theoretical
- Antiepileptics **(carbamazepine, fosphenytoin, phenobarbital, phenytoin, primidone)** decrease the exposure to antiepileptics **(tiagabine)**. Monitor and adjust **tiagabine** dose, p. 256. [Moderate] Study
- Antiepileptics **(fosphenytoin, phenytoin)** decrease the concentration of antiepileptics **(topiramate)** and antiepileptics **(topiramate)** increase the concentration of antiepileptics **(fosphenytoin, phenytoin)**. Monitor and adjust dose. [Moderate] Study
- Antiepileptics **(phenobarbital, primidone)** are predicted to decrease the concentration of antiepileptics **(topiramate)**. [Mild] Study
- Antiepileptics **(phenobarbital)** decrease the concentration of antiepileptics **(valproate)** and antiepileptics **(valproate)** increase the concentration of antiepileptics **(phenobarbital)**. Monitor and adjust dose. [Moderate] Study
- Antiepileptics **(topiramate)** increase the risk of toxicity when given with antiepileptics **(valproate)**. [Severe] Study
- Antiepileptics **(carbamazepine)** slightly to moderately decrease the concentration of antiepileptics **(zonisamide)** and antiepileptics **(zonisamide)** affect the concentration of antiepileptics **(carbamazepine)**. Monitor and adjust dose. [Moderate] Study
- Antiepileptics **(fosphenytoin, phenytoin)** slightly to moderately decrease the concentration of antiepileptics **(zonisamide)**. Monitor and adjust dose. [Moderate] Study
- Antiepileptics **(phenobarbital, primidone)** are predicted to decrease the concentration of antiepileptics **(zonisamide)**. Monitor and adjust dose. [Moderate] Study
- Antiepileptics **(topiramate)** potentially increase the risk of overheating and dehydration when given with antiepileptics **(zonisamide)**. Avoid in children. [Severe] Theoretical
- Antifungals, azoles **(itraconazole, ketoconazole, posaconazole, voriconazole)** are predicted to very slightly increase the exposure to **perampanel**. [Mild] Study
- Antifungals, azoles **(miconazole)** increase the risk of carbamazepine toxicity when given with **carbamazepine**. Monitor and adjust dose. [Severe] Anecdotal
- Antifungals, azoles **(miconazole)** increase the risk of phenytoin toxicity when given with **fosphenytoin**. Monitor and adjust dose. [Severe] Anecdotal
- Antifungals, azoles **(miconazole)** increase the risk of phenytoin toxicity when given with **phenytoin**. Monitor and adjust dose. [Severe] Anecdotal
- **Carbamazepine** is predicted to decrease the efficacy of antifungals, azoles **(fluconazole)** and antifungals, azoles **(fluconazole)** increase the concentration of **carbamazepine**. Avoid or monitor **carbamazepine** concentration and adjust dose accordingly, p. 234. [Severe] Theoretical
- Antifungals, azoles **(fluconazole)** increase the concentration of antiepileptics **(fosphenytoin, phenytoin)**. Monitor concentration and adjust dose. [Moderate] Study
- Antiepileptics **(carbamazepine, fosphenytoin, phenobarbital, phenytoin, primidone)** are predicted to decrease the exposure to antifungals, azoles **(isavuconazole)**. Avoid. [Severe] Study
- **Fosphenytoin** very markedly decreases the exposure to antifungals, azoles **(itraconazole)**. Avoid and for 14 days after stopping **fosphenytoin**. [Moderate] Study
- **Phenobarbital** decreases the concentration of antifungals, azoles **(itraconazole)**. Avoid and for 14 days after stopping **phenobarbital**. [Moderate] Study
- **Phenytoin** very markedly decreases the exposure to antifungals, azoles **(itraconazole)**. Avoid and for 14 days after stopping **phenytoin**. [Moderate] Study
- **Primidone** is predicted to decrease the concentration of antifungals, azoles **(itraconazole)**. [Moderate] Theoretical
- **Carbamazepine** is predicted to decrease the efficacy of antifungals, azoles **(itraconazole, voriconazole)** and antifungals, azoles **(itraconazole, voriconazole)** increase the concentration of **carbamazepine**. Avoid or adjust dose. [Moderate] Theoretical
- **Carbamazepine** is predicted to decrease the efficacy of antifungals, azoles **(ketoconazole)** and antifungals, azoles **(ketoconazole)** slightly increase the concentration of **carbamazepine**. Avoid or monitor **carbamazepine** concentration and adjust dose accordingly, p. 234. [Moderate] Study
- **Phenobarbital** is predicted to decrease the concentration of antifungals, azoles **(ketoconazole)**. Avoid. [Moderate] Study
- Antiepileptics **(fosphenytoin, phenytoin)** decrease the exposure to antifungals, azoles **(ketoconazole)**. Avoid. [Moderate] Study
- **Primidone** is predicted to decrease the concentration of antifungals, azoles **(ketoconazole, posaconazole)**. Avoid. [Moderate] Study
- **Carbamazepine** is predicted to decrease the efficacy of antifungals, azoles **(posaconazole)** and antifungals, azoles **(posaconazole)** increase the concentration of **carbamazepine**. Avoid. [Moderate] Theoretical
- **Phenobarbital** is predicted to decrease the concentration of antifungals, azoles **(posaconazole)**. Avoid. [Moderate] Study
- Antiepileptics **(fosphenytoin, phenytoin)** are predicted to decrease the exposure to antifungals, azoles **(posaconazole)**. Avoid. [Moderate] Study
- **Fosphenytoin** decreases the exposure to antifungals, azoles **(voriconazole)** and antifungals, azoles **(voriconazole)** increase the exposure to **fosphenytoin**. Avoid or adjust **voriconazole** dose and monitor phenytoin concentration, p. 468. [Moderate] Study
- **Phenytoin** decreases the exposure to antifungals, azoles **(voriconazole)** and antifungals, azoles **(voriconazole)** increase the exposure to **phenytoin**. Avoid or adjust **voriconazole** dose and monitor **phenytoin** concentration, p. 468, p. 249. [Moderate] Study
- Antiepileptics **(phenobarbital, primidone)** are predicted to decrease the concentration of antifungals, azoles **(voriconazole)**. Avoid. [Moderate] Theoretical
- Antihistamines, sedating **(hydroxyzine)** potentially increase the risk of overheating and dehydration when given with **zonisamide**. Avoid in children. [Severe] Theoretical
- Antiepileptics **(carbamazepine, fosphenytoin, phenobarbital, phenytoin, primidone)** are predicted to decrease the exposure to antimalarials **(artemether)** with lumefantrine. Avoid. [Severe] Study
- Antiepileptics **(carbamazepine, fosphenytoin, phenytoin)** might decrease the exposure to the active metabolite of antimalarials **(artesunate)**. Avoid. [Severe] Study
- Antimalarials **(pyrimethamine)** increase the risk of haematological toxicity when given with antiepileptics **(fosphenytoin, phenytoin)**. [Severe] Study
- Antimalarials **(pyrimethamine)** are predicted to increase the risk of haematological toxicity when given with antiepileptics **(phenobarbital, primidone)**. [Severe] Theoretical
- Antiepileptics **(carbamazepine, fosphenytoin, phenobarbital, phenytoin, primidone)** are predicted to decrease the concentration of antimalarials **(piperaquine)**. Avoid. [Moderate] Theoretical
- Antiepileptics **(carbamazepine, phenobarbital, primidone)** potentially increase the risk of toxicity when given with antimalarials **(quinine)**. [Unknown] Study
- Antiepileptics **(carbamazepine, fosphenytoin, phenobarbital, phenytoin, primidone)** are predicted to moderately decrease

A1 Interactions | **Appendix 1**

the exposure to atypical antipsychotics **(aripiprazole)**. Avoid or adjust dose—consult product literature. [Moderate] Study → Also see **TABLE 15** p. 1058 → Also see **TABLE 9** p. 1056

- Antiepileptics **(carbamazepine, fosphenytoin, phenobarbital, phenytoin, primidone)** are predicted to decrease the exposure to atypical antipsychotics **(cariprazine)**. Avoid. [Severe] Theoretical → Also see **TABLE 15** p. 1058 → Also see **TABLE 9** p. 1056
- **Carbamazepine** is predicted to increase the risk of myelosuppression when given with atypical antipsychotics **(clozapine)**. Avoid. [Severe] Anecdotal → Also see **TABLE 15** p. 1058
- **Valproate** has been reported to increase the risk of neutropenia and myocarditis when given with atypical antipsychotics **(clozapine)**. [Severe] Anecdotal → Also see **TABLE 15** p. 1058
- Antiepileptics **(fosphenytoin, phenobarbital, phenytoin, primidone)** are predicted to decrease the exposure to atypical antipsychotics **(clozapine)**. [Moderate] Anecdotal → Also see **TABLE 9** p. 1056
- Antiepileptics **(carbamazepine, fosphenytoin, phenobarbital, phenytoin, primidone)** are predicted to decrease the exposure to atypical antipsychotics **(lurasidone)**. Avoid. [Moderate] Study → Also see **TABLE 15** p. 1058 → Also see **TABLE 9** p. 1056
- **Carbamazepine** potentially decreases the exposure to atypical antipsychotics **(olanzapine)**. Monitor and adjust dose. [Moderate] Study → Also see **TABLE 15** p. 1058
- **Phenytoin** is predicted to decrease the exposure to atypical antipsychotics **(olanzapine)**. Monitor and adjust dose. [Moderate] Study → Also see **TABLE 9** p. 1056
- **Valproate** increases the risk of adverse effects when given with atypical antipsychotics **(olanzapine)**. [Severe] Study → Also see **TABLE 15** p. 1058
- **Valproate** slightly increases the exposure to atypical antipsychotics **(paliperidone)**. Adjust dose. [Moderate] Study → Also see **TABLE 15** p. 1058
- Antiepileptics **(carbamazepine, fosphenytoin, phenobarbital, phenytoin, primidone)** are predicted to decrease the exposure to atypical antipsychotics **(paliperidone)**. Monitor and adjust dose. [Severe] Study → Also see **TABLE 15** p. 1058 → Also see **TABLE 9** p. 1056
- **Valproate** potentially increases the risk of neutropenia when given with atypical antipsychotics **(quetiapine)**. [Moderate] Study → Also see **TABLE 15** p. 1058
- Antiepileptics **(carbamazepine, fosphenytoin, phenobarbital, phenytoin, primidone)** are predicted to decrease the exposure to atypical antipsychotics **(quetiapine)**. [Moderate] Study → Also see **TABLE 15** p. 1058 → Also see **TABLE 9** p. 1056
- Antiepileptics **(carbamazepine, fosphenytoin, phenobarbital, phenytoin, primidone)** are predicted to decrease the exposure to atypical antipsychotics **(risperidone)**. Adjust dose. [Moderate] Study → Also see **TABLE 15** p. 1058 → Also see **TABLE 9** p. 1056
- Antiepileptics **(carbamazepine, fosphenytoin, phenobarbital, phenytoin, primidone)** are predicted to decrease the exposure to **avacopan**. Avoid or monitor. [Severe] Study
- Antiepileptics **(carbamazepine, fosphenytoin, phenobarbital, phenytoin, primidone)** are predicted to decrease the exposure to **avapritinib**. Avoid. [Severe] Study
- Antiepileptics **(carbamazepine, fosphenytoin, phenobarbital, phenytoin, primidone)** are predicted to decrease the exposure to **axitinib**. Avoid or adjust dose. [Moderate] Study
- Antiepileptics **(carbamazepine, fosphenytoin, phenobarbital, phenytoin, primidone)** are predicted to decrease the exposure to **bazedoxifene**. [Moderate] Theoretical
- Antiepileptics **(carbamazepine, fosphenytoin, phenobarbital, phenytoin, primidone)** decrease the exposure to **bedaquiline**. Avoid. [Severe] Study
- Antiepileptics **(carbamazepine, fosphenytoin, phenobarbital, phenytoin, primidone)** are predicted to decrease the exposure to **belumosudil**. Adjust **belumosudil** dose, p. 650. [Severe] Study
- Antiepileptics **(carbamazepine, fosphenytoin, phenobarbital, phenytoin, primidone)** are predicted to decrease the exposure to benzodiazepines **(alprazolam)**. Adjust dose. [Moderate] Theoretical → Also see **TABLE 9** p. 1056
- **Stiripentol** increases the concentration of benzodiazepines **(clobazam)**. [Severe] Study
- **Sultiame** might increase the exposure to the active metabolite of benzodiazepines **(clobazam)**. [Moderate] Theoretical
- Benzodiazepines **(chlordiazepoxide)** affect the concentration of antiepileptics **(fosphenytoin, phenytoin)**. [Severe] Study → Also see **TABLE 9** p. 1056
- Benzodiazepines **(clobazam, clonazepam)** potentially affect the concentration of antiepileptics **(fosphenytoin, phenytoin)**. [Severe] Anecdotal → Also see **TABLE 9** p. 1056
- Benzodiazepines **(diazepam)** potentially affect the concentration of antiepileptics **(fosphenytoin, phenytoin)**. Monitor concentration and adjust dose. [Severe] Study → Also see **TABLE 9** p. 1056
- Antiepileptics **(carbamazepine, fosphenytoin, phenobarbital, phenytoin, primidone)** are predicted to decrease the exposure to benzodiazepines **(midazolam)**. Monitor and adjust dose. [Severe] Study → Also see **TABLE 9** p. 1056
- **Carbamazepine** is predicted to decrease the concentration of **berotralstat**. Avoid. [Severe] Theoretical
- Antiepileptics **(phenobarbital, primidone)** are predicted to decrease the exposure to beta blockers, non-selective **(carvedilol, labetalol)**. [Moderate] Theoretical
- Antiepileptics **(phenobarbital, primidone)** are predicted to decrease the exposure to beta blockers, non-selective **(propranolol)**. [Moderate] Study
- Antiepileptics **(phenobarbital, primidone)** are predicted to decrease the exposure to beta blockers, selective **(acebutolol, bisoprolol, metoprolol, nebivolol)**. [Moderate] Study
- Antiepileptics **(carbamazepine, fosphenytoin, phenobarbital, phenytoin, primidone)** are predicted to decrease the exposure to **bictegravir**. Avoid. [Moderate] Study
- **Oxcarbazepine** is predicted to decrease the exposure to **bictegravir**. Avoid. [Moderate] Theoretical
- **Bleomycin** -containing cytotoxic regimens might affect the concentration of antiepileptics **(fosphenytoin, phenytoin)**. Avoid. [Severe] Anecdotal
- Antiepileptics **(carbamazepine, fosphenytoin, phenobarbital, phenytoin, primidone)** slightly decrease the exposure to **bortezomib**. Avoid. [Severe] Study → Also see **TABLE 10** p. 1056
- Antiepileptics **(carbamazepine, fosphenytoin, phenobarbital, phenytoin, primidone)** are predicted to very markedly decrease the exposure to **bosutinib**. Avoid. [Severe] Study
- Antiepileptics **(carbamazepine, fosphenytoin, phenobarbital, phenytoin, primidone)** are predicted to decrease the exposure to **brigatinib**. Avoid. [Severe] Study
- **Bulevirtide** is predicted to increase the exposure to **carbamazepine**. [Moderate] Theoretical
- Antiepileptics **(carbamazepine, fosphenytoin, phenobarbital, phenytoin, primidone)** are predicted to markedly decrease the exposure to **bupropion**. [Severe] Study
- **Valproate** increases the exposure to **bupropion**. [Severe] Study
- Antiepileptics **(carbamazepine, fosphenytoin, phenobarbital, phenytoin, primidone)** are predicted to decrease the exposure to **buspirone**. Use with caution and adjust dose. [Severe] Study
- Antiepileptics **(carbamazepine, fosphenytoin, oxcarbazepine, phenobarbital, phenytoin, primidone)** might decrease the concentration of **cabotegravir**. Avoid. [Severe] Theoretical
- Antiepileptics **(carbamazepine, fosphenytoin, phenobarbital, phenytoin, primidone)** moderately decrease the exposure to **cabozantinib**. Avoid. [Moderate] Study
- Antiepileptics **(fosphenytoin, phenytoin)** are predicted to moderately increase the clearance of **caffeine citrate**. Monitor and adjust dose. [Moderate] Study
- Calcium-channel blockers **(diltiazem)** increase the concentration of **carbamazepine** and **carbamazepine** is predicted to decrease the exposure to calcium-channel blockers **(diltiazem)**. Monitor concentration and adjust dose. [Severe] Anecdotal
- Calcium-channel blockers **(verapamil)** increase the concentration of **carbamazepine** and **carbamazepine** is predicted to decrease the exposure to calcium-channel blockers **(verapamil)**. [Severe] Anecdotal
- Antiepileptics **(carbamazepine, fosphenytoin, phenobarbital, phenytoin, primidone)** are predicted to decrease the exposure to calcium-channel blockers **(amlodipine, felodipine, lacidipine, lercanidipine, nicardipine, nifedipine, nimodipine)**. Monitor and adjust dose. [Moderate] Study

Antiepileptics (continued)

- Antiepileptics **(phenobarbital, primidone)** are predicted to decrease the exposure to calcium-channel blockers **(diltiazem, verapamil)**. Severe Study
- Calcium-channel blockers **(diltiazem, verapamil)** potentially increase the concentration of antiepileptics **(fosphenytoin, phenytoin)** and antiepileptics **(fosphenytoin, phenytoin)** are predicted to decrease the exposure to calcium-channel blockers **(diltiazem, verapamil)**. Severe Study
- **Valproate** increases the exposure to calcium-channel blockers **(nimodipine)**. Adjust dose. Moderate Study
- Antiepileptics **(carbamazepine, fosphenytoin, phenobarbital, phenytoin, primidone)** are predicted to decrease the exposure to **cannabidiol**. Adjust dose. Moderate Study → Also see TABLE 9 p. 1056
- **Cannabidiol** increases the risk of increased ALT concentrations when given with **valproate**. Avoid or adjust dose. Severe Study
- **Capecitabine** increases the concentration of antiepileptics **(fosphenytoin, phenytoin)**. Severe Anecdotal
- Antiepileptics **(carbamazepine, fosphenytoin, phenobarbital, phenytoin, primidone)** are predicted to decrease the exposure to **capivasertib**. Avoid. Moderate Study
- **Carbapenems** decrease the concentration of **valproate**. Avoid. Severe Anecdotal
- Antiepileptics **(carbamazepine, fosphenytoin, phenytoin)** are predicted to decrease the concentration of **caspofungin**. Adjust **caspofungin** dose, p. 460. Moderate Theoretical
- **Cenobamate** might increase the exposure to antiepileptics **(fosphenytoin, primidone)**. Moderate Theoretical → Also see TABLE 9 p. 1056
- **Cenobamate** slightly increases the exposure to antiepileptics **(phenobarbital, phenytoin)**. Monitor and adjust dose. Moderate Study → Also see TABLE 9 p. 1056
- **Cenobamate** is predicted to decrease the concentration of **lamotrigine** and **lamotrigine** might affect the efficacy of **cenobamate**. Adjust dose. Moderate Study → Also see TABLE 9 p. 1056
- Antiepileptics **(carbamazepine, fosphenytoin, phenobarbital, phenytoin, primidone)** are predicted to decrease the exposure to **ceritinib**. Avoid. Severe Study
- **Ceritinib** is predicted to very slightly increase the exposure to **perampanel**. Mild Study
- Antiepileptics **(phenobarbital, primidone)** are predicted to affect the efficacy of **chenodeoxycholic acid**. Monitor and adjust dose. Moderate Theoretical
- Antiepileptics **(phenobarbital, primidone)** decrease the concentration of **chloramphenicol**. Moderate Study
- Intravenous **chloramphenicol** increases the concentration of antiepileptics **(fosphenytoin, phenytoin)** and antiepileptics **(fosphenytoin, phenytoin)** affect the concentration of intravenous **chloramphenicol**. Monitor concentration and adjust dose. Severe Study
- **Phenobarbital** decreases the effects of **cholic acid**. Avoid. Moderate Study
- Antiepileptics **(carbamazepine, fosphenytoin, phenobarbital, phenytoin, primidone)** decrease the concentration of **ciclosporin**. Severe Study
- **Oxcarbazepine** decreases the concentration of **ciclosporin**. Severe Anecdotal
- Antiepileptics **(carbamazepine, fosphenytoin, phenobarbital, phenytoin, primidone)** are predicted to alter the effects of **cilostazol**. Moderate Theoretical
- Antiepileptics **(carbamazepine, fosphenytoin, phenobarbital, phenytoin, primidone)** are predicted to decrease the exposure to **cinacalcet**. Monitor and adjust dose. Moderate Study
- **Carbamazepine** is predicted to increase the risk of haematological toxicity when given with oral **cladribine**. Moderate Theoretical
- Antiepileptics **(carbamazepine, fosphenytoin, phenobarbital, phenytoin, primidone)** decrease the exposure to **clomethiazole**. Monitor and adjust dose. Moderate Study → Also see TABLE 9 p. 1056
- Antiepileptics **(carbamazepine, fosphenytoin, phenobarbital, phenytoin, primidone)** are predicted to decrease the exposure to **cobicistat**. Avoid. Severe Study
- Antiepileptics **(eslicarbazepine, oxcarbazepine)** are predicted to decrease the concentration of **cobicistat**. Severe Theoretical
- **Cobicistat** is predicted to very slightly increase the exposure to **perampanel**. Mild Study
- Antiepileptics **(carbamazepine, fosphenytoin, phenobarbital, phenytoin, primidone)** are predicted to decrease the exposure to **cobimetinib**. Avoid. Severe Theoretical
- **Carbamazepine** is predicted to decrease the exposure to **colchicine**. Moderate Theoretical
- Antiepileptics **(carbamazepine, eslicarbazepine, fosphenytoin, oxcarbazepine, perampanel, phenobarbital, phenytoin, primidone, rufinamide, topiramate)** are predicted to decrease the efficacy of **combined hormonal contraceptives**. For CoSRH guidance, see Contraceptives, interactions p. 614. Severe Study
- **Combined hormonal contraceptives** alter the exposure to **lamotrigine** and **lamotrigine** might decrease the efficacy of **combined hormonal contraceptives**. Adjust dose. Moderate Study
- Antiepileptics **(carbamazepine, fosphenytoin, phenobarbital, phenytoin, primidone)** are predicted to decrease the exposure to corticosteroids **(budesonide, deflazacort, dexamethasone, fludrocortisone, hydrocortisone, methylprednisolone, prednisolone, triamcinolone)**. Monitor and adjust dose. Moderate Study
- Antiepileptics **(carbamazepine, fosphenytoin, phenobarbital, phenytoin, primidone)** are predicted to decrease the exposure to corticosteroids **(fluticasone)**. Unknown Theoretical
- Antiepileptics **(fosphenytoin, phenytoin)** are predicted to alter the anticoagulant effect of **coumarins**. Moderate Anecdotal
- Antiepileptics **(phenobarbital, primidone)** decrease the anticoagulant effect of **coumarins**. Monitor INR and adjust dose. Moderate Study
- **Carbamazepine** decreases the effects of **coumarins**. Monitor and adjust dose. Severe Study
- Antiepileptics **(carbamazepine, fosphenytoin, phenobarbital, phenytoin, primidone)** are predicted to markedly decrease the exposure to **crizotinib**. Avoid. Severe Study
- Antiepileptics **(carbamazepine, fosphenytoin, phenobarbital, phenytoin, primidone)** are predicted to decrease the exposure to **dabrafenib**. Avoid. Moderate Theoretical
- Antiepileptics **(carbamazepine, fosphenytoin, phenobarbital, phenytoin, primidone)** are predicted to decrease the exposure to **daridorexant**. Severe Study → Also see TABLE 9 p. 1056
- Antiepileptics **(carbamazepine, fosphenytoin, phenobarbital, phenytoin, primidone)** are predicted to decrease the exposure to **darifenacin**. Moderate Theoretical
- Antiepileptics **(carbamazepine, fosphenytoin, phenobarbital, phenytoin, primidone)** are predicted to markedly decrease the exposure to **dasatinib**. Avoid. Severe Study
- Antiepileptics **(carbamazepine, fosphenytoin, phenobarbital, phenytoin, primidone)** are predicted to slightly decrease the exposure to **delamanid**. Avoid. Moderate Study
- **Lamotrigine** is predicted to increase the risk of hyponatraemia when given with **desmopressin**. Severe Theoretical
- Antiepileptics **(carbamazepine, eslicarbazepine, fosphenytoin, oxcarbazepine, perampanel, phenobarbital, phenytoin, primidone, rufinamide, topiramate)** are predicted to decrease the efficacy of **desogestrel**. For CoSRH guidance, see Contraceptives, interactions p. 614. Severe Theoretical
- **Desogestrel** is predicted to increase the exposure to **lamotrigine** and **lamotrigine** might decrease the effects of **desogestrel**. For CoSRH guidance, see Contraceptives, interactions p. 614. Moderate Study
- Antiepileptics **(carbamazepine, fosphenytoin, phenobarbital, phenytoin, primidone)** are predicted to decrease the exposure to **deutivacaftor**. Avoid. Severe Theoretical
- **Diazoxide** decreases the concentration of antiepileptics **(fosphenytoin, phenytoin)** and antiepileptics **(fosphenytoin, phenytoin)** are predicted to decrease the effects of **diazoxide**. Monitor concentration and adjust dose. Moderate Anecdotal
- Antiepileptics **(carbamazepine, fosphenytoin, phenobarbital, phenytoin, primidone)** are predicted to markedly decrease the exposure to **dienogest**. Severe Study
- Antiepileptics **(fosphenytoin, phenytoin)** are predicted to decrease the concentration of **digoxin**. Moderate Anecdotal

- Antiepileptics **(carbamazepine, fosphenytoin, phenobarbital, phenytoin, primidone)** are predicted to decrease the exposure to dipeptidylpeptidase-4 inhibitors **(linagliptin)**. Moderate Study
- Antiepileptics **(carbamazepine, fosphenytoin, phenobarbital, phenytoin, primidone)** are predicted to moderately decrease the exposure to dipeptidylpeptidase-4 inhibitors **(saxagliptin)**. Moderate Study
- **Disulfiram** increases the concentration of antiepileptics **(fosphenytoin, phenytoin)**. Monitor concentration and adjust dose. Severe Study
- Antiepileptics **(fosphenytoin, phenobarbital, phenytoin, primidone)** are predicted to decrease the exposure to **dolutegravir**. Adjust **dolutegravir** dose, p. 508. Severe Study
- **Carbamazepine** decreases the exposure to **dolutegravir**. Adjust **dolutegravir** dose, p. 508. Severe Study
- **Oxcarbazepine** is predicted to decrease the exposure to **dolutegravir**. Adjust **dolutegravir** dose, p. 508. Severe Theoretical
- Antiepileptics **(carbamazepine, fosphenytoin, phenobarbital, phenytoin, primidone)** are predicted to decrease the exposure to **dronabinol**. Avoid or adjust dose. Mild Study → Also see TABLE 9 p. 1056
- Antiepileptics **(carbamazepine, eslicarbazepine, fosphenytoin, oxcarbazepine, perampanel, phenobarbital, phenytoin, primidone, rufinamide, topiramate)** are predicted to decrease the efficacy of **drospirenone**. For CoSRH guidance, see Contraceptives, interactions p. 614. Severe Theoretical
- **Lamotrigine** might decrease the effects of **drospirenone**. For CoSRH guidance, see Contraceptives, interactions p. 614. Severe Theoretical
- Antiepileptics **(carbamazepine, fosphenytoin, phenobarbital, phenytoin, primidone)** are predicted to decrease the exposure to **elacestrant**. Avoid or adjust dose depending on duration—consult product literature. Severe Study
- Antiepileptics **(carbamazepine, fosphenytoin, phenobarbital, phenytoin, primidone)** are predicted to decrease the exposure to **elbasvir**. Avoid. Severe Study
- Antiepileptics **(carbamazepine, fosphenytoin, phenobarbital, phenytoin, primidone)** is predicted to decrease the exposure to **elexacaftor**. Avoid. Severe Theoretical
- Antiepileptics **(carbamazepine, fosphenytoin, phenobarbital, phenytoin, primidone)** are predicted to decrease the exposure to **eliglustat**. Avoid. Severe Study
- Antiepileptics **(carbamazepine, fosphenytoin, phenobarbital, phenytoin, primidone)** are predicted to decrease the concentration of **elvitegravir**. Avoid. Severe Study
- Antiepileptics **(carbamazepine, fosphenytoin, phenobarbital, phenytoin, primidone)** are predicted to decrease the exposure to **encorafenib**. Severe Theoretical
- **Encorafenib** is predicted to decrease the exposure to **perampanel**. Monitor and adjust dose. Moderate Study
- Antiepileptics **(carbamazepine, fosphenytoin, phenobarbital, phenytoin, primidone)** affect the exposure to endothelin receptor antagonists **(bosentan)**. Avoid. Severe Study
- Antiepileptics **(carbamazepine, fosphenytoin, phenobarbital, phenytoin, primidone)** are predicted to decrease the exposure to endothelin receptor antagonists **(macitentan)**. Avoid. Severe Study
- Antiepileptics **(carbamazepine, fosphenytoin, phenobarbital, phenytoin, primidone)** are predicted to decrease the exposure to the cytotoxic component of **enfortumab vedotin**. Moderate Theoretical
- **Enteral feeds** decrease the absorption of **phenytoin**. Severe Study
- Antiepileptics **(carbamazepine, fosphenytoin, phenobarbital, phenytoin, primidone)** are predicted to decrease the exposure to **entrectinib**. Avoid. Severe Study
- Antiepileptics **(carbamazepine, fosphenytoin, phenobarbital, phenytoin, primidone)** are predicted to decrease the exposure to **erdafitinib**. Avoid. Severe Study
- Antiepileptics **(carbamazepine, fosphenytoin, phenobarbital, phenytoin, primidone)** are predicted to decrease the exposure to **erlotinib**. Avoid or adjust dose—consult product literature. Severe Study
- **Eslicarbazepine** is predicted to decrease the exposure to **erlotinib**. Severe Theoretical
- **Oxcarbazepine** decreases the exposure to **erlotinib**. Severe Study
- Antiepileptics **(carbamazepine, fosphenytoin, phenobarbital, phenytoin, primidone)** are predicted to decrease the exposure to **esketamine**. Adjust dose. Moderate Study → Also see TABLE 9 p. 1056
- Antiepileptics **(carbamazepine, eslicarbazepine, fosphenytoin, oxcarbazepine, perampanel, phenobarbital, phenytoin, primidone, rufinamide, topiramate)** are predicted to decrease the efficacy of **estradiol**. Moderate Theoretical
- Antiepileptics **(carbamazepine, fosphenytoin, phenobarbital, phenytoin, primidone)** are predicted to decrease the exposure to **eszopiclone**. Adjust dose. Moderate Theoretical → Also see TABLE 9 p. 1056
- Antiepileptics **(carbamazepine, eslicarbazepine, fosphenytoin, oxcarbazepine, perampanel, phenobarbital, phenytoin, primidone, rufinamide, topiramate)** are predicted to decrease the efficacy of **etonogestrel**. For CoSRH guidance, see Contraceptives, interactions p. 614. Severe Theoretical
- **Lamotrigine** might decrease the effects of **etonogestrel**. For CoSRH guidance, see Contraceptives, interactions p. 614. Moderate Theoretical
- Antiepileptics **(carbamazepine, fosphenytoin, phenobarbital, phenytoin, primidone)** are predicted to decrease the efficacy of **etoposide**. Moderate Study
- Antiepileptics **(carbamazepine, fosphenytoin, phenobarbital, phenytoin, primidone)** are predicted to decrease the concentration of **everolimus**. Avoid or adjust dose. Severe Study
- Antiepileptics **(carbamazepine, fosphenytoin, phenobarbital, phenytoin, primidone)** moderately decrease the exposure to **exemestane**. Moderate Study
- **Carbamazepine** is predicted to decrease the exposure to factor XA inhibitors **(apixaban)**. Use with caution or avoid. Severe Study
- **Fosphenytoin** is predicted to decrease the exposure to factor XA inhibitors **(apixaban)**. Severe Study
- **Primidone** decreases the exposure to factor XA inhibitors **(apixaban)**. Severe Study
- Antiepileptics **(phenobarbital, phenytoin)** decrease the exposure to factor XA inhibitors **(apixaban)**. Use with caution or avoid. Severe Study
- **Carbamazepine** is predicted to decrease the exposure to factor XA inhibitors **(edoxaban)**. Severe Study
- Antiepileptics **(fosphenytoin, phenobarbital, phenytoin, primidone)** are predicted to decrease the exposure to factor XA inhibitors **(edoxaban)**. Severe Theoretical
- **Oxcarbazepine** decreases the exposure to factor XA inhibitors **(rivaroxaban)**. Severe Study
- Antiepileptics **(carbamazepine, fosphenytoin)** are predicted to decrease the exposure to factor XA inhibitors **(rivaroxaban)**. Avoid unless patient can be monitored for signs of thrombosis. Severe Study
- Antiepileptics **(phenobarbital, phenytoin, primidone)** decrease the exposure to factor XA inhibitors **(rivaroxaban)**. Avoid unless patient can be monitored for signs of thrombosis. Severe Study
- Antiepileptics **(carbamazepine, fosphenytoin, phenobarbital, phenytoin, primidone)** are predicted to decrease the exposure to **fedratinib**. Avoid. Moderate Study
- Antiepileptics **(fosphenytoin, phenobarbital, phenytoin, primidone)** are predicted to decrease the exposure to **fenfluramine**. Moderate Theoretical
- **Carbamazepine** is predicted to decrease the concentration of **fenfluramine**. Adjust dose. Moderate Theoretical
- **Stiripentol** (given with clobazam, and with or without valproate) modestly increases the exposure to **fenfluramine**. Adjust **fenfluramine** dose, p. 238. Severe Study
- Antiepileptics **(carbamazepine, fosphenytoin, phenobarbital, phenytoin, primidone)** are predicted to decrease the exposure to **fesoterodine**. Avoid. Moderate Study
- **Fluorouracil** increases the concentration of antiepileptics **(fosphenytoin, phenytoin)**. Monitor concentration and adjust dose. Severe Anecdotal
- **Folates** are predicted to decrease the concentration of antiepileptics **(fosphenytoin, phenobarbital, phenytoin, primidone)**. Monitor concentration and adjust dose. Severe Study

Antiepileptics (continued)

- **Phenytoin** might decrease the effects of **foslevodopa**. Moderate Theoretical → Also see **TABLE 9** p. 1056
- Antiepileptics **(carbamazepine, fosphenytoin, phenobarbital, phenytoin, primidone)** are predicted to decrease the exposure to **fostamatinib**. Avoid. Severe Study
- Antiepileptics **(carbamazepine, fosphenytoin, phenobarbital, phenytoin, primidone)** are predicted to decrease the exposure to the active metabolite of **fostemsavir**. Avoid. Severe Study
- Antiepileptics **(carbamazepine, fosphenytoin, phenobarbital, phenytoin, primidone)** are predicted to decrease the exposure to **fruquintinib**. Avoid. Moderate Study
- **Carbamazepine** is predicted to decrease the exposure to **futibatinib**. Avoid or adjust dose. Moderate Study
- Antiepileptics **(carbamazepine, fosphenytoin, phenobarbital, phenytoin, primidone)** are predicted to decrease the exposure to **gefitinib**. Avoid. Severe Study
- **Eslicarbazepine** is predicted to decrease the exposure to **gefitinib**. Moderate Theoretical
- **Oxcarbazepine** decreases the exposure to **gefitinib**. Severe Study
- Antiepileptics **(carbamazepine, phenytoin)** are predicted to decrease the exposure to **gilteritinib**. Avoid. Severe Study
- Antiepileptics **(carbamazepine, fosphenytoin, phenobarbital, phenytoin, primidone)** are predicted to decrease the exposure to **glasdegib**. Avoid. Severe Study
- Antiepileptics **(carbamazepine, fosphenytoin, phenobarbital, phenytoin, primidone)** are predicted to moderately decrease the exposure to **glecaprevir**. Avoid. Severe Study
- Antiepileptics **(eslicarbazepine, oxcarbazepine)** potentially decrease the exposure to **glecaprevir**. Avoid. Severe Theoretical
- **Valproate** potentially opposes the effects of **glycerol phenylbutyrate**. Moderate Theoretical
- **Grapefruit** juice slightly increases the exposure to **carbamazepine**. Monitor and adjust dose. Moderate Study
- Antiepileptics **(carbamazepine, fosphenytoin, phenobarbital, phenytoin, primidone)** are predicted to decrease the exposure to **grazoprevir**. Avoid. Severe Study
- Antiepileptics **(phenobarbital, primidone)** decrease the effects of **griseofulvin**. Moderate Study
- Antiepileptics **(carbamazepine, fosphenytoin, phenobarbital, phenytoin, primidone)** are predicted to decrease the concentration of **guanfacine**. Adjust **guanfacine** dose, p. 281. Moderate Study → Also see **TABLE 9** p. 1056
- **Oxcarbazepine** is predicted to decrease the concentration of **guanfacine**. Monitor and adjust **guanfacine** dose, p. 281. Moderate Theoretical
- **Guanfacine** increases the concentration of **valproate**. Monitor and adjust dose. Moderate Study
- H_2 receptor antagonists **(cimetidine)** transiently increase the concentration of **carbamazepine**. Monitor concentration and adjust dose. Moderate Study
- H_2 receptor antagonists **(cimetidine)** increase the concentration of antiepileptics **(fosphenytoin, phenytoin)**. Monitor concentration and adjust dose. Severe Study
- Antiepileptics **(carbamazepine, fosphenytoin, phenobarbital, phenytoin, primidone)** decrease the concentration of **haloperidol**. Adjust dose. Moderate Study → Also see **TABLE 15** p. 1058 → Also see **TABLE 9** p. 1056
- **Haloperidol** potentially increases the risk of overheating and dehydration when given with **zonisamide**. Avoid in children. Severe Theoretical
- **HIV-protease inhibitors** are predicted to increase the exposure to **carbamazepine** and **carbamazepine** is predicted to decrease the exposure to **HIV-protease inhibitors**. Monitor and adjust dose. Severe Theoretical
- HIV-protease inhibitors **(ritonavir)** decrease the exposure to **lamotrigine**. Severe Study
- HIV-protease inhibitors **(ritonavir)** are predicted to decrease the concentration of **valproate**. Severe Anecdotal → Also see **TABLE 1** p. 1053
- **HIV-protease inhibitors** are predicted to affect the exposure to antiepileptics **(fosphenytoin, phenytoin)** and antiepileptics **(fosphenytoin, phenytoin)** decrease the concentration of **HIV-protease inhibitors**. Severe Theoretical
- **HIV-protease inhibitors** are predicted to affect the concentration of antiepileptics **(phenobarbital, primidone)** and antiepileptics **(phenobarbital, primidone)** are predicted to decrease the concentration of **HIV-protease inhibitors**. Severe Theoretical
- **HIV-protease inhibitors** are predicted to very slightly increase the exposure to **perampanel**. Mild Study
- Antiepileptics **(carbamazepine, eslicarbazepine, fosphenytoin, oxcarbazepine, perampanel, phenobarbital, phenytoin, primidone, rufinamide, topiramate)** are predicted to decrease the effects of **hormone replacement therapy**. Moderate Anecdotal
- **Hormone replacement therapy** is predicted to alter the exposure to **lamotrigine**. Moderate Theoretical
- Antiepileptics **(carbamazepine, fosphenytoin, phenobarbital, phenytoin, primidone)** are predicted to decrease the exposure to **ibrutinib**. Avoid or monitor. Severe Study
- Antiepileptics **(carbamazepine, fosphenytoin, phenobarbital, phenytoin, primidone)** are predicted to decrease the exposure to **idelalisib**. Avoid. Severe Study
- **Idelalisib** is predicted to very slightly increase the exposure to **perampanel**. Mild Study
- Antiepileptics **(carbamazepine, fosphenytoin, oxcarbazepine, phenobarbital, phenytoin, primidone)** are predicted to decrease the exposure to **imatinib**. Avoid. Moderate Study
- **Eslicarbazepine** is predicted to decrease the exposure to **imatinib**. Moderate Theoretical
- **Topiramate** is predicted to decrease the exposure to **imatinib**. Moderate Study
- Antiepileptics **(carbamazepine, fosphenytoin, phenobarbital, phenytoin, primidone)** are predicted to decrease the exposure to **irinotecan**. Avoid. Severe Study
- Antiepileptics **(carbamazepine, fosphenytoin, phenobarbital, phenytoin, primidone)** are predicted to decrease the exposure to iron chelators **(deferasirox)**. Monitor serum ferritin and adjust dose. Moderate Theoretical
- Iron chelators **(dexrazoxane)** might decrease the absorption of antiepileptics **(fosphenytoin, phenytoin)**. Avoid. Severe Theoretical
- **Isoniazid** increases the concentration of antiepileptics **(fosphenytoin, phenytoin)**. Moderate Study → Also see **TABLE 10** p. 1056
- **Isoniazid** markedly increases the concentration of **carbamazepine** and **carbamazepine** increases the risk of hepatotoxicity when given with **isoniazid**. Monitor concentration and adjust dose. Severe Study
- Antiepileptics **(carbamazepine, fosphenytoin, phenobarbital, phenytoin, primidone)** are predicted to decrease the exposure to **ivabradine**. Adjust dose. Moderate Theoretical
- Antiepileptics **(carbamazepine, fosphenytoin, phenobarbital, phenytoin, primidone)** are predicted to decrease the exposure to **ivacaftor**. Avoid. Severe Study
- Antiepileptics **(carbamazepine, fosphenytoin, phenobarbital, primidone)** are predicted to decrease the exposure to **ivosidenib**. Avoid. Severe Theoretical
- **Ivosidenib** might decrease the exposure to **lamotrigine**. Avoid or monitor efficacy. Unknown Theoretical
- **Ivosidenib** is predicted to decrease the exposure to **perampanel**. Monitor and adjust dose. Moderate Study
- **Phenytoin** is predicted to decrease the exposure to **ivosidenib** and **ivosidenib** might decrease the exposure to **phenytoin**. Avoid. Severe Study
- Antiepileptics **(carbamazepine, fosphenytoin, phenobarbital, phenytoin, primidone)** are predicted to decrease the exposure to **ixazomib**. Avoid. Severe Study
- Antiepileptics **(carbamazepine, fosphenytoin, phenobarbital, phenytoin, primidone)** are predicted to decrease the exposure to **ketamine**. Adjust dose. Moderate Theoretical → Also see **TABLE 9** p. 1056
- Antiepileptics **(carbamazepine, fosphenytoin, phenobarbital, phenytoin, primidone)** are predicted to decrease the exposure to **lapatinib**. Avoid. Severe Study
- Antiepileptics **(carbamazepine, fosphenytoin, phenobarbital, phenytoin, primidone)** are predicted to moderately decrease the exposure to **larotrectinib**. Avoid. Moderate Study

- Antiepileptics **(carbamazepine, fosphenytoin, phenobarbital, phenytoin, primidone)** are predicted to decrease the exposure to **lazertinib**. Avoid. [Severe] Study
- Antiepileptics **(fosphenytoin, oxcarbazepine, phenobarbital, phenytoin, primidone)** are predicted to decrease the exposure to **ledipasvir**. Avoid. [Severe] Theoretical
- **Carbamazepine** is predicted to decrease the exposure to **ledipasvir**. Avoid. [Severe] Study
- Antiepileptics **(carbamazepine, fosphenytoin, phenobarbital, phenytoin, primidone)** are predicted to decrease the exposure to **lenacapavir**. Avoid. [Severe] Study
- **Oxcarbazepine** is predicted to decrease the exposure to **lenacapavir**. Avoid. [Severe] Theoretical
- Antiepileptics **(carbamazepine, fosphenytoin, phenobarbital, phenytoin, primidone)** are predicted to decrease the exposure to **leniolisib**. Avoid. [Severe] Theoretical
- Antiepileptics **(carbamazepine, phenobarbital, primidone)** are predicted to decrease the concentration of **letermovir**. [Moderate] Theoretical
- **Letermovir** is predicted to decrease the concentration of antiepileptics **(fosphenytoin, phenytoin)** and antiepileptics **(fosphenytoin, phenytoin)** are predicted to decrease the concentration of **letermovir**. [Moderate] Theoretical
- Antiepileptics **(fosphenytoin, phenytoin)** decrease the effects of **levodopa**. [Moderate] Study → Also see **TABLE 9** p. 1056
- Antiepileptics **(carbamazepine, eslicarbazepine, fosphenytoin, oxcarbazepine, perampanel, phenobarbital, phenytoin, primidone, rufinamide, topiramate)** are predicted to decrease the efficacy of some contraceptive methods containing **levonorgestrel**. For CoSRH guidance, see Contraceptives, interactions p. 614. [Severe] Theoretical
- **Lamotrigine** might decrease the effects of **levonorgestrel**. For CoSRH guidance, see Contraceptives, interactions p. 614. [Moderate] Theoretical
- Antiepileptics **(carbamazepine, oxcarbazepine)** are predicted to increase the risk of neurotoxicity when given with **lithium**. [Severe] Anecdotal
- Antiepileptics **(carbamazepine, fosphenytoin, phenobarbital, phenytoin, primidone)** are predicted to decrease the exposure to **lomitapide**. Monitor and adjust dose. [Moderate] Theoretical
- Antiepileptics **(fosphenytoin, phenytoin)** decrease the effects of loop diuretics **(furosemide)**. [Moderate] Study
- Antiepileptics **(carbamazepine, fosphenytoin, phenobarbital, phenytoin, primidone)** are predicted to decrease the exposure to **lorlatinib**. Avoid. [Severe] Study
- **Lumacaftor** is predicted to decrease the exposure to antiepileptics **(carbamazepine, fosphenytoin, phenobarbital, phenytoin, primidone)**. Avoid. [Severe] Theoretical
- **Lumacaftor** is predicted to decrease the exposure to **perampanel**. Monitor and adjust dose. [Moderate] Study
- Macrolides **(clarithromycin)** slightly increase the concentration of **carbamazepine**. Monitor concentration and adjust dose. [Severe] Study
- Macrolides **(clarithromycin)** are predicted to very slightly increase the exposure to **perampanel**. [Mild] Study
- Macrolides **(erythromycin)** markedly increase the concentration of **carbamazepine**. Monitor concentration and adjust dose. [Severe] Study
- Antiepileptics **(phenobarbital, primidone)** are predicted to increase the effects of **MAOIs, irreversible**. [Severe] Theoretical
- **Carbamazepine** is predicted to increase the risk of severe toxic reaction when given with **MAOIs, irreversible**. Avoid and for 14 days after stopping the MAOI. [Severe] Theoretical
- Antiepileptics **(carbamazepine, fosphenytoin, phenobarbital, phenytoin, primidone)** are predicted to decrease the exposure to **maraviroc**. Adjust dose. [Severe] Study
- Antiepileptics **(carbamazepine, fosphenytoin, phenobarbital, phenytoin, primidone)** are predicted to decrease the exposure to **maribavir**. Avoid or adjust **maribavir** dose. [Severe] Study
- Antiepileptics **(carbamazepine, fosphenytoin, phenobarbital, phenytoin, primidone)** are predicted to decrease the exposure to **mavacamten**. Monitor and adjust dose—consult product literature. [Severe] Theoretical
- Antiepileptics **(carbamazepine, fosphenytoin, phenobarbital, phenytoin, primidone)** are predicted to decrease the exposure to meglitinides **(repaglinide)**. Monitor blood glucose and adjust dose. [Moderate] Study
- **Phenytoin** is predicted to decrease the exposure to **melatonin**. [Moderate] Theoretical → Also see **TABLE 9** p. 1056
- **Sultiame** might increase the risk of lactic acidosis when given with **metformin**. [Severe] Theoretical
- **Levetiracetam** decreases the clearance of **methotrexate**. [Severe] Anecdotal
- **Methotrexate** might decrease the concentration of **valproate**. [Severe] Theoretical → Also see **TABLE 1** p. 1053
- **Carbamazepine** might decrease the concentration of **methylphenidate**. [Moderate] Anecdotal
- **Valproate** might enhance the effects of **methylphenidate**. [Severe] Anecdotal
- Antiepileptics **(phenobarbital, primidone)** are predicted to decrease the exposure to **metronidazole**. [Moderate] Study
- Antiepileptics **(fosphenytoin, phenobarbital, phenytoin, primidone)** are predicted to decrease the effects of **metyrapone**. Avoid. [Moderate] Study
- **Phenytoin** is predicted to increase the clearance of **mexiletine**. Monitor and adjust dose. [Moderate] Study
- Antiepileptics **(phenobarbital, primidone)** are predicted to decrease the exposure to **mianserin**. [Moderate] Study → Also see **TABLE 9** p. 1056
- **Carbamazepine** markedly decreases the exposure to **mianserin**. Adjust dose. [Moderate] Study
- Antiepileptics **(carbamazepine, fosphenytoin, phenobarbital, phenytoin, primidone)** are predicted to decrease the exposure to **midostaurin**. Avoid. [Severe] Study
- Antiepileptics **(carbamazepine, fosphenytoin, phenobarbital, phenytoin, primidone)** are predicted to decrease the exposure to **mifepristone**. Adjust **mifepristone** dose. [Severe] Study
- Antiepileptics **(carbamazepine, fosphenytoin, phenobarbital, phenytoin, primidone)** are predicted to decrease the exposure to mineralocorticoid receptor antagonists **(eplerenone)**. Avoid. [Moderate] Theoretical
- Antiepileptics **(carbamazepine, fosphenytoin, phenobarbital, phenytoin, primidone)** are predicted to decrease the exposure to mineralocorticoid receptor antagonists **(finerenone)**. Avoid. [Severe] Study
- Antiepileptics **(carbamazepine, fosphenytoin, phenobarbital, phenytoin, primidone)** are predicted to decrease the exposure to **mirtazapine**. Adjust dose. [Moderate] Study → Also see **TABLE 15** p. 1058 → Also see **TABLE 9** p. 1056
- **Mitotane** is predicted to decrease the exposure to **perampanel**. Monitor and adjust dose. [Moderate] Study
- Antiepileptics **(carbamazepine, phenobarbital, primidone)** are predicted to decrease the exposure to **modafinil**. [Mild] Theoretical
- Antiepileptics **(fosphenytoin, phenytoin)** are predicted to decrease the exposure to **modafinil** and **modafinil** is predicted to increase the concentration of antiepileptics **(fosphenytoin, phenytoin)**. Monitor concentration and adjust dose. [Moderate] Theoretical
- Monoclonal antibodies **(elranatamab)** might affect the exposure to **phenytoin**. Monitor and adjust dose. [Moderate] Theoretical
- **Carbamazepine** is predicted to decrease the effects of monoclonal antibodies **(brentuximab vedotin)**. [Severe] Theoretical
- Monoclonal antibodies **(tocilizumab)** are predicted to decrease the exposure to antiepileptics **(fosphenytoin, phenytoin)**. Monitor and adjust dose. [Moderate] Theoretical
- Antiepileptics **(carbamazepine, fosphenytoin, phenobarbital, phenytoin, primidone)** are predicted to decrease the exposure to monoclonal antibodies **(polatuzumab vedotin)**. [Moderate] Theoretical
- Antiepileptics **(carbamazepine, fosphenytoin, phenobarbital, phenytoin, primidone)** are predicted to decrease the exposure to the cytotoxic component of monoclonal antibodies **(trastuzumab emtansine)**. [Severe] Theoretical
- Antiepileptics **(carbamazepine, fosphenytoin, phenobarbital, phenytoin, primidone)** are predicted to decrease the exposure to **montelukast**. [Mild] Study
- Antiepileptics **(carbamazepine, fosphenytoin, phenobarbital, phenytoin, primidone)** are predicted to markedly decrease the exposure to **naldemedine**. Avoid. [Severe] Study

Antiepileptics (continued)

- Antiepileptics **(carbamazepine, fosphenytoin, phenobarbital, phenytoin, primidone)** are predicted to markedly decrease the exposure to **naloxegol**. Avoid. Moderate Study
- Antiepileptics **(carbamazepine, fosphenytoin, phenobarbital, phenytoin, primidone)** are predicted to decrease the exposure to **neratinib**. Avoid. Severe Study
- Antiepileptics **(carbamazepine, fosphenytoin, phenobarbital, phenytoin, primidone)** are predicted to markedly decrease the exposure to neurokinin-1 receptor antagonists **(aprepitant)**. Avoid. Moderate Study
- Antiepileptics **(carbamazepine, fosphenytoin, phenobarbital, phenytoin, primidone)** are predicted to decrease the exposure to neurokinin-1 receptor antagonists **(fosaprepitant)**. Avoid. Moderate Theoretical
- Antiepileptics **(carbamazepine, fosphenytoin, phenobarbital, phenytoin, primidone)** are predicted to decrease the exposure to neurokinin-1 receptor antagonists **(netupitant)**. Avoid. Severe Study
- **Carbamazepine** is predicted to decrease the effects of (but acute use increases the effects of) neuromuscular blocking drugs, non-depolarising **(atracurium, cisatracurium, pancuronium, rocuronium, vecuronium)**. Monitor and adjust dose. Moderate Study
- Antiepileptics **(fosphenytoin, phenytoin)** decrease the effects of (but acute use increases the effects of) neuromuscular blocking drugs, non-depolarising **(atracurium, cisatracurium, pancuronium, rocuronium, vecuronium)**. Moderate Study
- Antiepileptics **(carbamazepine, fosphenytoin, phenobarbital, phenytoin, primidone)** are predicted to moderately decrease the exposure to **nilotinib**. Avoid. Severe Study
- Antiepileptics **(phenobarbital, phenytoin)** are predicted to decrease the exposure to **nintedanib**. Severe Theoretical
- **Carbamazepine** is predicted to decrease the exposure to **nintedanib**. Moderate Study
- Antiepileptics **(carbamazepine, fosphenytoin, phenobarbital, phenytoin, primidone)** are predicted to decrease the exposure to **nirmatrelvir** boosted with ritonavir. Avoid. Severe Study
- **Nirmatrelvir** boosted with ritonavir is predicted to decrease the concentration of antiepileptics **(lamotrigine, valproate)**. Severe Theoretical
- Antiepileptics **(carbamazepine, fosphenytoin, phenobarbital, phenytoin, primidone)** are predicted to decrease the exposure to **nitisinone**. Adjust dose. Moderate Theoretical
- NNRTIs **(efavirenz)** are predicted to affect the efficacy of **primidone** and **primidone** is predicted to slightly decrease the exposure to NNRTIs **(efavirenz)**. Severe Theoretical
- NNRTIs **(nevirapine)** are predicted to decrease the concentration of antiepileptics **(carbamazepine, fosphenytoin, phenobarbital, phenytoin, primidone)** and antiepileptics **(carbamazepine, fosphenytoin, phenobarbital, phenytoin, primidone)** are predicted to decrease the concentration of NNRTIs **(nevirapine)**. Severe Study
- **Oxcarbazepine** is predicted to decrease the exposure to NNRTIs **(doravirine)**. Avoid. Severe Theoretical
- Antiepileptics **(carbamazepine, fosphenytoin, phenobarbital, phenytoin, primidone)** are predicted to decrease the exposure to NNRTIs **(doravirine)**. Avoid. Severe Study
- **Carbamazepine** slightly decreases the exposure to NNRTIs **(efavirenz)** and NNRTIs **(efavirenz)** slightly decrease the exposure to **carbamazepine**. Severe Study
- **Phenobarbital** is predicted to decrease the exposure to NNRTIs **(efavirenz)** and NNRTIs **(efavirenz)** affect the concentration of **phenobarbital**. Severe Theoretical
- Antiepileptics **(fosphenytoin, phenytoin)** slightly decrease the exposure to NNRTIs **(efavirenz)** and NNRTIs **(efavirenz)** affect the concentration of antiepileptics **(fosphenytoin, phenytoin)**. Severe Theoretical
- Antiepileptics **(carbamazepine, fosphenytoin, phenobarbital, phenytoin, primidone)** are predicted to decrease the exposure to NNRTIs **(etravirine)**. Avoid. Severe Theoretical
- **Oxcarbazepine** is predicted to decrease the concentration of NNRTIs **(rilpivirine)**. Avoid. Severe Theoretical
- Antiepileptics **(carbamazepine, fosphenytoin, phenobarbital, phenytoin, primidone)** markedly decrease the exposure to NNRTIs **(rilpivirine)**. Avoid. Severe Study
- Antiepileptics **(carbamazepine, eslicarbazepine, fosphenytoin, oxcarbazepine, perampanel, phenobarbital, phenytoin, primidone, rufinamide, topiramate)** are predicted to decrease the efficacy of some contraceptive methods containing **norethisterone**. For CoSRH guidance, see Contraceptives, interactions p. 614. Severe Anecdotal
- **Lamotrigine** might decrease the effects of **norethisterone**. For CoSRH guidance, see Contraceptives, interactions p. 614. Moderate Theoretical
- Antiepileptics **(carbamazepine, fosphenytoin, phenobarbital, phenytoin, primidone)** are predicted to decrease the exposure to NRTIs **(abacavir)**. Moderate Theoretical
- **Valproate** slightly increases the exposure to NRTIs **(zidovudine)**. Moderate Study → Also see TABLE 1 p. 1053
- Antiepileptics **(carbamazepine, fosphenytoin, phenobarbital, phenytoin, primidone)** are predicted to decrease the exposure to **olaparib**. Avoid. Moderate Theoretical
- Antiepileptics **(carbamazepine, fosphenytoin, phenobarbital, phenytoin, primidone)** are predicted to decrease the exposure to **omaveloxolone**. Avoid. Severe Study
- Antiepileptics **(carbamazepine, fosphenytoin, phenobarbital, phenytoin, primidone)** are predicted to decrease the exposure to opioids **(alfentanil, fentanyl)**. Moderate Study → Also see TABLE 9 p. 1056
- Antiepileptics **(carbamazepine, fosphenytoin, phenobarbital, phenytoin, primidone)** are predicted to decrease the exposure to opioids **(buprenorphine)**. Monitor and adjust dose. Moderate Theoretical → Also see TABLE 9 p. 1056
- Antiepileptics **(carbamazepine, fosphenytoin, phenobarbital, phenytoin, primidone)** decrease the exposure to opioids **(methadone)**. Monitor and adjust dose. Severe Study → Also see TABLE 9 p. 1056
- Antiepileptics **(carbamazepine, fosphenytoin, phenobarbital, phenytoin, primidone)** are predicted to decrease the exposure to opioids **(oxycodone)**. Monitor and adjust dose. Moderate Study → Also see TABLE 9 p. 1056
- **Carbamazepine** decreases the concentration of opioids **(tramadol)**. Adjust dose. Severe Study → Also see TABLE 15 p. 1058
- Antiepileptics **(carbamazepine, fosphenytoin, phenobarbital, phenytoin, primidone)** are predicted to decrease the exposure to **osilodrostat**. Moderate Theoretical
- Antiepileptics **(carbamazepine, fosphenytoin, phenobarbital, phenytoin, primidone)** are predicted to moderately decrease the exposure to **osimertinib**. Avoid. Moderate Study
- Antiepileptics **(carbamazepine, fosphenytoin, phenobarbital, phenytoin, primidone)** are predicted to moderately decrease the exposure to **ospemifene**. Moderate Study
- **Oxybutynin** potentially increases the risk of overheating and dehydration when given with **zonisamide**. Avoid in children. Severe Theoretical
- Antiepileptics **(carbamazepine, fosphenytoin, phenobarbital, phenytoin, primidone)** are predicted to decrease the exposure to **palbociclib**. Avoid. Severe Study
- Antiepileptics **(carbamazepine, fosphenytoin, phenobarbital, phenytoin, primidone)** are predicted to decrease the exposure to **panobinostat**. Avoid. Moderate Theoretical
- Antiepileptics **(carbamazepine, fosphenytoin, phenobarbital, phenytoin, primidone)** decrease the exposure to **paracetamol**. Moderate Study
- Antiepileptics **(carbamazepine, fosphenytoin, phenobarbital, phenytoin, primidone)** are predicted to decrease the exposure to **pazopanib**. Avoid. Severe Theoretical
- Antiepileptics **(carbamazepine, fosphenytoin, phenobarbital, phenytoin, primidone)** are predicted to decrease the exposure to **pemigatinib**. Avoid. Severe Study
- **Valproate** increases the risk of adverse effects when given with penicillins **(pivmecillinam)**. Avoid. Severe Anecdotal
- Phenothiazine antipsychotics **(chlorpromazine)** decrease the concentration of antiepileptics **(phenobarbital, primidone)** and antiepileptics **(phenobarbital, primidone)** decrease the concentration of phenothiazine antipsychotics **(chlorpromazine)**. Moderate Study → Also see TABLE 9 p. 1056

- Antiepileptics **(carbamazepine, fosphenytoin, phenobarbital, phenytoin, primidone)** moderately decrease the exposure to phosphodiesterase type-4 inhibitors **(apremilast)**. Avoid. Severe Study
- Antiepileptics **(carbamazepine, fosphenytoin, phenobarbital, phenytoin, primidone)** are predicted to decrease the exposure to phosphodiesterase type-4 inhibitors **(roflumilast)**. Avoid. Moderate Study
- Antiepileptics **(carbamazepine, fosphenytoin, phenobarbital, phenytoin, primidone)** are predicted to decrease the exposure to phosphodiesterase type-5 inhibitors **(avanafil, tadalafil)**. Avoid. Severe Study
- Antiepileptics **(carbamazepine, fosphenytoin, phenobarbital, phenytoin, primidone)** are predicted to decrease the exposure to phosphodiesterase type-5 inhibitors **(sildenafil, vardenafil)**. Moderate Theoretical
- Antiepileptics **(carbamazepine, fosphenytoin, phenobarbital, phenytoin, primidone)** are predicted to moderately to markedly decrease the exposure to **pibrentasvir**. Avoid. Severe Study
- Antiepileptics **(eslicarbazepine, oxcarbazepine)** potentially decrease the exposure to **pibrentasvir**. Avoid. Severe Theoretical
- Antiepileptics **(fosphenytoin, phenytoin)** are predicted to decrease the exposure to **pirfenidone**. Moderate Theoretical
- Antiepileptics **(carbamazepine, fosphenytoin, phenobarbital, phenytoin, primidone)** are predicted to decrease the exposure to **pirtobrutinib**. Avoid. Moderate Study
- Antiepileptics **(carbamazepine, fosphenytoin, phenobarbital, phenytoin, primidone)** are predicted to moderately decrease the exposure to **pitolisant**. Moderate Study
- Antiepileptics **(carbamazepine, fosphenytoin, phenobarbital, phenytoin, primidone)** are predicted to decrease the exposure to **ponatinib**. Avoid. Moderate Theoretical
- Antiepileptics **(carbamazepine, fosphenytoin, phenobarbital, phenytoin, primidone)** are predicted to decrease the exposure to **pralsetinib**. Avoid or adjust dose with potent CYP3A4 inducers—consult product literature. Moderate Study
- Antiepileptics **(carbamazepine, fosphenytoin, phenobarbital, phenytoin, primidone)** are predicted to markedly decrease the exposure to **praziquantel**. Avoid. Moderate Study
- Antiepileptics **(carbamazepine, phenobarbital, phenytoin, primidone)** are predicted to increase the risk of hypersensitivity reactions when given with **procarbazine**. Severe Anecdotal
- **Fosphenytoin** is predicted to increase the risk of hypersensitivity when given with **procarbazine**. Severe Anecdotal
- **Valproate** potentially increases the concentration of **propofol**. Adjust dose. Severe Theoretical
- **Sultiame** might increase the exposure to proton pump inhibitors **(omeprazole)**. Moderate Theoretical
- Quinolones **(ciprofloxacin)** affect the concentration of antiepileptics **(fosphenytoin, phenytoin)**. Monitor concentration and adjust dose. Severe Study
- Antiepileptics **(carbamazepine, fosphenytoin, phenobarbital, phenytoin, primidone)** are predicted to decrease the exposure to **quizartinib**. Avoid. Severe Study
- Antiepileptics **(carbamazepine, fosphenytoin, phenobarbital, phenytoin, primidone)** are predicted to affect the exposure to **raltegravir**. Use with caution or avoid. Moderate Theoretical
- Antiepileptics **(carbamazepine, fosphenytoin, phenobarbital, phenytoin, primidone)** are predicted to decrease the exposure to **ranolazine**. Avoid. Severe Study
- Antiepileptics **(carbamazepine, fosphenytoin, phenobarbital, phenytoin, primidone)** are predicted to decrease the exposure to **reboxetine**. Moderate Anecdotal
- Antiepileptics **(carbamazepine, fosphenytoin, phenobarbital, phenytoin, primidone)** are predicted to decrease the exposure to **regorafenib**. Avoid. Moderate Study
- Antiepileptics **(carbamazepine, phenobarbital, phenytoin)** are predicted to decrease the exposure to **relugolix**. Avoid or adjust dose depending on indication—consult product literature. Moderate Study
- Antiepileptics **(oxcarbazepine, topiramate)** are predicted to decrease the exposure to **relugolix**. Avoid. Moderate Theoretical
- Antiepileptics **(carbamazepine, fosphenytoin, phenobarbital, phenytoin, primidone)** are predicted to markedly decrease the exposure to **ribociclib**. Avoid. Severe Study
- Rifamycins **(rifampicin)** slightly decrease the exposure to **brivaracetam**. Adjust dose. Moderate Study
- Rifamycins **(rifampicin)** markedly increase the clearance of **lamotrigine**. Adjust **lamotrigine** dose, p. 243. Moderate Study
- Rifamycins **(rifampicin)** are predicted to decrease the exposure to **perampanel**. Monitor and adjust dose. Moderate Study
- Rifamycins **(rifampicin)** are predicted to decrease the concentration of **zonisamide**. Monitor and adjust dose. Moderate Theoretical
- Rifamycins **(rifampicin)** decrease the concentration of antiepileptics **(fosphenytoin, phenytoin)**. Use with caution and adjust dose. Moderate Study
- Antiepileptics **(phenobarbital, primidone)** are predicted to decrease the exposure to rifamycins **(rifampicin)** and rifamycins **(rifampicin)** are predicted to decrease the exposure to antiepileptics **(phenobarbital, primidone)**. Use with caution and adjust dose. Moderate Study
- Antiepileptics **(carbamazepine, fosphenytoin, phenobarbital, phenytoin, primidone)** are predicted to decrease the exposure to **rimegepant**. Avoid. Moderate Theoretical
- Antiepileptics **(carbamazepine, fosphenytoin, phenobarbital, phenytoin, primidone)** are predicted to decrease the exposure to **ripretinib**. Avoid or adjust dose—consult product literature. Severe Study
- **Rucaparib** is predicted to increase the exposure to **phenytoin**. Monitor and adjust dose. Moderate Study
- Antiepileptics **(carbamazepine, fosphenytoin, phenobarbital, phenytoin, primidone)** are predicted to decrease the exposure to **ruxolitinib**. Monitor and adjust dose. Moderate Study
- Antiepileptics **(carbamazepine, fosphenytoin, phenytoin)** are predicted to decrease the exposure to the active component of **sacituzumab govitecan**. Severe Theoretical
- Antiepileptics **(carbamazepine, fosphenytoin, phenytoin)** are predicted to decrease the exposure to the active metabolite of **selexipag**. Adjust dose. Moderate Study
- **Valproate** is predicted to increase the exposure to **selexipag**. Unknown Theoretical
- Antiepileptics **(carbamazepine, fosphenytoin, phenobarbital, phenytoin, primidone)** are predicted to decrease the exposure to **selpercatinib**. Avoid. Moderate Study
- Antiepileptics **(carbamazepine, fosphenytoin, phenobarbital, phenytoin, primidone)** are predicted to decrease the exposure to **selumetinib**. Avoid. Severe Study
- Antiepileptics **(carbamazepine, fosphenytoin, phenobarbital, phenytoin, primidone)** are predicted to decrease the exposure to **siponimod**. Manufacturer advises caution depending on genotype—consult product literature. Severe Study
- Antiepileptics **(carbamazepine, fosphenytoin, phenobarbital, phenytoin, primidone)** are predicted to decrease the concentration of **sirolimus**. Avoid or monitor and adjust dose. Severe Study
- **Phenytoin** is predicted to decrease the exposure to SNRIs **(duloxetine)**. Moderate Theoretical → Also see TABLE 9 p. 1056
- Antiepileptics **(carbamazepine, phenobarbital, phenytoin, primidone)** are predicted to decrease the exposure to sodium glucose co-transporter 2 inhibitors **(canagliflozin)**. Adjust **canagliflozin** dose. Moderate Study
- **Fosphenytoin** is predicted to decrease the exposure to sodium glucose co-transporter 2 inhibitors **(empagliflozin)**. Avoid or monitor diabetic control. Moderate Theoretical
- **Phenytoin** might decrease the exposure to sodium glucose co-transporter 2 inhibitors **(empagliflozin)**. Avoid or monitor diabetic control. Moderate Theoretical
- **Valproate** increases the exposure to **sodium oxybate**. Adjust **sodium oxybate** dose. Moderate Study
- **Valproate** potentially decreases the effects of **sodium phenylbutyrate**. Moderate Anecdotal
- Antiepileptics **(fosphenytoin, oxcarbazepine, phenobarbital, phenytoin, primidone)** are predicted to decrease the exposure to **sofosbuvir**. Avoid. Severe Theoretical
- **Carbamazepine** is predicted to decrease the exposure to **sofosbuvir**. Avoid. Severe Study

Antiepileptics (continued)
- Antiepileptics **(carbamazepine, fosphenytoin, phenobarbital, phenytoin, primidone)** are predicted to decrease the exposure to **solifenacin**. Moderate Theoretical
- **Somapacitan** might decrease the exposure to **carbamazepine**. Moderate Theoretical
- **Somatrogon** might decrease the exposure to **carbamazepine**. Moderate Theoretical
- Antiepileptics **(carbamazepine, eslicarbazepine, fosphenytoin, phenobarbital, phenytoin, primidone)** are predicted to decrease the exposure to **sorafenib**. Moderate Theoretical
- **Oxcarbazepine** is predicted to decrease the exposure to **sorafenib**. Moderate Study
- Antiepileptics **(carbamazepine, fosphenytoin, phenobarbital, phenytoin, primidone)** are predicted to decrease the exposure to **sotorasib**. Avoid. Severe Study
- Antiepileptics **(carbamazepine, fosphenytoin, phenobarbital, phenytoin, primidone)** are predicted to decrease the exposure to **sparsentan**. Avoid. Severe Theoretical
- **SSRIs (fluoxetine, fluvoxamine)** increase the exposure to **carbamazepine**. Adjust dose or monitor. Moderate Study → Also see TABLE 15 p. 1058
- **SSRIs (fluoxetine, fluvoxamine)** are predicted to increase the concentration of antiepileptics **(fosphenytoin, phenytoin)**. Monitor and adjust dose. Severe Anecdotal → Also see TABLE 9 p. 1056
- **SSRIs (sertraline)** potentially increase the risk of toxicity when given with antiepileptics **(fosphenytoin, phenytoin)**. Monitor concentration and adjust dose. Severe Anecdotal → Also see TABLE 9 p. 1056
- Antiepileptics **(fosphenytoin, phenytoin)** decrease the concentration of **SSRIs (paroxetine)**. Moderate Study → Also see TABLE 9 p. 1056
- **St John's wort** is predicted to decrease the concentration of antiepileptics **(fosphenytoin, phenobarbital, phenytoin, primidone)**. Avoid. Severe Theoretical
- **St John's wort** is predicted to decrease the exposure to **brivaracetam**. Moderate Theoretical
- **St John's wort** is predicted to decrease the concentration of **carbamazepine**. Monitor and adjust dose. Moderate Theoretical
- **St John's wort** is predicted to decrease the exposure to **perampanel**. Monitor and adjust dose. Moderate Theoretical
- **St John's wort** is predicted to decrease the exposure to **tiagabine**. Avoid. Mild Theoretical
- **Carbamazepine** is predicted to decrease the exposure to **statins (atorvastatin)**. Monitor and adjust dose. Moderate Study
- **Eslicarbazepine** is predicted to decrease the exposure to **statins (atorvastatin)**. Monitor and adjust dose. Moderate Theoretical
- **Phenytoin** moderately decreases the exposure to **statins (atorvastatin)**. Moderate Study
- **Oxcarbazepine** is predicted to decrease the exposure to **statins (atorvastatin, simvastatin)**. Moderate Theoretical
- Antiepileptics **(fosphenytoin, phenobarbital, primidone)** are predicted to decrease the exposure to **statins (atorvastatin, simvastatin)**. Moderate Study
- **Eslicarbazepine** decreases the exposure to **statins (rosuvastatin)**. Moderate Study
- **Phenytoin** is predicted to decrease the exposure to **statins (simvastatin)**. Moderate Study
- Antiepileptics **(carbamazepine, eslicarbazepine)** moderately decrease the exposure to **statins (simvastatin)**. Monitor and adjust dose. Moderate Study
- **Sulfonamides (sulfadiazine)** are predicted to increase the concentration of **fosphenytoin**. Monitor and adjust dose. Moderate Study
- **Sulfonamides (sulfadiazine)** increase the concentration of **phenytoin**. Monitor and adjust dose. Moderate Study
- Antiepileptics **(carbamazepine, fosphenytoin, phenobarbital, phenytoin, primidone)** are predicted to decrease the exposure to **sunitinib**. Avoid or adjust dose—consult product literature. Moderate Study
- Antiepileptics **(fosphenytoin, phenytoin)** increase the effects of **suxamethonium**. Moderate Study
- **Carbamazepine** increases the risk of prolonged neuromuscular blockade when given with **suxamethonium**. Moderate Study
- Antiepileptics **(carbamazepine, fosphenytoin, phenobarbital, phenytoin, primidone)** decrease the concentration of **tacrolimus**. Avoid or monitor and adjust dose. Severe Study
- **Tamoxifen** (high-dose) might increase the concentration of **fosphenytoin** and **fosphenytoin** might decrease the concentration of **tamoxifen** (high-dose). Severe Theoretical
- **Tamoxifen** (high-dose) might increase the concentration of **phenytoin** and **phenytoin** might decrease the concentration of **tamoxifen** (high-dose). Severe Anecdotal
- Antiepileptics **(carbamazepine, fosphenytoin, phenobarbital, phenytoin, primidone)** are predicted to decrease the exposure to **taxanes (cabazitaxel)**. Avoid. Moderate Study → Also see TABLE 10 p. 1056
- Antiepileptics **(carbamazepine, fosphenytoin, phenobarbital, phenytoin, primidone)** are predicted to decrease the exposure to **taxanes (docetaxel)**. Severe Theoretical → Also see TABLE 10 p. 1056
- Antiepileptics **(carbamazepine, fosphenytoin, phenobarbital, phenytoin, primidone)** are predicted to decrease the exposure to **taxanes (paclitaxel)**. Avoid. Severe Study → Also see TABLE 10 p. 1056
- **Tegafur** potentially increases the concentration of antiepileptics **(fosphenytoin, phenytoin)**. Monitor concentration and adjust dose. Severe Anecdotal
- Antiepileptics **(carbamazepine, fosphenytoin, phenobarbital, phenytoin, primidone)** are predicted to decrease the concentration of **temsirolimus**. Avoid. Severe Study
- Antiepileptics **(carbamazepine, fosphenytoin, oxcarbazepine, phenobarbital, phenytoin, primidone)** are predicted to decrease the exposure to **tenofovir alafenamide**. Avoid. Moderate Theoretical
- **Fosphenytoin** is predicted to decrease the concentration of **tetracyclines (doxycycline)**. Adjust dose. Moderate Theoretical
- Antiepileptics **(carbamazepine, phenobarbital, phenytoin, primidone)** decrease the concentration of **tetracyclines (doxycycline)**. Adjust dose. Moderate Study
- Antiepileptics **(carbamazepine, fosphenytoin, phenobarbital, phenytoin, primidone)** are predicted to decrease the exposure to **tetracyclines (eravacycline)**. Adjust **eravacycline** dose. Moderate Study
- Antiepileptics **(carbamazepine, fosphenytoin, phenobarbital, phenytoin, primidone)** are predicted to decrease the exposure to **tezacaftor**. Avoid. Severe Theoretical
- Antiepileptics **(fosphenytoin, phenytoin)** are predicted to decrease the exposure to **theophylline**. Adjust dose. Moderate Study
- Antiepileptics **(phenobarbital, primidone)** are predicted to increase the clearance of **theophylline**. Adjust dose. Moderate Theoretical
- **Carbamazepine** potentially increases the clearance of **theophylline** and **theophylline** decreases the exposure to **carbamazepine**. Adjust dose. Moderate Anecdotal
- **Stiripentol** is predicted to increase the exposure to **theophylline**. Avoid. Moderate Theoretical
- **Carbamazepine** is predicted to decrease the exposure to **thrombin inhibitors (dabigatran)**. Avoid. Severe Study
- Antiepileptics **(fosphenytoin, phenytoin)** are predicted to decrease the exposure to **thrombin inhibitors (dabigatran)**. Avoid. Severe Theoretical
- Antiepileptics **(fosphenytoin, phenytoin)** are predicted to increase the risk of hypothyroidism when given with **thyroid hormones**. Moderate Study
- Antiepileptics **(phenobarbital, primidone)** are predicted to decrease the effects of **thyroid hormones**. Moderate Theoretical
- **Carbamazepine** is predicted to increase the risk of hypothyroidism when given with **thyroid hormones**. Monitor and adjust dose. Moderate Study
- Antiepileptics **(carbamazepine, fosphenytoin, phenobarbital, phenytoin, primidone)** are predicted to markedly decrease the exposure to **ticagrelor**. Avoid. Severe Study
- Antiepileptics **(carbamazepine, fosphenytoin, phenobarbital, phenytoin, primidone)** are predicted to decrease the exposure to the cytotoxic component of **tisotumab vedotin**. Moderate Theoretical

- Antiepileptics **(carbamazepine, fosphenytoin, phenobarbital, phenytoin, primidone)** are predicted to decrease the exposure to **tivozanib**. Severe Study
- Antiepileptics **(fosphenytoin, phenytoin)** moderately decrease the exposure to **tizanidine**. Mild Study → Also see TABLE 9 p. 1056
- Antiepileptics **(carbamazepine, fosphenytoin, phenobarbital, phenytoin, primidone)** are predicted to decrease the exposure to **tofacitinib**. Avoid. Severe Study
- Antiepileptics **(carbamazepine, fosphenytoin, phenobarbital, phenytoin, primidone)** are predicted to decrease the exposure to **tolvaptan**. Use with caution or avoid depending on indication. Severe Study
- Antiepileptics **(fosphenytoin, phenytoin)** increase the clearance of **topotecan**. Moderate Study
- Antiepileptics **(carbamazepine, fosphenytoin, phenobarbital, phenytoin, primidone)** are predicted to decrease the exposure to **toremifene**. Adjust dose. Moderate Study
- Antiepileptics **(carbamazepine, fosphenytoin, phenobarbital, phenytoin, primidone)** are predicted to decrease the exposure to **trabectedin**. Avoid. Severe Theoretical
- **Carbamazepine** decreases the concentration of **trazodone**. Adjust dose. Moderate Anecdotal → Also see TABLE 15 p. 1058
- Antiepileptics **(carbamazepine, phenobarbital, phenytoin)** are predicted to decrease the exposure to **treprostinil**. Adjust dose. Mild Theoretical
- Antiepileptics **(phenobarbital, primidone)** are predicted to decrease the exposure to **tricyclic antidepressants**. Moderate Study → Also see TABLE 9 p. 1056
- **Carbamazepine** decreases the exposure to **tricyclic antidepressants**. Adjust dose. Moderate Study → Also see TABLE 15 p. 1058
- **Tricyclic antidepressants (clomipramine, imipramine)** potentially increase the risk of overheating and dehydration when given with **zonisamide**. Avoid in children. Severe Theoretical
- **Valproate** increases the concentration of **tricyclic antidepressants (nortriptyline)**. Severe Study → Also see TABLE 15 p. 1058
- **Trimethoprim** increases the concentration of antiepileptics **(fosphenytoin, phenytoin)**. Moderate Study
- Antiepileptics **(carbamazepine, fosphenytoin, phenobarbital, phenytoin, primidone)** are predicted to decrease the exposure to **tucatinib**. Avoid. Severe Study
- **Tucatinib** is predicted to very slightly increase the exposure to **perampanel**. Mild Study
- Antiepileptics **(carbamazepine, eslicarbazepine, fosphenytoin, oxcarbazepine, perampanel, phenobarbital, phenytoin, primidone, rufinamide, topiramate)** decrease the efficacy of **ulipristal**. Avoid and for 4 weeks after stopping the enzyme inducing drug. For CoSRH guidance, see Contraceptives, interactions p. 614. Severe Anecdotal
- Antiepileptics **(carbamazepine, fosphenytoin, phenobarbital, phenytoin, primidone)** are predicted to decrease the exposure to **upadacitinib**. Moderate Study
- Antiepileptics **(carbamazepine, fosphenytoin, phenobarbital, phenytoin, primidone)** are predicted to decrease the exposure to **vandetanib**. Avoid. Moderate Study
- Antiepileptics **(carbamazepine, fosphenytoin, phenobarbital, phenytoin, primidone)** are predicted to decrease the exposure to **vanzacaftor**. Avoid. Severe Theoretical
- **Carbamazepine** might enhance the antidiuretic effect of **vasopressin**. Moderate Theoretical
- Antiepileptics **(carbamazepine, fosphenytoin, phenobarbital, phenytoin, primidone)** are predicted to moderately decrease the exposure to **velpatasvir**. Avoid. Severe Study
- **Oxcarbazepine** is predicted to decrease the exposure to **velpatasvir**. Avoid. Severe Theoretical
- Antiepileptics **(carbamazepine, fosphenytoin, phenobarbital, phenytoin, primidone)** are predicted to decrease the exposure to **vemurafenib**. Avoid. Severe Study
- Antiepileptics **(carbamazepine, fosphenytoin, phenobarbital, phenytoin, primidone)** are predicted to decrease the exposure to **venetoclax**. Avoid. Severe Study
- Antiepileptics **(carbamazepine, fosphenytoin, phenobarbital, phenytoin, primidone)** are predicted to decrease the exposure to **vinca alkaloids (vinblastine, vincristine, vindesine)**. Severe Theoretical → Also see TABLE 15 p. 1058 → Also see TABLE 10 p. 1056
- Antiepileptics **(carbamazepine, fosphenytoin, phenobarbital, phenytoin, primidone)** are predicted to decrease the exposure to **vinca alkaloids (vinorelbine)**. Use with caution or avoid. Severe Theoretical → Also see TABLE 15 p. 1058 → Also see TABLE 10 p. 1056
- Antiepileptics **(carbamazepine, fosphenytoin, phenobarbital, phenytoin, primidone)** are predicted to decrease the exposure to **vismodegib**. Avoid. Moderate Theoretical
- Antiepileptics **(fosphenytoin, phenytoin)** decrease the effects of **vitamin D substances**. Moderate Study
- Antiepileptics **(phenobarbital, primidone)** are predicted to decrease the effects of **vitamin D substances**. Moderate Theoretical
- **Carbamazepine** is predicted to decrease the effects of **vitamin D substances**. Moderate Study
- Antiepileptics **(carbamazepine, fosphenytoin, phenobarbital, phenytoin, primidone)** are predicted to decrease the exposure to **voclosporin**. Avoid. Severe Study
- Antiepileptics **(phenobarbital, primidone)** potentially increase the risk of nephrotoxicity when given with **volatile halogenated anaesthetics (methoxyflurane)**. Avoid. Severe Theoretical → Also see TABLE 9 p. 1056
- **Vorasidenib** might decrease the concentration of antiepileptics **(carbamazepine, fosphenytoin, phenobarbital, valproate)**. Avoid. Severe Theoretical → Also see TABLE 1 p. 1053
- **Phenytoin** is predicted to decrease the exposure to **vorasidenib**. Avoid. Severe Theoretical
- Antiepileptics **(carbamazepine, fosphenytoin, phenobarbital, phenytoin, primidone)** are predicted to decrease the exposure to **vortioxetine**. Monitor and adjust dose. Moderate Study
- Antiepileptics **(carbamazepine, fosphenytoin, phenobarbital, phenytoin, primidone)** are predicted to decrease the concentration of **voxilaprevir**. Avoid. Severe Study
- **Oxcarbazepine** is predicted to decrease the concentration of **voxilaprevir**. Avoid. Severe Theoretical
- Antiepileptics **(carbamazepine, fosphenytoin, phenobarbital, phenytoin, primidone)** are predicted to decrease the exposure to **zanubrutinib**. Avoid. Severe Study
- **Carbamazepine** moderately decreases the exposure to **zolpidem**. Moderate Study
- Antiepileptics **(carbamazepine, fosphenytoin, phenobarbital, phenytoin, primidone)** are predicted to decrease the exposure to **zopiclone**. Adjust dose. Moderate Study → Also see TABLE 9 p. 1056

Antifungals, azoles → see TABLE 1 p. 1053 (hepatotoxicity), TABLE 7 p. 1055 (QT-interval prolongation)

clotrimazole · fluconazole · isavuconazole · itraconazole · ketoconazole · miconazole · posaconazole · voriconazole

- Since systemic absorption can follow topical application, the possibility of interactions with topical **clotrimazole** or topical **ketoconazole** should be borne in mind.
- In general, **fluconazole** interactions relate to multiple-dose treatment.
- The use of carbonated drinks, such as cola, improves **itraconazole**, **ketoconazole**, and **posaconazole** bioavailability.
- Interactions of **miconazole** apply to the oral gel formulation, as a sufficient quantity can be absorbed to cause systemic effects. Systemic absorption from intravaginal and topical formulations might also occur.

- Antifungals, azoles **(fluconazole, isavuconazole)** are predicted to increase the exposure to **abemaciclib**. Moderate Study
- Antifungals, azoles **(itraconazole, ketoconazole, posaconazole, voriconazole)** are predicted to increase the exposure to **abemaciclib**. Avoid or adjust dose—consult product literature. Severe Study
- **Fluconazole** is predicted to increase the exposure to **abrocitinib**. Adjust **abrocitinib** dose, p. 926. Severe Study
- Antifungals, azoles **(fluconazole, isavuconazole)** are predicted to increase the exposure to **acalabrutinib**. Avoid or monitor. Severe Study

Antifungals, azoles (continued)

- Antifungals, azoles **(itraconazole, ketoconazole, posaconazole, voriconazole)** are predicted to increase the exposure to **acalabrutinib**. Avoid. Severe Study
- Antifungals, azoles **(itraconazole, ketoconazole)** are predicted to increase the exposure to **afatinib**. Moderate Study
- **Alcohol** potentially causes a disulfiram-like reaction when given with **ketoconazole**. Avoid. Moderate Anecdotal
- **Itraconazole** markedly increases the exposure to **aliskiren**. Avoid. Severe Study
- **Ketoconazole** moderately increases the exposure to **aliskiren**. Moderate Study
- **Itraconazole** increases the risk of busulfan toxicity when given with alkylating agents **(busulfan)**. Monitor and adjust dose. Moderate Study
- **Miconazole** is predicted to increase the concentration of alkylating agents **(busulfan)**. Use with caution and adjust dose. Moderate Theoretical
- **Isavuconazole** is predicted to increase the exposure to alkylating agents **(cyclophosphamide)**. Moderate Study
- Antifungals, azoles **(itraconazole, ketoconazole, posaconazole, voriconazole)** are predicted to moderately increase the exposure to alpha blockers **(alfuzosin, tamsulosin)**. Use with caution or avoid. Moderate Study
- Antifungals, azoles **(itraconazole, ketoconazole, posaconazole, voriconazole)** are predicted to increase the exposure to alpha blockers **(doxazosin)**. Moderate Study
- Antifungals, azoles **(fluconazole, isavuconazole)** are predicted to increase the exposure to alpha blockers **(tamsulosin)**. Moderate Theoretical
- **Miconazole** potentially decreases the exposure to aminoglycosides **(tobramycin)**. Moderate Anecdotal
- Oral **antacids** decrease the absorption of oral **itraconazole** capsules. Manufacturer advises take 2 hours before or 1 hour after antacids. Moderate Study
- Oral **antacids** decrease the absorption of oral **ketoconazole**. Separate administration by at least 2 hours. Moderate Study
- Anti-androgens **(apalutamide, enzalutamide)** are predicted to decrease the exposure to **isavuconazole**. Avoid. Severe Study
- Antifungals, azoles **(itraconazole, ketoconazole, posaconazole, voriconazole)** are predicted to increase the exposure to anti-androgens **(apalutamide)**. Monitor and adjust dose. Mild Study → Also see TABLE 7 p. 1055
- **Itraconazole** slightly increases the exposure to anti-androgens **(darolutamide)**. Monitor and adjust dose. Moderate Study
- **Ketoconazole** is predicted to increase the exposure to anti-androgens **(darolutamide)**. Monitor and adjust dose. Moderate Theoretical
- Antiarrhythmics **(dronedarone)** are predicted to increase the exposure to **isavuconazole**. Moderate Theoretical
- **Itraconazole** is predicted to increase the exposure to antiarrhythmics **(amiodarone)**. Avoid. Severe Anecdotal → Also see TABLE 1 p. 1053
- Antifungals, azoles **(ketoconazole, voriconazole)** are predicted to increase the exposure to antiarrhythmics **(amiodarone)**. Avoid. Moderate Theoretical → Also see TABLE 1 p. 1053 → Also see TABLE 7 p. 1055
- **Miconazole** is predicted to increase the exposure to antiarrhythmics **(disopyramide)**. Use with caution and adjust dose. Severe Theoretical
- Antifungals, azoles **(itraconazole, ketoconazole, posaconazole, voriconazole)** are predicted to increase the exposure to antiarrhythmics **(disopyramide)**. Avoid. Severe Theoretical → Also see TABLE 7 p. 1055
- **Fluconazole** is predicted to increase the exposure to antiarrhythmics **(dronedarone)**. Severe Theoretical → Also see TABLE 7 p. 1055
- Antifungals, azoles **(itraconazole, ketoconazole, posaconazole, voriconazole)** very markedly increase the exposure to antiarrhythmics **(dronedarone)**. Avoid. Severe Study → Also see TABLE 7 p. 1055
- Antifungals, azoles **(fluconazole, isavuconazole)** are predicted to increase the exposure to antiarrhythmics **(propafenone)**. Monitor and adjust dose. Moderate Study
- Antifungals, azoles **(itraconazole, ketoconazole, posaconazole, voriconazole)** are predicted to increase the exposure to antiarrhythmics **(propafenone)**. Monitor and adjust dose. Severe Study
- Antifungals, azoles **(itraconazole, ketoconazole, posaconazole, voriconazole)** are predicted to increase the exposure to anticholinesterases, centrally acting **(galantamine)**. Monitor and adjust dose. Moderate Study
- Antiepileptics **(carbamazepine)** are predicted to decrease the efficacy of **fluconazole** and **fluconazole** increases the concentration of antiepileptics **(carbamazepine)**. Avoid or monitor **carbamazepine** concentration and adjust dose accordingly, p. 234. Severe Theoretical
- Antiepileptics **(carbamazepine)** are predicted to decrease the efficacy of **ketoconazole** and **ketoconazole** slightly increases the concentration of antiepileptics **(carbamazepine)**. Avoid or monitor **carbamazepine** concentration and adjust dose accordingly, p. 234. Moderate Study
- Antiepileptics **(carbamazepine)** are predicted to decrease the efficacy of **posaconazole** and **posaconazole** increases the concentration of antiepileptics **(carbamazepine)**. Avoid. Moderate Theoretical
- Antiepileptics **(carbamazepine, fosphenytoin, phenobarbital, phenytoin, primidone)** are predicted to decrease the exposure to **isavuconazole**. Avoid. Severe Study
- Antiepileptics **(fosphenytoin)** very markedly decrease the exposure to **itraconazole**. Avoid and for 14 days after stopping **fosphenytoin**. Moderate Study
- Antiepileptics **(fosphenytoin)** decrease the exposure to **voriconazole** and **voriconazole** increases the exposure to antiepileptics **(fosphenytoin)**. Avoid or adjust **voriconazole** dose and monitor phenytoin concentration, p. 468. Moderate Study
- Antiepileptics **(fosphenytoin, phenytoin)** decrease the exposure to **ketoconazole**. Avoid. Moderate Study
- Antiepileptics **(fosphenytoin, phenytoin)** are predicted to decrease the exposure to **posaconazole**. Avoid. Moderate Study
- Antiepileptics **(phenobarbital)** decrease the concentration of **itraconazole**. Avoid and for 14 days after stopping **phenobarbital**. Moderate Study
- Antiepileptics **(phenobarbital)** are predicted to decrease the concentration of **ketoconazole**. Avoid. Moderate Study
- Antiepileptics **(phenobarbital)** are predicted to decrease the concentration of **posaconazole**. Avoid. Moderate Study
- Antiepileptics **(phenobarbital, primidone)** are predicted to decrease the concentration of **voriconazole**. Avoid. Moderate Theoretical
- Antiepileptics **(phenytoin)** very markedly decrease the exposure to **itraconazole**. Avoid and for 14 days after stopping **phenytoin**. Moderate Study
- Antiepileptics **(phenytoin)** decrease the exposure to **voriconazole** and **voriconazole** increases the exposure to antiepileptics **(phenytoin)**. Avoid or adjust **voriconazole** dose and monitor **phenytoin** concentration, p. 468, p. 249. Moderate Study
- Antiepileptics **(primidone)** are predicted to decrease the concentration of **itraconazole**. Moderate Theoretical
- **Miconazole** increases the risk of carbamazepine toxicity when given with antiepileptics **(carbamazepine)**. Monitor and adjust dose. Severe Anecdotal
- **Miconazole** increases the risk of phenytoin toxicity when given with antiepileptics **(fosphenytoin)**. Monitor and adjust dose. Severe Anecdotal
- **Fluconazole** increases the concentration of antiepileptics **(fosphenytoin, phenytoin)**. Monitor concentration and adjust dose. Moderate Study
- Antiepileptics **(carbamazepine)** are predicted to decrease the efficacy of antifungals, azoles **(itraconazole, voriconazole)** and antifungals, azoles **(itraconazole, voriconazole)** increase the concentration of antiepileptics **(carbamazepine)**. Avoid or adjust dose. Moderate Theoretical
- Antiepileptics **(primidone)** are predicted to decrease the concentration of antifungals, azoles **(ketoconazole, posaconazole)**. Avoid. Moderate Study
- Antifungals, azoles **(itraconazole, ketoconazole, posaconazole, voriconazole)** are predicted to very slightly increase the exposure to antiepileptics **(perampanel)**. Mild Study

A1 Interactions | **Appendix 1**

- **Miconazole** increases the risk of phenytoin toxicity when given with antiepileptics **(phenytoin)**. Monitor and adjust dose. Severe Anecdotal
- Antifungals, azoles **(fluconazole)** are predicted to increase the exposure to antifungals, azoles **(isavuconazole)**. Severe Theoretical
- Antifungals, azoles **(itraconazole, ketoconazole, posaconazole, voriconazole)** are predicted to increase the exposure to antifungals, azoles **(isavuconazole)**. Avoid or monitor adverse effects. Severe Study
- **Miconazole** is predicted to increase the exposure to antihistamines, non-sedating **(mizolastine)**. Avoid. Moderate Theoretical
- Antifungals, azoles **(fluconazole, isavuconazole)** are predicted to increase the exposure to antihistamines, non-sedating **(mizolastine)**. Severe Theoretical
- Antifungals, azoles **(itraconazole, ketoconazole, posaconazole, voriconazole)** are predicted to increase the exposure to antihistamines, non-sedating **(mizolastine)**. Avoid. Severe Study
- Antifungals, azoles **(fluconazole, isavuconazole, itraconazole, ketoconazole, posaconazole, voriconazole)** are predicted to increase the exposure to antihistamines, non-sedating **(rupatadine)**. Avoid. Moderate Study
- **Ketoconazole** increases the exposure to antimalarials **(mefloquine)**. Moderate Study
- Antifungals, azoles **(fluconazole, itraconazole, posaconazole, voriconazole)** are predicted to increase the exposure to antimalarials **(mefloquine)**. Moderate Theoretical
- Antifungals, azoles **(fluconazole, isavuconazole, itraconazole, ketoconazole, posaconazole, voriconazole)** are predicted to increase the concentration of antimalarials **(piperaquine)**. Severe Study
- Antifungals, azoles **(itraconazole, ketoconazole, posaconazole, voriconazole)** are predicted to increase the exposure to **atogepant**. Adjust **atogepant** dose. Moderate Study
- Antifungals, azoles **(itraconazole, ketoconazole, posaconazole, voriconazole)** are predicted to slightly increase the exposure to atypical antipsychotics **(aripiprazole)**. Avoid or adjust dose—consult product literature. Moderate Study
- Antifungals, azoles **(fluconazole, isavuconazole)** are predicted to increase the exposure to atypical antipsychotics **(cariprazine)**. Monitor and adjust dose. Severe Study
- Antifungals, azoles **(itraconazole, ketoconazole, posaconazole, voriconazole)** are predicted to moderately increase the exposure to atypical antipsychotics **(cariprazine)**. Avoid. Severe Study
- Antifungals, azoles **(fluconazole, isavuconazole)** are predicted to increase the exposure to atypical antipsychotics **(lurasidone)**. Adjust **lurasidone** dose. Moderate Study
- Antifungals, azoles **(itraconazole, ketoconazole, posaconazole, voriconazole)** are predicted to increase the exposure to atypical antipsychotics **(lurasidone, quetiapine)**. Avoid. Severe Study
- Antifungals, azoles **(fluconazole, isavuconazole)** are predicted to increase the exposure to atypical antipsychotics **(quetiapine)**. Avoid. Moderate Study
- Antifungals, azoles **(itraconazole, ketoconazole, posaconazole, voriconazole)** are predicted to increase the exposure to atypical antipsychotics **(risperidone)**. Adjust dose. Moderate Study
- Antifungals, azoles **(itraconazole, ketoconazole, posaconazole, voriconazole)** are predicted to increase the exposure to **avacopan**. Severe Study
- Antifungals, azoles **(fluconazole, isavuconazole)** are predicted to increase the exposure to **avapritinib**. Avoid or adjust dose—consult product literature. Moderate Study
- Antifungals, azoles **(itraconazole, ketoconazole, posaconazole, voriconazole)** are predicted to increase the exposure to **avapritinib**. Avoid. Moderate Study
- Antifungals, azoles **(fluconazole, miconazole)** are predicted to increase the exposure to **avatrombopag**. Adjust **avatrombopag** dose with moderate CYP2C9 inhibitors in chronic immune thrombocytopenia. Moderate Study
- Antifungals, azoles **(fluconazole, isavuconazole)** are predicted to increase the exposure to **axitinib**. Moderate Study
- Antifungals, azoles **(itraconazole, ketoconazole, posaconazole, voriconazole)** are predicted to increase the exposure to **axitinib**. Avoid or adjust dose. Moderate Study
- Antifungals, azoles **(fluconazole, isavuconazole)** might increase the exposure to **bedaquiline**. Mild Theoretical → Also see TABLE 7 p. 1055
- Antifungals, azoles **(itraconazole, ketoconazole, posaconazole, voriconazole)** might increase the exposure to **bedaquiline**. Mild Study → Also see TABLE 7 p. 1055
- Antifungals, azoles **(fluconazole, voriconazole)** are predicted to increase the exposure to **belzutifan**. Monitor and adjust dose. Severe Theoretical
- **Miconazole** is predicted to increase the exposure to benzodiazepines **(alprazolam)**. Use with caution and adjust dose. Moderate Theoretical
- Antifungals, azoles **(fluconazole, isavuconazole)** are predicted to increase the exposure to benzodiazepines **(alprazolam)**. Severe Study
- Antifungals, azoles **(itraconazole, ketoconazole, posaconazole, voriconazole)** moderately increase the exposure to benzodiazepines **(alprazolam)**. Avoid. Moderate Study
- Antifungals, azoles **(fluconazole, voriconazole)** potentially increase the exposure to benzodiazepines **(clobazam)**. Adjust dose. Moderate Theoretical
- Antifungals, azoles **(fluconazole, voriconazole)** moderately increase the exposure to benzodiazepines **(diazepam)**. Monitor and adjust dose. Moderate Study
- **Miconazole** is predicted to increase the exposure to intravenous benzodiazepines **(midazolam)**. Use with caution and adjust dose. Moderate Theoretical
- **Miconazole** is predicted to increase the exposure to oral benzodiazepines **(midazolam)**. Avoid. Moderate Theoretical
- Antifungals, azoles **(fluconazole, isavuconazole)** are predicted to increase the exposure to benzodiazepines **(midazolam)**. Monitor adverse effects and adjust dose. Severe Study
- Antifungals, azoles **(itraconazole, ketoconazole, posaconazole, voriconazole)** are predicted to markedly to very markedly increase the exposure to benzodiazepines **(midazolam)**. Avoid or adjust dose. Severe Study
- **Berotralstat** is predicted to increase the exposure to **isavuconazole**. Moderate Theoretical
- Antifungals, azoles **(itraconazole, ketoconazole)** are predicted to increase the exposure to beta blockers, non-selective **(nadolol)**. Moderate Study
- Antifungals, azoles **(itraconazole, ketoconazole, posaconazole, voriconazole)** are predicted to increase the exposure to beta$_2$ agonists **(salmeterol)**. Avoid. Severe Study
- Antifungals, azoles **(itraconazole, ketoconazole, posaconazole, voriconazole)** slightly increase the exposure to **bortezomib**. Moderate Study
- Antifungals, azoles **(fluconazole, isavuconazole, itraconazole, ketoconazole, posaconazole, voriconazole)** are predicted to increase the exposure to **bosutinib**. Avoid or adjust dose. Severe Study → Also see TABLE 7 p. 1055
- Antifungals, azoles **(fluconazole, isavuconazole)** are predicted to increase the exposure to **brigatinib**. Moderate Study
- Antifungals, azoles **(itraconazole, ketoconazole, posaconazole, voriconazole)** are predicted to increase the exposure to **brigatinib**. Avoid or adjust dose—consult product literature. Severe Study
- **Isavuconazole** slightly increases the exposure to **bupropion**. Adjust dose. Moderate Study
- Antifungals, azoles **(fluconazole, isavuconazole)** are predicted to increase the exposure to **buspirone**. Use with caution and adjust dose. Moderate Study
- Antifungals, azoles **(itraconazole, ketoconazole, posaconazole, voriconazole)** are predicted to increase the exposure to **buspirone**. Adjust **buspirone** dose. Severe Study
- **Miconazole** is predicted to increase the concentration of **buspirone**. Use with caution and adjust dose. Moderate Theoretical
- Antifungals, azoles **(fluconazole, isavuconazole, itraconazole, ketoconazole, posaconazole, voriconazole)** are predicted to increase the exposure to **cabozantinib**. Moderate Study → Also see TABLE 7 p. 1055
- Calcium-channel blockers **(diltiazem, verapamil)** are predicted to increase the exposure to **isavuconazole**. Moderate Theoretical

Antifungals, azoles (continued)

- Antifungals, azoles **(fluconazole, isavuconazole)** are predicted to increase the exposure to calcium-channel blockers **(amlodipine, felodipine, lacidipine, lercanidipine, nicardipine, nifedipine, nimodipine)**. Monitor and adjust dose. [Moderate] Study
- **Miconazole** is predicted to increase the exposure to calcium-channel blockers **(amlodipine, felodipine, lacidipine, lercanidipine, nicardipine, nifedipine, nimodipine, verapamil)**. Use with caution and adjust dose. [Moderate] Theoretical
- Antifungals, azoles **(itraconazole, ketoconazole, posaconazole, voriconazole)** are predicted to increase the exposure to calcium-channel blockers **(amlodipine, felodipine, lacidipine, nicardipine, nifedipine, nimodipine)**. Monitor and adjust dose. [Moderate] Study
- **Miconazole** is predicted to increase the exposure to calcium-channel blockers **(diltiazem)**. [Moderate] Theoretical
- **Fluconazole** (high-dose) is predicted to increase the exposure to calcium-channel blockers **(diltiazem, verapamil)**. [Moderate] Theoretical
- Antifungals, azoles **(itraconazole, ketoconazole, posaconazole, voriconazole)** are predicted to increase the exposure to calcium-channel blockers **(diltiazem, verapamil)**. [Severe] Study
- Antifungals, azoles **(itraconazole, ketoconazole, posaconazole, voriconazole)** are predicted to markedly increase the exposure to calcium-channel blockers **(lercanidipine)**. Avoid. [Severe] Study
- Antifungals, azoles **(itraconazole, ketoconazole, posaconazole, voriconazole)** are predicted to increase the exposure to **cannabidiol**. Avoid or adjust dose. [Mild] Study
- **Fluconazole** is predicted to increase the exposure to **cannabidiol**. [Moderate] Theoretical
- Antifungals, azoles **(fluconazole, isavuconazole, itraconazole, ketoconazole, posaconazole, voriconazole)** are predicted to increase the exposure to **capivasertib**. Adjust dose. [Moderate] Study
- **Cenobamate** is predicted to decrease the exposure to **isavuconazole**. Avoid. [Severe] Theoretical
- Antifungals, azoles **(fluconazole, isavuconazole)** are predicted to increase the exposure to **ceritinib**. [Moderate] Study → Also see TABLE 7 p. 1055
- Antifungals, azoles **(itraconazole, voriconazole)** are predicted to increase the exposure to **ceritinib**. Avoid or adjust dose—consult product literature. [Severe] Study → Also see TABLE 7 p. 1055
- **Ceritinib** is predicted to increase the exposure to **isavuconazole**. Avoid or monitor adverse effects. [Severe] Study
- **Ketoconazole** moderately increases the exposure to **ceritinib**. Avoid or adjust dose—consult product literature. [Severe] Study
- Antifungals, azoles **(fluconazole, isavuconazole)** are predicted to increase the concentration of **ciclosporin**. [Severe] Study
- Antifungals, azoles **(itraconazole, ketoconazole, posaconazole, voriconazole)** increase the concentration of **ciclosporin**. [Severe] Study
- **Miconazole** increases the concentration of **ciclosporin**. Monitor and adjust dose. [Severe] Anecdotal
- Antifungals, azoles **(itraconazole, ketoconazole, posaconazole, voriconazole)** are predicted to moderately increase the exposure to **cilostazol**. Adjust **cilostazol** dose. [Moderate] Study
- **Fluconazole** is predicted to increase the exposure to **cilostazol**. Adjust **cilostazol** dose. [Moderate] Theoretical
- **Miconazole** is predicted to increase the exposure to **cilostazol**. Use with caution and adjust dose. [Moderate] Theoretical
- Antifungals, azoles **(itraconazole, ketoconazole, posaconazole, voriconazole)** are predicted to moderately increase the exposure to **cinacalcet**. Adjust dose. [Moderate] Study
- **Fluconazole** is predicted to decrease the efficacy of **clopidogrel**. Avoid. [Severe] Theoretical
- **Voriconazole** is predicted to decrease the efficacy of **clopidogrel**. Avoid. [Moderate] Study
- **Cobicistat** is predicted to increase the exposure to antifungals, azoles **(fluconazole, posaconazole)**. [Moderate] Theoretical
- **Cobicistat** is predicted to increase the exposure to **isavuconazole**. Avoid or monitor adverse effects. [Severe] Study
- **Cobicistat** is predicted to increase the exposure to **itraconazole**. Adjust **itraconazole** dose, p. 465. [Moderate] Theoretical
- **Cobicistat** is predicted to increase the exposure to **ketoconazole**. Adjust **ketoconazole** dose, p. 550. [Moderate] Theoretical
- **Cobicistat** is predicted to affect the exposure to **voriconazole**. Avoid. [Moderate] Theoretical
- Antifungals, azoles **(fluconazole, isavuconazole)** are predicted to increase the exposure to **cobimetinib**. [Severe] Study
- Antifungals, azoles **(itraconazole, ketoconazole, posaconazole, voriconazole)** are predicted to increase the exposure to **cobimetinib**. Avoid or monitor for toxicity. [Severe] Study
- **Miconazole** is predicted to increase the exposure to **cobimetinib**. [Severe] Theoretical
- Antifungals, azoles **(fluconazole, isavuconazole)** are predicted to increase the exposure to **colchicine**. Adjust **colchicine** dose with moderate CYP3A4 inhibitors, p. 637. [Severe] Study
- Antifungals, azoles **(itraconazole, ketoconazole, posaconazole, voriconazole)** are predicted to increase the exposure to **colchicine**. Avoid potent CYP3A4 inhibitors or adjust **colchicine** dose, p. 637. [Severe] Study
- Antifungals, azoles **(itraconazole, ketoconazole, posaconazole, voriconazole)** are predicted to increase the exposure to corticosteroids **(beclometasone)** (risk with beclometasone is likely to be lower than with other corticosteroids). [Moderate] Theoretical
- Antifungals, azoles **(itraconazole, ketoconazole, posaconazole, voriconazole)** are predicted to increase the exposure to corticosteroids **(betamethasone, budesonide, ciclesonide, deflazacort, dexamethasone, fludrocortisone, fluticasone, hydrocortisone, methylprednisolone, mometasone, prednisolone, triamcinolone)**. Avoid or monitor adverse effects. [Severe] Study
- **Miconazole** is predicted to increase the concentration of corticosteroids **(methylprednisolone)**. Monitor and adjust dose. [Moderate] Theoretical
- Antifungals, azoles **(fluconazole, isavuconazole)** are predicted to increase the exposure to corticosteroids **(methylprednisolone)**. Monitor and adjust dose. [Moderate] Study
- Antifungals, azoles **(itraconazole, ketoconazole, posaconazole, voriconazole)** are predicted to increase the exposure to corticosteroids **(vamorolone)**. Adjust dose. [Severe] Study
- **Fluconazole** increases the anticoagulant effect of **coumarins**. Monitor INR and adjust dose. [Severe] Study
- **Itraconazole** potentially increases the anticoagulant effect of **coumarins**. [Severe] Anecdotal
- **Ketoconazole** potentially increases the anticoagulant effect of coumarins **(warfarin)**. Monitor INR and adjust dose. [Severe] Anecdotal
- **Miconazole** greatly increases the anticoagulant effect of **coumarins**. MHRA advises avoid unless INR can be monitored closely; monitor for signs of bleeding. [Severe] Study
- **Voriconazole** increases the anticoagulant effect of **coumarins**. Monitor INR and adjust dose. [Moderate] Study
- Antifungals, azoles **(fluconazole, isavuconazole)** are predicted to increase the exposure to **crizotinib**. [Moderate] Study → Also see TABLE 7 p. 1055
- Antifungals, azoles **(itraconazole, ketoconazole, posaconazole, voriconazole)** are predicted to increase the exposure to **crizotinib**. Avoid. [Moderate] Study → Also see TABLE 7 p. 1055
- Antifungals, azoles **(fluconazole, isavuconazole)** are predicted to increase the exposure to **dabrafenib**. [Moderate] Study
- Antifungals, azoles **(itraconazole, ketoconazole, posaconazole, voriconazole)** are predicted to increase the exposure to **dabrafenib**. Use with caution or avoid. [Moderate] Study
- **Dabrafenib** is predicted to decrease the exposure to **isavuconazole**. Avoid. [Severe] Theoretical
- Antifungals, azoles **(fluconazole, isavuconazole)** are predicted to increase the exposure to **daridorexant**. Adjust **daridorexant** dose. [Severe] Study
- Antifungals, azoles **(itraconazole, ketoconazole, posaconazole, voriconazole)** are predicted to increase the exposure to **daridorexant**. Avoid. [Severe] Study
- Antifungals, azoles **(itraconazole, ketoconazole, posaconazole, voriconazole)** are predicted to markedly to very markedly increase the exposure to **darifenacin**. Avoid. [Severe] Study

- ▶ **Fluconazole** slightly increases the exposure to **darifenacin**. Moderate Study
- ▶ **Isavuconazole** is predicted to increase the exposure to **darifenacin**. Moderate Study
- ▶ Antifungals, azoles **(fluconazole, isavuconazole)** are predicted to increase the exposure to **dasatinib**. Severe Study → Also see TABLE 7 p. 1055
- ▶ Antifungals, azoles **(itraconazole, ketoconazole, posaconazole, voriconazole)** are predicted to increase the exposure to **dasatinib**. Avoid or adjust dose—consult product literature. Severe Study → Also see TABLE 7 p. 1055
- ▶ Antifungals, azoles **(itraconazole, ketoconazole, posaconazole, voriconazole)** very slightly increase the exposure to **delamanid**. Severe Study → Also see TABLE 7 p. 1055
- ▶ Antifungals, azoles **(fluconazole, isavuconazole, itraconazole, ketoconazole, posaconazole, voriconazole)** are predicted to increase the exposure to **deutivacaftor**. Adjust dose, see deutivacaftor with tezacaftor and vanzacaftor p. 218. Severe Study
- ▶ Antifungals, azoles **(fluconazole, isavuconazole)** are predicted to slightly increase the exposure to **dienogest**. Moderate Study
- ▶ Antifungals, azoles **(itraconazole, ketoconazole, posaconazole, voriconazole)** are predicted to moderately increase the exposure to **dienogest**. Moderate Study
- ▶ **Isavuconazole** slightly increases the exposure to **digoxin**. Monitor and adjust dose. Moderate Study
- ▶ **Itraconazole** increases the concentration of **digoxin**. Monitor and adjust dose. Severe Study
- ▶ **Ketoconazole** is predicted to increase the exposure to **digoxin**. Severe Study
- ▶ **Posaconazole** is predicted to increase the concentration of **digoxin**. Severe Study
- ▶ Antifungals, azoles **(fluconazole, isavuconazole)** are predicted to increase the exposure to dipeptidylpeptidase-4 inhibitors **(saxagliptin)**. Mild Study
- ▶ Antifungals, azoles **(itraconazole, ketoconazole, posaconazole, voriconazole)** are predicted to increase the exposure to dipeptidylpeptidase-4 inhibitors **(saxagliptin)**. Moderate Study
- ▶ Antifungals, azoles **(fluconazole, isavuconazole, itraconazole, ketoconazole, posaconazole, voriconazole)** are predicted to increase the exposure to **domperidone**. Avoid. Severe Study
- ▶ Antifungals, azoles **(fluconazole, isavuconazole)** are predicted to increase the exposure to dopamine receptor agonists **(bromocriptine)**. Severe Theoretical
- ▶ Antifungals, azoles **(itraconazole, ketoconazole, posaconazole, voriconazole)** increase the exposure to dopamine receptor agonists **(bromocriptine)**. Severe Study
- ▶ Antifungals, azoles **(fluconazole, isavuconazole, itraconazole, ketoconazole, posaconazole, voriconazole)** are predicted to increase the concentration of dopamine receptor agonists **(cabergoline)**. Moderate Anecdotal
- ▶ **Isavuconazole** is predicted to increase the exposure to dopamine receptor agonists **(pramipexole)**. Adjust dose. Moderate Study
- ▶ Antifungals, azoles **(itraconazole, ketoconazole, posaconazole, voriconazole)** are predicted to increase the exposure to **dronabinol**. Adjust dose. Mild Study
- ▶ Antifungals, azoles **(fluconazole, isavuconazole, itraconazole, posaconazole, voriconazole)** are predicted to increase the exposure to **drospirenone**. Severe Study
- ▶ **Ketoconazole** moderately increases the exposure to **drospirenone**. Severe Study
- ▶ Antifungals, azoles **(fluconazole, isavuconazole)** are predicted to moderately increase the exposure to **dutasteride**. Mild Study
- ▶ Antifungals, azoles **(itraconazole, ketoconazole, posaconazole, voriconazole)** are predicted to increase the exposure to **dutasteride**. Monitor adverse effects and adjust dose. Moderate Theoretical
- ▶ Antifungals, azoles **(fluconazole, isavuconazole)** are predicted to increase the exposure to **elacestrant**. Avoid moderate CYP3A4 inhibitors or adjust **elacestrant** dose. Severe Theoretical
- ▶ Antifungals, azoles **(itraconazole, ketoconazole, posaconazole, voriconazole)** are predicted to increase the exposure to **elacestrant**. Avoid potent CYP3A4 inhibitors or adjust **elacestrant** dose. Severe Study
- ▶ Antifungals, azoles **(fluconazole, isavuconazole)** are predicted to increase the exposure to **elexacaftor**. Adjust ivacaftor with tezacaftor and elexacaftor p. 220 dose with moderate CYP3A4 inhibitors. Severe Theoretical
- ▶ Antifungals, azoles **(itraconazole, ketoconazole, posaconazole, voriconazole)** are predicted to increase the exposure to **elexacaftor**. Adjust ivacaftor with tezacaftor and elexacaftor p. 220 dose with potent CYP3A4 inhibitors. Severe Study
- ▶ Antifungals, azoles **(fluconazole, isavuconazole, itraconazole, ketoconazole, posaconazole, voriconazole)** are predicted to increase the exposure to **eliglustat**. Avoid or adjust dose—consult product literature. Severe Study
- ▶ Antifungals, azoles **(fluconazole, isavuconazole)** are predicted to moderately increase the exposure to **encorafenib**. Moderate Study → Also see TABLE 7 p. 1055
- ▶ Antifungals, azoles **(itraconazole, ketoconazole, posaconazole, voriconazole)** are predicted to increase the exposure to **encorafenib**. Avoid or monitor. Severe Study → Also see TABLE 7 p. 1055
- ▶ **Encorafenib** is predicted to decrease the exposure to **isavuconazole**. Avoid. Severe Study
- ▶ Endothelin receptor antagonists **(bosentan)** are predicted to decrease the exposure to **isavuconazole**. Avoid. Severe Theoretical
- ▶ **Fluconazole** is predicted to increase the exposure to endothelin receptor antagonists **(bosentan)**. Avoid. Severe Study
- ▶ **Itraconazole** is predicted to increase the exposure to endothelin receptor antagonists **(bosentan)**. Moderate Theoretical
- ▶ **Ketoconazole** moderately increases the exposure to endothelin receptor antagonists **(bosentan)**. Moderate Study
- ▶ **Voriconazole** is predicted to increase the exposure to endothelin receptor antagonists **(bosentan)**. Avoid. Severe Theoretical
- ▶ Antifungals, azoles **(fluconazole, isavuconazole, miconazole)** are predicted to increase the exposure to endothelin receptor antagonists **(macitentan)**. Manufacturer advises caution depending on other drugs taken—consult product literature. Moderate Theoretical
- ▶ Antifungals, azoles **(itraconazole, ketoconazole, posaconazole, voriconazole)** are predicted to increase the exposure to endothelin receptor antagonists **(macitentan)**. Moderate Study
- ▶ Antifungals, azoles **(itraconazole, ketoconazole, posaconazole, voriconazole)** are predicted to increase the exposure to the cytotoxic component of **enfortumab vedotin**. Severe Theoretical
- ▶ Antifungals, azoles **(fluconazole, isavuconazole)** are predicted to increase the exposure to **entrectinib**. Avoid or adjust dose with moderate CYP3A4 inhibitors—consult product literature. Severe Theoretical → Also see TABLE 7 p. 1055
- ▶ Antifungals, azoles **(itraconazole, ketoconazole, posaconazole, voriconazole)** are predicted to increase the exposure to **entrectinib**. Avoid or adjust dose with potent CYP3A4 inhibitors—consult product literature. Severe Study → Also see TABLE 7 p. 1055
- ▶ Antifungals, azoles **(fluconazole, itraconazole, ketoconazole, miconazole, posaconazole, voriconazole)** are predicted to increase the exposure to **erdafitinib**. Adjust dose. Severe Study
- ▶ Antifungals, azoles **(fluconazole, isavuconazole)** are predicted to increase the risk of ergotism when given with **ergometrine**. Severe Theoretical
- ▶ Antifungals, azoles **(itraconazole, ketoconazole, posaconazole, voriconazole)** are predicted to increase the risk of ergotism when given with **ergometrine**. Avoid. Severe Theoretical
- ▶ **Miconazole** is predicted to increase the exposure to **ergometrine**. Avoid. Moderate Theoretical
- ▶ Antifungals, azoles **(fluconazole, isavuconazole)** are predicted to increase the exposure to **erlotinib**. Moderate Study
- ▶ Antifungals, azoles **(itraconazole, ketoconazole, posaconazole, voriconazole)** are predicted to increase the exposure to **erlotinib**. Use with caution and adjust dose. Severe Study
- ▶ Antifungals, azoles **(itraconazole, ketoconazole, posaconazole, voriconazole)** are predicted to increase the exposure to **esketamine**. Adjust dose. Moderate Study
- ▶ Antifungals, azoles **(itraconazole, ketoconazole, posaconazole, voriconazole)** are predicted to increase the exposure to

Antifungals, azoles (continued)
eszopiclone. Adjust **eszopiclone** dose; avoid in the elderly. [Moderate] Study

- Antifungals, azoles **(itraconazole, ketoconazole, posaconazole, voriconazole)** are predicted to increase the concentration of subdermal **etonogestrel**. [Moderate] Theoretical
- Antifungals, azoles **(isavuconazole, itraconazole, ketoconazole, posaconazole, voriconazole)** are predicted to increase the exposure to **etrasimod**. Avoid in poor CYP2C9 metabolisers. [Severe] Theoretical
- **Fluconazole** slightly increases the exposure to **etrasimod**. Avoid. [Severe] Study
- Antifungals, azoles **(fluconazole, isavuconazole)** are predicted to increase the concentration of **everolimus**. Avoid or adjust dose. [Moderate] Study
- Antifungals, azoles **(itraconazole, ketoconazole, posaconazole, voriconazole)** are predicted to increase the exposure to **everolimus**. Avoid. [Severe] Study
- **Itraconazole** is predicted to increase the exposure to **factor XA inhibitors (apixaban)**. Avoid. [Severe] Theoretical
- **Ketoconazole** moderately increases the exposure to **factor XA inhibitors (apixaban, rivaroxaban)**. Avoid. [Severe] Study
- Antifungals, azoles **(posaconazole, voriconazole)** are predicted to increase the exposure to **factor XA inhibitors (apixaban, rivaroxaban)**. Avoid. [Severe] Theoretical
- **Itraconazole** is predicted to increase the exposure to **factor XA inhibitors (edoxaban)**. [Severe] Theoretical
- **Ketoconazole** slightly increases the exposure to **factor XA inhibitors (edoxaban)**. Adjust **edoxaban** dose. [Severe] Study
- **Itraconazole** is predicted to increase the exposure to **factor XA inhibitors (rivaroxaban)**. Avoid. [Severe] Anecdotal
- Antifungals, azoles **(itraconazole, ketoconazole, posaconazole, voriconazole)** are predicted to increase the exposure to **fedratinib**. Adjust dose, but avoid depending on other drugs taken—consult product literature. [Moderate] Study
- **Fluconazole** is predicted to increase the exposure to **fedratinib**. Avoid. [Moderate] Theoretical
- **Isavuconazole** is predicted to increase the exposure to **fedratinib**. Monitor and adjust dose. [Moderate] Study
- Antifungals, azoles **(fluconazole, isavuconazole)** are predicted to increase the exposure to **fesoterodine**. Adjust **fesoterodine** dose with moderate CYP3A4 inhibitors in hepatic and renal impairment. [Mild] Study
- Antifungals, azoles **(itraconazole, ketoconazole, posaconazole, voriconazole)** are predicted to moderately increase the exposure to **fesoterodine**. Adjust **fesoterodine** dose with potent CYP3A4 inhibitors; avoid in hepatic and renal impairment. [Severe] Study
- Antifungals, azoles **(itraconazole, ketoconazole)** are predicted to increase the exposure to **fidaxomicin**. Avoid. [Moderate] Study
- Antifungals, azoles **(itraconazole, ketoconazole, posaconazole, voriconazole)** are predicted to increase the exposure to **fostamatinib**. Monitor adverse effects and adjust dose. [Moderate] Study
- Antifungals, azoles **(itraconazole, ketoconazole)** are predicted to increase the exposure to **futibatinib**. Avoid or adjust dose—consult product literature. [Moderate] Study
- Antifungals, azoles **(fluconazole, isavuconazole)** are predicted to increase the exposure to **gefitinib**. [Moderate] Study
- Antifungals, azoles **(itraconazole, ketoconazole, posaconazole, voriconazole)** are predicted to increase the exposure to **gefitinib**. [Severe] Study
- Antifungals, azoles **(itraconazole, ketoconazole, posaconazole, voriconazole)** are predicted to increase the exposure to **gilteritinib**. [Moderate] Study
- Antifungals, azoles **(itraconazole, ketoconazole, posaconazole, voriconazole)** are predicted to increase the exposure to **glasdegib**. Use with caution or avoid. [Severe] Study → Also see TABLE 7 p. 1055
- Antifungals, azoles **(itraconazole, ketoconazole, posaconazole, voriconazole)** are predicted to moderately to markedly increase the exposure to **grazoprevir**. Avoid. [Severe] Study
- Antifungals, azoles **(fluconazole, isavuconazole)** are predicted to increase the concentration of **guanfacine**. Adjust **guanfacine** dose, p. 281. [Moderate] Theoretical
- Antifungals, azoles **(itraconazole, ketoconazole, posaconazole, voriconazole)** are predicted to increase the exposure to **guanfacine**. Adjust **guanfacine** dose, p. 281. [Moderate] Study
- **H_2 receptor antagonists** are predicted to decrease the absorption of **itraconazole**. Administer **itraconazole** capsules with an acidic beverage. [Moderate] Study
- **H_2 receptor antagonists** are predicted to decrease the absorption of **ketoconazole**. Administer **ketoconazole** with an acidic beverage. [Moderate] Study
- **H_2 receptor antagonists** are predicted to decrease the exposure to **posaconazole**. Avoid use of posaconazole oral suspension. [Moderate] Study
- **Itraconazole** increases the concentration of **haloperidol**. [Moderate] Study
- **HIV-protease inhibitors** are predicted to increase the exposure to **isavuconazole**. Avoid or monitor adverse effects. [Severe] Study
- **HIV-protease inhibitors** are predicted to increase the exposure to **itraconazole**. Use with caution and adjust dose. [Severe] Study → Also see TABLE 1 p. 1053
- **HIV-protease inhibitors** are predicted to increase the exposure to **ketoconazole**. Use with caution and adjust dose. [Moderate] Study
- **Miconazole** is predicted to increase the concentration of **HIV-protease inhibitors**. Use with caution and adjust dose. [Moderate] Theoretical
- **Posaconazole** is predicted to increase the exposure to **HIV-protease inhibitors**. [Moderate] Study
- **HIV-protease inhibitors** are predicted to affect the exposure to **voriconazole** and **voriconazole** potentially affects the exposure to **HIV-protease inhibitors**. [Severe] Study → Also see TABLE 1 p. 1053
- Antifungals, azoles **(fluconazole, isavuconazole)** are predicted to increase the exposure to **ibrutinib**. Adjust dose with moderate CYP3A4 inhibitors—consult product literature. [Severe] Study
- Antifungals, azoles **(itraconazole, ketoconazole, posaconazole, voriconazole)** are predicted to increase the exposure to **ibrutinib**. Avoid or adjust dose with potent CYP3A4 inhibitors—consult product literature. [Severe] Study
- Antifungals, azoles **(itraconazole, voriconazole)** are predicted to increase the exposure to **idelalisib**. [Moderate] Theoretical
- **Idelalisib** is predicted to increase the exposure to **isavuconazole**. Avoid or monitor adverse effects. [Severe] Study
- **Ketoconazole** slightly increases the exposure to **idelalisib**. [Moderate] Study
- Antifungals, azoles **(itraconazole, ketoconazole, posaconazole, voriconazole)** are predicted to increase the exposure to **imatinib**. [Moderate] Study
- **Fluconazole** is predicted to increase the exposure to **imatinib**. [Moderate] Theoretical
- **Imatinib** is predicted to increase the exposure to **isavuconazole**. [Moderate] Theoretical
- Antifungals, azoles **(fluconazole, isavuconazole)** are predicted to increase the exposure to the active metabolite of **irinotecan**. [Moderate] Theoretical
- Antifungals, azoles **(itraconazole, ketoconazole, posaconazole, voriconazole)** are predicted to increase the exposure to the active metabolite of **irinotecan**. Avoid. [Severe] Study
- Antifungals, azoles **(fluconazole, isavuconazole)** are predicted to increase the exposure to **ivabradine**. Adjust **ivabradine** dose. [Severe] Theoretical
- Antifungals, azoles **(itraconazole, ketoconazole, posaconazole, voriconazole)** are predicted to increase the exposure to **ivabradine**. Avoid. [Severe] Study
- Antifungals, azoles **(fluconazole, isavuconazole)** are predicted to increase the exposure to **ivacaftor**. Adjust dose with moderate CYP3A4 inhibitors, see ivacaftor p. 219, tezacaftor with ivacaftor p. 223, and ivacaftor with tezacaftor and elexacaftor p. 220. [Moderate] Study
- Antifungals, azoles **(itraconazole, ketoconazole, posaconazole, voriconazole)** are predicted to increase the exposure to **ivacaftor**. Adjust dose with potent CYP3A4 inhibitors, see ivacaftor p. 219, lumacaftor with ivacaftor p. 222, tezacaftor with ivacaftor p. 223, and ivacaftor with tezacaftor and elexacaftor p. 220. [Severe] Study

- Antifungals, azoles **(fluconazole, isavuconazole, voriconazole)** are predicted to increase the exposure to **ivosidenib**. Monitor and adjust dose—consult product literature. Severe Study → Also see TABLE 7 p. 1055
- **Ivosidenib** is predicted to decrease the exposure to **isavuconazole**. Avoid. Severe Study
- **Itraconazole** moderately increases the exposure to **ivosidenib** and **ivosidenib** is predicted to decrease the exposure to **itraconazole**. Avoid or adjust dose—consult product literature. Severe Study
- **Ketoconazole** is predicted to increase the exposure to **ivosidenib** and **ivosidenib** is predicted to decrease the exposure to **ketoconazole**. Avoid or adjust dose—consult product literature. Severe Study
- Antifungals, azoles **(itraconazole, ketoconazole, posaconazole, voriconazole)** are predicted to increase the exposure to **ketamine**. Adjust dose. Moderate Theoretical
- **Lanthanum** is predicted to decrease the absorption of **ketoconazole**. Separate administration by at least 2 hours. Moderate Theoretical
- Antifungals, azoles **(fluconazole, isavuconazole)** are predicted to increase the exposure to **lapatinib**. Moderate Study → Also see TABLE 7 p. 1055
- Antifungals, azoles **(itraconazole, ketoconazole, posaconazole, voriconazole)** are predicted to increase the exposure to **lapatinib**. Avoid. Moderate Study → Also see TABLE 7 p. 1055
- Antifungals, azoles **(fluconazole, isavuconazole)** are predicted to increase the exposure to **larotrectinib**. Monitor and adjust dose. Moderate Theoretical
- Antifungals, azoles **(itraconazole, ketoconazole, posaconazole, voriconazole)** are predicted to moderately increase the exposure to **larotrectinib**. Avoid or adjust dose—consult product literature. Moderate Study
- Antifungals, azoles **(fluconazole, isavuconazole, itraconazole, ketoconazole, posaconazole, voriconazole)** are predicted to increase the exposure to **leniolisib**. Avoid. Moderate Study
- **Letermovir** is predicted to increase the exposure to **isavuconazole**. Moderate Theoretical
- **Letermovir** slightly decreases the exposure to **voriconazole**. Moderate Study
- Antifungals, azoles **(fluconazole, isavuconazole)** are predicted to increase the exposure to **lomitapide**. Avoid. Moderate Theoretical → Also see TABLE 1 p. 1053
- Antifungals, azoles **(itraconazole, ketoconazole, posaconazole, voriconazole)** are predicted to markedly increase the exposure to **lomitapide**. Avoid. Severe Study → Also see TABLE 1 p. 1053
- **Clotrimazole** is predicted to increase the exposure to **lomitapide**. Separate administration by 12 hours. Moderate Theoretical
- Antifungals, azoles **(itraconazole, ketoconazole, posaconazole, voriconazole)** are predicted to increase the exposure to **lorlatinib**. Avoid or adjust dose—consult product literature. Severe Study
- **Fluconazole** is predicted to increase the exposure to **lorlatinib**. Moderate Theoretical
- **Lorlatinib** is predicted to decrease the exposure to **isavuconazole**. Avoid. Severe Theoretical
- **Lumacaftor** is predicted to decrease the exposure to antifungals, azoles **(itraconazole, ketoconazole, posaconazole, voriconazole)**. Avoid or monitor efficacy. Moderate Theoretical
- **Lumacaftor** is predicted to decrease the exposure to **isavuconazole**. Avoid. Severe Study
- Macrolides **(clarithromycin)** are predicted to increase the exposure to **isavuconazole**. Avoid or monitor adverse effects. Severe Study
- Macrolides **(erythromycin)** are predicted to increase the exposure to **isavuconazole**. Moderate Theoretical
- Antifungals, azoles **(itraconazole, ketoconazole, voriconazole)** are predicted to markedly increase the exposure to **maraviroc**. Adjust dose. Severe Study
- Antifungals, azoles **(fluconazole, isavuconazole)** are predicted to increase the exposure to **mavacamten**. Adjust dose—consult product literature. Moderate Study
- Antifungals, azoles **(itraconazole, ketoconazole, posaconazole, voriconazole)** are predicted to increase the exposure to **mavacamten**. Avoid or monitor—consult product literature. Severe Study
- Antifungals, azoles **(itraconazole, ketoconazole, posaconazole, voriconazole)** are predicted to increase the concentration of intramuscular **medroxyprogesterone**. Moderate Theoretical
- **Isavuconazole** is predicted to increase the exposure to **metformin**. Use with caution and adjust dose. Moderate Study
- **Metoclopramide** potentially decreases the absorption of **posaconazole** oral suspension. Moderate Study
- Antifungals, azoles **(fluconazole, isavuconazole)** are predicted to increase the exposure to **midostaurin**. Moderate Theoretical
- Antifungals, azoles **(itraconazole, ketoconazole, posaconazole, voriconazole)** are predicted to increase the exposure to **midostaurin**. Avoid or monitor for toxicity. Severe Study
- **Posaconazole** is predicted to increase the exposure to **mifepristone**. Moderate Theoretical
- Antifungals, azoles **(fluconazole, isavuconazole)** are predicted to increase the exposure to mineralocorticoid receptor antagonists **(eplerenone)**. Adjust **eplerenone** dose. Severe Study
- Antifungals, azoles **(itraconazole, ketoconazole, posaconazole, voriconazole)** are predicted to markedly increase the exposure to mineralocorticoid receptor antagonists **(eplerenone)**. Avoid. Severe Study
- Antifungals, azoles **(fluconazole, isavuconazole)** are predicted to increase the exposure to mineralocorticoid receptor antagonists **(finerenone)**. Severe Study
- Antifungals, azoles **(itraconazole, ketoconazole, posaconazole, voriconazole)** are predicted to increase the exposure to mineralocorticoid receptor antagonists **(finerenone)**. Avoid. Severe Study
- Antifungals, azoles **(itraconazole, ketoconazole, posaconazole, voriconazole)** are predicted to increase the exposure to **mirabegron**. Adjust **mirabegron** dose in hepatic and renal impairment. Moderate Study
- Antifungals, azoles **(itraconazole, ketoconazole, posaconazole, voriconazole)** are predicted to increase the exposure to **mirtazapine**. Moderate Study
- **Mitotane** is predicted to decrease the exposure to **isavuconazole**. Avoid. Severe Study
- Antifungals, azoles **(itraconazole, ketoconazole, posaconazole, voriconazole)** are predicted to increase the exposure to **modafinil**. Mild Theoretical
- Monoclonal antibodies **(mosunetuzumab)** are predicted to transiently increase the exposure to **voriconazole**. Monitor and adjust dose. Moderate Theoretical
- Antifungals, azoles **(itraconazole, ketoconazole, posaconazole, voriconazole)** are predicted to increase the risk of neutropenia when given with monoclonal antibodies **(brentuximab vedotin)**. Monitor and adjust dose. Severe Study
- Antifungals, azoles **(itraconazole, ketoconazole, posaconazole, voriconazole)** are predicted to increase the exposure to monoclonal antibodies **(polatuzumab vedotin)**. Moderate Theoretical
- Antifungals, azoles **(itraconazole, ketoconazole, posaconazole, voriconazole)** are predicted to increase the exposure to the cytotoxic component of monoclonal antibodies **(trastuzumab emtansine)**. Avoid or monitor. Severe Theoretical
- **Isavuconazole** increases the exposure to **mycophenolate**. Moderate Study
- Antifungals, azoles **(fluconazole, isavuconazole)** are predicted to increase the exposure to **naldemedine**. Moderate Study
- Antifungals, azoles **(itraconazole, ketoconazole, posaconazole, voriconazole)** are predicted to increase the exposure to **naldemedine**. Avoid or monitor. Moderate Study
- Antifungals, azoles **(fluconazole, isavuconazole)** are predicted to increase the exposure to **naloxegol**. Adjust **naloxegol** dose and monitor adverse effects. Moderate Study
- Antifungals, azoles **(itraconazole, ketoconazole, posaconazole, voriconazole)** are predicted to markedly increase the exposure to **naloxegol**. Avoid. Severe Study
- Antifungals, azoles **(fluconazole, isavuconazole)** are predicted to increase the exposure to **neratinib**. Avoid moderate CYP3A4 inhibitors or adjust dose and monitor for gastrointestinal adverse effects—consult product literature. Severe Study → Also see TABLE 1 p. 1053

Antifungals, azoles (continued)

- Antifungals, azoles **(itraconazole, ketoconazole, posaconazole, voriconazole)** are predicted to increase the exposure to **neratinib**. Avoid or adjust dose with potent CYP3A4 inhibitors—consult product literature. [Severe] Study → Also see TABLE 1 p. 1053
- Neurokinin-1 receptor antagonists **(aprepitant)** are predicted to increase the exposure to **isavuconazole**. [Moderate] Theoretical
- Neurokinin-1 receptor antagonists **(netupitant)** are predicted to decrease the exposure to **isavuconazole**. [Moderate] Theoretical
- **Fluconazole** is predicted to increase the exposure to neurokinin-1 receptor antagonists **(aprepitant)**. [Moderate] Theoretical
- Antifungals, azoles **(itraconazole, ketoconazole, posaconazole, voriconazole)** are predicted to markedly increase the exposure to neurokinin-1 receptor antagonists **(aprepitant)**. [Moderate] Study
- Antifungals, azoles **(itraconazole, ketoconazole, posaconazole, voriconazole)** are predicted to increase the exposure to neurokinin-1 receptor antagonists **(fosaprepitant)**. [Moderate] Theoretical
- Antifungals, azoles **(itraconazole, ketoconazole, posaconazole, voriconazole)** are predicted to increase the exposure to neurokinin-1 receptor antagonists **(netupitant)**. [Moderate] Study
- Antifungals, azoles **(fluconazole, isavuconazole)** are predicted to increase the exposure to **nilotinib**. [Moderate] Study → Also see TABLE 7 p. 1055
- Antifungals, azoles **(itraconazole, ketoconazole, posaconazole, voriconazole)** are predicted to increase the exposure to **nilotinib**. Avoid. [Severe] Study → Also see TABLE 7 p. 1055
- Antifungals, azoles **(itraconazole, ketoconazole)** are predicted to increase the exposure to **nintedanib**. [Moderate] Study
- **Voriconazole** is predicted to increase the exposure to **nintedanib**. [Moderate] Theoretical
- **Nirmatrelvir** boosted with ritonavir is predicted to increase the concentration of **isavuconazole**. [Severe] Theoretical
- **Nirmatrelvir** boosted with ritonavir increases the exposure to **itraconazole**. [Severe] Study
- **Nirmatrelvir** boosted with ritonavir is predicted to increase the concentration of **ketoconazole**. Adjust dose. [Moderate] Theoretical
- **Nirmatrelvir** boosted with ritonavir is predicted to decrease the concentration of **voriconazole**. Avoid. [Severe] Theoretical
- Antifungals, azoles **(itraconazole, ketoconazole, posaconazole, voriconazole)** are predicted to increase the exposure to **nitisinone**. Adjust dose. [Moderate] Theoretical
- NNRTIs **(efavirenz)** slightly decrease the exposure to **itraconazole**. Avoid and for 14 days after stopping **efavirenz**. [Moderate] Study
- NNRTIs **(efavirenz)** moderately decrease the exposure to **ketoconazole**. [Severe] Study
- NNRTIs **(efavirenz)** slightly decrease the exposure to **posaconazole**. Avoid. [Moderate] Study
- NNRTIs **(efavirenz)** moderately decrease the exposure to **voriconazole** and **voriconazole** slightly increases the exposure to NNRTIs **(efavirenz)**. Adjust dose. [Severe] Study → Also see TABLE 7 p. 1055
- NNRTIs **(efavirenz, etravirine, nevirapine)** are predicted to decrease the exposure to **isavuconazole**. Avoid. [Severe] Theoretical
- NNRTIs **(nevirapine)** moderately decrease the exposure to **itraconazole**. Avoid and for 14 days after stopping **nevirapine**. [Moderate] Study → Also see TABLE 1 p. 1053
- NNRTIs **(nevirapine)** moderately decrease the exposure to **ketoconazole**. Avoid. [Severe] Study
- NNRTIs **(nevirapine)** are predicted to decrease the exposure to **voriconazole** and **voriconazole** increases the exposure to NNRTIs **(nevirapine)**. Monitor and adjust dose. [Severe] Theoretical → Also see TABLE 1 p. 1053
- **Fluconazole** slightly to moderately increases the exposure to NNRTIs **(nevirapine)**. [Moderate] Study → Also see TABLE 1 p. 1053
- **Fluconazole** slightly increases the exposure to NRTIs **(zidovudine)**. [Moderate] Study → Also see TABLE 1 p. 1053
- **Fluconazole** moderately increases the exposure to NSAIDs **(celecoxib)**. Adjust **celecoxib** dose. [Moderate] Study
- **Voriconazole** slightly increases the exposure to NSAIDs **(diclofenac)**. Monitor and adjust dose. [Moderate] Study
- **Voriconazole** moderately increases the exposure to NSAIDs **(ibuprofen)**. Adjust dose. [Moderate] Study
- **Fluconazole** increases the exposure to NSAIDs **(parecoxib)**. Monitor and adjust dose. [Moderate] Study
- Antifungals, azoles **(fluconazole, isavuconazole)** are predicted to increase the exposure to **olaparib**. Avoid or adjust dose with moderate CYP3A4 inhibitors—consult product literature. [Moderate] Theoretical
- Antifungals, azoles **(itraconazole, ketoconazole, posaconazole, voriconazole)** are predicted to increase the exposure to **olaparib**. Avoid or adjust dose with potent CYP3A4 inhibitors—consult product literature. [Moderate] Study
- Antifungals, azoles **(fluconazole, isavuconazole)** are predicted to increase the exposure to **omaveloxolone**. Avoid or adjust **omaveloxolone** dose, p. 755. [Moderate] Study
- Antifungals, azoles **(itraconazole, ketoconazole, posaconazole, voriconazole)** are predicted to increase the exposure to **omaveloxolone**. Avoid or adjust **omaveloxolone** dose, p. 755. [Severe] Study
- **Miconazole** is predicted to increase the exposure to opioids **(alfentanil)**. Use with caution and adjust dose. [Moderate] Theoretical
- Antifungals, azoles **(fluconazole, isavuconazole)** are predicted to increase the exposure to opioids **(alfentanil, buprenorphine, fentanyl, oxycodone)**. Monitor and adjust dose. [Moderate] Study
- Antifungals, azoles **(itraconazole, ketoconazole, posaconazole, voriconazole)** are predicted to increase the exposure to opioids **(alfentanil, buprenorphine, fentanyl, oxycodone)**. Monitor and adjust dose. [Severe] Study
- Antifungals, azoles **(itraconazole, ketoconazole, voriconazole)** are predicted to increase the exposure to opioids **(methadone)**. Adjust dose. [Severe] Theoretical → Also see TABLE 7 p. 1055
- Antifungals, azoles **(fluconazole, isavuconazole)** are predicted to increase the exposure to opioids **(methadone, sufentanil)**. [Moderate] Theoretical → Also see TABLE 7 p. 1055
- Antifungals, azoles **(itraconazole, ketoconazole, posaconazole, voriconazole)** are predicted to increase the exposure to opioids **(sufentanil)**. [Moderate] Study
- Antifungals, azoles **(itraconazole, ketoconazole, posaconazole, voriconazole)** are predicted to increase the exposure to **osilodrostat**. [Moderate] Theoretical → Also see TABLE 7 p. 1055
- Antifungals, azoles **(itraconazole, ketoconazole, posaconazole, voriconazole)** are predicted to increase the exposure to **ospemifene**. Avoid in poor CYP2C9 metabolisers. [Moderate] Study
- **Fluconazole** increases the exposure to **ospemifene**. Use with caution or avoid. [Moderate] Study
- Antifungals, azoles **(itraconazole, ketoconazole, posaconazole, voriconazole)** are predicted to increase the exposure to **oxybutynin**. [Mild] Study
- Antifungals, azoles **(itraconazole, ketoconazole, posaconazole, voriconazole)** are predicted to increase the exposure to **palbociclib**. Avoid or adjust dose—consult product literature. [Severe] Study
- Antifungals, azoles **(itraconazole, ketoconazole, posaconazole, voriconazole)** are predicted to increase the exposure to **panobinostat**. Adjust dose—consult product literature; in hepatic impairment avoid. [Moderate] Study → Also see TABLE 7 p. 1055
- Antifungals, azoles **(fluconazole, isavuconazole)** are predicted to increase the exposure to **pazopanib**. [Moderate] Study → Also see TABLE 7 p. 1055
- Antifungals, azoles **(itraconazole, ketoconazole, posaconazole, voriconazole)** are predicted to increase the exposure to **pazopanib**. Avoid or adjust dose—consult product literature. [Moderate] Study → Also see TABLE 7 p. 1055
- Antifungals, azoles **(fluconazole, isavuconazole)** are predicted to increase the exposure to **pemigatinib**. [Severe] Study
- Antifungals, azoles **(itraconazole, ketoconazole, posaconazole, voriconazole)** are predicted to increase the exposure to **pemigatinib**. Avoid or adjust dose—consult product literature. [Severe] Study
- Penicillins **(flucloxacillin)** (particularly high-dose) might greatly decrease the concentration of **isavuconazole**. [Moderate] Anecdotal

- Penicillins **(flucloxacillin)** (particularly high-dose) might greatly decrease the concentration of **posaconazole**. Moderate Study
- Penicillins **(flucloxacillin)** (particularly high-dose) might greatly decrease the concentration of **voriconazole**. Avoid or monitor. Moderate Study
- **Miconazole** greatly increases the anticoagulant effect of **phenindione**. Severe Theoretical
- Antifungals, azoles **(fluconazole, isavuconazole)** are predicted to increase the exposure to phosphodiesterase type-5 inhibitors **(avanafil)**. Adjust **avanafil** dose. Moderate Theoretical
- Antifungals, azoles **(itraconazole, ketoconazole, posaconazole, voriconazole)** are predicted to increase the exposure to phosphodiesterase type-5 inhibitors **(avanafil, vardenafil)**. Avoid. Severe Study → Also see **TABLE 7** p. 1055
- **Miconazole** is predicted to increase the exposure to phosphodiesterase type-5 inhibitors **(sildenafil)**. Use with caution and adjust dose. Severe Theoretical
- Antifungals, azoles **(fluconazole, isavuconazole)** are predicted to increase the exposure to phosphodiesterase type-5 inhibitors **(sildenafil)**. Monitor or adjust **sildenafil** dose with moderate CYP3A4 inhibitors, p. 139. Moderate Study
- Antifungals, azoles **(itraconazole, ketoconazole, posaconazole, voriconazole)** are predicted to increase the exposure to phosphodiesterase type-5 inhibitors **(sildenafil)**. Avoid potent CYP3A4 inhibitors or adjust **sildenafil** dose, p. 139. Severe Study
- Antifungals, azoles **(fluconazole, isavuconazole)** are predicted to increase the exposure to phosphodiesterase type-5 inhibitors **(tadalafil)**. Severe Theoretical
- Antifungals, azoles **(itraconazole, ketoconazole, posaconazole, voriconazole)** are predicted to increase the exposure to phosphodiesterase type-5 inhibitors **(tadalafil)**. Use with caution or avoid. Severe Study
- Antifungals, azoles **(fluconazole, isavuconazole)** are predicted to increase the exposure to phosphodiesterase type-5 inhibitors **(vardenafil)**. Adjust dose. Severe Theoretical → Also see **TABLE 7** p. 1055
- Antifungals, azoles **(fluconazole, isavuconazole)** are predicted to increase the exposure to **pimozide**. Avoid. Severe Theoretical → Also see **TABLE 7** p. 1055
- Antifungals, azoles **(itraconazole, ketoconazole, posaconazole, voriconazole)** are predicted to increase the exposure to **pimozide**. Avoid. Severe Study → Also see **TABLE 7** p. 1055
- **Miconazole** is predicted to increase the exposure to **pimozide**. Avoid. Moderate Theoretical
- **Pioglitazone** potentially decreases the exposure to **isavuconazole**. Use with caution or avoid. Moderate Theoretical
- Antifungals, azoles **(fluconazole, isavuconazole)** are predicted to increase the exposure to **ponatinib**. Moderate Study
- Antifungals, azoles **(itraconazole, ketoconazole, posaconazole, voriconazole)** are predicted to slightly increase the exposure to **ponatinib**. Monitor and adjust dose—consult product literature. Moderate Study
- Antifungals, azoles **(fluconazole, isavuconazole)** are predicted to increase the exposure to **pralsetinib**. Moderate Theoretical
- Antifungals, azoles **(itraconazole, ketoconazole, posaconazole, voriconazole)** are predicted to increase the exposure to **pralsetinib**. Avoid or adjust dose with potent CYP3A4 inhibitors—consult product literature. Moderate Study
- Antifungals, azoles **(itraconazole, ketoconazole, posaconazole, voriconazole)** are predicted to moderately increase the exposure to **praziquantel**. Mild Study
- Antifungals, azoles **(itraconazole, ketoconazole, posaconazole, voriconazole)** given with carbimazole are predicted to increase the exposure to **propiverine**. Adjust starting dose. Moderate Theoretical
- **Proton pump inhibitors** decrease the absorption of **itraconazole**. Administer itraconazole capsules with an acidic beverage. Moderate Study
- **Proton pump inhibitors** decrease the absorption of **ketoconazole**. Administer ketoconazole with an acidic beverage. Moderate Study
- **Proton pump inhibitors** decrease the absorption of **posaconazole** oral suspension. Avoid. Moderate Study
- **Voriconazole** increases the exposure to proton pump inhibitors **(esomeprazole, omeprazole)**. Adjust dose. Moderate Study
- Antifungals, azoles **(itraconazole, ketoconazole, posaconazole, voriconazole)** are predicted to increase the exposure to **quizartinib**. Adjust dose—consult product literature. Severe Study → Also see **TABLE 7** p. 1055
- Antifungals, azoles **(fluconazole, isavuconazole)** are predicted to increase the exposure to **ranolazine**. Severe Study → Also see **TABLE 7** p. 1055
- Antifungals, azoles **(itraconazole, ketoconazole, posaconazole, voriconazole)** are predicted to increase the exposure to **ranolazine**. Avoid. Severe Study → Also see **TABLE 7** p. 1055
- Antifungals, azoles **(itraconazole, ketoconazole, posaconazole, voriconazole)** are predicted to increase the exposure to **reboxetine**. Avoid. Moderate Study
- **Miconazole** is predicted to increase the concentration of **reboxetine**. Use with caution and adjust dose. Moderate Theoretical
- Antifungals, azoles **(fluconazole, isavuconazole)** are predicted to increase the exposure to **regorafenib**. Moderate Study
- Antifungals, azoles **(itraconazole, ketoconazole, posaconazole, voriconazole)** are predicted to increase the exposure to **regorafenib**. Avoid. Moderate Study
- Antifungals, azoles **(itraconazole, ketoconazole)** are predicted to increase the exposure to **relugolix**. Avoid or take relugolix first and separate administration by at least 6 hours. Moderate Study
- Antifungals, azoles **(fluconazole, itraconazole, ketoconazole, miconazole, posaconazole, voriconazole)** are predicted to increase the exposure to retinoids **(alitretinoin)**. Adjust **alitretinoin** dose. Moderate Theoretical
- **Posaconazole** is predicted to increase the risk of tretinoin toxicity when given with retinoids **(tretinoin)**. Monitor and adjust dose. Severe Theoretical
- Antifungals, azoles **(fluconazole, ketoconazole, voriconazole)** are predicted to increase the risk of tretinoin toxicity when given with retinoids **(tretinoin)**. Moderate Study
- Antifungals, azoles **(fluconazole, isavuconazole)** are predicted to increase the exposure to **ribociclib**. Moderate Study → Also see **TABLE 7** p. 1055
- Antifungals, azoles **(itraconazole, ketoconazole, posaconazole, voriconazole)** are predicted to increase the exposure to **ribociclib**. Avoid or adjust dose—consult product literature. Moderate Study → Also see **TABLE 7** p. 1055
- Rifamycins **(rifabutin)** are predicted to decrease the exposure to **isavuconazole**. Avoid. Severe Theoretical
- Rifamycins **(rifabutin)** decrease the concentration of **voriconazole** and **voriconazole** increases the concentration of rifamycins **(rifabutin)**. Avoid or adjust **voriconazole** dose, p. 468. Severe Study
- Rifamycins **(rifampicin)** slightly decrease the exposure to **fluconazole**. Adjust dose. Moderate Study
- Rifamycins **(rifampicin)** are predicted to decrease the exposure to **isavuconazole**. Avoid. Severe Study
- Rifamycins **(rifampicin)** markedly decrease the exposure to **itraconazole**. Avoid and for 14 days after stopping **rifampicin**. Moderate Study
- Rifamycins **(rifampicin)** markedly decrease the exposure to **ketoconazole** and **ketoconazole** potentially decreases the exposure to rifamycins **(rifampicin)**. Avoid. Moderate Study
- Rifamycins **(rifampicin)** are predicted to decrease the exposure to **posaconazole**. Avoid. Moderate Anecdotal
- Rifamycins **(rifampicin)** very markedly decrease the exposure to **voriconazole**. Avoid. Moderate Study
- **Fluconazole** increases the risk of uveitis when given with rifamycins **(rifabutin)**. Adjust dose. Severe Study
- **Ketoconazole** is predicted to increase the concentration of rifamycins **(rifabutin)** and rifamycins **(rifabutin)** are predicted to decrease the concentration of **ketoconazole**. Avoid. Severe Theoretical
- **Miconazole** is predicted to increase the concentration of rifamycins **(rifabutin)**. Use with caution and adjust dose. Moderate Theoretical
- Antifungals, azoles **(itraconazole, posaconazole)** increase the concentration of rifamycins **(rifabutin)** and rifamycins **(rifabutin)** decrease the concentration of antifungals, azoles **(itraconazole, posaconazole)**. Avoid. Severe Study

A1

Interactions | **Appendix 1**

Antifungals, azoles (continued)

- Antifungals, azoles **(fluconazole, isavuconazole)** are predicted to increase the exposure to **rimegepant**. Avoid another dose of rimegepant within 48 hours of concurrent use. [Moderate] Study
- Antifungals, azoles **(itraconazole, ketoconazole, posaconazole, voriconazole)** are predicted to increase the exposure to **rimegepant**. Avoid. [Moderate] Study
- Antifungals, azoles **(itraconazole, posaconazole)** are predicted to increase the exposure to **riociguat**. Adjust **riociguat** dose and monitor blood pressure. [Moderate] Theoretical
- **Ketoconazole** moderately increases the exposure to **riociguat**. Adjust **riociguat** dose and monitor blood pressure. [Moderate] Study
- Antifungals, azoles **(itraconazole, ketoconazole, posaconazole, voriconazole)** are predicted to increase the exposure to **ripretinib**. [Moderate] Theoretical
- Antifungals, azoles **(itraconazole, ketoconazole, posaconazole, voriconazole)** are predicted to increase the exposure to **ruxolitinib**. Adjust dose depending on indication and monitor adverse effects—consult product literature. [Moderate] Study
- **Fluconazole** moderately increases the exposure to **ruxolitinib**. Avoid or adjust dose and monitor adverse effects—consult product literature. [Moderate] Study
- **Isavuconazole** is predicted to increase the exposure to **ruxolitinib**. [Moderate] Study
- **Ketoconazole** is predicted to increase the exposure to the active component of **sacituzumab govitecan**. [Severe] Theoretical
- **Fluconazole** moderately increases the exposure to **seladelpar**. [Moderate] Study
- **Fluconazole** is predicted to increase the exposure to **selexipag**. [Unknown] Theoretical
- Antifungals, azoles **(fluconazole, isavuconazole)** are predicted to increase the exposure to **selpercatinib**. [Moderate] Study → Also see **TABLE 7** p. 1055
- Antifungals, azoles **(itraconazole, ketoconazole, posaconazole, voriconazole)** are predicted to increase the exposure to **selpercatinib**. Adjust dose—consult product literature. [Moderate] Study → Also see **TABLE 7** p. 1055
- Antifungals, azoles **(fluconazole, isavuconazole, itraconazole, ketoconazole, posaconazole, voriconazole)** are predicted to increase the exposure to **selumetinib**. Avoid or adjust dose—consult product literature. [Severe] Study
- Antifungals, azoles **(fluconazole, isavuconazole, miconazole)** are predicted to increase the exposure to **siponimod**. Avoid depending on other drugs taken—consult product literature. [Severe] Study
- Antifungals, azoles **(itraconazole, ketoconazole, posaconazole, voriconazole)** are predicted to increase the exposure to **siponimod**. Avoid depending on other drugs taken—consult product literature. [Severe] Theoretical
- Antifungals, azoles **(fluconazole, isavuconazole)** increase the concentration of **sirolimus**. Monitor and adjust dose. [Moderate] Study
- Antifungals, azoles **(itraconazole, ketoconazole, posaconazole, voriconazole)** are predicted to increase the concentration of **sirolimus**. Avoid or monitor and adjust dose. [Severe] Study
- **Miconazole** is predicted to increase the concentration of **sirolimus**. Monitor and adjust dose. [Moderate] Study
- Antifungals, azoles **(itraconazole, ketoconazole, posaconazole, voriconazole)** are predicted to increase the exposure to **SNRIs (venlafaxine)**. [Moderate] Study
- Oral **sodium bicarbonate** decreases the absorption of oral **ketoconazole**. [Moderate] Study
- **Sodium zirconium cyclosilicate** is predicted to decrease the exposure to **antifungals, azoles**. Separate administration by at least 2 hours. [Moderate] Theoretical
- Antifungals, azoles **(itraconazole, ketoconazole, posaconazole, voriconazole)** are predicted to increase the exposure to **solifenacin**. Adjust solifenacin p. 604 or tamsulosin with solifenacin dose; avoid in hepatic and renal impairment. [Severe] Study
- **Sotorasib** is predicted to decrease the exposure to **isavuconazole**. Avoid. [Severe] Theoretical
- Antifungals, azoles **(fluconazole, isavuconazole)** are predicted to increase the exposure to **sparsentan**. [Moderate] Study
- Antifungals, azoles **(itraconazole, ketoconazole, posaconazole, voriconazole)** are predicted to increase the exposure to **sparsentan**. Avoid. [Severe] Study
- **Voriconazole** is predicted to increase the exposure to **SSRIs (citalopram)**. [Severe] Theoretical → Also see **TABLE 7** p. 1055
- Antifungals, azoles **(fluconazole, isavuconazole)** are predicted to increase the exposure to **SSRIs (dapoxetine)**. Adjust **dapoxetine** dose with moderate CYP3A4 inhibitors. [Moderate] Theoretical
- Antifungals, azoles **(itraconazole, ketoconazole, posaconazole, voriconazole)** are predicted to moderately increase the exposure to **SSRIs (dapoxetine)**. Avoid potent CYP3A4 inhibitors or adjust **dapoxetine** dose. [Severe] Study
- Antifungals, azoles **(fluconazole, voriconazole)** are predicted to increase the exposure to **SSRIs (escitalopram)**. Use with caution and adjust dose. [Severe] Study → Also see **TABLE 7** p. 1055
- Antifungals, azoles **(fluconazole, isavuconazole)** are predicted to increase the exposure to **SSRIs (sertraline)**. [Moderate] Theoretical
- Antifungals, azoles **(itraconazole, ketoconazole, posaconazole, voriconazole)** are predicted to increase the exposure to **SSRIs (sertraline)**. Avoid. [Moderate] Theoretical
- **St John's wort** is predicted to decrease the exposure to **isavuconazole**. Avoid. [Severe] Theoretical
- **St John's wort** moderately decreases the exposure to **voriconazole**. Avoid. [Moderate] Study
- **Isavuconazole** slightly increases the exposure to **statins (atorvastatin)**. [Moderate] Study
- **Miconazole** (including the oral gel) might increase the exposure to **statins (atorvastatin)**. [Moderate] Theoretical
- Antifungals, azoles **(itraconazole, ketoconazole, posaconazole, voriconazole)** are predicted to increase the exposure to **statins (atorvastatin)**. Avoid or adjust dose and monitor rhabdomyolysis. [Severe] Study → Also see **TABLE 1** p. 1053
- **Fluconazole** is predicted to increase the exposure to **statins (atorvastatin, simvastatin)**. Monitor and adjust dose. [Severe] Anecdotal → Also see **TABLE 1** p. 1053
- Antifungals, azoles **(fluconazole, miconazole)** are predicted to increase the exposure to **statins (fluvastatin)**. [Moderate] Study → Also see **TABLE 1** p. 1053
- **Isavuconazole** is predicted to increase the exposure to **statins (fluvastatin, rosuvastatin)**. [Moderate] Theoretical
- **Isavuconazole** is predicted to increase the exposure to **statins (simvastatin)**. Monitor and adjust dose. [Severe] Theoretical
- **Miconazole** (including the oral gel) is predicted to increase the exposure to **statins (simvastatin)**. Avoid. [Severe] Anecdotal
- Antifungals, azoles **(itraconazole, ketoconazole, posaconazole, voriconazole)** are predicted to increase the exposure to **statins (simvastatin)**. Avoid. [Severe] Study → Also see **TABLE 1** p. 1053
- **Isavuconazole** is predicted to increase the exposure to **sulfasalazine**. [Moderate] Theoretical
- **Miconazole** is predicted to increase the exposure to **sulfonylureas (glibenclamide, tolbutamide)**. [Moderate] Anecdotal
- **Miconazole** is predicted to increase the exposure to **sulfonylureas (gliclazide)**. Avoid. [Moderate] Anecdotal
- **Miconazole** is predicted to increase the exposure to **sulfonylureas (glimepiride)**. [Moderate] Theoretical
- **Miconazole** is predicted to increase the exposure to **sulfonylureas (glipizide)**. Avoid. [Moderate] Theoretical
- **Voriconazole** is predicted to increase the concentration of **sulfonylureas**. Use with caution and adjust dose. [Moderate] Study
- Antifungals, azoles **(fluconazole, isavuconazole)** are predicted to increase the exposure to **sunitinib**. [Moderate] Study → Also see **TABLE 7** p. 1055
- Antifungals, azoles **(itraconazole, ketoconazole, posaconazole, voriconazole)** are predicted to increase the exposure to **sunitinib**. Avoid or adjust dose—consult product literature. [Moderate] Study → Also see **TABLE 7** p. 1055
- Antifungals, azoles **(itraconazole, ketoconazole, posaconazole, voriconazole)** are predicted to increase the concentration of **tacrolimus**. Avoid. If concurrent use is unavoidable—consult product literature. [Severe] Study
- **Fluconazole** increases the concentration of **tacrolimus**. Monitor and adjust dose. [Severe] Study
- **Isavuconazole** moderately increases the exposure to **tacrolimus**. Monitor and adjust dose. [Severe] Study

- **Miconazole** is predicted to increase the concentration of tacrolimus. Monitor and adjust dose. [Severe] Theoretical
- Antifungals, azoles **(itraconazole, ketoconazole)** are predicted to slightly increase the exposure to **talazoparib**. Avoid or adjust dose—consult product literature. [Severe] Study
- Antifungals, azoles **(fluconazole, isavuconazole)** are predicted to increase the exposure to taxanes **(cabazitaxel)**. [Moderate] Theoretical
- Antifungals, azoles **(itraconazole, ketoconazole, posaconazole, voriconazole)** are predicted to increase the exposure to taxanes **(cabazitaxel)**. Avoid or adjust dose—consult product literature. [Severe] Study
- **Miconazole** is predicted to increase the concentration of taxanes **(docetaxel)**. Use with caution and adjust dose. [Moderate] Theoretical
- Antifungals, azoles **(fluconazole, isavuconazole)** are predicted to increase the exposure to taxanes **(docetaxel)**. [Severe] Study
- Antifungals, azoles **(itraconazole, ketoconazole, posaconazole, voriconazole)** are predicted to increase the exposure to taxanes **(docetaxel)**. Avoid or adjust dose. [Severe] Study
- Antifungals, azoles **(fluconazole, isavuconazole, itraconazole, ketoconazole, posaconazole, voriconazole)** are predicted to increase the exposure to taxanes **(paclitaxel)**. [Moderate] Anecdotal
- Antifungals, azoles **(fluconazole, isavuconazole)** are predicted to increase the concentration of **temsirolimus**. Use with caution or avoid. [Moderate] Theoretical
- Antifungals, azoles **(itraconazole, ketoconazole, posaconazole, voriconazole)** are predicted to increase the concentration of **temsirolimus**. Avoid. [Severe] Theoretical
- Antifungals, azoles **(fluconazole, isavuconazole)** are predicted to increase the exposure to **tezacaftor**. Adjust dose with moderate CYP3A4 inhibitors, see tezacaftor with ivacaftor p. 223, ivacaftor with tezacaftor and elexacaftor p. 220, and deutivacaftor with tezacaftor and vanzacaftor p. 218. [Severe] Study
- Antifungals, azoles **(itraconazole, ketoconazole, posaconazole, voriconazole)** are predicted to increase the exposure to **tezacaftor**. Adjust dose with potent CYP3A4 inhibitors, see tezacaftor with ivacaftor p. 223, ivacaftor with tezacaftor and elexacaftor p. 220, and deutivacaftor with tezacaftor and vanzacaftor p. 218. [Severe] Study
- **Isavuconazole** is predicted to increase the exposure to thrombin inhibitors **(dabigatran)**. Monitor and adjust dose. [Moderate] Study
- Antifungals, azoles **(fluconazole, posaconazole)** are predicted to increase the exposure to thrombin inhibitors **(dabigatran)**. [Severe] Study
- Antifungals, azoles **(itraconazole, ketoconazole)** are predicted to increase the exposure to thrombin inhibitors **(dabigatran)**. Avoid. [Severe] Study
- Antifungals, azoles **(itraconazole, ketoconazole, posaconazole, voriconazole)** are predicted to markedly increase the exposure to **ticagrelor**. Avoid. [Severe] Study
- Antifungals, azoles **(itraconazole, ketoconazole)** might increase the exposure to **tigecycline**. [Mild] Anecdotal → Also see TABLE 1 p. 1053
- Antifungals, azoles **(itraconazole, ketoconazole, posaconazole, voriconazole)** are predicted to increase the exposure to the cytotoxic component of **tisotumab vedotin**. [Severe] Theoretical
- Antifungals, azoles **(itraconazole, ketoconazole, posaconazole, voriconazole)** are predicted to increase the exposure to **tofacitinib**. Adjust **tofacitinib** dose, p. 803. [Moderate] Study
- **Fluconazole** increases the exposure to **tofacitinib**. Adjust **tofacitinib** dose, p. 803. [Moderate] Study
- **Isavuconazole** given with a potent CYP2C19 inhibitor is predicted to increase the exposure to **tofacitinib**. Adjust **tofacitinib** dose, p. 803. [Moderate] Study
- Antifungals, azoles **(itraconazole, ketoconazole, posaconazole, voriconazole)** are predicted to increase the exposure to **tolterodine**. Avoid. [Severe] Study → Also see TABLE 7 p. 1055
- Antifungals, azoles **(fluconazole, isavuconazole)** are predicted to increase the exposure to **tolvaptan**. Manufacturer advises caution or adjust **tolvaptan** dose with moderate CYP3A4 inhibitors. [Moderate] Study
- Antifungals, azoles **(itraconazole, ketoconazole, posaconazole, voriconazole)** are predicted to increase the exposure to **tolvaptan**. Manufacturer advises caution or adjust **tolvaptan** dose with potent CYP3A4 inhibitors. [Severe] Study
- Antifungals, azoles **(itraconazole, ketoconazole)** are predicted to increase the exposure to **topotecan**. [Severe] Study
- **Isavuconazole** is predicted to increase the exposure to **topotecan**. [Moderate] Theoretical
- Antifungals, azoles **(itraconazole, ketoconazole, posaconazole, voriconazole)** are predicted to increase the exposure to **toremifene**. [Moderate] Theoretical → Also see TABLE 7 p. 1055
- Antifungals, azoles **(itraconazole, ketoconazole, posaconazole, voriconazole)** are predicted to increase the exposure to **trabectedin**. Avoid or adjust dose. [Severe] Theoretical → Also see TABLE 1 p. 1053
- Antifungals, azoles **(itraconazole, ketoconazole)** are predicted to increase the concentration of **trametinib**. [Moderate] Theoretical
- Antifungals, azoles **(fluconazole, isavuconazole)** are predicted to increase the exposure to **trazodone**. [Moderate] Theoretical
- Antifungals, azoles **(itraconazole, ketoconazole, posaconazole, voriconazole)** are predicted to moderately increase the exposure to **trazodone**. Avoid or adjust dose. [Moderate] Study
- Antifungals, azoles **(itraconazole, ketoconazole, posaconazole, voriconazole)** increase the exposure to triptans **(almotriptan)**. [Mild] Study
- Antifungals, azoles **(itraconazole, ketoconazole, posaconazole, voriconazole)** are predicted to markedly increase the exposure to triptans **(eletriptan)**. Avoid. [Severe] Study
- **Tucatinib** is predicted to increase the exposure to **isavuconazole**. Avoid or monitor adverse effects. [Severe] Study
- Antifungals, azoles **(fluconazole, isavuconazole, posaconazole)** are predicted to increase the exposure to **ulipristal**. Avoid when used for uterine fibroids. [Moderate] Study
- Antifungals, azoles **(itraconazole, ketoconazole, voriconazole)** are predicted to increase the exposure to **ulipristal**. Avoid when used for uterine fibroids. [Severe] Study
- Antifungals, azoles **(itraconazole, ketoconazole, posaconazole, voriconazole)** are predicted to increase the exposure to **upadacitinib**. Manufacturer advises caution or avoid, or adjust **upadacitinib** dose depending on indication, p. 927. [Severe] Study
- Antifungals, azoles **(fluconazole, isavuconazole, itraconazole, ketoconazole, posaconazole, voriconazole)** are predicted to increase the exposure to **vanzacaftor**. Adjust dose, see deutivacaftor with tezacaftor and vanzacaftor p. 218. [Severe] Study
- Antifungals, azoles **(fluconazole, isavuconazole, itraconazole, ketoconazole, posaconazole, voriconazole)** are predicted to increase the exposure to **vemurafenib**. [Severe] Theoretical → Also see TABLE 7 p. 1055
- Antifungals, azoles **(fluconazole, isavuconazole, itraconazole, ketoconazole, posaconazole, voriconazole)** are predicted to increase the exposure to **venetoclax**. Avoid or adjust dose—consult product literature. [Severe] Study
- Antifungals, azoles **(fluconazole, isavuconazole, itraconazole, ketoconazole, posaconazole, voriconazole)** are predicted to increase the exposure to **vinca alkaloids**. [Severe] Theoretical
- **Miconazole** is predicted to increase the concentration of **vinca alkaloids**. Use with caution and adjust dose. [Moderate] Theoretical
- Antifungals, azoles **(clotrimazole, ketoconazole)** are predicted to decrease the exposure to vitamin D substances **(colecalciferol)**. [Moderate] Theoretical
- Antifungals, azoles **(itraconazole, ketoconazole, posaconazole, voriconazole)** are predicted to increase the exposure to vitamin D substances **(paricalcitol)**. [Moderate] Study
- Antifungals, azoles **(fluconazole, isavuconazole)** are predicted to increase the exposure to **voclosporin**. Adjust **voclosporin** dose. [Severe] Study → Also see TABLE 7 p. 1055
- Antifungals, azoles **(itraconazole, ketoconazole, posaconazole, voriconazole)** are predicted to increase the exposure to **voclosporin**. Avoid. [Severe] Study → Also see TABLE 7 p. 1055
- Antifungals, azoles **(fluconazole, isavuconazole)** are predicted to increase the exposure to **zanubrutinib**. Avoid or adjust dose with moderate CYP3A4 inhibitors—consult product literature. [Severe] Study
- Antifungals, azoles **(itraconazole, ketoconazole, posaconazole, voriconazole)** are predicted to increase the exposure to

Antifungals, azoles (continued)
zanubrutinib. Avoid or adjust dose with potent CYP3A4 inhibitors—consult product literature. Moderate Study
- Antifungals, azoles **(fluconazole, isavuconazole)** are predicted to increase the exposure to **zopiclone**. Adjust dose. Moderate Study
- Antifungals, azoles **(itraconazole, ketoconazole, posaconazole, voriconazole)** are predicted to increase the exposure to **zopiclone**. Adjust dose. Moderate Theoretical

Antihistamines, non-sedating → see TABLE 7 p. 1055 (QT-interval prolongation)

acrivastine · azelastine · bilastine · cetirizine · desloratadine · fexofenadine · levocetirizine · loratadine · mizolastine · rupatadine

- Since systemic absorption can follow topical application, the possibility of interactions with topical **azelastine** should be borne in mind.
- Apple juice and orange juice decrease the exposure to **fexofenadine**.

- Oral **antacids** decrease the absorption of oral **fexofenadine**. Separate administration by 2 hours. Mild Study
- Anti-androgens **(apalutamide)** slightly decrease the exposure to **fexofenadine**. Mild Study
- Anti-androgens **(darolutamide)** are predicted to increase the concentration of **fexofenadine**. Moderate Theoretical
- Antiarrhythmics **(amiodarone)** are predicted to increase the exposure to **fexofenadine**. Moderate Study
- Antiarrhythmics **(dronedarone)** are predicted to increase the exposure to **rupatadine**. Avoid. Moderate Study
- Antiarrhythmics **(dronedarone)** are predicted to increase the exposure to antihistamines, non-sedating **(fexofenadine, mizolastine)**. Severe Theoretical
- Antifungals, azoles **(fluconazole, isavuconazole)** are predicted to increase the exposure to **mizolastine**. Severe Theoretical
- Antifungals, azoles **(fluconazole, isavuconazole, itraconazole, ketoconazole, posaconazole, voriconazole)** are predicted to increase the exposure to **rupatadine**. Avoid. Moderate Study
- Antifungals, azoles **(itraconazole, ketoconazole, posaconazole, voriconazole)** are predicted to increase the exposure to **mizolastine**. Avoid. Severe Study
- Antifungals, azoles **(miconazole)** are predicted to increase the exposure to **mizolastine**. Avoid. Moderate Theoretical
- **Belumosudil** is predicted to increase the exposure to **fexofenadine**. Avoid or adjust dose. Moderate Study
- **Berotralstat** is predicted to increase the exposure to **mizolastine**. Severe Theoretical
- **Berotralstat** is predicted to increase the exposure to **rupatadine**. Avoid. Moderate Study
- **Antihistamines, non-sedating** are predicted to decrease the effects of **betahistine**. Moderate Theoretical
- **Bulevirtide** is predicted to increase the exposure to **fexofenadine**. Avoid or monitor. Moderate Theoretical
- Calcium-channel blockers **(diltiazem, verapamil)** are predicted to increase the exposure to **mizolastine**. Severe Theoretical
- Calcium-channel blockers **(diltiazem, verapamil)** are predicted to increase the exposure to **rupatadine**. Avoid. Moderate Study
- **Ceritinib** is predicted to increase the exposure to **fexofenadine**. Moderate Theoretical
- **Ceritinib** is predicted to increase the exposure to **mizolastine**. Avoid. Severe Study
- **Ceritinib** is predicted to increase the exposure to **rupatadine**. Avoid. Moderate Study
- **Ciclosporin** is predicted to increase the exposure to **fexofenadine**. Moderate Theoretical
- **Cobicistat** is predicted to increase the exposure to **fexofenadine**. Moderate Theoretical
- **Cobicistat** is predicted to increase the exposure to **mizolastine**. Avoid. Severe Study
- **Cobicistat** is predicted to increase the exposure to **rupatadine**. Avoid. Moderate Study
- **Crizotinib** is predicted to increase the exposure to **mizolastine**. Severe Theoretical
- **Crizotinib** is predicted to increase the exposure to **rupatadine**. Avoid. Moderate Study
- **Danicopan** is predicted to increase the exposure to **fexofenadine**. Moderate Study
- **Elexacaftor** is predicted to increase the exposure to **fexofenadine**. Moderate Theoretical
- **Eliglustat** is predicted to increase the exposure to **fexofenadine**. Adjust dose. Moderate Study
- **Encorafenib** is predicted to increase the exposure to **fexofenadine**. Mild Study
- **Fedratinib** is predicted to increase the exposure to **mizolastine**. Severe Theoretical
- **Fedratinib** is predicted to increase the exposure to **rupatadine**. Avoid. Moderate Study
- Fibrates **(gemfibrozil)** are predicted to increase the exposure to **fexofenadine**. Moderate Theoretical
- **Glecaprevir** is predicted to increase the exposure to **fexofenadine**. Severe Theoretical
- **Grapefruit** juice slightly decreases the exposure to **bilastine**. Bilastine should be taken 1 hour before or 2 hours after **grapefruit**. Moderate Study
- **Grapefruit** juice increases the exposure to **rupatadine**. Avoid. Moderate Study
- HIV-protease inhibitors **(atazanavir)** boosted with ritonavir are predicted to increase the exposure to **fexofenadine**. Moderate Theoretical
- **HIV-protease inhibitors** are predicted to increase the exposure to **mizolastine**. Avoid. Severe Study
- **HIV-protease inhibitors** are predicted to increase the exposure to **rupatadine**. Avoid. Moderate Study
- **Idelalisib** is predicted to increase the exposure to **mizolastine**. Avoid. Severe Study
- **Idelalisib** is predicted to increase the exposure to **rupatadine**. Avoid. Moderate Study
- **Imatinib** is predicted to increase the exposure to **mizolastine**. Severe Theoretical
- **Imatinib** is predicted to increase the exposure to **rupatadine**. Avoid. Moderate Study
- **Ivosidenib** is predicted to alter the exposure to **fexofenadine**. Moderate Theoretical
- **Lapatinib** is predicted to increase the exposure to **fexofenadine**. Moderate Theoretical
- **Leflunomide** is predicted to increase the exposure to **fexofenadine**. Moderate Study
- **Leniolisib** is predicted to increase the exposure to **fexofenadine**. Avoid. Moderate Theoretical
- **Letermovir** is predicted to increase the concentration of **fexofenadine**. Moderate Theoretical
- **Letermovir** is predicted to increase the exposure to **mizolastine**. Severe Theoretical
- **Letermovir** is predicted to increase the exposure to **rupatadine**. Avoid. Moderate Study
- **Lorlatinib** decreases the exposure to **fexofenadine**. Moderate Study
- Macrolides **(clarithromycin)** are predicted to increase the exposure to **fexofenadine**. Moderate Theoretical
- Macrolides **(clarithromycin)** are predicted to increase the exposure to **mizolastine**. Avoid. Severe Study
- Macrolides **(clarithromycin, erythromycin)** are predicted to increase the exposure to **rupatadine**. Avoid. Moderate Study
- Macrolides **(erythromycin)** are predicted to increase the exposure to **mizolastine**. Severe Theoretical
- **MAOIs, irreversible** are predicted to increase the risk of antimuscarinic adverse effects when given with **antihistamines, non-sedating**. Avoid. Severe Theoretical
- **Mirabegron** is predicted to increase the exposure to **fexofenadine**. Mild Theoretical
- Neurokinin-1 receptor antagonists **(aprepitant, netupitant)** are predicted to increase the exposure to **mizolastine**. Severe Theoretical
- Neurokinin-1 receptor antagonists **(aprepitant, netupitant)** are predicted to increase the exposure to **rupatadine**. Avoid. Moderate Study
- **Nilotinib** is predicted to increase the exposure to **mizolastine**. Severe Theoretical
- **Nilotinib** is predicted to increase the exposure to **rupatadine**. Avoid. Moderate Study
- **Olaparib** might increase the exposure to **fexofenadine**. Moderate Theoretical

- **Osimertinib** is predicted to increase the exposure to **fexofenadine.** Moderate Study
- **Pibrentasvir** with glecaprevir is predicted to increase the exposure to **fexofenadine.** Moderate Study
- **Pitolisant** is predicted to decrease the exposure to **fexofenadine.** Mild Theoretical
- **Ranolazine** is predicted to increase the exposure to **fexofenadine.** Moderate Theoretical
- Rifamycins **(rifampicin)** are predicted to decrease the exposure to **bilastine.** Moderate Theoretical
- Rifamycins **(rifampicin)** increase the clearance of **fexofenadine.** Moderate Study
- **Roxadustat** is predicted to increase the exposure to **fexofenadine.** Monitor adverse effects and adjust dose. Moderate Study
- **Sparsentan** is predicted to increase the exposure to **fexofenadine.** Severe Theoretical
- Taxanes **(cabazitaxel)** are predicted to affect the exposure to **fexofenadine.** Manufacturer advises take 12 hours before or 3 hours after **cabazitaxel.** Moderate Theoretical
- **Teriflunomide** is predicted to increase the exposure to **fexofenadine.** Moderate Study
- **Tucatinib** is predicted to increase the exposure to **mizolastine.** Avoid. Severe Study
- **Tucatinib** is predicted to increase the exposure to **rupatadine.** Avoid. Moderate Study
- **Velpatasvir** is predicted to increase the exposure to **fexofenadine.** Severe Theoretical
- **Vemurafenib** is predicted to increase the exposure to **fexofenadine.** Use with caution and adjust dose. Severe Theoretical
- **Venetoclax** is predicted to increase the exposure to **fexofenadine.** Moderate Theoretical
- **Voclosporin** is predicted to increase the exposure to **fexofenadine.** Mild Theoretical
- **Voxilaprevir** with sofosbuvir and velpatasvir is predicted to increase the exposure to **fexofenadine.** Moderate Study

Antihistamines, sedating → see TABLE 7 p. 1055 (QT-interval prolongation), TABLE 8 p. 1055 (antimuscarinics), TABLE 9 p. 1056 (CNS effects)

alimemazine · antazoline · buclizine · chlorphenamine · cinnarizine · cyclizine · cyproheptadine · doxylamine · hydroxyzine · ketotifen · pizotifen · promethazine

ROUTE-SPECIFIC INFORMATION Since systemic absorption can follow topical application of **ketotifen**, the possibility of interactions should be borne in mind.

- **Hydroxyzine** potentially increases the risk of overheating and dehydration when given with antiepileptics **(zonisamide)**. Avoid in children. Severe Theoretical
- Atypical antipsychotics **(clozapine)** can cause constipation, as can antihistamines, sedating **(chlorphenamine, cyclizine, cyproheptadine, hydroxyzine, promethazine)**; concurrent use might increase the risk of developing intestinal obstruction. Severe Theoretical → Also see TABLE 8 p. 1055 → Also see TABLE 9 p. 1056
- **Antihistamines, sedating** are predicted to decrease the effects of **betahistine** Moderate Theoretical
- **Cyproheptadine** might decrease the efficacy of **fenfluramine**. Severe Theoretical
- **MAOIs, irreversible** are predicted to increase the risk of antimuscarinic adverse effects when given with **antihistamines, sedating**. Avoid. Severe Theoretical
- **Cyproheptadine** decreases the effects of **metyrapone**. Avoid. Moderate Study
- **Antihistamines, sedating** are predicted to decrease the efficacy of **pitolisant** Moderate Theoretical
- **Cyproheptadine** potentially decreases the effects of **SSRIs**. Moderate Anecdotal → Also see TABLE 9 p. 1056

Antimalarials → see TABLE 16 p. 1058 (ototoxicity), TABLE 7 p. 1055 (QT-interval prolongation)

artemether · artenimol · artesunate · atovaquone · chloroquine · lumefantrine · mefloquine · piperaquine · primaquine · proguanil · pyrimethamine · quinine

PHARMACOLOGY **Piperaquine** has a long half-life; there is a potential for drug interactions to occur for up to 3 months after treatment has been stopped.

- **Chloroquine** is predicted to decrease the effects of **agalsidase alfa**. Avoid. Moderate Theoretical
- **Chloroquine** is predicted to decrease the effects of **agalsidase beta**. Avoid. Moderate Theoretical
- Oral **antacids** are predicted to decrease the absorption of oral **chloroquine.** Separate administration by at least 4 hours. Moderate Theoretical
- Oral **antacids** are predicted to decrease the absorption of oral **proguanil.** Separate administration by at least 2 hours. Moderate Study
- Anti-androgens **(apalutamide, enzalutamide)** are predicted to decrease the exposure to **artemether** with lumefantrine. Avoid. Severe Study → Also see TABLE 7 p. 1055
- Anti-androgens **(apalutamide, enzalutamide)** are predicted to decrease the concentration of **piperaquine.** Avoid. Moderate Theoretical
- Antiarrhythmics **(dronedarone)** are predicted to increase the concentration of **piperaquine.** Severe Study
- Antiepileptics **(carbamazepine, fosphenytoin, phenobarbital, phenytoin, primidone)** are predicted to decrease the exposure to **artemether** with lumefantrine. Avoid. Severe Study
- Antiepileptics **(carbamazepine, fosphenytoin, phenobarbital, phenytoin, primidone)** are predicted to decrease the concentration of **piperaquine.** Avoid. Moderate Theoretical
- Antiepileptics **(carbamazepine, fosphenytoin, phenytoin)** might decrease the exposure to the active metabolite of **artesunate.** Avoid. Severe Study
- Antiepileptics **(carbamazepine, phenobarbital, primidone)** potentially increase the risk of toxicity when given with **quinine.** Unknown Study
- **Pyrimethamine** increases the risk of haematological toxicity when given with antiepileptics **(fosphenytoin, phenytoin)**. Severe Study
- **Pyrimethamine** is predicted to increase the risk of haematological toxicity when given with antiepileptics **(phenobarbital, primidone)**. Severe Theoretical
- Antifungals, azoles **(fluconazole, isavuconazole, itraconazole, ketoconazole, posaconazole, voriconazole)** are predicted to increase the concentration of **piperaquine.** Severe Study
- Antifungals, azoles **(fluconazole, itraconazole, posaconazole, voriconazole)** are predicted to increase the exposure to **mefloquine.** Moderate Theoretical
- Antifungals, azoles **(ketoconazole)** increase the exposure to **mefloquine.** Moderate Study
- Antimalarials **(proguanil)** are predicted to increase the risk of adverse effects when given with antimalarials **(pyrimethamine)**. Severe Theoretical
- **Axitinib** might increase the exposure to the active metabolite of **artesunate.** Avoid. Unknown Theoretical
- **Berotralstat** is predicted to increase the concentration of **piperaquine.** Severe Study
- **Mefloquine** is predicted to increase the risk of bradycardia when given with **beta blockers, non-selective**. Severe Theoretical
- **Mefloquine** is predicted to increase the risk of bradycardia when given with **beta blockers, selective**. Severe Theoretical
- Oral calcium compounds **(calcium carbonate)** might decrease the absorption of oral **chloroquine.** Separate administration by at least 4 hours. Moderate Study
- **Mefloquine** is predicted to increase the risk of bradycardia when given with **calcium-channel blockers**. Severe Theoretical
- Calcium-channel blockers **(diltiazem, verapamil)** are predicted to increase the concentration of **piperaquine.** Severe Study
- **Ceritinib** is predicted to increase the concentration of **piperaquine.** Severe Study
- **Cobicistat** is predicted to increase the concentration of **piperaquine.** Severe Study
- **Crizotinib** is predicted to increase the concentration of **piperaquine.** Severe Study
- **Mefloquine** is predicted to increase the risk of bradycardia when given with **digoxin**. Severe Theoretical

A1 Interactions | Appendix 1

Antimalarials (continued)
- **Quinine** increases the concentration of **digoxin**. Monitor and adjust **digoxin** dose, p. 91. Severe Anecdotal
- **Encorafenib** is predicted to decrease the exposure to **artemether** with lumefantrine. Avoid. Severe Study → Also see TABLE 7 p. 1055
- **Encorafenib** is predicted to decrease the concentration of **piperaquine**. Avoid. Moderate Theoretical
- **Fedratinib** is predicted to increase the concentration of **piperaquine**. Severe Study
- **Grapefruit** juice increases the exposure to **artemether**. Unknown Study
- **Grapefruit** juice is predicted to increase the concentration of **piperaquine**. Avoid. Moderate Theoretical
- H_2 receptor antagonists **(cimetidine)** decrease the clearance of **chloroquine**. Moderate Study
- H_2 receptor antagonists **(cimetidine)** slightly increase the exposure to **quinine**. Moderate Study
- HIV-protease inhibitors **(ritonavir)** slightly decrease the exposure to the active metabolite of **artesunate**. Avoid. Severe Study
- **HIV-protease inhibitors** decrease the exposure to **atovaquone**. Avoid if boosted with ritonavir. Moderate Study
- **HIV-protease inhibitors** are predicted to increase the concentration of **piperaquine**. Severe Study
- **HIV-protease inhibitors** are predicted to decrease the exposure to **proguanil**. Avoid. Moderate Study
- **HIV-protease inhibitors** are predicted to affect the exposure to **quinine**. Severe Study
- **Idelalisib** is predicted to increase the concentration of **piperaquine**. Severe Study
- **Imatinib** might increase the exposure to the active metabolite of **artesunate**. Avoid. Unknown Theoretical
- **Imatinib** is predicted to increase the concentration of **piperaquine**. Severe Study
- **Ivosidenib** is predicted to decrease the exposure to **artemether** with lumefantrine. Avoid. Severe Study → Also see TABLE 7 p. 1055
- **Ivosidenib** is predicted to decrease the concentration of **piperaquine**. Avoid. Moderate Theoretical
- Oral **kaolin** decreases the absorption of oral **chloroquine**. Separate administration by at least 4 hours. Moderate Study
- **Lanthanum** is predicted to decrease the absorption of **chloroquine**. Separate administration by at least 2 hours. Moderate Theoretical
- **Chloroquine** is predicted to decrease the exposure to **laronidase**. Avoid simultaneous administration. Severe Theoretical
- **Letermovir** is predicted to increase the concentration of **piperaquine**. Severe Study
- **Chloroquine** might decrease the efficacy of **live vaccines (cholera vaccine (live))**. Avoid for at least 10 days before **chloroquine**. Moderate Study
- **Lumacaftor** is predicted to decrease the exposure to **artemether** with lumefantrine. Avoid. Severe Study
- **Lumacaftor** is predicted to decrease the concentration of **piperaquine**. Avoid. Moderate Theoretical
- **Macrolides** might increase the risk of serious cardiovascular adverse effects when given with **chloroquine**. Severe Theoretical
- Macrolides **(clarithromycin, erythromycin)** are predicted to increase the concentration of **piperaquine**. Severe Study
- Oral **magnesium** trisilicate decreases the absorption of oral **chloroquine**. Separate administration by at least 4 hours. Moderate Study
- **Mepacrine** is predicted to increase the concentration of **primaquine**. Avoid. Moderate Theoretical
- **Pyrimethamine** is predicted to increase the exposure to **metformin**. Use with caution and adjust dose. Moderate Study
- **Pyrimethamine** is predicted to increase the risk of adverse effects when given with **methotrexate**. Severe Theoretical
- **Metoclopramide** decreases the concentration of **atovaquone**. Avoid. Moderate Study
- **Mitotane** is predicted to decrease the exposure to **artemether** with lumefantrine. Avoid. Severe Study
- **Mitotane** is predicted to decrease the concentration of **piperaquine**. Avoid. Moderate Theoretical
- Neurokinin-1 receptor antagonists **(aprepitant, netupitant)** are predicted to increase the concentration of **piperaquine**. Severe Study
- **Nilotinib** is predicted to increase the concentration of **piperaquine**. Severe Study
- **Nirmatrelvir** boosted with ritonavir is predicted to decrease the concentration of **atovaquone**. Moderate Theoretical
- NNRTIs **(efavirenz)** decrease the concentration of **artemether**. Severe Study → Also see TABLE 7 p. 1055
- NNRTIs **(efavirenz)** moderately decrease the exposure to **atovaquone**. Avoid. Moderate Study
- NNRTIs **(efavirenz)** decrease the concentration of **piperaquine**. Avoid. Moderate Study
- NNRTIs **(efavirenz)** affect the exposure to **proguanil**. Avoid. Moderate Study
- NNRTIs **(etravirine)** decrease the exposure to **artemether**. Moderate Study
- NNRTIs **(nevirapine)** moderately decrease the exposure to the active metabolite of **artesunate**. Avoid. Severe Study
- **Pyrimethamine** is predicted to increase the risk of adverse effects when given with NRTIs **(zidovudine)**. Severe Theoretical
- NSAIDs **(diclofenac)** might increase the exposure to the active metabolite of **artesunate**. Avoid. Unknown Theoretical
- **Pyrimethamine** is predicted to increase the risk of adverse effects when given with **pemetrexed**. Severe Theoretical
- **Chloroquine** is predicted to increase the risk of haematological toxicity when given with **penicillamine**. Avoid. Severe Theoretical
- **Chloroquine** moderately decreases the exposure to **praziquantel**. Use with caution and adjust dose. Moderate Study
- **Chloroquine** decreases the efficacy of **rabies vaccine** (intradermal). Avoid. Moderate Study
- **Chloroquine** might decrease the effects of **remdesivir**. Avoid. Moderate Theoretical
- Rifamycins **(rifabutin)** slightly decrease the exposure to **atovaquone**. Avoid. Moderate Study
- Rifamycins **(rifampicin)** are predicted to decrease the exposure to **artemether** with lumefantrine. Avoid. Severe Study
- Rifamycins **(rifampicin)** might decrease the exposure to the active metabolite of **artesunate**. Avoid. Severe Study
- Rifamycins **(rifampicin)** moderately decrease the exposure to **atovaquone** and **atovaquone** slightly increases the exposure to rifamycins **(rifampicin)**. Avoid. Moderate Study
- Rifamycins **(rifampicin)** moderately decrease the exposure to **mefloquine**. Severe Study
- Rifamycins **(rifampicin)** are predicted to decrease the concentration of **piperaquine**. Avoid. Moderate Theoretical
- Rifamycins **(rifampicin)** decrease the exposure to **quinine**. Severe Study
- **St John's wort** is predicted to decrease the concentration of **piperaquine**. Avoid. Moderate Theoretical
- **Pyrimethamine** increases the risk of adverse effects when given with **sulfonamides**. Severe Study
- **Tamoxifen** increases the risk of retinopathy when given with **chloroquine**. RCOphth guidance advises monitor. Severe Study
- Tetracyclines **(tetracycline)** decrease the concentration of **atovaquone**. Moderate Study
- **Pyrimethamine** increases the risk of adverse effects when given with **trimethoprim**. Severe Study
- **Tucatinib** is predicted to increase the concentration of **piperaquine**. Severe Study
- **Vandetanib** might increase the exposure to the active metabolite of **artesunate**. Avoid. Unknown Theoretical

Antithymocyte immunoglobulin (rabbit) → see immunoglobulins
Apalutamide → see anti-androgens
Apixaban → see factor XA inhibitors
Apomorphine → see dopamine receptor agonists
Apraclonidine → see TABLE 4 p. 1054 (bradycardia), TABLE 6 p. 1054 (hypotension), TABLE 9 p. 1056 (CNS effects)
- **Amfetamines** are predicted to decrease the effects of **apraclonidine**. Avoid. Severe Theoretical
- **Methylphenidate** is predicted to decrease the effects of **apraclonidine**. Avoid. Severe Theoretical
- **Sympathomimetics, inotropic** are predicted to decrease the effects of **apraclonidine**. Avoid. Severe Theoretical

- **Sympathomimetics, vasoconstrictor** are predicted to decrease the effects of **apraclonidine**. Avoid. Severe Theoretical

Apremilast → see phosphodiesterase type-4 inhibitors
Aprepitant → see neurokinin-1 receptor antagonists
Argatroban → see thrombin inhibitors
Aripiprazole → see atypical antipsychotics
Arsenic trioxide → see TABLE 12 p. 1057 (myelosuppression), TABLE 7 p. 1055 (QT-interval prolongation)
Artemether → see antimalarials
Artenimol → see antimalarials
Artesunate → see antimalarials

Asciminib
- **Asciminib** slightly to moderately increases the exposure to coumarins **(warfarin)**. Severe Theoretical
- **Asciminib** is predicted to increase the exposure to **digoxin**. Severe Theoretical
- **Asciminib** is predicted to increase the exposure to **everolimus**. Severe Theoretical
- **Asciminib** is predicted to increase the exposure to factor XA inhibitors **(edoxaban)**. Severe Theoretical
- **Asciminib** is predicted to increase the exposure to opioids **(alfentanil)**. Severe Theoretical
- **Asciminib** is predicted to increase the exposure to **sirolimus**. Severe Theoretical
- **Asciminib** is predicted to increase the exposure to **temsirolimus**. Severe Theoretical
- **Asciminib** is predicted to increase the exposure to thrombin inhibitors **(dabigatran)**. Severe Theoretical

Ascorbic acid
- **Ascorbic acid** is predicted to increase the risk of cardiovascular adverse effects when given with iron chelators **(deferiprone)**. Severe Theoretical
- **Ascorbic acid** might increase the risk of cardiovascular adverse effects when given with iron chelators **(desferrioxamine)**. Manufacturer advises caution or adjust ascorbic acid dose; monitor cardiac function and avoid concurrent use in those with cardiac failure. Severe Theoretical

Asenapine → see atypical antipsychotics
Asparaginase → see TABLE 3 p. 1053 (bleeding), TABLE 1 p. 1053 (hepatotoxicity), TABLE 12 p. 1057 (myelosuppression)
- **Asparaginase** is predicted to increase the risk of hepatotoxicity when given with **imatinib**. Severe Theoretical → Also see TABLE 3 p. 1053 → Also see TABLE 12 p. 1057
- **Asparaginase** affects the efficacy of **methotrexate**. Severe Anecdotal → Also see TABLE 1 p. 1053 → Also see TABLE 12 p. 1057
- **Asparaginase** potentially increases the risk of neurotoxicity when given with vinca alkaloids **(vincristine)**. **Vincristine** should be taken 3 to 24 hours before **asparaginase**. Severe Anecdotal → Also see TABLE 12 p. 1057

Aspirin → see TABLE 3 p. 1053 (bleeding), TABLE 2 p. 1053 (nephrotoxicity)
- **Acetazolamide** increases the risk of severe toxic reaction when given with **aspirin** (high-dose). Severe Study
- Oral **antacids** decrease the absorption of oral **aspirin** (high-dose). Moderate Study
- **Aspirin** (high-dose) is predicted to increase the risk of gastrointestinal irritation when given with bisphosphonates **(alendronate, ibandronate)**. Moderate Study
- **Aspirin** (high-dose) is predicted to increase the risk of renal impairment when given with bisphosphonates **(clodronate)**. Severe Theoretical
- **Corticosteroids** are predicted to decrease the concentration of **aspirin** (high-dose) and **aspirin** (high-dose) increases the risk of gastrointestinal bleeding when given with **corticosteroids**. Moderate Study
- **Aspirin** (high-dose) increases the risk of renal impairment when given with **daptomycin**. Moderate Theoretical
- **Aspirin** (high-dose) might cause ototoxicity, as can **drugs that cause ototoxicity** (see TABLE 16 p. 1058); concurrent use might increase the risk of developing this effect. Moderate Theoretical
- **Erlotinib** is predicted to increase the risk of gastrointestinal perforation when given with **aspirin** (high-dose). Severe Theoretical
- **Aspirin** (high-dose) increases the exposure to factor XA inhibitors **(edoxaban)**. Avoid. Severe Study → Also see TABLE 3 p. 1053
- **Aspirin** (high-dose) is predicted to increase the risk of gastrointestinal bleeds when given with iron chelators **(deferasirox)**. Severe Theoretical → Also see TABLE 2 p. 1053
- **Aspirin** might increase the risk of Reye's syndrome when given with live vaccines **(influenza vaccine (live))**. Avoid **aspirin** for 4 weeks after vaccination. Severe Theoretical
- **Aspirin** might increase the risk of Reye's syndrome when given with live vaccines **(varicella-zoster vaccine)**. Avoid **aspirin** for 6 weeks after vaccination. Severe Theoretical
- **Aspirin** (high-dose) is predicted to increase the risk of toxicity when given with **methotrexate**. Severe Study → Also see TABLE 2 p. 1053
- **Aspirin** is predicted to increase the risk of gastrointestinal perforation when given with **nicorandil**. Severe Theoretical
- NRTIs **(zidovudine)** increase the risk of haematological toxicity when given with **aspirin** (high-dose). Severe Study
- **Aspirin** (high-dose) potentially increases the exposure to **pemetrexed**. Use with caution or avoid. Severe Theoretical → Also see TABLE 2 p. 1053
- **Selumetinib** might increase the risk of bleeding when given with **aspirin**. Severe Theoretical
- **Aspirin** (high-dose) increases the risk of acute renal failure when given with **thiazide diuretics**. Severe Theoretical

Ataluren
- **Ataluren** is predicted to increase the risk of nephrotoxicity when given with intravenous **aminoglycosides**. Avoid. Severe Study
- Rifamycins **(rifampicin)** decrease the exposure to **ataluren**. Moderate Study

Atazanavir → see HIV-protease inhibitors
Atenolol → see beta blockers, selective
Atezolizumab → see monoclonal antibodies

Atogepant
- Angiotensin-II receptor antagonists **(telmisartan)** are predicted to increase the exposure to **atogepant**. Adjust **atogepant** dose. Moderate Theoretical
- Anti-androgens **(darolutamide)** are predicted to increase the exposure to **atogepant**. Adjust **atogepant** dose. Moderate Theoretical
- Antifungals, azoles **(itraconazole, ketoconazole, posaconazole, voriconazole)** are predicted to increase the exposure to **atogepant**. Adjust **atogepant** dose. Moderate Study
- **Cenobamate** is predicted to decrease the exposure to **atogepant**. Adjust dose. Moderate Theoretical
- **Ceritinib** is predicted to increase the exposure to **atogepant**. Adjust **atogepant** dose. Moderate Study
- **Ciclosporin** is predicted to increase the exposure to **atogepant**. Adjust **atogepant** dose. Moderate Theoretical
- **Cobicistat** is predicted to increase the exposure to **atogepant**. Adjust **atogepant** dose. Moderate Study
- **Eltrombopag** is predicted to increase the exposure to **atogepant**. Adjust **atogepant** dose. Moderate Theoretical
- Fibrates **(gemfibrozil)** are predicted to increase the exposure to **atogepant**. Adjust **atogepant** dose. Moderate Theoretical
- **HIV-protease inhibitors** are predicted to increase the exposure to **atogepant**. Adjust **atogepant** dose. Moderate Study
- **Idelalisib** is predicted to increase the exposure to **atogepant**. Adjust **atogepant** dose. Moderate Study
- **Leflunomide** is predicted to increase the exposure to **atogepant**. Adjust **atogepant** dose. Moderate Theoretical
- Macrolides **(clarithromycin)** are predicted to increase the exposure to **atogepant**. Adjust **atogepant** dose. Moderate Study
- Macrolides **(erythromycin)** are predicted to increase the exposure to **atogepant**. Adjust **atogepant** dose. Moderate Theoretical
- Rifamycins **(rifampicin)** (single-dose) increase the exposure to **atogepant**. Adjust **atogepant** dose. Moderate Study
- **Roxadustat** is predicted to increase the exposure to **atogepant**. Adjust **atogepant** dose. Moderate Theoretical
- **Teriflunomide** is predicted to increase the exposure to **atogepant**. Adjust **atogepant** dose. Moderate Theoretical

Atogepant (continued)
- **Tucatinib** is predicted to increase the exposure to **atogepant**. Adjust **atogepant** dose. Moderate Study
- **Velpatasvir** is predicted to increase the exposure to **atogepant**. Adjust **atogepant** dose. Moderate Theoretical
- **Voxilaprevir** is predicted to increase the exposure to **atogepant**. Adjust **atogepant** dose. Moderate Theoretical

Atomoxetine
- **Amfetamines** are predicted to increase the risk of adverse effects when given with **atomoxetine**. Severe Theoretical
- **Berotralstat** is predicted to increase the exposure to **atomoxetine**. Adjust dose. Moderate Study
- **Atomoxetine** is predicted to increase the risk of cardiovascular adverse effects when given with **beta$_2$ agonists** (high-dose). Moderate Study
- **Bupropion** is predicted to markedly increase the exposure to **atomoxetine**. Adjust dose. Severe Study
- **Cinacalcet** is predicted to markedly increase the exposure to **atomoxetine**. Adjust dose. Severe Study
- **Dacomitinib** is predicted to markedly increase the exposure to **atomoxetine**. Adjust dose. Severe Study
- **Eliglustat** is predicted to increase the exposure to **atomoxetine**. Adjust dose. Moderate Theoretical
- **Givosiran** is predicted to increase the exposure to **atomoxetine**. Use with caution and adjust dose. Moderate Study
- Interferons **(ropeginterferon alfa)** are predicted to increase the exposure to **atomoxetine**. Moderate Theoretical
- **MAOIs, irreversible** are predicted to increase the risk of adverse effects when given with **atomoxetine**. Avoid and for 2 weeks after stopping the MAOI. Severe Theoretical
- **Panobinostat** is predicted to increase the exposure to **atomoxetine**. Monitor and adjust dose. Severe Theoretical
- SSRIs **(fluoxetine, paroxetine)** are predicted to markedly increase the exposure to **atomoxetine**. Adjust dose. Severe Study
- **Terbinafine** is predicted to markedly increase the exposure to **atomoxetine**. Adjust dose. Severe Study

Atorvastatin → see statins

Atovaquone → see antimalarials

Atracurium → see neuromuscular blocking drugs, non-depolarising

Atropine → see **TABLE 8** p. 1055 (antimuscarinics)

ROUTE-SPECIFIC INFORMATION Since systemic absorption can follow topical application of **atropine**, the possibility of interactions should be borne in mind.

- Atypical antipsychotics **(clozapine)** can cause constipation, as can **atropine**; concurrent use might increase the risk of developing intestinal obstruction. Severe Theoretical → Also see **TABLE 8** p. 1055
- **Atropine** increases the risk of severe hypertension when given with sympathomimetics, vasoconstrictor **(phenylephrine)**. Severe Study

Atypical antipsychotics → see **TABLE 15** p. 1058 (hyponatraemia), **TABLE 6** p. 1054 (hypotension), **TABLE 7** p. 1055 (QT-interval prolongation), **TABLE 8** p. 1055 (antimuscarinics), **TABLE 9** p. 1056 (CNS effects)

amisulpride · aripiprazole · asenapine · cariprazine · clozapine · lurasidone · olanzapine · paliperidone · quetiapine · risperidone

- **Clozapine** and **olanzapine** dose adjustment might be necessary if smoking started or stopped during treatment.
- Avoid concomitant use of **clozapine** with drugs that have a substantial potential for causing agranulocytosis or a substantial potential to depress bone marrow function.

- **Clozapine** can cause constipation, as can **aclidinium**; concurrent use might increase the risk of developing intestinal obstruction. Severe Theoretical → Also see **TABLE 8** p. 1055
- Anti-androgens **(apalutamide, enzalutamide)** are predicted to moderately decrease the exposure to **aripiprazole**. Avoid or adjust dose—consult product literature. Moderate Study
- Anti-androgens **(apalutamide, enzalutamide)** are predicted to decrease the exposure to **cariprazine**. Avoid. Severe Theoretical
- Anti-androgens **(apalutamide, enzalutamide)** are predicted to decrease the exposure to **lurasidone**. Avoid. Moderate Study
- Anti-androgens **(apalutamide, enzalutamide)** are predicted to decrease the exposure to **paliperidone**. Monitor and adjust dose. Severe Study → Also see **TABLE 7** p. 1055
- Anti-androgens **(apalutamide, enzalutamide)** are predicted to decrease the exposure to **quetiapine**. Moderate Study
- Anti-androgens **(apalutamide, enzalutamide)** are predicted to decrease the exposure to **risperidone**. Adjust dose. Moderate Study
- Anti-androgens **(enzalutamide)** are predicted to decrease the exposure to **clozapine**. Moderate Theoretical
- Antiarrhythmics **(dronedarone)** are predicted to increase the exposure to **cariprazine**. Monitor and adjust dose. Severe Study
- Antiarrhythmics **(dronedarone)** are predicted to increase the exposure to **lurasidone**. Adjust **lurasidone** dose, p. 303. Moderate Study
- Antiarrhythmics **(dronedarone)** are predicted to increase the exposure to **quetiapine**. Avoid. Moderate Study
- **Clozapine** can cause constipation, as can antiarrhythmics **(disopyramide, propafenone)**; concurrent use might increase the risk of developing intestinal obstruction. Severe Theoretical → Also see **TABLE 8** p. 1055
- Antiepileptics **(carbamazepine)** are predicted to increase the risk of myelosuppression when given with **clozapine**. Avoid. Severe Anecdotal → Also see **TABLE 15** p. 1058
- Antiepileptics **(carbamazepine)** potentially decrease the exposure to **olanzapine**. Monitor and adjust dose. Moderate Study → Also see **TABLE 15** p. 1058
- Antiepileptics **(carbamazepine, fosphenytoin, phenobarbital, phenytoin, primidone)** are predicted to moderately decrease the exposure to **aripiprazole**. Avoid or adjust dose—consult product literature. Moderate Study → Also see **TABLE 15** p. 1058 → Also see **TABLE 9** p. 1056
- Antiepileptics **(carbamazepine, fosphenytoin, phenobarbital, phenytoin, primidone)** are predicted to decrease the exposure to **cariprazine**. Avoid. Severe Theoretical → Also see **TABLE 15** p. 1058 → Also see **TABLE 9** p. 1056
- Antiepileptics **(carbamazepine, fosphenytoin, phenobarbital, phenytoin, primidone)** are predicted to decrease the exposure to **lurasidone**. Avoid. Moderate Study → Also see **TABLE 15** p. 1058 → Also see **TABLE 9** p. 1056
- Antiepileptics **(carbamazepine, fosphenytoin, phenobarbital, phenytoin, primidone)** are predicted to decrease the exposure to **paliperidone**. Monitor and adjust dose. Severe Study → Also see **TABLE 15** p. 1058 → Also see **TABLE 9** p. 1056
- Antiepileptics **(carbamazepine, fosphenytoin, phenobarbital, phenytoin, primidone)** are predicted to decrease the exposure to **quetiapine**. Moderate Study → Also see **TABLE 15** p. 1058 → Also see **TABLE 9** p. 1056
- Antiepileptics **(carbamazepine, fosphenytoin, phenobarbital, phenytoin, primidone)** are predicted to decrease the exposure to **risperidone**. Adjust dose. Moderate Study → Also see **TABLE 15** p. 1058 → Also see **TABLE 9** p. 1056
- Antiepileptics **(fosphenytoin, phenobarbital, phenytoin, primidone)** are predicted to decrease the exposure to **clozapine**. Moderate Anecdotal → Also see **TABLE 9** p. 1056
- Antiepileptics **(phenytoin)** are predicted to decrease the exposure to **olanzapine**. Monitor and adjust dose. Moderate Study → Also see **TABLE 9** p. 1056
- Antiepileptics **(valproate)** have been reported to increase the risk of neutropenia and myocarditis when given with **clozapine**. Severe Anecdotal → Also see **TABLE 15** p. 1058
- Antiepileptics **(valproate)** increase the risk of adverse effects when given with **olanzapine**. Severe Study → Also see **TABLE 15** p. 1058
- Antiepileptics **(valproate)** slightly increase the exposure to **paliperidone**. Adjust dose. Moderate Study → Also see **TABLE 15** p. 1058
- Antiepileptics **(valproate)** potentially increase the risk of neutropenia when given with **quetiapine**. Moderate Study → Also see **TABLE 15** p. 1058
- Antifungals, azoles **(fluconazole, isavuconazole)** are predicted to increase the exposure to **cariprazine**. Monitor and adjust dose. Severe Study

- Antifungals, azoles **(fluconazole, isavuconazole)** are predicted to increase the exposure to **lurasidone**. Adjust **lurasidone** dose, p. 303. [Moderate] Study
- Antifungals, azoles **(fluconazole, isavuconazole)** are predicted to increase the exposure to **quetiapine**. Avoid. [Moderate] Study
- Antifungals, azoles **(itraconazole, ketoconazole, posaconazole, voriconazole)** are predicted to slightly increase the exposure to **aripiprazole**. Avoid or adjust dose—consult product literature. [Moderate] Study
- Antifungals, azoles **(itraconazole, ketoconazole, posaconazole, voriconazole)** are predicted to moderately increase the exposure to **cariprazine**. Avoid. [Severe] Study
- Antifungals, azoles **(itraconazole, ketoconazole, posaconazole, voriconazole)** are predicted to increase the exposure to **risperidone**. Adjust dose. [Moderate] Study
- Antifungals, azoles **(itraconazole, ketoconazole, posaconazole, voriconazole)** are predicted to increase the exposure to atypical antipsychotics **(lurasidone, quetiapine)**. Avoid. [Severe] Study
- **Clozapine** can cause constipation, as can antihistamines, sedating **(chlorphenamine, cyclizine, cyproheptadine, hydroxyzine, promethazine)**; concurrent use might increase the risk of developing intestinal obstruction. [Severe] Theoretical → Also see **TABLE 8** p. 1055 → Also see **TABLE 9** p. 1056
- **Clozapine** can cause constipation, as can **atropine**; concurrent use might increase the risk of developing intestinal obstruction. [Severe] Theoretical → Also see **TABLE 8** p. 1055
- Atypical antipsychotics **(clozapine)** can cause constipation, as can atypical antipsychotics **(olanzapine, quetiapine)**; concurrent use might increase the risk of developing intestinal obstruction. [Severe] Anecdotal → Also see **TABLE 15** p. 1058 → Also see **TABLE 6** p. 1054 → Also see **TABLE 8** p. 1055 → Also see **TABLE 9** p. 1056
- **Axitinib** is predicted to increase the exposure to atypical antipsychotics **(clozapine, olanzapine)**. [Moderate] Theoretical
- **Clozapine** can cause constipation, as can **baclofen**; concurrent use might increase the risk of developing intestinal obstruction. [Severe] Theoretical → Also see **TABLE 6** p. 1054 → Also see **TABLE 8** p. 1055 → Also see **TABLE 9** p. 1056
- **Clozapine** might increase the risk of respiratory depression and circulatory collapse when given with **benzodiazepines**. [Severe] Anecdotal → Also see **TABLE 9** p. 1056
- **Berotralstat** is predicted to increase the exposure to **cariprazine**. Monitor and adjust dose. [Severe] Study
- **Berotralstat** is predicted to increase the exposure to **quetiapine**. Avoid. [Moderate] Study
- **Bupropion** is predicted to moderately increase the exposure to **aripiprazole**. Avoid or adjust dose—consult product literature. [Moderate] Study
- **Bupropion** is predicted to increase the exposure to **clozapine**. Use with caution and adjust dose. [Severe] Study
- **Bupropion** is predicted to increase the exposure to **risperidone**. Adjust dose. [Moderate] Study
- Calcium-channel blockers **(diltiazem, verapamil)** are predicted to increase the exposure to **cariprazine**. Monitor and adjust dose. [Severe] Study → Also see **TABLE 6** p. 1054
- Calcium-channel blockers **(diltiazem, verapamil)** are predicted to increase the exposure to **lurasidone**. Adjust **lurasidone** dose, p. 303. [Moderate] Study → Also see **TABLE 6** p. 1054
- Calcium-channel blockers **(diltiazem, verapamil)** are predicted to increase the exposure to **quetiapine**. Avoid. [Moderate] Study → Also see **TABLE 6** p. 1054
- **Cenobamate** is predicted to decrease the exposure to **aripiprazole**. Avoid or adjust dose—consult product literature. [Moderate] Study → Also see **TABLE 9** p. 1056
- **Cenobamate** is predicted to decrease the exposure to **cariprazine**. Avoid. [Severe] Theoretical → Also see **TABLE 9** p. 1056
- **Cenobamate** is predicted to decrease the exposure to **lurasidone**. Monitor and adjust dose. [Moderate] Theoretical → Also see **TABLE 9** p. 1056
- **Cenobamate** is predicted to decrease the exposure to **quetiapine**. [Moderate] Study → Also see **TABLE 9** p. 1056
- **Ceritinib** is predicted to slightly increase the exposure to **aripiprazole**. Avoid or adjust dose—consult product literature. [Moderate] Study
- **Ceritinib** is predicted to increase the exposure to atypical antipsychotics **(lurasidone, quetiapine)**. Avoid. [Severe] Study
- **Ceritinib** is predicted to moderately increase the exposure to **cariprazine**. Avoid. [Severe] Study
- **Ceritinib** is predicted to increase the exposure to **risperidone**. Adjust dose. [Moderate] Study
- **Cinacalcet** is predicted to moderately increase the exposure to **aripiprazole**. Avoid or adjust dose—consult product literature. [Moderate] Study
- **Cinacalcet** is predicted to increase the exposure to **clozapine**. Use with caution and adjust dose. [Severe] Study
- **Cinacalcet** is predicted to increase the exposure to **risperidone**. Adjust dose. [Moderate] Study
- **Cobicistat** is predicted to slightly increase the exposure to **aripiprazole**. Avoid or adjust dose—consult product literature. [Moderate] Study
- **Cobicistat** is predicted to increase the exposure to atypical antipsychotics **(lurasidone, quetiapine)**. Avoid. [Severe] Study
- **Cobicistat** is predicted to moderately increase the exposure to **cariprazine**. Avoid. [Severe] Study
- **Cobicistat** is predicted to increase the exposure to **risperidone**. Adjust dose. [Moderate] Study
- **Combined hormonal contraceptives** increases the concentration of **clozapine**. Monitor adverse effects and adjust dose. [Severe] Study
- **Combined hormonal contraceptives** is predicted to increase the exposure to **olanzapine**. Adjust dose. [Moderate] Anecdotal
- **Crizotinib** is predicted to increase the exposure to **cariprazine**. Monitor and adjust dose. [Severe] Study
- **Crizotinib** is predicted to increase the exposure to **lurasidone**. Adjust **lurasidone** dose, p. 303. [Moderate] Study
- **Crizotinib** is predicted to increase the exposure to **quetiapine**. Avoid. [Moderate] Study
- **Clozapine** can cause constipation, as can **cyclopentolate**; concurrent use might increase the risk of developing intestinal obstruction. [Severe] Theoretical → Also see **TABLE 8** p. 1055
- **Dabrafenib** is predicted to decrease the exposure to **aripiprazole**. Avoid or adjust dose—consult product literature. [Moderate] Study
- **Dabrafenib** is predicted to decrease the exposure to **cariprazine**. Avoid. [Severe] Theoretical
- **Dabrafenib** is predicted to decrease the exposure to **lurasidone**. Monitor and adjust dose. [Moderate] Theoretical
- **Dabrafenib** is predicted to decrease the exposure to **quetiapine**. [Moderate] Study
- **Dacomitinib** is predicted to moderately increase the exposure to **aripiprazole**. Avoid or adjust dose—consult product literature. [Moderate] Study
- **Dacomitinib** is predicted to increase the exposure to **clozapine**. Use with caution and adjust dose. [Severe] Study
- **Dacomitinib** is predicted to increase the exposure to **risperidone**. Adjust dose. [Moderate] Study
- **Clozapine** can cause constipation, as can **darifenacin**; concurrent use might increase the risk of developing intestinal obstruction. [Severe] Theoretical → Also see **TABLE 8** p. 1055
- **Clozapine** can cause constipation, as can **dicycloverine**; concurrent use might increase the risk of developing intestinal obstruction. [Severe] Theoretical → Also see **TABLE 8** p. 1055
- **Clozapine** can cause constipation, as can **dimenhydrinate**; concurrent use might increase the risk of developing intestinal obstruction. [Severe] Theoretical → Also see **TABLE 8** p. 1055 → Also see **TABLE 9** p. 1056
- **Asenapine** is predicted to decrease the effects of **dopamine receptor agonists**. Adjust dose. [Moderate] Theoretical → Also see **TABLE 6** p. 1054 → Also see **TABLE 9** p. 1056
- Atypical antipsychotics **(amisulpride, olanzapine, paliperidone, quetiapine, risperidone)** are predicted to decrease the effects of **dopamine receptor agonists**. Avoid. [Moderate] Theoretical → Also see **TABLE 6** p. 1054 → Also see **TABLE 7** p. 1055 → Also see **TABLE 8** p. 1055 → Also see **TABLE 9** p. 1056
- Atypical antipsychotics **(aripiprazole, clozapine)** are predicted to decrease the effects of **dopamine receptor agonists**. [Moderate]

Atypical antipsychotics (continued)
Theoretical → Also see TABLE 6 p. 1054 → Also see TABLE 8 p. 1055 → Also see TABLE 9 p. 1056

- **Encorafenib** is predicted to moderately decrease the exposure to **aripiprazole**. Avoid or adjust dose—consult product literature. Moderate Study
- **Encorafenib** is predicted to decrease the exposure to **cariprazine**. Avoid. Severe Theoretical
- **Encorafenib** is predicted to decrease the exposure to **lurasidone**. Avoid. Moderate Study
- **Encorafenib** is predicted to decrease the exposure to **paliperidone**. Monitor and adjust dose. Severe Study → Also see TABLE 7 p. 1055
- **Encorafenib** is predicted to decrease the exposure to **quetiapine**. Moderate Study
- **Encorafenib** is predicted to decrease the exposure to **risperidone**. Adjust dose. Moderate Study
- Endothelin receptor antagonists **(bosentan)** are predicted to decrease the exposure to **aripiprazole**. Avoid or adjust dose—consult product literature. Moderate Study
- Endothelin receptor antagonists **(bosentan)** are predicted to decrease the exposure to **cariprazine**. Avoid. Severe Theoretical
- Endothelin receptor antagonists **(bosentan)** are predicted to decrease the exposure to **lurasidone**. Monitor and adjust dose. Moderate Theoretical
- Endothelin receptor antagonists **(bosentan)** are predicted to decrease the exposure to **quetiapine**. Moderate Study
- **Fedratinib** is predicted to increase the exposure to **cariprazine**. Monitor and adjust dose. Severe Study
- **Fedratinib** is predicted to increase the exposure to **quetiapine**. Avoid. Moderate Study
- **Clozapine** can cause constipation, as can **fesoterodine**; concurrent use might increase the risk of developing intestinal obstruction. Severe Theoretical → Also see TABLE 8 p. 1055
- **Clozapine** can cause constipation, as can **flavoxate**; concurrent use might increase the risk of developing intestinal obstruction. Severe Theoretical → Also see TABLE 8 p. 1055
- **Clozapine** can cause constipation, as can **flupentixol**; concurrent use might increase the risk of developing intestinal obstruction. Severe Theoretical → Also see TABLE 15 p. 1058 → Also see TABLE 6 p. 1054 → Also see TABLE 8 p. 1055 → Also see TABLE 9 p. 1056
- **Atypical antipsychotics** might decrease the effects of the active metabolite of **foslevodopa**. Severe Theoretical → Also see TABLE 6 p. 1054 → Also see TABLE 9 p. 1056
- **Givosiran** increases the concentration of **clozapine**. Monitor adverse effects and adjust dose. Severe Study
- **Givosiran** is predicted to increase the exposure to **olanzapine**. Adjust dose. Moderate Anecdotal
- **Clozapine** can cause constipation, as can **glycopyrronium**; concurrent use might increase the risk of developing intestinal obstruction. Severe Theoretical → Also see TABLE 8 p. 1055
- **Grapefruit** juice is predicted to increase the exposure to atypical antipsychotics **(lurasidone, quetiapine)**. Avoid. Severe Theoretical
- **Grapefruit** juice is predicted to increase the exposure to **cariprazine**. Avoid. Moderate Study
- **Clozapine** can cause constipation, as can **haloperidol**; concurrent use might increase the risk of developing intestinal obstruction. Severe Theoretical → Also see TABLE 15 p. 1058 → Also see TABLE 6 p. 1054 → Also see TABLE 8 p. 1055 → Also see TABLE 9 p. 1056
- **HIV-protease inhibitors** are predicted to slightly increase the exposure to **aripiprazole**. Avoid or adjust dose—consult product literature. Moderate Study
- **HIV-protease inhibitors** are predicted to moderately increase the exposure to **cariprazine**. Avoid. Severe Study
- HIV-protease inhibitors **(ritonavir)** are predicted to affect the exposure to **clozapine**. Avoid. Severe Theoretical
- HIV-protease inhibitors **(ritonavir)** are predicted to decrease the exposure to **olanzapine**. Monitor and adjust dose. Moderate Study
- **HIV-protease inhibitors** are predicted to increase the exposure to atypical antipsychotics **(lurasidone, quetiapine)**. Avoid. Severe Study
- **HIV-protease inhibitors** are predicted to increase the exposure to **risperidone**. Adjust dose. Moderate Study
- **Clozapine** can cause constipation, as can **homatropine**; concurrent use might increase the risk of developing intestinal obstruction. Severe Theoretical → Also see TABLE 8 p. 1055
- **Clozapine** can cause constipation, as can **hyoscine**; concurrent use might increase the risk of developing intestinal obstruction. Severe Theoretical → Also see TABLE 8 p. 1055
- **Idelalisib** is predicted to slightly increase the exposure to **aripiprazole**. Avoid or adjust dose—consult product literature. Moderate Study
- **Idelalisib** is predicted to increase the exposure to atypical antipsychotics **(lurasidone, quetiapine)**. Avoid. Severe Study
- **Idelalisib** is predicted to moderately increase the exposure to **cariprazine**. Avoid. Severe Study
- **Idelalisib** is predicted to increase the exposure to **risperidone**. Adjust dose. Moderate Study
- **Imatinib** is predicted to increase the exposure to **cariprazine**. Monitor and adjust dose. Severe Study
- **Imatinib** is predicted to increase the exposure to **lurasidone**. Adjust **lurasidone** dose, p. 303. Moderate Study
- **Imatinib** is predicted to increase the exposure to **quetiapine**. Avoid. Moderate Study
- Interferons **(ropeginterferon alfa)** are predicted to increase the exposure to **risperidone**. Moderate Theoretical
- **Clozapine** can cause constipation, as can **ipratropium**; concurrent use might increase the risk of developing intestinal obstruction. Severe Theoretical → Also see TABLE 8 p. 1055
- **Clozapine** can cause constipation, as can **iron**; concurrent use might increase the risk of developing intestinal obstruction. Severe Anecdotal
- Iron chelators **(deferasirox)** are predicted to increase the exposure to **clozapine**. Avoid. Moderate Theoretical
- **Ivosidenib** is predicted to moderately decrease the exposure to **aripiprazole**. Avoid or adjust dose—consult product literature. Moderate Study
- **Ivosidenib** is predicted to decrease the exposure to **cariprazine**. Avoid. Severe Theoretical
- **Ivosidenib** is predicted to decrease the exposure to **lurasidone**. Avoid. Moderate Study
- **Ivosidenib** is predicted to decrease the exposure to **paliperidone**. Monitor and adjust dose. Severe Study → Also see TABLE 7 p. 1055
- **Ivosidenib** is predicted to decrease the exposure to **quetiapine**. Moderate Study
- **Ivosidenib** is predicted to decrease the exposure to **risperidone**. Adjust dose. Moderate Study
- **Leflunomide** is predicted to decrease the exposure to **clozapine**. Moderate Theoretical
- **Leflunomide** is predicted to decrease the exposure to **olanzapine**. Monitor and adjust dose. Moderate Study
- **Leniolisib** is predicted to increase the exposure to **clozapine**. Avoid. Moderate Theoretical
- **Letermovir** is predicted to increase the exposure to **cariprazine**. Monitor and adjust dose. Severe Study
- **Letermovir** is predicted to increase the exposure to **quetiapine**. Avoid. Moderate Study
- **Amisulpride** is predicted to decrease the effects of **levodopa**. Avoid. Severe Theoretical → Also see TABLE 9 p. 1056
- **Asenapine** is predicted to decrease the effects of **levodopa**. Adjust dose. Severe Theoretical → Also see TABLE 6 p. 1054 → Also see TABLE 9 p. 1056
- Atypical antipsychotics **(aripiprazole, clozapine, lurasidone, paliperidone)** are predicted to decrease the effects of **levodopa**. Severe Theoretical → Also see TABLE 6 p. 1054 → Also see TABLE 9 p. 1056
- **Olanzapine** decreases the effects of **levodopa**. Avoid or monitor worsening parkinsonian symptoms. Severe Anecdotal → Also see TABLE 6 p. 1054 → Also see TABLE 9 p. 1056

- **Quetiapine** decreases the effects of **levodopa**. Severe Anecdotal → Also see **TABLE 6** p. 1054 → Also see **TABLE 9** p. 1056
- **Risperidone** is predicted to decrease the effects of **levodopa**. Avoid or adjust dose. Severe Anecdotal → Also see **TABLE 6** p. 1054 → Also see **TABLE 9** p. 1056
- Atypical antipsychotics **(quetiapine, risperidone)** potentially increase the risk of neurotoxicity when given with **lithium**. Severe Anecdotal
- **Clozapine** can cause constipation, as can **loperamide**; concurrent use might increase the risk of developing intestinal obstruction. Severe Anecdotal
- **Lorlatinib** is predicted to decrease the exposure to **aripiprazole**. Avoid or adjust dose—consult product literature. Moderate Study
- **Lorlatinib** is predicted to decrease the exposure to **cariprazine**. Avoid. Severe Theoretical
- **Lorlatinib** is predicted to decrease the exposure to **lurasidone**. Monitor and adjust dose. Moderate Theoretical
- **Lorlatinib** is predicted to decrease the exposure to **quetiapine**. Moderate Study
- **Clozapine** can cause constipation, as can **loxapine**; concurrent use might increase the risk of developing intestinal obstruction. Severe Theoretical → Also see **TABLE 15** p. 1058 → Also see **TABLE 6** p. 1054 → Also see **TABLE 8** p. 1055 → Also see **TABLE 9** p. 1056
- **Lumacaftor** is predicted to moderately decrease the exposure to **aripiprazole**. Avoid or adjust dose—consult product literature. Moderate Study
- **Lumacaftor** is predicted to decrease the exposure to **cariprazine**. Avoid. Severe Theoretical
- **Lumacaftor** is predicted to decrease the exposure to **lurasidone**. Avoid. Moderate Study
- **Lumacaftor** is predicted to decrease the exposure to **paliperidone**. Monitor and adjust dose. Severe Study
- **Lumacaftor** is predicted to decrease the exposure to **quetiapine**. Moderate Study
- **Lumacaftor** is predicted to decrease the exposure to **risperidone**. Adjust dose. Moderate Study
- Macrolides **(clarithromycin)** are predicted to slightly increase the exposure to **aripiprazole**. Avoid or adjust dose—consult product literature. Moderate Study
- Macrolides **(clarithromycin)** are predicted to moderately increase the exposure to **cariprazine**. Avoid. Severe Study
- Macrolides **(clarithromycin)** are predicted to increase the exposure to **risperidone**. Adjust dose. Moderate Study
- Macrolides **(erythromycin)** are predicted to increase the exposure to **cariprazine**. Monitor and adjust dose. Severe Study
- Macrolides **(erythromycin)** potentially increase the risk of toxicity when given with **clozapine**. Severe Anecdotal
- Macrolides **(erythromycin)** are predicted to increase the exposure to **lurasidone**. Adjust **lurasidone** dose, p. 303. Moderate Study
- Macrolides **(erythromycin)** are predicted to increase the exposure to **quetiapine**. Avoid. Moderate Study
- Macrolides **(clarithromycin)** are predicted to increase the exposure to atypical antipsychotics **(lurasidone, quetiapine)**. Avoid. Severe Study
- **Methylphenidate** might increase the risk of dyskinesias when given with **paliperidone**. Severe Theoretical
- **Methylphenidate** increases the risk of dyskinesias when given with **risperidone**. Severe Anecdotal
- **Mexiletine** increases the concentration of **clozapine**. Monitor adverse effects and adjust dose. Severe Study
- **Mexiletine** is predicted to increase the exposure to **olanzapine**. Adjust dose. Moderate Anecdotal
- **Mitotane** is predicted to moderately decrease the exposure to **aripiprazole**. Avoid or adjust dose—consult product literature. Moderate Study
- **Mitotane** is predicted to decrease the exposure to **cariprazine**. Avoid. Severe Theoretical
- **Mitotane** is predicted to decrease the exposure to **lurasidone**. Avoid. Moderate Study
- **Mitotane** is predicted to decrease the exposure to **paliperidone**. Monitor and adjust dose. Severe Study
- **Mitotane** is predicted to decrease the exposure to **quetiapine**. Moderate Study
- **Mitotane** is predicted to decrease the exposure to **risperidone**. Adjust dose. Moderate Study
- Neurokinin-1 receptor antagonists **(aprepitant, netupitant)** are predicted to increase the exposure to **cariprazine**. Monitor and adjust dose. Severe Study
- Neurokinin-1 receptor antagonists **(aprepitant, netupitant)** are predicted to increase the exposure to **lurasidone**. Adjust **lurasidone** dose, p. 303. Moderate Study
- Neurokinin-1 receptor antagonists **(aprepitant, netupitant)** are predicted to increase the exposure to **quetiapine**. Avoid. Moderate Study
- **Nilotinib** is predicted to increase the exposure to **cariprazine**. Monitor and adjust dose. Severe Study
- **Nilotinib** is predicted to increase the exposure to **lurasidone**. Adjust **lurasidone** dose, p. 303. Moderate Study
- **Nilotinib** is predicted to increase the exposure to **quetiapine**. Avoid. Moderate Study
- **Nirmatrelvir** boosted with ritonavir is predicted to increase the concentration of **aripiprazole**. Adjust dose. Moderate Theoretical
- **Nirmatrelvir** boosted with ritonavir is predicted to increase the concentration of atypical antipsychotics **(lurasidone, quetiapine)**. Avoid. Severe Theoretical
- **Nirmatrelvir** boosted with ritonavir is predicted to increase the concentration of **cariprazine**. Avoid. Moderate Theoretical
- **Nirmatrelvir** boosted with ritonavir is predicted to increase the concentration of **clozapine**. Avoid or adjust dose. Severe Theoretical
- **Nirmatrelvir** boosted with ritonavir is predicted to increase the concentration of **risperidone**. Severe Theoretical
- NNRTIs **(efavirenz, etravirine, nevirapine)** are predicted to decrease the exposure to **aripiprazole**. Avoid or adjust dose—consult product literature. Moderate Study
- NNRTIs **(efavirenz, etravirine, nevirapine)** are predicted to decrease the exposure to **cariprazine**. Avoid. Severe Theoretical
- NNRTIs **(efavirenz, etravirine, nevirapine)** are predicted to decrease the exposure to **lurasidone**. Monitor and adjust dose. Moderate Theoretical
- NNRTIs **(efavirenz, etravirine, nevirapine)** are predicted to decrease the exposure to **quetiapine**. Moderate Study
- **Olaparib** might alter the exposure to **quetiapine**. Moderate Theoretical
- **Clozapine** can cause constipation, as can **opioids**; concurrent use might increase the risk of developing intestinal obstruction. Severe Anecdotal → Also see **TABLE 15** p. 1058 → Also see **TABLE 9** p. 1056
- **Clozapine** can cause constipation, as can **orphenadrine**; concurrent use might increase the risk of developing intestinal obstruction. Severe Theoretical → Also see **TABLE 8** p. 1055 → Also see **TABLE 9** p. 1056
- **Osilodrostat** increases the concentration of **clozapine**. Monitor adverse effects and adjust dose. Severe Study
- **Osilodrostat** is predicted to increase the exposure to **olanzapine**. Adjust dose. Moderate Anecdotal
- **Clozapine** can cause constipation, as can **oxybutynin**; concurrent use might increase the risk of developing intestinal obstruction. Severe Theoretical → Also see **TABLE 8** p. 1055
- **Clozapine** can cause constipation, as can **phenothiazine antipsychotics** ; concurrent use might increase the risk of developing intestinal obstruction. Severe Theoretical → Also see **TABLE 15** p. 1058 → Also see **TABLE 6** p. 1054 → Also see **TABLE 8** p. 1055 → Also see **TABLE 9** p. 1056
- **Clozapine** can cause constipation, as can **pimozide**; concurrent use might increase the risk of developing intestinal obstruction. Severe Theoretical → Also see **TABLE 15** p. 1058 → Also see **TABLE 6** p. 1054 → Also see **TABLE 8** p. 1055 → Also see **TABLE 9** p. 1056
- **Clozapine** can cause constipation, as can **pridinol**; concurrent use might increase the risk of developing intestinal obstruction. Severe Theoretical → Also see **TABLE 8** p. 1055
- **Clozapine** can cause constipation, as can **procyclidine**; concurrent use might increase the risk of developing

Atypical antipsychotics (continued)
intestinal obstruction. Severe Theoretical → Also see TABLE 8 p. 1055 → Also see TABLE 9 p. 1056

- **Clozapine** can cause constipation, as can **propantheline**; concurrent use might increase the risk of developing intestinal obstruction. Severe Theoretical → Also see TABLE 8 p. 1055
- **Clozapine** can cause constipation, as can **propiverine**; concurrent use might increase the risk of developing intestinal obstruction. Severe Theoretical → Also see TABLE 8 p. 1055
- Quinolones **(ciprofloxacin)** increase the concentration of **clozapine**. Monitor adverse effects and adjust dose. Severe Study
- Quinolones **(ciprofloxacin)** are predicted to increase the exposure to **olanzapine**. Adjust dose. Moderate Anecdotal
- **Ribociclib** (high-dose) is predicted to increase the exposure to **quetiapine**. Avoid. Moderate Theoretical
- Rifamycins **(rifampicin)** are predicted to moderately decrease the exposure to **aripiprazole**. Avoid or adjust dose—consult product literature. Moderate Study
- Rifamycins **(rifampicin)** are predicted to decrease the exposure to **cariprazine**. Avoid. Severe Theoretical
- Rifamycins **(rifampicin)** decrease the exposure to **clozapine**. Severe Anecdotal
- Rifamycins **(rifampicin)** are predicted to decrease the exposure to **lurasidone**. Avoid. Moderate Study
- Rifamycins **(rifampicin)** are predicted to decrease the exposure to **olanzapine**. Monitor and adjust dose. Moderate Study
- Rifamycins **(rifampicin)** are predicted to decrease the exposure to **paliperidone**. Monitor and adjust dose. Severe Study
- Rifamycins **(rifampicin)** are predicted to decrease the exposure to **quetiapine**. Moderate Study
- Rifamycins **(rifampicin)** are predicted to decrease the exposure to **risperidone**. Adjust dose. Moderate Study
- **Rucaparib** increases the concentration of **clozapine**. Monitor adverse effects and adjust dose. Severe Study
- **Rucaparib** is predicted to increase the exposure to **olanzapine**. Adjust dose. Moderate Anecdotal
- **Clozapine** can cause constipation, as can **solifenacin**; concurrent use might increase the risk of developing intestinal obstruction. Severe Theoretical → Also see TABLE 8 p. 1055
- **Sotorasib** is predicted to decrease the exposure to **aripiprazole**. Avoid or adjust dose—consult product literature. Moderate Study
- **Sotorasib** is predicted to decrease the exposure to **cariprazine**. Avoid. Severe Theoretical
- **Sotorasib** is predicted to decrease the exposure to **lurasidone**. Monitor and adjust dose. Moderate Theoretical
- **Sotorasib** is predicted to decrease the exposure to **quetiapine**. Moderate Study
- SSRIs **(fluoxetine, paroxetine)** are predicted to moderately increase the exposure to **aripiprazole**. Avoid or adjust dose—consult product literature. Moderate Study → Also see TABLE 15 p. 1058 → Also see TABLE 9 p. 1056
- SSRIs **(fluoxetine, paroxetine)** are predicted to increase the exposure to **clozapine**. Use with caution and adjust dose. Severe Study → Also see TABLE 15 p. 1058 → Also see TABLE 9 p. 1056
- SSRIs **(fluoxetine, paroxetine)** are predicted to increase the exposure to **risperidone**. Adjust dose. Moderate Study → Also see TABLE 15 p. 1058 → Also see TABLE 9 p. 1056
- SSRIs **(fluvoxamine)** increase the exposure to **asenapine**. Moderate Study → Also see TABLE 15 p. 1058 → Also see TABLE 9 p. 1056
- SSRIs **(fluvoxamine)** increase the concentration of **clozapine**. Monitor adverse effects and adjust dose. Severe Study → Also see TABLE 15 p. 1058 → Also see TABLE 9 p. 1056
- SSRIs **(fluvoxamine)** moderately increase the exposure to **olanzapine**. Adjust dose. Severe Anecdotal → Also see TABLE 15 p. 1058 → Also see TABLE 9 p. 1056
- SSRIs **(paroxetine)** moderately increase the exposure to **asenapine**. Moderate Study → Also see TABLE 15 p. 1058 → Also see TABLE 9 p. 1056
- **St John's wort** is predicted to decrease the exposure to **aripiprazole**. Avoid or adjust dose—consult product literature. Moderate Study
- **St John's wort** is predicted to decrease the exposure to **cariprazine**. Avoid. Severe Theoretical
- **St John's wort** is predicted to decrease the exposure to **lurasidone**. Monitor and adjust dose. Moderate Theoretical
- **St John's wort** is predicted to decrease the exposure to **paliperidone**. Severe Theoretical
- **St John's wort** is predicted to decrease the exposure to **quetiapine**. Moderate Study
- **Sulfonamides** might increase the risk of neutropenia when given with **clozapine**. Avoid. Severe Theoretical
- **Terbinafine** is predicted to moderately increase the exposure to **aripiprazole**. Avoid or adjust dose—consult product literature. Moderate Study
- **Terbinafine** is predicted to increase the exposure to **clozapine**. Use with caution and adjust dose. Severe Study
- **Terbinafine** is predicted to increase the exposure to **risperidone**. Adjust dose. Moderate Study
- **Teriflunomide** is predicted to decrease the exposure to **clozapine**. Moderate Theoretical
- **Teriflunomide** is predicted to decrease the exposure to **olanzapine**. Monitor and adjust dose. Moderate Study
- **Clozapine** can cause constipation, as can **tiotropium**; concurrent use might increase the risk of developing intestinal obstruction. Severe Theoretical → Also see TABLE 8 p. 1055
- **Clozapine** can cause constipation, as can **tolterodine**; concurrent use might increase the risk of developing intestinal obstruction. Severe Theoretical → Also see TABLE 8 p. 1055
- **Clozapine** can cause constipation, as can **tricyclic antidepressants**; concurrent use might increase the risk of developing intestinal obstruction. Severe Theoretical → Also see TABLE 15 p. 1058 → Also see TABLE 6 p. 1054 → Also see TABLE 8 p. 1055 → Also see TABLE 9 p. 1056
- **Clozapine** can cause constipation, as can **trihexyphenidyl**; concurrent use might increase the risk of developing intestinal obstruction. Severe Theoretical → Also see TABLE 8 p. 1055 → Also see TABLE 9 p. 1056
- **Trimethoprim** might increase the risk of neutropenia when given with **clozapine**. Avoid. Severe Theoretical
- **Clozapine** can cause constipation, as can **tropicamide**; concurrent use might increase the risk of developing intestinal obstruction. Severe Theoretical → Also see TABLE 8 p. 1055
- **Clozapine** can cause constipation, as can **trospium**; concurrent use might increase the risk of developing intestinal obstruction. Severe Theoretical → Also see TABLE 8 p. 1055
- **Tucatinib** is predicted to slightly increase the exposure to **aripiprazole**. Avoid or adjust dose—consult product literature. Moderate Study
- **Tucatinib** is predicted to increase the exposure to atypical antipsychotics **(lurasidone, quetiapine)**. Avoid. Severe Study
- **Tucatinib** is predicted to moderately increase the exposure to **cariprazine**. Avoid. Severe Study
- **Tucatinib** is predicted to increase the exposure to **risperidone**. Adjust dose. Moderate Study
- **Clozapine** can cause constipation, as can **umeclidinium**; concurrent use might increase the risk of developing intestinal obstruction. Severe Theoretical → Also see TABLE 8 p. 1055
- **Clozapine** might decrease the antidiuretic and hypertensive effects of **vasopressin**. Moderate Theoretical
- **Vemurafenib** increases the concentration of **clozapine**. Monitor adverse effects and adjust dose. Severe Study
- **Vemurafenib** is predicted to increase the exposure to **olanzapine**. Adjust dose. Moderate Anecdotal
- **Clozapine** can cause constipation, as can **zuclopenthixol**; concurrent use might increase the risk of developing intestinal obstruction. Severe Theoretical → Also see TABLE 15 p. 1058 → Also see TABLE 6 p. 1054 → Also see TABLE 8 p. 1055 → Also see TABLE 9 p. 1056

Avacopan
- Anti-androgens **(apalutamide, enzalutamide)** are predicted to decrease the exposure to **avacopan**. Avoid or monitor. Severe Study
- Antiepileptics **(carbamazepine, fosphenytoin, phenobarbital, phenytoin, primidone)** are predicted to decrease the exposure to **avacopan**. Avoid or monitor. Severe Study
- Antifungals, azoles **(itraconazole, ketoconazole, posaconazole, voriconazole)** are predicted to increase the exposure to **avacopan**. Severe Study
- **Cenobamate** is predicted to decrease the exposure to **avacopan**. Severe Theoretical
- **Ceritinib** is predicted to increase the exposure to **avacopan**. Severe Study
- **Cobicistat** is predicted to increase the exposure to **avacopan**. Severe Study
- **Dabrafenib** is predicted to decrease the exposure to **avacopan**. Severe Theoretical
- **Encorafenib** is predicted to decrease the exposure to **avacopan**. Avoid or monitor. Severe Study
- Endothelin receptor antagonists **(bosentan)** are predicted to decrease the exposure to **avacopan**. Severe Theoretical
- **Grapefruit** and grapefruit juice is predicted to increase the exposure to **avacopan**. Avoid. Moderate Theoretical
- **HIV-protease inhibitors** are predicted to increase the exposure to **avacopan**. Severe Study
- **Idelalisib** is predicted to increase the exposure to **avacopan**. Severe Study
- **Ivosidenib** is predicted to decrease the exposure to **avacopan**. Avoid or monitor. Severe Study
- **Lorlatinib** is predicted to decrease the exposure to **avacopan**. Severe Theoretical
- **Lumacaftor** is predicted to decrease the exposure to **avacopan**. Avoid or monitor. Severe Study
- Macrolides **(clarithromycin)** are predicted to increase the exposure to **avacopan**. Severe Study
- **Mitotane** is predicted to decrease the exposure to **avacopan**. Avoid or monitor. Severe Study
- **Modafinil** is predicted to decrease the exposure to **avacopan**. Severe Theoretical
- NNRTIs **(efavirenz, etravirine, nevirapine)** are predicted to decrease the exposure to **avacopan**. Severe Theoretical
- Rifamycins **(rifampicin)** are predicted to decrease the exposure to **avacopan**. Avoid or monitor. Severe Study
- **Sotorasib** is predicted to decrease the exposure to **avacopan**. Severe Theoretical
- **St John's wort** is predicted to decrease the exposure to **avacopan**. Severe Theoretical
- **Avacopan** moderately increases the exposure to statins **(simvastatin)**. Adjust dose. Moderate Study
- **Tucatinib** is predicted to increase the exposure to **avacopan**. Severe Study

Avanafil → see phosphodiesterase type-5 inhibitors

Avapritinib
- Anti-androgens **(apalutamide, enzalutamide)** are predicted to decrease the exposure to **avapritinib**. Avoid. Severe Study
- Antiarrhythmics **(dronedarone)** are predicted to increase the exposure to **avapritinib**. Avoid or adjust dose—consult product literature. Moderate Study
- Antiepileptics **(carbamazepine, fosphenytoin, phenobarbital, phenytoin, primidone)** are predicted to decrease the exposure to **avapritinib**. Avoid. Severe Study
- Antifungals, azoles **(fluconazole, isavuconazole)** are predicted to increase the exposure to **avapritinib**. Avoid or adjust dose—consult product literature. Moderate Study
- Antifungals, azoles **(itraconazole, ketoconazole, posaconazole, voriconazole)** are predicted to increase the exposure to **avapritinib**. Avoid. Moderate Study
- **Berotralstat** is predicted to increase the exposure to **avapritinib**. Avoid or adjust dose—consult product literature. Moderate Study
- Calcium-channel blockers **(diltiazem, verapamil)** are predicted to increase the exposure to **avapritinib**. Avoid or adjust dose—consult product literature. Moderate Study
- **Cenobamate** is predicted to decrease the exposure to **avapritinib**. Avoid. Severe Study
- **Ceritinib** is predicted to increase the exposure to **avapritinib**. Avoid. Moderate Study
- **Cobicistat** is predicted to increase the exposure to **avapritinib**. Avoid. Moderate Study
- Corticosteroids **(dexamethasone)** are predicted to decrease the exposure to **avapritinib**. Avoid. Severe Theoretical
- **Crizotinib** is predicted to increase the exposure to **avapritinib**. Avoid or adjust dose—consult product literature. Moderate Study
- **Dabrafenib** is predicted to decrease the exposure to **avapritinib**. Avoid. Severe Study
- **Drugs that cause bleeding** (see TABLE 3 p. 1053) might increase the risk of bleeding when given with **avapritinib**. Severe Theoretical
- **Encorafenib** is predicted to decrease the exposure to **avapritinib**. Avoid. Severe Study
- Endothelin receptor antagonists **(bosentan)** are predicted to decrease the exposure to **avapritinib**. Avoid. Severe Study
- **Fedratinib** is predicted to increase the exposure to **avapritinib**. Avoid or adjust dose—consult product literature. Moderate Study
- **Grapefruit** juice is predicted to increase the exposure to **avapritinib**. Avoid. Moderate Theoretical
- **HIV-protease inhibitors** are predicted to increase the exposure to **avapritinib**. Avoid. Moderate Study
- **Idelalisib** is predicted to increase the exposure to **avapritinib**. Avoid. Moderate Study
- **Imatinib** is predicted to increase the exposure to **avapritinib**. Avoid or adjust dose—consult product literature. Moderate Study
- **Ivosidenib** is predicted to decrease the exposure to **avapritinib**. Avoid. Severe Study
- **Letermovir** is predicted to increase the exposure to **avapritinib**. Avoid or adjust dose—consult product literature. Moderate Study
- **Lorlatinib** is predicted to decrease the exposure to **avapritinib**. Avoid. Severe Study
- **Lumacaftor** is predicted to decrease the exposure to **avapritinib**. Avoid. Severe Study
- Macrolides **(clarithromycin)** are predicted to increase the exposure to **avapritinib**. Avoid. Moderate Study
- Macrolides **(erythromycin)** are predicted to increase the exposure to **avapritinib**. Avoid or adjust dose—consult product literature. Moderate Study
- **Mitotane** is predicted to decrease the exposure to **avapritinib**. Avoid. Severe Study
- **Modafinil** is predicted to decrease the exposure to **avapritinib**. Avoid. Severe Theoretical
- Neurokinin-1 receptor antagonists **(aprepitant, netupitant)** are predicted to increase the exposure to **avapritinib**. Avoid or adjust dose—consult product literature. Moderate Study
- **Nilotinib** is predicted to increase the exposure to **avapritinib**. Avoid or adjust dose—consult product literature. Moderate Study
- NNRTIs **(efavirenz, etravirine, nevirapine)** are predicted to decrease the exposure to **avapritinib**. Avoid. Severe Study
- Rifamycins **(rifampicin)** are predicted to decrease the exposure to **avapritinib**. Avoid. Severe Study
- **Sotorasib** is predicted to decrease the exposure to **avapritinib**. Avoid. Severe Study
- **St John's wort** is predicted to decrease the exposure to **avapritinib**. Avoid. Severe Study
- **Tucatinib** is predicted to increase the exposure to **avapritinib**. Avoid. Moderate Study

Avatrombopag
- Anti-androgens **(enzalutamide)** are predicted to decrease the exposure to **avatrombopag**. Adjust **avatrombopag** dose with moderate CYP2C9 inducers in chronic immune thrombocytopenia. Moderate Study
- Antiarrhythmics **(amiodarone)** are predicted to increase the exposure to **avatrombopag**. Adjust **avatrombopag** dose with moderate CYP2C9 inhibitors in chronic immune thrombocytopenia. Moderate Study

Avatrombopag (continued)
- Antifungals, azoles **(fluconazole, miconazole)** are predicted to increase the exposure to **avatrombopag**. Adjust **avatrombopag** dose with moderate CYP2C9 inhibitors in chronic immune thrombocytopenia. [Moderate] Study
- **Mifepristone** is predicted to increase the exposure to **avatrombopag**. [Moderate] Theoretical
- Rifamycins **(rifampicin)** are predicted to decrease the exposure to **avatrombopag**. Adjust **avatrombopag** dose with moderate CYP2C9 inducers in chronic immune thrombocytopenia. [Moderate] Study
- **Sparsentan** is predicted to decrease the exposure to **avatrombopag**. [Moderate] Theoretical

Avelumab → see monoclonal antibodies

Axitinib → see TABLE 3 p. 1053 (bleeding), TABLE 12 p. 1057 (myelosuppression)
- **Axitinib** is predicted to increase the exposure to **agomelatine**. [Moderate] Theoretical
- **Axitinib** is predicted to increase the exposure to **aminophylline**. [Moderate] Theoretical
- **Axitinib** is predicted to increase the exposure to anaesthetics, local **(ropivacaine)**. [Moderate] Theoretical
- Anti-androgens **(apalutamide, enzalutamide)** are predicted to decrease the exposure to **axitinib**. Avoid or adjust dose. [Moderate] Study
- Antiarrhythmics **(dronedarone)** are predicted to increase the exposure to **axitinib**. [Moderate] Study
- Antiepileptics **(carbamazepine, fosphenytoin, phenobarbital, phenytoin, primidone)** are predicted to decrease the exposure to **axitinib**. Avoid or adjust dose. [Moderate] Study
- Antifungals, azoles **(fluconazole, isavuconazole)** are predicted to increase the exposure to **axitinib**. [Moderate] Study
- Antifungals, azoles **(itraconazole, ketoconazole, posaconazole, voriconazole)** are predicted to increase the exposure to **axitinib**. Avoid or adjust dose. [Moderate] Study
- **Axitinib** might increase the exposure to the active metabolite of antimalarials **(artesunate)**. Avoid. [Unknown] Theoretical
- **Axitinib** is predicted to increase the exposure to atypical antipsychotics **(clozapine, olanzapine)**. [Moderate] Theoretical
- **Berotralstat** is predicted to increase the exposure to **axitinib**. [Moderate] Study
- Calcium-channel blockers **(diltiazem, verapamil)** are predicted to increase the exposure to **axitinib**. [Moderate] Study
- **Ceritinib** is predicted to increase the exposure to **axitinib**. Avoid or adjust dose. [Moderate] Study → Also see TABLE 12 p. 1057
- **Cobicistat** is predicted to increase the exposure to **axitinib**. Avoid or adjust dose. [Moderate] Study
- **Crizotinib** is predicted to increase the exposure to **axitinib**. [Moderate] Study
- **Dabrafenib** is predicted to decrease the exposure to **axitinib**. [Moderate] Study
- **Axitinib** is predicted to increase the exposure to dopamine receptor agonists **(ropinirole)**. [Moderate] Theoretical
- **Encorafenib** is predicted to decrease the exposure to **axitinib**. Avoid or adjust dose. [Moderate] Study
- Endothelin receptor antagonists **(bosentan)** are predicted to decrease the exposure to **axitinib**. [Moderate] Study
- **Fedratinib** is predicted to increase the exposure to **axitinib**. [Moderate] Study
- **Grapefruit** juice is predicted to increase the exposure to **axitinib**. [Moderate] Theoretical
- **HIV-protease inhibitors** are predicted to increase the exposure to **axitinib**. Avoid or adjust dose. [Moderate] Study
- **Idelalisib** is predicted to increase the exposure to **axitinib**. Avoid or adjust dose. [Moderate] Study
- **Imatinib** is predicted to increase the exposure to **axitinib**. [Moderate] Study → Also see TABLE 3 p. 1053 → Also see TABLE 12 p. 1057
- **Ivosidenib** is predicted to decrease the exposure to **axitinib**. Avoid or adjust dose. [Moderate] Study
- **Letermovir** is predicted to increase the exposure to **axitinib**. [Moderate] Study
- **Lumacaftor** is predicted to decrease the exposure to **axitinib**. Avoid or adjust dose. [Moderate] Study
- Macrolides **(clarithromycin)** are predicted to increase the exposure to **axitinib**. Avoid or adjust dose. [Moderate] Study
- Macrolides **(erythromycin)** are predicted to increase the exposure to **axitinib**. [Moderate] Study
- **Axitinib** is predicted to increase the exposure to MAO-B inhibitors **(rasagiline)**. [Moderate] Theoretical
- **Axitinib** is predicted to increase the exposure to **melatonin**. [Moderate] Theoretical
- **Mitotane** is predicted to decrease the exposure to **axitinib**. Avoid or adjust dose. [Moderate] Study → Also see TABLE 12 p. 1057
- Neurokinin-1 receptor antagonists **(aprepitant, netupitant)** are predicted to increase the exposure to **axitinib**. [Moderate] Study
- **Nilotinib** is predicted to increase the exposure to **axitinib**. [Moderate] Study → Also see TABLE 12 p. 1057
- NNRTIs **(efavirenz, nevirapine)** are predicted to decrease the exposure to **axitinib**. [Moderate] Study
- **Axitinib** is predicted to increase the exposure to **pirfenidone**. [Moderate] Theoretical
- Rifamycins **(rifampicin)** are predicted to decrease the exposure to **axitinib**. Avoid or adjust dose. [Moderate] Study
- **Axitinib** is predicted to increase the exposure to SNRIs **(duloxetine)**. [Moderate] Theoretical → Also see TABLE 3 p. 1053
- **St John's wort** is predicted to decrease the exposure to **axitinib**. Avoid or adjust dose. [Moderate] Study
- **Axitinib** is predicted to increase the exposure to **theophylline**. [Moderate] Theoretical
- **Axitinib** is predicted to increase the exposure to **tizanidine**. [Moderate] Theoretical
- **Tucatinib** is predicted to increase the exposure to **axitinib**. Avoid or adjust dose. [Moderate] Study

Azacitidine → see TABLE 12 p. 1057 (myelosuppression)
- **Cedazuridine** is predicted to increase the exposure to **azacitidine**. Avoid. [Moderate] Theoretical

Azathioprine → see TABLE 12 p. 1057 (myelosuppression)
- **ACE inhibitors** are predicted to increase the risk of anaemia and/or leucopenia when given with **azathioprine**. [Severe] Anecdotal
- **Allopurinol** potentially increases the risk of haematological toxicity when given with **azathioprine**. Adjust **azathioprine** dose, p. 638. [Severe] Study
- **Baricitinib** is predicted to enhance the risk of immunosuppression when given with **azathioprine**. [Severe] Theoretical
- **Azathioprine** decreases the anticoagulant effect of **coumarins**. [Moderate] Study
- **Febuxostat** is predicted to increase the exposure to **azathioprine**. Avoid. [Severe] Theoretical
- **Live vaccines** are predicted to increase the risk of generalised infection (possibly life-threatening) when given with **azathioprine** (high-dose). UKHSA advises avoid (refer to Green Book). [Severe] Theoretical
- **Trimethoprim** might increase the risk of haematological toxicity when given with **azathioprine** in renal transplant patients. [Severe] Anecdotal

Azelastine → see antihistamines, non-sedating

Azilsartan → see angiotensin-II receptor antagonists

Azithromycin → see macrolides

Bacillus Calmette-Guérin vaccine → see live vaccines

Baclofen → see TABLE 6 p. 1054 (hypotension), TABLE 8 p. 1055 (antimuscarinics), TABLE 9 p. 1056 (CNS effects)
- Atypical antipsychotics **(clozapine)** can cause constipation, as can **baclofen**; concurrent use might increase the risk of developing intestinal obstruction. [Severe] Theoretical → Also see TABLE 6 p. 1054 → Also see TABLE 8 p. 1055 → Also see TABLE 9 p. 1056
- **Baclofen** is predicted to increase the risk of adverse effects when given with **levodopa**. [Severe] Anecdotal → Also see TABLE 6 p. 1054 → Also see TABLE 9 p. 1056

Baloxavir marboxil
- Oral **aluminium hydroxide** might decrease the concentration of the active metabolite of oral **baloxavir marboxil**. [Severe] Theoretical
- Oral **antacids** might decrease the concentration of the active metabolite of oral **baloxavir marboxil**. Avoid. [Severe] Theoretical

- Oral **calcium compounds** might decrease the concentration of the active metabolite of oral **baloxavir marboxil**. Avoid. Severe Theoretical
- Oral **docusates** might decrease the concentration of the active metabolite of oral **baloxavir marboxil**. Severe Theoretical
- Oral **iron** might decrease the concentration of the active metabolite of oral **baloxavir marboxil**. Avoid. Severe Theoretical
- **Baloxavir marboxil** might decrease the efficacy of live vaccines **(influenza vaccine (live))**. Moderate Theoretical
- Oral **magnesium** might decrease the concentration of the active metabolite of oral **baloxavir marboxil**. Avoid. Severe Theoretical
- Oral **selenium** might decrease the concentration of the active metabolite of oral **baloxavir marboxil**. Avoid. Severe Theoretical
- Oral **sodium picosulfate** might decrease the concentration of the active metabolite of oral **baloxavir marboxil**. Severe Theoretical
- Oral **zinc** might decrease the concentration of the active metabolite of oral **baloxavir marboxil**. Avoid. Severe Theoretical

Balsalazide
- **Balsalazide** is predicted to decrease the concentration of **digoxin**. Moderate Theoretical

Baricitinib
- **Baricitinib** is predicted to enhance the risk of immunosuppression when given with **azathioprine**. Severe Theoretical
- **Baricitinib** is predicted to enhance the risk of immunosuppression when given with **ciclosporin**. Manufacturer advises caution or avoid—consult product literature. Severe Theoretical
- **Filgotinib** is predicted to increase the risk of immunosuppression when given with **baricitinib**. Avoid. Severe Theoretical
- **Leflunomide** is predicted to increase the exposure to **baricitinib**. Moderate Study
- **Live vaccines** are predicted to increase the risk of generalised infection (possibly life-threatening) when given with **baricitinib**. Avoid. Severe Theoretical
- **Baricitinib** is predicted to enhance the risk of immunosuppression when given with **methotrexate**. Severe Study
- **Nitisinone** is predicted to increase the exposure to **baricitinib**. Moderate Study
- **Baricitinib** is predicted to enhance the risk of immunosuppression when given with **tacrolimus**. Severe Theoretical
- **Teriflunomide** is predicted to increase the exposure to **baricitinib**. Moderate Study
- **Vadadustat** is predicted to increase the exposure to **baricitinib**. Moderate Study

Basiliximab → see monoclonal antibodies

Bazedoxifene
- Antiepileptics **(carbamazepine, fosphenytoin, phenobarbital, phenytoin, primidone)** are predicted to decrease the exposure to **bazedoxifene**. Moderate Theoretical
- Rifamycins **(rifampicin)** are predicted to decrease the exposure to **bazedoxifene**. Moderate Theoretical

Beclometasone → see corticosteroids

Bedaquiline → see TABLE 7 p. 1055 (QT-interval prolongation)
- Anti-androgens **(apalutamide, enzalutamide)** decrease the exposure to **bedaquiline**. Avoid. Severe Study → Also see TABLE 7 p. 1055
- Antiarrhythmics **(dronedarone)** might increase the exposure to **bedaquiline**. Mild Theoretical → Also see TABLE 7 p. 1055
- Antiepileptics **(carbamazepine, fosphenytoin, phenobarbital, phenytoin, primidone)** decrease the exposure to **bedaquiline**. Avoid. Severe Study
- Antifungals, azoles **(fluconazole, isavuconazole)** might increase the exposure to **bedaquiline**. Mild Theoretical → Also see TABLE 7 p. 1055
- Antifungals, azoles **(itraconazole, ketoconazole, posaconazole, voriconazole)** might increase the exposure to **bedaquiline**. Mild Study → Also see TABLE 7 p. 1055
- **Berotralstat** might increase the exposure to **bedaquiline**. Mild Theoretical
- Calcium-channel blockers **(diltiazem, verapamil)** might increase the exposure to **bedaquiline**. Mild Theoretical
- **Cenobamate** is predicted to decrease the exposure to **bedaquiline**. Avoid. Severe Study
- **Ceritinib** might increase the exposure to **bedaquiline**. Mild Study → Also see TABLE 7 p. 1055
- **Clofazimine** potentially increases the risk of QT-prolongation when given with **bedaquiline**. Severe Study
- **Cobicistat** might increase the exposure to **bedaquiline**. Mild Study
- **Crizotinib** might increase the exposure to **bedaquiline**. Mild Theoretical → Also see TABLE 7 p. 1055
- **Dabrafenib** is predicted to decrease the exposure to **bedaquiline**. Avoid. Severe Study
- **Encorafenib** decreases the exposure to **bedaquiline**. Avoid. Severe Study → Also see TABLE 7 p. 1055
- Endothelin receptor antagonists **(bosentan)** are predicted to decrease the exposure to **bedaquiline**. Avoid. Severe Study
- **Fedratinib** might increase the exposure to **bedaquiline**. Mild Theoretical
- **HIV-protease inhibitors** might increase the exposure to **bedaquiline**. Mild Study
- **Idelalisib** might increase the exposure to **bedaquiline**. Mild Study
- **Imatinib** might increase the exposure to **bedaquiline**. Mild Theoretical
- **Ivosidenib** decreases the exposure to **bedaquiline**. Avoid. Severe Study → Also see TABLE 7 p. 1055
- **Letermovir** might increase the exposure to **bedaquiline**. Mild Theoretical
- **Lorlatinib** is predicted to decrease the exposure to **bedaquiline**. Avoid. Severe Study
- **Lumacaftor** decreases the exposure to **bedaquiline**. Avoid. Severe Study
- Macrolides **(clarithromycin)** might increase the exposure to **bedaquiline**. Mild Study
- Macrolides **(erythromycin)** might increase the exposure to **bedaquiline**. Mild Theoretical → Also see TABLE 7 p. 1055
- **Mitotane** decreases the exposure to **bedaquiline**. Avoid. Severe Study
- Neurokinin-1 receptor antagonists **(aprepitant, netupitant)** might increase the exposure to **bedaquiline**. Mild Theoretical
- **Nilotinib** might increase the exposure to **bedaquiline**. Mild Theoretical → Also see TABLE 7 p. 1055
- **Nirmatrelvir** boosted with ritonavir is predicted to increase the concentration of **bedaquiline**. Avoid or monitor. Moderate Theoretical
- NNRTIs **(efavirenz, etravirine, nevirapine)** are predicted to decrease the exposure to **bedaquiline**. Avoid. Severe Study → Also see TABLE 7 p. 1055
- Quinolones **(ciprofloxacin)** might increase the exposure to **bedaquiline**. Mild Theoretical
- Rifamycins **(rifampicin)** decrease the exposure to **bedaquiline**. Avoid. Severe Study
- **Sotorasib** is predicted to decrease the exposure to **bedaquiline**. Avoid. Severe Study
- **St John's wort** is predicted to decrease the exposure to **bedaquiline**. Avoid. Severe Study
- **Tucatinib** might increase the exposure to **bedaquiline**. Mild Study

Bee venom extracts

GENERAL INFORMATION Desensitising vaccines should be avoided in patients taking beta-blockers (adrenaline might be ineffective in case of a hypersensitivity reaction) or ACE inhibitors (risk of severe anaphylactoid reactions).

Belatacept → see TABLE 12 p. 1057 (myelosuppression)
- **Live vaccines** are predicted to increase the risk of generalised infection (possibly life-threatening) when given with **belatacept**. UKHSA advises avoid (refer to Green Book). Severe Theoretical
- Monoclonal antibodies **(rozanolixizumab)** might decrease the concentration of **belatacept**. Avoid and for 2 weeks after stopping **rozanolixizumab**. Moderate Theoretical

Belimumab → see monoclonal antibodies

Belumosudil

- Antacids is predicted to decrease the exposure to **belumosudil**. Separate administration by 12 hours. [Moderate] Theoretical
- Anti-androgens (apalutamide, enzalutamide) are predicted to decrease the exposure to **belumosudil**. Adjust **belumosudil** dose, p. 650. [Severe] Study
- Antiepileptics (carbamazepine, fosphenytoin, phenobarbital, phenytoin, primidone) are predicted to decrease the exposure to **belumosudil**. Adjust **belumosudil** dose, p. 650. [Severe] Study
- **Belumosudil** is predicted to increase the exposure to antihistamines, non-sedating (fexofenadine). Avoid or adjust dose. [Moderate] Study
- Calcium compounds (calcium carbonate) -containing antacids are predicted to decrease the exposure to **belumosudil**. Separate administration by 12 hours. [Moderate] Theoretical
- **Belumosudil** might increase the exposure to digoxin. Avoid or adjust dose. [Moderate] Theoretical
- Encorafenib is predicted to decrease the exposure to **belumosudil**. Adjust **belumosudil** dose, p. 650. [Severe] Study
- **Belumosudil** is predicted to increase the exposure to endothelin receptor antagonists (bosentan). Avoid or adjust dose. [Moderate] Study
- **Belumosudil** might increase the exposure to everolimus. Avoid or adjust dose. [Moderate] Theoretical
- H_2 receptor antagonists are predicted to decrease the exposure to **belumosudil**. Separate administration by 12 hours. [Moderate] Theoretical
- Ivosidenib is predicted to decrease the exposure to **belumosudil**. Adjust **belumosudil** dose, p. 650. [Severe] Study
- Lumacaftor is predicted to decrease the exposure to **belumosudil**. Adjust **belumosudil** dose, p. 650. [Severe] Study
- **Belumosudil** is predicted to increase the exposure to meglitinides (repaglinide). Avoid or adjust dose. [Moderate] Study
- Mitotane is predicted to decrease the exposure to **belumosudil**. Adjust **belumosudil** dose, p. 650. [Severe] Study
- Proton pump inhibitors are predicted to decrease the exposure to **belumosudil**. Adjust **belumosudil** dose, p. 650. [Severe] Study
- **Belumosudil** is predicted to affect the exposure to raltegravir. [Moderate] Theoretical
- Rifamycins (rifampicin) are predicted to decrease the exposure to **belumosudil**. Adjust **belumosudil** dose, p. 650. [Severe] Study
- **Belumosudil** might increase the exposure to sirolimus. Avoid or adjust dose. [Moderate] Theoretical
- **Belumosudil** is predicted to increase the exposure to statins (atorvastatin, pravastatin, rosuvastatin, simvastatin). Avoid or adjust dose. [Moderate] Study
- **Belumosudil** is predicted to increase the exposure to statins (fluvastatin). Avoid or adjust dose. [Moderate] Theoretical
- **Belumosudil** is predicted to increase the exposure to sulfasalazine. Avoid or adjust dose. [Moderate] Theoretical
- **Belumosudil** is predicted to increase the exposure to sulfonylureas (glibenclamide). Avoid or adjust dose. [Moderate] Study
- **Belumosudil** might increase the exposure to talazoparib. Avoid or adjust dose. [Moderate] Theoretical
- **Belumosudil** is predicted to increase the exposure to taxanes (docetaxel, paclitaxel). Avoid or adjust dose. [Moderate] Study
- **Belumosudil** increases the exposure to thrombin inhibitors (dabigatran). Avoid or adjust dose. [Moderate] Study
- **Belumosudil** is predicted to increase the exposure to topotecan. Avoid or adjust dose. [Moderate] Theoretical

Belzutifan

- Antifungals, azoles (fluconazole, voriconazole) are predicted to increase the exposure to **belzutifan**. Monitor and adjust dose. [Severe] Theoretical
- **Belzutifan** is predicted to decrease the exposure to bosutinib. Avoid or adjust dose. [Severe] Theoretical
- Cenobamate is predicted to increase the exposure to **belzutifan**. Monitor and adjust dose. [Severe] Theoretical
- **Belzutifan** is predicted to decrease the exposure to cobimetinib. Avoid or adjust dose. [Severe] Theoretical
- **Belzutifan** might decrease the efficacy of combined hormonal contraceptives. Use additional contraceptive precautions. [Severe] Theoretical
- **Belzutifan** is predicted to decrease the exposure to dasatinib. Avoid or adjust dose. [Severe] Theoretical
- **Belzutifan** is predicted to decrease the exposure to everolimus. Avoid or adjust dose. [Severe] Theoretical
- Fedratinib is predicted to increase the exposure to **belzutifan**. Monitor and adjust dose. [Severe] Theoretical
- **Belzutifan** is predicted to decrease the exposure to ibrutinib. Avoid or adjust dose. [Severe] Theoretical
- **Belzutifan** is predicted to decrease the exposure to maraviroc. Avoid or adjust dose. [Severe] Theoretical
- Moclobemide is predicted to increase the exposure to **belzutifan**. Monitor and adjust dose. [Severe] Theoretical
- Proton pump inhibitors (esomeprazole, omeprazole) are predicted to increase the exposure to **belzutifan**. Monitor and adjust dose. [Severe] Theoretical
- **Belzutifan** is predicted to decrease the exposure to sirolimus. Avoid or adjust dose. [Severe] Theoretical
- SSRIs (fluoxetine, fluvoxamine) are predicted to increase the exposure to **belzutifan**. Monitor and adjust dose. [Severe] Theoretical
- **Belzutifan** is predicted to decrease the exposure to temsirolimus. Avoid or adjust dose. [Severe] Theoretical

Bemiparin → see low molecular-weight heparins

Bempedoic acid

- **Bempedoic acid** increases the exposure to statins (pravastatin). [Moderate] Study
- **Bempedoic acid** increases the exposure to statins (simvastatin). Adjust **simvastatin** dose, p. 156. [Moderate] Study

Bendamustine → see alkylating agents

Bendroflumethiazide → see thiazide diuretics

Benperidol → see TABLE 15 p. 1058 (hyponatraemia), TABLE 6 p. 1054 (hypotension), TABLE 9 p. 1056 (CNS effects)

- **Benperidol** is predicted to decrease the effects of dopamine receptor agonists. Avoid. [Moderate] Theoretical → Also see TABLE 6 p. 1054 → Also see TABLE 9 p. 1056
- **Benperidol** opposes the effects of the active metabolite of foslevodopa. [Severe] Theoretical → Also see TABLE 6 p. 1054 → Also see TABLE 9 p. 1056
- **Benperidol** is predicted to decrease the effects of levodopa. [Severe] Study → Also see TABLE 6 p. 1054 → Also see TABLE 9 p. 1056

Benzathine benzylpenicillin → see penicillins

Benzodiazepines → see TABLE 9 p. 1056 (CNS effects)

alprazolam · chlordiazepoxide · clobazam · clonazepam · diazepam · flurazepam · loprazolam · lorazepam · lormetazepam · midazolam · nitrazepam · oxazepam · remimazolam · temazepam

- Anti-androgens (apalutamide) are predicted to decrease the exposure to **diazepam**. Avoid or monitor. [Mild] Study
- Anti-androgens (apalutamide, enzalutamide) are predicted to decrease the exposure to **alprazolam**. Adjust dose. [Moderate] Theoretical
- Anti-androgens (apalutamide, enzalutamide) are predicted to decrease the exposure to **midazolam**. Monitor and adjust dose. [Severe] Study
- Anti-androgens (enzalutamide) are predicted to affect the exposure to **clonazepam**. Use with caution or avoid. [Moderate] Theoretical
- Antiarrhythmics (dronedarone) are predicted to increase the exposure to **alprazolam**. [Severe] Study
- Antiarrhythmics (dronedarone) are predicted to increase the exposure to **midazolam**. Monitor adverse effects and adjust dose. [Severe] Study
- Antiepileptics (carbamazepine, fosphenytoin, phenobarbital, phenytoin, primidone) are predicted to decrease the exposure to **alprazolam**. Adjust dose. [Moderate] Theoretical → Also see TABLE 9 p. 1056
- Antiepileptics (carbamazepine, fosphenytoin, phenobarbital, phenytoin, primidone) are predicted to decrease the exposure to **midazolam**. Monitor and adjust dose. [Severe] Study → Also see TABLE 9 p. 1056
- Antiepileptics (stiripentol) increase the concentration of **clobazam**. [Severe] Study
- Antiepileptics (sultiame) might increase the exposure to the active metabolite of **clobazam**. [Moderate] Theoretical

- **Chlordiazepoxide** affects the concentration of antiepileptics **(fosphenytoin, phenytoin)**. Severe Study → Also see **TABLE 9** p. 1056
- **Diazepam** potentially affects the concentration of antiepileptics **(fosphenytoin, phenytoin)**. Monitor concentration and adjust dose. Severe Study → Also see **TABLE 9** p. 1056
- Benzodiazepines **(clobazam, clonazepam)** potentially affect the concentration of antiepileptics **(fosphenytoin, phenytoin)**. Severe Anecdotal → Also see **TABLE 9** p. 1056
- Antifungals, azoles **(fluconazole, isavuconazole)** are predicted to increase the exposure to **alprazolam**. Severe Study
- Antifungals, azoles **(fluconazole, isavuconazole)** are predicted to increase the exposure to **midazolam**. Monitor adverse effects and adjust dose. Severe Study
- Antifungals, azoles **(fluconazole, voriconazole)** potentially increase the exposure to **clobazam**. Adjust dose. Moderate Theoretical
- Antifungals, azoles **(fluconazole, voriconazole)** moderately increase the exposure to **diazepam**. Monitor and adjust dose. Moderate Study
- Antifungals, azoles **(itraconazole, ketoconazole, posaconazole, voriconazole)** moderately increase the exposure to **alprazolam**. Avoid. Moderate Study
- Antifungals, azoles **(itraconazole, ketoconazole, posaconazole, voriconazole)** are predicted to markedly to very markedly increase the exposure to **midazolam**. Avoid or adjust dose. Severe Study
- Antifungals, azoles **(miconazole)** are predicted to increase the exposure to **alprazolam**. Use with caution and adjust dose. Moderate Theoretical
- Antifungals, azoles **(miconazole)** are predicted to increase the exposure to intravenous **midazolam**. Use with caution and adjust dose. Moderate Theoretical
- Antifungals, azoles **(miconazole)** are predicted to increase the exposure to oral **midazolam**. Avoid. Moderate Theoretical
- Atypical antipsychotics **(clozapine)** might increase the risk of respiratory depression and circulatory collapse when given with **benzodiazepines**. Severe Anecdotal → Also see **TABLE 9** p. 1056
- **Berotralstat** is predicted to increase the exposure to **alprazolam**. Severe Study
- **Berotralstat** is predicted to increase the exposure to **midazolam**. Monitor adverse effects and adjust dose. Severe Study
- **Bulevirtide** slightly increases the exposure to **midazolam**. Moderate Theoretical
- **Cabozantinib** is predicted to increase the exposure to **midazolam**. Moderate Theoretical
- Calcium-channel blockers **(diltiazem, verapamil)** are predicted to increase the exposure to **alprazolam**. Severe Study
- Calcium-channel blockers **(diltiazem, verapamil)** are predicted to increase the exposure to **midazolam**. Monitor adverse effects and adjust dose. Severe Study
- **Cannabidiol** increases the exposure to the active metabolite of **clobazam** and **clobazam** increases the exposure to the active metabolite of **cannabidiol**. Adjust dose. Moderate Study → Also see **TABLE 9** p. 1056
- **Cenobamate** potentially increases the exposure to **clobazam**. Adjust dose. Moderate Theoretical → Also see **TABLE 9** p. 1056
- **Cenobamate** moderately decreases the exposure to **midazolam**. Adjust dose. Moderate Study → Also see **TABLE 9** p. 1056
- **Ceritinib** moderately increases the exposure to **alprazolam**. Avoid. Moderate Study
- **Ceritinib** is predicted to markedly to very markedly increase the exposure to **midazolam**. Avoid or adjust dose. Severe Study
- **Cobicistat** moderately increases the exposure to **alprazolam**. Avoid. Moderate Study
- **Cobicistat** is predicted to markedly to very markedly increase the exposure to **midazolam**. Avoid or adjust dose. Severe Study
- **Crizotinib** is predicted to increase the exposure to **alprazolam**. Severe Study
- **Crizotinib** is predicted to increase the exposure to **midazolam**. Monitor adverse effects and adjust dose. Severe Study
- **Dabrafenib** decreases the exposure to **midazolam**. Monitor and adjust dose. Moderate Study
- **Encorafenib** is predicted to decrease the exposure to **alprazolam**. Adjust dose. Moderate Theoretical
- **Encorafenib** is predicted to decrease the exposure to **midazolam**. Monitor and adjust dose. Severe Study
- Endothelin receptor antagonists **(bosentan)** are predicted to decrease the concentration of **midazolam**. Monitor and adjust dose. Moderate Theoretical
- **Fedratinib** is predicted to increase the exposure to **alprazolam**. Severe Study
- **Fedratinib** potentially increases the exposure to **clobazam**. Adjust dose. Moderate Theoretical
- **Fedratinib** is predicted to increase the exposure to **midazolam**. Monitor adverse effects and adjust dose. Severe Study
- **Benzodiazepines** might decrease the effects of **foslevodopa**. Moderate Theoretical → Also see **TABLE 9** p. 1056
- **Givinostat** increases the exposure to **midazolam**. Moderate Study
- **HIV-protease inhibitors** moderately increase the exposure to **alprazolam**. Avoid. Moderate Study
- HIV-protease inhibitors **(ritonavir)** are predicted to increase the exposure to benzodiazepines **(diazepam, flurazepam)**. Avoid. Moderate Theoretical
- **HIV-protease inhibitors** are predicted to markedly to very markedly increase the exposure to **midazolam**. Avoid or adjust dose. Severe Study
- **Idelalisib** moderately increases the exposure to **alprazolam**. Avoid. Moderate Study
- **Idelalisib** is predicted to increase the exposure to benzodiazepines **(diazepam, flurazepam)**. Monitor and adjust dose. Moderate Theoretical
- **Idelalisib** is predicted to markedly to very markedly increase the exposure to **midazolam**. Avoid or adjust dose. Severe Study
- **Imatinib** is predicted to increase the exposure to **alprazolam**. Severe Study
- **Imatinib** is predicted to increase the exposure to **midazolam**. Monitor adverse effects and adjust dose. Severe Study
- **Ivosidenib** is predicted to decrease the exposure to **alprazolam**. Adjust dose. Moderate Theoretical
- **Ivosidenib** is predicted to decrease the exposure to **midazolam**. Monitor and adjust dose. Severe Study
- **Larotrectinib** slightly increases the exposure to **midazolam**. Use with caution and adjust dose. Mild Study
- **Lenacapavir** moderately increases the exposure to **midazolam**. Moderate Study
- **Letermovir** is predicted to increase the exposure to **alprazolam**. Severe Study
- **Letermovir** is predicted to increase the exposure to **midazolam**. Monitor adverse effects and adjust dose. Severe Study
- **Alprazolam** is predicted to increase the exposure to **lomitapide**. Separate administration by 12 hours. Moderate Theoretical
- **Lorlatinib** moderately decreases the exposure to **midazolam**. Avoid. Moderate Study
- **Lumacaftor** is predicted to decrease the exposure to **alprazolam**. Adjust dose. Moderate Theoretical
- **Lumacaftor** is predicted to decrease the exposure to **midazolam**. Monitor and adjust dose. Severe Study
- Macrolides **(clarithromycin)** moderately increase the exposure to **alprazolam**. Avoid. Moderate Study
- Macrolides **(clarithromycin)** are predicted to markedly to very markedly increase the exposure to **midazolam**. Avoid or adjust dose. Severe Study
- Macrolides **(erythromycin)** are predicted to increase the exposure to **alprazolam**. Severe Study
- Macrolides **(erythromycin)** are predicted to increase the exposure to **midazolam**. Monitor adverse effects and adjust dose. Severe Study
- **Mitotane** is predicted to decrease the exposure to **alprazolam**. Adjust dose. Moderate Theoretical
- **Mitotane** is predicted to decrease the exposure to **midazolam**. Monitor and adjust dose. Severe Study
- **Moclobemide** potentially increases the exposure to **clobazam**. Adjust dose. Moderate Theoretical
- Monoclonal antibodies **(tocilizumab)** are predicted to decrease the exposure to benzodiazepines **(alprazolam, diazepam, midazolam)**. Monitor and adjust dose. Moderate Theoretical

Benzodiazepines (continued)
- Neurokinin-1 receptor antagonists **(aprepitant, netupitant)** are predicted to increase the exposure to **alprazolam**. Severe Study
- Neurokinin-1 receptor antagonists **(aprepitant, netupitant)** are predicted to increase the exposure to **midazolam**. Monitor adverse effects and adjust dose. Severe Study
- Neurokinin-1 receptor antagonists **(fosaprepitant)** are predicted to increase the exposure to **alprazolam**. Moderate Study
- Neurokinin-1 receptor antagonists **(fosaprepitant)** slightly increase the exposure to **midazolam**. Moderate Study
- **Nilotinib** is predicted to increase the exposure to **alprazolam**. Severe Study
- **Nilotinib** is predicted to increase the exposure to **midazolam**. Monitor adverse effects and adjust dose. Severe Study
- **Nirmatrelvir** boosted with ritonavir is predicted to increase the concentration of **alprazolam**. Moderate Theoretical
- **Nirmatrelvir** boosted with ritonavir is predicted to increase the concentration of benzodiazepines **(clonazepam, diazepam, flurazepam)**. Monitor and adjust dose. Severe Theoretical
- **Nirmatrelvir** boosted with ritonavir very markedly increases the exposure to **midazolam**. Avoid or adjust dose. Severe Study
- NNRTIs **(efavirenz)** are predicted to alter the effects of **midazolam**. Avoid. Moderate Theoretical
- NNRTIs **(efavirenz, nevirapine)** are predicted to decrease the concentration of **alprazolam**. Moderate Theoretical
- NNRTIs **(etravirine)** have been reported to increase the concentration of **clobazam**. Moderate Anecdotal
- NNRTIs **(etravirine)** are predicted to increase the exposure to **diazepam**. Avoid. Severe Theoretical
- NNRTIs **(nevirapine)** are predicted to decrease the concentration of **clonazepam** and **clonazepam** is predicted to decrease the concentration of NNRTIs **(nevirapine)**. Moderate Theoretical
- NNRTIs **(nevirapine)** decrease the concentration of **midazolam**. Monitor and adjust dose. Moderate Study
- **Palbociclib** increases the exposure to **midazolam**. Moderate Study
- **Pirtobrutinib** slightly increases the exposure to oral **midazolam**. Avoid or monitor. Moderate Study
- Proton pump inhibitors **(esomeprazole, omeprazole)** potentially increase the exposure to **clobazam**. Adjust dose. Moderate Theoretical
- **Ribociclib** moderately increases the exposure to **midazolam**. Avoid. Moderate Study
- Rifamycins **(rifampicin)** are predicted to decrease the exposure to **alprazolam**. Adjust dose. Moderate Theoretical
- Rifamycins **(rifampicin)** are predicted to decrease the exposure to **chlordiazepoxide**. Moderate Theoretical
- Rifamycins **(rifampicin)** moderately decrease the exposure to **diazepam**. Avoid. Moderate Study
- Rifamycins **(rifampicin)** are predicted to decrease the exposure to **midazolam**. Monitor and adjust dose. Severe Study
- Rifamycins **(rifampicin)** increase the clearance of benzodiazepines **(lorazepam, nitrazepam)**. Moderate Study
- **Ritlecitinib** moderately increases the exposure to **midazolam**. Moderate Study
- **Rucaparib** slightly increases the exposure to **midazolam**. Monitor and adjust dose. Severe Study
- **Sotorasib** moderately decreases the exposure to **midazolam**. Moderate Study
- **Sparsentan** is predicted to decrease the exposure to **diazepam**. Moderate Theoretical
- SSRIs **(fluoxetine, fluvoxamine)** potentially increase the exposure to **clobazam**. Adjust dose. Moderate Theoretical → Also see TABLE 9 p. 1056
- SSRIs **(fluvoxamine)** moderately increase the exposure to **alprazolam**. Adjust dose. Moderate Study → Also see TABLE 9 p. 1056
- SSRIs **(fluvoxamine)** moderately increase the exposure to **diazepam**. Moderate Study → Also see TABLE 9 p. 1056
- **St John's wort** moderately decreases the exposure to **alprazolam**. Moderate Study
- **St John's wort** moderately decreases the exposure to **midazolam**. Monitor and adjust dose. Moderate Study
- **Telotristat ethyl** decreases the exposure to **midazolam**. Moderate Study
- **Tucatinib** moderately increases the exposure to **alprazolam**. Avoid. Moderate Study
- **Tucatinib** is predicted to markedly to very markedly increase the exposure to **midazolam**. Avoid or adjust dose. Severe Study
- **Vemurafenib** slightly to moderately decreases the exposure to **midazolam**. Moderate Study

Benzydamine → see NSAIDs

Benzylpenicillin → see penicillins

Berotralstat
- **Berotralstat** is predicted to increase the exposure to **abemaciclib**. Moderate Study
- **Berotralstat** is predicted to increase the exposure to **acalabrutinib**. Avoid or monitor. Severe Study
- **Berotralstat** is predicted to increase the exposure to alpha blockers **(tamsulosin)**. Moderate Theoretical
- **Berotralstat** is predicted to increase the exposure to antiarrhythmics **(propafenone)**. Monitor and adjust dose. Moderate Study
- Antiepileptics **(carbamazepine)** are predicted to decrease the concentration of **berotralstat**. Avoid. Severe Theoretical
- **Berotralstat** is predicted to increase the exposure to antifungals, azoles **(isavuconazole)**. Moderate Theoretical
- **Berotralstat** is predicted to increase the exposure to antihistamines, non-sedating **(mizolastine)**. Severe Theoretical
- **Berotralstat** is predicted to increase the exposure to antihistamines, non-sedating **(rupatadine)**. Avoid. Moderate Study
- **Berotralstat** is predicted to increase the concentration of antimalarials **(piperaquine)**. Severe Study
- **Berotralstat** is predicted to increase the exposure to **atomoxetine**. Adjust dose. Moderate Study
- **Berotralstat** is predicted to increase the exposure to atypical antipsychotics **(cariprazine)**. Monitor and adjust dose. Severe Study
- **Berotralstat** is predicted to increase the exposure to atypical antipsychotics **(quetiapine)**. Avoid. Moderate Study
- **Berotralstat** is predicted to increase the exposure to **avapritinib**. Avoid or adjust dose—consult product literature. Moderate Study
- **Berotralstat** is predicted to increase the exposure to **axitinib**. Moderate Study
- **Berotralstat** might increase the exposure to **bedaquiline**. Mild Theoretical
- **Berotralstat** is predicted to increase the exposure to benzodiazepines **(alprazolam)**. Severe Study
- **Berotralstat** is predicted to increase the exposure to benzodiazepines **(midazolam)**. Monitor adverse effects and adjust dose. Severe Study
- **Berotralstat** is predicted to increase the exposure to beta blockers, selective **(metoprolol)**. Moderate Study
- **Berotralstat** is predicted to increase the exposure to beta blockers, selective **(nebivolol)**. Adjust dose. Moderate Study
- **Berotralstat** is predicted to increase the exposure to **bosutinib**. Avoid or adjust dose. Severe Study
- **Berotralstat** is predicted to increase the exposure to **brigatinib**. Moderate Study
- **Berotralstat** is predicted to increase the exposure to **buspirone**. Use with caution and adjust dose. Moderate Study
- **Berotralstat** is predicted to increase the exposure to **cabozantinib**. Moderate Study
- **Berotralstat** is predicted to increase the exposure to calcium-channel blockers **(amlodipine, felodipine, lacidipine, lercanidipine, nicardipine, nifedipine, nimodipine)**. Monitor and adjust dose. Moderate Study
- **Berotralstat** is predicted to increase the exposure to **capivasertib**. Adjust dose. Moderate Study
- **Berotralstat** is predicted to increase the exposure to **ceritinib**. Moderate Study
- **Berotralstat** is predicted to increase the exposure to **cobimetinib**. Severe Study
- **Berotralstat** is predicted to increase the exposure to **colchicine**. Adjust **colchicine** dose with moderate CYP3A4 inhibitors, p. 637. Severe Study

- **Berotralstat** is predicted to increase the exposure to corticosteroids **(methylprednisolone)**. Monitor and adjust dose. [Moderate] Study
- **Berotralstat** is predicted to increase the exposure to **dabrafenib**. [Moderate] Study
- **Berotralstat** is predicted to increase the exposure to **daridorexant**. Adjust **daridorexant** dose. [Severe] Study
- **Berotralstat** is predicted to increase the exposure to **dasatinib**. [Severe] Study
- **Berotralstat** is predicted to increase the exposure to **deutivacaftor**. Adjust dose, see deutivacaftor with tezacaftor and vanzacaftor p. 218. [Severe] Study
- **Berotralstat** is predicted to slightly increase the exposure to **dienogest**. [Moderate] Study
- **Berotralstat** is predicted to increase the concentration of **digoxin**. Monitor and adjust dose. [Moderate] Study
- **Berotralstat** is predicted to increase the exposure to dipeptidylpeptidase-4 inhibitors **(saxagliptin)**. [Mild] Study
- **Berotralstat** is predicted to increase the exposure to **domperidone**. Avoid. [Severe] Study
- **Berotralstat** is predicted to increase the exposure to dopamine receptor agonists **(bromocriptine)**. [Severe] Theoretical
- **Berotralstat** is predicted to increase the exposure to **drospirenone**. [Severe] Study
- **Berotralstat** is predicted to moderately increase the exposure to **dutasteride**. [Mild] Study
- **Berotralstat** is predicted to increase the exposure to **elacestrant**. Avoid moderate CYP3A4 inhibitors or adjust **elacestrant** dose. [Severe] Theoretical
- **Berotralstat** is predicted to increase the exposure to **elexacaftor**. Adjust ivacaftor with tezacaftor and elexacaftor p. 220 dose with moderate CYP3A4 inhibitors. [Severe] Theoretical
- **Berotralstat** is predicted to increase the exposure to **eliglustat**. Avoid or adjust dose—consult product literature. [Severe] Study
- **Berotralstat** is predicted to moderately increase the exposure to **encorafenib**. [Moderate] Study
- **Berotralstat** is predicted to increase the exposure to endothelin receptor antagonists **(macitentan)**. Manufacturer advises caution depending on other drugs taken—consult product literature. [Moderate] Theoretical
- **Berotralstat** is predicted to increase the exposure to **entrectinib**. Avoid or adjust dose with moderate CYP3A4 inhibitors—consult product literature. [Severe] Theoretical
- **Berotralstat** is predicted to increase the risk of ergotism when given with **ergometrine**. [Severe] Theoretical
- **Berotralstat** is predicted to increase the exposure to **erlotinib**. [Moderate] Study
- **Berotralstat** is predicted to increase the exposure to **etrasimod**. Avoid in poor CYP2C9 metabolisers. [Severe] Theoretical
- **Berotralstat** is predicted to increase the concentration of **everolimus**. Avoid or adjust dose. [Moderate] Study
- **Berotralstat** is predicted to increase the exposure to **fedratinib**. Monitor and adjust dose. [Moderate] Study
- **Berotralstat** is predicted to increase the exposure to **fesoterodine**. Adjust **fesoterodine** dose with moderate CYP3A4 inhibitors in hepatic and renal impairment. [Mild] Study
- **Berotralstat** is predicted to increase the exposure to **gefitinib**. [Moderate] Study
- **Grapefruit** juice is predicted to increase the exposure to **berotralstat**. [Moderate] Theoretical
- **Berotralstat** is predicted to increase the concentration of **guanfacine**. Adjust **guanfacine** dose, p. 281. [Moderate] Theoretical
- **Berotralstat** is predicted to increase the exposure to **ibrutinib**. Adjust dose with moderate CYP3A4 inhibitors—consult product literature. [Severe] Study
- **Berotralstat** is predicted to increase the exposure to the active metabolite of **irinotecan**. [Moderate] Theoretical
- **Berotralstat** is predicted to increase the exposure to **ivacaftor**. Adjust dose with moderate CYP3A4 inhibitors, see ivacaftor p. 219, tezacaftor with ivacaftor p. 223, and ivacaftor with tezacaftor and elexacaftor p. 220. [Moderate] Study
- **Berotralstat** is predicted to increase the exposure to **ivosidenib**. Monitor and adjust dose—consult product literature. [Severe] Study
- **Berotralstat** is predicted to increase the exposure to **lapatinib**. [Moderate] Study
- **Berotralstat** is predicted to increase the exposure to **larotrectinib**. Monitor and adjust dose. [Moderate] Theoretical
- **Berotralstat** is predicted to increase the exposure to **leniolisib**. Avoid. [Moderate] Study
- **Berotralstat** is predicted to increase the exposure to **lomitapide**. Avoid. [Moderate] Theoretical
- **Lorlatinib** is predicted to decrease the concentration of **berotralstat**. Avoid. [Severe] Theoretical
- **Berotralstat** is predicted to increase the exposure to **mavacamten**. Adjust dose—consult product literature. [Moderate] Study
- **Berotralstat** is predicted to increase the exposure to **midostaurin**. [Moderate] Theoretical
- **Berotralstat** is predicted to increase the exposure to mineralocorticoid receptor antagonists **(eplerenone)**. Adjust **eplerenone** dose. [Severe] Study
- **Berotralstat** is predicted to increase the exposure to mineralocorticoid receptor antagonists **(finerenone)**. [Severe] Study
- **Berotralstat** is predicted to increase the exposure to **naldemedine**. [Moderate] Study
- **Berotralstat** is predicted to increase the exposure to **naloxegol**. Adjust **naloxegol** dose and monitor adverse effects. [Moderate] Study
- **Berotralstat** is predicted to increase the exposure to **neratinib**. Avoid moderate CYP3A4 inhibitors or adjust dose and monitor for gastrointestinal adverse effects—consult product literature. [Severe] Study
- **Berotralstat** is predicted to increase the exposure to **olaparib**. Avoid or adjust dose with moderate CYP3A4 inhibitors—consult product literature. [Moderate] Theoretical
- **Berotralstat** is predicted to increase the exposure to **omaveloxolone**. Avoid or adjust **omaveloxolone** dose, p. 755. [Moderate] Study
- **Berotralstat** is predicted to increase the exposure to opioids **(alfentanil, buprenorphine, fentanyl, oxycodone)**. Monitor and adjust dose. [Moderate] Study
- **Berotralstat** is predicted to increase the exposure to opioids **(methadone, sufentanil)**. [Moderate] Theoretical
- **Berotralstat** is predicted to increase the exposure to **pazopanib**. [Moderate] Study
- **Berotralstat** is predicted to increase the exposure to **pemigatinib**. [Severe] Study
- **Berotralstat** is predicted to increase the exposure to phosphodiesterase type-5 inhibitors **(avanafil)**. Adjust **avanafil** dose. [Moderate] Theoretical
- **Berotralstat** is predicted to increase the exposure to phosphodiesterase type-5 inhibitors **(sildenafil)**. Monitor or adjust **sildenafil** dose with moderate CYP3A4 inhibitors, p. 139. [Moderate] Study
- **Berotralstat** is predicted to increase the exposure to phosphodiesterase type-5 inhibitors **(tadalafil)**. [Severe] Theoretical
- **Berotralstat** is predicted to increase the exposure to phosphodiesterase type-5 inhibitors **(vardenafil)**. Adjust dose. [Severe] Theoretical
- **Berotralstat** is predicted to increase the exposure to **pimozide**. Avoid. [Severe] Theoretical
- **Berotralstat** is predicted to increase the exposure to **ponatinib**. [Moderate] Study
- **Berotralstat** is predicted to increase the exposure to **pralsetinib**. [Moderate] Theoretical
- **Berotralstat** is predicted to increase the exposure to **ranolazine**. [Severe] Study
- **Berotralstat** is predicted to increase the exposure to **regorafenib**. [Moderate] Study
- **Berotralstat** is predicted to increase the exposure to **ribociclib**. [Moderate] Study
- Rifamycins **(rifampicin)** are predicted to decrease the concentration of **berotralstat**. Avoid. [Severe] Theoretical
- **Berotralstat** is predicted to increase the exposure to **rimegepant**. Avoid another dose of rimegepant within 48 hours of concurrent use. [Moderate] Study
- **Berotralstat** is predicted to increase the exposure to **ruxolitinib**. [Moderate] Study

Berotralstat (continued)
- **Berotralstat** is predicted to increase the exposure to **selpercatinib**. Moderate Study
- **Berotralstat** is predicted to increase the exposure to **selumetinib**. Avoid or adjust dose—consult product literature. Severe Study
- **Berotralstat** is predicted to increase the exposure to **siponimod**. Avoid depending on other drugs taken—consult product literature. Severe Study
- **Berotralstat** increases the concentration of **sirolimus**. Monitor and adjust dose. Moderate Study
- **Berotralstat** is predicted to increase the exposure to **sparsentan**. Moderate Study
- **Berotralstat** is predicted to increase the exposure to SSRIs **(dapoxetine)**. Adjust **dapoxetine** dose with moderate CYP3A4 inhibitors. Moderate Theoretical
- **Berotralstat** is predicted to increase the exposure to SSRIs **(sertraline)**. Moderate Theoretical
- **St John's wort** is predicted to decrease the concentration of **berotralstat**. Avoid. Severe Theoretical
- **Berotralstat** is predicted to increase the exposure to **sunitinib**. Moderate Study
- **Berotralstat** is predicted to increase the concentration of **tacrolimus**. Monitor and adjust dose. Severe Theoretical
- **Berotralstat** is predicted to increase the concentration of **talazoparib**. Monitor and adjust dose. Moderate Study
- **Berotralstat** is predicted to increase the exposure to taxanes **(cabazitaxel)**. Moderate Theoretical
- **Berotralstat** is predicted to increase the exposure to taxanes **(docetaxel)**. Severe Study
- **Berotralstat** is predicted to increase the exposure to taxanes **(paclitaxel)**. Moderate Anecdotal
- **Berotralstat** is predicted to increase the exposure to **temsirolimus**. Use with caution or avoid. Moderate Study
- **Berotralstat** is predicted to increase the exposure to **tezacaftor**. Adjust dose with moderate CYP3A4 inhibitors, see tezacaftor with ivacaftor p. 223, ivacaftor with tezacaftor and elexacaftor p. 220, and deutivacaftor with tezacaftor and vanzacaftor p. 218. Severe Study
- **Berotralstat** is predicted to increase the exposure to **tolvaptan**. Manufacturer advises caution or adjust **tolvaptan** dose with moderate CYP3A4 inhibitors. Moderate Study
- **Berotralstat** is predicted to increase the exposure to **trazodone**. Moderate Theoretical
- **Berotralstat** is predicted to increase the exposure to **tricyclic antidepressants**. Monitor and adjust dose. Moderate Theoretical
- **Berotralstat** is predicted to increase the exposure to **vanzacaftor**. Adjust dose, see deutivacaftor with tezacaftor and vanzacaftor p. 218. Severe Study
- **Berotralstat** is predicted to increase the exposure to **vemurafenib**. Severe Theoretical
- **Berotralstat** is predicted to increase the exposure to **venetoclax**. Avoid or adjust dose—consult product literature. Severe Study
- **Berotralstat** is predicted to increase the exposure to **vinca alkaloids**. Severe Theoretical
- **Berotralstat** is predicted to increase the exposure to **voclosporin**. Adjust **voclosporin** dose. Severe Study
- **Berotralstat** is predicted to increase the exposure to **zanubrutinib**. Avoid or adjust dose with moderate CYP3A4 inhibitors—consult product literature. Severe Study
- **Berotralstat** is predicted to increase the exposure to **zopiclone**. Adjust dose. Moderate Study

Beta blockers, non-selective → see TABLE 4 p. 1054 (bradycardia), TABLE 6 p. 1054 (hypotension), TABLE 13 p. 1057 (increased serum potassium), TABLE 7 p. 1055 (QT-interval prolongation)

carvedilol · labetalol · levobunolol · nadolol · pindolol · propranolol · sotalol · timolol

ROUTE-SPECIFIC INFORMATION Since systemic absorption can follow topical application of **levobunolol** or **timolol**, the possibility of interactions should be borne in mind.

- **Beta blockers, non-selective** are predicted to increase the risk of bronchospasm when given with **aminophylline**. Avoid. Severe Theoretical
- Anti-androgens **(enzalutamide)** are predicted to affect the exposure to **propranolol**. Use with caution or avoid. Moderate Theoretical
- Antiarrhythmics **(amiodarone, disopyramide, dronedarone, flecainide, lidocaine)** are predicted to increase the risk of cardiovascular adverse effects when given with **beta blockers, non-selective**. Use with caution or avoid. Severe Study → Also see TABLE 4 p. 1054 → Also see TABLE 7 p. 1055
- Antiarrhythmics **(propafenone)** increase the risk of cardiovascular adverse effects when given with **propranolol**. Use with caution or avoid. Severe Study → Also see TABLE 4 p. 1054
- Antiarrhythmics **(propafenone)** are predicted to increase the exposure to **timolol** and **timolol** is predicted to increase the risk of cardiodepression when given with antiarrhythmics **(propafenone)**. Severe Anecdotal → Also see TABLE 4 p. 1054
- Antiarrhythmics **(propafenone)** are predicted to increase the risk of cardiovascular adverse effects when given with beta blockers, non-selective **(labetalol, levobunolol, nadolol, pindolol, sotalol)**. Use with caution or avoid. Severe Study → Also see TABLE 4 p. 1054
- Antiepileptics **(phenobarbital, primidone)** are predicted to decrease the exposure to **propranolol**. Moderate Study
- Antiepileptics **(phenobarbital, primidone)** are predicted to decrease the exposure to beta blockers, non-selective **(carvedilol, labetalol)**. Moderate Theoretical
- Antifungals, azoles **(itraconazole, ketoconazole)** are predicted to increase the exposure to **nadolol**. Moderate Study
- Antimalarials **(mefloquine)** are predicted to increase the risk of bradycardia when given with **beta blockers, non-selective**. Severe Theoretical
- Calcium-channel blockers **(diltiazem)** are predicted to increase the risk of cardiodepression when given with **beta blockers, non-selective**. Severe Study → Also see TABLE 4 p. 1054 → Also see TABLE 6 p. 1054
- Calcium-channel blockers **(verapamil)** increase the risk of cardiovascular adverse effects when given with **beta blockers, non-selective**. Avoid intravenous **verapamil**. Severe Study → Also see TABLE 4 p. 1054 → Also see TABLE 6 p. 1054
- **Chloroprocaine** is predicted to increase the risk of cardiovascular adverse effects when given with **sotalol**. Severe Theoretical
- **Ciclosporin** is predicted to increase the exposure to **nadolol**. Moderate Study
- **Dacomitinib** is predicted to markedly increase the exposure to **propranolol**. Avoid. Severe Study
- **Eliglustat** is predicted to increase the exposure to **propranolol**. Adjust dose. Moderate Study
- **Beta blockers, non-selective** are predicted to increase the risk of peripheral vasoconstriction when given with **ergometrine**. Severe Study
- **Carvedilol** is predicted to increase the exposure to **gilteritinib**. Moderate Theoretical
- HIV-protease inhibitors **(lopinavir, ritonavir)** are predicted to increase the exposure to **nadolol**. Moderate Study
- **Beta blockers, non-selective** are predicted to increase the risk of bradycardia when given with **lanreotide**. Moderate Theoretical
- **Lapatinib** is predicted to increase the exposure to **nadolol**. Moderate Study
- **Macrolides** are predicted to increase the exposure to **nadolol**. Moderate Study
- **Mavacamten** can cause negative inotropic effects, as can **beta blockers, non-selective**. Severe Theoretical
- **Mexiletine** potentially increases the risk of cardiovascular adverse effects when given with **beta blockers, non-selective**. Avoid or monitor. Severe Theoretical
- **Omega-3-acid ethyl esters** might enhance the blood pressure-lowering effects of **beta blockers, non-selective**. Moderate Study
- **Ranolazine** is predicted to increase the exposure to **nadolol**. Moderate Study
- **Carvedilol** is predicted to increase the exposure to **relugolix**. Avoid or take relugolix first and separate administration by at least 6 hours. Moderate Theoretical
- Rifamycins **(rifampicin)** moderately decrease the exposure to **carvedilol**. Moderate Study

- Rifamycins **(rifampicin)** decrease the exposure to **propranolol**. Monitor and adjust dose. Moderate Study
- SSRIs **(fluvoxamine)** moderately increase the concentration of **propranolol**. Moderate Study
- **Beta blockers, non-selective** increase the risk of hypertension and bradycardia when given with sympathomimetics, inotropic **(dobutamine)**. Severe Theoretical
- **Beta blockers, non-selective** are predicted to increase the risk of hypertension and bradycardia when given with sympathomimetics, vasoconstrictor **(adrenaline, noradrenaline)**. Severe Study
- **Carvedilol** causes a small increase in the bioavailability of **talazoparib**. Avoid or adjust dose—consult product literature. Moderate Study
- **Beta blockers, non-selective** are predicted to increase the risk of bronchospasm when given with **theophylline**. Avoid. Severe Theoretical
- **Propranolol** slightly to moderately increases the exposure to triptans **(rizatriptan)**. Adjust **rizatriptan** dose and separate administration by at least 2 hours. Moderate Study
- **Vemurafenib** is predicted to increase the exposure to **nadolol**. Moderate Study

Beta blockers, selective → see TABLE 4 p. 1054 (bradycardia), TABLE 6 p. 1054 (hypotension)

acebutolol · atenolol · betaxolol · bisoprolol · celiprolol · esmolol · landiolol · metoprolol · nebivolol

- Since systemic absorption can follow topical application of **betaxolol**, the possibility of interactions should be borne in mind.
- Orange juice greatly decreases the exposure to **celiprolol**.

- **Beta blockers, selective** are predicted to increase the risk of bronchospasm when given with **aminophylline**. Avoid. Severe Theoretical
- Anti-androgens **(abiraterone)** are predicted to increase the exposure to **metoprolol**. Moderate Study
- Anti-androgens **(enzalutamide)** are predicted to affect the exposure to **bisoprolol**. Use with caution or avoid. Moderate Theoretical
- Antiarrhythmics **(amiodarone, disopyramide, dronedarone, flecainide, lidocaine)** are predicted to increase the risk of cardiovascular adverse effects when given with **beta blockers, selective**. Use with caution or avoid. Severe Study → Also see TABLE 4 p. 1054
- Antiarrhythmics **(propafenone)** are predicted to increase the exposure to **metoprolol**. Moderate Study → Also see TABLE 4 p. 1054
- Antiarrhythmics **(propafenone)** are predicted to increase the exposure to **nebivolol** and **nebivolol** is predicted to increase the risk of cardiodepression when given with antiarrhythmics **(propafenone)**. Avoid. Severe Theoretical → Also see TABLE 4 p. 1054
- Antiarrhythmics **(propafenone)** are predicted to increase the risk of cardiovascular adverse effects when given with beta blockers, selective **(acebutolol, atenolol, betaxolol, bisoprolol, celiprolol, esmolol)**. Use with caution or avoid. Severe Study → Also see TABLE 4 p. 1054
- Antiepileptics **(phenobarbital, primidone)** are predicted to decrease the exposure to beta blockers, selective **(acebutolol, bisoprolol, metoprolol, nebivolol)**. Moderate Study
- Antimalarials **(mefloquine)** are predicted to increase the risk of bradycardia when given with **beta blockers, selective**. Severe Theoretical
- **Berotralstat** is predicted to increase the exposure to **metoprolol**. Moderate Study
- **Berotralstat** is predicted to increase the exposure to **nebivolol**. Adjust dose. Moderate Study
- **Bupropion** is predicted to increase the exposure to beta blockers, selective **(metoprolol, nebivolol)**. Moderate Study
- Calcium-channel blockers **(diltiazem)** are predicted to increase the risk of cardiodepression when given with **beta blockers, selective**. Avoid or monitor. Severe Study → Also see TABLE 4 p. 1054 → Also see TABLE 6 p. 1054
- Calcium-channel blockers **(verapamil)** increase the risk of cardiovascular adverse effects when given with **beta blockers, selective**. Use with caution or avoid. Severe Study → Also see TABLE 4 p. 1054 → Also see TABLE 6 p. 1054
- **Cinacalcet** is predicted to increase the exposure to beta blockers, selective **(metoprolol, nebivolol)**. Moderate Study
- **Dacomitinib** is predicted to increase the exposure to beta blockers, selective **(metoprolol, nebivolol)**. Moderate Study
- **Eliglustat** is predicted to increase the exposure to **metoprolol**. Adjust dose. Moderate Study
- **Beta blockers, selective** are predicted to increase the risk of peripheral vasoconstriction when given with **ergometrine**. Severe Study
- **Givosiran** is predicted to increase the exposure to **metoprolol**. Moderate Study
- **Givosiran** is predicted to increase the exposure to **nebivolol**. Use with caution and adjust dose. Moderate Study
- **Grapefruit** juice greatly decreases the exposure to **celiprolol**. Moderate Study
- HIV-protease inhibitors **(ritonavir)** are predicted to increase the exposure to **metoprolol**. Moderate Study
- Interferons **(ropeginterferon alfa)** are predicted to increase the exposure to **nebivolol**. Moderate Theoretical
- **Beta blockers, selective** are predicted to increase the risk of bradycardia when given with **lanreotide**. Moderate Theoretical
- **Mavacamten** can cause negative inotropic effects, as can **beta blockers, selective**. Severe Theoretical
- **Mexiletine** potentially increases the risk of cardiovascular adverse effects when given with **beta blockers, selective**. Avoid or monitor. Severe Theoretical
- **Mirabegron** is predicted to increase the exposure to **metoprolol**. Moderate Study
- **Omega-3-acid ethyl esters** might enhance the blood pressure-lowering effects of **beta blockers, selective**. Moderate Study
- **Panobinostat** is predicted to increase the exposure to **metoprolol**. Monitor and adjust dose. Moderate Theoretical
- **Panobinostat** is predicted to increase the exposure to **nebivolol**. Monitor and adjust dose. Mild Theoretical
- Rifamycins **(rifampicin)** moderately decrease the exposure to **celiprolol**. Moderate Study
- Rifamycins **(rifampicin)** slightly decrease the exposure to beta blockers, selective **(bisoprolol, metoprolol)**. Mild Study
- SNRIs **(duloxetine)** are predicted to increase the exposure to **metoprolol**. Moderate Study
- SSRIs **(fluoxetine, paroxetine)** are predicted to increase the exposure to beta blockers, selective **(metoprolol, nebivolol)**. Moderate Study
- **Suxamethonium** might increase the concentration of **landiolol** and **landiolol** might prolong the effects of **suxamethonium**. Moderate Study → Also see TABLE 4 p. 1054
- **Beta blockers, selective** increase the risk of hypertension and bradycardia when given with sympathomimetics, inotropic **(dobutamine)**. Moderate Theoretical
- **Beta blockers, selective** are predicted to increase the risk of hypertension and bradycardia when given with sympathomimetics, vasoconstrictor **(adrenaline, noradrenaline)**. Severe Study
- **Terbinafine** is predicted to increase the exposure to beta blockers, selective **(metoprolol, nebivolol)**. Moderate Study
- **Beta blockers, selective** are predicted to increase the risk of bronchospasm when given with **theophylline**. Avoid. Severe Theoretical
- **Vaborbactam** is predicted to increase the concentration of **metoprolol**. Unknown Theoretical

Beta$_2$ agonists → see TABLE 14 p. 1057 (reduced serum potassium)

formoterol · indacaterol · olodaterol · salbutamol · salmeterol · terbutaline · vilanterol

- Anti-androgens **(apalutamide)** are predicted to decrease the exposure to **salmeterol**. Avoid or monitor. Moderate Study
- Antifungals, azoles **(itraconazole, ketoconazole, posaconazole, voriconazole)** are predicted to increase the exposure to **salmeterol**. Avoid. Severe Study
- **Atomoxetine** is predicted to increase the risk of cardiovascular adverse effects when given with **beta$_2$ agonists** (high-dose). Moderate Study
- **Cenobamate** is predicted to decrease the exposure to **salmeterol**. Adjust dose. Moderate Theoretical

Beta$_2$ agonists (continued)
- **Ceritinib** is predicted to increase the exposure to **salmeterol**. Avoid. Severe Study
- **Cobicistat** is predicted to increase the exposure to **salmeterol**. Avoid. Severe Study
- **HIV-protease inhibitors** are predicted to increase the exposure to **salmeterol**. Avoid. Severe Study
- **Idelalisib** is predicted to increase the exposure to **salmeterol**. Avoid. Severe Study
- **Beta$_2$ agonists** are predicted to increase the risk of glaucoma when given with **ipratropium**. Moderate Anecdotal
- **Ivosidenib** might decrease the exposure to **salmeterol**. Avoid or monitor. Moderate Theoretical
- **Beta$_2$ agonists** are predicted to increase the risk of elevated blood pressure when given with **linezolid**. Avoid. Severe Theoretical
- Macrolides **(clarithromycin)** are predicted to increase the exposure to **salmeterol**. Avoid. Severe Study
- MAO-B inhibitors **(rasagiline, selegiline)** are predicted to increase the risk of severe hypertension when given with **beta$_2$ agonists**. Avoid. Severe Theoretical
- MAO-B inhibitors **(safinamide)** are predicted to increase the risk of severe hypertension when given with **beta$_2$ agonists**. Severe Theoretical
- **MAOIs, irreversible** are predicted to increase the risk of cardiovascular adverse effects when given with **beta$_2$ agonists**. Moderate Anecdotal
- Neurokinin-1 receptor antagonists **(aprepitant, netupitant)** are predicted to increase the exposure to **salmeterol**. Moderate Study
- **Nirmatrelvir** boosted with ritonavir is predicted to increase the concentration of **salmeterol**. Avoid. Severe Theoretical
- **Tucatinib** is predicted to increase the exposure to **salmeterol**. Avoid. Severe Study

Betahistine
- **Antihistamines, non-sedating** are predicted to decrease the effects of **betahistine**. Moderate Theoretical
- **Antihistamines, sedating** are predicted to decrease the effects of **betahistine**. Moderate Theoretical

Betamethasone → see corticosteroids
Betaxolol → see beta blockers, selective
Bevacizumab → see monoclonal antibodies
Bexarotene → see retinoids
Bezafibrate → see fibrates
Bicalutamide → see anti-androgens

Bictegravir
- Oral **antacids** decrease the exposure to oral **bictegravir**. Separate administration by at least 2 hours. Moderate Study
- Anti-androgens **(apalutamide, enzalutamide)** are predicted to decrease the exposure to **bictegravir**. Avoid. Moderate Study
- Antiepileptics **(carbamazepine, fosphenytoin, phenobarbital, phenytoin, primidone)** are predicted to decrease the exposure to **bictegravir**. Avoid. Moderate Study
- Antiepileptics **(oxcarbazepine)** are predicted to decrease the exposure to **bictegravir**. Avoid. Moderate Theoretical
- **Ciclosporin** is predicted to increase the exposure to **bictegravir**. Avoid or monitor. Moderate Theoretical
- **Encorafenib** is predicted to decrease the exposure to **bictegravir**. Avoid. Moderate Study
- HIV-protease inhibitors **(atazanavir)** moderately increase the exposure to **bictegravir**. Avoid. Moderate Study
- Oral **iron** decreases the exposure to oral **bictegravir**. Manufacturer advises bictegravir should be taken 2 hours before iron. Moderate Study
- **Ivosidenib** is predicted to decrease the exposure to **bictegravir**. Avoid. Moderate Study
- **Lumacaftor** is predicted to decrease the exposure to **bictegravir**. Avoid. Moderate Study
- **Bictegravir** slightly increases the exposure to **metformin**. Moderate Study
- **Mitotane** is predicted to decrease the exposure to **bictegravir**. Avoid. Moderate Study
- Rifamycins **(rifabutin)** slightly decrease the exposure to **bictegravir**. Avoid. Mild Study
- Rifamycins **(rifampicin)** are predicted to decrease the exposure to **bictegravir**. Avoid. Moderate Study
- **St John's wort** is predicted to decrease the exposure to **bictegravir**. Avoid. Moderate Theoretical
- **Sucralfate** is predicted to decrease the exposure to **bictegravir**. Avoid. Moderate Theoretical

Bilastine → see antihistamines, non-sedating
Bimekizumab → see monoclonal antibodies
Bismuth compounds → see TABLE 3 p. 1053 (bleeding)

bismuth subcitrate potassium · bismuth subsalicylate

- Oral **bismuth subsalicylate** greatly decreases the absorption of oral **tetracyclines**. Separate administration by at least 2 to 3 hours. Moderate Study

Bismuth subcitrate potassium → see bismuth compounds
Bismuth subsalicylate → see bismuth compounds
Bisoprolol → see beta blockers, selective
Bisphosphonates → see TABLE 2 p. 1053 (nephrotoxicity)

alendronate · clodronate · ibandronate · pamidronate · risedronate · zoledronate

- **Aminoglycosides** increase the risk of hypocalcaemia when given with **bisphosphonates**. Moderate Anecdotal → Also see TABLE 2 p. 1053
- Oral **antacids** decrease the absorption of oral **alendronate**. Manufacturer advises take at least 30 minutes before antacids. Moderate Study
- Oral **antacids** decrease the absorption of oral **clodronate**. Avoid antacids for 2 hours before or 1 hour after **clodronate**. Moderate Study
- Oral **antacids** are predicted to decrease the absorption of oral **ibandronate**. Avoid antacids for at least 6 hours before or 1 hour after **ibandronate**. Moderate Theoretical
- Oral **antacids** decrease the absorption of oral **risedronate**. Separate administration by at least 2 hours. Moderate Study
- **Aspirin** (high-dose) is predicted to increase the risk of gastrointestinal irritation when given with bisphosphonates **(alendronate, ibandronate)**. Moderate Study
- **Aspirin** (high-dose) is predicted to increase the risk of renal impairment when given with **clodronate**. Severe Theoretical
- Oral **calcium compounds** decrease the absorption of oral **alendronate**. **Alendronate** should be taken at least 30 minutes before calcium. Moderate Study
- Oral **calcium compounds** decrease the absorption of oral **clodronate**. Avoid **calcium compounds** for 2 hours before or 1 hour after **clodronate**. Moderate Study
- Oral **calcium compounds** are predicted to decrease the absorption of oral **ibandronate**. Avoid **calcium compounds** for at least 6 hours before or 1 hour after **ibandronate**. Moderate Theoretical
- Oral **calcium compounds** decrease the absorption of oral **risedronate**. Separate administration by at least 2 hours. Moderate Study
- Oral **iron** decreases the absorption of oral **clodronate**. **Clodronate** should be taken 1 hour before or 2 hours after iron. Moderate Study
- Oral **iron** is predicted to decrease the absorption of oral **ibandronate**. **Ibandronate** should be taken 1 hour before or 6 hours after iron. Moderate Theoretical
- Oral **iron** decreases the absorption of oral **risedronate**. Separate administration by at least 2 hours. Moderate Study
- **Bisphosphonates** are predicted to increase the risk of gastrointestinal bleeding when given with iron chelators **(deferasirox)**. Severe Theoretical → Also see TABLE 2 p. 1053
- Oral **magnesium** decreases the absorption of oral **alendronate**. Manufacturer advises take at least 30 minutes before magnesium. Moderate Study
- Oral **magnesium** decreases the absorption of oral **clodronate**. Avoid magnesium for 2 hours before or 1 hour after **clodronate**. Moderate Study
- Oral **magnesium** is predicted to decrease the absorption of oral **ibandronate**. Avoid for at least 6 hours before or 1 hour after **ibandronate**. Moderate Theoretical
- Oral **magnesium** decreases the absorption of oral **risedronate**. Separate administration by at least 2 hours. Moderate Study

- **NSAIDs** are predicted to increase the risk of gastrointestinal irritation when given with bisphosphonates **(alendronate, ibandronate)**. Moderate Study
- **NSAIDs** are predicted to increase the risk of renal impairment when given with **clodronate**. Moderate Study
- **Bisphosphonates** are predicted to decrease the effects of **parathyroid hormone**. Avoid. Moderate Study
- Oral **zinc** decreases the absorption of oral **alendronate**. **Alendronate** should be taken at least 30 minutes before **zinc**. Moderate Study
- Oral **zinc** decreases the absorption of oral **clodronate**. Avoid **zinc** for 2 hours before or 1 hour after **clodronate**. Moderate Study
- Oral **zinc** is predicted to decrease the absorption of oral **ibandronate**. Avoid **zinc** for at least 6 hours before or 1 hour after **ibandronate**. Moderate Theoretical
- Oral **zinc** decreases the absorption of oral **risedronate**. Separate administration by at least 2 hours. Moderate Study

Bivalirudin → see thrombin inhibitors

Bleomycin → see TABLE 12 p. 1057 (myelosuppression)

- **Bleomycin**-containing cytotoxic regimens might affect the concentration of antiepileptics **(fosphenytoin, phenytoin)**. Avoid. Severe Anecdotal
- **Filgrastim** might increase the risk of pulmonary toxicity when given with **bleomycin**. Severe Theoretical
- **Lenograstim** might increase the risk of pulmonary toxicity when given with **bleomycin**. Severe Theoretical
- **Lipegfilgrastim** might increase the risk of pulmonary toxicity when given with **bleomycin**. Severe Theoretical
- **Live vaccines** are predicted to increase the risk of generalised infection (possibly life-threatening) when given with **bleomycin**. UKHSA advises avoid (refer to Green Book). Severe Theoretical
- Monoclonal antibodies **(brentuximab vedotin)** increase the risk of pulmonary toxicity when given with **bleomycin**. Avoid. Severe Study → Also see TABLE 12 p. 1057
- **Pegfilgrastim** might increase the risk of pulmonary toxicity when given with **bleomycin**. Severe Theoretical
- Platinum compounds **(cisplatin)** increase the risk of pulmonary toxicity when given with **bleomycin**. Severe Study → Also see TABLE 12 p. 1057

Blinatumomab → see monoclonal antibodies

Bortezomib → see TABLE 6 p. 1054 (hypotension), TABLE 12 p. 1057 (myelosuppression), TABLE 10 p. 1056 (peripheral neuropathy)

- Anti-androgens **(apalutamide, enzalutamide)** slightly decrease the exposure to **bortezomib**. Avoid. Severe Study
- Antiepileptics **(carbamazepine, fosphenytoin, phenobarbital, phenytoin, primidone)** slightly decrease the exposure to **bortezomib**. Avoid. Severe Study → Also see TABLE 10 p. 1056
- Antifungals, azoles **(itraconazole, ketoconazole, posaconazole, voriconazole)** slightly increase the exposure to **bortezomib**. Moderate Study
- **Ceritinib** slightly increases the exposure to **bortezomib**. Moderate Study → Also see TABLE 12 p. 1057
- **Cobicistat** slightly increases the exposure to **bortezomib**. Moderate Study
- **Encorafenib** slightly decreases the exposure to **bortezomib**. Avoid. Severe Study
- **HIV-protease inhibitors** slightly increase the exposure to **bortezomib**. Moderate Study
- **Idelalisib** slightly increases the exposure to **bortezomib**. Moderate Study
- **Ivosidenib** slightly decreases the exposure to **bortezomib**. Avoid. Severe Study
- **Lumacaftor** slightly decreases the exposure to **bortezomib**. Avoid. Severe Study
- Macrolides **(clarithromycin)** slightly increase the exposure to **bortezomib**. Moderate Study
- **Mitotane** slightly decreases the exposure to **bortezomib**. Avoid. Severe Study → Also see TABLE 12 p. 1057
- Rifamycins **(rifampicin)** slightly decrease the exposure to **bortezomib**. Avoid. Severe Study
- **Tucatinib** slightly increases the exposure to **bortezomib**. Moderate Study

Bosentan → see endothelin receptor antagonists

Bosutinib → see TABLE 3 p. 1053 (bleeding), TABLE 12 p. 1057 (myelosuppression), TABLE 7 p. 1055 (QT-interval prolongation)

- Oral **antacids** are predicted to decrease the absorption of oral **bosutinib**. Manufacturer advises take at least 12 hours before antacids. Moderate Theoretical
- Anti-androgens **(apalutamide, enzalutamide)** are predicted to very markedly decrease the exposure to **bosutinib**. Avoid. Severe Study → Also see TABLE 7 p. 1055
- Antiarrhythmics **(dronedarone)** are predicted to increase the exposure to **bosutinib**. Avoid or adjust dose. Severe Study → Also see TABLE 7 p. 1055
- Antiepileptics **(carbamazepine, fosphenytoin, phenobarbital, phenytoin, primidone)** are predicted to very markedly decrease the exposure to **bosutinib**. Avoid. Severe Study
- Antifungals, azoles **(fluconazole, isavuconazole, itraconazole, ketoconazole, posaconazole, voriconazole)** are predicted to increase the exposure to **bosutinib**. Avoid or adjust dose. Severe Study → Also see TABLE 7 p. 1055
- **Belzutifan** is predicted to decrease the exposure to **bosutinib**. Avoid or adjust dose. Severe Theoretical
- **Berotralstat** is predicted to increase the exposure to **bosutinib**. Avoid or adjust dose. Severe Study
- Oral calcium compounds **(calcium carbonate)**-containing antacids are predicted to decrease the absorption of oral **bosutinib**. Manufacturer advises take at least 12 hours before antacids. Moderate Theoretical
- Calcium-channel blockers **(diltiazem, verapamil)** are predicted to increase the exposure to **bosutinib**. Avoid or adjust dose. Severe Study
- **Cenobamate** is predicted to decrease the exposure to **bosutinib**. Avoid. Severe Study
- **Ceritinib** is predicted to increase the exposure to **bosutinib**. Avoid or adjust dose. Severe Study → Also see TABLE 12 p. 1057 → Also see TABLE 7 p. 1055
- **Cobicistat** is predicted to increase the exposure to **bosutinib**. Avoid or adjust dose. Severe Study
- **Crizotinib** is predicted to increase the exposure to **bosutinib**. Avoid or adjust dose. Severe Study → Also see TABLE 7 p. 1055
- **Dabrafenib** is predicted to decrease the exposure to **bosutinib**. Avoid. Severe Study
- **Encorafenib** is predicted to very markedly decrease the exposure to **bosutinib**. Avoid. Severe Study → Also see TABLE 7 p. 1055
- Endothelin receptor antagonists **(bosentan)** are predicted to decrease the exposure to **bosutinib**. Avoid. Severe Study
- **Fedratinib** is predicted to increase the exposure to **bosutinib**. Avoid or adjust dose. Severe Study
- **Grapefruit** juice is predicted to increase the exposure to **bosutinib**. Avoid. Moderate Theoretical
- **H_2 receptor antagonists** are predicted to decrease the absorption of **bosutinib**. Moderate Theoretical
- **HIV-protease inhibitors** are predicted to increase the exposure to **bosutinib**. Avoid or adjust dose. Severe Study
- **Idelalisib** is predicted to increase the exposure to **bosutinib**. Avoid or adjust dose. Severe Study
- **Imatinib** is predicted to increase the exposure to **bosutinib**. Avoid or adjust dose. Severe Study → Also see TABLE 3 p. 1053 → Also see TABLE 12 p. 1057
- **Ivosidenib** is predicted to very markedly decrease the exposure to **bosutinib**. Avoid. Severe Study → Also see TABLE 7 p. 1055
- **Letermovir** is predicted to increase the exposure to **bosutinib**. Avoid or adjust dose. Severe Study
- **Lorlatinib** is predicted to decrease the exposure to **bosutinib**. Avoid. Severe Study
- **Lumacaftor** is predicted to very markedly decrease the exposure to **bosutinib**. Avoid. Severe Study
- Macrolides **(clarithromycin, erythromycin)** are predicted to increase the exposure to **bosutinib**. Avoid or adjust dose. Severe Study → Also see TABLE 7 p. 1055
- **Mitotane** is predicted to very markedly decrease the exposure to **bosutinib**. Avoid. Severe Study → Also see TABLE 12 p. 1057
- **Modafinil** is predicted to decrease the exposure to **bosutinib**. Avoid. Severe Theoretical

Bosutinib (continued)
- Neurokinin-1 receptor antagonists **(aprepitant, netupitant)** are predicted to increase the exposure to **bosutinib**. Avoid or adjust dose. Severe Study
- Neurokinin-1 receptor antagonists **(fosaprepitant)** are predicted to increase the exposure to **bosutinib**. Severe Theoretical
- **Nilotinib** is predicted to increase the exposure to **bosutinib**. Avoid or adjust dose. Severe Study → Also see TABLE 12 p. 1057 → Also see TABLE 7 p. 1055
- NNRTIs **(efavirenz, etravirine, nevirapine)** are predicted to decrease the exposure to **bosutinib**. Avoid. Severe Study → Also see TABLE 7 p. 1055
- **Pitolisant** is predicted to decrease the exposure to **bosutinib**. Avoid. Severe Theoretical
- **Proton pump inhibitors** are predicted to decrease the absorption of **bosutinib**. Moderate Study
- Rifamycins **(rifampicin)** are predicted to very markedly decrease the exposure to **bosutinib**. Avoid. Severe Study
- Oral **sodium bicarbonate**-containing antacids are predicted to decrease the absorption of oral **bosutinib**. Manufacturer advises take at least 12 hours before antacids. Moderate Theoretical
- **Sotorasib** is predicted to decrease the exposure to **bosutinib**. Avoid. Severe Study
- **St John's wort** is predicted to decrease the exposure to **bosutinib**. Avoid. Severe Study
- **Tucatinib** is predicted to increase the exposure to **bosutinib**. Avoid or adjust dose. Severe Study

Botulinum toxin type A → see botulinum toxins

Botulinum toxins

botulinum toxin type A

Bowel cleansing preparations

SEPARATION OF ADMINISTRATION Other oral drugs should not be taken 1 hour before, or after, administration of bowel cleansing preparations because absorption might be impaired. Consider withholding ACE inhibitors, angiotensin-II receptor antagonists, and NSAIDs on the day that bowel cleansing preparations are given and for up to 72 hours after the procedure. Also consider withholding diuretics on the day that bowel cleansing preparations are given.

Brentuximab vedotin → see monoclonal antibodies

Brigatinib → see TABLE 4 p. 1054 (bradycardia)
- Anti-androgens **(apalutamide, enzalutamide)** are predicted to decrease the exposure to **brigatinib**. Avoid. Severe Study
- Antiarrhythmics **(dronedarone)** are predicted to increase the exposure to **brigatinib**. Moderate Study → Also see TABLE 4 p. 1054
- Antiepileptics **(carbamazepine, fosphenytoin, phenobarbital, phenytoin, primidone)** are predicted to decrease the exposure to **brigatinib**. Avoid. Severe Study
- Antifungals, azoles **(fluconazole, isavuconazole)** are predicted to increase the exposure to **brigatinib**. Moderate Study
- Antifungals, azoles **(itraconazole, ketoconazole, posaconazole, voriconazole)** are predicted to increase the exposure to **brigatinib**. Avoid or adjust dose—consult product literature. Severe Study
- **Berotralstat** is predicted to increase the exposure to **brigatinib**. Moderate Study
- Calcium-channel blockers **(diltiazem, verapamil)** are predicted to increase the exposure to **brigatinib**. Moderate Study → Also see TABLE 4 p. 1054
- **Cenobamate** is predicted to decrease the exposure to **brigatinib**. Avoid or adjust dose—consult product literature. Moderate Study
- **Ceritinib** is predicted to increase the exposure to **brigatinib**. Avoid or adjust dose—consult product literature. Severe Study → Also see TABLE 4 p. 1054
- **Brigatinib** might decrease the exposure to **ciclosporin**. Avoid. Moderate Theoretical
- **Cobicistat** is predicted to increase the exposure to **brigatinib**. Avoid or adjust dose—consult product literature. Severe Study
- **Brigatinib** is predicted to decrease the exposure to **combined hormonal contraceptives**. Use additional contraceptive precautions. Severe Theoretical
- **Crizotinib** is predicted to increase the exposure to **brigatinib**. Moderate Study → Also see TABLE 4 p. 1054
- **Dabrafenib** is predicted to decrease the exposure to **brigatinib**. Avoid or adjust dose—consult product literature. Moderate Study
- **Encorafenib** is predicted to decrease the exposure to **brigatinib**. Avoid. Severe Study
- Endothelin receptor antagonists **(bosentan)** are predicted to decrease the exposure to **brigatinib**. Avoid or adjust dose—consult product literature. Moderate Study
- **Fedratinib** is predicted to increase the exposure to **brigatinib**. Moderate Study
- **Grapefruit** juice is predicted to increase the concentration of **brigatinib**. Avoid. Severe Study
- **HIV-protease inhibitors** are predicted to increase the exposure to **brigatinib**. Avoid or adjust dose—consult product literature. Severe Study
- **Idelalisib** is predicted to increase the exposure to **brigatinib**. Avoid or adjust dose—consult product literature. Severe Study
- **Imatinib** is predicted to increase the exposure to **brigatinib**. Moderate Study
- **Ivosidenib** is predicted to decrease the exposure to **brigatinib**. Avoid. Severe Study
- **Letermovir** is predicted to increase the exposure to **brigatinib**. Moderate Study
- **Lorlatinib** is predicted to decrease the exposure to **brigatinib**. Avoid or adjust dose—consult product literature. Moderate Study
- **Lumacaftor** is predicted to decrease the exposure to **brigatinib**. Avoid. Severe Study
- Macrolides **(clarithromycin)** are predicted to increase the exposure to **brigatinib**. Avoid or adjust dose—consult product literature. Severe Study
- Macrolides **(erythromycin)** are predicted to increase the exposure to **brigatinib**. Moderate Study
- **Mitotane** is predicted to decrease the exposure to **brigatinib**. Avoid. Severe Study
- **Modafinil** is predicted to decrease the exposure to **brigatinib**. Avoid or adjust dose—consult product literature. Moderate Theoretical
- Neurokinin-1 receptor antagonists **(aprepitant, netupitant)** are predicted to increase the exposure to **brigatinib**. Moderate Study
- **Nilotinib** is predicted to increase the exposure to **brigatinib**. Moderate Study
- NNRTIs **(efavirenz, etravirine, nevirapine)** are predicted to decrease the exposure to **brigatinib**. Avoid or adjust dose—consult product literature. Moderate Study
- **Brigatinib** potentially decreases the concentration of opioids **(alfentanil, fentanyl)**. Avoid. Moderate Theoretical → Also see TABLE 4 p. 1054
- Rifamycins **(rifampicin)** are predicted to decrease the exposure to **brigatinib**. Avoid. Severe Study
- **Brigatinib** potentially decreases the concentration of **sirolimus**. Avoid. Moderate Theoretical
- **Sotorasib** is predicted to decrease the exposure to **brigatinib**. Avoid or adjust dose—consult product literature. Moderate Study
- **St John's wort** is predicted to decrease the exposure to **brigatinib**. Avoid or adjust dose—consult product literature. Moderate Study
- **Brigatinib** potentially decreases the concentration of **tacrolimus**. Avoid. Moderate Theoretical
- **Tucatinib** is predicted to increase the exposure to **brigatinib**. Avoid or adjust dose—consult product literature. Severe Study

Brimonidine → see TABLE 4 p. 1054 (bradycardia), TABLE 6 p. 1054 (hypotension), TABLE 9 p. 1056 (CNS effects)

Brinzolamide

ROUTE-SPECIFIC INFORMATION Since systemic absorption can follow topical application of **brinzolamide**, the possibility of interactions should be borne in mind.

Brivaracetam → see antiepileptics

Brodalumab → see monoclonal antibodies

Bromfenac → see NSAIDs

Bromocriptine → see dopamine receptor agonists

Buclizine → see antihistamines, sedating
Budesonide → see corticosteroids
Bulevirtide
- Angiotensin-II receptor antagonists **(irbesartan)** are predicted to affect the efficacy of **bulevirtide**. Avoid. Severe Theoretical
- **Bulevirtide** is predicted to increase the exposure to angiotensin-II receptor antagonists **(olmesartan, telmisartan, valsartan)**. Avoid or monitor. Moderate Theoretical
- **Bulevirtide** is predicted to increase the exposure to antiepileptics **(carbamazepine)**. Moderate Theoretical
- **Bulevirtide** is predicted to increase the exposure to antihistamines, non-sedating **(fexofenadine)**. Avoid or monitor. Moderate Theoretical
- **Bulevirtide** slightly increases the exposure to benzodiazepines **(midazolam)**. Moderate Theoretical
- **Ciclosporin** is predicted to affect the efficacy of **bulevirtide** and **bulevirtide** is predicted to increase the exposure to **ciclosporin**. Avoid. Severe Theoretical
- **Bulevirtide** is predicted to increase the exposure to endothelin receptor antagonists **(bosentan)**. Avoid or monitor. Moderate Theoretical
- **Bulevirtide** is predicted to increase the exposure to **everolimus**. Moderate Theoretical
- **Ezetimibe** is predicted to affect the efficacy of **bulevirtide**. Avoid. Severe Theoretical
- **Bulevirtide** is predicted to increase the exposure to **glecaprevir**. Avoid or monitor. Moderate Theoretical
- **Bulevirtide** is predicted to increase the exposure to **grazoprevir**. Avoid or monitor. Moderate Theoretical
- HIV-protease inhibitors **(ritonavir)** are predicted to affect the efficacy of **bulevirtide**. Avoid. Severe Theoretical
- **Bulevirtide** is predicted to increase the exposure to meglitinides **(repaglinide)**. Avoid or monitor. Moderate Theoretical
- **Bulevirtide** is predicted to increase the exposure to opioids **(alfentanil)**. Moderate Theoretical
- **Bulevirtide** is predicted to increase the exposure to **sirolimus**. Moderate Theoretical
- **Bulevirtide** is predicted to increase the exposure to **statins**. Avoid or monitor. Moderate Theoretical
- **Sulfasalazine** is predicted to affect the efficacy of **bulevirtide**. Avoid. Severe Theoretical
- **Bulevirtide** is predicted to increase the exposure to sulfonylureas **(glibenclamide)**. Avoid or monitor. Moderate Theoretical
- **Bulevirtide** is predicted to increase the exposure to **tacrolimus**. Moderate Theoretical
- **Bulevirtide** is predicted to increase the exposure to taxanes **(docetaxel, paclitaxel)**. Avoid or monitor. Moderate Theoretical
- **Bulevirtide** is predicted to increase the exposure to **temsirolimus**. Moderate Theoretical
- **Bulevirtide** is predicted to increase the exposure to **thyroid hormones**. Avoid or monitor. Moderate Theoretical
- **Bulevirtide** is predicted to increase the exposure to **voxilaprevir**. Avoid or monitor. Moderate Theoretical

Bumetanide → see loop diuretics
Bupivacaine → see anaesthetics, local
Buprenorphine → see opioids
Bupropion
- **Bupropion** is predicted to increase the exposure to anticholinesterases, centrally acting **(galantamine)**. Monitor and adjust dose. Moderate Study
- Antiepileptics **(carbamazepine, fosphenytoin, phenobarbital, phenytoin, primidone)** are predicted to markedly decrease the exposure to **bupropion**. Severe Study
- Antiepileptics **(valproate)** increase the exposure to **bupropion**. Severe Study
- Antifungals, azoles **(isavuconazole)** slightly increase the exposure to **bupropion**. Adjust dose. Moderate Study
- **Bupropion** is predicted to markedly increase the exposure to **atomoxetine**. Adjust dose. Severe Study
- **Bupropion** is predicted to moderately increase the exposure to atypical antipsychotics **(aripiprazole)**. Avoid or adjust dose—consult product literature. Moderate Study
- **Bupropion** is predicted to increase the exposure to atypical antipsychotics **(clozapine)**. Use with caution and adjust dose. Severe Study
- **Bupropion** is predicted to increase the exposure to atypical antipsychotics **(risperidone)**. Adjust dose. Moderate Study
- **Bupropion** is predicted to increase the exposure to beta blockers, selective **(metoprolol, nebivolol)**. Moderate Study
- **Clopidogrel** slightly increases the exposure to **bupropion**. Moderate Study
- **Bupropion** is predicted to slightly increase the exposure to **darifenacin**. Mild Study
- **Bupropion** might decrease the exposure to **digoxin**. Severe Study
- **Bupropion** increases the risk of adverse effects when given with dopamine receptor agonists **(amantadine)**. Moderate Study
- **Bupropion** might enhance the risk of serotonin toxicity when given with **drugs that cause serotonin toxicity** (see TABLE 11 p. 1056). Severe Anecdotal
- **Bupropion** is predicted to increase the exposure to **eliglustat**. Avoid or adjust dose—consult product literature. Severe Study
- **Bupropion** is predicted to increase the exposure to **fenfluramine**. Moderate Study
- **Bupropion** is predicted to increase the exposure to **fesoterodine**. Use with caution and adjust dose. Mild Theoretical
- **Bupropion** is predicted to increase the exposure to **gefitinib**. Moderate Theoretical
- **HIV-protease inhibitors** are predicted to decrease the exposure to **bupropion**. Moderate Study
- **Bupropion** increases the risk of adverse effects when given with **levodopa**. Moderate Study
- **Bupropion** is predicted to increase the risk of intraoperative hypertension when given with **linezolid**. Severe Anecdotal
- **Lumacaftor** is predicted to decrease the exposure to **bupropion**. Adjust dose. Moderate Theoretical
- **Bupropion** is predicted to increase the risk of severe hypertension when given with **MAO-B inhibitors**. Avoid. Moderate Theoretical
- **Bupropion** is predicted to increase the risk of severe hypertension when given with **MAOIs, irreversible**. Avoid and for 14 days after stopping the MAOI. Severe Theoretical
- **Methylthioninium chloride** is predicted to increase the risk of severe hypertension when given with **bupropion**. Avoid. Severe Theoretical
- **Bupropion** is predicted to increase the exposure to **mexiletine**. Moderate Study
- **Midostaurin** moderately decreases the exposure to the active metabolite of **bupropion**. Moderate Study
- **Bupropion** is predicted to increase the risk of severe hypertension when given with **moclobemide**. Avoid. Severe Theoretical
- **Nirmatrelvir** boosted with ritonavir is predicted to decrease the concentration of **bupropion**. Moderate Theoretical
- NNRTIs **(efavirenz)** are predicted to decrease the exposure to **bupropion**. Moderate Study
- **Bupropion** is predicted to decrease the efficacy of opioids **(codeine)**. Moderate Theoretical
- **Bupropion** is predicted to decrease the efficacy of opioids **(tramadol)**. Severe Study
- **Bupropion** is predicted to moderately increase the exposure to **pitolisant**. Use with caution and adjust dose. Moderate Study
- Rifamycins **(rifampicin)** are predicted to decrease the exposure to **bupropion**. Moderate Study
- **Bupropion** is predicted to increase the exposure to SSRIs **(dapoxetine)**. Moderate Theoretical
- **Bupropion** is predicted to decrease the efficacy of **tamoxifen**. Avoid. Severe Study
- **Bupropion** is predicted to increase the exposure to the active metabolite of **tetrabenazine**. Moderate Study
- **Bupropion** is predicted to increase the exposure to **tricyclic antidepressants**. Monitor for toxicity and adjust dose. Severe Study
- **Vemurafenib** is predicted to decrease the concentration of **bupropion**. Moderate Theoretical
- **Bupropion** is predicted to increase the exposure to **vortioxetine**. Monitor and adjust dose. Moderate Study

Buspirone

- Anti-androgens (apalutamide, enzalutamide) are predicted to decrease the exposure to **buspirone**. Use with caution and adjust dose. Severe Study
- Antiarrhythmics (dronedarone) are predicted to increase the exposure to **buspirone**. Use with caution and adjust dose. Moderate Study
- Antiepileptics (carbamazepine, fosphenytoin, phenobarbital, phenytoin, primidone) are predicted to decrease the exposure to **buspirone**. Use with caution and adjust dose. Severe Study
- Antifungals, azoles (fluconazole, isavuconazole) are predicted to increase the exposure to **buspirone**. Use with caution and adjust dose. Moderate Study
- Antifungals, azoles (itraconazole, ketoconazole, posaconazole, voriconazole) are predicted to increase the exposure to **buspirone**. Adjust **buspirone** dose. Severe Study
- Antifungals, azoles (miconazole) are predicted to increase the concentration of **buspirone**. Use with caution and adjust dose. Moderate Theoretical
- **Berotralstat** is predicted to increase the exposure to **buspirone**. Use with caution and adjust dose. Moderate Study
- Calcium-channel blockers (diltiazem, verapamil) are predicted to increase the exposure to **buspirone**. Use with caution and adjust dose. Moderate Study
- **Cenobamate** is predicted to decrease the exposure to **buspirone**. Adjust dose. Moderate Theoretical
- **Ceritinib** is predicted to increase the exposure to **buspirone**. Adjust **buspirone** dose. Severe Study
- **Cobicistat** is predicted to increase the exposure to **buspirone**. Adjust **buspirone** dose. Severe Study
- **Crizotinib** is predicted to increase the exposure to **buspirone**. Use with caution and adjust dose. Moderate Study
- **Encorafenib** is predicted to decrease the exposure to **buspirone**. Use with caution and adjust dose. Severe Study
- **Fedratinib** is predicted to increase the exposure to **buspirone**. Use with caution and adjust dose. Moderate Study
- **Grapefruit** juice increases the exposure to **buspirone**. Avoid. Mild Study
- **HIV-protease inhibitors** are predicted to increase the exposure to **buspirone**. Adjust **buspirone** dose. Severe Study
- **Idelalisib** is predicted to increase the exposure to **buspirone**. Adjust **buspirone** dose. Severe Study
- **Imatinib** is predicted to increase the exposure to **buspirone**. Use with caution and adjust dose. Moderate Study
- **Ivosidenib** is predicted to decrease the exposure to **buspirone**. Use with caution and adjust dose. Severe Study
- **Letermovir** is predicted to increase the exposure to **buspirone**. Use with caution and adjust dose. Moderate Study
- **Buspirone** is predicted to increase the risk of elevated blood pressure when given with **linezolid**. Avoid. Severe Theoretical
- **Lumacaftor** is predicted to decrease the exposure to **buspirone**. Use with caution and adjust dose. Severe Study
- Macrolides (clarithromycin) are predicted to increase the exposure to **buspirone**. Adjust **buspirone** dose. Severe Study
- Macrolides (erythromycin) are predicted to increase the exposure to **buspirone**. Use with caution and adjust dose. Moderate Study
- **Buspirone** is predicted to increase the risk of elevated blood pressure when given with **MAOIs, irreversible**. Avoid. Severe Anecdotal
- **Mitotane** is predicted to decrease the exposure to **buspirone**. Use with caution and adjust dose. Severe Study
- Neurokinin-1 receptor antagonists (aprepitant, netupitant) are predicted to increase the exposure to **buspirone**. Use with caution and adjust dose. Moderate Study
- **Nilotinib** is predicted to increase the exposure to **buspirone**. Use with caution and adjust dose. Moderate Study
- **Nirmatrelvir** boosted with ritonavir is predicted to increase the concentration of **buspirone**. Monitor and adjust dose. Moderate Theoretical
- Rifamycins (rifampicin) are predicted to decrease the exposure to **buspirone**. Use with caution and adjust dose. Severe Study
- **Tucatinib** is predicted to increase the exposure to **buspirone**. Adjust **buspirone** dose. Severe Study

Busulfan → see alkylating agents

Cabazitaxel → see taxanes

Cabergoline → see dopamine receptor agonists

Cabotegravir

- Oral **antacids** are predicted to decrease the concentration of oral **cabotegravir**. Manufacturer advises take 4 hours before or 2 hours after antacids. Moderate Theoretical
- Antiepileptics (carbamazepine, fosphenytoin, oxcarbazepine, phenobarbital, phenytoin, primidone) might decrease the concentration of **cabotegravir**. Avoid. Severe Theoretical
- Oral calcium compounds (calcium carbonate) are predicted to decrease the concentration of oral **cabotegravir**. Manufacturer advises take 4 hours before or 2 hours after antacids. Moderate Theoretical
- Rifamycins (rifabutin) have been reported to cause a small decrease in the exposure to **cabotegravir**. Avoid intramuscular **cabotegravir** or adjust frequency—consult product literature, p. 506. Moderate Study
- Rifamycins (rifampicin) modestly decrease the exposure to **cabotegravir**. Avoid. Severe Study

Cabozantinib → see TABLE 12 p. 1057 (myelosuppression), TABLE 7 p. 1055 (QT-interval prolongation)

- Anti-androgens (apalutamide, enzalutamide) moderately decrease the exposure to **cabozantinib**. Avoid. Moderate Study → Also see TABLE 7 p. 1055
- Antiarrhythmics (dronedarone) are predicted to increase the exposure to **cabozantinib**. Moderate Study → Also see TABLE 7 p. 1055
- Antiepileptics (carbamazepine, fosphenytoin, phenobarbital, phenytoin, primidone) moderately decrease the exposure to **cabozantinib**. Avoid. Moderate Study
- Antifungals, azoles (fluconazole, isavuconazole, itraconazole, ketoconazole, posaconazole, voriconazole) are predicted to increase the exposure to **cabozantinib**. Moderate Study → Also see TABLE 7 p. 1055
- **Cabozantinib** is predicted to increase the exposure to benzodiazepines (midazolam). Moderate Theoretical
- **Berotralstat** is predicted to increase the exposure to **cabozantinib**. Moderate Study
- Calcium-channel blockers (diltiazem, verapamil) are predicted to increase the exposure to **cabozantinib**. Moderate Study
- **Cenobamate** is predicted to decrease the exposure to **cabozantinib**. Moderate Study
- **Ceritinib** is predicted to increase the exposure to **cabozantinib**. Moderate Study → Also see TABLE 12 p. 1057 → Also see TABLE 7 p. 1055
- **Cobicistat** is predicted to increase the exposure to **cabozantinib**. Moderate Study
- **Cabozantinib** might affect the effects of **combined hormonal contraceptives**. Use additional contraceptive precautions. Severe Theoretical
- **Crizotinib** is predicted to increase the exposure to **cabozantinib**. Moderate Study → Also see TABLE 7 p. 1055
- **Dabrafenib** is predicted to decrease the exposure to **cabozantinib**. Moderate Study
- **Drugs that cause bleeding** (see TABLE 3 p. 1053) cause bleeding, as can **cabozantinib**; concurrent use might increase the risk of developing this effect. Severe Theoretical
- **Encorafenib** moderately decreases the exposure to **cabozantinib**. Avoid. Moderate Study → Also see TABLE 7 p. 1055
- Endothelin receptor antagonists (bosentan) are predicted to decrease the exposure to **cabozantinib**. Moderate Study
- **Fedratinib** is predicted to increase the exposure to **cabozantinib**. Moderate Study
- **Grapefruit** juice is predicted to increase the exposure to **cabozantinib**. Moderate Theoretical
- **HIV-protease inhibitors** are predicted to increase the exposure to **cabozantinib**. Moderate Study
- **Idelalisib** is predicted to increase the exposure to **cabozantinib**. Moderate Study
- **Imatinib** is predicted to increase the exposure to **cabozantinib**. Moderate Study → Also see TABLE 12 p. 1057
- **Ivosidenib** moderately decreases the exposure to **cabozantinib**. Avoid. Moderate Study → Also see TABLE 7 p. 1055
- **Letermovir** is predicted to increase the exposure to **cabozantinib**. Moderate Study

- **Lorlatinib** is predicted to decrease the exposure to **cabozantinib**. Moderate Study
- **Lumacaftor** moderately decreases the exposure to **cabozantinib**. Avoid. Moderate Study
- Macrolides **(clarithromycin, erythromycin)** are predicted to increase the exposure to **cabozantinib**. Moderate Study → Also see TABLE 7 p. 1055
- **Mitotane** moderately decreases the exposure to **cabozantinib**. Avoid. Moderate Study → Also see TABLE 12 p. 1057
- Neurokinin-1 receptor antagonists **(aprepitant, netupitant)** are predicted to increase the exposure to **cabozantinib**. Moderate Study
- **Nilotinib** is predicted to increase the exposure to **cabozantinib**. Moderate Study → Also see TABLE 12 p. 1057 → Also see TABLE 7 p. 1055
- NNRTIs **(efavirenz, etravirine, nevirapine)** are predicted to decrease the exposure to **cabozantinib**. Moderate Study → Also see TABLE 7 p. 1055
- Rifamycins **(rifampicin)** moderately decrease the exposure to **cabozantinib**. Avoid. Moderate Study
- **Sotorasib** is predicted to decrease the exposure to **cabozantinib**. Moderate Study
- **St John's wort** is predicted to decrease the exposure to **cabozantinib**. Moderate Study
- **Tucatinib** is predicted to increase the exposure to **cabozantinib**. Moderate Study

Caffeine citrate
- **Caffeine citrate** decreases the efficacy of antiarrhythmics **(adenosine)**. Separate administration by 24 hours. Mild Study
- Antiepileptics **(fosphenytoin, phenytoin)** are predicted to moderately increase the clearance of **caffeine citrate**. Monitor and adjust dose. Moderate Study
- HIV-protease inhibitors **(ritonavir)** are predicted to moderately increase the clearance of **caffeine citrate**. Monitor and adjust dose. Moderate Study
- **Leflunomide** is predicted to moderately increase the clearance of **caffeine citrate**. Monitor and adjust dose. Moderate Study
- Rifamycins **(rifampicin)** are predicted to moderately increase the clearance of **caffeine citrate**. Monitor and adjust dose. Moderate Study
- SSRIs **(fluvoxamine)** markedly decrease the clearance of **caffeine citrate**. Monitor and adjust dose. Severe Study
- **Teriflunomide** is predicted to moderately increase the clearance of **caffeine citrate**. Monitor and adjust dose. Moderate Study
- **Caffeine citrate** decreases the clearance of **theophylline**. Moderate Study

Calcifediol → see vitamin D substances
Calcipotriol → see vitamin D substances
Calcitonins
- **Calcitonins** decrease the concentration of **lithium**. Adjust dose. Moderate Study

Calcitriol → see vitamin D substances
Calcium acetate → see calcium compounds
Calcium carbonate → see calcium compounds
Calcium chloride → see calcium compounds
Calcium compounds

calcium acetate · calcium carbonate · calcium chloride · calcium gluconate · calcium lactate · calcium phosphate

SEPARATION OF ADMINISTRATION **Calcium carbonate-containing antacids** should preferably not be taken at the same time as other drugs since they might impair absorption. **Antacids** might damage enteric coatings designed to prevent dissolution in the stomach.

- Oral **calcium compounds** decrease the absorption of oral alkylating agents **(estramustine)**. Severe Study
- Oral **calcium carbonate** might decrease the absorption of oral antimalarials **(chloroquine)**. Separate administration by at least 4 hours. Moderate Study
- Oral **calcium compounds** might decrease the concentration of the active metabolite of oral **baloxavir marboxil**. Avoid. Severe Theoretical
- **Calcium carbonate** -containing antacids is predicted to decrease the exposure to **belumosudil**. Separate administration by 12 hours. Moderate Theoretical
- Oral **calcium compounds** decrease the absorption of oral bisphosphonates **(alendronate)**. **Alendronate** should be taken at least 30 minutes before calcium. Moderate Study
- Oral **calcium compounds** decrease the absorption of oral bisphosphonates **(clodronate)**. Avoid **calcium compounds** for 2 hours before or 1 hour after **clodronate**. Moderate Study
- Oral **calcium compounds** are predicted to decrease the absorption of oral bisphosphonates **(ibandronate)**. Avoid **calcium compounds** for at least 6 hours before or 1 hour after **ibandronate**. Moderate Theoretical
- Oral **calcium compounds** decrease the absorption of oral bisphosphonates **(risedronate)**. Separate administration by at least 2 hours. Moderate Study
- Oral **calcium carbonate**-containing antacids are predicted to decrease the absorption of oral **bosutinib**. Manufacturer advises take at least 12 hours before antacids. Moderate Theoretical
- Oral **calcium carbonate** is predicted to decrease the concentration of oral **cabotegravir**. Manufacturer advises take 4 hours before or 2 hours after antacids. Moderate Theoretical
- Intravenous cephalosporins **(ceftriaxone)** increase the risk of cardio-respiratory arrest when given with intravenous **calcium compounds**. Avoid. Severe Anecdotal
- Oral **calcium carbonate** -containing antacids are predicted to decrease the exposure to oral **dasatinib**. Separate administration by at least 2 hours. Moderate Study
- Intravenous **calcium compounds** increase the effects of **digoxin**. Avoid. Moderate Anecdotal
- Oral **calcium compounds** decrease the absorption of oral **dolutegravir**. **Dolutegravir** should be taken 2 hours before or 6 hours after calcium. Moderate Study
- Oral **calcium compounds** decrease the absorption of oral **eltrombopag**. **Eltrombopag** should be taken 2 hours before or 4 hours after calcium. Severe Study
- Oral **calcium carbonate**-containing antacids are predicted to decrease the absorption of oral **erlotinib**. Manufacturer advises take 2 hours before or 4 hours after antacids. Moderate Theoretical
- Oral **calcium carbonate** -containing antacids are predicted to decrease the exposure to oral **gefitinib**. Moderate Theoretical
- Oral **calcium carbonate** might decrease the absorption of oral **hydroxychloroquine**. Moderate Theoretical
- Oral **calcium carbonate** decreases the absorption of oral **iron**. **Calcium carbonate** should be taken 1 hour before or 2 hours after iron. Moderate Study
- Oral **calcium carbonate**-containing antacids are predicted to decrease the absorption of oral **lapatinib**. Avoid. Moderate Theoretical
- Oral **calcium carbonate** -containing antacids are predicted to decrease the exposure to oral **ledipasvir**. Separate administration by 4 hours. Moderate Theoretical
- Oral **calcium carbonate** -containing antacids are predicted to decrease the exposure to oral **neratinib**. Separate administration by at least 3 hours. Mild Theoretical
- Oral **calcium carbonate** -containing antacids might affect the exposure to oral **nilotinib**. Separate administration by at least 2 hours. Moderate Study
- Oral **calcium carbonate** -containing antacids are predicted to decrease the exposure to oral NNRTIs **(rilpivirine)**. Manufacturer advises take 4 hours before or 2 hours after antacids. Severe Theoretical
- Oral **calcium carbonate** -containing antacids might decrease the absorption of oral **pazopanib**. Manufacturer advises take 1 hour before or 2 hours after antacids. Moderate Theoretical
- Oral **calcium compounds** decrease the absorption of oral quinolones **(ciprofloxacin)**. Separate administration by 2 hours. Moderate Study
- Oral **calcium carbonate** -containing antacids greatly decrease the exposure to oral **raltegravir** (high-dose). Avoid. Severe Study

A1 Interactions | Appendix 1

Calcium compounds (continued)

- Oral **calcium compounds** decrease the exposure to oral **roxadustat**. **Roxadustat** should be taken at least 1 hour after calcium. Moderate Study
- Oral **calcium carbonate** is predicted to decrease the exposure to oral **sotorasib**. Manufacturer advises take 4 hours before or 10 hours after antacids. Moderate Theoretical
- Oral **calcium compounds** decrease the absorption of oral **strontium**. Separate administration by 2 hours. Moderate Study
- Oral **calcium compounds** are predicted to decrease the absorption of oral **tetracyclines**. Separate administration by 2 to 3 hours. Moderate Theoretical
- **Thiazide diuretics** increase the risk of hypercalcaemia when given with **calcium compounds**. Severe Anecdotal
- Oral **calcium compounds** are predicted to decrease the absorption of oral thyroid hormones **(levothyroxine)**. Separate administration by at least 4 hours. Moderate Anecdotal
- **Calcium carbonate** -containing antacids might decrease the efficacy of **ulipristal** for emergency hormonal contraception. For CoSRH guidance, see Contraceptives, interactions p. 614. Unknown Theoretical
- Oral **calcium compounds** decrease the exposure to oral **vadadustat**. **Vadadustat** should be taken at least 1 hour before or 2 hours after calcium. Moderate Study
- Oral **calcium carbonate**-containing antacids are predicted to decrease the concentration of oral **velpatasvir**. Separate administration by 4 hours. Moderate Theoretical
- Oral **calcium compounds** decrease the absorption of oral **zinc**. Moderate Study

Calcium gluconate → see calcium compounds

Calcium lactate → see calcium compounds

Calcium phosphate → see calcium compounds

Calcium-channel blockers → see TABLE 4 p. 1054 (bradycardia), TABLE 6 p. 1054 (hypotension)

amlodipine · diltiazem · felodipine · lacidipine · lercanidipine · nicardipine · nifedipine · nimodipine · verapamil

- Calcium-channel blockers **(diltiazem, verapamil)** are predicted to increase the exposure to **abemaciclib**. Moderate Study
- Calcium-channel blockers **(diltiazem, verapamil)** are predicted to increase the exposure to **acalabrutinib**. Avoid or monitor. Severe Study
- **Verapamil** is predicted to increase the exposure to **afatinib**. Moderate Study
- **Verapamil** moderately increases the exposure to **aliskiren**. Moderate Study → Also see TABLE 6 p. 1054
- Calcium-channel blockers **(diltiazem, verapamil)** are predicted to increase the exposure to alpha blockers **(tamsulosin)**. Moderate Theoretical → Also see TABLE 6 p. 1054
- **Verapamil** moderately increases the exposure to anthracyclines **(doxorubicin)**. Moderate Study
- Anti-androgens **(apalutamide, enzalutamide)** are predicted to decrease the exposure to calcium-channel blockers **(amlodipine, felodipine, lacidipine, lercanidipine, nicardipine, nifedipine, nimodipine)**. Monitor and adjust dose. Moderate Study
- Anti-androgens **(enzalutamide)** are predicted to decrease the exposure to calcium-channel blockers **(diltiazem, verapamil)**. Severe Study
- Antiarrhythmics **(disopyramide)** are predicted to increase the risk of cardiodepression when given with **verapamil**. Severe Theoretical
- Antiarrhythmics **(dronedarone)** are predicted to increase the exposure to calcium-channel blockers **(amlodipine, felodipine, lacidipine, lercanidipine, nicardipine, nifedipine, nimodipine)**. Monitor and adjust dose. Moderate Study
- Antiarrhythmics **(amiodarone)** are predicted to increase the risk of cardiodepression when given with calcium-channel blockers **(diltiazem, verapamil)**. Avoid. Severe Theoretical → Also see TABLE 4 p. 1054
- Calcium-channel blockers **(diltiazem, verapamil)** increase the exposure to antiarrhythmics **(dronedarone)** and antiarrhythmics **(dronedarone)** increase the exposure to calcium-channel blockers **(diltiazem, verapamil)**. Moderate Study → Also see TABLE 4 p. 1054
- **Verapamil** increases the risk of cardiodepression when given with antiarrhythmics **(flecainide)**. Severe Anecdotal → Also see TABLE 4 p. 1054
- Calcium-channel blockers **(diltiazem, verapamil)** are predicted to increase the exposure to antiarrhythmics **(propafenone)**. Monitor and adjust dose. Moderate Study → Also see TABLE 4 p. 1054
- Antiepileptics **(valproate)** increase the exposure to **nimodipine**. Adjust dose. Moderate Study
- Antiepileptics **(carbamazepine, fosphenytoin, phenobarbital, phenytoin, primidone)** are predicted to decrease the exposure to calcium-channel blockers **(amlodipine, felodipine, lacidipine, lercanidipine, nicardipine, nifedipine, nimodipine)**. Monitor and adjust dose. Moderate Study
- **Diltiazem** increases the concentration of antiepileptics **(carbamazepine)** and antiepileptics **(carbamazepine)** are predicted to decrease the exposure to **diltiazem**. Monitor concentration and adjust dose. Severe Anecdotal
- **Verapamil** increases the concentration of antiepileptics **(carbamazepine)** and antiepileptics **(carbamazepine)** are predicted to decrease the exposure to **verapamil**. Severe Anecdotal
- Antiepileptics **(phenobarbital, primidone)** are predicted to decrease the exposure to calcium-channel blockers **(diltiazem, verapamil)**. Severe Study
- Calcium-channel blockers **(diltiazem, verapamil)** potentially increase the concentration of antiepileptics **(fosphenytoin, phenytoin)** and antiepileptics **(fosphenytoin, phenytoin)** are predicted to decrease the exposure to calcium-channel blockers **(diltiazem, verapamil)**. Severe Study
- Antifungals, azoles **(itraconazole, ketoconazole, posaconazole, voriconazole)** are predicted to markedly increase the exposure to **lercanidipine**. Avoid. Severe Study
- Antifungals, azoles **(miconazole)** are predicted to increase the exposure to **diltiazem**. Moderate Theoretical
- Antifungals, azoles **(fluconazole, isavuconazole)** are predicted to increase the exposure to calcium-channel blockers **(amlodipine, felodipine, lacidipine, lercanidipine, nicardipine, nifedipine, nimodipine)**. Monitor and adjust dose. Moderate Study
- Antifungals, azoles **(miconazole)** are predicted to increase the exposure to calcium-channel blockers **(amlodipine, felodipine, lacidipine, lercanidipine, nicardipine, nifedipine, nimodipine, verapamil)**. Use with caution and adjust dose. Moderate Theoretical
- Antifungals, azoles **(itraconazole, ketoconazole, posaconazole, voriconazole)** are predicted to increase the exposure to calcium-channel blockers **(amlodipine, felodipine, lacidipine, nicardipine, nifedipine, nimodipine)**. Monitor and adjust dose. Moderate Study
- Antifungals, azoles **(fluconazole)** (high-dose) are predicted to increase the exposure to calcium-channel blockers **(diltiazem, verapamil)**. Moderate Theoretical
- Antifungals, azoles **(itraconazole, ketoconazole, posaconazole, voriconazole)** are predicted to increase the exposure to calcium-channel blockers **(diltiazem, verapamil)**. Severe Study
- Calcium-channel blockers **(diltiazem, verapamil)** are predicted to increase the exposure to antifungals, azoles **(isavuconazole)**. Moderate Theoretical
- Calcium-channel blockers **(diltiazem, verapamil)** are predicted to increase the exposure to antihistamines, non-sedating **(mizolastine)**. Severe Theoretical
- Calcium-channel blockers **(diltiazem, verapamil)** are predicted to increase the exposure to antihistamines, non-sedating **(rupatadine)**. Avoid. Moderate Study
- Antimalarials **(mefloquine)** are predicted to increase the risk of bradycardia when given with **calcium-channel blockers**. Severe Theoretical
- Calcium-channel blockers **(diltiazem, verapamil)** are predicted to increase the concentration of antimalarials **(piperaquine)**. Severe Study
- Calcium-channel blockers **(diltiazem, verapamil)** are predicted to increase the exposure to atypical antipsychotics **(cariprazine)**. Monitor and adjust dose. Severe Study → Also see TABLE 6 p. 1054

- Calcium-channel blockers **(diltiazem, verapamil)** are predicted to increase the exposure to atypical antipsychotics **(lurasidone)**. Adjust **lurasidone** dose. Moderate Study → Also see **TABLE 6** p. 1054
- Calcium-channel blockers **(diltiazem, verapamil)** are predicted to increase the exposure to atypical antipsychotics **(quetiapine)**. Avoid. Moderate Study → Also see **TABLE 6** p. 1054
- Calcium-channel blockers **(diltiazem, verapamil)** are predicted to increase the exposure to **avapritinib**. Avoid or adjust dose—consult product literature. Moderate Study
- Calcium-channel blockers **(diltiazem, verapamil)** are predicted to increase the exposure to **axitinib**. Moderate Study
- Calcium-channel blockers **(diltiazem, verapamil)** might increase the exposure to **bedaquiline**. Mild Theoretical
- Calcium-channel blockers **(diltiazem, verapamil)** are predicted to increase the exposure to benzodiazepines **(alprazolam)**. Severe Study
- Calcium-channel blockers **(diltiazem, verapamil)** are predicted to increase the exposure to benzodiazepines **(midazolam)**. Monitor adverse effects and adjust dose. Severe Study
- **Berotralstat** is predicted to increase the exposure to calcium-channel blockers **(amlodipine, felodipine, lacidipine, lercanidipine, nicardipine, nifedipine, nimodipine)**. Monitor and adjust dose. Moderate Study
- **Diltiazem** is predicted to increase the risk of cardiodepression when given with **beta blockers, non-selective**. Severe Study → Also see **TABLE 4** p. 1054 → Also see **TABLE 6** p. 1054
- **Verapamil** increases the risk of cardiovascular adverse effects when given with **beta blockers, non-selective**. Avoid intravenous **verapamil**, p. 129. Severe Study → Also see **TABLE 4** p. 1054 → Also see **TABLE 6** p. 1054
- **Diltiazem** is predicted to increase the risk of cardiodepression when given with **beta blockers, selective**. Avoid or monitor. Severe Study → Also see **TABLE 4** p. 1054 → Also see **TABLE 6** p. 1054
- **Verapamil** increases the risk of cardiovascular adverse effects when given with **beta blockers, selective**. Use with caution or avoid. Severe Study → Also see **TABLE 4** p. 1054 → Also see **TABLE 6** p. 1054
- Calcium-channel blockers **(diltiazem, verapamil)** are predicted to increase the exposure to **bosutinib**. Avoid or adjust dose. Severe Study
- Calcium-channel blockers **(diltiazem, verapamil)** are predicted to increase the exposure to **brigatinib**. Moderate Study → Also see **TABLE 4** p. 1054
- Calcium-channel blockers **(diltiazem, verapamil)** are predicted to increase the exposure to **buspirone**. Use with caution and adjust dose. Moderate Study
- Calcium channel blockers **(diltiazem, verapamil)** are predicted to increase the exposure to **cabozantinib**. Moderate Study
- Calcium-channel blockers **(diltiazem)** are predicted to increase the exposure to calcium-channel blockers **(amlodipine)**. Monitor and adjust dose. Moderate Study → Also see **TABLE 6** p. 1054
- Calcium-channel blockers **(verapamil)** are predicted to increase the exposure to calcium-channel blockers **(amlodipine, felodipine, lacidipine, lercanidipine, nicardipine, nifedipine, nimodipine)**. Monitor and adjust dose. Moderate Study → Also see **TABLE 6** p. 1054
- Calcium-channel blockers **(diltiazem)** are predicted to increase the exposure to calcium-channel blockers **(felodipine, lacidipine, lercanidipine, nicardipine, nifedipine, nimodipine)**. Monitor and adjust dose. Moderate Study → Also see **TABLE 6** p. 1054
- Calcium-channel blockers **(diltiazem, verapamil)** are predicted to increase the exposure to **capivasertib**. Adjust dose. Moderate Study
- **Cenobamate** is predicted to decrease the exposure to calcium-channel blockers **(amlodipine, felodipine, lacidipine, lercanidipine, nicardipine, nifedipine, nimodipine)**. Monitor and adjust dose. Moderate Theoretical
- **Cenobamate** is predicted to decrease the exposure to calcium-channel blockers **(diltiazem, verapamil)**. Moderate Theoretical
- Calcium-channel blockers **(diltiazem, verapamil)** are predicted to increase the exposure to **ceritinib**. Moderate Study → Also see **TABLE 4** p. 1054
- **Ceritinib** is predicted to increase the exposure to calcium-channel blockers **(amlodipine, felodipine, lacidipine, nicardipine, nifedipine, nimodipine)**. Monitor and adjust dose. Moderate Study
- **Ceritinib** is predicted to increase the exposure to calcium-channel blockers **(diltiazem, verapamil)**. Severe Study → Also see **TABLE 4** p. 1054
- **Ceritinib** is predicted to markedly increase the exposure to **lercanidipine**. Avoid. Severe Study
- Calcium-channel blockers **(diltiazem, verapamil)** are predicted to increase the concentration of **ciclosporin**. Severe Study
- **Ciclosporin** moderately increases the exposure to **lercanidipine**. Use with caution or avoid. Severe Study
- **Nicardipine** increases the concentration of **ciclosporin**. Severe Study
- Calcium-channel blockers **(nifedipine, nimodipine)** might increase the exposure to **cladribine**. Avoid or adjust dose. Moderate Theoretical
- **Cobicistat** is predicted to increase the exposure to calcium-channel blockers **(amlodipine, felodipine, lacidipine, nicardipine, nifedipine, nimodipine)**. Monitor and adjust dose. Moderate Study
- **Cobicistat** is predicted to increase the exposure to calcium-channel blockers **(diltiazem, verapamil)**. Severe Study
- **Cobicistat** is predicted to markedly increase the exposure to **lercanidipine**. Avoid. Severe Study
- Calcium-channel blockers **(diltiazem, verapamil)** are predicted to increase the exposure to **cobimetinib**. Severe Study
- Calcium-channel blockers **(diltiazem, verapamil)** are predicted to increase the exposure to **colchicine**. Adjust **colchicine** dose with moderate CYP3A4 inhibitors, p. 637. Severe Study
- Calcium-channel blockers **(diltiazem, verapamil)** are predicted to increase the exposure to corticosteroids **(methylprednisolone)**. Monitor and adjust dose. Moderate Study
- Calcium-channel blockers **(diltiazem, verapamil)** are predicted to increase the exposure to **crizotinib**. Avoid. Moderate Study → Also see **TABLE 4** p. 1054
- **Crizotinib** is predicted to increase the exposure to calcium-channel blockers **(amlodipine, felodipine, lacidipine, lercanidipine, nicardipine, nifedipine, nimodipine)**. Monitor and adjust dose. Moderate Study
- Calcium-channel blockers **(diltiazem, verapamil)** are predicted to increase the exposure to **dabrafenib**. Moderate Study
- **Dabrafenib** is predicted to decrease the exposure to calcium-channel blockers **(amlodipine, felodipine, lacidipine, lercanidipine, nicardipine, nifedipine, nimodipine)**. Monitor and adjust dose. Moderate Theoretical
- **Dabrafenib** is predicted to decrease the exposure to calcium-channel blockers **(diltiazem, verapamil)**. Moderate Theoretical
- Intravenous **dantrolene** potentially increases the risk of acute hyperkalaemia and cardiovascular collapse when given with calcium-channel blockers **(diltiazem, verapamil)**. Avoid. Severe Anecdotal
- Calcium-channel blockers **(diltiazem, verapamil)** are predicted to increase the exposure to **daridorexant**. Adjust **daridorexant** dose. Severe Study
- **Diltiazem** is predicted to increase the exposure to **darifenacin**. Moderate Study
- **Verapamil** is predicted to increase the exposure to **darifenacin**. Avoid. Moderate Study
- Calcium-channel blockers **(diltiazem, verapamil)** are predicted to increase the exposure to **dasatinib**. Severe Study
- Calcium-channel blockers **(diltiazem, verapamil)** are predicted to increase the exposure to **deutivacaftor**. Adjust dose, see deutivacaftor with tezacaftor and vanzacaftor p. 218. Severe Study
- Calcium-channel blockers **(diltiazem, verapamil)** are predicted to slightly increase the exposure to **dienogest**. Moderate Study
- Calcium-channel blockers **(diltiazem, verapamil)** increase the concentration of **digoxin**. Monitor and adjust dose. Severe Study → Also see **TABLE 4** p. 1054
- Calcium-channel blockers **(diltiazem, verapamil)** are predicted to increase the exposure to dipeptidylpeptidase-4 inhibitors **(saxagliptin)**. Mild Study
- Calcium-channel blockers **(diltiazem, verapamil)** are predicted to increase the exposure to **domperidone**. Avoid. Severe Study

A1 Interactions | **Appendix 1**

Calcium-channel blockers (continued)

- Calcium-channel blockers **(diltiazem, verapamil)** are predicted to increase the exposure to dopamine receptor agonists **(bromocriptine)**. Severe Theoretical → Also see TABLE 6 p. 1054
- Calcium-channel blockers **(diltiazem, verapamil)** are predicted to increase the concentration of dopamine receptor agonists **(cabergoline)**. Moderate Anecdotal → Also see TABLE 6 p. 1054
- Calcium-channel blockers **(diltiazem, verapamil)** are predicted to increase the exposure to **drospirenone**. Severe Study
- Calcium-channel blockers **(diltiazem, verapamil)** are predicted to moderately increase the exposure to **dutasteride**. Mild Study
- Calcium-channel blockers **(diltiazem, verapamil)** are predicted to increase the exposure to **elacestrant**. Avoid moderate CYP3A4 inhibitors or adjust **elacestrant** dose. Severe Theoretical
- Calcium-channel blockers **(diltiazem, verapamil)** are predicted to increase the exposure to **elexacaftor**. Adjust ivacaftor with tezacaftor and elexacaftor p. 220 dose with moderate CYP3A4 inhibitors. Severe Theoretical
- Calcium-channel blockers **(diltiazem, verapamil)** are predicted to increase the exposure to **eliglustat**. Avoid or adjust dose—consult product literature. Severe Study
- Calcium-channel blockers **(diltiazem, verapamil)** are predicted to moderately increase the exposure to **encorafenib**. Moderate Study
- **Encorafenib** is predicted to decrease the exposure to calcium-channel blockers **(amlodipine, felodipine, lacidipine, lercanidipine, nicardipine, nifedipine, nimodipine)**. Monitor and adjust dose. Moderate Study
- Endothelin receptor antagonists **(bosentan)** are predicted to decrease the exposure to calcium-channel blockers **(amlodipine, felodipine, lacidipine, lercanidipine, nicardipine, nifedipine, nimodipine)**. Monitor and adjust dose. Moderate Theoretical
- Endothelin receptor antagonists **(bosentan)** are predicted to decrease the exposure to calcium-channel blockers **(diltiazem, verapamil)**. Moderate Theoretical
- Calcium-channel blockers **(diltiazem, verapamil)** are predicted to increase the exposure to endothelin receptor antagonists **(macitentan)**. Manufacturer advises caution depending on other drugs taken—consult product literature. Moderate Theoretical
- Calcium-channel blockers **(diltiazem, verapamil)** are predicted to increase the exposure to **entrectinib**. Avoid or adjust dose with moderate CYP3A4 inhibitors—consult product literature. Severe Theoretical
- Calcium-channel blockers **(diltiazem, verapamil)** are predicted to increase the risk of ergotism when given with **ergometrine**. Severe Theoretical
- Calcium-channel blockers **(diltiazem, verapamil)** are predicted to increase the exposure to **erlotinib**. Moderate Study
- Calcium-channel blockers **(diltiazem, verapamil)** are predicted to increase the exposure to **etrasimod**. Avoid in poor CYP2C9 metabolisers. Severe Theoretical → Also see TABLE 4 p. 1054
- Calcium-channel blockers **(diltiazem, verapamil)** are predicted to increase the concentration of **everolimus**. Avoid or adjust dose. Moderate Study
- **Verapamil** slightly increases the exposure to factor XA inhibitors **(edoxaban)**. Moderate Study
- **Verapamil** slightly increases the exposure to factor XA inhibitors **(rivaroxaban)**. Manufacturer advises caution in renal impairment. Moderate Study
- Calcium-channel blockers **(diltiazem, verapamil)** are predicted to increase the exposure to **fedratinib**. Monitor and adjust dose. Moderate Study
- **Fedratinib** is predicted to increase the exposure to calcium-channel blockers **(amlodipine, felodipine, lacidipine, lercanidipine, nicardipine, nifedipine, nimodipine)**. Monitor and adjust dose. Moderate Study
- Calcium-channel blockers **(diltiazem, verapamil)** are predicted to increase the exposure to **fesoterodine**. Adjust **fesoterodine** dose with moderate CYP3A4 inhibitors in hepatic and renal impairment. Mild Study
- **Verapamil** is predicted to increase the exposure to **fidaxomicin**. Avoid. Moderate Study
- **Diltiazem** is predicted to increase the exposure to **fostamatinib**. Monitor adverse effects and adjust dose. Moderate Theoretical
- Calcium-channel blockers **(diltiazem, verapamil)** are predicted to increase the exposure to **gefitinib**. Moderate Study
- **Verapamil** is predicted to increase the exposure to **gilteritinib**. Moderate Theoretical
- **Grapefruit** juice very slightly increases the exposure to **amlodipine**. Avoid. Mild Study
- **Grapefruit** juice increases the exposure to calcium-channel blockers **(nifedipine, verapamil)**. Avoid. Mild Study
- **Grapefruit** juice increases the exposure to **felodipine**. Avoid. Moderate Study
- **Grapefruit** juice is predicted to increase the exposure to **lercanidipine**. Avoid. Moderate Theoretical
- **Grapefruit** juice increases the exposure to **nicardipine**. Mild Study
- Calcium-channel blockers **(diltiazem, verapamil)** are predicted to increase the concentration of **guanfacine**. Adjust **guanfacine** dose, p. 281. Moderate Theoretical → Also see TABLE 6 p. 1054
- H_2 receptor antagonists **(cimetidine)** (high-dose) are predicted to increase the exposure to **lercanidipine**. Moderate Theoretical
- H_2 receptor antagonists **(cimetidine)** moderately increase the exposure to **nifedipine**. Monitor and adjust dose. Severe Study
- H_2 receptor antagonists **(cimetidine)** increase the exposure to **verapamil**. Moderate Study
- H_2 receptor antagonists **(cimetidine)** slightly increase the exposure to calcium-channel blockers **(diltiazem, nimodipine)**. Monitor and adjust dose. Moderate Study
- **HIV-protease inhibitors** are predicted to increase the exposure to calcium-channel blockers **(amlodipine, felodipine, lacidipine, nicardipine, nifedipine, nimodipine)**. Monitor and adjust dose. Moderate Study
- **HIV-protease inhibitors** are predicted to increase the exposure to calcium-channel blockers **(diltiazem, verapamil)**. Severe Study
- **HIV-protease inhibitors** are predicted to markedly increase the exposure to **lercanidipine**. Avoid. Severe Study
- Calcium-channel blockers **(diltiazem, verapamil)** are predicted to increase the exposure to **ibrutinib**. Adjust dose with moderate CYP3A4 inhibitors—consult product literature. Severe Study
- **Idelalisib** is predicted to increase the exposure to calcium-channel blockers **(amlodipine, felodipine, lacidipine, nicardipine, nifedipine, nimodipine)**. Monitor and adjust dose. Moderate Study
- **Idelalisib** is predicted to increase the exposure to calcium-channel blockers **(diltiazem, verapamil)**. Severe Study
- **Idelalisib** is predicted to markedly increase the exposure to **lercanidipine**. Avoid. Severe Study
- Calcium-channel blockers **(diltiazem, verapamil)** are predicted to increase the exposure to **imatinib**. Moderate Theoretical
- **Imatinib** is predicted to increase the exposure to calcium-channel blockers **(amlodipine, felodipine, lacidipine, lercanidipine, nicardipine, nifedipine, nimodipine)**. Monitor and adjust dose. Moderate Study
- Calcium-channel blockers **(diltiazem, verapamil)** are predicted to increase the exposure to the active metabolite of **irinotecan**. Moderate Theoretical
- Calcium-channel blockers **(diltiazem, verapamil)** are predicted to increase the exposure to **ivabradine**. Avoid. Moderate Study → Also see TABLE 4 p. 1054
- Calcium-channel blockers **(diltiazem, verapamil)** are predicted to increase the exposure to **ivacaftor**. Adjust dose with moderate CYP3A4 inhibitors, see ivacaftor p. 219, tezacaftor with ivacaftor p. 223, and ivacaftor with tezacaftor and elexacaftor p. 220. Moderate Study
- Calcium-channel blockers **(diltiazem, verapamil)** are predicted to increase the exposure to **ivosidenib**. Monitor and adjust dose—consult product literature. Severe Study
- **Ivosidenib** is predicted to decrease the exposure to calcium-channel blockers **(amlodipine, felodipine, lacidipine, lercanidipine, nicardipine, nifedipine, nimodipine)**. Monitor and adjust dose. Moderate Study
- Calcium-channel blockers **(diltiazem, verapamil)** are predicted to increase the exposure to **lapatinib**. Moderate Study
- Calcium-channel blockers **(diltiazem, verapamil)** are predicted to increase the exposure to **larotrectinib**. Monitor and adjust dose. Moderate Theoretical

- Calcium-channel blockers **(diltiazem, verapamil)** are predicted to increase the exposure to **leniolisib**. Avoid. Moderate Study
- **Letermovir** is predicted to increase the exposure to calcium-channel blockers **(amlodipine, felodipine, lacidipine, lercanidipine, nicardipine, nifedipine, nimodipine)**. Monitor and adjust dose. Moderate Study
- Calcium-channel blockers **(diltiazem, verapamil)** are predicted to increase the risk of neurotoxicity when given with **lithium**. Severe Anecdotal
- Calcium-channel blockers **(amlodipine, lacidipine)** are predicted to increase the exposure to **lomitapide**. Separate administration by 12 hours. Moderate Theoretical
- Calcium-channel blockers **(diltiazem, verapamil)** are predicted to increase the exposure to **lomitapide**. Avoid. Moderate Theoretical
- **Lorlatinib** is predicted to decrease the exposure to calcium-channel blockers **(amlodipine, felodipine, lacidipine, lercanidipine, nicardipine, nifedipine, nimodipine)**. Monitor and adjust dose. Moderate Theoretical
- **Lorlatinib** is predicted to decrease the exposure to calcium-channel blockers **(diltiazem, verapamil)**. Moderate Theoretical
- **Lumacaftor** is predicted to decrease the exposure to calcium-channel blockers **(amlodipine, felodipine, lacidipine, lercanidipine, nicardipine, nifedipine, nimodipine)**. Monitor and adjust dose. Moderate Study
- Macrolides **(clarithromycin)** are predicted to markedly increase the exposure to **lercanidipine**. Avoid. Severe Study
- Macrolides **(erythromycin)** are predicted to increase the exposure to **diltiazem**. Severe Theoretical
- Macrolides **(erythromycin)** are predicted to increase the exposure to **verapamil**. Severe Study
- Macrolides **(erythromycin)** are predicted to increase the exposure to calcium-channel blockers **(amlodipine, felodipine, lacidipine, lercanidipine, nicardipine, nifedipine, nimodipine)**. Monitor and adjust dose. Moderate Study
- Macrolides **(clarithromycin)** are predicted to increase the exposure to calcium-channel blockers **(amlodipine, felodipine, lacidipine, nicardipine, nifedipine, nimodipine)**. Monitor and adjust dose. Moderate Study
- Macrolides **(clarithromycin)** are predicted to increase the exposure to calcium-channel blockers **(diltiazem, verapamil)**. Severe Study
- Intravenous **magnesium** potentially increases the risk of hypotension when given with calcium-channel blockers **(amlodipine, felodipine, lacidipine, lercanidipine, nicardipine, nifedipine, nimodipine, verapamil)** in pregnant women. Severe Anecdotal
- Calcium-channel blockers **(diltiazem, verapamil)** are predicted to increase the exposure to **mavacamten**. Adjust dose—consult product literature. Moderate Study
- **Mexiletine** increases the risk of cardiovascular adverse effects when given with **diltiazem**. Avoid or monitor. Severe Theoretical
- **Mexiletine** potentially increases the risk of cardiovascular adverse effects when given with **verapamil**. Avoid or monitor. Severe Theoretical
- Calcium-channel blockers **(diltiazem, verapamil)** are predicted to increase the exposure to **midostaurin**. Moderate Theoretical
- Calcium-channel blockers **(diltiazem, verapamil)** are predicted to increase the exposure to mineralocorticoid receptor antagonists **(eplerenone)**. Adjust **eplerenone** dose. Severe Study → Also see **TABLE 6** p. 1054
- Calcium-channel blockers **(diltiazem, verapamil)** are predicted to increase the exposure to mineralocorticoid receptor antagonists **(finerenone)**. Severe Study → Also see **TABLE 6** p. 1054
- **Mitotane** is predicted to decrease the exposure to calcium-channel blockers **(amlodipine, felodipine, lacidipine, lercanidipine, nicardipine, nifedipine, nimodipine)**. Monitor and adjust dose. Moderate Study
- **Mitotane** is predicted to decrease the exposure to **diltiazem**. Severe Study
- Monoclonal antibodies **(tocilizumab)** are predicted to decrease the exposure to **calcium-channel blockers**. Monitor and adjust dose. Moderate Theoretical
- **Verapamil** increases the risk of neutropenia when given with monoclonal antibodies **(brentuximab vedotin)**. Monitor and adjust dose. Severe Theoretical
- Calcium-channel blockers **(diltiazem, verapamil)** are predicted to increase the exposure to **naldemedine**. Moderate Study
- Calcium-channel blockers **(diltiazem, verapamil)** are predicted to increase the exposure to **naloxegol**. Adjust **naloxegol** dose and monitor adverse effects. Moderate Study
- Calcium-channel blockers **(diltiazem, verapamil)** are predicted to increase the exposure to **neratinib**. Avoid moderate CYP3A4 inhibitors or adjust dose and monitor for gastrointestinal adverse effects—consult product literature. Severe Study
- Neurokinin-1 receptor antagonists **(aprepitant, netupitant)** are predicted to increase the exposure to calcium-channel blockers **(amlodipine, felodipine, lacidipine, lercanidipine, nicardipine, nifedipine, nimodipine)**. Monitor and adjust dose. Moderate Study
- Calcium-channel blockers **(diltiazem, verapamil)** are predicted to increase the exposure to neurokinin-1 receptor antagonists **(aprepitant)** and neurokinin-1 receptor antagonists **(aprepitant)** are predicted to increase the exposure to calcium-channel blockers **(diltiazem, verapamil)**. Moderate Study
- Calcium-channel blockers **(diltiazem, verapamil)** are predicted to increase the exposure to **nilotinib**. Moderate Theoretical
- **Nilotinib** is predicted to increase the exposure to calcium-channel blockers **(amlodipine, felodipine, lacidipine, lercanidipine, nicardipine, nifedipine, nimodipine)**. Monitor and adjust dose. Moderate Study
- **Verapamil** is predicted to increase the exposure to **nintedanib**. Moderate Study
- **Nirmatrelvir** boosted with ritonavir is predicted to increase the concentration of **calcium-channel blockers**. Severe Theoretical
- NNRTIs **(efavirenz, etravirine, nevirapine)** are predicted to decrease the exposure to calcium-channel blockers **(amlodipine, felodipine, lacidipine, lercanidipine, nicardipine, nifedipine, nimodipine)**. Monitor and adjust dose. Moderate Theoretical
- NNRTIs **(efavirenz, etravirine, nevirapine)** are predicted to decrease the exposure to calcium-channel blockers **(diltiazem, verapamil)**. Moderate Theoretical
- Calcium-channel blockers **(diltiazem, verapamil)** are predicted to increase the exposure to **olaparib**. Avoid or adjust dose with moderate CYP3A4 inhibitors—consult product literature. Moderate Theoretical
- Calcium-channel blockers **(diltiazem, verapamil)** are predicted to increase the exposure to **omaveloxolone**. Avoid or adjust **omaveloxolone** dose, p. 755. Moderate Study
- Calcium-channel blockers **(diltiazem, verapamil)** are predicted to increase the exposure to opioids **(alfentanil, buprenorphine, fentanyl, oxycodone)**. Monitor and adjust dose. Moderate Study → Also see **TABLE 4** p. 1054
- **Nicardipine** is predicted to increase the exposure to opioids **(fentanyl)**. Monitor and adjust dose. Moderate Theoretical
- Calcium-channel blockers **(diltiazem, verapamil)** are predicted to increase the exposure to opioids **(methadone, sufentanil)**. Moderate Theoretical → Also see **TABLE 4** p. 1054
- **Verapamil** is predicted to increase the exposure to **panobinostat**. Adjust dose. Moderate Theoretical
- Calcium-channel blockers **(diltiazem, verapamil)** are predicted to increase the exposure to **pazopanib**. Moderate Study
- Calcium-channel blockers **(diltiazem, verapamil)** are predicted to increase the exposure to **pemigatinib**. Severe Study
- Calcium-channel blockers **(diltiazem, verapamil)** are predicted to increase the exposure to phosphodiesterase type-5 inhibitors **(avanafil)**. Adjust **avanafil** dose. Moderate Theoretical → Also see **TABLE 6** p. 1054
- Calcium-channel blockers **(diltiazem, verapamil)** are predicted to increase the exposure to phosphodiesterase type-5 inhibitors **(sildenafil)**. Monitor or adjust **sildenafil** dose with moderate CYP3A4 inhibitors, p. 139. Moderate Study → Also see **TABLE 6** p. 1054
- Calcium-channel blockers **(diltiazem, verapamil)** are predicted to increase the exposure to phosphodiesterase type-5 inhibitors **(tadalafil)**. Severe Theoretical → Also see **TABLE 6** p. 1054
- Calcium-channel blockers **(diltiazem, verapamil)** are predicted to increase the exposure to phosphodiesterase type-5 inhibitors **(vardenafil)**. Adjust dose. Severe Theoretical → Also see **TABLE 6** p. 1054

Calcium-channel blockers (continued)

- Calcium-channel blockers **(diltiazem, verapamil)** are predicted to increase the exposure to pimozide. Avoid. Severe Theoretical → Also see TABLE 6 p. 1054
- Calcium-channel blockers **(diltiazem, verapamil)** are predicted to increase the exposure to ponatinib. Moderate Study
- Calcium-channel blockers **(diltiazem, verapamil)** are predicted to increase the exposure to pralsetinib. Moderate Theoretical
- Calcium-channel blockers **(diltiazem, verapamil)** are predicted to increase the exposure to ranolazine. Severe Study
- Calcium-channel blockers **(diltiazem, verapamil)** are predicted to increase the exposure to regorafenib. Moderate Study
- **Verapamil** is predicted to increase the exposure to relugolix. Avoid or take relugolix first and separate administration by at least 6 hours. Moderate Study
- Calcium-channel blockers **(diltiazem, verapamil)** are predicted to increase the exposure to ribociclib. Moderate Study
- Rifamycins **(rifampicin)** greatly decrease the exposure to **nifedipine**. Avoid. Severe Study
- Rifamycins **(rifampicin)** are predicted to decrease the exposure to calcium-channel blockers **(amlodipine, felodipine, lacidipine, lercanidipine, nicardipine, nimodipine)**. Monitor and adjust dose. Moderate Study
- Rifamycins **(rifampicin)** greatly decrease the exposure to calcium-channel blockers **(diltiazem, verapamil)**. Severe Study
- Calcium-channel blockers **(diltiazem, verapamil)** are predicted to increase the exposure to rimegepant. Avoid another dose of rimegepant within 48 hours of concurrent use. Moderate Study
- Calcium-channel blockers **(diltiazem, verapamil)** are predicted to increase the exposure to ruxolitinib. Moderate Study
- Calcium-channel blockers **(diltiazem, verapamil)** are predicted to increase the exposure to selpercatinib. Moderate Study
- Calcium-channel blockers **(diltiazem, verapamil)** are predicted to increase the exposure to selumetinib. Avoid or adjust dose—consult product literature. Severe Study
- Calcium-channel blockers **(diltiazem, verapamil)** are predicted to increase the exposure to siponimod. Avoid depending on other drugs taken—consult product literature. Severe Study → Also see TABLE 4 p. 1054
- Calcium-channel blockers **(diltiazem, verapamil)** increase the concentration of sirolimus. Monitor and adjust dose. Moderate Study
- **Sotorasib** is predicted to decrease the exposure to calcium-channel blockers **(amlodipine, felodipine, lacidipine, lercanidipine, nicardipine, nifedipine, nimodipine)**. Monitor and adjust dose. Moderate Theoretical
- **Sotorasib** is predicted to decrease the exposure to calcium-channel blockers **(diltiazem, verapamil)**. Moderate Theoretical
- Calcium-channel blockers **(diltiazem, verapamil)** are predicted to increase the exposure to sparsentan. Moderate Study → Also see TABLE 6 p. 1054
- Calcium-channel blockers **(diltiazem, verapamil)** are predicted to increase the exposure to SSRIs (dapoxetine). Adjust **dapoxetine** dose with moderate CYP3A4 inhibitors. Moderate Theoretical
- Calcium-channel blockers **(diltiazem, verapamil)** are predicted to increase the exposure to SSRIs **(sertraline)**. Moderate Theoretical
- **St John's wort** is predicted to decrease the exposure to calcium-channel blockers **(amlodipine, felodipine, lacidipine, lercanidipine, nifedipine, nimodipine)**. Monitor and adjust dose. Moderate Theoretical
- **St John's wort** is predicted to decrease the exposure to calcium-channel blockers **(diltiazem, verapamil)**. Moderate Theoretical
- **Diltiazem** slightly increases the exposure to statins **(atorvastatin)**. Monitor and adjust dose. Severe Study
- **Verapamil** is predicted to slightly to moderately increase the exposure to statins **(atorvastatin)**. Monitor and adjust dose. Severe Theoretical
- **Amlodipine** causes a small increase in the exposure to statins **(simvastatin)**. Adjust **simvastatin** dose, p. 156. Moderate Study
- Calcium-channel blockers **(diltiazem, verapamil)** moderately increase the exposure to statins **(simvastatin)**. Monitor and adjust dose. Severe Study
- Calcium-channel blockers **(diltiazem, verapamil)** are predicted to increase the exposure to sunitinib. Moderate Study
- **Diltiazem** increases the concentration of tacrolimus. Monitor and adjust dose. Severe Anecdotal
- **Nicardipine** potentially increases the concentration of tacrolimus. Monitor concentration and adjust dose. Severe Anecdotal
- **Verapamil** is predicted to increase the concentration of tacrolimus. Monitor and adjust dose. Severe Theoretical
- Calcium-channel blockers **(diltiazem, felodipine)** very slightly increase the exposure to talazoparib. Moderate Study
- **Verapamil** is predicted to slightly increase the exposure to talazoparib. Avoid or adjust dose—consult product literature. Severe Study
- Calcium-channel blockers **(diltiazem, verapamil)** are predicted to increase the exposure to taxanes **(cabazitaxel)**. Moderate Theoretical
- Calcium-channel blockers **(diltiazem, verapamil)** are predicted to increase the exposure to taxanes **(docetaxel)**. Severe Study
- Calcium-channel blockers **(diltiazem, verapamil)** are predicted to increase the exposure to taxanes **(paclitaxel)**. Moderate Anecdotal
- Calcium-channel blockers **(diltiazem, verapamil)** are predicted to increase the concentration of, and the risk of angioedema, when given with temsirolimus. Use with caution or avoid. Moderate Theoretical
- **Temsirolimus** is predicted to increase the risk of angioedema when given with calcium-channel blockers **(amlodipine, felodipine, lacidipine, lercanidipine, nicardipine, nifedipine, nimodipine)**. Moderate Theoretical
- Calcium-channel blockers **(diltiazem, verapamil)** are predicted to increase the exposure to tezacaftor. Adjust dose with moderate CYP3A4 inhibitors, see tezacaftor with ivacaftor p. 223, ivacaftor with tezacaftor and elexacaftor p. 220, and deutivacaftor with tezacaftor and vanzacaftor p. 218. Severe Study
- **Verapamil** increases the exposure to thrombin inhibitors **(dabigatran)**. Monitor and adjust dose. Severe Study
- **Verapamil** might increase the exposure to tigecycline. Mild Anecdotal
- Calcium-channel blockers **(diltiazem, verapamil)** given with a potent CYP2C19 inhibitor are predicted to increase the exposure to tofacitinib. Adjust **tofacitinib** dose, p. 803. Moderate Study
- Calcium-channel blockers **(diltiazem, verapamil)** are predicted to increase the exposure to tolvaptan. Manufacturer advises caution or adjust **tolvaptan** dose with moderate CYP3A4 inhibitors. Moderate Study
- **Verapamil** is predicted to increase the exposure to topotecan. Severe Study
- **Verapamil** is predicted to increase the concentration of trametinib. Moderate Theoretical
- Calcium-channel blockers **(diltiazem, verapamil)** are predicted to increase the exposure to trazodone. Moderate Theoretical
- **Tucatinib** is predicted to increase the exposure to calcium-channel blockers **(amlodipine, felodipine, lacidipine, nicardipine, nifedipine, nimodipine)**. Monitor and adjust dose. Moderate Study
- **Tucatinib** is predicted to increase the exposure to calcium-channel blockers **(diltiazem, verapamil)**. Severe Study
- **Tucatinib** is predicted to markedly increase the exposure to **lercanidipine**. Avoid. Severe Study
- Calcium-channel blockers **(diltiazem, verapamil)** are predicted to increase the exposure to ulipristal. Avoid when used for uterine fibroids. Moderate Study
- Calcium-channel blockers **(diltiazem, verapamil)** are predicted to increase the exposure to vanzacaftor. Adjust dose, see deutivacaftor with tezacaftor and vanzacaftor p. 218. Severe Study
- Calcium-channel blockers **(diltiazem, verapamil)** are predicted to increase the exposure to vemurafenib. Severe Theoretical
- Calcium-channel blockers **(diltiazem, verapamil)** are predicted to increase the exposure to venetoclax. Avoid or adjust dose—consult product literature. Severe Study
- Calcium-channel blockers **(diltiazem, verapamil)** are predicted to increase the exposure to vinca alkaloids. Severe Theoretical

- Calcium-channel blockers **(diltiazem, verapamil)** are predicted to increase the exposure to voclosporin. Adjust **voclosporin** dose. [Severe] Study
- Calcium-channel blockers **(diltiazem, verapamil)** are predicted to increase the exposure to **zanubrutinib**. Avoid or adjust dose with moderate CYP3A4 inhibitors—consult product literature. [Severe] Study
- Calcium-channel blockers **(diltiazem, verapamil)** are predicted to increase the exposure to **zopiclone**. Adjust dose. [Moderate] Study

Canagliflozin → see sodium glucose co-transporter 2 inhibitors

Canakinumab → see monoclonal antibodies

Candesartan → see angiotensin-II receptor antagonists

Cangrelor → see TABLE 3 p. 1053 (bleeding)

- **Selumetinib** might increase the risk of bleeding when given with **cangrelor**. [Severe] Theoretical

Cannabidiol → see TABLE 9 p. 1056 (CNS effects)

- Anti-androgens **(apalutamide, enzalutamide)** are predicted to decrease the exposure to **cannabidiol**. Adjust dose. [Moderate] Study
- Antiepileptics **(carbamazepine, fosphenytoin, phenobarbital, phenytoin, primidone)** are predicted to decrease the exposure to **cannabidiol**. Adjust dose. [Moderate] Study → Also see TABLE 9 p. 1056
- **Cannabidiol** increases the risk of increased ALT concentrations when given with antiepileptics **(valproate)**. Avoid or adjust dose. [Severe] Study
- Antifungals, azoles **(fluconazole)** are predicted to increase the exposure to **cannabidiol**. [Moderate] Theoretical
- Antifungals, azoles **(itraconazole, ketoconazole, posaconazole, voriconazole)** are predicted to increase the exposure to **cannabidiol**. Avoid or adjust dose. [Mild] Study
- **Cannabidiol** increases the exposure to the active metabolite of benzodiazepines **(clobazam)** and benzodiazepines **(clobazam)** increase the exposure to the active metabolite of **cannabidiol**. Adjust dose. [Moderate] Study → Also see TABLE 9 p. 1056
- **Ceritinib** is predicted to increase the exposure to **cannabidiol**. Avoid or adjust dose. [Mild] Study
- **Cannabidiol** is predicted to increase the concentration of **ciclosporin**. Monitor and adjust dose. [Severe] Theoretical
- **Cobicistat** is predicted to increase the exposure to **cannabidiol**. Avoid or adjust dose. [Mild] Study
- **Cannabidiol** is predicted to increase the exposure to **digoxin**. Monitor and adjust dose. [Moderate] Study
- **Encorafenib** is predicted to decrease the exposure to **cannabidiol**. Adjust dose. [Moderate] Study
- **Cannabidiol** moderately increases the exposure to **everolimus**. Monitor and adjust dose. [Moderate] Study
- **HIV-protease inhibitors** are predicted to increase the exposure to **cannabidiol**. Avoid or adjust dose. [Mild] Study
- **Idelalisib** is predicted to increase the exposure to **cannabidiol**. Avoid or adjust dose. [Mild] Study
- **Ivosidenib** is predicted to decrease the exposure to **cannabidiol**. Adjust dose. [Moderate] Study
- **Lumacaftor** is predicted to decrease the exposure to **cannabidiol**. Adjust dose. [Moderate] Study
- Macrolides **(clarithromycin)** are predicted to increase the exposure to **cannabidiol**. Avoid or adjust dose. [Mild] Study
- **Mitotane** is predicted to decrease the exposure to **cannabidiol**. Adjust dose. [Moderate] Study
- **Moclobemide** is predicted to increase the exposure to **cannabidiol**. [Moderate] Theoretical
- Proton pump inhibitors **(esomeprazole)** are predicted to increase the exposure to **cannabidiol**. [Moderate] Theoretical
- Rifamycins **(rifampicin)** are predicted to decrease the exposure to **cannabidiol**. Adjust dose. [Moderate] Study
- **Cannabidiol** is predicted to increase the exposure to **sirolimus**. Monitor and adjust dose. [Moderate] Study
- SSRIs **(fluoxetine, fluvoxamine)** are predicted to increase the exposure to **cannabidiol**. [Moderate] Theoretical → Also see TABLE 9 p. 1056
- **St John's wort** is predicted to decrease the exposure to **cannabidiol**. Adjust dose. [Mild] Study
- **Cannabidiol** is predicted to increase the concentration of **tacrolimus**. Monitor and adjust dose. [Moderate] Theoretical
- **Cannabidiol** is predicted to increase the exposure to **talazoparib**. Monitor and adjust dose. [Moderate] Study
- **Cannabidiol** is predicted to increase the exposure to taxanes **(paclitaxel)**. Monitor and adjust dose. [Moderate] Study
- **Tucatinib** is predicted to increase the exposure to **cannabidiol**. Avoid or adjust dose. [Mild] Study

Capecitabine → see TABLE 1 p. 1053 (hepatotoxicity), TABLE 12 p. 1057 (myelosuppression)

- **Allopurinol** is predicted to decrease the effects of **capecitabine**. Avoid. [Severe] Study
- **Capecitabine** increases the concentration of antiepileptics **(fosphenytoin, phenytoin)**. [Severe] Anecdotal
- **Capecitabine** increases the effects of **coumarins**. Monitor INR and adjust dose. [Severe] Anecdotal
- **Folates** are predicted to increase the risk of toxicity when given with **capecitabine**. [Severe] Anecdotal
- H_2 receptor antagonists **(cimetidine)** are predicted to slightly increase the exposure to **capecitabine**. [Severe] Theoretical
- **Live vaccines** are predicted to increase the risk of generalised infection (possibly life-threatening) when given with **capecitabine**. UKHSA advises avoid (refer to Green Book). [Severe] Theoretical
- **Metronidazole** is predicted to increase the risk of capecitabine toxicity when given with **capecitabine**. [Severe] Theoretical

Capivasertib

- Anti-androgens **(apalutamide, enzalutamide)** are predicted to decrease the exposure to **capivasertib**. Avoid. [Moderate] Study
- Antiarrhythmics **(dronedarone)** are predicted to increase the exposure to **capivasertib**. Adjust dose. [Moderate] Study
- Antiepileptics **(carbamazepine, fosphenytoin, phenobarbital, phenytoin, primidone)** are predicted to decrease the exposure to **capivasertib**. Avoid. [Moderate] Study
- Antifungals, azoles **(fluconazole, isavuconazole, itraconazole, ketoconazole, posaconazole, voriconazole)** are predicted to increase the exposure to **capivasertib**. Adjust dose. [Moderate] Study
- **Berotralstat** is predicted to increase the exposure to **capivasertib**. Adjust dose. [Moderate] Study
- Calcium-channel blockers **(diltiazem, verapamil)** are predicted to increase the exposure to **capivasertib**. Adjust dose. [Moderate] Study
- **Cenobamate** is predicted to decrease the exposure to **capivasertib**. Avoid. [Moderate] Study
- **Ceritinib** is predicted to increase the exposure to **capivasertib**. Adjust dose. [Moderate] Study
- **Ciclosporin** is predicted to increase the exposure to **capivasertib**. Adjust dose. [Moderate] Theoretical
- **Cobicistat** is predicted to increase the exposure to **capivasertib**. Adjust dose. [Moderate] Study
- **Crizotinib** is predicted to increase the exposure to **capivasertib**. Adjust dose. [Moderate] Study
- **Dabrafenib** is predicted to decrease the exposure to **capivasertib**. Avoid. [Moderate] Study
- **Encorafenib** is predicted to decrease the exposure to **capivasertib**. Avoid. [Moderate] Study
- Endothelin receptor antagonists **(bosentan)** are predicted to decrease the exposure to **capivasertib**. Avoid. [Moderate] Study
- **Fedratinib** is predicted to increase the exposure to **capivasertib**. Adjust dose. [Moderate] Study
- **Grapefruit** and grapefruit juice is predicted to increase the exposure to **capivasertib**. Adjust dose. [Moderate] Theoretical
- **HIV-protease inhibitors** are predicted to increase the exposure to **capivasertib**. Adjust dose. [Moderate] Study
- **Idelalisib** is predicted to increase the exposure to **capivasertib**. Adjust dose. [Moderate] Study
- **Imatinib** is predicted to increase the exposure to **capivasertib**. Adjust dose. [Moderate] Study
- **Ivosidenib** is predicted to decrease the exposure to **capivasertib**. Avoid. [Moderate] Study
- **Letermovir** is predicted to increase the exposure to **capivasertib**. Adjust dose. [Moderate] Study
- **Lorlatinib** is predicted to decrease the exposure to **capivasertib**. Avoid. [Moderate] Study
- **Lumacaftor** is predicted to decrease the exposure to **capivasertib**. Avoid. [Moderate] Study

Capivasertib (continued)

- Macrolides **(clarithromycin, erythromycin)** are predicted to increase the exposure to **capivasertib**. Adjust dose. Moderate Study
- **Mifepristone** is predicted to increase the exposure to **capivasertib**. Adjust dose. Moderate Theoretical
- **Mitotane** is predicted to decrease the exposure to **capivasertib**. Avoid. Moderate Study
- **Modafinil** is predicted to decrease the exposure to **capivasertib**. Avoid. Moderate Theoretical
- Neurokinin-1 receptor antagonists **(aprepitant, netupitant)** are predicted to increase the exposure to **capivasertib**. Adjust dose. Moderate Study
- **Nilotinib** is predicted to increase the exposure to **capivasertib**. Adjust dose. Moderate Study
- NNRTIs **(efavirenz, etravirine, nevirapine)** are predicted to decrease the exposure to **capivasertib**. Avoid. Moderate Study
- Quinolones **(ciprofloxacin)** are predicted to increase the exposure to **capivasertib**. Adjust dose. Moderate Theoretical
- **Ribociclib** is predicted to increase the exposure to **capivasertib**. Adjust dose. Moderate Theoretical
- Rifamycins **(rifabutin)** are predicted to decrease the exposure to **capivasertib**. Avoid. Moderate Theoretical
- Rifamycins **(rifampicin)** are predicted to decrease the exposure to **capivasertib**. Avoid. Moderate Study
- **Sotorasib** is predicted to decrease the exposure to **capivasertib**. Avoid. Moderate Study
- SSRIs **(fluvoxamine)** are predicted to increase the exposure to **capivasertib**. Adjust dose. Moderate Theoretical
- **St John's wort** is predicted to decrease the exposure to **capivasertib**. Avoid. Moderate Study
- **Telotristat ethyl** is predicted to decrease the exposure to **capivasertib**. Avoid. Moderate Theoretical
- **Tucatinib** is predicted to increase the exposure to **capivasertib**. Adjust dose. Moderate Study

Caplacizumab

- **Drugs that cause bleeding** (see TABLE 3 p. 1053) cause bleeding, as can **caplacizumab**; concurrent use might increase the risk of developing this effect. Severe Theoretical

Captopril → see ACE inhibitors

Carbamazepine → see antiepileptics

Carbapenems

ertapenem · imipenem · meropenem

- **Carbapenems** decrease the concentration of antiepileptics **(valproate)**. Avoid. Severe Anecdotal
- **Ganciclovir** is predicted to increase the risk of seizures when given with **imipenem**. Avoid. Severe Anecdotal
- **Valganciclovir** is predicted to increase the risk of seizures when given with **imipenem**. Avoid. Severe Anecdotal

Carbidopa

- Oral **iron** is predicted to decrease the exposure to oral **carbidopa**. Moderate Theoretical

Carbimazole

- **Carbimazole** affects the concentration of **digoxin**. Monitor and adjust dose. Moderate Theoretical
- **Carbimazole** decreases the effects of **metyrapone**. Avoid. Moderate Theoretical
- **Carbimazole** given with a potent CYP3A4 inhibitor is predicted to increase the exposure to **propiverine**. Adjust starting dose. Moderate Theoretical

Carboplatin → see platinum compounds

Carfilzomib → see TABLE 12 p. 1057 (myelosuppression)

- **Carfilzomib** potentially decreases the efficacy of **combined hormonal contraceptives**. Use additional contraceptive precautions. Severe Theoretical

Cariprazine → see atypical antipsychotics

Carmustine → see alkylating agents

Carvedilol → see beta blockers, non-selective

Caspofungin → see TABLE 1 p. 1053 (hepatotoxicity)

- Antiepileptics **(carbamazepine, fosphenytoin, phenytoin)** are predicted to decrease the concentration of **caspofungin**. Adjust **caspofungin** dose, p. 460. Moderate Theoretical
- **Ciclosporin** slightly increases the exposure to **caspofungin**. Severe Study
- Corticosteroids **(dexamethasone)** are predicted to decrease the concentration of **caspofungin**. Adjust **caspofungin** dose, p. 460. Moderate Theoretical
- NNRTIs **(efavirenz)** are predicted to decrease the concentration of **caspofungin**. Adjust dose. Moderate Study
- NNRTIs **(nevirapine)** are predicted to decrease the concentration of **caspofungin**. Adjust dose. Moderate Theoretical → Also see TABLE 1 p. 1053
- Rifamycins **(rifampicin)** decrease the concentration of **caspofungin**. Adjust **caspofungin** dose, p. 460. Moderate Study

Cedazuridine

- **Cedazuridine** is predicted to increase the exposure to **azacitidine**. Avoid. Moderate Theoretical
- **Cedazuridine** is predicted to increase the exposure to **cytarabine**. Avoid. Moderate Theoretical
- **Cedazuridine** is predicted to increase the exposure to **gemcitabine**. Avoid. Moderate Theoretical

Cefaclor → see cephalosporins

Cefadroxil → see cephalosporins

Cefalexin → see cephalosporins

Cefazolin → see cephalosporins

Cefepime → see cephalosporins

Cefiderocol → see cephalosporins

Cefixime → see cephalosporins

Cefotaxime → see cephalosporins

Cefoxitin → see cephalosporins

Cefradine → see cephalosporins

Ceftaroline → see cephalosporins

Ceftazidime → see cephalosporins

Ceftobiprole → see cephalosporins

Ceftolozane → see cephalosporins

Ceftriaxone → see cephalosporins

Cefuroxime → see cephalosporins

Celecoxib → see NSAIDs

Celiprolol → see beta blockers, selective

Cemiplimab → see monoclonal antibodies

Cenobamate → see TABLE 9 p. 1056 (CNS effects)

- **Cenobamate** is predicted to decrease the exposure to **acalabrutinib**. Adjust dose. Moderate Theoretical
- **Cenobamate** is predicted to decrease the exposure to anti-androgens **(darolutamide)**. Avoid. Moderate Theoretical
- **Cenobamate** might increase the exposure to antiepileptics **(fosphenytoin, primidone)**. Moderate Theoretical → Also see TABLE 9 p. 1056
- **Cenobamate** is predicted to decrease the concentration of antiepileptics **(lamotrigine)** and antiepileptics **(lamotrigine)** might affect the efficacy of **cenobamate**. Adjust dose. Moderate Study → Also see TABLE 9 p. 1056
- **Cenobamate** slightly increases the exposure to antiepileptics **(phenobarbital, phenytoin)**. Monitor and adjust dose. Moderate Study → Also see TABLE 9 p. 1056
- **Cenobamate** is predicted to decrease the exposure to antifungals, azoles **(isavuconazole)**. Avoid. Severe Theoretical
- **Cenobamate** is predicted to decrease the exposure to **atogepant**. Adjust dose. Moderate Theoretical
- **Cenobamate** is predicted to decrease the exposure to atypical antipsychotics **(aripiprazole)**. Avoid or adjust dose—consult product literature. Moderate Study → Also see TABLE 9 p. 1056
- **Cenobamate** is predicted to decrease the exposure to atypical antipsychotics **(cariprazine)**. Avoid. Severe Theoretical → Also see TABLE 9 p. 1056
- **Cenobamate** is predicted to decrease the exposure to atypical antipsychotics **(lurasidone)**. Monitor and adjust dose. Moderate Theoretical → Also see TABLE 9 p. 1056
- **Cenobamate** is predicted to decrease the exposure to atypical antipsychotics **(quetiapine)**. Moderate Study → Also see TABLE 9 p. 1056
- **Cenobamate** is predicted to decrease the exposure to **avacopan**. Severe Theoretical
- **Cenobamate** is predicted to decrease the exposure to **avapritinib**. Avoid. Severe Study
- **Cenobamate** is predicted to decrease the exposure to **bedaquiline**. Avoid. Severe Study
- **Cenobamate** is predicted to increase the exposure to **belzutifan**. Monitor and adjust dose. Severe Theoretical

- **Cenobamate** potentially increases the exposure to benzodiazepines **(clobazam)**. Adjust dose. [Moderate] Theoretical → Also see **TABLE 9** p. 1056
- **Cenobamate** moderately decreases the exposure to benzodiazepines **(midazolam)**. Adjust dose. [Moderate] Study → Also see **TABLE 9** p. 1056
- **Cenobamate** is predicted to decrease the exposure to beta$_2$ agonists **(salmeterol)**. Adjust dose. [Moderate] Theoretical
- **Cenobamate** is predicted to decrease the exposure to **bosutinib**. Avoid. [Severe] Study
- **Cenobamate** is predicted to decrease the exposure to **brigatinib**. Avoid or adjust dose—consult product literature. [Moderate] Study
- **Cenobamate** is predicted to decrease the exposure to **buspirone**. Adjust dose. [Moderate] Theoretical
- **Cenobamate** is predicted to decrease the exposure to **cabozantinib**. [Moderate] Study
- **Cenobamate** is predicted to decrease the exposure to calcium-channel blockers **(amlodipine, felodipine, lacidipine, lercanidipine, nicardipine, nifedipine, nimodipine)**. Monitor and adjust dose. [Moderate] Theoretical
- **Cenobamate** is predicted to decrease the exposure to calcium-channel blockers **(diltiazem, verapamil)**. [Moderate] Theoretical
- **Cenobamate** is predicted to decrease the exposure to **capivasertib**. Avoid. [Moderate] Study
- **Cenobamate** is predicted to decrease the efficacy of **clopidogrel**. Avoid. [Moderate] Study
- **Cenobamate** is predicted to decrease the exposure to **cobicistat**. Avoid. [Severe] Theoretical
- **Cenobamate** is predicted to decrease the exposure to **cobimetinib**. Avoid. [Severe] Theoretical
- **Cenobamate** might decrease the efficacy of oral **combined hormonal contraceptives**. Use additional contraceptive precautions. [Severe] Theoretical
- **Cenobamate** is predicted to decrease the exposure to oral corticosteroids **(budesonide)**. Adjust dose. [Moderate] Theoretical
- **Cenobamate** is predicted to decrease the exposure to corticosteroids **(fluticasone)**. Adjust dose. [Moderate] Theoretical
- **Cenobamate** is predicted to decrease the exposure to **crizotinib**. Avoid. [Severe] Study
- **Cenobamate** is predicted to decrease the exposure to **daridorexant**. [Severe] Study → Also see **TABLE 9** p. 1056
- **Cenobamate** is predicted to decrease the exposure to **darifenacin**. Adjust dose. [Moderate] Theoretical
- **Cenobamate** is predicted to decrease the exposure to **dasatinib**. [Severe] Study
- **Cenobamate** is predicted to decrease the exposure to **deutivacaftor**. Avoid. [Severe] Theoretical
- **Cenobamate** is predicted to decrease the exposure to **elacestrant**. Avoid or adjust dose depending on duration—consult product literature. [Severe] Theoretical
- **Cenobamate** is predicted to moderately decrease the exposure to **elbasvir**. Avoid. [Severe] Study
- **Cenobamate** is predicted to decrease the concentration of **elvitegravir**. Avoid. [Severe] Theoretical
- **Cenobamate** is predicted to decrease the exposure to **encorafenib**. [Moderate] Study
- **Cenobamate** is predicted to decrease the exposure to **entrectinib**. Avoid. [Moderate] Theoretical
- **Cenobamate** is predicted to decrease the exposure to **erdafitinib**. Adjust dose. [Moderate] Theoretical
- **Cenobamate** is predicted to decrease the exposure to **erlotinib**. [Severe] Study
- **Cenobamate** is predicted to decrease the concentration of **everolimus**. Avoid or adjust dose. [Severe] Study
- **Cenobamate** is predicted to decrease the exposure to **fedratinib**. Avoid. [Moderate] Study
- **Cenobamate** is predicted to decrease the exposure to **fruquintinib**. Avoid. [Moderate] Study
- **Cenobamate** is predicted to decrease the exposure to **gefitinib**. Avoid. [Severe] Study
- **Cenobamate** is predicted to decrease the exposure to **glasdegib**. Avoid or adjust dose—consult product literature. [Moderate] Theoretical
- **Cenobamate** is predicted to decrease the exposure to **glecaprevir**. Avoid. [Severe] Study
- **Cenobamate** is predicted to markedly decrease the exposure to **grazoprevir**. Avoid. [Severe] Study
- **Cenobamate** is predicted to decrease the concentration of **guanfacine**. Adjust dose. [Moderate] Theoretical → Also see **TABLE 9** p. 1056
- **Cenobamate** is predicted to decrease the exposure to **ibrutinib**. Adjust dose. [Moderate] Theoretical
- **Cenobamate** is predicted to decrease the exposure to **idelalisib**. Avoid. [Moderate] Theoretical
- **Cenobamate** is predicted to decrease the exposure to **imatinib**. [Moderate] Study
- **Cenobamate** is predicted to decrease the exposure to **ivacaftor**. Adjust dose. [Moderate] Theoretical
- **Cenobamate** is predicted to decrease the exposure to **ixazomib**. [Moderate] Theoretical
- **Cenobamate** is predicted to decrease the exposure to **lapatinib**. Avoid. [Severe] Study
- **Cenobamate** is predicted to decrease the exposure to **larotrectinib**. Avoid. [Moderate] Study
- **Cenobamate** is predicted to decrease the exposure to **lenacapavir**. Avoid. [Severe] Study
- **Cenobamate** is predicted to decrease the exposure to **leniolisib**. Avoid. [Severe] Theoretical
- **Cenobamate** is predicted to decrease the exposure to **lomitapide**. Adjust dose. [Moderate] Theoretical
- **Cenobamate** is predicted to decrease the exposure to **maraviroc**. Adjust dose. [Moderate] Theoretical
- **Cenobamate** is predicted to decrease the exposure to **mavacamten**. Monitor and adjust dose—consult product literature. [Severe] Theoretical
- **Cenobamate** is predicted to decrease the exposure to **mifepristone**. Adjust **mifepristone** dose. [Severe] Study
- **Cenobamate** is predicted to decrease the exposure to mineralocorticoid receptor antagonists **(eplerenone)**. Adjust dose. [Moderate] Theoretical
- **Cenobamate** is predicted to decrease the exposure to mineralocorticoid receptor antagonists **(finerenone)**. Avoid. [Severe] Study
- **Cenobamate** is predicted to decrease the exposure to **naloxegol**. Adjust dose. [Moderate] Theoretical
- **Cenobamate** is predicted to decrease the exposure to **neratinib**. Avoid. [Severe] Theoretical
- **Cenobamate** is predicted to decrease the exposure to neurokinin-1 receptor antagonists **(netupitant)**. [Moderate] Theoretical
- **Cenobamate** is predicted to decrease the exposure to **nilotinib**. Avoid. [Severe] Theoretical
- **Cenobamate** is predicted to decrease the exposure to NNRTIs **(rilpivirine)**. Avoid. [Severe] Theoretical
- **Cenobamate** is predicted to decrease the exposure to **olaparib**. Avoid. [Moderate] Theoretical
- **Cenobamate** is predicted to decrease the exposure to **omaveloxolone**. Avoid. [Severe] Study
- **Cenobamate** is predicted to decrease the exposure to opioids **(alfentanil)**. Adjust dose. [Moderate] Theoretical → Also see **TABLE 9** p. 1056
- **Cenobamate** decreases the exposure to opioids **(methadone)**. Monitor and adjust dose. [Severe] Study → Also see **TABLE 9** p. 1056
- **Cenobamate** is predicted to decrease the exposure to **ospemifene**. [Moderate] Study
- **Cenobamate** is predicted to decrease the exposure to **pazopanib**. [Severe] Study
- **Cenobamate** is predicted to decrease the exposure to phosphodiesterase type-5 inhibitors **(avanafil, sildenafil, vardenafil)**. Adjust dose. [Moderate] Theoretical
- **Cenobamate** is predicted to decrease the exposure to **pibrentasvir**. Avoid. [Severe] Study
- **Cenobamate** is predicted to decrease the exposure to **pirtobrutinib**. [Moderate] Theoretical
- **Cenobamate** is predicted to decrease the exposure to **ponatinib**. [Severe] Study
- **Cenobamate** is predicted to decrease the exposure to **pralsetinib**. [Moderate] Theoretical

Cenobamate (continued)
- **Cenobamate** moderately increases the exposure to proton pump inhibitors **(omeprazole)**. Adjust dose. Moderate Study
- **Cenobamate** is predicted to decrease the exposure to **quizartinib**. Avoid. Severe Study
- **Cenobamate** is predicted to decrease the exposure to **rimegepant**. Avoid. Moderate Theoretical
- **Cenobamate** is predicted to decrease the exposure to **ripretinib**. Avoid or adjust dose—consult product literature. Moderate Theoretical
- **Cenobamate** is predicted to decrease the exposure to **ruxolitinib**. Monitor and adjust dose. Moderate Study
- **Cenobamate** is predicted to decrease the exposure to **selumetinib**. Avoid. Severe Study
- **Cenobamate** is predicted to decrease the exposure to **siponimod**. Manufacturer advises caution depending on genotype—consult product literature. Moderate Theoretical
- **Cenobamate** is predicted to decrease the exposure to **sirolimus**. Adjust dose. Moderate Theoretical
- **Cenobamate** is predicted to decrease the exposure to **sorafenib**. Moderate Study
- **Cenobamate** is predicted to decrease the exposure to **sparsentan**. Avoid. Severe Theoretical
- **Cenobamate** is predicted to increase the exposure to SSRIs **(escitalopram)**. Use with caution and adjust dose. Severe Study → Also see **TABLE 9** p. 1056
- **Cenobamate** is predicted to decrease the exposure to statins **(atorvastatin, simvastatin)**. Moderate Study
- **Cenobamate** is predicted to decrease the exposure to **sunitinib**. Moderate Study
- **Cenobamate** is predicted to decrease the exposure to taxanes **(docetaxel)**. Severe Theoretical
- **Cenobamate** is predicted to decrease the exposure to taxanes **(paclitaxel)**. Avoid. Severe Study
- **Cenobamate** is predicted to decrease the concentration of **temsirolimus**. Avoid. Moderate Theoretical
- **Cenobamate** is predicted to decrease the exposure to **tezacaftor**. Avoid. Severe Theoretical
- **Cenobamate** is predicted to decrease the exposure to **ticagrelor**. Moderate Theoretical
- **Cenobamate** is predicted to decrease the exposure to **tofacitinib**. Severe Study
- **Cenobamate** is predicted to decrease the exposure to **tolvaptan**. Adjust dose. Moderate Theoretical
- **Cenobamate** is predicted to decrease the exposure to triptans **(eletriptan)**. Adjust dose. Moderate Theoretical
- **Cenobamate** is predicted to decrease the exposure to **vanzacaftor**. Avoid. Severe Theoretical
- **Cenobamate** is predicted to decrease the exposure to **velpatasvir**. Avoid. Moderate Theoretical
- **Cenobamate** is predicted to decrease the exposure to **venetoclax**. Avoid. Severe Study
- **Cenobamate** is predicted to decrease the exposure to **voclosporin**. Adjust dose. Moderate Theoretical
- **Cenobamate** is predicted to decrease the concentration of **voxilaprevir**. Avoid. Severe Theoretical
- **Cenobamate** is predicted to decrease the exposure to **zanubrutinib**. Avoid or adjust dose with moderate CYP3A4 inducers—consult product literature. Severe Theoretical

Cephalosporins → see **TABLE 2** p. 1053 (nephrotoxicity)

cefaclor · cefadroxil · cefalexin · cefazolin · cefepime · cefiderocol · cefixime · cefotaxime · cefoxitin · cefradine · ceftaroline · ceftazidime · ceftobiprole · ceftolozane · ceftriaxone · cefuroxime

ROUTE-SPECIFIC INFORMATION Interactions do not generally apply to topical use of **cefuroxime** unless specified.

- Intravenous **ceftriaxone** increases the risk of cardio-respiratory arrest when given with intravenous **calcium compounds**. Avoid. Severe Anecdotal
- Cephalosporins **(cefazolin, ceftriaxone)** potentially increase the risk of bleeding events when given with **coumarins**. Severe Anecdotal
- **Ceftobiprole** is predicted to increase the exposure to endothelin receptor antagonists **(bosentan)**. Moderate Theoretical
- **Ivosidenib** is predicted to increase the exposure to **cefaclor**. Use with caution or avoid. Moderate Theoretical
- **Leflunomide** is predicted to increase the exposure to **cefaclor**. Moderate Study
- **Nitisinone** is predicted to increase the exposure to **cefaclor**. Moderate Study
- Cephalosporins **(cefazolin, ceftriaxone)** potentially increase the risk of bleeding events when given with **phenindione**. Severe Anecdotal
- **Ceftobiprole** is predicted to increase the concentration of **statins**. Moderate Theoretical
- **Ceftobiprole** is predicted to increase the concentration of sulfonylureas **(glibenclamide)**. Moderate Theoretical
- **Teriflunomide** is predicted to increase the exposure to **cefaclor**. Moderate Study
- **Vadadustat** is predicted to increase the exposure to **cefaclor**. Monitor and adjust dose. Moderate Study

Ceritinib → see **TABLE 4** p. 1054 (bradycardia), **TABLE 12** p. 1057 (myelosuppression), **TABLE 7** p. 1055 (QT-interval prolongation)
- **Ceritinib** is predicted to increase the exposure to **abemaciclib**. Avoid or adjust dose—consult product literature. Severe Study
- **Ceritinib** is predicted to increase the exposure to **acalabrutinib**. Avoid. Severe Study
- **Ceritinib** is predicted to increase the exposure to **aliskiren**. Moderate Theoretical
- **Ceritinib** is predicted to moderately increase the exposure to alpha blockers **(alfuzosin, tamsulosin)**. Use with caution or avoid. Moderate Study
- **Ceritinib** is predicted to increase the exposure to alpha blockers **(doxazosin)**. Moderate Study
- Oral **antacids** are predicted to decrease the absorption of oral **ceritinib**. Separate administration by 2 hours. Moderate Theoretical
- Anti-androgens **(apalutamide, enzalutamide)** are predicted to decrease the exposure to **ceritinib**. Avoid. Severe Study → Also see **TABLE 7** p. 1055
- **Ceritinib** is predicted to increase the exposure to anti-androgens **(apalutamide)**. Monitor and adjust dose. Mild Study → Also see **TABLE 7** p. 1055
- Antiarrhythmics **(dronedarone)** are predicted to increase the exposure to **ceritinib**. Moderate Study → Also see **TABLE 4** p. 1054 → Also see **TABLE 7** p. 1055
- **Ceritinib** very markedly increases the exposure to antiarrhythmics **(dronedarone)**. Avoid. Severe Study → Also see **TABLE 4** p. 1054 → Also see **TABLE 7** p. 1055
- **Ceritinib** is predicted to increase the exposure to antiarrhythmics **(propafenone)**. Monitor and adjust dose. Severe Study → Also see **TABLE 4** p. 1054
- **Ceritinib** is predicted to increase the exposure to anticholinesterases, centrally acting **(galantamine)**. Monitor and adjust dose. Moderate Study → Also see **TABLE 4** p. 1054
- Antiepileptics **(carbamazepine, fosphenytoin, phenobarbital, phenytoin, primidone)** are predicted to decrease the exposure to **ceritinib**. Avoid. Severe Study
- **Ceritinib** is predicted to very slightly increase the exposure to antiepileptics **(perampanel)**. Mild Study
- Antifungals, azoles **(fluconazole, isavuconazole)** are predicted to increase the exposure to **ceritinib**. Moderate Study → Also see **TABLE 7** p. 1055
- Antifungals, azoles **(itraconazole, voriconazole)** are predicted to increase the exposure to **ceritinib**. Avoid or adjust dose—consult product literature. Severe Study → Also see **TABLE 7** p. 1055
- Antifungals, azoles **(ketoconazole)** moderately increase the exposure to **ceritinib**. Avoid or adjust dose—consult product literature. Severe Study
- **Ceritinib** is predicted to increase the exposure to antifungals, azoles **(isavuconazole)**. Avoid or monitor adverse effects. Severe Study
- **Ceritinib** is predicted to increase the exposure to antihistamines, non-sedating **(fexofenadine)**. Moderate Theoretical
- **Ceritinib** is predicted to increase the exposure to antihistamines, non-sedating **(mizolastine)**. Avoid. Severe Study
- **Ceritinib** is predicted to increase the exposure to antihistamines, non-sedating **(rupatadine)**. Avoid. Moderate Study

- **Ceritinib** is predicted to increase the concentration of antimalarials **(piperaquine)**. Severe Study
- **Ceritinib** is predicted to increase the exposure to **atogepant**. Adjust **atogepant** dose. Moderate Study
- **Ceritinib** is predicted to slightly increase the exposure to atypical antipsychotics **(aripiprazole)**. Avoid or adjust dose—consult product literature. Moderate Study
- **Ceritinib** is predicted to moderately increase the exposure to atypical antipsychotics **(cariprazine)**. Avoid. Severe Study
- **Ceritinib** is predicted to increase the exposure to atypical antipsychotics **(lurasidone, quetiapine)**. Avoid. Severe Study
- **Ceritinib** is predicted to increase the exposure to atypical antipsychotics **(risperidone)**. Adjust dose. Moderate Study
- **Ceritinib** is predicted to increase the exposure to **avacopan**. Severe Study
- **Ceritinib** is predicted to increase the exposure to **avapritinib**. Avoid. Moderate Study
- **Ceritinib** is predicted to increase the exposure to **axitinib**. Avoid or adjust dose. Moderate Study → Also see **TABLE 12** p. 1057
- **Ceritinib** might increase the exposure to **bedaquiline**. Mild Study → Also see **TABLE 7** p. 1055
- **Ceritinib** moderately increases the exposure to benzodiazepines **(alprazolam)**. Avoid. Moderate Study
- **Ceritinib** is predicted to markedly to very markedly increase the exposure to benzodiazepines **(midazolam)**. Avoid or adjust dose. Severe Study
- **Berotralstat** is predicted to increase the exposure to **ceritinib**. Moderate Study
- **Ceritinib** is predicted to increase the exposure to beta$_2$ agonists **(salmeterol)**. Avoid. Severe Study
- **Ceritinib** slightly increases the exposure to **bortezomib**. Moderate Study → Also see **TABLE 12** p. 1057
- **Ceritinib** is predicted to increase the exposure to **bosutinib**. Avoid or adjust dose. Severe Study → Also see **TABLE 12** p. 1057 → Also see **TABLE 7** p. 1055
- **Ceritinib** is predicted to increase the exposure to **brigatinib**. Avoid or adjust dose—consult product literature. Severe Study → Also see **TABLE 4** p. 1054
- **Ceritinib** is predicted to increase the exposure to **buspirone**. Adjust **buspirone** dose. Severe Study
- **Ceritinib** is predicted to increase the exposure to **cabozantinib**. Moderate Study → Also see **TABLE 12** p. 1057 → Also see **TABLE 7** p. 1055
- Calcium-channel blockers **(diltiazem, verapamil)** are predicted to increase the exposure to **ceritinib**. Moderate Study → Also see **TABLE 4** p. 1054
- **Ceritinib** is predicted to increase the exposure to calcium-channel blockers **(amlodipine, felodipine, lacidipine, nicardipine, nifedipine, nimodipine)**. Monitor and adjust dose. Moderate Study
- **Ceritinib** is predicted to increase the exposure to calcium-channel blockers **(diltiazem, verapamil)**. Severe Study → Also see **TABLE 4** p. 1054
- **Ceritinib** is predicted to markedly increase the exposure to calcium-channel blockers **(lercanidipine)**. Avoid. Severe Study
- **Ceritinib** is predicted to increase the exposure to **cannabidiol**. Avoid or adjust dose. Mild Study
- **Ceritinib** is predicted to increase the exposure to **capivasertib**. Adjust dose. Moderate Study
- **Ceritinib** increases the concentration of **ciclosporin**. Severe Study
- **Ceritinib** is predicted to moderately increase the exposure to **cilostazol**. Adjust **cilostazol** dose. Moderate Study
- **Ceritinib** is predicted to moderately increase the exposure to **cinacalcet**. Adjust dose. Moderate Study
- **Cobicistat** is predicted to increase the exposure to **ceritinib**. Avoid or adjust dose—consult product literature. Severe Study
- **Ceritinib** is predicted to increase the exposure to **cobimetinib**. Avoid or monitor for toxicity. Severe Study
- **Ceritinib** is predicted to increase the exposure to **colchicine**. Avoid potent CYP3A4 inhibitors or adjust **colchicine** dose, p. 637. Severe Study
- **Ceritinib** is predicted to increase the exposure to corticosteroids **(beclometasone)** (risk with beclometasone is likely to be lower than with other corticosteroids). Moderate Theoretical
- **Ceritinib** is predicted to increase the exposure to corticosteroids **(betamethasone, budesonide, ciclesonide, deflazacort, dexamethasone, fludrocortisone, fluticasone, hydrocortisone, methylprednisolone, mometasone, prednisolone, triamcinolone)**. Avoid or monitor adverse effects. Severe Study
- **Ceritinib** is predicted to increase the exposure to corticosteroids **(vamorolone)**. Adjust dose. Severe Study
- **Ceritinib** is predicted to increase the exposure to coumarins **(acenocoumarol)**. Severe Theoretical
- **Ceritinib** increases the exposure to coumarins **(warfarin)**. Avoid or monitor INR. Severe Study
- **Ceritinib** is predicted to increase the exposure to **crizotinib**. Avoid. Moderate Study → Also see **TABLE 4** p. 1054 → Also see **TABLE 7** p. 1055
- **Crizotinib** is predicted to increase the exposure to **ceritinib**. Moderate Study → Also see **TABLE 4** p. 1054 → Also see **TABLE 7** p. 1055
- **Dabrafenib** is predicted to decrease the exposure to **ceritinib**. Severe Study
- **Ceritinib** is predicted to increase the exposure to **dabrafenib**. Use with caution or avoid. Moderate Study
- **Ceritinib** is predicted to increase the exposure to **daridorexant**. Avoid. Severe Study
- **Ceritinib** is predicted to markedly to very markedly increase the exposure to **darifenacin**. Avoid. Severe Study
- **Ceritinib** is predicted to increase the exposure to **dasatinib**. Avoid or adjust dose—consult product literature. Severe Study → Also see **TABLE 12** p. 1057 → Also see **TABLE 7** p. 1055
- **Ceritinib** very slightly increases the exposure to **delamanid**. Severe Study → Also see **TABLE 7** p. 1055
- **Ceritinib** is predicted to increase the exposure to **deutivacaftor**. Adjust dose, see deutivacaftor with tezacaftor and vanzacaftor p. 218. Severe Study
- **Ceritinib** is predicted to moderately increase the exposure to **dienogest**. Moderate Study
- **Ceritinib** is predicted to increase the risk of bradycardia when given with **digoxin**. Avoid. Severe Theoretical → Also see **TABLE 4** p. 1054
- **Ceritinib** is predicted to increase the exposure to dipeptidylpeptidase-4 inhibitors **(saxagliptin)**. Moderate Study
- **Ceritinib** is predicted to increase the exposure to **domperidone**. Avoid. Severe Study
- **Ceritinib** increases the exposure to dopamine receptor agonists **(bromocriptine)**. Severe Study
- **Ceritinib** is predicted to increase the exposure to **dronabinol**. Adjust dose. Mild Study
- **Ceritinib** is predicted to increase the exposure to **dutasteride**. Monitor adverse effects and adjust dose. Moderate Theoretical
- **Ceritinib** is predicted to increase the exposure to **elacestrant**. Avoid potent CYP3A4 inhibitors or adjust **elacestrant** dose. Severe Study
- **Ceritinib** is predicted to increase the exposure to **elexacaftor**. Adjust ivacaftor with tezacaftor and elexacaftor p. 220 dose with potent CYP3A4 inhibitors. Severe Study
- **Ceritinib** is predicted to increase the exposure to **eliglustat**. Avoid or adjust dose—consult product literature. Severe Study
- **Encorafenib** is predicted to decrease the exposure to **ceritinib**. Avoid. Severe Study → Also see **TABLE 7** p. 1055
- **Ceritinib** is predicted to increase the exposure to **encorafenib**. Avoid or monitor. Severe Study → Also see **TABLE 7** p. 1055
- Endothelin receptor antagonists **(bosentan)** are predicted to decrease the exposure to **ceritinib**. Severe Study
- **Ceritinib** is predicted to increase the exposure to endothelin receptor antagonists **(macitentan)**. Moderate Study
- **Ceritinib** is predicted to increase the exposure to the cytotoxic component of **enfortumab vedotin**. Severe Theoretical
- **Ceritinib** is predicted to increase the exposure to **entrectinib**. Avoid or adjust dose with potent CYP3A4 inhibitors—consult product literature. Severe Study → Also see **TABLE 7** p. 1055
- **Ceritinib** is predicted to increase the exposure to **erdafitinib**. Adjust dose. Severe Study
- **Ceritinib** is predicted to increase the risk of ergotism when given with **ergometrine**. Avoid. Severe Theoretical
- **Ceritinib** is predicted to increase the exposure to **erlotinib**. Use with caution and adjust dose. Severe Study

Ceritinib (continued)
- **Ceritinib** is predicted to increase the exposure to **esketamine**. Adjust dose. Moderate Study
- **Ceritinib** is predicted to increase the exposure to **eszopiclone**. Adjust **eszopiclone** dose; avoid in the elderly. Moderate Study
- **Ceritinib** is predicted to increase the concentration of subdermal **etonogestrel**. Moderate Theoretical
- **Ceritinib** is predicted to increase the exposure to **etrasimod**. Avoid in poor CYP2C9 metabolisers. Severe Theoretical → Also see TABLE 4 p. 1054
- **Ceritinib** is predicted to increase the exposure to **everolimus**. Avoid. Severe Study
- **Ceritinib** is predicted to increase the exposure to factor XA inhibitors **(apixaban, edoxaban)**. Moderate Theoretical
- **Ceritinib** might increase the exposure to factor XA inhibitors **(rivaroxaban)**. Manufacturer advises caution in renal impairment. Moderate Theoretical
- **Ceritinib** is predicted to increase the exposure to **fedratinib**. Adjust dose, but avoid depending on other drugs taken—consult product literature. Moderate Study
- **Fedratinib** is predicted to increase the exposure to **ceritinib**. Moderate Study
- **Ceritinib** is predicted to moderately increase the exposure to **fesoterodine**. Adjust **fesoterodine** dose with potent CYP3A4 inhibitors; avoid in hepatic and renal impairment. Severe Study
- **Ceritinib** is predicted to increase the exposure to **fostamatinib**. Monitor adverse effects and adjust dose. Moderate Study
- **Ceritinib** is predicted to increase the exposure to **gefitinib**. Severe Study
- **Ceritinib** is predicted to increase the exposure to **gilteritinib**. Moderate Study
- **Ceritinib** is predicted to increase the exposure to **glasdegib**. Use with caution or avoid. Severe Study → Also see TABLE 7 p. 1055
- **Grapefruit** juice is predicted to increase the exposure to **ceritinib**. Avoid. Severe Theoretical
- **Ceritinib** is predicted to moderately to markedly increase the exposure to **grazoprevir**. Avoid. Severe Study
- **Ceritinib** is predicted to increase the exposure to **guanfacine**. Adjust **guanfacine** dose, p. 281. Moderate Study
- **H_2 receptor antagonists** are predicted to decrease the absorption of **ceritinib**. Moderate Theoretical
- HIV-protease inhibitors **(atazanavir, darunavir, lopinavir)** boosted with ritonavir are predicted to increase the exposure to **ceritinib**. Avoid or adjust dose—consult product literature. Severe Study
- HIV-protease inhibitors **(fosamprenavir, ritonavir)** are predicted to increase the exposure to **ceritinib**. Avoid or adjust dose—consult product literature. Severe Study
- **Ceritinib** is predicted to increase the exposure to **ibrutinib**. Avoid or adjust dose with potent CYP3A4 inhibitors—consult product literature. Severe Study → Also see TABLE 12 p. 1057
- **Idelalisib** is predicted to increase the exposure to **ceritinib**. Avoid or adjust dose—consult product literature. Severe Study
- **Ceritinib** is predicted to increase the exposure to **imatinib**. Moderate Study → Also see TABLE 12 p. 1057
- **Imatinib** is predicted to increase the exposure to **ceritinib**. Moderate Study → Also see TABLE 12 p. 1057
- **Ceritinib** is predicted to increase the exposure to the active metabolite of **irinotecan**. Avoid. Severe Study → Also see TABLE 12 p. 1057
- **Ceritinib** is predicted to increase the exposure to **ivabradine**. Avoid. Severe Study → Also see TABLE 4 p. 1054
- **Ceritinib** is predicted to increase the exposure to **ivacaftor**. Adjust dose with potent CYP3A4 inhibitors, see ivacaftor p. 219, lumacaftor with ivacaftor p. 222, tezacaftor with ivacaftor p. 223, and ivacaftor with tezacaftor and elexacaftor p. 220. Severe Study
- **Ivosidenib** is predicted to decrease the exposure to **ceritinib**. Avoid. Severe Study → Also see TABLE 7 p. 1055
- **Ceritinib** is predicted to increase the exposure to **ketamine**. Adjust dose. Moderate Theoretical
- **Lapatinib** is predicted to increase the exposure to **ceritinib**. Moderate Theoretical → Also see TABLE 7 p. 1055
- **Ceritinib** is predicted to increase the exposure to **lapatinib**. Avoid. Moderate Study → Also see TABLE 7 p. 1055
- **Ceritinib** is predicted to moderately increase the exposure to **larotrectinib**. Avoid or adjust dose—consult product literature. Moderate Study
- **Ceritinib** is predicted to increase the exposure to **leniolisib**. Avoid. Moderate Study
- **Letermovir** is predicted to increase the exposure to **ceritinib**. Moderate Study
- **Ceritinib** is predicted to markedly increase the exposure to **lomitapide**. Avoid. Severe Study
- **Ceritinib** is predicted to increase the exposure to **loperamide**. Moderate Theoretical
- **Ceritinib** is predicted to increase the exposure to **lorlatinib**. Avoid or adjust dose—consult product literature. Severe Study
- **Lumacaftor** is predicted to decrease the exposure to **ceritinib**. Avoid. Severe Study
- Macrolides **(clarithromycin)** are predicted to increase the exposure to **ceritinib**. Avoid or adjust dose—consult product literature. Severe Study
- Macrolides **(erythromycin)** are predicted to increase the exposure to **ceritinib**. Moderate Study → Also see TABLE 7 p. 1055
- **Ceritinib** is predicted to increase the exposure to **mavacamten**. Avoid or monitor—consult product literature. Severe Study
- **Ceritinib** is predicted to increase the concentration of intramuscular **medroxyprogesterone**. Moderate Theoretical
- **Ceritinib** is predicted to increase the exposure to **midostaurin**. Avoid or monitor for toxicity. Severe Study
- **Ceritinib** is predicted to markedly increase the exposure to mineralocorticoid receptor antagonists **(eplerenone)**. Avoid. Severe Study
- **Ceritinib** is predicted to increase the exposure to mineralocorticoid receptor antagonists **(finerenone)**. Avoid. Severe Study
- **Ceritinib** is predicted to increase the exposure to **mirabegron**. Adjust **mirabegron** dose in hepatic and renal impairment. Moderate Study
- **Ceritinib** is predicted to increase the exposure to **mirtazapine**. Moderate Study
- **Mitotane** is predicted to decrease the exposure to **ceritinib**. Avoid. Severe Study → Also see TABLE 12 p. 1057
- **Ceritinib** is predicted to increase the exposure to **modafinil**. Mild Theoretical
- **Ceritinib** is predicted to increase the risk of neutropenia when given with monoclonal antibodies **(brentuximab vedotin)**. Monitor and adjust dose. Severe Study → Also see TABLE 12 p. 1057
- **Ceritinib** is predicted to increase the exposure to monoclonal antibodies **(polatuzumab vedotin)**. Moderate Theoretical
- **Ceritinib** is predicted to increase the exposure to the cytotoxic component of monoclonal antibodies **(trastuzumab emtansine)**. Avoid or monitor. Severe Theoretical → Also see TABLE 12 p. 1057
- **Ceritinib** is predicted to increase the exposure to **naldemedine**. Avoid or monitor. Moderate Study
- **Ceritinib** is predicted to markedly increase the exposure to **naloxegol**. Avoid. Severe Study
- **Ceritinib** is predicted to increase the exposure to **neratinib**. Avoid or adjust dose with potent CYP3A4 inhibitors—consult product literature. Severe Study
- Neurokinin-1 receptor antagonists **(aprepitant, netupitant)** are predicted to increase the exposure to **ceritinib**. Moderate Study
- Neurokinin-1 receptor antagonists **(fosaprepitant)** are predicted to increase the exposure to **ceritinib**. Severe Theoretical
- **Ceritinib** is predicted to markedly increase the exposure to neurokinin-1 receptor antagonists **(aprepitant)**. Moderate Study
- **Ceritinib** is predicted to increase the exposure to neurokinin-1 receptor antagonists **(fosaprepitant)**. Moderate Theoretical
- **Ceritinib** is predicted to increase the exposure to neurokinin-1 receptor antagonists **(netupitant)**. Moderate Study
- **Ceritinib** is predicted to increase the exposure to **nilotinib**. Avoid. Severe Study → Also see TABLE 12 p. 1057 → Also see TABLE 7 p. 1055
- **Nilotinib** is predicted to increase the exposure to **ceritinib**. Moderate Study → Also see TABLE 12 p. 1057 → Also see TABLE 7 p. 1055
- **Nirmatrelvir** boosted with ritonavir is predicted to increase the concentration of **ceritinib**. Avoid or adjust dose—consult product literature. Severe Theoretical

- **Ceritinib** is predicted to increase the exposure to **nitisinone**. Adjust dose. Moderate Theoretical
- NNRTIs **(efavirenz, nevirapine)** are predicted to decrease the exposure to **ceritinib**. Severe Study → Also see **TABLE 7** p. 1055
- NNRTIs **(etravirine)** are predicted to decrease the exposure to **ceritinib**. Severe Theoretical
- **Ceritinib** is predicted to increase the exposure to NSAIDs **(celecoxib, diclofenac)**. Adjust dose. Moderate Theoretical
- **Ceritinib** is predicted to increase the exposure to **olaparib**. Avoid or adjust dose with potent CYP3A4 inhibitors—consult product literature. Moderate Study → Also see **TABLE 12** p. 1057
- **Ceritinib** is predicted to increase the exposure to **omaveloxolone**. Avoid or adjust **omaveloxolone** dose, p. 755. Severe Study
- **Ceritinib** is predicted to increase the exposure to opioids **(alfentanil, buprenorphine, fentanyl, oxycodone)**. Monitor and adjust dose. Severe Study → Also see **TABLE 4** p. 1054
- **Ceritinib** is predicted to increase the exposure to opioids **(sufentanil)**. Moderate Study → Also see **TABLE 4** p. 1054
- **Ceritinib** is predicted to increase the exposure to **osilodrostat**. Moderate Theoretical → Also see **TABLE 7** p. 1055
- **Ceritinib** is predicted to increase the exposure to **ospemifene**. Avoid in poor CYP2C9 metabolisers. Moderate Study
- **Ceritinib** is predicted to increase the exposure to **oxybutynin**. Mild Study
- **Ceritinib** is predicted to increase the exposure to **palbociclib**. Avoid or adjust dose—consult product literature. Severe Study → Also see **TABLE 12** p. 1057
- **Ceritinib** is predicted to increase the exposure to **panobinostat**. Adjust dose—consult product literature; in hepatic impairment avoid. Moderate Study → Also see **TABLE 12** p. 1057 → Also see **TABLE 7** p. 1055
- **Ceritinib** is predicted to increase the exposure to **pazopanib**. Avoid or adjust dose—consult product literature. Moderate Study → Also see **TABLE 7** p. 1055
- **Ceritinib** is predicted to increase the exposure to **pemigatinib**. Avoid or adjust dose—consult product literature. Severe Study
- **Ceritinib** is predicted to increase the exposure to **phenindione**. Severe Theoretical
- **Ceritinib** is predicted to increase the exposure to phosphodiesterase type-5 inhibitors **(avanafil, vardenafil)**. Avoid. Severe Study → Also see **TABLE 7** p. 1055
- **Ceritinib** is predicted to increase the exposure to phosphodiesterase type-5 inhibitors **(sildenafil)**. Avoid potent CYP3A4 inhibitors or adjust **sildenafil** dose, p. 139. Severe Study
- **Ceritinib** is predicted to increase the exposure to phosphodiesterase type-5 inhibitors **(tadalafil)**. Use with caution or avoid. Severe Study
- **Ceritinib** is predicted to increase the exposure to **pimozide**. Avoid. Severe Study → Also see **TABLE 7** p. 1055
- **Ceritinib** is predicted to slightly increase the exposure to **ponatinib**. Monitor and adjust dose—consult product literature. Moderate Study
- **Ceritinib** is predicted to increase the exposure to **pralsetinib**. Avoid or adjust dose with potent CYP3A4 inhibitors—consult product literature. Moderate Study
- **Ceritinib** is predicted to moderately increase the exposure to **praziquantel**. Mild Study
- **Ceritinib** given with carbimazole is predicted to increase the exposure to **propiverine**. Adjust starting dose. Moderate Theoretical
- **Proton pump inhibitors** are predicted to decrease the absorption of **ceritinib**. Moderate Theoretical
- **Ceritinib** is predicted to increase the exposure to **quizartinib**. Adjust dose—consult product literature. Severe Study → Also see **TABLE 7** p. 1055
- **Ceritinib** is predicted to increase the exposure to **ranolazine**. Avoid. Severe Study → Also see **TABLE 7** p. 1055
- **Ceritinib** is predicted to increase the exposure to **reboxetine**. Avoid. Moderate Study
- **Ceritinib** is predicted to increase the exposure to **regorafenib**. Avoid. Moderate Study → Also see **TABLE 12** p. 1057
- **Ceritinib** is predicted to increase the exposure to retinoids **(alitretinoin)**. Adjust **alitretinoin** dose. Moderate Theoretical
- **Ceritinib** is predicted to increase the exposure to **ribociclib**. Avoid or adjust dose—consult product literature. Moderate Study → Also see **TABLE 12** p. 1057 → Also see **TABLE 7** p. 1055
- Rifamycins **(rifampicin)** are predicted to decrease the exposure to **ceritinib**. Avoid. Severe Study
- **Ceritinib** is predicted to increase the exposure to **rimegepant**. Avoid. Moderate Study
- **Ceritinib** is predicted to increase the exposure to **ripretinib**. Moderate Theoretical
- **Ceritinib** is predicted to increase the exposure to **ruxolitinib**. Adjust dose depending on indication and monitor adverse effects—consult product literature. Moderate Study → Also see **TABLE 12** p. 1057
- **Ceritinib** is predicted to increase the exposure to **selpercatinib**. Adjust dose—consult product literature. Moderate Study → Also see **TABLE 7** p. 1055
- **Ceritinib** is predicted to increase the exposure to **selumetinib**. Avoid or adjust dose—consult product literature. Severe Study
- **Ceritinib** is predicted to increase the exposure to **siponimod**. Avoid depending on other drugs taken—consult product literature. Severe Theoretical → Also see **TABLE 4** p. 1054
- **Ceritinib** is predicted to increase the concentration of **sirolimus**. Avoid or monitor and adjust dose. Severe Study
- **Ceritinib** is predicted to increase the exposure to SNRIs **(venlafaxine)**. Moderate Study
- **Ceritinib** is predicted to increase the exposure to **solifenacin**. Adjust solifenacin p. 604 or tamsulosin with solifenacin dose; avoid in hepatic and renal impairment. Severe Study
- **Ceritinib** is predicted to increase the exposure to **sparsentan**. Avoid. Severe Study
- **Ceritinib** is predicted to moderately increase the exposure to SSRIs **(dapoxetine)**. Avoid potent CYP3A4 inhibitors or adjust **dapoxetine** dose. Severe Study
- **Ceritinib** is predicted to increase the exposure to SSRIs **(sertraline)**. Avoid. Moderate Theoretical
- **St John's wort** is predicted to decrease the exposure to **ceritinib**. Avoid. Severe Theoretical
- **Ceritinib** is predicted to increase the exposure to statins **(atorvastatin)**. Avoid or adjust dose and monitor rhabdomyolysis. Severe Study
- **Ceritinib** is predicted to increase the exposure to statins **(simvastatin)**. Avoid. Severe Study
- **Ceritinib** is predicted to increase the exposure to sulfonylureas **(glimepiride)**. Adjust dose. Moderate Theoretical
- **Ceritinib** is predicted to increase the exposure to **sunitinib**. Avoid or adjust dose—consult product literature. Moderate Study → Also see **TABLE 12** p. 1057 → Also see **TABLE 7** p. 1055
- **Ceritinib** is predicted to increase the concentration of **tacrolimus**. Avoid. If concurrent use is unavoidable—consult product literature. Severe Study
- **Ceritinib** is predicted to increase the exposure to taxanes **(cabazitaxel)**. Avoid or adjust dose—consult product literature. Severe Study → Also see **TABLE 12** p. 1057
- **Ceritinib** is predicted to increase the exposure to taxanes **(docetaxel)**. Avoid or adjust dose. Severe Study → Also see **TABLE 12** p. 1057
- **Ceritinib** is predicted to increase the exposure to taxanes **(paclitaxel)**. Moderate Anecdotal → Also see **TABLE 12** p. 1057
- **Ceritinib** is predicted to increase the concentration of **temsirolimus**. Avoid. Severe Theoretical → Also see **TABLE 12** p. 1057
- **Ceritinib** is predicted to increase the exposure to **tezacaftor**. Adjust dose with potent CYP3A4 inhibitors, see tezacaftor with ivacaftor p. 223, ivacaftor with tezacaftor and elexacaftor p. 220, and deutivacaftor with tezacaftor and vanzacaftor p. 218. Severe Study
- **Ceritinib** is predicted to increase the exposure to thrombin inhibitors **(dabigatran)**. Moderate Theoretical
- **Ceritinib** is predicted to markedly increase the exposure to **ticagrelor**. Avoid. Severe Study → Also see **TABLE 4** p. 1054
- **Ceritinib** is predicted to increase the exposure to the cytotoxic component of **tisotumab vedotin**. Severe Theoretical
- **Ceritinib** is predicted to increase the exposure to **tofacitinib**. Adjust **tofacitinib** dose, p. 803. Moderate Study
- **Ceritinib** is predicted to increase the exposure to **tolterodine**. Avoid. Severe Study → Also see **TABLE 7** p. 1055

Ceritinib (continued)
- **Ceritinib** is predicted to increase the exposure to **tolvaptan**. Manufacturer advises caution or adjust **tolvaptan** dose with potent CYP3A4 inhibitors. [Severe] Study
- **Ceritinib** is predicted to increase the exposure to **topotecan**. [Moderate] Theoretical → Also see TABLE 12 p. 1057
- **Ceritinib** is predicted to increase the exposure to **toremifene**. [Moderate] Theoretical → Also see TABLE 7 p. 1055
- **Ceritinib** is predicted to increase the exposure to **trabectedin**. Avoid or adjust dose. [Severe] Theoretical → Also see TABLE 12 p. 1057
- **Ceritinib** is predicted to moderately increase the exposure to **trazodone**. Avoid or adjust dose. [Moderate] Study
- **Ceritinib** increases the exposure to triptans **(almotriptan)**. [Mild] Study
- **Ceritinib** is predicted to markedly increase the exposure to triptans **(eletriptan)**. Avoid. [Severe] Study
- **Tucatinib** is predicted to increase the exposure to **ceritinib**. Avoid or adjust dose—consult product literature. [Severe] Study
- **Ceritinib** is predicted to increase the exposure to **upadacitinib**. Manufacturer advises caution or avoid, or adjust **upadacitinib** dose depending on indication, p. 927. [Severe] Study
- **Ceritinib** is predicted to increase the exposure to **vanzacaftor**. Adjust dose, see deutivacaftor with tezacaftor and vanzacaftor p. 218. [Severe] Study
- **Ceritinib** is predicted to increase the exposure to **vemurafenib**. [Severe] Theoretical → Also see TABLE 7 p. 1055
- **Ceritinib** is predicted to increase the exposure to **venetoclax**. Avoid or adjust dose—consult product literature. [Severe] Study
- **Ceritinib** is predicted to increase the exposure to **vinca alkaloids**. [Severe] Theoretical → Also see TABLE 12 p. 1057
- **Ceritinib** is predicted to increase the exposure to vitamin D substances **(paricalcitol)**. [Moderate] Study
- **Ceritinib** is predicted to increase the exposure to **voclosporin**. Avoid. [Severe] Study → Also see TABLE 7 p. 1055
- **Ceritinib** is predicted to increase the exposure to **zanubrutinib**. Avoid or adjust dose with potent CYP3A4 inhibitors—consult product literature. [Moderate] Study
- **Ceritinib** is predicted to increase the exposure to **zopiclone**. Adjust dose. [Moderate] Theoretical

Certolizumab pegol → see monoclonal antibodies
Cetirizine → see antihistamines, non-sedating
Cetuximab → see monoclonal antibodies
Chenodeoxycholic acid
- Oral **aluminium hydroxide** decreases the absorption of **chenodeoxycholic acid**. [Moderate] Study
- Antiepileptics **(phenobarbital, primidone)** are predicted to affect the efficacy of **chenodeoxycholic acid**. Monitor and adjust dose. [Moderate] Theoretical
- **Ciclosporin** is predicted to affect the efficacy of **chenodeoxycholic acid**. Monitor and adjust dose. [Moderate] Theoretical
- Oral **combined hormonal contraceptives** potentially decrease the efficacy of oral **chenodeoxycholic acid**. Avoid. [Moderate] Theoretical
- **Sirolimus** is predicted to affect the efficacy of **chenodeoxycholic acid**. Monitor and adjust dose. [Moderate] Theoretical

Chikungunya vaccine (live) → see live vaccines
Chloral hydrate → see TABLE 9 p. 1056 (CNS effects)
- Intravenous loop diuretics **(furosemide)** potentially increase the risk of sweating, variable blood pressure, and tachycardia when given after **chloral hydrate**. [Moderate] Anecdotal

Chlorambucil → see alkylating agents
Chloramphenicol

ROUTE-SPECIFIC INFORMATION Since systemic absorption can follow topical application, the possibility of interactions should be borne in mind.

- Antiepileptics **(phenobarbital, primidone)** decrease the concentration of **chloramphenicol**. [Moderate] Study
- Intravenous **chloramphenicol** increases the concentration of antiepileptics **(fosphenytoin, phenytoin)** and antiepileptics **(fosphenytoin, phenytoin)** affect the concentration of intravenous **chloramphenicol**. Monitor concentration and adjust dose. [Severe] Study
- **Chloramphenicol** potentially increases the anticoagulant effect of **coumarins**. [Moderate] Anecdotal
- **Chloramphenicol** is predicted to increase the exposure to **guanfacine**. Adjust **guanfacine** dose, p. 281. [Moderate] Theoretical
- **Chloramphenicol** decreases the efficacy of **iron**. [Moderate] Anecdotal
- Rifamycins **(rifampicin)** decrease the concentration of **chloramphenicol**. [Moderate] Study
- **Chloramphenicol** is predicted to increase the exposure to **sulfonylureas**. [Severe] Study
- **Chloramphenicol** increases the concentration of **tacrolimus**. [Severe] Study

Chlordiazepoxide → see benzodiazepines
Chlormethine

ROUTE-SPECIFIC INFORMATION Since systemic absorption can follow topical application, the possibility of interactions should be borne in mind.

Chloroprocaine
- **Chloroprocaine** is predicted to increase the risk of cardiovascular adverse effects when given with antiarrhythmics **(amiodarone, dronedarone, vernakalant)**. [Severe] Theoretical
- **Chloroprocaine** is predicted to increase the risk of cardiovascular adverse effects when given with beta blockers, non-selective **(sotalol)**. [Severe] Theoretical
- **Chloroprocaine** is predicted to decrease the effects of **sulfonamides**. Avoid. [Severe] Theoretical

Chloroquine → see antimalarials
Chlorothiazide → see thiazide diuretics
Chlorphenamine → see antihistamines, sedating
Chlorpromazine → see phenothiazine antipsychotics
Chlortalidone → see thiazide diuretics
Cholera vaccine (live) → see live vaccines
Cholic acid
- Oral **antacids** are predicted to decrease the absorption of oral **cholic acid**. Separate administration by 5 hours. [Mild] Theoretical
- Antiepileptics **(phenobarbital)** decrease the effects of **cholic acid**. Avoid. [Moderate] Study
- **Ciclosporin** affects the concentration of **cholic acid**. Avoid. [Moderate] Study

Choline salicylate
- **Corticosteroids** are predicted to decrease the concentration of **choline salicylate**. [Moderate] Study

Ciclesonide → see corticosteroids
Ciclosporin → see TABLE 2 p. 1053 (nephrotoxicity), TABLE 13 p. 1057 (increased serum potassium)

- Pomelo juice is predicted to increase ciclosporin exposure, and purple grape juice is predicted to decrease ciclosporin exposure.
- Since systemic absorption can follow topical application, the possibility of interactions should be borne in mind.

- **Abrocitinib** might increase the exposure to **ciclosporin**. [Moderate] Theoretical
- **Ciclosporin** is predicted to increase the exposure to **afatinib**. [Moderate] Study
- **Ciclosporin** markedly increases the exposure to **aliskiren**. Avoid. [Severe] Study → Also see TABLE 13 p. 1057
- **Ciclosporin** is predicted to increase the exposure to **alpelisib**. [Moderate] Theoretical
- **Ciclosporin** increases the concentration of anthracyclines **(daunorubicin, doxorubicin, epirubicin, idarubicin, mitoxantrone)**. [Severe] Study
- Anti-androgens **(apalutamide, enzalutamide)** decrease the concentration of **ciclosporin**. [Severe] Study
- Antiarrhythmics **(amiodarone)** increase the concentration of **ciclosporin**. Monitor concentration and adjust dose. [Severe] Study
- Antiarrhythmics **(dronedarone)** are predicted to increase the concentration of **ciclosporin**. [Severe] Study
- Antiepileptics **(carbamazepine, fosphenytoin, phenobarbital, phenytoin, primidone)** decrease the concentration of **ciclosporin**. [Severe] Study
- Antiepileptics **(oxcarbazepine)** decrease the concentration of **ciclosporin**. [Severe] Anecdotal

- Antifungals, azoles **(fluconazole, isavuconazole)** are predicted to increase the concentration of **ciclosporin**. Severe Study
- Antifungals, azoles **(itraconazole, ketoconazole, posaconazole, voriconazole)** increase the concentration of **ciclosporin**. Severe Study
- Antifungals, azoles **(miconazole)** increase the concentration of **ciclosporin**. Monitor and adjust dose. Severe Anecdotal
- **Ciclosporin** is predicted to increase the exposure to antihistamines, non-sedating **(fexofenadine)**. Moderate Theoretical
- **Ciclosporin** is predicted to increase the exposure to **atogepant**. Adjust **atogepant** dose. Moderate Theoretical
- **Baricitinib** is predicted to enhance the risk of immunosuppression when given with **ciclosporin**. Manufacturer advises caution or avoid—consult product literature. Severe Theoretical
- **Ciclosporin** is predicted to increase the exposure to beta blockers, non-selective **(nadolol)**. Moderate Study
- **Ciclosporin** is predicted to increase the exposure to **bictegravir**. Avoid or monitor. Moderate Theoretical
- **Brigatinib** might decrease the exposure to **ciclosporin**. Avoid. Moderate Theoretical
- **Ciclosporin** is predicted to affect the efficacy of **bulevirtide** and **bulevirtide** is predicted to increase the exposure to **ciclosporin**. Avoid. Severe Theoretical
- Calcium-channel blockers **(diltiazem, verapamil)** are predicted to increase the concentration of **ciclosporin**. Severe Study
- Calcium-channel blockers **(nicardipine)** increase the concentration of **ciclosporin**. Severe Study
- **Ciclosporin** moderately increases the exposure to calcium-channel blockers **(lercanidipine)**. Use with caution or avoid. Severe Study
- **Cannabidiol** is predicted to increase the concentration of **ciclosporin**. Monitor and adjust dose. Severe Theoretical
- **Ciclosporin** is predicted to increase the exposure to **capivasertib**. Adjust dose. Moderate Theoretical
- **Ciclosporin** slightly increases the exposure to **caspofungin**. Severe Study
- **Ceritinib** increases the concentration of **ciclosporin**. Severe Study
- **Ciclosporin** is predicted to affect the efficacy of **chenodeoxycholic acid**. Monitor and adjust dose. Moderate Theoretical
- **Ciclosporin** affects the concentration of **cholic acid**. Avoid. Moderate Study
- **Ciclosporin** is predicted to increase the exposure to **cladribine**. Avoid or adjust dose. Moderate Theoretical
- **Cobicistat** increases the concentration of **ciclosporin**. Severe Study
- **Ciclosporin** increases the exposure to **colchicine**. Avoid P-glycoprotein inhibitors or adjust **colchicine** dose, p. 637. Severe Study
- **Crizotinib** is predicted to increase the concentration of **ciclosporin**. Severe Study
- **Ciclosporin** is predicted to increase the risk of rhabdomyolysis when given with **daptomycin**. Severe Theoretical
- **Ciclosporin** is predicted to increase the exposure to **daridorexant**. Adjust **daridorexant** dose. Unknown Theoretical
- **Ciclosporin** is predicted to increase the exposure to **darifenacin**. Avoid. Moderate Theoretical
- **Ciclosporin** increases the concentration of **digoxin**. Monitor and adjust dose. Severe Theoretical
- **Ciclosporin** is predicted to increase the exposure to **elacestrant**. Avoid or adjust **elacestrant** dose. Severe Theoretical
- **Ciclosporin** causes a small decrease in the exposure to **eltrombopag**. Monitor platelet count and adjust dose. Moderate Study
- **Encorafenib** decreases the concentration of **ciclosporin**. Severe Study
- Endothelin receptor antagonists **(bosentan)** moderately decrease the exposure to **ciclosporin** and **ciclosporin** moderately increases the exposure to endothelin receptor antagonists **(bosentan)**. Avoid. Severe Study
- **Ciclosporin** moderately increases the exposure to endothelin receptor antagonists **(ambrisentan)**. Adjust **ambrisentan** dose and monitor, p. 138. Moderate Study
- **Ciclosporin** is predicted to increase the exposure to **erlotinib**. Moderate Theoretical
- **Ciclosporin** increases the exposure to **etoposide**. Monitor and adjust dose. Severe Study
- **Ciclosporin** moderately increases the exposure to **everolimus**. Avoid or adjust dose. Severe Study
- **Ciclosporin** moderately increases the exposure to **ezetimibe** and **ezetimibe** slightly increases the exposure to **ciclosporin**. Moderate Study
- **Ciclosporin** is predicted to increase the exposure to factor XA inhibitors **(apixaban)**. Moderate Theoretical
- **Ciclosporin** slightly increases the exposure to factor XA inhibitors **(edoxaban)**. Adjust **edoxaban** dose. Severe Study
- **Ciclosporin** slightly increases the exposure to factor XA inhibitors **(rivaroxaban)**. Manufacturer advises caution in renal impairment. Moderate Study
- Fibrates **(bezafibrate)** are predicted to increase the risk of nephrotoxicity when given with **ciclosporin**. Severe Theoretical
- Fibrates **(fenofibrate)** increase the risk of nephrotoxicity when given with **ciclosporin**. Severe Study
- **Ciclosporin** is predicted to increase the exposure to **fidaxomicin**. Avoid. Moderate Study
- **Filgotinib** is predicted to increase the risk of immunosuppression when given with **ciclosporin**. Avoid. Severe Theoretical
- **Ciclosporin** is predicted to increase the exposure to **gilteritinib**. Moderate Theoretical
- **Ciclosporin** increases the exposure to **glecaprevir**. Avoid or monitor. Severe Study
- **Glofitamab** might affect the exposure to **ciclosporin**. Moderate Theoretical
- **Grapefruit** juice increases the concentration of **ciclosporin**. Avoid. Severe Study
- **Ciclosporin** greatly increases the exposure to **grazoprevir**. Avoid. Severe Study
- H_2 receptor antagonists **(cimetidine)** increase the concentration of **ciclosporin**. Mild Study
- **HIV-protease inhibitors** increase the concentration of **ciclosporin**. Severe Study
- **Idelalisib** increases the concentration of **ciclosporin**. Severe Study
- **Imatinib** is predicted to increase the concentration of **ciclosporin**. Severe Study
- Iron chelators **(dexrazoxane)** might increase the risk of immunosuppression when given with **ciclosporin**. Severe Theoretical
- **Ivacaftor** is predicted to increase the exposure to **ciclosporin**. Moderate Theoretical
- **Ivosidenib** decreases the concentration of **ciclosporin**. Severe Study
- **Ciclosporin** is predicted to increase the exposure to **ivosidenib** and **ivosidenib** might decrease the exposure to **ciclosporin**. Monitor and adjust dose—consult product literature. Severe Study
- **Lanreotide** is predicted to decrease the absorption of oral **ciclosporin**. Adjust dose. Severe Theoretical
- **Ciclosporin** might increase the concentration of **lapatinib**. Severe Theoretical
- **Larotrectinib** is predicted to increase the exposure to **ciclosporin**. Use with caution and adjust dose. Mild Theoretical
- **Lazertinib** is predicted to increase the exposure to **ciclosporin**. Moderate Study
- **Letermovir** increases the exposure to **ciclosporin** and **ciclosporin** increases the exposure to **letermovir**. Monitor and adjust **letermovir** dose. Severe Study
- **Live vaccines** are predicted to increase the risk of generalised infection (possibly life-threatening) when given with **ciclosporin**. UKHSA advises avoid (refer to Green Book). Severe Theoretical
- **Ciclosporin** is predicted to increase the exposure to **lomitapide**. Separate administration by 12 hours. Moderate Theoretical
- **Lorlatinib** is predicted to decrease the exposure to **ciclosporin**. Avoid. Moderate Theoretical
- **Lumacaftor** decreases the concentration of **ciclosporin**. Severe Study

Interactions | **Appendix 1**

A1

Ciclosporin (continued)

- Macrolides **(clarithromycin)** increase the concentration of **ciclosporin.** Severe Study
- Macrolides **(erythromycin)** greatly increase the exposure to **ciclosporin.** Avoid or monitor. Severe Study
- **Maribavir** is predicted to increase the exposure to **ciclosporin.** Monitor and adjust dose. Severe Theoretical
- **Ciclosporin** moderately increases the exposure to meglitinides **(repaglinide).** Moderate Study
- **Metreleptin** might alter the exposure to **ciclosporin.** Monitor concentration and adjust dose. Severe Theoretical
- **Metronidazole** has been reported to increase the concentration of **ciclosporin.** Severe Anecdotal
- **Midostaurin** might increase the concentration of **ciclosporin.** Severe Anecdotal
- **Ciclosporin** is predicted to decrease the efficacy of **mifamurtide.** Avoid. Severe Theoretical
- **Mitotane** decreases the concentration of **ciclosporin.** Severe Study
- **Ciclosporin** is predicted to increase the exposure to **momelotinib.** Moderate Study
- Monoclonal antibodies **(blinatumomab, mosunetuzumab)** are predicted to transiently increase the exposure to **ciclosporin.** Monitor and adjust dose. Moderate Theoretical
- Monoclonal antibodies **(elranatamab)** might affect the exposure to **ciclosporin.** Monitor and adjust dose. Moderate Theoretical
- Monoclonal antibodies **(sarilumab)** potentially affect the exposure to **ciclosporin.** Monitor and adjust dose. Moderate Theoretical
- Monoclonal antibodies **(teclistamab)** might affect the exposure to **ciclosporin.** Moderate Theoretical
- Monoclonal antibodies **(tocilizumab)** are predicted to decrease the exposure to **ciclosporin.** Monitor and adjust dose. Moderate Theoretical
- **Ciclosporin** increases the risk of neutropenia when given with monoclonal antibodies **(brentuximab vedotin).** Monitor and adjust dose. Severe Theoretical
- **Ciclosporin** is predicted to increase the exposure to **naldemedine.** Moderate Study
- **Ciclosporin** is predicted to increase the exposure to **neratinib.** Avoid or adjust dose and monitor for gastrointestinal adverse effects—consult product literature. Severe Study
- Neurokinin-1 receptor antagonists **(aprepitant, netupitant)** are predicted to increase the concentration of **ciclosporin.** Severe Study
- **Nilotinib** is predicted to increase the concentration of **ciclosporin.** Severe Study
- **Ciclosporin** is predicted to increase the exposure to **nintedanib.** Moderate Study
- **Nirmatrelvir** boosted with ritonavir is predicted to increase the concentration of **ciclosporin.** Avoid—consult product literature. Severe Theoretical
- NNRTIs **(efavirenz)** decrease the concentration of **ciclosporin.** Monitor concentration and adjust dose. Moderate Study
- NNRTIs **(etravirine)** are predicted to decrease the exposure to **ciclosporin.** Moderate Theoretical
- NNRTIs **(nevirapine)** are predicted to decrease the concentration of **ciclosporin.** Moderate Study
- **Ciclosporin** increases the concentration of NSAIDs **(diclofenac).** Severe Study → Also see TABLE 2 p. 1053 → Also see TABLE 13 p. 1057
- **Octreotide** decreases the absorption of oral **ciclosporin.** Adjust **ciclosporin** dose, p. 640. Severe Anecdotal
- **Olaparib** might alter the exposure to **ciclosporin.** Moderate Theoretical
- **Ciclosporin** is predicted to increase the exposure to **omaveloxolone.** Avoid or adjust **omaveloxolone** dose, p. 755. Moderate Theoretical
- **Palbociclib** is predicted to increase the exposure to **ciclosporin.** Adjust dose. Moderate Theoretical
- **Ciclosporin** is predicted to increase the exposure to **panobinostat.** Adjust dose. Moderate Theoretical
- **Pasireotide** is predicted to decrease the absorption of oral **ciclosporin.** Adjust dose. Severe Theoretical
- **Pitolisant** is predicted to decrease the exposure to **ciclosporin.** Avoid. Severe Theoretical
- **Pralsetinib** might affect the exposure to **ciclosporin** and **ciclosporin** is predicted to increase the exposure to **pralsetinib.** Avoid. Moderate Theoretical
- **Ciclosporin** is predicted to increase the concentration of **ranolazine** and **ranolazine** is predicted to increase the concentration of **ciclosporin.** Moderate Theoretical
- **Ciclosporin** is predicted to increase the exposure to **relugolix.** Avoid or take relugolix first and separate administration by at least 6 hours. Moderate Study
- **Ribociclib** is predicted to increase the exposure to **ciclosporin.** Use with caution and adjust dose. Moderate Theoretical
- Rifamycins **(rifampicin)** decrease the concentration of **ciclosporin.** Severe Study → Also see TABLE 2 p. 1053
- **Ciclosporin** very markedly increases the exposure to **rifaximin.** Severe Study
- **Ciclosporin** slightly increases the exposure to **rimegepant.** Avoid another dose of rimegepant within 48 hours of concurrent use. Moderate Study
- **Ciclosporin** is predicted to increase the exposure to **riociguat.** Moderate Theoretical
- **Ritlecitinib** is predicted to increase the exposure to **ciclosporin** and **ciclosporin** is predicted to increase the risk of generalised infection (possibly life-threatening) when given with **ritlecitinib.** Avoid. Severe Theoretical
- **Rucaparib** is predicted to increase the exposure to **ciclosporin.** Monitor and adjust dose. Moderate Study
- **Ciclosporin** moderately increases the exposure to **seladelpar.** Moderate Study
- **Ciclosporin** moderately increases the exposure to **sirolimus.** Separate administration by 4 hours. Severe Study
- **Somapacitan** might decrease the exposure to **ciclosporin.** Severe Theoretical
- **Somatrogon** might decrease the exposure to **ciclosporin.** Severe Theoretical
- **Ciclosporin** slightly increases the exposure to **sparsentan.** Moderate Study → Also see TABLE 13 p. 1057
- **St John's wort** decreases the concentration of **ciclosporin.** Avoid. Moderate Study
- **Ciclosporin** markedly to very markedly increases the exposure to statins **(atorvastatin).** Avoid or adjust **atorvastatin** dose, p. 154. Severe Study
- **Ciclosporin** moderately increases the exposure to statins **(fluvastatin).** Severe Study
- **Ciclosporin** markedly to very markedly increases the exposure to statins **(pravastatin).** Adjust dose. Severe Study
- **Ciclosporin** markedly increases the exposure to statins **(rosuvastatin).** Avoid. Severe Study
- **Ciclosporin** markedly to very markedly increases the exposure to statins **(simvastatin).** Avoid. Severe Study
- **Ciclosporin** is predicted to increase the exposure to sulfonylureas **(glibenclamide)** and sulfonylureas **(glibenclamide)** might increase the exposure to **ciclosporin.** Monitor and adjust **ciclosporin** dose, p. 640. Moderate Study
- **Ciclosporin** increases the concentration of **tacrolimus.** Avoid. Severe Study → Also see TABLE 2 p. 1053 → Also see TABLE 13 p. 1057
- **Ciclosporin** is predicted to slightly increase the exposure to **talazoparib.** Avoid or adjust dose—consult product literature. Severe Study
- **Ciclosporin** increases the concentration of taxanes **(docetaxel)** (oral). Unknown Study
- **Ciclosporin** increases the concentration of taxanes **(paclitaxel).** Severe Study
- **Tebentafusp** is predicted to transiently increase the exposure to **ciclosporin.** Monitor and adjust dose. Moderate Theoretical
- **Ciclosporin** is predicted to increase the exposure to **tenofovir alafenamide.** Moderate Theoretical
- **Ciclosporin** is predicted to increase the exposure to **tenofovir disoproxil.** Moderate Theoretical → Also see TABLE 2 p. 1053
- Tetracyclines **(doxycycline)** are predicted to increase the concentration of **ciclosporin.** Severe Theoretical
- **Ciclosporin** is predicted to increase the exposure to thrombin inhibitors **(dabigatran).** Avoid. Severe Study
- **Ciclosporin** is predicted to increase the exposure to **ticagrelor.** Use with caution or avoid. Severe Study

- **Ciclosporin** might increase the exposure to **tigecycline** and **tigecycline** has been reported to increase the concentration of **ciclosporin**. Severe Anecdotal
- **Ciclosporin** increases the exposure to **tofacitinib**. Avoid. Severe Study
- **Ciclosporin** is predicted to increase the exposure to **topotecan**. Severe Study
- **Ciclosporin** is predicted to increase the concentration of **trametinib**. Moderate Theoretical
- **Tucatinib** increases the concentration of **ciclosporin**. Severe Study
- **Ursodeoxycholic acid** affects the concentration of **ciclosporin**. Use with caution and adjust dose. Severe Anecdotal
- **Ciclosporin** might affect the exposure to **vemurafenib**. Severe Theoretical
- **Ciclosporin** is predicted to increase the exposure to **venetoclax**. Avoid or monitor for toxicity. Severe Theoretical
- **Ciclosporin** might increase the exposure to **vinca alkaloids**. Severe Theoretical
- **Vitamin E substances** affect the exposure to **ciclosporin**. Moderate Study
- **Vorasidenib** might decrease the concentration of **ciclosporin**. Avoid. Severe Theoretical
- **Ciclosporin** increases the concentration of **voxilaprevir**. Avoid. Severe Study

Cidofovir → see TABLE 2 p. 1053 (nephrotoxicity)

Cilostazol → see TABLE 3 p. 1053 (bleeding)

GENERAL INFORMATION Concurrent use with 2 or more antiplatelets or anticoagulants is contra-indicated.

- Anti-androgens **(apalutamide, enzalutamide)** are predicted to alter the effects of **cilostazol**. Moderate Theoretical
- Antiepileptics **(carbamazepine, fosphenytoin, phenobarbital, phenytoin, primidone)** are predicted to alter the effects of **cilostazol**. Moderate Theoretical
- Antifungals, azoles **(fluconazole)** are predicted to increase the exposure to **cilostazol**. Adjust **cilostazol** dose. Moderate Theoretical
- Antifungals, azoles **(itraconazole, ketoconazole, posaconazole, voriconazole)** are predicted to moderately increase the exposure to **cilostazol**. Adjust **cilostazol** dose. Moderate Study
- Antifungals, azoles **(miconazole)** are predicted to increase the exposure to **cilostazol**. Use with caution and adjust dose. Moderate Theoretical
- **Ceritinib** is predicted to moderately increase the exposure to **cilostazol**. Adjust **cilostazol** dose. Moderate Study
- **Cilostazol** might increase the exposure to **cladribine**. Avoid or adjust dose. Moderate Theoretical
- **Cobicistat** is predicted to moderately increase the exposure to **cilostazol**. Adjust **cilostazol** dose. Moderate Study
- **Encorafenib** is predicted to alter the effects of **cilostazol**. Moderate Theoretical
- **HIV-protease inhibitors** are predicted to moderately increase the exposure to **cilostazol**. Adjust **cilostazol** dose. Moderate Study
- **Idelalisib** is predicted to moderately increase the exposure to **cilostazol**. Adjust **cilostazol** dose. Moderate Study
- **Ivosidenib** is predicted to alter the effects of **cilostazol**. Moderate Theoretical
- **Cilostazol** is predicted to increase the exposure to **lomitapide**. Separate administration by 12 hours. Moderate Theoretical
- **Lumacaftor** is predicted to alter the effects of **cilostazol**. Moderate Theoretical
- Macrolides **(clarithromycin)** are predicted to moderately increase the exposure to **cilostazol**. Adjust **cilostazol** dose. Moderate Study
- Macrolides **(erythromycin)** slightly increase the exposure to **cilostazol**. Adjust **cilostazol** dose. Moderate Study
- **Cilostazol** might increase the exposure to **metoclopramide**. Moderate Study
- **Mitotane** is predicted to alter the effects of **cilostazol**. Moderate Theoretical
- **Moclobemide** is predicted to increase the exposure to **cilostazol**. Moderate Theoretical
- **Nirmatrelvir** boosted with ritonavir is predicted to increase the concentration of **cilostazol**. Adjust dose. Moderate Theoretical
- Proton pump inhibitors **(esomeprazole)** are predicted to increase the exposure to **cilostazol**. Moderate Theoretical
- Proton pump inhibitors **(omeprazole)** are predicted to increase the exposure to **cilostazol**. Adjust **cilostazol** dose. Moderate Study
- Rifamycins **(rifampicin)** are predicted to alter the effects of **cilostazol**. Moderate Theoretical
- **Selumetinib** might increase the risk of bleeding when given with **cilostazol**. Severe Theoretical
- SSRIs **(fluoxetine, fluvoxamine)** are predicted to increase the exposure to **cilostazol**. Adjust **cilostazol** dose. Moderate Theoretical → Also see TABLE 3 p. 1053
- **St John's wort** is predicted to alter the effects of **cilostazol**. Moderate Theoretical
- **Cilostazol** is predicted to increase the exposure to statins **(atorvastatin)**. Moderate Theoretical
- **Cilostazol** slightly increases the exposure to statins **(simvastatin)**. Moderate Study
- **Tucatinib** is predicted to moderately increase the exposure to **cilostazol**. Adjust **cilostazol** dose. Moderate Study

Cimetidine → see H_2 receptor antagonists

Cinacalcet

FOOD AND LIFESTYLE Dose adjustment might be necessary if smoking started or stopped during treatment.

- Anti-androgens **(apalutamide, enzalutamide)** are predicted to decrease the exposure to **cinacalcet**. Monitor and adjust dose. Moderate Study
- **Cinacalcet** is predicted to increase the exposure to anticholinesterases, centrally acting **(galantamine)**. Monitor and adjust dose. Moderate Study
- Antiepileptics **(carbamazepine, fosphenytoin, phenobarbital, phenytoin, primidone)** are predicted to decrease the exposure to **cinacalcet**. Monitor and adjust dose. Moderate Study
- Antifungals, azoles **(itraconazole, ketoconazole, posaconazole, voriconazole)** are predicted to moderately increase the exposure to **cinacalcet**. Adjust dose. Moderate Study
- **Cinacalcet** is predicted to markedly increase the exposure to **atomoxetine**. Adjust dose. Severe Study
- **Cinacalcet** is predicted to moderately increase the exposure to atypical antipsychotics **(aripiprazole)**. Avoid or adjust dose—consult product literature. Moderate Study
- **Cinacalcet** is predicted to increase the exposure to atypical antipsychotics **(clozapine)**. Use with caution and adjust dose. Severe Study
- **Cinacalcet** is predicted to increase the exposure to atypical antipsychotics **(risperidone)**. Adjust dose. Moderate Study
- **Cinacalcet** is predicted to increase the exposure to beta blockers, selective **(metoprolol, nebivolol)**. Moderate Study
- **Ceritinib** is predicted to moderately increase the exposure to **cinacalcet**. Adjust dose. Moderate Study
- **Cobicistat** is predicted to moderately increase the exposure to **cinacalcet**. Adjust dose. Moderate Study
- **Cinacalcet** is predicted to slightly increase the exposure to **darifenacin**. Mild Study
- **Cinacalcet** might increase the risk of hypocalcaemia when given with **denosumab**. Severe Theoretical
- **Cinacalcet** is predicted to increase the exposure to **eliglustat**. Avoid or adjust dose—consult product literature. Severe Study
- **Encorafenib** is predicted to decrease the exposure to **cinacalcet**. Monitor and adjust dose. Moderate Study
- **Cinacalcet** increases the risk of hypocalcaemia when given with **etelcalcetide**. Avoid. Severe Theoretical
- **Cinacalcet** is predicted to increase the exposure to **fenfluramine**. Moderate Study
- **Cinacalcet** is predicted to increase the exposure to **fesoterodine**. Use with caution and adjust dose. Mild Theoretical
- **Cinacalcet** is predicted to increase the exposure to **gefitinib**. Moderate Theoretical
- **HIV-protease inhibitors** are predicted to moderately increase the exposure to **cinacalcet**. Adjust dose. Moderate Study
- **Idelalisib** is predicted to moderately increase the exposure to **cinacalcet**. Adjust dose. Moderate Study
- **Ivosidenib** is predicted to decrease the exposure to **cinacalcet**. Monitor and adjust dose. Moderate Study

A1 Interactions | Appendix 1

Cinacalcet (continued)
- **Lumacaftor** is predicted to decrease the exposure to **cinacalcet**. Monitor and adjust dose. [Moderate] Study
- Macrolides **(clarithromycin)** are predicted to moderately increase the exposure to **cinacalcet**. Adjust dose. [Moderate] Study
- **Cinacalcet** is predicted to increase the exposure to **mexiletine**. [Moderate] Study
- **Mitotane** is predicted to decrease the exposure to **cinacalcet**. Monitor and adjust dose. [Moderate] Study
- **Cinacalcet** is predicted to decrease the efficacy of opioids **(codeine)**. [Moderate] Theoretical
- **Cinacalcet** is predicted to decrease the efficacy of opioids **(tramadol)**. [Severe] Study
- **Cinacalcet** is predicted to moderately increase the exposure to **pitolisant**. Use with caution and adjust dose. [Moderate] Study
- Rifamycins **(rifampicin)** are predicted to decrease the exposure to **cinacalcet**. Monitor and adjust dose. [Moderate] Study
- SSRIs **(fluvoxamine)** are predicted to increase the exposure to **cinacalcet**. Adjust dose. [Moderate] Theoretical
- **Cinacalcet** is predicted to increase the exposure to SSRIs **(dapoxetine)**. [Moderate] Theoretical
- **Cinacalcet** is predicted to decrease the efficacy of **tamoxifen**. Avoid. [Severe] Study
- **Cinacalcet** is predicted to increase the exposure to the active metabolite of **tetrabenazine**. [Moderate] Study
- **Cinacalcet** is predicted to increase the exposure to **tricyclic antidepressants**. Monitor for toxicity and adjust dose. [Severe] Study
- **Tucatinib** is predicted to moderately increase the exposure to **cinacalcet**. Adjust dose. [Moderate] Study
- **Cinacalcet** is predicted to increase the exposure to **vortioxetine**. Monitor and adjust dose. [Moderate] Study

Cinnarizine → see antihistamines, sedating
Ciprofibrate → see fibrates
Ciprofloxacin → see quinolones
Cisatracurium → see neuromuscular blocking drugs, non-depolarising
Cisplatin → see platinum compounds
Citalopram → see SSRIs
Cladribine → see TABLE 12 p. 1057 (myelosuppression)

SEPARATION OF ADMINISTRATION Oral cladribine might affect the absorption of concurrently administered drugs—consider separating administration by at least 3 hours.

- Anti-androgens **(darolutamide)** are predicted to increase the exposure to **cladribine**. Avoid or adjust dose. [Moderate] Theoretical
- Antiepileptics **(carbamazepine)** are predicted to increase the risk of haematological toxicity when given with oral **cladribine**. [Moderate] Theoretical
- Calcium-channel blockers **(nifedipine, nimodipine)** might increase the exposure to **cladribine**. Avoid or adjust dose. [Moderate] Theoretical
- **Ciclosporin** is predicted to increase the exposure to **cladribine**. Avoid or adjust dose. [Moderate] Theoretical
- **Cilostazol** might increase the exposure to **cladribine**. Avoid or adjust dose. [Moderate] Theoretical
- **Dipyridamole** might increase the exposure to **cladribine**. [Moderate] Theoretical
- **Eltrombopag** is predicted to increase the exposure to **cladribine**. Avoid or adjust dose. [Moderate] Theoretical
- **Febuxostat** is predicted to increase the exposure to **cladribine**. Avoid or adjust dose. [Moderate] Theoretical
- **Fostamatinib** is predicted to increase the exposure to **cladribine**. Avoid or adjust dose. [Moderate] Theoretical
- HIV-protease inhibitors **(ritonavir)** might increase the exposure to **cladribine**. [Moderate] Theoretical
- **Leflunomide** is predicted to increase the exposure to **cladribine**. Avoid or adjust dose. [Moderate] Theoretical → Also see TABLE 12 p. 1057
- **Live vaccines** are predicted to increase the risk of generalised infection (possibly life-threatening) when given with **cladribine**. UKHSA advises avoid (refer to Green Book). [Severe] Theoretical
- NSAIDs **(sulindac)** might increase the exposure to **cladribine**. Avoid or adjust dose. [Moderate] Theoretical
- **Roxadustat** is predicted to increase the exposure to **cladribine**. Avoid or adjust dose. [Moderate] Theoretical
- **Teriflunomide** is predicted to increase the exposure to **cladribine**. Avoid or adjust dose. [Moderate] Theoretical
- **Vadadustat** is predicted to increase the exposure to **cladribine**. Avoid or adjust dose. [Moderate] Theoretical
- **Velpatasvir** is predicted to increase the exposure to **cladribine**. Avoid or adjust dose. [Moderate] Theoretical
- **Voxilaprevir** is predicted to increase the exposure to **cladribine**. Avoid or adjust dose. [Moderate] Theoretical

Clarithromycin → see macrolides
Clindamycin

ROUTE-SPECIFIC INFORMATION Since systemic absorption can follow topical application of **clindamycin**, the possibility of interactions should be borne in mind.

- **Clindamycin** increases the effects of **neuromuscular blocking drugs, non-depolarising**. [Severe] Anecdotal
- **Clindamycin** increases the effects of **suxamethonium**. [Severe] Anecdotal

Clobazam → see benzodiazepines
Clodronate → see bisphosphonates
Clofarabine → see TABLE 1 p. 1053 (hepatotoxicity), TABLE 12 p. 1057 (myelosuppression)
- **Live vaccines** are predicted to increase the risk of generalised infection (possibly life-threatening) when given with **clofarabine**. UKHSA advises avoid (refer to Green Book). [Severe] Theoretical

Clofazimine
- **Clofazimine** potentially increases the risk of QT-prolongation when given with **bedaquiline**. [Severe] Study

Clomethiazole → see TABLE 9 p. 1056 (CNS effects)
- **Alcohol** causes serious, potentially fatal, CNS depression when given with **clomethiazole**. Avoid. [Severe] Study → Also see TABLE 9 p. 1056
- Anti-androgens **(apalutamide, enzalutamide)** decrease the exposure to **clomethiazole**. Monitor and adjust dose. [Moderate] Study
- Antiepileptics **(carbamazepine, fosphenytoin, phenobarbital, phenytoin, primidone)** decrease the exposure to **clomethiazole**. Monitor and adjust dose. [Moderate] Study → Also see TABLE 9 p. 1056
- **Encorafenib** decreases the exposure to **clomethiazole**. Monitor and adjust dose. [Moderate] Study
- **Ivosidenib** decreases the exposure to **clomethiazole**. Monitor and adjust dose. [Moderate] Study
- **Lumacaftor** decreases the exposure to **clomethiazole**. Monitor and adjust dose. [Moderate] Study
- **Mitotane** decreases the exposure to **clomethiazole**. Monitor and adjust dose. [Moderate] Study
- Rifamycins **(rifampicin)** decrease the exposure to **clomethiazole**. Monitor and adjust dose. [Moderate] Study

Clomipramine → see tricyclic antidepressants
Clonazepam → see benzodiazepines
Clonidine → see TABLE 4 p. 1054 (bradycardia), TABLE 6 p. 1054 (hypotension), TABLE 9 p. 1056 (CNS effects)
- **Tricyclic antidepressants** decrease the antihypertensive effects of **clonidine**. Monitor and adjust dose. [Moderate] Anecdotal → Also see TABLE 6 p. 1054 → Also see TABLE 9 p. 1056

Clopidogrel → see TABLE 3 p. 1053 (bleeding)
- **Clopidogrel** is predicted to increase the exposure to anti-androgens **(apalutamide)** and anti-androgens **(apalutamide)** are predicted to increase the exposure to the active metabolite of **clopidogrel**. Avoid or monitor. [Moderate] Study
- **Clopidogrel** moderately increases the exposure to anti-androgens **(enzalutamide)**. Avoid or adjust **enzalutamide** dose. [Severe] Study
- Antifungals, azoles **(fluconazole)** are predicted to decrease the efficacy of **clopidogrel**. Avoid. [Severe] Theoretical
- Antifungals, azoles **(voriconazole)** are predicted to decrease the efficacy of **clopidogrel**. Avoid. [Moderate] Study
- **Clopidogrel** slightly increases the exposure to **bupropion**. [Moderate] Study
- **Cenobamate** is predicted to decrease the efficacy of **clopidogrel**. Avoid. [Moderate] Study

- Cobicistat is predicted to decrease the concentration of the active metabolite of **clopidogrel**. Avoid. [Severe] Theoretical
- **Clopidogrel** is predicted to increase the exposure to **dabrafenib**. [Moderate] Theoretical
- **Clopidogrel** are predicted to increases the exposure to **etrasimod**. Avoid in poor CYP2C9 metabolisers. [Severe] Theoretical
- **Fedratinib** is predicted to decrease the efficacy of **clopidogrel**. Avoid. [Moderate] Study
- **Grapefruit** juice markedly decreases the exposure to **clopidogrel**. [Severe] Study
- HIV-protease inhibitors **(ritonavir)** might decrease the efficacy of **clopidogrel**. Avoid. [Moderate] Theoretical
- **Clopidogrel** increases the exposure to meglitinides **(repaglinide)**. Avoid. [Severe] Study
- **Moclobemide** is predicted to decrease the efficacy of **clopidogrel**. Avoid. [Moderate] Study
- **Clopidogrel** is predicted to moderately increase the exposure to **montelukast**. [Moderate] Study
- **Nirmatrelvir** boosted with ritonavir is predicted to decrease the concentration of **clopidogrel**. [Severe] Theoretical
- **Clopidogrel** is predicted to increase the exposure to the active metabolites of **ozanimod**. [Moderate] Study
- **Clopidogrel** increases the exposure to **pioglitazone**. Monitor blood glucose and adjust dose. [Severe] Study
- Proton pump inhibitors **(esomeprazole, omeprazole)** are predicted to decrease the efficacy of **clopidogrel**. Avoid. [Moderate] Study
- **Clopidogrel** is predicted to increase the exposure to retinoids **(alitretinoin)**. Adjust **alitretinoin** dose. [Moderate] Theoretical
- Rifamycins **(rifampicin)** moderately increase the exposure to the active metabolite of **clopidogrel**. Avoid. [Moderate] Study
- **Clopidogrel** is predicted to increase the exposure to **roxadustat**. Monitor haemoglobin and adjust dose—consult product literature. [Moderate] Study
- **Clopidogrel** is predicted to increase the exposure to **selexipag**. Adjust **selexipag** dose. [Moderate] Study
- **Selumetinib** might increase the risk of bleeding when given with **clopidogrel**. [Severe] Theoretical
- SSRIs **(fluoxetine, fluvoxamine)** are predicted to decrease the efficacy of **clopidogrel**. Avoid. [Severe] Theoretical → Also see TABLE 3 p. 1053
- **Clopidogrel** increases the exposure to statins **(rosuvastatin)**. Adjust **rosuvastatin** dose, p. 155. [Moderate] Study
- **Clopidogrel** is predicted to increase the concentration of taxanes **(paclitaxel)**. [Severe] Anecdotal
- **Clopidogrel** is predicted to increase the exposure to **treprostinil**. Adjust dose. [Moderate] Theoretical → Also see TABLE 3 p. 1053
- **Clopidogrel** is predicted to increase the exposure to **tucatinib**. Avoid or adjust dose—consult product literature. [Severe] Study

Clotrimazole → see antifungals, azoles

Clozapine → see atypical antipsychotics

Cobicistat

- **Cobicistat** is predicted to increase the exposure to **abemaciclib**. Avoid or adjust dose—consult product literature. [Severe] Study
- **Cobicistat** is predicted to increase the exposure to **acalabrutinib**. Avoid. [Severe] Study
- **Cobicistat** is predicted to increase the exposure to **afatinib**. [Moderate] Study
- **Cobicistat** is predicted to increase the exposure to **aliskiren**. [Moderate] Study
- **Cobicistat** is predicted to moderately increase the exposure to alpha blockers **(alfuzosin, tamsulosin)**. Use with caution or avoid. [Moderate] Study
- **Cobicistat** is predicted to increase the exposure to alpha blockers **(doxazosin)**. [Moderate] Study
- Anti-androgens **(apalutamide, enzalutamide)** are predicted to decrease the exposure to **cobicistat**. Avoid. [Severe] Study
- **Cobicistat** is predicted to increase the exposure to anti-androgens **(apalutamide)**. Monitor and adjust dose. [Mild] Study
- **Cobicistat** potentially increases the concentration of antiarrhythmics **(amiodarone, disopyramide, flecainide, lidocaine)**. [Severe] Theoretical
- **Cobicistat** very markedly increases the exposure to antiarrhythmics **(dronedarone)**. Avoid. [Severe] Study
- **Cobicistat** is predicted to increase the exposure to antiarrhythmics **(propafenone)**. Monitor and adjust dose. [Severe] Study
- **Cobicistat** is predicted to increase the exposure to anticholinesterases, centrally acting **(galantamine)**. Monitor and adjust dose. [Moderate] Study
- Antiepileptics **(carbamazepine, fosphenytoin, phenobarbital, phenytoin, primidone)** are predicted to decrease the exposure to **cobicistat**. Avoid. [Severe] Study
- Antiepileptics **(eslicarbazepine, oxcarbazepine)** are predicted to decrease the concentration of **cobicistat**. [Severe] Theoretical
- **Cobicistat** is predicted to very slightly increase the exposure to antiepileptics **(perampanel)**. [Mild] Study
- **Cobicistat** is predicted to increase the exposure to antifungals, azoles **(fluconazole, posaconazole)**. [Moderate] Theoretical
- **Cobicistat** is predicted to increase the exposure to antifungals, azoles **(isavuconazole)**. Avoid or monitor adverse effects. [Severe] Study
- **Cobicistat** is predicted to increase the exposure to antifungals, azoles **(itraconazole)**. Adjust **itraconazole** dose, p. 465. [Moderate] Theoretical
- **Cobicistat** is predicted to increase the exposure to antifungals, azoles **(ketoconazole)**. Adjust **ketoconazole** dose, p. 550. [Moderate] Theoretical
- **Cobicistat** is predicted to affect the exposure to antifungals, azoles **(voriconazole)**. Avoid. [Moderate] Theoretical
- **Cobicistat** is predicted to increase the exposure to antihistamines, non-sedating **(fexofenadine)**. [Moderate] Theoretical
- **Cobicistat** is predicted to increase the exposure to antihistamines, non-sedating **(mizolastine)**. Avoid. [Severe] Study
- **Cobicistat** is predicted to increase the exposure to antihistamines, non-sedating **(rupatadine)**. Avoid. [Moderate] Study
- **Cobicistat** is predicted to increase the concentration of antimalarials **(piperaquine)**. [Severe] Study
- **Cobicistat** is predicted to increase the exposure to **atogepant**. Adjust **atogepant** dose. [Moderate] Study
- **Cobicistat** is predicted to slightly increase the exposure to atypical antipsychotics **(aripiprazole)**. Avoid or adjust dose—consult product literature. [Moderate] Study
- **Cobicistat** is predicted to moderately increase the exposure to atypical antipsychotics **(cariprazine)**. Avoid. [Severe] Study
- **Cobicistat** is predicted to increase the exposure to atypical antipsychotics **(lurasidone, quetiapine)**. Avoid. [Severe] Study
- **Cobicistat** is predicted to increase the exposure to atypical antipsychotics **(risperidone)**. Adjust dose. [Moderate] Study
- **Cobicistat** is predicted to increase the exposure to **avacopan**. [Severe] Study
- **Cobicistat** is predicted to increase the exposure to **avapritinib**. Avoid. [Moderate] Study
- **Cobicistat** is predicted to increase the exposure to **axitinib**. Avoid or adjust dose. [Moderate] Study
- **Cobicistat** might increase the exposure to **bedaquiline**. [Mild] Study
- **Cobicistat** moderately increases the exposure to benzodiazepines **(alprazolam)**. Avoid. [Moderate] Study
- **Cobicistat** is predicted to markedly to very markedly increase the exposure to benzodiazepines **(midazolam)**. Avoid or adjust dose. [Severe] Study
- **Cobicistat** is predicted to increase the exposure to $beta_2$ agonists **(salmeterol)**. Avoid. [Severe] Study
- **Cobicistat** slightly increases the exposure to **bortezomib**. [Moderate] Study
- **Cobicistat** is predicted to increase the exposure to **bosutinib**. Avoid or adjust dose. [Severe] Study
- **Cobicistat** is predicted to increase the exposure to **brigatinib**. Avoid or adjust dose—consult product literature. [Severe] Study
- **Cobicistat** is predicted to increase the exposure to **buspirone**. Adjust **buspirone** dose. [Severe] Study
- **Cobicistat** is predicted to increase the exposure to **cabozantinib**. [Moderate] Study
- **Cobicistat** is predicted to increase the exposure to calcium-channel blockers **(amlodipine, felodipine, lacidipine, nicardipine,**

Cobicistat (continued)
nifedipine, nimodipine). Monitor and adjust dose. Moderate Study

- **Cobicistat** is predicted to increase the exposure to calcium-channel blockers **(diltiazem, verapamil)**. Severe Study
- **Cobicistat** is predicted to markedly increase the exposure to calcium-channel blockers **(lercanidipine)**. Avoid. Severe Study
- **Cobicistat** is predicted to increase the exposure to **cannabidiol**. Avoid or adjust dose. Mild Study
- **Cobicistat** is predicted to increase the exposure to **capivasertib**. Adjust dose. Moderate Study
- **Cenobamate** is predicted to decrease the exposure to **cobicistat**. Avoid. Severe Theoretical
- **Cobicistat** is predicted to increase the exposure to **ceritinib**. Avoid or adjust dose—consult product literature. Severe Study
- **Cobicistat** increases the concentration of **ciclosporin**. Severe Study
- **Cobicistat** is predicted to moderately increase the exposure to **cilostazol**. Adjust **cilostazol** dose. Moderate Study
- **Cobicistat** is predicted to moderately increase the exposure to **cinacalcet**. Adjust dose. Moderate Study
- **Cobicistat** is predicted to decrease the concentration of the active metabolite of **clopidogrel**. Avoid. Severe Theoretical
- **Cobicistat** is predicted to increase the exposure to **cobimetinib**. Avoid or monitor for toxicity. Severe Study
- **Cobicistat** is predicted to increase the exposure to **colchicine**. Avoid potent CYP3A4 inhibitors or adjust **colchicine** dose, p. 637. Severe Study
- **Cobicistat** is predicted to decrease the efficacy of **combined hormonal contraceptives**. Avoid. Severe Study
- **Cobicistat** is predicted to increase the exposure to corticosteroids **(beclometasone)** (risk with beclometasone is likely to be lower than with other corticosteroids). Moderate Theoretical
- **Cobicistat** is predicted to increase the exposure to corticosteroids **(betamethasone, budesonide, ciclesonide, deflazacort, dexamethasone, fludrocortisone, fluticasone, hydrocortisone, methylprednisolone, mometasone, prednisolone, triamcinolone)**. Avoid or monitor adverse effects. Severe Study
- **Cobicistat** is predicted to increase the exposure to corticosteroids **(vamorolone)**. Adjust dose. Severe Study
- **Cobicistat** is predicted to affect the exposure to coumarins **(warfarin)**. Moderate Theoretical
- **Cobicistat** is predicted to increase the exposure to **crizotinib**. Avoid. Moderate Study
- **Dabrafenib** is predicted to decrease the exposure to **cobicistat**. Avoid. Severe Theoretical
- **Cobicistat** is predicted to increase the exposure to **dabrafenib**. Use with caution or avoid. Moderate Study
- **Cobicistat** is predicted to increase the exposure to **daridorexant**. Avoid. Severe Study
- **Cobicistat** is predicted to markedly to very markedly increase the exposure to **darifenacin**. Avoid. Severe Study
- **Cobicistat** is predicted to increase the exposure to **dasatinib**. Avoid or adjust dose—consult product literature. Severe Study
- **Cobicistat** very slightly increases the exposure to **delamanid**. Severe Study
- **Cobicistat** is predicted to increase the exposure to **deutivacaftor**. Adjust dose, see deutivacaftor with tezacaftor and vanzacaftor p. 218. Severe Study
- **Cobicistat** is predicted to moderately increase the exposure to **dienogest**. Moderate Study
- **Cobicistat** is predicted to increase the exposure to dipeptidylpeptidase-4 inhibitors **(saxagliptin)**. Moderate Study
- **Cobicistat** is predicted to increase the exposure to **domperidone**. Avoid. Severe Study
- **Cobicistat** increases the exposure to dopamine receptor agonists **(bromocriptine)**. Severe Study
- **Cobicistat** is predicted to increase the concentration of dopamine receptor agonists **(cabergoline)**. Moderate Anecdotal
- **Cobicistat** is predicted to increase the exposure to **dronabinol**. Adjust dose. Mild Study
- **Cobicistat** is predicted to increase the exposure to **drospirenone**. Severe Study
- **Cobicistat** is predicted to increase the exposure to **dutasteride**. Monitor adverse effects and adjust dose. Moderate Theoretical
- **Cobicistat** is predicted to increase the exposure to **elacestrant**. Avoid potent CYP3A4 inhibitors or adjust **elacestrant** dose. Severe Study
- **Cobicistat** is predicted to increase the exposure to **elexacaftor**. Adjust ivacaftor with tezacaftor and elexacaftor p. 220 dose with potent CYP3A4 inhibitors. Severe Study
- **Cobicistat** is predicted to increase the exposure to **eliglustat**. Avoid or adjust dose—consult product literature. Severe Study
- **Encorafenib** is predicted to decrease the exposure to **cobicistat**. Avoid. Severe Study
- **Cobicistat** is predicted to increase the exposure to **encorafenib**. Avoid or monitor. Severe Study
- Endothelin receptor antagonists **(bosentan)** are predicted to decrease the exposure to **cobicistat**. Avoid. Severe Theoretical
- **Cobicistat** is predicted to increase the exposure to endothelin receptor antagonists **(macitentan)**. Moderate Study
- **Cobicistat** is predicted to increase the exposure to the cytotoxic component of **enfortumab vedotin**. Severe Theoretical
- **Cobicistat** is predicted to increase the exposure to **entrectinib**. Avoid or adjust dose with potent CYP3A4 inhibitors—consult product literature. Severe Study
- **Cobicistat** is predicted to increase the exposure to **erdafitinib**. Adjust dose. Severe Study
- **Cobicistat** is predicted to increase the risk of ergotism when given with **ergometrine**. Avoid. Severe Theoretical
- **Cobicistat** is predicted to increase the exposure to **erlotinib**. Use with caution and adjust dose. Severe Study
- **Cobicistat** is predicted to increase the exposure to **esketamine**. Adjust dose. Moderate Study
- **Cobicistat** is predicted to increase the exposure to **eszopiclone**. Adjust **eszopiclone** dose; avoid in the elderly. Moderate Study
- **Cobicistat** is predicted to increase the concentration of subdermal **etonogestrel**. Moderate Theoretical
- **Cobicistat** is predicted to increase the exposure to **etrasimod**. Avoid in poor CYP2C9 metabolisers. Severe Theoretical
- **Cobicistat** is predicted to increase the exposure to **everolimus**. Avoid. Severe Study
- **Cobicistat** is predicted to increase the exposure to factor XA inhibitors **(apixaban, edoxaban, rivaroxaban)**. Avoid. Severe Theoretical
- **Cobicistat** is predicted to increase the exposure to **fedratinib**. Adjust dose, but avoid depending on other drugs taken—consult product literature. Moderate Study
- **Cobicistat** is predicted to moderately increase the exposure to **fesoterodine**. Adjust **fesoterodine** dose with potent CYP3A4 inhibitors; avoid in hepatic and renal impairment. Severe Study
- **Cobicistat** is predicted to increase the exposure to **fidaxomicin**. Avoid. Moderate Study
- **Cobicistat** is predicted to increase the exposure to **fostamatinib**. Monitor adverse effects and adjust dose. Moderate Study
- **Cobicistat** is predicted to increase the exposure to **futibatinib**. Avoid or adjust dose—consult product literature. Moderate Study
- **Cobicistat** is predicted to increase the exposure to **gefitinib**. Severe Study
- **Cobicistat** is predicted to increase the exposure to **gilteritinib**. Moderate Study
- **Cobicistat** is predicted to increase the exposure to **glasdegib**. Use with caution or avoid. Severe Study
- **Cobicistat** is predicted to moderately to markedly increase the exposure to **grazoprevir**. Avoid. Severe Study
- **Cobicistat** is predicted to increase the exposure to **guanfacine**. Adjust **guanfacine** dose, p. 281. Moderate Study
- **Cobicistat** is predicted to increase the exposure to **ibrutinib**. Avoid or adjust dose with potent CYP3A4 inhibitors—consult product literature. Severe Study
- **Cobicistat** is predicted to increase the exposure to **idelalisib**. Moderate Theoretical
- **Cobicistat** is predicted to increase the exposure to **imatinib**. Moderate Study
- **Cobicistat** is predicted to increase the exposure to the active metabolite of **irinotecan**. Avoid. Severe Study

- **Cobicistat** is predicted to increase the exposure to **ivabradine**. Avoid. [Severe] Study
- **Cobicistat** is predicted to increase the exposure to **ivacaftor**. Adjust dose with potent CYP3A4 inhibitors, see ivacaftor p. 219, lumacaftor with ivacaftor p. 222, tezacaftor with ivacaftor p. 223, and ivacaftor with tezacaftor and elexacaftor p. 220. [Severe] Study
- **Ivosidenib** is predicted to decrease the exposure to **cobicistat**. Avoid. [Severe] Study
- **Cobicistat** is predicted to increase the exposure to **ivosidenib**. Monitor and adjust dose—consult product literature. [Severe] Study
- **Cobicistat** is predicted to increase the exposure to **ketamine**. Adjust dose. [Moderate] Theoretical
- **Cobicistat** is predicted to increase the exposure to **lapatinib**. Avoid. [Moderate] Study
- **Cobicistat** is predicted to moderately increase the exposure to **larotrectinib**. Avoid or adjust dose—consult product literature. [Moderate] Study
- **Cobicistat** is predicted to increase the exposure to **leniolisib**. Avoid. [Moderate] Study
- **Cobicistat** is predicted to markedly increase the exposure to **lomitapide**. Avoid. [Severe] Study
- **Cobicistat** is predicted to increase the exposure to **lorlatinib**. Avoid or adjust dose—consult product literature. [Severe] Study
- **Lorlatinib** is predicted to decrease the exposure to **cobicistat**. Avoid. [Severe] Theoretical
- **Lumacaftor** is predicted to decrease the exposure to **cobicistat**. Avoid. [Severe] Study
- **Cobicistat** is predicted to increase the concentration of macrolides **(erythromycin)**. [Moderate] Theoretical
- **Cobicistat** markedly increases the exposure to **maraviroc**. Refer to specialist literature. [Severe] Study
- **Cobicistat** is predicted to increase the exposure to **mavacamten**. Avoid or monitor—consult product literature. [Severe] Study
- **Cobicistat** is predicted to increase the concentration of intramuscular **medroxyprogesterone**. [Moderate] Theoretical
- **Cobicistat** potentially increases the exposure to **mexiletine**. [Severe] Theoretical
- **Cobicistat** is predicted to increase the exposure to **midostaurin**. Avoid or monitor for toxicity. [Severe] Study
- **Cobicistat** is predicted to markedly increase the exposure to mineralocorticoid receptor antagonists **(eplerenone)**. Avoid. [Severe] Study
- **Cobicistat** is predicted to increase the exposure to mineralocorticoid receptor antagonists **(finerenone)**. Avoid. [Severe] Study
- **Cobicistat** is predicted to increase the exposure to **mirabegron**. Adjust **mirabegron** dose in hepatic and renal impairment. [Moderate] Study
- **Cobicistat** is predicted to increase the exposure to **mirtazapine**. [Moderate] Study
- **Mitotane** is predicted to decrease the exposure to **cobicistat**. Avoid. [Severe] Study
- **Cobicistat** is predicted to increase the exposure to **modafinil**. [Mild] Theoretical
- **Cobicistat** is predicted to increase the risk of neutropenia when given with monoclonal antibodies **(brentuximab vedotin)**. Monitor and adjust dose. [Severe] Study
- **Cobicistat** is predicted to increase the exposure to monoclonal antibodies **(polatuzumab vedotin)**. [Moderate] Theoretical
- **Cobicistat** is predicted to increase the exposure to the cytotoxic component of monoclonal antibodies **(trastuzumab emtansine)**. Avoid or monitor. [Severe] Theoretical
- **Cobicistat** is predicted to increase the exposure to **naldemedine**. Avoid or monitor. [Moderate] Study
- **Cobicistat** is predicted to markedly increase the exposure to **naloxegol**. Avoid. [Severe] Study
- **Cobicistat** is predicted to increase the exposure to **neratinib**. Avoid or adjust dose with potent CYP3A4 inhibitors—consult product literature. [Severe] Study
- **Cobicistat** is predicted to markedly increase the exposure to neurokinin-1 receptor antagonists **(aprepitant)**. [Moderate] Study
- **Cobicistat** is predicted to increase the exposure to neurokinin-1 receptor antagonists **(fosaprepitant)**. [Moderate] Theoretical
- **Cobicistat** is predicted to increase the exposure to neurokinin-1 receptor antagonists **(netupitant)**. [Moderate] Study
- **Cobicistat** is predicted to increase the exposure to **nilotinib**. Avoid. [Severe] Study
- **Cobicistat** is predicted to increase the exposure to **nintedanib**. [Moderate] Study
- **Cobicistat** is predicted to increase the exposure to **nitisinone**. Adjust dose. [Moderate] Theoretical
- NNRTIs **(efavirenz, etravirine, nevirapine)** are predicted to decrease the exposure to **cobicistat**. Avoid. [Severe] Theoretical
- **Cobicistat** is predicted to increase the exposure to **olaparib**. Avoid or adjust dose with potent CYP3A4 inhibitors—consult product literature. [Moderate] Study
- **Cobicistat** is predicted to increase the exposure to **omaveloxolone**. Avoid or adjust **omaveloxolone** dose, p. 755. [Severe] Study
- **Cobicistat** is predicted to increase the exposure to opioids **(alfentanil, buprenorphine, fentanyl, oxycodone)**. Monitor and adjust dose. [Severe] Study
- **Cobicistat** is predicted to increase the exposure to opioids **(sufentanil)**. [Moderate] Study
- **Cobicistat** is predicted to increase the exposure to **osilodrostat**. [Moderate] Theoretical
- **Cobicistat** is predicted to increase the exposure to **ospemifene**. Avoid in poor CYP2C9 metabolisers. [Moderate] Study
- **Cobicistat** is predicted to increase the exposure to **oxybutynin**. [Mild] Study
- **Cobicistat** is predicted to increase the exposure to **palbociclib**. Avoid or adjust dose—consult product literature. [Severe] Study
- **Cobicistat** is predicted to increase the exposure to **panobinostat**. Adjust dose—consult product literature; in hepatic impairment avoid. [Moderate] Study
- **Cobicistat** is predicted to increase the exposure to **pazopanib**. Avoid or adjust dose—consult product literature. [Moderate] Study
- **Cobicistat** is predicted to increase the exposure to **pemigatinib**. Avoid or adjust dose—consult product literature. [Severe] Study
- **Cobicistat** is predicted to increase the exposure to phosphodiesterase type-5 inhibitors **(avanafil, vardenafil)**. Avoid. [Severe] Study
- **Cobicistat** is predicted to increase the exposure to phosphodiesterase type-5 inhibitors **(sildenafil)**. Avoid potent CYP3A4 inhibitors or adjust **sildenafil** dose, p. 139. [Severe] Study
- **Cobicistat** is predicted to increase the exposure to phosphodiesterase type-5 inhibitors **(tadalafil)**. Use with caution or avoid. [Severe] Study
- **Cobicistat** is predicted to increase the exposure to **pimozide**. Avoid. [Severe] Study
- **Cobicistat** is predicted to slightly increase the exposure to **ponatinib**. Monitor and adjust dose—consult product literature. [Moderate] Study
- **Cobicistat** is predicted to increase the exposure to **pralsetinib**. Avoid or adjust dose with potent CYP3A4 inhibitors—consult product literature. [Moderate] Study
- **Cobicistat** is predicted to moderately increase the exposure to **praziquantel**. [Mild] Study
- **Cobicistat** given with carbimazole is predicted to increase the exposure to **propiverine**. Adjust starting dose. [Moderate] Theoretical
- **Cobicistat** is predicted to increase the exposure to **quizartinib**. Adjust dose—consult product literature. [Severe] Study
- **Cobicistat** is predicted to increase the exposure to **ranolazine**. Avoid. [Severe] Study
- **Cobicistat** is predicted to increase the exposure to **reboxetine**. Avoid. [Moderate] Study
- **Cobicistat** is predicted to increase the exposure to **regorafenib**. Avoid. [Moderate] Study
- **Cobicistat** is predicted to increase the exposure to **relugolix**. Avoid or take relugolix first and separate administration by at least 6 hours. [Moderate] Study
- **Cobicistat** is predicted to increase the exposure to retinoids **(alitretinoin)**. Adjust **alitretinoin** dose. [Moderate] Theoretical

Cobicistat (continued)
- **Cobicistat** is predicted to increase the exposure to **ribociclib.** Avoid or adjust dose—consult product literature. Moderate Study
- Rifamycins **(rifabutin)** decrease the concentration of **cobicistat** and **cobicistat** increases the exposure to rifamycins **(rifabutin).** Avoid or adjust dose. Severe Study
- Rifamycins **(rifampicin)** are predicted to decrease the exposure to **cobicistat.** Avoid. Severe Study
- **Cobicistat** is predicted to increase the exposure to **rimegepant.** Avoid. Moderate Study
- **Cobicistat** is predicted to increase the exposure to **ripretinib.** Moderate Theoretical
- **Cobicistat** is predicted to increase the exposure to **ruxolitinib.** Adjust dose depending on indication and monitor adverse effects—consult product literature. Moderate Study
- **Cobicistat** is predicted to increase the exposure to **selpercatinib.** Adjust dose—consult product literature. Moderate Study
- **Cobicistat** is predicted to increase the exposure to **selumetinib.** Avoid or adjust dose—consult product literature. Severe Study
- **Cobicistat** is predicted to increase the exposure to **siponimod.** Avoid depending on other drugs taken—consult product literature. Severe Theoretical
- **Cobicistat** is predicted to increase the concentration of **sirolimus.** Avoid or monitor and adjust dose. Severe Study
- **Cobicistat** is predicted to increase the exposure to SNRIs **(venlafaxine).** Moderate Study
- **Cobicistat** is predicted to increase the exposure to **solifenacin.** Adjust solifenacin p. 604 or tamsulosin with solifenacin dose; avoid in hepatic and renal impairment. Severe Study
- **Sotorasib** is predicted to decrease the exposure to **cobicistat.** Avoid. Severe Theoretical
- **Cobicistat** is predicted to increase the exposure to **sparsentan.** Avoid. Severe Study
- **Cobicistat** is predicted to increase the exposure to SSRIs **(citalopram, escitalopram, fluoxetine, fluvoxamine, paroxetine).** Monitor and adjust dose. Moderate Theoretical
- **Cobicistat** is predicted to moderately increase the exposure to SSRIs **(dapoxetine).** Avoid potent CYP3A4 inhibitors or adjust **dapoxetine** dose. Severe Study
- **Cobicistat** is predicted to increase the exposure to SSRIs **(sertraline).** Avoid. Moderate Theoretical
- **St John's wort** is predicted to decrease the exposure to **cobicistat.** Avoid. Severe Theoretical
- **Cobicistat** is predicted to increase the exposure to statins **(atorvastatin).** Avoid or adjust dose and monitor rhabdomyolysis. Severe Study
- **Cobicistat** is predicted to increase the exposure to statins **(simvastatin).** Avoid. Severe Study
- **Cobicistat** is predicted to increase the exposure to **sunitinib.** Avoid or adjust dose—consult product literature. Moderate Study
- **Cobicistat** is predicted to increase the concentration of **tacrolimus.** Avoid. If concurrent use is unavoidable—consult product literature. Severe Study
- **Cobicistat** is predicted to slightly increase the exposure to **talazoparib.** Avoid or adjust dose—consult product literature. Severe Study
- **Cobicistat** is predicted to increase the exposure to taxanes **(cabazitaxel).** Avoid or adjust dose—consult product literature. Severe Study
- **Cobicistat** is predicted to increase the exposure to taxanes **(docetaxel).** Avoid or adjust dose. Severe Study
- **Cobicistat** is predicted to increase the exposure to taxanes **(paclitaxel).** Moderate Anecdotal
- **Cobicistat** is predicted to increase the concentration of **temsirolimus.** Avoid. Severe Theoretical
- **Cobicistat** is predicted to increase the exposure to **tezacaftor.** Adjust dose with potent CYP3A4 inhibitors, see tezacaftor with ivacaftor p. 223, ivacaftor with tezacaftor and elexacaftor p. 220, and deutivacaftor with tezacaftor and vanzacaftor p. 218. Severe Study
- **Cobicistat** moderately increases the exposure to thrombin inhibitors **(dabigatran).** Avoid. Severe Study
- **Cobicistat** is predicted to markedly increase the exposure to **ticagrelor.** Avoid. Severe Study
- **Cobicistat** is predicted to increase the exposure to the cytotoxic component of **tisotumab vedotin.** Severe Theoretical
- **Cobicistat** is predicted to increase the exposure to **tofacitinib.** Adjust **tofacitinib** dose, p. 803. Moderate Study
- **Cobicistat** is predicted to increase the exposure to **tolterodine.** Avoid. Severe Study
- **Cobicistat** is predicted to increase the exposure to **tolvaptan.** Manufacturer advises caution or adjust **tolvaptan** dose with potent CYP3A4 inhibitors. Severe Study
- **Cobicistat** is predicted to increase the exposure to **topotecan.** Severe Study
- **Cobicistat** is predicted to increase the exposure to **toremifene.** Moderate Theoretical
- **Cobicistat** is predicted to increase the exposure to **trabectedin.** Avoid or adjust dose. Severe Theoretical
- **Cobicistat** is predicted to increase the concentration of **trametinib.** Moderate Theoretical
- **Cobicistat** is predicted to moderately increase the exposure to **trazodone.** Avoid or adjust dose. Moderate Study
- **Cobicistat** is predicted to slightly increase the exposure to **tricyclic antidepressants.** Mild Study
- **Cobicistat** increases the exposure to triptans **(almotriptan).** Mild Study
- **Cobicistat** is predicted to markedly increase the exposure to triptans **(eletriptan).** Avoid. Severe Study
- **Cobicistat** is predicted to increase the exposure to **ulipristal.** Avoid when used for uterine fibroids. Severe Study
- **Cobicistat** is predicted to increase the exposure to **upadacitinib.** Manufacturer advises caution or avoid, or adjust **upadacitinib** dose depending on indication, p. 927. Severe Study
- **Cobicistat** is predicted to increase the exposure to **vanzacaftor.** Adjust dose, see deutivacaftor with tezacaftor and vanzacaftor p. 218. Severe Study
- **Cobicistat** is predicted to increase the exposure to **vemurafenib.** Severe Theoretical
- **Cobicistat** is predicted to increase the exposure to **venetoclax.** Avoid or adjust dose—consult product literature. Severe Study
- **Cobicistat** is predicted to increase the exposure to **vinca alkaloids.** Severe Theoretical
- **Cobicistat** is predicted to increase the exposure to vitamin D substances **(paricalcitol).** Moderate Study
- **Cobicistat** is predicted to increase the exposure to **voclosporin.** Avoid. Severe Study
- **Cobicistat** is predicted to increase the exposure to **zanubrutinib.** Avoid or adjust dose with potent CYP3A4 inhibitors—consult product literature. Moderate Study
- **Cobicistat** is predicted to increase the exposure to **zopiclone.** Adjust dose. Moderate Theoretical

Cobimetinib
- Anti-androgens **(apalutamide, enzalutamide)** are predicted to decrease the exposure to **cobimetinib.** Avoid. Severe Theoretical
- Antiarrhythmics **(dronedarone)** are predicted to increase the exposure to **cobimetinib.** Severe Study
- Antiepileptics **(carbamazepine, fosphenytoin, phenobarbital, phenytoin, primidone)** are predicted to decrease the exposure to **cobimetinib.** Avoid. Severe Theoretical
- Antifungals, azoles **(fluconazole, isavuconazole)** are predicted to increase the exposure to **cobimetinib.** Severe Study
- Antifungals, azoles **(itraconazole, ketoconazole, posaconazole, voriconazole)** are predicted to increase the exposure to **cobimetinib.** Avoid or monitor for toxicity. Severe Study
- Antifungals, azoles **(miconazole)** are predicted to increase the exposure to **cobimetinib.** Severe Theoretical
- **Belzutifan** is predicted to decrease the exposure to **cobimetinib.** Avoid or adjust dose. Severe Theoretical
- **Berotralstat** is predicted to increase the exposure to **cobimetinib.** Severe Study
- Calcium-channel blockers **(diltiazem, verapamil)** are predicted to increase the exposure to **cobimetinib.** Severe Study
- **Cenobamate** is predicted to decrease the exposure to **cobimetinib.** Avoid. Severe Theoretical
- **Ceritinib** is predicted to increase the exposure to **cobimetinib.** Avoid or monitor for toxicity. Severe Study

- **Cobicistat** is predicted to increase the exposure to **cobimetinib.** Avoid or monitor for toxicity. [Severe] Study
- **Crizotinib** is predicted to increase the exposure to **cobimetinib.** [Severe] Study
- **Dabrafenib** is predicted to decrease the exposure to **cobimetinib.** Avoid. [Severe] Theoretical
- **Drugs that cause bleeding** (see TABLE 3 p. 1053) cause bleeding, as can **cobimetinib**; concurrent use might increase the risk of developing this effect. [Severe] Theoretical
- **Encorafenib** is predicted to decrease the exposure to **cobimetinib.** Avoid. [Severe] Theoretical
- Endothelin receptor antagonists **(bosentan)** are predicted to decrease the exposure to **cobimetinib.** Avoid. [Severe] Theoretical
- **Fedratinib** is predicted to increase the exposure to **cobimetinib.** [Severe] Study
- **Grapefruit** juice is predicted to increase the exposure to **cobimetinib.** Avoid. [Severe] Theoretical
- **HIV-protease inhibitors** are predicted to increase the exposure to **cobimetinib.** Avoid or monitor for toxicity. [Severe] Study
- **Idelalisib** is predicted to increase the exposure to **cobimetinib.** Avoid or monitor for toxicity. [Severe] Study
- **Imatinib** is predicted to increase the exposure to **cobimetinib.** [Severe] Study
- **Ivosidenib** is predicted to decrease the exposure to **cobimetinib.** Avoid. [Severe] Theoretical
- **Letermovir** is predicted to increase the exposure to **cobimetinib.** [Severe] Study
- **Lorlatinib** is predicted to decrease the exposure to **cobimetinib.** Avoid. [Severe] Theoretical
- **Lumacaftor** is predicted to decrease the exposure to **cobimetinib.** Avoid. [Severe] Theoretical
- Macrolides **(clarithromycin)** are predicted to increase the exposure to **cobimetinib.** Avoid or monitor for toxicity. [Severe] Study
- Macrolides **(erythromycin)** are predicted to increase the exposure to **cobimetinib.** [Severe] Study
- **Mitotane** is predicted to decrease the exposure to **cobimetinib.** Avoid. [Severe] Theoretical
- Neurokinin-1 receptor antagonists **(aprepitant, netupitant)** are predicted to increase the exposure to **cobimetinib.** [Severe] Study
- **Nilotinib** is predicted to increase the exposure to **cobimetinib.** [Severe] Study
- NNRTIs **(efavirenz, etravirine, nevirapine)** are predicted to decrease the exposure to **cobimetinib.** Avoid. [Severe] Theoretical
- Rifamycins **(rifampicin)** are predicted to decrease the exposure to **cobimetinib.** Avoid. [Severe] Theoretical
- **Sotorasib** is predicted to decrease the exposure to **cobimetinib.** Avoid. [Severe] Theoretical
- **St John's wort** is predicted to decrease the exposure to **cobimetinib.** Avoid. [Severe] Theoretical
- **Tucatinib** is predicted to increase the exposure to **cobimetinib.** Avoid or monitor for toxicity. [Severe] Study

Codeine → see opioids

Colchicine

- Anti-androgens **(apalutamide)** are predicted to decrease the exposure to **colchicine.** [Mild] Study
- Antiarrhythmics **(amiodarone)** are predicted to increase the exposure to **colchicine.** Avoid P-glycoprotein inhibitors or adjust **colchicine** dose, p. 637. [Severe] Theoretical
- Antiarrhythmics **(dronedarone)** are predicted to increase the exposure to **colchicine.** Adjust **colchicine** dose with moderate CYP3A4 inhibitors, p. 637. [Severe] Study
- Antiepileptics **(carbamazepine)** are predicted to decrease the exposure to **colchicine.** [Moderate] Theoretical
- Antifungals, azoles **(fluconazole, isavuconazole)** are predicted to increase the exposure to **colchicine.** Adjust **colchicine** dose with moderate CYP3A4 inhibitors, p. 637. [Severe] Study
- Antifungals, azoles **(itraconazole, ketoconazole, posaconazole, voriconazole)** are predicted to increase the exposure to **colchicine.** Avoid potent CYP3A4 inhibitors or adjust **colchicine** dose, p. 637. [Severe] Study
- **Berotralstat** is predicted to increase the exposure to **colchicine.** Adjust **colchicine** dose with moderate CYP3A4 inhibitors, p. 637. [Severe] Study
- Calcium-channel blockers **(diltiazem, verapamil)** are predicted to increase the exposure to **colchicine.** Adjust **colchicine** dose with moderate CYP3A4 inhibitors, p. 637. [Severe] Study
- **Ceritinib** is predicted to increase the exposure to **colchicine.** Avoid potent CYP3A4 inhibitors or adjust **colchicine** dose, p. 637. [Severe] Study
- **Ciclosporin** increases the exposure to **colchicine.** Avoid P-glycoprotein inhibitors or adjust **colchicine** dose, p. 637. [Severe] Study
- **Cobicistat** is predicted to increase the exposure to **colchicine.** Avoid potent CYP3A4 inhibitors or adjust **colchicine** dose, p. 637. [Severe] Study
- **Crizotinib** is predicted to increase the exposure to **colchicine.** Adjust **colchicine** dose with moderate CYP3A4 inhibitors, p. 637. [Severe] Study
- **Danicopan** is predicted to increase the exposure to **colchicine.** [Moderate] Study
- **Eliglustat** is predicted to increase the exposure to **colchicine.** Avoid or adjust **colchicine** dose, p. 637. [Severe] Theoretical
- **Erdafitinib** is predicted to increase the exposure to **colchicine.** Separate administration by at least 6 hours. [Moderate] Theoretical
- **Fedratinib** is predicted to increase the exposure to **colchicine.** Adjust **colchicine** dose with moderate CYP3A4 inhibitors, p. 637. [Severe] Study
- **Colchicine** increases the risk of rhabdomyolysis when given with **fibrates.** [Severe] Anecdotal
- **Glecaprevir** is predicted to increase the exposure to **colchicine.** Avoid P-glycoprotein inhibitors or adjust **colchicine** dose, p. 637. [Severe] Theoretical
- **Grapefruit** juice is predicted to increase the exposure to **colchicine.** Avoid. [Severe] Anecdotal
- **HIV-protease inhibitors** are predicted to increase the exposure to **colchicine.** Avoid potent CYP3A4 inhibitors or adjust **colchicine** dose, p. 637. [Severe] Study
- **Idelalisib** is predicted to increase the exposure to **colchicine.** Avoid potent CYP3A4 inhibitors or adjust **colchicine** dose, p. 637. [Severe] Study
- **Imatinib** is predicted to increase the exposure to **colchicine.** Adjust **colchicine** dose with moderate CYP3A4 inhibitors, p. 637. [Severe] Study
- **Ivosidenib** is predicted to alter the exposure to **colchicine.** [Moderate] Theoretical
- **Lapatinib** is predicted to increase the exposure to **colchicine.** Avoid P-glycoprotein inhibitors or adjust **colchicine** dose, p. 637. [Severe] Theoretical
- **Letermovir** is predicted to increase the exposure to **colchicine.** Adjust **colchicine** dose with moderate CYP3A4 inhibitors, p. 637. [Severe] Study
- **Lorlatinib** is predicted to decrease the exposure to **colchicine.** [Moderate] Theoretical
- Macrolides **(azithromycin)** are predicted to increase the exposure to **colchicine.** Avoid P-glycoprotein inhibitors or adjust **colchicine** dose, p. 637. [Severe] Theoretical
- Macrolides **(clarithromycin)** are predicted to increase the exposure to **colchicine.** Avoid potent CYP3A4 inhibitors or adjust **colchicine** dose, p. 637. [Severe] Study
- Macrolides **(erythromycin)** are predicted to increase the exposure to **colchicine.** Adjust **colchicine** dose with moderate CYP3A4 inhibitors, p. 637. [Severe] Study
- **Mirabegron** is predicted to increase the exposure to **colchicine.** [Mild] Theoretical
- Neurokinin-1 receptor antagonists **(aprepitant, netupitant)** are predicted to increase the exposure to **colchicine.** Adjust **colchicine** dose with moderate CYP3A4 inhibitors, p. 637. [Severe] Study
- **Nilotinib** is predicted to increase the exposure to **colchicine.** Adjust **colchicine** dose with moderate CYP3A4 inhibitors, p. 637. [Severe] Study
- **Nirmatrelvir** boosted with ritonavir is predicted to increase the concentration of **colchicine.** Avoid. [Severe] Theoretical
- **Olaparib** might increase the exposure to **colchicine.** [Moderate] Theoretical
- **Osimertinib** is predicted to increase the exposure to **colchicine.** [Moderate] Study

Colchicine (continued)

- **Pibrentasvir** with glecaprevir is predicted to increase the exposure to **colchicine**. Avoid P-glycoprotein inhibitors or adjust **colchicine** dose, p. 637. Severe Study
- **Pitolisant** is predicted to decrease the exposure to **colchicine**. Mild Theoretical
- **Ranolazine** is predicted to increase the exposure to **colchicine**. Avoid P-glycoprotein inhibitors or adjust **colchicine** dose, p. 637. Severe Theoretical
- Rifamycins **(rifampicin)** are predicted to decrease the exposure to **colchicine**. Moderate Theoretical
- **Ritlecitinib** is predicted to increase the exposure to **colchicine**. Adjust dose. Moderate Theoretical
- **Sparsentan** is predicted to increase the exposure to **colchicine**. Severe Theoretical
- **St John's wort** is predicted to decrease the exposure to **colchicine**. Moderate Theoretical
- **Colchicine** has been reported to cause rhabdomyolysis when given with **statins**. Severe Anecdotal
- **Tucatinib** is predicted to increase the exposure to **colchicine**. Avoid potent CYP3A4 inhibitors or adjust **colchicine** dose, p. 637. Severe Study
- **Velpatasvir** is predicted to increase the exposure to **colchicine**. Avoid P-glycoprotein inhibitors or adjust **colchicine** dose, p. 637. Severe Theoretical
- **Vemurafenib** is predicted to increase the exposure to **colchicine**. Avoid P-glycoprotein inhibitors or adjust **colchicine** dose, p. 637. Severe Theoretical
- **Venetoclax** is predicted to increase the exposure to **colchicine**. Avoid or adjust dose. Severe Study
- **Voxilaprevir** with sofosbuvir and velpatasvir is predicted to increase the exposure to **colchicine**. Avoid P-glycoprotein inhibitors or adjust **colchicine** dose, p. 637. Severe Theoretical

Colecalciferol → see vitamin D substances

Colesevelam

SEPARATION OF ADMINISTRATION Manufacturer advises take 4 hours before, or after, other drugs.

Colestyramine

SEPARATION OF ADMINISTRATION Manufacturer advises take other drugs at least 1 hour before, or 4 to 6 hours after, colestyramine.

Colistimethate → see TABLE 2 p. 1053 (nephrotoxicity), TABLE 16 p. 1058 (ototoxicity)

- **Colistimethate** might prolong the effects of **neuromuscular blocking drugs, non-depolarising**. Moderate Theoretical
- **Colistimethate** might prolong the effects of **suxamethonium**. Moderate Theoretical

Combined hormonal contraceptives

- **Combined hormonal contraceptives** is predicted to increase the exposure to **agomelatine**. Moderate Study
- **Combined hormonal contraceptives** is predicted to increase the exposure to **aminophylline**. Adjust dose. Moderate Theoretical
- **Combined hormonal contraceptives** is predicted to increase the exposure to anaesthetics, local **(ropivacaine)**. Moderate Theoretical
- **Combined hormonal contraceptives** is predicted to increase the exposure to **anagrelide**. Moderate Theoretical
- Antiepileptics **(carbamazepine, eslicarbazepine, fosphenytoin, oxcarbazepine, perampanel, phenobarbital, phenytoin, primidone, rufinamide, topiramate)** are predicted to decrease the efficacy of **combined hormonal contraceptives**. For CoSRH guidance, see Contraceptives, interactions p. 614. Severe Study
- **Combined hormonal contraceptives** alter the exposure to antiepileptics **(lamotrigine)** and antiepileptics **(lamotrigine)** might decrease the efficacy of **combined hormonal contraceptives**. Adjust dose. Moderate Study
- **Combined hormonal contraceptives** increases the concentration of atypical antipsychotics **(clozapine)**. Monitor adverse effects and adjust dose. Severe Study
- **Combined hormonal contraceptives** is predicted to increase the exposure to atypical antipsychotics **(olanzapine)**. Adjust dose. Moderate Anecdotal
- **Belzutifan** might decrease the efficacy of **combined hormonal contraceptives**. Use additional contraceptive precautions. Severe Theoretical
- **Brigatinib** is predicted to decrease the exposure to **combined hormonal contraceptives**. Use additional contraceptive precautions. Severe Theoretical
- **Cabozantinib** might affect the effects of **combined hormonal contraceptives**. Use additional contraceptive precautions. Severe Theoretical
- **Carfilzomib** potentially decreases the efficacy of **combined hormonal contraceptives**. Use additional contraceptive precautions. Severe Theoretical
- **Cenobamate** might decrease the efficacy of oral **combined hormonal contraceptives**. Use additional contraceptive precautions. Severe Theoretical
- Oral **combined hormonal contraceptives** potentially decrease the efficacy of oral **chenodeoxycholic acid**. Avoid. Moderate Theoretical
- **Cobicistat** is predicted to decrease the efficacy of **combined hormonal contraceptives**. Avoid. Severe Study
- **Cytisinicline** might decrease the efficacy of **combined hormonal contraceptives**. Use additional contraceptive precautions. Severe Theoretical
- **Dabrafenib** is predicted to decrease the efficacy of **combined hormonal contraceptives**. Use additional contraceptive precautions. Severe Theoretical
- **Combined hormonal contraceptives** is predicted to increase the exposure to dopamine receptor agonists **(ropinirole)**. Adjust dose. Moderate Study
- **Encorafenib** might decrease the efficacy of **combined hormonal contraceptives**. Use additional contraceptive precautions or alternative methods. Severe Theoretical
- Endothelin receptor antagonists **(bosentan)** are predicted to decrease the efficacy of **combined hormonal contraceptives**. For CoSRH guidance, see Contraceptives, interactions p. 614. Severe Study
- **Erdafitinib** might decrease the efficacy of **combined hormonal contraceptives**. Use alternative methods during treatment with, and for at least 28 days after stopping, **erdafitinib**. Severe Theoretical
- **Combined hormonal contraceptives** are predicted to increases the exposure to **erlotinib**. Monitor adverse effects and adjust dose. Moderate Study
- **Combined hormonal contraceptives** is predicted to increase the exposure to **fezolinetant**. Avoid. Moderate Study
- **Futibatinib** might decrease the efficacy of **combined hormonal contraceptives**. Use additional contraceptive precautions. Severe Theoretical
- **Combined hormonal contraceptives** containing ethinylestradiol can increase ALT concentrations when given with **glecaprevir** with pibrentasvir. Avoid. Severe Study
- Glucagon-like peptide-1 receptor agonists **(tirzepatide)** might affect the absorption of oral **combined hormonal contraceptives**. Manufacturer advises precautions for those who are overweight or obese. Moderate Study
- HIV-protease inhibitors **(atazanavir)** affect the exposure to **combined hormonal contraceptives**. Adjust dose. Severe Study
- HIV-protease inhibitors **(ritonavir)** are predicted to decrease the efficacy of **combined hormonal contraceptives**. For CoSRH guidance, see Contraceptives, interactions p. 614. Severe Study
- **Ivosidenib** might decrease the concentration of **combined hormonal contraceptives**. Use alternative methods during treatment with, and for at least 28 days after stopping, **ivosidenib**. Severe Theoretical
- **Larotrectinib** potentially decreases the efficacy of **combined hormonal contraceptives**. Use additional contraceptive precautions. Severe Theoretical
- **Combined hormonal contraceptives** are predicted to increase the risk of venous thromboembolism when given with **lenalidomide**. Avoid. Severe Theoretical
- Oral **combined hormonal contraceptives** slightly increase the exposure to **lomitapide**. Separate administration by 12 hours. Moderate Theoretical

A1 Interactions | Appendix 1

- **Lorlatinib** is predicted to decrease the exposure to **combined hormonal contraceptives.** Avoid. Moderate Theoretical
- **Combined hormonal contraceptives** is predicted to increase the exposure to **loxapine**. Avoid. Unknown Theoretical
- **Lumacaftor** is predicted to decrease the exposure to **combined hormonal contraceptives.** Use additional contraceptive precautions. Severe Theoretical
- **Combined hormonal contraceptives** slightly increases the exposure to MAO-B inhibitors **(rasagiline).** Moderate Study
- **Combined hormonal contraceptives** increase the exposure to MAO-B inhibitors **(selegiline).** Avoid. Severe Study
- **Mavacamten** is predicted to affect the efficacy of some **combined hormonal contraceptives.** Use additional contraceptive precautions. Severe Theoretical
- **Combined hormonal contraceptives** is predicted to increase the exposure to **melatonin.** Moderate Theoretical
- **Metreleptin** might decrease the efficacy of **combined hormonal contraceptives.** Use additional contraceptive precautions. Severe Theoretical
- **Combined hormonal contraceptives** decrease the effects of **metyrapone.** Avoid. Moderate Theoretical
- **Mitotane** might decrease the efficacy of **combined hormonal contraceptives.** Use alternative methods with, and until concentrations are undetectable after stopping, **mitotane.** Severe Theoretical
- **Modafinil** is predicted to decrease the efficacy of **combined hormonal contraceptives.** For CoSRH guidance, see Contraceptives, interactions p. 614. Severe Study
- **Momelotinib** might decrease the efficacy of **combined hormonal contraceptives.** Additional non-hormonal contraception should be used for 7 days following administration. Severe Theoretical
- Monoclonal antibodies **(sarilumab)** potentially decrease the exposure to **combined hormonal contraceptives.** Severe Theoretical
- **Neratinib** might affect the efficacy of **combined hormonal contraceptives.** Use additional contraceptive precautions. Severe Theoretical
- Neurokinin-1 receptor antagonists **(aprepitant, fosaprepitant)** are predicted to decrease the efficacy of **combined hormonal contraceptives.** For CoSRH guidance, see Contraceptives, interactions p. 614. Severe Study
- **Nirmatrelvir** boosted with ritonavir is predicted to decrease the concentration of **combined hormonal contraceptives** containing ethinylestradiol. Use additional contraceptive precautions. Moderate Theoretical
- NNRTIs **(efavirenz, nevirapine)** are predicted to decrease the efficacy of **combined hormonal contraceptives.** For CoSRH guidance, see Contraceptives, interactions p. 614. Severe Study
- NNRTIs **(etravirine)** might decrease the efficacy of **combined hormonal contraceptives.** Follow CoSRH guidance for enzyme inducers, see Contraceptives, interactions p. 614. Severe Theoretical
- NSAIDs **(etoricoxib)** increase the exposure to **combined hormonal contraceptives.** Moderate Study
- **Olaparib** potentially affects the efficacy of **combined hormonal contraceptives.** Use additional contraceptive precautions. Moderate Theoretical
- **Omaveloxolone** might decrease the efficacy of **combined hormonal contraceptives.** Avoid. Severe Theoretical
- **Combined hormonal contraceptives** potentially oppose the effects of **ospemifene.** Avoid. Severe Theoretical
- **Combined hormonal contraceptives** is predicted to increase the exposure to phenothiazine antipsychotics **(chlorpromazine).** Moderate Theoretical
- **Combined hormonal contraceptives** is predicted to increase the exposure to phosphodiesterase type-4 inhibitors **(roflumilast).** Moderate Theoretical
- **Combined hormonal contraceptives** containing ethinylestradiol can increase ALT concentrations when given with **pibrentasvir** with glecaprevir. Avoid. Severe Study
- **Combined hormonal contraceptives** is predicted to increase the exposure to **pirfenidone.** Use with caution and adjust dose. Moderate Study
- **Pitolisant** is predicted to decrease the efficacy of **combined hormonal contraceptives.** Avoid. Severe Theoretical
- **Combined hormonal contraceptives** are predicted to increase the risk of venous thromboembolism when given with **pomalidomide.** Avoid. Severe Theoretical
- **Ponatinib** might affect the effects of **combined hormonal contraceptives.** Avoid or use additional contraceptive precautions. Severe Theoretical
- **Pralsetinib** might decrease the efficacy of **combined hormonal contraceptives.** Avoid or use additional contraceptive precautions. Severe Theoretical
- **Combined hormonal contraceptives** potentially oppose the effects of **raloxifene.** Avoid. Severe Theoretical
- **Rifamycins** are predicted to decrease the efficacy of **combined hormonal contraceptives.** For CoSRH guidance, see Contraceptives, interactions p. 614. Severe Study
- **Combined hormonal contraceptives** is predicted to increase the exposure to **riluzole.** Moderate Theoretical
- **Combined hormonal contraceptives** containing ethinylestradiol can increase ALT concentrations when given with **sofosbuvir** with velpatasvir and voxilaprevir. Avoid. Severe Study
- **St John's wort** decreases the efficacy of **combined hormonal contraceptives.** MHRA advises avoid. For CoSRH guidance, see Contraceptives, interactions p. 614. Severe Anecdotal
- **Sugammadex** is predicted to decrease the exposure to **combined hormonal contraceptives.** Refer to patient information leaflet for missed pill advice. Severe Theoretical
- **Combined hormonal contraceptives** might exacerbate skin pigmentation when given with tetracyclines **(minocycline).** Moderate Anecdotal
- **Combined hormonal contraceptives** are predicted to increase the risk of venous thromboembolism when given with **thalidomide.** Avoid. Severe Study
- **Combined hormonal contraceptives** is predicted to increase the exposure to **theophylline.** Monitor and adjust dose. Moderate Theoretical
- **Combined hormonal contraceptives** increases the exposure to **tizanidine.** Avoid. Moderate Study
- **Combined hormonal contraceptives** is predicted to increase the exposure to triptans **(zolmitriptan).** Adjust **zolmitriptan** dose, p. 347. Moderate Theoretical
- **Combined hormonal contraceptives** might decrease the efficacy of **ulipristal** and **ulipristal** might decrease the efficacy of **combined hormonal contraceptives.** Avoid when used for uterine fibroids. For CoSRH guidance when used for emergency hormonal contraception, see Contraceptives, interactions p. 614. Severe Theoretical
- **Combined hormonal contraceptives** containing ethinylestradiol can increase ALT concentrations when given with **velpatasvir** with sofosbuvir and voxilaprevir. Avoid. Severe Study
- **Vemurafenib** might decrease the efficacy of **combined hormonal contraceptives.** Use additional contraceptive precautions. Severe Theoretical
- **Combined hormonal contraceptives** are predicted to increase the exposure to **vorasidenib** and **vorasidenib** might decrease the concentration of **combined hormonal contraceptives.** Avoid. Severe Theoretical
- **Combined hormonal contraceptives** containing ethinylestradiol can increase ALT concentrations when given with **voxilaprevir** with sofosbuvir and velpatasvir. Avoid. Severe Study

Corticosteroids → see TABLE 14 p. 1057 (reduced serum potassium)

beclometasone · betamethasone · budesonide · ciclesonide · deflazacort · dexamethasone · fludrocortisone · fluticasone · hydrocortisone · methylprednisolone · mometasone · prednisolone · triamcinolone · vamorolone

- With intravitreal use of **dexamethasone** in adults: caution with concurrent administration of anticoagulant or antiplatelet drugs—increased risk of haemorrhagic events.
- Interactions do not generally apply to corticosteroids (except **budesonide** and **fluticasone**) used for topical action (including inhalation) unless specified. However, as systemic absorption might occur with **hydrocortisone** *eye drops*, the possibility of interactions should be borne in mind.

Corticosteroids (continued)

- Oral antacids are predicted to decrease the absorption of oral **deflazacort**. Separate administration by 2 hours. Moderate Theoretical
- Oral antacids decrease the absorption of oral **dexamethasone**. Moderate Study
- Anti-androgens **(apalutamide, enzalutamide)** are predicted to decrease the exposure to **fluticasone**. Unknown Theoretical
- Anti-androgens **(apalutamide, enzalutamide)** are predicted to decrease the exposure to corticosteroids **(budesonide, deflazacort, dexamethasone, fludrocortisone, hydrocortisone, methylprednisolone, prednisolone, triamcinolone)**. Monitor and adjust dose. Moderate Study
- Antiarrhythmics **(dronedarone)** are predicted to increase the exposure to **methylprednisolone**. Monitor and adjust dose. Moderate Study
- Antiepileptics **(carbamazepine, fosphenytoin, phenobarbital, phenytoin, primidone)** are predicted to decrease the exposure to **fluticasone**. Unknown Theoretical
- Antiepileptics **(carbamazepine, fosphenytoin, phenobarbital, phenytoin, primidone)** are predicted to decrease the exposure to corticosteroids **(budesonide, deflazacort, dexamethasone, fludrocortisone, hydrocortisone, methylprednisolone, prednisolone, triamcinolone)**. Monitor and adjust dose. Moderate Study
- Antifungals, azoles **(fluconazole, isavuconazole)** are predicted to increase the exposure to **methylprednisolone**. Monitor and adjust dose. Moderate Study
- Antifungals, azoles **(itraconazole, ketoconazole, posaconazole, voriconazole)** are predicted to increase the exposure to **beclometasone** (risk with beclometasone is likely to be lower than with other corticosteroids). Moderate Theoretical
- Antifungals, azoles **(itraconazole, ketoconazole, posaconazole, voriconazole)** are predicted to increase the exposure to **vamorolone**. Adjust dose. Severe Study
- Antifungals, azoles **(miconazole)** are predicted to increase the concentration of **methylprednisolone**. Monitor and adjust dose. Moderate Theoretical
- Antifungals, azoles **(itraconazole, ketoconazole, posaconazole, voriconazole)** are predicted to increase the exposure to corticosteroids **(betamethasone, budesonide, ciclesonide, deflazacort, dexamethasone, fludrocortisone, fluticasone, hydrocortisone, methylprednisolone, mometasone, prednisolone, triamcinolone)**. Avoid or monitor adverse effects. Severe Study
- **Corticosteroids** are predicted to decrease the concentration of aspirin (high-dose) and aspirin (high-dose) increases the risk of gastrointestinal bleeding when given with **corticosteroids**. Moderate Study
- **Dexamethasone** is predicted to decrease the exposure to avapritinib. Avoid. Severe Theoretical
- **Berotralstat** is predicted to increase the exposure to **methylprednisolone**. Monitor and adjust dose. Moderate Study
- Calcium-channel blockers **(diltiazem, verapamil)** are predicted to increase the exposure to **methylprednisolone**. Monitor and adjust dose. Moderate Study
- **Dexamethasone** is predicted to decrease the concentration of caspofungin. Adjust **caspofungin** dose, p. 460. Moderate Theoretical
- **Cenobamate** is predicted to decrease the exposure to oral **budesonide**. Adjust dose. Moderate Theoretical
- **Cenobamate** is predicted to decrease the exposure to **fluticasone**. Adjust dose. Moderate Theoretical
- **Ceritinib** is predicted to increase the exposure to **beclometasone** (risk with beclometasone is likely to be lower than with other corticosteroids). Moderate Theoretical
- **Ceritinib** is predicted to increase the exposure to corticosteroids **(betamethasone, budesonide, ciclesonide, deflazacort, dexamethasone, fludrocortisone, fluticasone, hydrocortisone, methylprednisolone, mometasone, prednisolone, triamcinolone)**. Avoid or monitor adverse effects. Severe Study
- **Ceritinib** is predicted to increase the exposure to **vamorolone**. Adjust dose. Severe Study
- **Corticosteroids** are predicted to decrease the concentration of **choline salicylate**. Moderate Study
- **Cobicistat** is predicted to increase the exposure to **beclometasone** (risk with beclometasone is likely to be lower than with other corticosteroids). Moderate Theoretical
- **Cobicistat** is predicted to increase the exposure to corticosteroids **(betamethasone, budesonide, ciclesonide, deflazacort, dexamethasone, fludrocortisone, fluticasone, hydrocortisone, methylprednisolone, mometasone, prednisolone, triamcinolone)**. Avoid or monitor adverse effects. Severe Study
- **Cobicistat** is predicted to increase the exposure to **vamorolone**. Adjust dose. Severe Study
- **Corticosteroids** are predicted to increase the effects of **coumarins**. Moderate Study
- **Crizotinib** is predicted to increase the exposure to **methylprednisolone**. Monitor and adjust dose. Moderate Study
- **Corticosteroids** are predicted to increase the risk of digoxin toxicity when given with **digoxin**. Avoid. Severe Theoretical
- **Encorafenib** is predicted to decrease the exposure to corticosteroids **(budesonide, deflazacort, dexamethasone, fludrocortisone, hydrocortisone, methylprednisolone, prednisolone, triamcinolone)**. Monitor and adjust dose. Moderate Study
- **Encorafenib** is predicted to decrease the exposure to **fluticasone**. Unknown Theoretical
- **Erlotinib** is predicted to increase the risk of gastrointestinal perforation when given with **corticosteroids**. Severe Theoretical
- **Fedratinib** is predicted to increase the exposure to **methylprednisolone**. Monitor and adjust dose. Moderate Study
- **Corticosteroids** potentially oppose the effects of **glycerol phenylbutyrate**. Moderate Theoretical
- **Grapefruit** juice moderately increases the exposure to oral **budesonide**. Avoid. Moderate Study
- **HIV-protease inhibitors** are predicted to increase the exposure to **beclometasone** (risk with beclometasone is likely to be lower than with other corticosteroids). Moderate Theoretical
- **HIV-protease inhibitors** are predicted to increase the exposure to corticosteroids **(betamethasone, budesonide, ciclesonide, deflazacort, dexamethasone, fludrocortisone, fluticasone, hydrocortisone, methylprednisolone, mometasone, prednisolone, triamcinolone)**. Avoid or monitor adverse effects. Severe Study
- **HIV-protease inhibitors** are predicted to increase the exposure to **vamorolone**. Adjust dose. Severe Study
- **Idelalisib** is predicted to increase the exposure to **beclometasone** (risk with beclometasone is likely to be lower than with other corticosteroids). Moderate Theoretical
- **Idelalisib** is predicted to increase the exposure to corticosteroids **(betamethasone, budesonide, ciclesonide, deflazacort, dexamethasone, fludrocortisone, fluticasone, hydrocortisone, methylprednisolone, mometasone, prednisolone, triamcinolone)**. Avoid or monitor adverse effects. Severe Study
- **Idelalisib** is predicted to increase the exposure to **vamorolone**. Adjust dose. Severe Study
- **Imatinib** is predicted to increase the exposure to **methylprednisolone**. Monitor and adjust dose. Moderate Study
- **Corticosteroids** are predicted to increase the risk of gastrointestinal bleeding when given with iron chelators **(deferasirox)**. Severe Theoretical
- **Ivosidenib** is predicted to decrease the exposure to corticosteroids **(budesonide, deflazacort, dexamethasone, fludrocortisone, hydrocortisone, methylprednisolone, prednisolone, triamcinolone)**. Monitor and adjust dose. Moderate Study
- **Ivosidenib** is predicted to decrease the exposure to **fluticasone**. Unknown Theoretical
- **Lenacapavir** is predicted to increase the concentration of corticosteroids **(beclometasone, betamethasone, budesonide, deflazacort, fludrocortisone, fluticasone, hydrocortisone, methylprednisolone, prednisolone, triamcinolone)**. Adjust starting dose and monitor. Severe Theoretical
- **Dexamethasone** might affect the efficacy of **lenacapavir** and **lenacapavir** is predicted to increase the concentration of **dexamethasone**. Adjust starting dose and monitor, or consider alternatives. Severe Theoretical

- ▶ **Lenacapavir** is predicted to increase the exposure to **vamorolone**. Adjust starting dose and monitor. Severe Theoretical
- ▶ **Letermovir** is predicted to increase the exposure to **methylprednisolone**. Monitor and adjust dose. Moderate Study
- ▶ **Live vaccines** are predicted to increase the risk of generalised infection (possibly life-threatening) when given with **corticosteroids** (high-dose). UKHSA advises avoid (refer to Green Book). Severe Theoretical
- ▶ **Lumacaftor** is predicted to decrease the exposure to corticosteroids **(budesonide, deflazacort, dexamethasone, fludrocortisone, hydrocortisone, methylprednisolone, prednisolone, triamcinolone)**. Monitor and adjust dose. Moderate Study
- ▶ **Lumacaftor** is predicted to decrease the exposure to **fluticasone**. Unknown Theoretical
- ▶ Macrolides **(clarithromycin)** are predicted to increase the exposure to **beclometasone** (risk with beclometasone is likely to be lower than with other corticosteroids). Moderate Theoretical
- ▶ Macrolides **(clarithromycin)** are predicted to increase the exposure to **vamorolone**. Adjust dose. Severe Study
- ▶ Macrolides **(erythromycin)** are predicted to increase the exposure to **methylprednisolone**. Monitor and adjust dose. Moderate Study
- ▶ Macrolides **(clarithromycin)** are predicted to increase the exposure to corticosteroids **(betamethasone, budesonide, ciclesonide, deflazacort, dexamethasone, fludrocortisone, fluticasone, hydrocortisone, methylprednisolone, mometasone, prednisolone, triamcinolone)**. Avoid or monitor adverse effects. Severe Study
- ▶ **Corticosteroids** are predicted to decrease the efficacy of **mifamurtide**. Avoid. Severe Theoretical
- ▶ **Mifepristone** is predicted to decrease the efficacy of **corticosteroids**. Use with caution and adjust dose. Moderate Theoretical
- ▶ **Mitotane** is predicted to decrease the exposure to corticosteroids **(budesonide, deflazacort, dexamethasone, fludrocortisone, hydrocortisone, methylprednisolone, prednisolone, triamcinolone)**. Monitor and adjust dose. Moderate Study
- ▶ **Mitotane** is predicted to decrease the exposure to **fluticasone**. Unknown Theoretical
- ▶ **Corticosteroids** might affect the efficacy of monoclonal antibodies **(atezolizumab, pembrolizumab, serplulimab)**. Use with caution or avoid. Severe Theoretical
- ▶ Monoclonal antibodies **(tocilizumab)** are predicted to decrease the exposure to corticosteroids **(dexamethasone, methylprednisolone)**. Monitor and adjust dose. Moderate Theoretical
- ▶ **Corticosteroids** are predicted to increase the risk of immunosuppression when given with monoclonal antibodies **(dinutuximab)**. Avoid except in life-threatening situations. Severe Theoretical
- ▶ **Corticosteroids** might affect the efficacy of monoclonal antibodies **(ipilimumab, nivolumab)**. Use with caution or avoid. Severe Theoretical
- ▶ **Corticosteroids** might increase the risk of generalised infection (possibly life-threatening) when given with monoclonal antibodies **(natalizumab)**. Manufacturer advises short courses of corticosteroids can be taken. Severe Theoretical
- ▶ Neurokinin-1 receptor antagonists **(aprepitant)** moderately increase the exposure to **dexamethasone**. Monitor and adjust dose. Moderate Study
- ▶ Neurokinin-1 receptor antagonists **(aprepitant, netupitant)** are predicted to increase the exposure to oral **budesonide**. Moderate Study
- ▶ Neurokinin-1 receptor antagonists **(aprepitant, netupitant)** are predicted to increase the exposure to **fluticasone**. Moderate Study
- ▶ Neurokinin-1 receptor antagonists **(aprepitant, netupitant)** are predicted to increase the exposure to **methylprednisolone**. Monitor and adjust dose. Moderate Study
- ▶ Neurokinin-1 receptor antagonists **(netupitant)** moderately increase the exposure to **dexamethasone**. Adjust dose. Moderate Study
- ▶ **Corticosteroids** are predicted to decrease the effects of **neuromuscular blocking drugs, non-depolarising**. Severe Anecdotal
- ▶ **Corticosteroids** increase the risk of gastrointestinal perforation when given with **nicorandil**. Severe Anecdotal
- ▶ **Nilotinib** is predicted to increase the exposure to **methylprednisolone**. Monitor and adjust dose. Moderate Study
- ▶ **Nirmatrelvir** boosted with ritonavir is predicted to increase the concentration of **beclometasone** (risk with beclometasone is likely to be lower than with other corticosteroids). Moderate Theoretical
- ▶ **Nirmatrelvir** boosted with ritonavir is predicted to increase the concentration of corticosteroids **(betamethasone, budesonide, ciclesonide, deflazacort, dexamethasone, fluticasone, hydrocortisone, methylprednisolone, mometasone, prednisolone, triamcinolone)**. Avoid or monitor adverse effects and consider beclomethasone as an alternative. Severe Theoretical
- ▶ **Nirmatrelvir** boosted with ritonavir is predicted to increase the concentration of corticosteroids **(fludrocortisone, vamorolone)**. Avoid or monitor adverse effects. Severe Theoretical
- ▶ **Dexamethasone** is predicted to decrease the concentration of NNRTIs **(rilpivirine)**. Avoid multiple-dose dexamethasone. Severe Theoretical
- ▶ **NSAIDs** increase the risk of gastrointestinal bleeding when given with **corticosteroids**. Severe Study
- ▶ **Corticosteroids** are predicted to increase the effects of **phenindione**. Moderate Anecdotal
- ▶ **Dexamethasone** decreases the exposure to **praziquantel**. Moderate Study
- ▶ Rifamycins **(rifampicin)** are predicted to decrease the exposure to **fluticasone**. Unknown Theoretical
- ▶ Rifamycins **(rifampicin)** are predicted to decrease the exposure to corticosteroids **(budesonide, deflazacort, dexamethasone, fludrocortisone, hydrocortisone, methylprednisolone, prednisolone, triamcinolone)**. Monitor and adjust dose. Moderate Study
- ▶ **Corticosteroids** potentially decrease the effects of **sodium phenylbutyrate**. Moderate Theoretical
- ▶ **Corticosteroids** might decrease the efficacy of **somapacitan**. Monitor and adjust dose. Moderate Theoretical
- ▶ **Corticosteroids** might decrease the efficacy of **somatrogon**. Monitor and adjust dose. Moderate Theoretical
- ▶ **Corticosteroids** are predicted to decrease the effects of **somatropin**. Moderate Theoretical
- ▶ **Dexamethasone** is predicted to decrease the exposure to **sparsentan**. Avoid. Severe Theoretical
- ▶ **Corticosteroids** are predicted to decrease the effects of **suxamethonium**. Severe Anecdotal
- ▶ **Tucatinib** is predicted to increase the exposure to **beclometasone** (risk with beclometasone is likely to be lower than with other corticosteroids). Moderate Theoretical
- ▶ **Tucatinib** is predicted to increase the exposure to corticosteroids **(betamethasone, budesonide, ciclesonide, deflazacort, dexamethasone, fludrocortisone, fluticasone, hydrocortisone, methylprednisolone, mometasone, prednisolone, triamcinolone)**. Avoid or monitor adverse effects. Severe Study
- ▶ **Tucatinib** is predicted to increase the exposure to **vamorolone**. Adjust dose. Severe Study
- ▶ **Fludrocortisone** might enhance the antidiuretic effect of **vasopressin**. Moderate Theoretical

Coumarins → see TABLE 3 p. 1053 (bleeding)

acenocoumarol • warfarin

FOOD AND LIFESTYLE The effects of coumarins can be reduced or abolished by vitamin K, including that found in health foods, food supplements, enteral feeds, or large amounts of some green vegetables or green tea. Major changes in diet (especially involving salads and vegetables) and in alcohol consumption can affect anticoagulant control. Pomegranate juice is predicted to increase the INR in response to **acenocoumarol** and **warfarin**.

- **Alcohol** (in those who drink heavily) potentially decreases the anticoagulant effect of **coumarins**. [Severe] Study
- Amfetamines **(dexamfetamine)** might increase the anticoagulant effect of **coumarins**. Monitor INR and adjust dose. [Moderate] Theoretical
- Anti-androgens **(apalutamide)** are predicted to decrease the exposure to **coumarins**. Avoid or monitor. [Mild] Study
- Anti-androgens **(enzalutamide)** potentially decrease the exposure to **coumarins**. Avoid or adjust dose and monitor INR. [Severe] Study
- Antiarrhythmics **(amiodarone)** increase the anticoagulant effect of **coumarins**. [Severe] Study
- Antiarrhythmics **(dronedarone)** might increase the anticoagulant effect of **coumarins**. [Moderate] Anecdotal
- Antiarrhythmics **(propafenone)** increase the anticoagulant effect of **coumarins**. Monitor INR and adjust dose. [Moderate] Study
- Antiepileptics **(carbamazepine)** decrease the effects of **coumarins**. Monitor and adjust dose. [Severe] Study
- Antiepileptics **(fosphenytoin, phenytoin)** are predicted to alter the anticoagulant effect of **coumarins**. [Moderate] Anecdotal
- Antiepileptics **(phenobarbital, primidone)** decrease the anticoagulant effect of **coumarins**. Monitor INR and adjust dose. [Moderate] Study
- Antifungals, azoles **(fluconazole)** increase the anticoagulant effect of **coumarins**. Monitor INR and adjust dose. [Severe] Study
- Antifungals, azoles **(itraconazole)** potentially increase the anticoagulant effect of **coumarins**. [Severe] Anecdotal
- Antifungals, azoles **(ketoconazole)** potentially increase the anticoagulant effect of **warfarin**. Monitor INR and adjust dose. [Severe] Anecdotal
- Antifungals, azoles **(miconazole)** greatly increase the anticoagulant effect of **coumarins**. MHRA advises avoid unless INR can be monitored closely; monitor for signs of bleeding. [Severe] Study
- Antifungals, azoles **(voriconazole)** increase the anticoagulant effect of **coumarins**. Monitor INR and adjust dose. [Moderate] Study
- **Asciminib** slightly to moderately increases the exposure to **warfarin**. [Severe] Theoretical
- **Azathioprine** decreases the anticoagulant effect of **coumarins**. [Moderate] Study
- **Capecitabine** increases the effects of **coumarins**. Monitor INR and adjust dose. [Severe] Anecdotal
- Cephalosporins **(cefazolin, ceftriaxone)** potentially increase the risk of bleeding events when given with **coumarins**. [Severe] Anecdotal
- **Ceritinib** is predicted to increase the exposure to **acenocoumarol**. [Severe] Theoretical
- **Ceritinib** increases the exposure to **warfarin**. Avoid or monitor INR. [Severe] Study
- **Chloramphenicol** potentially increases the anticoagulant effect of **coumarins**. [Moderate] Anecdotal
- **Cobicistat** is predicted to affect the exposure to **warfarin**. [Moderate] Theoretical
- **Corticosteroids** are predicted to increase the effects of **coumarins**. [Moderate] Study
- **Cranberry** juice potentially increases the anticoagulant effect of **warfarin**. Avoid. [Severe] Anecdotal
- **Crizotinib** is predicted to increase the risk of bleeding events when given with **coumarins**. [Severe] Theoretical
- **Dabrafenib** is predicted to decrease the anticoagulant effect of **coumarins**. [Severe] Theoretical
- **Deutivacaftor** is predicted to increase the exposure to **warfarin**. [Moderate] Theoretical
- **Disulfiram** increases the anticoagulant effect of **coumarins**. Monitor and adjust dose. [Severe] Study
- **Donanemab** can increase the risk of brain haemorrhage when given with **coumarins**. Avoid. [Severe] Anecdotal
- **Elvitegravir** is predicted to decrease the anticoagulant effect of **coumarins**. [Moderate] Anecdotal
- Endothelin receptor antagonists **(bosentan)** decrease the anticoagulant effect of **coumarins**. [Moderate] Study
- **Enteral feeds** (vitamin-K containing) potentially decrease the anticoagulant effect of **coumarins**. [Severe] Anecdotal
- **Erlotinib** increases the anticoagulant effect of **coumarins**. [Severe] Anecdotal
- **Fibrates** are predicted to increase the anticoagulant effect of **coumarins**. Monitor INR and adjust dose. [Severe] Study
- **Fluorouracil** increases the anticoagulant effect of **coumarins**. [Severe] Anecdotal
- **Fostamatinib** might cause bleeding when given with **acenocoumarol**. [Moderate] Theoretical
- **Fostamatinib** might causes bleeding when given with **warfarin**. [Moderate] Theoretical
- **Gefitinib** is predicted to increase the anticoagulant effect of **coumarins**. [Severe] Anecdotal
- **Glofitamab** might affect the exposure to **warfarin**. [Moderate] Theoretical
- **Glucagon** increases the anticoagulant effect of **warfarin**. [Severe] Study
- Glucagon-like peptide-1 receptor agonists **(semaglutide)** might decrease the anticoagulant effect of **acenocoumarol**. [Severe] Anecdotal
- Glucagon-like peptide-1 receptor agonists **(tirzepatide)** might affect the absorption of **warfarin**. [Severe] Theoretical
- **Glucosamine** potentially decreases the anticoagulant effect of **acenocoumarol**. [Moderate] Anecdotal
- **Glucosamine** potentially increases the anticoagulant effect of **warfarin**. Avoid. [Moderate] Anecdotal
- **Griseofulvin** potentially decreases the anticoagulant effect of **coumarins**. [Moderate] Anecdotal
- H_2 receptor antagonists **(cimetidine)** increase the anticoagulant effect of **coumarins**. [Severe] Study
- **HIV-protease inhibitors** are predicted to affect the anticoagulant effect of **coumarins**. [Moderate] Study
- **Imatinib** is predicted to increase the risk of bleeding events when given with **coumarins**. [Severe] Theoretical → Also see TABLE 3 p. 1053
- **Ivacaftor** is predicted to increase the exposure to **warfarin**. [Moderate] Theoretical
- **Ivermectin** potentially increases the anticoagulant effect of **coumarins**. [Severe] Anecdotal
- **Ivosidenib** might decrease the exposure to **warfarin**. Avoid or monitor efficacy. [Unknown] Study
- **Lapatinib** is predicted to increase the risk of bleeding events when given with **coumarins**. [Severe] Theoretical
- **Lecanemab** can increase the risk of brain haemorrhage when given with **coumarins**. Avoid. [Severe] Anecdotal
- **Leflunomide** increases the anticoagulant effect of **coumarins**. [Severe] Anecdotal
- **Letermovir** is predicted to decrease the concentration of **warfarin**. Monitor and adjust dose. [Moderate] Theoretical
- **Lomitapide** increases the exposure to **warfarin**. Monitor INR and adjust dose. [Severe] Study
- **Lorlatinib** is predicted to decrease the exposure to **coumarins**. [Moderate] Theoretical
- Macrolides **(azithromycin)** might increase the risk of bleeding events when given with **coumarins**. [Severe] Anecdotal
- Macrolides **(clarithromycin, erythromycin)** increase the anticoagulant effect of **coumarins**. Monitor INR and adjust dose. [Severe] Anecdotal
- **Mercaptopurine** decreases the anticoagulant effect of **coumarins**. [Moderate] Anecdotal
- **Metreleptin** might alter the exposure to **warfarin**. Monitor INR and adjust dose. [Severe] Theoretical
- **Metronidazole** increases the anticoagulant effect of **coumarins**. Monitor INR and adjust dose. [Severe] Study
- **Mexiletine** potentially affects the exposure to **warfarin**. Avoid. [Unknown] Theoretical
- **Mifepristone** is predicted to increase the exposure to **warfarin**. [Moderate] Theoretical
- Monoclonal antibodies **(bimekizumab)** might affect the exposure to **warfarin**. [Moderate] Theoretical
- Monoclonal antibodies **(blinatumomab, mosunetuzumab)** are predicted to transiently increase the exposure to **warfarin**. Monitor and adjust dose. [Moderate] Theoretical

A1 Interactions | **Appendix 1**

- ▶ Monoclonal antibodies **(elranatamab)** might affect the exposure to **warfarin**. Monitor and adjust dose. Moderate Theoretical
- ▶ Monoclonal antibodies **(sarilumab)** potentially affect the exposure to **warfarin**. Monitor and adjust dose. Severe Theoretical
- ▶ Monoclonal antibodies **(tocilizumab)** are predicted to decrease the exposure to **warfarin**. Monitor and adjust dose. Moderate Theoretical
- ▶ **Coumarins** might increase the risk of gastrointestinal bleeding when given with monoclonal antibodies **(ipilimumab)**. Severe Theoretical
- ▶ Neurokinin-1 receptor antagonists **(aprepitant)** decrease the anticoagulant effect of **coumarins**. Moderate Study
- ▶ Neurokinin-1 receptor antagonists **(fosaprepitant)** are predicted to decrease the anticoagulant effect of **coumarins**. Moderate Theoretical
- ▶ **Nilotinib** is predicted to increase the risk of bleeding events when given with **coumarins**. Severe Theoretical
- ▶ **Nirmatrelvir** boosted with ritonavir is predicted to affect the concentration of **coumarins**. Moderate Theoretical
- ▶ **Nitisinone** is predicted to increase the exposure to **warfarin**. Moderate Study
- ▶ NNRTIs **(efavirenz)** are predicted to affect the concentration of **coumarins**. Adjust dose. Moderate Theoretical
- ▶ NNRTIs **(etravirine)** increase the anticoagulant effect of **coumarins**. Moderate Theoretical
- ▶ NNRTIs **(nevirapine)** potentially alter the anticoagulant effect of **coumarins**. Severe Anecdotal
- ▶ **Obeticholic acid** decreases the anticoagulant effect of **warfarin**. Severe Study
- ▶ Opioids **(tramadol)** might increase the anticoagulant effect of **acenocoumarol**. Severe Study
- ▶ Opioids **(tramadol)** have been reported to increase the anticoagulant effect of **warfarin**. Severe Anecdotal
- ▶ **Oritavancin** might increase the exposure to **warfarin**. Moderate Theoretical
- ▶ **Oxymetholone** increases the anticoagulant effect of **coumarins**. Severe Anecdotal
- ▶ **Paracetamol** increases the anticoagulant effect of **coumarins**. Moderate Study
- ▶ **Penicillins** potentially alter the anticoagulant effect of **coumarins**. Monitor INR and adjust dose. Severe Anecdotal
- ▶ **Pitolisant** is predicted to decrease the exposure to **warfarin**. Mild Theoretical
- ▶ **Pralsetinib** might affect the exposure to **warfarin**. Avoid. Moderate Theoretical
- ▶ **Quinolones** increase the anticoagulant effect of **coumarins**. Severe Anecdotal
- ▶ Rifamycins **(rifabutin)** might decrease the anticoagulant effect of **coumarins**. Moderate Theoretical
- ▶ Rifamycins **(rifampicin)** decrease the anticoagulant effect of **coumarins**. Severe Study
- ▶ **Rifaximin** might decrease the anticoagulant effect of **acenocoumarol**. Monitor INR and adjust dose. Severe Theoretical
- ▶ **Rifaximin** has been reported to decrease the anticoagulant effect of **warfarin**. Monitor INR and adjust dose. Severe Anecdotal
- ▶ **Rucaparib** slightly increases the exposure to **warfarin**. Monitor and adjust dose. Severe Study
- ▶ **Selumetinib** might increase the risk of bleeding when given with **coumarins**. Severe Theoretical
- ▶ **Sofosbuvir** might affect the anticoagulant effect of **coumarins**. Moderate Theoretical
- ▶ **Sparsentan** is predicted to decrease the exposure to **warfarin**. Moderate Theoretical
- ▶ **St John's wort** decreases the anticoagulant effect of **coumarins**. Avoid. Severe Anecdotal
- ▶ Statins **(fluvastatin, rosuvastatin)** increase the anticoagulant effect of **coumarins**. Monitor INR and adjust dose. Severe Study
- ▶ **Sucralfate** potentially decreases the effects of **warfarin**. Separate administration by 2 hours. Moderate Anecdotal
- ▶ Sulfonamides **(sulfadiazine)** are predicted to increase the anticoagulant effect of **coumarins**. Severe Theoretical
- ▶ Sulfonamides **(sulfamethoxazole)** increase the anticoagulant effect of **coumarins**. Severe Study
- ▶ **Tamoxifen** increases the anticoagulant effect of **coumarins**. Severe Study
- ▶ **Tebentafusp** is predicted to transiently increase the exposure to **warfarin**. Monitor and adjust dose. Moderate Theoretical
- ▶ **Tegafur** increases the anticoagulant effect of **coumarins**. Monitor INR and adjust dose. Severe Theoretical
- ▶ **Teriflunomide** affects the anticoagulant effect of **coumarins**. Severe Study
- ▶ **Tetracyclines** increase the anticoagulant effect of **coumarins**. Severe Anecdotal
- ▶ **Tigecycline** is predicted to alter the anticoagulant effect of **coumarins**. Moderate Anecdotal
- ▶ **Tofacitinib** is predicted to increase the risk of bleeding when given with **coumarins**. Severe Theoretical
- ▶ **Toremifene** is predicted to increase the anticoagulant effect of **coumarins**. Severe Theoretical
- ▶ **Trimethoprim** is predicted to increase the anticoagulant effect of **coumarins**. Severe Study
- ▶ **Vemurafenib** is predicted to increase the exposure to **coumarins**. Moderate Study
- ▶ **Venetoclax** slightly increases the exposure to **warfarin**. Moderate Study
- ▶ **Vorasidenib** might decrease the concentration of **warfarin**. Avoid. Severe Theoretical

Cranberry

- ▶ **Cranberry** juice potentially increases the anticoagulant effect of coumarins **(warfarin)**. Avoid. Severe Anecdotal

Crisantaspase → see TABLE 3 p. 1053 (bleeding), TABLE 1 p. 1053 (hepatotoxicity), TABLE 12 p. 1057 (myelosuppression)

- ▶ **Crisantaspase** is predicted to increase the risk of hepatotoxicity when given with **imatinib**. Severe Theoretical → Also see TABLE 3 p. 1053 → Also see TABLE 12 p. 1057
- ▶ **Crisantaspase** affects the efficacy of **methotrexate**. Severe Anecdotal → Also see TABLE 1 p. 1053 → Also see TABLE 12 p. 1057
- ▶ **Crisantaspase** potentially increases the risk of neurotoxicity when given with vinca alkaloids **(vincristine)**. **Vincristine** should be taken 3 to 24 hours before **crisantaspase**. Severe Anecdotal → Also see TABLE 12 p. 1057

Crizotinib → see TABLE 4 p. 1054 (bradycardia), TABLE 7 p. 1055 (QT-interval prolongation)

GENERAL INFORMATION Caution with concurrent use of drugs that cause gastrointestinal perforation—discontinue treatment if gastrointestinal perforation occurs.

- ▶ **Crizotinib** is predicted to increase the exposure to **abemaciclib**. Moderate Study
- ▶ **Crizotinib** is predicted to increase the exposure to **acalabrutinib**. Avoid or monitor. Severe Study
- ▶ **Crizotinib** is predicted to increase the exposure to alpha blockers **(tamsulosin)**. Moderate Theoretical
- ▶ Anti-androgens **(apalutamide, enzalutamide)** are predicted to markedly decrease the exposure to **crizotinib**. Avoid. Severe Study → Also see TABLE 7 p. 1055
- ▶ Antiarrhythmics **(dronedarone)** are predicted to increase the exposure to **crizotinib**. Moderate Study → Also see TABLE 4 p. 1054 → Also see TABLE 7 p. 1055
- ▶ **Crizotinib** is predicted to increase the exposure to antiarrhythmics **(propafenone)**. Monitor and adjust dose. Moderate Study → Also see TABLE 4 p. 1054
- ▶ Antiepileptics **(carbamazepine, fosphenytoin, phenobarbital, phenytoin, primidone)** are predicted to markedly decrease the exposure to **crizotinib**. Avoid. Severe Study
- ▶ Antifungals, azoles **(fluconazole, isavuconazole)** are predicted to increase the exposure to **crizotinib**. Moderate Study → Also see TABLE 7 p. 1055
- ▶ Antifungals, azoles **(itraconazole, ketoconazole, posaconazole, voriconazole)** are predicted to increase the exposure to **crizotinib**. Avoid. Moderate Study → Also see TABLE 7 p. 1055
- ▶ **Crizotinib** is predicted to increase the exposure to antihistamines, non-sedating **(mizolastine)**. Severe Theoretical
- ▶ **Crizotinib** is predicted to increase the exposure to antihistamines, non-sedating **(rupatadine)**. Avoid. Moderate Study
- ▶ **Crizotinib** is predicted to increase the concentration of antimalarials **(piperaquine)**. Severe Study

Crizotinib (continued)
- **Crizotinib** is predicted to increase the exposure to atypical antipsychotics **(cariprazine)**. Monitor and adjust dose. Severe Study
- **Crizotinib** is predicted to increase the exposure to atypical antipsychotics **(lurasidone)**. Adjust **lurasidone** dose. Moderate Study
- **Crizotinib** is predicted to increase the exposure to atypical antipsychotics **(quetiapine)**. Avoid. Moderate Study
- **Crizotinib** is predicted to increase the exposure to **avapritinib**. Avoid or adjust dose—consult product literature. Moderate Study
- **Crizotinib** is predicted to increase the exposure to **axitinib**. Moderate Study
- **Crizotinib** might increase the exposure to **bedaquiline**. Mild Theoretical → Also see **TABLE 7** p. 1055
- **Crizotinib** is predicted to increase the exposure to benzodiazepines **(alprazolam)**. Severe Study
- **Crizotinib** is predicted to increase the exposure to benzodiazepines **(midazolam)**. Monitor adverse effects and adjust dose. Severe Study
- **Crizotinib** is predicted to increase the exposure to **bosutinib**. Avoid or adjust dose. Severe Study → Also see **TABLE 7** p. 1055
- **Crizotinib** is predicted to increase the exposure to **brigatinib**. Moderate Study → Also see **TABLE 4** p. 1054
- **Crizotinib** is predicted to increase the exposure to **buspirone**. Use with caution and adjust dose. Moderate Study
- **Crizotinib** is predicted to increase the exposure to **cabozantinib**. Moderate Study → Also see **TABLE 7** p. 1055
- Calcium-channel blockers **(diltiazem, verapamil)** are predicted to increase the exposure to **crizotinib**. Avoid. Moderate Study → Also see **TABLE 4** p. 1054
- **Crizotinib** is predicted to increase the exposure to calcium-channel blockers **(amlodipine, felodipine, lacidipine, lercanidipine, nicardipine, nifedipine, nimodipine)**. Monitor and adjust dose. Moderate Study
- **Crizotinib** is predicted to increase the exposure to **capivasertib**. Adjust dose. Moderate Study
- **Cenobamate** is predicted to decrease the exposure to **crizotinib**. Avoid. Severe Study
- **Ceritinib** is predicted to increase the exposure to **crizotinib**. Avoid. Moderate Study → Also see **TABLE 4** p. 1054 → Also see **TABLE 7** p. 1055
- **Crizotinib** is predicted to increase the exposure to **ceritinib**. Moderate Study → Also see **TABLE 4** p. 1054 → Also see **TABLE 7** p. 1055
- **Crizotinib** is predicted to increase the concentration of **ciclosporin**. Severe Study
- **Cobicistat** is predicted to increase the exposure to **crizotinib**. Avoid. Moderate Study
- **Crizotinib** is predicted to increase the exposure to **cobimetinib**. Severe Study
- **Crizotinib** is predicted to increase the exposure to **colchicine**. Adjust **colchicine** dose with moderate CYP3A4 inhibitors, p. 637. Severe Study
- **Crizotinib** is predicted to increase the exposure to corticosteroids **(methylprednisolone)**. Monitor and adjust dose. Moderate Study
- **Crizotinib** is predicted to increase the risk of bleeding events when given with **coumarins**. Severe Theoretical
- **Dabrafenib** is predicted to decrease the exposure to **crizotinib**. Avoid. Severe Study
- **Crizotinib** is predicted to increase the exposure to **dabrafenib**. Moderate Study
- **Crizotinib** is predicted to increase the exposure to **daridorexant**. Adjust **daridorexant** dose. Severe Study
- **Crizotinib** is predicted to increase the exposure to **darifenacin**. Moderate Study
- **Crizotinib** is predicted to increase the exposure to **dasatinib**. Severe Study → Also see **TABLE 7** p. 1055
- **Crizotinib** is predicted to increase the exposure to **deutivacaftor**. Adjust dose, see deutivacaftor with tezacaftor and vanzacaftor p. 218. Severe Study
- **Crizotinib** is predicted to slightly increase the exposure to **dienogest**. Moderate Study
- **Crizotinib** is predicted to increase the exposure to dipeptidylpeptidase-4 inhibitors **(saxagliptin)**. Mild Study
- **Crizotinib** is predicted to increase the exposure to **domperidone**. Avoid. Severe Study
- **Crizotinib** is predicted to increase the exposure to dopamine receptor agonists **(bromocriptine)**. Severe Theoretical
- **Crizotinib** is predicted to increase the concentration of dopamine receptor agonists **(cabergoline)**. Moderate Anecdotal
- **Crizotinib** is predicted to increase the exposure to **drospirenone**. Severe Study
- **Crizotinib** is predicted to moderately increase the exposure to **dutasteride**. Mild Study
- **Crizotinib** is predicted to increase the exposure to **elacestrant**. Avoid moderate CYP3A4 inhibitors or adjust **elacestrant** dose. Severe Theoretical
- **Crizotinib** is predicted to increase the exposure to **elexacaftor**. Adjust ivacaftor with tezacaftor and elexacaftor p. 220 dose with moderate CYP3A4 inhibitors. Severe Theoretical
- **Crizotinib** is predicted to increase the exposure to **eliglustat**. Avoid or adjust dose—consult product literature. Severe Study
- **Encorafenib** is predicted to markedly decrease the exposure to **crizotinib**. Avoid. Severe Study → Also see **TABLE 7** p. 1055
- **Crizotinib** is predicted to moderately increase the exposure to **encorafenib**. Moderate Study → Also see **TABLE 7** p. 1055
- Endothelin receptor antagonists **(bosentan)** are predicted to decrease the exposure to **crizotinib**. Avoid. Severe Study
- **Crizotinib** is predicted to increase the exposure to endothelin receptor antagonists **(macitentan)**. Manufacturer advises caution depending on other drugs taken—consult product literature. Moderate Theoretical
- **Crizotinib** is predicted to increase the exposure to **entrectinib**. Avoid or adjust dose with moderate CYP3A4 inhibitors—consult product literature. Severe Theoretical → Also see **TABLE 7** p. 1055
- **Crizotinib** is predicted to increase the risk of ergotism when given with **ergometrine**. Severe Theoretical
- **Crizotinib** is predicted to increase the exposure to **erlotinib**. Moderate Study
- **Crizotinib** is predicted to increase the exposure to **etrasimod**. Avoid in poor CYP2C9 metabolisers. Severe Theoretical → Also see **TABLE 4** p. 1054
- **Crizotinib** is predicted to increase the concentration of **everolimus**. Avoid or adjust dose. Moderate Study
- **Crizotinib** is predicted to increase the exposure to **fedratinib**. Monitor and adjust dose. Moderate Study
- **Crizotinib** is predicted to increase the exposure to **fesoterodine**. Adjust **fesoterodine** dose with moderate CYP3A4 inhibitors in hepatic and renal impairment. Mild Study
- **Crizotinib** is predicted to increase the exposure to **gefitinib**. Moderate Study
- **Crizotinib** potentially decreases the exposure to **glecaprevir**. Avoid. Severe Theoretical
- **Grapefruit** juice is predicted to increase the exposure to **crizotinib**. Avoid. Moderate Theoretical
- **Crizotinib** is predicted to increase the concentration of **guanfacine**. Adjust **guanfacine** dose, p. 281. Moderate Theoretical
- **HIV-protease inhibitors** are predicted to increase the exposure to **crizotinib**. Avoid. Moderate Study
- **Crizotinib** is predicted to increase the exposure to **ibrutinib**. Adjust dose with moderate CYP3A4 inhibitors—consult product literature. Severe Study
- **Idelalisib** is predicted to increase the exposure to **crizotinib**. Avoid. Moderate Study
- **Imatinib** is predicted to increase the exposure to **crizotinib**. Moderate Study
- **Crizotinib** is predicted to increase the exposure to the active metabolite of **irinotecan**. Moderate Theoretical
- **Crizotinib** is predicted to increase the exposure to **ivabradine**. Adjust **ivabradine** dose. Severe Theoretical → Also see **TABLE 4** p. 1054
- **Crizotinib** is predicted to increase the exposure to **ivacaftor**. Adjust dose with moderate CYP3A4 inhibitors, see ivacaftor p. 219, tezacaftor with ivacaftor p. 223, and ivacaftor with tezacaftor and elexacaftor p. 220. Moderate Study

- **Crizotinib** is predicted to increase the exposure to **ivosidenib**. Monitor and adjust dose—consult product literature. Severe Study → Also see TABLE 7 p. 1055
- **Ivosidenib** is predicted to markedly decrease the exposure to **crizotinib**. Avoid. Severe Study → Also see TABLE 7 p. 1055
- **Crizotinib** is predicted to increase the exposure to **lapatinib**. Moderate Study → Also see TABLE 7 p. 1055
- **Crizotinib** is predicted to increase the exposure to **larotrectinib**. Monitor and adjust dose. Moderate Theoretical
- **Crizotinib** is predicted to increase the exposure to **leniolisib**. Avoid. Moderate Study
- **Letermovir** is predicted to increase the exposure to **crizotinib**. Moderate Study
- **Crizotinib** is predicted to increase the exposure to **lomitapide**. Avoid. Moderate Theoretical
- **Lorlatinib** is predicted to decrease the exposure to **crizotinib**. Avoid. Severe Study
- **Lumacaftor** is predicted to markedly decrease the exposure to **crizotinib**. Avoid. Severe Study
- Macrolides **(clarithromycin, erythromycin)** are predicted to increase the exposure to **crizotinib**. Avoid. Moderate Study → Also see TABLE 7 p. 1055
- **Crizotinib** is predicted to increase the exposure to **mavacamten**. Adjust dose—consult product literature. Moderate Study
- **Crizotinib** is predicted to increase the exposure to **midostaurin**. Moderate Theoretical
- **Crizotinib** is predicted to increase the exposure to mineralocorticoid receptor antagonists **(eplerenone)**. Adjust **eplerenone** dose. Severe Study
- **Crizotinib** is predicted to increase the exposure to mineralocorticoid receptor antagonists **(finerenone)**. Severe Study
- **Mitotane** is predicted to markedly decrease the exposure to **crizotinib**. Avoid. Severe Study
- **Crizotinib** is predicted to increase the exposure to **naldemedine**. Moderate Study
- **Crizotinib** is predicted to increase the exposure to **naloxegol**. Adjust **naloxegol** dose and monitor adverse effects. Moderate Study
- **Crizotinib** is predicted to increase the exposure to **neratinib**. Avoid moderate CYP3A4 inhibitors or adjust dose and monitor for gastrointestinal adverse effects—consult product literature. Severe Study
- Neurokinin-1 receptor antagonists **(netupitant)** are predicted to increase the exposure to **crizotinib**. Moderate Study
- NNRTIs **(efavirenz, etravirine, nevirapine)** are predicted to decrease the exposure to **crizotinib**. Avoid. Severe Study → Also see TABLE 7 p. 1055
- **Crizotinib** is predicted to increase the exposure to **olaparib**. Avoid or adjust dose with moderate CYP3A4 inhibitors—consult product literature. Moderate Theoretical
- **Crizotinib** is predicted to increase the exposure to **omaveloxolone**. Avoid or adjust **omaveloxolone** dose, p. 755. Moderate Study
- **Crizotinib** is predicted to increase the exposure to opioids **(alfentanil, buprenorphine, fentanyl, oxycodone)**. Monitor and adjust dose. Moderate Study → Also see TABLE 4 p. 1054
- **Crizotinib** is predicted to increase the exposure to opioids **(methadone, sufentanil)**. Moderate Theoretical → Also see TABLE 4 p. 1054 → Also see TABLE 7 p. 1055
- **Crizotinib** is predicted to increase the exposure to **pazopanib**. Moderate Study → Also see TABLE 7 p. 1055
- **Crizotinib** is predicted to increase the exposure to **pemigatinib**. Severe Study
- **Crizotinib** is predicted to increase the risk of bleeding events when given with **phenindione**. Severe Theoretical
- **Crizotinib** is predicted to increase the exposure to phosphodiesterase type-5 inhibitors **(avanafil)**. Adjust **avanafil** dose. Moderate Theoretical
- **Crizotinib** is predicted to increase the exposure to phosphodiesterase type-5 inhibitors **(sildenafil)**. Monitor or adjust **sildenafil** dose with moderate CYP3A4 inhibitors, p. 139. Moderate Study
- **Crizotinib** is predicted to increase the exposure to phosphodiesterase type-5 inhibitors **(tadalafil)**. Severe Theoretical
- **Crizotinib** is predicted to increase the exposure to phosphodiesterase type-5 inhibitors **(vardenafil)**. Adjust dose. Severe Theoretical → Also see TABLE 7 p. 1055
- **Crizotinib** potentially decreases the exposure to **pibrentasvir**. Avoid. Severe Theoretical
- **Crizotinib** is predicted to increase the exposure to **pimozide**. Avoid. Severe Theoretical → Also see TABLE 7 p. 1055
- **Pitolisant** is predicted to decrease the exposure to **crizotinib**. Avoid. Severe Theoretical
- **Crizotinib** is predicted to increase the exposure to **ponatinib**. Moderate Study
- **Crizotinib** is predicted to increase the exposure to **pralsetinib**. Moderate Theoretical
- **Crizotinib** is predicted to increase the exposure to **ranolazine**. Severe Study → Also see TABLE 7 p. 1055
- **Crizotinib** is predicted to increase the exposure to **regorafenib**. Moderate Study
- **Crizotinib** is predicted to increase the exposure to **ribociclib**. Moderate Study → Also see TABLE 7 p. 1055
- Rifamycins **(rifampicin)** are predicted to markedly decrease the exposure to **crizotinib**. Avoid. Severe Study
- **Crizotinib** is predicted to increase the exposure to **rimegepant**. Avoid another dose of rimegepant within 48 hours of concurrent use. Moderate Study
- **Crizotinib** is predicted to increase the exposure to **ruxolitinib**. Moderate Study
- **Crizotinib** is predicted to increase the exposure to **selpercatinib**. Moderate Study → Also see TABLE 7 p. 1055
- **Crizotinib** is predicted to increase the exposure to **selumetinib**. Avoid or adjust dose—consult product literature. Severe Study
- **Crizotinib** is predicted to increase the exposure to **siponimod**. Avoid depending on other drugs taken—consult product literature. Severe Study → Also see TABLE 4 p. 1054
- **Crizotinib** increases the concentration of **sirolimus**. Monitor and adjust dose. Moderate Study
- **Sotorasib** is predicted to decrease the exposure to **crizotinib**. Avoid. Severe Study
- **Crizotinib** is predicted to increase the exposure to **sparsentan**. Moderate Study
- **Crizotinib** is predicted to increase the exposure to SSRIs **(dapoxetine)**. Adjust **dapoxetine** dose with moderate CYP3A4 inhibitors. Moderate Theoretical
- **Crizotinib** is predicted to increase the exposure to SSRIs **(sertraline)**. Moderate Theoretical
- **St John's wort** is predicted to decrease the exposure to **crizotinib**. Avoid. Severe Study
- **Crizotinib** is predicted to increase the exposure to statins **(atorvastatin)**. Monitor and adjust dose. Moderate Theoretical
- **Crizotinib** is predicted to increase the exposure to statins **(pravastatin)**. Moderate Theoretical
- **Crizotinib** is predicted to increase the exposure to statins **(simvastatin)**. Monitor and adjust dose. Severe Theoretical
- **Crizotinib** is predicted to increase the exposure to **sunitinib**. Moderate Study → Also see TABLE 7 p. 1055
- **Crizotinib** is predicted to increase the concentration of **tacrolimus**. Monitor and adjust dose. Severe Theoretical
- **Crizotinib** is predicted to increase the exposure to taxanes **(cabazitaxel)**. Moderate Theoretical
- **Crizotinib** is predicted to increase the exposure to taxanes **(docetaxel)**. Severe Study
- **Crizotinib** is predicted to increase the exposure to taxanes **(paclitaxel)**. Moderate Anecdotal
- **Crizotinib** is predicted to increase the concentration of **temsirolimus**. Use with caution or avoid. Moderate Theoretical
- **Crizotinib** is predicted to increase the exposure to **tezacaftor**. Adjust dose with moderate CYP3A4 inhibitors, see tezacaftor with ivacaftor p. 223, ivacaftor with tezacaftor and elexacaftor p. 220, and deutivacaftor with tezacaftor and vanzacaftor p. 218. Severe Study
- **Crizotinib** given with a potent CYP2C19 inhibitor is predicted to increase the exposure to **tofacitinib**. Adjust **tofacitinib** dose, p. 803. Moderate Study
- **Crizotinib** is predicted to increase the exposure to **tolvaptan**. Manufacturer advises caution or adjust **tolvaptan** dose with moderate CYP3A4 inhibitors. Moderate Study

Crizotinib (continued)
- **Crizotinib** is predicted to increase the exposure to **trazodone**. Moderate Theoretical
- **Tucatinib** is predicted to increase the exposure to **crizotinib**. Avoid. Moderate Study
- **Crizotinib** is predicted to increase the exposure to **ulipristal**. Avoid when used for uterine fibroids. Moderate Study
- **Crizotinib** is predicted to increase the exposure to **vanzacaftor**. Adjust dose, see deutivacaftor with tezacaftor and vanzacaftor p. 218. Severe Study
- **Crizotinib** is predicted to increase the exposure to **vemurafenib**. Severe Theoretical → Also see **TABLE 7** p. 1055
- **Crizotinib** is predicted to increase the exposure to **venetoclax**. Avoid or adjust dose—consult product literature. Severe Study
- **Crizotinib** is predicted to increase the exposure to **vinca alkaloids**. Severe Theoretical
- **Crizotinib** is predicted to increase the exposure to **voclosporin**. Adjust **voclosporin** dose. Severe Study → Also see **TABLE 7** p. 1055
- **Crizotinib** is predicted to increase the exposure to **zanubrutinib**. Avoid or adjust dose with moderate CYP3A4 inhibitors—consult product literature. Severe Study
- **Crizotinib** is predicted to increase the exposure to **zopiclone**. Adjust dose. Moderate Study

Crovalimab
- **Crovalimab** increases the risk of hypersensitivity reactions when given with monoclonal antibodies **(eculizumab)**. Severe Study
- **Crovalimab** increases the risk of hypersensitivity reactions when given with **ravulizumab**. Severe Study

Cyclizine → see antihistamines, sedating

Cyclopentolate → see **TABLE 8** p. 1055 (antimuscarinics)
- Atypical antipsychotics **(clozapine)** can cause constipation, as can **cyclopentolate**; concurrent use might increase the risk of developing intestinal obstruction. Severe Theoretical → Also see **TABLE 8** p. 1055

Cyclophosphamide → see alkylating agents

Cycloserine
- **Cycloserine** increases the risk of CNS toxicity when given with **isoniazid**. Monitor and adjust dose. Moderate Study

Cyproheptadine → see antihistamines, sedating

Cyproterone → see anti-androgens

Cytarabine → see **TABLE 1** p. 1053 (hepatotoxicity), **TABLE 12** p. 1057 (myelosuppression), **TABLE 10** p. 1056 (peripheral neuropathy)
- **Cedazuridine** is predicted to increase the exposure to **cytarabine**. Avoid. Moderate Theoretical
- **Cytarabine** decreases the concentration of **flucytosine**. Avoid. Severe Study
- **Live vaccines** are predicted to increase the risk of generalised infection (possibly life-threatening) when given with **cytarabine**. UKHSA advises avoid (refer to Green Book). Severe Theoretical

Cytisinicline
- **Cytisinicline** might decrease the efficacy of **combined hormonal contraceptives**. Use additional contraceptive precautions. Severe Theoretical

Cytomegalovirus immunoglobulin → see immunoglobulins

Dabigatran → see thrombin inhibitors

Dabrafenib
- **Dabrafenib** is predicted to decrease the exposure to **acalabrutinib**. Severe Study
- Anti-androgens **(apalutamide, enzalutamide)** are predicted to decrease the exposure to **dabrafenib**. Avoid. Moderate Theoretical
- **Dabrafenib** is predicted to decrease the exposure to anti-androgens **(darolutamide)**. Avoid. Moderate Theoretical
- Antiarrhythmics **(dronedarone)** are predicted to increase the exposure to **dabrafenib**. Moderate Study
- Antiepileptics **(carbamazepine, fosphenytoin, phenobarbital, phenytoin, primidone)** are predicted to decrease the exposure to **dabrafenib**. Avoid. Moderate Theoretical
- Antifungals, azoles **(fluconazole, isavuconazole)** are predicted to increase the exposure to **dabrafenib**. Moderate Study
- Antifungals, azoles **(itraconazole, ketoconazole, posaconazole, voriconazole)** are predicted to increase the exposure to **dabrafenib**. Use with caution or avoid. Moderate Study
- **Dabrafenib** is predicted to decrease the exposure to antifungals, azoles **(isavuconazole)**. Avoid. Severe Theoretical
- **Dabrafenib** is predicted to decrease the exposure to atypical antipsychotics **(aripiprazole)**. Avoid or adjust dose—consult product literature. Moderate Study
- **Dabrafenib** is predicted to decrease the exposure to atypical antipsychotics **(cariprazine)**. Avoid. Severe Theoretical
- **Dabrafenib** is predicted to decrease the exposure to atypical antipsychotics **(lurasidone)**. Monitor and adjust dose. Moderate Theoretical
- **Dabrafenib** is predicted to decrease the exposure to atypical antipsychotics **(quetiapine)**. Moderate Study
- **Dabrafenib** is predicted to decrease the exposure to **avacopan**. Severe Theoretical
- **Dabrafenib** is predicted to decrease the exposure to **avapritinib**. Avoid. Severe Study
- **Dabrafenib** is predicted to decrease the exposure to **axitinib**. Moderate Study
- **Dabrafenib** is predicted to decrease the exposure to **bedaquiline**. Avoid. Severe Study
- **Dabrafenib** decreases the exposure to benzodiazepines **(midazolam)**. Monitor and adjust dose. Moderate Study
- **Berotralstat** is predicted to increase the exposure to **dabrafenib**. Moderate Study
- **Dabrafenib** is predicted to decrease the exposure to **bosutinib**. Avoid. Severe Study
- **Dabrafenib** is predicted to decrease the exposure to **brigatinib**. Avoid or adjust dose—consult product literature. Moderate Study
- **Dabrafenib** is predicted to decrease the exposure to **cabozantinib**. Moderate Study
- Calcium-channel blockers **(diltiazem, verapamil)** are predicted to increase the exposure to **dabrafenib**. Moderate Study
- **Dabrafenib** is predicted to decrease the exposure to calcium-channel blockers **(amlodipine, felodipine, lacidipine, lercanidipine, nicardipine, nifedipine, nimodipine)**. Monitor and adjust dose. Moderate Theoretical
- **Dabrafenib** is predicted to decrease the exposure to calcium-channel blockers **(diltiazem, verapamil)**. Moderate Theoretical
- **Dabrafenib** is predicted to decrease the exposure to **capivasertib**. Avoid. Moderate Study
- **Dabrafenib** is predicted to decrease the exposure to **ceritinib**. Severe Study
- **Ceritinib** is predicted to increase the exposure to **dabrafenib**. Use with caution or avoid. Moderate Study
- **Clopidogrel** is predicted to increase the exposure to **dabrafenib**. Moderate Theoretical
- **Dabrafenib** is predicted to decrease the exposure to **cobicistat**. Avoid. Severe Theoretical
- **Cobicistat** is predicted to increase the exposure to **dabrafenib**. Use with caution or avoid. Moderate Study
- **Dabrafenib** is predicted to decrease the exposure to **cobimetinib**. Avoid. Severe Theoretical
- **Dabrafenib** is predicted to decrease the efficacy of **combined hormonal contraceptives**. Use additional contraceptive precautions. Severe Theoretical
- **Dabrafenib** is predicted to decrease the anticoagulant effect of **coumarins**. Severe Theoretical
- **Dabrafenib** is predicted to decrease the exposure to **crizotinib**. Avoid. Severe Study
- **Crizotinib** is predicted to increase the exposure to **dabrafenib**. Moderate Study
- **Dabrafenib** is predicted to decrease the exposure to **daridorexant**. Severe Study
- **Dabrafenib** is predicted to decrease the exposure to **dasatinib**. Severe Study
- **Dabrafenib** is predicted to decrease the exposure to **deutivacaftor**. Avoid. Severe Theoretical
- **Dabrafenib** is predicted to decrease the exposure to **digoxin**. Moderate Theoretical
- **Dabrafenib** is predicted to decrease the exposure to **dolutegravir**. Severe Study
- **Dabrafenib** is predicted to decrease the exposure to **elacestrant**. Avoid or adjust dose depending on duration—consult product literature. Severe Theoretical

- **Dabrafenib** is predicted to moderately decrease the exposure to **elbasvir**. Avoid. [Severe] Study
- **Dabrafenib** is predicted to decrease the concentration of **elvitegravir**. Avoid. [Severe] Theoretical
- **Dabrafenib** is predicted to decrease the exposure to **encorafenib**. [Moderate] Study
- **Encorafenib** is predicted to decrease the exposure to **dabrafenib**. Avoid. [Moderate] Theoretical
- Endothelin receptor antagonists **(bosentan)** are predicted to decrease the exposure to **dabrafenib**. [Moderate] Study
- **Dabrafenib** is predicted to decrease the exposure to **entrectinib**. Avoid. [Moderate] Theoretical
- **Dabrafenib** is predicted to decrease the exposure to **erdafitinib**. Adjust dose. [Moderate] Theoretical
- **Dabrafenib** is predicted to decrease the exposure to **erlotinib**. [Severe] Study
- **Dabrafenib** is predicted to decrease the concentration of **everolimus**. Avoid or adjust dose. [Severe] Study
- **Fedratinib** is predicted to increase the exposure to **dabrafenib**. [Moderate] Study
- **Dabrafenib** is predicted to decrease the exposure to **fedratinib**. Avoid. [Moderate] Study
- Fibrates **(gemfibrozil)** are predicted to increase the exposure to **dabrafenib**. [Moderate] Theoretical
- **Dabrafenib** is predicted to decrease the exposure to **fruquintinib**. Avoid. [Moderate] Study
- **Dabrafenib** is predicted to decrease the exposure to **gefitinib**. Avoid. [Severe] Study
- **Dabrafenib** is predicted to decrease the exposure to **glasdegib**. Avoid or adjust dose—consult product literature. [Moderate] Theoretical
- **Dabrafenib** is predicted to decrease the exposure to **glecaprevir**. Avoid. [Severe] Study
- **Dabrafenib** is predicted to markedly decrease the exposure to **grazoprevir**. Avoid. [Severe] Study
- **Dabrafenib** is predicted to decrease the concentration of **guanfacine**. Adjust dose. [Moderate] Theoretical
- **HIV-protease inhibitors** are predicted to increase the exposure to **dabrafenib**. Use with caution or avoid. [Moderate] Study
- **Dabrafenib** is predicted to decrease the exposure to **ibrutinib**. Avoid or monitor. [Severe] Study
- **Idelalisib** is predicted to increase the exposure to **dabrafenib**. Use with caution or avoid. [Moderate] Study
- **Dabrafenib** is predicted to decrease the exposure to **idelalisib**. Avoid. [Moderate] Theoretical
- **Imatinib** is predicted to increase the exposure to **dabrafenib**. [Moderate] Study
- **Dabrafenib** is predicted to decrease the exposure to **imatinib**. [Moderate] Study
- **Dabrafenib** is predicted to decrease the exposure to **ivacaftor**. [Moderate] Study
- **Ivosidenib** is predicted to decrease the exposure to **dabrafenib**. Avoid. [Moderate] Theoretical
- **Dabrafenib** is predicted to decrease the exposure to **ixazomib**. [Moderate] Theoretical
- **Dabrafenib** is predicted to decrease the exposure to **lapatinib**. Avoid. [Severe] Study
- **Dabrafenib** is predicted to decrease the exposure to **larotrectinib**. Avoid. [Moderate] Study
- **Dabrafenib** is predicted to decrease the exposure to **lenacapavir**. Avoid. [Severe] Study
- **Dabrafenib** is predicted to decrease the exposure to **leniolisib**. Avoid. [Severe] Theoretical
- **Letermovir** is predicted to increase the exposure to **dabrafenib**. [Moderate] Study
- **Lumacaftor** is predicted to decrease the exposure to **dabrafenib**. Avoid. [Moderate] Theoretical
- Macrolides **(clarithromycin)** are predicted to increase the exposure to **dabrafenib**. Use with caution or avoid. [Moderate] Study
- Macrolides **(erythromycin)** are predicted to increase the exposure to **dabrafenib**. [Moderate] Study
- **Dabrafenib** is predicted to decrease the exposure to **maribavir**. Avoid or adjust **maribavir** dose. [Severe] Study
- **Dabrafenib** is predicted to decrease the exposure to **mavacamten**. Monitor and adjust dose—consult product literature. [Severe] Theoretical
- **Dabrafenib** is predicted to decrease the exposure to **midostaurin**. [Severe] Study
- **Dabrafenib** is predicted to decrease the exposure to **mifepristone**. Adjust **mifepristone** dose. [Severe] Study
- **Dabrafenib** is predicted to decrease the exposure to mineralocorticoid receptor antagonists **(finerenone)**. Avoid. [Severe] Study
- **Mitotane** is predicted to decrease the exposure to **dabrafenib**. Avoid. [Moderate] Theoretical
- **Dabrafenib** is predicted to decrease the exposure to **naloxegol**. [Moderate] Theoretical
- **Dabrafenib** is predicted to decrease the exposure to **neratinib**. Avoid. [Severe] Theoretical
- Neurokinin-1 receptor antagonists **(aprepitant, netupitant)** are predicted to increase the exposure to **dabrafenib**. [Moderate] Study
- **Dabrafenib** is predicted to decrease the exposure to neurokinin-1 receptor antagonists **(netupitant)**. [Moderate] Theoretical
- **Dabrafenib** is predicted to decrease the exposure to **nilotinib**. Avoid. [Severe] Theoretical
- **Nilotinib** is predicted to increase the exposure to **dabrafenib**. [Moderate] Study
- NNRTIs **(efavirenz, nevirapine)** are predicted to decrease the exposure to **dabrafenib**. [Moderate] Study
- **Dabrafenib** is predicted to decrease the exposure to NNRTIs **(doravirine)**. Avoid or adjust doravirine or lamivudine with tenofovir disoproxil and doravirine dose. [Severe] Theoretical
- **Dabrafenib** is predicted to decrease the exposure to NNRTIs **(rilpivirine)**. Avoid. [Severe] Theoretical
- **Dabrafenib** is predicted to decrease the exposure to **olaparib**. Avoid. [Moderate] Theoretical
- **Dabrafenib** is predicted to decrease the exposure to **omaveloxolone**. Avoid. [Severe] Study
- **Dabrafenib** decreases the exposure to opioids **(methadone)**. Monitor and adjust dose. [Severe] Study
- **Dabrafenib** is predicted to decrease the exposure to **osimertinib**. Use with caution or avoid. [Severe] Study
- **Dabrafenib** is predicted to decrease the exposure to **ospemifene**. [Moderate] Study
- **Dabrafenib** is predicted to decrease the exposure to **pazopanib**. [Severe] Study
- **Dabrafenib** is predicted to decrease the exposure to **pemigatinib**. Avoid or monitor. [Severe] Study
- **Dabrafenib** is predicted to decrease the exposure to **phenindione**. [Moderate] Study
- **Dabrafenib** is predicted to decrease the exposure to **pibrentasvir**. Avoid. [Severe] Study
- **Dabrafenib** is predicted to decrease the exposure to **pirtobrutinib**. [Moderate] Theoretical
- **Dabrafenib** is predicted to decrease the exposure to **ponatinib**. [Severe] Study
- **Dabrafenib** is predicted to decrease the exposure to **pralsetinib**. [Moderate] Theoretical
- **Dabrafenib** is predicted to decrease the exposure to **quizartinib**. Avoid. [Severe] Study
- **Dabrafenib** is predicted to decrease the exposure to **regorafenib**. [Severe] Study
- Rifamycins **(rifampicin)** are predicted to decrease the exposure to **dabrafenib**. Avoid. [Moderate] Theoretical
- **Dabrafenib** is predicted to decrease the exposure to **rimegepant**. Avoid. [Moderate] Theoretical
- **Dabrafenib** is predicted to decrease the exposure to **ripretinib**. Avoid or adjust dose—consult product literature. [Moderate] Theoretical
- **Dabrafenib** is predicted to decrease the exposure to **ruxolitinib**. Monitor and adjust dose. [Moderate] Study
- **Dabrafenib** is predicted to decrease the exposure to **selpercatinib**. [Moderate] Study
- **Dabrafenib** is predicted to decrease the exposure to **selumetinib**. Avoid. [Severe] Study

A1

Interactions | Appendix 1

Dabrafenib (continued)
- **Dabrafenib** is predicted to decrease the exposure to **siponimod**. Manufacturer advises caution depending on genotype—consult product literature. [Moderate] Theoretical
- **Dabrafenib** is predicted to decrease the exposure to **sorafenib**. [Moderate] Study
- **Dabrafenib** is predicted to decrease the exposure to **sparsentan**. Avoid. [Severe] Theoretical
- **St John's wort** is predicted to decrease the exposure to **dabrafenib**. Avoid. [Moderate] Study
- **Dabrafenib** is predicted to decrease the exposure to statins **(atorvastatin, simvastatin)**. [Moderate] Study
- **Dabrafenib** is predicted to decrease the exposure to **sunitinib**. [Moderate] Study
- **Dabrafenib** is predicted to decrease the exposure to **tacrolimus**. Monitor and adjust dose. [Moderate] Theoretical
- **Dabrafenib** is predicted to decrease the exposure to taxanes **(cabazitaxel)**. [Moderate] Theoretical
- **Dabrafenib** is predicted to decrease the exposure to taxanes **(docetaxel)**. [Severe] Theoretical
- **Dabrafenib** is predicted to decrease the exposure to taxanes **(paclitaxel)**. Avoid. [Severe] Study
- **Dabrafenib** is predicted to decrease the concentration of **temsirolimus**. Avoid. [Moderate] Theoretical
- **Dabrafenib** is predicted to decrease the exposure to **tezacaftor**. Avoid. [Severe] Theoretical
- **Dabrafenib** is predicted to decrease the exposure to **ticagrelor**. [Moderate] Theoretical
- **Dabrafenib** is predicted to decrease the exposure to **tofacitinib**. [Severe] Study
- **Tucatinib** is predicted to increase the exposure to **dabrafenib**. Use with caution or avoid. [Moderate] Study
- **Dabrafenib** is predicted to decrease the efficacy of **ulipristal**. Avoid and for 4 weeks after stopping **dabrafenib**. [Severe] Theoretical
- **Dabrafenib** is predicted to decrease the exposure to **vandetanib**. [Moderate] Study
- **Dabrafenib** is predicted to decrease the exposure to **vanzacaftor**. Avoid. [Severe] Theoretical
- **Dabrafenib** is predicted to decrease the exposure to **velpatasvir**. Avoid. [Moderate] Theoretical
- **Dabrafenib** is predicted to decrease the exposure to **vemurafenib**. [Severe] Study
- **Dabrafenib** is predicted to decrease the exposure to **venetoclax**. Avoid. [Severe] Study
- **Dabrafenib** is predicted to decrease the exposure to **voclosporin**. Avoid. [Severe] Theoretical
- **Dabrafenib** is predicted to decrease the concentration of **voxilaprevir**. Avoid. [Severe] Theoretical
- **Dabrafenib** is predicted to decrease the exposure to **zanubrutinib**. Avoid or adjust dose with moderate CYP3A4 inducers—consult product literature. [Severe] Theoretical

Dacarbazine → see alkylating agents

Dacomitinib
- **Dacomitinib** is predicted to increase the exposure to anticholinesterases, centrally acting **(galantamine)**. Monitor and adjust dose. [Moderate] Study
- **Dacomitinib** is predicted to markedly increase the exposure to **atomoxetine**. Adjust dose. [Severe] Study
- **Dacomitinib** is predicted to moderately increase the exposure to atypical antipsychotics **(aripiprazole)**. Avoid or adjust dose—consult product literature. [Moderate] Study
- **Dacomitinib** is predicted to increase the exposure to atypical antipsychotics **(clozapine)**. Use with caution and adjust dose. [Severe] Study
- **Dacomitinib** is predicted to increase the exposure to atypical antipsychotics **(risperidone)**. Adjust dose. [Moderate] Study
- **Dacomitinib** is predicted to markedly increase the exposure to beta blockers, non-selective **(propranolol)**. Avoid. [Severe] Study
- **Dacomitinib** is predicted to increase the exposure to beta blockers, selective **(metoprolol, nebivolol)**. [Moderate] Study
- **Dacomitinib** is predicted to slightly increase the exposure to **darifenacin**. [Mild] Study
- **Dacomitinib** is predicted to increase the exposure to **eliglustat**. Avoid or adjust dose—consult product literature. [Severe] Study
- **Dacomitinib** is predicted to increase the exposure to **fenfluramine**. [Moderate] Study
- **Dacomitinib** is predicted to increase the exposure to **fesoterodine**. Use with caution and adjust dose. [Mild] Theoretical
- **Dacomitinib** is predicted to increase the exposure to **gefitinib**. [Moderate] Theoretical
- **H_2 receptor antagonists** are predicted to decrease the concentration of **dacomitinib**. **Dacomitinib** should be taken 2 hours before or 10 hours after **H_2 receptor antagonists**. [Unknown] Theoretical
- **Dacomitinib** is predicted to increase the exposure to **mexiletine**. [Moderate] Study
- **Dacomitinib** is predicted to decrease the efficacy of opioids **(codeine)**. [Moderate] Theoretical
- **Dacomitinib** is predicted to decrease the efficacy of opioids **(tramadol)**. [Severe] Study
- **Dacomitinib** is predicted to moderately increase the exposure to **pitolisant**. Use with caution and adjust dose. [Moderate] Study
- **Proton pump inhibitors** are predicted to decrease the exposure to **dacomitinib**. Avoid. [Moderate] Study
- **Dacomitinib** is predicted to increase the exposure to the active component of **sacituzumab govitecan**. [Severe] Theoretical
- **Dacomitinib** is predicted to increase the exposure to SSRIs **(dapoxetine)**. [Moderate] Theoretical
- **Dacomitinib** is predicted to decrease the efficacy of **tamoxifen**. Avoid. [Severe] Study
- **Dacomitinib** is predicted to increase the exposure to the active metabolite of **tetrabenazine**. [Moderate] Study
- **Dacomitinib** is predicted to markedly increase the exposure to **tolterodine**. Avoid. [Severe] Study
- **Dacomitinib** is predicted to increase the exposure to **tricyclic antidepressants**. Monitor for toxicity and adjust dose. [Severe] Study
- **Dacomitinib** is predicted to increase the exposure to **vortioxetine**. Monitor and adjust dose. [Moderate] Study

Dactinomycin → see TABLE 1 p. 1053 (hepatotoxicity), TABLE 12 p. 1057 (myelosuppression)
- **Live vaccines** are predicted to increase the risk of generalised infection (possibly life-threatening) when given with **dactinomycin**. UKHSA advises avoid (refer to Green Book). [Severe] Theoretical

Dalteparin → see low molecular-weight heparins

Danaparoid → see TABLE 3 p. 1053 (bleeding)
- **Donanemab** can increase the risk of brain haemorrhage when given with **danaparoid**. Avoid. [Severe] Anecdotal
- **Lecanemab** can increase the risk of brain haemorrhage when given with **danaparoid**. Avoid. [Severe] Anecdotal
- Monoclonal antibodies **(ipilimumab)** might increase the risk of gastrointestinal bleeding when given with **danaparoid**. [Severe] Theoretical

Danicopan
- **Danicopan** is predicted to increase the exposure to **aliskiren**. [Moderate] Study
- **Danicopan** is predicted to increase the exposure to antihistamines, non-sedating **(fexofenadine)**. [Moderate] Study
- **Danicopan** is predicted to increase the exposure to **colchicine**. [Moderate] Study
- **Danicopan** is predicted to increase the exposure to **digoxin**. [Moderate] Study
- **Danicopan** is predicted to increase the exposure to **everolimus**. [Moderate] Study
- **Danicopan** is predicted to increase the exposure to factor XA inhibitors **(edoxaban)**. [Moderate] Study
- **Danicopan** is predicted to increase the exposure to **loperamide**. [Moderate] Study
- **Danicopan** is predicted to increase the exposure to **pralsetinib**. [Moderate] Study
- **Danicopan** is predicted to increase the exposure to **ranolazine**. [Moderate] Study
- **Danicopan** is predicted to increase the exposure to **rimegepant**. [Moderate] Study
- **Danicopan** is predicted to increase the exposure to **sirolimus**. [Moderate] Study
- **Danicopan** is predicted to increase the exposure to statins **(atorvastatin, fluvastatin, rosuvastatin)**. [Moderate] Study

- **Danicopan** is predicted to increase the exposure to **sulfasalazine**. Moderate Study
- **Danicopan** is predicted to increase the exposure to **tacrolimus**. Moderate Theoretical
- **Danicopan** is predicted to increase the exposure to **talazoparib**. Moderate Study
- **Danicopan** is predicted to increase the exposure to taxanes **(paclitaxel)**. Moderate Study
- **Danicopan** is predicted to increase the exposure to thrombin inhibitors **(dabigatran)**. Moderate Study
- **Danicopan** is predicted to increase the exposure to **topotecan**. Moderate Study

Dantrolene

- Intravenous **dantrolene** potentially increases the risk of acute hyperkalaemia and cardiovascular collapse when given with calcium-channel blockers **(diltiazem, verapamil)**. Avoid. Severe Anecdotal

Dapagliflozin → see sodium glucose co-transporter 2 inhibitors

Dapoxetine → see SSRIs

Dapsone

- **Rifamycins** decrease the exposure to **dapsone**. Moderate Study
- **Dapsone** increases the exposure to **trimethoprim** and **trimethoprim** increases the exposure to **dapsone**. Severe Study

Daptomycin

- **Aspirin** (high-dose) increases the risk of renal impairment when given with **daptomycin**. Moderate Theoretical
- **Ciclosporin** is predicted to increase the risk of rhabdomyolysis when given with **daptomycin**. Severe Theoretical
- **Fibrates** are predicted to increase the risk of rhabdomyolysis when given with **daptomycin**. Severe Theoretical
- **NSAIDs** increase the risk of renal impairment when given with **daptomycin**. Moderate Theoretical
- **Statins** are predicted to increase the risk of rhabdomyolysis when given with **daptomycin**. Severe Theoretical

Daratumumab → see monoclonal antibodies

Daridorexant → see TABLE 9 p. 1056 (CNS effects)

- Anti-androgens **(apalutamide, enzalutamide)** are predicted to decrease the exposure to **daridorexant**. Severe Study
- Antiarrhythmics **(dronedarone)** are predicted to increase the exposure to **daridorexant**. Adjust **daridorexant** dose. Severe Study
- Antiepileptics **(carbamazepine, fosphenytoin, phenobarbital, phenytoin, primidone)** are predicted to decrease the exposure to **daridorexant**. Severe Study → Also see TABLE 9 p. 1056
- Antifungals, azoles **(fluconazole, isavuconazole)** are predicted to increase the exposure to **daridorexant**. Adjust **daridorexant** dose. Severe Study
- Antifungals, azoles **(itraconazole, ketoconazole, posaconazole, voriconazole)** are predicted to increase the exposure to **daridorexant**. Avoid. Severe Study
- **Berotralstat** is predicted to increase the exposure to **daridorexant**. Adjust **daridorexant** dose. Severe Study
- Calcium-channel blockers **(diltiazem, verapamil)** are predicted to increase the exposure to **daridorexant**. Adjust **daridorexant** dose. Severe Study
- **Cenobamate** is predicted to decrease the exposure to **daridorexant**. Severe Study → Also see TABLE 9 p. 1056
- **Ceritinib** is predicted to increase the exposure to **daridorexant**. Avoid. Severe Study
- **Ciclosporin** is predicted to increase the exposure to **daridorexant**. Adjust **daridorexant** dose. Unknown Theoretical
- **Cobicistat** is predicted to increase the exposure to **daridorexant**. Avoid. Severe Study
- **Crizotinib** is predicted to increase the exposure to **daridorexant**. Adjust **daridorexant** dose. Severe Study
- **Dabrafenib** is predicted to decrease the exposure to **daridorexant**. Severe Study
- **Daridorexant** is predicted to increase the exposure to **digoxin**. Moderate Study
- **Encorafenib** is predicted to decrease the exposure to **daridorexant**. Severe Study
- Endothelin receptor antagonists **(bosentan)** are predicted to decrease the exposure to **daridorexant**. Severe Study
- **Daridorexant** is predicted to increase the exposure to **everolimus**. Moderate Study
- **Fedratinib** is predicted to increase the exposure to **daridorexant**. Adjust **daridorexant** dose. Severe Study
- **Grapefruit** and grapefruit juice is predicted to increase the exposure to **daridorexant**. Avoid **grapefruit** in the evening. Moderate Theoretical
- **HIV-protease inhibitors** are predicted to increase the exposure to **daridorexant**. Avoid. Severe Study
- **Idelalisib** is predicted to increase the exposure to **daridorexant**. Avoid. Severe Study
- **Imatinib** is predicted to increase the exposure to **daridorexant**. Adjust **daridorexant** dose. Severe Study
- **Ivosidenib** is predicted to decrease the exposure to **daridorexant**. Severe Study
- **Letermovir** is predicted to increase the exposure to **daridorexant**. Adjust **daridorexant** dose. Severe Study
- **Lorlatinib** is predicted to decrease the exposure to **daridorexant**. Severe Study
- **Lumacaftor** is predicted to decrease the exposure to **daridorexant**. Severe Study
- Macrolides **(clarithromycin)** are predicted to increase the exposure to **daridorexant**. Avoid. Severe Study
- Macrolides **(erythromycin)** are predicted to increase the exposure to **daridorexant**. Adjust **daridorexant** dose. Severe Study
- **Mitotane** is predicted to decrease the exposure to **daridorexant**. Severe Study
- Neurokinin-1 receptor antagonists **(aprepitant, netupitant)** are predicted to increase the exposure to **daridorexant**. Adjust **daridorexant** dose. Severe Study
- **Nilotinib** is predicted to increase the exposure to **daridorexant**. Adjust **daridorexant** dose. Severe Study
- NNRTIs **(efavirenz, etravirine, nevirapine)** are predicted to decrease the exposure to **daridorexant**. Severe Study
- Quinolones **(ciprofloxacin)** are predicted to increase the exposure to **daridorexant**. Adjust **daridorexant** dose. Moderate Theoretical
- Rifamycins **(rifampicin)** are predicted to decrease the exposure to **daridorexant**. Severe Study
- **Daridorexant** is predicted to increase the exposure to **sirolimus**. Moderate Study
- **Sotorasib** is predicted to decrease the exposure to **daridorexant**. Severe Study
- **St John's wort** is predicted to decrease the exposure to **daridorexant**. Severe Study
- **Daridorexant** is predicted to increase the exposure to **talazoparib**. Moderate Study
- **Daridorexant** is predicted to increase the exposure to taxanes **(paclitaxel)**. Moderate Study
- **Tucatinib** is predicted to increase the exposure to **daridorexant**. Avoid. Severe Study

Darifenacin → see TABLE 8 p. 1055 (antimuscarinics)

- Anti-androgens **(apalutamide, enzalutamide)** are predicted to decrease the exposure to **darifenacin**. Moderate Theoretical
- Antiarrhythmics **(dronedarone)** are predicted to increase the exposure to **darifenacin**. Moderate Study
- **Darifenacin** is predicted to increase the concentration of antiarrhythmics **(flecainide)**. Moderate Theoretical
- Antiepileptics **(carbamazepine, fosphenytoin, phenobarbital, phenytoin, primidone)** are predicted to decrease the exposure to **darifenacin**. Moderate Theoretical
- Antifungals, azoles **(fluconazole)** slightly increase the exposure to **darifenacin**. Moderate Study
- Antifungals, azoles **(isavuconazole)** are predicted to increase the exposure to **darifenacin**. Moderate Study
- Antifungals, azoles **(itraconazole, ketoconazole, posaconazole, voriconazole)** are predicted to markedly to very markedly increase the exposure to **darifenacin**. Avoid. Severe Study
- Atypical antipsychotics **(clozapine)** can cause constipation, as can **darifenacin**; concurrent use might increase the risk of developing intestinal obstruction. Severe Theoretical → Also see TABLE 8 p. 1055
- **Bupropion** is predicted to slightly increase the exposure to **darifenacin**. Mild Study
- Calcium-channel blockers **(diltiazem)** are predicted to increase the exposure to **darifenacin**. Moderate Study

Darifenacin (continued)
- Calcium-channel blockers **(verapamil)** are predicted to increase the exposure to **darifenacin**. Avoid. Moderate Study
- **Cenobamate** is predicted to decrease the exposure to **darifenacin**. Adjust dose. Moderate Theoretical
- **Ceritinib** is predicted to markedly to very markedly increase the exposure to **darifenacin**. Avoid. Severe Study
- **Ciclosporin** is predicted to increase the exposure to **darifenacin**. Avoid. Moderate Theoretical
- **Cinacalcet** is predicted to slightly increase the exposure to **darifenacin**. Mild Study
- **Cobicistat** is predicted to markedly to very markedly increase the exposure to **darifenacin**. Avoid. Severe Study
- **Crizotinib** is predicted to increase the exposure to **darifenacin**. Moderate Study
- **Dacomitinib** is predicted to slightly increase the exposure to **darifenacin**. Mild Study
- **Encorafenib** is predicted to decrease the exposure to **darifenacin**. Moderate Theoretical
- **Grapefruit** juice is predicted to increase the exposure to **darifenacin**. Moderate Study
- H_2 receptor antagonists **(cimetidine)** increase the exposure to **darifenacin**. Mild Study
- **HIV-protease inhibitors** are predicted to markedly to very markedly increase the exposure to **darifenacin**. Avoid. Severe Study
- **Idelalisib** is predicted to markedly to very markedly increase the exposure to **darifenacin**. Avoid. Severe Study
- **Imatinib** is predicted to increase the exposure to **darifenacin**. Moderate Study
- **Ivosidenib** is predicted to decrease the exposure to **darifenacin**. Moderate Theoretical
- **Letermovir** is predicted to increase the exposure to **darifenacin**. Moderate Study
- **Lumacaftor** is predicted to decrease the exposure to **darifenacin**. Moderate Theoretical
- Macrolides **(clarithromycin)** are predicted to markedly to very markedly increase the exposure to **darifenacin**. Avoid. Severe Study
- Macrolides **(erythromycin)** slightly increase the exposure to **darifenacin**. Moderate Study
- **Mitotane** is predicted to decrease the exposure to **darifenacin**. Moderate Theoretical
- Neurokinin-1 receptor antagonists **(aprepitant, netupitant)** are predicted to increase the exposure to **darifenacin**. Moderate Study
- **Nilotinib** is predicted to increase the exposure to **darifenacin**. Moderate Study
- **Nirmatrelvir** boosted with ritonavir is predicted to increase the concentration of **darifenacin**. Adjust dose. Severe Theoretical
- Rifamycins **(rifampicin)** are predicted to decrease the exposure to **darifenacin**. Moderate Theoretical
- SSRIs **(fluoxetine, paroxetine)** are predicted to slightly increase the exposure to **darifenacin**. Mild Study
- **St John's wort** is predicted to decrease the exposure to **darifenacin**. Moderate Theoretical
- **Terbinafine** is predicted to slightly increase the exposure to **darifenacin**. Mild Study
- Darifenacin (high-dose) is predicted to increase the exposure to **tricyclic antidepressants**. Moderate Study → Also see TABLE 8 p. 1055
- **Tucatinib** is predicted to markedly to very markedly increase the exposure to **darifenacin**. Avoid. Severe Study

Darolutamide → see anti-androgens

Darunavir → see HIV-protease inhibitors

Dasatinib → see TABLE 3 p. 1053 (bleeding), TABLE 12 p. 1057 (myelosuppression), TABLE 7 p. 1055 (QT-interval prolongation)
- Oral **antacids** decrease the absorption of oral **dasatinib**. Separate administration by at least 2 hours. Moderate Study
- Anti-androgens **(apalutamide, enzalutamide)** are predicted to markedly decrease the exposure to **dasatinib**. Avoid. Severe Study → Also see TABLE 7 p. 1055
- Antiarrhythmics **(dronedarone)** are predicted to increase the exposure to **dasatinib**. Severe Study → Also see TABLE 7 p. 1055
- Antiepileptics **(carbamazepine, fosphenytoin, phenobarbital, phenytoin, primidone)** are predicted to markedly decrease the exposure to **dasatinib**. Avoid. Severe Study
- Antifungals, azoles **(fluconazole, isavuconazole)** are predicted to increase the exposure to **dasatinib**. Severe Study → Also see TABLE 7 p. 1055
- Antifungals, azoles **(itraconazole, ketoconazole, posaconazole, voriconazole)** are predicted to increase the exposure to **dasatinib**. Avoid or adjust dose—consult product literature. Severe Study → Also see TABLE 7 p. 1055
- **Belzutifan** is predicted to decrease the exposure to **dasatinib**. Avoid or adjust dose. Severe Theoretical
- **Berotralstat** is predicted to increase the exposure to **dasatinib**. Severe Study
- Oral calcium compounds **(calcium carbonate)** -containing antacids are predicted to decrease the exposure to oral **dasatinib**. Separate administration by at least 2 hours. Moderate Study
- Calcium-channel blockers **(diltiazem, verapamil)** are predicted to increase the exposure to **dasatinib**. Severe Study
- **Cenobamate** is predicted to decrease the exposure to **dasatinib**. Severe Study
- **Ceritinib** is predicted to increase the exposure to **dasatinib**. Avoid or adjust dose—consult product literature. Severe Study → Also see TABLE 12 p. 1057 → Also see TABLE 7 p. 1055
- **Cobicistat** is predicted to increase the exposure to **dasatinib**. Avoid or adjust dose—consult product literature. Severe Study
- **Crizotinib** is predicted to increase the exposure to **dasatinib**. Severe Study → Also see TABLE 7 p. 1055
- **Dabrafenib** is predicted to decrease the exposure to **dasatinib**. Severe Study
- **Encorafenib** is predicted to markedly decrease the exposure to **dasatinib**. Avoid. Severe Study → Also see TABLE 7 p. 1055
- Endothelin receptor antagonists **(bosentan)** are predicted to decrease the exposure to **dasatinib**. Severe Study
- **Fedratinib** is predicted to increase the exposure to **dasatinib**. Severe Study
- **Grapefruit** juice is predicted to increase the exposure to **dasatinib**. Avoid. Moderate Theoretical
- **H_2 receptor antagonists** are predicted to decrease the exposure to **dasatinib**. Avoid. Moderate Study
- **HIV-protease inhibitors** are predicted to increase the exposure to **dasatinib**. Avoid or adjust dose—consult product literature. Severe Study
- **Idelalisib** is predicted to increase the exposure to **dasatinib**. Avoid or adjust dose—consult product literature. Severe Study
- **Imatinib** is predicted to increase the exposure to **dasatinib**. Severe Study → Also see TABLE 3 p. 1053 → Also see TABLE 12 p. 1057
- **Ivosidenib** is predicted to markedly decrease the exposure to **dasatinib**. Avoid. Severe Study → Also see TABLE 7 p. 1055
- **Letermovir** is predicted to increase the exposure to **dasatinib**. Severe Study
- **Lorlatinib** is predicted to decrease the exposure to **dasatinib**. Severe Study
- **Lumacaftor** is predicted to markedly decrease the exposure to **dasatinib**. Avoid. Severe Study
- Macrolides **(clarithromycin)** are predicted to increase the exposure to **dasatinib**. Avoid or adjust dose—consult product literature. Severe Study
- Macrolides **(erythromycin)** are predicted to increase the exposure to **dasatinib**. Severe Study → Also see TABLE 7 p. 1055
- **Mitotane** is predicted to markedly decrease the exposure to **dasatinib**. Avoid. Severe Study → Also see TABLE 12 p. 1057
- Neurokinin-1 receptor antagonists **(aprepitant, netupitant)** are predicted to increase the exposure to **dasatinib**. Severe Study
- **Nilotinib** is predicted to increase the exposure to **dasatinib**. Severe Study → Also see TABLE 12 p. 1057 → Also see TABLE 7 p. 1055
- **Nirmatrelvir** boosted with ritonavir is predicted to increase the concentration of **dasatinib**. Avoid. Severe Theoretical
- NNRTIs **(efavirenz, etravirine, nevirapine)** are predicted to decrease the exposure to **dasatinib**. Severe Study → Also see TABLE 7 p. 1055
- **Pitolisant** is predicted to decrease the exposure to **dasatinib**. Avoid. Severe Theoretical

- **Proton pump inhibitors** are predicted to decrease the exposure to **dasatinib**. Avoid. Severe Study
- Rifamycins **(rifampicin)** are predicted to markedly decrease the exposure to **dasatinib**. Avoid. Severe Study
- Oral **sodium bicarbonate** -containing antacids are predicted to decrease the exposure to oral **dasatinib**. Separate administration by at least 2 hours. Moderate Study
- **Sodium zirconium cyclosilicate** is predicted to decrease the exposure to **dasatinib**. Separate administration by at least 2 hours. Moderate Theoretical
- **Sotorasib** is predicted to decrease the exposure to **dasatinib**. Severe Study
- **St John's wort** is predicted to decrease the exposure to **dasatinib** Severe Study
- **Dasatinib** is predicted to increase the exposure to statins **(simvastatin)**. Moderate Theoretical
- **Tucatinib** is predicted to increase the exposure to **dasatinib**. Avoid or adjust dose—consult product literature. Severe Study

Daunorubicin → see anthracyclines

Decitabine → see TABLE 1 p. 1053 (hepatotoxicity), TABLE 12 p. 1057 (myelosuppression)

Deferasirox → see iron chelators

Deferiprone → see iron chelators

Deflazacort → see corticosteroids

Delafloxacin → see quinolones

Delamanid → see TABLE 7 p. 1055 (QT-interval prolongation)

- Anti-androgens **(apalutamide, enzalutamide)** are predicted to slightly decrease the exposure to **delamanid**. Avoid. Moderate Study → Also see TABLE 7 p. 1055
- Antiepileptics **(carbamazepine, fosphenytoin, phenobarbital, phenytoin, primidone)** are predicted to slightly decrease the exposure to **delamanid**. Avoid. Moderate Study
- Antifungals, azoles **(itraconazole, ketoconazole, posaconazole, voriconazole)** very slightly increase the exposure to **delamanid**. Severe Study → Also see TABLE 7 p. 1055
- **Ceritinib** very slightly increases the exposure to **delamanid**. Severe Study → Also see TABLE 7 p. 1055
- **Cobicistat** very slightly increases the exposure to **delamanid**. Severe Study
- **Encorafenib** is predicted to slightly decrease the exposure to **delamanid**. Avoid. Moderate Study → Also see TABLE 7 p. 1055
- **HIV-protease inhibitors** very slightly increase the exposure to **delamanid**. Severe Study
- **Idelalisib** very slightly increases the exposure to **delamanid**. Severe Study
- **Ivosidenib** is predicted to slightly decrease the exposure to **delamanid**. Avoid. Moderate Study → Also see TABLE 7 p. 1055
- **Lumacaftor** is predicted to slightly decrease the exposure to **delamanid**. Avoid. Moderate Study
- Macrolides **(clarithromycin)** very slightly increase the exposure to **delamanid**. Severe Study
- **Mitotane** is predicted to slightly decrease the exposure to **delamanid**. Avoid. Moderate Study
- **Nirmatrelvir** boosted with ritonavir is predicted to increase the concentration of **delamanid**. Severe Theoretical
- Rifamycins **(rifampicin)** are predicted to slightly decrease the exposure to **delamanid**. Avoid. Moderate Study
- **Tucatinib** very slightly increases the exposure to **delamanid**. Severe Study

Demeclocycline → see tetracyclines

Dengue vaccine → see live vaccines

Denosumab

- **Cinacalcet** might increase the risk of hypocalcaemia when given with **denosumab**. Severe Theoretical
- **Etelcalcetide** might increase the risk of hypocalcaemia when given with **denosumab**. Severe Theoretical

Desferrioxamine → see iron chelators

Desflurane → see volatile halogenated anaesthetics

Desloratadine → see antihistamines, non-sedating

Desmopressin → see TABLE 15 p. 1058 (hyponatraemia)

- Antiepileptics **(lamotrigine)** are predicted to increase the risk of hyponatraemia when given with **desmopressin**. Severe Theoretical
- **Loperamide** greatly increases the absorption of oral **desmopressin** (and possibly sublingual). Moderate Study
- Phenothiazine antipsychotics **(chlorpromazine)** are predicted to increase the risk of hyponatraemia when given with **desmopressin**. Severe Theoretical → Also see TABLE 15 p. 1058

Desogestrel

- Antiepileptics **(carbamazepine, eslicarbazepine, fosphenytoin, oxcarbazepine, perampanel, phenobarbital, phenytoin, primidone, rufinamide, topiramate)** are predicted to decrease the efficacy of **desogestrel**. For CoSRH guidance, see Contraceptives, interactions p. 614. Severe Theoretical
- **Desogestrel** is predicted to increase the exposure to antiepileptics **(lamotrigine)** and antiepileptics **(lamotrigine)** might decrease the effects of **desogestrel**. For CoSRH guidance, see Contraceptives, interactions p. 614. Moderate Study
- Endothelin receptor antagonists **(bosentan)** are predicted to decrease the efficacy of **desogestrel**. For CoSRH guidance, see Contraceptives, interactions p. 614. Severe Theoretical
- Glucagon-like peptide-1 receptor agonists **(tirzepatide)** might affect the absorption of **desogestrel**. Manufacturer advises precautions for those who are overweight or obese. Moderate Study
- HIV-protease inhibitors **(ritonavir)** are predicted to decrease the efficacy of **desogestrel**. For CoSRH guidance, see Contraceptives, interactions p. 614. Severe Theoretical
- **Lumacaftor** might decrease the efficacy of **desogestrel**. Use additional contraceptive precautions. Severe Theoretical
- **Modafinil** is predicted to decrease the efficacy of **desogestrel**. For CoSRH guidance, see Contraceptives, interactions p. 614. Severe Theoretical
- Neurokinin-1 receptor antagonists **(aprepitant, fosaprepitant)** are predicted to decrease the efficacy of **desogestrel**. For CoSRH guidance, see Contraceptives, interactions p. 614. Severe Theoretical
- NNRTIs **(efavirenz, nevirapine)** are predicted to decrease the efficacy of **desogestrel**. For CoSRH guidance, see Contraceptives, interactions p. 614. Severe Theoretical
- NNRTIs **(etravirine)** might decrease the efficacy of **desogestrel**. Follow CoSRH guidance for enzyme inducers, see Contraceptives, interactions p. 614. Severe Theoretical
- **Rifamycins** are predicted to decrease the efficacy of **desogestrel**. For CoSRH guidance, see Contraceptives, interactions p. 614. Severe Theoretical
- **St John's wort** is predicted to decrease the efficacy of **desogestrel**. MHRA advises avoid. For CoSRH guidance, see Contraceptives, interactions p. 614. Severe Theoretical
- **Sugammadex** is predicted to decrease the exposure to **desogestrel**. Refer to patient information leaflet for missed pill advice. Severe Theoretical
- **Desogestrel** might decrease the efficacy of **ulipristal** and **ulipristal** might decrease the efficacy of **desogestrel**. Avoid when used for uterine fibroids. For CoSRH guidance when used for emergency hormonal contraception, see Contraceptives, interactions p. 614. Severe Theoretical

Deucravacitinib

- **Live vaccines** are predicted to increase the risk of generalised infection (possibly life-threatening) when given with **deucravacitinib**. Avoid. Severe Theoretical

Deutivacaftor

- Anti-androgens **(apalutamide, enzalutamide)** are predicted to decrease the exposure to **deutivacaftor**. Avoid. Severe Theoretical
- Antiarrhythmics **(dronedarone)** are predicted to increase the exposure to **deutivacaftor**. Adjust dose, see deutivacaftor with tezacaftor and vanzacaftor p. 218. Severe Study
- Antiepileptics **(carbamazepine, fosphenytoin, phenobarbital, phenytoin, primidone)** are predicted to decrease the exposure to **deutivacaftor**. Avoid. Severe Theoretical
- Antifungals, azoles **(fluconazole, isavuconazole, itraconazole, ketoconazole, posaconazole, voriconazole)** are predicted to increase the exposure to **deutivacaftor**. Adjust dose, see deutivacaftor with tezacaftor and vanzacaftor p. 218. Severe Study
- **Berotralstat** is predicted to increase the exposure to **deutivacaftor**. Adjust dose, see deutivacaftor with tezacaftor and vanzacaftor p. 218. Severe Study

Deutivacaftor (continued)
- Calcium-channel blockers **(diltiazem, verapamil)** are predicted to increase the exposure to **deutivacaftor**. Adjust dose, see deutivacaftor with tezacaftor and vanzacaftor p. 218. Severe Study
- **Cenobamate** is predicted to decrease the exposure to **deutivacaftor**. Avoid. Severe Theoretical
- **Ceritinib** is predicted to increase the exposure to **deutivacaftor**. Adjust dose, see deutivacaftor with tezacaftor and vanzacaftor p. 218. Severe Study
- **Cobicistat** is predicted to increase the exposure to **deutivacaftor**. Adjust dose, see deutivacaftor with tezacaftor and vanzacaftor p. 218. Severe Study
- **Deutivacaftor** is predicted to increase the exposure to coumarins **(warfarin)**. Moderate Theoretical
- **Crizotinib** is predicted to increase the exposure to **deutivacaftor**. Adjust dose, see deutivacaftor with tezacaftor and vanzacaftor p. 218. Severe Study
- **Dabrafenib** is predicted to decrease the exposure to **deutivacaftor**. Avoid. Severe Theoretical
- **Deutivacaftor** is predicted to increase the exposure to **digoxin**. Moderate Theoretical
- **Encorafenib** is predicted to decrease the exposure to **deutivacaftor**. Avoid. Severe Theoretical
- Endothelin receptor antagonists **(bosentan)** are predicted to decrease the exposure to **deutivacaftor**. Avoid. Severe Theoretical
- **Deutivacaftor** is predicted to increase the exposure to **everolimus**. Moderate Theoretical
- **Fedratinib** is predicted to increase the exposure to **deutivacaftor**. Adjust dose, see deutivacaftor with tezacaftor and vanzacaftor p. 218. Severe Study
- **Grapefruit** is predicted to increase the exposure to **deutivacaftor**. Avoid. Moderate Theoretical
- **HIV-protease inhibitors** are predicted to increase the exposure to **deutivacaftor**. Adjust dose, see deutivacaftor with tezacaftor and vanzacaftor p. 218. Severe Study
- **Idelalisib** is predicted to increase the exposure to **deutivacaftor**. Adjust dose, see deutivacaftor with tezacaftor and vanzacaftor p. 218. Severe Study
- **Imatinib** is predicted to increase the exposure to **deutivacaftor**. Adjust dose, see deutivacaftor with tezacaftor and vanzacaftor p. 218. Severe Study
- **Ivosidenib** is predicted to decrease the exposure to **deutivacaftor**. Avoid. Severe Theoretical
- **Letermovir** is predicted to increase the exposure to **deutivacaftor**. Adjust dose, see deutivacaftor with tezacaftor and vanzacaftor p. 218. Severe Study
- **Lorlatinib** is predicted to decrease the exposure to **deutivacaftor**. Avoid. Severe Theoretical
- **Lumacaftor** is predicted to decrease the exposure to **deutivacaftor**. Avoid. Severe Theoretical
- Macrolides **(clarithromycin, erythromycin)** are predicted to increase the exposure to **deutivacaftor**. Adjust dose, see deutivacaftor with tezacaftor and vanzacaftor p. 218. Severe Study
- **Mitotane** is predicted to decrease the exposure to **deutivacaftor**. Avoid. Severe Theoretical
- Neurokinin-1 receptor antagonists **(aprepitant, netupitant)** are predicted to increase the exposure to **deutivacaftor**. Adjust dose, see deutivacaftor with tezacaftor and vanzacaftor p. 218. Severe Study
- **Nilotinib** is predicted to increase the exposure to **deutivacaftor**. Adjust dose, see deutivacaftor with tezacaftor and vanzacaftor p. 218. Severe Study
- NNRTIs **(efavirenz, etravirine, nevirapine)** are predicted to decrease the exposure to **deutivacaftor**. Avoid. Severe Theoretical
- Rifamycins **(rifampicin)** are predicted to decrease the exposure to **deutivacaftor**. Avoid. Severe Theoretical
- **Deutivacaftor** is predicted to increase the exposure to **sirolimus**. Moderate Theoretical
- **Sotorasib** is predicted to decrease the exposure to **deutivacaftor**. Avoid. Severe Theoretical
- **St John's wort** is predicted to decrease the exposure to **deutivacaftor**. Avoid. Severe Theoretical
- **Deutivacaftor** is predicted to increase the exposure to **talazoparib**. Moderate Theoretical
- **Deutivacaftor** is predicted to increase the exposure to taxanes **(paclitaxel)**. Moderate Theoretical
- **Tucatinib** is predicted to increase the exposure to **deutivacaftor**. Adjust dose, see deutivacaftor with tezacaftor and vanzacaftor p. 218. Severe Study

Dexamethasone → see corticosteroids

Dexamfetamine → see amfetamines

Dexketoprofen → see NSAIDs

Dexmedetomidine → see TABLE 9 p. 1056 (CNS effects)

Dexrazoxane → see iron chelators

Diamorphine → see opioids

Diazepam → see benzodiazepines

Diazoxide → see TABLE 6 p. 1054 (hypotension)
- **Diazoxide** decreases the concentration of antiepileptics **(fosphenytoin, phenytoin)** and antiepileptics **(fosphenytoin, phenytoin)** are predicted to decrease the effects of **diazoxide**. Monitor concentration and adjust dose. Moderate Anecdotal
- **Diazoxide** increases the risk of severe hypotension when given with **hydralazine**. Severe Study → Also see TABLE 6 p. 1054

Diclofenac → see NSAIDs

Dicycloverine → see TABLE 8 p. 1055 (antimuscarinics)
- Atypical antipsychotics **(clozapine)** can cause constipation, as can **dicycloverine**; concurrent use might increase the risk of developing intestinal obstruction. Severe Theoretical → Also see TABLE 8 p. 1055

Dienogest
- Anti-androgens **(apalutamide, enzalutamide)** are predicted to markedly decrease the exposure to **dienogest**. Severe Study
- Antiarrhythmics **(dronedarone)** are predicted to slightly increase the exposure to **dienogest**. Moderate Study
- Antiepileptics **(carbamazepine, fosphenytoin, phenobarbital, phenytoin, primidone)** are predicted to markedly decrease the exposure to **dienogest**. Severe Study
- Antifungals, azoles **(fluconazole, isavuconazole)** are predicted to slightly increase the exposure to **dienogest**. Moderate Study
- Antifungals, azoles **(itraconazole, ketoconazole, posaconazole, voriconazole)** are predicted to moderately increase the exposure to **dienogest**. Moderate Study
- **Berotralstat** is predicted to slightly increase the exposure to **dienogest**. Moderate Study
- Calcium-channel blockers **(diltiazem, verapamil)** are predicted to slightly increase the exposure to **dienogest**. Moderate Study
- **Ceritinib** is predicted to moderately increase the exposure to **dienogest**. Moderate Study
- **Cobicistat** is predicted to moderately increase the exposure to **dienogest**. Moderate Study
- **Crizotinib** is predicted to slightly increase the exposure to **dienogest**. Moderate Study
- **Encorafenib** is predicted to markedly decrease the exposure to **dienogest**. Severe Study
- **Fedratinib** is predicted to slightly increase the exposure to **dienogest**. Moderate Study
- **HIV-protease inhibitors** are predicted to moderately increase the exposure to **dienogest**. Moderate Study
- **Idelalisib** is predicted to moderately increase the exposure to **dienogest**. Moderate Study
- **Imatinib** is predicted to slightly increase the exposure to **dienogest**. Moderate Study
- **Ivosidenib** is predicted to markedly decrease the exposure to **dienogest**. Severe Study
- **Letermovir** is predicted to slightly increase the exposure to **dienogest**. Moderate Study
- **Lumacaftor** is predicted to markedly decrease the exposure to **dienogest**. Severe Study
- Macrolides **(clarithromycin)** are predicted to moderately increase the exposure to **dienogest**. Moderate Study
- Macrolides **(erythromycin)** are predicted to slightly increase the exposure to **dienogest**. Moderate Study
- **Mitotane** is predicted to markedly decrease the exposure to **dienogest**. Severe Study

- Neurokinin-1 receptor antagonists **(aprepitant, netupitant)** are predicted to slightly increase the exposure to **dienogest**. Moderate Study
- **Nilotinib** is predicted to slightly increase the exposure to **dienogest** Moderate Study
- Rifamycins **(rifampicin)** are predicted to markedly decrease the exposure to **dienogest**. Severe Study
- **Tucatinib** is predicted to moderately increase the exposure to **dienogest**. Moderate Study

Difelikefalin → see TABLE 9 p. 1056 (CNS effects)

Digoxin → see TABLE 4 p. 1054 (bradycardia)

- **Abrocitinib** might increase the exposure to **digoxin**. Moderate Theoretical
- **Acarbose** decreases the concentration of **digoxin**. Moderate Study
- **Aminoglycosides** might increase the concentration of **digoxin**. Monitor and adjust dose. Moderate Study
- Oral **antacids** decrease the absorption of oral **digoxin**. Separate administration by 2 hours. Mild Study
- Anti-androgens **(apalutamide)** are predicted to decrease the exposure to **digoxin**. Mild Study
- Anti-androgens **(enzalutamide)** are predicted to increase the exposure to **digoxin**. Use with caution or avoid. Moderate Theoretical
- Antiarrhythmics **(amiodarone, dronedarone)** are predicted to moderately increase the exposure to **digoxin**. Monitor and adjust **digoxin** dose, p. 91. Severe Study → Also see TABLE 4 p. 1054
- Antiarrhythmics **(propafenone)** increase the concentration of **digoxin**. Monitor and adjust dose. Severe Study → Also see TABLE 4 p. 1054
- Antiepileptics **(fosphenytoin, phenytoin)** are predicted to decrease the concentration of **digoxin**. Moderate Anecdotal
- Antifungals, azoles **(isavuconazole)** slightly increase the exposure to **digoxin**. Monitor and adjust dose. Moderate Study
- Antifungals, azoles **(itraconazole)** increase the concentration of **digoxin**. Monitor and adjust dose. Severe Study
- Antifungals, azoles **(ketoconazole)** are predicted to increase the exposure to **digoxin**. Severe Study
- Antifungals, azoles **(posaconazole)** are predicted to increase the concentration of **digoxin**. Severe Study
- Antimalarials **(mefloquine)** are predicted to increase the risk of bradycardia when given with **digoxin**. Severe Theoretical
- Antimalarials **(quinine)** increase the concentration of **digoxin**. Monitor and adjust **digoxin** dose, p. 91. Severe Anecdotal
- **Asciminib** is predicted to increase the exposure to **digoxin**. Severe Theoretical
- **Balsalazide** is predicted to decrease the concentration of **digoxin**. Moderate Theoretical
- **Belumosudil** might increase the exposure to **digoxin**. Avoid or adjust dose. Moderate Theoretical
- **Berotralstat** is predicted to increase the concentration of **digoxin**. Monitor and adjust dose. Moderate Study
- **Bupropion** might decrease the exposure to **digoxin**. Severe Study
- Intravenous **calcium compounds** increase the effects of **digoxin**. Avoid. Moderate Anecdotal
- Calcium-channel blockers **(diltiazem, verapamil)** increase the concentration of **digoxin**. Monitor and adjust dose. Severe Study → Also see TABLE 4 p. 1054
- **Cannabidiol** is predicted to increase the exposure to **digoxin**. Monitor and adjust dose. Moderate Study
- **Carbimazole** affects the concentration of **digoxin**. Monitor and adjust dose. Moderate Theoretical
- **Ceritinib** is predicted to increase the risk of bradycardia when given with **digoxin**. Avoid. Severe Theoretical → Also see TABLE 4 p. 1054
- **Ciclosporin** increases the concentration of **digoxin**. Monitor and adjust dose. Severe Theoretical
- **Corticosteroids** are predicted to increase the risk of digoxin toxicity when given with **digoxin**. Avoid. Severe Theoretical
- **Dabrafenib** is predicted to decrease the exposure to **digoxin**. Moderate Theoretical
- **Danicopan** is predicted to increase the exposure to **digoxin**. Moderate Study
- **Daridorexant** is predicted to increase the exposure to **digoxin**. Moderate Study
- **Deutivacaftor** is predicted to increase the exposure to **digoxin**. Moderate Theoretical
- **Drugs that reduce serum potassium** (see TABLE 14 p. 1057) are predicted to increase the risk of digoxin toxicity when given with **digoxin**. Severe Study
- **Eliglustat** increases the exposure to **digoxin**. Adjust dose. Moderate Study
- **Erdafitinib** is predicted to increase the exposure to **digoxin**. Separate administration by at least 6 hours. Moderate Theoretical
- **Glecaprevir** with pibrentasvir increases the exposure to **digoxin**. Moderate Study
- Glucagon-like peptide-1 receptor agonists **(tirzepatide)** might affect the absorption of **digoxin**. Moderate Theoretical
- HIV-protease inhibitors **(lopinavir)** boosted with ritonavir are predicted to increase the exposure to **digoxin**. Severe Theoretical
- HIV-protease inhibitors **(ritonavir)** increase the concentration of **digoxin**. Adjust dose and monitor concentration. Severe Study
- **Ibrutinib** might increase the exposure to **digoxin**. Separate administration by at least 6 hours. Moderate Theoretical
- **Ivacaftor** slightly increases the exposure to **digoxin**. Moderate Study
- **Ivosidenib** is predicted to alter the exposure to **digoxin**. Moderate Theoretical
- **Lapatinib** slightly increases the exposure to **digoxin**. Moderate Study
- **Ledipasvir** is predicted to increase the exposure to **digoxin**. Monitor and adjust dose. Moderate Theoretical
- **Lenacapavir** is predicted to increase the concentration of **digoxin**. Moderate Theoretical
- **Lomitapide** might increase the exposure to **digoxin**. Adjust dose. Moderate Theoretical
- **Lorlatinib** is predicted to decrease the exposure to **digoxin**. Moderate Study
- **Macrolides** increase the concentration of **digoxin**. Severe Anecdotal
- **Maribavir** very slightly increases the exposure to **digoxin**. Monitor and adjust dose. Moderate Study
- Mineralocorticoid receptor antagonists **(eplerenone)** very slightly increase the exposure to **digoxin**. Mild Study
- Mineralocorticoid receptor antagonists **(spironolactone)** increase the concentration of **digoxin**. Monitor and adjust dose. Moderate Study
- **Mirabegron** slightly increases the exposure to **digoxin**. Monitor concentration and adjust dose. Severe Study
- **Neomycin** decreases the concentration of **digoxin**. Moderate Study
- **Neratinib** slightly increases the exposure to **digoxin**. Moderate Study
- Neuromuscular blocking drugs, non-depolarising **(pancuronium)** are predicted to increase the risk of cardiovascular adverse effects when given with **digoxin**. Severe Anecdotal
- **Nirmatrelvir** boosted with ritonavir is predicted to increase the concentration of **digoxin**. Severe Theoretical
- NSAIDs **(indometacin)** increase the concentration of **digoxin**. Severe Study
- **Olaparib** might increase the exposure to **digoxin**. Moderate Theoretical
- **Osimertinib** is predicted to increase the exposure to **digoxin**. Moderate Study
- **Pemigatinib** might increase the exposure to **digoxin**. Separate administration by at least 6 hours. Moderate Theoretical
- **Penicillamine** potentially decreases the concentration of **digoxin**. Separate administration by 2 hours. Severe Anecdotal
- **Pibrentasvir** with glecaprevir increases the exposure to **digoxin**. Moderate Study
- **Pirtobrutinib** slightly increases the exposure to **digoxin**. Avoid or monitor. Moderate Study
- **Pitolisant** is predicted to decrease the exposure to **digoxin**. Mild Theoretical
- **Ranolazine** increases the concentration of **digoxin**. Moderate Study
- **Ribociclib** is predicted to increase the exposure to **digoxin**. Moderate Theoretical

Digoxin (continued)

- Rifamycins **(rifampicin)** decrease the concentration of **digoxin**. Moderate Study
- **Selpercatinib** is predicted to increase the exposure to **digoxin**. Moderate Study
- **Sotorasib** very slightly increases the exposure to **digoxin**. Avoid or adjust dose. Moderate Study
- **Sparsentan** is predicted to increase the exposure to **digoxin**. Severe Theoretical
- **St John's wort** decreases the concentration of **digoxin**. Avoid. Severe Anecdotal
- **Sucralfate** decreases the absorption of **digoxin**. Separate administration by 2 hours. Severe Anecdotal
- **Sulfasalazine** decreases the concentration of **digoxin**. Moderate Study
- **Suxamethonium** is predicted to increase the risk of cardiovascular adverse effects when given with **digoxin**. Severe Anecdotal → Also see **TABLE 4** p. 1054
- **Tepotinib** is predicted to increase the concentration of **digoxin**. Severe Study
- **Thyroid hormones** are predicted to affect the concentration of **digoxin**. Monitor and adjust dose. Moderate Theoretical
- **Ticagrelor** increases the concentration of **digoxin**. Moderate Study → Also see **TABLE 4** p. 1054
- **Tolvaptan** slightly increases the exposure to **digoxin**. Moderate Study
- **Trimethoprim** increases the concentration of **digoxin**. Moderate Study
- **Tucatinib** slightly increases the exposure to **digoxin**. Use with caution and adjust dose. Moderate Study
- **Vandetanib** very slightly increases the exposure to **digoxin**. Moderate Study
- **Velpatasvir** is predicted to increase the exposure to **digoxin**. Severe Study
- **Vemurafenib** slightly increases the exposure to **digoxin**. Use with caution and adjust dose. Severe Study
- **Venetoclax** increases the exposure to **digoxin**. Avoid or adjust dose. Severe Study
- **Vitamin D substances** are predicted to increase the risk of toxicity when given with **digoxin**. Severe Theoretical
- **Voclosporin** slightly increases the exposure to **digoxin**. Moderate Study
- **Voxilaprevir** with sofosbuvir and velpatasvir is predicted to increase the exposure to **digoxin**. Monitor and adjust dose. Severe Theoretical

Dihydrocodeine → see opioids

Diltiazem → see calcium-channel blockers

Dimenhydrinate → see **TABLE 8** p. 1055 (antimuscarinics), **TABLE 9** p. 1056 (CNS effects)

- Atypical antipsychotics **(clozapine)** can cause constipation, as can **dimenhydrinate**; concurrent use might increase the risk of developing intestinal obstruction. Severe Theoretical → Also see **TABLE 8** p. 1055 → Also see **TABLE 9** p. 1056

Dimethyl fumarate

- **Alcohol** (excessive consumption) potentially increases the risk of gastrointestinal adverse effects when given with **dimethyl fumarate**. Avoid. Moderate Theoretical
- **Live vaccines** are predicted to increase the risk of generalised infection (possibly life-threatening) when given with **dimethyl fumarate**. UKHSA advises avoid (refer to Green Book). Severe Theoretical

Dinutuximab → see monoclonal antibodies

Dipeptidylpeptidase-4 inhibitors

alogliptin · linagliptin · saxagliptin · sitagliptin · vildagliptin

- Anti-androgens **(apalutamide, enzalutamide)** are predicted to decrease the exposure to **linagliptin**. Moderate Study
- Anti-androgens **(apalutamide, enzalutamide)** are predicted to moderately decrease the exposure to **saxagliptin**. Moderate Study
- Antiarrhythmics **(dronedarone)** are predicted to increase the exposure to **saxagliptin**. Mild Study
- Antiepileptics **(carbamazepine, fosphenytoin, phenobarbital, phenytoin, primidone)** are predicted to decrease the exposure to **linagliptin**. Moderate Study
- Antiepileptics **(carbamazepine, fosphenytoin, phenobarbital, phenytoin, primidone)** are predicted to moderately decrease the exposure to **saxagliptin**. Moderate Study
- Antifungals, azoles **(fluconazole, isavuconazole)** are predicted to increase the exposure to **saxagliptin**. Mild Study
- Antifungals, azoles **(itraconazole, ketoconazole, posaconazole, voriconazole)** are predicted to increase the exposure to **saxagliptin**. Moderate Study
- **Berotralstat** is predicted to increase the exposure to **saxagliptin**. Mild Study
- Calcium-channel blockers **(diltiazem, verapamil)** are predicted to increase the exposure to **saxagliptin**. Mild Study
- **Ceritinib** is predicted to increase the exposure to **saxagliptin**. Moderate Study
- **Cobicistat** is predicted to increase the exposure to **saxagliptin**. Moderate Study
- **Crizotinib** is predicted to increase the exposure to **saxagliptin**. Mild Study
- **Encorafenib** is predicted to decrease the exposure to **linagliptin**. Moderate Study
- **Encorafenib** is predicted to moderately decrease the exposure to **saxagliptin**. Moderate Study
- **Fedratinib** is predicted to increase the exposure to **saxagliptin**. Mild Study
- **Fenfluramine** might decrease blood glucose concentrations when given with **dipeptidylpeptidase-4 inhibitors**. Moderate Theoretical
- **Grapefruit** juice is predicted to increase the exposure to **saxagliptin**. Mild Theoretical
- **HIV-protease inhibitors** are predicted to increase the exposure to **saxagliptin**. Moderate Study
- **Idelalisib** is predicted to increase the exposure to **saxagliptin**. Moderate Study
- **Imatinib** is predicted to increase the exposure to **saxagliptin**. Mild Study
- **Ivosidenib** is predicted to decrease the exposure to **linagliptin**. Moderate Study
- **Ivosidenib** is predicted to moderately decrease the exposure to **saxagliptin**. Moderate Study
- **Letermovir** is predicted to increase the exposure to **saxagliptin**. Mild Study
- **Linagliptin** is predicted to increase the exposure to **lomitapide**. Separate administration by 12 hours. Moderate Theoretical
- **Lumacaftor** is predicted to decrease the exposure to **linagliptin**. Moderate Study
- **Lumacaftor** is predicted to moderately decrease the exposure to **saxagliptin**. Moderate Study
- Macrolides **(clarithromycin)** are predicted to increase the exposure to **saxagliptin**. Moderate Study
- Macrolides **(erythromycin)** are predicted to increase the exposure to **saxagliptin**. Mild Study
- **Mitotane** is predicted to decrease the exposure to **linagliptin**. Moderate Study
- **Mitotane** is predicted to moderately decrease the exposure to **saxagliptin**. Moderate Study
- Neurokinin-1 receptor antagonists **(aprepitant, netupitant)** are predicted to increase the exposure to **saxagliptin**. Mild Study
- **Nilotinib** is predicted to increase the exposure to **saxagliptin**. Mild Study
- **Nirmatrelvir** boosted with ritonavir is predicted to increase the concentration of **saxagliptin**. Adjust dose. Moderate Theoretical
- Rifamycins **(rifampicin)** are predicted to decrease the exposure to **linagliptin**. Moderate Study
- Rifamycins **(rifampicin)** are predicted to moderately decrease the exposure to **saxagliptin**. Moderate Study
- **Selpercatinib** is predicted to increase the exposure to **saxagliptin**. Moderate Study
- **Somapacitan** might increase blood glucose concentrations, opposing the blood glucose-lowering effects of **dipeptidylpeptidase-4 inhibitors**. Adjust dose. Moderate Theoretical
- **Somatrogon** might increase blood glucose concentrations, opposing the blood glucose-lowering effects of **dipeptidylpeptidase-4 inhibitors**. Adjust dose. Moderate Theoretical

A1 Interactions | Appendix 1

- **Tucatinib** is predicted to increase the exposure to **saxagliptin**. Moderate Study
- **Vemurafenib** is predicted to increase the exposure to **sitagliptin**. Use with caution or avoid. Moderate Theoretical

Diphenoxylate → see opioids

Dipipanone → see opioids

Dipyridamole → see TABLE 3 p. 1053 (bleeding), TABLE 6 p. 1054 (hypotension)

- Oral **antacids** are predicted to decrease the absorption of oral **dipyridamole** (immediate release tablets). Moderate Theoretical
- **Dipyridamole** increases the exposure to antiarrhythmics **(adenosine)**. Avoid or adjust dose. Severe Study
- **Dipyridamole** might increase the exposure to **cladribine**. Moderate Theoretical
- **H_2 receptor antagonists** are predicted to decrease the absorption of **dipyridamole** (immediate release tablets). Moderate Theoretical
- **Proton pump inhibitors** are predicted to decrease the absorption of **dipyridamole** (immediate release tablets). Moderate Theoretical
- **Selumetinib** might increase the risk of bleeding when given with **dipyridamole**. Moderate Theoretical

Diroximel fumarate

- **Live vaccines** are predicted to increase the risk of generalised infection (possibly life-threatening) when given with **diroximel fumarate**. Use with caution or avoid. Severe Theoretical

Disopyramide → see antiarrhythmics

Disulfiram

- **Alcohol** causes an extremely unpleasant systemic reaction when given with **disulfiram**. Avoid for at least 24 hours before and up to 14 days after stopping treatment. Severe Study
- **Disulfiram** increases the concentration of antiepileptics **(fosphenytoin, phenytoin)**. Monitor concentration and adjust dose. Severe Study
- **Disulfiram** increases the anticoagulant effect of **coumarins**. Monitor and adjust dose. Severe Study
- **Methylphenidate** has been reported to cause psychotic symptoms when given with **disulfiram**. Severe Anecdotal
- **Disulfiram** increases the risk of acute psychoses when given with **metronidazole**. Severe Study
- **Disulfiram** is predicted to increase the anticoagulant effect of **phenindione**. Severe Theoretical

Dobutamine → see sympathomimetics, inotropic

Docetaxel → see taxanes

Docusates

ROUTE SPECIFIC INFORMATION Interactions do not generally apply to topical use of **docusates** unless specified.

- Oral **docusates** might decrease the concentration of the active metabolite of oral **baloxavir marboxil**. Severe Theoretical

Dolutegravir

- Oral **antacids** decrease the exposure to oral **dolutegravir**. Manufacturer advises take 2 hours before or 6 hours after antacids. Moderate Study
- Anti-androgens **(apalutamide, enzalutamide)** are predicted to decrease the exposure to **dolutegravir**. Severe Study
- Antiepileptics **(carbamazepine)** decrease the exposure to **dolutegravir**. Adjust **dolutegravir** dose, p. 508. Severe Study
- Antiepileptics **(fosphenytoin, phenobarbital, phenytoin, primidone)** are predicted to decrease the exposure to **dolutegravir**. Adjust **dolutegravir** dose, p. 508. Severe Study
- Antiepileptics **(oxcarbazepine)** are predicted to decrease the exposure to **dolutegravir**. Adjust **dolutegravir** dose, p. 508. Severe Theoretical
- Oral **calcium compounds** decrease the absorption of oral **dolutegravir**. **Dolutegravir** should be taken 2 hours before or 6 hours after calcium. Moderate Study
- **Dabrafenib** is predicted to decrease the exposure to **dolutegravir**. Severe Study
- **Dolutegravir** is predicted to increase the exposure to dopamine receptor agonists **(pramipexole)**. Adjust dose. Moderate Study
- **Encorafenib** is predicted to increase the exposure to **dolutegravir**. Moderate Theoretical
- Endothelin receptor antagonists **(bosentan)** are predicted to decrease the exposure to **dolutegravir**. Severe Study
- **Dolutegravir** might increase the concentration of **fampridine**. Avoid. Severe Theoretical
- HIV-protease inhibitors **(atazanavir)** (alone or boosted with ritonavir) slightly increase the exposure to **dolutegravir**. Adjust dose—consult product literature. Moderate Study
- HIV-protease inhibitors **(fosamprenavir)** boosted with ritonavir slightly decrease the exposure to **dolutegravir**. Avoid if resistant to HIV-integrase inhibitors. Severe Study
- Oral **iron** decreases the absorption of oral **dolutegravir**. **Dolutegravir** should be taken 2 hours before or 6 hours after iron. Moderate Study
- **Dolutegravir** is predicted to increase the exposure to **metformin**. Use with caution and adjust dose. Moderate Study
- **Mitotane** is predicted to decrease the exposure to **dolutegravir**. Severe Study
- NNRTIs **(efavirenz)** moderately decrease the exposure to **dolutegravir**. Adjust **dolutegravir** dose, p. 508. Severe Study
- NNRTIs **(etravirine)** moderately decrease the exposure to **dolutegravir**. Adjust **dolutegravir** dose unless given with atazanavir, darunavir, or lopinavir (all boosted with ritonavir), p. 508. Severe Study
- NNRTIs **(nevirapine)** are predicted to decrease the exposure to **dolutegravir**. Adjust **dolutegravir** dose, p. 508. Severe Study
- Rifamycins **(rifampicin)** moderately decrease the exposure to **dolutegravir**. Adjust **dolutegravir** dose, p. 508. Severe Study
- **St John's wort** is predicted to decrease the exposure to **dolutegravir**. Adjust **dolutegravir** dose, p. 508. Severe Study
- **Sucralfate** decreases the absorption of **dolutegravir**. Moderate Study

Domperidone → see TABLE 7 p. 1055 (QT-interval prolongation)

- Antiarrhythmics **(dronedarone)** are predicted to increase the exposure to **domperidone**. Avoid. Severe Study
- Antifungals, azoles **(fluconazole, isavuconazole, itraconazole, ketoconazole, posaconazole, voriconazole)** are predicted to increase the exposure to **domperidone**. Avoid. Severe Study
- **Berotralstat** is predicted to increase the exposure to **domperidone**. Avoid. Severe Study
- Calcium-channel blockers **(diltiazem, verapamil)** are predicted to increase the exposure to **domperidone**. Avoid. Severe Study
- **Ceritinib** is predicted to increase the exposure to **domperidone**. Avoid. Severe Study
- **Cobicistat** is predicted to increase the exposure to **domperidone**. Avoid. Severe Study
- **Crizotinib** is predicted to increase the exposure to **domperidone**. Avoid. Severe Study
- **Domperidone** is predicted to decrease the prolactin-lowering effect of dopamine receptor agonists **(bromocriptine, cabergoline)**. Moderate Theoretical
- **Fedratinib** is predicted to increase the exposure to **domperidone**. Avoid. Severe Study
- **HIV-protease inhibitors** are predicted to increase the exposure to **domperidone**. Avoid. Severe Study
- **Idelalisib** is predicted to increase the exposure to **domperidone**. Avoid. Severe Study
- **Imatinib** is predicted to increase the exposure to **domperidone**. Avoid. Severe Study
- **Letermovir** is predicted to increase the exposure to **domperidone**. Avoid. Severe Study
- Macrolides **(clarithromycin, erythromycin)** are predicted to increase the exposure to **domperidone**. Avoid. Severe Study
- Neurokinin-1 receptor antagonists **(aprepitant, netupitant)** are predicted to increase the exposure to **domperidone**. Avoid. Severe Study
- **Nilotinib** is predicted to increase the exposure to **domperidone**. Avoid. Severe Study
- **Tucatinib** is predicted to increase the exposure to **domperidone**. Avoid. Severe Study

Donanemab

- **Donanemab** might increase the risk of brain haemorrhage when given with **alteplase**. Avoid except in life-threatening situations. Severe Theoretical
- **Donanemab** can increase the risk of brain haemorrhage when given with **coumarins**. Avoid. Severe Anecdotal
- **Donanemab** can increase the risk of brain haemorrhage when given with **danaparoid**. Avoid. Severe Anecdotal

Donanemab (continued)

- **Donanemab** can increase the risk of brain haemorrhage when given with **factor XA inhibitors**. Avoid. Severe Anecdotal
- **Donanemab** can increase the risk of brain haemorrhage when given with **heparin**. Avoid. Severe Anecdotal
- **Donanemab** can increase the risk of brain haemorrhage when given with **low molecular-weight heparins**. Avoid. Severe Anecdotal
- **Donanemab** can increase the risk of brain haemorrhage when given with **phenindione**. Avoid. Severe Anecdotal
- **Donanemab** might increase the risk of brain haemorrhage when given with **streptokinase**. Avoid except in life-threatening situations. Severe Theoretical
- **Donanemab** might increase the risk of brain haemorrhage when given with **tenecteplase**. Avoid except in life-threatening situations. Severe Theoretical
- **Donanemab** can increase the risk of brain haemorrhage when given with **thrombin inhibitors**. Avoid. Severe Anecdotal
- **Donanemab** might increase the risk of brain haemorrhage when given with **urokinase**. Avoid except in life-threatening situations. Severe Theoretical

Donepezil → see anticholinesterases, centrally acting

Dopamine → see sympathomimetics, inotropic

Dopamine receptor agonists → see TABLE 6 p. 1054 (hypotension), TABLE 7 p. 1055 (QT-interval prolongation), TABLE 8 p. 1055 (antimuscarinics), TABLE 9 p. 1056 (CNS effects)

amantadine · apomorphine · bromocriptine · cabergoline · pramipexole · quinagolide · ropinirole · rotigotine

FOOD AND LIFESTYLE Dose adjustment might be necessary if smoking started or stopped during treatment with **ropinirole**.

- **Apomorphine** is predicted to increase the risk of severe hypotension when given with 5-HT3-receptor antagonists **(granisetron, palonosetron)**. Severe Theoretical
- **Apomorphine** increases the risk of severe hypotension when given with 5-HT3-receptor antagonists **(ondansetron)**. Avoid. Severe Study → Also see TABLE 7 p. 1055
- Antiarrhythmics **(dronedarone)** are predicted to increase the exposure to **bromocriptine**. Severe Theoretical
- Antiarrhythmics **(dronedarone)** are predicted to increase the concentration of **cabergoline**. Severe Anecdotal
- Antifungals, azoles **(fluconazole, isavuconazole)** are predicted to increase the exposure to **bromocriptine**. Severe Theoretical
- Antifungals, azoles **(fluconazole, isavuconazole, itraconazole, ketoconazole, posaconazole, voriconazole)** are predicted to increase the concentration of **cabergoline**. Moderate Anecdotal
- Antifungals, azoles **(isavuconazole)** are predicted to increase the exposure to **pramipexole**. Adjust dose. Moderate Study
- Antifungals, azoles **(itraconazole, ketoconazole, posaconazole, voriconazole)** increase the exposure to **bromocriptine**. Severe Study
- Atypical antipsychotics **(amisulpride, olanzapine, paliperidone, quetiapine, risperidone)** are predicted to decrease the effects of **dopamine receptor agonists**. Avoid. Moderate Theoretical → Also see TABLE 6 p. 1054 → Also see TABLE 7 p. 1055 → Also see TABLE 8 p. 1055 → Also see TABLE 9 p. 1056
- Atypical antipsychotics **(aripiprazole, clozapine)** are predicted to decrease the effects of **dopamine receptor agonists**. Moderate Theoretical → Also see TABLE 6 p. 1054 → Also see TABLE 8 p. 1055 → Also see TABLE 9 p. 1056
- Atypical antipsychotics **(asenapine)** are predicted to decrease the effects of **dopamine receptor agonists**. Adjust dose. Moderate Theoretical → Also see TABLE 6 p. 1054 → Also see TABLE 9 p. 1056
- **Axitinib** is predicted to increase the exposure to **ropinirole**. Moderate Theoretical
- **Benperidol** is predicted to decrease the effects of **dopamine receptor agonists**. Avoid. Moderate Theoretical → Also see TABLE 6 p. 1054 → Also see TABLE 9 p. 1056
- **Berotralstat** is predicted to increase the exposure to **bromocriptine**. Severe Theoretical
- **Bupropion** increases the risk of adverse effects when given with **amantadine**. Moderate Study
- Calcium-channel blockers **(diltiazem, verapamil)** are predicted to increase the exposure to **bromocriptine**. Severe Theoretical → Also see TABLE 6 p. 1054
- Calcium-channel blockers **(diltiazem, verapamil)** are predicted to increase the concentration of **cabergoline**. Moderate Anecdotal → Also see TABLE 6 p. 1054
- **Ceritinib** increases the exposure to **bromocriptine**. Severe Study
- **Cobicistat** increases the exposure to **bromocriptine**. Severe Study
- **Cobicistat** is predicted to increase the concentration of **cabergoline**. Moderate Anecdotal
- **Combined hormonal contraceptives** is predicted to increase the exposure to **ropinirole**. Adjust dose. Moderate Study
- **Crizotinib** is predicted to increase the exposure to **bromocriptine**. Severe Theoretical
- **Crizotinib** is predicted to increase the concentration of **cabergoline**. Moderate Anecdotal
- **Dolutegravir** is predicted to increase the exposure to **pramipexole**. Adjust dose. Moderate Study
- **Domperidone** is predicted to decrease the prolactin-lowering effect of dopamine receptor agonists **(bromocriptine, cabergoline)**. Moderate Theoretical
- Dopamine receptor agonists **(cabergoline)** are predicted to increase the risk of ergotism when given with dopamine receptor agonists **(bromocriptine)**. Avoid. Moderate Theoretical → Also see TABLE 6 p. 1054 → Also see TABLE 9 p. 1056
- Dopamine receptor agonists **(amantadine)** are predicted to increase the exposure to dopamine receptor agonists **(pramipexole)**. Adjust dose. Moderate Theoretical → Also see TABLE 6 p. 1054
- **Droperidol** is predicted to decrease the effects of **dopamine receptor agonists**. Avoid. Moderate Theoretical → Also see TABLE 6 p. 1054 → Also see TABLE 7 p. 1055 → Also see TABLE 9 p. 1056
- **Ergometrine** is predicted to increase the risk of ergotism when given with **cabergoline**. Avoid. Moderate Theoretical
- **Fedratinib** is predicted to increase the exposure to **bromocriptine**. Severe Theoretical
- **Flupentixol** is predicted to decrease the effects of **dopamine receptor agonists**. Avoid. Moderate Theoretical → Also see TABLE 6 p. 1054 → Also see TABLE 8 p. 1055 → Also see TABLE 9 p. 1056
- **Amantadine** might increase the adverse effects of **foslevodopa**. Adjust dose. Moderate Theoretical → Also see TABLE 6 p. 1054
- **Givosiran** is predicted to increase the exposure to **ropinirole**. Adjust dose. Moderate Study
- H_2 receptor antagonists **(cimetidine)** are predicted to increase the exposure to **pramipexole**. Adjust dose. Moderate Study
- **Haloperidol** is predicted to decrease the effects of **dopamine receptor agonists**. Avoid. Moderate Theoretical → Also see TABLE 6 p. 1054 → Also see TABLE 7 p. 1055 → Also see TABLE 8 p. 1055 → Also see TABLE 9 p. 1056
- **HIV-protease inhibitors** increase the exposure to **bromocriptine**. Severe Study
- **HIV-protease inhibitors** are predicted to increase the concentration of **cabergoline**. Moderate Anecdotal
- **Hormone replacement therapy** decreases the clearance of **ropinirole**. Monitor and adjust dose. Moderate Study
- **Idelalisib** increases the exposure to **bromocriptine**. Severe Study
- **Idelalisib** is predicted to increase the concentration of **cabergoline**. Moderate Anecdotal
- **Imatinib** is predicted to increase the exposure to **bromocriptine**. Severe Theoretical
- **Imatinib** is predicted to increase the concentration of **cabergoline**. Moderate Anecdotal
- **Letermovir** is predicted to increase the exposure to **bromocriptine**. Severe Theoretical
- **Loxapine** is predicted to decrease the effects of **dopamine receptor agonists**. Moderate Theoretical → Also see TABLE 6 p. 1054 → Also see TABLE 8 p. 1055 → Also see TABLE 9 p. 1056
- Macrolides **(clarithromycin)** increase the exposure to **bromocriptine**. Severe Study
- Macrolides **(clarithromycin, erythromycin)** are predicted to increase the concentration of **cabergoline**. Avoid. Severe Study
- Macrolides **(erythromycin)** are predicted to increase the exposure to **bromocriptine**. Severe Theoretical
- **Amantadine** increases the risk of CNS toxicity when given with **memantine**. Use with caution or avoid. Severe Theoretical
- **Memantine** is predicted to increase the effects of dopamine receptor agonists **(apomorphine, bromocriptine, cabergoline,**

A1 Interactions | Appendix 1

pramipexole, quinagolide, ropinirole, rotigotine). Moderate Theoretical
- **Metoclopramide** is predicted to decrease the effects of dopamine receptor agonists **(apomorphine, bromocriptine, cabergoline, pramipexole, quinagolide, ropinirole, rotigotine).** Avoid. Moderate Study
- **Mexiletine** is predicted to increase the exposure to **ropinirole.** Adjust dose. Moderate Study
- Neurokinin-1 receptor antagonists **(aprepitant, netupitant)** are predicted to increase the exposure to **bromocriptine.** Severe Theoretical
- Neurokinin-1 receptor antagonists **(aprepitant, netupitant)** are predicted to increase the concentration of **cabergoline.** Moderate Anecdotal
- **Nilotinib** is predicted to increase the exposure to **bromocriptine.** Severe Theoretical
- **Nilotinib** is predicted to increase the concentration of **cabergoline.** Moderate Anecdotal
- **Osilodrostat** is predicted to increase the exposure to **ropinirole.** Adjust dose. Moderate Study
- **Phenothiazine antipsychotics** are predicted to decrease the effects of **dopamine receptor agonists.** Avoid. Moderate Theoretical → Also see **TABLE 6** p. 1054 → Also see **TABLE 7** p. 1055 → Also see **TABLE 8** p. 1055 → Also see **TABLE 9** p. 1056
- **Pimozide** is predicted to decrease the effects of **dopamine receptor agonists.** Avoid. Moderate Theoretical → Also see **TABLE 6** p. 1054 → Also see **TABLE 7** p. 1055 → Also see **TABLE 8** p. 1055 → Also see **TABLE 9** p. 1056
- Quinolones **(ciprofloxacin)** are predicted to increase the exposure to **ropinirole.** Adjust dose. Moderate Study
- **Ranolazine** is predicted to increase the exposure to **pramipexole.** Adjust dose. Moderate Study
- **Rucaparib** is predicted to increase the exposure to **ropinirole.** Adjust dose. Moderate Study
- SSRIs **(fluvoxamine)** are predicted to increase the exposure to **ropinirole.** Adjust dose. Moderate Study → Also see **TABLE 9** p. 1056
- **Sulpiride** is predicted to decrease the effects of **dopamine receptor agonists.** Avoid. Moderate Theoretical → Also see **TABLE 6** p. 1054 → Also see **TABLE 9** p. 1056
- Sympathomimetics, vasoconstrictor **(isometheptene)** potentially increase the risk of adverse effects when given with **bromocriptine.** Avoid. Severe Anecdotal
- **Trimethoprim** is predicted to increase the exposure to **pramipexole.** Adjust dose. Moderate Study
- **Tucatinib** increases the exposure to **bromocriptine.** Severe Study
- **Vandetanib** is predicted to increase the exposure to **pramipexole.** Adjust dose. Moderate Study
- **Vemurafenib** is predicted to increase the exposure to **ropinirole.** Adjust dose. Moderate Study
- **Zuclopenthixol** is predicted to decrease the effects of **dopamine receptor agonists.** Avoid. Moderate Theoretical → Also see **TABLE 6** p. 1054 → Also see **TABLE 8** p. 1055 → Also see **TABLE 9** p. 1056

Doravirine → see NNRTIs

Dorzolamide

ROUTE-SPECIFIC INFORMATION Since systemic absorption can follow topical application of **dorzolamide**, the possibility of interactions should be borne in mind.

Dostarlimab → see monoclonal antibodies

Dosulepin → see tricyclic antidepressants

Doxapram
- **Aminophylline** increases the risk of agitation when given with **doxapram.** Moderate Study
- **MAOIs, irreversible** are predicted to increase the effects of **doxapram.** Moderate Theoretical
- **Theophylline** increases the risk of agitation when given with **doxapram.** Moderate Study

Doxazosin → see alpha blockers

Doxepin → see tricyclic antidepressants

Doxorubicin → see anthracyclines

Doxycycline → see tetracyclines

Doxylamine → see antihistamines, sedating

Dronabinol → see **TABLE 9** p. 1056 (CNS effects)
- Anti-androgens **(apalutamide, enzalutamide)** are predicted to decrease the exposure to **dronabinol.** Avoid or adjust dose. Mild Study
- Antiepileptics **(carbamazepine, fosphenytoin, phenobarbital, phenytoin, primidone)** are predicted to decrease the exposure to **dronabinol.** Avoid or adjust dose. Mild Study → Also see **TABLE 9** p. 1056
- Antifungals, azoles **(itraconazole, ketoconazole, posaconazole, voriconazole)** are predicted to increase the exposure to **dronabinol.** Adjust dose. Mild Study
- **Ceritinib** is predicted to increase the exposure to **dronabinol.** Adjust dose. Mild Study
- **Cobicistat** is predicted to increase the exposure to **dronabinol.** Adjust dose. Mild Study
- **Encorafenib** is predicted to decrease the exposure to **dronabinol.** Avoid or adjust dose. Mild Study
- **HIV-protease inhibitors** are predicted to increase the exposure to **dronabinol.** Adjust dose. Mild Study
- **Idelalisib** is predicted to increase the exposure to **dronabinol.** Adjust dose. Mild Study
- **Ivosidenib** is predicted to decrease the exposure to **dronabinol.** Avoid or adjust dose. Mild Study
- **Lumacaftor** is predicted to decrease the exposure to **dronabinol.** Avoid or adjust dose. Mild Study
- Macrolides **(clarithromycin)** are predicted to increase the exposure to **dronabinol.** Adjust dose. Mild Study
- **Mitotane** is predicted to decrease the exposure to **dronabinol.** Avoid or adjust dose. Mild Study
- Rifamycins **(rifampicin)** are predicted to decrease the exposure to **dronabinol.** Avoid or adjust dose. Mild Study
- **St John's wort** is predicted to decrease the exposure to **dronabinol.** Avoid or adjust dose. Mild Study
- **Tucatinib** is predicted to increase the exposure to **dronabinol.** Adjust dose. Mild Study

Dronedarone → see antiarrhythmics

Droperidol → see **TABLE 15** p. 1058 (hyponatraemia), **TABLE 6** p. 1054 (hypotension), **TABLE 7** p. 1055 (QT-interval prolongation), **TABLE 9** p. 1056 (CNS effects)
- **Droperidol** is predicted to decrease the effects of **dopamine receptor agonists.** Avoid. Moderate Theoretical → Also see **TABLE 6** p. 1054 → Also see **TABLE 7** p. 1055 → Also see **TABLE 9** p. 1056
- **Droperidol** opposes the effects of the active metabolite of **foslevodopa.** Severe Theoretical → Also see **TABLE 6** p. 1054 → Also see **TABLE 9** p. 1056
- **Droperidol** decreases the effects of **levodopa.** Severe Study → Also see **TABLE 6** p. 1054 → Also see **TABLE 9** p. 1056

Drospirenone → see **TABLE 13** p. 1057 (increased serum potassium)
- Antiarrhythmics **(dronedarone)** are predicted to increase the exposure to **drospirenone.** Severe Study
- Antiepileptics **(carbamazepine, eslicarbazepine, fosphenytoin, oxcarbazepine, perampanel, phenobarbital, phenytoin, primidone, rufinamide, topiramate)** are predicted to decrease the efficacy of **drospirenone.** For CoSRH guidance, see Contraceptives, interactions p. 614. Severe Theoretical
- Antiepileptics **(lamotrigine)** might decrease the effects of **drospirenone.** For CoSRH guidance, see Contraceptives, interactions p. 614. Severe Theoretical
- Antifungals, azoles **(fluconazole, isavuconazole, itraconazole, posaconazole, voriconazole)** are predicted to increase the exposure to **drospirenone.** Severe Study
- Antifungals, azoles **(ketoconazole)** moderately increase the exposure to **drospirenone.** Severe Study
- **Berotralstat** is predicted to increase the exposure to **drospirenone.** Severe Study
- Calcium-channel blockers **(diltiazem, verapamil)** are predicted to increase the exposure to **drospirenone.** Severe Study
- **Cobicistat** is predicted to increase the exposure to **drospirenone.** Severe Study
- **Crizotinib** is predicted to increase the exposure to **drospirenone.** Severe Study
- Endothelin receptor antagonists **(bosentan)** are predicted to decrease the efficacy of **drospirenone.** For CoSRH guidance, see Contraceptives, interactions p. 614. Severe Theoretical
- **Fedratinib** is predicted to increase the exposure to **drospirenone.** Severe Study

Drospirenone (continued)
- Glucagon-like peptide-1 receptor agonists **(tirzepatide)** might affect the absorption of **drospirenone**. Manufacturer advises precautions for those who are overweight or obese. Moderate Study
- HIV-protease inhibitors **(atazanavir, darunavir, fosamprenavir, lopinavir)** are predicted to increase the exposure to **drospirenone**. Severe Study
- HIV-protease inhibitors **(ritonavir)** are predicted to decrease the efficacy of **drospirenone**. For CoSRH guidance, see Contraceptives, interactions p. 614. Severe Theoretical
- **Idelalisib** is predicted to increase the exposure to **drospirenone**. Severe Study
- **Imatinib** is predicted to increase the exposure to **drospirenone**. Severe Study
- **Letermovir** is predicted to increase the exposure to **drospirenone**. Severe Study
- **Lumacaftor** is predicted to decrease the efficacy of **drospirenone**. Use additional contraceptive precautions. Severe Theoretical
- Macrolides **(clarithromycin, erythromycin)** are predicted to increase the exposure to **drospirenone**. Severe Study
- **Modafinil** is predicted to decrease the efficacy of **drospirenone**. For CoSRH guidance, see Contraceptives, interactions p. 614. Severe Theoretical
- Neurokinin-1 receptor antagonists **(aprepitant, fosaprepitant)** are predicted to decrease the efficacy of **drospirenone**. For CoSRH guidance, see Contraceptives, interactions p. 614. Severe Theoretical
- Neurokinin-1 receptor antagonists **(netupitant)** are predicted to increase the exposure to **drospirenone**. Severe Study
- **Nilotinib** is predicted to increase the exposure to **drospirenone**. Severe Study
- NNRTIs **(efavirenz, nevirapine)** are predicted to decrease the efficacy of **drospirenone**. For CoSRH guidance, see Contraceptives, interactions p. 614. Severe Theoretical
- NNRTIs **(etravirine)** might decrease the efficacy of **drospirenone**. Follow CoSRH guidance for enzyme inducers, see Contraceptives, interactions p. 614. Severe Theoretical
- **Rifamycins** are predicted to decrease the efficacy of **drospirenone**. For CoSRH guidance, see Contraceptives, interactions p. 614. Severe Theoretical
- **St John's wort** is predicted to decrease the efficacy of **drospirenone**. For CoSRH guidance, see Contraceptives, interactions p. 614. Severe Theoretical
- **Sugammadex** is predicted to decrease the exposure to **drospirenone**. Use additional contraceptive precautions. Severe Theoretical
- **Drospirenone** might decrease the efficacy of **ulipristal** and **ulipristal** might decrease the efficacy of **drospirenone**. Avoid when used for uterine fibroids. For CoSRH guidance when used for emergency hormonal contraception, see Contraceptives, interactions p. 614. Severe Theoretical

Drugs that cause bleeding
- **Drugs that cause bleeding** (see TABLE 3 p. 1053) might increase the risk of bleeding when given with **avapritinib**. Severe Theoretical
- **Drugs that cause bleeding** (see TABLE 3 p. 1053) cause bleeding, as can **cabozantinib**; concurrent use might increase the risk of developing this effect. Severe Theoretical
- **Drugs that cause bleeding** (see TABLE 3 p. 1053) cause bleeding, as can **caplacizumab**; concurrent use might increase the risk of developing this effect. Severe Theoretical
- **Drugs that cause bleeding** (see TABLE 3 p. 1053) cause bleeding, as can **cobimetinib**; concurrent use might increase the risk of developing this effect. Severe Theoretical
- **Drugs that cause bleeding** (see TABLE 3 p. 1053) cause bleeding, as can **inotersen**; concurrent use might increase the risk of developing this effect. Severe Theoretical
- **Drugs that cause bleeding** (see TABLE 3 p. 1053) cause bleeding, as can monoclonal antibodies **(bevacizumab, trastuzumab emtansine)**; concurrent use might increase the risk of developing this effect. Severe Theoretical
- **Drugs that cause bleeding** (see TABLE 3 p. 1053) cause bleeding, as can **ranibizumab**; concurrent use might increase the risk of developing this effect. Severe Theoretical
- **Drugs that cause bleeding** (see TABLE 3 p. 1053) cause bleeding, as can **ruxolitinib**; concurrent use might increase the risk of developing this effect. Severe Theoretical
- **Drugs that cause bleeding** (see TABLE 3 p. 1053) cause bleeding, as can **trametinib**; concurrent use might increase the risk of developing this effect. Severe Theoretical
- **Drugs that cause bleeding** (see TABLE 3 p. 1053) cause bleeding, as can **volanesorsen**; concurrent use might increase the risk of developing this effect. Avoid depending on platelet count—consult product literature. Severe Theoretical

Drugs that cause hepatotoxicity
- **Alcohol**-induced liver disease increases the risk of hepatotoxicity in those taking **drugs that cause hepatotoxicity** (see TABLE 1 p. 1053). Severe Theoretical
- **Drugs that cause hepatotoxicity** (see TABLE 1 p. 1053) might increase the risk of hepatotoxicity when given with **low molecular-weight heparins** (high-dose). Severe Theoretical

Drugs that cause ototoxicity
- **Aspirin** (high-dose) might cause ototoxicity, as can **drugs that cause ototoxicity** (see TABLE 16 p. 1058); concurrent use might increase the risk of developing this effect. Moderate Theoretical
- **NSAIDs** (high-dose) might cause ototoxicity, as can **drugs that cause ototoxicity** (see TABLE 16 p. 1058); concurrent use might increase the risk of developing this effect. Moderate Theoretical

Drugs that cause serotonin toxicity
- **Bupropion** might enhance the risk of serotonin toxicity when given with **drugs that cause serotonin toxicity** (see TABLE 11 p. 1056). Severe Anecdotal
- Opioids **(tapentadol)** are predicted to increase the risk of serotonin toxicity when given with **drugs that cause serotonin toxicity** (see TABLE 11 p. 1056). Severe Theoretical

Drugs that reduce serum potassium
- **Drugs that reduce serum potassium** (see TABLE 14 p. 1057) are predicted to increase the risk of digoxin toxicity when given with **digoxin**. Severe Study

Drugs with antimuscarinic effects
- **Drugs with antimuscarinic effects** (see TABLE 8 p. 1055) might decrease the absorption of **levodopa**. Moderate Theoretical

Dulaglutide → see glucagon-like peptide-1 receptor agonists
Duloxetine → see SNRIs
Dupilumab → see monoclonal antibodies

Dutasteride
- Antiarrhythmics **(dronedarone)** are predicted to moderately increase the exposure to **dutasteride**. Mild Study
- Antifungals, azoles **(fluconazole, isavuconazole)** are predicted to moderately increase the exposure to **dutasteride**. Mild Study
- Antifungals, azoles **(itraconazole, ketoconazole, posaconazole, voriconazole)** are predicted to increase the exposure to **dutasteride**. Monitor adverse effects and adjust dose. Moderate Theoretical
- **Berotralstat** is predicted to moderately increase the exposure to **dutasteride**. Mild Study
- Calcium-channel blockers **(diltiazem, verapamil)** are predicted to moderately increase the exposure to **dutasteride**. Mild Study
- **Ceritinib** is predicted to increase the exposure to **dutasteride**. Monitor adverse effects and adjust dose. Moderate Theoretical
- **Cobicistat** is predicted to increase the exposure to **dutasteride**. Monitor adverse effects and adjust dose. Moderate Theoretical
- **Crizotinib** is predicted to moderately increase the exposure to **dutasteride**. Mild Study
- **Fedratinib** is predicted to moderately increase the exposure to **dutasteride**. Mild Study
- **HIV-protease inhibitors** are predicted to increase the exposure to **dutasteride**. Monitor adverse effects and adjust dose. Moderate Theoretical
- **Idelalisib** is predicted to increase the exposure to **dutasteride**. Monitor adverse effects and adjust dose. Moderate Theoretical
- **Imatinib** is predicted to moderately increase the exposure to **dutasteride**. Mild Study
- **Letermovir** is predicted to moderately increase the exposure to **dutasteride**. Mild Study

- Macrolides (clarithromycin) are predicted to increase the exposure to dutasteride. Monitor adverse effects and adjust dose. Moderate Theoretical
- Macrolides (erythromycin) are predicted to moderately increase the exposure to dutasteride. Mild Study
- Neurokinin-1 receptor antagonists (aprepitant, netupitant) are predicted to moderately increase the exposure to dutasteride. Mild Study
- Nilotinib is predicted to moderately increase the exposure to dutasteride. Mild Study
- Tucatinib is predicted to increase the exposure to dutasteride. Monitor adverse effects and adjust dose. Moderate Theoretical

Eculizumab → see monoclonal antibodies

Edoxaban → see factor XA inhibitors

Efavirenz → see NNRTIs

Efgartigimod alfa
- Live vaccines might increase the risk of generalised infection (possibly life-threatening) when given with efgartigimod alfa. Avoid. Severe Theoretical

Elacestrant
- Anti-androgens (apalutamide, enzalutamide) are predicted to decrease the exposure to elacestrant. Avoid or adjust dose depending on duration—consult product literature. Severe Study
- Antiarrhythmics (dronedarone) are predicted to increase the exposure to elacestrant. Avoid moderate CYP3A4 inhibitors or adjust elacestrant dose. Severe Theoretical
- Antiepileptics (carbamazepine, fosphenytoin, phenobarbital, phenytoin, primidone) are predicted to decrease the exposure to elacestrant. Avoid or adjust dose depending on duration—consult product literature. Severe Study
- Antifungals, azoles (fluconazole, isavuconazole) are predicted to increase the exposure to elacestrant. Avoid moderate CYP3A4 inhibitors or adjust elacestrant dose. Severe Theoretical
- Antifungals, azoles (itraconazole, ketoconazole, posaconazole, voriconazole) are predicted to increase the exposure to elacestrant. Avoid potent CYP3A4 inhibitors or adjust elacestrant dose. Severe Study
- Berotralstat is predicted to increase the exposure to elacestrant. Avoid moderate CYP3A4 inhibitors or adjust elacestrant dose. Severe Theoretical
- Calcium-channel blockers (diltiazem, verapamil) are predicted to increase the exposure to elacestrant. Avoid moderate CYP3A4 inhibitors or adjust elacestrant dose. Severe Theoretical
- Cenobamate is predicted to decrease the exposure to elacestrant. Avoid or adjust dose depending on duration—consult product literature. Severe Theoretical
- Ceritinib is predicted to increase the exposure to elacestrant. Avoid potent CYP3A4 inhibitors or adjust elacestrant dose. Severe Study
- Ciclosporin is predicted to increase the exposure to elacestrant. Avoid or adjust elacestrant dose. Severe Theoretical
- Cobicistat is predicted to increase the exposure to elacestrant. Avoid potent CYP3A4 inhibitors or adjust elacestrant dose. Severe Study
- Crizotinib is predicted to increase the exposure to elacestrant. Avoid moderate CYP3A4 inhibitors or adjust elacestrant dose. Severe Theoretical
- Dabrafenib is predicted to decrease the exposure to elacestrant. Avoid or adjust dose depending on duration—consult product literature. Severe Theoretical
- Encorafenib is predicted to decrease the exposure to elacestrant. Avoid or adjust dose depending on duration—consult product literature. Severe Study
- Endothelin receptor antagonists (bosentan) are predicted to decrease the exposure to elacestrant. Avoid or adjust dose depending on duration—consult product literature. Severe Theoretical
- Fedratinib is predicted to increase the exposure to elacestrant. Avoid moderate CYP3A4 inhibitors or adjust elacestrant dose. Severe Theoretical
- Grapefruit is predicted to increase the exposure to elacestrant. Avoid. Moderate Theoretical
- HIV-protease inhibitors are predicted to increase the exposure to elacestrant. Avoid potent CYP3A4 inhibitors or adjust elacestrant dose. Severe Study
- Idelalisib is predicted to increase the exposure to elacestrant. Avoid potent CYP3A4 inhibitors or adjust elacestrant dose. Severe Study
- Imatinib is predicted to increase the exposure to elacestrant. Avoid moderate CYP3A4 inhibitors or adjust elacestrant dose. Severe Theoretical
- Ivosidenib is predicted to decrease the exposure to elacestrant. Avoid or adjust dose depending on duration—consult product literature. Severe Study
- Letermovir is predicted to increase the exposure to elacestrant. Avoid moderate CYP3A4 inhibitors or adjust elacestrant dose. Severe Theoretical
- Lorlatinib is predicted to decrease the exposure to elacestrant. Avoid or adjust dose depending on duration—consult product literature. Severe Theoretical
- Lumacaftor is predicted to decrease the exposure to elacestrant. Avoid or adjust dose depending on duration—consult product literature. Severe Study
- Macrolides (clarithromycin) are predicted to increase the exposure to elacestrant. Avoid potent CYP3A4 inhibitors or adjust elacestrant dose. Severe Study
- Macrolides (erythromycin) are predicted to increase the exposure to elacestrant. Avoid moderate CYP3A4 inhibitors or adjust elacestrant dose. Severe Theoretical
- Mitotane is predicted to decrease the exposure to elacestrant. Avoid or adjust dose depending on duration—consult product literature. Severe Study
- Neurokinin-1 receptor antagonists (aprepitant, netupitant) are predicted to increase the exposure to elacestrant. Avoid moderate CYP3A4 inhibitors or adjust elacestrant dose. Severe Theoretical
- Nilotinib is predicted to increase the exposure to elacestrant. Avoid moderate CYP3A4 inhibitors or adjust elacestrant dose. Severe Theoretical
- NNRTIs (efavirenz, etravirine, nevirapine) are predicted to decrease the exposure to elacestrant. Avoid or adjust dose depending on duration—consult product literature. Severe Theoretical
- Quinolones (ciprofloxacin) are predicted to increase the exposure to elacestrant. Avoid or adjust elacestrant dose. Severe Theoretical
- Rifamycins (rifampicin) are predicted to decrease the exposure to elacestrant. Avoid or adjust dose depending on duration—consult product literature. Severe Study
- Sotorasib is predicted to decrease the exposure to elacestrant. Avoid or adjust dose depending on duration—consult product literature. Severe Theoretical
- SSRIs (fluvoxamine) are predicted to increase the exposure to elacestrant. Avoid or adjust elacestrant dose. Severe Theoretical
- St John's wort is predicted to decrease the exposure to elacestrant. Avoid or adjust dose depending on duration—consult product literature. Severe Theoretical
- Tucatinib is predicted to increase the exposure to elacestrant. Avoid potent CYP3A4 inhibitors or adjust elacestrant dose. Severe Study

Elafibranor
- Elafibranor might increase the risk of muscle effects when given with statins. Severe Theoretical

Elbasvir
- Anti-androgens (apalutamide, enzalutamide) are predicted to decrease the exposure to elbasvir. Avoid. Severe Study
- Antiepileptics (carbamazepine, fosphenytoin, phenobarbital, phenytoin, primidone) are predicted to decrease the exposure to elbasvir. Avoid. Severe Study
- Cenobamate is predicted to moderately decrease the exposure to elbasvir. Avoid. Severe Study
- Dabrafenib is predicted to moderately decrease the exposure to elbasvir. Avoid. Severe Study
- Encorafenib is predicted to decrease the exposure to elbasvir. Avoid. Severe Study

Elbasvir (continued)
- Endothelin receptor antagonists **(bosentan)** are predicted to moderately decrease the exposure to **elbasvir**. Avoid. Severe Study
- **Ivosidenib** is predicted to decrease the exposure to **elbasvir**. Avoid. Severe Study
- **Lorlatinib** is predicted to moderately decrease the exposure to **elbasvir**. Avoid. Severe Study
- **Lumacaftor** is predicted to decrease the exposure to **elbasvir**. Avoid. Severe Study
- **Mitotane** is predicted to decrease the exposure to **elbasvir**. Avoid. Severe Study
- **Modafinil** is predicted to decrease the exposure to **elbasvir**. Avoid. Unknown Theoretical
- **Nirmatrelvir** boosted with ritonavir is predicted to increase the concentration of **elbasvir**. Severe Theoretical
- NNRTIs **(efavirenz, etravirine, nevirapine)** are predicted to moderately decrease the exposure to **elbasvir**. Avoid. Severe Study
- Rifamycins **(rifampicin)** are predicted to decrease the exposure to **elbasvir**. Avoid. Severe Study
- **Sotorasib** is predicted to moderately decrease the exposure to **elbasvir**. Avoid. Severe Study
- **St John's wort** is predicted to moderately decrease the exposure to **elbasvir**. Avoid. Severe Study
- **Elbasvir** with grazoprevir slightly increases the exposure to statins **(atorvastatin)**. Adjust **atorvastatin** dose, p. 154. Moderate Study
- **Elbasvir** with grazoprevir is predicted to increase the exposure to statins **(fluvastatin)**. Adjust **fluvastatin** dose, p. 155. Moderate Theoretical
- **Elbasvir** with grazoprevir moderately increases the exposure to statins **(rosuvastatin)**. Adjust **rosuvastatin** dose, p. 155. Moderate Study
- **Elbasvir** with grazoprevir is predicted to increase the exposure to statins **(simvastatin)**. Adjust **simvastatin** dose, p. 156. Moderate Theoretical
- **Elbasvir** is predicted to increase the concentration of **sunitinib**. Use with caution and adjust dose. Moderate Theoretical
- **Elbasvir** is predicted to increase the concentration of thrombin inhibitors **(dabigatran)**. Moderate Theoretical

Eletriptan → see triptans

Elexacaftor
- Anti-androgens **(apalutamide, enzalutamide)** is predicted to decrease the exposure to **elexacaftor**. Avoid. Severe Theoretical
- Antiarrhythmics **(dronedarone)** are predicted to increase the exposure to **elexacaftor**. Adjust ivacaftor with tezacaftor and elexacaftor p. 220 dose with moderate CYP3A4 inhibitors. Severe Theoretical
- Antiepileptics **(carbamazepine, fosphenytoin, phenobarbital, phenytoin, primidone)** is predicted to decrease the exposure to **elexacaftor**. Avoid. Severe Theoretical
- Antifungals, azoles **(fluconazole, isavuconazole)** are predicted to increase the exposure to **elexacaftor**. Adjust ivacaftor with tezacaftor and elexacaftor p. 220 dose with moderate CYP3A4 inhibitors. Severe Theoretical
- Antifungals, azoles **(itraconazole, ketoconazole, posaconazole, voriconazole)** are predicted to increase the exposure to **elexacaftor**. Adjust ivacaftor with tezacaftor and elexacaftor p. 220 dose with potent CYP3A4 inhibitors. Severe Study
- **Elexacaftor** is predicted to increase the exposure to antihistamines, non-sedating **(fexofenadine)**. Moderate Theoretical
- **Berotralstat** is predicted to increase the exposure to **elexacaftor**. Adjust ivacaftor with tezacaftor and elexacaftor p. 220 dose with moderate CYP3A4 inhibitors. Severe Theoretical
- Calcium-channel blockers **(diltiazem, verapamil)** are predicted to increase the exposure to **elexacaftor**. Adjust ivacaftor with tezacaftor and elexacaftor p. 220 dose with moderate CYP3A4 inhibitors. Severe Theoretical
- **Ceritinib** is predicted to increase the exposure to **elexacaftor**. Adjust ivacaftor with tezacaftor and elexacaftor p. 220 dose with potent CYP3A4 inhibitors. Severe Study
- **Cobicistat** is predicted to increase the exposure to **elexacaftor**. Adjust ivacaftor with tezacaftor and elexacaftor p. 220 dose with potent CYP3A4 inhibitors. Severe Study
- **Crizotinib** is predicted to increase the exposure to **elexacaftor**. Adjust ivacaftor with tezacaftor and elexacaftor p. 220 dose with moderate CYP3A4 inhibitors. Severe Theoretical
- **Encorafenib** is predicted to decreases the exposure to **elexacaftor**. Avoid. Severe Theoretical
- **Elexacaftor** is predicted to increase the exposure to endothelin receptor antagonists **(bosentan)**. Moderate Theoretical
- **Fedratinib** is predicted to increase the exposure to **elexacaftor**. Adjust ivacaftor with tezacaftor and elexacaftor p. 220 dose with moderate CYP3A4 inhibitors. Severe Theoretical
- **Grapefruit** juice is predicted to increase the exposure to **elexacaftor**. Avoid. Moderate Theoretical
- **HIV-protease inhibitors** are predicted to increase the exposure to **elexacaftor**. Adjust ivacaftor with tezacaftor and elexacaftor p. 220 dose with potent CYP3A4 inhibitors. Severe Study
- **Idelalisib** is predicted to increase the exposure to **elexacaftor**. Adjust ivacaftor with tezacaftor and elexacaftor p. 220 dose with potent CYP3A4 inhibitors. Severe Study
- **Imatinib** is predicted to increase the exposure to **elexacaftor**. Adjust ivacaftor with tezacaftor and elexacaftor p. 220 dose with moderate CYP3A4 inhibitors. Severe Theoretical
- **Ivosidenib** is predicted to decreases the exposure to **elexacaftor**. Avoid. Severe Theoretical
- **Letermovir** is predicted to increase the exposure to **elexacaftor**. Adjust ivacaftor with tezacaftor and elexacaftor p. 220 dose with moderate CYP3A4 inhibitors. Severe Theoretical
- **Lumacaftor** is predicted to decreases the exposure to **elexacaftor**. Avoid. Severe Theoretical
- Macrolides **(clarithromycin)** are predicted to increase the exposure to **elexacaftor**. Adjust ivacaftor with tezacaftor and elexacaftor p. 220 dose with potent CYP3A4 inhibitors. Severe Study
- Macrolides **(erythromycin)** are predicted to increase the exposure to **elexacaftor**. Adjust ivacaftor with tezacaftor and elexacaftor p. 220 dose with moderate CYP3A4 inhibitors. Severe Theoretical
- **Elexacaftor** is predicted to increase the exposure to meglitinides **(repaglinide)**. Moderate Theoretical
- **Mitotane** is predicted to decreases the exposure to **elexacaftor**. Avoid. Severe Theoretical
- Neurokinin-1 receptor antagonists **(aprepitant, netupitant)** are predicted to increase the exposure to **elexacaftor**. Adjust ivacaftor with tezacaftor and elexacaftor p. 220 dose with moderate CYP3A4 inhibitors. Severe Theoretical
- **Nilotinib** is predicted to increase the exposure to **elexacaftor**. Adjust ivacaftor with tezacaftor and elexacaftor p. 220 dose with moderate CYP3A4 inhibitors. Severe Theoretical
- **Nirmatrelvir** boosted with ritonavir is predicted to increase the concentration of **elexacaftor** with tezacaftor and ivacaftor. Adjust dose. Severe Theoretical
- Rifamycins **(rifabutin)** are predicted to decrease the exposure to **elexacaftor**. Avoid. Severe Theoretical
- Rifamycins **(rifampicin)** is predicted to decrease the exposure to **elexacaftor**. Avoid. Severe Theoretical
- **St John's wort** is predicted to decrease the exposure to **elexacaftor**. Avoid. Severe Theoretical
- **Elexacaftor** is predicted to increase the exposure to statins **(atorvastatin, pravastatin, rosuvastatin, simvastatin)**. Moderate Theoretical
- **Elexacaftor** is predicted to increase the exposure to sulfonylureas **(glibenclamide)**. Moderate Theoretical
- **Elexacaftor** is predicted to increase the exposure to taxanes **(docetaxel, paclitaxel)**. Moderate Theoretical
- **Tucatinib** is predicted to increase the exposure to **elexacaftor**. Adjust ivacaftor with tezacaftor and elexacaftor p. 220 dose with potent CYP3A4 inhibitors. Severe Study

Eliglustat
- **Eliglustat** is predicted to increase the exposure to **aliskiren**. Adjust dose. Moderate Study
- Anti-androgens **(abiraterone)** are predicted to increase the exposure to **eliglustat**. Avoid or adjust dose—consult product literature. Severe Study
- Anti-androgens **(apalutamide, enzalutamide)** are predicted to decrease the exposure to **eliglustat**. Avoid. Severe Study

- Antiarrhythmics **(dronedarone, propafenone)** are predicted to increase the exposure to **eliglustat**. Avoid or adjust dose—consult product literature. Severe Study
- Antiepileptics **(carbamazepine, fosphenytoin, phenobarbital, phenytoin, primidone)** are predicted to decrease the exposure to **eliglustat**. Avoid. Severe Study
- Antifungals, azoles **(fluconazole, isavuconazole, itraconazole, ketoconazole, posaconazole, voriconazole)** are predicted to increase the exposure to **eliglustat**. Avoid or adjust dose—consult product literature. Severe Study
- **Eliglustat** is predicted to increase the exposure to antihistamines, non-sedating **(fexofenadine)**. Adjust dose. Moderate Study
- **Eliglustat** is predicted to increase the exposure to **atomoxetine**. Adjust dose. Moderate Theoretical
- **Berotralstat** is predicted to increase the exposure to **eliglustat**. Avoid or adjust dose—consult product literature. Severe Study
- **Eliglustat** is predicted to increase the exposure to beta blockers, non-selective **(propranolol)**. Adjust dose. Moderate Study
- **Eliglustat** is predicted to increase the exposure to beta blockers, selective **(metoprolol)**. Adjust dose. Moderate Study
- **Bupropion** is predicted to increase the exposure to **eliglustat**. Avoid or adjust dose—consult product literature. Severe Study
- Calcium-channel blockers **(diltiazem, verapamil)** are predicted to increase the exposure to **eliglustat**. Avoid or adjust dose—consult product literature. Severe Study
- **Ceritinib** is predicted to increase the exposure to **eliglustat**. Avoid or adjust dose—consult product literature. Severe Study
- **Cinacalcet** is predicted to increase the exposure to **eliglustat**. Avoid or adjust dose—consult product literature. Severe Study
- **Cobicistat** is predicted to increase the exposure to **eliglustat**. Avoid or adjust dose—consult product literature. Severe Study
- **Eliglustat** is predicted to increase the exposure to **colchicine**. Avoid or adjust **colchicine** dose, p. 637. Severe Theoretical
- **Crizotinib** is predicted to increase the exposure to **eliglustat**. Avoid or adjust dose—consult product literature. Severe Study
- **Dacomitinib** is predicted to increase the exposure to **eliglustat**. Avoid or adjust dose—consult product literature. Severe Study
- **Eliglustat** increases the exposure to **digoxin**. Adjust dose. Moderate Study
- **Encorafenib** is predicted to decrease the exposure to **eliglustat**. Avoid. Severe Study
- Endothelin receptor antagonists **(bosentan)** are predicted to decrease the exposure to **eliglustat**. Moderate Theoretical
- **Eliglustat** is predicted to increase the exposure to **everolimus**. Adjust dose. Moderate Study
- **Eliglustat** is predicted to increase the exposure to factor XA inhibitors **(edoxaban)**. Adjust dose. Moderate Study
- **Fedratinib** is predicted to increase the exposure to **eliglustat**. Avoid or adjust dose—consult product literature. Severe Study
- **Givosiran** is predicted to increase the exposure to **eliglustat**. Use with caution and adjust dose. Moderate Study
- **Grapefruit** juice is predicted to increase the exposure to **eliglustat**. Avoid. Severe Theoretical
- **HIV-protease inhibitors** are predicted to increase the exposure to **eliglustat**. Avoid or adjust dose—consult product literature. Severe Study
- **Idelalisib** is predicted to increase the exposure to **eliglustat**. Avoid or adjust dose—consult product literature. Severe Study
- **Imatinib** is predicted to increase the exposure to **eliglustat**. Avoid or adjust dose—consult product literature. Severe Study
- Interferons **(ropeginterferon alfa)** are predicted to increase the exposure to **eliglustat**. Moderate Theoretical
- **Ivosidenib** is predicted to decrease the exposure to **eliglustat**. Avoid. Severe Study
- **Letermovir** is predicted to increase the exposure to **eliglustat**. Avoid or adjust dose—consult product literature. Severe Study
- **Eliglustat** is predicted to increase the exposure to **loperamide**. Adjust dose. Moderate Study
- **Lumacaftor** is predicted to decrease the exposure to **eliglustat**. Avoid. Severe Study
- Macrolides **(clarithromycin, erythromycin)** are predicted to increase the exposure to **eliglustat**. Avoid or adjust dose—consult product literature. Severe Study
- **Mirabegron** is predicted to increase the exposure to **eliglustat**. Avoid or adjust dose—consult product literature. Severe Study
- **Mitotane** is predicted to decrease the exposure to **eliglustat**. Avoid. Severe Study
- **Moclobemide** is predicted to increase the exposure to **eliglustat**. Avoid or adjust dose—consult product literature. Severe Theoretical
- Neurokinin-1 receptor antagonists **(aprepitant, netupitant)** are predicted to increase the exposure to **eliglustat**. Avoid or adjust dose—consult product literature. Severe Study
- **Nilotinib** is predicted to increase the exposure to **eliglustat**. Avoid or adjust dose—consult product literature. Severe Study
- NNRTIs **(efavirenz, etravirine, nevirapine)** are predicted to decrease the exposure to **eliglustat**. Moderate Theoretical
- **Eliglustat** is predicted to increase the exposure to **pralsetinib**. Adjust dose. Moderate Study
- Quinolones **(ciprofloxacin)** are predicted to increase the exposure to **eliglustat**. Avoid or adjust dose—consult product literature. Severe Theoretical
- **Eliglustat** is predicted to increase the exposure to **ranolazine**. Adjust dose. Moderate Study
- Rifamycins **(rifampicin)** are predicted to decrease the exposure to **eliglustat**. Avoid. Severe Study
- **Eliglustat** is predicted to increase the exposure to **rimegepant**. Adjust dose. Moderate Study
- **Eliglustat** is predicted to increase the exposure to **sirolimus**. Adjust dose. Moderate Study
- SNRIs **(duloxetine)** are predicted to increase the exposure to **eliglustat**. Avoid or adjust dose—consult product literature. Severe Study
- SSRIs **(fluoxetine, paroxetine)** are predicted to increase the exposure to **eliglustat**. Avoid or adjust dose—consult product literature. Severe Study
- **St John's wort** is predicted to increase the exposure to **eliglustat**. Avoid. Severe Study
- **Eliglustat** is predicted to increase the exposure to statins **(pravastatin)**. Adjust dose. Moderate Study
- **Eliglustat** is predicted to increase the exposure to **talazoparib**. Adjust dose. Moderate Study
- **Eliglustat** is predicted to increase the exposure to taxanes **(paclitaxel)**. Adjust dose. Moderate Study
- **Terbinafine** is predicted to increase the exposure to **eliglustat**. Avoid or adjust dose—consult product literature. Severe Study
- **Eliglustat** is predicted to increase the exposure to thrombin inhibitors **(dabigatran)**. Adjust dose. Moderate Study
- **Eliglustat** is predicted to increase the exposure to **tolterodine**. Adjust dose. Moderate Theoretical
- **Eliglustat** is predicted to increase the exposure to tricyclic antidepressants **(nortriptyline)**. Adjust dose. Moderate Theoretical
- **Tucatinib** is predicted to increase the exposure to **eliglustat**. Avoid or adjust dose—consult product literature. Severe Study

Elotuzumab → see monoclonal antibodies

Elranatamab → see monoclonal antibodies

Eltrombopag

- **Eltrombopag** is predicted to increase the exposure to **alpelisib**. Moderate Theoretical
- Oral **antacids** decrease the absorption of oral **eltrombopag**. Manufacturer advises take 2 hours before or 4 hours after antacids. Severe Study
- **Eltrombopag** is predicted to increase the exposure to atogepant. Adjust **atogepant** dose. Moderate Theoretical
- Oral **calcium compounds** decrease the absorption of oral **eltrombopag**. **Eltrombopag** should be taken 2 hours before or 4 hours after calcium. Severe Study
- **Ciclosporin** causes a small decrease in the exposure to **eltrombopag**. Monitor platelet count and adjust dose. Moderate Study
- **Eltrombopag** is predicted to increase the exposure to **cladribine**. Avoid or adjust dose. Moderate Theoretical
- **Eltrombopag** is predicted to increase the exposure to **grazoprevir**. Avoid. Severe Theoretical
- Oral **iron** is predicted to decrease the absorption of oral **eltrombopag**. **Eltrombopag** should be taken 2 hours before or 4 hours after iron. Severe Theoretical

Eltrombopag (continued)
- **Eltrombopag** is predicted to increase the concentration of **letermovir**. Moderate Study
- **Eltrombopag** is predicted to increase the concentration of **methotrexate**. Moderate Theoretical
- **Eltrombopag** is predicted to increase the exposure to **momelotinib**. Moderate Study
- Rifamycins **(rifampicin)** are predicted to decrease the exposure to **eltrombopag** and **eltrombopag** is predicted to increase the concentration of rifamycins **(rifampicin)**. Moderate Theoretical
- **Eltrombopag** is predicted to increase the exposure to **seladelpar**. Moderate Study
- Oral **selenium** is predicted to decrease the absorption of **eltrombopag**. **Eltrombopag** should be taken 2 hours before or 4 hours after **selenium**. Severe Theoretical
- SSRIs **(fluvoxamine)** are predicted to increase the exposure to **eltrombopag**. Moderate Theoretical
- **Eltrombopag** is predicted to increase the exposure to **statins**. Monitor and adjust dose. Moderate Study
- **Eltrombopag** is predicted to increase the exposure to **talazoparib**. Avoid or monitor. Moderate Theoretical
- **Eltrombopag** is predicted to increase the exposure to taxanes **(docetaxel, paclitaxel)**. Moderate Theoretical
- **Eltrombopag** is predicted to increase the exposure to **tenofovir alafenamide**. Moderate Theoretical
- **Eltrombopag** is predicted to increase the exposure to **tenofovir disoproxil**. Moderate Theoretical
- **Eltrombopag** is predicted to increase the exposure to **topotecan**. Moderate Theoretical
- **Eltrombopag** is predicted to increase the exposure to **venetoclax**. Avoid or monitor for toxicity. Severe Theoretical
- Oral **zinc** is predicted to decrease the absorption of **eltrombopag**. **Eltrombopag** should be taken 2 hours before or 4 hours after **zinc**. Severe Theoretical

Elvitegravir
- Oral **antacids** decrease the exposure to oral **elvitegravir**. Separate administration by at least 4 hours. Moderate Study
- Anti-androgens **(apalutamide, enzalutamide)** are predicted to decrease the concentration of **elvitegravir**. Avoid. Severe Study
- Antiepileptics **(carbamazepine, fosphenytoin, phenobarbital, phenytoin, primidone)** are predicted to decrease the concentration of **elvitegravir**. Avoid. Severe Study
- **Cenobamate** is predicted to decrease the concentration of **elvitegravir**. Avoid. Severe Theoretical
- **Elvitegravir** is predicted to decrease the anticoagulant effect of **coumarins**. Moderate Anecdotal
- **Dabrafenib** is predicted to decrease the concentration of **elvitegravir**. Avoid. Severe Theoretical
- **Encorafenib** is predicted to decrease the concentration of **elvitegravir**. Avoid. Severe Study
- Endothelin receptor antagonists **(bosentan)** are predicted to decrease the concentration of **elvitegravir**. Avoid. Severe Theoretical
- **Elvitegravir** markedly increases the exposure to **grazoprevir**. Avoid. Severe Study
- HIV-protease inhibitors **(atazanavir, lopinavir)** boosted with ritonavir increase the concentration of **elvitegravir**. Refer to specialist literature. Moderate Study
- **Ivosidenib** is predicted to decrease the concentration of **elvitegravir**. Avoid. Severe Study
- **Lorlatinib** is predicted to decrease the concentration of **elvitegravir**. Avoid. Severe Theoretical
- **Lumacaftor** is predicted to decrease the concentration of **elvitegravir**. Avoid. Severe Study
- **Elvitegravir** boosted with ritonavir is predicted to increase the exposure to **midostaurin**. Severe Theoretical
- **Mitotane** is predicted to decrease the concentration of **elvitegravir**. Avoid. Severe Study
- NNRTIs **(efavirenz, etravirine, nevirapine)** are predicted to decrease the concentration of **elvitegravir**. Avoid. Severe Theoretical
- Rifamycins **(rifampicin)** are predicted to decrease the concentration of **elvitegravir**. Avoid. Severe Study
- **Sotorasib** is predicted to decrease the concentration of **elvitegravir**. Avoid. Severe Theoretical
- **St John's wort** is predicted to decrease the concentration of **elvitegravir**. Avoid. Severe Theoretical

Empagliflozin → see sodium glucose co-transporter 2 inhibitors

Emtricitabine → see NRTIs

Enalapril → see ACE inhibitors

Encorafenib → see TABLE 7 p. 1055 (QT-interval prolongation)
- **Encorafenib** is predicted to decrease the exposure to 5-HT3-receptor antagonists **(ondansetron)**. Moderate Study → Also see TABLE 7 p. 1055
- **Encorafenib** is predicted to markedly decrease the exposure to **abemaciclib**. Avoid. Severe Study
- **Encorafenib** is predicted to decrease the exposure to **acalabrutinib**. Avoid. Severe Study
- **Encorafenib** is predicted to decrease the exposure to **alpelisib**. Avoid. Moderate Study
- Anti-androgens **(apalutamide, enzalutamide)** are predicted to decrease the exposure to **encorafenib**. Severe Theoretical → Also see TABLE 7 p. 1055
- **Encorafenib** is predicted to decrease the exposure to anti-androgens **(abiraterone)**. Avoid. Severe Study
- **Encorafenib** is predicted to decrease the exposure to anti-androgens **(darolutamide)**. Avoid. Moderate Study
- Antiarrhythmics **(dronedarone)** are predicted to moderately increase the exposure to **encorafenib**. Moderate Study → Also see TABLE 7 p. 1055
- **Encorafenib** is predicted to decrease the exposure to antiarrhythmics **(disopyramide, dronedarone)**. Avoid. Severe Study → Also see TABLE 7 p. 1055
- **Encorafenib** is predicted to decrease the efficacy of antiarrhythmics **(propafenone)**. Moderate Study
- **Encorafenib** is predicted to decrease the exposure to anticholinesterases, centrally acting **(donepezil)**. Mild Study
- Antiepileptics **(carbamazepine, fosphenytoin, phenobarbital, phenytoin, primidone)** are predicted to decrease the exposure to **encorafenib**. Severe Theoretical
- **Encorafenib** is predicted to decrease the exposure to antiepileptics **(perampanel)**. Monitor and adjust dose. Moderate Study
- Antifungals, azoles **(fluconazole, isavuconazole)** are predicted to moderately increase the exposure to **encorafenib**. Moderate Study → Also see TABLE 7 p. 1055
- Antifungals, azoles **(itraconazole, ketoconazole, posaconazole, voriconazole)** are predicted to increase the exposure to **encorafenib**. Avoid or monitor. Severe Study → Also see TABLE 7 p. 1055
- **Encorafenib** is predicted to decrease the exposure to antifungals, azoles **(isavuconazole)**. Avoid. Severe Study
- **Encorafenib** is predicted to increase the exposure to antihistamines, non-sedating **(fexofenadine)**. Mild Study
- **Encorafenib** is predicted to decrease the exposure to antimalarials **(artemether)** with lumefantrine. Avoid. Severe Study → Also see TABLE 7 p. 1055
- **Encorafenib** is predicted to decrease the concentration of antimalarials **(piperaquine)**. Avoid. Moderate Theoretical
- **Encorafenib** is predicted to moderately decrease the exposure to atypical antipsychotics **(aripiprazole)**. Avoid or adjust dose—consult product literature. Moderate Study
- **Encorafenib** is predicted to decrease the exposure to atypical antipsychotics **(cariprazine)**. Avoid. Severe Theoretical
- **Encorafenib** is predicted to decrease the exposure to atypical antipsychotics **(lurasidone)**. Avoid. Moderate Study
- **Encorafenib** is predicted to decrease the exposure to atypical antipsychotics **(paliperidone)**. Monitor and adjust dose. Severe Study → Also see TABLE 7 p. 1055
- **Encorafenib** is predicted to decrease the exposure to atypical antipsychotics **(quetiapine)**. Moderate Study
- **Encorafenib** is predicted to decrease the exposure to atypical antipsychotics **(risperidone)**. Adjust dose. Moderate Study
- **Encorafenib** is predicted to decrease the exposure to **avacopan**. Avoid or monitor. Severe Study
- **Encorafenib** is predicted to decrease the exposure to **avapritinib**. Avoid. Severe Study
- **Encorafenib** is predicted to decrease the exposure to **axitinib**. Avoid or adjust dose. Moderate Study

- **Encorafenib** decreases the exposure to **bedaquiline**. Avoid. [Severe] Study → Also see TABLE 7 p. 1055
- **Encorafenib** is predicted to decrease the exposure to **belumosudil**. Adjust **belumosudil** dose, p. 650. [Severe] Study
- **Encorafenib** is predicted to decrease the exposure to benzodiazepines **(alprazolam)**. Adjust dose. [Moderate] Theoretical
- **Encorafenib** is predicted to decrease the exposure to benzodiazepines **(midazolam)**. Monitor and adjust dose. [Severe] Study
- **Berotralstat** is predicted to moderately increase the exposure to **encorafenib**. [Moderate] Study
- **Encorafenib** is predicted to decrease the exposure to **bictegravir**. Avoid. [Moderate] Study
- **Encorafenib** slightly decreases the exposure to **bortezomib**. Avoid. [Severe] Study
- **Encorafenib** is predicted to very markedly decrease the exposure to **bosutinib**. Avoid. [Severe] Study → Also see TABLE 7 p. 1055
- **Encorafenib** is predicted to decrease the exposure to **brigatinib**. Avoid. [Severe] Study
- **Encorafenib** is predicted to decrease the exposure to **buspirone**. Use with caution and adjust dose. [Severe] Study
- **Encorafenib** moderately decreases the exposure to **cabozantinib**. Avoid. [Moderate] Study → Also see TABLE 7 p. 1055
- Calcium-channel blockers **(diltiazem, verapamil)** are predicted to moderately increase the exposure to **encorafenib**. [Moderate] Study
- **Encorafenib** is predicted to decrease the exposure to calcium-channel blockers **(amlodipine, felodipine, lacidipine, lercanidipine, nicardipine, nifedipine, nimodipine)**. Monitor and adjust dose. [Moderate] Study
- **Encorafenib** is predicted to decrease the exposure to **cannabidiol**. Adjust dose. [Moderate] Study
- **Encorafenib** is predicted to decrease the exposure to **capivasertib**. Avoid. [Moderate] Study
- **Cenobamate** is predicted to decrease the exposure to **encorafenib**. [Moderate] Study
- **Encorafenib** is predicted to decrease the exposure to **ceritinib**. Avoid. [Severe] Study → Also see TABLE 7 p. 1055
- **Ceritinib** is predicted to increase the exposure to **encorafenib**. Avoid or monitor. [Severe] Study → Also see TABLE 7 p. 1055
- **Encorafenib** decreases the concentration of **ciclosporin**. [Severe] Study
- **Encorafenib** is predicted to alter the effects of **cilostazol**. [Moderate] Theoretical
- **Encorafenib** is predicted to decrease the exposure to **cinacalcet**. Monitor and adjust dose. [Moderate] Study
- **Encorafenib** decreases the exposure to **clomethiazole**. Monitor and adjust dose. [Moderate] Study
- **Encorafenib** is predicted to decrease the exposure to **cobicistat**. Avoid. [Severe] Study
- **Cobicistat** is predicted to increase the exposure to **encorafenib**. Avoid or monitor. [Severe] Study
- **Encorafenib** is predicted to decrease the exposure to **cobimetinib**. Avoid. [Severe] Theoretical
- **Encorafenib** might decrease the efficacy of **combined hormonal contraceptives**. Use additional contraceptive precautions or alternative methods. [Severe] Theoretical
- **Encorafenib** is predicted to decrease the exposure to corticosteroids **(budesonide, deflazacort, dexamethasone, fludrocortisone, hydrocortisone, methylprednisolone, prednisolone, triamcinolone)**. Monitor and adjust dose. [Moderate] Study
- **Encorafenib** is predicted to decrease the exposure to corticosteroids **(fluticasone)**. [Unknown] Theoretical
- **Encorafenib** is predicted to markedly decrease the exposure to **crizotinib**. Avoid. [Severe] Study → Also see TABLE 7 p. 1055
- **Crizotinib** is predicted to moderately increase the exposure to **encorafenib**. [Moderate] Study → Also see TABLE 7 p. 1055
- **Dabrafenib** is predicted to decrease the exposure to **encorafenib**. [Moderate] Study
- **Encorafenib** is predicted to decrease the exposure to **dabrafenib**. Avoid. [Moderate] Theoretical
- **Encorafenib** is predicted to decrease the exposure to **daridorexant**. [Severe] Study
- **Encorafenib** is predicted to decrease the exposure to **darifenacin**. [Moderate] Theoretical
- **Encorafenib** is predicted to markedly decrease the exposure to **dasatinib**. Avoid. [Severe] Study → Also see TABLE 7 p. 1055
- **Encorafenib** is predicted to slightly decrease the exposure to **delamanid**. Avoid. [Moderate] Study → Also see TABLE 7 p. 1055
- **Encorafenib** is predicted to decrease the exposure to **deutivacaftor**. Avoid. [Severe] Theoretical
- **Encorafenib** is predicted to markedly decrease the exposure to **dienogest**. [Severe] Study
- **Encorafenib** is predicted to decrease the exposure to dipeptidylpeptidase-4 inhibitors **(linagliptin)**. [Moderate] Study
- **Encorafenib** is predicted to moderately decrease the exposure to dipeptidylpeptidase-4 inhibitors **(saxagliptin)**. [Moderate] Study
- **Encorafenib** is predicted to increase the exposure to **dolutegravir**. [Moderate] Theoretical
- **Encorafenib** is predicted to decrease the exposure to **dronabinol**. Avoid or adjust dose. [Mild] Study
- **Encorafenib** is predicted to decrease the exposure to **elacestrant**. Avoid or adjust dose depending on duration—consult product literature. [Severe] Study
- **Encorafenib** is predicted to decrease the exposure to **elbasvir**. Avoid. [Severe] Study
- **Encorafenib** is predicted to decreases the exposure to **elexacaftor**. Avoid. [Severe] Theoretical
- **Encorafenib** is predicted to decrease the exposure to **eliglustat**. Avoid. [Severe] Study
- **Encorafenib** is predicted to decrease the concentration of **elvitegravir**. Avoid. [Severe] Study
- Endothelin receptor antagonists **(bosentan)** are predicted to decrease the exposure to **encorafenib**. [Moderate] Study
- **Encorafenib** affects the exposure to endothelin receptor antagonists **(bosentan)**. Avoid. [Severe] Study
- **Encorafenib** is predicted to decrease the exposure to endothelin receptor antagonists **(macitentan)**. Avoid. [Severe] Study
- **Encorafenib** is predicted to decrease the exposure to the cytotoxic component of **enfortumab vedotin**. [Moderate] Theoretical
- **Encorafenib** is predicted to decrease the exposure to **entrectinib**. Avoid. [Severe] Study → Also see TABLE 7 p. 1055
- **Encorafenib** is predicted to decrease the exposure to **erdafitinib**. Avoid. [Severe] Study
- **Encorafenib** is predicted to decrease the exposure to **erlotinib**. Avoid or adjust dose—consult product literature. [Severe] Study
- **Encorafenib** is predicted to decrease the exposure to **esketamine**. Adjust dose. [Moderate] Study
- **Encorafenib** is predicted to decrease the exposure to **eszopiclone**. Adjust dose. [Moderate] Theoretical
- **Encorafenib** is predicted to decrease the concentration of **everolimus**. Avoid or adjust dose. [Severe] Study
- **Encorafenib** moderately decreases the exposure to **exemestane**. [Moderate] Study
- **Encorafenib** is predicted to decrease the exposure to factor XA inhibitors **(apixaban)**. [Moderate] Study
- **Encorafenib** is predicted to decrease the exposure to factor XA inhibitors **(rivaroxaban)**. Avoid unless patient can be monitored for signs of thrombosis. [Moderate] Study
- **Fedratinib** is predicted to moderately increase the exposure to **encorafenib**. [Moderate] Study
- **Encorafenib** is predicted to decrease the exposure to **fedratinib**. Avoid. [Moderate] Study
- **Encorafenib** is predicted to decrease the exposure to **fesoterodine**. Avoid. [Moderate] Study
- **Encorafenib** is predicted to decrease the exposure to **fostamatinib**. Avoid. [Severe] Study
- **Encorafenib** is predicted to decrease the exposure to the active metabolite of **fostemsavir**. Avoid. [Severe] Study
- **Encorafenib** is predicted to decrease the exposure to **fruquintinib**. Avoid. [Moderate] Study
- **Encorafenib** is predicted to decrease the exposure to **gefitinib**. Avoid. [Severe] Study
- **Encorafenib** is predicted to decrease the exposure to **glasdegib**. Avoid. [Severe] Study → Also see TABLE 7 p. 1055
- **Grapefruit** juice is predicted to increase the exposure to **encorafenib**. Avoid. [Moderate] Study

Encorafenib (continued)
- **Encorafenib** is predicted to decrease the exposure to **grazoprevir**. Avoid. Severe Study
- **Encorafenib** is predicted to decrease the concentration of **guanfacine**. Adjust **guanfacine** dose, p. 281. Moderate Study
- **Encorafenib** decreases the concentration of **haloperidol**. Adjust dose. Moderate Study → Also see TABLE 7 p. 1055
- **HIV-protease inhibitors** are predicted to increase the exposure to **encorafenib**. Avoid or monitor. Severe Study
- **Encorafenib** is predicted to decrease the exposure to **ibrutinib**. Avoid or monitor. Severe Study
- **Idelalisib** is predicted to increase the exposure to **encorafenib**. Avoid or monitor. Severe Study
- **Encorafenib** is predicted to decrease the exposure to **idelalisib**. Avoid. Severe Study
- **Encorafenib** is predicted to decrease the exposure to **imatinib**. Avoid. Moderate Study
- **Imatinib** is predicted to moderately increase the exposure to **encorafenib**. Moderate Study
- **Encorafenib** is predicted to decrease the exposure to **irinotecan**. Avoid. Severe Study
- **Encorafenib** is predicted to decrease the exposure to **ivabradine**. Adjust dose. Moderate Theoretical
- **Encorafenib** is predicted to decrease the exposure to **ivacaftor**. Avoid. Severe Study
- **Ivosidenib** is predicted to decrease the exposure to **encorafenib**. Severe Theoretical → Also see TABLE 7 p. 1055
- **Encorafenib** is predicted to decrease the exposure to **ixazomib**. Avoid. Severe Study
- **Encorafenib** is predicted to decrease the exposure to **ketamine**. Adjust dose. Moderate Theoretical
- **Encorafenib** is predicted to decrease the exposure to **lapatinib**. Avoid. Severe Study → Also see TABLE 7 p. 1055
- **Encorafenib** is predicted to moderately decrease the exposure to **larotrectinib**. Avoid. Moderate Study
- **Encorafenib** is predicted to decrease the exposure to **lazertinib**. Avoid. Severe Study
- **Encorafenib** is predicted to decrease the exposure to **lenacapavir**. Avoid. Severe Study
- **Encorafenib** is predicted to decrease the exposure to **leniolisib**. Avoid. Severe Theoretical
- **Letermovir** is predicted to moderately increase the exposure to **encorafenib**. Moderate Study
- **Encorafenib** is predicted to decrease the exposure to **lomitapide**. Monitor and adjust dose. Moderate Theoretical
- **Encorafenib** is predicted to decrease the exposure to **lorlatinib**. Avoid. Severe Study
- **Lorlatinib** is predicted to decrease the exposure to **encorafenib**. Moderate Study
- **Lumacaftor** is predicted to decrease the exposure to **encorafenib**. Severe Theoretical
- Macrolides **(clarithromycin)** are predicted to increase the exposure to **encorafenib**. Avoid or monitor. Severe Study
- Macrolides **(erythromycin)** are predicted to moderately increase the exposure to **encorafenib**. Moderate Study → Also see TABLE 7 p. 1055
- **Encorafenib** is predicted to decrease the exposure to **maraviroc**. Adjust dose. Severe Study
- **Encorafenib** is predicted to decrease the exposure to **mavacamten**. Monitor and adjust dose—consult product literature. Severe Theoretical
- **Encorafenib** is predicted to decrease the exposure to meglitinides **(repaglinide)**. Monitor blood glucose and adjust dose. Moderate Study
- **Encorafenib** is predicted to decrease the exposure to **midostaurin**. Avoid. Severe Study
- **Encorafenib** is predicted to decrease the exposure to **mifepristone**. Adjust **mifepristone** dose. Severe Study
- **Encorafenib** is predicted to decrease the exposure to mineralocorticoid receptor antagonists **(eplerenone)**. Avoid. Moderate Theoretical
- **Encorafenib** is predicted to decrease the exposure to mineralocorticoid receptor antagonists **(finerenone)**. Avoid. Severe Study
- **Encorafenib** is predicted to decrease the exposure to **mirtazapine**. Adjust dose. Moderate Study
- **Mitotane** is predicted to decrease the exposure to **encorafenib**. Severe Theoretical
- **Modafinil** slightly decreases the exposure to **encorafenib**. Moderate Study
- **Encorafenib** is predicted to decrease the exposure to monoclonal antibodies **(polatuzumab vedotin)**. Moderate Theoretical
- **Encorafenib** is predicted to decrease the exposure to the cytotoxic component of monoclonal antibodies **(trastuzumab emtansine)**. Severe Theoretical
- **Encorafenib** is predicted to decrease the exposure to **montelukast**. Mild Study
- **Encorafenib** is predicted to markedly decrease the exposure to **naldemedine**. Avoid. Severe Study
- **Encorafenib** is predicted to markedly decrease the exposure to **naloxegol**. Avoid. Moderate Study
- **Encorafenib** is predicted to decrease the exposure to **neratinib**. Avoid. Severe Study
- Neurokinin-1 receptor antagonists **(aprepitant, netupitant)** are predicted to moderately increase the exposure to **encorafenib**. Moderate Study
- **Encorafenib** is predicted to markedly decrease the exposure to neurokinin-1 receptor antagonists **(aprepitant)**. Avoid. Moderate Study
- **Encorafenib** is predicted to decrease the exposure to neurokinin-1 receptor antagonists **(fosaprepitant)**. Avoid. Moderate Theoretical
- **Encorafenib** is predicted to decrease the exposure to neurokinin-1 receptor antagonists **(netupitant)**. Avoid. Severe Study
- **Encorafenib** is predicted to moderately decrease the exposure to **nilotinib**. Avoid. Severe Study → Also see TABLE 7 p. 1055
- **Nilotinib** is predicted to moderately increase the exposure to **encorafenib**. Moderate Study → Also see TABLE 7 p. 1055
- **Nirmatrelvir** boosted with ritonavir is predicted to increase the concentration of **encorafenib**. Avoid or monitor. Severe Theoretical
- **Encorafenib** is predicted to decrease the exposure to **nirmatrelvir** boosted with ritonavir. Avoid. Severe Study
- **Encorafenib** is predicted to decrease the exposure to **nitisinone**. Adjust dose. Moderate Theoretical
- NNRTIs **(efavirenz, etravirine, nevirapine)** are predicted to decrease the exposure to **encorafenib**. Moderate Study → Also see TABLE 7 p. 1055
- **Encorafenib** is predicted to decrease the exposure to NNRTIs **(doravirine)**. Avoid. Severe Study
- **Encorafenib** is predicted to decrease the exposure to NNRTIs **(etravirine)**. Avoid. Severe Theoretical
- **Encorafenib** markedly decreases the exposure to NNRTIs **(rilpivirine)**. Avoid. Severe Study
- **Encorafenib** is predicted to decrease the exposure to **olaparib**. Avoid. Moderate Theoretical
- **Encorafenib** is predicted to decrease the exposure to **omaveloxolone**. Avoid. Severe Study
- **Encorafenib** is predicted to decrease the exposure to opioids **(alfentanil, fentanyl)**. Moderate Study
- **Encorafenib** is predicted to decrease the exposure to opioids **(buprenorphine)**. Monitor and adjust dose. Moderate Theoretical
- **Encorafenib** decreases the exposure to opioids **(methadone)**. Monitor and adjust dose. Severe Study → Also see TABLE 7 p. 1055
- **Encorafenib** is predicted to decrease the exposure to opioids **(oxycodone)**. Monitor and adjust dose. Moderate Study
- **Encorafenib** is predicted to decrease the exposure to **osilodrostat**. Moderate Theoretical → Also see TABLE 7 p. 1055
- **Encorafenib** is predicted to moderately decrease the exposure to **osimertinib**. Avoid. Moderate Study → Also see TABLE 7 p. 1055
- **Encorafenib** is predicted to moderately decrease the exposure to **ospemifene**. Moderate Study
- **Encorafenib** is predicted to decrease the exposure to **palbociclib**. Avoid. Severe Study
- **Encorafenib** is predicted to decrease the exposure to **panobinostat**. Avoid. Moderate Theoretical → Also see TABLE 7 p. 1055

- **Encorafenib** is predicted to decrease the exposure to **pazopanib**. Avoid. Severe Theoretical → Also see TABLE 7 p. 1055
- **Encorafenib** is predicted to decrease the exposure to **pemigatinib**. Avoid. Severe Study
- **Encorafenib** moderately decreases the exposure to phosphodiesterase type-4 inhibitors **(apremilast)**. Avoid. Severe Study
- **Encorafenib** is predicted to decrease the exposure to phosphodiesterase type-4 inhibitors **(roflumilast)**. Avoid. Moderate Study
- **Encorafenib** is predicted to decrease the exposure to phosphodiesterase type-5 inhibitors **(avanafil, tadalafil)**. Avoid. Severe Study
- **Encorafenib** is predicted to decrease the exposure to phosphodiesterase type-5 inhibitors **(sildenafil, vardenafil)**. Moderate Theoretical → Also see TABLE 7 p. 1055
- **Encorafenib** is predicted to moderately to markedly decrease the exposure to **pibrentasvir**. Avoid. Severe Study
- **Encorafenib** is predicted to decrease the exposure to **pirtobrutinib**. Avoid. Moderate Study
- **Encorafenib** is predicted to moderately decrease the exposure to **pitolisant**. Moderate Study
- **Encorafenib** is predicted to decrease the exposure to **ponatinib**. Avoid. Moderate Theoretical
- **Encorafenib** is predicted to decrease the exposure to **pralsetinib**. Avoid or adjust dose with potent CYP3A4 inducers—consult product literature. Moderate Study
- **Encorafenib** is predicted to markedly decrease the exposure to **praziquantel**. Avoid. Moderate Study
- **Encorafenib** is predicted to decrease the exposure to **quizartinib**. Avoid. Severe Study → Also see TABLE 7 p. 1055
- **Encorafenib** is predicted to increase the exposure to **raltegravir**. Moderate Theoretical
- **Encorafenib** is predicted to decrease the exposure to **ranolazine**. Avoid. Severe Study → Also see TABLE 7 p. 1055
- **Encorafenib** is predicted to decrease the exposure to **reboxetine**. Moderate Anecdotal
- **Encorafenib** is predicted to decrease the exposure to **regorafenib**. Avoid. Moderate Study
- **Encorafenib** is predicted to markedly decrease the exposure to **ribociclib**. Avoid. Severe Study → Also see TABLE 7 p. 1055
- Rifamycins **(rifampicin)** are predicted to decrease the exposure to **encorafenib**. Severe Theoretical
- **Encorafenib** is predicted to decrease the exposure to **rimegepant**. Avoid. Moderate Theoretical
- **Encorafenib** is predicted to decrease the exposure to **ripretinib**. Avoid or adjust dose—consult product literature. Severe Study
- **Encorafenib** is predicted to decrease the exposure to **ruxolitinib**. Monitor and adjust dose. Moderate Study
- **Encorafenib** is predicted to decrease the exposure to **selpercatinib**. Avoid. Moderate Study → Also see TABLE 7 p. 1055
- **Encorafenib** is predicted to decrease the exposure to **selumetinib**. Avoid. Severe Study
- **Encorafenib** is predicted to decrease the exposure to **siponimod**. Manufacturer advises caution depending on genotype—consult product literature. Severe Study
- **Encorafenib** is predicted to decrease the concentration of **sirolimus**. Avoid or monitor and adjust dose. Severe Study
- **Encorafenib** is predicted to decrease the exposure to **solifenacin**. Moderate Theoretical
- **Encorafenib** is predicted to decrease the exposure to **sorafenib**. Moderate Theoretical → Also see TABLE 7 p. 1055
- **Encorafenib** is predicted to decrease the exposure to **sotorasib**. Avoid. Severe Study
- **Sotorasib** is predicted to decrease the exposure to **encorafenib**. Moderate Study
- **Encorafenib** is predicted to decrease the exposure to **sparsentan**. Avoid. Severe Theoretical
- **St John's wort** is predicted to decrease the exposure to **encorafenib**. Severe Theoretical
- **Encorafenib** is predicted to increase the exposure to statins **(atorvastatin)**. Mild Theoretical
- **Encorafenib** is predicted to increase the exposure to statins **(fluvastatin, pravastatin)**. Mild Study
- **Encorafenib** is predicted to affect the exposure to statins **(simvastatin)**. Mild Theoretical
- **Encorafenib** is predicted to increase the exposure to **sulfasalazine**. Mild Study
- **Encorafenib** is predicted to increase the exposure to sulfonylureas **(glibenclamide)**. Mild Study
- **Encorafenib** is predicted to decrease the exposure to **sunitinib**. Avoid or adjust dose—consult product literature. Moderate Study → Also see TABLE 7 p. 1055
- **Encorafenib** decreases the concentration of **tacrolimus**. Avoid or monitor and adjust dose. Severe Study
- **Encorafenib** is predicted to decrease the exposure to taxanes **(cabazitaxel)**. Avoid. Moderate Study
- **Encorafenib** is predicted to decrease the exposure to taxanes **(docetaxel)**. Severe Theoretical
- **Encorafenib** is predicted to decrease the exposure to taxanes **(paclitaxel)**. Avoid. Severe Study
- **Encorafenib** is predicted to decrease the concentration of **temsirolimus**. Avoid. Severe Study
- **Encorafenib** is predicted to decrease the exposure to tetracyclines **(eravacycline)**. Adjust **eravacycline** dose. Moderate Study
- **Encorafenib** is predicted to decrease the exposure to **tezacaftor**. Avoid. Severe Theoretical
- **Encorafenib** is predicted to markedly decrease the exposure to **ticagrelor**. Avoid. Severe Study
- **Encorafenib** is predicted to decrease the exposure to the cytotoxic component of **tisotumab vedotin**. Moderate Theoretical
- **Encorafenib** is predicted to decrease the exposure to **tivozanib**. Severe Study
- **Encorafenib** is predicted to decrease the exposure to **tofacitinib**. Avoid. Severe Study
- **Encorafenib** is predicted to decrease the exposure to **tolvaptan**. Use with caution or avoid depending on indication. Severe Study
- **Encorafenib** is predicted to increase the effects of **topotecan**. Mild Study
- **Encorafenib** is predicted to decrease the exposure to **toremifene**. Adjust dose. Moderate Study → Also see TABLE 7 p. 1055
- **Encorafenib** is predicted to decrease the exposure to **trabectedin**. Avoid. Severe Theoretical
- **Encorafenib** is predicted to decrease the exposure to **tucatinib**. Avoid. Severe Study
- **Tucatinib** is predicted to increase the exposure to **encorafenib**. Avoid or monitor. Severe Study
- **Encorafenib** is predicted to decrease the exposure to **upadacitinib**. Moderate Study
- **Encorafenib** is predicted to decrease the exposure to **vandetanib**. Avoid. Moderate Study → Also see TABLE 7 p. 1055
- **Encorafenib** is predicted to decrease the exposure to **vanzacaftor**. Avoid. Severe Theoretical
- **Encorafenib** is predicted to moderately decrease the exposure to **velpatasvir**. Avoid. Severe Study
- **Encorafenib** is predicted to decrease the exposure to **vemurafenib**. Avoid. Severe Study → Also see TABLE 7 p. 1055
- **Encorafenib** is predicted to decrease the exposure to **venetoclax**. Avoid. Severe Study
- **Encorafenib** is predicted to decrease the exposure to vinca alkaloids **(vinblastine, vincristine, vindesine)**. Severe Theoretical
- **Encorafenib** is predicted to decrease the exposure to vinca alkaloids **(vinorelbine)**. Use with caution or avoid. Severe Theoretical
- **Encorafenib** is predicted to decrease the exposure to **vismodegib**. Avoid. Moderate Theoretical
- **Encorafenib** is predicted to decrease the exposure to **voclosporin**. Avoid. Severe Study → Also see TABLE 7 p. 1055
- **Encorafenib** is predicted to decrease the exposure to **vortioxetine**. Monitor and adjust dose. Moderate Study
- **Encorafenib** is predicted to decrease the concentration of **voxilaprevir**. Avoid. Severe Study
- **Encorafenib** is predicted to decrease the exposure to **zanubrutinib**. Avoid. Severe Study
- **Encorafenib** is predicted to decrease the exposure to **zopiclone**. Adjust dose. Moderate Study

Endothelin receptor antagonists

ambrisentan · bosentan · macitentan

- **Bosentan** is predicted to decrease the exposure to **acalabrutinib**. Severe Study
- Anti-androgens **(apalutamide, enzalutamide)** affect the exposure to **bosentan**. Avoid. Severe Study
- Anti-androgens **(apalutamide, enzalutamide)** are predicted to decrease the exposure to **macitentan**. Avoid. Severe Study
- **Bosentan** is predicted to decrease the efficacy of anti-androgens **(cyproterone)** with ethinylestradiol (co-cyprindiol). Use alternative methods during treatment with, and for 28 days after, the enzyme inducing drug is stopped. Severe Study
- **Bosentan** is predicted to decrease the exposure to anti-androgens **(darolutamide)**. Avoid. Moderate Theoretical
- Antiarrhythmics **(amiodarone, dronedarone)** are predicted to increase the exposure to **macitentan**. Manufacturer advises caution depending on other drugs taken—consult product literature. Moderate Theoretical
- **Bosentan** is predicted to decrease the exposure to antiarrhythmics **(dronedarone)**. Severe Theoretical
- Antiepileptics **(carbamazepine, fosphenytoin, phenobarbital, phenytoin, primidone)** affect the exposure to **bosentan**. Avoid. Severe Study
- Antiepileptics **(carbamazepine, fosphenytoin, phenobarbital, phenytoin, primidone)** are predicted to decrease the exposure to **macitentan**. Avoid. Severe Study
- Antifungals, azoles **(fluconazole)** are predicted to increase the exposure to **bosentan**. Avoid. Severe Study
- Antifungals, azoles **(fluconazole, isavuconazole, miconazole)** are predicted to increase the exposure to **macitentan**. Manufacturer advises caution depending on other drugs taken—consult product literature. Moderate Theoretical
- Antifungals, azoles **(itraconazole)** are predicted to increase the exposure to **bosentan**. Moderate Theoretical
- Antifungals, azoles **(itraconazole, ketoconazole, posaconazole, voriconazole)** are predicted to increase the exposure to **macitentan**. Moderate Study
- Antifungals, azoles **(ketoconazole)** moderately increase the exposure to **bosentan**. Moderate Study
- Antifungals, azoles **(voriconazole)** are predicted to increase the exposure to **bosentan**. Avoid. Severe Theoretical
- **Bosentan** is predicted to decrease the exposure to antifungals, azoles **(isavuconazole)**. Avoid. Severe Theoretical
- **Bosentan** is predicted to decrease the exposure to atypical antipsychotics **(aripiprazole)**. Avoid or adjust dose—consult product literature. Moderate Study
- **Bosentan** is predicted to decrease the exposure to atypical antipsychotics **(cariprazine)**. Avoid. Severe Theoretical
- **Bosentan** is predicted to decrease the exposure to atypical antipsychotics **(lurasidone)**. Monitor and adjust dose. Moderate Theoretical
- **Bosentan** is predicted to decrease the exposure to atypical antipsychotics **(quetiapine)**. Moderate Study
- **Bosentan** is predicted to decrease the exposure to **avacopan**. Severe Theoretical
- **Bosentan** is predicted to decrease the exposure to **avapritinib**. Avoid. Severe Study
- **Bosentan** is predicted to decrease the exposure to **axitinib**. Moderate Study
- **Bosentan** is predicted to decrease the exposure to **bedaquiline**. Avoid. Severe Study
- **Belumosudil** is predicted to increase the exposure to **bosentan**. Avoid or adjust dose. Moderate Study
- **Bosentan** is predicted to decrease the concentration of benzodiazepines **(midazolam)**. Monitor and adjust dose. Moderate Theoretical
- **Berotralstat** is predicted to increase the exposure to **macitentan**. Manufacturer advises caution depending on other drugs taken—consult product literature. Moderate Theoretical
- **Bosentan** is predicted to decrease the exposure to **bosutinib**. Avoid. Severe Study
- **Bosentan** is predicted to decrease the exposure to **brigatinib**. Avoid or adjust dose—consult product literature. Moderate Study
- **Bulevirtide** is predicted to increase the exposure to **bosentan**. Avoid or monitor. Moderate Theoretical
- **Bosentan** is predicted to decrease the exposure to **cabozantinib**. Moderate Study
- Calcium-channel blockers **(diltiazem, verapamil)** are predicted to increase the exposure to **macitentan**. Manufacturer advises caution depending on other drugs taken—consult product literature. Moderate Theoretical
- **Bosentan** is predicted to decrease the exposure to calcium-channel blockers **(amlodipine, felodipine, lacidipine, lercanidipine, nicardipine, nifedipine, nimodipine)**. Monitor and adjust dose. Moderate Theoretical
- **Bosentan** is predicted to decrease the exposure to calcium-channel blockers **(diltiazem, verapamil)**. Moderate Theoretical
- **Bosentan** is predicted to decrease the exposure to **capivasertib**. Avoid. Moderate Study
- Cephalosporins **(ceftobiprole)** are predicted to increase the exposure to **bosentan**. Moderate Theoretical
- **Bosentan** is predicted to decrease the exposure to **ceritinib**. Severe Study
- **Ceritinib** is predicted to increase the exposure to **macitentan**. Moderate Study
- **Ciclosporin** moderately increases the exposure to **ambrisentan**. Adjust **ambrisentan** dose and monitor, p. 138. Moderate Study
- **Bosentan** moderately decreases the exposure to **ciclosporin** and **ciclosporin** moderately increases the exposure to **bosentan**. Avoid. Severe Study
- **Bosentan** is predicted to decrease the exposure to **cobicistat**. Avoid. Severe Theoretical
- **Cobicistat** is predicted to increase the exposure to **macitentan**. Moderate Study
- **Bosentan** is predicted to decrease the exposure to **cobimetinib**. Avoid. Severe Theoretical
- **Bosentan** is predicted to decrease the efficacy of **combined hormonal contraceptives**. For CoSRH guidance, see Contraceptives, interactions p. 614. Severe Study
- **Bosentan** decreases the anticoagulant effect of **coumarins**. Moderate Study
- **Bosentan** is predicted to decrease the exposure to **crizotinib**. Avoid. Severe Study
- **Crizotinib** is predicted to increase the exposure to **macitentan**. Manufacturer advises caution depending on other drugs taken—consult product literature. Moderate Theoretical
- **Bosentan** is predicted to decrease the exposure to **dabrafenib**. Moderate Study
- **Bosentan** is predicted to decrease the exposure to **daridorexant**. Severe Study
- **Bosentan** is predicted to decrease the exposure to **dasatinib**. Severe Study
- **Bosentan** is predicted to decrease the efficacy of **desogestrel**. For CoSRH guidance, see Contraceptives, interactions p. 614. Severe Theoretical
- **Bosentan** is predicted to decrease the exposure to **deutivacaftor**. Avoid. Severe Theoretical
- **Bosentan** is predicted to decrease the exposure to **dolutegravir**. Severe Study
- **Bosentan** is predicted to decrease the efficacy of **drospirenone**. For CoSRH guidance, see Contraceptives, interactions p. 614. Severe Theoretical
- **Bosentan** is predicted to decrease the exposure to **elacestrant**. Avoid or adjust dose depending on duration—consult product literature. Severe Theoretical
- **Bosentan** is predicted to moderately decrease the exposure to **elbasvir**. Avoid. Severe Study
- **Elexacaftor** is predicted to increase the exposure to **bosentan**. Moderate Theoretical
- **Bosentan** is predicted to decrease the exposure to **eliglustat**. Moderate Theoretical
- **Bosentan** is predicted to decrease the concentration of **elvitegravir**. Avoid. Severe Theoretical
- **Encorafenib** affects the exposure to **bosentan**. Avoid. Severe Study
- **Bosentan** is predicted to decrease the exposure to **encorafenib**. Moderate Study

A1 Interactions | Appendix 1

- **Encorafenib** is predicted to decrease the exposure to **macitentan**. Avoid. Severe Study
- **Bosentan** is predicted to decrease the exposure to **entrectinib**. Avoid. Moderate Theoretical
- **Bosentan** is predicted to decrease the exposure to **erdafitinib**. Adjust dose. Moderate Theoretical
- **Bosentan** is predicted to decrease the exposure to **erlotinib**. Severe Study
- **Bosentan** is predicted to decrease the efficacy of **estradiol**. Moderate Theoretical
- **Bosentan** is predicted to decrease the efficacy of **etonogestrel**. For CoSRH guidance, see Contraceptives, interactions p. 614. Severe Theoretical
- **Bosentan** is predicted to decrease the concentration of **everolimus**. Avoid or adjust dose. Severe Study
- **Bosentan** is predicted to decrease the exposure to **fedratinib**. Avoid. Moderate Study
- **Fedratinib** is predicted to increase the exposure to **macitentan**. Manufacturer advises caution depending on other drugs taken—consult product literature. Moderate Theoretical
- **Bosentan** is predicted to decrease the exposure to **fruquintinib**. Avoid. Moderate Study
- **Bosentan** is predicted to decrease the exposure to **gefitinib**. Avoid. Severe Study
- **Bosentan** is predicted to decrease the exposure to **glasdegib**. Avoid or adjust dose—consult product literature. Moderate Theoretical
- **Bosentan** is predicted to decrease the exposure to **glecaprevir**. Avoid. Severe Study
- **Bosentan** is predicted to markedly decrease the exposure to **grazoprevir**. Avoid. Severe Study
- **Bosentan** is predicted to decrease the concentration of **guanfacine**. Adjust dose. Moderate Theoretical
- **HIV-protease inhibitors** are predicted to increase the exposure to **bosentan**. Severe Study
- **HIV-protease inhibitors** are predicted to increase the exposure to **macitentan**. Moderate Study
- **Bosentan** is predicted to decrease the effects of **hormone replacement therapy**. Moderate Anecdotal
- **Bosentan** is predicted to decrease the exposure to **ibrutinib**. Avoid or monitor. Severe Study
- **Bosentan** is predicted to decrease the exposure to **idelalisib**. Avoid. Moderate Theoretical
- **Idelalisib** is predicted to increase the exposure to **macitentan**. Moderate Study
- **Bosentan** is predicted to decrease the exposure to **imatinib**. Moderate Study
- **Imatinib** is predicted to increase the exposure to **macitentan**. Manufacturer advises caution depending on other drugs taken—consult product literature. Moderate Theoretical
- **Bosentan** is predicted to decrease the exposure to **ivacaftor**. Moderate Study
- **Ivosidenib** affects the exposure to **bosentan**. Avoid. Severe Study
- **Ivosidenib** is predicted to decrease the exposure to **macitentan**. Avoid. Severe Study
- **Bosentan** is predicted to decrease the exposure to **ixazomib**. Moderate Theoretical
- **Bosentan** is predicted to decrease the exposure to **lapatinib**. Avoid. Severe Study
- **Bosentan** is predicted to decrease the exposure to **larotrectinib**. Avoid. Moderate Study
- **Leflunomide** is predicted to increase the exposure to **bosentan**. Moderate Study
- **Bosentan** is predicted to decrease the exposure to **lenacapavir**. Avoid Severe Study
- **Bosentan** is predicted to decrease the exposure to **leniolisib**. Avoid Severe Theoretical
- **Leniolisib** is predicted to increase the exposure to **bosentan**. Avoid Moderate Theoretical
- **Letermovir** is predicted to increase the concentration of **bosentan**. Moderate Theoretical
- **Letermovir** is predicted to increase the exposure to **macitentan**. Manufacturer advises caution depending on other drugs taken—consult product literature. Moderate Theoretical
- **Bosentan** is predicted to decrease the efficacy of some contraceptive methods containing **levonorgestrel**. For CoSRH guidance, see Contraceptives, interactions p. 614. Severe Theoretical
- **Lumacaftor** affects the exposure to **bosentan**. Avoid. Severe Study
- **Lumacaftor** is predicted to decrease the exposure to **macitentan**. Avoid. Severe Study
- Macrolides **(clarithromycin)** are predicted to increase the exposure to **bosentan**. Moderate Theoretical
- Macrolides **(clarithromycin)** are predicted to increase the exposure to **macitentan**. Moderate Study
- Macrolides **(erythromycin)** are predicted to increase the exposure to **macitentan**. Manufacturer advises caution depending on other drugs taken—consult product literature. Moderate Theoretical
- **Bosentan** is predicted to decrease the exposure to **maraviroc**. Avoid. Moderate Theoretical
- **Bosentan** is predicted to decrease the exposure to **maribavir**. Avoid or adjust **maribavir** dose. Severe Study
- **Bosentan** is predicted to decrease the exposure to **mavacamten**. Monitor and adjust dose—consult product literature. Severe Theoretical
- **Bosentan** is predicted to decrease the exposure to **midostaurin** and **midostaurin** is predicted to increase the exposure to **bosentan**. Severe Study
- **Bosentan** is predicted to decrease the exposure to **mifepristone**. Adjust **mifepristone** dose. Severe Study
- **Bosentan** is predicted to decrease the exposure to mineralocorticoid receptor antagonists **(finerenone)**. Avoid. Severe Study
- **Mitotane** affects the exposure to **bosentan**. Avoid. Severe Study
- **Mitotane** is predicted to decrease the exposure to **macitentan**. Avoid. Severe Study
- **Bosentan** is predicted to decrease the exposure to **naloxegol**. Moderate Theoretical
- **Bosentan** is predicted to decrease the exposure to **neratinib**. Avoid. Severe Theoretical
- Neurokinin-1 receptor antagonists **(aprepitant, netupitant)** are predicted to increase the exposure to **macitentan**. Manufacturer advises caution depending on other drugs taken—consult product literature. Moderate Theoretical
- **Bosentan** is predicted to decrease the exposure to neurokinin-1 receptor antagonists **(aprepitant)**. Moderate Study
- **Bosentan** is predicted to decrease the exposure to neurokinin-1 receptor antagonists **(fosaprepitant, netupitant)**. Moderate Theoretical
- **Bosentan** is predicted to decrease the exposure to **nilotinib**. Avoid. Severe Theoretical
- **Nilotinib** is predicted to increase the exposure to **macitentan**. Manufacturer advises caution depending on other drugs taken—consult product literature. Moderate Theoretical
- **Nirmatrelvir** boosted with ritonavir is predicted to increase the concentration of **bosentan**. Severe Theoretical
- **Bosentan** is predicted to decrease the exposure to NNRTIs **(doravirine)**. Avoid or adjust doravirine or lamivudine with tenofovir disoproxil and doravirine dose. Severe Theoretical
- **Bosentan** is predicted to decrease the exposure to NNRTIs **(nevirapine)**. Severe Theoretical
- **Bosentan** is predicted to decrease the exposure to NNRTIs **(rilpivirine)**. Avoid. Severe Theoretical
- **Bosentan** is predicted to decrease the efficacy of some contraceptive methods containing **norethisterone**. For CoSRH guidance, see Contraceptives, interactions p. 614. Severe Anecdotal
- **Bosentan** is predicted to decrease the exposure to **olaparib**. Avoid. Moderate Theoretical
- **Bosentan** is predicted to decrease the exposure to **omaveloxolone**. Avoid. Severe Study
- **Bosentan** decreases the exposure to opioids **(methadone)**. Monitor and adjust dose. Severe Study
- **Bosentan** is predicted to decrease the exposure to **osimertinib**. Use with caution or avoid. Severe Study
- **Bosentan** is predicted to decrease the exposure to **ospemifene**. Moderate Study

Endothelin receptor antagonists (continued)
- **Bosentan** is predicted to decrease the exposure to **pazopanib**. Severe Study
- **Bosentan** is predicted to decrease the exposure to **pemigatinib**. Avoid or monitor. Severe Study
- **Bosentan** decreases the exposure to **phosphodiesterase type-5 inhibitors**. Moderate Study
- **Bosentan** is predicted to decrease the exposure to **pibrentasvir**. Avoid. Severe Study
- **Bosentan** is predicted to decrease the exposure to **pirtobrutinib**. Moderate Theoretical
- **Bosentan** is predicted to decrease the exposure to **ponatinib**. Severe Study
- **Bosentan** is predicted to decrease the exposure to **pralsetinib**. Moderate Theoretical
- **Bosentan** is predicted to decrease the exposure to **quizartinib**. Avoid. Severe Study
- **Bosentan** is predicted to decrease the exposure to **regorafenib**. Severe Study
- **Bosentan** is predicted to decrease the exposure to **ribociclib**. Moderate Study
- Rifamycins **(rifampicin)** transiently increase the exposure to **ambrisentan**. Moderate Study
- Rifamycins **(rifampicin)** affect the exposure to **bosentan**. Avoid. Severe Study
- Rifamycins **(rifampicin)** are predicted to decrease the exposure to **macitentan**. Avoid. Severe Study
- **Bosentan** is predicted to decrease the exposure to **rimegepant**. Avoid. Moderate Theoretical
- **Bosentan** is predicted to decrease the exposure to **ripretinib**. Avoid or adjust dose—consult product literature. Moderate Theoretical
- **Roxadustat** is predicted to increase the exposure to **bosentan**. Monitor adverse effects and adjust dose. Moderate Study
- **Bosentan** is predicted to decrease the exposure to **ruxolitinib**. Monitor and adjust dose. Moderate Study
- **Bosentan** is predicted to decrease the exposure to **selpercatinib**. Moderate Study
- **Bosentan** is predicted to decrease the exposure to **selumetinib**. Avoid. Severe Study
- **Bosentan** is predicted to decrease the exposure to **siponimod**. Manufacturer advises caution depending on genotype—consult product literature. Moderate Theoretical
- **Bosentan** is predicted to decrease the concentration of **sirolimus** and **sirolimus** potentially increases the concentration of **bosentan**. Avoid. Severe Theoretical
- **Bosentan** is predicted to decrease the exposure to **sorafenib**. Moderate Study
- **Bosentan** is predicted to decrease the exposure to **sparsentan**. Avoid. Severe Theoretical
- **St John's wort** is predicted to decrease the exposure to **bosentan**. Avoid. Moderate Theoretical
- **St John's wort** is predicted to decrease the exposure to **macitentan**. Avoid. Severe Theoretical
- **Bosentan** is predicted to decrease the exposure to statins **(atorvastatin, simvastatin)**. Moderate Study
- **Bosentan** increases the risk of hepatotoxicity when given with sulfonylureas **(glibenclamide)**. Avoid. Severe Study
- **Bosentan** is predicted to decrease the exposure to **sunitinib**. Moderate Study
- **Bosentan** is predicted to decrease the concentration of **tacrolimus** and **tacrolimus** potentially increases the concentration of **bosentan**. Avoid. Severe Theoretical
- **Bosentan** is predicted to decrease the exposure to taxanes **(cabazitaxel)**. Moderate Theoretical
- **Bosentan** is predicted to decrease the exposure to taxanes **(docetaxel)**. Severe Theoretical
- **Bosentan** is predicted to decrease the exposure to taxanes **(paclitaxel)**. Avoid. Severe Study
- **Bosentan** is predicted to decrease the concentration of **temsirolimus**. Avoid. Moderate Theoretical
- **Teriflunomide** is predicted to increase the exposure to **bosentan**. Moderate Study
- **Bosentan** is predicted to decrease the exposure to **tezacaftor**. Avoid. Severe Theoretical
- **Bosentan** is predicted to decrease the exposure to **ticagrelor**. Moderate Theoretical
- **Bosentan** is predicted to decrease the exposure to **tofacitinib**. Severe Study
- **Tucatinib** is predicted to increase the exposure to **macitentan**. Moderate Study
- **Bosentan** decreases the efficacy of **ulipristal**. Avoid and for 4 weeks after stopping the enzyme inducing drug. For CoSRH guidance, see Contraceptives, interactions p. 614. Severe Anecdotal
- **Bosentan** is predicted to decrease the exposure to **vandetanib**. Moderate Study
- **Bosentan** is predicted to decrease the exposure to **vanzacaftor**. Avoid. Severe Theoretical
- **Bosentan** is predicted to decrease the exposure to **velpatasvir**. Avoid. Moderate Theoretical
- **Vemurafenib** is predicted to increase the exposure to **ambrisentan**. Use with caution or avoid. Moderate Theoretical
- **Bosentan** is predicted to decrease the exposure to **vemurafenib**. Severe Study
- **Bosentan** is predicted to decrease the exposure to **venetoclax**. Avoid. Severe Study
- **Venetoclax** is predicted to increase the exposure to **bosentan**. Moderate Theoretical
- **Bosentan** is predicted to decrease the exposure to **voclosporin** and **voclosporin** is predicted to increase the concentration of **bosentan**. Avoid. Severe Theoretical
- **Bosentan** is predicted to decrease the concentration of **voxilaprevir**. Avoid. Severe Theoretical
- **Bosentan** is predicted to decrease the exposure to **zanubrutinib**. Avoid or adjust dose with moderate CYP3A4 inducers—consult product literature. Severe Theoretical

Enfortumab vedotin
- Anti-androgens **(apalutamide, enzalutamide)** are predicted to decrease the exposure to the cytotoxic component of **enfortumab vedotin**. Moderate Theoretical
- Antiepileptics **(carbamazepine, fosphenytoin, phenobarbital, phenytoin, primidone)** are predicted to decrease the exposure to the cytotoxic component of **enfortumab vedotin**. Moderate Theoretical
- Antifungals, azoles **(itraconazole, ketoconazole, posaconazole, voriconazole)** are predicted to increase the exposure to the cytotoxic component of **enfortumab vedotin**. Severe Theoretical
- **Ceritinib** is predicted to increase the exposure to the cytotoxic component of **enfortumab vedotin**. Severe Theoretical
- **Cobicistat** is predicted to increase the exposure to the cytotoxic component of **enfortumab vedotin**. Severe Theoretical
- **Encorafenib** is predicted to decrease the exposure to the cytotoxic component of **enfortumab vedotin**. Moderate Theoretical
- **HIV-protease inhibitors** are predicted to increase the exposure to the cytotoxic component of **enfortumab vedotin**. Severe Theoretical
- **Idelalisib** is predicted to increase the exposure to the cytotoxic component of **enfortumab vedotin**. Severe Theoretical
- **Ivosidenib** is predicted to decrease the exposure to the cytotoxic component of **enfortumab vedotin**. Moderate Theoretical
- **Lumacaftor** is predicted to decrease the exposure to the cytotoxic component of **enfortumab vedotin**. Moderate Theoretical
- Macrolides **(clarithromycin)** are predicted to increase the exposure to the cytotoxic component of **enfortumab vedotin**. Severe Theoretical
- **Mitotane** is predicted to decrease the exposure to the cytotoxic component of **enfortumab vedotin**. Moderate Theoretical
- Rifamycins **(rifampicin)** are predicted to decrease the exposure to the cytotoxic component of **enfortumab vedotin**. Moderate Theoretical
- **St John's wort** is predicted to decrease the exposure to the cytotoxic component of **enfortumab vedotin**. Moderate Theoretical
- **Tucatinib** is predicted to increase the exposure to the cytotoxic component of **enfortumab vedotin**. Severe Theoretical

Enfuvirtide → see TABLE 10 p. 1056 (peripheral neuropathy)

Enoxaparin → see low molecular-weight heparins

Entacapone

- **Entacapone** might increase the exposure to the active metabolite of **foslevodopa**. Adjust dose. [Moderate] Theoretical
- Oral **entacapone** is predicted to decrease the absorption of oral **iron**. Separate administration by at least 2 hours. [Moderate] Theoretical
- **Entacapone** is predicted to increase the risk of cardiovascular adverse effects when given with **isoprenaline**. [Moderate] Study
- **Entacapone** increases the exposure to **levodopa**. Monitor adverse effects and adjust dose. [Moderate] Study
- **Entacapone** is predicted to increase the risk of elevated blood pressure when given with **MAOIs, irreversible**. Avoid. [Severe] Theoretical
- **Entacapone** is predicted to increase the exposure to **methyldopa**. [Moderate] Theoretical
- **Entacapone** is predicted to increase the risk of cardiovascular adverse effects when given with **sympathomimetics, inotropic**. [Moderate] Theoretical
- **Entacapone** is predicted to increase the risk of cardiovascular adverse effects when given with sympathomimetics, vasoconstrictor **(adrenaline, noradrenaline)**. [Moderate] Study

Enteral feeds

- **Aluminium hydroxide** increases the risk of blocked enteral or nasogastric tubes when given with **enteral feeds**. [Moderate] Study
- **Enteral feeds** decrease the absorption of antiepileptics **(phenytoin)**. [Severe] Study
- **Enteral feeds** (vitamin-K containing) potentially decrease the anticoagulant effect of **coumarins**. [Severe] Anecdotal
- **Enteral feeds** (vitamin-K containing) potentially decrease the effects of **phenindione**. [Severe] Theoretical
- **Enteral feeds** decrease the exposure to quinolones **(ciprofloxacin)**. [Moderate] Study
- **Sucralfate** increases the risk of blocked enteral or nasogastric tubes when given with **enteral feeds**. Separate administration by 1 hour. [Moderate] Study
- **Enteral feeds** decrease the exposure to **theophylline**. [Moderate] Study

Entrectinib → see TABLE 7 p. 1055 (QT-interval prolongation)

FOOD AND LIFESTYLE Bitter (Seville) orange is predicted to increase the exposure to entrectinib; manufacturer advises avoid.

- Anti-androgens **(apalutamide, enzalutamide)** are predicted to decrease the exposure to **entrectinib**. Avoid. [Severe] Study → Also see TABLE 7 p. 1055
- Antiarrhythmics **(dronedarone)** are predicted to increase the exposure to **entrectinib**. Avoid or adjust dose with moderate CYP3A4 inhibitors—consult product literature. [Severe] Theoretical → Also see TABLE 7 p. 1055
- Antiepileptics **(carbamazepine, fosphenytoin, phenobarbital, phenytoin, primidone)** are predicted to decrease the exposure to **entrectinib**. Avoid. [Severe] Study
- Antifungals, azoles **(fluconazole, isavuconazole)** are predicted to increase the exposure to **entrectinib**. Avoid or adjust dose with moderate CYP3A4 inhibitors—consult product literature. [Severe] Theoretical → Also see TABLE 7 p. 1055
- Antifungals, azoles **(itraconazole, ketoconazole, posaconazole, voriconazole)** are predicted to increase the exposure to **entrectinib**. Avoid or adjust dose with potent CYP3A4 inhibitors—consult product literature. [Severe] Study → Also see TABLE 7 p. 1055
- **Berotralstat** is predicted to increase the exposure to **entrectinib**. Avoid or adjust dose with moderate CYP3A4 inhibitors—consult product literature. [Severe] Theoretical
- Calcium-channel blockers **(diltiazem, verapamil)** are predicted to increase the exposure to **entrectinib**. Avoid or adjust dose with moderate CYP3A4 inhibitors—consult product literature. [Severe] Theoretical
- **Cenobamate** is predicted to decrease the exposure to **entrectinib**. Avoid. [Moderate] Theoretical
- **Ceritinib** is predicted to increase the exposure to **entrectinib**. Avoid or adjust dose with potent CYP3A4 inhibitors—consult product literature. [Severe] Study → Also see TABLE 7 p. 1055
- **Cobicistat** is predicted to increase the exposure to **entrectinib**. Avoid or adjust dose with potent CYP3A4 inhibitors—consult product literature. [Severe] Study
- **Crizotinib** is predicted to increase the exposure to **entrectinib**. Avoid or adjust dose with moderate CYP3A4 inhibitors—consult product literature. [Severe] Theoretical → Also see TABLE 7 p. 1055
- **Dabrafenib** is predicted to decrease the exposure to **entrectinib**. Avoid. [Moderate] Theoretical
- **Encorafenib** is predicted to decrease the exposure to **entrectinib**. Avoid. [Severe] Study → Also see TABLE 7 p. 1055
- Endothelin receptor antagonists **(bosentan)** are predicted to decrease the exposure to **entrectinib**. Avoid. [Moderate] Theoretical
- **Fedratinib** is predicted to increase the exposure to **entrectinib**. Avoid or adjust dose with moderate CYP3A4 inhibitors—consult product literature. [Severe] Theoretical
- **Grapefruit** is predicted to increase the exposure to **entrectinib**. Avoid. [Severe] Theoretical
- **HIV-protease inhibitors** are predicted to increase the exposure to **entrectinib**. Avoid or adjust dose with potent CYP3A4 inhibitors—consult product literature. [Severe] Study
- **Idelalisib** is predicted to increase the exposure to **entrectinib**. Avoid or adjust dose with potent CYP3A4 inhibitors—consult product literature. [Severe] Study
- **Imatinib** is predicted to increase the exposure to **entrectinib**. Avoid or adjust dose with moderate CYP3A4 inhibitors—consult product literature. [Severe] Theoretical
- **Ivosidenib** is predicted to decrease the exposure to **entrectinib**. Avoid. [Severe] Study → Also see TABLE 7 p. 1055
- **Letermovir** is predicted to increase the exposure to **entrectinib**. Avoid or adjust dose with moderate CYP3A4 inhibitors—consult product literature. [Severe] Theoretical
- **Lorlatinib** is predicted to decrease the exposure to **entrectinib**. Avoid. [Moderate] Theoretical
- **Lumacaftor** is predicted to decrease the exposure to **entrectinib**. Avoid. [Severe] Study
- Macrolides **(clarithromycin)** are predicted to increase the exposure to **entrectinib**. Avoid or adjust dose with potent CYP3A4 inhibitors—consult product literature. [Severe] Study
- Macrolides **(erythromycin)** are predicted to increase the exposure to **entrectinib**. Avoid or adjust dose with moderate CYP3A4 inhibitors—consult product literature. [Severe] Theoretical → Also see TABLE 7 p. 1055
- **Entrectinib** is predicted to increase the exposure to **mavacamten**. Monitor and adjust dose—consult product literature. [Moderate] Theoretical
- **Mitotane** is predicted to decrease the exposure to **entrectinib**. Avoid. [Severe] Study
- Neurokinin-1 receptor antagonists **(aprepitant, netupitant)** are predicted to increase the exposure to **entrectinib**. Avoid or adjust dose with moderate CYP3A4 inhibitors—consult product literature. [Severe] Theoretical
- **Nilotinib** is predicted to increase the exposure to **entrectinib**. Avoid or adjust dose with moderate CYP3A4 inhibitors—consult product literature. [Severe] Theoretical → Also see TABLE 7 p. 1055
- NNRTIs **(efavirenz, etravirine, nevirapine)** are predicted to decrease the exposure to **entrectinib**. Avoid. [Moderate] Theoretical → Also see TABLE 7 p. 1055
- Rifamycins **(rifampicin)** are predicted to decrease the exposure to **entrectinib**. Avoid. [Severe] Study
- **Sotorasib** is predicted to decrease the exposure to **entrectinib**. Avoid. [Moderate] Theoretical
- **St John's wort** is predicted to decrease the exposure to **entrectinib**. Avoid. [Moderate] Theoretical
- **Tucatinib** is predicted to increase the exposure to **entrectinib**. Avoid or adjust dose with potent CYP3A4 inhibitors—consult product literature. [Severe] Study

Enzalutamide → see anti-androgens

Ephedrine → see sympathomimetics, vasoconstrictor

Epirubicin → see anthracyclines

Eplerenone → see mineralocorticoid receptor antagonists

Epoprostenol → see TABLE 3 p. 1053 (bleeding), TABLE 6 p. 1054 (hypotension)

Eprosartan → see angiotensin-II receptor antagonists
Eptifibatide → see TABLE 3 p. 1053 (bleeding)
Eravacycline → see tetracyclines
Erdafitinib

FOOD AND LIFESTYLE Avoid bitter (Seville) oranges as they might increase the exposure to erdafitinib.

- Anti-androgens **(apalutamide, enzalutamide)** are predicted to decrease the exposure to **erdafitinib**. Avoid. Severe Study
- Antiarrhythmics **(amiodarone)** are predicted to increase the exposure to **erdafitinib**. Adjust dose. Severe Study
- Antiepileptics **(carbamazepine, fosphenytoin, phenobarbital, phenytoin, primidone)** are predicted to decrease the exposure to **erdafitinib**. Avoid. Severe Study
- Antifungals, azoles **(fluconazole, itraconazole, ketoconazole, miconazole, posaconazole, voriconazole)** are predicted to increase the exposure to **erdafitinib**. Adjust dose. Severe Study
- **Cenobamate** is predicted to decrease the exposure to **erdafitinib**. Adjust dose. Moderate Theoretical
- **Ceritinib** is predicted to increase the exposure to **erdafitinib**. Adjust dose. Severe Study
- **Cobicistat** is predicted to increase the exposure to **erdafitinib**. Adjust dose. Severe Study
- **Erdafitinib** is predicted to increase the exposure to **colchicine**. Separate administration by at least 6 hours. Moderate Theoretical
- **Erdafitinib** might decrease the efficacy of **combined hormonal contraceptives**. Use alternative methods during treatment with, and for at least 28 days after stopping, **erdafitinib**. Severe Theoretical
- **Dabrafenib** is predicted to decrease the exposure to **erdafitinib**. Adjust dose. Moderate Theoretical
- **Erdafitinib** is predicted to increase the exposure to **digoxin**. Separate administration by at least 6 hours. Moderate Theoretical
- **Encorafenib** is predicted to decrease the exposure to **erdafitinib**. Avoid. Severe Study
- Endothelin receptor antagonists **(bosentan)** are predicted to decrease the exposure to **erdafitinib**. Adjust dose. Moderate Theoretical
- **Erdafitinib** is predicted to increase the exposure to **everolimus**. Separate administration by at least 6 hours. Moderate Theoretical
- **Erdafitinib** is predicted to increase the exposure to factor XA inhibitors **(apixaban)**. Separate administration by at least 6 hours. Moderate Theoretical
- **Grapefruit** is predicted to increase the exposure to **erdafitinib**. Avoid. Moderate Theoretical
- **HIV-protease inhibitors** are predicted to increase the exposure to **erdafitinib**. Adjust dose. Severe Study
- **Idelalisib** is predicted to increase the exposure to **erdafitinib**. Adjust dose. Severe Study
- **Ivosidenib** is predicted to decrease the exposure to **erdafitinib**. Avoid. Severe Study
- **Lorlatinib** is predicted to decrease the exposure to **erdafitinib**. Adjust dose. Moderate Theoretical
- **Lumacaftor** is predicted to decrease the exposure to **erdafitinib**. Avoid. Severe Study
- Macrolides **(clarithromycin)** are predicted to increase the exposure to **erdafitinib**. Adjust dose. Severe Study
- **Mitotane** is predicted to decrease the exposure to **erdafitinib**. Avoid. Severe Study
- **Modafinil** is predicted to decrease the exposure to **erdafitinib**. Adjust dose. Moderate Theoretical
- NNRTIs **(efavirenz, etravirine, nevirapine)** are predicted to decrease the exposure to **erdafitinib**. Adjust dose. Moderate Theoretical
- Rifamycins **(rifabutin)** are predicted to decrease the exposure to **erdafitinib**. Adjust dose. Moderate Theoretical
- Rifamycins **(rifampicin)** are predicted to decrease the exposure to **erdafitinib**. Avoid. Severe Study
- **Erdafitinib** is predicted to increase the exposure to **sirolimus**. Separate administration by at least 6 hours. Moderate Theoretical
- **Sotorasib** is predicted to decrease the exposure to **erdafitinib**. Adjust dose. Moderate Theoretical
- **St John's wort** is predicted to decrease the exposure to **erdafitinib**. Avoid. Moderate Study
- **Erdafitinib** is predicted to increase the exposure to **talazoparib**. Separate administration by at least 6 hours. Moderate Theoretical
- **Erdafitinib** is predicted to increase the exposure to taxanes **(paclitaxel)**. Separate administration by at least 6 hours. Moderate Theoretical
- **Telotristat ethyl** is predicted to decrease the exposure to **erdafitinib**. Adjust dose. Moderate Theoretical
- **Erdafitinib** is predicted to increase the exposure to thrombin inhibitors **(dabigatran)**. Separate administration by at least 6 hours. Moderate Theoretical
- **Tucatinib** is predicted to increase the exposure to **erdafitinib**. Adjust dose. Severe Study

Erenumab

GENERAL INFORMATION Caution on concurrent use of **erenumab** with drugs that cause constipation.

Ergocalciferol → see vitamin D substances
Ergometrine

- Antiarrhythmics **(dronedarone)** are predicted to increase the risk of ergotism when given with **ergometrine**. Severe Theoretical
- Antifungals, azoles **(fluconazole, isavuconazole)** are predicted to increase the risk of ergotism when given with **ergometrine**. Severe Theoretical
- Antifungals, azoles **(itraconazole, ketoconazole, posaconazole, voriconazole)** are predicted to increase the risk of ergotism when given with **ergometrine**. Avoid. Severe Theoretical
- Antifungals, azoles **(miconazole)** are predicted to increase the exposure to **ergometrine**. Avoid. Moderate Theoretical
- **Berotralstat** is predicted to increase the risk of ergotism when given with **ergometrine**. Severe Theoretical
- **Beta blockers, non-selective** are predicted to increase the risk of peripheral vasoconstriction when given with **ergometrine**. Severe Study
- **Beta blockers, selective** are predicted to increase the risk of peripheral vasoconstriction when given with **ergometrine**. Severe Study
- Calcium-channel blockers **(diltiazem, verapamil)** are predicted to increase the risk of ergotism when given with **ergometrine**. Severe Theoretical
- **Ceritinib** is predicted to increase the risk of ergotism when given with **ergometrine**. Avoid. Severe Theoretical
- **Cobicistat** is predicted to increase the risk of ergotism when given with **ergometrine**. Avoid. Severe Theoretical
- **Crizotinib** is predicted to increase the risk of ergotism when given with **ergometrine**. Severe Theoretical
- **Ergometrine** is predicted to increase the risk of ergotism when given with dopamine receptor agonists **(cabergoline)**. Avoid. Moderate Theoretical
- **Esketamine** is predicted to increase the risk of elevated blood pressure when given with **ergometrine**. Avoid. Severe Theoretical
- **Fedratinib** is predicted to increase the risk of ergotism when given with **ergometrine**. Severe Theoretical
- **Grapefruit** juice is predicted to increase the exposure to **ergometrine**. Severe Theoretical
- **HIV-protease inhibitors** are predicted to increase the risk of ergotism when given with **ergometrine**. Avoid. Severe Theoretical
- **Idelalisib** is predicted to increase the risk of ergotism when given with **ergometrine**. Avoid. Severe Theoretical
- **Imatinib** is predicted to increase the risk of ergotism when given with **ergometrine**. Severe Theoretical
- **Ketamine** is predicted to increase the risk of elevated blood pressure when given with **ergometrine**. Severe Theoretical
- **Letermovir** is predicted to increase the risk of ergotism when given with **ergometrine**. Severe Theoretical
- Macrolides **(clarithromycin)** are predicted to increase the risk of ergotism when given with **ergometrine**. Avoid. Severe Theoretical
- Macrolides **(erythromycin)** are predicted to increase the risk of ergotism when given with **ergometrine**. Severe Theoretical

- **Metronidazole** is predicted to increase the exposure to **ergometrine.** Severe Theoretical
- Neurokinin-1 receptor antagonists **(aprepitant, netupitant)** are predicted to increase the risk of ergotism when given with **ergometrine.** Severe Theoretical
- **Nilotinib** is predicted to increase the risk of ergotism when given with **ergometrine.** Severe Theoretical
- **Nirmatrelvir** boosted with ritonavir is predicted to increase the concentration of **ergometrine.** Avoid. Severe Theoretical
- **Olaparib** might alter the exposure to **ergometrine.** Moderate Theoretical
- **Ergometrine** potentially increases the risk of peripheral vasoconstriction when given with sympathomimetics, inotropic **(dopamine).** Avoid. Severe Anecdotal
- **Ergometrine** is predicted to increase the risk of peripheral vasoconstriction when given with sympathomimetics, vasoconstrictor **(noradrenaline).** Severe Anecdotal
- **Tucatinib** is predicted to increase the risk of ergotism when given with **ergometrine.** Avoid. Severe Theoretical

Eribulin → see TABLE 12 p. 1057 (myelosuppression), TABLE 10 p. 1056 (peripheral neuropathy), TABLE 7 p. 1055 (QT-interval prolongation)

Erlotinib

FOOD AND LIFESTYLE Dose adjustment may be necessary if smoking started or stopped during treatment.

- Oral **antacids** are predicted to decrease the absorption of oral **erlotinib.** Manufacturer advises take 2 hours before or 4 hours after antacids. Moderate Theoretical
- Anti-androgens **(apalutamide, enzalutamide)** are predicted to decrease the exposure to **erlotinib.** Avoid or adjust dose—consult product literature. Severe Study
- Antiarrhythmics **(amiodarone)** are predicted to increase the exposure to **erlotinib.** Moderate Theoretical
- Antiarrhythmics **(dronedarone)** are predicted to increase the exposure to **erlotinib.** Moderate Study
- Antiepileptics **(carbamazepine, fosphenytoin, phenobarbital, phenytoin, primidone)** are predicted to decrease the exposure to **erlotinib.** Avoid or adjust dose—consult product literature. Severe Study
- Antiepileptics **(eslicarbazepine)** are predicted to decrease the exposure to **erlotinib.** Severe Theoretical
- Antiepileptics **(oxcarbazepine)** decrease the exposure to **erlotinib.** Severe Study
- Antifungals, azoles **(fluconazole, isavuconazole)** are predicted to increase the exposure to **erlotinib.** Moderate Study
- Antifungals, azoles **(itraconazole, ketoconazole, posaconazole, voriconazole)** are predicted to increase the exposure to **erlotinib.** Use with caution and adjust dose. Severe Study
- **Erlotinib** is predicted to increase the risk of gastrointestinal perforation when given with **aspirin** (high-dose). Severe Theoretical
- **Berotralstat** is predicted to increase the exposure to **erlotinib.** Moderate Study
- Oral calcium compounds **(calcium carbonate)** -containing antacids are predicted to decrease the absorption of oral **erlotinib.** Manufacturer advises take 2 hours before or 4 hours after antacids. Moderate Theoretical
- Calcium-channel blockers **(diltiazem, verapamil)** are predicted to increase the exposure to **erlotinib.** Moderate Study
- **Cenobamate** is predicted to decrease the exposure to **erlotinib.** Severe Study
- **Ceritinib** is predicted to increase the exposure to **erlotinib.** Use with caution and adjust dose. Severe Study
- **Ciclosporin** is predicted to increase the exposure to **erlotinib.** Moderate Theoretical
- **Cobicistat** is predicted to increase the exposure to **erlotinib.** Use with caution and adjust dose. Severe Study
- **Combined hormonal contraceptives** are predicted to increases the exposure to **erlotinib.** Monitor adverse effects and adjust dose. Moderate Study
- **Erlotinib** is predicted to increase the risk of gastrointestinal perforation when given with **corticosteroids.** Severe Theoretical
- **Erlotinib** increases the anticoagulant effect of **coumarins.** Severe Anecdotal
- **Crizotinib** is predicted to increase the exposure to **erlotinib.** Moderate Study
- **Dabrafenib** is predicted to decrease the exposure to **erlotinib.** Severe Study
- **Encorafenib** is predicted to increase the exposure to **erlotinib.** Avoid or adjust dose—consult product literature. Severe Study
- Endothelin receptor antagonists **(bosentan)** are predicted to decrease the exposure to **erlotinib.** Severe Study
- **Fedratinib** is predicted to increase the exposure to **erlotinib.** Moderate Study
- **Givosiran** are predicted to increases the exposure to **erlotinib.** Monitor adverse effects and adjust dose. Moderate Study
- **Glecaprevir** is predicted to increase the exposure to **erlotinib.** Moderate Theoretical
- **Grapefruit** juice is predicted to increase the exposure to **erlotinib.** Moderate Theoretical
- **H_2 receptor antagonists** are predicted to decrease the exposure to **erlotinib.** Manufacturer advises take 2 hours before or 10 hours after **H_2 receptor antagonists.** Moderate Study
- **HIV-protease inhibitors** are predicted to increase the exposure to **erlotinib.** Use with caution and adjust dose. Severe Study
- **Idelalisib** is predicted to increase the exposure to **erlotinib.** Use with caution and adjust dose. Severe Study
- **Imatinib** is predicted to increase the exposure to **erlotinib.** Moderate Study
- **Ivosidenib** is predicted to decrease the exposure to **erlotinib.** Avoid or adjust dose—consult product literature. Severe Study
- **Lapatinib** is predicted to increase the exposure to **erlotinib.** Moderate Theoretical
- **Letermovir** is predicted to increase the exposure to **erlotinib.** Moderate Study
- **Lorlatinib** is predicted to decrease the exposure to **erlotinib.** Severe Study
- **Lumacaftor** is predicted to decrease the exposure to **erlotinib.** Avoid or adjust dose—consult product literature. Severe Study
- Macrolides **(azithromycin)** are predicted to increase the exposure to **erlotinib.** Moderate Theoretical
- Macrolides **(clarithromycin)** are predicted to increase the exposure to **erlotinib.** Use with caution and adjust dose. Severe Study
- Macrolides **(erythromycin)** are predicted to increase the exposure to **erlotinib.** Moderate Study
- **Mexiletine** are predicted to increases the exposure to **erlotinib.** Monitor adverse effects and adjust dose. Moderate Study
- **Mitotane** is predicted to decrease the exposure to **erlotinib.** Avoid or adjust dose—consult product literature. Severe Study
- Neurokinin-1 receptor antagonists **(aprepitant, netupitant)** are predicted to increase the exposure to **erlotinib.** Moderate Study
- **Nilotinib** is predicted to increase the exposure to **erlotinib.** Moderate Study
- NNRTIs **(efavirenz, etravirine, nevirapine)** are predicted to decrease the exposure to **erlotinib.** Severe Study
- **Erlotinib** is predicted to increase the risk of gastrointestinal perforation when given with **NSAIDs.** Severe Theoretical
- **Osilodrostat** are predicted to increases the exposure to **erlotinib.** Monitor adverse effects and adjust dose. Moderate Study
- **Erlotinib** is predicted to increase the risk of bleeding events when given with **phenindione.** Severe Theoretical
- **Pibrentasvir** is predicted to increase the exposure to **erlotinib.** Moderate Theoretical
- **Proton pump inhibitors** are predicted to decrease the exposure to **erlotinib.** Avoid. Moderate Study
- Quinolones **(ciprofloxacin)** are predicted to increase the exposure to **erlotinib.** Monitor adverse effects and adjust dose. Moderate Study
- **Ranolazine** is predicted to increase the exposure to **erlotinib.** Moderate Theoretical
- Rifamycins **(rifampicin)** are predicted to decrease the exposure to **erlotinib.** Avoid or adjust dose—consult product literature. Severe Study
- **Rucaparib** are predicted to increases the exposure to **erlotinib.** Monitor adverse effects and adjust dose. Moderate Study
- **Erlotinib** is predicted to increase the exposure to the active component of **sacituzumab govitecan.** Severe Theoretical

Erlotinib (continued)
- Oral sodium bicarbonate-containing antacids are predicted to decrease the absorption of oral **erlotinib**. Manufacturer advises take 2 hours before or 4 hours after antacids. [Moderate] Theoretical
- Sodium zirconium cyclosilicate is predicted to decrease the exposure to **erlotinib**. Separate administration by at least 2 hours. [Moderate] Theoretical
- Sotorasib is predicted to decrease the exposure to **erlotinib**. [Severe] Study
- SSRIs **(fluvoxamine)** are predicted to increase the exposure to **erlotinib**. Monitor adverse effects and adjust dose. [Moderate] Theoretical
- St John's wort is predicted to decrease the exposure to **erlotinib**. [Severe] Study
- Tucatinib is predicted to increase the exposure to **erlotinib**. Use with caution and adjust dose. [Severe] Study
- Velpatasvir is predicted to increase the exposure to **erlotinib**. [Moderate] Theoretical
- Vemurafenib are predicted to increases the exposure to **erlotinib**. Monitor adverse effects and adjust dose. [Moderate] Study
- Voxilaprevir is predicted to increase the exposure to **erlotinib**. [Moderate] Theoretical

Ertapenem → see carbapenems
Ertugliflozin → see sodium glucose co-transporter 2 inhibitors
Erythromycin → see macrolides
Escitalopram → see SSRIs
Esketamine → see TABLE 6 p. 1054 (hypotension), TABLE 9 p. 1056 (CNS effects)
- **Esketamine** is predicted to increase the risk of seizures when given with aminophylline. Avoid. [Severe] Theoretical
- Anti-androgens **(apalutamide, enzalutamide)** are predicted to decrease the exposure to **esketamine**. Adjust dose. [Moderate] Study
- Antiepileptics **(carbamazepine, fosphenytoin, phenobarbital, phenytoin, primidone)** are predicted to decrease the exposure to **esketamine**. Adjust dose. [Moderate] Study → Also see TABLE 9 p. 1056
- Antifungals, azoles **(itraconazole, ketoconazole, posaconazole, voriconazole)** are predicted to increase the exposure to **esketamine**. Adjust dose. [Moderate] Study
- Ceritinib is predicted to increase the exposure to **esketamine**. Adjust dose. [Moderate] Study
- Cobicistat is predicted to increase the exposure to **esketamine**. Adjust dose. [Moderate] Study
- Encorafenib is predicted to decrease the exposure to **esketamine**. Adjust dose. [Moderate] Study
- **Esketamine** is predicted to increase the risk of elevated blood pressure when given with ergometrine. Avoid. [Severe] Theoretical
- HIV-protease inhibitors are predicted to increase the exposure to **esketamine**. Adjust dose. [Moderate] Study
- Idelalisib is predicted to increase the exposure to **esketamine**. Adjust dose. [Moderate] Study
- Ivosidenib is predicted to decrease the exposure to **esketamine**. Adjust dose. [Moderate] Study
- Lumacaftor is predicted to decrease the exposure to **esketamine**. Adjust dose. [Moderate] Study
- Macrolides **(clarithromycin)** are predicted to increase the exposure to **esketamine**. Adjust dose. [Moderate] Study
- Mitotane is predicted to decrease the exposure to **esketamine**. Adjust dose. [Moderate] Study
- Rifamycins **(rifampicin)** are predicted to decrease the exposure to **esketamine**. Adjust dose. [Moderate] Study
- St John's wort moderately decreases the exposure to **esketamine**. Adjust dose. [Moderate] Study
- **Esketamine** is predicted to increase the risk of seizures when given with theophylline. Avoid. [Severe] Theoretical
- Tucatinib is predicted to increase the exposure to **esketamine**. Adjust dose. [Moderate] Study

Eslicarbazepine → see antiepileptics
Esmolol → see beta blockers, selective
Esomeprazole → see proton pump inhibitors

Estradiol
- Antiepileptics **(carbamazepine, eslicarbazepine, fosphenytoin, oxcarbazepine, perampanel, phenobarbital, phenytoin, primidone, rufinamide, topiramate)** are predicted to decrease the efficacy of **estradiol**. [Moderate] Theoretical
- Endothelin receptor antagonists **(bosentan)** are predicted to decrease the efficacy of **estradiol**. [Moderate] Theoretical
- HIV-protease inhibitors **(ritonavir)** are predicted to decrease the efficacy of **estradiol**. [Moderate] Theoretical
- Modafinil is predicted to decrease the efficacy of **estradiol**. [Moderate] Theoretical
- Neurokinin-1 receptor antagonists **(aprepitant, fosaprepitant)** are predicted to decrease the efficacy of **estradiol**. [Moderate] Theoretical
- NNRTIs **(efavirenz, nevirapine)** are predicted to decrease the efficacy of **estradiol**. [Moderate] Theoretical
- Rifamycins are predicted to decrease the efficacy of **estradiol**. [Moderate] Theoretical
- St John's wort is predicted to decrease the efficacy of **estradiol**. [Moderate] Theoretical

Estramustine → see alkylating agents
Eszopiclone → see TABLE 9 p. 1056 (CNS effects)
- Anti-androgens **(apalutamide, enzalutamide)** are predicted to decrease the exposure to **eszopiclone**. Adjust dose. [Moderate] Theoretical
- Antiepileptics **(carbamazepine, fosphenytoin, phenobarbital, phenytoin, primidone)** are predicted to decrease the exposure to **eszopiclone**. Adjust dose. [Moderate] Theoretical → Also see TABLE 9 p. 1056
- Antifungals, azoles **(itraconazole, ketoconazole, posaconazole, voriconazole)** are predicted to increase the exposure to **eszopiclone**. Adjust **eszopiclone** dose; avoid in the elderly. [Moderate] Study
- Ceritinib is predicted to increase the exposure to **eszopiclone**. Adjust **eszopiclone** dose; avoid in the elderly. [Moderate] Study
- Cobicistat is predicted to increase the exposure to **eszopiclone**. Adjust **eszopiclone** dose; avoid in the elderly. [Moderate] Study
- Encorafenib is predicted to decrease the exposure to **eszopiclone**. Adjust dose. [Moderate] Theoretical
- HIV-protease inhibitors are predicted to increase the exposure to **eszopiclone**. Adjust **eszopiclone** dose; avoid in the elderly. [Moderate] Study
- Idelalisib is predicted to increase the exposure to **eszopiclone**. Adjust **eszopiclone** dose; avoid in the elderly. [Moderate] Study
- Ivosidenib is predicted to decrease the exposure to **eszopiclone**. Adjust dose. [Moderate] Theoretical
- Lumacaftor is predicted to decrease the exposure to **eszopiclone**. Adjust dose. [Moderate] Theoretical
- Macrolides **(clarithromycin)** are predicted to increase the exposure to **eszopiclone**. Adjust **eszopiclone** dose; avoid in the elderly. [Moderate] Study
- Mitotane is predicted to decrease the exposure to **eszopiclone**. Adjust dose. [Moderate] Theoretical
- Rifamycins **(rifampicin)** are predicted to decrease the exposure to **eszopiclone**. Adjust dose. [Moderate] Theoretical
- St John's wort is predicted to decrease the exposure to **eszopiclone**. Adjust dose. [Moderate] Theoretical
- Tucatinib is predicted to increase the exposure to **eszopiclone**. Adjust **eszopiclone** dose; avoid in the elderly. [Moderate] Study

Etanercept
- Abatacept is predicted to increase the risk of generalised infection (possibly life-threatening) when given with **etanercept**. Avoid. [Severe] Theoretical
- Anakinra is predicted to increase the risk of generalised infection (possibly life-threatening) when given with **etanercept**. Avoid. [Severe] Theoretical
- Filgotinib is predicted to increase the risk of immunosuppression when given with **etanercept**. Avoid. [Severe] Theoretical
- Live vaccines are predicted to increase the risk of generalised infection (possibly life-threatening) when given with **etanercept**. UKHSA advises avoid (refer to Green Book). [Severe] Theoretical

▸ Monoclonal antibodies (rozanolixizumab) might decrease the concentration of **etanercept**. Avoid and for 2 weeks after stopping rozanolixizumab. Moderate Theoretical
▸ Monoclonal antibodies (sarilumab) might cause severe infection and neutropenia when given with **etanercept**. Severe Theoretical

Etelcalcetide
▸ Cinacalcet increases the risk of hypocalcaemia when given with **etelcalcetide**. Avoid. Severe Theoretical
▸ **Etelcalcetide** might increase the risk of hypocalcaemia when given with denosumab. Severe Theoretical

Ethambutol
▸ Isoniazid increases the risk of optic neuropathy when given with **ethambutol**. Severe Anecdotal

Ethinylestradiol
▸ Fostemsavir increases the concentration of **ethinylestradiol** from a combined hormonal contraceptive. Adjust dose—consult product literature. Severe Study
▸ **Ethinylestradiol** might increase ALT concentrations when given with glecaprevir with pibrentasvir. Avoid. Severe Study
▸ **Ethinylestradiol** might increase ALT concentrations when given with pibrentasvir with glecaprevir. Avoid. Severe Study
▸ **Ethinylestradiol** might increase ALT concentrations when given with sofosbuvir with velpatasvir and voxilaprevir. Avoid. Severe Study
▸ **Ethinylestradiol** might increase ALT concentrations when given with velpatasvir with sofosbuvir and voxilaprevir. Avoid. Severe Study
▸ **Ethinylestradiol** might increase ALT concentrations when given with voxilaprevir with sofosbuvir and velpatasvir. Avoid. Severe Study

Ethosuximide → see antiepileptics

Etodolac → see NSAIDs

Etomidate → see TABLE 6 p. 1054 (hypotension), TABLE 9 p. 1056 (CNS effects)

Etonogestrel
▸ Antiepileptics (carbamazepine, eslicarbazepine, fosphenytoin, oxcarbazepine, perampanel, phenobarbital, phenytoin, primidone, rufinamide, topiramate) are predicted to decrease the efficacy of **etonogestrel**. For CoSRH guidance, see Contraceptives, interactions p. 614. Severe Theoretical
▸ Antiepileptics (lamotrigine) might decrease the effects of **etonogestrel**. For CoSRH guidance, see Contraceptives, interactions p. 614. Moderate Theoretical
▸ Antifungals, azoles (itraconazole, ketoconazole, posaconazole, voriconazole) are predicted to increase the concentration of subdermal **etonogestrel**. Moderate Theoretical
▸ Ceritinib is predicted to increase the concentration of subdermal **etonogestrel**. Moderate Theoretical
▸ Cobicistat is predicted to increase the concentration of subdermal **etonogestrel**. Moderate Theoretical
▸ Endothelin receptor antagonists (bosentan) are predicted to decrease the efficacy of **etonogestrel**. For CoSRH guidance, see Contraceptives, interactions p. 614. Severe Theoretical
▸ HIV-protease inhibitors (ritonavir) are predicted to decrease the efficacy of **etonogestrel**. For CoSRH guidance, see Contraceptives, interactions p. 614. Severe Theoretical
▸ HIV-protease inhibitors are predicted to increase the concentration of subdermal **etonogestrel**. Moderate Theoretical
▸ Idelalisib is predicted to increase the concentration of subdermal **etonogestrel**. Moderate Theoretical
▸ Lumacaftor might decrease the efficacy of subdermal **etonogestrel**. Use additional contraceptive precautions. Severe Theoretical
▸ Macrolides (clarithromycin) are predicted to increase the concentration of subdermal **etonogestrel**. Moderate Theoretical
▸ Modafinil is predicted to decrease the efficacy of **etonogestrel**. For CoSRH guidance, see Contraceptives, interactions p. 614. Severe Theoretical
▸ Neurokinin-1 receptor antagonists (aprepitant, fosaprepitant) are predicted to decrease the efficacy of **etonogestrel**. For CoSRH guidance, see Contraceptives, interactions p. 614. Severe Theoretical
▸ NNRTIs (efavirenz, nevirapine) are predicted to decrease the efficacy of **etonogestrel**. For CoSRH guidance, see Contraceptives, interactions p. 614. Severe Theoretical
▸ NNRTIs (etravirine) might decrease the efficacy of **etonogestrel**. Follow CoSRH guidance for enzyme inducers, see Contraceptives, interactions p. 614. Severe Theoretical
▸ Rifamycins are predicted to decrease the efficacy of **etonogestrel**. For CoSRH guidance, see Contraceptives, interactions p. 614. Severe Theoretical
▸ St John's wort is predicted to decrease the efficacy of **etonogestrel**. MHRA advises avoid. For CoSRH guidance, see Contraceptives, interactions p. 614. Severe Theoretical
▸ Sugammadex is predicted to decrease the efficacy of **etonogestrel**. Use additional contraceptive precautions. Severe Theoretical
▸ Tucatinib is predicted to increase the concentration of subdermal **etonogestrel**. Moderate Theoretical
▸ **Etonogestrel** might decrease the efficacy of ulipristal and ulipristal might decrease the efficacy of **etonogestrel**. Avoid when used for uterine fibroids. For CoSRH guidance when used for emergency hormonal contraception, see Contraceptives, interactions p. 614. Severe Theoretical

Etoposide → see TABLE 12 p. 1057 (myelosuppression)
▸ Antiepileptics (carbamazepine, fosphenytoin, phenobarbital, phenytoin, primidone) are predicted to decrease the efficacy of **etoposide**. Moderate Study
▸ Ciclosporin increases the exposure to **etoposide**. Monitor and adjust dose. Severe Study
▸ Live vaccines are predicted to increase the risk of generalised infection (possibly life-threatening) when given with **etoposide**. UKHSA advises avoid (refer to Green Book). Severe Theoretical
▸ Neurokinin-1 receptor antagonists (netupitant) slightly increase the exposure to **etoposide**. Moderate Study

Etoricoxib → see NSAIDs

Etrasimod → see TABLE 4 p. 1054 (bradycardia), TABLE 7 p. 1055 (QT-interval prolongation)
▸ Anti-androgens (enzalutamide) are predicted to decrease the exposure to **etrasimod**. Avoid. Severe Theoretical
▸ Antiarrhythmics (dronedarone) are predicted to increase the exposure to **etrasimod**. Avoid in poor CYP2C9 metabolisers. Severe Theoretical → Also see TABLE 4 p. 1054
▸ Antifungals, azoles (fluconazole) slightly increase the exposure to **etrasimod**. Avoid. Severe Study
▸ Antifungals, azoles (isavuconazole, itraconazole, ketoconazole, posaconazole, voriconazole) are predicted to increase the exposure to **etrasimod**. Avoid in poor CYP2C9 metabolisers. Severe Theoretical
▸ Berotralstat is predicted to increase the exposure to **etrasimod**. Avoid in poor CYP2C9 metabolisers. Severe Theoretical
▸ Calcium-channel blockers (diltiazem, verapamil) are predicted to increase the exposure to **etrasimod**. Avoid in poor CYP2C9 metabolisers. Severe Theoretical → Also see TABLE 4 p. 1054
▸ Ceritinib is predicted to increase the exposure to **etrasimod**. Avoid in poor CYP2C9 metabolisers. Severe Theoretical → Also see TABLE 4 p. 1054
▸ Clopidogrel are predicted to increases the exposure to **etrasimod**. Avoid in poor CYP2C9 metabolisers. Severe Theoretical
▸ Cobicistat is predicted to increase the exposure to **etrasimod**. Avoid in poor CYP2C9 metabolisers. Severe Theoretical
▸ Crizotinib is predicted to increase the exposure to **etrasimod**. Avoid in poor CYP2C9 metabolisers. Severe Theoretical → Also see TABLE 4 p. 1054
▸ Fedratinib is predicted to increase the exposure to **etrasimod**. Avoid in poor CYP2C9 metabolisers. Severe Theoretical
▸ Fibrates (gemfibrozil) are predicted to increase the exposure to **etrasimod**. Avoid in poor CYP2C9 metabolisers. Severe Theoretical
▸ HIV-protease inhibitors are predicted to increase the exposure to **etrasimod**. Avoid in poor CYP2C9 metabolisers. Severe Theoretical
▸ Idelalisib is predicted to increase the exposure to **etrasimod**. Avoid in poor CYP2C9 metabolisers. Severe Theoretical
▸ Imatinib is predicted to increase the exposure to **etrasimod**. Avoid in poor CYP2C9 metabolisers. Severe Theoretical

Etrasimod (continued)

- Iron chelators **(deferasirox)** are predicted to increase the exposure to **etrasimod**. Avoid in poor CYP2C9 metabolisers. [Severe] Theoretical
- **Leflunomide** are predicted to increases the exposure to **etrasimod**. Avoid in poor CYP2C9 metabolisers. [Severe] Theoretical
- **Letermovir** is predicted to increase the exposure to **etrasimod**. Avoid in poor CYP2C9 metabolisers. [Severe] Theoretical
- **Live vaccines** might increase the risk of generalised infection (possibly life-threatening) when given with **etrasimod**. Avoid and for at least 4 weeks before and 2 weeks after stopping **etrasimod**. [Severe] Theoretical
- Macrolides **(clarithromycin, erythromycin)** are predicted to increase the exposure to **etrasimod**. Avoid in poor CYP2C9 metabolisers. [Severe] Theoretical
- Neurokinin-1 receptor antagonists **(aprepitant, netupitant)** are predicted to increase the exposure to **etrasimod**. Avoid in poor CYP2C9 metabolisers. [Severe] Theoretical
- **Nilotinib** is predicted to increase the exposure to **etrasimod**. Avoid in poor CYP2C9 metabolisers. [Severe] Theoretical
- Rifamycins **(rifampicin)** slightly decrease the exposure to **etrasimod**. Avoid. [Severe] Study
- **Teriflunomide** are predicted to increases the exposure to **etrasimod**. Avoid in poor CYP2C9 metabolisers. [Severe] Theoretical
- **Tucatinib** is predicted to increase the exposure to **etrasimod**. Avoid in poor CYP2C9 metabolisers. [Severe] Theoretical

Etravirine → see NNRTIs

Everolimus

- **Abrocitinib** might increase the exposure to **everolimus**. [Moderate] Theoretical
- **Everolimus** potentially increases the risk of angioedema when given with **ACE inhibitors**. [Severe] Anecdotal
- Anti-androgens **(apalutamide, enzalutamide)** are predicted to decrease the concentration of **everolimus**. Avoid or adjust dose. [Severe] Study
- Antiarrhythmics **(amiodarone)** are predicted to increase the exposure to **everolimus**. Monitor and adjust dose. [Severe] Study
- Antiarrhythmics **(dronedarone)** are predicted to increase the concentration of **everolimus**. Avoid or adjust dose. [Moderate] Study
- Antiepileptics **(carbamazepine, fosphenytoin, phenobarbital, phenytoin, primidone)** are predicted to decrease the concentration of **everolimus**. Avoid or adjust dose. [Severe] Study
- Antifungals, azoles **(fluconazole, isavuconazole)** are predicted to increase the concentration of **everolimus**. Avoid or adjust dose. [Moderate] Study
- Antifungals, azoles **(itraconazole, ketoconazole, posaconazole, voriconazole)** are predicted to increase the exposure to **everolimus**. Avoid. [Severe] Study
- **Asciminib** is predicted to increase the exposure to **everolimus**. [Severe] Theoretical
- **Belumosudil** might increase the exposure to **everolimus**. Avoid or adjust dose. [Moderate] Theoretical
- **Belzutifan** is predicted to decrease the exposure to **everolimus**. Avoid or adjust dose. [Severe] Theoretical
- **Berotralstat** is predicted to increase the concentration of **everolimus**. Avoid or adjust dose. [Moderate] Study
- **Bulevirtide** is predicted to increase the exposure to **everolimus**. [Moderate] Theoretical
- Calcium-channel blockers **(diltiazem, verapamil)** are predicted to increase the concentration of **everolimus**. Avoid or adjust dose. [Moderate] Study
- **Cannabidiol** moderately increases the exposure to **everolimus**. Monitor and adjust dose. [Moderate] Study
- **Cenobamate** is predicted to decrease the concentration of **everolimus**. Avoid or adjust dose. [Severe] Study
- **Ceritinib** is predicted to increase the exposure to **everolimus**. Avoid. [Severe] Study
- **Ciclosporin** moderately increases the exposure to **everolimus**. Avoid or adjust dose. [Severe] Study
- **Cobicistat** is predicted to increase the exposure to **everolimus**. Avoid. [Severe] Study
- **Crizotinib** is predicted to increase the concentration of **everolimus**. Avoid or adjust dose. [Moderate] Study
- **Dabrafenib** is predicted to decrease the concentration of **everolimus**. Avoid or adjust dose. [Severe] Study
- **Danicopan** is predicted to increase the exposure to **everolimus**. [Moderate] Study
- **Daridorexant** is predicted to increase the exposure to **everolimus**. [Moderate] Study
- **Deutivacaftor** is predicted to increase the exposure to **everolimus**. [Moderate] Theoretical
- **Eliglustat** is predicted to increase the exposure to **everolimus**. Adjust dose. [Moderate] Study
- **Encorafenib** is predicted to decrease the concentration of **everolimus**. Avoid or adjust dose. [Severe] Study
- Endothelin receptor antagonists **(bosentan)** are predicted to decrease the concentration of **everolimus**. Avoid or adjust dose. [Severe] Study
- **Erdafitinib** is predicted to increase the exposure to **everolimus**. Separate administration by at least 6 hours. [Moderate] Theoretical
- **Fedratinib** is predicted to increase the concentration of **everolimus**. Avoid or adjust dose. [Moderate] Study
- **Fostamatinib** is predicted to increase the exposure to **everolimus**. Monitor and adjust dose. [Moderate] Theoretical
- **Givinostat** might increase the exposure to **everolimus**. [Moderate] Study
- **Glecaprevir** is predicted to increase the exposure to **everolimus**. [Moderate] Study
- **Grapefruit** juice is predicted to increase the exposure to **everolimus**. Avoid. [Severe] Theoretical
- **HIV-protease inhibitors** are predicted to increase the exposure to **everolimus**. Avoid. [Severe] Study
- **Ibrutinib** might increase the exposure to **everolimus**. Separate administration by at least 6 hours. [Moderate] Theoretical
- **Idelalisib** is predicted to increase the exposure to **everolimus**. Avoid. [Severe] Study
- **Imatinib** is predicted to increase the concentration of **everolimus**. Avoid or adjust dose. [Moderate] Study
- **Ivacaftor** is predicted to increase the exposure to **everolimus**. [Moderate] Study
- **Ivosidenib** is predicted to decrease the concentration of **everolimus**. Avoid or adjust dose. [Severe] Study
- **Lapatinib** is predicted to increase the exposure to **everolimus**. [Moderate] Theoretical
- **Larotrectinib** is predicted to increase the exposure to **everolimus**. Use with caution and adjust dose. [Mild] Theoretical
- **Lazertinib** is predicted to increase the exposure to **everolimus**. [Moderate] Study
- **Letermovir** is predicted to increase the concentration of **everolimus**. Avoid or adjust dose. [Moderate] Study
- **Live vaccines** are predicted to increase the risk of generalised infection (possibly life-threatening) when given with **everolimus**. UKHSA advises avoid (refer to Green Book). [Severe] Theoretical
- **Everolimus** is predicted to increase the exposure to **lomitapide** and **lomitapide** might increase the exposure to **everolimus**. Adjust **everolimus** dose and separate administration by 12 hours, p. 689. [Moderate] Theoretical
- **Lorlatinib** is predicted to decrease the concentration of **everolimus**. Avoid or adjust dose. [Severe] Study
- **Lumacaftor** is predicted to decrease the concentration of **everolimus**. Avoid or adjust dose. [Severe] Study
- Macrolides **(clarithromycin)** are predicted to increase the exposure to **everolimus**. Avoid. [Severe] Study
- Macrolides **(erythromycin)** are predicted to increase the concentration of **everolimus**. Avoid or adjust dose. [Moderate] Study
- **Maribavir** increases the exposure to **everolimus**. Monitor and adjust dose. [Severe] Study
- **Everolimus** is predicted to increase the exposure to **mavacamten**. Monitor and adjust dose—consult product literature. [Moderate] Theoretical
- **Mifepristone** is predicted to increase the exposure to **everolimus**. [Severe] Theoretical

- **Mirabegron** is predicted to increase the exposure to **everolimus**. Mild Theoretical
- **Mitotane** is predicted to decrease the concentration of **everolimus**. Avoid or adjust dose. Severe Study
- **Neratinib** is predicted to increase the exposure to **everolimus**. Moderate Study
- Neurokinin-1 receptor antagonists **(aprepitant, netupitant)** are predicted to increase the concentration of **everolimus**. Avoid or adjust dose. Moderate Study
- **Nilotinib** is predicted to increase the concentration of **everolimus**. Avoid or adjust dose. Moderate Study
- **Nirmatrelvir** boosted with ritonavir is predicted to increase the concentration of **everolimus**. Avoid—consult product literature. Severe Theoretical
- NNRTIs **(efavirenz, etravirine, nevirapine)** are predicted to decrease the concentration of **everolimus**. Avoid or adjust dose. Severe Study
- **Olaparib** might increase the exposure to **everolimus**. Moderate Theoretical
- **Osimertinib** is predicted to increase the exposure to **everolimus**. Moderate Study
- **Palbociclib** is predicted to increase the exposure to **everolimus**. Adjust dose. Moderate Theoretical
- **Pemigatinib** might increase the exposure to **everolimus**. Separate administration by at least 6 hours. Moderate Theoretical
- Penicillins **(flucloxacillin)** (high-dose) might decrease the exposure to **everolimus**. Moderate Study
- **Pibrentasvir** with glecaprevir is predicted to increase the exposure to **everolimus**. Moderate Study
- **Pirtobrutinib** is predicted to increase the exposure to **everolimus**. Avoid or monitor. Moderate Theoretical
- **Pitolisant** is predicted to decrease the exposure to **everolimus**. Avoid. Severe Theoretical
- **Ribociclib** is predicted to increase the exposure to **everolimus**. Use with caution and adjust dose. Moderate Theoretical
- Rifamycins **(rifampicin)** are predicted to decrease the concentration of **everolimus**. Avoid or adjust dose. Severe Study
- **Ritlecitinib** is predicted to increase the exposure to **everolimus**. Adjust dose. Moderate Theoretical
- **Selpercatinib** is predicted to increase the exposure to **everolimus**. Avoid. Moderate Study
- **Sotorasib** is predicted to decrease the concentration of **everolimus**. Avoid or adjust dose. Severe Study
- **Sparsentan** is predicted to increase the exposure to **everolimus**. Severe Theoretical
- **St John's wort** is predicted to decrease the concentration of **everolimus**. Avoid or adjust dose. Severe Study
- **Tepotinib** is predicted to increase the concentration of **everolimus**. Severe Study
- **Tucatinib** is predicted to increase the exposure to **everolimus**. Avoid. Severe Study
- **Velpatasvir** is predicted to increase the exposure to **everolimus**. Severe Theoretical
- **Vemurafenib** is predicted to increase the exposure to **everolimus**. Use with caution and adjust dose. Severe Theoretical
- **Venetoclax** is predicted to increase the exposure to **everolimus**. Avoid or adjust dose. Severe Study
- **Voclosporin** is predicted to increase the exposure to **everolimus**. Moderate Study
- **Vorasidenib** might decrease the concentration of **everolimus**. Avoid. Severe Theoretical
- **Voxilaprevir** with sofosbuvir and velpatasvir is predicted to increase the exposure to **everolimus**. Severe Theoretical

Exemestane

- Anti-androgens **(apalutamide, enzalutamide)** moderately decrease the exposure to **exemestane**. Moderate Study
- Antiepileptics **(carbamazepine, fosphenytoin, phenobarbital, phenytoin, primidone)** moderately decrease the exposure to **exemestane**. Moderate Study
- **Encorafenib** moderately decreases the exposure to **exemestane**. Moderate Study
- **Ivosidenib** moderately decreases the exposure to **exemestane**. Moderate Study
- **Lumacaftor** moderately decreases the exposure to **exemestane**. Moderate Study
- **Mitotane** moderately decreases the exposure to **exemestane**. Moderate Study
- Rifamycins **(rifampicin)** moderately decrease the exposure to **exemestane**. Moderate Study
- **St John's wort** is predicted to decrease the exposure to **exemestane**. Moderate Theoretical

Ezetimibe

- **Ezetimibe** is predicted to affect the efficacy of **bulevirtide**. Avoid. Severe Theoretical
- **Ciclosporin** moderately increases the exposure to **ezetimibe** and **ezetimibe** slightly increases the exposure to **ciclosporin**. Moderate Study
- **Fibrates** are predicted to increase the risk of gallstones when given with **ezetimibe**. Severe Theoretical

Factor XA inhibitors → see TABLE 3 p. 1053 (bleeding)

apixaban · edoxaban · fondaparinux · rivaroxaban

- **Abrocitinib** might increase the exposure to **edoxaban**. Moderate Theoretical
- Anti-androgens **(apalutamide)** are predicted to decrease the exposure to **edoxaban**. Monitor and adjust dose. Moderate Study
- Anti-androgens **(apalutamide, enzalutamide)** are predicted to decrease the exposure to **apixaban**. Moderate Study
- Anti-androgens **(apalutamide, enzalutamide)** are predicted to decrease the exposure to **rivaroxaban**. Avoid unless patient can be monitored for signs of thrombosis. Moderate Study
- Antiarrhythmics **(amiodarone)** slightly increase the exposure to **edoxaban**. Severe Study
- Antiarrhythmics **(amiodarone)** might increase the exposure to **rivaroxaban**. Manufacturer advises caution in renal impairment. Moderate Study
- Antiarrhythmics **(amiodarone, dronedarone)** are predicted to increase the exposure to **apixaban**. Moderate Theoretical
- Antiarrhythmics **(dronedarone)** slightly increase the exposure to **edoxaban**. Adjust **edoxaban** dose. Severe Study
- Antiarrhythmics **(dronedarone)** might increase the exposure to **rivaroxaban**. Avoid. Moderate Study
- Antiepileptics **(carbamazepine)** are predicted to decrease the exposure to **apixaban**. Use with caution or avoid. Severe Study
- Antiepileptics **(carbamazepine)** are predicted to decrease the exposure to **edoxaban**. Severe Study
- Antiepileptics **(carbamazepine, fosphenytoin)** are predicted to decrease the exposure to **rivaroxaban**. Avoid unless patient can be monitored for signs of thrombosis. Severe Study
- Antiepileptics **(fosphenytoin)** are predicted to decrease the exposure to **apixaban**. Severe Study
- Antiepileptics **(fosphenytoin, phenobarbital, phenytoin, primidone)** are predicted to decrease the exposure to **edoxaban**. Severe Theoretical
- Antiepileptics **(oxcarbazepine)** decrease the exposure to **rivaroxaban**. Severe Study
- Antiepileptics **(phenobarbital, phenytoin)** decrease the exposure to **apixaban**. Use with caution or avoid. Severe Study
- Antiepileptics **(phenobarbital, phenytoin, primidone)** decrease the exposure to **rivaroxaban**. Avoid unless patient can be monitored for signs of thrombosis. Severe Study
- Antiepileptics **(primidone)** decrease the exposure to **apixaban**. Severe Study
- Antifungals, azoles **(itraconazole)** are predicted to increase the exposure to **apixaban**. Avoid. Severe Theoretical
- Antifungals, azoles **(itraconazole)** are predicted to increase the exposure to **edoxaban**. Severe Theoretical
- Antifungals, azoles **(itraconazole)** are predicted to increase the exposure to **rivaroxaban**. Avoid. Severe Anecdotal
- Antifungals, azoles **(ketoconazole)** slightly increase the exposure to **edoxaban**. Adjust **edoxaban** dose. Severe Study
- Antifungals, azoles **(ketoconazole)** moderately increase the exposure to factor XA inhibitors **(apixaban, rivaroxaban)**. Avoid. Severe Study
- Antifungals, azoles **(posaconazole, voriconazole)** are predicted to increase the exposure to factor XA inhibitors **(apixaban, rivaroxaban)**. Avoid. Severe Theoretical

Factor XA inhibitors (continued)
- **Asciminib** is predicted to increase the exposure to **edoxaban**. [Severe] Theoretical
- **Aspirin** (high-dose) increases the exposure to **edoxaban**. Avoid. [Severe] Study → Also see TABLE 3 p. 1053
- Calcium-channel blockers **(verapamil)** slightly increase the exposure to **edoxaban**. [Moderate] Study
- Calcium-channel blockers **(verapamil)** slightly increase the exposure to **rivaroxaban**. Manufacturer advises caution in renal impairment. [Moderate] Study
- **Ceritinib** is predicted to increase the exposure to factor XA inhibitors **(apixaban, edoxaban)**. [Moderate] Theoretical
- **Ceritinib** might increase the exposure to **rivaroxaban**. Manufacturer advises caution in renal impairment. [Moderate] Theoretical
- **Ciclosporin** is predicted to increase the exposure to **apixaban**. [Moderate] Theoretical
- **Ciclosporin** slightly increases the exposure to **edoxaban**. Adjust **edoxaban** dose. [Severe] Study
- **Ciclosporin** slightly increases the exposure to **rivaroxaban**. Manufacturer advises caution in renal impairment. [Moderate] Study
- **Cobicistat** is predicted to increase the exposure to factor XA inhibitors **(apixaban, edoxaban, rivaroxaban)**. Avoid. [Severe] Theoretical
- **Danicopan** is predicted to increase the exposure to **edoxaban**. [Moderate] Study
- **Donanemab** can increase the risk of brain haemorrhage when given with **factor XA inhibitors**. Avoid. [Severe] Anecdotal
- **Eliglustat** is predicted to increase the exposure to **edoxaban**. Adjust dose. [Moderate] Study
- **Encorafenib** is predicted to decrease the exposure to **apixaban**. [Moderate] Study
- **Encorafenib** is predicted to decrease the exposure to **rivaroxaban**. Avoid unless patient can be monitored for signs of thrombosis. [Moderate] Study
- **Erdafitinib** is predicted to increase the exposure to **apixaban**. Separate administration by at least 6 hours. [Moderate] Theoretical
- **Glecaprevir** is predicted to increase the exposure to **apixaban**. [Moderate] Theoretical
- **Glecaprevir** is predicted to increase the exposure to **edoxaban**. [Severe] Theoretical
- **Glecaprevir** might increase the exposure to **rivaroxaban**. Manufacturer advises caution in renal impairment. [Moderate] Theoretical
- HIV-protease inhibitors **(darunavir)** boosted with ritonavir or cobicistat increase the exposure to **apixaban**. Avoid. [Severe] Anecdotal
- HIV-protease inhibitors **(darunavir)** boosted with ritonavir increase the concentration of **edoxaban**. Monitor and adjust dose. [Severe] Anecdotal
- HIV-protease inhibitors **(darunavir)** boosted with ritonavir are predicted to increase the exposure to **rivaroxaban**. Avoid. [Severe] Anecdotal
- HIV-protease inhibitors **(fosamprenavir)** boosted with ritonavir are predicted to increase the exposure to **apixaban**. [Severe] Theoretical
- HIV-protease inhibitors **(fosamprenavir)** boosted with ritonavir are predicted to increase the exposure to **rivaroxaban**. Manufacturer advises caution in renal impairment. [Severe] Theoretical
- HIV-protease inhibitors **(lopinavir)** boosted with ritonavir increase the exposure to **apixaban**. Avoid. [Severe] Anecdotal
- HIV-protease inhibitors **(lopinavir)** boosted with ritonavir increase the exposure to **edoxaban**. Monitor and adjust dose. [Severe] Study
- HIV-protease inhibitors **(lopinavir)** boosted with ritonavir increase the exposure to **rivaroxaban**. Avoid. [Severe] Study
- HIV-protease inhibitors **(ritonavir)** are predicted to increase the exposure to **apixaban**. Avoid. [Severe] Theoretical
- HIV-protease inhibitors **(ritonavir)** are predicted to increase the exposure to **edoxaban**. Monitor and adjust dose. [Severe] Theoretical
- HIV-protease inhibitors **(ritonavir)** moderately increase the exposure to **rivaroxaban**. Avoid. [Severe] Study
- HIV-protease inhibitors **(atazanavir)** boosted with ritonavir are predicted to increase the exposure to factor XA inhibitors **(apixaban, rivaroxaban)**. Avoid. [Severe] Theoretical
- **Idelalisib** is predicted to increase the exposure to **apixaban**. [Moderate] Theoretical
- **Idelalisib** might increase the exposure to **rivaroxaban**. Manufacturer advises caution in renal impairment. [Moderate] Theoretical
- **Ivosidenib** is predicted to decrease the exposure to **apixaban**. [Moderate] Study
- **Ivosidenib** is predicted to alter the exposure to **edoxaban**. [Moderate] Theoretical
- **Ivosidenib** is predicted to decrease the exposure to **rivaroxaban**. Avoid unless patient can be monitored for signs of thrombosis. [Moderate] Study
- **Lapatinib** is predicted to increase the exposure to **apixaban**. [Moderate] Theoretical
- **Lapatinib** is predicted to slightly increase the exposure to **edoxaban**. [Severe] Theoretical
- **Lapatinib** might increase the exposure to **rivaroxaban**. Manufacturer advises caution in renal impairment. [Moderate] Theoretical
- **Lecanemab** can increase the risk of brain haemorrhage when given with **factor XA inhibitors**. Avoid. [Severe] Anecdotal
- **Lenacapavir** is predicted to increase the concentration of factor XA inhibitors **(edoxaban, rivaroxaban)**. Monitor and adjust dose. [Severe] Theoretical
- **Lorlatinib** is predicted to decrease the exposure to **apixaban**. Use with caution or avoid. [Severe] Study
- **Lorlatinib** is predicted to decrease the exposure to **edoxaban**. [Severe] Study
- **Lorlatinib** is predicted to decrease the exposure to **rivaroxaban**. Avoid unless patient can be monitored for signs of thrombosis. [Severe] Study
- **Lumacaftor** is predicted to decrease the exposure to **apixaban**. [Moderate] Study
- **Lumacaftor** is predicted to decrease the exposure to **rivaroxaban**. Avoid unless patient can be monitored for signs of thrombosis. [Moderate] Study
- Macrolides **(azithromycin)** are predicted to increase the exposure to **rivaroxaban**. Manufacturer advises caution in renal impairment. [Moderate] Theoretical
- Macrolides **(clarithromycin, erythromycin)** slightly increase the exposure to **rivaroxaban**. Manufacturer advises caution in renal impairment. [Moderate] Study
- Macrolides **(erythromycin)** are predicted to increase the exposure to **apixaban**. [Moderate] Theoretical
- Macrolides **(erythromycin)** slightly increase the exposure to **edoxaban**. Adjust **edoxaban** dose. [Moderate] Study
- Macrolides **(azithromycin)** are predicted to increase the exposure to factor XA inhibitors **(apixaban, edoxaban)**. [Moderate] Theoretical
- Macrolides **(clarithromycin)** slightly increase the exposure to factor XA inhibitors **(apixaban, edoxaban)**. [Moderate] Study
- **Mirabegron** is predicted to increase the exposure to **edoxaban**. [Mild] Theoretical
- **Mitotane** is predicted to decrease the exposure to **apixaban**. [Moderate] Study
- **Mitotane** is predicted to decrease the exposure to **rivaroxaban**. Avoid unless patient can be monitored for signs of thrombosis. [Moderate] Study
- **Factor XA inhibitors** might increase the risk of gastrointestinal bleeding when given with monoclonal antibodies **(ipilimumab)**. [Severe] Theoretical
- **Neratinib** is predicted to increase the exposure to **apixaban**. [Moderate] Theoretical
- **Nirmatrelvir** boosted with ritonavir is predicted to increase the concentration of factor XA inhibitors **(apixaban, rivaroxaban)**. Avoid. [Severe] Theoretical
- **Olaparib** might increase the exposure to **edoxaban**. [Moderate] Theoretical
- **Osimertinib** is predicted to increase the exposure to **edoxaban**. [Moderate] Study

- **Pibrentasvir** is predicted to increase the exposure to **apixaban**. Moderate Theoretical
- **Pibrentasvir** with glecaprevir is predicted to increase the exposure to **edoxaban**. Moderate Study
- **Pibrentasvir** might increase the exposure to **rivaroxaban**. Manufacturer advises caution in renal impairment. Moderate Theoretical
- **Pitolisant** is predicted to decrease the exposure to **edoxaban**. Mild Theoretical
- **Ranolazine** is predicted to increase the exposure to **apixaban**. Moderate Theoretical
- **Ranolazine** is predicted to slightly increase the exposure to **edoxaban**. Severe Theoretical
- **Ranolazine** might increase the exposure to **rivaroxaban**. Manufacturer advises caution in renal impairment. Moderate Theoretical
- Rifamycins **(rifampicin)** are predicted to decrease the exposure to **apixaban**. Use with caution or avoid. Severe Study
- Rifamycins **(rifampicin)** are predicted to decrease the exposure to **edoxaban**. Severe Study
- Rifamycins **(rifampicin)** are predicted to decrease the exposure to **rivaroxaban**. Avoid unless patient can be monitored for signs of thrombosis. Severe Study
- **Sparsentan** is predicted to increase the exposure to **edoxaban**. Severe Theoretical
- **St John's wort** is predicted to decrease the exposure to **apixaban**. Use with caution or avoid. Severe Study
- **St John's wort** is predicted to decrease the exposure to **edoxaban**. Severe Study
- **St John's wort** is predicted to decrease the exposure to **rivaroxaban**. Avoid unless patient can be monitored for signs of thrombosis. Severe Study
- **Tucatinib** is predicted to increase the exposure to **apixaban**. Moderate Theoretical
- **Tucatinib** might increase the exposure to **rivaroxaban**. Manufacturer advises caution in renal impairment. Moderate Theoretical
- **Vandetanib** is predicted to increase the exposure to **apixaban**. Moderate Theoretical
- **Velpatasvir** is predicted to increase the exposure to **apixaban**. Moderate Theoretical
- **Velpatasvir** is predicted to increase the exposure to **edoxaban**. Severe Theoretical
- **Velpatasvir** might increase the exposure to **rivaroxaban**. Manufacturer advises caution in renal impairment. Moderate Theoretical
- **Vemurafenib** is predicted to increase the exposure to **apixaban**. Moderate Theoretical
- **Vemurafenib** is predicted to increase the exposure to **edoxaban**. Severe Theoretical
- **Vemurafenib** might increase the exposure to **rivaroxaban**. Manufacturer advises caution in renal impairment. Moderate Theoretical
- **Venetoclax** is predicted to increase the exposure to factor XA inhibitors **(edoxaban, rivaroxaban)**. Avoid or adjust dose. Severe Study
- **Voxilaprevir** is predicted to increase the exposure to **apixaban**. Moderate Theoretical
- **Voxilaprevir** with sofosbuvir and velpatasvir is predicted to increase the concentration of **edoxaban**. Avoid. Severe Theoretical
- **Voxilaprevir** might increase the exposure to **rivaroxaban**. Manufacturer advises caution in renal impairment. Moderate Theoretical

Famotidine → see H_2 receptor antagonists

Fampridine

- **Dolutegravir** might increase the concentration of **fampridine**. Avoid. Severe Theoretical
- H_2 receptor antagonists **(cimetidine)** increase the concentration of **fampridine**. Avoid. Severe Theoretical

Febuxostat

- **Febuxostat** is predicted to increase the exposure to **alpelisib**. Moderate Theoretical
- **Febuxostat** is predicted to increase the exposure to **azathioprine**. Avoid. Severe Theoretical
- **Febuxostat** is predicted to increase the exposure to **cladribine**. Avoid or adjust dose. Moderate Theoretical
- **Febuxostat** is predicted to increase the exposure to **mercaptopurine**. Avoid. Severe Theoretical
- **Febuxostat** is predicted to increase the exposure to **seladelpar**. Moderate Study
- **Febuxostat** increases the exposure to statins **(rosuvastatin)**. Adjust **rosuvastatin** dose, p. 155. Moderate Study
- **Febuxostat** is predicted to increase the exposure to **tenofovir alafenamide**. Moderate Theoretical
- **Febuxostat** is predicted to increase the exposure to **tenofovir disoproxil**. Moderate Theoretical
- **Febuxostat** is predicted to increase the exposure to **topotecan**. Moderate Theoretical

Fedratinib

- **Fedratinib** is predicted to increase the exposure to **abemaciclib**. Moderate Study
- **Fedratinib** is predicted to increase the exposure to **acalabrutinib**. Avoid or monitor. Severe Study
- **Fedratinib** is predicted to increase the exposure to alpha blockers **(tamsulosin)**. Moderate Theoretical
- Anti-androgens **(apalutamide, enzalutamide)** are predicted to decrease the exposure to **fedratinib**. Avoid. Moderate Study
- Antiarrhythmics **(dronedarone)** are predicted to increase the exposure to **fedratinib**. Monitor and adjust dose. Moderate Study
- **Fedratinib** is predicted to increase the exposure to antiarrhythmics **(propafenone)**. Monitor and adjust dose. Moderate Study
- Antiepileptics **(carbamazepine, fosphenytoin, phenobarbital, phenytoin, primidone)** are predicted to decrease the exposure to **fedratinib**. Avoid. Moderate Study
- Antifungals, azoles **(fluconazole)** are predicted to increase the exposure to **fedratinib**. Avoid. Moderate Theoretical
- Antifungals, azoles **(isavuconazole)** are predicted to increase the exposure to **fedratinib**. Monitor and adjust dose. Moderate Study
- Antifungals, azoles **(itraconazole, ketoconazole, posaconazole, voriconazole)** are predicted to increase the exposure to **fedratinib**. Adjust dose, but avoid depending on other drugs taken—consult product literature. Moderate Study
- **Fedratinib** is predicted to increase the exposure to antihistamines, non-sedating **(mizolastine)**. Severe Theoretical
- **Fedratinib** is predicted to increase the exposure to antihistamines, non-sedating **(rupatadine)**. Avoid. Moderate Study
- **Fedratinib** is predicted to increase the concentration of antimalarials **(piperaquine)**. Severe Study
- **Fedratinib** is predicted to increase the exposure to atypical antipsychotics **(cariprazine)**. Monitor and adjust dose. Severe Study
- **Fedratinib** is predicted to increase the exposure to atypical antipsychotics **(quetiapine)**. Avoid. Moderate Study
- **Fedratinib** is predicted to increase the exposure to **avapritinib**. Avoid or adjust dose—consult product literature. Moderate Study
- **Fedratinib** is predicted to increase the exposure to **axitinib**. Moderate Study
- **Fedratinib** might increase the exposure to **bedaquiline**. Mild Theoretical
- **Fedratinib** is predicted to increase the exposure to **belzutifan**. Monitor and adjust dose. Severe Theoretical
- **Fedratinib** is predicted to increase the exposure to benzodiazepines **(alprazolam)**. Severe Study
- **Fedratinib** potentially increases the exposure to benzodiazepines **(clobazam)**. Adjust dose. Moderate Theoretical
- **Fedratinib** is predicted to increase the exposure to benzodiazepines **(midazolam)**. Monitor adverse effects and adjust dose. Severe Study
- **Berotralstat** is predicted to increase the exposure to **fedratinib**. Monitor and adjust dose. Moderate Study
- **Fedratinib** is predicted to increase the exposure to **bosutinib**. Avoid or adjust dose. Severe Study
- **Fedratinib** is predicted to increase the exposure to **brigatinib**. Moderate Study

Fedratinib (continued)

- **Fedratinib** is predicted to increase the exposure to **buspirone**. Use with caution and adjust dose. Moderate Study
- **Fedratinib** is predicted to increase the exposure to **cabozantinib**. Moderate Study
- Calcium-channel blockers **(diltiazem, verapamil)** are predicted to increase the exposure to **fedratinib**. Monitor and adjust dose. Moderate Study
- **Fedratinib** is predicted to increase the exposure to calcium-channel blockers **(amlodipine, felodipine, lacidipine, lercanidipine, nicardipine, nifedipine, nimodipine)**. Monitor and adjust dose. Moderate Study
- **Fedratinib** is predicted to increase the exposure to **capivasertib**. Adjust dose. Moderate Study
- **Cenobamate** is predicted to decrease the exposure to **fedratinib**. Avoid. Moderate Study
- **Ceritinib** is predicted to increase the exposure to **fedratinib**. Adjust dose, but avoid depending on other drugs taken—consult product literature. Moderate Study
- **Fedratinib** is predicted to increase the exposure to **ceritinib**. Moderate Study
- **Fedratinib** is predicted to decrease the efficacy of **clopidogrel**. Avoid. Moderate Study
- **Cobicistat** is predicted to increase the exposure to **fedratinib**. Adjust dose, but avoid depending on other drugs taken—consult product literature. Moderate Study
- **Fedratinib** is predicted to increase the exposure to **cobimetinib**. Severe Study
- **Fedratinib** is predicted to increase the exposure to **colchicine**. Adjust **colchicine** dose with moderate CYP3A4 inhibitors, p. 637. Severe Study
- **Fedratinib** is predicted to increase the exposure to corticosteroids **(methylprednisolone)**. Monitor and adjust dose. Moderate Study
- **Crizotinib** is predicted to increase the exposure to **fedratinib**. Monitor and adjust dose. Moderate Study
- **Fedratinib** is predicted to increase the exposure to **dabrafenib**. Moderate Study
- **Dabrafenib** is predicted to decrease the exposure to **fedratinib**. Avoid. Moderate Study
- **Fedratinib** is predicted to increase the exposure to **daridorexant**. Adjust **daridorexant** dose. Severe Study
- **Fedratinib** is predicted to increase the exposure to **dasatinib**. Severe Study
- **Fedratinib** is predicted to increase the exposure to **deutivacaftor**. Adjust dose, see deutivacaftor with tezacaftor and vanzacaftor p. 218. Severe Study
- **Fedratinib** is predicted to slightly increase the exposure to **dienogest**. Moderate Study
- **Fedratinib** is predicted to increase the exposure to dipeptidylpeptidase-4 inhibitors **(saxagliptin)**. Mild Study
- **Fedratinib** is predicted to increase the exposure to **domperidone**. Avoid. Severe Study
- **Fedratinib** is predicted to increase the exposure to dopamine receptor agonists **(bromocriptine)**. Severe Theoretical
- **Fedratinib** is predicted to increase the exposure to **drospirenone**. Severe Study
- **Fedratinib** is predicted to moderately increase the exposure to **dutasteride**. Mild Study
- **Fedratinib** is predicted to increase the exposure to **elacestrant**. Avoid moderate CYP3A4 inhibitors or adjust **elacestrant** dose. Severe Theoretical
- **Fedratinib** is predicted to increase the exposure to **elexacaftor**. Adjust ivacaftor with tezacaftor and elexacaftor p. 220 dose with moderate CYP3A4 inhibitors. Severe Theoretical
- **Fedratinib** is predicted to increase the exposure to **eliglustat**. Avoid or adjust dose—consult product literature. Severe Study
- **Fedratinib** is predicted to moderately increase the exposure to **encorafenib**. Moderate Study
- **Encorafenib** is predicted to decrease the exposure to **fedratinib**. Avoid. Moderate Study
- Endothelin receptor antagonists **(bosentan)** are predicted to decrease the exposure to **fedratinib**. Avoid. Moderate Study
- **Fedratinib** is predicted to increase the exposure to endothelin receptor antagonists **(macitentan)**. Manufacturer advises caution depending on other drugs taken—consult product literature. Moderate Theoretical
- **Fedratinib** is predicted to increase the exposure to **entrectinib**. Avoid or adjust dose with moderate CYP3A4 inhibitors—consult product literature. Severe Theoretical
- **Fedratinib** is predicted to increase the risk of ergotism when given with **ergometrine**. Severe Theoretical
- **Fedratinib** is predicted to increase the exposure to **erlotinib**. Moderate Study
- **Fedratinib** is predicted to increase the exposure to **etrasimod**. Avoid in poor CYP2C9 metabolisers. Severe Theoretical
- **Fedratinib** is predicted to increase the concentration of **everolimus**. Avoid or adjust dose. Moderate Study
- **Fedratinib** is predicted to increase the exposure to **fesoterodine**. Adjust **fesoterodine** dose with moderate CYP3A4 inhibitors in hepatic and renal impairment. Mild Study
- **Fedratinib** is predicted to increase the exposure to **gefitinib**. Moderate Study
- **Grapefruit** and grapefruit juice is predicted to increase the exposure to **fedratinib**. Avoid. Moderate Theoretical
- **Fedratinib** is predicted to increase the concentration of **guanfacine**. Adjust **guanfacine** dose, p. 281. Moderate Theoretical
- **HIV-protease inhibitors** are predicted to increase the exposure to **fedratinib**. Adjust dose, but avoid depending on other drugs taken—consult product literature. Moderate Study
- **Fedratinib** is predicted to increase the exposure to **ibrutinib**. Adjust dose with moderate CYP3A4 inhibitors—consult product literature. Severe Study
- **Idelalisib** is predicted to increase the exposure to **fedratinib**. Adjust dose, but avoid depending on other drugs taken—consult product literature. Moderate Study
- **Imatinib** is predicted to increase the exposure to **fedratinib**. Monitor and adjust dose. Moderate Study
- **Fedratinib** is predicted to increase the exposure to the active metabolite of **irinotecan**. Moderate Theoretical
- **Fedratinib** is predicted to increase the exposure to **ivacaftor**. Adjust dose with moderate CYP3A4 inhibitors, see ivacaftor p. 219, tezacaftor with ivacaftor p. 223, and ivacaftor with tezacaftor and elexacaftor p. 220. Moderate Study
- **Fedratinib** is predicted to increase the exposure to **ivosidenib**. Monitor and adjust dose—consult product literature. Severe Study
- **Ivosidenib** is predicted to decrease the exposure to **fedratinib**. Avoid. Moderate Study
- **Fedratinib** is predicted to increase the exposure to **lapatinib**. Moderate Study
- **Fedratinib** is predicted to increase the exposure to **larotrectinib**. Monitor and adjust dose. Moderate Theoretical
- **Fedratinib** is predicted to increase the exposure to **leniolisib**. Avoid. Moderate Study
- **Letermovir** is predicted to increase the exposure to **fedratinib**. Monitor and adjust dose. Moderate Study
- **Fedratinib** is predicted to increase the exposure to **lomitapide**. Avoid. Moderate Theoretical
- **Lorlatinib** is predicted to decrease the exposure to **fedratinib**. Avoid. Moderate Study
- **Lumacaftor** is predicted to decrease the exposure to **fedratinib**. Avoid. Moderate Study
- Macrolides **(clarithromycin)** are predicted to increase the exposure to **fedratinib**. Adjust dose, but avoid depending on other drugs taken—consult product literature. Moderate Study
- Macrolides **(erythromycin)** are predicted to increase the exposure to **fedratinib**. Monitor and adjust dose. Moderate Study
- **Fedratinib** is predicted to increase the exposure to **mavacamten**. Adjust dose—consult product literature. Moderate Study
- **Fedratinib** is predicted to increase the exposure to **midostaurin**. Moderate Theoretical
- **Fedratinib** is predicted to increase the exposure to mineralocorticoid receptor antagonists **(eplerenone)**. Adjust **eplerenone** dose. Severe Study
- **Fedratinib** is predicted to increase the exposure to mineralocorticoid receptor antagonists **(finerenone)**. Severe Study

- Mitotane is predicted to decrease the exposure to **fedratinib**. Avoid. Moderate Study
- **Fedratinib** is predicted to increase the exposure to **naldemedine**. Moderate Study
- **Fedratinib** is predicted to increase the exposure to **naloxegol**. Adjust **naloxegol** dose and monitor adverse effects. Moderate Study
- **Fedratinib** is predicted to increase the exposure to **neratinib**. Avoid moderate CYP3A4 inhibitors or adjust dose and monitor for gastrointestinal adverse effects—consult product literature. Severe Study
- Neurokinin-1 receptor antagonists **(aprepitant, netupitant)** are predicted to increase the exposure to **fedratinib**. Monitor and adjust dose. Moderate Study
- **Nilotinib** is predicted to increase the exposure to **fedratinib**. Monitor and adjust dose. Moderate Study
- NNRTIs **(efavirenz, etravirine, nevirapine)** are predicted to decrease the exposure to **fedratinib**. Avoid. Moderate Study
- **Fedratinib** is predicted to increase the exposure to **olaparib**. Avoid or adjust dose with moderate CYP3A4 inhibitors—consult product literature. Moderate Theoretical
- **Fedratinib** is predicted to increase the exposure to **omaveloxolone**. Avoid or adjust **omaveloxolone** dose, p. 755. Moderate Study
- **Fedratinib** is predicted to increase the exposure to opioids **(alfentanil, buprenorphine, fentanyl, oxycodone)**. Monitor and adjust dose. Moderate Study
- **Fedratinib** is predicted to increase the exposure to opioids **(methadone, sufentanil)**. Moderate Theoretical
- **Fedratinib** is predicted to increase the exposure to **pazopanib**. Moderate Study
- **Fedratinib** is predicted to increase the exposure to **pemigatinib**. Severe Study
- **Fedratinib** is predicted to increase the exposure to phosphodiesterase type-5 inhibitors **(avanafil)**. Adjust **avanafil** dose. Moderate Theoretical
- **Fedratinib** is predicted to increase the exposure to phosphodiesterase type-5 inhibitors **(sildenafil)**. Monitor or adjust **sildenafil** dose with moderate CYP3A4 inhibitors, p. 139. Moderate Study
- **Fedratinib** is predicted to increase the exposure to phosphodiesterase type-5 inhibitors **(tadalafil)**. Severe Theoretical
- **Fedratinib** is predicted to increase the exposure to phosphodiesterase type-5 inhibitors **(vardenafil)**. Adjust dose. Severe Theoretical
- **Fedratinib** is predicted to increase the exposure to **pimozide**. Avoid. Severe Theoretical
- **Fedratinib** is predicted to increase the exposure to **ponatinib**. Moderate Study
- **Fedratinib** is predicted to increase the exposure to **pralsetinib**. Moderate Theoretical
- **Fedratinib** moderately increases the exposure to proton pump inhibitors **(omeprazole)**. Monitor and adjust dose. Moderate Study
- **Fedratinib** is predicted to increase the exposure to **ranolazine**. Severe Study
- **Fedratinib** is predicted to increase the exposure to **regorafenib**. Moderate Study
- **Fedratinib** is predicted to increase the exposure to **ribociclib**. Moderate Study
- Rifamycins **(rifampicin)** are predicted to decrease the exposure to **fedratinib**. Avoid. Moderate Study
- **Fedratinib** is predicted to increase the exposure to **rimegepant**. Avoid another dose of rimegepant within 48 hours of concurrent use. Moderate Study
- **Fedratinib** is predicted to increase the exposure to **ruxolitinib**. Moderate Study
- **Fedratinib** is predicted to increase the exposure to **selpercatinib**. Moderate Study
- **Fedratinib** is predicted to increase the exposure to **selumetinib**. Avoid or adjust dose—consult product literature. Severe Study
- **Fedratinib** is predicted to increase the exposure to **siponimod**. Avoid depending on other drugs taken—consult product literature. Severe Study
- **Fedratinib** increases the concentration of **sirolimus**. Monitor and adjust dose. Moderate Study
- **Sotorasib** is predicted to decrease the exposure to **fedratinib**. Avoid. Moderate Study
- **Fedratinib** is predicted to increase the exposure to **sparsentan**. Moderate Study
- SSRIs **(fluoxetine)** are predicted to increase the exposure to **fedratinib**. Avoid depending on other drugs taken—consult product literature. Moderate Theoretical
- SSRIs **(fluvoxamine)** are predicted to increase the exposure to **fedratinib**. Avoid. Moderate Theoretical
- **Fedratinib** is predicted to increase the exposure to SSRIs **(dapoxetine)**. Adjust **dapoxetine** dose with moderate CYP3A4 inhibitors. Moderate Theoretical
- **Fedratinib** is predicted to increase the exposure to SSRIs **(escitalopram)**. Use with caution and adjust dose. Severe Study
- **Fedratinib** is predicted to increase the exposure to SSRIs **(sertraline)**. Moderate Theoretical
- **St John's wort** is predicted to decrease the exposure to **fedratinib**. Avoid. Moderate Study
- **Fedratinib** is predicted to increase the exposure to **sunitinib**. Moderate Study
- **Fedratinib** is predicted to increase the concentration of **tacrolimus**. Monitor and adjust dose. Severe Theoretical
- **Fedratinib** is predicted to increase the exposure to taxanes **(cabazitaxel)**. Moderate Theoretical
- **Fedratinib** is predicted to increase the exposure to taxanes **(docetaxel)**. Severe Study
- **Fedratinib** is predicted to increase the exposure to taxanes **(paclitaxel)**. Moderate Anecdotal
- **Fedratinib** is predicted to increase the exposure to **temsirolimus** (oral). Monitor and adjust dose. Moderate Theoretical
- **Fedratinib** is predicted to increase the exposure to **tezacaftor**. Adjust dose with moderate CYP3A4 inhibitors, see tezacaftor with ivacaftor p. 223, ivacaftor with tezacaftor and elexacaftor p. 220, and deutivacaftor with tezacaftor and vanzacaftor p. 218. Severe Study
- **Fedratinib** is predicted to increase the exposure to **tolvaptan**. Manufacturer advises caution or adjust **tolvaptan** dose with moderate CYP3A4 inhibitors. Moderate Study
- **Fedratinib** is predicted to increase the exposure to **trazodone**. Moderate Theoretical
- **Tucatinib** is predicted to increase the exposure to **fedratinib**. Adjust dose, but avoid depending on other drugs taken—consult product literature. Moderate Study
- **Fedratinib** is predicted to increase the exposure to **vanzacaftor**. Adjust dose, see deutivacaftor with tezacaftor and vanzacaftor p. 218. Severe Study
- **Fedratinib** is predicted to increase the exposure to **vemurafenib**. Severe Theoretical
- **Fedratinib** is predicted to increase the exposure to **venetoclax**. Avoid or adjust dose—consult product literature. Severe Study
- **Fedratinib** is predicted to increase the exposure to **vinca alkaloids**. Severe Theoretical
- **Fedratinib** is predicted to increase the exposure to **voclosporin**. Adjust **voclosporin** dose. Severe Study
- **Fedratinib** is predicted to increase the exposure to **zanubrutinib**. Avoid or adjust dose with moderate CYP3A4 inhibitors—consult product literature. Severe Study
- **Fedratinib** is predicted to increase the exposure to **zopiclone**. Adjust dose. Moderate Study

Felodipine → see calcium-channel blockers

Fenfluramine → see TABLE 11 p. 1056 (serotonin toxicity)

- **Fenfluramine** might decrease blood glucose concentrations when given with **acarbose**. Moderate Theoretical
- Anti-androgens **(apalutamide, enzalutamide)** are predicted to decrease the exposure to **fenfluramine**. Moderate Theoretical
- Antiepileptics **(carbamazepine)** are predicted to decrease the concentration of **fenfluramine**. Adjust dose. Moderate Theoretical
- Antiepileptics **(fosphenytoin, phenobarbital, phenytoin, primidone)** are predicted to decrease the exposure to **fenfluramine**. Moderate Theoretical

A1 Interactions | Appendix 1

Fenfluramine (continued)
- Antiepileptics **(stiripentol)** (given with clobazam, and with or without valproate) modestly increase the exposure to **fenfluramine**. Adjust **fenfluramine** dose, p. 238. Severe Study
- Antihistamines, sedating **(cyproheptadine)** might decrease the efficacy of **fenfluramine**. Severe Theoretical
- **Bupropion** is predicted to increase the exposure to **fenfluramine**. Moderate Study
- **Cinacalcet** is predicted to increase the exposure to **fenfluramine**. Moderate Study
- **Dacomitinib** is predicted to increase the exposure to **fenfluramine**. Moderate Study
- **Fenfluramine** might decrease blood glucose concentrations when given with **dipeptidylpeptidase-4 inhibitors**. Moderate Theoretical
- **Fenfluramine** might decrease blood glucose concentrations when given with **glucagon-like peptide-1 receptor agonists**. Moderate Theoretical
- **Fenfluramine** might decrease blood glucose concentrations when given with **insulin**. Moderate Theoretical
- **Fenfluramine** might decrease blood glucose concentrations when given with **meglitinides**. Moderate Theoretical
- **Fenfluramine** might decrease blood glucose concentrations when given with **metformin**. Moderate Theoretical
- **Mitotane** is predicted to decrease the exposure to **fenfluramine**. Moderate Theoretical
- **Fenfluramine** might decrease blood glucose concentrations when given with **pioglitazone**. Moderate Theoretical
- Rifamycins **(rifampicin)** are predicted to decrease the concentration of **fenfluramine**. Moderate Theoretical
- **Fenfluramine** might decrease blood glucose concentrations when given with **sodium glucose co-transporter 2 inhibitors**. Moderate Theoretical
- SSRIs **(fluoxetine, paroxetine)** are predicted to increase the exposure to **fenfluramine**. Moderate Study → Also see TABLE 11 p. 1056
- SSRIs **(fluvoxamine)** moderately increase the exposure to **fenfluramine**. Moderate Study → Also see TABLE 11 p. 1056
- **Fenfluramine** might decrease blood glucose concentrations when given with **sulfonylureas**. Moderate Theoretical
- **Terbinafine** is predicted to increase the exposure to **fenfluramine**. Moderate Study

Fenofibrate → see fibrates

Fentanyl → see opioids

Fesoterodine → see TABLE 8 p. 1055 (antimuscarinics)
- Anti-androgens **(apalutamide, enzalutamide)** are predicted to decrease the exposure to **fesoterodine**. Avoid. Moderate Study
- Antiarrhythmics **(dronedarone)** are predicted to increase the exposure to **fesoterodine**. Adjust **fesoterodine** dose with moderate CYP3A4 inhibitors in hepatic and renal impairment. Mild Study
- Antiepileptics **(carbamazepine, fosphenytoin, phenobarbital, phenytoin, primidone)** are predicted to decrease the exposure to **fesoterodine**. Avoid. Moderate Study
- Antifungals, azoles **(fluconazole, isavuconazole)** are predicted to increase the exposure to **fesoterodine**. Adjust **fesoterodine** dose with moderate CYP3A4 inhibitors in hepatic and renal impairment. Mild Study
- Antifungals, azoles **(itraconazole, ketoconazole, posaconazole, voriconazole)** are predicted to moderately increase the exposure to **fesoterodine**. Adjust **fesoterodine** dose with potent CYP3A4 inhibitors; avoid in hepatic and renal impairment. Severe Study
- Atypical antipsychotics **(clozapine)** can cause constipation, as can **fesoterodine**; concurrent use might increase the risk of developing intestinal obstruction. Severe Theoretical → Also see TABLE 8 p. 1055
- **Berotralstat** is predicted to increase the exposure to **fesoterodine**. Adjust **fesoterodine** dose with moderate CYP3A4 inhibitors in hepatic and renal impairment. Mild Study
- **Bupropion** is predicted to increase the exposure to **fesoterodine**. Use with caution and adjust dose. Mild Theoretical
- Calcium-channel blockers **(diltiazem, verapamil)** are predicted to increase the exposure to **fesoterodine**. Adjust **fesoterodine** dose with moderate CYP3A4 inhibitors in hepatic and renal impairment. Mild Study
- **Ceritinib** is predicted to moderately increase the exposure to **fesoterodine**. Adjust **fesoterodine** dose with potent CYP3A4 inhibitors; avoid in hepatic and renal impairment. Severe Study
- **Cinacalcet** is predicted to increase the exposure to **fesoterodine**. Use with caution and adjust dose. Mild Theoretical
- **Cobicistat** is predicted to moderately increase the exposure to **fesoterodine**. Adjust **fesoterodine** dose with potent CYP3A4 inhibitors; avoid in hepatic and renal impairment. Severe Study
- **Crizotinib** is predicted to increase the exposure to **fesoterodine**. Adjust **fesoterodine** dose with moderate CYP3A4 inhibitors in hepatic and renal impairment. Mild Study
- **Dacomitinib** is predicted to increase the exposure to **fesoterodine**. Use with caution and adjust dose. Mild Theoretical
- **Encorafenib** is predicted to decrease the exposure to **fesoterodine**. Avoid. Moderate Study
- **Fedratinib** is predicted to increase the exposure to **fesoterodine**. Adjust **fesoterodine** dose with moderate CYP3A4 inhibitors in hepatic and renal impairment. Mild Study
- **HIV-protease inhibitors** are predicted to moderately increase the exposure to **fesoterodine**. Adjust **fesoterodine** dose with potent CYP3A4 inhibitors; avoid in hepatic and renal impairment. Severe Study
- **Idelalisib** is predicted to moderately increase the exposure to **fesoterodine**. Adjust **fesoterodine** dose with potent CYP3A4 inhibitors; avoid in hepatic and renal impairment. Severe Study
- **Imatinib** is predicted to increase the exposure to **fesoterodine**. Adjust **fesoterodine** dose with moderate CYP3A4 inhibitors in hepatic and renal impairment. Mild Study
- **Ivosidenib** is predicted to decrease the exposure to **fesoterodine**. Avoid. Moderate Study
- **Letermovir** is predicted to increase the exposure to **fesoterodine**. Adjust **fesoterodine** dose with moderate CYP3A4 inhibitors in hepatic and renal impairment. Mild Study
- **Lumacaftor** is predicted to decrease the exposure to **fesoterodine**. Avoid. Moderate Study
- Macrolides **(clarithromycin)** are predicted to moderately increase the exposure to **fesoterodine**. Adjust **fesoterodine** dose with potent CYP3A4 inhibitors; avoid in hepatic and renal impairment. Severe Study
- Macrolides **(erythromycin)** are predicted to increase the exposure to **fesoterodine**. Adjust **fesoterodine** dose with moderate CYP3A4 inhibitors in hepatic and renal impairment. Mild Study
- **Mitotane** is predicted to decrease the exposure to **fesoterodine**. Avoid. Moderate Study
- Neurokinin-1 receptor antagonists **(aprepitant, netupitant)** are predicted to increase the exposure to **fesoterodine**. Adjust **fesoterodine** dose with moderate CYP3A4 inhibitors in hepatic and renal impairment. Mild Study
- **Nilotinib** is predicted to increase the exposure to **fesoterodine**. Adjust **fesoterodine** dose with moderate CYP3A4 inhibitors in hepatic and renal impairment. Mild Study
- Rifamycins **(rifampicin)** are predicted to decrease the exposure to **fesoterodine**. Avoid. Moderate Study
- SSRIs **(fluoxetine, paroxetine)** are predicted to increase the exposure to **fesoterodine**. Use with caution and adjust dose. Mild Theoretical
- **St John's wort** is predicted to decrease the exposure to **fesoterodine**. Avoid. Severe Theoretical
- **Terbinafine** is predicted to increase the exposure to **fesoterodine**. Use with caution and adjust dose. Mild Theoretical
- **Tucatinib** is predicted to moderately increase the exposure to **fesoterodine**. Adjust **fesoterodine** dose with potent CYP3A4 inhibitors; avoid in hepatic and renal impairment. Severe Study

Fexofenadine → see antihistamines, non-sedating

Fezolinetant
- **Combined hormonal contraceptives** is predicted to increase the exposure to **fezolinetant**. Avoid. Moderate Study
- **Givosiran** is predicted to increase the exposure to **fezolinetant**. Avoid. Moderate Study
- **Mexiletine** is predicted to increase the exposure to **fezolinetant**. Avoid. Moderate Study

- **Osilodrostat** is predicted to increase the exposure to **fezolinetant**. Avoid. Moderate Study
- Quinolones **(ciprofloxacin)** are predicted to increase the exposure to **fezolinetant**. Avoid. Moderate Study
- **Rucaparib** is predicted to increase the exposure to **fezolinetant**. Avoid. Moderate Study
- SSRIs **(fluvoxamine)** are predicted to increase the exposure to **fezolinetant**. Avoid. Moderate Study
- **Vemurafenib** is predicted to increase the exposure to **fezolinetant**. Avoid. Moderate Study

Fibrates

bezafibrate · ciprofibrate · fenofibrate · gemfibrozil

- **Acipimox** is predicted to increase the risk of rhabdomyolysis when given with **fibrates**. Severe Theoretical
- Oral **antacids** decrease the exposure to oral **gemfibrozil**. Moderate Study
- **Gemfibrozil** slightly increases the exposure to anti-androgens **(apalutamide)**. Mild Study
- **Gemfibrozil** moderately increases the exposure to anti-androgens **(enzalutamide)**. Avoid or adjust **enzalutamide** dose. Severe Study
- **Gemfibrozil** is predicted to increase the exposure to antihistamines, non-sedating **(fexofenadine)**. Moderate Theoretical
- **Gemfibrozil** is predicted to increase the exposure to **atogepant**. Adjust **atogepant** dose. Moderate Theoretical
- **Bezafibrate** is predicted to increase the risk of nephrotoxicity when given with **ciclosporin**. Severe Theoretical
- **Fenofibrate** increases the risk of nephrotoxicity when given with **ciclosporin**. Severe Study
- **Colchicine** increases the risk of rhabdomyolysis when given with **fibrates**. Severe Anecdotal
- **Fibrates** are predicted to increase the anticoagulant effect of **coumarins**. Monitor INR and adjust dose. Severe Study
- **Gemfibrozil** is predicted to increase the exposure to **dabrafenib**. Moderate Theoretical
- **Fibrates** are predicted to increase the risk of rhabdomyolysis when given with **daptomycin**. Severe Theoretical
- **Gemfibrozil** are predicted to increases the exposure to **etrasimod**. Avoid in poor CYP2C9 metabolisers. Severe Theoretical
- **Fibrates** are predicted to increase the risk of gallstones when given with **ezetimibe**. Severe Theoretical
- **Gemfibrozil** is predicted to increase the exposure to **grazoprevir**. Avoid. Severe Theoretical
- **Fibrates** are predicted to increase the risk of hypoglycaemia when given with **insulin**. Moderate Theoretical
- **Gemfibrozil** is predicted to increase the exposure to **irinotecan**. Avoid. Moderate Theoretical
- **Gemfibrozil** is predicted to increase the concentration of **letermovir**. Moderate Study
- **Gemfibrozil** increases the exposure to meglitinides **(repaglinide)**. Avoid. Severe Study
- **Gemfibrozil** is predicted to increase the exposure to **momelotinib**. Moderate Study
- **Gemfibrozil** is predicted to moderately increase the exposure to **montelukast**. Moderate Study
- **Gemfibrozil** is predicted to increase the exposure to the active metabolites of **ozanimod**. Moderate Study
- **Fibrates** are predicted to increase the anticoagulant effect of **phenindione**. Monitor INR and adjust dose. Severe Study
- **Gemfibrozil** increases the exposure to **pioglitazone**. Monitor blood glucose and adjust dose. Severe Study
- **Gemfibrozil** is predicted to increase the exposure to retinoids **(alitretinoin)**. Adjust **alitretinoin** dose. Moderate Theoretical
- **Gemfibrozil** increases the concentration of retinoids **(bexarotene)**. Avoid. Severe Study
- **Gemfibrozil** is predicted to increase the exposure to **roxadustat**. Monitor haemoglobin and adjust dose—consult product literature. Moderate Study
- **Gemfibrozil** increases the exposure to **selexipag**. Avoid. Severe Study
- **Ciprofibrate** increases the risk of rhabdomyolysis when given with statins **(atorvastatin)**. Avoid or adjust dose. Severe Study
- **Fenofibrate** increases the risk of rhabdomyolysis when given with statins **(atorvastatin)**. Monitor and adjust **fenofibrate** dose, p. 153. Severe Anecdotal
- **Gemfibrozil** causes a small increase in the exposure to statins **(atorvastatin)**. Avoid. Severe Study
- **Bezafibrate** increases the risk of rhabdomyolysis when given with statins **(atorvastatin, fluvastatin)**. Severe Study
- **Ciprofibrate** increases the risk of rhabdomyolysis when given with statins **(fluvastatin)**. Severe Study
- **Fenofibrate** is predicted to increase the risk of rhabdomyolysis when given with statins **(fluvastatin)**. Use with caution and adjust **fenofibrate** dose, p. 153. Severe Theoretical
- **Gemfibrozil** increases the risk of rhabdomyolysis when given with statins **(fluvastatin)**. Severe Anecdotal
- **Fenofibrate** is predicted to increase the risk of rhabdomyolysis when given with statins **(pravastatin)**. Avoid. Severe Theoretical
- **Gemfibrozil** modestly increases the exposure to statins **(pravastatin)**. Avoid or monitor. Severe Study
- Fibrates **(bezafibrate, ciprofibrate)** increase the risk of rhabdomyolysis when given with statins **(pravastatin)**. Avoid. Severe Study
- **Fenofibrate** increases the risk of rhabdomyolysis when given with statins **(rosuvastatin)**. Adjust **fenofibrate** and **rosuvastatin** doses, p. 153, p. 155. Severe Anecdotal
- **Gemfibrozil** causes a small increase in the exposure to statins **(rosuvastatin)**. Avoid or adjust **rosuvastatin** dose, p. 155. Severe Study
- Fibrates **(bezafibrate, ciprofibrate)** increase the risk of rhabdomyolysis when given with statins **(rosuvastatin)**. Adjust **rosuvastatin** dose, p. 155. Severe Study
- **Fenofibrate** increases the risk of rhabdomyolysis when given with statins **(simvastatin)**. Adjust **fenofibrate** dose, p. 153. Severe Anecdotal
- **Gemfibrozil** modestly increases the exposure to statins **(simvastatin)**. Avoid. Severe Anecdotal
- Fibrates **(bezafibrate, ciprofibrate)** increase the risk of rhabdomyolysis when given with statins **(simvastatin)**. Adjust **simvastatin** dose, p. 156. Severe Study
- **Fibrates** are predicted to increase the risk of hypoglycaemia when given with **sulfonylureas**. Moderate Theoretical
- **Gemfibrozil** is predicted to increase the exposure to taxanes **(docetaxel)**. Moderate Theoretical
- **Gemfibrozil** is predicted to increase the concentration of taxanes **(paclitaxel)**. Severe Anecdotal
- **Gemfibrozil** increases the exposure to **treprostinil**. Adjust dose. Moderate Study
- **Gemfibrozil** is predicted to increase the exposure to **tucatinib**. Avoid or adjust dose—consult product literature. Severe Study
- **Fibrates** are predicted to decrease the efficacy of **ursodeoxycholic acid**. Avoid. Severe Theoretical
- **Gemfibrozil** is predicted to increase the exposure to **vadadustat**. Moderate Theoretical

Fidaxomicin

- Antiarrhythmics **(amiodarone, dronedarone)** are predicted to increase the exposure to **fidaxomicin**. Avoid. Moderate Study
- Antifungals, azoles **(itraconazole, ketoconazole)** are predicted to increase the exposure to **fidaxomicin**. Avoid. Moderate Study
- Calcium-channel blockers **(verapamil)** are predicted to increase the exposure to **fidaxomicin**. Avoid. Moderate Study
- **Ciclosporin** is predicted to increase the exposure to **fidaxomicin**. Avoid. Moderate Study
- **Cobicistat** is predicted to increase the exposure to **fidaxomicin**. Avoid. Moderate Study
- **Glecaprevir** is predicted to increase the exposure to **fidaxomicin**. Avoid. Moderate Study
- HIV-protease inhibitors **(lopinavir, ritonavir)** are predicted to increase the exposure to **fidaxomicin**. Avoid. Moderate Study
- **Lapatinib** is predicted to increase the exposure to **fidaxomicin**. Avoid. Moderate Study
- **Macrolides** are predicted to increase the exposure to **fidaxomicin**. Avoid. Moderate Study
- **Pibrentasvir** is predicted to increase the exposure to **fidaxomicin**. Avoid. Moderate Study
- **Ranolazine** is predicted to increase the exposure to **fidaxomicin**. Avoid. Moderate Study

Fidaxomicin (continued)
- **Velpatasvir** is predicted to increase the exposure to **fidaxomicin**. Avoid. Moderate Study
- **Vemurafenib** is predicted to increase the exposure to **fidaxomicin**. Avoid. Moderate Study
- **Voxilaprevir** is predicted to increase the exposure to **fidaxomicin**. Avoid. Moderate Study

Filgotinib
- **Filgotinib** is predicted to increase the risk of immunosuppression when given with **abatacept**. Avoid. Severe Theoretical
- **Filgotinib** is predicted to increase the risk of immunosuppression when given with **anakinra**. Avoid. Severe Theoretical
- **Filgotinib** is predicted to increase the risk of immunosuppression when given with **baricitinib**. Avoid. Severe Theoretical
- **Filgotinib** is predicted to increase the risk of immunosuppression when given with **ciclosporin**. Avoid. Severe Theoretical
- **Filgotinib** is predicted to increase the risk of immunosuppression when given with **etanercept**. Avoid. Severe Theoretical
- **Live vaccines** are predicted to increase the risk of generalised infection (possibly life-threatening) when given with **filgotinib**. Avoid. Severe Theoretical
- **Filgotinib** is predicted to increase the risk of immunosuppression when given with monoclonal antibodies **(adalimumab, certolizumab pegol, golimumab, infliximab, rituximab, sarilumab, secukinumab, tocilizumab)**. Avoid. Severe Theoretical
- **Filgotinib** is predicted to increase the risk of immunosuppression when given with **tacrolimus**. Avoid. Severe Theoretical
- **Filgotinib** is predicted to increase the risk of immunosuppression when given with **tofacitinib**. Avoid. Severe Theoretical
- **Filgotinib** is predicted to increase the risk of immunosuppression when given with **upadacitinib**. Avoid. Severe Theoretical

Filgrastim
- **Filgrastim** might increase the risk of pulmonary toxicity when given with **bleomycin**. Severe Theoretical

Finerenone → see mineralocorticoid receptor antagonists

Fingolimod → see **TABLE 4** p. 1054 (bradycardia), **TABLE 7** p. 1055 (QT-interval prolongation)
- **Live vaccines** might increase the risk of generalised infection (possibly life-threatening) when given with **fingolimod**. UKHSA advises avoid (refer to Green Book). Severe Theoretical
- Monoclonal antibodies **(alemtuzumab)** are predicted to increase the risk of generalised infection (possibly life-threatening) when given with **fingolimod**. Avoid. Severe Theoretical
- **St John's wort** is predicted to decrease the exposure to **fingolimod**. Avoid. Moderate Theoretical

Flavoxate → see **TABLE 8** p. 1055 (antimuscarinics)
- Atypical antipsychotics **(clozapine)** can cause constipation, as can **flavoxate**; concurrent use might increase the risk of developing intestinal obstruction. Severe Theoretical → Also see **TABLE 8** p. 1055

Flecainide → see antiarrhythmics

Flucloxacillin → see penicillins

Fluconazole → see antifungals, azoles

Flucytosine
- **Amphotericin B** increases the risk of toxicity when given with **flucytosine**. Severe Study
- **Cytarabine** decreases the concentration of **flucytosine**. Avoid. Severe Study
- NRTIs **(zidovudine)** increase the risk of haematological toxicity when given with **flucytosine**. Monitor and adjust dose. Severe Theoretical

Fludarabine → see **TABLE 1** p. 1053 (hepatotoxicity), **TABLE 12** p. 1057 (myelosuppression)
- **Live vaccines** are predicted to increase the risk of generalised infection (possibly life-threatening) when given with **fludarabine**. UKHSA advises avoid (refer to Green Book). Severe Theoretical
- **Fludarabine** increases the risk of pulmonary toxicity when given with **pentostatin**. Avoid. Severe Study → Also see **TABLE 12** p. 1057

Fludrocortisone → see corticosteroids

Fluocinolone

ROUTE-SPECIFIC INFORMATION With intravitreal use of **fluocinolone** in adults: caution with concurrent administration of anticoagulant or antiplatelet drugs (higher incidence of conjunctival haemorrhage). Interactions do not generally apply to corticosteroids used for topical action unless specified.

Fluorouracil → see **TABLE 1** p. 1053 (hepatotoxicity), **TABLE 12** p. 1057 (myelosuppression)

ROUTE-SPECIFIC INFORMATION Since systemic absorption can follow topical application of **fluorouracil**, the possibility of interactions should be borne in mind.

- **Fluorouracil** increases the concentration of antiepileptics **(fosphenytoin, phenytoin)**. Monitor concentration and adjust dose. Severe Anecdotal
- **Fluorouracil** increases the anticoagulant effect of **coumarins**. Severe Anecdotal
- Folates **(folic acid)** are predicted to increase the risk of toxicity when given with **fluorouracil**. Avoid. Severe Theoretical
- Folates **(folinic acid)** are predicted to increase the risk of toxicity when given with **fluorouracil**. Monitor and adjust dose. Severe Theoretical
- H_2 receptor antagonists **(cimetidine)** slightly increase the exposure to **fluorouracil**. Severe Study
- **Live vaccines** are predicted to increase the risk of generalised infection (possibly life-threatening) when given with **fluorouracil**. UKHSA advises avoid (refer to Green Book). Severe Theoretical
- **Methotrexate** potentially increases the risk of a severe skin reaction when given with topical **fluorouracil**. Severe Anecdotal → Also see **TABLE 1** p. 1053 → Also see **TABLE 12** p. 1057
- **Metronidazole** increases the risk of toxicity when given with **fluorouracil**. Severe Study

Fluoxetine → see SSRIs

Flupentixol → see **TABLE 15** p. 1058 (hyponatraemia), **TABLE 6** p. 1054 (hypotension), **TABLE 8** p. 1055 (antimuscarinics), **TABLE 9** p. 1056 (CNS effects)
- Atypical antipsychotics **(clozapine)** can cause constipation, as can **flupentixol**; concurrent use might increase the risk of developing intestinal obstruction. Severe Theoretical → Also see **TABLE 15** p. 1058 → Also see **TABLE 6** p. 1054 → Also see **TABLE 8** p. 1055 → Also see **TABLE 9** p. 1056
- **Flupentixol** is predicted to decrease the effects of **dopamine receptor agonists**. Avoid. Moderate Theoretical → Also see **TABLE 6** p. 1054 → Also see **TABLE 8** p. 1055 → Also see **TABLE 9** p. 1056
- **Flupentixol** opposes the effects of the active metabolite of **foslevodopa**. Severe Theoretical → Also see **TABLE 6** p. 1054 → Also see **TABLE 9** p. 1056
- **Flupentixol** decreases the effects of **levodopa**. Avoid or monitor worsening parkinsonian symptoms. Severe Theoretical → Also see **TABLE 6** p. 1054 → Also see **TABLE 9** p. 1056

Flurazepam → see benzodiazepines

Flurbiprofen → see NSAIDs

Flutamide → see anti-androgens

Fluticasone → see corticosteroids

Fluvastatin → see statins

Fluvoxamine → see SSRIs

Folates

folic acid · folinic acid · levofolinic acid

- **Folates** are predicted to decrease the concentration of antiepileptics **(fosphenytoin, phenobarbital, phenytoin, primidone)**. Monitor concentration and adjust dose. Severe Study
- **Folates** are predicted to increase the risk of toxicity when given with **capecitabine**. Severe Anecdotal
- **Folic acid** is predicted to increase the risk of toxicity when given with **fluorouracil**. Avoid. Severe Theoretical

- **Folinic acid** is predicted to increase the risk of toxicity when given with **fluorouracil**. Monitor and adjust dose. [Severe] Theoretical
- **Glucarpidase** decreases the exposure to **folinic acid**. Separate administration by at least 2 hours. [Moderate] Study
- **Glucarpidase** might decrease the exposure to **levofolinic acid**. Separate administration by at least 2 hours. [Moderate] Theoretical
- **Folates** are predicted to alter the effects of **raltitrexed**. Avoid. [Moderate] Study
- **Sulfasalazine** is predicted to decrease the absorption of **folates**. [Moderate] Study
- **Folates** are predicted to increase the risk of toxicity when given with **tegafur**. [Severe] Theoretical

Folic acid → see folates
Folinic acid → see folates
Fondaparinux → see factor XA inhibitors
Formoterol → see beta$_2$ agonists
Fosamprenavir → see HIV-protease inhibitors
Fosaprepitant → see neurokinin-1 receptor antagonists
Foscarnet → see TABLE 2 p. 1053 (nephrotoxicity)

- **Foscarnet** increases the risk of hypocalcaemia when given with **pentamidine**. [Severe] Anecdotal → Also see TABLE 2 p. 1053
- **Foscarnet** might decrease the antidiuretic and hypertensive effects of **vasopressin**. [Moderate] Theoretical

Fosinopril → see ACE inhibitors
Foslevodopa → see TABLE 6 p. 1054 (hypotension), TABLE 9 p. 1056 (CNS effects)

- Antiepileptics **(phenytoin)** might decrease the effects of **foslevodopa**. [Moderate] Theoretical → Also see TABLE 9 p. 1056
- **Atypical antipsychotics** might decrease the effects of the active metabolite of **foslevodopa**. [Severe] Theoretical → Also see TABLE 6 p. 1054 → Also see TABLE 9 p. 1056
- **Benperidol** opposes the effects of the active metabolite of **foslevodopa**. [Severe] Theoretical → Also see TABLE 6 p. 1054 → Also see TABLE 9 p. 1056
- **Benzodiazepines** might decrease the effects of **foslevodopa**. [Moderate] Theoretical → Also see TABLE 9 p. 1056
- Dopamine receptor agonists **(amantadine)** might increase the adverse effects of **foslevodopa**. Adjust dose. [Moderate] Theoretical → Also see TABLE 6 p. 1054
- **Droperidol** opposes the effects of the active metabolite of **foslevodopa**. [Severe] Theoretical → Also see TABLE 6 p. 1054 → Also see TABLE 9 p. 1056
- **Entacapone** might increase the exposure to the active metabolite of **foslevodopa**. Adjust dose. [Moderate] Theoretical
- **Flupentixol** opposes the effects of the active metabolite of **foslevodopa**. [Severe] Theoretical → Also see TABLE 6 p. 1054 → Also see TABLE 9 p. 1056
- **Haloperidol** opposes the effects of the active metabolite of **foslevodopa**. [Severe] Theoretical → Also see TABLE 6 p. 1054 → Also see TABLE 9 p. 1056
- **Isoniazid** might decrease the effects of **foslevodopa**. [Moderate] Theoretical
- **Loxapine** opposes the effects of the active metabolite of **foslevodopa**. [Severe] Theoretical → Also see TABLE 6 p. 1054 → Also see TABLE 9 p. 1056
- **MAO-B inhibitors** are predicted to increase the dopaminergic effects of **foslevodopa**. Adjust dose. [Mild] Theoretical → Also see TABLE 6 p. 1054
- **MAOIs, irreversible** might cause a hypertensive crisis when given with **foslevodopa**. Avoid and for 14 days after stopping the MAOI. [Severe] Theoretical → Also see TABLE 6 p. 1054
- **Metoclopramide** might decrease the effects of **foslevodopa**. [Moderate] Theoretical
- **Moclobemide** might increase the adverse effects of **foslevodopa**. [Moderate] Theoretical
- **Opicapone** might increase the exposure to the active metabolite of **foslevodopa**. Adjust dose. [Moderate] Theoretical
- **Phenothiazine antipsychotics** oppose the effects of the active metabolite of **foslevodopa**. [Severe] Theoretical → Also see TABLE 6 p. 1054 → Also see TABLE 9 p. 1056
- **Pimozide** opposes the effects of the active metabolite of **foslevodopa**. [Severe] Theoretical → Also see TABLE 6 p. 1054 → Also see TABLE 9 p. 1056
- **Sulpiride** opposes the effects of the active metabolite of **foslevodopa**. [Severe] Theoretical → Also see TABLE 6 p. 1054 → Also see TABLE 9 p. 1056
- Sympathomimetics, vasoconstrictor **(adrenaline, noradrenaline)** might increase the cardiovascular adverse effects of the active metabolite of **foslevodopa**. [Moderate] Theoretical
- **Tolcapone** might increase the exposure to the active metabolite of **foslevodopa**. Adjust dose. [Moderate] Theoretical
- **Zuclopenthixol** opposes the effects of the active metabolite of **foslevodopa**. [Severe] Theoretical → Also see TABLE 6 p. 1054 → Also see TABLE 9 p. 1056

Fosphenytoin → see antiepileptics
Fostamatinib

- **Fostamatinib** is predicted to increase the exposure to **alpelisib**. [Moderate] Theoretical
- Anti-androgens **(apalutamide, enzalutamide)** are predicted to decrease the exposure to **fostamatinib**. Avoid. [Severe] Study
- Antiepileptics **(carbamazepine, fosphenytoin, phenobarbital, phenytoin, primidone)** are predicted to decrease the exposure to **fostamatinib**. Avoid. [Severe] Study
- Antifungals, azoles **(itraconazole, ketoconazole, posaconazole, voriconazole)** are predicted to increase the exposure to **fostamatinib**. Monitor adverse effects and adjust dose. [Moderate] Study
- Calcium-channel blockers **(diltiazem)** are predicted to increase the exposure to **fostamatinib**. Monitor adverse effects and adjust dose. [Moderate] Theoretical
- **Ceritinib** is predicted to increase the exposure to **fostamatinib**. Monitor adverse effects and adjust dose. [Moderate] Study
- **Fostamatinib** is predicted to increase the exposure to **cladribine**. Avoid or adjust dose. [Moderate] Theoretical
- **Cobicistat** is predicted to increase the exposure to **fostamatinib**. Monitor adverse effects and adjust dose. [Moderate] Study
- **Fostamatinib** might cause bleeding when given with coumarins **(acenocoumarol)**. [Moderate] Theoretical
- **Fostamatinib** might causes bleeding when given with coumarins **(warfarin)**. [Moderate] Theoretical
- **Encorafenib** is predicted to decrease the exposure to **fostamatinib**. Avoid. [Severe] Study
- **Fostamatinib** is predicted to increase the exposure to **everolimus**. Monitor and adjust dose. [Moderate] Theoretical
- **Grapefruit** juice is predicted to increase the exposure to **fostamatinib**. Monitor adverse effects and adjust dose. [Moderate] Theoretical
- **HIV-protease inhibitors** are predicted to increase the exposure to **fostamatinib**. Monitor adverse effects and adjust dose. [Moderate] Study
- **Idelalisib** is predicted to increase the exposure to **fostamatinib**. Monitor adverse effects and adjust dose. [Moderate] Study
- **Ivosidenib** is predicted to decrease the exposure to **fostamatinib**. Avoid. [Severe] Study
- **Lumacaftor** is predicted to decrease the exposure to **fostamatinib**. Avoid. [Severe] Study
- Macrolides **(clarithromycin)** are predicted to increase the exposure to **fostamatinib**. Monitor adverse effects and adjust dose. [Moderate] Study
- **Mitotane** is predicted to decrease the exposure to **fostamatinib**. Avoid. [Severe] Study
- **Nirmatrelvir** boosted with ritonavir is predicted to increase the concentration of **fostamatinib**. Monitor adverse effects and adjust dose. [Moderate] Theoretical
- **Fostamatinib** is predicted to increase the exposure to opioids **(alfentanil)**. Monitor and adjust dose. [Moderate] Theoretical
- **Fostamatinib** might cause bleeding when given with **phenindione**. [Moderate] Theoretical
- Rifamycins **(rifampicin)** are predicted to decrease the exposure to **fostamatinib**. Avoid. [Severe] Study
- **Fostamatinib** is predicted to increase the exposure to **seladelpar**. [Moderate] Study
- **Fostamatinib** is predicted to increase the exposure to **sirolimus**. Monitor and adjust dose. [Moderate] Theoretical
- **Fostamatinib** is predicted to increase the exposure to statins **(atorvastatin, fluvastatin)**. Monitor and adjust dose. [Moderate] Theoretical

Fostamatinib (continued)

- **Fostamatinib** moderately increases the exposure to statins **(rosuvastatin)**. Avoid or adjust **rosuvastatin** dose, p. 155. Moderate Study
- **Fostamatinib** slightly increases the exposure to statins **(simvastatin)**. Monitor adverse effects and adjust dose. Moderate Study
- **Fostamatinib** is predicted to increase the exposure to **sulfasalazine**. Monitor and adjust dose. Moderate Theoretical
- **Fostamatinib** is predicted to increase the exposure to **temsirolimus**. Monitor and adjust dose. Moderate Theoretical
- **Fostamatinib** is predicted to increase the concentration of **tenofovir alafenamide**. Moderate Theoretical
- **Fostamatinib** is predicted to increase the exposure to **tenofovir disoproxil**. Moderate Theoretical
- **Fostamatinib** is predicted to increase the exposure to **topotecan**. Monitor and adjust dose. Moderate Theoretical
- **Tucatinib** is predicted to increase the exposure to **fostamatinib**. Monitor adverse effects and adjust dose. Moderate Study

Fostemsavir

- Anti-androgens **(apalutamide, enzalutamide)** are predicted to decrease the exposure to the active metabolite of **fostemsavir**. Avoid. Severe Study
- Antiepileptics **(carbamazepine, fosphenytoin, phenobarbital, phenytoin, primidone)** are predicted to decrease the exposure to the active metabolite of **fostemsavir**. Avoid. Severe Study
- **Encorafenib** is predicted to decrease the exposure to the active metabolite of **fostemsavir**. Avoid. Severe Study
- **Fostemsavir** increases the concentration of **ethinylestradiol** from a combined hormonal contraceptive. Adjust dose—consult product literature. Severe Study
- **Fostemsavir** is predicted to increase the exposure to **grazoprevir**. Avoid. Severe Theoretical
- **Ivosidenib** is predicted to decrease the exposure to the active metabolite of **fostemsavir**. Avoid. Severe Study
- **Lumacaftor** is predicted to decrease the exposure to the active metabolite of **fostemsavir**. Avoid. Severe Study
- **Mitotane** is predicted to decrease the exposure to the active metabolite of **fostemsavir**. Avoid. Severe Study
- Rifamycins **(rifampicin)** are predicted to decrease the exposure to the active metabolite of **fostemsavir**. Avoid. Severe Study
- **St John's wort** is predicted to decrease the exposure to the active metabolite of **fostemsavir**. Avoid. Severe Study
- **Fostemsavir** is predicted to increase the exposure to statins **(atorvastatin, fluvastatin, simvastatin)**. Adjust starting dose and monitor. Severe Theoretical
- **Fostemsavir** increases the exposure to statins **(rosuvastatin)**. Adjust starting dose and monitor. Severe Study
- **Fostemsavir** is predicted to increase the exposure to **tenofovir alafenamide**. Adjust dose—consult product literature. Moderate Theoretical

Frovatriptan → see triptans

Fruquintinib

- Anti-androgens **(apalutamide, enzalutamide)** are predicted to decrease the exposure to **fruquintinib**. Avoid. Moderate Study
- Antiepileptics **(carbamazepine, fosphenytoin, phenobarbital, phenytoin, primidone)** are predicted to decrease the exposure to **fruquintinib**. Avoid. Moderate Study
- **Cenobamate** is predicted to decrease the exposure to **fruquintinib**. Avoid. Moderate Study
- **Dabrafenib** is predicted to decrease the exposure to **fruquintinib**. Avoid. Moderate Study
- **Encorafenib** is predicted to decrease the exposure to **fruquintinib**. Avoid. Moderate Study
- Endothelin receptor antagonists **(bosentan)** are predicted to decrease the exposure to **fruquintinib**. Avoid. Moderate Study
- **Ivosidenib** is predicted to decrease the exposure to **fruquintinib**. Avoid. Moderate Study
- **Lorlatinib** is predicted to decrease the exposure to **fruquintinib**. Avoid. Moderate Study
- **Lumacaftor** is predicted to decrease the exposure to **fruquintinib**. Avoid. Moderate Study
- **Mitotane** is predicted to decrease the exposure to **fruquintinib**. Avoid. Moderate Study
- NNRTIs **(efavirenz, etravirine, nevirapine)** are predicted to decrease the exposure to **fruquintinib**. Avoid. Moderate Study
- Rifamycins **(rifampicin)** are predicted to decrease the exposure to **fruquintinib**. Avoid. Moderate Study
- **Sotorasib** is predicted to decrease the exposure to **fruquintinib**. Avoid. Moderate Study
- **St John's wort** is predicted to decrease the exposure to **fruquintinib**. Avoid. Moderate Study

Furosemide → see loop diuretics

Fusidate

- **Nirmatrelvir** boosted with ritonavir is predicted to increase the concentration of **fusidate**. Avoid. Moderate Theoretical
- **Fusidate** has been reported to cause rhabdomyolysis when given with **statins**. Avoid. Severe Anecdotal

Futibatinib

- Antiepileptics **(carbamazepine)** are predicted to decrease the exposure to **futibatinib**. Avoid or adjust dose. Moderate Study
- Antifungals, azoles **(itraconazole, ketoconazole)** are predicted to increase the exposure to **futibatinib**. Avoid or adjust dose—consult product literature. Moderate Study
- **Cobicistat** is predicted to increase the exposure to **futibatinib**. Avoid or adjust dose—consult product literature. Moderate Study
- **Futibatinib** might decrease the efficacy of **combined hormonal contraceptives**. Use additional contraceptive precautions. Severe Theoretical
- HIV-protease inhibitors **(lopinavir)** boosted with ritonavir are predicted to increase the exposure to **futibatinib**. Avoid or adjust dose—consult product literature. Moderate Study
- HIV-protease inhibitors **(ritonavir)** are predicted to increase the exposure to **futibatinib**. Avoid or adjust dose—consult product literature. Moderate Study
- **Lorlatinib** is predicted to decrease the exposure to **futibatinib**. Avoid or adjust dose. Moderate Study
- Macrolides **(clarithromycin)** are predicted to increase the exposure to **futibatinib**. Avoid or adjust dose—consult product literature. Moderate Study
- Rifamycins **(rifampicin)** moderately decrease the exposure to **futibatinib**. Avoid or adjust dose. Moderate Study
- **St John's wort** is predicted to decrease the exposure to **futibatinib**. Avoid or adjust dose. Moderate Study

Gabapentin → see antiepileptics

Galantamine → see anticholinesterases, centrally acting

Ganciclovir → see TABLE 12 p. 1057 (myelosuppression), TABLE 2 p. 1053 (nephrotoxicity)

ROUTE-SPECIFIC INFORMATION Since systemic absorption can follow topical application, the possibility of interactions should be borne in mind.

- **Ganciclovir** is predicted to increase the risk of seizures when given with carbapenems **(imipenem)**. Avoid. Severe Anecdotal
- **Ivosidenib** is predicted to increase the exposure to **ganciclovir**. Use with caution or avoid. Moderate Theoretical
- **Leflunomide** is predicted to increase the exposure to **ganciclovir**. Moderate Study → Also see TABLE 12 p. 1057
- **Maribavir** might decrease the efficacy of **ganciclovir**. Avoid. Severe Theoretical
- **Mycophenolate** is predicted to increase the risk of haematological toxicity when given with **ganciclovir**. Moderate Theoretical
- **Nitisinone** is predicted to increase the exposure to **ganciclovir**. Moderate Study
- **Teriflunomide** is predicted to increase the exposure to **ganciclovir**. Moderate Study
- **Vadadustat** is predicted to increase the exposure to **ganciclovir**. Monitor and adjust dose. Moderate Study

Gefitinib

- Oral **antacids** are predicted to decrease the exposure to oral **gefitinib**. Moderate Theoretical
- Anti-androgens **(apalutamide, enzalutamide)** are predicted to decrease the exposure to **gefitinib**. Avoid. Severe Study
- Antiarrhythmics **(dronedarone)** are predicted to increase the exposure to **gefitinib**. Moderate Study
- Antiepileptics **(carbamazepine, fosphenytoin, phenobarbital, phenytoin, primidone)** are predicted to decrease the exposure to **gefitinib**. Avoid. Severe Study

- Antiepileptics **(eslicarbazepine)** are predicted to decrease the exposure to **gefitinib**. Moderate Theoretical
- Antiepileptics **(oxcarbazepine)** decrease the exposure to **gefitinib**. Severe Study
- Antifungals, azoles **(fluconazole, isavuconazole)** are predicted to increase the exposure to **gefitinib**. Moderate Study
- Antifungals, azoles **(itraconazole, ketoconazole, posaconazole, voriconazole)** are predicted to increase the exposure to **gefitinib**. Severe Study
- **Berotralstat** is predicted to increase the exposure to **gefitinib**. Moderate Study
- **Bupropion** is predicted to increase the exposure to **gefitinib**. Moderate Theoretical
- Oral calcium compounds **(calcium carbonate)** -containing antacids are predicted to decrease the exposure to oral **gefitinib**. Moderate Theoretical
- Calcium-channel blockers **(diltiazem, verapamil)** are predicted to increase the exposure to **gefitinib**. Moderate Study
- **Cenobamate** is predicted to decrease the exposure to **gefitinib**. Avoid. Severe Study
- **Ceritinib** is predicted to increase the exposure to **gefitinib**. Severe Study
- **Cinacalcet** is predicted to increase the exposure to **gefitinib**. Moderate Theoretical
- **Cobicistat** is predicted to increase the exposure to **gefitinib**. Severe Study
- **Gefitinib** is predicted to increase the anticoagulant effect of **coumarins**. Severe Anecdotal
- **Crizotinib** is predicted to increase the exposure to **gefitinib**. Moderate Study
- **Dabrafenib** is predicted to decrease the exposure to **gefitinib**. Avoid. Severe Study
- **Dacomitinib** is predicted to increase the exposure to **gefitinib**. Moderate Theoretical
- **Encorafenib** is predicted to decrease the exposure to **gefitinib**. Avoid. Severe Study
- Endothelin receptor antagonists **(bosentan)** are predicted to decrease the exposure to **gefitinib**. Avoid. Severe Study
- **Fedratinib** is predicted to increase the exposure to **gefitinib**. Moderate Study
- **H_2 receptor antagonists** are predicted to slightly to moderately decrease the exposure to **gefitinib**. Moderate Study
- **HIV-protease inhibitors** are predicted to increase the exposure to **gefitinib**. Severe Study
- **Idelalisib** is predicted to increase the exposure to **gefitinib**. Severe Study
- **Imatinib** is predicted to increase the exposure to **gefitinib**. Moderate Study
- **Ivosidenib** is predicted to decrease the exposure to **gefitinib**. Avoid. Severe Study
- **Letermovir** is predicted to increase the exposure to **gefitinib**. Moderate Study
- **Lorlatinib** is predicted to decrease the exposure to **gefitinib**. Avoid Severe Study
- **Lumacaftor** is predicted to decrease the exposure to **gefitinib**. Avoid Severe Study
- Macrolides **(clarithromycin)** are predicted to increase the exposure to **gefitinib**. Severe Study
- Macrolides **(erythromycin)** are predicted to increase the exposure to **gefitinib**. Moderate Study
- **Mitotane** is predicted to decrease the exposure to **gefitinib**. Avoid. Severe Study
- Neurokinin-1 receptor antagonists **(aprepitant, netupitant)** are predicted to increase the exposure to **gefitinib**. Moderate Study
- **Nilotinib** is predicted to increase the exposure to **gefitinib**. Moderate Study
- NNRTIs **(efavirenz, etravirine, nevirapine)** are predicted to decrease the exposure to **gefitinib**. Avoid. Severe Study
- **Gefitinib** is predicted to increase the risk of bleeding events when given with **phenindione**. Severe Theoretical
- **Proton pump inhibitors** are predicted to decrease the exposure to **gefitinib**. Severe Theoretical
- Rifamycins **(rifampicin)** are predicted to decrease the exposure to **gefitinib**. Avoid. Severe Study
- **Gefitinib** is predicted to increase the exposure to the active component of **sacituzumab govitecan**. Severe Theoretical
- Oral **sodium bicarbonate** -containing antacids are predicted to decrease the exposure to oral **gefitinib**. Moderate Theoretical
- **Sotorasib** is predicted to decrease the exposure to **gefitinib**. Avoid. Severe Study
- SSRIs **(fluoxetine, paroxetine)** are predicted to increase the exposure to **gefitinib**. Moderate Theoretical
- **St John's wort** is predicted to decrease the exposure to **gefitinib**. Avoid. Severe Study
- **Terbinafine** is predicted to increase the exposure to **gefitinib**. Moderate Theoretical
- **Tucatinib** is predicted to increase the exposure to **gefitinib**. Severe Study
- **Gefitinib** might affect the exposure to **vemurafenib**. Moderate Theoretical

Gemcitabine → see TABLE 1 p. 1053 (hepatotoxicity), TABLE 12 p. 1057 (myelosuppression)

- **Cedazuridine** is predicted to increase the exposure to **gemcitabine**. Avoid. Moderate Theoretical
- **Live vaccines** are predicted to increase the risk of generalised infection (possibly life-threatening) when given with **gemcitabine**. UKHSA advises avoid (refer to Green Book). Severe Theoretical

Gemfibrozil → see fibrates

Gemtuzumab ozogamicin → see TABLE 12 p. 1057 (myelosuppression)

Gentamicin → see aminoglycosides

Gilteritinib

- ACE inhibitors **(captopril)** are predicted to increase the exposure to **gilteritinib**. Moderate Theoretical
- Anti-androgens **(enzalutamide)** are predicted to increase the exposure to **gilteritinib**. Moderate Theoretical
- Antiarrhythmics **(amiodarone, dronedarone)** are predicted to increase the exposure to **gilteritinib**. Moderate Theoretical
- Antiepileptics **(carbamazepine, phenytoin)** are predicted to decrease the exposure to **gilteritinib**. Avoid. Severe Study
- Antifungals, azoles **(itraconazole, ketoconazole, posaconazole, voriconazole)** are predicted to increase the exposure to **gilteritinib**. Moderate Study
- Beta blockers, non-selective **(carvedilol)** are predicted to increase the exposure to **gilteritinib**. Moderate Theoretical
- Calcium-channel blockers **(verapamil)** are predicted to increase the exposure to **gilteritinib**. Moderate Theoretical
- **Ceritinib** is predicted to increase the exposure to **gilteritinib**. Moderate Study
- **Ciclosporin** is predicted to increase the exposure to **gilteritinib**. Moderate Theoretical
- **Cobicistat** is predicted to increase the exposure to **gilteritinib**. Moderate Study
- **HIV-protease inhibitors** are predicted to increase the exposure to **gilteritinib**. Moderate Study
- **Idelalisib** is predicted to increase the exposure to **gilteritinib**. Moderate Study
- **Ivacaftor** is predicted to increase the exposure to **gilteritinib**. Moderate Theoretical
- **Lapatinib** is predicted to increase the exposure to **gilteritinib**. Moderate Theoretical
- Macrolides **(azithromycin, erythromycin)** are predicted to increase the exposure to **gilteritinib**. Moderate Theoretical
- Macrolides **(clarithromycin)** are predicted to increase the exposure to **gilteritinib**. Moderate Study
- **Maribavir** is predicted to increase the exposure to **gilteritinib**. Moderate Theoretical
- **Neratinib** is predicted to increase the exposure to **gilteritinib**. Moderate Theoretical
- **Ranolazine** is predicted to increase the exposure to **gilteritinib**. Moderate Theoretical
- Rifamycins **(rifampicin)** moderately decrease the exposure to **gilteritinib**. Avoid. Severe Study
- **Rucaparib** is predicted to increase the exposure to **gilteritinib**. Moderate Theoretical
- **Gilteritinib** is predicted to decrease the efficacy of SSRIs **(escitalopram, fluoxetine, sertraline)**. Avoid. Moderate Theoretical

Gilteritinib (continued)
- **St John's wort** is predicted to decrease the exposure to **gilteritinib**. Avoid. Severe Study
- **Tucatinib** is predicted to increase the exposure to **gilteritinib**. Moderate Study
- **Vandetanib** is predicted to increase the exposure to **gilteritinib**. Moderate Theoretical
- **Vemurafenib** is predicted to increase the exposure to **gilteritinib**. Moderate Theoretical
- **Voclosporin** is predicted to increase the exposure to **gilteritinib**. Moderate Theoretical

Givinostat
- **Givinostat** increases the exposure to benzodiazepines **(midazolam)**. Moderate Study
- **Givinostat** might increase the exposure to **everolimus**. Moderate Study
- **Givinostat** might increase the exposure to **metformin**. Moderate Theoretical
- **Givinostat** might increase the exposure to opioids **(alfentanil)**. Moderate Study
- **Givinostat** might increase the exposure to phosphodiesterase type-5 inhibitors **(sildenafil)**. Moderate Study
- **Givinostat** might increase the exposure to **sirolimus**. Moderate Study
- **Givinostat** might increase the exposure to statins **(simvastatin)**. Moderate Study
- **Givinostat** might increase the exposure to **tacrolimus**. Moderate Study
- **Givinostat** might increase the exposure to **temsirolimus**. Moderate Study
- **Givinostat** might increase the exposure to triptans **(eletriptan)**. Moderate Study

Givosiran
- **Givosiran** is predicted to increase the exposure to **agomelatine**. Moderate Study
- **Givosiran** is predicted to increase the exposure to **aminophylline**. Adjust dose. Moderate Theoretical
- **Givosiran** is predicted to increase the exposure to anaesthetics, local **(ropivacaine)**. Moderate Theoretical
- **Givosiran** is predicted to increase the exposure to **anagrelide**. Moderate Theoretical
- **Givosiran** is predicted to increase the exposure to **atomoxetine**. Use with caution and adjust dose. Moderate Study
- **Givosiran** increases the concentration of atypical antipsychotics **(clozapine)**. Monitor adverse effects and adjust dose. Severe Study
- **Givosiran** is predicted to increase the exposure to atypical antipsychotics **(olanzapine)**. Adjust dose. Moderate Anecdotal
- **Givosiran** is predicted to increase the exposure to beta blockers, selective **(metoprolol)**. Moderate Study
- **Givosiran** is predicted to increase the exposure to beta blockers, selective **(nebivolol)**. Use with caution and adjust dose. Moderate Study
- **Givosiran** is predicted to increase the exposure to dopamine receptor agonists **(ropinirole)**. Adjust dose. Moderate Study
- **Givosiran** is predicted to increase the exposure to **eliglustat**. Use with caution and adjust dose. Moderate Study
- **Givosiran** are predicted to increases the exposure to **erlotinib**. Monitor adverse effects and adjust dose. Moderate Study
- **Givosiran** is predicted to increase the exposure to **fezolinetant**. Avoid. Moderate Study
- **Givosiran** is predicted to increase the exposure to **loxapine**. Avoid. Unknown Theoretical
- **Givosiran** slightly increases the exposure to MAO-B inhibitors **(rasagiline)**. Moderate Study
- **Givosiran** is predicted to increase the exposure to **mavacamten**. Monitor and adjust dose—consult product literature. Moderate Theoretical
- **Givosiran** is predicted to increase the exposure to **melatonin**. Moderate Theoretical
- **Givosiran** is predicted to increase the exposure to phenothiazine antipsychotics **(chlorpromazine)**. Moderate Theoretical
- **Givosiran** is predicted to increase the exposure to phosphodiesterase type-4 inhibitors **(roflumilast)**. Moderate Theoretical
- **Givosiran** is predicted to increase the exposure to **pirfenidone**. Use with caution and adjust dose. Moderate Study
- **Givosiran** is predicted to increase the exposure to **riluzole**. Moderate Theoretical
- **Givosiran** is predicted to increase the exposure to SNRIs **(duloxetine)**. Use with caution and adjust dose. Moderate Study
- **Givosiran** is predicted to increase the exposure to **theophylline**. Monitor and adjust dose. Moderate Theoretical
- **Givosiran** increases the exposure to **tizanidine**. Avoid. Moderate Study
- **Givosiran** is predicted to increase the exposure to triptans **(zolmitriptan)**. Adjust **zolmitriptan** dose, p. 347. Moderate Theoretical
- **Givosiran** is predicted to increase the exposure to **vorasidenib**. Avoid. Moderate Theoretical

Glasdegib → see TABLE 7 p. 1055 (QT-interval prolongation)
- Anti-androgens **(apalutamide, enzalutamide)** are predicted to decrease the exposure to **glasdegib**. Avoid. Severe Study → Also see TABLE 7 p. 1055
- Antiepileptics **(carbamazepine, fosphenytoin, phenobarbital, phenytoin, primidone)** are predicted to decrease the exposure to **glasdegib**. Avoid. Severe Study
- Antifungals, azoles **(itraconazole, ketoconazole, posaconazole, voriconazole)** are predicted to increase the exposure to **glasdegib**. Use with caution or avoid. Severe Study → Also see TABLE 7 p. 1055
- **Cenobamate** is predicted to decrease the exposure to **glasdegib**. Avoid or adjust dose—consult product literature. Moderate Theoretical
- **Ceritinib** is predicted to increase the exposure to **glasdegib**. Use with caution or avoid. Severe Study → Also see TABLE 7 p. 1055
- **Cobicistat** is predicted to increase the exposure to **glasdegib**. Use with caution or avoid. Severe Study
- **Dabrafenib** is predicted to decrease the exposure to **glasdegib**. Avoid or adjust dose—consult product literature. Moderate Theoretical
- **Encorafenib** is predicted to decrease the exposure to **glasdegib**. Avoid. Severe Study → Also see TABLE 7 p. 1055
- Endothelin receptor antagonists **(bosentan)** are predicted to decrease the exposure to **glasdegib**. Avoid or adjust dose—consult product literature. Moderate Theoretical
- **Grapefruit** juice is predicted to increase the exposure to **glasdegib**. Use with caution or avoid. Moderate Theoretical
- **HIV-protease inhibitors** are predicted to increase the exposure to **glasdegib**. Use with caution or avoid. Severe Study
- **Idelalisib** is predicted to increase the exposure to **glasdegib**. Use with caution or avoid. Severe Study
- **Ivosidenib** is predicted to decrease the exposure to **glasdegib**. Avoid. Severe Study → Also see TABLE 7 p. 1055
- **Lorlatinib** is predicted to decrease the exposure to **glasdegib**. Avoid or adjust dose—consult product literature. Moderate Theoretical
- **Lumacaftor** is predicted to decrease the exposure to **glasdegib**. Avoid. Severe Study
- Macrolides **(clarithromycin)** are predicted to increase the exposure to **glasdegib**. Use with caution or avoid. Severe Study
- **Mitotane** is predicted to decrease the exposure to **glasdegib**. Avoid. Severe Study
- **Modafinil** is predicted to decrease the exposure to **glasdegib**. Avoid or adjust dose—consult product literature. Moderate Theoretical
- NNRTIs **(efavirenz, etravirine, nevirapine)** are predicted to decrease the exposure to **glasdegib**. Avoid or adjust dose—consult product literature. Moderate Theoretical → Also see TABLE 7 p. 1055
- Rifamycins **(rifampicin)** are predicted to decrease the exposure to **glasdegib**. Avoid. Severe Study
- **Sotorasib** is predicted to decrease the exposure to **glasdegib**. Avoid or adjust dose—consult product literature. Moderate Theoretical
- **St John's wort** is predicted to decrease the exposure to **glasdegib**. Avoid or adjust dose—consult product literature. Moderate Theoretical
- **Tucatinib** is predicted to increase the exposure to **glasdegib**. Use with caution or avoid. Severe Study

Glecaprevir
- **Glecaprevir** is predicted to increase the exposure to **afatinib**. Moderate Study
- **Glecaprevir** is predicted to increase the exposure to **aliskiren**. Severe Theoretical
- Anti-androgens **(enzalutamide)** are predicted to greatly decrease the concentration of **glecaprevir**. Avoid. Severe Study
- Antiepileptics **(carbamazepine, fosphenytoin, phenobarbital, phenytoin, primidone)** are predicted to moderately decrease the exposure to **glecaprevir**. Avoid. Severe Study
- Antiepileptics **(eslicarbazepine, oxcarbazepine)** potentially decrease the exposure to **glecaprevir**. Avoid. Severe Theoretical
- **Glecaprevir** is predicted to increase the exposure to antihistamines, non-sedating **(fexofenadine)**. Severe Theoretical
- **Bulevirtide** is predicted to increase the exposure to **glecaprevir**. Avoid or monitor. Moderate Theoretical
- **Cenobamate** is predicted to decrease the exposure to **glecaprevir**. Avoid. Severe Study
- **Ciclosporin** increases the exposure to **glecaprevir**. Avoid or monitor. Severe Study
- **Glecaprevir** is predicted to increase the exposure to **colchicine**. Avoid P-glycoprotein inhibitors or adjust **colchicine** dose, p. 637. Severe Theoretical
- **Combined hormonal contraceptives** containing ethinylestradiol can increase ALT concentrations when given with **glecaprevir** with pibrentasvir. Avoid. Severe Study
- **Crizotinib** potentially decreases the exposure to **glecaprevir**. Avoid. Severe Theoretical
- **Dabrafenib** is predicted to decrease the exposure to **glecaprevir**. Avoid. Severe Study
- **Glecaprevir** with pibrentasvir increases the exposure to **digoxin**. Moderate Study
- Endothelin receptor antagonists **(bosentan)** are predicted to decrease the exposure to **glecaprevir**. Avoid. Severe Study
- **Glecaprevir** is predicted to increase the exposure to **erlotinib**. Moderate Theoretical
- **Ethinylestradiol** might increase ALT concentrations when given with **glecaprevir** with pibrentasvir. Avoid. Severe Study
- **Glecaprevir** is predicted to increase the exposure to **everolimus**. Moderate Study
- **Glecaprevir** is predicted to increase the exposure to factor XA inhibitors **(apixaban)**. Moderate Theoretical
- **Glecaprevir** is predicted to increase the exposure to factor XA inhibitors **(edoxaban)**. Severe Theoretical
- **Glecaprevir** might increase the exposure to factor XA inhibitors **(rivaroxaban)**. Manufacturer advises caution in renal impairment. Moderate Theoretical
- **Glecaprevir** is predicted to increase the exposure to **fidaxomicin**. Avoid. Moderate Study
- HIV-protease inhibitors **(atazanavir, darunavir, lopinavir)** boosted with ritonavir increase the exposure to **glecaprevir**. Avoid. Severe Study
- HIV-protease inhibitors **(ritonavir)** increase the exposure to **glecaprevir**. Avoid. Severe Study
- **Hormone replacement therapy** might increase ALT concentrations when given with **glecaprevir** with pibrentasvir. Manufacturer advises caution; avoid ethinylestradiol. Severe Theoretical
- **Glecaprevir** is predicted to increase the exposure to **loperamide**. Severe Theoretical
- **Lorlatinib** is predicted to decrease the exposure to **glecaprevir**. Avoid. Severe Study
- **Lumacaftor** potentially decreases the exposure to **glecaprevir**. Avoid. Severe Theoretical
- **Glecaprevir** is predicted to increase the exposure to **mavacamten**. Monitor and adjust dose—consult product literature. Moderate Theoretical
- **Mitotane** is predicted to greatly decrease the concentration of **glecaprevir**. Avoid. Severe Study
- **Glecaprevir** is predicted to increase the risk of neutropenia when given with monoclonal antibodies **(brentuximab vedotin)**. Monitor and adjust dose. Severe Theoretical
- **Glecaprevir** is predicted to increase the exposure to **neratinib**. Avoid or adjust dose and monitor for gastrointestinal adverse effects—consult product literature. Severe Study
- **Glecaprevir** is predicted to increase the exposure to **nintedanib**. Moderate Study
- **Nirmatrelvir** boosted with ritonavir is predicted to increase the concentration of **glecaprevir**. Avoid. Severe Theoretical
- NNRTIs **(efavirenz, etravirine, nevirapine)** are predicted to decrease the exposure to **glecaprevir**. Avoid. Severe Study
- **Glecaprevir** is predicted to increase the exposure to **pralsetinib**. Moderate Theoretical
- **Glecaprevir** is predicted to increase the exposure to **ranolazine**. Adjust dose. Severe Theoretical
- **Glecaprevir** is predicted to increase the exposure to **relugolix**. Avoid or take relugolix first and separate administration by at least 6 hours. Moderate Study
- Rifamycins **(rifampicin)** markedly affect the exposure to **glecaprevir**. Avoid. Severe Study
- **Glecaprevir** is predicted to increase the exposure to **rimegepant**. Avoid another dose of rimegepant within 48 hours of concurrent use. Moderate Theoretical
- **Glecaprevir** is predicted to increase the exposure to **sirolimus**. Severe Theoretical
- **Sotorasib** is predicted to decrease the exposure to **glecaprevir**. Avoid. Severe Study
- **St John's wort** is predicted to decrease the exposure to **glecaprevir**. Avoid. Severe Study
- **Glecaprevir** with pibrentasvir markedly increases the exposure to statins **(atorvastatin)**. Avoid. Severe Study
- **Glecaprevir** with pibrentasvir is predicted to increase the exposure to statins **(fluvastatin)**. Moderate Theoretical
- **Glecaprevir** with pibrentasvir moderately increases the exposure to statins **(pravastatin)**. Use with caution and adjust **pravastatin** dose. Moderate Study
- **Glecaprevir** with pibrentasvir moderately increases the exposure to statins **(rosuvastatin)**. Use with caution and adjust **rosuvastatin** dose, p. 155. Moderate Study
- **Glecaprevir** with pibrentasvir moderately increases the exposure to statins **(simvastatin)**. Avoid. Moderate Study
- **Glecaprevir** with pibrentasvir slightly increases the exposure to **tacrolimus**. Monitor and adjust dose. Mild Study
- **Glecaprevir** is predicted to slightly increase the exposure to **talazoparib**. Avoid or adjust dose—consult product literature. Severe Study
- **Glecaprevir** is predicted to increase the exposure to taxanes **(paclitaxel)**. Severe Theoretical
- **Glecaprevir** with pibrentasvir increases the exposure to thrombin inhibitors **(dabigatran)**. Avoid. Moderate Study
- **Glecaprevir** is predicted to increase the exposure to **topotecan**. Severe Study
- **Glecaprevir** is predicted to increase the concentration of **trametinib**. Moderate Theoretical

Glibenclamide → see sulfonylureas

Gliclazide → see sulfonylureas

Glimepiride → see sulfonylureas

Glipizide → see sulfonylureas

Glofitamab
- **Glofitamab** might affect the exposure to **ciclosporin**. Moderate Theoretical
- **Glofitamab** might affect the exposure to coumarins **(warfarin)**. Moderate Theoretical

Glucagon
- **Glucagon** increases the anticoagulant effect of coumarins **(warfarin)**. Severe Study

Glucagon-like peptide-1 receptor agonists

dulaglutide · liraglutide · semaglutide · tirzepatide

- **Tirzepatide** might affect the absorption of oral **combined hormonal contraceptives**. Manufacturer advises precautions for those who are overweight or obese. Moderate Study
- **Semaglutide** might decrease the anticoagulant effect of coumarins **(acenocoumarol)**. Severe Anecdotal
- **Tirzepatide** might affect the absorption of coumarins **(warfarin)**. Severe Theoretical
- **Tirzepatide** might affect the absorption of **desogestrel**. Manufacturer advises precautions for those who are overweight or obese. Moderate Study

Interactions | Appendix 1 A1

Glucagon-like peptide-1 receptor agonists (continued)
- **Tirzepatide** might affect the absorption of **digoxin**. Moderate Theoretical
- **Tirzepatide** might affect the absorption of **drospirenone**. Manufacturer advises precautions for those who are overweight or obese. Moderate Study
- **Fenfluramine** might decrease blood glucose concentrations when given with **glucagon-like peptide-1 receptor agonists**. Moderate Theoretical
- **Tirzepatide** might affect the absorption of oral **levonorgestrel**. Manufacturer advises precautions for those who are overweight or obese. Moderate Study
- Monoclonal antibodies **(rozanolixizumab)** might decrease the concentration of **dulaglutide**. Avoid and for 2 weeks after stopping **rozanolixizumab**. Moderate Theoretical
- **Tirzepatide** might affect the absorption of oral **norethisterone**. Manufacturer advises precautions for those who are overweight or obese. Moderate Study
- **Somapacitan** might increase blood glucose concentrations, opposing the blood glucose-lowering effects of **glucagon-like peptide-1 receptor agonists**. Adjust dose. Moderate Theoretical
- **Somatrogon** might increase blood glucose concentrations, opposing the blood glucose-lowering effects of **glucagon-like peptide-1 receptor agonists**. Adjust dose. Moderate Theoretical
- **Semaglutide** slightly increases the exposure to thyroid hormones **(levothyroxine)**. Moderate Study

Glucarpidase
- **Glucarpidase** decreases the exposure to folates **(folinic acid)**. Separate administration by at least 2 hours. Moderate Study
- **Glucarpidase** might decrease the exposure to folates **(levofolinic acid)**. Separate administration by at least 2 hours. Moderate Theoretical

Glucosamine
- **Glucosamine** potentially decreases the anticoagulant effect of coumarins **(acenocoumarol)**. Moderate Anecdotal
- **Glucosamine** potentially increases the anticoagulant effect of coumarins **(warfarin)**. Avoid. Moderate Anecdotal

Glycerol phenylbutyrate
- Antiepileptics **(valproate)** potentially oppose the effects of **glycerol phenylbutyrate**. Moderate Theoretical
- **Corticosteroids** potentially oppose the effects of **glycerol phenylbutyrate**. Moderate Theoretical
- **Haloperidol** potentially opposes the effects of **glycerol phenylbutyrate**. Moderate Theoretical

Glyceryl trinitrate → see nitrates

Glycopyrronium → see TABLE 8 p. 1055 (antimuscarinics)

ROUTE-SPECIFIC INFORMATION Since systemic absorption can follow topical application of **glycopyrronium**, the possibility of interactions should be borne in mind.

- Atypical antipsychotics **(clozapine)** can cause constipation, as can **glycopyrronium**; concurrent use might increase the risk of developing intestinal obstruction. Severe Theoretical → Also see TABLE 8 p. 1055

Golimumab → see monoclonal antibodies

Granisetron → see 5-HT3-receptor antagonists

Grapefruit
- **Grapefruit** juice is predicted to increase the exposure to **abemaciclib**. Avoid. Moderate Theoretical
- **Grapefruit** juice moderately decreases the exposure to **aliskiren**. Avoid. Severe Study
- **Grapefruit** juice increases the exposure to antiarrhythmics **(amiodarone)**. Avoid. Moderate Study
- **Grapefruit** juice moderately increases the exposure to antiarrhythmics **(dronedarone)**. Avoid. Severe Study
- **Grapefruit** juice increases the exposure to antiarrhythmics **(propafenone)**. Monitor and adjust dose. Moderate Study
- **Grapefruit** juice slightly increases the exposure to antiepileptics **(carbamazepine)**. Monitor and adjust dose. Moderate Study
- **Grapefruit** juice slightly decreases the exposure to antihistamines, non-sedating **(bilastine)**. **Bilastine** should be taken 1 hour before or 2 hours after **grapefruit**. Moderate Study
- **Grapefruit** juice increases the exposure to antihistamines, non-sedating **(rupatadine)**. Avoid. Moderate Study
- **Grapefruit** juice increases the exposure to antimalarials **(artemether)**. Unknown Study
- **Grapefruit** juice is predicted to increase the concentration of antimalarials **(piperaquine)**. Avoid. Moderate Theoretical
- **Grapefruit** juice is predicted to increase the exposure to atypical antipsychotics **(cariprazine)**. Avoid. Moderate Study
- **Grapefruit** juice is predicted to increase the exposure to atypical antipsychotics **(lurasidone, quetiapine)**. Avoid. Severe Theoretical
- **Grapefruit** and grapefruit juice is predicted to increase the exposure to **avacopan**. Avoid. Moderate Theoretical
- **Grapefruit** juice is predicted to increase the exposure to **avapritinib**. Avoid. Moderate Theoretical
- **Grapefruit** juice is predicted to increase the exposure to **axitinib**. Moderate Theoretical
- **Grapefruit** juice is predicted to increase the exposure to **berotralstat**. Moderate Theoretical
- **Grapefruit** juice greatly decreases the exposure to beta blockers, selective **(celiprolol)**. Moderate Study
- **Grapefruit** juice is predicted to increase the exposure to **bosutinib**. Avoid. Moderate Theoretical
- **Grapefruit** juice is predicted to increase the concentration of **brigatinib**. Avoid. Severe Study
- **Grapefruit** juice increases the exposure to **buspirone**. Avoid. Mild Study
- **Grapefruit** juice is predicted to increase the exposure to **cabozantinib**. Moderate Theoretical
- **Grapefruit** juice very slightly increases the exposure to calcium-channel blockers **(amlodipine)**. Avoid. Mild Study
- **Grapefruit** juice increases the exposure to calcium-channel blockers **(felodipine)**. Avoid. Moderate Study
- **Grapefruit** juice is predicted to increase the exposure to calcium-channel blockers **(lercanidipine)**. Avoid. Moderate Theoretical
- **Grapefruit** juice increases the exposure to calcium-channel blockers **(nicardipine)**. Mild Study
- **Grapefruit** juice increases the exposure to calcium-channel blockers **(nifedipine, verapamil)**. Avoid. Mild Study
- **Grapefruit** and grapefruit juice is predicted to increase the exposure to **capivasertib**. Adjust dose. Moderate Theoretical
- **Grapefruit** juice is predicted to increase the exposure to **ceritinib**. Avoid. Severe Theoretical
- **Grapefruit** juice increases the concentration of **ciclosporin**. Avoid. Severe Study
- **Grapefruit** juice markedly decreases the exposure to **clopidogrel**. Severe Study
- **Grapefruit** juice is predicted to increase the exposure to **cobimetinib**. Avoid. Severe Theoretical
- **Grapefruit** juice is predicted to increase the exposure to **colchicine**. Avoid. Severe Anecdotal
- **Grapefruit** juice moderately increases the exposure to oral corticosteroids **(budesonide)**. Avoid. Moderate Study
- **Grapefruit** juice is predicted to increase the exposure to **crizotinib**. Avoid. Moderate Theoretical
- **Grapefruit** and grapefruit juice is predicted to increase the exposure to **daridorexant**. Avoid **grapefruit** in the evening. Moderate Theoretical
- **Grapefruit** juice is predicted to increase the exposure to **darifenacin**. Moderate Study
- **Grapefruit** juice is predicted to increase the exposure to **dasatinib**. Avoid. Moderate Theoretical
- **Grapefruit** is predicted to increase the exposure to **deutivacaftor**. Avoid. Moderate Theoretical
- **Grapefruit** juice is predicted to increase the exposure to dipeptidylpeptidase-4 inhibitors **(saxagliptin)**. Mild Theoretical
- **Grapefruit** is predicted to increase the exposure to **elacestrant**. Avoid. Moderate Theoretical
- **Grapefruit** juice is predicted to increase the exposure to **elexacaftor**. Avoid. Moderate Theoretical
- **Grapefruit** juice is predicted to increase the exposure to **eliglustat**. Avoid. Severe Theoretical
- **Grapefruit** juice is predicted to increase the exposure to **encorafenib**. Avoid. Moderate Study

- **Grapefruit** is predicted to increase the exposure to **entrectinib**. Avoid. Severe Theoretical
- **Grapefruit** is predicted to increase the exposure to **erdafitinib**. Avoid. Moderate Theoretical
- **Grapefruit** juice is predicted to increase the exposure to **ergometrine**. Severe Theoretical
- **Grapefruit** juice is predicted to increase the exposure to **erlotinib**. Moderate Theoretical
- **Grapefruit** juice is predicted to increase the exposure to **everolimus**. Avoid. Severe Theoretical
- **Grapefruit** and grapefruit juice is predicted to increase the exposure to **fedratinib**. Avoid. Moderate Theoretical
- **Grapefruit** juice is predicted to increase the exposure to **fostamatinib**. Monitor adverse effects and adjust dose. Moderate Theoretical
- **Grapefruit** juice is predicted to increase the exposure to **glasdegib**. Use with caution or avoid. Moderate Theoretical
- **Grapefruit** juice is predicted to increase the exposure to **guanfacine**. Avoid. Moderate Theoretical
- **Grapefruit** juice is predicted to increase the exposure to **ibrutinib**. Avoid. Moderate Theoretical
- **Grapefruit** juice is predicted to increase the exposure to **imatinib**. Moderate Theoretical
- **Grapefruit** juice is predicted to increase the exposure to **ivabradine**. Avoid. Moderate Study
- **Grapefruit** juice is predicted to increase the exposure to **ivacaftor**. Avoid. Moderate Theoretical
- **Grapefruit** and grapefruit juice are predicted to increase the exposure to **ivosidenib**. Avoid. Moderate Study
- **Grapefruit** juice is predicted to increase the exposure to **lapatinib**. Avoid. Moderate Theoretical
- **Grapefruit** juice is predicted to increase the exposure to **larotrectinib**. Avoid. Moderate Theoretical
- **Grapefruit** juice is predicted to increase the exposure to **leniolisib**. Avoid. Moderate Theoretical
- **Grapefruit** juice is predicted to increase the exposure to **lomitapide**. Avoid. Mild Theoretical
- **Grapefruit** juice is predicted to increase the concentration of **lorlatinib**. Avoid. Moderate Theoretical
- **Grapefruit** is predicted to increase the exposure to **mavacamten**. Monitor and adjust dose—consult product literature. Moderate Theoretical
- **Grapefruit** juice is predicted to increase the exposure to **midostaurin**. Moderate Theoretical
- **Grapefruit** juice is predicted to increase the exposure to **mifepristone**. Moderate Theoretical
- **Grapefruit** and grapefruit juice is predicted to increase the exposure to mineralocorticoid receptor antagonists **(finerenone)**. Avoid. Moderate Theoretical
- **Grapefruit** juice is predicted to increase the exposure to **naldemedine**. Avoid or monitor. Moderate Theoretical
- **Grapefruit** juice is predicted to increase the exposure to **naloxegol**. Avoid. Moderate Theoretical
- **Grapefruit** juice is predicted to increase the exposure to **neratinib**. Avoid. Severe Theoretical
- **Grapefruit** juice is predicted to increase the exposure to **nilotinib**. Avoid. Severe Theoretical
- **Grapefruit** juice is predicted to increase the exposure to **olaparib**. Avoid. Moderate Theoretical
- **Grapefruit** juice is predicted to increase the exposure to **omaveloxolone**. Avoid. Moderate Theoretical
- **Grapefruit** juice is predicted to increase the exposure to **palbociclib**. Avoid. Severe Theoretical
- **Grapefruit** and grapefruit juice is predicted to increase the exposure to **panobinostat**. Avoid. Moderate Theoretical
- **Grapefruit** juice is predicted to increase the exposure to **pazopanib**. Avoid. Severe Theoretical
- **Grapefruit** and grapefruit juice is predicted to increase the exposure to **pemigatinib**. Avoid. Severe Study
- **Grapefruit** juice is predicted to increase the exposure to **phosphodiesterase type-5 inhibitors**. Use with caution or avoid. Moderate Study
- **Grapefruit** juice increases the exposure to **pimozide**. Avoid. Severe Theoretical
- **Grapefruit** juice is predicted to increase the exposure to **ponatinib**. Moderate Theoretical
- **Grapefruit** juice is predicted to increase the exposure to **pralsetinib**. Avoid. Moderate Study
- **Grapefruit** juice is predicted to increase the exposure to **praziquantel**. Moderate Study
- **Grapefruit** juice is predicted to increase the concentration of **ranolazine**. Avoid. Severe Theoretical
- **Grapefruit** juice is predicted to increase the exposure to **regorafenib**. Avoid. Moderate Theoretical
- **Grapefruit** juice is predicted to increase the exposure to **ribociclib**. Avoid. Moderate Theoretical
- **Grapefruit** juice is predicted to increase the exposure to **ripretinib**. Avoid. Mild Theoretical
- **Grapefruit** juice is predicted to increase the exposure to **ruxolitinib**. Severe Theoretical
- **Grapefruit** juice is predicted to increase the exposure to **selumetinib**. Avoid. Moderate Theoretical
- **Grapefruit** juice increases the concentration of **sirolimus**. Avoid. Moderate Study
- **Grapefruit** is predicted to increase the exposure to **sparsentan**. Avoid. Severe Theoretical
- **Grapefruit** juice moderately increases the exposure to SSRIs **(sertraline)**. Avoid. Moderate Study
- **Grapefruit** juice increases the exposure to statins **(atorvastatin)**. Mild Study
- **Grapefruit** juice increases the exposure to statins **(simvastatin)**. Avoid. Severe Study
- **Grapefruit** juice is predicted to increase the exposure to **sunitinib**. Avoid. Moderate Theoretical
- **Grapefruit** juice greatly increases the concentration of **tacrolimus**. Avoid. Severe Study
- **Grapefruit** juice is predicted to increase the concentration of **temsirolimus**. Use with caution or avoid. Moderate Theoretical
- **Grapefruit** juice is predicted to increase the exposure to **tezacaftor**. Avoid. Severe Study
- **Grapefruit** juice moderately increases the exposure to **ticagrelor**. Moderate Study
- **Grapefruit** juice increases the exposure to **tolvaptan**. Avoid. Moderate Study
- **Grapefruit** juice is predicted to increase the exposure to **ulipristal**. Avoid when used for uterine fibroids. Moderate Theoretical
- **Grapefruit** is predicted to increase the exposure to **upadacitinib**. Avoid. Moderate Theoretical
- **Grapefruit** is predicted to increase the exposure to **vanzacaftor**. Avoid. Moderate Theoretical
- **Grapefruit** juice is predicted to increase the exposure to **venetoclax**. Avoid. Severe Theoretical
- **Grapefruit** and grapefruit juice are predicted to increase the exposure to **voclosporin**. Avoid. Moderate Theoretical
- **Grapefruit** juice is predicted to increase the exposure to **zanubrutinib**. Moderate Theoretical

Grass pollen extracts

GENERAL INFORMATION Desensitising vaccines should be avoided in patients taking beta-blockers (adrenaline might be ineffective in case of a hypersensitivity reaction) or ACE inhibitors (risk of severe anaphylactoid reactions).

Grazoprevir

- Anti-androgens **(apalutamide, enzalutamide)** are predicted to decrease the exposure to **grazoprevir**. Avoid. Severe Study
- Anti-androgens **(darolutamide)** are predicted to increase the exposure to **grazoprevir**. Avoid. Severe Theoretical
- Antiarrhythmics **(amiodarone, dronedarone)** are predicted to increase the exposure to **grazoprevir**. Avoid. Severe Theoretical
- Antiepileptics **(carbamazepine, fosphenytoin, phenobarbital, phenytoin, primidone)** are predicted to decrease the exposure to **grazoprevir**. Avoid. Severe Study
- Antifungals, azoles **(itraconazole, ketoconazole, posaconazole, voriconazole)** are predicted to moderately to markedly increase the exposure to **grazoprevir**. Avoid. Severe Study
- **Bulevirtide** is predicted to increase the exposure to **grazoprevir**. Avoid or monitor. Moderate Theoretical
- **Cenobamate** is predicted to markedly decrease the exposure to **grazoprevir**. Avoid. Severe Study

Grazoprevir (continued)
- **Ceritinib** is predicted to moderately to markedly increase the exposure to **grazoprevir**. Avoid. Severe Study
- **Ciclosporin** greatly increases the exposure to **grazoprevir**. Avoid. Severe Study
- **Cobicistat** is predicted to moderately to markedly increase the exposure to **grazoprevir**. Avoid. Severe Study
- **Dabrafenib** is predicted to markedly decrease the exposure to **grazoprevir**. Avoid. Severe Study
- **Eltrombopag** is predicted to increase the exposure to **grazoprevir**. Avoid. Severe Theoretical
- **Elvitegravir** markedly increases the exposure to **grazoprevir**. Avoid. Severe Study
- **Encorafenib** is predicted to decrease the exposure to **grazoprevir**. Avoid. Severe Study
- Endothelin receptor antagonists **(bosentan)** are predicted to markedly decrease the exposure to **grazoprevir**. Avoid. Severe Study
- Fibrates **(gemfibrozil)** are predicted to increase the exposure to **grazoprevir**. Avoid. Severe Theoretical
- **Fostemsavir** is predicted to increase the exposure to **grazoprevir**. Avoid. Severe Theoretical
- **HIV-protease inhibitors** are predicted to moderately to markedly increase the exposure to **grazoprevir**. Avoid. Severe Study
- **Idelalisib** is predicted to moderately to markedly increase the exposure to **grazoprevir**. Avoid. Severe Study
- **Ivosidenib** is predicted to decrease the exposure to **grazoprevir**. Avoid. Severe Study
- **Lapatinib** is predicted to increase the exposure to **grazoprevir**. Avoid. Severe Theoretical
- **Leflunomide** is predicted to increase the exposure to **grazoprevir**. Avoid. Severe Theoretical
- **Lorlatinib** is predicted to markedly decrease the exposure to **grazoprevir**. Avoid. Severe Study
- **Lumacaftor** is predicted to decrease the exposure to **grazoprevir**. Avoid. Severe Study
- Macrolides **(azithromycin, erythromycin)** are predicted to increase the exposure to **grazoprevir**. Avoid. Severe Theoretical
- Macrolides **(clarithromycin)** are predicted to moderately to markedly increase the exposure to **grazoprevir**. Avoid. Severe Study
- **Mitotane** is predicted to decrease the exposure to **grazoprevir**. Avoid. Severe Study
- **Modafinil** is predicted to decrease the exposure to **grazoprevir**. Avoid. Severe Theoretical
- **Nirmatrelvir** boosted with ritonavir is predicted to increase the concentration of **grazoprevir**. Severe Theoretical
- NNRTIs **(efavirenz, etravirine, nevirapine)** are predicted to markedly decrease the exposure to **grazoprevir**. Avoid. Severe Study
- **Pibrentasvir** is predicted to increase the exposure to **grazoprevir**. Avoid. Severe Theoretical
- **Ranolazine** is predicted to increase the exposure to **grazoprevir**. Avoid. Severe Theoretical
- Rifamycins **(rifampicin)** are predicted to decrease the exposure to **grazoprevir**. Avoid. Severe Study
- **Roxadustat** is predicted to increase the exposure to **grazoprevir**. Avoid. Severe Theoretical
- **Sotorasib** is predicted to markedly decrease the exposure to **grazoprevir**. Avoid. Severe Study
- **St John's wort** is predicted to markedly decrease the exposure to **grazoprevir**. Avoid. Severe Study
- **Grazoprevir** moderately increases the exposure to statins **(atorvastatin)**. Adjust **atorvastatin** dose, p. 154. Moderate Study
- **Grazoprevir** with elbasvir is predicted to increase the exposure to statins **(fluvastatin)**. Adjust **fluvastatin** dose, p. 155. Moderate Theoretical
- **Grazoprevir** with elbasvir moderately increases the exposure to statins **(rosuvastatin)**. Adjust **rosuvastatin** dose, p. 155. Moderate Study
- **Grazoprevir** with elbasvir is predicted to increase the exposure to statins **(simvastatin)**. Adjust **simvastatin** dose, p. 156. Moderate Theoretical
- **Grazoprevir** is predicted to increase the concentration of **sunitinib**. Use with caution and adjust dose. Moderate Theoretical
- **Grazoprevir** increases the exposure to **tacrolimus**. Moderate Study
- **Teriflunomide** is predicted to increase the exposure to **grazoprevir**. Avoid. Severe Theoretical
- **Tucatinib** is predicted to moderately to markedly increase the exposure to **grazoprevir**. Avoid. Severe Study
- **Velpatasvir** is predicted to increase the exposure to **grazoprevir**. Avoid. Severe Theoretical
- **Vemurafenib** is predicted to increase the exposure to **grazoprevir**. Avoid. Severe Theoretical
- **Voxilaprevir** increases the exposure to **grazoprevir**. Avoid. Severe Theoretical

Griseofulvin

ROUTE-SPECIFIC INFORMATION Interactions do not generally apply to topical use unless specified.

- **Alcohol** potentially causes a disulfiram-like reaction when given with **griseofulvin**. Moderate Anecdotal
- Antiepileptics **(phenobarbital, primidone)** decrease the effects of **griseofulvin**. Moderate Study
- **Griseofulvin** potentially decreases the anticoagulant effect of **coumarins**. Moderate Anecdotal

Guanfacine → see TABLE 6 p. 1054 (hypotension), TABLE 9 p. 1056 (CNS effects)
- Anti-androgens **(apalutamide, enzalutamide)** are predicted to decrease the concentration of **guanfacine**. Adjust **guanfacine** dose, p. 281. Moderate Study
- Antiarrhythmics **(dronedarone)** are predicted to increase the concentration of **guanfacine**. Adjust **guanfacine** dose, p. 281. Moderate Theoretical
- Antiepileptics **(carbamazepine, fosphenytoin, phenobarbital, phenytoin, primidone)** are predicted to decrease the concentration of **guanfacine**. Adjust **guanfacine** dose, p. 281. Moderate Study → Also see TABLE 9 p. 1056
- Antiepileptics **(oxcarbazepine)** are predicted to decrease the concentration of **guanfacine**. Monitor and adjust **guanfacine** dose, p. 281. Moderate Theoretical
- **Guanfacine** increases the concentration of antiepileptics **(valproate)**. Monitor and adjust dose. Moderate Study
- Antifungals, azoles **(fluconazole, isavuconazole)** are predicted to increase the concentration of **guanfacine**. Adjust **guanfacine** dose, p. 281. Moderate Theoretical
- Antifungals, azoles **(itraconazole, ketoconazole, posaconazole, voriconazole)** are predicted to increase the exposure to **guanfacine**. Adjust **guanfacine** dose, p. 281. Moderate Study
- **Berotralstat** is predicted to increase the concentration of **guanfacine**. Adjust **guanfacine** dose, p. 281. Moderate Theoretical
- Calcium-channel blockers **(diltiazem, verapamil)** are predicted to increase the concentration of **guanfacine**. Adjust **guanfacine** dose, p. 281. Moderate Theoretical → Also see TABLE 6 p. 1054
- **Cenobamate** is predicted to decrease the concentration of **guanfacine**. Adjust dose. Moderate Theoretical → Also see TABLE 9 p. 1056
- **Ceritinib** is predicted to increase the exposure to **guanfacine**. Adjust **guanfacine** dose, p. 281. Moderate Study
- **Chloramphenicol** is predicted to increase the exposure to **guanfacine**. Adjust **guanfacine** dose, p. 281. Moderate Theoretical
- **Cobicistat** is predicted to increase the exposure to **guanfacine**. Adjust **guanfacine** dose, p. 281. Moderate Study
- **Crizotinib** is predicted to increase the concentration of **guanfacine**. Adjust **guanfacine** dose, p. 281. Moderate Theoretical
- **Dabrafenib** is predicted to decrease the concentration of **guanfacine**. Adjust dose. Moderate Theoretical
- **Encorafenib** is predicted to decrease the concentration of **guanfacine**. Adjust **guanfacine** dose, p. 281. Moderate Study
- Endothelin receptor antagonists **(bosentan)** are predicted to decrease the concentration of **guanfacine**. Adjust dose. Moderate Theoretical
- **Fedratinib** is predicted to increase the concentration of **guanfacine**. Adjust **guanfacine** dose, p. 281. Moderate Theoretical
- **Grapefruit** juice is predicted to increase the exposure to **guanfacine**. Avoid. Moderate Theoretical

- **HIV-protease inhibitors** are predicted to increase the exposure to **guanfacine**. Adjust **guanfacine** dose, p. 281. Moderate Study
- **Idelalisib** is predicted to increase the exposure to **guanfacine**. Adjust **guanfacine** dose, p. 281. Moderate Study
- **Imatinib** is predicted to increase the concentration of **guanfacine**. Adjust **guanfacine** dose, p. 281. Moderate Theoretical
- **Ivosidenib** is predicted to decrease the concentration of **guanfacine**. Adjust **guanfacine** dose, p. 281. Moderate Study
- **Letermovir** is predicted to increase the concentration of **guanfacine**. Adjust **guanfacine** dose, p. 281. Moderate Theoretical
- **Lorlatinib** is predicted to decrease the concentration of **guanfacine**. Adjust dose. Moderate Theoretical
- **Lumacaftor** is predicted to decrease the concentration of **guanfacine**. Adjust **guanfacine** dose, p. 281. Moderate Study
- Macrolides **(clarithromycin)** are predicted to increase the exposure to **guanfacine**. Adjust **guanfacine** dose, p. 281. Moderate Study
- Macrolides **(erythromycin)** are predicted to increase the concentration of **guanfacine**. Adjust **guanfacine** dose, p. 281. Moderate Theoretical
- **Guanfacine** is predicted to increase the concentration of **metformin**. Moderate Theoretical
- **Mitotane** is predicted to decrease the concentration of **guanfacine**. Adjust **guanfacine** dose, p. 281. Moderate Study
- Neurokinin-1 receptor antagonists **(aprepitant, netupitant)** are predicted to increase the concentration of **guanfacine**. Adjust **guanfacine** dose, p. 281. Moderate Theoretical
- Neurokinin-1 receptor antagonists **(fosaprepitant)** are predicted to increase the concentration of **guanfacine**. Moderate Theoretical
- **Nilotinib** is predicted to increase the concentration of **guanfacine**. Adjust **guanfacine** dose, p. 281. Moderate Theoretical
- NNRTIs **(efavirenz, etravirine, nevirapine)** are predicted to decrease the concentration of **guanfacine**. Adjust dose. Moderate Theoretical
- Quinolones **(ciprofloxacin)** are predicted to increase the concentration of **guanfacine**. Adjust **guanfacine** dose, p. 281. Moderate Theoretical
- Rifamycins **(rifampicin)** are predicted to decrease the concentration of **guanfacine**. Adjust **guanfacine** dose, p. 281. Moderate Study
- **Sotorasib** is predicted to decrease the concentration of **guanfacine**. Adjust dose. Moderate Theoretical
- **St John's wort** is predicted to decrease the concentration of **guanfacine**. Adjust dose. Moderate Theoretical
- **Tucatinib** is predicted to increase the exposure to **guanfacine**. Adjust **guanfacine** dose, p. 281. Moderate Study

Guselkumab → see monoclonal antibodies

H_2 receptor antagonists

cimetidine · famotidine · nizatidine

- **Cimetidine** decreases the clearance of **albendazole**. Moderate Study
- **Cimetidine** increases the concentration of **aminophylline**. Adjust dose. Severe Study
- **Cimetidine** slightly increases the exposure to anthracyclines **(epirubicin)**. Avoid. Moderate Study
- **Cimetidine** increases the exposure to antiarrhythmics **(amiodarone)**. Moderate Study
- **Cimetidine** slightly increases the exposure to antiarrhythmics **(flecainide)**. Monitor and adjust dose. Mild Study
- **Cimetidine** increases the exposure to antiarrhythmics **(lidocaine)**. Monitor and adjust dose. Moderate Study
- **Cimetidine** is predicted to increase the exposure to antiarrhythmics **(propafenone)**. Monitor and adjust dose. Moderate Theoretical
- **Cimetidine** transiently increases the concentration of antiepileptics **(carbamazepine)**. Monitor concentration and adjust dose. Moderate Study
- **Cimetidine** increases the concentration of antiepileptics **(fosphenytoin, phenytoin)**. Monitor concentration and adjust dose. Severe Study
- **H_2 receptor antagonists** are predicted to decrease the absorption of antifungals, azoles **(itraconazole)**. Administer **itraconazole** capsules with an acidic beverage. Moderate Study
- **H_2 receptor antagonists** are predicted to decrease the absorption of antifungals, azoles **(ketoconazole)**. Administer **ketoconazole** with an acidic beverage. Moderate Study
- **H_2 receptor antagonists** are predicted to decrease the exposure to antifungals, azoles **(posaconazole)**. Avoid use of posaconazole oral suspension. Moderate Study
- **Cimetidine** decreases the clearance of antimalarials **(chloroquine)**. Moderate Study
- **Cimetidine** slightly increases the exposure to antimalarials **(quinine)**. Moderate Study
- **H_2 receptor antagonists** are predicted to decrease the exposure to **belumosudil**. Separate administration by 12 hours. Moderate Theoretical
- **H_2 receptor antagonists** are predicted to decrease the absorption of **bosutinib**. Moderate Theoretical
- **Cimetidine** slightly increases the exposure to calcium-channel blockers **(diltiazem, nimodipine)**. Monitor and adjust dose. Moderate Study
- **Cimetidine** (high-dose) is predicted to increase the exposure to calcium-channel blockers **(lercanidipine)**. Moderate Theoretical
- **Cimetidine** moderately increases the exposure to calcium-channel blockers **(nifedipine)**. Monitor and adjust dose. Severe Study
- **Cimetidine** increases the exposure to calcium-channel blockers **(verapamil)**. Moderate Study
- **Cimetidine** is predicted to slightly increase the exposure to **capecitabine**. Severe Theoretical
- **H_2 receptor antagonists** are predicted to decrease the absorption of **ceritinib**. Moderate Theoretical
- **Cimetidine** increases the concentration of **ciclosporin**. Mild Study
- **Cimetidine** increases the anticoagulant effect of **coumarins**. Severe Study
- **H_2 receptor antagonists** are predicted to decrease the concentration of **dacomitinib**. **Dacomitinib** should be taken 2 hours before or 10 hours after **H_2 receptor antagonists**. Unknown Theoretical
- **Cimetidine** increases the exposure to **darifenacin**. Mild Study
- **H_2 receptor antagonists** are predicted to decrease the exposure to **dasatinib**. Avoid. Moderate Study
- **H_2 receptor antagonists** are predicted to decrease the absorption of **dipyridamole** (immediate release tablets). Moderate Theoretical
- **Cimetidine** is predicted to increase the exposure to dopamine receptor agonists **(pramipexole)**. Adjust dose. Moderate Study
- **H_2 receptor antagonists** are predicted to decrease the exposure to **erlotinib**. Manufacturer advises take 2 hours before or 10 hours after **H_2 receptor antagonists**. Moderate Study
- **Cimetidine** increases the concentration of **fampridine**. Avoid. Severe Theoretical
- **Cimetidine** slightly increases the exposure to **fluorouracil**. Severe Study
- **H_2 receptor antagonists** are predicted to slightly to moderately decrease the exposure to **gefitinib**. Moderate Study
- **H_2 receptor antagonists** decrease the exposure to HIV-protease inhibitors **(atazanavir)**. Monitor and adjust dose. Moderate Study
- **Cimetidine** is predicted to decrease the clearance of **hydroxychloroquine**. Moderate Theoretical
- **Ivosidenib** is predicted to increase the exposure to H_2 receptor antagonists **(cimetidine, famotidine)**. Use with caution or avoid. Moderate Theoretical
- **H_2 receptor antagonists** are predicted to decrease the absorption of **lapatinib**. Avoid. Moderate Theoretical
- **H_2 receptor antagonists** are predicted to decrease the exposure to **ledipasvir**. Adjust dose, see ledipasvir with sofosbuvir p. 495. Moderate Study
- **Leflunomide** is predicted to increase the exposure to **famotidine**. Moderate Study
- **Cimetidine** is predicted to increase the exposure to **lomitapide**. Separate administration by 12 hours. Mild Theoretical
- **Cimetidine** slightly increases the exposure to macrolides **(erythromycin)**. Moderate Study
- **Cimetidine** is predicted to increase the exposure to **mavacamten**. Monitor and adjust dose—consult product literature. Moderate Theoretical

H_2 receptor antagonists (continued)

- **Cimetidine** increases the concentration of **mebendazole**. [Moderate] Study
- **Cimetidine** is predicted to increase the exposure to **metformin**. Use with caution and adjust dose. [Moderate] Study
- **Cimetidine** slightly increases the exposure to **mirtazapine**. Use with caution and adjust dose. [Moderate] Theoretical
- **Cimetidine** increases the exposure to **moclobemide**. Adjust **moclobemide** dose. [Mild] Study
- **H_2 receptor antagonists** are predicted to decrease the exposure to **neratinib**. Manufacturer advises take 2 hours before or 10 hours after **H_2 receptor antagonists**. [Severe] Study
- **H_2 receptor antagonists** might affect the absorption of **nilotinib**. **H_2 receptor antagonists** should be taken 10 hours before or 2 hours after **nilotinib**. [Mild] Theoretical
- **Nitisinone** is predicted to increase the exposure to **famotidine**. [Moderate] Study
- **H_2 receptor antagonists** are predicted to decrease the exposure to NNRTIs **(rilpivirine)**. **H_2 receptor antagonists** should be taken 12 hours before or 4 hours after **rilpivirine**. [Severe] Study
- **Cimetidine** increases the concentration of opioids **(alfentanil)**. Use with caution and adjust dose. [Severe] Study
- **Cimetidine** might increase the exposure to opioids **(fentanyl)**. Monitor and adjust dose. [Moderate] Study
- **H_2 receptor antagonists** are predicted to decrease the exposure to **pazopanib**. Manufacturer advises take 2 hours before or 10 hours after **H_2 receptor antagonists**. [Moderate] Theoretical
- **Cimetidine** increases the exposure to **phenindione**. [Severe] Anecdotal
- **Cimetidine** slightly increases the exposure to phosphodiesterase type-4 inhibitors **(roflumilast)**. [Moderate] Study
- **Cimetidine** moderately increases the exposure to **praziquantel**. [Moderate] Study
- **Cimetidine** is predicted to increase the exposure to **ruxolitinib**. [Moderate] Theoretical
- **H_2 receptor antagonists** are predicted to decrease the exposure to **selpercatinib**. Manufacturer advises take 2 hours before or 10 hours after **H_2 receptor antagonists**. [Moderate] Study
- **Cimetidine** slightly increases the exposure to SNRIs **(venlafaxine)**. [Mild] Study
- **H_2 receptor antagonists** potentially decrease the exposure to **sofosbuvir**. Adjust dose, see ledipasvir with sofosbuvir p. 495, sofosbuvir with velpatasvir p. 496, and sofosbuvir with velpatasvir and voxilaprevir. [Moderate] Study
- **H_2 receptor antagonists** are predicted to decrease the exposure to **sotorasib**. Manufacturer advises give **sotorasib** with an acidic beverage or use an antacid. [Moderate] Study
- **Cimetidine** slightly increases the exposure to SSRIs **(citalopram, escitalopram)**. Adjust dose. [Moderate] Study
- **Cimetidine** slightly increases the exposure to SSRIs **(paroxetine, sertraline)**. [Moderate] Study
- **Cimetidine** is predicted to increase the risk of toxicity when given with **tegafur**. [Severe] Theoretical
- **Teriflunomide** is predicted to increase the exposure to **famotidine**. [Moderate] Study
- **Cimetidine** increases the concentration of **theophylline**. Adjust dose. [Severe] Study
- **Cimetidine** increases the exposure to **tricyclic antidepressants**. [Moderate] Study
- **Cimetidine** slightly increases the exposure to triptans **(zolmitriptan)**. Adjust **zolmitriptan** dose, p. 347. [Mild] Study
- **H_2 receptor antagonists** might decrease the efficacy of **ulipristal** for emergency hormonal contraception. For CoSRH guidance, see Contraceptives, interactions p. 614. [Unknown] Theoretical
- **Vadadustat** is predicted to increase the exposure to **famotidine**. Monitor and adjust dose. [Moderate] Study
- **H_2 receptor antagonists** are predicted to decrease the concentration of **velpatasvir**. Adjust dose, see sofosbuvir with velpatasvir p. 496. [Moderate] Study

Haloperidol → see TABLE 15 p. 1058 (hyponatraemia), TABLE 6 p. 1054 (hypotension), TABLE 7 p. 1055 (QT-interval prolongation), TABLE 8 p. 1055 (antimuscarinics), TABLE 9 p. 1056 (CNS effects)

FOOD AND LIFESTYLE Dose adjustment might be necessary if smoking started or stopped during treatment.

- Anti-androgens **(apalutamide, enzalutamide)** decrease the concentration of **haloperidol**. Adjust dose. [Moderate] Study → Also see TABLE 7 p. 1055
- Antiepileptics **(carbamazepine, fosphenytoin, phenobarbital, phenytoin, primidone)** decrease the concentration of **haloperidol**. Adjust dose. [Moderate] Study → Also see TABLE 15 p. 1058 → Also see TABLE 9 p. 1056
- **Haloperidol** potentially increases the risk of overheating and dehydration when given with antiepileptics **(zonisamide)**. Avoid in children. [Severe] Theoretical
- Antifungals, azoles **(itraconazole)** increase the concentration of **haloperidol**. [Moderate] Study
- Atypical antipsychotics **(clozapine)** can cause constipation, as can **haloperidol**; concurrent use might increase the risk of developing intestinal obstruction. [Severe] Theoretical → Also see TABLE 15 p. 1058 → Also see TABLE 6 p. 1054 → Also see TABLE 8 p. 1055 → Also see TABLE 9 p. 1056
- **Haloperidol** is predicted to decrease the effects of **dopamine receptor agonists**. Avoid. [Moderate] Theoretical → Also see TABLE 6 p. 1054 → Also see TABLE 7 p. 1055 → Also see TABLE 8 p. 1055 → Also see TABLE 9 p. 1056
- **Encorafenib** decreases the concentration of **haloperidol**. Adjust dose. [Moderate] Study → Also see TABLE 7 p. 1055
- **Haloperidol** opposes the effects of the active metabolite of **foslevodopa**. [Severe] Theoretical → Also see TABLE 6 p. 1054 → Also see TABLE 9 p. 1056
- **Haloperidol** potentially opposes the effects of **glycerol phenylbutyrate**. [Moderate] Theoretical
- HIV-protease inhibitors **(ritonavir)** are predicted to increase the exposure to **haloperidol**. [Severe] Theoretical
- **Ivosidenib** decreases the concentration of **haloperidol**. Adjust dose. [Moderate] Study → Also see TABLE 7 p. 1055
- **Haloperidol** decreases the effects of **levodopa**. [Severe] Study → Also see TABLE 6 p. 1054 → Also see TABLE 9 p. 1056
- **Lumacaftor** decreases the concentration of **haloperidol**. Adjust dose. [Moderate] Study
- **Mitotane** decreases the concentration of **haloperidol**. Adjust dose. [Moderate] Study
- **Nirmatrelvir** boosted with ritonavir is predicted to increase the concentration of **haloperidol**. [Severe] Theoretical
- Rifamycins **(rifampicin)** decrease the concentration of **haloperidol**. Adjust dose. [Moderate] Study
- SNRIs **(venlafaxine)** slightly increase the exposure to **haloperidol**. [Severe] Study → Also see TABLE 15 p. 1058 → Also see TABLE 9 p. 1056
- **Haloperidol** potentially decreases the effects of **sodium phenylbutyrate**. [Moderate] Anecdotal
- SSRIs **(fluoxetine)** increase the concentration of **haloperidol**. Adjust dose. [Moderate] Anecdotal → Also see TABLE 15 p. 1058 → Also see TABLE 9 p. 1056
- SSRIs **(fluvoxamine)** increase the concentration of **haloperidol**. Adjust dose. [Moderate] Study → Also see TABLE 15 p. 1058 → Also see TABLE 9 p. 1056
- **Haloperidol** might enhance the antidiuretic and hypertensive effects of **vasopressin**. [Moderate] Theoretical

Heparin → see TABLE 3 p. 1053 (bleeding), TABLE 1 p. 1053 (hepatotoxicity), TABLE 13 p. 1057 (increased serum potassium)

- **Andexanet alfa** has been reported to affect the anticoagulant effect of **heparin**. Avoid. [Severe] Anecdotal
- **Donanemab** can increase the risk of brain haemorrhage when given with **heparin**. Avoid. [Severe] Anecdotal
- **Lecanemab** can increase the risk of brain haemorrhage when given with **heparin**. Avoid. [Severe] Anecdotal
- **Heparin** might increase the risk of gastrointestinal bleeding when given with monoclonal antibodies **(ipilimumab)**. [Severe] Theoretical
- **Oritavancin** might cause a falsely elevated aPTT when given with **heparin**. Avoid and for 120 hours after stopping **oritavancin**. [Severe] Theoretical
- **Heparin** might decrease the antidiuretic effect of **vasopressin**. [Moderate] Theoretical

Hepatitis B immunoglobulin → see immunoglobulins

HIV-protease inhibitors → see TABLE 1 p. 1053 (hepatotoxicity)

atazanavir · darunavir · fosamprenavir · lopinavir · ritonavir

GENERAL INFORMATION Caution on concurrent use of **atazanavir, lopinavir with ritonavir,** or **ritonavir** with drugs that prolong the PR interval.

- **HIV-protease inhibitors** are predicted to increase the exposure to **abemaciclib**. Avoid or adjust dose—consult product literature. Severe Study
- **HIV-protease inhibitors** are predicted to increase the exposure to **acalabrutinib**. Avoid. Severe Study
- HIV-protease inhibitors **(lopinavir, ritonavir)** are predicted to increase the exposure to **afatinib**. Moderate Study
- **Ritonavir** is predicted to decrease the exposure to **agomelatine**. Moderate Theoretical
- **Ritonavir** decreases the exposure to **albendazole**. Moderate Study
- **Ritonavir** is predicted to increase the exposure to **aliskiren**. Moderate Theoretical
- **HIV-protease inhibitors** are predicted to moderately increase the exposure to alpha blockers **(alfuzosin, tamsulosin)**. Use with caution or avoid. Moderate Study
- **HIV-protease inhibitors** are predicted to increase the exposure to alpha blockers **(doxazosin)**. Moderate Study
- **Ritonavir** is predicted to increase the exposure to **amfetamines**. Severe Theoretical
- **Ritonavir** decreases the exposure to **aminophylline**. Adjust dose. Moderate Study
- **Ritonavir** is predicted to decrease the exposure to anaesthetics, local **(ropivacaine)**. Moderate Theoretical
- Oral **antacids** are predicted to decrease the absorption of oral **atazanavir**. Manufacturer advises take 2 hours before or 1 hour after antacids. Severe Theoretical
- Anti-androgens **(enzalutamide)** are predicted to affect the exposure to **ritonavir**. Use with caution or avoid. Moderate Theoretical
- **HIV-protease inhibitors** are predicted to increase the exposure to anti-androgens **(apalutamide)**. Monitor and adjust dose. Mild Study
- **Ritonavir** is predicted to decrease the efficacy of anti-androgens **(cyproterone)** with ethinylestradiol (co-cyprindiol). Use alternative methods during treatment with, and for 28 days after, the enzyme inducing drug is stopped. Severe Study
- HIV-protease inhibitors **(lopinavir, ritonavir)** are predicted to increase the exposure to anti-androgens **(darolutamide)**. Monitor and adjust dose. Moderate Theoretical
- **HIV-protease inhibitors** are predicted to increase the exposure to antiarrhythmics **(amiodarone)**. Avoid. Severe Theoretical → Also see TABLE 1 p. 1053
- **HIV-protease inhibitors** are predicted to increase the exposure to antiarrhythmics **(disopyramide)**. Severe Theoretical
- **HIV-protease inhibitors** very markedly increase the exposure to antiarrhythmics **(dronedarone)**. Avoid. Severe Study
- **Ritonavir** is predicted to increase the exposure to antiarrhythmics **(flecainide)**. Avoid or monitor adverse effects. Severe Theoretical
- **HIV-protease inhibitors** are predicted to increase the exposure to antiarrhythmics **(lidocaine)**. Avoid. Severe Study
- **HIV-protease inhibitors** are predicted to increase the exposure to antiarrhythmics **(propafenone)**. Monitor and adjust dose. Severe Study
- **HIV-protease inhibitors** are predicted to increase the exposure to anticholinesterases, centrally acting **(galantamine)**. Monitor and adjust dose. Moderate Study
- **HIV-protease inhibitors** are predicted to increase the exposure to antiepileptics **(carbamazepine)** and antiepileptics **(carbamazepine)** are predicted to decrease the exposure to **HIV-protease inhibitors**. Monitor and adjust dose. Severe Theoretical
- **HIV-protease inhibitors** are predicted to affect the exposure to antiepileptics **(fosphenytoin, phenytoin)** and antiepileptics **(fosphenytoin, phenytoin)** decrease the concentration of **HIV-protease inhibitors**. Severe Theoretical
- **Ritonavir** decreases the exposure to antiepileptics **(lamotrigine)**. Severe Study
- **HIV-protease inhibitors** are predicted to very slightly increase the exposure to antiepileptics **(perampanel)**. Mild Study
- **HIV-protease inhibitors** are predicted to affect the concentration of antiepileptics **(phenobarbital, primidone)** and antiepileptics **(phenobarbital, primidone)** are predicted to decrease the concentration of **HIV-protease inhibitors**. Severe Theoretical
- **Ritonavir** is predicted to decrease the concentration of antiepileptics **(valproate)**. Severe Anecdotal → Also see TABLE 1 p. 1053
- Antifungals, azoles **(miconazole)** are predicted to increase the concentration of **HIV-protease inhibitors**. Use with caution and adjust dose. Moderate Theoretical
- Antifungals, azoles **(posaconazole)** are predicted to increase the exposure to **HIV-protease inhibitors**. Moderate Study
- **HIV-protease inhibitors** are predicted to increase the exposure to antifungals, azoles **(isavuconazole)**. Avoid or monitor adverse effects. Severe Study
- **HIV-protease inhibitors** are predicted to increase the exposure to antifungals, azoles **(itraconazole)**. Use with caution and adjust dose. Severe Study → Also see TABLE 1 p. 1053
- **HIV-protease inhibitors** are predicted to increase the exposure to antifungals, azoles **(ketoconazole)**. Use with caution and adjust dose. Moderate Study
- **HIV-protease inhibitors** are predicted to affect the exposure to antifungals, azoles **(voriconazole)** and antifungals, azoles **(voriconazole)** potentially affect the exposure to **HIV-protease inhibitors**. Severe Study → Also see TABLE 1 p. 1053
- **Atazanavir** boosted with ritonavir is predicted to increase the exposure to antihistamines, non-sedating **(fexofenadine)**. Moderate Theoretical
- **HIV-protease inhibitors** are predicted to increase the exposure to antihistamines, non-sedating **(mizolastine)**. Avoid. Severe Study
- **HIV-protease inhibitors** are predicted to increase the exposure to antihistamines, non-sedating **(rupatadine)**. Avoid. Moderate Study
- **Ritonavir** slightly decreases the exposure to the active metabolite of antimalarials **(artesunate)**. Avoid. Severe Study
- **HIV-protease inhibitors** decrease the exposure to antimalarials **(atovaquone)**. Avoid if boosted with ritonavir. Moderate Study
- **HIV-protease inhibitors** are predicted to increase the concentration of antimalarials **(piperaquine)**. Severe Study
- **HIV-protease inhibitors** are predicted to decrease the exposure to antimalarials **(proguanil)**. Avoid. Moderate Study
- **HIV-protease inhibitors** are predicted to affect the exposure to antimalarials **(quinine)**. Severe Study
- **HIV-protease inhibitors** are predicted to increase the exposure to **atogepant**. Adjust **atogepant** dose. Moderate Study
- **HIV-protease inhibitors** are predicted to slightly increase the exposure to atypical antipsychotics **(aripiprazole)**. Avoid or adjust dose—consult product literature. Moderate Study
- **HIV-protease inhibitors** are predicted to moderately increase the exposure to atypical antipsychotics **(cariprazine)**. Avoid. Severe Study
- **Ritonavir** is predicted to affect the exposure to atypical antipsychotics **(clozapine)**. Avoid. Severe Theoretical
- **HIV-protease inhibitors** are predicted to increase the exposure to atypical antipsychotics **(lurasidone, quetiapine)**. Avoid. Severe Study
- **Ritonavir** is predicted to decrease the exposure to atypical antipsychotics **(olanzapine)**. Monitor and adjust dose. Moderate Study
- **HIV-protease inhibitors** are predicted to increase the exposure to atypical antipsychotics **(risperidone)**. Adjust dose. Moderate Study
- **HIV-protease inhibitors** are predicted to increase the exposure to **avacopan**. Severe Study
- **HIV-protease inhibitors** are predicted to increase the exposure to **avapritinib**. Avoid. Moderate Study
- **HIV-protease inhibitors** are predicted to increase the exposure to **axitinib**. Avoid or adjust dose. Moderate Study
- **HIV-protease inhibitors** might increase the exposure to **bedaquiline**. Mild Study
- **HIV-protease inhibitors** moderately increase the exposure to benzodiazepines **(alprazolam)**. Avoid. Moderate Study

HIV-protease inhibitors (continued)
- **Ritonavir** is predicted to increase the exposure to benzodiazepines **(diazepam, flurazepam)**. Avoid. Moderate Theoretical
- **HIV-protease inhibitors** are predicted to markedly to very markedly increase the exposure to benzodiazepines **(midazolam)**. Avoid or adjust dose. Severe Study
- HIV-protease inhibitors **(lopinavir, ritonavir)** are predicted to increase the exposure to beta blockers, non-selective **(nadolol)**. Moderate Study
- **Ritonavir** is predicted to increase the exposure to beta blockers, selective **(metoprolol)**. Moderate Study
- **HIV-protease inhibitors** are predicted to increase the exposure to beta$_2$ agonists **(salmeterol)**. Avoid. Severe Study
- **Atazanavir** moderately increases the exposure to **bictegravir**. Avoid. Moderate Study
- **HIV-protease inhibitors** slightly increase the exposure to **bortezomib**. Moderate Study
- **HIV-protease inhibitors** are predicted to increase the exposure to **bosutinib**. Avoid or adjust dose. Severe Study
- **HIV-protease inhibitors** are predicted to increase the exposure to **brigatinib**. Avoid or adjust dose—consult product literature. Severe Study
- **Ritonavir** is predicted to affect the efficacy of **bulevirtide**. Avoid. Severe Theoretical
- **HIV-protease inhibitors** are predicted to decrease the exposure to **bupropion**. Moderate Study
- **HIV-protease inhibitors** are predicted to increase the exposure to **buspirone**. Adjust **buspirone** dose. Severe Study
- **HIV-protease inhibitors** are predicted to increase the exposure to **cabozantinib**. Moderate Study
- **Ritonavir** is predicted to moderately increase the clearance of **caffeine citrate**. Monitor and adjust dose. Moderate Study
- **HIV-protease inhibitors** are predicted to increase the exposure to calcium-channel blockers **(amlodipine, felodipine, lacidipine, nicardipine, nifedipine, nimodipine)**. Monitor and adjust dose. Moderate Study
- **HIV-protease inhibitors** are predicted to increase the exposure to calcium-channel blockers **(diltiazem, verapamil)**. Severe Study
- **HIV-protease inhibitors** are predicted to markedly increase the exposure to calcium-channel blockers **(lercanidipine)**. Avoid. Severe Study
- **HIV-protease inhibitors** are predicted to increase the exposure to **cannabidiol**. Avoid or adjust dose. Mild Study
- **HIV-protease inhibitors** are predicted to increase the exposure to **capivasertib**. Adjust dose. Moderate Study
- HIV-protease inhibitors **(atazanavir, darunavir, lopinavir)** boosted with ritonavir are predicted to increase the exposure to **ceritinib**. Avoid or adjust dose—consult product literature. Severe Study
- HIV-protease inhibitors **(fosamprenavir, ritonavir)** are predicted to increase the exposure to **ceritinib**. Avoid or adjust dose—consult product literature. Severe Study
- **HIV-protease inhibitors** increase the concentration of **ciclosporin**. Severe Study
- **HIV-protease inhibitors** are predicted to moderately increase the exposure to **cilostazol**. Adjust **cilostazol** dose. Moderate Study
- **HIV-protease inhibitors** are predicted to moderately increase the exposure to **cinacalcet**. Adjust dose. Moderate Study
- **Ritonavir** might increase the exposure to **cladribine**. Moderate Theoretical
- **Ritonavir** might decrease the efficacy of **clopidogrel**. Avoid. Moderate Theoretical
- **HIV-protease inhibitors** are predicted to increase the exposure to **cobimetinib**. Avoid or monitor for toxicity. Severe Study
- **HIV-protease inhibitors** are predicted to increase the exposure to **colchicine**. Avoid potent CYP3A4 inhibitors or adjust **colchicine** dose, p. 637. Severe Study
- **Atazanavir** affects the exposure to **combined hormonal contraceptives**. Adjust dose. Severe Study
- **Ritonavir** is predicted to decrease the efficacy of **combined hormonal contraceptives**. For CoSRH guidance, see Contraceptives, interactions p. 614. Severe Study
- **HIV-protease inhibitors** are predicted to increase the exposure to corticosteroids **(beclometasone)** (risk with beclometasone is likely to be lower than with other corticosteroids). Moderate Theoretical
- **HIV-protease inhibitors** are predicted to increase the exposure to corticosteroids **(betamethasone, budesonide, ciclesonide, deflazacort, dexamethasone, fludrocortisone, fluticasone, hydrocortisone, methylprednisolone, mometasone, prednisolone, triamcinolone)**. Avoid or monitor adverse effects. Severe Study
- **HIV-protease inhibitors** are predicted to increase the exposure to corticosteroids **(vamorolone)**. Adjust dose. Severe Study
- **HIV-protease inhibitors** are predicted to affect the anticoagulant effect of **coumarins**. Moderate Study
- **HIV-protease inhibitors** are predicted to increase the exposure to **crizotinib**. Avoid. Moderate Study
- **HIV-protease inhibitors** are predicted to increase the exposure to **dabrafenib**. Use with caution or avoid. Moderate Study
- **HIV-protease inhibitors** are predicted to increase the exposure to **daridorexant**. Avoid. Severe Study
- **HIV-protease inhibitors** are predicted to markedly to very markedly increase the exposure to **darifenacin**. Avoid. Severe Study
- **HIV-protease inhibitors** are predicted to increase the exposure to **dasatinib**. Avoid or adjust dose—consult product literature. Severe Study
- **HIV-protease inhibitors** very slightly increase the exposure to **delamanid**. Severe Study
- **Ritonavir** is predicted to decrease the efficacy of **desogestrel**. For CoSRH guidance, see Contraceptives, interactions p. 614. Severe Theoretical
- **HIV-protease inhibitors** are predicted to increase the exposure to **deutivacaftor**. Adjust dose, see deutivacaftor with tezacaftor and vanzacaftor p. 218. Severe Study
- **HIV-protease inhibitors** are predicted to moderately increase the exposure to **dienogest**. Moderate Study
- **Lopinavir** boosted with ritonavir is predicted to increase the exposure to **digoxin**. Severe Theoretical
- **Ritonavir** increases the concentration of **digoxin**. Adjust dose and monitor concentration. Severe Study
- **HIV-protease inhibitors** are predicted to increase the exposure to dipeptidylpeptidase-4 inhibitors **(saxagliptin)**. Moderate Study
- **Atazanavir** (alone or boosted with ritonavir) slightly increases the exposure to **dolutegravir**. Adjust dose—consult product literature. Moderate Study
- **Fosamprenavir** boosted with ritonavir slightly decreases the exposure to **dolutegravir**. Avoid if resistant to HIV-integrase inhibitors. Severe Study
- **HIV-protease inhibitors** are predicted to increase the exposure to **domperidone**. Avoid. Severe Study
- **HIV-protease inhibitors** increase the exposure to dopamine receptor agonists **(bromocriptine)**. Severe Study
- **HIV-protease inhibitors** are predicted to increase the concentration of dopamine receptor agonists **(cabergoline)**. Moderate Anecdotal
- **HIV-protease inhibitors** are predicted to increase the exposure to **dronabinol**. Adjust dose. Mild Study
- HIV-protease inhibitors **(atazanavir, darunavir, fosamprenavir, lopinavir)** are predicted to increase the exposure to **drospirenone**. Severe Study
- **Ritonavir** is predicted to decrease the efficacy of **drospirenone**. For CoSRH guidance, see Contraceptives, interactions p. 614. Severe Theoretical
- **HIV-protease inhibitors** are predicted to increase the exposure to **dutasteride**. Monitor adverse effects and adjust dose. Moderate Theoretical
- **HIV-protease inhibitors** are predicted to increase the exposure to **elacestrant**. Avoid potent CYP3A4 inhibitors or adjust **elacestrant** dose. Severe Study
- **HIV-protease inhibitors** are predicted to increase the exposure to **elexacaftor**. Adjust ivacaftor with tezacaftor and elexacaftor p. 220 dose with potent CYP3A4 inhibitors. Severe Study

- **HIV-protease inhibitors** are predicted to increase the exposure to **eliglustat**. Avoid or adjust dose—consult product literature. [Severe] Study
- HIV-protease inhibitors **(atazanavir, lopinavir)** boosted with ritonavir increase the concentration of **elvitegravir**. Refer to specialist literature. [Moderate] Study
- **HIV-protease inhibitors** are predicted to increase the exposure to **encorafenib**. Avoid or monitor. [Severe] Study
- **HIV-protease inhibitors** are predicted to increase the exposure to endothelin receptor antagonists **(bosentan)**. [Severe] Study
- **HIV-protease inhibitors** are predicted to increase the exposure to endothelin receptor antagonists **(macitentan)**. [Moderate] Study
- **HIV-protease inhibitors** are predicted to increase the exposure to the cytotoxic component of **enfortumab vedotin**. [Severe] Theoretical
- **HIV-protease inhibitors** are predicted to increase the exposure to **entrectinib**. Avoid or adjust dose with potent CYP3A4 inhibitors—consult product literature. [Severe] Study
- **HIV-protease inhibitors** are predicted to increase the exposure to **erdafitinib**. Adjust dose. [Severe] Study
- **HIV-protease inhibitors** are predicted to increase the risk of ergotism when given with **ergometrine**. Avoid. [Severe] Theoretical
- **HIV-protease inhibitors** are predicted to increase the exposure to **erlotinib**. Use with caution and adjust dose. [Severe] Study
- **HIV-protease inhibitors** are predicted to increase the exposure to **esketamine**. Adjust dose. [Moderate] Study
- **Ritonavir** is predicted to decrease the efficacy of **estradiol**. [Moderate] Theoretical
- **HIV-protease inhibitors** are predicted to increase the exposure to **eszopiclone**. Adjust **eszopiclone** dose; avoid in the elderly. [Moderate] Study
- **HIV-protease inhibitors** are predicted to increase the concentration of subdermal **etonogestrel**. [Moderate] Theoretical
- **Ritonavir** is predicted to decrease the efficacy of **etonogestrel**. For CoSRH guidance, see Contraceptives, interactions p. 614. [Severe] Theoretical
- **HIV-protease inhibitors** are predicted to increase the exposure to **etrasimod**. Avoid in poor CYP2C9 metabolisers. [Severe] Theoretical
- **HIV-protease inhibitors** are predicted to increase the exposure to **everolimus**. Avoid. [Severe] Study
- **Darunavir** boosted with ritonavir or cobicistat increases the exposure to factor XA inhibitors **(apixaban)**. Avoid. [Severe] Anecdotal
- **Fosamprenavir** boosted with ritonavir is predicted to increase the exposure to factor XA inhibitors **(apixaban)**. [Severe] Theoretical
- **Lopinavir** boosted with ritonavir increases the exposure to factor XA inhibitors **(apixaban)**. Avoid. [Severe] Anecdotal
- **Ritonavir** is predicted to increase the exposure to factor XA inhibitors **(apixaban)**. Avoid. [Severe] Theoretical
- **Atazanavir** boosted with ritonavir is predicted to increase the exposure to factor XA inhibitors **(apixaban, rivaroxaban)**. Avoid. [Severe] Theoretical
- **Darunavir** boosted with ritonavir increases the concentration of factor XA inhibitors **(edoxaban)**. Monitor and adjust dose. [Severe] Anecdotal
- **Lopinavir** boosted with ritonavir increases the exposure to factor XA inhibitors **(edoxaban)**. Monitor and adjust dose. [Severe] Study
- **Ritonavir** is predicted to increase the exposure to factor XA inhibitors **(edoxaban)**. Monitor and adjust dose. [Severe] Theoretical
- **Darunavir** boosted with ritonavir is predicted to increase the exposure to factor XA inhibitors **(rivaroxaban)**. Avoid. [Severe] Anecdotal
- **Fosamprenavir** boosted with ritonavir is predicted to increase the exposure to factor XA inhibitors **(rivaroxaban)**. Manufacturer advises caution in renal impairment. [Severe] Theoretical
- **Lopinavir** boosted with ritonavir increases the exposure to factor XA inhibitors **(rivaroxaban)**. Avoid. [Severe] Study
- **Ritonavir** moderately increases the exposure to factor XA inhibitors **(rivaroxaban)**. Avoid. [Severe] Study
- **HIV-protease inhibitors** are predicted to increase the exposure to **fedratinib**. Adjust dose, but avoid depending on other drugs taken—consult product literature. [Moderate] Study
- **HIV-protease inhibitors** are predicted to moderately increase the exposure to **fesoterodine**. Adjust **fesoterodine** dose with potent CYP3A4 inhibitors; avoid in hepatic and renal impairment. [Severe] Study
- HIV-protease inhibitors **(lopinavir, ritonavir)** are predicted to increase the exposure to **fidaxomicin**. Avoid. [Moderate] Study
- **HIV-protease inhibitors** are predicted to increase the exposure to **fostamatinib**. Monitor adverse effects and adjust dose. [Moderate] Study
- **Lopinavir** boosted with ritonavir is predicted to increase the exposure to **futibatinib**. Avoid or adjust dose—consult product literature. [Moderate] Study
- **Ritonavir** is predicted to increase the exposure to **futibatinib**. Avoid or adjust dose—consult product literature. [Moderate] Study
- **HIV-protease inhibitors** are predicted to increase the exposure to **gefitinib**. [Severe] Study
- **HIV-protease inhibitors** are predicted to increase the exposure to **gilteritinib**. [Moderate] Study
- **HIV-protease inhibitors** are predicted to increase the exposure to **glasdegib**. Use with caution or avoid. [Severe] Study
- HIV-protease inhibitors **(atazanavir, darunavir, lopinavir)** boosted with ritonavir increase the exposure to **glecaprevir**. Avoid. [Severe] Study
- **Ritonavir** increases the exposure to **glecaprevir**. Avoid. [Severe] Study
- **HIV-protease inhibitors** are predicted to moderately to markedly increase the exposure to **grazoprevir**. Avoid. [Severe] Study
- **HIV-protease inhibitors** are predicted to increase the exposure to **guanfacine**. Adjust **guanfacine** dose, p. 281. [Moderate] Study
- H_2 **receptor antagonists** decrease the exposure to **atazanavir**. Monitor and adjust dose. [Moderate] Study
- **Ritonavir** is predicted to increase the exposure to **haloperidol**. [Severe] Theoretical
- **Ritonavir** is predicted to decrease the effects of **hormone replacement therapy**. [Moderate] Anecdotal
- **HIV-protease inhibitors** are predicted to increase the exposure to **ibrutinib**. Avoid or adjust dose with potent CYP3A4 inhibitors—consult product literature. [Severe] Study
- HIV-protease inhibitors **(atazanavir, darunavir, fosamprenavir, lopinavir)** boosted with ritonavir are predicted to increase the exposure to **idelalisib**. [Moderate] Theoretical
- **Ritonavir** is predicted to increase the exposure to **idelalisib**. [Moderate] Theoretical
- **HIV-protease inhibitors** are predicted to increase the exposure to **imatinib**. [Moderate] Study
- **HIV-protease inhibitors** are predicted to increase the exposure to the active metabolite of **irinotecan**. Avoid. [Severe] Study
- **Ritonavir** is predicted to decrease the exposure to iron chelators **(deferasirox)**. Monitor serum ferritin and adjust dose. [Moderate] Theoretical
- **HIV-protease inhibitors** are predicted to increase the exposure to **ivabradine**. Avoid. [Severe] Study
- **HIV-protease inhibitors** are predicted to increase the exposure to **ivacaftor**. Adjust dose with potent CYP3A4 inhibitors, see ivacaftor p. 219, lumacaftor with ivacaftor p. 222, tezacaftor with ivacaftor p. 223, and ivacaftor with tezacaftor and elexacaftor p. 220. [Severe] Study
- **HIV-protease inhibitors** are predicted to increase the exposure to **ivosidenib**. Monitor and adjust dose—consult product literature. [Severe] Study
- **HIV-protease inhibitors** are predicted to increase the exposure to **ketamine**. Adjust dose. [Moderate] Theoretical
- **HIV-protease inhibitors** are predicted to increase the exposure to **lapatinib**. Avoid. [Moderate] Study
- **HIV-protease inhibitors** are predicted to moderately increase the exposure to **larotrectinib**. Avoid or adjust dose—consult product literature. [Moderate] Study
- **Atazanavir** moderately increases the exposure to **lenacapavir**. Avoid. [Severe] Study

HIV-protease inhibitors (continued)
- **HIV-protease inhibitors** are predicted to increase the exposure to **leniolisib**. Avoid. [Moderate] Study
- HIV-protease inhibitors **(atazanavir, lopinavir)** boosted with ritonavir are predicted to increase the concentration of **letermovir**. [Moderate] Study
- **Ritonavir** is predicted to decrease the concentration of **letermovir**. [Moderate] Theoretical
- **Ritonavir** is predicted to decrease the efficacy of some contraceptive methods containing **levonorgestrel**. For CoSRH guidance, see Contraceptives, interactions p. 614. [Severe] Theoretical
- **HIV-protease inhibitors** are predicted to markedly increase the exposure to **lomitapide**. Avoid. [Severe] Study → Also see TABLE 1 p. 1053
- **HIV-protease inhibitors** are predicted to increase the exposure to **lorlatinib**. Avoid or adjust dose—consult product literature. [Severe] Study
- **Atazanavir** is predicted to increase the exposure to macrolides **(clarithromycin)**. Adjust dose in renal impairment. [Severe] Study
- **Ritonavir** increases the exposure to macrolides **(clarithromycin)**. Adjust dose in renal impairment. [Severe] Study
- HIV-protease inhibitors **(darunavir, fosamprenavir, lopinavir)** boosted with ritonavir are predicted to increase the exposure to macrolides **(clarithromycin)**. Adjust dose in renal impairment. [Severe] Study
- **HIV-protease inhibitors** are predicted to increase the exposure to macrolides **(erythromycin)**. [Severe] Theoretical
- **Atazanavir** moderately to markedly increases the exposure to **maraviroc**. Refer to specialist literature. [Severe] Study
- **Darunavir** boosted with ritonavir markedly increases the exposure to **maraviroc**. Refer to specialist literature. [Severe] Study
- **Maraviroc** potentially decreases the exposure to **fosamprenavir** and **fosamprenavir** potentially decreases the exposure to **maraviroc**. Avoid. [Severe] Study
- **Lopinavir** boosted with ritonavir moderately increases the exposure to **maraviroc**. Refer to specialist literature. [Severe] Study
- **Ritonavir** markedly increases the exposure to **maraviroc**. Refer to specialist literature. [Severe] Study
- **HIV-protease inhibitors** are predicted to increase the exposure to **mavacamten**. Avoid or monitor—consult product literature. [Severe] Study
- **HIV-protease inhibitors** are predicted to increase the concentration of intramuscular **medroxyprogesterone**. [Moderate] Theoretical
- **Ritonavir** is predicted to decrease the exposure to **melatonin**. [Moderate] Theoretical
- **Ritonavir** is predicted to increase the clearance of **mexiletine**. Monitor and adjust dose. [Moderate] Study
- **HIV-protease inhibitors** are predicted to increase the exposure to **midostaurin**. Avoid or monitor for toxicity. [Severe] Study
- **HIV-protease inhibitors** are predicted to markedly increase the exposure to mineralocorticoid receptor antagonists **(eplerenone)**. Avoid. [Severe] Study
- **HIV-protease inhibitors** are predicted to increase the exposure to mineralocorticoid receptor antagonists **(finerenone)**. Avoid. [Severe] Study
- **HIV-protease inhibitors** are predicted to increase the exposure to **mirabegron**. Adjust **mirabegron** dose in hepatic and renal impairment. [Moderate] Study
- **HIV-protease inhibitors** are predicted to increase the exposure to **mirtazapine**. [Moderate] Study
- **HIV-protease inhibitors** are predicted to increase the exposure to **modafinil**. [Mild] Theoretical
- HIV-protease inhibitors **(atazanavir, lopinavir)** are predicted to increase the exposure to **momelotinib**. [Moderate] Study
- **HIV-protease inhibitors** are predicted to increase the risk of neutropenia when given with monoclonal antibodies **(brentuximab vedotin)**. Monitor and adjust dose. [Severe] Study
- **HIV-protease inhibitors** are predicted to increase the exposure to monoclonal antibodies **(polatuzumab vedotin)**. [Moderate] Theoretical
- **HIV-protease inhibitors** are predicted to increase the exposure to the cytotoxic component of monoclonal antibodies **(trastuzumab emtansine)**. Avoid or monitor. [Severe] Theoretical
- **HIV-protease inhibitors** are predicted to increase the exposure to **naldemedine**. Avoid or monitor. [Moderate] Study
- **HIV-protease inhibitors** are predicted to markedly increase the exposure to **naloxegol**. Avoid. [Severe] Study
- **HIV-protease inhibitors** are predicted to increase the exposure to **neratinib**. Avoid or adjust dose with potent CYP3A4 inhibitors—consult product literature. [Severe] Study → Also see TABLE 1 p. 1053
- **HIV-protease inhibitors** are predicted to markedly increase the exposure to neurokinin-1 receptor antagonists **(aprepitant)**. [Moderate] Study
- **HIV-protease inhibitors** are predicted to increase the exposure to neurokinin-1 receptor antagonists **(fosaprepitant)**. [Moderate] Theoretical
- **HIV-protease inhibitors** are predicted to increase the exposure to neurokinin-1 receptor antagonists **(netupitant)**. [Moderate] Study
- **HIV-protease inhibitors** are predicted to increase the exposure to **nilotinib**. Avoid. [Severe] Study
- HIV-protease inhibitors **(atazanavir, darunavir, fosamprenavir)** boosted with ritonavir are predicted to increase the exposure to **nintedanib**. [Moderate] Theoretical
- HIV-protease inhibitors **(lopinavir, ritonavir)** are predicted to increase the exposure to **nintedanib**. [Moderate] Study
- **Nirmatrelvir** boosted with ritonavir is predicted to increase the concentration of HIV-protease inhibitors **(atazanavir, darunavir, fosamprenavir, lopinavir)**. [Moderate] Theoretical
- **HIV-protease inhibitors** are predicted to increase the exposure to **nitisinone**. Adjust dose. [Moderate] Theoretical
- NNRTIs **(efavirenz)** decrease the exposure to **HIV-protease inhibitors**. Refer to specialist literature. [Severe] Study
- NNRTIs **(etravirine)** increase the exposure to **fosamprenavir** boosted with ritonavir. Refer to specialist literature. [Moderate] Study
- NNRTIs **(nevirapine)** decrease the exposure to **HIV-protease inhibitors**. Refer to specialist literature. [Moderate] Study → Also see TABLE 1 p. 1053
- **Ritonavir** is predicted to decrease the efficacy of some contraceptive methods containing **norethisterone**. For CoSRH guidance, see Contraceptives, interactions p. 614. [Severe] Anecdotal
- **HIV-protease inhibitors** are predicted to increase the exposure to **olaparib**. Avoid or adjust dose with potent CYP3A4 inhibitors—consult product literature. [Moderate] Study
- **HIV-protease inhibitors** are predicted to increase the exposure to **omaveloxolone**. Avoid or adjust **omaveloxolone** dose, p. 755. [Severe] Study
- **HIV-protease inhibitors** are predicted to increase the exposure to opioids **(alfentanil, buprenorphine, fentanyl, oxycodone)**. Monitor and adjust dose. [Severe] Study
- **HIV-protease inhibitors** boosted with ritonavir are predicted to decrease the exposure to opioids **(methadone)**. [Moderate] Study
- **Ritonavir** is predicted to decrease the concentration of opioids **(morphine)**. [Moderate] Theoretical
- **Ritonavir** increases the risk of CNS toxicity when given with opioids **(pethidine)**. Avoid. [Severe] Study
- **HIV-protease inhibitors** are predicted to increase the exposure to opioids **(sufentanil)**. [Moderate] Study
- **HIV-protease inhibitors** are predicted to increase the exposure to **osilodrostat**. [Moderate] Theoretical
- **HIV-protease inhibitors** are predicted to increase the exposure to **ospemifene**. Avoid in poor CYP2C9 metabolisers. [Moderate] Study
- **HIV-protease inhibitors** are predicted to increase the exposure to **oxybutynin**. [Mild] Study
- **HIV-protease inhibitors** are predicted to increase the exposure to **palbociclib**. Avoid or adjust dose—consult product literature. [Severe] Study
- **HIV-protease inhibitors** are predicted to increase the exposure to **panobinostat**. Adjust dose—consult product literature; in hepatic impairment avoid. [Moderate] Study

- **HIV-protease inhibitors** are predicted to increase the exposure to **pazopanib**. Avoid or adjust dose—consult product literature. Moderate Study
- **HIV-protease inhibitors** are predicted to increase the exposure to **pemigatinib**. Avoid or adjust dose—consult product literature. Severe Study
- **HIV-protease inhibitors** are predicted to increase the exposure to phosphodiesterase type-5 inhibitors **(avanafil, vardenafil)**. Avoid. Severe Study
- **HIV-protease inhibitors** are predicted to increase the exposure to phosphodiesterase type-5 inhibitors **(sildenafil)**. Avoid potent CYP3A4 inhibitors or adjust **sildenafil** dose, p. 139. Severe Study
- **HIV-protease inhibitors** are predicted to increase the exposure to phosphodiesterase type-5 inhibitors **(tadalafil)**. Use with caution or avoid. Severe Study
- HIV-protease inhibitors **(atazanavir, lopinavir)** boosted with ritonavir increase the exposure to **pibrentasvir**. Avoid. Severe Study
- **Ritonavir** potentially increases the exposure to **pibrentasvir**. Severe Theoretical
- **HIV-protease inhibitors** are predicted to increase the exposure to **pimozide**. Avoid. Severe Study
- **Ritonavir** is predicted to decrease the exposure to **pirfenidone**. Moderate Theoretical
- **HIV-protease inhibitors** are predicted to slightly increase the exposure to **ponatinib**. Monitor and adjust dose—consult product literature. Moderate Study
- **HIV-protease inhibitors** are predicted to increase the exposure to **pralsetinib**. Avoid or adjust dose with potent CYP3A4 inhibitors—consult product literature. Moderate Study
- **HIV-protease inhibitors** are predicted to moderately increase the exposure to **praziquantel**. Mild Study
- **HIV-protease inhibitors** given with carbimazole are predicted to increase the exposure to **propiverine**. Adjust starting dose. Moderate Theoretical
- **Proton pump inhibitors** decrease the exposure to **atazanavir**. Avoid or adjust dose. Severe Study
- **HIV-protease inhibitors** are predicted to increase the exposure to **quizartinib**. Adjust dose—consult product literature. Severe Study
- **Atazanavir** increases the exposure to **raltegravir** (high-dose). Avoid. Moderate Study
- **Darunavir** increases the risk of rash when given with **raltegravir**. Moderate Study
- **Fosamprenavir** boosted with ritonavir decreases the exposure to **raltegravir** and **raltegravir** decreases the exposure to **fosamprenavir** boosted with ritonavir. Avoid. Severe Study
- **HIV-protease inhibitors** are predicted to increase the exposure to **ranolazine**. Avoid. Severe Study
- **HIV-protease inhibitors** are predicted to increase the exposure to **reboxetine**. Avoid. Moderate Study
- **HIV protease inhibitors** are predicted to increase the exposure to **regorafenib**. Avoid. Moderate Study
- HIV protease inhibitors **(lopinavir, ritonavir)** are predicted to increase the exposure to **relugolix**. Avoid or take relugolix first and separate administration by at least 6 hours. Moderate Study
- **HIV-protease inhibitors** are predicted to increase the exposure to retinoids **(alitretinoin)**. Adjust **alitretinoin** dose. Moderate Theoretical
- **HIV-protease inhibitors** are predicted to increase the exposure to **ribociclib**. Avoid or adjust dose—consult product literature. Moderate Study
- Rifamycins **(rifampicin)** slightly decrease the exposure to **ritonavir**. Severe Study
- Rifamycins **(rifampicin)** are predicted to moderately to markedly decrease the exposure to HIV-protease inhibitors **(atazanavir, darunavir, fosamprenavir, lopinavir)**. Avoid. Severe Study
- **Ritonavir** markedly increases the exposure to rifamycins **(rifabutin)**. Avoid or adjust dose. Severe Study
- HIV-protease inhibitors **(atazanavir, darunavir, fosamprenavir, lopinavir)** boosted with ritonavir increase the exposure to rifamycins **(rifabutin)**. Monitor and adjust dose. Severe Study
- **HIV-protease inhibitors** are predicted to increase the exposure to **rimegepant**. Avoid. Moderate Study
- **Ritonavir** is predicted to increase the exposure to **riociguat**. Adjust dose and monitor blood pressure. Moderate Theoretical
- **HIV-protease inhibitors** are predicted to increase the exposure to **ripretinib**. Moderate Theoretical
- **HIV-protease inhibitors** are predicted to increase the exposure to **ruxolitinib**. Adjust dose depending on indication and monitor adverse effects—consult product literature. Moderate Study
- **HIV-protease inhibitors** are predicted to decrease the exposure to the active component of **sacituzumab govitecan**. Severe Theoretical
- **HIV-protease inhibitors** are predicted to increase the exposure to **selpercatinib**. Adjust dose—consult product literature. Moderate Study
- **HIV-protease inhibitors** are predicted to increase the exposure to **selumetinib**. Avoid or adjust dose—consult product literature. Severe Study
- **HIV-protease inhibitors** are predicted to increase the exposure to **siponimod**. Avoid depending on other drugs taken—consult product literature. Severe Theoretical
- **HIV-protease inhibitors** are predicted to increase the concentration of **sirolimus**. Avoid or monitor and adjust dose. Severe Study
- **Ritonavir** is predicted to decrease the exposure to SNRIs **(duloxetine)**. Moderate Theoretical
- **HIV-protease inhibitors** are predicted to increase the exposure to SNRIs **(venlafaxine)**. Moderate Study
- **Ritonavir** is predicted to decrease the exposure to sodium glucose co-transporter 2 inhibitors **(canagliflozin)**. Adjust **canagliflozin** dose. Moderate Study
- **Sodium zirconium cyclosilicate** is predicted to decrease the exposure to **HIV-protease inhibitors**. Separate administration by at least 2 hours. Moderate Theoretical
- **HIV-protease inhibitors** are predicted to increase the exposure to **solifenacin**. Adjust solifenacin p. 604 or tamsulosin with solifenacin dose; avoid in hepatic and renal impairment. Severe Study
- **HIV-protease inhibitors** are predicted to increase the exposure to **sparsentan**. Avoid. Severe Study
- **HIV-protease inhibitors** are predicted to moderately increase the exposure to SSRIs **(dapoxetine)**. Avoid potent CYP3A4 inhibitors or adjust **dapoxetine** dose. Severe Study
- **HIV-protease inhibitors** are predicted to increase the exposure to SSRIs **(sertraline)**. Avoid. Moderate Theoretical
- **St John's wort** is predicted to decrease the exposure to **HIV-protease inhibitors**. Avoid. Severe Study
- **HIV-protease inhibitors** are predicted to increase the exposure to statins **(atorvastatin)**. Avoid or adjust dose and monitor rhabdomyolysis. Severe Study → Also see TABLE 1 p. 1053
- **HIV-protease inhibitors** might affect the exposure to statins **(pravastatin)**. Moderate Study → Also see TABLE 1 p. 1053
- **Fosamprenavir** is predicted to increase the exposure to statins **(rosuvastatin)**. Use with caution and adjust dose. Severe Study
- HIV-protease inhibitors **(atazanavir, lopinavir)** boosted with ritonavir moderately increase the exposure to statins **(rosuvastatin)**. Avoid or adjust **rosuvastatin** dose, p. 155. Severe Study
- HIV-protease inhibitors **(darunavir, ritonavir)** are predicted to increase the exposure to statins **(rosuvastatin)**. Avoid or adjust dose. Severe Study → Also see TABLE 1 p. 1053
- **HIV-protease inhibitors** are predicted to increase the exposure to statins **(simvastatin)**. Avoid. Severe Study → Also see TABLE 1 p. 1053
- HIV-protease inhibitors **(atazanavir, lopinavir)** boosted with ritonavir are predicted to increase the exposure to sulfonylureas **(glibenclamide)**. Moderate Theoretical
- **HIV-protease inhibitors** are predicted to increase the exposure to **sunitinib**. Avoid or adjust dose—consult product literature. Moderate Study
- **HIV-protease inhibitors** are predicted to increase the concentration of **tacrolimus**. Avoid. If concurrent use is unavoidable—consult product literature. Severe Study
- **Darunavir** is predicted to increase the exposure to **talazoparib**. Avoid or adjust dose—consult product literature. Moderate Theoretical

HIV-protease inhibitors (continued)

- HIV-protease inhibitors **(lopinavir, ritonavir)** are predicted to slightly increase the exposure to **talazoparib**. Avoid or adjust dose—consult product literature. Severe Study
- **HIV-protease inhibitors** are predicted to increase the exposure to taxanes **(cabazitaxel)**. Avoid or adjust dose—consult product literature. Severe Study
- **HIV-protease inhibitors** are predicted to increase the exposure to taxanes **(docetaxel)**. Avoid or adjust dose. Severe Study
- **HIV-protease inhibitors** are predicted to increase the exposure to taxanes **(paclitaxel)**. Moderate Anecdotal
- **HIV-protease inhibitors** are predicted to increase the concentration of **temsirolimus**. Avoid. Severe Theoretical
- HIV-protease inhibitors **(atazanavir, darunavir, lopinavir)** increase the exposure to **tenofovir alafenamide**. Avoid or adjust dose. Moderate Study
- HIV-protease inhibitors **(atazanavir, darunavir, lopinavir)** are predicted to increase the risk of renal impairment when given with **tenofovir disoproxil**. Severe Anecdotal
- **HIV-protease inhibitors** are predicted to increase the exposure to **tezacaftor**. Adjust dose with potent CYP3A4 inhibitors, see tezacaftor with ivacaftor p. 223, ivacaftor with tezacaftor and elexacaftor p. 220, and deutivacaftor with tezacaftor and vanzacaftor p. 218. Severe Study
- **Ritonavir** is predicted to decrease the exposure to **theophylline**. Adjust dose. Moderate Study
- **Fosamprenavir** boosted with ritonavir is predicted to increase the exposure to thrombin inhibitors **(dabigatran)**. Avoid. Severe Theoretical
- **Ritonavir** is predicted to increase the exposure to thrombin inhibitors **(dabigatran)**. Avoid. Severe Study
- HIV-protease inhibitors **(atazanavir, darunavir, lopinavir)** boosted with ritonavir are predicted to increase the exposure to thrombin inhibitors **(dabigatran)**. Avoid. Severe Anecdotal
- **Ritonavir** decreases the concentration of thyroid hormones **(levothyroxine)**. MHRA advises monitor TSH for at least one month after starting or stopping ritonavir. Moderate Anecdotal
- **HIV-protease inhibitors** are predicted to markedly increase the exposure to **ticagrelor**. Avoid. Severe Study
- HIV-protease inhibitors **(lopinavir, ritonavir)** might increase the exposure to **tigecycline**. Mild Anecdotal → Also see TABLE 1 p. 1053
- **HIV-protease inhibitors** are predicted to increase the exposure to the cytotoxic component of **tisotumab vedotin**. Severe Theoretical
- **Ritonavir** moderately decreases the exposure to **tizanidine**. Mild Study
- **HIV-protease inhibitors** are predicted to increase the exposure to **tofacitinib**. Adjust **tofacitinib** dose, p. 803. Moderate Study
- **HIV-protease inhibitors** are predicted to increase the exposure to **tolterodine**. Avoid. Severe Study
- **HIV-protease inhibitors** are predicted to increase the exposure to **tolvaptan**. Manufacturer advises caution or adjust **tolvaptan** dose with potent CYP3A4 inhibitors. Severe Study
- HIV-protease inhibitors **(lopinavir, ritonavir)** are predicted to increase the exposure to **topotecan**. Severe Study
- **HIV-protease inhibitors** are predicted to increase the exposure to **toremifene**. Moderate Theoretical
- **HIV-protease inhibitors** are predicted to increase the exposure to **trabectedin**. Avoid or adjust dose. Severe Theoretical → Also see TABLE 1 p. 1053
- HIV-protease inhibitors **(lopinavir, ritonavir)** are predicted to increase the concentration of **trametinib**. Moderate Theoretical
- **HIV-protease inhibitors** are predicted to moderately increase the exposure to **trazodone**. Avoid or adjust dose. Moderate Study
- **Ritonavir** is predicted to increase the exposure to **tricyclic antidepressants**. Moderate Theoretical
- **HIV-protease inhibitors** increase the exposure to triptans **(almotriptan)**. Mild Study
- **HIV-protease inhibitors** are predicted to markedly increase the exposure to triptans **(eletriptan)**. Avoid. Severe Study
- HIV-protease inhibitors **(atazanavir, darunavir, fosamprenavir, lopinavir)** boosted with ritonavir are predicted to increase the exposure to **ulipristal**. Avoid when used for uterine fibroids. Severe Study
- **Ritonavir** decreases the efficacy of **ulipristal**. Avoid and for 4 weeks after stopping the enzyme inducing drug. For CoSRH guidance, see Contraceptives, interactions p. 614. Severe Anecdotal
- **HIV-protease inhibitors** are predicted to increase the exposure to **upadacitinib**. Manufacturer advises caution or avoid, or adjust **upadacitinib** dose depending on indication, p. 927. Severe Study
- **HIV-protease inhibitors** are predicted to increase the exposure to **vanzacaftor**. Adjust dose, see deutivacaftor with tezacaftor and vanzacaftor p. 218. Severe Study
- **HIV-protease inhibitors** are predicted to increase the exposure to **vemurafenib**. Severe Theoretical
- **HIV-protease inhibitors** are predicted to increase the exposure to **venetoclax**. Avoid or adjust dose—consult product literature. Severe Study
- **HIV-protease inhibitors** are predicted to increase the exposure to **vinca alkaloids**. Severe Theoretical
- **HIV-protease inhibitors** are predicted to increase the exposure to vitamin D substances **(paricalcitol)**. Moderate Study
- **HIV-protease inhibitors** are predicted to increase the exposure to **voclosporin**. Avoid. Severe Study
- **Ritonavir** is predicted to decrease the exposure to **vorasidenib**. Avoid. Severe Theoretical → Also see TABLE 1 p. 1053
- **Atazanavir** boosted with ritonavir increases the concentration of **voxilaprevir**. Avoid. Severe Study
- **Lopinavir** boosted with ritonavir is predicted to increase the concentration of **voxilaprevir**. Avoid. Severe Theoretical
- **HIV-protease inhibitors** are predicted to increase the exposure to **zanubrutinib**. Avoid or adjust dose with potent CYP3A4 inhibitors—consult product literature. Moderate Study
- **HIV-protease inhibitors** are predicted to increase the exposure to **zopiclone**. Adjust dose. Moderate Theoretical

Homatropine → see TABLE 8 p. 1055 (antimuscarinics)

- Atypical antipsychotics **(clozapine)** can cause constipation, as can **homatropine**; concurrent use might increase the risk of developing intestinal obstruction. Severe Theoretical → Also see TABLE 8 p. 1055

Hormone replacement therapy

- Antiepileptics **(carbamazepine, eslicarbazepine, fosphenytoin, oxcarbazepine, perampanel, phenobarbital, phenytoin, primidone, rufinamide, topiramate)** are predicted to decrease the effects of **hormone replacement therapy**. Moderate Anecdotal
- **Hormone replacement therapy** is predicted to alter the exposure to antiepileptics **(lamotrigine)**. Moderate Theoretical
- **Hormone replacement therapy** decreases the clearance of dopamine receptor agonists **(ropinirole)**. Monitor and adjust dose. Moderate Study
- Endothelin receptor antagonists **(bosentan)** are predicted to decrease the effects of **hormone replacement therapy**. Moderate Anecdotal
- **Hormone replacement therapy** might increase ALT concentrations when given with **glecaprevir** with pibrentasvir. Manufacturer advises caution; avoid ethinylestradiol. Severe Theoretical
- HIV-protease inhibitors **(ritonavir)** are predicted to decrease the effects of **hormone replacement therapy**. Moderate Anecdotal
- **Hormone replacement therapy** is predicted to increase the risk of venous thromboembolism when given with **lenalidomide**. Moderate Theoretical
- **Hormone replacement therapy** is predicted to increase the exposure to MAO-B inhibitors **(selegiline)**. Avoid. Moderate Study
- **Modafinil** is predicted to decrease the effects of **hormone replacement therapy**. Moderate Anecdotal
- Neurokinin-1 receptor antagonists **(aprepitant, fosaprepitant)** are predicted to decrease the effects of **hormone replacement therapy**. Moderate Anecdotal
- NNRTIs **(efavirenz, nevirapine)** are predicted to decrease the effects of **hormone replacement therapy**. Moderate Anecdotal
- NSAIDs **(etoricoxib)** increase the exposure to **hormone replacement therapy**. Moderate Study
- **Hormone replacement therapy** potentially opposes the effects of **ospemifene**. Avoid. Severe Theoretical
- **Hormone replacement therapy** might increase ALT

concentrations when given with **pibrentasvir** with glecaprevir. Manufacturer advises caution; avoid ethinylestradiol. [Severe] Theoretical

- **Hormone replacement therapy** is predicted to increase the risk of venous thromboembolism when given with **pomalidomide**. [Severe] Theoretical
- **Hormone replacement therapy** potentially opposes the effects of **raloxifene**. Avoid. [Severe] Theoretical
- **Rifamycins** are predicted to decrease the effects of **hormone replacement therapy**. [Moderate] Anecdotal
- **Hormone replacement therapy** might increase ALT concentrations when given with **sofosbuvir** with velpatasvir and voxilaprevir. Manufacturer advises caution; avoid ethinylestradiol. [Severe] Theoretical
- **St John's wort** is predicted to decrease the efficacy of **hormone replacement therapy**. [Moderate] Theoretical
- **Hormone replacement therapy** is predicted to increase the risk of venous thromboembolism when given with **thalidomide**. [Severe] Theoretical
- Oral **hormone replacement therapy** is predicted to decrease the effects of **thyroid hormones**. [Moderate] Theoretical
- **Hormone replacement therapy** might increase ALT concentrations when given with **velpatasvir** with sofosbuvir and voxilaprevir. Manufacturer advises caution; avoid ethinylestradiol. [Severe] Theoretical
- **Hormone replacement therapy** might increase ALT concentrations when given with **voxilaprevir** with sofosbuvir and velpatasvir. Manufacturer advises caution; avoid ethinylestradiol. [Severe] Theoretical

House-dust mite extracts

GENERAL INFORMATION Desensitising vaccines should be avoided in patients taking beta-blockers (adrenaline might be ineffective in case of a hypersensitivity reaction) or ACE inhibitors (risk of severe anaphylactoid reactions).

Hydralazine → see TABLE 6 p. 1054 (hypotension)

- **Diazoxide** increases the risk of severe hypotension when given with **hydralazine**. [Severe] Study → Also see TABLE 6 p. 1054

Hydrochlorothiazide → see thiazide diuretics

Hydrocortisone → see corticosteroids

Hydroflumethiazide → see thiazide diuretics

Hydromorphone → see opioids

Hydroxycarbamide → see TABLE 12 p. 1057 (myelosuppression)

- **Live vaccines** are predicted to increase the risk of generalised infection (possibly life-threatening) when given with **hydroxycarbamide**. UKHSA advises avoid (refer to Green Book). [Severe] Theoretical

Hydroxychloroquine → see TABLE 16 p. 1058 (ototoxicity), TABLE 7 p. 1055 (QT-interval prolongation)

- **Hydroxychloroquine** is predicted to decrease the effects of **agalsidase alfa**. [Moderate] Theoretical
- **Hydroxychloroquine** is predicted to decrease the exposure to **agalsidase beta**. [Moderate] Theoretical
- Oral **antacids** are predicted to decrease the absorption of oral **hydroxychloroquine**. Separate administration by at least 4 hours. [Moderate] Theoretical
- Oral **calcium compounds (calcium carbonate)** might decrease the absorption of oral **hydroxychloroquine**. [Moderate] Theoretical
- H_2-**receptor antagonists (cimetidine)** are predicted to decrease the clearance of **hydroxychloroquine**. [Moderate] Theoretical
- Oral **kaolin** is predicted to decrease the absorption of oral **hydroxychloroquine**. [Moderate] Theoretical
- **Lanthanum** is predicted to decrease the absorption of **hydroxychloroquine**. Separate administration by at least 2 hours. [Moderate] Theoretical
- **Hydroxychloroquine** is predicted to decrease the exposure to **laronidase**. Avoid simultaneous administration. [Severe] Theoretical
- **Macrolides** might increase the risk of serious cardiovascular adverse effects when given with **hydroxychloroquine**. [Severe] Theoretical → Also see TABLE 7 p. 1055
- Oral **magnesium** trisilicate is predicted to decrease the absorption of oral **hydroxychloroquine**. [Moderate] Theoretical
- **Hydroxychloroquine** is predicted to increase the risk of haematological toxicity when given with **penicillamine**. Avoid. [Severe] Theoretical
- **Hydroxychloroquine** is predicted to decrease efficacy **rabies vaccine**. [Moderate] Theoretical
- **Hydroxychloroquine** might decrease the effects of **remdesivir**. Avoid. [Moderate] Theoretical
- **Tamoxifen** increases the risk of retinopathy when given with **hydroxychloroquine**. RCOphth guidance advises monitor. [Severe] Study

Hydroxyzine → see antihistamines, sedating

Hyoscine → see TABLE 8 p. 1055 (antimuscarinics)

- **Atypical antipsychotics (clozapine)** can cause constipation, as can **hyoscine**; concurrent use might increase the risk of developing intestinal obstruction. [Severe] Theoretical → Also see TABLE 8 p. 1055

Ibandronate → see bisphosphonates

Ibrutinib → see TABLE 3 p. 1053 (bleeding), TABLE 12 p. 1057 (myelosuppression)

FOOD AND LIFESTYLE Avoid food or drink containing bitter (Seville) oranges as they are predicted to increase the exposure to ibrutinib.

- **Anti-androgens (apalutamide, enzalutamide)** are predicted to decrease the exposure to **ibrutinib**. Avoid or monitor. [Severe] Study
- **Antiarrhythmics (amiodarone)** are predicted to increase the exposure to **ibrutinib**. Adjust dose—consult product literature. [Severe] Theoretical
- **Antiarrhythmics (dronedarone)** are predicted to increase the exposure to **ibrutinib**. Adjust dose with moderate CYP3A4 inhibitors—consult product literature. [Severe] Study
- **Antiepileptics (carbamazepine, fosphenytoin, phenobarbital, phenytoin, primidone)** are predicted to decrease the exposure to **ibrutinib**. Avoid or monitor. [Severe] Study
- **Antifungals, azoles (fluconazole, isavuconazole)** are predicted to increase the exposure to **ibrutinib**. Adjust dose with moderate CYP3A4 inhibitors—consult product literature. [Severe] Study
- **Antifungals, azoles (itraconazole, ketoconazole, posaconazole, voriconazole)** are predicted to increase the exposure to **ibrutinib**. Avoid or adjust dose with potent CYP3A4 inhibitors—consult product literature. [Severe] Study
- **Belzutifan** is predicted to decrease the exposure to **ibrutinib**. Avoid or adjust dose. [Severe] Theoretical
- **Berotralstat** is predicted to increase the exposure to **ibrutinib**. Adjust dose with moderate CYP3A4 inhibitors—consult product literature. [Severe] Study
- **Calcium-channel blockers (diltiazem, verapamil)** are predicted to increase the exposure to **ibrutinib**. Adjust dose with moderate CYP3A4 inhibitors—consult product literature. [Severe] Study
- **Cenobamate** is predicted to decrease the exposure to **ibrutinib**. Adjust dose. [Moderate] Theoretical
- **Ceritinib** is predicted to increase the exposure to **ibrutinib**. Avoid or adjust dose with potent CYP3A4 inhibitors—consult product literature. [Severe] Study → Also see TABLE 12 p. 1057
- **Cobicistat** is predicted to increase the exposure to **ibrutinib**. Avoid or adjust dose with potent CYP3A4 inhibitors—consult product literature. [Severe] Study
- **Crizotinib** is predicted to increase the exposure to **ibrutinib**. Adjust dose with moderate CYP3A4 inhibitors—consult product literature. [Severe] Study
- **Dabrafenib** is predicted to decrease the exposure to **ibrutinib**. Avoid or monitor. [Severe] Study
- **Ibrutinib** might increase the exposure to **digoxin**. Separate administration by at least 6 hours. [Moderate] Theoretical
- **Encorafenib** is predicted to decrease the exposure to **ibrutinib**. Avoid or monitor. [Severe] Study
- **Endothelin receptor antagonists (bosentan)** are predicted to decrease the exposure to **ibrutinib**. Avoid or monitor. [Severe] Study
- **Ibrutinib** might increase the exposure to **everolimus**. Separate administration by at least 6 hours. [Moderate] Theoretical
- **Fedratinib** is predicted to increase the exposure to **ibrutinib**. Adjust dose with moderate CYP3A4 inhibitors—consult product literature. [Severe] Study
- **Grapefruit** juice is predicted to increase the exposure to **ibrutinib**. Avoid. [Moderate] Theoretical

Ibrutinib (continued)

- **HIV-protease inhibitors** are predicted to increase the exposure to **ibrutinib**. Avoid or adjust dose with potent CYP3A4 inhibitors—consult product literature. Severe Study
- **Idelalisib** is predicted to increase the exposure to **ibrutinib**. Avoid or adjust dose with potent CYP3A4 inhibitors—consult product literature. Severe Study
- **Imatinib** is predicted to increase the exposure to **ibrutinib**. Adjust dose with moderate CYP3A4 inhibitors—consult product literature. Severe Study → Also see TABLE 3 p. 1053 → Also see TABLE 12 p. 1057
- **Ivosidenib** is predicted to decrease the exposure to **ibrutinib**. Avoid or monitor. Severe Study
- **Letermovir** is predicted to increase the exposure to **ibrutinib**. Adjust dose with moderate CYP3A4 inhibitors—consult product literature. Severe Study
- **Lumacaftor** is predicted to decrease the exposure to **ibrutinib**. Avoid or monitor. Severe Study
- Macrolides **(clarithromycin)** are predicted to increase the exposure to **ibrutinib**. Avoid or adjust dose with potent CYP3A4 inhibitors—consult product literature. Severe Study
- Macrolides **(erythromycin)** are predicted to increase the exposure to **ibrutinib**. Adjust dose with moderate CYP3A4 inhibitors—consult product literature. Severe Study
- **Mitotane** is predicted to decrease the exposure to **ibrutinib**. Avoid or monitor. Severe Study → Also see TABLE 12 p. 1057
- Neurokinin-1 receptor antagonists **(aprepitant, netupitant)** are predicted to increase the exposure to **ibrutinib**. Adjust dose with moderate CYP3A4 inhibitors—consult product literature. Severe Study
- Neurokinin-1 receptor antagonists **(fosaprepitant)** are predicted to slightly increase the exposure to **ibrutinib**. Moderate Theoretical
- **Nilotinib** is predicted to increase the exposure to **ibrutinib**. Adjust dose with moderate CYP3A4 inhibitors—consult product literature. Severe Study → Also see TABLE 12 p. 1057
- **Nirmatrelvir** boosted with ritonavir is predicted to increase the concentration of **ibrutinib**. Avoid or adjust dose—consult product literature. Severe Theoretical
- NNRTIs **(efavirenz, etravirine, nevirapine)** are predicted to decrease the exposure to **ibrutinib**. Avoid or monitor. Severe Study
- Quinolones **(ciprofloxacin)** are predicted to increase the exposure to **ibrutinib**. Adjust dose—consult product literature. Severe Theoretical
- Rifamycins **(rifampicin)** are predicted to decrease the exposure to **ibrutinib**. Avoid or monitor. Severe Study
- **Ibrutinib** might increase the exposure to **sirolimus**. Separate administration by at least 6 hours. Moderate Theoretical
- **St John's wort** is predicted to decrease the exposure to **ibrutinib**. Avoid. Severe Theoretical
- **Ibrutinib** might increase the exposure to **talazoparib**. Separate administration by at least 6 hours. Moderate Theoretical → Also see TABLE 12 p. 1057
- **Ibrutinib** might increase the exposure to taxanes **(paclitaxel)**. Separate administration by at least 6 hours. Moderate Theoretical → Also see TABLE 12 p. 1057
- **Tucatinib** is predicted to increase the exposure to **ibrutinib**. Avoid or adjust dose with potent CYP3A4 inhibitors—consult product literature. Severe Study

Ibuprofen → see NSAIDs

Icatibant

- **ACE inhibitors** are predicted to decrease the efficacy of **icatibant** and **icatibant** is predicted to decrease the efficacy of **ACE inhibitors**. Avoid. Moderate Theoretical

Icosapent → see TABLE 3 p. 1053 (bleeding)

Idarubicin → see anthracyclines

Idelalisib

- **Idelalisib** is predicted to increase the exposure to **abemaciclib**. Avoid or adjust dose—consult product literature. Severe Study
- **Idelalisib** is predicted to increase the exposure to **acalabrutinib**. Avoid. Severe Study
- **Idelalisib** is predicted to moderately increase the exposure to alpha blockers **(alfuzosin, tamsulosin)**. Use with caution or avoid. Moderate Study
- **Idelalisib** is predicted to increase the exposure to alpha blockers **(doxazosin)**. Moderate Study
- Anti-androgens **(apalutamide, enzalutamide)** are predicted to decrease the exposure to **idelalisib**. Avoid. Severe Study
- **Idelalisib** is predicted to increase the exposure to anti-androgens **(apalutamide)**. Monitor and adjust dose. Mild Study
- **Idelalisib** is predicted to increase the exposure to antiarrhythmics **(amiodarone)**. Avoid. Moderate Theoretical
- **Idelalisib** very markedly increases the exposure to antiarrhythmics **(dronedarone)**. Avoid. Severe Study
- **Idelalisib** is predicted to increase the exposure to antiarrhythmics **(propafenone)**. Monitor and adjust dose. Severe Study
- **Idelalisib** is predicted to increase the exposure to anticholinesterases, centrally acting **(galantamine)**. Monitor and adjust dose. Moderate Study
- Antiepileptics **(carbamazepine, fosphenytoin, phenobarbital, phenytoin, primidone)** are predicted to decrease the exposure to **idelalisib**. Avoid. Severe Study
- **Idelalisib** is predicted to very slightly increase the exposure to antiepileptics **(perampanel)**. Mild Study
- Antifungals, azoles **(itraconazole, voriconazole)** are predicted to increase the exposure to **idelalisib**. Moderate Theoretical
- Antifungals, azoles **(ketoconazole)** slightly increase the exposure to **idelalisib**. Moderate Study
- **Idelalisib** is predicted to increase the exposure to antifungals, azoles **(isavuconazole)**. Avoid or monitor adverse effects. Severe Study
- **Idelalisib** is predicted to increase the exposure to antihistamines, non-sedating **(mizolastine)**. Avoid. Severe Study
- **Idelalisib** is predicted to increase the exposure to antihistamines, non-sedating **(rupatadine)**. Avoid. Moderate Study
- **Idelalisib** is predicted to increase the concentration of antimalarials **(piperaquine)**. Severe Study
- **Idelalisib** is predicted to increase the exposure to **atogepant**. Adjust **atogepant** dose. Moderate Study
- **Idelalisib** is predicted to slightly increase the exposure to atypical antipsychotics **(aripiprazole)**. Avoid or adjust dose—consult product literature. Moderate Study
- **Idelalisib** is predicted to moderately increase the exposure to atypical antipsychotics **(cariprazine)**. Avoid. Severe Study
- **Idelalisib** is predicted to increase the exposure to atypical antipsychotics **(lurasidone, quetiapine)**. Avoid. Severe Study
- **Idelalisib** is predicted to increase the exposure to atypical antipsychotics **(risperidone)**. Adjust dose. Moderate Study
- **Idelalisib** is predicted to increase the exposure to **avacopan**. Severe Study
- **Idelalisib** is predicted to increase the exposure to **avapritinib**. Avoid. Moderate Study
- **Idelalisib** is predicted to increase the exposure to **axitinib**. Avoid or adjust dose. Moderate Study
- **Idelalisib** might increase the exposure to **bedaquiline**. Mild Study
- **Idelalisib** moderately increases the exposure to benzodiazepines **(alprazolam)**. Avoid. Moderate Study
- **Idelalisib** is predicted to increase the exposure to benzodiazepines **(diazepam, flurazepam)**. Monitor and adjust dose. Moderate Theoretical
- **Idelalisib** is predicted to markedly to very markedly increase the exposure to benzodiazepines **(midazolam)**. Avoid or adjust dose. Severe Study
- **Idelalisib** is predicted to increase the exposure to beta$_2$ agonists **(salmeterol)**. Avoid. Severe Study
- **Idelalisib** slightly increases the exposure to **bortezomib**. Moderate Study
- **Idelalisib** is predicted to increase the exposure to **bosutinib**. Avoid or adjust dose. Severe Study
- **Idelalisib** is predicted to increase the exposure to **brigatinib**. Avoid or adjust dose—consult product literature. Severe Study
- **Idelalisib** is predicted to increase the exposure to **buspirone**. Adjust **buspirone** dose. Severe Study
- **Idelalisib** is predicted to increase the exposure to **cabozantinib**. Moderate Study
- **Idelalisib** is predicted to increase the exposure to calcium-channel blockers **(amlodipine, felodipine, lacidipine, nicardipine,**

nifedipine, nimodipine). Monitor and adjust dose. Moderate Study
- Idelalisib is predicted to increase the exposure to calcium-channel blockers **(diltiazem, verapamil)**. Severe Study
- **Idelalisib** is predicted to markedly increase the exposure to calcium-channel blockers **(lercanidipine)**. Avoid. Severe Study
- **Idelalisib** is predicted to increase the exposure to **cannabidiol**. Avoid or adjust dose. Mild Study
- **Idelalisib** is predicted to increase the exposure to **capivasertib**. Adjust dose. Moderate Study
- **Cenobamate** is predicted to decrease the exposure to **idelalisib**. Avoid. Moderate Theoretical
- **Idelalisib** is predicted to increase the exposure to **ceritinib**. Avoid or adjust dose—consult product literature. Severe Study
- **Idelalisib** increases the concentration of **ciclosporin**. Severe Study
- **Idelalisib** is predicted to moderately increase the exposure to **cilostazol**. Adjust **cilostazol** dose. Moderate Study
- **Idelalisib** is predicted to moderately increase the exposure to **cinacalcet**. Adjust dose. Moderate Study
- **Cobicistat** is predicted to increase the exposure to **idelalisib**. Moderate Theoretical
- **Idelalisib** is predicted to increase the exposure to **cobimetinib**. Avoid or monitor for toxicity. Severe Study
- **Idelalisib** is predicted to increase the exposure to **colchicine**. Avoid potent CYP3A4 inhibitors or adjust **colchicine** dose, p. 637. Severe Study
- **Idelalisib** is predicted to increase the exposure to corticosteroids **(beclometasone)** (risk with beclometasone is likely to be lower than with other corticosteroids). Moderate Theoretical
- **Idelalisib** is predicted to increase the exposure to corticosteroids **(betamethasone, budesonide, ciclesonide, deflazacort, dexamethasone, fludrocortisone, fluticasone, hydrocortisone, methylprednisolone, mometasone, prednisolone, triamcinolone)**. Avoid or monitor adverse effects. Severe Study
- **Idelalisib** is predicted to increase the exposure to corticosteroids **(vamorolone)**. Adjust dose. Severe Study
- **Idelalisib** is predicted to increase the exposure to **crizotinib**. Avoid. Moderate Study
- **Idelalisib** is predicted to increase the exposure to **dabrafenib**. Use with caution or avoid. Moderate Study
- **Dabrafenib** is predicted to decrease the exposure to **idelalisib**. Avoid. Moderate Theoretical
- **Idelalisib** is predicted to increase the exposure to **daridorexant**. Avoid. Severe Study
- **Idelalisib** is predicted to markedly to very markedly increase the exposure to **darifenacin**. Avoid. Severe Study
- **Idelalisib** is predicted to increase the exposure to **dasatinib**. Avoid or adjust dose—consult product literature. Severe Study
- **Idelalisib** very slightly increases the exposure to **delamanid**. Severe Study
- **Idelalisib** is predicted to increase the exposure to **deutivacaftor**. Adjust dose, see deutivacaftor with tezacaftor and vanzacaftor p. 218. Severe Study
- **Idelalisib** is predicted to moderately increase the exposure to **dienogest**. Moderate Study
- **Idelalisib** is predicted to increase the exposure to dipeptidylpeptidase-4 inhibitors **(saxagliptin)**. Moderate Study
- **Idelalisib** is predicted to increase the exposure to **domperidone**. Avoid. Severe Study
- **Idelalisib** increases the exposure to dopamine receptor agonists **(bromocriptine)**. Severe Study
- **Idelalisib** is predicted to increase the concentration of dopamine receptor agonists **(cabergoline)**. Moderate Anecdotal
- **Idelalisib** is predicted to increase the exposure to **dronabinol**. Adjust dose. Mild Study
- **Idelalisib** is predicted to increase the exposure to **drospirenone**. Severe Study
- **Idelalisib** is predicted to increase the exposure to **dutasteride**. Monitor adverse effects and adjust dose. Moderate Theoretical
- **Idelalisib** is predicted to increase the exposure to **elacestrant**. Avoid potent CYP3A4 inhibitors or adjust **elacestrant** dose. Severe Study
- **Idelalisib** is predicted to increase the exposure to **elexacaftor**. Adjust ivacaftor with tezacaftor and elexacaftor p. 220 dose with potent CYP3A4 inhibitors. Severe Study
- **Idelalisib** is predicted to increase the exposure to **eliglustat**. Avoid or adjust dose—consult product literature. Severe Study
- **Idelalisib** is predicted to increase the exposure to **encorafenib**. Avoid or monitor. Severe Study
- **Encorafenib** is predicted to decrease the exposure to **idelalisib**. Avoid. Severe Study
- Endothelin receptor antagonists **(bosentan)** are predicted to decrease the exposure to **idelalisib**. Avoid. Moderate Theoretical
- **Idelalisib** is predicted to increase the exposure to endothelin receptor antagonists **(macitentan)**. Moderate Study
- **Idelalisib** is predicted to increase the exposure to the cytotoxic component of **enfortumab vedotin**. Severe Theoretical
- **Idelalisib** is predicted to increase the exposure to **entrectinib**. Avoid or adjust dose with potent CYP3A4 inhibitors—consult product literature. Severe Study
- **Idelalisib** is predicted to increase the exposure to **erdafitinib**. Adjust dose. Severe Study
- **Idelalisib** is predicted to increase the risk of ergotism when given with **ergometrine**. Avoid. Severe Theoretical
- **Idelalisib** is predicted to increase the exposure to **erlotinib**. Use with caution and adjust dose. Severe Study
- **Idelalisib** is predicted to increase the exposure to **esketamine**. Adjust dose. Moderate Study
- **Idelalisib** is predicted to increase the exposure to **eszopiclone**. Adjust **eszopiclone** dose; avoid in the elderly. Moderate Study
- **Idelalisib** is predicted to increase the concentration of subdermal **etonogestrel**. Moderate Theoretical
- **Idelalisib** is predicted to increase the exposure to **etrasimod**. Avoid in poor CYP2C9 metabolisers. Severe Theoretical
- **Idelalisib** is predicted to increase the exposure to **everolimus**. Avoid. Severe Study
- **Idelalisib** is predicted to increase the exposure to factor XA inhibitors **(apixaban)**. Moderate Theoretical
- **Idelalisib** might increase the exposure to factor XA inhibitors **(rivaroxaban)**. Manufacturer advises caution in renal impairment. Moderate Theoretical
- **Idelalisib** is predicted to increase the exposure to **fedratinib**. Adjust dose, but avoid depending on other drugs taken—consult product literature. Moderate Study
- **Idelalisib** is predicted to moderately increase the exposure to **fesoterodine**. Adjust **fesoterodine** dose with potent CYP3A4 inhibitors; avoid in hepatic and renal impairment. Severe Study
- **Idelalisib** is predicted to increase the exposure to **fostamatinib**. Monitor adverse effects and adjust dose. Moderate Study
- **Idelalisib** is predicted to increase the exposure to **gefitinib**. Severe Study
- **Idelalisib** is predicted to increase the exposure to **gilteritinib**. Moderate Study
- **Idelalisib** is predicted to increase the exposure to **glasdegib**. Use with caution or avoid. Severe Study
- **Idelalisib** is predicted to moderately to markedly increase the exposure to **grazoprevir**. Avoid. Severe Study
- **Idelalisib** is predicted to increase the exposure to **guanfacine**. Adjust **guanfacine** dose, p. 281. Moderate Study
- HIV-protease inhibitors **(atazanavir, darunavir, fosamprenavir, lopinavir)** boosted with ritonavir are predicted to increase the exposure to **idelalisib**. Moderate Theoretical
- HIV-protease inhibitors **(ritonavir)** are predicted to increase the exposure to **idelalisib**. Moderate Theoretical
- **Idelalisib** is predicted to increase the exposure to **ibrutinib**. Avoid or adjust dose with potent CYP3A4 inhibitors—consult product literature. Severe Study
- **Idelalisib** is predicted to increase the exposure to **imatinib**. Moderate Study
- **Idelalisib** is predicted to increase the exposure to the active metabolite of **irinotecan**. Avoid. Severe Study
- **Idelalisib** is predicted to increase the exposure to **ivabradine**. Avoid. Severe Study
- **Idelalisib** is predicted to increase the exposure to **ivacaftor**. Adjust dose with potent CYP3A4 inhibitors, see ivacaftor p. 219, lumacaftor with ivacaftor p. 222, tezacaftor with

Idelalisib (continued)
ivacaftor p. 223, and ivacaftor with tezacaftor and elexacaftor p. 220. Severe Study
- Idelalisib is predicted to increase the exposure to **ivosidenib**. Monitor and adjust dose—consult product literature. Severe Study
- **Ivosidenib** is predicted to decrease the exposure to **idelalisib**. Avoid. Severe Study
- **Idelalisib** is predicted to increase the exposure to **ketamine**. Adjust dose. Moderate Theoretical
- **Idelalisib** is predicted to increase the exposure to **lapatinib**. Avoid. Moderate Study
- **Idelalisib** is predicted to moderately increase the exposure to **larotrectinib**. Avoid or adjust dose—consult product literature. Moderate Study
- **Idelalisib** is predicted to increase the exposure to **leniolisib**. Avoid. Moderate Study
- **Idelalisib** is predicted to markedly increase the exposure to **lomitapide**. Avoid. Severe Study
- **Idelalisib** is predicted to increase the exposure to **lorlatinib**. Avoid or adjust dose—consult product literature. Severe Study
- **Lorlatinib** is predicted to decrease the exposure to **idelalisib**. Avoid. Moderate Theoretical
- **Lumacaftor** is predicted to decrease the exposure to **idelalisib**. Avoid. Severe Study
- **Macrolides** are predicted to increase the exposure to **idelalisib**. Moderate Theoretical
- **Idelalisib** markedly increases the exposure to **maraviroc**. Adjust dose. Severe Theoretical
- **Maribavir** is predicted to increase the exposure to **idelalisib**. Moderate Theoretical
- **Idelalisib** is predicted to increase the exposure to **mavacamten**. Avoid or monitor—consult product literature. Severe Study
- **Idelalisib** is predicted to increase the concentration of intramuscular **medroxyprogesterone**. Moderate Theoretical
- **Idelalisib** is predicted to increase the exposure to **midostaurin**. Avoid or monitor for toxicity. Severe Study
- **Idelalisib** is predicted to markedly increase the exposure to mineralocorticoid receptor antagonists **(eplerenone)**. Avoid. Severe Study
- **Idelalisib** is predicted to increase the exposure to mineralocorticoid receptor antagonists **(finerenone)**. Avoid. Severe Study
- **Idelalisib** is predicted to increase the exposure to **mirabegron**. Adjust **mirabegron** dose in hepatic and renal impairment. Moderate Study
- **Idelalisib** is predicted to increase the exposure to **mirtazapine**. Moderate Study
- **Mitotane** is predicted to decrease the exposure to **idelalisib**. Avoid. Severe Study
- **Idelalisib** is predicted to increase the exposure to **modafinil**. Mild Theoretical
- **Idelalisib** is predicted to increase the risk of neutropenia when given with monoclonal antibodies **(brentuximab vedotin)**. Monitor and adjust dose. Severe Study
- **Idelalisib** is predicted to increase the exposure to monoclonal antibodies **(polatuzumab vedotin)**. Moderate Theoretical
- **Idelalisib** is predicted to increase the exposure to the cytotoxic component of monoclonal antibodies **(trastuzumab emtansine)**. Avoid or monitor. Severe Theoretical
- **Idelalisib** is predicted to increase the exposure to **naldemedine**. Avoid or monitor. Moderate Study
- **Idelalisib** is predicted to markedly increase the exposure to **naloxegol**. Avoid. Severe Study
- **Idelalisib** is predicted to increase the exposure to **neratinib**. Avoid or adjust dose with potent CYP3A4 inhibitors—consult product literature. Severe Study
- **Idelalisib** is predicted to markedly increase the exposure to neurokinin-1 receptor antagonists **(aprepitant)**. Moderate Study
- **Idelalisib** is predicted to increase the exposure to neurokinin-1 receptor antagonists **(fosaprepitant)**. Moderate Theoretical
- **Idelalisib** is predicted to increase the exposure to neurokinin-1 receptor antagonists **(netupitant)**. Moderate Study
- **Idelalisib** is predicted to increase the exposure to **nilotinib**. Avoid. Severe Study
- **Idelalisib** is predicted to increase the exposure to **nitisinone**. Adjust dose. Moderate Theoretical
- NNRTIs **(efavirenz, etravirine, nevirapine)** are predicted to decrease the exposure to **idelalisib**. Avoid. Moderate Theoretical
- **Idelalisib** is predicted to increase the exposure to **olaparib**. Avoid or adjust dose with potent CYP3A4 inhibitors—consult product literature. Moderate Study
- **Idelalisib** is predicted to increase the exposure to **omaveloxolone**. Avoid or adjust **omaveloxolone** dose, p. 755. Severe Study
- **Idelalisib** is predicted to increase the exposure to opioids **(alfentanil, buprenorphine, fentanyl, oxycodone)**. Monitor and adjust dose. Severe Study
- **Idelalisib** is predicted to increase the exposure to opioids **(methadone)**. Severe Theoretical
- **Idelalisib** is predicted to increase the exposure to opioids **(sufentanil)**. Moderate Study
- **Idelalisib** is predicted to increase the exposure to **osilodrostat**. Moderate Theoretical
- **Idelalisib** is predicted to increase the exposure to **ospemifene**. Avoid in poor CYP2C9 metabolisers. Moderate Study
- **Idelalisib** is predicted to increase the exposure to **oxybutynin**. Mild Study
- **Idelalisib** is predicted to increase the exposure to **palbociclib**. Avoid or adjust dose—consult product literature. Severe Study
- **Idelalisib** is predicted to increase the exposure to **panobinostat**. Adjust dose—consult product literature; in hepatic impairment avoid. Moderate Study
- **Idelalisib** is predicted to increase the exposure to **pazopanib**. Avoid or adjust dose—consult product literature. Moderate Study
- **Idelalisib** is predicted to increase the exposure to **pemigatinib**. Avoid or adjust dose—consult product literature. Severe Study
- **Idelalisib** is predicted to increase the exposure to phosphodiesterase type-5 inhibitors **(avanafil, vardenafil)**. Avoid. Severe Study
- **Idelalisib** is predicted to increase the exposure to phosphodiesterase type-5 inhibitors **(sildenafil)**. Avoid potent CYP3A4 inhibitors or adjust **sildenafil** dose, p. 139. Severe Study
- **Idelalisib** is predicted to increase the exposure to phosphodiesterase type-5 inhibitors **(tadalafil)**. Use with caution or avoid. Severe Study
- **Idelalisib** is predicted to increase the exposure to **pimozide**. Avoid. Severe Study
- **Idelalisib** is predicted to slightly increase the exposure to **ponatinib**. Monitor and adjust dose—consult product literature. Moderate Study
- **Idelalisib** is predicted to increase the exposure to **pralsetinib**. Avoid or adjust dose with potent CYP3A4 inhibitors—consult product literature. Moderate Study
- **Idelalisib** is predicted to moderately increase the exposure to **praziquantel**. Mild Study
- **Idelalisib** given with carbimazole is predicted to increase the exposure to **propiverine**. Adjust starting dose. Moderate Theoretical
- **Idelalisib** is predicted to increase the exposure to **quizartinib**. Adjust dose—consult product literature. Severe Study
- **Idelalisib** is predicted to increase the exposure to **ranolazine**. Avoid. Severe Study
- **Idelalisib** is predicted to increase the exposure to **reboxetine**. Avoid. Moderate Study
- **Idelalisib** is predicted to increase the exposure to **regorafenib**. Avoid. Moderate Study
- **Idelalisib** is predicted to increase the exposure to retinoids **(alitretinoin)**. Adjust **alitretinoin** dose. Moderate Theoretical
- **Idelalisib** is predicted to increase the exposure to **ribociclib**. Avoid or adjust dose—consult product literature. Moderate Study
- Rifamycins **(rifampicin)** are predicted to decrease the exposure to **idelalisib**. Avoid. Severe Study
- **Idelalisib** is predicted to increase the exposure to **rimegepant**. Avoid. Moderate Study
- **Idelalisib** is predicted to increase the exposure to **ripretinib**. Avoid. Moderate Theoretical

A1 Interactions | Appendix 1

- ▸ **Rucaparib** is predicted to increase the exposure to **idelalisib**. Moderate Theoretical
- ▸ **Idelalisib** is predicted to increase the exposure to **ruxolitinib**. Adjust dose depending on indication and monitor adverse effects—consult product literature. Moderate Study
- ▸ **Idelalisib** is predicted to increase the exposure to **selpercatinib**. Adjust dose—consult product literature. Moderate Study
- ▸ **Idelalisib** is predicted to increase the exposure to **selumetinib**. Avoid or adjust dose—consult product literature. Severe Study
- ▸ **Idelalisib** is predicted to increase the exposure to **siponimod**. Avoid depending on other drugs taken—consult product literature. Severe Theoretical
- ▸ **Idelalisib** is predicted to increase the concentration of **sirolimus**. Avoid or monitor and adjust dose. Severe Study
- ▸ **Idelalisib** is predicted to increase the exposure to SNRIs **(venlafaxine)**. Moderate Study
- ▸ **Idelalisib** is predicted to increase the exposure to **solifenacin**. Adjust solifenacin p. 604 or tamsulosin with solifenacin dose; avoid in hepatic and renal impairment. Severe Study
- ▸ **Sotorasib** is predicted to decrease the exposure to **idelalisib**. Avoid. Moderate Theoretical
- ▸ **Idelalisib** is predicted to increase the exposure to **sparsentan**. Avoid. Severe Study
- ▸ **Idelalisib** is predicted to moderately increase the exposure to SSRIs **(dapoxetine)**. Avoid potent CYP3A4 inhibitors or adjust **dapoxetine** dose. Severe Study
- ▸ **Idelalisib** is predicted to increase the exposure to SSRIs **(sertraline)**. Avoid. Moderate Theoretical
- ▸ **St John's wort** is predicted to decrease the exposure to **idelalisib**. Avoid. Moderate Theoretical
- ▸ **Idelalisib** is predicted to increase the exposure to statins **(atorvastatin)**. Avoid or adjust dose and monitor rhabdomyolysis. Severe Study
- ▸ **Idelalisib** is predicted to increase the exposure to statins **(simvastatin)**. Avoid. Severe Study
- ▸ **Idelalisib** is predicted to increase the exposure to **sunitinib**. Avoid or adjust dose—consult product literature. Moderate Study
- ▸ **Idelalisib** is predicted to increase the concentration of **tacrolimus**. Avoid. If concurrent use is unavoidable—consult product literature. Severe Study
- ▸ **Idelalisib** is predicted to increase the exposure to taxanes **(cabazitaxel)**. Avoid or adjust dose—consult product literature. Severe Study
- ▸ **Idelalisib** is predicted to increase the exposure to taxanes **(docetaxel)**. Avoid or adjust dose. Severe Study
- ▸ **Idelalisib** is predicted to increase the exposure to taxanes **(paclitaxel)**. Moderate Anecdotal
- ▸ **Idelalisib** is predicted to increase the concentration of **temsirolimus**. Avoid. Severe Theoretical
- ▸ **Idelalisib** is predicted to increase the exposure to **tezacaftor**. Adjust dose with potent CYP3A4 inhibitors, see tezacaftor with ivacaftor p. 223, ivacaftor with tezacaftor and elexacaftor p. 220, and deutivacaftor with tezacaftor and vanzacaftor p. 218. Severe Study
- ▸ **Idelalisib** is predicted to markedly increase the exposure to **ticagrelor**. Avoid. Severe Study
- ▸ **Idelalisib** is predicted to increase the exposure to the cytotoxic component of **tisotumab vedotin**. Severe Theoretical
- ▸ **Idelalisib** is predicted to increase the exposure to **tofacitinib**. Adjust **tofacitinib** dose, p. 803. Moderate Study
- ▸ **Idelalisib** is predicted to increase the exposure to **tolterodine**. Avoid. Severe Study
- ▸ **Idelalisib** is predicted to increase the exposure to **tolvaptan**. Manufacturer advises caution or adjust **tolvaptan** dose with potent CYP3A4 inhibitors. Severe Study
- ▸ **Idelalisib** is predicted to increase the exposure to **toremifene**. Moderate Theoretical
- ▸ **Idelalisib** is predicted to increase the exposure to **trabectedin**. Avoid or adjust dose. Severe Theoretical
- ▸ **Idelalisib** is predicted to moderately increase the exposure to **trazodone**. Avoid or adjust dose. Moderate Study
- ▸ **Idelalisib** increases the exposure to triptans **(almotriptan)**. Mild Study
- ▸ **Idelalisib** is predicted to markedly increase the exposure to triptans **(eletriptan)**. Avoid. Severe Study
- ▸ **Tucatinib** is predicted to increase the exposure to **idelalisib**. Moderate Theoretical
- ▸ **Idelalisib** is predicted to increase the exposure to **ulipristal**. Avoid when used for uterine fibroids. Severe Study
- ▸ **Idelalisib** is predicted to increase the exposure to **upadacitinib**. Manufacturer advises caution or avoid, or adjust **upadacitinib** dose depending on indication, p. 927. Severe Study
- ▸ **Vandetanib** is predicted to increase the exposure to **idelalisib**. Moderate Theoretical
- ▸ **Idelalisib** is predicted to increase the exposure to **vanzacaftor**. Adjust dose, see deutivacaftor with tezacaftor and vanzacaftor p. 218. Severe Study
- ▸ **Idelalisib** is predicted to increase the exposure to **vemurafenib**. Severe Theoretical
- ▸ **Idelalisib** is predicted to increase the exposure to **venetoclax**. Avoid or adjust dose—consult product literature. Severe Study
- ▸ **Idelalisib** is predicted to increase the exposure to **vinca alkaloids**. Severe Theoretical
- ▸ **Idelalisib** is predicted to increase the exposure to vitamin D substances **(paricalcitol)**. Moderate Study
- ▸ **Idelalisib** is predicted to increase the exposure to **voclosporin**. Avoid. Severe Study
- ▸ **Idelalisib** is predicted to increase the exposure to **zanubrutinib**. Avoid or adjust dose with potent CYP3A4 inhibitors—consult product literature. Moderate Study
- ▸ **Idelalisib** is predicted to increase the exposure to **zolpidem**. Monitor and adjust dose. Moderate Theoretical
- ▸ **Idelalisib** is predicted to increase the exposure to **zopiclone**. Adjust dose. Moderate Theoretical

Ifosfamide → see alkylating agents

Iloprost → see TABLE 3 p. 1053 (bleeding), TABLE 6 p. 1054 (hypotension)

Imatinib → see TABLE 3 p. 1053 (bleeding), TABLE 12 p. 1057 (myelosuppression)

- ▸ **Imatinib** is predicted to increase the exposure to **abemaciclib**. Moderate Study
- ▸ **Imatinib** is predicted to increase the exposure to **acalabrutinib**. Avoid or monitor. Severe Study → Also see TABLE 3 p. 1053
- ▸ **Imatinib** is predicted to increase the exposure to alpha blockers **(tamsulosin)**. Moderate Theoretical
- ▸ Anti-androgens **(apalutamide, enzalutamide)** are predicted to decrease the exposure to **imatinib**. Avoid. Moderate Study
- ▸ **Imatinib** is predicted to increase the exposure to antiarrhythmics **(dronedarone)**. Severe Theoretical
- ▸ **Imatinib** is predicted to increase the exposure to antiarrhythmics **(propafenone)**. Monitor and adjust dose. Moderate Study
- ▸ Antiepileptics **(carbamazepine, fosphenytoin, oxcarbazepine, phenobarbital, phenytoin, primidone)** are predicted to decrease the exposure to **imatinib**. Avoid. Moderate Study
- ▸ Antiepileptics **(eslicarbazepine)** are predicted to decrease the exposure to **imatinib**. Moderate Theoretical
- ▸ Antiepileptics **(topiramate)** are predicted to decrease the exposure to **imatinib**. Moderate Study
- ▸ Antifungals, azoles **(fluconazole)** are predicted to increase the exposure to **imatinib**. Moderate Theoretical
- ▸ Antifungals, azoles **(itraconazole, ketoconazole, posaconazole, voriconazole)** are predicted to increase the exposure to **imatinib**. Moderate Study
- ▸ **Imatinib** is predicted to increase the exposure to antifungals, azoles **(isavuconazole)**. Moderate Theoretical
- ▸ **Imatinib** is predicted to increase the exposure to antihistamines, non-sedating **(mizolastine)**. Severe Theoretical
- ▸ **Imatinib** is predicted to increase the exposure to antihistamines, non-sedating **(rupatadine)**. Avoid. Moderate Study
- ▸ **Imatinib** might increase the exposure to the active metabolite of antimalarials **(artesunate)**. Avoid. Unknown Theoretical
- ▸ **Imatinib** is predicted to increase the concentration of antimalarials **(piperaquine)**. Severe Study
- ▸ **Asparaginase** is predicted to increase the risk of hepatotoxicity when given with **imatinib**. Severe Theoretical → Also see TABLE 3 p. 1053 → Also see TABLE 12 p. 1057

Imatinib (continued)

- **Imatinib** is predicted to increase the exposure to atypical antipsychotics **(cariprazine)**. Monitor and adjust dose. Severe Study
- **Imatinib** is predicted to increase the exposure to atypical antipsychotics **(lurasidone)**. Adjust **lurasidone** dose. Moderate Study
- **Imatinib** is predicted to increase the exposure to atypical antipsychotics **(quetiapine)**. Avoid. Moderate Study
- **Imatinib** is predicted to increase the exposure to **avapritinib**. Avoid or adjust dose—consult product literature. Moderate Study
- **Imatinib** is predicted to increase the exposure to **axitinib**. Moderate Study → Also see **TABLE 3** p. 1053 → Also see **TABLE 12** p. 1057
- **Imatinib** might increase the exposure to **bedaquiline**. Mild Theoretical
- **Imatinib** is predicted to increase the exposure to benzodiazepines **(alprazolam)**. Severe Study
- **Imatinib** is predicted to increase the exposure to benzodiazepines **(midazolam)**. Monitor adverse effects and adjust dose. Severe Study
- **Imatinib** is predicted to increase the exposure to **bosutinib**. Avoid or adjust dose. Severe Study → Also see **TABLE 3** p. 1053 → Also see **TABLE 12** p. 1057
- **Imatinib** is predicted to increase the exposure to **brigatinib**. Moderate Study
- **Imatinib** is predicted to increase the exposure to **buspirone**. Use with caution and adjust dose. Moderate Study
- **Imatinib** is predicted to increase the exposure to **cabozantinib**. Moderate Study → Also see **TABLE 12** p. 1057
- Calcium-channel blockers **(diltiazem, verapamil)** are predicted to increase the exposure to **imatinib**. Moderate Theoretical
- **Imatinib** is predicted to increase the exposure to calcium-channel blockers **(amlodipine, felodipine, lacidipine, lercanidipine, nicardipine, nifedipine, nimodipine)**. Monitor and adjust dose. Moderate Study
- **Imatinib** is predicted to increase the exposure to **capivasertib**. Adjust dose. Moderate Study
- **Cenobamate** is predicted to decrease the exposure to **imatinib**. Moderate Study
- **Ceritinib** is predicted to increase the exposure to **imatinib**. Moderate Study → Also see **TABLE 12** p. 1057
- **Imatinib** is predicted to increase the exposure to **ceritinib**. Moderate Study → Also see **TABLE 12** p. 1057
- **Imatinib** is predicted to increase the concentration of **ciclosporin**. Severe Study
- **Cobicistat** is predicted to increase the exposure to **imatinib**. Moderate Study
- **Imatinib** is predicted to increase the exposure to **cobimetinib**. Severe Study
- **Imatinib** is predicted to increase the exposure to **colchicine**. Adjust **colchicine** dose with moderate CYP3A4 inhibitors, p. 637. Severe Study
- **Imatinib** is predicted to increase the exposure to corticosteroids **(methylprednisolone)**. Monitor and adjust dose. Moderate Study
- **Imatinib** is predicted to increase the risk of bleeding events when given with **coumarins**. Severe Theoretical → Also see **TABLE 3** p. 1053
- **Crisantaspase** is predicted to increase the risk of hepatotoxicity when given with **imatinib**. Severe Theoretical → Also see **TABLE 3** p. 1053 → Also see **TABLE 12** p. 1057
- **Imatinib** is predicted to increase the exposure to **crizotinib**. Moderate Study
- **Imatinib** is predicted to increase the exposure to **dabrafenib**. Moderate Study
- **Dabrafenib** is predicted to decrease the exposure to **imatinib**. Moderate Study
- **Imatinib** is predicted to increase the exposure to **daridorexant**. Adjust **daridorexant** dose. Severe Study
- **Imatinib** is predicted to increase the exposure to **darifenacin**. Moderate Study
- **Imatinib** is predicted to increase the exposure to **dasatinib**. Severe Study → Also see **TABLE 3** p. 1053 → Also see **TABLE 12** p. 1057
- **Imatinib** is predicted to increase the exposure to **deutivacaftor**. Adjust dose, see deutivacaftor with tezacaftor and vanzacaftor p. 218. Severe Study
- **Imatinib** is predicted to slightly increase the exposure to **dienogest**. Moderate Study
- **Imatinib** is predicted to increase the exposure to dipeptidylpeptidase-4 inhibitors **(saxagliptin)**. Mild Study
- **Imatinib** is predicted to increase the exposure to **domperidone**. Avoid. Severe Study
- **Imatinib** is predicted to increase the exposure to dopamine receptor agonists **(bromocriptine)**. Severe Theoretical
- **Imatinib** is predicted to increase the concentration of dopamine receptor agonists **(cabergoline)**. Moderate Anecdotal
- **Imatinib** is predicted to increase the exposure to **drospirenone**. Severe Study
- **Imatinib** is predicted to moderately increase the exposure to **dutasteride**. Mild Study
- **Imatinib** is predicted to increase the exposure to **elacestrant**. Avoid moderate CYP3A4 inhibitors or adjust **elacestrant** dose. Severe Theoretical
- **Imatinib** is predicted to increase the exposure to **elexacaftor**. Adjust ivacaftor with tezacaftor and elexacaftor p. 220 dose with moderate CYP3A4 inhibitors. Severe Theoretical
- **Imatinib** is predicted to increase the exposure to **eliglustat**. Avoid or adjust dose—consult product literature. Severe Study
- **Encorafenib** is predicted to decrease the exposure to **imatinib**. Avoid. Moderate Study
- **Imatinib** is predicted to moderately increase the exposure to **encorafenib**. Moderate Study
- Endothelin receptor antagonists **(bosentan)** are predicted to decrease the exposure to **imatinib**. Moderate Study
- **Imatinib** is predicted to increase the exposure to endothelin receptor antagonists **(macitentan)**. Manufacturer advises caution depending on other drugs taken—consult product literature. Moderate Theoretical
- **Imatinib** is predicted to increase the exposure to **entrectinib**. Avoid or adjust dose with moderate CYP3A4 inhibitors—consult product literature. Severe Theoretical
- **Imatinib** is predicted to increase the risk of ergotism when given with **ergometrine**. Severe Theoretical
- **Imatinib** is predicted to increase the exposure to **erlotinib**. Moderate Study
- **Imatinib** is predicted to increase the exposure to **etrasimod**. Avoid in poor CYP2C9 metabolisers. Severe Theoretical
- **Imatinib** is predicted to increase the concentration of **everolimus**. Avoid or adjust dose. Moderate Study
- **Imatinib** is predicted to increase the exposure to **fedratinib**. Monitor and adjust dose. Moderate Study
- **Imatinib** is predicted to increase the exposure to **fesoterodine**. Adjust **fesoterodine** dose with moderate CYP3A4 inhibitors in hepatic and renal impairment. Mild Study
- **Imatinib** is predicted to increase the exposure to **gefitinib**. Moderate Study
- **Grapefruit** juice is predicted to increase the exposure to **imatinib**. Moderate Theoretical
- **Imatinib** is predicted to increase the concentration of **guanfacine**. Adjust **guanfacine** dose, p. 281. Moderate Theoretical
- **HIV-protease inhibitors** are predicted to increase the exposure to **imatinib**. Moderate Study
- **Imatinib** is predicted to increase the exposure to **ibrutinib**. Adjust dose with moderate CYP3A4 inhibitors—consult product literature. Severe Study → Also see **TABLE 3** p. 1053 → Also see **TABLE 12** p. 1057
- **Idelalisib** is predicted to increase the exposure to **imatinib**. Moderate Study
- **Imatinib** is predicted to increase the exposure to the active metabolite of **irinotecan**. Moderate Theoretical → Also see **TABLE 12** p. 1057
- **Imatinib** is predicted to increase the exposure to **ivabradine**. Adjust **ivabradine** dose. Severe Theoretical
- **Imatinib** is predicted to increase the exposure to **ivacaftor**. Adjust dose with moderate CYP3A4 inhibitors, see ivacaftor p. 219, tezacaftor with ivacaftor p. 223, and ivacaftor with tezacaftor and elexacaftor p. 220. Moderate Study

- **Imatinib** is predicted to increase the exposure to **ivosidenib.** Monitor and adjust dose—consult product literature. Severe Study
- **Ivosidenib** is predicted to decrease the exposure to **imatinib.** Avoid. Moderate Study
- **Imatinib** is predicted to increase the exposure to **lapatinib.** Moderate Study
- **Imatinib** is predicted to increase the exposure to **larotrectinib.** Monitor and adjust dose. Moderate Theoretical
- **Imatinib** is predicted to increase the exposure to **leniolisib.** Avoid. Moderate Study
- **Letermovir** is predicted to increase the exposure to **imatinib.** Moderate Study
- **Imatinib** is predicted to increase the exposure to **lomitapide.** Avoid. Moderate Theoretical
- **Lorlatinib** is predicted to decrease the exposure to **imatinib.** Moderate Study
- **Lumacaftor** is predicted to decrease the exposure to **imatinib.** Avoid. Moderate Study
- Macrolides **(clarithromycin)** are predicted to increase the exposure to **imatinib.** Moderate Study
- Macrolides **(erythromycin)** are predicted to increase the exposure to **imatinib.** Moderate Theoretical
- **Imatinib** is predicted to increase the exposure to **mavacamten.** Adjust dose—consult product literature. Moderate Study
- **Imatinib** might affect the clearance of **methotrexate** (particularly high-dose). Severe Theoretical → Also see **TABLE 12** p. 1057
- **Imatinib** is predicted to increase the exposure to **midostaurin.** Moderate Theoretical
- **Imatinib** is predicted to increase the exposure to mineralocorticoid receptor antagonists **(eplerenone).** Adjust **eplerenone** dose. Severe Study
- **Imatinib** is predicted to increase the exposure to mineralocorticoid receptor antagonists **(finerenone).** Severe Study
- **Mitotane** is predicted to decrease the exposure to **imatinib.** Avoid. Moderate Study → Also see **TABLE 12** p. 1057
- **Imatinib** is predicted to increase the exposure to **naldemedine.** Moderate Study
- **Imatinib** is predicted to increase the exposure to **naloxegol.** Adjust **naloxegol** dose and monitor adverse effects. Moderate Study
- **Imatinib** is predicted to increase the exposure to **neratinib.** Avoid moderate CYP3A4 inhibitors or adjust dose and monitor for gastrointestinal adverse effects—consult product literature. Severe Study
- Neurokinin-1 receptor antagonists **(aprepitant, netupitant)** are predicted to increase the exposure to **imatinib.** Moderate Theoretical
- **Nilotinib** is predicted to increase the exposure to **imatinib.** Moderate Study → Also see **TABLE 12** p. 1057
- NNRTIs **(efavirenz, etravirine, nevirapine)** are predicted to decrease the exposure to **imatinib.** Moderate Study
- **Imatinib** is predicted to increase the exposure to **olaparib.** Avoid or adjust dose with moderate CYP3A4 inhibitors—consult product literature. Moderate Theoretical → Also see **TABLE 12** p. 1057
- **Imatinib** is predicted to increase the exposure to **omaveloxolone.** Avoid or adjust **omaveloxolone** dose, p. 755. Moderate Study
- **Imatinib** is predicted to increase the exposure to opioids **(alfentanil, buprenorphine, fentanyl, oxycodone).** Monitor and adjust dose. Moderate Study
- **Imatinib** is predicted to increase the exposure to opioids **(methadone, sufentanil).** Moderate Theoretical
- **Imatinib** increases the risk of hepatotoxicity when given with **paracetamol.** Severe Anecdotal
- **Imatinib** is predicted to increase the exposure to **pazopanib.** Moderate Study → Also see **TABLE 3** p. 1053
- **Pegaspargase** is predicted to increase the risk of hepatotoxicity when given with **imatinib.** Severe Theoretical → Also see **TABLE 3** p. 1053 → Also see **TABLE 12** p. 1057
- **Imatinib** is predicted to increase the exposure to **pemigatinib.** Severe Study
- **Imatinib** is predicted to increase the risk of bleeding events when given with **phenindione.** Severe Theoretical → Also see **TABLE 3** p. 1053
- **Imatinib** is predicted to increase the exposure to phosphodiesterase type-5 inhibitors **(avanafil).** Adjust **avanafil** dose. Moderate Theoretical
- **Imatinib** is predicted to increase the exposure to phosphodiesterase type-5 inhibitors **(sildenafil).** Monitor or adjust **sildenafil** dose with moderate CYP3A4 inhibitors, p. 139. Moderate Study
- **Imatinib** is predicted to increase the exposure to phosphodiesterase type-5 inhibitors **(tadalafil).** Severe Theoretical
- **Imatinib** is predicted to increase the exposure to phosphodiesterase type-5 inhibitors **(vardenafil).** Adjust dose. Severe Theoretical
- **Imatinib** is predicted to increase the exposure to **pimozide.** Avoid. Severe Theoretical
- **Imatinib** is predicted to increase the exposure to **ponatinib.** Moderate Study → Also see **TABLE 3** p. 1053
- **Imatinib** is predicted to increase the exposure to **pralsetinib.** Moderate Theoretical
- **Imatinib** is predicted to increase the exposure to **ranolazine.** Severe Study
- **Imatinib** is predicted to increase the exposure to **regorafenib.** Moderate Study → Also see **TABLE 3** p. 1053 → Also see **TABLE 12** p. 1057
- **Imatinib** is predicted to increase the exposure to **ribociclib.** Moderate Study → Also see **TABLE 12** p. 1057
- Rifamycins **(rifampicin)** are predicted to decrease the exposure to **imatinib.** Avoid. Moderate Study
- **Imatinib** is predicted to increase the exposure to **rimegepant.** Avoid another dose of rimegepant within 48 hours of concurrent use. Moderate Study
- **Imatinib** is predicted to increase the exposure to **ruxolitinib.** Moderate Study → Also see **TABLE 12** p. 1057
- **Imatinib** is predicted to increase the exposure to **selpercatinib.** Moderate Study
- **Imatinib** is predicted to increase the exposure to **selumetinib.** Avoid or adjust dose—consult product literature. Severe Study
- **Imatinib** is predicted to increase the exposure to **siponimod.** Avoid depending on other drugs taken—consult product literature. Severe Study
- **Imatinib** increases the concentration of **sirolimus.** Monitor and adjust dose. Moderate Study
- **Sotorasib** is predicted to decrease the exposure to **imatinib.** Moderate Study
- **Imatinib** is predicted to increase the exposure to **sparsentan.** Moderate Study
- **Imatinib** is predicted to increase the exposure to SSRIs **(dapoxetine).** Adjust **dapoxetine** dose with moderate CYP3A4 inhibitors. Moderate Theoretical → Also see **TABLE 3** p. 1053
- **Imatinib** is predicted to increase the exposure to SSRIs **(sertraline).** Moderate Theoretical → Also see **TABLE 3** p. 1053
- **St John's wort** is predicted to decrease the exposure to **imatinib.** Moderate Study
- **Imatinib** is predicted to increase the exposure to statins **(atorvastatin).** Monitor and adjust dose. Severe Theoretical
- **Imatinib** moderately increases the exposure to statins **(simvastatin).** Monitor and adjust dose. Severe Study
- **Imatinib** is predicted to increase the exposure to **sunitinib.** Moderate Study → Also see **TABLE 3** p. 1053 → Also see **TABLE 12** p. 1057
- **Imatinib** increases the concentration of **tacrolimus.** Monitor and adjust dose. Severe Study
- **Imatinib** is predicted to increase the exposure to taxanes **(cabazitaxel).** Moderate Theoretical → Also see **TABLE 12** p. 1057
- **Imatinib** is predicted to increase the exposure to taxanes **(docetaxel).** Severe Study → Also see **TABLE 12** p. 1057
- **Imatinib** is predicted to increase the exposure to taxanes **(paclitaxel).** Moderate Anecdotal → Also see **TABLE 12** p. 1057
- **Tedizolid** is predicted to increase the exposure to **imatinib.** Avoid. Moderate Theoretical
- **Imatinib** is predicted to increase the concentration of **temsirolimus.** Use with caution or avoid. Moderate Theoretical → Also see **TABLE 12** p. 1057

Imatinib (continued)

- **Imatinib** is predicted to increase the exposure to **tezacaftor**. Adjust dose with moderate CYP3A4 inhibitors, see tezacaftor with ivacaftor p. 223, ivacaftor with tezacaftor and elexacaftor p. 220, and deutivacaftor with tezacaftor and vanzacaftor p. 218. Severe Study
- **Imatinib** causes hypothyroidism when given with thyroid hormones **(levothyroxine)** in thyroidectomy patients. Moderate Study
- **Imatinib** given with a potent CYP2C19 inhibitor is predicted to increase the exposure to **tofacitinib**. Adjust **tofacitinib** dose, p. 803. Moderate Study
- **Imatinib** is predicted to increase the exposure to **tolvaptan**. Manufacturer advises caution or adjust **tolvaptan** dose with moderate CYP3A4 inhibitors. Moderate Study
- **Imatinib** is predicted to increase the exposure to **trazodone**. Moderate Theoretical
- **Tucatinib** is predicted to increase the exposure to **imatinib**. Moderate Study
- **Imatinib** is predicted to increase the exposure to **ulipristal**. Avoid when used for uterine fibroids. Moderate Study
- **Imatinib** is predicted to increase the exposure to **vanzacaftor**. Adjust dose, see deutivacaftor with tezacaftor and vanzacaftor p. 218. Severe Study
- **Imatinib** is predicted to increase the exposure to **vemurafenib**. Severe Theoretical
- **Imatinib** is predicted to increase the exposure to **venetoclax**. Avoid or adjust dose—consult product literature. Severe Study
- **Imatinib** is predicted to increase the exposure to **vinca alkaloids**. Severe Theoretical → Also see TABLE 12 p. 1057
- **Imatinib** is predicted to increase the exposure to **voclosporin**. Adjust **voclosporin** dose. Severe Study
- **Imatinib** is predicted to increase the exposure to **zanubrutinib**. Avoid or adjust dose with moderate CYP3A4 inhibitors—consult product literature. Severe Study → Also see TABLE 3 p. 1053
- **Imatinib** is predicted to increase the exposure to **zopiclone**. Adjust dose. Moderate Study

Imidapril → see ACE inhibitors

Imipenem → see carbapenems

Imipramine → see tricyclic antidepressants

Immunoglobulins

Anti-D immunoglobulins · antithymocyte immunoglobulin (rabbit) · cytomegalovirus immunoglobulin · hepatitis B immunoglobulin · normal immunoglobulin · rabies immunoglobulin · tetanus immunoglobulin · varicella-zoster immunoglobulin

- **Immunoglobulins** are predicted to decrease the efficacy of live vaccines **(chikungunya vaccine (live), cholera vaccine (live), dengue vaccine, influenza vaccine (live), measles, mumps, and rubella vaccine, rotavirus vaccine, typhoid vaccine (live), varicella-zoster vaccine)**. Avoid and for 3 months after stopping **immunoglobulins**. Moderate Theoretical
- **Loop diuretics** are predicted to increase the risk of adverse effects when given with **cytomegalovirus immunoglobulin**. Avoid. Moderate Theoretical
- **Loop diuretics** might increase the risk of adverse effects when given with immunoglobulins **(hepatitis B immunoglobulin, normal immunoglobulin)**. Avoid. Moderate Theoretical
- Monoclonal antibodies **(rozanolixizumab)** might decrease the concentration of **immunoglobulins**. Avoid and for 2 weeks after stopping **rozanolixizumab**. Moderate Theoretical
- **Normal immunoglobulin** is predicted to alter the effects of monoclonal antibodies **(dinutuximab)**. Avoid. Severe Theoretical

Indacaterol → see beta$_2$ agonists

Indapamide → see thiazide diuretics

Indometacin → see NSAIDs

Indoramin → see alpha blockers

Infliximab → see monoclonal antibodies

Influenza vaccine (live) → see live vaccines

Inotersen → see TABLE 2 p. 1053 (nephrotoxicity)

- **Drugs that cause bleeding** (see TABLE 3 p. 1053) cause bleeding, as can **inotersen**; concurrent use might increase the risk of developing this effect. Severe Theoretical

Inotuzumab ozogamicin → see monoclonal antibodies

Insulin

- **Fenfluramine** might decrease blood glucose concentrations when given with **insulin**. Moderate Theoretical
- **Fibrates** are predicted to increase the risk of hypoglycaemia when given with **insulin**. Moderate Theoretical
- Macrolides **(clarithromycin)** have been reported to cause hypoglycaemia when given with **insulin**. Severe Anecdotal
- **Metreleptin** is predicted to increase the risk of hypoglycaemia when given with **insulin**. Monitor blood glucose and adjust dose. Severe Theoretical
- **Somapacitan** might increase blood glucose concentrations, opposing the blood glucose-lowering effects of **insulin**. Adjust dose. Moderate Theoretical
- **Somatrogon** might increase blood glucose concentrations, opposing the blood glucose-lowering effects of **insulin**. Adjust dose. Moderate Theoretical

Interferon beta → see interferons

Interferons → see TABLE 12 p. 1057 (myelosuppression)

interferon beta · peginterferon alfa · ropeginterferon alfa

- **Interferons** are predicted to slightly increase the exposure to **aminophylline**. Adjust dose. Moderate Theoretical
- **Ropeginterferon alfa** is predicted to increase the exposure to **atomoxetine**. Moderate Theoretical
- **Ropeginterferon alfa** is predicted to increase the exposure to atypical antipsychotics **(risperidone)**. Moderate Theoretical
- **Ropeginterferon alfa** is predicted to increase the exposure to beta blockers, selective **(nebivolol)**. Moderate Theoretical
- **Ropeginterferon alfa** is predicted to increase the exposure to **eliglustat**. Moderate Theoretical
- **Ropeginterferon alfa** is predicted to increase the exposure to opioids **(methadone)**. Moderate Theoretical
- **Interferons** slightly increase the exposure to **theophylline**. Adjust dose. Moderate Study
- **Ropeginterferon alfa** is predicted to increase the exposure to **vortioxetine**. Moderate Theoretical

Ipilimumab → see monoclonal antibodies

Ipratropium → see TABLE 8 p. 1055 (antimuscarinics)

- Atypical antipsychotics **(clozapine)** can cause constipation, as can **ipratropium**; concurrent use might increase the risk of developing intestinal obstruction. Severe Theoretical → Also see TABLE 8 p. 1055
- **Beta$_2$ agonists** are predicted to increase the risk of glaucoma when given with **ipratropium**. Moderate Anecdotal

Iptacopan

- Rifamycins **(rifampicin)** are predicted to decrease the exposure to **iptacopan**. Avoid or monitor. Moderate Theoretical

Irbesartan → see angiotensin-II receptor antagonists

Irinotecan → see TABLE 12 p. 1057 (myelosuppression)

- Anti-androgens **(apalutamide, enzalutamide)** are predicted to decrease the exposure to **irinotecan**. Avoid. Severe Study
- Antiarrhythmics **(dronedarone)** are predicted to increase the exposure to the active metabolite of **irinotecan**. Moderate Theoretical
- Antiepileptics **(carbamazepine, fosphenytoin, phenobarbital, phenytoin, primidone)** are predicted to decrease the exposure to **irinotecan**. Avoid. Severe Study
- Antifungals, azoles **(fluconazole, isavuconazole)** are predicted to increase the exposure to the active metabolite of **irinotecan**. Moderate Theoretical
- Antifungals, azoles **(itraconazole, ketoconazole, posaconazole, voriconazole)** are predicted to increase the exposure to the active metabolite of **irinotecan**. Avoid. Severe Study
- **Berotralstat** is predicted to increase the exposure to the active metabolite of **irinotecan**. Moderate Theoretical
- Calcium-channel blockers **(diltiazem, verapamil)** are predicted to increase the exposure to the active metabolite of **irinotecan**. Moderate Theoretical
- **Ceritinib** is predicted to increase the exposure to the active metabolite of **irinotecan**. Avoid. Severe Study → Also see TABLE 12 p. 1057
- **Cobicistat** is predicted to increase the exposure to the active metabolite of **irinotecan**. Avoid. Severe Study
- **Crizotinib** is predicted to increase the exposure to the active metabolite of **irinotecan**. Moderate Theoretical

- **Encorafenib** is predicted to decrease the exposure to **irinotecan**. Avoid. Severe Study
- **Fedratinib** is predicted to increase the exposure to the active metabolite of **irinotecan**. Moderate Theoretical
- Fibrates **(gemfibrozil)** are predicted to increase the exposure to **irinotecan**. Avoid. Moderate Theoretical
- **HIV-protease inhibitors** are predicted to increase the exposure to the active metabolite of **irinotecan**. Avoid. Severe Study
- **Idelalisib** is predicted to increase the exposure to the active metabolite of **irinotecan**. Avoid. Severe Study
- **Imatinib** is predicted to increase the exposure to the active metabolite of **irinotecan**. Moderate Theoretical → Also see **TABLE 12** p. 1057
- **Ivosidenib** is predicted to decrease the exposure to **irinotecan**. Avoid. Severe Study
- **Lapatinib** increases the exposure to the active metabolite of **irinotecan**. Monitor adverse effects and adjust dose. Severe Study
- **Letermovir** is predicted to increase the exposure to the active metabolite of **irinotecan**. Moderate Theoretical
- **Live vaccines** are predicted to increase the risk of generalised infection (possibly life-threatening) when given with **irinotecan**. UKHSA advises avoid (refer to Green Book). Severe Theoretical
- **Lumacaftor** is predicted to decrease the exposure to **irinotecan**. Avoid. Severe Study
- Macrolides **(clarithromycin)** are predicted to increase the exposure to the active metabolite of **irinotecan**. Avoid. Severe Study
- Macrolides **(erythromycin)** are predicted to increase the exposure to the active metabolite of **irinotecan**. Moderate Theoretical
- **Mitotane** is predicted to decrease the exposure to **irinotecan**. Avoid Severe Study → Also see **TABLE 12** p. 1057
- Neurokinin-1 receptor antagonists **(aprepitant, fosaprepitant)** are predicted to increase the exposure to intravenous **irinotecan**. Severe Theoretical
- Neurokinin-1 receptor antagonists **(netupitant)** are predicted to increase the exposure to **irinotecan**. Moderate Study
- **Irinotecan** is predicted to decrease the effects of **neuromuscular blocking drugs, non-depolarising**. Moderate Theoretical
- **Nilotinib** is predicted to increase the exposure to the active metabolite of **irinotecan**. Moderate Theoretical → Also see **TABLE 12** p. 1057
- **Pitolisant** is predicted to decrease the exposure to **irinotecan**. Mild Theoretical
- Rifamycins **(rifampicin)** are predicted to decrease the exposure to **irinotecan**. Avoid. Severe Study
- **St John's wort** slightly decreases the exposure to **irinotecan**. Avoid. Severe Study
- **Irinotecan** is predicted to increase the risk of prolonged neuromuscular blockade when given with **suxamethonium**. Moderate Theoretical
- **Tucatinib** is predicted to increase the exposure to the active metabolite of **irinotecan**. Avoid. Severe Study

Iron

- Oral **antacids** decrease the absorption of oral **iron**. Manufacturer advises iron should be taken 1 hour before or 2 hours after antacids. Moderate Study
- Atypical antipsychotics **(clozapine)** can cause constipation, as can **iron**; concurrent use might increase the risk of developing intestinal obstruction. Severe Anecdotal
- Oral **iron** might decrease the concentration of the active metabolite of oral **baloxavir marboxil**. Avoid. Severe Theoretical
- Oral **iron** decreases the exposure to oral **bictegravir**. Manufacturer advises bictegravir should be taken 2 hours before iron. Moderate Study
- Oral **iron** decreases the absorption of oral bisphosphonates **(clodronate)**. **Clodronate** should be taken 1 hour before or 2 hours after iron. Moderate Study
- Oral **iron** is predicted to decrease the absorption of oral bisphosphonates **(ibandronate)**. **Ibandronate** should be taken 1 hour before or 6 hours after iron. Moderate Theoretical
- Oral **iron** decreases the absorption of oral bisphosphonates **(risedronate)**. Separate administration by at least 2 hours. Moderate Study
- Oral calcium compounds **(calcium carbonate)** decrease the absorption of oral **iron**. **Calcium carbonate** should be taken 1 hour before or 2 hours after iron. Moderate Study
- Oral **iron** is predicted to decrease the exposure to oral **carbidopa**. Moderate Theoretical
- **Chloramphenicol** decreases the efficacy of **iron**. Moderate Anecdotal
- Oral **iron** decreases the absorption of oral **dolutegravir**. **Dolutegravir** should be taken 2 hours before or 6 hours after iron. Moderate Study
- Oral **iron** is predicted to decrease the absorption of oral **eltrombopag**. **Eltrombopag** should be taken 2 hours before or 4 hours after iron. Severe Theoretical
- Oral **entacapone** is predicted to decrease the absorption of oral **iron**. Separate administration by at least 2 hours. Moderate Theoretical
- Oral **iron** is predicted to decrease the absorption of oral iron chelators **(deferiprone)**. Moderate Theoretical
- Oral **iron** decreases the absorption of oral **levodopa**. Moderate Study
- Oral **iron** decreases the effects of oral **methyldopa**. Moderate Study
- Oral **iron** is predicted to decrease the absorption of oral **penicillamine**. Separate administration by at least 2 hours. Mild Study
- Oral **iron** decreases the exposure to oral **quinolones**. Separate administration by at least 2 hours. Moderate Study
- Oral **iron** is predicted to decrease the exposure to oral **raltegravir**. Separate administration by at least 2 hours. Moderate Theoretical
- Oral **iron** might decrease the exposure to oral **roxadustat**. **Roxadustat** should be taken at least 1 hour after iron. Mild Theoretical
- Oral **iron** decreases the absorption of oral **tetracyclines**. **Tetracyclines** should be taken 2 to 3 hours after iron. Moderate Study
- Oral **iron** decreases the absorption of oral thyroid hormones **(levothyroxine)**. Separate administration by at least 4 hours. Moderate Study
- Oral **trientine** potentially decreases the absorption of oral **iron**. Moderate Theoretical
- Oral **iron** decreases the exposure to oral **vadadustat**. **Vadadustat** should be taken 1 hour before iron. Moderate Study
- Oral **zinc** is predicted to decrease the efficacy of oral **iron** and oral **iron** is predicted to decrease the efficacy of oral **zinc**. Moderate Study

Iron chelators → see **TABLE 12** p. 1057 (myelosuppression), **TABLE 2** p. 1053 (nephrotoxicity)

deferasirox · deferiprone · desferrioxamine · dexrazoxane

- **Deferasirox** has been reported to increase the exposure to alkylating agents **(busulfan)**. Monitor and adjust dose. Unknown Anecdotal
- **Aluminium hydroxide** is predicted to decrease the exposure to **deferasirox**. Avoid. Moderate Theoretical
- **Aluminium hydroxide** is predicted to decrease the absorption of **deferiprone**. Avoid. Moderate Theoretical
- **Deferasirox** is predicted to increase the exposure to **aminophylline**. Avoid. Moderate Theoretical
- Antiepileptics **(carbamazepine, fosphenytoin, phenobarbital, phenytoin, primidone)** are predicted to decrease the exposure to **deferasirox**. Monitor serum ferritin and adjust dose. Moderate Theoretical
- **Dexrazoxane** might decrease the absorption of antiepileptics **(fosphenytoin, phenytoin)**. Avoid. Severe Theoretical
- **Ascorbic acid** is predicted to increase the risk of cardiovascular adverse effects when given with **deferiprone**. Severe Theoretical
- **Ascorbic acid** might increase the risk of cardiovascular adverse effects when given with **desferrioxamine**. Manufacturer advises caution or adjust ascorbic acid dose; monitor cardiac function and avoid concurrent use in those with cardiac failure. Severe Theoretical

Iron chelators (continued)

- **Aspirin** (high-dose) is predicted to increase the risk of gastrointestinal bleeds when given with **deferasirox**. Severe Theoretical → Also see TABLE 2 p. 1053
- **Deferasirox** is predicted to increase the exposure to atypical antipsychotics **(clozapine)**. Avoid. Moderate Theoretical
- **Bisphosphonates** are predicted to increase the risk of gastrointestinal bleeding when given with **deferasirox**. Severe Theoretical → Also see TABLE 2 p. 1053
- **Dexrazoxane** might increase the risk of immunosuppression when given with **ciclosporin**. Severe Theoretical
- **Corticosteroids** are predicted to increase the risk of gastrointestinal bleeding when given with **deferasirox**. Severe Theoretical
- **Deferasirox** are predicted to increases the exposure to **etrasimod**. Avoid in poor CYP2C9 metabolisers. Severe Theoretical
- HIV-protease inhibitors **(ritonavir)** are predicted to decrease the exposure to **deferasirox**. Monitor serum ferritin and adjust dose. Moderate Theoretical
- Oral **iron** is predicted to decrease the absorption of oral **deferiprone**. Moderate Theoretical
- **Live vaccines** are predicted to increase the risk of generalised infection (possibly life-threatening) when given with **dexrazoxane**. Avoid. Severe Theoretical
- **Deferasirox** moderately increases the exposure to meglitinides **(repaglinide)**. Avoid. Moderate Study
- **Deferasirox** is predicted to increase the exposure to **montelukast**. Moderate Theoretical
- **NSAIDs** are predicted to increase the risk of gastrointestinal bleeding when given with **deferasirox**. Severe Theoretical → Also see TABLE 2 p. 1053
- NSAIDs **(diclofenac)** are predicted to increase the exposure to **deferiprone**. Moderate Theoretical
- **Deferasirox** is predicted to increase the exposure to **pioglitazone**. Moderate Study
- Rifamycins **(rifampicin)** are predicted to decrease the exposure to **deferasirox**. Monitor serum ferritin and adjust dose. Moderate Study → Also see TABLE 2 p. 1053
- **Deferasirox** is predicted to increase the exposure to **selexipag**. Adjust **selexipag** dose. Moderate Study
- **Dexrazoxane** might increase the risk of immunosuppression when given with **tacrolimus**. Severe Theoretical
- **Deferasirox** is predicted to increase the concentration of taxanes **(paclitaxel)**. Severe Anecdotal
- **Deferasirox** increases the exposure to **theophylline**. Avoid. Moderate Study
- **Deferasirox** is predicted to increase the exposure to **tizanidine**. Avoid. Moderate Theoretical
- **Deferasirox** is predicted to increase the exposure to **treprostinil**. Adjust dose. Moderate Theoretical
- **Deferasirox** is predicted to increase the exposure to **tucatinib**. Moderate Theoretical
- Oral **zinc** is predicted to decrease the absorption of oral **deferiprone**. Moderate Theoretical

Isavuconazole → see antifungals, azoles

Isocarboxazid → see MAOIs, irreversible

Isoflurane → see volatile halogenated anaesthetics

Isometheptene → see sympathomimetics, vasoconstrictor

Isoniazid → see TABLE 1 p. 1053 (hepatotoxicity), TABLE 10 p. 1056 (peripheral neuropathy)

> **FOOD AND LIFESTYLE** Avoid tyramine-rich foods (such as mature cheeses, salami, pickled herring, *Bovril*®, *Oxo*®, *Marmite*® or any similar meat or yeast extract or fermented soya bean extract, and some beers, lagers or wines) or histamine-rich foods (such as very mature cheese or fish from the scromboid family (e.g. tuna, mackerel, salmon)) with **isoniazid**, as tachycardia, palpitation, hypotension, flushing, headache, dizziness, and sweating reported.

- **Isoniazid** is predicted to affect the clearance of **aminophylline**. Severe Theoretical
- **Isoniazid** markedly increases the concentration of antiepileptics **(carbamazepine)** and antiepileptics **(carbamazepine)** increase the risk of hepatotoxicity when given with **isoniazid**. Monitor concentration and adjust dose. Severe Study
- **Isoniazid** increases the concentration of antiepileptics **(fosphenytoin, phenytoin)**. Moderate Study → Also see TABLE 10 p. 1056
- **Cycloserine** increases the risk of CNS toxicity when given with **isoniazid**. Monitor and adjust dose. Moderate Study
- **Isoniazid** increases the risk of optic neuropathy when given with **ethambutol**. Severe Anecdotal
- **Isoniazid** might decrease the effects of **foslevodopa**. Moderate Theoretical
- **Isoniazid** decreases the effects of **levodopa**. Moderate Study
- **Isoniazid** is predicted to increase the exposure to **lomitapide**. Separate administration by 12 hours. Unknown Theoretical → Also see TABLE 1 p. 1053
- **Isoniazid** is predicted to increase the exposure to **mavacamten**. Monitor and adjust dose—consult product literature. Moderate Theoretical
- **Isoniazid** is predicted to affect the clearance of **theophylline**. Severe Anecdotal
- **Isoniazid** potentially increases the risk of nephrotoxicity when given with volatile halogenated anaesthetics **(methoxyflurane)**. Avoid. Severe Theoretical
- **Isoniazid** might increase the risk of sevoflurane toxicity when given with volatile halogenated anaesthetics **(sevoflurane)**. Avoid **isoniazid** from 1 week before, until 15 days after, surgery. Moderate Theoretical

Isoprenaline → see TABLE 14 p. 1057 (reduced serum potassium)

- **Entacapone** is predicted to increase the risk of cardiovascular adverse effects when given with **isoprenaline**. Moderate Study
- **Opicapone** is predicted to increase the risk of cardiovascular adverse effects when given with **isoprenaline**. Moderate Theoretical
- **Tolcapone** is predicted to increase the risk of cardiovascular adverse effects when given with **isoprenaline**. Moderate Theoretical

Isosorbide dinitrate → see nitrates

Isosorbide mononitrate → see nitrates

Isotretinoin → see retinoids

Itraconazole → see antifungals, azoles

Ivabradine → see TABLE 4 p. 1054 (bradycardia), TABLE 7 p. 1055 (QT-interval prolongation)

- Anti-androgens **(apalutamide, enzalutamide)** are predicted to decrease the exposure to **ivabradine**. Adjust dose. Moderate Theoretical
- Antiarrhythmics **(dronedarone)** are predicted to increase the exposure to **ivabradine**. Adjust **ivabradine** dose. Severe Theoretical → Also see TABLE 4 p. 1054
- Antiepileptics **(carbamazepine, fosphenytoin, phenobarbital, phenytoin, primidone)** are predicted to decrease the exposure to **ivabradine**. Adjust dose. Moderate Theoretical
- Antifungals, azoles **(fluconazole, isavuconazole)** are predicted to increase the exposure to **ivabradine**. Adjust **ivabradine** dose. Severe Theoretical
- Antifungals, azoles **(itraconazole, ketoconazole, posaconazole, voriconazole)** are predicted to increase the exposure to **ivabradine**. Avoid. Severe Study
- Calcium-channel blockers **(diltiazem, verapamil)** are predicted to increase the exposure to **ivabradine**. Avoid. Moderate Study → Also see TABLE 4 p. 1054
- **Ceritinib** is predicted to increase the exposure to **ivabradine**. Avoid. Severe Study → Also see TABLE 4 p. 1054
- **Cobicistat** is predicted to increase the exposure to **ivabradine**. Avoid. Severe Study
- **Crizotinib** is predicted to increase the exposure to **ivabradine**. Adjust **ivabradine** dose. Severe Theoretical → Also see TABLE 4 p. 1054
- **Encorafenib** is predicted to decrease the exposure to **ivabradine**. Adjust dose. Moderate Theoretical
- **Grapefruit** juice is predicted to increase the exposure to **ivabradine**. Avoid. Moderate Study
- **HIV-protease inhibitors** are predicted to increase the exposure to **ivabradine**. Avoid. Severe Study
- **Idelalisib** is predicted to increase the exposure to **ivabradine**. Avoid. Severe Study
- **Imatinib** is predicted to increase the exposure to **ivabradine**. Adjust **ivabradine** dose. Severe Theoretical

- **Ivosidenib** is predicted to decrease the exposure to **ivabradine**. Adjust dose. [Moderate] Theoretical
- **Lumacaftor** is predicted to decrease the exposure to **ivabradine**. Adjust dose. [Moderate] Theoretical
- Macrolides **(clarithromycin)** are predicted to increase the exposure to **ivabradine**. Avoid. [Severe] Study
- Macrolides **(erythromycin)** are predicted to increase the exposure to **ivabradine**. Avoid. [Severe] Theoretical
- **Mitotane** is predicted to decrease the exposure to **ivabradine**. Adjust dose. [Moderate] Theoretical
- Neurokinin-1 receptor antagonists **(aprepitant, netupitant)** are predicted to increase the exposure to **ivabradine**. Adjust **ivabradine** dose. [Severe] Theoretical
- **Nilotinib** is predicted to increase the exposure to **ivabradine**. Adjust **ivabradine** dose. [Severe] Theoretical
- **Nirmatrelvir** boosted with ritonavir is predicted to increase the concentration of **ivabradine**. Avoid. [Severe] Theoretical
- Rifamycins **(rifampicin)** are predicted to decrease the exposure to **ivabradine**. Adjust dose. [Moderate] Theoretical
- **St John's wort** decreases the exposure to **ivabradine**. Avoid. [Moderate] Study
- **Tucatinib** is predicted to increase the exposure to **ivabradine**. Avoid. [Severe] Study

Ivacaftor

FOOD AND LIFESTYLE Food or drinks containing bitter (Seville) oranges are predicted to increase the exposure to ivacaftor.

- Anti-androgens **(apalutamide, enzalutamide)** are predicted to decrease the exposure to **ivacaftor**. Avoid. [Severe] Study
- Antiarrhythmics **(dronedarone)** are predicted to increase the exposure to **ivacaftor**. Adjust dose with moderate CYP3A4 inhibitors, see ivacaftor p. 219, tezacaftor with ivacaftor p. 223, and ivacaftor with tezacaftor and elexacaftor p. 220. [Moderate] Study
- Antiepileptics **(carbamazepine, fosphenytoin, phenobarbital, phenytoin, primidone)** are predicted to decrease the exposure to **ivacaftor**. Avoid. [Severe] Study
- Antifungals, azoles **(fluconazole, isavuconazole)** are predicted to increase the exposure to **ivacaftor**. Adjust dose with moderate CYP3A4 inhibitors, see ivacaftor p. 219, tezacaftor with ivacaftor p. 223, and ivacaftor with tezacaftor and elexacaftor p. 220. [Moderate] Study
- Antifungals, azoles **(itraconazole, ketoconazole, posaconazole, voriconazole)** are predicted to increase the exposure to **ivacaftor**. Adjust dose with potent CYP3A4 inhibitors, see ivacaftor p. 219, lumacaftor with ivacaftor p. 222, tezacaftor with ivacaftor p. 223, and ivacaftor with tezacaftor and elexacaftor p. 220. [Severe] Study
- **Berotralstat** is predicted to increase the exposure to **ivacaftor**. Adjust dose with moderate CYP3A4 inhibitors, see ivacaftor p. 219, tezacaftor with ivacaftor p. 223, and ivacaftor with tezacaftor and elexacaftor p. 220. [Moderate] Study
- Calcium-channel blockers **(diltiazem, verapamil)** are predicted to increase the exposure to **ivacaftor**. Adjust dose with moderate CYP3A4 inhibitors, see ivacaftor p. 219, tezacaftor with ivacaftor p. 223, and ivacaftor with tezacaftor and elexacaftor p. 220. [Moderate] Study
- **Cenobamate** is predicted to decrease the exposure to **ivacaftor**. Adjust dose. [Moderate] Theoretical
- **Ceritinib** is predicted to increase the exposure to **ivacaftor**. Adjust dose with potent CYP3A4 inhibitors, see ivacaftor p. 219, lumacaftor with ivacaftor p. 222, tezacaftor with ivacaftor p. 223, and ivacaftor with tezacaftor and elexacaftor p. 220. [Severe] Study
- **Ivacaftor** is predicted to increase the exposure to **ciclosporin**. [Moderate] Theoretical
- **Cobicistat** is predicted to increase the exposure to **ivacaftor**. Adjust dose with potent CYP3A4 inhibitors, see ivacaftor p. 219, lumacaftor with ivacaftor p. 222, tezacaftor with ivacaftor p. 223, and ivacaftor with tezacaftor and elexacaftor p. 220. [Severe] Study
- **Ivacaftor** is predicted to increase the exposure to **coumarins (warfarin)**. [Moderate] Theoretical
- **Crizotinib** is predicted to increase the exposure to **ivacaftor**. Adjust dose with moderate CYP3A4 inhibitors, see ivacaftor p. 219, tezacaftor with ivacaftor p. 223, and ivacaftor with tezacaftor and elexacaftor p. 220. [Moderate] Study
- **Dabrafenib** is predicted to decrease the exposure to **ivacaftor**. [Moderate] Study
- **Ivacaftor** slightly increases the exposure to **digoxin**. [Moderate] Study
- **Encorafenib** is predicted to decrease the exposure to **ivacaftor**. Avoid. [Severe] Study
- Endothelin receptor antagonists **(bosentan)** are predicted to decrease the exposure to **ivacaftor**. [Moderate] Study
- **Ivacaftor** is predicted to increase the exposure to **everolimus**. [Moderate] Study
- **Fedratinib** is predicted to increase the exposure to **ivacaftor**. Adjust dose with moderate CYP3A4 inhibitors, see ivacaftor p. 219, tezacaftor with ivacaftor p. 223, and ivacaftor with tezacaftor and elexacaftor p. 220. [Moderate] Study
- **Ivacaftor** is predicted to increase the exposure to **gilteritinib**. [Moderate] Theoretical
- **Grapefruit** juice is predicted to increase the exposure to **ivacaftor**. Avoid. [Moderate] Theoretical
- **HIV-protease inhibitors** are predicted to increase the exposure to **ivacaftor**. Adjust dose with potent CYP3A4 inhibitors, see ivacaftor p. 219, lumacaftor with ivacaftor p. 222, tezacaftor with ivacaftor p. 223, and ivacaftor with tezacaftor and elexacaftor p. 220. [Severe] Study
- **Idelalisib** is predicted to increase the exposure to **ivacaftor**. Adjust dose with potent CYP3A4 inhibitors, see ivacaftor p. 219, lumacaftor with ivacaftor p. 222, tezacaftor with ivacaftor p. 223, and ivacaftor with tezacaftor and elexacaftor p. 220. [Severe] Study
- **Imatinib** is predicted to increase the exposure to **ivacaftor**. Adjust dose with moderate CYP3A4 inhibitors, see ivacaftor p. 219, tezacaftor with ivacaftor p. 223, and ivacaftor with tezacaftor and elexacaftor p. 220. [Moderate] Study
- **Ivosidenib** is predicted to decrease the exposure to **ivacaftor**. Avoid. [Severe] Study
- **Letermovir** is predicted to increase the exposure to **ivacaftor**. Adjust dose with moderate CYP3A4 inhibitors, see ivacaftor p. 219, tezacaftor with ivacaftor p. 223, and ivacaftor with tezacaftor and elexacaftor p. 220. [Moderate] Study
- **Ivacaftor** is predicted to increase the exposure to **lomitapide**. Separate administration by 12 hours. [Moderate] Theoretical
- **Lumacaftor** is predicted to decrease the exposure to **ivacaftor**. Avoid. [Severe] Study
- Macrolides **(clarithromycin)** are predicted to increase the exposure to **ivacaftor**. Adjust dose with potent CYP3A4 inhibitors, see ivacaftor p. 219, lumacaftor with ivacaftor p. 222, tezacaftor with ivacaftor p. 223, and ivacaftor with tezacaftor and elexacaftor p. 220. [Severe] Study
- Macrolides **(erythromycin)** are predicted to increase the exposure to **ivacaftor**. Adjust dose with moderate CYP3A4 inhibitors, see ivacaftor p. 219, tezacaftor with ivacaftor p. 223, and ivacaftor with tezacaftor and elexacaftor p. 220. [Moderate] Study
- **Ivacaftor** is predicted to increase the exposure to **mavacamten**. Monitor and adjust dose—consult product literature. [Moderate] Theoretical
- **Mitotane** is predicted to decrease the exposure to **ivacaftor**. Avoid. [Severe] Study
- Neurokinin-1 receptor antagonists **(aprepitant, netupitant)** are predicted to increase the exposure to **ivacaftor**. Adjust dose with moderate CYP3A4 inhibitors, see ivacaftor p. 219, tezacaftor with ivacaftor p. 223, and ivacaftor with tezacaftor and elexacaftor p. 220. [Moderate] Study
- **Nilotinib** is predicted to increase the exposure to **ivacaftor**. Adjust dose with moderate CYP3A4 inhibitors, see ivacaftor p. 219, tezacaftor with ivacaftor p. 223, and ivacaftor with tezacaftor and elexacaftor p. 220. [Moderate] Study
- **Nirmatrelvir** boosted with ritonavir is predicted to increase the concentration of **ivacaftor**. Adjust dose. [Severe] Theoretical
- NNRTIs **(efavirenz, nevirapine)** are predicted to decrease the exposure to **ivacaftor**. [Moderate] Study
- Rifamycins **(rifampicin)** are predicted to decrease the exposure to **ivacaftor**. Avoid. [Severe] Study

Ivacaftor (continued)
- **Ivacaftor** is predicted to increase the exposure to **sirolimus**. Moderate Study
- **St John's wort** is predicted to decrease the exposure to **ivacaftor**. Avoid. Severe Study
- **Ivacaftor** is predicted to increase the exposure to **tacrolimus**. Moderate Theoretical
- **Ivacaftor** is predicted to increase the exposure to **talazoparib**. Moderate Study
- **Ivacaftor** is predicted to increase the exposure to taxanes **(paclitaxel)**. Moderate Study
- **Ivacaftor** might increase the exposure to **tigecycline**. Mild Anecdotal
- **Tucatinib** is predicted to increase the exposure to **ivacaftor**. Adjust dose with potent CYP3A4 inhibitors, see ivacaftor p. 219, lumacaftor with ivacaftor p. 222, tezacaftor with ivacaftor p. 223, and ivacaftor with tezacaftor and elexacaftor p. 220. Severe Study
- **Ivacaftor** is predicted to increase the exposure to **venetoclax**. Avoid or monitor for toxicity. Severe Theoretical
- **Ivacaftor** might increase the exposure to **vinca alkaloids**. Severe Theoretical

Ivermectin

ROUTE-SPECIFIC INFORMATION Since systemic absorption can follow topical application, the possibility of interactions should be borne in mind.

- **Ivermectin** potentially increases the anticoagulant effect of **coumarins**. Severe Anecdotal
- **Levamisole** increases the exposure to **ivermectin**. Moderate Study

Ivosidenib → see TABLE 7 p. 1055 (QT-interval prolongation)
- **Ivosidenib** is predicted to decrease the exposure to 5-HT3-receptor antagonists **(ondansetron)**. Moderate Study → Also see TABLE 7 p. 1055
- **Ivosidenib** is predicted to markedly decrease the exposure to **abemaciclib**. Avoid. Severe Study
- **Ivosidenib** is predicted to decrease the exposure to **acalabrutinib**. Avoid. Severe Study
- **Ivosidenib** is predicted to alter the exposure to **aliskiren**. Moderate Theoretical
- **Ivosidenib** might decrease the exposure to alkylating agents **(cyclophosphamide, ifosfamide)**. Avoid or monitor efficacy. Unknown Theoretical
- **Ivosidenib** is predicted to decrease the exposure to **alpelisib**. Avoid. Moderate Study
- Anti-androgens **(apalutamide, enzalutamide)** are predicted to decrease the exposure to **ivosidenib**. Avoid. Severe Theoretical → Also see TABLE 7 p. 1055
- **Ivosidenib** is predicted to decrease the exposure to anti-androgens **(abiraterone)**. Avoid. Severe Study
- **Ivosidenib** is predicted to decrease the exposure to anti-androgens **(darolutamide)**. Avoid. Moderate Study
- Antiarrhythmics **(dronedarone)** are predicted to increase the exposure to **ivosidenib**. Monitor and adjust dose—consult product literature. Severe Study → Also see TABLE 7 p. 1055
- **Ivosidenib** is predicted to decrease the exposure to antiarrhythmics **(disopyramide, dronedarone)**. Avoid. Severe Study → Also see TABLE 7 p. 1055
- **Ivosidenib** is predicted to decrease the efficacy of antiarrhythmics **(propafenone)**. Moderate Study
- **Ivosidenib** is predicted to decrease the exposure to anticholinesterases, centrally acting **(donepezil)**. Mild Study
- Antiepileptics **(carbamazepine, fosphenytoin, phenobarbital, primidone)** are predicted to decrease the exposure to **ivosidenib**. Avoid. Severe Theoretical
- Antiepileptics **(phenytoin)** are predicted to decrease the exposure to **ivosidenib** and **ivosidenib** might decrease the exposure to antiepileptics **(phenytoin)**. Avoid. Severe Study
- **Ivosidenib** might decrease the exposure to antiepileptics **(lamotrigine)**. Avoid or monitor efficacy. Unknown Theoretical
- **Ivosidenib** is predicted to decrease the exposure to antiepileptics **(perampanel)**. Monitor and adjust dose. Moderate Study
- Antifungals, azoles **(fluconazole, isavuconazole, voriconazole)** are predicted to increase the exposure to **ivosidenib**. Monitor and adjust dose—consult product literature. Severe Study → Also see TABLE 7 p. 1055
- Antifungals, azoles **(itraconazole)** moderately increase the exposure to **ivosidenib** and **ivosidenib** is predicted to decrease the exposure to antifungals, azoles **(itraconazole)**. Avoid or adjust dose—consult product literature. Severe Study
- Antifungals, azoles **(ketoconazole)** are predicted to increase the exposure to **ivosidenib** and **ivosidenib** is predicted to decrease the exposure to antifungals, azoles **(ketoconazole)**. Avoid or adjust dose—consult product literature. Severe Study
- **Ivosidenib** is predicted to decrease the exposure to antifungals, azoles **(isavuconazole)**. Avoid. Severe Study
- **Ivosidenib** is predicted to alter the exposure to antihistamines, non-sedating **(fexofenadine)**. Moderate Theoretical
- **Ivosidenib** is predicted to decrease the exposure to antimalarials **(artemether)** with lumefantrine. Avoid. Severe Study → Also see TABLE 7 p. 1055
- **Ivosidenib** is predicted to decrease the concentration of antimalarials **(piperaquine)**. Avoid. Moderate Theoretical
- **Ivosidenib** is predicted to moderately decrease the exposure to atypical antipsychotics **(aripiprazole)**. Avoid or adjust dose—consult product literature. Moderate Study
- **Ivosidenib** is predicted to decrease the exposure to atypical antipsychotics **(cariprazine)**. Avoid. Severe Theoretical
- **Ivosidenib** is predicted to decrease the exposure to atypical antipsychotics **(lurasidone)**. Avoid. Moderate Study
- **Ivosidenib** is predicted to decrease the exposure to atypical antipsychotics **(paliperidone)**. Monitor and adjust dose. Severe Study → Also see TABLE 7 p. 1055
- **Ivosidenib** is predicted to decrease the exposure to atypical antipsychotics **(quetiapine)**. Moderate Study
- **Ivosidenib** is predicted to decrease the exposure to atypical antipsychotics **(risperidone)**. Adjust dose. Moderate Study
- **Ivosidenib** is predicted to decrease the exposure to **avacopan**. Avoid or monitor. Severe Study
- **Ivosidenib** is predicted to decrease the exposure to **avapritinib**. Avoid. Severe Study
- **Ivosidenib** is predicted to decrease the exposure to **axitinib**. Avoid or adjust dose. Moderate Study
- **Ivosidenib** decreases the exposure to **bedaquiline**. Avoid. Severe Study → Also see TABLE 7 p. 1055
- **Ivosidenib** is predicted to decrease the exposure to **belumosudil**. Adjust **belumosudil** dose, p. 650. Severe Study
- **Ivosidenib** is predicted to decrease the exposure to benzodiazepines **(alprazolam)**. Adjust dose. Moderate Theoretical
- **Ivosidenib** is predicted to decrease the exposure to benzodiazepines **(midazolam)**. Monitor and adjust dose. Severe Study
- **Berotralstat** is predicted to increase the exposure to **ivosidenib**. Monitor and adjust dose—consult product literature. Severe Study
- **Ivosidenib** might decrease the exposure to $beta_2$ agonists **(salmeterol)**. Avoid or monitor. Moderate Theoretical
- **Ivosidenib** is predicted to decrease the exposure to **bictegravir**. Avoid. Moderate Study
- **Ivosidenib** slightly decreases the exposure to **bortezomib**. Avoid. Severe Study
- **Ivosidenib** is predicted to very markedly decrease the exposure to **bosutinib**. Avoid. Severe Study → Also see TABLE 7 p. 1055
- **Ivosidenib** is predicted to decrease the exposure to **brigatinib**. Avoid. Severe Study
- **Ivosidenib** is predicted to decrease the exposure to **buspirone**. Use with caution and adjust dose. Severe Study
- **Ivosidenib** moderately decreases the exposure to **cabozantinib**. Avoid. Moderate Study → Also see TABLE 7 p. 1055
- Calcium-channel blockers **(diltiazem, verapamil)** are predicted to increase the exposure to **ivosidenib**. Monitor and adjust dose—consult product literature. Severe Study
- **Ivosidenib** is predicted to decrease the exposure to calcium-channel blockers **(amlodipine, felodipine, lacidipine, lercanidipine, nicardipine, nifedipine, nimodipine)**. Monitor and adjust dose. Moderate Study
- **Ivosidenib** is predicted to decrease the exposure to **cannabidiol**. Adjust dose. Moderate Study

- **Ivosidenib** is predicted to decrease the exposure to **capivasertib**. Avoid. [Moderate] Study
- **Ivosidenib** is predicted to increase the exposure to cephalosporins **(cefaclor)**. Use with caution or avoid. [Moderate] Theoretical
- **Ivosidenib** is predicted to decrease the exposure to **ceritinib**. Avoid. [Severe] Study → Also see **TABLE 7** p. 1055
- **Ivosidenib** decreases the concentration of **ciclosporin**. [Severe] Study
- **Ciclosporin** is predicted to increase the exposure to **ivosidenib** and **ivosidenib** might decrease the exposure to **ciclosporin**. Monitor and adjust dose—consult product literature. [Severe] Study
- **Ivosidenib** is predicted to alter the effects of **cilostazol**. [Moderate] Theoretical
- **Ivosidenib** is predicted to decrease the exposure to **cinacalcet**. Monitor and adjust dose. [Moderate] Study
- **Ivosidenib** decreases the exposure to **clomethiazole**. Monitor and adjust dose. [Moderate] Study
- **Ivosidenib** is predicted to decrease the exposure to **cobicistat**. Avoid. [Severe] Study
- **Cobicistat** is predicted to increase the exposure to **ivosidenib**. Monitor and adjust dose—consult product literature. [Severe] Study
- **Ivosidenib** is predicted to decrease the exposure to **cobimetinib**. Avoid. [Severe] Theoretical
- **Ivosidenib** is predicted to alter the exposure to **colchicine**. [Moderate] Theoretical
- **Ivosidenib** might decrease the concentration of **combined hormonal contraceptives**. Use alternative methods during treatment with, and for at least 28 days after stopping, **ivosidenib**. [Severe] Theoretical
- **Ivosidenib** is predicted to decrease the exposure to corticosteroids **(budesonide, deflazacort, dexamethasone, fludrocortisone, hydrocortisone, methylprednisolone, prednisolone, triamcinolone)**. Monitor and adjust dose. [Moderate] Study
- **Ivosidenib** is predicted to decrease the exposure to corticosteroids **(fluticasone)**. [Unknown] Theoretical
- **Ivosidenib** might decrease the exposure to coumarins **(warfarin)**. Avoid or monitor efficacy. [Unknown] Study
- **Crizotinib** is predicted to increase the exposure to **ivosidenib**. Monitor and adjust dose—consult product literature. [Severe] Study → Also see **TABLE 7** p. 1055
- **Ivosidenib** is predicted to markedly decrease the exposure to **crizotinib**. Avoid. [Severe] Study → Also see **TABLE 7** p. 1055
- **Ivosidenib** is predicted to decrease the exposure to **dabrafenib**. Avoid. [Moderate] Theoretical
- **Ivosidenib** is predicted to decrease the exposure to **daridorexant**. [Severe] Study
- **Ivosidenib** is predicted to decrease the exposure to **darifenacin**. [Moderate] Theoretical
- **Ivosidenib** is predicted to markedly decrease the exposure to **dasatinib**. Avoid. [Severe] Study → Also see **TABLE 7** p. 1055
- **Ivosidenib** is predicted to slightly decrease the exposure to **delamanid**. Avoid. [Moderate] Study → Also see **TABLE 7** p. 1055
- **Ivosidenib** is predicted to decrease the exposure to **deutivacaftor**. Avoid. [Severe] Theoretical
- **Ivosidenib** is predicted to markedly decrease the exposure to **dienogest**. [Severe] Study
- **Ivosidenib** is predicted to alter the exposure to **digoxin**. [Moderate] Theoretical
- **Ivosidenib** is predicted to decrease the exposure to dipeptidylpeptidase-4 inhibitors **(linagliptin)**. [Moderate] Study
- **Ivosidenib** is predicted to moderately decrease the exposure to dipeptidylpeptidase-4 inhibitors **(saxagliptin)**. [Moderate] Study
- **Ivosidenib** is predicted to decrease the exposure to **dronabinol**. Avoid or adjust dose. [Mild] Study
- **Ivosidenib** is predicted to decrease the exposure to **elacestrant**. Avoid or adjust dose depending on duration—consult product literature. [Severe] Study
- **Ivosidenib** is predicted to decrease the exposure to **elbasvir**. Avoid. [Severe] Study
- **Ivosidenib** is predicted to decreases the exposure to **elexacaftor**. Avoid. [Severe] Theoretical
- **Ivosidenib** is predicted to decrease the exposure to **eliglustat**. Avoid. [Severe] Study
- **Ivosidenib** is predicted to decrease the concentration of **elvitegravir**. Avoid. [Severe] Study
- **Ivosidenib** is predicted to decrease the exposure to **encorafenib**. [Severe] Theoretical → Also see **TABLE 7** p. 1055
- **Ivosidenib** affects the exposure to endothelin receptor antagonists **(bosentan)**. Avoid. [Severe] Study
- **Ivosidenib** is predicted to decrease the exposure to endothelin receptor antagonists **(macitentan)**. Avoid. [Severe] Study
- **Ivosidenib** is predicted to decrease the exposure to the cytotoxic component of **enfortumab vedotin**. [Moderate] Theoretical
- **Ivosidenib** is predicted to decrease the exposure to **entrectinib**. Avoid. [Severe] Study → Also see **TABLE 7** p. 1055
- **Ivosidenib** is predicted to decrease the exposure to **erdafitinib**. Avoid. [Severe] Study
- **Ivosidenib** is predicted to decrease the exposure to **erlotinib**. Avoid or adjust dose—consult product literature. [Severe] Study
- **Ivosidenib** is predicted to decrease the exposure to **esketamine**. Adjust dose. [Moderate] Study
- **Ivosidenib** is predicted to decrease the exposure to **eszopiclone**. Adjust dose. [Moderate] Theoretical
- **Ivosidenib** is predicted to decrease the concentration of **everolimus**. Avoid or adjust dose. [Severe] Study
- **Ivosidenib** moderately decreases the exposure to **exemestane**. [Moderate] Study
- **Ivosidenib** is predicted to decrease the exposure to factor XA inhibitors **(apixaban)**. [Moderate] Study
- **Ivosidenib** is predicted to alter the exposure to factor XA inhibitors **(edoxaban)**. [Moderate] Theoretical
- **Ivosidenib** is predicted to decrease the exposure to factor XA inhibitors **(rivaroxaban)**. Avoid unless patient can be monitored for signs of thrombosis. [Moderate] Study
- **Fedratinib** is predicted to increase the exposure to **ivosidenib**. Monitor and adjust dose—consult product literature. [Severe] Study
- **Ivosidenib** is predicted to decrease the exposure to **fedratinib**. Avoid. [Moderate] Study
- **Ivosidenib** is predicted to decrease the exposure to **fesoterodine**. Avoid. [Moderate] Study
- **Ivosidenib** is predicted to decrease the exposure to **fostamatinib**. Avoid. [Severe] Study
- **Ivosidenib** is predicted to decrease the exposure to the active metabolite of **fostemsavir**. Avoid. [Severe] Study
- **Ivosidenib** is predicted to decrease the exposure to **fruquintinib**. Avoid. [Moderate] Study
- **Ivosidenib** is predicted to increase the exposure to **ganciclovir**. Use with caution or avoid. [Moderate] Theoretical
- **Ivosidenib** is predicted to decrease the exposure to **gefitinib**. Avoid. [Severe] Study
- **Ivosidenib** is predicted to decrease the exposure to **glasdegib**. Avoid. [Severe] Study → Also see **TABLE 7** p. 1055
- **Grapefruit** and grapefruit juice are predicted to increase the exposure to **ivosidenib**. Avoid. [Moderate] Study
- **Ivosidenib** is predicted to decrease the exposure to **grazoprevir**. Avoid. [Severe] Study
- **Ivosidenib** is predicted to decrease the concentration of **guanfacine**. Adjust **guanfacine** dose, p. 281. [Moderate] Study
- **Ivosidenib** is predicted to increase the exposure to H_2 receptor antagonists **(cimetidine, famotidine)**. Use with caution or avoid. [Moderate] Theoretical
- **Ivosidenib** decreases the concentration of **haloperidol**. Adjust dose. [Moderate] Study → Also see **TABLE 7** p. 1055
- **HIV-protease inhibitors** are predicted to increase the exposure to **ivosidenib**. Monitor and adjust dose—consult product literature. [Severe] Study
- **Ivosidenib** is predicted to decrease the exposure to **ibrutinib**. Avoid or monitor. [Severe] Study
- **Idelalisib** is predicted to increase the exposure to **ivosidenib**. Monitor and adjust dose—consult product literature. [Severe] Study
- **Ivosidenib** is predicted to decrease the exposure to **idelalisib**. Avoid. [Severe] Study

Ivosidenib (continued)
- **Imatinib** is predicted to increase the exposure to **ivosidenib**. Monitor and adjust dose—consult product literature. Severe Study
- **Ivosidenib** is predicted to decrease the exposure to **imatinib**. Avoid. Moderate Study
- **Ivosidenib** is predicted to decrease the exposure to **irinotecan**. Avoid. Severe Study
- **Ivosidenib** is predicted to decrease the exposure to **ivabradine**. Adjust dose. Moderate Theoretical
- **Ivosidenib** is predicted to decrease the exposure to **ivacaftor**. Avoid. Severe Study
- **Ivosidenib** is predicted to decrease the exposure to **ixazomib**. Avoid. Severe Study
- **Ivosidenib** is predicted to decrease the exposure to **ketamine**. Adjust dose. Moderate Theoretical
- **Ivosidenib** is predicted to decrease the exposure to **lapatinib**. Avoid. Severe Study → Also see TABLE 7 p. 1055
- **Ivosidenib** is predicted to moderately decrease the exposure to **larotrectinib**. Avoid. Moderate Study
- **Ivosidenib** is predicted to decrease the exposure to **lazertinib**. Avoid. Severe Study
- **Ivosidenib** is predicted to decrease the exposure to **lenacapavir**. Avoid. Severe Study
- **Ivosidenib** is predicted to decrease the exposure to **leniolisib**. Avoid. Severe Theoretical
- **Letermovir** is predicted to increase the exposure to **ivosidenib**. Monitor and adjust dose—consult product literature. Severe Study
- **Ivosidenib** is predicted to decrease the exposure to **lomitapide**. Monitor and adjust dose. Moderate Theoretical
- **Ivosidenib** is predicted to increase the exposure to loop diuretics **(furosemide)**. Manufacturer advises caution or avoid—consult product literature. Moderate Theoretical
- **Ivosidenib** is predicted to alter the exposure to **loperamide**. Moderate Theoretical
- **Ivosidenib** is predicted to decrease the exposure to **lorlatinib**. Avoid. Severe Study
- Macrolides **(clarithromycin, erythromycin)** are predicted to increase the exposure to **ivosidenib**. Monitor and adjust dose—consult product literature. Severe Study → Also see TABLE 7 p. 1055
- **Ivosidenib** is predicted to decrease the exposure to **maraviroc**. Adjust dose. Severe Study
- **Ivosidenib** is predicted to decrease the exposure to **mavacamten**. Monitor and adjust dose—consult product literature. Severe Theoretical
- **Ivosidenib** is predicted to decrease the exposure to meglitinides **(repaglinide)**. Monitor blood glucose and adjust dose. Moderate Study
- **Ivosidenib** is predicted to increase the exposure to **methotrexate**. Use with caution or avoid. Moderate Theoretical
- **Ivosidenib** is predicted to decrease the exposure to **midostaurin**. Avoid. Severe Study
- **Ivosidenib** is predicted to decrease the exposure to **mifepristone**. Adjust **mifepristone** dose. Severe Study
- **Ivosidenib** is predicted to decrease the exposure to mineralocorticoid receptor antagonists **(eplerenone)**. Avoid. Moderate Theoretical
- **Ivosidenib** is predicted to decrease the exposure to mineralocorticoid receptor antagonists **(finerenone)**. Avoid. Severe Study
- **Ivosidenib** is predicted to decrease the exposure to **mirtazapine**. Adjust dose. Moderate Study
- **Mitotane** is predicted to decrease the exposure to **ivosidenib**. Avoid. Severe Theoretical
- **Ivosidenib** is predicted to decrease the exposure to monoclonal antibodies **(polatuzumab vedotin)**. Moderate Theoretical
- **Ivosidenib** is predicted to decrease the exposure to the cytotoxic component of monoclonal antibodies **(trastuzumab emtansine)**. Severe Theoretical
- **Ivosidenib** is predicted to decrease the exposure to **montelukast**. Mild Study
- **Ivosidenib** is predicted to markedly decrease the exposure to **naldemedine**. Avoid. Severe Study
- **Ivosidenib** is predicted to markedly decrease the exposure to **naloxegol**. Avoid. Moderate Study
- **Ivosidenib** is predicted to decrease the exposure to **neratinib**. Avoid. Severe Study
- Neurokinin-1 receptor antagonists **(aprepitant, netupitant)** are predicted to increase the exposure to **ivosidenib**. Monitor and adjust dose—consult product literature. Severe Study
- **Ivosidenib** is predicted to markedly decrease the exposure to neurokinin-1 receptor antagonists **(aprepitant)**. Avoid. Moderate Study
- **Ivosidenib** is predicted to decrease the exposure to neurokinin-1 receptor antagonists **(fosaprepitant)**. Avoid. Moderate Theoretical
- **Ivosidenib** is predicted to decrease the exposure to neurokinin-1 receptor antagonists **(netupitant)**. Avoid. Severe Study
- **Nilotinib** is predicted to increase the exposure to **ivosidenib**. Monitor and adjust dose—consult product literature. Severe Study → Also see TABLE 7 p. 1055
- **Ivosidenib** is predicted to moderately decrease the exposure to **nilotinib**. Avoid. Severe Study → Also see TABLE 7 p. 1055
- **Nirmatrelvir** boosted with ritonavir is predicted to increase the concentration of **ivosidenib**. Monitor and adjust dose—consult product literature. Severe Theoretical
- **Ivosidenib** is predicted to decrease the exposure to **nirmatrelvir** boosted with ritonavir. Avoid. Severe Study
- **Ivosidenib** is predicted to decrease the exposure to **nitisinone**. Adjust dose. Moderate Theoretical
- **Ivosidenib** is predicted to decrease the exposure to NNRTIs **(doravirine)**. Avoid. Severe Study
- **Ivosidenib** is predicted to decrease the exposure to NNRTIs **(etravirine)**. Avoid. Severe Theoretical
- **Ivosidenib** markedly decreases the exposure to NNRTIs **(rilpivirine)**. Avoid. Severe Study
- **Ivosidenib** is predicted to decrease the exposure to **olaparib**. Avoid. Moderate Theoretical
- **Ivosidenib** is predicted to decrease the exposure to **omaveloxolone**. Avoid. Severe Study
- **Ivosidenib** is predicted to decrease the exposure to opioids **(alfentanil, fentanyl)**. Moderate Study
- **Ivosidenib** is predicted to decrease the exposure to opioids **(buprenorphine)**. Monitor and adjust dose. Moderate Theoretical
- **Ivosidenib** decreases the exposure to opioids **(methadone)**. Monitor and adjust dose. Severe Study → Also see TABLE 7 p. 1055
- **Ivosidenib** is predicted to decrease the exposure to opioids **(oxycodone)**. Monitor and adjust dose. Moderate Study
- **Ivosidenib** is predicted to increase the exposure to the active metabolite of **oseltamivir**. Use with caution or avoid. Moderate Theoretical
- **Ivosidenib** is predicted to decrease the exposure to **osilodrostat**. Moderate Theoretical → Also see TABLE 7 p. 1055
- **Ivosidenib** is predicted to moderately decrease the exposure to **osimertinib**. Avoid. Moderate Study → Also see TABLE 7 p. 1055
- **Ivosidenib** is predicted to moderately decrease the exposure to **ospemifene**. Moderate Study
- **Ivosidenib** is predicted to decrease the exposure to **palbociclib**. Avoid. Severe Study
- **Ivosidenib** is predicted to decrease the exposure to **panobinostat**. Avoid. Moderate Theoretical → Also see TABLE 7 p. 1055
- **Ivosidenib** is predicted to decrease the exposure to **pazopanib**. Avoid. Severe Theoretical → Also see TABLE 7 p. 1055
- **Ivosidenib** is predicted to decrease the exposure to **pemigatinib**. Avoid. Severe Study
- **Ivosidenib** is predicted to increase the exposure to penicillins **(benzylpenicillin)**. Use with caution or avoid. Moderate Theoretical
- **Ivosidenib** moderately decreases the exposure to phosphodiesterase type-4 inhibitors **(apremilast)**. Avoid. Severe Study
- **Ivosidenib** is predicted to decrease the exposure to phosphodiesterase type-4 inhibitors **(roflumilast)**. Avoid. Moderate Study
- **Ivosidenib** is predicted to decrease the exposure to phosphodiesterase type-5 inhibitors **(avanafil, tadalafil)**. Avoid. Severe Study

- **Ivosidenib** is predicted to decrease the exposure to phosphodiesterase type-5 inhibitors **(sildenafil, vardenafil)**. [Moderate] Theoretical → Also see TABLE 7 p. 1055
- **Ivosidenib** is predicted to moderately to markedly decrease the exposure to **pibrentasvir**. Avoid. [Severe] Study
- **Ivosidenib** might decrease the exposure to **pimozide**. Avoid or monitor efficacy. [Moderate] Theoretical → Also see TABLE 7 p. 1055
- **Ivosidenib** might decrease the exposure to **pioglitazone**. Avoid or monitor efficacy. [Unknown] Study
- **Ivosidenib** is predicted to decrease the exposure to **pirtobrutinib**. Avoid. [Moderate] Study
- **Ivosidenib** is predicted to moderately decrease the exposure to **pitolisant**. [Moderate] Study
- **Ivosidenib** is predicted to decrease the exposure to **ponatinib**. Avoid. [Moderate] Theoretical
- **Ivosidenib** is predicted to decrease the exposure to **pralsetinib**. Avoid or adjust dose with potent CYP3A4 inducers—consult product literature. [Moderate] Study
- **Ivosidenib** is predicted to markedly decrease the exposure to **praziquantel**. Avoid. [Moderate] Study
- **Ivosidenib** might decrease the exposure to proton pump inhibitors **(omeprazole)**. Avoid or monitor efficacy. [Unknown] Theoretical
- **Ivosidenib** is predicted to decrease the exposure to **quizartinib**. Avoid. [Severe] Study → Also see TABLE 7 p. 1055
- **Ivosidenib** might decrease the exposure to **raltegravir**. Avoid or monitor efficacy. [Unknown] Theoretical
- **Ivosidenib** is predicted to decrease the exposure to **ranolazine**. Avoid. [Severe] Study → Also see TABLE 7 p. 1055
- **Ivosidenib** is predicted to decrease the exposure to **reboxetine**. [Moderate] Anecdotal
- **Ivosidenib** is predicted to decrease the exposure to **regorafenib**. Avoid. [Moderate] Study
- **Ivosidenib** is predicted to markedly decrease the exposure to **ribociclib**. Avoid. [Severe] Study → Also see TABLE 7 p. 1055
- Rifamycins **(rifampicin)** are predicted to decrease the exposure to **ivosidenib**. Avoid. [Severe] Theoretical
- **Ivosidenib** is predicted to decrease the exposure to **rimegepant**. Avoid. [Moderate] Theoretical
- **Ivosidenib** is predicted to decrease the exposure to **ripretinib**. Avoid or adjust dose—consult product literature. [Severe] Study
- **Ivosidenib** is predicted to decrease the exposure to **ruxolitinib**. Monitor and adjust dose. [Moderate] Study
- **Ivosidenib** is predicted to decrease the exposure to **selpercatinib**. Avoid. [Moderate] Study → Also see TABLE 7 p. 1055
- **Ivosidenib** is predicted to decrease the exposure to **selumetinib**. Avoid. [Severe] Study
- **Ivosidenib** is predicted to decrease the exposure to **siponimod**. Manufacturer advises caution depending on genotype—consult product literature. [Severe] Study
- **Ivosidenib** is predicted to decrease the concentration of **sirolimus**. Avoid or monitor and adjust dose. [Severe] Study
- **Ivosidenib** is predicted to decrease the exposure to **solifenacin**. [Moderate] Theoretical
- **Ivosidenib** is predicted to decrease the exposure to **sorafenib**. [Moderate] Theoretical → Also see TABLE 7 p. 1055
- **Ivosidenib** is predicted to decrease the exposure to **sotorasib**. Avoid. [Severe] Study
- **Ivosidenib** is predicted to decrease the exposure to **sparsentan**. Avoid. [Severe] Theoretical
- **St John's wort** is predicted to decreases the exposure to **ivosidenib**. Avoid. [Moderate] Theoretical
- **Ivosidenib** is predicted to increase the exposure to statins **(atorvastatin, pravastatin, rosuvastatin)**. Use with caution or avoid. [Unknown] Theoretical
- **Ivosidenib** might affect the exposure to statins **(simvastatin)**. Avoid or monitor. [Moderate] Theoretical
- **Ivosidenib** is predicted to decrease the exposure to **sunitinib**. Avoid or adjust dose—consult product literature. [Moderate] Study → Also see TABLE 7 p. 1055
- **Ivosidenib** decreases the concentration of **tacrolimus**. Avoid or monitor and adjust dose. [Severe] Study
- **Ivosidenib** is predicted to alter the exposure to **talazoparib**. [Moderate] Theoretical
- **Ivosidenib** is predicted to decrease the exposure to taxanes **(cabazitaxel)**. Avoid. [Moderate] Study
- **Ivosidenib** is predicted to decrease the exposure to taxanes **(docetaxel)**. [Severe] Theoretical
- **Ivosidenib** is predicted to decrease the exposure to taxanes **(paclitaxel)**. Avoid. [Severe] Study
- **Ivosidenib** is predicted to decrease the concentration of **temsirolimus**. Avoid. [Severe] Study
- **Ivosidenib** is predicted to decrease the exposure to tetracyclines **(eravacycline)**. Adjust **eravacycline** dose. [Moderate] Study
- **Ivosidenib** is predicted to decrease the exposure to **tezacaftor**. Avoid. [Severe] Theoretical
- **Ivosidenib** is predicted to alter the exposure to thrombin inhibitors **(dabigatran)**. Avoid. [Moderate] Theoretical
- **Ivosidenib** is predicted to markedly decrease the exposure to **ticagrelor**. Avoid. [Severe] Study
- **Ivosidenib** is predicted to decrease the exposure to the cytotoxic component of **tisotumab vedotin**. [Moderate] Theoretical
- **Ivosidenib** is predicted to decrease the exposure to **tivozanib**. [Severe] Study
- **Ivosidenib** is predicted to decrease the exposure to **tofacitinib**. Avoid. [Severe] Study
- **Ivosidenib** is predicted to decrease the exposure to **tolvaptan**. Use with caution or avoid depending on indication. [Severe] Study
- **Ivosidenib** is predicted to decrease the exposure to **toremifene**. Adjust dose. [Moderate] Study → Also see TABLE 7 p. 1055
- **Ivosidenib** is predicted to decrease the exposure to **trabectedin**. Avoid. [Severe] Theoretical
- **Ivosidenib** might decrease the exposure to triptans **(eletriptan)**. Avoid or monitor. [Moderate] Theoretical
- **Ivosidenib** is predicted to decrease the exposure to **tucatinib**. Avoid. [Severe] Study
- **Ivosidenib** is predicted to decrease the exposure to **upadacitinib**. [Moderate] Study
- **Ivosidenib** is predicted to decrease the exposure to **vandetanib**. Avoid. [Moderate] Study → Also see TABLE 7 p. 1055
- **Ivosidenib** is predicted to decrease the exposure to **vanzacaftor**. Avoid. [Severe] Theoretical
- **Ivosidenib** is predicted to moderately decrease the exposure to **velpatasvir**. Avoid. [Severe] Study
- **Ivosidenib** is predicted to decrease the exposure to **vemurafenib**. Avoid. [Severe] Study → Also see TABLE 7 p. 1055
- **Ivosidenib** is predicted to decrease the exposure to **venetoclax**. Avoid. [Severe] Study
- **Ivosidenib** is predicted to decrease the exposure to vinca alkaloids **(vinblastine, vincristine, vindesine)**. [Severe] Theoretical
- **Ivosidenib** is predicted to decrease the exposure to vinca alkaloids **(vinorelbine)**. Use with caution or avoid. [Severe] Theoretical
- **Ivosidenib** is predicted to decrease the exposure to **vismodegib**. Avoid. [Moderate] Theoretical
- **Ivosidenib** is predicted to decrease the exposure to **voclosporin**. Avoid. [Severe] Study → Also see TABLE 7 p. 1055
- **Ivosidenib** is predicted to decrease the exposure to **vortioxetine**. Monitor and adjust dose. [Moderate] Study
- **Ivosidenib** is predicted to decrease the concentration of **voxilaprevir**. Avoid. [Severe] Study
- **Ivosidenib** is predicted to decrease the exposure to **zanubrutinib**. Avoid. [Severe] Study
- **Ivosidenib** is predicted to decrease the exposure to **zopiclone**. Adjust dose. [Moderate] Study

Ixazomib

- Anti-androgens **(apalutamide, enzalutamide)** are predicted to decrease the exposure to **ixazomib**. Avoid. [Severe] Study
- Antiepileptics **(carbamazepine, fosphenytoin, phenobarbital, phenytoin, primidone)** are predicted to decrease the exposure to **ixazomib**. Avoid. [Severe] Study
- **Cenobamate** is predicted to decrease the exposure to **ixazomib**. [Moderate] Theoretical
- **Dabrafenib** is predicted to decrease the exposure to **ixazomib**. [Moderate] Theoretical
- **Encorafenib** is predicted to decrease the exposure to **ixazomib**. Avoid. [Severe] Study

Ixazomib (continued)
- Endothelin receptor antagonists **(bosentan)** are predicted to decrease the exposure to **ixazomib**. Moderate Theoretical
- **Ivosidenib** is predicted to decrease the exposure to **ixazomib**. Avoid. Severe Study
- **Lorlatinib** is predicted to decrease the exposure to **ixazomib**. Moderate Theoretical
- **Lumacaftor** is predicted to decrease the exposure to **ixazomib**. Avoid. Severe Study
- **Mitotane** is predicted to decrease the exposure to **ixazomib**. Avoid. Severe Study
- NNRTIs **(efavirenz, etravirine, nevirapine)** are predicted to decrease the exposure to **ixazomib**. Moderate Theoretical
- Rifamycins **(rifampicin)** are predicted to decrease the exposure to **ixazomib**. Avoid. Severe Study
- **Sotorasib** is predicted to decrease the exposure to **ixazomib**. Moderate Theoretical
- **St John's wort** is predicted to decrease the exposure to **ixazomib**. Avoid. Severe Theoretical

Ixekizumab → see monoclonal antibodies

Kaolin
- Oral **kaolin** decreases the absorption of oral antimalarials **(chloroquine)**. Separate administration by at least 4 hours. Moderate Study
- Oral **kaolin** is predicted to decrease the absorption of oral **hydroxychloroquine**. Moderate Theoretical
- Oral **kaolin** is predicted to decrease the absorption of oral **tetracyclines**. Moderate Theoretical

Ketamine → see TABLE 6 p. 1054 (hypotension), TABLE 9 p. 1056 (CNS effects)
- Anti-androgens **(apalutamide, enzalutamide)** are predicted to decrease the exposure to **ketamine**. Adjust dose. Moderate Theoretical
- Antiepileptics **(carbamazepine, fosphenytoin, phenobarbital, phenytoin, primidone)** are predicted to decrease the exposure to **ketamine**. Adjust dose. Moderate Theoretical → Also see TABLE 9 p. 1056
- Antifungals, azoles **(itraconazole, ketoconazole, posaconazole, voriconazole)** are predicted to increase the exposure to **ketamine**. Adjust dose. Moderate Theoretical
- **Ceritinib** is predicted to increase the exposure to **ketamine**. Adjust dose. Moderate Theoretical
- **Cobicistat** is predicted to increase the exposure to **ketamine**. Adjust dose. Moderate Theoretical
- **Encorafenib** is predicted to decrease the exposure to **ketamine**. Adjust dose. Moderate Theoretical
- **Ketamine** is predicted to increase the risk of elevated blood pressure when given with **ergometrine**. Severe Theoretical
- **HIV-protease inhibitors** are predicted to increase the exposure to **ketamine**. Adjust dose. Moderate Theoretical
- **Idelalisib** is predicted to increase the exposure to **ketamine**. Adjust dose. Moderate Theoretical
- **Ivosidenib** is predicted to decrease the exposure to **ketamine**. Adjust dose. Moderate Theoretical
- **Lumacaftor** is predicted to decrease the exposure to **ketamine**. Adjust dose. Moderate Theoretical
- Macrolides **(clarithromycin)** are predicted to increase the exposure to **ketamine**. Adjust dose. Moderate Theoretical
- **Memantine** is predicted to increase the risk of CNS adverse effects when given with **ketamine**. Avoid. Severe Theoretical
- **Mitotane** is predicted to decrease the exposure to **ketamine**. Adjust dose. Moderate Theoretical
- Rifamycins **(rifampicin)** are predicted to decrease the exposure to **ketamine**. Adjust dose. Moderate Theoretical
- **St John's wort** is predicted to decrease the exposure to **ketamine**. Adjust dose. Moderate Theoretical
- **Tucatinib** is predicted to increase the exposure to **ketamine**. Adjust dose. Moderate Theoretical

Ketoconazole → see antifungals, azoles

Ketoprofen → see NSAIDs

Ketorolac → see NSAIDs

Ketotifen → see antihistamines, sedating

Labetalol → see beta blockers, non-selective

Lacidipine → see calcium-channel blockers

Lacosamide → see antiepileptics

Lamivudine → see NRTIs

Lamotrigine → see antiepileptics

Landiolol → see beta blockers, selective

Lanreotide
- **Beta blockers, non-selective** are predicted to increase the risk of bradycardia when given with **lanreotide**. Moderate Theoretical
- **Beta blockers, selective** are predicted to increase the risk of bradycardia when given with **lanreotide**. Moderate Theoretical
- **Lanreotide** is predicted to decrease the absorption of oral **ciclosporin**. Adjust dose. Severe Theoretical

Lansoprazole → see proton pump inhibitors

Lanthanum
- **Lanthanum** is predicted to decrease the absorption of antifungals, azoles **(ketoconazole)**. Separate administration by at least 2 hours. Moderate Theoretical
- **Lanthanum** is predicted to decrease the absorption of antimalarials **(chloroquine)**. Separate administration by at least 2 hours. Moderate Theoretical
- **Lanthanum** is predicted to decrease the absorption of **hydroxychloroquine**. Separate administration by at least 2 hours. Moderate Theoretical
- **Lanthanum** moderately decreases the exposure to **quinolones**. **Quinolones** should be taken 2 hours before or 4 hours after **lanthanum**. Moderate Study
- Oral **lanthanum** might decrease the absorption of oral **tetracyclines**. Separate administration by 2 hours. Moderate Theoretical
- **Lanthanum** decreases the absorption of **thyroid hormones**. Separate administration by 2 hours. Moderate Study
- Oral **lanthanum** is predicted to decrease the exposure to oral **vadadustat**. Manufacturer advises take at least 1 hour before or 2 hours after **lanthanum**. Moderate Theoretical

Lapatinib → see TABLE 7 p. 1055 (QT-interval prolongation)
- **Lapatinib** is predicted to increase the exposure to **afatinib**. Moderate Study
- **Lapatinib** is predicted to increase the exposure to **aliskiren**. Moderate Theoretical
- **Lapatinib** is predicted to increase the exposure to **alpelisib**. Moderate Theoretical
- Oral **antacids** is predicted to decrease the absorption of oral **lapatinib**. Avoid. Moderate Theoretical
- Anti-androgens **(apalutamide, enzalutamide)** are predicted to decrease the exposure to **lapatinib**. Avoid. Severe Study → Also see TABLE 7 p. 1055
- Antiarrhythmics **(dronedarone)** are predicted to increase the exposure to **lapatinib**. Moderate Study → Also see TABLE 7 p. 1055
- Antiepileptics **(carbamazepine, fosphenytoin, phenobarbital, phenytoin, primidone)** are predicted to decrease the exposure to **lapatinib**. Avoid. Severe Study
- Antifungals, azoles **(fluconazole, isavuconazole)** are predicted to increase the exposure to **lapatinib**. Moderate Study → Also see TABLE 7 p. 1055
- Antifungals, azoles **(itraconazole, ketoconazole, posaconazole, voriconazole)** are predicted to increase the exposure to **lapatinib**. Avoid. Moderate Study → Also see TABLE 7 p. 1055
- **Lapatinib** is predicted to increase the exposure to antihistamines, non-sedating **(fexofenadine)**. Moderate Theoretical
- **Berotralstat** is predicted to increase the exposure to **lapatinib**. Moderate Study
- **Lapatinib** is predicted to increase the exposure to beta blockers, non-selective **(nadolol)**. Moderate Study
- Oral calcium compounds **(calcium carbonate)** -containing antacids are predicted to decrease the absorption of oral **lapatinib**. Avoid. Moderate Theoretical
- Calcium-channel blockers **(diltiazem, verapamil)** are predicted to increase the exposure to **lapatinib**. Moderate Study
- **Cenobamate** is predicted to decrease the exposure to **lapatinib**. Avoid. Severe Study
- **Lapatinib** is predicted to increase the exposure to **ceritinib**. Moderate Theoretical → Also see TABLE 7 p. 1055
- **Ceritinib** is predicted to increase the exposure to **lapatinib**. Avoid. Moderate Study → Also see TABLE 7 p. 1055
- **Ciclosporin** might increase the concentration of **lapatinib**. Severe Theoretical

- Cobicistat is predicted to increase the exposure to **lapatinib**. Avoid. Moderate Study
- **Lapatinib** is predicted to increase the exposure to colchicine. Avoid P-glycoprotein inhibitors or adjust **colchicine** dose, p. 637. Severe Theoretical
- **Lapatinib** is predicted to increase the risk of bleeding events when given with coumarins. Severe Theoretical
- Crizotinib is predicted to increase the exposure to **lapatinib**. Moderate Study → Also see TABLE 7 p. 1055
- Dabrafenib is predicted to decrease the exposure to **lapatinib**. Avoid. Severe Study
- **Lapatinib** slightly increases the exposure to digoxin. Moderate Study
- Encorafenib is predicted to decrease the exposure to **lapatinib**. Avoid. Severe Study → Also see TABLE 7 p. 1055
- Endothelin receptor antagonists (bosentan) are predicted to decrease the exposure to **lapatinib**. Avoid. Severe Study
- **Lapatinib** is predicted to increase the exposure to erlotinib. Moderate Theoretical
- **Lapatinib** is predicted to increase the exposure to everolimus. Moderate Theoretical
- **Lapatinib** is predicted to increase the exposure to factor XA inhibitors (apixaban). Moderate Theoretical
- **Lapatinib** is predicted to slightly increase the exposure to factor XA inhibitors (edoxaban). Severe Theoretical
- **Lapatinib** might increase the exposure to factor XA inhibitors (rivaroxaban). Manufacturer advises caution in renal impairment. Moderate Theoretical
- Fedratinib is predicted to increase the exposure to **lapatinib**. Moderate Study
- **Lapatinib** is predicted to increase the exposure to fidaxomicin. Avoid. Moderate Study
- **Lapatinib** is predicted to increase the exposure to gilteritinib. Moderate Theoretical
- Grapefruit juice is predicted to increase the exposure to **lapatinib**. Avoid. Moderate Theoretical
- **Lapatinib** is predicted to increase the exposure to grazoprevir. Avoid. Severe Theoretical
- H_2 receptor antagonists are predicted to decrease the absorption of **lapatinib**. Avoid. Moderate Theoretical
- HIV-protease inhibitors are predicted to increase the exposure to **lapatinib**. Avoid. Moderate Study
- Idelalisib is predicted to increase the exposure to **lapatinib**. Avoid. Moderate Study
- Imatinib is predicted to increase the exposure to **lapatinib**. Moderate Study
- **Lapatinib** increases the exposure to the active metabolite of irinotecan. Monitor adverse effects and adjust dose. Severe Study
- Ivosidenib is predicted to decrease the exposure to **lapatinib**. Avoid. Severe Study → Also see TABLE 7 p. 1055
- Letermovir is predicted to increase the exposure to **lapatinib**. Moderate Study
- **Lapatinib** is predicted to increase the exposure to lomitapide. Separate administration by 12 hours. Mild Theoretical
- **Lapatinib** is predicted to increase the exposure to loperamide. Moderate Theoretical
- Lorlatinib is predicted to decrease the exposure to **lapatinib**. Avoid. Severe Study
- Lumacaftor is predicted to decrease the exposure to **lapatinib**. Avoid. Severe Study
- Macrolides (clarithromycin) are predicted to increase the exposure to **lapatinib**. Avoid. Moderate Study
- Macrolides (erythromycin) are predicted to increase the exposure to **lapatinib**. Moderate Study → Also see TABLE 7 p. 1055
- **Lapatinib** is predicted to increase the exposure to mavacamten. Monitor and adjust dose—consult product literature. Moderate Theoretical
- Mitotane is predicted to decrease the exposure to **lapatinib**. Avoid. Severe Study
- **Lapatinib** increases the risk of neutropenia when given with monoclonal antibodies (brentuximab vedotin). Monitor and adjust dose. Severe Theoretical
- Neurokinin-1 receptor antagonists (aprepitant, netupitant) are predicted to increase the exposure to **lapatinib**. Moderate Study
- Nilotinib is predicted to increase the exposure to **lapatinib**. Moderate Study → Also see TABLE 7 p. 1055
- **Lapatinib** is predicted to increase the exposure to nintedanib. Moderate Study
- NNRTIs (efavirenz, etravirine, nevirapine) are predicted to decrease the exposure to **lapatinib**. Avoid. Severe Study → Also see TABLE 7 p. 1055
- **Lapatinib** is predicted to increase the exposure to panobinostat. Adjust dose. Moderate Theoretical → Also see TABLE 7 p. 1055
- **Lapatinib** increases the exposure to pazopanib. Avoid. Severe Study → Also see TABLE 7 p. 1055
- **Lapatinib** is predicted to increase the risk of bleeding events when given with phenindione. Severe Theoretical
- Pitolisant is predicted to decrease the exposure to **lapatinib**. Avoid. Severe Theoretical
- **Lapatinib** is predicted to increase the exposure to pralsetinib. Moderate Theoretical
- **Lapatinib** is predicted to increase the exposure to ranolazine. Moderate Theoretical → Also see TABLE 7 p. 1055
- **Lapatinib** is predicted to increase the exposure to relugolix. Avoid or take relugolix first and separate administration by at least 6 hours. Moderate Study
- Rifamycins (rifampicin) are predicted to decrease the exposure to **lapatinib**. Avoid. Severe Study
- **Lapatinib** is predicted to increase the exposure to rimegepant. Avoid another dose of rimegepant within 48 hours of concurrent use. Moderate Theoretical
- **Lapatinib** is predicted to increase the exposure to the active component of sacituzumab govitecan. Severe Theoretical
- **Lapatinib** is predicted to increase the exposure to sirolimus. Moderate Theoretical
- Oral sodium bicarbonate-containing antacids are predicted to decrease the absorption of oral **lapatinib**. Avoid. Moderate Theoretical
- Sotorasib is predicted to decrease the exposure to **lapatinib**. Avoid. Severe Study
- St John's wort is predicted to decrease the exposure to **lapatinib**. Avoid. Severe Study
- **Lapatinib** is predicted to slightly increase the exposure to talazoparib. Avoid or adjust dose—consult product literature. Severe Study
- **Lapatinib** slightly increases the exposure to taxanes (paclitaxel). Severe Study
- Tedizolid is predicted to increase the exposure to **lapatinib**. Avoid. Moderate Theoretical
- **Lapatinib** is predicted to increase the exposure to thrombin inhibitors (dabigatran). Severe Theoretical
- **Lapatinib** might increase the exposure to tigecycline. Mild Anecdotal
- **Lapatinib** is predicted to increase the exposure to topotecan. Severe Study
- **Lapatinib** is predicted to increase the concentration of trametinib. Moderate Theoretical
- Tucatinib is predicted to increase the exposure to **lapatinib**. Avoid. Moderate Study
- **Lapatinib** is predicted to increase the exposure to venetoclax. Avoid or monitor for toxicity. Severe Theoretical
- **Lapatinib** might increase the exposure to vinca alkaloids. Severe Theoretical

Laronidase

- Antimalarials (chloroquine) are predicted to decrease the exposure to **laronidase**. Avoid simultaneous administration. Severe Theoretical
- Hydroxychloroquine is predicted to decrease the exposure to **laronidase**. Avoid simultaneous administration. Severe Theoretical

Larotrectinib

- Anti-androgens (apalutamide, enzalutamide) are predicted to moderately decrease the exposure to **larotrectinib**. Avoid. Moderate Study
- Antiarrhythmics (dronedarone) are predicted to increase the exposure to **larotrectinib**. Monitor and adjust dose. Moderate Theoretical

Larotrectinib (continued)

- Antiepileptics **(carbamazepine, fosphenytoin, phenobarbital, phenytoin, primidone)** are predicted to moderately decrease the exposure to **larotrectinib**. Avoid. [Moderate] Study
- Antifungals, azoles **(fluconazole, isavuconazole)** are predicted to increase the exposure to **larotrectinib**. Monitor and adjust dose. [Moderate] Theoretical
- Antifungals, azoles **(itraconazole, ketoconazole, posaconazole, voriconazole)** are predicted to moderately increase the exposure to **larotrectinib**. Avoid or adjust dose—consult product literature. [Moderate] Study
- **Larotrectinib** slightly increases the exposure to benzodiazepines **(midazolam)**. Use with caution and adjust dose. [Mild] Study
- **Berotralstat** is predicted to increase the exposure to **larotrectinib**. Monitor and adjust dose. [Moderate] Theoretical
- Calcium-channel blockers **(diltiazem, verapamil)** are predicted to increase the exposure to **larotrectinib**. Monitor and adjust dose. [Moderate] Theoretical
- **Cenobamate** is predicted to decrease the exposure to **larotrectinib**. Avoid. [Moderate] Study
- **Ceritinib** is predicted to moderately increase the exposure to **larotrectinib**. Avoid or adjust dose—consult product literature. [Moderate] Study
- **Larotrectinib** is predicted to increase the exposure to **ciclosporin**. Use with caution and adjust dose. [Mild] Theoretical
- **Cobicistat** is predicted to moderately increase the exposure to **larotrectinib**. Avoid or adjust dose—consult product literature. [Moderate] Study
- **Larotrectinib** potentially decreases the efficacy of **combined hormonal contraceptives**. Use additional contraceptive precautions. [Severe] Theoretical
- **Crizotinib** is predicted to increase the exposure to **larotrectinib**. Monitor and adjust dose. [Moderate] Theoretical
- **Dabrafenib** is predicted to decrease the exposure to **larotrectinib**. Avoid. [Moderate] Study
- **Encorafenib** is predicted to moderately decrease the exposure to **larotrectinib**. Avoid. [Moderate] Study
- Endothelin receptor antagonists **(bosentan)** are predicted to decrease the exposure to **larotrectinib**. Avoid. [Moderate] Study
- **Larotrectinib** is predicted to increase the exposure to **everolimus**. Use with caution and adjust dose. [Mild] Theoretical
- **Fedratinib** is predicted to increase the exposure to **larotrectinib**. Monitor and adjust dose. [Moderate] Theoretical
- **Grapefruit** juice is predicted to increase the exposure to **larotrectinib**. Avoid. [Moderate] Theoretical
- **HIV-protease inhibitors** are predicted to moderately increase the exposure to **larotrectinib**. Avoid or adjust dose—consult product literature. [Moderate] Study
- **Idelalisib** is predicted to moderately increase the exposure to **larotrectinib**. Avoid or adjust dose—consult product literature. [Moderate] Study
- **Imatinib** is predicted to increase the exposure to **larotrectinib**. Monitor and adjust dose. [Moderate] Theoretical
- **Ivosidenib** is predicted to moderately decrease the exposure to **larotrectinib**. Avoid. [Moderate] Study
- **Letermovir** is predicted to increase the exposure to **larotrectinib**. Monitor and adjust dose. [Moderate] Theoretical
- **Lorlatinib** is predicted to decrease the exposure to **larotrectinib**. Avoid. [Moderate] Study
- **Lumacaftor** is predicted to moderately decrease the exposure to **larotrectinib**. Avoid. [Moderate] Study
- Macrolides **(clarithromycin)** are predicted to moderately increase the exposure to **larotrectinib**. Avoid or adjust dose—consult product literature. [Moderate] Study
- Macrolides **(erythromycin)** are predicted to increase the exposure to **larotrectinib**. Monitor and adjust dose. [Moderate] Theoretical
- **Larotrectinib** is predicted to increase the exposure to **mavacamten**. Monitor and adjust dose—consult product literature. [Moderate] Theoretical
- **Mitotane** is predicted to moderately decrease the exposure to **larotrectinib**. Avoid. [Moderate] Study
- Neurokinin-1 receptor antagonists **(aprepitant, netupitant)** are predicted to increase the exposure to **larotrectinib**. Monitor and adjust dose. [Moderate] Theoretical
- **Nilotinib** is predicted to increase the exposure to **larotrectinib**. Monitor and adjust dose. [Moderate] Theoretical
- NNRTIs **(efavirenz, etravirine, nevirapine)** are predicted to decrease the exposure to **larotrectinib**. Avoid. [Moderate] Study
- **Larotrectinib** is predicted to increase the exposure to opioids **(alfentanil, fentanyl)**. Use with caution and adjust dose. [Mild] Theoretical
- **Larotrectinib** is predicted to increase the exposure to **pimozide**. Use with caution and adjust dose. [Mild] Theoretical
- Rifamycins **(rifampicin)** are predicted to moderately decrease the exposure to **larotrectinib**. Avoid. [Moderate] Study
- **Larotrectinib** is predicted to increase the exposure to **sirolimus**. Use with caution and adjust dose. [Mild] Theoretical
- **Sotorasib** is predicted to decrease the exposure to **larotrectinib**. Avoid. [Moderate] Study
- **St John's wort** is predicted to decrease the exposure to **larotrectinib**. Avoid. [Moderate] Study
- **Larotrectinib** is predicted to increase the exposure to **tacrolimus**. Use with caution and adjust dose. [Mild] Theoretical
- **Larotrectinib** is predicted to increase the exposure to **temsirolimus**. Use with caution and adjust dose. [Mild] Theoretical
- **Tucatinib** is predicted to moderately increase the exposure to **larotrectinib**. Avoid or adjust dose—consult product literature. [Moderate] Study

Lazertinib

- Anti-androgens **(apalutamide, enzalutamide)** are predicted to decrease the exposure to **lazertinib**. Avoid. [Severe] Study
- Antiepileptics **(carbamazepine, fosphenytoin, phenobarbital, phenytoin, primidone)** are predicted to decrease the exposure to **lazertinib**. Avoid. [Severe] Study
- **Lazertinib** is predicted to increase the exposure to **ciclosporin**. [Moderate] Study
- **Encorafenib** is predicted to decrease the exposure to **lazertinib**. Avoid. [Severe] Study
- **Lazertinib** is predicted to increase the exposure to **everolimus**. [Moderate] Study
- **Ivosidenib** is predicted to decrease the exposure to **lazertinib**. Avoid. [Severe] Study
- **Lumacaftor** is predicted to decrease the exposure to **lazertinib**. Avoid. [Severe] Study
- **Mitotane** is predicted to decrease the exposure to **lazertinib**. Avoid. [Severe] Study
- **Lazertinib** is predicted to increase the exposure to opioids **(alfentanil)**. [Moderate] Study
- **Lazertinib** is predicted to increase the exposure to **pimozide**. [Moderate] Study
- Rifamycins **(rifampicin)** are predicted to decrease the exposure to **lazertinib**. Avoid. [Severe] Study
- **Lazertinib** is predicted to increase the exposure to **sirolimus**. [Moderate] Study
- **St John's wort** is predicted to decrease the exposure to **lazertinib**. Avoid. [Severe] Study
- **Lazertinib** moderately increases the exposure to statins **(rosuvastatin)**. [Moderate] Study
- **Lazertinib** is predicted to increase the exposure to **tacrolimus**. [Moderate] Study
- **Lazertinib** is predicted to increase the exposure to **temsirolimus**. [Moderate] Study

Lebrikizumab → see monoclonal antibodies

Lecanemab

- **Lecanemab** might increase the risk of brain haemorrhage when given with **alteplase**. Avoid except in life-threatening situations. [Severe] Theoretical
- **Lecanemab** can increase the risk of brain haemorrhage when given with **coumarins**. Avoid. [Severe] Anecdotal
- **Lecanemab** can increase the risk of brain haemorrhage when given with **danaparoid**. Avoid. [Severe] Anecdotal
- **Lecanemab** can increase the risk of brain haemorrhage when given with **factor XA inhibitors**. Avoid. [Severe] Anecdotal
- **Lecanemab** can increase the risk of brain haemorrhage when given with **heparin**. Avoid. [Severe] Anecdotal
- **Lecanemab** can increase the risk of brain haemorrhage when given with **low molecular-weight heparins**. Avoid. [Severe] Anecdotal

- **Lecanemab** can increase the risk of brain haemorrhage when given with **phenindione.** Avoid. Severe Anecdotal
- **Lecanemab** might increase the risk of brain haemorrhage when given with **streptokinase.** Avoid except in life-threatening situations. Severe Theoretical
- **Lecanemab** might increase the risk of brain haemorrhage when given with **tenecteplase.** Avoid except in life-threatening situations. Severe Theoretical
- **Lecanemab** can increase the risk of brain haemorrhage when given with **thrombin inhibitors**. Avoid. Severe Anecdotal
- **Lecanemab** might increase the risk of brain haemorrhage when given with **urokinase.** Avoid except in life-threatening situations. Severe Theoretical

Ledipasvir

- Oral antacids are predicted to decrease the exposure to oral **ledipasvir**. Separate administration by 4 hours. Moderate Theoretical
- **Ledipasvir** increases the risk of severe bradycardia or heart block when given with antiarrhythmics **(amiodarone).** Refer to specialist literature. Severe Anecdotal
- Antiepileptics **(carbamazepine)** are predicted to decrease the exposure to **ledipasvir.** Avoid. Severe Study
- Antiepileptics **(fosphenytoin, oxcarbazepine, phenobarbital, phenytoin, primidone)** are predicted to decrease the exposure to **ledipasvir.** Avoid. Severe Theoretical
- Oral calcium compounds **(calcium carbonate)** -containing antacids are predicted to decrease the exposure to oral **ledipasvir.** Separate administration by 4 hours. Moderate Theoretical
- **Ledipasvir** is predicted to increase the exposure to **digoxin.** Monitor and adjust dose. Moderate Theoretical
- **H_2 receptor antagonists** are predicted to decrease the exposure to **ledipasvir.** Adjust dose, see ledipasvir with sofosbuvir p. 495. Moderate Study
- **Lorlatinib** is predicted to decrease the exposure to **ledipasvir.** Avoid. Severe Study
- **Proton pump inhibitors** are predicted to decrease the exposure to **ledipasvir.** Adjust dose, see ledipasvir with sofosbuvir p. 495. Moderate Theoretical
- Rifamycins **(rifabutin)** are predicted to decrease the exposure to **ledipasvir.** Avoid. Severe Theoretical
- Rifamycins **(rifampicin)** are predicted to decrease the exposure to **ledipasvir.** Avoid. Severe Study
- **Sodium zirconium cyclosilicate** is predicted to decrease the exposure to **ledipasvir.** Separate administration by at least 2 hours. Moderate Theoretical
- **St John's wort** is predicted to decrease the exposure to **ledipasvir.** Avoid. Severe Study
- **Ledipasvir** with sofosbuvir is predicted to increase the exposure to statins **(atorvastatin).** Monitor and adjust dose. Moderate Anecdotal
- **Ledipasvir** with sofosbuvir is predicted to increase the exposure to statins **(fluvastatin, pravastatin, simvastatin).** Monitor and adjust dose. Moderate Theoretical
- **Ledipasvir** with sofosbuvir is predicted to increase the exposure to statins **(rosuvastatin).** Avoid. Severe Theoretical
- **Ledipasvir** with sofosbuvir slightly increases the exposure to **tenofovir disoproxil.** Moderate Study
- **Ledipasvir** is predicted to increase the exposure to thrombin inhibitors **(dabigatran).** Moderate Theoretical

Leflunomide → see TABLE 12 p. 1057 (myelosuppression), TABLE 10 p. 1056 (peripheral neuropathy)

PHARMACOLOGY Leflunomide has a long half-life; washout procedure recommended before switching to other DMARDs (consult product literature).

- **Leflunomide** is predicted to decrease the exposure to **agomelatine.** Moderate Theoretical
- **Leflunomide** is predicted to increase the exposure to **alpelisib.** Moderate Theoretical
- **Leflunomide** decreases the exposure to **aminophylline.** Adjust dose. Moderate Study
- **Leflunomide** is predicted to decrease the exposure to anaesthetics, local **(ropivacaine).** Moderate Theoretical
- **Leflunomide** is predicted to increase the exposure to anthracyclines **(daunorubicin, doxorubicin, mitoxantrone).** Moderate Theoretical → Also see TABLE 12 p. 1057
- **Leflunomide** is predicted to increase the exposure to antihistamines, non-sedating **(fexofenadine).** Moderate Study
- **Leflunomide** is predicted to increase the exposure to **atogepant.** Adjust **atogepant** dose. Moderate Theoretical
- **Leflunomide** is predicted to decrease the exposure to atypical antipsychotics **(clozapine).** Moderate Theoretical
- **Leflunomide** is predicted to decrease the exposure to atypical antipsychotics **(olanzapine).** Monitor and adjust dose. Moderate Study
- **Leflunomide** is predicted to increase the exposure to **baricitinib.** Moderate Study
- **Leflunomide** is predicted to moderately increase the clearance of **caffeine citrate.** Monitor and adjust dose. Moderate Study
- **Leflunomide** is predicted to increase the exposure to cephalosporins **(cefaclor).** Moderate Study
- **Leflunomide** is predicted to increase the exposure to **cladribine.** Avoid or adjust dose. Moderate Theoretical → Also see TABLE 12 p. 1057
- **Leflunomide** increases the anticoagulant effect of **coumarins.** Severe Anecdotal
- **Leflunomide** is predicted to increase the exposure to endothelin receptor antagonists **(bosentan).** Moderate Study
- **Leflunomide** are predicted to increases the exposure to **etrasimod.** Avoid in poor CYP2C9 metabolisers. Severe Theoretical
- **Leflunomide** is predicted to increase the exposure to **ganciclovir.** Moderate Study → Also see TABLE 12 p. 1057
- **Leflunomide** is predicted to increase the exposure to **grazoprevir.** Avoid. Severe Theoretical
- **Leflunomide** is predicted to increase the exposure to H_2 receptor antagonists **(famotidine).** Moderate Study
- **Leflunomide** is predicted to increase the concentration of **letermovir.** Moderate Study
- **Live vaccines** are predicted to increase the risk of generalised infection (possibly life-threatening) when given with **leflunomide.** UKHSA advises avoid (refer to Green Book). Severe Theoretical
- **Leflunomide** is predicted to increase the exposure to loop diuretics **(furosemide).** Moderate Study
- **Leflunomide** is predicted to increase the exposure to meglitinides **(repaglinide).** Moderate Study
- **Leflunomide** is predicted to decrease the exposure to **melatonin.** Moderate Theoretical
- **Leflunomide** is predicted to increase the exposure to **methotrexate.** Avoid. Severe Study → Also see TABLE 12 p. 1057
- **Leflunomide** is predicted to increase the clearance of **mexiletine.** Monitor and adjust dose. Moderate Study
- **Leflunomide** is predicted to increase the exposure to **momelotinib.** Moderate Study
- **Leflunomide** is predicted to increase the exposure to **montelukast.** Moderate Theoretical
- **Leflunomide** is predicted to increase the exposure to NRTIs **(zidovudine).** Moderate Theoretical
- **Leflunomide** is predicted to increase the exposure to NSAIDs **(indometacin, ketoprofen).** Moderate Theoretical
- **Leflunomide** is predicted to increase the exposure to **oseltamivir.** Moderate Study
- **Leflunomide** is predicted to increase the exposure to penicillins **(benzylpenicillin).** Moderate Study
- **Leflunomide** is predicted to increase the exposure to **pioglitazone.** Moderate Study
- **Leflunomide** is predicted to decrease the exposure to **pirfenidone.** Moderate Theoretical
- **Leflunomide** is predicted to increase the exposure to quinolones **(ciprofloxacin).** Moderate Theoretical
- Rifamycins **(rifampicin)** might affect the exposure to **leflunomide.** Moderate Theoretical
- **Leflunomide** is predicted to increase the exposure to **roxadustat.** Monitor haemoglobin and adjust dose—consult product literature. Moderate Study
- **Leflunomide** is predicted to increase the exposure to **seladelpar.** Moderate Study

Leflunomide (continued)
- **Leflunomide** is predicted to increase the exposure to **selexipag**. Adjust **selexipag** dose. Moderate Study
- **Leflunomide** is predicted to decrease the exposure to SNRIs **(duloxetine)**. Moderate Theoretical
- **Leflunomide** is predicted to increase the exposure to statins **(atorvastatin, fluvastatin, pravastatin, simvastatin)**. Moderate Study
- **Leflunomide** is predicted to increase the exposure to statins **(rosuvastatin)**. Adjust **rosuvastatin** dose, p. 155. Moderate Study
- **Leflunomide** is predicted to increase the exposure to **sulfasalazine**. Moderate Study → Also see TABLE 12 p. 1057
- **Leflunomide** is predicted to increase the exposure to sulfonylureas **(glibenclamide)**. Moderate Study
- **Leflunomide** is predicted to increase the exposure to **talazoparib**. Avoid or monitor. Moderate Theoretical → Also see TABLE 12 p. 1057
- **Leflunomide** is predicted to increase the exposure to taxanes **(docetaxel)**. Moderate Study → Also see TABLE 12 p. 1057 → Also see TABLE 10 p. 1056
- **Leflunomide** is predicted to increase the concentration of taxanes **(paclitaxel)**. Severe Anecdotal → Also see TABLE 12 p. 1057 → Also see TABLE 10 p. 1056
- **Leflunomide** is predicted to increase the exposure to **tenofovir alafenamide**. Moderate Theoretical
- **Leflunomide** is predicted to increase the exposure to **tenofovir disoproxil**. Moderate Theoretical
- **Leflunomide** is predicted to decrease the exposure to **theophylline**. Adjust dose. Moderate Study
- **Leflunomide** moderately decreases the exposure to **tizanidine**. Mild Study
- **Leflunomide** is predicted to increase the exposure to **topotecan**. Moderate Study → Also see TABLE 12 p. 1057
- **Leflunomide** is predicted to increase the exposure to **tucatinib**. Moderate Theoretical
- **Leflunomide** is predicted to increase the exposure to **vadadustat**. Moderate Study
- **Leflunomide** is predicted to increase the exposure to **venetoclax**. Avoid or monitor for toxicity. Severe Theoretical
- **Leflunomide** is predicted to decrease the exposure to **vorasidenib**. Avoid. Severe Theoretical

Lenacapavir
- Anti-androgens **(apalutamide, enzalutamide)** are predicted to decrease the exposure to **lenacapavir**. Avoid. Severe Study
- Antiepileptics **(carbamazepine, fosphenytoin, phenobarbital, phenytoin, primidone)** are predicted to decrease the exposure to **lenacapavir**. Avoid. Severe Study
- Antiepileptics **(oxcarbazepine)** are predicted to decrease the exposure to **lenacapavir**. Avoid. Severe Theoretical
- **Lenacapavir** moderately increases the exposure to benzodiazepines **(midazolam)**. Moderate Study
- **Cenobamate** is predicted to decrease the exposure to **lenacapavir**. Avoid. Severe Study
- Corticosteroids **(dexamethasone)** might affect the efficacy of **lenacapavir** and **lenacapavir** is predicted to increase the concentration of corticosteroids **(dexamethasone)**. Adjust starting dose and monitor, or consider alternatives. Severe Theoretical
- **Lenacapavir** is predicted to increase the concentration of corticosteroids **(beclometasone, betamethasone, budesonide, deflazacort, fludrocortisone, fluticasone, hydrocortisone, methylprednisolone, prednisolone, triamcinolone)**. Adjust starting dose and monitor. Severe Theoretical
- **Lenacapavir** is predicted to increase the exposure to corticosteroids **(vamorolone)**. Adjust starting dose and monitor. Severe Theoretical
- **Dabrafenib** is predicted to decrease the exposure to **lenacapavir**. Avoid. Severe Study
- **Lenacapavir** is predicted to increase the concentration of **digoxin**. Moderate Theoretical
- **Encorafenib** is predicted to decrease the exposure to **lenacapavir**. Avoid. Severe Study
- Endothelin receptor antagonists **(bosentan)** are predicted to decrease the exposure to **lenacapavir**. Avoid. Severe Study
- **Lenacapavir** is predicted to increase the concentration of factor XA inhibitors **(edoxaban, rivaroxaban)**. Monitor and adjust dose. Severe Theoretical
- HIV-protease inhibitors **(atazanavir)** moderately increase the exposure to **lenacapavir**. Avoid. Severe Study
- **Ivosidenib** is predicted to decrease the exposure to **lenacapavir**. Avoid. Severe Study
- **Lorlatinib** is predicted to decrease the exposure to **lenacapavir**. Avoid. Severe Study
- **Lumacaftor** is predicted to decrease the exposure to **lenacapavir**. Avoid. Severe Study
- **Mitotane** is predicted to decrease the exposure to **lenacapavir**. Avoid. Severe Study
- **Lenacapavir** is predicted to increase the concentration of **naloxegol**. Moderate Theoretical
- NNRTIs **(efavirenz, etravirine, nevirapine)** are predicted to decrease the exposure to **lenacapavir**. Avoid. Severe Study
- **Lenacapavir** is predicted to affect the concentration of opioids **(buprenorphine, methadone)**. Moderate Theoretical
- **Lenacapavir** is predicted to increase the concentration of phosphodiesterase type-5 inhibitors **(sildenafil)**. Adjust starting dose for erectile dysfunction. Severe Theoretical
- **Lenacapavir** is predicted to increase the concentration of phosphodiesterase type-5 inhibitors **(tadalafil)**. Avoid or adjust dose depending on indication—consult product literature. Severe Theoretical
- **Lenacapavir** is predicted to increase the concentration of phosphodiesterase type-5 inhibitors **(vardenafil)**. Adjust dose for erectile dysfunction. Severe Theoretical
- Rifamycins **(rifabutin)** are predicted to decrease the exposure to **lenacapavir**. Avoid. Severe Theoretical
- Rifamycins **(rifampicin)** are predicted to decrease the exposure to **lenacapavir**. Avoid. Severe Study
- **Sotorasib** is predicted to decrease the exposure to **lenacapavir**. Avoid. Severe Study
- **St John's wort** is predicted to decrease the exposure to **lenacapavir**. Avoid. Severe Study
- **Lenacapavir** is predicted to increase the concentration of statins **(simvastatin)**. Adjust starting dose and monitor. Moderate Theoretical
- **Lenacapavir** is predicted to increase the concentration of thrombin inhibitors **(dabigatran)**. Monitor and adjust dose. Severe Theoretical

Lenalidomide → see TABLE 1 p. 1053 (hepatotoxicity), TABLE 12 p. 1057 (myelosuppression), TABLE 10 p. 1056 (peripheral neuropathy)
- **Combined hormonal contraceptives** are predicted to increase the risk of venous thromboembolism when given with **lenalidomide**. Avoid. Severe Theoretical
- **Hormone replacement therapy** is predicted to increase the risk of venous thromboembolism when given with **lenalidomide**. Moderate Theoretical

Leniolisib
- Anti-androgens **(apalutamide, enzalutamide)** are predicted to decrease the exposure to **leniolisib**. Avoid. Severe Theoretical
- Antiarrhythmics **(dronedarone)** are predicted to increase the exposure to **leniolisib**. Avoid. Moderate Study
- Antiepileptics **(carbamazepine, fosphenytoin, phenobarbital, phenytoin, primidone)** are predicted to decrease the exposure to **leniolisib**. Avoid. Severe Theoretical
- Antifungals, azoles **(fluconazole, isavuconazole, itraconazole, ketoconazole, posaconazole, voriconazole)** are predicted to increase the exposure to **leniolisib**. Avoid. Moderate Study
- **Leniolisib** is predicted to increase the exposure to antihistamines, non-sedating **(fexofenadine)**. Avoid. Moderate Theoretical
- **Leniolisib** is predicted to increase the exposure to atypical antipsychotics **(clozapine)**. Avoid. Moderate Theoretical
- **Berotralstat** is predicted to increase the exposure to **leniolisib**. Avoid. Moderate Study
- Calcium-channel blockers **(diltiazem, verapamil)** are predicted to increase the exposure to **leniolisib**. Avoid. Moderate Study
- **Cenobamate** is predicted to decrease the exposure to **leniolisib**. Avoid. Severe Theoretical

- Ceritinib is predicted to increase the exposure to **leniolisib**. Avoid. [Moderate] Study
- **Cobicistat** is predicted to increase the exposure to **leniolisib**. Avoid. [Moderate] Study
- **Crizotinib** is predicted to increase the exposure to **leniolisib**. Avoid. [Moderate] Study
- **Dabrafenib** is predicted to decrease the exposure to **leniolisib**. Avoid. [Severe] Theoretical
- **Encorafenib** is predicted to decrease the exposure to **leniolisib**. Avoid. [Severe] Theoretical
- Endothelin receptor antagonists **(bosentan)** are predicted to decrease the exposure to **leniolisib**. Avoid. [Severe] Theoretical
- **Leniolisib** is predicted to increase the exposure to endothelin receptor antagonists **(bosentan)**. Avoid. [Moderate] Theoretical
- **Fedratinib** is predicted to increase the exposure to **leniolisib**. Avoid. [Moderate] Study
- **Grapefruit** juice is predicted to increase the exposure to **leniolisib**. Avoid. [Moderate] Theoretical
- **HIV-protease inhibitors** are predicted to increase the exposure to **leniolisib**. Avoid. [Moderate] Study
- **Idelalisib** is predicted to increase the exposure to **leniolisib**. Avoid. [Moderate] Study
- **Imatinib** is predicted to increase the exposure to **leniolisib**. Avoid. [Moderate] Study
- **Ivosidenib** is predicted to decrease the exposure to **leniolisib**. Avoid. [Severe] Theoretical
- **Letermovir** is predicted to increase the exposure to **leniolisib**. Avoid. [Moderate] Study
- **Lorlatinib** is predicted to decrease the exposure to **leniolisib**. Avoid. [Severe] Theoretical
- **Lumacaftor** is predicted to decrease the exposure to **leniolisib**. Avoid. [Severe] Theoretical
- Macrolides **(clarithromycin, erythromycin)** are predicted to increase the exposure to **leniolisib**. Avoid. [Moderate] Study
- **Leniolisib** is predicted to increase the exposure to meglitinides **(repaglinide)**. Avoid. [Moderate] Theoretical
- **Leniolisib** is predicted to increase the exposure to **melatonin**. Avoid. [Moderate] Theoretical
- **Mitotane** is predicted to decrease the exposure to **leniolisib**. Avoid. [Severe] Theoretical
- **Modafinil** is predicted to decrease the exposure to **leniolisib**. Avoid. [Severe] Theoretical
- Neurokinin-1 receptor antagonists **(aprepitant, netupitant)** are predicted to increase the exposure to **leniolisib**. Avoid. [Moderate] Study
- **Nilotinib** is predicted to increase the exposure to **leniolisib**. Avoid. [Moderate] Study
- NNRTIs **(efavirenz, etravirine, nevirapine)** are predicted to decrease the exposure to **leniolisib**. Avoid. [Severe] Theoretical
- Rifamycins **(rifampicin)** are predicted to decrease the exposure to **leniolisib**. Avoid. [Severe] Theoretical
- **Leniolisib** is predicted to increase the exposure to SNRIs **(duloxetine)**. Avoid. [Moderate] Theoretical
- **Sotorasib** is predicted to decrease the exposure to **leniolisib**. Avoid. [Severe] Theoretical
- **St John's wort** is predicted to decrease the exposure to **leniolisib**. Avoid. [Severe] Theoretical
- **Leniolisib** is predicted to increase the exposure to **statins**. Avoid. [Moderate] Theoretical
- **Leniolisib** is predicted to increase the exposure to **sulfasalazine**. Avoid. [Moderate] Theoretical
- **Leniolisib** is predicted to increase the exposure to sulfonylureas **(glibenclamide)**. Avoid. [Moderate] Theoretical
- **Leniolisib** is predicted to increase the exposure to taxanes **(docetaxel, paclitaxel)**. Avoid. [Moderate] Theoretical
- **Leniolisib** is predicted to increase the exposure to **theophylline**. Avoid. [Moderate] Theoretical
- **Leniolisib** is predicted to increase the exposure to **tizanidine**. Avoid. [Moderate] Theoretical
- **Leniolisib** is predicted to increase the exposure to **topotecan**. Avoid. [Moderate] Theoretical
- **Tucatinib** is predicted to increase the exposure to **leniolisib**. Avoid. [Moderate] Study

Lenograstim

- **Lenograstim** might increase the risk of pulmonary toxicity when given with **bleomycin**. [Severe] Theoretical

Lenvatinib → see TABLE 3 p. 1053 (bleeding), TABLE 7 p. 1055 (QT-interval prolongation)

Lercanidipine → see calcium-channel blockers

Letermovir

- **Letermovir** is predicted to increase the exposure to **abemaciclib**. [Moderate] Study
- **Letermovir** is predicted to increase the exposure to **acalabrutinib**. Avoid or monitor. [Severe] Study
- **Letermovir** is predicted to increase the exposure to alpha blockers **(tamsulosin)**. [Moderate] Theoretical
- **Letermovir** is predicted to increase the concentration of antiarrhythmics **(amiodarone)**. [Moderate] Theoretical
- **Letermovir** is predicted to increase the exposure to antiarrhythmics **(propafenone)**. Monitor and adjust dose. [Moderate] Study
- Antiepileptics **(carbamazepine, phenobarbital, primidone)** are predicted to decrease the concentration of **letermovir**. [Moderate] Theoretical
- **Letermovir** is predicted to decrease the concentration of antiepileptics **(fosphenytoin, phenytoin)** and antiepileptics **(fosphenytoin, phenytoin)** are predicted to decrease the concentration of **letermovir**. [Moderate] Theoretical
- **Letermovir** is predicted to increase the exposure to antifungals, azoles **(isavuconazole)**. [Moderate] Theoretical
- **Letermovir** slightly decreases the exposure to antifungals, azoles **(voriconazole)**. [Moderate] Study
- **Letermovir** is predicted to increase the concentration of antihistamines, non-sedating **(fexofenadine)**. [Moderate] Theoretical
- **Letermovir** is predicted to increase the exposure to antihistamines, non-sedating **(mizolastine)**. [Severe] Theoretical
- **Letermovir** is predicted to increase the exposure to antihistamines, non-sedating **(rupatadine)**. Avoid. [Moderate] Study
- **Letermovir** is predicted to increase the concentration of antimalarials **(piperaquine)**. [Severe] Study
- **Letermovir** is predicted to increase the exposure to atypical antipsychotics **(cariprazine)**. Monitor and adjust dose. [Severe] Study
- **Letermovir** is predicted to increase the exposure to atypical antipsychotics **(quetiapine)**. Avoid. [Moderate] Study
- **Letermovir** is predicted to increase the exposure to **avapritinib**. Avoid or adjust dose—consult product literature. [Moderate] Study
- **Letermovir** is predicted to increase the exposure to **axitinib**. [Moderate] Study
- **Letermovir** might increase the exposure to **bedaquiline**. [Mild] Theoretical
- **Letermovir** is predicted to increase the exposure to benzodiazepines **(alprazolam)**. [Severe] Study
- **Letermovir** is predicted to increase the exposure to benzodiazepines **(midazolam)**. Monitor adverse effects and adjust dose. [Severe] Study
- **Letermovir** is predicted to increase the exposure to **bosutinib**. Avoid or adjust dose. [Severe] Study
- **Letermovir** is predicted to increase the exposure to **brigatinib**. [Moderate] Study
- **Letermovir** is predicted to increase the exposure to **buspirone**. Use with caution and adjust dose. [Moderate] Study
- **Letermovir** is predicted to increase the exposure to **cabozantinib**. [Moderate] Study
- **Letermovir** is predicted to increase the exposure to calcium-channel blockers **(amlodipine, felodipine, lacidipine, lercanidipine, nicardipine, nifedipine, nimodipine)**. Monitor and adjust dose. [Moderate] Study
- **Letermovir** is predicted to increase the exposure to **capivasertib**. Adjust dose. [Moderate] Study
- **Letermovir** is predicted to increase the exposure to **ceritinib**. [Moderate] Study
- **Letermovir** increases the exposure to **ciclosporin** and **ciclosporin** increases the exposure to **letermovir**. Monitor and adjust **letermovir** dose. [Severe] Study
- **Letermovir** is predicted to increase the exposure to **cobimetinib**. [Severe] Study

Letermovir (continued)

- **Letermovir** is predicted to increase the exposure to **colchicine**. Adjust **colchicine** dose with moderate CYP3A4 inhibitors, p. 637. [Severe] Study
- **Letermovir** is predicted to increase the exposure to corticosteroids **(methylprednisolone)**. Monitor and adjust dose. [Moderate] Study
- **Letermovir** is predicted to decrease the concentration of coumarins **(warfarin)**. Monitor and adjust dose. [Moderate] Theoretical
- **Letermovir** is predicted to increase the exposure to **crizotinib**. [Moderate] Study
- **Letermovir** is predicted to increase the exposure to **dabrafenib**. [Moderate] Study
- **Letermovir** is predicted to increase the exposure to **daridorexant**. Adjust **daridorexant** dose. [Severe] Study
- **Letermovir** is predicted to increase the exposure to **darifenacin**. [Moderate] Study
- **Letermovir** is predicted to increase the exposure to **dasatinib**. [Severe] Study
- **Letermovir** is predicted to increase the exposure to **deutivacaftor**. Adjust dose, see deutivacaftor with tezacaftor and vanzacaftor p. 218. [Severe] Study
- **Letermovir** is predicted to slightly increase the exposure to **dienogest**. [Moderate] Study
- **Letermovir** is predicted to increase the exposure to dipeptidylpeptidase-4 inhibitors **(saxagliptin)**. [Mild] Study
- **Letermovir** is predicted to increase the exposure to **domperidone**. Avoid. [Severe] Study
- **Letermovir** is predicted to increase the exposure to dopamine receptor agonists **(bromocriptine)**. [Severe] Theoretical
- **Letermovir** is predicted to increase the exposure to **drospirenone**. [Severe] Study
- **Letermovir** is predicted to moderately increase the exposure to **dutasteride**. [Mild] Study
- **Letermovir** is predicted to increase the exposure to **elacestrant**. Avoid moderate CYP3A4 inhibitors or adjust **elacestrant** dose. [Severe] Theoretical
- **Letermovir** is predicted to increase the exposure to **elexacaftor**. Adjust ivacaftor with tezacaftor and elexacaftor p. 220 dose with moderate CYP3A4 inhibitors. [Severe] Theoretical
- **Letermovir** is predicted to increase the exposure to **eliglustat**. Avoid or adjust dose—consult product literature. [Severe] Study
- **Eltrombopag** is predicted to increase the concentration of **letermovir**. [Moderate] Study
- **Letermovir** is predicted to moderately increase the exposure to **encorafenib**. [Moderate] Study
- **Letermovir** is predicted to increase the concentration of endothelin receptor antagonists **(bosentan)**. [Moderate] Theoretical
- **Letermovir** is predicted to increase the exposure to endothelin receptor antagonists **(macitentan)**. Manufacturer advises caution depending on other drugs taken—consult product literature. [Moderate] Theoretical
- **Letermovir** is predicted to increase the exposure to **entrectinib**. Avoid or adjust dose with moderate CYP3A4 inhibitors—consult product literature. [Severe] Theoretical
- **Letermovir** is predicted to increase the risk of ergotism when given with **ergometrine**. [Severe] Theoretical
- **Letermovir** is predicted to increase the exposure to **erlotinib**. [Moderate] Study
- **Letermovir** is predicted to increase the exposure to **etrasimod**. Avoid in poor CYP2C9 metabolisers. [Severe] Theoretical
- **Letermovir** is predicted to increase the concentration of **everolimus**. Avoid or adjust dose. [Moderate] Study
- **Letermovir** is predicted to increase the exposure to **fedratinib**. Monitor and adjust dose. [Moderate] Study
- **Letermovir** is predicted to increase the exposure to **fesoterodine**. Adjust **fesoterodine** dose with moderate CYP3A4 inhibitors in hepatic and renal impairment. [Mild] Study
- Fibrates **(gemfibrozil)** are predicted to increase the concentration of **letermovir**. [Moderate] Study
- **Letermovir** is predicted to increase the exposure to **gefitinib**. [Moderate] Study
- **Letermovir** is predicted to increase the concentration of **guanfacine**. Adjust **guanfacine** dose, p. 281. [Moderate] Theoretical
- HIV-protease inhibitors **(atazanavir, lopinavir)** boosted with ritonavir are predicted to increase the concentration of **letermovir**. [Moderate] Study
- HIV-protease inhibitors **(ritonavir)** are predicted to decrease the concentration of **letermovir**. [Moderate] Theoretical
- **Letermovir** is predicted to increase the exposure to **ibrutinib**. Adjust dose with moderate CYP3A4 inhibitors—consult product literature. [Severe] Study
- **Letermovir** is predicted to increase the exposure to **imatinib**. [Moderate] Study
- **Letermovir** is predicted to increase the exposure to the active metabolite of **irinotecan**. [Moderate] Theoretical
- **Letermovir** is predicted to increase the exposure to **ivacaftor**. Adjust dose with moderate CYP3A4 inhibitors, see ivacaftor p. 219, tezacaftor with ivacaftor p. 223, and ivacaftor with tezacaftor and elexacaftor p. 220. [Moderate] Study
- **Letermovir** is predicted to increase the exposure to **ivosidenib**. Monitor and adjust dose—consult product literature. [Severe] Study
- **Letermovir** is predicted to increase the exposure to **lapatinib**. [Moderate] Study
- **Letermovir** is predicted to increase the exposure to **larotrectinib**. Monitor and adjust dose. [Moderate] Theoretical
- **Leflunomide** is predicted to increase the concentration of **letermovir**. [Moderate] Study
- **Letermovir** is predicted to increase the exposure to **leniolisib**. Avoid. [Moderate] Study
- **Letermovir** is predicted to increase the exposure to **lomitapide**. Avoid. [Moderate] Theoretical
- Macrolides **(clarithromycin, erythromycin)** are predicted to increase the concentration of **letermovir**. [Moderate] Study
- **Letermovir** is predicted to increase the exposure to **mavacamten**. Adjust dose—consult product literature. [Moderate] Study
- **Letermovir** is predicted to increase the concentration of meglitinides **(repaglinide)**. Avoid. [Moderate] Theoretical
- **Letermovir** is predicted to increase the exposure to **midostaurin**. [Moderate] Theoretical
- **Letermovir** is predicted to increase the exposure to mineralocorticoid receptor antagonists **(eplerenone)**. Adjust **eplerenone** dose. [Severe] Study
- **Letermovir** is predicted to increase the exposure to mineralocorticoid receptor antagonists **(finerenone)**. [Severe] Study
- **Modafinil** is predicted to decrease the concentration of **letermovir**. [Moderate] Theoretical
- **Letermovir** is predicted to increase the exposure to **naldemedine**. [Moderate] Study
- **Letermovir** is predicted to increase the exposure to **naloxegol**. Adjust **naloxegol** dose and monitor adverse effects. [Moderate] Study
- **Letermovir** is predicted to increase the exposure to **neratinib**. Avoid moderate CYP3A4 inhibitors or adjust dose and monitor for gastrointestinal adverse effects—consult product literature. [Severe] Study
- **Letermovir** is predicted to increase the exposure to **nilotinib**. [Moderate] Study
- NNRTIs **(efavirenz)** are predicted to decrease the concentration of **letermovir**. [Moderate] Theoretical
- NNRTIs **(etravirine)** are predicted to decrease the exposure to **letermovir**. [Moderate] Theoretical
- **Letermovir** is predicted to increase the exposure to **olaparib**. Avoid or adjust dose with moderate CYP3A4 inhibitors—consult product literature. [Moderate] Theoretical
- **Letermovir** is predicted to increase the exposure to **omaveloxolone**. Avoid or adjust **omaveloxolone** dose, p. 755. [Moderate] Study
- **Letermovir** is predicted to increase the exposure to opioids **(alfentanil, buprenorphine, fentanyl, oxycodone)**. Monitor and adjust dose. [Moderate] Study
- **Letermovir** is predicted to increase the exposure to opioids **(methadone, sufentanil)**. [Moderate] Theoretical
- **Letermovir** is predicted to increase the exposure to **pazopanib**. [Moderate] Study
- **Letermovir** is predicted to increase the exposure to **pemigatinib**. [Severe] Study

- **Letermovir** is predicted to increase the exposure to phosphodiesterase type-5 inhibitors **(avanafil)**. Adjust **avanafil** dose. Moderate Theoretical
- **Letermovir** is predicted to increase the exposure to phosphodiesterase type-5 inhibitors **(sildenafil)**. Monitor or adjust **sildenafil** dose with moderate CYP3A4 inhibitors, p. 139. Moderate Study
- **Letermovir** is predicted to increase the exposure to phosphodiesterase type-5 inhibitors **(tadalafil)**. Severe Theoretical
- **Letermovir** is predicted to increase the exposure to phosphodiesterase type-5 inhibitors **(vardenafil)**. Adjust dose. Severe Theoretical
- **Letermovir** is predicted to increase the exposure to **pimozide**. Avoid. Severe Theoretical
- **Letermovir** is predicted to increase the exposure to **ponatinib**. Moderate Study
- **Letermovir** is predicted to increase the exposure to **pralsetinib**. Moderate Theoretical
- **Letermovir** is predicted to increase the exposure to **ranolazine**. Severe Study
- **Letermovir** is predicted to increase the exposure to **regorafenib**. Moderate Study
- **Letermovir** is predicted to increase the exposure to **ribociclib**. Moderate Study
- Rifamycins **(rifabutin)** are predicted to decrease the concentration of **letermovir**. Moderate Theoretical
- Rifamycins **(rifampicin)** are predicted to affect the concentration of **letermovir**. Severe Theoretical
- **Letermovir** is predicted to increase the exposure to **rimegepant**. Avoid another dose of rimegepant within 48 hours of concurrent use. Moderate Study
- **Letermovir** is predicted to increase the exposure to **ruxolitinib**. Moderate Study
- **Letermovir** is predicted to increase the exposure to **selpercatinib**. Moderate Study
- **Letermovir** is predicted to increase the exposure to **selumetinib**. Avoid or adjust dose—consult product literature. Severe Study
- **Letermovir** is predicted to increase the exposure to **siponimod**. Avoid depending on other drugs taken—consult product literature. Severe Study
- **Letermovir** increases the concentration of **sirolimus**. Monitor and adjust dose. Moderate Study
- **Letermovir** is predicted to increase the exposure to **sparsentan**. Moderate Study
- **Letermovir** is predicted to increase the exposure to SSRIs **(dapoxetine)**. Adjust **dapoxetine** dose with moderate CYP3A4 inhibitors. Moderate Theoretical
- **Letermovir** is predicted to increase the exposure to SSRIs **(sertraline)**. Moderate Theoretical
- **St John's wort** is predicted to decrease the concentration of **letermovir**. Moderate Theoretical
- **Letermovir** moderately increases the exposure to statins **(atorvastatin)**. Avoid or adjust **atorvastatin** dose, p. 154. Severe Study
- **Letermovir** is predicted to increase the exposure to statins **(fluvastatin)**. Monitor and adjust dose. Moderate Theoretical
- **Letermovir** is predicted to increase the exposure to statins **(pravastatin)**. Avoid or adjust dose. Moderate Theoretical
- **Letermovir** is predicted to increase the exposure to statins **(rosuvastatin, simvastatin)**. Avoid. Severe Study
- **Letermovir** is predicted to increase the concentration of sulfonylureas **(glibenclamide)**. Moderate Theoretical
- **Letermovir** is predicted to increase the exposure to **sunitinib**. Moderate Study
- **Letermovir** moderately increases the exposure to **tacrolimus**. Monitor and adjust dose. Severe Study
- **Letermovir** is predicted to increase the exposure to taxanes **(cabazitaxel)**. Moderate Theoretical
- **Letermovir** is predicted to increase the exposure to taxanes **(docetaxel)**. Severe Study
- **Letermovir** is predicted to increase the exposure to taxanes **(paclitaxel)**. Moderate Anecdotal
- **Teriflunomide** is predicted to increase the concentration of **letermovir**. Moderate Study
- **Letermovir** is predicted to increase the exposure to **tezacaftor**. Adjust dose with moderate CYP3A4 inhibitors, see tezacaftor with ivacaftor p. 223, ivacaftor with tezacaftor and elexacaftor p. 220, and deutivacaftor with tezacaftor and vanzacaftor p. 218. Severe Study
- **Letermovir** is predicted to decrease the concentration of thrombin inhibitors **(dabigatran)**. Avoid. Severe Theoretical
- **Letermovir** given with a potent CYP2C19 inhibitor is predicted to increase the exposure to **tofacitinib**. Adjust **tofacitinib** dose, p. 803. Moderate Study
- **Letermovir** is predicted to increase the exposure to **tolvaptan**. Manufacturer advises caution or adjust **tolvaptan** dose with moderate CYP3A4 inhibitors. Moderate Study
- **Letermovir** is predicted to increase the exposure to **trazodone**. Moderate Theoretical
- **Letermovir** is predicted to increase the exposure to **ulipristal**. Avoid when used for uterine fibroids. Moderate Study
- **Letermovir** is predicted to increase the exposure to **vanzacaftor**. Adjust dose, see deutivacaftor with tezacaftor and vanzacaftor p. 218. Severe Study
- **Letermovir** is predicted to increase the exposure to **vemurafenib**. Severe Theoretical
- **Letermovir** is predicted to increase the exposure to **venetoclax**. Avoid or adjust dose—consult product literature. Severe Study
- **Letermovir** is predicted to increase the exposure to **vinca alkaloids**. Severe Theoretical
- **Letermovir** is predicted to increase the exposure to **voclosporin**. Adjust **voclosporin** dose. Severe Study
- **Letermovir** is predicted to increase the exposure to **zanubrutinib**. Avoid or adjust dose with moderate CYP3A4 inhibitors—consult product literature. Severe Study
- **Letermovir** is predicted to increase the exposure to **zopiclone**. Adjust dose. Moderate Study

Levamisole
- **Albendazole** slightly decreases the exposure to **levamisole** and **levamisole** moderately decreases the exposure to **albendazole**. Moderate Study
- **Alcohol** potentially causes a disulfiram-like reaction when given with **levamisole**. Moderate Study
- **Levamisole** increases the exposure to **ivermectin**. Moderate Study

Levetiracetam → see antiepileptics
Levobunolol → see beta blockers, non-selective
Levobupivacaine → see anaesthetics, local
Levocetirizine → see antihistamines, non-sedating
Levodopa → see TABLE 6 p. 1054 (hypotension), TABLE 9 p. 1056 (CNS effects)
- Antiepileptics **(fosphenytoin, phenytoin)** decrease the effects of **levodopa**. Moderate Study → Also see TABLE 9 p. 1056
- Atypical antipsychotics **(amisulpride)** are predicted to decrease the effects of **levodopa**. Avoid. Severe Theoretical → Also see TABLE 9 p. 1056
- Atypical antipsychotics **(aripiprazole, clozapine, lurasidone, paliperidone)** are predicted to decrease the effects of **levodopa**. Severe Theoretical → Also see TABLE 6 p. 1054 → Also see TABLE 9 p. 1056
- Atypical antipsychotics **(asenapine)** are predicted to decrease the effects of **levodopa**. Adjust dose. Severe Theoretical → Also see TABLE 6 p. 1054 → Also see TABLE 9 p. 1056
- Atypical antipsychotics **(olanzapine)** decrease the effects of **levodopa**. Avoid or monitor worsening parkinsonian symptoms. Severe Anecdotal → Also see TABLE 6 p. 1054 → Also see TABLE 9 p. 1056
- Atypical antipsychotics **(quetiapine)** decrease the effects of **levodopa**. Severe Anecdotal → Also see TABLE 6 p. 1054 → Also see TABLE 9 p. 1056
- Atypical antipsychotics **(risperidone)** are predicted to decrease the effects of **levodopa**. Avoid or adjust dose. Severe Anecdotal → Also see TABLE 6 p. 1054 → Also see TABLE 9 p. 1056
- **Baclofen** is predicted to increase the risk of adverse effects when given with **levodopa**. Severe Anecdotal → Also see TABLE 6 p. 1054 → Also see TABLE 9 p. 1056
- **Benperidol** is predicted to decrease the effects of **levodopa**. Severe Study → Also see TABLE 6 p. 1054 → Also see TABLE 9 p. 1056

Levodopa (continued)

- **Bupropion** increases the risk of adverse effects when given with **levodopa**. Moderate Study
- **Droperidol** decreases the effects of **levodopa**. Severe Study → Also see **TABLE 6** p. 1054 → Also see **TABLE 9** p. 1056
- **Drugs with antimuscarinic effects** (see **TABLE 8** p. 1055) might decrease the absorption of **levodopa**. Moderate Theoretical
- **Entacapone** increases the exposure to **levodopa**. Monitor adverse effects and adjust dose. Moderate Study
- **Flupentixol** decreases the effects of **levodopa**. Avoid or monitor worsening parkinsonian symptoms. Severe Theoretical → Also see **TABLE 6** p. 1054 → Also see **TABLE 9** p. 1056
- **Haloperidol** decreases the effects of **levodopa**. Severe Study → Also see **TABLE 6** p. 1054 → Also see **TABLE 9** p. 1056
- Oral **iron** decreases the absorption of oral **levodopa**. Moderate Study
- **Isoniazid** decreases the effects of **levodopa**. Moderate Study
- **Levodopa** is predicted to increase the risk of elevated blood pressure when given with **linezolid**. Avoid. Severe Theoretical
- **Loxapine** is predicted to decrease the effects of **levodopa**. Severe Theoretical → Also see **TABLE 6** p. 1054 → Also see **TABLE 9** p. 1056
- **MAO-B inhibitors** are predicted to increase the effects of **levodopa**. Adjust dose. Mild Study → Also see **TABLE 6** p. 1054
- **Levodopa** increases the risk of a hypertensive crisis when given with **MAOIs, irreversible**. Avoid and for 14 days after stopping the MAOI. Severe Study → Also see **TABLE 6** p. 1054
- **Memantine** is predicted to increase the effects of **levodopa**. Moderate Theoretical
- **Metoclopramide** decreases the effects of **levodopa**. Avoid. Moderate Study
- **Levodopa** increases the risk of adverse effects when given with **moclobemide**. Moderate Study
- **Opicapone** increases the exposure to **levodopa**. Adjust dose. Moderate Study
- **Phenothiazine antipsychotics** decrease the effects of **levodopa**. Avoid or monitor worsening parkinsonian symptoms. Severe Study → Also see **TABLE 6** p. 1054 → Also see **TABLE 9** p. 1056
- **Pimozide** decreases the effects of **levodopa**. Severe Theoretical → Also see **TABLE 6** p. 1054 → Also see **TABLE 9** p. 1056
- **Sulpiride** is predicted to decrease the effects of **levodopa**. Avoid. Severe Theoretical → Also see **TABLE 6** p. 1054 → Also see **TABLE 9** p. 1056
- **Tetrabenazine** is predicted to decrease the effects of **levodopa**. Use with caution or avoid. Moderate Theoretical → Also see **TABLE 9** p. 1056
- **Tolcapone** increases the exposure to **levodopa**. Monitor and adjust dose. Moderate Study
- **Tryptophan** greatly decreases the concentration of **levodopa**. Moderate Study
- **Zuclopenthixol** is predicted to decrease the effects of **levodopa**. Avoid or monitor worsening parkinsonian symptoms. Severe Theoretical → Also see **TABLE 6** p. 1054 → Also see **TABLE 9** p. 1056

Levofloxacin → see quinolones

Levofolinic acid → see folates

Levomepromazine → see phenothiazine antipsychotics

Levonorgestrel

- Antiepileptics **(carbamazepine, eslicarbazepine, fosphenytoin, oxcarbazepine, perampanel, phenobarbital, phenytoin, primidone, rufinamide, topiramate)** are predicted to decrease the efficacy of some contraceptive methods containing **levonorgestrel**. For CoSRH guidance, see Contraceptives, interactions p. 614. Severe Theoretical
- Antiepileptics **(lamotrigine)** might decrease the effects of **levonorgestrel**. For CoSRH guidance, see Contraceptives, interactions p. 614. Moderate Theoretical
- Endothelin receptor antagonists **(bosentan)** are predicted to decrease the efficacy of some contraceptive methods containing **levonorgestrel**. For CoSRH guidance, see Contraceptives, interactions p. 614. Severe Theoretical
- Glucagon-like peptide-1 receptor agonists **(tirzepatide)** might affect the absorption of oral **levonorgestrel**. Manufacturer advises precautions for those who are overweight or obese. Moderate Study
- HIV-protease inhibitors **(ritonavir)** are predicted to decrease the efficacy of some contraceptive methods containing **levonorgestrel**. For CoSRH guidance, see Contraceptives, interactions p. 614. Severe Theoretical
- **Lumacaftor** is predicted to decrease the efficacy of **levonorgestrel**. Use additional contraceptive precautions. Severe Theoretical
- **Modafinil** is predicted to decrease the efficacy of some contraceptive methods containing **levonorgestrel**. For CoSRH guidance, see Contraceptives, interactions p. 614. Severe Theoretical
- Neurokinin-1 receptor antagonists **(aprepitant, fosaprepitant)** are predicted to decrease the efficacy of some contraceptive methods containing **levonorgestrel**. For CoSRH guidance, see Contraceptives, interactions p. 614. Severe Theoretical
- NNRTIs **(efavirenz, nevirapine)** are predicted to decrease the efficacy of some contraceptive methods containing **levonorgestrel**. For CoSRH guidance, see Contraceptives, interactions p. 614. Severe Theoretical
- NNRTIs **(etravirine)** might decrease the efficacy of some contraceptive methods containing **levonorgestrel**. Follow CoSRH guidance for enzyme inducers, see Contraceptives, interactions p. 614. Severe Theoretical
- **Rifamycins** are predicted to decrease the efficacy of some contraceptive methods containing **levonorgestrel**. For CoSRH guidance, see Contraceptives, interactions p. 614. Severe Theoretical
- **St John's wort** is predicted to decrease the efficacy of **levonorgestrel**. MHRA advises avoid. For CoSRH guidance, see Contraceptives, interactions p. 614. Severe Theoretical
- **Sugammadex** is predicted to decrease the exposure to **levonorgestrel**. Use additional contraceptive precautions. Severe Theoretical
- **Levonorgestrel** might decrease the efficacy of **ulipristal** and **ulipristal** might decrease the efficacy of **levonorgestrel**. Avoid. For CoSRH guidance, see Contraceptives, interactions p. 614. Severe Theoretical

Levothyroxine → see thyroid hormones

Lidocaine → see antiarrhythmics

Linagliptin → see dipeptidylpeptidase-4 inhibitors

Linezolid → see **TABLE 11** p. 1056 (serotonin toxicity)

FOOD AND LIFESTYLE Patients taking linezolid should avoid consuming large amounts of tyramine-rich foods (such as mature cheese, salami, pickled herring, *Bovril*®, *Oxo*®, *Marmite*® or any similar meat or yeast extract or fermented soya bean extract, and some beers, lagers or wines).

- **Beta$_2$ agonists** are predicted to increase the risk of elevated blood pressure when given with **linezolid**. Avoid. Severe Theoretical
- **Bupropion** is predicted to increase the risk of intraoperative hypertension when given with **linezolid**. Severe Anecdotal
- **Buspirone** is predicted to increase the risk of elevated blood pressure when given with **linezolid**. Avoid. Severe Theoretical
- **Levodopa** is predicted to increase the risk of elevated blood pressure when given with **linezolid**. Avoid. Severe Theoretical
- Macrolides **(clarithromycin)** increase the exposure to **linezolid**. Moderate Anecdotal
- MAO-B inhibitors **(rasagiline, selegiline)** are predicted to increase the risk of adverse effects when given with **linezolid**. Avoid and for 14 days after stopping the MAOI. Severe Theoretical
- MAO-B inhibitors **(safinamide)** are predicted to increase the risk of adverse effects when given with **linezolid**. Avoid and for 1 week after stopping **safinamide**. Severe Theoretical
- **MAOIs, irreversible** are predicted to increase the risk of adverse effects when given with **linezolid**. Avoid and for 14 days after stopping the MAOI. Severe Theoretical → Also see **TABLE 11** p. 1056
- **Methylphenidate** might increase the risk of elevated blood pressure when given with **linezolid**. Avoid. Severe Theoretical
- **Moclobemide** is predicted to increase the risk of adverse effects when given with **linezolid**. Avoid and for 14 days after stopping **moclobemide**. Severe Theoretical → Also see **TABLE 11** p. 1056
- **Ozanimod** might increase the risk of a hypertensive crisis when given with **linezolid**. Avoid. Severe Theoretical

- **Reboxetine** is predicted to increase the risk of a hypertensive crisis when given with **linezolid**. Avoid. Severe Theoretical
- Rifamycins **(rifampicin)** slightly decrease the exposure to **linezolid**. Moderate Study
- **Sympathomimetics, inotropic** are predicted to increase the risk of elevated blood pressure when given with **linezolid**. Avoid. Severe Theoretical
- Sympathomimetics, vasoconstrictor **(adrenaline, ephedrine, isometheptene, noradrenaline, phenylephrine)** are predicted to increase the risk of elevated blood pressure when given with **linezolid**. Avoid. Severe Theoretical
- Sympathomimetics, vasoconstrictor **(midodrine)** might increase the risk of a hypertensive crisis when given with **linezolid**. Avoid. Severe Theoretical
- Sympathomimetics, vasoconstrictor **(pseudoephedrine)** increase the risk of elevated blood pressure when given with **linezolid**. Avoid. Severe Study

Linzagolix
- **Linzagolix** slightly increases the exposure to meglitinides **(repaglinide)**. Avoid. Mild Study
- **Linzagolix** is predicted to increase the exposure to **sorafenib**. Avoid. Mild Theoretical
- **Linzagolix** is predicted to increase the exposure to taxanes **(paclitaxel)**. Avoid. Mild Theoretical

Liothyronine → see thyroid hormones

Lipegfilgrastim
- **Lipegfilgrastim** might increase the risk of pulmonary toxicity when given with **bleomycin**. Severe Theoretical

Liraglutide → see glucagon-like peptide-1 receptor agonists

Lisdexamfetamine → see amfetamines

Lisinopril → see ACE inhibitors

Lithium → see TABLE 2 p. 1053 (nephrotoxicity)
- **ACE inhibitors** are predicted to increase the concentration of **lithium**. Monitor and adjust dose. Severe Anecdotal → Also see TABLE 2 p. 1053
- **Acetazolamide** alters the concentration of **lithium**. Severe Anecdotal
- **Aminophylline** is predicted to decrease the concentration of **lithium**. Moderate Theoretical
- **Angiotensin-II receptor antagonists** potentially increase the concentration of **lithium**. Avoid or monitor. Severe Anecdotal
- Antiepileptics **(carbamazepine, oxcarbazepine)** are predicted to increase the risk of neurotoxicity when given with **lithium**. Severe Anecdotal
- Atypical antipsychotics **(quetiapine, risperidone)** potentially increase the risk of neurotoxicity when given with **lithium**. Severe Anecdotal
- **Calcitonins** decrease the concentration of **lithium**. Adjust dose. Moderate Study
- Calcium-channel blockers **(diltiazem, verapamil)** are predicted to increase the risk of neurotoxicity when given with **lithium**. Severe Anecdotal
- **Loop diuretics** increase the concentration of **lithium**. Monitor and adjust dose. Severe Study
- **Methyldopa** increases the risk of neurotoxicity when given with **lithium**. Severe Anecdotal
- **Metronidazole** is predicted to increase the concentration of **lithium**. Avoid or adjust dose. Severe Anecdotal
- **Mexiletine** potentially affects the exposure to **lithium**. Avoid. Unknown Theoretical
- Mineralocorticoid receptor antagonists **(eplerenone)** potentially increase the concentration of **lithium**. Avoid. Moderate Theoretical
- Mineralocorticoid receptor antagonists **(spironolactone)** potentially increase the concentration of **lithium**. Moderate Study
- **NSAIDs** increase the concentration of **lithium**. Monitor and adjust dose. Severe Study → Also see TABLE 2 p. 1053
- **Phenothiazine antipsychotics** potentially increase the risk of neurotoxicity when given with **lithium**. Severe Anecdotal
- Potassium-sparing diuretics **(triamterene)** potentially increase the clearance of **lithium**. Moderate Study
- **Sodium bicarbonate** decreases the concentration of **lithium**. Severe Anecdotal
- **Sparsentan** might increase the concentration of **lithium**. Severe Theoretical
- **Sulpiride** potentially increases the risk of neurotoxicity when given with **lithium**. Severe Anecdotal
- **Tetracyclines** are predicted to increase the risk of lithium toxicity when given with **lithium**. Avoid or adjust dose. Severe Anecdotal
- **Theophylline** is predicted to decrease the concentration of **lithium**. Monitor concentration and adjust dose. Moderate Anecdotal
- **Thiazide diuretics** increase the concentration of **lithium**. Avoid or adjust dose and monitor concentration. Severe Study
- **Tricyclic antidepressants** potentially increase the risk of neurotoxicity when given with **lithium**. Severe Anecdotal
- **Lithium** might decrease the antidiuretic and hypertensive effects of **vasopressin**. Moderate Theoretical
- **Zuclopenthixol** potentially increases the risk of neurotoxicity when given with **lithium**. Severe Anecdotal

Live vaccines

Bacillus Calmette-Guérin vaccine · chikungunya vaccine (live) · cholera vaccine (live) · dengue vaccine · influenza vaccine (live) · measles, mumps, and rubella vaccine · rotavirus vaccine · typhoid vaccine (live) · varicella-zoster vaccine · yellow fever vaccine

- Antibacterials might decrease the efficacy **cholera vaccine (live)**. Avoid concurrent use with, for 14 days before, and for 10 days after, giving cholera vaccine (live).
- **Typhoid vaccine (live)** is inactivated by concurrent administration of antibacterials or antimalarials: antibacterials should be avoided for 3 days before and after live typhoid vaccination; *mefloquine* should be avoided for at least 12 hours before or after live typhoid vaccination; for other antimalarials live typhoid vaccine vaccination should be completed at least 3 days before the first dose of the antimalarial (except proguanil hydrochloride with atovaquone, which can be given concurrently).

- **Live vaccines** are predicted to increase the risk of generalised infection (possibly life-threatening) when given with **abatacept**. UKHSA advises avoid (refer to Green Book). Severe Theoretical
- **Live vaccines** are predicted to increase the risk of generalised infection (possibly life-threatening) when given with **abrocitinib**. Avoid. Severe Theoretical
- **Live vaccines** are predicted to increase the risk of generalised infection (possibly life-threatening) when given with **alkylating agents**. UKHSA advises avoid (refer to Green Book). Severe Theoretical
- **Live vaccines** are predicted to increase the risk of generalised infection (possibly life-threatening) when given with **amsacrine**. UKHSA advises avoid (refer to Green Book). Severe Theoretical
- **Live vaccines** are predicted to increase the risk of generalised infection (possibly life-threatening) when given with **anakinra**. UKHSA advises avoid (refer to Green Book). Severe Theoretical
- **Live vaccines** are predicted to increase the risk of generalised infection (possibly life-threatening) when given with **anthracyclines**. UKHSA advises avoid (refer to Green Book). Severe Theoretical
- Antimalarials **(chloroquine)** might decrease the efficacy of **cholera vaccine (live)**. Avoid for at least 10 days before **chloroquine**. Moderate Study
- **Aspirin** might increase the risk of Reye's syndrome when given with **influenza vaccine (live)**. Avoid **aspirin** for 4 weeks after vaccination. Severe Theoretical
- **Aspirin** might increase the risk of Reye's syndrome when given with **varicella-zoster vaccine**. Avoid **aspirin** for 6 weeks after vaccination. Severe Theoretical
- **Live vaccines** are predicted to increase the risk of generalised infection (possibly life-threatening) when given with **azathioprine** (high-dose). UKHSA advises avoid (refer to Green Book). Severe Theoretical
- **Baloxavir marboxil** might decrease the efficacy of **influenza vaccine (live)**. Moderate Theoretical

Live vaccines (continued)
- **Live vaccines** are predicted to increase the risk of generalised infection (possibly life-threatening) when given with **baricitinib**. Avoid. Severe Theoretical
- **Live vaccines** are predicted to increase the risk of generalised infection (possibly life-threatening) when given with **belatacept**. UKHSA advises avoid (refer to Green Book). Severe Theoretical
- **Live vaccines** are predicted to increase the risk of generalised infection (possibly life-threatening) when given with **bleomycin**. UKHSA advises avoid (refer to Green Book). Severe Theoretical
- **Live vaccines** are predicted to increase the risk of generalised infection (possibly life-threatening) when given with **capecitabine**. UKHSA advises avoid (refer to Green Book). Severe Theoretical
- **Live vaccines** are predicted to increase the risk of generalised infection (possibly life-threatening) when given with **ciclosporin**. UKHSA advises avoid (refer to Green Book). Severe Theoretical
- **Live vaccines** are predicted to increase the risk of generalised infection (possibly life-threatening) when given with **cladribine**. UKHSA advises avoid (refer to Green Book). Severe Theoretical
- **Live vaccines** are predicted to increase the risk of generalised infection (possibly life-threatening) when given with **clofarabine**. UKHSA advises avoid (refer to Green Book). Severe Theoretical
- **Live vaccines** are predicted to increase the risk of generalised infection (possibly life-threatening) when given with **corticosteroids** (high-dose). UKHSA advises avoid (refer to Green Book). Severe Theoretical
- **Live vaccines** are predicted to increase the risk of generalised infection (possibly life-threatening) when given with **cytarabine**. UKHSA advises avoid (refer to Green Book). Severe Theoretical
- **Live vaccines** are predicted to increase the risk of generalised infection (possibly life-threatening) when given with **dactinomycin**. UKHSA advises avoid (refer to Green Book). Severe Theoretical
- **Live vaccines** are predicted to increase the risk of generalised infection (possibly life-threatening) when given with **deucravacitinib**. Avoid. Severe Theoretical
- **Live vaccines** are predicted to increase the risk of generalised infection (possibly life-threatening) when given with **dimethyl fumarate**. UKHSA advises avoid (refer to Green Book). Severe Theoretical
- **Live vaccines** are predicted to increase the risk of generalised infection (possibly life-threatening) when given with **diroximel fumarate**. Use with caution or avoid. Severe Theoretical
- **Live vaccines** might increase the risk of generalised infection (possibly life-threatening) when given with **efgartigimod alfa**. Avoid. Severe Theoretical
- **Live vaccines** are predicted to increase the risk of generalised infection (possibly life-threatening) when given with **etanercept**. UKHSA advises avoid (refer to Green Book). Severe Theoretical
- **Live vaccines** are predicted to increase the risk of generalised infection (possibly life-threatening) when given with **etoposide**. UKHSA advises avoid (refer to Green Book). Severe Theoretical
- **Live vaccines** might increase the risk of generalised infection (possibly life-threatening) when given with **etrasimod**. Avoid and for at least 4 weeks before and 2 weeks after stopping **etrasimod**. Severe Theoretical
- **Live vaccines** are predicted to increase the risk of generalised infection (possibly life-threatening) when given with **everolimus**. UKHSA advises avoid (refer to Green Book). Severe Theoretical
- **Live vaccines** are predicted to increase the risk of generalised infection (possibly life-threatening) when given with **filgotinib**. Avoid. Severe Theoretical
- **Live vaccines** might increase the risk of generalised infection (possibly life-threatening) when given with **fingolimod**. UKHSA advises avoid (refer to Green Book). Severe Theoretical
- **Live vaccines** are predicted to increase the risk of generalised infection (possibly life-threatening) when given with **fludarabine**. UKHSA advises avoid (refer to Green Book). Severe Theoretical
- **Live vaccines** are predicted to increase the risk of generalised infection (possibly life-threatening) when given with **fluorouracil**. UKHSA advises avoid (refer to Green Book). Severe Theoretical
- **Live vaccines** are predicted to increase the risk of generalised infection (possibly life-threatening) when given with **gemcitabine**. UKHSA advises avoid (refer to Green Book). Severe Theoretical
- **Live vaccines** are predicted to increase the risk of generalised infection (possibly life-threatening) when given with **hydroxycarbamide**. UKHSA advises avoid (refer to Green Book). Severe Theoretical
- **Immunoglobulins** are predicted to decrease the efficacy of live vaccines **(chikungunya vaccine (live), cholera vaccine (live), dengue vaccine, influenza vaccine (live), measles, mumps, and rubella vaccine, rotavirus vaccine, typhoid vaccine (live), varicella-zoster vaccine)**. Avoid and for 3 months after stopping **immunoglobulins**. Moderate Theoretical
- **Live vaccines** are predicted to increase the risk of generalised infection (possibly life-threatening) when given with **irinotecan**. UKHSA advises avoid (refer to Green Book). Severe Theoretical
- **Live vaccines** are predicted to increase the risk of generalised infection (possibly life-threatening) when given with iron chelators **(dexrazoxane)**. Avoid. Severe Theoretical
- **Live vaccines** are predicted to increase the risk of generalised infection (possibly life-threatening) when given with **leflunomide**. UKHSA advises avoid (refer to Green Book). Severe Theoretical
- **Live vaccines** are predicted to increase the risk of generalised infection (possibly life-threatening) when given with **mercaptopurine** (high-dose). UKHSA advises avoid (refer to Green Book). Severe Theoretical
- **Live vaccines** are predicted to increase the risk of generalised infection (possibly life-threatening) when given with **methotrexate** (high-dose). UKHSA advises avoid (refer to Green Book). Severe Theoretical
- **Live vaccines** are predicted to increase the risk of generalised infection (possibly life-threatening) when given with **mitomycin**. UKHSA advises avoid (refer to Green Book). Severe Theoretical
- **Live vaccines** are predicted to increase the risk of generalised infection (possibly life-threatening) when given with monoclonal antibodies **(adalimumab, alemtuzumab, atezolizumab, avelumab, basiliximab, belimumab, bevacizumab, bimekizumab, blinatumomab, brentuximab vedotin, brodalumab, canakinumab, cemiplimab, certolizumab pegol, cetuximab, daratumumab, dinutuximab, dostarlimab, dupilumab, eculizumab, elotuzumab, elranatamab, golimumab, guselkumab, infliximab, inotuzumab ozogamicin, ipilimumab, ixekizumab, lebrikizumab, loncastuximab tesirine, mirikizumab, mogamulizumab, mosunetuzumab, natalizumab, nemolizumab, nivolumab, obinutuzumab, ocrelizumab, ofatumumab, panitumumab, pembrolizumab, pertuzumab, polatuzumab vedotin, ramucirumab, risankizumab, rituximab, rozanolixizumab, sarilumab, satralizumab, secukinumab, serplulimab, siltuximab, spesolimab, tafasitamab, teclistamab, teplizumab, tezepelumab, tildrakizumab, tocilizumab, tralokinumab, trastuzumab, trastuzumab deruxtecan, trastuzumab emtansine, ublituximab, ustekinumab, vedolizumab)**. UKHSA advises avoid (refer to Green Book). Severe Theoretical
- **Live vaccines** are predicted to increase the risk of generalised infection (possibly life-threatening) when given with **mycophenolate**. UKHSA advises avoid (refer to Green Book). Severe Theoretical
- **Oseltamivir** might decrease the efficacy of **influenza vaccine (live)**. Moderate Theoretical

- **Live vaccines** might increase the risk of generalised infection (possibly life-threatening) when given with **ozanimod**. Avoid and for 3 months after stopping **ozanimod**. Severe Theoretical
- **Live vaccines** are predicted to increase the risk of generalised infection (possibly life-threatening) when given with **pemetrexed**. UKHSA advises avoid (refer to Green Book). Severe Theoretical
- **Live vaccines** are predicted to increase the risk of generalised infection (possibly life-threatening) when given with **platinum compounds**. UKHSA advises avoid (refer to Green Book). Severe Theoretical
- **Live vaccines** might increase the risk of generalised infection (possibly life-threatening) when given with **ponesimod**. Avoid and for 1 week after stopping **ponesimod**. Severe Theoretical
- **Live vaccines** are predicted to increase the risk of generalised infection (possibly life-threatening) when given with **procarbazine**. UKHSA advises avoid (refer to Green Book). Severe Theoretical
- **Live vaccines** are predicted to increase the risk of generalised infection (possibly life-threatening) when given with **raltitrexed**. UKHSA advises avoid (refer to Green Book). Severe Theoretical
- **Live vaccines** are predicted to increase the risk of generalised infection (possibly life-threatening) when given with **ritlecitinib**. Avoid. Severe Theoretical
- **Live vaccines** might increase the risk of generalised infection (possibly life-threatening) when given with **siponimod**. Avoid and for 4 weeks after stopping **siponimod**. Severe Theoretical
- **Live vaccines** are predicted to increase the risk of generalised infection (possibly life-threatening) when given with **sirolimus**. UKHSA advises avoid (refer to Green Book). Severe Theoretical
- **Live vaccines** are predicted to increase the risk of generalised infection (possibly life-threatening) when given with **streptozocin**. UKHSA advises avoid (refer to Green Book). Severe Theoretical
- **Live vaccines** are predicted to increase the risk of generalised infection (possibly life-threatening) when given with **tacrolimus**. UKHSA advises avoid (refer to Green Book). Severe Theoretical
- **Live vaccines** are predicted to increase the risk of generalised infection (possibly life-threatening) when given with taxanes **(docetaxel, paclitaxel)**. UKHSA advises avoid (refer to Green Book). Severe Theoretical
- **Live vaccines** are predicted to increase the risk of generalised infection (possibly life-threatening) when given with **tegafur**. UKHSA advises avoid (refer to Green Book). Severe Theoretical
- **Live vaccines** are predicted to increase the risk of generalised infection (possibly life-threatening) when given with **temsirolimus**. UKHSA advises avoid (refer to Green Book). Severe Theoretical
- **Live vaccines** are predicted to increase the risk of generalised infection (possibly life-threatening) when given with **teriflunomide**. UKHSA advises avoid (refer to Green Book). Severe Theoretical
- **Live vaccines** are predicted to increase the risk of generalised infection (possibly life-threatening) when given with **tioguanine**. UKHSA advises avoid (refer to Green Book). Severe Theoretical
- **Live vaccines** potentially increase the risk of generalised infection (possibly life-threatening) when given with **tofacitinib**. Avoid. Severe Theoretical
- **Live vaccines** are predicted to increase the risk of generalised infection (possibly life-threatening) when given with **topotecan**. UKHSA advises avoid (refer to Green Book). Severe Theoretical
- **Live vaccines** are predicted to increase the risk of generalised infection (possibly life-threatening) when given with **trabectedin**. UKHSA advises avoid (refer to Green Book). Severe Theoretical
- **Live vaccines** are predicted to increase the risk of generalised infection (possibly life-threatening) when given with **upadacitinib**. Avoid. Severe Theoretical
- **Venetoclax** potentially decreases the efficacy of **live vaccines**. Avoid. Severe Theoretical
- **Live vaccines** are predicted to increase the risk of generalised infection (possibly life-threatening) when given with **vinca alkaloids**. UKHSA advises avoid (refer to Green Book). Severe Theoretical
- **Live vaccines** are predicted to increase the risk of generalised infection (possibly life-threatening) when given with **voclosporin**. UKHSA advises avoid (refer to Green Book). Severe Theoretical
- **Zanamivir** might decrease the efficacy of **influenza vaccine (live)**. Moderate Theoretical

Lofepramine → see tricyclic antidepressants

Lofexidine → see TABLE 6 p. 1054 (hypotension), TABLE 9 p. 1056 (CNS effects)

Lomitapide → see TABLE 1 p. 1053 (hepatotoxicity)

FOOD AND LIFESTYLE Bitter (Seville) orange is predicted to increase the exposure to lomitapide; separate administration by 12 hours.

- Anti-androgens **(apalutamide, enzalutamide)** are predicted to decrease the exposure to **lomitapide**. Monitor and adjust dose. Moderate Theoretical
- Anti-androgens **(bicalutamide)** are predicted to increase the exposure to **lomitapide**. Separate administration by 12 hours. Moderate Theoretical
- Antiarrhythmics **(amiodarone)** are predicted to increase the exposure to **lomitapide**. Separate administration by 12 hours. Moderate Theoretical → Also see TABLE 1 p. 1053
- Antiarrhythmics **(dronedarone)** are predicted to increase the exposure to **lomitapide**. Avoid. Moderate Theoretical
- Antiepileptics **(carbamazepine, fosphenytoin, phenobarbital, phenytoin, primidone)** are predicted to decrease the exposure to **lomitapide**. Monitor and adjust dose. Moderate Theoretical
- Antifungals, azoles **(clotrimazole)** are predicted to increase the exposure to **lomitapide**. Separate administration by 12 hours. Moderate Theoretical
- Antifungals, azoles **(fluconazole, isavuconazole)** are predicted to increase the exposure to **lomitapide**. Avoid. Moderate Theoretical → Also see TABLE 1 p. 1053
- Antifungals, azoles **(itraconazole, ketoconazole, posaconazole, voriconazole)** are predicted to markedly increase the exposure to **lomitapide**. Avoid. Severe Study → Also see TABLE 1 p. 1053
- Benzodiazepines **(alprazolam)** are predicted to increase the exposure to **lomitapide**. Separate administration by 12 hours. Moderate Theoretical
- **Berotralstat** is predicted to increase the exposure to **lomitapide**. Avoid. Moderate Theoretical
- Calcium-channel blockers **(amlodipine, lacidipine)** are predicted to increase the exposure to **lomitapide**. Separate administration by 12 hours. Moderate Theoretical
- Calcium-channel blockers **(diltiazem, verapamil)** are predicted to increase the exposure to **lomitapide**. Avoid. Moderate Theoretical
- **Cenobamate** is predicted to decrease the exposure to **lomitapide**. Adjust dose. Moderate Theoretical
- **Ceritinib** is predicted to markedly increase the exposure to **lomitapide**. Avoid. Severe Study
- **Ciclosporin** is predicted to increase the exposure to **lomitapide**. Separate administration by 12 hours. Moderate Theoretical
- **Cilostazol** is predicted to increase the exposure to **lomitapide**. Separate administration by 12 hours. Moderate Theoretical
- **Cobicistat** is predicted to markedly increase the exposure to **lomitapide**. Avoid. Severe Study
- Oral **combined hormonal contraceptives** slightly increase the exposure to **lomitapide**. Separate administration by 12 hours. Moderate Theoretical
- **Lomitapide** increases the exposure to coumarins **(warfarin)**. Monitor INR and adjust dose. Severe Study
- **Crizotinib** is predicted to increase the exposure to **lomitapide**. Avoid. Moderate Theoretical
- **Lomitapide** might increase the exposure to **digoxin**. Adjust dose. Moderate Theoretical
- Dipeptidylpeptidase-4 inhibitors **(linagliptin)** are predicted to increase the exposure to **lomitapide**. Separate administration by 12 hours. Moderate Theoretical
- **Encorafenib** is predicted to decrease the exposure to **lomitapide**. Monitor and adjust dose. Moderate Theoretical

Lomitapide (continued)
- **Everolimus** is predicted to increase the exposure to **lomitapide** and **lomitapide** might increase the exposure to **everolimus**. Adjust **everolimus** dose and separate administration by 12 hours, p. 689. [Moderate] Theoretical
- **Fedratinib** is predicted to increase the exposure to **lomitapide**. Avoid. [Moderate] Theoretical
- **Grapefruit** juice is predicted to increase the exposure to **lomitapide**. Avoid. [Mild] Theoretical
- H_2 receptor antagonists **(cimetidine)** are predicted to increase the exposure to **lomitapide**. Separate administration by 12 hours. [Mild] Theoretical
- **HIV-protease inhibitors** are predicted to markedly increase the exposure to **lomitapide**. Avoid. [Severe] Study → Also see TABLE 1 p. 1053
- **Idelalisib** is predicted to markedly increase the exposure to **lomitapide**. Avoid. [Severe] Study
- **Imatinib** is predicted to increase the exposure to **lomitapide**. Avoid. [Moderate] Theoretical
- **Isoniazid** is predicted to increase the exposure to **lomitapide**. Separate administration by 12 hours. [Unknown] Theoretical → Also see TABLE 1 p. 1053
- **Ivacaftor** is predicted to increase the exposure to **lomitapide**. Separate administration by 12 hours. [Moderate] Theoretical
- **Ivosidenib** is predicted to decrease the exposure to **lomitapide**. Monitor and adjust dose. [Moderate] Theoretical
- **Lapatinib** is predicted to increase the exposure to **lomitapide**. Separate administration by 12 hours. [Mild] Theoretical
- **Letermovir** is predicted to increase the exposure to **lomitapide**. Avoid. [Moderate] Theoretical
- **Lumacaftor** is predicted to decrease the exposure to **lomitapide**. Monitor and adjust dose. [Moderate] Theoretical
- Macrolides **(azithromycin)** are predicted to increase the exposure to **lomitapide**. Separate administration by 12 hours. [Moderate] Theoretical
- Macrolides **(clarithromycin)** are predicted to markedly increase the exposure to **lomitapide**. Avoid. [Severe] Study
- Macrolides **(erythromycin)** are predicted to increase the exposure to **lomitapide**. Avoid. [Moderate] Theoretical
- **Lomitapide** is predicted to increase the exposure to **mavacamten**. Monitor and adjust dose—consult product literature. [Moderate] Theoretical
- **Mitotane** is predicted to decrease the exposure to **lomitapide**. Monitor and adjust dose. [Moderate] Theoretical
- Neurokinin-1 receptor antagonists **(aprepitant, netupitant)** are predicted to increase the exposure to **lomitapide**. Avoid. [Moderate] Theoretical
- Neurokinin-1 receptor antagonists **(fosaprepitant)** are predicted to increase the exposure to **lomitapide**. Separate administration by 12 hours. [Mild] Theoretical
- **Nilotinib** is predicted to increase the exposure to **lomitapide**. Avoid. [Moderate] Theoretical
- **Nirmatrelvir** boosted with ritonavir is predicted to increase the concentration of **lomitapide**. Avoid. [Severe] Theoretical
- **Pazopanib** is predicted to increase the exposure to **lomitapide**. Separate administration by 12 hours. [Mild] Theoretical
- **Peppermint** oil is predicted to increase the exposure to **lomitapide**. Separate administration by 12 hours. [Moderate] Theoretical
- **Propiverine** is predicted to increase the exposure to **lomitapide**. Separate administration by 12 hours. [Moderate] Theoretical
- **Ranolazine** is predicted to increase the exposure to **lomitapide**. Separate administration by 12 hours. [Mild] Theoretical
- Rifamycins **(rifampicin)** are predicted to decrease the exposure to **lomitapide**. Monitor and adjust dose. [Moderate] Theoretical
- **Lomitapide** might increase the exposure to **sirolimus**. Adjust dose. [Moderate] Theoretical
- SSRIs **(fluoxetine)** are predicted to increase the exposure to **lomitapide**. Separate administration by 12 hours. [Unknown] Theoretical
- SSRIs **(fluvoxamine)** are predicted to increase the exposure to **lomitapide**. Separate administration by 12 hours. [Mild] Theoretical
- **Lomitapide** increases the exposure to statins **(atorvastatin)**. Adjust **lomitapide** dose or separate administration by 12 hours. [Mild] Study → Also see TABLE 1 p. 1053
- **Lomitapide** increases the exposure to statins **(simvastatin)**. Monitor and adjust **simvastatin** dose, p. 156. [Moderate] Study → Also see TABLE 1 p. 1053
- **Tacrolimus** is predicted to increase the exposure to **lomitapide**. Separate administration by 12 hours. [Moderate] Theoretical
- **Lomitapide** might increase the exposure to **talazoparib**. Adjust dose. [Moderate] Theoretical
- **Lomitapide** might increase the exposure to taxanes **(paclitaxel)**. Adjust dose. [Moderate] Theoretical
- **Ticagrelor** is predicted to increase the exposure to **lomitapide**. Separate administration by 12 hours. [Moderate] Theoretical
- **Tolvaptan** is predicted to increase the exposure to **lomitapide**. Separate administration by 12 hours. [Moderate] Theoretical
- **Tucatinib** is predicted to markedly increase the exposure to **lomitapide**. Avoid. [Severe] Study

Lomustine → see alkylating agents

Loncastuximab tesirine → see monoclonal antibodies

Loop diuretics → see TABLE 15 p. 1058 (hyponatraemia), TABLE 6 p. 1054 (hypotension), TABLE 16 p. 1058 (ototoxicity), TABLE 14 p. 1057 (reduced serum potassium)

bumetanide · furosemide · torasemide

- **Aliskiren** slightly decreases the exposure to **furosemide**. [Moderate] Study → Also see TABLE 6 p. 1054
- **Loop diuretics** increase the risk of nephrotoxicity when given with **aminoglycosides**. Avoid. [Moderate] Study → Also see TABLE 16 p. 1058
- Antiepileptics **(fosphenytoin, phenytoin)** decrease the effects of **furosemide**. [Moderate] Study
- Intravenous **furosemide** potentially increases the risk of sweating, variable blood pressure, and tachycardia when given after **chloral hydrate**. [Moderate] Anecdotal
- **Loop diuretics** are predicted to increase the risk of adverse effects when given with immunoglobulins **(cytomegalovirus immunoglobulin)**. Avoid. [Moderate] Theoretical
- **Loop diuretics** might increase the risk of adverse effects when given with immunoglobulins **(hepatitis B immunoglobulin, normal immunoglobulin)**. Avoid. [Moderate] Theoretical
- **Ivosidenib** is predicted to increase the exposure to **furosemide**. Manufacturer advises caution or avoid—consult product literature. [Moderate] Theoretical
- **Leflunomide** is predicted to increase the exposure to **furosemide**. [Moderate] Study
- **Loop diuretics** increase the concentration of **lithium**. Monitor and adjust dose. [Severe] Study
- **Nitisinone** is predicted to increase the exposure to **furosemide**. [Moderate] Study
- **Reboxetine** is predicted to increase the risk of hypokalaemia when given with **loop diuretics**. [Moderate] Theoretical
- **Selpercatinib** is predicted to increase the exposure to **torasemide**. Avoid. [Severe] Study
- **Teriflunomide** is predicted to increase the exposure to **furosemide**. [Moderate] Study
- **Furosemide** might slightly decrease the clearance of **treprostinil**. [Unknown] Theoretical → Also see TABLE 6 p. 1054
- **Vadadustat** increases the exposure to **furosemide**. Monitor and adjust dose. [Moderate] Study

Loperamide
- Anti-androgens **(apalutamide)** are predicted to decrease the exposure to **loperamide**. Monitor and adjust dose. [Moderate] Study
- Antiarrhythmics **(dronedarone)** are predicted to increase the exposure to **loperamide**. [Severe] Theoretical
- Atypical antipsychotics **(clozapine)** can cause constipation, as can **loperamide**; concurrent use might increase the risk of developing intestinal obstruction. [Severe] Anecdotal
- **Ceritinib** is predicted to increase the exposure to **loperamide**. [Moderate] Theoretical
- **Danicopan** is predicted to increase the exposure to **loperamide**. [Moderate] Study
- **Loperamide** greatly increases the absorption of oral **desmopressin** (and possibly sublingual). [Moderate] Study

A1 Interactions | Appendix 1

- **Eliglustat** is predicted to increase the exposure to **loperamide**. Adjust dose. Moderate Study
- **Glecaprevir** is predicted to increase the exposure to **loperamide**. Severe Theoretical
- **Ivosidenib** is predicted to alter the exposure to **loperamide**. Moderate Theoretical
- **Lapatinib** is predicted to increase the exposure to **loperamide**. Moderate Theoretical
- **Lorlatinib** is predicted to decrease the exposure to **loperamide**. Moderate Study
- **Mifepristone** is predicted to increase the exposure to **loperamide**. Moderate Theoretical
- **Mirabegron** is predicted to increase the exposure to **loperamide**. Mild Theoretical
- **Olaparib** might increase the exposure to **loperamide**. Moderate Theoretical
- **Opicapone** is predicted to increase the exposure to **loperamide**. Avoid. Moderate Study
- **Osimertinib** is predicted to increase the exposure to **loperamide**. Moderate Study
- **Pibrentasvir** with glecaprevir is predicted to increase the exposure to **loperamide**. Moderate Study
- **Pitolisant** is predicted to decrease the exposure to **loperamide**. Mild Theoretical
- **Sparsentan** is predicted to increase the exposure to **loperamide**. Severe Theoretical
- **Velpatasvir** is predicted to increase the exposure to **loperamide**. Severe Theoretical
- **Vemurafenib** might increase the exposure to **loperamide**. Use with caution and adjust dose. Moderate Theoretical
- **Voxilaprevir** with sofosbuvir and velpatasvir is predicted to increase the exposure to **loperamide**. Severe Theoretical

Lopinavir → see HIV-protease inhibitors

Loprazolam → see benzodiazepines

Loratadine → see antihistamines, non-sedating

Lorazepam → see benzodiazepines

Lorlatinib

- **Lorlatinib** is predicted to decrease the exposure to **afatinib**. Moderate Study
- **Lorlatinib** decreases the exposure to **aliskiren**. Moderate Study
- Anti-androgens **(apalutamide, enzalutamide)** are predicted to decrease the exposure to **lorlatinib**. Avoid. Severe Study
- **Lorlatinib** is predicted to decrease the exposure to anti-androgens **(darolutamide)**. Avoid. Moderate Theoretical
- Antiepileptics **(carbamazepine, fosphenytoin, phenobarbital, phenytoin, primidone)** are predicted to decrease the exposure to **lorlatinib**. Avoid. Severe Study
- Antifungals, azoles **(fluconazole)** are predicted to increase the exposure to **lorlatinib**. Moderate Theoretical
- Antifungals, azoles **(itraconazole, ketoconazole, posaconazole, voriconazole)** are predicted to increase the exposure to **lorlatinib**. Avoid or adjust dose—consult product literature. Severe Study
- **Lorlatinib** is predicted to decrease the exposure to antifungals, azoles **(isavuconazole)**. Avoid. Severe Theoretical
- **Lorlatinib** decreases the exposure to antihistamines, non-sedating **(fexofenadine)**. Moderate Study
- **Lorlatinib** is predicted to decrease the exposure to atypical antipsychotics **(aripiprazole)**. Avoid or adjust dose—consult product literature. Moderate Study
- **Lorlatinib** is predicted to decrease the exposure to atypical antipsychotics **(cariprazine)**. Avoid. Severe Theoretical
- **Lorlatinib** is predicted to decrease the exposure to atypical antipsychotics **(lurasidone)**. Monitor and adjust dose. Moderate Theoretical
- **Lorlatinib** is predicted to decrease the exposure to atypical antipsychotics **(quetiapine)**. Moderate Study
- **Lorlatinib** is predicted to decrease the exposure to **avacopan**. Severe Theoretical
- **Lorlatinib** is predicted to decrease the exposure to **avapritinib**. Avoid. Severe Study
- **Lorlatinib** is predicted to decrease the exposure to **bedaquiline**. Avoid. Severe Study
- **Lorlatinib** moderately decreases the exposure to benzodiazepines **(midazolam)**. Avoid. Moderate Study
- **Lorlatinib** is predicted to decrease the concentration of **berotralstat**. Avoid. Severe Theoretical
- **Lorlatinib** is predicted to decrease the exposure to **bosutinib**. Avoid. Severe Study
- **Lorlatinib** is predicted to decrease the exposure to **brigatinib**. Avoid or adjust dose—consult product literature. Moderate Study
- **Lorlatinib** is predicted to decrease the exposure to **cabozantinib**. Moderate Study
- **Lorlatinib** is predicted to decrease the exposure to calcium-channel blockers **(amlodipine, felodipine, lacidipine, lercanidipine, nicardipine, nifedipine, nimodipine)**. Monitor and adjust dose. Moderate Theoretical
- **Lorlatinib** is predicted to decrease the exposure to calcium-channel blockers **(diltiazem, verapamil)**. Moderate Theoretical
- **Lorlatinib** is predicted to decrease the exposure to **capivasertib**. Avoid. Moderate Study
- **Ceritinib** is predicted to increase the exposure to **lorlatinib**. Avoid or adjust dose—consult product literature. Severe Study
- **Lorlatinib** is predicted to decrease the exposure to **ciclosporin**. Avoid. Moderate Theoretical
- **Cobicistat** is predicted to increase the exposure to **lorlatinib**. Avoid or adjust dose—consult product literature. Severe Study
- **Lorlatinib** is predicted to decrease the exposure to **cobicistat**. Avoid. Severe Theoretical
- **Lorlatinib** is predicted to decrease the exposure to **cobimetinib**. Avoid. Severe Theoretical
- **Lorlatinib** is predicted to decrease the exposure to **colchicine**. Moderate Theoretical
- **Lorlatinib** is predicted to decrease the exposure to **combined hormonal contraceptives**. Avoid. Moderate Theoretical
- **Lorlatinib** is predicted to decrease the exposure to **coumarins**. Moderate Theoretical
- **Lorlatinib** is predicted to decrease the exposure to **crizotinib**. Avoid. Severe Study
- **Lorlatinib** is predicted to decrease the exposure to **daridorexant**. Severe Study
- **Lorlatinib** is predicted to decrease the exposure to **dasatinib**. Severe Study
- **Lorlatinib** is predicted to decrease the exposure to **deutivacaftor**. Avoid. Severe Theoretical
- **Lorlatinib** is predicted to decrease the exposure to **digoxin**. Moderate Study
- **Lorlatinib** is predicted to decrease the exposure to **elacestrant**. Avoid or adjust dose depending on duration—consult product literature. Severe Theoretical
- **Lorlatinib** is predicted to moderately decrease the exposure to **elbasvir**. Avoid. Severe Study
- **Lorlatinib** is predicted to decrease the concentration of **elvitegravir**. Avoid. Severe Theoretical
- **Encorafenib** is predicted to decrease the exposure to **lorlatinib**. Avoid. Severe Study
- **Lorlatinib** is predicted to decrease the exposure to **encorafenib**. Moderate Study
- **Lorlatinib** is predicted to decrease the exposure to **entrectinib**. Avoid. Moderate Theoretical
- **Lorlatinib** is predicted to decrease the exposure to **erdafitinib**. Adjust dose. Moderate Theoretical
- **Lorlatinib** is predicted to decrease the exposure to **erlotinib**. Severe Study
- **Lorlatinib** is predicted to decrease the concentration of **everolimus**. Avoid or adjust dose. Severe Study
- **Lorlatinib** is predicted to decrease the exposure to factor XA inhibitors **(apixaban)**. Use with caution or avoid. Severe Study
- **Lorlatinib** is predicted to decrease the exposure to factor XA inhibitors **(edoxaban)**. Severe Study
- **Lorlatinib** is predicted to decrease the exposure to factor XA inhibitors **(rivaroxaban)**. Avoid unless patient can be monitored for signs of thrombosis. Severe Study
- **Lorlatinib** is predicted to decrease the exposure to **fedratinib**. Avoid. Moderate Study
- **Lorlatinib** is predicted to decrease the exposure to **fruquintinib**. Avoid. Moderate Study
- **Lorlatinib** is predicted to decrease the exposure to **futibatinib**. Avoid or adjust dose. Moderate Study

Lorlatinib (continued)

- Lorlatinib is predicted to decrease the exposure to gefitinib. Avoid. Severe Study
- Lorlatinib is predicted to decrease the exposure to glasdegib. Avoid or adjust dose—consult product literature. Moderate Theoretical
- Lorlatinib is predicted to decrease the exposure to glecaprevir. Avoid. Severe Study
- Grapefruit juice is predicted to increase the concentration of lorlatinib. Avoid. Moderate Theoretical
- Lorlatinib is predicted to markedly decrease the exposure to grazoprevir. Avoid. Severe Study
- Lorlatinib is predicted to decrease the concentration of guanfacine. Adjust dose. Moderate Theoretical
- HIV-protease inhibitors are predicted to increase the exposure to lorlatinib. Avoid or adjust dose—consult product literature. Severe Study
- Idelalisib is predicted to increase the exposure to lorlatinib. Avoid or adjust dose—consult product literature. Severe Study
- Lorlatinib is predicted to decrease the exposure to idelalisib. Avoid. Moderate Theoretical
- Lorlatinib is predicted to decrease the exposure to imatinib. Moderate Study
- Ivosidenib is predicted to decrease the exposure to lorlatinib. Avoid. Severe Study
- Lorlatinib is predicted to decrease the exposure to ixazomib. Moderate Theoretical
- Lorlatinib is predicted to decrease the exposure to lapatinib. Avoid. Severe Study
- Lorlatinib is predicted to decrease the exposure to larotrectinib. Avoid. Moderate Study
- Lorlatinib is predicted to decrease the exposure to ledipasvir. Avoid. Severe Study
- Lorlatinib is predicted to decrease the exposure to lenacapavir. Avoid. Severe Study
- Lorlatinib is predicted to decrease the exposure to leniolisib. Avoid. Severe Theoretical
- Lorlatinib is predicted to decrease the exposure to loperamide. Moderate Study
- Lumacaftor is predicted to decrease the exposure to lorlatinib. Avoid. Severe Study
- Macrolides (clarithromycin) are predicted to increase the exposure to lorlatinib. Avoid or adjust dose—consult product literature. Severe Study
- Lorlatinib is predicted to decrease the exposure to mavacamten. Monitor and adjust dose—consult product literature. Severe Theoretical
- Lorlatinib is predicted to decrease the exposure to mifepristone. Adjust mifepristone dose. Severe Study
- Lorlatinib is predicted to decrease the exposure to mineralocorticoid receptor antagonists (finerenone). Avoid. Severe Study
- Mitotane is predicted to decrease the exposure to lorlatinib. Avoid. Severe Study
- Lorlatinib is predicted to decrease the exposure to naloxegol. Moderate Theoretical
- Lorlatinib is predicted to decrease the exposure to neratinib. Avoid. Severe Theoretical
- Lorlatinib is predicted to decrease the exposure to neurokinin-1 receptor antagonists (netupitant). Moderate Theoretical
- Lorlatinib is predicted to decrease the exposure to nilotinib. Avoid. Severe Theoretical
- Lorlatinib is predicted to decrease the exposure to nintedanib. Moderate Study
- Lorlatinib is predicted to decrease the exposure to NNRTIs (rilpivirine). Avoid. Severe Theoretical
- Lorlatinib is predicted to decrease the exposure to olaparib. Avoid. Moderate Theoretical
- Lorlatinib is predicted to decrease the exposure to omaveloxolone. Avoid. Severe Study
- Lorlatinib is predicted to decrease the exposure to opioids (alfentanil, fentanyl). Avoid. Moderate Theoretical
- Lorlatinib decreases the exposure to opioids (methadone). Monitor and adjust dose. Severe Study
- Lorlatinib is predicted to decrease the exposure to ospemifene. Moderate Study
- Lorlatinib is predicted to decrease the exposure to pazopanib. Severe Study
- Lorlatinib is predicted to decrease the exposure to pemigatinib. Avoid or monitor. Severe Study
- Lorlatinib is predicted to decrease the exposure to pibrentasvir. Avoid. Severe Study
- Lorlatinib is predicted to decrease the exposure to pimozide. Avoid. Moderate Theoretical
- Lorlatinib is predicted to decrease the exposure to pirtobrutinib. Moderate Theoretical
- Lorlatinib is predicted to decrease the exposure to ponatinib. Severe Study
- Lorlatinib is predicted to decrease the exposure to pralsetinib. Moderate Theoretical
- Lorlatinib is predicted to decrease the exposure to quizartinib. Avoid. Severe Study
- Lorlatinib is predicted to decrease the exposure to ranolazine. Moderate Theoretical
- Rifamycins (rifampicin) are predicted to decrease the exposure to lorlatinib. Avoid. Severe Study
- Lorlatinib is predicted to decrease the exposure to rimegepant. Avoid. Moderate Theoretical
- Lorlatinib is predicted to decrease the exposure to ripretinib. Avoid or adjust dose—consult product literature. Moderate Theoretical
- Lorlatinib is predicted to decrease the exposure to ruxolitinib. Monitor and adjust dose. Moderate Study
- Lorlatinib is predicted to decrease the exposure to selpercatinib. Moderate Study
- Lorlatinib is predicted to decrease the exposure to selumetinib. Avoid. Severe Study
- Lorlatinib is predicted to decrease the exposure to siponimod. Manufacturer advises caution depending on genotype—consult product literature. Moderate Theoretical
- Lorlatinib is predicted to decrease the exposure to sirolimus. Avoid. Moderate Theoretical
- Lorlatinib is predicted to decrease the exposure to sofosbuvir. Avoid. Severe Study
- Lorlatinib is predicted to decrease the exposure to sorafenib. Moderate Study
- Lorlatinib is predicted to decrease the exposure to sparsentan. Avoid. Severe Theoretical
- St John's wort is predicted to decrease the exposure to lorlatinib. Avoid. Severe Theoretical
- Lorlatinib is predicted to decrease the exposure to statins (atorvastatin, simvastatin). Moderate Study
- Lorlatinib is predicted to decrease the exposure to sunitinib. Moderate Study
- Lorlatinib is predicted to decrease the exposure to tacrolimus. Avoid. Moderate Theoretical
- Lorlatinib is predicted to decrease the exposure to talazoparib. Moderate Study
- Lorlatinib is predicted to decrease the exposure to taxanes (docetaxel). Severe Theoretical
- Lorlatinib is predicted to decrease the exposure to taxanes (paclitaxel). Avoid. Severe Study
- Lorlatinib is predicted to decrease the concentration of temsirolimus. Avoid. Moderate Theoretical
- Lorlatinib is predicted to decrease the exposure to tenofovir alafenamide. Avoid. Moderate Theoretical
- Lorlatinib is predicted to decrease the exposure to tezacaftor. Avoid. Severe Theoretical
- Lorlatinib is predicted to decrease the exposure to thrombin inhibitors (dabigatran). Avoid. Severe Study
- Lorlatinib is predicted to decrease the exposure to ticagrelor. Moderate Theoretical
- Lorlatinib is predicted to decrease the exposure to tofacitinib. Severe Study
- Tucatinib is predicted to increase the exposure to lorlatinib. Avoid or adjust dose—consult product literature. Severe Study
- Lorlatinib is predicted to decrease the exposure to vanzacaftor. Avoid. Severe Theoretical

- **Lorlatinib** is predicted to decrease the exposure to **velpatasvir**. Avoid. Moderate Theoretical
- **Lorlatinib** is predicted to decrease the exposure to **venetoclax**. Avoid. Severe Study
- **Lorlatinib** is predicted to decrease the concentration of **voxilaprevir**. Avoid. Severe Theoretical
- **Lorlatinib** is predicted to decrease the exposure to **zanubrutinib**. Avoid or adjust dose with moderate CYP3A4 inducers—consult product literature. Severe Theoretical

Lormetazepam → see benzodiazepines

Losartan → see angiotensin-II receptor antagonists

Low molecular-weight heparins → see TABLE 3 p. 1053 (bleeding), TABLE 13 p. 1057 (increased serum potassium)

bemiparin · dalteparin · enoxaparin · tinzaparin

- **Andexanet alfa** is predicted to affect the anticoagulant effect of **low molecular-weight heparins**. Avoid. Severe Theoretical
- **Donanemab** can increase the risk of brain haemorrhage when given with **low molecular-weight heparins**. Avoid. Severe Anecdotal
- **Drugs that cause hepatotoxicity** (see TABLE 1 p. 1053) might increase the risk of hepatotoxicity when given with **low molecular-weight heparins** (high-dose). Severe Theoretical
- **Lecanemab** can increase the risk of brain haemorrhage when given with **low molecular-weight heparins**. Avoid. Severe Anecdotal
- **Low molecular-weight heparins** might increase the risk of gastrointestinal bleeding when given with monoclonal antibodies **(ipilimumab)**. Severe Theoretical

Loxapine → see TABLE 15 p. 1058 (hyponatraemia), TABLE 6 p. 1054 (hypotension), TABLE 8 p. 1055 (antimuscarinics), TABLE 9 p. 1056 (CNS effects)

- Atypical antipsychotics **(clozapine)** can cause constipation, as can **loxapine**; concurrent use might increase the risk of developing intestinal obstruction. Severe Theoretical → Also see TABLE 15 p. 1058 → Also see TABLE 6 p. 1054 → Also see TABLE 8 p. 1055 → Also see TABLE 9 p. 1056
- **Combined hormonal contraceptives** is predicted to increase the exposure to **loxapine**. Avoid. Unknown Theoretical
- **Loxapine** is predicted to decrease the effects of **dopamine receptor agonists**. Moderate Theoretical → Also see TABLE 6 p. 1054 → Also see TABLE 8 p. 1055 → Also see TABLE 9 p. 1056
- **Loxapine** opposes the effects of the active metabolite of **foslevodopa**. Severe Theoretical → Also see TABLE 6 p. 1054 → Also see TABLE 9 p. 1056
- **Givosiran** is predicted to increase the exposure to **loxapine**. Avoid. Unknown Theoretical
- **Loxapine** is predicted to decrease the effects of **levodopa**. Severe Theoretical → Also see TABLE 6 p. 1054 → Also see TABLE 9 p. 1056
- **Mexiletine** is predicted to increase the exposure to **loxapine**. Avoid. Unknown Theoretical
- **Osilodrostat** is predicted to increase the exposure to **loxapine**. Avoid. Unknown Theoretical
- Quinolones **(ciprofloxacin)** are predicted to increase the exposure to **loxapine**. Avoid. Unknown Theoretical
- **Rucaparib** is predicted to increase the exposure to **loxapine**. Avoid Unknown Theoretical
- SSRIs **(fluvoxamine)** are predicted to increase the exposure to **loxapine**. Avoid. Unknown Theoretical → Also see TABLE 15 p. 1058 → Also see TABLE 9 p. 1056
- **Vemurafenib** is predicted to increase the exposure to **loxapine**. Avoid. Unknown Theoretical

Lumacaftor

- **Lumacaftor** is predicted to decrease the exposure to 5-HT3-receptor antagonists **(ondansetron)**. Moderate Study
- **Lumacaftor** is predicted to markedly decrease the exposure to **abemaciclib**. Avoid. Severe Study
- **Lumacaftor** is predicted to decrease the exposure to **acalabrutinib**. Avoid. Severe Study
- **Lumacaftor** is predicted to decrease the exposure to **alpelisib**. Avoid. Moderate Study
- **Lumacaftor** is predicted to decrease the exposure to anti-androgens **(abiraterone)**. Avoid. Severe Study
- **Lumacaftor** is predicted to decrease the exposure to anti-androgens **(darolutamide)**. Avoid. Moderate Study
- **Lumacaftor** is predicted to decrease the exposure to antiarrhythmics **(disopyramide, dronedarone)**. Avoid. Severe Study
- **Lumacaftor** is predicted to decrease the efficacy of antiarrhythmics **(propafenone)**. Moderate Study
- **Lumacaftor** is predicted to decrease the exposure to anticholinesterases, centrally acting **(donepezil)**. Mild Study
- **Lumacaftor** is predicted to decrease the exposure to antiepileptics **(carbamazepine, fosphenytoin, phenobarbital, phenytoin, primidone)**. Avoid. Severe Theoretical
- **Lumacaftor** is predicted to decrease the exposure to antiepileptics **(perampanel)**. Monitor and adjust dose. Moderate Study
- **Lumacaftor** is predicted to decrease the exposure to antifungals, azoles **(isavuconazole)**. Avoid. Severe Study
- **Lumacaftor** is predicted to decrease the exposure to antifungals, azoles **(itraconazole, ketoconazole, posaconazole, voriconazole)**. Avoid or monitor efficacy. Moderate Theoretical
- **Lumacaftor** is predicted to decrease the exposure to antimalarials **(artemether)** with lumefantrine. Avoid. Severe Study
- **Lumacaftor** is predicted to decrease the concentration of antimalarials **(piperaquine)**. Avoid. Moderate Theoretical
- **Lumacaftor** is predicted to moderately decrease the exposure to atypical antipsychotics **(aripiprazole)**. Avoid or adjust dose—consult product literature. Moderate Study
- **Lumacaftor** is predicted to decrease the exposure to atypical antipsychotics **(cariprazine)**. Avoid. Severe Theoretical
- **Lumacaftor** is predicted to decrease the exposure to atypical antipsychotics **(lurasidone)**. Avoid. Moderate Study
- **Lumacaftor** is predicted to decrease the exposure to atypical antipsychotics **(paliperidone)**. Monitor and adjust dose. Severe Study
- **Lumacaftor** is predicted to decrease the exposure to atypical antipsychotics **(quetiapine)**. Moderate Study
- **Lumacaftor** is predicted to decrease the exposure to atypical antipsychotics **(risperidone)**. Adjust dose. Moderate Study
- **Lumacaftor** is predicted to decrease the exposure to **avacopan**. Avoid or monitor. Severe Study
- **Lumacaftor** is predicted to decrease the exposure to **avapritinib**. Avoid. Severe Study
- **Lumacaftor** is predicted to decrease the exposure to **axitinib**. Avoid or adjust dose. Moderate Study
- **Lumacaftor** decreases the exposure to **bedaquiline**. Avoid. Severe Study
- **Lumacaftor** is predicted to decrease the exposure to **belumosudil**. Adjust **belumosudil** dose, p. 650. Severe Study
- **Lumacaftor** is predicted to decrease the exposure to benzodiazepines **(alprazolam)**. Adjust dose. Moderate Theoretical
- **Lumacaftor** is predicted to decrease the exposure to benzodiazepines **(midazolam)**. Monitor and adjust dose. Severe Study
- **Lumacaftor** is predicted to decrease the exposure to **bictegravir**. Avoid. Moderate Study
- **Lumacaftor** slightly decreases the exposure to **bortezomib**. Avoid. Severe Study
- **Lumacaftor** is predicted to very markedly decrease the exposure to **bosutinib**. Avoid. Severe Study
- **Lumacaftor** is predicted to decrease the exposure to **brigatinib**. Avoid. Severe Study
- **Lumacaftor** is predicted to decrease the exposure to **bupropion**. Adjust dose. Moderate Theoretical
- **Lumacaftor** is predicted to decrease the exposure to **buspirone**. Use with caution and adjust dose. Severe Study
- **Lumacaftor** moderately decreases the exposure to **cabozantinib**. Avoid. Moderate Study
- **Lumacaftor** is predicted to decrease the exposure to calcium-channel blockers **(amlodipine, felodipine, lacidipine, lercanidipine, nicardipine, nifedipine, nimodipine)**. Monitor and adjust dose. Moderate Study
- **Lumacaftor** is predicted to decrease the exposure to **cannabidiol**. Adjust dose. Moderate Study
- **Lumacaftor** is predicted to decrease the exposure to **capivasertib**. Avoid. Moderate Study

Lumacaftor (continued)
- **Lumacaftor** is predicted to decrease the exposure to **ceritinib**. Avoid. Severe Study
- **Lumacaftor** decreases the concentration of **ciclosporin**. Severe Study
- **Lumacaftor** is predicted to alter the effects of **cilostazol**. Moderate Theoretical
- **Lumacaftor** is predicted to decrease the exposure to **cinacalcet**. Monitor and adjust dose. Moderate Study
- **Lumacaftor** decreases the exposure to **clomethiazole**. Monitor and adjust dose. Moderate Study
- **Lumacaftor** is predicted to decrease the exposure to **cobicistat**. Avoid. Severe Study
- **Lumacaftor** is predicted to decrease the exposure to **cobimetinib**. Avoid. Severe Theoretical
- **Lumacaftor** is predicted to decrease the exposure to **combined hormonal contraceptives**. Use additional contraceptive precautions. Severe Theoretical
- **Lumacaftor** is predicted to decrease the exposure to corticosteroids **(budesonide, deflazacort, dexamethasone, fludrocortisone, hydrocortisone, methylprednisolone, prednisolone, triamcinolone)**. Monitor and adjust dose. Moderate Study
- **Lumacaftor** is predicted to decrease the exposure to corticosteroids **(fluticasone)**. Unknown Theoretical
- **Lumacaftor** is predicted to markedly decrease the exposure to **crizotinib**. Avoid. Severe Study
- **Lumacaftor** is predicted to decrease the exposure to **dabrafenib**. Avoid. Moderate Theoretical
- **Lumacaftor** is predicted to decrease the exposure to **daridorexant**. Severe Study
- **Lumacaftor** is predicted to decrease the exposure to **darifenacin**. Moderate Theoretical
- **Lumacaftor** is predicted to markedly decrease the exposure to **dasatinib**. Avoid. Severe Study
- **Lumacaftor** is predicted to slightly decrease the exposure to **delamanid**. Avoid. Moderate Study
- **Lumacaftor** might decrease the efficacy of **desogestrel**. Use additional contraceptive precautions. Severe Theoretical
- **Lumacaftor** is predicted to decrease the exposure to **deutivacaftor**. Avoid. Severe Theoretical
- **Lumacaftor** is predicted to markedly decrease the exposure to **dienogest**. Severe Study
- **Lumacaftor** is predicted to decrease the exposure to dipeptidylpeptidase-4 inhibitors **(linagliptin)**. Moderate Study
- **Lumacaftor** is predicted to moderately decrease the exposure to dipeptidylpeptidase-4 inhibitors **(saxagliptin)**. Moderate Study
- **Lumacaftor** is predicted to decrease the exposure to **dronabinol**. Avoid or adjust dose. Mild Study
- **Lumacaftor** is predicted to decrease the efficacy of **drospirenone**. Use additional contraceptive precautions. Severe Theoretical
- **Lumacaftor** is predicted to decrease the exposure to **elacestrant**. Avoid or adjust dose depending on duration—consult product literature. Severe Study
- **Lumacaftor** is predicted to decrease the exposure to **elbasvir**. Avoid. Severe Study
- **Lumacaftor** is predicted to decreases the exposure to **elexacaftor**. Avoid. Severe Theoretical
- **Lumacaftor** is predicted to decrease the exposure to **eliglustat**. Avoid. Severe Study
- **Lumacaftor** is predicted to decrease the concentration of **elvitegravir**. Avoid. Severe Study
- **Lumacaftor** is predicted to decrease the exposure to **encorafenib**. Severe Theoretical
- **Lumacaftor** affects the exposure to endothelin receptor antagonists **(bosentan)**. Avoid. Severe Study
- **Lumacaftor** is predicted to decrease the exposure to endothelin receptor antagonists **(macitentan)**. Avoid. Severe Study
- **Lumacaftor** is predicted to decrease the exposure to the cytotoxic component of **enfortumab vedotin**. Moderate Theoretical
- **Lumacaftor** is predicted to decrease the exposure to **entrectinib**. Avoid. Severe Study
- **Lumacaftor** is predicted to decrease the exposure to **erdafitinib**. Avoid. Severe Study
- **Lumacaftor** is predicted to decrease the exposure to **erlotinib**. Avoid or adjust dose—consult product literature. Severe Study
- **Lumacaftor** is predicted to decrease the exposure to **esketamine**. Adjust dose. Moderate Study
- **Lumacaftor** is predicted to decrease the exposure to **eszopiclone**. Adjust dose. Moderate Theoretical
- **Lumacaftor** might decrease the efficacy of subdermal **etonogestrel**. Use additional contraceptive precautions. Severe Theoretical
- **Lumacaftor** is predicted to decrease the concentration of **everolimus**. Avoid or adjust dose. Severe Study
- **Lumacaftor** moderately decreases the exposure to **exemestane**. Moderate Study
- **Lumacaftor** is predicted to decrease the exposure to factor XA inhibitors **(apixaban)**. Moderate Study
- **Lumacaftor** is predicted to decrease the exposure to factor XA inhibitors **(rivaroxaban)**. Avoid unless patient can be monitored for signs of thrombosis. Moderate Study
- **Lumacaftor** is predicted to decrease the exposure to **fedratinib**. Avoid. Moderate Study
- **Lumacaftor** is predicted to decrease the exposure to **fesoterodine**. Avoid. Moderate Study
- **Lumacaftor** is predicted to decrease the exposure to **fostamatinib**. Avoid. Severe Study
- **Lumacaftor** is predicted to decrease the exposure to the active metabolite of **fostemsavir**. Avoid. Severe Study
- **Lumacaftor** is predicted to decrease the exposure to **fruquintinib**. Avoid. Moderate Study
- **Lumacaftor** is predicted to decrease the exposure to **gefitinib**. Avoid. Severe Study
- **Lumacaftor** is predicted to decrease the exposure to **glasdegib**. Avoid. Severe Study
- **Lumacaftor** potentially decreases the exposure to **glecaprevir**. Avoid. Severe Theoretical
- **Lumacaftor** is predicted to decrease the exposure to **grazoprevir**. Avoid. Severe Study
- **Lumacaftor** is predicted to decrease the concentration of **guanfacine**. Adjust **guanfacine** dose, p. 281. Moderate Study
- **Lumacaftor** decreases the concentration of **haloperidol**. Adjust dose. Moderate Study
- **Lumacaftor** is predicted to decrease the exposure to **ibrutinib**. Avoid or monitor. Severe Study
- **Lumacaftor** is predicted to decrease the exposure to **idelalisib**. Avoid. Severe Study
- **Lumacaftor** is predicted to decrease the exposure to **imatinib**. Avoid. Moderate Study
- **Lumacaftor** is predicted to decrease the exposure to **irinotecan**. Avoid. Severe Study
- **Lumacaftor** is predicted to decrease the exposure to **ivabradine**. Adjust dose. Moderate Theoretical
- **Lumacaftor** is predicted to decrease the exposure to **ivacaftor**. Avoid. Severe Study
- **Lumacaftor** is predicted to decrease the exposure to **ixazomib**. Avoid. Severe Study
- **Lumacaftor** is predicted to decrease the exposure to **ketamine**. Adjust dose. Moderate Theoretical
- **Lumacaftor** is predicted to decrease the exposure to **lapatinib**. Avoid. Severe Study
- **Lumacaftor** is predicted to moderately decrease the exposure to **larotrectinib**. Avoid. Moderate Study
- **Lumacaftor** is predicted to decrease the exposure to **lazertinib**. Avoid. Severe Study
- **Lumacaftor** is predicted to decrease the exposure to **lenacapavir**. Avoid. Severe Study
- **Lumacaftor** is predicted to decrease the exposure to **leniolisib**. Avoid. Severe Theoretical
- **Lumacaftor** is predicted to decrease the efficacy of **levonorgestrel**. Use additional contraceptive precautions. Severe Theoretical
- **Lumacaftor** is predicted to decrease the exposure to **lomitapide**. Monitor and adjust dose. Moderate Theoretical
- **Lumacaftor** is predicted to decrease the exposure to **lorlatinib**. Avoid. Severe Study

- **Lumacaftor** is predicted to decrease the exposure to macrolides **(clarithromycin, erythromycin)**. Moderate Theoretical
- **Lumacaftor** is predicted to decrease the exposure to **maraviroc**. Adjust dose. Severe Study
- **Lumacaftor** is predicted to decrease the exposure to **mavacamten**. Monitor and adjust dose—consult product literature. Severe Theoretical
- **Lumacaftor** is predicted to decrease the exposure to meglitinides **(repaglinide)**. Monitor blood glucose and adjust dose. Moderate Study
- **Lumacaftor** is predicted to decrease the exposure to **midostaurin**. Avoid. Severe Study
- **Lumacaftor** is predicted to decrease the exposure to **mifepristone**. Adjust **mifepristone** dose. Severe Study
- **Lumacaftor** is predicted to decrease the exposure to mineralocorticoid receptor antagonists **(eplerenone)**. Avoid. Moderate Theoretical
- **Lumacaftor** is predicted to decrease the exposure to mineralocorticoid receptor antagonists **(finerenone)**. Avoid. Severe Study
- **Lumacaftor** is predicted to decrease the exposure to **mirtazapine**. Adjust dose. Moderate Study
- **Lumacaftor** is predicted to decrease the exposure to monoclonal antibodies **(polatuzumab vedotin)**. Moderate Theoretical
- **Lumacaftor** is predicted to decrease the exposure to the cytotoxic component of monoclonal antibodies **(trastuzumab emtansine)**. Severe Theoretical
- **Lumacaftor** is predicted to decrease the exposure to **montelukast**. Mild Study
- **Lumacaftor** is predicted to markedly decrease the exposure to **naldemedine**. Avoid. Severe Study
- **Lumacaftor** is predicted to markedly decrease the exposure to **naloxegol**. Avoid. Moderate Study
- **Lumacaftor** is predicted to decrease the exposure to **neratinib**. Avoid. Severe Study
- **Lumacaftor** is predicted to markedly decrease the exposure to neurokinin-1 receptor antagonists **(aprepitant)**. Avoid. Moderate Study
- **Lumacaftor** is predicted to decrease the exposure to neurokinin-1 receptor antagonists **(fosaprepitant)**. Avoid. Moderate Theoretical
- **Lumacaftor** is predicted to decrease the exposure to neurokinin-1 receptor antagonists **(netupitant)**. Avoid. Severe Study
- **Lumacaftor** is predicted to moderately decrease the exposure to **nilotinib**. Avoid. Severe Study
- **Lumacaftor** is predicted to decrease the exposure to **nirmatrelvir** boosted with ritonavir. Avoid. Severe Study
- **Lumacaftor** is predicted to decrease the exposure to **nitisinone**. Adjust dose. Moderate Theoretical
- **Lumacaftor** is predicted to decrease the exposure to NNRTIs **(doravirine)**. Avoid. Severe Study
- **Lumacaftor** is predicted to decrease the exposure to NNRTIs **(etravirine)**. Avoid. Severe Theoretical
- **Lumacaftor** markedly decreases the exposure to NNRTIs **(rilpivirine)**. Avoid. Severe Study
- **Lumacaftor** might decrease the efficacy of **norethisterone**. Use additional contraceptive precautions. Severe Theoretical
- **Lumacaftor** is predicted to decrease the exposure to **olaparib**. Avoid. Moderate Theoretical
- **Lumacaftor** is predicted to decrease the exposure to **omaveloxolone**. Avoid. Severe Study
- **Lumacaftor** is predicted to decrease the exposure to opioids **(alfentanil, fentanyl)**. Moderate Study
- **Lumacaftor** is predicted to decrease the exposure to opioids **(buprenorphine)**. Monitor and adjust dose. Moderate Theoretical
- **Lumacaftor** decreases the exposure to opioids **(methadone)**. Monitor and adjust dose. Severe Study
- **Lumacaftor** is predicted to decrease the exposure to opioids **(oxycodone)**. Monitor and adjust dose. Moderate Study
- **Lumacaftor** is predicted to decrease the exposure to **osilodrostat**. Moderate Theoretical
- **Lumacaftor** is predicted to moderately decrease the exposure to **osimertinib**. Avoid. Moderate Study
- **Lumacaftor** is predicted to moderately decrease the exposure to **ospemifene**. Moderate Study
- **Lumacaftor** is predicted to decrease the exposure to **palbociclib**. Avoid. Severe Study
- **Lumacaftor** is predicted to decrease the exposure to **panobinostat**. Avoid. Moderate Theoretical
- **Lumacaftor** is predicted to decrease the exposure to **pazopanib**. Avoid. Severe Theoretical
- **Lumacaftor** is predicted to decrease the exposure to **pemigatinib**. Avoid. Severe Study
- **Lumacaftor** moderately decreases the exposure to phosphodiesterase type-4 inhibitors **(apremilast)**. Avoid. Severe Study
- **Lumacaftor** is predicted to decrease the exposure to phosphodiesterase type-4 inhibitors **(roflumilast)**. Avoid. Moderate Study
- **Lumacaftor** is predicted to decrease the exposure to phosphodiesterase type-5 inhibitors **(avanafil, tadalafil)**. Avoid. Severe Study
- **Lumacaftor** is predicted to decrease the exposure to phosphodiesterase type-5 inhibitors **(sildenafil, vardenafil)**. Moderate Theoretical
- **Lumacaftor** is predicted to moderately to markedly decrease the exposure to **pibrentasvir**. Avoid. Severe Study
- **Lumacaftor** is predicted to decrease the exposure to **pirtobrutinib**. Avoid. Moderate Study
- **Lumacaftor** is predicted to moderately decrease the exposure to **pitolisant**. Moderate Study
- **Lumacaftor** is predicted to decrease the exposure to **ponatinib**. Avoid. Moderate Theoretical
- **Lumacaftor** is predicted to decrease the exposure to **pralsetinib**. Avoid or adjust dose with potent CYP3A4 inducers—consult product literature. Moderate Study
- **Lumacaftor** is predicted to markedly decrease the exposure to **praziquantel**. Avoid. Moderate Study
- **Lumacaftor** is predicted to decrease the exposure to **quizartinib**. Avoid. Severe Study
- **Lumacaftor** is predicted to decrease the exposure to **ranolazine**. Avoid. Severe Study
- **Lumacaftor** is predicted to decrease the exposure to **reboxetine**. Moderate Anecdotal
- **Lumacaftor** is predicted to decrease the exposure to **regorafenib**. Avoid. Moderate Study
- **Lumacaftor** is predicted to markedly decrease the exposure to **ribociclib**. Avoid. Severe Study
- **Lumacaftor** is predicted to decrease the exposure to rifamycins **(rifabutin)**. Adjust dose. Moderate Theoretical
- **Lumacaftor** is predicted to decrease the exposure to **rimegepant**. Avoid. Moderate Theoretical
- **Lumacaftor** is predicted to decrease the exposure to **ripretinib**. Avoid or adjust dose—consult product literature. Severe Study
- **Lumacaftor** is predicted to decrease the exposure to **ruxolitinib**. Monitor and adjust dose. Moderate Study
- **Lumacaftor** is predicted to decrease the exposure to **selpercatinib**. Avoid. Moderate Study
- **Lumacaftor** is predicted to decrease the exposure to **selumetinib**. Avoid. Severe Study
- **Lumacaftor** is predicted to decrease the exposure to **siponimod**. Manufacturer advises caution depending on genotype—consult product literature. Severe Study
- **Lumacaftor** is predicted to decrease the concentration of **sirolimus**. Avoid or monitor and adjust dose. Severe Study
- **Lumacaftor** is predicted to decrease the exposure to **solifenacin**. Moderate Theoretical
- **Lumacaftor** is predicted to decrease the exposure to **sorafenib**. Moderate Theoretical
- **Lumacaftor** is predicted to decrease the exposure to **sotorasib**. Avoid. Severe Study
- **Lumacaftor** is predicted to decrease the exposure to **sparsentan**. Avoid. Severe Theoretical
- **Lumacaftor** is predicted to decrease the exposure to **sunitinib**. Avoid or adjust dose—consult product literature. Moderate Study
- **Lumacaftor** decreases the concentration of **tacrolimus**. Avoid or monitor and adjust dose. Severe Study

Lumacaftor (continued)

- **Lumacaftor** is predicted to decrease the exposure to taxanes **(cabazitaxel)**. Avoid. Moderate Study
- **Lumacaftor** is predicted to decrease the exposure to taxanes **(docetaxel)**. Severe Theoretical
- **Lumacaftor** is predicted to decrease the exposure to taxanes **(paclitaxel)**. Avoid. Severe Study
- **Lumacaftor** is predicted to decrease the concentration of **temsirolimus**. Avoid. Severe Study
- **Lumacaftor** is predicted to decrease the exposure to tetracyclines **(eravacycline)**. Adjust **eravacycline** dose. Moderate Study
- **Lumacaftor** is predicted to decrease the exposure to **tezacaftor**. Avoid. Severe Theoretical
- **Lumacaftor** is predicted to markedly decrease the exposure to **ticagrelor**. Avoid. Severe Study
- **Lumacaftor** is predicted to decrease the exposure to the cytotoxic component of **tisotumab vedotin**. Moderate Theoretical
- **Lumacaftor** is predicted to decrease the exposure to **tivozanib**. Severe Study
- **Lumacaftor** is predicted to decrease the exposure to **tofacitinib**. Avoid. Severe Study
- **Lumacaftor** is predicted to decrease the exposure to **tolvaptan**. Use with caution or avoid depending on indication. Severe Study
- **Lumacaftor** is predicted to decrease the exposure to **toremifene**. Adjust dose. Moderate Study
- **Lumacaftor** is predicted to decrease the exposure to **trabectedin**. Avoid. Severe Theoretical
- **Lumacaftor** is predicted to decrease the exposure to **tucatinib**. Avoid. Severe Study
- **Lumacaftor** is predicted to decrease the efficacy of **ulipristal**. Use additional contraceptive precautions. Severe Theoretical
- **Lumacaftor** is predicted to decrease the exposure to **upadacitinib**. Moderate Study
- **Lumacaftor** is predicted to decrease the exposure to **vandetanib**. Avoid. Moderate Study
- **Lumacaftor** is predicted to decrease the exposure to **vanzacaftor**. Avoid. Severe Theoretical
- **Lumacaftor** is predicted to moderately decrease the exposure to **velpatasvir**. Avoid. Severe Study
- **Lumacaftor** is predicted to decrease the exposure to **vemurafenib**. Avoid. Severe Study
- **Lumacaftor** is predicted to decrease the exposure to **venetoclax**. Avoid. Severe Study
- **Lumacaftor** is predicted to decrease the exposure to vinca alkaloids **(vinblastine, vincristine, vindesine)**. Severe Theoretical
- **Lumacaftor** is predicted to decrease the exposure to vinca alkaloids **(vinorelbine)**. Use with caution or avoid. Severe Theoretical
- **Lumacaftor** is predicted to decrease the exposure to **vismodegib**. Avoid. Moderate Theoretical
- **Lumacaftor** is predicted to decrease the exposure to **voclosporin**. Avoid. Severe Study
- **Lumacaftor** is predicted to decrease the exposure to **vortioxetine**. Monitor and adjust dose. Moderate Study
- **Lumacaftor** is predicted to decrease the concentration of **voxilaprevir**. Avoid. Severe Study
- **Lumacaftor** is predicted to decrease the exposure to **zanubrutinib**. Avoid. Severe Study
- **Lumacaftor** is predicted to decrease the exposure to **zopiclone**. Adjust dose. Moderate Study

Lumefantrine → see antimalarials

Lurasidone → see atypical antipsychotics

Lymecycline → see tetracyclines

Macitentan → see endothelin receptor antagonists

Macrogol 3350

SEPARATION OF ADMINISTRATION Macrogol-containing preparations have been reported to decrease the efficacy of some drugs (such as antiepileptics) when given concurrently. Some manufacturers advise that other oral drugs should be avoided for 1 hour before, or 1 hour after, macrogol-containing preparations.

Macrolides → see TABLE 7 p. 1055 (QT-interval prolongation)

azithromycin · clarithromycin · erythromycin

- Interactions do not generally apply to topical use of **azithromycin** unless specified.
- Since systemic absorption can follow topical application of **erythromycin**, the possibility of interactions should be borne in mind.

- **Clarithromycin** is predicted to increase the exposure to **abemaciclib**. Avoid or adjust dose—consult product literature. Severe Study
- **Erythromycin** is predicted to increase the exposure to **abemaciclib**. Moderate Study
- **Clarithromycin** is predicted to increase the exposure to **acalabrutinib**. Avoid. Severe Study
- **Erythromycin** is predicted to increase the exposure to **acalabrutinib**. Avoid or monitor. Severe Study
- **Macrolides** are predicted to increase the exposure to **afatinib**. Moderate Study
- **Azithromycin** is predicted to increase the exposure to **aliskiren**. Moderate Theoretical
- Macrolides **(clarithromycin, erythromycin)** are predicted to increase the exposure to **aliskiren**. Moderate Study
- **Clarithromycin** is predicted to moderately increase the exposure to alpha blockers **(alfuzosin, tamsulosin)**. Use with caution or avoid. Moderate Study
- **Clarithromycin** is predicted to increase the exposure to alpha blockers **(doxazosin)**. Moderate Study
- **Erythromycin** is predicted to increase the exposure to alpha blockers **(tamsulosin)**. Moderate Theoretical
- **Azithromycin** is predicted to increase the exposure to **aminophylline**. Moderate Theoretical
- **Clarithromycin** is predicted to increase the exposure to **aminophylline**. Adjust dose. Moderate Theoretical
- **Aminophylline** is predicted to decrease the exposure to **erythromycin**. Adjust dose. Severe Study
- Anti-androgens **(enzalutamide)** are predicted to affect the exposure to **clarithromycin**. Use with caution or avoid. Moderate Theoretical
- **Clarithromycin** is predicted to increase the exposure to anti-androgens **(apalutamide)**. Monitor and adjust dose. Mild Study
- **Clarithromycin** is predicted to increase the exposure to anti-androgens **(darolutamide)**. Monitor and adjust dose. Moderate Theoretical
- **Clarithromycin** is predicted to increase the exposure to antiarrhythmics **(amiodarone)**. Avoid. Moderate Theoretical
- **Clarithromycin** very markedly increases the exposure to antiarrhythmics **(dronedarone)**. Avoid. Severe Study
- **Erythromycin** is predicted to moderately increase the exposure to antiarrhythmics **(dronedarone)**. Avoid. Severe Theoretical → Also see TABLE 7 p. 1055
- Macrolides **(clarithromycin, erythromycin)** are predicted to increase the exposure to antiarrhythmics **(lidocaine)**. Moderate Theoretical
- **Clarithromycin** is predicted to increase the exposure to antiarrhythmics **(propafenone)**. Monitor and adjust dose. Severe Study
- **Erythromycin** is predicted to increase the exposure to antiarrhythmics **(propafenone)**. Monitor and adjust dose. Moderate Study
- **Clarithromycin** is predicted to increase the exposure to anticholinesterases, centrally acting **(galantamine)**. Monitor and adjust dose. Moderate Study
- **Clarithromycin** slightly increases the concentration of antiepileptics **(carbamazepine)**. Monitor concentration and adjust dose. Severe Study
- **Erythromycin** markedly increases the concentration of antiepileptics **(carbamazepine)**. Monitor concentration and adjust dose. Severe Study
- **Clarithromycin** is predicted to very slightly increase the exposure to antiepileptics **(perampanel)**. Mild Study
- **Clarithromycin** is predicted to increase the exposure to antifungals, azoles **(isavuconazole)**. Avoid or monitor adverse effects. Severe Study

- **Erythromycin** is predicted to increase the exposure to antifungals, azoles **(isavuconazole)**. Moderate Theoretical
- **Clarithromycin** is predicted to increase the exposure to antihistamines, non-sedating **(fexofenadine)**. Moderate Theoretical
- **Clarithromycin** is predicted to increase the exposure to antihistamines, non-sedating **(mizolastine)**. Avoid. Severe Study
- **Erythromycin** is predicted to increase the exposure to antihistamines, non-sedating **(mizolastine)**. Severe Theoretical
- Macrolides **(clarithromycin, erythromycin)** are predicted to increase the exposure to antihistamines, non-sedating **(rupatadine)**. Avoid. Moderate Study
- **Macrolides** might increase the risk of serious cardiovascular adverse effects when given with antimalarials **(chloroquine)**. Severe Theoretical
- Macrolides **(clarithromycin, erythromycin)** are predicted to increase the concentration of antimalarials **(piperaquine)**. Severe Study
- **Clarithromycin** is predicted to increase the exposure to **atogepant**. Adjust **atogepant** dose. Moderate Study
- **Erythromycin** is predicted to increase the exposure to **atogepant**. Adjust **atogepant** dose. Moderate Theoretical
- **Clarithromycin** is predicted to slightly increase the exposure to atypical antipsychotics **(aripiprazole)**. Avoid or adjust dose—consult product literature. Moderate Study
- **Clarithromycin** is predicted to moderately increase the exposure to atypical antipsychotics **(cariprazine)**. Avoid. Severe Study
- **Erythromycin** is predicted to increase the exposure to atypical antipsychotics **(cariprazine)**. Monitor and adjust dose. Severe Study
- **Erythromycin** potentially increases the risk of toxicity when given with atypical antipsychotics **(clozapine)**. Severe Anecdotal
- **Erythromycin** is predicted to increase the exposure to atypical antipsychotics **(lurasidone)**. Adjust **lurasidone** dose. Moderate Study
- **Clarithromycin** is predicted to increase the exposure to atypical antipsychotics **(lurasidone, quetiapine)**. Avoid. Severe Study
- **Erythromycin** is predicted to increase the exposure to atypical antipsychotics **(quetiapine)**. Avoid. Moderate Study
- **Clarithromycin** is predicted to increase the exposure to atypical antipsychotics **(risperidone)**. Adjust dose. Moderate Study
- **Clarithromycin** is predicted to increase the exposure to **avacopan**. Severe Study
- **Clarithromycin** is predicted to increase the exposure to **avapritinib**. Avoid. Moderate Study
- **Erythromycin** is predicted to increase the exposure to **avapritinib**. Avoid or adjust dose—consult product literature. Moderate Study
- **Clarithromycin** is predicted to increase the exposure to **axitinib**. Avoid or adjust dose. Moderate Study
- **Erythromycin** is predicted to increase the exposure to **axitinib**. Moderate Study
- **Clarithromycin** might increase the exposure to **bedaquiline**. Mild Study
- **Erythromycin** might increase the exposure to **bedaquiline**. Mild Theoretical → Also see TABLE 7 p. 1055
- **Clarithromycin** moderately increases the exposure to benzodiazepines **(alprazolam)**. Avoid. Moderate Study
- **Erythromycin** is predicted to increase the exposure to benzodiazepines **(alprazolam)**. Severe Study
- **Clarithromycin** is predicted to markedly to very markedly increase the exposure to benzodiazepines **(midazolam)**. Avoid or adjust dose. Severe Study
- **Erythromycin** is predicted to increase the exposure to benzodiazepines **(midazolam)**. Monitor adverse effects and adjust dose. Severe Study
- **Macrolides** are predicted to increase the exposure to beta blockers, non-selective **(nadolol)**. Moderate Study
- **Clarithromycin** is predicted to increase the exposure to beta$_2$ agonists **(salmeterol)**. Avoid. Severe Study
- **Clarithromycin** slightly increases the exposure to **bortezomib**. Moderate Study
- Macrolides **(clarithromycin, erythromycin)** are predicted to increase the exposure to **bosutinib**. Avoid or adjust dose. Severe Study → Also see TABLE 7 p. 1055
- **Clarithromycin** is predicted to increase the exposure to **brigatinib**. Avoid or adjust dose—consult product literature. Severe Study
- **Erythromycin** is predicted to increase the exposure to **brigatinib**. Moderate Study
- **Clarithromycin** is predicted to increase the exposure to **buspirone**. Adjust **buspirone** dose. Severe Study
- **Erythromycin** is predicted to increase the exposure to **buspirone**. Use with caution and adjust dose. Moderate Study
- Macrolides **(clarithromycin, erythromycin)** are predicted to increase the exposure to **cabozantinib**. Moderate Study → Also see TABLE 7 p. 1055
- **Erythromycin** is predicted to increase the exposure to calcium-channel blockers **(amlodipine, felodipine, lacidipine, lercanidipine, nicardipine, nifedipine, nimodipine)**. Monitor and adjust dose. Moderate Study
- **Clarithromycin** is predicted to increase the exposure to calcium-channel blockers **(amlodipine, felodipine, lacidipine, nicardipine, nifedipine, nimodipine)**. Monitor and adjust dose. Moderate Study
- **Erythromycin** is predicted to increase the exposure to calcium-channel blockers **(diltiazem)**. Severe Theoretical
- **Clarithromycin** is predicted to increase the exposure to calcium-channel blockers **(diltiazem, verapamil)**. Severe Study
- **Clarithromycin** is predicted to markedly increase the exposure to calcium-channel blockers **(lercanidipine)**. Avoid. Severe Study
- **Erythromycin** is predicted to increase the exposure to calcium-channel blockers **(verapamil)**. Severe Study
- **Clarithromycin** is predicted to increase the exposure to **cannabidiol**. Avoid or adjust dose. Mild Study
- Macrolides **(clarithromycin, erythromycin)** are predicted to increase the exposure to **capivasertib**. Adjust dose. Moderate Study
- **Clarithromycin** is predicted to increase the exposure to **ceritinib**. Avoid or adjust dose—consult product literature. Severe Study
- **Erythromycin** is predicted to increase the exposure to **ceritinib**. Moderate Study → Also see TABLE 7 p. 1055
- **Clarithromycin** increases the concentration of **ciclosporin**. Severe Study
- **Erythromycin** greatly increases the exposure to **ciclosporin**. Avoid or monitor. Severe Study
- **Clarithromycin** is predicted to moderately increase the exposure to **cilostazol**. Adjust **cilostazol** dose. Moderate Study
- **Erythromycin** slightly increases the exposure to **cilostazol**. Adjust **cilostazol** dose. Moderate Study
- **Clarithromycin** is predicted to moderately increase the exposure to **cinacalcet**. Adjust dose. Moderate Study
- **Cobicistat** is predicted to increase the concentration of **erythromycin**. Moderate Theoretical
- **Clarithromycin** is predicted to increase the exposure to **cobimetinib**. Avoid or monitor for toxicity. Severe Study
- **Erythromycin** is predicted to increase the exposure to **cobimetinib**. Severe Study
- **Azithromycin** is predicted to increase the exposure to **colchicine**. Avoid P-glycoprotein inhibitors or adjust **colchicine** dose, p. 637. Severe Theoretical
- **Clarithromycin** is predicted to increase the exposure to **colchicine**. Avoid potent CYP3A4 inhibitors or adjust **colchicine** dose, p. 637. Severe Study
- **Erythromycin** is predicted to increase the exposure to **colchicine**. Adjust **colchicine** dose with moderate CYP3A4 inhibitors, p. 637. Severe Study
- **Clarithromycin** is predicted to increase the exposure to corticosteroids **(beclometasone)** (risk with beclometasone is likely to be lower than with other corticosteroids). Moderate Theoretical
- **Clarithromycin** is predicted to increase the exposure to corticosteroids **(betamethasone, budesonide, ciclesonide, deflazacort, dexamethasone, fludrocortisone, fluticasone, hydrocortisone, methylprednisolone, mometasone, prednisolone, triamcinolone)**. Avoid or monitor adverse effects. Severe Study

A1 Interactions | Appendix 1

Macrolides (continued)

- **Erythromycin** is predicted to increase the exposure to corticosteroids **(methylprednisolone)**. Monitor and adjust dose. [Moderate] Study
- **Clarithromycin** is predicted to increase the exposure to corticosteroids **(vamorolone)**. Adjust dose. [Severe] Study
- **Azithromycin** might increase the risk of bleeding events when given with **coumarins**. [Severe] Anecdotal
- Macrolides **(clarithromycin, erythromycin)** increase the anticoagulant effect of **coumarins**. Monitor INR and adjust dose. [Severe] Anecdotal
- Macrolides **(clarithromycin, erythromycin)** are predicted to increase the exposure to **crizotinib**. Avoid. [Moderate] Study → Also see TABLE 7 p. 1055
- **Clarithromycin** is predicted to increase the exposure to **dabrafenib**. Use with caution or avoid. [Moderate] Study
- **Erythromycin** is predicted to increase the exposure to **dabrafenib**. [Moderate] Study
- **Clarithromycin** is predicted to increase the exposure to **daridorexant**. Avoid. [Severe] Study
- **Erythromycin** is predicted to increase the exposure to **daridorexant**. Adjust **daridorexant** dose. [Severe] Study
- **Clarithromycin** is predicted to markedly to very markedly increase the exposure to **darifenacin**. Avoid. [Severe] Study
- **Erythromycin** slightly increases the exposure to **darifenacin**. [Moderate] Study
- **Clarithromycin** is predicted to increase the exposure to **dasatinib**. Avoid or adjust dose—consult product literature. [Severe] Study
- **Erythromycin** is predicted to increase the exposure to **dasatinib**. [Severe] Study → Also see TABLE 7 p. 1055
- **Clarithromycin** very slightly increases the exposure to **delamanid**. [Severe] Study
- Macrolides **(clarithromycin, erythromycin)** are predicted to increase the exposure to **deutivacaftor**. Adjust dose, see deutivacaftor with tezacaftor and vanzacaftor p. 218. [Severe] Study
- **Clarithromycin** is predicted to moderately increase the exposure to **dienogest**. [Moderate] Study
- **Erythromycin** is predicted to slightly increase the exposure to **dienogest**. [Moderate] Study
- **Macrolides** increase the concentration of **digoxin**. [Severe] Anecdotal
- **Clarithromycin** is predicted to increase the exposure to dipeptidylpeptidase-4 inhibitors **(saxagliptin)**. [Moderate] Study
- **Erythromycin** is predicted to increase the exposure to dipeptidylpeptidase-4 inhibitors **(saxagliptin)**. [Mild] Study
- Macrolides **(clarithromycin, erythromycin)** are predicted to increase the exposure to **domperidone**. Avoid. [Severe] Study
- **Clarithromycin** increases the exposure to dopamine receptor agonists **(bromocriptine)**. [Severe] Study
- **Erythromycin** is predicted to increase the exposure to dopamine receptor agonists **(bromocriptine)**. [Severe] Theoretical
- Macrolides **(clarithromycin, erythromycin)** are predicted to increase the concentration of dopamine receptor agonists **(cabergoline)**. Avoid. [Severe] Study
- **Clarithromycin** is predicted to increase the exposure to **dronabinol**. Adjust dose. [Mild] Study
- Macrolides **(clarithromycin, erythromycin)** are predicted to increase the exposure to **drospirenone**. [Severe] Study
- **Clarithromycin** is predicted to increase the exposure to **dutasteride**. Monitor adverse effects and adjust dose. [Moderate] Theoretical
- **Erythromycin** is predicted to moderately increase the exposure to **dutasteride**. [Mild] Study
- **Clarithromycin** is predicted to increase the exposure to **elacestrant**. Avoid potent CYP3A4 inhibitors or adjust **elacestrant** dose. [Severe] Study
- **Erythromycin** is predicted to increase the exposure to **elacestrant**. Avoid moderate CYP3A4 inhibitors or adjust **elacestrant** dose. [Severe] Theoretical
- **Clarithromycin** is predicted to increase the exposure to **elexacaftor**. Adjust ivacaftor with tezacaftor and elexacaftor p. 220 dose with potent CYP3A4 inhibitors. [Severe] Study
- **Erythromycin** is predicted to increase the exposure to **elexacaftor**. Adjust ivacaftor with tezacaftor and elexacaftor p. 220 dose with moderate CYP3A4 inhibitors. [Severe] Theoretical
- Macrolides **(clarithromycin, erythromycin)** are predicted to increase the exposure to **eliglustat**. Avoid or adjust dose—consult product literature. [Severe] Study
- **Clarithromycin** is predicted to increase the exposure to **encorafenib**. Avoid or monitor. [Severe] Study
- **Erythromycin** is predicted to moderately increase the exposure to **encorafenib**. [Moderate] Study → Also see TABLE 7 p. 1055
- **Clarithromycin** is predicted to increase the exposure to endothelin receptor antagonists **(bosentan)**. [Moderate] Theoretical
- **Clarithromycin** is predicted to increase the exposure to endothelin receptor antagonists **(macitentan)**. [Moderate] Study
- **Erythromycin** is predicted to increase the exposure to endothelin receptor antagonists **(macitentan)**. Manufacturer advises caution depending on other drugs taken—consult product literature. [Moderate] Theoretical
- **Clarithromycin** is predicted to increase the exposure to the cytotoxic component of **enfortumab vedotin**. [Severe] Theoretical
- **Clarithromycin** is predicted to increase the exposure to **entrectinib**. Avoid or adjust dose with potent CYP3A4 inhibitors—consult product literature. [Severe] Study
- **Erythromycin** is predicted to increase the exposure to **entrectinib**. Avoid or adjust dose with moderate CYP3A4 inhibitors—consult product literature. [Severe] Theoretical → Also see TABLE 7 p. 1055
- **Clarithromycin** is predicted to increase the exposure to **erdafitinib**. Adjust dose. [Severe] Study
- **Clarithromycin** is predicted to increase the risk of ergotism when given with **ergometrine**. Avoid. [Severe] Theoretical
- **Erythromycin** is predicted to increase the risk of ergotism when given with **ergometrine**. [Severe] Theoretical
- **Azithromycin** is predicted to increase the exposure to **erlotinib**. [Moderate] Theoretical
- **Clarithromycin** is predicted to increase the exposure to **erlotinib**. Use with caution and adjust dose. [Severe] Study
- **Erythromycin** is predicted to increase the exposure to **erlotinib**. [Moderate] Study
- **Clarithromycin** is predicted to increase the exposure to **esketamine**. Adjust dose. [Moderate] Study
- **Clarithromycin** is predicted to increase the exposure to **eszopiclone**. Adjust **eszopiclone** dose; avoid in the elderly. [Moderate] Study
- **Clarithromycin** is predicted to increase the concentration of subdermal **etonogestrel**. [Moderate] Theoretical
- Macrolides **(clarithromycin, erythromycin)** are predicted to increase the exposure to **etrasimod**. Avoid in poor CYP2C9 metabolisers. [Severe] Theoretical
- **Clarithromycin** is predicted to increase the exposure to **everolimus**. Avoid. [Severe] Study
- **Erythromycin** is predicted to increase the concentration of **everolimus**. Avoid or adjust dose. [Moderate] Study
- **Erythromycin** is predicted to increase the exposure to factor XA inhibitors **(apixaban)**. [Moderate] Theoretical
- **Azithromycin** is predicted to increase the exposure to factor XA inhibitors **(apixaban, edoxaban)**. [Moderate] Theoretical
- **Clarithromycin** slightly increases the exposure to factor XA inhibitors **(apixaban, edoxaban)**. [Moderate] Study
- **Erythromycin** slightly increases the exposure to factor XA inhibitors **(edoxaban)**. Adjust **edoxaban** dose. [Moderate] Study
- **Azithromycin** is predicted to increase the exposure to factor XA inhibitors **(rivaroxaban)**. Manufacturer advises caution in renal impairment. [Moderate] Theoretical
- Macrolides **(clarithromycin, erythromycin)** slightly increase the exposure to factor XA inhibitors **(rivaroxaban)**. Manufacturer advises caution in renal impairment. [Moderate] Study
- **Clarithromycin** is predicted to increase the exposure to **fedratinib**. Adjust dose, but avoid depending on other drugs taken—consult product literature. [Moderate] Study
- **Erythromycin** is predicted to increase the exposure to **fedratinib**. Monitor and adjust dose. [Moderate] Study
- **Clarithromycin** is predicted to moderately increase the exposure to **fesoterodine**. Adjust **fesoterodine** dose with potent

CYP3A4 inhibitors; avoid in hepatic and renal impairment. [Severe] Study
- **Erythromycin** is predicted to increase the exposure to **fesoterodine**. Adjust **fesoterodine** dose with moderate CYP3A4 inhibitors in hepatic and renal impairment. [Mild] Study
- **Macrolides** are predicted to increase the exposure to **fidaxomicin**. Avoid. [Moderate] Study
- **Clarithromycin** is predicted to increase the exposure to **fostamatinib**. Monitor adverse effects and adjust dose. [Moderate] Study
- **Clarithromycin** is predicted to increase the exposure to **futibatinib**. Avoid or adjust dose—consult product literature. [Moderate] Study
- **Clarithromycin** is predicted to increase the exposure to **gefitinib**. [Severe] Study
- **Erythromycin** is predicted to increase the exposure to **gefitinib**. [Moderate] Study
- **Clarithromycin** is predicted to increase the exposure to **gilteritinib**. [Moderate] Study
- Macrolides **(azithromycin, erythromycin)** are predicted to increase the exposure to **gilteritinib**. [Moderate] Theoretical
- **Clarithromycin** is predicted to increase the exposure to **glasdegib**. Use with caution or avoid. [Severe] Study
- **Clarithromycin** is predicted to moderately to markedly increase the exposure to **grazoprevir**. Avoid. [Severe] Study
- Macrolides **(azithromycin, erythromycin)** are predicted to increase the exposure to **grazoprevir**. Avoid. [Severe] Theoretical
- **Clarithromycin** is predicted to increase the exposure to **guanfacine**. Adjust **guanfacine** dose, p. 281. [Moderate] Study
- **Erythromycin** is predicted to increase the concentration of **guanfacine**. Adjust **guanfacine** dose, p. 281. [Moderate] Theoretical
- H_2 receptor antagonists **(cimetidine)** slightly increase the exposure to **erythromycin**. [Moderate] Study
- HIV-protease inhibitors **(atazanavir)** are predicted to increase the exposure to **clarithromycin**. Adjust dose in renal impairment. [Severe] Study
- HIV-protease inhibitors **(darunavir, fosamprenavir, lopinavir)** boosted with ritonavir are predicted to increase the exposure to **clarithromycin**. Adjust dose in renal impairment. [Severe] Study
- HIV-protease inhibitors **(ritonavir)** increase the exposure to **clarithromycin**. Adjust dose in renal impairment. [Severe] Study
- **HIV-protease inhibitors** are predicted to increase the exposure to **erythromycin**. [Severe] Theoretical
- **Macrolides** might increase the risk of serious cardiovascular adverse effects when given with **hydroxychloroquine**. [Severe] Theoretical → Also see TABLE 7 p. 1055
- **Clarithromycin** is predicted to increase the exposure to **ibrutinib**. Avoid or adjust dose with potent CYP3A4 inhibitors—consult product literature. [Severe] Study
- **Erythromycin** is predicted to increase the exposure to **ibrutinib**. Adjust dose with moderate CYP3A4 inhibitors—consult product literature. [Severe] Study
- **Macrolides** are predicted to increase the exposure to **idelalisib**. [Moderate] Theoretical
- **Clarithromycin** is predicted to increase the exposure to **imatinib**. [Moderate] Study
- **Erythromycin** is predicted to increase the exposure to **imatinib**. [Moderate] Theoretical
- **Clarithromycin** has been reported to cause hypoglycaemia when given with **insulin**. [Severe] Anecdotal
- **Clarithromycin** is predicted to increase the exposure to the active metabolite of **irinotecan**. Avoid. [Severe] Study
- **Erythromycin** is predicted to increase the exposure to the active metabolite of **irinotecan**. [Moderate] Theoretical
- **Clarithromycin** is predicted to increase the exposure to **ivabradine**. Avoid. [Severe] Study
- **Erythromycin** is predicted to increase the exposure to **ivabradine**. Avoid. [Severe] Theoretical
- **Clarithromycin** is predicted to increase the exposure to **ivacaftor**. Adjust dose with potent CYP3A4 inhibitors, see ivacaftor p. 219, lumacaftor with ivacaftor p. 222, tezacaftor with ivacaftor p. 223, and ivacaftor with tezacaftor and elexacaftor p. 220. [Severe] Study
- **Erythromycin** is predicted to increase the exposure to **ivacaftor**. Adjust dose with moderate CYP3A4 inhibitors, see ivacaftor p. 219, tezacaftor with ivacaftor p. 223, and ivacaftor with tezacaftor and elexacaftor p. 220. [Moderate] Study
- Macrolides **(clarithromycin, erythromycin)** are predicted to increase the exposure to **ivosidenib**. Monitor and adjust dose—consult product literature. [Severe] Study → Also see TABLE 7 p. 1055
- **Clarithromycin** is predicted to increase the exposure to **ketamine**. Adjust dose. [Moderate] Theoretical
- **Clarithromycin** is predicted to increase the exposure to **lapatinib**. Avoid. [Moderate] Study
- **Erythromycin** is predicted to increase the exposure to **lapatinib**. [Moderate] Study → Also see TABLE 7 p. 1055
- **Clarithromycin** is predicted to moderately increase the exposure to **larotrectinib**. Avoid or adjust dose—consult product literature. [Moderate] Study
- **Erythromycin** is predicted to increase the exposure to **larotrectinib**. Monitor and adjust dose. [Moderate] Theoretical
- Macrolides **(clarithromycin, erythromycin)** are predicted to increase the exposure to **leniolisib**. Avoid. [Moderate] Study
- Macrolides **(clarithromycin, erythromycin)** are predicted to increase the concentration of **letermovir**. [Moderate] Study
- **Clarithromycin** increases the exposure to **linezolid**. [Moderate] Anecdotal
- **Azithromycin** is predicted to increase the exposure to **lomitapide**. Separate administration by 12 hours. [Moderate] Theoretical
- **Clarithromycin** is predicted to markedly increase the exposure to **lomitapide**. Avoid. [Severe] Study
- **Erythromycin** is predicted to increase the exposure to **lomitapide**. Avoid. [Moderate] Theoretical
- **Clarithromycin** is predicted to increase the exposure to **lorlatinib**. Avoid or adjust dose—consult product literature. [Severe] Study
- **Lumacaftor** is predicted to decrease the exposure to macrolides **(clarithromycin, erythromycin)**. [Moderate] Theoretical
- **Clarithromycin** is predicted to markedly increase the exposure to **maraviroc**. Adjust dose. [Severe] Study
- **Clarithromycin** is predicted to increase the exposure to **mavacamten**. Avoid or monitor—consult product literature. [Severe] Study
- **Erythromycin** is predicted to increase the exposure to **mavacamten**. Adjust dose—consult product literature. [Moderate] Study
- **Clarithromycin** is predicted to increase the concentration of intramuscular **medroxyprogesterone**. [Moderate] Theoretical
- **Clarithromycin** might cause hypoglycaemia when given with meglitinides **(repaglinide)**. [Moderate] Anecdotal
- **Clarithromycin** is predicted to increase the exposure to **midostaurin**. Avoid or monitor for toxicity. [Severe] Study
- **Erythromycin** is predicted to increase the exposure to **midostaurin**. [Moderate] Theoretical
- **Clarithromycin** is predicted to markedly increase the exposure to mineralocorticoid receptor antagonists **(eplerenone)**. Avoid. [Severe] Study
- **Erythromycin** is predicted to increase the exposure to mineralocorticoid receptor antagonists **(eplerenone)**. Adjust **eplerenone** dose. [Severe] Study
- **Clarithromycin** is predicted to increase the exposure to mineralocorticoid receptor antagonists **(finerenone)**. Avoid. [Severe] Study
- **Erythromycin** is predicted to increase the exposure to mineralocorticoid receptor antagonists **(finerenone)**. [Severe] Study
- **Clarithromycin** is predicted to increase the exposure to **mirabegron**. Adjust **mirabegron** dose in hepatic and renal impairment. [Moderate] Study
- **Clarithromycin** is predicted to increase the exposure to **mirtazapine**. [Moderate] Study
- **Clarithromycin** is predicted to increase the exposure to **modafinil**. [Mild] Theoretical
- Macrolides **(clarithromycin, erythromycin)** are predicted to increase the exposure to **momelotinib**. [Moderate] Study

Macrolides (continued)
- **Azithromycin** is predicted to increase the risk of neutropenia when given with monoclonal antibodies **(brentuximab vedotin)**. Monitor and adjust dose. Severe Theoretical
- **Clarithromycin** is predicted to increase the risk of neutropenia when given with monoclonal antibodies **(brentuximab vedotin)**. Monitor and adjust dose. Severe Study
- **Erythromycin** increases the risk of neutropenia when given with monoclonal antibodies **(brentuximab vedotin)**. Monitor and adjust dose. Severe Theoretical
- **Clarithromycin** is predicted to increase the exposure to monoclonal antibodies **(polatuzumab vedotin)**. Moderate Theoretical
- **Clarithromycin** is predicted to increase the exposure to the cytotoxic component of monoclonal antibodies **(trastuzumab emtansine)**. Avoid or monitor. Severe Theoretical
- **Clarithromycin** is predicted to increase the exposure to **naldemedine**. Avoid or monitor. Moderate Study
- Macrolides **(azithromycin, erythromycin)** are predicted to increase the exposure to **naldemedine**. Moderate Study
- **Clarithromycin** is predicted to markedly increase the exposure to **naloxegol**. Avoid. Severe Study
- **Erythromycin** is predicted to increase the exposure to **naloxegol**. Adjust **naloxegol** dose and monitor adverse effects. Moderate Study
- **Azithromycin** is predicted to increase the exposure to **neratinib**. Avoid or adjust dose and monitor for gastrointestinal adverse effects—consult product literature. Severe Study
- **Clarithromycin** is predicted to increase the exposure to **neratinib**. Avoid or adjust dose with potent CYP3A4 inhibitors—consult product literature. Severe Study
- **Erythromycin** is predicted to increase the exposure to **neratinib**. Avoid moderate CYP3A4 inhibitors or adjust dose and monitor for gastrointestinal adverse effects—consult product literature. Severe Study
- **Clarithromycin** is predicted to markedly increase the exposure to neurokinin-1 receptor antagonists **(aprepitant)**. Moderate Study
- **Erythromycin** is predicted to increase the exposure to neurokinin-1 receptor antagonists **(aprepitant)**. Moderate Study
- **Clarithromycin** is predicted to increase the exposure to neurokinin-1 receptor antagonists **(fosaprepitant)**. Moderate Theoretical
- **Clarithromycin** is predicted to increase the exposure to neurokinin-1 receptor antagonists **(netupitant)**. Moderate Study
- **Clarithromycin** is predicted to increase the exposure to **nilotinib**. Avoid. Severe Study
- **Erythromycin** is predicted to increase the exposure to **nilotinib**. Moderate Study → Also see TABLE 7 p. 1055
- **Macrolides** are predicted to increase the exposure to **nintedanib**. Moderate Study
- **Nirmatrelvir** boosted with ritonavir is predicted to increase the concentration of **clarithromycin**. Monitor; adjust dose in renal impairment. Moderate Theoretical
- **Nirmatrelvir** boosted with ritonavir is predicted to increase the concentration of **erythromycin**. Moderate Theoretical
- **Clarithromycin** is predicted to increase the exposure to **nitisinone**. Adjust dose. Moderate Theoretical
- NNRTIs **(efavirenz, nevirapine)** decrease the exposure to **clarithromycin**. Moderate Study
- NNRTIs **(etravirine)** decrease the exposure to **clarithromycin** and **clarithromycin** slightly increases the exposure to NNRTIs **(etravirine)**. Severe Study
- **Erythromycin** is predicted to increase the exposure to NNRTIs **(nevirapine)**. Moderate Theoretical
- **Clarithromycin** decreases the absorption of NRTIs **(zidovudine)**. Separate administration by 4 hours. Moderate Study
- **Clarithromycin** is predicted to increase the exposure to **olaparib**. Avoid or adjust dose with potent CYP3A4 inhibitors—consult product literature. Moderate Study
- **Erythromycin** is predicted to increase the exposure to **olaparib**. Avoid or adjust dose with moderate CYP3A4 inhibitors—consult product literature. Moderate Theoretical
- **Clarithromycin** is predicted to increase the exposure to **omaveloxolone**. Avoid or adjust **omaveloxolone** dose, p. 755. Severe Study
- **Erythromycin** is predicted to increase the exposure to **omaveloxolone**. Avoid or adjust **omaveloxolone** dose, p. 755. Moderate Study
- **Clarithromycin** is predicted to increase the exposure to opioids **(alfentanil, buprenorphine, fentanyl, oxycodone)**. Monitor and adjust dose. Severe Study
- **Erythromycin** is predicted to increase the exposure to opioids **(alfentanil, buprenorphine, fentanyl, oxycodone)**. Monitor and adjust dose. Moderate Study
- **Clarithromycin** is predicted to increase the concentration of opioids **(methadone)**. Severe Theoretical
- **Erythromycin** is predicted to increase the exposure to opioids **(methadone, sufentanil)**. Moderate Theoretical → Also see TABLE 7 p. 1055
- **Clarithromycin** is predicted to increase the exposure to opioids **(sufentanil)**. Moderate Study
- **Clarithromycin** is predicted to increase the exposure to **osilodrostat**. Moderate Theoretical
- **Clarithromycin** is predicted to increase the exposure to **ospemifene**. Avoid in poor CYP2C9 metabolisers. Moderate Study
- **Clarithromycin** is predicted to increase the exposure to **oxybutynin**. Mild Study
- **Clarithromycin** is predicted to increase the exposure to **palbociclib**. Avoid or adjust dose—consult product literature. Severe Study
- **Clarithromycin** is predicted to increase the exposure to **panobinostat**. Adjust dose—consult product literature; in hepatic impairment avoid. Moderate Study
- Macrolides **(azithromycin, erythromycin)** are predicted to increase the exposure to **panobinostat**. Adjust dose. Moderate Theoretical → Also see TABLE 7 p. 1055
- **Clarithromycin** is predicted to increase the exposure to **pazopanib**. Avoid or adjust dose—consult product literature. Moderate Study
- **Erythromycin** is predicted to increase the exposure to **pazopanib**. Moderate Study → Also see TABLE 7 p. 1055
- **Clarithromycin** is predicted to increase the exposure to **pemigatinib**. Avoid or adjust dose—consult product literature. Severe Study
- **Erythromycin** is predicted to increase the exposure to **pemigatinib**. Severe Study
- **Azithromycin** might increase the risk of bleeding events when given with **phenindione**. Severe Theoretical
- **Erythromycin** is predicted to increase the exposure to phosphodiesterase type-5 inhibitors **(avanafil)**. Adjust **avanafil** dose. Moderate Theoretical
- **Clarithromycin** is predicted to increase the exposure to phosphodiesterase type-5 inhibitors **(avanafil, vardenafil)**. Avoid. Severe Study
- **Clarithromycin** is predicted to increase the exposure to phosphodiesterase type-5 inhibitors **(sildenafil)**. Avoid potent CYP3A4 inhibitors or adjust **sildenafil** dose, p. 139. Severe Study
- **Erythromycin** is predicted to increase the exposure to phosphodiesterase type-5 inhibitors **(sildenafil)**. Monitor or adjust **sildenafil** dose with moderate CYP3A4 inhibitors, p. 139. Moderate Study
- **Clarithromycin** is predicted to increase the exposure to phosphodiesterase type-5 inhibitors **(tadalafil)**. Use with caution or avoid. Severe Study
- **Erythromycin** is predicted to increase the exposure to phosphodiesterase type-5 inhibitors **(tadalafil)**. Severe Theoretical
- **Erythromycin** is predicted to increase the exposure to phosphodiesterase type-5 inhibitors **(vardenafil)**. Adjust dose. Severe Theoretical → Also see TABLE 7 p. 1055
- **Clarithromycin** is predicted to increase the exposure to **pimozide**. Avoid. Severe Study
- **Erythromycin** is predicted to increase the exposure to **pimozide**. Avoid. Severe Theoretical → Also see TABLE 7 p. 1055
- **Clarithromycin** might cause hypoglycaemia when given with **pioglitazone**. Moderate Theoretical

- **Clarithromycin** is predicted to slightly increase the exposure to **ponatinib**. Monitor and adjust dose—consult product literature. Moderate Study
- **Erythromycin** is predicted to increase the exposure to **ponatinib**. Moderate Study
- **Clarithromycin** is predicted to increase the exposure to **pralsetinib**. Avoid or adjust dose with potent CYP3A4 inhibitors—consult product literature. Moderate Study
- Macrolides **(azithromycin, erythromycin)** are predicted to increase the exposure to **pralsetinib**. Moderate Theoretical
- **Clarithromycin** is predicted to moderately increase the exposure to **praziquantel**. Mild Study
- **Clarithromycin** given with carbimazole is predicted to increase the exposure to **propiverine**. Adjust starting dose. Moderate Theoretical
- **Clarithromycin** is predicted to increase the exposure to **quizartinib**. Adjust dose—consult product literature. Severe Study
- **Clarithromycin** is predicted to increase the exposure to **ranolazine**. Avoid. Severe Study
- **Erythromycin** is predicted to increase the exposure to **ranolazine**. Severe Study → Also see TABLE 7 p. 1055
- **Clarithromycin** is predicted to increase the exposure to **reboxetine**. Avoid. Moderate Study
- **Clarithromycin** is predicted to increase the exposure to **regorafenib**. Avoid. Moderate Study
- **Erythromycin** is predicted to increase the exposure to **regorafenib**. Moderate Study
- **Macrolides** are predicted to increase the exposure to **relugolix**. Avoid or take relugolix first and separate administration by at least 6 hours. Moderate Study
- **Clarithromycin** is predicted to increase the exposure to retinoids **(alitretinoin)**. Adjust **alitretinoin** dose. Moderate Theoretical
- **Clarithromycin** is predicted to increase the exposure to **ribociclib**. Avoid or adjust dose—consult product literature. Moderate Study
- **Erythromycin** is predicted to increase the exposure to **ribociclib**. Moderate Study → Also see TABLE 7 p. 1055
- Rifamycins **(rifabutin)** have been reported to cause neutropenia when given with **azithromycin**. Severe Study
- Rifamycins **(rifabutin)** decrease the concentration of **clarithromycin** and **clarithromycin** increases the concentration of rifamycins **(rifabutin)**. Monitor and adjust dose. Severe Study
- Rifamycins **(rifampicin)** greatly decrease the concentration of **clarithromycin**. Severe Study
- **Erythromycin** is predicted to increase the concentration of rifamycins **(rifabutin)** and rifamycins **(rifabutin)** are predicted to decrease the concentration of **erythromycin**. Monitor and adjust dose. Severe Theoretical
- **Azithromycin** is predicted to increase the exposure to **rimegepant**. Avoid another dose of rimegepant within 48 hours of concurrent use. Moderate Theoretical
- **Clarithromycin** is predicted to increase the exposure to **rimegepant**. Avoid. Moderate Study
- **Erythromycin** is predicted to increase the exposure to **rimegepant**. Avoid another dose of rimegepant within 48 hours of concurrent use. Moderate Study
- Macrolides **(clarithromycin, erythromycin)** are predicted to increase the exposure to **ripretinib**. Moderate Theoretical
- **Clarithromycin** is predicted to increase the exposure to **ruxolitinib**. Adjust dose depending on indication and monitor adverse effects—consult product literature. Moderate Study
- **Erythromycin** slightly increases the exposure to **ruxolitinib**. Mild Study
- **Clarithromycin** is predicted to increase the exposure to **selpercatinib**. Adjust dose—consult product literature. Moderate Study
- **Erythromycin** is predicted to increase the exposure to **selpercatinib**. Moderate Study → Also see TABLE 7 p. 1055
- Macrolides **(clarithromycin, erythromycin)** are predicted to increase the exposure to **selumetinib**. Avoid or adjust dose—consult product literature. Severe Study
- **Clarithromycin** is predicted to increase the exposure to **siponimod**. Avoid depending on other drugs taken—consult product literature. Severe Theoretical
- **Erythromycin** is predicted to increase the exposure to **siponimod**. Avoid depending on other drugs taken—consult product literature. Severe Study
- **Clarithromycin** is predicted to increase the concentration of **sirolimus**. Avoid or monitor and adjust dose. Severe Study
- **Erythromycin** increases the concentration of **sirolimus**. Monitor and adjust dose. Moderate Study
- **Clarithromycin** is predicted to increase the exposure to SNRIs **(venlafaxine)**. Moderate Study
- **Clarithromycin** is predicted to increase the exposure to **solifenacin**. Adjust solifenacin p. 604 or tamsulosin with solifenacin dose; avoid in hepatic and renal impairment. Severe Study
- **Clarithromycin** is predicted to increase the exposure to **sparsentan**. Avoid. Severe Study
- **Erythromycin** is predicted to increase the exposure to **sparsentan**. Moderate Study
- **Clarithromycin** is predicted to moderately increase the exposure to SSRIs **(dapoxetine)**. Avoid potent CYP3A4 inhibitors or adjust **dapoxetine** dose. Severe Study
- **Erythromycin** is predicted to increase the exposure to SSRIs **(dapoxetine)**. Adjust **dapoxetine** dose with moderate CYP3A4 inhibitors. Moderate Theoretical
- **Clarithromycin** is predicted to increase the exposure to SSRIs **(sertraline)**. Avoid. Moderate Theoretical
- **Erythromycin** is predicted to increase the exposure to SSRIs **(sertraline)**. Moderate Theoretical
- **Clarithromycin** is predicted to increase the exposure to statins **(atorvastatin)**. Avoid or adjust dose and monitor rhabdomyolysis. Severe Study
- **Erythromycin** slightly increases the exposure to statins **(atorvastatin)**. Monitor and adjust dose. Severe Study
- **Clarithromycin** moderately increases the exposure to statins **(pravastatin)**. Severe Study
- **Erythromycin** slightly increases the exposure to statins **(pravastatin)**. Severe Study
- **Clarithromycin** is predicted to increase the exposure to statins **(simvastatin)**. Avoid. Severe Study
- **Erythromycin** markedly increases the exposure to statins **(simvastatin)**. Avoid. Severe Study
- **Clarithromycin** might increase the exposure to **sulfonylureas**. Moderate Theoretical
- **Clarithromycin** is predicted to increase the exposure to **sunitinib**. Avoid or adjust dose—consult product literature. Moderate Study
- **Erythromycin** is predicted to increase the exposure to **sunitinib**. Moderate Study → Also see TABLE 7 p. 1055
- **Clarithromycin** is predicted to increase the concentration of **tacrolimus**. Avoid. If concurrent use is unavoidable—consult product literature. Severe Study
- **Erythromycin** increases the concentration of **tacrolimus**. Avoid. If concurrent use is unavoidable—consult product literature. Severe Anecdotal
- **Macrolides** are predicted to slightly increase the exposure to **talazoparib**. Avoid or adjust dose—consult product literature. Severe Study
- **Clarithromycin** is predicted to increase the exposure to taxanes **(cabazitaxel)**. Avoid or adjust dose—consult product literature. Severe Study
- **Erythromycin** is predicted to increase the exposure to taxanes **(cabazitaxel)**. Moderate Theoretical
- **Clarithromycin** is predicted to increase the exposure to taxanes **(docetaxel)**. Avoid or adjust dose. Severe Study
- **Erythromycin** is predicted to increase the exposure to taxanes **(docetaxel)**. Severe Study
- **Azithromycin** is predicted to increase the exposure to taxanes **(paclitaxel)**. Moderate Theoretical
- Macrolides **(clarithromycin, erythromycin)** are predicted to increase the exposure to taxanes **(paclitaxel)**. Moderate Anecdotal
- **Clarithromycin** is predicted to increase the concentration of **temsirolimus**. Avoid. Severe Theoretical

Macrolides (continued)
- **Erythromycin** is predicted to increase the concentration of **temsirolimus**. Use with caution or avoid. Moderate Theoretical
- **Clarithromycin** is predicted to increase the exposure to **tezacaftor**. Adjust dose with potent CYP3A4 inhibitors, see tezacaftor with ivacaftor p. 223, ivacaftor with tezacaftor and elexacaftor p. 220, and deutivacaftor with tezacaftor and vanzacaftor p. 218. Severe Study
- **Erythromycin** is predicted to increase the exposure to **tezacaftor**. Adjust dose with moderate CYP3A4 inhibitors, see tezacaftor with ivacaftor p. 223, ivacaftor with tezacaftor and elexacaftor p. 220, and deutivacaftor with tezacaftor and vanzacaftor p. 218. Severe Study
- **Erythromycin** decreases the clearance of **theophylline** and **theophylline** potentially decreases the clearance of **erythromycin**. Adjust dose. Severe Study
- Macrolides **(azithromycin, clarithromycin)** are predicted to increase the exposure to **theophylline**. Adjust dose. Moderate Anecdotal
- **Clarithromycin** increases the exposure to thrombin inhibitors **(dabigatran)**. Moderate Study
- Macrolides **(azithromycin, erythromycin)** are predicted to increase the exposure to thrombin inhibitors **(dabigatran)**. Severe Theoretical
- **Azithromycin** is predicted to increase the exposure to **ticagrelor**. Use with caution or avoid. Severe Study
- **Clarithromycin** is predicted to markedly increase the exposure to **ticagrelor**. Avoid. Severe Study
- **Macrolides** might increase the exposure to **tigecycline**. Mild Anecdotal
- **Clarithromycin** is predicted to increase the exposure to the cytotoxic component of **tisotumab vedotin**. Severe Theoretical
- **Clarithromycin** is predicted to increase the exposure to **tofacitinib**. Adjust **tofacitinib** dose, p. 803. Moderate Study
- **Erythromycin** given with a potent CYP2C19 inhibitor is predicted to increase the exposure to **tofacitinib**. Adjust **tofacitinib** dose, p. 803. Moderate Study
- **Clarithromycin** is predicted to increase the exposure to **tolterodine**. Avoid. Severe Study
- **Clarithromycin** is predicted to increase the exposure to **tolvaptan**. Manufacturer advises caution or adjust **tolvaptan** dose with potent CYP3A4 inhibitors. Severe Study
- **Erythromycin** is predicted to increase the exposure to **tolvaptan**. Manufacturer advises caution or adjust **tolvaptan** dose with moderate CYP3A4 inhibitors. Moderate Study
- **Macrolides** are predicted to increase the exposure to **topotecan**. Severe Study
- **Clarithromycin** is predicted to increase the exposure to **toremifene**. Moderate Theoretical
- **Clarithromycin** is predicted to increase the exposure to **trabectedin**. Avoid or adjust dose. Severe Theoretical
- **Macrolides** are predicted to increase the concentration of **trametinib**. Moderate Theoretical
- **Clarithromycin** is predicted to moderately increase the exposure to **trazodone**. Avoid or adjust dose. Moderate Study
- **Erythromycin** is predicted to increase the exposure to **trazodone**. Moderate Theoretical
- **Clarithromycin** increases the exposure to triptans **(almotriptan)**. Mild Study
- **Clarithromycin** is predicted to markedly increase the exposure to triptans **(eletriptan)**. Avoid. Severe Study
- **Erythromycin** moderately increases the exposure to triptans **(eletriptan)**. Avoid. Moderate Study
- **Clarithromycin** is predicted to increase the exposure to **ulipristal**. Avoid when used for uterine fibroids. Severe Study
- **Erythromycin** moderately increases the exposure to **ulipristal**. Avoid when used for uterine fibroids. Moderate Study
- **Clarithromycin** is predicted to increase the exposure to **upadacitinib**. Manufacturer advises caution or avoid, or adjust **upadacitinib** dose depending on indication, p. 927. Severe Study
- Macrolides **(clarithromycin, erythromycin)** are predicted to increase the exposure to **vanzacaftor**. Adjust dose, see deutivacaftor with tezacaftor and vanzacaftor p. 218. Severe Study
- Macrolides **(clarithromycin, erythromycin)** are predicted to increase the exposure to **vemurafenib**. Severe Theoretical → Also see TABLE 7 p. 1055
- Macrolides **(clarithromycin, erythromycin)** are predicted to increase the exposure to **venetoclax**. Avoid or adjust dose—consult product literature. Severe Study
- **Azithromycin** might increase the exposure to **vinca alkaloids**. Severe Theoretical
- Macrolides **(clarithromycin, erythromycin)** are predicted to increase the exposure to **vinca alkaloids**. Severe Theoretical
- **Clarithromycin** is predicted to increase the exposure to vitamin D substances **(paricalcitol)**. Moderate Study
- **Clarithromycin** is predicted to increase the exposure to **voclosporin**. Avoid. Severe Study
- **Erythromycin** is predicted to increase the exposure to **voclosporin**. Adjust **voclosporin** dose. Severe Study → Also see TABLE 7 p. 1055
- **Clarithromycin** is predicted to increase the exposure to **zanubrutinib**. Avoid or adjust dose with potent CYP3A4 inhibitors—consult product literature. Moderate Study
- **Erythromycin** is predicted to increase the exposure to **zanubrutinib**. Avoid or adjust dose with moderate CYP3A4 inhibitors—consult product literature. Severe Study
- **Clarithromycin** is predicted to increase the exposure to **zopiclone**. Adjust dose. Moderate Theoretical
- **Erythromycin** is predicted to increase the exposure to **zopiclone**. Adjust dose. Moderate Study

Magnesium

SEPARATION OF ADMINISTRATION **Magnesium-containing antacids** and other **oral magnesium preparations** should preferably not be taken at the same time as other drugs since they might impair absorption; some manufacturers suggest separating administration by several hours. **Magnesium-containing antacids** might damage enteric coatings designed to prevent dissolution in the stomach.

- Oral **magnesium** trisilicate decreases the absorption of oral antimalarials **(chloroquine)**. Separate administration by at least 4 hours. Moderate Study
- Oral **magnesium** might decrease the concentration of the active metabolite of oral **baloxavir marboxil**. Avoid. Severe Theoretical
- Oral **magnesium** decreases the absorption of oral bisphosphonates **(alendronate)**. Manufacturer advises take at least 30 minutes before magnesium. Moderate Study
- Oral **magnesium** decreases the absorption of oral bisphosphonates **(clodronate)**. Avoid magnesium for 2 hours before or 1 hour after **clodronate**. Moderate Study
- Oral **magnesium** is predicted to decrease the absorption of oral bisphosphonates **(ibandronate)**. Avoid for at least 6 hours before or 1 hour after **ibandronate**. Moderate Theoretical
- Oral **magnesium** decreases the absorption of oral bisphosphonates **(risedronate)**. Separate administration by at least 2 hours. Moderate Study
- Intravenous **magnesium** potentially increases the risk of hypotension when given with calcium-channel blockers **(amlodipine, felodipine, lacidipine, lercanidipine, nicardipine, nifedipine, nimodipine, verapamil)** in pregnant women. Severe Anecdotal
- Oral **magnesium** trisilicate is predicted to decrease the absorption of oral **hydroxychloroquine**. Moderate Theoretical
- Intravenous **magnesium** increases the effects of **neuromuscular blocking drugs, non-depolarising**. Moderate Study
- Oral **magnesium** trisilicate decreases the absorption of oral **nitrofurantoin**. Moderate Study
- Oral **magnesium** might decrease the exposure to oral **roxadustat**. Manufacturer advises take at least 1 hour after magnesium. Moderate Theoretical
- Intravenous **magnesium** is predicted to increase the effects of **suxamethonium**. Moderate Study
- Oral **magnesium** is predicted to decrease the exposure to oral **vadadustat**. Manufacturer advises take at least 1 hour before or 2 hours after magnesium. Moderate Theoretical

Mannitol → see TABLE 15 p. 1058 (hyponatraemia)

MAO-B inhibitors → see TABLE 4 p. 1054 (bradycardia), TABLE 6 p. 1054 (hypotension)

rasagiline · safinamide · selegiline

FOOD AND LIFESTYLE Hypertension is predicted to occur when high-dose **selegiline** is taken with tyramine-rich foods (such as mature cheese, salami, pickled herring, *Bovril*®, *Oxo*®, *Marmite*® or any similar meat or yeast extract or fermented soya bean extract, and some beers, lagers or wines).

- MAO-B inhibitors **(rasagiline, selegiline)** are predicted to increase the risk of severe hypertension when given with **amfetamines**. Avoid. [Severe] Theoretical
- **Safinamide** is predicted to increase the risk of severe hypertension when given with **amfetamines**. [Severe] Theoretical
- **Axitinib** is predicted to increase the exposure to **rasagiline**. [Moderate] Theoretical
- MAO-B inhibitors **(rasagiline, selegiline)** are predicted to increase the risk of severe hypertension when given with **beta$_2$ agonists**. Avoid. [Severe] Theoretical
- **Safinamide** is predicted to increase the risk of severe hypertension when given with **beta$_2$ agonists**. [Severe] Theoretical
- **Bupropion** is predicted to increase the risk of severe hypertension when given with **MAO-B inhibitors**. Avoid. [Moderate] Theoretical
- **Combined hormonal contraceptives** slightly increases the exposure to **rasagiline**. [Moderate] Study
- **Combined hormonal contraceptives** increase the exposure to **selegiline**. Avoid. [Severe] Study
- **MAO-B inhibitors** are predicted to increase the dopaminergic effects of **foslevodopa**. Adjust dose. [Mild] Theoretical → Also see TABLE 6 p. 1054
- **Givosiran** slightly increases the exposure to **rasagiline**. [Moderate] Study
- **Hormone replacement therapy** is predicted to increase the exposure to **selegiline**. Avoid. [Moderate] Study
- **MAO-B inhibitors** are predicted to increase the effects of **levodopa**. Adjust dose. [Mild] Study → Also see TABLE 6 p. 1054
- MAO-B inhibitors **(rasagiline, selegiline)** are predicted to increase the risk of adverse effects when given with **linezolid**. Avoid and for 14 days after stopping the MAOI. [Severe] Theoretical
- **Safinamide** is predicted to increase the risk of adverse effects when given with **linezolid**. Avoid and for 1 week after stopping **safinamide**. [Severe] Theoretical
- MAO-B inhibitors **(rasagiline, selegiline)** are predicted to increase the risk of adverse effects when given with **MAOIs, irreversible**. Avoid and for 14 days after stopping the MAOI. [Severe] Theoretical → Also see TABLE 6 p. 1054
- **Safinamide** is predicted to increase the risk of adverse effects when given with **MAOIs, irreversible**. Avoid and for 1 week after stopping **safinamide**. [Severe] Theoretical
- **Rasagiline** is predicted to increase the risk of a hypertensive crisis when given with **methylphenidate**. Avoid. [Severe] Theoretical
- **Selegiline** might increase the risk of a hypertensive crisis when given with **methylphenidate**. Avoid. [Severe] Theoretical
- **Mexiletine** slightly increases the exposure to **rasagiline**. [Moderate] Study
- **Moclobemide** is predicted to increase the effects of MAO-B inhibitors **(rasagiline, selegiline)**. Avoid. [Severe] Theoretical
- **Moclobemide** is predicted to increase the risk of adverse effects when given with **safinamide**. Avoid and for 1 week after stopping **safinamide**. [Severe] Theoretical
- **Rasagiline** is predicted to increase the risk of adverse effects when given with opioids **(pethidine)**. Avoid and for 14 days after stopping **rasagiline**. [Severe] Theoretical
- **Safinamide** is predicted to increase the risk of adverse effects when given with opioids **(pethidine)**. Avoid and for 1 week after stopping **safinamide**. [Severe] Theoretical
- **Selegiline** increases the risk of adverse effects when given with opioids **(pethidine)**. Avoid. [Severe] Anecdotal
- **Osilodrostat** slightly increases the exposure to **rasagiline**. [Moderate] Study
- **Ozanimod** might increase the risk of a hypertensive crisis when given with **MAO-B inhibitors** and **MAO-B inhibitors** might decrease the exposure to the active metabolites of **ozanimod**. Avoid. [Severe] Theoretical → Also see TABLE 4 p. 1054
- Quinolones **(ciprofloxacin)** slightly increase the exposure to **rasagiline**. [Moderate] Study
- **Reboxetine** is predicted to increase the risk of a hypertensive crisis when given with MAO-B inhibitors **(rasagiline, selegiline)**. Avoid. [Severe] Theoretical
- **Rucaparib** slightly increases the exposure to **rasagiline**. [Moderate] Study
- **Solriamfetol** is predicted to increase the risk of a hypertensive crisis when given with **MAO-B inhibitors**. Avoid and for 14 days after stopping **MAO-B inhibitors**. [Severe] Theoretical
- **Sympathomimetics, inotropic** are predicted to increase the risk of a hypertensive crisis when given with **MAO-B inhibitors**. Avoid. [Severe] Anecdotal
- **Sympathomimetics, vasoconstrictor** are predicted to increase the risk of a hypertensive crisis when given with **MAO-B inhibitors**. Avoid. [Severe] Anecdotal
- **Tetrabenazine** potentially increases the risk of CNS excitation and hypertension when given with **MAO-B inhibitors**. [Severe] Theoretical
- **Vemurafenib** slightly increases the exposure to **rasagiline**. [Moderate] Study

MAOIs, irreversible → see TABLE 6 p. 1054 (hypotension), TABLE 11 p. 1056 (serotonin toxicity)

isocarboxazid · phenelzine · tranylcypromine

FOOD AND LIFESTYLE Potentially life-threatening hypertensive crisis can develop in those taking MAOIs who eat tyramine-rich food (such as mature cheese, salami, pickled herring, *Bovril*®, *Oxo*®, *Marmite*® or any similar meat or yeast extract or fermented soya bean extract, and some beers, lagers or wines) or foods containing dopa (such as broad bean pods). Avoid tyramine-rich or dopa-rich food or drinks with, or for 2 to 3 weeks after stopping, the MAOI.

- **MAOIs, irreversible** are predicted to increase the effects of alpha blockers **(indoramin)**. Avoid. [Severe] Theoretical → Also see TABLE 6 p. 1054
- **Amfetamines** are predicted to increase the risk of a hypertensive crisis when given with **MAOIs, irreversible**. Avoid and for 14 days after stopping the MAOI. [Severe] Anecdotal → Also see TABLE 11 p. 1056
- Antiepileptics **(carbamazepine)** are predicted to increase the risk of severe toxic reaction when given with **MAOIs, irreversible**. Avoid and for 14 days after stopping the MAOI. [Severe] Theoretical
- Antiepileptics **(phenobarbital, primidone)** are predicted to increase the effects of **MAOIs, irreversible**. [Severe] Theoretical
- **MAOIs, irreversible** are predicted to increase the risk of antimuscarinic adverse effects when given with **antihistamines, non-sedating**. Avoid. [Severe] Theoretical
- **MAOIs, irreversible** are predicted to increase the risk of antimuscarinic adverse effects when given with **antihistamines, sedating**. Avoid. [Severe] Theoretical
- **MAOIs, irreversible** are predicted to increase the risk of adverse effects when given with **atomoxetine**. Avoid and for 2 weeks after stopping the MAOI. [Severe] Theoretical
- **MAOIs, irreversible** are predicted to increase the risk of cardiovascular adverse effects when given with **beta$_2$ agonists**. [Moderate] Anecdotal
- **Bupropion** is predicted to increase the risk of severe hypertension when given with **MAOIs, irreversible**. Avoid and for 14 days after stopping the MAOI. [Severe] Theoretical
- **Buspirone** is predicted to increase the risk of elevated blood pressure when given with **MAOIs, irreversible**. Avoid. [Severe] Anecdotal
- **MAOIs, irreversible** are predicted to increase the effects of **doxapram**. [Moderate] Theoretical
- **Entacapone** is predicted to increase the risk of elevated blood pressure when given with **MAOIs, irreversible**. Avoid. [Severe] Theoretical
- **MAOIs, irreversible** might cause a hypertensive crisis when given with **foslevodopa**. Avoid and for 14 days after stopping the MAOI. [Severe] Theoretical → Also see TABLE 6 p. 1054

MAOIs, irreversible (continued)
- **Levodopa** increases the risk of a hypertensive crisis when given with **MAOIs, irreversible**. Avoid and for 14 days after stopping the MAOI. Severe Study → Also see **TABLE 6** p. 1054
- **MAOIs, irreversible** are predicted to increase the risk of adverse effects when given with **linezolid**. Avoid and for 14 days after stopping the MAOI. Severe Theoretical → Also see **TABLE 11** p. 1056
- MAO-B inhibitors **(rasagiline, selegiline)** are predicted to increase the risk of adverse effects when given with **MAOIs, irreversible**. Avoid and for 14 days after stopping the MAOI. Severe Theoretical → Also see **TABLE 6** p. 1054
- MAO-B inhibitors **(safinamide)** are predicted to increase the risk of adverse effects when given with **MAOIs, irreversible**. Avoid and for 1 week after stopping **safinamide**. Severe Theoretical
- **MAOIs, irreversible** are predicted to alter the antihypertensive effects of **methyldopa**. Avoid. Severe Theoretical → Also see **TABLE 6** p. 1054
- **Methylphenidate** causes a hypertensive crisis when given with **MAOIs, irreversible**. Avoid and for 14 days after stopping the MAOI. Severe Theoretical
- **Mianserin** is predicted to increase the risk of toxicity when given with **MAOIs, irreversible**. Avoid and for 14 days after stopping the MAOI. Severe Theoretical
- **Nefopam** is predicted to increase the risk of serious elevations in blood pressure when given with **MAOIs, irreversible**. Avoid. Severe Theoretical
- **Opicapone** is predicted to increase the risk of elevated blood pressure when given with **MAOIs, irreversible**. Avoid. Severe Theoretical
- **Opioids** are predicted to increase the risk of CNS excitation or depression when given with **MAOIs, irreversible**. Avoid. Severe Study → Also see **TABLE 11** p. 1056
- **Ozanimod** might increase the risk of a hypertensive crisis when given with **MAOIs, irreversible**. Avoid. Severe Theoretical
- MAOIs, irreversible **(isocarboxazid, phenelzine)** are predicted to increase the risk of neuroleptic malignant syndrome when given with **phenothiazine antipsychotics**. Severe Theoretical → Also see **TABLE 6** p. 1054
- **Tranylcypromine** is predicted to increase the risk of neuroleptic malignant syndrome when given with **phenothiazine antipsychotics**. Avoid. Severe Theoretical → Also see **TABLE 6** p. 1054
- **Reboxetine** is predicted to increase the risk of a hypertensive crisis when given with **MAOIs, irreversible**. Avoid. Severe Theoretical
- **Solriamfetol** is predicted to increase the risk of a hypertensive crisis when given with **MAOIs, irreversible**. Avoid and for 14 days after stopping the MAOI. Severe Theoretical
- **Sympathomimetics, inotropic** are predicted to increase the risk of a hypertensive crisis when given with **MAOIs, irreversible**. Avoid and for 14 days after stopping the MAOI. Severe Theoretical
- **Sympathomimetics, vasoconstrictor** are predicted to increase the risk of a hypertensive crisis when given with **MAOIs, irreversible**. Avoid and for 14 days after stopping the MAOI. Severe Study
- **Tetrabenazine** potentially increases the risk of CNS excitation and hypertension when given with **MAOIs, irreversible**. Avoid and for 14 days after stopping the MAOI. Severe Theoretical
- **Tolcapone** is predicted to increase the effects of **MAOIs, irreversible**. Avoid. Severe Theoretical
- **Tricyclic antidepressants** are predicted to increase the risk of severe toxic reaction when given with **MAOIs, irreversible**. Avoid and for 14 days after stopping the MAOI. Severe Theoretical → Also see **TABLE 6** p. 1054 → Also see **TABLE 11** p. 1056
- **MAOIs, irreversible** are predicted to increase the exposure to triptans **(rizatriptan, sumatriptan)**. Avoid and for 14 days after stopping the MAOI. Severe Theoretical
- **MAOIs, irreversible** are predicted to increase the exposure to triptans **(zolmitriptan)**. Severe Theoretical
- **Tryptophan** increases the risk of adverse effects when given with **MAOIs, irreversible**. Severe Anecdotal → Also see **TABLE 11** p. 1056

Maraviroc
- Anti-androgens **(apalutamide, enzalutamide)** are predicted to decrease the exposure to **maraviroc**. Adjust dose. Severe Study
- Antiepileptics **(carbamazepine, fosphenytoin, phenobarbital, phenytoin, primidone)** are predicted to decrease the exposure to **maraviroc**. Adjust dose. Severe Study
- Antifungals, azoles **(itraconazole, ketoconazole, voriconazole)** are predicted to markedly increase the exposure to **maraviroc**. Adjust dose. Severe Study
- **Belzutifan** is predicted to decrease the exposure to **maraviroc**. Avoid or adjust dose. Severe Theoretical
- **Cenobamate** is predicted to decrease the exposure to **maraviroc**. Adjust dose. Moderate Theoretical
- **Cobicistat** markedly increases the exposure to **maraviroc**. Refer to specialist literature. Severe Study
- **Encorafenib** is predicted to decrease the exposure to **maraviroc**. Adjust dose. Severe Study
- Endothelin receptor antagonists **(bosentan)** are predicted to decrease the exposure to **maraviroc**. Avoid. Moderate Theoretical
- HIV-protease inhibitors **(atazanavir)** moderately to markedly increase the exposure to **maraviroc**. Refer to specialist literature. Severe Study
- HIV-protease inhibitors **(darunavir)** boosted with ritonavir markedly increase the exposure to **maraviroc**. Refer to specialist literature. Severe Study
- HIV-protease inhibitors **(lopinavir)** boosted with ritonavir moderately increase the exposure to **maraviroc**. Refer to specialist literature. Severe Study
- HIV-protease inhibitors **(ritonavir)** markedly increase the exposure to **maraviroc**. Refer to specialist literature. Severe Study
- **Maraviroc** potentially decreases the exposure to HIV-protease inhibitors **(fosamprenavir)** and HIV-protease inhibitors **(fosamprenavir)** potentially decrease the exposure to **maraviroc**. Avoid. Severe Study
- **Idelalisib** markedly increases the exposure to **maraviroc**. Adjust dose. Severe Theoretical
- **Ivosidenib** is predicted to decrease the exposure to **maraviroc**. Adjust dose. Severe Study
- **Lumacaftor** is predicted to decrease the exposure to **maraviroc**. Adjust dose. Severe Study
- Macrolides **(clarithromycin)** are predicted to markedly increase the exposure to **maraviroc**. Adjust dose. Severe Study
- **Mitotane** is predicted to decrease the exposure to **maraviroc**. Adjust dose. Severe Study
- Neurokinin-1 receptor antagonists **(aprepitant, netupitant)** are predicted to increase the exposure to **maraviroc**. Moderate Study
- **Nirmatrelvir** boosted with ritonavir is predicted to increase the concentration of **maraviroc**. Refer to specialist literature. Severe Theoretical
- NNRTIs **(efavirenz)** decrease the exposure to **maraviroc**. Refer to specialist literature. Severe Theoretical
- NNRTIs **(etravirine)** slightly decrease the exposure to **maraviroc**. Refer to specialist literature. Moderate Study
- Rifamycins **(rifampicin)** are predicted to decrease the exposure to **maraviroc**. Adjust dose. Severe Study
- **St John's wort** is predicted to decrease the exposure to **maraviroc**. Avoid. Severe Theoretical
- **Vemurafenib** is predicted to increase the exposure to **maraviroc**. Use with caution or avoid. Moderate Theoretical

Maribavir
- Anti-androgens **(apalutamide, enzalutamide)** are predicted to decrease the exposure to **maribavir**. Avoid or adjust **maribavir** dose. Severe Study
- Antiepileptics **(carbamazepine, fosphenytoin, phenobarbital, phenytoin, primidone)** are predicted to decrease the exposure to **maribavir**. Avoid or adjust **maribavir** dose. Severe Study
- **Maribavir** is predicted to increase the exposure to **ciclosporin**. Monitor and adjust dose. Severe Theoretical
- **Dabrafenib** is predicted to decrease the exposure to **maribavir**. Avoid or adjust **maribavir** dose. Severe Study
- **Maribavir** very slightly increases the exposure to **digoxin**. Monitor and adjust dose. Moderate Study

- Endothelin receptor antagonists **(bosentan)** are predicted to decrease the exposure to **maribavir**. Avoid or adjust **maribavir** dose. [Severe] Study
- **Maribavir** increases the exposure to **everolimus**. Monitor and adjust dose. [Severe] Study
- **Maribavir** might decrease the efficacy of **ganciclovir**. Avoid. [Severe] Theoretical
- **Maribavir** is predicted to increase the exposure to **gilteritinib**. [Moderate] Theoretical
- **Maribavir** is predicted to increase the exposure to **idelalisib**. [Moderate] Theoretical
- **Mitotane** is predicted to decrease the exposure to **maribavir**. Avoid or adjust **maribavir** dose. [Severe] Study
- NNRTIs **(efavirenz, nevirapine)** are predicted to decrease the exposure to **maribavir**. Avoid or adjust **maribavir** dose. [Severe] Study
- NNRTIs **(etravirine)** are predicted to decrease the exposure to **maribavir**. Avoid or adjust **maribavir** dose. [Severe] Theoretical
- Rifamycins **(rifabutin)** are predicted to decrease the exposure to **maribavir**. Avoid. [Severe] Theoretical
- Rifamycins **(rifampicin)** are predicted to decrease the exposure to **maribavir**. Avoid. [Severe] Study
- **Maribavir** is predicted to increase the exposure to **sirolimus**. Monitor and adjust dose. [Severe] Study
- **St John's wort** is predicted to decrease the exposure to **maribavir**. Avoid. [Severe] Study
- **Maribavir** is predicted to increase the exposure to statins **(rosuvastatin)**. [Moderate] Theoretical
- **Maribavir** is predicted to slightly increase the exposure to **tacrolimus**. Monitor and adjust dose. [Severe] Study
- **Maribavir** is predicted to increase the exposure to taxanes **(paclitaxel)**. Use with caution and adjust dose. [Unknown] Study
- **Maribavir** is predicted to decrease the exposure to **theophylline**. Avoid. [Mild] Theoretical
- **Maribavir** is predicted to increase the exposure to thrombin inhibitors **(dabigatran)**. [Moderate] Study
- **Maribavir** is predicted to decrease the exposure to **tizanidine**. Avoid. [Mild] Theoretical
- **Maribavir** might decrease the efficacy of **valganciclovir**. Avoid. [Severe] Theoretical

Mavacamten

- Anti-androgens **(apalutamide, enzalutamide)** are predicted to decrease the exposure to **mavacamten**. Monitor and adjust dose—consult product literature. [Severe] Theoretical
- Antiarrhythmics **(amiodarone)** are predicted to increase the exposure to **mavacamten**. Monitor and adjust dose—consult product literature. [Moderate] Theoretical
- Antiarrhythmics **(dronedarone)** are predicted to increase the exposure to **mavacamten**. Adjust dose—consult product literature. [Moderate] Study
- Antiepileptics **(carbamazepine, fosphenytoin, phenobarbital, phenytoin, primidone)** are predicted to decrease the exposure to **mavacamten**. Monitor and adjust dose—consult product literature. [Severe] Theoretical
- Antifungals, azoles **(fluconazole, isavuconazole)** are predicted to increase the exposure to **mavacamten**. Adjust dose—consult product literature. [Moderate] Study
- Antifungals, azoles **(itraconazole, ketoconazole, posaconazole, voriconazole)** are predicted to increase the exposure to **mavacamten**. Avoid or monitor—consult product literature. [Severe] Study
- **Berotralstat** is predicted to increase the exposure to **mavacamten**. Adjust dose—consult product literature. [Moderate] Study
- **Mavacamten** can cause negative inotropic effects, as can **beta blockers, non-selective**. [Severe] Theoretical
- **Mavacamten** can cause negative inotropic effects, as can **beta blockers, selective**. [Severe] Theoretical
- Calcium-channel blockers **(diltiazem, verapamil)** are predicted to increase the exposure to **mavacamten**. Adjust dose—consult product literature. [Moderate] Study
- **Cenobamate** is predicted to decrease the exposure to **mavacamten**. Monitor and adjust dose—consult product literature. [Severe] Theoretical
- **Ceritinib** is predicted to increase the exposure to **mavacamten**. Avoid or monitor—consult product literature. [Severe] Study
- **Cobicistat** is predicted to increase the exposure to **mavacamten**. Avoid or monitor—consult product literature. [Severe] Study
- **Mavacamten** is predicted to affect the efficacy of some **combined hormonal contraceptives**. Use additional contraceptive precautions. [Severe] Theoretical
- **Crizotinib** is predicted to increase the exposure to **mavacamten**. Adjust dose—consult product literature. [Moderate] Study
- **Dabrafenib** is predicted to decrease the exposure to **mavacamten**. Monitor and adjust dose—consult product literature. [Severe] Theoretical
- **Encorafenib** is predicted to decrease the exposure to **mavacamten**. Monitor and adjust dose—consult product literature. [Severe] Theoretical
- Endothelin receptor antagonists **(bosentan)** are predicted to decrease the exposure to **mavacamten**. Monitor and adjust dose—consult product literature. [Severe] Theoretical
- **Entrectinib** is predicted to increase the exposure to **mavacamten**. Monitor and adjust dose—consult product literature. [Moderate] Theoretical
- **Everolimus** is predicted to increase the exposure to **mavacamten**. Monitor and adjust dose—consult product literature. [Moderate] Theoretical
- **Fedratinib** is predicted to increase the exposure to **mavacamten**. Adjust dose—consult product literature. [Moderate] Study
- **Givosiran** is predicted to increase the exposure to **mavacamten**. Monitor and adjust dose—consult product literature. [Moderate] Theoretical
- **Glecaprevir** is predicted to increase the exposure to **mavacamten**. Monitor and adjust dose—consult product literature. [Moderate] Theoretical
- **Grapefruit** is predicted to increase the exposure to **mavacamten**. Monitor and adjust dose—consult product literature. [Moderate] Theoretical
- H_2 receptor antagonists **(cimetidine)** are predicted to increase the exposure to **mavacamten**. Monitor and adjust dose—consult product literature. [Moderate] Theoretical
- **HIV-protease inhibitors** are predicted to increase the exposure to **mavacamten**. Avoid or monitor—consult product literature. [Severe] Study
- **Idelalisib** is predicted to increase the exposure to **mavacamten**. Avoid or monitor—consult product literature. [Severe] Study
- **Imatinib** is predicted to increase the exposure to **mavacamten**. Adjust dose—consult product literature. [Moderate] Study
- **Isoniazid** is predicted to increase the exposure to **mavacamten**. Monitor and adjust dose—consult product literature. [Moderate] Theoretical
- **Ivacaftor** is predicted to increase the exposure to **mavacamten**. Monitor and adjust dose—consult product literature. [Moderate] Theoretical
- **Ivosidenib** is predicted to decrease the exposure to **mavacamten**. Monitor and adjust dose—consult product literature. [Severe] Theoretical
- **Lapatinib** is predicted to increase the exposure to **mavacamten**. Monitor and adjust dose—consult product literature. [Moderate] Theoretical
- **Larotrectinib** is predicted to increase the exposure to **mavacamten**. Monitor and adjust dose—consult product literature. [Moderate] Theoretical
- **Letermovir** is predicted to increase the exposure to **mavacamten**. Adjust dose—consult product literature. [Moderate] Study
- **Lomitapide** is predicted to increase the exposure to **mavacamten**. Monitor and adjust dose—consult product literature. [Moderate] Theoretical
- **Lorlatinib** is predicted to decrease the exposure to **mavacamten**. Monitor and adjust dose—consult product literature. [Severe] Theoretical
- **Lumacaftor** is predicted to decrease the exposure to **mavacamten**. Monitor and adjust dose—consult product literature. [Severe] Theoretical

Mavacamten (continued)

- Macrolides **(clarithromycin)** are predicted to increase the exposure to **mavacamten**. Avoid or monitor—consult product literature. Severe Study
- Macrolides **(erythromycin)** are predicted to increase the exposure to **mavacamten**. Adjust dose—consult product literature. Moderate Study
- **Mitotane** is predicted to decrease the exposure to **mavacamten**. Monitor and adjust dose—consult product literature. Severe Theoretical
- **Moclobemide** is predicted to increase the exposure to **mavacamten**. Adjust dose—consult product literature. Severe Theoretical
- **Modafinil** is predicted to increase the exposure to **mavacamten**. Monitor and adjust dose—consult product literature. Moderate Theoretical
- Neurokinin-1 receptor antagonists **(aprepitant, netupitant)** are predicted to increase the exposure to **mavacamten**. Adjust dose—consult product literature. Moderate Study
- Neurokinin-1 receptor antagonists **(fosaprepitant)** are predicted to increase the exposure to **mavacamten**. Monitor and adjust dose—consult product literature. Moderate Theoretical
- **Nilotinib** is predicted to increase the exposure to **mavacamten**. Adjust dose—consult product literature. Moderate Study
- NNRTIs **(efavirenz, etravirine, nevirapine)** are predicted to decrease the exposure to **mavacamten**. Monitor and adjust dose—consult product literature. Severe Theoretical
- **Osilodrostat** is predicted to increase the exposure to **mavacamten**. Monitor and adjust dose—consult product literature. Moderate Theoretical
- **Pazopanib** is predicted to increase the exposure to **mavacamten**. Monitor and adjust dose—consult product literature. Moderate Theoretical
- Proton pump inhibitors **(esomeprazole, omeprazole)** are predicted to increase the exposure to **mavacamten**. Adjust dose—consult product literature. Severe Theoretical
- Proton pump inhibitors **(pantoprazole)** might increase the exposure to **mavacamten**. Monitor and adjust dose—consult product literature. Moderate Theoretical
- **Ranolazine** is predicted to increase the exposure to **mavacamten**. Monitor and adjust dose—consult product literature. Moderate Theoretical
- Rifamycins **(rifampicin)** are predicted to decrease the exposure to **mavacamten**. Monitor and adjust dose—consult product literature. Severe Theoretical
- **Rucaparib** is predicted to increase the exposure to **mavacamten**. Monitor and adjust dose—consult product literature. Moderate Theoretical
- **Selpercatinib** is predicted to increase the exposure to **mavacamten**. Monitor and adjust dose—consult product literature. Moderate Theoretical
- **Sotorasib** is predicted to decrease the exposure to **mavacamten**. Monitor and adjust dose—consult product literature. Severe Theoretical
- SSRIs **(fluoxetine)** are predicted to increase the exposure to **mavacamten**. Adjust dose—consult product literature. Severe Theoretical
- SSRIs **(fluvoxamine)** are predicted to increase the exposure to **mavacamten**. Monitor and adjust dose—consult product literature. Moderate Theoretical
- **St John's wort** is predicted to decrease the exposure to **mavacamten**. Monitor and adjust dose—consult product literature. Severe Theoretical
- **Tucatinib** is predicted to increase the exposure to **mavacamten**. Avoid or monitor—consult product literature. Severe Study

Measles, mumps, and rubella vaccine → see live vaccines

Mebendazole

- H_2 receptor antagonists **(cimetidine)** increase the concentration of **mebendazole**. Moderate Study
- **Metronidazole** might cause a severe skin reaction, as can **mebendazole**. Avoid. Severe Anecdotal

Medroxyprogesterone

- Antifungals, azoles **(itraconazole, ketoconazole, posaconazole, voriconazole)** are predicted to increase the concentration of intramuscular **medroxyprogesterone**. Moderate Theoretical
- **Ceritinib** is predicted to increase the concentration of intramuscular **medroxyprogesterone**. Moderate Theoretical
- **Cobicistat** is predicted to increase the concentration of intramuscular **medroxyprogesterone**. Moderate Theoretical
- **HIV-protease inhibitors** are predicted to increase the concentration of intramuscular **medroxyprogesterone**. Moderate Theoretical
- **Idelalisib** is predicted to increase the concentration of intramuscular **medroxyprogesterone**. Moderate Theoretical
- Macrolides **(clarithromycin)** are predicted to increase the concentration of intramuscular **medroxyprogesterone**. Moderate Theoretical
- **Sugammadex** is predicted to decrease the exposure to **medroxyprogesterone**. Use additional contraceptive precautions. Severe Theoretical
- **Tucatinib** is predicted to increase the concentration of intramuscular **medroxyprogesterone**. Moderate Theoretical
- **Medroxyprogesterone** might decrease the efficacy of **ulipristal** and **ulipristal** might decrease the efficacy of **medroxyprogesterone**. Avoid when used for uterine fibroids. For CoSRH guidance when used for emergency hormonal contraception, see Contraceptives, interactions p. 614. Severe Theoretical

Mefenamic acid → see NSAIDs

Mefloquine → see antimalarials

Meglitinides

repaglinide

- Anti-androgens **(abiraterone)** are predicted to increase the exposure to **repaglinide**. Moderate Anecdotal
- Anti-androgens **(apalutamide, enzalutamide)** are predicted to decrease the exposure to **repaglinide**. Monitor blood glucose and adjust dose. Moderate Study
- Anti-androgens **(darolutamide)** are predicted to increase the concentration of **repaglinide**. Moderate Theoretical
- Antiepileptics **(carbamazepine, fosphenytoin, phenobarbital, phenytoin, primidone)** are predicted to decrease the exposure to **repaglinide**. Monitor blood glucose and adjust dose. Moderate Study
- **Belumosudil** is predicted to increase the exposure to **repaglinide**. Avoid or adjust dose. Moderate Study
- **Bulevirtide** is predicted to increase the exposure to **repaglinide**. Avoid or monitor. Moderate Theoretical
- **Ciclosporin** moderately increases the exposure to **repaglinide**. Moderate Study
- **Clopidogrel** increases the exposure to **repaglinide**. Avoid. Severe Study
- **Elexacaftor** is predicted to increase the exposure to **repaglinide**. Moderate Theoretical
- **Encorafenib** is predicted to decrease the exposure to **repaglinide**. Monitor blood glucose and adjust dose. Moderate Study
- **Fenfluramine** might decrease blood glucose concentrations when given with **meglitinides**. Moderate Theoretical
- Fibrates **(gemfibrozil)** increase the exposure to **repaglinide**. Avoid. Severe Study
- Iron chelators **(deferasirox)** moderately increase the exposure to **repaglinide**. Avoid. Moderate Study
- **Ivosidenib** is predicted to decrease the exposure to **repaglinide**. Monitor blood glucose and adjust dose. Moderate Study
- **Leflunomide** is predicted to increase the exposure to **repaglinide**. Moderate Study
- **Leniolisib** is predicted to increase the exposure to **repaglinide**. Avoid. Moderate Theoretical
- **Letermovir** is predicted to increase the concentration of **repaglinide**. Avoid. Moderate Theoretical
- **Linzagolix** slightly increases the exposure to **repaglinide**. Avoid. Mild Study
- **Lumacaftor** is predicted to decrease the exposure to **repaglinide**. Monitor blood glucose and adjust dose. Moderate Study
- Macrolides **(clarithromycin)** might cause hypoglycaemia when given with **repaglinide**. Moderate Anecdotal
- **Mifepristone** is predicted to increase the exposure to **repaglinide**. Moderate Theoretical

Interactions | Appendix 1 A1

- **Mitotane** is predicted to decrease the exposure to **repaglinide**. Monitor blood glucose and adjust dose. Moderate Study
- **Opicapone** is predicted to increase the exposure to **repaglinide**. Avoid. Moderate Study
- **Pirtobrutinib** moderately increases the exposure to **repaglinide**. Moderate Study
- **Pitolisant** is predicted to decrease the exposure to **repaglinide**. Mild Theoretical
- Rifamycins **(rifampicin)** are predicted to decrease the exposure to **repaglinide**. Monitor blood glucose and adjust dose. Moderate Study
- **Roxadustat** is predicted to increase the exposure to **repaglinide**. Monitor adverse effects and adjust dose. Moderate Study
- **Selpercatinib** increases the exposure to **repaglinide**. Avoid. Moderate Study
- **Somapacitan** might increase blood glucose concentrations, opposing the blood glucose-lowering effects of **meglitinides**. Adjust dose. Moderate Theoretical
- **Somatrogon** might increase blood glucose concentrations, opposing the blood glucose-lowering effects of **meglitinides**. Adjust dose. Moderate Theoretical
- Taxanes **(cabazitaxel)** are predicted to affect the exposure to **repaglinide**. Manufacturer advises take 12 hours before or 3 hours after **cabazitaxel**. Moderate Theoretical
- **Teriflunomide** is predicted to increase the exposure to **repaglinide**. Moderate Study
- **Trimethoprim** slightly increases the exposure to **repaglinide**. Avoid or monitor blood glucose. Moderate Study
- **Velpatasvir** is predicted to increase the exposure to **repaglinide**. Moderate Study
- **Venetoclax** is predicted to increase the exposure to **repaglinide**. Moderate Theoretical
- **Voclosporin** is predicted to increase the concentration of **repaglinide**. Moderate Theoretical
- **Voxilaprevir** with sofosbuvir and velpatasvir is predicted to increase the exposure to **repaglinide**. Moderate Study

Melatonin → see TABLE 9 p. 1056 (CNS effects)

- Antiepileptics **(phenytoin)** are predicted to decrease the exposure to **melatonin**. Moderate Theoretical → Also see TABLE 9 p. 1056
- **Axitinib** is predicted to increase the exposure to **melatonin**. Moderate Theoretical
- **Combined hormonal contraceptives** is predicted to increase the exposure to **melatonin**. Moderate Theoretical
- **Givosiran** is predicted to increase the exposure to **melatonin**. Moderate Theoretical
- HIV-protease inhibitors **(ritonavir)** are predicted to decrease the exposure to **melatonin**. Moderate Theoretical
- **Leflunomide** is predicted to decrease the exposure to **melatonin**. Moderate Theoretical
- **Leniolisib** is predicted to increase the exposure to **melatonin**. Avoid. Moderate Theoretical
- **Mexiletine** is predicted to increase the exposure to **melatonin**. Moderate Theoretical
- **Osilodrostat** is predicted to increase the exposure to **melatonin**. Moderate Theoretical
- Quinolones **(ciprofloxacin)** are predicted to increase the exposure to **melatonin**. Moderate Theoretical
- Rifamycins **(rifampicin)** are predicted to decrease the exposure to **melatonin**. Moderate Theoretical
- **Rucaparib** is predicted to increase the exposure to **melatonin**. Moderate Theoretical
- SSRIs **(fluvoxamine)** very markedly increase the exposure to **melatonin**. Avoid. Severe Study → Also see TABLE 9 p. 1056
- **Teriflunomide** is predicted to decrease the exposure to **melatonin**. Moderate Theoretical
- **Vemurafenib** is predicted to increase the exposure to **melatonin**. Moderate Theoretical

Meloxicam → see NSAIDs

Melphalan → see alkylating agents

Memantine

- Dopamine receptor agonists **(amantadine)** increase the risk of CNS toxicity when given with **memantine**. Use with caution or avoid. Severe Theoretical
- **Memantine** is predicted to increase the effects of dopamine receptor agonists **(apomorphine, bromocriptine, cabergoline, pramipexole, quinagolide, ropinirole, rotigotine)**. Moderate Theoretical
- **Memantine** is predicted to increase the risk of CNS adverse effects when given with **ketamine**. Avoid. Severe Theoretical
- **Memantine** is predicted to increase the effects of **levodopa**. Moderate Theoretical

Mepacrine

- **Mepacrine** is predicted to increase the concentration of antimalarials **(primaquine)**. Avoid. Moderate Theoretical

Mepivacaine → see anaesthetics, local

Meptazinol → see opioids

Mercaptopurine → see TABLE 1 p. 1053 (hepatotoxicity), TABLE 12 p. 1057 (myelosuppression)

- **Allopurinol** potentially increases the risk of haematological toxicity when given with **mercaptopurine**. Adjust **mercaptopurine** dose, p. 671. Severe Study
- **Mercaptopurine** decreases the anticoagulant effect of **coumarins**. Moderate Anecdotal
- **Febuxostat** is predicted to increase the exposure to **mercaptopurine**. Avoid. Severe Theoretical
- **Live vaccines** are predicted to increase the risk of generalised infection (possibly life-threatening) when given with **mercaptopurine** (high-dose). UKHSA advises avoid (refer to Green Book). Severe Theoretical
- **Trimethoprim** might increase the risk of haematological toxicity when given with **mercaptopurine** in renal transplant patients. Severe Theoretical

Meropenem → see carbapenems

Mesalazine → see TABLE 2 p. 1053 (nephrotoxicity)

ROUTE-SPECIFIC INFORMATION The manufacturers of some mesalazine gastro-resistant and modified-release medicines (*Asacol MR* tablets, *Ipocol*, *Salofalk* granules) suggest that preparations that lower stool pH (e.g. lactulose) might prevent the release of mesalazine.

Metaraminol → see sympathomimetics, vasoconstrictor

Metformin

- **Alcohol** (excessive consumption) potentially increases the risk of lactic acidosis when given with **metformin**. Avoid excessive alcohol consumption. Moderate Theoretical
- Antiepileptics **(sultiame)** might increase the risk of lactic acidosis when given with **metformin**. Severe Theoretical
- Antifungals, azoles **(isavuconazole)** are predicted to increase the exposure to **metformin**. Use with caution and adjust dose. Moderate Study
- Antimalarials **(pyrimethamine)** are predicted to increase the exposure to **metformin**. Use with caution and adjust dose. Moderate Study
- **Bictegravir** slightly increases the exposure to **metformin**. Moderate Study
- **Dolutegravir** is predicted to increase the exposure to **metformin**. Use with caution and adjust dose. Moderate Study
- **Fenfluramine** might decrease blood glucose concentrations when given with **metformin**. Moderate Theoretical
- **Givinostat** might increase the exposure to **metformin**. Moderate Theoretical
- **Guanfacine** is predicted to increase the concentration of **metformin**. Moderate Theoretical
- H_2 receptor antagonists **(cimetidine)** are predicted to increase the exposure to **metformin**. Use with caution and adjust dose. Moderate Study
- **Mexiletine** is predicted to affect the exposure to **metformin**. Unknown Theoretical
- **Pitolisant** is predicted to increase the exposure to **metformin**. Mild Theoretical
- **Ranolazine** is predicted to increase the exposure to **metformin**. Use with caution and adjust dose. Moderate Study
- **Ribociclib** is predicted to increase the exposure to **metformin**. Moderate Theoretical
- **Risdiplam** is predicted to increase the concentration of **metformin**. Monitor and adjust dose. Moderate Theoretical
- **Somapacitan** might increase blood glucose concentrations, opposing the blood glucose-lowering effects of **metformin**. Adjust dose. Moderate Theoretical

Metformin (continued)
- **Somatrogon** might increase blood glucose concentrations, opposing the blood glucose-lowering effects of **metformin**. Adjust dose. [Moderate] Theoretical
- **Trimethoprim** is predicted to increase the exposure to **metformin**. Use with caution and adjust dose. [Moderate] Study
- **Vandetanib** is predicted to increase the exposure to **metformin**. Use with caution and adjust dose. [Moderate] Study

Methadone → see opioids

Methenamine
- **Acetazolamide** is predicted to decrease the efficacy of **methenamine**. Avoid. [Moderate] Theoretical
- **Potassium citrate** is predicted to decrease the efficacy of **methenamine**. Avoid. [Moderate] Theoretical
- **Sodium bicarbonate** is predicted to decrease the efficacy of **methenamine**. Avoid. [Moderate] Theoretical
- **Sodium citrate** is predicted to decrease the efficacy of **methenamine**. Avoid. [Moderate] Theoretical
- **Methenamine** might increase the risk of crystalluria when given with **sulfasalazine**. Avoid. [Severe] Theoretical
- **Methenamine** might increase the risk of crystalluria when given with **sulfonamides**. Avoid. [Severe] Theoretical
- Thiazide diuretics **(metolazone)** are predicted to decrease the efficacy of **methenamine**. [Moderate] Theoretical

Methocarbamol → see TABLE 9 p. 1056 (CNS effects)

Methotrexate → see TABLE 1 p. 1053 (hepatotoxicity), TABLE 12 p. 1057 (myelosuppression), TABLE 2 p. 1053 (nephrotoxicity)
- **Acetazolamide** increases the urinary excretion of **methotrexate**. [Moderate] Study
- **Methotrexate** is predicted to decrease the clearance of **aminophylline**. [Moderate] Theoretical
- Anti-androgens **(apalutamide)** are predicted to decrease the exposure to **methotrexate**. [Mild] Study
- Anti-androgens **(darolutamide)** are predicted to increase the concentration of **methotrexate**. [Moderate] Theoretical
- Antiepileptics **(levetiracetam)** decrease the clearance of **methotrexate**. [Severe] Anecdotal
- **Methotrexate** might decrease the concentration of antiepileptics **(valproate)**. [Severe] Theoretical → Also see TABLE 1 p. 1053
- Antimalarials **(pyrimethamine)** are predicted to increase the risk of adverse effects when given with **methotrexate**. [Severe] Theoretical
- **Asparaginase** affects the efficacy of **methotrexate**. [Severe] Anecdotal → Also see TABLE 1 p. 1053 → Also see TABLE 12 p. 1057
- **Aspirin** (high-dose) is predicted to increase the risk of toxicity when given with **methotrexate**. [Severe] Study → Also see TABLE 2 p. 1053
- **Baricitinib** is predicted to enhance the risk of immunosuppression when given with **methotrexate**. [Severe] Study
- **Crisantaspase** affects the efficacy of **methotrexate**. [Severe] Anecdotal → Also see TABLE 1 p. 1053 → Also see TABLE 12 p. 1057
- **Eltrombopag** is predicted to increase the concentration of **methotrexate**. [Moderate] Theoretical
- **Methotrexate** potentially increases the risk of a severe skin reaction when given with topical **fluorouracil**. [Severe] Anecdotal → Also see TABLE 1 p. 1053 → Also see TABLE 12 p. 1057
- **Imatinib** might affect the clearance of **methotrexate** (particularly high-dose). [Severe] Theoretical → Also see TABLE 12 p. 1057
- **Ivosidenib** is predicted to increase the exposure to **methotrexate**. Use with caution or avoid. [Moderate] Theoretical
- **Leflunomide** is predicted to increase the exposure to **methotrexate**. Avoid. [Severe] Study → Also see TABLE 12 p. 1057
- **Live vaccines** are predicted to increase the risk of generalised infection (possibly life-threatening) when given with **methotrexate** (high-dose). UKHSA advises avoid (refer to Green Book). [Severe] Theoretical
- **Nitisinone** is predicted to increase the exposure to **methotrexate**. [Moderate] Study
- **Nitrous oxide** potentially increases the risk of methotrexate toxicity when given with **methotrexate**. Avoid. [Severe] Study
- **NSAIDs** are predicted to increase the risk of toxicity when given with **methotrexate** (particularly high-dose). [Severe] Study → Also see TABLE 2 p. 1053
- **Pegaspargase** affects the efficacy of **methotrexate**. [Severe] Anecdotal → Also see TABLE 1 p. 1053 → Also see TABLE 12 p. 1057
- **Penicillins** are predicted to increase the risk of toxicity when given with **methotrexate**. [Severe] Anecdotal
- **Pirtobrutinib** is predicted to increase the exposure to **methotrexate**. [Moderate] Theoretical
- **Potassium aminobenzoate** increases the concentration of **methotrexate**. [Moderate] Theoretical
- **Proton pump inhibitors** decrease the clearance of **methotrexate** (high-dose). Use with caution or avoid. [Severe] Study
- Quinolones **(ciprofloxacin)** potentially increase the risk of toxicity when given with **methotrexate**. [Severe] Anecdotal
- **Regorafenib** is predicted to increase the exposure to **methotrexate**. [Moderate] Theoretical → Also see TABLE 12 p. 1057
- Retinoids **(acitretin)** are predicted to increase the concentration of **methotrexate**. Avoid. [Moderate] Anecdotal → Also see TABLE 1 p. 1053
- **Methotrexate** is predicted to decrease the efficacy of **sapropterin**. [Moderate] Theoretical
- **Sulfonamides** are predicted to increase the exposure to **methotrexate**. Use with caution or avoid. [Severe] Theoretical
- **Tedizolid** is predicted to increase the exposure to **methotrexate**. Avoid. [Moderate] Theoretical
- **Methotrexate** is predicted to increase the risk of toxicity when given with **tegafur**. [Severe] Theoretical → Also see TABLE 12 p. 1057
- **Teriflunomide** is predicted to increase the exposure to **methotrexate**. [Moderate] Study
- **Methotrexate** decreases the clearance of **theophylline**. [Moderate] Study
- **Trimethoprim** increases the risk of haematological side-effects (sometimes fatal) when given with **methotrexate**. Avoid. See methotrexate p. 672 for further information. [Severe] Anecdotal → Also see TABLE 2 p. 1053
- **Vadadustat** is predicted to increase the exposure to **methotrexate**. Monitor and adjust dose. [Moderate] Study

Methoxyflurane → see volatile halogenated anaesthetics

Methyldopa → see TABLE 6 p. 1054 (hypotension)
- **Entacapone** is predicted to increase the exposure to **methyldopa**. [Moderate] Theoretical
- Oral **iron** decreases the effects of oral **methyldopa**. [Moderate] Study
- **Methyldopa** increases the risk of neurotoxicity when given with **lithium**. [Severe] Anecdotal
- **MAOIs, irreversible** are predicted to alter the antihypertensive effects of **methyldopa**. Avoid. [Severe] Theoretical → Also see TABLE 6 p. 1054
- **Methyldopa** might enhance the antidiuretic and hypertensive effects of **vasopressin**. [Moderate] Theoretical

Methylphenidate
- **Alcohol** might increase the concentration of **methylphenidate**. Avoid. [Moderate] Study
- Antiepileptics **(carbamazepine)** might decrease the concentration of **methylphenidate**. [Moderate] Anecdotal
- Antiepileptics **(valproate)** might enhance the effects of **methylphenidate**. [Severe] Anecdotal
- **Methylphenidate** is predicted to decrease the effects of **apraclonidine**. Avoid. [Severe] Theoretical
- **Methylphenidate** might increase the risk of dyskinesias when given with atypical antipsychotics **(paliperidone)**. [Severe] Theoretical
- **Methylphenidate** increases the risk of dyskinesias when given with atypical antipsychotics **(risperidone)**. [Severe] Anecdotal
- **Methylphenidate** has been reported to cause psychotic symptoms when given with **disulfiram**. [Severe] Anecdotal
- **Methylphenidate** might increase the risk of elevated blood pressure when given with **linezolid**. Avoid. [Severe] Theoretical
- MAO-B inhibitors **(rasagiline)** are predicted to increase the risk of a hypertensive crisis when given with **methylphenidate**. Avoid. [Severe] Theoretical
- MAO-B inhibitors **(selegiline)** might increase the risk of a hypertensive crisis when given with **methylphenidate**. Avoid. [Severe] Theoretical

- **Methylphenidate** causes a hypertensive crisis when given with **MAOIs, irreversible**. Avoid and for 14 days after stopping the MAOI. Severe Theoretical
- **Methylphenidate** is predicted to cause a hypertensive crisis when given with **methylthioninium chloride**. Severe Theoretical
- **Methylphenidate** is predicted to cause a hypertensive crisis when given with **moclobemide**. Severe Theoretical
- **Nirmatrelvir** boosted with ritonavir is predicted to increase the concentration of **methylphenidate**. Severe Theoretical
- **Methylphenidate** is predicted to increase the risk of a hypertensive crisis when given with **ozanimod**. Severe Theoretical
- **Methylphenidate** might increase the concentration of **tricyclic antidepressants**. Use with caution and adjust dose. Moderate Study
- **Methylphenidate** might increase the risk of hypertension and arrhythmias when given with **volatile halogenated anaesthetics**. Avoid **methylphenidate** on day of surgery, p. 277. Severe Theoretical

Methylprednisolone → see corticosteroids

Methylthioninium chloride → see TABLE 11 p. 1056 (serotonin toxicity)

- **Methylthioninium chloride** is predicted to increase the risk of severe hypertension when given with **bupropion**. Avoid. Severe Theoretical
- **Methylphenidate** is predicted to cause a hypertensive crisis when given with **methylthioninium chloride**. Severe Theoretical

Metoclopramide

- **Metoclopramide** potentially decreases the absorption of antifungals, azoles **(posaconazole)** oral suspension. Moderate Study
- **Metoclopramide** decreases the concentration of antimalarials **(atovaquone)**. Avoid. Moderate Study
- **Cilostazol** might increase the exposure to **metoclopramide**. Moderate Study
- **Metoclopramide** is predicted to decrease the effects of dopamine receptor agonists **(apomorphine, bromocriptine, cabergoline, pramipexole, quinagolide, ropinirole, rotigotine)**. Avoid. Moderate Study
- **Metoclopramide** might decrease the effects of **foslevodopa**. Moderate Theoretical
- **Metoclopramide** decreases the effects of **levodopa**. Avoid. Moderate Study
- **Metoclopramide** is predicted to increase the effects of **neuromuscular blocking drugs, non-depolarising**. Moderate Theoretical
- **Metoclopramide** increases the effects of **suxamethonium**. Moderate Study

Metolazone → see thiazide diuretics

Metoprolol → see beta blockers, selective

Metreleptin

- **Metreleptin** might alter the exposure to **aminophylline**. Severe Theoretical
- **Metreleptin** might alter the exposure to **ciclosporin**. Monitor concentration and adjust dose. Severe Theoretical
- **Metreleptin** might decrease the efficacy of **combined hormonal contraceptives**. Use additional contraceptive precautions. Severe Theoretical
- **Metreleptin** might alter the exposure to coumarins **(warfarin)**. Monitor INR and adjust dose. Severe Theoretical
- **Metreleptin** is predicted to increase the risk of hypoglycaemia when given with **insulin**. Monitor blood glucose and adjust dose. Severe Theoretical
- **Metreleptin** is predicted to increase the risk of hypoglycaemia when given with **sulfonylureas**. Monitor blood glucose and adjust dose. Severe Theoretical
- **Metreleptin** might alter the exposure to **theophylline**. Monitor concentration and adjust dose. Severe Theoretical

Metronidazole → see TABLE 10 p. 1056 (peripheral neuropathy)

ROUTE-SPECIFIC INFORMATION Since systemic absorption can follow topical application, the possibility of interactions should be borne in mind.

- **Alcohol** potentially causes a disulfiram-like reaction when given with **metronidazole**. Avoid for at least 48 hours after stopping treatment. Moderate Study
- **Metronidazole** increases the risk of toxicity when given with alkylating agents **(busulfan)** (high-dose). Severe Study
- Antiepileptics **(phenobarbital, primidone)** are predicted to decrease the exposure to **metronidazole**. Moderate Study
- **Metronidazole** is predicted to increase the risk of capecitabine toxicity when given with **capecitabine**. Severe Theoretical
- **Metronidazole** has been reported to increase the concentration of **ciclosporin**. Severe Anecdotal
- **Metronidazole** increases the anticoagulant effect of **coumarins**. Monitor INR and adjust dose. Severe Study
- **Disulfiram** increases the risk of acute psychoses when given with **metronidazole**. Severe Study
- **Metronidazole** is predicted to increase the exposure to **ergometrine**. Severe Theoretical
- **Metronidazole** increases the risk of toxicity when given with **fluorouracil**. Severe Study
- **Metronidazole** is predicted to increase the concentration of **lithium**. Avoid or adjust dose. Severe Anecdotal
- **Metronidazole** might cause a severe skin reaction, as can **mebendazole**. Avoid. Severe Anecdotal
- **Metronidazole** decreases the exposure to **mycophenolate**. Moderate Anecdotal
- **Metronidazole** has been reported to increase the concentration of **tacrolimus**. Severe Anecdotal

Metyrapone

- Antiepileptics **(fosphenytoin, phenobarbital, phenytoin, primidone)** are predicted to decrease the effects of **metyrapone**. Avoid. Moderate Study
- Antihistamines, sedating **(cyproheptadine)** decrease the effects of **metyrapone**. Avoid. Moderate Study
- **Carbimazole** decreases the effects of **metyrapone**. Avoid. Moderate Theoretical
- **Combined hormonal contraceptives** decrease the effects of **metyrapone**. Avoid. Moderate Theoretical
- Phenothiazine antipsychotics **(chlorpromazine)** decrease the effects of **metyrapone**. Avoid. Moderate Theoretical
- **Propylthiouracil** is predicted to decrease the effects of **metyrapone**. Avoid. Moderate Theoretical
- Tricyclic antidepressants **(amitriptyline)** decrease the effects of **metyrapone**. Avoid. Moderate Theoretical

Mexiletine

FOOD AND LIFESTYLE Dose adjustment might be necessary if smoking started or stopped during treatment.

- **Mexiletine** is predicted to increase the exposure to **agomelatine**. Moderate Study
- **Mexiletine** is predicted to increase the exposure to **aminophylline**. Adjust dose. Moderate Theoretical
- **Mexiletine** is predicted to increase the exposure to anaesthetics, local **(ropivacaine)**. Moderate Theoretical
- **Mexiletine** is predicted to increase the exposure to **anagrelide**. Moderate Theoretical
- **Mexiletine** is predicted to increase the risk of torsade de pointes when given with **antiarrhythmics**. Avoid. Severe Theoretical
- Antiepileptics **(phenytoin)** are predicted to increase the clearance of **mexiletine**. Monitor and adjust dose. Moderate Study
- **Mexiletine** increases the concentration of atypical antipsychotics **(clozapine)**. Monitor adverse effects and adjust dose. Severe Study
- **Mexiletine** is predicted to increase the exposure to atypical antipsychotics **(olanzapine)**. Adjust dose. Moderate Anecdotal
- **Mexiletine** potentially increases the risk of cardiovascular adverse effects when given with **beta blockers, non-selective**. Avoid or monitor. Severe Theoretical
- **Mexiletine** potentially increases the risk of cardiovascular adverse effects when given with **beta blockers, selective**. Avoid or monitor. Severe Theoretical
- **Bupropion** is predicted to increase the exposure to **mexiletine**. Moderate Study
- **Mexiletine** increases the risk of cardiovascular adverse effects when given with calcium-channel blockers **(diltiazem)**. Avoid or monitor. Severe Theoretical

Mexiletine (continued)
- **Mexiletine** potentially increases the risk of cardiovascular adverse effects when given with calcium-channel blockers **(verapamil)**. Avoid or monitor. Severe Theoretical
- **Cinacalcet** is predicted to increase the exposure to **mexiletine**. Moderate Study
- **Cobicistat** potentially increases the exposure to **mexiletine**. Severe Theoretical
- **Mexiletine** potentially affects the exposure to coumarins **(warfarin)**. Avoid. Unknown Theoretical
- **Dacomitinib** is predicted to increase the exposure to **mexiletine**. Moderate Study
- **Mexiletine** is predicted to increase the exposure to dopamine receptor agonists **(ropinirole)**. Adjust dose. Moderate Study
- **Mexiletine** are predicted to increases the exposure to **erlotinib**. Monitor adverse effects and adjust dose. Moderate Study
- **Mexiletine** is predicted to increase the exposure to **fezolinetant**. Avoid. Moderate Study
- HIV-protease inhibitors **(ritonavir)** are predicted to increase the clearance of **mexiletine**. Monitor and adjust dose. Moderate Study
- **Leflunomide** is predicted to increase the clearance of **mexiletine**. Monitor and adjust dose. Moderate Study
- **Mexiletine** potentially affects the exposure to **lithium**. Avoid. Unknown Theoretical
- **Mexiletine** is predicted to increase the exposure to **loxapine**. Avoid. Unknown Theoretical
- **Mexiletine** slightly increases the exposure to MAO-B inhibitors **(rasagiline)**. Moderate Study
- **Mexiletine** is predicted to increase the exposure to **melatonin**. Moderate Theoretical
- **Mexiletine** is predicted to affect the exposure to **metformin**. Unknown Theoretical
- **Opioids** potentially decrease the absorption of oral **mexiletine**. Moderate Study
- **Mexiletine** is predicted to increase the exposure to phenothiazine antipsychotics **(chlorpromazine)**. Moderate Theoretical
- **Mexiletine** is predicted to increase the exposure to phosphodiesterase type-4 inhibitors **(roflumilast)**. Moderate Theoretical
- **Mexiletine** is predicted to increase the exposure to **pirfenidone**. Use with caution and adjust dose. Moderate Study
- Rifamycins **(rifampicin)** are predicted to increase the clearance of **mexiletine**. Monitor and adjust dose. Moderate Study
- **Mexiletine** is predicted to increase the exposure to **riluzole**. Moderate Theoretical
- **Mexiletine** is predicted to increase the exposure to SNRIs **(duloxetine)**. Moderate Theoretical
- SSRIs **(fluoxetine, fluvoxamine, paroxetine)** are predicted to increase the exposure to **mexiletine**. Moderate Study
- **Terbinafine** is predicted to increase the exposure to **mexiletine**. Moderate Study
- **Teriflunomide** is predicted to increase the clearance of **mexiletine**. Monitor and adjust dose. Moderate Study
- **Mexiletine** is predicted to increase the exposure to **theophylline**. Monitor and adjust dose. Moderate Theoretical
- **Mexiletine** increases the exposure to **tizanidine**. Avoid. Moderate Study
- **Mexiletine** is predicted to increase the exposure to triptans **(zolmitriptan)**. Adjust **zolmitriptan** dose, p. 347. Moderate Theoretical
- **Mexiletine** is predicted to increase the exposure to **vorasidenib**. Avoid. Moderate Theoretical

Mianserin → see TABLE 9 p. 1056 (CNS effects)
- Antiepileptics **(carbamazepine)** markedly decrease the exposure to **mianserin**. Adjust dose. Moderate Study
- Antiepileptics **(phenobarbital, primidone)** are predicted to decrease the exposure to **mianserin**. Moderate Study → Also see TABLE 9 p. 1056
- **Mianserin** is predicted to increase the risk of toxicity when given with **MAOIs, irreversible**. Avoid and for 14 days after stopping the MAOI. Severe Theoretical
- **Mianserin** is predicted to increase the risk of toxicity when given with **moclobemide**. Avoid and for 1 week after stopping **mianserin**. Severe Theoretical
- **Mianserin** is predicted to decrease the efficacy of **pitolisant**. Moderate Theoretical
- **Mianserin** decreases the effects of sympathomimetics, vasoconstrictor **(ephedrine)**. Severe Anecdotal

Micafungin → see TABLE 1 p. 1053 (hepatotoxicity)
- **Micafungin** slightly increases the exposure to **amphotericin B**. Avoid or monitor toxicity. Moderate Study

Miconazole → see antifungals, azoles

Midazolam → see benzodiazepines

Midodrine → see sympathomimetics, vasoconstrictor

Midostaurin
- Anti-androgens **(apalutamide, enzalutamide)** are predicted to decrease the exposure to **midostaurin**. Avoid. Severe Study
- Antiarrhythmics **(dronedarone)** are predicted to increase the exposure to **midostaurin**. Moderate Theoretical
- Antiepileptics **(carbamazepine, fosphenytoin, phenobarbital, phenytoin, primidone)** are predicted to decrease the exposure to **midostaurin**. Avoid. Severe Study
- Antifungals, azoles **(fluconazole, isavuconazole)** are predicted to increase the exposure to **midostaurin**. Moderate Theoretical
- Antifungals, azoles **(itraconazole, ketoconazole, posaconazole, voriconazole)** are predicted to increase the exposure to **midostaurin**. Avoid or monitor for toxicity. Severe Study
- **Berotralstat** is predicted to increase the exposure to **midostaurin**. Moderate Theoretical
- **Midostaurin** moderately decreases the exposure to the active metabolite of **bupropion**. Moderate Study
- Calcium-channel blockers **(diltiazem, verapamil)** are predicted to increase the exposure to **midostaurin**. Moderate Theoretical
- **Ceritinib** is predicted to increase the exposure to **midostaurin**. Avoid or monitor for toxicity. Severe Study
- **Midostaurin** might increase the concentration of **ciclosporin**. Severe Anecdotal
- **Cobicistat** is predicted to increase the exposure to **midostaurin**. Avoid or monitor for toxicity. Severe Study
- **Crizotinib** is predicted to increase the exposure to **midostaurin**. Moderate Theoretical
- **Dabrafenib** is predicted to decrease the exposure to **midostaurin**. Severe Study
- **Elvitegravir** boosted with ritonavir is predicted to increase the exposure to **midostaurin**. Severe Theoretical
- **Encorafenib** is predicted to decrease the exposure to **midostaurin**. Avoid. Severe Study
- Endothelin receptor antagonists **(bosentan)** are predicted to decrease the exposure to **midostaurin** and **midostaurin** is predicted to increase the exposure to endothelin receptor antagonists **(bosentan)**. Severe Study
- **Fedratinib** is predicted to increase the exposure to **midostaurin**. Moderate Theoretical
- **Grapefruit** juice is predicted to increase the exposure to **midostaurin**. Moderate Theoretical
- **HIV-protease inhibitors** are predicted to increase the exposure to **midostaurin**. Avoid or monitor for toxicity. Severe Study
- **Idelalisib** is predicted to increase the exposure to **midostaurin**. Avoid or monitor for toxicity. Severe Study
- **Imatinib** is predicted to increase the exposure to **midostaurin**. Moderate Theoretical
- **Ivosidenib** is predicted to decrease the exposure to **midostaurin**. Avoid. Severe Study
- **Letermovir** is predicted to increase the exposure to **midostaurin**. Moderate Theoretical
- **Lumacaftor** is predicted to decrease the exposure to **midostaurin**. Avoid. Severe Study
- Macrolides **(clarithromycin)** are predicted to increase the exposure to **midostaurin**. Avoid or monitor for toxicity. Severe Study
- Macrolides **(erythromycin)** are predicted to increase the exposure to **midostaurin**. Moderate Theoretical
- **Mitotane** is predicted to decrease the exposure to **midostaurin**. Avoid. Severe Study

A1 Interactions | Appendix 1

- Neurokinin-1 receptor antagonists **(aprepitant, netupitant)** are predicted to increase the exposure to **midostaurin.** Moderate Theoretical
- **Nilotinib** is predicted to increase the exposure to **midostaurin.** Moderate Theoretical
- NNRTIs **(efavirenz, etravirine, nevirapine)** are predicted to decrease the exposure to **midostaurin.** Severe Study
- Rifamycins **(rifampicin)** are predicted to decrease the exposure to **midostaurin.** Avoid. Severe Study
- **St John's wort** is predicted to decrease the exposure to **midostaurin.** Avoid. Severe Theoretical
- **Tucatinib** is predicted to increase the exposure to **midostaurin.** Avoid or monitor for toxicity. Severe Study

Mifamurtide → see TABLE 12 p. 1057 (myelosuppression)

- **Ciclosporin** is predicted to decrease the efficacy of **mifamurtide.** Avoid. Severe Theoretical
- **Corticosteroids** are predicted to decrease the efficacy of **mifamurtide.** Avoid. Severe Theoretical
- **NSAIDs** (high-dose) are predicted to decrease the efficacy of **mifamurtide.** Avoid. Severe Theoretical
- **Pimecrolimus** is predicted to decrease the efficacy of **mifamurtide.** Avoid. Severe Theoretical
- **Sirolimus** is predicted to decrease the efficacy of **mifamurtide.** Avoid. Severe Theoretical
- **Tacrolimus** is predicted to affect the efficacy of **mifamurtide.** Avoid. Severe Theoretical

Mifepristone

- Anti-androgens **(apalutamide, enzalutamide)** are predicted to decrease the exposure to **mifepristone.** Adjust **mifepristone** dose. Severe Study
- Antiepileptics **(carbamazepine, fosphenytoin, phenobarbital, phenytoin, primidone)** are predicted to decrease the exposure to **mifepristone.** Adjust **mifepristone** dose. Severe Study
- Antifungals, azoles **(posaconazole)** are predicted to increase the exposure to **mifepristone.** Moderate Theoretical
- **Mifepristone** is predicted to increase the exposure to **avatrombopag.** Moderate Theoretical
- **Mifepristone** is predicted to increase the exposure to **capivasertib.** Adjust dose. Moderate Theoretical
- **Cenobamate** is predicted to decrease the exposure to **mifepristone.** Adjust **mifepristone** dose. Severe Study
- **Mifepristone** is predicted to decrease the efficacy of **corticosteroids.** Use with caution and adjust dose. Moderate Theoretical
- **Mifepristone** is predicted to increase the exposure to coumarins **(warfarin).** Moderate Theoretical
- **Dabrafenib** is predicted to decrease the exposure to **mifepristone.** Adjust **mifepristone** dose. Severe Study
- **Encorafenib** is predicted to decrease the exposure to **mifepristone.** Adjust **mifepristone** dose. Severe Study
- Endothelin receptor antagonists **(bosentan)** are predicted to decrease the exposure to **mifepristone.** Adjust **mifepristone** dose. Severe Study
- **Mifepristone** is predicted to increase the exposure to **everolimus.** Severe Theoretical
- **Grapefruit** juice is predicted to increase the exposure to **mifepristone.** Moderate Theoretical
- **Ivosidenib** is predicted to decrease the exposure to **mifepristone.** Adjust **mifepristone** dose. Severe Study
- **Mifepristone** is predicted to increase the exposure to **loperamide.** Moderate Theoretical
- **Lorlatinib** is predicted to decrease the exposure to **mifepristone.** Adjust **mifepristone** dose. Severe Study
- **Lumacaftor** is predicted to decrease the exposure to **mifepristone.** Adjust **mifepristone** dose. Severe Study
- **Mifepristone** is predicted to increase the exposure to meglitinides **(repaglinide).** Moderate Theoretical
- **Mitotane** is predicted to decrease the exposure to **mifepristone.** Adjust **mifepristone** dose. Severe Study
- **Mifepristone** is predicted to increase the exposure to **montelukast.** Moderate Theoretical
- NNRTIs **(efavirenz, etravirine, nevirapine)** are predicted to decrease the exposure to **mifepristone.** Adjust **mifepristone** dose. Severe Study
- **Mifepristone** is predicted to increase the exposure to opioids **(alfentanil).** Severe Theoretical
- **Mifepristone** is predicted to increase the exposure to **pioglitazone.** Moderate Theoretical
- Rifamycins **(rifampicin)** are predicted to decrease the exposure to **mifepristone.** Adjust **mifepristone** dose. Severe Study
- **Mifepristone** might increase the exposure to **seladelpar.** Moderate Study
- **Mifepristone** is predicted to increase the exposure to **siponimod.** Moderate Theoretical
- **Mifepristone** is predicted to increase the exposure to **sirolimus.** Severe Theoretical
- **Sotorasib** is predicted to decrease the exposure to **mifepristone.** Adjust **mifepristone** dose. Severe Study
- **St John's wort** is predicted to decrease the exposure to **mifepristone.** Adjust **mifepristone** dose. Severe Study
- **Mifepristone** moderately increases the exposure to statins **(fluvastatin).** Moderate Study
- **Mifepristone** very markedly increases the exposure to statins **(simvastatin).** Severe Study
- **Mifepristone** is predicted to increase the exposure to sulfonylureas **(glimepiride, tolbutamide).** Moderate Theoretical
- **Mifepristone** is predicted to increase the exposure to **temsirolimus.** Severe Theoretical

Mineralocorticoid receptor antagonists → see TABLE 6 p. 1054 (hypotension), TABLE 13 p. 1057 (increased serum potassium)

eplerenone · finerenone · spironolactone

- Anti-androgens **(apalutamide, enzalutamide)** are predicted to decrease the exposure to **eplerenone.** Avoid. Moderate Theoretical
- Anti-androgens **(apalutamide, enzalutamide)** are predicted to decrease the exposure to **finerenone.** Avoid. Severe Study
- **Spironolactone** might oppose the effects of anti-androgens **(abiraterone).** Avoid. Severe Anecdotal
- Antiarrhythmics **(amiodarone)** are predicted to increase the exposure to **eplerenone.** Adjust **eplerenone** dose. Severe Theoretical
- Antiarrhythmics **(dronedarone)** are predicted to increase the exposure to **eplerenone.** Adjust **eplerenone** dose. Severe Study
- Antiarrhythmics **(dronedarone)** are predicted to increase the exposure to **finerenone.** Severe Study
- Antiepileptics **(carbamazepine, fosphenytoin, phenobarbital, phenytoin, primidone)** are predicted to decrease the exposure to **eplerenone.** Avoid. Moderate Theoretical
- Antiepileptics **(carbamazepine, fosphenytoin, phenobarbital, phenytoin, primidone)** are predicted to decrease the exposure to **finerenone.** Avoid. Severe Study
- Antifungals, azoles **(fluconazole, isavuconazole)** are predicted to increase the exposure to **eplerenone.** Adjust **eplerenone** dose. Severe Study
- Antifungals, azoles **(fluconazole, isavuconazole)** are predicted to increase the exposure to **finerenone.** Severe Study
- Antifungals, azoles **(itraconazole, ketoconazole, posaconazole, voriconazole)** are predicted to markedly increase the exposure to **eplerenone.** Avoid. Severe Study
- Antifungals, azoles **(itraconazole, ketoconazole, posaconazole, voriconazole)** are predicted to increase the exposure to **finerenone.** Avoid. Severe Study
- **Berotralstat** is predicted to increase the exposure to **eplerenone.** Adjust **eplerenone** dose. Severe Study
- **Berotralstat** is predicted to increase the exposure to **finerenone.** Severe Study
- Calcium-channel blockers **(diltiazem, verapamil)** are predicted to increase the exposure to **eplerenone.** Adjust **eplerenone** dose. Severe Study → Also see TABLE 6 p. 1054
- Calcium-channel blockers **(diltiazem, verapamil)** are predicted to increase the exposure to **finerenone.** Severe Study → Also see TABLE 6 p. 1054
- **Cenobamate** is predicted to decrease the exposure to **eplerenone.** Adjust dose. Moderate Theoretical
- **Cenobamate** is predicted to decrease the exposure to **finerenone.** Avoid. Severe Study
- **Ceritinib** is predicted to markedly increase the exposure to **eplerenone.** Avoid. Severe Study

Mineralocorticoid receptor antagonists (continued)

- **Ceritinib** is predicted to increase the exposure to **finerenone**. Avoid. Severe Study
- **Cobicistat** is predicted to markedly increase the exposure to **eplerenone**. Avoid. Severe Study
- **Cobicistat** is predicted to increase the exposure to **finerenone**. Avoid. Severe Study
- **Crizotinib** is predicted to increase the exposure to **eplerenone**. Adjust **eplerenone** dose. Severe Study
- **Crizotinib** is predicted to increase the exposure to **finerenone**. Severe Study
- **Dabrafenib** is predicted to decrease the exposure to **finerenone**. Avoid. Severe Study
- **Eplerenone** very slightly increases the exposure to **digoxin**. Mild Study
- **Spironolactone** increases the concentration of **digoxin**. Monitor and adjust dose. Moderate Study
- **Encorafenib** is predicted to decrease the exposure to **eplerenone**. Avoid. Moderate Theoretical
- **Encorafenib** is predicted to decrease the exposure to **finerenone**. Avoid. Severe Study
- Endothelin receptor antagonists **(bosentan)** are predicted to decrease the exposure to **finerenone**. Avoid. Severe Study
- **Fedratinib** is predicted to increase the exposure to **eplerenone**. Adjust **eplerenone** dose. Severe Study
- **Fedratinib** is predicted to increase the exposure to **finerenone**. Severe Study
- **Grapefruit** and grapefruit juice is predicted to increase the exposure to **finerenone**. Avoid. Moderate Theoretical
- **HIV-protease inhibitors** are predicted to markedly increase the exposure to **eplerenone**. Avoid. Severe Study
- **HIV-protease inhibitors** are predicted to increase the exposure to **finerenone**. Avoid. Severe Study
- **Idelalisib** is predicted to markedly increase the exposure to **eplerenone**. Avoid. Severe Study
- **Idelalisib** is predicted to increase the exposure to **finerenone**. Avoid. Severe Study
- **Imatinib** is predicted to increase the exposure to **eplerenone**. Adjust **eplerenone** dose. Severe Study
- **Imatinib** is predicted to increase the exposure to **finerenone**. Severe Study
- **Ivosidenib** is predicted to decrease the exposure to **eplerenone**. Avoid. Moderate Theoretical
- **Ivosidenib** is predicted to decrease the exposure to **finerenone**. Avoid. Severe Study
- **Letermovir** is predicted to increase the exposure to **eplerenone**. Adjust **eplerenone** dose. Severe Study
- **Letermovir** is predicted to increase the exposure to **finerenone**. Severe Study
- **Eplerenone** potentially increases the concentration of **lithium**. Avoid. Moderate Theoretical
- **Spironolactone** potentially increases the concentration of **lithium**. Moderate Study
- **Lorlatinib** is predicted to decrease the exposure to **finerenone**. Avoid. Severe Study
- **Lumacaftor** is predicted to decrease the exposure to **eplerenone**. Avoid. Moderate Theoretical
- **Lumacaftor** is predicted to decrease the exposure to **finerenone**. Avoid. Severe Study
- Macrolides **(clarithromycin)** are predicted to markedly increase the exposure to **eplerenone**. Avoid. Severe Study
- Macrolides **(clarithromycin)** are predicted to increase the exposure to **finerenone**. Avoid. Severe Study
- Macrolides **(erythromycin)** are predicted to increase the exposure to **eplerenone**. Adjust **eplerenone** dose. Severe Study
- Macrolides **(erythromycin)** are predicted to increase the exposure to **finerenone**. Severe Study
- **Mitotane** is predicted to decrease the exposure to **eplerenone**. Avoid. Moderate Theoretical
- **Mitotane** is predicted to decrease the exposure to **finerenone**. Avoid. Severe Study
- **Spironolactone** is predicted to decrease the effects of **mitotane**. Avoid. Severe Anecdotal
- Neurokinin-1 receptor antagonists **(aprepitant, netupitant)** are predicted to increase the exposure to **eplerenone**. Adjust **eplerenone** dose. Severe Study
- Neurokinin-1 receptor antagonists **(aprepitant, netupitant)** are predicted to increase the exposure to **finerenone**. Severe Study
- **Nilotinib** is predicted to increase the exposure to **eplerenone**. Adjust **eplerenone** dose. Severe Study
- **Nilotinib** is predicted to increase the exposure to **finerenone**. Severe Study
- **Nirmatrelvir** boosted with ritonavir is predicted to increase the concentration of mineralocorticoid receptor antagonists **(eplerenone, finerenone)**. Avoid. Severe Theoretical
- NNRTIs **(efavirenz, etravirine, nevirapine)** are predicted to decrease the exposure to **finerenone**. Avoid. Severe Study
- Rifamycins **(rifampicin)** are predicted to decrease the exposure to **eplerenone**. Avoid. Moderate Theoretical
- Rifamycins **(rifampicin)** are predicted to decrease the exposure to **finerenone**. Avoid. Severe Study
- **Sotorasib** is predicted to decrease the exposure to **finerenone**. Avoid. Severe Study
- **St John's wort** is predicted to slightly decrease the exposure to **eplerenone**. Avoid. Moderate Study
- **St John's wort** is predicted to decrease the exposure to **finerenone**. Avoid. Severe Study
- **Tucatinib** is predicted to markedly increase the exposure to **eplerenone**. Avoid. Severe Study
- **Tucatinib** is predicted to increase the exposure to **finerenone**. Avoid. Severe Study

Minocycline → see tetracyclines

Minoxidil → see TABLE 6 p. 1054 (hypotension)

ROUTE-SPECIFIC INFORMATION Since systemic absorption can follow topical application, the possibility of interactions should be borne in mind.

Mirabegron

- **Mirabegron** is predicted to increase the exposure to **aliskiren**. Mild Theoretical
- Antifungals, azoles **(itraconazole, ketoconazole, posaconazole, voriconazole)** are predicted to increase the exposure to **mirabegron**. Adjust **mirabegron** dose in hepatic and renal impairment. Moderate Study
- **Mirabegron** is predicted to increase the exposure to antihistamines, non-sedating **(fexofenadine)**. Mild Theoretical
- **Mirabegron** is predicted to increase the exposure to beta blockers, selective **(metoprolol)**. Moderate Study
- **Ceritinib** is predicted to increase the exposure to **mirabegron**. Adjust **mirabegron** dose in hepatic and renal impairment. Moderate Study
- **Cobicistat** is predicted to increase the exposure to **mirabegron**. Adjust **mirabegron** dose in hepatic and renal impairment. Moderate Study
- **Mirabegron** is predicted to increase the exposure to **colchicine**. Mild Theoretical
- **Mirabegron** slightly increases the exposure to **digoxin**. Monitor concentration and adjust dose. Severe Study
- **Mirabegron** is predicted to increase the exposure to **eliglustat**. Avoid or adjust dose—consult product literature. Severe Study
- **Mirabegron** is predicted to increase the exposure to **everolimus**. Mild Theoretical
- **Mirabegron** is predicted to increase the exposure to factor XA inhibitors **(edoxaban)**. Mild Theoretical
- **HIV-protease inhibitors** are predicted to increase the exposure to **mirabegron**. Adjust **mirabegron** dose in hepatic and renal impairment. Moderate Study
- **Idelalisib** is predicted to increase the exposure to **mirabegron**. Adjust **mirabegron** dose in hepatic and renal impairment. Moderate Study
- **Mirabegron** is predicted to increase the exposure to **loperamide**. Mild Theoretical
- Macrolides **(clarithromycin)** are predicted to increase the exposure to **mirabegron**. Adjust **mirabegron** dose in hepatic and renal impairment. Moderate Study
- **Mirabegron** is predicted to increase the exposure to **sirolimus**. Mild Theoretical
- **Mirabegron** is predicted to increase the exposure to taxanes **(paclitaxel)**. Mild Theoretical

- **Mirabegron** is predicted to increase the exposure to thrombin inhibitors **(dabigatran)**. Severe Theoretical
- **Tucatinib** is predicted to increase the exposure to **mirabegron**. Adjust **mirabegron** dose in hepatic and renal impairment. Moderate Study

Mirikizumab → see monoclonal antibodies

Mirtazapine → see TABLE 15 p. 1058 (hyponatraemia), TABLE 9 p. 1056 (CNS effects)

- Anti-androgens **(apalutamide, enzalutamide)** are predicted to decrease the exposure to **mirtazapine**. Adjust dose. Moderate Study
- Antiepileptics **(carbamazepine, fosphenytoin, phenobarbital, phenytoin, primidone)** are predicted to decrease the exposure to **mirtazapine**. Adjust dose. Moderate Study → Also see TABLE 15 p. 1058 → Also see TABLE 9 p. 1056
- Antifungals, azoles **(itraconazole, ketoconazole, posaconazole, voriconazole)** are predicted to increase the exposure to **mirtazapine**. Moderate Study
- **Ceritinib** is predicted to increase the exposure to **mirtazapine**. Moderate Study
- **Cobicistat** is predicted to increase the exposure to **mirtazapine**. Moderate Study
- **Encorafenib** is predicted to decrease the exposure to **mirtazapine**. Adjust dose. Moderate Study
- H_2 receptor antagonists **(cimetidine)** slightly increase the exposure to **mirtazapine**. Use with caution and adjust dose. Moderate Theoretical
- **HIV-protease inhibitors** are predicted to increase the exposure to **mirtazapine**. Moderate Study
- **Idelalisib** is predicted to increase the exposure to **mirtazapine**. Moderate Study
- **Ivosidenib** is predicted to decrease the exposure to **mirtazapine**. Adjust dose. Moderate Study
- **Lumacaftor** is predicted to decrease the exposure to **mirtazapine**. Adjust dose. Moderate Study
- Macrolides **(clarithromycin)** are predicted to increase the exposure to **mirtazapine**. Moderate Study
- **Mitotane** is predicted to decrease the exposure to **mirtazapine**. Adjust dose. Moderate Study
- **Mirtazapine** is predicted to decrease the efficacy of **pitolisant**. Moderate Theoretical
- Rifamycins **(rifampicin)** are predicted to decrease the exposure to **mirtazapine**. Adjust dose. Moderate Study
- **Tucatinib** is predicted to increase the exposure to **mirtazapine**. Moderate Study

Misoprostol

- **Misoprostol** can cause uterine contractions, as can **oxytocin**; concurrent use might increase the risk of developing this effect. Avoid and for 4 hours after stopping **misoprostol**. Severe Theoretical

Mitomycin → see TABLE 12 p. 1057 (myelosuppression)

- **Live vaccines** are predicted to increase the risk of generalised infection (possibly life-threatening) when given with **mitomycin**. UKHSA advises avoid (refer to Green Book). Severe Theoretical

Mitotane → see TABLE 12 p. 1057 (myelosuppression)

- **Mitotane** is predicted to decrease the exposure to 5-HT3-receptor antagonists **(ondansetron)**. Moderate Study
- **Mitotane** is predicted to markedly decrease the exposure to **abemaciclib**. Avoid. Severe Study
- **Mitotane** is predicted to decrease the exposure to **acalabrutinib**. Avoid. Severe Study
- **Mitotane** is predicted to decrease the exposure to **alpelisib**. Avoid. Moderate Study
- **Mitotane** is predicted to decrease the exposure to anti-androgens **(abiraterone)**. Avoid. Severe Study
- **Mitotane** is predicted to decrease the exposure to anti-androgens **(darolutamide)**. Avoid. Moderate Study
- **Mitotane** is predicted to decrease the exposure to antiarrhythmics **(disopyramide, dronedarone)**. Avoid. Severe Study
- **Mitotane** is predicted to decrease the efficacy of antiarrhythmics **(propafenone)**. Moderate Study
- **Mitotane** is predicted to decrease the exposure to anticholinesterases, centrally acting **(donepezil)**. Mild Study
- **Mitotane** is predicted to decrease the exposure to antiepileptics **(perampanel)**. Monitor and adjust dose. Moderate Study
- **Mitotane** is predicted to decrease the exposure to antifungals, azoles **(isavuconazole)**. Avoid. Severe Study
- **Mitotane** is predicted to decrease the exposure to antimalarials **(artemether)** with lumefantrine. Avoid. Severe Study
- **Mitotane** is predicted to decrease the concentration of antimalarials **(piperaquine)**. Avoid. Moderate Theoretical
- **Mitotane** is predicted to moderately decrease the exposure to atypical antipsychotics **(aripiprazole)**. Avoid or adjust dose—consult product literature. Moderate Study
- **Mitotane** is predicted to decrease the exposure to atypical antipsychotics **(cariprazine)**. Avoid. Severe Theoretical
- **Mitotane** is predicted to decrease the exposure to atypical antipsychotics **(lurasidone)**. Avoid. Moderate Study
- **Mitotane** is predicted to decrease the exposure to atypical antipsychotics **(paliperidone)**. Monitor and adjust dose. Severe Study
- **Mitotane** is predicted to decrease the exposure to atypical antipsychotics **(quetiapine)**. Moderate Study
- **Mitotane** is predicted to decrease the exposure to atypical antipsychotics **(risperidone)**. Adjust dose. Moderate Study
- **Mitotane** is predicted to decrease the exposure to **avacopan**. Avoid or monitor. Severe Study
- **Mitotane** is predicted to decrease the exposure to **avapritinib**. Avoid. Severe Study
- **Mitotane** is predicted to decrease the exposure to **axitinib**. Avoid or adjust dose. Moderate Study → Also see TABLE 12 p. 1057
- **Mitotane** decreases the exposure to **bedaquiline**. Avoid. Severe Study
- **Mitotane** is predicted to decrease the exposure to **belumosudil**. Adjust **belumosudil** dose, p. 650. Severe Study
- **Mitotane** is predicted to decrease the exposure to benzodiazepines **(alprazolam)**. Adjust dose. Moderate Theoretical
- **Mitotane** is predicted to decrease the exposure to benzodiazepines **(midazolam)**. Monitor and adjust dose. Severe Study
- **Mitotane** is predicted to decrease the exposure to **bictegravir**. Avoid. Moderate Study
- **Mitotane** slightly decreases the exposure to **bortezomib**. Avoid. Severe Study → Also see TABLE 12 p. 1057
- **Mitotane** is predicted to very markedly decrease the exposure to **bosutinib**. Avoid. Severe Study → Also see TABLE 12 p. 1057
- **Mitotane** is predicted to decrease the exposure to **brigatinib**. Avoid. Severe Study
- **Mitotane** is predicted to decrease the exposure to **buspirone**. Use with caution and adjust dose. Severe Study
- **Mitotane** moderately decreases the exposure to **cabozantinib**. Avoid. Moderate Study → Also see TABLE 12 p. 1057
- **Mitotane** is predicted to decrease the exposure to calcium-channel blockers **(amlodipine, felodipine, lacidipine, lercanidipine, nicardipine, nifedipine, nimodipine)**. Monitor and adjust dose. Moderate Study
- **Mitotane** is predicted to decrease the exposure to calcium-channel blockers **(diltiazem)**. Severe Study
- **Mitotane** is predicted to decrease the exposure to **cannabidiol**. Adjust dose. Moderate Study
- **Mitotane** is predicted to decrease the exposure to **capivasertib**. Avoid. Moderate Study
- **Mitotane** is predicted to decrease the exposure to **ceritinib**. Avoid. Severe Study → Also see TABLE 12 p. 1057
- **Mitotane** decreases the concentration of **ciclosporin**. Severe Study
- **Mitotane** is predicted to alter the effects of **cilostazol**. Moderate Theoretical
- **Mitotane** is predicted to decrease the exposure to **cinacalcet**. Monitor and adjust dose. Moderate Study
- **Mitotane** decreases the exposure to **clomethiazole**. Monitor and adjust dose. Moderate Study
- **Mitotane** is predicted to decrease the exposure to **cobicistat**. Avoid. Severe Study
- **Mitotane** is predicted to decrease the exposure to **cobimetinib**. Avoid. Severe Theoretical
- **Mitotane** might decrease the efficacy of **combined hormonal contraceptives**. Use alternative methods with, and until

Mitotane (continued)
concentrations are undetectable after stopping, **mitotane**. Severe Theoretical

- **Mitotane** is predicted to decrease the exposure to corticosteroids **(budesonide, deflazacort, dexamethasone, fludrocortisone, hydrocortisone, methylprednisolone, prednisolone, triamcinolone)**. Monitor and adjust dose. Moderate Study
- **Mitotane** is predicted to decrease the exposure to corticosteroids **(fluticasone)**. Unknown Theoretical
- **Mitotane** is predicted to markedly decrease the exposure to **crizotinib**. Avoid. Severe Study
- **Mitotane** is predicted to decrease the exposure to **dabrafenib**. Avoid. Moderate Theoretical
- **Mitotane** is predicted to decrease the exposure to **daridorexant**. Severe Study
- **Mitotane** is predicted to decrease the exposure to **darifenacin**. Moderate Theoretical
- **Mitotane** is predicted to markedly decrease the exposure to **dasatinib**. Avoid. Severe Study → Also see TABLE 12 p. 1057
- **Mitotane** is predicted to slightly decrease the exposure to **delamanid**. Avoid. Moderate Study
- **Mitotane** is predicted to decrease the exposure to **deutivacaftor**. Avoid. Severe Theoretical
- **Mitotane** is predicted to markedly decrease the exposure to **dienogest**. Severe Study
- **Mitotane** is predicted to decrease the exposure to dipeptidylpeptidase-4 inhibitors **(linagliptin)**. Moderate Study
- **Mitotane** is predicted to moderately decrease the exposure to dipeptidylpeptidase-4 inhibitors **(saxagliptin)**. Moderate Study
- **Mitotane** is predicted to decrease the exposure to **dolutegravir**. Severe Study
- **Mitotane** is predicted to decrease the exposure to **dronabinol**. Avoid or adjust dose. Mild Study
- **Mitotane** is predicted to decrease the exposure to **elacestrant**. Avoid or adjust dose depending on duration—consult product literature. Severe Study
- **Mitotane** is predicted to decrease the exposure to **elbasvir**. Avoid. Severe Study
- **Mitotane** is predicted to decreases the exposure to **elexacaftor**. Avoid. Severe Theoretical
- **Mitotane** is predicted to decrease the exposure to **eliglustat**. Avoid. Severe Study
- **Mitotane** is predicted to decrease the concentration of **elvitegravir**. Avoid. Severe Study
- **Mitotane** is predicted to decrease the exposure to **encorafenib**. Severe Theoretical
- **Mitotane** affects the exposure to endothelin receptor antagonists **(bosentan)**. Avoid. Severe Study
- **Mitotane** is predicted to decrease the exposure to endothelin receptor antagonists **(macitentan)**. Avoid. Severe Study
- **Mitotane** is predicted to decrease the exposure to the cytotoxic component of **enfortumab vedotin**. Moderate Theoretical
- **Mitotane** is predicted to decrease the exposure to **entrectinib**. Avoid. Severe Study
- **Mitotane** is predicted to decrease the exposure to **erdafitinib**. Avoid. Severe Study
- **Mitotane** is predicted to decrease the exposure to **erlotinib**. Avoid or adjust dose—consult product literature. Severe Study
- **Mitotane** is predicted to decrease the exposure to **esketamine**. Adjust dose. Moderate Study
- **Mitotane** is predicted to decrease the exposure to **eszopiclone**. Adjust dose. Moderate Theoretical
- **Mitotane** is predicted to decrease the concentration of **everolimus**. Avoid or adjust dose. Severe Study
- **Mitotane** moderately decreases the exposure to **exemestane**. Moderate Study
- **Mitotane** is predicted to decrease the exposure to factor XA inhibitors **(apixaban)**. Moderate Study
- **Mitotane** is predicted to decrease the exposure to factor XA inhibitors **(rivaroxaban)**. Avoid unless patient can be monitored for signs of thrombosis. Moderate Study
- **Mitotane** is predicted to decrease the exposure to **fedratinib**. Avoid. Moderate Study
- **Mitotane** is predicted to decrease the exposure to **fenfluramine**. Moderate Theoretical
- **Mitotane** is predicted to decrease the exposure to **fesoterodine**. Avoid. Moderate Study
- **Mitotane** is predicted to decrease the exposure to **fostamatinib**. Avoid. Severe Study
- **Mitotane** is predicted to decrease the exposure to the active metabolite of **fostemsavir**. Avoid. Severe Study
- **Mitotane** is predicted to decrease the exposure to **fruquintinib**. Avoid. Moderate Study
- **Mitotane** is predicted to decrease the exposure to **gefitinib**. Avoid. Severe Study
- **Mitotane** is predicted to decrease the exposure to **glasdegib**. Avoid. Severe Study
- **Mitotane** is predicted to greatly decrease the concentration of **glecaprevir**. Avoid. Severe Study
- **Mitotane** is predicted to decrease the exposure to **grazoprevir**. Avoid. Severe Study
- **Mitotane** is predicted to decrease the concentration of **guanfacine**. Adjust **guanfacine** dose, p. 281. Moderate Study
- **Mitotane** decreases the concentration of **haloperidol**. Adjust dose. Moderate Study
- **Mitotane** is predicted to decrease the exposure to **ibrutinib**. Avoid or monitor. Severe Study → Also see TABLE 12 p. 1057
- **Mitotane** is predicted to decrease the exposure to **idelalisib**. Avoid. Severe Study
- **Mitotane** is predicted to decrease the exposure to **imatinib**. Avoid. Moderate Study → Also see TABLE 12 p. 1057
- **Mitotane** is predicted to decrease the exposure to **irinotecan**. Avoid. Severe Study → Also see TABLE 12 p. 1057
- **Mitotane** is predicted to decrease the exposure to **ivabradine**. Adjust dose. Moderate Theoretical
- **Mitotane** is predicted to decrease the exposure to **ivacaftor**. Avoid. Severe Study
- **Mitotane** is predicted to decrease the exposure to **ivosidenib**. Avoid. Severe Theoretical
- **Mitotane** is predicted to decrease the exposure to **ixazomib**. Avoid. Severe Study
- **Mitotane** is predicted to decrease the exposure to **ketamine**. Adjust dose. Moderate Theoretical
- **Mitotane** is predicted to decrease the exposure to **lapatinib**. Avoid. Severe Study
- **Mitotane** is predicted to moderately decrease the exposure to **larotrectinib**. Avoid. Moderate Study
- **Mitotane** is predicted to decrease the exposure to **lazertinib**. Avoid. Severe Study
- **Mitotane** is predicted to decrease the exposure to **lenacapavir**. Avoid. Severe Study
- **Mitotane** is predicted to decrease the exposure to **leniolisib**. Avoid. Severe Theoretical
- **Mitotane** is predicted to decrease the exposure to **lomitapide**. Monitor and adjust dose. Moderate Theoretical
- **Mitotane** is predicted to decrease the exposure to **lorlatinib**. Avoid. Severe Study
- **Mitotane** is predicted to decrease the exposure to **maraviroc**. Adjust dose. Severe Study
- **Mitotane** is predicted to decrease the exposure to **maribavir**. Avoid or adjust **maribavir** dose. Severe Study
- **Mitotane** is predicted to decrease the exposure to **mavacamten**. Monitor and adjust dose—consult product literature. Severe Theoretical
- **Mitotane** is predicted to decrease the exposure to meglitinides **(repaglinide)**. Monitor blood glucose and adjust dose. Moderate Study
- **Mitotane** is predicted to decrease the exposure to **midostaurin**. Avoid. Severe Study
- **Mitotane** is predicted to decrease the exposure to **mifepristone**. Adjust **mifepristone** dose. Severe Study
- Mineralocorticoid receptor antagonists **(spironolactone)** are predicted to decrease the effects of **mitotane**. Avoid. Severe Anecdotal
- **Mitotane** is predicted to decrease the exposure to mineralocorticoid receptor antagonists **(eplerenone)**. Avoid. Moderate Theoretical

- **Mitotane** is predicted to decrease the exposure to mineralocorticoid receptor antagonists **(finerenone)**. Avoid. Severe Study
- **Mitotane** is predicted to decrease the exposure to **mirtazapine**. Adjust dose. Moderate Study
- **Mitotane** is predicted to decrease the exposure to monoclonal antibodies **(polatuzumab vedotin)**. Moderate Theoretical
- **Mitotane** is predicted to decrease the exposure to the cytotoxic component of monoclonal antibodies **(trastuzumab emtansine)**. Severe Theoretical → Also see **TABLE 12** p. 1057
- **Mitotane** is predicted to decrease the exposure to **montelukast**. Mild Study
- **Mitotane** is predicted to markedly decrease the exposure to **naldemedine**. Avoid. Severe Study
- **Mitotane** is predicted to markedly decrease the exposure to **naloxegol**. Avoid. Moderate Study
- **Mitotane** is predicted to decrease the exposure to **neratinib**. Avoid. Severe Study
- **Mitotane** is predicted to markedly decrease the exposure to neurokinin-1 receptor antagonists **(aprepitant)**. Avoid. Moderate Study
- **Mitotane** is predicted to decrease the exposure to neurokinin-1 receptor antagonists **(fosaprepitant)**. Avoid. Moderate Theoretical
- **Mitotane** is predicted to decrease the exposure to neurokinin-1 receptor antagonists **(netupitant)**. Avoid. Severe Study
- **Mitotane** is predicted to moderately decrease the exposure to **nilotinib**. Avoid. Severe Study → Also see **TABLE 12** p. 1057
- **Mitotane** is predicted to decrease the exposure to **nirmatrelvir** boosted with ritonavir. Avoid. Severe Study
- **Mitotane** is predicted to decrease the exposure to **nitisinone**. Adjust dose. Moderate Theoretical
- **Mitotane** is predicted to decrease the exposure to NNRTIs **(doravirine)**. Avoid. Severe Study
- **Mitotane** is predicted to decrease the exposure to NNRTIs **(etravirine)**. Avoid. Severe Theoretical
- **Mitotane** is predicted to decrease the exposure to NNRTIs **(nevirapine)**. Severe Theoretical
- **Mitotane** markedly decreases the exposure to NNRTIs **(rilpivirine)**. Avoid. Severe Study
- **Mitotane** is predicted to decrease the exposure to **olaparib**. Avoid. Moderate Theoretical → Also see **TABLE 12** p. 1057
- **Mitotane** is predicted to decrease the exposure to **omaveloxolone**. Avoid. Severe Study
- **Mitotane** is predicted to decrease the exposure to opioids **(alfentanil, fentanyl)**. Moderate Study
- **Mitotane** is predicted to decrease the exposure to opioids **(buprenorphine)**. Monitor and adjust dose. Moderate Theoretical
- **Mitotane** decreases the exposure to opioids **(methadone)**. Monitor and adjust dose. Severe Study
- **Mitotane** is predicted to decrease the exposure to opioids **(oxycodone)**. Monitor and adjust dose. Moderate Study
- **Mitotane** is predicted to decrease the exposure to **osilodrostat**. Moderate Theoretical
- **Mitotane** is predicted to moderately decrease the exposure to **osimertinib**. Avoid. Moderate Study
- **Mitotane** is predicted to moderately decrease the exposure to **ospemifene**. Moderate Study
- **Mitotane** is predicted to decrease the exposure to **palbociclib**. Avoid. Severe Study → Also see **TABLE 12** p. 1057
- **Mitotane** is predicted to decrease the exposure to **panobinostat**. Avoid. Moderate Theoretical → Also see **TABLE 12** p. 1057
- **Mitotane** is predicted to decrease the exposure to **pazopanib**. Avoid. Severe Theoretical
- **Mitotane** is predicted to decrease the exposure to **pemigatinib**. Avoid. Severe Study
- **Mitotane** moderately decreases the exposure to phosphodiesterase type-4 inhibitors **(apremilast)**. Avoid. Severe Study
- **Mitotane** is predicted to decrease the exposure to phosphodiesterase type-4 inhibitors **(roflumilast)**. Avoid. Moderate Study
- **Mitotane** is predicted to decrease the exposure to phosphodiesterase type-5 inhibitors **(avanafil, tadalafil)**. Avoid. Severe Study
- **Mitotane** is predicted to decrease the exposure to phosphodiesterase type-5 inhibitors **(sildenafil, vardenafil)**. Moderate Theoretical
- **Mitotane** is predicted to moderately to markedly decrease the exposure to **pibrentasvir**. Avoid. Severe Study
- **Mitotane** is predicted to decrease the exposure to **pirtobrutinib**. Avoid. Moderate Study
- **Mitotane** is predicted to moderately decrease the exposure to **pitolisant**. Moderate Study
- **Mitotane** is predicted to decrease the exposure to **ponatinib**. Avoid. Moderate Theoretical
- **Mitotane** is predicted to decrease the exposure to **pralsetinib**. Avoid or adjust dose with potent CYP3A4 inducers—consult product literature. Moderate Study
- **Mitotane** is predicted to markedly decrease the exposure to **praziquantel**. Avoid. Moderate Study
- **Mitotane** is predicted to decrease the exposure to **quizartinib**. Avoid. Severe Study
- **Mitotane** is predicted to decrease the exposure to **ranolazine**. Avoid. Severe Study
- **Mitotane** is predicted to decrease the exposure to **reboxetine**. Moderate Anecdotal
- **Mitotane** is predicted to decrease the exposure to **regorafenib**. Avoid. Moderate Study → Also see **TABLE 12** p. 1057
- **Mitotane** is predicted to markedly decrease the exposure to **ribociclib**. Avoid. Severe Study → Also see **TABLE 12** p. 1057
- **Mitotane** is predicted to decrease the exposure to **rimegepant**. Avoid. Moderate Theoretical
- **Mitotane** is predicted to decrease the exposure to **ripretinib**. Avoid or adjust dose—consult product literature. Severe Study
- **Mitotane** is predicted to decrease the exposure to **ruxolitinib**. Monitor and adjust dose. Moderate Study → Also see **TABLE 12** p. 1057
- **Mitotane** is predicted to decrease the exposure to **selpercatinib**. Avoid. Moderate Study
- **Mitotane** is predicted to decrease the exposure to **selumetinib**. Avoid. Severe Study
- **Mitotane** is predicted to decrease the exposure to **siponimod**. Manufacturer advises caution depending on genotype—consult product literature. Severe Study
- **Mitotane** is predicted to decrease the concentration of **sirolimus**. Avoid or monitor and adjust dose. Severe Study
- **Mitotane** is predicted to decrease the exposure to **solifenacin**. Moderate Theoretical
- **Mitotane** is predicted to decrease the exposure to **sorafenib**. Moderate Theoretical → Also see **TABLE 12** p. 1057
- **Mitotane** is predicted to decrease the exposure to **sotorasib**. Avoid. Severe Study
- **Mitotane** is predicted to decrease the exposure to **sparsentan**. Avoid. Severe Theoretical
- **Mitotane** is predicted to decrease the exposure to statins **(atorvastatin, simvastatin)**. Moderate Study
- **Mitotane** is predicted to decrease the exposure to **sunitinib**. Avoid or adjust dose—consult product literature. Moderate Study → Also see **TABLE 12** p. 1057
- **Mitotane** decreases the concentration of **tacrolimus**. Avoid or monitor and adjust dose. Severe Study
- **Mitotane** is predicted to decrease the exposure to taxanes **(cabazitaxel)**. Avoid. Moderate Study → Also see **TABLE 12** p. 1057
- **Mitotane** is predicted to decrease the exposure to taxanes **(docetaxel)**. Severe Theoretical → Also see **TABLE 12** p. 1057
- **Mitotane** is predicted to decrease the exposure to taxanes **(paclitaxel)**. Avoid. Severe Study → Also see **TABLE 12** p. 1057
- **Mitotane** is predicted to decrease the concentration of **temsirolimus**. Avoid. Severe Study → Also see **TABLE 12** p. 1057
- **Mitotane** is predicted to decrease the exposure to tetracyclines **(eravacycline)**. Adjust **eravacycline** dose. Moderate Study
- **Mitotane** is predicted to decrease the exposure to **tezacaftor**. Avoid. Severe Theoretical
- **Mitotane** is predicted to markedly decrease the exposure to **ticagrelor**. Avoid. Severe Study
- **Mitotane** is predicted to decrease the exposure to the cytotoxic component of **tisotumab vedotin**. Moderate Theoretical
- **Mitotane** is predicted to decrease the exposure to **tivozanib**. Severe Study

Mitotane (continued)
- **Mitotane** is predicted to decrease the exposure to **tofacitinib**. Avoid. Severe Study
- **Mitotane** is predicted to decrease the exposure to **tolvaptan**. Use with caution or avoid depending on indication. Severe Study
- **Mitotane** is predicted to decrease the exposure to **toremifene**. Adjust dose. Moderate Study
- **Mitotane** is predicted to decrease the exposure to **trabectedin**. Avoid. Severe Theoretical → Also see **TABLE 12** p. 1057
- **Mitotane** is predicted to decrease the exposure to **tucatinib**. Avoid. Severe Study
- **Mitotane** is predicted to decrease the efficacy of **ulipristal**. Avoid and for 4 weeks after stopping **mitotane**. Severe Theoretical
- **Mitotane** is predicted to decrease the exposure to **upadacitinib**. Moderate Study
- **Mitotane** is predicted to decrease the exposure to **vandetanib**. Avoid. Moderate Study
- **Mitotane** is predicted to decrease the exposure to **vanzacaftor**. Avoid. Severe Theoretical
- **Mitotane** is predicted to moderately decrease the exposure to **velpatasvir**. Avoid. Severe Study
- **Mitotane** is predicted to decrease the exposure to **vemurafenib**. Avoid. Severe Study
- **Mitotane** is predicted to decrease the exposure to **venetoclax**. Avoid. Severe Study
- **Mitotane** is predicted to decrease the exposure to vinca alkaloids **(vinblastine, vincristine, vindesine)**. Severe Theoretical → Also see **TABLE 12** p. 1057
- **Mitotane** is predicted to decrease the exposure to vinca alkaloids **(vinorelbine)**. Use with caution or avoid. Severe Theoretical → Also see **TABLE 12** p. 1057
- **Mitotane** is predicted to decrease the exposure to **vismodegib**. Avoid. Moderate Theoretical
- **Mitotane** is predicted to decrease the exposure to **voclosporin**. Avoid. Severe Study
- **Mitotane** is predicted to decrease the exposure to **vortioxetine**. Monitor and adjust dose. Moderate Study
- **Mitotane** is predicted to decrease the concentration of **voxilaprevir**. Avoid. Severe Study
- **Mitotane** is predicted to decrease the exposure to **zanubrutinib**. Avoid. Severe Study
- **Mitotane** is predicted to decrease the exposure to **zopiclone**. Adjust dose. Moderate Study

Mitoxantrone → see anthracyclines
Mivacurium → see neuromuscular blocking drugs, non-depolarising
Mizolastine → see antihistamines, non-sedating
Moclobemide → see **TABLE 11** p. 1056 (serotonin toxicity)

FOOD AND LIFESTYLE Moclobemide is claimed to cause less potentiation of the pressor effect of tyramine than the traditional (irreversible) MAOIs, but patients should avoid consuming large amounts of tyramine-rich foods (such as mature cheese, salami, pickled herring, *Bovril*®, *Oxo*®, *Marmite*® or any similar meat or yeast extract or fermented soya bean extract, and some beers, lagers or wines).

- **Amfetamines** are predicted to increase the risk of a hypertensive crisis when given with **moclobemide**. Avoid. Severe Theoretical → Also see **TABLE 11** p. 1056
- Anti-androgens **(apalutamide)** are predicted to decrease the exposure to **moclobemide**. Avoid or monitor. Mild Study
- **Moclobemide** is predicted to increase the exposure to **belzutifan**. Monitor and adjust dose. Severe Theoretical
- **Moclobemide** potentially increases the exposure to benzodiazepines **(clobazam)**. Adjust dose. Moderate Theoretical
- **Bupropion** is predicted to increase the risk of severe hypertension when given with **moclobemide**. Avoid. Severe Theoretical
- **Moclobemide** is predicted to increase the exposure to **cannabidiol**. Moderate Theoretical
- **Moclobemide** is predicted to increase the exposure to **cilostazol**. Moderate Theoretical
- **Moclobemide** is predicted to decrease the efficacy of **clopidogrel**. Avoid. Moderate Study
- **Moclobemide** is predicted to increase the exposure to **eliglustat**. Avoid or adjust dose—consult product literature. Severe Theoretical
- **Moclobemide** might increase the adverse effects of **foslevodopa**. Moderate Theoretical
- H_2 receptor antagonists **(cimetidine)** increase the exposure to **moclobemide**. Adjust **moclobemide** dose. Mild Study
- **Levodopa** increases the risk of adverse effects when given with **moclobemide**. Moderate Study
- **Moclobemide** is predicted to increase the risk of adverse effects when given with **linezolid**. Avoid and for 14 days after stopping **moclobemide**. Severe Theoretical → Also see **TABLE 11** p. 1056
- **Moclobemide** is predicted to increase the effects of MAO-B inhibitors **(rasagiline, selegiline)**. Avoid. Severe Theoretical
- **Moclobemide** is predicted to increase the risk of adverse effects when given with MAO-B inhibitors **(safinamide)**. Avoid and for 1 week after stopping **safinamide**. Severe Theoretical
- **Moclobemide** is predicted to increase the exposure to **mavacamten**. Adjust dose—consult product literature. Severe Theoretical
- **Methylphenidate** is predicted to cause a hypertensive crisis when given with **moclobemide**. Severe Theoretical
- **Mianserin** is predicted to increase the risk of toxicity when given with **moclobemide**. Avoid and for 1 week after stopping **mianserin**. Severe Theoretical
- **Opicapone** is predicted to increase the risk of elevated blood pressure when given with **moclobemide**. Avoid. Severe Theoretical
- **Moclobemide** might cause serotonin toxicity, as can opioids **(tramadol)**; concurrent use might increase the risk of developing this effect. Avoid. Severe Anecdotal → Also see **TABLE 11** p. 1056
- **Ozanimod** might increase the risk of a hypertensive crisis when given with **moclobemide**. Avoid. Severe Theoretical
- **Moclobemide** increases the risk of adverse effects when given with phenothiazine antipsychotics **(levomepromazine)**. Moderate Study
- **Reboxetine** is predicted to increase the risk of a hypertensive crisis when given with **moclobemide**. Avoid. Severe Theoretical
- **Moclobemide** is predicted to increase the exposure to **selumetinib**. Avoid or adjust dose—consult product literature. Severe Theoretical
- **Sparsentan** is predicted to decrease the exposure to **moclobemide**. Moderate Theoretical
- **Moclobemide** is predicted to increase the exposure to SSRIs **(escitalopram)**. Use with caution and adjust dose. Severe Study → Also see **TABLE 11** p. 1056
- **Moclobemide** might cause serotonin toxicity, as can **St John's wort**; concurrent use might increase the risk of developing this effect. Avoid. Severe Theoretical → Also see **TABLE 11** p. 1056
- Sympathomimetics, vasoconstrictor **(ephedrine, isometheptene, phenylephrine, pseudoephedrine)** are predicted to increase the risk of a hypertensive crisis when given with **moclobemide**. Avoid. Severe Study
- **Tetrabenazine** potentially increases the risk of CNS excitation and hypertension when given with **moclobemide**. Severe Theoretical
- **Tricyclic antidepressants** are predicted to increase the risk of severe toxic reaction when given with **moclobemide**. Avoid. Severe Theoretical → Also see **TABLE 11** p. 1056
- **Moclobemide** slightly increases the exposure to triptans **(almotriptan)**. Avoid. Severe Study
- **Moclobemide** increases the concentration of triptans **(eletriptan, frovatriptan, naratriptan)**. Avoid. Severe Study
- **Moclobemide** moderately increases the exposure to triptans **(rizatriptan, sumatriptan)**. Avoid. Severe Study
- **Moclobemide** slightly increases the exposure to triptans **(zolmitriptan)**. Avoid or adjust **zolmitriptan** dose, p. 347. Severe Study

Modafinil
- **Modafinil** is predicted to decrease the efficacy of anti-androgens **(cyproterone)** with ethinylestradiol (co-cyprindiol). Use alternative methods during treatment with, and for 28 days after, the enzyme inducing drug is stopped. Severe Study

- Antiepileptics **(carbamazepine, phenobarbital, primidone)** are predicted to decrease the exposure to **modafinil**. Mild Theoretical
- Antiepileptics **(fosphenytoin, phenytoin)** are predicted to decrease the exposure to **modafinil** and **modafinil** is predicted to increase the concentration of antiepileptics **(fosphenytoin, phenytoin)**. Monitor concentration and adjust dose. Moderate Theoretical
- Antifungals, azoles **(itraconazole, ketoconazole, posaconazole, voriconazole)** are predicted to increase the exposure to **modafinil**. Mild Theoretical
- **Modafinil** is predicted to decrease the exposure to **avacopan**. Severe Theoretical
- **Modafinil** is predicted to decrease the exposure to **avapritinib**. Avoid. Severe Theoretical
- **Modafinil** is predicted to decrease the exposure to **bosutinib**. Avoid. Severe Theoretical
- **Modafinil** is predicted to decrease the exposure to **brigatinib**. Avoid or adjust dose—consult product literature. Moderate Theoretical
- **Modafinil** is predicted to decrease the exposure to **capivasertib**. Avoid. Moderate Theoretical
- **Ceritinib** is predicted to increase the exposure to **modafinil**. Mild Theoretical
- **Cobicistat** is predicted to increase the exposure to **modafinil**. Mild Theoretical
- **Modafinil** is predicted to decrease the efficacy of **combined hormonal contraceptives**. For CoSRH guidance, see Contraceptives, interactions p. 614. Severe Study
- **Modafinil** is predicted to decrease the efficacy of **desogestrel**. For CoSRH guidance, see Contraceptives, interactions p. 614. Severe Theoretical
- **Modafinil** is predicted to decrease the efficacy of **drospirenone**. For CoSRH guidance, see Contraceptives, interactions p. 614. Severe Theoretical
- **Modafinil** is predicted to decrease the exposure to **elbasvir**. Avoid. Unknown Theoretical
- **Modafinil** slightly decreases the exposure to **encorafenib**. Moderate Study
- **Modafinil** is predicted to decrease the exposure to **erdafitinib**. Adjust dose. Moderate Theoretical
- **Modafinil** is predicted to decrease the efficacy of **estradiol**. Moderate Theoretical
- **Modafinil** is predicted to decrease the efficacy of **etonogestrel**. For CoSRH guidance, see Contraceptives, interactions p. 614. Severe Theoretical
- **Modafinil** is predicted to decrease the exposure to **glasdegib**. Avoid or adjust dose—consult product literature. Moderate Theoretical
- **Modafinil** is predicted to decrease the exposure to **grazoprevir**. Avoid. Severe Theoretical
- **HIV-protease inhibitors** are predicted to increase the exposure to **modafinil**. Mild Theoretical
- **Modafinil** is predicted to decrease the effects of **hormone replacement therapy**. Moderate Anecdotal
- **Idelalisib** is predicted to increase the exposure to **modafinil**. Mild Theoretical
- **Modafinil** is predicted to decrease the exposure to **leniolisib**. Avoid. Severe Theoretical
- **Modafinil** is predicted to decrease the concentration of **letermovir**. Moderate Theoretical
- **Modafinil** is predicted to decrease the efficacy of some contraceptive methods containing **levonorgestrel**. For CoSRH guidance, see Contraceptives, interactions p. 614. Severe Theoretical
- Macrolides **(clarithromycin)** are predicted to increase the exposure to **modafinil**. Mild Theoretical
- **Modafinil** is predicted to increase the exposure to **mavacamten**. Monitor and adjust dose—consult product literature. Moderate Theoretical
- **Modafinil** is predicted to decrease the exposure to NNRTIs **(doravirine)**. Avoid or adjust doravirine or lamivudine with tenofovir disoproxil and doravirine dose. Severe Theoretical
- **Modafinil** is predicted to decrease the efficacy of some contraceptive methods containing **norethisterone**. For CoSRH guidance, see Contraceptives, interactions p. 614. Severe Anecdotal
- **Modafinil** is predicted to decrease the exposure to **osimertinib**. Use with caution or avoid. Severe Theoretical
- Rifamycins **(rifampicin)** are predicted to decrease the exposure to **modafinil**. Moderate Theoretical
- **Modafinil** is predicted to decrease the exposure to **sofosbuvir**. Avoid. Severe Theoretical
- **Tucatinib** is predicted to increase the exposure to **modafinil**. Mild Theoretical
- **Modafinil** decreases the efficacy of **ulipristal**. Avoid and for 4 weeks after stopping the enzyme inducing drug. For CoSRH guidance, see Contraceptives, interactions p. 614. Severe Anecdotal
- **Modafinil** is predicted to decrease the exposure to **velpatasvir**. Avoid. Severe Theoretical
- **Modafinil** is predicted to decrease the concentration of **voxilaprevir**. Avoid. Severe Theoretical
- **Modafinil** is predicted to decrease the exposure to **zanubrutinib**. Avoid. Moderate Theoretical

Mogamulizumab → see monoclonal antibodies

Momelotinib

- Anti-androgens **(darolutamide)** are predicted to increase the exposure to **momelotinib**. Moderate Study
- **Ciclosporin** is predicted to increase the exposure to **momelotinib**. Moderate Study
- **Momelotinib** might decrease the efficacy of **combined hormonal contraceptives**. Additional non-hormonal contraception should be used for 7 days following administration. Severe Theoretical
- **Eltrombopag** is predicted to increase the exposure to **momelotinib**. Moderate Study
- Fibrates **(gemfibrozil)** are predicted to increase the exposure to **momelotinib**. Moderate Study
- HIV-protease inhibitors **(atazanavir, lopinavir)** are predicted to increase the exposure to **momelotinib**. Moderate Study
- **Leflunomide** is predicted to increase the exposure to **momelotinib**. Moderate Study
- Macrolides **(clarithromycin, erythromycin)** are predicted to increase the exposure to **momelotinib**. Moderate Study
- Rifamycins **(rifampicin)** are predicted to increase the exposure to **momelotinib**. Moderate Study
- **Roxadustat** is predicted to increase the exposure to **momelotinib**. Moderate Study
- **Momelotinib** increases the exposure to statins **(rosuvastatin)**. Moderate Study
- **Teriflunomide** is predicted to increase the exposure to **momelotinib**. Moderate Study
- **Velpatasvir** is predicted to increase the exposure to **momelotinib**. Moderate Study
- **Voxilaprevir** is predicted to increase the exposure to **momelotinib**. Moderate Study

Mometasone → see corticosteroids

Monoclonal antibodies → see TABLE 12 p. 1057 (myelosuppression), TABLE 10 p. 1056 (peripheral neuropathy), TABLE 7 p. 1055 (QT-interval prolongation)

adalimumab · alemtuzumab · atezolizumab · avelumab · basiliximab · belimumab · bevacizumab · bimekizumab · blinatumomab · brentuximab vedotin · brodalumab · canakinumab · cemiplimab · certolizumab pegol · cetuximab · daratumumab · dinutuximab · dostarlimab · dupilumab · eculizumab · elotuzumab · elranatamab · golimumab · guselkumab · infliximab · inotuzumab ozogamicin · ipilimumab · ixekizumab · lebrikizumab · loncastuximab tesirine · mirikizumab · mogamulizumab · mosunetuzumab · natalizumab · nemolizumab · nivolumab · obinutuzumab · ocrelizumab · ofatumumab · panitumumab · pembrolizumab · pertuzumab · polatuzumab vedotin · ramucirumab · risankizumab · rituximab · rozanolixizumab · sarilumab · satralizumab · secukinumab · serplulimab · siltuximab · spesolimab · tafasitamab · teclistamab · teplizumab · tezepelumab · tildrakizumab · tocilizumab · tralokinumab · trastuzumab · trastuzumab deruxtecan · trastuzumab emtansine · ublituximab · ustekinumab · vedolizumab

- **Certolizumab pegol** is predicted to increase the risk of generalised infection (possibly life-threatening) when given with **abatacept**. Avoid. Severe Theoretical

Monoclonal antibodies (continued)

- **Abatacept** is predicted to increase the risk of generalised infection (possibly life-threatening) when given with monoclonal antibodies **(adalimumab, golimumab, infliximab)**. Avoid. Severe Theoretical
- **Rozanolixizumab** might decrease the concentration of **abatacept**. Avoid and for 2 weeks after stopping **rozanolixizumab**. Moderate Theoretical
- **Rozanolixizumab** might decrease the concentration of **aflibercept**. Avoid and for 2 weeks after stopping **rozanolixizumab**. Moderate Theoretical
- **Blinatumomab** is predicted to transiently increase the exposure to **aminophylline**. Monitor and adjust dose. Moderate Theoretical
- **Sarilumab** potentially affects the exposure to **aminophylline**. Monitor and adjust dose. Moderate Theoretical
- **Tocilizumab** is predicted to decrease the exposure to **aminophylline**. Monitor and adjust dose. Moderate Theoretical
- **Certolizumab pegol** is predicted to increase the risk of generalised infection (possibly life-threatening) when given with **anakinra**. Avoid. Severe Theoretical
- **Anakinra** is predicted to increase the risk of generalised infection (possibly life-threatening) when given with **golimumab**. Avoid. Severe Theoretical
- **Anthracyclines** are predicted to increase the risk of cardiotoxicity when given with monoclonal antibodies **(trastuzumab, trastuzumab emtansine)**. Avoid. Severe Theoretical → Also see TABLE 12 p. 1057
- **Anthracyclines** are predicted to increase the risk of cardiotoxicity when given with **trastuzumab deruxtecan**. Severe Theoretical → Also see TABLE 12 p. 1057
- Anti-androgens **(apalutamide, enzalutamide)** are predicted to decrease the exposure to **polatuzumab vedotin**. Moderate Theoretical
- Anti-androgens **(apalutamide, enzalutamide)** are predicted to decrease the exposure to the cytotoxic component of **trastuzumab emtansine**. Severe Theoretical
- Antiarrhythmics **(amiodarone)** are predicted to increase the risk of neutropenia when given with **brentuximab vedotin**. Monitor and adjust dose. Severe Theoretical → Also see TABLE 10 p. 1056
- Antiarrhythmics **(dronedarone)** increase the risk of neutropenia when given with **brentuximab vedotin**. Monitor and adjust dose. Severe Theoretical
- Antiepileptics **(carbamazepine)** are predicted to decrease the effects of **brentuximab vedotin**. Severe Theoretical
- Antiepileptics **(carbamazepine, fosphenytoin, phenobarbital, phenytoin, primidone)** are predicted to decrease the exposure to **polatuzumab vedotin**. Moderate Theoretical
- Antiepileptics **(carbamazepine, fosphenytoin, phenobarbital, phenytoin, primidone)** are predicted to decrease the exposure to the cytotoxic component of **trastuzumab emtansine**. Severe Theoretical
- **Tocilizumab** is predicted to decrease the exposure to antiepileptics **(fosphenytoin, phenytoin)**. Monitor and adjust dose. Moderate Theoretical
- **Elranatamab** might affect the exposure to antiepileptics **(phenytoin)**. Monitor and adjust dose. Moderate Theoretical
- Antifungals, azoles **(itraconazole, ketoconazole, posaconazole, voriconazole)** are predicted to increase the risk of neutropenia when given with **brentuximab vedotin**. Monitor and adjust dose. Severe Study
- Antifungals, azoles **(itraconazole, ketoconazole, posaconazole, voriconazole)** are predicted to increase the exposure to **polatuzumab vedotin**. Moderate Theoretical
- Antifungals, azoles **(itraconazole, ketoconazole, posaconazole, voriconazole)** are predicted to increase the exposure to the cytotoxic component of **trastuzumab emtansine**. Avoid or monitor. Severe Theoretical
- **Mosunetuzumab** is predicted to transiently increase the exposure to antifungals, azoles **(voriconazole)**. Monitor and adjust dose. Moderate Theoretical
- **Rozanolixizumab** might decrease the concentration of **belatacept**. Avoid and for 2 weeks after stopping **rozanolixizumab**. Moderate Theoretical
- **Tocilizumab** is predicted to decrease the exposure to benzodiazepines **(alprazolam, diazepam, midazolam)**. Monitor and adjust dose. Moderate Theoretical
- **Brentuximab vedotin** increases the risk of pulmonary toxicity when given with **bleomycin**. Avoid. Severe Study → Also see TABLE 12 p. 1057
- Calcium-channel blockers **(verapamil)** increase the risk of neutropenia when given with **brentuximab vedotin**. Monitor and adjust dose. Severe Theoretical
- **Tocilizumab** is predicted to decrease the exposure to **calcium-channel blockers**. Monitor and adjust dose. Moderate Theoretical
- **Ceritinib** is predicted to increase the risk of neutropenia when given with **brentuximab vedotin**. Monitor and adjust dose. Severe Study → Also see TABLE 12 p. 1057
- **Ceritinib** is predicted to increase the exposure to **polatuzumab vedotin**. Moderate Theoretical
- **Ceritinib** is predicted to increase the exposure to the cytotoxic component of **trastuzumab emtansine**. Avoid or monitor. Severe Theoretical → Also see TABLE 12 p. 1057
- **Ciclosporin** increases the risk of neutropenia when given with **brentuximab vedotin**. Monitor and adjust dose. Severe Theoretical
- **Elranatamab** might affect the exposure to **ciclosporin**. Monitor and adjust dose. Moderate Theoretical
- Monoclonal antibodies **(blinatumomab, mosunetuzumab)** are predicted to transiently increase the exposure to **ciclosporin**. Monitor and adjust dose. Moderate Theoretical
- **Sarilumab** potentially affects the exposure to **ciclosporin**. Monitor and adjust dose. Moderate Theoretical
- **Teclistamab** might affect the exposure to **ciclosporin**. Moderate Theoretical
- **Tocilizumab** is predicted to decrease the exposure to **ciclosporin**. Monitor and adjust dose. Moderate Theoretical
- **Cobicistat** is predicted to increase the risk of neutropenia when given with **brentuximab vedotin**. Monitor and adjust dose. Severe Study
- **Cobicistat** is predicted to increase the exposure to **polatuzumab vedotin**. Moderate Theoretical
- **Cobicistat** is predicted to increase the exposure to the cytotoxic component of **trastuzumab emtansine**. Avoid or monitor. Severe Theoretical
- **Sarilumab** potentially decreases the exposure to **combined hormonal contraceptives**. Severe Theoretical
- **Corticosteroids** are predicted to increase the risk of immunosuppression when given with **dinutuximab**. Avoid except in life-threatening situations. Severe Theoretical
- **Corticosteroids** might affect the efficacy of monoclonal antibodies **(atezolizumab, pembrolizumab, serplulimab)**. Use with caution or avoid. Severe Theoretical
- **Corticosteroids** might affect the efficacy of monoclonal antibodies **(ipilimumab, nivolumab)**. Use with caution or avoid. Severe Theoretical
- **Corticosteroids** might increase the risk of generalised infection (possibly life-threatening) when given with **natalizumab**. Manufacturer advises short courses of corticosteroids can be taken. Severe Theoretical
- **Tocilizumab** is predicted to decrease the exposure to corticosteroids **(dexamethasone, methylprednisolone)**. Monitor and adjust dose. Moderate Theoretical
- **Bimekizumab** might affect the exposure to coumarins **(warfarin)**. Moderate Theoretical
- **Elranatamab** might affect the exposure to coumarins **(warfarin)**. Monitor and adjust dose. Moderate Theoretical
- **Coumarins** might increase the risk of gastrointestinal bleeding when given with **ipilimumab**. Severe Theoretical
- **Sarilumab** potentially affects the exposure to coumarins **(warfarin)**. Monitor and adjust dose. Severe Theoretical
- **Tocilizumab** is predicted to decrease the exposure to coumarins **(warfarin)**. Monitor and adjust dose. Moderate Theoretical
- Monoclonal antibodies **(blinatumomab, mosunetuzumab)** are predicted to transiently increase the exposure to coumarins **(warfarin)**. Monitor and adjust dose. Moderate Theoretical
- **Crovalimab** increases the risk of hypersensitivity reactions when given with **eculizumab**. Severe Study

- **Ipilimumab** might increase the risk of gastrointestinal bleeding when given with **danaparoid**. Severe Theoretical
- **Drugs that cause bleeding** (see TABLE 3 p. 1053) cause bleeding, as can monoclonal antibodies **(bevacizumab, trastuzumab emtansine)**; concurrent use might increase the risk of developing this effect. Severe Theoretical
- **Encorafenib** is predicted to decrease the exposure to **polatuzumab vedotin**. Moderate Theoretical
- **Encorafenib** is predicted to decrease the exposure to the cytotoxic component of **trastuzumab emtansine**. Severe Theoretical
- **Rozanolixizumab** might decrease the concentration of **etanercept**. Avoid and for 2 weeks after stopping **rozanolixizumab**. Moderate Theoretical
- **Sarilumab** might cause severe infection and neutropenia when given with **etanercept**. Severe Theoretical
- **Factor XA inhibitors** might increase the risk of gastrointestinal bleeding when given with **ipilimumab**. Severe Theoretical
- **Filgotinib** is predicted to increase the risk of immunosuppression when given with monoclonal antibodies **(adalimumab, certolizumab pegol, golimumab, infliximab, rituximab, sarilumab, secukinumab, tocilizumab)**. Avoid. Severe Theoretical
- **Alemtuzumab** is predicted to increase the risk of generalised infection (possibly life-threatening) when given with **fingolimod**. Avoid. Severe Theoretical
- **Glecaprevir** is predicted to increase the risk of neutropenia when given with **brentuximab vedotin**. Monitor and adjust dose. Severe Theoretical
- **Rozanolixizumab** might decrease the concentration of glucagon-like peptide-1 receptor agonists **(dulaglutide)**. Avoid and for 2 weeks after stopping **rozanolixizumab**. Moderate Theoretical
- **Heparin** might increase the risk of gastrointestinal bleeding when given with **ipilimumab**. Severe Theoretical
- **HIV-protease inhibitors** are predicted to increase the risk of neutropenia when given with **brentuximab vedotin**. Monitor and adjust dose. Severe Study
- **HIV-protease inhibitors** are predicted to increase the exposure to **polatuzumab vedotin**. Moderate Theoretical
- **HIV-protease inhibitors** are predicted to increase the exposure to the cytotoxic component of **trastuzumab emtansine**. Avoid or monitor. Severe Theoretical
- **Idelalisib** is predicted to increase the risk of neutropenia when given with **brentuximab vedotin**. Monitor and adjust dose. Severe Study
- **Idelalisib** is predicted to increase the exposure to **polatuzumab vedotin**. Moderate Theoretical
- **Idelalisib** is predicted to increase the exposure to the cytotoxic component of **trastuzumab emtansine**. Avoid or monitor. Severe Theoretical
- Immunoglobulins **(normal immunoglobulin)** are predicted to alter the effects of **dinutuximab**. Avoid. Severe Theoretical
- **Rozanolixizumab** might decrease the concentration of **immunoglobulins**. Avoid and for 2 weeks after stopping **rozanolixizumab**. Moderate Theoretical
- **Ivosidenib** is predicted to decrease the exposure to **polatuzumab vedotin**. Moderate Theoretical
- **Ivosidenib** is predicted to decrease the exposure to the cytotoxic component of **trastuzumab emtansine**. Severe Theoretical
- **Lapatinib** increases the risk of neutropenia when given with **brentuximab vedotin**. Monitor and adjust dose. Severe Theoretical
- **Live vaccines** are predicted to increase the risk of generalised infection (possibly life-threatening) when given with monoclonal antibodies **(adalimumab, alemtuzumab, atezolizumab, avelumab, basiliximab, belimumab, bevacizumab, bimekizumab, blinatumomab, brentuximab vedotin, brodalumab, canakinumab, cemiplimab, certolizumab pegol, cetuximab, daratumumab, dinutuximab, dostarlimab, dupilumab, eculizumab, elotuzumab, elranatamab, golimumab, guselkumab, infliximab, inotuzumab ozogamicin, ipilimumab, ixekizumab, lebrikizumab, loncastuximab tesirine, mirikizumab, mogamulizumab, mosunetuzumab, natalizumab, nemolizumab, nivolumab, obinutuzumab, ocrelizumab, ofatumumab, panitumumab, pembrolizumab, pertuzumab, polatuzumab vedotin, ramucirumab, risankizumab, rituximab, rozanolixizumab, sarilumab, satralizumab, secukinumab, serplulimab, siltuximab, spesolimab, tafasitamab, teclistamab, teplizumab, tezepelumab, tildrakizumab, tocilizumab, tralokinumab, trastuzumab, trastuzumab deruxtecan, trastuzumab emtansine, ublituximab, ustekinumab, vedolizumab)**. UKHSA advises avoid (refer to Green Book). Severe Theoretical
- **Low molecular-weight heparins** might increase the risk of gastrointestinal bleeding when given with **ipilimumab**. Severe Theoretical
- **Lumacaftor** is predicted to decrease the exposure to **polatuzumab vedotin**. Moderate Theoretical
- **Lumacaftor** is predicted to decrease the exposure to the cytotoxic component of **trastuzumab emtansine**. Severe Theoretical
- Macrolides **(azithromycin)** are predicted to increase the risk of neutropenia when given with **brentuximab vedotin**. Monitor and adjust dose. Severe Theoretical
- Macrolides **(clarithromycin)** are predicted to increase the risk of neutropenia when given with **brentuximab vedotin**. Monitor and adjust dose. Severe Study
- Macrolides **(clarithromycin)** are predicted to increase the exposure to **polatuzumab vedotin**. Moderate Theoretical
- Macrolides **(clarithromycin)** are predicted to increase the exposure to the cytotoxic component of **trastuzumab emtansine**. Avoid or monitor. Severe Theoretical
- Macrolides **(erythromycin)** increase the risk of neutropenia when given with **brentuximab vedotin**. Monitor and adjust dose. Severe Theoretical
- **Mitotane** is predicted to decrease the exposure to **polatuzumab vedotin**. Moderate Theoretical
- **Mitotane** is predicted to decrease the exposure to the cytotoxic component of **trastuzumab emtansine**. Severe Theoretical → Also see TABLE 12 p. 1057
- Monoclonal antibodies **(sarilumab)** might cause severe infection and neutropenia when given with monoclonal antibodies **(adalimumab, certolizumab pegol, infliximab)**. Severe Theoretical
- Monoclonal antibodies **(sarilumab)** might cause the risk of severe infection and neutropenia when given with monoclonal antibodies **(golimumab)**. Severe Theoretical
- **Alemtuzumab** is predicted to increase the risk of generalised infection (possibly life-threatening) when given with **ozanimod**. Avoid. Severe Theoretical
- **Phenindione** might increase the risk of gastrointestinal bleeding when given with **ipilimumab**. Severe Theoretical
- **Pibrentasvir** is predicted to increase the risk of neutropenia when given with **brentuximab vedotin**. Monitor and adjust dose. Severe Theoretical
- **Alemtuzumab** is predicted to increase the risk of generalised infection (possibly life-threatening) when given with **ponesimod**. Severe Theoretical
- **Ranolazine** increases the risk of neutropenia when given with **brentuximab vedotin**. Monitor and adjust dose. Severe Theoretical
- Rifamycins **(rifampicin)** decrease the effects of **brentuximab vedotin**. Severe Study
- Rifamycins **(rifampicin)** are predicted to decrease the exposure to **polatuzumab vedotin**. Moderate Theoretical
- Rifamycins **(rifampicin)** are predicted to decrease the exposure to the cytotoxic component of **trastuzumab emtansine**. Severe Theoretical
- **Rozanolixizumab** might decrease the concentration of **romiplostim**. Avoid and for 2 weeks after stopping **rozanolixizumab**. Moderate Theoretical
- **Alemtuzumab** is predicted to increase the risk of generalised infection (possibly life-threatening) when given with **siponimod**. Avoid. Severe Theoretical
- **Elranatamab** might affect the exposure to **sirolimus**. Monitor and adjust dose. Moderate Theoretical
- **Sarilumab** potentially affects the exposure to **sirolimus**. Monitor and adjust dose. Moderate Theoretical

Monoclonal antibodies (continued)
- **Sarilumab** is predicted to decrease the exposure to statins (atorvastatin, simvastatin). Moderate Study
- **Tocilizumab** is predicted to decrease the exposure to statins (atorvastatin, simvastatin). Monitor and adjust dose. Moderate Study
- **Sarilumab** potentially affects the exposure to tacrolimus. Monitor and adjust dose. Moderate Theoretical
- **Blinatumomab** is predicted to transiently increase the exposure to theophylline. Monitor and adjust dose. Moderate Theoretical
- **Sarilumab** potentially affects the exposure to theophylline. Monitor and adjust dose. Moderate Theoretical
- **Tocilizumab** is predicted to decrease the exposure to theophylline. Monitor and adjust dose. Moderate Theoretical
- Thrombin inhibitors might increase the risk of gastrointestinal bleeding when given with **ipilimumab**. Severe Theoretical
- Tucatinib is predicted to increase the risk of neutropenia when given with **brentuximab vedotin**. Monitor and adjust dose. Severe Study
- Tucatinib is predicted to increase the exposure to **polatuzumab vedotin**. Moderate Theoretical
- Tucatinib is predicted to increase the exposure to the cytotoxic component of **trastuzumab emtansine**. Avoid or monitor. Severe Theoretical
- Velpatasvir is predicted to increase the risk of neutropenia when given with **brentuximab vedotin**. Monitor and adjust dose. Severe Theoretical
- Vemurafenib increases the risk of neutropenia when given with **brentuximab vedotin**. Monitor and adjust dose. Severe Theoretical
- **Ipilimumab** might increase the risk of hepatotoxicity when given with vemurafenib. Avoid. Severe Study
- Voxilaprevir is predicted to increase the risk of neutropenia when given with **brentuximab vedotin**. Monitor and adjust dose. Severe Theoretical

Montelukast
- Anti-androgens (apalutamide, enzalutamide) are predicted to decrease the exposure to **montelukast**. Mild Study
- Antiepileptics (carbamazepine, fosphenytoin, phenobarbital, phenytoin, primidone) are predicted to decrease the exposure to **montelukast**. Mild Study
- Clopidogrel is predicted to moderately increase the exposure to **montelukast**. Moderate Study
- Encorafenib is predicted to decrease the exposure to **montelukast**. Mild Study
- Fibrates (gemfibrozil) are predicted to moderately increase the exposure to **montelukast**. Moderate Study
- Iron chelators (deferasirox) are predicted to increase the exposure to **montelukast**. Moderate Theoretical
- Ivosidenib is predicted to decrease the exposure to **montelukast**. Mild Study
- Leflunomide is predicted to increase the exposure to **montelukast**. Moderate Theoretical
- Lumacaftor is predicted to decrease the exposure to **montelukast**. Mild Study
- Mifepristone is predicted to increase the exposure to **montelukast**. Moderate Theoretical
- Mitotane is predicted to decrease the exposure to **montelukast**. Mild Study
- Opicapone is predicted to increase the exposure to **montelukast**. Avoid. Moderate Study
- Pirtobrutinib is predicted to increase the exposure to **montelukast**. Moderate Theoretical
- Rifamycins (rifampicin) are predicted to decrease the exposure to **montelukast**. Mild Study
- Selpercatinib is predicted to increase the exposure to **montelukast**. Avoid. Moderate Study
- Teriflunomide is predicted to increase the exposure to **montelukast**. Moderate Theoretical

Morphine → see opioids
Mosunetuzumab → see monoclonal antibodies
Moxifloxacin → see quinolones
Moxonidine → see TABLE 6 p. 1054 (hypotension), TABLE 9 p. 1056 (CNS effects)
- Tricyclic antidepressants are predicted to decrease the effects of **moxonidine**. Avoid. Moderate Theoretical → Also see TABLE 6 p. 1054 → Also see TABLE 9 p. 1056

Mycophenolate
- **Mycophenolate** is predicted to increase the risk of haematological toxicity when given with aciclovir. Moderate Theoretical
- Oral antacids decrease the exposure to oral **mycophenolate**. Moderate Study
- Antifungals, azoles (isavuconazole) increase the exposure to **mycophenolate**. Moderate Study
- **Mycophenolate** is predicted to increase the risk of haematological toxicity when given with ganciclovir. Moderate Theoretical
- Live vaccines are predicted to increase the risk of generalised infection (possibly life-threatening) when given with **mycophenolate**. UKHSA advises avoid (refer to Green Book). Severe Theoretical
- Metronidazole decreases the exposure to **mycophenolate**. Moderate Anecdotal
- Rifamycins (rifampicin) decrease the concentration of **mycophenolate**. Monitor and adjust dose. Severe Study
- **Mycophenolate** is predicted to increase the risk of haematological toxicity when given with valaciclovir. Moderate Theoretical
- **Mycophenolate** is predicted to increase the risk of haematological toxicity when given with valganciclovir. Moderate Theoretical

Nabilone → see TABLE 9 p. 1056 (CNS effects)
- **Nabilone** is predicted to increase the risk of cardiovascular adverse effects when given with amfetamines. Severe Theoretical

Nabumetone → see NSAIDs
Nadolol → see beta blockers, non-selective
Naldemedine
- Anti-androgens (apalutamide, enzalutamide) are predicted to markedly decrease the exposure to **naldemedine**. Avoid. Severe Study
- Antiarrhythmics (amiodarone, dronedarone) are predicted to increase the exposure to **naldemedine**. Moderate Study
- Antiepileptics (carbamazepine, fosphenytoin, phenobarbital, phenytoin, primidone) are predicted to markedly decrease the exposure to **naldemedine**. Avoid. Severe Study
- Antifungals, azoles (fluconazole, isavuconazole) are predicted to increase the exposure to **naldemedine**. Moderate Study
- Antifungals, azoles (itraconazole, ketoconazole, posaconazole, voriconazole) are predicted to increase the exposure to **naldemedine**. Avoid or monitor. Moderate Study
- Berotralstat is predicted to increase the exposure to **naldemedine**. Moderate Study
- Calcium-channel blockers (diltiazem, verapamil) are predicted to increase the exposure to **naldemedine**. Moderate Study
- Ceritinib is predicted to increase the exposure to **naldemedine**. Avoid or monitor. Moderate Study
- Ciclosporin is predicted to increase the exposure to **naldemedine**. Moderate Study
- Cobicistat is predicted to increase the exposure to **naldemedine**. Avoid or monitor. Moderate Study
- Crizotinib is predicted to increase the exposure to **naldemedine**. Moderate Study
- Encorafenib is predicted to markedly decrease the exposure to **naldemedine**. Avoid. Severe Study
- Fedratinib is predicted to increase the exposure to **naldemedine**. Moderate Study
- Grapefruit juice is predicted to increase the exposure to **naldemedine**. Avoid or monitor. Moderate Theoretical
- HIV-protease inhibitors are predicted to increase the exposure to **naldemedine**. Avoid or monitor. Moderate Study
- Idelalisib is predicted to increase the exposure to **naldemedine**. Avoid or monitor. Moderate Study
- Imatinib is predicted to increase the exposure to **naldemedine**. Moderate Study
- Ivosidenib is predicted to markedly decrease the exposure to **naldemedine**. Avoid. Severe Study

- **Letermovir** is predicted to increase the exposure to **naldemedine**. [Moderate] Study
- **Lumacaftor** is predicted to markedly decrease the exposure to **naldemedine**. Avoid. [Severe] Study
- Macrolides **(azithromycin, erythromycin)** are predicted to increase the exposure to **naldemedine**. [Moderate] Study
- Macrolides **(clarithromycin)** are predicted to increase the exposure to **naldemedine**. Avoid or monitor. [Moderate] Study
- **Mitotane** is predicted to markedly decrease the exposure to **naldemedine**. Avoid. [Severe] Study
- Neurokinin-1 receptor antagonists **(aprepitant, netupitant)** are predicted to increase the exposure to **naldemedine**. [Moderate] Study
- **Nilotinib** is predicted to increase the exposure to **naldemedine**. [Moderate] Study
- **Ranolazine** is predicted to increase the exposure to **naldemedine**. [Moderate] Study
- Rifamycins **(rifampicin)** are predicted to markedly decrease the exposure to **naldemedine**. Avoid. [Severe] Study
- **St John's wort** is predicted to decrease the exposure to **naldemedine**. Avoid. [Severe] Study
- **Tucatinib** is predicted to increase the exposure to **naldemedine**. Avoid or monitor. [Moderate] Study
- **Vemurafenib** is predicted to increase the exposure to **naldemedine**. [Moderate] Study

Nalmefene
- **Nalmefene** is predicted to decrease the efficacy of **opioids**. Avoid except in an emergency situation—consult product literature. [Severe] Theoretical

Naloxegol
- Anti-androgens **(apalutamide, enzalutamide)** are predicted to markedly decrease the exposure to **naloxegol**. Avoid. [Moderate] Study
- Antiarrhythmics **(dronedarone)** are predicted to increase the exposure to **naloxegol**. Adjust **naloxegol** dose and monitor adverse effects. [Moderate] Study
- Antiepileptics **(carbamazepine, fosphenytoin, phenobarbital, phenytoin, primidone)** are predicted to markedly decrease the exposure to **naloxegol**. Avoid. [Moderate] Study
- Antifungals, azoles **(fluconazole, isavuconazole)** are predicted to increase the exposure to **naloxegol**. Adjust **naloxegol** dose and monitor adverse effects. [Moderate] Study
- Antifungals, azoles **(itraconazole, ketoconazole, posaconazole, voriconazole)** are predicted to markedly increase the exposure to **naloxegol**. Avoid. [Severe] Study
- **Berotralstat** is predicted to increase the exposure to **naloxegol**. Adjust **naloxegol** dose and monitor adverse effects. [Moderate] Study
- Calcium-channel blockers **(diltiazem, verapamil)** are predicted to increase the exposure to **naloxegol**. Adjust **naloxegol** dose and monitor adverse effects. [Moderate] Study
- **Cenobamate** is predicted to decrease the exposure to **naloxegol**. Adjust dose. [Moderate] Theoretical
- **Ceritinib** is predicted to markedly increase the exposure to **naloxegol**. Avoid. [Severe] Study
- **Cobicistat** is predicted to markedly increase the exposure to **naloxegol**. Avoid. [Severe] Study
- **Crizotinib** is predicted to increase the exposure to **naloxegol**. Adjust **naloxegol** dose and monitor adverse effects. [Moderate] Study
- **Dabrafenib** is predicted to decrease the exposure to **naloxegol**. [Moderate] Theoretical
- **Encorafenib** is predicted to markedly decrease the exposure to **naloxegol**. Avoid. [Moderate] Study
- Endothelin receptor antagonists **(bosentan)** are predicted to decrease the exposure to **naloxegol**. [Moderate] Theoretical
- **Fedratinib** is predicted to increase the exposure to **naloxegol**. Adjust **naloxegol** dose and monitor adverse effects. [Moderate] Study
- **Grapefruit** juice is predicted to increase the exposure to **naloxegol**. Avoid. [Moderate] Theoretical
- **HIV-protease inhibitors** are predicted to markedly increase the exposure to **naloxegol**. Avoid. [Severe] Study
- **Idelalisib** is predicted to markedly increase the exposure to **naloxegol**. Avoid. [Severe] Study
- **Imatinib** is predicted to increase the exposure to **naloxegol**. Adjust **naloxegol** dose and monitor adverse effects. [Moderate] Study
- **Ivosidenib** is predicted to markedly decrease the exposure to **naloxegol**. Avoid. [Moderate] Study
- **Lenacapavir** is predicted to increase the concentration of **naloxegol**. [Moderate] Theoretical
- **Letermovir** is predicted to increase the exposure to **naloxegol**. Adjust **naloxegol** dose and monitor adverse effects. [Moderate] Study
- **Lorlatinib** is predicted to decrease the exposure to **naloxegol**. [Moderate] Theoretical
- **Lumacaftor** is predicted to markedly decrease the exposure to **naloxegol**. Avoid. [Moderate] Study
- Macrolides **(clarithromycin)** are predicted to markedly increase the exposure to **naloxegol**. Avoid. [Severe] Study
- Macrolides **(erythromycin)** are predicted to increase the exposure to **naloxegol**. Adjust **naloxegol** dose and monitor adverse effects. [Moderate] Study
- **Mitotane** is predicted to markedly decrease the exposure to **naloxegol**. Avoid. [Moderate] Study
- Neurokinin-1 receptor antagonists **(aprepitant, netupitant)** are predicted to increase the exposure to **naloxegol**. Adjust **naloxegol** dose and monitor adverse effects. [Moderate] Study
- **Nilotinib** is predicted to increase the exposure to **naloxegol**. Adjust **naloxegol** dose and monitor adverse effects. [Moderate] Study
- **Nirmatrelvir** boosted with ritonavir is predicted to increase the concentration of **naloxegol**. Avoid. [Severe] Theoretical
- NNRTIs **(efavirenz, etravirine, nevirapine)** are predicted to decrease the exposure to **naloxegol**. [Moderate] Theoretical
- Rifamycins **(rifampicin)** are predicted to markedly decrease the exposure to **naloxegol**. Avoid. [Moderate] Study
- **Sotorasib** is predicted to decrease the exposure to **naloxegol**. [Moderate] Theoretical
- **St John's wort** is predicted to decrease the exposure to **naloxegol**. Avoid. [Moderate] Theoretical
- **Tucatinib** is predicted to markedly increase the exposure to **naloxegol**. Avoid. [Severe] Study

Naltrexone
- **Naltrexone** is predicted to decrease the efficacy of **opioids**. Avoid except in an emergency situation—consult product literature. [Severe] Theoretical

Naproxen → see NSAIDs
Naratriptan → see triptans
Natalizumab → see monoclonal antibodies
Nebivolol → see beta blockers, selective

Nefopam
- **Nefopam** is predicted to increase the risk of serious elevations in blood pressure when given with **MAOIs, irreversible**. Avoid. [Severe] Theoretical

Nelarabine → see TABLE 1 p. 1053 (hepatotoxicity), TABLE 12 p. 1057 (myelosuppression)
Nemolizumab → see monoclonal antibodies
Neomycin → see TABLE 2 p. 1053 (nephrotoxicity), TABLE 16 p. 1058 (ototoxicity)

ROUTE-SPECIFIC INFORMATION Since systemic absorption can follow topical application of **neomycin**, the possibility of interactions should be borne in mind.

- **Neomycin** decreases the concentration of **digoxin**. [Moderate] Study
- **Neomycin** might prolong the effects of **neuromuscular blocking drugs, non-depolarising**. [Severe] Theoretical
- **Neomycin** moderately decreases the exposure to **sorafenib**. [Moderate] Study
- **Neomycin** might prolong the effects of **suxamethonium**. [Severe] Theoretical

Neostigmine → see TABLE 4 p. 1054 (bradycardia)
- **Aminoglycosides** are predicted to decrease the effects of **neostigmine**. [Moderate] Theoretical

Nepafenac → see NSAIDs

A1 Interactions | Appendix 1

Neratinib → see TABLE 1 p. 1053 (hepatotoxicity)

FOOD AND LIFESTYLE Avoid pomegranate, and pomegranate juice, as it might increase the concentration of neratinib.

- Oral **antacids** are predicted to decrease the exposure to oral **neratinib**. Separate administration by at least 3 hours. [Mild] Theoretical
- Anti-androgens **(apalutamide, enzalutamide)** are predicted to decrease the exposure to **neratinib**. Avoid. [Severe] Study
- Antiarrhythmics **(amiodarone)** are predicted to increase the exposure to **neratinib**. Avoid or adjust dose and monitor for gastrointestinal adverse effects—consult product literature. [Severe] Study → Also see TABLE 1 p. 1053
- Antiarrhythmics **(dronedarone)** are predicted to increase the exposure to **neratinib**. Avoid moderate CYP3A4 inhibitors or adjust dose and monitor for gastrointestinal adverse effects—consult product literature. [Severe] Study
- Antiepileptics **(carbamazepine, fosphenytoin, phenobarbital, phenytoin, primidone)** are predicted to decrease the exposure to **neratinib**. Avoid. [Severe] Study
- Antifungals, azoles **(fluconazole, isavuconazole)** are predicted to increase the exposure to **neratinib**. Avoid moderate CYP3A4 inhibitors or adjust dose and monitor for gastrointestinal adverse effects—consult product literature. [Severe] Study → Also see TABLE 1 p. 1053
- Antifungals, azoles **(itraconazole, ketoconazole, posaconazole, voriconazole)** are predicted to increase the exposure to **neratinib**. Avoid or adjust dose with potent CYP3A4 inhibitors—consult product literature. [Severe] Study → Also see TABLE 1 p. 1053
- **Berotralstat** is predicted to increase the exposure to **neratinib**. Avoid moderate CYP3A4 inhibitors or adjust dose and monitor for gastrointestinal adverse effects—consult product literature. [Severe] Study
- Oral calcium compounds **(calcium carbonate)** -containing antacids are predicted to decrease the exposure to oral **neratinib**. Separate administration by at least 3 hours. [Mild] Theoretical
- Calcium-channel blockers **(diltiazem, verapamil)** are predicted to increase the exposure to **neratinib**. Avoid moderate CYP3A4 inhibitors or adjust dose and monitor for gastrointestinal adverse effects—consult product literature. [Severe] Study
- **Cenobamate** is predicted to decrease the exposure to **neratinib**. Avoid. [Severe] Theoretical
- **Ceritinib** is predicted to increase the exposure to **neratinib**. Avoid or adjust dose with potent CYP3A4 inhibitors—consult product literature. [Severe] Study
- **Ciclosporin** is predicted to increase the exposure to **neratinib**. Avoid or adjust dose and monitor for gastrointestinal adverse effects—consult product literature. [Severe] Study
- **Cobicistat** is predicted to increase the exposure to **neratinib**. Avoid or adjust dose with potent CYP3A4 inhibitors—consult product literature. [Severe] Study
- **Neratinib** might affect the efficacy of **combined hormonal contraceptives**. Use additional contraceptive precautions. [Severe] Theoretical
- **Crizotinib** is predicted to increase the exposure to **neratinib**. Avoid moderate CYP3A4 inhibitors or adjust dose and monitor for gastrointestinal adverse effects—consult product literature. [Severe] Study
- **Dabrafenib** is predicted to decrease the exposure to **neratinib**. Avoid. [Severe] Theoretical
- **Neratinib** slightly increases the exposure to **digoxin**. [Moderate] Study
- **Encorafenib** is predicted to decrease the exposure to **neratinib**. Avoid. [Severe] Study
- Endothelin receptor antagonists **(bosentan)** are predicted to decrease the exposure to **neratinib**. Avoid. [Severe] Theoretical
- **Neratinib** is predicted to increase the exposure to **everolimus**. [Moderate] Study
- **Neratinib** is predicted to increase the exposure to factor XA inhibitors **(apixaban)**. [Moderate] Theoretical
- **Fedratinib** is predicted to increase the exposure to **neratinib**. Avoid moderate CYP3A4 inhibitors or adjust dose and monitor for gastrointestinal adverse effects—consult product literature. [Severe] Study
- **Neratinib** is predicted to increase the exposure to **gilteritinib**. [Moderate] Theoretical
- **Glecaprevir** is predicted to increase the exposure to **neratinib**. Avoid or adjust dose and monitor for gastrointestinal adverse effects—consult product literature. [Severe] Study
- **Grapefruit** juice is predicted to increase the exposure to **neratinib**. Avoid. [Severe] Theoretical
- **H_2 receptor antagonists** are predicted to decrease the exposure to **neratinib**. Manufacturer advises take 2 hours before or 10 hours after **H_2 receptor antagonists**. [Severe] Study
- **HIV-protease inhibitors** are predicted to increase the exposure to **neratinib**. Avoid or adjust dose with potent CYP3A4 inhibitors—consult product literature. [Severe] Study → Also see TABLE 1 p. 1053
- **Idelalisib** is predicted to increase the exposure to **neratinib**. Avoid or adjust dose with potent CYP3A4 inhibitors—consult product literature. [Severe] Study
- **Imatinib** is predicted to increase the exposure to **neratinib**. Avoid moderate CYP3A4 inhibitors or adjust dose and monitor for gastrointestinal adverse effects—consult product literature. [Severe] Study
- **Ivosidenib** is predicted to decrease the exposure to **neratinib**. Avoid. [Severe] Study
- **Letermovir** is predicted to increase the exposure to **neratinib**. Avoid moderate CYP3A4 inhibitors or adjust dose and monitor for gastrointestinal adverse effects—consult product literature. [Severe] Study
- **Lorlatinib** is predicted to decrease the exposure to **neratinib**. Avoid. [Severe] Theoretical
- **Lumacaftor** is predicted to decrease the exposure to **neratinib**. Avoid. [Severe] Study
- Macrolides **(azithromycin)** are predicted to increase the exposure to **neratinib**. Avoid or adjust dose and monitor for gastrointestinal adverse effects—consult product literature. [Severe] Study
- Macrolides **(clarithromycin)** are predicted to increase the exposure to **neratinib**. Avoid or adjust dose with potent CYP3A4 inhibitors—consult product literature. [Severe] Study
- Macrolides **(erythromycin)** are predicted to increase the exposure to **neratinib**. Avoid moderate CYP3A4 inhibitors or adjust dose and monitor for gastrointestinal adverse effects—consult product literature. [Severe] Study
- **Mitotane** is predicted to decrease the exposure to **neratinib**. Avoid. [Severe] Study
- Neurokinin-1 receptor antagonists **(aprepitant, netupitant)** are predicted to increase the exposure to **neratinib**. Avoid moderate CYP3A4 inhibitors or adjust dose and monitor for gastrointestinal adverse effects—consult product literature. [Severe] Study
- **Nilotinib** is predicted to increase the exposure to **neratinib**. Avoid moderate CYP3A4 inhibitors or adjust dose and monitor for gastrointestinal adverse effects—consult product literature. [Severe] Study
- **Nirmatrelvir** boosted with ritonavir is predicted to increase the concentration of **neratinib**. Avoid. [Severe] Theoretical
- NNRTIs **(efavirenz, etravirine, nevirapine)** are predicted to decrease the exposure to **neratinib**. Avoid. [Severe] Theoretical → Also see TABLE 1 p. 1053
- **Pibrentasvir** is predicted to increase the exposure to **neratinib**. Avoid or adjust dose and monitor for gastrointestinal adverse effects—consult product literature. [Severe] Study
- **Proton pump inhibitors** are predicted to decrease the exposure to **neratinib**. Avoid. [Severe] Study
- **Ranolazine** is predicted to increase the exposure to **neratinib**. Avoid or adjust dose and monitor for gastrointestinal adverse effects—consult product literature. [Severe] Study
- Rifamycins **(rifampicin)** are predicted to decrease the exposure to **neratinib**. Avoid. [Severe] Study
- **Neratinib** is predicted to increase the exposure to the active component of **sacituzumab govitecan**. [Severe] Theoretical
- **Neratinib** is predicted to increase the exposure to **sirolimus**. [Moderate] Study

- Oral sodium bicarbonate -containing antacids are predicted to decrease the exposure to oral **neratinib**. Separate administration by at least 3 hours. Mild Theoretical
- **Sotorasib** is predicted to decrease the exposure to **neratinib**. Avoid. Severe Theoretical → Also see TABLE 1 p. 1053
- **St John's wort** is predicted to decrease the exposure to **neratinib**. Avoid. Severe Theoretical
- **Neratinib** is predicted to increase the exposure to **talazoparib**. Moderate Study
- **Neratinib** is predicted to increase the exposure to taxanes **(paclitaxel)**. Moderate Study
- **Neratinib** might increase the exposure to **tigecycline**. Mild Anecdotal → Also see TABLE 1 p. 1053
- **Tucatinib** is predicted to increase the exposure to **neratinib**. Avoid or adjust dose with potent CYP3A4 inhibitors—consult product literature. Severe Study
- **Velpatasvir** is predicted to increase the exposure to **neratinib**. Avoid or adjust dose and monitor for gastrointestinal adverse effects—consult product literature. Severe Study
- **Vemurafenib** is predicted to increase the exposure to **neratinib**. Avoid or adjust dose and monitor for gastrointestinal adverse effects—consult product literature. Severe Study
- **Neratinib** is predicted to increase the exposure to **venetoclax**. Avoid or monitor for toxicity. Severe Theoretical
- **Neratinib** might increase the exposure to **vinca alkaloids**. Severe Theoretical
- **Voxilaprevir** is predicted to increase the exposure to **neratinib**. Avoid or adjust dose and monitor for gastrointestinal adverse effects—consult product literature. Severe Study

Netilmicin → see aminoglycosides

Netupitant → see neurokinin-1 receptor antagonists

Neurokinin-1 receptor antagonists

aprepitant · fosaprepitant · netupitant

- Neurokinin-1 receptor antagonists **(aprepitant, netupitant)** are predicted to increase the exposure to **abemaciclib**. Moderate Study
- Neurokinin-1 receptor antagonists **(aprepitant, netupitant)** are predicted to increase the exposure to **acalabrutinib**. Avoid or monitor. Severe Study
- **Netupitant** very slightly increases the exposure to alkylating agents **(cyclophosphamide)**. Moderate Study
- **Netupitant** is predicted to increase the exposure to alkylating agents **(ifosfamide)**. Moderate Study
- Neurokinin-1 receptor antagonists **(aprepitant, fosaprepitant)** are predicted to increase the exposure to alkylating agents **(ifosfamide)**. Severe Theoretical
- Neurokinin-1 receptor antagonists **(aprepitant, netupitant)** are predicted to increase the exposure to alpha blockers **(tamsulosin)**. Moderate Theoretical
- Anti-androgens **(apalutamide, enzalutamide)** are predicted to markedly decrease the exposure to **aprepitant**. Avoid. Moderate Study
- Anti-androgens **(apalutamide, enzalutamide)** are predicted to decrease the exposure to **fosaprepitant**. Avoid. Moderate Theoretical
- Anti-androgens **(apalutamide, enzalutamide)** are predicted to decrease the exposure to **netupitant**. Avoid. Severe Study
- Neurokinin-1 receptor antagonists **(aprepitant, fosaprepitant)** are predicted to decrease the efficacy of anti-androgens **(cyproterone)** with ethinylestradiol (co-cyprindiol). Use alternative methods during treatment with, and for 28 days after, the enzyme inducing drug is stopped. Severe Study
- **Aprepitant** increases the exposure to antiarrhythmics **(dronedarone)**. Severe Theoretical
- Neurokinin-1 receptor antagonists **(aprepitant, netupitant)** are predicted to increase the exposure to antiarrhythmics **(propafenone)**. Monitor and adjust dose. Moderate Study
- Antiepileptics **(carbamazepine, fosphenytoin, phenobarbital, phenytoin, primidone)** are predicted to markedly decrease the exposure to **aprepitant**. Avoid. Moderate Study
- Antiepileptics **(carbamazepine, fosphenytoin, phenobarbital, phenytoin, primidone)** are predicted to decrease the exposure to **fosaprepitant**. Avoid. Moderate Theoretical
- Antiepileptics **(carbamazepine, fosphenytoin, phenobarbital, phenytoin, primidone)** are predicted to decrease the exposure to **netupitant**. Avoid. Severe Study
- Antifungals, azoles **(fluconazole)** are predicted to increase the exposure to **aprepitant**. Moderate Theoretical
- Antifungals, azoles **(itraconazole, ketoconazole, posaconazole, voriconazole)** are predicted to markedly increase the exposure to **aprepitant**. Moderate Study
- Antifungals, azoles **(itraconazole, ketoconazole, posaconazole, voriconazole)** are predicted to increase the exposure to **fosaprepitant**. Moderate Theoretical
- Antifungals, azoles **(itraconazole, ketoconazole, posaconazole, voriconazole)** are predicted to increase the exposure to **netupitant**. Moderate Study
- **Aprepitant** is predicted to increase the exposure to antifungals, azoles **(isavuconazole)**. Moderate Theoretical
- **Netupitant** is predicted to decrease the exposure to antifungals, azoles **(isavuconazole)**. Moderate Theoretical
- Neurokinin-1 receptor antagonists **(aprepitant, netupitant)** are predicted to increase the exposure to antihistamines, non-sedating **(mizolastine)**. Severe Theoretical
- Neurokinin-1 receptor antagonists **(aprepitant, netupitant)** are predicted to increase the exposure to antihistamines, non-sedating **(rupatadine)**. Avoid. Moderate Study
- Neurokinin-1 receptor antagonists **(aprepitant, netupitant)** are predicted to increase the concentration of antimalarials **(piperaquine)**. Severe Study
- Neurokinin-1 receptor antagonists **(aprepitant, netupitant)** are predicted to increase the exposure to atypical antipsychotics **(cariprazine)**. Monitor and adjust dose. Severe Study
- Neurokinin-1 receptor antagonists **(aprepitant, netupitant)** are predicted to increase the exposure to atypical antipsychotics **(lurasidone)**. Adjust **lurasidone** dose. Moderate Study
- Neurokinin-1 receptor antagonists **(aprepitant, netupitant)** are predicted to increase the exposure to atypical antipsychotics **(quetiapine)**. Avoid. Moderate Study
- Neurokinin-1 receptor antagonists **(aprepitant, netupitant)** are predicted to increase the exposure to **avapritinib**. Avoid or adjust dose—consult product literature. Moderate Study
- Neurokinin-1 receptor antagonists **(aprepitant, netupitant)** are predicted to increase the exposure to **axitinib**. Moderate Study
- Neurokinin-1 receptor antagonists **(aprepitant, netupitant)** might increase the exposure to **bedaquiline**. Mild Theoretical
- **Fosaprepitant** is predicted to increase the exposure to benzodiazepines **(alprazolam)**. Moderate Study
- Neurokinin-1 receptor antagonists **(aprepitant, netupitant)** are predicted to increase the exposure to benzodiazepines **(alprazolam)**. Severe Study
- **Fosaprepitant** slightly increases the exposure to benzodiazepines **(midazolam)**. Moderate Study
- Neurokinin-1 receptor antagonists **(aprepitant, netupitant)** are predicted to increase the exposure to benzodiazepines **(midazolam)**. Monitor adverse effects and adjust dose. Severe Study
- Neurokinin-1 receptor antagonists **(aprepitant, netupitant)** are predicted to increase the exposure to beta$_2$ agonists **(salmeterol)**. Moderate Study
- **Fosaprepitant** is predicted to increase the exposure to **bosutinib**. Severe Theoretical
- Neurokinin-1 receptor antagonists **(aprepitant, netupitant)** are predicted to increase the exposure to **bosutinib**. Avoid or adjust dose. Severe Study
- Neurokinin-1 receptor antagonists **(aprepitant, netupitant)** are predicted to increase the exposure to **brigatinib**. Moderate Study
- Neurokinin-1 receptor antagonists **(aprepitant, netupitant)** are predicted to increase the exposure to **buspirone**. Use with caution and adjust dose. Moderate Study
- Neurokinin-1 receptor antagonists **(aprepitant, netupitant)** are predicted to increase the exposure to **cabozantinib**. Moderate Study
- Calcium-channel blockers **(diltiazem, verapamil)** are predicted to increase the exposure to **aprepitant** and **aprepitant** is predicted to increase the exposure to calcium-channel blockers **(diltiazem, verapamil)**. Moderate Study

Neurokinin-1 receptor antagonists (continued)
- ▶ Neurokinin-1 receptor antagonists **(aprepitant, netupitant)** are predicted to increase the exposure to calcium-channel blockers **(amlodipine, felodipine, lacidipine, lercanidipine, nicardipine, nifedipine, nimodipine)**. Monitor and adjust dose. Moderate Study
- ▶ Neurokinin-1 receptor antagonists **(aprepitant, netupitant)** are predicted to increase the exposure to **capivasertib**. Adjust dose. Moderate Study
- ▶ **Cenobamate** is predicted to decrease the exposure to **netupitant**. Moderate Theoretical
- ▶ **Ceritinib** is predicted to markedly increase the exposure to **aprepitant**. Moderate Study
- ▶ **Fosaprepitant** is predicted to increase the exposure to **ceritinib**. Severe Theoretical
- ▶ **Ceritinib** is predicted to increase the exposure to **fosaprepitant**. Moderate Theoretical
- ▶ **Ceritinib** is predicted to increase the exposure to **netupitant**. Moderate Study
- ▶ Neurokinin-1 receptor antagonists **(aprepitant, netupitant)** are predicted to increase the exposure to **ceritinib**. Moderate Study
- ▶ Neurokinin-1 receptor antagonists **(aprepitant, netupitant)** are predicted to increase the concentration of **ciclosporin**. Severe Study
- ▶ **Cobicistat** is predicted to markedly increase the exposure to **aprepitant**. Moderate Study
- ▶ **Cobicistat** is predicted to increase the exposure to **fosaprepitant**. Moderate Theoretical
- ▶ **Cobicistat** is predicted to increase the exposure to **netupitant**. Moderate Study
- ▶ Neurokinin-1 receptor antagonists **(aprepitant, netupitant)** are predicted to increase the exposure to **cobimetinib**. Severe Study
- ▶ Neurokinin-1 receptor antagonists **(aprepitant, netupitant)** are predicted to increase the exposure to **colchicine**. Adjust **colchicine** dose with moderate CYP3A4 inhibitors, p. 637. Severe Study
- ▶ Neurokinin-1 receptor antagonists **(aprepitant, fosaprepitant)** are predicted to decrease the efficacy of **combined hormonal contraceptives**. For CoSRH guidance, see Contraceptives, interactions p. 614. Severe Study
- ▶ Neurokinin-1 receptor antagonists **(aprepitant, netupitant)** are predicted to increase the exposure to oral corticosteroids **(budesonide)**. Moderate Study
- ▶ **Aprepitant** moderately increases the exposure to corticosteroids **(dexamethasone)**. Monitor and adjust dose. Moderate Study
- ▶ **Netupitant** moderately increases the exposure to corticosteroids **(dexamethasone)**. Adjust dose. Moderate Study
- ▶ Neurokinin-1 receptor antagonists **(aprepitant, netupitant)** are predicted to increase the exposure to corticosteroids **(fluticasone)**. Moderate Study
- ▶ Neurokinin-1 receptor antagonists **(aprepitant, netupitant)** are predicted to increase the exposure to corticosteroids **(methylprednisolone)**. Monitor and adjust dose. Moderate Study
- ▶ **Aprepitant** decreases the anticoagulant effect of **coumarins**. Moderate Study
- ▶ **Fosaprepitant** is predicted to decrease the anticoagulant effect of **coumarins**. Moderate Theoretical
- ▶ **Netupitant** is predicted to increase the exposure to **crizotinib**. Moderate Study
- ▶ **Dabrafenib** is predicted to decrease the exposure to **netupitant**. Moderate Theoretical
- ▶ Neurokinin-1 receptor antagonists **(aprepitant, netupitant)** are predicted to increase the exposure to **dabrafenib**. Moderate Study
- ▶ Neurokinin-1 receptor antagonists **(aprepitant, netupitant)** are predicted to increase the exposure to **daridorexant**. Adjust **daridorexant** dose. Severe Study
- ▶ Neurokinin-1 receptor antagonists **(aprepitant, netupitant)** are predicted to increase the exposure to **darifenacin**. Moderate Study
- ▶ Neurokinin-1 receptor antagonists **(aprepitant, netupitant)** are predicted to increase the exposure to **dasatinib**. Severe Study
- ▶ Neurokinin-1 receptor antagonists **(aprepitant, fosaprepitant)** are predicted to decrease the efficacy of **desogestrel**. For CoSRH guidance, see Contraceptives, interactions p. 614. Severe Theoretical
- ▶ Neurokinin-1 receptor antagonists **(aprepitant, netupitant)** are predicted to increase the exposure to **deutivacaftor**. Adjust dose, see deutivacaftor with tezacaftor and vanzacaftor p. 218. Severe Study
- ▶ Neurokinin-1 receptor antagonists **(aprepitant, netupitant)** are predicted to slightly increase the exposure to **dienogest**. Moderate Study
- ▶ Neurokinin-1 receptor antagonists **(aprepitant, netupitant)** are predicted to increase the exposure to dipeptidylpeptidase-4 inhibitors **(saxagliptin)**. Mild Study
- ▶ Neurokinin-1 receptor antagonists **(aprepitant, netupitant)** are predicted to increase the exposure to **domperidone**. Avoid. Severe Study
- ▶ Neurokinin-1 receptor antagonists **(aprepitant, netupitant)** are predicted to increase the exposure to dopamine receptor agonists **(bromocriptine)**. Severe Theoretical
- ▶ Neurokinin-1 receptor antagonists **(aprepitant, netupitant)** are predicted to increase the concentration of dopamine receptor agonists **(cabergoline)**. Moderate Anecdotal
- ▶ **Netupitant** is predicted to increase the exposure to **drospirenone**. Severe Study
- ▶ Neurokinin-1 receptor antagonists **(aprepitant, fosaprepitant)** are predicted to decrease the efficacy of **drospirenone**. For CoSRH guidance, see Contraceptives, interactions p. 614. Severe Theoretical
- ▶ Neurokinin-1 receptor antagonists **(aprepitant, netupitant)** are predicted to moderately increase the exposure to **dutasteride**. Mild Study
- ▶ Neurokinin-1 receptor antagonists **(aprepitant, netupitant)** are predicted to increase the exposure to **elacestrant**. Avoid moderate CYP3A4 inhibitors or adjust **elacestrant** dose. Severe Theoretical
- ▶ Neurokinin-1 receptor antagonists **(aprepitant, netupitant)** are predicted to increase the exposure to **elexacaftor**. Adjust ivacaftor with tezacaftor and elexacaftor p. 220 dose with moderate CYP3A4 inhibitors. Severe Theoretical
- ▶ Neurokinin-1 receptor antagonists **(aprepitant, netupitant)** are predicted to increase the exposure to **eliglustat**. Avoid or adjust dose—consult product literature. Severe Study
- ▶ **Encorafenib** is predicted to markedly decrease the exposure to **aprepitant**. Avoid. Moderate Study
- ▶ **Encorafenib** is predicted to decrease the exposure to **fosaprepitant**. Avoid. Moderate Theoretical
- ▶ **Encorafenib** is predicted to decrease the exposure to **netupitant**. Avoid. Severe Study
- ▶ Neurokinin-1 receptor antagonists **(aprepitant, netupitant)** are predicted to moderately increase the exposure to **encorafenib**. Moderate Study
- ▶ Endothelin receptor antagonists **(bosentan)** are predicted to decrease the exposure to **aprepitant**. Moderate Study
- ▶ Endothelin receptor antagonists **(bosentan)** are predicted to decrease the exposure to neurokinin-1 receptor antagonists **(fosaprepitant, netupitant)**. Moderate Theoretical
- ▶ Neurokinin-1 receptor antagonists **(aprepitant, netupitant)** are predicted to increase the exposure to endothelin receptor antagonists **(macitentan)**. Manufacturer advises caution depending on other drugs taken—consult product literature. Moderate Theoretical
- ▶ Neurokinin-1 receptor antagonists **(aprepitant, netupitant)** are predicted to increase the exposure to **entrectinib**. Avoid or adjust dose with moderate CYP3A4 inhibitors—consult product literature. Severe Theoretical
- ▶ Neurokinin-1 receptor antagonists **(aprepitant, netupitant)** are predicted to increase the risk of ergotism when given with **ergometrine**. Severe Theoretical
- ▶ Neurokinin-1 receptor antagonists **(aprepitant, netupitant)** are predicted to increase the exposure to **erlotinib**. Moderate Study
- ▶ Neurokinin-1 receptor antagonists **(aprepitant, fosaprepitant)** are predicted to decrease the efficacy of **estradiol**. Moderate Theoretical
- ▶ Neurokinin-1 receptor antagonists **(aprepitant, fosaprepitant)** are predicted to decrease the efficacy of **etonogestrel**. For CoSRH

guidance, see Contraceptives, interactions p. 614. Severe Theoretical

- **Netupitant** slightly increases the exposure to **etoposide**. Moderate Study
- Neurokinin-1 receptor antagonists **(aprepitant, netupitant)** are predicted to increase the exposure to **etrasimod**. Avoid in poor CYP2C9 metabolisers. Severe Theoretical
- Neurokinin-1 receptor antagonists **(aprepitant, netupitant)** are predicted to increase the concentration of **everolimus**. Avoid or adjust dose. Moderate Study
- Neurokinin-1 receptor antagonists **(aprepitant, netupitant)** are predicted to increase the exposure to **fedratinib**. Monitor and adjust dose. Moderate Study
- Neurokinin-1 receptor antagonists **(aprepitant, netupitant)** are predicted to increase the exposure to **fesoterodine**. Adjust **fesoterodine** dose with moderate CYP3A4 inhibitors in hepatic and renal impairment. Mild Study
- Neurokinin-1 receptor antagonists **(aprepitant, netupitant)** are predicted to increase the exposure to **gefitinib**. Moderate Study
- **Fosaprepitant** is predicted to increase the concentration of **guanfacine**. Moderate Theoretical
- Neurokinin-1 receptor antagonists **(aprepitant, netupitant)** are predicted to increase the concentration of **guanfacine**. Adjust **guanfacine** dose, p. 281. Moderate Theoretical
- **HIV-protease inhibitors** are predicted to markedly increase the exposure to **aprepitant**. Moderate Study
- **HIV-protease inhibitors** are predicted to increase the exposure to **fosaprepitant**. Moderate Theoretical
- **HIV-protease inhibitors** are predicted to increase the exposure to **netupitant**. Moderate Study
- Neurokinin-1 receptor antagonists **(aprepitant, fosaprepitant)** are predicted to decrease the effects of **hormone replacement therapy**. Moderate Anecdotal
- **Fosaprepitant** is predicted to slightly increase the exposure to **ibrutinib**. Moderate Theoretical
- Neurokinin-1 receptor antagonists **(aprepitant, netupitant)** are predicted to increase the exposure to **ibrutinib**. Adjust dose with moderate CYP3A4 inhibitors—consult product literature. Severe Study
- **Idelalisib** is predicted to markedly increase the exposure to **aprepitant**. Moderate Study
- **Idelalisib** is predicted to increase the exposure to **fosaprepitant**. Moderate Theoretical
- **Idelalisib** is predicted to increase the exposure to **netupitant**. Moderate Study
- Neurokinin-1 receptor antagonists **(aprepitant, netupitant)** are predicted to increase the exposure to **imatinib**. Moderate Theoretical
- **Netupitant** is predicted to increase the exposure to **irinotecan**. Moderate Study
- Neurokinin-1 receptor antagonists **(aprepitant, fosaprepitant)** are predicted to increase the exposure to intravenous **irinotecan**. Severe Theoretical
- Neurokinin-1 receptor antagonists **(aprepitant, netupitant)** are predicted to increase the exposure to **ivabradine**. Adjust **ivabradine** dose. Severe Theoretical
- Neurokinin-1 receptor antagonists **(aprepitant, netupitant)** are predicted to increase the exposure to **ivacaftor**. Adjust dose with moderate CYP3A4 inhibitors, see ivacaftor p. 219, tezacaftor with ivacaftor p. 223, and ivacaftor with tezacaftor and elexacaftor p. 220. Moderate Study
- **Ivosidenib** is predicted to markedly decrease the exposure to **aprepitant**. Avoid. Moderate Study
- **Ivosidenib** is predicted to decrease the exposure to **fosaprepitant**. Avoid. Moderate Theoretical
- **Ivosidenib** is predicted to decrease the exposure to **netupitant**. Avoid. Severe Study
- Neurokinin-1 receptor antagonists **(aprepitant, netupitant)** are predicted to increase the exposure to **ivosidenib**. Monitor and adjust dose—consult product literature. Severe Study
- Neurokinin-1 receptor antagonists **(aprepitant, netupitant)** are predicted to increase the exposure to **lapatinib**. Moderate Study
- Neurokinin-1 receptor antagonists **(aprepitant, netupitant)** are predicted to increase the exposure to **larotrectinib**. Monitor and adjust dose. Moderate Theoretical
- Neurokinin-1 receptor antagonists **(aprepitant, netupitant)** are predicted to increase the exposure to **leniolisib**. Avoid. Moderate Study
- Neurokinin-1 receptor antagonists **(aprepitant, fosaprepitant)** are predicted to decrease the efficacy of some contraceptive methods containing **levonorgestrel**. For CoSRH guidance, see Contraceptives, interactions p. 614. Severe Theoretical
- **Fosaprepitant** is predicted to increase the exposure to **lomitapide**. Separate administration by 12 hours. Mild Theoretical
- Neurokinin-1 receptor antagonists **(aprepitant, netupitant)** are predicted to increase the exposure to **lomitapide**. Avoid. Moderate Theoretical
- **Lorlatinib** is predicted to decrease the exposure to **netupitant**. Moderate Theoretical
- **Lumacaftor** is predicted to markedly decrease the exposure to **aprepitant**. Avoid. Moderate Study
- **Lumacaftor** is predicted to decrease the exposure to **fosaprepitant**. Avoid. Moderate Theoretical
- **Lumacaftor** is predicted to decrease the exposure to **netupitant**. Avoid. Severe Study
- **Macrolides (clarithromycin)** are predicted to markedly increase the exposure to **aprepitant**. Moderate Study
- **Macrolides (clarithromycin)** are predicted to increase the exposure to **fosaprepitant**. Moderate Theoretical
- **Macrolides (clarithromycin)** are predicted to increase the exposure to **netupitant**. Moderate Study
- **Macrolides (erythromycin)** are predicted to increase the exposure to **aprepitant**. Moderate Study
- Neurokinin-1 receptor antagonists **(aprepitant, netupitant)** are predicted to increase the exposure to **maraviroc**. Moderate Study
- **Fosaprepitant** is predicted to increase the exposure to **mavacamten**. Monitor and adjust dose—consult product literature. Moderate Theoretical
- Neurokinin-1 receptor antagonists **(aprepitant, netupitant)** are predicted to increase the exposure to **mavacamten**. Adjust dose—consult product literature. Moderate Study
- Neurokinin-1 receptor antagonists **(aprepitant, netupitant)** are predicted to increase the exposure to **midostaurin**. Moderate Theoretical
- Neurokinin-1 receptor antagonists **(aprepitant, netupitant)** are predicted to increase the exposure to **mineralocorticoid receptor antagonists (eplerenone)**. Adjust **eplerenone** dose. Severe Study
- Neurokinin-1 receptor antagonists **(aprepitant, netupitant)** are predicted to increase the exposure to **mineralocorticoid receptor antagonists (finerenone)**. Severe Study
- **Mitotane** is predicted to markedly decrease the exposure to **aprepitant**. Avoid. Moderate Study
- **Mitotane** is predicted to decrease the exposure to **fosaprepitant**. Avoid. Moderate Theoretical
- **Mitotane** is predicted to decrease the exposure to **netupitant**. Avoid. Severe Study
- Neurokinin-1 receptor antagonists **(aprepitant, netupitant)** are predicted to increase the exposure to **naldemedine**. Moderate Study
- Neurokinin-1 receptor antagonists **(aprepitant, netupitant)** are predicted to increase the exposure to **naloxegol**. Adjust **naloxegol** dose and monitor adverse effects. Moderate Study
- Neurokinin-1 receptor antagonists **(aprepitant, netupitant)** are predicted to increase the exposure to **neratinib**. Avoid moderate CYP3A4 inhibitors or adjust dose and monitor for gastrointestinal adverse effects—consult product literature. Severe Study
- Neurokinin-1 receptor antagonists **(aprepitant, netupitant)** are predicted to increase the exposure to **nilotinib**. Moderate Study
- **NNRTIs (efavirenz, etravirine, nevirapine)** are predicted to decrease the exposure to **aprepitant**. Moderate Study
- **NNRTIs (etravirine)** are predicted to decrease the exposure to **netupitant**. Moderate Theoretical
- **NNRTIs (efavirenz, nevirapine)** are predicted to decrease the exposure to neurokinin-1 receptor antagonists **(fosaprepitant, netupitant)**. Moderate Theoretical
- Neurokinin-1 receptor antagonists **(aprepitant, fosaprepitant)** are predicted to decrease the efficacy of some contraceptive

Neurokinin-1 receptor antagonists (continued)
methods containing **norethisterone**. For CoSRH guidance, see Contraceptives, interactions p. 614. Severe Anecdotal
- Neurokinin-1 receptor antagonists **(aprepitant, netupitant)** are predicted to increase the exposure to **olaparib**. Avoid or adjust dose with moderate CYP3A4 inhibitors—consult product literature. Moderate Theoretical
- Neurokinin-1 receptor antagonists **(aprepitant, netupitant)** are predicted to increase the exposure to **omaveloxolone**. Avoid or adjust **omaveloxolone** dose, p. 755. Moderate Study
- Neurokinin-1 receptor antagonists **(aprepitant, netupitant)** are predicted to increase the exposure to opioids **(alfentanil, buprenorphine, fentanyl, oxycodone)**. Monitor and adjust dose. Moderate Study
- Neurokinin-1 receptor antagonists **(aprepitant, netupitant)** are predicted to increase the exposure to opioids **(methadone, sufentanil)**. Moderate Theoretical
- Neurokinin-1 receptor antagonists **(aprepitant, netupitant)** are predicted to increase the exposure to **pazopanib**. Moderate Study
- Neurokinin-1 receptor antagonists **(aprepitant, netupitant)** are predicted to increase the exposure to **pemigatinib**. Severe Study
- Neurokinin-1 receptor antagonists **(aprepitant, netupitant)** are predicted to increase the exposure to phosphodiesterase type-5 inhibitors **(avanafil)**. Adjust **avanafil** dose. Moderate Theoretical
- Neurokinin-1 receptor antagonists **(aprepitant, netupitant)** are predicted to increase the exposure to phosphodiesterase type-5 inhibitors **(sildenafil)**. Monitor or adjust **sildenafil** dose with moderate CYP3A4 inhibitors, p. 139. Moderate Study
- Neurokinin-1 receptor antagonists **(aprepitant, netupitant)** are predicted to increase the exposure to phosphodiesterase type-5 inhibitors **(tadalafil)**. Severe Theoretical
- Neurokinin-1 receptor antagonists **(aprepitant, netupitant)** are predicted to increase the exposure to phosphodiesterase type-5 inhibitors **(vardenafil)**. Adjust dose. Severe Theoretical
- **Neurokinin-1 receptor antagonists** are predicted to increase the exposure to **pimozide**. Avoid. Severe Theoretical
- Neurokinin-1 receptor antagonists **(aprepitant, netupitant)** are predicted to increase the exposure to **ponatinib**. Moderate Study
- Neurokinin-1 receptor antagonists **(aprepitant, netupitant)** are predicted to increase the exposure to **pralsetinib**. Moderate Theoretical
- Neurokinin-1 receptor antagonists **(aprepitant, netupitant)** are predicted to increase the exposure to **ranolazine**. Severe Study
- Neurokinin-1 receptor antagonists **(aprepitant, netupitant)** are predicted to increase the exposure to **regorafenib**. Moderate Study
- Neurokinin-1 receptor antagonists **(aprepitant, netupitant)** are predicted to increase the exposure to **ribociclib**. Moderate Study
- Rifamycins **(rifampicin)** are predicted to markedly decrease the exposure to **aprepitant**. Avoid. Moderate Study
- Rifamycins **(rifampicin)** are predicted to decrease the exposure to **fosaprepitant**. Avoid. Moderate Theoretical
- Rifamycins **(rifampicin)** are predicted to decrease the exposure to **netupitant**. Avoid. Severe Study
- Neurokinin-1 receptor antagonists **(aprepitant, netupitant)** are predicted to increase the exposure to **rimegepant**. Avoid another dose of rimegepant within 48 hours of concurrent use. Moderate Study
- Neurokinin-1 receptor antagonists **(aprepitant, netupitant)** are predicted to increase the exposure to **ruxolitinib**. Moderate Study
- Neurokinin-1 receptor antagonists **(aprepitant, netupitant)** are predicted to increase the exposure to **selpercatinib**. Moderate Study
- Neurokinin-1 receptor antagonists **(aprepitant, netupitant)** are predicted to increase the exposure to **selumetinib**. Avoid or adjust dose—consult product literature. Severe Study
- Neurokinin-1 receptor antagonists **(aprepitant, netupitant)** are predicted to increase the exposure to **siponimod**. Avoid depending on other drugs taken—consult product literature. Severe Study
- Neurokinin-1 receptor antagonists **(aprepitant, netupitant)** increase the concentration of **sirolimus**. Monitor and adjust dose. Moderate Study
- **Sotorasib** is predicted to decrease the exposure to **netupitant**. Moderate Theoretical
- Neurokinin-1 receptor antagonists **(aprepitant, netupitant)** are predicted to increase the exposure to **sparsentan**. Moderate Study
- Neurokinin-1 receptor antagonists **(aprepitant, netupitant)** are predicted to increase the exposure to SSRIs **(dapoxetine)**. Adjust **dapoxetine** dose with moderate CYP3A4 inhibitors. Moderate Theoretical
- Neurokinin-1 receptor antagonists **(aprepitant, netupitant)** are predicted to increase the exposure to SSRIs **(sertraline)**. Moderate Theoretical
- **St John's wort** is predicted to decrease the exposure to **netupitant**. Moderate Theoretical
- **St John's wort** is predicted to decrease the exposure to neurokinin-1 receptor antagonists **(aprepitant, fosaprepitant)**. Avoid. Moderate Theoretical
- Neurokinin-1 receptor antagonists **(aprepitant, netupitant)** are predicted to increase the exposure to statins **(atorvastatin, simvastatin)**. Monitor and adjust dose. Severe Theoretical
- Neurokinin-1 receptor antagonists **(aprepitant, netupitant)** are predicted to increase the exposure to **sunitinib**. Moderate Study
- **Aprepitant** increases the concentration of **tacrolimus**. Monitor and adjust dose. Severe Study
- **Netupitant** is predicted to increase the concentration of **tacrolimus**. Monitor and adjust dose. Severe Theoretical
- Neurokinin-1 receptor antagonists **(aprepitant, netupitant)** are predicted to increase the exposure to taxanes **(cabazitaxel)**. Moderate Theoretical
- Neurokinin-1 receptor antagonists **(aprepitant, netupitant)** are predicted to increase the exposure to taxanes **(docetaxel)**. Severe Study
- Neurokinin-1 receptor antagonists **(aprepitant, netupitant)** are predicted to increase the exposure to taxanes **(paclitaxel)**. Moderate Anecdotal
- Neurokinin-1 receptor antagonists **(aprepitant, netupitant)** are predicted to increase the concentration of **temsirolimus**. Use with caution or avoid. Moderate Theoretical
- Neurokinin-1 receptor antagonists **(aprepitant, netupitant)** are predicted to increase the exposure to **tezacaftor**. Adjust dose with moderate CYP3A4 inhibitors, see tezacaftor with ivacaftor p. 223, ivacaftor with tezacaftor and elexacaftor p. 220, and deutivacaftor with tezacaftor and vanzacaftor p. 218. Severe Study
- Neurokinin-1 receptor antagonists **(aprepitant, netupitant)** given with a potent CYP2C19 inhibitor are predicted to increase the exposure to **tofacitinib**. Adjust **tofacitinib** dose, p. 803. Moderate Study
- Neurokinin-1 receptor antagonists **(aprepitant, netupitant)** are predicted to increase the exposure to **tolvaptan**. Manufacturer advises caution or adjust **tolvaptan** dose with moderate CYP3A4 inhibitors. Moderate Study
- Neurokinin-1 receptor antagonists **(aprepitant, netupitant)** are predicted to increase the exposure to **trazodone**. Moderate Theoretical
- Neurokinin-1 receptor antagonists **(aprepitant, netupitant)** are predicted to increase the exposure to triptans **(eletriptan)**. Moderate Study
- **Tucatinib** is predicted to markedly increase the exposure to **aprepitant**. Moderate Study
- **Tucatinib** is predicted to increase the exposure to **fosaprepitant**. Moderate Theoretical
- **Tucatinib** is predicted to increase the exposure to **netupitant**. Moderate Study
- **Netupitant** is predicted to increase the exposure to **ulipristal**. Avoid when used for uterine fibroids. Moderate Study
- Neurokinin-1 receptor antagonists **(aprepitant, fosaprepitant)** decrease the efficacy of **ulipristal**. Avoid and for 4 weeks after stopping the enzyme inducing drug. For CoSRH guidance, see Contraceptives, interactions p. 614. Severe Anecdotal
- Neurokinin-1 receptor antagonists **(aprepitant, netupitant)** are predicted to increase the exposure to **vanzacaftor**. Adjust dose, see deutivacaftor with tezacaftor and vanzacaftor p. 218. Severe Study

- Neurokinin-1 receptor antagonists **(aprepitant, netupitant)** are predicted to increase the exposure to **vemurafenib**. Severe Theoretical
- Neurokinin-1 receptor antagonists **(aprepitant, netupitant)** are predicted to increase the exposure to **venetoclax**. Avoid or adjust dose—consult product literature. Severe Study
- **Neurokinin-1 receptor antagonists** are predicted to increase the exposure to **vinca alkaloids**. Severe Theoretical
- Neurokinin-1 receptor antagonists **(aprepitant, netupitant)** are predicted to increase the exposure to **voclosporin**. Adjust **voclosporin** dose. Severe Study
- Neurokinin-1 receptor antagonists **(aprepitant, netupitant)** are predicted to increase the exposure to **zanubrutinib**. Avoid or adjust dose with moderate CYP3A4 inhibitors—consult product literature. Severe Study
- Neurokinin-1 receptor antagonists **(aprepitant, netupitant)** are predicted to increase the exposure to **zopiclone**. Adjust dose. Moderate Study

Neuromuscular blocking drugs, non-depolarising

atracurium · cisatracurium · mivacurium · pancuronium · rocuronium · vecuronium

- **Aminoglycosides** might prolong the effects of **neuromuscular blocking drugs, non-depolarising**. Severe Theoretical
- **Anticholinesterases, centrally acting** are predicted to decrease the effects of **neuromuscular blocking drugs, non-depolarising**. Moderate Theoretical
- Antiepileptics **(carbamazepine)** are predicted to decrease the effects of (but acute use increases the effects of) neuromuscular blocking drugs, non-depolarising **(atracurium, cisatracurium, pancuronium, rocuronium, vecuronium)**. Monitor and adjust dose. Moderate Study
- Antiepileptics **(fosphenytoin, phenytoin)** decrease the effects of (but acute use increases the effects of) neuromuscular blocking drugs, non-depolarising **(atracurium, cisatracurium, pancuronium, rocuronium, vecuronium)**. Moderate Study
- **Clindamycin** increases the effects of **neuromuscular blocking drugs, non-depolarising**. Severe Anecdotal
- **Colistimethate** might prolong the effects of **neuromuscular blocking drugs, non-depolarising**. Moderate Theoretical
- **Corticosteroids** are predicted to decrease the effects of **neuromuscular blocking drugs, non-depolarising**. Severe Anecdotal
- **Pancuronium** is predicted to increase the risk of cardiovascular adverse effects when given with **digoxin**. Severe Anecdotal
- **Irinotecan** is predicted to decrease the effects of **neuromuscular blocking drugs, non-depolarising**. Moderate Theoretical
- Intravenous **magnesium** increases the effects of **neuromuscular blocking drugs, non-depolarising**. Moderate Study
- **Metoclopramide** is predicted to increase the effects of **neuromuscular blocking drugs, non-depolarising**. Moderate Theoretical
- **Neomycin** might prolong the effects of **neuromuscular blocking drugs, non-depolarising**. Severe Theoretical
- Penicillins **(piperacillin)** increase the effects of **neuromuscular blocking drugs, non-depolarising**. Moderate Study
- **Polymyxin b** might prolong the effects of **neuromuscular blocking drugs, non-depolarising**. Severe Theoretical
- **SSRIs** potentially increase the risk of prolonged neuromuscular blockade when given with **mivacurium**. Unknown Theoretical

Nevirapine → see NNRTIs

Nicardipine → see calcium-channel blockers

Nicorandil → see TABLE 6 p. 1054 (hypotension)

- **Aspirin** is predicted to increase the risk of gastrointestinal perforation when given with **nicorandil**. Severe Theoretical
- **Corticosteroids** increase the risk of gastrointestinal perforation when given with **nicorandil**. Severe Anecdotal
- **Nicorandil** is predicted to increase the risk of gastrointestinal perforation when given with **NSAIDs**. Severe Theoretical
- **Nicorandil** is predicted to increase the risk of hypotension when given with **phosphodiesterase type-5 inhibitors**. Avoid. Severe Theoretical → Also see TABLE 6 p. 1054

Nicotinic acid → see TABLE 3 p. 1053 (bleeding), TABLE 1 p. 1053 (hepatotoxicity)

- **Nicotinic acid** might increase the risk of rhabdomyolysis when given with **statins**. Use with caution or avoid. Severe Theoretical → Also see TABLE 1 p. 1053

Nifedipine → see calcium-channel blockers

Nilotinib → see TABLE 12 p. 1057 (myelosuppression), TABLE 7 p. 1055 (QT-interval prolongation)

- **Nilotinib** is predicted to increase the exposure to **abemaciclib**. Moderate Study
- **Nilotinib** is predicted to increase the exposure to **acalabrutinib**. Avoid or monitor. Severe Study
- **Nilotinib** is predicted to increase the exposure to alpha blockers **(tamsulosin)**. Moderate Theoretical
- Oral **antacids** might affect the absorption of oral **nilotinib**. Separate administration by at least 2 hours. Moderate Theoretical
- Anti-androgens **(apalutamide, enzalutamide)** are predicted to moderately decrease the exposure to **nilotinib**. Avoid. Severe Study → Also see TABLE 7 p. 1055
- **Nilotinib** is predicted to increase the exposure to antiarrhythmics **(propafenone)**. Monitor and adjust dose. Moderate Study
- Antiepileptics **(carbamazepine, fosphenytoin, phenobarbital, phenytoin, primidone)** are predicted to moderately decrease the exposure to **nilotinib**. Avoid. Severe Study
- Antifungals, azoles **(fluconazole, isavuconazole)** are predicted to increase the exposure to **nilotinib**. Moderate Study → Also see TABLE 7 p. 1055
- Antifungals, azoles **(itraconazole, ketoconazole, posaconazole, voriconazole)** are predicted to increase the exposure to **nilotinib**. Avoid. Severe Study → Also see TABLE 7 p. 1055
- **Nilotinib** is predicted to increase the exposure to antihistamines, non-sedating **(mizolastine)**. Severe Theoretical
- **Nilotinib** is predicted to increase the exposure to antihistamines, non-sedating **(rupatadine)**. Avoid. Moderate Study
- **Nilotinib** is predicted to increase the concentration of antimalarials **(piperaquine)**. Severe Study
- **Nilotinib** is predicted to increase the exposure to atypical antipsychotics **(cariprazine)**. Monitor and adjust dose. Severe Study
- **Nilotinib** is predicted to increase the exposure to atypical antipsychotics **(lurasidone)**. Adjust **lurasidone** dose. Moderate Study
- **Nilotinib** is predicted to increase the exposure to atypical antipsychotics **(quetiapine)**. Avoid. Moderate Study
- **Nilotinib** is predicted to increase the exposure to **avapritinib**. Avoid or adjust dose—consult product literature. Moderate Study
- **Nilotinib** is predicted to increase the exposure to **axitinib**. Moderate Study → Also see TABLE 12 p. 1057
- **Nilotinib** might increase the exposure to **bedaquiline**. Mild Theoretical → Also see TABLE 7 p. 1055
- **Nilotinib** is predicted to increase the exposure to benzodiazepines **(alprazolam)**. Severe Study
- **Nilotinib** is predicted to increase the exposure to benzodiazepines **(midazolam)**. Monitor adverse effects and adjust dose. Severe Study
- **Nilotinib** is predicted to increase the exposure to **bosutinib**. Avoid or adjust dose. Severe Study → Also see TABLE 12 p. 1057 → Also see TABLE 7 p. 1055
- **Nilotinib** is predicted to increase the exposure to **brigatinib**. Moderate Study
- **Nilotinib** is predicted to increase the exposure to **buspirone**. Use with caution and adjust dose. Moderate Study
- **Nilotinib** is predicted to increase the exposure to **cabozantinib**. Moderate Study → Also see TABLE 12 p. 1057 → Also see TABLE 7 p. 1055
- Oral calcium compounds **(calcium carbonate)** -containing antacids might affect the exposure to oral **nilotinib**. Separate administration by at least 2 hours. Moderate Study
- Calcium-channel blockers **(diltiazem, verapamil)** are predicted to increase the exposure to **nilotinib**. Moderate Theoretical
- **Nilotinib** is predicted to increase the exposure to calcium-channel blockers **(amlodipine, felodipine, lacidipine, lercanidipine, nicardipine, nifedipine, nimodipine)**. Monitor and adjust dose. Moderate Study

Nilotinib (continued)
- **Nilotinib** is predicted to increase the exposure to **capivasertib**. Adjust dose. [Moderate] Study
- **Cenobamate** is predicted to decrease the exposure to **nilotinib**. Avoid. [Severe] Theoretical
- **Ceritinib** is predicted to increase the exposure to **nilotinib**. Avoid. [Severe] Study → Also see TABLE 12 p. 1057 → Also see TABLE 7 p. 1055
- **Nilotinib** is predicted to increase the exposure to **ceritinib**. [Moderate] Study → Also see TABLE 12 p. 1057 → Also see TABLE 7 p. 1055
- **Nilotinib** is predicted to increase the concentration of **ciclosporin**. [Severe] Study
- **Cobicistat** is predicted to increase the exposure to **nilotinib**. Avoid. [Severe] Study
- **Nilotinib** is predicted to increase the exposure to **cobimetinib**. [Severe] Study
- **Nilotinib** is predicted to increase the exposure to **colchicine**. Adjust **colchicine** dose with moderate CYP3A4 inhibitors, p. 637. [Severe] Study
- **Nilotinib** is predicted to increase the exposure to corticosteroids **(methylprednisolone)**. Monitor and adjust dose. [Moderate] Study
- **Nilotinib** is predicted to increase the risk of bleeding events when given with **coumarins**. [Severe] Theoretical
- **Dabrafenib** is predicted to decrease the exposure to **nilotinib**. Avoid. [Severe] Theoretical
- **Nilotinib** is predicted to increase the exposure to **dabrafenib**. [Moderate] Study
- **Nilotinib** is predicted to increase the exposure to **daridorexant**. Adjust **daridorexant** dose. [Severe] Study
- **Nilotinib** is predicted to increase the exposure to **darifenacin**. [Moderate] Study
- **Nilotinib** is predicted to increase the exposure to **dasatinib**. [Severe] Study → Also see TABLE 12 p. 1057 → Also see TABLE 7 p. 1055
- **Nilotinib** is predicted to increase the exposure to **deutivacaftor**. Adjust dose, see deutivacaftor with tezacaftor and vanzacaftor p. 218. [Severe] Study
- **Nilotinib** is predicted to slightly increase the exposure to **dienogest**. [Moderate] Study
- **Nilotinib** is predicted to increase the exposure to dipeptidylpeptidase-4 inhibitors **(saxagliptin)**. [Mild] Study
- **Nilotinib** is predicted to increase the exposure to **domperidone**. Avoid. [Severe] Study
- **Nilotinib** is predicted to increase the exposure to dopamine receptor agonists **(bromocriptine)**. [Severe] Theoretical
- **Nilotinib** is predicted to increase the concentration of dopamine receptor agonists **(cabergoline)**. [Moderate] Anecdotal
- **Nilotinib** is predicted to increase the exposure to **drospirenone**. [Severe] Study
- **Nilotinib** is predicted to moderately increase the exposure to **dutasteride**. [Mild] Study
- **Nilotinib** is predicted to increase the exposure to **elacestrant**. Avoid moderate CYP3A4 inhibitors or adjust **elacestrant** dose. [Severe] Theoretical
- **Nilotinib** is predicted to increase the exposure to **elexacaftor**. Adjust ivacaftor with tezacaftor and elexacaftor p. 220 dose with moderate CYP3A4 inhibitors. [Severe] Theoretical
- **Nilotinib** is predicted to increase the exposure to **eliglustat**. Avoid or adjust dose—consult product literature. [Severe] Study
- **Encorafenib** is predicted to moderately decrease the exposure to **nilotinib**. Avoid. [Severe] Study → Also see TABLE 7 p. 1055
- **Nilotinib** is predicted to moderately increase the exposure to **encorafenib**. [Moderate] Study → Also see TABLE 7 p. 1055
- Endothelin receptor antagonists **(bosentan)** are predicted to decrease the exposure to **nilotinib**. Avoid. [Severe] Theoretical
- **Nilotinib** is predicted to increase the exposure to endothelin receptor antagonists **(macitentan)**. Manufacturer advises caution depending on other drugs taken—consult product literature. [Moderate] Theoretical
- **Nilotinib** is predicted to increase the exposure to **entrectinib**. Avoid or adjust dose with moderate CYP3A4 inhibitors—consult product literature. [Severe] Theoretical → Also see TABLE 7 p. 1055
- **Nilotinib** is predicted to increase the risk of ergotism when given with **ergometrine**. [Severe] Theoretical
- **Nilotinib** is predicted to increase the exposure to **erlotinib**. [Moderate] Study
- **Nilotinib** is predicted to increase the exposure to **etrasimod**. Avoid in poor CYP2C9 metabolisers. [Severe] Theoretical
- **Nilotinib** is predicted to increase the concentration of **everolimus**. Avoid or adjust dose. [Moderate] Study
- **Nilotinib** is predicted to increase the exposure to **fedratinib**. Monitor and adjust dose. [Moderate] Study
- **Nilotinib** is predicted to increase the exposure to **fesoterodine**. Adjust **fesoterodine** dose with moderate CYP3A4 inhibitors in hepatic and renal impairment. [Mild] Study
- **Nilotinib** is predicted to increase the exposure to **gefitinib**. [Moderate] Study
- **Grapefruit** juice is predicted to increase the exposure to **nilotinib**. Avoid. [Severe] Theoretical
- **Nilotinib** is predicted to increase the concentration of **guanfacine**. Adjust **guanfacine** dose, p. 281. [Moderate] Theoretical
- H_2 **receptor antagonists** might affect the absorption of **nilotinib**. H_2 **receptor antagonists** should be taken 10 hours before or 2 hours after **nilotinib**. [Mild] Theoretical
- **HIV-protease inhibitors** are predicted to increase the exposure to **nilotinib**. Avoid. [Severe] Study
- **Nilotinib** is predicted to increase the exposure to **ibrutinib**. Adjust dose with moderate CYP3A4 inhibitors—consult product literature. [Severe] Study → Also see TABLE 12 p. 1057
- **Idelalisib** is predicted to increase the exposure to **nilotinib**. Avoid. [Severe] Study
- **Nilotinib** is predicted to increase the exposure to **imatinib**. [Moderate] Study → Also see TABLE 12 p. 1057
- **Nilotinib** is predicted to increase the exposure to the active metabolite of **irinotecan**. [Moderate] Theoretical → Also see TABLE 12 p. 1057
- **Nilotinib** is predicted to increase the exposure to **ivabradine**. Adjust **ivabradine** dose. [Severe] Theoretical
- **Nilotinib** is predicted to increase the exposure to **ivacaftor**. Adjust dose with moderate CYP3A4 inhibitors, see ivacaftor p. 219, tezacaftor with ivacaftor p. 223, and ivacaftor with tezacaftor and elexacaftor p. 220. [Moderate] Study
- **Nilotinib** is predicted to increase the exposure to **ivosidenib**. Monitor and adjust dose—consult product literature. [Severe] Study → Also see TABLE 7 p. 1055
- **Ivosidenib** is predicted to moderately decrease the exposure to **nilotinib**. Avoid. [Severe] Study → Also see TABLE 7 p. 1055
- **Nilotinib** is predicted to increase the exposure to **lapatinib**. [Moderate] Study → Also see TABLE 7 p. 1055
- **Nilotinib** is predicted to increase the exposure to **larotrectinib**. Monitor and adjust dose. [Moderate] Theoretical
- **Nilotinib** is predicted to increase the exposure to **leniolisib**. Avoid. [Moderate] Study
- **Letermovir** is predicted to increase the exposure to **nilotinib**. [Moderate] Study
- **Nilotinib** is predicted to increase the exposure to **lomitapide**. Avoid. [Moderate] Theoretical
- **Lorlatinib** is predicted to decrease the exposure to **nilotinib**. Avoid. [Severe] Theoretical
- **Lumacaftor** is predicted to moderately decrease the exposure to **nilotinib**. Avoid. [Severe] Study
- Macrolides **(clarithromycin)** are predicted to increase the exposure to **nilotinib**. Avoid. [Severe] Study
- Macrolides **(erythromycin)** are predicted to increase the exposure to **nilotinib**. [Moderate] Study → Also see TABLE 7 p. 1055
- **Nilotinib** is predicted to increase the exposure to **mavacamten**. Adjust dose—consult product literature. [Moderate] Study
- **Nilotinib** is predicted to increase the exposure to **midostaurin**. [Moderate] Theoretical
- **Nilotinib** is predicted to increase the exposure to mineralocorticoid receptor antagonists **(eplerenone)**. Adjust **eplerenone** dose. [Severe] Study
- **Nilotinib** is predicted to increase the exposure to mineralocorticoid receptor antagonists **(finerenone)**. [Severe] Study
- **Mitotane** is predicted to moderately decrease the exposure to **nilotinib**. Avoid. [Severe] Study → Also see TABLE 12 p. 1057
- **Nilotinib** is predicted to increase the exposure to **naldemedine**. [Moderate] Study

Interactions | **Appendix 1** A1

- **Nilotinib** is predicted to increase the exposure to **naloxegol**. Adjust **naloxegol** dose and monitor adverse effects. Moderate Study
- **Nilotinib** is predicted to increase the exposure to **neratinib**. Avoid moderate CYP3A4 inhibitors or adjust dose and monitor for gastrointestinal adverse effects—consult product literature. Severe Study
- Neurokinin-1 receptor antagonists **(aprepitant, netupitant)** are predicted to increase the exposure to **nilotinib**. Moderate Study
- **Nirmatrelvir** boosted with ritonavir is predicted to increase the concentration of **nilotinib**. Avoid. Severe Theoretical
- NNRTIs **(efavirenz, etravirine, nevirapine)** are predicted to decrease the exposure to **nilotinib**. Avoid. Severe Theoretical → Also see **TABLE 7** p. 1055
- **Nilotinib** is predicted to increase the exposure to **olaparib**. Avoid or adjust dose with moderate CYP3A4 inhibitors—consult product literature. Moderate Theoretical → Also see **TABLE 12** p. 1057
- **Nilotinib** is predicted to increase the exposure to **omaveloxolone**. Avoid or adjust **omaveloxolone** dose, p. 755. Moderate Study
- **Nilotinib** is predicted to increase the exposure to opioids **(alfentanil, buprenorphine, fentanyl, oxycodone)**. Monitor and adjust dose. Moderate Study
- **Nilotinib** is predicted to increase the exposure to opioids **(methadone, sufentanil)**. Moderate Theoretical → Also see **TABLE 7** p. 1055
- **Nilotinib** is predicted to increase the exposure to **pazopanib**. Moderate Study → Also see **TABLE 7** p. 1055
- **Nilotinib** is predicted to increase the exposure to **pemigatinib**. Severe Study
- **Nilotinib** is predicted to increase the risk of bleeding events when given with **phenindione**. Severe Theoretical
- **Nilotinib** is predicted to increase the exposure to phosphodiesterase type-5 inhibitors **(avanafil)**. Adjust **avanafil** dose. Moderate Theoretical
- **Nilotinib** is predicted to increase the exposure to phosphodiesterase type-5 inhibitors **(sildenafil)**. Monitor or adjust **sildenafil** dose with moderate CYP3A4 inhibitors, p. 139. Moderate Study
- **Nilotinib** is predicted to increase the exposure to phosphodiesterase type-5 inhibitors **(tadalafil)**. Severe Theoretical
- **Nilotinib** is predicted to increase the exposure to phosphodiesterase type-5 inhibitors **(vardenafil)**. Adjust dose. Severe Theoretical → Also see **TABLE 7** p. 1055
- **Nilotinib** is predicted to increase the exposure to **pimozide**. Avoid. Severe Theoretical → Also see **TABLE 7** p. 1055
- **Pitolisant** is predicted to decrease the exposure to **nilotinib**. Avoid. Severe Theoretical
- **Nilotinib** is predicted to increase the exposure to **ponatinib**. Moderate Study
- **Nilotinib** is predicted to increase the exposure to **pralsetinib**. Moderate Theoretical
- **Nilotinib** is predicted to increase the exposure to **ranolazine**. Severe Study → Also see **TABLE 7** p. 1055
- **Nilotinib** is predicted to increase the exposure to **regorafenib**. Moderate Study → Also see **TABLE 12** p. 1057
- **Nilotinib** is predicted to increase the exposure to **ribociclib**. Moderate Study → Also see **TABLE 12** p. 1057 → Also see **TABLE 7** p. 1055
- Rifamycins **(rifampicin)** are predicted to moderately decrease the exposure to **nilotinib**. Avoid. Severe Study
- **Nilotinib** is predicted to increase the exposure to **rimegepant**. Avoid another dose of rimegepant within 48 hours of concurrent use. Moderate Study
- **Nilotinib** is predicted to increase the exposure to **ruxolitinib**. Moderate Study → Also see **TABLE 12** p. 1057
- **Nilotinib** is predicted to increase the exposure to **selpercatinib**. Moderate Study → Also see **TABLE 7** p. 1055
- **Nilotinib** is predicted to increase the exposure to **selumetinib**. Avoid or adjust dose—consult product literature. Severe Study
- **Nilotinib** is predicted to increase the exposure to **siponimod**. Avoid depending on other drugs taken—consult product literature. Severe Study
- **Nilotinib** increases the concentration of **sirolimus**. Monitor and adjust dose. Moderate Study
- Oral **sodium bicarbonate**-containing antacids might affect the exposure to oral **nilotinib**. Separate administration by at least 2 hours. Moderate Study
- **Sodium zirconium cyclosilicate** is predicted to decrease the exposure to **nilotinib**. Separate administration by at least 2 hours. Moderate Theoretical
- **Sotorasib** is predicted to decrease the exposure to **nilotinib**. Avoid. Severe Theoretical
- **Nilotinib** is predicted to increase the exposure to **sparsentan**. Moderate Study
- **Nilotinib** is predicted to increase the exposure to SSRIs **(dapoxetine)**. Adjust **dapoxetine** dose with moderate CYP3A4 inhibitors. Moderate Theoretical
- **Nilotinib** is predicted to increase the exposure to SSRIs **(sertraline)**. Moderate Theoretical
- **St John's wort** is predicted to decrease the exposure to **nilotinib**. Avoid. Severe Theoretical
- **Nilotinib** is predicted to increase the exposure to statins **(atorvastatin)**. Monitor and adjust dose. Moderate Theoretical
- **Nilotinib** is predicted to increase the exposure to statins **(simvastatin)**. Monitor and adjust dose. Severe Theoretical
- **Nilotinib** is predicted to increase the exposure to **sunitinib**. Moderate Study → Also see **TABLE 12** p. 1057 → Also see **TABLE 7** p. 1055
- **Nilotinib** is predicted to increase the concentration of **tacrolimus**. Monitor and adjust dose. Severe Theoretical
- **Nilotinib** is predicted to increase the exposure to taxanes **(cabazitaxel)**. Moderate Theoretical → Also see **TABLE 12** p. 1057
- **Nilotinib** is predicted to increase the exposure to taxanes **(docetaxel)**. Severe Study → Also see **TABLE 12** p. 1057
- **Nilotinib** is predicted to increase the exposure to taxanes **(paclitaxel)**. Moderate Anecdotal → Also see **TABLE 12** p. 1057
- **Nilotinib** is predicted to increase the concentration of **temsirolimus**. Use with caution or avoid. Moderate Theoretical → Also see **TABLE 12** p. 1057
- **Nilotinib** is predicted to increase the exposure to **tezacaftor**. Adjust dose with moderate CYP3A4 inhibitors, see tezacaftor with ivacaftor p. 223, ivacaftor with tezacaftor and elexacaftor p. 220, and deutivacaftor with tezacaftor and vanzacaftor p. 218. Severe Study
- **Nilotinib** given with a potent CYP2C19 inhibitor is predicted to increase the exposure to **tofacitinib**. Adjust **tofacitinib** dose, p. 803. Moderate Study
- **Nilotinib** is predicted to increase the exposure to **tolvaptan**. Manufacturer advises caution or adjust **tolvaptan** dose with moderate CYP3A4 inhibitors. Moderate Study
- **Nilotinib** is predicted to increase the exposure to **trazodone**. Moderate Theoretical
- **Tucatinib** is predicted to increase the exposure to **nilotinib**. Avoid. Severe Study
- **Nilotinib** is predicted to increase the exposure to **ulipristal**. Avoid when used for uterine fibroids. Moderate Study
- **Nilotinib** is predicted to increase the exposure to **vanzacaftor**. Adjust dose, see deutivacaftor with tezacaftor and vanzacaftor p. 218. Severe Study
- **Nilotinib** is predicted to increase the exposure to **vemurafenib**. Severe Theoretical → Also see **TABLE 7** p. 1055
- **Nilotinib** is predicted to increase the exposure to **venetoclax**. Avoid or adjust dose—consult product literature. Severe Study
- **Nilotinib** is predicted to increase the exposure to **vinca alkaloids**. Severe Theoretical → Also see **TABLE 12** p. 1057
- **Nilotinib** is predicted to increase the exposure to **voclosporin**. Adjust **voclosporin** dose. Severe Study → Also see **TABLE 7** p. 1055
- **Nilotinib** is predicted to increase the exposure to **zanubrutinib**. Avoid or adjust dose with moderate CYP3A4 inhibitors—consult product literature. Severe Study
- **Nilotinib** is predicted to increase the exposure to **zopiclone**. Adjust dose. Moderate Study

Nimodipine → see calcium-channel blockers

Nintedanib → see **TABLE 3** p. 1053 (bleeding)

- Antiarrhythmics **(amiodarone, dronedarone)** are predicted to increase the exposure to **nintedanib**. Moderate Study

Nintedanib (continued)
- Antiepileptics **(carbamazepine)** are predicted to decrease the exposure to **nintedanib.** Moderate Study
- Antiepileptics **(phenobarbital, phenytoin)** are predicted to decrease the exposure to **nintedanib.** Severe Theoretical
- Antifungals, azoles **(itraconazole, ketoconazole)** are predicted to increase the exposure to **nintedanib.** Moderate Study
- Antifungals, azoles **(voriconazole)** are predicted to increase the exposure to **nintedanib.** Moderate Theoretical
- Calcium-channel blockers **(verapamil)** are predicted to increase the exposure to **nintedanib.** Moderate Study
- **Ciclosporin** is predicted to increase the exposure to **nintedanib.** Moderate Study
- **Cobicistat** is predicted to increase the exposure to **nintedanib.** Moderate Study
- **Glecaprevir** is predicted to increase the exposure to **nintedanib.** Moderate Study
- HIV-protease inhibitors **(atazanavir, darunavir, fosamprenavir)** boosted with ritonavir are predicted to increase the exposure to **nintedanib.** Moderate Theoretical
- HIV-protease inhibitors **(lopinavir, ritonavir)** are predicted to increase the exposure to **nintedanib.** Moderate Study
- **Lapatinib** is predicted to increase the exposure to **nintedanib.** Moderate Study
- **Lorlatinib** is predicted to decrease the exposure to **nintedanib.** Moderate Study
- **Macrolides** are predicted to increase the exposure to **nintedanib.** Moderate Study
- **Pibrentasvir** is predicted to increase the exposure to **nintedanib.** Moderate Study
- **Ranolazine** is predicted to increase the exposure to **nintedanib.** Moderate Study
- Rifamycins **(rifampicin)** are predicted to decrease the exposure to **nintedanib.** Moderate Study
- **St John's wort** is predicted to decrease the exposure to **nintedanib.** Moderate Study
- **Velpatasvir** is predicted to increase the exposure to **nintedanib.** Moderate Study
- **Vemurafenib** is predicted to increase the exposure to **nintedanib.** Moderate Study
- **Voxilaprevir** is predicted to increase the exposure to **nintedanib.** Moderate Study

Niraparib → see TABLE 12 p. 1057 (myelosuppression)

Nirmatrelvir
- **Nirmatrelvir** boosted with ritonavir is predicted to increase the concentration of **abemaciclib.** Avoid or adjust dose—consult product literature. Severe Theoretical
- **Nirmatrelvir** boosted with ritonavir is predicted to increase the concentration of **afatinib.** Moderate Theoretical
- **Nirmatrelvir** boosted with ritonavir is predicted to increase the concentration of **aliskiren.** Avoid. Severe Theoretical
- **Nirmatrelvir** boosted with ritonavir is predicted to increase the concentration of alpha blockers **(alfuzosin, tamsulosin).** Avoid. Severe Theoretical
- **Nirmatrelvir** boosted with ritonavir is predicted to increase the concentration of **amfetamines.** Severe Theoretical
- **Nirmatrelvir** boosted with ritonavir is predicted to decrease the concentration of **aminophylline.** Adjust dose. Moderate Theoretical
- Anti-androgens **(apalutamide, enzalutamide)** are predicted to decrease the exposure to **nirmatrelvir** boosted with ritonavir. Avoid. Severe Study
- **Nirmatrelvir** boosted with ritonavir is predicted to increase the concentration of antiarrhythmics **(amiodarone, dronedarone, flecainide, propafenone).** Avoid. Severe Theoretical
- **Nirmatrelvir** boosted with ritonavir is predicted to increase the concentration of antiarrhythmics **(disopyramide, lidocaine).** Severe Theoretical
- Antiepileptics **(carbamazepine, fosphenytoin, phenobarbital, phenytoin, primidone)** are predicted to decrease the exposure to **nirmatrelvir** boosted with ritonavir. Avoid. Severe Study
- **Nirmatrelvir** boosted with ritonavir is predicted to decrease the concentration of antiepileptics **(lamotrigine, valproate).** Severe Theoretical
- **Nirmatrelvir** boosted with ritonavir is predicted to increase the concentration of antifungals, azoles **(isavuconazole).** Severe Theoretical
- **Nirmatrelvir** boosted with ritonavir increases the exposure to antifungals, azoles **(itraconazole).** Severe Study
- **Nirmatrelvir** boosted with ritonavir is predicted to increase the concentration of antifungals, azoles **(ketoconazole).** Adjust dose. Moderate Theoretical
- **Nirmatrelvir** boosted with ritonavir is predicted to decrease the concentration of antifungals, azoles **(voriconazole).** Avoid. Severe Theoretical
- **Nirmatrelvir** boosted with ritonavir is predicted to decrease the concentration of antimalarials **(atovaquone).** Moderate Theoretical
- **Nirmatrelvir** boosted with ritonavir is predicted to increase the concentration of atypical antipsychotics **(aripiprazole).** Adjust dose. Moderate Theoretical
- **Nirmatrelvir** boosted with ritonavir is predicted to increase the concentration of atypical antipsychotics **(cariprazine).** Avoid. Moderate Theoretical
- **Nirmatrelvir** boosted with ritonavir is predicted to increase the concentration of atypical antipsychotics **(clozapine).** Avoid or adjust dose. Severe Theoretical
- **Nirmatrelvir** boosted with ritonavir is predicted to increase the concentration of atypical antipsychotics **(lurasidone, quetiapine).** Avoid. Severe Theoretical
- **Nirmatrelvir** boosted with ritonavir is predicted to increase the concentration of atypical antipsychotics **(risperidone).** Severe Theoretical
- **Nirmatrelvir** boosted with ritonavir is predicted to increase the concentration of **bedaquiline.** Avoid or monitor. Moderate Theoretical
- **Nirmatrelvir** boosted with ritonavir is predicted to increase the concentration of benzodiazepines **(alprazolam).** Moderate Theoretical
- **Nirmatrelvir** boosted with ritonavir is predicted to increase the concentration of benzodiazepines **(clonazepam, diazepam, flurazepam).** Monitor and adjust dose. Severe Theoretical
- **Nirmatrelvir** boosted with ritonavir very markedly increases the exposure to benzodiazepines **(midazolam).** Avoid or adjust dose. Severe Study
- **Nirmatrelvir** boosted with ritonavir is predicted to increase the concentration of beta$_2$ agonists **(salmeterol).** Avoid. Severe Theoretical
- **Nirmatrelvir** boosted with ritonavir is predicted to decrease the concentration of **bupropion.** Moderate Theoretical
- **Nirmatrelvir** boosted with ritonavir is predicted to increase the concentration of **buspirone.** Monitor and adjust dose. Moderate Theoretical
- **Nirmatrelvir** boosted with ritonavir is predicted to increase the concentration of **calcium-channel blockers.** Severe Theoretical
- **Nirmatrelvir** boosted with ritonavir is predicted to increase the concentration of **ceritinib.** Avoid or adjust dose—consult product literature. Severe Theoretical
- **Nirmatrelvir** boosted with ritonavir is predicted to increase the concentration of **ciclosporin.** Avoid—consult product literature. Severe Theoretical
- **Nirmatrelvir** boosted with ritonavir is predicted to increase the concentration of **cilostazol.** Adjust dose. Moderate Theoretical
- **Nirmatrelvir** boosted with ritonavir is predicted to decrease the concentration of **clopidogrel.** Severe Theoretical
- **Nirmatrelvir** boosted with ritonavir is predicted to increase the concentration of **colchicine.** Avoid. Severe Theoretical
- **Nirmatrelvir** boosted with ritonavir is predicted to decrease the concentration of **combined hormonal contraceptives** containing ethinylestradiol. Use additional contraceptive precautions. Moderate Theoretical
- **Nirmatrelvir** boosted with ritonavir is predicted to increase the concentration of corticosteroids **(beclometasone)** (risk with beclometasone is likely to be lower than with other corticosteroids). Moderate Theoretical
- **Nirmatrelvir** boosted with ritonavir is predicted to increase the concentration of corticosteroids **(betamethasone, budesonide, ciclesonide, deflazacort, dexamethasone, fluticasone, hydrocortisone, methylprednisolone, mometasone,**

prednisolone, triamcinolone). Avoid or monitor adverse effects and consider beclomethasone as an alternative. Severe Theoretical
- **Nirmatrelvir** boosted with ritonavir is predicted to increase the concentration of corticosteroids **(fludrocortisone, vamorolone)**. Avoid or monitor adverse effects. Severe Theoretical
- **Nirmatrelvir** boosted with ritonavir is predicted to affect the concentration of **coumarins**. Moderate Theoretical
- **Nirmatrelvir** boosted with ritonavir is predicted to increase the concentration of **darifenacin**. Adjust dose. Severe Theoretical
- **Nirmatrelvir** boosted with ritonavir is predicted to increase the concentration of **dasatinib**. Avoid. Severe Theoretical
- **Nirmatrelvir** boosted with ritonavir is predicted to increase the concentration of **delamanid**. Severe Theoretical
- **Nirmatrelvir** boosted with ritonavir is predicted to increase the concentration of **digoxin**. Severe Theoretical
- **Nirmatrelvir** boosted with ritonavir is predicted to increase the concentration of dipeptidylpeptidase-4 inhibitors **(saxagliptin)**. Adjust dose. Moderate Theoretical
- **Nirmatrelvir** boosted with ritonavir is predicted to increase the concentration of **elbasvir**. Severe Theoretical
- **Nirmatrelvir** boosted with ritonavir is predicted to increase the concentration of **elexacaftor** with tezacaftor and ivacaftor. Adjust dose. Severe Theoretical
- **Nirmatrelvir** boosted with ritonavir is predicted to increase the concentration of **encorafenib**. Avoid or monitor. Severe Theoretical
- **Encorafenib** is predicted to decrease the exposure to **nirmatrelvir** boosted with ritonavir. Avoid. Severe Study
- **Nirmatrelvir** boosted with ritonavir is predicted to increase the concentration of endothelin receptor antagonists **(bosentan)**. Severe Theoretical
- **Nirmatrelvir** boosted with ritonavir is predicted to increase the concentration of **ergometrine**. Avoid. Severe Theoretical
- **Nirmatrelvir** boosted with ritonavir is predicted to increase the concentration of **everolimus**. Avoid—consult product literature. Severe Theoretical
- **Nirmatrelvir** boosted with ritonavir is predicted to increase the concentration of factor XA inhibitors **(apixaban, rivaroxaban)**. Avoid. Severe Theoretical
- **Nirmatrelvir** boosted with ritonavir is predicted to increase the concentration of **fostamatinib**. Monitor adverse effects and adjust dose. Moderate Theoretical
- **Nirmatrelvir** boosted with ritonavir is predicted to increase the concentration of **fusidate**. Avoid. Moderate Theoretical
- **Nirmatrelvir** boosted with ritonavir is predicted to increase the concentration of **glecaprevir**. Avoid. Severe Theoretical
- **Nirmatrelvir** boosted with ritonavir is predicted to increase the concentration of **grazoprevir**. Severe Theoretical
- **Nirmatrelvir** boosted with ritonavir is predicted to increase the concentration of **haloperidol**. Severe Theoretical
- **Nirmatrelvir** boosted with ritonavir is predicted to increase the concentration of HIV-protease inhibitors **(atazanavir, darunavir, fosamprenavir, lopinavir)**. Moderate Theoretical
- **Nirmatrelvir** boosted with ritonavir is predicted to increase the concentration of **ibrutinib**. Avoid or adjust dose—consult product literature. Severe Theoretical
- **Nirmatrelvir** boosted with ritonavir is predicted to increase the concentration of **ivabradine**. Avoid. Severe Theoretical
- **Nirmatrelvir** boosted with ritonavir is predicted to increase the concentration of **ivacaftor**. Adjust dose. Severe Theoretical
- **Nirmatrelvir** boosted with ritonavir is predicted to increase the concentration of **ivosidenib**. Monitor and adjust dose—consult product literature. Severe Theoretical
- **Ivosidenib** is predicted to decrease the exposure to **nirmatrelvir** boosted with ritonavir. Avoid. Severe Study
- **Nirmatrelvir** boosted with ritonavir is predicted to increase the concentration of **lomitapide**. Avoid. Severe Theoretical
- **Lumacaftor** is predicted to decrease the exposure to **nirmatrelvir** boosted with ritonavir. Avoid. Severe Study
- **Nirmatrelvir** boosted with ritonavir is predicted to increase the concentration of macrolides **(clarithromycin)**. Monitor; adjust dose in renal impairment. Moderate Theoretical
- **Nirmatrelvir** boosted with ritonavir is predicted to increase the concentration of macrolides **(erythromycin)**. Moderate Theoretical
- **Nirmatrelvir** boosted with ritonavir is predicted to increase the concentration of **maraviroc**. Refer to specialist literature. Severe Theoretical
- **Nirmatrelvir** boosted with ritonavir is predicted to increase the concentration of **methylphenidate**. Severe Theoretical
- **Nirmatrelvir** boosted with ritonavir is predicted to increase the concentration of mineralocorticoid receptor antagonists **(eplerenone, finerenone)**. Avoid. Severe Theoretical
- **Mitotane** is predicted to decrease the exposure to **nirmatrelvir** boosted with ritonavir. Avoid. Severe Study
- **Nirmatrelvir** boosted with ritonavir is predicted to increase the concentration of **naloxegol**. Avoid. Severe Theoretical
- **Nirmatrelvir** boosted with ritonavir is predicted to increase the concentration of **neratinib**. Avoid. Severe Theoretical
- **Nirmatrelvir** boosted with ritonavir is predicted to increase the concentration of **nilotinib**. Avoid. Severe Theoretical
- **Nirmatrelvir** boosted with ritonavir is predicted to increase the concentration of NNRTIs **(efavirenz, nevirapine)**. Moderate Theoretical
- **Nirmatrelvir** boosted with ritonavir is predicted to increase the concentration of opioids **(buprenorphine)**. Monitor and adjust dose. Moderate Theoretical
- **Nirmatrelvir** boosted with ritonavir is predicted to increase the concentration of opioids **(fentanyl, oxycodone, pethidine)**. Severe Theoretical
- **Nirmatrelvir** boosted with ritonavir is predicted to decrease the concentration of opioids **(methadone)**. Adjust dose. Moderate Theoretical
- **Nirmatrelvir** boosted with ritonavir is predicted to decrease the concentration of opioids **(morphine)**. Moderate Theoretical
- **Nirmatrelvir** boosted with ritonavir is predicted to affect the concentration of **phenindione**. Moderate Theoretical
- **Nirmatrelvir** boosted with ritonavir is predicted to increase the concentration of phosphodiesterase type-5 inhibitors **(avanafil, vardenafil)**. Avoid. Severe Theoretical
- **Nirmatrelvir** boosted with ritonavir is predicted to increase the concentration of phosphodiesterase type-5 inhibitors **(sildenafil, tadalafil)**. Avoid or adjust dose—consult product literature. Severe Theoretical
- **Nirmatrelvir** boosted with ritonavir is predicted to increase the concentration of **pibrentasvir**. Avoid. Severe Theoretical
- **Nirmatrelvir** boosted with ritonavir is predicted to increase the concentration of **pimozide**. Avoid. Severe Theoretical
- **Nirmatrelvir** boosted with ritonavir is predicted to increase the concentration of **ranolazine**. Avoid. Severe Theoretical
- Rifamycins **(rifampicin)** are predicted to decrease the exposure to **nirmatrelvir** boosted with ritonavir. Avoid. Severe Study
- **Nirmatrelvir** boosted with ritonavir is predicted to increase the concentration of rifamycins **(rifabutin)**. Adjust dose. Severe Theoretical
- **Nirmatrelvir** boosted with ritonavir is predicted to increase the concentration of **rimegepant**. Avoid. Severe Theoretical
- **Nirmatrelvir** boosted with ritonavir is predicted to increase the concentration of **riociguat**. Adjust dose. Moderate Theoretical
- **Nirmatrelvir** boosted with ritonavir is predicted to increase the concentration of **sirolimus**. Avoid—consult product literature. Severe Theoretical
- **Nirmatrelvir** boosted with ritonavir is predicted to increase the concentration of **sofosbuvir** with velpatasvir and voxilaprevir. Severe Theoretical
- **St John's wort** is predicted to decrease the exposure to **nirmatrelvir** boosted with ritonavir. Avoid. Severe Theoretical
- **Nirmatrelvir** boosted with ritonavir is predicted to increase the concentration of statins **(atorvastatin, rosuvastatin)**. Adjust dose. Severe Theoretical
- **Nirmatrelvir** boosted with ritonavir is predicted to increase the concentration of statins **(simvastatin)**. Avoid. Severe Theoretical
- **Nirmatrelvir** boosted with ritonavir is predicted to increase the concentration of **tacrolimus**. Avoid—consult product literature. Severe Theoretical
- **Nirmatrelvir** boosted with ritonavir is predicted to increase the exposure to **temsirolimus**. Avoid—consult product literature. Severe Theoretical

Nirmatrelvir (continued)
- **Nirmatrelvir** boosted with ritonavir is predicted to increase the concentration of **tezacaftor** with ivacaftor. Adjust dose. [Severe] Theoretical
- **Nirmatrelvir** boosted with ritonavir is predicted to decrease the concentration of **theophylline**. Adjust dose. [Moderate] Theoretical
- **Nirmatrelvir** boosted with ritonavir moderately increases the exposure to thrombin inhibitors **(dabigatran)**. Avoid. [Severe] Study
- **Nirmatrelvir** boosted with ritonavir might decrease the efficacy of thyroid hormones **(levothyroxine)**. [Moderate] Theoretical
- **Nirmatrelvir** boosted with ritonavir is predicted to increase the concentration of **ticagrelor**. Avoid. [Severe] Theoretical
- **Nirmatrelvir** boosted with ritonavir is predicted to increase the concentration of **tofacitinib**. Adjust dose. [Severe] Theoretical
- **Nirmatrelvir** boosted with ritonavir is predicted to increase the concentration of **tolvaptan**. Avoid. [Severe] Theoretical
- **Nirmatrelvir** boosted with ritonavir is predicted to increase the concentration of **trazodone**. [Moderate] Theoretical
- **Nirmatrelvir** boosted with ritonavir is predicted to increase the concentration of **tricyclic antidepressants**. [Moderate] Theoretical
- **Nirmatrelvir** boosted with ritonavir is predicted to increase the concentration of triptans **(eletriptan)**. Avoid. [Severe] Theoretical
- **Nirmatrelvir** boosted with ritonavir is predicted to increase the concentration of **upadacitinib**. Adjust dose. [Severe] Theoretical
- **Nirmatrelvir** boosted with ritonavir is predicted to increase the concentration of **velpatasvir** with sofosbuvir and voxilaprevir. [Severe] Theoretical
- **Nirmatrelvir** boosted with ritonavir is predicted to increase the concentration of **venetoclax**. Avoid or adjust dose—consult product literature. [Severe] Theoretical
- **Nirmatrelvir** boosted with ritonavir is predicted to increase the concentration of vinca alkaloids **(vinblastine, vincristine)**. [Severe] Theoretical
- **Nirmatrelvir** boosted with ritonavir is predicted to increase the concentration of **voclosporin**. Avoid. [Severe] Theoretical
- **Nirmatrelvir** boosted with ritonavir is predicted to increase the concentration of **voxilaprevir** with sofosbuvir and velpatasvir. [Severe] Theoretical
- **Nirmatrelvir** boosted with ritonavir is predicted to increase the concentration of **zolpidem**. [Severe] Theoretical

Nitisinone
- Anti-androgens **(apalutamide, enzalutamide)** are predicted to decrease the exposure to **nitisinone**. Adjust dose. [Moderate] Theoretical
- Antiepileptics **(carbamazepine, fosphenytoin, phenobarbital, phenytoin, primidone)** are predicted to decrease the exposure to **nitisinone**. Adjust dose. [Moderate] Theoretical
- Antifungals, azoles **(itraconazole, ketoconazole, posaconazole, voriconazole)** are predicted to increase the exposure to **nitisinone**. Adjust dose. [Moderate] Theoretical
- **Nitisinone** is predicted to increase the exposure to **baricitinib**. [Moderate] Study
- **Nitisinone** is predicted to increase the exposure to cephalosporins **(cefaclor)**. [Moderate] Study
- **Ceritinib** is predicted to increase the exposure to **nitisinone**. Adjust dose. [Moderate] Theoretical
- **Cobicistat** is predicted to increase the exposure to **nitisinone**. Adjust dose. [Moderate] Theoretical
- **Nitisinone** is predicted to increase the exposure to coumarins **(warfarin)**. [Moderate] Study
- **Encorafenib** is predicted to decrease the exposure to **nitisinone**. Adjust dose. [Moderate] Theoretical
- **Nitisinone** is predicted to increase the exposure to **ganciclovir**. [Moderate] Study
- **Nitisinone** is predicted to increase the exposure to H_2 receptor antagonists **(famotidine)**. [Moderate] Study
- **HIV-protease inhibitors** are predicted to increase the exposure to **nitisinone**. Adjust dose. [Moderate] Theoretical
- **Idelalisib** is predicted to increase the exposure to **nitisinone**. Adjust dose. [Moderate] Theoretical
- **Ivosidenib** is predicted to decrease the exposure to **nitisinone**. Adjust dose. [Moderate] Theoretical
- **Nitisinone** is predicted to increase the exposure to loop diuretics **(furosemide)**. [Moderate] Study
- **Lumacaftor** is predicted to decrease the exposure to **nitisinone**. Adjust dose. [Moderate] Theoretical
- Macrolides **(clarithromycin)** are predicted to increase the exposure to **nitisinone**. Adjust dose. [Moderate] Theoretical
- **Nitisinone** is predicted to increase the exposure to **methotrexate**. [Moderate] Study
- **Mitotane** is predicted to decrease the exposure to **nitisinone**. Adjust dose. [Moderate] Theoretical
- **Nitisinone** is predicted to increase the exposure to NSAIDs **(celecoxib)**. [Moderate] Study
- **Nitisinone** is predicted to increase the exposure to **oseltamivir**. [Moderate] Study
- **Nitisinone** is predicted to increase the exposure to penicillins **(benzylpenicillin)**. [Moderate] Study
- **Nitisinone** is predicted to increase the exposure to quinolones **(ciprofloxacin)**. [Moderate] Study
- Rifamycins **(rifampicin)** are predicted to decrease the exposure to **nitisinone**. Adjust dose. [Moderate] Theoretical
- **Nitisinone** is predicted to increase the exposure to sulfonylureas **(glimepiride, tolbutamide)**. [Moderate] Study
- **Nitisinone** is predicted to increase the exposure to **tenofovir alafenamide**. [Moderate] Study
- **Nitisinone** is predicted to increase the exposure to **tenofovir disoproxil**. [Moderate] Study
- **Tucatinib** is predicted to increase the exposure to **nitisinone**. Adjust dose. [Moderate] Theoretical

Nitrates → see TABLE 6 p. 1054 (hypotension)

glyceryl trinitrate · isosorbide dinitrate · isosorbide mononitrate

PHARMACOLOGY Drugs with antimuscarinic effects can cause dry mouth, which can reduce the effectiveness of sublingual glyceryl trinitrate tablets.

- **Acetylcysteine** might increase the vasodilatory effects of **glyceryl trinitrate**. [Moderate] Theoretical
- **Nitrates** potentially increase the risk of hypotension when given with **phosphodiesterase type-5 inhibitors**. Avoid. [Severe] Study → Also see TABLE 6 p. 1054

Nitrazepam → see benzodiazepines

Nitrofurantoin → see TABLE 10 p. 1056 (peripheral neuropathy)
- **Acetazolamide** might decrease the efficacy of **nitrofurantoin**. [Unknown] Theoretical
- Oral **magnesium** trisilicate decreases the absorption of oral **nitrofurantoin**. [Moderate] Study
- **Potassium citrate** might decrease the efficacy of **nitrofurantoin**. [Unknown] Theoretical
- **Sodium bicarbonate** might decrease the efficacy of **nitrofurantoin**. [Unknown] Theoretical
- **Sodium citrate** might decrease the efficacy of **nitrofurantoin**. [Unknown] Theoretical

Nitroprusside → see TABLE 6 p. 1054 (hypotension)

Nitrous oxide → see TABLE 6 p. 1054 (hypotension), TABLE 9 p. 1056 (CNS effects)
- **Nitrous oxide** potentially increases the risk of methotrexate toxicity when given with **methotrexate**. Avoid. [Severe] Study

Nivolumab → see monoclonal antibodies

Nizatidine → see H_2 receptor antagonists

NNRTIs → see TABLE 1 p. 1053 (hepatotoxicity), TABLE 7 p. 1055 (QT-interval prolongation)

doravirine · efavirenz · etravirine · nevirapine · rilpivirine

- **Efavirenz** is predicted to decrease the exposure to **abrocitinib**. Avoid. [Moderate] Theoretical
- NNRTIs **(efavirenz, nevirapine)** are predicted to decrease the exposure to **acalabrutinib**. [Severe] Study
- Oral **antacids** are predicted to decrease the exposure to oral **rilpivirine**. Manufacturer advises take 4 hours before or 2 hours after antacids. [Severe] Theoretical
- Anti-androgens **(apalutamide, enzalutamide)** are predicted to decrease the exposure to **doravirine**. Avoid. [Severe] Study
- Anti-androgens **(apalutamide, enzalutamide)** are predicted to decrease the exposure to **etravirine**. Avoid. [Severe] Theoretical
- Anti-androgens **(apalutamide, enzalutamide)** are predicted to decrease the exposure to **nevirapine**. [Severe] Study

- Anti-androgens **(apalutamide, enzalutamide)** markedly decrease the exposure to **rilpivirine**. Avoid. Severe Study
- NNRTIs **(efavirenz, nevirapine)** are predicted to decrease the efficacy of anti-androgens **(cyproterone)** with ethinylestradiol (co-cyprindiol). Use alternative methods during treatment with, and for 28 days after, the enzyme inducing drug is stopped. Severe Study
- NNRTIs **(efavirenz, etravirine, nevirapine)** are predicted to decrease the exposure to anti-androgens **(darolutamide)**. Avoid. Moderate Theoretical
- NNRTIs **(efavirenz, etravirine, nevirapine)** are predicted to decrease the exposure to antiarrhythmics **(dronedarone)**. Severe Theoretical → Also see TABLE 7 p. 1055
- Antiepileptics **(carbamazepine)** slightly decrease the exposure to **efavirenz** and **efavirenz** slightly decreases the exposure to antiepileptics **(carbamazepine)**. Severe Study
- Antiepileptics **(carbamazepine, fosphenytoin, phenobarbital, phenytoin, primidone)** are predicted to decrease the exposure to **doravirine**. Avoid. Severe Study
- Antiepileptics **(carbamazepine, fosphenytoin, phenobarbital, phenytoin, primidone)** are predicted to decrease the exposure to **etravirine**. Avoid. Severe Theoretical
- Antiepileptics **(carbamazepine, fosphenytoin, phenobarbital, phenytoin, primidone)** markedly decrease the exposure to **rilpivirine**. Avoid. Severe Study
- Antiepileptics **(fosphenytoin, phenytoin)** slightly decrease the exposure to **efavirenz** and **efavirenz** affects the concentration of antiepileptics **(fosphenytoin, phenytoin)**. Severe Theoretical
- Antiepileptics **(oxcarbazepine)** are predicted to decrease the exposure to **doravirine**. Avoid. Severe Theoretical
- Antiepileptics **(oxcarbazepine)** are predicted to decrease the concentration of **rilpivirine**. Avoid. Severe Theoretical
- Antiepileptics **(phenobarbital)** are predicted to decrease the exposure to **efavirenz** and **efavirenz** affects the concentration of antiepileptics **(phenobarbital)**. Severe Theoretical
- **Nevirapine** is predicted to decrease the concentration of antiepileptics **(carbamazepine, fosphenytoin, phenobarbital, phenytoin, primidone)** and antiepileptics **(carbamazepine, fosphenytoin, phenobarbital, phenytoin, primidone)** are predicted to decrease the concentration of **nevirapine**. Severe Study
- **Efavirenz** is predicted to affect the efficacy of antiepileptics **(primidone)** and antiepileptics **(primidone)** are predicted to slightly decrease the exposure to **efavirenz**. Severe Theoretical
- Antifungals, azoles **(fluconazole)** slightly to moderately increase the exposure to **nevirapine**. Moderate Study → Also see TABLE 1 p. 1053
- NNRTIs **(efavirenz, etravirine, nevirapine)** are predicted to decrease the exposure to antifungals, azoles **(isavuconazole)**. Avoid. Severe Theoretical
- **Efavirenz** slightly decreases the exposure to antifungals, azoles **(itraconazole)**. Avoid and for 14 days after stopping **efavirenz**. Moderate Study
- **Nevirapine** moderately decreases the exposure to antifungals, azoles **(itraconazole)**. Avoid and for 14 days after stopping **nevirapine**. Moderate Study → Also see TABLE 1 p. 1053
- **Efavirenz** moderately decreases the exposure to antifungals, azoles **(ketoconazole)**. Severe Study
- **Nevirapine** moderately decreases the exposure to antifungals, azoles **(ketoconazole)**. Avoid. Severe Study
- **Efavirenz** slightly decreases the exposure to antifungals, azoles **(posaconazole)**. Avoid. Moderate Study
- **Efavirenz** moderately decreases the exposure to antifungals, azoles **(voriconazole)** and antifungals, azoles **(voriconazole)** slightly increase the exposure to **efavirenz**. Adjust dose. Severe Study → Also see TABLE 7 p. 1055
- **Nevirapine** is predicted to decrease the exposure to antifungals, azoles **(voriconazole)** and antifungals, azoles **(voriconazole)** increase the exposure to **nevirapine**. Monitor and adjust dose. Severe Theoretical → Also see TABLE 1 p. 1053
- **Efavirenz** decreases the concentration of antimalarials **(artemether)**. Severe Study → Also see TABLE 7 p. 1055
- **Etravirine** decreases the exposure to antimalarials **(artemether)**. Moderate Study
- **Nevirapine** moderately decreases the exposure to the active metabolite of antimalarials **(artesunate)**. Avoid. Severe Study
- **Efavirenz** moderately decreases the exposure to antimalarials **(atovaquone)**. Avoid. Moderate Study
- **Efavirenz** decreases the concentration of antimalarials **(piperaquine)**. Avoid. Moderate Study
- **Efavirenz** affects the exposure to antimalarials **(proguanil)**. Avoid. Moderate Study
- NNRTIs **(efavirenz, etravirine, nevirapine)** are predicted to decrease the exposure to atypical antipsychotics **(aripiprazole)**. Avoid or adjust dose—consult product literature. Moderate Study
- NNRTIs **(efavirenz, etravirine, nevirapine)** are predicted to decrease the exposure to atypical antipsychotics **(cariprazine)**. Avoid. Severe Theoretical
- NNRTIs **(efavirenz, etravirine, nevirapine)** are predicted to decrease the exposure to atypical antipsychotics **(lurasidone)**. Monitor and adjust dose. Moderate Theoretical
- NNRTIs **(efavirenz, etravirine, nevirapine)** are predicted to decrease the exposure to atypical antipsychotics **(quetiapine)**. Moderate Study
- NNRTIs **(efavirenz, etravirine, nevirapine)** are predicted to decrease the exposure to **avacopan**. Severe Theoretical
- NNRTIs **(efavirenz, etravirine, nevirapine)** are predicted to decrease the exposure to **avapritinib**. Avoid. Severe Study
- NNRTIs **(efavirenz, nevirapine)** are predicted to decrease the exposure to **axitinib**. Moderate Study
- NNRTIs **(efavirenz, etravirine, nevirapine)** are predicted to decrease the exposure to **bedaquiline**. Avoid. Severe Study → Also see TABLE 7 p. 1055
- NNRTIs **(efavirenz, nevirapine)** are predicted to decrease the concentration of benzodiazepines **(alprazolam)**. Moderate Theoretical
- **Etravirine** has been reported to increase the concentration of benzodiazepines **(clobazam)**. Moderate Anecdotal
- **Nevirapine** is predicted to decrease the concentration of benzodiazepines **(clonazepam)** and benzodiazepines **(clonazepam)** are predicted to decrease the concentration of **nevirapine**. Moderate Theoretical
- **Etravirine** is predicted to increase the exposure to benzodiazepines **(diazepam)**. Avoid. Severe Theoretical
- **Efavirenz** is predicted to alter the effects of benzodiazepines **(midazolam)**. Avoid. Moderate Theoretical
- **Nevirapine** decreases the concentration of benzodiazepines **(midazolam)**. Monitor and adjust dose. Moderate Study
- NNRTIs **(efavirenz, etravirine, nevirapine)** are predicted to decrease the exposure to **bosutinib**. Avoid. Severe Study → Also see TABLE 7 p. 1055
- NNRTIs **(efavirenz, etravirine, nevirapine)** are predicted to decrease the exposure to **brigatinib**. Avoid or adjust dose—consult product literature. Moderate Study
- **Efavirenz** is predicted to decrease the exposure to **bupropion**. Moderate Study
- NNRTIs **(efavirenz, etravirine, nevirapine)** are predicted to decrease the exposure to **cabozantinib**. Moderate Study → Also see TABLE 7 p. 1055
- Oral calcium compounds **(calcium carbonate)** -containing antacids are predicted to decrease the exposure to oral **rilpivirine**. Manufacturer advises take 4 hours before or 2 hours after antacids. Severe Theoretical
- NNRTIs **(efavirenz, etravirine, nevirapine)** are predicted to decrease the exposure to calcium-channel blockers **(amlodipine, felodipine, lacidipine, lercanidipine, nicardipine, nifedipine, nimodipine)**. Monitor and adjust dose. Moderate Theoretical
- NNRTIs **(efavirenz, etravirine, nevirapine)** are predicted to decrease the exposure to calcium-channel blockers **(diltiazem, verapamil)**. Moderate Theoretical
- NNRTIs **(efavirenz, etravirine, nevirapine)** are predicted to decrease the exposure to **capivasertib**. Avoid. Moderate Study
- **Efavirenz** is predicted to decrease the concentration of **caspofungin**. Adjust dose. Moderate Study
- **Nevirapine** is predicted to decrease the concentration of **caspofungin**. Adjust dose. Moderate Theoretical → Also see TABLE 1 p. 1053

NNRTIs (continued)

- **Cenobamate** is predicted to decrease the exposure to **rilpivirine**. Avoid. Severe Theoretical
- **Etravirine** is predicted to decrease the exposure to **ceritinib**. Severe Theoretical
- NNRTIs **(efavirenz, nevirapine)** are predicted to decrease the exposure to **ceritinib**. Severe Study → Also see TABLE 7 p. 1055
- **Efavirenz** decreases the concentration of **ciclosporin**. Monitor concentration and adjust dose. Moderate Study
- **Etravirine** is predicted to decrease the exposure to **ciclosporin**. Moderate Theoretical
- **Nevirapine** is predicted to decrease the concentration of **ciclosporin**. Moderate Study
- NNRTIs **(efavirenz, etravirine, nevirapine)** are predicted to decrease the exposure to **cobicistat**. Avoid. Severe Theoretical
- NNRTIs **(efavirenz, etravirine, nevirapine)** are predicted to decrease the exposure to **cobimetinib**. Avoid. Severe Theoretical
- **Etravirine** might decrease the efficacy of **combined hormonal contraceptives**. Follow CoSRH guidance for enzyme inducers, see Contraceptives, interactions p. 614. Severe Theoretical
- NNRTIs **(efavirenz, nevirapine)** are predicted to decrease the efficacy of **combined hormonal contraceptives**. For CoSRH guidance, see Contraceptives, interactions p. 614. Severe Study
- Corticosteroids **(dexamethasone)** are predicted to decrease the concentration of **rilpivirine**. Avoid multiple-dose dexamethasone. Severe Theoretical
- **Efavirenz** is predicted to affect the concentration of **coumarins**. Adjust dose. Moderate Theoretical
- **Etravirine** increases the anticoagulant effect of **coumarins**. Moderate Theoretical
- **Nevirapine** potentially alters the anticoagulant effect of **coumarins**. Severe Anecdotal
- NNRTIs **(efavirenz, etravirine, nevirapine)** are predicted to decrease the exposure to **crizotinib**. Avoid. Severe Study → Also see TABLE 7 p. 1055
- **Dabrafenib** is predicted to decrease the exposure to **doravirine**. Avoid or adjust doravirine or lamivudine with tenofovir disoproxil and doravirine dose. Severe Theoretical
- NNRTIs **(efavirenz, nevirapine)** are predicted to decrease the exposure to **dabrafenib**. Moderate Study
- **Dabrafenib** is predicted to decrease the exposure to **rilpivirine**. Avoid. Severe Theoretical
- NNRTIs **(efavirenz, etravirine, nevirapine)** are predicted to decrease the exposure to **daridorexant**. Severe Study
- NNRTIs **(efavirenz, etravirine, nevirapine)** are predicted to decrease the exposure to **dasatinib**. Severe Study → Also see TABLE 7 p. 1055
- **Etravirine** might decrease the efficacy of **desogestrel**. Follow CoSRH guidance for enzyme inducers, see Contraceptives, interactions p. 614. Severe Theoretical
- NNRTIs **(efavirenz, nevirapine)** are predicted to decrease the efficacy of **desogestrel**. For CoSRH guidance, see Contraceptives, interactions p. 614. Severe Theoretical
- NNRTIs **(efavirenz, etravirine, nevirapine)** are predicted to decrease the exposure to **deutivacaftor**. Avoid. Severe Theoretical
- **Efavirenz** moderately decreases the exposure to **dolutegravir**. Adjust **dolutegravir** dose, p. 508. Severe Study
- **Etravirine** moderately decreases the exposure to **dolutegravir**. Adjust **dolutegravir** dose unless given with atazanavir, darunavir, or lopinavir (all boosted with ritonavir), p. 508. Severe Study
- **Nevirapine** is predicted to decrease the exposure to **dolutegravir**. Adjust **dolutegravir** dose, p. 508. Severe Study
- **Etravirine** might decrease the efficacy of **drospirenone**. Follow CoSRH guidance for enzyme inducers, see Contraceptives, interactions p. 614. Severe Theoretical
- NNRTIs **(efavirenz, nevirapine)** are predicted to decrease the efficacy of **drospirenone**. For CoSRH guidance, see Contraceptives, interactions p. 614. Severe Theoretical
- NNRTIs **(efavirenz, etravirine, nevirapine)** are predicted to decrease the exposure to **elacestrant**. Avoid or adjust dose depending on duration—consult product literature. Severe Theoretical
- NNRTIs **(efavirenz, etravirine, nevirapine)** are predicted to moderately decrease the exposure to **elbasvir**. Avoid. Severe Study
- NNRTIs **(efavirenz, etravirine, nevirapine)** are predicted to decrease the exposure to **eliglustat**. Moderate Theoretical
- NNRTIs **(efavirenz, etravirine, nevirapine)** are predicted to decrease the concentration of **elvitegravir**. Avoid. Severe Theoretical
- **Encorafenib** is predicted to decrease the exposure to **doravirine**. Avoid. Severe Study
- **Encorafenib** is predicted to decrease the exposure to **etravirine**. Avoid. Severe Theoretical
- NNRTIs **(efavirenz, etravirine, nevirapine)** are predicted to decrease the exposure to **encorafenib**. Moderate Study → Also see TABLE 7 p. 1055
- **Encorafenib** markedly decreases the exposure to **rilpivirine**. Avoid. Severe Study
- Endothelin receptor antagonists **(bosentan)** are predicted to decrease the exposure to **doravirine**. Avoid or adjust doravirine or lamivudine with tenofovir disoproxil and doravirine dose. Severe Theoretical
- Endothelin receptor antagonists **(bosentan)** are predicted to decrease the exposure to **nevirapine**. Severe Theoretical
- Endothelin receptor antagonists **(bosentan)** are predicted to decrease the exposure to **rilpivirine**. Avoid. Severe Theoretical
- NNRTIs **(efavirenz, etravirine, nevirapine)** are predicted to decrease the exposure to **entrectinib**. Avoid. Moderate Theoretical → Also see TABLE 7 p. 1055
- NNRTIs **(efavirenz, etravirine, nevirapine)** are predicted to decrease the exposure to **erdafitinib**. Adjust dose. Moderate Theoretical
- NNRTIs **(efavirenz, etravirine, nevirapine)** are predicted to decrease the exposure to **erlotinib**. Severe Study
- NNRTIs **(efavirenz, nevirapine)** are predicted to decrease the efficacy of **estradiol**. Moderate Theoretical
- **Etravirine** might decrease the efficacy of **etonogestrel**. Follow CoSRH guidance for enzyme inducers, see Contraceptives, interactions p. 614. Severe Theoretical
- NNRTIs **(efavirenz, nevirapine)** are predicted to decrease the efficacy of **etonogestrel**. For CoSRH guidance, see Contraceptives, interactions p. 614. Severe Theoretical
- NNRTIs **(efavirenz, etravirine, nevirapine)** are predicted to decrease the concentration of **everolimus**. Avoid or adjust dose. Severe Study
- NNRTIs **(efavirenz, etravirine, nevirapine)** are predicted to decrease the exposure to **fedratinib**. Avoid. Moderate Study
- NNRTIs **(efavirenz, etravirine, nevirapine)** are predicted to decrease the exposure to **fruquintinib**. Avoid. Moderate Study
- NNRTIs **(efavirenz, etravirine, nevirapine)** are predicted to decrease the exposure to **gefitinib**. Avoid. Severe Study
- NNRTIs **(efavirenz, etravirine, nevirapine)** are predicted to decrease the exposure to **glasdegib**. Avoid or adjust dose—consult product literature. Moderate Theoretical → Also see TABLE 7 p. 1055
- NNRTIs **(efavirenz, etravirine, nevirapine)** are predicted to decrease the exposure to **glecaprevir**. Avoid. Severe Study
- NNRTIs **(efavirenz, etravirine, nevirapine)** are predicted to markedly decrease the exposure to **grazoprevir**. Avoid. Severe Study
- NNRTIs **(efavirenz, etravirine, nevirapine)** are predicted to decrease the concentration of **guanfacine**. Adjust dose. Moderate Theoretical
- H_2 **receptor antagonists** are predicted to decrease the exposure to **rilpivirine**. H_2 **receptor antagonists** should be taken 12 hours before or 4 hours after **rilpivirine**. Severe Study
- **Efavirenz** decreases the exposure to **HIV-protease inhibitors**. Refer to specialist literature. Severe Study
- **Etravirine** increases the exposure to HIV-protease inhibitors **(fosamprenavir)** boosted with ritonavir. Refer to specialist literature. Moderate Study
- **Nevirapine** decreases the exposure to **HIV-protease inhibitors**. Refer to specialist literature. Moderate Study → Also see TABLE 1 p. 1053
- NNRTIs **(efavirenz, nevirapine)** are predicted to decrease the effects of **hormone replacement therapy**. Moderate Anecdotal

- NNRTIs **(efavirenz, etravirine, nevirapine)** are predicted to decrease the exposure to **ibrutinib**. Avoid or monitor. Severe Study
- NNRTIs **(efavirenz, etravirine, nevirapine)** are predicted to decrease the exposure to **idelalisib**. Avoid. Moderate Theoretical
- NNRTIs **(efavirenz, etravirine, nevirapine)** are predicted to decrease the exposure to **imatinib**. Moderate Study
- NNRTIs **(efavirenz, nevirapine)** are predicted to decrease the exposure to **ivacaftor**. Moderate Study
- **Ivosidenib** is predicted to decrease the exposure to **doravirine**. Avoid. Severe Study
- **Ivosidenib** is predicted to decrease the exposure to **etravirine**. Avoid. Severe Theoretical
- **Ivosidenib** markedly decreases the exposure to **rilpivirine**. Avoid. Severe Study
- NNRTIs **(efavirenz, etravirine, nevirapine)** are predicted to decrease the exposure to **ixazomib**. Moderate Theoretical
- NNRTIs **(efavirenz, etravirine, nevirapine)** are predicted to decrease the exposure to **lapatinib**. Avoid. Severe Study → Also see TABLE 7 p. 1055
- NNRTIs **(efavirenz, etravirine, nevirapine)** are predicted to decrease the exposure to **larotrectinib**. Avoid. Moderate Study
- NNRTIs **(efavirenz, etravirine, nevirapine)** are predicted to decrease the exposure to **lenacapavir**. Avoid. Severe Study
- NNRTIs **(efavirenz, etravirine, nevirapine)** are predicted to decrease the exposure to **leniolisib**. Avoid. Severe Theoretical
- **Efavirenz** is predicted to decrease the concentration of **letermovir**. Moderate Theoretical
- **Etravirine** is predicted to decrease the exposure to **letermovir**. Moderate Theoretical
- **Etravirine** might decrease the efficacy of some contraceptive methods containing **levonorgestrel**. Follow CoSRH guidance for enzyme inducers, see Contraceptives, interactions p. 614. Severe Theoretical
- NNRTIs **(efavirenz, nevirapine)** are predicted to decrease the efficacy of some contraceptive methods containing **levonorgestrel**. For CoSRH guidance, see Contraceptives, interactions p. 614. Severe Theoretical
- **Lorlatinib** is predicted to decrease the exposure to **rilpivirine**. Avoid. Severe Theoretical
- **Lumacaftor** is predicted to decrease the exposure to **doravirine**. Avoid. Severe Study
- **Lumacaftor** is predicted to decrease the exposure to **etravirine**. Avoid. Severe Theoretical
- **Lumacaftor** markedly decreases the exposure to **rilpivirine**. Avoid. Severe Study
- Macrolides **(erythromycin)** are predicted to increase the exposure to **nevirapine**. Moderate Theoretical
- **Etravirine** decreases the exposure to macrolides **(clarithromycin)** and macrolides **(clarithromycin)** slightly increase the exposure to **etravirine**. Severe Study
- NNRTIs **(efavirenz, nevirapine)** decrease the exposure to macrolides **(clarithromycin)**. Moderate Study
- **Efavirenz** decreases the exposure to **maraviroc**. Refer to specialist literature. Severe Theoretical
- **Etravirine** slightly decreases the exposure to **maraviroc**. Refer to specialist literature. Moderate Study
- **Etravirine** is predicted to decrease the exposure to **maribavir**. Avoid or adjust **maribavir** dose. Severe Theoretical
- NNRTIs **(efavirenz, nevirapine)** are predicted to decrease the exposure to **maribavir**. Avoid or adjust **maribavir** dose. Severe Study
- NNRTIs **(efavirenz, etravirine, nevirapine)** are predicted to decrease the exposure to **mavacamten**. Monitor and adjust dose—consult product literature. Severe Theoretical
- NNRTIs **(efavirenz, etravirine, nevirapine)** are predicted to decrease the exposure to **midostaurin**. Severe Study
- NNRTIs **(efavirenz, etravirine, nevirapine)** are predicted to decrease the exposure to **mifepristone**. Adjust **mifepristone** dose. Severe Study
- NNRTIs **(efavirenz, etravirine, nevirapine)** are predicted to decrease the exposure to mineralocorticoid receptor antagonists **(finerenone)**. Avoid. Severe Study
- **Mitotane** is predicted to decrease the exposure to **doravirine**. Avoid. Severe Study
- **Mitotane** is predicted to decrease the exposure to **etravirine**. Avoid. Severe Theoretical
- **Mitotane** is predicted to decrease the exposure to **nevirapine**. Severe Theoretical
- **Mitotane** markedly decreases the exposure to **rilpivirine**. Avoid. Severe Study
- **Modafinil** is predicted to decrease the exposure to **doravirine**. Avoid or adjust doravirine or lamivudine with tenofovir disoproxil and doravirine dose. Severe Theoretical
- NNRTIs **(efavirenz, etravirine, nevirapine)** are predicted to decrease the exposure to **naloxegol**. Moderate Theoretical
- NNRTIs **(efavirenz, etravirine, nevirapine)** are predicted to decrease the exposure to **neratinib**. Avoid. Severe Theoretical → Also see TABLE 1 p. 1053
- NNRTIs **(efavirenz, etravirine, nevirapine)** are predicted to decrease the exposure to neurokinin-1 receptor antagonists **(aprepitant)**. Moderate Study
- NNRTIs **(efavirenz, nevirapine)** are predicted to decrease the exposure to neurokinin-1 receptor antagonists **(fosaprepitant, netupitant)**. Moderate Theoretical
- **Etravirine** is predicted to decrease the exposure to neurokinin-1 receptor antagonists **(netupitant)**. Moderate Theoretical
- NNRTIs **(efavirenz, etravirine, nevirapine)** are predicted to decrease the exposure to **nilotinib**. Avoid. Severe Theoretical → Also see TABLE 7 p. 1055
- **Nirmatrelvir** boosted with ritonavir is predicted to increase the concentration of NNRTIs **(efavirenz, nevirapine)**. Moderate Theoretical
- NNRTIs **(efavirenz, nevirapine)** are predicted to decrease the exposure to NNRTIs **(doravirine)**. Avoid or adjust doravirine or lamivudine with tenofovir disoproxil and doravirine dose. Severe Theoretical
- NNRTIs **(etravirine)** are predicted to decrease the exposure to NNRTIs **(doravirine)**. Avoid. Severe Theoretical
- NNRTIs **(nevirapine)** decrease the concentration of NNRTIs **(efavirenz)**. Avoid. Severe Study
- NNRTIs **(efavirenz, etravirine, nevirapine)** are predicted to decrease the exposure to NNRTIs **(rilpivirine)**. Avoid. Severe Theoretical
- **Etravirine** might decrease the efficacy of some contraceptive methods containing **norethisterone**. Follow CoSRH guidance for enzyme inducers, see Contraceptives, interactions p. 614. Severe Theoretical
- NNRTIs **(efavirenz, nevirapine)** are predicted to decrease the efficacy of some contraceptive methods containing **norethisterone**. For CoSRH guidance, see Contraceptives, interactions p. 614. Severe Anecdotal
- **Nevirapine** is predicted to slightly decrease the exposure to NRTIs **(zidovudine)**. Refer to specialist literature. Severe Theoretical → Also see TABLE 1 p. 1053
- NNRTIs **(efavirenz, etravirine, nevirapine)** are predicted to decrease the exposure to **olaparib**. Avoid. Moderate Theoretical
- NNRTIs **(efavirenz, etravirine, nevirapine)** are predicted to decrease the exposure to **omaveloxolone**. Avoid. Severe Study
- **Efavirenz** moderately decreases the exposure to opioids **(buprenorphine)**. Adjust dose. Moderate Study
- NNRTIs **(efavirenz, etravirine, nevirapine)** decrease the exposure to opioids **(methadone)**. Monitor and adjust dose. Severe Study → Also see TABLE 7 p. 1055
- **Etravirine** is predicted to decrease the exposure to **osimertinib**. Use with caution or avoid. Severe Theoretical
- NNRTIs **(efavirenz, nevirapine)** are predicted to decrease the exposure to **osimertinib**. Use with caution or avoid. Severe Study → Also see TABLE 7 p. 1055
- NNRTIs **(efavirenz, etravirine, nevirapine)** are predicted to decrease the exposure to **ospemifene**. Moderate Study
- NNRTIs **(efavirenz, etravirine, nevirapine)** are predicted to decrease the exposure to **pazopanib**. Severe Study → Also see TABLE 7 p. 1055
- **Efavirenz** is predicted to decrease the exposure to **pemigatinib** and **pemigatinib** might decrease the exposure to **efavirenz**. Avoid or monitor. Severe Study
- NNRTIs **(etravirine, nevirapine)** are predicted to decrease the exposure to **pemigatinib**. Avoid or monitor. Severe Study

NNRTIs (continued)
- **Etravirine** moderately decreases the exposure to **phosphodiesterase type-5 inhibitors**. Adjust dose. Moderate Study
- NNRTIs **(efavirenz, nevirapine)** are predicted to decrease the exposure to **phosphodiesterase type-5 inhibitors**. Moderate Theoretical → Also see TABLE 7 p. 1055
- NNRTIs **(efavirenz, etravirine, nevirapine)** are predicted to decrease the exposure to **pibrentasvir**. Avoid. Severe Study
- NNRTIs **(efavirenz, etravirine, nevirapine)** are predicted to decrease the exposure to **pirtobrutinib**. Moderate Theoretical
- **Pitolisant** is predicted to decrease the exposure to **efavirenz**. Mild Theoretical
- NNRTIs **(efavirenz, etravirine, nevirapine)** are predicted to decrease the exposure to **ponatinib**. Severe Study
- NNRTIs **(efavirenz, nevirapine)** are predicted to decrease the exposure to **pralsetinib**. Moderate Theoretical
- **Proton pump inhibitors** are predicted to decrease the exposure to oral **rilpivirine**. Avoid. Severe Study
- NNRTIs **(efavirenz, etravirine, nevirapine)** are predicted to decrease the exposure to **quizartinib**. Avoid. Severe Study → Also see TABLE 7 p. 1055
- NNRTIs **(efavirenz, etravirine, nevirapine)** are predicted to decrease the exposure to **regorafenib**. Severe Study
- **Efavirenz** is predicted to decrease the exposure to **relugolix**. Avoid or adjust dose depending on indication—consult product literature. Moderate Study
- NNRTIs **(efavirenz, etravirine, nevirapine)** are predicted to decrease the exposure to **ribociclib**. Moderate Study → Also see TABLE 7 p. 1055
- Rifamycins **(rifabutin)** moderately decrease the exposure to **doravirine**. Adjust doravirine or lamivudine with tenofovir disoproxil and doravirine dose. Moderate Study
- Rifamycins **(rifabutin)** decrease the exposure to **etravirine**. Moderate Study
- Rifamycins **(rifabutin)** modestly decrease the exposure to **rilpivirine**. Avoid or adjust dose—consult product literature. Severe Study
- Rifamycins **(rifampicin)** are predicted to decrease the exposure to **doravirine**. Avoid. Severe Study
- Rifamycins **(rifampicin)** slightly decrease the exposure to **efavirenz**. Adjust dose. Severe Study
- Rifamycins **(rifampicin)** are predicted to decrease the exposure to **etravirine**. Avoid. Severe Theoretical
- Rifamycins **(rifampicin)** decrease the concentration of **nevirapine**. Avoid. Severe Study
- Rifamycins **(rifampicin)** markedly decrease the exposure to **rilpivirine**. Avoid. Severe Study
- **Efavirenz** slightly decreases the exposure to rifamycins **(rifabutin)**. Adjust dose. Severe Study
- NNRTIs **(efavirenz, etravirine, nevirapine)** are predicted to decrease the exposure to **rimegepant**. Avoid. Moderate Theoretical
- NNRTIs **(efavirenz, etravirine, nevirapine)** are predicted to decrease the exposure to **ripretinib**. Avoid or adjust dose—consult product literature. Moderate Theoretical
- NNRTIs **(efavirenz, etravirine, nevirapine)** are predicted to decrease the exposure to **ruxolitinib**. Monitor and adjust dose. Moderate Study
- NNRTIs **(efavirenz, etravirine, nevirapine)** are predicted to decrease the exposure to **selpercatinib**. Moderate Study → Also see TABLE 7 p. 1055
- NNRTIs **(efavirenz, etravirine, nevirapine)** are predicted to decrease the exposure to **selumetinib**. Avoid. Severe Study
- NNRTIs **(efavirenz, etravirine, nevirapine)** are predicted to decrease the exposure to **siponimod**. Manufacturer advises caution depending on genotype—consult product literature. Moderate Theoretical
- **Doravirine** is predicted to decrease the exposure to **sirolimus**. Monitor **sirolimus** concentration and adjust dose, p. 641. Moderate Theoretical
- **Etravirine** is predicted to decrease the exposure to **sirolimus**. Monitor and adjust dose. Moderate Study
- NNRTIs **(efavirenz, nevirapine)** are predicted to decrease the concentration of **sirolimus**. Monitor and adjust dose. Moderate Theoretical
- Oral **sodium bicarbonate** -containing antacids are predicted to decrease the exposure to oral **rilpivirine**. Manufacturer advises take 4 hours before or 2 hours after antacids. Severe Theoretical
- **Efavirenz** is predicted to decrease the exposure to sodium glucose co-transporter 2 inhibitors **(canagliflozin)**. Adjust **canagliflozin** dose. Moderate Study
- **Sodium zirconium cyclosilicate** is predicted to decrease the exposure to **rilpivirine**. Separate administration by at least 2 hours. Moderate Theoretical
- NNRTIs **(efavirenz, etravirine, nevirapine)** are predicted to decrease the exposure to **sorafenib**. Moderate Study → Also see TABLE 7 p. 1055
- **Sotorasib** is predicted to decrease the exposure to **rilpivirine**. Avoid. Severe Theoretical
- NNRTIs **(efavirenz, etravirine, nevirapine)** are predicted to decrease the exposure to **sparsentan**. Avoid. Severe Theoretical
- **St John's wort** is predicted to decrease the exposure to NNRTIs **(doravirine, rilpivirine)**. Avoid. Severe Theoretical
- **St John's wort** is predicted to decrease the concentration of NNRTIs **(efavirenz, nevirapine)**. Avoid. Severe Theoretical
- NNRTIs **(efavirenz, etravirine, nevirapine)** are predicted to decrease the exposure to statins **(atorvastatin, simvastatin)**. Moderate Study → Also see TABLE 1 p. 1053
- **Etravirine** is predicted to increase the exposure to statins **(fluvastatin)**. Adjust dose. Severe Theoretical
- NNRTIs **(efavirenz, etravirine, nevirapine)** are predicted to decrease the exposure to **sunitinib**. Moderate Study → Also see TABLE 7 p. 1055
- **Doravirine** is predicted to decrease the exposure to **tacrolimus**. Monitor **tacrolimus** concentration and adjust dose, p. 642. Moderate Theoretical
- **Etravirine** is predicted to decrease the exposure to **tacrolimus**. Monitor and adjust dose. Moderate Theoretical
- NNRTIs **(efavirenz, nevirapine)** are predicted to decrease the concentration of **tacrolimus**. Monitor and adjust dose. Moderate Theoretical
- NNRTIs **(efavirenz, etravirine, nevirapine)** are predicted to decrease the exposure to taxanes **(cabazitaxel)**. Moderate Theoretical
- NNRTIs **(efavirenz, etravirine, nevirapine)** are predicted to decrease the exposure to taxanes **(docetaxel)**. Severe Theoretical
- NNRTIs **(efavirenz, etravirine, nevirapine)** are predicted to decrease the exposure to taxanes **(paclitaxel)**. Avoid. Severe Study
- **Telotristat ethyl** is predicted to decrease the exposure to **doravirine**. Avoid or adjust doravirine or lamivudine with tenofovir disoproxil and doravirine dose. Severe Theoretical
- NNRTIs **(efavirenz, etravirine, nevirapine)** are predicted to decrease the concentration of **temsirolimus**. Avoid. Moderate Theoretical
- NNRTIs **(efavirenz, etravirine, nevirapine)** are predicted to decrease the exposure to **tezacaftor**. Avoid. Severe Theoretical
- NNRTIs **(efavirenz, etravirine, nevirapine)** are predicted to decrease the exposure to **ticagrelor**. Moderate Theoretical
- NNRTIs **(efavirenz, etravirine, nevirapine)** are predicted to decrease the exposure to **tofacitinib**. Severe Study
- **Etravirine** might decrease the efficacy of **ulipristal**. Avoid and for 4 weeks after stopping the enzyme inducing drug. For CoSRH guidance, see Contraceptives, interactions p. 614. Severe Theoretical
- NNRTIs **(efavirenz, nevirapine)** decrease the efficacy of **ulipristal**. Avoid and for 4 weeks after stopping the enzyme inducing drug. For CoSRH guidance, see Contraceptives, interactions p. 614. Severe Anecdotal
- NNRTIs **(efavirenz, etravirine, nevirapine)** are predicted to decrease the exposure to **vandetanib**. Moderate Study → Also see TABLE 7 p. 1055
- NNRTIs **(efavirenz, etravirine, nevirapine)** are predicted to decrease the exposure to **vanzacaftor**. Avoid. Severe Theoretical
- NNRTIs **(efavirenz, etravirine, nevirapine)** are predicted to decrease the exposure to **velpatasvir**. Avoid. Moderate Theoretical

- NNRTIs (efavirenz, etravirine, nevirapine) are predicted to decrease the exposure to vemurafenib. Severe Study → Also see TABLE 7 p. 1055
- NNRTIs (efavirenz, etravirine, nevirapine) are predicted to decrease the exposure to venetoclax. Avoid. Severe Study
- NNRTIs (efavirenz, etravirine, nevirapine) are predicted to decrease the exposure to voclosporin. Avoid. Severe Theoretical → Also see TABLE 7 p. 1055
- NNRTIs (efavirenz, etravirine, nevirapine) are predicted to decrease the concentration of voxilaprevir. Avoid. Severe Theoretical
- NNRTIs (efavirenz, etravirine, nevirapine) are predicted to decrease the exposure to zanubrutinib. Avoid or adjust dose with moderate CYP3A4 inducers—consult product literature. Severe Theoretical

Noradrenaline → see sympathomimetics, vasoconstrictor

Norethisterone

- Antiepileptics (carbamazepine, eslicarbazepine, fosphenytoin, oxcarbazepine, perampanel, phenobarbital, phenytoin, primidone, rufinamide, topiramate) are predicted to decrease the efficacy of some contraceptive methods containing norethisterone. For CoSRH guidance, see Contraceptives, interactions p. 614. Severe Anecdotal
- Antiepileptics (lamotrigine) might decrease the effects of norethisterone. For CoSRH guidance, see Contraceptives, interactions p. 614. Moderate Theoretical
- Endothelin receptor antagonists (bosentan) are predicted to decrease the efficacy of some contraceptive methods containing norethisterone. For CoSRH guidance, see Contraceptives, interactions p. 614. Severe Anecdotal
- Glucagon-like peptide-1 receptor agonists (tirzepatide) might affect the absorption of oral norethisterone. Manufacturer advises precautions for those who are overweight or obese. Moderate Study
- HIV-protease inhibitors (ritonavir) are predicted to decrease the efficacy of some contraceptive methods containing norethisterone. For CoSRH guidance, see Contraceptives, interactions p. 614. Severe Anecdotal
- Lumacaftor might decrease the efficacy of norethisterone. Use additional contraceptive precautions. Severe Theoretical
- Modafinil is predicted to decrease the efficacy of some contraceptive methods containing norethisterone. For CoSRH guidance, see Contraceptives, interactions p. 614. Severe Anecdotal
- Neurokinin-1 receptor antagonists (aprepitant, fosaprepitant) are predicted to decrease the efficacy of some contraceptive methods containing norethisterone. For CoSRH guidance, see Contraceptives, interactions p. 614. Severe Anecdotal
- NNRTIs (efavirenz, nevirapine) are predicted to decrease the efficacy of some contraceptive methods containing norethisterone. For CoSRH guidance, see Contraceptives, interactions p. 614. Severe Anecdotal
- NNRTIs (etravirine) might decrease the efficacy of some contraceptive methods containing norethisterone. Follow CoSRH guidance for enzyme inducers, see Contraceptives, interactions p. 614. Severe Theoretical
- Rifamycins are predicted to decrease the efficacy of some contraceptive methods containing norethisterone. For CoSRH guidance, see Contraceptives, interactions p. 614. Severe Anecdotal
- St John's wort is predicted to decrease the efficacy of norethisterone. MHRA advises avoid. For CoSRH guidance, see Contraceptives, interactions p. 614. Severe Anecdotal
- Sugammadex is predicted to decrease the exposure to norethisterone. Use additional contraceptive precautions. Severe Theoretical
- Norethisterone might decrease the efficacy of ulipristal and ulipristal might decrease the efficacy of norethisterone. Avoid when used for uterine fibroids. For CoSRH guidance when used for emergency hormonal contraception, see Contraceptives, interactions p. 614. Severe Theoretical

Normal immunoglobulin → see immunoglobulins

Nortriptyline → see tricyclic antidepressants

NRTIs → see TABLE 1 p. 1053 (hepatotoxicity), TABLE 10 p. 1056 (peripheral neuropathy)

abacavir · emtricitabine · lamivudine · zidovudine

- Antiepileptics (carbamazepine, fosphenytoin, phenobarbital, phenytoin, primidone) are predicted to decrease the exposure to abacavir. Moderate Theoretical
- Antiepileptics (valproate) slightly increase the exposure to zidovudine. Moderate Study → Also see TABLE 1 p. 1053
- Antifungals, azoles (fluconazole) slightly increase the exposure to zidovudine. Moderate Study → Also see TABLE 1 p. 1053
- Antimalarials (pyrimethamine) are predicted to increase the risk of adverse effects when given with zidovudine. Severe Theoretical
- Zidovudine increases the risk of haematological toxicity when given with aspirin (high-dose). Severe Study
- Zidovudine increases the risk of haematological toxicity when given with flucytosine. Monitor and adjust dose. Severe Theoretical
- Leflunomide is predicted to increase the exposure to zidovudine. Moderate Theoretical
- Macrolides (clarithromycin) decrease the absorption of zidovudine. Separate administration by 4 hours. Moderate Study
- NNRTIs (nevirapine) are predicted to slightly decrease the exposure to zidovudine. Refer to specialist literature. Severe Theoretical → Also see TABLE 1 p. 1053
- NRTIs (zidovudine) increase the risk of toxicity when given with NRTIs (lamivudine). Severe Anecdotal
- Zidovudine increases the risk of haematological toxicity when given with NSAIDs. Severe Study
- Ribavirin increases the risk of anaemia and/or leucopenia when given with zidovudine. Avoid. Severe Study
- Abacavir might increase the exposure to riociguat. Adjust dose and monitor blood pressure. Moderate Study
- Teriflunomide is predicted to increase the exposure to zidovudine. Moderate Theoretical
- Trimethoprim slightly increases the exposure to lamivudine. Moderate Study
- Vadadustat is predicted to increase the exposure to zidovudine. Monitor and adjust dose. Moderate Study

NSAIDs → see TABLE 3 p. 1053 (bleeding), TABLE 15 p. 1058 (hyponatraemia), TABLE 2 p. 1053 (nephrotoxicity), TABLE 13 p. 1057 (increased serum potassium)

aceclofenac · benzydamine · bromfenac · celecoxib · dexketoprofen · diclofenac · etodolac · etoricoxib · flurbiprofen · ibuprofen · indometacin · ketoprofen · ketorolac · mefenamic acid · meloxicam · nabumetone · naproxen · nepafenac · parecoxib · phenazone · piroxicam · sulindac · tenoxicam · tiaprofenic acid · tolfenamic acid

ROUTE-SPECIFIC INFORMATION Since systemic absorption can follow topical application of NSAIDs, the possibility of interactions should be borne in mind.

- Celecoxib is predicted to increase the exposure to antiarrhythmics (flecainide, propafenone). Monitor and adjust dose. Moderate Theoretical
- Antifungals, azoles (fluconazole) moderately increase the exposure to celecoxib. Adjust celecoxib dose. Moderate Study
- Antifungals, azoles (fluconazole) increase the exposure to parecoxib. Monitor and adjust dose. Moderate Study
- Antifungals, azoles (voriconazole) slightly increase the exposure to diclofenac. Monitor and adjust dose. Moderate Study
- Antifungals, azoles (voriconazole) moderately increase the exposure to ibuprofen. Adjust dose. Moderate Study
- Diclofenac might increase the exposure to the active metabolite of antimalarials (artesunate). Avoid. Unknown Theoretical
- NSAIDs are predicted to increase the risk of gastrointestinal irritation when given with bisphosphonates (alendronate, ibandronate). Moderate Study
- NSAIDs are predicted to increase the risk of renal impairment when given with bisphosphonates (clodronate). Moderate Study
- Ceritinib is predicted to increase the exposure to NSAIDs (celecoxib, diclofenac). Adjust dose. Moderate Theoretical
- Ciclosporin increases the concentration of diclofenac. Severe Study → Also see TABLE 2 p. 1053 → Also see TABLE 13 p. 1057
- Sulindac might increase the exposure to cladribine. Avoid or adjust dose. Moderate Theoretical

NSAIDs (continued)
- **Etoricoxib** increases the exposure to **combined hormonal contraceptives.** Moderate Study
- **NSAIDs** increase the risk of gastrointestinal bleeding when given with **corticosteroids.** Severe Study
- **NSAIDs** increase the risk of renal impairment when given with **daptomycin.** Moderate Theoretical
- **Indometacin** increases the concentration of **digoxin.** Severe Study
- **NSAIDs** (high-dose) might cause ototoxicity, as can **drugs that cause ototoxicity** (see TABLE 16 p. 1058); concurrent use might increase the risk of developing this effect. Moderate Theoretical
- **Erlotinib** is predicted to increase the risk of gastrointestinal perforation when given with **NSAIDs.** Severe Theoretical
- **Etoricoxib** increases the exposure to **hormone replacement therapy.** Moderate Study
- **NSAIDs** are predicted to increase the risk of gastrointestinal bleeding when given with iron chelators **(deferasirox).** Severe Theoretical → Also see TABLE 2 p. 1053
- **Diclofenac** is predicted to increase the exposure to iron chelators **(deferiprone).** Moderate Theoretical
- **Leflunomide** is predicted to increase the exposure to NSAIDs **(indometacin, ketoprofen).** Moderate Theoretical
- **NSAIDs** increase the concentration of **lithium.** Monitor and adjust dose. Severe Study → Also see TABLE 2 p. 1053
- **NSAIDs** are predicted to increase the risk of toxicity when given with **methotrexate** (particularly high-dose). Severe Study → Also see TABLE 2 p. 1053
- **NSAIDs** (high-dose) are predicted to decrease the efficacy of **mifamurtide.** Avoid. Severe Theoretical
- **Nicorandil** is predicted to increase the risk of gastrointestinal perforation when given with **NSAIDs.** Severe Theoretical
- **Nitisinone** is predicted to increase the exposure to **celecoxib.** Moderate Study
- NRTIs **(zidovudine)** increase the risk of haematological toxicity when given with **NSAIDs.** Severe Study
- **NSAIDs** are predicted to increase the exposure to **pemetrexed.** Use with caution or avoid. Severe Theoretical → Also see TABLE 2 p. 1053
- **NSAIDs** potentially increase the risk of seizures when given with **quinolones.** Severe Theoretical
- **Mefenamic acid** is predicted to increase the exposure to **regorafenib.** Avoid. Moderate Theoretical → Also see TABLE 3 p. 1053
- Rifamycins **(rifampicin)** moderately decrease the exposure to NSAIDs **(celecoxib, diclofenac, etoricoxib).** Moderate Study → Also see TABLE 2 p. 1053
- **Sparsentan** is predicted to decrease the exposure to NSAIDs **(celecoxib, ibuprofen).** Moderate Theoretical → Also see TABLE 13 p. 1057
- **Teriflunomide** is predicted to increase the exposure to NSAIDs **(indometacin, ketoprofen).** Moderate Theoretical
- **NSAIDs** increase the risk of acute renal failure when given with **thiazide diuretics.** Severe Theoretical → Also see TABLE 15 p. 1058
- **Indometacin** might prolong the antidiuretic effect of **vasopressin.** Moderate Study

Obeticholic acid
- **Obeticholic acid** decreases the anticoagulant effect of coumarins **(warfarin).** Severe Study
- **Obeticholic acid** is predicted to increase the exposure to **theophylline.** Severe Theoretical
- **Obeticholic acid** is predicted to increase the exposure to **tizanidine.** Severe Theoretical

Obinutuzumab → see monoclonal antibodies

Ocrelizumab → see monoclonal antibodies

Octreotide
- **Octreotide** decreases the absorption of oral **ciclosporin.** Adjust ciclosporin dose, p. 640. Severe Anecdotal
- **Octreotide** (short-acting) decreases the exposure to **telotristat ethyl. Telotristat ethyl** should be taken at least 30 minutes before **octreotide.** Moderate Study

Ofatumumab → see monoclonal antibodies

Ofloxacin → see quinolones

Olanzapine → see atypical antipsychotics

Olaparib → see TABLE 12 p. 1057 (myelosuppression)

FOOD AND LIFESTYLE Bitter (Seville) orange is predicted to increase the exposure to olaparib.

- **Olaparib** might increase the exposure to **aliskiren.** Moderate Theoretical
- Anti-androgens **(apalutamide, enzalutamide)** are predicted to decrease the exposure to **olaparib.** Avoid. Moderate Theoretical
- Antiarrhythmics **(dronedarone)** are predicted to increase the exposure to **olaparib.** Avoid or adjust dose with moderate CYP3A4 inhibitors—consult product literature. Moderate Theoretical
- Antiepileptics **(carbamazepine, fosphenytoin, phenobarbital, phenytoin, primidone)** are predicted to decrease the exposure to **olaparib.** Avoid. Moderate Theoretical
- Antifungals, azoles **(fluconazole, isavuconazole)** are predicted to increase the exposure to **olaparib.** Avoid or adjust dose with moderate CYP3A4 inhibitors—consult product literature. Moderate Theoretical
- Antifungals, azoles **(itraconazole, ketoconazole, posaconazole, voriconazole)** are predicted to increase the exposure to **olaparib.** Avoid or adjust dose with potent CYP3A4 inhibitors—consult product literature. Moderate Study
- **Olaparib** might increase the exposure to antihistamines, non-sedating **(fexofenadine).** Moderate Theoretical
- **Olaparib** might alter the exposure to atypical antipsychotics **(quetiapine).** Moderate Theoretical
- **Berotralstat** is predicted to increase the exposure to **olaparib.** Avoid or adjust dose with moderate CYP3A4 inhibitors—consult product literature. Moderate Theoretical
- Calcium-channel blockers **(diltiazem, verapamil)** are predicted to increase the exposure to **olaparib.** Avoid or adjust dose with moderate CYP3A4 inhibitors—consult product literature. Moderate Theoretical
- **Cenobamate** is predicted to decrease the exposure to **olaparib.** Avoid. Moderate Theoretical
- **Ceritinib** is predicted to increase the exposure to **olaparib.** Avoid or adjust dose with potent CYP3A4 inhibitors—consult product literature. Moderate Study → Also see TABLE 12 p. 1057
- **Olaparib** might alter the exposure to **ciclosporin.** Moderate Theoretical
- **Cobicistat** is predicted to increase the exposure to **olaparib.** Avoid or adjust dose with potent CYP3A4 inhibitors—consult product literature. Moderate Study
- **Olaparib** might increase the exposure to **colchicine.** Moderate Theoretical
- **Olaparib** potentially affects the efficacy of **combined hormonal contraceptives.** Use additional contraceptive precautions. Moderate Theoretical
- **Crizotinib** is predicted to increase the exposure to **olaparib.** Avoid or adjust dose with moderate CYP3A4 inhibitors—consult product literature. Moderate Theoretical
- **Dabrafenib** is predicted to decrease the exposure to **olaparib.** Avoid. Moderate Theoretical
- **Olaparib** might increase the exposure to **digoxin.** Moderate Theoretical
- **Encorafenib** is predicted to decrease the exposure to **olaparib.** Avoid. Moderate Theoretical
- Endothelin receptor antagonists **(bosentan)** are predicted to decrease the exposure to **olaparib.** Avoid. Moderate Theoretical
- **Olaparib** might alter the exposure to **ergometrine.** Moderate Theoretical
- **Olaparib** might increase the exposure to **everolimus.** Moderate Theoretical
- **Olaparib** might increase the exposure to factor XA inhibitors **(edoxaban).** Moderate Theoretical
- **Fedratinib** is predicted to increase the exposure to **olaparib.** Avoid or adjust dose with moderate CYP3A4 inhibitors—consult product literature. Moderate Theoretical
- **Grapefruit** juice is predicted to increase the exposure to **olaparib.** Avoid. Moderate Theoretical
- **HIV-protease inhibitors** are predicted to increase the exposure to **olaparib.** Avoid or adjust dose with potent CYP3A4 inhibitors—consult product literature. Moderate Study

- **Idelalisib** is predicted to increase the exposure to **olaparib**. Avoid or adjust dose with potent CYP3A4 inhibitors—consult product literature. [Moderate] Study
- **Imatinib** is predicted to increase the exposure to **olaparib**. Avoid or adjust dose with moderate CYP3A4 inhibitors—consult product literature. [Moderate] Theoretical → Also see TABLE 12 p. 1057
- **Ivosidenib** is predicted to decrease the exposure to **olaparib**. Avoid. [Moderate] Theoretical
- **Letermovir** is predicted to increase the exposure to **olaparib**. Avoid or adjust dose with moderate CYP3A4 inhibitors—consult product literature. [Moderate] Theoretical
- **Olaparib** might increase the exposure to **loperamide**. [Moderate] Theoretical
- **Lorlatinib** is predicted to decrease the exposure to **olaparib**. Avoid. [Moderate] Theoretical
- **Lumacaftor** is predicted to decrease the exposure to **olaparib**. Avoid. [Moderate] Theoretical
- Macrolides **(clarithromycin)** are predicted to increase the exposure to **olaparib**. Avoid or adjust dose with potent CYP3A4 inhibitors—consult product literature. [Moderate] Study
- Macrolides **(erythromycin)** are predicted to increase the exposure to **olaparib**. Avoid or adjust dose with moderate CYP3A4 inhibitors—consult product literature. [Moderate] Theoretical
- **Mitotane** is predicted to decrease the exposure to **olaparib**. Avoid. [Moderate] Theoretical → Also see TABLE 12 p. 1057
- Neurokinin-1 receptor antagonists **(aprepitant, netupitant)** are predicted to increase the exposure to **olaparib**. Avoid or adjust dose with moderate CYP3A4 inhibitors—consult product literature. [Moderate] Theoretical
- **Nilotinib** is predicted to increase the exposure to **olaparib**. Avoid or adjust dose with moderate CYP3A4 inhibitors—consult product literature. [Moderate] Theoretical → Also see TABLE 12 p. 1057
- NNRTIs **(efavirenz, etravirine, nevirapine)** are predicted to decrease the exposure to **olaparib**. Avoid. [Moderate] Theoretical
- **Olaparib** might alter the exposure to opioids **(alfentanil)**. [Moderate] Theoretical
- **Olaparib** might alter the exposure to **pimozide**. [Moderate] Theoretical
- **Olaparib** might increase the exposure to **pralsetinib**. [Moderate] Theoretical
- **Olaparib** might increase the exposure to **ranolazine**. [Moderate] Theoretical
- Rifamycins **(rifampicin)** are predicted to decrease the exposure to **olaparib**. Avoid. [Moderate] Theoretical
- **Olaparib** might increase the exposure to **rimegepant**. [Moderate] Theoretical
- **Olaparib** might increase the exposure to **sirolimus**. [Moderate] Theoretical
- **Sotorasib** is predicted to decrease the exposure to **olaparib**. Avoid. [Moderate] Theoretical
- **St John's wort** is predicted to decrease the exposure to **olaparib**. Avoid. [Moderate] Theoretical
- **Olaparib** is predicted to increase the exposure to **statins**. [Moderate] Theoretical
- **Olaparib** might alter the exposure to **tacrolimus**. [Moderate] Theoretical
- **Olaparib** might increase the exposure to **talazoparib**. [Moderate] Theoretical → Also see TABLE 12 p. 1057
- **Olaparib** might increase the exposure to taxanes **(paclitaxel)**. [Moderate] Theoretical → Also see TABLE 12 p. 1057
- **Olaparib** might alter the exposure to **temsirolimus**. [Moderate] Theoretical → Also see TABLE 12 p. 1057
- **Olaparib** might increase the exposure to thrombin inhibitors **(dabigatran)**. [Moderate] Theoretical
- **Tucatinib** is predicted to increase the exposure to **olaparib**. Avoid or adjust dose with potent CYP3A4 inhibitors—consult product literature. [Moderate] Study

Olmesartan → see angiotensin-II receptor antagonists

Olodaterol → see beta$_2$ agonists

Omaveloxolone

- Anti-androgens **(apalutamide, enzalutamide)** are predicted to decrease the exposure to **omaveloxolone**. Avoid. [Severe] Study
- Antiarrhythmics **(dronedarone)** are predicted to increase the exposure to **omaveloxolone**. Avoid or adjust **omaveloxolone** dose, p. 755. [Moderate] Study
- Antiepileptics **(carbamazepine, fosphenytoin, phenobarbital, phenytoin, primidone)** are predicted to decrease the exposure to **omaveloxolone**. Avoid. [Severe] Study
- Antifungals, azoles **(fluconazole, isavuconazole)** are predicted to increase the exposure to **omaveloxolone**. Avoid or adjust **omaveloxolone** dose, p. 755. [Moderate] Study
- Antifungals, azoles **(itraconazole, ketoconazole, posaconazole, voriconazole)** are predicted to increase the exposure to **omaveloxolone**. Avoid or adjust **omaveloxolone** dose, p. 755. [Severe] Study
- **Berotralstat** is predicted to increase the exposure to **omaveloxolone**. Avoid or adjust **omaveloxolone** dose, p. 755. [Moderate] Study
- Calcium-channel blockers **(diltiazem, verapamil)** are predicted to increase the exposure to **omaveloxolone**. Avoid or adjust **omaveloxolone** dose, p. 755. [Moderate] Study
- **Cenobamate** is predicted to decrease the exposure to **omaveloxolone**. Avoid. [Severe] Study
- **Ceritinib** is predicted to increase the exposure to **omaveloxolone**. Avoid or adjust **omaveloxolone** dose, p. 755. [Severe] Study
- **Ciclosporin** is predicted to increase the exposure to **omaveloxolone**. Avoid or adjust **omaveloxolone** dose, p. 755. [Moderate] Theoretical
- **Cobicistat** is predicted to increase the exposure to **omaveloxolone**. Avoid or adjust **omaveloxolone** dose, p. 755. [Severe] Study
- **Omaveloxolone** might decrease the efficacy of **combined hormonal contraceptives**. Avoid. [Severe] Theoretical
- **Crizotinib** is predicted to increase the exposure to **omaveloxolone**. Avoid or adjust **omaveloxolone** dose, p. 755. [Moderate] Study
- **Dabrafenib** is predicted to decrease the exposure to **omaveloxolone**. Avoid. [Severe] Study
- **Encorafenib** is predicted to decrease the exposure to **omaveloxolone**. Avoid. [Severe] Study
- Endothelin receptor antagonists **(bosentan)** are predicted to decrease the exposure to **omaveloxolone**. Avoid. [Severe] Study
- **Fedratinib** is predicted to increase the exposure to **omaveloxolone**. Avoid or adjust **omaveloxolone** dose, p. 755. [Moderate] Study
- **Grapefruit** juice is predicted to increase the exposure to **omaveloxolone**. Avoid. [Moderate] Theoretical
- **HIV-protease inhibitors** are predicted to increase the exposure to **omaveloxolone**. Avoid or adjust **omaveloxolone** dose, p. 755. [Severe] Study
- **Idelalisib** is predicted to increase the exposure to **omaveloxolone**. Avoid or adjust **omaveloxolone** dose, p. 755. [Severe] Study
- **Imatinib** is predicted to increase the exposure to **omaveloxolone**. Avoid or adjust **omaveloxolone** dose, p. 755. [Moderate] Study
- **Ivosidenib** is predicted to decrease the exposure to **omaveloxolone**. Avoid. [Severe] Study
- **Letermovir** is predicted to increase the exposure to **omaveloxolone**. Avoid or adjust **omaveloxolone** dose, p. 755. [Moderate] Study
- **Lorlatinib** is predicted to decrease the exposure to **omaveloxolone**. Avoid. [Severe] Study
- **Lumacaftor** is predicted to decrease the exposure to **omaveloxolone**. Avoid. [Severe] Study
- Macrolides **(clarithromycin)** are predicted to increase the exposure to **omaveloxolone**. Avoid or adjust **omaveloxolone** dose, p. 755. [Severe] Study
- Macrolides **(erythromycin)** are predicted to increase the exposure to **omaveloxolone**. Avoid or adjust **omaveloxolone** dose, p. 755. [Moderate] Study
- **Mitotane** is predicted to decrease the exposure to **omaveloxolone**. Avoid. [Severe] Study
- Neurokinin-1 receptor antagonists **(aprepitant, netupitant)** are predicted to increase the exposure to **omaveloxolone**. Avoid or adjust **omaveloxolone** dose, p. 755. [Moderate] Study

Omaveloxolone (continued)
- **Nilotinib** is predicted to increase the exposure to **omaveloxolone**. Avoid or adjust **omaveloxolone** dose, p. 755. Moderate Study
- NNRTIs **(efavirenz, etravirine, nevirapine)** are predicted to decrease the exposure to **omaveloxolone**. Avoid. Severe Study
- Quinolones **(ciprofloxacin)** are predicted to increase the exposure to **omaveloxolone**. Avoid or adjust **omaveloxolone** dose, p. 755. Moderate Theoretical
- Rifamycins **(rifampicin)** are predicted to decrease the exposure to **omaveloxolone**. Avoid. Severe Study
- **Sotorasib** is predicted to decrease the exposure to **omaveloxolone**. Avoid. Severe Study
- SSRIs **(fluvoxamine)** are predicted to increase the exposure to **omaveloxolone**. Avoid or adjust **omaveloxolone** dose, p. 755. Moderate Theoretical
- **St John's wort** is predicted to decrease the exposure to **omaveloxolone**. Avoid. Severe Study
- **Tucatinib** is predicted to increase the exposure to **omaveloxolone**. Avoid or adjust **omaveloxolone** dose, p. 755. Severe Study

Omega-3-acid ethyl esters → see TABLE 3 p. 1053 (bleeding)
- **Omega-3-acid ethyl esters** might enhance the blood pressure-lowering effects of **beta blockers, non-selective**. Moderate Study
- **Omega-3-acid ethyl esters** might enhance the blood pressure-lowering effects of **beta blockers, selective**. Moderate Study

Omeprazole → see proton pump inhibitors

Ondansetron → see 5-HT3-receptor antagonists

Opicapone
- **Opicapone** might increase the exposure to the active metabolite of **foslevodopa**. Adjust dose. Moderate Theoretical
- **Opicapone** is predicted to increase the risk of cardiovascular adverse effects when given with **isoprenaline**. Moderate Theoretical
- **Opicapone** increases the exposure to **levodopa**. Adjust dose. Moderate Study
- **Opicapone** is predicted to increase the exposure to **loperamide**. Avoid. Moderate Study
- **Opicapone** is predicted to increase the risk of elevated blood pressure when given with **MAOIs, irreversible**. Avoid. Severe Theoretical
- **Opicapone** is predicted to increase the exposure to meglitinides **(repaglinide)**. Avoid. Moderate Study
- **Opicapone** is predicted to increase the risk of elevated blood pressure when given with **moclobemide**. Avoid. Severe Theoretical
- **Opicapone** is predicted to increase the exposure to **montelukast**. Avoid. Moderate Study
- **Opicapone** is predicted to increase the exposure to **pioglitazone**. Avoid. Moderate Study
- **Opicapone** is predicted to increase the risk of cardiovascular adverse effects when given with **sympathomimetics, inotropic**. Severe Theoretical
- **Opicapone** is predicted to increase the risk of cardiovascular adverse effects when given with sympathomimetics, vasoconstrictor **(adrenaline, noradrenaline)**. Severe Theoretical

Opioids → see TABLE 4 p. 1054 (bradycardia), TABLE 15 p. 1058 (hyponatraemia), TABLE 11 p. 1056 (serotonin toxicity), TABLE 7 p. 1055 (QT-interval prolongation), TABLE 9 p. 1056 (CNS effects)

alfentanil · buprenorphine · codeine · diamorphine · dihydrocodeine · diphenoxylate · dipipanone · fentanyl · hydromorphone · meptazinol · methadone · morphine · oxycodone · pentazocine · pethidine · remifentanil · sufentanil · tapentadol · tramadol

- **Alcohol** causes rapid release of opioids **(hydromorphone, morphine)** from extended-release preparations. Avoid. Severe Study → Also see TABLE 9 p. 1056
- Anti-androgens **(apalutamide, enzalutamide)** are predicted to decrease the exposure to **buprenorphine**. Monitor and adjust dose. Moderate Theoretical
- Anti-androgens **(apalutamide, enzalutamide)** decrease the exposure to **methadone**. Monitor and adjust dose. Severe Study → Also see TABLE 7 p. 1055
- Anti-androgens **(apalutamide, enzalutamide)** are predicted to decrease the exposure to **oxycodone**. Monitor and adjust dose. Moderate Study
- Anti-androgens **(enzalutamide)** are predicted to affect the exposure to **tramadol**. Use with caution or avoid. Moderate Theoretical
- Anti-androgens **(apalutamide, enzalutamide)** are predicted to decrease the exposure to opioids **(alfentanil, fentanyl)**. Moderate Study
- Antiarrhythmics **(amiodarone)** are predicted to increase the concentration of **fentanyl**. Monitor and adjust dose. Moderate Theoretical → Also see TABLE 4 p. 1054
- Antiarrhythmics **(dronedarone)** are predicted to increase the exposure to opioids **(alfentanil, buprenorphine, fentanyl, oxycodone)**. Monitor and adjust dose. Moderate Study → Also see TABLE 4 p. 1054
- Antiarrhythmics **(dronedarone)** are predicted to increase the exposure to opioids **(methadone, sufentanil)**. Moderate Theoretical → Also see TABLE 4 p. 1054 → Also see TABLE 7 p. 1055
- Antiepileptics **(carbamazepine)** decrease the concentration of **tramadol**. Adjust dose. Severe Study → Also see TABLE 15 p. 1058
- Antiepileptics **(carbamazepine, fosphenytoin, phenobarbital, phenytoin, primidone)** are predicted to decrease the exposure to **buprenorphine**. Monitor and adjust dose. Moderate Theoretical → Also see TABLE 9 p. 1056
- Antiepileptics **(carbamazepine, fosphenytoin, phenobarbital, phenytoin, primidone)** decrease the exposure to **methadone**. Monitor and adjust dose. Severe Study → Also see TABLE 9 p. 1056
- Antiepileptics **(carbamazepine, fosphenytoin, phenobarbital, phenytoin, primidone)** are predicted to decrease the exposure to **oxycodone**. Monitor and adjust dose. Moderate Study → Also see TABLE 9 p. 1056
- Antiepileptics **(carbamazepine, fosphenytoin, phenobarbital, phenytoin, primidone)** are predicted to decrease the exposure to opioids **(alfentanil, fentanyl)**. Moderate Study → Also see TABLE 9 p. 1056
- Antifungals, azoles **(itraconazole, ketoconazole, posaconazole, voriconazole)** are predicted to increase the exposure to **sufentanil**. Moderate Study
- Antifungals, azoles **(itraconazole, ketoconazole, voriconazole)** are predicted to increase the exposure to **methadone**. Adjust dose. Severe Theoretical → Also see TABLE 7 p. 1055
- Antifungals, azoles **(miconazole)** are predicted to increase the exposure to **alfentanil**. Use with caution and adjust dose. Moderate Theoretical
- Antifungals, azoles **(fluconazole, isavuconazole)** are predicted to increase the exposure to opioids **(alfentanil, buprenorphine, fentanyl, oxycodone)**. Monitor and adjust dose. Moderate Study
- Antifungals, azoles **(itraconazole, ketoconazole, posaconazole, voriconazole)** are predicted to increase the exposure to opioids **(alfentanil, buprenorphine, fentanyl, oxycodone)**. Monitor and adjust dose. Severe Study
- Antifungals, azoles **(fluconazole, isavuconazole)** are predicted to increase the exposure to opioids **(methadone, sufentanil)**. Moderate Theoretical → Also see TABLE 7 p. 1055
- **Asciminib** is predicted to increase the exposure to **alfentanil**. Severe Theoretical
- Atypical antipsychotics **(clozapine)** can cause constipation, as can **opioids**; concurrent use might increase the risk of developing intestinal obstruction. Severe Anecdotal → Also see TABLE 15 p. 1058 → Also see TABLE 9 p. 1056
- **Berotralstat** is predicted to increase the exposure to opioids **(alfentanil, buprenorphine, fentanyl, oxycodone)**. Monitor and adjust dose. Moderate Study
- **Berotralstat** is predicted to increase the exposure to opioids **(methadone, sufentanil)**. Moderate Theoretical
- **Brigatinib** potentially decreases the concentration of opioids **(alfentanil, fentanyl)**. Avoid. Moderate Theoretical → Also see TABLE 4 p. 1054
- **Bulevirtide** is predicted to increase the exposure to **alfentanil**. Moderate Theoretical
- **Bupropion** is predicted to decrease the efficacy of **codeine**. Moderate Theoretical
- **Bupropion** is predicted to decrease the efficacy of **tramadol**. Severe Study
- Calcium-channel blockers **(nicardipine)** are predicted to increase the exposure to **fentanyl**. Monitor and adjust dose. Moderate Theoretical

- Calcium-channel blockers **(diltiazem, verapamil)** are predicted to increase the exposure to opioids **(alfentanil, buprenorphine, fentanyl, oxycodone)**. Monitor and adjust dose. [Moderate] Study → Also see TABLE 4 p. 1054
- Calcium-channel blockers **(diltiazem, verapamil)** are predicted to increase the exposure to opioids **(methadone, sufentanil)**. [Moderate] Theoretical → Also see TABLE 4 p. 1054
- **Cenobamate** is predicted to decrease the exposure to **alfentanil**. Adjust dose. [Moderate] Theoretical → Also see TABLE 9 p. 1056
- **Cenobamate** decreases the exposure to **methadone**. Monitor and adjust dose. [Severe] Study → Also see TABLE 9 p. 1056
- **Ceritinib** is predicted to increase the exposure to opioids **(alfentanil, buprenorphine, fentanyl, oxycodone)**. Monitor and adjust dose. [Severe] Study → Also see TABLE 4 p. 1054
- **Ceritinib** is predicted to increase the exposure to **sufentanil**. [Moderate] Study → Also see TABLE 4 p. 1054
- **Cinacalcet** is predicted to decrease the efficacy of **codeine**. [Moderate] Theoretical
- **Cinacalcet** is predicted to decrease the efficacy of **tramadol**. [Severe] Study
- **Cobicistat** is predicted to increase the exposure to opioids **(alfentanil, buprenorphine, fentanyl, oxycodone)**. Monitor and adjust dose. [Severe] Study
- **Cobicistat** is predicted to increase the exposure to **sufentanil**. [Moderate] Study
- **Tramadol** might increase the anticoagulant effect of coumarins **(acenocoumarol)**. [Severe] Study
- **Tramadol** has been reported to increase the anticoagulant effect of coumarins **(warfarin)**. [Severe] Anecdotal
- **Crizotinib** is predicted to increase the exposure to opioids **(alfentanil, buprenorphine, fentanyl, oxycodone)**. Monitor and adjust dose. [Moderate] Study → Also see TABLE 4 p. 1054
- **Crizotinib** is predicted to increase the exposure to opioids **(methadone, sufentanil)**. [Moderate] Theoretical → Also see TABLE 4 p. 1054 → Also see TABLE 7 p. 1055
- **Dabrafenib** decreases the exposure to **methadone**. Monitor and adjust dose. [Severe] Study
- **Dacomitinib** is predicted to decrease the efficacy of **codeine**. [Moderate] Theoretical
- **Dacomitinib** is predicted to decrease the efficacy of **tramadol**. [Severe] Study
- **Tapentadol** is predicted to increase the risk of serotonin toxicity when given with **drugs that cause serotonin toxicity** (see TABLE 11 p. 1056). [Severe] Theoretical
- **Encorafenib** is predicted to decrease the exposure to **buprenorphine**. Monitor and adjust dose. [Moderate] Theoretical
- **Encorafenib** decreases the exposure to **methadone**. Monitor and adjust dose. [Severe] Study → Also see TABLE 7 p. 1055
- **Encorafenib** is predicted to decrease the exposure to opioids **(alfentanil, fentanyl)**. [Moderate] Study
- **Encorafenib** is predicted to decrease the exposure to **oxycodone**. Monitor and adjust dose. [Moderate] Study
- Endothelin receptor antagonists **(bosentan)** decrease the exposure to **methadone**. Monitor and adjust dose. [Severe] Study
- **Fedratinib** is predicted to increase the exposure to opioids **(alfentanil, buprenorphine, fentanyl, oxycodone)**. Monitor and adjust dose. [Moderate] Study
- **Fedratinib** is predicted to increase the exposure to opioids **(methadone, sufentanil)**. [Moderate] Theoretical
- **Fostamatinib** is predicted to increase the exposure to **alfentanil**. Monitor and adjust dose. [Moderate] Theoretical
- **Givinostat** might increase the exposure to **alfentanil**. [Moderate] Study
- H_2 receptor antagonists **(cimetidine)** increase the concentration of **alfentanil**. Use with caution and adjust dose. [Severe] Study
- H_2 receptor antagonists **(cimetidine)** might increase the exposure to **fentanyl**. Monitor and adjust dose. [Moderate] Study
- **HIV-protease inhibitors** boosted with ritonavir are predicted to decrease the exposure to **methadone**. [Moderate] Study
- HIV-protease inhibitors **(ritonavir)** are predicted to decrease the concentration of **morphine**. [Moderate] Theoretical
- HIV-protease inhibitors **(ritonavir)** increase the risk of CNS toxicity when given with **pethidine**. Avoid. [Severe] Study
- **HIV-protease inhibitors** are predicted to increase the exposure to opioids **(alfentanil, buprenorphine, fentanyl, oxycodone)**. Monitor and adjust dose. [Severe] Study
- **HIV-protease inhibitors** are predicted to increase the exposure to **sufentanil**. [Moderate] Study
- **Idelalisib** is predicted to increase the exposure to **methadone**. [Severe] Theoretical
- **Idelalisib** is predicted to increase the exposure to opioids **(alfentanil, buprenorphine, fentanyl, oxycodone)**. Monitor and adjust dose. [Severe] Study
- **Idelalisib** is predicted to increase the exposure to **sufentanil**. [Moderate] Study
- **Imatinib** is predicted to increase the exposure to opioids **(alfentanil, buprenorphine, fentanyl, oxycodone)**. Monitor and adjust dose. [Moderate] Study
- **Imatinib** is predicted to increase the exposure to opioids **(methadone, sufentanil)**. [Moderate] Theoretical
- Interferons **(ropeginterferon alfa)** are predicted to increase the exposure to **methadone**. [Moderate] Theoretical
- **Ivosidenib** is predicted to decrease the exposure to **buprenorphine**. Monitor and adjust dose. [Moderate] Theoretical
- **Ivosidenib** decreases the exposure to **methadone**. Monitor and adjust dose. [Severe] Study → Also see TABLE 7 p. 1055
- **Ivosidenib** is predicted to decrease the exposure to opioids **(alfentanil, fentanyl)**. [Moderate] Study
- **Ivosidenib** is predicted to decrease the exposure to **oxycodone**. Monitor and adjust dose. [Moderate] Study
- **Larotrectinib** is predicted to increase the exposure to opioids **(alfentanil, fentanyl)**. Use with caution and adjust dose. [Mild] Theoretical
- **Lazertinib** is predicted to increase the exposure to **alfentanil**. [Moderate] Study
- **Lenacapavir** is predicted to affect the concentration of opioids **(buprenorphine, methadone)**. [Moderate] Theoretical
- **Letermovir** is predicted to increase the exposure to opioids **(alfentanil, buprenorphine, fentanyl, oxycodone)**. Monitor and adjust dose. [Moderate] Study
- **Letermovir** is predicted to increase the exposure to opioids **(methadone, sufentanil)**. [Moderate] Theoretical
- **Lorlatinib** decreases the exposure to **methadone**. Monitor and adjust dose. [Severe] Study
- **Lorlatinib** is predicted to decrease the exposure to opioids **(alfentanil, fentanyl)**. Avoid. [Moderate] Theoretical
- **Lumacaftor** is predicted to decrease the exposure to **buprenorphine**. Monitor and adjust dose. [Moderate] Theoretical
- **Lumacaftor** decreases the exposure to **methadone**. Monitor and adjust dose. [Severe] Study
- **Lumacaftor** is predicted to decrease the exposure to opioids **(alfentanil, fentanyl)**. [Moderate] Study
- **Lumacaftor** is predicted to decrease the exposure to **oxycodone**. Monitor and adjust dose. [Moderate] Study
- Macrolides **(clarithromycin)** are predicted to increase the concentration of **methadone**. [Severe] Theoretical
- Macrolides **(clarithromycin)** are predicted to increase the exposure to **sufentanil**. [Moderate] Study
- Macrolides **(clarithromycin)** are predicted to increase the exposure to opioids **(alfentanil, buprenorphine, fentanyl, oxycodone)**. Monitor and adjust dose. [Severe] Study
- Macrolides **(erythromycin)** are predicted to increase the exposure to opioids **(alfentanil, buprenorphine, fentanyl, oxycodone)**. Monitor and adjust dose. [Moderate] Study
- Macrolides **(erythromycin)** are predicted to increase the exposure to opioids **(methadone, sufentanil)**. [Moderate] Theoretical → Also see TABLE 7 p. 1055
- MAO-B inhibitors **(rasagiline)** are predicted to increase the risk of adverse effects when given with **pethidine**. Avoid and for 14 days after stopping **rasagiline**. [Severe] Theoretical
- MAO-B inhibitors **(safinamide)** are predicted to increase the risk of adverse effects when given with **pethidine**. Avoid and for 1 week after stopping **safinamide**. [Severe] Theoretical
- MAO-B inhibitors **(selegiline)** increase the risk of adverse effects when given with **pethidine**. Avoid. [Severe] Anecdotal
- **Opioids** are predicted to increase the risk of CNS excitation or depression when given with **MAOIs, irreversible**. Avoid. [Severe] Study → Also see TABLE 11 p. 1056

Opioids (continued)
- **Opioids** potentially decrease the absorption of oral **mexiletine**. Moderate Study
- **Mifepristone** is predicted to increase the exposure to **alfentanil**. Severe Theoretical
- **Mitotane** is predicted to decrease the exposure to **buprenorphine**. Monitor and adjust dose. Moderate Theoretical
- **Mitotane** decreases the exposure to **methadone**. Monitor and adjust dose. Severe Study
- **Mitotane** is predicted to decrease the exposure to opioids **(alfentanil, fentanyl)**. Moderate Study
- **Mitotane** is predicted to decrease the exposure to **oxycodone**. Monitor and adjust dose. Moderate Study
- **Moclobemide** might cause serotonin toxicity, as can **tramadol**; concurrent use might increase the risk of developing this effect. Avoid. Severe Anecdotal → Also see TABLE 11 p. 1056
- **Nalmefene** is predicted to decrease the efficacy of **opioids**. Avoid except in an emergency situation—consult product literature. Severe Theoretical
- **Naltrexone** is predicted to decrease the efficacy of **opioids**. Avoid except in an emergency situation—consult product literature. Severe Theoretical
- Neurokinin-1 receptor antagonists **(aprepitant, netupitant)** are predicted to increase the exposure to opioids **(alfentanil, buprenorphine, fentanyl, oxycodone)**. Monitor and adjust dose. Moderate Study
- Neurokinin-1 receptor antagonists **(aprepitant, netupitant)** are predicted to increase the exposure to opioids **(methadone, sufentanil)**. Moderate Theoretical
- **Nilotinib** is predicted to increase the exposure to opioids **(alfentanil, buprenorphine, fentanyl, oxycodone)**. Monitor and adjust dose. Moderate Study
- **Nilotinib** is predicted to increase the exposure to opioids **(methadone, sufentanil)**. Moderate Theoretical → Also see TABLE 7 p. 1055
- **Nirmatrelvir** boosted with ritonavir is predicted to increase the concentration of **buprenorphine**. Monitor and adjust dose. Moderate Theoretical
- **Nirmatrelvir** boosted with ritonavir is predicted to decrease the concentration of **methadone**. Adjust dose. Moderate Theoretical
- **Nirmatrelvir** boosted with ritonavir is predicted to decrease the concentration of **morphine**. Moderate Theoretical
- **Nirmatrelvir** boosted with ritonavir is predicted to increase the concentration of opioids **(fentanyl, oxycodone, pethidine)**. Severe Theoretical
- NNRTIs **(efavirenz)** moderately decrease the exposure to **buprenorphine**. Adjust dose. Moderate Study
- NNRTIs **(efavirenz, etravirine, nevirapine)** decrease the exposure to **methadone**. Monitor and adjust dose. Severe Study → Also see TABLE 7 p. 1055
- **Olaparib** might alter the exposure to **alfentanil**. Moderate Theoretical
- Opioids **(buprenorphine)** are predicted to increase the risk of opiate withdrawal when given with opioids **(alfentanil)**. Severe Theoretical → Also see TABLE 9 p. 1056
- Opioids **(meptazinol)** are predicted to increase the risk of opiate withdrawal when given with opioids **(alfentanil, codeine, diamorphine, dihydrocodeine, dipipanone, fentanyl, hydromorphone)**. Severe Theoretical → Also see TABLE 9 p. 1056
- Opioids **(pentazocine)** are predicted to increase the risk of opiate withdrawal when given with opioids **(alfentanil, codeine, diamorphine, dihydrocodeine, dipipanone, fentanyl, hydromorphone, methadone, morphine, oxycodone)**. Severe Theoretical → Also see TABLE 11 p. 1056 → Also see TABLE 9 p. 1056
- Opioids **(buprenorphine)** are predicted to increase the risk of opiate withdrawal when given with opioids **(codeine, diamorphine, dihydrocodeine, dipipanone, fentanyl, hydromorphone, methadone, morphine, oxycodone, pethidine, remifentanil, sufentanil, tapentadol, tramadol)**. Severe Theoretical → Also see TABLE 9 p. 1056
- Opioids **(meptazinol)** are predicted to increase the risk of opiate withdrawal when given with opioids **(methadone, morphine, oxycodone, pethidine, remifentanil, sufentanil, tapentadol, tramadol)**. Severe Theoretical → Also see TABLE 9 p. 1056
- Opioids **(pentazocine)** are predicted to increase the risk of opiate withdrawal when given with opioids **(pethidine, remifentanil, tapentadol, tramadol)**. Severe Theoretical → Also see TABLE 11 p. 1056 → Also see TABLE 9 p. 1056
- Opioids **(pentazocine)** are predicted to increase the risk of opiate withdrawal when given with opioids **(sufentanil)**. Severe Anecdotal → Also see TABLE 9 p. 1056
- **Opioids** might increase the risk of adverse effects when given with **ozanimod**. Severe Theoretical → Also see TABLE 4 p. 1054
- **Palbociclib** is predicted to increase the exposure to opioids **(alfentanil, fentanyl)**. Adjust dose. Moderate Theoretical
- **Pemigatinib** might decrease the exposure to **methadone**. Moderate Theoretical
- **Tramadol** might increase the anticoagulant effect of **phenindione**. Severe Anecdotal
- **Pirtobrutinib** is predicted to increase the exposure to **alfentanil**. Avoid or monitor. Moderate Theoretical
- **Pitolisant** is predicted to decrease the exposure to **morphine**. Mild Theoretical
- **Ribociclib** is predicted to increase the exposure to opioids **(alfentanil, fentanyl)**. Use with caution and adjust dose. Moderate Theoretical
- Rifamycins **(rifampicin)** are predicted to decrease the exposure to **buprenorphine**. Monitor and adjust dose. Moderate Theoretical
- Rifamycins **(rifampicin)** decrease the exposure to **methadone**. Monitor and adjust dose. Severe Study
- Rifamycins **(rifampicin)** are predicted to decrease the exposure to **oxycodone**. Monitor and adjust dose. Moderate Study
- Rifamycins **(rifampicin)** are predicted to decrease the exposure to opioids **(alfentanil, fentanyl)**. Moderate Study
- Rifamycins **(rifampicin)** decrease the exposure to opioids **(codeine, morphine)**. Moderate Study
- **Ritlecitinib** is predicted to increase the exposure to **alfentanil**. Moderate Theoretical
- **Rucaparib** is predicted to increase the exposure to opioids **(alfentanil, fentanyl)**. Monitor and adjust dose. Moderate Study
- **Selpercatinib** is predicted to increase the exposure to opioids **(alfentanil, buprenorphine)**. Avoid. Moderate Study
- **Sotorasib** is predicted to decrease the exposure to **alfentanil**. Avoid or adjust dose. Moderate Theoretical
- **Sotorasib** decreases the exposure to **methadone**. Monitor and adjust dose. Severe Study
- SSRIs **(fluoxetine, paroxetine)** are predicted to decrease the efficacy of **codeine**. Moderate Theoretical → Also see TABLE 9 p. 1056
- SSRIs **(fluoxetine, paroxetine)** are predicted to decrease the efficacy of **tramadol**. Severe Study → Also see TABLE 15 p. 1058 → Also see TABLE 11 p. 1056 → Also see TABLE 9 p. 1056
- **St John's wort** decreases the exposure to **methadone**. Monitor and adjust dose. Severe Study → Also see TABLE 11 p. 1056
- **St John's wort** moderately decreases the exposure to **oxycodone**. Adjust dose. Moderate Study
- **Terbinafine** is predicted to decrease the efficacy of **codeine**. Moderate Theoretical
- **Terbinafine** is predicted to decrease the efficacy of **tramadol**. Severe Study
- **Tucatinib** is predicted to increase the exposure to opioids **(alfentanil, buprenorphine, fentanyl, oxycodone)**. Monitor and adjust dose. Severe Study
- **Tucatinib** is predicted to increase the exposure to **sufentanil**. Moderate Study
- **Vorasidenib** might decrease the concentration of opioids **(alfentanil, fentanyl)**. Avoid. Severe Theoretical

Opium → see interactions of codeine and morphine under opioids

Oritavancin
- **Oritavancin** might increase the exposure to coumarins **(warfarin)**. Moderate Theoretical
- **Oritavancin** might cause a falsely elevated aPTT when given with **heparin**. Avoid and for 120 hours after stopping **oritavancin**. Severe Theoretical

Orlistat

SEPARATION OF ADMINISTRATION Orlistat might affect the absorption of concurrently administered oral drugs—consider separating administration. Particular care should be taken with antiepileptics, antiretrovirals, oral contraceptives, and drugs that have a narrow therapeutic index.

Orphenadrine → see TABLE 8 p. 1055 (antimuscarinics), TABLE 9 p. 1056 (CNS effects)
- Atypical antipsychotics (**clozapine**) can cause constipation, as can **orphenadrine**; concurrent use might increase the risk of developing intestinal obstruction. Severe Theoretical → Also see TABLE 8 p. 1055 → Also see TABLE 9 p. 1056

Oseltamivir
- **Ivosidenib** is predicted to increase the exposure to the active metabolite of **oseltamivir**. Use with caution or avoid. Moderate Theoretical
- **Leflunomide** is predicted to increase the exposure to **oseltamivir**. Moderate Study
- **Oseltamivir** might decrease the efficacy of live vaccines (**influenza vaccine (live)**). Moderate Theoretical
- **Nitisinone** is predicted to increase the exposure to **oseltamivir**. Moderate Study
- **Teriflunomide** is predicted to increase the exposure to **oseltamivir**. Moderate Study
- **Vadadustat** is predicted to increase the exposure to the active metabolite of **oseltamivir**. Monitor and adjust dose. Moderate Study

Osilodrostat → see TABLE 7 p. 1055 (QT-interval prolongation)
- **Osilodrostat** is predicted to increase the exposure to **agomelatine**. Moderate Study
- **Osilodrostat** is predicted to increase the exposure to **aminophylline**. Adjust dose. Moderate Theoretical
- **Osilodrostat** is predicted to increase the exposure to anaesthetics, local (**ropivacaine**). Moderate Theoretical
- **Osilodrostat** is predicted to increase the exposure to **anagrelide**. Moderate Theoretical → Also see TABLE 7 p. 1055
- Anti-androgens (**apalutamide, enzalutamide**) are predicted to decrease the exposure to **osilodrostat**. Moderate Theoretical → Also see TABLE 7 p. 1055
- Antiepileptics (**carbamazepine, fosphenytoin, phenobarbital, phenytoin, primidone**) are predicted to decrease the exposure to **osilodrostat**. Moderate Theoretical
- Antifungals, azoles (**itraconazole, ketoconazole, posaconazole, voriconazole**) are predicted to increase the exposure to **osilodrostat**. Moderate Theoretical → Also see TABLE 7 p. 1055
- **Osilodrostat** increases the concentration of atypical antipsychotics (**clozapine**). Monitor adverse effects and adjust dose. Severe Study
- **Osilodrostat** is predicted to increase the exposure to atypical antipsychotics (**olanzapine**). Adjust dose. Moderate Anecdotal
- **Ceritinib** is predicted to increase the exposure to **osilodrostat**. Moderate Theoretical → Also see TABLE 7 p. 1055
- **Cobicistat** is predicted to increase the exposure to **osilodrostat**. Moderate Theoretical
- **Osilodrostat** is predicted to increase the exposure to dopamine receptor agonists (**ropinirole**). Adjust dose. Moderate Study
- **Encorafenib** is predicted to decrease the exposure to **osilodrostat**. Moderate Theoretical → Also see TABLE 7 p. 1055
- **Osilodrostat** are predicted to increases the exposure to **erlotinib**. Monitor adverse effects and adjust dose. Moderate Study
- **Osilodrostat** is predicted to increase the exposure to **fezolinetant**. Avoid. Moderate Study
- **HIV-protease inhibitors** are predicted to increase the exposure to **osilodrostat**. Moderate Theoretical
- **Idelalisib** is predicted to increase the exposure to **osilodrostat**. Moderate Theoretical
- **Ivosidenib** is predicted to decrease the exposure to **osilodrostat**. Moderate Theoretical → Also see TABLE 7 p. 1055
- **Osilodrostat** is predicted to increase the exposure to **loxapine**. Avoid. Unknown Theoretical
- **Lumacaftor** is predicted to decrease the exposure to **osilodrostat**. Moderate Theoretical
- Macrolides (**clarithromycin**) are predicted to increase the exposure to **osilodrostat**. Moderate Theoretical
- **Osilodrostat** slightly increases the exposure to MAO-B inhibitors (**rasagiline**). Moderate Study
- **Osilodrostat** is predicted to increase the exposure to **mavacamten**. Monitor and adjust dose—consult product literature. Moderate Theoretical
- **Osilodrostat** is predicted to increase the exposure to **melatonin**. Moderate Theoretical
- **Mitotane** is predicted to decrease the exposure to **osilodrostat**. Moderate Theoretical
- **Osilodrostat** is predicted to increase the exposure to phenothiazine antipsychotics (**chlorpromazine**). Moderate Theoretical → Also see TABLE 7 p. 1055
- **Osilodrostat** is predicted to increase the exposure to phosphodiesterase type-4 inhibitors (**roflumilast**). Moderate Theoretical
- **Osilodrostat** is predicted to increase the exposure to **pirfenidone**. Use with caution and adjust dose. Moderate Study
- Rifamycins (**rifampicin**) are predicted to decrease the exposure to **osilodrostat**. Moderate Theoretical
- **Osilodrostat** is predicted to increase the exposure to **riluzole**. Moderate Theoretical
- **Osilodrostat** is predicted to increase the exposure to SNRIs (**duloxetine**). Moderate Theoretical
- **Osilodrostat** is predicted to increase the exposure to **theophylline**. Monitor and adjust dose. Moderate Theoretical
- **Osilodrostat** increases the exposure to **tizanidine**. Avoid. Moderate Study
- **Osilodrostat** is predicted to increase the exposure to triptans (**zolmitriptan**). Adjust **zolmitriptan** dose, p. 347. Moderate Theoretical
- **Tucatinib** is predicted to increase the exposure to **osilodrostat**. Moderate Theoretical
- **Osilodrostat** is predicted to increase the exposure to **vorasidenib**. Avoid. Moderate Theoretical

Osimertinib → see TABLE 7 p. 1055 (QT-interval prolongation)
- **Osimertinib** is predicted to increase the exposure to **aliskiren**. Moderate Study
- Anti-androgens (**apalutamide, enzalutamide**) are predicted to moderately decrease the exposure to **osimertinib**. Avoid. Moderate Study → Also see TABLE 7 p. 1055
- Antiepileptics (**carbamazepine, fosphenytoin, phenobarbital, phenytoin, primidone**) are predicted to moderately decrease the exposure to **osimertinib**. Avoid. Moderate Study
- **Osimertinib** is predicted to increase the exposure to antihistamines, non-sedating (**fexofenadine**). Moderate Study
- **Osimertinib** is predicted to increase the exposure to **colchicine**. Moderate Study
- **Dabrafenib** is predicted to decrease the exposure to **osimertinib**. Use with caution or avoid. Severe Study
- **Osimertinib** is predicted to increase the exposure to **digoxin**. Moderate Study
- **Encorafenib** is predicted to moderately decrease the exposure to **osimertinib**. Avoid. Moderate Study → Also see TABLE 7 p. 1055
- Endothelin receptor antagonists (**bosentan**) are predicted to decrease the exposure to **osimertinib**. Use with caution or avoid. Severe Study
- **Osimertinib** is predicted to increase the exposure to **everolimus**. Moderate Study
- **Osimertinib** is predicted to increase the exposure to factor XA inhibitors (**edoxaban**). Moderate Study
- **Ivosidenib** is predicted to moderately decrease the exposure to **osimertinib**. Avoid. Moderate Study → Also see TABLE 7 p. 1055
- **Osimertinib** is predicted to increase the exposure to **loperamide**. Moderate Study
- **Lumacaftor** is predicted to moderately decrease the exposure to **osimertinib**. Avoid. Moderate Study
- **Mitotane** is predicted to moderately decrease the exposure to **osimertinib**. Avoid. Moderate Study
- **Modafinil** is predicted to decrease the exposure to **osimertinib**. Use with caution or avoid. Severe Theoretical
- NNRTIs (**efavirenz, nevirapine**) are predicted to decrease the exposure to **osimertinib**. Use with caution or avoid. Severe Study → Also see TABLE 7 p. 1055
- NNRTIs (**etravirine**) are predicted to decrease the exposure to **osimertinib**. Use with caution or avoid. Severe Theoretical
- **Osimertinib** is predicted to increase the exposure to **pralsetinib**. Moderate Study

A1 Interactions | Appendix 1

Osimertinib (continued)
- **Osimertinib** is predicted to increase the exposure to **ranolazine**. [Moderate] Study → Also see TABLE 7 p. 1055
- Rifamycins **(rifampicin)** are predicted to moderately decrease the exposure to **osimertinib**. Avoid. [Moderate] Study
- **Osimertinib** is predicted to increase the exposure to **rimegepant**. [Moderate] Study
- **Osimertinib** is predicted to increase the exposure to the active component of **sacituzumab govitecan**. [Severe] Theoretical
- **Osimertinib** is predicted to increase the exposure to **sirolimus**. [Moderate] Study
- **St John's wort** is predicted to decrease the exposure to **osimertinib**. Avoid. [Severe] Study
- **Osimertinib** causes a small increase in the exposure to statins **(rosuvastatin)**. [Severe] Study
- **Osimertinib** is predicted to increase the exposure to **talazoparib**. [Moderate] Study
- **Osimertinib** is predicted to increase the exposure to taxanes **(paclitaxel)**. [Moderate] Study
- **Osimertinib** is predicted to increase the exposure to thrombin inhibitors **(dabigatran)**. [Moderate] Study

Ospemifene
- Anti-androgens **(apalutamide, enzalutamide)** are predicted to moderately decrease the exposure to **ospemifene**. [Moderate] Study
- Antiepileptics **(carbamazepine, fosphenytoin, phenobarbital, phenytoin, primidone)** are predicted to moderately decrease the exposure to **ospemifene**. [Moderate] Study
- Antifungals, azoles **(fluconazole)** increase the exposure to **ospemifene**. Use with caution or avoid. [Moderate] Study
- Antifungals, azoles **(itraconazole, ketoconazole, posaconazole, voriconazole)** are predicted to increase the exposure to **ospemifene**. Avoid in poor CYP2C9 metabolisers. [Moderate] Study
- **Cenobamate** is predicted to decrease the exposure to **ospemifene**. [Moderate] Study
- **Ceritinib** is predicted to increase the exposure to **ospemifene**. Avoid in poor CYP2C9 metabolisers. [Moderate] Study
- **Cobicistat** is predicted to increase the exposure to **ospemifene**. Avoid in poor CYP2C9 metabolisers. [Moderate] Study
- **Combined hormonal contraceptives** potentially oppose the effects of **ospemifene**. Avoid. [Severe] Theoretical
- **Dabrafenib** is predicted to decrease the exposure to **ospemifene**. [Moderate] Study
- **Encorafenib** is predicted to moderately decrease the exposure to **ospemifene**. [Moderate] Study
- Endothelin receptor antagonists **(bosentan)** are predicted to decrease the exposure to **ospemifene**. [Moderate] Study
- **HIV-protease inhibitors** are predicted to increase the exposure to **ospemifene**. Avoid in poor CYP2C9 metabolisers. [Moderate] Study
- **Hormone replacement therapy** potentially opposes the effects of **ospemifene**. Avoid. [Severe] Theoretical
- **Idelalisib** is predicted to increase the exposure to **ospemifene**. Avoid in poor CYP2C9 metabolisers. [Moderate] Study
- **Ivosidenib** is predicted to moderately decrease the exposure to **ospemifene**. [Moderate] Study
- **Lorlatinib** is predicted to decrease the exposure to **ospemifene**. [Moderate] Study
- **Lumacaftor** is predicted to moderately decrease the exposure to **ospemifene**. [Moderate] Study
- Macrolides **(clarithromycin)** are predicted to increase the exposure to **ospemifene**. Avoid in poor CYP2C9 metabolisers. [Moderate] Study
- **Mitotane** is predicted to moderately decrease the exposure to **ospemifene**. [Moderate] Study
- NNRTIs **(efavirenz, etravirine, nevirapine)** are predicted to decrease the exposure to **ospemifene**. [Moderate] Study
- Rifamycins **(rifampicin)** are predicted to moderately decrease the exposure to **ospemifene**. [Moderate] Study
- **Sotorasib** is predicted to decrease the exposure to **ospemifene**. [Moderate] Study
- **St John's wort** is predicted to decrease the exposure to **ospemifene**. [Moderate] Study
- **Tucatinib** is predicted to increase the exposure to **ospemifene**. Avoid in poor CYP2C9 metabolisers. [Moderate] Study

Oxaliplatin → see platinum compounds
Oxandrolone → see TABLE 1 p. 1053 (hepatotoxicity)
Oxazepam → see benzodiazepines
Oxcarbazepine → see antiepileptics
Oxybuprocaine → see anaesthetics, local
Oxybutynin → see TABLE 8 p. 1055 (antimuscarinics)
- **Oxybutynin** potentially increases the risk of overheating and dehydration when given with antiepileptics **(zonisamide)**. Avoid in children. [Severe] Theoretical
- Antifungals, azoles **(itraconazole, ketoconazole, posaconazole, voriconazole)** are predicted to increase the exposure to **oxybutynin**. [Mild] Study
- Atypical antipsychotics **(clozapine)** can cause constipation, as can **oxybutynin**; concurrent use might increase the risk of developing intestinal obstruction. [Severe] Theoretical → Also see TABLE 8 p. 1055
- **Ceritinib** is predicted to increase the exposure to **oxybutynin**. [Mild] Study
- **Cobicistat** is predicted to increase the exposure to **oxybutynin**. [Mild] Study
- **HIV-protease inhibitors** are predicted to increase the exposure to **oxybutynin**. [Mild] Study
- **Idelalisib** is predicted to increase the exposure to **oxybutynin**. [Mild] Study
- Macrolides **(clarithromycin)** are predicted to increase the exposure to **oxybutynin**. [Mild] Study
- **Tucatinib** is predicted to increase the exposure to **oxybutynin**. [Mild] Study

Oxycodone → see opioids
Oxymetholone → see TABLE 1 p. 1053 (hepatotoxicity)
- **Oxymetholone** increases the anticoagulant effect of **coumarins**. [Severe] Anecdotal
- **Oxymetholone** increases the anticoagulant effect of **phenindione**. [Severe] Anecdotal

Oxytetracycline → see tetracyclines
Oxytocin → see TABLE 15 p. 1058 (hyponatraemia)
- **Misoprostol** can cause uterine contractions, as can **oxytocin**; concurrent use might increase the risk of developing this effect. Avoid and for 4 hours after stopping **misoprostol**. [Severe] Theoretical

Ozanimod → see TABLE 4 p. 1054 (bradycardia), TABLE 7 p. 1055 (QT-interval prolongation)

FOOD AND LIFESTYLE Tyramine-rich foods might increase the risk of hypertensive crisis when given ozanimod.

- **Clopidogrel** is predicted to increase the exposure to the active metabolites of **ozanimod**. [Moderate] Study
- Fibrates **(gemfibrozil)** are predicted to increase the exposure to the active metabolites of **ozanimod**. [Moderate] Study
- **Ozanimod** might increase the risk of a hypertensive crisis when given with **linezolid**. Avoid. [Severe] Theoretical
- **Live vaccines** might increase the risk of generalised infection (possibly life-threatening) when given with **ozanimod**. Avoid and for 3 months after stopping **ozanimod**. [Severe] Theoretical
- **Ozanimod** might increase the risk of a hypertensive crisis when given with **MAO-B inhibitors** and **MAO-B inhibitors** might decrease the exposure to the active metabolites of **ozanimod**. Avoid. [Severe] Theoretical → Also see TABLE 4 p. 1054
- **Ozanimod** might increase the risk of a hypertensive crisis when given with **MAOIs, irreversible**. Avoid. [Severe] Theoretical
- **Methylphenidate** is predicted to increase the risk of a hypertensive crisis when given with **ozanimod**. [Severe] Theoretical
- **Ozanimod** might increase the risk of a hypertensive crisis when given with **moclobemide**. Avoid. [Severe] Theoretical
- Monoclonal antibodies **(alemtuzumab)** are predicted to increase the risk of generalised infection (possibly life-threatening) when given with **ozanimod**. Avoid. [Severe] Theoretical
- **Opioids** might increase the risk of adverse effects when given with **ozanimod**. [Severe] Theoretical → Also see TABLE 4 p. 1054
- Rifamycins **(rifampicin)** moderately decrease the exposure to the active metabolites of **ozanimod**. Avoid. [Moderate] Study
- SNRIs **(duloxetine)** might increase the risk of adverse effects when given with **ozanimod**. [Severe] Theoretical

- **SSRIs** might increase the risk of adverse effects when given with **ozanimod**. Severe Theoretical
- **Sympathomimetics, vasoconstrictor** might increase the risk of a hypertensive crisis when given with **ozanimod**. Severe Theoretical
- **Tricyclic antidepressants** might increase the risk of adverse effects when given with **ozanimod**. Severe Theoretical

Paclitaxel → see taxanes

Palbociclib → see TABLE 12 p. 1057 (myelosuppression)

- Anti-androgens **(apalutamide, enzalutamide)** are predicted to decrease the exposure to **palbociclib**. Avoid. Severe Study
- Antiepileptics **(carbamazepine, fosphenytoin, phenobarbital, phenytoin, primidone)** are predicted to decrease the exposure to **palbociclib**. Avoid. Severe Study
- Antifungals, azoles **(itraconazole, ketoconazole, posaconazole, voriconazole)** are predicted to increase the exposure to **palbociclib**. Avoid or adjust dose—consult product literature. Severe Study
- **Palbociclib** increases the exposure to benzodiazepines **(midazolam)**. Moderate Study
- **Ceritinib** is predicted to increase the exposure to **palbociclib**. Avoid or adjust dose—consult product literature. Severe Study → Also see TABLE 12 p. 1057
- **Palbociclib** is predicted to increase the exposure to **ciclosporin**. Adjust dose. Moderate Theoretical
- **Cobicistat** is predicted to increase the exposure to **palbociclib**. Avoid or adjust dose—consult product literature. Severe Study
- **Encorafenib** is predicted to decrease the exposure to **palbociclib**. Avoid. Severe Study
- **Palbociclib** is predicted to increase the exposure to **everolimus**. Adjust dose. Moderate Theoretical
- **Grapefruit** juice is predicted to increase the exposure to **palbociclib**. Avoid. Severe Theoretical
- **HIV-protease inhibitors** are predicted to increase the exposure to **palbociclib**. Avoid or adjust dose—consult product literature. Severe Study
- **Idelalisib** is predicted to increase the exposure to **palbociclib**. Avoid or adjust dose—consult product literature. Severe Study
- **Ivosidenib** is predicted to decrease the exposure to **palbociclib**. Avoid. Severe Study
- **Lumacaftor** is predicted to decrease the exposure to **palbociclib**. Avoid. Severe Study
- Macrolides **(clarithromycin)** are predicted to increase the exposure to **palbociclib**. Avoid or adjust dose—consult product literature. Severe Study
- **Mitotane** is predicted to decrease the exposure to **palbociclib**. Avoid. Severe Study → Also see TABLE 12 p. 1057
- **Palbociclib** is predicted to increase the exposure to opioids **(alfentanil, fentanyl)**. Adjust dose. Moderate Theoretical
- **Palbociclib** is predicted to increase the exposure to **pimozide**. Adjust dose. Moderate Theoretical
- Rifamycins **(rifampicin)** are predicted to decrease the exposure to **palbociclib**. Avoid. Severe Study
- **Palbociclib** is predicted to increase the exposure to **sirolimus**. Adjust dose. Moderate Theoretical
- **St John's wort** is predicted to decrease the exposure to **palbociclib**. Avoid. Severe Theoretical
- **Palbociclib** is predicted to increase the exposure to **tacrolimus**. Adjust dose. Moderate Theoretical
- **Tucatinib** is predicted to increase the exposure to **palbociclib**. Avoid or adjust dose—consult product literature. Severe Study

Paliperidone → see atypical antipsychotics

Palonosetron → see 5-HT3-receptor antagonists

Pamidronate → see bisphosphonates

Pancreatin

- **Pancreatin** is predicted to decrease the effects of **acarbose**. Avoid. Moderate Theoretical

Pancuronium → see neuromuscular blocking drugs, non-depolarising

Panitumumab → see monoclonal antibodies

Panobinostat → see TABLE 12 p. 1057 (myelosuppression), TABLE 7 p. 1055 (QT-interval prolongation)

FOOD AND LIFESTYLE Avoid pomegranate, pomegranate juice, and star fruit as they are predicted to increase panobinostat exposure.

- Anti-androgens **(apalutamide, enzalutamide)** are predicted to decrease the exposure to **panobinostat**. Avoid. Moderate Theoretical → Also see TABLE 7 p. 1055
- Antiarrhythmics **(amiodarone, dronedarone)** are predicted to increase the exposure to **panobinostat**. Adjust dose. Moderate Theoretical → Also see TABLE 7 p. 1055
- Antiepileptics **(carbamazepine, fosphenytoin, phenobarbital, phenytoin, primidone)** are predicted to decrease the exposure to **panobinostat**. Avoid. Moderate Theoretical
- Antifungals, azoles **(itraconazole, ketoconazole, posaconazole, voriconazole)** are predicted to increase the exposure to **panobinostat**. Adjust dose—consult product literature; in hepatic impairment avoid. Moderate Study → Also see TABLE 7 p. 1055
- **Panobinostat** is predicted to increase the exposure to **atomoxetine**. Monitor and adjust dose. Severe Theoretical
- **Panobinostat** is predicted to increase the exposure to beta blockers, selective **(metoprolol)**. Monitor and adjust dose. Moderate Theoretical
- **Panobinostat** is predicted to increase the exposure to beta blockers, selective **(nebivolol)**. Monitor and adjust dose. Mild Theoretical
- Calcium-channel blockers **(verapamil)** are predicted to increase the exposure to **panobinostat**. Adjust dose. Moderate Theoretical
- **Ceritinib** is predicted to increase the exposure to **panobinostat**. Adjust dose—consult product literature; in hepatic impairment avoid. Moderate Study → Also see TABLE 12 p. 1057 → Also see TABLE 7 p. 1055
- **Ciclosporin** is predicted to increase the exposure to **panobinostat**. Adjust dose. Moderate Theoretical
- **Cobicistat** is predicted to increase the exposure to **panobinostat**. Adjust dose—consult product literature; in hepatic impairment avoid. Moderate Study
- **Encorafenib** is predicted to decrease the exposure to **panobinostat**. Avoid. Moderate Theoretical → Also see TABLE 7 p. 1055
- **Grapefruit** and grapefruit juice is predicted to increase the exposure to **panobinostat**. Avoid. Moderate Theoretical
- **HIV-protease inhibitors** are predicted to increase the exposure to **panobinostat**. Adjust dose—consult product literature; in hepatic impairment avoid. Moderate Study
- **Idelalisib** is predicted to increase the exposure to **panobinostat**. Adjust dose—consult product literature; in hepatic impairment avoid. Moderate Study
- **Ivosidenib** is predicted to decrease the exposure to **panobinostat**. Avoid. Moderate Theoretical → Also see TABLE 7 p. 1055
- **Lapatinib** is predicted to increase the exposure to **panobinostat**. Adjust dose. Moderate Theoretical → Also see TABLE 7 p. 1055
- **Lumacaftor** is predicted to decrease the exposure to **panobinostat**. Avoid. Moderate Theoretical
- Macrolides **(azithromycin, erythromycin)** are predicted to increase the exposure to **panobinostat**. Adjust dose. Moderate Theoretical → Also see TABLE 7 p. 1055
- Macrolides **(clarithromycin)** are predicted to increase the exposure to **panobinostat**. Adjust dose—consult product literature; in hepatic impairment avoid. Moderate Study
- **Mitotane** is predicted to decrease the exposure to **panobinostat**. Avoid. Moderate Theoretical → Also see TABLE 12 p. 1057
- **Panobinostat** is predicted to increase the exposure to **pimozide**. Avoid. Severe Theoretical → Also see TABLE 7 p. 1055
- **Ranolazine** is predicted to increase the exposure to **panobinostat**. Adjust dose. Moderate Theoretical → Also see TABLE 7 p. 1055
- Rifamycins **(rifampicin)** are predicted to decrease the exposure to **panobinostat**. Avoid. Moderate Theoretical
- **St John's wort** is predicted to decrease the exposure to **panobinostat**. Avoid. Moderate Theoretical
- **Tucatinib** is predicted to increase the exposure to **panobinostat**. Adjust dose—consult product literature; in hepatic impairment avoid. Moderate Study

Panobinostat (continued)
- ▶ **Vemurafenib** is predicted to increase the exposure to **panobinostat**. Adjust dose. Moderate Theoretical → Also see TABLE 7 p. 1055

Pantoprazole → see proton pump inhibitors

Paracetamol → see TABLE 1 p. 1053 (hepatotoxicity)
- ▶ **Alcohol** (in those who drink heavily) causes severe liver damage when given with **paracetamol**. Severe Study
- ▶ **Paracetamol** is predicted to decrease the clearance of alkylating agents **(busulfan)**. Moderate Theoretical
- ▶ Antiepileptics **(carbamazepine, fosphenytoin, phenobarbital, phenytoin, primidone)** decrease the exposure to **paracetamol**. Moderate Study
- ▶ **Paracetamol** increases the anticoagulant effect of **coumarins**. Moderate Study
- ▶ **Imatinib** increases the risk of hepatotoxicity when given with **paracetamol**. Severe Anecdotal
- ▶ **Paracetamol** has been reported to cause high anion gap metabolic acidosis when given with penicillins **(flucloxacillin)**. Severe Anecdotal
- ▶ **Paracetamol** is predicted to increase the anticoagulant effect of **phenindione**. Severe Theoretical
- ▶ **Pitolisant** is predicted to decrease the exposure to **paracetamol**. Mild Theoretical
- ▶ Rifamycins **(rifampicin)** decrease the exposure to **paracetamol**. Moderate Study

Paraldehyde → see antiepileptics

Parathyroid hormone
- ▶ **Bisphosphonates** are predicted to decrease the effects of **parathyroid hormone**. Avoid. Moderate Study

Parecoxib → see NSAIDs

Paricalcitol → see vitamin D substances

Paroxetine → see SSRIs

Pasireotide → see TABLE 4 p. 1054 (bradycardia), TABLE 7 p. 1055 (QT-interval prolongation)
- ▶ **Pasireotide** is predicted to decrease the absorption of oral **ciclosporin**. Adjust dose. Severe Theoretical

Patiromer

SEPARATION OF ADMINISTRATION Manufacturer advises take 3 hours before, or after, other drugs.

Pazopanib → see TABLE 3 p. 1053 (bleeding), TABLE 7 p. 1055 (QT-interval prolongation)
- ▶ Oral **antacids** are predicted to decrease the absorption of oral **pazopanib**. Manufacturer advises take 1 hour before or 2 hours after antacids. Moderate Theoretical
- ▶ Anti-androgens **(apalutamide, enzalutamide)** are predicted to decrease the exposure to **pazopanib**. Avoid. Severe Theoretical → Also see TABLE 7 p. 1055
- ▶ Antiarrhythmics **(dronedarone)** are predicted to increase the exposure to **pazopanib**. Moderate Study → Also see TABLE 7 p. 1055
- ▶ Antiepileptics **(carbamazepine, fosphenytoin, phenobarbital, phenytoin, primidone)** are predicted to decrease the exposure to **pazopanib**. Avoid. Severe Theoretical
- ▶ Antifungals, azoles **(fluconazole, isavuconazole)** are predicted to increase the exposure to **pazopanib**. Moderate Study → Also see TABLE 7 p. 1055
- ▶ Antifungals, azoles **(itraconazole, ketoconazole, posaconazole, voriconazole)** are predicted to increase the exposure to **pazopanib**. Avoid or adjust dose—consult product literature. Moderate Study → Also see TABLE 7 p. 1055
- ▶ **Berotralstat** is predicted to increase the exposure to **pazopanib**. Moderate Study
- ▶ Oral calcium compounds **(calcium carbonate)**-containing antacids might decrease the absorption of oral **pazopanib**. Manufacturer advises take 1 hour before or 2 hours after antacids. Moderate Theoretical
- ▶ Calcium-channel blockers **(diltiazem, verapamil)** are predicted to increase the exposure to **pazopanib**. Moderate Study
- ▶ **Cenobamate** is predicted to decrease the exposure to **pazopanib**. Severe Study
- ▶ **Ceritinib** is predicted to increase the exposure to **pazopanib**. Avoid or adjust dose—consult product literature. Moderate Study → Also see TABLE 7 p. 1055
- ▶ **Cobicistat** is predicted to increase the exposure to **pazopanib**. Avoid or adjust dose—consult product literature. Moderate Study
- ▶ **Crizotinib** is predicted to increase the exposure to **pazopanib**. Moderate Study → Also see TABLE 7 p. 1055
- ▶ **Dabrafenib** is predicted to decrease the exposure to **pazopanib**. Severe Study
- ▶ **Encorafenib** is predicted to decrease the exposure to **pazopanib**. Avoid. Severe Theoretical → Also see TABLE 7 p. 1055
- ▶ Endothelin receptor antagonists **(bosentan)** are predicted to decrease the exposure to **pazopanib**. Severe Study
- ▶ **Fedratinib** is predicted to increase the exposure to **pazopanib**. Moderate Study
- ▶ **Grapefruit** juice is predicted to increase the exposure to **pazopanib**. Avoid. Severe Theoretical
- ▶ **H_2 receptor antagonists** are predicted to decrease the exposure to **pazopanib**. Manufacturer advises take 2 hours before or 10 hours after **H_2 receptor antagonists**. Moderate Theoretical
- ▶ **HIV-protease inhibitors** are predicted to increase the exposure to **pazopanib**. Avoid or adjust dose—consult product literature. Moderate Study
- ▶ **Idelalisib** is predicted to increase the exposure to **pazopanib**. Avoid or adjust dose—consult product literature. Moderate Study
- ▶ **Imatinib** is predicted to increase the exposure to **pazopanib**. Moderate Study → Also see TABLE 3 p. 1053
- ▶ **Ivosidenib** is predicted to decrease the exposure to **pazopanib**. Avoid. Severe Theoretical → Also see TABLE 7 p. 1055
- ▶ **Lapatinib** increases the exposure to **pazopanib**. Avoid. Severe Study → Also see TABLE 7 p. 1055
- ▶ **Letermovir** is predicted to increase the exposure to **pazopanib**. Moderate Study
- ▶ **Pazopanib** is predicted to increase the exposure to **lomitapide**. Separate administration by 12 hours. Mild Theoretical
- ▶ **Lorlatinib** is predicted to decrease the exposure to **pazopanib**. Severe Study
- ▶ **Lumacaftor** is predicted to decrease the exposure to **pazopanib**. Avoid. Severe Theoretical
- ▶ Macrolides **(clarithromycin)** are predicted to increase the exposure to **pazopanib**. Avoid or adjust dose—consult product literature. Moderate Study
- ▶ Macrolides **(erythromycin)** are predicted to increase the exposure to **pazopanib**. Moderate Study → Also see TABLE 7 p. 1055
- ▶ **Pazopanib** is predicted to increase the exposure to **mavacamten**. Monitor and adjust dose—consult product literature. Moderate Theoretical
- ▶ **Mitotane** is predicted to decrease the exposure to **pazopanib**. Avoid. Severe Theoretical
- ▶ Neurokinin-1 receptor antagonists **(aprepitant, netupitant)** are predicted to increase the exposure to **pazopanib**. Moderate Study
- ▶ **Nilotinib** is predicted to increase the exposure to **pazopanib**. Moderate Study → Also see TABLE 7 p. 1055
- ▶ NNRTIs **(efavirenz, etravirine, nevirapine)** are predicted to decrease the exposure to **pazopanib**. Severe Study → Also see TABLE 7 p. 1055
- ▶ **Pazopanib** is predicted to increase the risk of bleeding events when given with **phenindione**. Severe Theoretical → Also see TABLE 3 p. 1053
- ▶ **Proton pump inhibitors** are predicted to decrease the exposure to **pazopanib**. Avoid or administer concurrently without food. Moderate Study
- ▶ Rifamycins **(rifampicin)** are predicted to decrease the exposure to **pazopanib**. Avoid. Severe Theoretical
- ▶ Oral **sodium bicarbonate**-containing antacids might decrease the absorption of oral **pazopanib**. Manufacturer advises take 1 hour before or 2 hours after antacids. Moderate Theoretical
- ▶ **Sotorasib** is predicted to decrease the exposure to **pazopanib**. Severe Study
- ▶ **St John's wort** is predicted to decrease the exposure to **pazopanib**. Severe Study
- ▶ **Pazopanib** might affect the exposure to statins **(atorvastatin, pravastatin, rosuvastatin)**. Moderate Theoretical
- ▶ **Pazopanib** might cause increased ALT concentrations when given with statins **(simvastatin)**. Moderate Study

- **Tucatinib** is predicted to increase the exposure to **pazopanib**. Avoid or adjust dose—consult product literature. Moderate Study

Peanut protein

GENERAL INFORMATION Desensitising vaccines should be avoided in patients taking beta-blockers (adrenaline might be ineffective in case of a hypersensitivity reaction) or ACE inhibitors (risk of severe anaphylactoid reactions).

Pegaspargase → see TABLE 3 p. 1053 (bleeding), TABLE 1 p. 1053 (hepatotoxicity), TABLE 12 p. 1057 (myelosuppression)

- **Pegaspargase** is predicted to increase the risk of hepatotoxicity when given with **imatinib**. Severe Theoretical → Also see TABLE 3 p. 1053 → Also see TABLE 12 p. 1057
- **Pegaspargase** affects the efficacy of **methotrexate**. Severe Anecdotal → Also see TABLE 1 p. 1053 → Also see TABLE 12 p. 1057
- **Pegaspargase** potentially increases the risk of neurotoxicity when given with vinca alkaloids **(vincristine)**. **Vincristine** should be taken 3 to 24 hours before **pegaspargase**. Severe Anecdotal → Also see TABLE 12 p. 1057

Pegfilgrastim

- **Pegfilgrastim** might increase the risk of pulmonary toxicity when given with **bleomycin**. Severe Theoretical

Peginterferon alfa → see interferons

Pembrolizumab → see monoclonal antibodies

Pemetrexed → see TABLE 1 p. 1053 (hepatotoxicity), TABLE 12 p. 1057 (myelosuppression), TABLE 2 p. 1053 (nephrotoxicity)

- Antimalarials **(pyrimethamine)** are predicted to increase the risk of adverse effects when given with **pemetrexed**. Severe Theoretical
- **Aspirin** (high-dose) potentially increases the exposure to **pemetrexed**. Use with caution or avoid. Severe Theoretical → Also see TABLE 2 p. 1053
- **Live vaccines** are predicted to increase the risk of generalised infection (possibly life-threatening) when given with **pemetrexed**. UKHSA advises avoid (refer to Green Book). Severe Theoretical
- **NSAIDs** are predicted to increase the exposure to **pemetrexed**. Use with caution or avoid. Severe Theoretical → Also see TABLE 2 p. 1053

Pemigatinib

- **Pemigatinib** might increase the exposure to the active metabolite of alkylating agents **(cyclophosphamide)**. Moderate Theoretical
- **Pemigatinib** might decrease the exposure to alkylating agents **(ifosfamide)**. Moderate Theoretical
- Anti-androgens **(apalutamide, enzalutamide)** are predicted to decrease the exposure to **pemigatinib**. Avoid. Severe Study
- Antiarrhythmics **(dronedarone)** are predicted to increase the exposure to **pemigatinib**. Severe Study
- Antiepileptics **(carbamazepine, fosphenytoin, phenobarbital, phenytoin, primidone)** are predicted to decrease the exposure to **pemigatinib**. Avoid. Severe Study
- Antifungals, azoles **(fluconazole, isavuconazole)** are predicted to increase the exposure to **pemigatinib**. Severe Study
- Antifungals, azoles **(itraconazole, ketoconazole, posaconazole, voriconazole)** are predicted to increase the exposure to **pemigatinib**. Avoid or adjust dose—consult product literature. Severe Study
- **Berotralstat** is predicted to increase the exposure to **pemigatinib**. Severe Study
- Calcium-channel blockers **(diltiazem, verapamil)** are predicted to increase the exposure to **pemigatinib**. Severe Study
- **Ceritinib** is predicted to increase the exposure to **pemigatinib**. Avoid or adjust dose—consult product literature. Severe Study
- **Cobicistat** is predicted to increase the exposure to **pemigatinib**. Avoid or adjust dose—consult product literature. Severe Study
- **Crizotinib** is predicted to increase the exposure to **pemigatinib**. Severe Study
- **Dabrafenib** is predicted to decrease the exposure to **pemigatinib**. Avoid or monitor. Severe Study
- **Pemigatinib** might increase the exposure to **digoxin**. Separate administration by at least 6 hours. Moderate Theoretical
- **Encorafenib** is predicted to decrease the exposure to **pemigatinib**. Avoid. Severe Study
- Endothelin receptor antagonists **(bosentan)** are predicted to decrease the exposure to **pemigatinib**. Avoid or monitor. Severe Study
- **Pemigatinib** might increase the exposure to **everolimus**. Separate administration by at least 6 hours. Moderate Theoretical
- **Fedratinib** is predicted to increase the exposure to **pemigatinib**. Severe Study
- **Grapefruit** and grapefruit juice is predicted to increase the exposure to **pemigatinib**. Avoid. Severe Study
- **HIV-protease inhibitors** are predicted to increase the exposure to **pemigatinib**. Avoid or adjust dose—consult product literature. Severe Study
- **Idelalisib** is predicted to increase the exposure to **pemigatinib**. Avoid or adjust dose—consult product literature. Severe Study
- **Imatinib** is predicted to increase the exposure to **pemigatinib**. Severe Study
- **Ivosidenib** is predicted to decrease the exposure to **pemigatinib**. Avoid. Severe Study
- **Letermovir** is predicted to increase the exposure to **pemigatinib**. Severe Study
- **Lorlatinib** is predicted to decrease the exposure to **pemigatinib**. Avoid or monitor. Severe Study
- **Lumacaftor** is predicted to decrease the exposure to **pemigatinib**. Avoid. Severe Study
- Macrolides **(clarithromycin)** are predicted to increase the exposure to **pemigatinib**. Avoid or adjust dose—consult product literature. Severe Study
- Macrolides **(erythromycin)** are predicted to increase the exposure to **pemigatinib**. Severe Study
- **Mitotane** is predicted to decrease the exposure to **pemigatinib**. Avoid. Severe Study
- Neurokinin-1 receptor antagonists **(aprepitant, netupitant)** are predicted to increase the exposure to **pemigatinib**. Severe Study
- **Nilotinib** is predicted to increase the exposure to **pemigatinib**. Severe Study
- NNRTIs **(efavirenz)** are predicted to decrease the exposure to **pemigatinib** and **pemigatinib** might decrease the exposure to NNRTIs **(efavirenz)**. Avoid or monitor. Severe Study
- NNRTIs **(etravirine, nevirapine)** are predicted to decrease the exposure to **pemigatinib**. Avoid or monitor. Severe Study
- **Pemigatinib** might decrease the exposure to opioids **(methadone)**. Moderate Theoretical
- **Pemigatinib** is predicted to increase the risk of hyperphosphataemia when given with **phosphate**. Moderate Theoretical
- **Proton pump inhibitors** have been reported to decrease the exposure to **pemigatinib**. Avoid. Severe Anecdotal
- Rifamycins **(rifampicin)** are predicted to decrease the exposure to **pemigatinib**. Avoid. Severe Study
- **Pemigatinib** might increase the exposure to **sirolimus**. Separate administration by at least 6 hours. Moderate Theoretical
- **Sotorasib** is predicted to decrease the exposure to **pemigatinib**. Avoid or monitor. Severe Study
- **St John's wort** is predicted to decrease the exposure to **pemigatinib**. Avoid. Severe Study
- **Pemigatinib** might increase the exposure to **talazoparib**. Separate administration by at least 6 hours. Moderate Theoretical
- **Pemigatinib** might increase the exposure to taxanes **(paclitaxel)**. Separate administration by at least 6 hours. Moderate Theoretical
- **Tucatinib** is predicted to increase the exposure to **pemigatinib**. Avoid or adjust dose—consult product literature. Severe Study

Penicillamine

- Oral **antacids** decrease the absorption of oral **penicillamine**. Separate administration by 2 hours. Mild Study
- Antimalarials **(chloroquine)** are predicted to increase the risk of haematological toxicity when given with **penicillamine**. Avoid. Severe Theoretical
- **Penicillamine** potentially decreases the concentration of **digoxin**. Separate administration by 2 hours. Severe Anecdotal

Penicillamine (continued)

- **Hydroxychloroquine** is predicted to increase the risk of haematological toxicity when given with **penicillamine**. Avoid. Severe Theoretical
- Oral **iron** is predicted to decrease the absorption of oral **penicillamine**. Separate administration by at least 2 hours. Mild Study
- **Zinc** is predicted to decrease the absorption of **penicillamine**. Mild Theoretical

Penicillins

amoxicillin · ampicillin · benzathine benzylpenicillin · benzylpenicillin · flucloxacillin · phenoxymethylpenicillin · piperacillin · pivmecillinam · temocillin

- **Allopurinol** increases the risk of skin rash when given with penicillins **(amoxicillin, ampicillin)**. Moderate Study
- Antiepileptics **(valproate)** increase the risk of adverse effects when given with **pivmecillinam**. Avoid. Severe Anecdotal
- **Flucloxacillin** (particularly high-dose) might greatly decrease the concentration of antifungals, azoles **(isavuconazole)**. Moderate Anecdotal
- **Flucloxacillin** (particularly high-dose) might greatly decrease the concentration of antifungals, azoles **(posaconazole)**. Moderate Study
- **Flucloxacillin** (particularly high-dose) might greatly decrease the concentration of antifungals, azoles **(voriconazole)**. Avoid or monitor. Moderate Study
- **Penicillins** potentially alter the anticoagulant effect of **coumarins**. Monitor INR and adjust dose. Severe Anecdotal
- **Flucloxacillin** (high-dose) might decrease the exposure to **everolimus**. Moderate Study
- **Ivosidenib** is predicted to increase the exposure to **benzylpenicillin**. Use with caution or avoid. Moderate Theoretical
- **Leflunomide** is predicted to increase the exposure to **benzylpenicillin**. Moderate Study
- **Penicillins** are predicted to increase the risk of toxicity when given with **methotrexate**. Severe Anecdotal
- **Piperacillin** increases the effects of **neuromuscular blocking drugs, non-depolarising**. Moderate Study
- **Nitisinone** is predicted to increase the exposure to **benzylpenicillin**. Moderate Study
- **Paracetamol** has been reported to cause high anion gap metabolic acidosis when given with **flucloxacillin**. Severe Anecdotal
- **Penicillins** are predicted to increase the risk of bleeding events when given with **phenindione**. Severe Theoretical
- **Piperacillin** increases the effects of **suxamethonium**. Moderate Study
- **Flucloxacillin** (high-dose) might decrease the exposure to **tacrolimus**. Moderate Study
- **Teriflunomide** is predicted to increase the exposure to **benzylpenicillin**. Moderate Study
- **Benzylpenicillin** is predicted to increase the exposure to **vadadustat** and **vadadustat** is predicted to increase the exposure to **benzylpenicillin**. Moderate Study

Pentamidine → see TABLE 2 p. 1053 (nephrotoxicity), TABLE 7 p. 1055 (QT-interval prolongation), TABLE 13 p. 1057 (increased serum potassium)

- **Foscarnet** increases the risk of hypocalcaemia when given with **pentamidine**. Severe Anecdotal → Also see TABLE 2 p. 1053
- **Pentamidine** might enhance the antidiuretic and hypertensive effects of **vasopressin**. Moderate Theoretical

Pentazocine → see opioids

Pentosan → see TABLE 3 p. 1053 (bleeding)

Pentostatin → see TABLE 12 p. 1057 (myelosuppression)

- Alkylating agents **(cyclophosphamide)** (high-dose) increase the risk of toxicity when given with **pentostatin**. Avoid. Severe Anecdotal → Also see TABLE 12 p. 1057
- **Fludarabine** increases the risk of pulmonary toxicity when given with **pentostatin**. Avoid. Severe Study → Also see TABLE 12 p. 1057

Pentoxifylline

- **Pentoxifylline** is predicted to increase the concentration of **aminophylline**. Use with caution or avoid. Severe Theoretical
- Quinolones **(ciprofloxacin)** very slightly increase the exposure to **pentoxifylline**. Moderate Study
- SSRIs **(fluvoxamine)** are predicted to increase the exposure to **pentoxifylline**. Moderate Theoretical
- **Pentoxifylline** increases the concentration of **theophylline**. Monitor and adjust dose. Severe Study

Peppermint

- **Peppermint** oil is predicted to increase the exposure to **lomitapide**. Separate administration by 12 hours. Moderate Theoretical

Perampanel → see antiepileptics

Pericyazine → see phenothiazine antipsychotics

Perindopril → see ACE inhibitors

Pertuzumab → see monoclonal antibodies

Pethidine → see opioids

Phenazone → see NSAIDs

Phenelzine → see MAOIs, irreversible

Phenindione → see TABLE 3 p. 1053 (bleeding)

FOOD AND LIFESTYLE The effects of phenindione can be reduced or abolished by vitamin K, including that found in health foods, food supplements, enteral feeds, or large amounts of some green vegetables or green tea. Major changes in diet (especially involving salads and vegetables) and in alcohol consumption can affect anticoagulant control.

- Antiarrhythmics **(dronedarone)** might increase the anticoagulant effect of **phenindione**. Moderate Anecdotal
- Antiarrhythmics **(propafenone)** are predicted to increase the anticoagulant effect of **phenindione**. Monitor and adjust dose. Moderate Theoretical
- Antifungals, azoles **(miconazole)** greatly increase the anticoagulant effect of **phenindione**. Severe Theoretical
- Cephalosporins **(cefazolin, ceftriaxone)** potentially increase the risk of bleeding events when given with **phenindione**. Severe Anecdotal
- **Ceritinib** is predicted to increase the exposure to **phenindione**. Severe Theoretical
- **Corticosteroids** are predicted to increase the effects of **phenindione**. Moderate Anecdotal
- **Crizotinib** is predicted to increase the risk of bleeding events when given with **phenindione**. Severe Theoretical
- **Dabrafenib** is predicted to decrease the exposure to **phenindione**. Moderate Study
- **Disulfiram** is predicted to increase the anticoagulant effect of **phenindione**. Severe Theoretical
- **Donanemab** can increase the risk of brain haemorrhage when given with **phenindione**. Avoid. Severe Anecdotal
- **Enteral feeds** (vitamin-K containing) potentially decrease the effects of **phenindione**. Severe Theoretical
- **Erlotinib** is predicted to increase the risk of bleeding events when given with **phenindione**. Severe Theoretical
- **Fibrates** are predicted to increase the anticoagulant effect of **phenindione**. Monitor INR and adjust dose. Severe Study
- **Fostamatinib** might cause bleeding when given with **phenindione**. Moderate Theoretical
- **Gefitinib** is predicted to increase the risk of bleeding events when given with **phenindione**. Severe Theoretical
- H_2 receptor antagonists **(cimetidine)** increase the exposure to **phenindione**. Severe Anecdotal
- **Imatinib** is predicted to increase the risk of bleeding events when given with **phenindione**. Severe Theoretical → Also see TABLE 3 p. 1053
- **Lapatinib** is predicted to increase the risk of bleeding events when given with **phenindione**. Severe Theoretical
- **Lecanemab** can increase the risk of brain haemorrhage when given with **phenindione**. Avoid. Severe Anecdotal
- Macrolides **(azithromycin)** might increase the risk of bleeding events when given with **phenindione**. Severe Theoretical
- **Phenindione** might increase the risk of gastrointestinal bleeding when given with monoclonal antibodies **(ipilimumab)**. Severe Theoretical
- **Nilotinib** is predicted to increase the risk of bleeding events when given with **phenindione**. Severe Theoretical
- **Nirmatrelvir** boosted with ritonavir is predicted to affect the concentration of **phenindione**. Moderate Theoretical
- Opioids **(tramadol)** might increase the anticoagulant effect of **phenindione**. Severe Anecdotal

- **Oxymetholone** increases the anticoagulant effect of **phenindione**. Severe Anecdotal
- **Paracetamol** is predicted to increase the anticoagulant effect of **phenindione**. Severe Theoretical
- **Pazopanib** is predicted to increase the risk of bleeding events when given with **phenindione**. Severe Theoretical → Also see TABLE 3 p. 1053
- **Penicillins** are predicted to increase the risk of bleeding events when given with **phenindione**. Severe Theoretical
- **Selumetinib** might increase the risk of bleeding when given with **phenindione**. Severe Theoretical
- **Sofosbuvir** might affect the anticoagulant effect of **phenindione**. Moderate Theoretical
- Statins **(rosuvastatin)** are predicted to increase the anticoagulant effect of **phenindione**. Monitor INR and adjust dose. Severe Theoretical
- **Tetracyclines** are predicted to increase the anticoagulant effect of **phenindione**. Severe Theoretical
- **Tigecycline** is predicted to increase the anticoagulant effect of **phenindione**. Severe Theoretical
- **Tofacitinib** is predicted to increase the risk of bleeding when given with **phenindione**. Severe Theoretical
- **Vemurafenib** is predicted to increase the exposure to **phenindione**. Moderate Study

Phenobarbital → see antiepileptics

Phenothiazine antipsychotics → see TABLE 15 p. 1058 (hyponatraemia), TABLE 6 p. 1054 (hypotension), TABLE 7 p. 1055 (QT-interval prolongation), TABLE 8 p. 1055 (antimuscarinics), TABLE 9 p. 1056 (CNS effects)

chlorpromazine · levomepromazine · pericyazine · prochlorperazine · promazine · trifluoperazine

FOOD AND LIFESTYLE **Chlorpromazine** dose adjustment might be necessary if smoking started or stopped during treatment.

- **Phenothiazine antipsychotics** are predicted to decrease the effects of **amfetamines** and **amfetamines** are predicted to decrease the effects of **phenothiazine antipsychotics**. Moderate Study
- Oral **antacids** decrease the absorption of oral **phenothiazine antipsychotics**. Moderate Anecdotal
- **Chlorpromazine** decreases the concentration of antiepileptics **(phenobarbital, primidone)** and antiepileptics **(phenobarbital, primidone)** decrease the concentration of **chlorpromazine**. Moderate Study → Also see TABLE 9 p. 1056
- Atypical antipsychotics **(clozapine)** can cause constipation, as can **phenothiazine antipsychotics**; concurrent use might increase the risk of developing intestinal obstruction. Severe Theoretical → Also see TABLE 15 p. 1058 → Also see TABLE 6 p. 1054 → Also see TABLE 8 p. 1055 → Also see TABLE 9 p. 1056
- **Combined hormonal contraceptives** is predicted to increase the exposure to **chlorpromazine**. Moderate Theoretical
- **Chlorpromazine** is predicted to increase the risk of hyponatraemia when given with **desmopressin**. Severe Theoretical → Also see TABLE 15 p. 1058
- **Phenothiazine antipsychotics** are predicted to decrease the effects of **dopamine receptor agonists**. Avoid. Moderate Theoretical → Also see TABLE 6 p. 1054 → Also see TABLE 7 p. 1055 → Also see TABLE 8 p. 1055 → Also see TABLE 9 p. 1056
- **Phenothiazine antipsychotics** oppose the effects of the active metabolite of **foslevodopa**. Severe Theoretical → Also see TABLE 6 p. 1054 → Also see TABLE 9 p. 1056
- **Givosiran** is predicted to increase the exposure to **chlorpromazine**. Moderate Theoretical
- **Phenothiazine antipsychotics** decrease the effects of **levodopa**. Avoid or monitor worsening parkinsonism symptoms. Severe Study → Also see TABLE 6 p. 1054 → Also see TABLE 9 p. 1056
- **Phenothiazine antipsychotics** potentially increase the risk of neurotoxicity when given with **lithium**. Severe Anecdotal
- MAOIs, irreversible **(isocarboxazid, phenelzine)** are predicted to increase the risk of neuroleptic malignant syndrome when given with **phenothiazine antipsychotics**. Severe Theoretical → Also see TABLE 6 p. 1054
- MAOIs, irreversible **(tranylcypromine)** are predicted to increase the risk of neuroleptic malignant syndrome when given with **phenothiazine antipsychotics**. Avoid. Severe Theoretical → Also see TABLE 6 p. 1054
- **Chlorpromazine** decreases the effects of **metyrapone**. Avoid. Moderate Theoretical
- **Mexiletine** is predicted to increase the exposure to **chlorpromazine**. Moderate Theoretical
- **Moclobemide** increases the risk of adverse effects when given with **levomepromazine**. Moderate Study
- **Osilodrostat** is predicted to increase the exposure to **chlorpromazine**. Moderate Theoretical → Also see TABLE 7 p. 1055
- Quinolones **(ciprofloxacin)** are predicted to increase the exposure to **chlorpromazine**. Moderate Theoretical
- **Rucaparib** is predicted to increase the exposure to **chlorpromazine**. Moderate Theoretical
- SSRIs **(fluvoxamine)** are predicted to increase the exposure to **chlorpromazine**. Moderate Theoretical → Also see TABLE 15 p. 1058 → Also see TABLE 9 p. 1056
- **Vemurafenib** is predicted to increase the exposure to **chlorpromazine**. Moderate Theoretical → Also see TABLE 7 p. 1055

Phenoxymethylpenicillin → see penicillins

Phenylephrine → see sympathomimetics, vasoconstrictor

Phenytoin → see antiepileptics

Phosphate

- **Pemigatinib** is predicted to increase the risk of hyperphosphataemia when given with **phosphate**. Moderate Theoretical

Phosphodiesterase type-4 inhibitors

apremilast · roflumilast

- **Aminophylline** is predicted to slightly increase the exposure to **roflumilast**. Avoid. Moderate Theoretical
- Anti-androgens **(apalutamide, enzalutamide)** moderately decrease the exposure to **apremilast**. Avoid. Severe Study
- Anti-androgens **(apalutamide, enzalutamide)** are predicted to decrease the exposure to **roflumilast**. Avoid. Moderate Study
- Antiepileptics **(carbamazepine, fosphenytoin, phenobarbital, phenytoin, primidone)** moderately decrease the exposure to **apremilast**. Avoid. Severe Study
- Antiepileptics **(carbamazepine, fosphenytoin, phenobarbital, phenytoin, primidone)** are predicted to decrease the exposure to **roflumilast**. Avoid. Moderate Study
- **Combined hormonal contraceptives** is predicted to increase the exposure to **roflumilast**. Moderate Theoretical
- **Encorafenib** moderately decreases the exposure to **apremilast**. Avoid. Severe Study
- **Encorafenib** is predicted to decrease the exposure to **roflumilast**. Avoid. Moderate Study
- **Givosiran** is predicted to increase the exposure to **roflumilast**. Moderate Theoretical
- H_2 receptor antagonists **(cimetidine)** slightly increase the exposure to **roflumilast**. Moderate Study
- **Ivosidenib** moderately decreases the exposure to **apremilast**. Avoid. Severe Study
- **Ivosidenib** is predicted to decrease the exposure to **roflumilast**. Avoid. Moderate Study
- **Lumacaftor** moderately decreases the exposure to **apremilast**. Avoid. Severe Study
- **Lumacaftor** is predicted to decrease the exposure to **roflumilast**. Avoid. Moderate Study
- **Mexiletine** is predicted to increase the exposure to **roflumilast**. Moderate Theoretical
- **Mitotane** moderately decreases the exposure to **apremilast**. Avoid. Severe Study
- **Mitotane** is predicted to decrease the exposure to **roflumilast**. Avoid. Moderate Study
- **Osilodrostat** is predicted to increase the exposure to **roflumilast**. Moderate Theoretical
- Quinolones **(ciprofloxacin)** are predicted to increase the exposure to **roflumilast**. Moderate Theoretical
- Rifamycins **(rifampicin)** moderately decrease the exposure to **apremilast**. Avoid. Severe Study
- Rifamycins **(rifampicin)** are predicted to decrease the exposure to **roflumilast**. Avoid. Moderate Study
- **Rucaparib** is predicted to increase the exposure to **roflumilast**. Moderate Theoretical

Phosphodiesterase type-4 inhibitors (continued)
- SSRIs **(fluvoxamine)** are predicted to increase the exposure to **roflumilast**. Moderate Study
- **St John's wort** is predicted to decrease the exposure to **apremilast**. Avoid. Severe Theoretical
- **Theophylline** is predicted to slightly increase the exposure to **roflumilast**. Avoid. Moderate Theoretical
- **Vemurafenib** is predicted to increase the exposure to **roflumilast**. Moderate Theoretical

Phosphodiesterase type-5 inhibitors → see TABLE 6 p. 1054 (hypotension), TABLE 7 p. 1055 (QT-interval prolongation)

avanafil · sildenafil · tadalafil · vardenafil

- **Alpha blockers** cause significant hypotensive effects when given with **phosphodiesterase type-5 inhibitors.** Patient should be stabilised on first drug then second drug should be added at the lowest recommended dose. Severe Study → Also see TABLE 6 p. 1054
- Anti-androgens **(apalutamide, enzalutamide)** are predicted to decrease the exposure to phosphodiesterase type-5 inhibitors **(avanafil, tadalafil)**. Avoid. Severe Study
- Anti-androgens **(apalutamide, enzalutamide)** are predicted to decrease the exposure to phosphodiesterase type-5 inhibitors **(sildenafil, vardenafil)**. Moderate Theoretical → Also see TABLE 7 p. 1055
- Antiarrhythmics **(dronedarone)** are predicted to increase the exposure to **avanafil**. Adjust **avanafil** dose. Moderate Theoretical
- Antiarrhythmics **(dronedarone)** are predicted to increase the exposure to **sildenafil**. Monitor or adjust **sildenafil** dose with moderate CYP3A4 inhibitors, p. 139. Moderate Study
- Antiarrhythmics **(dronedarone)** are predicted to increase the exposure to **tadalafil**. Severe Theoretical
- Antiarrhythmics **(dronedarone)** are predicted to increase the exposure to **vardenafil**. Adjust dose. Severe Theoretical → Also see TABLE 7 p. 1055
- Antiepileptics **(carbamazepine, fosphenytoin, phenobarbital, phenytoin, primidone)** are predicted to decrease the exposure to phosphodiesterase type-5 inhibitors **(avanafil, tadalafil)**. Avoid. Severe Study
- Antiepileptics **(carbamazepine, fosphenytoin, phenobarbital, phenytoin, primidone)** are predicted to decrease the exposure to phosphodiesterase type-5 inhibitors **(sildenafil, vardenafil)**. Moderate Theoretical
- Antifungals, azoles **(fluconazole, isavuconazole)** are predicted to increase the exposure to **avanafil**. Adjust **avanafil** dose. Moderate Theoretical
- Antifungals, azoles **(fluconazole, isavuconazole)** are predicted to increase the exposure to **sildenafil**. Monitor or adjust **sildenafil** dose with moderate CYP3A4 inhibitors, p. 139. Moderate Study
- Antifungals, azoles **(fluconazole, isavuconazole)** are predicted to increase the exposure to **tadalafil**. Severe Theoretical
- Antifungals, azoles **(fluconazole, isavuconazole)** are predicted to increase the exposure to **vardenafil**. Adjust dose. Severe Theoretical → Also see TABLE 7 p. 1055
- Antifungals, azoles **(itraconazole, ketoconazole, posaconazole, voriconazole)** are predicted to increase the exposure to **sildenafil**. Avoid potent CYP3A4 inhibitors or adjust **sildenafil** dose, p. 139. Severe Study
- Antifungals, azoles **(itraconazole, ketoconazole, posaconazole, voriconazole)** are predicted to increase the exposure to **tadalafil**. Use with caution or avoid. Severe Study
- Antifungals, azoles **(miconazole)** are predicted to increase the exposure to **sildenafil**. Use with caution and adjust dose. Severe Theoretical
- Antifungals, azoles **(itraconazole, ketoconazole, posaconazole, voriconazole)** are predicted to increase the exposure to phosphodiesterase type-5 inhibitors **(avanafil, vardenafil)**. Avoid. Severe Study → Also see TABLE 7 p. 1055
- **Berotralstat** is predicted to increase the exposure to **avanafil**. Adjust **avanafil** dose. Moderate Theoretical
- **Berotralstat** is predicted to increase the exposure to **sildenafil**. Monitor or adjust **sildenafil** dose with moderate CYP3A4 inhibitors, p. 139. Moderate Study
- **Berotralstat** is predicted to increase the exposure to **tadalafil**. Severe Theoretical
- **Berotralstat** is predicted to increase the exposure to **vardenafil**. Adjust dose. Severe Theoretical
- Calcium-channel blockers **(diltiazem, verapamil)** are predicted to increase the exposure to **avanafil**. Adjust **avanafil** dose. Moderate Theoretical → Also see TABLE 6 p. 1054
- Calcium-channel blockers **(diltiazem, verapamil)** are predicted to increase the exposure to **sildenafil**. Monitor or adjust **sildenafil** dose with moderate CYP3A4 inhibitors, p. 139. Moderate Study → Also see TABLE 6 p. 1054
- Calcium-channel blockers **(diltiazem, verapamil)** are predicted to increase the exposure to **tadalafil**. Severe Theoretical → Also see TABLE 6 p. 1054
- Calcium-channel blockers **(diltiazem, verapamil)** are predicted to increase the exposure to **vardenafil**. Adjust dose. Severe Theoretical → Also see TABLE 6 p. 1054
- **Cenobamate** is predicted to decrease the exposure to phosphodiesterase type-5 inhibitors **(avanafil, sildenafil, vardenafil)**. Adjust dose. Moderate Theoretical
- **Ceritinib** is predicted to increase the exposure to phosphodiesterase type-5 inhibitors **(avanafil, vardenafil)**. Avoid. Severe Study → Also see TABLE 7 p. 1055
- **Ceritinib** is predicted to increase the exposure to **sildenafil**. Avoid potent CYP3A4 inhibitors or adjust **sildenafil** dose, p. 139. Severe Study
- **Ceritinib** is predicted to increase the exposure to **tadalafil**. Use with caution or avoid. Severe Study
- **Cobicistat** is predicted to increase the exposure to phosphodiesterase type-5 inhibitors **(avanafil, vardenafil)**. Avoid. Severe Study
- **Cobicistat** is predicted to increase the exposure to **sildenafil**. Avoid potent CYP3A4 inhibitors or adjust **sildenafil** dose, p. 139. Severe Study
- **Cobicistat** is predicted to increase the exposure to **tadalafil**. Use with caution or avoid. Severe Study
- **Crizotinib** is predicted to increase the exposure to **avanafil**. Adjust **avanafil** dose. Moderate Theoretical
- **Crizotinib** is predicted to increase the exposure to **sildenafil**. Monitor or adjust **sildenafil** dose with moderate CYP3A4 inhibitors, p. 139. Moderate Study
- **Crizotinib** is predicted to increase the exposure to **tadalafil**. Severe Theoretical
- **Crizotinib** is predicted to increase the exposure to **vardenafil**. Adjust dose. Severe Theoretical → Also see TABLE 7 p. 1055
- **Encorafenib** is predicted to decrease the exposure to phosphodiesterase type-5 inhibitors **(avanafil, tadalafil)**. Avoid. Severe Study
- **Encorafenib** is predicted to decrease the exposure to phosphodiesterase type-5 inhibitors **(sildenafil, vardenafil)**. Moderate Theoretical → Also see TABLE 7 p. 1055
- Endothelin receptor antagonists **(bosentan)** decrease the exposure to **phosphodiesterase type-5 inhibitors.** Moderate Study
- **Fedratinib** is predicted to increase the exposure to **avanafil**. Adjust **avanafil** dose. Moderate Theoretical
- **Fedratinib** is predicted to increase the exposure to **sildenafil**. Monitor or adjust **sildenafil** dose with moderate CYP3A4 inhibitors, p. 139. Moderate Study
- **Fedratinib** is predicted to increase the exposure to **tadalafil**. Severe Theoretical
- **Fedratinib** is predicted to increase the exposure to **vardenafil**. Adjust dose. Severe Theoretical
- **Givinostat** might increase the exposure to **sildenafil**. Moderate Study
- **Grapefruit** juice is predicted to increase the exposure to **phosphodiesterase type-5 inhibitors**. Use with caution or avoid. Moderate Study
- **HIV-protease inhibitors** are predicted to increase the exposure to phosphodiesterase type-5 inhibitors **(avanafil, vardenafil)**. Avoid. Severe Study
- **HIV-protease inhibitors** are predicted to increase the exposure to **sildenafil**. Avoid potent CYP3A4 inhibitors or adjust **sildenafil** dose, p. 139. Severe Study
- **HIV-protease inhibitors** are predicted to increase the exposure to **tadalafil**. Use with caution or avoid. Severe Study

- **Idelalisib** is predicted to increase the exposure to phosphodiesterase type-5 inhibitors **(avanafil, vardenafil)**. Avoid. Severe Study
- **Idelalisib** is predicted to increase the exposure to **sildenafil**. Avoid potent CYP3A4 inhibitors or adjust **sildenafil** dose, p. 139. Severe Study
- **Idelalisib** is predicted to increase the exposure to **tadalafil**. Use with caution or avoid. Severe Study
- **Imatinib** is predicted to increase the exposure to **avanafil**. Adjust **avanafil** dose. Moderate Theoretical
- **Imatinib** is predicted to increase the exposure to **sildenafil**. Monitor or adjust **sildenafil** dose with moderate CYP3A4 inhibitors, p. 139. Moderate Study
- **Imatinib** is predicted to increase the exposure to **tadalafil**. Severe Theoretical
- **Imatinib** is predicted to increase the exposure to **vardenafil**. Adjust dose. Severe Theoretical
- **Ivosidenib** is predicted to decrease the exposure to phosphodiesterase type-5 inhibitors **(avanafil, tadalafil)**. Avoid. Severe Study
- **Ivosidenib** is predicted to decrease the exposure to phosphodiesterase type-5 inhibitors **(sildenafil, vardenafil)**. Moderate Theoretical → Also see TABLE 7 p. 1055
- **Lenacapavir** is predicted to increase the concentration of **sildenafil**. Adjust starting dose for erectile dysfunction. Severe Theoretical
- **Lenacapavir** is predicted to increase the concentration of **tadalafil**. Avoid or adjust dose depending on indication—consult product literature. Severe Theoretical
- **Lenacapavir** is predicted to increase the concentration of **vardenafil**. Adjust dose for erectile dysfunction. Severe Theoretical
- **Letermovir** is predicted to increase the exposure to **avanafil**. Adjust **avanafil** dose. Moderate Theoretical
- **Letermovir** is predicted to increase the exposure to **sildenafil**. Monitor or adjust **sildenafil** dose with moderate CYP3A4 inhibitors, p. 139. Moderate Study
- **Letermovir** is predicted to increase the exposure to **tadalafil**. Severe Theoretical
- **Letermovir** is predicted to increase the exposure to **vardenafil**. Adjust dose. Severe Theoretical
- **Lumacaftor** is predicted to decrease the exposure to phosphodiesterase type-5 inhibitors **(avanafil, tadalafil)**. Avoid. Severe Study
- **Lumacaftor** is predicted to decrease the exposure to phosphodiesterase type-5 inhibitors **(sildenafil, vardenafil)**. Moderate Theoretical
- Macrolides **(clarithromycin)** are predicted to increase the exposure to **sildenafil**. Avoid potent CYP3A4 inhibitors or adjust **sildenafil** dose, p. 139. Severe Study
- Macrolides **(clarithromycin)** are predicted to increase the exposure to **tadalafil**. Use with caution or avoid. Severe Study
- Macrolides **(erythromycin)** are predicted to increase the exposure to **avanafil**. Adjust **avanafil** dose. Moderate Theoretical
- Macrolides **(erythromycin)** are predicted to increase the exposure to **sildenafil**. Monitor or adjust **sildenafil** dose with moderate CYP3A4 inhibitors, p. 139. Moderate Study
- Macrolides **(erythromycin)** are predicted to increase the exposure to **tadalafil**. Severe Theoretical
- Macrolides **(erythromycin)** are predicted to increase the exposure to **vardenafil**. Adjust dose. Severe Theoretical → Also see TABLE 7 p. 1055
- Macrolides **(clarithromycin)** are predicted to increase the exposure to phosphodiesterase type-5 inhibitors **(avanafil, vardenafil)**. Avoid. Severe Study
- **Mitotane** is predicted to decrease the exposure to phosphodiesterase type-5 inhibitors **(avanafil, tadalafil)**. Avoid. Severe Study
- **Mitotane** is predicted to decrease the exposure to phosphodiesterase type-5 inhibitors **(sildenafil, vardenafil)**. Moderate Theoretical
- Neurokinin-1 receptor antagonists **(aprepitant, netupitant)** are predicted to increase the exposure to **avanafil**. Adjust **avanafil** dose. Moderate Theoretical
- Neurokinin-1 receptor antagonists **(aprepitant, netupitant)** are predicted to increase the exposure to **sildenafil**. Monitor or adjust **sildenafil** dose with moderate CYP3A4 inhibitors, p. 139. Moderate Study
- Neurokinin-1 receptor antagonists **(aprepitant, netupitant)** are predicted to increase the exposure to **tadalafil**. Severe Theoretical
- Neurokinin-1 receptor antagonists **(aprepitant, netupitant)** are predicted to increase the exposure to **vardenafil**. Adjust dose. Severe Theoretical
- **Nicorandil** is predicted to increase the risk of hypotension when given with **phosphodiesterase type-5 inhibitors**. Avoid. Severe Theoretical → Also see TABLE 6 p. 1054
- **Nilotinib** is predicted to increase the exposure to **avanafil**. Adjust **avanafil** dose. Moderate Theoretical
- **Nilotinib** is predicted to increase the exposure to **sildenafil**. Monitor or adjust **sildenafil** dose with moderate CYP3A4 inhibitors, p. 139. Moderate Study
- **Nilotinib** is predicted to increase the exposure to **tadalafil**. Severe Theoretical
- **Nilotinib** is predicted to increase the exposure to **vardenafil**. Adjust dose. Severe Theoretical → Also see TABLE 7 p. 1055
- **Nirmatrelvir** boosted with ritonavir is predicted to increase the concentration of phosphodiesterase type-5 inhibitors **(avanafil, vardenafil)**. Avoid. Severe Theoretical
- **Nirmatrelvir** boosted with ritonavir is predicted to increase the concentration of phosphodiesterase type-5 inhibitors **(sildenafil, tadalafil)**. Avoid or adjust dose—consult product literature. Severe Theoretical
- **Nitrates** potentially increase the risk of hypotension when given with **phosphodiesterase type-5 inhibitors**. Avoid. Severe Study → Also see TABLE 6 p. 1054
- NNRTIs **(efavirenz, nevirapine)** are predicted to decrease the exposure to **phosphodiesterase type-5 inhibitors**. Moderate Theoretical → Also see TABLE 7 p. 1055
- NNRTIs **(etravirine)** moderately decrease the exposure to **phosphodiesterase type-5 inhibitors**. Adjust dose. Moderate Study
- Quinolones **(ciprofloxacin)** moderately increase the exposure to **sildenafil**. Moderate Theoretical
- **Ribociclib** is predicted to increase the exposure to **sildenafil**. Avoid. Moderate Theoretical
- Rifamycins **(rifampicin)** are predicted to decrease the exposure to phosphodiesterase type-5 inhibitors **(avanafil, tadalafil)**. Avoid. Severe Study
- Rifamycins **(rifampicin)** are predicted to decrease the exposure to phosphodiesterase type-5 inhibitors **(sildenafil, vardenafil)**. Moderate Theoretical
- **Phosphodiesterase type-5 inhibitors** are predicted to increase the risk of hypotension when given with **sapropterin**. Moderate Theoretical → Also see TABLE 6 p. 1054
- **St John's wort** is predicted to decrease the exposure to **phosphodiesterase type-5 inhibitors**. Moderate Theoretical
- **Tucatinib** is predicted to increase the exposure to phosphodiesterase type-5 inhibitors **(avanafil, vardenafil)**. Avoid. Severe Study
- **Tucatinib** is predicted to increase the exposure to **sildenafil**. Avoid potent CYP3A4 inhibitors or adjust **sildenafil** dose, p. 139. Severe Study
- **Tucatinib** is predicted to increase the exposure to **tadalafil**. Use with caution or avoid. Severe Study

Pibrentasvir

- **Pibrentasvir** is predicted to increase the exposure to **afatinib**. Moderate Study
- **Pibrentasvir** with glecaprevir is predicted to increase the exposure to **aliskiren**. Moderate Study
- Anti-androgens **(apalutamide, enzalutamide)** are predicted to moderately to markedly decrease the exposure to **pibrentasvir**. Avoid. Severe Study
- Antiepileptics **(carbamazepine, fosphenytoin, phenobarbital, phenytoin, primidone)** are predicted to moderately to markedly decrease the exposure to **pibrentasvir**. Avoid. Severe Study
- Antiepileptics **(eslicarbazepine, oxcarbazepine)** potentially decrease the exposure to **pibrentasvir**. Avoid. Severe Theoretical

Pibrentasvir (continued)

- **Pibrentasvir** with glecaprevir is predicted to increase the exposure to antihistamines, non-sedating **(fexofenadine)**. Moderate Study
- **Cenobamate** is predicted to decrease the exposure to **pibrentasvir**. Avoid. Severe Study
- **Pibrentasvir** with glecaprevir is predicted to increase the exposure to **colchicine**. Avoid P-glycoprotein inhibitors or adjust **colchicine** dose, p. 637. Severe Study
- **Combined hormonal contraceptives** containing ethinylestradiol can increase ALT concentrations when given with **pibrentasvir** with glecaprevir. Avoid. Severe Study
- **Crizotinib** potentially decreases the exposure to **pibrentasvir**. Avoid. Severe Theoretical
- **Dabrafenib** is predicted to decrease the exposure to **pibrentasvir**. Avoid. Severe Study
- **Pibrentasvir** with glecaprevir increases the exposure to **digoxin**. Moderate Study
- **Encorafenib** is predicted to moderately to markedly decrease the exposure to **pibrentasvir**. Avoid. Severe Study
- Endothelin receptor antagonists **(bosentan)** are predicted to decrease the exposure to **pibrentasvir**. Avoid. Severe Study
- **Pibrentasvir** is predicted to increase the exposure to **erlotinib**. Moderate Theoretical
- **Ethinylestradiol** might increase ALT concentrations when given with **pibrentasvir** with glecaprevir. Avoid. Severe Study
- **Pibrentasvir** with glecaprevir is predicted to increase the exposure to **everolimus**. Moderate Study
- **Pibrentasvir** is predicted to increase the exposure to factor XA inhibitors **(apixaban)**. Moderate Theoretical
- **Pibrentasvir** with glecaprevir is predicted to increase the exposure to factor XA inhibitors **(edoxaban)**. Moderate Study
- **Pibrentasvir** might increase the exposure to factor XA inhibitors **(rivaroxaban)**. Manufacturer advises caution in renal impairment. Moderate Theoretical
- **Pibrentasvir** is predicted to increase the exposure to **fidaxomicin**. Avoid. Moderate Study
- **Pibrentasvir** is predicted to increase the exposure to **grazoprevir**. Avoid. Severe Theoretical
- HIV-protease inhibitors **(atazanavir, lopinavir)** boosted with ritonavir increase the exposure to **pibrentasvir**. Avoid. Severe Study
- HIV-protease inhibitors **(ritonavir)** potentially increase the exposure to **pibrentasvir**. Severe Theoretical
- **Hormone replacement therapy** might increase ALT concentrations when given with **pibrentasvir** with glecaprevir. Manufacturer advises caution; avoid ethinylestradiol. Severe Theoretical
- **Ivosidenib** is predicted to moderately to markedly decrease the exposure to **pibrentasvir**. Avoid. Severe Study
- **Pibrentasvir** with glecaprevir is predicted to increase the exposure to **loperamide**. Moderate Study
- **Lorlatinib** is predicted to decrease the exposure to **pibrentasvir**. Avoid. Severe Study
- **Lumacaftor** is predicted to moderately to markedly decrease the exposure to **pibrentasvir**. Avoid. Severe Study
- **Mitotane** is predicted to moderately to markedly decrease the exposure to **pibrentasvir**. Avoid. Severe Study
- **Pibrentasvir** is predicted to increase the risk of neutropenia when given with monoclonal antibodies **(brentuximab vedotin)**. Monitor and adjust dose. Severe Theoretical
- **Pibrentasvir** is predicted to increase the exposure to **neratinib**. Avoid or adjust dose and monitor for gastrointestinal adverse effects—consult product literature. Severe Study
- **Pibrentasvir** is predicted to increase the exposure to **nintedanib**. Moderate Study
- **Nirmatrelvir** boosted with ritonavir is predicted to increase the concentration of **pibrentasvir**. Avoid. Severe Theoretical
- NNRTIs **(efavirenz, etravirine, nevirapine)** are predicted to decrease the exposure to **pibrentasvir**. Avoid. Severe Study
- **Pibrentasvir** is predicted to increase the exposure to **pralsetinib**. Moderate Theoretical
- **Pibrentasvir** is predicted to increase the exposure to **relugolix**. Avoid or take relugolix first and separate administration by at least 6 hours. Moderate Study
- Rifamycins **(rifampicin)** are predicted to moderately to markedly decrease the exposure to **pibrentasvir**. Avoid. Severe Study
- **Pibrentasvir** is predicted to increase the exposure to **rimegepant**. Avoid another dose of rimegepant within 48 hours of concurrent use. Moderate Theoretical
- **Pibrentasvir** with glecaprevir is predicted to increase the exposure to **sirolimus**. Moderate Study
- **Sotorasib** is predicted to decrease the exposure to **pibrentasvir**. Avoid. Severe Study
- **St John's wort** is predicted to decrease the exposure to **pibrentasvir**. Avoid. Severe Study
- **Pibrentasvir** with glecaprevir markedly increases the exposure to statins **(atorvastatin)**. Avoid. Severe Study
- **Pibrentasvir** with glecaprevir is predicted to increase the exposure to statins **(fluvastatin)**. Moderate Theoretical
- **Pibrentasvir** with glecaprevir moderately increases the exposure to statins **(pravastatin)**. Use with caution and adjust **pravastatin** dose. Moderate Study
- **Pibrentasvir** with glecaprevir moderately increases the exposure to statins **(rosuvastatin)**. Use with caution and adjust **rosuvastatin** dose, p. 155. Moderate Study
- **Pibrentasvir** with glecaprevir moderately increases the exposure to statins **(simvastatin)**. Avoid. Moderate Study
- **Pibrentasvir** with glecaprevir slightly increases the exposure to **tacrolimus**. Monitor and adjust dose. Mild Study
- **Pibrentasvir** is predicted to slightly increase the exposure to **talazoparib**. Avoid or adjust dose—consult product literature. Severe Study
- **Pibrentasvir** with glecaprevir is predicted to increase the exposure to taxanes **(paclitaxel)**. Moderate Study
- **Pibrentasvir** with glecaprevir increases the exposure to thrombin inhibitors **(dabigatran)**. Avoid. Moderate Study
- **Pibrentasvir** is predicted to increase the exposure to **topotecan**. Severe Study
- **Pibrentasvir** is predicted to increase the concentration of **trametinib**. Moderate Theoretical

Pilocarpine

ROUTE-SPECIFIC INFORMATION Since systemic absorption can follow topical application, the possibility of interactions should be borne in mind.

Pimecrolimus

- **Alcohol** increases the risk of facial flushing and skin irritation when given with topical **pimecrolimus**. Moderate Study
- **Pimecrolimus** is predicted to decrease the efficacy of **mifamurtide**. Avoid. Severe Theoretical

Pimozide → see **TABLE 15** p. 1058 (hyponatraemia), **TABLE 6** p. 1054 (hypotension), **TABLE 7** p. 1055 (QT-interval prolongation), **TABLE 8** p. 1055 (antimuscarinics), **TABLE 9** p. 1056 (CNS effects)

- Antiarrhythmics **(dronedarone)** are predicted to increase the exposure to **pimozide**. Avoid. Severe Theoretical → Also see **TABLE 7** p. 1055
- Antifungals, azoles **(fluconazole, isavuconazole)** are predicted to increase the exposure to **pimozide**. Avoid. Severe Theoretical → Also see **TABLE 7** p. 1055
- Antifungals, azoles **(itraconazole, ketoconazole, posaconazole, voriconazole)** are predicted to increase the exposure to **pimozide**. Avoid. Severe Study → Also see **TABLE 7** p. 1055
- Antifungals, azoles **(miconazole)** are predicted to increase the exposure to **pimozide**. Avoid. Moderate Theoretical
- Atypical antipsychotics **(clozapine)** can cause constipation, as can **pimozide**; concurrent use might increase the risk of developing intestinal obstruction. Severe Theoretical → Also see **TABLE 15** p. 1058 → Also see **TABLE 6** p. 1054 → Also see **TABLE 8** p. 1055 → Also see **TABLE 9** p. 1056
- **Berotralstat** is predicted to increase the exposure to **pimozide**. Avoid. Severe Theoretical
- Calcium-channel blockers **(diltiazem, verapamil)** are predicted to increase the exposure to **pimozide**. Avoid. Severe Theoretical → Also see **TABLE 6** p. 1054
- **Ceritinib** is predicted to increase the exposure to **pimozide**. Avoid. Severe Study → Also see **TABLE 7** p. 1055
- **Cobicistat** is predicted to increase the exposure to **pimozide**. Avoid. Severe Study

- **Crizotinib** is predicted to increase the exposure to **pimozide**. Avoid. [Severe] Theoretical → Also see **TABLE 7** p. 1055
- **Pimozide** is predicted to decrease the effects of **dopamine receptor agonists**. Avoid. [Moderate] Theoretical → Also see **TABLE 6** p. 1054 → Also see **TABLE 7** p. 1055 → Also see **TABLE 8** p. 1055 → Also see **TABLE 9** p. 1056
- **Fedratinib** is predicted to increase the exposure to **pimozide**. Avoid. [Severe] Theoretical
- **Pimozide** opposes the effects of the active metabolite of **foslevodopa**. [Severe] Theoretical → Also see **TABLE 6** p. 1054 → Also see **TABLE 9** p. 1056
- **Grapefruit** juice increases the exposure to **pimozide**. Avoid. [Severe] Theoretical
- **HIV-protease inhibitors** are predicted to increase the exposure to **pimozide**. Avoid. [Severe] Study
- **Idelalisib** is predicted to increase the exposure to **pimozide**. Avoid. [Severe] Study
- **Imatinib** is predicted to increase the exposure to **pimozide**. Avoid. [Severe] Theoretical
- **Ivosidenib** might decrease the exposure to **pimozide**. Avoid or monitor efficacy. [Moderate] Theoretical → Also see **TABLE 7** p. 1055
- **Larotrectinib** is predicted to increase the exposure to **pimozide**. Use with caution and adjust dose. [Mild] Theoretical
- **Lazertinib** is predicted to increase the exposure to **pimozide**. [Moderate] Study
- **Letermovir** is predicted to increase the exposure to **pimozide**. Avoid. [Severe] Theoretical
- **Pimozide** decreases the effects of **levodopa**. [Severe] Theoretical → Also see **TABLE 6** p. 1054 → Also see **TABLE 9** p. 1056
- **Lorlatinib** is predicted to decrease the exposure to **pimozide**. Avoid. [Moderate] Theoretical
- Macrolides **(clarithromycin)** are predicted to increase the exposure to **pimozide**. Avoid. [Severe] Study
- Macrolides **(erythromycin)** are predicted to increase the exposure to **pimozide**. Avoid. [Severe] Theoretical → Also see **TABLE 7** p. 1055
- **Neurokinin-1 receptor antagonists** are predicted to increase the exposure to **pimozide**. Avoid. [Severe] Theoretical
- **Nilotinib** is predicted to increase the exposure to **pimozide**. Avoid. [Severe] Theoretical → Also see **TABLE 7** p. 1055
- **Nirmatrelvir** boosted with ritonavir is predicted to increase the concentration of **pimozide**. Avoid. [Severe] Theoretical
- **Olaparib** might alter the exposure to **pimozide**. [Moderate] Theoretical
- **Palbociclib** is predicted to increase the exposure to **pimozide**. Adjust dose. [Moderate] Theoretical
- **Panobinostat** is predicted to increase the exposure to **pimozide**. Avoid. [Severe] Theoretical → Also see **TABLE 7** p. 1055
- **Pitolisant** is predicted to decrease the exposure to **pimozide**. Avoid. [Severe] Theoretical
- **Ribociclib** (high-dose) is predicted to increase the exposure to **pimozide**. Avoid. [Moderate] Theoretical → Also see **TABLE 7** p. 1055
- **Ritlecitinib** is predicted to increase the exposure to **pimozide**. [Moderate] Theoretical
- **Rucaparib** is predicted to increase the exposure to **pimozide**. Monitor and adjust dose. [Moderate] Study
- **Tucatinib** is predicted to increase the exposure to **pimozide**. Avoid. [Severe] Study
- **Vorasidenib** might decrease the concentration of **pimozide**. Avoid. [Severe] Theoretical

Pindolol → see beta blockers, non-selective

Pioglitazone

- Anti-androgens **(abiraterone)** slightly increase the exposure to **pioglitazone**. [Moderate] Study
- **Pioglitazone** potentially decreases the exposure to antifungals, azoles **(isavuconazole)**. Use with caution or avoid. [Moderate] Theoretical
- **Clopidogrel** increases the exposure to **pioglitazone**. Monitor blood glucose and adjust dose. [Severe] Study
- **Fenfluramine** might decrease blood glucose concentrations when given with **pioglitazone**. [Moderate] Theoretical
- Fibrates **(gemfibrozil)** increase the exposure to **pioglitazone**. Monitor blood glucose and adjust dose. [Severe] Study
- Iron chelators **(deferasirox)** are predicted to increase the exposure to **pioglitazone**. [Moderate] Study
- **Ivosidenib** might decrease the exposure to **pioglitazone**. Avoid or monitor efficacy. [Unknown] Study
- **Leflunomide** is predicted to increase the exposure to **pioglitazone**. [Moderate] Study
- Macrolides **(clarithromycin)** might cause hypoglycaemia when given with **pioglitazone**. [Moderate] Theoretical
- **Mifepristone** is predicted to increase the exposure to **pioglitazone**. [Moderate] Theoretical
- **Opicapone** is predicted to increase the exposure to **pioglitazone**. Avoid. [Moderate] Study
- **Pirtobrutinib** is predicted to increase the exposure to **pioglitazone**. [Moderate] Theoretical
- Rifamycins **(rifampicin)** moderately decrease the exposure to **pioglitazone**. Monitor and adjust dose. [Moderate] Study
- **Somapacitan** might increase blood glucose concentrations, opposing the blood glucose-lowering effects of **pioglitazone**. Adjust dose. [Moderate] Theoretical
- **Somatrogon** might increase blood glucose concentrations, opposing the blood glucose-lowering effects of **pioglitazone**. Adjust dose. [Moderate] Theoretical
- **St John's wort** slightly decreases the exposure to **pioglitazone**. [Mild] Study
- **Teriflunomide** is predicted to increase the exposure to **pioglitazone**. [Moderate] Study

Piperacillin → see penicillins

Piperaquine → see antimalarials

Pirfenidone

FOOD AND LIFESTYLE Smoking increases pirfenidone clearance; patients should be encouraged to stop smoking before and during treatment with pirfenidone.

- Antiepileptics **(fosphenytoin, phenytoin)** are predicted to decrease the exposure to **pirfenidone**. [Moderate] Theoretical
- **Axitinib** is predicted to increase the exposure to **pirfenidone**. [Moderate] Theoretical
- **Combined hormonal contraceptives** is predicted to increase the exposure to **pirfenidone**. Use with caution and adjust dose. [Moderate] Study
- **Givosiran** is predicted to increase the exposure to **pirfenidone**. Use with caution and adjust dose. [Moderate] Study
- HIV-protease inhibitors **(ritonavir)** are predicted to decrease the exposure to **pirfenidone**. [Moderate] Theoretical
- **Leflunomide** is predicted to decrease the exposure to **pirfenidone**. [Moderate] Theoretical
- **Mexiletine** is predicted to increase the exposure to **pirfenidone**. Use with caution and adjust dose. [Moderate] Study
- **Osilodrostat** is predicted to increase the exposure to **pirfenidone**. Use with caution and adjust dose. [Moderate] Study
- Quinolones **(ciprofloxacin)** are predicted to increase the exposure to **pirfenidone**. Use with caution and adjust dose. [Moderate] Study
- Rifamycins **(rifampicin)** are predicted to decrease the exposure to **pirfenidone**. Avoid. [Moderate] Theoretical
- **Ritlecitinib** is predicted to increase the exposure to **pirfenidone**. Adjust dose. [Moderate] Theoretical
- **Rucaparib** is predicted to increase the exposure to **pirfenidone**. Use with caution and adjust dose. [Moderate] Study
- SSRIs **(fluvoxamine)** are predicted to moderately increase the exposure to **pirfenidone**. Avoid. [Moderate] Study
- **Teriflunomide** is predicted to decrease the exposure to **pirfenidone**. [Moderate] Theoretical
- **Vemurafenib** is predicted to increase the exposure to **pirfenidone**. Use with caution and adjust dose. [Moderate] Study

Piroxicam → see NSAIDs

Pirtobrutinib

- **Pirtobrutinib** is predicted to increase the exposure to anthracyclines **(mitoxantrone)**. [Moderate] Theoretical
- Anti-androgens **(apalutamide, enzalutamide)** are predicted to decrease the exposure to **pirtobrutinib**. Avoid. [Moderate] Study
- Antiepileptics **(carbamazepine, fosphenytoin, phenobarbital, phenytoin, primidone)** are predicted to decrease the exposure to **pirtobrutinib**. Avoid. [Moderate] Study
- **Pirtobrutinib** slightly increases the exposure to oral benzodiazepines **(midazolam)**. Avoid or monitor. [Moderate] Study
- **Cenobamate** is predicted to decrease the exposure to **pirtobrutinib**. [Moderate] Theoretical

Pirtobrutinib (continued)
- **Dabrafenib** is predicted to decrease the exposure to **pirtobrutinib**. Moderate Theoretical
- **Pirtobrutinib** slightly increases the exposure to **digoxin**. Avoid or monitor. Moderate Study
- **Encorafenib** is predicted to decrease the exposure to **pirtobrutinib**. Avoid. Moderate Study
- Endothelin receptor antagonists **(bosentan)** are predicted to decrease the exposure to **pirtobrutinib**. Moderate Theoretical
- **Pirtobrutinib** is predicted to increase the exposure to **everolimus**. Avoid or monitor. Moderate Theoretical
- **Ivosidenib** is predicted to decrease the exposure to **pirtobrutinib**. Avoid. Moderate Study
- **Lorlatinib** is predicted to decrease the exposure to **pirtobrutinib**. Moderate Theoretical
- **Lumacaftor** is predicted to decrease the exposure to **pirtobrutinib**. Avoid. Moderate Study
- **Pirtobrutinib** moderately increases the exposure to meglitinides **(repaglinide)**. Moderate Study
- **Pirtobrutinib** is predicted to increase the exposure to **methotrexate**. Moderate Theoretical
- **Mitotane** is predicted to decrease the exposure to **pirtobrutinib**. Avoid. Moderate Study
- **Pirtobrutinib** is predicted to increase the exposure to **montelukast**. Moderate Theoretical
- NNRTIs **(efavirenz, etravirine, nevirapine)** are predicted to decrease the exposure to **pirtobrutinib**. Moderate Theoretical
- **Pirtobrutinib** is predicted to increase the exposure to opioids **(alfentanil)**. Avoid or monitor. Moderate Theoretical
- **Pirtobrutinib** is predicted to increase the exposure to **pioglitazone**. Moderate Theoretical
- Rifamycins **(rifampicin)** are predicted to decrease the exposure to **pirtobrutinib**. Avoid. Moderate Study
- **Pirtobrutinib** is predicted to increase the exposure to **selexipag**. Moderate Theoretical
- **Pirtobrutinib** is predicted to increase the exposure to **sirolimus**. Avoid or monitor. Moderate Theoretical
- **Sotorasib** is predicted to decrease the exposure to **pirtobrutinib**. Moderate Theoretical
- **St John's wort** is predicted to decrease the exposure to **pirtobrutinib**. Moderate Theoretical
- **Pirtobrutinib** is predicted to increase the exposure to statins **(atorvastatin, fluvastatin, rosuvastatin)**. Moderate Theoretical
- **Pirtobrutinib** is predicted to increase the exposure to **sulfasalazine**. Moderate Theoretical
- **Pirtobrutinib** is predicted to increase the exposure to **talazoparib**. Avoid or monitor. Moderate Theoretical
- **Pirtobrutinib** is predicted to increase the exposure to taxanes **(paclitaxel)**. Avoid or monitor. Moderate Theoretical
- **Pirtobrutinib** is predicted to increase the exposure to **temsirolimus**. Avoid or monitor. Moderate Theoretical
- **Pirtobrutinib** is predicted to increase the exposure to thrombin inhibitors **(dabigatran)**. Avoid or monitor. Moderate Theoretical
- **Pirtobrutinib** is predicted to increase the exposure to **topotecan**. Moderate Theoretical

Pitolisant
- **Pitolisant** is predicted to decrease the exposure to **aliskiren**. Mild Theoretical
- Anti-androgens **(apalutamide, enzalutamide)** are predicted to moderately decrease the exposure to **pitolisant**. Moderate Study
- Antiepileptics **(carbamazepine, fosphenytoin, phenobarbital, phenytoin, primidone)** are predicted to moderately decrease the exposure to **pitolisant**. Moderate Study
- **Pitolisant** is predicted to decrease the exposure to antihistamines, non-sedating **(fexofenadine)**. Mild Theoretical
- **Antihistamines, sedating** are predicted to decrease the efficacy of **pitolisant**. Moderate Theoretical
- **Pitolisant** is predicted to decrease the exposure to **bosutinib**. Avoid. Severe Theoretical
- **Bupropion** is predicted to moderately increase the exposure to **pitolisant**. Use with caution and adjust dose. Moderate Study
- **Pitolisant** is predicted to decrease the exposure to **ciclosporin**. Avoid. Severe Theoretical
- **Cinacalcet** is predicted to moderately increase the exposure to **pitolisant**. Use with caution and adjust dose. Moderate Study
- **Pitolisant** is predicted to decrease the exposure to **colchicine**. Mild Theoretical
- **Pitolisant** is predicted to decrease the efficacy of **combined hormonal contraceptives**. Avoid. Severe Theoretical
- **Pitolisant** is predicted to decrease the exposure to coumarins **(warfarin)**. Mild Theoretical
- **Pitolisant** is predicted to decrease the exposure to **crizotinib**. Avoid. Severe Theoretical
- **Dacomitinib** is predicted to moderately increase the exposure to **pitolisant**. Use with caution and adjust dose. Moderate Study
- **Pitolisant** is predicted to decrease the exposure to **dasatinib**. Avoid. Severe Theoretical
- **Pitolisant** is predicted to decrease the exposure to **digoxin**. Mild Theoretical
- **Encorafenib** is predicted to moderately decrease the exposure to **pitolisant**. Moderate Study
- **Pitolisant** is predicted to decrease the exposure to **everolimus**. Avoid. Severe Theoretical
- **Pitolisant** is predicted to decrease the exposure to factor XA inhibitors **(edoxaban)**. Mild Theoretical
- **Pitolisant** is predicted to decrease the exposure to **irinotecan**. Mild Theoretical
- **Ivosidenib** is predicted to moderately decrease the exposure to **pitolisant**. Moderate Study
- **Pitolisant** is predicted to decrease the exposure to **lapatinib**. Avoid. Severe Theoretical
- **Pitolisant** is predicted to decrease the exposure to **loperamide**. Mild Theoretical
- **Lumacaftor** is predicted to moderately decrease the exposure to **pitolisant**. Moderate Study
- **Pitolisant** is predicted to decrease the exposure to meglitinides **(repaglinide)**. Mild Theoretical
- **Pitolisant** is predicted to increase the exposure to **metformin**. Mild Theoretical
- **Mianserin** is predicted to decrease the efficacy of **pitolisant**. Moderate Theoretical
- **Mirtazapine** is predicted to decrease the efficacy of **pitolisant**. Moderate Theoretical
- **Mitotane** is predicted to moderately decrease the exposure to **pitolisant**. Moderate Study
- **Pitolisant** is predicted to decrease the exposure to **nilotinib**. Avoid. Severe Theoretical
- **Pitolisant** is predicted to decrease the exposure to NNRTIs **(efavirenz)**. Mild Theoretical
- **Pitolisant** is predicted to decrease the exposure to opioids **(morphine)**. Mild Theoretical
- **Pitolisant** is predicted to decrease the exposure to **paracetamol**. Mild Theoretical
- **Pitolisant** is predicted to decrease the exposure to **pimozide**. Avoid. Severe Theoretical
- Rifamycins **(rifampicin)** are predicted to moderately decrease the exposure to **pitolisant**. Moderate Study
- **Pitolisant** is predicted to decrease the exposure to **sirolimus**. Avoid. Severe Theoretical
- SNRIs **(duloxetine)** are predicted to increase the exposure to **pitolisant**. Use with caution and adjust dose. Moderate Study
- SNRIs **(venlafaxine)** are predicted to increase the exposure to **pitolisant**. Use with caution and adjust dose. Mild Theoretical
- SSRIs **(fluoxetine, paroxetine)** are predicted to moderately increase the exposure to **pitolisant**. Use with caution and adjust dose. Moderate Study
- **St John's wort** is predicted to decrease the exposure to **pitolisant**. Monitor and adjust dose. Moderate Theoretical
- **Pitolisant** is predicted to decrease the exposure to **tacrolimus**. Avoid. Severe Theoretical
- **Pitolisant** is predicted to decrease the exposure to taxanes **(docetaxel)**. Avoid. Severe Theoretical
- **Pitolisant** is predicted to decrease the exposure to taxanes **(paclitaxel)**. Mild Theoretical
- **Pitolisant** is predicted to decrease the exposure to **temsirolimus**. Avoid. Severe Theoretical
- **Terbinafine** is predicted to moderately increase the exposure to **pitolisant**. Use with caution and adjust dose. Moderate Study
- **Pitolisant** is predicted to decrease the exposure to thrombin inhibitors **(dabigatran)**. Mild Theoretical

- **Tricyclic antidepressants** are predicted to decrease the efficacy of **pitolisant**. Mild Theoretical

Pivmecillinam → see penicillins

Pixantrone → see anthracyclines

Pizotifen → see antihistamines, sedating

Platinum compounds → see TABLE 15 p. 1058 (hyponatraemia), TABLE 12 p. 1057 (myelosuppression), TABLE 2 p. 1053 (nephrotoxicity), TABLE 16 p. 1058 (ototoxicity), TABLE 10 p. 1056 (peripheral neuropathy)

carboplatin · cisplatin · oxaliplatin

- **Cisplatin** increases the risk of pulmonary toxicity when given with **bleomycin**. Severe Study → Also see TABLE 12 p. 1057
- **Live vaccines** are predicted to increase the risk of generalised infection (possibly life-threatening) when given with **platinum compounds**. UKHSA advises avoid (refer to Green Book). Severe Theoretical

Polatuzumab vedotin → see monoclonal antibodies

Polymyxin b

ROUTE-SPECIFIC INFORMATION Since systemic absorption can follow topical application of **polymyxin B**, the possibility of interactions should be borne in mind.

- **Polymyxin b** might prolong the effects of **neuromuscular blocking drugs, non-depolarising**. Severe Theoretical
- **Polymyxin b** might prolong the effects of **suxamethonium**. Severe Theoretical

Polystyrene sulfonate

SEPARATION OF ADMINISTRATION Manufacturers advise take other drugs at least 3 hours before or after calcium- or sodium-polystyrene sulfonate; a 6-hour separation should be considered in gastroparesis.

- Oral **antacids** increase the risk of metabolic alkalosis when given with oral **polystyrene sulfonate**. Severe Anecdotal

Pomalidomide → see TABLE 1 p. 1053 (hepatotoxicity), TABLE 12 p. 1057 (myelosuppression), TABLE 10 p. 1056 (peripheral neuropathy)

- **Combined hormonal contraceptives** are predicted to increase the risk of venous thromboembolism when given with **pomalidomide**. Avoid. Severe Theoretical
- **Hormone replacement therapy** is predicted to increase the risk of venous thromboembolism when given with **pomalidomide**. Severe Theoretical
- Quinolones **(ciprofloxacin)** are predicted to increase the exposure to **pomalidomide**. Adjust dose—consult product literature. Moderate Theoretical
- SSRIs **(fluvoxamine)** moderately increase the exposure to **pomalidomide**. Adjust dose—consult product literature. Moderate Study

Ponatinib → see TABLE 3 p. 1053 (bleeding)

- Anti-androgens **(apalutamide, enzalutamide)** are predicted to decrease the exposure to **ponatinib**. Avoid. Moderate Theoretical
- Antiarrhythmics **(dronedarone)** are predicted to increase the exposure to **ponatinib**. Moderate Study
- Antiepileptics **(carbamazepine, fosphenytoin, phenobarbital, phenytoin, primidone)** are predicted to decrease the exposure to **ponatinib**. Avoid. Moderate Theoretical
- Antifungals, azoles **(fluconazole, isavuconazole)** are predicted to increase the exposure to **ponatinib**. Moderate Study
- Antifungals, azoles **(itraconazole, ketoconazole, posaconazole, voriconazole)** are predicted to slightly increase the exposure to **ponatinib**. Monitor and adjust dose—consult product literature. Moderate Study
- **Berotralstat** is predicted to increase the exposure to **ponatinib**. Moderate Study
- Calcium-channel blockers **(diltiazem, verapamil)** are predicted to increase the exposure to **ponatinib**. Moderate Study
- **Cenobamate** is predicted to decrease the exposure to **ponatinib**. Severe Study
- **Ceritinib** is predicted to slightly increase the exposure to **ponatinib**. Monitor and adjust dose—consult product literature. Moderate Study
- **Cobicistat** is predicted to slightly increase the exposure to **ponatinib**. Monitor and adjust dose—consult product literature. Moderate Study
- **Ponatinib** might affect the effects of **combined hormonal contraceptives**. Avoid or use additional contraceptive precautions. Severe Theoretical
- **Crizotinib** is predicted to increase the exposure to **ponatinib**. Moderate Study
- **Dabrafenib** is predicted to decrease the exposure to **ponatinib**. Severe Study
- **Encorafenib** is predicted to decrease the exposure to **ponatinib**. Avoid. Moderate Theoretical
- Endothelin receptor antagonists **(bosentan)** are predicted to decrease the exposure to **ponatinib**. Severe Study
- **Fedratinib** is predicted to increase the exposure to **ponatinib**. Moderate Study
- **Grapefruit** juice is predicted to increase the exposure to **ponatinib**. Moderate Theoretical
- **HIV-protease inhibitors** are predicted to slightly increase the exposure to **ponatinib**. Monitor and adjust dose—consult product literature. Moderate Study
- **Idelalisib** is predicted to slightly increase the exposure to **ponatinib**. Monitor and adjust dose—consult product literature. Moderate Study
- **Imatinib** is predicted to increase the exposure to **ponatinib**. Moderate Study → Also see TABLE 3 p. 1053
- **Ivosidenib** is predicted to decrease the exposure to **ponatinib**. Avoid. Moderate Theoretical
- **Letermovir** is predicted to increase the exposure to **ponatinib**. Moderate Study
- **Lorlatinib** is predicted to decrease the exposure to **ponatinib**. Severe Study
- **Lumacaftor** is predicted to decrease the exposure to **ponatinib**. Avoid. Moderate Theoretical
- Macrolides **(clarithromycin)** are predicted to slightly increase the exposure to **ponatinib**. Monitor and adjust dose—consult product literature. Moderate Study
- Macrolides **(erythromycin)** are predicted to increase the exposure to **ponatinib**. Moderate Study
- **Mitotane** is predicted to decrease the exposure to **ponatinib**. Avoid. Moderate Theoretical
- Neurokinin-1 receptor antagonists **(aprepitant, netupitant)** are predicted to increase the exposure to **ponatinib**. Moderate Study
- **Nilotinib** is predicted to increase the exposure to **ponatinib**. Moderate Study
- NNRTIs **(efavirenz, etravirine, nevirapine)** are predicted to decrease the exposure to **ponatinib**. Severe Study
- Rifamycins **(rifampicin)** are predicted to decrease the exposure to **ponatinib**. Avoid. Moderate Theoretical
- **Sotorasib** is predicted to decrease the exposure to **ponatinib**. Severe Study
- **St John's wort** is predicted to decrease the exposure to **ponatinib**. Avoid. Severe Theoretical
- **Tucatinib** is predicted to slightly increase the exposure to **ponatinib**. Monitor and adjust dose—consult product literature. Moderate Study

Ponesimod → see TABLE 4 p. 1054 (bradycardia), TABLE 7 p. 1055 (QT-interval prolongation)

- ▸ **Live vaccines** might increase the risk of generalised infection (possibly life-threatening) when given with **ponesimod**. Avoid and for 1 week after stopping **ponesimod**. Severe Theoretical
- Monoclonal antibodies **(alemtuzumab)** are predicted to increase the risk of generalised infection (possibly life-threatening) when given with **ponesimod**. Severe Theoretical

Posaconazole → see antifungals, azoles

Potassium aminobenzoate → see TABLE 13 p. 1057 (increased serum potassium)

- **Potassium aminobenzoate** increases the concentration of **methotrexate**. Moderate Theoretical
- **Potassium aminobenzoate** is predicted to affect the efficacy of **sulfonamides**. Avoid. Severe Theoretical

Potassium canrenoate → see TABLE 13 p. 1057 (increased serum potassium)

Potassium chloride → see TABLE 13 p. 1057 (increased serum potassium)

Potassium citrate

- **Potassium citrate** is predicted to decrease the efficacy of methenamine. Avoid. [Moderate] Theoretical
- **Potassium citrate** might decrease the efficacy of nitrofurantoin. [Unknown] Theoretical
- **Potassium citrate** increases the risk of adverse effects when given with sucralfate. Avoid. [Moderate] Theoretical

Potassium-sparing diuretics → see TABLE 15 p. 1058 (hyponatraemia), TABLE 13 p. 1057 (increased serum potassium)

amiloride · triamterene

- **Triamterene** potentially increases the clearance of lithium. [Moderate] Study

Pralsetinib

FOOD AND LIFESTYLE Bitter (Seville) orange is predicted to increase the exposure to pralsetinib. Avoid.

- Anti-androgens (apalutamide, enzalutamide) are predicted to decrease the exposure to **pralsetinib**. Avoid or adjust dose with potent CYP3A4 inducers—consult product literature. [Moderate] Study
- Antiarrhythmics (amiodarone, dronedarone) are predicted to increase the exposure to **pralsetinib**. [Moderate] Theoretical
- Antiepileptics (carbamazepine, fosphenytoin, phenobarbital, phenytoin, primidone) are predicted to decrease the exposure to **pralsetinib**. Avoid or adjust dose with potent CYP3A4 inducers—consult product literature. [Moderate] Study
- Antifungals, azoles (fluconazole, isavuconazole) are predicted to increase the exposure to **pralsetinib**. [Moderate] Theoretical
- Antifungals, azoles (itraconazole, ketoconazole, posaconazole, voriconazole) are predicted to increase the exposure to **pralsetinib**. Avoid or adjust dose with potent CYP3A4 inhibitors—consult product literature. [Moderate] Study
- Berotralstat is predicted to increase the exposure to **pralsetinib**. [Moderate] Theoretical
- Calcium-channel blockers (diltiazem, verapamil) are predicted to increase the exposure to **pralsetinib**. [Moderate] Theoretical
- Cenobamate is predicted to decrease the exposure to **pralsetinib**. [Moderate] Theoretical
- Ceritinib is predicted to increase the exposure to **pralsetinib**. Avoid or adjust dose with potent CYP3A4 inhibitors—consult product literature. [Moderate] Study
- **Pralsetinib** might affect the exposure to ciclosporin and ciclosporin is predicted to increase the exposure to **pralsetinib**. Avoid. [Moderate] Theoretical
- Cobicistat is predicted to increase the exposure to **pralsetinib**. Avoid or adjust dose with potent CYP3A4 inhibitors—consult product literature. [Moderate] Study
- **Pralsetinib** might decrease the efficacy of combined hormonal contraceptives. Avoid or use additional contraceptive precautions. [Severe] Theoretical
- **Pralsetinib** might affect the exposure to coumarins (warfarin). Avoid. [Moderate] Theoretical
- Crizotinib is predicted to increase the exposure to **pralsetinib**. [Moderate] Theoretical
- Dabrafenib is predicted to decrease the exposure to **pralsetinib**. [Moderate] Theoretical
- Danicopan is predicted to increase the exposure to **pralsetinib**. [Moderate] Study
- Eliglustat is predicted to increase the exposure to **pralsetinib**. Adjust dose. [Moderate] Study
- Encorafenib is predicted to decrease the exposure to **pralsetinib**. Avoid or adjust dose with potent CYP3A4 inducers—consult product literature. [Moderate] Study
- Endothelin receptor antagonists (bosentan) are predicted to decrease the exposure to **pralsetinib**. [Moderate] Theoretical
- Fedratinib is predicted to increase the exposure to **pralsetinib**. [Moderate] Theoretical
- Glecaprevir is predicted to increase the exposure to **pralsetinib**. [Moderate] Theoretical
- Grapefruit juice is predicted to increase the exposure to **pralsetinib**. Avoid. [Moderate] Study
- HIV-protease inhibitors are predicted to increase the exposure to **pralsetinib**. Avoid or adjust dose with potent CYP3A4 inhibitors—consult product literature. [Moderate] Study
- Idelalisib is predicted to increase the exposure to **pralsetinib**. Avoid or adjust dose with potent CYP3A4 inhibitors—consult product literature. [Moderate] Study
- Imatinib is predicted to increase the exposure to **pralsetinib**. [Moderate] Theoretical
- Ivosidenib is predicted to decrease the exposure to **pralsetinib**. Avoid or adjust dose with potent CYP3A4 inducers—consult product literature. [Moderate] Study
- Lapatinib is predicted to increase the exposure to **pralsetinib**. [Moderate] Theoretical
- Letermovir is predicted to increase the exposure to **pralsetinib**. [Moderate] Theoretical
- Lorlatinib is predicted to decrease the exposure to **pralsetinib**. [Moderate] Theoretical
- Lumacaftor is predicted to decrease the exposure to **pralsetinib**. Avoid or adjust dose with potent CYP3A4 inducers—consult product literature. [Moderate] Study
- Macrolides (azithromycin, erythromycin) are predicted to increase the exposure to **pralsetinib**. [Moderate] Theoretical
- Macrolides (clarithromycin) are predicted to increase the exposure to **pralsetinib**. Avoid or adjust dose with potent CYP3A4 inhibitors—consult product literature. [Moderate] Study
- Mitotane is predicted to decrease the exposure to **pralsetinib**. Avoid or adjust dose with potent CYP3A4 inducers—consult product literature. [Moderate] Study
- Neurokinin-1 receptor antagonists (aprepitant, netupitant) are predicted to increase the exposure to **pralsetinib**. [Moderate] Theoretical
- Nilotinib is predicted to increase the exposure to **pralsetinib**. [Moderate] Theoretical
- NNRTIs (efavirenz, nevirapine) are predicted to decrease the exposure to **pralsetinib**. [Moderate] Theoretical
- Olaparib might increase the exposure to **pralsetinib**. [Moderate] Theoretical
- Osimertinib is predicted to increase the exposure to **pralsetinib**. [Moderate] Study
- Pibrentasvir is predicted to increase the exposure to **pralsetinib**. [Moderate] Theoretical
- Ranolazine is predicted to increase the exposure to **pralsetinib**. [Moderate] Theoretical
- Rifamycins (rifabutin) are predicted to decrease the exposure to **pralsetinib**. Avoid or adjust dose—consult product literature. [Moderate] Study
- Rifamycins (rifampicin) are predicted to decrease the exposure to **pralsetinib**. Avoid or adjust dose with potent CYP3A4 inducers—consult product literature. [Moderate] Study
- Sotorasib is predicted to decrease the exposure to **pralsetinib**. [Moderate] Theoretical
- Sparsentan is predicted to increase the exposure to **pralsetinib**. [Severe] Theoretical
- St John's wort is predicted to decrease the exposure to **pralsetinib**. Avoid or adjust dose—consult product literature. [Moderate] Study
- **Pralsetinib** might affect the exposure to taxanes (paclitaxel). Avoid. [Moderate] Theoretical
- Tucatinib is predicted to increase the exposure to **pralsetinib**. Avoid or adjust dose with potent CYP3A4 inhibitors—consult product literature. [Moderate] Study
- Velpatasvir is predicted to increase the exposure to **pralsetinib**. [Moderate] Theoretical
- Vemurafenib is predicted to increase the exposure to **pralsetinib**. [Moderate] Theoretical
- Voxilaprevir is predicted to increase the exposure to **pralsetinib**. [Moderate] Theoretical

Pramipexole → see dopamine receptor agonists

Prasugrel → see TABLE 3 p. 1053 (bleeding)

- Selumetinib might increase the risk of bleeding when given with **prasugrel**. [Severe] Theoretical

Pravastatin → see statins

Praziquantel

- Anti-androgens (apalutamide, enzalutamide) are predicted to markedly decrease the exposure to **praziquantel**. Avoid. [Moderate] Study

- Antiepileptics **(carbamazepine, fosphenytoin, phenobarbital, phenytoin, primidone)** are predicted to markedly decrease the exposure to **praziquantel**. Avoid. Moderate Study
- Antifungals, azoles **(itraconazole, ketoconazole, posaconazole, voriconazole)** are predicted to moderately increase the exposure to **praziquantel**. Mild Study
- Antimalarials **(chloroquine)** moderately decrease the exposure to **praziquantel**. Use with caution and adjust dose. Moderate Study
- **Ceritinib** is predicted to moderately increase the exposure to **praziquantel**. Mild Study
- **Cobicistat** is predicted to moderately increase the exposure to **praziquantel**. Mild Study
- Corticosteroids **(dexamethasone)** decrease the exposure to **praziquantel**. Moderate Study
- **Encorafenib** is predicted to markedly decrease the exposure to **praziquantel**. Avoid. Moderate Study
- **Grapefruit** juice is predicted to increase the exposure to **praziquantel**. Moderate Study
- H_2 receptor antagonists **(cimetidine)** moderately increase the exposure to **praziquantel**. Moderate Study
- **HIV-protease inhibitors** are predicted to moderately increase the exposure to **praziquantel**. Mild Study
- **Idelalisib** is predicted to moderately increase the exposure to **praziquantel**. Mild Study
- **Ivosidenib** is predicted to markedly decrease the exposure to **praziquantel**. Avoid. Moderate Study
- **Lumacaftor** is predicted to markedly decrease the exposure to **praziquantel**. Avoid. Moderate Study
- Macrolides **(clarithromycin)** are predicted to moderately increase the exposure to **praziquantel**. Mild Study
- **Mitotane** is predicted to markedly decrease the exposure to **praziquantel**. Avoid. Moderate Study
- Rifamycins **(rifampicin)** are predicted to markedly decrease the exposure to **praziquantel**. Avoid. Moderate Study
- **Tucatinib** is predicted to moderately increase the exposure to **praziquantel**. Mild Study

Prazosin → see alpha blockers
Prednisolone → see corticosteroids
Pregabalin → see antiepileptics
Pridinol → see TABLE 8 p. 1055 (antimuscarinics)

- Atypical antipsychotics **(clozapine)** can cause constipation, as can **pridinol**; concurrent use might increase the risk of developing intestinal obstruction. Severe Theoretical → Also see TABLE 8 p. 1055

Prilocaine → see anaesthetics, local
Primaquine → see antimalarials
Primidone → see antiepileptics
Procarbazine → see TABLE 12 p. 1057 (myelosuppression)

FOOD AND LIFESTYLE Procarbazine is a mild monoamine-oxidase inhibitor and might rarely interact with tyramine-rich foods (such as mature cheese, salami, pickled herring, *Bovril*®, *Oxo*®, *Marmite*® or any similar meat or yeast extract or fermented soya bean extract, and some beers, lagers or wines).

- **Alcohol** potentially causes a disulfiram-like reaction when given with **procarbazine**. Moderate Anecdotal
- Antiepileptics **(carbamazepine, phenobarbital, phenytoin, primidone)** are predicted to increase the risk of hypersensitivity reactions when given with **procarbazine**. Severe Anecdotal
- Antiepileptics **(fosphenytoin)** are predicted to increase the risk of hypersensitivity when given with **procarbazine**. Severe Anecdotal
- **Live vaccines** are predicted to increase the risk of generalised infection (possibly life-threatening) when given with **procarbazine**. UKHSA advises avoid (refer to Green Book). Severe Theoretical

Prochlorperazine → see phenothiazine antipsychotics
Procyclidine → see TABLE 8 p. 1055 (antimuscarinics), TABLE 9 p. 1056 (CNS effects)

- Atypical antipsychotics **(clozapine)** can cause constipation, as can **procyclidine**; concurrent use might increase the risk of developing intestinal obstruction. Severe Theoretical → Also see TABLE 8 p. 1055 → Also see TABLE 9 p. 1056
- SSRIs **(paroxetine)** slightly increase the exposure to **procyclidine**. Monitor and adjust dose. Moderate Study → Also see TABLE 9 p. 1056

Proguanil → see antimalarials
Promazine → see phenothiazine antipsychotics
Promethazine → see antihistamines, sedating
Propafenone → see antiarrhythmics
Propantheline → see TABLE 8 p. 1055 (antimuscarinics)

- Atypical antipsychotics **(clozapine)** can cause constipation, as can **propantheline**; concurrent use might increase the risk of developing intestinal obstruction. Severe Theoretical → Also see TABLE 8 p. 1055

Propiverine → see TABLE 8 p. 1055 (antimuscarinics)

- Antifungals, azoles **(itraconazole, ketoconazole, posaconazole, voriconazole)** given with carbimazole are predicted to increase the exposure to **propiverine**. Adjust starting dose. Moderate Theoretical
- Atypical antipsychotics **(clozapine)** can cause constipation, as can **propiverine**; concurrent use might increase the risk of developing intestinal obstruction. Severe Theoretical → Also see TABLE 8 p. 1055
- **Carbimazole** given with a potent CYP3A4 inhibitor is predicted to increase the exposure to **propiverine**. Adjust starting dose. Moderate Theoretical
- **Ceritinib** given with carbimazole is predicted to increase the exposure to **propiverine**. Adjust starting dose. Moderate Theoretical
- **Cobicistat** given with carbimazole is predicted to increase the exposure to **propiverine**. Adjust starting dose. Moderate Theoretical
- **HIV-protease inhibitors** given with carbimazole are predicted to increase the exposure to **propiverine**. Adjust starting dose. Moderate Theoretical
- **Idelalisib** given with carbimazole is predicted to increase the exposure to **propiverine**. Adjust starting dose. Moderate Theoretical
- **Propiverine** is predicted to increase the exposure to **lomitapide**. Separate administration by 12 hours. Moderate Theoretical
- Macrolides **(clarithromycin)** given with carbimazole are predicted to increase the exposure to **propiverine**. Adjust starting dose. Moderate Theoretical
- **Tucatinib** given with carbimazole is predicted to increase the exposure to **propiverine**. Adjust starting dose. Moderate Theoretical

Propofol → see TABLE 4 p. 1054 (bradycardia), TABLE 6 p. 1054 (hypotension), TABLE 9 p. 1056 (CNS effects)

- Antiepileptics **(valproate)** potentially increase the concentration of **propofol**. Adjust dose. Severe Theoretical
- **Propofol** is predicted to increase the exposure to the active component of **sacituzumab govitecan**. Severe Theoretical

Propranolol → see beta blockers, non-selective
Propylthiouracil

- **Propylthiouracil** is predicted to decrease the effects of **metyrapone**. Avoid. Moderate Theoretical

Proton pump inhibitors

esomeprazole · lansoprazole · omeprazole · pantoprazole · rabeprazole

- **Pantoprazole** is predicted to increase the exposure to **alpelisib**. Moderate Theoretical
- Anti-androgens **(apalutamide)** markedly decrease the exposure to **omeprazole**. Avoid or monitor. Moderate Study
- Anti-androgens **(apalutamide)** are predicted to decrease the exposure to proton pump inhibitors **(lansoprazole, rabeprazole)**. Avoid or monitor. Mild Study
- Antiepileptics **(sultiame)** might increase the exposure to **omeprazole**. Moderate Theoretical
- Antifungals, azoles **(voriconazole)** increase the exposure to proton pump inhibitors **(esomeprazole, omeprazole)**. Adjust dose. Moderate Study
- **Proton pump inhibitors** decrease the absorption of antifungals, azoles **(itraconazole)**. Administer itraconazole capsules with an acidic beverage. Moderate Study

Proton pump inhibitors (continued)
- **Proton pump inhibitors** decrease the absorption of antifungals, azoles **(ketoconazole)**. Administer ketoconazole with an acidic beverage. Moderate Study
- **Proton pump inhibitors** decrease the absorption of antifungals, azoles **(posaconazole)** oral suspension. Avoid. Moderate Study
- **Proton pump inhibitors** are predicted to decrease the exposure to **belumosudil**. Adjust **belumosudil** dose, p. 650. Severe Study
- Proton pump inhibitors **(esomeprazole, omeprazole)** are predicted to increase the exposure to **belzutifan**. Monitor and adjust dose. Severe Theoretical
- Proton pump inhibitors **(esomeprazole, omeprazole)** potentially increase the exposure to benzodiazepines **(clobazam)**. Adjust dose. Moderate Theoretical
- **Proton pump inhibitors** are predicted to decrease the absorption of **bosutinib**. Moderate Study
- **Esomeprazole** is predicted to increase the exposure to **cannabidiol**. Moderate Theoretical
- **Cenobamate** moderately increases the exposure to **omeprazole**. Adjust dose. Moderate Study
- **Proton pump inhibitors** are predicted to decrease the absorption of **ceritinib**. Moderate Theoretical
- **Esomeprazole** is predicted to increase the exposure to **cilostazol**. Moderate Theoretical
- **Omeprazole** is predicted to increase the exposure to **cilostazol**. Adjust **cilostazol** dose. Moderate Study
- Proton pump inhibitors **(esomeprazole, omeprazole)** are predicted to decrease the efficacy of **clopidogrel**. Avoid. Moderate Study
- **Proton pump inhibitors** are predicted to decrease the exposure to **dacomitinib**. Avoid. Moderate Study
- **Proton pump inhibitors** are predicted to decrease the exposure to **dasatinib**. Avoid. Severe Study
- **Proton pump inhibitors** are predicted to decrease the absorption of **dipyridamole** (immediate release tablets). Moderate Theoretical
- **Proton pump inhibitors** are predicted to decrease the exposure to **erlotinib**. Avoid. Moderate Study
- **Fedratinib** moderately increases the exposure to **omeprazole**. Monitor and adjust dose. Moderate Study
- **Proton pump inhibitors** are predicted to decrease the exposure to **gefitinib**. Severe Theoretical
- **Proton pump inhibitors** decrease the exposure to HIV-protease inhibitors **(atazanavir)**. Avoid or adjust dose. Severe Study
- **Ivosidenib** might decrease the exposure to **omeprazole**. Avoid or monitor efficacy. Unknown Theoretical
- **Proton pump inhibitors** are predicted to decrease the exposure to **ledipasvir**. Adjust dose, see ledipasvir with sofosbuvir p. 495. Moderate Theoretical
- **Pantoprazole** might increase the exposure to **mavacamten**. Monitor and adjust dose—consult product literature. Moderate Theoretical
- Proton pump inhibitors **(esomeprazole, omeprazole)** are predicted to increase the exposure to **mavacamten**. Adjust dose—consult product literature. Severe Theoretical
- **Proton pump inhibitors** decrease the clearance of **methotrexate** (high-dose). Use with caution or avoid. Severe Study
- **Proton pump inhibitors** are predicted to decrease the exposure to **neratinib**. Avoid. Severe Study
- **Proton pump inhibitors** are predicted to decrease the exposure to oral NNRTIs **(rilpivirine)**. Avoid. Severe Study
- **Proton pump inhibitors** are predicted to decrease the exposure to **pazopanib**. Avoid or administer concurrently without food. Moderate Study
- **Proton pump inhibitors** have been reported to decrease the exposure to **pemigatinib**. Avoid. Severe Anecdotal
- **Proton pump inhibitors** are predicted to decrease the exposure to **selpercatinib**. Manufacturer advises take with food. Moderate Study
- Proton pump inhibitors **(esomeprazole, omeprazole)** are predicted to increase the exposure to **selumetinib**. Avoid or adjust dose—consult product literature. Severe Theoretical
- **Proton pump inhibitors** potentially decrease the exposure to **sofosbuvir**. Adjust dose, see ledipasvir with sofosbuvir p. 495, sofosbuvir with velpatasvir p. 496, and sofosbuvir with velpatasvir and voxilaprevir. Moderate Study
- **Proton pump inhibitors** are predicted to decrease the exposure to **sotorasib**. Manufacturer advises give **sotorasib** with an acidic beverage or use an antacid. Moderate Study
- **Sparsentan** is predicted to decrease the exposure to proton pump inhibitors **(lansoprazole, omeprazole, rabeprazole)**. Moderate Theoretical
- **Esomeprazole** increases the exposure to SSRIs **(citalopram)**. Monitor and adjust dose. Severe Theoretical
- **Omeprazole** moderately increases the exposure to SSRIs **(citalopram)**. Monitor and adjust dose. Severe Study
- Proton pump inhibitors **(esomeprazole, omeprazole)** are predicted to increase the exposure to SSRIs **(escitalopram)**. Use with caution and adjust dose. Severe Study
- **Esomeprazole** might increase the concentration of SSRIs **(sertraline)**. Moderate Study
- **Proton pump inhibitors** might decrease the efficacy of **ulipristal** for emergency hormonal contraception. For CoSRH guidance, see Contraceptives, interactions p. 614. Unknown Theoretical
- **Proton pump inhibitors** are predicted to decrease the concentration of **velpatasvir**. Adjust dose, see sofosbuvir with velpatasvir p. 496. Moderate Study
- **Proton pump inhibitors** are predicted to decrease the exposure to **voxilaprevir**. Adjust dose, see sofosbuvir with velpatasvir and voxilaprevir. Moderate Study

Proxymetacaine → see anaesthetics, local
Pseudoephedrine → see sympathomimetics, vasoconstrictor
Pyrazinamide → see TABLE 1 p. 1053 (hepatotoxicity)
- **Allopurinol** is predicted to increase the risk of hyperuricaemia when given with **pyrazinamide**. Moderate Theoretical

Pyridostigmine → see TABLE 4 p. 1054 (bradycardia)
- **Aminoglycosides** are predicted to decrease the effects of **pyridostigmine**. Moderate Theoretical

Pyrimethamine → see antimalarials
Quetiapine → see atypical antipsychotics
Quinagolide → see dopamine receptor agonists
Quinapril → see ACE inhibitors
Quinine → see antimalarials
Quinolones → see TABLE 7 p. 1055 (QT-interval prolongation)

ciprofloxacin · delafloxacin · levofloxacin · moxifloxacin · ofloxacin

- Avoid concurrent administration of dairy products and mineral-fortified drinks with *oral* **ciprofloxacin** due to reduced exposure.
- Since systemic absorption can follow topical application of **ciprofloxacin**, **levofloxacin**, or **ofloxacin**, the possibility of interactions should be borne in mind.
- Interactions do not generally apply to topical use of **moxifloxacin** unless specified.

- **Ciprofloxacin** is predicted to increase the exposure to **agomelatine**. Moderate Study
- **Ciprofloxacin** is predicted to increase the exposure to **aminophylline**. Adjust dose. Moderate Theoretical
- **Ciprofloxacin** is predicted to increase the exposure to anaesthetics, local **(ropivacaine)**. Moderate Theoretical
- **Ciprofloxacin** is predicted to increase the exposure to **anagrelide**. Moderate Theoretical
- Oral **antacids** decrease the absorption of oral **quinolones**. Manufacturer advises take 2 hours before or 4 hours after antacids. Moderate Study
- **Ciprofloxacin** slightly increases the exposure to antiarrhythmics **(lidocaine)**. Mild Study
- **Ciprofloxacin** affects the concentration of antiepileptics **(fosphenytoin, phenytoin)**. Monitor concentration and adjust dose. Severe Study
- **Ciprofloxacin** increases the concentration of atypical antipsychotics **(clozapine)**. Monitor adverse effects and adjust dose. Severe Study
- **Ciprofloxacin** is predicted to increase the exposure to atypical antipsychotics **(olanzapine)**. Adjust dose. Moderate Anecdotal
- **Ciprofloxacin** might increase the exposure to **bedaquiline**. Mild Theoretical

- Oral **calcium compounds** decrease the absorption of oral **ciprofloxacin**. Separate administration by 2 hours. [Moderate] Study
- **Ciprofloxacin** is predicted to increase the exposure to **capivasertib**. Adjust dose. [Moderate] Theoretical
- **Quinolones** increase the anticoagulant effect of **coumarins**. [Severe] Anecdotal
- **Ciprofloxacin** is predicted to increase the exposure to **daridorexant**. Adjust **daridorexant** dose. [Moderate] Theoretical
- **Ciprofloxacin** is predicted to increase the exposure to dopamine receptor agonists **(ropinirole)**. Adjust dose. [Moderate] Study
- **Ciprofloxacin** is predicted to increase the exposure to **elacestrant**. Avoid or adjust **elacestrant** dose. [Severe] Theoretical
- **Ciprofloxacin** is predicted to increase the exposure to **eliglustat**. Avoid or adjust dose—consult product literature. [Severe] Theoretical
- **Enteral feeds** decrease the exposure to **ciprofloxacin**. [Moderate] Study
- **Ciprofloxacin** are predicted to increases the exposure to **erlotinib**. Monitor adverse effects and adjust dose. [Moderate] Study
- **Ciprofloxacin** is predicted to increase the exposure to **fezolinetant**. Avoid. [Moderate] Study
- **Ciprofloxacin** is predicted to increase the concentration of **guanfacine**. Adjust **guanfacine** dose, p. 281. [Moderate] Theoretical
- **Ciprofloxacin** is predicted to increase the exposure to **ibrutinib**. Adjust dose—consult product literature. [Severe] Theoretical
- Oral **iron** decreases the exposure to oral **quinolones**. Separate administration by at least 2 hours. [Moderate] Study
- **Lanthanum** moderately decreases the exposure to **quinolones**. **Quinolones** should be taken 2 hours before or 4 hours after **lanthanum**. [Moderate] Study
- **Leflunomide** is predicted to increase the exposure to **ciprofloxacin**. [Moderate] Theoretical
- **Ciprofloxacin** is predicted to increase the exposure to **loxapine**. Avoid. [Unknown] Theoretical
- **Ciprofloxacin** slightly increases the exposure to MAO-B inhibitors **(rasagiline)**. [Moderate] Study
- **Ciprofloxacin** is predicted to increase the exposure to **melatonin**. [Moderate] Theoretical
- **Ciprofloxacin** potentially increases the risk of toxicity when given with **methotrexate**. [Severe] Anecdotal
- **Nitisinone** is predicted to increase the exposure to **ciprofloxacin**. [Moderate] Study
- **NSAIDs** potentially increase the risk of seizures when given with **quinolones**. [Severe] Theoretical
- **Ciprofloxacin** is predicted to increase the exposure to **omaveloxolone**. Avoid or adjust **omaveloxolone** dose, p. 755. [Moderate] Theoretical
- **Ciprofloxacin** very slightly increases the exposure to **pentoxifylline**. [Moderate] Study
- **Ciprofloxacin** is predicted to increase the exposure to phenothiazine antipsychotics **(chlorpromazine)**. [Moderate] Theoretical
- **Ciprofloxacin** is predicted to increase the exposure to phosphodiesterase type-4 inhibitors **(roflumilast)**. [Moderate] Theoretical
- **Ciprofloxacin** moderately increases the exposure to phosphodiesterase type-5 inhibitors **(sildenafil)**. [Moderate] Theoretical
- **Ciprofloxacin** is predicted to increase the exposure to **pirfenidone**. Use with caution and adjust dose. [Moderate] Study
- **Ciprofloxacin** is predicted to increase the exposure to **pomalidomide**. Adjust dose—consult product literature. [Moderate] Theoretical
- **Ciprofloxacin** is predicted to increase the exposure to **riluzole**. [Moderate] Theoretical
- **Ciprofloxacin** is predicted to increase the exposure to **ruxolitinib**. [Moderate] Theoretical
- **Ciprofloxacin** is predicted to increase the exposure to SNRIs **(duloxetine)**. Avoid. [Moderate] Theoretical
- **Strontium** is predicted to decrease the absorption of **quinolones**. Avoid. [Moderate] Theoretical
- **Sucralfate** decreases the exposure to **quinolones**. Separate administration by 2 hours. [Moderate] Study
- **Teriflunomide** is predicted to increase the exposure to **ciprofloxacin**. [Moderate] Theoretical
- **Ciprofloxacin** is predicted to increase the exposure to **theophylline**. Monitor and adjust dose. [Moderate] Theoretical
- **Ciprofloxacin** increases the exposure to **tizanidine**. Avoid. [Moderate] Study
- **Ciprofloxacin** is predicted to increase the exposure to **tolvaptan**. Use with caution and adjust **tolvaptan** dose. [Moderate] Theoretical
- **Ciprofloxacin** is predicted to increase the exposure to triptans **(zolmitriptan)**. Adjust **zolmitriptan** dose, p. 347. [Moderate] Theoretical
- **Vadadustat** is predicted to increase the exposure to **ciprofloxacin**. Monitor and adjust dose. [Moderate] Study
- **Ciprofloxacin** is predicted to increase the exposure to **venetoclax**. Avoid or adjust dose—consult product literature. [Severe] Theoretical
- **Ciprofloxacin** moderately increases the exposure to **vorasidenib**. Avoid. [Moderate] Study
- **Ciprofloxacin** is predicted to increase the exposure to **zanubrutinib**. Avoid or adjust dose—consult product literature. [Severe] Theoretical
- **Zinc** is predicted to decrease the exposure to **quinolones**. Separate administration by 2 hours. [Moderate] Study

Quizartinib → see TABLE 7 p. 1055 (QT-interval prolongation)

- Anti-androgens **(apalutamide, enzalutamide)** are predicted to decrease the exposure to **quizartinib**. Avoid. [Severe] Study → Also see TABLE 7 p. 1055
- Antiepileptics **(carbamazepine, fosphenytoin, phenobarbital, phenytoin, primidone)** are predicted to decrease the exposure to **quizartinib**. Avoid. [Severe] Study
- Antifungals, azoles **(itraconazole, ketoconazole, posaconazole, voriconazole)** are predicted to increase the exposure to **quizartinib**. Adjust dose—consult product literature. [Severe] Study → Also see TABLE 7 p. 1055
- **Cenobamate** is predicted to decrease the exposure to **quizartinib**. Avoid. [Severe] Study
- **Ceritinib** is predicted to increase the exposure to **quizartinib**. Adjust dose—consult product literature. [Severe] Study → Also see TABLE 7 p. 1055
- **Cobicistat** is predicted to increase the exposure to **quizartinib**. Adjust dose—consult product literature. [Severe] Study
- **Dabrafenib** is predicted to decrease the exposure to **quizartinib**. Avoid. [Severe] Study
- **Encorafenib** is predicted to decrease the exposure to **quizartinib**. Avoid. [Severe] Study → Also see TABLE 7 p. 1055
- Endothelin receptor antagonists **(bosentan)** are predicted to decrease the exposure to **quizartinib**. Avoid. [Severe] Study
- **HIV-protease inhibitors** are predicted to increase the exposure to **quizartinib**. Adjust dose—consult product literature. [Severe] Study
- **Idelalisib** is predicted to increase the exposure to **quizartinib**. Adjust dose—consult product literature. [Severe] Study
- **Ivosidenib** is predicted to decrease the exposure to **quizartinib**. Avoid. [Severe] Study → Also see TABLE 7 p. 1055
- **Lorlatinib** is predicted to decrease the exposure to **quizartinib**. Avoid. [Severe] Study
- **Lumacaftor** is predicted to decrease the exposure to **quizartinib**. Avoid. [Severe] Study
- Macrolides **(clarithromycin)** are predicted to increase the exposure to **quizartinib**. Adjust dose—consult product literature. [Severe] Study
- **Mitotane** is predicted to decrease the exposure to **quizartinib**. Avoid. [Severe] Study
- NNRTIs **(efavirenz, etravirine, nevirapine)** are predicted to decrease the exposure to **quizartinib**. Avoid. [Severe] Study → Also see TABLE 7 p. 1055
- Rifamycins **(rifampicin)** are predicted to decrease the exposure to **quizartinib**. Avoid. [Severe] Study
- **Sotorasib** is predicted to decrease the exposure to **quizartinib**. Avoid. [Severe] Study
- **St John's wort** is predicted to decrease the exposure to **quizartinib**. Avoid. [Severe] Study
- **Tucatinib** is predicted to increase the exposure to **quizartinib**. Adjust dose—consult product literature. [Severe] Study

Rabeprazole → see proton pump inhibitors
Rabies immunoglobulin → see immunoglobulins
Rabies vaccine
- Antimalarials (chloroquine) decrease the efficacy of rabies vaccine (intradermal). Avoid. Moderate Study
- Hydroxychloroquine is predicted to decrease efficacy rabies vaccine. Moderate Theoretical

Raloxifene
- Combined hormonal contraceptives potentially oppose the effects of raloxifene. Avoid. Severe Theoretical
- Hormone replacement therapy potentially opposes the effects of raloxifene. Avoid. Severe Theoretical

Raltegravir
- Oral antacids decrease the exposure to oral raltegravir. Avoid. Moderate Study
- Antiepileptics (carbamazepine, fosphenytoin, phenobarbital, phenytoin, primidone) are predicted to affect the exposure to raltegravir. Use with caution or avoid. Moderate Theoretical
- Belumosudil is predicted to affect the exposure to raltegravir. Moderate Theoretical
- Oral calcium compounds (calcium carbonate) -containing antacids greatly decrease the exposure to oral raltegravir (high-dose). Avoid. Severe Study
- Encorafenib is predicted to increase the exposure to raltegravir. Moderate Theoretical
- HIV-protease inhibitors (atazanavir) increase the exposure to raltegravir (high-dose). Avoid. Moderate Study
- HIV-protease inhibitors (darunavir) increase the risk of rash when given with raltegravir. Moderate Study
- HIV-protease inhibitors (fosamprenavir) boosted with ritonavir decrease the exposure to raltegravir and raltegravir decreases the exposure to HIV-protease inhibitors (fosamprenavir) boosted with ritonavir. Avoid. Severe Study
- Oral iron is predicted to decrease the exposure to oral raltegravir. Separate administration by at least 2 hours. Moderate Theoretical
- Ivosidenib might decrease the exposure to raltegravir. Avoid or monitor efficacy. Unknown Theoretical
- Rifamycins (rifampicin) slightly decrease the exposure to raltegravir. Avoid or adjust dose—consult product literature. Moderate Study
- Sodium zirconium cyclosilicate is predicted to decrease the exposure to raltegravir. Separate administration by at least 2 hours. Moderate Theoretical

Raltitrexed → see TABLE 12 p. 1057 (myelosuppression)
- Folates are predicted to alter the effects of raltitrexed. Avoid. Moderate Study
- Live vaccines are predicted to increase the risk of generalised infection (possibly life-threatening) when given with raltitrexed. UKHSA advises avoid (refer to Green Book). Severe Theoretical

Ramipril → see ACE inhibitors
Ramucirumab → see monoclonal antibodies
Ranibizumab
- Drugs that cause bleeding (see TABLE 3 p. 1053) cause bleeding, as can ranibizumab; concurrent use might increase the risk of developing this effect. Severe Theoretical

Ranolazine → see TABLE 7 p. 1055 (QT-interval prolongation)
- Ranolazine is predicted to increase the exposure to afatinib. Moderate Study
- Ranolazine is predicted to increase the exposure to aliskiren. Moderate Theoretical
- Anti-androgens (apalutamide, enzalutamide) are predicted to decrease the exposure to ranolazine. Avoid. Severe Study → Also see TABLE 7 p. 1055
- Antiarrhythmics (dronedarone) are predicted to increase the exposure to ranolazine. Severe Study → Also see TABLE 7 p. 1055
- Antiepileptics (carbamazepine, fosphenytoin, phenobarbital, phenytoin, primidone) are predicted to decrease the exposure to ranolazine. Avoid. Severe Study
- Antifungals, azoles (fluconazole, isavuconazole) are predicted to increase the exposure to ranolazine. Severe Study → Also see TABLE 7 p. 1055
- Antifungals, azoles (itraconazole, ketoconazole, posaconazole, voriconazole) are predicted to increase the exposure to ranolazine. Avoid. Severe Study → Also see TABLE 7 p. 1055
- Ranolazine is predicted to increase the exposure to antihistamines, non-sedating (fexofenadine). Moderate Theoretical
- Berotralstat is predicted to increase the exposure to ranolazine. Severe Study
- Ranolazine is predicted to increase the exposure to beta blockers, non-selective (nadolol). Moderate Study
- Calcium-channel blockers (diltiazem, verapamil) are predicted to increase the exposure to ranolazine. Severe Study
- Ceritinib is predicted to increase the exposure to ranolazine. Avoid. Severe Study → Also see TABLE 7 p. 1055
- Ciclosporin is predicted to increase the concentration of ranolazine and ranolazine is predicted to increase the concentration of ciclosporin. Moderate Theoretical
- Cobicistat is predicted to increase the exposure to ranolazine. Avoid. Severe Study
- Ranolazine is predicted to increase the exposure to colchicine. Avoid P-glycoprotein inhibitors or adjust colchicine dose, p. 637. Severe Theoretical
- Crizotinib is predicted to increase the exposure to ranolazine. Severe Study → Also see TABLE 7 p. 1055
- Danicopan is predicted to increase the exposure to ranolazine. Moderate Study
- Ranolazine increases the concentration of digoxin. Moderate Study
- Ranolazine is predicted to increase the exposure to dopamine receptor agonists (pramipexole). Adjust dose. Moderate Study
- Eliglustat is predicted to increase the exposure to ranolazine. Adjust dose. Moderate Study
- Encorafenib is predicted to decrease the exposure to ranolazine. Avoid. Severe Study → Also see TABLE 7 p. 1055
- Ranolazine is predicted to increase the exposure to erlotinib. Moderate Theoretical
- Ranolazine is predicted to increase the exposure to factor XA inhibitors (apixaban). Moderate Theoretical
- Ranolazine is predicted to slightly increase the exposure to factor XA inhibitors (edoxaban). Severe Theoretical
- Ranolazine might increase the exposure to factor XA inhibitors (rivaroxaban). Manufacturer advises caution in renal impairment. Moderate Theoretical
- Fedratinib is predicted to increase the exposure to ranolazine. Severe Study
- Ranolazine is predicted to increase the exposure to fidaxomicin. Avoid. Moderate Study
- Ranolazine is predicted to increase the exposure to gilteritinib. Moderate Theoretical
- Glecaprevir is predicted to increase the exposure to ranolazine. Adjust dose. Severe Theoretical
- Grapefruit juice is predicted to increase the concentration of ranolazine. Avoid. Severe Theoretical
- Ranolazine is predicted to increase the exposure to grazoprevir. Avoid. Severe Theoretical
- HIV-protease inhibitors are predicted to increase the exposure to ranolazine. Avoid. Severe Study
- Idelalisib is predicted to increase the exposure to ranolazine. Avoid. Severe Study
- Imatinib is predicted to increase the exposure to ranolazine. Severe Study
- Ivosidenib is predicted to decrease the exposure to ranolazine. Avoid. Severe Study → Also see TABLE 7 p. 1055
- Lapatinib is predicted to increase the exposure to ranolazine. Moderate Theoretical → Also see TABLE 7 p. 1055
- Letermovir is predicted to increase the exposure to ranolazine. Severe Study
- Ranolazine is predicted to increase the exposure to lomitapide. Separate administration by 12 hours. Mild Theoretical
- Lorlatinib is predicted to decrease the exposure to ranolazine. Moderate Theoretical
- Lumacaftor is predicted to decrease the exposure to ranolazine. Avoid. Severe Study
- Macrolides (clarithromycin) are predicted to increase the exposure to ranolazine. Avoid. Severe Study

A1 Interactions | Appendix 1

- Macrolides **(erythromycin)** are predicted to increase the exposure to **ranolazine**. Severe Study → Also see TABLE 7 p. 1055
- **Ranolazine** is predicted to increase the exposure to **mavacamten**. Monitor and adjust dose—consult product literature. Moderate Theoretical
- **Ranolazine** is predicted to increase the exposure to **metformin**. Use with caution and adjust dose. Moderate Study
- **Mitotane** is predicted to decrease the exposure to **ranolazine**. Avoid. Severe Study
- **Ranolazine** increases the risk of neutropenia when given with monoclonal antibodies **(brentuximab vedotin)**. Monitor and adjust dose. Severe Theoretical
- **Ranolazine** is predicted to increase the exposure to **naldemedine**. Moderate Study
- **Ranolazine** is predicted to increase the exposure to **neratinib**. Avoid or adjust dose and monitor for gastrointestinal adverse effects—consult product literature. Severe Study
- Neurokinin-1 receptor antagonists **(aprepitant, netupitant)** are predicted to increase the exposure to **ranolazine**. Severe Study
- **Nilotinib** is predicted to increase the exposure to **ranolazine**. Severe Study → Also see TABLE 7 p. 1055
- **Ranolazine** is predicted to increase the exposure to **nintedanib**. Moderate Study
- **Nirmatrelvir** boosted with ritonavir is predicted to increase the concentration of **ranolazine**. Avoid. Severe Theoretical
- **Olaparib** might increase the exposure to **ranolazine**. Moderate Theoretical
- **Osimertinib** is predicted to increase the exposure to **ranolazine**. Moderate Study → Also see TABLE 7 p. 1055
- **Ranolazine** is predicted to increase the exposure to **panobinostat**. Adjust dose. Moderate Theoretical → Also see TABLE 7 p. 1055
- **Ranolazine** is predicted to increase the exposure to **pralsetinib**. Moderate Theoretical
- **Ranolazine** is predicted to increase the exposure to **relugolix**. Avoid or take relugolix first and separate administration by at least 6 hours. Moderate Study
- Rifamycins **(rifampicin)** are predicted to decrease the exposure to **ranolazine**. Avoid. Severe Study
- **Ranolazine** is predicted to increase the exposure to **rimegepant**. Avoid another dose of rimegepant within 48 hours of concurrent use. Moderate Theoretical
- **Sparsentan** is predicted to increase the exposure to **ranolazine**. Severe Theoretical
- **St John's wort** is predicted to decrease the exposure to **ranolazine**. Avoid. Severe Study
- **Ranolazine** is predicted to increase the exposure to statins **(atorvastatin)**. Moderate Theoretical
- **Ranolazine** slightly increases the exposure to statins **(simvastatin)**. Adjust **simvastatin** dose, p. 156. Moderate Study
- **Ranolazine** increases the concentration of **tacrolimus**. Adjust dose. Severe Anecdotal
- **Ranolazine** is predicted to slightly increase the exposure to **talazoparib**. Avoid or adjust dose—consult product literature. Severe Study
- **Ranolazine** is predicted to increase the exposure to taxanes **(paclitaxel)**. Severe Theoretical
- **Ranolazine** is predicted to increase the exposure to thrombin inhibitors **(dabigatran)**. Severe Theoretical
- **Ranolazine** is predicted to increase the exposure to **ticagrelor**. Use with caution or avoid. Severe Study
- **Ranolazine** might increase the exposure to **tigecycline**. Mild Anecdotal
- **Ranolazine** is predicted to increase the exposure to **topotecan**. Severe Study
- **Ranolazine** is predicted to increase the concentration of **trametinib**. Moderate Theoretical
- **Tucatinib** is predicted to increase the exposure to **ranolazine**. Avoid. Severe Study
- **Vemurafenib** might increase the exposure to **ranolazine**. Use with caution or avoid. Moderate Theoretical → Also see TABLE 7 p. 1055
- **Ranolazine** is predicted to increase the exposure to **venetoclax**. Avoid or monitor for toxicity. Severe Theoretical
- **Ranolazine** might increase the exposure to **vinca alkaloids**. Severe Theoretical
- **Voxilaprevir** with sofosbuvir and velpatasvir is predicted to increase the exposure to **ranolazine**. Adjust dose. Severe Theoretical

Rasagiline → see MAO-B inhibitors

Ravulizumab
- **Crovalimab** increases the risk of hypersensitivity reactions when given with **ravulizumab**. Severe Study

Reboxetine
- Anti-androgens **(apalutamide, enzalutamide)** are predicted to decrease the exposure to **reboxetine**. Moderate Anecdotal
- Antiepileptics **(carbamazepine, fosphenytoin, phenobarbital, phenytoin, primidone)** are predicted to decrease the exposure to **reboxetine**. Moderate Anecdotal
- Antifungals, azoles **(itraconazole, ketoconazole, posaconazole, voriconazole)** are predicted to increase the exposure to **reboxetine**. Avoid. Moderate Study
- Antifungals, azoles **(miconazole)** are predicted to increase the concentration of **reboxetine**. Use with caution and adjust dose. Moderate Theoretical
- **Ceritinib** is predicted to increase the exposure to **reboxetine**. Avoid. Moderate Study
- **Cobicistat** is predicted to increase the exposure to **reboxetine**. Avoid. Moderate Study
- **Encorafenib** is predicted to decrease the exposure to **reboxetine**. Moderate Anecdotal
- **HIV-protease inhibitors** are predicted to increase the exposure to **reboxetine**. Avoid. Moderate Study
- **Idelalisib** is predicted to increase the exposure to **reboxetine**. Avoid. Moderate Study
- **Ivosidenib** is predicted to decrease the exposure to **reboxetine**. Moderate Anecdotal
- **Reboxetine** is predicted to increase the risk of a hypertensive crisis when given with **linezolid**. Avoid. Severe Theoretical
- **Reboxetine** is predicted to increase the risk of hypokalaemia when given with **loop diuretics**. Moderate Theoretical
- **Lumacaftor** is predicted to decrease the exposure to **reboxetine**. Moderate Anecdotal
- Macrolides **(clarithromycin)** are predicted to increase the exposure to **reboxetine**. Avoid. Moderate Study
- **Reboxetine** is predicted to increase the risk of a hypertensive crisis when given with MAO-B inhibitors **(rasagiline, selegiline)**. Avoid. Severe Theoretical
- **Reboxetine** is predicted to increase the risk of a hypertensive crisis when given with **MAOIs, irreversible**. Avoid. Severe Theoretical
- **Mitotane** is predicted to decrease the exposure to **reboxetine**. Moderate Anecdotal
- **Reboxetine** is predicted to increase the risk of a hypertensive crisis when given with **moclobemide**. Avoid. Severe Theoretical
- Rifamycins **(rifampicin)** are predicted to decrease the exposure to **reboxetine**. Moderate Anecdotal
- **Reboxetine** is predicted to increase the risk of hypokalaemia when given with **thiazide diuretics**. Moderate Anecdotal
- **Tucatinib** is predicted to increase the exposure to **reboxetine**. Avoid. Moderate Study

Regorafenib → see TABLE 3 p. 1053 (bleeding), TABLE 12 p. 1057 (myelosuppression)
- Anti-androgens **(apalutamide, enzalutamide)** are predicted to decrease the exposure to **regorafenib**. Avoid. Moderate Study
- Antiarrhythmics **(dronedarone)** are predicted to increase the exposure to **regorafenib**. Moderate Study
- Antiepileptics **(carbamazepine, fosphenytoin, phenobarbital, phenytoin, primidone)** are predicted to decrease the exposure to **regorafenib**. Avoid. Moderate Study
- Antifungals, azoles **(fluconazole, isavuconazole)** are predicted to increase the exposure to **regorafenib**. Moderate Study
- Antifungals, azoles **(itraconazole, ketoconazole, posaconazole, voriconazole)** are predicted to increase the exposure to **regorafenib**. Avoid. Moderate Study
- **Berotralstat** is predicted to increase the exposure to **regorafenib**. Moderate Study
- Calcium-channel blockers **(diltiazem, verapamil)** are predicted to increase the exposure to **regorafenib**. Moderate Study

Regorafenib (continued)
- **Ceritinib** is predicted to increase the exposure to **regorafenib**. Avoid. Moderate Study → Also see TABLE 12 p. 1057
- **Cobicistat** is predicted to increase the exposure to **regorafenib**. Avoid. Moderate Study
- **Crizotinib** is predicted to increase the exposure to **regorafenib**. Moderate Study
- **Dabrafenib** is predicted to decrease the exposure to **regorafenib**. Severe Study
- **Encorafenib** is predicted to decrease the exposure to **regorafenib**. Avoid. Moderate Study
- Endothelin receptor antagonists **(bosentan)** are predicted to decrease the exposure to **regorafenib**. Severe Study
- **Fedratinib** is predicted to increase the exposure to **regorafenib**. Moderate Study
- **Grapefruit** juice is predicted to increase the exposure to **regorafenib**. Avoid. Moderate Theoretical
- **HIV-protease inhibitors** are predicted to increase the exposure to **regorafenib**. Avoid. Moderate Study
- **Idelalisib** is predicted to increase the exposure to **regorafenib**. Avoid. Moderate Study
- **Imatinib** is predicted to increase the exposure to **regorafenib**. Moderate Study → Also see TABLE 3 p. 1053 → Also see TABLE 12 p. 1057
- **Ivosidenib** is predicted to decrease the exposure to **regorafenib**. Avoid. Moderate Study
- **Letermovir** is predicted to increase the exposure to **regorafenib**. Moderate Study
- **Lumacaftor** is predicted to decrease the exposure to **regorafenib**. Avoid. Moderate Study
- Macrolides **(clarithromycin)** are predicted to increase the exposure to **regorafenib**. Avoid. Moderate Study
- Macrolides **(erythromycin)** are predicted to increase the exposure to **regorafenib**. Moderate Study
- **Regorafenib** is predicted to increase the exposure to **methotrexate**. Moderate Theoretical → Also see TABLE 12 p. 1057
- **Mitotane** is predicted to decrease the exposure to **regorafenib**. Avoid. Moderate Study → Also see TABLE 12 p. 1057
- Neurokinin-1 receptor antagonists **(aprepitant, netupitant)** are predicted to increase the exposure to **regorafenib**. Moderate Study
- **Nilotinib** is predicted to increase the exposure to **regorafenib**. Moderate Study → Also see TABLE 12 p. 1057
- NNRTIs **(efavirenz, etravirine, nevirapine)** are predicted to decrease the exposure to **regorafenib**. Severe Study
- NSAIDs **(mefenamic acid)** are predicted to increase the exposure to **regorafenib**. Avoid. Moderate Theoretical → Also see TABLE 3 p. 1053
- Rifamycins **(rifampicin)** are predicted to decrease the exposure to **regorafenib**. Avoid. Moderate Study
- **Regorafenib** is predicted to increase the exposure to the active component of **sacituzumab govitecan**. Severe Theoretical
- **St John's wort** is predicted to decrease the exposure to **regorafenib**. Avoid. Severe Study
- **Regorafenib** is predicted to increase the exposure to statins **(atorvastatin, fluvastatin)**. Moderate Study
- **Regorafenib** moderately increases the exposure to statins **(rosuvastatin)**. Avoid or adjust **rosuvastatin** dose, p. 155. Moderate Study
- **Regorafenib** is predicted to increase the exposure to **sulfasalazine**. Moderate Study → Also see TABLE 12 p. 1057
- **Regorafenib** is predicted to increase the exposure to **topotecan**. Moderate Study → Also see TABLE 12 p. 1057
- **Tucatinib** is predicted to increase the exposure to **regorafenib**. Avoid. Moderate Study

Relugolix
- Aminoglycosides **(gentamicin)** are predicted to increase the exposure to **relugolix**. Avoid or take relugolix first and separate administration by at least 6 hours. Moderate Theoretical
- Anti-androgens **(apalutamide)** are predicted to decrease the exposure to **relugolix**. Avoid or adjust dose depending on indication—consult product literature. Moderate Study
- Antiarrhythmics **(amiodarone, dronedarone)** are predicted to increase the exposure to **relugolix**. Avoid or take relugolix first and separate administration by at least 6 hours. Moderate Study
- Antiarrhythmics **(propafenone)** are predicted to increase the exposure to **relugolix**. Avoid or take relugolix first and separate administration by at least 6 hours. Moderate Theoretical
- Antiepileptics **(carbamazepine, phenobarbital, phenytoin)** are predicted to decrease the exposure to **relugolix**. Avoid or adjust dose depending on indication—consult product literature. Moderate Study
- Antiepileptics **(oxcarbazepine, topiramate)** are predicted to decrease the exposure to **relugolix**. Avoid. Moderate Theoretical
- Antifungals, azoles **(itraconazole, ketoconazole)** are predicted to increase the exposure to **relugolix**. Avoid or take relugolix first and separate administration by at least 6 hours. Moderate Study
- Beta blockers, non-selective **(carvedilol)** are predicted to increase the exposure to **relugolix**. Avoid or take relugolix first and separate administration by at least 6 hours. Moderate Theoretical
- Calcium-channel blockers **(verapamil)** are predicted to increase the exposure to **relugolix**. Avoid or take relugolix first and separate administration by at least 6 hours. Moderate Study
- **Ciclosporin** is predicted to increase the exposure to **relugolix**. Avoid or take relugolix first and separate administration by at least 6 hours. Moderate Study
- **Cobicistat** is predicted to increase the exposure to **relugolix**. Avoid or take relugolix first and separate administration by at least 6 hours. Moderate Study
- **Glecaprevir** is predicted to increase the exposure to **relugolix**. Avoid or take relugolix first and separate administration by at least 6 hours. Moderate Study
- HIV-protease inhibitors **(lopinavir, ritonavir)** are predicted to increase the exposure to **relugolix**. Avoid or take relugolix first and separate administration by at least 6 hours. Moderate Study
- **Lapatinib** is predicted to increase the exposure to **relugolix**. Avoid or take relugolix first and separate administration by at least 6 hours. Moderate Study
- **Macrolides** are predicted to increase the exposure to **relugolix**. Avoid or take relugolix first and separate administration by at least 6 hours. Moderate Study
- NNRTIs **(efavirenz)** are predicted to decrease the exposure to **relugolix**. Avoid or adjust dose depending on indication—consult product literature. Moderate Study
- **Pibrentasvir** is predicted to increase the exposure to **relugolix**. Avoid or take relugolix first and separate administration by at least 6 hours. Moderate Study
- **Ranolazine** is predicted to increase the exposure to **relugolix**. Avoid or take relugolix first and separate administration by at least 6 hours. Moderate Study
- **Rifamycins** are predicted to decrease the exposure to **relugolix**. Avoid or adjust dose depending on indication—consult product literature. Moderate Study
- **St John's wort** is predicted to decrease the exposure to **relugolix**. Avoid or adjust dose depending on indication—consult product literature. Moderate Study
- Tetracyclines **(tetracycline)** are predicted to increase the exposure to **relugolix**. Avoid or take relugolix first and separate administration by at least 6 hours. Moderate Theoretical
- **Velpatasvir** is predicted to increase the exposure to **relugolix**. Avoid or take relugolix first and separate administration by at least 6 hours. Moderate Study
- **Vemurafenib** is predicted to increase the exposure to **relugolix**. Avoid or take relugolix first and separate administration by at least 6 hours. Moderate Study
- **Voxilaprevir** is predicted to increase the exposure to **relugolix**. Avoid or take relugolix first and separate administration by at least 6 hours. Moderate Study

Remdesivir
- Antimalarials **(chloroquine)** might decrease the effects of **remdesivir**. Avoid. Moderate Theoretical
- **Hydroxychloroquine** might decrease the effects of **remdesivir**. Avoid. Moderate Theoretical

Remifentanil → see opioids

Interactions | Appendix 1 A1

Remimazolam → see benzodiazepines
Repaglinide → see meglitinides
Retigabine → see antiepileptics
Retinoids → see **TABLE 1** p. 1053 (hepatotoxicity), **TABLE 12** p. 1057 (myelosuppression)

acitretin · adapalene · alitretinoin · bexarotene · isotretinoin · tretinoin

- Avoid concomitant use of keratolytics in patients taking **acitretin** or **isotretinoin**.
- Since systemic absorption can follow topical application of **isotretinoin** or **tretinoin**, the possibility of interactions should be borne in mind.

- **Alcohol** potentially increases the concentration of **acitretin**. Avoid and for 2 months after stopping **acitretin**. [Moderate] Study
- Antiarrhythmics **(amiodarone)** are predicted to increase the exposure to **alitretinoin**. Adjust **alitretinoin** dose. [Moderate] Theoretical
- Antifungals, azoles **(fluconazole, itraconazole, ketoconazole, miconazole, posaconazole, voriconazole)** are predicted to increase the exposure to **alitretinoin**. Adjust **alitretinoin** dose. [Moderate] Theoretical
- Antifungals, azoles **(fluconazole, ketoconazole, voriconazole)** are predicted to increase the risk of tretinoin toxicity when given with **tretinoin**. [Moderate] Study
- Antifungals, azoles **(posaconazole)** are predicted to increase the risk of tretinoin toxicity when given with **tretinoin**. Monitor and adjust dose. [Severe] Theoretical
- **Ceritinib** is predicted to increase the exposure to **alitretinoin**. Adjust **alitretinoin** dose. [Moderate] Theoretical
- **Clopidogrel** is predicted to increase the exposure to **alitretinoin**. Adjust **alitretinoin** dose. [Moderate] Theoretical
- **Cobicistat** is predicted to increase the exposure to **alitretinoin**. Adjust **alitretinoin** dose. [Moderate] Theoretical
- Fibrates **(gemfibrozil)** are predicted to increase the exposure to **alitretinoin**. Adjust **alitretinoin** dose. [Moderate] Theoretical
- Fibrates **(gemfibrozil)** increase the concentration of **bexarotene**. Avoid. [Severe] Study
- **HIV-protease inhibitors** are predicted to increase the exposure to **alitretinoin**. Adjust **alitretinoin** dose. [Moderate] Theoretical
- **Idelalisib** is predicted to increase the exposure to **alitretinoin**. Adjust **alitretinoin** dose. [Moderate] Theoretical
- Macrolides **(clarithromycin)** are predicted to increase the exposure to **alitretinoin**. Adjust **alitretinoin** dose. [Moderate] Theoretical
- **Acitretin** is predicted to increase the concentration of **methotrexate**. Avoid. [Moderate] Anecdotal → Also see **TABLE 1** p. 1053
- Retinoids **(acitretin, alitretinoin, isotretinoin, tretinoin)** increase the risk of benign intracranial hypertension when given with **tetracyclines**. Avoid. [Severe] Anecdotal → Also see **TABLE 1** p. 1053
- Retinoids **(acitretin, alitretinoin, isotretinoin, tretinoin)** increase the risk of benign intracranial hypertension when given with **tigecycline**. Avoid. [Severe] Anecdotal → Also see **TABLE 1** p. 1053
- **Tucatinib** is predicted to increase the exposure to **alitretinoin**. Adjust **alitretinoin** dose. [Moderate] Theoretical
- **Bexarotene** is predicted to increase the risk of toxicity when given with **vitamin A**. Adjust dose. [Moderate] Theoretical → Also see **TABLE 1** p. 1053
- Retinoids **(acitretin, alitretinoin, isotretinoin)** are predicted to increase the risk of vitamin A toxicity when given with **vitamin A**. Avoid. [Severe] Theoretical → Also see **TABLE 1** p. 1053
- **Tretinoin** is predicted to increase the risk of vitamin A toxicity when given with **vitamin A**. Avoid. [Severe] Study

Ribavirin
- **Ribavirin** increases the risk of anaemia and/or leucopenia when given with NRTIs **(zidovudine)**. Avoid. [Severe] Study

Ribociclib → see **TABLE 12** p. 1057 (myelosuppression), **TABLE 7** p. 1055 (QT-interval prolongation)

FOOD AND LIFESTYLE Avoid concomitant use of pomegranate or pomegranate juice as it is predicted to increase ribociclib exposure.

- **Ribociclib** (high-dose) is predicted to increase the exposure to alpha blockers **(alfuzosin)**. Avoid. [Moderate] Theoretical
- Anti-androgens **(apalutamide, enzalutamide)** are predicted to markedly decrease the exposure to **ribociclib**. Avoid. [Severe] Study → Also see **TABLE 7** p. 1055
- Antiarrhythmics **(dronedarone)** are predicted to increase the exposure to **ribociclib**. [Moderate] Study → Also see **TABLE 7** p. 1055
- **Ribociclib** (high-dose) is predicted to increase the exposure to antiarrhythmics **(amiodarone)**. Avoid. [Moderate] Theoretical → Also see **TABLE 7** p. 1055
- Antiepileptics **(carbamazepine, fosphenytoin, phenobarbital, phenytoin, primidone)** are predicted to markedly decrease the exposure to **ribociclib**. Avoid. [Severe] Study
- Antifungals, azoles **(fluconazole, isavuconazole)** are predicted to increase the exposure to **ribociclib**. [Moderate] Study → Also see **TABLE 7** p. 1055
- Antifungals, azoles **(itraconazole, ketoconazole, posaconazole, voriconazole)** are predicted to increase the exposure to **ribociclib**. Avoid or adjust dose—consult product literature. [Moderate] Study → Also see **TABLE 7** p. 1055
- **Ribociclib** (high-dose) is predicted to increase the exposure to atypical antipsychotics **(quetiapine)**. Avoid. [Moderate] Theoretical
- **Ribociclib** moderately increases the exposure to benzodiazepines **(midazolam)**. Avoid. [Moderate] Study
- **Berotralstat** is predicted to increase the exposure to **ribociclib**. [Moderate] Study
- Calcium-channel blockers **(diltiazem, verapamil)** are predicted to increase the exposure to **ribociclib**. [Moderate] Study
- **Ribociclib** is predicted to increase the exposure to **capivasertib**. Adjust dose. [Moderate] Theoretical
- **Ceritinib** is predicted to increase the exposure to **ribociclib**. Avoid or adjust dose—consult product literature. [Moderate] Study → Also see **TABLE 12** p. 1057 → Also see **TABLE 7** p. 1055
- **Ribociclib** is predicted to increase the exposure to **ciclosporin**. Use with caution and adjust dose. [Moderate] Theoretical
- **Cobicistat** is predicted to increase the exposure to **ribociclib**. Avoid or adjust dose—consult product literature. [Moderate] Study
- **Crizotinib** is predicted to increase the exposure to **ribociclib**. [Moderate] Study → Also see **TABLE 7** p. 1055
- **Ribociclib** is predicted to increase the exposure to **digoxin**. [Moderate] Theoretical
- **Encorafenib** is predicted to markedly decrease the exposure to **ribociclib**. Avoid. [Severe] Study → Also see **TABLE 7** p. 1055
- Endothelin receptor antagonists **(bosentan)** are predicted to decrease the exposure to **ribociclib**. [Moderate] Study
- **Ribociclib** is predicted to increase the exposure to **everolimus**. Use with caution and adjust dose. [Moderate] Theoretical
- **Fedratinib** is predicted to increase the exposure to **ribociclib**. [Moderate] Study
- **Grapefruit** juice is predicted to increase the exposure to **ribociclib**. Avoid. [Moderate] Theoretical
- **HIV-protease inhibitors** are predicted to increase the exposure to **ribociclib**. Avoid or adjust dose—consult product literature. [Moderate] Study
- **Idelalisib** is predicted to increase the exposure to **ribociclib**. Avoid or adjust dose—consult product literature. [Moderate] Study
- **Imatinib** is predicted to increase the exposure to **ribociclib**. [Moderate] Study → Also see **TABLE 12** p. 1057
- **Ivosidenib** is predicted to markedly decrease the exposure to **ribociclib**. Avoid. [Severe] Study → Also see **TABLE 7** p. 1055
- **Letermovir** is predicted to increase the exposure to **ribociclib**. [Moderate] Study
- **Lumacaftor** is predicted to markedly decrease the exposure to **ribociclib**. Avoid. [Severe] Study
- Macrolides **(clarithromycin)** are predicted to increase the exposure to **ribociclib**. Avoid or adjust dose—consult product literature. [Moderate] Study
- Macrolides **(erythromycin)** are predicted to increase the exposure to **ribociclib**. [Moderate] Study → Also see **TABLE 7** p. 1055
- **Ribociclib** is predicted to increase the exposure to **metformin**. [Moderate] Theoretical
- **Mitotane** is predicted to markedly decrease the exposure to **ribociclib**. Avoid. [Severe] Study → Also see **TABLE 12** p. 1057
- Neurokinin-1 receptor antagonists **(aprepitant, netupitant)** are predicted to increase the exposure to **ribociclib**. [Moderate] Study

Ribociclib (continued)
- **Nilotinib** is predicted to increase the exposure to **ribociclib**. [Moderate] Study → Also see TABLE 12 p. 1057 → Also see TABLE 7 p. 1055
- NNRTIs **(efavirenz, etravirine, nevirapine)** are predicted to decrease the exposure to **ribociclib**. [Moderate] Study → Also see TABLE 7 p. 1055
- **Ribociclib** is predicted to increase the exposure to opioids **(alfentanil, fentanyl)**. Use with caution and adjust dose. [Moderate] Theoretical
- **Ribociclib** is predicted to increase the exposure to phosphodiesterase type-5 inhibitors **(sildenafil)**. Avoid. [Moderate] Theoretical
- **Ribociclib** (high-dose) is predicted to increase the exposure to **pimozide**. Avoid. [Moderate] Theoretical → Also see TABLE 7 p. 1055
- Rifamycins **(rifampicin)** are predicted to markedly decrease the exposure to **ribociclib**. Avoid. [Severe] Study
- **Ribociclib** is predicted to increase the exposure to **sirolimus**. Use with caution and adjust dose. [Moderate] Theoretical
- **St John's wort** is predicted to decrease the exposure to **ribociclib**. Avoid. [Severe] Study
- **Ribociclib** is predicted to increase the exposure to statins **(pravastatin, rosuvastatin)**. [Moderate] Theoretical
- **Ribociclib** (high-dose) is predicted to increase the exposure to statins **(simvastatin)**. Avoid. [Moderate] Theoretical
- **Ribociclib** is predicted to increase the exposure to **tacrolimus**. Use with caution and adjust dose. [Moderate] Theoretical
- **Tucatinib** is predicted to increase the exposure to **ribociclib**. Avoid or adjust dose—consult product literature. [Moderate] Study

Rifabutin → see rifamycins

Rifampicin → see rifamycins

Rifamycins → see TABLE 2 p. 1053 (nephrotoxicity)

rifabutin · rifampicin

GENERAL INFORMATION Although some manufacturers class rifabutin as a potent inducer of CYP3A4, clinical data suggests it is potentially a weak inducer, and therefore the BNF does not extrapolate the interactions of potent CYP3A4 inducers to rifabutin. For those who wish to err on the side of caution, see the interactions of rifampicin but bear in mind other mechanisms might be involved.

- **Rifampicin** is predicted to decrease the exposure to 5-HT3-receptor antagonists **(ondansetron)**. [Moderate] Study
- **Rifampicin** is predicted to markedly decrease the exposure to **abemaciclib**. Avoid. [Severe] Study
- **Rifampicin** is predicted to decrease the exposure to **abrocitinib**. Avoid. [Moderate] Study
- **Rifampicin** is predicted to decrease the exposure to **acalabrutinib**. Avoid. [Severe] Study
- **Rifampicin** is predicted to decrease the exposure to **afatinib**. [Moderate] Study
- **Rifampicin** is predicted to decrease the exposure to **agomelatine**. [Moderate] Theoretical
- **Rifampicin** decreases the exposure to **aliskiren**. [Moderate] Study
- **Rifampicin** is predicted to decrease the exposure to **alpelisib**. Avoid. [Moderate] Study
- **Rifampicin** decreases the exposure to **aminophylline**. Adjust dose. [Moderate] Study
- **Rifampicin** is predicted to decrease the exposure to anaesthetics, local **(ropivacaine)**. [Moderate] Theoretical
- Oral **antacids** decrease the absorption of oral **rifampicin**. Manufacturer advises take 1 hour before antacids. [Moderate] Study
- **Rifampicin** is predicted to decrease the exposure to anti-androgens **(abiraterone)**. Avoid. [Severe] Study
- **Rifamycins** are predicted to decrease the efficacy of anti-androgens **(cyproterone)** with ethinylestradiol (co-cyprindiol). Use alternative methods during treatment with, and for 28 days after, the enzyme inducing drug is stopped. [Severe] Study
- **Rifampicin** is predicted to decrease the exposure to anti-androgens **(darolutamide)**. Avoid. [Moderate] Study
- **Rifampicin** is predicted to decrease the exposure to antiarrhythmics **(disopyramide, dronedarone)**. Avoid. [Severe] Study
- **Rifampicin** is predicted to decrease the efficacy of antiarrhythmics **(propafenone)**. [Moderate] Study
- **Rifampicin** is predicted to decrease the exposure to anticholinesterases, centrally acting **(donepezil)**. [Mild] Study
- Antiepileptics **(phenobarbital, primidone)** are predicted to decrease the exposure to **rifampicin** and **rifampicin** is predicted to decrease the exposure to antiepileptics **(phenobarbital, primidone)**. Use with caution and adjust dose. [Moderate] Study
- **Rifampicin** slightly decreases the exposure to antiepileptics **(brivaracetam)**. Adjust dose. [Moderate] Study
- **Rifampicin** decreases the concentration of antiepileptics **(fosphenytoin, phenytoin)**. Use with caution and adjust dose. [Moderate] Study
- **Rifampicin** markedly increases the clearance of antiepileptics **(lamotrigine)**. Adjust **lamotrigine** dose, p. 243. [Moderate] Study
- **Rifampicin** is predicted to decrease the exposure to antiepileptics **(perampanel)**. Monitor and adjust dose. [Moderate] Study
- **Rifampicin** is predicted to decrease the concentration of antiepileptics **(zonisamide)**. Monitor and adjust dose. [Moderate] Theoretical
- Antifungals, azoles **(fluconazole)** increase the risk of uveitis when given with **rifabutin**. Adjust dose. [Severe] Study
- Antifungals, azoles **(itraconazole, posaconazole)** increase the concentration of **rifabutin** and **rifabutin** decreases the concentration of antifungals, azoles **(itraconazole, posaconazole)**. Avoid. [Severe] Study
- Antifungals, azoles **(ketoconazole)** are predicted to increase the concentration of **rifabutin** and **rifabutin** is predicted to decrease the concentration of antifungals, azoles **(ketoconazole)**. Avoid. [Severe] Theoretical
- Antifungals, azoles **(miconazole)** are predicted to increase the concentration of **rifabutin**. Use with caution and adjust dose. [Moderate] Theoretical
- **Rifampicin** slightly decreases the exposure to antifungals, azoles **(fluconazole)**. Adjust dose. [Moderate] Study
- **Rifabutin** is predicted to decrease the exposure to antifungals, azoles **(isavuconazole)**. Avoid. [Severe] Theoretical
- **Rifampicin** is predicted to decrease the exposure to antifungals, azoles **(isavuconazole)**. Avoid. [Severe] Study
- **Rifampicin** markedly decreases the exposure to antifungals, azoles **(itraconazole)**. Avoid and for 14 days after stopping **rifampicin**. [Moderate] Study
- **Rifampicin** markedly decreases the exposure to antifungals, azoles **(ketoconazole)** and antifungals, azoles **(ketoconazole)** potentially decrease the exposure to **rifampicin**. Avoid. [Moderate] Study
- **Rifampicin** is predicted to decrease the exposure to antifungals, azoles **(posaconazole)**. Avoid. [Moderate] Anecdotal
- **Rifabutin** decreases the concentration of antifungals, azoles **(voriconazole)** and antifungals, azoles **(voriconazole)** increase the concentration of **rifabutin**. Avoid or adjust **voriconazole** dose, p. 468. [Severe] Study
- **Rifampicin** very markedly decreases the exposure to antifungals, azoles **(voriconazole)**. Avoid. [Moderate] Study
- **Rifampicin** is predicted to decrease the exposure to antihistamines, non-sedating **(bilastine)**. [Moderate] Theoretical
- **Rifampicin** increases the clearance of antihistamines, non-sedating **(fexofenadine)**. [Moderate] Study
- **Rifampicin** is predicted to decrease the exposure to antimalarials **(artemether)** with lumefantrine. Avoid. [Severe] Study
- **Rifampicin** might decrease the exposure to the active metabolite of antimalarials **(artesunate)**. Avoid. [Severe] Study
- **Rifabutin** slightly decreases the exposure to antimalarials **(atovaquone)**. Avoid. [Moderate] Study
- **Rifampicin** moderately decreases the exposure to antimalarials **(atovaquone)** and antimalarials **(atovaquone)** slightly increase the exposure to **rifampicin**. Avoid. [Moderate] Study
- **Rifampicin** moderately decreases the exposure to antimalarials **(mefloquine)**. [Severe] Study

- **Rifampicin** is predicted to decrease the concentration of antimalarials **(piperaquine)**. Avoid. Moderate Theoretical
- **Rifampicin** decreases the exposure to antimalarials **(quinine)**. Severe Study
- **Rifampicin** decreases the exposure to **ataluren**. Moderate Study
- **Rifampicin** (single-dose) increases the exposure to **atogepant**. Adjust **atogepant** dose. Moderate Study
- **Rifampicin** is predicted to moderately decrease the exposure to atypical antipsychotics **(aripiprazole)**. Avoid or adjust dose—consult product literature. Moderate Study
- **Rifampicin** is predicted to decrease the exposure to atypical antipsychotics **(cariprazine)**. Avoid. Severe Theoretical
- **Rifampicin** decreases the exposure to atypical antipsychotics **(clozapine)**. Severe Anecdotal
- **Rifampicin** is predicted to decrease the exposure to atypical antipsychotics **(lurasidone)**. Avoid. Moderate Study
- **Rifampicin** is predicted to decrease the exposure to atypical antipsychotics **(olanzapine)**. Monitor and adjust dose. Moderate Study
- **Rifampicin** is predicted to decrease the exposure to atypical antipsychotics **(paliperidone)**. Monitor and adjust dose. Severe Study
- **Rifampicin** is predicted to decrease the exposure to atypical antipsychotics **(quetiapine)**. Moderate Study
- **Rifampicin** is predicted to decrease the exposure to atypical antipsychotics **(risperidone)**. Adjust dose. Moderate Study
- **Rifampicin** is predicted to decrease the exposure to **avacopan**. Avoid or monitor. Severe Study
- **Rifampicin** is predicted to decrease the exposure to **avapritinib**. Avoid. Severe Study
- **Rifampicin** is predicted to decrease the exposure to **avatrombopag**. Adjust **avatrombopag** dose with moderate CYP2C9 inducers in chronic immune thrombocytopenia. Moderate Study
- **Rifampicin** is predicted to decrease the exposure to **axitinib**. Avoid or adjust dose. Moderate Study
- **Rifampicin** is predicted to decrease the exposure to **bazedoxifene**. Moderate Theoretical
- **Rifampicin** decreases the exposure to **bedaquiline**. Avoid. Severe Study
- **Rifampicin** is predicted to decrease the exposure to **belumosudil**. Adjust **belumosudil** dose, p. 650. Severe Study
- **Rifampicin** is predicted to decrease the exposure to benzodiazepines **(alprazolam)**. Adjust dose. Moderate Theoretical
- **Rifampicin** is predicted to decrease the exposure to benzodiazepines **(chlordiazepoxide)**. Moderate Theoretical
- **Rifampicin** moderately decreases the exposure to benzodiazepines **(diazepam)**. Avoid. Moderate Study
- **Rifampicin** increases the clearance of benzodiazepines **(lorazepam, nitrazepam)**. Moderate Study
- **Rifampicin** is predicted to decrease the exposure to benzodiazepines **(midazolam)**. Monitor and adjust dose. Severe Study
- **Rifampicin** is predicted to decrease the concentration of **berotralstat**. Avoid. Severe Theoretical
- **Rifampicin** moderately decreases the exposure to beta blockers, non-selective **(carvedilol)**. Moderate Study
- **Rifampicin** decreases the exposure to beta blockers, non-selective **(propranolol)**. Monitor and adjust dose. Moderate Study
- **Rifampicin** slightly decreases the exposure to beta blockers, selective **(bisoprolol, metoprolol)**. Mild Study
- **Rifampicin** moderately decreases the exposure to beta blockers, selective **(celiprolol)**. Moderate Study
- **Rifabutin** slightly decreases the exposure to **bictegravir**. Avoid. Mild Study
- **Rifampicin** is predicted to decrease the exposure to **bictegravir**. Avoid. Moderate Study
- **Rifampicin** slightly decreases the exposure to **bortezomib**. Avoid. Severe Study
- **Rifampicin** is predicted to very markedly decrease the exposure to **bosutinib**. Avoid. Severe Study
- **Rifampicin** is predicted to decrease the exposure to **brigatinib**. Avoid. Severe Study
- **Rifampicin** is predicted to decrease the exposure to **bupropion**. Moderate Study
- **Rifampicin** is predicted to decrease the exposure to **buspirone**. Use with caution and adjust dose. Severe Study
- **Rifabutin** has been reported to cause a small decrease in the exposure to **cabotegravir**. Avoid intramuscular **cabotegravir** or adjust frequency—consult product literature, p. 506. Moderate Study
- **Rifampicin** modestly decreases the exposure to **cabotegravir**. Avoid. Severe Study
- **Rifampicin** moderately decreases the exposure to **cabozantinib**. Avoid. Moderate Study
- **Rifampicin** is predicted to moderately increase the clearance of **caffeine citrate**. Monitor and adjust dose. Moderate Study
- **Rifampicin** is predicted to decrease the exposure to calcium-channel blockers **(amlodipine, felodipine, lacidipine, lercanidipine, nicardipine, nimodipine)**. Monitor and adjust dose. Moderate Study
- **Rifampicin** greatly decreases the exposure to calcium-channel blockers **(diltiazem, verapamil)**. Severe Study
- **Rifampicin** greatly decreases the exposure to calcium-channel blockers **(nifedipine)**. Avoid. Severe Study
- **Rifampicin** is predicted to decrease the exposure to **cannabidiol**. Adjust dose. Moderate Study
- **Rifabutin** is predicted to decrease the exposure to **capivasertib**. Avoid. Moderate Theoretical
- **Rifampicin** is predicted to decrease the exposure to **capivasertib**. Avoid. Moderate Study
- **Rifampicin** decreases the concentration of **caspofungin**. Adjust **caspofungin** dose, p. 460. Moderate Study
- **Rifampicin** is predicted to decrease the exposure to **ceritinib**. Avoid. Severe Study
- **Rifampicin** decreases the concentration of **chloramphenicol**. Moderate Study
- **Rifampicin** decreases the concentration of **ciclosporin**. Severe Study → Also see TABLE 2 p. 1053
- **Rifampicin** is predicted to alter the effects of **cilostazol**. Moderate Theoretical
- **Rifampicin** is predicted to decrease the exposure to **cinacalcet**. Monitor and adjust dose. Moderate Study
- **Rifampicin** decreases the exposure to **clomethiazole**. Monitor and adjust dose. Moderate Study
- **Rifampicin** moderately increases the exposure to the active metabolite of **clopidogrel**. Avoid. Moderate Study
- **Rifabutin** decreases the concentration of **cobicistat** and **cobicistat** increases the exposure to **rifabutin**. Avoid or adjust dose. Severe Study
- **Rifampicin** is predicted to decrease the exposure to **cobicistat**. Avoid. Severe Study
- **Rifampicin** is predicted to decrease the exposure to **cobimetinib**. Avoid. Severe Theoretical
- **Rifampicin** is predicted to decrease the exposure to **colchicine**. Moderate Theoretical
- **Rifamycins** are predicted to decrease the efficacy of **combined hormonal contraceptives**. For CoSRH guidance, see Contraceptives, interactions p. 614. Severe Study
- **Rifampicin** is predicted to decrease the exposure to corticosteroids **(budesonide, deflazacort, dexamethasone, fludrocortisone, hydrocortisone, methylprednisolone, prednisolone, triamcinolone)**. Monitor and adjust dose. Moderate Study
- **Rifampicin** is predicted to decrease the exposure to corticosteroids **(fluticasone)**. Unknown Theoretical
- **Rifabutin** might decrease the anticoagulant effect of **coumarins**. Moderate Theoretical
- **Rifampicin** decreases the anticoagulant effect of **coumarins**. Severe Study
- **Rifampicin** is predicted to markedly decrease the exposure to **crizotinib**. Avoid. Severe Study
- **Rifampicin** is predicted to decrease the exposure to **dabrafenib**. Avoid. Moderate Theoretical
- **Rifamycins** decrease the exposure to **dapsone**. Moderate Study
- **Rifampicin** is predicted to decrease the exposure to **daridorexant**. Severe Study
- **Rifampicin** is predicted to decrease the exposure to **darifenacin**. Moderate Theoretical

Rifamycins (continued)
- **Rifampicin** is predicted to markedly decrease the exposure to **dasatinib**. Avoid. Severe Study
- **Rifampicin** is predicted to slightly decrease the exposure to **delamanid**. Avoid. Moderate Study
- **Rifamycins** are predicted to decrease the efficacy of **desogestrel**. For CoSRH guidance, see Contraceptives, interactions p. 614. Severe Theoretical
- **Rifampicin** is predicted to decrease the exposure to **deutivacaftor**. Avoid. Severe Theoretical
- **Rifampicin** is predicted to markedly decrease the exposure to **dienogest**. Severe Study
- **Rifampicin** decreases the concentration of **digoxin**. Moderate Study
- **Rifampicin** is predicted to decrease the exposure to dipeptidylpeptidase-4 inhibitors **(linagliptin)**. Moderate Study
- **Rifampicin** is predicted to moderately decrease the exposure to dipeptidylpeptidase-4 inhibitors **(saxagliptin)**. Moderate Study
- **Rifampicin** moderately decreases the exposure to **dolutegravir**. Adjust **dolutegravir** dose, p. 508. Severe Study
- **Rifampicin** is predicted to decrease the exposure to **dronabinol**. Avoid or adjust dose. Mild Study
- **Rifamycins** are predicted to decrease the efficacy of **drospirenone**. For CoSRH guidance, see Contraceptives, interactions p. 614. Severe Theoretical
- **Rifampicin** is predicted to decrease the exposure to **elacestrant**. Avoid or adjust dose depending on duration—consult product literature. Severe Study
- **Rifampicin** is predicted to decrease the exposure to **elbasvir**. Avoid. Severe Study
- **Rifabutin** is predicted to decrease the exposure to **elexacaftor**. Avoid. Severe Theoretical
- **Rifampicin** is predicted to decreases the exposure to **elexacaftor**. Avoid. Severe Theoretical
- **Rifampicin** is predicted to decrease the exposure to **eliglustat**. Avoid. Severe Study
- **Rifampicin** is predicted to decrease the exposure to **eltrombopag** and **eltrombopag** is predicted to increase the concentration of **rifampicin**. Moderate Theoretical
- **Rifampicin** is predicted to decrease the concentration of **elvitegravir**. Avoid. Severe Study
- **Rifampicin** is predicted to decrease the exposure to **encorafenib**. Severe Theoretical
- **Rifampicin** transiently increases the exposure to endothelin receptor antagonists **(ambrisentan)**. Moderate Study
- **Rifampicin** affects the exposure to endothelin receptor antagonists **(bosentan)**. Avoid. Severe Study
- **Rifampicin** is predicted to decrease the exposure to endothelin receptor antagonists **(macitentan)**. Avoid. Severe Study
- **Rifampicin** is predicted to decrease the exposure to the cytotoxic component of **enfortumab vedotin**. Moderate Theoretical
- **Rifampicin** is predicted to decrease the exposure to **entrectinib**. Avoid. Severe Study
- **Rifabutin** is predicted to decrease the exposure to **erdafitinib**. Adjust dose. Moderate Theoretical
- **Rifampicin** is predicted to decrease the exposure to **erdafitinib**. Avoid. Severe Study
- **Rifampicin** is predicted to decrease the exposure to **erlotinib**. Avoid or adjust dose—consult product literature. Severe Study
- **Rifampicin** is predicted to decrease the exposure to **esketamine**. Adjust dose. Moderate Study
- **Rifamycins** are predicted to decrease the efficacy of **estradiol**. Moderate Theoretical
- **Rifampicin** is predicted to decrease the exposure to **eszopiclone**. Adjust dose. Moderate Theoretical
- **Rifamycins** are predicted to decrease the efficacy of **etonogestrel**. For CoSRH guidance, see Contraceptives, interactions p. 614. Severe Theoretical
- **Rifampicin** slightly decreases the exposure to **etrasimod**. Avoid. Severe Study
- **Rifampicin** is predicted to decrease the concentration of **everolimus**. Avoid or adjust dose. Severe Study
- **Rifampicin** moderately decreases the exposure to **exemestane**. Moderate Study
- **Rifampicin** is predicted to decrease the exposure to factor XA inhibitors **(apixaban)**. Use with caution or avoid. Severe Study
- **Rifampicin** is predicted to decrease the exposure to factor XA inhibitors **(edoxaban)**. Severe Study
- **Rifampicin** is predicted to decrease the exposure to factor XA inhibitors **(rivaroxaban)**. Avoid unless patient can be monitored for signs of thrombosis. Severe Study
- **Rifampicin** is predicted to decrease the exposure to **fedratinib**. Avoid. Moderate Study
- **Rifampicin** is predicted to decrease the concentration of **fenfluramine**. Moderate Theoretical
- **Rifampicin** is predicted to decrease the exposure to **fesoterodine**. Avoid. Moderate Study
- **Rifampicin** is predicted to decrease the exposure to **fostamatinib**. Avoid. Severe Study
- **Rifampicin** is predicted to decrease the exposure to the active metabolite of **fostemsavir**. Avoid. Severe Study
- **Rifampicin** is predicted to decrease the exposure to **fruquintinib**. Avoid. Moderate Study
- **Rifampicin** moderately decreases the exposure to **futibatinib**. Avoid or adjust dose. Moderate Study
- **Rifampicin** is predicted to decrease the exposure to **gefitinib**. Avoid. Severe Study
- **Rifampicin** moderately decreases the exposure to **gilteritinib**. Avoid. Severe Study
- **Rifampicin** is predicted to decrease the exposure to **glasdegib**. Avoid. Severe Study
- **Rifampicin** markedly affects the exposure to **glecaprevir**. Avoid. Severe Study
- **Rifampicin** is predicted to decrease the exposure to **grazoprevir**. Avoid. Severe Study
- **Rifampicin** is predicted to decrease the concentration of **guanfacine**. Adjust **guanfacine** dose, p. 281. Moderate Study
- **Rifampicin** decreases the concentration of **haloperidol**. Adjust dose. Moderate Study
- HIV-protease inhibitors **(atazanavir, darunavir, fosamprenavir, lopinavir)** boosted with ritonavir increase the exposure to **rifabutin**. Monitor and adjust dose. Severe Study
- HIV-protease inhibitors **(ritonavir)** markedly increase the exposure to **rifabutin**. Avoid or adjust dose. Severe Study
- **Rifampicin** is predicted to moderately to markedly decrease the exposure to HIV-protease inhibitors **(atazanavir, darunavir, fosamprenavir, lopinavir)**. Avoid. Severe Study
- **Rifampicin** slightly decreases the exposure to HIV-protease inhibitors **(ritonavir)**. Severe Study
- **Rifamycins** are predicted to decrease the effects of **hormone replacement therapy**. Moderate Anecdotal
- **Rifampicin** is predicted to decrease the exposure to **ibrutinib**. Avoid or monitor. Severe Study
- **Rifampicin** is predicted to decrease the exposure to **idelalisib**. Avoid. Severe Study
- **Rifampicin** is predicted to decrease the exposure to **imatinib**. Avoid. Moderate Study
- **Rifampicin** is predicted to decrease the exposure to **iptacopan**. Avoid or monitor. Moderate Theoretical
- **Rifampicin** is predicted to decrease the exposure to **irinotecan**. Avoid. Severe Study
- **Rifampicin** is predicted to decrease the exposure to iron chelators **(deferasirox)**. Monitor serum ferritin and adjust dose. Moderate Study → Also see TABLE 2 p. 1053
- **Rifampicin** is predicted to decrease the exposure to **ivabradine**. Adjust dose. Moderate Theoretical
- **Rifampicin** is predicted to decrease the exposure to **ivacaftor**. Avoid. Severe Study
- **Rifampicin** is predicted to decrease the exposure to **ivosidenib**. Avoid. Severe Theoretical
- **Rifampicin** is predicted to decrease the exposure to **ixazomib**. Avoid. Severe Study
- **Rifampicin** is predicted to decrease the exposure to **ketamine**. Adjust dose. Moderate Theoretical
- **Rifampicin** is predicted to decrease the exposure to **lapatinib**. Avoid. Severe Study
- **Rifampicin** is predicted to moderately decrease the exposure to **larotrectinib**. Avoid. Moderate Study

- **Rifampicin** is predicted to decrease the exposure to **lazertinib**. Avoid. Severe Study
- **Rifabutin** is predicted to decrease the exposure to **ledipasvir**. Avoid. Severe Theoretical
- **Rifampicin** is predicted to decrease the exposure to **ledipasvir**. Avoid. Severe Study
- **Rifampicin** might affect the exposure to **leflunomide**. Moderate Theoretical
- **Rifabutin** is predicted to decrease the exposure to **lenacapavir**. Avoid. Severe Theoretical
- **Rifampicin** is predicted to decrease the exposure to **lenacapavir**. Avoid. Severe Study
- **Rifampicin** is predicted to decrease the exposure to **leniolisib**. Avoid. Severe Theoretical
- **Rifabutin** is predicted to decrease the concentration of **letermovir**. Moderate Theoretical
- **Rifampicin** is predicted to affect the concentration of **letermovir**. Severe Theoretical
- **Rifamycins** are predicted to decrease the efficacy of some contraceptive methods containing **levonorgestrel**. For CoSRH guidance, see Contraceptives, interactions p. 614. Severe Theoretical
- **Rifampicin** slightly decreases the exposure to **linezolid**. Moderate Study
- **Rifampicin** is predicted to decrease the exposure to **lomitapide**. Monitor and adjust dose. Moderate Theoretical
- **Rifampicin** is predicted to decrease the exposure to **lorlatinib**. Avoid. Severe Study
- **Lumacaftor** is predicted to decrease the exposure to **rifabutin**. Adjust dose. Moderate Theoretical
- Macrolides **(erythromycin)** are predicted to increase the concentration of **rifabutin** and **rifabutin** is predicted to decrease the concentration of macrolides **(erythromycin)**. Monitor and adjust dose. Severe Theoretical
- **Rifabutin** has been reported to cause neutropenia when given with macrolides **(azithromycin)**. Severe Study
- **Rifabutin** decreases the concentration of macrolides **(clarithromycin)** and macrolides **(clarithromycin)** increase the concentration of **rifabutin**. Monitor and adjust dose. Severe Study
- **Rifampicin** greatly decreases the concentration of macrolides **(clarithromycin)**. Severe Study
- **Rifampicin** is predicted to decrease the exposure to **maraviroc**. Adjust dose. Severe Study
- **Rifabutin** is predicted to decrease the exposure to **maribavir**. Avoid. Severe Theoretical
- **Rifampicin** is predicted to decrease the exposure to **maribavir**. Avoid. Severe Study
- **Rifampicin** is predicted to decrease the exposure to **mavacamten**. Monitor and adjust dose—consult product literature. Severe Theoretical
- **Rifampicin** is predicted to decrease the exposure to meglitinides **(repaglinide)**. Monitor blood glucose and adjust dose. Moderate Study
- **Rifampicin** is predicted to decrease the exposure to **melatonin**. Moderate Theoretical
- **Rifampicin** is predicted to increase the clearance of **mexiletine**. Monitor and adjust dose. Moderate Study
- **Rifampicin** is predicted to decrease the exposure to **midostaurin**. Avoid. Severe Study
- **Rifampicin** is predicted to decrease the exposure to **mifepristone**. Adjust **mifepristone** dose. Severe Study
- **Rifampicin** is predicted to decrease the exposure to mineralocorticoid receptor antagonists **(eplerenone)**. Avoid. Moderate Theoretical
- **Rifampicin** is predicted to decrease the exposure to mineralocorticoid receptor antagonists **(finerenone)**. Avoid. Severe Study
- **Rifampicin** is predicted to decrease the exposure to **mirtazapine**. Adjust dose. Moderate Study
- **Rifampicin** is predicted to decrease the exposure to **modafinil**. Moderate Theoretical
- **Rifampicin** is predicted to increase the exposure to **momelotinib**. Moderate Study
- **Rifampicin** decreases the effects of monoclonal antibodies **(brentuximab vedotin)**. Severe Study
- **Rifampicin** is predicted to decrease the exposure to monoclonal antibodies **(polatuzumab vedotin)**. Moderate Theoretical
- **Rifampicin** is predicted to decrease the exposure to the cytotoxic component of monoclonal antibodies **(trastuzumab emtansine)**. Severe Theoretical
- **Rifampicin** is predicted to decrease the exposure to **montelukast**. Mild Study
- **Rifampicin** decreases the concentration of **mycophenolate**. Monitor and adjust dose. Severe Study
- **Rifampicin** is predicted to markedly decrease the exposure to **naldemedine**. Avoid. Severe Study
- **Rifampicin** is predicted to markedly decrease the exposure to **naloxegol**. Avoid. Moderate Study
- **Rifampicin** is predicted to decrease the exposure to **neratinib**. Avoid. Severe Study
- **Rifampicin** is predicted to markedly decrease the exposure to neurokinin-1 receptor antagonists **(aprepitant)**. Avoid. Moderate Study
- **Rifampicin** is predicted to decrease the exposure to neurokinin-1 receptor antagonists **(fosaprepitant)**. Avoid. Moderate Theoretical
- **Rifampicin** is predicted to decrease the exposure to neurokinin-1 receptor antagonists **(netupitant)**. Avoid. Severe Study
- **Rifampicin** is predicted to moderately decrease the exposure to **nilotinib**. Avoid. Severe Study
- **Rifampicin** is predicted to decrease the exposure to **nintedanib**. Moderate Study
- **Nirmatrelvir** boosted with ritonavir is predicted to increase the concentration of **rifabutin**. Adjust dose. Severe Theoretical
- **Rifampicin** is predicted to decrease the exposure to **nirmatrelvir** boosted with ritonavir. Avoid. Severe Study
- **Rifampicin** is predicted to decrease the exposure to **nitisinone**. Adjust dose. Moderate Theoretical
- NNRTIs **(efavirenz)** slightly decrease the exposure to **rifabutin**. Adjust dose. Severe Study
- **Rifabutin** moderately decreases the exposure to NNRTIs **(doravirine)**. Adjust doravirine or lamivudine with tenofovir disoproxil and doravirine dose. Moderate Study
- **Rifampicin** is predicted to decrease the exposure to NNRTIs **(doravirine)**. Avoid. Severe Study
- **Rifampicin** slightly decreases the exposure to NNRTIs **(efavirenz)**. Adjust dose. Severe Study
- **Rifabutin** decreases the exposure to NNRTIs **(etravirine)**. Moderate Study
- **Rifampicin** is predicted to decrease the exposure to NNRTIs **(etravirine)**. Avoid. Severe Theoretical
- **Rifampicin** decreases the concentration of NNRTIs **(nevirapine)**. Avoid. Severe Study
- **Rifabutin** modestly decreases the exposure to NNRTIs **(rilpivirine)**. Avoid or adjust dose—consult product literature. Severe Study
- **Rifampicin** markedly decreases the exposure to NNRTIs **(rilpivirine)**. Avoid. Severe Study
- **Rifamycins** are predicted to decrease the efficacy of some contraceptive methods containing **norethisterone**. For CoSRH guidance, see Contraceptives, interactions p. 614. Severe Anecdotal
- **Rifampicin** moderately decreases the exposure to NSAIDs **(celecoxib, diclofenac, etoricoxib)**. Moderate Study → Also see TABLE 2 p. 1053
- **Rifampicin** is predicted to decrease the exposure to **olaparib**. Avoid. Moderate Theoretical
- **Rifampicin** is predicted to decrease the exposure to **omaveloxolone**. Avoid. Severe Study
- **Rifampicin** is predicted to decrease the exposure to opioids **(alfentanil, fentanyl)**. Moderate Study
- **Rifampicin** is predicted to decrease the exposure to opioids **(buprenorphine)**. Monitor and adjust dose. Moderate Theoretical
- **Rifampicin** decreases the exposure to opioids **(codeine, morphine)**. Moderate Study
- **Rifampicin** decreases the exposure to opioids **(methadone)**. Monitor and adjust dose. Severe Study
- **Rifampicin** is predicted to decrease the exposure to opioids **(oxycodone)**. Monitor and adjust dose. Moderate Study

Rifamycins (continued)
- **Rifampicin** is predicted to decrease the exposure to **osilodrostat**. [Moderate] Theoretical
- **Rifampicin** is predicted to moderately decrease the exposure to **osimertinib**. Avoid. [Moderate] Study
- **Rifampicin** is predicted to moderately decrease the exposure to **ospemifene**. [Moderate] Study
- **Rifampicin** moderately decreases the exposure to the active metabolites of **ozanimod**. Avoid. [Moderate] Study
- **Rifampicin** is predicted to decrease the exposure to **palbociclib**. Avoid. [Severe] Study
- **Rifampicin** is predicted to decrease the exposure to **panobinostat**. Avoid. [Moderate] Theoretical
- **Rifampicin** decreases the exposure to **paracetamol**. [Moderate] Study
- **Rifampicin** is predicted to decrease the exposure to **pazopanib**. Avoid. [Severe] Theoretical
- **Rifampicin** is predicted to decrease the exposure to **pemigatinib**. Avoid. [Severe] Study
- **Rifampicin** moderately decreases the exposure to phosphodiesterase type-4 inhibitors **(apremilast)**. Avoid. [Severe] Study
- **Rifampicin** is predicted to decrease the exposure to phosphodiesterase type-4 inhibitors **(roflumilast)**. Avoid. [Moderate] Study
- **Rifampicin** is predicted to decrease the exposure to phosphodiesterase type-5 inhibitors **(avanafil, tadalafil)**. Avoid. [Severe] Study
- **Rifampicin** is predicted to decrease the exposure to phosphodiesterase type-5 inhibitors **(sildenafil, vardenafil)**. [Moderate] Theoretical
- **Rifampicin** is predicted to moderately to markedly decrease the exposure to **pibrentasvir**. Avoid. [Severe] Study
- **Rifampicin** moderately decreases the exposure to **pioglitazone**. Monitor and adjust dose. [Moderate] Study
- **Rifampicin** is predicted to decrease the exposure to **pirfenidone**. Avoid. [Moderate] Theoretical
- **Rifampicin** is predicted to decrease the exposure to **pirtobrutinib**. Avoid. [Moderate] Study
- **Rifampicin** is predicted to moderately decrease the exposure to **pitolisant**. [Moderate] Study
- **Rifampicin** is predicted to decrease the exposure to **ponatinib**. Avoid. [Moderate] Theoretical
- **Rifabutin** is predicted to decrease the exposure to **pralsetinib**. Avoid or adjust dose—consult product literature. [Moderate] Study
- **Rifampicin** is predicted to decrease the exposure to **pralsetinib**. Avoid or adjust dose with potent CYP3A4 inducers—consult product literature. [Moderate] Study
- **Rifampicin** is predicted to markedly decrease the exposure to **praziquantel**. Avoid. [Moderate] Study
- **Rifampicin** is predicted to decrease the exposure to **quizartinib**. Avoid. [Severe] Study
- **Rifampicin** slightly decreases the exposure to **raltegravir**. Avoid or adjust dose—consult product literature. [Moderate] Study
- **Rifampicin** is predicted to decrease the exposure to **ranolazine**. Avoid. [Severe] Study
- **Rifampicin** is predicted to decrease the exposure to **reboxetine**. [Moderate] Anecdotal
- **Rifampicin** is predicted to decrease the exposure to **regorafenib**. Avoid. [Moderate] Study
- **Rifamycins** are predicted to decrease the exposure to **relugolix**. Avoid or adjust dose depending on indication—consult product literature. [Moderate] Study
- **Rifampicin** is predicted to markedly decrease the exposure to **ribociclib**. Avoid. [Severe] Study
- **Rifampicin** is predicted to decrease the exposure to **rimegepant**. Avoid. [Moderate] Theoretical
- **Rifampicin** is predicted to decrease the exposure to **ripretinib**. Avoid or adjust dose—consult product literature. [Severe] Study
- **Rifampicin** might decrease the exposure to **roxadustat**. Monitor haemoglobin and adjust dose—consult product literature. [Moderate] Theoretical
- **Rifabutin** is predicted to decrease the exposure to **ruxolitinib**. Monitor and adjust dose. [Moderate] Theoretical
- **Rifampicin** is predicted to decrease the exposure to **ruxolitinib**. Monitor and adjust dose. [Moderate] Study
- **Rifampicin** is predicted to decrease the exposure to the active component of **sacituzumab govitecan**. [Severe] Theoretical
- **Rifampicin** moderately decreases the exposure to the active metabolite of **selexipag**. Adjust dose. [Moderate] Study
- **Rifampicin** is predicted to decrease the exposure to **selpercatinib**. Avoid. [Moderate] Study
- **Rifampicin** is predicted to decrease the exposure to **selumetinib**. Avoid. [Severe] Study
- **Rifampicin** is predicted to decrease the exposure to **siponimod**. Manufacturer advises caution depending on genotype—consult product literature. [Severe] Study
- **Rifampicin** is predicted to decrease the concentration of **sirolimus**. Avoid or monitor and adjust dose. [Severe] Study
- **Rifampicin** is predicted to decrease the exposure to SNRIs **(duloxetine)**. [Moderate] Theoretical
- **Rifampicin** moderately decreases the exposure to sodium glucose co-transporter 2 inhibitors **(canagliflozin)**. Adjust **canagliflozin** dose. [Moderate] Study
- **Rifampicin** might decrease the exposure to sodium glucose co-transporter 2 inhibitors **(empagliflozin)**. Avoid or monitor diabetic control. [Moderate] Theoretical
- **Rifampicin** is predicted to decrease the exposure to **sofosbuvir**. Avoid. [Severe] Study
- **Rifampicin** is predicted to decrease the exposure to **solifenacin**. [Moderate] Theoretical
- **Rifampicin** is predicted to decrease the exposure to **sorafenib**. [Moderate] Theoretical
- **Rifampicin** is predicted to decrease the exposure to **sotorasib**. Avoid. [Severe] Study
- **Rifampicin** is predicted to decrease the exposure to **sparsentan**. Avoid. [Severe] Theoretical
- **Rifampicin** is predicted to decrease the exposure to SSRIs **(citalopram, sertraline)**. [Moderate] Anecdotal
- **Rifampicin** markedly decreases the exposure to statins **(atorvastatin)**. Manufacturer advises take both drugs at the same time. [Moderate] Study
- **Rifampicin** moderately decreases the exposure to statins **(fluvastatin)**. Monitor and adjust dose. [Moderate] Study
- **Rifampicin** very markedly decreases the exposure to statins **(simvastatin)**. [Moderate] Study
- **Rifampicin** is predicted to decrease the exposure to **sulfonylureas**. [Moderate] Study
- **Rifampicin** is predicted to decrease the exposure to **sunitinib**. Avoid or adjust dose—consult product literature. [Moderate] Study
- **Rifampicin** decreases the concentration of **tacrolimus**. Avoid or monitor and adjust dose. [Severe] Study → Also see **TABLE 2** p. 1053
- **Rifampicin** markedly decreases the exposure to **tamoxifen**. [Unknown] Study
- **Rifabutin** is predicted to decrease the exposure to taxanes **(cabazitaxel)**. Avoid. [Moderate] Theoretical
- **Rifampicin** is predicted to decrease the exposure to taxanes **(cabazitaxel)**. Avoid. [Moderate] Study
- **Rifampicin** is predicted to decrease the exposure to taxanes **(docetaxel)**. [Severe] Theoretical
- **Rifampicin** is predicted to decrease the exposure to taxanes **(paclitaxel)**. Avoid. [Severe] Study
- **Rifampicin** is predicted to decrease the concentration of **temsirolimus**. Avoid. [Severe] Study
- **Rifamycins** are predicted to decrease the exposure to **tenofovir alafenamide**. Avoid. [Moderate] Theoretical
- **Rifampicin** decreases the exposure to **terbinafine**. Adjust dose. [Moderate] Study
- **Rifampicin** might affect the exposure to **teriflunomide**. [Moderate] Theoretical
- **Rifampicin** modestly decreases the exposure to tetracyclines **(doxycycline)**. Adjust dose. [Moderate] Study
- **Rifampicin** is predicted to decrease the exposure to tetracyclines **(eravacycline)**. Adjust **eravacycline** dose. [Moderate] Study

- **Rifamycins** are predicted to decrease the exposure to **tezacaftor**. Avoid. [Severe] Theoretical
- **Rifampicin** is predicted to decrease the exposure to **theophylline**. Adjust dose. [Moderate] Study
- **Rifampicin** is predicted to decrease the exposure to thrombin inhibitors **(dabigatran)**. Avoid. [Severe] Study
- **Rifampicin** is predicted to markedly decrease the exposure to **ticagrelor**. Avoid. [Severe] Study
- **Rifampicin** is predicted to decrease the exposure to the cytotoxic component of **tisotumab vedotin**. [Moderate] Theoretical
- **Rifampicin** is predicted to decrease the exposure to **tivozanib**. [Severe] Study
- **Rifampicin** moderately decreases the exposure to **tizanidine**. [Mild] Study
- **Rifampicin** is predicted to decrease the exposure to **tofacitinib**. Avoid. [Severe] Study
- **Rifampicin** is predicted to decrease the exposure to **tolvaptan**. Use with caution or avoid depending on indication. [Severe] Study
- **Rifampicin** is predicted to decrease the exposure to **toremifene**. Adjust dose. [Moderate] Study
- **Rifampicin** is predicted to decrease the exposure to **trabectedin**. Avoid. [Severe] Theoretical
- **Rifampicin** slightly decreases the exposure to **treprostinil**. Adjust dose. [Mild] Study
- **Rifampicin** decreases the exposure to **trimethoprim**. [Moderate] Study → Also see TABLE 2 p. 1053
- **Rifampicin** is predicted to decrease the exposure to **tucatinib**. Avoid. [Severe] Study
- **Rifamycins** decrease the efficacy of **ulipristal**. Avoid and for 4 weeks after stopping the enzyme inducing drug. For CoSRH guidance, see Contraceptives, interactions p. 614. [Severe] Anecdotal
- **Rifampicin** is predicted to decrease the exposure to **upadacitinib**. [Moderate] Study
- **Rifampicin** is predicted to increase the exposure to **vadadustat**. [Moderate] Theoretical
- **Rifampicin** is predicted to decrease the exposure to **vandetanib**. Avoid. [Moderate] Study
- **Rifampicin** is predicted to decrease the exposure to **vanzacaftor**. Avoid. [Severe] Theoretical
- **Rifabutin** is predicted to decrease the exposure to **velpatasvir**. Avoid. [Severe] Theoretical
- **Rifampicin** is predicted to moderately decrease the exposure to **velpatasvir**. Avoid. [Severe] Study
- **Rifampicin** is predicted to decrease the exposure to **vemurafenib**. Avoid. [Severe] Study
- **Rifampicin** is predicted to decrease the exposure to **venetoclax**. Avoid. [Severe] Study
- **Rifampicin** is predicted to decrease the exposure to vinca alkaloids **(vinblastine, vincristine, vindesine)**. [Severe] Theoretical
- **Rifampicin** is predicted to decrease the exposure to vinca alkaloids **(vinorelbine)**. Use with caution or avoid. [Severe] Theoretical
- **Rifampicin** is predicted to decrease the exposure to **vismodegib**. Avoid. [Moderate] Theoretical
- **Rifampicin** is predicted to decrease the exposure to **voclosporin**. Avoid. [Severe] Study → Also see TABLE 2 p. 1053
- **Rifampicin** potentially increases the risk of nephrotoxicity when given with volatile halogenated anaesthetics **(methoxyflurane)**. Avoid. [Severe] Theoretical
- **Rifampicin** is predicted to decrease the exposure to **vorasidenib**. Avoid. [Severe] Theoretical
- **Rifampicin** is predicted to decrease the exposure to **vortioxetine**. Monitor and adjust dose. [Moderate] Study
- **Rifabutin** is predicted to decrease the concentration of **voxilaprevir**. Avoid. [Severe] Theoretical
- **Rifampicin** is predicted to decrease the concentration of **voxilaprevir**. Avoid. [Severe] Study
- **Rifampicin** is predicted to decrease the exposure to **zanubrutinib**. Avoid. [Severe] Study
- **Rifampicin** moderately decreases the exposure to **zolpidem**. [Moderate] Study
- **Rifampicin** is predicted to decrease the exposure to **zopiclone**. Adjust dose. [Moderate] Study

Rifaximin

- **Ciclosporin** very markedly increases the exposure to **rifaximin**. [Severe] Study
- **Rifaximin** might decrease the anticoagulant effect of coumarins **(acenocoumarol)**. Monitor INR and adjust dose. [Severe] Theoretical
- **Rifaximin** has been reported to decrease the anticoagulant effect of coumarins **(warfarin)**. Monitor INR and adjust dose. [Severe] Anecdotal

Rilpivirine → see NNRTIs

Riluzole

FOOD AND LIFESTYLE Charcoal-grilled foods are predicted to decrease the exposure to riluzole.

- **Combined hormonal contraceptives** is predicted to increase the exposure to **riluzole**. [Moderate] Theoretical
- **Givosiran** is predicted to increase the exposure to **riluzole**. [Moderate] Theoretical
- **Mexiletine** is predicted to increase the exposure to **riluzole**. [Moderate] Theoretical
- **Osilodrostat** is predicted to increase the exposure to **riluzole**. [Moderate] Theoretical
- Quinolones **(ciprofloxacin)** are predicted to increase the exposure to **riluzole**. [Moderate] Theoretical
- **Rucaparib** is predicted to increase the exposure to **riluzole**. [Moderate] Theoretical
- SSRIs **(fluvoxamine)** are predicted to increase the exposure to **riluzole**. [Moderate] Theoretical
- **Vemurafenib** is predicted to increase the exposure to **riluzole**. [Moderate] Theoretical

Rimegepant

- Anti-androgens **(apalutamide, enzalutamide)** are predicted to decrease the exposure to **rimegepant**. Avoid. [Moderate] Theoretical
- Antiarrhythmics **(amiodarone)** are predicted to increase the exposure to **rimegepant**. Avoid another dose of rimegepant within 48 hours of concurrent use. [Moderate] Theoretical
- Antiarrhythmics **(dronedarone)** are predicted to increase the exposure to **rimegepant**. Avoid another dose of rimegepant within 48 hours of concurrent use. [Moderate] Study
- Antiepileptics **(carbamazepine, fosphenytoin, phenobarbital, phenytoin, primidone)** are predicted to decrease the exposure to **rimegepant**. Avoid. [Moderate] Theoretical
- Antifungals, azoles **(fluconazole, isavuconazole)** are predicted to increase the exposure to **rimegepant**. Avoid another dose of rimegepant within 48 hours of concurrent use. [Moderate] Study
- Antifungals, azoles **(itraconazole, ketoconazole, posaconazole, voriconazole)** are predicted to increase the exposure to **rimegepant**. Avoid. [Moderate] Study
- **Berotralstat** is predicted to increase the exposure to **rimegepant**. Avoid another dose of rimegepant within 48 hours of concurrent use. [Moderate] Study
- Calcium-channel blockers **(diltiazem, verapamil)** are predicted to increase the exposure to **rimegepant**. Avoid another dose of rimegepant within 48 hours of concurrent use. [Moderate] Study
- **Cenobamate** is predicted to decrease the exposure to **rimegepant**. Avoid. [Moderate] Theoretical
- **Ceritinib** is predicted to increase the exposure to **rimegepant**. Avoid. [Moderate] Study
- **Ciclosporin** slightly increases the exposure to **rimegepant**. Avoid another dose of rimegepant within 48 hours of concurrent use. [Moderate] Study
- **Cobicistat** is predicted to increase the exposure to **rimegepant**. Avoid. [Moderate] Study
- **Crizotinib** is predicted to increase the exposure to **rimegepant**. Avoid another dose of rimegepant within 48 hours of concurrent use. [Moderate] Study
- **Dabrafenib** is predicted to decrease the exposure to **rimegepant**. Avoid. [Moderate] Theoretical
- **Danicopan** is predicted to increase the exposure to **rimegepant**. [Moderate] Study
- **Eliglustat** is predicted to increase the exposure to **rimegepant**. Adjust dose. [Moderate] Study
- **Encorafenib** is predicted to decrease the exposure to **rimegepant**. Avoid. [Moderate] Theoretical

Rimegepant (continued)

- Endothelin receptor antagonists **(bosentan)** are predicted to decrease the exposure to **rimegepant**. Avoid. Moderate Theoretical
- **Fedratinib** is predicted to increase the exposure to **rimegepant**. Avoid another dose of rimegepant within 48 hours of concurrent use. Moderate Study
- **Glecaprevir** is predicted to increase the exposure to **rimegepant**. Avoid another dose of rimegepant within 48 hours of concurrent use. Moderate Theoretical
- **HIV-protease inhibitors** are predicted to increase the exposure to **rimegepant**. Avoid. Moderate Study
- **Idelalisib** is predicted to increase the exposure to **rimegepant**. Avoid. Moderate Study
- **Imatinib** is predicted to increase the exposure to **rimegepant**. Avoid another dose of rimegepant within 48 hours of concurrent use. Moderate Study
- **Ivosidenib** is predicted to decrease the exposure to **rimegepant**. Avoid. Moderate Theoretical
- **Lapatinib** is predicted to increase the exposure to **rimegepant**. Avoid another dose of rimegepant within 48 hours of concurrent use. Moderate Theoretical
- **Letermovir** is predicted to increase the exposure to **rimegepant**. Avoid another dose of rimegepant within 48 hours of concurrent use. Moderate Study
- **Lorlatinib** is predicted to decrease the exposure to **rimegepant**. Avoid. Moderate Theoretical
- **Lumacaftor** is predicted to decrease the exposure to **rimegepant**. Avoid. Moderate Theoretical
- Macrolides **(azithromycin)** are predicted to increase the exposure to **rimegepant**. Avoid another dose of rimegepant within 48 hours of concurrent use. Moderate Theoretical
- Macrolides **(clarithromycin)** are predicted to increase the exposure to **rimegepant**. Avoid. Moderate Study
- Macrolides **(erythromycin)** are predicted to increase the exposure to **rimegepant**. Avoid another dose of rimegepant within 48 hours of concurrent use. Moderate Study
- **Mitotane** is predicted to decrease the exposure to **rimegepant**. Avoid. Moderate Theoretical
- Neurokinin-1 receptor antagonists **(aprepitant, netupitant)** are predicted to increase the exposure to **rimegepant**. Avoid another dose of rimegepant within 48 hours of concurrent use. Moderate Study
- **Nilotinib** is predicted to increase the exposure to **rimegepant**. Avoid another dose of rimegepant within 48 hours of concurrent use. Moderate Study
- **Nirmatrelvir** boosted with ritonavir is predicted to increase the concentration of **rimegepant**. Avoid. Severe Theoretical
- NNRTIs **(efavirenz, etravirine, nevirapine)** are predicted to decrease the exposure to **rimegepant**. Avoid. Moderate Theoretical
- **Olaparib** might increase the exposure to **rimegepant**. Moderate Theoretical
- **Osimertinib** is predicted to increase the exposure to **rimegepant**. Moderate Study
- **Pibrentasvir** is predicted to increase the exposure to **rimegepant**. Avoid another dose of rimegepant within 48 hours of concurrent use. Moderate Theoretical
- **Ranolazine** is predicted to increase the exposure to **rimegepant**. Avoid another dose of rimegepant within 48 hours of concurrent use. Moderate Theoretical
- Rifamycins **(rifampicin)** are predicted to decrease the exposure to **rimegepant**. Avoid. Moderate Theoretical
- **Sotorasib** is predicted to decrease the exposure to **rimegepant**. Avoid. Moderate Theoretical
- **Sparsentan** is predicted to increase the exposure to **rimegepant**. Severe Theoretical
- **St John's wort** is predicted to decrease the exposure to **rimegepant**. Avoid. Moderate Theoretical
- **Tucatinib** is predicted to increase the exposure to **rimegepant**. Avoid. Moderate Study
- **Velpatasvir** is predicted to increase the exposure to **rimegepant**. Avoid another dose of rimegepant within 48 hours of concurrent use. Moderate Theoretical
- **Vemurafenib** is predicted to increase the exposure to **rimegepant**. Avoid another dose of rimegepant within 48 hours of concurrent use. Moderate Theoretical
- **Voxilaprevir** with sofosbuvir and velpatasvir is predicted to increase the exposure to **rimegepant**. Avoid another dose of rimegepant within 48 hours of concurrent use. Moderate Theoretical

Riociguat → see TABLE 6 p. 1054 (hypotension)

FOOD AND LIFESTYLE Dose adjustment might be necessary if smoking is started or stopped during treatment.

- Oral **antacids** decrease the exposure to oral **riociguat**. Manufacturer advises take 1 hour before or 2 hours after antacids. Mild Study
- Antifungals, azoles **(itraconazole, posaconazole)** are predicted to increase the exposure to **riociguat**. Adjust **riociguat** dose and monitor blood pressure. Moderate Theoretical
- Antifungals, azoles **(ketoconazole)** moderately increase the exposure to **riociguat**. Adjust **riociguat** dose and monitor blood pressure. Moderate Study
- **Ciclosporin** is predicted to increase the exposure to **riociguat**. Moderate Theoretical
- HIV-protease inhibitors **(ritonavir)** are predicted to increase the exposure to **riociguat**. Adjust dose and monitor blood pressure. Moderate Theoretical
- **Nirmatrelvir** boosted with ritonavir is predicted to increase the concentration of **riociguat**. Adjust dose. Moderate Theoretical
- NRTIs **(abacavir)** might increase the exposure to **riociguat**. Adjust dose and monitor blood pressure. Moderate Study

Ripretinib

- Anti-androgens **(apalutamide, enzalutamide)** are predicted to decrease the exposure to **ripretinib**. Avoid or adjust dose—consult product literature. Severe Study
- Antiepileptics **(carbamazepine, fosphenytoin, phenobarbital, phenytoin, primidone)** are predicted to decrease the exposure to **ripretinib**. Avoid or adjust dose—consult product literature. Severe Study
- Antifungals, azoles **(itraconazole, ketoconazole, posaconazole, voriconazole)** are predicted to increase the exposure to **ripretinib**. Moderate Theoretical
- **Cenobamate** is predicted to decrease the exposure to **ripretinib**. Avoid or adjust dose—consult product literature. Moderate Theoretical
- **Ceritinib** is predicted to increase the exposure to **ripretinib**. Moderate Theoretical
- **Cobicistat** is predicted to increase the exposure to **ripretinib**. Moderate Theoretical
- **Dabrafenib** is predicted to decrease the exposure to **ripretinib**. Avoid or adjust dose—consult product literature. Moderate Theoretical
- **Encorafenib** is predicted to decrease the exposure to **ripretinib**. Avoid or adjust dose—consult product literature. Severe Study
- Endothelin receptor antagonists **(bosentan)** are predicted to decrease the exposure to **ripretinib**. Avoid or adjust dose—consult product literature. Moderate Theoretical
- **Grapefruit** juice is predicted to increase the exposure to **ripretinib**. Avoid. Mild Theoretical
- **HIV-protease inhibitors** are predicted to increase the exposure to **ripretinib**. Moderate Theoretical
- **Idelalisib** is predicted to increase the exposure to **ripretinib**. Moderate Theoretical
- **Ivosidenib** is predicted to decrease the exposure to **ripretinib**. Avoid or adjust dose—consult product literature. Severe Study
- **Lorlatinib** is predicted to decrease the exposure to **ripretinib**. Avoid or adjust dose—consult product literature. Moderate Theoretical
- **Lumacaftor** is predicted to decrease the exposure to **ripretinib**. Avoid or adjust dose—consult product literature. Severe Study
- Macrolides **(clarithromycin, erythromycin)** are predicted to increase the exposure to **ripretinib**. Moderate Theoretical
- **Mitotane** is predicted to decrease the exposure to **ripretinib**. Avoid or adjust dose—consult product literature. Severe Study
- NNRTIs **(efavirenz, etravirine, nevirapine)** are predicted to decrease the exposure to **ripretinib**. Avoid or adjust dose—consult product literature. Moderate Theoretical

- Rifamycins (rifampicin) are predicted to decrease the exposure to ripretinib. Avoid or adjust dose—consult product literature. [Severe] Study
- Sotorasib is predicted to decrease the exposure to ripretinib. Avoid or adjust dose—consult product literature. [Moderate] Theoretical
- St John's wort is predicted to decrease the exposure to ripretinib. Avoid or adjust dose—consult product literature. [Moderate] Theoretical
- Tucatinib is predicted to increase the exposure to ripretinib. [Moderate] Theoretical

Risankizumab → see monoclonal antibodies

Risdiplam

- Risdiplam is predicted to increase the concentration of metformin. Monitor and adjust dose. [Moderate] Theoretical

Risedronate → see bisphosphonates

Risperidone → see atypical antipsychotics

Ritlecitinib

- Ritlecitinib moderately increases the exposure to benzodiazepines (midazolam). [Moderate] Study
- Ritlecitinib is predicted to increase the exposure to ciclosporin and ciclosporin is predicted to increase the risk of generalised infection (possibly life-threatening) when given with ritlecitinib. Avoid. [Severe] Theoretical
- Ritlecitinib is predicted to increase the exposure to colchicine. Adjust dose. [Moderate] Theoretical
- Ritlecitinib is predicted to increase the exposure to everolimus. Adjust dose. [Moderate] Theoretical
- Live vaccines are predicted to increase the risk of generalised infection (possibly life-threatening) when given with ritlecitinib. Avoid. [Severe] Theoretical
- Ritlecitinib is predicted to increase the exposure to opioids (alfentanil). [Moderate] Theoretical
- Ritlecitinib is predicted to increase the exposure to pimozide. [Moderate] Theoretical
- Ritlecitinib is predicted to increase the exposure to pirfenidone. Adjust dose. [Moderate] Theoretical
- Ritlecitinib is predicted to increase the exposure to sirolimus. Adjust dose. [Moderate] Theoretical
- Ritlecitinib is predicted to increase the exposure to tacrolimus. Adjust dose. [Moderate] Theoretical
- Ritlecitinib is predicted to increase the exposure to temsirolimus. [Moderate] Theoretical
- Ritlecitinib is predicted to increase the exposure to theophylline. Adjust dose. [Moderate] Theoretical
- Ritlecitinib is predicted to increase the exposure to tizanidine. [Moderate] Theoretical

Ritonavir → see HIV-protease inhibitors

Rituximab → see monoclonal antibodies

Rivaroxaban → see factor XA inhibitors

Rivastigmine → see anticholinesterases, centrally acting

Rizatriptan → see triptans

Rocuronium → see neuromuscular blocking drugs, non-depolarising

Roflumilast → see phosphodiesterase type-4 inhibitors

Romiplostim

- Monoclonal antibodies (rozanolixizumab) might decrease the concentration of romiplostim. Avoid and for 2 weeks after stopping rozanolixizumab. [Moderate] Theoretical

Ropeginterferon alfa → see interferons

Ropinirole → see dopamine receptor agonists

Ropivacaine → see anaesthetics, local

Rosuvastatin → see statins

Rotavirus vaccine → see live vaccines

Rotigotine → see dopamine receptor agonists

Roxadustat

- Roxadustat is predicted to increase the exposure to alpelisib. [Moderate] Theoretical
- Oral aluminium hydroxide might decrease the exposure to oral roxadustat. Manufacturer advises take at least 1 hour after aluminium-containing products. [Moderate] Theoretical
- Oral antacids might decrease the exposure to oral roxadustat. Manufacturer advises take at least 1 hour after antacids. [Moderate] Theoretical
- Roxadustat is predicted to increase the exposure to antihistamines, non-sedating (fexofenadine). Monitor adverse effects and adjust dose. [Moderate] Study
- Roxadustat is predicted to increase the exposure to atogepant. Adjust atogepant dose. [Moderate] Theoretical
- Oral calcium compounds decrease the exposure to oral roxadustat. Roxadustat should be taken at least 1 hour after calcium. [Moderate] Study
- Roxadustat is predicted to increase the exposure to cladribine. Avoid or adjust dose. [Moderate] Theoretical
- Clopidogrel is predicted to increase the exposure to roxadustat. Monitor haemoglobin and adjust dose—consult product literature. [Moderate] Study
- Roxadustat is predicted to increase the exposure to endothelin receptor antagonists (bosentan). Monitor adverse effects and adjust dose. [Moderate] Study
- Fibrates (gemfibrozil) are predicted to increase the exposure to roxadustat. Monitor haemoglobin and adjust dose—consult product literature. [Moderate] Study
- Roxadustat is predicted to increase the exposure to grazoprevir. Avoid. [Severe] Theoretical
- Oral iron might decrease the exposure to oral roxadustat. Roxadustat should be taken at least 1 hour after iron. [Mild] Theoretical
- Leflunomide is predicted to increase the exposure to roxadustat. Monitor haemoglobin and adjust dose—consult product literature. [Moderate] Study
- Oral magnesium might decrease the exposure to oral roxadustat. Manufacturer advises take at least 1 hour after magnesium. [Moderate] Theoretical
- Roxadustat is predicted to increase the exposure to meglitinides (repaglinide). Monitor adverse effects and adjust dose. [Moderate] Study
- Roxadustat is predicted to increase the exposure to momelotinib. [Moderate] Study
- Rifamycins (rifampicin) might decrease the exposure to roxadustat. Monitor haemoglobin and adjust dose—consult product literature. [Moderate] Theoretical
- Oral sevelamer decreases the exposure to oral roxadustat. Roxadustat should be taken at least 1 hour after sevelamer. [Moderate] Study
- Roxadustat is predicted to increase the exposure to statins (atorvastatin, pravastatin, rosuvastatin, simvastatin). Monitor adverse effects and adjust dose. [Moderate] Study
- Roxadustat might increase the exposure to statins (fluvastatin). Monitor adverse effects and adjust dose. [Moderate] Theoretical
- Roxadustat might increase the exposure to sulfasalazine. Monitor adverse effects and adjust dose. [Moderate] Theoretical
- Roxadustat is predicted to increase the exposure to sulfonylureas (glibenclamide). Monitor adverse effects and adjust dose. [Moderate] Study
- Roxadustat is predicted to increase the exposure to taxanes (docetaxel, paclitaxel). Monitor adverse effects and adjust dose. [Moderate] Study
- Roxadustat is predicted to increase the exposure to tenofovir alafenamide. [Moderate] Theoretical
- Roxadustat is predicted to increase the exposure to tenofovir disoproxil. [Moderate] Theoretical
- Teriflunomide is predicted to increase the exposure to roxadustat. Monitor haemoglobin and adjust dose—consult product literature. [Moderate] Study
- Roxadustat might increase the exposure to topotecan. Monitor adverse effects and adjust dose. [Moderate] Theoretical
- Vadadustat is predicted to increase the exposure to roxadustat. Monitor haemoglobin and adjust dose—consult product literature. [Moderate] Study

Rozanolixizumab → see monoclonal antibodies

Rucaparib → see TABLE 12 p. 1057 (myelosuppression)

- Rucaparib is predicted to increase the exposure to agomelatine. [Moderate] Study
- Rucaparib is predicted to increase the exposure to aminophylline. Adjust dose. [Moderate] Theoretical
- Rucaparib is predicted to increase the exposure to anaesthetics, local (ropivacaine). [Moderate] Theoretical

Rucaparib (continued)
- **Rucaparib** is predicted to increase the exposure to **anagrelide**. Moderate Theoretical
- **Rucaparib** is predicted to increase the exposure to antiepileptics **(phenytoin)**. Monitor and adjust dose. Moderate Study
- **Rucaparib** increases the concentration of atypical antipsychotics **(clozapine)**. Monitor adverse effects and adjust dose. Severe Study
- **Rucaparib** is predicted to increase the exposure to atypical antipsychotics **(olanzapine)**. Adjust dose. Moderate Anecdotal
- **Rucaparib** slightly increases the exposure to benzodiazepines **(midazolam)**. Monitor and adjust dose. Severe Study
- **Rucaparib** is predicted to increase the exposure to **ciclosporin**. Monitor and adjust dose. Moderate Study
- **Rucaparib** slightly increases the exposure to coumarins **(warfarin)**. Monitor and adjust dose. Severe Study
- **Rucaparib** is predicted to increase the exposure to dopamine receptor agonists **(ropinirole)**. Adjust dose. Moderate Study
- **Rucaparib** are predicted to increases the exposure to **erlotinib**. Monitor adverse effects and adjust dose. Moderate Study
- **Rucaparib** is predicted to increase the exposure to **fezolinetant**. Avoid. Moderate Study
- **Rucaparib** is predicted to increase the exposure to **gilteritinib**. Moderate Theoretical
- **Rucaparib** is predicted to increase the exposure to **idelalisib**. Moderate Theoretical
- **Rucaparib** is predicted to increase the exposure to **loxapine**. Avoid. Unknown Theoretical
- **Rucaparib** slightly increases the exposure to MAO-B inhibitors **(rasagiline)**. Moderate Study
- **Rucaparib** is predicted to increase the exposure to **mavacamten**. Monitor and adjust dose—consult product literature. Moderate Theoretical
- **Rucaparib** is predicted to increase the exposure to **melatonin**. Moderate Theoretical
- **Rucaparib** is predicted to increase the exposure to opioids **(alfentanil, fentanyl)**. Monitor and adjust dose. Moderate Study
- **Rucaparib** is predicted to increase the exposure to phenothiazine antipsychotics **(chlorpromazine)**. Moderate Theoretical
- **Rucaparib** is predicted to increase the exposure to phosphodiesterase type-4 inhibitors **(roflumilast)**. Moderate Theoretical
- **Rucaparib** is predicted to increase the exposure to **pimozide**. Monitor and adjust dose. Moderate Study
- **Rucaparib** is predicted to increase the exposure to **pirfenidone**. Use with caution and adjust dose. Moderate Study
- **Rucaparib** is predicted to increase the exposure to **riluzole**. Moderate Theoretical
- **Rucaparib** is predicted to increase the exposure to **sirolimus**. Monitor and adjust dose. Moderate Study
- **Rucaparib** is predicted to increase the exposure to SNRIs **(duloxetine)**. Monitor and adjust dose. Moderate Study
- **Rucaparib** is predicted to increase the exposure to **tacrolimus**. Monitor and adjust dose. Moderate Study
- **Rucaparib** is predicted to increase the exposure to **theophylline**. Monitor and adjust dose. Moderate Theoretical
- **Rucaparib** increases the exposure to **tizanidine**. Avoid. Moderate Study
- **Rucaparib** is predicted to increase the exposure to triptans **(zolmitriptan)**. Adjust **zolmitriptan** dose, p. 347. Moderate Theoretical
- **Rucaparib** might increase the exposure to **vinca alkaloids**. Severe Theoretical → Also see TABLE 12 p. 1057
- **Rucaparib** is predicted to increase the exposure to **vorasidenib**. Avoid. Moderate Theoretical

Rufinamide → see antiepileptics
Rupatadine → see antihistamines, non-sedating
Ruxolitinib → see TABLE 12 p. 1057 (myelosuppression)
- Anti-androgens **(apalutamide, enzalutamide)** are predicted to decrease the exposure to **ruxolitinib**. Monitor and adjust dose. Moderate Study
- Antiarrhythmics **(dronedarone)** are predicted to increase the exposure to **ruxolitinib**. Moderate Study
- Antiepileptics **(carbamazepine, fosphenytoin, phenobarbital, phenytoin, primidone)** are predicted to decrease the exposure to **ruxolitinib**. Monitor and adjust dose. Moderate Study
- Antifungals, azoles **(fluconazole)** moderately increase the exposure to **ruxolitinib**. Avoid or adjust dose and monitor adverse effects—consult product literature. Moderate Study
- Antifungals, azoles **(isavuconazole)** are predicted to increase the exposure to **ruxolitinib**. Moderate Study
- Antifungals, azoles **(itraconazole, ketoconazole, posaconazole, voriconazole)** are predicted to increase the exposure to **ruxolitinib**. Adjust dose depending on indication and monitor adverse effects—consult product literature. Moderate Study
- **Berotralstat** is predicted to increase the exposure to **ruxolitinib**. Moderate Study
- Calcium-channel blockers **(diltiazem, verapamil)** are predicted to increase the exposure to **ruxolitinib**. Moderate Study
- **Cenobamate** is predicted to decrease the exposure to **ruxolitinib**. Monitor and adjust dose. Moderate Study
- **Ceritinib** is predicted to increase the exposure to **ruxolitinib**. Adjust dose depending on indication and monitor adverse effects—consult product literature. Moderate Study → Also see TABLE 12 p. 1057
- **Cobicistat** is predicted to increase the exposure to **ruxolitinib**. Adjust dose depending on indication and monitor adverse effects—consult product literature. Moderate Study
- **Crizotinib** is predicted to increase the exposure to **ruxolitinib**. Moderate Study
- **Dabrafenib** is predicted to decrease the exposure to **ruxolitinib**. Monitor and adjust dose. Moderate Study
- **Drugs that cause bleeding** (see TABLE 3 p. 1053) cause bleeding, as can **ruxolitinib**; concurrent use might increase the risk of developing this effect. Severe Theoretical
- **Encorafenib** is predicted to decrease the exposure to **ruxolitinib**. Monitor and adjust dose. Moderate Study
- Endothelin receptor antagonists **(bosentan)** are predicted to decrease the exposure to **ruxolitinib**. Monitor and adjust dose. Moderate Study
- **Fedratinib** is predicted to increase the exposure to **ruxolitinib**. Moderate Study
- **Grapefruit** juice is predicted to increase the exposure to **ruxolitinib**. Severe Theoretical
- H_2 receptor antagonists **(cimetidine)** are predicted to increase the exposure to **ruxolitinib**. Moderate Theoretical
- **HIV-protease inhibitors** are predicted to increase the exposure to **ruxolitinib**. Adjust dose depending on indication and monitor adverse effects—consult product literature. Moderate Study
- **Idelalisib** is predicted to increase the exposure to **ruxolitinib**. Adjust dose depending on indication and monitor adverse effects—consult product literature. Moderate Study
- **Imatinib** is predicted to increase the exposure to **ruxolitinib**. Moderate Study → Also see TABLE 12 p. 1057
- **Ivosidenib** is predicted to decrease the exposure to **ruxolitinib**. Monitor and adjust dose. Moderate Study
- **Letermovir** is predicted to increase the exposure to **ruxolitinib**. Moderate Study
- **Lorlatinib** is predicted to decrease the exposure to **ruxolitinib**. Monitor and adjust dose. Moderate Study
- **Lumacaftor** is predicted to decrease the exposure to **ruxolitinib**. Monitor and adjust dose. Moderate Study
- Macrolides **(clarithromycin)** are predicted to increase the exposure to **ruxolitinib**. Adjust dose depending on indication and monitor adverse effects—consult product literature. Moderate Study
- Macrolides **(erythromycin)** slightly increase the exposure to **ruxolitinib**. Mild Study
- **Mitotane** is predicted to decrease the exposure to **ruxolitinib**. Monitor and adjust dose. Moderate Study → Also see TABLE 12 p. 1057
- Neurokinin-1 receptor antagonists **(aprepitant, netupitant)** are predicted to increase the exposure to **ruxolitinib**. Moderate Study
- **Nilotinib** is predicted to increase the exposure to **ruxolitinib**. Moderate Study → Also see TABLE 12 p. 1057

- NNRTIs **(efavirenz, etravirine, nevirapine)** are predicted to decrease the exposure to **ruxolitinib**. Monitor and adjust dose. [Moderate] Study
- Quinolones **(ciprofloxacin)** are predicted to increase the exposure to **ruxolitinib**. [Moderate] Theoretical
- Rifamycins **(rifabutin)** are predicted to decrease the exposure to **ruxolitinib**. Monitor and adjust dose. [Moderate] Theoretical
- Rifamycins **(rifampicin)** are predicted to decrease the exposure to **ruxolitinib**. Monitor and adjust dose. [Moderate] Study
- **Sotorasib** is predicted to decrease the exposure to **ruxolitinib**. Monitor and adjust dose. [Moderate] Study
- **St John's wort** is predicted to decrease the exposure to **ruxolitinib**. Monitor and adjust dose. [Moderate] Study
- **Tucatinib** is predicted to increase the exposure to **ruxolitinib**. Adjust dose depending on indication and monitor adverse effects—consult product literature. [Moderate] Study

Sacituzumab govitecan
- **Afatinib** is predicted to increase the exposure to the active component of **sacituzumab govitecan**. [Severe] Theoretical
- Antiepileptics **(carbamazepine, fosphenytoin, phenytoin)** are predicted to decrease the exposure to the active component of **sacituzumab govitecan**. [Severe] Theoretical
- Antifungals, azoles **(ketoconazole)** are predicted to increase the exposure to the active component of **sacituzumab govitecan**. [Severe] Theoretical
- **Dacomitinib** is predicted to increase the exposure to the active component of **sacituzumab govitecan**. [Severe] Theoretical
- **Erlotinib** is predicted to increase the exposure to the active component of **sacituzumab govitecan**. [Severe] Theoretical
- **Gefitinib** is predicted to increase the exposure to the active component of **sacituzumab govitecan**. [Severe] Theoretical
- **HIV-protease inhibitors** are predicted to decrease the exposure to the active component of **sacituzumab govitecan**. [Severe] Theoretical
- **Lapatinib** is predicted to increase the exposure to the active component of **sacituzumab govitecan**. [Severe] Theoretical
- **Neratinib** is predicted to increase the exposure to the active component of **sacituzumab govitecan**. [Severe] Theoretical
- **Osimertinib** is predicted to increase the exposure to the active component of **sacituzumab govitecan**. [Severe] Theoretical
- **Propofol** is predicted to increase the exposure to the active component of **sacituzumab govitecan**. [Severe] Theoretical
- **Regorafenib** is predicted to increase the exposure to the active component of **sacituzumab govitecan**. [Severe] Theoretical
- Rifamycins **(rifampicin)** are predicted to decrease the exposure to the active component of **sacituzumab govitecan**. [Severe] Theoretical
- **Sorafenib** is predicted to increase the exposure to the active component of **sacituzumab govitecan**. [Severe] Theoretical
- **Vandetanib** is predicted to increase the exposure to the active component of **sacituzumab govitecan**. [Severe] Theoretical

Sacubitril → see TABLE 6 p. 1054 (hypotension)
- **Sacubitril** with valsartan increases the exposure to statins **(atorvastatin)**. [Moderate] Study

Safinamide → see MAO-B inhibitors

Salbutamol → see beta$_2$ agonists

Salmeterol → see beta$_2$ agonists

Sapropterin → see TABLE 6 p. 1054 (hypotension)
- **Methotrexate** is predicted to decrease the efficacy of **sapropterin**. [Moderate] Theoretical
- **Phosphodiesterase type-5 inhibitors** are predicted to increase the risk of hypotension when given with **sapropterin**. [Moderate] Theoretical → Also see TABLE 6 p. 1054
- **Trimethoprim** is predicted to decrease the efficacy of **sapropterin**. [Moderate] Theoretical

Sarilumab → see monoclonal antibodies

Satralizumab → see monoclonal antibodies

Saxagliptin → see dipeptidylpeptidase-4 inhibitors

Secukinumab → see monoclonal antibodies

Seladelpar
- Anti-androgens **(darolutamide)** are predicted to increase the exposure to **seladelpar**. [Moderate] Study
- Antifungals, azoles **(fluconazole)** moderately increase the exposure to **seladelpar**. [Moderate] Study
- **Ciclosporin** moderately increases the exposure to **seladelpar**. [Moderate] Study
- **Eltrombopag** is predicted to increase the exposure to **seladelpar**. [Moderate] Study
- **Febuxostat** is predicted to increase the exposure to **seladelpar**. [Moderate] Study
- **Fostamatinib** is predicted to increase the exposure to **seladelpar**. [Moderate] Study
- **Leflunomide** is predicted to increase the exposure to **seladelpar**. [Moderate] Study
- **Mifepristone** might increase the exposure to **seladelpar**. [Moderate] Study
- **Teriflunomide** is predicted to increase the exposure to **seladelpar**. [Moderate] Study
- **Velpatasvir** is predicted to increase the exposure to **seladelpar**. [Moderate] Study
- **Voxilaprevir** is predicted to increase the exposure to **seladelpar**. [Moderate] Study

Selegiline → see MAO-B inhibitors

Selenium

ROUTE-SPECIFIC INFORMATION Interactions do not generally apply to topical use unless specified.

- Oral **selenium** might decrease the concentration of the active metabolite of oral **baloxavir marboxil**. Avoid. [Severe] Theoretical
- Oral **selenium** is predicted to decrease the absorption of **eltrombopag**. **Eltrombopag** should be taken 2 hours before or 4 hours after **selenium**. [Severe] Theoretical

Selexipag
- Antiepileptics **(carbamazepine, fosphenytoin, phenytoin)** are predicted to decrease the exposure to the active metabolite of **selexipag**. Adjust dose. [Moderate] Study
- Antiepileptics **(valproate)** are predicted to increase the exposure to **selexipag**. [Unknown] Theoretical
- Antifungals, azoles **(fluconazole)** are predicted to increase the exposure to **selexipag**. [Unknown] Theoretical
- **Clopidogrel** is predicted to increase the exposure to **selexipag**. Adjust **selexipag** dose. [Moderate] Study
- Fibrates **(gemfibrozil)** increase the exposure to **selexipag**. Avoid. [Severe] Study
- Iron chelators **(deferasirox)** are predicted to increase the exposure to **selexipag**. Adjust **selexipag** dose. [Moderate] Study
- **Leflunomide** is predicted to increase the exposure to **selexipag**. Adjust **selexipag** dose. [Moderate] Study
- **Pirtobrutinib** is predicted to increase the exposure to **selexipag**. [Moderate] Theoretical
- Rifamycins **(rifampicin)** moderately decrease the exposure to the active metabolite of **selexipag**. Adjust dose. [Moderate] Study
- **Selpercatinib** is predicted to increase the exposure to **selexipag**. Avoid. [Moderate] Study
- **Teriflunomide** is predicted to increase the exposure to **selexipag**. Adjust **selexipag** dose. [Moderate] Study

Selpercatinib → see TABLE 7 p. 1055 (QT-interval prolongation)
- **Antacids** are predicted to decrease the exposure to **selpercatinib**. [Moderate] Theoretical
- Anti-androgens **(apalutamide, enzalutamide)** are predicted to decrease the exposure to **selpercatinib**. Avoid. [Moderate] Study → Also see TABLE 7 p. 1055
- Antiarrhythmics **(dronedarone)** are predicted to increase the exposure to **selpercatinib**. [Moderate] Study → Also see TABLE 7 p. 1055
- Antiepileptics **(carbamazepine, fosphenytoin, phenobarbital, phenytoin, primidone)** are predicted to decrease the exposure to **selpercatinib**. Avoid. [Moderate] Study
- Antifungals, azoles **(fluconazole, isavuconazole)** are predicted to increase the exposure to **selpercatinib**. [Moderate] Study → Also see TABLE 7 p. 1055
- Antifungals, azoles **(itraconazole, ketoconazole, posaconazole, voriconazole)** are predicted to increase the exposure to **selpercatinib**. Adjust dose—consult product literature. [Moderate] Study → Also see TABLE 7 p. 1055
- **Berotralstat** is predicted to increase the exposure to **selpercatinib**. [Moderate] Study
- Calcium-channel blockers **(diltiazem, verapamil)** are predicted to increase the exposure to **selpercatinib**. [Moderate] Study

Selpercatinib (continued)
- **Ceritinib** is predicted to increase the exposure to **selpercatinib**. Adjust dose—consult product literature. Moderate Study → Also see TABLE 7 p. 1055
- **Cobicistat** is predicted to increase the exposure to **selpercatinib**. Adjust dose—consult product literature. Moderate Study
- **Crizotinib** is predicted to increase the exposure to **selpercatinib**. Moderate Study → Also see TABLE 7 p. 1055
- **Dabrafenib** is predicted to decrease the exposure to **selpercatinib**. Moderate Study
- **Selpercatinib** is predicted to increase the exposure to **digoxin**. Moderate Study
- **Selpercatinib** is predicted to increase the exposure to dipeptidylpeptidase-4 inhibitors **(saxagliptin)**. Moderate Study
- **Encorafenib** is predicted to decrease the exposure to **selpercatinib**. Avoid. Moderate Study → Also see TABLE 7 p. 1055
- Endothelin receptor antagonists **(bosentan)** are predicted to decrease the exposure to **selpercatinib**. Moderate Study
- **Selpercatinib** is predicted to increase the exposure to **everolimus**. Avoid. Moderate Study
- **Fedratinib** is predicted to increase the exposure to **selpercatinib**. Moderate Study
- **H_2 receptor antagonists** are predicted to decrease the exposure to **selpercatinib**. Manufacturer advises take 2 hours before or 10 hours after **H_2 receptor antagonists**. Moderate Study
- **HIV-protease inhibitors** are predicted to increase the exposure to **selpercatinib**. Adjust dose—consult product literature. Moderate Study
- **Idelalisib** is predicted to increase the exposure to **selpercatinib**. Adjust dose—consult product literature. Moderate Study
- **Imatinib** is predicted to increase the exposure to **selpercatinib**. Moderate Study
- **Ivosidenib** is predicted to decrease the exposure to **selpercatinib**. Avoid. Moderate Study → Also see TABLE 7 p. 1055
- **Letermovir** is predicted to increase the exposure to **selpercatinib**. Moderate Study
- **Selpercatinib** is predicted to increase the exposure to loop diuretics **(torasemide)**. Avoid. Severe Study
- **Lorlatinib** is predicted to decrease the exposure to **selpercatinib**. Moderate Study
- **Lumacaftor** is predicted to decrease the exposure to **selpercatinib**. Avoid. Moderate Study
- Macrolides **(clarithromycin)** are predicted to increase the exposure to **selpercatinib**. Adjust dose—consult product literature. Moderate Study
- Macrolides **(erythromycin)** are predicted to increase the exposure to **selpercatinib**. Moderate Study → Also see TABLE 7 p. 1055
- **Selpercatinib** is predicted to increase the exposure to **mavacamten**. Monitor and adjust dose—consult product literature. Moderate Theoretical
- **Selpercatinib** increases the exposure to meglitinides **(repaglinide)**. Avoid. Moderate Study
- **Mitotane** is predicted to decrease the exposure to **selpercatinib**. Avoid. Moderate Study
- **Selpercatinib** is predicted to increase the exposure to **montelukast**. Avoid. Moderate Study
- Neurokinin-1 receptor antagonists **(aprepitant, netupitant)** are predicted to increase the exposure to **selpercatinib**. Moderate Study
- **Nilotinib** is predicted to increase the exposure to **selpercatinib**. Moderate Study → Also see TABLE 7 p. 1055
- NNRTIs **(efavirenz, etravirine, nevirapine)** are predicted to decrease the exposure to **selpercatinib**. Moderate Study → Also see TABLE 7 p. 1055
- **Selpercatinib** is predicted to increase the exposure to opioids **(alfentanil, buprenorphine)**. Avoid. Moderate Study
- **Proton pump inhibitors** are predicted to decrease the exposure to **selpercatinib**. Manufacturer advises take with food. Moderate Study
- Rifamycins **(rifampicin)** are predicted to decrease the exposure to **selpercatinib**. Avoid. Moderate Study
- **Selpercatinib** is predicted to increase the exposure to **selexipag**. Avoid. Moderate Study
- **Selpercatinib** is predicted to increase the exposure to **sirolimus**. Avoid. Moderate Study
- **Selpercatinib** is predicted to increase the exposure to **sorafenib**. Avoid. Severe Study → Also see TABLE 7 p. 1055
- **Sotorasib** is predicted to decrease the exposure to **selpercatinib**. Moderate Study
- **St John's wort** is predicted to decrease the exposure to **selpercatinib**. Avoid. Moderate Study
- **Selpercatinib** is predicted to increase the exposure to **talazoparib**. Moderate Study
- **Selpercatinib** is predicted to increase the exposure to **temsirolimus**. Avoid. Moderate Study
- **Selpercatinib** slightly increases the exposure to thrombin inhibitors **(dabigatran)**. Moderate Study
- **Tucatinib** is predicted to increase the exposure to **selpercatinib**. Adjust dose—consult product literature. Moderate Study

Selumetinib
- Anti-androgens **(apalutamide, enzalutamide)** are predicted to decrease the exposure to **selumetinib**. Avoid. Severe Study
- Antiarrhythmics **(dronedarone)** are predicted to increase the exposure to **selumetinib**. Avoid or adjust dose—consult product literature. Severe Study
- Antiepileptics **(carbamazepine, fosphenytoin, phenobarbital, phenytoin, primidone)** are predicted to decrease the exposure to **selumetinib**. Avoid. Severe Study
- Antifungals, azoles **(fluconazole, isavuconazole, itraconazole, ketoconazole, posaconazole, voriconazole)** are predicted to increase the exposure to **selumetinib**. Avoid or adjust dose—consult product literature. Severe Study
- **Selumetinib** might increase the risk of bleeding when given with **aspirin**. Severe Theoretical
- **Berotralstat** is predicted to increase the exposure to **selumetinib**. Avoid or adjust dose—consult product literature. Severe Study
- Calcium-channel blockers **(diltiazem, verapamil)** are predicted to increase the exposure to **selumetinib**. Avoid or adjust dose—consult product literature. Severe Study
- **Selumetinib** might increase the risk of bleeding when given with **cangrelor**. Severe Theoretical
- **Cenobamate** is predicted to decrease the exposure to **selumetinib**. Avoid. Severe Study
- **Ceritinib** is predicted to increase the exposure to **selumetinib**. Avoid or adjust dose—consult product literature. Severe Study
- **Selumetinib** might increase the risk of bleeding when given with **cilostazol**. Severe Theoretical
- **Selumetinib** might increase the risk of bleeding when given with **clopidogrel**. Severe Theoretical
- **Cobicistat** is predicted to increase the exposure to **selumetinib**. Avoid or adjust dose—consult product literature. Severe Study
- **Selumetinib** might increase the risk of bleeding when given with **coumarins**. Severe Theoretical
- **Crizotinib** is predicted to increase the exposure to **selumetinib**. Avoid or adjust dose—consult product literature. Severe Study
- **Dabrafenib** is predicted to decrease the exposure to **selumetinib**. Avoid. Severe Study
- **Selumetinib** might increase the risk of bleeding when given with **dipyridamole**. Moderate Theoretical
- **Encorafenib** is predicted to decrease the exposure to **selumetinib**. Avoid. Severe Study
- Endothelin receptor antagonists **(bosentan)** are predicted to decrease the exposure to **selumetinib**. Avoid. Severe Study
- **Fedratinib** is predicted to increase the exposure to **selumetinib**. Avoid or adjust dose—consult product literature. Severe Study
- **Grapefruit** juice is predicted to increase the exposure to **selumetinib**. Avoid. Moderate Theoretical
- **HIV-protease inhibitors** are predicted to increase the exposure to **selumetinib**. Avoid or adjust dose—consult product literature. Severe Study
- **Idelalisib** is predicted to increase the exposure to **selumetinib**. Avoid or adjust dose—consult product literature. Severe Study
- **Imatinib** is predicted to increase the exposure to **selumetinib**. Avoid or adjust dose—consult product literature. Severe Study
- **Ivosidenib** is predicted to decrease the exposure to **selumetinib**. Avoid. Severe Study

- ▸ **Letermovir** is predicted to increase the exposure to **selumetinib**. Avoid or adjust dose—consult product literature. [Severe] Study
- ▸ **Lorlatinib** is predicted to decrease the exposure to **selumetinib**. Avoid. [Severe] Study
- ▸ **Lumacaftor** is predicted to decrease the exposure to **selumetinib**. Avoid. [Severe] Study
- ▸ Macrolides **(clarithromycin, erythromycin)** are predicted to increase the exposure to **selumetinib**. Avoid or adjust dose—consult product literature. [Severe] Study
- ▸ **Mitotane** is predicted to decrease the exposure to **selumetinib**. Avoid. [Severe] Study
- ▸ **Moclobemide** is predicted to increase the exposure to **selumetinib**. Avoid or adjust dose—consult product literature. [Severe] Theoretical
- ▸ Neurokinin-1 receptor antagonists **(aprepitant, netupitant)** are predicted to increase the exposure to **selumetinib**. Avoid or adjust dose—consult product literature. [Severe] Study
- ▸ **Nilotinib** is predicted to increase the exposure to **selumetinib**. Avoid or adjust dose—consult product literature. [Severe] Study
- ▸ NNRTIs **(efavirenz, etravirine, nevirapine)** are predicted to decrease the exposure to **selumetinib**. Avoid. [Severe] Study
- ▸ **Selumetinib** might increase the risk of bleeding when given with **phenindione**. [Severe] Theoretical
- ▸ **Selumetinib** might increase the risk of bleeding when given with **prasugrel**. [Severe] Theoretical
- ▸ Proton pump inhibitors **(esomeprazole, omeprazole)** are predicted to increase the exposure to **selumetinib**. Avoid or adjust dose—consult product literature. [Severe] Theoretical
- ▸ Rifamycins **(rifampicin)** are predicted to decrease the exposure to **selumetinib**. Avoid. [Severe] Study
- ▸ **Sotorasib** is predicted to decrease the exposure to **selumetinib**. Avoid [Severe] Study
- ▸ SSRIs **(fluoxetine)** are predicted to increase the exposure to **selumetinib**. Avoid or adjust dose—consult product literature. [Severe] Theoretical
- ▸ SSRIs **(fluvoxamine)** are predicted to increase the exposure to **selumetinib**. Avoid or monitor—consult product literature. [Severe] Theoretical
- ▸ **St John's wort** is predicted to decrease the exposure to **selumetinib**. Avoid. [Severe] Study
- ▸ **Selumetinib** might increase the risk of bleeding when given with **ticagrelor**. [Severe] Theoretical
- ▸ **Tucatinib** is predicted to increase the exposure to **selumetinib**. Avoid or adjust dose—consult product literature. [Severe] Study
- ▸ **Vitamin E substances** might increase the risk of bleeding when given with **selumetinib**. Avoid. [Severe] Theoretical

Semaglutide → see glucagon-like peptide-1 receptor agonists

Serplulimab → see monoclonal antibodies

Sertraline → see SSRIs

Sevelamer

SEPARATION OF ADMINISTRATION Drugs for which a reduction in bioavailability could be clinically important should be administered at least 1 hour before, or 3 hours after, sevelamer; alternatively consider monitoring blood concentrations.

- ▸ Oral **sevelamer** decreases the exposure to oral **roxadustat**. **Roxadustat** should be taken at least 1 hour after **sevelamer**. [Moderate] Study
- ▸ Oral **sevelamer** decreases the exposure to oral **vadadustat**. Manufacturer advises take at least 1 hour before or 2 hours after **sevelamer**. [Moderate] Study

Sevoflurane → see volatile halogenated anaesthetics

Sildenafil → see phosphodiesterase type-5 inhibitors

Siltuximab → see monoclonal antibodies

Simvastatin → see statins

Siponimod → see **TABLE 4** p. 1054 (bradycardia), **TABLE 7** p. 1055 (QT-interval prolongation)

- ▸ Anti-androgens **(apalutamide, enzalutamide)** are predicted to decrease the exposure to **siponimod**. Manufacturer advises caution depending on genotype—consult product literature. [Severe] Study
- ▸ Antiarrhythmics **(amiodarone, dronedarone)** are predicted to increase the exposure to **siponimod**. Avoid depending on other drugs taken—consult product literature. [Severe] Study → Also see **TABLE 4** p. 1054
- ▸ Antiepileptics **(carbamazepine, fosphenytoin, phenobarbital, phenytoin, primidone)** are predicted to decrease the exposure to **siponimod**. Manufacturer advises caution depending on genotype—consult product literature. [Severe] Study
- ▸ Antifungals, azoles **(fluconazole, isavuconazole, miconazole)** are predicted to increase the exposure to **siponimod**. Avoid depending on other drugs taken—consult product literature. [Severe] Study
- ▸ Antifungals, azoles **(itraconazole, ketoconazole, posaconazole, voriconazole)** are predicted to increase the exposure to **siponimod**. Avoid depending on other drugs taken—consult product literature. [Severe] Theoretical
- ▸ **Berotralstat** is predicted to increase the exposure to **siponimod**. Avoid depending on other drugs taken—consult product literature. [Severe] Study
- ▸ Calcium-channel blockers **(diltiazem, verapamil)** are predicted to increase the exposure to **siponimod**. Avoid depending on other drugs taken—consult product literature. [Severe] Study → Also see **TABLE 4** p. 1054
- ▸ **Cenobamate** is predicted to decrease the exposure to **siponimod**. Manufacturer advises caution depending on genotype—consult product literature. [Moderate] Theoretical
- ▸ **Ceritinib** is predicted to increase the exposure to **siponimod**. Avoid depending on other drugs taken—consult product literature. [Severe] Theoretical → Also see **TABLE 4** p. 1054
- ▸ **Cobicistat** is predicted to increase the exposure to **siponimod**. Avoid depending on other drugs taken—consult product literature. [Severe] Theoretical
- ▸ **Crizotinib** is predicted to increase the exposure to **siponimod**. Avoid depending on other drugs taken—consult product literature. [Severe] Study → Also see **TABLE 4** p. 1054
- ▸ **Dabrafenib** is predicted to decrease the exposure to **siponimod**. Manufacturer advises caution depending on genotype—consult product literature. [Moderate] Theoretical
- ▸ **Encorafenib** is predicted to decrease the exposure to **siponimod**. Manufacturer advises caution depending on genotype—consult product literature. [Severe] Study
- ▸ Endothelin receptor antagonists **(bosentan)** are predicted to decrease the exposure to **siponimod**. Manufacturer advises caution depending on genotype—consult product literature. [Moderate] Theoretical
- ▸ **Fedratinib** is predicted to increase the exposure to **siponimod**. Avoid depending on other drugs taken—consult product literature. [Severe] Study
- ▸ **HIV-protease inhibitors** are predicted to increase the exposure to **siponimod**. Avoid depending on other drugs taken—consult product literature. [Severe] Theoretical
- ▸ **Idelalisib** is predicted to increase the exposure to **siponimod**. Avoid depending on other drugs taken—consult product literature. [Severe] Theoretical
- ▸ **Imatinib** is predicted to increase the exposure to **siponimod**. Avoid depending on other drugs taken—consult product literature. [Severe] Study
- ▸ **Ivosidenib** is predicted to decrease the exposure to **siponimod**. Manufacturer advises caution depending on genotype—consult product literature. [Severe] Study
- ▸ **Letermovir** is predicted to increase the exposure to **siponimod**. Avoid depending on other drugs taken—consult product literature. [Severe] Study
- ▸ **Live vaccines** might increase the risk of generalised infection (possibly life-threatening) when given with **siponimod**. Avoid and for 4 weeks after stopping **siponimod**. [Severe] Theoretical
- ▸ **Lorlatinib** is predicted to decrease the exposure to **siponimod**. Manufacturer advises caution depending on genotype—consult product literature. [Moderate] Theoretical
- ▸ **Lumacaftor** is predicted to decrease the exposure to **siponimod**. Manufacturer advises caution depending on genotype—consult product literature. [Severe] Study
- ▸ Macrolides **(clarithromycin)** are predicted to increase the exposure to **siponimod**. Avoid depending on other drugs taken—consult product literature. [Severe] Theoretical

Siponimod (continued)

- Macrolides **(erythromycin)** are predicted to increase the exposure to **siponimod**. Avoid depending on other drugs taken—consult product literature. Severe Study
- **Mifepristone** is predicted to increase the exposure to **siponimod**. Moderate Theoretical
- **Mitotane** is predicted to decrease the exposure to **siponimod**. Manufacturer advises caution depending on genotype—consult product literature. Severe Study
- Monoclonal antibodies **(alemtuzumab)** are predicted to increase the risk of generalised infection (possibly life-threatening) when given with **siponimod**. Avoid. Severe Theoretical
- Neurokinin-1 receptor antagonists **(aprepitant, netupitant)** are predicted to increase the exposure to **siponimod**. Avoid depending on other drugs taken—consult product literature. Severe Study
- **Nilotinib** is predicted to increase the exposure to **siponimod**. Avoid depending on other drugs taken—consult product literature. Severe Study
- NNRTIs **(efavirenz, etravirine, nevirapine)** are predicted to decrease the exposure to **siponimod**. Manufacturer advises caution depending on genotype—consult product literature. Moderate Theoretical
- Rifamycins **(rifampicin)** are predicted to decrease the exposure to **siponimod**. Manufacturer advises caution depending on genotype—consult product literature. Severe Study
- **Sotorasib** is predicted to decrease the exposure to **siponimod**. Manufacturer advises caution depending on genotype—consult product literature. Moderate Theoretical
- **Sparsentan** is predicted to decrease the exposure to **siponimod**. Moderate Theoretical
- **St John's wort** is predicted to decrease the exposure to **siponimod**. Manufacturer advises caution depending on genotype—consult product literature. Moderate Theoretical
- **Tucatinib** is predicted to increase the exposure to **siponimod**. Avoid depending on other drugs taken—consult product literature. Severe Theoretical

Sirolimus

- **Abrocitinib** might increase the exposure to **sirolimus**. Moderate Theoretical
- Anti-androgens **(apalutamide, enzalutamide)** are predicted to decrease the concentration of **sirolimus**. Avoid or monitor and adjust dose. Severe Study
- Antiarrhythmics **(amiodarone)** are predicted to increase the concentration of **sirolimus**. Severe Anecdotal
- Antiarrhythmics **(dronedarone)** increase the concentration of **sirolimus**. Monitor and adjust dose. Moderate Study
- Antiepileptics **(carbamazepine, fosphenytoin, phenobarbital, phenytoin, primidone)** are predicted to decrease the concentration of **sirolimus**. Avoid or monitor and adjust dose. Severe Study
- Antifungals, azoles **(fluconazole, isavuconazole)** increase the concentration of **sirolimus**. Monitor and adjust dose. Moderate Study
- Antifungals, azoles **(itraconazole, ketoconazole, posaconazole, voriconazole)** are predicted to increase the concentration of **sirolimus**. Avoid or monitor and adjust dose. Severe Study
- Antifungals, azoles **(miconazole)** are predicted to increase the concentration of **sirolimus**. Monitor and adjust dose. Moderate Study
- **Asciminib** is predicted to increase the exposure to **sirolimus**. Severe Theoretical
- **Belumosudil** might increase the exposure to **sirolimus**. Avoid or adjust dose. Moderate Theoretical
- **Belzutifan** is predicted to decrease the exposure to **sirolimus**. Avoid or adjust dose. Severe Theoretical
- **Berotralstat** increases the concentration of **sirolimus**. Monitor and adjust dose. Moderate Study
- **Brigatinib** potentially decreases the concentration of **sirolimus**. Avoid. Moderate Theoretical
- **Bulevirtide** is predicted to increase the exposure to **sirolimus**. Moderate Theoretical
- Calcium-channel blockers **(diltiazem, verapamil)** increase the concentration of **sirolimus**. Monitor and adjust dose. Moderate Study
- **Cannabidiol** is predicted to increase the exposure to **sirolimus**. Monitor and adjust dose. Moderate Study
- **Cenobamate** is predicted to decrease the exposure to **sirolimus**. Adjust dose. Moderate Theoretical
- **Ceritinib** is predicted to increase the concentration of **sirolimus**. Avoid or monitor and adjust dose. Severe Study
- **Sirolimus** is predicted to affect the efficacy of **chenodeoxycholic acid**. Monitor and adjust dose. Moderate Theoretical
- **Ciclosporin** moderately increases the exposure to **sirolimus**. Separate administration by 4 hours. Severe Study
- **Cobicistat** is predicted to increase the concentration of **sirolimus**. Avoid or monitor and adjust dose. Severe Study
- **Crizotinib** increases the concentration of **sirolimus**. Monitor and adjust dose. Moderate Study
- **Danicopan** is predicted to increase the exposure to **sirolimus**. Moderate Study
- **Daridorexant** is predicted to increase the exposure to **sirolimus**. Moderate Study
- **Deutivacaftor** is predicted to increase the exposure to **sirolimus**. Moderate Theoretical
- **Eliglustat** is predicted to increase the exposure to **sirolimus**. Adjust dose. Moderate Study
- **Encorafenib** is predicted to decrease the concentration of **sirolimus**. Avoid or monitor and adjust dose. Severe Study
- Endothelin receptor antagonists **(bosentan)** are predicted to decrease the concentration of **sirolimus** and **sirolimus** potentially increases the concentration of endothelin receptor antagonists **(bosentan)**. Avoid. Severe Theoretical
- **Erdafitinib** is predicted to increase the exposure to **sirolimus**. Separate administration by at least 6 hours. Moderate Theoretical
- **Fedratinib** increases the concentration of **sirolimus**. Monitor and adjust dose. Moderate Study
- **Fostamatinib** is predicted to increase the exposure to **sirolimus**. Monitor and adjust dose. Moderate Theoretical
- **Givinostat** might increase the exposure to **sirolimus**. Moderate Study
- **Glecaprevir** is predicted to increase the exposure to **sirolimus**. Severe Theoretical
- **Grapefruit** juice increases the concentration of **sirolimus**. Avoid. Moderate Study
- **HIV-protease inhibitors** are predicted to increase the concentration of **sirolimus**. Avoid or monitor and adjust dose. Severe Study
- **Ibrutinib** might increase the exposure to **sirolimus**. Separate administration by at least 6 hours. Moderate Theoretical
- **Idelalisib** is predicted to increase the concentration of **sirolimus**. Avoid or monitor and adjust dose. Severe Study
- **Imatinib** increases the concentration of **sirolimus**. Monitor and adjust dose. Moderate Study
- **Ivacaftor** is predicted to increase the exposure to **sirolimus**. Moderate Study
- **Ivosidenib** is predicted to decrease the concentration of **sirolimus**. Avoid or monitor and adjust dose. Severe Study
- **Lapatinib** is predicted to increase the exposure to **sirolimus**. Moderate Theoretical
- **Larotrectinib** is predicted to increase the exposure to **sirolimus**. Use with caution and adjust dose. Mild Theoretical
- **Lazertinib** is predicted to increase the exposure to **sirolimus**. Moderate Study
- **Letermovir** increases the concentration of **sirolimus**. Monitor and adjust dose. Moderate Study
- **Live vaccines** are predicted to increase the risk of generalised infection (possibly life-threatening) when given with **sirolimus**. UKHSA advises avoid (refer to Green Book). Severe Theoretical
- **Lomitapide** might increase the exposure to **sirolimus**. Adjust dose. Moderate Theoretical
- **Lorlatinib** is predicted to decrease the exposure to **sirolimus**. Avoid. Moderate Theoretical
- **Lumacaftor** is predicted to decrease the concentration of **sirolimus**. Avoid or monitor and adjust dose. Severe Study
- Macrolides **(clarithromycin)** are predicted to increase the concentration of **sirolimus**. Avoid or monitor and adjust dose. Severe Study

- Macrolides **(erythromycin)** increase the concentration of **sirolimus**. Monitor and adjust dose. Moderate Study
- **Maribavir** is predicted to increase the exposure to **sirolimus**. Monitor and adjust dose. Severe Study
- **Sirolimus** is predicted to decrease the efficacy of **mifamurtide**. Avoid. Severe Theoretical
- **Mifepristone** is predicted to increase the exposure to **sirolimus**. Severe Theoretical
- **Mirabegron** is predicted to increase the exposure to **sirolimus**. Mild Theoretical
- **Mitotane** is predicted to decrease the concentration of **sirolimus**. Avoid or monitor and adjust dose. Severe Study
- Monoclonal antibodies **(elranatamab)** might affect the exposure to **sirolimus**. Monitor and adjust dose. Moderate Theoretical
- Monoclonal antibodies **(sarilumab)** potentially affect the exposure to **sirolimus**. Monitor and adjust dose. Moderate Theoretical
- **Neratinib** is predicted to increase the exposure to **sirolimus**. Moderate Study
- Neurokinin-1 receptor antagonists **(aprepitant, netupitant)** increase the concentration of **sirolimus**. Monitor and adjust dose. Moderate Study
- **Nilotinib** increases the concentration of **sirolimus**. Monitor and adjust dose. Moderate Study
- **Nirmatrelvir** boosted with ritonavir is predicted to increase the concentration of **sirolimus**. Avoid—consult product literature. Severe Theoretical
- NNRTIs **(doravirine)** are predicted to decrease the exposure to **sirolimus**. Monitor **sirolimus** concentration and adjust dose, p. 641. Moderate Theoretical
- NNRTIs **(efavirenz, nevirapine)** are predicted to decrease the concentration of **sirolimus**. Monitor and adjust dose. Moderate Theoretical
- NNRTIs **(etravirine)** are predicted to decrease the exposure to **sirolimus**. Monitor and adjust dose. Moderate Study
- **Olaparib** might increase the exposure to **sirolimus**. Moderate Theoretical
- **Osimertinib** is predicted to increase the exposure to **sirolimus**. Moderate Study
- **Palbociclib** is predicted to increase the exposure to **sirolimus**. Adjust dose. Moderate Theoretical
- **Pemigatinib** might increase the exposure to **sirolimus**. Separate administration by at least 6 hours. Moderate Theoretical
- **Pibrentasvir** with glecaprevir is predicted to increase the exposure to **sirolimus**. Moderate Study
- **Pirtobrutinib** is predicted to increase the exposure to **sirolimus**. Avoid or monitor. Moderate Theoretical
- **Pitolisant** is predicted to decrease the exposure to **sirolimus**. Avoid. Severe Theoretical
- **Ribociclib** is predicted to increase the exposure to **sirolimus**. Use with caution and adjust dose. Moderate Theoretical
- Rifamycins **(rifampicin)** are predicted to decrease the concentration of **sirolimus**. Avoid or monitor and adjust dose. Severe Study
- **Ritlecitinib** is predicted to increase the exposure to **sirolimus**. Adjust dose. Moderate Theoretical
- **Rucaparib** is predicted to increase the exposure to **sirolimus**. Monitor and adjust dose. Moderate Study
- **Selpercatinib** is predicted to increase the exposure to **sirolimus**. Avoid. Moderate Study
- **Sotorasib** is predicted to decrease the exposure to **sirolimus**. Avoid or adjust dose. Severe Theoretical
- **Sparsentan** is predicted to increase the exposure to **sirolimus**. Severe Theoretical
- **St John's wort** is predicted to decrease the concentration of **sirolimus**. Monitor and adjust dose. Severe Theoretical
- **Sirolimus** is predicted to decrease the concentration of **tacrolimus** and **tacrolimus** increases the exposure to **sirolimus**. Severe Study
- **Tarlatamab** might affect the exposure to **sirolimus**. Monitor and adjust dose. Moderate Theoretical
- **Tepotinib** is predicted to increase the concentration of **sirolimus**. Severe Study
- **Tucatinib** is predicted to increase the concentration of **sirolimus**. Avoid or monitor and adjust dose. Severe Study
- **Velpatasvir** is predicted to increase the exposure to **sirolimus**. Severe Theoretical
- **Vemurafenib** is predicted to increase the exposure to **sirolimus**. Use with caution and adjust dose. Severe Theoretical
- **Venetoclax** is predicted to increase the exposure to **sirolimus**. Avoid or adjust dose. Severe Study
- **Voclosporin** is predicted to increase the exposure to **sirolimus**. Moderate Study
- **Vorasidenib** might decrease the concentration of **sirolimus**. Avoid. Severe Theoretical
- **Voxilaprevir** with sofosbuvir and velpatasvir is predicted to increase the exposure to **sirolimus**. Severe Theoretical

Sitagliptin → see dipeptidylpeptidase-4 inhibitors

SNRIs → see **TABLE 3** p. 1053 (bleeding), **TABLE 15** p. 1058 (hyponatraemia), **TABLE 11** p. 1056 (serotonin toxicity), **TABLE 9** p. 1056 (CNS effects)

duloxetine · venlafaxine

- Antiepileptics **(phenytoin)** are predicted to decrease the exposure to **duloxetine**. Moderate Theoretical → Also see **TABLE 9** p. 1056
- Antifungals, azoles **(itraconazole, ketoconazole, posaconazole, voriconazole)** are predicted to increase the exposure to **venlafaxine**. Moderate Study
- **Axitinib** is predicted to increase the exposure to **duloxetine**. Moderate Theoretical → Also see **TABLE 3** p. 1053
- **Duloxetine** is predicted to increase the exposure to beta blockers, selective **(metoprolol)**. Moderate Study
- **Ceritinib** is predicted to increase the exposure to **venlafaxine**. Moderate Study
- **Cobicistat** is predicted to increase the exposure to **venlafaxine**. Moderate Study
- **Duloxetine** is predicted to increase the exposure to **eliglustat**. Avoid or adjust dose—consult product literature. Severe Study
- **Givosiran** is predicted to increase the exposure to **duloxetine**. Use with caution and adjust dose. Moderate Study
- H_2 receptor antagonists **(cimetidine)** slightly increase the exposure to **venlafaxine**. Mild Study
- **Venlafaxine** slightly increases the exposure to **haloperidol**. Severe Study → Also see **TABLE 15** p. 1058 → Also see **TABLE 9** p. 1056
- HIV-protease inhibitors **(ritonavir)** are predicted to decrease the exposure to **duloxetine**. Moderate Theoretical
- **HIV-protease inhibitors** are predicted to increase the exposure to **venlafaxine**. Moderate Study
- **Idelalisib** is predicted to increase the exposure to **venlafaxine**. Moderate Study
- **Leflunomide** is predicted to decrease the exposure to **duloxetine**. Moderate Theoretical
- **Leniolisib** is predicted to increase the exposure to **duloxetine**. Avoid. Moderate Theoretical
- Macrolides **(clarithromycin)** are predicted to increase the exposure to **venlafaxine**. Moderate Study
- **Mexiletine** is predicted to increase the exposure to **duloxetine**. Moderate Theoretical
- **Osilodrostat** is predicted to increase the exposure to **duloxetine**. Moderate Theoretical
- **Duloxetine** might increase the risk of adverse effects when given with **ozanimod**. Severe Theoretical
- **Duloxetine** is predicted to increase the exposure to **pitolisant**. Use with caution and adjust dose. Moderate Study
- **Venlafaxine** is predicted to increase the exposure to **pitolisant**. Use with caution and adjust dose. Mild Theoretical
- Quinolones **(ciprofloxacin)** are predicted to increase the exposure to **duloxetine**. Avoid. Moderate Theoretical
- Rifamycins **(rifampicin)** are predicted to decrease the exposure to **duloxetine**. Moderate Theoretical
- **Rucaparib** is predicted to increase the exposure to **duloxetine**. Monitor and adjust dose. Moderate Study
- SSRIs **(fluvoxamine)** markedly increase the exposure to **duloxetine**. Avoid. Severe Study → Also see **TABLE 3** p. 1053 → Also see **TABLE 15** p. 1058 → Also see **TABLE 11** p. 1056 → Also see **TABLE 9** p. 1056
- **Tacrolimus** potentially increases the risk of serotonin toxicity when given with **venlafaxine**. Severe Anecdotal

SNRIs (continued)
- **Teriflunomide** is predicted to decrease the exposure to **duloxetine.** Moderate Theoretical
- **Tucatinib** is predicted to increase the exposure to **venlafaxine.** Moderate Study
- **Vaborbactam** is predicted to increase the concentration of **venlafaxine.** Unknown Theoretical
- **Vemurafenib** is predicted to increase the exposure to **duloxetine.** Use with caution or avoid. Moderate Theoretical

Sodium bicarbonate

ROUTE-SPECIFIC INFORMATION Interactions do not generally apply to topical use of **sodium bicarbonate** unless specified.

- Oral **sodium bicarbonate** decreases the absorption of oral antifungals, azoles **(ketoconazole)**. Moderate Study
- Oral **sodium bicarbonate** -containing antacids are predicted to decrease the absorption of oral **bosutinib**. Manufacturer advises take at least 12 hours before antacids. Moderate Theoretical
- Oral **sodium bicarbonate** -containing antacids are predicted to decrease the exposure to oral **dasatinib**. Separate administration by at least 2 hours. Moderate Study
- Oral **sodium bicarbonate** -containing antacids are predicted to decrease the absorption of oral **erlotinib**. Manufacturer advises take 2 hours before or 4 hours after antacids. Moderate Theoretical
- Oral **sodium bicarbonate** -containing antacids are predicted to decrease the exposure to oral **gefitinib**. Moderate Theoretical
- Oral **sodium bicarbonate** -containing antacids are predicted to decrease the absorption of oral **lapatinib**. Avoid. Moderate Theoretical
- **Sodium bicarbonate** decreases the concentration of **lithium**. Severe Anecdotal
- **Sodium bicarbonate** is predicted to decrease the efficacy of **methenamine**. Avoid. Moderate Theoretical
- Oral **sodium bicarbonate** -containing antacids are predicted to decrease the exposure to oral **neratinib**. Separate administration by at least 3 hours. Mild Theoretical
- Oral **sodium bicarbonate** -containing antacids might affect the exposure to oral **nilotinib**. Separate administration by at least 2 hours. Moderate Study
- **Sodium bicarbonate** might decrease the efficacy of **nitrofurantoin**. Unknown Theoretical
- Oral **sodium bicarbonate** -containing antacids are predicted to decrease the exposure to oral NNRTIs **(rilpivirine)**. Manufacturer advises take 4 hours before or 2 hours after antacids. Severe Theoretical
- Oral **sodium bicarbonate** -containing antacids might decrease the absorption of oral **pazopanib**. Manufacturer advises take 1 hour before or 2 hours after antacids. Moderate Theoretical
- Oral **sodium bicarbonate** is predicted to decrease the exposure to oral **sotorasib**. Manufacturer advises take 4 hours before or 10 hours after antacids. Moderate Theoretical

Sodium citrate
- **Sodium citrate** is predicted to decrease the efficacy of **methenamine**. Avoid. Moderate Theoretical
- **Sodium citrate** might decrease the efficacy of **nitrofurantoin**. Unknown Theoretical
- **Sodium citrate** is predicted to increase the risk of adverse effects when given with **sucralfate**. Avoid. Moderate Theoretical

Sodium glucose co-transporter 2 inhibitors → see TABLE 6 p. 1054 (hypotension)

canagliflozin · dapagliflozin · empagliflozin · ertugliflozin

- Antiepileptics **(carbamazepine, phenobarbital, phenytoin, primidone)** are predicted to decrease the exposure to **canagliflozin**. Adjust **canagliflozin** dose. Moderate Study
- Antiepileptics **(fosphenytoin)** are predicted to decrease the exposure to **empagliflozin**. Avoid or monitor diabetic control. Moderate Theoretical
- Antiepileptics **(phenytoin)** might decrease the exposure to **empagliflozin**. Avoid or monitor diabetic control. Moderate Theoretical
- **Fenfluramine** might decrease blood glucose concentrations when given with **sodium glucose co-transporter 2 inhibitors**. Moderate Theoretical
- HIV-protease inhibitors **(ritonavir)** are predicted to decrease the exposure to **canagliflozin**. Adjust **canagliflozin** dose. Moderate Study
- NNRTIs **(efavirenz)** are predicted to decrease the exposure to **canagliflozin**. Adjust **canagliflozin** dose. Moderate Study
- Rifamycins **(rifampicin)** moderately decrease the exposure to **canagliflozin**. Adjust **canagliflozin** dose. Moderate Study
- Rifamycins **(rifampicin)** might decrease the exposure to **empagliflozin**. Avoid or monitor diabetic control. Moderate Theoretical
- **Somapacitan** might increase blood glucose concentrations, opposing the blood glucose-lowering effects of **sodium glucose co-transporter 2 inhibitors**. Adjust dose. Moderate Theoretical
- **Somatrogon** might increase blood glucose concentrations, opposing the blood glucose-lowering effects of **sodium glucose co-transporter 2 inhibitors**. Adjust dose. Moderate Theoretical
- **St John's wort** is predicted to decrease the exposure to **canagliflozin**. Adjust **canagliflozin** dose. Moderate Study
- **Empagliflozin** has been reported to increase the risk of muscle effects when given after statins **(atorvastatin)**. Moderate Anecdotal

Sodium oxybate → see TABLE 6 p. 1054 (hypotension), TABLE 9 p. 1056 (CNS effects)
- Antiepileptics **(valproate)** increase the exposure to **sodium oxybate**. Adjust **sodium oxybate** dose. Moderate Study

Sodium phenylbutyrate
- Antiepileptics **(valproate)** potentially decrease the effects of **sodium phenylbutyrate**. Moderate Anecdotal
- **Corticosteroids** potentially decrease the effects of **sodium phenylbutyrate**. Moderate Theoretical
- **Haloperidol** potentially decreases the effects of **sodium phenylbutyrate**. Moderate Anecdotal

Sodium picosulfate
- Oral **sodium picosulfate** might decrease the concentration of the active metabolite of oral **baloxavir marboxil**. Severe Theoretical

Sodium zirconium cyclosilicate
- **Sodium zirconium cyclosilicate** is predicted to decrease the exposure to **antifungals, azoles**. Separate administration by at least 2 hours. Moderate Theoretical
- **Sodium zirconium cyclosilicate** is predicted to decrease the exposure to **dasatinib**. Separate administration by at least 2 hours. Moderate Theoretical
- **Sodium zirconium cyclosilicate** is predicted to decrease the exposure to **erlotinib**. Separate administration by at least 2 hours. Moderate Theoretical
- **Sodium zirconium cyclosilicate** is predicted to decrease the exposure to **HIV-protease inhibitors**. Separate administration by at least 2 hours. Moderate Theoretical
- **Sodium zirconium cyclosilicate** is predicted to decrease the exposure to **ledipasvir**. Separate administration by at least 2 hours. Moderate Theoretical
- **Sodium zirconium cyclosilicate** is predicted to decrease the exposure to **nilotinib**. Separate administration by at least 2 hours. Moderate Theoretical
- **Sodium zirconium cyclosilicate** is predicted to decrease the exposure to NNRTIs **(rilpivirine)**. Separate administration by at least 2 hours. Moderate Theoretical
- **Sodium zirconium cyclosilicate** is predicted to decrease the exposure to **raltegravir**. Separate administration by at least 2 hours. Moderate Theoretical

Sofosbuvir
- **Sofosbuvir** is predicted to increase the risk of severe bradycardia or heart block when given with antiarrhythmics **(amiodarone)**. Refer to specialist literature. Severe Anecdotal
- Antiepileptics **(carbamazepine)** are predicted to decrease the exposure to **sofosbuvir**. Avoid. Severe Study
- Antiepileptics **(fosphenytoin, oxcarbazepine, phenobarbital, phenytoin, primidone)** are predicted to decrease the exposure to **sofosbuvir**. Avoid. Severe Theoretical
- **Combined hormonal contraceptives** containing ethinylestradiol can increase ALT concentrations when given with **sofosbuvir** with velpatasvir and voxilaprevir. Avoid. Severe Study
- **Sofosbuvir** might affect the anticoagulant effect of **coumarins**. Moderate Theoretical

- **Ethinylestradiol** might increase ALT concentrations when given with **sofosbuvir** with velpatasvir and voxilaprevir. Avoid. [Severe] Study
- **H₂ receptor antagonists** potentially decrease the exposure to **sofosbuvir**. Adjust dose, see ledipasvir with sofosbuvir p. 495, sofosbuvir with velpatasvir p. 496, and sofosbuvir with velpatasvir and voxilaprevir. [Moderate] Study
- **Hormone replacement therapy** might increase ALT concentrations when given with **sofosbuvir** with velpatasvir and voxilaprevir. Manufacturer advises caution; avoid ethinylestradiol. [Severe] Theoretical
- **Lorlatinib** is predicted to decrease the exposure to **sofosbuvir**. Avoid. [Severe] Study
- **Modafinil** is predicted to decrease the exposure to **sofosbuvir**. Avoid. [Severe] Theoretical
- **Nirmatrelvir** boosted with ritonavir is predicted to increase the concentration of **sofosbuvir** with velpatasvir and voxilaprevir. [Severe] Theoretical
- **Sofosbuvir** might affect the anticoagulant effect of **phenindione**. [Moderate] Theoretical
- **Proton pump inhibitors** potentially decrease the exposure to **sofosbuvir**. Adjust dose, see ledipasvir with sofosbuvir p. 495, sofosbuvir with velpatasvir p. 496, and sofosbuvir with velpatasvir and voxilaprevir. [Moderate] Study
- Rifamycins **(rifampicin)** are predicted to decrease the exposure to **sofosbuvir**. Avoid. [Severe] Study
- **St John's wort** is predicted to decrease the exposure to **sofosbuvir**. Avoid. [Severe] Study

Solifenacin → see TABLE 8 p. 1055 (antimuscarinics)

- Anti-androgens **(apalutamide, enzalutamide)** are predicted to decrease the exposure to **solifenacin**. [Moderate] Theoretical
- Antiepileptics **(carbamazepine, fosphenytoin, phenobarbital, phenytoin, primidone)** are predicted to decrease the exposure to **solifenacin**. [Moderate] Theoretical
- Antifungals, azoles **(itraconazole, ketoconazole, posaconazole, voriconazole)** are predicted to increase the exposure to **solifenacin**. Adjust solifenacin p. 604 or tamsulosin with solifenacin dose; avoid in hepatic and renal impairment. [Severe] Study
- Atypical antipsychotics **(clozapine)** can cause constipation, as can **solifenacin**; concurrent use might increase the risk of developing intestinal obstruction. [Severe] Theoretical → Also see TABLE 8 p. 1055
- **Ceritinib** is predicted to increase the exposure to **solifenacin**. Adjust solifenacin p. 604 or tamsulosin with solifenacin dose; avoid in hepatic and renal impairment. [Severe] Study
- **Cobicistat** is predicted to increase the exposure to **solifenacin**. Adjust solifenacin p. 604 or tamsulosin with solifenacin dose; avoid in hepatic and renal impairment. [Severe] Study
- **Encorafenib** is predicted to decrease the exposure to **solifenacin**. [Moderate] Theoretical
- **HIV-protease inhibitors** are predicted to increase the exposure to **solifenacin**. Adjust solifenacin p. 604 or tamsulosin with solifenacin dose; avoid in hepatic and renal impairment. [Severe] Study
- **Idelalisib** is predicted to increase the exposure to **solifenacin**. Adjust solifenacin p. 604 or tamsulosin with solifenacin dose; avoid in hepatic and renal impairment. [Severe] Study
- **Ivosidenib** is predicted to decrease the exposure to **solifenacin**. [Moderate] Theoretical
- **Lumacaftor** is predicted to decrease the exposure to **solifenacin**. [Moderate] Theoretical
- Macrolides **(clarithromycin)** are predicted to increase the exposure to **solifenacin**. Adjust solifenacin p. 604 or tamsulosin with solifenacin dose; avoid in hepatic and renal impairment. [Severe] Study
- **Mitotane** is predicted to decrease the exposure to **solifenacin**. [Moderate] Theoretical
- Rifamycins **(rifampicin)** are predicted to decrease the exposure to **solifenacin**. [Moderate] Theoretical
- **Tucatinib** is predicted to increase the exposure to **solifenacin**. Adjust solifenacin p. 604 or tamsulosin with solifenacin dose; avoid in hepatic and renal impairment. [Severe] Study

Solriamfetol

- **Solriamfetol** is predicted to increase the risk of a hypertensive crisis when given with **MAO-B inhibitors**. Avoid and for 14 days after stopping **MAO-B inhibitors**. [Severe] Theoretical
- **Solriamfetol** is predicted to increase the risk of a hypertensive crisis when given with **MAOIs, irreversible**. Avoid and for 14 days after stopping the MAOI. [Severe] Theoretical

Somapacitan

- **Somapacitan** might increase blood glucose concentrations, opposing the blood glucose-lowering effects of **acarbose**. Adjust dose. [Moderate] Theoretical
- **Somapacitan** might decrease the exposure to antiepileptics **(carbamazepine)**. [Moderate] Theoretical
- **Somapacitan** might decrease the exposure to **ciclosporin**. [Severe] Theoretical
- **Corticosteroids** might decrease the efficacy of **somapacitan**. Monitor and adjust dose. [Moderate] Theoretical
- **Somapacitan** might increase blood glucose concentrations, opposing the blood glucose-lowering effects of **dipeptidylpeptidase-4 inhibitors**. Adjust dose. [Moderate] Theoretical
- **Somapacitan** might increase blood glucose concentrations, opposing the blood glucose-lowering effects of **glucagon-like peptide-1 receptor agonists**. Adjust dose. [Moderate] Theoretical
- **Somapacitan** might increase blood glucose concentrations, opposing the blood glucose-lowering effects of **insulin**. Adjust dose. [Moderate] Theoretical
- **Somapacitan** might increase blood glucose concentrations, opposing the blood glucose-lowering effects of **meglitinides**. Adjust dose. [Moderate] Theoretical
- **Somapacitan** might increase blood glucose concentrations, opposing the blood glucose-lowering effects of **metformin**. Adjust dose. [Moderate] Theoretical
- **Somapacitan** might increase blood glucose concentrations, opposing the blood glucose-lowering effects of **pioglitazone**. Adjust dose. [Moderate] Theoretical
- **Somapacitan** might increase blood glucose concentrations, opposing the blood glucose-lowering effects of **sodium glucose co-transporter 2 inhibitors**. Adjust dose. [Moderate] Theoretical
- **Somapacitan** might increase blood glucose concentrations, opposing the blood glucose-lowering effects of **sulfonylureas**. Adjust dose. [Moderate] Theoretical
- **Somapacitan** might decrease the concentration of **testosterone**. [Moderate] Theoretical
- **Somapacitan** might affect the efficacy of **thyroid hormones**. Monitor and adjust dose. [Moderate] Theoretical

Somatrogon

- **Somatrogon** might increase blood glucose concentrations, opposing the blood glucose-lowering effects of **acarbose**. Adjust dose. [Moderate] Theoretical
- **Somatrogon** might decrease the exposure to antiepileptics **(carbamazepine)**. [Moderate] Theoretical
- **Somatrogon** might decrease the exposure to **ciclosporin**. [Severe] Theoretical
- **Corticosteroids** might decrease the efficacy of **somatrogon**. Monitor and adjust dose. [Moderate] Theoretical
- **Somatrogon** might increase blood glucose concentrations, opposing the blood glucose-lowering effects of **dipeptidylpeptidase-4 inhibitors**. Adjust dose. [Moderate] Theoretical
- **Somatrogon** might increase blood glucose concentrations, opposing the blood glucose-lowering effects of **glucagon-like peptide-1 receptor agonists**. Adjust dose. [Moderate] Theoretical
- **Somatrogon** might increase blood glucose concentrations, opposing the blood glucose-lowering effects of **insulin**. Adjust dose. [Moderate] Theoretical
- **Somatrogon** might increase blood glucose concentrations, opposing the blood glucose-lowering effects of **meglitinides**. Adjust dose. [Moderate] Theoretical
- **Somatrogon** might increase blood glucose concentrations, opposing the blood glucose-lowering effects of **metformin**. Adjust dose. [Moderate] Theoretical
- **Somatrogon** might increase blood glucose concentrations, opposing the blood glucose-lowering effects of **pioglitazone**. Adjust dose. [Moderate] Theoretical

Somatrogon (continued)
- **Somatrogon** might increase blood glucose concentrations, opposing the blood glucose-lowering effects of **sodium glucose co-transporter 2 inhibitors**. Adjust dose. [Moderate] Theoretical
- **Somatrogon** might increase blood glucose concentrations, opposing the blood glucose-lowering effects of **sulfonylureas**. Adjust dose. [Moderate] Theoretical
- **Somatrogon** might decrease the concentration of **testosterone**. [Moderate] Theoretical
- **Somatrogon** might affect the efficacy of **thyroid hormones**. Adjust dose. [Moderate] Theoretical

Somatropin
- **Corticosteroids** are predicted to decrease the effects of **somatropin**. [Moderate] Theoretical

Sorafenib → see TABLE 3 p. 1053 (bleeding), TABLE 12 p. 1057 (myelosuppression), TABLE 7 p. 1055 (QT-interval prolongation)
- Anti-androgens **(apalutamide, enzalutamide)** are predicted to decrease the exposure to **sorafenib**. [Moderate] Theoretical → Also see TABLE 7 p. 1055
- Antiepileptics **(carbamazepine, eslicarbazepine, fosphenytoin, phenobarbital, phenytoin, primidone)** are predicted to decrease the exposure to **sorafenib**. [Moderate] Theoretical
- Antiepileptics **(oxcarbazepine)** are predicted to decrease the exposure to **sorafenib**. [Moderate] Study
- **Cenobamate** is predicted to decrease the exposure to **sorafenib**. [Moderate] Study
- **Dabrafenib** is predicted to decrease the exposure to **sorafenib**. [Moderate] Study
- **Encorafenib** is predicted to decrease the exposure to **sorafenib**. [Moderate] Theoretical → Also see TABLE 7 p. 1055
- Endothelin receptor antagonists **(bosentan)** are predicted to decrease the exposure to **sorafenib**. [Moderate] Study
- **Ivosidenib** is predicted to decrease the exposure to **sorafenib**. [Moderate] Theoretical → Also see TABLE 7 p. 1055
- **Linzagolix** is predicted to increase the exposure to **sorafenib**. Avoid. [Mild] Theoretical
- **Lorlatinib** is predicted to decrease the exposure to **sorafenib**. [Moderate] Study
- **Lumacaftor** is predicted to decrease the exposure to **sorafenib**. [Moderate] Theoretical
- **Mitotane** is predicted to decrease the exposure to **sorafenib**. [Moderate] Theoretical → Also see TABLE 12 p. 1057
- **Neomycin** moderately decreases the exposure to **sorafenib**. [Moderate] Study
- NNRTIs **(efavirenz, etravirine, nevirapine)** are predicted to decrease the exposure to **sorafenib**. [Moderate] Study → Also see TABLE 7 p. 1055
- Rifamycins **(rifampicin)** are predicted to decrease the exposure to **sorafenib**. [Moderate] Theoretical
- **Sorafenib** is predicted to increase the exposure to the active component of **sacituzumab govitecan**. [Severe] Theoretical
- **Selpercatinib** is predicted to increase the exposure to **sorafenib**. Avoid. [Severe] Study → Also see TABLE 7 p. 1055
- **Sotorasib** is predicted to decrease the exposure to **sorafenib**. [Moderate] Study
- **St John's wort** is predicted to decrease the exposure to **sorafenib**. [Moderate] Study

Sotalol → see beta blockers, non-selective

Sotorasib → see TABLE 1 p. 1053 (hepatotoxicity)
- Oral **antacids** are predicted to decrease the exposure to oral **sotorasib**. Manufacturer advises take 4 hours before or 10 hours after antacids. [Moderate] Theoretical
- Anti-androgens **(apalutamide, enzalutamide)** are predicted to decrease the exposure to **sotorasib**. Avoid. [Severe] Study
- **Sotorasib** is predicted to decrease the exposure to anti-androgens **(darolutamide)**. Avoid. [Moderate] Theoretical
- Antiepileptics **(carbamazepine, fosphenytoin, phenobarbital, phenytoin, primidone)** are predicted to decrease the exposure to **sotorasib**. Avoid. [Severe] Study
- **Sotorasib** is predicted to decrease the exposure to antifungals, azoles **(isavuconazole)**. Avoid. [Severe] Theoretical
- **Sotorasib** is predicted to decrease the exposure to atypical antipsychotics **(aripiprazole)**. Avoid or adjust dose—consult product literature. [Moderate] Study
- **Sotorasib** is predicted to decrease the exposure to atypical antipsychotics **(cariprazine)**. Avoid. [Severe] Theoretical
- **Sotorasib** is predicted to decrease the exposure to atypical antipsychotics **(lurasidone)**. Monitor and adjust dose. [Moderate] Theoretical
- **Sotorasib** is predicted to decrease the exposure to atypical antipsychotics **(quetiapine)**. [Moderate] Study
- **Sotorasib** is predicted to decrease the exposure to **avacopan**. [Severe] Theoretical
- **Sotorasib** is predicted to decrease the exposure to **avapritinib**. Avoid. [Severe] Study
- **Sotorasib** is predicted to decrease the exposure to **bedaquiline**. Avoid. [Severe] Study
- **Sotorasib** moderately decreases the exposure to benzodiazepines **(midazolam)**. [Moderate] Study
- **Sotorasib** is predicted to decrease the exposure to **bosutinib**. Avoid. [Severe] Study
- **Sotorasib** is predicted to decrease the exposure to **brigatinib**. Avoid or adjust dose—consult product literature. [Moderate] Study
- **Sotorasib** is predicted to decrease the exposure to **cabozantinib**. [Moderate] Study
- Oral calcium compounds **(calcium carbonate)** are predicted to decrease the exposure to oral **sotorasib**. Manufacturer advises take 4 hours before or 10 hours after antacids. [Moderate] Theoretical
- **Sotorasib** is predicted to decrease the exposure to calcium-channel blockers **(amlodipine, felodipine, lacidipine, lercanidipine, nicardipine, nifedipine, nimodipine)**. Monitor and adjust dose. [Moderate] Theoretical
- **Sotorasib** is predicted to decrease the exposure to calcium-channel blockers **(diltiazem, verapamil)**. [Moderate] Theoretical
- **Sotorasib** is predicted to decrease the exposure to **capivasertib**. Avoid. [Moderate] Study
- **Sotorasib** is predicted to decrease the exposure to **cobicistat**. Avoid. [Severe] Theoretical
- **Sotorasib** is predicted to decrease the exposure to **cobimetinib**. Avoid. [Severe] Theoretical
- **Sotorasib** is predicted to decrease the exposure to **crizotinib**. Avoid. [Severe] Study
- **Sotorasib** is predicted to decrease the exposure to **daridorexant**. [Severe] Study
- **Sotorasib** is predicted to decrease the exposure to **dasatinib**. [Severe] Study
- **Sotorasib** is predicted to decrease the exposure to **deutivacaftor**. Avoid. [Severe] Theoretical
- **Sotorasib** very slightly increases the exposure to **digoxin**. Avoid or adjust dose. [Moderate] Study
- **Sotorasib** is predicted to decrease the exposure to **elacestrant**. Avoid or adjust dose depending on duration—consult product literature. [Severe] Theoretical
- **Sotorasib** is predicted to moderately decrease the exposure to **elbasvir**. Avoid. [Severe] Study
- **Sotorasib** is predicted to decrease the concentration of **elvitegravir**. Avoid. [Severe] Theoretical
- **Encorafenib** is predicted to decrease the exposure to **sotorasib**. Avoid. [Severe] Study
- **Sotorasib** is predicted to decrease the exposure to **encorafenib**. [Moderate] Study
- **Sotorasib** is predicted to decrease the exposure to **entrectinib**. Avoid. [Moderate] Theoretical
- **Sotorasib** is predicted to decrease the exposure to **erdafitinib**. Adjust dose. [Moderate] Theoretical
- **Sotorasib** is predicted to decrease the exposure to **erlotinib**. [Severe] Study
- **Sotorasib** is predicted to decrease the concentration of **everolimus**. Avoid or adjust dose. [Severe] Study
- **Sotorasib** is predicted to decrease the exposure to **fedratinib**. Avoid. [Moderate] Study
- **Sotorasib** is predicted to decrease the exposure to **fruquintinib**. Avoid. [Moderate] Study
- **Sotorasib** is predicted to decrease the exposure to **gefitinib**. Avoid. [Severe] Study

A1 Interactions | Appendix 1

- **Sotorasib** is predicted to decrease the exposure to **glasdegib**. Avoid or adjust dose—consult product literature. Moderate Theoretical
- **Sotorasib** is predicted to decrease the exposure to **glecaprevir**. Avoid. Severe Study
- **Sotorasib** is predicted to markedly decrease the exposure to **grazoprevir**. Avoid. Severe Study
- **Sotorasib** is predicted to decrease the concentration of **guanfacine**. Adjust dose. Moderate Theoretical
- **H_2 receptor antagonists** are predicted to decrease the exposure to **sotorasib**. Manufacturer advises give **sotorasib** with an acidic beverage or use an antacid. Moderate Study
- **Sotorasib** is predicted to decrease the exposure to **idelalisib**. Avoid. Moderate Theoretical
- **Sotorasib** is predicted to decrease the exposure to **imatinib**. Moderate Study
- **Ivosidenib** is predicted to decrease the exposure to **sotorasib**. Avoid. Severe Study
- **Sotorasib** is predicted to decrease the exposure to **ixazomib**. Moderate Theoretical
- **Sotorasib** is predicted to decrease the exposure to **lapatinib**. Avoid. Severe Study
- **Sotorasib** is predicted to decrease the exposure to **larotrectinib**. Avoid. Moderate Study
- **Sotorasib** is predicted to decrease the exposure to **lenacapavir**. Avoid. Severe Study
- **Sotorasib** is predicted to decrease the exposure to **leniolisib**. Avoid. Severe Theoretical
- **Lumacaftor** is predicted to decrease the exposure to **sotorasib**. Avoid. Severe Study
- **Sotorasib** is predicted to decrease the exposure to **mavacamten**. Monitor and adjust dose—consult product literature. Severe Theoretical
- **Sotorasib** is predicted to decrease the exposure to **mifepristone**. Adjust **mifepristone** dose. Severe Study
- **Sotorasib** is predicted to decrease the exposure to mineralocorticoid receptor antagonists **(finerenone)**. Avoid. Severe Study
- **Mitotane** is predicted to decrease the exposure to **sotorasib**. Avoid. Severe Study
- **Sotorasib** is predicted to decrease the exposure to **naloxegol**. Moderate Theoretical
- **Sotorasib** is predicted to decrease the exposure to **neratinib**. Avoid. Severe Theoretical → Also see **TABLE 1** p. 1053
- **Sotorasib** is predicted to decrease the exposure to neurokinin-1 receptor antagonists **(netupitant)**. Moderate Theoretical
- **Sotorasib** is predicted to decrease the exposure to **nilotinib**. Avoid. Severe Theoretical
- **Sotorasib** is predicted to decrease the exposure to NNRTIs **(rilpivirine)**. Avoid. Severe Theoretical
- **Sotorasib** is predicted to decrease the exposure to **olaparib**. Avoid. Moderate Theoretical
- **Sotorasib** is predicted to decrease the exposure to **omaveloxolone**. Avoid. Severe Study
- **Sotorasib** is predicted to decrease the exposure to opioids **(alfentanil)**. Avoid or adjust dose. Moderate Theoretical
- **Sotorasib** decreases the exposure to opioids **(methadone)**. Monitor and adjust dose. Severe Study
- **Sotorasib** is predicted to decrease the exposure to **ospemifene**. Moderate Study
- **Sotorasib** is predicted to decrease the exposure to **pazopanib**. Severe Study
- **Sotorasib** is predicted to decrease the exposure to **pemigatinib**. Avoid or monitor. Severe Study
- **Sotorasib** is predicted to decrease the exposure to **pibrentasvir**. Avoid. Severe Study
- **Sotorasib** is predicted to decrease the exposure to **pirtobrutinib**. Moderate Theoretical
- **Sotorasib** is predicted to decrease the exposure to **ponatinib**. Severe Study
- **Sotorasib** is predicted to decrease the exposure to **pralsetinib**. Moderate Theoretical
- **Proton pump inhibitors** are predicted to decrease the exposure to **sotorasib**. Manufacturer advises give **sotorasib** with an acidic beverage or use an antacid. Moderate Study
- **Sotorasib** is predicted to decrease the exposure to **quizartinib**. Avoid. Severe Study
- Rifamycins **(rifampicin)** are predicted to decrease the exposure to **sotorasib**. Avoid. Severe Study
- **Sotorasib** is predicted to decrease the exposure to **rimegepant**. Avoid. Moderate Theoretical
- **Sotorasib** is predicted to decrease the exposure to **ripretinib**. Avoid or adjust dose—consult product literature. Moderate Theoretical
- **Sotorasib** is predicted to decrease the exposure to **ruxolitinib**. Monitor and adjust dose. Moderate Study
- **Sotorasib** is predicted to decrease the exposure to **selpercatinib**. Moderate Study
- **Sotorasib** is predicted to decrease the exposure to **selumetinib**. Avoid. Severe Study
- **Sotorasib** is predicted to decrease the exposure to **siponimod**. Manufacturer advises caution depending on genotype—consult product literature. Moderate Theoretical
- **Sotorasib** is predicted to decrease the exposure to **sirolimus**. Avoid or adjust dose. Severe Theoretical
- Oral **sodium bicarbonate** is predicted to decrease the exposure to oral **sotorasib**. Manufacturer advises take 4 hours before or 10 hours after antacids. Moderate Theoretical
- **Sotorasib** is predicted to decrease the exposure to **sorafenib**. Moderate Study
- **Sotorasib** is predicted to decrease the exposure to **sparsentan**. Avoid. Severe Theoretical
- **Sotorasib** is predicted to decrease the exposure to statins **(atorvastatin, simvastatin)**. Moderate Study → Also see **TABLE 1** p. 1053
- **Sotorasib** is predicted to increase the exposure to statins **(fluvastatin, rosuvastatin)**. Monitor and adjust dose. Moderate Study → Also see **TABLE 1** p. 1053
- **Sotorasib** is predicted to increase the exposure to **sulfasalazine**. Monitor and adjust dose. Moderate Study
- **Sotorasib** is predicted to decrease the exposure to **sunitinib**. Moderate Study
- **Sotorasib** is predicted to decrease the exposure to **tacrolimus**. Monitor and adjust dose. Severe Theoretical
- **Sotorasib** is predicted to decrease the exposure to taxanes **(docetaxel)**. Severe Theoretical
- **Sotorasib** is predicted to decrease the exposure to taxanes **(paclitaxel)**. Avoid. Severe Study
- **Sotorasib** is predicted to decrease the concentration of **temsirolimus**. Avoid. Moderate Theoretical
- **Sotorasib** is predicted to decrease the exposure to **tezacaftor**. Avoid. Severe Theoretical
- **Sotorasib** is predicted to decrease the exposure to **ticagrelor**. Moderate Theoretical
- **Sotorasib** is predicted to decrease the exposure to **tofacitinib**. Severe Study
- **Sotorasib** is predicted to decrease the exposure to **vanzacaftor**. Avoid. Severe Theoretical
- **Sotorasib** is predicted to decrease the exposure to **velpatasvir**. Avoid. Moderate Theoretical
- **Sotorasib** is predicted to decrease the exposure to **venetoclax**. Avoid. Severe Study
- **Sotorasib** is predicted to decrease the concentration of **voxilaprevir**. Avoid. Severe Theoretical
- **Sotorasib** is predicted to decrease the exposure to **zanubrutinib**. Avoid or adjust dose with moderate CYP3A4 inducers—consult product literature. Severe Theoretical

Sparsentan → see **TABLE 6** p. 1054 (hypotension), **TABLE 13** p. 1057 (increased serum potassium)

- **Sparsentan** is predicted to increase the exposure to **aliskiren**. Avoid. Severe Theoretical → Also see **TABLE 6** p. 1054 → Also see **TABLE 13** p. 1057
- Anti-androgens **(apalutamide, enzalutamide)** are predicted to decrease the exposure to **sparsentan**. Avoid. Severe Theoretical
- Antiarrhythmics **(dronedarone)** are predicted to increase the exposure to **sparsentan**. Moderate Study
- Antiepileptics **(carbamazepine, fosphenytoin, phenobarbital, phenytoin, primidone)** are predicted to decrease the exposure to **sparsentan**. Avoid. Severe Theoretical

Sparsentan (continued)
- Antifungals, azoles **(fluconazole, isavuconazole)** are predicted to increase the exposure to **sparsentan**. Moderate Study
- Antifungals, azoles **(itraconazole, ketoconazole, posaconazole, voriconazole)** are predicted to increase the exposure to **sparsentan**. Avoid. Severe Study
- **Sparsentan** is predicted to increase the exposure to antihistamines, non-sedating **(fexofenadine)**. Severe Theoretical
- **Sparsentan** is predicted to decrease the exposure to **avatrombopag**. Moderate Theoretical
- **Sparsentan** is predicted to increase the exposure to benzodiazepines **(diazepam)**. Moderate Theoretical
- **Berotralstat** is predicted to increase the exposure to **sparsentan**. Moderate Study
- Calcium-channel blockers **(diltiazem, verapamil)** are predicted to increase the exposure to **sparsentan**. Moderate Study → Also see TABLE 6 p. 1054
- **Cenobamate** is predicted to decrease the exposure to **sparsentan**. Avoid. Severe Theoretical
- **Ceritinib** is predicted to increase the exposure to **sparsentan**. Avoid. Severe Study
- **Ciclosporin** slightly increases the exposure to **sparsentan**. Moderate Study → Also see TABLE 13 p. 1057
- **Cobicistat** is predicted to increase the exposure to **sparsentan**. Avoid. Severe Study
- **Sparsentan** is predicted to increase the exposure to **colchicine**. Severe Theoretical
- Corticosteroids **(dexamethasone)** are predicted to decrease the exposure to **sparsentan**. Avoid. Severe Theoretical
- **Sparsentan** is predicted to decrease the exposure to coumarins **(warfarin)**. Moderate Theoretical
- **Crizotinib** is predicted to increase the exposure to **sparsentan**. Moderate Study
- **Dabrafenib** is predicted to decrease the exposure to **sparsentan**. Avoid. Severe Theoretical
- **Sparsentan** is predicted to increase the exposure to **digoxin**. Severe Theoretical
- **Encorafenib** is predicted to decrease the exposure to **sparsentan**. Avoid. Severe Theoretical
- Endothelin receptor antagonists **(bosentan)** are predicted to decrease the exposure to **sparsentan**. Avoid. Severe Theoretical
- **Sparsentan** is predicted to increase the exposure to **everolimus**. Severe Theoretical
- **Sparsentan** is predicted to increase the exposure to factor XA inhibitors **(edoxaban)**. Severe Theoretical
- **Fedratinib** is predicted to increase the exposure to **sparsentan**. Moderate Study
- **Grapefruit** is predicted to increase the exposure to **sparsentan**. Avoid. Severe Theoretical
- **HIV-protease inhibitors** are predicted to increase the exposure to **sparsentan**. Avoid. Severe Study
- **Idelalisib** is predicted to increase the exposure to **sparsentan**. Avoid. Severe Study
- **Imatinib** is predicted to increase the exposure to **sparsentan**. Moderate Study
- **Ivosidenib** is predicted to decrease the exposure to **sparsentan**. Avoid. Severe Theoretical
- **Letermovir** is predicted to increase the exposure to **sparsentan**. Moderate Study
- **Sparsentan** might increase the concentration of **lithium**. Severe Theoretical
- **Sparsentan** is predicted to increase the exposure to **loperamide**. Severe Theoretical
- **Lorlatinib** is predicted to decrease the exposure to **sparsentan**. Avoid. Severe Theoretical
- **Lumacaftor** is predicted to decrease the exposure to **sparsentan**. Avoid. Severe Theoretical
- Macrolides **(clarithromycin)** are predicted to increase the exposure to **sparsentan**. Avoid. Severe Study
- Macrolides **(erythromycin)** are predicted to increase the exposure to **sparsentan**. Moderate Study
- **Mitotane** is predicted to decrease the exposure to **sparsentan**. Avoid. Severe Theoretical
- **Sparsentan** is predicted to decrease the exposure to **moclobemide**. Moderate Theoretical
- Neurokinin-1 receptor antagonists **(aprepitant, netupitant)** are predicted to increase the exposure to **sparsentan**. Moderate Study
- **Nilotinib** is predicted to increase the exposure to **sparsentan**. Moderate Study
- NNRTIs **(efavirenz, etravirine, nevirapine)** are predicted to decrease the exposure to **sparsentan**. Avoid. Severe Theoretical
- **Sparsentan** is predicted to decrease the exposure to NSAIDs **(celecoxib, ibuprofen)**. Moderate Theoretical → Also see TABLE 13 p. 1057
- **Sparsentan** is predicted to increase the exposure to **pralsetinib**. Severe Theoretical
- **Sparsentan** is predicted to decrease the exposure to proton pump inhibitors **(lansoprazole, omeprazole, rabeprazole)**. Moderate Theoretical
- **Sparsentan** is predicted to increase the exposure to **ranolazine**. Severe Theoretical
- Rifamycins **(rifampicin)** are predicted to decrease the exposure to **sparsentan**. Avoid. Severe Theoretical
- **Sparsentan** is predicted to increase the exposure to **rimegepant**. Severe Theoretical
- **Sparsentan** is predicted to decrease the exposure to **siponimod**. Moderate Theoretical
- **Sparsentan** is predicted to increase the exposure to **sirolimus**. Severe Theoretical
- **Sotorasib** is predicted to decrease the exposure to **sparsentan**. Avoid. Severe Theoretical
- **Sparsentan** is predicted to decrease the exposure to SSRIs **(citalopram)**. Moderate Theoretical
- **St John's wort** is predicted to decrease the exposure to **sparsentan**. Avoid. Severe Theoretical
- **Sparsentan** is predicted to increase the exposure to statins **(atorvastatin, fluvastatin, rosuvastatin)**. Moderate Theoretical
- **Sparsentan** is predicted to increase the exposure to **sulfasalazine**. Moderate Theoretical
- **Sparsentan** is predicted to decrease the exposure to sulfonylureas **(glimepiride, tolbutamide)**. Moderate Theoretical
- **Sparsentan** is predicted to increase the exposure to **talazoparib**. Severe Theoretical
- **Sparsentan** is predicted to increase the exposure to taxanes **(paclitaxel)**. Severe Theoretical
- **Sparsentan** is predicted to increase the exposure to thrombin inhibitors **(dabigatran)**. Severe Theoretical
- **Sparsentan** is predicted to increase the exposure to **topotecan**. Moderate Theoretical
- **Tucatinib** is predicted to increase the exposure to **sparsentan**. Avoid. Severe Study

Spesolimab → see monoclonal antibodies

Spironolactone → see mineralocorticoid receptor antagonists

SSRIs → see TABLE 3 p. 1053 (bleeding), TABLE 15 p. 1058 (hyponatraemia), TABLE 11 p. 1056 (serotonin toxicity), TABLE 7 p. 1055 (QT-interval prolongation), TABLE 9 p. 1056 (CNS effects)

citalopram · dapoxetine · escitalopram · fluoxetine · fluvoxamine · paroxetine · sertraline

- SSRIs **(fluoxetine, fluvoxamine)** are predicted to increase the exposure to **abrocitinib**. Adjust **abrocitinib** dose, p. 926. Severe Study
- **Fluvoxamine** very markedly increases the exposure to **agomelatine**. Avoid. Severe Study → Also see TABLE 9 p. 1056
- SSRIs **(fluoxetine, paroxetine)** are predicted to increase the exposure to **amfetamines**. Severe Theoretical → Also see TABLE 11 p. 1056
- **Fluvoxamine** moderately to markedly increases the exposure to **aminophylline**. Avoid. Severe Study
- **Fluvoxamine** decreases the clearance of anaesthetics, local **(ropivacaine)**. Avoid prolonged use. Moderate Study
- **Fluvoxamine** is predicted to increase the exposure to **anagrelide**. Moderate Theoretical → Also see TABLE 3 p. 1053
- Anti-androgens **(apalutamide)** are predicted to decrease the exposure to **citalopram**. Avoid or monitor. Mild Study → Also see TABLE 7 p. 1055
- Antiarrhythmics **(dronedarone)** are predicted to increase the exposure to **dapoxetine**. Adjust **dapoxetine** dose with moderate CYP3A4 inhibitors. Moderate Theoretical

- Antiarrhythmics **(dronedarone)** are predicted to increase the exposure to **sertraline**. Moderate Theoretical
- Antiarrhythmics **(dronedarone)** are predicted to increase the exposure to SSRIs **(citalopram, escitalopram, fluoxetine, fluvoxamine, paroxetine)**. Severe Theoretical → Also see **TABLE 7** p. 1055
- **Fluvoxamine** is predicted to increase the exposure to antiarrhythmics **(propafenone)**. Monitor and adjust dose. Moderate Study
- SSRIs **(fluoxetine, paroxetine)** are predicted to increase the exposure to anticholinesterases, centrally acting **(galantamine)**. Monitor and adjust dose. Moderate Study
- Antiepileptics **(fosphenytoin, phenytoin)** decrease the concentration of **paroxetine**. Moderate Study → Also see **TABLE 9** p. 1056
- SSRIs **(fluoxetine, fluvoxamine)** increase the exposure to antiepileptics **(carbamazepine)**. Adjust dose or monitor. Moderate Study → Also see **TABLE 15** p. 1058
- **Sertraline** potentially increases the risk of toxicity when given with antiepileptics **(fosphenytoin, phenytoin)**. Monitor concentration and adjust dose. Severe Anecdotal → Also see **TABLE 9** p. 1056
- SSRIs **(fluoxetine, fluvoxamine)** are predicted to increase the concentration of antiepileptics **(fosphenytoin, phenytoin)**. Monitor and adjust dose. Severe Anecdotal → Also see **TABLE 9** p. 1056
- Antifungals, azoles **(fluconazole, isavuconazole)** are predicted to increase the exposure to **dapoxetine**. Adjust **dapoxetine** dose with moderate CYP3A4 inhibitors. Moderate Theoretical
- Antifungals, azoles **(fluconazole, isavuconazole)** are predicted to increase the exposure to **sertraline**. Moderate Theoretical
- Antifungals, azoles **(fluconazole, voriconazole)** are predicted to increase the exposure to **escitalopram**. Use with caution and adjust dose. Severe Study → Also see **TABLE 7** p. 1055
- Antifungals, azoles **(itraconazole, ketoconazole, posaconazole, voriconazole)** are predicted to moderately increase the exposure to **dapoxetine**. Avoid potent CYP3A4 inhibitors or adjust **dapoxetine** dose. Severe Study
- Antifungals, azoles **(itraconazole, ketoconazole, posaconazole, voriconazole)** are predicted to increase the exposure to **sertraline**. Avoid. Moderate Theoretical
- Antifungals, azoles **(voriconazole)** are predicted to increase the exposure to **citalopram**. Severe Theoretical → Also see **TABLE 7** p. 1055
- Antihistamines, sedating **(cyproheptadine)** potentially decrease the effects of **SSRIs**. Moderate Anecdotal → Also see **TABLE 9** p. 1056
- SSRIs **(fluoxetine, paroxetine)** are predicted to markedly increase the exposure to **atomoxetine**. Adjust dose. Severe Study
- SSRIs **(fluoxetine, paroxetine)** are predicted to moderately increase the exposure to atypical antipsychotics **(aripiprazole)**. Avoid or adjust dose—consult product literature. Moderate Study → Also see **TABLE 15** p. 1058 → Also see **TABLE 9** p. 1056
- **Fluvoxamine** increases the exposure to atypical antipsychotics **(asenapine)**. Moderate Study → Also see **TABLE 15** p. 1058 → Also see **TABLE 9** p. 1056
- **Paroxetine** moderately increases the exposure to atypical antipsychotics **(asenapine)**. Moderate Study → Also see **TABLE 15** p. 1058 → Also see **TABLE 9** p. 1056
- **Fluvoxamine** increases the concentration of atypical antipsychotics **(clozapine)**. Monitor adverse effects and adjust dose. Severe Study → Also see **TABLE 15** p. 1058 → Also see **TABLE 9** p. 1056
- SSRIs **(fluoxetine, paroxetine)** are predicted to increase the exposure to atypical antipsychotics **(clozapine)**. Use with caution and adjust dose. Severe Study → Also see **TABLE 15** p. 1058 → Also see **TABLE 9** p. 1056
- **Fluvoxamine** moderately increases the exposure to atypical antipsychotics **(olanzapine)**. Adjust dose. Severe Anecdotal → Also see **TABLE 15** p. 1058 → Also see **TABLE 9** p. 1056
- SSRIs **(fluoxetine, paroxetine)** are predicted to increase the exposure to atypical antipsychotics **(risperidone)**. Adjust dose. Moderate Study → Also see **TABLE 15** p. 1058 → Also see **TABLE 9** p. 1056
- SSRIs **(fluoxetine, fluvoxamine)** are predicted to increase the exposure to **belzutifan**. Monitor and adjust dose. Severe Theoretical
- **Fluvoxamine** moderately increases the exposure to benzodiazepines **(alprazolam)**. Adjust dose. Moderate Study → Also see **TABLE 9** p. 1056
- SSRIs **(fluoxetine, fluvoxamine)** potentially increase the exposure to benzodiazepines **(clobazam)**. Adjust dose. Moderate Theoretical → Also see **TABLE 9** p. 1056
- **Fluvoxamine** moderately increases the exposure to benzodiazepines **(diazepam)**. Moderate Study → Also see **TABLE 9** p. 1056
- **Berotralstat** is predicted to increase the exposure to **dapoxetine**. Adjust **dapoxetine** dose with moderate CYP3A4 inhibitors. Moderate Theoretical
- **Berotralstat** is predicted to increase the exposure to **sertraline**. Moderate Theoretical
- **Fluvoxamine** moderately increases the concentration of beta blockers, non-selective **(propranolol)**. Moderate Study
- SSRIs **(fluoxetine, paroxetine)** are predicted to increase the exposure to beta blockers, selective **(metoprolol, nebivolol)**. Moderate Study
- **Bupropion** is predicted to increase the exposure to **dapoxetine**. Moderate Theoretical
- **Fluvoxamine** markedly decreases the clearance of **caffeine citrate**. Monitor and adjust dose. Severe Study
- Calcium-channel blockers **(diltiazem, verapamil)** are predicted to increase the exposure to **dapoxetine**. Adjust **dapoxetine** dose with moderate CYP3A4 inhibitors. Moderate Theoretical
- Calcium-channel blockers **(diltiazem, verapamil)** are predicted to increase the exposure to **sertraline**. Moderate Theoretical
- SSRIs **(fluoxetine, fluvoxamine)** are predicted to increase the exposure to **cannabidiol**. Moderate Theoretical → Also see **TABLE 9** p. 1056
- **Fluvoxamine** is predicted to increase the exposure to **capivasertib**. Adjust dose. Moderate Theoretical
- **Cenobamate** is predicted to increase the exposure to **escitalopram**. Use with caution and adjust dose. Severe Study → Also see **TABLE 9** p. 1056
- **Ceritinib** is predicted to moderately increase the exposure to **dapoxetine**. Avoid potent CYP3A4 inhibitors or adjust **dapoxetine** dose. Severe Study
- **Ceritinib** is predicted to increase the exposure to **sertraline**. Avoid. Moderate Theoretical
- SSRIs **(fluoxetine, fluvoxamine)** are predicted to increase the exposure to **cilostazol**. Adjust **cilostazol** dose. Moderate Theoretical → Also see **TABLE 3** p. 1053
- **Cinacalcet** is predicted to increase the exposure to **dapoxetine**. Moderate Theoretical
- **Fluvoxamine** is predicted to increase the exposure to **cinacalcet**. Adjust dose. Moderate Theoretical
- SSRIs **(fluoxetine, fluvoxamine)** are predicted to decrease the efficacy of **clopidogrel**. Avoid. Severe Theoretical → Also see **TABLE 3** p. 1053
- **Cobicistat** is predicted to moderately increase the exposure to **dapoxetine**. Avoid potent CYP3A4 inhibitors or adjust **dapoxetine** dose. Severe Study
- **Cobicistat** is predicted to increase the exposure to **sertraline**. Avoid. Moderate Theoretical
- **Cobicistat** is predicted to increase the exposure to SSRIs **(citalopram, escitalopram, fluoxetine, fluvoxamine, paroxetine)**. Monitor and adjust dose. Moderate Theoretical
- **Crizotinib** is predicted to increase the exposure to **dapoxetine**. Adjust **dapoxetine** dose with moderate CYP3A4 inhibitors. Moderate Theoretical
- **Crizotinib** is predicted to increase the exposure to **sertraline**. Moderate Theoretical
- **Dacomitinib** is predicted to increase the exposure to **dapoxetine**. Moderate Theoretical
- SSRIs **(fluoxetine, paroxetine)** are predicted to slightly increase the exposure to **darifenacin**. Mild Study
- **Fluvoxamine** is predicted to increase the exposure to dopamine receptor agonists **(ropinirole)**. Adjust dose. Moderate Study → Also see **TABLE 9** p. 1056

A1

Interactions | **Appendix 1**

SSRIs (continued)

- **Fluvoxamine** is predicted to increase the exposure to **elacestrant**. Avoid or adjust **elacestrant** dose. [Severe] Theoretical
- SSRIs **(fluoxetine, paroxetine)** are predicted to increase the exposure to **eliglustat**. Avoid or adjust dose—consult product literature. [Severe] Study
- **Fluvoxamine** is predicted to increase the exposure to **eltrombopag**. [Moderate] Theoretical
- **Fluvoxamine** is predicted to increase the exposure to **erlotinib**. Monitor adverse effects and adjust dose. [Moderate] Theoretical
- **Fedratinib** is predicted to increase the exposure to **dapoxetine**. Adjust **dapoxetine** dose with moderate CYP3A4 inhibitors. [Moderate] Theoretical
- **Fedratinib** is predicted to increase the exposure to **escitalopram**. Use with caution and adjust dose. [Severe] Study
- **Fluoxetine** is predicted to increase the exposure to **fedratinib**. Avoid depending on other drugs taken—consult product literature. [Moderate] Theoretical
- **Fluvoxamine** is predicted to increase the exposure to **fedratinib**. Avoid. [Moderate] Theoretical
- **Fedratinib** is predicted to increase the exposure to **sertraline**. [Moderate] Theoretical
- **Fluvoxamine** moderately increases the exposure to **fenfluramine**. [Moderate] Study → Also see **TABLE 11** p. 1056
- SSRIs **(fluoxetine, paroxetine)** are predicted to increase the exposure to **fenfluramine**. [Moderate] Study → Also see **TABLE 11** p. 1056
- SSRIs **(fluoxetine, paroxetine)** are predicted to increase the exposure to **fesoterodine**. Use with caution and adjust dose. [Mild] Theoretical
- **Fluvoxamine** is predicted to increase the exposure to **fezolinetant**. Avoid. [Moderate] Study
- SSRIs **(fluoxetine, paroxetine)** are predicted to increase the exposure to **gefitinib**. [Moderate] Theoretical
- **Gilteritinib** is predicted to decrease the efficacy of SSRIs **(escitalopram, fluoxetine, sertraline)**. Avoid. [Moderate] Theoretical
- **Grapefruit** juice moderately increases the exposure to **sertraline**. Avoid. [Moderate] Study
- H_2 receptor antagonists **(cimetidine)** slightly increase the exposure to SSRIs **(citalopram, escitalopram)**. Adjust dose. [Moderate] Study
- H_2 receptor antagonists **(cimetidine)** slightly increase the exposure to SSRIs **(paroxetine, sertraline)**. [Moderate] Study
- **Fluoxetine** increases the concentration of **haloperidol**. Adjust dose. [Moderate] Anecdotal → Also see **TABLE 15** p. 1058 → Also see **TABLE 9** p. 1056
- **Fluvoxamine** increases the concentration of **haloperidol**. Adjust dose. [Moderate] Study → Also see **TABLE 15** p. 1058 → Also see **TABLE 9** p. 1056
- **HIV-protease inhibitors** are predicted to moderately increase the exposure to **dapoxetine**. Avoid potent CYP3A4 inhibitors or adjust **dapoxetine** dose. [Severe] Study
- **HIV-protease inhibitors** are predicted to increase the exposure to **sertraline**. Avoid. [Moderate] Theoretical
- **Idelalisib** is predicted to moderately increase the exposure to **dapoxetine**. Avoid potent CYP3A4 inhibitors or adjust **dapoxetine** dose. [Severe] Study
- **Idelalisib** is predicted to increase the exposure to **sertraline**. Avoid. [Moderate] Theoretical
- **Imatinib** is predicted to increase the exposure to **dapoxetine**. Adjust **dapoxetine** dose with moderate CYP3A4 inhibitors. [Moderate] Theoretical → Also see **TABLE 3** p. 1053
- **Imatinib** is predicted to increase the exposure to **sertraline**. [Moderate] Theoretical → Also see **TABLE 3** p. 1053
- **Letermovir** is predicted to increase the exposure to **dapoxetine**. Adjust **dapoxetine** dose with moderate CYP3A4 inhibitors. [Moderate] Theoretical
- **Letermovir** is predicted to increase the exposure to **sertraline**. [Moderate] Theoretical
- **Fluoxetine** is predicted to increase the exposure to **lomitapide**. Separate administration by 12 hours. [Unknown] Theoretical
- **Fluvoxamine** is predicted to increase the exposure to **lomitapide**. Separate administration by 12 hours. [Mild] Theoretical
- **Fluvoxamine** is predicted to increase the exposure to **loxapine**. Avoid. [Unknown] Theoretical → Also see **TABLE 15** p. 1058 → Also see **TABLE 9** p. 1056
- Macrolides **(clarithromycin)** are predicted to moderately increase the exposure to **dapoxetine**. Avoid potent CYP3A4 inhibitors or adjust **dapoxetine** dose. [Severe] Study
- Macrolides **(clarithromycin)** are predicted to increase the exposure to **sertraline**. Avoid. [Moderate] Theoretical
- Macrolides **(erythromycin)** are predicted to increase the exposure to **dapoxetine**. Adjust **dapoxetine** dose with moderate CYP3A4 inhibitors. [Moderate] Theoretical
- Macrolides **(erythromycin)** are predicted to increase the exposure to **sertraline**. [Moderate] Theoretical
- **Fluoxetine** is predicted to increase the exposure to **mavacamten**. Adjust dose—consult product literature. [Severe] Theoretical
- **Fluvoxamine** is predicted to increase the exposure to **mavacamten**. Monitor and adjust dose—consult product literature. [Moderate] Theoretical
- **Fluvoxamine** very markedly increases the exposure to **melatonin**. Avoid. [Severe] Study → Also see **TABLE 9** p. 1056
- SSRIs **(fluoxetine, fluvoxamine, paroxetine)** are predicted to increase the exposure to **mexiletine**. [Moderate] Study
- **Moclobemide** is predicted to increase the exposure to **escitalopram**. Use with caution and adjust dose. [Severe] Study → Also see **TABLE 11** p. 1056
- Neurokinin-1 receptor antagonists **(aprepitant, netupitant)** are predicted to increase the exposure to **dapoxetine**. Adjust **dapoxetine** dose with moderate CYP3A4 inhibitors. [Moderate] Theoretical
- Neurokinin-1 receptor antagonists **(aprepitant, netupitant)** are predicted to increase the exposure to **sertraline**. [Moderate] Theoretical
- **SSRIs** potentially increase the risk of prolonged neuromuscular blockade when given with neuromuscular blocking drugs, non-depolarising **(mivacurium)**. [Unknown] Theoretical
- **Nilotinib** is predicted to increase the exposure to **dapoxetine**. Adjust **dapoxetine** dose with moderate CYP3A4 inhibitors. [Moderate] Theoretical
- **Nilotinib** is predicted to increase the exposure to **sertraline**. [Moderate] Theoretical
- **Fluvoxamine** is predicted to increase the exposure to **omaveloxolone**. Avoid or adjust **omaveloxolone** dose, p. 755. [Moderate] Theoretical
- SSRIs **(fluoxetine, paroxetine)** are predicted to decrease the efficacy of opioids **(codeine)**. [Moderate] Theoretical → Also see **TABLE 9** p. 1056
- SSRIs **(fluoxetine, paroxetine)** are predicted to decrease the efficacy of opioids **(tramadol)**. [Severe] Study → Also see **TABLE 15** p. 1058 → Also see **TABLE 11** p. 1056 → Also see **TABLE 9** p. 1056
- **SSRIs** might increase the risk of adverse effects when given with **ozanimod**. [Severe] Theoretical
- **Fluvoxamine** is predicted to increase the exposure to **pentoxifylline**. [Moderate] Theoretical
- **Fluvoxamine** is predicted to increase the exposure to phenothiazine antipsychotics **(chlorpromazine)**. [Moderate] Theoretical → Also see **TABLE 15** p. 1058 → Also see **TABLE 9** p. 1056
- **Fluvoxamine** is predicted to increase the exposure to phosphodiesterase type-4 inhibitors **(roflumilast)**. [Moderate] Study
- **Fluvoxamine** is predicted to moderately increase the exposure to **pirfenidone**. Avoid. [Moderate] Study
- SSRIs **(fluoxetine, paroxetine)** are predicted to moderately increase the exposure to **pitolisant**. Use with caution and adjust dose. [Moderate] Study
- **Fluvoxamine** moderately increases the exposure to **pomalidomide**. Adjust dose—consult product literature. [Moderate] Study
- **Paroxetine** slightly increases the exposure to **procyclidine**. Monitor and adjust dose. [Moderate] Study → Also see **TABLE 9** p. 1056
- Proton pump inhibitors **(esomeprazole)** increase the exposure to **citalopram**. Monitor and adjust dose. [Severe] Theoretical
- Proton pump inhibitors **(esomeprazole)** might increase the concentration of **sertraline**. [Moderate] Study

Interactions | **Appendix 1**

A1

- Proton pump inhibitors **(esomeprazole, omeprazole)** are predicted to increase the exposure to **escitalopram**. Use with caution and adjust dose. [Severe] Study
- Proton pump inhibitors **(omeprazole)** moderately increase the exposure to **citalopram**. Monitor and adjust dose. [Severe] Study
- Rifamycins **(rifampicin)** are predicted to decrease the exposure to SSRIs **(citalopram, sertraline)**. [Moderate] Anecdotal
- **Fluvoxamine** is predicted to increase the exposure to **riluzole**. [Moderate] Theoretical
- **Fluoxetine** is predicted to increase the exposure to **selumetinib**. Avoid or adjust dose—consult product literature. [Severe] Theoretical
- **Fluvoxamine** is predicted to increase the exposure to **selumetinib**. Avoid or monitor—consult product literature. [Severe] Theoretical
- **Fluvoxamine** markedly increases the exposure to SNRIs **(duloxetine)**. Avoid. [Severe] Study → Also see **TABLE 3** p. 1053 → Also see **TABLE 15** p. 1058 → Also see **TABLE 11** p. 1056 → Also see **TABLE 9** p. 1056
- **Sparsentan** is predicted to decrease the exposure to **citalopram**. [Moderate] Theoretical
- SSRIs **(fluvoxamine)** are predicted to increase the exposure to SSRIs **(citalopram)**. Monitor and adjust dose. [Severe] Anecdotal → Also see **TABLE 3** p. 1053 → Also see **TABLE 15** p. 1058 → Also see **TABLE 11** p. 1056 → Also see **TABLE 9** p. 1056
- SSRIs **(fluoxetine, paroxetine)** are predicted to increase the exposure to SSRIs **(dapoxetine)**. [Moderate] Theoretical → Also see **TABLE 3** p. 1053 → Also see **TABLE 11** p. 1056 → Also see **TABLE 9** p. 1056
- SSRIs **(fluoxetine, fluvoxamine)** are predicted to increase the exposure to SSRIs **(escitalopram)**. Use with caution and adjust dose. [Severe] Study → Also see **TABLE 3** p. 1053 → Also see **TABLE 15** p. 1058 → Also see **TABLE 11** p. 1056 → Also see **TABLE 9** p. 1056
- **SSRIs** potentially increase the risk of prolonged neuromuscular blockade when given with **suxamethonium**. [Unknown] Theoretical
- **Fluvoxamine** very slightly increases the exposure to **talazoparib**. [Moderate] Study
- SSRIs **(fluoxetine, paroxetine)** are predicted to decrease the efficacy of **tamoxifen**. Avoid. [Severe] Study
- **Terbinafine** is predicted to increase the exposure to **fluoxetine**. Adjust dose. [Moderate] Theoretical
- **Terbinafine** moderately increases the exposure to **paroxetine**. [Moderate] Study
- **Terbinafine** is predicted to increase the exposure to SSRIs **(citalopram, dapoxetine, escitalopram, fluvoxamine, sertraline)**. [Moderate] Theoretical
- SSRIs **(fluoxetine, paroxetine)** are predicted to increase the exposure to the active metabolite of **tetrabenazine**. [Moderate] Study → Also see **TABLE 9** p. 1056
- **Fluvoxamine** moderately to markedly increases the exposure to **theophylline**. Avoid. [Severe] Study
- **Fluvoxamine** very markedly increases the exposure to **tizanidine**. Avoid. [Severe] Study → Also see **TABLE 9** p. 1056
- SSRIs **(fluoxetine, fluvoxamine)** given with a moderate CYP3A4 inhibitor are predicted to increase the exposure to **tofacitinib**. Adjust **tofacitinib** dose, p. 803. [Moderate] Study
- SSRIs **(fluoxetine, paroxetine)** are predicted to increase the exposure to **tricyclic antidepressants**. Monitor for toxicity and adjust dose. [Severe] Study → Also see **TABLE 15** p. 1058 → Also see **TABLE 11** p. 1056 → Also see **TABLE 9** p. 1056
- **Fluvoxamine** increases the exposure to tricyclic antidepressants **(amitriptyline, imipramine)**. Adjust dose. [Severe] Study → Also see **TABLE 15** p. 1058 → Also see **TABLE 11** p. 1056 → Also see **TABLE 9** p. 1056
- **Fluvoxamine** markedly increases the exposure to tricyclic antidepressants **(clomipramine)**. Adjust dose. [Severe] Study → Also see **TABLE 15** p. 1058 → Also see **TABLE 11** p. 1056 → Also see **TABLE 9** p. 1056
- **Fluvoxamine** increases the concentration of triptans **(frovatriptan)**. [Severe] Study
- **Fluvoxamine** is predicted to increase the exposure to triptans **(zolmitriptan)**. Adjust **zolmitriptan** dose, p. 347. [Severe] Theoretical
- **Tucatinib** is predicted to moderately increase the exposure to **dapoxetine**. Avoid potent CYP3A4 inhibitors or adjust **dapoxetine** dose. [Severe] Study
- **Tucatinib** is predicted to increase the exposure to **sertraline**. Avoid. [Moderate] Theoretical
- **SSRIs** might enhance the antidiuretic and hypertensive effects of **vasopressin**. [Moderate] Theoretical
- **Fluvoxamine** is predicted to increase the exposure to **vorasidenib**. Avoid. [Moderate] Study
- SSRIs **(fluoxetine, paroxetine)** are predicted to increase the exposure to **vortioxetine**. Monitor and adjust dose. [Moderate] Study → Also see **TABLE 3** p. 1053 → Also see **TABLE 11** p. 1056

St John's wort → see **TABLE 11** p. 1056 (serotonin toxicity)

- **St John's wort** is predicted to decrease the exposure to **abemaciclib**. Avoid. [Severe] Study
- **St John's wort** is predicted to decrease the exposure to **acalabrutinib**. Avoid. [Severe] Study
- **St John's wort** is predicted to decrease the exposure to **afatinib**. [Moderate] Study
- **St John's wort** decreases the exposure to **aliskiren**. [Moderate] Study
- **St John's wort** is predicted to decrease the concentration of **aminophylline**. [Severe] Theoretical
- **St John's wort** is predicted to decrease the efficacy of anti-androgens **(cyproterone)** with ethinylestradiol (co-cyprindiol). Use alternative methods during treatment with, and for 28 days after, the enzyme inducing drug is stopped. [Severe] Study
- **St John's wort** is predicted to decrease the exposure to anti-androgens **(darolutamide)**. Avoid. [Moderate] Theoretical
- **St John's wort** is predicted to decrease the exposure to antiarrhythmics **(dronedarone)**. Avoid. [Severe] Theoretical
- **St John's wort** is predicted to decrease the exposure to antiepileptics **(brivaracetam)**. [Moderate] Theoretical
- **St John's wort** is predicted to decrease the concentration of antiepileptics **(carbamazepine)**. Monitor and adjust dose. [Moderate] Theoretical
- **St John's wort** is predicted to decrease the concentration of antiepileptics **(fosphenytoin, phenobarbital, phenytoin, primidone)**. Avoid. [Severe] Theoretical
- **St John's wort** is predicted to decrease the exposure to antiepileptics **(perampanel)**. Monitor and adjust dose. [Moderate] Theoretical
- **St John's wort** is predicted to decrease the exposure to antiepileptics **(tiagabine)**. Avoid. [Mild] Theoretical
- **St John's wort** is predicted to decrease the exposure to antifungals, azoles **(isavuconazole)**. Avoid. [Severe] Theoretical
- **St John's wort** moderately decreases the exposure to antifungals, azoles **(voriconazole)**. Avoid. [Moderate] Study
- **St John's wort** is predicted to decrease the concentration of antimalarials **(piperaquine)**. Avoid. [Moderate] Theoretical
- **St John's wort** is predicted to decrease the exposure to atypical antipsychotics **(aripiprazole)**. Avoid or adjust dose—consult product literature. [Moderate] Study
- **St John's wort** is predicted to decrease the exposure to atypical antipsychotics **(cariprazine)**. Avoid. [Severe] Theoretical
- **St John's wort** is predicted to decrease the exposure to atypical antipsychotics **(lurasidone)**. Monitor and adjust dose. [Moderate] Theoretical
- **St John's wort** is predicted to decrease the exposure to atypical antipsychotics **(paliperidone)**. [Severe] Theoretical
- **St John's wort** is predicted to decrease the exposure to atypical antipsychotics **(quetiapine)**. [Moderate] Study
- **St John's wort** is predicted to decrease the exposure to **avacopan**. [Severe] Theoretical
- **St John's wort** is predicted to decrease the exposure to **avapritinib**. Avoid. [Severe] Study
- **St John's wort** is predicted to decrease the exposure to **axitinib**. Avoid or adjust dose. [Moderate] Study
- **St John's wort** is predicted to decrease the exposure to **bedaquiline**. Avoid. [Severe] Study
- **St John's wort** moderately decreases the exposure to benzodiazepines **(alprazolam)**. [Moderate] Study

St John's wort (continued)

- **St John's wort** moderately decreases the exposure to benzodiazepines **(midazolam)**. Monitor and adjust dose. Moderate Study
- **St John's wort** is predicted to decrease the concentration of **berotralstat**. Avoid. Severe Theoretical
- **St John's wort** is predicted to decrease the exposure to **bictegravir**. Avoid. Moderate Theoretical
- **St John's wort** is predicted to decrease the exposure to **bosutinib**. Avoid. Severe Study
- **St John's wort** is predicted to decrease the exposure to **brigatinib**. Avoid or adjust dose—consult product literature. Moderate Study
- **St John's wort** is predicted to decrease the exposure to **cabozantinib**. Moderate Study
- **St John's wort** is predicted to decrease the exposure to calcium-channel blockers **(amlodipine, felodipine, lacidipine, lercanidipine, nicardipine, nifedipine, nimodipine)**. Monitor and adjust dose. Moderate Theoretical
- **St John's wort** is predicted to decrease the exposure to calcium-channel blockers **(diltiazem, verapamil)**. Moderate Theoretical
- **St John's wort** is predicted to decrease the exposure to **cannabidiol**. Adjust dose. Mild Study
- **St John's wort** is predicted to decrease the exposure to **capivasertib**. Avoid. Moderate Study
- **St John's wort** is predicted to decrease the exposure to **ceritinib**. Avoid. Severe Theoretical
- **St John's wort** decreases the concentration of **ciclosporin**. Avoid. Moderate Study
- **St John's wort** is predicted to alter the effects of **cilostazol**. Moderate Theoretical
- **St John's wort** is predicted to decrease the exposure to **cobicistat**. Avoid. Severe Theoretical
- **St John's wort** is predicted to decrease the exposure to **cobimetinib**. Avoid. Severe Theoretical
- **St John's wort** is predicted to decrease the exposure to **colchicine**. Moderate Theoretical
- **St John's wort** decreases the efficacy of **combined hormonal contraceptives**. MHRA advises avoid. For CoSRH guidance, see Contraceptives, interactions p. 614. Severe Anecdotal
- **St John's wort** decreases the anticoagulant effect of **coumarins**. Avoid. Severe Anecdotal
- **St John's wort** is predicted to decrease the exposure to **crizotinib**. Avoid. Severe Study
- **St John's wort** is predicted to decrease the exposure to **dabrafenib**. Avoid. Moderate Study
- **St John's wort** is predicted to decrease the exposure to **daridorexant**. Severe Study
- **St John's wort** is predicted to decrease the exposure to **darifenacin**. Moderate Theoretical
- **St John's wort** is predicted to decrease the exposure to **dasatinib**. Severe Study
- **St John's wort** is predicted to decrease the efficacy of **desogestrel**. MHRA advises avoid. For CoSRH guidance, see Contraceptives, interactions p. 614. Severe Theoretical
- **St John's wort** is predicted to decrease the exposure to **deutivacaftor**. Avoid. Severe Theoretical
- **St John's wort** decreases the concentration of **digoxin**. Avoid. Severe Anecdotal
- **St John's wort** is predicted to decrease the exposure to **dolutegravir**. Adjust **dolutegravir** dose, p. 508. Severe Study
- **St John's wort** is predicted to decrease the exposure to **dronabinol**. Avoid or adjust dose. Mild Study
- **St John's wort** is predicted to decrease the efficacy of **drospirenone**. For CoSRH guidance, see Contraceptives, interactions p. 614. Severe Theoretical
- **St John's wort** is predicted to decrease the exposure to **elacestrant**. Avoid or adjust dose depending on duration—consult product literature. Severe Theoretical
- **St John's wort** is predicted to moderately decrease the exposure to **elbasvir**. Avoid. Severe Study
- **St John's wort** is predicted to decrease the exposure to **elexacaftor**. Avoid. Severe Theoretical
- **St John's wort** is predicted to increase the exposure to **eliglustat**. Avoid. Severe Study
- **St John's wort** is predicted to decrease the concentration of **elvitegravir**. Avoid. Severe Theoretical
- **St John's wort** is predicted to decrease the exposure to **encorafenib**. Severe Theoretical
- **St John's wort** is predicted to decrease the exposure to endothelin receptor antagonists **(bosentan)**. Avoid. Moderate Theoretical
- **St John's wort** is predicted to decrease the exposure to endothelin receptor antagonists **(macitentan)**. Avoid. Severe Theoretical
- **St John's wort** is predicted to decrease the exposure to the cytotoxic component of **enfortumab vedotin**. Moderate Theoretical
- **St John's wort** is predicted to decrease the exposure to **entrectinib**. Avoid. Moderate Theoretical
- **St John's wort** is predicted to decrease the exposure to **erdafitinib**. Avoid. Moderate Study
- **St John's wort** is predicted to decrease the exposure to **erlotinib**. Severe Study
- **St John's wort** moderately decreases the exposure to **esketamine**. Adjust dose. Moderate Study
- **St John's wort** is predicted to decrease the efficacy of **estradiol**. Moderate Theoretical
- **St John's wort** is predicted to decrease the exposure to **eszopiclone**. Adjust dose. Moderate Theoretical
- **St John's wort** is predicted to decrease the efficacy of **etonogestrel**. MHRA advises avoid. For CoSRH guidance, see Contraceptives, interactions p. 614. Severe Theoretical
- **St John's wort** is predicted to decrease the concentration of **everolimus**. Avoid or adjust dose. Severe Study
- **St John's wort** is predicted to decrease the exposure to **exemestane**. Moderate Theoretical
- **St John's wort** is predicted to decrease the exposure to factor XA inhibitors **(apixaban)**. Use with caution or avoid. Severe Study
- **St John's wort** is predicted to decrease the exposure to factor XA inhibitors **(edoxaban)**. Severe Study
- **St John's wort** is predicted to decrease the exposure to factor XA inhibitors **(rivaroxaban)**. Avoid unless patient can be monitored for signs of thrombosis. Severe Study
- **St John's wort** is predicted to decrease the exposure to **fedratinib**. Avoid. Moderate Study
- **St John's wort** is predicted to decrease the exposure to **fesoterodine**. Avoid. Severe Theoretical
- **St John's wort** is predicted to decrease the exposure to **fingolimod**. Avoid. Moderate Theoretical
- **St John's wort** is predicted to decrease the exposure to the active metabolite of **fostemsavir**. Avoid. Severe Study
- **St John's wort** is predicted to decrease the exposure to **fruquintinib**. Avoid. Moderate Study
- **St John's wort** is predicted to decrease the exposure to **futibatinib**. Avoid or adjust dose. Moderate Study
- **St John's wort** is predicted to decrease the exposure to **gefitinib**. Avoid. Severe Study
- **St John's wort** is predicted to decrease the exposure to **gilteritinib**. Avoid. Severe Study
- **St John's wort** is predicted to decrease the exposure to **glasdegib**. Avoid or adjust dose—consult product literature. Moderate Theoretical
- **St John's wort** is predicted to decrease the exposure to **glecaprevir**. Avoid. Severe Study
- **St John's wort** is predicted to markedly decrease the exposure to **grazoprevir**. Avoid. Severe Study
- **St John's wort** is predicted to decrease the concentration of **guanfacine**. Adjust dose. Moderate Theoretical
- **St John's wort** is predicted to decrease the exposure to **HIV-protease inhibitors**. Avoid. Severe Study
- **St John's wort** is predicted to decrease the efficacy of **hormone replacement therapy**. Moderate Theoretical
- **St John's wort** is predicted to decrease the exposure to **ibrutinib**. Avoid. Severe Theoretical
- **St John's wort** is predicted to decrease the exposure to **idelalisib**. Avoid. Moderate Theoretical
- **St John's wort** is predicted to decrease the exposure to **imatinib**. Moderate Study

- **St John's wort** slightly decreases the exposure to **irinotecan**. Avoid. Severe Study
- **St John's wort** decreases the exposure to **ivabradine**. Avoid. Moderate Study
- **St John's wort** is predicted to decrease the exposure to **ivacaftor**. Avoid. Severe Study
- **St John's wort** is predicted to decreases the exposure to **ivosidenib**. Avoid. Moderate Theoretical
- **St John's wort** is predicted to decrease the exposure to **ixazomib**. Avoid. Severe Theoretical
- **St John's wort** is predicted to decrease the exposure to **ketamine**. Adjust dose. Moderate Theoretical
- **St John's wort** is predicted to decrease the exposure to **lapatinib**. Avoid. Severe Study
- **St John's wort** is predicted to decrease the exposure to **larotrectinib**. Avoid. Moderate Study
- **St John's wort** is predicted to decrease the exposure to **lazertinib**. Avoid. Severe Study
- **St John's wort** is predicted to decrease the exposure to **ledipasvir**. Avoid. Severe Study
- **St John's wort** is predicted to decrease the exposure to **lenacapavir**. Avoid. Severe Study
- **St John's wort** is predicted to decrease the exposure to **leniolisib**. Avoid. Severe Theoretical
- **St John's wort** is predicted to decrease the concentration of **letermovir**. Moderate Theoretical
- **St John's wort** is predicted to decrease the efficacy of **levonorgestrel**. MHRA advises avoid. For CoSRH guidance, see Contraceptives, interactions p. 614. Severe Theoretical
- **St John's wort** is predicted to decrease the exposure to **lorlatinib**. Avoid. Severe Theoretical
- **St John's wort** is predicted to decrease the exposure to **maraviroc**. Avoid. Severe Theoretical
- **St John's wort** is predicted to decrease the exposure to **maribavir**. Avoid. Severe Study
- **St John's wort** is predicted to decrease the exposure to **mavacamten**. Monitor and adjust dose—consult product literature. Severe Theoretical
- **St John's wort** is predicted to decrease the exposure to **midostaurin**. Avoid. Severe Theoretical
- **St John's wort** is predicted to decrease the exposure to **mifepristone**. Adjust **mifepristone** dose. Severe Study
- **St John's wort** is predicted to slightly decrease the exposure to mineralocorticoid receptor antagonists **(eplerenone)**. Avoid. Moderate Study
- **St John's wort** is predicted to decrease the exposure to mineralocorticoid receptor antagonists **(finerenone)**. Avoid. Severe Study
- **Moclobemide** might cause serotonin toxicity, as can **St John's wort**; concurrent use might increase the risk of developing this effect. Avoid. Severe Theoretical → Also see TABLE 11 p. 1056
- **St John's wort** is predicted to decrease the exposure to **naldemedine**. Avoid. Severe Study
- **St John's wort** is predicted to decrease the exposure to **naloxegol**. Avoid. Moderate Theoretical
- **St John's wort** is predicted to decrease the exposure to **neratinib**. Avoid. Severe Theoretical
- **St John's wort** is predicted to decrease the exposure to neurokinin-1 receptor antagonists **(aprepitant, fosaprepitant)**. Avoid. Moderate Theoretical
- **St John's wort** is predicted to decrease the exposure to neurokinin-1 receptor antagonists **(netupitant)**. Moderate Theoretical
- **St John's wort** is predicted to decrease the exposure to **nilotinib**. Avoid. Severe Theoretical
- **St John's wort** is predicted to decrease the exposure to **nintedanib**. Moderate Study
- **St John's wort** is predicted to decrease the exposure to **nirmatrelvir** boosted with ritonavir. Avoid. Severe Theoretical
- **St John's wort** is predicted to decrease the exposure to NNRTIs **(doravirine, rilpivirine)**. Avoid. Severe Theoretical
- **St John's wort** is predicted to decrease the concentration of NNRTIs **(efavirenz, nevirapine)**. Avoid. Severe Theoretical
- **St John's wort** is predicted to decrease the efficacy of **norethisterone**. MHRA advises avoid. For CoSRH guidance, see Contraceptives, interactions p. 614. Severe Anecdotal
- **St John's wort** is predicted to decrease the exposure to **olaparib**. Avoid. Moderate Theoretical
- **St John's wort** is predicted to decrease the exposure to **omaveloxolone**. Avoid. Severe Study
- **St John's wort** decreases the exposure to opioids **(methadone)**. Monitor and adjust dose. Severe Study → Also see TABLE 11 p. 1056
- **St John's wort** moderately decreases the exposure to opioids **(oxycodone)**. Adjust dose. Moderate Study
- **St John's wort** is predicted to decrease the exposure to **osimertinib**. Avoid. Severe Study
- **St John's wort** is predicted to decrease the exposure to **ospemifene**. Moderate Study
- **St John's wort** is predicted to decrease the exposure to **palbociclib**. Avoid. Severe Theoretical
- **St John's wort** is predicted to decrease the exposure to **panobinostat**. Avoid. Moderate Theoretical
- **St John's wort** is predicted to decrease the exposure to **pazopanib**. Severe Study
- **St John's wort** is predicted to decrease the exposure to **pemigatinib**. Avoid. Severe Study
- **St John's wort** is predicted to decrease the exposure to phosphodiesterase type-4 inhibitors **(apremilast)**. Avoid. Severe Theoretical
- **St John's wort** is predicted to decrease the exposure to **phosphodiesterase type-5 inhibitors**. Moderate Theoretical
- **St John's wort** is predicted to decrease the exposure to **pibrentasvir**. Avoid. Severe Study
- **St John's wort** slightly decreases the exposure to **pioglitazone**. Mild Study
- **St John's wort** is predicted to decrease the exposure to **pirtobrutinib**. Moderate Theoretical
- **St John's wort** is predicted to decrease the exposure to **pitolisant**. Monitor and adjust dose. Moderate Theoretical
- **St John's wort** is predicted to decrease the exposure to **ponatinib**. Avoid. Severe Theoretical
- **St John's wort** is predicted to decrease the exposure to **pralsetinib**. Avoid or adjust dose—consult product literature. Moderate Study
- **St John's wort** is predicted to decrease the exposure to **quizartinib**. Avoid. Severe Study
- **St John's wort** is predicted to decrease the exposure to **ranolazine**. Avoid. Severe Study
- **St John's wort** is predicted to decrease the exposure to **regorafenib**. Avoid. Severe Study
- **St John's wort** is predicted to decrease the exposure to **relugolix**. Avoid or adjust dose depending on indication—consult product literature. Moderate Study
- **St John's wort** is predicted to decrease the exposure to **ribociclib**. Avoid. Severe Study
- **St John's wort** is predicted to decrease the exposure to **rimegepant**. Avoid. Moderate Theoretical
- **St John's wort** is predicted to decrease the exposure to **ripretinib**. Avoid or adjust dose—consult product literature. Moderate Theoretical
- **St John's wort** is predicted to decrease the exposure to **ruxolitinib**. Monitor and adjust dose. Moderate Study
- **St John's wort** is predicted to decrease the exposure to **selpercatinib**. Avoid. Moderate Study
- **St John's wort** is predicted to decrease the exposure to **selumetinib**. Avoid. Severe Study
- **St John's wort** is predicted to decrease the exposure to **siponimod**. Manufacturer advises caution depending on genotype—consult product literature. Moderate Theoretical
- **St John's wort** is predicted to decrease the concentration of **sirolimus**. Monitor and adjust dose. Severe Theoretical
- **St John's wort** is predicted to decrease the exposure to sodium glucose co-transporter 2 inhibitors **(canagliflozin)**. Adjust **canagliflozin** dose. Moderate Study
- **St John's wort** is predicted to decrease the exposure to **sofosbuvir**. Avoid. Severe Study
- **St John's wort** is predicted to decrease the exposure to **sorafenib**. Moderate Study

A1

Interactions | **Appendix 1**

St John's wort (continued)

- **St John's wort** is predicted to decrease the exposure to **sparsentan**. Avoid. Severe Theoretical
- **St John's wort** is predicted to decrease the exposure to statins **(atorvastatin, simvastatin)**. Moderate Study
- **St John's wort** is predicted to decrease the exposure to **sunitinib**. Moderate Study
- **St John's wort** decreases the concentration of **tacrolimus**. Avoid. Severe Study
- **St John's wort** is predicted to decrease the exposure to taxanes **(cabazitaxel)**. Avoid. Severe Theoretical
- **St John's wort** is predicted to decrease the exposure to taxanes **(docetaxel)**. Severe Theoretical
- **St John's wort** is predicted to decrease the exposure to taxanes **(paclitaxel)**. Avoid. Severe Study
- **St John's wort** is predicted to decrease the concentration of **temsirolimus**. Avoid. Moderate Theoretical
- **St John's wort** is predicted to decrease the exposure to **tenofovir alafenamide**. Avoid. Moderate Theoretical
- **St John's wort** is predicted to decrease the exposure to tetracyclines **(eravacycline)**. Adjust **eravacycline** dose. Moderate Theoretical
- **St John's wort** is predicted to decrease the exposure to **tezacaftor**. Avoid. Severe Theoretical
- **St John's wort** potentially decreases the exposure to **theophylline**. Severe Anecdotal
- **St John's wort** is predicted to decrease the exposure to thrombin inhibitors **(dabigatran)**. Avoid. Severe Study
- **St John's wort** is predicted to decrease the exposure to **ticagrelor**. Moderate Theoretical
- **St John's wort** is predicted to decrease the exposure to **tivozanib**. Avoid. Severe Study
- **St John's wort** is predicted to decrease the exposure to **tofacitinib**. Severe Study
- **St John's wort** is predicted to decrease the exposure to **tolvaptan**. Avoid. Moderate Theoretical
- **St John's wort** is predicted to decrease the exposure to **topotecan**. Severe Theoretical
- **St John's wort** is predicted to decrease the exposure to **treprostinil**. Adjust dose. Mild Theoretical
- **St John's wort** is predicted to decrease the exposure to **tucatinib**. Avoid. Severe Theoretical
- **St John's wort** is predicted to decrease the efficacy of **ulipristal**. For CoSRH guidance, see Contraceptives, interactions p. 614. Severe Anecdotal
- **St John's wort** is predicted to decrease the exposure to **vandetanib**. Avoid. Severe Study
- **St John's wort** is predicted to decrease the exposure to **vanzacaftor**. Avoid. Severe Theoretical
- **St John's wort** is predicted to decrease the exposure to **velpatasvir**. Avoid. Moderate Theoretical
- **St John's wort** is predicted to decrease the exposure to **vemurafenib**. Avoid. Severe Study
- **St John's wort** is predicted to decrease the exposure to **venetoclax**. Avoid. Severe Study
- **St John's wort** is predicted to decrease the exposure to **vinca alkaloids**. Severe Theoretical
- **St John's wort** is predicted to decrease the exposure to **vismodegib**. Avoid. Moderate Theoretical
- **St John's wort** is predicted to decrease the exposure to **voclosporin**. Avoid. Severe Theoretical
- **St John's wort** has been reported to cause severe hypotension when given with **volatile halogenated anaesthetics**. Severe Theoretical
- **St John's wort** is predicted to decrease the concentration of **voxilaprevir**. Avoid. Severe Theoretical
- **St John's wort** is predicted to decrease the exposure to **zanubrutinib**. Avoid or adjust dose with moderate CYP3A4 inducers—consult product literature. Severe Theoretical

Statins → see TABLE 1 p. 1053 (hepatotoxicity)

atorvastatin · fluvastatin · pravastatin · rosuvastatin · simvastatin

- **Acipimox** is predicted to increase the risk of rhabdomyolysis when given with **statins**. Severe Theoretical
- **Atorvastatin** slightly to moderately increases the exposure to **aliskiren**. Moderate Study
- Oral **antacids** decrease the absorption of oral **rosuvastatin**. Separate administration by 2 hours. Moderate Study
- Anti-androgens **(apalutamide)** are predicted to decrease the exposure to **atorvastatin**. Moderate Study
- Anti-androgens **(apalutamide)** are predicted to decrease the exposure to **fluvastatin**. Monitor and adjust dose. Mild Theoretical
- Anti-androgens **(apalutamide)** are predicted to decrease the exposure to **pravastatin**. Mild Study
- Anti-androgens **(apalutamide)** slightly decrease the exposure to **rosuvastatin**. Mild Study
- Anti-androgens **(apalutamide)** are predicted to decrease the exposure to **simvastatin**. Avoid or monitor. Moderate Study
- Anti-androgens **(darolutamide)** markedly increase the exposure to **rosuvastatin**. Avoid or adjust **rosuvastatin** dose, p. 155. Severe Study
- Anti-androgens **(darolutamide)** are predicted to increase the exposure to statins **(atorvastatin, fluvastatin)**. Avoid. Severe Theoretical
- Anti-androgens **(enzalutamide)** are predicted to decrease the exposure to statins **(atorvastatin, simvastatin)**. Moderate Study
- Anti-androgens **(darolutamide)** are predicted to increase the concentration of statins **(pravastatin, simvastatin)**. Moderate Theoretical
- Antiarrhythmics **(amiodarone)** are predicted to increase the exposure to **atorvastatin**. Monitor and adjust dose. Moderate Theoretical → Also see TABLE 1 p. 1053
- Antiarrhythmics **(amiodarone)** are predicted to increase the exposure to **fluvastatin**. Moderate Study → Also see TABLE 1 p. 1053
- Antiarrhythmics **(amiodarone)** increase the exposure to **simvastatin**. Adjust **simvastatin** dose, p. 156. Severe Study → Also see TABLE 1 p. 1053
- Antiarrhythmics **(dronedarone)** slightly increase the exposure to **atorvastatin**. Monitor and adjust dose. Severe Study
- Antiarrhythmics **(dronedarone)** slightly increase the exposure to **rosuvastatin**. Adjust dose. Severe Study
- Antiarrhythmics **(dronedarone)** moderately increase the exposure to **simvastatin**. Monitor and adjust dose. Severe Study
- Antiepileptics **(carbamazepine)** are predicted to decrease the exposure to **atorvastatin**. Monitor and adjust dose. Moderate Study
- Antiepileptics **(carbamazepine, eslicarbazepine)** moderately decrease the exposure to **simvastatin**. Monitor and adjust dose. Moderate Study
- Antiepileptics **(eslicarbazepine)** are predicted to decrease the exposure to **atorvastatin**. Monitor and adjust dose. Moderate Theoretical
- Antiepileptics **(eslicarbazepine)** decrease the exposure to **rosuvastatin**. Moderate Study
- Antiepileptics **(phenytoin)** moderately decrease the exposure to **atorvastatin**. Moderate Study
- Antiepileptics **(phenytoin)** are predicted to decrease the exposure to **simvastatin**. Moderate Study
- Antiepileptics **(fosphenytoin, phenobarbital, primidone)** are predicted to decrease the exposure to statins **(atorvastatin, simvastatin)**. Moderate Study
- Antiepileptics **(oxcarbazepine)** are predicted to decrease the exposure to statins **(atorvastatin, simvastatin)**. Moderate Theoretical
- Antifungals, azoles **(fluconazole, miconazole)** are predicted to increase the exposure to **fluvastatin**. Moderate Study → Also see TABLE 1 p. 1053
- Antifungals, azoles **(isavuconazole)** slightly increase the exposure to **atorvastatin**. Moderate Study
- Antifungals, azoles **(isavuconazole)** are predicted to increase the exposure to **simvastatin**. Monitor and adjust dose. Severe Theoretical
- Antifungals, azoles **(itraconazole, ketoconazole, posaconazole, voriconazole)** are predicted to increase the exposure to **atorvastatin**. Avoid or adjust dose and monitor rhabdomyolysis. Severe Study → Also see TABLE 1 p. 1053
- Antifungals, azoles **(itraconazole, ketoconazole, posaconazole, voriconazole)** are predicted to increase the exposure to **simvastatin**. Avoid. Severe Study → Also see TABLE 1 p. 1053

- Antifungals, azoles **(miconazole)** (including the oral gel) might increase the exposure to **atorvastatin**. Moderate Theoretical
- Antifungals, azoles **(miconazole)** (including the oral gel) are predicted to increase the exposure to **simvastatin**. Avoid. Severe Anecdotal
- Antifungals, azoles **(fluconazole)** are predicted to increase the exposure to statins **(atorvastatin, simvastatin)**. Monitor and adjust dose. Severe Anecdotal → Also see TABLE 1 p. 1053
- Antifungals, azoles **(isavuconazole)** are predicted to increase the exposure to statins **(fluvastatin, rosuvastatin)**. Moderate Theoretical
- **Avacopan** moderately increases the exposure to **simvastatin**. Adjust dose. Moderate Study
- **Belumosudil** is predicted to increase the exposure to **fluvastatin**. Avoid or adjust dose. Moderate Theoretical
- **Belumosudil** is predicted to increase the exposure to statins **(atorvastatin, pravastatin, rosuvastatin, simvastatin)**. Avoid or adjust dose. Moderate Study
- **Bempedoic acid** increases the exposure to **pravastatin**. Moderate Study
- **Bempedoic acid** increases the exposure to **simvastatin**. Adjust **simvastatin** dose, p. 156. Moderate Study
- **Bulevirtide** is predicted to increase the exposure to **statins**. Avoid or monitor. Moderate Theoretical
- Calcium channel blockers **(amlodipine)** cause a small increase in the exposure to **simvastatin**. Adjust **simvastatin** dose, p. 156. Moderate Study
- Calcium-channel blockers **(diltiazem)** slightly increase the exposure to **atorvastatin**. Monitor and adjust dose. Severe Study
- Calcium-channel blockers **(diltiazem, verapamil)** moderately increase the exposure to **simvastatin**. Monitor and adjust dose. Severe Study
- Calcium-channel blockers **(verapamil)** are predicted to slightly to moderately increase the exposure to **atorvastatin**. Monitor and adjust dose. Severe Theoretical
- **Cenobamate** is predicted to decrease the exposure to statins **(atorvastatin, simvastatin)**. Moderate Study
- Cephalosporins **(ceftobiprole)** are predicted to increase the concentration of **statins**. Moderate Theoretical
- **Ceritinib** is predicted to increase the exposure to **atorvastatin**. Avoid or adjust dose and monitor rhabdomyolysis. Severe Study
- **Ceritinib** is predicted to increase the exposure to **simvastatin**. Avoid. Severe Study
- **Ciclosporin** markedly to very markedly increases the exposure to **atorvastatin**. Avoid or adjust **atorvastatin** dose, p. 154. Severe Study
- **Ciclosporin** moderately increases the exposure to **fluvastatin**. Severe Study
- **Ciclosporin** markedly to very markedly increases the exposure to **pravastatin**. Adjust dose. Severe Study
- **Ciclosporin** markedly increases the exposure to **rosuvastatin**. Avoid. Severe Study
- **Ciclosporin** markedly to very markedly increases the exposure to **simvastatin**. Avoid. Severe Study
- **Cilostazol** is predicted to increase the exposure to **atorvastatin**. Moderate Theoretical
- **Cilostazol** slightly increases the exposure to **simvastatin**. Moderate Study
- **Clopidogrel** increases the exposure to **rosuvastatin**. Adjust **rosuvastatin** dose, p. 155. Moderate Study
- **Cobicistat** is predicted to increase the exposure to **atorvastatin**. Avoid or adjust dose and monitor rhabdomyolysis. Severe Study
- **Cobicistat** is predicted to increase the exposure to **simvastatin**. Avoid. Severe Study
- **Colchicine** has been reported to cause rhabdomyolysis when given with **statins**. Severe Anecdotal
- **Statins (fluvastatin, rosuvastatin)** increase the anticoagulant effect of **coumarins**. Monitor INR and adjust dose. Severe Study
- **Crizotinib** is predicted to increase the exposure to **atorvastatin**. Monitor and adjust dose. Moderate Theoretical
- **Crizotinib** is predicted to increase the exposure to **pravastatin**. Moderate Theoretical
- **Crizotinib** is predicted to increase the exposure to **simvastatin**. Monitor and adjust dose. Severe Theoretical
- **Dabrafenib** is predicted to decrease the exposure to statins **(atorvastatin, simvastatin)**. Moderate Study
- **Danicopan** is predicted to increase the exposure to statins **(atorvastatin, fluvastatin, rosuvastatin)**. Moderate Study
- **Statins** are predicted to increase the risk of rhabdomyolysis when given with **daptomycin**. Severe Theoretical
- **Dasatinib** is predicted to increase the exposure to **simvastatin**. Moderate Theoretical
- **Elafibranor** might increase the risk of muscle effects when given with **statins**. Severe Theoretical
- **Elbasvir** with grazoprevir slightly increases the exposure to **atorvastatin**. Adjust **atorvastatin** dose, p. 154. Moderate Study
- **Elbasvir** with grazoprevir is predicted to increase the exposure to **fluvastatin**. Adjust **fluvastatin** dose, p. 155. Moderate Theoretical
- **Elbasvir** with grazoprevir moderately increases the exposure to **rosuvastatin**. Adjust **rosuvastatin** dose, p. 155. Moderate Study
- **Elbasvir** with grazoprevir is predicted to increase the exposure to **simvastatin**. Adjust **simvastatin** dose, p. 156. Moderate Theoretical
- **Elexacaftor** is predicted to increase the exposure to statins **(atorvastatin, pravastatin, rosuvastatin, simvastatin)**. Moderate Theoretical
- **Eliglustat** is predicted to increase the exposure to **pravastatin**. Adjust dose. Moderate Study
- **Eltrombopag** is predicted to increase the exposure to **statins**. Monitor and adjust dose. Moderate Study
- **Encorafenib** is predicted to increase the exposure to **atorvastatin**. Mild Theoretical
- **Encorafenib** is predicted to affect the exposure to **simvastatin**. Mild Theoretical
- **Encorafenib** is predicted to increase the exposure to statins **(fluvastatin, pravastatin)**. Mild Study
- Endothelin receptor antagonists **(bosentan)** are predicted to decrease the exposure to statins **(atorvastatin, simvastatin)**. Moderate Study
- **Febuxostat** increases the exposure to **rosuvastatin**. Adjust **rosuvastatin** dose, p. 155. Moderate Study
- Fibrates **(bezafibrate, ciprofibrate)** increase the risk of rhabdomyolysis when given with **pravastatin**. Avoid. Severe Study
- Fibrates **(bezafibrate, ciprofibrate)** increase the risk of rhabdomyolysis when given with **rosuvastatin**. Adjust **rosuvastatin** dose, p. 155. Severe Study
- Fibrates **(bezafibrate, ciprofibrate)** increase the risk of rhabdomyolysis when given with **simvastatin**. Adjust **simvastatin** dose, p. 156. Severe Study
- Fibrates **(ciprofibrate)** increase the risk of rhabdomyolysis when given with **atorvastatin**. Avoid or adjust dose. Severe Study
- Fibrates **(ciprofibrate)** increase the risk of rhabdomyolysis when given with **fluvastatin**. Severe Study
- Fibrates **(fenofibrate)** increase the risk of rhabdomyolysis when given with **atorvastatin**. Monitor and adjust **fenofibrate** dose, p. 153. Severe Anecdotal
- Fibrates **(fenofibrate)** are predicted to increase the risk of rhabdomyolysis when given with **fluvastatin**. Use with caution and adjust **fenofibrate** dose, p. 153. Severe Theoretical
- Fibrates **(fenofibrate)** are predicted to increase the risk of rhabdomyolysis when given with **pravastatin**. Avoid. Severe Theoretical
- Fibrates **(fenofibrate)** increase the risk of rhabdomyolysis when given with **rosuvastatin**. Adjust **fenofibrate and rosuvastatin** doses, p. 153, p. 155. Severe Anecdotal
- Fibrates **(fenofibrate)** increase the risk of rhabdomyolysis when given with **simvastatin**. Adjust **fenofibrate** dose, p. 153. Severe Anecdotal
- Fibrates **(gemfibrozil)** cause a small increase in the exposure to **atorvastatin**. Avoid. Severe Study
- Fibrates **(gemfibrozil)** increase the risk of rhabdomyolysis when given with **fluvastatin**. Severe Anecdotal
- Fibrates **(gemfibrozil)** modestly increase the exposure to **pravastatin**. Avoid or monitor. Severe Study

Statins (continued)
- Fibrates **(gemfibrozil)** cause a small increase in the exposure to **rosuvastatin**. Avoid or adjust **rosuvastatin** dose, p. 155. Severe Study
- Fibrates **(gemfibrozil)** modestly increase the exposure to **simvastatin**. Avoid. Severe Anecdotal
- Fibrates **(bezafibrate)** increase the risk of rhabdomyolysis when given with statins **(atorvastatin, fluvastatin)**. Severe Study
- **Fostamatinib** moderately increases the exposure to **rosuvastatin**. Avoid or adjust **rosuvastatin** dose, p. 155. Moderate Study
- **Fostamatinib** slightly increases the exposure to **simvastatin**. Monitor adverse effects and adjust dose. Moderate Study
- **Fostamatinib** is predicted to increase the exposure to statins **(atorvastatin, fluvastatin)**. Monitor and adjust dose. Moderate Theoretical
- **Fostemsavir** increases the exposure to **rosuvastatin**. Adjust starting dose and monitor. Severe Study
- **Fostemsavir** is predicted to increase the exposure to statins **(atorvastatin, fluvastatin, simvastatin)**. Adjust starting dose and monitor. Severe Theoretical
- **Fusidate** has been reported to cause rhabdomyolysis when given with **statins**. Avoid. Severe Anecdotal
- **Givinostat** might increase the exposure to **simvastatin**. Moderate Study
- **Glecaprevir** with pibrentasvir markedly increases the exposure to **atorvastatin**. Avoid. Severe Study
- **Glecaprevir** with pibrentasvir is predicted to increase the exposure to **fluvastatin**. Moderate Theoretical
- **Glecaprevir** with pibrentasvir moderately increases the exposure to **pravastatin**. Use with caution and adjust **pravastatin** dose, p. 155. Moderate Study
- **Glecaprevir** with pibrentasvir moderately increases the exposure to **rosuvastatin**. Use with caution and adjust **rosuvastatin** dose, p. 155. Moderate Study
- **Glecaprevir** with pibrentasvir moderately increases the exposure to **simvastatin**. Avoid. Moderate Study
- **Grapefruit** juice increases the exposure to **atorvastatin**. Mild Study
- **Grapefruit** juice increases the exposure to **simvastatin**. Avoid. Severe Study
- **Grazoprevir** moderately increases the exposure to **atorvastatin**. Adjust **atorvastatin** dose, p. 154. Moderate Study
- **Grazoprevir** with elbasvir is predicted to increase the exposure to **fluvastatin**. Adjust **fluvastatin** dose, p. 155. Moderate Theoretical
- **Grazoprevir** with elbasvir moderately increases the exposure to **rosuvastatin**. Adjust **rosuvastatin** dose, p. 155. Moderate Study
- **Grazoprevir** with elbasvir is predicted to increase the exposure to **simvastatin**. Adjust **simvastatin** dose, p. 156. Moderate Theoretical
- **HIV-protease inhibitors** are predicted to increase the exposure to **atorvastatin**. Avoid or adjust dose and monitor rhabdomyolysis. Severe Study → Also see **TABLE 1** p. 1053
- **HIV-protease inhibitors** might affect the exposure to **pravastatin**. Moderate Study → Also see **TABLE 1** p. 1053
- HIV-protease inhibitors **(atazanavir, lopinavir)** boosted with ritonavir moderately increase the exposure to **rosuvastatin**. Avoid or adjust **rosuvastatin** dose, p. 155. Severe Study
- HIV-protease inhibitors **(darunavir, ritonavir)** are predicted to increase the exposure to **rosuvastatin**. Avoid or adjust dose. Severe Study → Also see **TABLE 1** p. 1053
- HIV-protease inhibitors **(fosamprenavir)** are predicted to increase the exposure to **rosuvastatin**. Use with caution and adjust dose. Severe Study
- **HIV-protease inhibitors** are predicted to increase the exposure to **simvastatin**. Avoid. Severe Study → Also see **TABLE 1** p. 1053
- **Idelalisib** is predicted to increase the exposure to **atorvastatin**. Avoid or adjust dose and monitor rhabdomyolysis. Severe Study
- **Idelalisib** is predicted to increase the exposure to **simvastatin**. Avoid. Severe Study
- **Imatinib** is predicted to increase the exposure to **atorvastatin**. Monitor and adjust dose. Severe Theoretical
- **Imatinib** moderately increases the exposure to **simvastatin**. Monitor and adjust dose. Severe Study
- **Ivosidenib** might affect the exposure to **simvastatin**. Avoid or monitor. Moderate Theoretical
- **Ivosidenib** is predicted to increase the exposure to statins **(atorvastatin, pravastatin, rosuvastatin)**. Use with caution or avoid. Unknown Theoretical
- **Lazertinib** moderately increases the exposure to **rosuvastatin**. Moderate Study
- **Ledipasvir** with sofosbuvir is predicted to increase the exposure to **atorvastatin**. Monitor and adjust dose. Moderate Anecdotal
- **Ledipasvir** with sofosbuvir is predicted to increase the exposure to **rosuvastatin**. Avoid. Severe Theoretical
- **Ledipasvir** with sofosbuvir is predicted to increase the exposure to statins **(fluvastatin, pravastatin, simvastatin)**. Monitor and adjust dose. Moderate Theoretical
- **Leflunomide** is predicted to increase the exposure to **rosuvastatin**. Adjust **rosuvastatin** dose, p. 155. Moderate Study
- **Leflunomide** is predicted to increase the exposure to statins **(atorvastatin, fluvastatin, pravastatin, simvastatin)**. Moderate Study
- **Lenacapavir** is predicted to increase the concentration of **simvastatin**. Adjust starting dose and monitor. Moderate Theoretical
- **Leniolisib** is predicted to increase the exposure to **statins**. Avoid. Moderate Theoretical
- **Letermovir** moderately increases the exposure to **atorvastatin**. Avoid or adjust **atorvastatin** dose, p. 154. Severe Study
- **Letermovir** is predicted to increase the exposure to **fluvastatin**. Monitor and adjust dose. Moderate Theoretical
- **Letermovir** is predicted to increase the exposure to **pravastatin**. Avoid or adjust dose. Moderate Theoretical
- **Letermovir** is predicted to increase the exposure to statins **(rosuvastatin, simvastatin)**. Avoid. Severe Study
- **Lomitapide** increases the exposure to **atorvastatin**. Adjust **lomitapide** dose or separate administration by 12 hours. Mild Study → Also see **TABLE 1** p. 1053
- **Lomitapide** increases the exposure to **simvastatin**. Monitor and adjust **simvastatin** dose, p. 156. Moderate Study → Also see **TABLE 1** p. 1053
- **Lorlatinib** is predicted to decrease the exposure to statins **(atorvastatin, simvastatin)**. Moderate Study
- Macrolides **(clarithromycin)** are predicted to increase the exposure to **atorvastatin**. Avoid or adjust dose and monitor rhabdomyolysis. Severe Study
- Macrolides **(clarithromycin)** moderately increase the exposure to **pravastatin**. Severe Study
- Macrolides **(clarithromycin)** are predicted to increase the exposure to **simvastatin**. Avoid. Severe Study
- Macrolides **(erythromycin)** slightly increase the exposure to **atorvastatin**. Monitor and adjust dose. Severe Study
- Macrolides **(erythromycin)** slightly increase the exposure to **pravastatin**. Severe Study
- Macrolides **(erythromycin)** markedly increase the exposure to **simvastatin**. Avoid. Severe Study
- **Maribavir** is predicted to increase the exposure to **rosuvastatin**. Moderate Theoretical
- **Mifepristone** moderately increases the exposure to **fluvastatin**. Moderate Study
- **Mifepristone** very markedly increases the exposure to **simvastatin**. Severe Study
- **Mitotane** is predicted to decrease the exposure to statins **(atorvastatin, simvastatin)**. Moderate Study
- **Momelotinib** increases the exposure to **rosuvastatin**. Moderate Study
- Monoclonal antibodies **(sarilumab)** are predicted to decrease the exposure to statins **(atorvastatin, simvastatin)**. Moderate Study
- Monoclonal antibodies **(tocilizumab)** are predicted to decrease the exposure to statins **(atorvastatin, simvastatin)**. Monitor and adjust dose. Moderate Study
- Neurokinin-1 receptor antagonists **(aprepitant, netupitant)** are predicted to increase the exposure to statins **(atorvastatin, simvastatin)**. Monitor and adjust dose. Severe Theoretical

- **Nicotinic acid** might increase the risk of rhabdomyolysis when given with **statins**. Use with caution or avoid. Severe Theoretical → Also see TABLE 1 p. 1053
- **Nilotinib** is predicted to increase the exposure to **atorvastatin**. Monitor and adjust dose. Moderate Theoretical
- **Nilotinib** is predicted to increase the exposure to **simvastatin**. Monitor and adjust dose. Severe Theoretical
- **Nirmatrelvir** boosted with ritonavir is predicted to increase the concentration of **simvastatin**. Avoid. Severe Theoretical
- **Nirmatrelvir** boosted with ritonavir is predicted to increase the concentration of statins **(atorvastatin, rosuvastatin)**. Adjust dose. Severe Theoretical
- NNRTIs **(etravirine)** are predicted to increase the exposure to **fluvastatin**. Adjust dose. Severe Theoretical
- NNRTIs **(efavirenz, etravirine, nevirapine)** are predicted to decrease the exposure to statins **(atorvastatin, simvastatin)**. Moderate Study → Also see TABLE 1 p. 1053
- **Olaparib** is predicted to increase the exposure to **statins**. Moderate Theoretical
- **Osimertinib** causes a small increase in the exposure to **rosuvastatin**. Severe Study
- **Pazopanib** might cause increased ALT concentrations when given with **simvastatin**. Moderate Study
- **Pazopanib** might affect the exposure to statins **(atorvastatin, pravastatin, rosuvastatin)**. Moderate Theoretical
- **Rosuvastatin** is predicted to increase the anticoagulant effect of **phenindione**. Monitor INR and adjust dose. Severe Theoretical
- **Pibrentasvir** with glecaprevir markedly increases the exposure to **atorvastatin**. Avoid. Severe Study
- **Pibrentasvir** with glecaprevir is predicted to increase the exposure to **fluvastatin**. Moderate Theoretical
- **Pibrentasvir** with glecaprevir moderately increases the exposure to **pravastatin**. Use with caution and adjust **pravastatin** dose, p. 155. Moderate Study
- **Pibrentasvir** with glecaprevir moderately increases the exposure to **rosuvastatin**. Use with caution and adjust **rosuvastatin** dose, p. 155. Moderate Study
- **Pibrentasvir** with glecaprevir moderately increases the exposure to **simvastatin**. Avoid. Moderate Study
- **Pirtobrutinib** is predicted to increase the exposure to statins **(atorvastatin, fluvastatin, rosuvastatin)**. Moderate Theoretical
- **Ranolazine** is predicted to increase the exposure to **atorvastatin**. Moderate Theoretical
- **Ranolazine** slightly increases the exposure to **simvastatin**. Adjust **simvastatin** dose, p. 156. Moderate Study
- **Regorafenib** moderately increases the exposure to **rosuvastatin**. Avoid or adjust **rosuvastatin** dose, p. 155. Moderate Study
- **Regorafenib** is predicted to increase the exposure to statins **(atorvastatin, fluvastatin)**. Moderate Study
- **Ribociclib** (high-dose) is predicted to increase the exposure to **simvastatin**. Avoid. Moderate Theoretical
- **Ribociclib** is predicted to increase the exposure to statins **(pravastatin, rosuvastatin)**. Moderate Theoretical
- Rifamycins **(rifampicin)** markedly decrease the exposure to **atorvastatin**. Manufacturer advises take both drugs at the same time. Moderate Study
- Rifamycins **(rifampicin)** moderately decrease the exposure to **fluvastatin**. Monitor and adjust dose. Moderate Study
- Rifamycins **(rifampicin)** very markedly decrease the exposure to **simvastatin**. Moderate Study
- **Roxadustat** might increase the exposure to **fluvastatin**. Monitor adverse effects and adjust dose. Moderate Theoretical
- **Roxadustat** is predicted to increase the exposure to statins **(atorvastatin, pravastatin, rosuvastatin, simvastatin)**. Monitor adverse effects and adjust dose. Moderate Study
- **Sacubitril** with valsartan increases the exposure to **atorvastatin**. Moderate Study
- Sodium glucose co-transporter 2 inhibitors **(empagliflozin)** have been reported to increase the risk of muscle effects when given after **atorvastatin**. Moderate Anecdotal
- **Sotorasib** is predicted to decrease the exposure to statins **(atorvastatin, simvastatin)**. Moderate Study → Also see TABLE 1 p. 1053
- **Sotorasib** is predicted to increase the exposure to statins **(fluvastatin, rosuvastatin)**. Monitor and adjust dose. Moderate Study → Also see TABLE 1 p. 1053
- **Sparsentan** is predicted to increase the exposure to statins **(atorvastatin, fluvastatin, rosuvastatin)**. Moderate Theoretical
- **St John's wort** is predicted to decrease the exposure to statins **(atorvastatin, simvastatin)**. Moderate Study
- **Fluvastatin** slightly increases the exposure to sulfonylureas **(glibenclamide)**. Mild Study
- **Tafamidis** slightly increases the exposure to **rosuvastatin**. Severe Study
- **Atorvastatin** very slightly increases the exposure to **talazoparib**. Moderate Study
- Taxanes **(cabazitaxel)** are predicted to affect the exposure to statins **(atorvastatin, pravastatin, rosuvastatin, simvastatin)**. Manufacturer advises take 12 hours before or 3 hours after **cabazitaxel**. Moderate Theoretical
- **Tedizolid** is predicted to increase the exposure to statins **(atorvastatin, fluvastatin, rosuvastatin)**. Avoid. Moderate Study
- **Teriflunomide** moderately increases the exposure to **rosuvastatin**. Adjust **rosuvastatin** dose, p. 155. Moderate Study
- **Teriflunomide** is predicted to increase the exposure to statins **(atorvastatin, fluvastatin, pravastatin, simvastatin)**. Moderate Study
- **Ticagrelor** slightly to moderately increases the exposure to **simvastatin**. Adjust **simvastatin** dose, p. 156. Moderate Study
- **Tucatinib** is predicted to increase the exposure to **atorvastatin**. Avoid or adjust dose and monitor rhabdomyolysis. Severe Study
- **Tucatinib** is predicted to increase the exposure to **simvastatin**. Avoid. Severe Study
- **Vadadustat** increases the exposure to **simvastatin**. Monitor and adjust dose. Moderate Study
- **Vadadustat** is predicted to increase the exposure to statins **(atorvastatin, fluvastatin, rosuvastatin)**. Monitor and adjust dose. Moderate Study
- **Velpatasvir** with sofosbuvir slightly increases the exposure to **atorvastatin**. Severe Study
- **Velpatasvir** moderately increases the exposure to **rosuvastatin**. Avoid or adjust **rosuvastatin** dose, p. 155. Severe Study
- **Velpatasvir** with sofosbuvir is predicted to increase the exposure to statins **(fluvastatin, simvastatin)**. Monitor adverse effects and adjust dose. Severe Theoretical
- **Venetoclax** is predicted to increase the exposure to **atorvastatin**. Moderate Study
- **Venetoclax** is predicted to increase the exposure to statins **(fluvastatin, pravastatin, rosuvastatin, simvastatin)**. Moderate Theoretical
- **Voclosporin** is predicted to increase the concentration of statins **(atorvastatin, pravastatin, rosuvastatin, simvastatin)**. Moderate Theoretical
- **Voxilaprevir** with sofosbuvir and velpatasvir is predicted to increase the exposure to **atorvastatin**. Adjust **atorvastatin** dose, p. 154. Moderate Theoretical
- **Voxilaprevir** with sofosbuvir and velpatasvir moderately increases the exposure to **pravastatin**. Monitor and adjust **pravastatin** dose, p. 155. Moderate Study
- **Voxilaprevir** with sofosbuvir and velpatasvir markedly increases the exposure to **rosuvastatin**. Avoid. Severe Study
- **Voxilaprevir** with sofosbuvir and velpatasvir is predicted to increase the exposure to statins **(fluvastatin, simvastatin)**. Avoid. Moderate Theoretical

Stiripentol → see antiepileptics

Streptokinase → see TABLE 3 p. 1053 (bleeding)

- **Donanemab** might increase the risk of brain haemorrhage when given with **streptokinase**. Avoid except in life-threatening situations. Severe Theoretical
- **Lecanemab** might increase the risk of brain haemorrhage when given with **streptokinase**. Avoid except in life-threatening situations. Severe Theoretical

Streptomycin → see aminoglycosides

Streptozocin → see TABLE 1 p. 1053 (hepatotoxicity), TABLE 12 p. 1057 (myelosuppression), TABLE 2 p. 1053 (nephrotoxicity)

- **Live vaccines** are predicted to increase the risk of generalised infection (possibly life-threatening) when given with

A1 Interactions | Appendix 1

streptozocin. UKHSA advises avoid (refer to Green Book). [Severe] Theoretical

Strontium
- Oral **antacids** decrease the absorption of oral **strontium**. Separate administration by 2 hours. [Moderate] Study
- Oral **calcium compounds** decrease the absorption of oral **strontium**. Separate administration by 2 hours. [Moderate] Study
- **Strontium** is predicted to decrease the absorption of **quinolones**. Avoid. [Moderate] Theoretical
- **Strontium** is predicted to decrease the absorption of **tetracyclines**. Avoid. [Moderate] Theoretical

Sucralfate
- **Sucralfate** is predicted to decrease the exposure to **bictegravir**. Avoid. [Moderate] Theoretical
- **Sucralfate** potentially decreases the effects of **coumarins (warfarin)**. Separate administration by 2 hours. [Moderate] Anecdotal
- **Sucralfate** decreases the absorption of **digoxin**. Separate administration by 2 hours. [Severe] Anecdotal
- **Sucralfate** decreases the absorption of **dolutegravir**. [Moderate] Study
- **Sucralfate** increases the risk of blocked enteral or nasogastric tubes when given with **enteral feeds**. Separate administration by 1 hour. [Moderate] Study
- **Potassium citrate** increases the risk of adverse effects when given with **sucralfate**. Avoid. [Moderate] Theoretical
- **Sucralfate** decreases the exposure to **quinolones**. Separate administration by 2 hours. [Moderate] Study
- **Sodium citrate** is predicted to increase the risk of adverse effects when given with **sucralfate**. Avoid. [Moderate] Theoretical
- **Sucralfate** decreases the absorption of **sulpiride**. Separate administration by 2 hours. [Moderate] Study
- Oral **sucralfate** might decrease the absorption of oral **tetracyclines**. [Moderate] Theoretical
- **Sucralfate** potentially decreases the absorption of **theophylline**. Separate administration by at least 2 hours. [Moderate] Study
- **Sucralfate** decreases the absorption of **thyroid hormones (levothyroxine)**. Separate administration by at least 4 hours. [Moderate] Study
- **Sucralfate** is predicted to decrease the absorption of **tricyclic antidepressants**. [Moderate] Study

Sucroferric oxyhydroxide → see interactions of iron

Sufentanil → see opioids

Sugammadex
- **Sugammadex** is predicted to decrease the exposure to **combined hormonal contraceptives**. Refer to patient information leaflet for missed pill advice. [Severe] Theoretical
- **Sugammadex** is predicted to decrease the exposure to **desogestrel**. Refer to patient information leaflet for missed pill advice. [Severe] Theoretical
- **Sugammadex** is predicted to decrease the exposure to **drospirenone**. Use additional contraceptive precautions. [Severe] Theoretical
- **Sugammadex** is predicted to decrease the efficacy of **etonogestrel**. Use additional contraceptive precautions. [Severe] Theoretical
- **Sugammadex** is predicted to decrease the exposure to **levonorgestrel**. Use additional contraceptive precautions. [Severe] Theoretical
- **Sugammadex** is predicted to decrease the exposure to **medroxyprogesterone**. Use additional contraceptive precautions. [Severe] Theoretical
- **Sugammadex** is predicted to decrease the exposure to **norethisterone**. Use additional contraceptive precautions. [Severe] Theoretical

Sulfadiazine → see sulfonamides

Sulfadiazine silver

PHARMACOLOGY Silver might inactivate enzymatic debriding agents—concurrent use might not be appropriate.

Sulfamethoxazole → see sulfonamides

Sulfasalazine → see TABLE 12 p. 1057 (myelosuppression), TABLE 2 p. 1053 (nephrotoxicity)
- **Anti-androgens (apalutamide)** are predicted to decrease the exposure to **sulfasalazine**. [Mild] Study
- **Anti-androgens (darolutamide)** are predicted to increase the exposure to **sulfasalazine**. Avoid. [Severe] Theoretical
- **Antifungals, azoles (isavuconazole)** are predicted to increase the exposure to **sulfasalazine**. [Moderate] Theoretical
- **Belumosudil** is predicted to increase the exposure to **sulfasalazine**. Avoid or adjust dose. [Moderate] Theoretical
- **Sulfasalazine** is predicted to affect the efficacy of **bulevirtide**. Avoid. [Severe] Theoretical
- **Danicopan** is predicted to increase the exposure to **sulfasalazine**. [Moderate] Study
- **Sulfasalazine** decreases the concentration of **digoxin**. [Moderate] Study
- **Encorafenib** is predicted to increase the exposure to **sulfasalazine**. [Mild] Study
- **Sulfasalazine** is predicted to decrease the absorption of **folates**. [Moderate] Study
- **Fostamatinib** is predicted to increase the exposure to **sulfasalazine**. Monitor and adjust dose. [Moderate] Theoretical
- **Leflunomide** is predicted to increase the exposure to **sulfasalazine**. [Moderate] Study → Also see TABLE 12 p. 1057
- **Leniolisib** is predicted to increase the exposure to **sulfasalazine**. Avoid. [Moderate] Theoretical
- **Methenamine** might increase the risk of crystalluria when given with **sulfasalazine**. Avoid. [Severe] Theoretical
- **Pirtobrutinib** is predicted to increase the exposure to **sulfasalazine**. [Moderate] Theoretical
- **Regorafenib** is predicted to increase the exposure to **sulfasalazine**. [Moderate] Study → Also see TABLE 12 p. 1057
- **Roxadustat** might increase the exposure to **sulfasalazine**. Monitor adverse effects and adjust dose. [Moderate] Theoretical
- **Sotorasib** is predicted to increase the exposure to **sulfasalazine**. Monitor and adjust dose. [Moderate] Study
- **Sparsentan** is predicted to increase the exposure to **sulfasalazine**. [Moderate] Theoretical
- **Tedizolid** is predicted to increase the exposure to **sulfasalazine**. Avoid. [Moderate] Study
- **Teriflunomide** is predicted to increase the exposure to **sulfasalazine**. [Moderate] Study
- **Vadadustat** is predicted to increase the exposure to **sulfasalazine**. Monitor and adjust dose. [Moderate] Study
- **Velpatasvir** is predicted to increase the exposure to **sulfasalazine**. [Moderate] Theoretical
- **Venetoclax** is predicted to increase the exposure to **sulfasalazine**. [Moderate] Theoretical
- **Voclosporin** is predicted to increase the concentration of **sulfasalazine**. [Moderate] Theoretical → Also see TABLE 2 p. 1053
- **Voxilaprevir** is predicted to increase the concentration of **sulfasalazine**. Avoid. [Severe] Theoretical

Sulfonamides

sulfadiazine · sulfamethoxazole

- **Sulfadiazine** is predicted to increase the concentration of **antiepileptics (fosphenytoin)**. Monitor and adjust dose. [Moderate] Study
- **Sulfadiazine** increases the concentration of **antiepileptics (phenytoin)**. Monitor and adjust dose. [Moderate] Study
- **Antimalarials (pyrimethamine)** increase the risk of adverse effects when given with **sulfonamides**. [Severe] Study
- **Sulfonamides** might increase the risk of neutropenia when given with **atypical antipsychotics (clozapine)**. Avoid. [Severe] Theoretical
- **Chloroprocaine** is predicted to decrease the effects of **sulfonamides**. Avoid. [Severe] Theoretical
- **Sulfadiazine** is predicted to increase the anticoagulant effect of **coumarins**. [Severe] Theoretical
- **Sulfamethoxazole** increases the anticoagulant effect of **coumarins**. [Severe] Study
- **Methenamine** might increase the risk of crystalluria when given with **sulfonamides**. Avoid. [Severe] Theoretical
- **Sulfonamides** are predicted to increase the exposure to **methotrexate**. Use with caution or avoid. [Severe] Theoretical
- **Potassium aminobenzoate** is predicted to affect the efficacy of **sulfonamides**. Avoid. [Severe] Theoretical
- **Sulfonamides** are predicted to increase the exposure to **sulfonylureas**. [Moderate] Study

- **Sulfonamides** are predicted to increase the effects of **thiopental**. [Moderate] Theoretical

Sulfonylureas

glibenclamide · gliclazide · glimepiride · glipizide · tolbutamide

- Anti-androgens **(apalutamide)** are predicted to decrease the exposure to **glibenclamide**. Monitor and adjust dose. [Mild] Theoretical
- Anti-androgens **(darolutamide)** are predicted to increase the concentration of **glibenclamide**. [Moderate] Theoretical
- Antiarrhythmics **(amiodarone)** are predicted to increase the exposure to **sulfonylureas**. [Moderate] Theoretical
- Antifungals, azoles **(miconazole)** are predicted to increase the exposure to **gliclazide**. Avoid. [Moderate] Anecdotal
- Antifungals, azoles **(miconazole)** are predicted to increase the exposure to **glimepiride**. [Moderate] Theoretical
- Antifungals, azoles **(miconazole)** are predicted to increase the exposure to **glipizide**. Avoid. [Moderate] Theoretical
- Antifungals, azoles **(voriconazole)** are predicted to increase the concentration of **sulfonylureas**. Use with caution and adjust dose. [Moderate] Study
- Antifungals, azoles **(miconazole)** are predicted to increase the exposure to sulfonylureas **(glibenclamide, tolbutamide)**. [Moderate] Anecdotal
- **Belumosudil** is predicted to increase the exposure to **glibenclamide**. Avoid or adjust dose. [Moderate] Study
- **Bulevirtide** is predicted to increase the exposure to **glibenclamide**. Avoid or monitor. [Moderate] Theoretical
- Cephalosporins **(ceftobiprole)** are predicted to increase the concentration of **glibenclamide**. [Moderate] Theoretical
- **Ceritinib** is predicted to increase the exposure to **glimepiride**. Adjust dose. [Moderate] Theoretical
- **Chloramphenicol** is predicted to increase the exposure to **sulfonylureas**. [Severe] Study
- **Ciclosporin** is predicted to increase the exposure to **glibenclamide** and **glibenclamide** might increase the exposure to **ciclosporin**. Monitor and adjust **ciclosporin** dose, p. 640. [Moderate] Study
- **Elexacaftor** is predicted to increase the exposure to **glibenclamide**. [Moderate] Theoretical
- **Encorafenib** is predicted to increase the exposure to **glibenclamide**. [Mild] Study
- Endothelin receptor antagonists **(bosentan)** increase the risk of hepatotoxicity when given with **glibenclamide**. Avoid. [Severe] Study
- **Fenfluramine** might decrease blood glucose concentrations when given with **sulfonylureas**. [Moderate] Theoretical
- **Fibrates** are predicted to increase the risk of hypoglycaemia when given with **sulfonylureas**. [Moderate] Theoretical
- HIV-protease inhibitors **(atazanavir, lopinavir)** boosted with ritonavir are predicted to increase the exposure to **glibenclamide**. [Moderate] Theoretical
- **Leflunomide** is predicted to increase the exposure to **glibenclamide**. [Moderate] Study
- **Leniolisib** is predicted to increase the exposure to **glibenclamide**. Avoid. [Moderate] Theoretical
- **Letermovir** is predicted to increase the concentration of **glibenclamide**. [Moderate] Theoretical
- Macrolides **(clarithromycin)** might increase the exposure to **sulfonylureas**. [Moderate] Theoretical
- **Metreleptin** is predicted to increase the risk of hypoglycaemia when given with **sulfonylureas**. Monitor blood glucose and adjust dose. [Severe] Theoretical
- **Mifepristone** is predicted to increase the exposure to sulfonylureas **(glimepiride, tolbutamide)**. [Moderate] Theoretical
- **Nitisinone** is predicted to increase the exposure to sulfonylureas **(glimepiride, tolbutamide)**. [Moderate] Study
- Rifamycins **(rifampicin)** are predicted to decrease the exposure to **sulfonylureas**. [Moderate] Study
- **Roxadustat** is predicted to increase the exposure to **glibenclamide**. Monitor adverse effects and adjust dose. [Moderate] Study
- **Somapacitan** might increase blood glucose concentrations, opposing the blood glucose-lowering effects of **sulfonylureas**. Adjust dose. [Moderate] Theoretical
- **Somatrogon** might increase blood glucose concentrations, opposing the blood glucose-lowering effects of **sulfonylureas**. Adjust dose. [Moderate] Theoretical
- **Sparsentan** is predicted to decrease the exposure to sulfonylureas **(glimepiride, tolbutamide)**. [Moderate] Theoretical
- Statins **(fluvastatin)** slightly increase the exposure to **glibenclamide**. [Mild] Study
- **Sulfonamides** are predicted to increase the exposure to **sulfonylureas**. [Moderate] Study
- Taxanes **(cabazitaxel)** are predicted to affect the exposure to **glibenclamide**. Manufacturer advises take 12 hours before or 3 hours after **cabazitaxel**. [Moderate] Theoretical
- **Teriflunomide** is predicted to increase the exposure to **glibenclamide**. [Moderate] Study
- **Velpatasvir** is predicted to increase the exposure to **glibenclamide**. [Moderate] Study
- **Venetoclax** is predicted to increase the exposure to **glibenclamide**. [Moderate] Theoretical
- **Voclosporin** is predicted to increase the concentration of **glibenclamide**. [Moderate] Theoretical
- **Voxilaprevir** with sofosbuvir and velpatasvir is predicted to increase the exposure to **glibenclamide**. [Moderate] Study

Sulindac → see NSAIDs

Sulpiride → see **TABLE 15** p. 1058 (hyponatraemia), **TABLE 6** p. 1054 (hypotension), **TABLE 9** p. 1056 (CNS effects)

- Oral **antacids** decrease the absorption of oral **sulpiride**. Separate administration by 2 hours. [Moderate] Study
- **Sulpiride** is predicted to decrease the effects of **dopamine receptor agonists**. Avoid. [Moderate] Theoretical → Also see **TABLE 6** p. 1054 → Also see **TABLE 9** p. 1056
- **Sulpiride** opposes the effects of the active metabolite of **foslevodopa**. [Severe] Theoretical → Also see **TABLE 6** p. 1054 → Also see **TABLE 9** p. 1056
- **Sulpiride** is predicted to decrease the effects of **levodopa**. Avoid. [Severe] Theoretical → Also see **TABLE 6** p. 1054 → Also see **TABLE 9** p. 1056
- **Sulpiride** potentially increases the risk of neurotoxicity when given with **lithium**. [Severe] Anecdotal
- **Sucralfate** decreases the absorption of **sulpiride**. Separate administration by 2 hours. [Moderate] Study

Sultiame → see antiepileptics

Sumatriptan → see triptans

Sunitinib → see **TABLE 3** p. 1053 (bleeding), **TABLE 12** p. 1057 (myelosuppression), **TABLE 7** p. 1055 (QT-interval prolongation)

- Anti-androgens **(apalutamide, enzalutamide)** are predicted to decrease the exposure to **sunitinib**. Avoid or adjust dose—consult product literature. [Moderate] Study → Also see **TABLE 7** p. 1055
- Antiarrhythmics **(dronedarone)** are predicted to increase the exposure to **sunitinib**. [Moderate] Study → Also see **TABLE 7** p. 1055
- Antiepileptics **(carbamazepine, fosphenytoin, phenobarbital, phenytoin, primidone)** are predicted to decrease the exposure to **sunitinib**. Avoid or adjust dose—consult product literature. [Moderate] Study
- Antifungals, azoles **(fluconazole, isavuconazole)** are predicted to increase the exposure to **sunitinib**. [Moderate] Study → Also see **TABLE 7** p. 1055
- Antifungals, azoles **(itraconazole, ketoconazole, posaconazole, voriconazole)** are predicted to increase the exposure to **sunitinib**. Avoid or adjust dose—consult product literature. [Moderate] Study → Also see **TABLE 7** p. 1055
- **Berotralstat** is predicted to increase the exposure to **sunitinib**. [Moderate] Study
- Calcium-channel blockers **(diltiazem, verapamil)** are predicted to increase the exposure to **sunitinib**. [Moderate] Study
- **Cenobamate** is predicted to decrease the exposure to **sunitinib**. [Moderate] Study
- **Ceritinib** is predicted to increase the exposure to **sunitinib**. Avoid or adjust dose—consult product literature. [Moderate] Study → Also see **TABLE 12** p. 1057 → Also see **TABLE 7** p. 1055
- **Cobicistat** is predicted to increase the exposure to **sunitinib**. Avoid or adjust dose—consult product literature. [Moderate] Study
- **Crizotinib** is predicted to increase the exposure to **sunitinib**. [Moderate] Study → Also see **TABLE 7** p. 1055

Sunitinib (continued)

- Dabrafenib is predicted to decrease the exposure to sunitinib. Moderate Study
- Elbasvir is predicted to increase the concentration of sunitinib. Use with caution and adjust dose. Moderate Theoretical
- Encorafenib is predicted to decrease the exposure to sunitinib. Avoid or adjust dose—consult product literature. Moderate Study → Also see TABLE 7 p. 1055
- Endothelin receptor antagonists (bosentan) are predicted to decrease the exposure to sunitinib. Moderate Study
- Fedratinib is predicted to increase the exposure to sunitinib. Moderate Study
- Grapefruit juice is predicted to increase the exposure to sunitinib. Avoid. Moderate Theoretical
- Grazoprevir is predicted to increase the concentration of sunitinib. Use with caution and adjust dose. Moderate Theoretical
- HIV-protease inhibitors are predicted to increase the exposure to sunitinib. Avoid or adjust dose—consult product literature. Moderate Study
- Idelalisib is predicted to increase the exposure to sunitinib. Avoid or adjust dose—consult product literature. Moderate Study
- Imatinib is predicted to increase the exposure to sunitinib. Moderate Study → Also see TABLE 3 p. 1053 → Also see TABLE 12 p. 1057
- Ivosidenib is predicted to decrease the exposure to sunitinib. Avoid or adjust dose—consult product literature. Moderate Study → Also see TABLE 7 p. 1055
- Letermovir is predicted to increase the exposure to sunitinib. Moderate Study
- Lorlatinib is predicted to decrease the exposure to sunitinib. Moderate Study
- Lumacaftor is predicted to decrease the exposure to sunitinib. Avoid or adjust dose—consult product literature. Moderate Study
- Macrolides (clarithromycin) are predicted to increase the exposure to sunitinib. Avoid or adjust dose—consult product literature. Moderate Study
- Macrolides (erythromycin) are predicted to increase the exposure to sunitinib. Moderate Study → Also see TABLE 7 p. 1055
- Mitotane is predicted to decrease the exposure to sunitinib. Avoid or adjust dose—consult product literature. Moderate Study → Also see TABLE 12 p. 1057
- Neurokinin-1 receptor antagonists (aprepitant, netupitant) are predicted to increase the exposure to sunitinib. Moderate Study
- Nilotinib is predicted to increase the exposure to sunitinib. Moderate Study → Also see TABLE 12 p. 1057 → Also see TABLE 7 p. 1055
- NNRTIs (efavirenz, etravirine, nevirapine) are predicted to decrease the exposure to sunitinib. Moderate Study → Also see TABLE 7 p. 1055
- Rifamycins (rifampicin) are predicted to decrease the exposure to sunitinib. Avoid or adjust dose—consult product literature. Moderate Study
- Sotorasib is predicted to decrease the exposure to sunitinib. Moderate Study
- St John's wort is predicted to decrease the exposure to sunitinib. Moderate Study
- Sunitinib has been reported to cause hypothyroidism when given with thyroid hormones (levothyroxine). Moderate Anecdotal
- Tucatinib is predicted to increase the exposure to sunitinib. Avoid or adjust dose—consult product literature. Moderate Study

Suxamethonium → see TABLE 4 p. 1054 (bradycardia), TABLE 13 p. 1057 (increased serum potassium)

- Alkylating agents (cyclophosphamide) increase the risk of prolonged neuromuscular blockade when given with suxamethonium. Moderate Study
- Aminoglycosides might prolong the effects of suxamethonium. Severe Theoretical
- Antiarrhythmics (lidocaine) are predicted to increase the effects of suxamethonium. Moderate Study
- Anticholinesterases, centrally acting increase the effects of suxamethonium. Moderate Theoretical → Also see TABLE 4 p. 1054
- Antiepileptics (carbamazepine) increase the risk of prolonged neuromuscular blockade when given with suxamethonium. Moderate Study
- Antiepileptics (fosphenytoin, phenytoin) increase the effects of suxamethonium. Moderate Study
- Suxamethonium might increase the concentration of beta blockers, selective (landiolol) and beta blockers, selective (landiolol) might prolong the effects of suxamethonium. Moderate Study → Also see TABLE 4 p. 1054
- Clindamycin increases the effects of suxamethonium. Severe Anecdotal
- Colistimethate might prolong the effects of suxamethonium. Moderate Theoretical
- Corticosteroids are predicted to decrease the effects of suxamethonium. Severe Anecdotal
- Suxamethonium is predicted to increase the risk of cardiovascular adverse effects when given with digoxin. Severe Anecdotal → Also see TABLE 4 p. 1054
- Irinotecan is predicted to increase the risk of prolonged neuromuscular blockade when given with suxamethonium. Moderate Theoretical
- Intravenous magnesium is predicted to increase the effects of suxamethonium. Moderate Study
- Metoclopramide increases the effects of suxamethonium. Moderate Study
- Neomycin might prolong the effects of suxamethonium. Severe Theoretical
- Penicillins (piperacillin) increase the effects of suxamethonium. Moderate Study
- Polymyxin b might prolong the effects of suxamethonium. Severe Theoretical
- SSRIs potentially increase the risk of prolonged neuromuscular blockade when given with suxamethonium. Unknown Theoretical

Sympathomimetics, inotropic

dobutamine · dopamine

- Sympathomimetics, inotropic are predicted to decrease the effects of apraclonidine. Avoid. Severe Theoretical
- Beta blockers, non-selective increase the risk of hypertension and bradycardia when given with dobutamine. Severe Theoretical
- Beta blockers, selective increase the risk of hypertension and bradycardia when given with dobutamine. Moderate Theoretical
- Entacapone is predicted to increase the risk of cardiovascular adverse effects when given with sympathomimetics, inotropic. Moderate Theoretical
- Ergometrine potentially increases the risk of peripheral vasoconstriction when given with dopamine. Avoid. Severe Anecdotal
- Sympathomimetics, inotropic are predicted to increase the risk of elevated blood pressure when given with linezolid. Avoid. Severe Theoretical
- Sympathomimetics, inotropic are predicted to increase the risk of a hypertensive crisis when given with MAO-B inhibitors. Avoid. Severe Anecdotal
- Sympathomimetics, inotropic are predicted to increase the risk of a hypertensive crisis when given with MAOIs, irreversible. Avoid and for 14 days after stopping the MAOI. Severe Theoretical
- Opicapone is predicted to increase the risk of cardiovascular adverse effects when given with sympathomimetics, inotropic. Severe Theoretical
- Tolcapone is predicted to increase the risk of cardiovascular adverse effects when given with sympathomimetics, inotropic. Moderate Theoretical

Sympathomimetics, vasoconstrictor

adrenaline · ephedrine · isometheptene · metaraminol · midodrine · noradrenaline · phenylephrine · pseudoephedrine · xylometazoline

ROUTE-SPECIFIC INFORMATION Since systemic absorption can follow topical application of **phenylephrine** or **xylometazoline**, the possibility of interactions should be borne in mind.

- **Ephedrine** increases the risk of adverse effects when given with **aminophylline**. Avoid in children. [Moderate] Study
- **Sympathomimetics, vasoconstrictor** are predicted to decrease the effects of **apraclonidine**. Avoid. [Severe] Theoretical
- **Atropine** increases the risk of severe hypertension when given with **phenylephrine**. [Severe] Study
- **Beta blockers, non-selective** are predicted to increase the risk of hypertension and bradycardia when given with sympathomimetics, vasoconstrictor **(adrenaline, noradrenaline)**. [Severe] Study
- **Beta blockers, selective** are predicted to increase the risk of hypertension and bradycardia when given with sympathomimetics, vasoconstrictor **(adrenaline, noradrenaline)**. [Severe] Study
- **Isometheptene** potentially increases the risk of adverse effects when given with dopamine receptor agonists **(bromocriptine)**. Avoid. [Severe] Anecdotal
- **Entacapone** is predicted to increase the risk of cardiovascular adverse effects when given with sympathomimetics, vasoconstrictor **(adrenaline, noradrenaline)**. [Moderate] Study
- **Ergometrine** is predicted to increase the risk of peripheral vasoconstriction when given with **noradrenaline**. [Severe] Anecdotal
- Sympathomimetics, vasoconstrictor **(adrenaline, noradrenaline)** might increase the cardiovascular adverse effects of the active metabolite of **foslevodopa**. [Moderate] Theoretical
- **Midodrine** might increase the risk of a hypertensive crisis when given with **linezolid**. Avoid. [Severe] Theoretical
- **Pseudoephedrine** increases the risk of elevated blood pressure when given with **linezolid**. Avoid. [Severe] Study
- Sympathomimetics, vasoconstrictor **(adrenaline, ephedrine, isometheptene, noradrenaline, phenylephrine)** are predicted to increase the risk of elevated blood pressure when given with **linezolid**. Avoid. [Severe] Theoretical
- **Sympathomimetics, vasoconstrictor** are predicted to increase the risk of a hypertensive crisis when given with **MAO-B inhibitors**. Avoid. [Severe] Anecdotal
- **Sympathomimetics, vasoconstrictor** are predicted to increase the risk of a hypertensive crisis when given with **MAOIs, irreversible**. Avoid and for 14 days after stopping the MAOI. [Severe] Study
- **Mianserin** decreases the effects of **ephedrine**. [Severe] Anecdotal
- Sympathomimetics, vasoconstrictor **(ephedrine, isometheptene, phenylephrine, pseudoephedrine)** are predicted to increase the risk of a hypertensive crisis when given with **moclobemide**. Avoid. [Severe] Study
- **Opicapone** is predicted to increase the risk of cardiovascular adverse effects when given with sympathomimetics, vasoconstrictor **(adrenaline, noradrenaline)**. [Severe] Theoretical
- **Sympathomimetics, vasoconstrictor** might increase the risk of a hypertensive crisis when given with **ozanimod**. [Severe] Theoretical
- **Ephedrine** increases the risk of adverse effects when given with **theophylline**. Avoid in children. [Moderate] Study
- **Tolcapone** is predicted to increase the effects of sympathomimetics, vasoconstrictor **(adrenaline, noradrenaline)**. [Moderate] Theoretical
- **Tricyclic antidepressants** are predicted to decrease the effects of **ephedrine**. Avoid. [Severe] Study
- **Tricyclic antidepressants** increase the effects of sympathomimetics, vasoconstrictor **(adrenaline, noradrenaline, phenylephrine)**. Avoid. [Severe] Study
- **Adrenaline** might increase the hypertensive effect of **vasopressin**. [Moderate] Theoretical
- **Noradrenaline** might affect the hypertensive effect of **vasopressin**. [Moderate] Theoretical
- Volatile halogenated anaesthetics **(sevoflurane)** can cause hypertension, as can **ephedrine**. Avoid **ephedrine** for several days before surgery. [Severe] Theoretical
- Volatile halogenated anaesthetics **(sevoflurane)** can cause hypertension, as can **pseudoephedrine**. Avoid **pseudoephedrine** for several days before surgery. [Severe] Theoretical
- Volatile halogenated anaesthetics **(sevoflurane)** can cause hypertension, as can **xylometazoline**. Avoid **xylometazoline** for several days before surgery. [Severe] Theoretical

Tacalcitol → see vitamin D substances

Tacrolimus → see TABLE 2 p. 1053 (nephrotoxicity), TABLE 13 p. 1057 (increased serum potassium)

> - Pomelo and pomegranate juices might greatly increase the concentration of tacrolimus.
> - Since systemic absorption can follow topical application, the possibility of interactions should be borne in mind.

- **Tacrolimus** is predicted to increase the exposure to **afatinib**. [Moderate] Theoretical
- **Alcohol** increases the risk of facial flushing and skin irritation when given with topical **tacrolimus**. [Moderate] Study
- Anti-androgens **(apalutamide, enzalutamide)** decrease the concentration of **tacrolimus**. Avoid or monitor and adjust dose. [Severe] Study
- Antiarrhythmics **(amiodarone)** are predicted to increase the concentration of **tacrolimus**. [Severe] Anecdotal
- Antiarrhythmics **(dronedarone)** are predicted to increase the concentration of **tacrolimus**. Monitor and adjust dose. [Severe] Theoretical
- Antiepileptics **(carbamazepine, fosphenytoin, phenobarbital, phenytoin, primidone)** decrease the concentration of **tacrolimus**. Avoid or monitor and adjust dose. [Severe] Study
- Antifungals, azoles **(fluconazole)** increase the concentration of **tacrolimus**. Monitor and adjust dose. [Severe] Study
- Antifungals, azoles **(isavuconazole)** moderately increase the exposure to **tacrolimus**. Monitor and adjust dose. [Severe] Study
- Antifungals, azoles **(itraconazole, ketoconazole, posaconazole, voriconazole)** are predicted to increase the concentration of **tacrolimus**. Avoid. If concurrent use is unavoidable—consult product literature. [Severe] Study
- Antifungals, azoles **(miconazole)** are predicted to increase the concentration of **tacrolimus**. Monitor and adjust dose. [Severe] Theoretical
- **Baricitinib** is predicted to enhance the risk of immunosuppression when given with **tacrolimus**. [Severe] Theoretical
- **Berotralstat** is predicted to increase the concentration of **tacrolimus**. Monitor and adjust dose. [Severe] Theoretical
- **Brigatinib** potentially decreases the concentration of **tacrolimus**. Avoid. [Moderate] Theoretical
- **Bulevirtide** is predicted to increase the exposure to **tacrolimus**. [Moderate] Theoretical
- Calcium-channel blockers **(diltiazem)** increase the concentration of **tacrolimus**. Monitor and adjust dose. [Severe] Anecdotal
- Calcium-channel blockers **(nicardipine)** potentially increase the concentration of **tacrolimus**. Monitor concentration and adjust dose. [Severe] Anecdotal
- Calcium-channel blockers **(verapamil)** are predicted to increase the concentration of **tacrolimus**. Monitor and adjust dose. [Severe] Theoretical
- **Cannabidiol** is predicted to increase the concentration of **tacrolimus**. Monitor and adjust dose. [Moderate] Theoretical
- **Ceritinib** is predicted to increase the concentration of **tacrolimus**. Avoid. If concurrent use is unavoidable—consult product literature. [Severe] Study
- **Chloramphenicol** increases the concentration of **tacrolimus**. [Severe] Study
- **Ciclosporin** increases the concentration of **tacrolimus**. Avoid. [Severe] Study → Also see TABLE 2 p. 1053 → Also see TABLE 13 p. 1057
- **Cobicistat** is predicted to increase the concentration of **tacrolimus**. Avoid. If concurrent use is unavoidable—consult product literature. [Severe] Study
- **Crizotinib** is predicted to increase the concentration of **tacrolimus**. Monitor and adjust dose. [Severe] Theoretical
- **Dabrafenib** is predicted to decrease the exposure to **tacrolimus**. Monitor and adjust dose. [Moderate] Theoretical
- **Danicopan** is predicted to increase the exposure to **tacrolimus**. [Moderate] Theoretical
- **Encorafenib** decreases the concentration of **tacrolimus**. Avoid or monitor and adjust dose. [Severe] Study
- Endothelin receptor antagonists **(bosentan)** are predicted to decrease the concentration of **tacrolimus** and **tacrolimus** potentially increases the concentration of endothelin receptor antagonists **(bosentan)**. Avoid. [Severe] Theoretical

Tacrolimus (continued)
- **Fedratinib** is predicted to increase the concentration of **tacrolimus**. Monitor and adjust dose. Severe Theoretical
- **Filgotinib** is predicted to increase the risk of immunosuppression when given with **tacrolimus**. Avoid. Severe Theoretical
- **Givinostat** might increase the exposure to **tacrolimus**. Moderate Study
- **Glecaprevir** with pibrentasvir slightly increases the exposure to **tacrolimus**. Monitor and adjust dose. Mild Study
- **Grapefruit** juice greatly increases the concentration of **tacrolimus**. Avoid. Severe Study
- **Grazoprevir** increases the exposure to **tacrolimus**. Moderate Study
- **HIV-protease inhibitors** are predicted to increase the concentration of **tacrolimus**. Avoid. If concurrent use is unavoidable—consult product literature. Severe Study
- **Idelalisib** is predicted to increase the concentration of **tacrolimus**. Avoid. If concurrent use is unavoidable—consult product literature. Severe Study
- **Imatinib** increases the concentration of **tacrolimus**. Monitor and adjust dose. Severe Study
- Iron chelators **(dexrazoxane)** might increase the risk of immunosuppression when given with **tacrolimus**. Severe Theoretical
- **Ivacaftor** is predicted to increase the exposure to **tacrolimus**. Moderate Theoretical
- **Ivosidenib** decreases the concentration of **tacrolimus**. Avoid or monitor and adjust dose. Severe Study
- **Larotrectinib** is predicted to increase the exposure to **tacrolimus**. Use with caution and adjust dose. Mild Theoretical
- **Lazertinib** is predicted to increase the exposure to **tacrolimus**. Moderate Study
- **Letermovir** moderately increases the exposure to **tacrolimus**. Monitor and adjust dose. Severe Study
- **Live vaccines** are predicted to increase the risk of generalised infection (possibly life-threatening) when given with **tacrolimus**. UKHSA advises avoid (refer to Green Book). Severe Theoretical
- **Tacrolimus** is predicted to increase the exposure to **lomitapide**. Separate administration by 12 hours. Moderate Theoretical
- **Lorlatinib** is predicted to decrease the exposure to **tacrolimus**. Avoid. Moderate Theoretical
- **Lumacaftor** decreases the concentration of **tacrolimus**. Avoid or monitor and adjust dose. Severe Study
- Macrolides **(clarithromycin)** are predicted to increase the concentration of **tacrolimus**. Avoid. If concurrent use is unavoidable—consult product literature. Severe Study
- Macrolides **(erythromycin)** increase the concentration of **tacrolimus**. Avoid. If concurrent use is unavoidable—consult product literature. Severe Anecdotal
- **Maribavir** is predicted to slightly increase the exposure to **tacrolimus**. Monitor and adjust dose. Severe Study
- **Metronidazole** has been reported to increase the concentration of **tacrolimus**. Severe Anecdotal
- **Tacrolimus** is predicted to affect the efficacy of **mifamurtide**. Avoid. Severe Theoretical
- **Mitotane** decreases the concentration of **tacrolimus**. Avoid or monitor and adjust dose. Severe Study
- Monoclonal antibodies **(sarilumab)** potentially affect the exposure to **tacrolimus**. Monitor and adjust dose. Moderate Theoretical
- Neurokinin-1 receptor antagonists **(aprepitant)** increase the concentration of **tacrolimus**. Monitor and adjust dose. Severe Study
- Neurokinin-1 receptor antagonists **(netupitant)** are predicted to increase the concentration of **tacrolimus**. Monitor and adjust dose. Severe Theoretical
- **Nilotinib** is predicted to increase the concentration of **tacrolimus**. Monitor and adjust dose. Severe Theoretical
- **Nirmatrelvir** boosted with ritonavir is predicted to increase the concentration of **tacrolimus**. Avoid—consult product literature. Severe Theoretical
- NNRTIs **(doravirine)** are predicted to decrease the exposure to **tacrolimus**. Monitor **tacrolimus** concentration and adjust dose, p. 642. Moderate Theoretical
- NNRTIs **(efavirenz, nevirapine)** are predicted to decrease the concentration of **tacrolimus**. Monitor and adjust dose. Moderate Theoretical
- NNRTIs **(etravirine)** are predicted to decrease the exposure to **tacrolimus**. Monitor and adjust dose. Moderate Theoretical
- **Olaparib** might alter the exposure to **tacrolimus**. Moderate Theoretical
- **Palbociclib** is predicted to increase the exposure to **tacrolimus**. Adjust dose. Moderate Theoretical
- Penicillins **(flucloxacillin)** (high-dose) might decrease the exposure to **tacrolimus**. Moderate Study
- **Pibrentasvir** with glecaprevir slightly increases the exposure to **tacrolimus**. Monitor and adjust dose. Mild Study
- **Pitolisant** is predicted to decrease the exposure to **tacrolimus**. Avoid. Severe Theoretical
- **Ranolazine** increases the concentration of **tacrolimus**. Adjust dose. Severe Anecdotal
- **Ribociclib** is predicted to increase the exposure to **tacrolimus**. Use with caution and adjust dose. Moderate Theoretical
- Rifamycins **(rifampicin)** decrease the concentration of **tacrolimus**. Avoid or monitor and adjust dose. Severe Study → Also see TABLE 2 p. 1053
- **Ritlecitinib** is predicted to increase the exposure to **tacrolimus**. Adjust dose. Moderate Theoretical
- **Rucaparib** is predicted to increase the exposure to **tacrolimus**. Monitor and adjust dose. Moderate Study
- **Sirolimus** is predicted to decrease the concentration of **tacrolimus** and **tacrolimus** increases the exposure to **sirolimus**. Severe Study
- **Tacrolimus** potentially increases the risk of serotonin toxicity when given with SNRIs **(venlafaxine)**. Severe Anecdotal
- **Sotorasib** is predicted to decrease the exposure to **tacrolimus**. Monitor and adjust dose. Severe Theoretical
- **St John's wort** decreases the concentration of **tacrolimus**. Avoid. Severe Study
- **Tarlatamab** might affect the exposure to **tacrolimus**. Monitor and adjust dose. Moderate Theoretical
- **Tacrolimus** is predicted to increase the exposure to thrombin inhibitors **(dabigatran)**. Avoid. Severe Theoretical
- **Tigecycline** has been reported to increase the concentration of **tacrolimus**. Severe Anecdotal
- **Tacrolimus** increases the exposure to **tofacitinib**. Avoid. Severe Study
- **Tucatinib** is predicted to increase the concentration of **tacrolimus**. Avoid. If concurrent use is unavoidable—consult product literature. Severe Study
- **Vorasidenib** might decrease the concentration of **tacrolimus**. Avoid. Severe Theoretical

Tadalafil → see phosphodiesterase type-5 inhibitors

Tafamidis
- **Tafamidis** slightly increases the exposure to statins **(rosuvastatin)**. Severe Study

Tafasitamab → see monoclonal antibodies

Talazoparib → see TABLE 12 p. 1057 (myelosuppression)
- Anti-androgens **(apalutamide)** are predicted to decrease the exposure to **talazoparib**. Monitor and adjust dose. Moderate Study
- Anti-androgens **(enzalutamide)** moderately increase the exposure to **talazoparib**. Adjust starting dose. Moderate Study
- Antiarrhythmics **(amiodarone, dronedarone)** are predicted to slightly increase the exposure to **talazoparib**. Avoid or adjust dose—consult product literature. Severe Study
- Antiarrhythmics **(propafenone)** are predicted to increase the exposure to **talazoparib**. Avoid or adjust dose—consult product literature. Moderate Theoretical
- Antifungals, azoles **(itraconazole, ketoconazole)** are predicted to slightly increase the exposure to **talazoparib**. Avoid or adjust dose—consult product literature. Severe Study
- **Belumosudil** might increase the exposure to **talazoparib**. Avoid or adjust dose. Moderate Theoretical
- **Berotralstat** is predicted to increase the concentration of **talazoparib**. Monitor and adjust dose. Moderate Study

- Beta blockers, non-selective (carvedilol) cause a small increase in the bioavailability of **talazoparib**. Avoid or adjust dose—consult product literature. Moderate Study
- Calcium-channel blockers (diltiazem, felodipine) very slightly increase the exposure to **talazoparib**. Moderate Study
- Calcium-channel blockers (verapamil) are predicted to slightly increase the exposure to **talazoparib**. Avoid or adjust dose—consult product literature. Severe Study
- **Cannabidiol** is predicted to increase the exposure to **talazoparib**. Monitor and adjust dose. Moderate Study
- **Ciclosporin** is predicted to slightly increase the exposure to **talazoparib**. Avoid or adjust dose—consult product literature. Severe Study
- **Cobicistat** is predicted to slightly increase the exposure to **talazoparib**. Avoid or adjust dose—consult product literature. Severe Study
- **Danicopan** is predicted to increase the exposure to **talazoparib**. Moderate Study
- **Daridorexant** is predicted to increase the exposure to **talazoparib**. Moderate Study
- **Deutivacaftor** is predicted to increase the exposure to **talazoparib**. Moderate Theoretical
- **Eliglustat** is predicted to increase the exposure to **talazoparib**. Adjust dose. Moderate Study
- **Eltrombopag** is predicted to increase the exposure to **talazoparib**. Avoid or monitor. Moderate Theoretical
- **Erdafitinib** is predicted to increase the exposure to **talazoparib**. Separate administration by at least 6 hours. Moderate Theoretical
- **Glecaprevir** is predicted to slightly increase the exposure to **talazoparib**. Avoid or adjust dose—consult product literature. Severe Study
- HIV-protease inhibitors (darunavir) are predicted to increase the exposure to **talazoparib**. Avoid or adjust dose—consult product literature. Moderate Theoretical
- HIV-protease inhibitors (lopinavir, ritonavir) are predicted to slightly increase the exposure to **talazoparib**. Avoid or adjust dose—consult product literature. Severe Study
- **Ibrutinib** might increase the exposure to **talazoparib**. Separate administration by at least 6 hours. Moderate Theoretical → Also see TABLE 12 p. 1057
- **Ivacaftor** is predicted to increase the exposure to **talazoparib**. Moderate Study
- **Ivosidenib** is predicted to alter the exposure to **talazoparib**. Moderate Theoretical
- **Lapatinib** is predicted to slightly increase the exposure to **talazoparib**. Avoid or adjust dose—consult product literature. Severe Study
- **Leflunomide** is predicted to increase the exposure to **talazoparib**. Avoid or monitor. Moderate Theoretical → Also see TABLE 12 p. 1057
- **Lomitapide** might increase the exposure to **talazoparib**. Adjust dose. Moderate Theoretical
- **Lorlatinib** is predicted to decrease the exposure to **talazoparib**. Moderate Study
- **Macrolides** are predicted to slightly increase the exposure to **talazoparib**. Avoid or adjust dose—consult product literature. Severe Study
- **Neratinib** is predicted to increase the exposure to **talazoparib**. Moderate Study
- **Olaparib** might increase the exposure to **talazoparib**. Moderate Theoretical → Also see TABLE 12 p. 1057
- **Osimertinib** is predicted to increase the exposure to **talazoparib**. Moderate Study
- **Pemigatinib** might increase the exposure to **talazoparib**. Separate administration by at least 6 hours. Moderate Theoretical
- **Pibrentasvir** is predicted to slightly increase the exposure to **talazoparib**. Avoid or adjust dose—consult product literature. Severe Study
- **Pirtobrutinib** is predicted to increase the exposure to **talazoparib**. Avoid or monitor. Moderate Theoretical
- **Ranolazine** is predicted to slightly increase the exposure to **talazoparib**. Avoid or adjust dose—consult product literature. Severe Study
- **Selpercatinib** is predicted to increase the exposure to **talazoparib**. Moderate Study
- **Sparsentan** is predicted to increase the exposure to **talazoparib**. Severe Theoretical
- SSRIs (fluvoxamine) very slightly increase the exposure to **talazoparib**. Moderate Study
- Statins (atorvastatin) very slightly increase the exposure to **talazoparib**. Moderate Study
- **Tepotinib** is predicted to increase the concentration of **talazoparib**. Severe Study
- **Teriflunomide** is predicted to increase the exposure to **talazoparib**. Avoid or monitor. Moderate Theoretical
- **Tucatinib** is predicted to increase the exposure to **talazoparib**. Use with caution and adjust dose. Moderate Theoretical
- **Velpatasvir** is predicted to slightly increase the exposure to **talazoparib**. Avoid or adjust dose—consult product literature. Severe Study
- **Vemurafenib** is predicted to slightly increase the exposure to **talazoparib**. Avoid or adjust dose—consult product literature. Severe Study
- **Voclosporin** is predicted to increase the exposure to **talazoparib**. Moderate Study
- **Voxilaprevir** is predicted to slightly increase the exposure to **talazoparib**. Avoid or adjust dose—consult product literature. Severe Study

Tamoxifen

- **Tamoxifen** (high-dose) might increase the concentration of antiepileptics (fosphenytoin) and antiepileptics (fosphenytoin) might decrease the concentration of **tamoxifen** (high-dose). Severe Theoretical
- **Tamoxifen** (high-dose) might increase the concentration of antiepileptics (phenytoin) and antiepileptics (phenytoin) might decrease the concentration of **tamoxifen** (high-dose). Severe Anecdotal
- **Tamoxifen** increases the risk of retinopathy when given with antimalarials (chloroquine). RCOphth guidance advises monitor. Severe Study
- **Bupropion** is predicted to decrease the efficacy of **tamoxifen**. Avoid. Severe Study
- **Cinacalcet** is predicted to decrease the efficacy of **tamoxifen**. Avoid. Severe Study
- **Tamoxifen** increases the anticoagulant effect of **coumarins**. Severe Study
- **Dacomitinib** is predicted to decrease the efficacy of **tamoxifen**. Avoid. Severe Study
- **Tamoxifen** increases the risk of retinopathy when given with **hydroxychloroquine**. RCOphth guidance advises monitor. Severe Study
- Rifamycins (rifampicin) markedly decrease the exposure to **tamoxifen**. Unknown Study
- SSRIs (fluoxetine, paroxetine) are predicted to decrease the efficacy of **tamoxifen**. Avoid. Severe Study
- **Terbinafine** is predicted to decrease the efficacy of **tamoxifen**. Avoid. Severe Study
- **Vorasidenib** might decrease the concentration of **tamoxifen**. Avoid. Severe Theoretical

Tamsulosin → see alpha blockers

Tapentadol → see opioids

Tarlatamab

- **Tarlatamab** might affect the exposure to **sirolimus**. Monitor and adjust dose. Moderate Theoretical
- **Tarlatamab** might affect the exposure to **tacrolimus**. Monitor and adjust dose. Moderate Theoretical

Taxanes → see TABLE 12 p. 1057 (myelosuppression), TABLE 10 p. 1056 (peripheral neuropathy)

cabazitaxel · docetaxel · paclitaxel

- **Cabazitaxel** is predicted to affect the exposure to angiotensin-II receptor antagonists (valsartan). Manufacturer advises take 12 hours before or 3 hours after **cabazitaxel**. Moderate Theoretical
- Anti-androgens (apalutamide, enzalutamide) are predicted to decrease the exposure to **cabazitaxel**. Avoid. Moderate Study
- Anti-androgens (apalutamide, enzalutamide) are predicted to decrease the exposure to **docetaxel**. Severe Theoretical

A1 Interactions | Appendix 1

Taxanes (continued)

- Anti-androgens **(apalutamide, enzalutamide)** are predicted to decrease the exposure to **paclitaxel**. Avoid. Severe Study
- Anti-androgens **(darolutamide)** are predicted to increase the exposure to **paclitaxel**. Severe Theoretical
- Antiarrhythmics **(amiodarone)** are predicted to increase the exposure to **paclitaxel**. Severe Theoretical → Also see TABLE 10 p. 1056
- Antiarrhythmics **(dronedarone)** are predicted to increase the exposure to **cabazitaxel**. Moderate Theoretical
- Antiarrhythmics **(dronedarone)** are predicted to increase the exposure to **docetaxel**. Severe Study
- Antiarrhythmics **(dronedarone)** are predicted to increase the exposure to **paclitaxel**. Moderate Anecdotal
- Antiepileptics **(carbamazepine, fosphenytoin, phenobarbital, phenytoin, primidone)** are predicted to decrease the exposure to **cabazitaxel**. Avoid. Moderate Study → Also see TABLE 10 p. 1056
- Antiepileptics **(carbamazepine, fosphenytoin, phenobarbital, phenytoin, primidone)** are predicted to decrease the exposure to **docetaxel**. Severe Theoretical → Also see TABLE 10 p. 1056
- Antiepileptics **(carbamazepine, fosphenytoin, phenobarbital, phenytoin, primidone)** are predicted to decrease the exposure to **paclitaxel**. Avoid. Severe Study → Also see TABLE 10 p. 1056
- Antifungals, azoles **(fluconazole, isavuconazole)** are predicted to increase the exposure to **cabazitaxel**. Moderate Theoretical
- Antifungals, azoles **(fluconazole, isavuconazole)** are predicted to increase the exposure to **docetaxel**. Severe Study
- Antifungals, azoles **(fluconazole, isavuconazole, itraconazole, ketoconazole, posaconazole, voriconazole)** are predicted to increase the exposure to **paclitaxel**. Moderate Anecdotal
- Antifungals, azoles **(itraconazole, ketoconazole, posaconazole, voriconazole)** are predicted to increase the exposure to **cabazitaxel**. Avoid or adjust dose—consult product literature. Severe Study
- Antifungals, azoles **(itraconazole, ketoconazole, posaconazole, voriconazole)** are predicted to increase the exposure to **docetaxel**. Avoid or adjust dose. Severe Study
- Antifungals, azoles **(miconazole)** are predicted to increase the concentration of **docetaxel**. Use with caution and adjust dose. Moderate Theoretical
- **Cabazitaxel** is predicted to affect the exposure to antihistamines, non-sedating **(fexofenadine)**. Manufacturer advises take 12 hours before or 3 hours after **cabazitaxel**. Moderate Theoretical
- **Belumosudil** is predicted to increase the exposure to taxanes **(docetaxel, paclitaxel)**. Avoid or adjust dose. Moderate Study
- **Berotralstat** is predicted to increase the exposure to **cabazitaxel**. Moderate Theoretical
- **Berotralstat** is predicted to increase the exposure to **docetaxel**. Severe Study
- **Berotralstat** is predicted to increase the exposure to **paclitaxel**. Moderate Anecdotal
- **Bulevirtide** is predicted to increase the exposure to taxanes **(docetaxel, paclitaxel)**. Avoid or monitor. Moderate Theoretical
- Calcium-channel blockers **(diltiazem, verapamil)** are predicted to increase the exposure to **cabazitaxel**. Moderate Theoretical
- Calcium-channel blockers **(diltiazem, verapamil)** are predicted to increase the exposure to **docetaxel**. Severe Study
- Calcium-channel blockers **(diltiazem, verapamil)** are predicted to increase the exposure to **paclitaxel**. Moderate Anecdotal
- **Cannabidiol** is predicted to increase the exposure to **paclitaxel**. Monitor and adjust dose. Moderate Study
- **Cenobamate** is predicted to decrease the exposure to **docetaxel**. Severe Theoretical
- **Cenobamate** is predicted to decrease the exposure to **paclitaxel**. Avoid. Severe Study
- **Ceritinib** is predicted to increase the exposure to **cabazitaxel**. Avoid or adjust dose—consult product literature. Severe Study → Also see TABLE 12 p. 1057
- **Ceritinib** is predicted to increase the exposure to **docetaxel**. Avoid or adjust dose. Severe Study → Also see TABLE 12 p. 1057
- **Ceritinib** is predicted to increase the exposure to **paclitaxel**. Moderate Anecdotal → Also see TABLE 12 p. 1057
- **Ciclosporin** increases the concentration of **docetaxel** (oral). Unknown Study
- **Ciclosporin** increases the concentration of **paclitaxel**. Severe Study
- **Clopidogrel** is predicted to increase the concentration of **paclitaxel**. Severe Anecdotal
- **Cobicistat** is predicted to increase the exposure to **cabazitaxel**. Avoid or adjust dose—consult product literature. Severe Study
- **Cobicistat** is predicted to increase the exposure to **docetaxel**. Avoid or adjust dose. Severe Study
- **Cobicistat** is predicted to increase the exposure to **paclitaxel**. Moderate Anecdotal
- **Crizotinib** is predicted to increase the exposure to **cabazitaxel**. Moderate Theoretical
- **Crizotinib** is predicted to increase the exposure to **docetaxel**. Severe Study
- **Crizotinib** is predicted to increase the exposure to **paclitaxel**. Moderate Anecdotal
- **Dabrafenib** is predicted to decrease the exposure to **cabazitaxel**. Moderate Theoretical
- **Dabrafenib** is predicted to decrease the exposure to **docetaxel**. Severe Theoretical
- **Dabrafenib** is predicted to decrease the exposure to **paclitaxel**. Avoid. Severe Study
- **Danicopan** is predicted to increase the exposure to **paclitaxel**. Moderate Study
- **Daridorexant** is predicted to increase the exposure to **paclitaxel**. Moderate Study
- **Deutivacaftor** is predicted to increase the exposure to **paclitaxel**. Moderate Theoretical
- **Elexacaftor** is predicted to increase the exposure to taxanes **(docetaxel, paclitaxel)**. Moderate Theoretical
- **Eliglustat** is predicted to increase the exposure to **paclitaxel**. Adjust dose. Moderate Study
- **Eltrombopag** is predicted to increase the exposure to taxanes **(docetaxel, paclitaxel)**. Moderate Theoretical
- **Encorafenib** is predicted to decrease the exposure to **cabazitaxel**. Avoid. Moderate Study
- **Encorafenib** is predicted to decrease the exposure to **docetaxel**. Severe Theoretical
- **Encorafenib** is predicted to decrease the exposure to **paclitaxel**. Avoid. Severe Study
- Endothelin receptor antagonists **(bosentan)** are predicted to decrease the exposure to **cabazitaxel**. Moderate Theoretical
- Endothelin receptor antagonists **(bosentan)** are predicted to decrease the exposure to **docetaxel**. Severe Theoretical
- Endothelin receptor antagonists **(bosentan)** are predicted to decrease the exposure to **paclitaxel**. Avoid. Severe Study
- **Erdafitinib** is predicted to increase the exposure to **paclitaxel**. Separate administration by at least 6 hours. Moderate Theoretical
- **Fedratinib** is predicted to increase the exposure to **cabazitaxel**. Moderate Theoretical
- **Fedratinib** is predicted to increase the exposure to **docetaxel**. Severe Study
- **Fedratinib** is predicted to increase the exposure to **paclitaxel**. Moderate Anecdotal
- Fibrates **(gemfibrozil)** are predicted to increase the exposure to **docetaxel**. Moderate Theoretical
- Fibrates **(gemfibrozil)** are predicted to increase the concentration of **paclitaxel**. Severe Anecdotal
- **Glecaprevir** is predicted to increase the exposure to **paclitaxel**. Severe Theoretical
- **HIV-protease inhibitors** are predicted to increase the exposure to **cabazitaxel**. Avoid or adjust dose—consult product literature. Severe Study
- **HIV-protease inhibitors** are predicted to increase the exposure to **docetaxel**. Avoid or adjust dose. Severe Study
- **HIV-protease inhibitors** are predicted to increase the exposure to **paclitaxel**. Moderate Anecdotal
- **Ibrutinib** might increase the exposure to **paclitaxel**. Separate administration by at least 6 hours. Moderate Theoretical → Also see TABLE 12 p. 1057
- **Idelalisib** is predicted to increase the exposure to **cabazitaxel**. Avoid or adjust dose—consult product literature. Severe Study
- **Idelalisib** is predicted to increase the exposure to **docetaxel**. Avoid or adjust dose. Severe Study

- **Idelalisib** is predicted to increase the exposure to **paclitaxel**. [Moderate] Anecdotal
- **Imatinib** is predicted to increase the exposure to **cabazitaxel**. [Moderate] Theoretical → Also see TABLE 12 p. 1057
- **Imatinib** is predicted to increase the exposure to **docetaxel**. [Severe] Study → Also see TABLE 12 p. 1057
- **Imatinib** is predicted to increase the exposure to **paclitaxel**. [Moderate] Anecdotal → Also see TABLE 12 p. 1057
- Iron chelators **(deferasirox)** are predicted to increase the concentration of **paclitaxel**. [Severe] Anecdotal
- **Ivacaftor** is predicted to increase the exposure to **paclitaxel**. [Moderate] Study
- **Ivosidenib** is predicted to decrease the exposure to **cabazitaxel**. Avoid. [Moderate] Study
- **Ivosidenib** is predicted to decrease the exposure to **docetaxel**. [Severe] Theoretical
- **Ivosidenib** is predicted to decrease the exposure to **paclitaxel**. Avoid. [Severe] Study
- **Lapatinib** slightly increases the exposure to **paclitaxel**. [Severe] Study
- **Leflunomide** is predicted to increase the exposure to **docetaxel**. [Moderate] Study → Also see TABLE 12 p. 1057 → Also see TABLE 10 p. 1056
- **Leflunomide** is predicted to increase the concentration of **paclitaxel**. [Severe] Anecdotal → Also see TABLE 12 p. 1057 → Also see TABLE 10 p. 1056
- **Leniolisib** is predicted to increase the exposure to taxanes **(docetaxel, paclitaxel)**. Avoid. [Moderate] Theoretical
- **Letermovir** is predicted to increase the exposure to **cabazitaxel**. [Moderate] Theoretical
- **Letermovir** is predicted to increase the exposure to **docetaxel**. [Severe] Study
- **Letermovir** is predicted to increase the exposure to **paclitaxel**. [Moderate] Anecdotal
- **Linzagolix** is predicted to increase the exposure to **paclitaxel**. Avoid. [Mild] Theoretical
- **Live vaccines** are predicted to increase the risk of generalised infection (possibly life-threatening) when given with taxanes **(docetaxel, paclitaxel)**. UKHSA advises avoid (refer to Green Book). [Severe] Theoretical
- **Lomitapide** might increase the exposure to **paclitaxel**. Adjust dose. [Moderate] Theoretical
- **Lorlatinib** is predicted to decrease the exposure to **docetaxel**. [Severe] Theoretical
- **Lorlatinib** is predicted to decrease the exposure to **paclitaxel**. Avoid. [Severe] Study
- **Lumacaftor** is predicted to decrease the exposure to **cabazitaxel**. Avoid. [Moderate] Study
- **Lumacaftor** is predicted to decrease the exposure to **docetaxel**. [Severe] Theoretical
- **Lumacaftor** is predicted to decrease the exposure to **paclitaxel**. Avoid. [Severe] Study
- Macrolides **(azithromycin)** are predicted to increase the exposure to **paclitaxel**. [Moderate] Theoretical
- Macrolides **(clarithromycin)** are predicted to increase the exposure to **cabazitaxel**. Avoid or adjust dose—consult product literature. [Severe] Study
- Macrolides **(clarithromycin)** are predicted to increase the exposure to **docetaxel**. Avoid or adjust dose. [Severe] Study
- Macrolides **(clarithromycin, erythromycin)** are predicted to increase the exposure to **paclitaxel**. [Moderate] Anecdotal
- Macrolides **(erythromycin)** are predicted to increase the exposure to **cabazitaxel**. [Moderate] Theoretical
- Macrolides **(erythromycin)** are predicted to increase the exposure to **docetaxel**. [Severe] Study
- **Maribavir** is predicted to increase the exposure to **paclitaxel**. Use with caution and adjust dose. [Unknown] Study
- **Cabazitaxel** is predicted to affect the exposure to meglitinides **(repaglinide)**. Manufacturer advises take 12 hours before or 3 hours after **cabazitaxel**. [Moderate] Theoretical
- **Mirabegron** is predicted to increase the exposure to **paclitaxel**. [Mild] Theoretical
- **Mitotane** is predicted to decrease the exposure to **cabazitaxel**. Avoid. [Moderate] Study → Also see TABLE 12 p. 1057
- **Mitotane** is predicted to decrease the exposure to **docetaxel**. [Severe] Theoretical → Also see TABLE 12 p. 1057
- **Mitotane** is predicted to decrease the exposure to **paclitaxel**. Avoid. [Severe] Study → Also see TABLE 12 p. 1057
- **Neratinib** is predicted to increase the exposure to **paclitaxel**. [Moderate] Study
- Neurokinin-1 receptor antagonists **(aprepitant, netupitant)** are predicted to increase the exposure to **cabazitaxel**. [Moderate] Theoretical
- Neurokinin-1 receptor antagonists **(aprepitant, netupitant)** are predicted to increase the exposure to **docetaxel**. [Severe] Study
- Neurokinin-1 receptor antagonists **(aprepitant, netupitant)** are predicted to increase the exposure to **paclitaxel**. [Moderate] Anecdotal
- **Nilotinib** is predicted to increase the exposure to **cabazitaxel**. [Moderate] Theoretical → Also see TABLE 12 p. 1057
- **Nilotinib** is predicted to increase the exposure to **docetaxel**. [Severe] Study → Also see TABLE 12 p. 1057
- **Nilotinib** is predicted to increase the exposure to **paclitaxel**. [Moderate] Anecdotal → Also see TABLE 12 p. 1057
- NNRTIs **(efavirenz, etravirine, nevirapine)** are predicted to decrease the exposure to **cabazitaxel**. [Moderate] Theoretical
- NNRTIs **(efavirenz, etravirine, nevirapine)** are predicted to decrease the exposure to **docetaxel**. [Severe] Theoretical
- NNRTIs **(efavirenz, etravirine, nevirapine)** are predicted to decrease the exposure to **paclitaxel**. Avoid. [Severe] Study
- **Olaparib** might increase the exposure to **paclitaxel**. [Moderate] Theoretical → Also see TABLE 12 p. 1057
- **Osimertinib** is predicted to increase the exposure to **paclitaxel**. [Moderate] Study
- **Pemigatinib** might increase the exposure to **paclitaxel**. Separate administration by at least 6 hours. [Moderate] Theoretical
- **Pibrentasvir** with glecaprevir is predicted to increase the exposure to **paclitaxel**. [Moderate] Study
- **Pirtobrutinib** is predicted to increase the exposure to **paclitaxel**. Avoid or monitor. [Moderate] Theoretical
- **Pitolisant** is predicted to decrease the exposure to **docetaxel**. Avoid. [Severe] Theoretical
- **Pitolisant** is predicted to decrease the exposure to **paclitaxel**. [Mild] Theoretical
- **Pralsetinib** might affect the exposure to **paclitaxel**. Avoid. [Moderate] Theoretical
- **Ranolazine** is predicted to increase the exposure to **paclitaxel**. [Severe] Theoretical
- Rifamycins **(rifabutin)** are predicted to decrease the exposure to **cabazitaxel**. Avoid. [Moderate] Theoretical
- Rifamycins **(rifampicin)** are predicted to decrease the exposure to **cabazitaxel**. Avoid. [Moderate] Study
- Rifamycins **(rifampicin)** are predicted to decrease the exposure to **docetaxel**. [Severe] Theoretical
- Rifamycins **(rifampicin)** are predicted to decrease the exposure to **paclitaxel**. Avoid. [Severe] Study
- **Roxadustat** is predicted to increase the exposure to taxanes **(docetaxel, paclitaxel)**. Monitor adverse effects and adjust dose. [Moderate] Study
- **Sotorasib** is predicted to decrease the exposure to **docetaxel**. [Severe] Theoretical
- **Sotorasib** is predicted to decrease the exposure to **paclitaxel**. Avoid. [Severe] Study
- **Sparsentan** is predicted to increase the exposure to **paclitaxel**. [Severe] Theoretical
- **St John's wort** is predicted to decrease the exposure to **cabazitaxel**. Avoid. [Severe] Theoretical
- **St John's wort** is predicted to decrease the exposure to **docetaxel**. [Severe] Theoretical
- **St John's wort** is predicted to decrease the exposure to **paclitaxel**. Avoid. [Severe] Study
- **Cabazitaxel** is predicted to affect the exposure to statins **(atorvastatin, pravastatin, rosuvastatin, simvastatin)**. Manufacturer advises take 12 hours before or 3 hours after **cabazitaxel**. [Moderate] Theoretical
- **Cabazitaxel** is predicted to affect the exposure to sulfonylureas **(glibenclamide)**. Manufacturer advises take 12 hours before or 3 hours after **cabazitaxel**. [Moderate] Theoretical

Taxanes (continued)
- **Tepotinib** is predicted to increase the concentration of **paclitaxel.** Severe Study
- **Teriflunomide** is predicted to increase the exposure to **docetaxel.** Moderate Study → Also see TABLE 10 p. 1056
- **Teriflunomide** is predicted to increase the concentration of **paclitaxel.** Severe Anecdotal → Also see TABLE 10 p. 1056
- **Tucatinib** is predicted to increase the exposure to **cabazitaxel.** Avoid or adjust dose—consult product literature. Severe Study
- **Tucatinib** is predicted to increase the exposure to **docetaxel.** Avoid or adjust dose. Severe Study
- **Tucatinib** is predicted to increase the exposure to **paclitaxel.** Moderate Anecdotal
- **Velpatasvir** is predicted to increase the exposure to **docetaxel.** Moderate Study
- **Velpatasvir** is predicted to increase the exposure to **paclitaxel.** Severe Theoretical
- **Vemurafenib** is predicted to increase the exposure to **paclitaxel.** Use with caution and adjust dose. Severe Theoretical
- **Voclosporin** is predicted to increase the exposure to **paclitaxel.** Moderate Study
- **Voxilaprevir** with sofosbuvir and velpatasvir is predicted to increase the exposure to taxanes **(docetaxel, paclitaxel).** Moderate Study

Tebentafusp
- **Tebentafusp** is predicted to transiently increase the exposure to **ciclosporin.** Monitor and adjust dose. Moderate Theoretical
- **Tebentafusp** is predicted to transiently increase the exposure to coumarins **(warfarin).** Monitor and adjust dose. Moderate Theoretical

Teclistamab → see monoclonal antibodies

Tedizolid
- **Tedizolid** is predicted to increase the exposure to **imatinib.** Avoid. Moderate Theoretical
- **Tedizolid** is predicted to increase the exposure to **lapatinib.** Avoid. Moderate Theoretical
- **Tedizolid** is predicted to increase the exposure to **methotrexate.** Avoid. Moderate Theoretical
- **Tedizolid** is predicted to increase the exposure to statins **(atorvastatin, fluvastatin, rosuvastatin).** Avoid. Moderate Study
- **Tedizolid** is predicted to increase the exposure to **sulfasalazine.** Avoid. Moderate Study
- **Tedizolid** is predicted to increase the exposure to **topotecan.** Avoid. Moderate Study

Tegafur → see TABLE 12 p. 1057 (myelosuppression)
- **Tegafur** potentially increases the concentration of antiepileptics **(fosphenytoin, phenytoin).** Monitor concentration and adjust dose. Severe Anecdotal
- **Tegafur** increases the anticoagulant effect of **coumarins.** Monitor INR and adjust dose. Severe Theoretical
- **Folates** are predicted to increase the risk of toxicity when given with **tegafur.** Severe Theoretical
- H_2 receptor antagonists **(cimetidine)** are predicted to increase the risk of toxicity when given with **tegafur.** Severe Theoretical
- **Live vaccines** are predicted to increase the risk of generalised infection (possibly life-threatening) when given with **tegafur.** UKHSA advises avoid (refer to Green Book). Severe Theoretical
- **Methotrexate** is predicted to increase the risk of toxicity when given with **tegafur.** Severe Theoretical → Also see TABLE 12 p. 1057

Teicoplanin

GENERAL INFORMATION If other nephrotoxic or neurotoxic drugs are given, monitor renal and auditory function on prolonged administration.

Telmisartan → see angiotensin-II receptor antagonists

Telotristat ethyl
- **Telotristat ethyl** decreases the exposure to benzodiazepines **(midazolam).** Moderate Study
- **Telotristat ethyl** is predicted to decrease the exposure to **capivasertib.** Avoid. Moderate Theoretical
- **Telotristat ethyl** is predicted to decrease the exposure to **erdafitinib.** Adjust dose. Moderate Theoretical
- **Telotristat ethyl** is predicted to decrease the exposure to NNRTIs **(doravirine).** Avoid or adjust doravirine or lamivudine with tenofovir disoproxil and doravirine dose. Severe Theoretical
- **Octreotide** (short-acting) decreases the exposure to **telotristat ethyl. Telotristat ethyl** should be taken at least 30 minutes before **octreotide.** Moderate Study

Temazepam → see benzodiazepines

Temocillin → see penicillins

Temozolomide → see alkylating agents

Temsirolimus → see TABLE 12 p. 1057 (myelosuppression)
- **ACE inhibitors** are predicted to increase the risk of angioedema when given with **temsirolimus.** Moderate Theoretical
- Anti-androgens **(apalutamide, enzalutamide)** are predicted to decrease the concentration of **temsirolimus.** Avoid. Severe Study
- Antiarrhythmics **(dronedarone)** are predicted to increase the concentration of **temsirolimus.** Use with caution or avoid. Moderate Theoretical
- Antiepileptics **(carbamazepine, fosphenytoin, phenobarbital, phenytoin, primidone)** are predicted to decrease the concentration of **temsirolimus.** Avoid. Severe Study
- Antifungals, azoles **(fluconazole, isavuconazole)** are predicted to increase the concentration of **temsirolimus.** Use with caution or avoid. Moderate Theoretical
- Antifungals, azoles **(itraconazole, ketoconazole, posaconazole, voriconazole)** are predicted to increase the concentration of **temsirolimus.** Avoid. Severe Theoretical
- **Asciminib** is predicted to increase the exposure to **temsirolimus.** Severe Theoretical
- **Belzutifan** is predicted to decrease the exposure to **temsirolimus.** Avoid or adjust dose. Severe Theoretical
- **Berotralstat** is predicted to increase the exposure to **temsirolimus.** Use with caution or avoid. Moderate Study
- **Bulevirtide** is predicted to increase the exposure to **temsirolimus.** Moderate Theoretical
- Calcium-channel blockers **(diltiazem, verapamil)** are predicted to increase the concentration of, and the risk of angioedema, when given with **temsirolimus.** Use with caution or avoid. Moderate Theoretical
- **Temsirolimus** is predicted to increase the risk of angioedema when given with calcium-channel blockers **(amlodipine, felodipine, lacidipine, lercanidipine, nicardipine, nifedipine, nimodipine).** Moderate Theoretical
- **Cenobamate** is predicted to decrease the concentration of **temsirolimus.** Avoid. Moderate Theoretical
- **Ceritinib** is predicted to increase the concentration of **temsirolimus.** Avoid. Severe Theoretical → Also see TABLE 12 p. 1057
- **Cobicistat** is predicted to increase the concentration of **temsirolimus.** Avoid. Severe Theoretical
- **Crizotinib** is predicted to increase the concentration of **temsirolimus.** Use with caution or avoid. Moderate Theoretical
- **Dabrafenib** is predicted to decrease the concentration of **temsirolimus.** Avoid. Moderate Theoretical
- **Encorafenib** is predicted to decrease the concentration of **temsirolimus.** Avoid. Severe Study
- Endothelin receptor antagonists **(bosentan)** are predicted to decrease the concentration of **temsirolimus.** Avoid. Moderate Theoretical
- **Fedratinib** is predicted to increase the exposure to **temsirolimus** (oral). Monitor and adjust dose. Moderate Theoretical
- **Fostamatinib** is predicted to increase the exposure to **temsirolimus.** Monitor and adjust dose. Moderate Theoretical
- **Givinostat** might increase the exposure to **temsirolimus.** Moderate Study
- **Grapefruit** juice is predicted to increase the concentration of **temsirolimus.** Use with caution or avoid. Moderate Theoretical
- **HIV-protease inhibitors** are predicted to increase the concentration of **temsirolimus.** Avoid. Severe Theoretical
- **Idelalisib** is predicted to increase the concentration of **temsirolimus.** Avoid. Severe Theoretical
- **Imatinib** is predicted to increase the concentration of **temsirolimus.** Use with caution or avoid. Moderate Theoretical → Also see TABLE 12 p. 1057
- **Ivosidenib** is predicted to decrease the concentration of **temsirolimus.** Avoid. Severe Study
- **Larotrectinib** is predicted to increase the exposure to **temsirolimus.** Use with caution and adjust dose. Mild Theoretical

- **Lazertinib** is predicted to increase the exposure to **temsirolimus.** Moderate Study
- **Live vaccines** are predicted to increase the risk of generalised infection (possibly life-threatening) when given with **temsirolimus.** UKHSA advises avoid (refer to Green Book). Severe Theoretical
- **Lorlatinib** is predicted to decrease the concentration of **temsirolimus.** Avoid. Moderate Theoretical
- **Lumacaftor** is predicted to decrease the concentration of **temsirolimus.** Avoid. Severe Study
- Macrolides **(clarithromycin)** are predicted to increase the concentration of **temsirolimus.** Avoid. Severe Theoretical
- Macrolides **(erythromycin)** are predicted to increase the concentration of **temsirolimus.** Use with caution or avoid. Moderate Theoretical
- **Mifepristone** is predicted to increase the exposure to **temsirolimus.** Severe Theoretical
- **Mitotane** is predicted to decrease the concentration of **temsirolimus.** Avoid. Severe Study → Also see TABLE 12 p. 1057
- Neurokinin-1 receptor antagonists **(aprepitant, netupitant)** are predicted to increase the concentration of **temsirolimus.** Use with caution or avoid. Moderate Theoretical
- **Nilotinib** is predicted to increase the concentration of **temsirolimus.** Use with caution or avoid. Moderate Theoretical → Also see TABLE 12 p. 1057
- **Nirmatrelvir** boosted with ritonavir is predicted to increase the exposure to **temsirolimus.** Avoid—consult product literature. Severe Theoretical
- NNRTIs **(efavirenz, etravirine, nevirapine)** are predicted to decrease the concentration of **temsirolimus.** Avoid. Moderate Theoretical
- **Olaparib** might alter the exposure to **temsirolimus.** Moderate Theoretical → Also see TABLE 12 p. 1057
- **Pirtobrutinib** is predicted to increase the exposure to **temsirolimus.** Avoid or monitor. Moderate Theoretical
- **Pitolisant** is predicted to decrease the exposure to **temsirolimus.** Avoid. Severe Theoretical
- Rifamycins **(rifampicin)** are predicted to decrease the concentration of **temsirolimus.** Avoid. Severe Study
- **Ritlecitinib** is predicted to increase the exposure to **temsirolimus.** Moderate Theoretical
- **Selpercatinib** is predicted to increase the exposure to **temsirolimus.** Avoid. Moderate Study
- **Sotorasib** is predicted to decrease the concentration of **temsirolimus.** Avoid. Moderate Theoretical
- **St John's wort** is predicted to decrease the concentration of **temsirolimus.** Avoid. Moderate Theoretical
- **Tucatinib** is predicted to increase the concentration of **temsirolimus.** Avoid. Severe Theoretical
- **Vorasidenib** might decrease the concentration of **temsirolimus.** Avoid. Severe Theoretical

Tenecteplase → see TABLE 3 p. 1053 (bleeding)

- **Donanemab** might increase the risk of brain haemorrhage when given with **tenecteplase.** Avoid except in life-threatening situations. Severe Theoretical
- **Lecanemab** might increase the risk of brain haemorrhage when given with **tenecteplase.** Avoid except in life-threatening situations. Severe Theoretical

Tenofovir alafenamide

- Anti-androgens **(darolutamide)** are predicted to increase the exposure to **tenofovir alafenamide.** Moderate Theoretical
- Antiepileptics **(carbamazepine, fosphenytoin, oxcarbazepine, phenobarbital, phenytoin, primidone)** are predicted to decrease the exposure to **tenofovir alafenamide.** Avoid. Moderate Theoretical
- **Ciclosporin** is predicted to increase the exposure to **tenofovir alafenamide.** Moderate Theoretical
- **Eltrombopag** is predicted to increase the exposure to **tenofovir alafenamide.** Moderate Theoretical
- **Febuxostat** is predicted to increase the exposure to **tenofovir alafenamide.** Moderate Theoretical
- **Fostamatinib** is predicted to increase the concentration of **tenofovir alafenamide.** Moderate Theoretical
- **Fostemsavir** is predicted to increase the exposure to **tenofovir alafenamide.** Adjust dose—consult product literature. Moderate Theoretical
- HIV-protease inhibitors **(atazanavir, darunavir, lopinavir)** increase the exposure to **tenofovir alafenamide.** Avoid or adjust dose. Moderate Study
- **Leflunomide** is predicted to increase the exposure to **tenofovir alafenamide.** Moderate Theoretical
- **Lorlatinib** is predicted to decrease the exposure to **tenofovir alafenamide.** Avoid. Moderate Theoretical
- **Nitisinone** is predicted to increase the exposure to **tenofovir alafenamide.** Moderate Study
- **Rifamycins** are predicted to decrease the exposure to **tenofovir alafenamide.** Avoid. Moderate Theoretical
- **Roxadustat** is predicted to increase the exposure to **tenofovir alafenamide.** Moderate Theoretical
- **St John's wort** is predicted to decrease the exposure to **tenofovir alafenamide.** Avoid. Moderate Theoretical
- **Teriflunomide** is predicted to increase the exposure to **tenofovir alafenamide.** Moderate Theoretical
- **Vadadustat** is predicted to increase the exposure to **tenofovir alafenamide.** Moderate Theoretical

Tenofovir disoproxil → see TABLE 2 p. 1053 (nephrotoxicity)

- Anti-androgens **(darolutamide)** are predicted to increase the exposure to **tenofovir disoproxil.** Moderate Theoretical
- **Ciclosporin** is predicted to increase the exposure to **tenofovir disoproxil.** Moderate Theoretical → Also see TABLE 2 p. 1053
- **Eltrombopag** is predicted to increase the exposure to **tenofovir disoproxil.** Moderate Theoretical
- **Febuxostat** is predicted to increase the exposure to **tenofovir disoproxil.** Moderate Theoretical
- **Fostamatinib** is predicted to increase the exposure to **tenofovir disoproxil.** Moderate Theoretical
- HIV-protease inhibitors **(atazanavir, darunavir, lopinavir)** are predicted to increase the risk of renal impairment when given with **tenofovir disoproxil.** Severe Anecdotal
- **Ledipasvir** with sofosbuvir slightly increases the exposure to **tenofovir disoproxil.** Moderate Study
- **Leflunomide** is predicted to increase the exposure to **tenofovir disoproxil.** Moderate Theoretical
- **Nitisinone** is predicted to increase the exposure to **tenofovir disoproxil.** Moderate Study
- **Roxadustat** is predicted to increase the exposure to **tenofovir disoproxil.** Moderate Theoretical
- **Teriflunomide** is predicted to increase the exposure to **tenofovir disoproxil.** Moderate Theoretical
- **Vadadustat** is predicted to increase the exposure to **tenofovir disoproxil.** Moderate Theoretical
- **Velpatasvir** is predicted to increase the exposure to **tenofovir disoproxil.** Moderate Theoretical
- **Voxilaprevir** is predicted to increase the exposure to **tenofovir disoproxil.** Moderate Theoretical

Tenoxicam → see NSAIDs

Teplizumab → see monoclonal antibodies

Tepotinib

- **Tepotinib** is predicted to increase the concentration of **digoxin.** Severe Study
- **Tepotinib** is predicted to increase the concentration of **everolimus.** Severe Study
- **Tepotinib** is predicted to increase the concentration of **sirolimus.** Severe Study
- **Tepotinib** is predicted to increase the concentration of **talazoparib.** Severe Study
- **Tepotinib** is predicted to increase the concentration of taxanes **(paclitaxel).** Severe Study

Teprotumumab → see TABLE 16 p. 1058 (ototoxicity)

Terazosin → see alpha blockers

Terbinafine

ROUTE-SPECIFIC INFORMATION Since systemic absorption can follow topical application, the possibility of interactions should be borne in mind.

- **Terbinafine** is predicted to increase the exposure to anticholinesterases, centrally acting **(galantamine).** Monitor and adjust dose. Moderate Study

Terbinafine (continued)
- **Terbinafine** is predicted to markedly increase the exposure to **atomoxetine**. Adjust dose. Severe Study
- **Terbinafine** is predicted to moderately increase the exposure to atypical antipsychotics **(aripiprazole)**. Avoid or adjust dose—consult product literature. Moderate Study
- **Terbinafine** is predicted to increase the exposure to atypical antipsychotics **(clozapine)**. Use with caution and adjust dose. Severe Study
- **Terbinafine** is predicted to increase the exposure to atypical antipsychotics **(risperidone)**. Adjust dose. Moderate Study
- **Terbinafine** is predicted to increase the exposure to beta blockers, selective **(metoprolol, nebivolol)**. Moderate Study
- **Terbinafine** is predicted to slightly increase the exposure to **darifenacin**. Mild Study
- **Terbinafine** is predicted to increase the exposure to **eliglustat**. Avoid or adjust dose—consult product literature. Severe Study
- **Terbinafine** is predicted to increase the exposure to **fenfluramine**. Moderate Study
- **Terbinafine** is predicted to increase the exposure to **fesoterodine**. Use with caution and adjust dose. Mild Theoretical
- **Terbinafine** is predicted to increase the exposure to **gefitinib**. Moderate Theoretical
- **Terbinafine** is predicted to increase the exposure to **mexiletine**. Moderate Study
- **Terbinafine** is predicted to decrease the efficacy of opioids **(codeine)**. Moderate Theoretical
- **Terbinafine** is predicted to decrease the efficacy of opioids **(tramadol)**. Severe Study
- **Terbinafine** is predicted to moderately increase the exposure to **pitolisant**. Use with caution and adjust dose. Moderate Study
- Rifamycins **(rifampicin)** decrease the exposure to **terbinafine**. Adjust dose. Moderate Study
- **Terbinafine** is predicted to increase the exposure to SSRIs **(citalopram, dapoxetine, escitalopram, fluvoxamine, sertraline)**. Moderate Theoretical
- **Terbinafine** is predicted to increase the exposure to SSRIs **(fluoxetine)**. Adjust dose. Moderate Theoretical
- **Terbinafine** moderately increases the exposure to SSRIs **(paroxetine)**. Moderate Study
- **Terbinafine** is predicted to decrease the efficacy of **tamoxifen**. Avoid. Severe Study
- **Terbinafine** is predicted to increase the exposure to the active metabolite of **tetrabenazine**. Moderate Study
- **Terbinafine** is predicted to increase the exposure to **tricyclic antidepressants**. Monitor for toxicity and adjust dose. Severe Study
- **Terbinafine** is predicted to increase the exposure to **vortioxetine**. Monitor and adjust dose. Moderate Study

Terbutaline → see beta$_2$ agonists

Teriflunomide → see TABLE 10 p. 1056 (peripheral neuropathy)
- **Teriflunomide** is predicted to decrease the exposure to **agomelatine**. Moderate Theoretical
- **Teriflunomide** is predicted to increase the exposure to **alpelisib**. Moderate Theoretical
- **Teriflunomide** decreases the exposure to **aminophylline**. Adjust dose. Moderate Study
- **Teriflunomide** is predicted to decrease the exposure to anaesthetics, local **(ropivacaine)**. Moderate Theoretical
- **Teriflunomide** is predicted to increase the exposure to anthracyclines **(daunorubicin, doxorubicin, mitoxantrone)**. Moderate Theoretical
- **Teriflunomide** is predicted to increase the exposure to antihistamines, non-sedating **(fexofenadine)**. Moderate Study
- **Teriflunomide** is predicted to increase the exposure to **atogepant**. Adjust **atogepant** dose. Moderate Theoretical
- **Teriflunomide** is predicted to decrease the exposure to atypical antipsychotics **(clozapine)**. Moderate Theoretical
- **Teriflunomide** is predicted to decrease the exposure to atypical antipsychotics **(olanzapine)**. Monitor and adjust dose. Moderate Study
- **Teriflunomide** is predicted to increase the exposure to **baricitinib**. Moderate Study
- **Teriflunomide** is predicted to moderately increase the clearance of **caffeine citrate**. Monitor and adjust dose. Moderate Study
- **Teriflunomide** is predicted to increase the exposure to cephalosporins **(cefaclor)**. Moderate Study
- **Teriflunomide** is predicted to increase the exposure to **cladribine**. Avoid or adjust dose. Moderate Theoretical
- **Teriflunomide** affects the anticoagulant effect of **coumarins**. Severe Study
- **Teriflunomide** is predicted to increase the exposure to endothelin receptor antagonists **(bosentan)**. Moderate Study
- **Teriflunomide** are predicted to increases the exposure to **etrasimod**. Avoid in poor CYP2C9 metabolisers. Severe Theoretical
- **Teriflunomide** is predicted to increase the exposure to **ganciclovir**. Moderate Study
- **Teriflunomide** is predicted to increase the exposure to **grazoprevir**. Avoid. Severe Theoretical
- **Teriflunomide** is predicted to increase the exposure to H_2 receptor antagonists **(famotidine)**. Moderate Study
- **Teriflunomide** is predicted to increase the concentration of **letermovir**. Moderate Study
- **Live vaccines** are predicted to increase the risk of generalised infection (possibly life-threatening) when given with **teriflunomide**. UKHSA advises avoid (refer to Green Book). Severe Theoretical
- **Teriflunomide** is predicted to increase the exposure to loop diuretics **(furosemide)**. Moderate Study
- **Teriflunomide** is predicted to increase the exposure to meglitinides **(repaglinide)**. Moderate Study
- **Teriflunomide** is predicted to decrease the exposure to **melatonin**. Moderate Theoretical
- **Teriflunomide** is predicted to increase the exposure to **methotrexate**. Moderate Study
- **Teriflunomide** is predicted to increase the clearance of **mexiletine**. Monitor and adjust dose. Moderate Study
- **Teriflunomide** is predicted to increase the exposure to **momelotinib**. Moderate Study
- **Teriflunomide** is predicted to increase the exposure to **montelukast**. Moderate Theoretical
- **Teriflunomide** is predicted to increase the exposure to NRTIs **(zidovudine)**. Moderate Theoretical
- **Teriflunomide** is predicted to increase the exposure to NSAIDs **(indometacin, ketoprofen)**. Moderate Theoretical
- **Teriflunomide** is predicted to increase the exposure to **oseltamivir**. Moderate Study
- **Teriflunomide** is predicted to increase the exposure to penicillins **(benzylpenicillin)**. Moderate Study
- **Teriflunomide** is predicted to increase the exposure to **pioglitazone**. Moderate Study
- **Teriflunomide** is predicted to decrease the exposure to **pirfenidone**. Moderate Theoretical
- **Teriflunomide** is predicted to increase the exposure to quinolones **(ciprofloxacin)**. Moderate Theoretical
- Rifamycins **(rifampicin)** might affect the exposure to **teriflunomide**. Moderate Theoretical
- **Teriflunomide** is predicted to increase the exposure to **roxadustat**. Monitor haemoglobin and adjust dose—consult product literature. Moderate Study
- **Teriflunomide** is predicted to increase the exposure to **seladelpar**. Moderate Study
- **Teriflunomide** is predicted to increase the exposure to **selexipag**. Adjust **selexipag** dose. Moderate Study
- **Teriflunomide** is predicted to decrease the exposure to SNRIs **(duloxetine)**. Moderate Theoretical
- **Teriflunomide** is predicted to increase the exposure to statins **(atorvastatin, fluvastatin, pravastatin, simvastatin)**. Moderate Study
- **Teriflunomide** moderately increases the exposure to statins **(rosuvastatin)**. Adjust **rosuvastatin** dose, p. 155. Moderate Study
- **Teriflunomide** is predicted to increase the exposure to **sulfasalazine**. Moderate Study
- **Teriflunomide** is predicted to increase the exposure to sulfonylureas **(glibenclamide)**. Moderate Study

A1 Interactions | **Appendix 1**

- **Teriflunomide** is predicted to increase the exposure to talazoparib. Avoid or monitor. [Moderate] Theoretical
- **Teriflunomide** is predicted to increase the exposure to taxanes (docetaxel). [Moderate] Study → Also see TABLE 10 p. 1056
- **Teriflunomide** is predicted to increase the concentration of taxanes (paclitaxel). [Severe] Anecdotal → Also see TABLE 10 p. 1056
- **Teriflunomide** is predicted to increase the exposure to tenofovir alafenamide. [Moderate] Theoretical
- **Teriflunomide** is predicted to increase the exposure to tenofovir disoproxil. [Moderate] Theoretical
- **Teriflunomide** is predicted to decrease the exposure to theophylline. Adjust dose. [Moderate] Study
- **Teriflunomide** moderately decreases the exposure to tizanidine. [Mild] Study
- **Teriflunomide** is predicted to increase the exposure to topotecan. [Moderate] Study
- **Teriflunomide** is predicted to increase the exposure to tucatinib. [Moderate] Theoretical
- **Teriflunomide** is predicted to increase the exposure to vadadustat. [Moderate] Study
- **Teriflunomide** is predicted to increase the exposure to venetoclax. Avoid or monitor for toxicity. [Severe] Theoretical
- **Teriflunomide** is predicted to decrease the exposure to vorasidenib. Avoid. [Severe] Theoretical

Testosterone → see TABLE 1 p. 1053 (hepatotoxicity)

- Somapacitan might decrease the concentration of **testosterone**. [Moderate] Theoretical
- Somatrogon might decrease the concentration of **testosterone**. [Moderate] Theoretical

Tetanus immunoglobulin → see immunoglobulins

Tetrabenazine → see TABLE 7 p. 1055 (QT-interval prolongation), TABLE 9 p. 1056 (CNS effects)

- Bupropion is predicted to increase the exposure to the active metabolite of **tetrabenazine**. [Moderate] Study
- Cinacalcet is predicted to increase the exposure to the active metabolite of **tetrabenazine**. [Moderate] Study
- Dacomitinib is predicted to increase the exposure to the active metabolite of **tetrabenazine**. [Moderate] Study
- **Tetrabenazine** is predicted to decrease the effects of levodopa. Use with caution or avoid. [Moderate] Theoretical → Also see TABLE 9 p. 1056
- **Tetrabenazine** potentially increases the risk of CNS excitation and hypertension when given with MAO-B inhibitors. [Severe] Theoretical
- **Tetrabenazine** potentially increases the risk of CNS excitation and hypertension when given with MAOIs, irreversible. Avoid and for 14 days after stopping the MAOI. [Severe] Theoretical
- **Tetrabenazine** potentially increases the risk of CNS excitation and hypertension when given with moclobemide. [Severe] Theoretical
- SSRIs (fluoxetine, paroxetine) are predicted to increase the exposure to the active metabolite of **tetrabenazine**. [Moderate] Study → Also see TABLE 9 p. 1056
- Terbinafine is predicted to increase the exposure to the active metabolite of **tetrabenazine**. [Moderate] Study

Tetracaine → see anaesthetics, local

Tetracycline → see tetracyclines

Tetracyclines → see TABLE 1 p. 1053 (hepatotoxicity)

demeclocycline · doxycycline · eravacycline · lymecycline · minocycline · oxytetracycline · tetracycline

- Dairy products decrease the absorption of **demeclocycline** and **oxytetracycline**.
- Interactions do not generally apply to topical use of **oxytetracycline** unless specified.
- Dairy products decrease the exposure to **tetracycline**—manufacturer advises take 1 hour before or 2 hours after dairy products.

- Oral ACE inhibitors (quinapril) (magnesium carbonate-containing forms) might decrease the absorption of oral **tetracyclines**. Avoid. [Moderate] Study
- Oral antacids greatly decrease the absorption of oral **tetracyclines**. Separate administration by 2 to 3 hours. [Moderate] Study
- Anti-androgens (apalutamide, enzalutamide) are predicted to decrease the exposure to **eravacycline**. Adjust **eravacycline** dose. [Moderate] Study
- Anti-androgens (enzalutamide) are predicted to affect the exposure to **doxycycline**. Use with caution or avoid. [Moderate] Theoretical
- Antiepileptics (carbamazepine, fosphenytoin, phenobarbital, phenytoin, primidone) are predicted to decrease the exposure to **eravacycline**. Adjust **eravacycline** dose. [Moderate] Study
- Antiepileptics (carbamazepine, phenobarbital, phenytoin, primidone) decrease the concentration of **doxycycline**. Adjust dose. [Moderate] Study
- Antiepileptics (fosphenytoin) are predicted to decrease the concentration of **doxycycline**. Adjust dose. [Moderate] Theoretical
- **Tetracycline** decreases the concentration of antimalarials (atovaquone). [Moderate] Study
- Oral bismuth compounds (bismuth subsalicylate) greatly decrease the absorption of oral **tetracyclines**. Separate administration by at least 2 to 3 hours. [Moderate] Study
- Oral calcium compounds are predicted to decrease the absorption of oral **tetracyclines**. Separate administration by 2 to 3 hours. [Moderate] Theoretical
- **Doxycycline** is predicted to increase the concentration of ciclosporin. [Severe] Theoretical
- Combined hormonal contraceptives might exacerbate skin pigmentation when given with **minocycline**. [Moderate] Anecdotal
- **Tetracyclines** increase the anticoagulant effect of coumarins. [Severe] Anecdotal
- Encorafenib is predicted to decrease the exposure to **eravacycline**. Adjust **eravacycline** dose. [Moderate] Study
- Oral iron decreases the absorption of oral **tetracyclines**. **Tetracyclines** should be taken 2 to 3 hours after iron. [Moderate] Study
- Ivosidenib is predicted to decrease the exposure to **eravacycline**. Adjust **eravacycline** dose. [Moderate] Study
- Oral kaolin is predicted to decrease the absorption of oral **tetracyclines**. [Moderate] Theoretical
- Oral lanthanum might decrease the absorption of oral **tetracyclines**. Separate administration by 2 hours. [Moderate] Theoretical
- **Tetracyclines** are predicted to increase the risk of lithium toxicity when given with lithium. Avoid or adjust dose. [Severe] Anecdotal
- Lumacaftor is predicted to decrease the exposure to **eravacycline**. Adjust **eravacycline** dose. [Moderate] Study
- Mitotane is predicted to decrease the exposure to **eravacycline**. Adjust **eravacycline** dose. [Moderate] Study
- **Tetracyclines** are predicted to increase the anticoagulant effect of phenindione. [Severe] Theoretical
- **Tetracycline** is predicted to increase the exposure to relugolix. Avoid or take relugolix first and separate administration by at least 6 hours. [Moderate] Theoretical
- Retinoids (acitretin, alitretinoin, isotretinoin, tretinoin) increase the risk of benign intracranial hypertension when given with **tetracyclines**. Avoid. [Severe] Anecdotal → Also see TABLE 1 p. 1053
- Rifamycins (rifampicin) modestly decrease the exposure to **doxycycline**. Adjust dose. [Moderate] Study
- Rifamycins (rifampicin) are predicted to decrease the exposure to **eravacycline**. Adjust **eravacycline** dose. [Moderate] Study
- St John's wort is predicted to decrease the exposure to **eravacycline**. Adjust **eravacycline** dose. [Moderate] Theoretical
- Strontium is predicted to decrease the absorption of **tetracyclines**. Avoid. [Moderate] Theoretical
- Oral sucralfate might decrease the absorption of oral **tetracyclines**. [Moderate] Theoretical
- **Demeclocycline** might decrease the antidiuretic and hypertensive effects of vasopressin. [Moderate] Theoretical
- Volatile halogenated anaesthetics (methoxyflurane) might increase the risk of nephrotoxicity when given with **tetracycline**. [Severe] Anecdotal
- Oral zinc is predicted to decrease the absorption of **tetracyclines**. Separate administration by 2 to 3 hours. [Moderate] Theoretical

Tezacaftor

FOOD AND LIFESTYLE Bitter (Seville) oranges might increase the exposure to tezacaftor.

- Anti-androgens **(apalutamide, enzalutamide)** are predicted to decrease the exposure to **tezacaftor**. Avoid. Severe Theoretical
- Antiarrhythmics **(dronedarone)** are predicted to increase the exposure to **tezacaftor**. Adjust dose with moderate CYP3A4 inhibitors, see tezacaftor with ivacaftor p. 223, ivacaftor with tezacaftor and elexacaftor p. 220, and deutivacaftor with tezacaftor and vanzacaftor p. 218. Severe Study
- Antiepileptics **(carbamazepine, fosphenytoin, phenobarbital, phenytoin, primidone)** are predicted to decrease the exposure to **tezacaftor**. Avoid. Severe Theoretical
- Antifungals, azoles **(fluconazole, isavuconazole)** are predicted to increase the exposure to **tezacaftor**. Adjust dose with moderate CYP3A4 inhibitors, see tezacaftor with ivacaftor p. 223, ivacaftor with tezacaftor and elexacaftor p. 220, and deutivacaftor with tezacaftor and vanzacaftor p. 218. Severe Study
- Antifungals, azoles **(itraconazole, ketoconazole, posaconazole, voriconazole)** are predicted to increase the exposure to **tezacaftor**. Adjust dose with potent CYP3A4 inhibitors, see tezacaftor with ivacaftor p. 223, ivacaftor with tezacaftor and elexacaftor p. 220, and deutivacaftor with tezacaftor and vanzacaftor p. 218. Severe Study
- **Berotralstat** is predicted to increase the exposure to **tezacaftor**. Adjust dose with moderate CYP3A4 inhibitors, see tezacaftor with ivacaftor p. 223, ivacaftor with tezacaftor and elexacaftor p. 220, and deutivacaftor with tezacaftor and vanzacaftor p. 218. Severe Study
- Calcium-channel blockers **(diltiazem, verapamil)** are predicted to increase the exposure to **tezacaftor**. Adjust dose with moderate CYP3A4 inhibitors, see tezacaftor with ivacaftor p. 223, ivacaftor with tezacaftor and elexacaftor p. 220, and deutivacaftor with tezacaftor and vanzacaftor p. 218. Severe Study
- **Cenobamate** is predicted to decrease the exposure to **tezacaftor**. Avoid. Severe Theoretical
- **Ceritinib** is predicted to increase the exposure to **tezacaftor**. Adjust dose with potent CYP3A4 inhibitors, see tezacaftor with ivacaftor p. 223, ivacaftor with tezacaftor and elexacaftor p. 220, and deutivacaftor with tezacaftor and vanzacaftor p. 218. Severe Study
- **Cobicistat** is predicted to increase the exposure to **tezacaftor**. Adjust dose with potent CYP3A4 inhibitors, see tezacaftor with ivacaftor p. 223, ivacaftor with tezacaftor and elexacaftor p. 220, and deutivacaftor with tezacaftor and vanzacaftor p. 218. Severe Study
- **Crizotinib** is predicted to increase the exposure to **tezacaftor**. Adjust dose with moderate CYP3A4 inhibitors, see tezacaftor with ivacaftor p. 223, ivacaftor with tezacaftor and elexacaftor p. 220, and deutivacaftor with tezacaftor and vanzacaftor p. 218. Severe Study
- **Dabrafenib** is predicted to decrease the exposure to **tezacaftor**. Avoid. Severe Theoretical
- **Encorafenib** is predicted to decrease the exposure to **tezacaftor**. Avoid. Severe Theoretical
- Endothelin receptor antagonists **(bosentan)** are predicted to decrease the exposure to **tezacaftor**. Avoid. Severe Theoretical
- **Fedratinib** is predicted to increase the exposure to **tezacaftor**. Adjust dose with moderate CYP3A4 inhibitors, see tezacaftor with ivacaftor p. 223, ivacaftor with tezacaftor and elexacaftor p. 220, and deutivacaftor with tezacaftor and vanzacaftor p. 218. Severe Study
- **Grapefruit** juice is predicted to increase the exposure to **tezacaftor**. Avoid. Severe Study
- **HIV-protease inhibitors** are predicted to increase the exposure to **tezacaftor**. Adjust dose with potent CYP3A4 inhibitors, see tezacaftor with ivacaftor p. 223, ivacaftor with tezacaftor and elexacaftor p. 220, and deutivacaftor with tezacaftor and vanzacaftor p. 218. Severe Study
- **Idelalisib** is predicted to increase the exposure to **tezacaftor**. Adjust dose with potent CYP3A4 inhibitors, see tezacaftor with ivacaftor p. 223, ivacaftor with tezacaftor and elexacaftor p. 220, and deutivacaftor with tezacaftor and vanzacaftor p. 218. Severe Study
- **Imatinib** is predicted to increase the exposure to **tezacaftor**. Adjust dose with moderate CYP3A4 inhibitors, see tezacaftor with ivacaftor p. 223, ivacaftor with tezacaftor and elexacaftor p. 220, and deutivacaftor with tezacaftor and vanzacaftor p. 218. Severe Study
- **Ivosidenib** is predicted to decrease the exposure to **tezacaftor**. Avoid. Severe Theoretical
- **Letermovir** is predicted to increase the exposure to **tezacaftor**. Adjust dose with moderate CYP3A4 inhibitors, see tezacaftor with ivacaftor p. 223, ivacaftor with tezacaftor and elexacaftor p. 220, and deutivacaftor with tezacaftor and vanzacaftor p. 218. Severe Study
- **Lorlatinib** is predicted to decrease the exposure to **tezacaftor**. Avoid. Severe Theoretical
- **Lumacaftor** is predicted to decrease the exposure to **tezacaftor**. Avoid. Severe Theoretical
- Macrolides **(clarithromycin)** are predicted to increase the exposure to **tezacaftor**. Adjust dose with potent CYP3A4 inhibitors, see tezacaftor with ivacaftor p. 223, ivacaftor with tezacaftor and elexacaftor p. 220, and deutivacaftor with tezacaftor and vanzacaftor p. 218. Severe Study
- Macrolides **(erythromycin)** are predicted to increase the exposure to **tezacaftor**. Adjust dose with moderate CYP3A4 inhibitors, see tezacaftor with ivacaftor p. 223, ivacaftor with tezacaftor and elexacaftor p. 220, and deutivacaftor with tezacaftor and vanzacaftor p. 218. Severe Study
- **Mitotane** is predicted to decrease the exposure to **tezacaftor**. Avoid. Severe Theoretical
- Neurokinin-1 receptor antagonists **(aprepitant, netupitant)** are predicted to increase the exposure to **tezacaftor**. Adjust dose with moderate CYP3A4 inhibitors, see tezacaftor with ivacaftor p. 223, ivacaftor with tezacaftor and elexacaftor p. 220, and deutivacaftor with tezacaftor and vanzacaftor p. 218. Severe Study
- **Nilotinib** is predicted to increase the exposure to **tezacaftor**. Adjust dose with moderate CYP3A4 inhibitors, see tezacaftor with ivacaftor p. 223, ivacaftor with tezacaftor and elexacaftor p. 220, and deutivacaftor with tezacaftor and vanzacaftor p. 218. Severe Study
- **Nirmatrelvir** boosted with ritonavir is predicted to increase the concentration of **tezacaftor** with ivacaftor. Adjust dose. Severe Theoretical
- NNRTIs **(efavirenz, etravirine, nevirapine)** are predicted to decrease the exposure to **tezacaftor**. Avoid. Severe Theoretical
- **Rifamycins** are predicted to decrease the exposure to **tezacaftor**. Avoid. Severe Theoretical
- **Sotorasib** is predicted to decrease the exposure to **tezacaftor**. Avoid. Severe Theoretical
- **St John's wort** is predicted to decrease the exposure to **tezacaftor**. Avoid. Severe Theoretical
- **Tucatinib** is predicted to increase the exposure to **tezacaftor**. Adjust dose with potent CYP3A4 inhibitors, see tezacaftor with ivacaftor p. 223, ivacaftor with tezacaftor and elexacaftor p. 220, and deutivacaftor with tezacaftor and vanzacaftor p. 218. Severe Study

Tezepelumab → see monoclonal antibodies

Thalidomide → see TABLE 4 p. 1054 (bradycardia), TABLE 1 p. 1053 (hepatotoxicity), TABLE 12 p. 1057 (myelosuppression), TABLE 10 p. 1056 (peripheral neuropathy), TABLE 9 p. 1056 (CNS effects)

- **Combined hormonal contraceptives** are predicted to increase the risk of venous thromboembolism when given with **thalidomide**. Avoid. Severe Study
- **Hormone replacement therapy** is predicted to increase the risk of venous thromboembolism when given with **thalidomide**. Severe Theoretical

Theophylline → see TABLE 14 p. 1057 (reduced serum potassium)

FOOD AND LIFESTYLE Smoking can increase theophylline clearance and increased doses of theophylline are therefore required; dose adjustments are likely to be necessary if smoking started or stopped during treatment.

- **Aciclovir** is predicted to increase the exposure to **theophylline**. Monitor and adjust dose. Severe Theoretical

- **Theophylline** decreases the efficacy of antiarrhythmics **(adenosine)**. Separate administration by 24 hours. [Mild] Study
- Antiepileptics **(carbamazepine)** potentially increase the clearance of **theophylline** and **theophylline** decreases the exposure to antiepileptics **(carbamazepine)**. Adjust dose. [Moderate] Anecdotal
- Antiepileptics **(fosphenytoin, phenytoin)** are predicted to decrease the exposure to **theophylline**. Adjust dose. [Moderate] Study
- Antiepileptics **(phenobarbital, primidone)** are predicted to increase the clearance of **theophylline**. Adjust dose. [Moderate] Theoretical
- Antiepileptics **(stiripentol)** are predicted to increase the exposure to **theophylline**. Avoid. [Moderate] Theoretical
- **Axitinib** is predicted to increase the exposure to **theophylline**. [Moderate] Theoretical
- **Beta blockers, non-selective** are predicted to increase the risk of bronchospasm when given with **theophylline**. Avoid. [Severe] Theoretical
- **Beta blockers, selective** are predicted to increase the risk of bronchospasm when given with **theophylline**. Avoid. [Severe] Theoretical
- **Caffeine citrate** decreases the clearance of **theophylline**. [Moderate] Study
- **Combined hormonal contraceptives** is predicted to increase the exposure to **theophylline**. Monitor and adjust dose. [Moderate] Theoretical
- **Theophylline** increases the risk of agitation when given with **doxapram**. [Moderate] Study
- **Enteral feeds** decrease the exposure to **theophylline**. [Moderate] Study
- **Esketamine** is predicted to increase the risk of seizures when given with **theophylline**. Avoid. [Severe] Theoretical
- **Givosiran** is predicted to increase the exposure to **theophylline**. Monitor and adjust dose. [Moderate] Theoretical
- H_2 receptor antagonists **(cimetidine)** increase the concentration of **theophylline**. Adjust dose. [Severe] Study
- HIV protease inhibitors **(ritonavir)** are predicted to decrease the exposure to **theophylline**. Adjust dose. [Moderate] Study
- **Interferons** slightly increase the exposure to **theophylline**. Adjust dose. [Moderate] Study
- Iron chelators **(deferasirox)** increase the exposure to **theophylline**. Avoid. [Moderate] Study
- **Isoniazid** is predicted to affect the clearance of **theophylline**. [Severe] Anecdotal
- **Leflunomide** is predicted to decrease the exposure to **theophylline**. Adjust dose. [Moderate] Study
- **Leniolisib** is predicted to increase the exposure to **theophylline**. Avoid. [Moderate] Theoretical
- **Theophylline** is predicted to decrease the concentration of **lithium**. Monitor concentration and adjust dose. [Moderate] Anecdotal
- Macrolides **(azithromycin, clarithromycin)** are predicted to increase the exposure to **theophylline**. Adjust dose. [Moderate] Anecdotal
- Macrolides **(erythromycin)** decrease the clearance of **theophylline** and **theophylline** potentially decreases the clearance of macrolides **(erythromycin)**. Adjust dose. [Severe] Study
- **Maribavir** is predicted to decrease the exposure to **theophylline**. Avoid. [Mild] Theoretical
- **Methotrexate** decreases the clearance of **theophylline**. [Moderate] Study
- **Metreleptin** might alter the exposure to **theophylline**. Monitor concentration and adjust dose. [Severe] Theoretical
- **Mexiletine** is predicted to increase the exposure to **theophylline**. Monitor and adjust dose. [Moderate] Theoretical
- Monoclonal antibodies **(blinatumomab)** are predicted to transiently increase the exposure to **theophylline**. Monitor and adjust dose. [Moderate] Theoretical
- Monoclonal antibodies **(sarilumab)** potentially affect the exposure to **theophylline**. Monitor and adjust dose. [Moderate] Theoretical
- Monoclonal antibodies **(tocilizumab)** are predicted to decrease the exposure to **theophylline**. Monitor and adjust dose. [Moderate] Theoretical
- **Nirmatrelvir** boosted with ritonavir is predicted to decrease the concentration of **theophylline**. Adjust dose. [Moderate] Theoretical
- **Obeticholic acid** is predicted to increase the exposure to **theophylline**. [Severe] Theoretical
- **Osilodrostat** is predicted to increase the exposure to **theophylline**. Monitor and adjust dose. [Moderate] Theoretical
- **Pentoxifylline** increases the concentration of **theophylline**. Monitor and adjust dose. [Severe] Study
- **Theophylline** is predicted to slightly increase the exposure to phosphodiesterase type-4 inhibitors **(roflumilast)**. Avoid. [Moderate] Theoretical
- Quinolones **(ciprofloxacin)** are predicted to increase the exposure to **theophylline**. Monitor and adjust dose. [Moderate] Theoretical
- Rifamycins **(rifampicin)** are predicted to decrease the exposure to **theophylline**. Adjust dose. [Moderate] Study
- **Ritlecitinib** is predicted to increase the exposure to **theophylline**. Adjust dose. [Moderate] Theoretical
- **Rucaparib** is predicted to increase the exposure to **theophylline**. Monitor and adjust dose. [Moderate] Theoretical
- SSRIs **(fluvoxamine)** moderately to markedly increase the exposure to **theophylline**. Avoid. [Severe] Study
- **St John's wort** potentially decreases the exposure to **theophylline**. [Severe] Anecdotal
- **Sucralfate** potentially decreases the absorption of **theophylline**. Separate administration by at least 2 hours. [Moderate] Study
- Sympathomimetics, vasoconstrictor **(ephedrine)** increase the risk of adverse effects when given with **theophylline**. Avoid in children. [Moderate] Study
- **Teriflunomide** is predicted to decrease the exposure to **theophylline**. Adjust dose. [Moderate] Study
- **Valaciclovir** is predicted to increase the exposure to **theophylline**. [Severe] Theoretical
- **Vemurafenib** is predicted to increase the exposure to **theophylline**. Monitor and adjust dose. [Moderate] Theoretical

Thiazide diuretics → see TABLE 15 p. 1058 (hyponatraemia), TABLE 6 p. 1054 (hypotension), TABLE 14 p. 1057 (reduced serum potassium)

bendroflumethiazide · chlorothiazide · chlortalidone · hydrochlorothiazide · hydroflumethiazide · indapamide · metolazone · xipamide

- **Thiazide diuretics** are predicted to increase the risk of hypersensitivity reactions when given with **allopurinol**. [Severe] Theoretical
- **Aspirin** (high-dose) increases the risk of acute renal failure when given with **thiazide diuretics**. [Severe] Theoretical
- **Thiazide diuretics** increase the risk of hypercalcaemia when given with **calcium compounds**. [Severe] Anecdotal
- **Thiazide diuretics** increase the concentration of **lithium**. Avoid or adjust dose and monitor concentration. [Severe] Study
- **Metolazone** is predicted to decrease the efficacy of **methenamine**. [Moderate] Theoretical
- **NSAIDs** increase the risk of acute renal failure when given with **thiazide diuretics**. [Severe] Theoretical → Also see TABLE 15 p. 1058
- **Reboxetine** is predicted to increase the risk of hypokalaemia when given with **thiazide diuretics**. [Moderate] Anecdotal
- **Thiazide diuretics** are predicted to increase the risk of hypercalcaemia when given with **toremifene**. [Severe] Theoretical
- **Thiazide diuretics** increase the risk of hypercalcaemia when given with **vitamin D substances** (high-dose). [Moderate] Theoretical

Thiopental → see TABLE 6 p. 1054 (hypotension), TABLE 9 p. 1056 (CNS effects)

- **Sulfonamides** are predicted to increase the effects of **thiopental**. [Moderate] Theoretical
- **Tricyclic antidepressants** increase the risk of cardiac arrhythmias and hypotension when given with **thiopental**. [Moderate] Study → Also see TABLE 6 p. 1054 → Also see TABLE 9 p. 1056

Thiotepa → see alkylating agents

A1 Interactions | Appendix 1

Thrombin inhibitors → see TABLE 3 p. 1053 (bleeding)

argatroban · bivalirudin · dabigatran

- **Abrocitinib** slightly increases the exposure to **dabigatran**. Moderate Study
- Anti-androgens **(apalutamide)** are predicted to decrease the exposure to **dabigatran**. Mild Study
- Antiarrhythmics **(amiodarone)** increase the exposure to **dabigatran**. Monitor and adjust dose. Severe Study
- Antiarrhythmics **(dronedarone)** moderately increase the exposure to **dabigatran**. Avoid. Severe Study
- Antiepileptics **(carbamazepine)** are predicted to decrease the exposure to **dabigatran**. Avoid. Severe Study
- Antiepileptics **(fosphenytoin, phenytoin)** are predicted to decrease the exposure to **dabigatran**. Avoid. Severe Theoretical
- Antifungals, azoles **(fluconazole, posaconazole)** are predicted to increase the exposure to **dabigatran**. Severe Study
- Antifungals, azoles **(isavuconazole)** are predicted to increase the exposure to **dabigatran**. Monitor and adjust dose. Moderate Study
- Antifungals, azoles **(itraconazole, ketoconazole)** are predicted to increase the exposure to **dabigatran**. Avoid. Severe Study
- **Asciminib** is predicted to increase the exposure to **dabigatran**. Severe Theoretical
- **Belumosudil** increases the exposure to **dabigatran**. Avoid or adjust dose. Moderate Study
- Calcium-channel blockers **(verapamil)** increase the exposure to **dabigatran**. Monitor and adjust dose. Severe Study
- **Ceritinib** is predicted to increase the exposure to **dabigatran**. Moderate Theoretical
- **Ciclosporin** is predicted to increase the exposure to **dabigatran**. Avoid. Severe Study
- **Cobicistat** moderately increases the exposure to **dabigatran**. Avoid. Severe Study
- **Danicopan** is predicted to increase the exposure to **dabigatran**. Moderate Study
- **Donanemab** can increase the risk of brain haemorrhage when given with **thrombin inhibitors**. Avoid. Severe Anecdotal
- **Elbasvir** is predicted to increase the concentration of **dabigatran**. Moderate Theoretical
- **Eliglustat** is predicted to increase the exposure to **dabigatran**. Adjust dose. Moderate Study
- **Erdafitinib** is predicted to increase the exposure to **dabigatran**. Separate administration by at least 6 hours. Moderate Theoretical
- **Glecaprevir** with pibrentasvir increases the exposure to **dabigatran**. Avoid. Moderate Study
- HIV-protease inhibitors **(atazanavir, darunavir, lopinavir)** boosted with ritonavir are predicted to increase the exposure to **dabigatran**. Avoid. Severe Anecdotal
- HIV-protease inhibitors **(fosamprenavir)** boosted with ritonavir are predicted to increase the exposure to **dabigatran**. Avoid. Severe Theoretical
- HIV-protease inhibitors **(ritonavir)** are predicted to increase the exposure to **dabigatran**. Avoid. Severe Study
- **Ivosidenib** is predicted to alter the exposure to **dabigatran**. Avoid. Moderate Theoretical
- **Lapatinib** is predicted to increase the exposure to **dabigatran**. Severe Theoretical
- **Lecanemab** can increase the risk of brain haemorrhage when given with **thrombin inhibitors**. Avoid. Severe Anecdotal
- **Ledipasvir** is predicted to increase the exposure to **dabigatran**. Moderate Theoretical
- **Lenacapavir** is predicted to increase the concentration of **dabigatran**. Monitor and adjust dose. Severe Theoretical
- **Letermovir** is predicted to decrease the concentration of **dabigatran**. Avoid. Severe Theoretical
- **Lorlatinib** is predicted to decrease the exposure to **dabigatran**. Avoid. Severe Study
- Macrolides **(azithromycin, erythromycin)** are predicted to increase the exposure to **dabigatran**. Severe Theoretical
- Macrolides **(clarithromycin)** increase the exposure to **dabigatran**. Moderate Study
- **Maribavir** is predicted to increase the exposure to **dabigatran**. Moderate Study
- **Mirabegron** is predicted to increase the exposure to **dabigatran**. Severe Theoretical
- **Thrombin inhibitors** might increase the risk of gastrointestinal bleeding when given with monoclonal antibodies **(ipilimumab)**. Severe Theoretical
- **Nirmatrelvir** boosted with ritonavir moderately increases the exposure to **dabigatran**. Avoid. Severe Study
- **Olaparib** might increase the exposure to **dabigatran**. Moderate Theoretical
- **Osimertinib** is predicted to increase the exposure to **dabigatran**. Moderate Study
- **Pibrentasvir** with glecaprevir increases the exposure to **dabigatran**. Avoid. Moderate Study
- **Pirtobrutinib** is predicted to increase the exposure to **dabigatran**. Avoid or monitor. Moderate Theoretical
- **Pitolisant** is predicted to decrease the exposure to **dabigatran**. Mild Theoretical
- **Ranolazine** is predicted to increase the exposure to **dabigatran**. Severe Theoretical
- Rifamycins **(rifampicin)** are predicted to decrease the exposure to **dabigatran**. Avoid. Severe Study
- **Selpercatinib** slightly increases the exposure to **dabigatran**. Moderate Study
- **Sparsentan** is predicted to increase the exposure to **dabigatran**. Severe Theoretical
- **St John's wort** is predicted to decrease the exposure to **dabigatran**. Avoid. Severe Study
- **Tacrolimus** is predicted to increase the exposure to **dabigatran**. Avoid. Severe Theoretical
- **Ticagrelor** increases the exposure to **dabigatran**. Monitor and adjust dose. Severe Study → Also see TABLE 3 p. 1053
- **Velpatasvir** increases the exposure to **dabigatran**. Avoid. Severe Study
- **Vemurafenib** is predicted to increase the exposure to **dabigatran**. Monitor and adjust dose. Severe Theoretical
- **Venetoclax** is predicted to increase the exposure to **dabigatran**. Avoid or adjust dose. Severe Study
- **Voclosporin** is predicted to increase the exposure to **dabigatran**. Mild Theoretical
- **Voxilaprevir** with sofosbuvir and velpatasvir increases the concentration of **dabigatran**. Avoid. Severe Study

Thyroid hormones

levothyroxine · liothyronine

FOOD AND LIFESTYLE Food, including dietary fibre, milk, soya products, and coffee, might decrease the absorption of levothyroxine.

- Oral **antacids** are predicted to decrease the absorption of oral **levothyroxine**. Separate administration by at least 4 hours. Moderate Anecdotal
- Anti-androgens **(apalutamide)** potentially decrease the exposure to **levothyroxine**. Mild Theoretical
- Anti-androgens **(enzalutamide)** are predicted to affect the exposure to **levothyroxine**. Use with caution or avoid. Moderate Theoretical
- Antiarrhythmics **(amiodarone)** are predicted to increase the risk of thyroid dysfunction when given with **thyroid hormones**. Avoid. Moderate Study
- Antiepileptics **(carbamazepine)** are predicted to increase the risk of hypothyroidism when given with **thyroid hormones**. Monitor and adjust dose. Moderate Study
- Antiepileptics **(fosphenytoin, phenytoin)** are predicted to increase the risk of hypothyroidism when given with **thyroid hormones**. Moderate Study
- Antiepileptics **(phenobarbital, primidone)** are predicted to decrease the effects of **thyroid hormones**. Moderate Theoretical
- **Bulevirtide** is predicted to increase the exposure to **thyroid hormones**. Avoid or monitor. Moderate Theoretical
- Oral **calcium compounds** are predicted to decrease the absorption of oral **levothyroxine**. Separate administration by at least 4 hours. Moderate Anecdotal
- **Thyroid hormones** are predicted to affect the concentration of **digoxin**. Monitor and adjust dose. Moderate Theoretical
- Glucagon-like peptide-1 receptor agonists **(semaglutide)** slightly increase the exposure to **levothyroxine**. Moderate Study

- HIV-protease inhibitors **(ritonavir)** decrease the concentration of **levothyroxine**. MHRA advises monitor TSH for at least one month after starting or stopping ritonavir. [Moderate] Anecdotal
- Oral **hormone replacement therapy** is predicted to decrease the effects of **thyroid hormones**. [Moderate] Theoretical
- **Imatinib** causes hypothyroidism when given with **levothyroxine** in thyroidectomy patients. [Moderate] Study
- Oral **iron** decreases the absorption of oral **levothyroxine**. Separate administration by at least 4 hours. [Moderate] Study
- **Lanthanum** decreases the absorption of **thyroid hormones**. Separate administration by 2 hours. [Moderate] Study
- **Nirmatrelvir** boosted with ritonavir might decrease the efficacy of **levothyroxine**. [Moderate] Theoretical
- **Somapacitan** might affect the efficacy of **thyroid hormones**. Monitor and adjust dose. [Moderate] Theoretical
- **Somatrogon** might affect the efficacy of **thyroid hormones**. Adjust dose. [Moderate] Theoretical
- **Sucralfate** decreases the absorption of **levothyroxine**. Separate administration by at least 4 hours. [Moderate] Study
- **Sunitinib** has been reported to cause hypothyroidism when given with **levothyroxine**. [Moderate] Anecdotal

Tiagabine → see antiepileptics

Tiaprofenic acid → see NSAIDs

Ticagrelor → see TABLE 3 p. 1053 (bleeding), TABLE 4 p. 1054 (bradycardia)

- Anti-androgens **(apalutamide, enzalutamide)** are predicted to markedly decrease the exposure to **ticagrelor**. Avoid. [Severe] Study
- Antiarrhythmics **(amiodarone)** are predicted to increase the exposure to **ticagrelor**. Use with caution or avoid. [Severe] Study → Also see TABLE 4 p. 1054
- Antiepileptics **(carbamazepine, fosphenytoin, phenobarbital, phenytoin, primidone)** are predicted to markedly decrease the exposure to **ticagrelor**. Avoid. [Severe] Study
- Antifungals, azoles **(itraconazole, ketoconazole, posaconazole, voriconazole)** are predicted to markedly increase the exposure to **ticagrelor**. Avoid. [Severe] Study
- **Cenobamate** is predicted to decrease the exposure to **ticagrelor**. [Moderate] Theoretical
- **Ceritinib** is predicted to markedly increase the exposure to **ticagrelor**. Avoid. [Severe] Study → Also see TABLE 4 p. 1054
- **Ciclosporin** is predicted to increase the exposure to **ticagrelor**. Use with caution or avoid. [Severe] Study
- **Cobicistat** is predicted to markedly increase the exposure to **ticagrelor**. Avoid. [Severe] Study
- **Dabrafenib** is predicted to decrease the exposure to **ticagrelor**. [Moderate] Theoretical
- **Ticagrelor** increases the concentration of **digoxin**. [Moderate] Study → Also see TABLE 4 p. 1054
- **Encorafenib** is predicted to markedly decrease the exposure to **ticagrelor**. Avoid. [Severe] Study
- Endothelin receptor antagonists **(bosentan)** are predicted to decrease the exposure to **ticagrelor**. [Moderate] Theoretical
- **Grapefruit** juice moderately increases the exposure to **ticagrelor**. [Moderate] Study
- **HIV-protease inhibitors** are predicted to markedly increase the exposure to **ticagrelor**. Avoid. [Severe] Study
- **Idelalisib** is predicted to markedly increase the exposure to **ticagrelor**. Avoid. [Severe] Study
- **Ivosidenib** is predicted to markedly decrease the exposure to **ticagrelor**. Avoid. [Severe] Study
- **Ticagrelor** is predicted to increase the exposure to **lomitapide**. Separate administration by 12 hours. [Moderate] Theoretical
- **Lorlatinib** is predicted to decrease the exposure to **ticagrelor**. [Moderate] Theoretical
- **Lumacaftor** is predicted to markedly decrease the exposure to **ticagrelor**. Avoid. [Severe] Study
- Macrolides **(azithromycin)** are predicted to increase the exposure to **ticagrelor**. Use with caution or avoid. [Severe] Study
- Macrolides **(clarithromycin)** are predicted to markedly increase the exposure to **ticagrelor**. Avoid. [Severe] Study
- **Mitotane** is predicted to markedly decrease the exposure to **ticagrelor**. Avoid. [Severe] Study
- **Nirmatrelvir** boosted with ritonavir is predicted to increase the concentration of **ticagrelor**. Avoid. [Severe] Theoretical
- NNRTIs **(efavirenz, etravirine, nevirapine)** are predicted to decrease the exposure to **ticagrelor**. [Moderate] Theoretical
- **Ranolazine** is predicted to increase the exposure to **ticagrelor**. Use with caution or avoid. [Severe] Study
- Rifamycins **(rifampicin)** are predicted to markedly decrease the exposure to **ticagrelor**. Avoid. [Severe] Study
- **Selumetinib** might increase the risk of bleeding when given with **ticagrelor**. [Severe] Theoretical
- **Sotorasib** is predicted to decrease the exposure to **ticagrelor**. [Moderate] Theoretical
- **St John's wort** is predicted to decrease the exposure to **ticagrelor**. [Moderate] Theoretical
- **Ticagrelor** slightly to moderately increases the exposure to statins **(simvastatin)**. Adjust **simvastatin** dose, p. 156. [Moderate] Study
- **Ticagrelor** increases the exposure to thrombin inhibitors **(dabigatran)**. Monitor and adjust dose. [Severe] Study → Also see TABLE 3 p. 1053
- **Tucatinib** is predicted to markedly increase the exposure to **ticagrelor**. Avoid. [Severe] Study
- **Vemurafenib** is predicted to increase the exposure to **ticagrelor**. Use with caution or avoid. [Severe] Study

Tigecycline → see TABLE 1 p. 1053 (hepatotoxicity)

- Antiarrhythmics **(amiodarone, dronedarone)** might increase the exposure to **tigecycline**. [Mild] Anecdotal → Also see TABLE 1 p. 1053
- Antifungals, azoles **(itraconazole, ketoconazole)** might increase the exposure to **tigecycline**. [Mild] Anecdotal → Also see TABLE 1 p. 1053
- Calcium-channel blockers **(verapamil)** might increase the exposure to **tigecycline**. [Mild] Anecdotal
- **Ciclosporin** might increase the exposure to **tigecycline** and **tigecycline** has been reported to increase the concentration of **ciclosporin**. [Severe] Anecdotal
- **Tigecycline** is predicted to alter the anticoagulant effect of **coumarins**. [Moderate] Anecdotal
- HIV-protease inhibitors **(lopinavir, ritonavir)** might increase the exposure to **tigecycline**. [Mild] Anecdotal → Also see TABLE 1 p. 1053
- **Ivacaftor** might increase the exposure to **tigecycline**. [Mild] Anecdotal
- **Lapatinib** might increase the exposure to **tigecycline**. [Mild] Anecdotal
- **Macrolides** might increase the exposure to **tigecycline**. [Mild] Anecdotal
- **Neratinib** might increase the exposure to **tigecycline**. [Mild] Anecdotal → Also see TABLE 1 p. 1053
- **Tigecycline** is predicted to increase the anticoagulant effect of **phenindione**. [Severe] Theoretical
- **Ranolazine** might increase the exposure to **tigecycline**. [Mild] Anecdotal
- Retinoids **(acitretin, alitretinoin, isotretinoin, tretinoin)** increase the risk of benign intracranial hypertension when given with **tigecycline**. Avoid. [Severe] Anecdotal → Also see TABLE 1 p. 1053
- **Tigecycline** has been reported to increase the concentration of **tacrolimus**. [Severe] Anecdotal
- **Vandetanib** might increase the exposure to **tigecycline**. [Mild] Anecdotal
- **Vemurafenib** might increase the exposure to **tigecycline**. [Mild] Anecdotal

Tildrakizumab → see monoclonal antibodies

Timolol → see beta blockers, non-selective

Tinzaparin → see low molecular-weight heparins

Tioguanine → see TABLE 1 p. 1053 (hepatotoxicity), TABLE 12 p. 1057 (myelosuppression)

- **Live vaccines** are predicted to increase the risk of generalised infection (possibly life-threatening) when given with **tioguanine**. UKHSA advises avoid (refer to Green Book). [Severe] Theoretical

Tiotropium → see TABLE 8 p. 1055 (antimuscarinics)

- Atypical antipsychotics **(clozapine)** can cause constipation, as can **tiotropium**; concurrent use might increase the risk of developing intestinal obstruction. [Severe] Theoretical → Also see TABLE 8 p. 1055

Tirofiban → see TABLE 3 p. 1053 (bleeding)

Tirzepatide → see glucagon-like peptide-1 receptor agonists

A1

Interactions | Appendix 1

Tisotumab vedotin
- Anti-androgens **(apalutamide, enzalutamide)** are predicted to decrease the exposure to the cytotoxic component of **tisotumab vedotin.** [Moderate] Theoretical
- Antiepileptics **(carbamazepine, fosphenytoin, phenobarbital, phenytoin, primidone)** are predicted to decrease the exposure to the cytotoxic component of **tisotumab vedotin.** [Moderate] Theoretical
- Antifungals, azoles **(itraconazole, ketoconazole, posaconazole, voriconazole)** are predicted to increase the exposure to the cytotoxic component of **tisotumab vedotin.** [Severe] Theoretical
- **Ceritinib** is predicted to increase the exposure to the cytotoxic component of **tisotumab vedotin.** [Severe] Theoretical
- **Cobicistat** is predicted to increase the exposure to the cytotoxic component of **tisotumab vedotin.** [Severe] Theoretical
- **Encorafenib** is predicted to decrease the exposure to the cytotoxic component of **tisotumab vedotin.** [Moderate] Theoretical
- **HIV-protease inhibitors** are predicted to increase the exposure to the cytotoxic component of **tisotumab vedotin.** [Severe] Theoretical
- **Idelalisib** is predicted to increase the exposure to the cytotoxic component of **tisotumab vedotin.** [Severe] Theoretical
- **Ivosidenib** is predicted to decrease the exposure to the cytotoxic component of **tisotumab vedotin.** [Moderate] Theoretical
- **Lumacaftor** is predicted to decrease the exposure to the cytotoxic component of **tisotumab vedotin.** [Moderate] Theoretical
- Macrolides **(clarithromycin)** are predicted to increase the exposure to the cytotoxic component of **tisotumab vedotin.** [Severe] Theoretical
- **Mitotane** is predicted to decrease the exposure to the cytotoxic component of **tisotumab vedotin.** [Moderate] Theoretical
- Rifamycins **(rifampicin)** are predicted to decrease the exposure to the cytotoxic component of **tisotumab vedotin.** [Moderate] Theoretical
- **Tucatinib** is predicted to increase the exposure to the cytotoxic component of **tisotumab vedotin.** [Severe] Theoretical

Tivozanib
- Anti-androgens **(apalutamide, enzalutamide)** are predicted to decrease the exposure to **tivozanib.** [Severe] Study
- Antiepileptics **(carbamazepine, fosphenytoin, phenobarbital, phenytoin, primidone)** are predicted to decrease the exposure to **tivozanib.** [Severe] Study
- **Encorafenib** is predicted to decrease the exposure to **tivozanib.** [Severe] Study
- **Ivosidenib** is predicted to decrease the exposure to **tivozanib.** [Severe] Study
- **Lumacaftor** is predicted to decrease the exposure to **tivozanib.** [Severe] Study
- **Mitotane** is predicted to decrease the exposure to **tivozanib.** [Severe] Study
- Rifamycins **(rifampicin)** are predicted to decrease the exposure to **tivozanib.** [Severe] Study
- **St John's wort** is predicted to decrease the exposure to **tivozanib.** Avoid. [Severe] Study

Tizanidine → see TABLE 4 p. 1054 (bradycardia), TABLE 6 p. 1054 (hypotension), TABLE 9 p. 1056 (CNS effects)
- Antiepileptics **(fosphenytoin, phenytoin)** moderately decrease the exposure to **tizanidine.** [Mild] Study → Also see TABLE 9 p. 1056
- **Axitinib** is predicted to increase the exposure to **tizanidine.** [Moderate] Theoretical
- **Combined hormonal contraceptives** increases the exposure to **tizanidine.** Avoid. [Moderate] Study
- **Givosiran** increases the exposure to **tizanidine.** Avoid. [Moderate] Study
- HIV-protease inhibitors **(ritonavir)** moderately decrease the exposure to **tizanidine.** [Mild] Study
- Iron chelators **(deferasirox)** are predicted to increase the exposure to **tizanidine.** Avoid. [Moderate] Theoretical
- **Leflunomide** moderately decreases the exposure to **tizanidine.** [Mild] Study
- **Leniolisib** is predicted to increase the exposure to **tizanidine.** Avoid. [Moderate] Theoretical
- **Maribavir** is predicted to decrease the exposure to **tizanidine.** Avoid. [Mild] Theoretical
- **Mexiletine** increases the exposure to **tizanidine.** Avoid. [Moderate] Study
- **Obeticholic acid** is predicted to increase the exposure to **tizanidine.** [Severe] Theoretical
- **Osilodrostat** increases the exposure to **tizanidine.** Avoid. [Moderate] Study
- Quinolones **(ciprofloxacin)** increase the exposure to **tizanidine.** Avoid. [Moderate] Study
- Rifamycins **(rifampicin)** moderately decrease the exposure to **tizanidine.** [Mild] Study
- **Ritlecitinib** is predicted to increase the exposure to **tizanidine.** [Moderate] Theoretical
- **Rucaparib** increases the exposure to **tizanidine.** Avoid. [Moderate] Study
- SSRIs **(fluvoxamine)** very markedly increase the exposure to **tizanidine.** Avoid. [Severe] Study → Also see TABLE 9 p. 1056
- **Teriflunomide** moderately decreases the exposure to **tizanidine.** [Mild] Study
- **Vemurafenib** increases the exposure to **tizanidine.** Avoid. [Moderate] Study

Tobramycin → see aminoglycosides
Tocilizumab → see monoclonal antibodies

Tofacitinib
- Anti-androgens **(apalutamide, enzalutamide)** are predicted to decrease the exposure to **tofacitinib.** Avoid. [Severe] Study
- Antiarrhythmics **(dronedarone)** given with a potent CYP2C19 inhibitor are predicted to increase the exposure to **tofacitinib.** Adjust **tofacitinib** dose, p. 803. [Moderate] Study
- Antiepileptics **(carbamazepine, fosphenytoin, phenobarbital, phenytoin, primidone)** are predicted to decrease the exposure to **tofacitinib.** Avoid. [Severe] Study
- Antifungals, azoles **(fluconazole)** increase the exposure to **tofacitinib.** Adjust **tofacitinib** dose, p. 803. [Moderate] Study
- Antifungals, azoles **(isavuconazole)** given with a potent CYP2C19 inhibitor are predicted to increase the exposure to **tofacitinib.** Adjust **tofacitinib** dose, p. 803. [Moderate] Study
- Antifungals, azoles **(itraconazole, ketoconazole, posaconazole, voriconazole)** are predicted to increase the exposure to **tofacitinib.** Adjust **tofacitinib** dose, p. 803. [Moderate] Study
- Calcium-channel blockers **(diltiazem, verapamil)** given with a potent CYP2C19 inhibitor are predicted to increase the exposure to **tofacitinib.** Adjust **tofacitinib** dose, p. 803. [Moderate] Study
- **Cenobamate** is predicted to decrease the exposure to **tofacitinib.** [Severe] Study
- **Ceritinib** is predicted to increase the exposure to **tofacitinib.** Adjust **tofacitinib** dose, p. 803. [Moderate] Study
- **Ciclosporin** increases the exposure to **tofacitinib.** Avoid. [Severe] Study
- **Cobicistat** is predicted to increase the exposure to **tofacitinib.** Adjust **tofacitinib** dose, p. 803. [Moderate] Study
- **Tofacitinib** is predicted to increase the risk of bleeding when given with **coumarins.** [Severe] Theoretical
- **Crizotinib** given with a potent CYP2C19 inhibitor is predicted to increase the exposure to **tofacitinib.** Adjust **tofacitinib** dose, p. 803. [Moderate] Study
- **Dabrafenib** is predicted to decrease the exposure to **tofacitinib.** [Severe] Study
- **Encorafenib** is predicted to decrease the exposure to **tofacitinib.** Avoid. [Severe] Study
- Endothelin receptor antagonists **(bosentan)** are predicted to decrease the exposure to **tofacitinib.** [Severe] Study
- **Filgotinib** is predicted to increase the risk of immunosuppression when given with **tofacitinib.** Avoid. [Severe] Theoretical
- **HIV-protease inhibitors** are predicted to increase the exposure to **tofacitinib.** Adjust **tofacitinib** dose, p. 803. [Moderate] Study
- **Idelalisib** is predicted to increase the exposure to **tofacitinib.** Adjust **tofacitinib** dose, p. 803. [Moderate] Study
- **Imatinib** given with a potent CYP2C19 inhibitor is predicted to increase the exposure to **tofacitinib.** Adjust **tofacitinib** dose, p. 803. [Moderate] Study
- **Ivosidenib** is predicted to decrease the exposure to **tofacitinib.** Avoid. [Severe] Study

- **Letermovir** given with a potent CYP2C19 inhibitor is predicted to increase the exposure to **tofacitinib**. Adjust **tofacitinib** dose, p. 803. Moderate Study
- **Live vaccines** potentially increase the risk of generalised infection (possibly life-threatening) when given with **tofacitinib**. Avoid. Severe Theoretical
- **Lorlatinib** is predicted to decrease the exposure to **tofacitinib**. Severe Study
- **Lumacaftor** is predicted to decrease the exposure to **tofacitinib**. Avoid. Severe Study
- Macrolides **(clarithromycin)** are predicted to increase the exposure to **tofacitinib**. Adjust **tofacitinib** dose, p. 803. Moderate Study
- Macrolides **(erythromycin)** given with a potent CYP2C19 inhibitor are predicted to increase the exposure to **tofacitinib**. Adjust **tofacitinib** dose, p. 803. Moderate Study
- **Mitotane** is predicted to decrease the exposure to **tofacitinib**. Avoid. Severe Study
- Neurokinin-1 receptor antagonists **(aprepitant, netupitant)** given with a potent CYP2C19 inhibitor are predicted to increase the exposure to **tofacitinib**. Adjust **tofacitinib** dose, p. 803. Moderate Study
- **Nilotinib** given with a potent CYP2C19 inhibitor is predicted to increase the exposure to **tofacitinib**. Adjust **tofacitinib** dose, p. 803. Moderate Study
- **Nirmatrelvir** boosted with ritonavir is predicted to increase the concentration of **tofacitinib**. Adjust dose. Severe Theoretical
- NNRTIs **(efavirenz, etravirine, nevirapine)** are predicted to decrease the exposure to **tofacitinib**. Severe Study
- **Tofacitinib** is predicted to increase the risk of bleeding when given with **phenindione**. Severe Theoretical
- Rifamycins **(rifampicin)** are predicted to decrease the exposure to **tofacitinib**. Avoid. Severe Study
- **Sotorasib** is predicted to decrease the exposure to **tofacitinib**. Severe Study
- SSRIs **(fluoxetine, fluvoxamine)** given with a moderate CYP3A4 inhibitor are predicted to increase the exposure to **tofacitinib**. Adjust **tofacitinib** dose, p. 803. Moderate Study
- **St John's wort** is predicted to decrease the exposure to **tofacitinib**. Severe Study
- **Tacrolimus** increases the exposure to **tofacitinib**. Avoid. Severe Study
- **Tucatinib** is predicted to increase the exposure to **tofacitinib**. Adjust **tofacitinib** dose, p. 803. Moderate Study

Tolbutamide → see sulfonylureas

Tolcapone
- **Tolcapone** might increase the exposure to the active metabolite of **foslevodopa**. Adjust dose. Moderate Theoretical
- **Tolcapone** is predicted to increase the risk of cardiovascular adverse effects when given with **isoprenaline**. Moderate Theoretical
- **Tolcapone** increases the exposure to **levodopa**. Monitor and adjust dose. Moderate Study
- **Tolcapone** is predicted to increase the effects of **MAOIs, irreversible**. Avoid. Severe Theoretical
- **Tolcapone** is predicted to increase the risk of cardiovascular adverse effects when given with **sympathomimetics, inotropic**. Moderate Theoretical
- **Tolcapone** is predicted to increase the effects of sympathomimetics, vasoconstrictor **(adrenaline, noradrenaline)**. Moderate Theoretical

Tolfenamic acid → see NSAIDs

Tolterodine → see TABLE 7 p. 1055 (QT-interval prolongation), TABLE 8 p. 1055 (antimuscarinics)
- Antifungals, azoles **(itraconazole, ketoconazole, posaconazole, voriconazole)** are predicted to increase the exposure to **tolterodine**. Avoid. Severe Study → Also see TABLE 7 p. 1055
- Atypical antipsychotics **(clozapine)** can cause constipation, as can **tolterodine**; concurrent use might increase the risk of developing intestinal obstruction. Severe Theoretical → Also see TABLE 8 p. 1055
- **Ceritinib** is predicted to increase the exposure to **tolterodine**. Avoid. Severe Study → Also see TABLE 7 p. 1055
- **Cobicistat** is predicted to increase the exposure to **tolterodine**. Avoid. Severe Study
- **Dacomitinib** is predicted to markedly increase the exposure to **tolterodine**. Avoid. Severe Study
- **Eliglustat** is predicted to increase the exposure to **tolterodine**. Adjust dose. Moderate Theoretical
- **HIV-protease inhibitors** are predicted to increase the exposure to **tolterodine**. Avoid. Severe Study
- **Idelalisib** is predicted to increase the exposure to **tolterodine**. Avoid. Severe Study
- Macrolides **(clarithromycin)** are predicted to increase the exposure to **tolterodine**. Avoid. Severe Study
- **Tucatinib** is predicted to increase the exposure to **tolterodine**. Avoid. Severe Study

Tolvaptan → see TABLE 13 p. 1057 (increased serum potassium)

GENERAL INFORMATION Avoid concurrent use of drugs that increase serum-sodium concentrations.

- Anti-androgens **(apalutamide, enzalutamide)** are predicted to decrease the exposure to **tolvaptan**. Use with caution or avoid depending on indication. Severe Study
- Antiarrhythmics **(dronedarone)** are predicted to increase the exposure to **tolvaptan**. Manufacturer advises caution or adjust **tolvaptan** dose with moderate CYP3A4 inhibitors. Moderate Study
- Antiepileptics **(carbamazepine, fosphenytoin, phenobarbital, phenytoin, primidone)** are predicted to decrease the exposure to **tolvaptan**. Use with caution or avoid depending on indication. Severe Study
- Antifungals, azoles **(fluconazole, isavuconazole)** are predicted to increase the exposure to **tolvaptan**. Manufacturer advises caution or adjust **tolvaptan** dose with moderate CYP3A4 inhibitors. Moderate Study
- Antifungals, azoles **(itraconazole, ketoconazole, posaconazole, voriconazole)** are predicted to increase the exposure to **tolvaptan**. Manufacturer advises caution or adjust **tolvaptan** dose with potent CYP3A4 inhibitors. Severe Study
- **Berotralstat** is predicted to increase the exposure to **tolvaptan**. Manufacturer advises caution or adjust **tolvaptan** dose with moderate CYP3A4 inhibitors. Moderate Study
- Calcium-channel blockers **(diltiazem, verapamil)** are predicted to increase the exposure to **tolvaptan**. Manufacturer advises caution or adjust **tolvaptan** dose with moderate CYP3A4 inhibitors. Moderate Study
- **Cenobamate** is predicted to decrease the exposure to **tolvaptan**. Adjust dose. Moderate Theoretical
- **Ceritinib** is predicted to increase the exposure to **tolvaptan**. Manufacturer advises caution or adjust **tolvaptan** dose with potent CYP3A4 inhibitors. Severe Study
- **Cobicistat** is predicted to increase the exposure to **tolvaptan**. Manufacturer advises caution or adjust **tolvaptan** dose with potent CYP3A4 inhibitors. Severe Study
- **Crizotinib** is predicted to increase the exposure to **tolvaptan**. Manufacturer advises caution or adjust **tolvaptan** dose with moderate CYP3A4 inhibitors. Moderate Study
- **Tolvaptan** slightly increases the exposure to **digoxin**. Moderate Study
- **Encorafenib** is predicted to decrease the exposure to **tolvaptan**. Use with caution or avoid depending on indication. Severe Study
- **Fedratinib** is predicted to increase the exposure to **tolvaptan**. Manufacturer advises caution or adjust **tolvaptan** dose with moderate CYP3A4 inhibitors. Moderate Study
- **Grapefruit** juice increases the exposure to **tolvaptan**. Avoid. Moderate Study
- **HIV-protease inhibitors** are predicted to increase the exposure to **tolvaptan**. Manufacturer advises caution or adjust **tolvaptan** dose with potent CYP3A4 inhibitors. Severe Study
- **Idelalisib** is predicted to increase the exposure to **tolvaptan**. Manufacturer advises caution or adjust **tolvaptan** dose with potent CYP3A4 inhibitors. Severe Study
- **Imatinib** is predicted to increase the exposure to **tolvaptan**. Manufacturer advises caution or adjust **tolvaptan** dose with moderate CYP3A4 inhibitors. Moderate Study
- **Ivosidenib** is predicted to decrease the exposure to **tolvaptan**. Use with caution or avoid depending on indication. Severe Study

Tolvaptan (continued)
- **Letermovir** is predicted to increase the exposure to **tolvaptan**. Manufacturer advises caution or adjust **tolvaptan** dose with moderate CYP3A4 inhibitors. Moderate Study
- **Tolvaptan** is predicted to increase the exposure to **lomitapide**. Separate administration by 12 hours. Moderate Theoretical
- **Lumacaftor** is predicted to decrease the exposure to **tolvaptan**. Use with caution or avoid depending on indication. Severe Study
- Macrolides **(clarithromycin)** are predicted to increase the exposure to **tolvaptan**. Manufacturer advises caution or adjust **tolvaptan** dose with potent CYP3A4 inhibitors. Severe Study
- Macrolides **(erythromycin)** are predicted to increase the exposure to **tolvaptan**. Manufacturer advises caution or adjust **tolvaptan** dose with moderate CYP3A4 inhibitors. Moderate Study
- **Mitotane** is predicted to decrease the exposure to **tolvaptan**. Use with caution or avoid depending on indication. Severe Study
- Neurokinin-1 receptor antagonists **(aprepitant, netupitant)** are predicted to increase the exposure to **tolvaptan**. Manufacturer advises caution or adjust **tolvaptan** dose with moderate CYP3A4 inhibitors. Moderate Study
- **Nilotinib** is predicted to increase the exposure to **tolvaptan**. Manufacturer advises caution or adjust **tolvaptan** dose with moderate CYP3A4 inhibitors. Moderate Study
- **Nirmatrelvir** boosted with ritonavir is predicted to increase the concentration of **tolvaptan**. Avoid. Severe Theoretical
- Quinolones **(ciprofloxacin)** are predicted to increase the exposure to **tolvaptan**. Use with caution and adjust **tolvaptan** dose. Moderate Theoretical
- Rifamycins **(rifampicin)** are predicted to decrease the exposure to **tolvaptan**. Use with caution or avoid depending on indication. Severe Study
- **St John's wort** is predicted to decrease the exposure to **tolvaptan**. Avoid. Moderate Theoretical
- **Tucatinib** is predicted to increase the exposure to **tolvaptan**. Manufacturer advises caution or adjust **tolvaptan** dose with potent CYP3A4 inhibitors. Severe Study

Topiramate → see antiepileptics

Topotecan → see TABLE 12 p. 1057 (myelosuppression)
- Anti-androgens **(apalutamide)** are predicted to decrease the exposure to **topotecan**. Monitor and adjust dose. Moderate Theoretical
- Anti-androgens **(darolutamide)** are predicted to increase the exposure to **topotecan**. Avoid. Severe Theoretical
- Antiarrhythmics **(amiodarone, dronedarone)** are predicted to increase the exposure to **topotecan**. Severe Study
- Antiepileptics **(fosphenytoin, phenytoin)** increase the clearance of **topotecan**. Moderate Study
- Antifungals, azoles **(isavuconazole)** are predicted to increase the exposure to **topotecan**. Moderate Theoretical
- Antifungals, azoles **(itraconazole, ketoconazole)** are predicted to increase the exposure to **topotecan**. Severe Study
- **Belumosudil** is predicted to increase the exposure to **topotecan**. Avoid or adjust dose. Moderate Theoretical
- Calcium-channel blockers **(verapamil)** are predicted to increase the exposure to **topotecan**. Severe Study
- **Ceritinib** is predicted to increase the exposure to **topotecan**. Moderate Theoretical → Also see TABLE 12 p. 1057
- **Ciclosporin** is predicted to increase the exposure to **topotecan**. Severe Study
- **Cobicistat** is predicted to increase the exposure to **topotecan**. Severe Study
- **Danicopan** is predicted to increase the exposure to **topotecan**. Moderate Study
- **Eltrombopag** is predicted to increase the exposure to **topotecan**. Moderate Theoretical
- **Encorafenib** is predicted to increase the effects of **topotecan**. Mild Study
- **Febuxostat** is predicted to increase the exposure to **topotecan**. Moderate Theoretical
- **Fostamatinib** is predicted to increase the exposure to **topotecan**. Monitor and adjust dose. Moderate Theoretical
- **Glecaprevir** is predicted to increase the exposure to **topotecan**. Severe Study
- HIV-protease inhibitors **(lopinavir, ritonavir)** are predicted to increase the exposure to **topotecan**. Severe Study
- **Lapatinib** is predicted to increase the exposure to **topotecan**. Severe Study
- **Leflunomide** is predicted to increase the exposure to **topotecan**. Moderate Study → Also see TABLE 12 p. 1057
- **Leniolisib** is predicted to increase the exposure to **topotecan**. Avoid. Moderate Theoretical
- **Live vaccines** are predicted to increase the risk of generalised infection (possibly life-threatening) when given with **topotecan**. UKHSA advises avoid (refer to Green Book). Severe Theoretical
- **Macrolides** are predicted to increase the exposure to **topotecan**. Severe Study
- **Pibrentasvir** is predicted to increase the exposure to **topotecan**. Severe Study
- **Pirtobrutinib** is predicted to increase the exposure to **topotecan**. Moderate Theoretical
- **Ranolazine** is predicted to increase the exposure to **topotecan**. Severe Study
- **Regorafenib** is predicted to increase the exposure to **topotecan**. Moderate Study → Also see TABLE 12 p. 1057
- **Roxadustat** might increase the exposure to **topotecan**. Monitor adverse effects and adjust dose. Moderate Theoretical
- **Sparsentan** is predicted to increase the exposure to **topotecan**. Moderate Theoretical
- **St John's wort** is predicted to decrease the exposure to **topotecan**. Severe Theoretical
- **Tedizolid** is predicted to increase the exposure to **topotecan**. Avoid. Moderate Study
- **Teriflunomide** is predicted to increase the exposure to **topotecan**. Moderate Study
- **Vadadustat** is predicted to increase the exposure to **topotecan**. Monitor and adjust dose. Moderate Study
- **Velpatasvir** is predicted to increase the exposure to **topotecan**. Severe Study
- **Vemurafenib** is predicted to increase the exposure to **topotecan**. Severe Study
- **Venetoclax** is predicted to increase the exposure to **topotecan**. Moderate Theoretical
- **Voxilaprevir** is predicted to increase the exposure to **topotecan**. Severe Study

Torasemide → see loop diuretics

Toremifene → see TABLE 7 p. 1055 (QT-interval prolongation)
- Anti-androgens **(apalutamide, enzalutamide)** are predicted to decrease the exposure to **toremifene**. Adjust dose. Moderate Study → Also see TABLE 7 p. 1055
- Antiepileptics **(carbamazepine, fosphenytoin, phenobarbital, phenytoin, primidone)** are predicted to decrease the exposure to **toremifene**. Adjust dose. Moderate Study
- Antifungals, azoles **(itraconazole, ketoconazole, posaconazole, voriconazole)** are predicted to increase the exposure to **toremifene**. Moderate Theoretical → Also see TABLE 7 p. 1055
- **Ceritinib** is predicted to increase the exposure to **toremifene**. Moderate Theoretical → Also see TABLE 7 p. 1055
- **Cobicistat** is predicted to increase the exposure to **toremifene**. Moderate Theoretical
- **Toremifene** is predicted to increase the anticoagulant effect of **coumarins**. Severe Theoretical
- **Encorafenib** is predicted to decrease the exposure to **toremifene**. Adjust dose. Moderate Study → Also see TABLE 7 p. 1055
- **HIV-protease inhibitors** are predicted to increase the exposure to **toremifene**. Moderate Theoretical
- **Idelalisib** is predicted to increase the exposure to **toremifene**. Moderate Theoretical
- **Ivosidenib** is predicted to decrease the exposure to **toremifene**. Adjust dose. Moderate Study → Also see TABLE 7 p. 1055
- **Lumacaftor** is predicted to decrease the exposure to **toremifene**. Adjust dose. Moderate Study
- Macrolides **(clarithromycin)** are predicted to increase the exposure to **toremifene**. Moderate Theoretical

- **Mitotane** is predicted to decrease the exposure to **toremifene**. Adjust dose. Moderate Study
- Rifamycins (rifampicin) are predicted to decrease the exposure to **toremifene**. Adjust dose. Moderate Study
- **Thiazide diuretics** are predicted to increase the risk of hypercalcaemia when given with **toremifene**. Severe Theoretical
- **Tucatinib** is predicted to increase the exposure to **toremifene**. Moderate Theoretical

Trabectedin → see TABLE 1 p. 1053 (hepatotoxicity), TABLE 12 p. 1057 (myelosuppression)
- Anti-androgens (apalutamide, enzalutamide) are predicted to decrease the exposure to **trabectedin**. Avoid. Severe Theoretical
- Antiepileptics (carbamazepine, fosphenytoin, phenobarbital, phenytoin, primidone) are predicted to decrease the exposure to **trabectedin**. Avoid. Severe Theoretical
- Antifungals, azoles (itraconazole, ketoconazole, posaconazole, voriconazole) are predicted to increase the exposure to **trabectedin**. Avoid or adjust dose. Severe Theoretical → Also see TABLE 1 p. 1053
- **Ceritinib** is predicted to increase the exposure to **trabectedin**. Avoid or adjust dose. Severe Theoretical → Also see TABLE 12 p. 1057
- **Cobicistat** is predicted to increase the exposure to **trabectedin**. Avoid or adjust dose. Severe Theoretical
- **Encorafenib** is predicted to decrease the exposure to **trabectedin**. Avoid. Severe Theoretical
- **HIV-protease inhibitors** are predicted to increase the exposure to **trabectedin**. Avoid or adjust dose. Severe Theoretical → Also see TABLE 1 p. 1053
- **Idelalisib** is predicted to increase the exposure to **trabectedin**. Avoid or adjust dose. Severe Theoretical
- **Ivosidenib** is predicted to decrease the exposure to **trabectedin**. Avoid. Severe Theoretical
- **Live vaccines** are predicted to increase the risk of generalised infection (possibly life-threatening) when given with **trabectedin**. UKHSA advises avoid (refer to Green Book). Severe Theoretical
- **Lumacaftor** is predicted to decrease the exposure to **trabectedin**. Avoid. Severe Theoretical
- Macrolides (clarithromycin) are predicted to increase the exposure to **trabectedin**. Avoid or adjust dose. Severe Theoretical
- **Mitotane** is predicted to decrease the exposure to **trabectedin**. Avoid. Severe Theoretical → Also see TABLE 12 p. 1057
- Rifamycins (rifampicin) are predicted to decrease the exposure to **trabectedin**. Avoid. Severe Theoretical
- **Tucatinib** is predicted to increase the exposure to **trabectedin**. Avoid or adjust dose. Severe Theoretical

Tralokinumab → see monoclonal antibodies

Tramadol → see opioids

Trametinib
- Antiarrhythmics (amiodarone, dronedarone) are predicted to increase the concentration of **trametinib**. Moderate Theoretical
- Antifungals, azoles (itraconazole, ketoconazole) are predicted to increase the concentration of **trametinib**. Moderate Theoretical
- Calcium-channel blockers (verapamil) are predicted to increase the concentration of **trametinib**. Moderate Theoretical
- **Ciclosporin** is predicted to increase the concentration of **trametinib**. Moderate Theoretical
- **Cobicistat** is predicted to increase the concentration of **trametinib**. Moderate Theoretical
- **Drugs that cause bleeding** (see TABLE 3 p. 1053) cause bleeding, as can **trametinib**; concurrent use might increase the risk of developing this effect. Severe Theoretical
- **Glecaprevir** is predicted to increase the concentration of **trametinib**. Moderate Theoretical
- HIV-protease inhibitors (lopinavir, ritonavir) are predicted to increase the concentration of **trametinib**. Moderate Theoretical
- **Lapatinib** is predicted to increase the concentration of **trametinib**. Moderate Theoretical
- **Macrolides** are predicted to increase the concentration of **trametinib**. Moderate Theoretical
- **Pibrentasvir** is predicted to increase the concentration of **trametinib**. Moderate Theoretical
- **Ranolazine** is predicted to increase the concentration of **trametinib**. Moderate Theoretical
- **Velpatasvir** is predicted to increase the concentration of **trametinib**. Moderate Theoretical
- **Vemurafenib** is predicted to increase the concentration of **trametinib**. Moderate Theoretical
- **Voxilaprevir** is predicted to increase the concentration of **trametinib**. Moderate Theoretical

Trandolapril → see ACE inhibitors

Tranylcypromine → see MAOIs, irreversible

Trastuzumab → see monoclonal antibodies

Trastuzumab deruxtecan → see monoclonal antibodies

Trastuzumab emtansine → see monoclonal antibodies

Trazodone → see TABLE 15 p. 1058 (hyponatraemia), TABLE 11 p. 1056 (serotonin toxicity), TABLE 9 p. 1056 (CNS effects)
- Antiarrhythmics (dronedarone) are predicted to increase the exposure to **trazodone**. Moderate Theoretical
- Antiepileptics (carbamazepine) decrease the concentration of **trazodone**. Adjust dose. Moderate Anecdotal → Also see TABLE 15 p. 1058
- Antifungals, azoles (fluconazole, isavuconazole) are predicted to increase the exposure to **trazodone**. Moderate Theoretical
- Antifungals, azoles (itraconazole, ketoconazole, posaconazole, voriconazole) are predicted to moderately increase the exposure to **trazodone**. Avoid or adjust dose. Moderate Study
- **Berotralstat** is predicted to increase the exposure to **trazodone**. Moderate Theoretical
- Calcium-channel blockers (diltiazem, verapamil) are predicted to increase the exposure to **trazodone**. Moderate Theoretical
- **Ceritinib** is predicted to moderately increase the exposure to **trazodone**. Avoid or adjust dose. Moderate Study
- **Cobicistat** is predicted to moderately increase the exposure to **trazodone**. Avoid or adjust dose. Moderate Study
- **Crizotinib** is predicted to increase the exposure to **trazodone**. Moderate Theoretical
- **Fedratinib** is predicted to increase the exposure to **trazodone**. Moderate Theoretical
- **HIV-protease inhibitors** are predicted to moderately increase the exposure to **trazodone**. Avoid or adjust dose. Moderate Study
- **Idelalisib** is predicted to moderately increase the exposure to **trazodone**. Avoid or adjust dose. Moderate Study
- **Imatinib** is predicted to increase the exposure to **trazodone**. Moderate Theoretical
- **Letermovir** is predicted to increase the exposure to **trazodone**. Moderate Theoretical
- Macrolides (clarithromycin) are predicted to moderately increase the exposure to **trazodone**. Avoid or adjust dose. Moderate Study
- Macrolides (erythromycin) are predicted to increase the exposure to **trazodone**. Moderate Theoretical
- Neurokinin-1 receptor antagonists (aprepitant, netupitant) are predicted to increase the exposure to **trazodone**. Moderate Theoretical
- **Nilotinib** is predicted to increase the exposure to **trazodone**. Moderate Theoretical
- **Nirmatrelvir** boosted with ritonavir is predicted to increase the concentration of **trazodone**. Moderate Theoretical
- **Tucatinib** is predicted to moderately increase the exposure to **trazodone**. Avoid or adjust dose. Moderate Study

Tree pollen extracts

GENERAL INFORMATION Desensitising vaccines should be avoided in patients taking beta-blockers (adrenaline might be ineffective in case of a hypersensitivity reaction) or ACE inhibitors (risk of severe anaphylactoid reactions).

Treosulfan → see alkylating agents

Treprostinil → see TABLE 3 p. 1053 (bleeding), TABLE 6 p. 1054 (hypotension)
- Antiepileptics (carbamazepine, phenobarbital, phenytoin) are predicted to decrease the exposure to **treprostinil**. Adjust dose. Mild Theoretical
- **Clopidogrel** is predicted to increase the exposure to **treprostinil**. Adjust dose. Moderate Theoretical → Also see TABLE 3 p. 1053

Treprostinil (continued)
- Fibrates **(gemfibrozil)** increase the exposure to **treprostinil**. Adjust dose. [Moderate] Study
- Iron chelators **(deferasirox)** are predicted to increase the exposure to **treprostinil**. Adjust dose. [Moderate] Theoretical
- Loop diuretics **(furosemide)** might slightly decrease the clearance of **treprostinil**. [Unknown] Theoretical → Also see TABLE 6 p. 1054
- Rifamycins **(rifampicin)** slightly decrease the exposure to **treprostinil**. Adjust dose. [Mild] Study
- **St John's wort** is predicted to decrease the exposure to **treprostinil**. Adjust dose. [Mild] Theoretical
- **Trimethoprim** is predicted to increase the exposure to **treprostinil**. Adjust dose. [Moderate] Theoretical

Tretinoin → see retinoids
Triamcinolone → see corticosteroids
Triamterene → see potassium-sparing diuretics
Tricyclic antidepressants → see TABLE 15 p. 1058 (hyponatraemia), TABLE 6 p. 1054 (hypotension), TABLE 11 p. 1056 (serotonin toxicity), TABLE 7 p. 1055 (QT-interval prolongation), TABLE 8 p. 1055 (antimuscarinics), TABLE 9 p. 1056 (CNS effects)

amitriptyline · clomipramine · dosulepin · doxepin · imipramine · lofepramine · nortriptyline · trimipramine

ROUTE-SPECIFIC INFORMATION Since systemic absorption can follow topical application, the possibility of interactions of topical **doxepin** should be borne in mind.

- Antiarrhythmics **(dronedarone)** are predicted to increase the exposure to **tricyclic antidepressants**. Avoid. [Severe] Theoretical → Also see TABLE 7 p. 1055
- Antiarrhythmics **(propafenone)** are predicted to increase the concentration of **tricyclic antidepressants**. [Moderate] Theoretical → Also see TABLE 8 p. 1055
- Antiepileptics **(carbamazepine)** decrease the exposure to **tricyclic antidepressants**. Adjust dose. [Moderate] Study → Also see TABLE 15 p. 1058
- Antiepileptics **(phenobarbital, primidone)** are predicted to decrease the exposure to **tricyclic antidepressants**. [Moderate] Study → Also see TABLE 9 p. 1056
- Antiepileptics **(valproate)** increase the concentration of **nortriptyline**. [Severe] Study → Also see TABLE 15 p. 1058
- Tricyclic antidepressants **(clomipramine, imipramine)** potentially increase the risk of overheating and dehydration when given with antiepileptics **(zonisamide)**. Avoid in children. [Severe] Theoretical
- Atypical antipsychotics **(clozapine)** can cause constipation, as can **tricyclic antidepressants** ; concurrent use might increase the risk of developing intestinal obstruction. [Severe] Theoretical → Also see TABLE 15 p. 1058 → Also see TABLE 6 p. 1054 → Also see TABLE 8 p. 1055 → Also see TABLE 9 p. 1056
- **Berotralstat** is predicted to increase the exposure to **tricyclic antidepressants**. Monitor and adjust dose. [Moderate] Theoretical
- **Bupropion** is predicted to increase the exposure to **tricyclic antidepressants**. Monitor for toxicity and adjust dose. [Severe] Study
- **Cinacalcet** is predicted to increase the exposure to **tricyclic antidepressants**. Monitor for toxicity and adjust dose. [Severe] Study
- **Tricyclic antidepressants** decrease the antihypertensive effects of **clonidine**. Monitor and adjust dose. [Moderate] Anecdotal → Also see TABLE 6 p. 1054 → Also see TABLE 9 p. 1056
- **Cobicistat** is predicted to slightly increase the exposure to **tricyclic antidepressants**. [Mild] Study
- **Dacomitinib** is predicted to increase the exposure to **tricyclic antidepressants**. Monitor for toxicity and adjust dose. [Severe] Study
- **Darifenacin** (high-dose) is predicted to increase the exposure to **tricyclic antidepressants**. [Moderate] Study → Also see TABLE 8 p. 1055
- **Eliglustat** is predicted to increase the exposure to **nortriptyline**. Adjust dose. [Moderate] Theoretical
- H_2 receptor antagonists **(cimetidine)** increase the exposure to **tricyclic antidepressants**. [Moderate] Study
- HIV-protease inhibitors **(ritonavir)** are predicted to increase the exposure to **tricyclic antidepressants**. [Moderate] Theoretical
- **Tricyclic antidepressants** potentially increase the risk of neurotoxicity when given with **lithium**. [Severe] Anecdotal
- **Tricyclic antidepressants** are predicted to increase the risk of severe toxic reaction when given with **MAOIs, irreversible**. Avoid and for 14 days after stopping the MAOI. [Severe] Theoretical → Also see TABLE 6 p. 1054 → Also see TABLE 11 p. 1056
- **Methylphenidate** might increase the concentration of **tricyclic antidepressants**. Use with caution and adjust dose. [Moderate] Study
- **Amitriptyline** decreases the effects of **metyrapone**. Avoid. [Moderate] Theoretical
- **Tricyclic antidepressants** are predicted to increase the risk of severe toxic reaction when given with **moclobemide**. Avoid. [Severe] Theoretical → Also see TABLE 11 p. 1056
- **Tricyclic antidepressants** are predicted to decrease the effects of **moxonidine**. Avoid. [Moderate] Theoretical → Also see TABLE 6 p. 1054 → Also see TABLE 9 p. 1056
- **Nirmatrelvir** boosted with ritonavir is predicted to increase the concentration of **tricyclic antidepressants**. [Moderate] Theoretical
- **Tricyclic antidepressants** might increase the risk of adverse effects when given with **ozanimod**. [Severe] Theoretical
- **Tricyclic antidepressants** are predicted to decrease the efficacy of **pitolisant**. [Mild] Theoretical
- SSRIs **(fluoxetine, paroxetine)** are predicted to increase the exposure to **tricyclic antidepressants**. Monitor for toxicity and adjust dose. [Severe] Study → Also see TABLE 15 p. 1058 → Also see TABLE 11 p. 1056 → Also see TABLE 9 p. 1056
- SSRIs **(fluvoxamine)** markedly increase the exposure to **clomipramine**. Adjust dose. [Severe] Study → Also see TABLE 15 p. 1058 → Also see TABLE 11 p. 1056 → Also see TABLE 9 p. 1056
- SSRIs **(fluvoxamine)** increase the exposure to tricyclic antidepressants **(amitriptyline, imipramine)**. Adjust dose. [Severe] Study → Also see TABLE 15 p. 1058 → Also see TABLE 11 p. 1056 → Also see TABLE 9 p. 1056
- **Sucralfate** is predicted to decrease the absorption of **tricyclic antidepressants**. [Moderate] Study
- **Tricyclic antidepressants** increase the effects of sympathomimetics, vasoconstrictor **(adrenaline, noradrenaline, phenylephrine)**. Avoid. [Severe] Study
- **Tricyclic antidepressants** are predicted to decrease the effects of sympathomimetics, vasoconstrictor **(ephedrine)**. Avoid. [Severe] Study
- **Terbinafine** is predicted to increase the exposure to **tricyclic antidepressants**. Monitor for toxicity and adjust dose. [Severe] Study
- **Tricyclic antidepressants** increase the risk of cardiac arrhythmias and hypotension when given with **thiopental**. [Moderate] Study → Also see TABLE 6 p. 1054 → Also see TABLE 9 p. 1056
- **Tricyclic antidepressants** might enhance the antidiuretic and hypertensive effects of **vasopressin**. [Moderate] Theoretical
- **Vorasidenib** might decrease the concentration of tricyclic antidepressants **(amitriptyline, dosulepin, imipramine, trimipramine)**. Avoid. [Severe] Theoretical

Trientine
- Oral **trientine** potentially decreases the absorption of oral **iron**. [Moderate] Theoretical
- **Trientine** potentially decreases the absorption of **zinc**. [Moderate] Theoretical

Trifluoperazine → see phenothiazine antipsychotics
Trihexyphenidyl → see TABLE 8 p. 1055 (antimuscarinics), TABLE 9 p. 1056 (CNS effects)
- Atypical antipsychotics **(clozapine)** can cause constipation, as can **trihexyphenidyl**; concurrent use might increase the risk of developing intestinal obstruction. [Severe] Theoretical → Also see TABLE 8 p. 1055 → Also see TABLE 9 p. 1056

Trimethoprim → see TABLE 2 p. 1053 (nephrotoxicity), TABLE 13 p. 1057 (increased serum potassium)
- **Trimethoprim** increases the concentration of antiepileptics **(fosphenytoin, phenytoin)**. [Moderate] Study
- Antimalarials **(pyrimethamine)** increase the risk of adverse effects when given with **trimethoprim**. [Severe] Study
- **Trimethoprim** might increase the risk of neutropenia when given with atypical antipsychotics **(clozapine)**. Avoid. [Severe] Theoretical

- **Trimethoprim** might increase the risk of haematological toxicity when given with **azathioprine** in renal transplant patients. Severe Anecdotal
- **Trimethoprim** is predicted to increase the anticoagulant effect of **coumarins**. Severe Study
- **Dapsone** increases the exposure to **trimethoprim** and **trimethoprim** increases the exposure to **dapsone**. Severe Study
- **Trimethoprim** increases the concentration of **digoxin**. Moderate Study
- **Trimethoprim** is predicted to increase the exposure to dopamine receptor agonists **(pramipexole)**. Adjust dose. Moderate Study
- **Trimethoprim** slightly increases the exposure to meglitinides **(repaglinide)**. Avoid or monitor blood glucose. Moderate Study
- **Trimethoprim** might increase the risk of haematological toxicity when given with **mercaptopurine** in renal transplant patients. Severe Theoretical
- **Trimethoprim** is predicted to increase the exposure to **metformin**. Use with caution and adjust dose. Moderate Study
- **Trimethoprim** increases the risk of haematological side-effects (sometimes fatal) when given with **methotrexate**. Avoid. See methotrexate p. 672 for further information. Severe Anecdotal → Also see TABLE 2 p. 1053
- **Trimethoprim** slightly increases the exposure to NRTIs **(lamivudine)**. Moderate Study
- Rifamycins **(rifampicin)** decrease the exposure to **trimethoprim**. Moderate Study → Also see TABLE 2 p. 1053
- **Trimethoprim** is predicted to decrease the efficacy of **sapropterin**. Moderate Theoretical
- **Trimethoprim** is predicted to increase the exposure to **treprostinil**. Adjust dose. Moderate Theoretical

Trimipramine → see tricyclic antidepressants

Triptans

almotriptan · eletriptan · frovatriptan · naratriptan · rizatriptan · sumatriptan · zolmitriptan

- Anti-androgens **(enzalutamide)** are predicted to decrease the exposure to **eletriptan**. Severe Study
- Antifungals, azoles **(itraconazole, ketoconazole, posaconazole, voriconazole)** increase the exposure to **almotriptan**. Mild Study
- Antifungals, azoles **(itraconazole, ketoconazole, posaconazole, voriconazole)** are predicted to markedly increase the exposure to **eletriptan**. Avoid. Severe Study
- Beta blockers, non-selective **(propranolol)** slightly to moderately increase the exposure to **rizatriptan**. Adjust **rizatriptan** dose and separate administration by at least 2 hours. Moderate Study
- **Cenobamate** is predicted to decrease the exposure to **eletriptan**. Adjust dose. Moderate Theoretical
- **Ceritinib** increases the exposure to **almotriptan**. Mild Study
- **Ceritinib** is predicted to markedly increase the exposure to **eletriptan**. Avoid. Severe Study
- **Cobicistat** increases the exposure to **almotriptan**. Mild Study
- **Cobicistat** is predicted to markedly increase the exposure to **eletriptan**. Avoid. Severe Study
- **Combined hormonal contraceptives** is predicted to increase the exposure to **zolmitriptan**. Adjust **zolmitriptan** dose, p. 347. Moderate Theoretical
- **Givinostat** might increase the exposure to **eletriptan**. Moderate Study
- **Givosiran** is predicted to increase the exposure to **zolmitriptan**. Adjust **zolmitriptan** dose, p. 347. Moderate Theoretical
- H_2 receptor antagonists **(cimetidine)** slightly increase the exposure to **zolmitriptan**. Adjust **zolmitriptan** dose, p. 347. Mild Study
- **HIV-protease inhibitors** increase the exposure to **almotriptan**. Mild Study
- **HIV-protease inhibitors** are predicted to markedly increase the exposure to **eletriptan**. Avoid. Severe Study
- **Idelalisib** increases the exposure to **almotriptan**. Mild Study
- **Idelalisib** is predicted to markedly increase the exposure to **eletriptan**. Avoid. Severe Study
- **Ivosidenib** might decrease the exposure to **eletriptan**. Avoid or monitor. Moderate Theoretical
- Macrolides **(clarithromycin)** increase the exposure to **almotriptan**. Mild Study
- Macrolides **(clarithromycin)** are predicted to markedly increase the exposure to **eletriptan**. Avoid. Severe Study
- Macrolides **(erythromycin)** moderately increase the exposure to **eletriptan**. Avoid. Moderate Study
- **MAOIs, irreversible** are predicted to increase the exposure to triptans **(rizatriptan, sumatriptan)**. Avoid and for 14 days after stopping the MAOI. Severe Theoretical
- **MAOIs, irreversible** are predicted to increase the exposure to **zolmitriptan**. Severe Theoretical
- **Mexiletine** is predicted to increase the exposure to **zolmitriptan**. Adjust **zolmitriptan** dose, p. 347. Moderate Theoretical
- **Moclobemide** slightly increases the exposure to **almotriptan**. Avoid. Severe Study
- **Moclobemide** increases the concentration of triptans **(eletriptan, frovatriptan, naratriptan)**. Avoid. Severe Study
- **Moclobemide** moderately increases the exposure to triptans **(rizatriptan, sumatriptan)**. Avoid. Severe Study
- **Moclobemide** slightly increases the exposure to **zolmitriptan**. Avoid or adjust **zolmitriptan** dose, p. 347. Severe Study
- Neurokinin-1 receptor antagonists **(aprepitant, netupitant)** are predicted to increase the exposure to **eletriptan**. Moderate Study
- **Nirmatrelvir** boosted with ritonavir is predicted to increase the concentration of **eletriptan**. Avoid. Severe Theoretical
- **Osilodrostat** is predicted to increase the exposure to **zolmitriptan**. Adjust **zolmitriptan** dose, p. 347. Moderate Theoretical
- Quinolones **(ciprofloxacin)** are predicted to increase the exposure to **zolmitriptan**. Adjust **zolmitriptan** dose, p. 347. Moderate Theoretical
- **Rucaparib** is predicted to increase the exposure to **zolmitriptan**. Adjust **zolmitriptan** dose, p. 347. Moderate Theoretical
- SSRIs **(fluvoxamine)** increase the concentration of **frovatriptan**. Severe Study
- SSRIs **(fluvoxamine)** are predicted to increase the exposure to **zolmitriptan**. Adjust **zolmitriptan** dose, p. 347. Severe Theoretical
- **Tucatinib** increases the exposure to **almotriptan**. Mild Study
- **Tucatinib** is predicted to markedly increase the exposure to **eletriptan**. Avoid. Severe Study
- **Vemurafenib** is predicted to increase the exposure to **zolmitriptan**. Adjust **zolmitriptan** dose, p. 347. Moderate Theoretical

Tropicamide → see TABLE 8 p. 1055 (antimuscarinics)

- Atypical antipsychotics **(clozapine)** can cause constipation, as can **tropicamide**; concurrent use might increase the risk of developing intestinal obstruction. Severe Theoretical → Also see TABLE 8 p. 1055

Trospium → see TABLE 8 p. 1055 (antimuscarinics)

- Atypical antipsychotics **(clozapine)** can cause constipation, as can **trospium**; concurrent use might increase the risk of developing intestinal obstruction. Severe Theoretical → Also see TABLE 8 p. 1055

Tryptophan → see TABLE 11 p. 1056 (serotonin toxicity)

- **Tryptophan** greatly decreases the concentration of **levodopa**. Moderate Study
- **Tryptophan** increases the risk of adverse effects when given with **MAOIs, irreversible**. Severe Anecdotal → Also see TABLE 11 p. 1056

Tucatinib

- **Tucatinib** is predicted to increase the exposure to **abemaciclib**. Avoid or adjust dose—consult product literature. Severe Study
- **Tucatinib** is predicted to increase the exposure to **acalabrutinib**. Avoid. Severe Study
- **Tucatinib** is predicted to moderately increase the exposure to alpha blockers **(alfuzosin, tamsulosin)**. Use with caution or avoid. Moderate Study
- **Tucatinib** is predicted to increase the exposure to alpha blockers **(doxazosin)**. Moderate Study
- Anti-androgens **(apalutamide, enzalutamide)** are predicted to decrease the exposure to **tucatinib**. Avoid. Severe Study
- **Tucatinib** is predicted to increase the exposure to anti-androgens **(apalutamide)**. Monitor and adjust dose. Mild Study

Tucatinib (continued)
- **Tucatinib** very markedly increases the exposure to antiarrhythmics **(dronedarone)**. Avoid. Severe Study
- **Tucatinib** is predicted to increase the exposure to antiarrhythmics **(propafenone)**. Monitor and adjust dose. Severe Study
- **Tucatinib** is predicted to increase the exposure to anticholinesterases, centrally acting **(galantamine)**. Monitor and adjust dose. Moderate Study
- Antiepileptics **(carbamazepine, fosphenytoin, phenobarbital, phenytoin, primidone)** are predicted to decrease the exposure to **tucatinib**. Avoid. Severe Study
- **Tucatinib** is predicted to very slightly increase the exposure to antiepileptics **(perampanel)**. Mild Study
- **Tucatinib** is predicted to increase the exposure to antifungals, azoles **(isavuconazole)**. Avoid or monitor adverse effects. Severe Study
- **Tucatinib** is predicted to increase the exposure to antihistamines, non-sedating **(mizolastine)**. Avoid. Severe Study
- **Tucatinib** is predicted to increase the exposure to antihistamines, non-sedating **(rupatadine)**. Avoid. Moderate Study
- **Tucatinib** is predicted to increase the concentration of antimalarials **(piperaquine)**. Severe Study
- **Tucatinib** is predicted to increase the exposure to **atogepant**. Adjust **atogepant** dose. Moderate Study
- **Tucatinib** is predicted to slightly increase the exposure to atypical antipsychotics **(aripiprazole)**. Avoid or adjust dose—consult product literature. Moderate Study
- **Tucatinib** is predicted to moderately increase the exposure to atypical antipsychotics **(cariprazine)**. Avoid. Severe Study
- **Tucatinib** is predicted to increase the exposure to atypical antipsychotics **(lurasidone, quetiapine)**. Avoid. Severe Study
- **Tucatinib** is predicted to increase the exposure to atypical antipsychotics **(risperidone)**. Adjust dose. Moderate Study
- **Tucatinib** is predicted to increase the exposure to **avacopan**. Severe Study
- **Tucatinib** is predicted to increase the exposure to **avapritinib**. Avoid. Moderate Study
- **Tucatinib** is predicted to increase the exposure to **axitinib**. Avoid or adjust dose. Moderate Study
- **Tucatinib** might increase the exposure to **bedaquiline**. Mild Study
- **Tucatinib** moderately increases the exposure to benzodiazepines **(alprazolam)**. Avoid. Moderate Study
- **Tucatinib** is predicted to markedly to very markedly increase the exposure to benzodiazepines **(midazolam)**. Avoid or adjust dose. Severe Study
- **Tucatinib** is predicted to increase the exposure to beta$_2$ agonists **(salmeterol)**. Avoid. Severe Study
- **Tucatinib** slightly increases the exposure to **bortezomib**. Moderate Study
- **Tucatinib** is predicted to increase the exposure to **bosutinib**. Avoid or adjust dose. Severe Study
- **Tucatinib** is predicted to increase the exposure to **brigatinib**. Avoid or adjust dose—consult product literature. Severe Study
- **Tucatinib** is predicted to increase the exposure to **buspirone**. Adjust **buspirone** dose. Severe Study
- **Tucatinib** is predicted to increase the exposure to **cabozantinib**. Moderate Study
- **Tucatinib** is predicted to increase the exposure to calcium-channel blockers **(amlodipine, felodipine, lacidipine, nicardipine, nifedipine, nimodipine)**. Monitor and adjust dose. Moderate Study
- **Tucatinib** is predicted to increase the exposure to calcium-channel blockers **(diltiazem, verapamil)**. Severe Study
- **Tucatinib** is predicted to markedly increase the exposure to calcium-channel blockers **(lercanidipine)**. Avoid. Severe Study
- **Tucatinib** is predicted to increase the exposure to **cannabidiol**. Avoid or adjust dose. Mild Study
- **Tucatinib** is predicted to increase the exposure to **capivasertib**. Adjust dose. Moderate Study
- **Tucatinib** is predicted to increase the exposure to **ceritinib**. Avoid or adjust dose—consult product literature. Severe Study
- **Tucatinib** increases the concentration of **ciclosporin**. Severe Study
- **Tucatinib** is predicted to moderately increase the exposure to **cilostazol**. Adjust **cilostazol** dose. Moderate Study
- **Tucatinib** is predicted to moderately increase the exposure to **cinacalcet**. Adjust dose. Moderate Study
- **Clopidogrel** is predicted to increase the exposure to **tucatinib**. Avoid or adjust dose—consult product literature. Severe Study
- **Tucatinib** is predicted to increase the exposure to **cobimetinib**. Avoid or monitor for toxicity. Severe Study
- **Tucatinib** is predicted to increase the exposure to **colchicine**. Avoid potent CYP3A4 inhibitors or adjust **colchicine** dose, p. 637. Severe Study
- **Tucatinib** is predicted to increase the exposure to corticosteroids **(beclometasone)** (risk with beclometasone is likely to be lower than with other corticosteroids). Moderate Theoretical
- **Tucatinib** is predicted to increase the exposure to corticosteroids **(betamethasone, budesonide, ciclesonide, deflazacort, dexamethasone, fludrocortisone, fluticasone, hydrocortisone, methylprednisolone, mometasone, prednisolone, triamcinolone)**. Avoid or monitor adverse effects. Severe Study
- **Tucatinib** is predicted to increase the exposure to corticosteroids **(vamorolone)**. Adjust dose. Severe Study
- **Tucatinib** is predicted to increase the exposure to **crizotinib**. Avoid. Moderate Study
- **Tucatinib** is predicted to increase the exposure to **dabrafenib**. Use with caution or avoid. Moderate Study
- **Tucatinib** is predicted to increase the exposure to **daridorexant**. Avoid. Severe Study
- **Tucatinib** is predicted to markedly to very markedly increase the exposure to **darifenacin**. Avoid. Severe Study
- **Tucatinib** is predicted to increase the exposure to **dasatinib**. Avoid or adjust dose—consult product literature. Severe Study
- **Tucatinib** very slightly increases the exposure to **delamanid**. Severe Study
- **Tucatinib** is predicted to increase the exposure to **deutivacaftor**. Adjust dose, see deutivacaftor with tezacaftor and vanzacaftor p. 218. Severe Study
- **Tucatinib** is predicted to moderately increase the exposure to **dienogest**. Moderate Study
- **Tucatinib** slightly increases the exposure to **digoxin**. Use with caution and adjust dose. Moderate Study
- **Tucatinib** is predicted to increase the exposure to dipeptidylpeptidase-4 inhibitors **(saxagliptin)**. Moderate Study
- **Tucatinib** is predicted to increase the exposure to **domperidone**. Avoid. Severe Study
- **Tucatinib** increases the exposure to dopamine receptor agonists **(bromocriptine)**. Severe Study
- **Tucatinib** is predicted to increase the exposure to **dronabinol**. Adjust dose. Mild Study
- **Tucatinib** is predicted to increase the exposure to **dutasteride**. Monitor adverse effects and adjust dose. Moderate Theoretical
- **Tucatinib** is predicted to increase the exposure to **elacestrant**. Avoid potent CYP3A4 inhibitors or adjust **elacestrant** dose. Severe Study
- **Tucatinib** is predicted to increase the exposure to **elexacaftor**. Adjust ivacaftor with tezacaftor and elexacaftor p. 220 dose with potent CYP3A4 inhibitors. Severe Study
- **Tucatinib** is predicted to increase the exposure to **eliglustat**. Avoid or adjust dose—consult product literature. Severe Study
- **Encorafenib** is predicted to decrease the exposure to **tucatinib**. Avoid. Severe Study
- **Tucatinib** is predicted to increase the exposure to **encorafenib**. Avoid or monitor. Severe Study
- **Tucatinib** is predicted to increase the exposure to endothelin receptor antagonists **(macitentan)**. Moderate Study
- **Tucatinib** is predicted to increase the exposure to the cytotoxic component of **enfortumab vedotin**. Severe Theoretical
- **Tucatinib** is predicted to increase the exposure to **entrectinib**. Avoid or adjust dose with potent CYP3A4 inhibitors—consult product literature. Severe Study
- **Tucatinib** is predicted to increase the exposure to **erdafitinib**. Adjust dose. Severe Study
- **Tucatinib** is predicted to increase the risk of ergotism when given with **ergometrine**. Avoid. Severe Theoretical

- **Tucatinib** is predicted to increase the exposure to **erlotinib**. Use with caution and adjust dose. Severe Study
- **Tucatinib** is predicted to increase the exposure to **esketamine**. Adjust dose. Moderate Study
- **Tucatinib** is predicted to increase the exposure to **eszopiclone**. Adjust **eszopiclone** dose; avoid in the elderly. Moderate Study
- **Tucatinib** is predicted to increase the concentration of subdermal **etonogestrel**. Moderate Theoretical
- **Tucatinib** is predicted to increase the exposure to **etrasimod**. Avoid in poor CYP2C9 metabolisers. Severe Theoretical
- **Tucatinib** is predicted to increase the exposure to **everolimus**. Avoid. Severe Study
- **Tucatinib** is predicted to increase the exposure to factor XA inhibitors **(apixaban)**. Moderate Theoretical
- **Tucatinib** might increase the exposure to factor XA inhibitors **(rivaroxaban)**. Manufacturer advises caution in renal impairment. Moderate Theoretical
- **Tucatinib** is predicted to increase the exposure to **fedratinib**. Adjust dose, but avoid depending on other drugs taken—consult product literature. Moderate Study
- **Tucatinib** is predicted to moderately increase the exposure to **fesoterodine**. Adjust **fesoterodine** dose with potent CYP3A4 inhibitors; avoid in hepatic and renal impairment. Severe Study
- Fibrates **(gemfibrozil)** are predicted to increase the exposure to **tucatinib**. Avoid or adjust dose—consult product literature. Severe Study
- **Tucatinib** is predicted to increase the exposure to **fostamatinib**. Monitor adverse effects and adjust dose. Moderate Study
- **Tucatinib** is predicted to increase the exposure to **gefitinib**. Severe Study
- **Tucatinib** is predicted to increase the exposure to **gilteritinib**. Moderate Study
- **Tucatinib** is predicted to increase the exposure to **glasdegib**. Use with caution or avoid. Severe Study
- **Tucatinib** is predicted to moderately to markedly increase the exposure to **grazoprevir**. Avoid. Severe Study
- **Tucatinib** is predicted to increase the exposure to **guanfacine**. Adjust **guanfacine** dose, p. 281. Moderate Study
- **Tucatinib** is predicted to increase the exposure to **ibrutinib**. Avoid or adjust dose with potent CYP3A4 inhibitors—consult product literature. Severe Study
- **Tucatinib** is predicted to increase the exposure to **idelalisib**. Moderate Theoretical
- **Tucatinib** is predicted to increase the exposure to **imatinib**. Moderate Study
- **Tucatinib** is predicted to increase the exposure to the active metabolite of **irinotecan**. Avoid. Severe Study
- Iron chelators **(deferasirox)** are predicted to increase the exposure to **tucatinib**. Moderate Theoretical
- **Tucatinib** is predicted to increase the exposure to **ivabradine**. Avoid. Severe Study
- **Tucatinib** is predicted to increase the exposure to **ivacaftor**. Adjust dose with potent CYP3A4 inhibitors, see ivacaftor p. 219, lumacaftor with ivacaftor p. 222, tezacaftor with ivacaftor p. 223, and ivacaftor with tezacaftor and elexacaftor p. 220. Severe Study
- **Ivosidenib** is predicted to decrease the exposure to **tucatinib**. Avoid. Severe Study
- **Tucatinib** is predicted to increase the exposure to **ketamine**. Adjust dose. Moderate Theoretical
- **Tucatinib** is predicted to increase the exposure to **lapatinib**. Avoid. Moderate Study
- **Tucatinib** is predicted to moderately increase the exposure to **larotrectinib**. Avoid or adjust dose—consult product literature. Moderate Study
- **Leflunomide** is predicted to increase the exposure to **tucatinib**. Moderate Theoretical
- **Tucatinib** is predicted to increase the exposure to **leniolisib**. Avoid. Moderate Study
- **Tucatinib** is predicted to markedly increase the exposure to **lomitapide**. Avoid. Severe Study
- **Tucatinib** is predicted to increase the exposure to **lorlatinib**. Avoid or adjust dose—consult product literature. Severe Study
- **Lumacaftor** is predicted to decrease the exposure to **tucatinib**. Avoid. Severe Study
- **Tucatinib** is predicted to increase the exposure to **mavacamten**. Avoid or monitor—consult product literature. Severe Study
- **Tucatinib** is predicted to increase the concentration of intramuscular **medroxyprogesterone**. Moderate Theoretical
- **Tucatinib** is predicted to increase the exposure to **midostaurin**. Avoid or monitor for toxicity. Severe Study
- **Tucatinib** is predicted to markedly increase the exposure to mineralocorticoid receptor antagonists **(eplerenone)**. Avoid. Severe Study
- **Tucatinib** is predicted to increase the exposure to mineralocorticoid receptor antagonists **(finerenone)**. Avoid. Severe Study
- **Tucatinib** is predicted to increase the exposure to **mirabegron**. Adjust **mirabegron** dose in hepatic and renal impairment. Moderate Study
- **Tucatinib** is predicted to increase the exposure to **mirtazapine**. Moderate Study
- **Mitotane** is predicted to decrease the exposure to **tucatinib**. Avoid. Severe Study
- **Tucatinib** is predicted to increase the exposure to **modafinil**. Mild Theoretical
- **Tucatinib** is predicted to increase the risk of neutropenia when given with monoclonal antibodies **(brentuximab vedotin)**. Monitor and adjust dose. Severe Study
- **Tucatinib** is predicted to increase the exposure to monoclonal antibodies **(polatuzumab vedotin)**. Moderate Theoretical
- **Tucatinib** is predicted to increase the exposure to the cytotoxic component of monoclonal antibodies **(trastuzumab emtansine)**. Avoid or monitor. Severe Theoretical
- **Tucatinib** is predicted to increase the exposure to **naldemedine**. Avoid or monitor. Moderate Study
- **Tucatinib** is predicted to markedly increase the exposure to **naloxegol**. Avoid. Severe Study
- **Tucatinib** is predicted to increase the exposure to **neratinib**. Avoid or adjust dose with potent CYP3A4 inhibitors—consult product literature. Severe Study
- **Tucatinib** is predicted to markedly increase the exposure to neurokinin-1 receptor antagonists **(aprepitant)**. Moderate Study
- **Tucatinib** is predicted to increase the exposure to neurokinin-1 receptor antagonists **(fosaprepitant)**. Moderate Theoretical
- **Tucatinib** is predicted to increase the exposure to neurokinin-1 receptor antagonists **(netupitant)**. Moderate Study
- **Tucatinib** is predicted to increase the exposure to **nilotinib**. Avoid. Severe Study
- **Tucatinib** is predicted to increase the exposure to **nitisinone**. Adjust dose. Moderate Theoretical
- **Tucatinib** is predicted to increase the exposure to **olaparib**. Avoid or adjust dose with potent CYP3A4 inhibitors—consult product literature. Moderate Study
- **Tucatinib** is predicted to increase the exposure to **omaveloxolone**. Avoid or adjust **omaveloxolone** dose, p. 755. Severe Study
- **Tucatinib** is predicted to increase the exposure to opioids **(alfentanil, buprenorphine, fentanyl, oxycodone)**. Monitor and adjust dose. Severe Study
- **Tucatinib** is predicted to increase the exposure to opioids **(sufentanil)**. Moderate Study
- **Tucatinib** is predicted to increase the exposure to **osilodrostat**. Moderate Theoretical
- **Tucatinib** is predicted to increase the exposure to **ospemifene**. Avoid in poor CYP2C9 metabolisers. Moderate Study
- **Tucatinib** is predicted to increase the exposure to **oxybutynin**. Mild Study
- **Tucatinib** is predicted to increase the exposure to **palbociclib**. Avoid or adjust dose—consult product literature. Severe Study
- **Tucatinib** is predicted to increase the exposure to **panobinostat**. Adjust dose—consult product literature; in hepatic impairment avoid. Moderate Study
- **Tucatinib** is predicted to increase the exposure to **pazopanib**. Avoid or adjust dose—consult product literature. Moderate Study
- **Tucatinib** is predicted to increase the exposure to **pemigatinib**. Avoid or adjust dose—consult product literature. Severe Study

Tucatinib (continued)
- **Tucatinib** is predicted to increase the exposure to phosphodiesterase type-5 inhibitors **(avanafil, vardenafil)**. Avoid. [Severe] Study
- **Tucatinib** is predicted to increase the exposure to phosphodiesterase type-5 inhibitors **(sildenafil)**. Avoid potent CYP3A4 inhibitors or adjust **sildenafil** dose, p. 139. [Severe] Study
- **Tucatinib** is predicted to increase the exposure to phosphodiesterase type-5 inhibitors **(tadalafil)**. Use with caution or avoid. [Severe] Study
- **Tucatinib** is predicted to increase the exposure to **pimozide**. Avoid. [Severe] Study
- **Tucatinib** is predicted to slightly increase the exposure to **ponatinib**. Monitor and adjust dose—consult product literature. [Moderate] Study
- **Tucatinib** is predicted to increase the exposure to **pralsetinib**. Avoid or adjust dose with potent CYP3A4 inhibitors—consult product literature. [Moderate] Study
- **Tucatinib** is predicted to moderately increase the exposure to **praziquantel**. [Mild] Study
- **Tucatinib** given with carbimazole is predicted to increase the exposure to **propiverine**. Adjust starting dose. [Moderate] Theoretical
- **Tucatinib** is predicted to increase the exposure to **quizartinib**. Adjust dose—consult product literature. [Severe] Study
- **Tucatinib** is predicted to increase the exposure to **ranolazine**. Avoid. [Severe] Study
- **Tucatinib** is predicted to increase the exposure to **reboxetine**. Avoid. [Moderate] Study
- **Tucatinib** is predicted to increase the exposure to **regorafenib**. Avoid. [Moderate] Study
- **Tucatinib** is predicted to increase the exposure to retinoids **(alitretinoin)**. Adjust **alitretinoin** dose. [Moderate] Theoretical
- **Tucatinib** is predicted to increase the exposure to **ribociclib**. Avoid or adjust dose—consult product literature. [Moderate] Study
- Rifamycins **(rifampicin)** are predicted to decrease the exposure to **tucatinib**. Avoid. [Severe] Study
- **Tucatinib** is predicted to increase the exposure to **rimegepant**. Avoid. [Moderate] Study
- **Tucatinib** is predicted to increase the exposure to **ripretinib**. [Moderate] Theoretical
- **Tucatinib** is predicted to increase the exposure to **ruxolitinib**. Adjust dose depending on indication and monitor adverse effects—consult product literature. [Moderate] Study
- **Tucatinib** is predicted to increase the exposure to **selpercatinib**. Adjust dose—consult product literature. [Moderate] Study
- **Tucatinib** is predicted to increase the exposure to **selumetinib**. Avoid or adjust dose—consult product literature. [Severe] Study
- **Tucatinib** is predicted to increase the exposure to **siponimod**. Avoid depending on other drugs taken—consult product literature. [Severe] Theoretical
- **Tucatinib** is predicted to increase the concentration of **sirolimus**. Avoid or monitor and adjust dose. [Severe] Study
- **Tucatinib** is predicted to increase the exposure to SNRIs **(venlafaxine)**. [Moderate] Study
- **Tucatinib** is predicted to increase the exposure to **solifenacin**. Adjust solifenacin p. 604 or tamsulosin with solifenacin dose; avoid in hepatic and renal impairment. [Severe] Study
- **Tucatinib** is predicted to increase the exposure to **sparsentan**. Avoid. [Severe] Study
- **Tucatinib** is predicted to moderately increase the exposure to SSRIs **(dapoxetine)**. Avoid potent CYP3A4 inhibitors or adjust **dapoxetine** dose. [Severe] Study
- **Tucatinib** is predicted to increase the exposure to SSRIs **(sertraline)**. Avoid. [Moderate] Theoretical
- **St John's wort** is predicted to decrease the exposure to **tucatinib**. Avoid. [Severe] Theoretical
- **Tucatinib** is predicted to increase the exposure to statins **(atorvastatin)**. Avoid or adjust dose and monitor rhabdomyolysis. [Severe] Study
- **Tucatinib** is predicted to increase the exposure to statins **(simvastatin)**. Avoid. [Severe] Study
- **Tucatinib** is predicted to increase the exposure to **sunitinib**. Avoid or adjust dose—consult product literature. [Moderate] Study
- **Tucatinib** is predicted to increase the concentration of **tacrolimus**. Avoid. If concurrent use is unavoidable—consult product literature. [Severe] Study
- **Tucatinib** is predicted to increase the exposure to **talazoparib**. Use with caution and adjust dose. [Moderate] Theoretical
- **Tucatinib** is predicted to increase the exposure to taxanes **(cabazitaxel)**. Avoid or adjust dose—consult product literature. [Severe] Study
- **Tucatinib** is predicted to increase the exposure to taxanes **(docetaxel)**. Avoid or adjust dose. [Severe] Study
- **Tucatinib** is predicted to increase the exposure to taxanes **(paclitaxel)**. [Moderate] Anecdotal
- **Tucatinib** is predicted to increase the concentration of **temsirolimus**. Avoid. [Severe] Theoretical
- **Teriflunomide** is predicted to increase the exposure to **tucatinib**. [Moderate] Theoretical
- **Tucatinib** is predicted to increase the exposure to **tezacaftor**. Adjust dose with potent CYP3A4 inhibitors, see tezacaftor with ivacaftor p. 223, ivacaftor with tezacaftor and elexacaftor p. 220, and deutivacaftor with tezacaftor and vanzacaftor p. 218. [Severe] Study
- **Tucatinib** is predicted to markedly increase the exposure to **ticagrelor**. Avoid. [Severe] Study
- **Tucatinib** is predicted to increase the exposure to the cytotoxic component of **tisotumab vedotin**. [Severe] Theoretical
- **Tucatinib** is predicted to increase the exposure to **tofacitinib**. Adjust **tofacitinib** dose, p. 803. [Moderate] Study
- **Tucatinib** is predicted to increase the exposure to **tolterodine**. Avoid. [Severe] Study
- **Tucatinib** is predicted to increase the exposure to **tolvaptan**. Manufacturer advises caution or adjust **tolvaptan** dose with potent CYP3A4 inhibitors. [Severe] Study
- **Tucatinib** is predicted to increase the exposure to **toremifene**. [Moderate] Theoretical
- **Tucatinib** is predicted to increase the exposure to **trabectedin**. Avoid or adjust dose. [Severe] Theoretical
- **Tucatinib** is predicted to moderately increase the exposure to **trazodone**. Avoid or adjust dose. [Moderate] Study
- **Tucatinib** increases the exposure to triptans **(almotriptan)**. [Mild] Study
- **Tucatinib** is predicted to markedly increase the exposure to triptans **(eletriptan)**. Avoid. [Severe] Study
- **Tucatinib** is predicted to increase the exposure to **upadacitinib**. Manufacturer advises caution or avoid, or adjust **upadacitinib** dose depending on indication, p. 927. [Severe] Study
- **Tucatinib** is predicted to increase the exposure to **vanzacaftor**. Adjust dose, see deutivacaftor with tezacaftor and vanzacaftor p. 218. [Severe] Study
- **Tucatinib** is predicted to increase the exposure to **vemurafenib**. [Severe] Theoretical
- **Tucatinib** is predicted to increase the exposure to **venetoclax**. Avoid or adjust dose—consult product literature. [Severe] Study
- **Tucatinib** is predicted to increase the exposure to **vinca alkaloids**. [Severe] Theoretical
- **Tucatinib** is predicted to increase the exposure to vitamin D substances **(paricalcitol)**. [Moderate] Study
- **Tucatinib** is predicted to increase the exposure to **voclosporin**. Avoid. [Severe] Study
- **Tucatinib** is predicted to increase the exposure to **zanubrutinib**. Avoid or adjust dose with potent CYP3A4 inhibitors—consult product literature. [Moderate] Study
- **Tucatinib** is predicted to increase the exposure to **zopiclone**. Adjust dose. [Moderate] Theoretical

Typhoid vaccine (live) → see live vaccines

Ublituximab → see monoclonal antibodies

Ulipristal
- **Antacids** might decrease the efficacy of **ulipristal** for emergency hormonal contraception. For CoSRH guidance, see Contraceptives, interactions p. 614. [Unknown] Theoretical
- Anti-androgens **(apalutamide)** are predicted to decrease the efficacy of **ulipristal**. Avoid and for 4 weeks after stopping **apalutamide**. [Severe] Theoretical

A1 Interactions | **Appendix 1**

- Anti-androgens **(enzalutamide)** are predicted to decrease the efficacy of **ulipristal**. Avoid and for 4 weeks after stopping **enzalutamide**. [Severe] Theoretical
- Antiarrhythmics **(dronedarone)** are predicted to increase the exposure to **ulipristal**. Avoid when used for uterine fibroids. [Moderate] Study
- Antiepileptics **(carbamazepine, eslicarbazepine, fosphenytoin, oxcarbazepine, perampanel, phenobarbital, phenytoin, primidone, rufinamide, topiramate)** decrease the efficacy of **ulipristal**. Avoid and for 4 weeks after stopping the enzyme inducing drug. For CoSRH guidance, see Contraceptives, interactions p. 614. [Severe] Anecdotal
- Antifungals, azoles **(fluconazole, isavuconazole, posaconazole)** are predicted to increase the exposure to **ulipristal**. Avoid when used for uterine fibroids. [Moderate] Study
- Antifungals, azoles **(itraconazole, ketoconazole, voriconazole)** are predicted to increase the exposure to **ulipristal**. Avoid when used for uterine fibroids. [Severe] Study
- Calcium compounds **(calcium carbonate)** -containing antacids might decrease the efficacy of **ulipristal** for emergency hormonal contraception. For CoSRH guidance, see Contraceptives, interactions p. 614. [Unknown] Theoretical
- Calcium-channel blockers **(diltiazem, verapamil)** are predicted to increase the exposure to **ulipristal**. Avoid when used for uterine fibroids. [Moderate] Study
- **Cobicistat** is predicted to increase the exposure to **ulipristal**. Avoid when used for uterine fibroids. [Severe] Study
- **Combined hormonal contraceptives** might decrease the efficacy of **ulipristal** and **ulipristal** might decrease the efficacy of **combined hormonal contraceptives**. Avoid when used for uterine fibroids. For CoSRH guidance when used for emergency hormonal contraception, see Contraceptives, interactions p. 614. [Severe] Theoretical
- **Crizotinib** is predicted to increase the exposure to **ulipristal**. Avoid when used for uterine fibroids. [Moderate] Study
- **Dabrafenib** is predicted to decrease the efficacy of **ulipristal**. Avoid and for 4 weeks after stopping **dabrafenib**. [Severe] Theoretical
- **Desogestrel** might decrease the efficacy of **ulipristal** and **ulipristal** might decrease the efficacy of **desogestrel**. Avoid when used for uterine fibroids. For CoSRH guidance when used for emergency hormonal contraception, see Contraceptives, interactions p. 614. [Severe] Theoretical
- **Drospirenone** might decrease the efficacy of **ulipristal** and **ulipristal** might decrease the efficacy of **drospirenone**. Avoid when used for uterine fibroids. For CoSRH guidance when used for emergency hormonal contraception, see Contraceptives, interactions p. 614. [Severe] Theoretical
- Endothelin receptor antagonists **(bosentan)** decrease the efficacy of **ulipristal**. Avoid and for 4 weeks after stopping the enzyme inducing drug. For CoSRH guidance, see Contraceptives, interactions p. 614. [Severe] Anecdotal
- **Etonogestrel** might decrease the efficacy of **ulipristal** and **ulipristal** might decrease the efficacy of **etonogestrel**. Avoid when used for uterine fibroids. For CoSRH guidance when used for emergency hormonal contraception, see Contraceptives, interactions p. 614. [Severe] Theoretical
- **Grapefruit juice** is predicted to increase the exposure to **ulipristal**. Avoid when used for uterine fibroids. [Moderate] Theoretical
- **H_2 receptor antagonists** might decrease the efficacy of **ulipristal** for emergency hormonal contraception. For CoSRH guidance, see Contraceptives, interactions p. 614. [Unknown] Theoretical
- HIV-protease inhibitors **(atazanavir, darunavir, fosamprenavir, lopinavir)** boosted with ritonavir are predicted to increase the exposure to **ulipristal**. Avoid when used for uterine fibroids. [Severe] Study
- HIV-protease inhibitors **(ritonavir)** decrease the efficacy of **ulipristal**. Avoid and for 4 weeks after stopping the enzyme inducing drug. For CoSRH guidance, see Contraceptives, interactions p. 614. [Severe] Anecdotal
- **Idelalisib** is predicted to increase the exposure to **ulipristal**. Avoid when used for uterine fibroids. [Severe] Study
- **Imatinib** is predicted to increase the exposure to **ulipristal**. Avoid when used for uterine fibroids. [Moderate] Study
- **Letermovir** is predicted to increase the exposure to **ulipristal**. Avoid when used for uterine fibroids. [Moderate] Study
- **Levonorgestrel** might decrease the efficacy of **ulipristal** and **ulipristal** might decrease the efficacy of **levonorgestrel**. Avoid. For CoSRH guidance, see Contraceptives, interactions p. 614. [Severe] Theoretical
- **Lumacaftor** is predicted to decrease the efficacy of **ulipristal**. Use additional contraceptive precautions. [Severe] Theoretical
- Macrolides **(clarithromycin)** are predicted to increase the exposure to **ulipristal**. Avoid when used for uterine fibroids. [Severe] Study
- Macrolides **(erythromycin)** moderately increase the exposure to **ulipristal**. Avoid when used for uterine fibroids. [Moderate] Study
- **Medroxyprogesterone** might decrease the efficacy of **ulipristal** and **ulipristal** might decrease the efficacy of **medroxyprogesterone**. Avoid when used for uterine fibroids. For CoSRH guidance when used for emergency hormonal contraception, see Contraceptives, interactions p. 614. [Severe] Theoretical
- **Mitotane** is predicted to decrease the efficacy of **ulipristal**. Avoid and for 4 weeks after stopping **mitotane**. [Severe] Theoretical
- **Modafinil** decreases the efficacy of **ulipristal**. Avoid and for 4 weeks after stopping the enzyme inducing drug. For CoSRH guidance, see Contraceptives, interactions p. 614. [Severe] Anecdotal
- Neurokinin-1 receptor antagonists **(aprepitant, fosaprepitant)** decrease the efficacy of **ulipristal**. Avoid and for 4 weeks after stopping the enzyme inducing drug. For CoSRH guidance, see Contraceptives, interactions p. 614. [Severe] Anecdotal
- Neurokinin-1 receptor antagonists **(netupitant)** are predicted to increase the exposure to **ulipristal**. Avoid when used for uterine fibroids. [Moderate] Study
- **Nilotinib** is predicted to increase the exposure to **ulipristal**. Avoid when used for uterine fibroids. [Moderate] Study
- NNRTIs **(efavirenz, nevirapine)** decrease the efficacy of **ulipristal**. Avoid and for 4 weeks after stopping the enzyme inducing drug. For CoSRH guidance, see Contraceptives, interactions p. 614. [Severe] Anecdotal
- NNRTIs **(etravirine)** might decrease the efficacy of **ulipristal**. Avoid and for 4 weeks after stopping the enzyme inducing drug. For CoSRH guidance, see Contraceptives, interactions p. 614. [Severe] Theoretical
- **Norethisterone** might decrease the efficacy of **ulipristal** and **ulipristal** might decrease the efficacy of **norethisterone**. Avoid when used for uterine fibroids. For CoSRH guidance when used for emergency hormonal contraception, see Contraceptives, interactions p. 614. [Severe] Theoretical
- **Proton pump inhibitors** might decrease the efficacy of **ulipristal** for emergency hormonal contraception. For CoSRH guidance, see Contraceptives, interactions p. 614. [Unknown] Theoretical
- **Rifamycins** decrease the efficacy of **ulipristal**. Avoid and for 4 weeks after stopping the enzyme inducing drug. For CoSRH guidance, see Contraceptives, interactions p. 614. [Severe] Anecdotal
- **St John's wort** is predicted to decrease the efficacy of **ulipristal**. For CoSRH guidance, see Contraceptives, interactions p. 614. [Severe] Anecdotal

Umeclidinium → see TABLE 8 p. 1055 (antimuscarinics)

- Atypical antipsychotics **(clozapine)** can cause constipation, as can **umeclidinium**; concurrent use might increase the risk of developing intestinal obstruction. [Severe] Theoretical → Also see TABLE 8 p. 1055

Upadacitinib

- Anti-androgens **(apalutamide, enzalutamide)** are predicted to decrease the exposure to **upadacitinib**. [Moderate] Study
- Antiepileptics **(carbamazepine, fosphenytoin, phenobarbital, phenytoin, primidone)** are predicted to decrease the exposure to **upadacitinib**. [Moderate] Study
- Antifungals, azoles **(itraconazole, ketoconazole, posaconazole, voriconazole)** are predicted to increase the exposure to **upadacitinib**. Manufacturer advises caution or avoid, or adjust **upadacitinib** dose depending on indication, p. 927. [Severe] Study

Upadacitinib (continued)
- **Ceritinib** is predicted to increase the exposure to **upadacitinib**. Manufacturer advises caution or avoid, or adjust **upadacitinib** dose depending on indication, p. 927. Severe Study
- **Cobicistat** is predicted to increase the exposure to **upadacitinib**. Manufacturer advises caution or avoid, or adjust **upadacitinib** dose depending on indication, p. 927. Severe Study
- **Encorafenib** is predicted to decrease the exposure to **upadacitinib**. Moderate Study
- **Filgotinib** is predicted to increase the risk of immunosuppression when given with **upadacitinib**. Avoid. Severe Theoretical
- **Grapefruit** is predicted to increase the exposure to **upadacitinib**. Avoid. Moderate Theoretical
- **HIV-protease inhibitors** are predicted to increase the exposure to **upadacitinib**. Manufacturer advises caution or avoid, or adjust **upadacitinib** dose depending on indication, p. 927. Severe Study
- **Idelalisib** is predicted to increase the exposure to **upadacitinib**. Manufacturer advises caution or avoid, or adjust **upadacitinib** dose depending on indication, p. 927. Severe Study
- **Ivosidenib** is predicted to decrease the exposure to **upadacitinib**. Moderate Study
- **Live vaccines** are predicted to increase the risk of generalised infection (possibly life-threatening) when given with **upadacitinib**. Avoid. Severe Theoretical
- **Lumacaftor** is predicted to decrease the exposure to **upadacitinib**. Moderate Study
- Macrolides **(clarithromycin)** are predicted to increase the exposure to **upadacitinib**. Manufacturer advises caution or avoid, or adjust **upadacitinib** dose depending on indication, p. 927. Severe Study
- **Mitotane** is predicted to decrease the exposure to **upadacitinib**. Moderate Study
- **Nirmatrelvir** boosted with ritonavir is predicted to increase the concentration of **upadacitinib**. Adjust dose. Severe Theoretical
- Rifamycins **(rifampicin)** are predicted to decrease the exposure to **upadacitinib**. Moderate Study
- **Tucatinib** is predicted to increase the exposure to **upadacitinib**. Manufacturer advises caution or avoid, or adjust **upadacitinib** dose depending on indication, p. 927. Severe Study

Urokinase → see TABLE 3 p. 1053 (bleeding)
- **Donanemab** might increase the risk of brain haemorrhage when given with **urokinase**. Avoid except in life-threatening situations. Severe Theoretical
- **Lecanemab** might increase the risk of brain haemorrhage when given with **urokinase**. Avoid except in life-threatening situations. Severe Theoretical

Ursodeoxycholic acid
- Oral **antacids** are predicted to decrease the absorption of oral **ursodeoxycholic acid**. Separate administration by 2 hours. Moderate Theoretical
- **Ursodeoxycholic acid** affects the concentration of **ciclosporin**. Use with caution and adjust dose. Severe Anecdotal
- **Fibrates** are predicted to decrease the efficacy of **ursodeoxycholic acid**. Avoid. Severe Theoretical

Ustekinumab → see monoclonal antibodies

Vaborbactam
- **Vaborbactam** is predicted to increase the concentration of beta blockers, selective **(metoprolol)**. Unknown Theoretical
- **Vaborbactam** is predicted to increase the concentration of SNRIs **(venlafaxine)**. Unknown Theoretical

Vadadustat
- **Vadadustat** is predicted to increase the exposure to **alpelisib**. Moderate Theoretical
- Oral **aluminium hydroxide** is predicted to decrease the exposure to oral **vadadustat**. Manufacturer advises take at least 1 hour before or 2 hours after aluminium-containing products. Moderate Theoretical
- **Vadadustat** is predicted to increase the exposure to angiotensin-II receptor antagonists **(olmesartan)**. Monitor and adjust dose. Moderate Study
- Oral **antacids** is predicted to decrease the exposure to oral **vadadustat**. Manufacturer advises take at least 1 hour before or 2 hours after antacids. Moderate Theoretical
- **Vadadustat** is predicted to increase the exposure to **baricitinib**. Moderate Study
- Oral **calcium compounds** decrease the exposure to oral **vadadustat**. **Vadadustat** should be taken at least 1 hour before or 2 hours after calcium. Moderate Study
- **Vadadustat** is predicted to increase the exposure to cephalosporins **(cefaclor)**. Monitor and adjust dose. Moderate Study
- **Vadadustat** is predicted to increase the exposure to **cladribine**. Avoid or adjust dose. Moderate Theoretical
- Fibrates **(gemfibrozil)** are predicted to increase the exposure to **vadadustat**. Moderate Theoretical
- **Vadadustat** is predicted to increase the exposure to **ganciclovir**. Monitor and adjust dose. Moderate Study
- **Vadadustat** is predicted to increase the exposure to H_2 receptor antagonists **(famotidine)**. Monitor and adjust dose. Moderate Study
- Oral **iron** decreases the exposure to oral **vadadustat**. **Vadadustat** should be taken 1 hour before iron. Moderate Study
- Oral **lanthanum** is predicted to decrease the exposure to oral **vadadustat**. Manufacturer advises take at least 1 hour before or 2 hours after **lanthanum**. Moderate Theoretical
- **Leflunomide** is predicted to increase the exposure to **vadadustat**. Moderate Study
- **Vadadustat** increases the exposure to loop diuretics **(furosemide)**. Monitor and adjust dose. Moderate Study
- Oral **magnesium** is predicted to decrease the exposure to oral **vadadustat**. Manufacturer advises take at least 1 hour before or 2 hours after magnesium. Moderate Theoretical
- **Vadadustat** is predicted to increase the exposure to **methotrexate**. Monitor and adjust dose. Moderate Study
- **Vadadustat** is predicted to increase the exposure to NRTIs **(zidovudine)**. Monitor and adjust dose. Moderate Study
- **Vadadustat** is predicted to increase the exposure to the active metabolite of **oseltamivir**. Monitor and adjust dose. Moderate Study
- Penicillins **(benzylpenicillin)** are predicted to increase the exposure to **vadadustat** and **vadadustat** is predicted to increase the exposure to penicillins **(benzylpenicillin)**. Moderate Study
- **Vadadustat** is predicted to increase the exposure to quinolones **(ciprofloxacin)**. Monitor and adjust dose. Moderate Study
- Rifamycins **(rifampicin)** are predicted to increase the exposure to **vadadustat**. Moderate Theoretical
- **Vadadustat** is predicted to increase the exposure to **roxadustat**. Monitor haemoglobin and adjust dose—consult product literature. Moderate Study
- Oral **sevelamer** decreases the exposure to oral **vadadustat**. Manufacturer advises take at least 1 hour before or 2 hours after **sevelamer**. Moderate Study
- **Vadadustat** is predicted to increase the exposure to statins **(atorvastatin, fluvastatin, rosuvastatin)**. Monitor and adjust dose. Moderate Study
- **Vadadustat** increases the exposure to statins **(simvastatin)**. Monitor and adjust dose. Moderate Study
- **Vadadustat** is predicted to increase the exposure to **sulfasalazine**. Monitor and adjust dose. Moderate Study
- **Vadadustat** is predicted to increase the exposure to **tenofovir alafenamide**. Moderate Theoretical
- **Vadadustat** is predicted to increase the exposure to **tenofovir disoproxil**. Moderate Theoretical
- **Teriflunomide** is predicted to increase the exposure to **vadadustat**. Moderate Study
- **Vadadustat** is predicted to increase the exposure to **topotecan**. Monitor and adjust dose. Moderate Study

Valaciclovir → see TABLE 2 p. 1053 (nephrotoxicity)
- **Valaciclovir** is predicted to increase the exposure to **aminophylline**. Severe Anecdotal
- **Mycophenolate** is predicted to increase the risk of haematological toxicity when given with **valaciclovir**. Moderate Theoretical
- **Valaciclovir** is predicted to increase the exposure to **theophylline**. Severe Theoretical

Valganciclovir → see TABLE 12 p. 1057 (myelosuppression), TABLE 2 p. 1053 (nephrotoxicity)

- **Valganciclovir** is predicted to increase the risk of seizures when given with carbapenems **(imipenem)**. Avoid. [Severe] Anecdotal
- **Maribavir** might decrease the efficacy of **valganciclovir**. Avoid. [Severe] Theoretical
- **Mycophenolate** is predicted to increase the risk of haematological toxicity when given with **valganciclovir**. [Moderate] Theoretical

Valproate → see antiepileptics
Valsartan → see angiotensin-II receptor antagonists
Vamorolone → see corticosteroids
Vancomycin → see TABLE 2 p. 1053 (nephrotoxicity), TABLE 16 p. 1058 (ototoxicity)
Vandetanib → see TABLE 7 p. 1055 (QT-interval prolongation)

- Anti-androgens **(apalutamide, enzalutamide)** are predicted to decrease the exposure to **vandetanib**. Avoid. [Moderate] Study → Also see TABLE 7 p. 1055
- Antiepileptics **(carbamazepine, fosphenytoin, phenobarbital, phenytoin, primidone)** are predicted to decrease the exposure to **vandetanib**. Avoid. [Moderate] Study
- **Vandetanib** might increase the exposure to the active metabolite of antimalarials **(artesunate)**. Avoid. [Unknown] Theoretical
- **Dabrafenib** is predicted to decrease the exposure to **vandetanib**. [Moderate] Study
- **Vandetanib** very slightly increases the exposure to **digoxin**. [Moderate] Study
- **Vandetanib** is predicted to increase the exposure to dopamine receptor agonists **(pramipexole)**. Adjust dose. [Moderate] Study
- **Encorafenib** is predicted to decrease the exposure to **vandetanib**. Avoid. [Moderate] Study → Also see TABLE 7 p. 1055
- Endothelin receptor antagonists **(bosentan)** are predicted to decrease the exposure to **vandetanib**. [Moderate] Study
- **Vandetanib** is predicted to increase the exposure to factor XA inhibitors **(apixaban)**. [Moderate] Theoretical
- **Vandetanib** is predicted to increase the exposure to **gilteritinib**. [Moderate] Theoretical
- **Vandetanib** is predicted to increase the exposure to **idelalisib**. [Moderate] Theoretical
- **Ivosidenib** is predicted to decrease the exposure to **vandetanib**. Avoid. [Moderate] Study → Also see TABLE 7 p. 1055
- **Lumacaftor** is predicted to decrease the exposure to **vandetanib**. Avoid. [Moderate] Study
- **Vandetanib** is predicted to increase the exposure to **metformin**. Use with caution and adjust dose. [Moderate] Study
- **Mitotane** is predicted to decrease the exposure to **vandetanib**. Avoid. [Moderate] Study
- NNRTIs **(efavirenz, etravirine, nevirapine)** are predicted to decrease the exposure to **vandetanib**. [Moderate] Study → Also see TABLE 7 p. 1055
- Rifamycins **(rifampicin)** are predicted to decrease the exposure to **vandetanib**. Avoid. [Moderate] Study
- **Vandetanib** is predicted to increase the exposure to the active component of **sacituzumab govitecan**. [Severe] Theoretical
- **St John's wort** is predicted to decrease the exposure to **vandetanib**. Avoid. [Severe] Study
- **Vandetanib** might increase the exposure to **tigecycline**. [Mild] Anecdotal
- **Vandetanib** might increase the exposure to **vinca alkaloids**. [Severe] Theoretical

Vanzacaftor

- Anti-androgens **(apalutamide, enzalutamide)** are predicted to decrease the exposure to **vanzacaftor**. Avoid. [Severe] Theoretical
- Antiarrhythmics **(dronedarone)** are predicted to increase the exposure to **vanzacaftor**. Adjust dose, see deutivacaftor with tezacaftor and vanzacaftor p. 218. [Severe] Study
- Antiepileptics **(carbamazepine, fosphenytoin, phenobarbital, phenytoin, primidone)** are predicted to decrease the exposure to **vanzacaftor**. Avoid. [Severe] Theoretical
- Antifungals, azoles **(fluconazole, isavuconazole, itraconazole, ketoconazole, posaconazole, voriconazole)** are predicted to increase the exposure to **vanzacaftor**. Adjust dose, see deutivacaftor with tezacaftor and vanzacaftor p. 218. [Severe] Study
- **Berotralstat** is predicted to increase the exposure to **vanzacaftor**. Adjust dose, see deutivacaftor with tezacaftor and vanzacaftor p. 218. [Severe] Study
- Calcium-channel blockers **(diltiazem, verapamil)** are predicted to increase the exposure to **vanzacaftor**. Adjust dose, see deutivacaftor with tezacaftor and vanzacaftor p. 218. [Severe] Study
- **Cenobamate** is predicted to decrease the exposure to **vanzacaftor**. Avoid. [Severe] Theoretical
- **Ceritinib** is predicted to increase the exposure to **vanzacaftor**. Adjust dose, see deutivacaftor with tezacaftor and vanzacaftor p. 218. [Severe] Study
- **Cobicistat** is predicted to increase the exposure to **vanzacaftor**. Adjust dose, see deutivacaftor with tezacaftor and vanzacaftor p. 218. [Severe] Study
- **Crizotinib** is predicted to increase the exposure to **vanzacaftor**. Adjust dose, see deutivacaftor with tezacaftor and vanzacaftor p. 218. [Severe] Study
- **Dabrafenib** is predicted to decrease the exposure to **vanzacaftor**. Avoid. [Severe] Theoretical
- **Encorafenib** is predicted to decrease the exposure to **vanzacaftor**. Avoid. [Severe] Theoretical
- Endothelin receptor antagonists **(bosentan)** are predicted to decrease the exposure to **vanzacaftor**. Avoid. [Severe] Theoretical
- **Fedratinib** is predicted to increase the exposure to **vanzacaftor**. Adjust dose, see deutivacaftor with tezacaftor and vanzacaftor p. 218. [Severe] Study
- **Grapefruit** is predicted to increase the exposure to **vanzacaftor**. Avoid. [Moderate] Theoretical
- **HIV-protease inhibitors** are predicted to increase the exposure to **vanzacaftor**. Adjust dose, see deutivacaftor with tezacaftor and vanzacaftor p. 218. [Severe] Study
- **Idelalisib** is predicted to increase the exposure to **vanzacaftor**. Adjust dose, see deutivacaftor with tezacaftor and vanzacaftor p. 218. [Severe] Study
- **Imatinib** is predicted to increase the exposure to **vanzacaftor**. Adjust dose, see deutivacaftor with tezacaftor and vanzacaftor p. 218. [Severe] Study
- **Ivosidenib** is predicted to decrease the exposure to **vanzacaftor**. Avoid. [Severe] Theoretical
- **Letermovir** is predicted to increase the exposure to **vanzacaftor**. Adjust dose, see deutivacaftor with tezacaftor and vanzacaftor p. 218. [Severe] Study
- **Lorlatinib** is predicted to decrease the exposure to **vanzacaftor**. Avoid. [Severe] Theoretical
- **Lumacaftor** is predicted to decrease the exposure to **vanzacaftor**. Avoid. [Severe] Theoretical
- Macrolides **(clarithromycin, erythromycin)** are predicted to increase the exposure to **vanzacaftor**. Adjust dose, see deutivacaftor with tezacaftor and vanzacaftor p. 218. [Severe] Study
- **Mitotane** is predicted to decrease the exposure to **vanzacaftor**. Avoid. [Severe] Theoretical
- Neurokinin-1 receptor antagonists **(aprepitant, netupitant)** are predicted to increase the exposure to **vanzacaftor**. Adjust dose, see deutivacaftor with tezacaftor and vanzacaftor p. 218. [Severe] Study
- **Nilotinib** is predicted to increase the exposure to **vanzacaftor**. Adjust dose, see deutivacaftor with tezacaftor and vanzacaftor p. 218. [Severe] Study
- NNRTIs **(efavirenz, etravirine, nevirapine)** are predicted to decrease the exposure to **vanzacaftor**. Avoid. [Severe] Theoretical
- Rifamycins **(rifampicin)** are predicted to decrease the exposure to **vanzacaftor**. Avoid. [Severe] Theoretical
- **Sotorasib** is predicted to decrease the exposure to **vanzacaftor**. Avoid. [Severe] Theoretical
- **St John's wort** is predicted to decrease the exposure to **vanzacaftor**. Avoid. [Severe] Theoretical
- **Tucatinib** is predicted to increase the exposure to **vanzacaftor**. Adjust dose, see deutivacaftor with tezacaftor and vanzacaftor p. 218. [Severe] Study

Vardenafil → see phosphodiesterase type-5 inhibitors
Varicella-zoster immunoglobulin → see immunoglobulins
Varicella-zoster vaccine → see live vaccines

Vasopressin
- ACE inhibitors **(enalapril)** might enhance the antidiuretic and hypertensive effects of **vasopressin.** Moderate Theoretical
- **Alcohol** might decrease the antidiuretic effect of **vasopressin.** Moderate Theoretical
- Alkylating agents **(cyclophosphamide, ifosfamide)** might enhance the antidiuretic and hypertensive effects of **vasopressin.** Moderate Theoretical
- Antiepileptics **(carbamazepine)** might enhance the antidiuretic effect of **vasopressin.** Moderate Theoretical
- Atypical antipsychotics **(clozapine)** might decrease the antidiuretic and hypertensive effects of **vasopressin.** Moderate Theoretical
- Corticosteroids **(fludrocortisone)** might enhance the antidiuretic effect of **vasopressin.** Moderate Theoretical
- **Foscarnet** might decrease the antidiuretic and hypertensive effects of **vasopressin.** Moderate Theoretical
- **Haloperidol** might enhance the antidiuretic and hypertensive effects of **vasopressin.** Moderate Theoretical
- **Heparin** might decrease the antidiuretic effect of **vasopressin.** Moderate Theoretical
- **Lithium** might decrease the antidiuretic and hypertensive effects of **vasopressin.** Moderate Theoretical
- **Methyldopa** might enhance the antidiuretic and hypertensive effects of **vasopressin.** Moderate Theoretical
- NSAIDs **(indometacin)** might prolong the antidiuretic effect of **vasopressin.** Moderate Study
- **Pentamidine** might enhance the antidiuretic and hypertensive effects of **vasopressin.** Moderate Theoretical
- **SSRIs** might enhance the antidiuretic and hypertensive effects of **vasopressin.** Moderate Theoretical
- Sympathomimetics, vasoconstrictor **(adrenaline)** might increase the hypertensive effect of **vasopressin.** Moderate Theoretical
- Sympathomimetics, vasoconstrictor **(noradrenaline)** might affect the hypertensive effect of **vasopressin.** Moderate Theoretical
- Tetracyclines **(demeclocycline)** might decrease the antidiuretic and hypertensive effects of **vasopressin.** Moderate Theoretical
- **Tricyclic antidepressants** might enhance the antidiuretic and hypertensive effects of **vasopressin.** Moderate Theoretical
- Vinca alkaloids **(vincristine)** might enhance the antidiuretic and hypertensive effects of **vasopressin.** Moderate Theoretical

Vecuronium → see neuromuscular blocking drugs, non-depolarising

Vedolizumab → see monoclonal antibodies

Velpatasvir
- **Velpatasvir** is predicted to increase the exposure to **afatinib.** Moderate Study
- **Velpatasvir** is predicted to increase the exposure to **aliskiren.** Severe Theoretical
- **Velpatasvir** is predicted to increase the exposure to **alpelisib.** Moderate Theoretical
- Oral **antacids** are predicted to decrease the concentration of oral **velpatasvir**. Separate administration by 4 hours. Moderate Theoretical
- Anti-androgens **(apalutamide, enzalutamide)** are predicted to moderately decrease the exposure to **velpatasvir**. Avoid. Severe Study
- Antiarrhythmics **(amiodarone)** are predicted to increase the concentration of **velpatasvir**. Avoid or monitor. Moderate Theoretical
- Antiepileptics **(carbamazepine, fosphenytoin, phenobarbital, phenytoin, primidone)** are predicted to moderately decrease the exposure to **velpatasvir**. Avoid. Severe Study
- Antiepileptics **(oxcarbazepine)** are predicted to decrease the exposure to **velpatasvir**. Avoid. Severe Theoretical
- **Velpatasvir** is predicted to increase the exposure to antihistamines, non-sedating **(fexofenadine).** Severe Theoretical
- **Velpatasvir** is predicted to increase the exposure to **atogepant.** Adjust **atogepant** dose. Moderate Theoretical
- Oral calcium compounds **(calcium carbonate)**-containing antacids are predicted to decrease the concentration of oral **velpatasvir**. Separate administration by 4 hours. Moderate Theoretical
- **Cenobamate** is predicted to decrease the exposure to **velpatasvir**. Avoid. Moderate Theoretical
- **Velpatasvir** is predicted to increase the exposure to **cladribine.** Avoid or adjust dose. Moderate Theoretical
- **Velpatasvir** is predicted to increase the exposure to **colchicine.** Avoid P-glycoprotein inhibitors or adjust **colchicine** dose, p. 637. Severe Theoretical
- **Combined hormonal contraceptives** containing ethinylestradiol can increase ALT concentrations when given with **velpatasvir** with sofosbuvir and voxilaprevir. Avoid. Severe Study
- **Dabrafenib** is predicted to decrease the exposure to **velpatasvir**. Avoid. Moderate Theoretical
- **Velpatasvir** is predicted to increase the exposure to **digoxin.** Severe Study
- **Encorafenib** is predicted to moderately decrease the exposure to **velpatasvir**. Avoid. Severe Study
- Endothelin receptor antagonists **(bosentan)** are predicted to decrease the exposure to **velpatasvir**. Avoid. Moderate Theoretical
- **Velpatasvir** is predicted to increase the exposure to **erlotinib.** Moderate Theoretical
- **Ethinylestradiol** might increase ALT concentrations when given with **velpatasvir** with sofosbuvir and voxilaprevir. Avoid. Severe Study
- **Velpatasvir** is predicted to increase the exposure to **everolimus.** Severe Theoretical
- **Velpatasvir** is predicted to increase the exposure to factor XA inhibitors **(apixaban).** Moderate Theoretical
- **Velpatasvir** is predicted to increase the exposure to factor XA inhibitors **(edoxaban).** Severe Theoretical
- **Velpatasvir** might increase the exposure to factor XA inhibitors **(rivaroxaban).** Manufacturer advises caution in renal impairment. Moderate Theoretical
- **Velpatasvir** is predicted to increase the exposure to **fidaxomicin.** Avoid. Moderate Study
- **Velpatasvir** is predicted to increase the exposure to **grazoprevir.** Avoid. Severe Theoretical
- **H_2 receptor antagonists** are predicted to decrease the concentration of **velpatasvir**. Adjust dose, see sofosbuvir with velpatasvir p. 496. Moderate Study
- **Hormone replacement therapy** might increase ALT concentrations when given with **velpatasvir** with sofosbuvir and voxilaprevir. Manufacturer advises caution; avoid ethinylestradiol. Severe Theoretical
- **Ivosidenib** is predicted to moderately decrease the exposure to **velpatasvir**. Avoid. Severe Study
- **Velpatasvir** is predicted to increase the exposure to **loperamide.** Severe Theoretical
- **Lorlatinib** is predicted to decrease the exposure to **velpatasvir**. Avoid. Moderate Theoretical
- **Lumacaftor** is predicted to moderately decrease the exposure to **velpatasvir**. Avoid. Severe Study
- **Velpatasvir** is predicted to increase the exposure to meglitinides **(repaglinide).** Moderate Study
- **Mitotane** is predicted to moderately decrease the exposure to **velpatasvir**. Avoid. Severe Study
- **Modafinil** is predicted to decrease the exposure to **velpatasvir**. Avoid. Severe Theoretical
- **Velpatasvir** is predicted to increase the exposure to **momelotinib.** Moderate Study
- **Velpatasvir** is predicted to increase the risk of neutropenia when given with monoclonal antibodies **(brentuximab vedotin).** Monitor and adjust dose. Severe Theoretical
- **Velpatasvir** is predicted to increase the exposure to **neratinib.** Avoid or adjust dose and monitor for gastrointestinal adverse effects—consult product literature. Severe Study
- **Velpatasvir** is predicted to increase the exposure to **nintedanib.** Moderate Study
- **Nirmatrelvir** boosted with ritonavir is predicted to increase the concentration of **velpatasvir** with sofosbuvir and voxilaprevir. Severe Theoretical
- NNRTIs **(efavirenz, etravirine, nevirapine)** are predicted to decrease the exposure to **velpatasvir**. Avoid. Moderate Theoretical
- **Velpatasvir** is predicted to increase the exposure to **pralsetinib.** Moderate Theoretical

- **Proton pump inhibitors** are predicted to decrease the concentration of **velpatasvir**. Adjust dose, see sofosbuvir with velpatasvir p. 496. Moderate Study
- **Velpatasvir** is predicted to increase the exposure to **relugolix**. Avoid or take relugolix first and separate administration by at least 6 hours. Moderate Study
- Rifamycins **(rifabutin)** are predicted to decrease the exposure to **velpatasvir**. Avoid. Severe Theoretical
- Rifamycins **(rifampicin)** are predicted to moderately decrease the exposure to **velpatasvir**. Avoid. Severe Study
- **Velpatasvir** is predicted to increase the exposure to **rimegepant**. Avoid another dose of rimegepant within 48 hours of concurrent use. Moderate Theoretical
- **Velpatasvir** is predicted to increase the exposure to **seladelpar**. Moderate Study
- **Velpatasvir** is predicted to increase the exposure to **sirolimus**. Severe Theoretical
- **Sotorasib** is predicted to decrease the exposure to **velpatasvir**. Avoid. Moderate Theoretical
- **St John's wort** is predicted to decrease the exposure to **velpatasvir**. Avoid. Moderate Theoretical
- **Velpatasvir** with sofosbuvir slightly increases the exposure to statins **(atorvastatin)**. Severe Study
- **Velpatasvir** with sofosbuvir is predicted to increase the exposure to statins **(fluvastatin, simvastatin)**. Monitor adverse effects and adjust dose. Severe Theoretical
- **Velpatasvir** moderately increases the exposure to statins **(rosuvastatin)**. Avoid or adjust **rosuvastatin** dose, p. 155. Severe Study
- **Velpatasvir** is predicted to increase the exposure to **sulfasalazine**. Moderate Theoretical
- **Velpatasvir** is predicted to increase the exposure to sulfonylureas **(glibenclamide)**. Moderate Study
- **Velpatasvir** is predicted to slightly increase the exposure to **talazoparib**. Avoid or adjust dose—consult product literature. Severe Study
- **Velpatasvir** is predicted to increase the exposure to taxanes **(docetaxel)**. Moderate Study
- **Velpatasvir** is predicted to increase the exposure to taxanes **(paclitaxel)**. Severe Theoretical
- **Velpatasvir** is predicted to increase the exposure to **tenofovir disoproxil**. Moderate Theoretical
- **Velpatasvir** increases the exposure to thrombin inhibitors **(dabigatran)**. Avoid. Severe Study
- **Velpatasvir** is predicted to increase the exposure to **topotecan**. Severe Study
- **Velpatasvir** is predicted to increase the concentration of **trametinib**. Moderate Theoretical

Vemurafenib → see TABLE 7 p. 1055 (QT-interval prolongation)

- **Vemurafenib** is predicted to increase the exposure to **afatinib**. Moderate Study
- **Vemurafenib** is predicted to increase the exposure to **agomelatine**. Moderate Study
- **Vemurafenib** is predicted to increase the exposure to **aliskiren**. Use with caution and adjust dose. Moderate Theoretical
- **Vemurafenib** is predicted to increase the exposure to **aminophylline**. Adjust dose. Moderate Theoretical
- **Vemurafenib** is predicted to increase the exposure to anaesthetics, local **(ropivacaine)**. Moderate Theoretical
- **Vemurafenib** is predicted to increase the exposure to **anagrelide**. Moderate Theoretical → Also see TABLE 7 p. 1055
- Anti-androgens **(apalutamide, enzalutamide)** are predicted to decrease the exposure to **vemurafenib**. Avoid. Severe Study → Also see TABLE 7 p. 1055
- Antiarrhythmics **(dronedarone)** are predicted to increase the exposure to **vemurafenib**. Severe Theoretical → Also see TABLE 7 p. 1055
- Antiepileptics **(carbamazepine, fosphenytoin, phenobarbital, phenytoin, primidone)** are predicted to decrease the exposure to **vemurafenib**. Avoid. Severe Study
- Antifungals, azoles **(fluconazole, isavuconazole, itraconazole, ketoconazole, posaconazole, voriconazole)** are predicted to increase the exposure to **vemurafenib**. Severe Theoretical → Also see TABLE 7 p. 1055
- **Vemurafenib** is predicted to increase the exposure to antihistamines, non-sedating **(fexofenadine)**. Use with caution and adjust dose. Severe Theoretical
- **Vemurafenib** increases the concentration of atypical antipsychotics **(clozapine)**. Monitor adverse effects and adjust dose. Severe Study
- **Vemurafenib** is predicted to increase the exposure to atypical antipsychotics **(olanzapine)**. Adjust dose. Moderate Anecdotal
- **Vemurafenib** slightly to moderately decreases the exposure to benzodiazepines **(midazolam)**. Moderate Study
- **Berotralstat** is predicted to increase the exposure to **vemurafenib**. Severe Theoretical
- **Vemurafenib** is predicted to increase the exposure to beta blockers, non-selective **(nadolol)**. Moderate Study
- **Vemurafenib** is predicted to decrease the concentration of **bupropion**. Moderate Theoretical
- Calcium-channel blockers **(diltiazem, verapamil)** are predicted to increase the exposure to **vemurafenib**. Severe Theoretical
- **Ceritinib** is predicted to increase the exposure to **vemurafenib**. Severe Theoretical → Also see TABLE 7 p. 1055
- **Ciclosporin** might affect the exposure to **vemurafenib**. Severe Theoretical
- **Cobicistat** is predicted to increase the exposure to **vemurafenib**. Severe Theoretical
- **Vemurafenib** is predicted to increase the exposure to **colchicine**. Avoid P-glycoprotein inhibitors or adjust **colchicine** dose, p. 637. Severe Theoretical
- **Vemurafenib** might decrease the efficacy of **combined hormonal contraceptives**. Use additional contraceptive precautions. Severe Theoretical
- **Vemurafenib** is predicted to increase the exposure to **coumarins**. Moderate Study
- **Crizotinib** is predicted to increase the exposure to **vemurafenib**. Severe Theoretical → Also see TABLE 7 p. 1055
- **Dabrafenib** is predicted to decrease the exposure to **vemurafenib**. Severe Study
- **Vemurafenib** slightly increases the exposure to **digoxin**. Use with caution and adjust dose. Severe Study
- **Vemurafenib** is predicted to increase the exposure to dipeptidylpeptidase-4 inhibitors **(sitagliptin)**. Use with caution or avoid. Moderate Theoretical
- **Vemurafenib** is predicted to increase the exposure to dopamine receptor agonists **(ropinirole)**. Adjust dose. Moderate Study
- **Encorafenib** is predicted to decrease the exposure to **vemurafenib**. Avoid. Severe Study → Also see TABLE 7 p. 1055
- Endothelin receptor antagonists **(bosentan)** are predicted to decrease the exposure to **vemurafenib**. Severe Study
- **Vemurafenib** is predicted to increase the exposure to endothelin receptor antagonists **(ambrisentan)**. Use with caution or avoid. Moderate Theoretical
- **Vemurafenib** are predicted to increases the exposure to **erlotinib**. Monitor adverse effects and adjust dose. Moderate Study
- **Vemurafenib** is predicted to increase the exposure to **everolimus**. Use with caution and adjust dose. Severe Theoretical
- **Vemurafenib** is predicted to increase the exposure to factor XA inhibitors **(apixaban)**. Moderate Theoretical
- **Vemurafenib** is predicted to increase the exposure to factor XA inhibitors **(edoxaban)**. Severe Theoretical
- **Vemurafenib** might increase the exposure to factor XA inhibitors **(rivaroxaban)**. Manufacturer advises caution in renal impairment. Moderate Theoretical
- **Fedratinib** is predicted to increase the exposure to **vemurafenib**. Severe Theoretical
- **Vemurafenib** is predicted to increase the exposure to **fezolinetant**. Avoid. Moderate Study
- **Vemurafenib** is predicted to increase the exposure to **fidaxomicin**. Avoid. Moderate Study
- **Gefitinib** might affect the exposure to **vemurafenib**. Moderate Theoretical
- **Vemurafenib** is predicted to increase the exposure to **gilteritinib**. Moderate Theoretical
- **Vemurafenib** is predicted to increase the exposure to **grazoprevir**. Avoid. Severe Theoretical

Vemurafenib (continued)
- HIV-protease inhibitors are predicted to increase the exposure to **vemurafenib**. Severe Theoretical
- Idelalisib is predicted to increase the exposure to **vemurafenib**. Severe Theoretical
- Imatinib is predicted to increase the exposure to **vemurafenib**. Severe Theoretical
- Ivosidenib is predicted to decrease the exposure to **vemurafenib**. Avoid. Severe Study → Also see TABLE 7 p. 1055
- Letermovir is predicted to increase the exposure to **vemurafenib**. Severe Theoretical
- **Vemurafenib** might increase the exposure to loperamide. Use with caution and adjust dose. Moderate Theoretical
- **Vemurafenib** is predicted to increase the exposure to loxapine. Avoid. Unknown Theoretical
- Lumacaftor is predicted to decrease the exposure to **vemurafenib**. Avoid. Severe Study
- Macrolides (clarithromycin, erythromycin) are predicted to increase the exposure to **vemurafenib**. Severe Theoretical → Also see TABLE 7 p. 1055
- **Vemurafenib** slightly increases the exposure to MAO-B inhibitors (rasagiline). Moderate Study
- **Vemurafenib** is predicted to increase the exposure to maraviroc. Use with caution or avoid. Moderate Theoretical
- **Vemurafenib** is predicted to increase the exposure to melatonin. Moderate Theoretical
- Mitotane is predicted to decrease the exposure to **vemurafenib**. Avoid. Severe Study
- Monoclonal antibodies (ipilimumab) might increase the risk of hepatotoxicity when given with **vemurafenib**. Avoid. Severe Study
- **Vemurafenib** increases the risk of neutropenia when given with monoclonal antibodies (brentuximab vedotin). Monitor and adjust dose. Severe Theoretical
- **Vemurafenib** is predicted to increase the exposure to naldemedine. Moderate Study
- **Vemurafenib** is predicted to increase the exposure to neratinib. Avoid or adjust dose and monitor for gastrointestinal adverse effects—consult product literature. Severe Study
- Neurokinin-1 receptor antagonists (aprepitant, netupitant) are predicted to increase the exposure to **vemurafenib**. Severe Theoretical
- Nilotinib is predicted to increase the exposure to **vemurafenib**. Severe Theoretical → Also see TABLE 7 p. 1055
- **Vemurafenib** is predicted to increase the exposure to nintedanib. Moderate Study
- NNRTIs (efavirenz, etravirine, nevirapine) are predicted to decrease the exposure to **vemurafenib**. Severe Study → Also see TABLE 7 p. 1055
- **Vemurafenib** is predicted to increase the exposure to panobinostat. Adjust dose. Moderate Theoretical → Also see TABLE 7 p. 1055
- **Vemurafenib** is predicted to increase the exposure to phenindione. Moderate Study
- **Vemurafenib** is predicted to increase the exposure to phenothiazine antipsychotics (chlorpromazine). Moderate Theoretical → Also see TABLE 7 p. 1055
- **Vemurafenib** is predicted to increase the exposure to phosphodiesterase type-4 inhibitors (roflumilast). Moderate Theoretical
- **Vemurafenib** is predicted to increase the exposure to pirfenidone. Use with caution and adjust dose. Moderate Study
- **Vemurafenib** is predicted to increase the exposure to pralsetinib. Moderate Theoretical
- **Vemurafenib** might increase the exposure to ranolazine. Use with caution or avoid. Moderate Theoretical → Also see TABLE 7 p. 1055
- **Vemurafenib** is predicted to increase the exposure to relugolix. Avoid or take relugolix first and separate administration by at least 6 hours. Moderate Study
- Rifamycins (rifampicin) are predicted to decrease the exposure to **vemurafenib**. Avoid. Severe Study
- **Vemurafenib** is predicted to increase the exposure to riluzole. Moderate Theoretical
- **Vemurafenib** is predicted to increase the exposure to rimegepant. Avoid another dose of rimegepant within 48 hours of concurrent use. Moderate Theoretical
- **Vemurafenib** is predicted to increase the exposure to sirolimus. Use with caution and adjust dose. Severe Theoretical
- **Vemurafenib** is predicted to increase the exposure to SNRIs (duloxetine). Use with caution or avoid. Moderate Theoretical
- St John's wort is predicted to decrease the exposure to **vemurafenib**. Avoid. Severe Study
- **Vemurafenib** is predicted to slightly increase the exposure to talazoparib. Avoid or adjust dose—consult product literature. Severe Study
- **Vemurafenib** is predicted to increase the exposure to taxanes (paclitaxel). Use with caution and adjust dose. Severe Theoretical
- **Vemurafenib** is predicted to increase the exposure to theophylline. Monitor and adjust dose. Moderate Theoretical
- **Vemurafenib** is predicted to increase the exposure to thrombin inhibitors (dabigatran). Monitor and adjust dose. Severe Theoretical
- **Vemurafenib** is predicted to increase the exposure to ticagrelor. Use with caution or avoid. Severe Study
- **Vemurafenib** might increase the exposure to tigecycline. Mild Anecdotal
- **Vemurafenib** increases the exposure to tizanidine. Avoid. Moderate Study
- **Vemurafenib** is predicted to increase the exposure to topotecan. Severe Study
- **Vemurafenib** is predicted to increase the concentration of trametinib. Moderate Theoretical
- **Vemurafenib** is predicted to increase the exposure to triptans (zolmitriptan). Adjust **zolmitriptan** dose, p. 347. Moderate Theoretical
- Tucatinib is predicted to increase the exposure to **vemurafenib**. Severe Theoretical
- **Vemurafenib** is predicted to increase the exposure to venetoclax. Avoid or monitor for toxicity. Severe Theoretical
- **Vemurafenib** might increase the exposure to vinca alkaloids. Severe Theoretical
- **Vemurafenib** is predicted to increase the exposure to vorasidenib. Avoid. Moderate Theoretical

Venetoclax

FOOD AND LIFESTYLE Avoid bitter (Seville) orange and star fruit as they might increase the exposure to venetoclax.

- Anti-androgens (apalutamide, enzalutamide) are predicted to decrease the exposure to **venetoclax**. Avoid. Severe Study
- Antiarrhythmics (amiodarone) are predicted to increase the exposure to **venetoclax**. Avoid or monitor for toxicity. Severe Theoretical
- Antiarrhythmics (dronedarone) are predicted to increase the exposure to **venetoclax**. Avoid or adjust dose—consult product literature. Severe Study
- Antiepileptics (carbamazepine, fosphenytoin, phenobarbital, phenytoin, primidone) are predicted to decrease the exposure to **venetoclax**. Avoid. Severe Study
- Antifungals, azoles (fluconazole, isavuconazole, itraconazole, ketoconazole, posaconazole, voriconazole) are predicted to increase the exposure to **venetoclax**. Avoid or adjust dose—consult product literature. Severe Study
- **Venetoclax** is predicted to increase the exposure to antihistamines, non-sedating (fexofenadine). Moderate Theoretical
- Berotralstat is predicted to increase the exposure to **venetoclax**. Avoid or adjust dose—consult product literature. Severe Study
- Calcium-channel blockers (diltiazem, verapamil) are predicted to increase the exposure to **venetoclax**. Avoid or adjust dose—consult product literature. Severe Study
- Cenobamate is predicted to decrease the exposure to **venetoclax**. Avoid. Severe Study
- Ceritinib is predicted to increase the exposure to **venetoclax**. Avoid or adjust dose—consult product literature. Severe Study
- Ciclosporin is predicted to increase the exposure to **venetoclax**. Avoid or monitor for toxicity. Severe Theoretical
- Cobicistat is predicted to increase the exposure to **venetoclax**. Avoid or adjust dose—consult product literature. Severe Study

A1 Interactions | Appendix 1

- **Venetoclax** is predicted to increase the exposure to **colchicine**. Avoid or adjust dose. Severe Study
- **Venetoclax** slightly increases the exposure to coumarins **(warfarin)**. Moderate Study
- **Crizotinib** is predicted to increase the exposure to **venetoclax**. Avoid or adjust dose—consult product literature. Severe Study
- **Dabrafenib** is predicted to decrease the exposure to **venetoclax**. Avoid. Severe Study
- **Venetoclax** increases the exposure to **digoxin**. Avoid or adjust dose. Severe Study
- **Eltrombopag** is predicted to increase the exposure to **venetoclax**. Avoid or monitor for toxicity. Severe Theoretical
- **Encorafenib** is predicted to decrease the exposure to **venetoclax**. Avoid. Severe Study
- Endothelin receptor antagonists **(bosentan)** are predicted to decrease the exposure to **venetoclax**. Avoid. Severe Study
- **Venetoclax** is predicted to increase the exposure to endothelin receptor antagonists **(bosentan)**. Moderate Theoretical
- **Venetoclax** is predicted to increase the exposure to **everolimus**. Avoid or adjust dose. Severe Study
- **Venetoclax** is predicted to increase the exposure to factor XA inhibitors **(edoxaban, rivaroxaban)**. Avoid or adjust dose. Severe Study
- **Fedratinib** is predicted to increase the exposure to **venetoclax**. Avoid or adjust dose—consult product literature. Severe Study
- **Grapefruit** juice is predicted to increase the exposure to **venetoclax**. Avoid. Severe Theoretical
- **HIV-protease inhibitors** are predicted to increase the exposure to **venetoclax**. Avoid or adjust dose—consult product literature. Severe Study
- **Idelalisib** is predicted to increase the exposure to **venetoclax**. Avoid or adjust dose—consult product literature. Severe Study
- **Imatinib** is predicted to increase the exposure to **venetoclax**. Avoid or adjust dose—consult product literature. Severe Study
- **Ivacaftor** is predicted to increase the exposure to **venetoclax**. Avoid or monitor for toxicity. Severe Theoretical
- **Ivosidenib** is predicted to decrease the exposure to **venetoclax**. Avoid. Severe Study
- **Lapatinib** is predicted to increase the exposure to **venetoclax**. Avoid or monitor for toxicity. Severe Theoretical
- **Leflunomide** is predicted to increase the exposure to **venetoclax**. Avoid or monitor for toxicity. Severe Theoretical
- **Letermovir** is predicted to increase the exposure to **venetoclax**. Avoid or adjust dose—consult product literature. Severe Study
- **Venetoclax** potentially decreases the efficacy of **live vaccines**. Avoid. Severe Theoretical
- **Lorlatinib** is predicted to decrease the exposure to **venetoclax**. Avoid. Severe Study
- **Lumacaftor** is predicted to decrease the exposure to **venetoclax**. Avoid. Severe Study
- Macrolides **(clarithromycin, erythromycin)** are predicted to increase the exposure to **venetoclax**. Avoid or adjust dose—consult product literature. Severe Study
- **Venetoclax** is predicted to increase the exposure to meglitinides **(repaglinide)**. Moderate Theoretical
- **Mitotane** is predicted to decrease the exposure to **venetoclax**. Avoid. Severe Study
- **Neratinib** is predicted to increase the exposure to **venetoclax**. Avoid or monitor for toxicity. Severe Theoretical
- Neurokinin-1 receptor antagonists **(aprepitant, netupitant)** are predicted to increase the exposure to **venetoclax**. Avoid or adjust dose—consult product literature. Severe Study
- **Nilotinib** is predicted to increase the exposure to **venetoclax**. Avoid or adjust dose—consult product literature. Severe Study
- **Nirmatrelvir** boosted with ritonavir is predicted to increase the concentration of **venetoclax**. Avoid or adjust dose—consult product literature. Severe Theoretical
- NNRTIs **(efavirenz, etravirine, nevirapine)** are predicted to decrease the exposure to **venetoclax**. Avoid. Severe Study
- Quinolones **(ciprofloxacin)** are predicted to increase the exposure to **venetoclax**. Avoid or adjust dose—consult product literature. Severe Theoretical
- **Ranolazine** is predicted to increase the exposure to **venetoclax**. Avoid or monitor for toxicity. Severe Theoretical
- Rifamycins **(rifampicin)** are predicted to decrease the exposure to **venetoclax**. Avoid. Severe Study
- **Venetoclax** is predicted to increase the exposure to **sirolimus**. Avoid or adjust dose. Severe Study
- **Sotorasib** is predicted to decrease the exposure to **venetoclax**. Avoid. Severe Study
- **St John's wort** is predicted to decrease the exposure to **venetoclax**. Avoid. Severe Study
- **Venetoclax** is predicted to increase the exposure to statins **(atorvastatin)**. Moderate Study
- **Venetoclax** is predicted to increase the exposure to statins **(fluvastatin, pravastatin, rosuvastatin, simvastatin)**. Moderate Theoretical
- **Venetoclax** is predicted to increase the exposure to **sulfasalazine**. Moderate Theoretical
- **Venetoclax** is predicted to increase the exposure to sulfonylureas **(glibenclamide)**. Moderate Theoretical
- **Teriflunomide** is predicted to increase the exposure to **venetoclax**. Avoid or monitor for toxicity. Severe Theoretical
- **Venetoclax** is predicted to increase the exposure to thrombin inhibitors **(dabigatran)**. Avoid or adjust dose. Severe Study
- **Venetoclax** is predicted to increase the exposure to **topotecan**. Moderate Theoretical
- **Tucatinib** is predicted to increase the exposure to **venetoclax**. Avoid or adjust dose—consult product literature. Severe Study
- **Vemurafenib** is predicted to increase the exposure to **venetoclax**. Avoid or monitor for toxicity. Severe Theoretical

Venlafaxine → see SNRIs

Verapamil → see calcium-channel blockers

Vericiguat → see TABLE 6 p. 1054 (hypotension)

Vernakalant → see antiarrhythmics

Verteporfin

GENERAL INFORMATION Caution on concurrent use with other photosensitising drugs.

Vigabatrin → see antiepileptics

Vilanterol → see $beta_2$ agonists

Vildagliptin → see dipeptidylpeptidase-4 inhibitors

Vinblastine → see vinca alkaloids

Vinca alkaloids → see TABLE 15 p. 1058 (hyponatraemia), TABLE 12 p. 1057 (myelosuppression), TABLE 16 p. 1058 (ototoxicity), TABLE 10 p. 1056 (peripheral neuropathy)

vinblastine · vincristine · vindesine · vinorelbine

- Anti-androgens **(apalutamide, enzalutamide)** are predicted to decrease the exposure to **vinorelbine**. Use with caution or avoid. Severe Theoretical
- Anti-androgens **(apalutamide, enzalutamide)** are predicted to decrease the exposure to vinca alkaloids **(vinblastine, vincristine, vindesine)**. Severe Theoretical
- Antiarrhythmics **(amiodarone)** might increase the exposure to **vinca alkaloids**. Severe Theoretical → Also see TABLE 10 p. 1056
- Antiarrhythmics **(dronedarone)** are predicted to increase the exposure to **vinca alkaloids**. Severe Theoretical
- Antiepileptics **(carbamazepine, fosphenytoin, phenobarbital, phenytoin, primidone)** are predicted to decrease the exposure to **vinorelbine**. Use with caution or avoid. Severe Theoretical → Also see TABLE 15 p. 1058 → Also see TABLE 10 p. 1056
- Antiepileptics **(carbamazepine, fosphenytoin, phenobarbital, phenytoin, primidone)** are predicted to decrease the exposure to vinca alkaloids **(vinblastine, vincristine, vindesine)**. Severe Theoretical → Also see TABLE 15 p. 1058 → Also see TABLE 10 p. 1056
- Antifungals, azoles **(fluconazole, isavuconazole, itraconazole, ketoconazole, posaconazole, voriconazole)** are predicted to increase the exposure to **vinca alkaloids**. Severe Theoretical
- Antifungals, azoles **(miconazole)** are predicted to increase the concentration of **vinca alkaloids**. Use with caution and adjust dose. Moderate Theoretical
- **Asparaginase** potentially increases the risk of neurotoxicity when given with **vincristine**. **Vincristine** should be taken 3 to 24 hours before **asparaginase**. Severe Anecdotal → Also see TABLE 12 p. 1057
- **Berotralstat** is predicted to increase the exposure to **vinca alkaloids**. Severe Theoretical
- Calcium-channel blockers **(diltiazem, verapamil)** are predicted to increase the exposure to **vinca alkaloids**. Severe Theoretical

Vinca alkaloids (continued)
- **Ceritinib** is predicted to increase the exposure to **vinca alkaloids.** Severe Theoretical → Also see TABLE 12 p. 1057
- **Ciclosporin** might increase the exposure to **vinca alkaloids.** Severe Theoretical
- **Cobicistat** is predicted to increase the exposure to **vinca alkaloids.** Severe Theoretical
- **Crisantaspase** potentially increases the risk of neurotoxicity when given with **vincristine. Vincristine** should be taken 3 to 24 hours before **crisantaspase.** Severe Anecdotal → Also see TABLE 12 p. 1057
- **Crizotinib** is predicted to increase the exposure to **vinca alkaloids.** Severe Theoretical
- **Encorafenib** is predicted to decrease the exposure to vinca alkaloids **(vinblastine, vincristine, vindesine).** Severe Theoretical
- **Encorafenib** is predicted to decrease the exposure to **vinorelbine.** Use with caution or avoid. Severe Theoretical
- **Fedratinib** is predicted to increase the exposure to **vinca alkaloids.** Severe Theoretical
- **HIV-protease inhibitors** are predicted to increase the exposure to **vinca alkaloids.** Severe Theoretical
- **Idelalisib** is predicted to increase the exposure to **vinca alkaloids.** Severe Theoretical
- **Imatinib** is predicted to increase the exposure to **vinca alkaloids.** Severe Theoretical → Also see TABLE 12 p. 1057
- **Ivacaftor** might increase the exposure to **vinca alkaloids.** Severe Theoretical
- **Ivosidenib** is predicted to decrease the exposure to vinca alkaloids **(vinblastine, vincristine, vindesine).** Severe Theoretical
- **Ivosidenib** is predicted to decrease the exposure to **vinorelbine.** Use with caution or avoid. Severe Theoretical
- **Lapatinib** might increase the exposure to **vinca alkaloids.** Severe Theoretical
- **Letermovir** is predicted to increase the exposure to **vinca alkaloids.** Severe Theoretical
- **Live vaccines** are predicted to increase the risk of generalised infection (possibly life-threatening) when given with **vinca alkaloids.** UKHSA advises avoid (refer to Green Book). Severe Theoretical
- **Lumacaftor** is predicted to decrease the exposure to vinca alkaloids **(vinblastine, vincristine, vindesine).** Severe Theoretical
- **Lumacaftor** is predicted to decrease the exposure to **vinorelbine.** Use with caution or avoid. Severe Theoretical
- Macrolides **(azithromycin)** might increase the exposure to **vinca alkaloids.** Severe Theoretical
- Macrolides **(clarithromycin, erythromycin)** are predicted to increase the exposure to **vinca alkaloids.** Severe Theoretical
- **Mitotane** is predicted to decrease the exposure to vinca alkaloids **(vinblastine, vincristine, vindesine).** Severe Theoretical → Also see TABLE 12 p. 1057
- **Mitotane** is predicted to decrease the exposure to **vinorelbine.** Use with caution or avoid. Severe Theoretical → Also see TABLE 12 p. 1057
- **Neratinib** might increase the exposure to **vinca alkaloids.** Severe Theoretical
- **Neurokinin-1 receptor antagonists** are predicted to increase the exposure to **vinca alkaloids.** Severe Theoretical
- **Nilotinib** is predicted to increase the exposure to **vinca alkaloids.** Severe Theoretical → Also see TABLE 12 p. 1057
- **Nirmatrelvir** boosted with ritonavir is predicted to increase the concentration of vinca alkaloids **(vinblastine, vincristine).** Severe Theoretical
- **Pegaspargase** potentially increases the risk of neurotoxicity when given with **vincristine. Vincristine** should be taken 3 to 24 hours before **pegaspargase.** Severe Anecdotal → Also see TABLE 12 p. 1057
- **Ranolazine** might increase the exposure to **vinca alkaloids.** Severe Theoretical
- Rifamycins **(rifampicin)** are predicted to decrease the exposure to **vinorelbine.** Use with caution or avoid. Severe Theoretical
- Rifamycins **(rifampicin)** are predicted to decrease the exposure to vinca alkaloids **(vinblastine, vincristine, vindesine).** Severe Theoretical
- **Rucaparib** might increase the exposure to **vinca alkaloids.** Severe Theoretical → Also see TABLE 12 p. 1057
- **St John's wort** is predicted to decrease the exposure to **vinca alkaloids.** Severe Theoretical
- **Tucatinib** is predicted to increase the exposure to **vinca alkaloids.** Severe Theoretical
- **Vandetanib** might increase the exposure to **vinca alkaloids.** Severe Theoretical
- **Vincristine** might enhance the antidiuretic and hypertensive effects of **vasopressin.** Moderate Theoretical
- **Vemurafenib** might increase the exposure to **vinca alkaloids.** Severe Theoretical

Vincristine → see vinca alkaloids
Vindesine → see vinca alkaloids
Vinorelbine → see vinca alkaloids

Vismodegib
- Anti-androgens **(apalutamide, enzalutamide)** are predicted to decrease the exposure to **vismodegib.** Avoid. Moderate Theoretical
- Antiepileptics **(carbamazepine, fosphenytoin, phenobarbital, phenytoin, primidone)** are predicted to decrease the exposure to **vismodegib.** Avoid. Moderate Theoretical
- **Encorafenib** is predicted to decrease the exposure to **vismodegib.** Avoid. Moderate Theoretical
- **Ivosidenib** is predicted to decrease the exposure to **vismodegib.** Avoid. Moderate Theoretical
- **Lumacaftor** is predicted to decrease the exposure to **vismodegib.** Avoid. Moderate Theoretical
- **Mitotane** is predicted to decrease the exposure to **vismodegib.** Avoid. Moderate Theoretical
- Rifamycins **(rifampicin)** are predicted to decrease the exposure to **vismodegib.** Avoid. Moderate Theoretical
- **St John's wort** is predicted to decrease the exposure to **vismodegib.** Avoid. Moderate Theoretical

Vitamin A → see TABLE 1 p. 1053 (hepatotoxicity)
- Retinoids **(acitretin, alitretinoin, isotretinoin)** are predicted to increase the risk of vitamin A toxicity when given with **vitamin A.** Avoid. Severe Theoretical → Also see TABLE 1 p. 1053
- Retinoids **(bexarotene)** are predicted to increase the risk of toxicity when given with **vitamin A.** Adjust dose. Moderate Theoretical → Also see TABLE 1 p. 1053
- Retinoids **(tretinoin)** are predicted to increase the risk of vitamin A toxicity when given with **vitamin A.** Avoid. Severe Study

Vitamin D substances

alfacalcidol · calcifediol · calcipotriol · calcitriol · colecalciferol · ergocalciferol · paricalcitol · tacalcitol

ROUTE-SPECIFIC INFORMATION Since systemic absorption can follow topical application, the possibility of interactions with topical **calcitriol** should be borne in mind.

- Antiepileptics **(carbamazepine)** are predicted to decrease the effects of **vitamin D substances.** Moderate Study
- Antiepileptics **(fosphenytoin, phenytoin)** decrease the effects of **vitamin D substances.** Moderate Study
- Antiepileptics **(phenobarbital, primidone)** are predicted to decrease the effects of **vitamin D substances.** Moderate Theoretical
- Antifungals, azoles **(clotrimazole, ketoconazole)** are predicted to decrease the exposure to **colecalciferol.** Moderate Theoretical
- Antifungals, azoles **(itraconazole, ketoconazole, posaconazole, voriconazole)** are predicted to increase the exposure to **paricalcitol.** Moderate Study
- **Ceritinib** is predicted to increase the exposure to **paricalcitol.** Moderate Study
- **Cobicistat** is predicted to increase the exposure to **paricalcitol.** Moderate Study
- **Vitamin D substances** are predicted to increase the risk of toxicity when given with **digoxin.** Severe Theoretical
- **HIV-protease inhibitors** are predicted to increase the exposure to **paricalcitol.** Moderate Study
- **Idelalisib** is predicted to increase the exposure to **paricalcitol.** Moderate Study
- Macrolides **(clarithromycin)** are predicted to increase the exposure to **paricalcitol.** Moderate Study

- **Thiazide diuretics** increase the risk of hypercalcaemia when given with **vitamin D substances** (high-dose). Moderate Theoretical
- **Tucatinib** is predicted to increase the exposure to **paricalcitol**. Moderate Study

Vitamin E substances

- **Vitamin E substances** affect the exposure to **ciclosporin**. Moderate Study
- **Vitamin E substances** might increase the risk of bleeding when given with **selumetinib**. Avoid. Severe Theoretical

Voclosporin → see TABLE 2 p. 1053 (nephrotoxicity), TABLE 13 p. 1057 (increased serum potassium), TABLE 7 p. 1055 (QT-interval prolongation)

- Anti-androgens **(apalutamide, enzalutamide)** are predicted to decrease the exposure to **voclosporin**. Avoid. Severe Study → Also see TABLE 7 p. 1055
- Antiarrhythmics **(dronedarone)** are predicted to increase the exposure to **voclosporin**. Adjust **voclosporin** dose. Severe Study → Also see TABLE 7 p. 1055
- Antiepileptics **(carbamazepine, fosphenytoin, phenobarbital, phenytoin, primidone)** are predicted to decrease the exposure to **voclosporin**. Avoid. Severe Study
- Antifungals, azoles **(fluconazole, isavuconazole)** are predicted to increase the exposure to **voclosporin**. Adjust **voclosporin** dose. Severe Study → Also see TABLE 7 p. 1055
- Antifungals, azoles **(itraconazole, ketoconazole, posaconazole, voriconazole)** are predicted to increase the exposure to **voclosporin**. Avoid. Severe Study → Also see TABLE 7 p. 1055
- **Voclosporin** is predicted to increase the exposure to antihistamines, non-sedating **(fexofenadine)**. Mild Theoretical
- **Berotralstat** is predicted to increase the exposure to **voclosporin**. Adjust **voclosporin** dose. Severe Study
- Calcium-channel blockers **(diltiazem, verapamil)** are predicted to increase the exposure to **voclosporin**. Adjust **voclosporin** dose. Severe Study
- **Cenobamate** is predicted to decrease the exposure to **voclosporin**. Adjust dose. Moderate Theoretical
- **Ceritinib** is predicted to increase the exposure to **voclosporin**. Avoid. Severe Study → Also see TABLE 7 p. 1055
- **Cobicistat** is predicted to increase the exposure to **voclosporin**. Avoid. Severe Study
- **Crizotinib** is predicted to increase the exposure to **voclosporin**. Adjust **voclosporin** dose. Severe Study → Also see TABLE 7 p. 1055
- **Dabrafenib** is predicted to decrease the exposure to **voclosporin**. Avoid. Severe Theoretical
- **Voclosporin** slightly increases the exposure to **digoxin**. Moderate Study
- **Encorafenib** is predicted to decrease the exposure to **voclosporin**. Avoid. Severe Study → Also see TABLE 7 p. 1055
- Endothelin receptor antagonists **(bosentan)** are predicted to decrease the exposure to **voclosporin** and **voclosporin** is predicted to increase the concentration of endothelin receptor antagonists **(bosentan)**. Avoid. Severe Theoretical
- **Voclosporin** is predicted to increase the exposure to **everolimus**. Moderate Study
- **Fedratinib** is predicted to increase the exposure to **voclosporin**. Adjust **voclosporin** dose. Severe Study
- **Voclosporin** is predicted to increase the exposure to **gilteritinib**. Moderate Theoretical
- **Grapefruit** and grapefruit juice are predicted to increase the exposure to **voclosporin**. Avoid. Moderate Theoretical
- **HIV-protease inhibitors** are predicted to increase the exposure to **voclosporin**. Avoid. Severe Study
- **Idelalisib** is predicted to increase the exposure to **voclosporin**. Avoid. Severe Study
- **Imatinib** is predicted to increase the exposure to **voclosporin**. Adjust **voclosporin** dose. Severe Study
- **Ivosidenib** is predicted to decrease the exposure to **voclosporin**. Avoid. Severe Study → Also see TABLE 7 p. 1055
- **Letermovir** is predicted to increase the exposure to **voclosporin**. Adjust **voclosporin** dose. Severe Study
- **Live vaccines** are predicted to increase the risk of generalised infection (possibly life-threatening) when given with **voclosporin**. UKHSA advises avoid (refer to Green Book). Severe Theoretical
- **Lumacaftor** is predicted to decrease the exposure to **voclosporin**. Avoid. Severe Study
- Macrolides **(clarithromycin)** are predicted to increase the exposure to **voclosporin**. Avoid. Severe Study
- Macrolides **(erythromycin)** are predicted to increase the exposure to **voclosporin**. Adjust **voclosporin** dose. Severe Study → Also see TABLE 7 p. 1055
- **Voclosporin** is predicted to increase the concentration of meglitinides **(repaglinide)**. Moderate Theoretical
- **Mitotane** is predicted to decrease the exposure to **voclosporin**. Avoid. Severe Study
- Neurokinin-1 receptor antagonists **(aprepitant, netupitant)** are predicted to increase the exposure to **voclosporin**. Adjust **voclosporin** dose. Severe Study
- **Nilotinib** is predicted to increase the exposure to **voclosporin**. Adjust **voclosporin** dose. Severe Study → Also see TABLE 7 p. 1055
- **Nirmatrelvir** boosted with ritonavir is predicted to increase the concentration of **voclosporin**. Avoid. Severe Theoretical
- NNRTIs **(efavirenz, etravirine, nevirapine)** are predicted to decrease the exposure to **voclosporin**. Avoid. Severe Theoretical → Also see TABLE 7 p. 1055
- Rifamycins **(rifampicin)** are predicted to decrease the exposure to **voclosporin**. Avoid. Severe Study → Also see TABLE 2 p. 1053
- **Voclosporin** is predicted to increase the exposure to **sirolimus**. Moderate Study
- **St John's wort** is predicted to decrease the exposure to **voclosporin**. Avoid. Severe Theoretical
- **Voclosporin** is predicted to increase the concentration of statins **(atorvastatin, pravastatin, rosuvastatin, simvastatin)**. Moderate Theoretical
- **Voclosporin** is predicted to increase the concentration of **sulfasalazine**. Moderate Theoretical → Also see TABLE 2 p. 1053
- **Voclosporin** is predicted to increase the concentration of sulfonylureas **(glibenclamide)**. Moderate Theoretical
- **Voclosporin** is predicted to increase the exposure to **talazoparib**. Moderate Study
- **Voclosporin** is predicted to increase the exposure to taxanes **(paclitaxel)**. Moderate Study
- **Voclosporin** is predicted to increase the exposure to thrombin inhibitors **(dabigatran)**. Mild Theoretical
- **Tucatinib** is predicted to increase the exposure to **voclosporin**. Avoid. Severe Study

Volanesorsen

- **Drugs that cause bleeding** (see TABLE 3 p. 1053) cause bleeding, as can **volanesorsen**; concurrent use might increase the risk of developing this effect. Avoid depending on platelet count—consult product literature. Severe Theoretical

Volatile halogenated anaesthetics → see TABLE 6 p. 1054 (hypotension), TABLE 7 p. 1055 (QT-interval prolongation), TABLE 9 p. 1056 (CNS effects)

desflurane · isoflurane · methoxyflurane · sevoflurane

- **Sevoflurane** can cause hypertension, as can **amfetamines**. Avoid **amfetamines** for several days before surgery. Severe Theoretical
- Antiepileptics **(phenobarbital, primidone)** potentially increase the risk of nephrotoxicity when given with **methoxyflurane**. Avoid. Severe Theoretical → Also see TABLE 9 p. 1056
- **Isoniazid** potentially increases the risk of nephrotoxicity when given with **methoxyflurane**. Avoid. Severe Theoretical
- **Isoniazid** might increase the risk of sevoflurane toxicity when given with **sevoflurane**. Avoid **isoniazid** from 1 week before, until 15 days after, surgery. Moderate Theoretical
- **Methylphenidate** might increase the risk of hypertension and arrhythmias when given with **volatile halogenated anaesthetics**. Avoid **methylphenidate** on day of surgery, p. 277. Severe Theoretical
- Rifamycins **(rifampicin)** potentially increase the risk of nephrotoxicity when given with **methoxyflurane**. Avoid. Severe Theoretical
- **St John's wort** has been reported to cause severe hypotension when given with **volatile halogenated anaesthetics**. Severe Theoretical
- **Sevoflurane** can cause hypertension, as can sympathomimetics, vasoconstrictor **(ephedrine)**. Avoid **ephedrine** for several days before surgery. Severe Theoretical

Volatile halogenated anaesthetics (continued)
- **Sevoflurane** can cause hypertension, as can sympathomimetics, vasoconstrictor **(pseudoephedrine)**. Avoid **pseudoephedrine** for several days before surgery. Severe Theoretical
- **Sevoflurane** can cause hypertension, as can sympathomimetics, vasoconstrictor **(xylometazoline)**. Avoid **xylometazoline** for several days before surgery. Severe Theoretical
- **Methoxyflurane** might increase the risk of nephrotoxicity when given with tetracyclines **(tetracycline)**. Severe Anecdotal

Vorasidenib → see TABLE 1 p. 1053 (hepatotoxicity)

FOOD AND LIFESTYLE Smoking can decrease the concentration of vorasidenib; manufacturer advises avoid concurrent use.

- **Vorasidenib** might decrease the concentration of alkylating agents **(ifosfamide)**. Avoid. Severe Theoretical
- Antiepileptics **(phenytoin)** are predicted to decrease the exposure to **vorasidenib**. Avoid. Severe Theoretical
- **Vorasidenib** might decrease the concentration of antiepileptics **(carbamazepine, fosphenytoin, phenobarbital, valproate)**. Avoid. Severe Theoretical → Also see TABLE 1 p. 1053
- **Vorasidenib** might decrease the concentration of **ciclosporin**. Avoid. Severe Theoretical
- **Combined hormonal contraceptives** are predicted to increase the exposure to **vorasidenib** and **vorasidenib** might decrease the concentration of **combined hormonal contraceptives**. Avoid. Severe Theoretical
- **Vorasidenib** might decrease the concentration of coumarins **(warfarin)**. Avoid. Severe Theoretical
- **Vorasidenib** might decrease the concentration of **everolimus**. Avoid. Severe Theoretical
- **Givosiran** is predicted to increase the exposure to **vorasidenib**. Avoid. Moderate Theoretical
- HIV-protease inhibitors **(ritonavir)** are predicted to decrease the exposure to **vorasidenib**. Avoid. Severe Theoretical → Also see TABLE 1 p. 1053
- **Leflunomide** is predicted to decrease the exposure to **vorasidenib**. Avoid. Severe Theoretical
- **Mexiletine** is predicted to increase the exposure to **vorasidenib**. Avoid. Moderate Theoretical
- **Vorasidenib** might decrease the concentration of opioids **(alfentanil, fentanyl)**. Avoid. Severe Theoretical
- **Osilodrostat** is predicted to increase the exposure to **vorasidenib**. Avoid. Moderate Theoretical
- **Vorasidenib** might decrease the concentration of **pimozide**. Avoid. Severe Theoretical
- Quinolones **(ciprofloxacin)** moderately increase the exposure to **vorasidenib**. Avoid. Moderate Study
- Rifamycins **(rifampicin)** are predicted to decrease the exposure to **vorasidenib**. Avoid. Severe Theoretical
- **Rucaparib** is predicted to increase the exposure to **vorasidenib**. Avoid. Moderate Theoretical
- **Vorasidenib** might decrease the concentration of **sirolimus**. Avoid. Severe Theoretical
- SSRIs **(fluvoxamine)** are predicted to increase the exposure to **vorasidenib**. Avoid. Moderate Study
- **Vorasidenib** might decrease the concentration of **tacrolimus**. Avoid. Severe Theoretical
- **Vorasidenib** might decrease the concentration of **tamoxifen**. Avoid. Severe Theoretical
- **Vorasidenib** might decrease the concentration of **temsirolimus**. Avoid. Severe Theoretical
- **Teriflunomide** is predicted to decrease the exposure to **vorasidenib**. Avoid. Severe Theoretical
- **Vorasidenib** might decrease the concentration of tricyclic antidepressants **(amitriptyline, dosulepin, imipramine, trimipramine)**. Avoid. Severe Theoretical
- **Vemurafenib** is predicted to increase the exposure to **vorasidenib**. Avoid. Moderate Theoretical

Voriconazole → see antifungals, azoles

Vortioxetine → see TABLE 3 p. 1053 (bleeding), TABLE 11 p. 1056 (serotonin toxicity)
- Anti-androgens **(apalutamide, enzalutamide)** are predicted to decrease the exposure to **vortioxetine**. Monitor and adjust dose. Moderate Study
- Antiepileptics **(carbamazepine, fosphenytoin, phenobarbital, phenytoin, primidone)** are predicted to decrease the exposure to **vortioxetine**. Monitor and adjust dose. Moderate Study
- **Bupropion** is predicted to increase the exposure to **vortioxetine**. Monitor and adjust dose. Moderate Study
- **Cinacalcet** is predicted to increase the exposure to **vortioxetine**. Monitor and adjust dose. Moderate Study
- **Dacomitinib** is predicted to increase the exposure to **vortioxetine**. Monitor and adjust dose. Moderate Study
- **Encorafenib** is predicted to decrease the exposure to **vortioxetine**. Monitor and adjust dose. Moderate Study
- Interferons **(ropeginterferon alfa)** are predicted to increase the exposure to **vortioxetine**. Moderate Theoretical
- **Ivosidenib** is predicted to decrease the exposure to **vortioxetine**. Monitor and adjust dose. Moderate Study
- **Lumacaftor** is predicted to decrease the exposure to **vortioxetine**. Monitor and adjust dose. Moderate Study
- **Mitotane** is predicted to decrease the exposure to **vortioxetine**. Monitor and adjust dose. Moderate Study
- Rifamycins **(rifampicin)** are predicted to decrease the exposure to **vortioxetine**. Monitor and adjust dose. Moderate Study
- SSRIs **(fluoxetine, paroxetine)** are predicted to increase the exposure to **vortioxetine**. Monitor and adjust dose. Moderate Study → Also see TABLE 3 p. 1053 → Also see TABLE 11 p. 1056
- **Terbinafine** is predicted to increase the exposure to **vortioxetine**. Monitor and adjust dose. Moderate Study

Voxilaprevir
- **Voxilaprevir** is predicted to increase the exposure to **afatinib**. Moderate Study
- **Voxilaprevir** with sofosbuvir and velpatasvir is predicted to increase the exposure to **aliskiren**. Severe Theoretical
- **Voxilaprevir** is predicted to increase the exposure to **alpelisib**. Moderate Theoretical
- Anti-androgens **(apalutamide, enzalutamide)** are predicted to decrease the concentration of **voxilaprevir**. Avoid. Severe Study
- Antiepileptics **(carbamazepine, fosphenytoin, phenobarbital, phenytoin, primidone)** are predicted to decrease the concentration of **voxilaprevir**. Avoid. Severe Study
- Antiepileptics **(oxcarbazepine)** are predicted to decrease the concentration of **voxilaprevir**. Avoid. Severe Theoretical
- **Voxilaprevir** with sofosbuvir and velpatasvir is predicted to increase the exposure to antihistamines, non-sedating **(fexofenadine)**. Moderate Study
- **Voxilaprevir** is predicted to increase the exposure to **atogepant**. Adjust **atogepant** dose. Moderate Theoretical
- **Bulevirtide** is predicted to increase the exposure to **voxilaprevir**. Avoid or monitor. Moderate Theoretical
- **Cenobamate** is predicted to decrease the concentration of **voxilaprevir**. Avoid. Severe Theoretical
- **Ciclosporin** increases the concentration of **voxilaprevir**. Avoid. Severe Study
- **Voxilaprevir** is predicted to increase the exposure to **cladribine**. Avoid or adjust dose. Moderate Theoretical
- **Voxilaprevir** with sofosbuvir and velpatasvir is predicted to increase the exposure to **colchicine**. Avoid P-glycoprotein inhibitors or adjust **colchicine** dose, p. 637. Severe Theoretical
- **Combined hormonal contraceptives** containing ethinylestradiol can increase ALT concentrations when given with **voxilaprevir** with sofosbuvir and velpatasvir. Avoid. Severe Study
- **Dabrafenib** is predicted to decrease the concentration of **voxilaprevir**. Avoid. Severe Theoretical
- **Voxilaprevir** with sofosbuvir and velpatasvir is predicted to increase the exposure to **digoxin**. Monitor and adjust dose. Severe Theoretical
- **Encorafenib** is predicted to decrease the concentration of **voxilaprevir**. Avoid. Severe Study
- Endothelin receptor antagonists **(bosentan)** are predicted to decrease the concentration of **voxilaprevir**. Avoid. Severe Theoretical
- **Voxilaprevir** is predicted to increase the exposure to **erlotinib**. Moderate Theoretical
- **Ethinylestradiol** might increase ALT concentrations when given with **voxilaprevir** with sofosbuvir and velpatasvir. Avoid. Severe Study

- **Voxilaprevir** with sofosbuvir and velpatasvir is predicted to increase the exposure to **everolimus**. Severe Theoretical
- **Voxilaprevir** is predicted to increase the exposure to factor XA inhibitors **(apixaban)**. Moderate Theoretical
- **Voxilaprevir** with sofosbuvir and velpatasvir is predicted to increase the concentration of factor XA inhibitors **(edoxaban)**. Avoid. Severe Theoretical
- **Voxilaprevir** might increase the exposure to factor XA inhibitors **(rivaroxaban)**. Manufacturer advises caution in renal impairment. Moderate Theoretical
- **Voxilaprevir** is predicted to increase the exposure to **fidaxomicin**. Avoid. Moderate Study
- **Voxilaprevir** increases the exposure to **grazoprevir**. Avoid. Severe Theoretical
- HIV-protease inhibitors **(atazanavir)** boosted with ritonavir increase the concentration of **voxilaprevir**. Avoid. Severe Study
- HIV-protease inhibitors **(lopinavir)** boosted with ritonavir are predicted to increase the concentration of **voxilaprevir**. Avoid. Severe Theoretical
- **Hormone replacement therapy** might increase ALT concentrations when given with **voxilaprevir** with sofosbuvir and velpatasvir. Manufacturer advises caution; avoid ethinylestradiol. Severe Theoretical
- **Ivosidenib** is predicted to decrease the concentration of **voxilaprevir**. Avoid. Severe Study
- **Voxilaprevir** with sofosbuvir and velpatasvir is predicted to increase the exposure to **loperamide**. Severe Theoretical
- **Lorlatinib** is predicted to decrease the concentration of **voxilaprevir**. Avoid. Severe Theoretical
- **Lumacaftor** is predicted to decrease the concentration of **voxilaprevir**. Avoid. Severe Study
- **Voxilaprevir** with sofosbuvir and velpatasvir is predicted to increase the exposure to meglitinides **(repaglinide)**. Moderate Study
- **Mitotane** is predicted to decrease the concentration of **voxilaprevir**. Avoid. Severe Study
- **Modafinil** is predicted to decrease the concentration of **voxilaprevir**. Avoid. Severe Theoretical
- **Voxilaprevir** is predicted to increase the exposure to **momelotinib**. Moderate Study
- **Voxilaprevir** is predicted to increase the risk of neutropenia when given with monoclonal antibodies **(brentuximab vedotin)**. Monitor and adjust dose. Severe Theoretical
- **Voxilaprevir** is predicted to increase the exposure to **neratinib**. Avoid or adjust dose and monitor for gastrointestinal adverse effects—consult product literature. Severe Study
- **Voxilaprevir** is predicted to increase the exposure to **nintedanib**. Moderate Study
- **Nirmatrelvir** boosted with ritonavir is predicted to increase the concentration of **voxilaprevir** with sofosbuvir and velpatasvir. Severe Theoretical
- NNRTIs **(efavirenz, etravirine, nevirapine)** are predicted to decrease the concentration of **voxilaprevir**. Avoid. Severe Theoretical
- **Voxilaprevir** is predicted to increase the exposure to **pralsetinib**. Moderate Theoretical
- **Proton pump inhibitors** are predicted to decrease the exposure to **voxilaprevir**. Adjust dose, see sofosbuvir with velpatasvir and voxilaprevir. Moderate Study
- **Voxilaprevir** with sofosbuvir and velpatasvir is predicted to increase the exposure to **ranolazine**. Adjust dose. Severe Theoretical
- **Voxilaprevir** is predicted to increase the exposure to **relugolix**. Avoid or take relugolix first and separate administration by at least 6 hours. Moderate Study
- Rifamycins **(rifabutin)** are predicted to decrease the concentration of **voxilaprevir**. Avoid. Severe Theoretical
- Rifamycins **(rifampicin)** are predicted to decrease the concentration of **voxilaprevir**. Avoid. Severe Study
- **Voxilaprevir** with sofosbuvir and velpatasvir is predicted to increase the exposure to **rimegepant**. Avoid another dose of rimegepant within 48 hours of concurrent use. Moderate Theoretical
- **Voxilaprevir** is predicted to increase the exposure to **seladelpar**. Moderate Study
- **Voxilaprevir** with sofosbuvir and velpatasvir is predicted to increase the exposure to **sirolimus**. Severe Theoretical
- **Sotorasib** is predicted to decrease the concentration of **voxilaprevir**. Avoid. Severe Theoretical
- **St John's wort** is predicted to decrease the concentration of **voxilaprevir**. Avoid. Severe Theoretical
- **Voxilaprevir** with sofosbuvir and velpatasvir is predicted to increase the exposure to statins **(atorvastatin)**. Adjust **atorvastatin** dose, p. 154. Moderate Theoretical
- **Voxilaprevir** with sofosbuvir and velpatasvir is predicted to increase the exposure to statins **(fluvastatin, simvastatin)**. Avoid. Moderate Theoretical
- **Voxilaprevir** with sofosbuvir and velpatasvir moderately increases the exposure to statins **(pravastatin)**. Monitor and adjust **pravastatin** dose. Moderate Study
- **Voxilaprevir** with sofosbuvir and velpatasvir markedly increases the exposure to statins **(rosuvastatin)**. Avoid. Severe Study
- **Voxilaprevir** is predicted to increase the concentration of **sulfasalazine**. Avoid. Severe Theoretical
- **Voxilaprevir** with sofosbuvir and velpatasvir is predicted to increase the exposure to sulfonylureas **(glibenclamide)**. Moderate Study
- **Voxilaprevir** is predicted to slightly increase the exposure to **talazoparib**. Avoid or adjust dose—consult product literature. Severe Study
- **Voxilaprevir** with sofosbuvir and velpatasvir is predicted to increase the exposure to taxanes **(docetaxel, paclitaxel)**. Moderate Study
- **Voxilaprevir** is predicted to increase the exposure to **tenofovir disoproxil**. Moderate Theoretical
- **Voxilaprevir** with sofosbuvir and velpatasvir increases the concentration of thrombin inhibitors **(dabigatran)**. Avoid. Severe Study
- **Voxilaprevir** is predicted to increase the exposure to **topotecan**. Severe Study
- **Voxilaprevir** is predicted to increase the concentration of **trametinib**. Moderate Theoretical

Warfarin → see coumarins

Wasp venom extracts

GENERAL INFORMATION Desensitising vaccines should be avoided in patients taking beta-blockers (adrenaline might be ineffective in case of a hypersensitivity reaction) or ACE inhibitors (risk of severe anaphylactoid reactions).

Xipamide → see thiazide diuretics

Xylometazoline → see sympathomimetics, vasoconstrictor

Yellow fever vaccine → see live vaccines

Zanamivir

- **Zanamivir** might decrease the efficacy of live vaccines **(influenza vaccine (live))**. Moderate Theoretical

Zanubrutinib → see TABLE 3 p. 1053 (bleeding)

FOOD AND LIFESTYLE Bitter (Seville) orange is predicted to increase the exposure to zanubrutinib.

- Anti-androgens **(apalutamide, enzalutamide)** are predicted to decrease the exposure to **zanubrutinib**. Avoid. Severe Study
- Antiarrhythmics **(dronedarone)** are predicted to increase the exposure to **zanubrutinib**. Avoid or adjust dose with moderate CYP3A4 inhibitors—consult product literature. Severe Study
- Antiepileptics **(carbamazepine, fosphenytoin, phenobarbital, phenytoin, primidone)** are predicted to decrease the exposure to **zanubrutinib**. Avoid. Severe Study
- Antifungals, azoles **(fluconazole, isavuconazole)** are predicted to increase the exposure to **zanubrutinib**. Avoid or adjust dose with moderate CYP3A4 inhibitors—consult product literature. Severe Study
- Antifungals, azoles **(itraconazole, ketoconazole, posaconazole, voriconazole)** are predicted to increase the exposure to **zanubrutinib**. Avoid or adjust dose with potent CYP3A4 inhibitors—consult product literature. Moderate Study
- **Berotralstat** is predicted to increase the exposure to **zanubrutinib**. Avoid or adjust dose with moderate CYP3A4 inhibitors—consult product literature. Severe Study
- Calcium-channel blockers **(diltiazem, verapamil)** are predicted to increase the exposure to **zanubrutinib**. Avoid or adjust dose

Zanubrutinib (continued)
with moderate CYP3A4 inhibitors—consult product literature. Severe Study
- **Cenobamate** is predicted to decrease the exposure to **zanubrutinib**. Avoid or adjust dose with moderate CYP3A4 inducers—consult product literature. Severe Theoretical
- **Ceritinib** is predicted to increase the exposure to **zanubrutinib**. Avoid or adjust dose with potent CYP3A4 inhibitors—consult product literature. Moderate Study
- **Cobicistat** is predicted to increase the exposure to **zanubrutinib**. Avoid or adjust dose with potent CYP3A4 inhibitors—consult product literature. Moderate Study
- **Crizotinib** is predicted to increase the exposure to **zanubrutinib**. Avoid or adjust dose with moderate CYP3A4 inhibitors—consult product literature. Severe Study
- **Dabrafenib** is predicted to decrease the exposure to **zanubrutinib**. Avoid or adjust dose with moderate CYP3A4 inducers—consult product literature. Severe Theoretical
- **Encorafenib** is predicted to decrease the exposure to **zanubrutinib**. Avoid. Severe Study
- Endothelin receptor antagonists **(bosentan)** are predicted to decrease the exposure to **zanubrutinib**. Avoid or adjust dose with moderate CYP3A4 inducers—consult product literature. Severe Theoretical
- **Fedratinib** is predicted to increase the exposure to **zanubrutinib**. Avoid or adjust dose with moderate CYP3A4 inhibitors—consult product literature. Severe Study
- **Grapefruit** juice is predicted to increase the exposure to **zanubrutinib**. Moderate Theoretical
- **HIV-protease inhibitors** are predicted to increase the exposure to **zanubrutinib**. Avoid or adjust dose with potent CYP3A4 inhibitors—consult product literature. Moderate Study
- **Idelalisib** is predicted to increase the exposure to **zanubrutinib**. Avoid or adjust dose with potent CYP3A4 inhibitors—consult product literature. Moderate Study
- **Imatinib** is predicted to increase the exposure to **zanubrutinib**. Avoid or adjust dose with moderate CYP3A4 inhibitors—consult product literature. Severe Study → Also see TABLE 3 p. 1053
- **Ivosidenib** is predicted to decrease the exposure to **zanubrutinib**. Avoid. Severe Study
- **Letermovir** is predicted to increase the exposure to **zanubrutinib**. Avoid or adjust dose with moderate CYP3A4 inhibitors—consult product literature. Severe Study
- **Lorlatinib** is predicted to decrease the exposure to **zanubrutinib**. Avoid or adjust dose with moderate CYP3A4 inducers—consult product literature. Severe Theoretical
- **Lumacaftor** is predicted to decrease the exposure to **zanubrutinib**. Avoid. Severe Study
- Macrolides **(clarithromycin)** are predicted to increase the exposure to **zanubrutinib**. Avoid or adjust dose with potent CYP3A4 inhibitors—consult product literature. Moderate Study
- Macrolides **(erythromycin)** are predicted to increase the exposure to **zanubrutinib**. Avoid or adjust dose with moderate CYP3A4 inhibitors—consult product literature. Severe Study
- **Mitotane** is predicted to decrease the exposure to **zanubrutinib**. Avoid. Severe Study
- **Modafinil** is predicted to decrease the exposure to **zanubrutinib**. Avoid. Moderate Theoretical
- Neurokinin-1 receptor antagonists **(aprepitant, netupitant)** are predicted to increase the exposure to **zanubrutinib**. Avoid or adjust dose with moderate CYP3A4 inhibitors—consult product literature. Severe Study
- **Nilotinib** is predicted to increase the exposure to **zanubrutinib**. Avoid or adjust dose with moderate CYP3A4 inhibitors—consult product literature. Severe Study
- NNRTIs **(efavirenz, etravirine, nevirapine)** are predicted to decrease the exposure to **zanubrutinib**. Avoid or adjust dose with moderate CYP3A4 inducers—consult product literature. Severe Theoretical
- Quinolones **(ciprofloxacin)** are predicted to increase the exposure to **zanubrutinib**. Avoid or adjust dose—consult product literature. Severe Theoretical
- Rifamycins **(rifampicin)** are predicted to decrease the exposure to **zanubrutinib**. Avoid. Severe Study
- **Sotorasib** is predicted to decrease the exposure to **zanubrutinib**. Avoid or adjust dose with moderate CYP3A4 inducers—consult product literature. Severe Theoretical
- **St John's wort** is predicted to decrease the exposure to **zanubrutinib**. Avoid or adjust dose with moderate CYP3A4 inducers—consult product literature. Severe Theoretical
- **Tucatinib** is predicted to increase the exposure to **zanubrutinib**. Avoid or adjust dose with potent CYP3A4 inhibitors—consult product literature. Moderate Study

Zidovudine → see NRTIs

Zinc

ROUTE-SPECIFIC INFORMATION Interactions do not generally apply to topical use unless specified.

- Oral **zinc** might decrease the concentration of the active metabolite of oral **baloxavir marboxil**. Avoid. Severe Theoretical
- Oral **zinc** decreases the absorption of oral bisphosphonates **(alendronate)**. **Alendronate** should be taken at least 30 minutes before **zinc**. Moderate Study
- Oral **zinc** decreases the absorption of oral bisphosphonates **(clodronate)**. Avoid **zinc** for 2 hours before or 1 hour after **clodronate**. Moderate Study
- Oral **zinc** is predicted to decrease the absorption of oral bisphosphonates **(ibandronate)**. Avoid **zinc** for at least 6 hours before or 1 hour after **ibandronate**. Moderate Theoretical
- Oral **zinc** decreases the absorption of oral bisphosphonates **(risedronate)**. Separate administration by at least 2 hours. Moderate Study
- Oral **calcium compounds** decrease the absorption of oral **zinc**. Moderate Study
- Oral **zinc** is predicted to decrease the absorption of **eltrombopag**. **Eltrombopag** should be taken 2 hours before or 4 hours after **zinc**. Severe Theoretical
- Oral **zinc** is predicted to decrease the efficacy of oral **iron** and oral **iron** is predicted to decrease the efficacy of oral **zinc**. Moderate Study
- Oral **zinc** is predicted to decrease the absorption of oral iron chelators **(deferiprone)**. Moderate Theoretical
- **Zinc** is predicted to decrease the absorption of **penicillamine**. Mild Theoretical
- **Zinc** is predicted to decrease the exposure to **quinolones**. Separate administration by 2 hours. Moderate Study
- Oral **zinc** is predicted to decrease the absorption of **tetracyclines**. Separate administration by 2 to 3 hours. Moderate Theoretical
- **Trientine** potentially decreases the absorption of **zinc**. Moderate Theoretical

Zoledronate → see bisphosphonates

Zolmitriptan → see triptans

Zolpidem → see TABLE 9 p. 1056 (CNS effects)
- Anti-androgens **(enzalutamide)** are predicted to affect the exposure to **zolpidem**. Use with caution or avoid. Moderate Theoretical
- Antiepileptics **(carbamazepine)** moderately decrease the exposure to **zolpidem**. Moderate Study
- **Idelalisib** is predicted to increase the exposure to **zolpidem**. Monitor and adjust dose. Moderate Theoretical
- **Nirmatrelvir** boosted with ritonavir is predicted to increase the concentration of **zolpidem**. Severe Theoretical
- Rifamycins **(rifampicin)** moderately decrease the exposure to **zolpidem**. Moderate Study

Zonisamide → see antiepileptics

Zopiclone → see TABLE 9 p. 1056 (CNS effects)
- Anti-androgens **(apalutamide, enzalutamide)** are predicted to decrease the exposure to **zopiclone**. Adjust dose. Moderate Study
- Antiarrhythmics **(dronedarone)** are predicted to increase the exposure to **zopiclone**. Adjust dose. Moderate Study
- Antiepileptics **(carbamazepine, fosphenytoin, phenobarbital, phenytoin, primidone)** are predicted to decrease the exposure to **zopiclone**. Adjust dose. Moderate Study → Also see TABLE 9 p. 1056
- Antifungals, azoles **(fluconazole, isavuconazole)** are predicted to increase the exposure to **zopiclone**. Adjust dose. Moderate Study

- Antifungals, azoles **(itraconazole, ketoconazole, posaconazole, voriconazole)** are predicted to increase the exposure to **zopiclone**. Adjust dose. [Moderate] Theoretical
- **Berotralstat** is predicted to increase the exposure to **zopiclone**. Adjust dose. [Moderate] Study
- Calcium-channel blockers **(diltiazem, verapamil)** are predicted to increase the exposure to **zopiclone**. Adjust dose. [Moderate] Study
- **Ceritinib** is predicted to increase the exposure to **zopiclone**. Adjust dose. [Moderate] Theoretical
- **Cobicistat** is predicted to increase the exposure to **zopiclone**. Adjust dose. [Moderate] Theoretical
- **Crizotinib** is predicted to increase the exposure to **zopiclone**. Adjust dose. [Moderate] Study
- **Encorafenib** is predicted to decrease the exposure to **zopiclone**. Adjust dose. [Moderate] Study
- **Fedratinib** is predicted to increase the exposure to **zopiclone**. Adjust dose. [Moderate] Study
- **HIV-protease inhibitors** are predicted to increase the exposure to **zopiclone**. Adjust dose. [Moderate] Theoretical
- **Idelalisib** is predicted to increase the exposure to **zopiclone**. Adjust dose. [Moderate] Theoretical
- **Imatinib** is predicted to increase the exposure to **zopiclone**. Adjust dose. [Moderate] Study
- **Ivosidenib** is predicted to decrease the exposure to **zopiclone**. Adjust dose. [Moderate] Study
- **Letermovir** is predicted to increase the exposure to **zopiclone**. Adjust dose. [Moderate] Study
- **Lumacaftor** is predicted to decrease the exposure to **zopiclone**. Adjust dose. [Moderate] Study
- Macrolides **(clarithromycin)** are predicted to increase the exposure to **zopiclone**. Adjust dose. [Moderate] Theoretical
- Macrolides **(erythromycin)** are predicted to increase the exposure to **zopiclone**. Adjust dose. [Moderate] Study
- **Mitotane** is predicted to decrease the exposure to **zopiclone**. Adjust dose. [Moderate] Study
- Neurokinin-1 receptor antagonists **(aprepitant, netupitant)** are predicted to increase the exposure to **zopiclone**. Adjust dose. [Moderate] Study
- **Nilotinib** is predicted to increase the exposure to **zopiclone**. Adjust dose. [Moderate] Study
- Rifamycins **(rifampicin)** are predicted to decrease the exposure to **zopiclone**. Adjust dose. [Moderate] Study
- **Tucatinib** is predicted to increase the exposure to **zopiclone**. Adjust dose. [Moderate] Theoretical

Zuclopenthixol → see TABLE 15 p. 1058 (hyponatraemia), TABLE 6 p. 1054 (hypotension), TABLE 8 p. 1055 (antimuscarinics), TABLE 9 p. 1056 (CNS effects)

- Atypical antipsychotics **(clozapine)** can cause constipation, as can **zuclopenthixol**; concurrent use might increase the risk of developing intestinal obstruction. [Severe] Theoretical → Also see TABLE 15 p. 1058 → Also see TABLE 6 p. 1054 → Also see TABLE 8 p. 1055 → Also see TABLE 9 p. 1056
- **Zuclopenthixol** is predicted to decrease the effects of **dopamine receptor agonists**. Avoid. [Moderate] Theoretical → Also see TABLE 6 p. 1054 → Also see TABLE 8 p. 1055 → Also see TABLE 9 p. 1056
- **Zuclopenthixol** opposes the effects of the active metabolite of **foslevodopa**. [Severe] Theoretical → Also see TABLE 6 p. 1054 → Also see TABLE 9 p. 1056
- **Zuclopenthixol** is predicted to decrease the effects of **levodopa**. Avoid or monitor worsening parkinsonian symptoms. [Severe] Theoretical → Also see TABLE 6 p. 1054 → Also see TABLE 9 p. 1056
- **Zuclopenthixol** potentially increases the risk of neurotoxicity when given with **lithium**. [Severe] Anecdotal

Appendix 2
Borderline substances

CONTENTS

In certain conditions some foods (and toilet preparations) have characteristics of drugs and the Advisory Committee on Borderline Substances (ACBS) advises as to the circumstances in which such substances may be regarded as drugs. Prescriptions issued in accordance with the Committee's advice and endorsed 'ACBS' will normally not be investigated.

Information

General Practitioners are reminded that the ACBS recommends products on the basis that they may be regarded as drugs for the management of specified conditions. Doctors should satisfy themselves that the products can safely be prescribed, that patients are adequately monitored and that, where necessary, expert hospital supervision is available.

Foods which may be prescribed on FP10, GP10 (Scotland), or WP10 (Wales)

All the food products listed in this appendix have ACBS approval. The clinical condition for which the product has been approved is included with each entry.

Note Foods included in this appendix may contain cariogenic sugars and patients should be advised to take appropriate oral hygiene measures.

Enteral feeds and oral nutritional supplements

For most enteral feeds and oral nutritional supplements, the main source of **carbohydrate** is either maltodextrin or glucose syrup; other carbohydrate sources include fructose, hydrolysed corn starch, and sucrose. Products containing residual lactose (less than 1 g lactose/100 mL formula) are described as 'clinically lactose-free' or 'lactose-free' by some manufacturers. The presence of lactose (including residual lactose) is indicated in the relevant entry. The primary sources of **protein** or **amino acids** are included with each product entry. The **fat** or **oil** content is derived from a variety of sources such as vegetables, soya bean, corn, palm nuts, and seeds; where the fat content is derived from animal or fish sources, this information is included in the relevant product entry. The presence of medium chain triglycerides (MCT) is also noted where the quantity exceeds 30% of the fat content.

Enteral feeds and oral nutritional supplements can contain varying amounts of **vitamins**, **minerals**, and **trace elements**—the manufacturer's product literature should be consulted for more detailed information. Products containing vitamin K may affect the INR in patients receiving warfarin.
The suitability of food products for patients requiring a vegan, kosher, halal, or other compliant diet should be confirmed with individual manufacturers.
Note Feeds containing more than 6 g/100 mL protein or 2 g/100 mL fibre should be avoided in children unless recommended by an appropriate specialist or dietician.

Nutritional values

Representative values for enteral feeds and oral nutritional supplements are included where nutritional values vary between flavour or pack size, and are usually based on neutral or vanilla flavour.
For details of all presentations of a product range, consult product literature.

Other conditions for which ACBS products can be prescribed

Clinical conditions for which the ACBS has approved toilet preparations.

Dermatitis, Eczema and Pruritus
See Emollient and barrier preparations p. 888
Disfiguring skin lesions (birthmarks, mutilating lesions, scars, vitiligo)
See Camouflages p. 946
Disinfectants (antiseptics)
See Skin cleansers, antiseptics and desloughing agents p. 943
Photodermatoses (skin protection in)
See Sunscreen p. 947

Paediatric ACBS indications: Disease-related malnutrition, intractable malabsorption, growth failure, pre-operative preparation of malnourished patients, dysphagia, short-bowel syndrome, bowel fistula
Standard ACBS indications: Disease-related malnutrition, intractable malabsorption, pre-operative preparation of malnourished patients, dysphagia, proven inflammatory bowel disease, following total gastrectomy, short-bowel syndrome, bowel fistula

Table 1 Enteral nutrition

Tube feeds: Additional protein fortifiers

1 kcal/mL higher protein

Product	Formulation	Energy	Protein	Carbohydrate	Fat	Fibre	Special Characteristics	ACBS Indications	Presentation & Flavour
Nutrison® Protein Shot (Nutricia Ltd)	Liquid (tube feed) per 100 mL	480 kJ (113 kcal)	27.5 g whey protein hydrolysate	0.6 g	0.1 g	Nil	Contains beef derivatives, residual lactose	Disease related malnutrition for tube fed patients with increased protein requirements.	Nutrison Protein Shot liquid: 240 ml = £9.77
Not suitable for use in child under 3 years									
ProSource® TF (Nutrinovo Ltd)	Liquid (tube feed) per 100 mL	373 kJ (98 kcal)	24.4 g collagen protein, protein equivalent (amino acids)	2.2 g (sugars Nil)	Less than 1 g	Less than 1 g	Contains bovine derivatives. Gluten-free, lactose-free	Hypoproteinaemia.	ProSource TF liquid 45ml sachets: 100 sachet = £164.21
Not recommended for child under 3 years									
ProSource® TF ENFit (Nutrinovo Ltd)	Liquid (tube feed) per 100 mL	530 kJ (127 kcal)	33.3 g collagen protein, protein equivalent (amino acids)	0.55 g (sugars 0.55 g)	0.2 g	0.33 g	Contains bovine derivatives. Gluten-free, lactose-free	Hypoproteinaemia.	ProSource TF ENFit liquid 60ml sachets: 50 sachet = £139.27
Not recommended for child under 3 years									

2 kcal/mL higher protein

Product	Formulation	Energy	Protein	Carbohydrate	Fat	Fibre	Special Characteristics	ACBS Indications	Presentation & Flavour
ProSource® TF plant (Nutrinovo Ltd)	Liquid (tube feed) per 100 mL	837 kJ (200 kcal)	33 g pea protein hydrolysate	12 g (sugars less than 1 g)	1.1 g	1.5 g	Gluten-free, lactose-free	Hypoproteinaemia.	ProSource TF plant liquid 45ml sachets: 50 sachet = £124.95
Not recommended for child under 3 years									

Tube feeds: Critically ill

1.5 kcal/mL peptide based, higher protein

Product	Formulation	Energy	Protein	Carbohydrate	Fat	Fibre	Special Characteristics	ACBS Indications	Presentation & Flavour
Peptamen® AF (Nestle Health Science)	Liquid (tube feed) per 100 mL	638 kJ (152 kcal)	9.4 g whey protein	14 g (sugars 1.4 g)	6.5 g (MCT 52 %)	Nil	Contains fish oil, residual lactose, soya. Gluten-free	Borderline substances standard ACBS indications p. 1375 except dysphagia.	Peptamen AF liquid: 500 ml = £11.45
Suitable for over 3 years									

Tube feeds: Impaired gastro-intestinal function or malabsorption

Less than 1 kcal/mL peptide based

Product	Formulation	Energy	Protein	Carbohydrate	Fat	Fibre	Special Characteristics	ACBS Indications	Presentation & Flavour
Peptamen® Junior 0.6 (Nestle Health Science)	Liquid (tube feed) per 100 mL	254 kJ (60 kcal)	2.3 g whey protein	6.8 g (sugars 1.5 g)	2.5 g (MCT 36%)	0.8 g	Contains fish oil, residual lactose, soya. Gluten-free	Disease-related malnutrition in patients with malabsorption and/or maldigestion who have reduced energy requirements.	Peptamen Junior 0.6 liquid: 500 ml = £9.49
Not suitable for use in child under 1 year									

1 to less than 1.5 kcal/mL peptide based

Product	Formulation	Energy	Protein	Carbohydrate	Fat	Fibre	Special Characteristics	ACBS Indications	Presentation & Flavour
Nutrini® Peptisorb (Nutricia Ltd)	Liquid (tube feed) per 100 mL	419 kJ (100 kcal)	2.8 g whey protein hydrolysate	13.6 g (sugars 0.43 g)	3.9 g (MCT 46 %)	Nil	Contains residual lactose, soya. Gluten-free	Borderline substances standard ACBS indications p. 1375 and growth failure.	Nutrini Peptisorb liquid: 500 ml = £17.52
Not suitable for use in child under 1 year; not recommended for child over 6 years									
Nutrison® Peptisorb (Nutricia Ltd)	Liquid (tube feed) per 100 mL	425 kJ (100 kcal)	4 g whey protein hydrolysate	17.6 g (sugars 1.7 g)	1.7 g (MCT 47 %)	Nil	Contains residual lactose, soya. Gluten-free	Borderline substances standard ACBS indications p. 1375; also growth failure.	Nutrison Peptisorb liquid: 500 ml = £12.71
Not suitable for use in child under 1 year; not recommended for child 1-6 years									
PaediaSure® Peptide tube feed (Abbott Laboratories Ltd)	Liquid (tube feed) per 100 mL	420 kJ (100 kcal)	3 g caseinates, whey protein hydrolysate	13 g (sugars 2.7 g)	4 (MCT 46%) g	Nil	Contains residual lactose, soya. Gluten-free	Borderline substances standard ACBS indications p. 1375; also growth failure.	PaediaSure Peptide tube feed liquid: 500 ml = £17.58
Not suitable for use in child under 1 year; suitable for child 1-10 years or 8-30 kg									
Peptamen® HN (Nestle Health Science)	Liquid (sip or tube feed) per 100 mL	559 kJ (133 kcal)	6.6 g whey protein hydrolysate	16 g (sugars 1.4 g)	4.9 g (MCT 69%)	Nil	Contains meat derivatives, residual lactose, soya. Gluten-free	Impaired gastrointestinal function, short bowel syndrome, intractable malabsorption, proven inflammatory bowel disease and bowel fistula or with higher nutritional requirements.	Peptamen HN liquid: 500 ml = £10.48; 1000 ml = £19.66
Not suitable for use in child under 3 years									
Peptamen® Junior Liquid (Nestle Health Science)	Liquid (tube feed) per 100 mL	420 kJ (100 kcal)	3 g whey protein hydrolysate	13 g (sugars 2.5 g)	4 g (MCT 60%)	less than 1 g	Contains residual lactose, soya. Gluten-free	Short-bowel syndrome, intractable malabsorption, proven inflammatory bowel disease, bowel fistulae.	Peptamen Junior liquid: 500 ml = £9.73
Not suitable for use in child under 1 year; not recommended for child over 10 years									
Peptamen® Junior PHGG (Nestle Health Science)	Liquid (tube feed) per 100 mL	518 kJ (124 kcal)	3.6 g whey protein	15.0 g (sugars 3.0 g)	5.2 g (MCT 54%)	1.2 g	Contains fish oil, residual lactose, soya lecithin. Gluten-free	Short bowel syndrome, intractable malabsorption, proven inflammatory bowel disease and bowel fistulae.	Peptamen Junior PHGG tube feed liquid: 500 ml = £8.86
Suitable for child 1-10 years									
Peptamen® tube feed (Nestle Health Science)	Liquid (sip or tube feed) per 100 mL	421 kJ (100 kcal)	4 g whey protein	13 g (sugars 0.48 g)	3.7 g (MCT 70 %)	Nil	Contains residual lactose, soya. Gluten-free	Short bowel syndrome, intractable malabsorption, proven inflammatory bowel disease, bowel fistulae.	Peptamen tube feed liquid unflavoured: 500 ml = £9.74; 1000 ml = £18.28
Not suitable for use in child under 3 years; not recommended for child under 5 years									

1 to less than 1.5 kcal/mL peptide based (product list continued)

Product	Formulation	Energy	Protein	Carbohydrate	Fat	Fibre	Special Characteristics	ACBS Indications	Presentation & Flavour
Survimed® OPD HN (Fresenius Kabi Ltd)	Liquid (tube feed) per 100 mL	560 kJ (133 kcal)	6.7 g whey protein hydrolysate	18.3 g (sugars 1.33 g)	3.7 g (MCT 52%)	Less than or equal to 0.1 g	Contains fish oil, residual lactose. Gluten-free	Borderline substances standard ACBS indications p. 1375; also haemodialysis and continuous ambulatory peritoneal dialysis.	Survimed OPD HN liquid: 500 ml = £10.15
Not suitable for use in child under 3 years; use with caution in child under 6 years									
Survimed® OPD tube feed (Fresenius Kabi Ltd)	Liquid (tube feed) per 100 mL	420 kJ (100 kcal)	4.5 g whey protein hydrolysate	14.3 g (sugars 1.1 g)	2.8 g (MCT 51%)	Less than or equal to 0.1 g	Contains fish oil, residual lactose. Gluten-free	Borderline substances standard ACBS indications p. 1375	Survimed OPD tube feed liquid: 500 ml = £10.47; 1000 ml = £19.81
Not suitable for use in child under 3 years; use with caution in child under 6 years									

1.5 kcal/mL or more peptide based

Product	Formulation	Energy	Protein	Carbohydrate	Fat	Fibre	Special Characteristics	ACBS Indications	Presentation & Flavour
Nutrini® Peptisorb Energy (Nutricia Ltd)	Liquid (tube feed) per 100 mL	630 kJ (150 kcal)	4.2 g whey protein hydrolysate	18.6 g (sugars 0.4 g)	6.6 g (MCT 52%)	Less than 0.5 g	Contains fish oil, residual lactose, soya. Gluten-free	Borderline substances paediatric ACBS indications p. 1375; also proven inflammatory bowel disease and following total gastrectomy.	Nutrini Peptisorb Energy liquid: 500 ml = £17.53
Not suitable for use in child under 1 year; not suitable for use in child over 6 years									
Nutrison® Peptisorb Plus HEHP (Nutricia Ltd)	Liquid (tube feed) per 100 ml	631 kJ (150 kcal)	7.5 g whey protein hydrolysate	18.7 g (sugars 1.4 g)	5 g (MCT 60%)	Less than 0.5 g	Contains residual lactose, soya. Gluten-free	Borderline substances standard ACBS indications p. 1375 except dysphagia.	Nutrison Peptisorb Plus HEHP liquid: 500 ml = £12.66; 1000 ml = £23.83
Not suitable for use in child under 1 year; not recommended for child 1-6 years									
Peptamen® Junior Advance (Nestle Health Science)	Liquid (tube feed) per 100 mL	632 kJ (151 kcal)	4.5 g whey protein hydrolysate	18 g (sugars 2.1 g)	6.6 g (MCT 61%)	0.7 g	Contains fish oil, residual lactose, soya. Gluten-free.	Short-bowel syndrome, intractable malabsorption, proven inflammatory bowel disease, bowel fistula.	Peptamen Junior Advance liquid: 500 ml = £11.11
Not suitable for use in child under 1 year, not recommended for child over 10 years									

Tube feeds: Non-milk based feeds

1 kcal/mL soya based

Product	Formulation	Energy	Protein	Carbohydrate	Fat	Fibre	Special Characteristics	ACBS Indications	Presentation & Flavour
Nutrison® PlantBased Soya (Nutricia Ltd)	Liquid (tube feed) per 100 mL	420 kJ (100 kcal)	4 g soya protein	12.3 g (sugars 0.97 g)	3.9 g	Nil	Contains residual lactose, soya. Gluten-free	Borderline substances standard ACBS indications p. 1375; also cow's milk protein and lactose intolerance.	Nutrison PlantBased Soya liquid: 1000 ml = £17.45
Not suitable for use in child under 3 years; use with caution in child over 3 years									

1 kcal/mL soya based with fibre

Product	Formulation	Energy	Protein	Carbohydrate	Fat	Fibre	Special Characteristics	ACBS Indications	Presentation & Flavour
Fresubin® Soya Fibre (Fresenius Kabi Ltd)	Liquid (tube feed) per 100 mL	420 kJ (100 kcal)	3.8 g soya protein	12.1 g (sugars 4.1 g)	3.6 g	2 g	Contains fish oil, soya. Gluten-free, lactose-free	Borderline substances standard ACBS indications p. 1375 except dysphagia. Also cow's milk protein intolerance, lactose intolerance.	Fresubin Soya Fibre liquid: 500 ml = £7.15
Not suitable for use in child under 3 years; use with caution in child under 6 years									
Nutrison® PlantBased Soya Multi Fibre (Nutricia Ltd)	Liquid (tube feed) per 100 mL	430 kJ (103 kcal)	4 g soya protein	12.3 g (sugars 0.7 g)	3.9 g	1.5 g	Contains residual lactose, soya. Gluten-free	Borderline substances standard ACBS indications p. 1375; also cows' milk protein and lactose intolerance.	Nutrison PlantBased Soya Multi Fibre liquid: 1500 ml = £29.02
Not suitable for use in child under 3 years; use with caution in child over 3 years									

Tube feeds: Standard feeds

Less than 1 kcal/mL with fibre

Product	Formulation	Energy	Protein	Carbohydrate	Fat	Fibre	Special Characteristics	ACBS Indications	Presentation & Flavour
Nutrini® Low Energy Multifibre (Nutricia Ltd)	Liquid (tube feed) per 100 mL	320 kJ (76 kcal)	2 g caseinates, whey protein	9.3 g (sugars 0.6 g)	3.3 g	0.7 g	Contains fish oil, residual lactose, soya. Gluten-free	Borderline substances paediatric ACBS indications p. 1375 except bowel fistula; also total gastrectomy.	Nutrini Low Energy Multifibre liquid: 200 ml = £4.31; 500 ml = £11.00
Not suitable for use in child under 1 year; not recommended for child over 6 years									

Less than 1 kcal/mL with fibre, higher protein

Product	Formulation	Energy	Protein	Carbohydrate	Fat	Fibre	Special Characteristics	ACBS Indications	Presentation & Flavour
Nutrison® 800 Complete Multi Fibre (Nutricia Ltd)	Liquid (tube feed) per 100 mL	345 kJ (83 kcal)	5.5 g caseinate, pea, soya, whey proteins	8.8 g (sugars 0.6 g)	2.5 g	1.5 g	Contains fish oil, residual lactose, soya. Gluten-free	Borderline substances standard ACBS indications p. 1375 except bowel fistula.	Nutrison 800 Complete Multi Fibre liquid: 1000 ml = £17.16
Not suitable for use in child under 6 years; not recommended for child under 12 years									

1 to less than 1.5 kcal/mL

Product	Formulation	Energy	Protein	Carbohydrate	Fat	Fibre	Special Characteristics	ACBS Indications	Presentation & Flavour
Frebini® Original (Fresenius Kabi Ltd)	Liquid (tube feed) per 100 mL	420 kJ (100 kcal)	2.5 g milk protein	12.5 g (sugars 0.9 g)	4.4 g	Nil	Contains fish oil, residual lactose, soya. Gluten-free	Borderline substances standard ACBS indications p. 1375 and growth failure.	Frebini Original liquid: 500 ml = £9.73
Not suitable for use in child under 1 year or in adults; not recommended for child over 10 years									
Fresubin® Original tube feed (Fresenius Kabi Ltd)	Liquid (tube feed) per 100 mL	420 kJ (100 kcal)	3.8 g milk, soya proteins	13.8 g (sugars 0.85 g)	3.4 g	Nil	Contains fish oil, residual lactose, soya. Gluten-free	Borderline substances standard ACBS indications p. 1375; also Refsum's Disease.	Fresubin Original tube feed liquid: 500 ml = £7.04; 1000 ml = £11.92; 1500 ml = £18.46
Not suitable for use in child under 3 years; use with caution in child under 6 years									
Infatrini® tube feed (Nutricia Ltd)	Liquid (tube feed) per 100 mL	418 kJ (100 kcal)	2.6 g cow's milk, whey protein	10.2 g (sugars 5.9 g)	5.3 g	0.57 g	Contains fish oil, lactose, soya. Gluten-free	Disease-related malnutrition, malabsorption, and growth failure.	Infatrini tube feed liquid: 500 ml = £9.74
Suitable for child from birth to 18 months or less than 9 kg									

1 to less than 1.5 kcal/mL (product list continued)

Product	Formulation	Energy	Protein	Carbohydrate	Fat	Fibre	Special Characteristics	ACBS Indications	Presentation & Flavour
Nutrini® (Nutricia Ltd)	Liquid (tube feed) per 100 mL	420 kJ (100 kcal)	2.7 g caseinate, whey protein	12.3 g (sugars 0.8 g)	4.4 g	Nil	Contains fish oil, residual lactose, soya. Gluten-free	Borderline substances paediatric ACBS indications p. 1375.	Nutrini liquid: 200 ml = £4.49; 500 ml = £11.20
Not suitable for use in child under 1 year; not recommended for child over 6 years									
Nutrison® (Nutricia Ltd)	Liquid (tube feed) per 100 mL	420 kJ (100 kcal)	4 g cow's milk, pea, soya, whey proteins	12.4 g (sugars 0.81 g)	3.9 g	Nil	Contains fish oil, residual lactose, soya. Gluten-free	Borderline substances standard ACBS indications p. 1375.	Nutrison liquid: 500 ml = £8.06; 1000 ml = £14.17; 1500 ml = £21.28
Not suitable for use in child under 3 years; use with caution in child over 3 years									
PaediaSure® tube feed (Abbott Laboratories Ltd)	Liquid (tube feed) per 100 mL	422 kJ (101 kcal)	2.8 g caseinate, milk protein isolate, whey protein	11.16 g (sugars 3.7 g)	4.98 g	Nil	Contains residual lactose, soya. Gluten-free	Borderline substances paediatric ACBS indications p. 1375.	PaediaSure tube feed liquid: 500 ml = £11.26
Not suitable for use in child under 1 year; suitable for child 1-10 years or 8-30 kg									
Tentrini® (Nutricia Ltd)	Liquid (tube feed) per 100 mL	420 kJ (100 kcal)	3.3 g caseinates, whey protein	12.3 g (sugars 0.8 g)	4.2 g	Nil	Contains fish oil, residual lactose, soya. Gluten-free	Borderline substances paediatric ACBS indications p. 1375; also inflammatory bowel disease and total gastrectomy.	Tentrini liquid: 500 ml = £9.87
Not suitable for use in child under 1 year; not recommended for child under 6 years, not recommended for child over 12 years									

1 to less than 1.5 kcal/mL higher protein

Product	Formulation	Energy	Protein	Carbohydrate	Fat	Fibre	Special Characteristics	ACBS Indications	Presentation & Flavour
Nutrison® Protein Plus (Nutricia Ltd)	Liquid (tube feed) per 100 mL	525 kJ (125 kcal)	6.3 g caseinates, pea, soya, whey proteins	14.2 g (sugars 0.9 g)	4.9 g	Less than 0.1 g	Contains fish oil, residual lactose, soya. Gluten-free	Disease related malnutrition.	Nutrison Protein Plus liquid: 500 ml = £8.70; 1000 ml = £16.84
Not suitable for use in child under 1 year; not recommended for child 1–6 years									

1 to less than 1.5 kcal/mL with fibre

Product	Formulation	Energy	Protein	Carbohydrate	Fat	Fibre	Special Characteristics	ACBS Indications	Presentation & Flavour
Compleat® 1.1 (Nestle Health Science)	Liquid (tube feed) per 100 mL	461 kJ (110 kcal)	4.4 g chicken, milk proteins	14 g (sugars 1.4 g)	3.7 g	1.4 g	Contains fish oil, meat derivatives, residual lactose. Gluten-free	Borderline substances standard ACBS indications p. 1375; also feeding intolerance, and developmental disabilities.	Compleat 1.1 tube feed liquid: 1000 ml = £14.38
Suitable from 3 years									
Compleat® Paediatric (Nestle Health Science)	Liquid (tube feed) per 100 mL	492 kJ (117 kcal)	3.6 g chicken, milk proteins	14 g (sugars 1.3 g)	5 g	1 g	Contains fish oil, meat derivatives, residual lactose. Gluten-free	Borderline substances standard ACBS indications p. 1375; also feeding intolerance, and developmental disabilities.	Compleat: paediatric (SimpLink) 250 ml = £4.17; paediatric 500 ml = £8.88
Suitable from 1 year									

Frebini® Original Fibre (Fresenius Kabi Ltd)	Liquid (tube feed) **per 100 mL**	420 kJ (100 kcal)	2.5 g milk protein	12.1 g (sugars 0.9 g)	4.5 g	0.8 g	Contains fish oil, residual lactose, soya. Gluten-free	Borderline substances paediatric ACBS indications p. 1375; also proven inflammatory bowel disease, and following total gastrectomy.	Frebini Original Fibre liquid: 500 ml = £10.81
Not suitable for use in child under 1 year or in adults; not recommended for child over 10 years									
Fresubin® 1500 Complete (Fresenius Kabi Ltd)	Liquid (tube feed) **per 100 mL**	420 kJ (100 kcal)	3.8 g milk, soya proteins	13 g (sugars 0.9 g)	3.4 g	1.5 g	Contains fish oil, residual lactose, soya. Gluten-free	Borderline substances standard ACBS indications p. 1375 except bowel fistula and pre-operative preparation of malnourished patients.	Fresubin 1500 Complete liquid: 1.5 litre = £20.64
Not suitable for use in child under 3 years; use with caution in child under 6 years									
Fresubin® Original Fibre (Fresenius Kabi Ltd)	Liquid (tube feed) **per 100 mL**	420 kJ (100 kcal)	3.8 g milk, soya proteins	13.0 g (sugars 0.9 g)	3.4 g	1.5 g	Contains fish oil, residual lactose, soya. Gluten-free	Borderline substances standard ACBS indications p. 1375 except bowel fistula and pre-operative preparation of malnourished patients.	Fresubin Original Fibre liquid: 500 ml = £7.16; 1000 ml = £13.78
Not suitable for use in child under 3 years; use with caution in child under 6 years									
Nutrini® Multifibre (Nutricia Ltd)	Liquid (tube feed) **per 100 mL**	425 kJ (101 kcal)	2.7 g caseinates, whey protein	12.3 g (sugars 0.8 g)	4.4 g	0.8 g	Contains fish oil, residual lactose, soya. Gluten-free	Borderline substances paediatric ACBS indications p. 1375; also proven inflammatory bowel disease, following total gastrectomy.	Nutrini Multifibre liquid: 200 ml = £4.97; 500 ml = £12.42
Not suitable for use in child under 1 year, not suitable for use in child over 6 years									
Nutrison® Multi Fibre (Nutricia Ltd)	Liquid (tube feed) **per 100 mL**	433 kJ (103 kcal)	4 g caseinate, pea, soya, whey proteins	12.3 g (sugars 0.88 g)	3.9 g	1.5 g	Contains fish oil, residual lactose, soya. Gluten-free	Borderline substances standard ACBS indications p. 1375.	Nutrison Multi Fibre liquid: 500 ml = £8.72; 1000 ml = £16.40; 1500 ml = £24.59
Not suitable for use in child under 3 years; use with caution in child over 3 years									
PaediaSure® Fibre tube feed (Abbott Laboratories Ltd)	Liquid (tube feed) **per 100 mL**	424 kJ (101 kcal)	2.8 g caseinates, whey protein	10.9 g (sugars 3.75 g)	4.98 g	0.73 g	Contains residual lactose, soya. Gluten-free	Borderline substances paediatric ACBS indications p. 1375.	PaediaSure fibre tube feed liquid: 500 ml = £12.51
Not suitable for use in child under 1 year; suitable for child 1-10 years or 8-30 kg									
Tentrini® Multifibre (Nutricia Ltd)	Liquid (tube feed) **per 100 mL**	430 kJ (102 kcal)	3.3 g caseinates, whey protein	12.3 g (sugars 0.8 g)	4.2 g	1.1 g	Contains fish oil, residual lactose, soya	Borderline substances paediatric ACBS indications p. 1375 except bowel fistula; also inflammatory bowel disease, and total gastrectomy.	Tentrini Multifibre liquid: 500 ml = £10.88
Not suitable for use in child under 1 year; not recommended for child 1-6 years, not recommended for child over 12 years									

1 to less than 1.5 kcal/mL with fibre, higher protein

Product	Formulation	Energy	Protein	Carbohydrate	Fat	Fibre	Special Characteristics	ACBS Indications	Presentation & Flavour
Fresubin® 1000 Complete (Fresenius Kabi Ltd)	Liquid (tube feed) **per 100 mL**	418 kJ (100 kcal)	5.5 g milk protein	12.5 g (sugars 1.1 g)	2.7 g	2 g	Contains fish oil, residual lactose, soya lecithin. Gluten-free	Borderline substances standard ACBS indications p. 1375	Fresubin 1000 Complete liquid: 1 litre = £14.88
Not suitable for use in child under 3 years; use with caution in child under 6 years									

1 to less than 1.5 kcal/mL with fibre, higher protein (product list continued)

Product	Formulation	Energy	Protein	Carbohydrate	Fat	Fibre	Special Characteristics	ACBS Indications	Presentation & Flavour
Fresubin® 1200 Complete (Fresenius Kabi Ltd)	Liquid (tube feed) per 100 mL	504 kJ (120 kcal)	6 g milk protein	14 g (sugars 1.17 g)	4.1 g	2 g	Contains fish oil, residual lactose, soya lecithin. Gluten-free	Borderline substances standard ACBS indications p. 1375 except dysphagia.	Fresubin 1200 Complete liquid: 1 litre = £17.45
Not suitable for use in child under 3 years; use with caution in child under 6 years									
Fresubin® 1800 Complete (Fresenius Kabi Ltd)	Liquid (tube feed) per 100 mL	504 kJ (120 kcal)	6 g milk protein	14 g (sugars 1.17 g)	4.1 g	2 g	Contains fish oil, residual lactose, soya lecithin. Gluten-free	Borderline substances standard ACBS indications p. 1375 except dysphagia.	Fresubin 1800 Complete liquid: 1.5 litre = £18.55
Not suitable for use in child under 3 years; use with caution in child under 6 years									
Nutrison® 1000 Complete Multi Fibre (Nutricia Ltd)	Liquid (tube feed) per 100 mL	440 kJ (104 kcal)	5.5 g caseinate, pea, soya, whey proteins	11.3 g (sugars 0.8 g)	3.7 g	2 g	Contains fish oil, residual lactose, soya. Gluten-free	Disease related malnutrition in patients with low energy and/or low fluid requirements.	Nutrison 1000 Complete Multi Fibre liquid: 1000 ml = £18.22
Not suitable for use in child under 1 year; not recommended for child under 12 years									
Nutrison® 1200 Complete Multi Fibre (Nutricia Ltd)	Liquid (tube feed) per 100 mL	525 kJ (124 kcal)	5.5 g caseinates, pea, soya, whey proteins	15 g (sugars 1 g)	4.3 g	2 g	Contains fish oil, residual lactose, soya. Gluten-free	Borderline substances standard ACBS indications p. 1375 except bowel fistula.	Nutrison 1200 Complete Multi Fibre liquid: 1000 ml = £19.26; 1500 ml = £28.94
Not suitable for use in child under 1 year; not recommended for child under 12 years									
Nutrison® Protein Plus Multifibre (Nutricia Ltd)	Liquid (tube feed) per 100 mL	535 kJ (128 kcal)	6.3 g caseinates, pea, soya, whey proteins	14.1 g (sugars 1 g)	4.9 g	1.5 g	Contains fish oil, residual lactose, soya. Gluten-free	Disease related malnutrition.	Nutrison Protein Plus Multifibre liquid: 500 ml = £9.66; 1000 ml = £18.77
Not suitable for use in child under 1 year; not recommended in child 1-6 years									

1.5 to less than 2 kcal/mL

Product	Formulation	Energy	Protein	Carbohydrate	Fat	Fibre	Special Characteristics	ACBS Indications	Presentation & Flavour
Frebini® Energy tube feed (Fresenius Kabi Ltd)	Liquid (tube feed) per 100 mL	630 kJ (150 kcal)	3.8 g milk protein	18.7 g (sugars 2.5 g)	6.7 g	Nil	Contains fish oil, residual lactose, soya. Gluten-free	Borderline substances standard ACBS indications p. 1375; also growth failure.	Frebini Energy liquid unflavoured: 500 ml = £12.22
Not suitable for use in child under 1 year or in adults; not recommended for child over 10 years									
Fresubin® Energy tube feed (Fresenius Kabi Ltd)	Liquid (tube feed) per 100 mL	630 kJ (150 kcal)	5.6 g milk protein, whey protein	18.8 g (sugars 1.15 g)	5.8 g	Nil	Contains fish oil, residual lactose, soya. Gluten-free	Borderline substances standard ACBS indications p. 1375.	Fresubin Energy tube feed liquid unflavoured: 500 ml = £7.57; 1000 ml = £14.46; 1500 ml = £22.25
Not suitable for use in child under 3 years; use with caution in child under 6 years									

Nutrini® Energy (Nutricia Ltd)	Liquid (tube feed) per 100 mL	630 kJ (150 kcal)	4 g caseinates, whey protein	18.5 g (sugars 1.1 g)	6.7 g	Nil	Contains fish oil, residual lactose, soya. Gluten-free	Borderline substances paediatric ACBS indications p. 1375; also patients with proven inflammatory bowel disease, following total gastrectomy.	Nutrini Energy liquid: 200 ml = £5.48; 500 ml = £14.07
Not suitable for use in child under 1 year; not suitable for use in child over 6 years									
Nutrison® Energy (Nutricia Ltd)	Liquid (tube feed) per 100 mL	630 kJ (150 kcal)	6 g caseinate, pea, soya, whey proteins	18.5 g (sugars 1.2 g)	5.8 g	Nil	Contains fish oil, residual lactose, soya. Gluten-free	Borderline substances standard ACBS indications p. 1375.	Nutrison Energy liquid: 500 ml = £9.41; 1000 ml = £17.67; 1500 ml = £26.48
Not suitable for use in child under 3 years; use with caution in child over 3 years									
PaediaSure® Plus tube feed (Abbott Laboratories Ltd)	Liquid (tube feed) per 100 mL	628 kJ (150 kcal)	4.2 g caseinates, whey protein	16.7 g (sugars 2.2 g)	7.47 g	Nil	Contains residual lactose, soya. Gluten-free	Borderline substances paediatric ACBS indications p. 1375.	PaediaSure Plus tube feed liquid: 500 ml = £14.15
Not suitable for use in child under 1 year; suitable for child 1-10 years or 8-30 kg									
Tentrini® Energy (Nutricia Ltd)	Liquid (tube feed) per 100 mL	630 kJ (150 kcal)	4.8 g caseinate, whey protein	18.5 g (sugars 1.1 g)	6.3 g	Nil	Contains fish oil, residual lactose, soya. Gluten-free	Borderline substances paediatric ACBS indications p. 1375; also inflammatory bowel disease and total gastrectomy.	Tentrini Energy liquid: 500 ml = £12.21
Not suitable for use in child under 1 year; not recommended for child under 7 years, not recommended for child over 12 years									

1.5 to less than 2 kcal/mL higher protein

Product	Formulation	Energy	Protein	Carbohydrate	Fat	Fibre	Special Characteristics	ACBS Indications	Presentation & Flavour
Fresubin® HP Energy (Fresenius Kabi Ltd)	Liquid (tube feed) per 100 mL	630 kJ (150 kcal)	7.5 g milk protein	17 g (sugars 1 g)	5.8 g (MCT 57 %)	Nil	Contains fish oil, residual lactose, soya. Gluten-free	Borderline substances standard ACBS indications p. 1375; also CAPD and haemodialysis.	Fresubin HP Energy liquid: 500 ml = £7.96; 1000 ml = £14.98
Not suitable for use in child under 1 year; use with caution in child under 6 years									
Nutrison® Bolus Energy HP (Nutricia Ltd)	Liquid (tube feed) per 100 mL	672 kJ (160 kcal)	8 g caseinate, whey protein	18.1 g (sugars 5.8 g)	6.2 g	Nil	Contains fish oil, residual lactose, soya lecithin. Gluten-free	Borderline substances standard ACBS indications p. 1375.	Nutrison Bolus Energy HP liquid: 250 ml = £4.33
Not suitable for use in child under 3 years; use with caution in child over 3 years									
Nutrison® Protein Plus Energy (Nutricia Ltd)	Liquid (tube feed) per 100 mL	630 kJ (150 kcal)	7.5 g caseinates, pea, soya, whey proteins	16.9 g (sugars 3.3 g)	5.8 g	Less than 0.1 g	Contains fish oil, residual lactose, soya. Gluten-free	Borderline substances standard ACBS indications p. 1375.	Nutrison Protein Plus Energy liquid: 500 ml = £9.41; 1000 ml = £17.69
Not suitable for use in child under 1 year; not recommended for child 1-6 years									

1.5 to less than 2 kcal/mL with fibre

Product	Formulation	Energy	Protein	Carbohydrate	Fat	Fibre	Special Characteristics	ACBS Indications	Presentation & Flavour
Frebini® Energy Fibre tube feed (Fresenius Kabi Ltd)	Liquid (tube feed) per 100 mL	630 kJ (150 kcal)	3.8 g milk protein	18.1 g (sugars 2.5 g)	6.67 g	1.1 g	Contains fish oil, residual lactose, soya. Gluten-free	Borderline substances standard ACBS indications p. 1375 and growth failure.	Frebini Energy Fibre tube feed liquid unflavoured: 500 ml = £12.21
Not suitable for use in child under 1 year; not recommended for child over 10 years									

1.5 to less than 2 kcal/mL with fibre (product list continued)

Product	Formulation	Energy	Protein	Carbohydrate	Fat	Fibre	Special Characteristics	ACBS Indications	Presentation & Flavour
Fresubin® 2250 Complete (Fresenius Kabi Ltd)	Liquid (tube feed) per 100 mL	630 kJ (150 kcal)	5.6 g milk, soya proteins	18 g (sugars 1.2 g)	5.8 g	1.5 g	Contains fish oil, residual lactose, soya. Gluten-free	Borderline substances standard ACBS indications p. 1375	Fresubin 2250 Complete liquid: 1.5 litre = £22.48
Not suitable for use in child under 3 years; not recommended for child under 6 years									
Fresubin® Energy Fibre tube feed (Fresenius Kabi Ltd)	Liquid (tube feed) per 100 mL	630 kJ (150 kcal)	5.6 g milk, soya proteins	18.8 g (sugars 1.2 g)	5.8 g	1.5 g	Contains fish oil, residual lactose, soya. Gluten-free	Borderline substances standard ACBS indications p. 1375.	Fresubin Energy Fibre tube feed liquid unflavoured: 500 ml = £8.11; 1000 ml = £15.59
Not suitable for use in child under 3 years; use with caution in child under 6 years									
Nutrini® Energy Multifibre (Nutricia Ltd)	Liquid (tube feed) per 100 mL	635 kJ (151 kcal)	4 g caseinates, whey protein	18.5 g (sugars 1.1 g)	6.7 g	0.8 g	Contains fish oil, residual lactose, soya. Gluten-free	Borderline substances paediatric ACBS indications p. 1375 except bowel fistula; also total gastrectomy.	Nutrini Energy Multifibre liquid: 200 ml = £5.79; 500 ml = £14.54
Not suitable for use in child under 1 year; not suitable for use in child over 6 years									
Nutrison® Energy Multi Fibre (Nutricia Ltd)	Liquid (tube feed) per 100 mL	643 kJ (153 kcal)	6 g caseinates, pea, soya, whey proteins	18.4 g (sugars 2.6 g)	5.8 g	1.5 g	Contains fish oil, residual lactose, soya. Gluten-free	Borderline substances standard ACBS indications p. 1375.	Nutrison Energy Multi Fibre liquid: 500 ml = £10.43; 1000 ml = £19.63; 1500 ml = £30.30
Not suitable for use in child under 3 years; use with caution in child over 3 years									
Nutrison® Energy Multi Fibre Vanilla (Nutricia Ltd)	Liquid (tube feed) per 100 mL	645 kJ (154 kcal)	6 g milk protein	18.4 g (sugars 6.8 g)	5.8 g	2.2 g	Contains residual lactose, soya. Gluten-free	Borderline substances standard ACBS indications p. 1375.	Nutrison Energy Multi Fibre Vanilla liquid: 200 ml = £3.50
Not suitable for use in child under 3 years; not recommended for child under 6 years									
PaediaSure® Plus fibre tube feed (Abbott Laboratories Ltd)	Liquid (tube feed) per 100 mL	635 kJ (152 kcal)	4.2 g caseinates, whey protein	16.39 g (sugars 2.2 g)	7.47 g	1.1 g	Contains residual lactose, soya. Gluten-free	Borderline substances paediatric ACBS indications p. 1375.	PaediaSure Plus fibre tube feed liquid: 500 ml = £14.60
Not suitable for use in child under 1 year; suitable for child 1-10 years or 8-30 kg									
Tentrini® Energy Multifibre (Nutricia Ltd)	Liquid (tube feed) per 100 mL	640 kJ (152 kcal)	4.8 g caseinate, whey protein	18.5 g (sugars 1.1 g)	6.3 g	1.1 g	Contains fish oil, residual lactose, soya. Gluten-free	Borderline substances paediatric ACBS indications p. 1375 except bowel fistula; also inflammatory bowel disease and total gastrectomy.	Tentrini Energy Multifibre liquid: 500 ml = £13.43
Not suitable for use in child under 1 year; not recommended for child under 6 years									

1.5 to less than 2 kcal/mL with fibre, higher protein

Product	Formulation	Energy	Protein	Carbohydrate	Fat	Fibre	Special Characteristics	ACBS Indications	Presentation & Flavour
Fresubin® HP Energy Fibre (Fresenius Kabi Ltd)	Liquid (tube feed) per 100 mL	630 kJ (150 kcal)	7.5 g milk protein	16.2 g (sugars 1.11 g)	5.8 g (MCT 57%)	1.5 g	Contains fish oil, residual lactose, soya. Gluten-free	Borderline substances standard ACBS indications p. 1375 except dysphagia. Also CAPD and haemodialysis.	Fresubin HP Energy Fibre liquid: 500 ml = £8.67; 1000 ml = £16.52
Not suitable for use in child under 3 years; use with caution in child under 6 years									

Product	Formulation	Energy	Protein	Carbohydrate	Fat	Fibre	Special Characteristics	ACBS Indications	Presentation & Flavour
Fresubin® Plant Based tube feed (Fresenius Kabi Ltd)	Liquid (tube feed) per 100 mL	630 kJ (150 kcal)	7.5 g soya protein	16.1 g (sugars 6.3 g)	5.7 g	2.3 g	Contains soya. Gluten and lactose-free	Borderline substances standard ACBS indications p. 1375	Fresubin Plant-Based tube feed liquid: 500 ml = £8.67

Not suitable for use in child under 3 years; use with caution in child under 6 years

2 kcal/mL or more higher protein

Product	Formulation	Energy	Protein	Carbohydrate	Fat	Fibre	Special Characteristics	ACBS Indications	Presentation & Flavour
Fresubin® 2kcal HP (Fresenius Kabi Ltd)	Liquid (tube feed) per 100 mL	838 kJ (200 kcal)	10 g milk protein	18 g (sugars 2.7 g)	10 g	Nil	Contains fish oil, residual lactose, soya lecithin. Gluten-free	Disease-related malnutrition requiring a high energy and protein supply within a low volume, including patients with chronic diseases e.g. cancer, cardiac failure, COPD, renal and liver disease.	Fresubin 2kcal HP tube liquid feed: 500 ml = £10.11

Not suitable for use in child under 3 years; use with caution in child under 6 years

2 kcal/mL or more with fibre, higher protein

Product	Formulation	Energy	Protein	Carbohydrate	Fat	Fibre	Special Characteristics	ACBS Indications	Presentation & Flavour
Fresubin® 2kcal HP Fibre (Fresenius Kabi Ltd)	Liquid (tube feed) per 100 mL	840 kJ (200 kcal)	10 g milk protein	16.7 g (sugars 2.53 g)	10 g	1.5 g	Contains fish oil, residual lactose, soya lecithin. Gluten-free	Disease-related malnutrition requiring a high energy and protein supply within a low volume, including patients with chronic diseases e.g. cancer, cardiac failure, COPD, renal and liver disease.	Fresubin 2kcal HP Fibre tube feed liquid: 500 ml = £11.99

Not suitable for use in child under 3 years; use with caution in child under 6 years

Product	Formulation	Energy	Protein	Carbohydrate	Fat	Fibre	Special Characteristics	ACBS Indications	Presentation & Flavour
Nutrison® PlantBased 2kcal HP Multi Fibre (Nutricia Ltd)	Liquid (tube feed) per 100 mL	839 kJ (200 kcal)	10 g pea protein isolate, soya protein	18.5 g sugars (1.3 g)	9.3 g	1.5 g	Contains residual lactose, soya. Gluten-free	Borderline substances standard ACBS indications p. 1375	Nutrison PlantBased 2kcal HP Multi Fibre liquid: 500 ml = £13.19

Not suitable for use in child under 3 years; use with caution in child 3-17 years

Table 2 Oral nutrition

Oral nutritional supplements: Cancer (ready to serve)

1.5 kcal/mL milkshake

Product	Formulation	Energy	Protein	Carbohydrate	Fat	Fibre	Special Characteristics	ACBS Indications	Presentation & Flavour
Supportan® (Fresenius Kabi Ltd)	Liquid (sip feed) per 100 mL	630 kJ (150 kcal)	10 g milk protein	11.6 g sucrose (sugars 7.5 g)	6.7 g	1.5 g	Contains fish oil, residual lactose, soya lecithin. Gluten-free Minerals/100 mL: Na 2.1 mmol K 3.3 mmol Ca 5.1 mmol P 3.9 mmol	Patients with pancreatic cancer or patients with lung cancer undergoing chemotherapy.	Supportan drink tropical fruits: 800 ml = £16.18

Not suitable for use in child under 3 years; use with caution in child under 6 years

Oral nutritional supplements: Dysphagia (ready to serve)

1.3 kcal/g dessert style (fruit based)

Product	Formulation	Energy	Protein	Carbohydrate	Fat	Fibre	Special Characteristics	ACBS Indications	Presentation & Flavour
Nutilis® Fruit Dessert Level 4 (Nutricia Ltd)	Semi-solid per 100 g	575 kJ (137 kcal)	6.9 g whey protein isolate	17 g (sugars 11.5 g)	4 g	2.6 g	Contains residual lactose, soya. Gluten-free	Borderline substances standard ACBS indications p. 1375 except bowel fistula; also CAPD, haemodialysis.	Nutilis Fruit Dessert Level 4: apple 450 gram = £10.52; strawberry 450 gram = £10.52

Not suitable for use in child under 3 years; not recommended for child under 6 years

1.5 kcal/mL milkshake higher protein, pre-thickened

Product	Formulation	Energy	Protein	Carbohydrate	Fat	Fibre	Special Characteristics	ACBS Indications	Presentation & Flavour
Fresubin® Thickened (Fresenius Kabi Ltd)	Liquid (sip feed) per 100 mL	630 kJ (150 kcal)	10 g milk protein	12 g sucrose (sugars 7.3 g)	6.7 g	0.83 g	Contains soya lecithin, residual lactose. Gluten-free	Dysphagia or disease-related malnutrition.	Fresubin Thickened Level 2: wild strawberry 800 ml = £10.87; vanilla 800 ml = £10.87; Fresubin Thickened Level 3: wild strawberry 800 ml = £10.87; vanilla 800 ml = £10.87

Not suitable for use in child under 3 years; use with caution in child under 6 years

2.4 kcal/g dessert style (milk based)

Product	Formulation	Energy	Protein	Carbohydrate	Fat	Fibre	Special Characteristics	ACBS Indications	Presentation & Flavour
Nutilis® Complete Creme Level 3 (Nutricia Ltd)	Semi-solid per 100 g	1030 kJ (245 kcal)	9.6 g milk protein	29.1 g (sugars 11.8 g)	9.4 g	3.2 g	Contains residual lactose, soya. Gluten-free	Borderline substances standard ACBS indications p. 1375.	Nutilis Complete Creme Level 3 custard: chocolate 500 gram = £11.99; vanilla 500 gram = £11.99; strawberry 500 gram = £11.99

Not suitable for use in child under 3 years; not recommended for child under 6 years

2.4 kcal/mL milkshake lower volume

Product	Formulation	Energy	Protein	Carbohydrate	Fat	Fibre	Special Characteristics	ACBS Indications	Presentation & Flavour
Nutilis® Complete Drink Level 3 (Nutricia Ltd)	Liquid (sip feed) per 100 mL	1025 kJ (245 kcal)	9.6 g caseinates, milk proteins	29.1 g (sugars 5.4 g)	9.3 g	3.2 g	Contains residual lactose, soya. Gluten-free	Borderline substances standard ACBS indications p. 1375	Nutilis Complete Drink Level 3 liquid: mango & passionfruit 500 ml = £11.99; strawberry 500 ml = £11.99; chocolate 500 ml = £11.99; vanilla 500 ml = £11.99; lemon tea 500 ml = £11.99

Not suitable for use in child under 3 years; not recommended for child under 6 years

Oral nutritional supplements: Impaired gastro-intestinal function or malabsorption (powder)

4.4 kcal/g amino acid based with MCT

Product	Formulation	Energy	Protein	Carbohydrate	Fat	Fibre	Special Characteristics	ACBS Indications	Presentation & Flavour
Emsogen® (Nutricia Ltd)	Powder per 100 g	1839 kJ (438 kcal)	12.5 g protein equivalent (essential and nonessential amino acids)	60 g (sugars 7.9 g)	16.4 g (MCT 83 %)	Nil		Short-bowel syndrome, intractable malabsorption, proven inflammatory bowel disease, bowel fistula.	Emsogen powder unflavoured: 100 gram = £11.54

Standard dilution (20% w/v) of powder provides: protein 2.5 g, carbohydrate 12 g, fat 3.3 g, energy 368 kJ (88 kcal)/100 mL
Not suitable for use in child under 1 year; use with caution in child under 5 years

4.4 kcal/g juice style

Product	Formulation	Energy	Protein	Carbohydrate	Fat	Fibre	Special Characteristics	ACBS Indications	Presentation & Flavour
Elemental 028® Extra powder (Nutricia Ltd)	Powder per 100 g	1871 kJ (443 kcal)	12.5 g protein equivalent (essential and nonessential amino acids)	59 g (sugars 5.3 g)	17.5 g (MCT 35%)	Nil	Contains residual lactose. Gluten-free	Short bowel syndrome, intractable malabsorption, proven inflammatory bowel disease, bowel fistulae.	Elemental 028 Extra powder: orange 100 gram = £11.21; plain 100 gram = £11.21; banana 100 gram = £11.21

Standard dilution (20% w/v) of powder provides: protein 2.5 g, carbohydrate 11.8 g, fat 3.5 g, energy 374 kJ (89 kcal)/100 mL
Not suitable for use in child under 1 year; use with caution in child under 5 years

4.6 kcal/g peptide based formula

Product	Formulation	Energy	Protein	Carbohydrate	Fat	Fibre	Special Characteristics	ACBS Indications	Presentation & Flavour
Peptamen® Junior powder (Nestle Health Science)	Powder per 100 g	1948 kJ (463 kcal)	13.7 g whey protein	62.8 g (sugars 15 g)	17.5 g (MCT 53 %)	Nil	Contains residual lactose, soya. Gluten-free	Short bowel syndrome, intractable malabsorption, proven inflammatory bowel disease, bowel fistulae.	Peptamen Junior powder: 400 gram = £25.53

Powder 55 g reconstituted with 215 ml water provides: protein 7.6 g, carbohydrate 34.8 g, fat 9.7 g, energy 1071 kJ (257 kcal)
Not suitable for use in child under 1 year; not recommended for child over 10 years

5 kcal/g milkshake

Product	Formulation	Energy	Protein	Carbohydrate	Fat	Fibre	Special Characteristics	ACBS Indications	Presentation & Flavour
Modulen IBD® (Nestle Health Science)	Powder per 100 g	2066 kJ (493 kcal)	17.5 g casein	54 g (sugars 21 g)	23 g	Nil	Contains residual lactose, soya. Gluten-free	Sole source of nutrition during active phase of Crohn's disease, and nutritional support during remission phase for malnourished patients.	Modulen IBD powder: 350 gram = £17.82

Standard dilution (20 % w/v) of powder provides: protein 3.5 g, carbohydrate 11 g, fat 4.6 g, energy 413 kJ (99 kcal)/100 mL
Not suitable for use in child under 1 year; use with caution in child under 5 years

Oral nutritional supplements: Impaired gastro-intestinal function or malabsorption (ready to serve)

0.9 kcal/mL juice style

Product	Formulation	Energy	Protein	Carbohydrate	Fat	Fibre	Special Characteristics	ACBS Indications	Presentation & Flavour
Elemental 028® Extra liquid (Nutricia Ltd)	Liquid (sip feed) per 100 mL	360 kJ (86 kcal)	2.5 g protein equivalent (essential and nonessential amino acids)	11 g (sugars 4.7 g)	3.5 g (MCT 35%)	Nil	Gluten-free, lactose-free	Short bowel syndrome, intractable malabsorption, proven inflammatory bowel disease, bowel fistulae.	Elemental 028 Extra liquid: summer fruits 250 ml = £5.74; orange & pineapple 250 ml = £5.74; grapefruit 250 ml = £5.74
Not suitable for use in child under 1 year; not recommended for child 1-5 years									

1 kcal/mL milkshake

Product	Formulation	Energy	Protein	Carbohydrate	Fat	Fibre	Special Characteristics	ACBS Indications	Presentation & Flavour
PaediaSure® Peptide (Abbott Laboratories Ltd)	Liquid (sip feed) per 100 mL	420 kJ (100 kcal)	3 g caseinates, whey protein hydrolysate	13 g (sugars 2.7 g)	4 (MCT 46%) g	Nil	Contains residual lactose, soya. Gluten-free	Borderline substances standard ACBS indications p. 1375; also growth failure.	PaediaSure Peptide liquid: 200 ml = £6.31
Not suitable for use in child under 1 year									
Peptamen® (Nestle Health Science)	Liquid (sip feed) per 100 mL	421 kJ (100 kcal)	4 g whey protein	12.7 g (sugars 3.3 g)	3.7 g (MCT 68 %)	Nil	Contains residual lactose, soya	Short bowel syndrome, intractable malabsorption, proven inflammatory bowel disease, bowel fistulae.	Peptamen liquid vanilla: 800 ml = £17.35
Not suitable for use in child under 3 years; not recommended for child under 5 years									
Survimed® OPD (Fresenius Kabi Ltd)	Liquid (sip feed) per 100 mL	420 kJ (100 kcal)	4.65 g whey protein hydrolysate	14.1 g (sugars 5 g)	2.8 g (MCT 48%)	Less than 0.1 g	Contains residual lactose. Gluten-free	Borderline substances standard ACBS indications p. 1375	Survimed OPD liquid: 800 ml = £15.27
Not suitable for use in child under 3 years; use with caution in child under 6 years									

1.5 kcal/mL milkshake

Product	Formulation	Energy	Protein	Carbohydrate	Fat	Fibre	Special Characteristics	ACBS Indications	Presentation & Flavour
Peptamen® Junior 1.5 (Nestle Health Science)	Liquid (sip feed) per 100 mL	632 kJ (151 kcal)	4.5 g whey protein	18 g (sugars 4.3 g)	6.6 g (MCT 61%)	0.7 g	Contains fish oil, residual lactose, soya. Gluten-free	Disease related malnutrition in patients with short bowel syndrome, intractable malabsorption, proven inflammatory bowel disease, bowel fistulae.	Peptamen Junior 1.5 liquid vanilla: 800 ml = £20.70
Not suitable for use in child under 1 year; not recommended for child over 15 years									

1.5 kcal/mL milkshake higher protein, higher energy

Product	Formulation	Energy	Protein	Carbohydrate	Fat	Fibre	Special Characteristics	ACBS Indications	Presentation & Flavour
Peptisip Energy HP (Nutricia Ltd)	Liquid (sip feed) per 100 mL	634 kJ (150 kcal)	7.5 g whey protein hydrolysate	18.8 g (sugars 4.1 g)	5 g (MCT 60 %)	0.28 g	Contains residual lactose, soya lecithin	Disease-related malnutrition in patients with malabsorption and/or maldigestion.	Peptisip Energy HP liquid: 200 ml = £4.10
Not suitable for use in child under 3 years; use with caution in child 3-6 years									

Product	Formulation	Energy	Protein	Carbohydrate	Fat	Fibre	Special Characteristics	ACBS Indications	Presentation & Flavour
Survimed® OPD 1.5kcal (Fresenius Kabi Ltd)	Liquid (sip feed) per 100 mL	630 kJ (150 kcal)	7.5 g whey protein hydrolysate	20.6 g (sugars 7.4 g)	4.2 g (MCT 50%)	Less than 0.1 g	Contains residual lactose. Gluten-free	Borderline substances standard ACBS indications p. 1375 except dysphagia.	Survimed OPD 1.5kcal drink: vanilla 200 ml = £3.82; cappuccino 200 ml = £3.82

Not suitable for use in child under 3 years; use with caution in child under 6 years

Oral nutritional supplements: Liver failure (powder)

4.7 kcal/g formula

Product	Formulation	Energy	Protein	Carbohydrate	Fat	Fibre	Special Characteristics	ACBS Indications	Presentation & Flavour
Heparon Junior® (Nutricia Ltd)	Standard dilution (18% w/v) of powder per 100 mL	357 kJ (85 kcal)	2.2 g whey protein	10 g (sugars 3.4 g)	4 g (MCT 50%)	0.5 g	Contains fish oil, lactose Electrolytes/100 mL: Na^+ 0.77 mmol K^+ 2.25 mmol Ca^{2+} 2.43 mmol P^+ 1.68 mmol	Acute and chronic liver failure.	Heparon Junior powder: 400 gram = £34.00

Powder provides: protein 12 g, carbohydrate 55.7 g, fat 22 g, energy 1985 kJ (474 kcal)/100 g

Oral nutritional supplements: Renal failure (powder)

3.7 kcal/g energy and protein fortifier

Product	Formulation	Energy	Protein	Carbohydrate	Fat	Fibre	Special Characteristics	ACBS Indications	Presentation & Flavour
Renapro® (Stanningley Pharma Ltd)	Powder per 100 g	1611 kJ (385 kcal)	90 g whey protein	3.4 g	1 g	Nil	Gluten-free Minerals/100 g: Na 300 mg K 310 mg Ca 340 mg P 140 mg	Dialysis and hypoproteinaemia.	Renapro powder 20g sachets: 30 sachet = £69.60

Powder 20 g reconstituted with 60-100 mL cold water provides: protein 18 g, carbohydrate 0.7 g, fat less than 0.2 g, energy 322 kJ (77 kcal)
Not suitable for use in child under 1 year

4.8 kcal/g milk replacer

Product	Formulation	Energy	Protein	Carbohydrate	Fat	Fibre	Special Characteristics	ACBS Indications	Presentation & Flavour
Renamil® (Stanningley Pharma Ltd)	Powder per 100 g	2012 kJ (479 kcal)	5 g milk protein, whey protein isolate	71.2 g (sugars 6.8 g)	19.3 g	Nil	Contains lactose, soya. Gluten-free Minerals/100 mL: Na 3 mmol K 0.1 mmol Ca 3.7 mmol P 0.8 mmol	Chronic renal failure.	Renamil powder 100g sachets: 10 sachet = £33.15

Not suitable for use in child under 1 year

5 kcal/g high energy, low protein formula

Product	Formulation	Energy	Protein	Carbohydrate	Fat	Fibre	Special Characteristics	ACBS Indications	Presentation & Flavour
Renastart® (Vitaflo International Ltd)	Standard dilution (20%) of powder per 100 mL	419 kJ (100 kcal)	1.5 g caseinates, whey protein	12.6 g (sugars 1.3 g)	4.8 g	Nil	Contains lactose Minerals/100 mL: Na 2.1 mmol K 0.6 mmol Ca 0.6 mmol P 0.6 mmol	Renal failure.	Renastart powder: 400 gram = £43.44

Powder provides: protein 7.5 g, carbohydrate 62.5 g, fat 24 g, energy 2078 kJ (496 kcal)/100 g.
Not recommended for child over 10 years

5 kcal/g formula

Product	Formulation	Energy	Protein	Carbohydrate	Fat	Fibre	Special Characteristics	ACBS Indications	Presentation & Flavour
Kindergen® (Nutricia Ltd)	Standard dilution (20% w/v) of powder per 100 mL	418 kJ (100 kcal)	1.5 g whey protein	11.6 g (sugars 1.6 g)	5.2 g	0.6 g	Contains fish oil, residual lactose, soya Minerals/100 mL Na 2 mmol K 0.6 mmol Ca 1.2 mmol P 0.7 mmol	Children with chronic renal failure receiving peritoneal rapid overnight dialysis.	Kindergen powder: 400 gram = £45.62

Powder provides: protein 7.5 g, carbohydrate 57.6 g, fat 25.9 g, energy 2083 kJ (498 kcal)/100 g

Oral nutritional supplements: Renal failure (ready to serve)

2 kcal/mL milkshake lower volume

Product	Formulation	Energy	Protein	Carbohydrate	Fat	Fibre	Special Characteristics	ACBS Indications	Presentation & Flavour
Renastep® (Vitaflo International Ltd)	Liquid (sip or tube feed) per 100 mL	836 kJ (200 kcal)	4 g milk protein	21 g (sugars 3.4 g)	11.1 g	Nil	Contains fish oil Minerals/100 mL: Na 3.6 mmol K 0.9 mmol Ca 1.2 mmol P 1.1 mmol	Renal failure.	Renastep liquid: 125 ml = £6.77

Not suitable for use in child under 3 years

Product	Formulation	Energy	Protein	Carbohydrate	Fat	Fibre	Special Characteristics	ACBS Indications	Presentation & Flavour
Renilon® 7.5 (Nutricia Ltd)	Liquid (sip feed) per 100 mL	835 kJ (199 kcal)	7.3 g milk protein	20 g (sugars 4.8 g)	10 g	Nil	Contains residual lactose, soya Minerals/100 mL: Na 2.7 mmol K 0.9 mmol Ca less than 0.27 mmol P less than 0.29 mmol	Borderline substances standard ACBS indications p. 1375 except dysphagia.	Renilon 7.5 liquid: caramel 500 ml = £14.00; apricot 500 ml = £14.00

Not suitable for use in child under 3 years; not recommended for child under 6 years

Oral nutritional supplements: Standard feeds (powder)

1 - 2.2 kcal/mL soup

Product	Formulation	Energy	Protein	Carbohydrate	Fat	Fibre	Special Characteristics	ACBS Indications	Presentation & Flavour
Aymes® ActaSolve Savoury (Aymes International Ltd)	Powder per 100 g	1844 kJ (438 kcal)	15.9 g milk protein	60.3 g (sugars 11.9-22.6 g)	14.7 g	0.5 g	Contains celery (vegetable flavour only), lactose, meat derivatives (chicken flavour only). Gluten-free	Borderline substances standard ACBS indications p. 1375 except dysphagia.	Aymes ActaSolve Savoury Starter Pack powder: 3 sachet = £2.89; Aymes ActaSolve Savoury powder 57g sachets: chicken 7 sachet = £6.75; potato & leek 7 sachet = £6.75; vegetable 7 sachet = £6.75

Powder 57 g reconstituted with 200 mL water provides: protein 9.1 g, carbohydrate 34.4 g, fat 8.4 g, energy 1051 kJ (250 kcal)
Not suitable for use in child under 3 years; use with caution in child under 6 years

1.4 - 1.6 kcal/mL milkshake

Product	Formulation	Energy	Protein	Carbohydrate	Fat	Fibre	Special Characteristics	ACBS Indications	Presentation & Flavour
Aymes® Actajuni Shake (Aymes International Ltd)	Powder per 100 g	2112 kJ (504 kcal)	14 g milk protein	53.9 g (sugars 20.5-22.3 g)	25.7 g	0.1 g	Contains soya. Gluten-free	Disease-related malnutrition and growth failure.	Aymes ActaJuni Shake Starter Pack powder: 5 sachet = £7.03; Aymes Actajuni Shake powder 57g sachets: banana milkshake 7 sachet = £9.84; simply neutral 7 sachet = £9.84; smooth vanilla 7 sachet = £9.84; classic chocolate 7 sachet = £9.84; strawberry burst 7 sachet = £9.84

Powder 57 g reconstituted with 150 mL water provides: protein 8 g, carbohydrate 30.7 g, fat 14.7 g, energy 1204 kJ (288 kcal)
Suitable for child 3-10 years and/or weighing up to 35 kg; not suitable for infants

Product	Formulation	Energy	Protein	Carbohydrate	Fat	Fibre	Special Characteristics	ACBS Indications	Presentation & Flavour
Aymes® Shake (Aymes International Ltd)	Powder per 100 g	1871 kJ (445 kcal)	21 g milk protein	57 g (sugars 31.5 g)	14.8 g	0.2 g	Contains lactose, soya. Gluten-free	Borderline substances standard ACBS indications p. 1375	Aymes Shake powder: banana 1600 gram = £16.08; chocolate 1600 gram = £16.08; neutral 1600 gram = £16.08; strawberry 1600 gram = £16.08; vanilla 1600 gram = £16.08; Aymes Shake Starter Pack powder: 6 sachet = £4.61; Aymes Shake powder 57g sachets: banana 7 sachet = £4.02; ginger 7 sachet = £4.02; chocolate 7 sachet = £4.02; vanilla 7 sachet = £4.02; strawberry 7 sachet = £4.02; neutral 7 sachet = £4.02

Powder 57 g reconstituted with 200 mL whole milk provides: protein 19 g, carbohydrate 42 g, fat 15.8 g, energy 1618 kJ (383 kcal)
Not suitable for use in child under 3 years; use with caution in child under 6 years

1.4 - 1.6 kcal/mL milkshake (product list continued)

Product	Formulation	Energy	Protein	Carbohydrate	Fat	Fibre	Special Characteristics	ACBS Indications	Presentation & Flavour
Complan® Shake (Nutricia Ltd)	Powder per 100 g	1862 kJ (442 kcal)	15.4 g cow's milk	61.8 g (sugars 31.8 g)	14.9 g	Nil	Contains lactose. Gluten-free	Borderline substances standard ACBS indications p. 1375.	Complan Shake Starter Pack sachets: 5 sachet = £3.84; Complan Shake oral powder 57g sachets: vanilla 4 sachet = £2.20; strawberry 4 sachet = £2.20; chocolate 4 sachet = £2.20; milk 4 sachet = £2.20; banana 4 sachet = £2.20
Powder 57 g reconstituted with 200 mL whole milk provides: protein 15.8 g, carbohydrate 44.7 g, fat 15.9 g, energy 1605kJ (381 kcal) Not suitable for use in child under 3 years; use with caution in child 3-6 years									
EnergieShake® Powder (Anaiah Healthcare PVT Ltd)	Powder per 100 g	1849 kJ (439 kcal)	16.5 g milk protein	62.1 g (sugars 26.8 g)	13.9 g	Less than 1 g	Contains lactose, soya	Borderline substances standard ACBS indications p. 1375.	EnergieShake Powder Starter Pack oral powder sachets: 285 gram = £2.88; EnergieShake Powder oral powder 57g sachets: neutral 4 sachet = £1.76; 7 sachet = £3.08; banana 4 sachet = £1.76; 7 sachet = £3.08; strawberry 4 sachet = £1.76; 7 sachet = £3.08; chocolate 4 sachet = £1.76; 7 sachet = £3.08; vanilla 4 sachet = £1.76; 7 sachet = £3.08
Powder 57 g reconstituted with 200 mL water provides: protein 9.4 g, carbohydrate 35.4 g, fat 7.9 g, energy 1054 kJ (250 kcal) Not recommended for use in child under 6 years									
Foodlink® Complete (Nualtra Ltd)	Powder per 100 g	1869 kJ (444 kcal)	21 g milk protein	56 g (sugars 43 g)	15 g	Nil	Contains lactose, soya. Gluten-free	Borderline substances standard ACBS indications p. 1375	Foodlink Complete powder: banana 1596 gram = £16.24; chocolate 1596 gram = £16.24; natural 1596 gram = £16.24; strawberry 1596 gram = £16.24; vanilla 1596 gram = £16.24; Foodlink Complete Starter Pack powder: 5 sachet = £4.80; Foodlink Complete powder 57g sachets: chocolate 7 sachet = £4.06; vanilla 7 sachet = £4.06; natural 7 sachet = £4.06; strawberry 7 sachet = £4.06; banana 7 sachet = £4.06
Powder 57 g reconstituted with 200 ml whole milk provides: protein 19 g, carbohydrate 41 g, fat 16 g, energy 1611 kJ (383 kcal) Not suitable for use in child under 3 years; not recommended in child 3-6 years									

1.5 kcal/mL smoothie

Product	Formulation	Energy	Protein	Carbohydrate	Fat	Fibre	Special Characteristics	ACBS Indications	Presentation & Flavour
Aymes® ActaSolve Smoothie (Aymes International Ltd)	Powder per 100 g	1892 kJ (450 kcal)	16.2 g soya protein isolate	62.8 g (sugars 24.8 g)	14.6 g	0.7 g	Contains soya. Gluten-free	Borderline substances standard ACBS indications p. 1375 except dysphagia.	Aymes ActaSolve Smoothie Starter Pack powder: 4 sachet = £5.93; Aymes ActaSolve Smoothie powder 66g sachets: strawberry & cranberry 7 sachet = £7.56; pineapple 7 sachet = £7.56; peach 7 sachet = £7.56; mango 7 sachet = £7.56
Powder 66 g reconstituted with 150ml water provides: protein 10.7 g, carbohydrate 41.5 g, fat 9.7 g, energy 1249 kJ (297 kcal) Not suitable for use in child under 3 years; use with caution in child under 6 years									
Foodlink® Smoothie (Nualtra Ltd)	Powder per 100 g	1810 kJ (435 kcal)	15 g soya protein isolate	69 g (sugars 24 g)	11 g	Nil	Contains soya. Gluten-free, lactose-free	Disease-related malnutrition.	Foodlink Smoothie Starter Pack sachets: 4 sachet = £4.80; Foodlink Smoothie powder 66g sachets: orange & mango 7 sachet = £7.77; tropical 7 sachet = £7.77; red berry 7 sachet = £7.77; peach 7 sachet = £7.77
Powder 66 g reconstituted with 150 mL water provides: protein 10 g, carbohydrate 45 g, fat 7 g, energy 1195 kJ (287 kcal) Not suitable for use in child under 3 years; use with caution in child under 6 years									

1.6 kcal/mL milkshake with fibre

Product	Formulation	Energy	Protein	Carbohydrate	Fat	Fibre	Special Characteristics	ACBS Indications	Presentation & Flavour
Aymes® Actasolve Shake Fibre (Aymes International Ltd)	Powder per 100 g	1793 kJ (427 kcal)	21 g milk protein	48.1 g (sugars 34.2 g)	14.8 g	8.8 g	Contains lactose, soya. Gluten-free	Borderline substances standard ACBS indications p. 1375 except dysphagia.	Aymes Actasolve Shake Fibre Starter Pack powder: 5 sachet = £4.53; Aymes Actasolve Shake Fibre powder 57g sachets: classic chocolate 7 sachet = £6.35; smooth vanilla 7 sachet = £6.35; strawberry burst 7 sachet = £6.35; banana milkshake 7 sachet = £6.35; simply neutral 7 sachet = £6.35
Powder 57 g reconstituted with 200 mL whole milk provides: protein 19 g, carbohydrate 36.9 g, fat 15.8 g, energy 1573 kJ (375 kcal) Not suitable for use in child under 3 years; use with caution in child under 6 years									
Foodlink® Complete with Fibre (Nualtra Ltd)	Powder per 100 g	1779 kJ (423 kcal)	19 g milk, soya proteins	52 g (sugars 40 g)	14 g	7.2 g	Contains lactose, soya. Gluten-free	Borderline substances standard ACBS indications p. 1375	Foodlink Complete powder with fibre 63g sachets: strawberry 7 sachet = £7.16; chocolate 7 sachet = £7.16; banana 7 sachet = £7.16; vanilla 7 sachet = £7.16; natural 7 sachet = £7.16; Foodlink Complete powder with fibre Starter Pack: 5 sachet = £5.32
Powder 63 g reconstituted with 200 ml whole milk provides: protein 19 g, carbohydrate 42 g, fat 16 g, energy 1667 kJ (397 kcal) Not suitable for use in child under 3 years; not recommended for child 3-6 years									

2 kcal/mL milkshake higher volume, higher energy

Product	Formulation	Energy	Protein	Carbohydrate	Fat	Fibre	Special Characteristics	ACBS Indications	Presentation & Flavour
Aymes® ActaSolve High Energy (Aymes International Ltd)	Powder per 100 g	2105 kJ (503 kcal)	4.8 g milk protein	63.8 g (sugar 22.5 g)	25.3 g	0.40 g	Contains lactose, soya. Gluten-free	Borderline substances standard ACBS indications p. 1375 except dysphagia.	Aymes ActaSolve High Energy Starter Pack powder: 4 sachet = £8.96; Aymes ActaSolve High Energy powder 85g sachets: vanilla 6 sachet = £9.62; banana 6 sachet = £9.62; chocolate 6 sachet = £9.62; strawberry 6 sachet = £9.62
Powder 85 g reconstituted with 240 ml whole milk provides: protein 12.3 g, carbohydrate 65.6 g, fat 30.4 g, energy 2451 kJ (586 kcal) Not suitable for use in child under 3 years; use with caution in child under 6 years									
Calshake® powder (Fresenius Kabi Ltd)	Powder per 100 g	2086 kJ (497 kcal)	2.4 g milk protein	71.1 g dextrose and maltodextrin (sugars 10.1 g)	22.6 g	Nil	Contains lactose. Gluten-free.	Disease related malnutrition, malabsorption states or other conditions requiring fortification with a fat/carbohydrate supplement.	Calshake powder 87g sachets: neutral 7 sachet = £21.83; vanilla 7 sachet = £21.83; strawberry 7 sachet = £21.83; banana 7 sachet = £21.83; Calshake powder 90g sachets chocolate: 7 sachet = £21.83
Powder 87 g reconstituted with 240 mL whole milk provides: protein 3.3 g, carbohydrate 23.4 g, fat 9 g, energy 787 kJ (188 kcal)/100 mL Not suitable for use in child under 3 years; use with caution in child under 6 years									
Enshake® (Abbott Laboratories Ltd)	Powder per 100 g	1902 kJ (452 kcal)	8.4 g caseinate, milk, soya protein isolates	69.5 g 67.4 g corn syrup (sugars 11 g)	15.6 g	Nil	Contains residual lactose, soya. Gluten-free	Disease-related malnutrition, malabsorption states or other conditions requiring fortification with a fat/carbohydrate supplement.	Enshake oral powder 96.5g sachets: strawberry 6 sachet = £22.92; vanilla 6 sachet = £22.92; banana 6 sachet = £22.92; chocolate 6 sachet = £22.92
Powder 96.5 g reconstituted with 240 mL whole milk provides: protein 16 g, carbohydrate 78.9 g, fat 24.7 g, energy 2528 kJ (602 kcal) Not suitable for use in child under 1 year; not recommended for use in children									
Foodlink® Extra (Nualtra Ltd)	Powder per 100 g	2186 kJ (523 kcal)	4.9 g milk protein	60 g (sugars 15 g)	30 g	Nil	Contains lactose. Gluten-free	Disease-related malnutrition.	Foodlink Extra Starter Pack sachets: 4 sachet = £6.89; Foodlink Extra powder 85g sachets: strawberry 7 sachet = £11.20; banana 7 sachet = £11.20; vanilla 7 sachet = £11.20; chocolate 7 sachet = £11.20
Powder 85 g reconstituted with 240 mL whole milk provides: protein 13 g, carbohydrate 62 g, fat 35 g, energy 2513 kJ (601 kcal) Not suitable for use in child under 3 years; use with caution in child under 6 years									
Scandishake® Mix (Nutricia Ltd)	Powder per 100 g	2120 kJ (507 kcal)	4.8 g caseinates	67 g (sugars 20.5 g)	24.5 g	Nil	Contains lactose, soya.	Disease-related malnutrition, malabsorption states or other conditions requiring fortification with a fat / carbohydrate supplement.	Scandishake Mix oral powder 85g sachets: unflavoured 6 sachet = £22.32; caramel 6 sachet = £22.32; vanilla 6 sachet = £22.32; chocolate 6 sachet = £22.32; strawberry 6 sachet = £22.32; banana 6 sachet = £22.32
Powder 85 g reconstituted with 240 mL whole milk provides: protein 12.1 g, carbohydrate 68.2 g, fat 29.6 g, energy 2460 kJ (587 kcal) Not suitable for use in child under 3 years									

2.3 - 2.4 kcal/mL milkshake lower volume

Product	Formulation	Energy	Protein	Carbohydrate	Fat	Fibre	Special Characteristics	ACBS Indications	Presentation & Flavour
Aymes® Shake Compact (Aymes International Ltd)	Powder per 100 g	1862 kJ (442 kcal)	15.5 g milk protein	61.7 g (sugars 35 g)	14.8 g	0.2 g	Contains lactose, soya. Gluten-free	Borderline substances standard ACBS indications p. 1375 except dysphagia.	Aymes Shake Compact Starter Pack powder: 6 sachet = £4.61; Aymes Shake Compact powder 57g sachets: chocolate 7 sachet = £4.02; ginger 7 sachet = £4.02; neutral 7 sachet = £4.02; vanilla 7 sachet = £4.02; strawberry 7 sachet = £4.02; banana 7 sachet = £4.02
Powder 57 g reconstituted with 100 ml milk provides: protein 12.2 g, carbohydrate 39.7 g, fat 12.4 g, energy 1343 kJ (320 kcal) Not suitable for child under 1 year, not recommended for child under 6 years									
Foodlink® Complete Compact (Nualtra Ltd)	Powder per 100 g	1869 kJ (444 kcal)	21 g milk protein	56 g (sugars 43 g)	15 g	Nil	Contains lactose, soya. Gluten-free	Disease-related malnutrition.	Foodlink Complete Compact Starter Pack sachets: 5 sachet = £4.80; Foodlink Complete Compact powder 57g sachets: strawberry 7 sachet = £4.06; vanilla 7 sachet = £4.06; banana 7 sachet = £4.06; natural 7 sachet = £4.06; chocolate 7 sachet = £4.06
Powder 57 g reconstituted with 100 ml whole milk provides: protein 15 g, carbohydrate 37 g, fat 12 g, energy 1338 kJ (318 kcal) Not suitable for use in children under 3 years; not recommended for child 3-6 years									

2.4 kcal/mL milkshake lower volume, higher protein

Product	Formulation	Energy	Protein	Carbohydrate	Fat	Fibre	Special Characteristics	ACBS Indications	Presentation & Flavour
Aymes® Actasolve Protein Compact (Aymes International Ltd)	Powder per 100 g	1843 kJ (437 kcal)	29.7 g milk, soya proteins	53.2 g (sugars 22.1 g)	11.6 g	0.40 g	Contains soya. Gluten-free	Borderline substances standard ACBS indications p. 1375 except dysphagia.	Aymes ActaSolve Protein Compact Starter Pack powder: 5 sachet = £6.06; Aymes Actasolve Protein Compact powder 57g sachets: simply neutral 7 sachet = £8.49; classic chocolate 7 sachet = £8.49; strawberry burst 7 sachet = £8.49; smooth vanilla 7 sachet = £8.49; banana milkshake 7 sachet = £8.49
Powder 57 g reconstituted with 100 mL whole milk provides: protein 20.4 g, carbohydrate 35.1 g, fat 10.3 g, energy 1326 kJ (315 kcal) Not suitable for use in child under 3 years; use with caution in child under 6 years									

2.6 kcal/g dessert style (milk based)

Product	Formulation	Energy	Protein	Carbohydrate	Fat	Fibre	Special Characteristics	ACBS Indications	Presentation & Flavour
Aymes® ActaSolve Delight (Aymes International Ltd)	Powder per 100 g	1857 kJ (441 kcal)	15.2 g milk protein	62 g (sugars 38.6 g)	14.5 g	0.9 g	Contains lactose, soya	Borderline substances standard ACBS indications p. 1375 except dysphagia.	Aymes ActaSolve Delight Starter Pack powder: 3 sachet = £4.32; Aymes ActaSolve Delight powder 57g sachets: butterscotch 7 sachet = £8.35; mixed berries 7 sachet = £8.35; lemon 7 sachet = £8.35
Powder 57 g reconstituted with 75 ml milk provides: protein 11.2 g, carbohydrate 38.7 g, fat 11.3 g, energy 1270 kJ (302 kcal) Not suitable for use in child under 1 year, not recommended for child under 6 years									

Oral nutritional supplements: Standard feeds (ready to serve)

1 kcal/mL milkshake lower energy with fibre

Product	Formulation	Energy	Protein	Carbohydrate	Fat	Fibre	Special Characteristics	ACBS Indications	Presentation & Flavour
Fortini® 1.0 Multi Fibre (Nutricia Ltd)	Liquid (sip feed) per 100 mL	420 kJ (100 kcal)	2.4 g caseinates	11.8 g (sugars 4.7 g)	4.5 g	1.5 g	Contains residual lactose, soya. Gluten-free	Disease-related malnutrition, growth failure.	Fortini 1.0 Multi Fibre liquid: strawberry 200 ml = £3.96; vanilla 200 ml = £3.96; chocolate 200 ml = £3.96; banana 200 ml = £3.96
Not suitable for use in child under 1 year									
PaediaSure® Fibre (Abbott Laboratories Ltd)	Liquid (sip feed) per 100 mL	424 kJ (101 kcal)	2.8 g caseinates, whey protein	10.9 g (sugars 3.8 g)	5 g	0.7 g	Contains residual lactose, soya. Gluten-free	Borderline substances paediatric ACBS indications p. 1375.	PaediaSure fibre liquid: vanilla 200 ml = £4.25; strawberry 200 ml = £4.25; banana 200 ml = £4.25
Not suitable for use in child under 1 year; not recommended for child over 10 years									

1 - 1.3 kcal/mL milkshake lower energy

Product	Formulation	Energy	Protein	Carbohydrate	Fat	Fibre	Special Characteristics	ACBS Indications	Presentation & Flavour
Fresubin® Original (Fresenius Kabi Ltd)	Liquid (sip feed) per 100 mL	420 kJ (100 kcal)	3.8 g milk, soya proteins	13.8 g (sugars 3.5 g)	3.4 g	Nil	Contains residual lactose, soya. Gluten-free	Borderline substances standard ACBS indications p. 1375; also Refsum's Disease.	Fresubin Original drink vanilla: 200 ml = £3.31
Not suitable for use in child under 3 years; use with caution in child under 6 years									
PaediaSure® (Abbott Laboratories Ltd)	Liquid (sip feed) per 100 mL	422 kJ (101 kcal)	2.8 g caseinate, milk protein isolate, whey protein	11.16 g (sugars 3.7 g)	4.98 g	Nil	Contains residual lactose, soya. Gluten-free	Borderline substances paediatric ACBS indications p. 1375.	PaediaSure liquid: vanilla 200 ml = £4.04; strawberry 200 ml = £4.04; chocolate 200 ml = £4.04; banana 200 ml = £4.04
Not suitable for use in child under 1 year; suitable for child 1-10 years or 8-30 kg; chocolate flavour suitable for child 3-10 years or 12-30 kg									

1.4 - 2 kcal/g dessert style (milk based)

Product	Formulation	Energy	Protein	Carbohydrate	Fat	Fibre	Special Characteristics	ACBS Indications	Presentation & Flavour
Aymes® Actagain Creme (Aymes International Ltd)	Semi-solid per 100 g	632 kJ (150 kcal)	7.5 g milk protein	19 g (sugars 8.1 g)	4.9 g	Nil	Contains residual lactose. Gluten-free.	Borderline substances standard ACBS indications p. 1375 except dysphagia.	Aymes Actagain Creme Starter Pack dessert: 500 gram = £6.28; Aymes Actagain Creme dessert: smooth vanilla 500 gram = £6.41; creamy caramel 500 gram = £6.41; classic chocolate 500 gram = £6.41; nutty chocolate 500 gram = £6.41
Not suitable for use in child under 3 years; use with caution in child under 6 years									
EnergieShake® dessert (Anaiah Healthcare PVT Ltd)	Semi-solid per 100 g	632 kJ (150 kcal)	7.5 g caseinates, milk protein isolate	19 g (sugars 8.1 g)	4.9 g	Nil	Contains residual lactose. Gluten-free	Borderline substances standard ACBS indications p. 1375 except dysphagia.	EnergieShake dessert: caramel 375 gram = £3.30; chocolate 375 gram = £3.30
Not suitable for use in child under 3 years									

Forticreme® Complete (Nutricia Ltd)	Semi-solid per 100 g	675 kJ (160 kcal)	9.5 g milk proteins	19.2 g (sugars 10.6 g)	5 g	Less than 0.5 g	Contains residual lactose. Gluten-free	Borderline substances standard ACBS indications p. 1375; also continuous ambulatory peritoneal dialysis (CAPD), haemodialysis.	Forticreme Complete dessert: banana 500 gram = £9.20; vanilla 500 gram = £9.20; forest fruits 500 gram = £9.20; chocolate 500 gram = £9.20
Not suitable for use in child under 3 years; not recommended for child under 6 years									
Fortini® Creamy Fruit Multi Fibre (Nutricia Ltd)	Semi-solid per 100 g	630 kJ (150 kcal)	3.5 g whey protein	19.4 g (sugars 11.7 g)	6.1 g	1.9 g	Contains lactose, soya. Gluten-free	Disease-related malnutrition, growth failure.	Fortini Creamy Fruit Multi Fibre: summer fruit 400 gram = £10.86; berry fruit 400 gram = £10.86
Not suitable for use in child under 1 year									
Fresubin® 2kcal Creme (Fresenius Kabi Ltd)	Semi-solid per 100 g	840 kJ (200 kcal)	10 g milk protein	22.5 g sucrose (sugars 13.4 g)	7.8 g	Nil	Contains residual lactose, soya	Borderline substances standard ACBS indications p. 1375, continuous ambulatory peritoneal dialysis (CAPD) and haemodialysis.	Fresubin 2kcal Creme dessert: chocolate 500 gram = £8.40; vanilla 500 gram = £8.40; wild strawberry 500 gram = £8.40; praline 500 gram = £8.40; cappuccino 500 gram = £8.40
Not suitable for use in child under 3 years; not recommended for child under 6 years									
Fresubin® YOcrème (Fresenius Kabi Ltd)	Semi-solid per 100 g	630 kJ (150 kcal)	7.5 g milk, whey proteins	19.3 g sucrose (sugars 17.4 g)	4.7 g	0.4 g	Contains lactose, soya lecithin. Gluten-free	Patients with or at risk of malnutrition in particular with increased energy or protein needs or dysphagia.	Fresubin YOcreme dessert: raspberry 500 gram = £11.11; lemon 500 gram = £11.11; biscuit 500 gram = £11.11; apricot-peach 500 gram = £11.11
Not suitable for use in child under 3 years; use with caution in child under 6 years									
Nutricrem® (Nualtra Ltd)	Semi-solid per 100 g	756 kJ (180 kcal)	10 g caseinates, milk protein, soya protein	18.8 g (sugars 9.7 g)	7.2 g	Nil	Contains residual lactose, soya. Gluten-free	Borderline substances standard ACBS indications p. 1375.	Nutricrem Starter Pack dessert: 500 gram = £9.56; Nutricrem dessert: vanilla 500 gram = £9.90; chocolate orange 500 gram = £9.90; mint chocolate 500 gram = £9.90; strawberry 500 gram = £9.90
Not suitable for use in child under 3 years; not recommended for child under 6 years									

1.5 kcal/mL juice style

Product	Formulation	Energy	Protein	Carbohydrate	Fat	Fibre	Special Characteristics	ACBS Indications	Presentation & Flavour
Altrajuce® (Nualtra Ltd)	Liquid (sip feed) per 100 mL	636 kJ (150 kcal)	3.9 g milk protein	33.5 g (sugars 13.5 g)	Nil	Nil	Contains residual lactose. Gluten-free	Borderline substances standard ACBS indications p. 1375 except dysphagia.	Altrajuce Starter Pack liquid: 800 ml = £9.60; Altrajuce liquid: apple 200 ml = £1.97; orange 200 ml = £1.97; blackcurrant 200 ml = £1.97; strawberry 200 ml = £1.97
Not suitable for use in child under 3 years; not recommended for child under 6 years									

1.5 kcal/mL juice style (product list continued)

Product	Formulation	Energy	Protein	Carbohydrate	Fat	Fibre	Special Characteristics	ACBS Indications	Presentation & Flavour
Aymes® Actagain Juce (Aymes International Ltd)	Liquid (sip feed) **per 100 mL**	638 kJ (150 kcal)	5 g milk protein	32.5 g (sugars 13.5 g)	Nil	Nil	Gluten-free	Borderline substances standard ACBS indications p. 1375 except dysphagia.	Aymes Actagain Juce Starter Pack liquid: 1000 ml = £9.50; Aymes Actagain Juce liquid berry medley: 200 ml = £1.80; Aymes Actagain Juce liquid exotic fruit: 200 ml = £1.80; Aymes Actagain Juce liquid juicy peach: 200 ml = £1.80; Aymes Actagain Juce liquid juicy apple: 200 ml = £1.80; Aymes Actagain Juce liquid zesty orange: 200 ml = £1.80
Not suitable for use in child under 6 years; use with caution in child under 11 years									
Ensure® Plus Juce (Abbott Laboratories Ltd)	Liquid (sip or tube feed) **per 100 mL**	638 kJ (150 kcal)	4.8 g whey protein isolate	32.7 g (sugars 9.4 g)	Nil	Nil	Contains residual lactose. Gluten-free	Borderline substances standard ACBS indications p. 1375	Ensure Plus Juce Starter Pack liquid: 1320 ml = £10.80; Ensure Plus Juce liquid: peach 220 ml = £1.80; fruit punch 220 ml = £1.80; lemon & lime 220 ml = £1.80; apple 220 ml = £1.80; orange 220 ml = £1.80; strawberry 220 ml = £1.80
Not suitable for use in child under 1 year; use with caution in child under 5 years									
Fortijuce® (Nutricia Ltd)	Liquid (sip feed) **per 100 mL**	635 kJ (150 kcal)	3.9 g milk protein	33.5 g (sugars 13.1 g)	Nil	Nil	Contains residual lactose. Gluten-free	Borderline substances standard ACBS indications p. 1375; except dysphagia.	Fortijuce Starter Pack liquid: 800 ml = £7.20; Fortijuce liquid: tropical 200 ml = £1.80; lemon 200 ml = £1.80; orange 200 ml = £1.80; apple 200 ml = £1.80; strawberry 200 ml = £1.80
Not suitable for use in child under 1 year; not recommended for child 1-5 years									
Fresubin® Jucy (Fresenius Kabi Ltd)	Liquid (sip feed) **per 100 mL**	630 kJ (150 kcal)	4 g whey protein	33.5 g (sugars 8 g)	Nil	Nil	Contains residual lactose. Gluten-free	Borderline substances standard ACBS indications p. 1375; also CAPD and haemodialysis.	Fresubin Jucy drink: starter pack 1200 ml = £12.45; pineapple 800 ml = £7.57; apple 800 ml = £7.57; orange 800 ml = £7.57; cherry 800 ml = £7.57; blackcurrant 800 ml = £7.57
Not suitable for use in child under 3 years; use with caution in child under 6 years									
PaediaSure® Plus Juce (Abbott Laboratories Ltd)	Liquid (sip feed) **per 100 mL**	638 kJ (150 kcal)	4.20 g whey protein isolate	33.3 g (sugars 10.4 g)	Nil	Nil	Contains residual lactose. Gluten-free	Disease-related malnutrition and, or growth failure.	PaediaSure Plus Juce liquid: apple 200 ml = £5.19; very berry 200 ml = £5.19
Not recommended for child under 1 year									

1.5 kcal/mL milkshake

Product	Formulation	Energy	Protein	Carbohydrate	Fat	Fibre	Special Characteristics	ACBS Indications	Presentation & Flavour
Altraplen® Energy (Nualtra Ltd)	Liquid (sip feed) per 100 mL	640 kJ (150 kcal)	6 g milk protein	18.5 g (sugars 6.5 g)	5.8 g	Nil	Gluten-free	Disease related malnutrition.	Altraplen Energy Starter Pack liquid: 800 ml = £5.09; Altraplen Energy liquid: banana 200 ml = £0.99; chocolate 200 ml = £0.99; vanilla 200 ml = £0.99; strawberry 200 ml = £0.99
Not suitable for use in child under 3 years; not recommended for child 3-6 years									
Aymes® Actagain 1.5 Complete (Aymes International Ltd)	Liquid (sip feed) per 100 mL	630 kJ (150 kcal)	7 g milk protein	17 g (sugars 6.8 g)	6 g	Nil	Contains residual lactose. Gluten-free	Borderline substances standard ACBS indications p. 1375.	Aymes Actagain 1.5 Complete Starter Pack liquid: 800 ml = £4.88; Aymes Actagain 1.5 Complete liquid: banana milkshake 200 ml = £0.99; strawberry burst 200 ml = £0.99; double chocolate 200 ml = £0.99; smooth vanilla 200 ml = £0.99
Not suitable for use in child under 3 years; not suitable as a sole source of nutrition in child under 11 years									
Aymes® Actagain 1.5 Plant Powered (Aymes International Ltd)	Liquid (sip feed) per 100 mL	631 kJ (150 kcal)	6.7 g faba protein isolate	17 g (sugars 4.3 g)	6 g	0.1 g	Gluten-free, lactose-free	Borderline substances standard ACBS indications p. 1375 except dysphagia.	Aymes Actagain 1.5 Plant Powered Starter Pack liquid: 600 ml = £4.62; Aymes Actagain 1.5 Plant Powered liquid: cafe latte 200 ml = £1.54; salted caramel 200 ml = £1.54; madagascan vanilla 200 ml = £1.54
Not suitable for use in child under 3 years; use with caution in child over 3 years									
Aymes® ActaJuni (Aymes International Ltd)	Liquid (sip feed) per 100 mL	630 kJ (150 kcal)	4 g milk proteins	17.8 g sugars (3.5 g)	7 g	0.6 g	Contains residual lactose. Gluten-free	Disease-related malnutrition.	Aymes ActaJuni Starter Pack liquid: 600 ml = £7.87; Aymes ActaJuni liquid: chocolate 200 ml = £2.62; strawberry 200 ml = £2.62; vanilla 200 ml = £2.62
Suitable for child 1-10 years; not suitable for use in child under 1 year; use with caution in child under 10 years									
EnergieShake® Complete 1.5kcal (Anaiah Healthcare PVT Ltd)	Liquid (sip feed) per 100 mL	630 kJ (150 kcal)	6 g milk proteins	18 g (sugars 6.5 g)	6 g	Nil	Contains lactose, soya. Gluten-free	Borderline substances standard ACBS indications p. 1375, CAPD and haemodialysis.	EnergieShake Complete 1.5kcal liquid: chocolate 200 ml = £0.89; vanilla 200 ml = £0.89; strawberry 200 ml = £0.89; banana 200 ml = £0.89
Not suitable for use in child under 3 years; not recommended for child under 11 years									
Fortini® (Nutricia Ltd)	Liquid (sip feed) per 100 mL	630 kJ (150 kcal)	3.3 g caseinates	18.8 g (sugars 7.4 g)	6.8 g	Nil	Contains residual lactose, soya. Gluten-free	Disease-related malnutrition, growth failure.	Fortini liquid: vanilla 200 ml = £5.15; strawberry 200 ml = £5.15
Not suitable for use in child under 1 year									
Fortisip® Bottle (Nutricia Ltd)	Liquid (sip feed) per 100 mL	625 kJ (150 kcal)	5.9 g milk proteins	18.4 g (sugars 6.7 g)	5.8 g	Nil	Contains residual lactose, soya.	Borderline substances standard ACBS indications p. 1375	Fortisip Bottle: banana 200 ml = £1.50; vanilla 200 ml = £1.50; chocolate 200 ml = £1.50; strawberry 200 ml = £1.50; neutral 200 ml = £1.50
Not suitable for use in child under 3 years									

1.5 kcal/mL milkshake (product list continued)

Product	Formulation	Energy	Protein	Carbohydrate	Fat	Fibre	Special Characteristics	ACBS Indications	Presentation & Flavour
Fortisip® PlantBased 1.5kcal (Nutricia Ltd)	Liquid (sip feed) per 100 mL	630 kJ (150 kcal)	6.0 g pea protein isolate, soy protein isolate	18.6 g (sugars 9.4 g)	5.8 g	0.05 g	Contains soya. Lactose-free	Borderline substances standard ACBS indications p. 1375 except dysphagia.	Fortisip PlantBased 1.5kcal liquid: mango passionfruit 200 ml = £1.60; mocha 200 ml = £1.60
Not suitable for use in child under 3 years; use with caution in child over 3 years									
Frebini® Energy Drink (Fresenius Kabi Ltd)	Liquid (sip feed) per 100 mL	630 kJ (150 kcal)	3.8 g milk protein	18.7 g (sugars 4.5 g)	6.7 g	Nil	Contains soya, residual lactose. Gluten-free	Borderline substances standard ACBS indications p. 1375 and growth failure.	Frebini Energy Drink: banana 200 ml = £4.32; strawberry 200 ml = £4.32
Not suitable for use in child under 1 year or in adults; not recommended for child over 10 years									
Fresubin® Energy (Fresenius Kabi Ltd)	Liquid (sip feed) per 100 mL	630 kJ (150 kcal)	5.6 g milk protein	18.8 g (sugars 3.9-6.3 g)	5.8 g	Nil	Contains residual lactose, soya lecithin. Gluten-free	Borderline substances standard ACBS indications p. 1375.	Fresubin Energy liquid: tropical fruits 200 ml = £1.53; blackcurrant 200 ml = £1.53; cappuccino 200 ml = £1.53; chocolate 200 ml = £1.53; strawberry 200 ml = £1.53; vanilla 200 ml = £1.53; banana 200 ml = £1.53
Not suitable for use in child under 3 years; use with caution in child under 6 years									
Fresubin® Plant-Based drink (Fresenius Kabi Ltd)	Liquid (sip feed) per 100 mL	630 kJ (150 kcal)	7.5 g soya protein	16.1 g sugars (6.3 g)	5.7 g	2.3 g	Contains soya. Gluten-free, lactose-free	Borderline substances standard ACBS indications p. 1375	Fresubin Plant-Based drink: 200 ml = £1.60
Not suitable for use in child under 3 years; use with caution in child under 6 years									
PaediaSure® Plus (Abbott Laboratories Ltd)	Liquid (sip feed) per 100 mL	628-632 kJ (150-151 kcal)	4.2 g caseinates, whey protein	16.7 g (sugars 2.2-5.5 g)	7.5 g	Nil	Contains residual lactose, soya. Gluten-free	Borderline substances paediatric ACBS indications p. 1375.	PaediaSure Plus liquid: strawberry 200 ml = £5.23; unflavoured 200 ml = £5.23; vanilla 200 ml = £5.23; banana 200 ml = £5.23
Not suitable for use in child under 1 year; not recommended for child over 10 years									
Resource® Junior (Nestle Health Science)	Liquid (sip feed) per 100 mL	637 kJ (152 kcal)	3 g milk protein	21 g (sugars 5.2 g)	6.2 g	Nil	Contains residual lactose. Gluten-free	Borderline substances standard ACBS indications p. 1375.	Resource Junior complete sip feed: vanilla 200 ml = £2.92; strawberry 200 ml = £2.92
Suitable for child 1-10 years; not suitable for use in child under 1 year									

1.5 kcal/mL smoothie

Product	Formulation	Energy	Protein	Carbohydrate	Fat	Fibre	Special Characteristics	ACBS Indications	Presentation & Flavour
Fortini® Smoothie Multi Fibre (Nutricia Ltd)	Liquid (sip feed) per 100 mL	625 kJ (150 kcal)	3.4 g whey protein	19 g (sugars 11.5 g)	6.4 g	1.4 g	Contains residual lactose, soya. Gluten-free	Disease-related malnutrition, growth failure.	Fortini Smoothie Multi Fibre liquid: summer fruit 200 ml = £5.40; berry fruit 200 ml = £5.40
Not suitable for use in child under 1 year									

1.5 kcal/mL yoghurt style drink

Product	Formulation	Energy	Protein	Carbohydrate	Fat	Fibre	Special Characteristics	ACBS Indications	Presentation & Flavour
Fresubin® YoDrink (Fresenius Kabi Ltd)	Liquid (sip feed) per 100 mL	630 kJ (150 kcal)	7.5 g milk, whey proteins	19.5 g sucrose (sugars 15.4 g)	4.7 g	0.1 g	Contains lactose, soya. Gluten-free	Dietary management of patients with or at risk of malnutrition who are not able to meet their nutritional requirements from ordinary foods alone. Includes elderly patients, patients with chronic wasting disease (cancer, HIV/AIDS), peri-operative patients, further patients with evidence based indication for oral nutritional supplementation (eg pre- and post-organ transplantation, inflammatory bowel disease).	Fresubin YoDrink: apricot-peach 200 ml = £1.92; lemon 200 ml = £1.92; raspberry 200 ml = £1.92

Not suitable for use in child under 3 years; not recommended for child under 6 years

1.5 - 1.6 kcal/mL milkshake higher protein

Product	Formulation	Energy	Protein	Carbohydrate	Fat	Fibre	Special Characteristics	ACBS Indications	Presentation & Flavour
Altraplen® Protein (Nualtra Ltd)	Liquid (sip feed) per 100 mL	632 kJ (150 kcal)	10 g milk, soya proteins	15 g (sugars 4.6 g)	5.6 g	Nil	Contains residual lactose, soya. Gluten-free	Borderline substances standard ACBS indications p. 1375.	Altraplen Protein Starter Pack liquid: 400 ml = £4.80; Altraplen Protein liquid: strawberry 800 ml = £9.94; vanilla 800 ml = £9.94
Not suitable for use in child under 3 years; not recommended for child under 6 years									
Fortisip® Extra (Nutricia Ltd)	Liquid (sip feed) per 100 mL	670 kJ (159 kcal)	9.8 g milk proteins	18.1 g (sugars 9 g)	5.3 g	Nil	Contains lactose, soya. Gluten-free	Borderline substances standard ACBS indications p. 1375	Fortisip Extra liquid: vanilla 200 ml = £1.65; strawberry 200 ml = £1.65
Not suitable for use in child under 3 years									
Fresubin® Protein Energy (Fresenius Kabi Ltd)	Liquid (sip feed) per 100 mL	630 kJ (150 kcal)	10 g milk protein	12.4 g maltodextrin and sucrose (sugars 6.5-7.4 g)	6.7 g	Nil	Contains residual lactose, soya lecithin. Gluten-free	Borderline substances standard ACBS indications p. 1375; also CAPD, haemodialysis.	Fresubin Protein Energy drink: wild strawberry 200 ml = £2.45; cappuccino 200 ml = £2.45; chocolate 200 ml = £2.45; vanilla 200 ml = £2.45; tropical fruits 200 ml = £2.45

Not suitable for use in child under 3 years; use with caution in child under 6 years

1.5 - 1.6 kcal/mL milkshake with fibre

Product	Formulation	Energy	Protein	Carbohydrate	Fat	Fibre	Special Characteristics	ACBS Indications	Presentation & Flavour
Fortini® Multi Fibre (Nutricia Ltd)	Liquid (sip feed) per 100 mL	640 kJ (153 kcal)	3.3 g caseinates	18.8 g (sugars 7.4 g)	6.8 g	1.5 g	Contains residual lactose, soya. Gluten-free	Disease-related malnutrition, growth failure.	Fortini Multi Fibre liquid: unflavoured 200 ml = £5.40; chocolate 200 ml = £5.40; banana 200 ml = £5.40; vanilla 200 ml = £5.40; strawberry 200 ml = £5.40

Not suitable for use in child under 1 year

1.5 - 1.6 kcal/mL milkshake with fibre (product list continued)

Product	Formulation	Energy	Protein	Carbohydrate	Fat	Fibre	Special Characteristics	ACBS Indications	Presentation & Flavour
Frebini® Energy Fibre (Fresenius Kabi Ltd)	Liquid (sip feed) per 100 mL	630 kJ (150 kcal)	3.8 g milk protein	18.1 g (sugars 4.5 g)	6.7 g	1.1 g	Contains residual lactose, soya. Gluten-free	Borderline substances paediatric ACBS indications p. 1375; also proven inflammatory bowel disease and following total gastrectomy.	Frebini Energy Fibre liquid: chocolate 200 ml = £4.40; vanilla 200 ml = £4.40
Not suitable for use in child under 1 year or in adults; not recommended for child over 10 years									
Fresubin® Energy Fibre (Fresenius Kabi Ltd)	Liquid (sip feed) per 100 mL	630 kJ (150 kcal)	5.6 g milk protein	17.8 g (sugars 5-6.4 g)	5.8 g	2 g	Contains residual lactose, soya lecithin. Gluten-free	Borderline substances standard ACBS indications p. 1375.	Fresubin Energy Fibre liquid: strawberry 200 ml = £2.76; chocolate 200 ml = £2.76; caramel 200 ml = £2.76; vanilla 200 ml = £2.76; cherry 200 ml = £2.76; banana 200 ml = £2.76
Not suitable for use in child under 3 years; use with caution in child under 6 years									
PaediaSure® Plus Fibre (Abbott Laboratories Ltd)	Liquid (sip feed) per 100 mL	635 kJ (152 kcal)	4.2 g caseinates, milk protein, whey protein	16.4 g (sugars 5.5-6.0 g)	7.47 g	1.1 g	Contains residual lactose, soya. Gluten-free	Borderline substances paediatric ACBS indications p. 1375.	PaediaSure Plus fibre Starter Pack liquid: 800 ml = £20.32; PaediaSure Plus fibre liquid: banana 200 ml = £5.65; vanilla 200 ml = £5.65; 400 ml = ; strawberry 200 ml = £5.65; chocolate 200 ml = £5.65
Not suitable for use in child under 1 year; suitable for child 1-10 years or 8-30 kg; chocolate flavour suitable for child 3-10 years or 12-30 kg									

1.6 kcal/g dessert style (fruit based)

Product	Formulation	Energy	Protein	Carbohydrate	Fat	Fibre	Special Characteristics	ACBS Indications	Presentation & Flavour
Fresubin® Dessert Fruit Puree (Fresenius Kabi Ltd)	Semi-solid per 100 g	670 kJ (160 kcal)	7 g whey protein	18.7 g sucrose (sugars 16.2 g)	5.6 g	3.5 g	Contains residual lactose, soya lecithin. Gluten-free	Borderline substances standard ACBS indications p. 1375 except intractable malabsorption.	Fresubin Dessert Fruit Puree: 500 gram = £11.23
Not suitable for use in child under 3 years; use with caution in child under 6 years									

2 kcal/mL milkshake higher protein, higher energy with fibre

Product	Formulation	Energy	Protein	Carbohydrate	Fat	Fibre	Special Characteristics	ACBS Indications	Presentation & Flavour
Aymes® Actagain 2.0 Fibre (Aymes International Ltd)	Liquid (sip feed) per 100 mL	855 kJ (204 kcal)	10 g milk protein	21.5 g (sugars 7.5 g)	8.1 g	2.5 g	Contains residual lactose, soya. Gluten-free	Borderline substances standard ACBS indications p. 1375 except dysphagia.	Aymes Actagain 2.0 Fibre Starter Pack liquid: 600 ml = £6.45; Aymes Actagain 2.0 Fibre liquid: strawberry burst 200 ml = £2.18; smooth vanilla 200 ml = £2.18; cafe latte 200 ml = £2.18
Not suitable for use in child under 6 years; use with caution in child under 11 years									
Fresubin® 2kcal Fibre (Fresenius Kabi Ltd)	Liquid (sip feed) per 100 mL	840 kJ (200 kcal)	10 g milk protein	21.8 g (sugars 3.3-5.9 g)	7.8 g	1.5 g	Contains residual lactose, soya lecithin. Gluten-free	Borderline substances standard ACBS indications p. 1375; also CAPD, haemodialysis.	Fresubin 2kcal Fibre drink: vanilla 200 ml = £2.50; chocolate 200 ml = £2.50; lemon 200 ml = £2.50; apricot-peach 200 ml = £2.50; neutral 200 ml = £2.50; cappuccino 200 ml = £2.50
Not suitable for use in child under 3 years; use with caution in child under 6 years									

Resource® 2.0 Fibre (Nestle Health Science)	Liquid (sip or tube feed) per 100 mL	835 kJ (200 kcal)	9 g milk protein	20 g (sugars 6 g)	8.7 g	2.5 g	Contains residual lactose. Gluten-free	Borderline substances standard ACBS indications p. 1375.	Resource Fibre 2.0 liquid: strawberry 200 ml = £2.68; vanilla 200 ml = £2.68
Not suitable for use in child under 6 years; use with caution in child under 10 years									

2 - 2.4 kcal/mL milkshake higher protein, higher energy

Product	Formulation	Energy	Protein	Carbohydrate	Fat	Fibre	Special Characteristics	ACBS Indications	Presentation & Flavour
Aymes® Actagain 2.0 (Aymes International Ltd)	Liquid (sip feed) **per 100 mL**	857 kJ (200 kcal)	10 g milk protein	23 g (sugars 7.5 g)	8 g	Nil	Contains residual lactose. Gluten-free	Borderline substances standard ACBS indications p. 1375 except dysphagia.	Aymes Actagain 2.0 Starter Pack liquid: 1200 ml = £13.12; Aymes Actagain 2.0 liquid: neutral 200 ml = £2.18; cafe latte 200 ml = £2.18; smooth vanilla 200 ml = £2.18; golden apricot 200 ml = £2.18; dulce de leche 200 ml = £2.18; berry medley 200 ml = £2.18
Not suitable for use in child under 6 years; use with caution in child under 11 years									
Aymes® Actagain 2.4 (Aymes International Ltd)	Liquid (sip feed) **per 100 mL**	1008 kJ (240 kcal)	9.6 g milk protein	29 g (sugars 8 g)	9.6 g	Nil	Contains residual lactose. Gluten-free	Borderline substances standard ACBS indications p. 1375 except dysphagia.	Aymes Actagain 2.4 Starter Pack liquid: 600 ml = £5.39; Aymes Actagain 2.4 liquid: banana milkshake 200 ml = £1.79; smooth vanilla 200 ml = £1.79; strawberry burst 200 ml = £1.79
Not suitable for use in child under 6 years; use with caution in child under 11 years									
EnergieShake® 2.0kcal (Anaiah Healthcare PVT Ltd)	Liquid (sip feed) **per 100 mL**	840 kJ (200 kcal)	9.6 g milk protein	21.7 g (sugars 10.1 g)	8.2 g	Nil	Contains residual lactose. Gluten-free	Borderline substances standard ACBS indications p. 1375; also CAPD and haemodialysis.	EnergieShake 2.0kcal liquid: strawberry 200 ml = £1.52; banana 200 ml = £1.52; vanilla 200 ml = £1.52
Not suitable for use in child under 6 years; not recommended for child 6-11 years									
Fortisip® 2kcal (Nutricia Ltd)	Liquid (sip feed) **per 100 mL**	839 kJ (201 kcal)	10.1 g milk proteins	20.6 g (sugars 15.4 g)	8.6 g	Nil	Contains residual lactose, soya.	Borderline substances standard ACBS indications p. 1375 except dysphagia; also CAPD and haemodialysis.	Fortisip 2kcal liquid: vanilla 200 ml = £2.50; strawberry 200 ml = £2.50; forest fruit 200 ml = £2.50; chocolate-caramel 200 ml = £2.50; mocha 200 ml = £2.50
Not suitable for use in child under 3 years; use with caution in child 3-6 years									
Fortisip® PlantBased 2kcal (Nutricia Ltd)	Liquid (sip feed) **per 100 mL**	840 kJ (200 kcal)	10 g pea protein isolate, soy protein isolate	22.5 g (sugars 6.5 g)	7.8 g	Nil	Contains soya. Gluten-free, residual lactose	Borderline substances standard ACBS indications p. 1375 except dysphagia.	Fortisip PlantBased 2kcal liquid: pea mint 200 ml = £2.50; tropical 200 ml = £2.50; cafe latte 200 ml = £2.50; pumpkin carrot ginger 200 ml = £2.50
Not suitable for use in child under 3 years; use with caution in child over 3 years									

2 - 2.4 kcal/mL milkshake higher protein, higher energy (product list continued)

Product	Formulation	Energy	Protein	Carbohydrate	Fat	Fibre	Special Characteristics	ACBS Indications	Presentation & Flavour
Fresubin® 2kcal (Fresenius Kabi Ltd)	Liquid (sip feed) per 100 mL	840 kJ (200 kcal)	10 g milk protein	22.5 g (sugars 3.2-5.8 g)	7.8 g	Nil	Contains residual lactose, soya. Gluten-free	Borderline substances standard ACBS indications p. 1375; also CAPD, haemodialysis.	Fresubin 2kcal drink: toffee 200 ml = £2.40; cappuccino 200 ml = £2.40; vanilla 200 ml = £2.40; apricot-peach 200 ml = £2.40; neutral 200 ml = £2.40; fruits of the forest 200 ml = £2.40
Not suitable for use in child under 3 years; use with caution in child under 6 years									

2 - 2.4 kcal/mL milkshake lower volume

Product	Formulation	Energy	Protein	Carbohydrate	Fat	Fibre	Special Characteristics	ACBS Indications	Presentation & Flavour
Altraplen® Compact (Nualtra Ltd)	Liquid (sip feed) per 100 mL	1008 kJ (240 kcal)	9.6 g milk, soya proteins	28.8 g (sugars 11.6 g)	9.6 g	Nil	Contains residual lactose, soya. Gluten-free	Borderline substances standard ACBS indications p. 1375.	Altraplen Compact Starter Pack liquid: 500 ml = £8.60; Altraplen Compact liquid: vanilla 500 ml = £6.40; hazel chocolate 500 ml = £6.40; banana 500 ml = £6.40; strawberry 500 ml = £6.40
Not suitable for use in child under 3 years; not recommended for child under 6 years									
Fortisip® Compact (Nutricia Ltd)	Liquid (sip feed) per 100 mL	1010 kJ (240 kcal)	9.6 g milk proteins	29.6 g (sugars 15.5 g)	9.3 g	Nil	Contains residual lactose, soya	Borderline substances standard ACBS indications p. 1375 except dysphagia.	Fortisip Compact Starter Pack liquid: 750 ml = £9.60; Fortisip Compact liquid: strawberry 500 ml = £6.40; mocha 500 ml = £6.40; neutral 500 ml = £6.40; chocolate 500 ml = £6.40; banana 500 ml = £6.40; vanilla 500 ml = £6.40
Not suitable for use in child under 3 years; use with caution in child 3-6 years									
Fresubin® 2kcal Mini (Fresenius Kabi Ltd)	Liquid (sip feed) per 100 mL	840 kJ (200 kcal)	10 g milk protein	22.5 g (sugars 5.3-5.8 g)	7.8 g	Nil	Contains residual lactose, soya lecithin. Gluten-free	Borderline substances standard ACBS indications p. 1375; also CAPD, haemodialysis.	Fresubin 2kcal Mini drink: vanilla 500 ml = £5.80; fruits of the forest 500 ml = £5.80; apricot-peach 500 ml = £5.80
Not suitable for use in child under 3 years; use with caution in child under 6 years									
PaediaSure® Compact (Abbott Laboratories Ltd)	Liquid (sip feed) per 100 mL	1007 kJ (240 kcal)	6.72 g caseinates, milk protein, protein equivalent (amino acids)	26.2 g corn syrup (sugars 4.3 g)	11.9 g	0.73 g	Contains lactose, soya. Gluten-free	Disease-related malnutrition.	PaediaSure Compact Starter Pack liquid: 500 ml = £18.13; PaediaSure Compact liquid: vanilla 500 ml = £20.14; banana 500 ml = £20.14; strawberry 500 ml = £20.14
Not suitable for use in child under 1 year; suitable for child 1-10 years or 8-30 kg									

2 - 2.4 kcal/mL milkshake lower volume with fibre

Product	Formulation	Energy	Protein	Carbohydrate	Fat	Fibre	Special Characteristics	ACBS Indications	Presentation & Flavour
Altrini Compact® Fibre (Nualtra Ltd)	Liquid (sip feed) per 100 mL	1008 kJ (240 kcal)	6 g milk protein	35.2 g sugars (7.5 g)	8 g	1.4 g	Contains residual lactose, soya. Gluten-free	Disease-related malnutrition.	Altrini Compact Fibre liquid: strawberry 500 ml = £14.00; vanilla 500 ml = £14.00
Suitable for child 1-10 years; not suitable for use in child under 1 year									

Product	Formulation	Energy	Protein	Carbohydrate	Fat	Fibre	Special Characteristics	ACBS Indications	Presentation & Flavour
Fortini® Compact Multi Fibre (Nutricia Ltd)	Liquid (sip feed) per 100 mL	1006 kJ (240 kcal)	5.7 g milk protein	28.5 g (sugars 14.9 g)	10.9 g	2.4 g	Contains residual lactose, soya. Gluten-free	Disease-related malnutrition, growth failure.	Fortini Compact Multi Fibre liquid: strawberry 125 ml = £4.85; neutral 125 ml = £4.85; chocolate-caramel 125 ml = £4.85
Not suitable for use in child under 1 year									
Fortisip® Compact Fibre (Nutricia Ltd)	Liquid (sip feed) per 100 mL	1007 kJ (240 kcal)	9.5 g cow's milk	25.4 g (sugars 13.4 g)	10.4 g	3.6 g	Contains residual lactose, soya	Borderline substances standard ACBS indications p. 1375 except dysphagia.	Fortisip Compact Fibre liquid: vanilla 500 ml = £11.96; strawberry 500 ml = £11.96; mocha 500 ml = £11.96
Not suitable for use in child under 3 years; use with caution in child 3-6 years									
Fresubin® 2kcal Fibre Mini (Fresenius Kabi Ltd)	Liquid (sip feed) per 100 mL	840 kJ (200 kcal)	10 g milk protein	21.8 g (sugars 5.9 g)	7.8 g	1.5 g	Contains residual lactose, soya lecithin. Gluten-free	Borderline substances standard ACBS indications p. 1375; also CAPD, haemodialysis.	Fresubin 2kcal Fibre Mini drink: vanilla 500 ml = £6.24; chocolate 500 ml = £6.24
Not suitable for use in child under 3 years; use with caution in child under 6 years									

2.4 kcal/mL milkshake higher volume

Product	Formulation	Energy	Protein	Carbohydrate	Fat	Fibre	Special Characteristics	ACBS Indications	Presentation & Flavour
Altraplen® Compact Daily (Nualtra Ltd)	Liquid (sip feed) per 100 mL	1008 kJ (240 kcal)	9.6 g milk protein, soya protein	28.8 g (sugars 11.3 g)	9.6 g	Nil	Contains residual lactose, soya. Gluten-free	Disease related malnutrition.	Altraplen Compact Daily Starter Pack liquid: 1000 ml = £7.16; Altraplen Compact Daily liquid: strawberry 250 ml = £1.60; vanilla 250 ml = £1.60; banana 250 ml = £1.60
Not suitable for use in child under 3 years; use with caution in child under 6 years									
Aymes® Actagain 2.4 Daily (Aymes International Ltd)	Liquid (sip feed) per 100 mL	1008 kJ (240 kcal)	9.6 g milk protein	29 g (sugars 8 g)	9.6 g	Nil	Contains residual lactose. Gluten-free	Borderline substances standard ACBS indications p. 1375 except dysphagia.	Aymes Actagain 2.4 Daily Starter Pack liquid: 750 ml = £4.80; Aymes Actagain 2.4 Daily liquid: smooth vanilla 250 ml = £1.60; banana milkshake 250 ml = £1.60; strawberry burst 250 ml = £1.60
Not suitable for use in child under 6 years; use with caution in child under 11 years									

2.4 kcal/mL milkshake lower volume, higher protein

Product	Formulation	Energy	Protein	Carbohydrate	Fat	Fibre	Special Characteristics	ACBS Indications	Presentation & Flavour
Fortisip® Compact Protein (Nutricia Ltd)	Liquid (sip feed) per 100 mL	1029 kJ (245 kcal)	14.6 g milk proteins	25.1 g (sugars 13.7 g)	9.6 g	Nil	Contains residual lactose, soya. Gluten-free	Borderline substances standard ACBS indications p. 1375 except dysphagia.	Fortisip Compact Protein Starter Pack liquid: 1000 ml = £21.60; Fortisip Compact Protein liquid: banana 500 ml = £10.80; strawberry 500 ml = £10.80; peach & mango 500 ml = £10.80; cool red fruits 500 ml = £10.80; mocha 500 ml = £10.80; neutral 500 ml = £10.80; vanilla 500 ml = £10.80; berries 500 ml = £10.80; hot tropical ginger 500 ml = £10.80
Not suitable for use in child under 6 years; use with caution in child 6-10 years									

2.4 kcal/mL milkshake lower volume, higher protein (product list continued)

Product	Formulation	Energy	Protein	Carbohydrate	Fat	Fibre	Special Characteristics	ACBS Indications	Presentation & Flavour
Fresubin® 3.2kcal (Fresenius Kabi Ltd)	Liquid (sip feed) per 100 mL	1344 kJ (320 kcal)	16 g collagen, milk proteins	28 g (sugars 11 g)	16 g	0.4 g	Contains residual lactose, soya lecithin. Gluten-free	Borderline substances standard ACBS indications p. 1375.	Fresubin 3.2kcal drink: mango 500 ml = £10.24; vanilla-caramel 500 ml = £10.24; hazelnut 500 ml = £10.24; cappuccino 500 ml = £10.24
Not suitable for use in child under 3 years; use with caution in child under 6 years									
Fresubin® Pro Compact (Fresenius Kabi Ltd)	Liquid (sip feed) per 100 mL	1008 kJ (240 kcal)	14.4 g milk protein	24 g (sugars 3.9 g)	9.4 g	Nil	Contains residual lactose, soya lecithin. Gluten-free	Borderline substances standard ACBS indications p. 1375 except dysphagia.	Fresubin Pro Compact drink: cappuccino 125 ml = £1.69; neutral 125 ml = £1.69; hazelnut 125 ml = £1.69; vanilla 125 ml = £1.69; apricot-peach 125 ml = £1.69
Not suitable for use in child under 7 years; use with caution in child under 10 years									

Table 3 Infant nutrition

Condition specific infant formula

Cow's milk protein allergy: Extensively hydrolysed formula

Product	Formulation	Energy	Protein	Carbohydrate	Fat	Fibre	Special Characteristics	ACBS Indications	Presentation & Flavour
Aptamil Pepti® 1 (Nutricia Ltd)	Standard dilution (13.64 % w/v) of powder per 100 mL	276 kJ (66 kcal)	1.6 g whey hydrolysate	7.1 g (sugars 3.5 g)	3.4 g	0.5 g	Contains fish oil, lactose	Established cows' milk allergy with/without proven secondary lactose intolerance.	Aptamil Pepti 1 powder: 400 gram = £10.98; 800 gram = £21.97
Powder provides: protein 11.6 g, carbohydrate 51.8 g, fat 24.7 g, energy 2024 kJ (484 kcal)/100 g.									
Aptamil Pepti® 2 (Nutricia Ltd)	Standard dilution (14.43 % w/v) of powder per 100 mL	285 kJ (68 kcal)	1.6 g whey protein hydrolysate	7.8 g (sugars 3.6 g)	3.2 g	0.6 g	Contains fish oil, lactose	Established cows' milk allergy.	Aptamil Pepti 2 powder: 400 gram = £10.98; 800 gram = £21.97
Powder provides: protein 11.4 g, carbohydrate 54.3 g, fat 22.3 g, energy 1974 kJ (471 kcal)/100 g. Not suitable for use in child under 6 months									
Aptamil® Pepti Syneo (Nutricia Ltd)	Standard dilution (13.7 % w/v) of powder per 100 mL	276 kJ (66 kcal)	1.6 g whey protein hydrolysate	7.1 g (sugars 3.5 g)	3.4 g	0.6 g	Contains fish oil, lactose	Cow's milk protein allergy.	Aptamil Pepti Syneo powder: 400 gram = £10.98; 800 gram = £21.97
Powder provides: protein 11.6 g, carbohydrate 51.7 g, fat 24.7 g, energy 2023 kJ (483 kcal)/100 g									
Arize (Abbott Laboratories Ltd)	Standard dilution (13.5 % w/v) of powder per 100 mL	287 kJ (68 kcal)	2 g rice protein hydrolysate	7.3 g (sugars 1.4 g)	3.4 g (MCT 30.6%)	0.02 g	Contains residual lactose, soya oil. Gluten-free	Cow's milk protein allergy and other conditions where an extensively hydrolysed formula is indicated.	Arize powder: 400 gram = £15.89
Powder provides: protein 15 g, carbohydrate 54 g, fat 9.8 g, energy 2125 kJ (508 kcal)/100 g									

Nutramigen 1 with LGG® (Reckitt Benckiser Healthcare (UK) Ltd)	Standard dilution (13.5 % w/v) of powder per 100 mL	284 kJ (68 kcal)	1.88 g casein hydrolysate	7.4 g (sugars 0.77 g)	3.4 g	Nil	Contains soya oil. Lactose-free	Cow's milk allergy with / or without lactose intolerance.	Nutramigen 1 with LGG powder: 400 gram = £12.92

Powder provides: protein 14 g, carbohydrate 55 g, fat 25 g, energy 2098 kJ (501 kcal)/100 g.
Suitable for child from birth to 6 months

Nutramigen 2 with LGG® (Reckitt Benckiser Healthcare (UK) Ltd)	Standard dilution (13.5 % w/v) of powder per 100 mL	285 kJ (68 kcal)	1.68 g casein hydrolysate	7.7 g (sugars 3.5 g)	3.4 g	Nil	Contains soya oil. Lactose-free	Cow's milk allergy with / or without lactose intolerance.	Nutramigen 2 with LGG powder: 400 gram = £12.92

Powder provides: protein 12.5 g, carbohydrate 57 g, fat 25 g, energy 2107 kJ (503 kcal)/100 g.
Suitable from 6 months

SMA Althera® (Nestle Health Science)	Standard dilution (13.2% w/v) of powder per 100 mL	280 kJ (67 kcal)	1.7 g whey protein	7.3 g lactose (sugars 4.0 g)	3.4 g	Nil	Contains lactose. Gluten-free	Dietary management of cows' milk protein allergy and/or multiple food protein allergies.	SMA Althera powder: 400 gram = £11.04

Powder provides: protein 12.5 g, carbohydrate 55.5 g, fat 26 g, energy 2118 kJ (506 kcal)/100 g
Not recommended for child over 3 years

Cow's milk protein allergy with impaired gastro-intestinal function or malabsorption: Extensively hydrolysed formula with MCT

Product	Formulation	Energy	Protein	Carbohydrate	Fat	Fibre	Special Characteristics	ACBS Indications	Presentation & Flavour
Aptamil Pepti-Junior® (Nutricia Ltd)	Standard dilution (13.4 % w/v) of powder per 100 mL	276 kJ (66 kcal)	1.8 g whey protein	7.2 g (sugars 1.1 g)	3.4 g (MCT 50%)	Nil	Contains fish oil, residual lactose	Disaccharide and/or whole protein intolerance, or where amino acids and peptides are indicated in conjunction with MCT.	Aptamil Pepti-Junior powder: 450 gram = £19.45

Powder provides: protein 13.3 g, carbohydrate 53.5 g, fat 25.2 g, energy 2063 kJ (493 kcal)/100 g

Cow's milk protein allergy with impaired gastro-intestinal function or malabsorption and faltering growth: Extensively hydrolysed formula, high energy

Product	Formulation	Energy	Protein	Carbohydrate	Fat	Fibre	Special Characteristics	ACBS Indications	Presentation & Flavour
Infatrini® Peptisorb (Nutricia Ltd)	Liquid (sip or tube feed) per 100 mL	418 kJ (100 kcal)	2.6 g whey protein hydrolysate	10.2 g (sugars 2.7 g)	5.4 g (MCT 52%)	Nil	Contains fish oil, residual lactose. Gluten-free	Disease-related malnutrition, intractable malabsorption, inflammatory bowel disease, short bowel syndrome, bowel fistulae and intolerance to whole protein feeds.	Infatrini Peptisorb liquid: 200 ml = £5.46

Not recommended for child over 18 months

Disorders of calcium metabolism: Low calcium infant formula

Product	Formulation	Energy	Protein	Carbohydrate	Fat	Fibre	Special Characteristics	ACBS Indications	Presentation & Flavour
Locasol® (Nutricia Ltd)	Standard dilution (13.1% w/v) of powder per 100 mL	278 kJ (66 kcal)	1.9 g caseinates, whey protein	7 g (sugars 6.9 g)	3.4 g	Nil	Contains lactose	Calcium intolerance.	Locasol powder: 400 gram = £36.69

Powder provides: protein 14.6 g, carbohydrate 53.7 g, fat 26.1 g, energy 2125 kJ (508 kcal)/100 g

Faltering growth: High energy infant formula

Product	Formulation	Energy	Protein	Carbohydrate	Fat	Fibre	Special Characteristics	ACBS Indications	Presentation & Flavour
Infatrini® (Nutricia Ltd)	Liquid (sip or tube feed) per 100 mL	418 kJ (100 kcal)	2.6 g milk, whey proteins	10.2 g (sugars 5.9 g)	5.3 g	0.6 g	Contains fish oil, lactose, soya. Gluten-free	Disease-related malnutrition, malabsorption, and growth failure.	Infatrini liquid: 125 ml = £1.99; 200 ml = £3.18
Not recommended for child over 18 months									
Similac® High Energy (Abbott Laboratories Ltd)	Liquid (sip or tube feed) per 100 mL	419 kJ (100 kcal)	2.6 g milk, whey proteins	10.1 g (sugars 5.5 g)	5.4 g	0.4 g	Contains lactose, soya. Gluten-free	Patients who have faltering growth, increased energy requirements and/or require a fluid restriction.	Similac High Energy liquid: 200 ml = £3.63
Not recommended for child over 18 months									
SMA High Energy® (SMA Nutrition)	Liquid per 100 mL	418 kJ (100 kcal)	2.6 g whey protein	10 g (sugars 6.7 g)	5.5 g	Nil	Contains fish oil, lactose	Disease-related malnutrition, malabsorption and growth failure in infancy.	SMA High Energy liquid: 200 ml = £2.43
Not recommended for child over 18 months									

Lactose intolerance: Lactose-free formula

Product	Formulation	Energy	Protein	Carbohydrate	Fat	Fibre	Special Characteristics	ACBS Indications	Presentation & Flavour
SMA LF® (SMA Nutrition)	Standard dilution (13.3% w/v) of powder per 100 mL	281 kJ (67 kcal)	1.6 g casein, whey protein	7.6 g (sugars 1.1 g)	3.4 g	Nil	Contains fish oil, residual lactose, soya	Proven lactose intolerance.	SMA LF powder: 400 gram = £6.46
Powder provides: protein 11.7 g, carbohydrate 56.7 g, fat 25.5 g, energy 2106 kJ (503 kcal)/100 g Not recommended for child over 18 months									

Severe cow's milk protein allergy or multiple food allergies: Amino acid formula

Product	Formulation	Energy	Protein	Carbohydrate	Fat	Fibre	Special Characteristics	ACBS Indications	Presentation & Flavour
EleCare® (Abbott Laboratories Ltd)	Standard dilution (13 % w/v) of powder per 100 mL	283 kJ (68 kcal)	1.8 g protein equivalent (amino acids)	7.2 g (sugars 0.6 g)	3.3 g	0.02 g	Contains residual lactose, soya. Gluten-free	Cow's milk allergy, severe and/or multiple food allergies or other conditions where an amino acid-based formula is indicated.	EleCare powder: 400 gram = £23.92
Powder provides: protein 14 g, carbohydrate 55.1 g, fat 25.3 g, energy 2171 kJ (519 kcal)/100 g.									
Neocate® LCP (Nutricia Ltd)	Standard dilution (13.5% w/v) of powder per 100 mL	278 kJ (67 kcal)	1.8 g protein equivalent (amino acids)	7.1 g (sugars 0.62 g)	3.5 g	Nil		Cow's milk allergy, multiple food protein allergies and other conditions where an elemental diet is recommended.	Neocate LCP powder: 420 gram = £25.56
Powder provides: protein 13.3 g, carbohydrate 52.5 g, fat 25.6 g, energy 2062 kJ (493 kcal)/100 g.									
Neocate® Syneo (Nutricia Ltd)	Standard dilution (14.4%) of powder per 100ml	286 kJ (68 kcal)	1.9 g protein equivalent (amino acids)	7.2 g (sugars 0.67 g)	3.4 g (MCT 33%)	0.64 g		Cow's milk allergy, multiple food protein allergies and other conditions requiring an amino acid-based diet.	Neocate Syneo powder: 400 gram = £25.56
Powder provides: protein 13.2 g, carbohydrate 50.2 g, fat 23.6 g, energy 1985 kJ (474 kcal)/100 g. Suitable for infants from birth; not suitable for use in premature infants									

Nutramigen® PurAmino (Reckitt Benckiser Healthcare (UK) Ltd)	Standard dilution (13.2 %) of powder per 100 ml	285 kJ (68 kcal)	1.88 g	6.9 g (sugars 0.55 g)	3.7 g	Nil	Contains soya oil. Lactose-free	Severe cow's milk allergy and multiple food intolerance. Suitable for other indications requiring an elemental diet.	Nutramigen PurAmino powder: 400 gram = £22.98
Powder provides: protein 14.3 g, carbohydrate 52 g, fat 28 g, energy 2140 kJ (510 kcal)/100 g.									
SMA Alfamino® (Nestle Health Science)	Standard dilution (13.3 % w/v) of powder per 100 mL	278 kJ (66 kcal)	1.8 g protein equivalent (essential and non-essential amino acids)	7.5 g (sugars 0.5 g)	3.3 g	Nil	Gluten-free, lactose-free	Dietary management of cows' milk allergy and/or multiple food allergies and other conditions where an amino acid formula is recommended.	SMA Alfamino powder: 400 gram = £25.73
Powder provides: protein 13 g, carbohydrate 56.3 g, fat 24.6 g, energy 2093 kJ (500 kcal)/100 g Not recommended for child over 3 years									

Significant reflux: Pre-thickened formula

Product	Formulation	Energy	Protein	Carbohydrate	Fat	Fibre	Special Characteristics	ACBS Indications	Presentation & Flavour
SMA® Anti-Reflux (SMA Nutrition)	Standard dilution (13% w/v) of powder per 100 mL	280 kJ (67 kcal)	1.3 g whey protein	7.8 g (sugars 4.9 g)	3.4 g	0.065 g	Contains fish oil, lactose	Significant reflux (regurgitation). Not to be used in conjunction with any other thickener or antacid products.	SMA Anti-Reflux powder: 800 gram = £9.43
Powder provides: protein 9.8 g, carbohydrate 60 g, fat 26 g, energy 2150 kJ (514 kcal)/100 g Not recommended for child over 1 year									

Condition specific follow-on formula

Cow's milk protein allergy: Extensively hydrolysed formula

Product	Formulation	Energy	Protein	Carbohydrate	Fat	Fibre	Special Characteristics	ACBS Indications	Presentation & Flavour
Nutramigen 3 with LGG® (Reckitt Benckiser Healthcare (UK) Ltd)	Standard dilution (13.5 % w/v) of powder per 100 ml	280 kJ (68 kcal)	1.55 g casein hydrolysate	7.7 g (sugars: 3.5 g)	3.4 g	Nil	Contains soya oil. Lactose-free	Cow's milk protein allergy.	Nutramigen 3 with LGG powder: 400 gram = £12.92
Powder provides: protein 11.5 g, carbohydrate 57 g, fat 25 g, energy 2100 kJ (500 kcal)/100 g Suitable from 1 year									

Cow's milk protein allergy with impaired gastro-intestinal function or malabsorption: Amino acid products

Product	Formulation	Energy	Protein	Carbohydrate	Fat	Fibre	Special Characteristics	ACBS Indications	Presentation & Flavour
Neocate® Junior (Nutricia Ltd)	Standard dilution (21.1 %) of powder per 100ml	420 kJ (100 kcal)	2.8 g protein equivalent (amino acids)	12 g (sugars 1.1 g)	4.6 g (MCT 35%)	Nil		Proven whole protein allergy, short bowel syndrome, intractable malabsorption and other gastrointestinal disorders where an amino acid diet is recommended.	Neocate Junior powder: strawberry 400 gram = £39.61; vanilla 400 gram = £39.61; unflavoured 400 gram = £39.61
Powder provides: protein 13.3 g, carbohydrate 56 g, fat 22 g, energy 1992 kJ (475 kcal)/100 g. Not suitable for use in child under 1 year									

Cow's milk protein allergy with impaired gastro-intestinal function or malabsorption: Amino acid products (product list continued)

Product	Formulation	Energy	Protein	Carbohydrate	Fat	Fibre	Special Characteristics	ACBS Indications	Presentation & Flavour
Neocate® Spoon (Nutricia Ltd)	Powder per 100 g	1981 kJ (472 kcal)	8.2 g protein equivalent (amino acids)	67.4 g (sugars 12.3 g)	18.8 g	Nil		Cow's milk allergy, multiple food protein allergy and other conditions requiring an amino acid-based food.	Neocate Spoon powder 37g sachets: 15 sachet = £61.35
Powder 37 g reconstituted with 60 ml water provides: protein 3 g, carbohydrate 24.9 g, fat 7 g, energy 733 kJ (175 kcal) Not suitable for use in child under 6 months									

Infant formula additive

Lactose intolerance: Lactase

Product	Formulation	Energy	Protein	Carbohydrate	Fat	Fibre	Special Characteristics	ACBS Indications	Presentation & Flavour
Care® Co-Lactase (Thornton & Ross Ltd)	Liquid per 100 g	923 kJ (223 kcal)	4.2 g	52 g (sugars Nil)	Nil	Nil		For transient lactase deficiency.	Care Co-Lactase infant drops: 10 ml = £7.24
Colief® (Crosscare Ltd)	Liquid per 100 g	886 kJ (211 kcal)	4.8 g	47.9 g	Nil	Nil		For transient lactase deficiency.	Colief 50,000units/g infant drops: 7 ml = £8.40

Preterm infant formula

Infants born before 34 weeks gestation, weighing less than 2 kg, and not breastfed

Product	Formulation	Energy	Protein	Carbohydrate	Fat	Fibre	Special Characteristics	ACBS Indications	Presentation & Flavour
Nutriprem® 2 Liquid (Nutricia Ltd)	Liquid (sip feed) per 100 mL	301 kJ (72 kcal)	2 g casein, whey protein	7.2 g lactose (sugars 6 g)	3.8 g	0.6 g	Contains egg, fish oil, lactose, soya	Catch-up growth in pre-term infants (ie less than 35 weeks at birth) and small for gestational age infants, until 6 months corrected age.	Nutriprem 2 liquid: 200 ml = £2.33
Not suitable for use in child over 6 months corrected age									
Nutriprem® 2 Powder (Nutricia Ltd)	Standard dilution (14.7% w/v) of powder per 100 mL	301 kJ (72 kcal)	2 g casein, whey protein	7.2 g lactose (sugars 6 g)	3.8 g	0.6 g	Contains egg, fish oil, lactose, soya	Catch-up growth in pre-term infants (ie less than 35 weeks at birth) and small for gestational age infants, until 6 months corrected age.	Nutriprem 2 powder: 800 gram = £14.02
Powder provides: protein 13.5 g, carbohydrate 49.1 g, fat 25.9 g, energy 2052 kJ (490 kcal)/100 g Not suitable for use in child over 6 months corrected age									
SMA Gold Prem® 2 liquid (SMA Nutrition)	Liquid (sip feed) per 100 mL	306 kJ (73 kcal)	2 g whey protein	7.7 g lactose (sugars 5.5 g)	3.8 g	Nil	Contains fish oil, lactose	Preterm and low birthweight infants.	SMA Gold Prem 2 liquid: 200 ml = £2.25
SMA Gold Prem® 2 powder (SMA Nutrition)	Standard dilution (14 % w/v) of powder per 100 mL	306 kJ (73 kcal)	2 g whey protein	7.7 g (sugars 5.5 g)	3.8 g	Nil	Contains fish oil, lactose	Preterm and low birthweight infants.	SMA Gold Prem 2 powder: 800 gram = £13.62
Powder provides: protein 14 g, carbohydrate 53 g, fat 26 g, energy 2123 kJ (507 kcal)/100 g									

Preterm human milk fortifier

Infants born before 34 weeks gestation, weighing less than 1.5 kg, and breastfed

Product	Formulation	Energy	Protein	Carbohydrate	Fat	Fibre	Special Characteristics	ACBS Indications	Presentation & Flavour
Nutriprem® Human Milk Fortifier (Nutricia Ltd)	Powder per 100 g	1800 kJ (400 kcal)	33 g casein hydrolysate, whey protein hydrolysate	37 g (sugars 2 g)	18 g	Nil	Contains egg, fish oil, residual lactose	Preterm and low birthweight infants.	Nutriprem Human Milk Fortifier oral powder 1g sachets: 50 sachet = £10.97
Powder 4 g reconstituted with 100 ml human milk provides: protein 2.92 g, carbohydrate 8.8 g, fat 4.2 g, energy 353 kJ (84 kcal)									
SMA Gold Prem® Breast Milk fortifier (SMA Nutrition)	Powder per 100 g	1800 kJ (430 kcal)	36 g whey protein hydrolysate	32 g	18 g (MCT 56 %)	Nil	Contains fish oil, residual lactose	Preterm and low birthweight infants.	SMA Gold Prem Breast Milk fortifier 1g powder sachets: 72 sachet = £15.31
Powder 4 g reconstituted with 100 ml human milk provides: protein 2.54 g, carbohydrate 7.58 g, fat 4.32 g, energy 352 kJ (84 kcal)									

Table 4 Energy, protein, and fibre fortifiers

Energy (carbohydrate) fortifiers

Product	Formulation	Energy	Protein	Carbohydrate	Fat	Fibre	Special Characteristics	ACBS Indications	Presentation & Flavour
Duocal® Super Soluble (Nutricia Ltd)	Powder per 100 g	2061 kJ (492 kcal)	Nil	72.7 g (sugars 6.5 g)	22.3 g (MCT 38 %)	Nil		Disease related malnutrition, malabsorption states or other conditions requiring fortification with a fat/carbohydrate supplement.	Duocal Super Soluble powder: 400 gram = £28.39
Maxijul® Super Soluble (Nutricia Ltd)	Powder per 100 g	1615 kJ (380 kcal)	Nil	95 g (sugars 8.6 g)	Nil	Nil	Gluten-free, lactose-free	Disease-related malnutrition, malabsorption states or other conditions requiring fortification with a high or readily available carbohydrate supplement.	Maxijul Super Soluble: powder 132g sachets 4 sachet = £10.04; powder 200 gram = £4.05; 25000 gram = £244.47
Polycal® liquid (Nutricia Ltd)	Liquid (sip feed) per 100 mL	1050 kJ (247 kcal)	Nil	61.9 g (sugars 12.2 g)	Nil	Nil		Disease related malnutrition, malabsorption states or other conditions requiring fortification with a high or readily available carbohydrate supplement.	Polycal liquid neutral: 200 ml = £2.77
Not suitable for use in child under 3 years									
Polycal® powder (Nutricia Ltd)	Powder per 100 g	1630 kJ (384 kcal)	Nil	96 g (sugars 6 g)	Nil	Nil		Disease-related malnutrition, malabsorption states or other conditions requiring fortification with a high or readily available carbohydrate supplement.	Polycal powder: 400 gram = £7.02
Not suitable for infants; use with caution in child 1-6 years									
Vitajoule® (Vitaflo International Ltd)	Powder per 100 g	1615 kJ (380 kcal)	Nil	95 g (sugars 9 g)	Nil	Nil		Disease related malnutrition, malabsorption states, other conditions requiring fortification with carbohydrate and as a carbohydrate source in modular feeds.	Vitajoule powder: 500 gram = £7.17
Suitable from birth									

Energy (fat) fortifiers

Product	Formulation	Energy	Protein	Carbohydrate	Fat	Fibre	Special Characteristics	ACBS Indications	Presentation & Flavour
Calogen® (Nutricia Ltd)	Liquid (sip or tube feed) **per 100 mL**	1850 kJ (450 kcal)	Nil	0.1 g (sugars Nil)	50 g	Nil		Disease-related malnutrition, malabsorption states, or other conditions requiring fortification with a high fat supplement, with or without fluid and electrolyte restrictions.	Calogen emulsion: strawberry 200 ml = £7.14; neutral 200 ml = £7.14
Use with caution in child under 6 years; strawberry flavour not suitable for child under 3 years									
Fresubin® 5kcal shot (Fresenius Kabi Ltd)	Liquid (sip feed) **per 100 mL**	2100 kJ (500 kcal)	Nil	4 g sucrose (sugars 4 g)	53.8 g	0.4 g	Gluten-free, lactose-free	Disease related malnutrition malabsorption states or other conditions requiring fortification with a high fat supplement with or without fluid or electrolyte restrictions.	Fresubin 5kcal shot drink: neutral 480 ml = £14.20; lemon 480 ml = £14.20
Not suitable for use in child under 3 years									

Energy and protein fortifiers

Product	Formulation	Energy	Protein	Carbohydrate	Fat	Fibre	Special Characteristics	ACBS Indications	Presentation & Flavour
Altrashot® (Nualtra Ltd)	Liquid (sip feed) **per 100 mL**	1451 kJ (350 kcal)	5 g milk protein isolate	17 g (sugars 6.1 g)	29.1 g	Nil	Contains residual lactose. Gluten-free	Disease-related malnutrition.	Altrashot 120ml bottles: vanilla 4 bottle = £12.53; neutral 4 bottle = £11.80; strawberry 4 bottle = £12.53; Altrashot Starter Pack liquid: 2 bottle = £6.24
Not suitable for use in child under 3 years; not recommended for child under 6 years									
Calogen® Extra (Nutricia Ltd)	Liquid (sip or tube feed) **per 100 mL**	1650 kJ (400 kcal)	5 g caseinates, whey protein hydrolysate	4.5 g (sugars 3.5 g)	40.3 g	Nil	Contains residual lactose. Gluten-free	Disease related malnutrition, malabsorption states or other conditions requiring fortification with a high fat supplement with or without fluid restriction.	Calogen Extra Shots emulsion: strawberry 240 ml = £7.50; neutral 240 ml = £7.50; Calogen Extra emulsion: strawberry 200 ml = £6.29; neutral 200 ml = £6.29
Not suitable for use in child under 3 years; use with caution in child 3-6 years									
MCTprocal® (Vitaflo International Ltd)	Powder **per 100 g**	2907 kJ (703 kcal)	12.2 g caseinates	20.6 g (sugars 3.1 g)	63.5 g (MCT 96%)	Nil	Contains residual lactose	Disorders of long chain fatty acid oxidation, fat malabsorption and other disorders requiring a low LCT, high MCT supplement.	MCTprocal oral powder 16g sachets: 30 sachet = £39.11
Powder 16 g provides: protein 2 g, carbohydrate 3.3 g, fat 10 g, energy 465 kJ (112 kcal) Suitable from 3 years									
Pro-Cal® powder (Vitaflo International Ltd)	Powder **per 100 g**	2744 kJ (662 kcal)	13.5 g milk protein	26 g (sugars 20 g)	56 g	Nil	Contains residual lactose. Gluten-free	Disease-related malnutrition, malabsorption states or other conditions requiring fortification with a fat / carbohydrate supplement (with protein).	Pro-Cal powder: 510 gram = £24.13; 1500 gram = £49.21; 12500 gram = £350.05; Pro-Cal powder: 15g sachets 30 sachet = £31.03; starter pack 8 sachet = £8.20
Powder 15 g reconstituted with 100 ml water provides: protein 2 g, carbohydrate 3.9 g, fat 8.4 g, energy 412 kJ (100 kcal) Suitable from 3 years									

Pro-Cal® Shot (Vitaflo International Ltd)	Liquid (sip feed) **per 100 mL**	1385 kJ (334 kcal)	6.7 g caseinates, milk protein	13.4 g lactose (sugars 13.3 g)	28.2 g	Nil	Contains lactose, soya. Gluten-free	Disease-related malnutrition, malabsorption states or other conditions requiring fortification with a fat/carbohydrate supplement (with protein).	Pro-Cal: shot starter pack 360 ml = £11.42; shot banana 720 ml = £22.88; shot neutral 720 ml = £22.88; shot strawberry 720 ml = £22.88
Suitable from 3 years									

Energy and higher protein fortifiers

Product	Formulation	Energy	Protein	Carbohydrate	Fat	Fibre	Special Characteristics	ACBS Indications	Presentation & Flavour
Altrapro (Nualtra Ltd)	Liquid (sip feed) **per 100 mL**	574 kJ (135 kcal)	33.3 g milk protein	0.09 g (sugars 0.03 g)	0.04 g	Nil	Gluten-free, lactose-free	Disease-related malnutrition in patients with higher protein needs.	Altrapro liquid: lemon & lime 60 ml = £1.75; berry 60 ml = £1.75
Not suitable for use in child under 3 years; use with caution in child under 6 years									
Aymes® Actagain Protein Shot (Aymes International Ltd)	Liquid (sip or tube feed) **per 100 mL**	644 kJ (154 kcal)	37 g collagen protein	2 g fructose (sugars 2 g)	Nil	Nil	Contains bovine derivatives. Gluten-free, lactose-free	Hypoproteinaemia.	Aymes Actagain Protein: Shot Starter Pack 240 ml = £7.00; Shot tropical fruit 60 ml = £1.75; Shot mixed berry 60 ml = £1.75
Not suitable for use in child under 3 years; use with caution in child under 7 years									
ProSource® 20 (Nutrinovo Ltd)	Liquid (sip and tube feed) **per 100 mL**	628 kJ (150 kcal)	33.3 g collagen protein, whey protein isolate	3.33 g (sugars Nil)	Nil	Nil	Contains beef derivatives, residual lactose. Gluten-free	Hypoproteinaemia.	ProSource 20 liquid: orange & pineapple 60 ml = £2.32; red berry 60 ml = £2.32; blackcurrant 60 ml = £2.32
Not recommended for child under 3 years									
ProSource® liquid (Nutrinovo Ltd)	Liquid (sip or tube feed) **per 100 mL**	1400 kJ (333 kcal)	33.3 g collagen protein, whey protein isolate	50 g (sugars 26.7 g)	Less than 1 g	Less than 1 g	Contains residual lactose, porcine derivatives. Gluten-free	Biochemically proven hypoproteinaemia.	ProSource liquid 30ml sachets: orange creme 100 sachet = £152.84; neutral 100 sachet = £152.84; citrus berry 100 sachet = £152.84
Not recommended for child under 3 years									
ProSource® Plus (Nutrinovo Ltd)	Liquid (sip and tube feed) **per 100 mL**	1400 kJ (333 kcal)	50 g collagen protein, whey protein isolate	36.7 g sucrose (sugars 33.3 g)	Less than 1 g	Less than 1 g	Contains porcine derivatives, residual lactose. Gluten-free	Hypoproteinaemia.	ProSource Plus liquid 30ml sachets: orange creme 50 sachet = £102.45; 100 sachet = £204.89; neutral 50 sachet = £102.45; 100 sachet = £204.89; citrus berry 50 sachet = £102.45; 100 sachet = £204.89; ProSource Plus liquid citrus berry: 887 ml = £58.70; neutral: 887 ml = £58.70; orange creme: 887 ml = £58.70
Not recommended for child under 3 years									
Protifar® (Nutricia Ltd)	Powder **per 100 g**	1560 kJ (368 kcal)	87.2 g cow's milk	1.5 g	1.6 g	Nil	Contains lactose, soya. Gluten-free	Hypoproteinaemia.	Protifar powder: 225 gram = £14.30
Powder 2.5 g (scoop) provides: protein 2.2 g, carbohydrate 0.04 g, fat 0.04 g, energy 39 kJ (9 kcal) Not suitable for use in child under 3 years									

Energy and higher protein fortifiers (product list continued)

Product	Formulation	Energy	Protein	Carbohydrate	Fat	Fibre	Special Characteristics	ACBS Indications	Presentation & Flavour
Renapro® Shot (Stanningley Pharma Ltd)	Liquid (sip or tube feed) **per 100 mL**	711 kJ (167 kcal)	33 g collagen protein	4.9 g fructose (sugars 4.9 g)	Less than 0.5 g	Nil	Contains beef derivatives. Gluten-free, lactose-free	Hypoproteinaemia.	Renapro Shot 60ml bottles: wild berry 30 bottle = £69.60; apple 30 bottle = £69.60; pineapple & coconut 30 bottle = £69.60; cola 30 bottle = £69.60; peach 30 bottle = £69.60

Not suitable for use in child under 3 years

Higher protein fortifiers

Product	Formulation	Energy	Protein	Carbohydrate	Fat	Fibre	Special Characteristics	ACBS Indications	Presentation & Flavour
ProSource® jelly (Nutrinovo Ltd)	Semi-solid **per 100 mL**	315 kJ (75 kcal)	16.9 g collagen protein, whey protein isolate	Less than 1 g	Nil	Less than 1 g	Contains porcine derivatives, residual lactose. Gluten-free	Hypoproteinaemia.	ProSource jelly: blackcurrant 118 ml = £2.77; orange 118 ml = £2.77; lime 118 ml = £2.77; fruit punch 118 ml = £2.77

Not recommended for child under 3 years

Fibre fortifiers

Product	Formulation	Energy	Protein	Carbohydrate	Fat	Fibre	Special Characteristics	ACBS Indications	Presentation & Flavour
HyFiber® (Nutrinovo Ltd)	Liquid (sip or tube feed) **per 100 mL**	484 kJ (119 kcal)	Nil	10.4 g (sugars 10.4 g)	Nil	39 g	Gluten-free, lactose-free	Bowel transit disorders.	HyFiber: liquid 887 ml = £34.11; liquid 30ml sachets 100 sachet = £116.55
Not recommended for child under 3 years									
Optifibre® (Nestle Health Science)	Powder **per 100 g**	816 kJ (202 kcal)	Less than 1.5 g	6 g partially hydrolysed guar gum (sugars 6 g)	Nil	86 g	Contains residual lactose. Gluten-free	Borderline substances standard ACBS indications p. 1375 except dysphagia.	Optifibre: powder 5g sachets 16 sachet = £5.95; powder 250 gram = £14.70

Not suitable for use in child under 5 years

Flavour additives

Flavour additive powders

FlavourPac®

▸ For use with Vitaflo's inborn error range of protein substitutes. Not suitable for use in child under 3 years.

POWDER

FlavourPac oral powder 4g sachets blackcurrant (Vitaflo International Ltd)
30 sachet (ACBS) • NHS indicative price = £22.68

FlavourPac oral powder 4g sachets orange (Vitaflo International Ltd)
30 sachet (ACBS) • NHS indicative price = £22.68

FlavourPac oral powder 4g sachets raspberry (Vitaflo International Ltd)
30 sachet (ACBS) • NHS indicative price = £22.68

FlavourPac oral powder 4g sachets tropical (Vitaflo International Ltd)
30 sachet (ACBS) • NHS indicative price = £22.68

Nutricia Flavour Modjul®

▸ For use with a range of unflavoured amino acid and peptide based foods for special medical purposes. Not suitable for use in child under 6 months.

POWDER

Nutricia Flavour Modjul powder blackcurrant (Nutricia Ltd)
100 gram (ACBS) • NHS indicative price = £19.10

Nutricia Flavour Modjul powder orange (Nutricia Ltd)
100 gram (ACBS) • NHS indicative price = £19.10

Nutricia Flavour Modjul powder pineapple (Nutricia Ltd)
100 gram (ACBS) • NHS indicative price = £19.10

Foods for special diets

Gluten-free foods

ACBS indications: coeliac disease and dermatitis herpetiformis.

Bread

Genius® Loaves

GLUTEN-FREE

Genius gluten free multi seeded farmhouse loaf (Genius Foods Ltd)
550 gram (ACBS) • NHS indicative price = £5.06

Genius gluten free soft brown farmhouse loaf (Genius Foods Ltd)
550 gram (ACBS) • NHS indicative price = £5.11

Genius gluten free soft white farmhouse loaf (Genius Foods Ltd)
550 gram (ACBS) • NHS indicative price = £5.12

Glutafin® Loaves

GLUTEN-FREE

Glutafin gluten free fibre loaf sliced (Dr Schar UK Ltd)
300 gram (ACBS) • NHS indicative price = £3.47

Glutafin gluten free high fibre loaf sliced (Dr Schar UK Ltd)
350 gram (ACBS) • NHS indicative price = £4.04

Glutafin gluten free white loaf sliced (Dr Schar UK Ltd)
300 gram (ACBS) • NHS indicative price = £3.47

Glutafin® Select Loaves

GLUTEN-FREE

Glutafin gluten free Select fibre loaf sliced (Dr Schar UK Ltd)
400 gram (ACBS) • NHS indicative price = £4.13

Glutafin gluten free Select fresh brown loaf sliced (Dr Schar UK Ltd)
400 gram (ACBS) • NHS indicative price = £4.20

Glutafin gluten free Select fresh white loaf sliced (Dr Schar UK Ltd)
400 gram (ACBS) • NHS indicative price = £4.20

Glutafin gluten free Select seeded loaf sliced (Dr Schar UK Ltd)
400 gram (ACBS) • NHS indicative price = £4.47

Glutafin gluten free Select white loaf sliced (Dr Schar UK Ltd)
400 gram (ACBS) • NHS indicative price = £4.13

Juvela® Loaf

GLUTEN-FREE

Juvela gluten free fibre loaf sliced (Juvela Ltd)
400 gram (ACBS) • NHS indicative price = £4.22

Juvela gluten free fibre loaf unsliced (Juvela Ltd)
400 gram (ACBS) • NHS indicative price = £4.22

Juvela gluten free fresh fibre loaf sliced (Juvela Ltd)
400 gram (ACBS) • NHS indicative price = £4.22

Juvela gluten free fresh white loaf sliced (Juvela Ltd)
400 gram (ACBS) • NHS indicative price = £4.22

Juvela gluten free loaf sliced (Juvela Ltd)
400 gram (ACBS) • NHS indicative price = £4.22

Juvela gluten free loaf unsliced (Juvela Ltd)
400 gram (ACBS) • NHS indicative price = £4.22

Juvela gluten free part baked fibre loaf (Juvela Ltd)
400 gram (ACBS) • NHS indicative price = £4.63

Juvela gluten free part baked loaf (Juvela Ltd)
400 gram (ACBS) • NHS indicative price = £4.63

Warburtons® Bread

GLUTEN-FREE

Warburtons gluten free brown bread sliced (Warburtons Ltd)
400 gram (ACBS) • NHS indicative price = £3.34

Warburtons gluten free white bread sliced (Warburtons Ltd)
400 gram (ACBS) • NHS indicative price = £3.34

Flour type mixes

Finax® Flour mixes

GLUTEN-FREE

Finax gluten free coarse flour mix (Drossa (London) Ltd)
900 gram (ACBS) • NHS indicative price = £9.97

Finax gluten free fibre bread mix (Drossa (London) Ltd)
1000 gram (ACBS) • NHS indicative price = £11.92

Finax gluten free flour mix (Drossa (London) Ltd)
900 gram (ACBS) • NHS indicative price = £9.97

Glutafin® Flour mixes

GLUTEN-FREE

Glutafin gluten free bread mix (Dr Schar UK Ltd)
500 gram (ACBS) • NHS indicative price = £8.02

Glutafin gluten free fibre bread mix (Dr Schar UK Ltd)
500 gram (ACBS) • NHS indicative price = £8.02

Glutafin gluten free multipurpose white mix (Dr Schar UK Ltd)
500 gram (ACBS) • NHS indicative price = £8.02

Glutafin gluten free wheat free fibre mix (Dr Schar UK Ltd)
500 gram (ACBS) • NHS indicative price = £8.02

Glutafin® Select Flour mix

GLUTEN-FREE

Glutafin gluten free Select bread mix (Dr Schar UK Ltd)
500 gram (ACBS) • NHS indicative price = £8.02

Glutafin gluten free Select multipurpose fibre mix (Dr Schar UK Ltd)
500 gram (ACBS) • NHS indicative price = £8.02

Glutafin gluten free Select multipurpose white mix (Dr Schar UK Ltd)
500 gram (ACBS) • NHS indicative price = £8.02

Juvela® Flour mixes

GLUTEN-FREE

Juvela gluten free fibre mix (Juvela Ltd)
500 gram (ACBS) • NHS indicative price = £8.50

Juvela gluten free harvest mix (Juvela Ltd)
500 gram (ACBS) • NHS indicative price = £8.50

Juvela gluten free mix (Juvela Ltd)
500 gram (ACBS) • NHS indicative price = £8.50

Rolls and baguettes

Glutafin® Rolls and baguettes

GLUTEN-FREE

Glutafin gluten free 4 white rolls (Dr Schar UK Ltd)
200 gram (ACBS) • NHS indicative price = £4.43

Glutafin gluten free baguettes (Dr Schar UK Ltd)
350 gram (ACBS) • NHS indicative price = £4.22

Glutafin gluten free fresh white rolls (Dr Schar UK Ltd)
260 gram (ACBS) • NHS indicative price = £4.07

Glutafin gluten free part baked 2 long white rolls (Dr Schar UK Ltd)
150 gram (ACBS) • NHS indicative price = £3.38

Glutafin gluten free part baked 4 fibre rolls (Dr Schar UK Ltd)
200 gram (ACBS) • NHS indicative price = £4.43

Glutafin gluten free part baked 4 white rolls (Dr Schar UK Ltd)
200 gram (ACBS) • NHS indicative price = £4.43

Juvela® Rolls
GLUTEN-FREE

Juvela gluten free bread rolls (Juvela Ltd)
425 gram (ACBS) • NHS indicative price = £5.77

Juvela gluten free fibre bread rolls (Juvela Ltd)
425 gram (ACBS) • NHS indicative price = £5.77

Juvela gluten free fresh fibre rolls (Juvela Ltd)
425 gram (ACBS) • NHS indicative price = £5.40

Juvela gluten free fresh white rolls (Juvela Ltd)
425 gram (ACBS) • NHS indicative price = £5.40

Juvela gluten free part baked fibre bread rolls (Juvela Ltd)
375 gram (ACBS) • NHS indicative price = £5.77

Juvela gluten free part baked white bread rolls (Juvela Ltd)
375 gram (ACBS) • NHS indicative price = £5.77

Warburtons® Rolls
GLUTEN-FREE

Warburtons gluten free brown rolls (Warburtons Ltd)
232 gram (ACBS) • NHS indicative price = £2.80

Warburtons gluten free white rolls (Warburtons Ltd)
232 gram (ACBS) • NHS indicative price = £2.80

Low-protein foods

ACBS indications: inherited metabolic disorders, renal or liver failure, requiring a low-protein diet.

Bread, rolls, and baguettes

Juvela® Bread and rolls
LOW-PROTEIN

Juvela low protein bread rolls (Juvela Ltd)
350 gram (ACBS) • NHS indicative price = £5.66

Juvela low protein loaf sliced (Juvela Ltd)
400 gram (ACBS) • NHS indicative price = £4.63

Mevalia® Bread and rolls
LOW-PROTEIN

Mevalia low protein ciabattine (Vitaflo International Ltd)
260 gram (ACBS) • NHS indicative price = £4.73

Mevalia low protein pan carre (Vitaflo International Ltd)
300 gram (ACBS) • NHS indicative price = £3.46

Mevalia low protein pane casereccio (Vitaflo International Ltd)
220 gram (ACBS) • NHS indicative price = £3.06

Promin® Bread and rolls
LOW-PROTEIN

Promin low protein breadcrumbs (Firstplay Dietary Foods Ltd)
300 gram (ACBS) • NHS indicative price = £8.30

Promin low protein croutons 40g sachets (Firstplay Dietary Foods Ltd)
4 sachet (ACBS) • NHS indicative price = £8.00

Promin low protein farmhouse loaf (Firstplay Dietary Foods Ltd)
400 gram (ACBS) • NHS indicative price = £4.84

Promin low protein fresh baked bread buns (Firstplay Dietary Foods Ltd)
450 gram (ACBS) • NHS indicative price = £6.95

Promin low protein fresh baked bread sliced (Firstplay Dietary Foods Ltd)
800 gram (ACBS) • NHS indicative price = £9.00

Promin low protein fresh baked brown bread sliced (Firstplay Dietary Foods Ltd)
400 gram (ACBS) • NHS indicative price = £4.25

Breakfast cereals

Loprofin® Cereals
LOW-PROTEIN

Loprofin low protein breakfast flakes chocolate (Nutricia Ltd)
375 gram (ACBS) • NHS indicative price = £11.83

Loprofin low protein breakfast flakes strawberry (Nutricia Ltd)
375 gram (ACBS) • NHS indicative price = £11.83

Loprofin low protein breakfast loops (Nutricia Ltd)
375 gram (ACBS) • NHS indicative price = £12.26

Promin® Cereals
LOW-PROTEIN

Promin low protein cereal chocolate (Firstplay Dietary Foods Ltd)
340 gram (ACBS) • NHS indicative price = £8.75

Promin low protein hot breakfast powder 56g sachets original (Firstplay Dietary Foods Ltd)
6 sachet (ACBS) • NHS indicative price = £10.95

Promin low protein hot breakfast powder 57g sachets apple & cinnamon (Firstplay Dietary Foods Ltd)
6 sachet (ACBS) • NHS indicative price = £10.95

Promin low protein hot breakfast powder 57g sachets banana (Firstplay Dietary Foods Ltd)
6 sachet (ACBS) • NHS indicative price = £10.95

Promin low protein hot breakfast powder 57g sachets chocolate (Firstplay Dietary Foods Ltd)
6 sachet (ACBS) • NHS indicative price = £10.95

Cake, confectionery, and sweet biscuits

metaX Sweet biscuits
LOW-PROTEIN

metaX low protein lemon wafers (metaX Institut fuer Diaetetik GmbH)
100 gram (ACBS) • NHS indicative price = £5.65

Mevalia® Cake, confectionery, and sweet biscuits
LOW-PROTEIN

Mevalia low protein chocotino bars (Vitaflo International Ltd)
100 gram (ACBS) • NHS indicative price = £6.88

Mevalia low protein cookies (Vitaflo International Ltd)
200 gram (ACBS) • NHS indicative price = £9.41

Mevalia low protein frollini biscuits (Vitaflo International Ltd)
200 gram (ACBS) • NHS indicative price = £10.35

Mevalia low protein fruit bar (Vitaflo International Ltd)
125 gram (ACBS) • NHS indicative price = £6.59

Promin® Cake, confectionery, and sweet biscuits
LOW-PROTEIN

Promin low protein 40g breakfast bars apple & cinnamon (Firstplay Dietary Foods Ltd)
6 pack (ACBS) • NHS indicative price = £13.15

Promin low protein 40g breakfast bars banana (Firstplay Dietary Foods Ltd)
6 pack (ACBS) • NHS indicative price = £13.15

Promin low protein 40g breakfast bars chocolate & cranberry (Firstplay Dietary Foods Ltd)
6 pack (ACBS) • NHS indicative price = £13.15

Promin low protein 40g breakfast bars cranberry (Firstplay Dietary Foods Ltd)
6 pack (ACBS) • NHS indicative price = £13.15

Promin low protein fresh baked fruit loaf (Firstplay Dietary Foods Ltd)
800 gram (ACBS) • NHS indicative price = £7.95

Taranis® Cake, confectionery, and sweet biscuits
LOW-PROTEIN

Taranis low protein apricot cake (Lactalis Nutrition Sante)
240 gram (ACBS) • NHS indicative price = £7.05

Taranis low protein biscuits with caramel shards (Lactalis Nutrition Sante)
120 gram (ACBS) • NHS indicative price = £6.00

Taranis low protein chocolate chip biscuits (Lactalis Nutrition Sante)
120 gram (ACBS) • NHS indicative price = £6.20

Taranis low protein chocolate chip cookies (Lactalis Nutrition Sante)
160 gram (ACBS) • NHS indicative price = £12.15

Taranis low protein lemon cake (Lactalis Nutrition Sante)
240 gram (ACBS) · NHS indicative price = £7.05

Taranis low protein raspberry shortbread biscuits (Lactalis Nutrition Sante)
120 gram (ACBS) · NHS indicative price = £6.20

Taranis low protein shortbread biscuits (Lactalis Nutrition Sante)
120 gram (ACBS) · NHS indicative price = £5.50

VitaBite ® Confectionery
LOW-PROTEIN

VitaBite bar (Vitaflo International Ltd)
175 gram (ACBS) · NHS indicative price = £14.14

Cake and flour type mixes

Fate ® Cake and flour type mixes
LOW-PROTEIN

Fate low protein all purpose mix (Fate Special Foods)
500 gram (ACBS) · NHS indicative price = £8.96

Fate low protein chocolate cake mix (Fate Special Foods)
500 gram (ACBS) · NHS indicative price = £8.96

Fate low protein plain cake mix (Fate Special Foods)
500 gram (ACBS) · NHS indicative price = £8.96

Juvela ® Low Protein flour mixes
LOW-PROTEIN

Juvela low protein mix (Juvela Ltd)
500 gram (ACBS) · NHS indicative price = £9.53

Loprofin ® Cake and flour type mixes
LOW-PROTEIN

Loprofin low protein chocolate flavour cake mix (Nutricia Ltd)
500 gram (ACBS) · NHS indicative price = £13.23

Loprofin low protein mix (Nutricia Ltd)
500 gram (ACBS) · NHS indicative price = £12.32

Mevalia ® Cake and flour type mixes
LOW-PROTEIN

Mevalia low protein bread mix (Vitaflo International Ltd)
500 gram (ACBS) · NHS indicative price = £8.40

Promin ® Cake and flour type mixes
LOW-PROTEIN

Promin low protein all purpose baking mix (Firstplay Dietary Foods Ltd)
1000 gram (ACBS) · NHS indicative price = £15.50

Promin low protein chocolate cake mix (Firstplay Dietary Foods Ltd)
500 gram (ACBS) · NHS indicative price = £7.45

Promin low protein classic cake mix (Firstplay Dietary Foods Ltd)
500 gram (ACBS) · NHS indicative price = £7.45

Promin low protein potato cake mix (Firstplay Dietary Foods Ltd)
300 gram (ACBS) · NHS indicative price = £7.45

Promin low protein sweet pancake mix (Firstplay Dietary Foods Ltd)
300 gram (ACBS) · NHS indicative price = £4.80

Taranis ® Cake and flour type mixes
LOW-PROTEIN

Taranis low protein natural cake mix (Lactalis Nutrition Sante)
300 gram (ACBS) · NHS indicative price = £5.15

Taranis low protein pancakes and waffles mix (Lactalis Nutrition Sante)
300 gram (ACBS) · NHS indicative price = £5.15

Desserts

Promin ® Desserts
LOW-PROTEIN

Promin low protein dessert 36.5g sachets caramel (Firstplay Dietary Foods Ltd)
6 sachet (ACBS) · NHS indicative price = £8.60

Promin low protein dessert 36.5g sachets chocolate & banana (Firstplay Dietary Foods Ltd)
6 sachet (ACBS) · NHS indicative price = £8.60

Promin low protein dessert 36.5g sachets custard (Firstplay Dietary Foods Ltd)
6 sachet (ACBS) · NHS indicative price = £8.60

Promin low protein dessert 36.5g sachets strawberry & vanilla (Firstplay Dietary Foods Ltd)
6 sachet (ACBS) · NHS indicative price = £8.60

Promin low protein imitation rice pudding 69g sachets apple (Firstplay Dietary Foods Ltd)
4 sachet (ACBS) · NHS indicative price = £8.75

Promin low protein imitation rice pudding 69g sachets banana (Firstplay Dietary Foods Ltd)
4 sachet (ACBS) · NHS indicative price = £8.75

Promin low protein imitation rice pudding 69g sachets original (Firstplay Dietary Foods Ltd)
4 sachet (ACBS) · NHS indicative price = £8.75

Promin low protein imitation rice pudding 69g sachets strawberry (Firstplay Dietary Foods Ltd)
4 sachet (ACBS) · NHS indicative price = £8.75

Taranis ® Pause Desserts
LOW-PROTEIN

Taranis Pause low protein dessert caramel (Lactalis Nutrition Sante)
500 gram (ACBS) · NHS indicative price = £12.80

Taranis Pause low protein dessert strawberry (Lactalis Nutrition Sante)
500 gram (ACBS) · NHS indicative price = £12.80

YoguMaxx ® Dessert
LOW-PROTEIN

YoguMaxx low protein instant powder (Firstplay Dietary Foods Ltd)
400 gram (ACBS) · NHS indicative price = £20.45

Egg replacers

Loprofin ® Egg replacers
LOW-PROTEIN

Loprofin low protein egg replacer (Nutricia Ltd)
500 gram (ACBS) · NHS indicative price = £23.00

Loprofin low protein egg white replacer (Nutricia Ltd)
100 gram (ACBS) · NHS indicative price = £14.77

Promin ® Egg replacer
LOW-PROTEIN

Promin low protein scrambled egg & omelette mix (Firstplay Dietary Foods Ltd)
500 gram (ACBS) · NHS indicative price = £11.20

Meat and fish replacers

Meta Healthcare low protein chicken substitute
LOW-PROTEIN

Meta Healthcare low protein chicken substitute (Meta Healthcare Ltd)
250 gram (ACBS) · NHS indicative price = £15.37

Meta Healthcare low protein meat substitute
LOW-PROTEIN

Meta Healthcare low protein meat substitute (Meta Healthcare Ltd)
250 gram (ACBS) · NHS indicative price = £17.14

Promin ® Meat replacers
LOW-PROTEIN

Promin low protein burger mix 62g sachets lamb & mint (Firstplay Dietary Foods Ltd)
4 sachet (ACBS) · NHS indicative price = £17.70

Promin low protein burger mix 62g sachets original (Firstplay Dietary Foods Ltd)
4 sachet (ACBS) · NHS indicative price = £17.70

Promin low protein chicken burger mix 62g sachets (Firstplay Dietary Foods Ltd)
4 sachet (ACBS) · NHS indicative price = £15.85

Promin low protein sausage mix 30g sachets apple & sage (Firstplay Dietary Foods Ltd)
4 sachet (ACBS) · NHS indicative price = £9.95

Promin low protein sausage mix 30g sachets original (Firstplay Dietary Foods Ltd)
4 sachet (ACBS) · NHS indicative price = £9.95

Promin low protein sausage mix 30g sachets tomato & basil (Firstplay Dietary Foods Ltd)
4 sachet (ACBS) · NHS indicative price = £9.95

Taranis® Fish substitute
LOW-PROTEIN

Taranis low protein fish substitute (Lactalis Nutrition Sante)
248 gram (ACBS) · NHS indicative price = £14.95

Milk replacers

Loprofin® Drinks
LOW-PROTEIN

Loprofin drink LQ (Nutricia Ltd)
200 ml (ACBS) · NHS indicative price = £1.08

Loprofin SNO-PRO drink (Nutricia Ltd)
200 ml (ACBS) · NHS indicative price = £1.83

ProZero® Drink
LOW-PROTEIN

ProZero liquid chocolate (Vitaflo International Ltd)
250 ml (ACBS) · NHS indicative price = £2.35

ProZero liquid unflavoured (Vitaflo International Ltd)
250 ml (ACBS) · NHS indicative price = £2.35 | 1000 ml (ACBS) · NHS indicative price = £9.46

Taranis® Milk substitutes
LOW-PROTEIN

Taranis Dalia low protein milk (Lactalis Nutrition Sante)
200 ml (ACBS) · NHS indicative price = £1.39

Taranis low protein Dalia milk substitute powder (Lactalis Nutrition Sante)
400 gram (ACBS) · NHS indicative price = £9.90

Pasta and pizza bases

Loprofin® Pasta
LOW-PROTEIN

Loprofin low protein pasta animal shapes (Nutricia Ltd)
500 gram (ACBS) · NHS indicative price = £12.59

Loprofin low protein pasta fusilli (Nutricia Ltd)
500 gram (ACBS) · NHS indicative price = £13.04

Loprofin low protein pasta lasagne (Nutricia Ltd)
250 gram (ACBS) · NHS indicative price = £6.35

Loprofin low protein pasta macaroni (Nutricia Ltd)
250 gram (ACBS) · NHS indicative price = £6.27

Loprofin low protein pasta penne (Nutricia Ltd)
500 gram (ACBS) · NHS indicative price = £13.04

Loprofin low protein pasta spaghetti (Nutricia Ltd)
500 gram (ACBS) · NHS indicative price = £13.04

Loprofin low protein pasta tagliatelle (Nutricia Ltd)
250 gram (ACBS) · NHS indicative price = £6.27

Mevalia® Pasta and pizza bases
LOW-PROTEIN

Mevalia low protein fusilli (Vitaflo International Ltd)
500 gram (ACBS) · NHS indicative price = £8.81

Mevalia low protein pasta ditali (Vitaflo International Ltd)
500 gram (ACBS) · NHS indicative price = £8.81

Mevalia low protein penne (Vitaflo International Ltd)
500 gram (ACBS) · NHS indicative price = £8.81

Mevalia low protein pizza base (Vitaflo International Ltd)
340 gram (ACBS) · NHS indicative price = £8.32

Mevalia low protein spaghetti (Vitaflo International Ltd)
500 gram (ACBS) · NHS indicative price = £8.82

Promin® Pasta
LOW-PROTEIN

Promin low protein lasagne sheets (Firstplay Dietary Foods Ltd)
200 gram (ACBS) · NHS indicative price = £3.70

Promin low protein pastameal (Firstplay Dietary Foods Ltd)
500 gram (ACBS) · NHS indicative price = £8.60

Promin low protein pasta alphabets (Firstplay Dietary Foods Ltd)
500 gram (ACBS) · NHS indicative price = £8.60

Promin low protein pasta flat noodles (Firstplay Dietary Foods Ltd)
500 gram (ACBS) · NHS indicative price = £8.35

Promin low protein pasta macaroni (Firstplay Dietary Foods Ltd)
500 gram (ACBS) · NHS indicative price = £8.60

Promin low protein pasta shells (Firstplay Dietary Foods Ltd)
500 gram (ACBS) · NHS indicative price = £8.60

Promin low protein pasta short cut spaghetti (Firstplay Dietary Foods Ltd)
500 gram (ACBS) · NHS indicative price = £8.60

Promin low protein pasta spirals (Firstplay Dietary Foods Ltd)
500 gram (ACBS) · NHS indicative price = £8.60

Promin low protein tricolour pasta alphabets (Firstplay Dietary Foods Ltd)
500 gram (ACBS) · NHS indicative price = £8.60

Promin low protein tricolour pasta shells (Firstplay Dietary Foods Ltd)
500 gram (ACBS) · NHS indicative price = £8.60

Promin low protein tricolour pasta spirals (Firstplay Dietary Foods Ltd)
500 gram (ACBS) · NHS indicative price = £8.60

Ready meals

Promin® Ready meals
LOW-PROTEIN

Promin low protein Mac Pot cheese (Firstplay Dietary Foods Ltd)
244 gram (ACBS) · NHS indicative price = £25.50

Promin low protein Mac Pot tomato (Firstplay Dietary Foods Ltd)
244 gram (ACBS) · NHS indicative price = £25.50

Promin low protein pasta in sauce 66g sachets cheese & broccoli (Firstplay Dietary Foods Ltd)
4 sachet (ACBS) · NHS indicative price = £10.35

Promin low protein pasta in sauce 72g sachets tomato, pepper & herb (Firstplay Dietary Foods Ltd)
4 sachet (ACBS) · NHS indicative price = £11.55

Promin low protein pasta spirals in Moroccan type sauce 72g sachets (Firstplay Dietary Foods Ltd)
4 sachet (ACBS) · NHS indicative price = £11.55

Promin low protein potato pot with croutons cabbage & bacon (Firstplay Dietary Foods Ltd)
200 gram (ACBS) · NHS indicative price = £22.60

Promin low protein potato pot with croutons onion (Firstplay Dietary Foods Ltd)
200 gram (ACBS) · NHS indicative price = £22.60

Promin low protein potato pot with croutons sausage (Firstplay Dietary Foods Ltd)
200 gram (ACBS) · NHS indicative price = £22.60

Promin low protein X-Pot all day scramble (Firstplay Dietary Foods Ltd)
240 gram (ACBS) · NHS indicative price = £28.20

Promin low protein X-Pot beef & tomato (Firstplay Dietary Foods Ltd)
240 gram (ACBS) · NHS indicative price = £28.20

Promin low protein X-Pot chip shop curry (Firstplay Dietary Foods Ltd)
240 gram (ACBS) · NHS indicative price = £28.20

Promin low protein X-Pot rogan style curry (Firstplay Dietary Foods Ltd)
240 gram (ACBS) · NHS indicative price = £28.20

Rice and cous cous replacers

Loprofin® Rice replacer
LOW-PROTEIN

Loprofin low protein rice replacer (Nutricia Ltd)
500 gram (ACBS) · NHS indicative price = £12.68

Mevalia® Rice replacer
LOW-PROTEIN

Mevalia low protein rice replacer (Vitaflo International Ltd)
400 gram (ACBS) · NHS indicative price = £7.26

Promin® Rice and cous cous replacers
LOW-PROTEIN

Promin low protein cous cous (Firstplay Dietary Foods Ltd)
500 gram (ACBS) · NHS indicative price = £8.60

Promin low protein imitation rice (Firstplay Dietary Foods Ltd)
500 gram (ACBS) · NHS indicative price = £8.60

Taranis® Rice replacer
LOW-PROTEIN

Taranis low protein risotto substitute (Lactalis Nutrition Sante)
1200 gram (ACBS) · NHS indicative price = £33.20

Sauces

Promin® Sauce mix
LOW-PROTEIN

Promin low protein cheese sauce mix (Firstplay Dietary Foods Ltd)
225 gram (ACBS) · NHS indicative price = £6.95

Savoury biscuits and snacks

Loprofin® Savoury biscuits and snacks
LOW-PROTEIN

Loprofin low protein crackers (Nutricia Ltd)
150 gram (ACBS) · NHS indicative price = £5.34

Loprofin low protein herb crackers (Nutricia Ltd)
150 gram (ACBS) · NHS indicative price = £5.34

Meta Healthcare low protein pizza crackers
LOW-PROTEIN

Meta Healthcare low protein pizza crackers (Meta Healthcare Ltd)
100 gram (ACBS) · NHS indicative price = £3.18

Meta Healthcare low protein salty sticks
LOW-PROTEIN

Meta Healthcare low protein salty sticks (Meta Healthcare Ltd)
150 gram (ACBS) · NHS indicative price = £4.77

Promin® Savoury biscuits and snacks
LOW-PROTEIN

Promin low protein Snax (Firstplay Dietary Foods Ltd)
12 sachet (ACBS) · NHS indicative price = £14.75

Promin low protein Snax cheese & onion 25g sachets (Firstplay Dietary Foods Ltd)
3 sachet · No NHS indicative price available | 12 sachet (ACBS) · NHS indicative price = £14.75

Promin low protein Snax jalapeno 25g sachets (Firstplay Dietary Foods Ltd)
3 sachet · No NHS indicative price available | 12 sachet (ACBS) · NHS indicative price = £14.75

Promin low protein Snax ready salted 25g sachets (Firstplay Dietary Foods Ltd)
3 sachet · No NHS indicative price available | 12 sachet (ACBS) · NHS indicative price = £14.75

Promin low protein Snax salt & vinegar 25g sachets (Firstplay Dietary Foods Ltd)
3 sachet · No NHS indicative price available | 12 sachet (ACBS) · NHS indicative price = £14.75

Vitaflo Choices® Snacks
LOW-PROTEIN

Vitaflo Choices mini crackers (Vitaflo International Ltd)
40 gram (ACBS) · NHS indicative price = £1.37

Soups

Promin® Soups
LOW-PROTEIN

Promin low protein soup with croutons oral powder 28g sachets creamy chicken (Firstplay Dietary Foods Ltd)
4 sachet (ACBS) · NHS indicative price = £6.95

Promin low protein soup with croutons oral powder 23g sachets creamy tomato (Firstplay Dietary Foods Ltd)
4 sachet (ACBS) · NHS indicative price = £6.95

Promin low protein soup with croutons oral powder 28g sachets minestrone (Firstplay Dietary Foods Ltd)
4 sachet (ACBS) · NHS indicative price = £6.95

Promin low protein soup with croutons oral powder 23g sachets pea and mint (Firstplay Dietary Foods Ltd)
4 sachet (ACBS) · NHS indicative price = £6.95

Spreads

Meta Healthcare low protein hazelnut spread
LOW-PROTEIN

Meta Healthcare low protein hazelnut spread (Meta Healthcare Ltd)
300 gram (ACBS) · NHS indicative price = £12.72

Taranis® Spreads
LOW-PROTEIN

Taranis low protein hazelnut spread (Lactalis Nutrition Sante)
230 gram (ACBS) · NHS indicative price = £10.40

Ketogenic diet

Medium chain triglycerides (MCT) liquid

K.Quik®
▸ Ketogenic diet or conditions requiring a source of MCT. Suitable from 3 years.
LIQUID (SIP FEED), medium chain triglycerides (MCT) 20 g, energy 777 kJ (189 kcal)/100 mL.

K.Quik liquid (Vitaflo International Ltd)
225 ml (ACBS) · NHS indicative price = £5.24

K.Vita®
▸ For the dietary management of drug resistant epilepsy. Suitable from 3 years.
LIQUID (SIP OR TUBE FEED), medium chain triglycerides (MCT) 33.5 g, energy 1265 kJ (308 kcal)/100 mL.

K.Vita liquid (Vitaflo International Ltd)
120 ml (ACBS) · NHS indicative price = £19.34

Kanso® MCT Oil 100%
▸ Intractable epilepsy, pyruvate dehydrogenase deficiency, glucose transporter type 1 deficiency syndrome and other conditions where a ketogenic diet is indicated.
LIQUID, medium chain triglycerides (MCT) 91 g, energy 3367 kJ (819 kcal)/100 mL.

Kanso MCT Oil 100% liquid (Dr Schar UK Ltd)
500 ml (ACBS) · NHS indicative price = £17.30

Liquigen®
▸ Steatorrhoea associated with cystic fibrosis of the pancreas, intestinal lymphangiectasia, surgery of the intestine, chronic liver disease, liver cirrhosis, other proven malabsorption syndromes, a ketogenic diet in the management of epilepsy and in type 1 hyperlipoproteinaemia.
LIQUID (SIP OR TUBE FEED), medium chain triglycerides (MCT) 49.1 g, energy 1865 kJ (454 kcal)/100 mL.

Liquigen emulsion (Nutricia Ltd)
250 ml (ACBS) · NHS indicative price = £14.54

MCT Oil
▸ Steatorrhoea associated with cystic fibrosis of the pancreas, intestinal lymphangiectasia, surgery of the intestine, chronic liver disease, liver cirrhosis, other proven malabsorption syndromes, in a ketogenic diet in the management of epilepsy and in type 1 hyperlipoproteinaemia.
LIQUID, medium chain triglycerides (MCT) 95 g, energy 3515 kJ (855 kcal)/100 mL.

MCT oil (Nutricia Ltd)
500 ml (ACBS) · NHS indicative price = £23.05

Powder

KetoCal® 3:1
▸ Drug resistant epilepsy and/or other conditions for which a ketogenic diet is indicated.
POWDER, protein 15.4 g, carbohydrate 7.2 g, fat 68.6 g, fibre Nil, energy 2935 kJ (711 kcal)/100 g.

KetoCal 3:1 powder (Nutricia Ltd)
300 gram (ACBS) · NHS indicative price = £46.34

KetoCal® 4:1
▸ For use as part of the ketogenic diet in the management of epilepsy resistant to drug therapy. Only to be prescribed on the advice of a secondary care physician with experience of the ketogenic diet. Suitable from 1 year.
POWDER, protein 14.4 g, carbohydrate 2.9 g, fat 69.2 g, fibre 5.4 g, energy 2897 kJ (703 kcal)/100 g.

KetoCal 4:1 powder unflavoured (Nutricia Ltd)
300 gram (ACBS) • NHS indicative price = £47.87

KetoCal 4:1 powder vanilla (Nutricia Ltd)
300 gram (ACBS) • NHS indicative price = £47.87

Ready to serve

K.Flo ® 4:1

▸ Epilepsy, neurometabolic disorders (e.g. glut 1 deficiency syndrome) and other conditions requiring a ketogenic diet. Suitable from 3 years.
LIQUID (SIP OR TUBE FEED), protein 3.4 g, carbohydrate 0.35 g, fat 14.7 g, fibre 1.4 g, energy 619 kJ (150 kcal)/100 mL.

K.Flo liquid (Vitaflo International Ltd)
250 ml (ACBS) • NHS indicative price = £7.88

K.Yo ® 3:1

▸ Epilepsy in a ketogenic diet, glut 1 deficiency syndrome or other conditions requiring a ketogenic diet. Suitable from 3 years.
SEMI-SOLID, protein 8 g, carbohydrate 1.5 g, fat 30 g, fibre Nil, energy 1272 kJ (308 kcal)/100 g.

K.Yo semi-solid food 100g pots berry (Vitaflo International Ltd)
4 pot (ACBS) • NHS indicative price = £37.16 | 36 pot (ACBS) • NHS indicative price = £250.88

K.Yo semi-solid food 100g pots chocolate (Vitaflo International Ltd)
4 pot (ACBS) • NHS indicative price = £38.81 | 36 pot (ACBS) • NHS indicative price = £262.04

K.Yo semi-solid food 100g pots vanilla (Vitaflo International Ltd)
4 pot (ACBS) • NHS indicative price = £38.81 | 36 pot (ACBS) • NHS indicative price = £262.04

KetoCal ® 2.5:1 LQ

▸ Drug resistant epilepsy or other conditions for which the ketogenic diet is indicated. Only to be prescribed on the advice of a specialist with experience of the ketogenic diet. Not suitable for use in child under 8 years.
LIQUID (SIP OR TUBE FEED), protein 4.5 g, carbohydrate 1.1 g, fat 14.3 g, fibre 1.1 g, energy 637 kJ (153 kcal)/100 mL.

KetoCal 2.5:1LQ liquid (Nutricia Ltd)
200 ml (ACBS) • NHS indicative price = £6.79

KetoCal ® 4:1 LQ

▸ Drug resistant epilepsy or other conditions for which a ketogenic diet is indicated. Suitable from 1 year.
LIQUID (SIP OR TUBE FEED), protein 3.09 g, carbohydrate 0.61 g, fat 14.8 g, fibre 1.12 g, energy 620 kJ (150 kcal)/100 mL.

KetoCal 4:1LQ liquid unflavoured (Nutricia Ltd)
200 ml (ACBS) • NHS indicative price = £6.43

KetoCal 4:1LQ liquid vanilla (Nutricia Ltd)
200 ml (ACBS) • NHS indicative price = £6.43

KetoVie ® 4:1

▸ Intractable epilepsy and other conditions where a ketogenic diet is indicated. Not suitable for use in child under 3 years.
LIQUID (SIP OR TUBE FEED), protein 3.4 g, carbohydrate 0.2 g, fat 14 g, fibre 1.8 g, energy 602 kJ (144 kcal)/100 mL.

KetoVie 4:1 liquid chocolate (Cambrooke UK Ltd)
250 ml (ACBS) • NHS indicative price = £7.83

KetoVie 4:1 liquid vanilla (Cambrooke UK Ltd)
250 ml (ACBS) • NHS indicative price = £7.83

KetoVie ® 4:1 Plant-Based Protein

▸ Intractable epilepsy and other conditions where a ketogenic diet is indicated. Not suitable for use in child under 3 years.
LIQUID (SIP OR TUBE FEED), protein 3.4 g, carbohydrate 0.2 g, fat 14 g, fibre 1.8 g, energy 619 kJ (148 kcal)/100 mL.

KetoVie 4:1 Plant-Based Protein liquid (Cambrooke UK Ltd)
250 ml (ACBS) • NHS indicative price = £8.28

KetoVie ® Peptide 4:1

▸ Intractable epilepsy and other conditions where a ketogenic diet is indicated. Not suitable for use in child under 3 years.
LIQUID (SIP OR TUBE FEED), protein 3.2 g, carbohydrate 0.33 g, fat 15 g, fibre 1.1 g, energy 632 kJ (151 kcal)/100 mL.

KetoVie Peptide 4:1 liquid (Cambrooke UK Ltd)
250 ml (ACBS) • NHS indicative price = £7.58

Specialist food replacers

Kanso ® 4.8:1 DeliMCT CacaoBar

▸ Intractable epilepsy when following a ketogenic diet, pyruvate dehydrogenase deficiency, glucose transporter type 1 deficiency syndrome or other conditions requiring a ketogenic diet. Suitable from 3 years.
SOLID, protein 7.1 g, carbohydrate 15.4 g, fat 55.4 g (MCT 38 %), fibre 18.9 g, energy 2394 kJ (582 kcal)/100 g.

Kanso DeliMCT CacaoBar (Dr Schar UK Ltd)
100 gram (ACBS) • NHS indicative price = £6.32

KetoClassic ® 3:1 Bar

▸ Intractable epilepsy, pyruvate dehydrogenase deficiency, glucose transporter type 1 deficiency and other conditions where a ketogenic diet is indicated. Suitable from 3 years.
SOLID, protein 10.8 g, carbohydrate 3.3 g, fat 43.6 g, fibre 28.7 g, energy 2082 kJ (498 kcal)/100 g.

KetoClassic 3:1 Bar (KetoCare Foods Ltd)
420 gram (ACBS) • NHS indicative price = £30.38

KetoClassic ® 3:1 Bisk

▸ Intractable epilepsy, pyruvate dehydrogenase deficiency, glucose transporter type 1 deficiency and other conditions where a ketogenic diet is indicated. Suitable from 3 years.
SOLID, protein 10.7 g, carbohydrate 4.6 g, fat 47.1 g, fibre 23.3 g, energy 2206 kJ (534 kcal)/100 g.

KetoClassic 3:1 Bisk (KetoCare Foods Ltd)
420 gram (ACBS) • NHS indicative price = £29.71

KetoClassic ® 3:1 Breakfast Muesli

▸ Intractable epilepsy, pyruvate dehydrogenase deficiency, glucose transporter type 1 deficiency and other conditions where a ketogenic diet is indicated. Suitable from 3 years.
SOLID, protein 11 g, carbohydrate 7.5 g, fat 57.1 g, fibre 17.5 g, energy 2569 kJ (623 kcal)/100 g.

KetoClassic 3:1 Breakfast muesli (KetoCare Foods Ltd)
600 gram (ACBS) • NHS indicative price = £50.36

KetoClassic ® 3:1 Breakfast Porridge

▸ Intractable epilepsy, pyruvate dehydrogenase deficiency, glucose transporter type 1 deficiency and other conditions where a ketogenic diet is indicated. Suitable from 3 years.
SOLID, protein 11.7 g, carbohydrate 7.8 g, fat 59.1 g, fibre 16.7 g, energy 2649 kJ (643 kcal)/100 g.

KetoClassic 3:1 Breakfast porridge (KetoCare Foods Ltd)
600 gram (ACBS) • NHS indicative price = £50.36

KetoClassic ® 3:1 Meal

▸ Intractable epilepsy, pyruvate dehydrogenase deficiency, glucose transporter type 1 deficiency and other conditions where a ketogenic diet is indicated. Suitable from 3 years.
SEMI-SOLID, protein 5.1-5.2 g, carbohydrate 2-3.7 g, fat 21.7-26.7 g, fibre 0.4-6 g, energy 936-1182 kJ (224-287 kcal)/100 g.

KetoClassic 3:1 Meal bolognese 130g pouches (KetoCare Foods Ltd)
14 pouch (ACBS) • NHS indicative price = £109.54

KetoClassic 3:1 Meal chicken 135g pouches (KetoCare Foods Ltd)
14 pouch (ACBS) • NHS indicative price = £110.86

KetoClassic ® 3:1 Savoury Bread

▸ Intractable epilepsy, pyruvate dehydrogenase deficiency, glucose transporter type 1 deficiency and other conditions where a ketogenic diet is indicated. Suitable from 3 years.
SOLID, protein 9 g, carbohydrate 7.3 g, fat 48.7 g, fibre 13.7 g, energy 2190 kJ (531 kcal)/100 g.

KetoClassic 3:1 Savoury meal (KetoCare Foods Ltd)
840 gram (ACBS) • NHS indicative price = £62.53

KetoVie ® 4:1 Kwik Mix

▸ Intractable epilepsy and other conditions where a ketogenic diet is indicated. Suitable from 3 years.
POWDER, protein 5.1 g, carbohydrate 5.8 g, fat 44 g, fibre 36 g, energy 2122 kJ (507 kcal)/100 g.

KetoVie Kwik Mix baking mix (Cambrooke UK Ltd)
680 gram (ACBS) • NHS indicative price = £43.83

Nutritional products for inherited metabolic disorders

Glucose plus galactose intolerance

Carbohydrate supplements

Galactomin 19 ®

▶ Nutritional supplement for the dietary management of glucose plus galactose intolerance. Includes added vitamins A, B, C, D, E and K.

POWDER, protein 14.6 g, carbohydrate 49.7 g, fat 30.8 g, energy 2233 kJ (534 kcal)/100 g.

Galactomin 19 powder (Nutricia Ltd)
400 gram (ACBS) · NHS indicative price = £69.46

Glutaric aciduria type 1

5 g protein equivalent

GA amino5 ®

▶ Nutritional supplement for the dietary management of glutaric aciduria type 1 (GA1).

POWDER, protein equivalent 83 g, carbohydrate Nil, fat Nil, energy 1411 kJ (332 kcal)/100 g

GA amino5 oral powder 6g sachets (Vitaflo International Ltd)
30 sachet (ACBS) · NHS indicative price = £166.26

GA explore5 ®

▶ Nutritional supplement for the dietary management of glutaric aciduria type 1. Suitable for child 6 months to 5 years. Includes added vitamins A, B, C, D, E and K.

POWDER protein equivalent 40 g, carbohydrate 42 g, fat 1.5 g, energy 1450 kJ (342 kcal)/100 g.

GA explore5 oral powder 12.5g sachets (Vitaflo International Ltd)
30 sachet (ACBS) · NHS indicative price = £185.92

10 g protein equivalent

GA gel ®

▶ Nutritional supplement for dietary management of type 1 glutaric aciduria. Suitable for child 6 months to 10 years. Includes added vitamins A, B, C, D, E and K.

POWDER, protein equivalent 41.7 g, carbohydrate 42.9 g, fat 0.05 g, energy 1440 kJ (339 kcal)/100 g.

GA gel oral powder 24g sachets (Vitaflo International Ltd)
30 sachet (ACBS) · NHS indicative price = £350.30

GA1 Anamix ® **Junior**

▶ Nutritional supplement for the dietary management of glutaric aciduria type 1. Suitable for child 1-10 years. Includes added vitamins A, B, C, D, E and K.

POWDER, protein 28 g, carbohydrate 30 g, fat 12.5 g, fibre 11.2 g, energy 1538 kJ (367 kcal)/100 g.

GA1 Anamix Junior oral powder 18g sachets (Nutricia Ltd)
30 sachet (ACBS) · NHS indicative price = £184.50

15 g protein equivalent

GA express ® **plus 15**

▶ Nutritional supplement for the dietary management of glutaric aciduria type 1 (GA1). Suitable from 3 years. Includes added vitamins A, B, C, D, E and K.

POWDER, protein equivalent 60 g, carbohydrate 14 g, fat 2.2 g, energy 1339 kJ (316 kcal)/100 g.

GA express plus 15 oral powder 25g sachets (Vitaflo International Ltd)
30 sachet (ACBS) · NHS indicative price = £534.15

Powder protein source

XLYS TRY Glutaridon ®

▶ Nutritional supplement for the dietary management of type 1 glutaric aciduria.

POWDER, protein 79 g, carbohydrate 4 g, fat Nil, energy 1411 kJ (332 kcal)/100 g.

XLYS TRY Glutaridon powder (Nutricia Ltd)
500 gram (ACBS) · NHS indicative price = £292.32

Infant formula protein source

GA1 Anamix ® **Infant**

▶ Nutritional supplement for the dietary management of proven glutaric aciduria type 1. Suitable for child from birth to 3 years. Includes added vitamins A, B, C, D, E and K.

POWDER, protein 13.1 g, carbohydrate 50.1 g, fat 23 g, fibre 3.7 g, energy 1950 kJ (466 kcal)/100 g.

GA1 Anamix Infant powder (Nutricia Ltd)
400 gram (ACBS) · NHS indicative price = £59.55

Glycogen storage disease

Slow-release carbohydrate supplements

Glycosade ®

▶ Nutritional supplement for the dietary management of hepatic glycogen storage disease. Unflavoured suitable from 2 years; lemon flavour suitable from 3 years.

POWDER, protein Nil, carbohydrate 88 g, fat Nil, energy 1496 kJ (352 kcal)/100 g

Glycosade oral powder 60g sachets lemon (Vitaflo International Ltd)
30 sachet (ACBS) · NHS indicative price = £184.00

Glycosade oral powder 60g sachets unflavoured (Vitaflo International Ltd)
30 sachet (ACBS) · NHS indicative price = £184.00

Homocystinuria

5 g protein equivalent

HCU explore5 ®

▶ Nutritional supplement for the dietary management of homocystinuria. Suitable for child from 6 months to 5 years. Includes added vitamins A, B, C, D, E and K.

POWDER, protein equivalent 40 g, carbohydrate 42 g, fat 1.5 g, energy 1450 kJ (342 kcal)/100 g.

HCU explore5 oral powder 12.5g sachets (Vitaflo International Ltd)
30 sachet (ACBS) · NHS indicative price = £185.92

10 g protein equivalent

HCU Anamix ® **Junior**

▶ Nutritional supplement for the dietary management of homocystinuria. Suitable for child 1-10 years. Includes added vitamins A, B, C, D, E and K.

POWDER, protein 28 g, carbohydrate 32 g, fat 12.5 g, energy 1572 kJ (375 kcal)/100 g.

HCU Anamix Junior oral powder 36g sachets (Nutricia Ltd)
30 sachet (ACBS) · NHS indicative price = £369.60

HCU cooler ® **10**

▶ Nutritional supplement for the dietary management of homocystinuria. Suitable from 3 years. Includes added vitamins A, B, C, D, E and K.

LIQUID, protein equivalent 11.5 g, carbohydrate 5.1 g, fat 0.9 g, energy 316 kJ (75 kcal)/100 mL.

HCU red cooler10 liquid (Vitaflo International Ltd)
87 ml (ACBS) · NHS indicative price = £11.16

HCU gel ®

▶ Nutritional supplement for the dietary management of homocystinuria. Suitable for child from 6 months to 10 years. Includes added vitamins A, B, C, D, E and K.

POWDER, protein equivalent 41.7 g, carbohydrate 42.9 g, fat 0.1 g, energy 1440 kJ (339 kcal)/100 g.

HCU gel oral powder 24g sachets (Vitaflo International Ltd)
30 sachet (ACBS) · NHS indicative price = £350.22

HCU Lophlex ® **LQ 10**

▶ Nutritional supplement for the dietary management of proven homocystinuria. Suitable from 4 years. Includes added vitamins A, B, C, D, E and K.

LIQUID, protein 16 g, carbohydrate 7 g, fat 0.35 g, energy 407 kJ (96 kcal)/100 mL.

HCU Lophlex LQ 10 liquid (Nutricia Ltd)
62.5 ml (ACBS) · NHS indicative price = £12.20

15 g protein equivalent

HCU cooler ® 15

▸ Nutritional supplement for the dietary management of homocystinuria. Suitable from 3 years. Includes added vitamins A, B, C, D, E and K.
LIQUID, protein equivalent 11.5 g, carbohydrate 5.1 g, fat 0.9 g, energy 316 kJ (75 kcal)/100 ml.

HCU orange cooler15 liquid (Vitaflo International Ltd)
130 ml (ACBS) · NHS indicative price = £18.46

HCU red cooler15 liquid (Vitaflo International Ltd)
130 ml (ACBS) · NHS indicative price = £18.46

HCU express ® 15

▸ Nutritional supplement for the dietary management of homocystinuria. Suitable from 8 years. Includes added vitamins A, B, C, D, E and K.
POWDER, protein equivalent 60 g, carbohydrate 13.7 g, fat 0.2 g, energy 1260 kJ (297 kcal)/100 g.

HCU express15 oral powder 25g sachets (Vitaflo International Ltd)
30 sachet (ACBS) · NHS indicative price = £544.02

20 g protein equivalent

HCU cooler ® 20

▸ Nutritional supplement for the dietary management of homocystinuria. Suitable from 3 years. Includes added vitamins A, B, C, D, E and K.
LIQUID, protein equivalent 11.5 g, carbohydrate 5.1 g, fat 0.9 g, energy 316 kJ (75 kcal)/100 mL.

HCU red cooler20 liquid (Vitaflo International Ltd)
174 ml (ACBS) · NHS indicative price = £23.34

HCU Lophlex ®

▸ Nutritional supplement for the dietary management of homocystinuria. Suitable from 3 years. Includes added vitamins A, B, C, D, E and K.
POWDER, protein 68.9 g, carbohydrate 13.4 g, fat 1.4 g, energy 1430 kJ (338 kcal)/100 g.

HCU Lophlex powder 29g sachets (Nutricia Ltd)
30 sachet (ACBS) · NHS indicative price = £677.40

HCU Lophlex ® LQ 20

▸ Nutritional supplement for the dietary management of proven homocystinuria. Suitable from 4 years. Includes added vitamins A, B, C, D, E and K.
LIQUID, protein 16 g, carbohydrate 7 g, fat 0.35 g, energy 407 kJ (96 kcal)/100 mL.

HCU Lophlex LQ 20 liquid (Nutricia Ltd)
125 ml (ACBS) · NHS indicative price = £25.17

HCU-LV ®

▸ Nutritional supplement for the dietary management of hypermethioninaemia or vitamin B6 non-responsive homocystinuria. Suitable from 8 years. Includes added vitamins A, B, C, D, E and K.
POWDER, protein 72 g, carbohydrate 5 g, fat 0.7 g, energy 1335 kJ (314 kcal)/100 g.

HCU-LV oral powder 27.8g sachets tropical (Nutricia Ltd)
30 sachet (ACBS) · NHS indicative price = £774.00

Powder protein source

HCU Maxamum ®

▸ Nutritional supplement for the dietary management of hypermethioninaemia, homocystinuria. Suitable from 8 years. Includes added vitamins A, B, C, D, E and K.
POWDER, protein 39 g, carbohydrate 34 g, fat less than 0.5 g, energy 1260 kJ (297 kcal)/100 g.

HCU Maxamum powder (Nutricia Ltd)
500 gram (ACBS) · NHS indicative price = £247.34

Infant formula protein source

HCU Anamix ® Infant

▸ Nutritional supplement for the dietary management of proven vitamin B6 non-responsive homocystinuria or hypermethioninaemia. Suitable for child from birth to 3 years. Includes added vitamins A, B C, D, E and K.
POWDER, protein equivalent (essential and non-essential amino acids) 13.1 g, carbohydrate 50.1 g, fat 23 g, energy 1950 kJ (466 kcal)/100 g.

HCU Anamix Infant powder (Nutricia Ltd)
400 gram (ACBS) · NHS indicative price = £59.55

Homocystinuria or hypermethioninaemia

Powder protein source

XMET Homidon ®

▸ Nutritional supplement for the dietary management of homocystinuria or hypermethioninaemia.
POWDER, protein 77 g, carbohydrate 4.5 g, fat Nil, energy 1386 kJ (326 kcal)/100 g.

XMET Homidon powder (Nutricia Ltd)
500 gram (ACBS) · NHS indicative price = £292.32

Hyperlysinaemia

Infant formula protein source

HYPER LYS Anamix ® Infant

▸ Nutritional supplement for the dietary management of hyperlysinaemia. Suitable for child from birth to 3 years. Includes added vitamins A, B, C, D, E and K.
POWDER, protein 13.1 g, carbohydrate 50.1 g, fat 23.0 g, fibre 3.7 g, energy 1950 kJ (466 kcal)/100 g.

HYPER LYS Anamix Infant powder (Nutricia Ltd)
400 gram (ACBS) · NHS indicative price = £59.55

Isovaleric acidaemia

Powder protein source

IVA Anamix ® Junior

▸ Nutritional supplement for the dietary management of proven isovaleric acidaemia. Suitable for child 1-10 years. Includes added vitamins A, B, C, D, E and K.
POWDER, protein 28 g, carbohydrate 30 g, fat 12.5 g, fibre 11.2 g, energy 1538 kJ (367 kcal)/100 g.

IVA Anamix Junior powder (Nutricia Ltd)
400 gram (ACBS) · NHS indicative price = £132.82

Infant formula protein source

IVA Anamix ® Infant

▸ Nutritional supplement for the dietary management of proven isovaleric acidaemia or other proven disorders of leucine metabolism. Suitable for child from birth to 3 years. Includes added vitamins A, B, C, D, E and K.
POWDER, protein 13.1 g, carbohydrate 50.1 g, fat 23 g, fibre 3.7 g, energy 1950 kJ (466 kcal)/100 g.

IVA Anamix Infant powder (Nutricia Ltd)
400 gram (ACBS) · NHS indicative price = £59.55

Lipid metabolism disorders

Infant formula MCT fat source

Lipistart ®

▸ Nutritional supplement for the dietary management of fat malabsorption, long chain fatty acid oxidation disorders and disorders requiring management using a high MCT, low LCT formula. Includes added vitamins A, B, C, D, E and K. Suitable for child from birth to 10 years.
POWDER, protein 12 g, carbohydrate 58 g, fat 21 g, energy 1967 kJ (469 kcal)/100 g.

Lipistart powder (Vitaflo International Ltd)
400 gram (ACBS) · NHS indicative price = £31.90

Monogen ®

▸ For the dietary management of disorders requiring a low LCT, high MCT intake, such as long chain fatty acid oxidation defects (long chain acyl CoA dehydrogenase deficiency (LCAD) and carnitine palmitoyl transferase deficiency (CPTD)), primary and secondary lipoprotein lipase deficiency (hyperlipoproteinaemia

type 1), chylothorax and lymphangiectasia. Includes added vitamins A, B, C, D, E and K.
POWDER, protein 12.8 g, carbohydrate 68.6 g, fat 12.9 g, energy 1859 kJ (441 kcal)/100 g.

Monogen powder (Nutricia Ltd)
400 gram (ACBS) • NHS indicative price = £31.87

Maple syrup urine disease

5 g protein equivalent

MSUD amino5®
▸ Nutritional supplement for the dietary management of maple syrup urine disease (MSUD).
POWDER, protein equivalent 83 g, carbohydrate Nil, fat Nil, energy 1411 kJ (332 kcal)/100 g

MSUD amino5 oral powder 6g sachets (Vitaflo International Ltd)
30 sachet (ACBS) • NHS indicative price = £166.33

MSUD explore5®
▸ Nutritional supplement for the dietary management of maple syrup urine disease. Suitable for child 6 months to 5 years.
POWDERprotein 40g, carbohydrate 42g, fat 1.5g, energy 1450 kJ (342 kcal)/100g.

MSUD explore5 oral powder 12.5g sachets (Vitaflo International Ltd)
30 sachet (ACBS) • NHS indicative price = £185.92

10 g protein equivalent

MSUD Anamix® Junior
▸ Nutritional supplement for the dietary management of maple syrup urine disease. Suitable for child 1–10 years. Includes added vitamins A, B, C, D, E and K.
POWDER, protein equivalent (essential and non-essential amino acids) 28 g, carbohydrate 32 g, fat 12.5 g, energy 1572 kJ (375 kcal)/100 g.

MSUD Anamix Junior oral powder 36g sachets (Nutricia Ltd)
30 sachet (ACBS) • NHS indicative price = £325.80

MSUD Anamix® Junior LQ
▸ Nutritional supplement for the dietary management of maple syrup urine disease. Suitable for child from 1 year. Includes added vitamins A, B, C, D, E and K.
LIQUID, protein equivalent (essential and non-essential amino acids) 8 g, carbohydrate 7 g, fat 3.8 g, fibre 0.25 g, energy 396 kJ (94 kcal)/100 mL.

MSUD Anamix Junior LQ liquid (Nutricia Ltd)
125 ml (ACBS) • NHS indicative price = £13.60

MSUD cooler® 10
▸ Nutritional supplement for the dietary management of maple syrup urine disease. Suitable from 3 years. Includes added vitamins A, B, C, D, E and K.
LIQUID, protein equivalent 11.5 g, carbohydrate 5.1 g, fat 0.9 g, energy 316 kJ (75 kcal)/100 mL.

MSUD red cooler10 liquid (Vitaflo International Ltd)
87 ml (ACBS) • NHS indicative price = £11.16

MSUD gel®
▸ Nutritional supplement for the dietary management of maple syrup urine disease. Suitable for child 1–10 years. Includes added vitamins A, B, C, D, E and K.
POWDER, protein equivalent 41.7 g, carbohydrate 42.9 g, fat 0.05 g, energy 1440 kJ (339 kcal)/100 g..

MSUD gel 24g sachets (Vitaflo International Ltd)
30 sachet (ACBS) • NHS indicative price = £354.33

MSUD Lophlex® LQ 10
▸ Nutritional supplement for the dietary management of maple syrup urine disease. Includes added vitamins A, B, C, D, E and K.
LIQUID, protein 16 g, carbohydrate 7 g, fat 0.35 g, energy 407 kJ (96 kcal)/100 mL.

MSUD Lophlex LQ 10 liquid (Nutricia Ltd)
62.5 ml (ACBS) • NHS indicative price = £12.20

15 g protein equivalent

MSUD cooler® 15
▸ Nutritional supplement for the dietary management of maple syrup urine disease. Suitable from 3 years. Includes added vitamins A, B, C, D, E and K.
LIQUID, protein equivalent 11.5 g, carbohydrate 5.1 g, fat 0.9 g, energy 316 kJ (75 kcal)/100 mL.

MSUD orange cooler15 liquid (Vitaflo International Ltd)
130 ml (ACBS) • NHS indicative price = £18.46

MSUD red cooler15 liquid (Vitaflo International Ltd)
130 ml (ACBS) • NHS indicative price = £18.46

MSUD express® 15
▸ Nutritional supplement for the dietary management of maple syrup urine disease. Suitable from 8 years. Includes added vitamins A, B, C, D, E, K.
POWDER, protein equivalent 60 g, carbohydrate 13.7 g, fat 0.2 g, energy 1260 kJ (297 kcal)/100 g.

MSUD express15 oral powder 25g sachets (Vitaflo International Ltd)
30 sachet (ACBS) • NHS indicative price = £544.02

20 g protein equivalent

MSUD cooler® 20
▸ Nutritional supplement for the dietary management of maple syrup urine disease. Suitable from 3 years. Includes added vitamins A, B, C, D, E and K.
LIQUID, protein equivalent 11.5 g, carbohydrate 5.1 g, fat 0.9 g, energy 316 kJ (75 kcal)/100 mL.

MSUD red cooler20 liquid (Vitaflo International Ltd)
174 ml (ACBS) • NHS indicative price = £23.34

MSUD Lophlex®
▸ Nutritional supplement for the dietary management of maple syrup urine disease. Suitable from 3 years. Includes added vitamins A, B, C, D, E and K.
POWDER, protein 71.4 g, carbohydrate 15 g, fat 1.5 g, energy 1530 kJ (355 kcal)/100 g.

MSUD Lophlex powder 28g sachets (Nutricia Ltd)
30 sachet (ACBS) • NHS indicative price = £677.40

MSUD Lophlex® LQ 20
▸ Nutritional supplement for the dietary management of maple syrup urine disease. Includes added vitamins A, B, C, D, E and K.
LIQUID, protein 16 g, carbohydrate 7 g, fat 0.35 g, energy 407 kJ (96 kcal)/100 mL.

MSUD Lophlex LQ 20 liquid (Nutricia Ltd)
125 ml (ACBS) • NHS indicative price = £25.17

Powder protein source

MSUD Aid III®
▸ Nutritional supplement for the dietary management of maple syrup urine disease (MSUD) and related conditions when it is necessary to limit the intake of branched chain amino acids.
POWDER, protein 77 g, carbohydrate 4.5 g, fat Nil, energy 1386 kJ (326 kcal)/100 g.

MSUD Aid 111 powder (Nutricia Ltd)
500 gram (ACBS) • NHS indicative price = £292.32

MSUD Maxamum®
▸ Nutritional supplement for the dietary management of maple syrup urine disease. Suitable from 8 years. Includes added vitamins A, B, C, D, E and K.
POWDER, protein equivalent (essential and non-essential amino acids) 39 g, carbohydrate 34 g, fat less than 0.5 g, energy 1260 kJ (297 kcal)/100 g.

MSUD Maxamum powder orange (Nutricia Ltd)
500 gram (ACBS) • NHS indicative price = £247.34

MSUD Maxamum powder unflavoured (Nutricia Ltd)
500 gram (ACBS) • NHS indicative price = £247.34

Infant formula protein source

MSUD Anamix ® Infant

▸ Nutritional supplement for the dietary management of proven maple syrup urine disease. Suitable for child from birth to 3 years. Contains added vitamins A, B, C, D E and K.
POWDER, protein 13.1 g, carbohydrate 50.1 g, fat 23 g, energy 1950 kJ (466 kcal)/100 g.

MSUD Anamix Infant powder (Nutricia Ltd)
400 gram (ACBS) · NHS indicative price = £59.55

Methylmalonic or propionic acidaemia

5 g protein equivalent

MMA/PA amino5 ®

▸ Nutritional supplement for the dietary management of the organic acidaemias, methylmalonic acidaemia (MMA) and the propionic acidaemia (PA).
POWDER, protein equivalent 83 g, carbohydrate Nil, fat Nil, energy 1411 kJ (332 kcal)/100 g

MMA / PA amino5 oral powder 6g sachets (Vitaflo International Ltd)
30 sachet (ACBS) · NHS indicative price = £166.33

MMA/PA Anamix ® Junior

▸ Nutritional supplement for the dietary management of proven methylmalonic acidaemia or propionic acidaemia. Suitable for child 1-10 years. Includes added vitamins A, B, C, D, E and K.
POWDER, protein 28 g, carbohydrate 30 g, fat 12.5 g, energy 1538 kJ (367 kcal)/100 g.

MMA / PA Anamix Junior oral powder 18g sachets (Nutricia Ltd)
30 sachet (ACBS) · NHS indicative price = £184.80

MMA/PA explore5 ®

▸ Nutritional supplement for the dietary management of methylmalonic or propionic acidaemia. Suitable for child from 6 months to 5 years. Includes added vitamins A, B, C, D, E and K.
POWDER, protein equivalent 40 g, carbohydrate 42 g, fat 1.5 g, energy 1450 kJ (342 kcal)/100 g.

MMA / PA explore5 oral powder 12.5g sachets (Vitaflo International Ltd)
30 sachet (ACBS) · NHS indicative price = £182.00

Powder protein source

MMA/PA Maxamum ®

▸ Nutritional supplement for the dietary management of methylmalonic acidaemia or propionic acidaemia. Suitable from 8 years. Includes added vitamins A, B, C, D, E and K.
POWDER, protein 39 g, carbohydrate 34 g, fat less than 0.5 g, energy 1260 kJ (297 kcal)/100 g.

MMA / PA Maxamum powder (Nutricia Ltd)
500 gram (ACBS) · NHS indicative price = £247.34

XMTVI Asadon ®

▸ Nutritional supplement for the dietary management of methylmalonic acidaemia or propionic acidaemia.
POWDER, protein 77 g, carbohydrate 4.5 g, fat Nil, energy 1386 kJ (326 kcal)/100 g.

XMTVI Asadon powder (Nutricia Ltd)
200 gram (ACBS) · NHS indicative price = £116.93

Infant formula protein source

MMA/PA Anamix ® Infant

▸ Nutritional supplement for the dietary management of proven methylmalonic acidaemia or propionic acidaemia. Suitable for child from birth to 3 years. Includes added vitamins A, B, C, D, E and K.
POWDER, protein 13.1 g, carbohydrate 50.1 g, fat 23 g, energy 1950 kJ (466 kcal)/100 g.

MMA / PA Anamix Infant powder (Nutricia Ltd)
400 gram (ACBS) · NHS indicative price = £59.55

Non-specific inherited metabolic disorders

Energy (carbohydrate) fortifiers

S.O.S. ®

▸ Nutritional supplement for the dietary management of inherited metabolic disorders.
POWDER, protein Nil, carbohydrate 95 g, fat Nil, energy 1615 kJ (380 kcal)/100 g.

S.O.S10 oral powder 21g sachets (Vitaflo International Ltd)
30 sachet (ACBS) · NHS indicative price = £23.02

S.O.S15 oral powder 31g sachets (Vitaflo International Ltd)
30 sachet (ACBS) · NHS indicative price = £27.20

S.O.S20 oral powder 42g sachets (Vitaflo International Ltd)
30 sachet (ACBS) · NHS indicative price = £36.88

S.O.S25 oral powder 52g sachets (Vitaflo International Ltd)
30 sachet (ACBS) · NHS indicative price = £45.60

Energy (carbohydrate and fat) fortifiers

Basecal200 ®

▸ Nutritional supplement for the dietary management of inborn errors of protein metabolism requiring a low protein diet. Suitable from 3 years. Includes added vitamins A, B, C, D, E and K.
POWDER, protein equivalent Nil, carbohydrate 69.8 g, fat 20.7 g, energy 1952 kJ (465 kcal)/100 g.

Basecal200 oral powder 43g sachets (Vitaflo International Ltd)
30 sachet (ACBS) · NHS indicative price = £112.25

Essential fatty acid supplements

KeyOmega ®

▸ Nutritional supplement for the dietary management of inborn errors of metabolism. Includes added vitamin C.
POWDER, protein 4.4 g, carbohydrate 70 g, fat 19 g, energy 1999 kJ (476 kcal)/100 g.

KeyOmega oral powder 4g sachets (Vitaflo International Ltd)
30 sachet (ACBS) · NHS indicative price = £65.81

Single L-amino acid supplements

Cystine500 ®

▸ Nutritional supplement for the dietary management of inborn errors of amino acid metabolism. Suitable from 3 years.
POWDER, protein equivalent 11.6 g, carbohydrate 82.5 g, fat Nil, energy 1600 kJ (376 kcal)/100 g.

Cystine500 oral powder sachets (Vitaflo International Ltd)
30 sachet (ACBS) · NHS indicative price = £88.93

Isoleucine50 ®

▸ Nutritional supplement for the dietary management of inborn errors of amino acid metabolism.
POWDER, protein equivalent 1 g, carbohydrate 95 g, fat Nil, energy 1632 kJ (384 kcal)/100 g.

Isoleucine50 oral powder 4g sachets (Vitaflo International Ltd)
30 sachet (ACBS) · NHS indicative price = £88.93

L-Tyrosine

▸ Nutritional supplement for the dietary management of maternal phenylketonuria in patients with low plasma tyrosine levels.
POWDER, protein 90.1 g, carbohydrate Nil, fat Nil, energy 1532 kJ (360 kcal)/100 g.

L-Tyrosine powder (Nutricia Ltd)
100 gram (ACBS) · NHS indicative price = £34.41

Leucine100 ®

▸ Nutritional supplement for the dietary management of inborn errors of amino acid metabolism.
POWDER, protein equivalent 2.2 g, carbohydrate 92.5 g, fat Nil, energy 1610 kJ (379 kcal)/100 g.

Leucine100 oral powder sachets (Vitaflo International Ltd)
30 sachet (ACBS) · NHS indicative price = £88.93

Phenylalanine50 ®

▸ Nutritional supplement for the dietary management of inborn errors of amino acid metabolism.

POWDER, protein equivalent 1.1 g, carbohydrate 95 g, fat Nil, energy 1634 kJ (384 kcal)/100 g.

Phenylalanine50 oral powder sachets (Vitaflo International Ltd)
30 sachet (ACBS) • NHS indicative price = £86.35

Tyrosine1000®
▸ Nutritional supplement for the dietary management of inborn errors of amino acid metabolism. Not suitable for use in child under 3 years.
POWDER, protein equivalent 22.5 g, carbohydrate 72.5 g, fat Nil, energy 1615 kJ (380 kcal)/100 g.

Tyrosine1000 oral powder 4g sachets (Vitaflo International Ltd)
30 sachet (ACBS) • NHS indicative price = £7.92

Valine50®
▸ Nutritional supplement for the dietary management of inborn errors of amino acid metabolism.
POWDER, protein equivalent 1 g, carbohydrate 95 g, fat Nil, energy 1632 kJ (384 kcal)/100 g.

Valine50 oral powder 4g sachets (Vitaflo International Ltd)
30 sachet (ACBS) • NHS indicative price = £88.93

Phenylketonuria

5 g protein equivalent

PKU Anamix® First Spoon
▸ Nutritional supplement for the dietary management of proven phenylketonuria. Suitable for child from 6 months to 5 years. Includes added vitamins A, B, C, D, E and K.
POWDER, protein 40 g, carbohydrate 38.4 g, fat 1.15 g, energy 1377 kJ (324 kcal)/100 g.

PKU Anamix First Spoon oral powder 12.5g sachets (Nutricia Ltd)
30 sachet (ACBS) • NHS indicative price = £134.10

PKU explore® 5
▸ Nutritional supplement for the dietary management of phenylketonuria. Suitable for child from 6 months to 5 years. Includes added vitamins A, B, C, D, E and K.
POWDER, protein 40 g, carbohydrate 42 g, fat 1.5 g, energy 1450 kJ (342 kcal)/100 g.

PKU explore5 oral powder 12.5g sachets (Vitaflo International Ltd)
30 sachet (ACBS) • NHS indicative price = £133.25

PKU GoLike® Bar 5
▸ Nutritional supplement for the dietary management of phenylketonuria. Suitable from 3 years.
SOLID, protein equivalent (amino acids) 17 g, carbohydrate 50 g, fat Nil, energy 1170 kJ (275 kcal)/100 g.

PKU GoLike Bar 5 30g bars (Nutrinovo Ltd)
40 bar (ACBS) • NHS indicative price = £152.00

10 g GMP protein equivalent

Glytactin® Build 10
▸ Nutritional supplement for the dietary management of phenylketonuria. Suitable from 3 years. Includes added vitamins A, B, C, D, E and K.
POWDER, protein equivalent 67 g, carbohydrate 2.4 g, fat 4.2 g, energy 1400 kJ (335 kcal)/100 g.

Glytactin Build 10 oral powder 16g sachets (Cambrooke UK Ltd)
30 sachet (ACBS) • NHS indicative price = £238.79

PKU GMPro®
▸ Nutritional supplement for the dietary management of phenylketonuria. Suitable from 3 years; use with caution in child 3–6 years. Includes added vitamins A, B, C, D, E and K.
POWDER, protein 30 g, carbohydrate 37.5 g, fat 11.7 g, energy 1616 kJ (384 kcal)/100 g.

PKU GMPro oral powder 33.3g sachets (Nutricia Ltd)
16 sachet (ACBS) • NHS indicative price = £127.68

PKU GMPro® LQ
▸ Nutritional supplement for the dietary management of phenylketonuria. Suitable from 3 years; use with caution in child 3–6 years. Includes added vitamins A, B C, D, E and K.
LIQUID, protein equivalent 4 g, carbohydrate 3.4 g, fat 1.6 g, energy 188 kJ (45 kcal)/100 mL

PKU GMPro LQ liquid (Nutricia Ltd)
250 ml (ACBS) • NHS indicative price = £7.99

PKU GMPro® Mix-In
▸ Nutritional supplement for the dietary management of phenylketonuria. Not suitable for use in child under 3 years.
POWDER, protein 80 g, carbohydrate 3.4 g, fat nil, energy 1418 kJ (334 kcal)/100 g.

PKU GMPro Mix-In oral powder 12.5g sachets (Nutricia Ltd)
30 sachet (ACBS) • NHS indicative price = £195.90

10 g protein equivalent

Mevalia® PKU Motion 10
▸ Nutritional supplement for the dietary management of phenylketonuria. Suitable from 3 years. Includes added vitamins A, B, C, D, E and K.
LIQUID, protein equivalent 14 g, carbohydrate 5 g, fat Nil, energy 328 kJ (77 kcal)/100 mL.

Mevalia PKU Motion 10 liquid red fruits (Vitaflo International Ltd)
70 ml (ACBS) • NHS indicative price = £5.65

Mevalia PKU Motion 10 liquid tropical (Vitaflo International Ltd)
70 ml (ACBS) • NHS indicative price = £5.65

Phlexy-10® drink mix
▸ Nutritional supplement for the dietary management of phenylketonuria. Suitable from 1 year.
POWDER, protein 41.7 g, carbohydrate 44 g, fat Nil, energy 1456 kJ (343 kcal)/100 g.

Phlexy-10 drink mix 20g sachets apple & blackcurrant (Nutricia Ltd)
30 sachet (ACBS) • NHS indicative price = £194.70

Phlexy-10 drink mix 20g sachets citrus burst (Nutricia Ltd)
30 sachet (ACBS) • NHS indicative price = £194.70

Phlexy-10 drink mix 20g sachets tropical surprise (Nutricia Ltd)
30 sachet (ACBS) • NHS indicative price = £194.70

PKU Anamix® Junior
▸ Nutritional supplement for the dietary management of phenylketonuria. Suitable for child 1-10 years. Includes added vitamins A, B, C, D, E and K.
POWDER, protein 28 g, carbohydrate 32 g, fat 12.5 g, energy 1572 kJ (375 kcal)/100 g.

PKU Anamix Junior powder 36g sachets berry (Nutricia Ltd)
30 sachet (ACBS) • NHS indicative price = £191.70

PKU Anamix Junior powder 36g sachets chocolate (Nutricia Ltd)
30 sachet (ACBS) • NHS indicative price = £191.70

PKU Anamix Junior powder 36g sachets neutral (Nutricia Ltd)
30 sachet (ACBS) • NHS indicative price = £191.70

PKU Anamix Junior powder 36g sachets orange (Nutricia Ltd)
30 sachet (ACBS) • NHS indicative price = £191.70

PKU Anamix Junior powder 36g sachets vanilla (Nutricia Ltd)
30 sachet (ACBS) • NHS indicative price = £191.70

PKU Anamix® Junior LQ
▸ Nutritional supplement for the dietary management of phenylketonuria. Suitable for child 1-10 years. Includes added vitamins A, B, C, D, E, K.
LIQUID, protein 8 g, carbohydrate 7 g, fat 3.8 g, fibre 0.3 g, energy 396 kJ (94 kcal)/100 mL.

PKU Anamix Junior LQ liquid berry (Nutricia Ltd)
125 ml (ACBS) • NHS indicative price = £8.51

PKU Anamix Junior LQ liquid orange (Nutricia Ltd)
125 ml (ACBS) • NHS indicative price = £8.51

PKU cooler® 10
▸ Nutritional supplement for the dietary management of phenylketonuria. Suitable from 3 years. Includes added vitamins A, B, C, D, E and K.
LIQUID, protein equivalent 11.5 g, carbohydrate 5.1 g, fat 0.9 g, energy 316 kJ (75 kcal)/100 mL.

PKU orange cooler10 liquid (Vitaflo International Ltd)
87 ml (ACBS) • NHS indicative price = £7.50

PKU purple cooler10 liquid (Vitaflo International Ltd)
87 ml (ACBS) • NHS indicative price = £7.50

PKU red cooler10 liquid (Vitaflo International Ltd)
87 ml (ACBS) · NHS indicative price = £7.50

PKU white cooler10 liquid (Vitaflo International Ltd)
87 ml (ACBS) · NHS indicative price = £7.50

PKU yellow cooler10 liquid (Vitaflo International Ltd)
87 ml (ACBS) · NHS indicative price = £7.50

PKU explore® 10
▸ Nutritional supplement for the dietary management of phenylketonuria. Suitable for child 1-5 years. Includes added vitamins A, B, C, D, E and K.
POWDER, protein 40 g, carbohydrate 39 g, fat 1.5 g, energy 1399 kJ (330 kcal)/100 g.

PKU explore10 oral powder 25g sachets orange (Vitaflo International Ltd)
30 sachet (ACBS) · NHS indicative price = £266.60

PKU explore10 oral powder 25g sachets raspberry (Vitaflo International Ltd)
30 sachet (ACBS) · NHS indicative price = £266.60

PKU GoLike® Bar 10
▸ Nutritional supplement for the dietary management of phenylketonuria. Suitable from 3 years.
SOLID, protein equivalent (amino acids) 17 g, carbohydrate 53 g, fat Nil, energy 1236 kJ (292 kcal)/100 g.

PKU GoLike Bar 10 60g bars (Nutrinovo Ltd)
20 bar (ACBS) · NHS indicative price = £152.00

PKU Lophlex® LQ 10
▸ Nutritional supplement for the dietary management of proven phenylketonuria. Suitable from 4 years. Includes added vitamins A, B, C, D, E and K.
LIQUID, protein 16 g, carbohydrate 7 g, fat Nil, energy 391 kJ (92 kcal)/100 mL.

PKU Lophlex LQ 10 liquid berry (Nutricia Ltd)
62.5 ml (ACBS) · NHS indicative price = £7.66

PKU Lophlex LQ 10 liquid juicy berries (Nutricia Ltd)
62.5 ml (ACBS) · NHS indicative price = £7.66

PKU Lophlex LQ 10 liquid juicy citrus (Nutricia Ltd)
62.5 ml (ACBS) · NHS indicative price = £7.66

PKU Lophlex LQ 10 liquid juicy orange (Nutricia Ltd)
62.5 ml (ACBS) · NHS indicative price = £7.66

PKU Lophlex LQ 10 liquid juicy tropical (Nutricia Ltd)
62.5 ml (ACBS) · NHS indicative price = £7.66

PKU squeezie®
▸ Nutritional supplement for the dietary management of phenylketonuria. Suitable for child from 6 months to 10 years. Includes added vitamins A, B, C, D, E and K.
LIQUID, protein equivalent 12 g, carbohydrate 26 g, fat 0.6 g, energy 668 kJ (157 kcal)/100 g.

PKU squeezie liquid 85g pouches (Vitaflo International Ltd)
30 pouch (ACBS) · NHS indicative price = £218.09

XPhe® jump 10
▸ Nutritional supplement for the dietary management of phenylketonuria (PKU) or hyperphenylalaninemia (HPA). Suitable from 3 years. Includes added vitamins A, B, C, D, E and K.
LIQUID, protein equivalent 16 g, carbohydrate 9 g, fat less than 0.1 g, energy 376 kJ (89 kcal)/100 mL.

XPhe jump 10 liquid cola (metaX Institut fuer Diatetik GmbH)
63 ml (ACBS) · NHS indicative price = £4.94

XPhe jump 10 liquid neutral (metaX Institut fuer Diatetik GmbH)
63 ml (ACBS) · NHS indicative price = £4.94

XPhe jump 10 liquid orange (metaX Institut fuer Diatetik GmbH)
63 ml (ACBS) · NHS indicative price = £4.94

XPhe jump 10 liquid tropical (metaX Institut fuer Diatetik GmbH)
63 ml (ACBS) · NHS indicative price = £4.94

XPhe jump 10 liquid vanilla (metaX Institut fuer Diatetik GmbH)
63 ml (ACBS) · NHS indicative price = £4.94

XPhe jump 10 liquid wild berries (metaX Institut fuer Diatetik GmbH)
63 ml (ACBS) · NHS indicative price = £4.94

15 g GMP protein equivalent

Glytactin® Complete 15
▸ Nutritional supplement for the dietary management of phenylketonuria. Suitable from 3 years. Includes added vitamins A, B, C, D, E and K.
SOLID, protein equivalent 19 g, carbohydrate 43 g, fat 15 g, energy 1705 kJ (407 kcal)/100 g.

Glytactin Complete 15 81g bars peanut butter (Cambrooke UK Ltd)
7 bar (ACBS) · NHS indicative price = £83.49

Glytactin® RTD 15
▸ Nutritional supplement for the dietary management of phenylketonuria. Suitable for over 3 years. Includes added vitamins A, B, C, D, E and K.
LIQUID, protein equivalent 6 g, carbohydrate 9.2 g, fat 2 g, energy 335 kJ (80 kcal)/100 mL.

Glytactin RTD 15 liquid chocolate (Cambrooke UK Ltd)
250 ml (ACBS) · NHS indicative price = £11.93

Glytactin RTD 15 liquid original (Cambrooke UK Ltd)
250 ml (ACBS) · NHS indicative price = £11.93

Glytactin® RTD Lite 15
▸ Nutritional supplement for the dietary management of phenylketonuria. Suitable for over 3 years. Includes added vitamins A, B, C, D, E and K.
LIQUID, protein 6 g, carbohydrate 3 g, fat 1.4 g, energy 201 kJ (48 kcal)/100 mL.

Glytactin RTD Lite 15 liquid coffee mocha (Cambrooke UK Ltd)
250 ml (ACBS) · NHS indicative price = £12.05

Glytactin RTD Lite 15 liquid vanilla (Cambrooke UK Ltd)
250 ml (ACBS) · NHS indicative price = £12.05

PKU sphere® 15
▸ Nutritional supplement for the dietary management of phenylketonuria. Suitable from 4 years. Includes added vitamins A, B, C, D, E and K.
POWDER, protein 56 g, carbohydrate 18 g, fat 4.7 g, energy 1432 kJ (338 kcal)/100 g.

PKU sphere15 oral powder 27g sachets chocolate (Vitaflo International Ltd)
30 sachet (ACBS) · NHS indicative price = £362.86

PKU sphere15 oral powder 27g sachets red berry (Vitaflo International Ltd)
30 sachet (ACBS) · NHS indicative price = £362.86

PKU sphere15 oral powder 27g sachets vanilla (Vitaflo International Ltd)
30 sachet (ACBS) · NHS indicative price = £362.86

15 g protein equivalent

PKU Air® 15
▸ Nutritional supplement for the dietary management of phenylketonuria. Suitable from 3 years. Includes added vitamins A, B, C, D, E and K.
LIQUID, protein equivalent 11.5 g, carbohydrate 1.5 g, fat 0.6 g, energy 243 kJ (57 kcal)/100 mL.

PKU Air15 gold liquid (Vitaflo International Ltd)
130 ml (ACBS) · NHS indicative price = £10.80

PKU Air15 green liquid (Vitaflo International Ltd)
130 ml (ACBS) · NHS indicative price = £10.80

PKU Air15 red liquid (Vitaflo International Ltd)
130 ml (ACBS) · NHS indicative price = £10.80

PKU Air15 white liquid (Vitaflo International Ltd)
130 ml (ACBS) · NHS indicative price = £10.80

PKU Air15 yellow liquid (Vitaflo International Ltd)
130 ml (ACBS) · NHS indicative price = £10.80

PKU cooler® 15
▸ Nutritional supplement for the dietary management of phenylketonuria. Suitable from 3 years. Includes added vitamins A, B, C, D, E and K.
LIQUID, protein equivalent 11.5 g, carbohydrate 5.1 g, fat 0.9 g, energy 316 kJ (75 kcal)/100 mL.

PKU orange cooler15 liquid (Vitaflo International Ltd)
130 ml (ACBS) · NHS indicative price = £11.18

PKU purple cooler15 liquid (Vitaflo International Ltd)
130 ml (ACBS) • NHS indicative price = £11.18

PKU red cooler15 liquid (Vitaflo International Ltd)
130 ml (ACBS) • NHS indicative price = £11.18

PKU white cooler15 liquid (Vitaflo International Ltd)
130 ml (ACBS) • NHS indicative price = £11.18

PKU yellow cooler15 liquid (Vitaflo International Ltd)
130 ml (ACBS) • NHS indicative price = £11.18

PKU express ® plus15

▸ Nutritional supplement for the dietary management of phenylketonuria. Suitable from 3 years. Includes added vitamins A, B, C, D, E and K.

POWDER, protein equivalent 60 g, carbohydrate 14 g, fat 2.2 g, energy 1339 kJ (316 kcal)/100 g.

PKU express plus15 powder 25g sachets lemon (Vitaflo International Ltd)
30 sachet (ACBS) • NHS indicative price = £323.52

PKU express plus15 powder 25g sachets orange (Vitaflo International Ltd)
30 sachet (ACBS) • NHS indicative price = £323.52

PKU express plus15 powder 25g sachets raspberry (Vitaflo International Ltd)
30 sachet (ACBS) • NHS indicative price = £309.74

PKU express plus15 powder 25g sachets tropical (Vitaflo International Ltd)
30 sachet (ACBS) • NHS indicative price = £323.52

PKU express plus15 powder 25g sachets unflavoured (Vitaflo International Ltd)
30 sachet (ACBS) • NHS indicative price = £323.52

PKU GoLike ® Plus 3-16

▸ Nutritional supplement for the dietary management of phenylketonuria. Suitable for child 3–16 years. Includes added vitamins A, B, C, D, E and K.

GRANULES, protein equivalent 62.2 g, carbohydrate 4.3 g, fat Nil, energy 1187 kJ (280 kcal)/100 g.

PKU GoLike Plus 3-16 oral powder 24g sachets (Nutrinovo Ltd)
30 sachet (ACBS) • NHS indicative price = £289.15

20 g GMP protein equivalent

PKU GMPro ® Ultra

▸ Nutritional supplement for the dietary management of phenylketonuria. Suitable from 3 years; use with caution in child 3–6 years. Includes added vitamins A, B, C, D, E and K.

POWDER, protein 60 g, carbohydrate 14.7 g, fat 2.2 g, energy 1356 kJ (320 kcal)/100 g.

PKU GMPro Ultra oral powder 33.4g sachets lemonade (Nutricia Ltd)
30 sachet (ACBS) • NHS indicative price = £392.40

PKU GMPro Ultra oral powder 33.4g sachets vanilla (Nutricia Ltd)
30 sachet (ACBS) • NHS indicative price = £392.40

PKU sphere ® 20

▸ Nutritional supplement for the dietary management of phenylketonuria. Suitable from 4 years. Includes added vitamins A, B, C, D, E and K.

POWDER, protein 56 g, carbohydrate 18 g, fat 4.7 g, energy 1432 kJ (338 kcal)/100 g.

PKU sphere20 oral powder 35g sachets banana (Vitaflo International Ltd)
30 sachet (ACBS) • NHS indicative price = £512.82

PKU sphere20 oral powder 35g sachets chocolate (Vitaflo International Ltd)
30 sachet (ACBS) • NHS indicative price = £512.82

PKU sphere20 oral powder 35g sachets lemon (Vitaflo International Ltd)
30 sachet (ACBS) • NHS indicative price = £512.82

PKU sphere20 oral powder 35g sachets red berry (Vitaflo International Ltd)
30 sachet (ACBS) • NHS indicative price = £512.82

PKU sphere20 oral powder 35g sachets vanilla (Vitaflo International Ltd)
30 sachet (ACBS) • NHS indicative price = £512.82

PKU sphere ® 20 liquid

▸ Nutritional supplement for the dietary management of phenylketonuria. Suitable from 3 years. Includes added vitamins A, B, C, D, E and K.

LIQUID, protein 8.4 g, carbohydrate 2.8 g, fat 0.5 g, energy 209 kJ (50 kcal)/100 mL.

PKU sphere20 liquid banana (Vitaflo International Ltd)
237 ml (ACBS) • NHS indicative price = £16.16

PKU sphere20 liquid chocolate (Vitaflo International Ltd)
237 ml (ACBS) • NHS indicative price = £16.16

PKU sphere20 liquid vanilla (Vitaflo International Ltd)
237 ml (ACBS) • NHS indicative price = £16.16

20 g protein equivalent

Easiphen ®

▸ Nutritional supplement for the dietary management of phenylketonuria. Suitable from 8 years. Includes added vitamins A, B, C, D, E and K.

LIQUID, protein equivalent 6.7 g, carbohydrate 5.1 g, fat 2 g, energy 275 kJ (65 kcal)/100 mL

Easiphen liquid (Nutricia Ltd)
250 ml (ACBS) • NHS indicative price = £14.66

Glytactin ® Build 20/20

▸ Nutritional supplement for the dietary management of phenylketonuria. Suitable from 3 years. Includes added vitamins A, B, C, D, E and K.

POWDER, protein equivalent 67 g, carbohydrate 2.4 g, fat 4.2 g, energy 1400 kJ (335 kcal)/100 g.

Glytactin Build 20/20 oral powder 32g sachets chocolate (Cambrooke UK Ltd)
30 sachet (ACBS) • NHS indicative price = £469.94

Glytactin Build 20/20 oral powder 30g sachets neutral (Cambrooke UK Ltd)
30 sachet (ACBS) • NHS indicative price = £477.15

Glytactin Build 20/20 oral powder 31g sachets raspberry lemonade (Cambrooke UK Ltd)
30 sachet (ACBS) • NHS indicative price = £469.94

Glytactin Build 20/20 oral powder 31.2g sachets smooth (Cambrooke UK Ltd)
30 sachet (ACBS) • NHS indicative price = £469.94

Glytactin Build 20/20 oral powder 33g sachets vanilla (Cambrooke UK Ltd)
30 sachet (ACBS) • NHS indicative price = £469.94

Mevalia ® PKU Motion 20

▸ Nutritional supplement for the dietary management of phenylketonuria. Suitable from 3 years. Includes added vitamins A, B, C, D, E and K.

LIQUID, protein equivalent 14 g, carbohydrate 5 g, fat Nil, energy 328 kJ (77 kcal)/100 mL.

Mevalia PKU Motion 20 liquid red fruits (Vitaflo International Ltd)
140 ml (ACBS) • NHS indicative price = £11.31

Mevalia PKU Motion 20 liquid tropical (Vitaflo International Ltd)
140 ml (ACBS) • NHS indicative price = £11.31

PKU Air ® 20

▸ Nutritional supplement for the dietary management of phenylketonuria. Suitable from 3 years. Includes added vitamins A, B, C, D, E and K.

LIQUID, protein equivalent 11.5 g, carbohydrate 1.5 g, fat 0.6 g, energy 243 kJ (57 kcal)/100 mL.

PKU Air20 gold liquid (Vitaflo International Ltd)
174 ml (ACBS) • NHS indicative price = £14.48

PKU Air20 green liquid (Vitaflo International Ltd)
174 ml (ACBS) • NHS indicative price = £14.48

PKU Air20 red liquid (Vitaflo International Ltd)
174 ml (ACBS) • NHS indicative price = £14.48

PKU Air20 white liquid (Vitaflo International Ltd)
174 ml (ACBS) • NHS indicative price = £14.48

PKU Air20 yellow liquid (Vitaflo International Ltd)
174 ml (ACBS) • NHS indicative price = £14.48

PKU cooler® 20

▸ Nutritional supplement for the dietary management of phenylketonuria. Suitable from 3 years. Includes added vitamins A, B, C, D, E and K.

LIQUID, protein equivalent 11.5 g, carbohydrate 5.1 g, fat 0.9 g, energy 316 kJ (75 kcal)/100 mL.

PKU orange cooler20 liquid (Vitaflo International Ltd)
174 ml (ACBS) · NHS indicative price = £15.04

PKU purple cooler20 liquid (Vitaflo International Ltd)
174 ml (ACBS) · NHS indicative price = £15.04

PKU red cooler20 liquid (Vitaflo International Ltd)
174 ml (ACBS) · NHS indicative price = £15.04

PKU white cooler20 liquid (Vitaflo International Ltd)
174 ml (ACBS) · NHS indicative price = £15.04

PKU yellow cooler20 liquid (Vitaflo International Ltd)
174 ml (ACBS) · NHS indicative price = £15.04

PKU express® plus20

▸ Nutritional supplement for the dietary management of phenylketonuria. Suitable from 3 years. Includes added vitamins A, B, C, D, E and K.

POWDER, protein equivalent 60 g, carbohydrate 14 g, fat 2.2 g, energy 1339 kJ (316 kcal)/100 g.

PKU express plus20 powder 34g sachets lemon (Vitaflo International Ltd)
30 sachet (ACBS) · NHS indicative price = £431.36

PKU express plus20 powder 34g sachets orange (Vitaflo International Ltd)
30 sachet (ACBS) · NHS indicative price = £431.36

PKU express plus20 powder 34g sachets raspberry (Vitaflo International Ltd)
30 sachet (ACBS) · NHS indicative price = £412.99

PKU express plus20 powder 34g sachets tropical (Vitaflo International Ltd)
30 sachet (ACBS) · NHS indicative price = £431.36

PKU express plus20 powder 34g sachets unflavoured (Vitaflo International Ltd)
30 sachet (ACBS) · NHS indicative price = £431.36

PKU Lophlex®

▸ Nutritional supplement for the dietary management of proven phenylketonuria. Not suitable for use in child under 3 years. Includes added vitamins A, B, C, D, E and K.

POWDER, protein 71.4 g, carbohydrate 13.6 g, fat 1.5 g, energy 1487 kJ (350 kcal)/100 g.

PKU Lophlex powder 28g sachets berries (Nutricia Ltd)
30 sachet (ACBS) · NHS indicative price = £429.30

PKU Lophlex powder 28g sachets neutral (Nutricia Ltd)
30 sachet (ACBS) · NHS indicative price = £429.30

PKU Lophlex powder 28g sachets orange (Nutricia Ltd)
30 sachet (ACBS) · NHS indicative price = £429.30

PKU Lophlex® LQ 20

▸ Nutritional supplement for the dietary management of proven phenylketonuria. Suitable from 4 years. Includes added vitamins A, B, C, D, E and K.

LIQUID, protein 16 g, carbohydrate 7 g, fat Nil, energy 391 kJ (92 kcal)/100 mL.

PKU Lophlex LQ 20 liquid berry (Nutricia Ltd)
125 ml (ACBS) · NHS indicative price = £15.31

PKU Lophlex LQ 20 liquid juicy berries (Nutricia Ltd)
125 ml (ACBS) · NHS indicative price = £15.31

PKU Lophlex LQ 20 liquid juicy citrus (Nutricia Ltd)
125 ml (ACBS) · NHS indicative price = £15.31

PKU Lophlex LQ 20 liquid juicy orange (Nutricia Ltd)
125 ml (ACBS) · NHS indicative price = £15.31

PKU Lophlex LQ 20 liquid juicy tropical (Nutricia Ltd)
125 ml (ACBS) · NHS indicative price = £15.31

PKU Lophlex LQ 20 liquid orange (Nutricia Ltd)
125 ml (ACBS) · NHS indicative price = £15.31

PKU Lophlex® Select 20

▸ Nutritional supplement for the dietary management of phenylketonuria. Suitable from 4 years. Includes added vitamins A, B, C, D, E and K.

LIQUID, protein 16 g, carbohydrate 4.1 g, fat 0.3 g, energy 342 kJ (81.7 kcal)/100 mL.

PKU Lophlex Select 20 liquid (Nutricia Ltd)
125 ml (ACBS) · NHS indicative price = £13.56

PKU Lophlex® Sensation 20

▸ Nutritional supplement for the dietary management of phenylketonuria. Suitable from 4 years. Includes added vitamins A, B, C, D, E and K.

SEMI-SOLID, protein 18.3 g, carbohydrate 18.5 g, fat 0.34 g, energy 648 kJ (152 kcal)/100 g.

PKU Lophlex Sensation 20 berries (Nutricia Ltd)
327 gram (ACBS) · NHS indicative price = £48.93

PKU Maxamum® sachets

▸ Nutritional supplement for the dietary management of phenylketonuria. Suitable from 8 years. Includes added vitamins A, B, C, D, E and K.

POWDER, protein 39 g, carbohydrate 34 g, fat less than 0.5 g, energy 1260 kJ (297 kcal)/100 g.

PKU Maxamum oral powder 50g sachets orange (Nutricia Ltd)
30 sachet (ACBS) · NHS indicative price = £409.50

PKU Maxamum oral powder 50g sachets unflavoured (Nutricia Ltd)
30 sachet (ACBS) · NHS indicative price = £409.50

PKU Synergy®

▸ Nutritional supplement for the dietary management of phenylketonuria and hyperphenylalaninaemia. Suitable from 10 years. Includes added vitamins A, B, C, D, E and K.

POWDER, protein equivalent 60.6 g, carbohydrate 10.7 g, fat 1 g, energy 1238 kJ (296 kcal)/100 g.

PKU Synergy oral powder 33g sachets (Nutricia Ltd)
30 sachet (ACBS) · NHS indicative price = £471.30

XPhe® jump 20

▸ Nutritional supplement for the dietary management of phenylketonuria (PKU) or hyperphenylalaninemia (HPA). Suitable from 3 years. Includes added vitamins A, B, C, D, E and K.

LIQUID, protein equivalent 16 g, carbohydrate 9 g, fat less than 0.1 g, energy 376 kJ (89 kcal)/100 mL.

XPhe jump 20 liquid cola (metaX Institut fuer Diaetetik GmbH)
125 ml (ACBS) · NHS indicative price = £9.85

XPhe jump 20 liquid neutral (metaX Institut fuer Diaetetik GmbH)
125 ml (ACBS) · NHS indicative price = £9.85

XPhe jump 20 liquid orange (metaX Institut fuer Diaetetik GmbH)
125 ml (ACBS) · NHS indicative price = £9.85

XPhe jump 20 liquid tropical (metaX Institut fuer Diaetetik GmbH)
125 ml (ACBS) · NHS indicative price = £9.85

XPhe jump 20 liquid vanilla (metaX Institut fuer Diaetetik GmbH)
125 ml (ACBS) · NHS indicative price = £9.85

XPhe jump 20 liquid wild berries (metaX Institut fuer Diaetetik GmbH)
125 ml (ACBS) · NHS indicative price = £9.85

Powder protein source

PK Aid 4®

▸ Nutritional supplement for the dietary management of phenylketonuria.

POWDER, protein 79 g, carbohydrate 4.5 g, fat Nil, energy 1420 kJ (334 kcal)/100 g.

PK Aid 4 powder (Nutricia Ltd)
500 gram (ACBS) · NHS indicative price = £217.68

PKU Maxamum®

▸ Nutritional supplement for the dietary management of phenylketonuria. Suitable from 8 years. Includes added vitamins A, B, C, D, E and K.

POWDER, protein 39 g, carbohydrate 34 g, fat less than 0.5 g, energy 1260 kJ (297 kcal)/100 g.

PKU Maxamum powder orange (Nutricia Ltd)
500 gram (ACBS) · NHS indicative price = £136.77

PKU Maxamum powder unflavoured (Nutricia Ltd)
500 gram (ACBS) · NHS indicative price = £136.77

Infant formula protein source

PKU Anamix® Infant
▸ Nutritional supplement for the dietary management of proven phenylketonuria. Suitable for child from birth to 3 years. Includes added vitamins A, B, C, D, E and K.
POWDER, protein 13.1 g, carbohydrate 50.1 g, fat 23 g, fibre 3.7 g, energy 1950 kJ (466 kcal)/100 g.

PKU Anamix Infant powder (Nutricia Ltd)
400 gram (ACBS) · NHS indicative price = £50.72

PKU start®
▸ Nutritional supplement for the dietary management of phenylketonuria. Includes added vitamins A, B, C, D, E and K.
POWDER, protein equivalent 14.3 g, carbohydrate 51 g, fat 25 g, energy 2035 kJ (486 kcal)/100 g.

PKU start powder (Vitaflo International Ltd)
400 gram (ACBS) · NHS indicative price = £57.54

Tablet protein source

Phlexy-10® tablets
▸ Nutritional supplement for the dietary management of phenylketonuria. Suitable from 8 years.
SOLID, protein 56.4 g, carbohydrate 4.4 g, fat 2.6 g, energy 1310 kJ (307 kcal)/100 g.

Phlexy-10 tablets (Nutricia Ltd)
75 tablet (ACBS) · NHS indicative price = £42.41

PKU Easy® microtabs
▸ Nutritional supplement for the dietary management of phenylketonuria. Suitable from 8 years.
SOLID, protein equivalent (essential and non-essential amino acids) 70.8 g, carbohydrate 13 g, fat 3.6 g, energy 1678 kJ (396 kcal)/100 g.

PKU Easy microtabs (Galen Ltd)
440 gram (ACBS) · NHS indicative price = £235.12

XPhe® minis
▸ Nutritional supplement for the dietary management of phenylketonuria and hyperphenylalaninemia. Suitable from 7 years. Includes added vitamins A, B, C, D, E and K.
SOLID, protein 62 g, carbohydrate nil, fat 2 g, energy 1175 kJ (278 kcal)/100 g.

XPhe minis tablets (metaX Institut fuer Diaetetik GmbH)
720 tablet (ACBS) · NHS indicative price = £170.35

Pyridoxine-dependent epilepsy

5 g protein equivalent

PDE reach® 5
▸ Nutritional supplement for the dietary management of pyridoxine-dependent epilepsy. Suitable from 1 year. Includes added vitamins A, B, C, D, E and K.
POWDER, protein equivalent 28 g, carbohydrate 58 g, fat 0.4 g, energy 1477 kJ (348 kcal)/100 g.

PDE reach5 oral powder 18g sachets (Vitaflo International Ltd)
30 sachet (ACBS) · NHS indicative price = £178.00

Sucrase-isomaltase deficiency

Carbohydrate supplements

Glucose powder
▸ For use as an energy supplement in sucrose-isomaltase deficiency.
POWDER, contains dextrose monohydrate.

Glucose powder for oral use BP 1980 (Thornton & Ross Ltd)
500 gram (ACBS) · NHS indicative price = £2.41 · Drug Tariff (Part VIIIA Category C) price = £2.41

Tyrosinaemia

5 g protein equivalent

TYR explore® 5
▸ Nutritional supplement for the dietary management of tyrosinaemia. Suitable for child from 6 months to 5 years. Contains added vitamins A, B, C, D, E and K.
POWDER, protein 40 g, carbohydrate 42 g, fat 1.5 g, energy 1450 kJ (342 kcal)/100 g.

TYR explore5 oral powder 12.5g sachets (Vitaflo International Ltd)
30 sachet (ACBS) · NHS indicative price = £185.92

10 g protein equivalent

TYR Anamix® Junior
▸ Nutritional supplement for the dietary management of proven tyrosinaemia. Suitable for child 1–10 years. Includes added vitamins A, B, C, D, E and K.
POWDER, protein 28 g, carbohydrate 32 g, fat 12.5 g, energy 1572 kJ (375 kcal)/100 g.

TYR Anamix Junior oral powder 36g sachets (Nutricia Ltd)
30 sachet (ACBS) · NHS indicative price = £324.30

TYR Anamix® Junior LQ
▸ Nutritional supplement for the dietary management of tyrosinaemia type 1 (when nitisinone (NTBC) is used, see nitisinone p. 762), type II, and type III. Suitable from 1 year. Includes added vitamins A, B, C, D, E and K.
LIQUID, protein 8 g, carbohydrate 7 g, fat 3.8 g, energy 398 kJ (95 kcal)/100 mL.

TYR Anamix Junior LQ liquid (Nutricia Ltd)
125 ml (ACBS) · NHS indicative price = £14.15

TYR cooler® 10
▸ Nutritional supplement for the dietary management of tyrosinaemia. Suitable from 3 years. Includes added vitamins A, B, C, D, E and K.
LIQUID, protein equivalent 11.5 g, carbohydrate 5.1 g, fat 0.9 g, energy 316 kJ (75 kcal)/100 mL.

TYR red cooler10 liquid (Vitaflo International Ltd)
87 ml (ACBS) · NHS indicative price = £11.16

TYR gel®
▸ Nutritional supplement for the dietary management of tyrosinaemia. Suitable for child 1–10 years. Includes added vitamins A, B, C, D, E and K.
POWDER, protein equivalent 41.7 g, carbohydrate 42.9 g, fat 0.05 g, energy 1440 kJ (339 kcal)/100 g.

TYR gel oral powder 24g sachets (Vitaflo International Ltd)
30 sachet (ACBS) · NHS indicative price = £350.22

TYR Lophlex® LQ 10
▸ Nutritional supplement for the dietary management of proven tyrosinaemia. Includes added vitamins A, B, C, D, E and K.
LIQUID, protein 16 g, carbohydrate 7 g, fat 0.35 g, energy 407 kJ (96 kcal)/100 mL.

TYR Lophlex LQ 10 liquid (Nutricia Ltd)
62.5 ml (ACBS) · NHS indicative price = £12.20

15 g protein equivalent

TYR cooler® 15
▸ Nutritional supplement for the dietary management of tyrosinaemia. Suitable from 3 years. Includes added vitamins A, B, C, D, E and K.
LIQUID, protein equivalent 11.5 g, carbohydrate 5.1 g, fat 0.9 g, energy 316 kJ (75 kcal)/100 mL.

TYR orange cooler15 liquid (Vitaflo International Ltd)
130 ml (ACBS) · NHS indicative price = £18.46

TYR red cooler15 liquid (Vitaflo International Ltd)
130 ml (ACBS) · NHS indicative price = £18.46

TYR express® 15
▸ Nutritional supplement for the dietary management of tyrosinaemia. Suitable from 8 years. Includes added vitamins A, B, C, D, E and K.
POWDER, protein equivalent 60 g, carbohydrate 13.7 g, fat 0.2 g, energy 1260 kJ (297 kcal)/100 g.

TYR express15 oral powder 25g sachets (Vitaflo International Ltd)
30 sachet (ACBS) · NHS indicative price = £544.02

20 g GMP protein equivalent

TYR sphere® 20
▸ Nutritional supplement for the dietary management of tyrosinaemia. Suitable from 3 years. Includes added vitamins A, B, C, D, E and K.
POWDER, protein 56 g, carbohydrate 17 g, fat 4.7 g, energy 1415 kJ (335 kcal)/100 g.

TYR sphere20 oral powder 35g sachets red berry (Vitaflo International Ltd)
30 sachet (ACBS) · NHS indicative price = £742.01

TYR sphere20 oral powder 35g sachets vanilla (Vitaflo International Ltd)
30 sachet (ACBS) · NHS indicative price = £742.01

20 g protein equivalent

TYR cooler® 20
▸ Nutritional supplement in the dietary management of tyrosinaemia. Suitable from 3 years. Includes added vitamins A, B, C, D, E and K.
LIQUID, protein equivalent 11.5 g, carbohydrate 5.1 g, fat 0.9 g, energy 316 kJ (75 kcal)/100 mL.

TYR red cooler20 liquid (Vitaflo International Ltd)
174 ml (ACBS) · NHS indicative price = £23.34

TYR express® 20
▸ Nutritional supplement for the dietary management of tyrosinaemia. Suitable from 8 years. Includes added vitamins A, B, C, D, E and K.
POWDER, protein equivalent 60 g, carbohydrate 13.7 g, fat 0.2 g, energy 1260 kJ (297 kcal)/100 g.

TYR express20 oral powder 34g sachets (Vitaflo International Ltd)
30 sachet (ACBS) · NHS indicative price = £702.86

TYR Lophlex®
▸ Nutritional supplement for the dietary management of tyrosinaemia. Suitable from 3 years. Includes added vitamins A, B, C, D, E and K.
POWDER, protein 71.4 g, carbohydrate 13.7 g, fat 1.5 g, energy 1488 kJ (350 kcal)/100 g.

TYR Lophlex powder 28g sachets (Nutricia Ltd)
30 sachet (ACBS) · NHS indicative price = £677.40

TYR Lophlex® LQ 20
▸ Nutritional supplement for the dietary management of proven tyrosinaemia. Includes added vitamins A, B, C, D, E and K.
LIQUID, protein 16 g, carbohydrate 7 g, fat 0.35 g, energy 407 kJ (96 kcal)/100 mL.

TYR Lophlex LQ 20 liquid (Nutricia Ltd)
125 ml (ACBS) · NHS indicative price = £25.17

Powder protein source

XPHEN TYR Tyrosidon®
▸ Nutritional supplement for the dietary management of tyrosinaemia where plasma methionine levels are normal.
POWDER, protein 77 g, carbohydrate 4.5 g, fat Nil, energy 1386 kJ (326 kcal)/100 g.

XPHEN TYR Tyrosidon Free AA Mix powder (Nutricia Ltd)
500 gram (ACBS) · NHS indicative price = £292.32

Infant formula protein source

TYR Anamix® Infant
▸ Nutritional supplement for the dietary management of proven tyrosinaemia when plasma methionine is normal. Suitable for child from birth to 3 years. Includes added vitamins A, B, C, D, E and K.
POWDER, protein 13.1 g, carbohydrate 50.1 g, fat 23 g, energy 1950 kJ (466 kcal)/100 g.

TYR Anamix Infant powder (Nutricia Ltd)
400 gram (ACBS) · NHS indicative price = £59.55

Tablet protein source

TYR Easy®
▸ Nutritional supplement for the dietary management of tyrosinaemia. Suitable from 8 years.
SOLID, protein equivalent 73.0 g, carbohydrate 8.7 g, fat 3.2 g, energy 1703 kJ (402 kcal)/100 g.

TYR Easy tablets (Galen Ltd)
462 tablet (ACBS) · NHS indicative price = £384.57

Urea cycle disorders

5 g protein equivalent

EAA® Supplement
▸ Nutritional supplement for the dietary management of disorders of protein metabolism including urea cycle disorders. Suitable from 3 years. Includes added vitamins A, B, C, D, E and K.
POWDER, protein equivalent 40 g, carbohydrate 26 g, fat 0.1 g, energy 1126 kJ (265 kcal)/100 g.

EAA Supplement oral powder 12.5g sachets (Vitaflo International Ltd)
30 sachet (ACBS) · NHS indicative price = £201.39

UCD amino5®
▸ Nutritional supplement for the dietary management of urea cycle disorders (UCD).
POWDER, protein equivalent 75.4 g, carbohydrate Nil, fat Nil, energy 1282 kJ (302 kcal)/100 g.

UCD amino5 oral powder 6.6g sachets (Vitaflo International Ltd)
30 sachet (ACBS) · NHS indicative price = £166.33

Powder protein source

Dialamine®
▸ Nutritional supplement for oral feeding where essential amino acid supplements are required, for example chronic renal failure, hypoproteinaemia, wound fistula leakage with excessive protein loss, conditions requiring a controlled nitrogen intake and haemodialysis. Suitable from 6 months. Includes added vitamin C.
POWDER, protein 25 g, carbohydrate 65 g, fat Nil, energy 1530 kJ (360 kcal)/100 g.

Dialamine powder (Nutricia Ltd)
400 gram (ACBS) · NHS indicative price = £115.39

Thickeners and pre-thickened drinks

Thickeners: gum based powder

Instant Carobel®
▸ For thickening of liquids or foods in the treatment of vomiting.
POWDER, contains maltodextrin, carob bean gum, calcium carbonate, iron sulfate, zinc sulfate. Contains residual lactose.

Instant Carobel powder (Nutricia Ltd)
135 gram (ACBS) · NHS indicative price = £4.10

Nutilis® Clear
▸ For thickening of liquids or foods in dysphagia. Not suitable for use in child under 3 years.
POWDER, contains guar gum, maltodextrin, xanthan gum. Gluten-free, lactose-free.

Nutilis Clear powder (Nutricia Ltd)
175 gram (ACBS) · NHS indicative price = £11.00

Nutilis Clear powder 1.25g sachets (Nutricia Ltd)
50 sachet (ACBS) · NHS indicative price = £14.50

Osmosip® Clear and Thick Instant Thickener
▸ For thickening of liquids or foods in dysphagia. Not suitable for use in child under 3 years.
POWDER, contains maltodextrin (corn, potato), potassium chloride, xanthan gum. Gluten-free.

Osmosip Clear & Thick Instant Thickener powder (Spectral Pharmaceuticals Ltd)
133 gram (ACBS) · NHS indicative price = £3.95

Resource ® ThickenUp ® Clear

▶ For thickening of liquids or foods in dysphagia. Not suitable for use in child under 3 years.
POWDER contains maltodextrin (corn, potato), potassium chloride, residual lactose (tin only), xanthan gum. Gluten-free.

Resource ThickenUp Clear powder (Nestle Health Science)
215 gram (ACBS) · NHS indicative price = £15.27

Resource ThickenUp Clear powder 1.2g sachets (Nestle Health Science)
24 sachet (ACBS) · NHS indicative price = £5.28

Swalloweze ® Clear Instant Food & Fluid Thickener

▶ For thickening of liquids or foods in dysphagia. Not suitable for use in child under 3 years.
POWDER, contains erythritol (E968), maltodextrin, xanthan gum (E415). Gluten-free, lactose-free.

Swalloweze Clear Instant Food & Fluid Thickener powder (Nualtra Ltd)
165 gram (ACBS) · NHS indicative price = £5.50

Swalloweze Clear Instant Food & Fluid Thickener powder 1.6g sachets (Nualtra Ltd)
48 sachet (ACBS) · NHS indicative price = £9.60

Thick and Easy ® Clear

▶ For thickening of liquids or foods in dysphagia. Not suitable for use in child under 3 years.
POWDER, contains maltodextrin, xanthan gum, carrageenan, erythritol. Gluten-free, lactose-free.

Thick & Easy Clear powder (Fresenius Kabi Ltd)
126 gram (ACBS) · NHS indicative price = £6.69

Thickeners: starch based powder

Thick and Easy ® Original

▶ For thickening of liquids or foods in dysphagia. Not suitable for use in child under 3 years.
POWDER, contains maltodextrin, modified maize starch (E1442). Gluten-free, lactose-free.

Thick & Easy Original powder (Fresenius Kabi Ltd)
225 gram (ACBS) · NHS indicative price = £6.27 | 4540 gram (ACBS) · NHS indicative price = £131.73

Thixo-D ® Original

▶ For thickening of liquids or foods in dysphagia. Not recommended for child under 1 year.
POWDER, contains modified maize starch. Gluten-free, lactose-free.

Thixo-D Original powder (Ecogreen Technologies Ltd)
375 gram (ACBS) · NHS indicative price = £9.05

Vitamin and mineral supplements

Cystic fibrosis

DEKAs ® Essential capsules

▶ Vitamin supplement in cystic fibrosis on the specific recommendation of a cystic fibrosis specialist. Suitable from 4 years.
CAPSULES, containing vitamins A, D, E and K.

DEKAs Essential capsules (Alveolus Biomedical B.V.)
60 capsule (ACBS) · NHS indicative price = £41.92

DEKAs ® Plus chewable tablets

▶ Vitamin and mineral supplement in cystic fibrosis on the specific recommendation of a cystic fibrosis specialist. Suitable from 4 years.
CHEWABLE TABLETS, containing vitamins A, B, C, D, E and K, minerals, and trace elements.

DEKAs Plus chewable tablets (Alveolus Biomedical B.V.)
60 tablet (ACBS) · NHS indicative price = £48.87

DEKAs ® Plus liquid

▶ Vitamin and mineral supplement in cystic fibrosis on the specific recommendation of a cystic fibrosis specialist. Suitable for child 0 to 10 years.
LIQUID, containing vitamins A, B, C, D, E and K, minerals, and trace elements.

DEKAs Plus liquid (Alveolus Biomedical B.V.)
60 ml (ACBS) · NHS indicative price = £38.16

DEKAs ® Plus softgels capsules

▶ Vitamin and mineral supplement in cystic fibrosis on the specific recommendation of a cystic fibrosis specialist. Suitable from 10 years.
CAPSULES, containing vitamins A, B, C, D, E and K, minerals, and trace elements.

DEKAs Plus softgels capsules (Alveolus Biomedical B.V.)
60 capsule (ACBS) · NHS indicative price = £48.87

Paravit ®-CF capsules

▶ Vitamin supplement in cystic fibrosis on the specific recommendation of a cystic fibrosis specialist. Suitable from 3 years.
CAPSULES, containing vitamins A, D, E and K.

Paravit-CF capsules (Nordic Pharma Ltd)
60 capsule (ACBS) · NHS indicative price = £44.95

Paravit ®-CF liquid

▶ Vitamin supplement in cystic fibrosis on the specific recommendation of a cystic fibrosis specialist.
LIQUID, containing vitamins A, D, E and K.

Paravit-CF liquid (Nordic Pharma Ltd)
7 ml (ACBS) · NHS indicative price = £35.60

Paravit ®-Mod capsules

▶ Vitamin supplement in cystic fibrosis on the specific recommendation of a cystic fibrosis specialist. Suitable from 3 years.
CAPSULES, containing vitamins A, D, E and K.

Paravit-Mod capsules (Nordic Pharma Ltd)
60 capsule (ACBS) · NHS indicative price = £43.75

Paravit ®-Mod liquid

▶ Vitamin supplement in cystic fibrosis on the specific recommendation of a cystic fibrosis specialist.
LIQUID, containing vitamins A, D, E and K.

Paravit-Mod liquid (Nordic Pharma Ltd)
7 ml (ACBS) · NHS indicative price = £34.67

Restrictive therapeutic diet

Energivit ®

▶ Additional energy, vitamins, minerals, and trace elements for infants following a protein-restricted diet. Suitable from birth.
POWDER, containing vitamins A, B, C, D, E and K, minerals, and trace elements.
Powder also provides: protein Nil, carbohydrate 66.9 g, fat 25 g, energy 2059 kJ (492 kcal)/100 g. Standard dilution (15% w/v) of powder provides: protein Nil, carbohydrate 10 g, fat 3.8 g, energy 309 kJ (74 kcal)/100 mL.

Energivit powder (Nutricia Ltd)
400 gram (ACBS) · NHS indicative price = £34.52

FruitiVits ®

▶ Vitamin and mineral supplement in restrictive therapeutic diets. Suitable for child 3 to 10 years.
POWDER, containing vitamins A, B, C, D, E and K, minerals, and trace elements.
Powder also provides: protein Nil, carbohydrate 8.3 g, fat Nil, energy 168 kJ (40 kcal)/100 g. Powder 6 g reconstituted with 60 mL water provides: protein Nil, carbohydrate 0.5 g, fat Nil, energy 10 kJ (2.4 kcal)

FruitiVits oral powder 6g sachets (Vitaflo International Ltd)
30 sachet (ACBS) · NHS indicative price = £105.86

Paediatric Seravit ®

▶ Vitamin and mineral supplement in restrictive therapeutic diets. Suitable for infants and children (pineapple flavour not suitable for children under 3 years because of sweeteners).
POWDER, containing vitamins A, B, C, D, E and K, minerals, and trace elements.
Powder also provides: protein Nil, carbohydrate 75 g, fat Nil, energy 1246 kJ (293 kcal)/100 g. Powder 15 g reconstituted with

75 mL water provides: protein Nil, carbohydrate 11.3 g, fat Nil, energy 187 kJ (44 kcal)

Seravit Paediatric powder pineapple (Nutricia Ltd)
200 gram (ACBS) · NHS indicative price = £29.98

Seravit Paediatric powder unflavoured (Nutricia Ltd)
200 gram (ACBS) · NHS indicative price = £28.11

Phlexy-Vits ® powder

▸ Vitamin and mineral supplement in phenylketonuria and similar amino acid abnormalities. Suitable from 11 years.
POWDER, containing vitamins A, B, C, D, E and K, minerals, and trace elements.
Powder also provides: protein 0.3 g, carbohydrate 0.5 g, fat Nil, energy 63 kJ (15 kcal)/100 g. Powder 7 g sachet provides: protein 0.02 g, carbohydrate 0.04 g, fat Nil, energy 4 kJ (1 kcal)

Phlexy-Vits powder 7g sachets (Nutricia Ltd)
30 sachet (ACBS) · NHS indicative price = £107.70

Phlexy-Vits ® tablets

▸ Vitamin and mineral supplement in phenylketonuria and similar amino acid abnormalities. Suitable from 11 years.
TABLETS, containing vitamins A, B, C, D, E and K, minerals, and trace elements.

Phlexy-Vits tablets (Nutricia Ltd)
180 tablet (ACBS) · NHS indicative price = £124.24

Appendix 3
Cautionary and advisory labels for dispensed medicines

Guidance for cautionary and advisory labels

Medicinal forms within BNF Publications include code numbers of the cautionary labels that pharmacists are recommended to add when dispensing. It is also expected that pharmacists will counsel patients and carers when necessary.

Counselling needs to be related to the age, experience, background, and understanding of the individual patient or carer. The pharmacist should ensure understanding of how to take or use the medicine and how to follow the correct dosage schedule. Any effects of the medicine on co-ordination, performance of skilled tasks (e.g. driving or work), any foods or medicines to be avoided, and what to do if a dose is missed should also be explained. Other matters, such as the possibility of staining of the clothes or skin, or discolouration of urine or stools by a medicine should also be mentioned.

For some medicines there is a special need for counselling, such as an unusual method or time of administration or a potential interaction with a common food or domestic remedy, and this should be mentioned where necessary.

Original packs

Most preparations are dispensed in unbroken original packs that include further advice for the patient in the form of patient information leaflets. The advice in patient information leaflets may be less appropriate when the medicine is for a child, particularly for unlicensed medicines or indications. Pharmacists should explain discrepancies to carers, if necessary. The patient information leaflet should only be withheld in exceptional circumstances because it contains other information that should be provided. Label 10 may be of value where appropriate. More general leaflets advising on the administration of preparations such as eye drops, eye ointments, inhalers, and suppositories are also available.

Scope of labels

In general no label recommendations have been made for injections on the assumption that they will be administered by a healthcare professional or a well-instructed patient. The labelling is not exhaustive and pharmacists are recommended to use their professional discretion in labelling new preparations and those for which no labels are shown.

Individual labelling advice is not given on the administration of the large variety of antacids. In the absence of instructions from the prescriber, and if on enquiry the patient has had no verbal instructions, the directions given under 'Dose' should be used on the label.

It is recognised that there may be occasions when pharmacists will use their knowledge and professional discretion and decide to omit one or more of the recommended labels for a particular patient. In this case counselling is of the utmost importance. There may also be an occasion when a prescriber does not wish additional cautionary labels to be used, in which case the prescription should be endorsed 'NCL' (no cautionary labels). The exact wording that is required instead should then be specified on the prescription.

Pharmacists label medicines with various wordings in addition to those directions specified on the prescription. Such labels include 'Shake the bottle', 'For external use only', and 'Store in a cool place', as well as 'Discard.... days after opening' and 'Do not use after....', which apply particularly to antibiotic mixtures, diluted liquid and topical preparations, and to eye-drops. Although not listed in BNFC these labels should continue to be used when appropriate; indeed, 'For external use only' is a legal requirement on external liquid preparations, while 'Keep out of the reach of children' is a legal requirement on all dispensed medicines. Care should be taken not to obscure other relevant information with adhesive labelling.

It is the usual practice for patients to take standard tablets with water or other liquid and for this reason no separate label has been recommended.

The label wordings recommended by BNFC apply to medicines dispensed against a prescription. Children and carers should be aware that a dispensed medicine should never be taken by, or shared with, anyone other than for whom the prescriber intended it. Therefore, BNFC does not include warnings against the use of a dispensed medicine by persons other than for whom it was specifically prescribed.

The label or labels for each preparation are recommended after careful consideration of the information available. However, it is recognised that in some cases this information may be either incomplete or open to a different interpretation. BNFC will therefore be grateful to receive any constructive comments on the labelling suggested for any preparation.

Recommended label wordings

For BNFC 2011–2012, a revised set of cautionary and advisory labels were introduced. All of the existing labels were user-tested, and the revised wording selected reflects terminology that is better understood by patients.

Wordings which can be given as separate warnings are labels 1–19, 29–30, and 32. Wordings which can be incorporated in an appropriate position in the directions for dosage or administration are labels 21–28. A label has been omitted for number 20; labels 31 and 33 no longer apply to any medicines in BNFC and have therefore been deleted.

If separate labels are used it is recommended that the wordings be used without modification.

Welsh labels

Comprehensive Welsh translations are available for each cautionary and advisory label.

Labels

1 Warning: This medicine may make you sleepy

Rhybudd: Gall y feddyginiaeth hon eich gwneud yn gysglyd

To be used on *preparations for children* containing antihistamines, or other preparations given to children where the warnings of label 2 on driving or alcohol would not be appropriate.

2 Warning: This medicine may make you sleepy. If this happens, do not drive or use tools or machines. Do not drink alcohol

Rhybudd: Gall y feddyginiaeth hon eich gwneud yn gysglyd. Peidiwch â gyrru, defnyddio offer llaw neu beiriannau os yw hyn yn digwydd. Peidiwch ag yfed alcohol

To be used on *preparations for adults that can cause drowsiness*, thereby affecting coordination and the ability to drive and operate hazardous machinery; label 1 is more appropriate for children. *It is an offence to drive while under the influence of drink or drugs.*

Some of these preparations only cause drowsiness in the first few days of treatment and some only cause drowsiness in higher doses.

In such cases the patient should be told that the advice applies until the effects have worn off. However many of these preparations can produce a slowing of reaction time and a loss of mental concentration that can have the same effects as drowsiness.

Patients who are parents or carers of babies aged up to 12 months should be counselled on the risks of co-sleeping (sleeping with a baby on a bed, sofa, chair, etc.); for further information on safer sleeping and co-sleeping, see the Lullaby Trust at: https://www.lullabytrust.org.uk/baby-safety/safer-sleep-information/co-sleeping/.

Avoidance of alcoholic drink is recommended because the effects of CNS depressants are enhanced by alcohol. Strict prohibition however could lead to some patients not taking the medicine. Pharmacists should therefore explain the risk and encourage compliance, particularly in patients who may think they already tolerate the effects of alcohol (see also label 3). Queries from patients with epilepsy regarding fitness to drive should be referred back to the patient's doctor.

Side-effects unrelated to drowsiness that may affect a patient's ability to drive or operate machinery safely include *blurred vision, dizziness, or nausea*. In general, no label has been recommended to cover these cases, but the patient should be suitably counselled.

3 Warning: This medicine may make you sleepy. If this happens, do not drive or use tools or machines

Rhybudd: Gall y feddyginiaeth hon eich gwneud yn gysglyd. Peidiwch â gyrru, defnyddio offer llaw neu beiriannau os yw hyn yn digwydd

To be used on *preparations containing monoamine-oxidase inhibitors*; the warning to avoid alcohol and dealcoholised (low alcohol) drink is covered by the patient information leaflet.

Also to be used as an *alternative to label 2* when alcohol is not an issue.

See label 2 notes (above) for further information on warnings relevant to the use of this label.

4 Warning: Do not drink alcohol

Rhybudd: Peidiwch ag yfed alcohol

To be used on *preparations where a reaction such as flushing may occur if alcohol is taken* (e.g. metronidazole). Alcohol may also enhance the hypoglycaemia produced by some oral antidiabetic drugs but routine application of a warning label is not considered necessary.

Patients should be advised not to drink alcohol for as long as they are receiving/using a course of medication, and in some cases for a period of time after the course is finished.

5 Do not take indigestion remedies 2 hours before or after you take this medicine

Peidiwch â chymryd meddyginiaethau camdreuliad 2 awr cyn neu ar ôl y feddyginiaeth hon

To be used with label 25 on *preparations coated to resist gastric acid* (e.g. enteric-coated tablets). This is to avoid the possibility of premature dissolution of the coating in the presence of an alkaline pH.

Label 5 also applies to drugs such as gabapentin *where the absorption is significantly affected by antacids*. Pharmacists will be aware (from a knowledge of physiology) that the usual time during which indigestion remedies should be avoided is at least 2 hours before and after the majority of medicines have been taken; when a manufacturer advises a different time period, this can be followed, and should be explained to the patient.

6 Do not take indigestion remedies, or medicines containing iron or zinc, 2 hours before or after you take this medicine

Peidiwch â chymryd meddyginiaethau camdreuliad neu feddyginiaethau sy'n cynnwys haearn neu sinc, 2 awr cyn neu ar ôl y feddyginiaeth hon

To be used on *preparations containing ofloxacin and some other quinolones, doxycycline, lymecycline, minocycline, and penicillamine*. These drugs chelate calcium, iron, and zinc and are less well absorbed when taken with calcium-containing antacids or preparations containing iron or zinc. Pharmacists will be aware (from a knowledge of physiology) that these incompatible preparations should be taken at least 2 hours apart for the majority of medicines; when a manufacturer advises a different time period, this can be followed, and should be explained to the patient.

7 Do not take milk, indigestion remedies, or medicines containing iron or zinc, 2 hours before or after you take this medicine

Peidiwch â chymryd llaeth, meddyginiaethau camdreuliad, neu feddyginiaeth sy'n cynnwys haearn neu sinc, 2 awr cyn neu ar ôl cymryd y feddyginiaeth hon

To be used on *preparations containing ciprofloxacin, norfloxacin, or tetracyclines that chelate calcium, iron, magnesium, and zinc,* and are thus less available for absorption. Pharmacists will be aware (from a knowledge of physiology) that these incompatible preparations should be taken at least 2 hours apart for the majority of medicines; when a manufacturer advises a different time period, this can be followed, and should be explained to the patient. Doxycycline, lymecycline, and minocycline are less liable to form chelates and therefore only require label 6 (see above).

8 Warning: Do not stop taking this medicine unless your doctor tells you to stop

Rhybudd: Peidiwch â stopio cymryd y feddyginiaeth hon, oni bai fod eich meddyg yn dweud wrthych am stopio

To be used on *preparations that contain a drug which is required to be taken over long periods without the patient necessarily perceiving any benefit* (e.g. antituberculous drugs).

Also to be used on *preparations that contain a drug whose withdrawal is likely to be a particular hazard* (e.g. clonidine for hypertension). Label 10 (see below) is more appropriate for corticosteroids.

9 Space the doses evenly throughout the day. Keep taking this medicine until the course is finished, unless you are told to stop

Gadewch yr un faint o amser rhwng pob dôs yn ystod y dydd. Parhewch i gymryd y feddyginiaeth nes bod y cyfan wedi'i orffen, oni bai eich bod yn cael cyngor i stopio

To be used on *preparations where a course of treatment should be completed* to reduce the incidence of relapse or failure of treatment.

The preparations are antimicrobial drugs given by mouth. Very occasionally, some may have severe side-effects (e.g. diarrhoea in patients receiving clindamycin) and in such cases the patient may need to be advised of reasons for stopping treatment quickly and returning to the doctor.

The pharmacist should omit the first sentence of the label for antimicrobial drugs that are given once daily, and the patient should be suitably counselled.

10 Warning: Read the additional information given with this medicine

Rhybudd: Darllenwch y wybodaeth ychwanegol gyda'r feddyginiaeth hon

To be used particularly on *preparations containing anticoagulants, lithium, and oral corticosteroids*. The appropriate treatment card should be given to the patient and any necessary explanations given.

This label may also be used on other preparations to remind the patient of the instructions that have been given.

11 Protect your skin from sunlight—even on a bright but cloudy day. Do not use sunbeds

Diogelwch eich croen rhag golau'r haul, hyd yn oed ar ddiwrnod braf ond cymylog. Peidiwch â defnyddio gwely haul

To be used on *preparations that may cause phototoxic or photoallergic reactions* if the patient is exposed to ultraviolet radiation. Exposure to high intensity ultraviolet radiation from sunray lamps and sunbeds is particularly likely to cause reactions.

12 Do not take anything containing aspirin while taking this medicine

Peidiwch â chymryd unrhyw beth sy'n cynnwys aspirin gyda'r feddyginiaeth hon

To be used on *preparations containing sulfinpyrazone* whose activity is reduced by aspirin.

Label 12 should not be used for anticoagulants since label 10 is more appropriate.

13 Dissolve or mix with water before taking

Gadewch i doddi mewn dŵr cyn ei gymryd

To be used on *preparations that are intended to be dissolved in water* (e.g. soluble tablets) or *mixed with water* (e.g. powders, granules) before use. In a few cases other liquids such as fruit juice or milk may be used.

14 This medicine may colour your urine. This is harmless

Gall y feddyginiaeth hon liwio eich dŵr. Nid yw hyn yn arwydd o ddrwg

To be used on *preparations that may cause the patient's urine to turn an unusual colour*. These include triamterene (blue under some lights), levodopa (dark reddish), and rifampicin (red).

15 Caution: flammable. Keep your body away from fire or flames after you have put on the medicine

Rhybudd: Fflamadwy. Ar ôl rhoi'r feddyginiaeth ymlaen, cadwch yn glir o dân neu fflamau

To be used on *preparations containing sufficient flammable solvent to render them flammable if exposed to a naked flame*.

16 Dissolve the tablet under your tongue—do not swallow. Store the tablets in this bottle with the cap tightly closed. Get a new supply 8 weeks after opening

Rhowch y dabled i doddi dan eich tafod - peidiwch â'i lyncu. Cadwch y tabledi yn y botel yma gyda'r caead wedi'i gau yn dynn. Gofynnwch am dabledi newydd 8 wythnos ar ôl ei hagor

To be used on *glyceryl trinitrate tablets* to remind the patient not to transfer the tablets to plastic or less suitable containers.

17 Do not take more than... in 24 hours

Peidiwch â chymryd mwy na... mewn 24 awr

To be used on *preparations for the treatment of acute migraine* except those containing ergotamine, for which label 18 is used. The dose form should be specified, e.g. tablets or capsules.

It may also be used on preparations for which no dose has been specified by the prescriber.

18 Do not take more than... in 24 hours. Also, do not take more than... in any one week

Peidiwch â chymryd mwy na... mewn 24 awr. Hefyd, peidiwch â chymryd mwy na... mewn wythnos

To be used on preparations containing ergotamine. The dose form should be specified, e.g. tablets or suppositories.

19 Warning: This medicine makes you sleepy. If you still feel sleepy the next day, do not drive or use tools or machines. Do not drink alcohol

Rhybudd: Bydd y feddyginiaeth hon yn eich gwneud yn gysglyd. Os ydych yn dal i deimlo'n gysglyd drannoeth, peidiwch â gyrru, defnyddio offer llaw neu beiriannau. Peidiwch ag yfed alcohol

To be used on *preparations containing hypnotics (or some other drugs with sedative effects) prescribed to be taken at night*. On the rare occasions when hypnotics are prescribed for daytime administration (e.g. nitrazepam in epilepsy), this label would clearly not be appropriate. Also to be used as an *alternative to the label 2 wording* (the choice being at the discretion of the pharmacist) *for anxiolytics prescribed to be taken at night*.

It is hoped that this wording will convey adequately the problem of residual morning sedation after taking 'sleeping tablets'.

See label 2 notes (above) for further information on warnings relevant to the use of this label.

21 Take with or just after food, or a meal

Cymerwch gyda neu ar ôl bwyd

To be used on *preparations that are liable to cause gastric irritation, or those that are better absorbed with food*.

Patients should be advised that a *small amount of food is sufficient*.

22 Take 30 to 60 minutes before food

Cymerwch 30 i 60 munud cyn bwyd

To be used on some preparations *whose absorption is thereby improved*.

Most oral antibacterials require label 23 instead (see below).

23 Take this medicine when your stomach is empty. This means an hour before food or 2 hours after food

Cymerwch y feddyginiaeth hon ar stumog wag. Mae hyn yn golygu awr cyn, neu 2 awr ar ôl bwyd

To be used on *oral antibacterials whose absorption may be reduced by the presence of food and acid in the stomach*.

Patients should be advised that food must be avoided for 2 hours before **and** an hour after taking each dose.

24 Suck or chew this medicine

Bydd angen cnoi neu sugno'r feddyginiaeth hon

To be used on *preparations that should be sucked or chewed*.

The pharmacist should use discretion as to which of these words is appropriate.

25 Swallow this medicine whole. Do not chew or crush

Llyncwch yn gyfan. Peidiwch â chnoi neu falu'n fân

To be used on *preparations that are enteric-coated or designed for modified-release*.

Also to be used on *preparations that taste very unpleasant or may damage the mouth* if not swallowed whole.

Patients should be advised (where relevant) that some modified-release preparations can be broken in half, but that the halved tablet should still be swallowed whole, and not chewed or crushed.

26 Dissolve this medicine under your tongue

Gadewch i'r feddyginiaeth hon doddi o dan y tafod

To be used on *preparations designed for sublingual use*. Patients should be advised to hold under the tongue and avoid swallowing until dissolved. The buccal mucosa between the gum and cheek is occasionally specified by the prescriber.

27 Take with a full glass of water

Cymerwch gyda llond gwydr o ddŵr

To be used on *preparations that should be well diluted* (e.g. chloral hydrate), *where a high fluid intake is required* (e.g. sulfonamides), or *where water is required to aid the action* (e.g. methylcellulose). The patient should be advised that 'a full glass' means at least 150 mL. In most cases fruit juice, tea, or coffee may be used.

28 Spread thinly on the affected skin only

Taenwch yn denau ar y croen sydd wedi'i effeithio yn unig

To be used on *external preparations* that should be applied sparingly (e.g. corticosteroids, dithranol).

29 Do not take more than 2 at any one time. Do not take more than 8 in 24 hours

Peidiwch â chymryd mwy na 2 ar unrhyw un adeg. Peidiwch â chymryd mwy nag 8 mewn 24 awr

To be used on containers of dispensed *solid dose preparations containing paracetamol for adults when the instruction on the label indicates that the dose can be taken on an 'as required' basis*. The dose form should be specified, e.g. tablets or capsules.

This label has been introduced because of the serious consequences of overdosage with paracetamol.

30 Contains paracetamol. Do not take anything else containing paracetamol while taking this medicine. Talk to a doctor at once if you take too much of this medicine, even if you feel well

Yn cynnwys paracetamol. Peidiwch â chymryd unrhyw beth arall sy'n cynnwys paracetamol tra'n cymryd y feddyginiaeth hon. Siaradwch gyda'ch meddyg ar unwaith os ydych yn cymryd gormod, hyd yn oed os ydych yn teimlo'n iawn

To be used on all containers of dispensed *preparations containing paracetamol*.

32 Contains aspirin. Do not take anything else containing aspirin while taking this medicine

Yn cynnwys aspirin. Peidiwch â chymryd unrhyw beth arall sy'n cynnwys aspirin tra'n cymryd y feddyginiaeth hon

To be used on containers of dispensed *preparations containing aspirin when the name on the label does not include the word 'aspirin'*.

Dental Practitioners' Formulary

List of Dental Preparations

The following list has been approved by the appropriate Secretaries of State, and the preparations therein may be prescribed by dental practitioners on form FP10D (GP14 in Scotland, WP10D in Wales).

Licensed **sugar-free** versions, where available, are preferred.

Licensed **alcohol-free** mouthwashes, where available, are preferred.

Aciclovir Cream, BP
Aciclovir Oral Suspension, BP, 200 mg/5 mL
Aciclovir Tablets, BP, 200 mg
Aciclovir Tablets, BP, 800 mg
Amoxicillin Capsules, BP
Amoxicillin Oral Powder, DPF
Amoxicillin Oral Suspension, BP
Artificial Saliva Gel, DPF
Artificial Saliva Oral Spray, DPF
Artificial Saliva Pastilles, DPF
Artificial Saliva Protective Spray, DPF
Artificial Saliva Substitutes as listed below (to be prescribed only for indications approved by ACBS (patients suffering from dry mouth as a result of having or, having undergone, radiotherapy or sicca syndrome):
BioXtra® Gel Mouthspray
Glandosane®
Saliveze®
Artificial Saliva Substitute Spray, DPF
Aspirin Tablets, Dispersible, BP
Azithromycin Capsules, 250 mg, DPF
Azithromycin Oral Suspension, 200 mg/5 mL, DPF
Azithromycin Tablets, 250 mg, DPF
Azithromycin Tablets, 500 mg, DPF
Beclometasone Pressurised Inhalation, BP, 50 micrograms/metered inhalation, CFC-free, as:
Clenil Modulite®
Benzydamine Mouthwash, BP 0.15%
Benzydamine Oromucosal Spray, BP 0.15%
Betamethasone Soluble Tablets, 500 micrograms, DPF
Carbamazepine Tablets, BP
Cefalexin Capsules, BP
Cefalexin Oral Suspension, BP
Cefalexin Tablets, BP
Cefradine Capsules, BP
Cetirizine Oral Solution, BP, 5 mg/5 mL
Cetirizine Tablets, BP, 10 mg
Chlorhexidine Gluconate Gel, BP
Chlorhexidine Mouthwash, BP
Chlorhexidine Oral Spray, DPF
Chlorphenamine Oral Solution, BP
Chlorphenamine Tablets, BP
Choline Salicylate Dental Gel, BP
Clarithromycin Oral Suspension, 125 mg/5 mL, DPF
Clarithromycin Oral Suspension, 250 mg/5 mL, DPF
Clarithromycin Tablets, BP
Clindamycin Capsules, BP
Co-amoxiclav Tablets, BP, 250/125 (amoxicillin 250 mg as trihydrate, clavulanic acid 125 mg as potassium salt)
Co-amoxiclav Oral Suspension, BP, 125/31 (amoxicillin 125 mg as trihydrate, clavulanic acid 31.25 mg as potassium salt)/5 mL
Co-amoxiclav Oral Suspension, BP, 250/62 (amoxicillin 250 mg as trihydrate, clavulanic acid 62.5 mg as potassium salt)/5 mL
Diazepam Oral Solution, BP, 2 mg/5 mL
Diazepam Tablets, BP
Diclofenac Sodium Tablets, Gastro-resistant, BP
Dihydrocodeine Tablets, BP, 30 mg
Doxycycline Tablets, Dispersible, BP
Doxycycline Capsules, BP, 100 mg
Doxycycline Tablets, 20 mg, DPF
Ephedrine Nasal Drops, BP
Erythromycin Ethyl Succinate Oral Suspension, BP
Erythromycin Ethyl Succinate Tablets, BP
Erythromycin Stearate Tablets, BP
Erythromycin Tablets, Gastro-resistant, BP
Fluconazole Capsules, 50 mg, DPF
Fluconazole Oral Suspension, 50 mg/5 mL, DPF
Hydrocortisone Cream, BP, 1%
Hydrocortisone Oromucosal Tablets, BP
Hydrogen Peroxide Mouthwash, BP, 6%
Ibuprofen Oral Suspension, BP, sugar-free
Ibuprofen Tablets, BP
Lansoprazole Capsules, Gastro-resistant, BP
Lidocaine Ointment, BP, 5%
Lidocaine Spray 10%, DPF
Loratadine Syrup, 5 mg/5 mL, DPF
Loratadine Tablets, BP, 10 mg
Menthol and Eucalyptus Inhalation, BP 1980
Metronidazole Oral Suspension, BP
Metronidazole Tablets, BP
Miconazole Cream, BP
Miconazole Oromucosal Gel, BP
Miconazole and Hydrocortisone Cream, BP
Miconazole and Hydrocortisone Ointment, BP
Nystatin Oral Suspension, BP
Omeprazole Capsules, Gastro-resistant, BP
Oxytetracycline Tablets, BP
Paracetamol Oral Suspension, BP
Paracetamol Tablets, BP
Paracetamol Tablets, Soluble, BP
Phenoxymethylpenicillin Oral Solution, BP
Phenoxymethylpenicillin Tablets, BP
Promethazine Hydrochloride Tablets, BP
Promethazine Oral Solution, BP
Saliva Stimulating Tablets, DPF
Sodium Chloride Mouthwash, Compound, BP
Sodium Fluoride Mouthwash, BP
Sodium Fluoride Oral Drops, BP
Sodium Fluoride Tablets, BP
Sodium Fluoride Toothpaste 0.619%, DPF
Sodium Fluoride Toothpaste 1.1%, DPF
Sodium Fusidate Ointment, BP
Temazepam Oral Solution, BP
Temazepam Tablets, BP
Tetracycline Tablets, BP

Preparations in this list which are not included in the BP or BPC are described under Details of DPF preparations.

For details of preparations that can be prescribed, see individual entries under the relevant drug monographs throughout the BNF publications.

Details of DPF preparations

Preparations on the List of Dental Preparations which are specified as DPF are described as follows in the DPF. Although brand names have sometimes been included for identification purposes preparations on the list should be prescribed by non-proprietary name.

Amoxicillin Oral Powder
amoxicillin (as trihydrate) 3 g sachet

Artificial Saliva Gel
(proprietary products: *BioXtra Dry Mouth Oral Gel*; *Oralieve Moisturising Mouth Gel*) consists of lactoperoxidase, lactoferrin, glucose oxidase, xylitol, and other ingredients, in a gel basis

Artificial Saliva Oral Spray
(proprietary products: *Xerotin*) consists of water, sorbitol, carmellose (carboxymethylcellulose), potassium chloride, sodium chloride, potassium phosphate, magnesium chloride, calcium chloride and other ingredients, pH neutral

Artificial Saliva Pastilles
(proprietary product: *Salivix*), consists of acacia, malic acid, and other ingredients

Artificial Saliva Protective Spray
(proprietary product: *Aequasyal*) consists of oxidised glycerol triesters, silicon dioxide, flavouring agents, aspartame

Artificial Saliva Substitute Spray
(proprietary product: *AS Saliva Orthana Spray*) consists of mucin, methylparaben, benzalkonium chloride, EDTA, xylitol, peppermint oil, spearmint oil, mineral salts

Azithromycin Capsules
azithromycin 250 mg

Azithromycin Oral Suspension 200 mg/5 mL
azithromycin 200 mg/5 mL when reconstituted with water

Azithromycin Tablets
azithromycin 250 mg and 500 mg

Betamethasone Soluble Tablets 500 micrograms
betamethasone (as sodium phosphate) 500 micrograms

Chlorhexidine Oral Spray
(proprietary product: *Corsodyl Oral Spray*), chlorhexidine gluconate 0.2%

Clarithromycin Oral Suspension 125 mg/5 mL
clarithromycin 125 mg/5 mL when reconstituted with water

Clarithromycin Oral Suspension 250 mg/5 mL
clarithromycin 250 mg/5 mL when reconstituted with water

Doxycycline Tablets 20 mg
(proprietary product: *Periostat*), doxycycline (as hyclate) 20 mg

Fluconazole Capsules 50 mg
fluconazole 50 mg

Fluconazole Oral Suspension 50 mg/5 mL
(proprietary product: *Diflucan*), fluconazole 50 mg/5 mL when reconstituted with water

Lidocaine Spray 10%
(proprietary product: *Xylocaine Spray*), lidocaine 10% supplying 10 mg lidocaine/spray

Loratadine Syrup 5 mg/5 mL
loratadine 5 mg/5 mL

Saliva Stimulating Tablets
(proprietary product: *SST*), citric acid, malic acid and other ingredients in a sorbitol base

Sodium Fluoride Toothpaste 0.619%
(proprietary product: *Duraphat '2800 ppm' Toothpaste*), sodium fluoride 0.619%

Sodium Fluoride Toothpaste 1.1%
(proprietary product: *Duraphat '5000 ppm' Toothpaste*), sodium fluoride 1.1%

Approved list for prescribing by Community Practitioner Nurse Prescribers (NPF)

Nurse Prescribers' Formulary for Community Practitioners

List of preparations approved by the Secretary of State which may be prescribed on form FP10P (form HS21(N) in Northern Ireland, form GP10(N) in Scotland, forms WP10CN and WP10PN in Wales) by Nurses for National Health Service patients.

Community practitioners who have completed the necessary training may only prescribe items appearing in the nurse prescribers' list set out below. Community Practitioner Nurse Prescribers are recommended to prescribe generically, except where this would not be clinically appropriate or where there is no approved generic name.

This list is for reference only; see BNF for full prescribing information.

Medicinal Preparations

Preparations on this list which are not included in the BP or BPC are described under Details of NPF preparations.

- Almond Oil Ear Drops, BP
- Arachis Oil Enema, NPF
- Aspirin Tablets, Dispersible, 300 mg, BP (max. 96 tablets; max. pack size 32 tablets)
- Bisacodyl Suppositories, BP (includes 5-mg and 10-mg strengths)
- Bisacodyl Tablets, BP
- Catheter Maintenance Solution, Sodium Chloride, NPF
- Catheter Maintenance Solution, 'Solution G', NPF
- Catheter Maintenance Solution, 'Solution R', NPF
- Chlorhexidine Gluconate Alcoholic Solutions containing at least 0.05%
- Chlorhexidine Gluconate Aqueous Solutions containing at least 0.05%
- Choline Salicylate Dental Gel, BP
- Clotrimazole Cream 1%, BP
- Co-danthramer Capsules, NPF
- Co-danthramer Capsules, Strong, NPF
- Co-danthramer Oral Suspension, NPF
- Co-danthramer Oral Suspension, Strong, NPF
- Co-danthrusate Capsules, BP
- Co-danthrusate Oral Suspension, NPF
- Crotamiton Cream, BP
- Crotamiton Lotion, BP
- Dimeticone barrier creams containing at least 10%
- Dimeticone Lotion, NPF
- Docusate Capsules, BP
- Docusate Enema, NPF
- Docusate Oral Solution, BP
- Docusate Oral Solution, Paediatric, BP
- Econazole Cream 1%, BP
- Emollients as listed below:
  - Aquadrate® 10% w/w Cream
  - Arachis Oil, BP
  - Balneum® Plus Cream
  - Cetraben® Emollient Cream
  - Dermamist®
  - Diprobase® Cream
  - Diprobase® Ointment
  - Doublebase®
  - Doublebase® Dayleve Gel
  - E45® Cream
  - E45® Itch Relief Cream
  - Emulsifying Ointment, BP
  - Eucerin® Intensive 10% w/w Urea Treatment Cream
  - Eucerin® Intensive 10% w/w Urea Treatment Lotion
  - Hydromol® Cream
  - Hydromol® Intensive
  - Hydrous Ointment, BP
  - Lipobase®
  - Liquid and White Soft Paraffin Ointment, NPF
  - Neutrogena® Norwegian Formula Dermatological Cream
  - Nutraplus® Cream
  - Oilatum® Cream
  - Oilatum® Junior Cream
  - Paraffin, White Soft, BP
  - Paraffin, Yellow Soft, BP
  - Ultrabase®
  - Unguentum M®
- Emollient bath and shower preparations as listed below:
  - Aqueous Cream, BP
  - Balneum® (except pack sizes that are not to be prescribed under the NHS (see Part XVIIIA of the Drug Tariff, Part XI of the Northern Ireland Drug Tariff))
  - Balneum Plus® Bath Oil (except pack sizes that are not to be prescribed under the NHS (see Part XVIIIA of the Drug Tariff, Part XI of the Northern Ireland Drug Tariff))
  - Cetraben® Emollient Bath Additive
  - Dermalo® Bath Emollient
  - Doublebase® Emollient Bath Additive
  - Doublebase® Emollient Shower Gel
  - Doublebase® Emollient Wash Gel
  - Hydromol® Bath and Shower Emollient
  - Oilatum® Emollient
  - Oilatum® Gel
  - Oilatum® Junior Bath Additive
  - Zerolatum® Emollient Medicinal Bath Oil
- Folic Acid Tablets 400 micrograms, BP
- Glycerol Suppositories, BP
- Ibuprofen Oral Suspension, BP (except for indications and doses that are prescription-only)
- Ibuprofen Tablets, BP (except for indications and doses that are prescription-only)
- Ispaghula Husk Granules, BP
- Ispaghula Husk Granules, Effervescent, BP
- Ispaghula Husk Oral Powder, BP
- Lactulose Solution, BP
- Lidocaine Ointment, BP
- Lidocaine and Chlorhexidine Gel, BP
- Macrogol Oral Liquid, Compound, NPF
- Macrogol Oral Powder, Compound, NPF
- Macrogol Oral Powder, Compound, Half-strength, NPF
- Magnesium Hydroxide Mixture, BP
- Magnesium Sulfate Paste, BP
- Malathion aqueous lotions containing at least 0.5%
- Mebendazole Oral Suspension, NPF
- Mebendazole Tablets, NPF
- Methylcellulose Tablets, BP [discontinued]
- Miconazole Cream 2%, BP
- Miconazole Oromucosal Gel, BP

- Mouthwash Solution-tablets, NPF
- Nicotine Inhalation Cartridge for Oromucosal Use, NPF
- Nicotine Lozenge, NPF
- Nicotine Medicated Chewing Gum, NPF
- Nicotine Nasal Spray, NPF
- Nicotine Oral Spray, NPF
- Nicotine Sublingual Tablets, NPF
- Nicotine Transdermal Patches, NPF
- Nystatin Oral Suspension, BP
- Olive Oil Ear Drops, BP
- Paracetamol Oral Suspension, BP (includes 120 mg/5 mL and 250 mg/5 mL strengths—both of which are available as sugar-free formulations)
- Paracetamol Tablets, BP (max. 96 tablets; max. pack size 32 tablets)
- Paracetamol Tablets, Soluble, BP (max. 96 tablets; max. pack size 32 tablets)
- Permethrin Cream, NPF
- Phosphates Enema, BP
- Povidone–Iodine Solution, BP
- Senna Oral Solution, NPF
- Senna Tablets, BP
- Senna and Ispaghula Granules, NPF
- Sodium Chloride Solution, Sterile, BP
- Sodium Citrate Compound Enema, NPF
- Sodium Picosulfate Capsules, NPF
- Sodium Picosulfate Elixir, NPF
- Spermicidal contraceptives as listed below:
  - Gygel® Contraceptive Jelly
- Sterculia Granules, NPF
- Sterculia and Frangula Granules, NPF
- Titanium Ointment, BP
- Water for Injections, BP
- Zinc and Castor Oil Ointment, BP
- Zinc Oxide and Dimeticone Spray, NPF
- Zinc Oxide Impregnated Medicated Bandage, NPF
- Zinc Oxide Impregnated Medicated Stocking, NPF
- Zinc Paste Bandage, BP 1993
- Zinc Paste and Ichthammol Bandage, BP 1993

Appliances and Reagents (including Wound Management Products)

Community Practitioner Nurse Prescribers in England, Wales and Northern Ireland can prescribe any appliance or reagent in the relevant Drug Tariff. In the Scottish Drug Tariff, Appliances and Reagents which may **not** be prescribed by Nurses are annotated **Nx**.

Appliances (including Contraceptive Devices) as listed in Part IXA of the Drug Tariff (Part III of the Northern Ireland Drug Tariff, Part 3 (Appliances) and Part 2 (Dressings) of the Scottish Drug Tariff). (Where it is not appropriate for nurse prescribers in family planning clinics to prescribe contraceptive devices using form FP10(P) (forms WP10CN and WP10PN in Wales), they may prescribe using the same system as doctors in the clinic.)

Incontinence Appliances as listed in Part IXB of the Drug Tariff (Part III of the Northern Ireland Drug Tariff, Part 5 of the Scottish Drug Tariff).

Stoma Appliances and Associated Products as listed in Part IXC of the Drug Tariff (Part III of the Northern Ireland Drug Tariff, Part 6 of the Scottish Drug Tariff).

Chemical Reagents as listed in Part IXR of the Drug Tariff (Part II of the Northern Ireland Drug Tariff, Part 9 of the Scottish Drug Tariff).

The Drug Tariffs can be accessed online at:

National Health Service Drug Tariff for England and Wales: www.nhsbsa.nhs.uk/pharmacies-gp-practices-and-appliance-contractors/drug-tariff

Health and Personal Social Services for Northern Ireland Drug Tariff: bso.hscni.net/directorates/operations/family-practitioner-services/pharmacy/contractor-information/drug-tariff-and-related-materials/drug-tariff-2/

Scottish Drug Tariff: publichealthscotland.scot/resources-and-tools/medical-practice-and-pharmaceuticals/scottish-drug-tariff/

Details of NPF preparations

Preparations on the Nurse Prescribers' Formulary which are not included in the BP or BPC are described as follows in the Nurse Prescribers' Formulary. Although brand names have sometimes been included for identification purposes, it is recommended that non-proprietary names should be used for prescribing medicinal preparations in the NPF except where a non-proprietary name is not available.

- **Arachis oil enema**
  - arachis oil 100%
- **Catheter maintenance solution, sodium chloride**
  - (proprietary products: *OptiFlo S; Uro-Tainer Sodium Chloride; Uriflex-S*), sodium chloride 0.9%
- **Catheter maintenance solution, 'Solution G'**
  - (proprietary products: *OptiFlo G; Uro-Tainer Suby G; Uriflex G*), citric acid 3.23%, magnesium oxide 0.38%, sodium bicarbonate 0.7%, disodium edetate 0.01%
- **Catheter maintenance solution, 'Solution R'**
  - (proprietary products: *OptiFlo R; Uro-Tainer Solutio R; Uriflex R*), citric acid 6%, gluconolactone 0.6%, magnesium carbonate 2.8%, disodium edetate 0.01%
- **Chlorhexidine gluconate alcoholic solutions**
  - (proprietary products: *ChloraPrep; Hydrex Solution; Hydrex spray*), chlorhexidine gluconate in alcoholic solution
- **Chlorhexidine gluconate aqueous solutions**
  - (proprietary product: *Unisept*), chlorhexidine gluconate in aqueous solution
- **Co-danthramer capsules** PoM
  - co-danthramer 25/200 (dantron 25 mg, poloxamer '188' 200 mg)
- **Co-danthramer capsules, strong** PoM
  - co-danthramer 37.5/500 (dantron 37.5 mg, poloxamer '188' 500 mg)
- **Co-danthramer oral suspension** PoM
  - co-danthramer 25/200 in 5 mL (dantron 25 mg, poloxamer '188' 200 mg/5 mL)
- **Co-danthramer oral suspension, strong** PoM
  - co-danthramer 75/1000 in 5 mL (dantron 75 mg, poloxamer '188' 1 g/5 mL)
- **Co-danthrusate oral suspension** PoM
  - (proprietary product: *Normax*), co-danthrusate 50/60 (dantron 50 mg, docusate sodium 60 mg/5 mL)
- **Dimeticone barrier creams**
  - (proprietary products *Conotrane Cream*, dimeticone '350' 22%; *Siopel Barrier Cream*, dimeticone '1000' 10%), dimeticone 10–22%
- **Dimeticone lotion**
  - (proprietary product: *Hedrin*), dimeticone 4%
- **Docusate enema**
  - (proprietary product: *Norgalax Micro-enema*), docusate sodium 120 mg in 10 g
- **Liquid and white soft paraffin ointment**
  - liquid paraffin 50%, white soft paraffin 50%
- **Macrogol oral liquid, compound**
  - (proprietary product: *Movicol Liquid*), macrogol '3350' (polyethylene glycol '3350') 13.125 g, sodium bicarbonate 178.5 mg, sodium chloride 350.7 mg, potassium chloride 46.6 mg/25 mL
- **Macrogol oral powder, compound**
  - (proprietary products: *Laxido Orange, Molaxole, Movicol*), macrogol '3350' (polyethylene glycol '3350') 13.125 g, sodium bicarbonate 178.5 mg, sodium chloride 350.7 mg, potassium chloride 46.6 mg/sachet; (amount of potassium chloride varies according to flavour of *Movicol*® as follows: plain-flavour (sugar-free) = 50.2 mg/sachet; lime and lemon flavour = 46.6 mg/sachet; chocolate flavour = 31.7 mg/sachet. 1 sachet when reconstituted with 125 mL water provides K^+ 5.4 mmol/litre)

- **Macrogol oral powder, compound, half-strength**
  - (proprietary product: *Movicol-Half*), macrogol '3350' (polyethylene glycol '3350') 6.563 g, sodium bicarbonate 89.3 g, sodium chloride 175.4 mg, potassium chloride 23.3 mg/sachet
- **Malathion aqueous lotions**
  - (proprietary products: *Derbac-M Liquid*), malathion 0.5% in an aqueous basis
- **Mebendazole oral suspension** PoM
  - (proprietary product: *Vermox*), mebendazole 100 mg/5 mL
- **Mebendazole tablets** PoM
  - (proprietary products: *Ovex, Vermox*), mebendazole 100 mg (can be supplied for oral use in the treatment of enterobiasis in adults and children over 2 years provided its container or package is labelled to show a max. single dose of 100 mg and it is supplied in a container or package containing not more than 800 mg)
- **Mouthwash solution-tablets**
  - consist of tablets which may contain antimicrobial, colouring and flavouring agents in a suitable soluble effervescent basis to make a mouthwash
- **Nicotine inhalation cartridge for oromucosal use**
  - (proprietary products: *NicAssist Inhalator, Nicorette Inhalator*), nicotine 15 mg (for use with inhalation mouthpiece; to be prescribed as either a starter pack (6 cartridges with inhalator device and holder) or refill pack (42 cartridges with inhalator device)
- **Nicotine lozenge**
  - nicotine (as bitartrate) 1 mg or 2 mg (proprietary product: *Nicorette Mint Lozenge, Nicotinell Mint Lozenge*), or nicotine (as resinate) 1.5 mg, 2 mg, or 4 mg (proprietary product: *NiQuitin Lozenges, NiQuitin Minis, NiQuitin Pre-quit*)
- **Nicotine medicated chewing gum**
  - (proprietary products: *NicAssist Gum, Nicorette Gum, Nicotinell Gum, NiQuitin Gum*), nicotine 2 mg or 4 mg
- **Nicotine nasal spray**
  - (proprietary product: *NicAssist Nasal Spray, Nicorette Nasal Spray*), nicotine 500 micrograms/metered spray
- **Nicotine oral spray**
  - (proprietary product: *Nicorette Quickmist*), nicotine 1 mg/metered spray
- **Nicotine sublingual tablets**
  - (proprietary product: *NicAssist Microtab, Nicorette Microtab*), nicotine (as a cyclodextrin complex) 2 mg (to be prescribed as either a starter pack (2 × 15-tablet discs with dispenser) or refill pack (7 × 15-tablet discs))
- **Nicotine transdermal patches**
  - releasing in each 16 hours, nicotine approx. 5 mg, 10 mg, or 15 mg (proprietary products: *Boots NicAssist Patch, Nicorette Patch*), or releasing in each 16 hours approx. 10 mg, 15 mg, or 25 mg (proprietary products: *NicAssist Translucent Patch, Nicorette Invisi Patch*), or releasing in each 24 hours nicotine approx. 7 mg, 14 mg, or 21 mg (proprietary products: *Nicopatch, Nicotinell TTS, NiQuitin, NiQuitin Clear*) (prescriber should specify the brand to be dispensed)
- **Permethrin cream**
  - (proprietary product: *Lyclear Dermal Cream*), permethrin 5%
- **Senna oral solution**
  - (proprietary product: *Senokot Syrup*), sennosides 7.5 mg/5 mL
- **Senna and ispaghula granules**
  - (proprietary product: *Manevac Granules*), senna fruit 12.4%, ispaghula 54.2%
- **Sodium citrate compound enema**
  - (proprietary products: *Micolette Micro-enema; Micralax Micro-enema; Relaxit Micro-enema*), sodium citrate 450 mg with glycerol, sorbitol and an anionic surfactant
- **Sodium picosulfate capsules**
  - (proprietary products: *Dulcolax Perles*), sodium picosulfate 2.5 mg
- **Sodium picosulfate elixir**
  - (proprietary product: *Dulcolax Liquid*), sodium picosulfate 5 mg/5 mL
- **Sterculia granules**
  - (proprietary product: *Normacol Granules*), sterculia 62%
- **Sterculia and frangula granules**
  - (proprietary product: *Normacol Plus Granules*), sterculia 62%, frangula (standardised) 8%
- **Zinc oxide and dimeticone spray**
  - (proprietary product: *Sprilon*), dimeticone 1.04%, zinc oxide 12.5% in a pressurised aerosol unit
- **Zinc oxide impregnated medicated bandage**
  - (proprietary product: *Steripaste*), sterile cotton bandage impregnated with paste containing zinc oxide 15%
- **Zinc oxide impregnated medicated stocking**
  - (proprietary product: *Zipzoc*), sterile rayon stocking impregnated with ointment containing zinc oxide 20%

Non-medical prescribing

Overview

A range of non-medical healthcare professionals can prescribe medicines for patients as either Independent or Supplementary Prescribers.

Independent prescribers are practitioners responsible and accountable for the assessment of patients with previously undiagnosed or diagnosed conditions and for decisions about the clinical management required, including prescribing. They are recommended to prescribe generically, except where this would not be clinically appropriate or where there is no approved non-proprietary name.

Supplementary prescribing is a partnership between an independent prescriber (a doctor or a dentist) and a supplementary prescriber to implement an agreed Clinical Management Plan for an individual patient with that patient's agreement.

Independent and Supplementary Prescribers are identified by an annotation next to their name in the relevant professional register.

Information and guidance on non-medical prescribing is available on the Department of Health website at www.dh.gov.uk/health/2012/04/prescribing-change.

For information on the mixing of medicines by Independent and Supplementary Prescribers, see *Mixing of medicines prior to administration in clinical practice: medical and non-medical prescribing*, National Prescribing Centre, May 2010 (available at www.gov.uk/government/publications/mixing-of-medicines-prior-to-administration-in-clinical-practice-medical-and-non-medical-prescribing).

For information on the supply and administration of medicines to groups of patients using Patient Group Directions see Guidance on prescribing p. 1.

In order to protect patient safety, the initial prescribing and supply of medicines prescribed should normally remain separate functions performed by separate healthcare professionals.

Nurses

Nurse Independent Prescribers (formerly known as Extended Formulary Nurse Prescribers) are able to prescribe any medicine for any medical condition. Unlicensed medicines are excluded from the Nurse Prescribing Formulary in Scotland.

Nurse Independent Prescribers are able to prescribe, administer, and give directions for the administration of Schedule 2, 3, 4, and 5 Controlled Drugs. This extends to diamorphine hydrochloride p. 332, dipipanone, or cocaine for treating organic disease or injury, but not for treating addiction.

Nurse Independent Prescribers must work within their own level of professional competence and expertise.

The Approved list for prescribing by Community Practitioner Nurse Prescribers (NPF) p. 1439 for Community Practitioners provides information on prescribing.

Pharmacists

Pharmacist Independent Prescribers can prescribe any medicine for any medical condition. This includes unlicensed medicines, subject to accepted clinical good practice.

They are also able to prescribe, administer, and give directions for the administration of Schedule 2, 3, 4, and 5 Controlled Drugs. This extends to diamorphine hydrochloride p. 332, dipipanone, or cocaine for treating organic disease or injury, but not for treating addiction.

Pharmacist Independent Prescribers must work within their own level of professional competence and expertise.

Physiotherapists

Physiotherapist Independent Prescribers can prescribe any medicine for any medical condition. This includes "off-label" medicines subject to accepted clinical good practice. They are also allowed to prescribe the following Controlled Drugs: oral or injectable morphine p. 338, transdermal fentanyl p. 334 and oral diazepam p. 270, dihydrocodeine tartrate p. 333, lorazepam p. 272, oxycodone hydrochloride p. 340 or temazepam p. 1024.

Physiotherapist Independent Prescribers must work within their own level of professional competence and expertise.

Therapeutic radiographers

Therapeutic Radiographer Independent Prescribers can prescribe any medicine for any medical condition. This includes "off-label" medicines subject to accepted clinical good practice. Prescribing of Controlled Drugs is subject to legislative changes. Therapeutic Radiographer Independent Prescribers must work within their own level of professional competence and expertise.

Optometrists

Optometrist Independent Prescribers can prescribe any licensed medicine for ocular conditions affecting the eye and the tissues surrounding the eye, except Controlled Drugs or medicines for parenteral administration. Optometrist Independent Prescribers must work within their own level of professional competence and expertise.

Podiatrists

Podiatrist Independent Prescribers can prescribe any medicine for any medical condition. This includes "off-label" medicines subject to accepted clinical good practice. They are also allowed to prescribe the following Controlled Drugs for oral administration: diazepam p. 270, dihydrocodeine tartrate p. 333, lorazepam p. 272 and temazepam p. 1024.

Podiatrist Independent Prescribers must work within their own level of professional competence and expertise.

Paramedics

Paramedic Independent Prescribers can prescribe any medicine for any medical condition. This includes "off-label" medicines subject to accepted clinical good practice. Prescribing of Controlled Drugs is subject to legislative changes. Paramedic Independent Prescribers must work within their own level of professional competence and expertise.

Further Information

For further details about the different types of prescribers, see *Medicines, Ethics and Practice*, London, Pharmaceutical Press (always consult latest edition).

Index of manufacturers

The following is an alphabetical list of manufacturers and other companies referenced in BNF Publications, with their medicines information or general contact details. For information on 'special-order' manufacturers and specialist importing companies see Special-order manufacturers p. 1448.

3M Health Care Ltd, Tel: 01509 611611

AAH Pharmaceuticals Ltd, Tel: 03445 612 266

A. Menarini Farmaceutica Internazionale SRL, Tel: 0800 0858678, menarini@medinformation.co.uk

A1 Pharmaceuticals, Tel: 01708 528900, enquiries@a1plc.co.uk

Abbott Healthcare Products Ltd, Tel: 0800 1701177, ukabbottnutrition@abbott.com

AbbVie Ltd, Tel: 01628 561092, ukmedinfo@abbvie.com

Accord Healthcare Ltd, Tel: 01271 385257, medinfo@accord-healthcare.com

Advanced Medical Solutions Ltd, Tel: 01606 863500

Advancis Medical, Tel: 01623 751500

Advanz Pharma, Tel: 08700 703033, medicalinformation@advanzpharma.com

AFT Pharma UK Ltd, Tel: 0203 6707602, customer.service@aftpharm.com

AgaMatrix Europe Ltd, Tel: 0800 0931812, info@agamatrix.co.uk

Agepha Pharma s.r.o., Tel: +42 1692054363, office@agepha.com

Aguettant Ltd, Tel: 01275 463691, info@aguettant.co.uk

AJ Vaccines, Tel: +45 7229 7000, ajvaccines@ajvaccines.com

Alan Pharmaceuticals, Tel: 020 72842887, info@alanpharmaceuticals.com

Alcon Eye Care Ltd, Tel: 0345 2669363, gb.medicaldepartment@alcon.com

Alexion Pharma UK Ltd, Tel: 0800 028 4394, medinfo.EMEA@alexion.com

Alimera Sciences Ltd, Tel: 0800 0191253, medicalinformation@alimerasciences.com

Alissa Healthcare Research Ltd, Tel: 01489 564069, enquiries@alissahealthcare.com

ALK-Abello Ltd, Tel: 0118 9037940, info@uk.alk-abello.com

Allergan Ltd, Tel: 01628 494026, UK_MedInfo@Allergan.com

Allergy Therapeutics (UK) Ltd, Tel: 01903 844702, infoservices@allergytherapeutics.com

Alliance Pharmaceuticals Ltd, Tel: 01249 466966, medinfo@alliancepharma.co.uk

Almirall Ltd, Tel: 0800 0087399, Almirall@EU.ProPharmaGroup.com

Almus Pharmaceuticals Ltd, Tel: 0800 9177983, med.info@almus.co.uk

Alnylam UK Ltd, Tel: 0800 1412569, medinfo@alnylam.com

Altacor Ltd, Tel: 01182 210150, info@altacor-pharma.com

Alturix Ltd, Tel: 0845 5191609, medinfo@alturix.com

Alveolus Biomedical B.V., Tel: 07879 427173, info@alveolus.nl

Ambe Ltd, Tel: 01732 760900, info@ambemedical.com

Amgen Ltd, Tel: 01223 436441, gbinfoline@amgen.com

Amicus Therapeutics UK Ltd, Tel: 0808 2346864, PhV.Migalastat_SO@Quintiles.com

AMO UK Ltd, Tel: 01344 864042, crc@its.jnj.com

Amring Pharmaceuticals Ltd, Tel: +33 1 58 28 16 80, infomed.france@amringpharma.com

Amryt Pharma, Tel: 01604 549952, medinfo@amrytpharma.com

AOP Orphan Pharmaceuticals AG, Tel: 0121 2624119, office.uk@aoporphan.com

Aristo Pharma Ltd, Tel: 01353 887100, contactus@aristo-pharma.co.uk

Arjun Products Ltd, Tel: 0800 0157806, info@arjunproducts.co.uk

Ascot Laboratories Ltd, Tel: 01923 711971, specials@ascotpharma.com

Aspar Pharmaceuticals Ltd, Tel: 020 82059846, info@aspar.co.uk

Aspen Pharma Trading Ltd, Tel: 0800 0087392, aspenmedinfo@professionalinformation.co.uk

Aspire Pharma Ltd, Tel: 01730 231148, medinfo@aspirepharma.co.uk

Astellas Pharma Ltd, Tel: 0800 7835018, medinfo.gb@astellas.com

AstraZeneca UK Ltd, Tel: 0800 7830033, medical.informationuk@astrazeneca.com

Atnahs Pharma UK Ltd, Tel: 01279 406759, atnahspv@diamondpharmaservices.com

Axunio Pharma GmbH, Tel: + 49 40 38 02 32 14, medinfo@axunio.eu

AYMES International Ltd, Tel: 0845 6805496, info@aymes.com

B. Braun Medical Ltd, Tel: 0800 298 0299, medinfo.bbmuk@bbraun.com

B. Braun Melsungen AG, Tel: +49 5661 710, info@bbraun.com

Bard Ltd, Tel: 01293 527888, customer.services@crbard.com

Bausch & Lomb UK Ltd, Tel: 0800 041 8721, UKMedInformation@bausch.com

Baxter Healthcare Ltd, Tel: 01635 206345, medinfo_uki@baxter.com

Bayer Plc, Tel: 0118 206 3116, medical.information@bayer.co.uk

BBI Healthcare Ltd, Tel: 01656 868930, info@bbihealthcare.com

Becton, Dickinson UK Ltd, Tel: 0800 0437 546, SafetyInformation@bd.com

Beiersdorf UK Ltd, Tel: 0121 329 8800

Bell, Sons & Co (Druggists) Ltd, Tel: 0151 4221200, Med-info@bells-healthcare.com

Besins Healthcare (UK) Ltd, Tel: 01748 828 789, besins@eu.propharmagroup.com

BHR Pharmaceuticals Ltd, Tel: 02476 377210

BIAL Pharma UK Ltd, Tel: 01753 916010, medinfo.uk@bial.com

Bio Med Sciences, Tel: +1 610 5303193, info@silon.com

Bio Products Laboratory Ltd, Tel: 020 89572255, medinfo@bpl.co.uk

BioCare Ltd, Tel: 01214 338702, clinicalnutrition@biocare.co.uk

Bio-Diagnostics Ltd, Tel: 01684 592262, enquiries@bio-diagnostics.co.uk

Biogen Idec Ltd, Tel: 0800 0087401, MedInfoUKI@biogen.com

Biolitec Pharma Ltd, Tel: +49 3641 5195330, medinfo@biolitecpharma.com

BioMarin Europe Ltd, Tel: 0845 0177013, medinfoeu@bmrn.com

Bioprojet UK Ltd, Tel: 01722 742900, medicalinformation@bioprojet.uk

Bio-Tech Pharmacal Inc, Tel: +1 800 3451199, customerservice@bio-tech-pharm.com

Biotest (UK) Ltd, Tel: 0845 241 3090, medinfo.uk@grifols.com

Blackrock Pharmaceuticals Ltd, Tel: 0115 9890841, safety.uk@lambda-cro.com

Blueprint Medicines (UK) Ltd, Tel: +31 85 064 4001, medinfoeurope@blueprintmedicines.com

BOC Ltd, Tel: 0800 136603, healthcare.home-uk@boc.com

Boehringer Ingelheim Ltd, Tel: 01344 742579, medinfo@bra.boehringer-ingelheim.com

Bowmed Ibisqus Ltd, Tel: 01483 212151, medinfo@bowmed.com

Brancaster Pharma Ltd, Tel: 01737 243407, safety@brancasterpharma.com

Bray Group Ltd, Tel: 01367 240736, info@bray-healthcare.com

Bristol Laboratories Ltd, Tel: 01442 200922, info@bristol-labs.co.uk

Bristol-Myers Squibb Pharmaceuticals Ltd, Tel: 0800 7311736, medical.information@bms.com

Britannia Pharmaceuticals Ltd, Tel: 0808 196 8585, medinfo@britannia-pharm.com

Brown & Burk UK Ltd, Tel: 0203 384 7188, bbukqa@bbukltd.com

BSN Medical Ltd, Tel: 01482 670100, orders.uk@bsnmedical.com

C D Medical Ltd, Tel: 01942 813933

Cambridge Healthcare Supplies Ltd, Tel: 0330 1359434, medinfo@cambridge-healthcare.co.uk

Cambridge Sensors Ltd, Tel: 0800 0883920, info@microdotcs.com

Cambrooke Therapeutics, Tel: 0161 9627377, Tel: 07950 716133, ukinfo@cambrooke.com

Camurus AB, medicalinfo@camurus.com

CD Pharma Srl, Tel: +39 02 43980539, info@cdpharmagroup.one

Celltrion Healthcare UK Ltd, Tel: 01753 983500, UKMedical@celltrionhc.com

Chemidex Pharma Ltd, Tel: 01784 477167, info@chemidex.co.uk

Chiesi Ltd, Tel: 01748 827 271, medinfo.uk@chiesi.com

Chugai Pharma UK Ltd, Tel: 020 89875600, medinfo@chugai-pharm.co.uk

Church & Dwight UK Ltd, Tel: 0800 0281454, AESIP@sipdrugsafety.com

Cipla EU Ltd, Tel: 0800 0472144, Drugsafety@cipla.com

Clement Clarke International Ltd, Tel: 01279 414969, resp@clement-clarke.com

Clinigen Healthcare Ltd, Tel: 01932 824 026, medicalinformation@clinigengroup.com

CliniMed Ltd, Tel: 0808 1596017, info@clinimed.co.uk

Clinisupplies Ltd, Tel: 020 88634168, info@clinisupplies.co.uk

Clovis Oncology UK Ltd, Tel: 0330 1004723, medinfo.GB@clovisoncology.com

CNX Therapeutics Ltd, Tel: 0207 821 2840, medinfo@cnx-therapeutics.com

Colgate-Palmolive (UK) Ltd, Tel: 00800 32132132

Colonis Pharma Ltd, Tel: 01892 739403, medinfo@colonis.co.uk

Coloplast Ltd, Tel: 0800 374654, hcp@coloplastcharter.co.uk

Combe International Ltd, care@combe.co.uk

Consilient Health Ltd, Tel: 020 37511888, drugsafety@consilienthealth.com

ConvaTec Ltd, Tel: 0800 289738, wound.webcare@convatec.com

Correvio UK Ltd, Tel: +41 848 007870, medinfo@correvio.com

Covidien (UK) Commercial Ltd, Tel: 0203 0271757, email.csUK@covidien.com

Cox Pharmaceuticals Ltd, Tel: 01614 655237, cox.pharmaceutical@redlinepv.co.uk

Crawford Healthcare Ltd, Tel: 01565 654920, customercomments@acelity.com

Crescent Pharma Ltd, Tel: 01256 772730, info@crescentpharma.com

CSL Behring UK Ltd, Tel: 01444 447405, medinfo@cslbehring.com

CST Pharma Ltd, enquiry@cstpharma.co.uk

Cubic Pharmaceuticals Ltd, Tel: 01634 726628, orders@cubicpharmacy.co.uk

Curaprox (UK) Ltd, Tel: 01480 862084, contact@curaprox.co.uk

Cytoplan Ltd, nutrition@cytoplan.co.uk

Daiichi Sankyo UK Ltd, Tel: 0800 0285122, medinfo@daiichi-sankyo.co.uk

Dawa Ltd, Tel: 020 8423 3800, info@drugsrus.co.uk

Dendron Ltd, Tel: 01923 204492, customerdesk@dddltd.co.uk

Dentsply Ltd, Tel: 01932 838338, UKD-CustomerServices@dentsplysirona.com

Derma UK Ltd, Tel: 0191 3759020, info@dermauk.co.uk

Dermacea Ltd, Tel: 01562 884898, info@skinniesuk.com

Dermal Laboratories Ltd, Tel: 01462 458866, info@dermal.co.uk

Dermatonics Ltd, Tel: 01480 462910, sales@dermatonics.co.uk

Desitin Pharma Ltd, Tel: 01908 488817, medinfo@desitin.co.uk

Dexcel-Pharma Ltd, Tel: 01748 828784, Dexcel@EU.ProPharmaGroup.com

DHP Healthcare Ltd, Tel: 0330 1359 454, dhphealthcare@redlinepv.co.uk

Dr. Falk Pharma UK Ltd, Tel: 07765 004275, office@drfalkpharma.co.uk

Dr Reddy's Laboratories (UK) Ltd, Tel: 01748 828873, drreddysGB@EU.ProPharmaGroup.com

Dr Schär Ltd (UK), Tel: 0800 1615838, foodservice.it@drschaer.com

Dreamskin Health Ltd, Tel: 01707 260505

Drossa Ltd, Tel: 020 3393 0859

Dunelm Pharmaceuticals Ltd, Tel: 0800 0614116

Durbin Plc, Tel: 020 88696500, products@durbin.co.uk

E Sallis Ltd, Tel: 0115 9787841, info@sallis.co.uk

Easigrip Ltd, Tel: 01926 497108, info@easigrip.co.uk

Ecogreen Technologies Ltd, brian@ecogreentechnologies.co.uk

Ecolab Healthcare Division, Tel: 0113 2322480, info.healthcare@ecolab.co.uk

Eisai Ltd, Tel: 0845 6761400, EUMedInfo@eisai.net

Eli Lilly and Company Ltd, Tel: 01256 315000, ukmedinfo@lilly.com

Emergent BioSolutions UK, Tel: 0800 088 5449, MedicalInformation@ebsi.com

Endo Ventures Ltd, Tel: 0800 0698421, medinfoEU@endo.com

Ennogen Healthcare Ltd, Tel: 01322 629220, info@ennogen.com

Ennogen Pharma Ltd, Tel: 01322 629220, info@ennogen.com

Entra Health Systems, Tel: +1 619 6846232, info@entrahealth.com

Espère Healthcare Ltd, Tel: 01462 346100, info@esperehealth.co.uk

Essential Pharmaceuticals Ltd, Tel: 01784 477167, info@essentialpharmaceuticals.com

Essential-Healthcare Ltd, Tel: 01277 286199, info@essential-healthcare.co.uk

Ethicon Ltd, Tel: +1 877 3844266, customersupport@eesus.jnj.com

Ethypharm UK Ltd, Tel: 01277 266600, medinfo@martindalepharma.co.uk

Eumedica Pharmaceuticals, Tel: +32 64 448859, MIR@eumedica.com

Eurocept International bv, Tel: +31 35 5283957, regulatory@eurocept.nl

EUSA Pharma Ltd, Tel: 0330 5001155, medicalinformation-uk@eusapharma.com

Ever Pharma UK Ltd, Tel: 0800 254 0174

Evolan Pharma AB, Tel: +46 8 54496030, info@evolan.se

Farla Medical Ltd, Tel: 0345 1935193, sales@farla.co.uk

Farmigea S.p.A., Tel: 01942 367516, info@farmigea.co.uk

Fate Special Foods, Tel: 01384 233230, admin@fatespecialfoods.com

FDC International Ltd, fdcil@btconnect.com

Ferndale Pharmaceuticals Ltd, Tel: 01937 541122, info@ferndalepharma.co.uk

Ferring Pharmaceuticals Ltd, Tel: 0800 1114125, medical.uk@ferring.com

Firstplay Dietary Foods Ltd, Tel: 0161 4804602, info@prominpku.com

Flamingo Pharma (UK) Ltd, Tel: 07733 522465, Richard.eggleston@flamingopharma.co.uk

Flen Health UK Ltd, Tel: 0207 8725460, info@flenhealth.com

Flexipharm Austrading Ltd, Tel: 01628 958001, medinfo@cambreg.co.uk

Flynn Pharma Ltd, Tel: 01438 727822, medinfo@flynnpharma.com

Fontus Health Ltd, Tel: 0121 6614615, Medinfo.uk@fontushealth.com

Ford Medical Associates Ltd, Tel: 01233 633224, enquiries@fordmedical.co.uk

Forum Health Products Ltd, Tel: 01737 857700

Fresenius Kabi Ltd, Tel: 01928 533 575, Medical.Information-UK@fresenius-kabi.com

Fyne Dynamics Ltd, Tel: 01279 423423

Galderma (UK) Ltd, Tel: 01923 208950, info.uk@galderma.com

Galen Ltd, Tel: 028 38334974, customer.services@galen-pharma.com

Galpharm International Ltd, Tel: 0203 598 9603, UKLOcustomerservice@perrigo.com

Galvany Pharma Ltd, Tel: 01438 310048, information@galvanypharma.com

Gedeon Richter (UK) Ltd, Tel: 0207 6048806, medinfo.uk@gedeonrichter.eu

Geistlich Sons Ltd, Tel: 0161 4902038, info@geistlich.co.uk

Genesis Pharmaceuticals Ltd, Tel: 020 72010400, info@genesis-pharma.com

Genus Pharmaceuticals Ltd, Tel: 01484 848164, thorntonross@medinformation.co.uk

Gilead Sciences International Ltd, Tel: 08000 113700, ukmedinfo@gilead.com

G.L. Pharma UK Ltd, Tel: 01353 882875, pv@gl-pharma.co.uk

GlaxoSmithKline Consumer Healthcare, Tel: 0800 7838881, customer.relations@gsk.com

GlaxoSmithKline UK Ltd, Tel: 0800 221441, ukmedinfo@gsk.com

Glenmark Pharmaceuticals Europe Ltd, Tel: 0800 4580383, Medical_information@glenmarkpharma.com

Glenwood GmbH, Tel: +49 89 18935363, info@glenwood.de

GlucoRx Ltd, Tel: 01483 755133, info@glucorx.co.uk

Gluten Free Foods Ltd, Tel: 0208 9534444, info@glutenfree-foods.co.uk

G.R. Lane Health Products Ltd, Tel: 01452 524012, info@laneshealth.com

Grifols UK Ltd, Tel: 01223 395700, medinfo.uk@grifols.com

Grünenthal Ltd, Tel: 0870 3518960, medicalinformationuk@grunenthal.com

GW Pharma Ltd, Tel: 01223 238170, medinfo@gwpharm.com

H&R Healthcare Ltd, Tel: 01482 631606, customerservices@hrhealthcare.co.uk

Hameln pharma Ltd, Tel: 01452 621661, drugsafety@hameln.co.uk

HBS Healthcare Ltd, Tel: 01480 279481, mi@hbshealthcare.com

Healthcare Pharma Ltd, Tel: 01233 822 297, mi@healthcarepharma.co.uk

Health+Plus Ltd, Tel: 01323 872277, contact@healthplus.co.uk

HEC Pharm GmbH, Tel: +49 (0) 30 330 077 21, medinfo@hecpharm.de

Hennig Arzneimittel GmbH & Co. KG, info@hennig-am.de

Henry Schein Ltd, Tel: 0800 0304169, info@henryscheinmedical.co.uk

Hero UK Ltd, Tel: 0800 7831992, info@juvela.co.uk

HFA Healthcare Products Ltd, Tel: 0844 3358270, uk@movianto.com

Higher Nature Ltd, technicalsupport@highernature.com

Hope Pharmaceuticals Ltd, questions@hopepharm.com

HRA Pharma UK Ltd, Tel: 0800 9179548, med.info.uk@hra-pharma.com

Huntleigh Healthcare Ltd, Tel: 029 20485885

Huxley Europe Ltd, Tel: 0161 7730485

Ideal Medical Solutions Ltd, Tel: 020 8773784-4, info@ideal-ms.com

Immedica Pharma AB, Tel: +46 (0)8 533 39 500, medicalinfo@immedica.com

Inceptua AB, Tel: +49 30 1202 1381, Inceptua.mi@primevigilance.com

Incyte Biosciences UK Ltd, Tel: 00800 00027423, eumedinfo@incyte.com

Indivior UK Ltd, Tel: +1 800 27081901, PatientSafetyROW@indivior.com

INFAI UK Ltd, Tel: 01904 435228, info@infai.co.uk

infirst Healthcare Ltd, Tel: 0808 2810143, medinfo@infirst.co.uk

Innovative Solutions UK Ltd, Tel: 01706 746713, keeley@pureglutenfree.co.uk

Insight Medical Products Ltd, Tel: 01666 500055, info@insightmedical.net

Ipca Laboratories UK Ltd, Tel: 01332 959126, ipca@callisto-consulting.co.uk

Ipsen Ltd, Tel: 01753 627777, medinfo.uk-ie@ipsen.com

J M Loveridge Ltd, Tel: 01264 367610

Janssen-Cilag Ltd, Tel: 0800 7318450, medinfo@janssen-cilag.co.uk

Jazz Pharmaceuticals UK, Tel: 0808 189 0387, Medinfo-uk@jazzpharma.com

Johnson & Johnson Ltd, Tel: 01344 864042, crc@its.jnj.com

JR Biomedical Ltd, Tel: 01745 535207, help@jrbiomedical.com

Juvela (Hero UK) Ltd, Tel: 0800 7831992, info@juvela.co.uk

Karo Pharma, Tel: 0808 1894327, Medinfo@karopharma.com

KCI Medical Ltd, Tel: 0800 9808880, UKCUSTSERV@kci-medical.com

Kent Pharmaceuticals Ltd, Tel: 01233 506574, medical@athlone-laboratories.com

Kestrel Ophthalmics Ltd, Tel: 01202 696963, info@kestrelophthalmics.co.uk

KetoCare Foods Ltd, info@ketocarefoods.com

Key Pharmaceuticals Ltd, Tel: 01487 840917, PV@keypharma.co.uk

KL Pharmaceuticals Ltd, Tel: 01294 215951, enquiries@klpharm.co.uk

Kora Healthcare, Tel: 0845 3038631, medinfo@korahealthcare.com

Krka UK Ltd, Tel: 07572 410 233, info.uk@krka.biz

Kyowa Kirin Ltd, Tel: 01896 664000, medinfo@kyowakirin.com

L&R Medical UK Ltd, Tel: 01283 576800, customersolutions@uk.lrmed.com

Laboratoires CTRS, Tel: +33 1 41220970, ctrs@ctrs.fr

Lactalis Nutrition Santé, Tel: +33 2 9492000, info@lns-privatelabel.com

L.D. Collins & Co. Ltd, Tel: 02071 298660, medicalinfo@ldcollins.com

Leadiant Biosciences Ltd, Tel: 08000 431 268, medical.information@leadiantcorp.wpengine.com

LEO Pharma, Tel: 01844 347333, medical-info.uk@leo-pharma.com

Leyden Delta B.V., Tel: 0207 3655 842, Medical.information@leydendelta.nl

LFB Biopharmaceuticals Ltd, Tel: +33 (0) 1 69 82 70 04, infomed@lfb.fr

LifeScan, Tel: +1 800 227 8862, customercare@LifeScan.co.uk

Lipomed GmbH, Tel: +41 61 7020200, lipomed@lipomed.com

Logixx Pharma Solutions Ltd, Tel: 0330 1359 454, mi@logixxpharma.com

Lohmann & Rauscher, Tel: +49 2634 990, info@de.LRmed.com

Lundbeck Ltd, Tel: 01908 638972, ukmedicalinformation@lundbeck.com

Lupin Healthcare (UK) Ltd, Tel: 01565 751 378, UKMedical@lupin.com

Luye Pharma Ltd, safety@luyepharma.co.uk

M & A Pharmachem Ltd, Tel: 01942 852085, safety@mapharmachem.co.uk

Macleods Pharma UK Ltd, Tel: 0800 023 6165, safety@macleodspharma.com

Manuka Medical Ltd, Tel: +1 615 6567852, supportUSA@manukamed.com

Manx Healthcare Ltd, Tel: 01926 482511, info@manxhealthcare.co.uk

Marlborough Pharmaceuticals Ltd, Tel: 01268 594777, info@atnahs.com

Martindale Pharmaceuticals Ltd, Tel: 01277 266600, medinfo@ethypharm.com

Masters Pharmaceuticals Ltd, Tel: 020 369 59305, pv-uk@addmedica.com

McNeil Products Ltd, Tel: 01344 864042, crc@its.jnj.com

Meadow Laboratories Ltd, enquiries@meadowlabs.co.uk

MeCoBo Ltd, Tel: 0844 8001705, enquiries@mecobo.com

Meda Pharmaceuticals Ltd, Tel: 01748 828810, meda@professionalinformation.co.uk

medac UK, Tel: 01786 458086, info@medacpharma.co.uk

Medical Developments UK Ltd, Tel: 01279 504055, info@medicaldev.co.uk

Medicareplus International Ltd, Tel: 020 88108811, info@medicareplus.co.uk

Medicom Healthcare Ltd, Tel: 01489 574119, info@medicomhealthcare.com

Medihealth (Northern) Ltd, Tel: 0800 633 5977

Medreich Plc, info@medreich.co.uk

Merck Serono Ltd, Tel: 020 88187373, medinfo.uk@merckgroup.com

Merck Sharp & Dohme Ltd, Tel: 0208 1548000, medicalinformationuk@msd.com

Merz Pharma UK Ltd, Tel: 0333 2004143, medical.information@merz.com

Mibe Pharma UK Ltd, Tel: 020 387 07504

Millpledge Healthcare, Tel: 01777 708440, sales@millpledge.com

Milpharm Ltd, Tel: 0208 8458811, medinfo@aurobindo.com

Mitsubishi Tanabe Pharma Europe Ltd, Tel: 0207 3829000, medinfo@mitsubishi-pharma.eu

Mölnlycke Health Care Ltd, Tel: 01908 355200

Morningside Healthcare Ltd, Tel: 0116 478 0322, medicalenquiry@morningsidehealthcare.com

Nagor Ltd, Tel: 01236 780780, enquiries@nagor.com

Napp Pharmaceuticals Ltd, Tel: 01223 424444, medicalinformationuk@napp.co.uk

Neoceuticals Ltd, Tel: 01748 828865, neoceuticals@professionalinformation.co.uk

Neomedic Ltd, Tel: 01923 836379, marketing@neomedic.co.uk

Neon Diagnostics Ltd, Tel: 01376 500720

Neon Healthcare Ltd, Tel: 01992 926330, office@neonhealthcare.com

Nestlé Health Science, Tel: 00800 68874846, nestlehealthcarenutrition@uk.nestle.com

Neuraxpharm UK Ltd, Tel: 07508 844 104

Niche Generics Ltd, Tel: +353526126960, info@nichegenerics.com

Nipro Diagnostics (UK) Ltd, Tel: 0800 0858808, diagnostics-uk@nipro-group.com

Noden Pharma DAC, Tel: 0800 783 8918, Medinfo@nodenpharma.com

Nordic Pharma Ltd, Tel: 0800 1218924, nordic@professionalinformation.co.uk

Norgine Pharmaceuticals Ltd, Tel: 01895 826600, medinfo@norgine.com

Northumbria Pharma Ltd, Tel: 01740 618611, ukmedinfo@northumbriapharma.com

Nova Laboratories Ltd, Tel: 08707 120655, Novalabsgb@EU.propharmagroup.com

Novartis Pharmaceuticals UK Ltd, Tel: 01276 698370, medinfo.uk@novartis.com

Novo Nordisk Ltd, Tel: 0800 023 2573, CustomerCare@novonordisk.com

nSPIRE Health Ltd, Tel: 01992 526300, info@nspirehealth.com

Nualtra Ltd, Tel: 0118 4532853, support@nualtra.co.uk

Nutraconcepts Ltd, Tel: 0800 1123085, info@nutraconcepts.com

Nutri Advanced Ltd, Tel: 0800 0435777, advice@nutriadvanced.co.uk

Nutricia, Tel: 01225 751098, resourcecentre@nutricia.com

Nutrinovo Ltd, Tel: 01304 829068, info@nutrinovo.com

OakMed Ltd, Tel: 01604 586529, info@oakmed.co.uk

Octapharma Ltd, Tel: 0161 837 3781, medinfo.uk@octapharma.com

Omega Pharma Ltd, Tel: 0203 5989603, UKLOcustomerservice@perrigo.com

Oralieve UK, Tel: 01582 439122, hello@oralieve.co.uk

Orexigen Therapeutics Ireland Ltd, Tel: 0800 0516402, currax.mi@primevigilance.com

Organon Pharma (UK) Ltd, Tel: 0208 159 3593, medicalinformationuk@organon.com

Orion Pharma (UK) Ltd, Tel: 01635 520300, uk.medicalinformation@orionpharma.com

Typharm Ltd, Tel: 02037 694160, medinfo@typharm.com

UCB Pharma Ltd, Tel: 01753 777100, UCBCaresUK@ucb.com

Ultrapharm Ltd, Tel: 01495 765570, info@ultrapharm.eu

Unilever UK Home & Personal Care, Tel: 01372 945001

Univar Solutions B.V., Prescription.Medicines@UnivarSolutions.com

Upjohn UK Ltd, Tel: 01304 616 161

Urgo Ltd, Tel: 01509 502051, woundcare@uk.urgo.com

Valneva UK Ltd, Tel: 01506 446608, medinfo@valneva.com

Vega Nutritionals Ltd, Tel: 01639 825107, info@vegavitamins.co.uk

Veriton Pharma Ltd, Tel: 01932 690325, centralmedicalinformation@veritonpharma.com

Vertex Pharmaceuticals (UK) Ltd, Tel: 01923 437672, vertexmedicalinfo@vrtx.com

Vianex S.A., pvvnx@vianex.gr

Viatris UK Healthcare Ltd, Tel: 0170 785 3000, reception@viatris.com

Vifor Pharma UK Ltd, Tel: 01276 853633, medicalinfo_UK@viforpharma.com

ViiV Healthcare UK Ltd, Tel: 020 83806200

Visufarma UK Ltd, Tel: 0113 4680661, UKMedicalinformation@VISUfarma.com

Vitaflo International Ltd, Tel: 0151 7099020, vitaflo@vitaflo.co.uk

Vitalograph Ltd, Tel: 01280 827110

Vygoris Ltd, Tel: 01223 395 301, safety@productlife-group.com

Wallace, Cameron & Company Ltd, Tel: 01698 354600, sales@wallacecameron.com

Wallace Manufacturing Chemists Ltd, Tel: 01235 538700

Warburtons, Tel: 0800 243684, customercare@warburtons.co.uk

Waymade Healthcare Plc, Tel: 01268 535200, info@waymade.co.uk

Welland Medical Ltd, Tel: 01293 615455, info@wellandmedical.com

Williams Medical Supplies Ltd, Tel: 01685 846666, medicalservices@wms.co.uk

Wockhardt UK Ltd, Tel: 01978 661261

Wyvern Medical Ltd, Tel: 01264 332172, info@wyvernmedical.co.uk

Xellia Pharmaceuticals ApS, Tel: +48 226604571, safety@xellia.com

Xiromed, Tel: +1 844 947 6633

Zambon UK Ltd, Tel: 0800 0288942, infouk@zambongroup.com

Zentiva, Tel: 0800 0902408, UKMedInfo@zentiva.com

Zeroderma Ltd, Tel: 01484 848164, thorntonross@medinformation.co.uk

Special-order manufacturers

Unlicensed medicines are available from 'special-order' manufacturers and specialist-importing companies; the MHRA maintains a register of these companies at www.gov.uk/government/publications/human-and-veterinary-medicines-register-of-licensed-manufacturing-sites.

Licensed **hospital manufacturing units** also manufacture 'special-order' products as unlicensed medicines, the principal NHS units are listed below. A database (*Pro-File*; www.pro-file.nhs.uk) provides information on medicines manufactured in the NHS; access is restricted to NHS pharmacy staff.

The Association of Pharmaceutical Specials Manufacturers may also be able to provide further information about commercial companies (www.apsm-uk.com).

The MHRA recommends that an unlicensed medicine should only be used when a patient has special requirements that cannot be met by use of a licensed medicine.

As well as being available direct from the hospital manufacturer(s) concerned, many NHS-manufactured Specials may be bought from the Oxford Pharmacy Store, owned and operated by Oxford Health NHS Foundation Trust.

England

London

Barts Health NHS Trust

T. Patel, Head of Pharmacy, Shared Services
Pharmacy Technical Services Unit
First Floor, Pathology and Pharmacy Building
80 Newark Street
London
E1 2ES
(020) 3246 0397 (order/enquiry)
tejal.patel5@nhs.net

Guy's and St. Thomas' NHS Foundation Trust

Mr P. Forsey, Associate Chief Pharmacist
Guy's and St. Thomas' NHS Foundation Trust
Guy's Hospital
Pharmacy Department
Great Maze Pond
London
SE1 9RT
(020) 7188 4992 (order)
(020) 7188 5003 (enquiry)
Fax: (020) 7188 5013
paul.forsey@gstt.nhs.uk

London North West Healthcare NHS Trust

Mr K. Wong,
London North West Healthcare NHS Trust
Pharmacy Technical Services Department
Northwick Park Hospital
Watford Road
Harrow
Middlesex
HA1 3UJ
(020) 8869 2295 (order/enquiry)
Fax: (020) 8869 2370
LNWH-tr.nphmanufacturing@nhs.net (enquiry)
kwong@nhs.net

Royal Free London NHS Foundation Trust

Mr M. Baker, Head of Pharmacy Manufacturing Unit
Royal Free Specials Pharmaceuticals
Royal Free London NHS Foundation Trust
Pond Street
Hampstead
London
NW3 2QG
(020) 7830 2424 (order/enquiry)
rf.specials@nhs.net (order/enquiry)
marc.baker@nhs.net

St George's Healthcare NHS Trust

Mr V. Kumar, Chief Pharmacist
St George's University Hospitals
NHS Foundation Trust
Ground Floor, Lanesborough Wing
Blackshaw Road
London
SW17 0QT
(020) 8725 1378
vinodh.kumar@stgeorges.nhs.uk

University College Hospital NHS Foundation Trust

Mr T. Murphy, Production Manager
University College Hospital
235 Euston Road
London
NW1 2BU
(020) 7380 9723 (order)
(020) 7380 9472 (enquiry)
Fax: (020) 7380 9726
tony.murphy@uclh.nhs.uk

Midlands and Eastern

Barking, Havering and Redbridge University Trust

Mr N. Fisher, Senior Principal Pharmacist
Queen's Hospital
Pharmacy Department
Romford
Essex
RM7 0AG
(01708) 435 463 (order)
(01708) 435 042 (enquiry)
neil.fisher@bhrhospitals.nhs.uk

Burton Hospitals NHS Foundation Trust

Mr D. Raynor, Head of Pharmacy Manufacturing Unit
Queens Hospital
Burton Hospitals NHS Foundation Trust
Pharmacy Manufacturing Unit
Belvedere Road
Burton-on-Trent
DE13 0RB
(01283) 511 511 ext: 5275 (order/enquiry)
Fax: (01283) 593 036
david.raynor@burtonft.nhs.uk

East Suffolk and North Essex NHS Foundation Trust (Colchester site)

Mr S. Pullen, Head of Pharmacy Production
Colchester Hospital
Pharmacy Manufacturing Unit
Turner Road
Colchester
Essex
CO4 5JL
(01206) 742 007 (order)
(01206) 744 208 (enquiry)
Pharmacy.Stores@esneft.nhs.uk (order)
PSU.Enquiries@esneft.nhs.uk (enquiry)

East Suffolk and North Essex NHS Foundation Trust (Ipswich site)

Mr B. Tabrizi, Deputy Head of Production
Ipswich Hospital
Pharmacy Manufacturing Unit
Heath Road
Ipswich
Suffolk
IP4 5PD
(01473) 703 440 (order)
(01473) 703 603 (enquiry)
pharmacy.manufacture@esneft.nhs.uk (order/enquiry)
behnam.tabrizi@esneft.nhs.uk

Nottingham University Hospitals NHS Trust

Mr J. Graham, Senior Pharmacist, Production
Queens Medical Centre Campus
Pharmacy Production
Derby Road
Nottingham
NG7 2UH
(0115) 924 9924 ext: 87516 (order/enquiry)
jeff.graham@nuh.nhs.uk

North East

The Newcastle upon Tyne Hospitals NHS Foundation Trust

Mr Y. Hunter-Blair, Production Manager
Royal Victoria Infirmary
Newcastle Specials
Pharmacy Production Unit
Queen Victoria Road
Newcastle-upon-Tyne
NE1 4LP
(0191) 282 0395 (order)
(0191) 282 0389 (enquiry)
Fax: (0191) 282 0469
yan.hunter-blair@nuth.nhs.uk

North West

Preston Pharmaceuticals

J. Parrington, Head of Production
Preston Pharmaceuticals
Pharmacy Manufacturing Unit
Royal Preston Hospital
Sharoe Green Lane
Fulwood
Preston
PR2 9HT
(01772) 523 617 (order/enquiry)
prestonpharmaceuticals@lthtr.nhs.uk (order/enquiry)
janet.parrington@lthtr.nhs.uk

Stockport Pharmaceuticals

Mr A. Singleton, Head of Production
Stepping Hill Hospital
Stockport NHS Foundation Trust
Stockport Pharmaceuticals
Poplar Grove
Stockport
SK2 7JE
(0161) 419 5666 (order/enquiry)
Fax: (0161) 419 5426
sppu.orders@stockport.nhs.uk
andrew.singleton@stockport.nhs.uk

South

Portsmouth Hospitals University NHS Trust

Mr R. Lucas, Quality Assurance Manager
Portsmouth Hospitals University NHS Trust
Pharmacy Manufacturing Unit
Unit D2, Railway Triangle
Walton Road
Farlington
Portsmouth
PO6 1TF
(02392) 389 078 (order/enquiry)
PMU.office@porthosp.nhs.uk (order)
robert.lucas@porthosp.nhs.uk

South West

Torbay Pharmaceuticals

Mr L. Rudd, Commercial Strategy Director
Torbay and South Devon NHS Foundation Trust
Torbay Pharmaceuticals
Wilkins Drive
Paignton
TQ4 7FG
(01803) 664 707 (order/enquiry)
Fax: (01803) 231 121
torbaypharmaceuticals@nhs.net
leon.rudd@nhs.net

Yorkshire

Calderdale and Huddersfield NHS Foundation Trust

Dr B. Grewal, Managing Director
Calderdale and Huddersfield NHS Foundation Trust
Huddersfield Pharmacy Specials
Gate 2 - Acre Mills, School Street West
Huddersfield
HD3 3ET
(01484) 355 388 (order/enquiry)
hps.orders@cht.nhs.uk

Northern Ireland

Victoria Pharmaceuticals

Mr S. Cameron, Production Manager - Pharmacy
Victoria Pharmaceuticals
Royal Hospitals
Plenum Building
Grosvenor Road
Belfast
BT12 6BA
(028) 9615 1000 (order/enquiry)
samuel.cameron@belfasttrust.hscni.net

Scotland

NHS Scotland Pharmaceutical 'Specials' Service

Mr S. Bath, Production Manager
Ninewells Hospital
James Arrott Drive
Dundee
DD2 1UB
(01382) 496702 (order/enquiry)
(01382) 496730 (technical enquiry)
Fax: (01382) 496703 (order)
tay.pssoffice@nhs.scot (order/enquiry)
simond.bath@nhs.scot (technical enquiry)

Wales

Cardiff and Vale University Health Board

Ms A. Jones, Principal Pharmacist - Head of Technical Services
Cardiff and Vale University Health Board
20 Fieldway
Cardiff
CF14 4HY
(029) 2184 8120 (order/enquiry)
Fax: (029) 2184 8130
contact@smpu.co.uk

Index

A

INDEX

D

H

U

V

Recommended wording of cautionary and advisory labels

For details including Welsh Language translation see p. 1433

1 **Warning: This medicine may make you sleepy**

2 **Warning: This medicine may make you sleepy. If this happens, do not drive or use tools or machines. Do not drink alcohol**

3 **Warning: This medicine may make you sleepy. If this happens, do not drive or use tools or machines**

4 **Warning: Do not drink alcohol**

5 **Do not take indigestion remedies 2 hours before or after you take this medicine**

6 **Do not take indigestion remedies, or medicines containing iron or zinc, 2 hours before or after you take this medicine**

7 **Do not take milk, indigestion remedies, or medicines containing iron or zinc, 2 hours before or after you take this medicine**

8 **Warning: Do not stop taking this medicine unless your doctor tells you to stop**

9 **Space the doses evenly throughout the day. Keep taking this medicine until the course is finished, unless you are told to stop**

10 **Warning: Read the additional information given with this medicine**

11 **Protect your skin from sunlight—even on a bright but cloudy day. Do not use sunbeds**

12 **Do not take anything containing aspirin while taking this medicine**

13 **Dissolve or mix with water before taking**

14 **This medicine may colour your urine. This is harmless**

15 **Caution: flammable. Keep your body away from fire or flames after you have put on the medicine**

16 **Dissolve the tablet under your tongue—do not swallow. Store the tablets in this bottle with the cap tightly closed. Get a new supply 8 weeks after opening**

17 **Do not take more than... in 24 hours**

18 **Do not take more than... in 24 hours. Also, do not take more than... in any one week**

19 **Warning: This medicine makes you sleepy. If you still feel sleepy the next day, do not drive or use tools or machines. Do not drink alcohol**

21 **Take with or just after food, or a meal**

22 **Take 30 to 60 minutes before food**

23 **Take this medicine when your stomach is empty. This means an hour before food or 2 hours after food**

24 **Suck or chew this medicine**

25 **Swallow this medicine whole. Do not chew or crush**

26 **Dissolve this medicine under your tongue**

27 **Take with a full glass of water**

28 **Spread thinly on the affected skin only**

29 **Do not take more than 2 at any one time. Do not take more than 8 in 24 hours**

30 **Contains paracetamol. Do not take anything else containing paracetamol while taking this medicine. Talk to a doctor at once if you take too much of this medicine, even if you feel well**

32 **Contains aspirin. Do not take anything else containing aspirin while taking this medicine**

Approximate Conversions and Units

Conversion of pounds to kilograms

lb	kg
1	0.45
2	0.91
3	1.36
4	1.81
5	2.27
6	2.72
7	3.18
8	3.63
9	4.08
10	4.54
11	4.99
12	5.44
13	5.90
14	6.35

Conversion of stones to kilograms

stones	kg
1	6.35
2	12.70
3	19.05
4	25.40
5	31.75
6	38.10
7	44.45
8	50.80
9	57.15
10	63.50
11	69.85
12	76.20
13	82.55
14	88.90
15	95.25

Conversion from millilitres to fluid ounces

mL	fl oz
50	1.8
100	3.5
150	5.3
200	7.0
500	17.6
1000	35.2

Length

1 metre (m) = 1000 millimetres (mm)
1 centimetre (cm) = 10 mm
1 inch (in) = 25.4 mm
1 foot (ft) = 12 inches
12 inches = 304.8 mm

Mass

1 kilogram (kg) = 1000 grams (g)
1 gram (g) = 1000 milligrams (mg)
1 milligram (mg) = 1000 micrograms
1 microgram = 1000 nanograms
1 nanogram = 1000 picograms

Volume

1 litre = 1000 millilitres (mL)
1 millilitre (1 mL) = 1000 microlitres
1 pint ≈ 568 mL

Other units

1 kilocalorie (kcal) = 4186.8 joules (J)
1000 kilocalories (kcal) = 4.1868 megajoules (MJ)
1 megajoule (MJ) = 238.8 kilocalories (kcal)
1 millimetre of mercury (mmHg) = 133.3 pascals (Pa)
1 kilopascal (kPa) = 7.5 mmHg (pressure)

Plasma-drug concentrations

Plasma-drug concentrations in BNF Publications are expressed in mass units per litre (e.g. mg/litre). The approximate equivalent in terms of amount of substance units (e.g. micromol/litre) is given in brackets.

Prescribing for children: weight, height, and sex

The table below shows the **mean values** for weight, height and sex by age; these values have been derived from the UK-WHO growth charts 2009 and UK 1990 standard centile charts, by extrapolating the 50th centile, and may be used to calculate doses in the absence of actual measurements. However, the child's actual weight and height might vary considerably from the values in the table and it is important to see the child to ensure that the value chosen is appropriate. In most cases the child's actual measurement should be obtained as soon as possible and the dose re-calculated.

Age	Weight (kg)	Height (cm)
Full-term neonate	3.5	51
1 month	4.3	55
2 months	5.4	58
3 months	6.1	61
4 months	6.7	63
6 months	7.6	67
1 year	9	75
3 years	14	96
5 years	18	109
7 years	23	122
10 years	32	138
12 years	39	149
14 year old boy	49	163
14 year old girl	50	159
Adult male	68	176
Adult female	58	164

Abbreviations and Symbols

Internationally recognised units and symbols are used in BNF Publications where possible.

ACBS Advisory Committee on Borderline Substances, *see* Borderline Substances
ACE Angiotensin-converting enzyme
ADHD Attention deficit hyperactivity disorder
AIDS Acquired immunodeficiency syndrome
approx. approximately
AV atrioventricular
AWMSG All Wales Medicines Strategy Group
BAN British Approved Name
BMI body mass index
BP British Pharmacopoeia 2013, unless otherwise stated
BPC British Pharmaceutical Codex 1973 and Supplement 1976, unless otherwise stated
BRCA breast cancer gene
CAPD Continuous ambulatory peritoneal dialysis
CD1 preparation in Schedule 1 of the Misuse of Drugs Regulations 2001 (and subsequent amendments). For regulations *see* Controlled drugs and drug dependence p. 8.
CD2 preparation in Schedule 2 of the Misuse of Drugs Regulations 2001 (and subsequent amendments). For regulations *see* Controlled drugs and drug dependence p. 8.
CD3 preparation in Schedule 3 of the Misuse of Drugs Regulations 2001 (and subsequent amendments). For regulations *see* Controlled drugs and drug dependence p. 8.
CD4-1 preparation in Schedule 4 (Part I) of the Misuse of Drugs Regulations 2001 (and subsequent amendments). For regulations *see* Controlled drugs and drug dependence p. 8.
CD4-2 preparation in Schedule 4 (Part II) of the Misuse of Drugs Regulations 2001 (and subsequent amendments). For regulations *see* Controlled drugs and drug dependence p. 8.
CD5 preparation in Schedule 5 of the Misuse of Drugs Regulations 2001 (and subsequent amendments). For regulations *see* Controlled drugs and drug dependence p. 8.
CHM Commission on Human Medicines
CHMP Committee for Medicinal Products for Human Use
CNS central nervous system
CoSRH College of Sexual and Reproductive Healthcare (formerly Faculty of Sexual and Reproductive Healthcare (FSRH))
CSM Committee on Safety of Medicines (now subsumed under Commission on Human Medicines)
d. c. direct current
DMARD Disease-modifying antirheumatic drug
DPF Dental Practitioners' Formulary
DT Drug Tariff price
e/c enteric-coated (termed gastro-resistant in BP)
ECG electrocardiogram
EEG electro-encephalogram
eGFR estimated glomerular filtration rate, *see* Prescribing in renal impairment p. 16
EMA European Medicines Agency
FSRH Faculty of Sexual and Reproductive Healthcare
G6PD glucose 6-phosphate dehydrogenase
GSL general sales list
HDL-cholesterol high-density lipoprotein cholesterol
HIV Human immunodeficiency virus
HRT Hormone replacement therapy
i/m intramuscular
i/v intravenous
INR international normalised ratio
JCVI Joint Committee on Vaccination and Immunisation
LDL-cholesterol low-density lipoprotein cholesterol
MAO Monoamine-oxidase inhibitor
max. maximum
MHRA Medicines and Healthcare products Regulatory Agency
NCL no cautionary labels (prescription endorsement made by prescriber when recommended cautionary labels are not required)
NHS National Health Service
NICE National Institute for Health and Care Excellence
NPF Nurse Prescribers' Formulary
NSAID Non-steroidal anti-inflammatory drug
NSTEMI non-ST-segment elevation myocardial infarction
P pharmacy only medicine
PARP poly (ADP-ribose) polymerase
PGD patient group direction
PHE Public Health England (formerly Health Protection Agency (HPA))
PoM prescription-only medicine, *see* Fig. 1 *How to use BNF Publications*
® registered trade mark
rINN Recommended International Non-proprietary Name
RSV respiratory syncytial virus
SF sugar-free
SIGN Scottish Intercollegiate Guidelines Network
SLS Selected List Scheme
SMC Scottish Medicines Consortium
SPC Summary of Product Characteristics
spp. species
SSRI Selective serotonin reuptake inhibitor
STEMI ST-segment elevation myocardial infarction
UK United Kingdom
UKHSA United Kingdom Health Security Agency (formerly Public Health England (PHE))
Units for SI units *see* Prescription writing p. 4
WHO World Health Organization
▼ limited experience of the use of this product and the MHRA requests that all suspected adverse reactions should be reported, *see* Adverse reactions to drugs p. 11
(drug-class symbol) drug-class monograph, *see* How to use BNF Publications, p. xi
1234 drug monograph has a corresponding drug-class monograph; the page number of the class monograph is indicated within the tab, *see* How to use BNF Publications, p. xi
EvGr precedes evidence graded content, *see* How BNF Publications are constructed p. viii
A to E symbols will be displayed – grades reflect the strengths of recommendations in evidence graded content, see How BNF Publications are constructed p. viii
M indicates manufacturer information, see How BNF Publications are constructed p. viii
(no price symbol) no price available

Latin abbreviations

Directions should be in English without abbreviation. However, Latin abbreviations have been used when prescribing.

The following is a list of appropriate abbreviations. It should be noted that the English version is not always an exact translation.

a. c. = ante cibum (before food)
b. d. = bis die (twice daily)
o. d. = omni die (every day)
o. m. = omni mane (every morning)
o. n. = omni nocte (every night)
p. c. = post cibum (after food)
p. r. n. = pro re nata (when required)
q. d. s. = quater die sumendum (to be taken four times daily)
q. q. h. = quarta quaque hora (every four hours)
stat = immediately
t. d. s. = ter die sumendum (to be taken three times daily)
t.i.d. = ter in die (three times daily)

E numbers

The following is a list of common E numbers and the inactive ingredients to which they correspond.

E102	Tartrazine
E104	Quinoline Yellow
E110	Sunset Yellow FCF
E123	Amaranth
E124	Ponceau 4R
E127	Erythrosine BS
E132	Indigo Carmine
E142	Green S
E171	Titanium Dioxide
E172	Iron oxides, iron hydroxides
E200	Sorbic Acid
E211	Sodium Benzoate
E223	Sodium Metabisulfite
E320	Butylated Hydroxyanisole
E321	Butylated Hydroxytoluene
E322	Lecithins
E420	Sorbitol
E421	Mannitol
E422	Glycerol
E901	Beeswax (white and yellow)
E1520	Propylene Glycol

Body Surface Area in Children

Body-weight under 40 kg

Body-weight (kg)	Surface area (m^2)
1	0.10
1.5	0.13
2	0.16
2.5	0.19
3	0.21
3.5	0.24
4	0.26
4.5	0.28
5	0.30
5.5	0.32
6	0.34
6.5	0.36
7	0.38
7.5	0.40
8	0.42
8.5	0.44
9	0.46
9.5	0.47
10	0.49
11	0.53
12	0.56
13	0.59
14	0.62
15	0.65
16	0.68

Body-weight (kg)	Surface area (m^2)
17	0.71
18	0.74
19	0.77
20	0.79
21	0.82
22	0.85
23	0.87
24	0.90
25	0.92
26	0.95
27	0.97
28	1.0
29	1.0
30	1.1
31	1.1
32	1.1
33	1.1
34	1.1
35	1.2
36	1.2
37	1.2
38	1.2
39	1.3
40	1.3

Values are calculated using the Boyd equation

Note Height is not required to estimate body surface using these tables

Body Surface Area in Children

Body-weight over 40 kg

Body-weight (kg)	Surface area (m²)	Body-weight (kg)	Surface area (m²)
41	1.3	66	1.8
42	1.3	67	1.8
43	1.3	68	1.8
44	1.4	69	1.8
45	1.4	70	1.9
46	1.4	71	1.9
47	1.4	72	1.9
48	1.4	73	1.9
49	1.5	74	1.9
50	1.5	75	1.9
51	1.5	76	2.0
52	1.5	77	2.0
53	1.5	78	2.0
54	1.6	79	2.0
55	1.6	80	2.0
56	1.6	81	2.0
57	1.6	82	2.1
58	1.6	83	2.1
59	1.7	84	2.1
60	1.7	85	2.1
61	1.7	86	2.1
62	1.7	87	2.1
63	1.7	88	2.2
64	1.7	89	2.2
65	1.8	90	2.2

Values are calculated using the Boyd equation

Note Height is not required to estimate body surface using these tables

Medical emergencies in the community

16-Dec-2024

Overview

Drug treatment outlined below is intended for use by appropriately qualified healthcare professionals. Only drugs that are used for immediate relief are shown; advice on supporting care is not given. Where the child's condition requires investigation and further treatment, the child should be transferred to hospital promptly.

Airways disease, obstructive

▶ **ASTHMA: ACUTE**

EvGr Emergency asthma consultations should be regarded as being for severe acute asthma until shown otherwise. Children with features of severe or life-threatening acute asthma, and children who fail to respond adequately at any time should be referred to hospital immediately. Acute asthma in children aged under 2 years should be managed in hospital. (A)

High-flow **oxygen** should be given if available (via tight-fitting face mask in children) to achieve and maintain an SpO_2 level of 94-98%.

▶ EITHER **Salbutamol aerosol inhaler** **p. 181** (100 micrograms/dose inhaler)

BY INHALATION OF AEROSOL VIA A SPACER (AND A CLOSE-FITTING FACE MASK IF CHILD UNDER 3 YEARS)

- Child 1-17 years: 100 micrograms every 0.5–1 minute for up to 10 doses; each dose is to be inhaled separately; repeat every 10–20 minutes or when required

▶ OR **Salbutamol dry powder inhaler** (100 micrograms/dose inhaler, 200 micrograms/dose inhaler)

BY INHALATION OF DRY POWDER

- Child 6-17 years: 100 micrograms every 0.5–1 minute for up to 10 doses, *or alternatively* 200 micrograms every 0.5–1 minute for up to 5 doses; each dose is to be inhaled separately; repeat every 10–20 minutes or when required

▶ OR **Salbutamol nebuliser solution** (1 mg/mL, 2 mg/mL)

BY INHALATION OF NEBULISED SOLUTION (VIA OXYGEN-DRIVEN NEBULISER IF AVAILABLE)

- Child 6-17 years: 2.5 mg; repeat every 20–30 minutes or when required
- Child 6-17 years: 2.5–5 mg; repeat every 20–30 minutes or when required

▶ OR **Terbutaline sulfate nebuliser solution** **p. 183** (2.5 mg/mL)

BY INHALATION OF NEBULISED SOLUTION (VIA OXYGEN-DRIVEN NEBULISER IF AVAILABLE)

- Child 4 years and below: 5 mg every 20–30 minutes or as necessary
- Child 5-11 years: 5–10 mg every 20–30 minutes or as necessary
- Child 12-17 years: 10 mg every 20–30 minutes or as necessary

▶ PLUS **(in all cases)**

▶ EITHER **Prednisolone tablets** **p. 548** **(*or* prednisolone soluble tablets)** (5 mg)

BY MOUTH

- Child 11 years and below: 1–2 mg/kg (max. 40 mg) once daily for up to 3 days or longer if necessary; if child has been taking an oral corticosteroid for more than a few days, give prednisolone 2 mg/kg (max. 60 mg) once daily
- Child 12-17 years: 40–50 mg once daily for at least 5 days

▶ OR **Hydrocortisone** **p. 544** **(preferably as sodium succinate)**

BY INTRAVENOUS INJECTION

- Child 17 years and below: 4 mg/kg (max. 100 mg) every 6 hours until conversion to oral prednisolone is possible; alternative dose if weight unavailable:
  - Child 1 year and below: 25 mg
  - Child 2-4 years: 50 mg
  - Child 5-17 years: 100 mg

Monitor response 15 to 30 minutes after nebulisation; if any signs of acute asthma persist, arrange hospital admission. While awaiting ambulance, repeat **nebulised beta$_2$ agonist** (as above) and give with

Ipratropium bromide nebuliser solution **p. 177** (250 micrograms/mL)

BY INHALATION OF NEBULISED SOLUTION (VIA OXYGEN-DRIVEN NEBULISER IF AVAILABLE)

- Child 11 years and below: 250 micrograms, repeated every 20–30 minutes for the first 2 hours, then every 4–6 hours as necessary
- Child 12-17 years: 500 micrograms every 4–6 hours as necessary

▶ **CROUP**

Dexamethasone oral solution **p. 543** (2 mg/5 mL)

BY MOUTH

- Child 1 month-2 years: 150 micrograms/kg as a single dose

Anaphylaxis

▶ **ANAPHYLAXIS**

Adrenaline injection **p. 159** (1 mg/mL (1 in 1000))

BY INTRAMUSCULAR INJECTION

- Child up to 6 months: 100–150 micrograms (0.1–0.15 mL), repeated after 5 minutes if necessary
- Child 6 months-5 years: 150 micrograms (0.15 mL), repeated after 5 minutes if necessary
- Child 6-11 years: 300 micrograms (0.3 mL), repeated after 5 minutes if necessary
- Child 12-17 years: 500 micrograms (0.5 mL), repeated after 5 minutes if necessary; 300 micrograms (0.3 mL) should be given if child is small or prepubertal

If life-threatening features persist, further doses of intramuscular adrenaline can be given every 5 minutes until specialist critical care available.

High-flow **oxygen** should be given as soon as available. For guidance on other treatment that may be used for the management of anaphylaxis, *see* Antihistamines, allergen immunotherapy and allergic emergencies p. 199.

Bacterial disease

▶ **SUSPECTED MENINGOCOCCAL DISEASE, AND SUSPECTED BACTERIAL MENINGITIS (WHERE THERE IS LIKELY TO BE A CLINICALLY SIGNIFICANT DELAY IN TRANSFER TO HOSPITAL).**

NOTE Administer a single dose before urgent transfer to hospital, unless this will delay transfer.

Benzylpenicillin sodium injection **p. 415** (600 mg, 1.2 g)

BY INTRAVENOUS INJECTION (OR BY INTRAMUSCULAR INJECTION IF VENOUS ACCESS NOT AVAILABLE)

- Child 1 month-11 months: 300 mg
- Child 1-9 years: 600 mg
- Child 10-17 years: 1.2 g

▸ OR **Ceftriaxone injection p. 391** (250 mg, 1 g, 2 g)

BY DEEP INTRAMUSCULAR INJECTION

- Child 1 month: 250 mg
- Child 2-11 months: 500 mg
- Child 1-4 years: 1 g
- Child 5-8 years: 1.5 g
- Child 9-11 years: 2 g

BY INTRAVENOUS INJECTION OR BY DEEP INTRAMUSCULAR INJECTION

- Child 12-17 years: 2 g

Do not administer antibacterial treatment outside of hospital if history of severe allergy to a beta-lactam antibacterial.
See also Central nervous system infections, antibacterial therapy p. 365.

▸ **SUSPECTED MENINGOCOCCAL DISEASE**
Benzylpenicillin sodium injection (600 mg, 1.2 g)

BY INTRAVENOUS INJECTION (OR BY INTRAMUSCULAR INJECTION IF VENOUS ACCESS NOT AVAILABLE)

- Neonate: 300 mg

NOTE Administer a single dose before urgent transfer to hospital, unless this will delay transfer. See also Neonatal infection, antibacterial therapy p. 369.

Hypoglycaemia

▸ **DIABETIC HYPOGLYCAEMIA**
Fast-acting carbohydrate (glucose p. 730 is preferred)

CHILD UP TO 5 YEARS

BY MOUTH

- 5 g (20 mL *Lift*® (previously *Glucojuice*®) oral glucose liquid *or* 1.5 glucose tablets *or* half a tube of glucose 40% oral gel *or* 1 teaspoonful of sugar dissolved in an appropriate volume of water), repeated after 15 minutes if necessary

Or by buccal administration [in conscious but uncooperative children]

- 5 g (half a tube of glucose 40% oral gel), repeated after 15 minutes if necessary

CHILD 5-11 YEARS

BY MOUTH

- 10 g (40 mL *Lift*® (previously *Glucojuice*®) oral glucose liquid *or* 3 glucose tablets *or* 1 tube of glucose 40% oral gel *or* 2 teaspoonfuls of sugar dissolved in an appropriate volume of water), repeated after 15 minutes if necessary

Or by buccal administration [in conscious but uncooperative children]

- 10 g (1 tube of glucose 40% oral gel), repeated after 15 minutes if necessary

CHILD 12-17 YEARS

BY MOUTH

- 15 g (60 mL *Lift*® (previously *Glucojuice*®) oral glucose liquid *or* 4 glucose tablets *or* 1.5 tubes of glucose 40% oral gel *or* 3 teaspoonfuls of sugar dissolved in an appropriate volume of water), repeated after 15 minutes if necessary

Or by buccal administration [in conscious but uncooperative children]

- 15 g (1.5 tubes of glucose 40% oral gel), repeated after 15 minutes if necessary

NOTE Examples of glucose preparations which can be used to give oral doses are based on the use of oral liquid containing glucose 250 mg/mL and tablets containing glucose 4 g per tablet. Buccal dosing is based on tubes of 40% oral gel containing glucose 10 g per tube.

▸ OR **if hypoglycaemia unresponsive *or* if oral route cannot be used**

Glucagon injection p. 579 (*GlucaGen*® 1 mg/mL)

BY INTRAMUSCULAR INJECTION

- Child 8 years and below or body-weight up to 25 kg: 500 micrograms (0.5 mL)
- Child 9-17 years or body-weight 25 kg and over: 1 mg (1 mL)

▸ OR **if hypoglycaemia prolonged *or* unresponsive to glucagon after 10 minutes**

Glucose intravenous infusion (10%) p. 730

BY INTRAVENOUS INJECTION INTO LARGE VEIN

- Child 1 month-17 years 5 ml/kg (glucose 500 mg/kg)

Seizures

▸ **CONVULSIVE (INCLUDING FEBRILE) SEIZURES LASTING 5 MINUTES OR LONGER, OR RECURRENT SEIZURES WITHOUT RECOVERY IN BETWEEN**

▸ EITHER **Diazepam rectal solution p. 270** (2 mg/mL, 4 mg/mL)

BY RECTUM

- Neonate: 1.25–2.5 mg, repeated once after 5–10 minutes if necessary
- Child 1 month-1 year: 5 mg, repeated once after 5–10 minutes if necessary
- Child 2-11 years: 5–10 mg, repeated once after 5–10 minutes if necessary
- Child 12-17 years: 10–20 mg, repeated once after 5–10 minutes if necessary

▸ OR **Midazolam oromucosal solution p. 273**

BY BUCCAL ADMINISTRATION

- Neonate: 300 micrograms/kg, repeated once after 5–10 minutes if necessary [unlicensed]
- Child 1-2 months: 300 micrograms/kg (max. 2.5 mg), repeated once after 5–10 minutes if necessary [unlicensed]
- Child 3 months-11 months: 2.5 mg, repeated once after 5–10 minutes if necessary
- Child 1-4 years: 5 mg, repeated once after 5–10 minutes if necessary
- Child 5-9 years: 7.5 mg, repeated once after 5–10 minutes if necessary
- Child 10-17 years: 10 mg, repeated once after 5–10 minutes if necessary

Newborn Life Support Algorithm

Newborn life support

(Antenatal counselling)
Team briefing and equipment check

Birth
Start clock

Delay cord clamping. Stimulate. Thermal care.

Assess
Breathing, heart rate

Ensure an open airway

Breathing inadequate

- Give 5 inflation breaths – 30 cm H_2O, air, look for chest rise
- PEEP 5–6 cm H_2O, if possible
- SpO_2 +/- ECG monitoring

Reassess heart rate and chest rise

Chest moving

- Start ventilation breaths (30 min^{-1})

Chest not moving

- Check mask, head and jaw position
- 2 person support
- Consider:
  - SGA
  - ↑Inflation pressures
  - Suction
  - Tracheal tube
- **Repeat 5 inflation breaths**

Reassess heart rate and chest rise

Once chest is moving continue ventilation breaths

If heart rate is < 60 min^{-1} after 30 seconds of ventilation breaths
15 cycles of 3 chest compressions : 1 ventilation

- Synchronise chest compressions and ventilation
- 100% Oxygen
- Consider SGA or intubation
- Reassess heart rate/chest rise every 30 seconds

If the heart rate remains < 60 min^{-1}

- Continue chest compressions
- Vascular access
- Consider drugs and intravascular volume
- Check blood glucose
- Consider other factors – hypovolaemia, pneumothorax, congenital abnormality

Update parents, complete records and debrief team

Approx 60 s

Keep baby warm

Is help needed?

Preterm < 32 weeks

Place undried body in a plastic bag + radiant heat

If breathing consider:

- CPAP 5–8 cm H_2O
- $\geq$ 30% FiO_2

If not breathing:

- Initial PIP 25 cm H_2O
- Peep 6 cm H_2O
- $\geq$ 30% FiO_2

Acceptable pre-ductal SpO_2	
3 min	70–75%
5 min	80–85%
10 min	85–95%
Titrate O_2 to achieve target SpO_2	

Reproduced with the kind permission of the Resuscitation Council (UK) from Resuscitation Guidelines, 2025

Paediatric Basic Life Support Algorithm

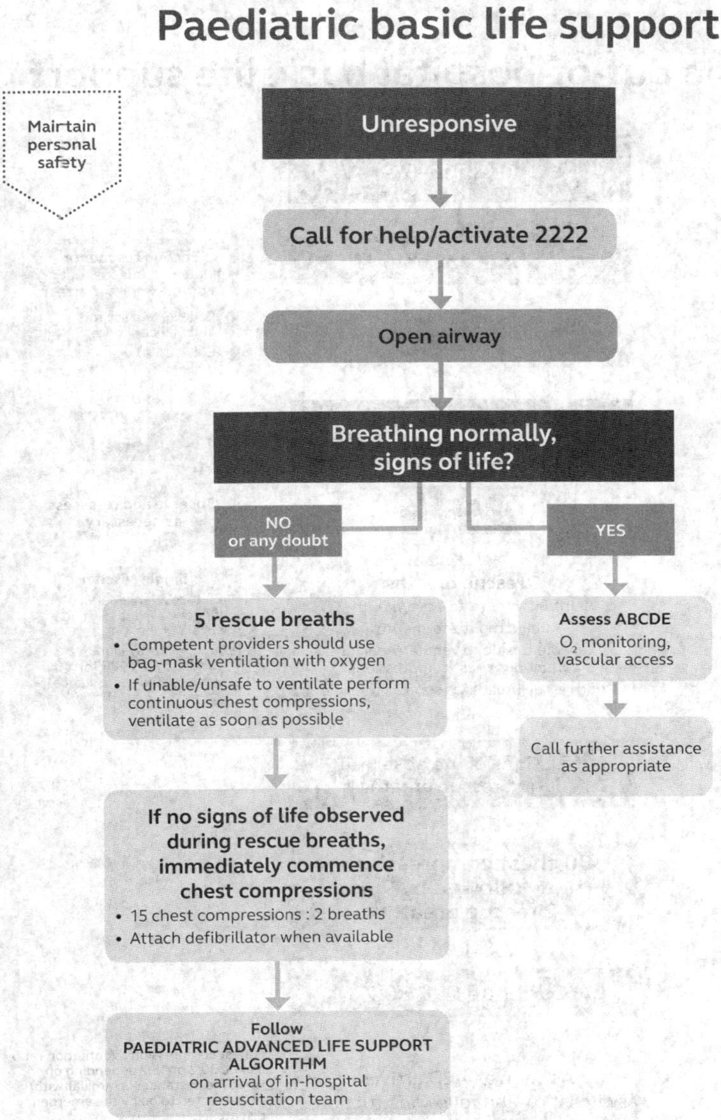

Paediatric Out-of-Hospital Basic Life Support Algorithm

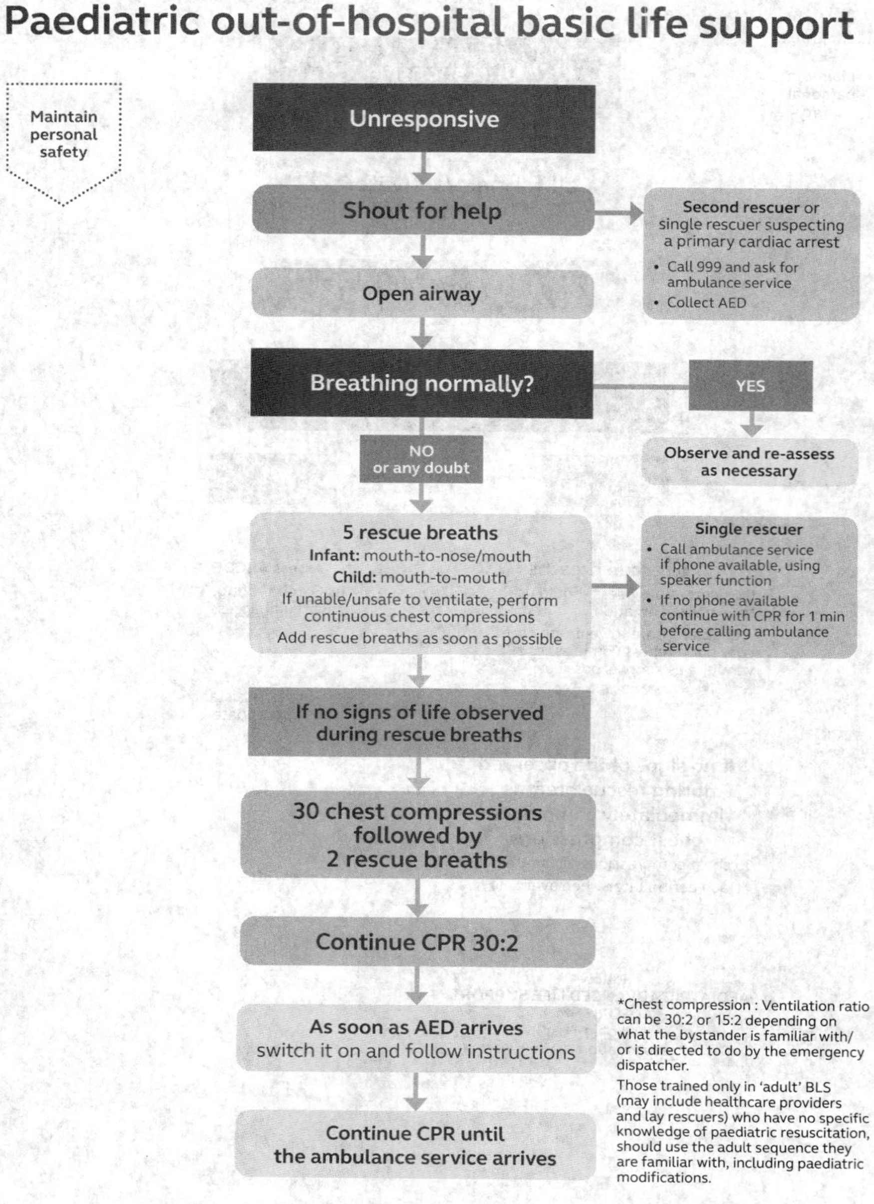

Reproduced with the kind permission of the Resuscitation Council (UK) from Resuscitation Guidelines, 2025